ANDERSON'S PATHOLOGY

ANDERSON'S PATHOLOGY

TENTH EDITION

Edited by:

Ivan Damjanov, M.D., Ph.D.
Professor and Chairman
Department of Pathology
University of Kansas School of Medicine
University of Kansas Medical Center
Kansas City, Kansas

■

James Linder, M.D.
Professor and Vice-Chairman
Department of Pathology and Microbiology
Associate Dean
College of Medicine
University of Nebraska Medical Center
Omaha, Nebraska

with 3366 illustrations, 1927 in color
Mary Jean McFadden
Illustrator

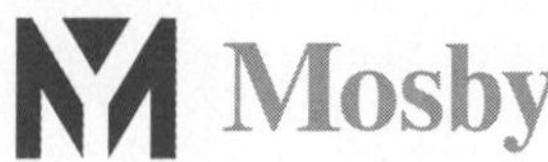

St. Louis Baltimore Boston Carlsbad Chicago Naples New York Philadelphia Portland
London Madrid Mexico City Singapore Sydney Tokyo Toronto Wiesbaden

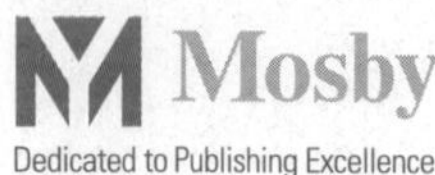

Dedicated to Publishing Excellence

A Times Mirror Company

Publisher: Anne S. Patterson
Senior Managing Editor: Lynne Gery
Project Manager: Dana Peick
Production Editor: Stavra Demetrulias
Manuscript Editor: Carl Masthay
Designer: Amy Buxton
Manufacturing Supervisor: Betty Richmond

TENTH EDITION

Printed in the United States of America
Composition by Clarinda Company
Color Separation by Color Dot Graphics, Inc.
Printing/binding by Von Hoffman Press, Inc.

Mosby-Year Book, Inc.
11830 Westline Industrial Drive
St. Louis, Missouri 63146

International Standard Book Number 0–8016–7236–8

95 96 97 98 99 / 9 8 7 6 5 4 3 2 1

Contributors

Nabil A. Abaza, D.M.D, Ph.D.
Professor of Pathology and Laboratory Medicine, and Professor of Oral and Maxillofacial Surgery, Medical College of Pennsylvania and Hahnemann University; Clinical Professor of Oral and Maxillofacial Surgery, School of Dental Medicine, University of Pennsylvania, Philadelphia, Pennsylvania
Chapter 50 Mouth, Teeth, and Pharynx

Jorge Albores-Saavedra, M.D.
Professor of Pathology, and Director, Division of Anatomic Pathology, University of Texas Southwestern Medical Center; Director, Division of Anatomic Pathology, Parkland Memorial Hospital, Dallas, Texas
Chapter 58 Gallbladder and Extrahepatic Biliary Ducts

D. Craig Allred, M.D.
Professor of Pathology, University of Texas Health Science Center at San Antonio, San Antonio, Texas
Chapter 70 Breast

Peter S. Amenta, M.D., Ph.D.
Associate Professor of Clinical Pathology and Chief of Pathology Service, Robert Wood Johnson Medical School and Robert Wood Johnson University Hospital, New Brunswick/Piscataway, New Jersey
Chapter 19 Repair and Regeneration

Mahul B. Amin, M.D.
Senior Staff, Department of Pathology and Bone and Joint Centre, Henry Ford Hospital, Detroit; Assistant Professor of Pathology, Case Western Reserve University School of Medicine, Cleveland, Ohio, and Clinical Assistant Professor of Pathology, Wayne State University School of Medicine, Detroit, Michigan
Chapter 67 Male Reproductive System

Robert E. Anderson, M.D.
Professor, Department of Laboratory Medicine and Pathology, University of Minnesota Medical School, Minneapolis, Minnesota
Chapter 23 Radiation Injury

Douglas C. Anthony, M.D., Ph.D.
Assistant Professor of Pathology, Harvard Medical School; Director of Neuropathology, Children's Hospital; Neuropathologist, Brigham and Women's Hospital, Boston, Massachusetts
Chapter 78 Peripheral Nervous System

Alberto G. Ayala, M.D.
Professor of Pathology, Deputy Chairman, and Director of Surgical Pathology, University of Texas, M.D. Anderson Cancer Center, Houston, Texas
Chapter 73 Bone Tumors

Shelina Babul, B.Sc.
Research and Education Coordinator, Cardiovascular Research Laboratory, Department of Pathology and Laboratory Medicine, St. Paul's Hospital, Vancouver, British Columbia, Canada
Chapter 2 Autopsy

Adam Bagg, M.D.
Assistant Professor of Pathology and Medicine, Director of Hematopathology, and Director, Hematology Laboratory, Georgetown University Medical Center, Washington, D.C.
Chapter 11 Diagnostic Molecular Pathology

Lewis A. Barness, M.D.
Professor of Pediatrics, University of South Florida College of Medicine and Emeritus Professor of Pediatrics, University of Wisconsin, Madison, Wisconsin
Chapter 14 Metabolic Diseases

Jay H. Beckstead, M.D.
Professor of Pathology, Oregon Health Sciences University, Portland, Oregon
Chapter 9 Histochemistry

Dwight A. Bellinger, D.V.M., Ph.D.
Associate Professor of Laboratory Animal Medicine and Pathology, University of North Carolina School of Medicine, Chapel Hill, North Carolina
Chapter 22 Hemostasis and Thrombosis

Morgan Berthrong, M.D.
Director Emeritus, Department of Pathology, Penrose/St. Francis Health Care System, Colorado Springs, Colorado; Professor Emeritus, Department of Pathology, University of Colorado School of Medicine, Denver, Colorado, and University of New Mexico School of Medicine, Albuquerque, New Mexico
Chapter 23 Radiation Injury

Nathan D. Bills, Ph.D.
Adjunct Assistant Professor of Pathology and Microbiology, University of Nebraska Medical Center, Omaha, Nebraska
Chapter 31 Nutritional Deprivation Diseases

David G. Bostwick, M.D.
Professor of Pathology and Consultant in Pathology, Department of Laboratory Medicine and Pathology, Mayo Medical School and Mayo Clinic, Rochester, Minnesota
Chapter 67 Male Reproductive System

Julia A. Bridge, M.D.
Associate Professor of Pathology and Microbiology, Pediatrics, and Orthopaedic Surgery; Director of Fragile X DNA Laboratory; Associate Director of Clinical Cytogenetics, University of Nebraska Medical Center, Omaha, Nebraska
Chapter 12 Cytogenetics

Richard D. Brunning, M.D.
Professor of Laboratory Medicine and Pathology, University of Minnesota Medical School; Head, Hematopathology Laboratory, University of Minnesota Hospital, Minneapolis, Minnesota
Chapter 41 Blood and Bone Marrow

David J. Bylund, M.D.
Adjunct Assistant Member, Department of Molecular and Experimental Medicine, The Scripps Research Institute, La Jolla; Director, Scripps Reference Laboratory, San Diego, California
Chapter 26 Autoimmunity and Autoimmune Diseases

Maria Luisa Carcangiu, M.D.
Associate Professor of Pathology and Obstetrics and Gynecology, Yale University School of Medicine and Yale New Haven Hospital, New Haven, Connecticut
Chapter 61 Thyroid Gland

John L. Carey III, M.D.
Division Head, Immunopathology, Henry Ford Health Care Corporation,

Farmington Hills, Michigan
Chapter 13 Flow and Imaging Cytometry

Wing (John) C. Chan, M.B., B.S., M.D.
Professor, Department of Pathology and Microbiology, University of Nebraska Medical Center, Omaha, Nebraska
Chapter 42 Lymph Nodes

Francis W. Chandler, D.V.M., Ph.D.
Professor, Department of Pathology, Medical College of Georgia, Augusta, Georgia
Chapter 37 Fungal Diseases

Gregorio Chejfec, M.D.
Professor of Pathology, Loyola University of Chicago, Stritch School of Medicine; Director, Anatomic Pathology, Loyola University Medical Center, Maywood; Chief, Pathology and Laboratory Medicine Service, Hines Veterans Administration Hospital, Hines, Illinois
Chapter 52 Esophagus

Stephen W. Chensue, M.D., Ph.D.
Associate Professor of Pathology, University of Michigan Medical School; Staff Pathologist, Veterans Affairs Medical Center, Ann Arbor, Michigan
Chapter 18 Inflammation

Arthur H. Cohen, M.D.
Professor of Pathology and Medicine, University of California, Los Angeles, School of Medicine; Attending Pathologist, Cedars-Sinai Medical Center, Los Angeles, California
Chapter 65 Kidney

Samuel M. Cohen, M.D., Ph.D.
Professor and Chairman, Department of Pathology and Microbiology, and Professor, Eppley Institute for Research in Cancer and Allied Diseases, University of Nebraska Medical Center, Omaha, Nebraska
Chapter 66 Lower Urinary Tract

Félix Contreras, M.D.
Professor of Pathology, Universidad Autónoma; Chairman, Department of Pathology, La Paz Hospital, Madrid, Spain
Chapter 71 Skin

Jeffrey Cossman, M.D.
Oscar Benwood Hunter Professor and Chairman, Department of Pathology, Georgetown University Medical Center; Pathologist-in-Chief, Georgetown University Hospital, Washington, D.C.
Chapter 11 Diagnostic Molecular Pathology

Richard J. Cote, M.D.
Associate Professor of Pathology, University of Southern California School of Medicine; Attending Pathologist, Kenneth Norris Jr. Comprehensive Cancer Center, Los Angeles, California
Chapter 8 Immunohistochemistry and Related Marking Techniques

John E. Craighead, M.D.
Professor of Pathology, University of Vermont College of Medicine; Attending Pathologist, Fletcher Allen Health Care, Burlington, Vermont
Chapter 49 Lung

Ivan Damjanov, M.D., Ph.D.
Professor and Chairman, Department of Pathology, University of Kansas Medical Center, Kansas City, Kansas
Chapter 32 Pathology of Obesity
Chapter 54 Small Intestine
Chapter 67 Male Reproductive System
Appendix-Table of Normal Values

Michael J. Davies, M.D.
Professor of Cardiovascular Pathology, University of London; Honorary Consultant, St. George's Hospital, London, United Kingdom
Chapter 45 Heart Disease in the Adult

Stephen J. DeArmond, M.D., Ph.D.
Professor of Pathology (Neuropathology) and Neurology, University of California, San Francisco, School of Medicine, San Francisco General Hospital, and San Francisco Veterans Administration Hospital, San Francisco, California
Chapter 40 Prions

Ronald A. DeLellis, M.D.
Professor of Pathology, Tufts University School of Medicine; Senior Pathologist, New England Medical Center, Boston, Massachusetts
Chapter 61 Thyroid Gland

J. Stephen Dumler, M.D.
Assistant Professor of Pathology, University of Maryland School of Medicine; Associate Director of Clinical Microbiology, University of Maryland Medical Center, Baltimore, Maryland
Chapter 35 Rickettsial and Chlamydial Diseases

Ralph C. Eagle, Jr., M.D.
Professor of Ophthalmology, Jefferson Medical College of Thomas Jefferson University; Director, Department of Pathology, Wills Eye Hospital, Philadelphia, Pennsylvania
Chapter 79 Eye and Ocular Adnexa

John N. Eble, M.D.
Professor of Pathology and of Experimental Oncology, Indiana University School of Medicine; Chief Pathologist, Richard L. Roudebush Veterans Affairs Medical Center, Indianapolis, Indiana
Chapter 65 Kidney

Jesse E. Edwards, M.D.
Clinical Professor of Pathology, University of Minnesota Medical School, Minneapolis; Senior Consultant, Registry of Cardiovascular Disease, United Hospital, St. Paul., Minnesota
Chapter 21 Circulatory Disturbances

William D. Edwards, M.D.
Professor of Pathology, Mayo Medical School and Mayo Graduate School of Medicine; Consultant, Division of Anatomic Pathology, and Clinical Appointment, Division of Cardiology, Mayo Clinic, Rochester, Minnesota
Chapter 46 Congenital Heart Disease

Samir K. El-Mofty, D.M.D., Ph.D.
Professor of Oral Pathology, Associate Professor of Pathology and Otolaryngology, Washington University School of Medicine; Attending Medical Staff, Barnes Hospital, Jewish Hospital, and St. Louis Children's Hospital; Consultant Pathologist, Veterans Administration Hospital, St. Louis, Missouri
Chapter 50 Mouth, Teeth, and Pharynx
Chapter 51 Salivary Glands

Luis F. Fajardo M.D.
Professor of Pathology, Stanford University School of Medicine, Stanford; Chief of Pathology and Laboratory Medicine, Veterans Affairs Medical Center, Palo Alto, California
Chapter 23 Radiation Injury

Lorraine A. Fitzpatrick, M.D.
Professor of Medicine, Consultant in Endocrinology and Metabolism, and Director, Bone Histomorphometry Laboratory, Mayo Clinic and Mayo Foundation, Rochester, Minnesota
Chapter 74 Metabolic and Nontumorous Bone Disorders

Howard S. Fox, M.D., Ph.D.
Assistant Member, Department of Neuropharmacology, The Scripps Research Institute, and Consultant, Department of Pathology, Scripps Clinic Medical Group, La Jolla; Assay Development, Scripps Reference Laboratory, San Diego, California
Chapter 26 Autoimmunity and Autoimmune Diseases

Stephen A. Geller, M.D.
Chairman, Department of Pathology and Laboratory Medicine, Cedars-Sinai Medical Center, and Professor, Department of Pathology and Laboratory Medicine, University of California, Los Angeles,

School of Medicine, Los Angeles, California
Chapter 28 Acquired Immunodeficiency Syndrome (AIDS)

Robert M. Genta, M.D.
Associate Professor of Pathology, Medicine, and Microbiology and Immunology, Baylor College of Medicine, Houston, Texas
Chapter 53 Stomach and Duodenum

Allen R. Gibbs, T.D., M.B., Ch.B., FRCPath
Consultant Pathologist, Llandough Hospital, Penarth; Honorary Clinical Teacher, University of Wales College of Medicine, Cardiff, United Kingdom
Chapter 49 Lung

Enid Gilbert-Barness, M.D.
Professor of Pathology and Pediatrics, University of South Florida College of Medicine, Tampa, Florida; Professor Emeritus of Pathology and Pediatrics; Distinguished Medical Alumni Professor Emeritus, University of Wisconsin Medical School, Madison, Wisconsin
Chapter 14 Metabolic Diseases

Douglas R. Gnepp, M.D.
Professor of Pathology, Rhode Island Hospital, and Brown University School of Medicine, Providence, Rhode Island
Chapter 51 Salivary Glands

John R. Goldblum, M.D.
Staff Pathologist, Cleveland Clinic Foundation, Cleveland, Ohio
Chapter 55 Appendix

Neal S. Goldstein, M.D.
Anatomic Pathologist, William Beaumont Hospital, Royal Oak, Michigan
Chapter 44 Thymus and Mediastinum

John G. Gruhn, M.D.
Associate Professor of Pathology, Rush Medical College, Chicago, Illinois
Chapter 63 Adrenal Glands

Yezid Gutierrez, M.D.
Associate Professor of Pathology, Institute of Pathology, Case Western Reserve University School of Medicine; Adjunct Staff, Department of Microbiology, Cleveland Clinic Foundation, Cleveland, Ohio
Chapter 38 Protozoal Diseases
Chapter 39 Metazoan Diseases

Sheryl Haggerty, Ph.D.
Assistant Professor, Department of Pathology and Microbiology, University of Nebraska Medical Center, Omaha, Nebraska; American Foundation for AIDS Research Scholar
Chapter 36 Viral Diseases

Christopher J. Harrison, M.D.
Associate Professor of Pediatrics and Medical Microbiology, Creighton University School of Medicine; Associate Professor of Pediatrics, and Clinical Staff, University of Nebraska Medical Center; Hospital Epidemiologist and Active Staff, Children's Hospital; Active Staff, St. Joseph Hospital, Omaha, Nebraska
Chapter 36 Viral Diseases

Reid R. Heffner, Jr., M.D.
Professor and Associate Chairman, Department of Pathology, State University of New York at Buffalo School of Medicine and Biomedical Sciences, Buffalo, New York
Chapter 76 Skeletal Muscle

Philipp U. Heitz, M.D.
Professor and Chairman, Department of Pathology, University of Zürich, Zürich, Switzerland
Chapter 64 Diabetes and Endocrine Pancreas

Steven H. Hinrichs, M.D.
Associate Professor, Department of Pathology and Microbiology, Department of Orthopaedic Surgery, and Eppley Research Institute; Director of Virology and Director of Molecular Diagnostics, University of Nebraska Medical Center; Associate Faculty, Pediatric Infectious Disease, Creighton University School of Medicine, Omaha, Nebraska
Chapter 15 Molecular Basis of Human Disease
Chapter 36 Viral Diseases

Charles S. Hirsch, M.D.
Professor and Chairman, Department of Forensic Medicine, and Professor, Department of Pathology, New York University School of Medicine; Chief Medical Examiner, City of New York, New York
Chapter 5 Forensic Pathology

Dikran S. Horoupian, M.D.
Professor, Department of Pathology; and Director, Neuropathology Division, Stanford University School of Medicine, Stanford, California
Chapter 77 Central Nervous System

Eva Horvath, Ph.D.
Associate Professor of Pathology, St. Michaels Hospital, University of Toronto Faculty of Medicine, Toronto, Ontario, Canada
Chapter 60 Pituitary Gland

Aubrey J. Hough, Jr., M.D.
Professor and Chairman, Department of Pathology, University of Arkansas College of Medicine, Little Rock, Arkansas
Chapter 75 Joints

Kamal G. Ishak, M.D., Ph.D.
Chairman, Department of Hepatic and Gastrointestinal Pathology, Armed Forces Institute of Pathology, Washington, D.C.; Clinical Professor of Pathology, Uniformed Services University for the Health Sciences and Medical Care, Bethesda, Maryland; Professorial Lecturer, Mount Sinai School of Medicine, New York, New York
Chapter 57 Liver

J. Charles Jennette, M.D.
Professor of Pathology and Medicine, and Director, Nephropathology Laboratory, University of North Carolina School of Medicine, Chapel Hill, North Carolina
Chapter 47 Vascular System

Jose Jessurun, M.D.
Associate Professor of Pathology, University of Minnesota Medical School, Minneapolis, Minnesota
Chapter 58 Gallbladder and Extrahepatic Biliary Ducts

Sonny L. Johansson, M.D., Ph.D
Professor and Director of Anatomic Pathology, Department of Pathology and Microbiology, and Professor, Eppley Institute for Research in Cancer and Allied Diseases, University of Nebraska Medical Center, Omaha, Nebraska
Chapter 66 Lower Urinary Tract

William W. Johnston, M.D.
Professor of Pathology, Chief, Division of Anatomic Pathology, and Head, Section of Cytopathology, Duke University School of Medicine, Durham, North Carolina
Chapter 4 Cytopathology

Vijay V. Joshi, M.D., FRCPath
Professor of Pathology and Clinical Professor of Pediatrics, East Carolina University School of Medicine, Greenville, North Carolina; Consultant in Pediatric Pathology, Beth Israel Medical Center, New York, New York
Chapter 28 Acquired Immunodeficiency Syndrome (AIDS)

Dagmar K. Kalousek, M.D., FRCPC, FCCMG
Professor of Pathology, The University of British Columbia Faculty of Medicine; Director of Cellular Pathology Program, Department of Pathology, B.C. Children's Hospital, Vancouver, British Columbia, Canada
Chapter 16 Developmental Pathology

David G. Kaufman, M.D., Ph.D.
Professor of Pathology, University of North Carolina School of Medicine,

Chapel Hill, North Carolina
Chapter 17 Cell Injury and Cellular Adaptations

James K. Kelly, M.B.
Chief, Anatomical Pathology, Greater Victoria Hospital Society, Victoria, British Columbia, Canada
Chapter 56 Large Intestine and Anus

Thomas Kirchner, M.D.
Professor and Chairman, Institute of Pathology, University of Erlangen, Erlangen, Germany
Chapter 44 Thymus and Mediastinum

Robert Kisilevsky, M.D., Ph.D., FRCPC
Professor, Departments of Pathology and Biochemistry, Queen's University Faculty of Medicine; Attending Staff, Departments of Pathology, Kingston General and Hotel Dieu Hospitals, Kingston, Ontario, Canada
Chapter 20 Amyloidosis

John M. Kissane, M.D.
Professor of Pathology and of Pediatrics, Washington University School of Medicine; Pathologist, Barnes and Affiliated Hospitals, Children's Hospital, and Jewish Hospital, St. Louis, Missouri
Chapter 33 Bacterial Diseases

Gordon K. Klintworth, M.D., Ph.D.
Professor of Pathology, Joseph A.C. Wadsworth Research Professor of Ophthalmology, and Director of Research, Duke University Eye Center, Durham, North Carolina
Chapter 79 Eye and Ocular Adnexa

Günter Klöppel, M.D., Ph.D.
Professor and Director, Department of Pathology, University of Kiel, Kiel, Germany
Chapter 64 Diabetes and Endocrine Pancreas

Paul Komminoth, M.D.
Department of Pathology, University of Zürich, Zürich, Switzerland
Chapter 64 Diabetes and Endocrine Pancreas

Kalman Kovacs, M.D., Ph.D., D.Sc., FRCPC, FCAF, FRC(Path)
Professor, Department of Pathology, St. Michaels Hospital, University of Toronto Faculty of Medicine, Toronto, Ontario, Canada
Chapter 60 Pituitary Gland

Charles Kuhn III, M.D.
Professor of Pathology, Brown University Program in Medicine, Providence, Rhode Island; Pathologist-in-Chief, Memorial Hospital of Rhode Island, Pawtucket, Rhode Island
Chapter 49 Lung

Ernest E. Lack, M.D.
Professor of Pathology and Director of Anatomic Pathology, Georgetown University School of Medicine, Washington, D.C.
Chapter 63 Adrenal Glands

Benjamin Landing, M.D.
Professor Emeritus, Pathology and Pediatrics, University of Southern California School of Medicine; Research Pathologist, Children's Hospital of Los Angeles, Los Angeles, California
Chapter 14 Metabolic Diseases

Russell M. Lebovitz, M.D., Ph.D.
Assistant Professor, Departments of Pathology and Cell Biology, Baylor College of Medicine, Houston, Texas
Chapter 24 Neoplasia

Juan Lechago, M.D., Ph.D.
Professor of Pathology, Baylor College of Medicine; Director, Surgical Pathology, The Methodist Hospital, Houston, Texas
Chapter 53 Stomach and Duodenum

Michael W. Lieberman, M.D., Ph.D.
The W. L. Moody Jr. Professor and Chairman, Department of Pathology, Baylor College of Medicine, Houston, Texas
Chapter 24 Neoplasia

James Linder, M.D.
Professor and Vice-Chairman, Department of Pathology and Microbiology, University of Nebraska Medical Center, Omaha, Nebraska
Chapter 4 Cytopathology
Chapter 6 Informatics

Craig E. Litz, M.D.
Associate Professor, Department of Laboratory Medicine and Pathology, University of Minnesota Medical School, Minneapolis, Minnesota
Chapter 41 Blood and Bone Marrow

Ricardo V. Lloyd, M.D., Ph.D.
Professor of Pathology and Senior Associate Consultant, Mayo Clinic and Mayo Foundation, Rochester, Minnesota
Chapter 60 Pituitary Gland

Daniel S. Longnecker, M.D.
Professor, Department of Pathology, Dartmouth Medical School, Hanover, and Dartmouth-Hitchcock Medical Center, Lebanon, New Hampshire
Chapter 59 Pancreas

Bruce Mackay, M.D., Ph.D.
Professor of Pathology, University of Texas, M.D. Anderson Cancer Center, Houston, Texas
Chapter 7 Electron Microscopy

Alberto Marchevsky, M.D.
Clinical Professor of Pathology, University of California, Los Angeles, School of Medicine; Director, Division of Anatomic Pathology, Cedars-Sinai Medical Center, Los Angeles, California
Chapter 44 Thymus and Mediastinum

Rodney S. Markin, M.D., Ph.D.
Professor of Pathology and Microbiology and of Surgery, Department of Pathology and Microbiology, University of Nebraska Medical Center, Omaha, Nebraska
Chapter 6 Informatics
Chapter 57 Liver

Antonio Martinez-Hernandez, M.D.
Professor, Department of Pathology, University of Tennessee College of Medicine; Chief, Pathology and Laboratory Medicine Service, Veterans Affairs Medical Center, Memphis, Tennessee
Chapter 19 Repair and Regeneration

Alexander Marx, M.D.
Lecturer in Pathology, University of Würzburg, Würzburg, Germany
Chapter 44 Thymus and Mediastinum

John S. McClure, M.D.
Pathologist, Unity Hospital, Allina Laboratories, Fridley, Minnesota
Chapter 41 Blood and Bone Marrow

Miles M. McFarland, M.D.
Clinical Assistant Professor of Pathology, Medical College of Pennsylvania and Hahnemann University, Philadelphia, Pennsylvania
Chapter 50 Mouth, Teeth, and Pharnyx

Bruce M. McManus, M.D., Ph.D.
Professor and Head, Department of Pathology and Laboratory Medicine, University of British Columbia Faculty of Medicine; Chairman, Department of Pathology and Laboratory Medicine, St. Paul's Hospital, Vancouver, British Columbia, Canada
Chapter 2 Autopsy
Chapter 30 Pathology of Prosthetic Materials and Devices
Chapter 45 Heart Disease in the Adult

Neil Scott McNutt, M.D.
Professor of Pathology, Cornell University Medical Center; Director,

Dermatopathology Division, Department of Pathology, Cornell University Medical Center and The New York Hospital; Consultant in Pathology, Memorial Sloan-Kettering Cancer Center, New York, New York
Chapter 71 Skin

Wayne M. Meyers, M.D., Ph.D.
Chief, Mycobacteriology Branch, Armed Forces Institute of Pathology, Washington D.C.; Research Affiliate, Tulane University, New Orleans, Louisiana
Chapter 34 Mycobacterial Diseases

Leslie Michaels, M.D., FRCPath, FRCPC
Professor Emeritus, University of London; Department of Histopathology, UCL Medical School, London, United Kingdom
Chapter 80 Ear

Markku Miettinen, M.D.
Associate Professor of Pathology, Jefferson Medical College of Thomas Jefferson University; Attending Pathologist, Thomas Jefferson University Hospital, Philadelphia, Pennsylvania
Chapter 72 Soft Tissue Tumors

Stacey E. Mills, M.D.
Professor of Pathology and Associate Director of Surgical Pathology, University of Virginia Health Sciences Center, Charlottesville, Virginia
Chapter 3 Surgical Pathology

Sean Moore M.B., B.Ch., FRCPC
Professor of Pathology, McGill University Faculty of Medicine; Consultant Pathologist, Royal Victoria Hospital, Montreal, Quebec, Canada
Chapter 47 Vascular System

Hans Konrad Mueller-Hermelink, M.D.
Professor and Chairman, Institute of Pathology, University of Würzburg, Würzburg, Germany
Chapter 44 Thymus and Mediastinum

Robert M. Nakamura, M.D.
Chairman Emeritus, Department of Pathology, Scripps Clinic and Research Foundation, La Jolla, California
Chapter 26 Autoimmunity and Autoimmune Diseases

Cynthia C. Nast, M.D.
Associate Professor of Pathology, University of California, Los Angeles, School of Medicine; Associate Pathologist, Cedars-Sinai Medical Center, Los Angeles, California
Chapter 65 Kidney

Richard S. Neiman, M.D.
Professor of Pathology and Laboratory Medicine and of Medicine; Director of Hematopathology, Department of Pathology and Laboratory Medicine, Indiana University Medical Center, Indianapolis, Indiana
Chapter 43 Spleen

Christian Nezelof, M.D.
Professor Emeritus d'Anatomie Pathologique, Faculté de Médecine de Paris, Consultant Pathologist, Hôpital Saint-Vincent de Paul, Paris, France
Chapter 1 The History of Pathology: An Overview
Chapter 27 Primary Immunodeficiencies

Gerard J. Nuovo, M.D.
Associate Professor of Pathology and Obstetrics and Gynecology, State University of New York at Stony Brook, Stony Brook, New York
Chapter 10 In Situ Hybridization

Attilio Orazi, M.D.
Associate Professor of Pathology and Laboratory Medicine, Indiana University School of Medicine; Director of Immunohistochemistry, Indiana University Medical Center, Indianapolis, Indiana
Chapter 43 Spleen

Nelson G. Ordóñez, M.D.
Professor of Pathology, Director of Immunocytochemistry Section, University of Texas, M.D. Anderson Cancer Center, Houston, Texas
Chapter 7 Electron Microscopy

David A. Owen, M.B., B.Ch., FRCPath, FRCPC
Professor of Pathology, University of British Columbia Faculty of Medicine; Head, Division of Anatomical Pathology, Vancouver Hospital and Health Sciences Centre, Vancouver, B.C., Canada
Chapter 56 Large Intestine and Anus

Robert E. Petras, M.D.
Chairman, Department of Anatomic Pathology, The Cleveland Clinic Foundation, Cleveland, Ohio
Chapter 55 Appendix

Edwina J. Popek, D.O.
Assistant Professor of Pathology, Baylor College of Medicine; Perinatal and Placental Pathologist, Texas Children's Hospital, Houston, Texas
Chapter 69 Placenta

James M. Powers, M.D.
Professor of Pathology and Neurology, Associate Chair for Education, and Director, Neuropathology Unit, University of Rochester, Rochester, New York
Chapter 77 Central Nervous System

Jaime Prat, M.D., FRCPath
Professor of Pathology, Autonomous University of Barcelona; Director, Department of Pathology, Hospital de la Santa Creu i Sant Pau, Barcelona, Spain
Chapter 68 Female Reproductive System

Stanley B. Prusiner, M.D.
Professor of Neurology and of Biochemistry and Biophysics, University of California, San Francisco, School of Medicine, San Francisco, California
Chapter 40 Prions

Stanley J. Radio, M.D.
Associate Professor of Pathology and Director, Cytology and Cardiovascular Registry, Department of Pathology and Microbiology, University of Nebraska Medical Center, Omaha, Nebraska
Chapter 29 Transplantation Pathology
Chapter 30 Pathology of Prosthetic Materials and Devices

Juhani Rapola, M.D.
Chief of Pathology Unit, Children's Hospital, University of Helsinki, Helsinki, Finland
Chapter 14 Metabolic Diseases

A. Kevin Raymond, M.D.
Associate Professor of Pathology, University of Texas, M.D. Anderson Cancer Center, Houston, Texas
Chapter 73 Bone Tumors

Robert L. Reddick, M.D.
Brinkhous Professor of Pathology, University of North Carolina School of Medicine, Chapel Hill, North Carolina
Chapter 22 Hemostasis and Thrombosis

Janardan K. Reddy, M.D.
Magerstadt Professor and Chairman, Department of Pathology, Northwestern University Medical School; Attending Pathologist, Northwestern Memorial Hospital, Chicago Illinois
Chapter 17 Cell Injury

Jae Y. Ro, M.D., Ph.D.
Professor of Pathology, University of Texas, M.D. Anderson Cancer Center, Houston, Texas
Chapter 73 Bone Tumors

Seymour Rosen, M.D.
Director of Surgical Pathology and Senior Pathologist, Department of Pathology, Beth Israel Hospital; Professor of Pathology, Harvard Medical School, Boston, Massachusetts
Chapter 47 Vascular System

Sanford I. Roth, M.D.
Professor of Pathology, Northwestern University Medical School; Attending Pathologist, Northwestern Memorial Hospital, Chicago, Illinois
Chapter 62 Parathyroid Glands

Jürgen Roth, M.D., Ph.D.
Professor of Cell and Molecular Pathology, Division of Cell and Molecular Pathology, Department of Pathology, University of Zürich, Zürich, Switzerland
Chapter 64 Diabetes and Endocrine Pancreas

Jonathan W. Said, M.D.
Professor of Pathology, University of California, Los Angeles, School of Medicine; Associate Pathologist, Cedars-Sinai Medical Center, Los Angeles, California
Chapter 28 Acquired Immunodeficiency Syndrome (AIDS)

Carolyn M. Salafia, M.D.
Associate Professor of Pathology and of Obstetrics and Gynecology, Georgetown University Medical Center, Washington, D.C.; Section Head, Perinatal Pathology, Perinatology Research Faculty, National Institute of Child Health and Human Development, Bethesda, Maryland
Chapter 69 Placenta

George E. Sale, M.D.
Professor of Pathology, University of Washington School of Medicine; Member and Pathology Program Head, Fred Hutchinson Cancer Research Center, Seattle, Washington
Chapter 29 Transplantation Pathology

Avery A. Sandberg, M.D., D.Sc.
Senior Medical Director, Genetrix, Inc., and Vice-President and Director of Cancer Center, Southwest Biomedical Research Institute, Scottsdale; Senior Clinical Lecturer, University of Arizona College of Medicine, Tucson, Arizona
Chapter 12 Cytogenetics

Gail M. Schauer, M.D.
Clinical Assistant Professor, Departments of Pathology and Obstetrics and Gynecology, The Ohio State University College of Medicine; Director, Autopsy Service, Columbus Children's Hospital, Columbus, Ohio
Chapter 16 Developmental Pathology

Bertram Schnitzer, M.D.
Professor of Pathology and Director of Hematopathology, University of Michigan Medical Center, Ann Arbor, Michigan
Chapter 42 Lymph Nodes

Sydney S. Schochet, Jr., M.D.
Professor of Pathology, Neurology and Neurosurgery, West Virginia University School of Medicine, Morgantown, West Virginia
Chapter 76 Skeletal Muscle

Thomas A. Seemayer, M.D.
Professor of Pathology and Microbiology and of Pediatrics, University of Nebraska Medical Center, Omaha, Nebraska; Adjunct Professor of Pathology, McGill University Faculty of Medicine, Montreal, Quebec, Canada
Chapter 1 The History of Pathology: An Overview
Chapter 27 Primary Immunodeficiencies

Stewart Sell, M.D.
Professor, Department of Pathology and Laboratory Medicine, University of Texas Medical School, Houston, Texas
Chapter 25 Immunopathologic Mechanisms

Francis E. Sharkey, M.D.
Associate Professor of Pathology, University of Texas Health Science Center; Consulting Pathologist, Audie Murphy Memorial Veterans Administration Hospital, San Antonio, Texas
Chapter 70 Breast

Herschel Sidransky, M.D.
Professor and Chairman, Department of Pathology, George Washington University Medical Center, Washington, D.C.
Chapter 31 Nutritional Deprivation Diseases

Jerome H. Smith, M.S., M.Sc. Hyg., M.D.
Professor and Director of Pathology Education, Department of Pathology, University of Texas Medical Branch, Galveston, Texas
Chapter 39 Metazoan Diseases

Bruce R. Smoller, M.D.
Associate Professor of Pathology and Dermatology, Stanford University Medical Center; Director, Dermatopathology, Stanford University Hospital, Stanford, California
Chapter 71 Skin

Dale C. Snover, M.D.
Professor and Director of Anatomic Pathology, Department of Laboratory Medicine and Pathology, University of Minnesota Medical School, Minneapolis, Minnesota
Chapter 29 Transplantation Pathology

Lucia Stefaneanu, Ph.D.
Assistant Professor of Pathology, St. Michaels Hospital, University of Toronto Faculty of Medicine, Toronto, Ontario, Canada
Chapter 60 Pituitary Gland

Jerome B. Taxy, M.D.
Associate Pathologist, Lutheran General Hospital, Park Ridge, Illinois; Clinical Associate Professor of Pathology, Northwestern University Medical School, Chicago, Illinois
Chapter 48 Upper Respiratory Tract

Clive R. Taylor, M.A., M.D., D. Phil, FRCPath
Professor and Chair, Department of Pathology and Laboratory Medicine University of Southern California School of Medicine; Director of Laboratories, Los Angeles County-University of Southern California Medical Center, University Hospital, and Norris Cancer Hospital and Research Institute, Los Angeles, California
Chapter 8 Immunohistochemistry and Related Marking Techniques

Jack L. Titus, M.D., Ph.D.
Clinical Professor of Laboratory Medicine and Pathology, University of Minnesota Medical School, Minneapolis; Director, Registry of Cardiovascular Diseases, United Hospital, St. Paul, Minnesota
Chapter 21 Circulatory Disturbances

Monica D. Traystman, Ph.D.
Assistant Professor of Pathology and Microbiology and Pediatrics; Eppley Research Institute, University of Nebraska Medical Center, Omaha, Nebraska
Chapter 15 Molecular Basis of Human Disease

Robert L. Trelstad, M.D.
Professor and Chairman, Department of Pathology, Robert Wood Johnson Medical School, New Brunswick/Piscataway, New Jersey
Chapter 19 Repair and Regeneration

Philip T. Valente, M.D.
Associate Professor of Pathology and of Obstetrics and Gynecology, University of Texas Health Science Center at San Antonio; Director of Cytology, University Hospital and Audie Murphy Veterans Administration Hospital, San Antonio, Texas
Chapter 70 Breast

F. Stephen Vogel, M.D.
Professor of Pathology, Emeritus, Duke University School of Medicine, Durham, North Carolina; Clinical Professor of Pathology, Medical College of Georgia, Augusta, Georgia
Chapter 78 Peripheral Nervous System

Franz von Lichtenberg, M.D.
Professor of Pathology, Emeritus, Harvard Medical School; Senior Pathologist, Brigham and Women's Hospital, Boston, Massachusetts
Chapter 38 Protozoal Diseases

David H. Walker, M.D.
Professor and Chairman, Department of Pathology, University of Texas

Medical Branch; Director, Center for Tropical Diseases, Galveston, Texas
Chapter 35 Rickettsial and Chlamydial Diseases

Peter A. Ward, M.D.
Godfrey D. Stobbe Professor and Chairman, Department of Pathology, University of Michigan Medical School and Hospitals, Ann Arbor, Michigan
Chapter 18 Inflammation

John C. Watts, M.D.
Chief, Surgical Pathology, Department of Anatomic Pathology, William Beaumont Hospital, Royal Oak, Michigan, Clinical Associate Professor of Pathology, Wayne State University School of Medicine, Detroit, Michigan
Chapter 37 Fungal Diseases

David S. Weinberg, M.D., Ph.D.
Associate Professor of Pathology, Harvard Medical School; Pathologist, and Medical Director, Hematology Laboratory, Brigham and Women's Hospital, Boston, Massachusetts
Chapter 13 Flow and Imaging Cytometry

Lawrence M. Weiss, M.D.
Director of Surgical Pathology, Department of Pathology, City of Hope National Medical Center, Duarte, California
Chapter 42 Lymph Nodes

Sharon W. Weiss, M.D.
James French Professor of Pathology and Director of Anatomic Pathology, University of Michigan Hospitals, Ann Arbor, Michigan
Chapter 72 Soft Tissue Tumors

William W. West, M.D.
Associate Professor of Pathology, University of Nebraska School of Medicine; Pathologist in Chief, Veterans Administration Hospital, Omaha, Nebraska
Chapter 49 Lung

Mark R. Wick, M.D.
Professor of Pathology and Director of Surgical Pathology, Washington University School of Medicine; Associate Director of Anatomic Pathology, Washington University Medical Center, St. Louis, Missouri
Chapter 3 Surgical Pathology

Washington C. Winn, Jr., M.D., M.B.A.
Professor of Pathology, University of Vermont College of Medicine; Director, Clinical Microbiology, Department of Pathology and Laboratory Medicine, Fletcher Allen Health Care, Burlington, Vermont
Chapter 33 Bacterial Diseases

James L. Wisecarver, M.D., Ph.D.
Associate Professor, Department of Pathology and Microbiology, and Medical Director, Transplant Immunology Laboratory, University of Nebraska Medical Center, Omaha, Nebraska
Chapter 25 Immunopathologic Mechanisms

Gail L. Woods, M.D.
Professor of Pathology with joint appointmnents in Internal Medicine and Microbiology and Immunology, University of Texas Medical Branch, Galveston, Texas
Chapter 34 Mycobacterial Diseases

Anjana V. Yeldandi, M.D.
Assistant Professor of Pathology, Northwestern University Medical School; Staff Pathologist, Veterans Administration Lakeside Hospital, and Attending Pathologist, Northwestern Memorial Hospital, Chicago, Illinois
Chapter 17 Cell Injury and Cellular Adaptations

Iain D. Young, M.D., C.M., FRCPC
Associate Professor of Pathology, Queen's University Faculty of Medicine; Attending Staff, Departments of Pathology, Kingston General and Hotel Dieu Hospitals, Kingston, Ontario, Canada
Chapter 20 Amyloidosis

Ross E. Zumwalt, M.D.
Professor of Pathology, University of New Mexico School of Medicine; Chief Medical Investigator, State of New Mexico, Albuquerque, New Mexico
Chapter 5 Forensic Pathology

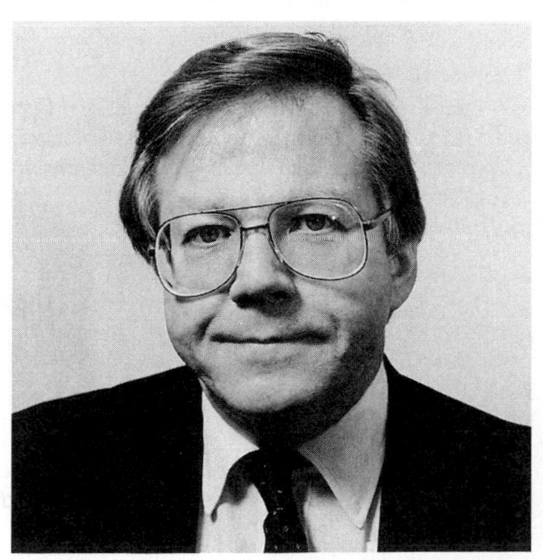

David T. Purtilo, M.D.
1939-1992

"The only solid piece of scientific truth about which I feel totally confident is that we are profoundly ignorant about nature. . . It is this sudden confrontation with the depth and scope of ignorance that represents the most significant contribution of twentieth-century science to the human intellect"

—Lewis Thomas (1913-1993), *The Medusa and the Snail,* The Viking Press, 1979, New York

This book is dedicated to David T. Purtilo, M.D., friend and mentor of pathologists throughout the world, in the spirit of bridging the ignorance that we face in our struggle to understand, diagnose, and treat disease.

Preface

The first edition of *Anderson's Pathology* appeared in 1948. As the first modern multiauthored textbook of pathology, it was enthusiastically greeted and almost immediately adopted as the standard textbook for graduate and postgraduate medical education. Generations of physicians grew up on *Anderson's Pathology,* and many of them still practice medicine remembering fondly the book that has introduced them to clinical medicine. During the next 40-plus years, the book saw eight editions published, the first six of which were edited by Dr. W.A.D. Anderson. For the seventh edition Dr. John M. Kissane became the co-editor and after Dr. Anderson's death on January 20, 1986, Dr. Kissane prepared the ninth edition. The baton has been passed now to us.

Few textbooks have names as resonant as *Anderson's Pathology.* It was thus with considerable trepidation that we accepted the publisher's invitation to devise a major revision of this venerable textbook and redesign it for the new generations of physicians who will be practicing in the 21st century. At the end of the project we are, nevertheless, pleased that we undertook it. On behalf of all our contributors we are proud to present the 10th edition, confident that it will herald a new era in the history of this textbook.

In order to restore the luster and popularity of the original edition, we had to make some drastic changes, both in the content and in the design. First of all, we expanded the text. This was achieved by increasing the number of pages and by a more judicious use of space. The number of chapters was increased from 42 in the ninth edition to 80 in the tenth edition. The group of outstanding contributors was increased proportionally, from 58 to 170. With this redesign we were in a position to give every contributor a smaller and presumably more manageable task. The contributors were asked, in turn, to provide more details and cover the assigned topics in greater depth. For example, alimentary tract pathology, which previously was presented in a single chapter, is now subdivided into five smaller chapters, and hematopathology has been subdivided into three chapters.

The first chapter deals with the history of pathology: we are standing on the shoulders of our predecessors and we thought that new generations of physicians should know that they are not working in a vacuum but are continuing in the tradition of true giants. The subsequent chapters deal with techniques that are essential for the practice of pathology. It would be inconceivable to study modern pathology without a solid understanding of these techniques. We also believe that the study of pathology requires solid understanding of basic pathologic processes, which are discussed in considerable detail.

The diseases that affect the entire body and those that have a common cause or pathogenesis have been grouped together. Although these chapters were conceived as overviews in which not all the diseases could be discussed at extreme length, they still provide a solid foundation—a starting point from which the interested physician can proceed further. Nevertheless, we feel that there are few books like this one, in which one will find a general overview of the pathology of Mendelian disorders and a description of a rare disease such as hyperpipecolicacidemia in the same subdivision.

The last part of Volume One and all of Volume Two are devoted to diseases of organ systems. In addition to lesions seen by the surgical pathologist, these chapters deal also with "medical" diseases. Whenever it was appropriate the specific diseases were discussed in terms of their etiology, pathogenesis, and clinical significance. Numerous tables, diagrams, and black and white or color photographs were included as a supplement to enhance the message of the written text.

In contrast to previous editions, which were illustrated almost exclusively with black and white photographs, this edition contains many color illustrations. To make the material more readable and esthetically pleasing, the text has been enhanced by a four-color design. We anticipate that the colors will break the monotony, highlight the salient features, and enable the reader to grasp the visually enhanced message more efficiently. Two-color computer-generated graphic illustrations have been designed with the same aim in mind.

By design the tenth edition of *Anderson's Pathology* is a detailed book. Obviously it is too big for sophomore medical students, although we assume that some students looking for a good reference text might buy it as a source book and a "companion for life." We anticipate that the primary users of the book will be residents in pathology and related disciplines, and practicing pathologists. Specifically, we had in mind residents looking for a comprehensive textbook of pathology that is "one notch higher" than their sophomore pathology textbook. We hope that they will use this book as their primary text while preparing for the specialty boards, but also annotate it and keep it handy as they enter pathology practice. Practicing pathologists will find in it authoritative reviews of new information. They could use it also as a quick reference or a guide for more detailed reading. Educators who want to be one step ahead of their students should find in it enough material to enliven their lectures or seminars. Finally, although we do not expect our clinical colleagues to read it cover to cover, we hope that they will find it useful for consultation and reference.

The electronic media revolution has had a major impact on our thinking and has changed both our way of life and how we practice pathology. To meet the requirements of new generations of pathologists more comfortable with computers than books, we will produce a CD-ROM version of *Anderson's Pathology.* Like the Habsburg king, Charles V of Austria, who was known in Spain as Carlos I, the first CD-ROM version will also be known under two names, depending on the constituents who are using it. Since history does not teach us how to prognosticate, we do not know which dynastic branch will survive longer. We hope that both the printed and the electronic version will have their own followers. We are very eager to learn which format will be more popular.

We hope that the readers will react favorably to our team effort. To produce an even better book in the next edition we are soliciting comments and criticism from the readers. We can be reached via the internet at **idamjano@kumc.wpo.ukans.edu** and **jlinder@unmc.edu.** We are asking not only for creative suggestions for revisions but also entries and references that could help us in updating the text. We are inviting all pathologists to keep us informed of their important new publications and encourage them to deposit the references of their papers, along with a brief descriptor, into our e-mail bags. Furthermore, we are inviting junior (and not so junior) pathologists who would like to be considered as contributors for future editions of the textbook to send us their credentials.

We are pleased that so many outstanding pathologists agreed to share their time and expertise in completing this tenth edition. Without their dedication, this book would not exist. Our thanks are directed also to the publisher and especially Susan Gay, Lynne Gery, Stavra Demetrulias, and Dana Peick.

The support we received at our respective insitutions and from our families was invaluable. Judith Russell and Sandra Dixon-Ross deserve all the credit for the work done at Thomas Jefferson University, Philadelphia, where the entire project was conceived and begun. Cynthia Van Derbur has our thanks for the work done at the University of Kansas Medical Center. I (ID) thank also my wife, Andrea Damjanov, for her encouragement, dedication, and understanding, even when I did not deserve it.

At the University of Nebraska Medical Center our sincere thanks go to Valerie Gunderson, who provided the major organizational support for the textbook in addition to typing many of the chapters, proofreading, and extensive correspondence with contributors. I (JL) thank Samuel M. Cohen, M.D., Ph.D., Chairman of the Department of Pathology and Microbiology, and Harold M. Maurer, M.D., Dean of the College of Medicine, for providing an atmosphere that allowed us to complete a project of this scope. The project would not have been possible without the support of faculty and resident colleagues at the University of Nebraska Medical Center, particularly Dr. Thomas Seemayer, who provided invaluable guidance on many chapters. Finally, I thank my wife, Wendy Linder, M.D., and our children, Emily, Kari, and Eric Linder, for their patience and support.

Ivan Damjanov
James Linder

Contents

VOLUME ONE

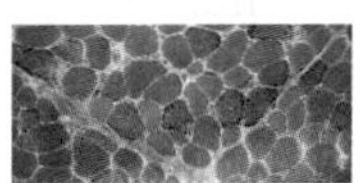

PART ONE METHODS IN PATHOLOGY

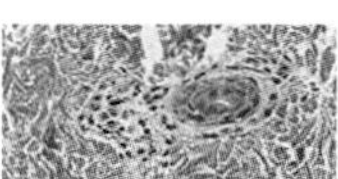

PART TWO SYSTEMIC PATHOLOGY

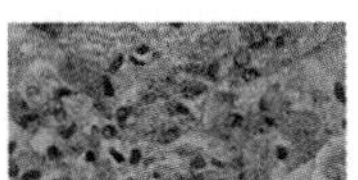

PART THREE INFECTIOUS DISEASES

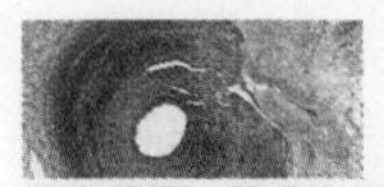

PART FOUR DISEASES OF THE BLOOD, HEART, AND LUNGS

VOLUME TWO

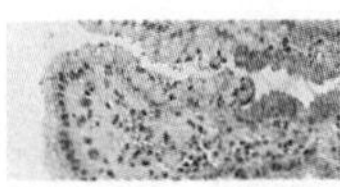

PART FIVE DISEASES OF THE DIGESTIVE SYSTEM

ANDERSON'S PATHOLOGY

Part Five

DISEASES OF THE DIGESTIVE SYSTEM

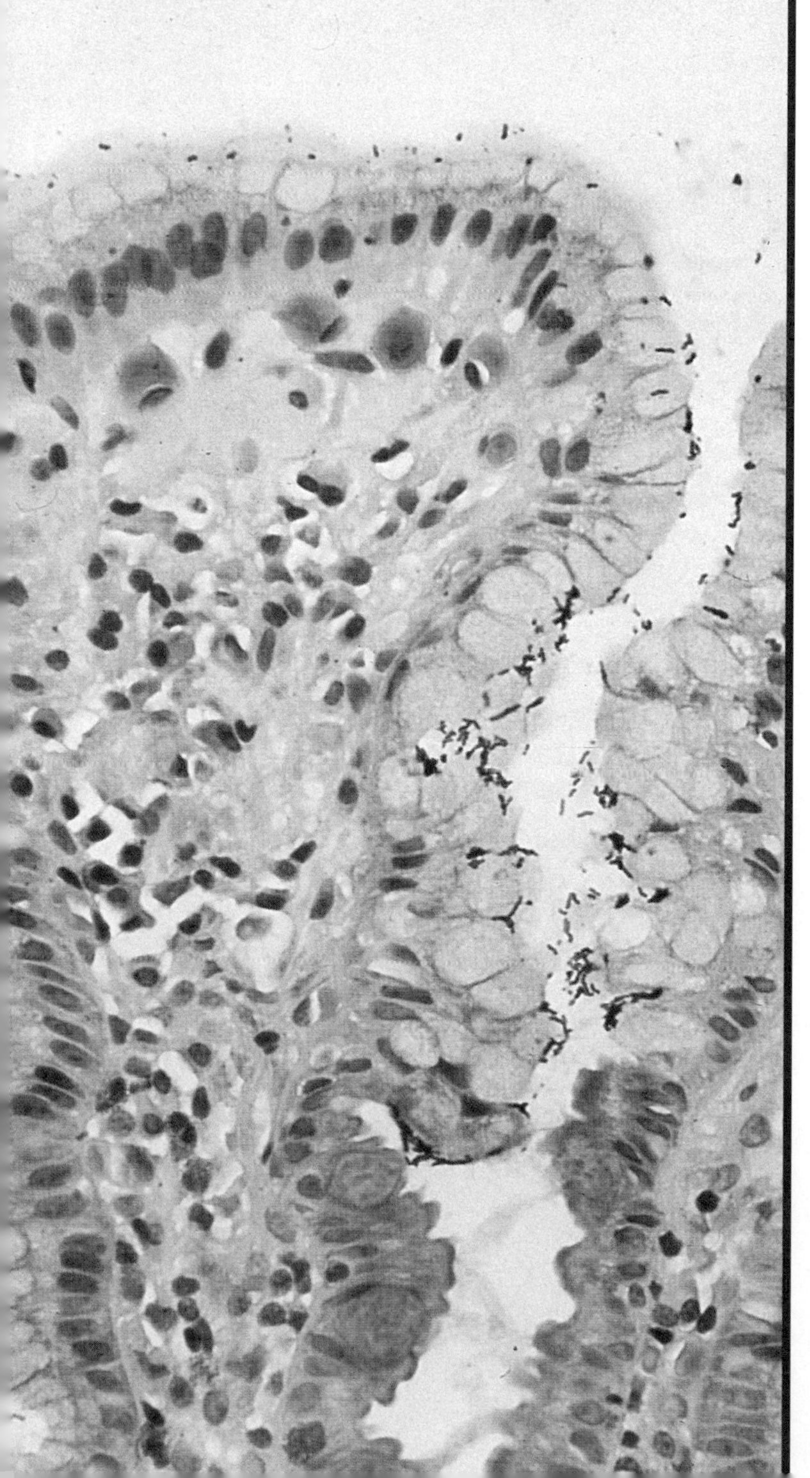

50 Mouth, Teeth, and Pharynx

Miles McFarland
Nabil A. Abaza
Samir El-Mofty

The diseases of the mouth and teeth require an understanding of the unique features of this region. Many of the terms are unique to this region, are confusing, and sound similar, and odontogenic lesions are unlike those in other sites. Interpretation of small mucosal biopsy specimens often requires clinical information that may be omitted on the submission slip. Specific diagnosis of cysts and tumors of the jawbones often also requires radiologic correlation. General pathologists are rarely exposed to oral lesions, most of which are examined by oral pathologists. Because of all these reasons, oral pathology is often intimidating to general pathologists. For more details on this subject, the reader is referred to several recent pathology texts, atlases, and chapters dealing with oral and pharyngeal anomalies and diseases.[1-13]

NORMAL DEVELOPMENT AND STRUCTURE

Orofacial development

The lower face forms mostly from processes developing out of the first branchial (mandibular) arch. In the first month of embryonic development, an invagination of ectoderm develops between the two lateral maxillary processes and cephalad to the mandibular processes. This stomodeal pit deepens to form the primitive oral cavity, the stomodeum. The posterior wall of the stomodeum meets the anterior end of the foregut tube, and after rupture of the buccopharyngeal membrane, they communicate. The mucosa of the mouth, the salivary glands, and the enamel of the teeth derive from ectoderm, whereas the mucosa of the pharynx derives from endoderm.[14-16]

By the end of the fourth week of development, the ectoderm over the forebrain thickens to form bilateral nasal placodes. During the next week, ectomesenchymal proliferation under each placode produces elevations, the medial and lateral nasal processes. Over the next 2 weeks, the medial nasal processes merge with each other to begin forming the middle upper lip (philtrum), middle upper jaw, and the primary palate (the anteromedial portion of the future hard palate). The nasal processes also merge with the more lateral maxillary processes of the first branchial arch. The maxillary processes will form the remaining upper lip, upper jaw, and secondary palate (the lateral and posterior portions of the future hard palate). Folds of tissue from the maxillary processes grow downward on either side of the tongue to form the palatine processes separating the oral and pharyngeal cavities. The palatine processes then fuse superiorly to form the posterior portion of the secondary palate. By the twelfth week of development, the secondary palate has fused with the primary palate anteriorly and the nasal septum above, to form separate oral and dual nasal chambers.[17]

The mandibular processes of the first branchial arch merge in the midline to begin forming the lower jaw, lip, and related structures. In the fourth week of development there is a focal median elevation on the floor of the primitive pharynx, anterior to the thyroid anlage. This anterior median elevation is the tuberculum impar. The anterior two thirds of the tongue develops from swellings that arise on each side of the tuberculum impar, but the posterior third of the tongue develops from a midline elevation, just posterior to the thyroid anlage. This posterior elevation, the hypobranchial eminence, derives from the second and third branchial arches and will also give rise to the epiglottis. Thus the tongue derives from the first three branchial arches.

At the end of the first month of development, the thyroid anlage begins as a thickening in the median floor of the primitive pharynx. This thickening forms an outpouching, the thyroid diverticulum. The thyroid descends into the neck as the head and tongue grow, passing just ventral to the developing hyoid bone and larynx. For a time, the developing thyroid remains connected to the tongue by a narrow tube, the thyroglossal duct, the lingual opening of which is the foramen cecum. By 7 weeks the superior portion of the thyroglossal duct has usually degenerated and disappeared, but the inferior portion often persists as the pyramidal lobe of the thyroid. The *foramen cecum* also persists as a small blind pit in the dorsal midline of the tongue.

Around the fourth week of development, an outpouching of ectoderm in the dorsal roof of the primitive oral cavity, called *Rathke's pouch,* extends toward the brain. By the fifth week it meets a ventral extension from the diencephalon, the infundibulum. Thus the anterior lobe of the pituitary gland (the adenohypophysis) derives from oral ectoderm.

It was formerly believed that fusion of the embryonic processes often entrapped rests of nonodontogenic epithelium, which later (infrequently) developed into epithelial cysts within the bone or parosteal tissues of the jaws. This theory about the origin of so-called fissural cysts is now in disrepute. However, failure of fusion leads to cleft lip, cleft palate, or other defects.

Tooth development and structure

Morphodifferentiation phase

During the sixth week of embryonic life, formation of the primary (deciduous) teeth begins, and tooth formation will continue until about 17 years of age, when the third molars erupt. The first phase of tooth development is that of morphodifferentiation. The oral epithelium in the maxillary and mandibular processes proliferates and then extends into the primitive mesenchyme where the primary teeth are destined to grow. These *dental lamina* are induced to proliferate focally and thicken by the adjacent mesenchymal cells within the future alveolar ridges *(bud stage).* Tooth development begins first in the mandible and then the maxilla, proceeding from front to back (Fig. 50-1).

The foremost epithelial cells in the dental lamina form a cap-shaped structure, the primitive enamel organ *(cap stage).* As this cap expands to resemble a bell, the ectodermal cells differentiate into three layers *(bell stage):* a peripheral layer of palisaded, cuboidal cells (external enamel epithelium), a middle, loosely arranged network of epithelial cells within a mucopolysaccharide-rich matrix (stellate reticulum), and an inner layer of columnar cells (internal enamel epithelium). The cells of the internal enamel epithelium will become

STAGES OF TOOTH DEVELOPMENT

Morphodifferentiation phase
Bud stage
Cap stage
Bell stage
Histodifferentiation phase

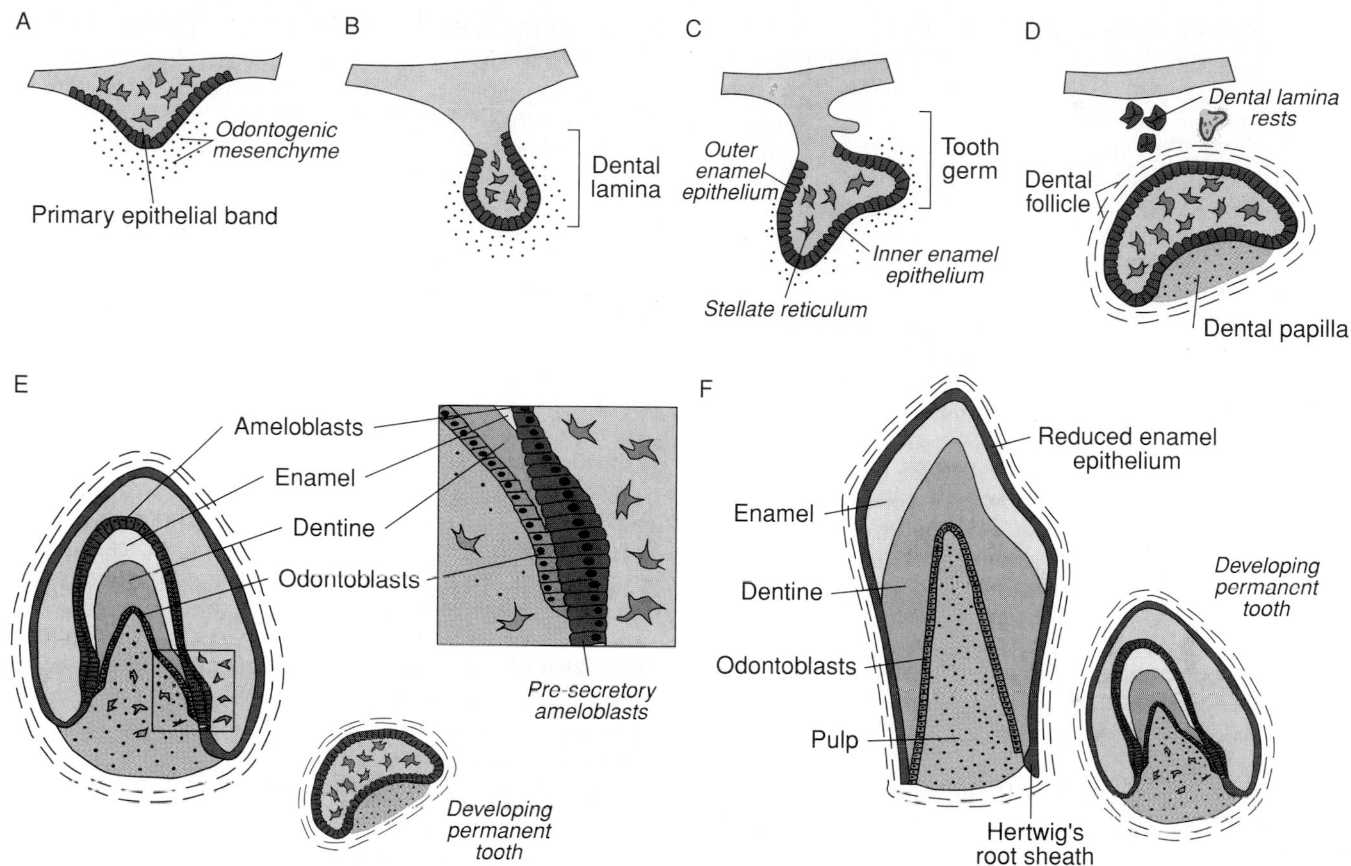

Fig. 50-1 **A,** By 6 weeks in utero horseshoe-shaped thickenings within the ectoderm covering the maxillary and mandibular processes give rise to the primary epithelial bands. **B,** The primary epithelial bands grow inward to produce the dental lamina, which gives rise to the dentition. Localized proliferation within the dental lamina leads to the formation of a series of epithelial ingrowths, the tooth germs. **C,** The tooth germ develops into a cap-shaped structure comprising an inner and outer layer of regular cuboidal epithelial cells, the inner and outer enamel epithelia. Sandwiched between the two layers is the stellate reticulum, which comprises loosely packed epithelial cells with prominent desmosomal junctions. **D,** As the tooth germ develops, the odontogenic mesenchyme related to the concavity of the cap becomes densely cellular and forms the dental papilla, which eventually gives rise to the dental pulp. The odontogenic mesenchyme immediately surrounding the tooth germ is known as the dental follicle, and this eventually gives rise to the supporting tissues of the tooth, including cementum and periodontal ligament. **E,** Regional differences in growth pressure cause folding of the inner enamel epithelium, and the tooth germ becomes bell shaped. The cuboidal cells of inner enamel epithelium elongate and their nuclei become aligned adjacent to the stellate reticulum (reversed polarity). Concomitantly, subjacent cells in the dental papilla line up below the inner enamel epithelium and differentiate into odontoblasts, which start to elaborate dentine matrix. Dentine formation induces the cells of the inner enamel epithelium to mature into ameloblasts, which start to move away from the dentine, secreting enamel matrix as they go. **F,** As the ameloblasts move toward the outer enamel epithelium, the stellate reticulum atrophies, and eventually the inner and outer enamel epithelia meet and combine to form the reduced enamel epithelium. Although enamel is confined to the crown, odontogenic epithelium is required to initiate dentine formation in the root. Cells derived from the reduced enamel epithelium proliferate downwards, forming Hertwig's root sheath, which induces dentine formation and maps out the form of the root. Once the root sheath has begun dentine formation it atrophies, leaving behind it isolated epithelial islands, the cell rests of Malassez. (From Tinkler S: The jaws. In McGee JO'D, Isaacson PG, Wright NA, editors: *The Oxford textbook of pathology of systems,* vol 2, Oxford, 1992, Oxford University Press.)

ameloblasts and produce the enamel covering the crown of the tooth. The mesenchyme contained within the bell-shaped enamel organ will become the dental papilla, from which the odontoblasts (producers of dentin) and the central pulp will arise. The mesenchyme around the enlarging tooth germ is compressed to form a dental sac or follicle that surrounds the tooth.

During this bell stage of odontogenesis, some ectodermal cells extend lingually from the outer epithelial cell layer of the enamel organ to become the dental lamina anlage for the successional permanent teeth, and some cells extend posteriorly to form the anlage for the nonsuccessional permanent molar teeth. In the late bell stage, a fourth layer of flattened cells, the stratum intermedium, forms between the stellate reticulum and the internal enamel epithelium. That strand of ectoderm from which the tooth developed, the dental lamina, breaks up as the hard tissues of the teeth form, leaving nests of odontogenic epithelium (the epithelial rests of Serres).

Histodifferentiation phase

The next phase of tooth development is that of histodifferentiation, the time of which varies for the different teeth. The ameloblasts mature and induce maturation of the contiguous mesenchymal cells (within the dental papilla) into odontoblasts. The odontoblasts produce dentinal matrix, which in turn induces the ameloblasts to begin producing enamel matrix. Hertwig's epithelial root sheath forms where the inner and outer layers of odontogenic epithelium meet at the "rim" of the bell-shaped tooth germ. This epithelium promotes root dentin formation by inducing odontoblast formation but does not produce enamel. After root dentinogenesis begins, the root sheath epithelium breaks up, leaving epithelial rests of Malassez entrapped within the developing periodontium.

Mesenchymal cells in the dental sac adjacent to the dentin differentiate into cementoblasts and produce bonelike cementum over the newly formed dentin. More peripheral mesenchymal cells become osteoblasts and help form the alveolar bone to support and cradle the teeth. Connective tissue fibers from the dental sac, known as "Sharpey's fibers," become embedded in the forming cementum and bone around the roots, mineralize, and form the periodontal ligament, anchoring the tooth to the surrounding alveolar bone.

Although root dentinogenesis continues, the enamel organ regresses to become a thin layer, the reduced enamel epithelium. Before the tooth erupts, this epithelium (which covers and formed the enamel, to which it is still attached) fuses with the overlying epithelium at the gingival crest. The incisal edge or the cuspal surface of the tooth then penetrates these epithelia to erupt into the oral cavity. After the enamel organ is destroyed, no more enamel can be produced.

Except for the ectodermally derived enamel, the tooth structures arise from the mesenchyme in the maxillary and mandibular processes. This oral mesoderm is believed to be of neural crest origin and is also described as neuroectoderm or ectomesenchyme.

The dental lamina remains active for about 5 years before it breaks up. Rests of odontogenic epithelium (the rests of Serres from the dental lamina, the rests of Malassez from the epithelial root sheath, and residues of the enamel organs) remain within the jaws and gingivae. Infrequently, they give rise to odontogenic cysts and tumors, which are unique to this part of the body. The specialized odontogenic mesoderm may also, on occasion, form tumors that are specific for the jaws.

Structure of erupted teeth

There are normally 20 *deciduous* (primary) *teeth,* which have all erupted by 3 years of age. The *permanent* (secondary) *teeth* begin to erupt at about 6 years of age, and the deciduous teeth are usually gone by about 13 years of age. By age 14 the permanent teeth have all erupted, though the third molars ("wisdom teeth") may erupt later or become impacted within the jaw. There are 32 permanent teeth, which are, from front to back: central incisor, lateral incisor, canine, first and second premolars, and first through third molars (four of each).[18]

Teeth have three parts. The *crown* of an erupted tooth is the part covered with enamel and projecting into the oral cavity. The *root* of the tooth is the part covered with cementum and embedded in the periodontium. The *neck* is the constricted portion of the tooth at the junction of crown and root, where the tooth emerges above the gingival line. Prominent projections on the occlusal surface of the crown are cusps. The tip (deepest part) of the tooth root or roots is the apex. Teeth can be identified by their shape and the number of cusps and roots present.

The mature tooth has a myxomatous core, the *pulp,* with vessels and nerves. The pulp is surrounded by a zone of odontoblasts. Surrounding both pulp and odontoblasts is *dentin,* which composes most of the tooth. Dentin is characterized by dentinal tubules that contain the long cellular processes of the odontoblasts. The dentin of the crown is covered by *enamel.* Enamel is the hardest material in the body, composed almost entirely of hydroxyapatite arranged in tightly packed hexagonal rods (being mostly mineral, mature enamel rarely survives decalcification and is infrequently seen in histologic sections). The dentin of the root is covered by bonelike *cementum,* which is attached to the alveolar bone by the connective tissue fibers of the periodontal ligament.

Periodontium refers to the structures that support the teeth: gingiva, periodontal ligament, cementum, and alveolar bone.[19] The alveolar bone is the ridge on the maxilla and the mandible in which the teeth are embedded. In the maxilla, there may be little bone separating the teeth and maxillary sinuses.

Structure of the mouth (oral cavity) and pharynx

Anatomy of the mouth

The anterior wall of the oral cavity is formed by the lips and oral orifice (encircled by the labial vermilion border). The superior border (roof) of the mouth is the hard palate. The inner (buccal) surface of the cheeks forms the lateral walls. The floor of the oral cavity is the anterior two thirds of the tongue. Posteriorly, the oral cavity is divided from the oropharynx at the fauces (from the Latin faux, a 'gorge' or 'narrow pass'). The faucial opening is defined by the arch formed where the hard and soft palates join above and by the line formed by the circumvallate papillae of the tongue below. Two vertical bands of muscle, like paired columns on each side of the fauces, are the tonsillar pillars.

Projecting into the mouth are the alveolar ridges (with gingivae and teeth) and tongue. The labial sulcus (buccal sulcus) is the gutter separating the alveolar ridges from the lips and cheeks. The lingual frenulum is a vertical fold of tissue on the ventral surface of the tongue. On either side of the frenulum is a small eminence, the sublingual caruncle. The duct of each submandibular gland (Wharton's duct) and the ducts of each major sublingual gland empty into the mouth through separate openings on the sublingual caruncles. The ducts of the parotid glands (Stensen's duct) drain into the mouth through an opening lateral to each second upper molar. The space posterior to the last molars is the retromolar trigone.

Histology of the mouth

The skin of the external lips transforms to the stratified squamous mucosa of the oral cavity at the vermilion border. There are three types of oral mucosae. The *lining mucosa* (buccal, labial, and alveolar mucosae, and mucosae of the soft palate, floor of the mouth, and ventral surface of tongue) is mostly nonkeratinized with broad rete ridges overlying vascular fibrous tissue. The dorsal surface of the tongue is covered by *specialized mucosa,* adapted for taste and mastication. It has a thick parakeratotic stratified squamous epithelium with many areas of specialization (filiform, fungiform, circumvallate and foliate papillae, and associated taste buds). The *masticatory mucosa* of the hard palate and contiguous gingiva is orthokeratinized or parakeratinized with prominent rete ridges and little submucosa. Increased orthokeratosis and parakeratosis and prominent rete ridges (acanthosis) often develop in areas of chronic irritation or inflammation (from ill-fitting dentures, cheek biting, tobacco use, and so forth).

The keratinized gingival mucosa (gum) surrounds each tooth where it leaves its bony socket and extends over the alveolar ridge to merge with the alveolar mucosa. A small sulcus lies between the tooth and the bulk of the gingiva that, under ideal conditions, is less than 1 mm deep. The mucosa of this gingival sulcus is generally thin and nonkeratinized.

Melanocytes are normally present in oral mucosa but are often inconspicuous on hematoxylin and eosin–stained sections where they appear as clear cells between the basal squamous cells. They are better demonstrated on silver stains or with S-100 antibody staining, where their dendritic shape can be appreciated. Melanocytes derive from neuroectodermal cells that migrate to the oral epithelium during embryonic life, similar to skin melanocytes.

The submucosa of the mouth contains variable numbers of minor salivary glands, generally mucus secreting but also of serous type. The hard palate and tongue are particularly rich in mucous glands. The submucosa of the sulcal gingival mucosa often contains chronic inflammatory cells, dense fibrous tissue (extensions of the periodontal ligaments), and rests of odontogenic epithelium. The deeper tissues of the mouth elsewhere often contain skeletal muscle fibers (the orbicularis oris muscle of the lips, the buccinator muscle fibers of the cheeks, and the muscle of the tongue) and sometimes adipose tissue. The deep tissue of the hard palate is bone and periosteum.

Anatomy of the pharynx

The pharynx is divided into three parts: the nasopharynx, oropharynx, and the hypopharynx. The oropharynx is separated from the nasopharynx above by the soft palate, but the oropharynx is continuous with the hypopharynx below, and their separation is demarcated by the plane of the epiglottic tip.[20]

Anteriorly the *nasopharynx* communicates with the nasal cavity through the posterior nares (choanae). Superiorly and posteriorly the nasopharynx is defined by the base of the skull (sphenoid and occipital bones) and laterally by the temporal bones (through which the eustachian tubes pass). The floor (or trap door) of the nasopharynx is the mobile soft palate (which opens during breathing and closes during swallowing and speaking).

The soft palate is also the roof of the *oropharynx*. Anterior to the oropharynx is the opening to the mouth (fauces) above and the posterior aspect of the tongue below. The epiglottis is the anterior floor of the oropharynx and demarcates where the hypopharynx begins, behind it. Thus the oropharynx is the crossing point for the respiratory and digestive passageways, and food and fluid are kept out of the nasal and bronchial passages by the twin closing of the soft palate and epiglottis during swallowing.

The *hypopharynx* is shaped somewhat like a funnel but is indented anteriorly by the larynx. The lateral recesses of the hypopharynx, which partially embrace the intrusive larynx, are the piriform sinuses. Lateral to the piriform sinuses is cervical soft tissue containing the common carotid artery. The wide part of the funnel opens into the oropharynx above, and the narrow part of the funnel empties into the esophagus below (this separation is at the level of the inferior pharyngeal constrictor muscle).

The *parapharyngeal space* lies beyond the lateral submucosa of the pharynx. This "space" is composed of loose connective tissue containing the internal carotid artery, internal jugular vein, cranial nerves IX to XII, cervical sympathetic chain, vagal and carotid bodies, and lymph nodes. Lateral to the parapharyngeal space are the mandibular ramus, pterygoid lamina, and deep lobe of the parotid gland. The *retropharyngeal space* is a thin layer of loose connective tissue between the posterior walls of the oropharynx and hypopharynx in front and the prevertebral fascia behind.

Histology of the pharynx

The mucosa of the oropharynx and hypopharynx is covered by nonkeratinized stratified squamous epithelium (keratinization may occur in areas of chronic irritation). The anterior wall and the roof of the nasopharynx are mostly surfaced by respiratory epithelium, which abruptly or gradually gives way to the nonkeratinized stratified squamous epithelium lining the remaining nasopharynx (sometimes the respiratory and squamous epithelium are separated by intermediate epithelium, blending features of both).

The submucosa of the pharynx is composed of connective tissue rich in blood vessels, lymphatic vessels, seromucinous glands, and lymphoid tissue. Scattered about the submucosa of the nasopharynx are aggregates of lymphoid tissue, the pharyngeal tonsil (adenoid). Between the tonsillar pillars of the fauces lie the relatively large palatine tonsils (often simply referred to as "tonsils"). The palatine tonsils have invaginations of the surface epithelium, the tonsillar crypts, which occasionally contain *Actinomyces* colonies. The base of the tongue also has abundant lymphoid tissue, the lingual tonsil, and there are patches of lymphoid tissue in the oropharynx and hypopharynx. Together, the pharyngeal, palatine, and lingual tonsils form a discontinuous band of lymphoid tissue encircling the aerodigestive passageways, known as *Waldeyer's ring*. The tonsils are generally more prominent in children.

DEVELOPMENTAL ANOMALIES

Common variations

Fordyce's granules (Fordyce's spots)

Intraoral sebaceous glands, particularly common near the angles of the mouth, open directly onto the mucosal surface of the lips and appear white. These are benign and common but are occasionally mistaken for more significant lesions and biopsies are performed.

Physiologic and racial mucosal pigmentation

The degree of oral pigmentation is related to age and racial skin pigmentation. There is little oral pigmentation at birth, and most is deposited during the first decade of life. Nearly all blacks have oral pigmentation, followed in decreasing frequency by Asians, those of Mediterranean background, and northern Europeans. This physiologic pigmentation predominantly involves the lips and gingivae and is symmetric and persistent. The appearance is usually characteristic but occasionally may be difficult to distinguish from smoker's melanosis, Peutz-Jeghers syndrome, or Addison's disease. Disorders of oral mucosal pigmentation are discussed later in this chapter.

Leukoedema

Symmetric, gray-white areas on the buccal mucosa are found in half of black children, 90% of black adults, and occasionally in white adults. The cause of this asymptomatic condition is unknown. The condition is usually not examined through biopsy, but the histologic features show epithelial parakeratosis and acanthosis, with pronounced intracellular edema (causing enlargement, cytoplasmic clearing, and nuclear pyknosis) of the spinous cells. There is no inflammation, no increased malignant potential, and no need for therapy. The significance of this condition is that it should not be confused with leukoplakia (discussed later) or white sponge nevus.

Hairy tongue

Hairy tongue is a clinically descriptive term for a condition in which there is hypertrophy of the filiform papillae on the dorsal surface of the tongue, with accumulation of bacteria, fungi, keratin, and foreign debris. The color varies from white to tan to dark, depending on the contents of this coating (such as keratin, tobacco residues, products of chromogenic bacteria, and dietary pigments). Hairy tongue is more of an unsightly or disconcerting overgrowth than a disease, and individuals with this condition are usually asymptomatic (infrequently the papillae are so long as to cause a tickling or gagging sensation). Although usually idiopathic, it may occur after use of antibiotics, systemic corticosteroids, or local radiation therapy. The condition is benign, gradually disappearing in most people after discontinuation of any predisposing agents and attention to proper oral hygiene.

Cleft lip and palate

Facial cleft problems are a common type of developmental anomaly,[21] ranging from 1 in 250 births in Native Americans, to 1 in 800 births in whites, to 1 in 2500 births in blacks. About 20% of cases are associated with other anomalies or syndromes (there are over 200 cleft syndromes). When one parent has a cleft, the risk of his or her child having a cleft is about 10%. Clefts result from failure of the facial processes to fuse at about the seventh week in utero. They are more common in males than females (3:2), are more often unilateral than bilateral (8:1), and are more common on the left than on the right (2:1).

Clefts usually involve the upper lip (harelip) and range from a shallow notch to a deep gap extending to the nasal cavity. About half of cleft lips are associated with cleft palate. Clefts where the primary and secondary palates fuse interfere with the development of the lateral incisor, usually leading to a missing maxillary lateral incisor. Cleft lip and palate with micrognathia are orofacial features of trisomy 13 (Patau's syndrome), which also includes abnormalities of brain, heart, viscera, genitalia, and hand development.

Palatal clefts range in severity from minor (cleft uvula, submucous cleft) to large defects interfering with sucking and swallowing. Cleft (bifid) uvula is fairly common and usually insignificant. Submucous clefts may not be noticed unless associated with speech impairment. Cleft palate without cleft lip is more common in females. Isolated cleft palate is associated with Down and Pierre Robin syndromes.[12]

Down syndrome (trisomy 21) has numerous oral manifestations, both developmental anomalies and those attributable to immune deficits: short or cleft palate, maxillary hypoplasia, macroglossia, abnormalities of lingual papillae and tooth development, periodontal disease, acute ulcerative gingivitis, and candidiasis.[22]

Pierre Robin syndrome is characterized by cleft palate, small mandible (micrognathia), a small, posteriorly displaced tongue (microglossia with glossoptosis) leading to respiratory difficulties, and abnormalities of the larynx. Pierre Robin syndrome may be associated with an autosomal recessive defect in type II collagen synthesis (Stickler syndrome), with fetal alcohol, methadone, and hydantoin syndromes, with mental retardation, or with heart anomalies.

Anomalies of teeth

Positioning. The most common problem of tooth development is poor positioning; the teeth are not straight, do not properly appose their neighbors, or do not meet their counterparts in the other jaw *(malocclusion)*. This problem can be cosmetic or interfere with mastication and is corrected by orthodontic treatments such as braces. Another common problem is that of third molars becoming impacted within the alveolar bone, preventing eruption, interfering with the position of the other molar teeth, and occasionally becoming infected. These impacted molars are excised, often being broken up in the process of removal.

Number. Complete absence of teeth (total anodontia) is rare and usually associated with congenital ectodermal dysplasia. The absence of one or more teeth (hypodontia) is often familial. One or more supernumerary teeth (hyperdontia) sometimes occur, usually one or a pair of small mesiodentes posterior to the maxillary incisors, where they can interfere with the position and eruption of the normal teeth. Occasionally, there are extra molars, posterior to the third molars.

Eruption. About 1 in 2000 infants is born with teeth (natal teeth), which may lacerate the infant's tongue, detach and be aspirated, or cause maternal discomfort during breast feeding. Delays in eruption may result from many causes including impaction and cretinism.

Size. Abnormalities of a tooth's size (macrodontia and microdontia) occur occasionally. Rarely, all the teeth are too large or too small.

Shape. Misshapen teeth occasionally occur. The lateral maxillary incisors may be pegshaped. Congenital syphilis results in screwdriver-shaped incisors and other abnormalities of tooth formation (to be discussed later). Rarely, teeth are fused. The crown may be finely nodular, like a raspberry. Roots may be deformed or branch abnormally.

Enamel formation. The disturbances in enamel formation may involve one or all of the teeth. The enamel may have pits or pearls. Enamel hypoplasia results in pits and fissures in the crown. Factors disrupting enamel formation include nutritional deficiencies (such as rickets), infectious diseases (such as measles, congenital syphilis, infection of a deciduous precursor), endocrine disturbances (such as hypoparathyroidism, pseudohypoparathyroidism), and tetracycline. *Amelogenesis imperfecta* is a rare autosomal dominant disorder in which the enamel is soft, yellow-brown, and hypocalcified. *Enamel pearls* are spherical masses of enamel attached to a tooth, which are formed by aberrant ameloblasts.

Dentinogenesis. In rickets, the dentin is hypocalcified with wide predentin seams analogous to the wide osteoid seams in the newly formed osteomalacic bone. *Dentinogenesis imperfecta,* a rare (1 in 8000 persons), autosomal dominant disorder occasionally seen in white children, is characterized by opalescent, undermineralized dentin causing brown to blue teeth. The enamel is normally formed, but the attachment with the dentin is poor, and it fractures off quickly to expose short brown stumps of dentin. *Radicular dentin dysplasia* is characterized by normal-appearing crowns over rootless and pulpless teeth.

Coloration. Teeth are often discolored by *exogenous stains* that can be removed by abrasives. Common examples in adults include staining caused by tobacco use, tea, coffee, and other substances in the diet. In children, thin lines of brown or black may form along the gingival border of teeth, as a result of chromogenic bacteria in dental plaque. Green, yellow, or orange stains may also occur.

Endogenous (or *intrinsic*) *stains* occur during tooth development and are attributable to deposition of substances from the blood; these substances are incorporated within the enamel, not just on the tooth surface. The best known example of endogenous staining is the discoloration produced by tetracycline. At first the erupted teeth will be bright yellow and will fluoresce with ultraviolet light. With time, the tetracycline oxidizes and the enamel changes color to gray or brown with loss of fluorescence. Remember that tetracycline usually does not cause tooth discoloration in children and that the staining is related to the patient's age and the dosage and duration of drug administration.

Severe erythroblastosis fetalis may cause green or bluish-black discoloration of the deciduous teeth. Maternal antibodies against Rh+ fetal red blood cells cross the placenta and cause intravascular hemolysis in the fetus. The released hemoglobin breakdown products (such as bilirubin) are incorporated into the developing teeth. Severe congenital liver disease can cause green to yellow-brown discoloration of teeth attributable to deposition of bilirubin. Congenital porphyria can lead to red or brown teeth that fluoresce with ultraviolet light because of the deposition of porphyrin.

Anomalies of the tongue

Enlarged tongue (macroglossia). Congenital enlargement of the tongue is usually caused by a vascular malformation (lymphangioma or hemangioma). Muscular hypertrophy, congenital neurofibromatosis, Down syndrome, congenital hypothyroidism, and numerous other conditions can cause congenital enlargement. Enlargement of half of the tongue as a result of one-sided muscular hypertrophy is associated with *congenital hemifacial hypertrophy* (unilateral enlargement of teeth, bones of the head, and lingual papillae may also be present). Causes of tongue enlargement in adults include myxedema, acromegaly, tumor, and amyloidosis.

Cleft tongue. Cleft tongue is a rare congenital anomaly, a defect in the first branchial arch in which the lateral portions of the tongue fail to fuse.

Microglossia and aglossia. Microglossia and aglossia are rare congenital anomalies often associated with other defects. Atrophy of the tongue in adults may be unilateral or bilateral, occurring after hypoglossal nerve damage caused by inflammation or trauma.

Fissured tongue. Approximately 1% of children have fissured tongue, but it may appear after puberty. Also called "scrotal" or plicated tongue, it has little significance except that it is associated with several other conditions. Fissured tongue is commonly present with *erythema migrans* (also known as "migratory glossitis" or "geographic tongue"), in which the filiform papillae focally desquamate to form irregular smooth pink areas surrounded by a yellow-white border. Fissured tongue is one feature of the *Melkersson-Rosenthal syndrome* (also including facial paralysis, facial swelling, and plicated oral mucosal swelling). Fissured tongue has a higher incidence with Down's syndrome and psoriasis.

Lingual thyroid. During embryonic development, the thyroid anlage originates from the posterior tongue (at the site of the foramen cecum in adults) from where it tracks down to its normal position in the anterior neck. The thyroglossal tract then atrophies, but occasional remnants undergo cystic enlargement. Rarely these remnants become infected, or enlarged and hyperfunctional. The midline of the upper neck is a much more common site for this to occur, but, very rarely, cystic tract remnants or thyroid tissue masses occur in the tongue. The cystic rests are usually lined by squamous epithelium, but ciliated columnar epithelium may also be present. Reddish thyroid tissue is sometimes visible on the posterior area of the tongue, but the amount of thyroid tissue varies.

Anomalies of the pharynx and tonsils

Branchial fistula is a rare communication between the skin on the side of the neck and a tonsillar crypt, resulting from persistence of the second branchial groove and second pharyngeal pouch.

X-linked (Bruton's) agammaglobulinemia is attributable to a defect in B-cell differentiation.[23] Mature B cells are usually absent, and so there is *hypoplasia of the lymphoid tissue* of the pharynx and intestinal sites. This disorder has an incidence of 1 in 100,000 and affects boys, beginning in infancy.[24]

Anomalies of the jaws

Prognathism (also known as "exognathia" or "prognathia") is abnormal protrusion of the mandible and may be developmental or acquired (as in acromegaly). *Hypognathism* (also known as "hypognathia") is abnormal recession of the mandible relative to the maxilla and is usually developmental or occurs after bone resorption in edentulous individuals. These conditions may cause malocclusion of the teeth as well as cosmetic concern, but surgical reconstruction has made great strides, even in severe cases.

Benign bony overgrowths (exostoses) may occur on the palate or lingual aspect of the mandible and are referred to as *torus palatinus* and *torus mandibularis,* respectively. Palatal tori form a midline nodule or ridge, whereas mandibular tori often form a shelf or are lobulated. Tori are usually asymptomatic and are discovered incidentally.

INFECTIOUS DISEASES

Infectious diseases of the oral cavity and pharynx are very common, particularly pharyngitis. Pharyngitis (sore throat) is most common in children but annually accounts for approximately 40 million visits by adults to physicians in the United States. Pharyngitis is most often attributable to viruses, followed by bacteria (most often streptococci) and rarely (usually as opportunists) fungi (Table 50-1). *Streptococcus pyogenes* is the most important cause of pharyngitis because of the possibility of serious complications. In most cases, it is difficult to distinguish clinically between viral and bacterial pharyngitis; the severity of symptoms and the presence of exudate are not very reliable indicators. (Pharyngitis is further discussed below, by etiologic agent.)

Table 50-1 Infectious causes of pharyngitis

Class of agent	Specific examples
Viruses	Adenoviruses
	Rhinoviruses
	Enteroviruses (including Coxsackieviruses)
	Influenzaviruses
	Parainfluenza viruses
	Respiratory syncytial viruses
	Coronaviruses
	Echoviruses
	Herpes simplex type I
	Epstein-Barr virus
Bacteria	Streptococci (groups A, C, and G)
	Corynebacterium diphtheriae
	Mycoplasma pneumoniae
	Neisseria gonorrhoeae
	Treponema pallidum
	Haemophilus influenzae
	Miscellaneous oral commensals
Fungi	*Candida albicans*

Acute infections of the upper respiratory tract (rhinitis, oropharyngitis, tonsillitis, sinusitis, laryngitis, and bronchitis) may occur together or sequentially, and the site of predominant symptoms and clinical findings determines the specific diagnosis. Acute otitis media is usually attributable to extension of infection from the nose and nasopharynx and is a common complication in children.

Bacterial infections

Bacterial pharyngitis. Approximately 15% to 20% of all pharyngeal infections are caused by beta-hemolytic streptococci. Group A beta-hemolytic streptococci *(S. pyogenes)* frequently cause a pharyngitis (called "strep throat") that is easily spread by respiratory droplets, often from asymptomatic nasal carriers. Any age is susceptible, but infection is most common in children between 5 and 15 years of age. Infection is heralded by abrupt onset of sore throat and fever, sometimes with pain on swallowing, headache, malaise, and anorexia. The throat is red and swollen. The tonsils are enlarged and often covered by gray or yellow exudate. The appearance is not characteristic unless the tonsillar pillars and soft palate are red with petechiae. Painful anterior cervical lymphadenopathy is a common finding. Confirmation of diagnosis is by throat culture or more recently developed rapid immunoassays.

Treatment is penicillin and analgesia. Complications of untreated or inadequately treated strep throat are divided into suppurative and nonsuppurative. Suppurative complications include perinasal sinusitis, otitis media, mastoiditis, and, less commonly, peritonsillar abscess, lymphadenitis, and bacteremia. Nonsuppurative complications include rheumatic fever and poststreptococcal glomerulonephritis.

Erythrogenic toxin-producing streptococci can cause *scarlet fever* in nonimmunized patients (usually in children with no prior exposure). The erythematous rash usually appears within a few days of the onset of sore throat, starting in the neck and upper trunk, and progressing peripherally. The enanthema of scarlet fever involves the tongue (raspberry or strawberry tongue). Other bacteria causing pharyngitis include group C and group G streptococci, *Neisseria gonorrhoeae, Treponema pallidum, Corynebacterium diphtheriae,* and *Mycoplasma pneumoniae*. In immunosuppressed patients, oral commensals may cause infection. *Haemophilus influenzae* may colonize the pharynx and rarely causes a painful, nonexudative pharyngitis. In most cases, the etiologic agent (whether bacterial or viral) cannot be identified clinically, and so culture (or one of several specific tests) is used when this determination is clinically desirable. Noninfectious causes of pharyngitis include allergies, postnasal discharge, pollutants, smoking, and other irritants.

Acute tonsillitis. Most common in children, exudative infection of the tonsils is usually attributable to beta-hemolytic streptococci, pneumococcus, *H. influenzae,* or respiratory viruses. Transmission is primarily by droplets. There is rapid onset of fever, with increasing sore throat, odynophagia, and sometimes a sensation of fullness in the throat. Nasal symptoms (obstruction, discharge) and systemic symptoms (malaise, chills, arthralgia, myalgia) may also be present. The breath may be foul. The enlarged, erythematous tonsils have a white-yellow exudate. The lingual tonsils and adenoids may be similarly affected, and reactive lymphoid hyperplasia of the latter may block the eustachian tube and lead to otitis media. The pharynx is also inflamed, and there may be cervical lymphadenopathy and leukocytosis.

Treatment is antibiotics after culturing the exudate. Culture may dictate a change in the initial antibiotic coverage and helps to exclude diphtheria. Inadequately treated tonsillitis may lead to tonsillar ulceration, peritonsillar abscess (quinsy), or parapharyngeal cellulitis.

Recurrent tonsillitis. Repeated infections can lead to enlargement of the tonsils and possible airway obstruction. Tonsillectomy may benefit selected patients.

"Chronic tonsillitis" is a term used by many pathologists in referring to lymphoid hyperplasia of surgically removed tonsils. Because this lymphoid hyperplasia is very common and probably the normal condition in children, this term may be inappropriate.

Diphtheria. Caused by the toxigenic, pleomorphic, gram-positive bacillus *Corynebacterium diphtheriae,* diphtheria is now infrequently reported. It is spread by respiratory droplets, by cutaneous lesions, or on fomites. Symptoms are nonspecific and include gradual onset of sore throat (which is not usually severe), a mild fever, and progressive systemic symptoms of nausea, vomiting, and headache. The tonsils and pharynx are inflamed and covered by an adherent gray membrane. When the membrane is rubbed off by a culture swab, the pharyngeal mucosa bleeds and has a musty odor. Other signs typically include mildly elevated temperature, tachycardia, and anterior cervical lymphadenopathy. Hoarseness and croupy cough indicate laryngeal involvement. Stain of the lesional smear supports the diagnosis, but confirmation by culture and toxigenic assay is necessary.

Although diphtherial infection of the skin, anterior nares, and middle ear is often mild, nonspecific, and undiagnosed, rapid diagnosis of pharyngeal diphtheria with isolation and immediate initiation of treatment is important. The necrotizing mucositis can extend into the larynx or bronchi, and the necrotic-inflammatory membrane may cause airway obstruction with stridor and cyanosis. Some *C. diphtheriae* produce a phage-mediated exotoxin that can lead to systemic complications (vascular collapse, myocarditis with arrhythmias, and neuritis with cranial and peripheral nerve paralysis). Rarely, *C. diphtheriae* are invasive, causing bacteremia, sepsis, and endocarditis. Treatment includes (1) prevention of complications such as airway obstruction, (2) diphtheria antitoxin in patients who are not hypersensitive, and (3) antibiotics. Note that diphtheria vaccine induces antibodies against the exotoxin but does not prevent *C. diphtheriae* infection.

Anaerobic bacteria. Normally present in the mouth, anaerobes play an important role in tooth infections (plaque, caries, root canal infection), periodontal infections (gingivitis, periapical abscess, osteomyelitis of the jaws), acute necrotizing ulcerative gingivitis (ANUG), noma, and infections occurring after head and neck surgery. These oral commensals include peptostreptococci, fusobacteria, and *Bacteroides* (usually not *B. fragilis*) species.

Acute necrotizing ulcerative gingivitis (Vincent's disease, fusospirochetosis). The cause of the rare condition acute necrotizing ulcerative gingivitis (ANUG) is only partly understood but does not appear to be contagious. Emotional stress, smoking, and Down's syndrome are predisposing factors that may suppress host immune mechanisms, permitting infection of the gingiva by organisms normally present there, including *Bacteroides intermedius*, fusiform bacteria (such as *Fusobacterium necrophorum*) and a spirochete, *Borrelia vincentii*. The age range is generally 15 to 30 years, though it also occurs in African children. ANUG is also associated with human immunodeficiency virus (HIV) infection where it can appear gradually or suddenly.[25]

Gingival necrosis starts between the teeth (in the interdental papillae) and rapidly extends to the free gingival margin and the entire gum. Rarely, ANUG extends to the fauces, the mucosa of the soft palate and tonsils (Vincent's angina, membranous tonsillitis), and the patient has sore throat. The necrotic mucosa ulcerates, and the patient has fetid breath and local discomfort, sometimes with concurrent mild fever and lymphadenopathy. The ulcers are covered by a pseudomembrane of fibrinoinflammatory exudate, necrotic debris, and bacteria. Adjacent teeth often have calculus deposits.

The vernacular term "trench mouth" derives from the frequency of this condition in the trenches at the front lines in World War I but is also used for other vesicular and ulcerative lesions, including herpetic stomatitis, herpangina, bullous pemphigoid, and erosive gingival lichen planus. Herpetic stomatitis is usually in younger patients, has a prodromal fever, and involves other areas of the oral mucosa. Bullous pemphigoid and lichen planus occur in older patients and have bullae and white striae, respectively.

Treatment of ANUG involves debridement of the necrotic tissue followed by hydrogen peroxide gargles, antibiotics, daily brushing, and scrupulous cleaning between the teeth. Relief is usually rapid, but healing of the ulcerated gingiva takes months. Antibiotics are reserved for acutely ill patients. Proper oral hygiene and discontinuance of tobacco use are recommended to prevent recurrence.

Syphilis. Oral lesions caused by *Treponema pallidum* occur in congenital syphilis and in all stages of acquired syphilis. Biopsies of oral lesions are rare and not specific; diagnosis is generally made on clinical appearance, serologic tests, and occasionally on smears.

Oral manifestations of congenital syphilis are now rare because of prenatal screening. Mucocutaneous lesions similar to those of secondary acquired syphilis may be noted at birth. Rhagades (fine radiating scars or fissures) about the mouth occur infrequently, and gummas occur rarely after congenital syphilis. Syphilitic infection of the developing bones can cause short maxilla and high palatal arch. Infection of the developing permanent teeth causes Hutchinson incisors (notched incisors or small, sharp, widely separated incisors resembling the ends of screwdrivers) and mulberry molars (berrylike malformation of the first molars caused by nodular overgrowth of the enamel over small cusps). Note that the primary dentition is not a consideration with syphilis because early infection is fatal to the fetus.

The primary lesion of acquired syphilis, the *chancre*, occurs at the site of inoculation, which, in the mouth, is usually the lips or tongue. The chancre is a painless, slightly firm nodule with focal ulceration and may resemble a cancer. Regional lymphadenopathy is common, and the lesion usually heals within a few months.

Oral mucosal lesions of secondary (disseminated) untreated syphilis occur less often than the skin lesions. The characteristic oral lesion is the mucous patch, a round erosion that is a few centimeters in diameter, is covered by a thin yellowish-gray exudate, and has an erythematous rim. Mucous patches may form confluent serpiginous ("snail-track") ulcers. Patients may have sore throat as a result of pharyngotonsillitis. Oral condylomata lata (elevated broad-based plaques) have also been described in secondary syphilis.

After the lesions of secondary syphilis heal, the untreated patient enters a latent phase that lasts for years. The characteristic but now very rare oral lesions of the tertiary (late) stage of syphilis are the gumma and syphilitic glossitis. Oral gummas, necrotic granulomas that may ulcerate, usually occur in the palate or tongue. Large or multiple gummas can perforate the hard palate or distort the tongue. Syphilitic glossitis, a generalized inflammation of the tongue with mucosal atrophy, is a putative risk factor for the development of squamous cancer of the mouth (this is a historical association that has been questioned because syphilis was formerly treated with arsenical agents known to be carcinogens).

Gonorrhea. Infection by *Neisseria gonorrhoeae* is usually transmitted by orogenital contact. Symptoms and signs of oropharyngeal infection are variable and nonspecific. Patients are usually asymptomatic but may have a sore throat or a burning sensation. The lesions are usually erythematous or ulcerated (less commonly exudative or vesicular) and are more likely to involve pharyngeal mucosa, which appears to be less resistant, than to involve oral mucosa.

Granuloma inguinale. The granulomatous-ulcerative lesions of granuloma inguinale, which are attributable to genital-oral transmission of *Calymmatobacterium granulomatis*, are rarely seen in the mouth.[26]

Actinomycosis. *Actinomyces israelii* is a normal oral saprophyte. Grossly or microscopically visible *Actinomyces* colonies, known as sulfur granules, are frequently seen when one is examining tonsillectomy specimens.[27] Rarely, they are associated with small erosions of the tonsillar crypt epithelium with neutrophilic exudation. *Actinomyces* organisms can cause disease if they penetrate a mucosal barrier, as with cervicofacial actinomycosis (described below) or abdominal actinomycosis, or are aspirated, as with thoracic actinomycosis.

Cervicofacial actinomycosis starts as a painless swelling over the mandible (rarely the maxilla) that progresses to induration of the skin and soft tissues, with draining sinuses in which sulfur granules can be seen. Microscopy reveals granulomas and suppuration with scattered colonies of radiating filamentous bacteria. Cervicofacial actinomycosis is associated with periodontal disease, tooth extraction, gingival surgery, or trauma. Localized infection then spreads to the oral mucous membranes and hence to the soft tissues and skin of the face and the neck. The jawbones are rarely involved. Other Actinomyces species and *Nocardia asteroides* sometimes cause clinically similar infections.

Tuberculosis. Oral lesions attributable to *Mycobacterium tuberculosis* are very rare. Oral tuberculosis is usually attributed to implantation of organisms during chronic coughing by patients with unsuspected or untreated active pulmonary infection. The typical lesion is a stellate or irregular ulcer, most often near the dorsal midline of the tongue. Lips and palate are less common sites. The ulcer may be painful or painless. Sometimes it is nodular, resembling a cancer. Biopsy of the lesion shows granulomas, but caseation and stainable organisms may be sparse. Diagnosis is usually confirmed by chest x-ray film and sputum examination.

Noma (cancrum oris, gangrenous stomatitis). Noma (from the Greek for 'eating sores'), or gangrene of the mouth, is rare except in underdeveloped countries where it primarily occurs in children who are malnourished or debilitated by severe disease. Typically, it begins as a small infected vesicle or ulcer on the gingiva that becomes necrotic. Unchecked, the infection spreads to the lips, buccal mucosa, the deep tissues of the face, and the jawbones. The infected, necrotic tissues become blackened with disfigurement, possible perforation through the cheeks, pneumonia, sepsis, and death. Various bacteria, including *Treponema vincentii* and *Bacteroides melaninogenicus,* have been implicated.

Fungal infections

Most fungal infections in the mouth are attributable to *Candida* species. The remaining fungal infections can be broadly classified as deep or opportunistic.

Deep fungal infections generally represent oral dissemination by sputum or blood from a pulmonary source and often manifest as chronic, nonhealing ulcers. *Histoplasma capsulatum, Coccidioides immitis, Blastomyces dermatitidis,* and *Cryptococcus neoformans* are the most common agents. Biopsy or culture is generally required for diagnosis. The biopsy specimen shows granulomatous inflammation, sometimes with suppuration and pseudoepitheliomatous hyperplasia (particularly with blastomycosis). Fungal stains (such as Gomori's methenamine silver) may facilitate recognition of the organism, including mucicarmine stain for encapsulated cryptococci.

Opportunistic infections of the oral cavity and pharynx occur when systemic health, particularly the immune system, is compromised. *Candida* species are the most common cause of oral mycosis and are associated with immunosuppression and numerous other conditions (Table 50-2). Poorly controlled diabetics may become infected with *Mucor* and *Rhizopus* species, from bread mold or decaying fruit and vegetables. These infections, referred to as phycomycosis or mucormycosis, usually cause pain, swelling, and ulceration in the nasal cavity and paranasal sinuses but can also involve the oropharynx and rarely cause palatal perforation. Identification is by biopsy or culture. Biopsy shows acute and chronic inflammation, and there is often necrosis because these fungi are angiocentric and angiodestructive. The broad, nonseptate hyphae, branching at right angles, are easy to identify with hematoxylin and eosin (H&E) stain.

Table 50-2 Risk factors for oral candidiasis

General cause	Specific examples
Immature immune system	Prematurity Neonates, young infants
Compromised immune system	HIV infection/AIDS Cancer chemotherapy and radiation therapy Therapy to prevent transplant rejection Debilitated, elderly patients Leukemia or advanced malignancy Corticosteroid therapy Malabsorption and malnutrition Primary immunodeficiency
Inherited conditions	Familial chronic mucocutaneous syndromes (immune defects are variable or ill defined)
Altered oral microflora	Antibiotics, particularly broad spectrum Poor oral hygiene Xerostomia (saliva is antimicrobial)
Endocrine disorders	Poorly controlled diabetes mellitus Pregnancy Endocrine candidiasis syndrome
Miscellaneous	Denture use (most common cause in adults) Iron deficiency

Candidiasis (Moniliasis)

Infection by *Candida* species is usually attributable to *Candida albicans,* but other species (that is, *C. tropicalis, C. pseudotropicalis, C. krusei*) sometimes cause oral infection. Diseases attributable to *C. albicans* are difficult to study because it is present in the mouths of over half of asymptomatic people and may be present with other conditions. The relationship between the commensal and pathogenic states of *C. albicans* is complex, involving both local (such as dentures, oral hygiene, perturbation of the normal oral microflora by antibiotics) and systemic (such as endocrine milieu, immunocompetence) factors.

There are numerous manifestations of oral candidiasis, which are described by their location and clinical appearance (Table 50-3). *Acute candidal infection* can cause a loosely adherent, white pseudomembrane (thrush), which must be distinguished from leukoplakia. However, *chronic candidal infection* may manifest as leukoplakia. Some lesions are erythematous, papillary, or ulcerated. Chronic candidiasis causes squamous proliferation and has been suggested as contributing to the development of squamous carcinoma (*C. albicans* produces a carcinogen, *N*-nitrosobenzylmethylamine).

This fungus is dimorphic at body temperature, and the yeast forms (about 2 to 5 μm in diameter, smaller than red blood cells) and pseudohyphae are easy to recognize in cytologic preparations because the organisms favor the superficial portion of the epithelium. Biopsies may be necessary for chronic lesions to distinguish candidal infection from a lesion that is superficially colonized with candidal organisms. H&E stain is often sufficient to demonstrate *Candida* species if there are numerous typical organisms, but fungal stains are more sensitive. If only a few yeast are identified on the surface of a lesion, they may be commensals.

Treatment of candidiasis is with antifungal preparations like nystatin mouthwash. The prognosis is excellent if the underlying condition can be rectified.

Thrush. Also known as "pseudomembranous candidiasis," thrush is very common in patients with HIV infection or who are being treated for cancer with chemotherapy and radiation therapy. Infection is sometimes seen in neonates or young infants (who have incompletely developed immune systems) and debilitated, elderly patients. Symptoms range from minimal to severe burning and tenderness. The pseudomembrane is creamy and easily wiped off to expose an erythematous, eroded, tender mucosa (Fig. 50-2). Lesions are often multiple. The location is usually the buccal mucosa, oropharynx, and lateral edges of the tongue's dorsum. The white pseudomembrane is composed of fungal organisms, squamous cells, keratin debris, inflammatory cells, bacteria, and fibrinous exudate (unlike the gray pseudomembrane of diphtheria that is mostly necrotic slough).

Denture-induced stomatis (denture sore mouth). The common condition denture-induced stomatitis in denture wearers is usually seen on the palate in women. Tight-fitting dentures may prevent the normal exposure of the underlying mucosa to saliva, with its antimicrobial properties, and candidiasis develops (candidiasis associated with xerostomia is presumably attributable to the same mechanism of action). Ill-fitting dentures and failure to remove them at night are also contributory. The area of mucosal erythema and edema corresponds to the covering denture. Although usually asymptomatic, it may prevent proper denture function and lead to angular stomatitis (see below). Microscopy shows *Candida* organisms and inflamed acanthotic epithelium (the leukoplakia or papillary hyperplasia seen with other types of chronic candidiasis is not seen in this condition, possibly why it is inaccurately referred to as "chronic atrophic candidiasis").

Angular stomatitis (angular cheilitis, perlèche). Angular stomatitis is often associated with intraoral candidiasis, especially in patients who have deep grooves at the angles of the mouth or lick their lips. Therefore this condition is most commonly seen in elderly patients with candidal denture stomatitis whose sagging facial tissues permit exposure of the skin to infected saliva. A similar condition, seen in chronic lip lickers with oral candidiasis, is called *circumoral candidal dermatitis*. Angular stomatitis caused by *Candida* organisms must be differentiated from that of iron deficiency (with which it may be related) and that of *Staphylococcus aureus*.

Candidal leukoplakia (chronic hypertrophic candidiasis). The plaque in the condition candidal leukoplakia is tightly adherent, unlike the pseudomembrane of thrush. The cause of this usually asymptomatic condition is unknown. Candidal leukoplakia usually involves healthy middle-aged adults and may be associated with heavy cigarette use. When the midline

Table 50-3 Classification of oral candidiasis*

Intraoral
Thrush (pseudomembranous candidiasis)
Acute (immunocompetent individuals)
Chronic (immunosuppressed individuals)
Chronic oral candidiasis (nonthrush)
Denture stomatitis (denture sore mouth)
Candidal leukoplakia (chronic hypertrophic candidiasis)
Median rhomboid glossitis
Inflammatory papillary hyperplasia
Erythematous
Intraoral and extraoral
Chronic mucocutaneous candidiasis
Familial localized (limited) type
Diffuse type (usually sporadic, few familial cases)
Endocrine candidiasis syndromes
Late onset type (thymoma, myasthenia gravis, and so forth)
Lips (These forms are usually a complication of intraoral candidiasis)
Angular stomatitis (angular cheilitis, angular perlèche)
Circumoral candidal dermatitis

*Any of the three major categories may be seen in immunosuppressed individuals, often with chronic, refractory, multifocal, and sometimes severe manifestations.

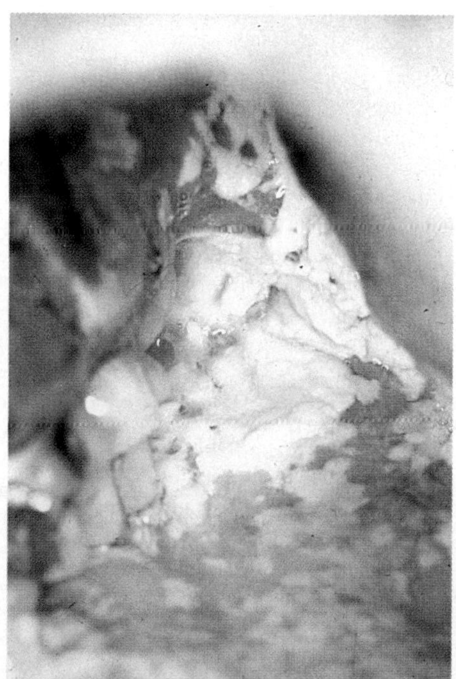

Fig. 50-2 Pseudomembranous candidal infection in an HIV-seropositive patient. Notice the yellowish creamy color.

dorsum of the tongue is involved, there is often a lozenge-shaped area of depapillation referred to as *median rhomboid glossitis* (this condition was formerly believed to be a developmental anomaly). *Inflammatory papillary hyperplasia* usually occurs on the hard palatal mucosa, predominantly beneath complete maxillary dentures (this condition, which may be associated with candidal infection, is discussed later).

Chronic mucocutaneous candidiasis. There are several variants of chronic mucocutaneous candidiasis, most of which have an early age of onset. The oral lesions in these syndromes are similar to the above-described types of candidiasis (though one variant has more extensive oral involvement). These conditions are distinguished by extraoral candidal involvement and other extraoral clinical findings. Although HIV infection and other causes (congenital, acquired, and iatrogenic) of severe immunodeficiency are associated with chronic mucocutaneous candidiasis, an immune defect is not evident in all cases.

The *diffuse type of mucocutaneous candidiasis* is the most severe variant and is generally sporadic. There is severe candidiasis of skin, nails, and mucous (such as oral, vaginal, conjunctival) membranes, as well as bacterial infections of the skin and respiratory tract. This type was formerly called "candidal granuloma" because of the disfiguring epithelial overgrowths, particularly on the face and scalp (this *Candida*-associated epithelial hyperplasia is analogous to the oral mucosal hyperplasia seen in other forms of chronic candidiasis). It is associated with iron-deficiency anemia, and many patients have defective cell-mediated immunity (either diffuse or a specific defect for *C. albicans*).

Familial (limited) mucocutaneous candidiasis usually begins in infancy with thrush, which evolves into chronic leukoplakic candidiasis. Dermal or ungual infection may occur later but is almost always mild. This condition is usually autosomal recessive and is associated with sideropenia. Treatment with iron improves the response to antifungal therapy. Defects in immunity are variable and often unclear, and many patients have no detectable defect.

Many patients with chronic mucocutaneous candidiasis have endocrine disorders, and several *endocrine candidiasis syndromes* have been described. The most common association is with hypoparathyroidism. One cause of this association is *DiGeorge's syndrome* (defective development of third and fourth branchial pouches leading to hypoplasia or aplasia of the thymus and parathyroid glands and other anomalies). Chronic mucocutaneous candidiasis and hypoparathyroidism are also part of *type I polyendocrinopathy syndrome* (which also includes Addison's disease and other endocrine disturbances). Organ-specific antibodies are often present in this autosomal recessive syndrome. Candidiasis is usually mild and often begins in childhood, frequently preceding manifestations of endocrinopathy by several years.

A fourth, rare variant, *late-onset mucocutaneous candidiasis,* is associated with thymoma, myasthenia gravis, pure red blood cell aplasia, and defective cell-mediated immunity.

Viral infections

Viral pharyngitis. Adenoviruses, picornaviruses (rhinoviruses and enteroviruses), myxoviruses (influenza, parainfluenza, and respiratory syncytial viruses), coronaviruses, and herpes simplex type I are causes of viral pharyngitis with scratchy or sore throat. Odynophagia is infrequent with viral pharyngitis. Hoarseness, cough, and rhinitis occur with infection of other sites. Malaise and fever are more common with influenza and adenovirus infections. The mucosa of the pharynx is erythematous and swollen and usually without exudate (though exudate may be seen with adenovirus, herpes, and infectious mononucleosis, as well as streptococcal pharyngitis). Many of these viruses are very contagious, and infection is spread by person-to-person contact, aerosols, or fomites. Treatment is directed toward alleviating systems of this common, vexing, but self-limited condition.

A common manifestation of *infectious mononucleosis* is sore throat. The Epstein-Barr virus (EBV) first infects pharyngeal epithelial cells and then spreads to the mucosal B-lymphocytes (these are the only cell types that carry the EBV receptor, which is also the receptor for the C3b fragment of complement). The B-lymphocytes circulate throughout the body, accounting for the systemic systems of fatigue, malaise, and fever. The tonsils and pharynx are inflamed with a gray exudate, and physical examination will often reveal cervical lymphadenopathy, hepatosplenomegaly, and diffuse rash. Enlarged tonsils and small petechiae on the palate may also be present. Enlargement of the lymphoid tissues is attributable to both follicular hyperplasia and the reaction from activated, atypical-appearing T-lymphocytes.

Herpangina. Coxsackievirus A (occasionally coxsackievirus B or echovirus) causes an acute pharyngitis. Rapid onset of sore throat is accompanied by odynophagia, fever, and lymphadenopathy, usually in children between 3 and 10 years of age. Examination of the soft palate and adjacent pharynx reveals several small herpetic vesicles or ulcers surrounded by erythema (vesicular enanthema).

Herpetic gingivostomatitis. Herpetic gingivostomatitis is a common affliction, usually caused by herpes simplex type I, or rarely type II. Formerly more often found in children, it is now seen as often in adults, but the overall incidence is decreasing. The primary infection is often subclinical. Symptomatic primary cases are characterized by painful vesicles on the oropharyngeal mucosa, lips, and gingivae, with cervical lymphadenopathy and fever. Oral vesicles are more likely to rupture than pharyngeal ones. Microscopy reveals intraepithelial vesicles and squamous cells exhibiting herpetic cytopathic effect (multinucleate giant cells with crowded nuclei containing eosinophilic inclusion bodies or glassy chromatin), but the vesicles are often inflamed and eroded. The oral lesions and symptoms are more severe than those of herpangina and are sometimes misdiagnosed as ANUG (Table 50-4). Lesions typically heal within 2 weeks, but almost a third of patients have recurrences.[28]

Recurrent herpes simplex (herpes labialis) usually involves the vermilion border of the lips or adjacent skin and often has a neuralgic prodrome of soreness or paresthesia. Oral vesicles and ulcers may also be present. The herpesvirus is present in the trigeminal ganglia in latent form but can be reactivated by many stimuli, including febrile illnesses (herpes labialis is commonly known as "cold sores," or "fever blisters"), stress, orofacial trauma, or bright sunlight.

Hand-foot-and-mouth disease (vesicular stomatitis with exanthema). Hand-foot-and -mouth disease is a common but usually mild infection in young children. It often occurs in the summer and early fall, both as sporadic cases or epidemics. It is usually caused by coxsackieviruses A, particularly type A16. Symptoms are usually mild and include low-grade fever,

Table 50-4 Common causes of stomatitis*

Class of agent	Specific examples	Comments
Viruses	Herpesvirus	Usually type I
	Coxsackievirus	Herpangina, usually type A
Fungi	*Candida albicans*	Thrush and other conditions
Unknown	Lichen planus	

*See also Table 50-6 for vesiculobullous lesions and Table 50-8 for ulcerative conditions.

anorexia, malaise, and a sore mouth. The oral mucosa and lips have erythematous macules, progressing to vesicles and ulcers, resembling herpetic stomatitis. A vesicular rash on the distal extremities (exanthema) often accompanies the enanthema, except in adults. This condition is mild and self-limited, and laboratory confirmation or treatment is usually unnecessary.

Measles. Koplik's spots are small prodromal spots with a punctate, blue-white center surrounded by an erythematous rim, which occur on the labial and buccal mucosa 1 to 2 days before the skin rash of measles.

OSTEOMYELITIS

Osteomyelitis of the jaws differs from osteomyelitis of the long bones in several ways: it is usually a localized condition associated with periodontal infection, it usually involves otherwise healthy adults who have little or no systemic symptoms, and it is often caused by anaerobes (Table 50-5).

Acute suppurative osteomyelitis

Acute suppurative osteomyelitis most often occurs in adult males who present with fever, severe jaw pain, and swelling, sometimes with anesthesia of the lip (from involvement of the inferior alveolar nerve). Grossly, there are signs of inflammation, sometimes with drainage of pus from sinus tracts or next to a tooth. After the first week, radiographs show lytic bone destruction, with residual radiopaque sequestra. Later, periosteal bone formation is evident. Biopsy allows identification of the organism by culture, and histologic testing demonstrates bony destruction with neutrophilic exudate in the marrow and adjacent bone remodeling. The infection is often intractable, with widespread involvement of the bone and occasional extensive necrosis of overlying soft tissues.

About one half of cases are attributable to aerobic bacteria (especially staphylococcal and gram-negative species) and the remaining cases are caused by anaerobes, particularly *Bacteroides* species, fusobacteria, and anaerobic cocci.[29] Although the route of entry is often not identified, many cases are attributed to spread from periodontal infection. Jaw fracture or penetrating injury (such as bullet wound, surgery) may also cause acute osteomyelitis, but these wounds are treated with debridement and antibiotics to prevent this complication. Osteomyelitis of the jaws rarely occurs by spread of infection from adjacent soft tissues or hematogenously.

Table 50-5 Classification of osteomyelitis of jaws

Acute suppurative
Chronic suppurative
Without prior acute osteomyelitis (primary)
With prior acute osteomyelitis (secondary)
Chronic nonsuppurative
Focal sclerosing (condensing)
Diffuse sclerosing
With proliferative periostitis (Garré's)
Actinomycotic
Syphilitic
Tuberculous
Sterile (such as radiation osteonecrosis)

Chronic osteomyelitis

Chronic suppurative infection of the jawbones occurs after inadequately treated acute osteomyelitis (secondary osteomyelitis), or it may occur without any evident acute phase (primary osteomyelitis). Chronic suppurative osteomyelitis has a more insidious onset than acute osteomyelitis, with jaw tenderness and fistulas.

Chronic osteomyelitis of the jaws may occur with tuberculosis, syphilis, and actinomycosis but is a rare complication of these diseases.

Two other types of chronic osteomyelitis, which are unique to the jaws, are associated with pronounced bony sclerosis. *Chronic focal sclerosing osteomyelitis (condensing osteitis)* appears to be a pronounced bony reaction to periapical infection. Patients are usually less than 20 years old, and a carious, nonvital mandibular first permanent molar is usually involved. The lesion may be painless or mildly painful. X-ray films show a radiopaque area around one or both roots surrounded by intact, densely sclerotic bone. Microscopy reveals dense compact bone with scant fibrotic interstitial tissue containing a few lymphocytes.

Diffuse sclerosing osteomyelitis is also characterized by a pronounced bony reaction to periodontal infection but occurs in patients with widespread periodontitis, and therefore is more extensive. It usually involves elderly blacks, who may be dentate or edentulous. Lesions may be asymptomatic, but exacerbations can cause vague pain and an unpleasant taste. Fistulas with drainage may be seen during these acute exacerbations. Radiographs show diffuse or nodular sclerosis, often bilateral, of mandible or maxilla. The appearance on biopsy is fairly similar to chronic focal sclerosing osteomyelitis (see above), though neutrophils may be seen with acute exacerbations.

Chronic osteomyelitis with proliferative periostitis (Garré's osteomyelitis) is an unusual variant of osteomyelitis with a prominent periosteal reaction.[30]

INFLAMMATORY DISEASES OF SKIN AND ORAL MUCOSA

Vesiculobullous diseases

Biopsies are frequently used to distinguish these conditions (Table 50-6) because pemphigus vulgaris and erythema multiforme may be lethal. The biopsy specimen is preferably taken from the margin of an intact vesicle (blister). The biopsy specimen is then halved so that one part can be submitted for routine histologic examination, and the other half can be frozen for immunofluorescent examination.

Pemphigus vulgaris. Circulating autoantibodies against the intercellular attachments in the squamous epithelium possibly activate proteases, leading to acantholysis and the vesicle formation in this condition. Pemphigus vulgaris usually affects middle-aged women, and the mouth is often the first site of involvement. The oral vesicles are fragile and easily disrupted, appearing as nonspecific erosions or large areas of epithelial sloughing. Spread to the skin follows in time and can lead to extensive, potentially life-threatening bullous formation.

Small, intact vesicles are preferable for biopsy, but the characteristic histologic appearance of acantholytic, suprabasilar vesicles can often be seen in the intact skin at the edges of the erosions. Direct immunofluorescence on frozen biopsy sections of intact mucosa will demonstrate IgG along the margins of epithelial cells. Indirect immunofluorescence of normal mucosa treated with patient's serum often demonstrates circulating antibodies to intercellular attachments but is usually unnecessary. Early diagnosis of severe cases is important, so that immunosuppressive treatment is not delayed.

Mucous membrane pemphigoid (cicatricial or ocular pemphigoid). Mucous membrane pemphigoid is another mucocutaneous bullous disease that appears to be immunologically mediated, this time by immunoglobulins (especially IgG) and C3 at the basement membrane. Mucous membrane pemphigoid tends to be more indolent and to involve older women (in their 60s and 70s) than pemphigus vulgaris. The gingivae are often involved by mucous membrane pemphigoid but generally spared by pemphigus vulgaris.

The separation of the epithelium in bullous pemphigoid occurs under the basal cell layer. Immunofluorescence often shows IgG and C3 in the basement membrane, but circulating antibodies are usually undetectable. From this description, it is clear than mucous membrane pemphigoid is similar to bullous pemphigoid. However, the former predominantly involves the oral and ocular mucosa (with lesser involvement of esophagus, larynx, and skin), whereas the latter predominantly involves the skin, with only rare oral lesions. Scarring in the mouth is rare, but eye involvement by mucous membrane pemphigoid can lead to blindness. Treatment is with topical corticosteroids.

Bullous erythema multiforme. In the condition bullous erythema multiforme, usually affecting young males, there are extensive, ill-defined oral erosions, often with swelling, bleeding, and crusting of the lips. The mouth may be the only site of involvement. Fever, lymphadenopathy, skin lesions (such as "target lesions," diffuse erythema, bullae), ocular lesions (especially conjunctivitis), genital ulcers, and renal involvement may also occur, and *Stevens-Johnson syndrome* is a term often used for severe manifestations of bullous erythema multiforme. The condition often recurs and may lead to death or blindness.

The cause is unknown but may be immunologically mediated. Bullous erythema multiforme has followed infections and certain drugs (especially sulfonamides), but often no precipitating event is identified. Histologic examination shows vesicular degeneration of the epithelium with scattered necrotic keratinocytes. Epithelial necrosis and detachment can follow. There is a brisk mononuclear cell infiltrate near the base of the epithelium and around blood vessels, without frank vasculitis. Sometimes the histologic changes are nonspecific. Immunofluorescence is reported to show immunoglobulin and C3 deposition in blood vessels, of unclear significance in the absence of vasculitis.

Lichen planus

Oral lichen planus is a common, often asymptomatic, chronic condition that usually affects women in middle age or older. Patients are often described as nervous and high strung. It is similar to lichen planus of the skin but frequently occurs without skin involvement. The cause is unknown and controversial, but it appears to be a T-cell–mediated cellular reaction to oral epithelium.[31-36] Some drugs (such as gold salts) and graft-versus-host disease can elicit a lichen planus reaction.[37]

The most common oral manifestation is that of radiating white or gray, velvety, threadlike papules in a linear, annular, or retiform arrangement forming lacy patches, rings, and streaks. The lesions are symmetrically distributed over both sides of the buccal mucosa. The dorsal area of the tongue is the next most common site, but lesions in this site are more variable. Lips and palate may also be involved. Plaques, erythematous atrophic areas, and erosions are sometimes seen. The erosions may be covered by fibrinous exudate. The striae are asymptomatic, but the erosive areas may cause discomfort.

The clinical picture is usually characteristic, and biopsy is unnecessary. When biopsy is performed, it is often done on

Table 50-6 Causes of vesiculobullous lesions in the mouth*

Class of agent	Specific examples	Comments
Virus	Herpetic stomatitis	Herpes simplex virus
	Chickenpox/herpes zoster	Varicella virus
	Herpangina	Coxsackievirus, usually type A
	Hand-foot-and-mouth disease	
Autoimmunity(?)	Pemphigus	Oral lesion may precede skin
	Bullous pemphigoid	Oral lesion may precede skin
	Dermatitis herpetiformis	
Other	Erythema multiforme/Stevens-Johnson syndrome	
	Epidermolysis bullosa	May occur after dental trauma; associated with malformed teeth
	Allergic reactions	

*Vesiculobullous diseases may ulcerate, and ulcerative lesions should be included in the differential diagnosis of such vesiculobullous lesions in the mouth (see Table 50-8).

atypical lesions, and the microscopic appearance may be nonspecific. The microscopic appearance of the typical striate lesions and plaques corresponds to the classic pattern of the skin: (1) hyperorthokeratosis or parakeratosis, (2) "saw-toothed acanthosis," (3) degenerate cells (Civatte bodies) in the epithelium, (4) liquefactive degeneration of the basal cell layer, and (5) a dense, bandlike, subepithelial, mononuclear cell infiltrate. Microscopy of the atrophic lesions shows a thinned epithelium with a flattened base and denser mononuclear cell infiltrate. The microscopic appearance of the erosions is nonspecific, though the intact epithelium at the margins may be more characteristic.

Desquamative lesions of lichen planus may sometimes be confused with the above-described vesiculobullous diseases. Occasionally, lesions of lichen planus resemble those of systemic lupus erythematosus (SLE) or dysplastic/malignant epithelial lesions. There is a possible mildly increased incidence of oral cancer with lichen planus, particularly squamous carcinoma arising in long-standing erosive lesions.[38-43]

SYSTEMIC DISEASES INVOLVING THE MOUTH

Acquired immunodeficiency syndrome

Oral lesions are a prominent and often early sign in patients with HIV-related diseases (Table 50-7). Refractory candidiasis is present in most patients, often as the first manifestation of immunodeficiency. Thrush (pseudomembranous candidiasis) in these patients is usually found on the palatal and buccal mucosae (Fig. 50-2). White lesions of hyperplastic candidiasis, which cannot be scraped off like the lesions of thrush, are usually found on the posterior part of the buccal mucosa, sometimes the palatal mucosa. Asymptomatic erythematous lesions of candidiasis sometimes occur on the palatal and lingual mucosa of HIV-infected patients who have not yet developed the acquired immunodeficiency syndrome (AIDS).

Patients with AIDS have an increased risk for other bacterial, fungal, and viral infections of the mouth. Dental caries and gingivitis may be quite troublesome. Acute necrotizing ulcerative gingivitis, now rare in developed countries, should prompt the clinician to consider that the patient may have AIDS.

The oral lesions of herpes simplex infections in patients with AIDS are often multiple, deeper, and more painful, heal slower, and are more widely distributed compared with herpetic lesions in immunocompetent individuals. Unusual appearances, such as linear fissures on the tongue, have been described.[44]

Hairy leukoplakia is a common, often early and relatively specific sign of immunodeficiency, particularly in HIV-positive male homosexuals. It represents a squamous hyperplasia that appears to be induced by EBV, possibly acting in concert with human papillomavirus or *Candida,* in a patient whose immune system has been compromised by HIV infection. EBV has been demonstrated in squamous cells within this lesion by DNA hybridization, immunohistology for viral antigens, and electron microscopy.[45]

Hairy leukoplakia is asymptomatic but is sometimes discovered by the patient. The appearance of the lesions varies. The most characteristic lesions are bilateral, soft, white, hairy excrescences on the lateral margins of the tongue. However, lesions can be unilateral, corrugated, or smooth, or occur elsewhere on the tongue or oral mucosa (a corrugated surface is more common than a hairy surface). Lesions may sometimes resemble other types of leukoplakia (idiopathic, tobacco use, lichen planus, chronic hyperplastic candidiasis). Although the name is similar, it is unrelated to and does not clinically resemble hairy tongue (discussed earlier in this chapter).

Microscopically, hairy leukoplakia shows:

1. Squamous hyperplasia
2. Hyperparakeratosis, often with surface ridges or projections
3. Candidal forms in the superficial layers of the epithelium
4. Ballooning degeneration and perinuclear clearing (koilocytosis) in the spiny cell layer,
5. Sparse subepithelial inflammatory cell infiltrate.

Treatment is usually unnecessary. Recognition of hairy leukoplakia is important because it is a sign that a patient is probably infected with HIV and is likely to develop AIDS within the next few months or years.

Oral lesions of Kaposi's sarcoma often occur in patients with AIDS (Fig. 50-3). Although the mouth may be the presenting site, skin lesions are usually found first. The palate is the most common site in the mouth, and Kaposi's sarcoma may resemble other common oral lesions (such as pyogenic granulomas).

Table 50-7 Oral manifestations of AIDS

Secondary infections	
Fungal	Candidiasis
	Chronic thrush
	Hyperplastic
	Erythematous
	Angular cheilitis
	Mucocutaneous
	Histoplasmosis
	Cryptococcosis
Bacterial	Increased risk of dental caries and periodontitis
	Acute necrotizing ulcerative gingivitis
	Mycobacterial infection (such as *M. tuberculosis, M. avium–intracellulare)*
	Gram-negative bacteria (such as *Klebsiella pneumoniae*)
	Submandibular cellulitis
Viral	Herpetic stomatitis
	Cytomegalovirus
	Hairy leukoplakia
	Herpes zoster
	Human papillomavirus (condyloma acuminatum)
	Focal epithelial hyperplasia
Tumors	Kaposi's sarcoma
	Squamous cell carcinoma
	Non-Hodgkin's lymphoma
Miscellaneous	Recurrent aphthous ulcers
	Progressive necrotizing ulceration
	Delayed wound healing
	Xerostomia
	Benign lymphoepithelial cysts of salivary glands

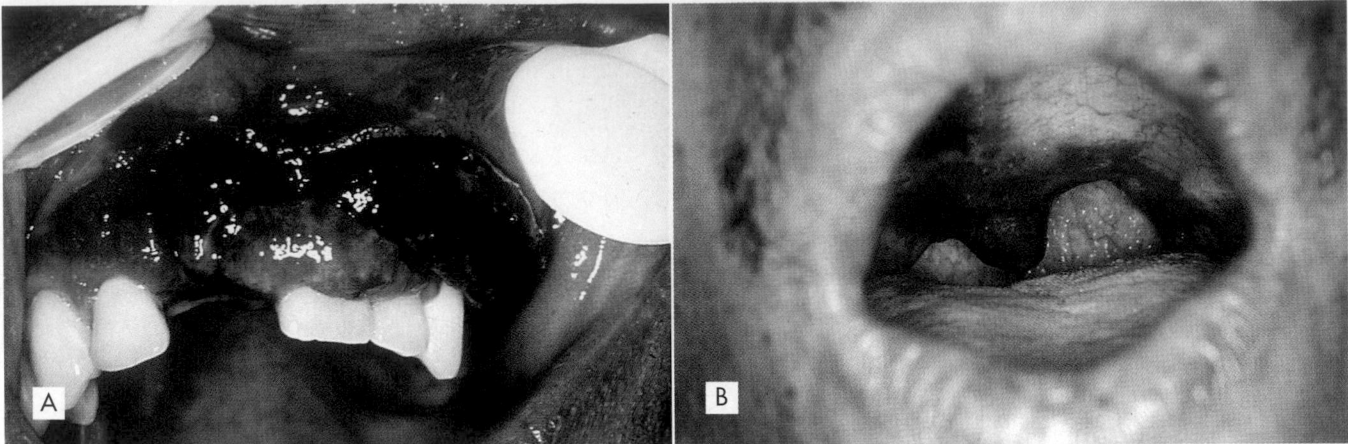

Fig. 50-3 Multifocal presence of Kaposi's sarcoma in anterior maxilla, **A,** and the soft palate, **B,** of an HIV infected patient.

Sjögren's syndrome

The autoimmune disorder Sjögren's syndrome, which involves the eyes, the salivary glands, and the mouth, is associated with a host of other autoimmune disorders and is discussed more broadly elsewhere, particularly in Chapter 51. This section concentrates on the oral manifestations of Sjögren's syndrome. The mouth and pharynx feel dry, and the patient may complain of dysphagia and dysphonia. Examination reveals angular cheilitis and dry, cracked skin on the lips. The oral mucosa is atrophic and shiny. The saliva is thick and ropy. Because saliva is necessary for dental hygiene, dental caries may become widespread.

There are many other causes of decreased saliva and dry mouth (xerostomia), including medications (such as phenothiazines, tricyclic antidepressants, antihistamines), cervicofacial irradiation, megaloblastic anemia, sarcoid, and dehydration.

Systemic lupus erythematosus

There are numerous oral manifestations of systemic lupus erythematosus (SLE).[46] Up to 30% of patients have Sjögren's syndrome. From 10% to 25% of patients with SLE have painless superficial ulcers, erythematous patches, or white keratotic lesions, most commonly on the palate. Edema and petechiae may also be seen on the oral mucosa, and there may be a scaly crust on the lips. A mucosal biopsy specimen shows an interface mucositis with vacuolization of basal keratinocytes, patchy thickening of the basement membrane, and scattered chronic inflammatory cell infiltrates. Although the biopsy specimen may show only nonspecific lymphocyte infiltrates, immunofluorescence of oral lesions demonstrates immunoglobulin and complement deposition, analogous to the skin.

Progressive systemic sclerosis (scleroderma)

Progressive systemic sclerosis can cause constriction of the mouth aperture and radial furrows in the lips, giving the mouth a pursed look. As the lips become immobile and the mouth aperture shrinks, food intake and chewing become difficult (trismus). The oral mucosa is pale and rigid. The tongue may lose mobility. As the disease progresses, there may be tongue atrophy and bony resorption. X-ray films reveal widening of the periodontal ligaments in over half of patients.

Crohn's disease

Crohn's disease occasionally affects the lips and oral mucous membranes, more commonly in males. Involvement of the mouth may be concurrent with gastrointestinal (GI) manifestations, precede them, or be the only manifestation of the disease. Signs include cobblestone-like hyperplasia of the buccal mucosa, swelling and cracking of the lips, oral ulcers (usually in the mucobuccal fold), and aphthous ulcers on the palate. A biopsy specimen may show only nonspecific chronic inflammation, but when it shows noncaseating granulomas, the diagnosis of Crohn's disease can be made if sarcoid and tuberculosis can be excluded.[47]

Behçet's syndrome

Oral ulcers, genital ulcers, and ocular lesions (particularly uveitis) compose this syndrome, but manifestations vary widely. This condition usually afflicts young males and is more common in Turkey and Japan. Disorders of other sites often occur (such as nervous system, skin, joints, GI tract, kidneys), and so classification is difficult and distinction from other multisystem disorders (such as ulcerative colitis) is sometimes problematical. Various immunologic abnormalities have been reported but have not yet explained the cause of this syndrome or suggested a specific therapy.

The oral ulcers are seen in 90% of patients with Behçet's syndrome and resemble recurrent aphthous ulcers, described below. Recurrent aphthous ulcers is a very common condition, however, and is only rarely followed by the other signs of Behçet's syndrome.

Gardner's syndrome

Gardner's syndrome is an autosomal dominant disorder associated with a mutation on chromosome 5. There is a variety of abnormalities, but the classic tetrad is (1) multiple adenomatous polyps in the small and large intestines, (2) osteomas of jaws, skull, and facial bones, (3) fibromas of soft tissues, and (4) epidermal and trichilemmal cysts of the skin. Expression of these abnormalities varies among affected individuals.

When present with Gardner's syndrome, the osteoma often forms a mass at the angle of the mandible. Another site of involvement is the alveolar bone, where there may be loosening of teeth, unerupted teeth, supernumerary teeth, multiple odontomas, and other dental abnormalities. Osteomas may also occur in the paranasal sinuses, on the inner and outer tables of the skull bones, and in the long bones. The presence of multiple osteomas should alert the clinician to the possibility of Gardner's syndrome because patients with this syndrome need to be investigated for intestinal tumors.[48]

Wegener's granulomatosis

Wegener's granulomatosis is a necrotizing, granulomatosis vasculitis that classically involves the upper respiratory tract, lungs, and kidneys. Diagnosis is usually made by biopsy of one of these sites (though the characteristic granulomas and vasculitis may be hard to demonstrate) and by elevated serum antineutrophil cytoplasmic antibodies. Oral lesions can be seen early in the disease[49] and include mucosal ulcers, a destructive periodontitis, and failure of extraction wounds to heal. Diffuse gingival hyperplasia with petechiae has occasionally been reported and seems to be characteristic of this disease.[50]

Langerhans' cell histiocytosis (histiocytosis X)

The idiopathic condition Langerhans' cell histiocytosis is characterized by a proliferation of large cells resembling Langerhans' cells of the skin.[51] Children and young adults are usually affected, with a male preponderance. Lesions may occur in the bones, lungs, skin, or any site, and lesions of the head and neck are very common. Langerhans' cell histiocytosis (LCH) can present with oral lesions. Loosening or even exfoliation of teeth, caused by involvement of the alveolar bone (particularly of the mandible), is relatively common. Lesions start in the marrow but can perforate the cortex and extend into the gingiva. X-ray films show teeth surrounded by radiolucent areas so that the teeth appear to "float in space." Sharply defined, lytic lesions can occur elsewhere in the jawbones. The gingival tissues can be inflamed, hyperplastic, and ulcerate. Cervical lymphadenopathy and otitis media are other manifestations of LCH.

Microscopy shows the proliferation of Langerhans' cells. These cells are large with indistinct cell borders, abundant pale cytoplasm, and oval to reniform, vesicular nuclei. They stain with S-100 antigen, and ultrastructural analysis reveals Birbeck granules in the cytoplasm. Langerhans' cells are associated with variable numbers of eosinophils and other inflammatory cells.

Lesions of the jawbones can usually be treated with surgical curettage, with sacrifice of involved teeth. The prognosis for localized LCH (as opposed to the acute disseminated form in infants known as Letterer-Siwe disease) is excellent, but new lesions may occur.[52]

Sarcoid (sarcoidosis)

Oral manifestations of sarcoid usually occur after this condition is diagnosed; they are rarely presenting features of this disease. There may be a rash and nodules on the face and lips. Oral mucosal lesions are similar but less common. These firm, painless nodules are dark red or brown. They vary in size and number and may be discrete or confluent. Ulceration is uncommon. The nodules occur anywhere in the mouth but especially on the lips, gingivae, hard palate, and buccal mucosa. Microscopy shows typical small, compact, noncaseating granulomas. Sarcoid involvement of salivary and lacrimal glands is rare but can mimic Sjögren's syndrome, with gland swelling, dry eyes, and xerostomia. The combination of uveitis, parotid gland enlargement, fever, and facial paralysis with sarcoid is called *uveoparotid fever* or *Heerfordt's syndrome*.

OTHER INFLAMMATORY, REACTIVE, OR ULCERATIVE CONDITIONS OF THE MOUTH

Recurrent aphthous ulcers (canker sores, aphthous stomatitis)

The affliction *recurrent aphthous ulcers* was described by Hippocrates in about 400 B.C., but its cause is still unknown. Approximately 10% to 20% of people have had recurrent aphthae, making it the most common disease of the oral mucosa. This condition is characterized by recurrent shallow ulcers (aphthae) that may be single or multiple. The lesions develop initially between 10 and 30 years of age, in individuals who are otherwise healthy. Women are more commonly affected than men, and nonsmokers more commonly than smokers.[53]

Early lesions are associated with a burning sensation and can be intensely painful. The aphthae last from 1 to 3 weeks. Subsequent episodes vary in frequency, separated by intervals of weeks, months, or years, but the condition eventually spontaneously disappears in most people.

Despite considerable investigation, the pathogenesis of the lesions is unknown. The ulcers tend to occur in association with mechanical trauma, physical or emotional stress, and use of certain food products.[54] Other possible associations include nutritional deficiency, hormonal changes (particularly in females), and hypersensitivity to microorganisms.[55] Recent studies have suggested that there are immunologic abnormalities in patients who are prone to develop aphthous ulcers: in particular, a decrease in helper T-cell to suppresser T-cell ratios in the peripheral blood of patients with aphthae as compared to controls.[56,57]

The ulcers usually occur on the unattached oral mucosa, particularly that of the lip, cheek, tongue, and floor of the mouth. The ulcers are shallow, round, or oval, and vary in size but are usually less than 1 cm in diameter. The surface of the ulcers is covered with yellowish-grayish, fibrinous material. The ulcer margins are well defined and characteristically surrounded by an erythematous halo. Microscopically, the ulcer is covered by fibrinopurulent exudate and necrotic tissue. The underlying inflammatory infiltrate is composed of neutrophils (which predominate superficially) and mononuclear cells. Accessory salivary gland tissue is commonly found in the area of the ulcer, and this typically shows periductal and perialveolar inflammation and fibrosis. The lesions heal without scar formation.

The patient generally has no other symptoms, signs, or laboratory findings. History excludes ulcers caused by biting or dentures. Treatment is analgesia and prevention of secondary infection, but the ulcer will usually heal on its own in a few weeks. Frequently recurring cases may require prednisone to interrupt the cycle. Ulcers persisting more than three weeks may be attributable to other conditions (such as syphilis, cancer) and should be investigated.

Although recurrent aphthous ulcers usually are found in otherwise healthy people, they are also part of Behçet's and Reiter's syndromes and are occasionally seen with Crohn's disease. Aphthae have also been described with nutritional deficiencies in patients with subclinical GI diseases (such as celiac and inflammatory bowel diseases). Severe aphthae may be seen in the mouth and oropharynx of HIV-positive patients.[58] See Table 50-8 for various causes of oral ulcers.

Fibrous hyperplasia (epulis fissuratum)

Fibrous hyperplasia is a common fibrosing reaction to chronic irritation from ill-fitting dentures. "Epulis fissuratum" is an outdated synonym. This fibrous overgrowth of the oral mucosa reacting to chronic trauma is not limited to dentures, and focal nodules may form at other sites of chronic mechanical trauma that are referred to as *fibromas* (discussed later in this chapter).

Fibrous hyperplasia presents as single or multiple folds of redundant mucosa, usually on the alveolar ridge and oral sulci along the denture flange. The hyperplastic tissue is firm and shows normal mucosal color. Ulcers may be present at the base of the fold next to the denture. Microscopically, the lesion is covered with surface squamous epithelium, which may be hyperorthokeratotic or parakeratotic. The rete ridges are usually elongated. The lamina propria is composed of dense bundles of collagen fibers with few fibroblasts and blood vessels. Inflammatory cell infiltrates can be focally present, particularly around the ulcerated areas.

Because this is essentially a hypertrophic scar, better-fitting dentures will not suffice to correct this condition, and surgical removal may be necessary.

Inflammatory papillary hyperplasia (palatal papillomatosis)

Inflammatory papillary hyperplasia is a distinctive variant of fibrous hyperplasia of the oral mucosa. It occurs predominantly but not exclusively in the hard palate under a full maxillary denture. Old, ill-fitting dentures and poor oral hygiene contribute to the development of this lesion. An etiologic relationship to *Candida albicans* has been suggested, but organisms are not commonly identified in this lesion.[59,60]

Clinically, there are numerous, closely arranged papillary projections that involve a large part of the surface of the palate. They can be edematous, or erythematous, or have a normal mucosal color. Microscopically the lesion is composed of numerous small papillary projections covered with parakeratotic and occasionally orthokeratotic stratified squamous epithelium (Fig. 50-4). The epithelium often shows pseudoepitheliomatous hyperplasia. The supporting fibrous connective tissue cores usually contain an inflammatory cell infiltrate.

Inflammatory papillary hyperplasia has no known neoplastic potential. However, it must be distinguished from verrucous carcinoma. In inflammatory papillary hyperplasia, the epithelium does not extend deeply into the underlying stroma, keratinization is not pronounced, and keratin plugging is not evident.

Generalized gingival hyperplasia

The most common cause of generalized gingival enlargement is *generalized fibrous hyperplasia*. Diffuse enlargement of the gingivae caused by fibrous overgrowth can vary considerably in severity. In more severe cases, the crowns of the teeth are totally covered by hyperplastic gingiva. Usually the gingival hyperplasia appears to be an exaggerated reaction to chronic irritation from plaque and bacteria.

Phenytoin (Dilantin) therapy has for many years been known to cause generalized fibrous hyperplasia of the gums in many patients. More recently, other drugs have been observed to have a similar effect, including cyclosporin A and nifedipine. Generalized fibrous hyperplasia of the gingiva can also occur in childhood, where it can be isolated, hereditary (hereditary gingival fibromatosis), or one part of a syndrome (such as Zimmermann-Laband syndrome).

Table 50-8 Causes of mouth ulcers*

Class of agent	Specific examples	Comments
Bacteria	Tuberculosis	Infrequent complication
	Syphilis	Chancres and gummas may ulcerate
	Acute necrotizing ulcerative gingivitis	Miscellaneous bacterial commensals cultured Stress, tobacco use, etc. are also implicated
	Noma (gangrenous stomatitis)	Rare in developed countries
Fungi	Candidal infection	
Viruses	Herpes stomatitis	
	Herpes zoster (shingles)	
Neoplasms	Squamous carcinoma	
	Lymphomas and leukemias	
	Melanoma	
Miscellaneous	Traumatic ulcer	Biting, ill-fitting dentures
Unknown	Recurrent aphthous ulcers	Usually occur alone but are occasionally associated with Behçet's & Reiter's syndromes and other conditions
	Erosive lichen planus	Skin lesions may be absent
	Crohn's disease	Infrequent
	Behçet's syndrome	
	Reiter's syndrome	
	Necrotizing sialoadenitis	
	Eosinophilic ulcer	

*Vesiculobullous diseases may ulcerate and should be included in the differential diagnosis of ulcerated lesion in the mouth (see Table 50-6).

Clinically, it presents as diffuse enlargement of the gingivae, which become swollen and rounded and later might become lobulated. The gums become firm and resilient, with little tendency to bleed. Microscopy shows sparsely vascular fibrous connective tissue with thick, dense, interlacing bundles of collagen fibers. Characteristically, the surface epithelium is thick, and the rete ridges are elongated and slender, acquiring a "test-tube" appearance.

Surgical reduction can be performed when the hyperplastic gingival tissue becomes esthetically objectionable. Rigorous oral hygiene and control of bacterial plaque and dental calculus are helpful in reducing the progression of hyperplasia.[61]

Occasionally, generalized gingival hyperplasia may have other causes, most notably leukemic infiltration (especially acute monocytic leukemia).

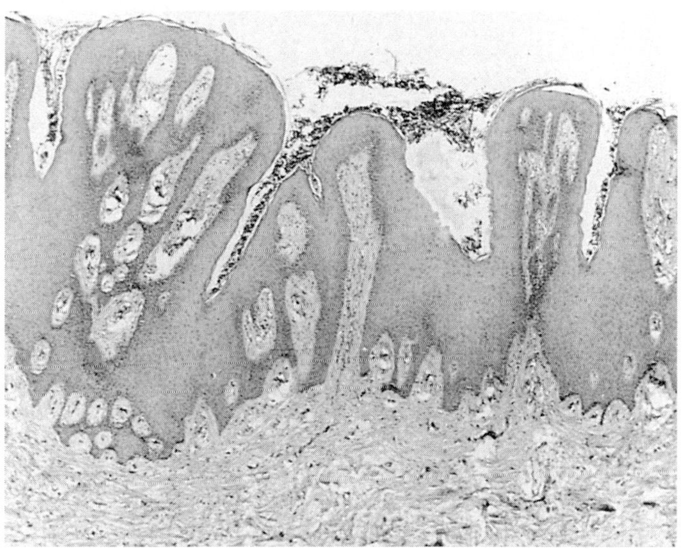

Fig. 50-4 Inflammatory papillary hyperplasia with numerous papillary squamous epithelial projections and inflammatory cell infiltrate of the submucosa.

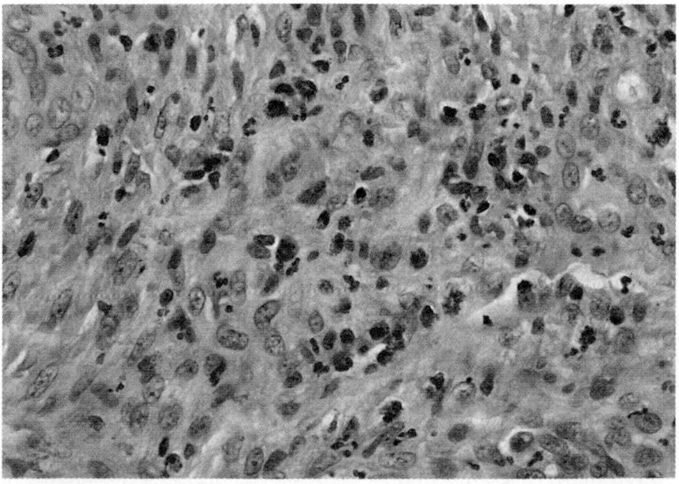

Fig. 50-5 Eosinophilic ulcer of oral mucosa. Photomicrograph of an incisional biopsy specimen of the lesion showing the infiltration of inflammatory cells, in particular eosinophils and large mononuclear cells.

Eosinophilic ulcer of the oral mucosa (traumatic eosinophilic granuloma)

Eosinophilic ulcer of the oral mucosa is a benign self-healing lesion, unrelated to eosinophilic granuloma of LCH. It usually presents as a well-defined ulcer on the lateral or ventral surface of the tongue. It can resemble squamous carcinoma clinically and lymphoma microscopically. The lesion sometimes appears as a raised, white or red induration before it ulcerates. It is painless, affecting older adults in their sixth and seventh decades.[62,63]

Microscopy shows a polymorphous inflammatory cell infiltrate extending deeply into the submucosa and between muscle fibers (Fig. 50-5). Eosinophils and large mononuclear cells usually predominate. The mononuclear cells have pale nuclei and show mitotic activity that may be pronounced. Lymphocytes, plasma cells, macrophages, and neutrophils are present in varying numbers in different lesions.

The cause is unknown but, based on clinical and experimental evidence, trauma may have an etiologic role. More recent immunohistochemical observations[64] suggest a role for T-cell immunity in the pathogenesis of this lesion. The large mononuclear cells with pale nuclei are believed to be derived from myofibroblasts. The polymorphic nature of the cellular infiltrate and the immunohistochemical phenotype of the large mononuclear cells help to distinguish eosinophilic ulcer from lymphoma of the oral mucosa.

Eosinophilic ulcer of the oral mucosa resolves spontaneously even without surgical intervention. However, multiple synchronous and metachronous lesions at different sites in the mouth have been reported.[65]

Necrotizing sialometaplasia

Necrotizing sialometaplasia most commonly presents with the sudden onset of a sharply demarcated ulcer, usually on the hard palate of adult males. Symptoms are generally mild if one considers the appearance of the lesion. The importance of this benign, self-healing ulcer is that it may be mistaken, both clinically and microscopically, for squamous or mucoepidermoid carcinoma.[66] Necrotizing sialometaplasia is further discussed in Chapter 51.

DISORDERS OF MUCOSAL PIGMENTATION

Endogenous (melanin) pigmentation

Oral melanotic macule (oral focal melanosis). Oral melanotic macules are nonspecific descriptive terms for a flat area of hyperpigmentation that may be attributable to many conditions, including physiologic or racial variation, freckling, lentigo, postinflammatory hyperpigmentation, smoker's melanosis, and so forth. When melanotic macules are prominent in the mouth or on the lips, Peutz-Jeghers syndrome and Addison's disease should be considered. Darkening of the mucosa may also be idiopathic or associated with nonmelanotic lesions (such as hemangioma, hematoma, amalgam tattoo).

Ephelides (freckles). Ephelides are occasionally seen in the mouth, especially on the lips, but are much less common than those of the skin.

Nevi. Lentigines and melanocytic nevi, so common on the skin, are rare in the oral cavity.[67] The blue nevus is also rarely found in this location. Melanoma and melanotic neuroectodermal tumor of infancy are discussed later.

Inflammatory hyperpigmentation. As in the skin, chronic inflammation (such as lichen planus) can sometimes cause darker pigmentation. With postinflammatory hyperpigmentation, the pigmentation persists long after the inflammation has subsided, and most of the pigment is present in stromal macrophages (melanophages).

Smoker's melanosis. Smoker's melanosis appears to be attributable to a property of tobacco smoke that stimulates melanocytes (smokeless tobacco is not associated with this condition). Females, especially those using oral contraceptives, are more commonly affected. The degree of pigmentation is related to the duration and amount of smoking, but when one considers the prevalence of smoking, this condition is surprisingly uncommon. When present, the pigmentation is usually found on the anterior labial aspect of the gingivae in cigarette smokers, and the palatal or buccal mucosa in pipe smokers. The melanin in smoker's melanosis is deposited in basal keratinocytes near the stimulated melanocytes. The pigmentation may take years to resolve after smoking is discontinued.

Systemic disorders. The hyperpigmentation of Peutz-Jeghers syndrome is often characteristic, but the oral hyperpigmentation of the other disorders may be subtle and difficult to distinguish without knowledge of the pattern of skin pigmentation and other manifestations of the syndromes.

Pigmentation of the perioral skin and mucosa of the mouth is an early sign of Peutz-Jeghers syndrome, though the intestinal polyps are more significant clinically. The pigmentation varies from ephelides to brown-black macules but can be distinguished from other conditions because the pigmentation of Peutz-Jeghers syndrome develops in infancy or childhood, is darker than most ephelides, and involves other unusual locations (such as nasal, conjunctival, and rectal mucosa).[68] The pigmentation on the facial skin may fade but not the mucosal pigmentation. The lower lip and buccal mucosa are the most common intraoral sites.

The skin hyperpigmentation of Addison's disease is sometimes accompanied by hyperpigmentation of oral mucosa, which may be an early sign. Ephelides or larger brown-black patches may occur on the buccal mucosa, tongue, lips, and gingivae, resembling the pattern of pigmentation commonly seen in dark-skinned races. When Addison's disease is part of multiple endocrine neoplasia syndrome type 1, there may also be white lesions of chronic mucocutaneous candidiasis.[69]

Intraoral pigmented macules may also be present with Albright's syndrome and neurofibromatosis.

Exogenous pigmentation

Amalgam tattoo (focal argyrosis). Amalgam tattoo is the most common pigmentation of oral mucosa and is attributable to iatrogenic implantation of amalgam particles during procedures involving teeth restored with amalgam alloy.[70] The lesions are gray, flat, and painless. This appearance and the distribution of pigment on the gingiva, buccal mucosa, or the floor of mouth or palate near the area of the restored tooth, is usually adequate for diagnosis. Rarely, an amalgam tattoo may be biopsied because of unexpected location (such as the lips), the presence of another nearby lesion, to exclude melanoma and so forth. Microscopy shows brown or black particles of varying size in the fibrous tissue and around blood vessels (Fig. 50-6). Lymphocytes, macrophages, and multinucleate giant cells may be present, but there is usually little or no inflammatory reaction.

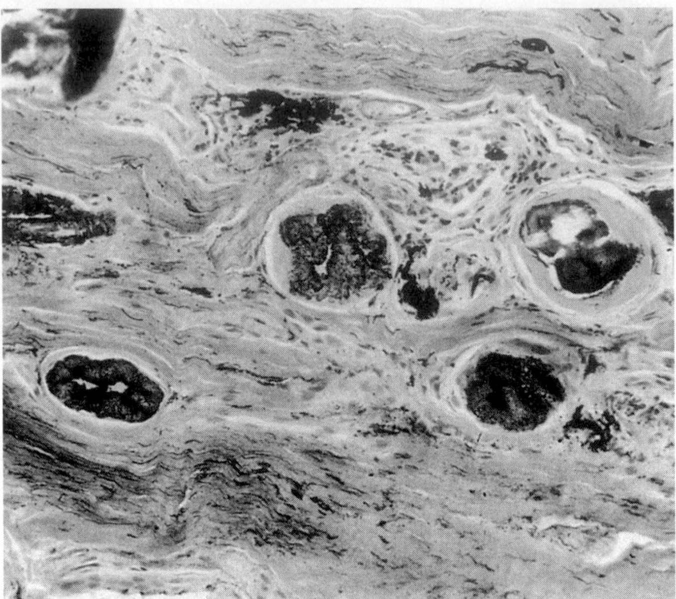

Fig. 50-6 Photomicrograph of amalgam tattoo showing the dark metal granules in both the fibrous tissue and the walls of blood vessels.

Heavy-metal pigmentation. Arsenic, bismuth, lead, and mercury have been described as causing pigmentation of oral mucosa, particularly along the gingival margins. The heavy metals react with sulfides in the dental plaque to form a gray to black line along the gingival margin. Historically, this was attributable to occupational exposure to metal vapors or to medication with arsenic and bismuth compounds. *Cis*-platinum (cisplatin) has also been reported as causing a similar line along the gingival margin.

Drug-associated hyperpigmentation

In addition to the heavy-metal medications just discussed, there are several drugs associated with hyperpigmentation. Phenothiazines and antimalarials may produce diffuse oral hyperpigmentation. Minocycline (used to treat acne) may cause focal hyperpigmentation. Cyclophosphamide and azidothymidine (AZT) can also cause oral hyperpigmentation.

BENIGN EPITHELIAL PROLIFERATIONS

Oral papillomas

Squamous papilloma. Squamous papilloma is the most common oral neoplasm. The cause of this benign tumor is believed to be viral but is yet unproved (human papillomavirus, HPV, has been identified in many but not all lesions). It affects all ages but is usually seen in adults. The squamous papilloma presents as a painless, exophytic mass with a warty or papillary surface. It is usually less than 1 cm in diameter but may measure up to 3 cm. The color varies from pink to white, depending on the degree of keratinization. It is usually single but may be multiple. Preferred sites are the palate, tongue, gingivae, and lips.

Microscopy shows papillary projections composed of a stratified squamous epithelial lining around a relatively scant fibrovascular core.[71] The papillary projections may branch. The squamous epithelium is hyperplastic, with varying amounts of keratinization or parakeratosis. There may be ulceration, superficial candidal colonization, or inflammation. Squamous cell atypia or basal epithelial hyperplasia occasionally occur, but dysplasia is rare. Recurrences of squamous papilloma are infrequent and usually occur after incomplete excision.

Clinically and histologically the differential diagnosis of solitary (or a few) papillary lesions in the mouth also includes warts, verruciform xanthoma (discussed later in this chapter), warty dyskeratoma, verrucous carcinoma, and papillary growth in a squamous carcinoma.[72] The differential diagnosis of numerous papillary lesions includes upper aerodigestive (juvenile laryngeal) papillomatosis, florid oral papillomatosis, inflammatory papillary hyperplasia, follicular keratosis, and focal epithelial hyperplasia (Heck's disease).[73,74]

Verruca vulgaris. Verruca vulgaris (common wart) uncommonly involves the mouth, usually on the lips in children, who may autoinoculate the virus from a cutaneous lesion. When the large basophilic inclusions seen in cutaneous lesions are inapparent, microscopic distinction from other papillomas is difficult or impossible.

Condyloma acuminatum. Condyloma acuminatum (genital wart) can also involve the mouth, either singly or multiply. Without the typical parakeratosis and koilocytic atypia of the genital lesions, condyloma acuminatum may be impossible to distinguish histologically from other squamous papillomas (with which it may be related anyway). The presence of genital lesions, in situ DNA hybridization, and other markers for HPV infection may be useful for diagnosis, if necessary.

Upper aerodigestive (juvenile laryngeal) *papillomatosis* is attributable to infection of the baby by HPV. (usually types 6 and 11) from the mother. There are multiple lesions, predominantly in the larynx, but the mouth can also be involved.

Inflammatory papillary hyperplasia (palatal papillomatosis). Inflammatory papillary hyperplasia, a common, benign, reactive condition on the palate of denture-wearers (which grossly is more nodular or cobblestone-like than papillary), is discussed earlier in this chapter.

Pseudoepitheliomatous hyperplasia (pseudocarcinomatous hyperplasia)

Chronic inflammation as a result of numerous conditions causes hyperplasia of squamous epithelium and irregular elongation of the epithelial rete. Infrequently this acanthosis can mimic squamous carcinoma, particularly when (1) the retia are deep and jagged, (2) the squamous epithelium exhibits considerable inflammatory or regenerative atypia, (3) the reaction in the stroma resembles tumor-associated desmoplasia and inflammatory response, and (4) the biopsy section is too small or poorly oriented. The squamous epithelium over granular cell tumors also may show hyperplasia, which is occasionally pronounced. If the cause of the epithelial proliferation is treated, the pseudoepitheliomatous hyperplasia resolves.

When presented with such a case, careful attention to the cytologic criteria for malignancy, exclusion of benign conditions that could be responsible for the reaction, more extensive sampling of the lesion, and clinical correlation are recommended.

PREMALIGNANT LESIONS AND CONDITIONS

Premalignant lesions are morphologically altered areas of a tissue in which cancer is more likely to occur than in its apparently normal counterpart. Leukoplakia, erythroplakia, and reverse smoker's palate are precancerous lesions that occur in the oral mucosa (the first two of which also occur in other sites). A premalignant condition is defined as a generalized state or a disease that is associated with an increased risk of subsequently developing cancer. Examples include syphilis, sideropenic dysphagia, submucosal fibrosis, lichen planus, epidermolysis bullosa hereditaria, and xeroderma pigmentosum.[75-78]

Premalignant lesions

Leukoplakia. Leukoplakia is a clinical term for a white patch or plaque occurring on the surface of a mucous membrane (as on the epithelium of the mouth, larynx, esophagus, or genital tract). In the mouth, the term *leukoplakia* is more narrowly defined to include only those white patches or plaques that will not rub off (to exclude pseudomembranous candidiasis) and that are not clinically or histologically attributable to another oral disease[79,80] (Table 50-9).

The incidence of leukoplakia has ranged from 1% to 6% in large series of oral surgical pathology specimens from different parts of the world, but its prevalence is more difficult to estimate. Although tobacco use (smoking or chewing), alcohol abuse, dental restorations (either by friction or by the galvanic action induced when dissimilar metals are used), and overzealous tooth brushing have been implicated as contributing factors, many patients have no identifiable cause.

Leukoplakia is considered to be premalignant, since about 6% of leukoplakic lesions will have carcinoma found on the first biopsy specimen, and about 4% of benign lesions will subsequently undergo malignant transformation. Interestingly the incidence of malignant transformation of oral leukoplakia is higher in nonsmokers than in smokers (the biologic basis of this observation still eludes explanation).

Leukoplakia chiefly occurs in the fifth to seventh decades of life and is slightly more common in males. The lesion may be asymptomatic or sensed as a rough area in the mouth. It can occur in any area of the oral cavity, but the mandibular and buccal mucosa are the most common sites. Certain sites of

Table 50-9 Chronic white lesions of oropharyngeal mucosa

Benign	Fordyce's spots White hairy tongue Geographic tongue Candidiasis (premalignant?) Lupus erythematosus (premalignant?) Leukoedema White sponge nevus Epstein's pearls (newborns)
Premalignant and malignant	Oral lichen planus Leukoplakia with or without dysplasia Keratinizing squamous cell carcinoma

leukoplakia are at increased risk for dysplasia and squamous carcinoma: the floor of the mouth, the ventrolateral surface of the tongue, and the lips.

Leukoplakic lesions may be localized or diffuse. They vary from nonpalpable, faintly translucent areas to thick, fissured, indurated lesions. The surface is often finely wrinkled or "shriveled" and may feel rough. Some lesions are smooth, deeply fissured, or verrucous. The lesions do not have to be white: some are gray, yellow-white, or, in smokers, brown-yellow. Based on the appearance, some workers subclassify leukoplakic lesions (such as homogeneous, speckled, nodular types) (Fig. 50-7, *A*)

Lesions with small red granular areas and indefinite margins are more worrisome for dysplasia and cancer, and fissured and thickened leukoplakic lesions may be more likely to become malignant, but there is no reliable clinical sign or symptom that allows one to predict premalignant or early malignant change. Therefore, biopsy is mandatory. Large lesions that are not excised require multiple, repeated biopsies. Lasers are emerging as a method to eradicate large lesions without scarring.

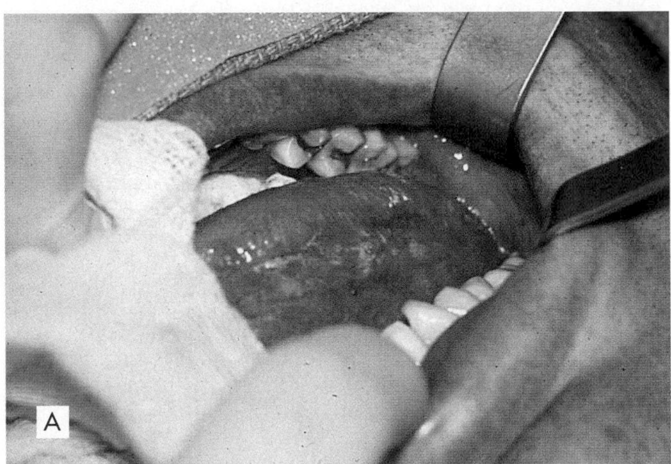

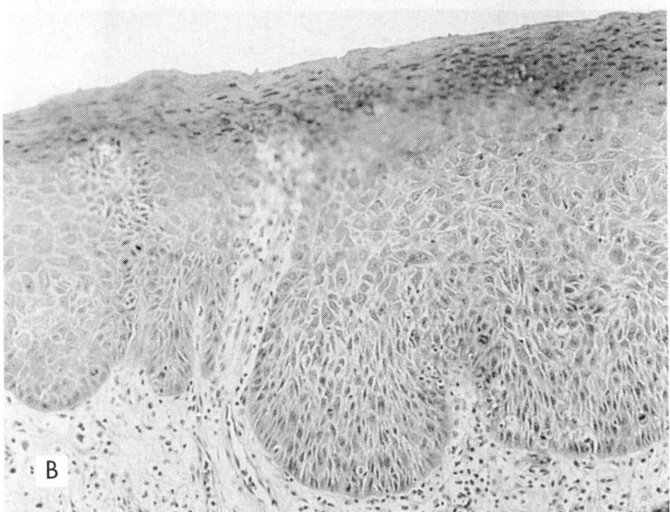

Fig. 50-7 **A,** Speckled erythroplakia of the ventrolateral border of the tongue of a 35-year-old nonsmoking man. **B,** Severe dysplasia with its associated intraepithelial hyperchromatism and disturbance of maturation of the mucosa. In other areas hyperkeratosis, hyperparakeratosis, and acanthosis were seen.

The biopsy of the lesion will show varying degrees of surface keratinization: hyperorthokeratosis, parakeratosis, or (occasionally) parakeratotic cells with atypical nuclear features. The lesions often exhibit acanthosis, and less commonly contain dysplasia or carcinoma (either in situ or invasive). Since leukoplakic lesions have variable histologic findings, of varying significance, it is widely recommended that *leukoplakia* be used only as a convenient clinical term to refer to white lesions (as defined above) and not be used as a histologic diagnosis. To have a histopathologic term for the commonly occurring leukoplakic lesions that do not contain dysplasia or cancer, some workers refer to them as *keratoses.*

In Waldron and Shafer's monumental study of 3256 oral leukoplakias,[81] 80.1% were combinations of hyperorthokeratosis, hyperparakeratosis, and acanthosis without atypia; 12.2% of biopsy specimens showed mild to moderate epithelial dysplasia; 4% revealed severe epithelial dysplasia (Fig. 50-7) or carcinoma in situ; and 3.1% of specimens were diagnosed as showing infiltrating squamous carcinoma. The authors used the following microscopic criteria for epithelial dysplasia:

1. Irregular epithelial stratification
2. Hyperplasia of the basal layer
3. Drop-shaped rete processes
4. Keratinization of single cells or cell groups in the prickle layer
5. Loss of intercellular adherence
6. Increased mitotic activity with occasional abnormal mitotic spindles
7. Increased nuclear-cytoplasmic ratio
8. Loss of polarity of basal cells
9. Cellular pleomorphism
10. Enlarged or multiple nucleoli

The microscopic features of clinical leukoplakia show a range of microscopic changes, reaching even invasive squamous carcinoma. The progression or regression of these lesions has not been studied as well as squamous epithelial lesions of the female genital tract, but it appears that severely dysplastic lesions and squamous carcinoma in situ are unlikely to regress spontaneously.[82-84] There is interest in studying biologic modifiers to prevent development of cancer in patients with leukoplakia.[85]

Erythroplakia (erythroplasia of Queyrat). In recent years, emphasis has been placed on the recognition of ery-

Table 50-10 **Chronic red lesions of oropharyngeal mucosa**

Benign	Hemangioma
	Chronic gingivitis
	Eosinophilic granuloma
	Peripheral giant cell granuloma
	Pyogenic granuloma
	Median rhomboid glossitis
	Chronic candidiasis
Premalignant/malignant	Sideropenic dysphagia
	Erythroplakia and squamous carcinoma
	Lymphoma and leukemia
	Kaposi's sarcoma

throplakia because it so frequently proves to be squamous dysplasia or early carcinoma on biopsy. It was originally described by Queyrat in 1911 as a lesion occurring on the glans penis of an elderly syphilitic person.[86] Since then, similar lesions have been described as occurring on the vulva and oral mucosa in patients who are not syphilitic. To correspond with *leukoplakia,* the term *erythroplakia* has replaced *erythroplasia.* In comparison, erythroplakia is much less common than leukoplakia but is much more likely to be severe dysplasia or cancer.

The World Health Organization's definition of erythroplakia is widely accepted: "lesions of the oral mucosa that present as bright red, velvety plaques which cannot be characterized clinically or pathologically as being due to any other condition."[87] Therefore the clinical diagnosis of erythroplakia is one of exclusion, since many oral conditions produce a "red" lesion (Table 50-10). As for leukoplakia, the definition of erythroplakia does not indicate a histologic diagnosis, but almost all erythroplakic lesions will prove to be squamous dysplasia or carcinoma on biopsy. The risk factors for erythroplakia are the same as for squamous carcinoma.

Erythroplakia has no sex predilection and is most commonly seen in the sixth to seventh decades of life. The most common sites are the floor of the mouth, the soft palate–anterior pillar–retromolar complex, and the ventrolateral border of the posterior two thirds of the tongue (these three sites are also high-risk areas for invasive squamous carcinomas).[88]

Most lesions of erythroplakia are asymptomatic, uniformly bright red, and velvety patches, but occasionally the surface is nodular or there are white or yellow spots of keratinization on a red background (Fig. 50-8, *A*). Lesions that are mixtures of white areas (resembling leukoplakia) and red areas are sometimes referred to as "speckled erythroplakia" (this term is preferred to "speckled leukoplakia" because the lesions that contain red patches have a high incidence of malignancy) (Fig. 50-8, *A*).

Microscopy of erythroplakic lesions will reveal invasive squamous carcinoma, carcinoma in situ, or severe dysplasia in about 90% of biopsy specimens. The remaining 10% of cases generally show mild or moderate dysplasia. The invasive squamous cell carcinoma in an erythroplakic lesion can range from well to poorly differentiated but is usually superficial and often multifocal. Microscopy also clarifies the reasons for the redness; the subepithelial connective tissue papillae extend high into the epithelium and contain prominent, dilated capillaries; and the overlying epithelium is thin and exhibits little keratinization.[89-91]

Because of the high likelihood that a lesion is carcinoma, management of erythroplakia is by complete excision and thorough pathologic examination.

Reverse smoker's palate. As mentioned above, tobacco use contributes to the development of some cases of oral leukoplakia. In India, the habit of reverse smoking (with the lit end of the cigarette held in the mouth) causes palatal keratosis, umbilicated excrescences, ulcerations, and white and red areas. The characteristic histologic features of this lesion are hyperorthokeratosis and squamous epithelial hyperplasia, but squamous dysplasia and carcinoma have developed when patients were followed for 10 years.[92,93]

Precancerous conditions

Sideropenic dysphagia (Paterson-Kelly syndrome, Plummer-Vinson syndrome). Sideropenic dysphagia is a manifestation of iron-deficiency anemia, with dysphagia, glossitis, and pharyngoesophageal ulcers. The syndrome occurs chiefly in women in their fourth and fifth decades of life. In addition to signs and symptoms of iron-deficiency anemia (such as fatigue, a lemon-tinted pallor to the skin, and nail changes), there are cracks or fissures at the corners of the mouth, a smooth, red, painful tongue with atrophy of the filiform, and later the fungiform papillae, leukoplakia, and dysphagia resulting from an esophageal stricture or web. Patients with

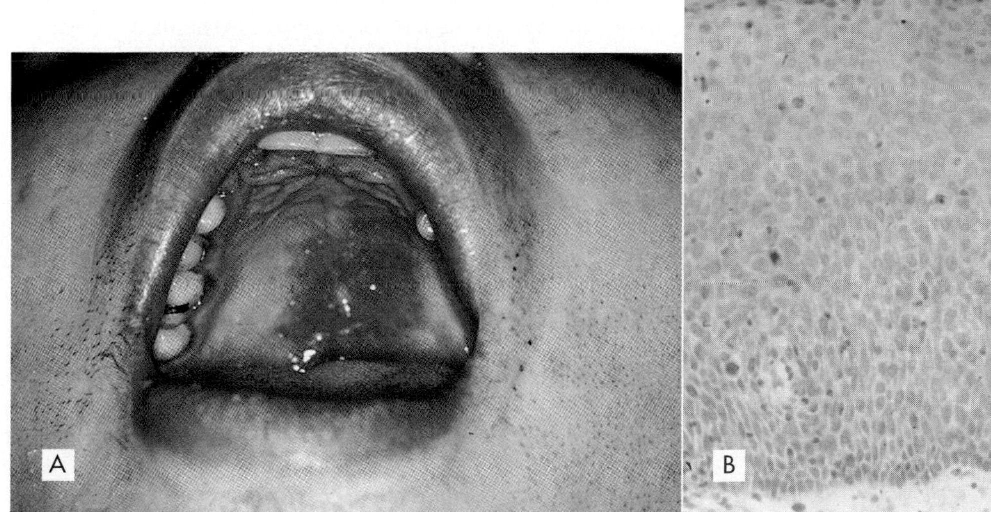

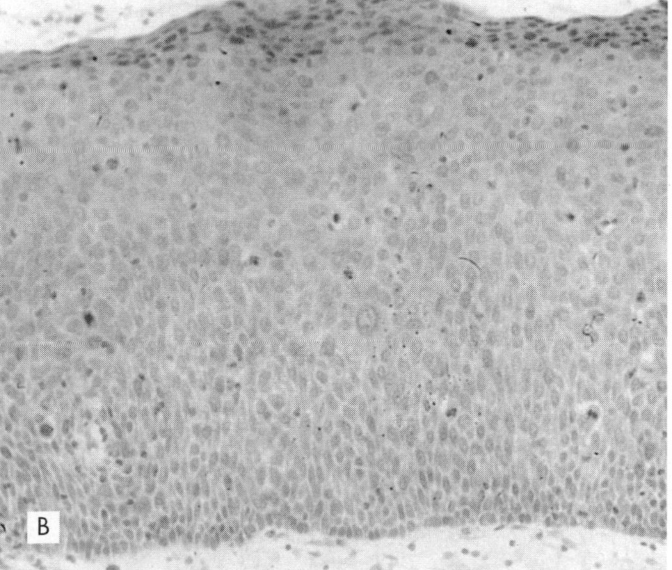

Fig. 50-8 **A,** A red lesion of the hard palate of a 30-year-old man who is known to smoke. No apparent cause of the redness was elicited. **B,** Carcinoma in situ with complete loss of the maturation sequence and frequent mitoses in the upper strata of the epithelium.

sideropenic dysphagia are at increased risk for cancer of the oral cavity, hypopharynx, and upper esophagus.[94,95]

Oral submucous fibrosis (oral submucosal fibrosis). Oral submucous fibrosis is an insidious chronic disease that is most common in people from Southeast Asia and is rare in this hemisphere. Dietary factors, particularly chronic betel (areca) nut chewing and chillies (a strongly irritating spice commonly used in India), are implicated in its pathogenesis. It begins as a subepithelial inflammatory reaction followed by fibroelastic change in the lamina propria, epithelial atrophy, and dense collagen deposition in the submucosa. The progressive fibrosis can involve any area of the oral cavity and sometimes the pharynx. Eventually, there is loss of mobility, trismus, and the inability to eat. This disease is suspected of predisposing patients to oral carcinoma.[96,97]

PRIMARY EPITHELIAL CANCERS

Carcinomas account for 96% of all oral cancers, of which squamous cancer is the most common type.[98] Salivary gland carcinomas are described in Chapter 51.

Squamous cell carcinoma (epidermoid carcinoma)

Etiology and risk factors. The genetic basis for oral and pharyngeal carcinomas has not been as thoroughly worked out as that for colon and breast carcinomas, but information is beginning to develop. Deletions of chromosomes 3p and 18q, nonrandom deletions and rearrangements of other chromosomes, p53 mutations, amplification and overexpression of the epidermal growth factor receptor, and amplification of oncogenes have been described.[99]

Of all the factors believed to cause oral and pharyngeal cancer, tobacco use and alcohol consumption, alone or in combination, are the major offenders.[100-106] All forms of tobacco use (cigarette, pipe, cigar, smokeless) are associated with oral and pharyngeal cancer, and the risk increases with dose and duration.[107] Numerous carcinogens have been isolated from tobacco, including various aromatic hydrocarbons and nitrosamines.

As early as 1957, a study implicated alcohol consumption as a risk factor for oral cancer, but the mechanisms underlying this association remain poorly understood.[108,109] The dehydrating and irritating effects of alcohol on the mucosa, its potential role as a solvent for carcinogens, presence of carcinogens in alcoholic beverages, and liver-mediated cellular changes are among the proposed theories. Commonly, heavy drinkers also smoke, and a synergistic relationship between tobacco and alcohol abuse has been shown for oral and pharyngeal carcinoma.[110,111] Some but not all studies have linked use of mouthwash (which generally contains alcohol) with an increased risk of oral and pharyngeal cancer.[112-117]

The possible role of oncogenic viruses in causing some forms of oral and pharyngeal cancer is being investigated. EBV has been linked to Burkitt's lymphoma and nasopharyngeal carcinoma but not to oral squamous cell carcinoma.[118-120] Cytomegalovirus has been linked to Kaposi's sarcoma.[121] Some types of HPV are associated with upper aerodigestive tract papillomas and squamous cell carcinomas, including verrucous carcinoma.[122-124] Herpes simplex virus has also been suggested as being related to lip cancer, though this association is tentative.[125]

Ultraviolet rays and tobacco use are the major causes of carcinomas of the lips. The role of poor oral hygiene and chronic irritation (as from ill-fitting dental restorations, hot or spicy foods) in the development of oral carcinoma is unclear and doubtful. They may act as promoters (by causing inflammation and cell proliferation) rather than initiators (that is, mutagens). An association between oral cancer and chronic syphilis or candidal infection has been suggested but is tenuous (see discussions of these organisms earlier in this chapter). Iron deficiency (with sideropenic dysphagia) is the only nutritional deficiency with a widely accepted link to oral carcinoma.

Epidemiology. In 1996, an estimated 29,600 individuals in the United States will be diagnosed with cancer of the oral cavity and pharynx: 19,800 males and 9800 females.[126] This accounts for 3% of potentially life-threatening cancers (excluding basal cell and squamous cell carcinomas of the skin and in situ carcinomas) diagnosed in males and 2% of those diagnosed in females. Over 90% of oral and pharyngeal cancers are squamous cell carcinoma. The typical patient with oral or pharyngeal squamous cancer is a male over 50 years of age who drinks alcohol and uses tobacco.

From 1973 to 1987, the incidence of oral cancer declined by 0.4% per year, except in black males, in whom it increased by 0.7% per year. The incidence of pharyngeal cancer has risen for the overall population (1% increase per year), largely because of the increase of 6% per year in black males.[127] The mortalities for cancer of the oral cavity and pharynx are greater in males than in females and in blacks than in whites. Although the overall 5-year relative survival rate is 53%, the rate among blacks is only 31%.[128]

Site. Squamous cell carcinoma can occur anywhere on the oral and pharyngeal mucosa, but certain sites are more frequent. In the oral cavity, tongue cancer accounts for almost 30% of cases, followed by lip (17.4%) and floor of mouth (16.4%). The mortality from squamous carcinoma also varies by site in the mouth, with the lowest mortality from lip cancer and the highest for cancer of the tongue. Cancers in the oral cavity are almost three times more likely to be localized at the time of diagnosis than pharyngeal cancers (47% versus 17%).

Clinical Features. The most common presenting symptoms and signs of squamous cell carcinoma of the oral cavity and pharynx are listed in Table 50-11.[129]

Advanced or widely metastatic oral and pharyngeal cancer can also present with nonspecific wasting symptoms (such as cachexia, rapid weight loss), or signs and symptoms from metastases to remote sites (most frequently lung, liver, and bones).

Pathology. The gross appearance reflects the clinical presentation of the cancer. The cut surface of the tumor is usually white or tan-white, sometimes with areas of necrosis or hemorrhage (Fig. 50-9). The cancer usually has irregular borders.

The microscopic features are similar to squamous cell carcinomas arising in other mucosal sites. Dysplastic squamous epithelium or in situ carcinoma may be seen at the edges of early lesions. Infiltration of the stroma is signified by an increase in tumor cell size and pleomorphism, by irregularity and loss of definition of the epitheliostromal junction, by stromal desmoplasia, and generally by increased inflammation. Larger tumors ulcerate, become necrotic, and invade adjacent structures. High mitotic activity, infiltrative borders, lymphatic and blood vessel invasion indicate aggressive cancers.

Table 50-11 Signs and symptoms of squamous cell carcinoma of oral cavity and pharynx

- A mucosal ulcer with rolled margins and indurated bed, or ulcer extending into muscle or jawbones
- An exophytic growth where the majority of the tumor mass extends beyond its base
- An endophytic growth with fixation to underlying organs or tissues (such as bone)
- A lesion that does not heal (usually painless at first; excruciating pain often signifies invasion of nerve fibers)
- Painless lymphadenopathy, with large or firm lymph nodes caused by metastatic cancer (with time, the lymph nodes can become fixed to adjacent tissues because of extranodal invasion)
- Painless trismus (limitation of mouth opening) unassociated with infection can occur when carcinoma in the posterior portion of the tongue or floor of mouth invades the masticatory muscles, particularly the internal pterygoid
- Erythroplakia
- Leukoplakia, particularly involving tongue, floor of mouth, and lips
- Loosening of teeth not explained by periodontal disease (indicating possible gingival or alveolar mucosal carcinoma)
- Unilateral nasal stuffiness or discharge, unilateral swelling or bulging of the maxillary alveolar ridge, palate, mucobuccal fold or face inferior and lateral to the eye (these may indicate an advanced carcinoma of the maxillary antrum)
- Sore throat, hoarseness, dysphagia, sensation of a mass in the throat, hemoptysis, sharp pain referred to the ipsilateral ear, face, or neck, and pain on tongue movement (these are symptoms associated with pharyngeal carcinoma)

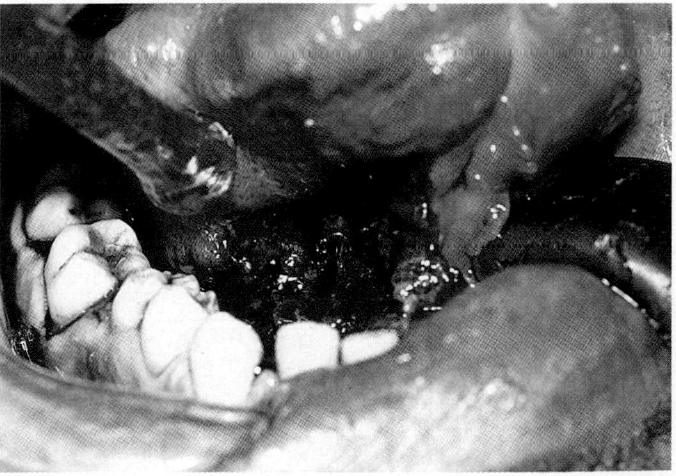

Fig. 50-9 Advanced oral squamous cell carcinoma. Notice the large malignant ulcer with considerable necrosis and hemorrhage of the anterior floor of the mouth.

Well-differentiated (grade 1) cancers form broad bands and nests of cells, usually with rounded contours. There may be "maturation" of cancer cells from the periphery of the bands and nests toward the center, mimicking normal squamous epithelium. The cancer cells generally have abundant eosinophilic cytoplasm, intercellular bridges, and prominent keratinization (either as single cells or keratin pearls). Nuclear atypia and mitotic activity are more restrained than in more poorly differentiated lesions.

The cells in moderately differentiated (grade 2) carcinomas still resemble squamous epithelial cells, but there is less evidence of squamous differentiation (that is, less maturation toward the centers of nests, scantier cytoplasm, fewer intercellular bridges, and less keratinization than those in grade I carcinomas). Cancer cell groups are more irregular and infiltrative, individual cells vary more in size and shape, nuclei are more pleomorphic and hyperchromatic, and mitotic spindles are more frequent and more often abnormal.

The cells of poorly differentiated (grade 3) squamous cell carcinomas bear little resemblance to their cell of origin. The cancer forms snaky cords and irregular nests of poorly cohesive cells. Keratinization is infrequent, particularly in the form of well-developed keratin pearls. Cellular pleomorphism, nuclear atypia, and mitotic rates are all greatly increased. Bizarre tumor giant cells and mitotic spindles may be prominent. The cancer cells at the periphery of the tumor are more infiltrative than in better-differentiated carcinomas. Sometimes, the cancer cells show mixed patterns of differentiation (such as abundant keratinization but with very bizarre nuclei and frequent mitoses). Other poorly differentiated squamous carcinomas are composed of sheets of uniform cells (small cell, large cell, or spindle cell types; these variants are discussed later).

Within a single tumor, the degree of differentiation may vary from one area to another. Since the overall grade is dictated by the least differentiated area, the pathologist should routinely sample several areas.

Special diagnostic techniques. Although light microscopic examination of routinely stained tissue samples is the cornerstone for the diagnosis of squamous carcinomas, immunohistochemistry and ultrastructural analysis are very useful when faced with anaplastic cancers of uncertain type or lineage. Poorly differentiated squamous carcinoma cells have few tonofilament bundles and rare primitive junctional complexes, but squamous differentiation may be indicated by electron microscopic demonstration of curvilinear tonofibril bundles.[130]

Cytokeratin is an excellent marker for epithelial differentiation.[131] Nineteen subclasses of keratins have been characterized, with different profiles in different types of epithelia.[132-135] These subclasses can be identified with monoclonal antibodies. For example, normal cornified squamous epithelium expresses keratin subclasses 1 and 10 in the upper layers, whereas normal noncornified oral epithelium expresses keratins 4 and 13. Well-differentiated oral squamous carcinomas express these keratin subclasses. Less differentiated carcinomas tend to express keratins 8 and 18. In anaplastic carcinomas, keratins 5 or 14, favor the diagnosis of squamous carcinoma over adenocarcinoma.[136]

Exfoliative cytologic features of surface scrapings from oral mucosal lesions can indicate dysplastic or neoplastic changes.[137] However, this technique has limited value because (1) the major dysplastic alterations in leukoplakia occur in the subcornified layers of epithelium and few, if any, of the dysplastic cells may appear at the keratotic surface, and (2) biopsies are easy to perform with a diagnostic reliability of close to 100%, whereas the exfoliative cytology yield for oral squamous carcinoma is only 86%.[138]

Fine-needle aspiration biopsy (FNAB), however, is becoming an important modality in the diagnosis of cervical lymph node metastases. FNAB can be performed easily in an outpatient setting and provides a quick, inexpensive, reliable diagnosis.[139] It should be stressed that FNAB is only one part of the integrated work-up of such lesions.

Prognostic factors. The survival rates for oral and pharyngeal carcinomas depend primarily on several factors: (1) the stage of the cancer, (2) the site of the primary tumor, (3) the adequacy of initial treatment, (4) patient's performance status, and (5) the histologic grade of the malignancy.[140,141] Secondary factors include the patient's continued smoking and alcohol consumption and predisposition to developing multiple oral malignancies.

The stage of oral and pharyngeal carcinoma is assigned by using the TNM classification when the cancer is first diagnosed. This classification takes into account the size and local spread of the primary tumor (T), regional lymph node spread (N), and distant metastases (M).[142] Using this system, stage I carcinomas are up to 2 cm in greatest diameter; stage II carcinomas are larger, up to 4 cm in diameter; stage III carcinomas are greater than 4 cm in diameter, or have a single homolateral lymph node involved (less than 3 cm in diameter); and stage IV carcinomas invade adjacent structures (such as skin, cortical bone, deep structures), exhibit more extensive lymph node involvement by cancer, or have distant metastases.

In addition to providing the information necessary to arrive at the correct stage, the pathologist should (where possible) describe the tumor grade; depth of tumor invasion; involvement of adjacent structures; the contours of the tumor margins (rounded versus infiltrative); presence of perineural, lymphatic, or blood vessel invasion; and relationship of the cancer to the resection margins. Description of the lymph nodes should involve counts of involved and total lymph nodes (including their sites when possible), size of the largest involved lymph node, and presence of extranodal cancer extension.[143]

Most oral and pharyngeal cancers are localized or regional at the time of diagnosis (38% and 41%, respectively). The 5-year relative survival rates for oral and pharyngeal cancers are 75% for localized cases, 41% for regional cases, and 18% for cases with distant metastases at presentation.

Although the diagnosis and staging of oral and pharyngeal carcinomas are primarily arrived at by clinical examination and biopsy, imaging has assumed an important role in the assessment of depth of invasion, involvement of deep structures, regional lymph nodes, and possible metastatic sites.[144-147]

Routes of spread. Oral and pharyngeal carcinomas spread primarily by local extension and lymphatic dissemination. Although hematogenous spread is less common, it is important in the spread of cancer to remote sites.

Adipose tissue and skeletal muscle offer little resistance to local cancer invasion, but periosteum initially resists. With time, the periosteum and bone cortex are breached, and the marrow is invaded. Lymphatic spread to regional lymph nodes is a common occurrence, found in up to 50% of cases, and is often the first indication of cancer.[148] The likelihood of lymph node involvement correlates with (1) tumor size and depth of invasion, (2) primary tumor site (increased risk of lymph node metastases with more posterior sites), and (3) tumor grade.[149,150] Lungs, bone, and liver are the most common sites of distant metastases from oral and pharyngeal carcinomas, which eventually occur in 11% to 25% of patients.[151,152]

Therapy. Surgery, radiation, and chemotherapy (alone or in combination) are the currently used modalities for oral and pharyngeal cancers. Surgery or radiation therapy, or both, are used with curative intent for localized cancers or cancers with regional spread. Chemotherapy is commonly accepted for palliation of patients with recurrent or metastatic disease, but an expanded role is being investigated with protocols for induction chemotherapy, organ preservation, concurrent use with radiation therapy, and chemosuppression of premalignant lesions.[153-157]

Unfortunately, these therapies cause considerable morbidity, and failure rates are still high. Surgery often requires sacrifice of cosmetically or functionally important structures such as lip, tongue, mandible, and occasionally the eye. Radiation therapy is associated with mucositis, xerostomia (secondary to injury of salivary glands), loss of taste, alopecia, osteonecrosis, rampant tooth caries, and transverse myelitis of the spinal cord. Chemotherapy toxicities include nausea, vomiting, oral and gastrointestinal ulcers, and complications of bone marrow suppression.

The patients should be closely followed for recurrences and second primary cancers (usually in the respiratory or upper digestive tracts), which occur at an annual rate of 3% to 7% per year, with an excess mortality of 5.2% per year.[158,159]

Variants of squamous cell carcinoma

The light microscopic diagnosis of squamous cell carcinomas is generally straightforward when the biopsy is of adequate size and well oriented, but there are exceptions. Some well-differentiated cancers may be difficult to distinguish from benign proliferations. Some poorly differentiated histologic variants of squamous carcinoma may be confused with other cancers, particularly when there is little keratinization. Recognition of these aberrant patterns—together with more extensive tumor sampling or judicious use of adjunctive techniques (such as special stains, immunohistochemistry, electron microscopy)—may clarify ambiguous cases.

Poorly differentiated variants. *Nonkeratinizing squamous cell carcinomas* composed predominantly of large round cells with large vesicular nuclei may be difficult to distinguish from melanoma, large cell lymphomas, rhabdomyosarcoma, or other anaplastic cancers. In some cancers, particularly in the nasopharynx, there is no light microscopic evidence of squamous differentiation, and the cancer is termed *undifferentiated carcinoma.* In some undifferentiated carcinomas, the cancer cells are accompanied by numerous lymphocytes (which may almost obscure the cancer cells), a pattern known as *lymphoepithelioma* but more properly referred to as *lymphocyte-rich carcinoma,* to indicate that it is not a lymphoma.

The *basaloid squamous carcinoma* is a variant composed of small cancer cells that may be difficult to distinguish from lymphoma, neuroendocrine carcinomas (including metastatic oat cell carcinoma), and basaloid adenoid cystic carcinoma.[160] The *spindle cell carcinoma* variant resembles sarcomas.[161] *Adenosquamous carcinomas* may be difficult to distinguish from high-grade mucoepidermoid carcinoma of the salivary gland.[162]

Papillary squamous carcinoma. Some squamous carcinomas are predominantly exophytic growths, with the formation of papillary fronds.[163] Difficulty with these papillary squamous carcinomas occurs in recognizing if there is stromal invasion and in distinguishing them from other lesions such as squamous papillomas and verrucous carcinoma.

Verrucous carcinoma. Verrucous carcinoma is best described as an uncommon "low-grade" variant of well differentiated squamous carcinoma, which occurs in the oral cavity, larynx, nasal fossae, esophagus, penis, anorectal region, scrotum, vulva, vagina, uterine cervix, and skin. In the oral cavity, verrucous carcinoma is most commonly found in the mandibular sulcus and the alveolar mucosa of the mandibular ridge.[164,165] It is strongly associated with chewing tobacco and snuff use, and there is a possible association with HPV.[166]

Verrucous carcinoma is estimated to represent less than 5% of all oral cancers. It occurs in elderly patients and has a male predominance. The neoplasm appears to evolve indolently in an area of leukoplakia. It is predominantly exophytic with a finely nodular or papillary surface. It may grow to a large size by lateral spread before it involves deep underlying structures. Regardless of its size and depth of penetration, it maintains a well-differentiated morphology. At diagnosis, there may be tender and enlarged regional lymph nodes, but these are generally reactive. Regional lymph node metastases are rare, and distant metastases have not been reported.

The microscopic features of verrucous carcinoma include (1) a thick, orderly layer of proliferating squamous epithelium with little cellular atypia, mitotic activity, or other characteristics of malignancy; (2) a verrucous surface with cleftlike spaces covered by parakeratinized cells extending deep into the lesion; (3) a rounded contour to the epithelial extensions at the advancing growth margin, with a well-defined carcinoma-stroma junction; and (4) a brisk chronic inflammatory cell response in the underlying connective tissue (Fig. 50-10). The histologic features appear deceptively harmless, particularly in small, superficial, or badly oriented biopsy specimens, and this cancer can be underdiagnosed as benign epithelial hyperplasia, keratosis, squamous papilloma, or keratoacanthoma.

From this discussion, it should be clear that this entity should be recognized for two reasons: (1) it should not be mistaken for a benign epithelial proliferation, and (2) it carries the most favorable prognosis of all forms of buccal carcinoma.[167] It is treated surgically, and recurrences follow incomplete excision. Although controversial, some believe that radiation therapy may lead to transformation of verrucous carcinoma into a poorly differentiated squamous cell carcinoma.

Nasopharyngeal carcinoma. Squamous cell carcinoma arising in the nasopharynx has several features that distinguish it from those of the mouth and oropharynx: its epidemiology, its presentation, its preference for undifferentiated and lymphocyte-rich histologic patterns, and its therapy.[168,169]

Nasopharyngeal carcinoma is very rare in the United States but accounts for 18% of all cancers in China. The incidence decreases in Chinese who emigrate to low-risk areas but still remains higher than in non-Chinese. Nasopharyngeal carcinoma is associated with the HLA-A2 histocompatibility locus, as well as with elevated EBV antibody titers. These cancers often present with nasal and ear symptoms (such as nasal discharge, bleeding or obstruction, otalgia, loss of hearing), headache, or cervical mass (from lymph node metastasis).

These cancers are classified as undifferentiated (most common), keratinizing or nonkeratinizing (least common) types. Keratinizing squamous carcinomas can be of any histologic grade. The nonkeratinizing carcinoma is essentially a squamous carcinoma whose microscopic appearance resembles high-grade urothelial carcinoma, with multiple layers of elongated cells. The cells in undifferentiated carcinomas may have a large cell, clear cell, or spindle cell morphology, but they tend to grow in patternless syncytia, to have large vesicular nuclei, and to elicit no desmoplastic stromal response. Lymphocyte-rich infiltrates are particularly common in the undifferentiated type.

Because of the difficult location and advanced stage of these cancers, primary treatment is radiation therapy. Interestingly, undifferentiated carcinomas have the best response to radiation and the best 5-year survival rate.

Melanoma

Primary malignant melanoma of the oral mucosa constitutes 0.2% to 2% of all melanomas in the United States, but 8% to 25% in Japan.[170,171] Over 80% of these lesions arise on the palate or maxillary alveolar mucosa. Oral melanomas usually arise in patients over 50 years of age, sometimes from a preexisting melanosis or nevus.[172-174] The lesions are variably colored, have irregular borders, and may be macular, papular, or ulcerated.

Both nodular and superficial spreading types occur, though the majority show microscopic features resembling acral-lentiginous melanoma of the skin. The biology of oral melanomas has not been as widely studied as those of the skin, and contemporary surgical pathology concepts about cutaneous melanomas have not been widely applied to oral melanomas. Most reports indicate a very poor prognosis for oral melanomas with about 5% of the patients surviving. However, most tumors are advanced when first detected.[175,176]

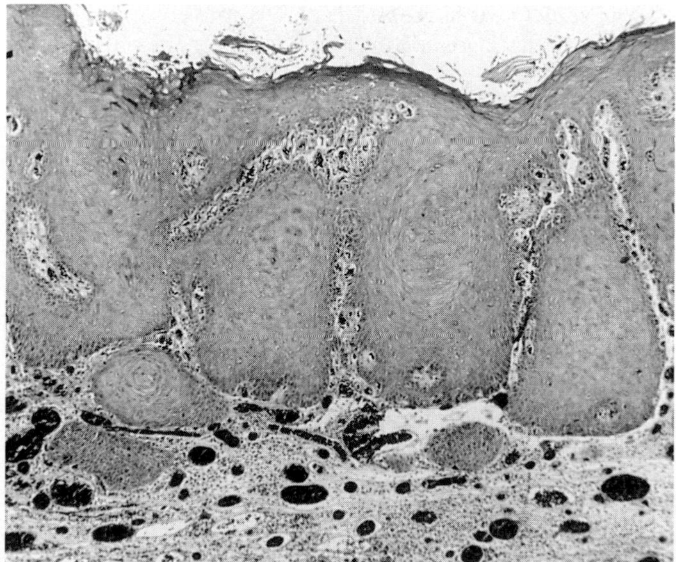

Fig. 50-10 Verrucous carcinoma showing rounded contour of neoplastic epithelium and groups of tumor cells extending from it into the underlying connective tissue.

CYSTS OF THE MUCOUS MEMBRANES AND SOFT TISSUES

Mucoceles are usually not true cysts but are briefly discussed below because they are so common in the mouth and the terminology is confusing (oral mucoceles are further discussed in Chapter 51). The other cysts discussed in this section are rare, except for the gingival cysts of infants. Intraosseous cysts (jaw cysts) are discussed in a later section of this chapter.

The mucocele and most gingival cysts of adults are acquired cysts. The remaining cysts described in this section are considered to be developmental.

Cysts of the gingiva

Gingival cyst of infants (dental lamina cyst of the newborn). Gingival cysts of infants are usually small, white or yellow nodules or cysts seen along the alveolar ridges of newborns. They may be solitary or multiple.[177] These asymptomatic gingival cysts are very common but rarely large enough to be obvious. Microscopy shows a thin epithelial lining of stratified squamous cells with flattened basal cells, parakeratinized surface cells, and keratin in the lumen. These gingival cysts are believed to arise from the rests of Serres (epithelial remnants of the dental lamina). Treatment is unnecessary because they generally rupture spontaneously and heal by 3 months of age.

Similar cysts are found in the superficial mucosa along the midpalate or the junction of hard and soft palates. These cysts, called *Epstein's pearls,* are nonodontogenic but have an identical gross and microscopic appearance and the same clinical course.[178]

Gingival cyst of adults. A gingival cyst of adults presents as a small, painless nodule on the gingiva. Except for the location, it can clinically resemble a mucocele. It is infrequent, particularly in comparison with gingival cysts of infants. Some gingival cysts in adults appear to arise from cystic degeneration of the rests of Serres, whereas others may arise from traumatic epithelial inclusions.[179] Simple excision is curative.

Nasolabial (nasoalveolar) cyst. The rare nasolabial cyst is found in the soft tissue on the alveolar process near the base of the nostril. It may erode into the outer surface of the bone but does not occur within the bone; therefore the alternative name *nasoalveolar cyst* is inaccurate. This cyst is believed to arise from the nasolacrimal duct or embryonic rests persisting after formation of the duct.[180]

The predominant complaint is of soft-tissue swelling, often near the canines. There may be discomfort or nasal stuffiness. Middle-aged females are predominantly affected. The cyst lining is usually pseudostratified columnar cells with numerous goblet cells, but cuboidal and stratified squamous epithelium may also be present. There is a fibrous capsule around the cyst. Treatment is simple excision.

Nongingival mucosal and soft-tissue cysts

Mucoceles. Mucocele is a descriptive clinical term for cysts or cystlike lesions resulting from mucus accumulation. By far the most common intraoral mucocele is the *mucus extravasation* type of mucocele (usually referred to simply as mucocele). In this type of mucocele, traumatic rupture of a minor salivary gland duct leads to spillage of mucus that elicits a granulation tissue reaction and a modest inflammatory response in the surrounding tissue. The consequent mass is a mucus extravasation cavity, not a true cyst. This lesion is common on the lower lip (because of lip biting and other trauma) but can occur elsewhere in the oral mucosa.

Much less common than the mucus extravasation mucocele is the *mucus retention cyst,* caused by salivary duct blockage and accumulation of mucin within the dilated duct. This is a true cyst, lined by salivary duct epithelium. *Ranula* is a clinical term for mucoceles in the floor of the mouth (of either mucus retention or extravasation type). Ranula is usually associated with a sublingual salivary gland duct, occasionally a submandibular gland duct.

Note that mucoceles also occur within the maxillary sinuses where they are attributable to accumulation of mucus produced by the sinus lining mucosa, not mucus from the salivary glands as with the intraoral mucoceles.

Lymphoepithelial cyst. A lymphoepithelial cyst occurs more often in the lateral aspects of the neck where it is usually called a branchial (cleft) cyst. The most common intraoral location is laterally on the floor of the mouth, followed by the tongue. The cyst is usually asymptomatic and is discovered incidentally or when it becomes infected. The lymphoepithelial cyst is lined by stratified squamous epithelium, pseudstratified respiratory-like epithelium, or both.[181] The fibrous cyst capsule contains lymphoid aggregates, often with germinal centers.

Dermoid cyst. The mouth is an unusual site for dermoid cysts. The most frequent intraoral location is the floor of the mouth, usually in or near the midline. It presents as a painless, slowly growing, fluctuant mass that can interfere with tongue function. Microscopically, it resembles dermoid cysts of the skin and elsewhere.

Thyroglossal duct cyst. A thyroglossal duct cyst usually occurs in the superior midline of the neck but can occur in the tongue (see the discussion of anomalies of the tongue, earlier in this chapter).

NONEPITHELIAL TUMORS AND TUMORLIKE LESIONS OF THE MUCOUS MEMBRANES AND SOFT TISSUES

Benign lesions

Fibroma (irritation fibroma, focal fibrous hyperplasia). In the oral cavity, the term *fibroma* is used for focal fibrous hyperplasia. This is a very common lesion, which is probably stimulated by constant local irritation (such as cheek biting). It can occur at any age but is usually detected in the third to fifth decades of life. The most common sites are the lateral border of the tongue, buccal and labial mucosa, and the gingival margin.[182]

The fibroma is usually slow growing and painless. It is dome shaped, either sessile or pedunculated, and varies from soft to firm. The lesion may be lighter than the adjacent mucosa because of decreased vascularity. The covering mucosa may appear normal, keratotic, or ulcerated. Oral fibroma does not usually exceed 1 cm in diameter but can occasionally grow to several centimeters.

Microscopy shows a fibrous nodule projecting above the surrounding mucosal surface. The covering epithelium may be thin and stretched. The connective tissue of the nodule is usually hypocellular and is composed of interlacing dense collagen bundles and fibroblasts. Increased vascularity and inflammatory cells are present in some cases.

Usually the diagnosis of fibroma is not difficult. Occasionally, pyogenic granulomas is a diagnostic considerations, but these are more vascular. Fibromas seldom recur after simple excision.

Fibroma may occur on the gingiva and should be distinguished from other polypoid gingival lesions such as the *peripheral ossifying fibroma* (which contains calcium deposits, globular cementum-like particles, osteoid or bone), the *peripheral odontogenic fibroma* (which contains odontogenic epithelium), and[183] the *peripheral giant cell granuloma* (which contains multinucleate giant cells. These lesions are further discussed in the section on odontogenic tumors.

Note that the nonspecific term *epulis* is still sometimes used for these and other gingival masses but should be avoided by pathologists unless the type of lesion is specified.

Pyogenic granuloma (granuloma pyogenicum, lobular capillary hemangioma). A pyogenic granuloma is neither pyogenic nor granulomatous but is presumed to be hyperplastic granulation tissue.[184] The adjective "pyogenic," as used here, should be interpreted as meaning caused by an inflammatory stimulation and not suppurative.

Even though the stimulus that engenders a pyogenic granuloma is not always known, infection and trauma are postulated as the causes. Hormonal stimulation has been implicated in causing a variant of pyogenic granuloma that occurs during pregnancy, *granuloma gravidarum.*[185] Pyogenic granulomas are viewed by some as being hemangiomas.

In the mouth, the most common site is the gingival margin followed by the lip and tongue (Fig. 50-11, *A*). The lesion presents as a purple-red, painless, polypoid mass that can be sessile or pedunculated. It is usually friable and hemorrhagic. The surface may be ulcerated and covered with fibrinous material. The size varies from a few millimeters to a few centimeters. The rate of growth of pyogenic granuloma is sometimes alarmingly rapid. The lesion can occur at any age and is more common in females. On the gingiva, pyogenic granuloma may be mistaken for peripheral giant cell granuloma. Fibromas form similar masses but are usually firmer and pale.

Microscopically, the covering epithelium is usually atrophic or ulcerated. The pyogenic granuloma contains prominent blood vessels in a lobular growth pattern (each lobule is composed of a central larger vessel surrounded by con geries of small capillaries) (Fig. 50-11, *B*). The stroma is fibromyxoid or edematous, or both. Acute and chronic inflammatory cells are common, especially in ulcerated lesions, near the surface. Mitotic activity in both endothelial cells and stromal fibroblasts can be brisk, especially in secondarily inflamed lesions. The histologic appearance of pyogenic granuloma is generally characteristic, but more fibrotic, senescent examples may overlap the appearance of fibromas.

Recurrence of pyogenic granuloma after surgical excision can be as frequent as 16%, occasionally with an alarming growth rate.[186] Granuloma gravidarum regresses dramatically after parturition.

Peripheral ossifying fibroma. A peripheral ossifying fibroma is a calcifying or ossifying fibrous nodule on the gingival margin. It appears to develop from the periodontal ligament. Although the peripheral ossifying fibroma can occur at any age, it is somewhat more common in children and young adults. There is a slight female bias. Clinically, the lesion presents as a painless, usually small, pedunculated, or sessile nodule on the gingival margin, anterior to the molar area. It occurs with equal freqency in the maxilla and the mandible. The color of the lesion might be slightly erythematous or similar to normal gingiva.

Histologically, the epithelium over the lesion is more frequently ulcerated than intact. The tumor is composed of very cellular connective tissue with plump fibroblasts in a delicate fibrillar stroma. Blood vessels are not prominent. The distinctive feature is the presence of calcified structures, which might be in the form of granular dystrophic calcifications, globular cementumlike particles, or interconnecting trabeculas of bone and osteoid. The frequency and relative proportions of these calcified structures varies between lesions, and some lesions are almost totally calcified.

Adequate treatment requires excision of the lesion at its origin on the surface of the root, but extraction of the involved tooth is not usually needed. Recurrence after simple excision is common; rates of 16% to 20% have been reported.[187]

Peripheral giant cell granuloma. A peripheral giant cell granuloma is an unusual gingival lesion that is histologically

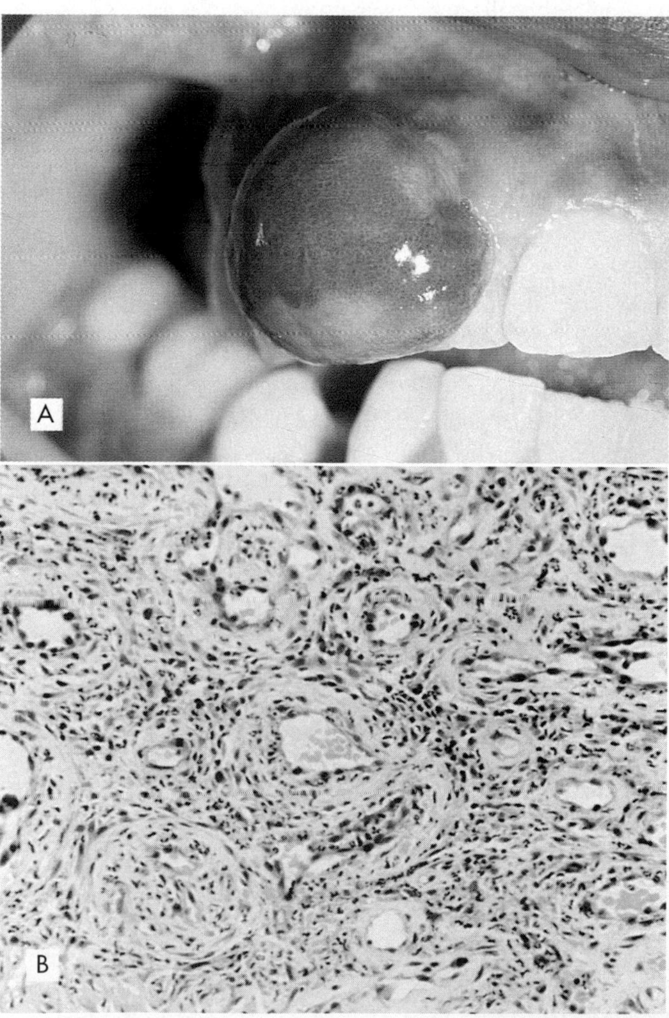

Fig. 50-11 **A,** Large purple-red pyogenic granuloma attached to the gingiva of the anterior maxilla of a young man. **B,** Photomicrograph shows prominent blood vessels and edematous fibromyxoid stroma. The covering epithelium was ulcerated.

identical to the *central giant cell granuloma* (in oral pathology, "peripheral" refers to the soft tissues of the gingiva and "central" to intraosseous lesions of the jaws). This lesion can occur at any age (average age is 30 years), and females are affected twice as frequently as males.[188,189] Clinically, it usually forms a mass on the gingival margin or alveolar mucosa anterior to the molars, slightly more commonly on the mandible than the maxilla. It can occasionally develop on the alveolar mucosa of an edentulous individual.

The peripheral giant cell granuloma is usually dark red or purplish, often hemorrhagic and ulcerated, and either pedunculated or sessile (Fig. 50-12). It rarely exceeds 2 cm in diameter. Larger lesions may cause superficial erosion of the alveolar bone or cupping of the alveolar ridge when examined radiographically. Grossly, it resembles a pyogenic granuloma. The distinguishing histologic features are the presence of aggregates of osteoclastlike giant cells dispersed in a vascular stroma with delicate fibers investing plump fibroblastic cells showing phenotypic similarity to myofibroblasts.[190] Much of the lesion contains blood-filled sinusoidal spaces, with capillaries present at the periphery. Histiocytic mononuclear cells are present and are believed to be precursors for the giant cells.[191] Metaplastic osteoid and bone and variable numbers of inflammatory cells may also be present.

It is treated by surgical excision. Recurrence may follow incomplete removal. Peripheral giant cell granuloma has been reported in association with hyperparathyroidism, which is interesting because it also microscopically resembles the brown tumor of bone in that entity.[192]

Verruciform xanthoma. A verruciform xanthoma is a benign lesion of the skin and mucosa that was first reported in the oral cavity by Schafer in 1971.[193] It resembles a squamous papilloma, but none of the human papillomaviruses tested has so far been detected in the lesions.[194,195] Several other pathogenetic theories have been proposed including lipid storage disease,[196] fatty degeneration of epithelial cells,[197] and immunologic disorders.

In the mouth, the most frequent sites are the gingivae and alveolar ridge. About 75% of the patients are in the fifth to seventh decades of life, and there is a predilection for females. This warty lesion is usually less than 2 cm, white to red, and occasionally multiple. Occasionally it is flat. Microscopically, parakeratin covers the rough verrucous surface. Invaginating crypts may extend deep into the epithelium with parakeratin plugging. There is acanthosis with uniform elongation of the rete ridges (Fig. 50-13). Numerous foamy xanthomatous cells fill the connective tissue papillae, extending downward only to the tips of the rete ridges. No recurrences have been reported after conservative excision.

Schwannoma, neurofibroma. Neurilemoma (schwannoma) and neurofibroma of the oral cavity are usually on the tongue, presenting as a submucosal nodule. They are similar to their counterparts in the skin and other sites. With neurofibromatosis, multiple neoplasms may be present, usually as discrete tumors, but occasionally as diffuse or plexiform lesions.[198] Diffuse neurofibromatosis is a rare cause of macroglossia.

Neuroma. Traumatic neuroma is a reactive overgrowth of nerves and fibrous tissue at the proximal end of a crushed or severed peripheral nerve.[199] A history of tooth extraction or prior soft-tissue trauma can usually be elicited. The lesion usually appears as a nodule having normal surface coloration. The most common sites are the mental foramen area, lower lip, and tongue, though any area of the oral mucosa may be involved. Microscopically, these lesions resemble those seen elsewhere on the body.

Multiple mucosal neuromas are noticed on the lips, tongue, and buccal mucosa in multiple endocrine adenomatosis type III (multiple mucosal neuroma syndrome), together with medullary thyroid carcinoma, pheochromocytoma, and other conditions.[200,201] Mucosal neuromas are generally small and discrete and may also be found on the conjunctiva and larynx and along the intestinal tract. Microscopy shows benign proliferations of nerves and fibrous tissue. They may resemble neurofibromatosis but should be distinguished because of the

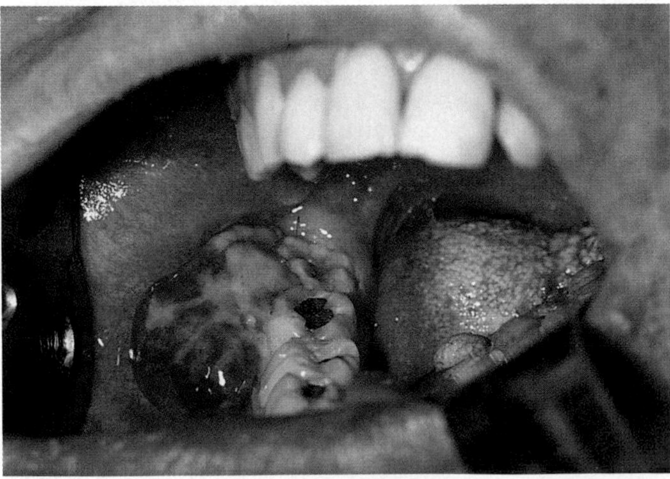

Fig. 50-12 Dark red and purplish peripheral giant cell granuloma. The lesion bled easily with slight manipulation and at surgery was found to be a pedunculated mass attached to the cervical gingiva of the mandibular right second molar with a small stalk.

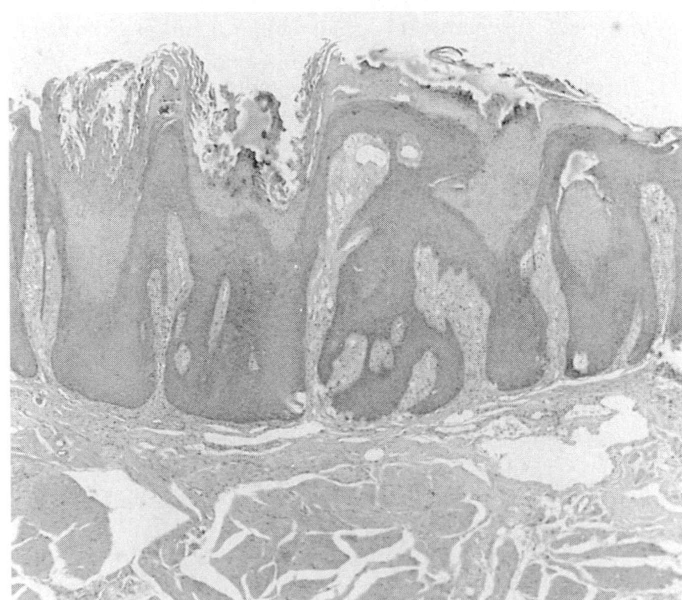

Fig. 50-13 Verruciform xanthoma. Notice the surface parakeratin, the uniform elongation of the rete, and acanthosis. The connective tissue between epithelial ridges contains pale xanthomatous cells.

other, more clinically significant components of these two syndromes.

Granular cell tumor. Described by Abrikossoff in 1926, it was initially assumed to be of striated muscle origin and was known for many years as granular cell myoblastoma. The histogenesis of this neoplasm has been the subject of considerable controversy, but most investigators now believe it to be of neural origin. Electron microscopic and immunohistochemical investigations have added support to the neural (Schwann cell) theory of origin. The tumor cells stain positively for neural markers, including S-100 protein, Leu 7, and myelin basic protein.[202-204]

Granular cell tumor originates in a variety of tissues, especially the skin and mucous membranes. About 20% arise in the tongue. There appears to be no age preference in adults, but the lesion is rare in children. The lesion is more common in women. In the oral cavity, the tumor presents as a firm, painless, submucosal nodule.

Microscopically it is distinctive (Fig. 50-14), consisting of large, uniform, polyhedral cells with acidophilic granular cytoplasm (ultrastructural studies have demonstrated that the granules are autophagic lysosomes). The granular cell nucleus is small, hyperchromatic, and centrally to eccentrically located. The tumor cells form sheets, nests, and cords. Although the granular cell tumor is almost always benign, it may be infiltrative. Mitoses are rare. Occasionally the overlying epithelium exhibits pseudoepitheliomatous hyperplasia, and this can be so pronounced in tongue lesions that it is mistaken for squamous carcinoma.

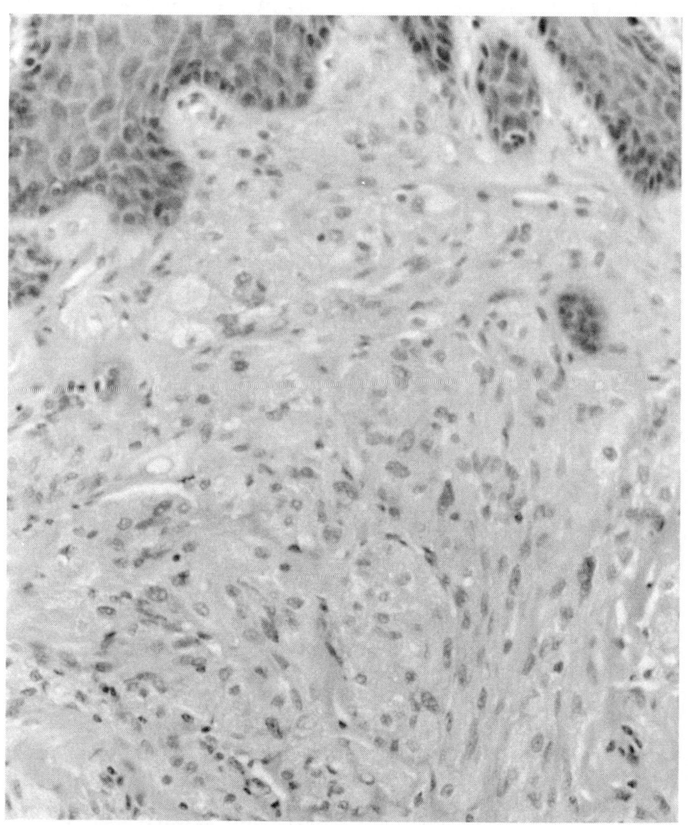

Fig. 50-14 Granular cell tumor. The tumor is composed of large cells with acidophilic granular cytoplasm.

Treatment is excision; recurrence may follow incomplete removal. About 10% of granular cell tumors are multiple. *Malignant granular cell tumors* are exceedingly rare and are characterized by high mitotic activity, necrosis, cellular and nuclear pleomorphism, macronucleoli, and metastases.

Congenital epulis (gingival granular cell tumor of the newborn). The gingival lesion congenital epulis microscopically and ultrastructurally resembles the granular cell tumor but is believed to be histogenetically unrelated.[205,206] Affecting female infants much more often than males, it forms a polyp near the incisor area (it is twice as common on the upper gingiva as on the lower gingiva). It is benign and rarely multiple and does not recur after simple excision.[207]

Hemangioma and other vascular lesions. The hemangioma (strawberry nevus) is the most common tumor in infancy and childhood, the majority of which occur on the skin and mucous membranes of the head and neck.[208] They are common in the oral mucosa and are usually found soon after birth or during infancy. Oral hemangiomas are usually of capillary type and are infrequently of cavernous type but occasionally are composed of both types. Early hemangiomas are cellular and typically grow rapidly over several months before stabilizing and then regressing over a few years. Clinically the hemangioma is red or purplish and blanches on pressure.

Intravascular papillary endothelial hyperplasia may occur within a pyogenic granuloma, hemangioma, dilated blood vessel, or other vascular lesion. Endothelial cellularity and nuclear atypia within these lesions can be alarming, but they should not be confused with angiosarcoma. The location of the lesion within a vascular structure and the presence of hyalinized cores within the papillae are important diagnostic features.[209]

Hemangiopericytoma[210] and glomangioma[211] are rarely encountered in the oral cavity. These show histologic features identical to their counterparts in other anatomic sites.

Hereditary hemorrhagic telangiectasia (Osler-Rendu-Weber disease) is manifested by numerous small (0.5 to 3 mm diameter) spiderlike angiomas of the face, nares, lips, tongue, oral mucosa and elsewhere. Nasal mucosal involvement results in frequent epistaxis, usually noted at puberty. Bleeding is also common from the upper and lower digestive tract, causing iron-deficiency anemia. This rare condition is autosomal dominant. Microscopically the individual lesion is a superficial blood vessel surrounded by abnormal elastic fibers that permit dilatation.[212]

Encephalofacial angiomatosis (Sturge-Weber syndrome) consists of superficial and deep-seated hemangiomas, usually on the upper two thirds or half of the face, associated with leptomeningeal angiomas, cerebral calcifications, seizures, glaucoma, and mental retardation. There are many clinical variations.[212] Vascular lesions may involve the buccal mucosa and gingiva.

Lymphangiomas are usually found at birth in the head and neck region. They can cause enlargement of the tongue (macroglossia) or lip (macrocheilia).[213]

Lipoma. Lipomas are uncommon in the mouth and pharynx and are most frequent in the cheeks, tongue, and oral floor. There is no sex predilection.[214,215]

Leiomyoma. Leiomyomas infrequently occur in the mouth. Most cases have been found in the tongue or lower lip. Any age may be affected, and they present as slow-growing submucosal masses. Both the typical solid form and the vascular form (angioleiomyoma), the latter presumably derived from smooth muscle in the walls of blood vessels, have been reported.[216] Microscopically, the spindle cells may resemble schwannoma and other mesenchymal neoplasms but immunohistochemical staining for smooth muscle antigens (such as desmin, actin) can resolve this problem. Epithelioid leiomyoma of the oral cavity has also been reported.[217] Mitoses and nuclear atypia should suggest the possibility of malignancy (that is, leiomyosarcoma). Leiomyomas are benign and should not recur after simple excision.

Rhabdomyoma. A rhabdomyoma is a very rare benign tumor. Most oral lesions occur in the floor of the mouth, tongue, or soft palate. The tumor is found in males about twice as often as females. Children or adults can be affected, with most patients over 40 years of age. Histologically, the tumor is composed of large polyhedral cells with granular cytoplasm and occasional cross striations, resembling mature skeletal muscle fibers.[218] The fetal type of rhabdomyoma is composed of elongated cells with fewer cross striations, possibly causing confusion with rhabdomyosarcoma (discussed below).

Soft-tissue osteoma and chondroma (choristoma). Small, circumscribed tumorlike lesions composed of mature laminated bone (osteoma) or mature cartilage (chondroma) may be rarely encountered in the oral cavity, mostly in the tongue. Chondromas are usually located on the lateral border and ventral surface of the tongue, whereas osteomas are seen mostly on the posterior dorsum in the region of the circumvallate papillae.[219]

Malignant tumors

Lymphoma. Non-Hodgkin's lymphoma (NHL) is the third most common form of oral cancer, though it is very infrequent when compared with squamous cell carcinoma and carcinomas of salivary gland origin. After Waldeyer's ring, the palate, vestibular mucosa, and gingiva are the most common sites of extranodal lymphomas of the oral soft tissue. At diagnosis, most patients are over 50 years of age. A painless submucosal mass, which may have a reddish or purplish coloration, is the typical clinical presentation. Although all histologic subtypes of NHL may be encountered, diffuse small cleaved cell and large cell types are the most common.[220-223] Cases of low-grade NHL may be difficult to distinguish from benign lymphoid hyperplasia, and high-grade NHL may be difficult to distinguish from undifferentiated carcinoma or melanoma.

Hodgkin's lymphoma is very rare in the oral cavity but may involve the tonsils.[224]

Soft-tissue sarcomas. About 10% to 15% of soft-tissue sarcomas involve the head and neck.[225] Almost every type of soft-tissue sarcoma may occur in the oral soft tissue, but all are uncommon.[226] Histologically, these tumors resemble their counterparts in other sites.

Rhabdomyosarcoma accounts for about 45% of head and neck sarcomas. Oral rhabdomyosarcoma most commonly occurs on the soft palate or cheek.[227] Most patients are under 10 years of age, and the majority are of the embryonal histologic subtype.

DISEASES OF TEETH AND THEIR SUPPORTING STRUCTURES

Dental caries and periodontal disease are universal problems. These two diseases are major concerns of public health policy around the world. The prevention, diagnosis, treatment, and management of their sequelae constitute a significant proportion of the practice of dentistry and its subspecialities. A brief consideration of both diseases is provided here, but voluminous details are available in specialized textbooks.[228-230]

Dental caries

Based on extensive epidemiologic studies and germ-free animal experimentation, microbes are known to be the cause of this progressive destruction of calcified dental tissues. Over 200 species of bacteria and some fungi have been implicated, but the most common offender is *Streptococcus mutans*.[231,232]

Central to the pathogenesis of dental caries and periodontal disease is the formation of dental *plaque*. Plaque is a film on the surface of an erupted tooth composed of organic matrix with embedded microorganisms and food debris. Plaque thickness, composition, and rate of formation vary between individuals. If the plaque is left undisturbed, it calcifies and is referred to as "calculus," or "tartar." Calculus *per se* is not directly implicated in disease but acts as a nidus for further plaque accumulation.

For dental caries to develop from a plaque, the appropriate microorganisms need to be present on a susceptible tooth surface, with access to suitable substrates (such as trapped food, salivary glycoproteins) for an adequate time. Initially, cocci predominate in the plaque and produce extracellular matrix. This matrix is then colonized by other bacteria, including filamentous organisms and anaerobes. Organic acids and enzymes produced by the microorganisms cause decalcification, proteolysis, and slow, progressive decay of the tooth, starting with the covering enamel. If unchecked, the infection penetrates the dentin and destroys the pulp (Fig. 50-15).

Several factors influence the risk of dental caries:

1. Microorganisms are essential for formation of caries.
2. Regular brushing and flossing prevent accumulation of food debris, reducing the incidence of caries and their sequelae.
3. Sugar promotes dental caries, since bacteria metabolize carbohydrates. The stickiness of the dental plaque is caused by dextran, which is a product of sucrose fermentation by *Streptococcus mutans*.
4. Adherent plaque cannot be removed by brushing, but periodic mechanical removal of the plaque (scaling) by the dentist or dental hygienist decreases the incidence of caries.
5. Fluoride ingested or locally applied to tooth surfaces is an effective preventive agent. It has weak bactericidal action and, more importantly, it makes the enamel more resistant to bacterial degradation (by changing the composition of enamel from hydroxyapatite to fluorapatite).
6. Saliva has a mechanical cleansing action and contains bactericidal substances such as lysozyme and IgA. When salivary flow is decreased, as with Sjögren's syndrome or salivary gland irradiation, there is a pronounced increase in the incidence of dental caries.

Early dental caries appear as white spots, usually in enamel located at contact points between adjacent teeth, in pits and fissures on the crown, and near the gingival margin on the tooth surface. Acidity with demineralization of the enamel seems to be important in the early stage of caries formation. Once the lesion reaches dentin, cavitation in the enamel

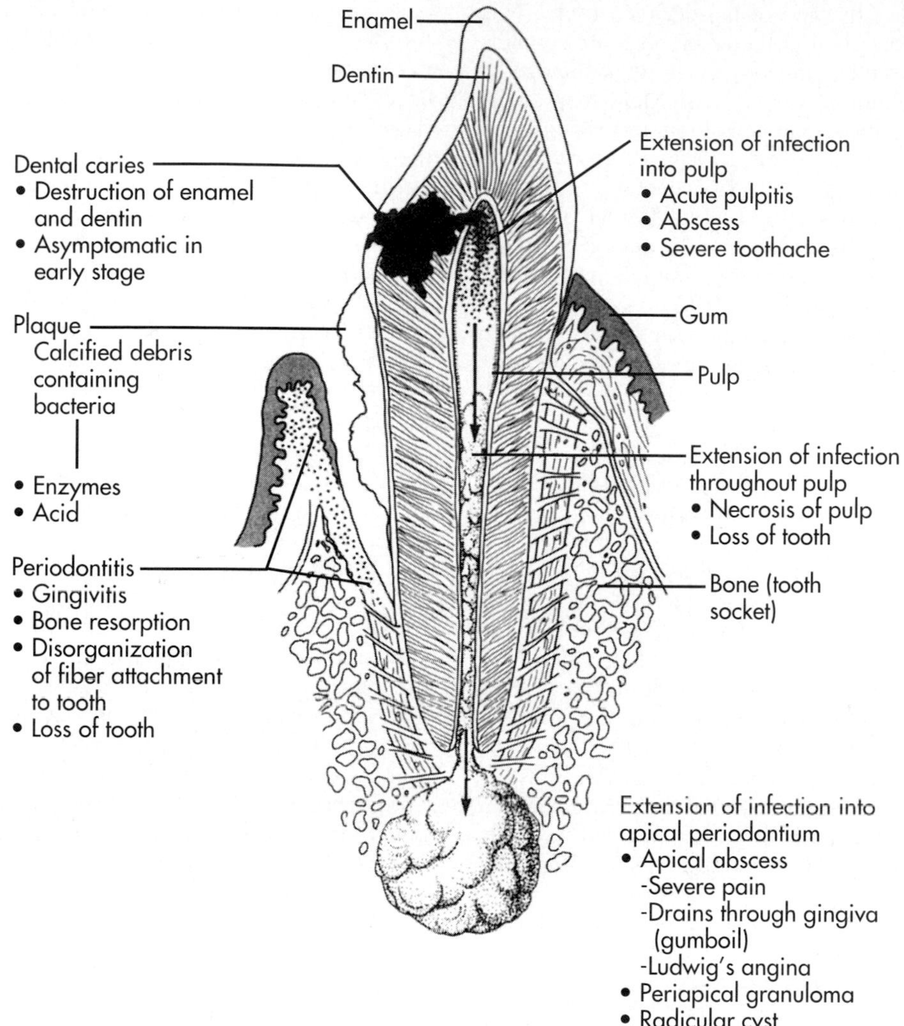

Fig. 50-15 Diagram of dental caries, periodontitis, and their sequelae. (From Chandrasoma P, Taylor CR: *Concise pathology,* Norwalk, Conn, 1991, Appleton & Lange.)

occurs. The *tooth cavity* is saucer-shaped or conical, with its base at the external surface of the tooth.

After the carious cavity reaches the dentinoenamel junction, the infection can rapidly extend laterally along this interface. Since dentin is traversed by the cell processes of the odontoblasts (whose bodies form the outer boundaries of the dental pulp), extension of caries to the dentin evokes a reaction in the dentin-pulp complex. The odontoblasts react by depositing dentin on the walls of the dentinal tubules and by forming irregular secondary dentin in an attempt to wall off the infection. If untreated, the infection invades and spreads along the dentinal tubules. Further progression causes destruction of the dentinal tubules, and the organisms invade the intertubular dentin, with dentinal softening, liquefaction, and formation of transverse clefts. Proteolytic enzymes produced by the bacteria are believed to play a major role in the spread of the lesion at this stage.

In patients who have periodontal disease (see below), *root caries* can also develop. Root caries, or caries of cementum, are believed to be initiated by filamentous microorganisms (in contrast to the cocci initiating coronal caries). *Streptococcus salivarius* may also be important in the initiation of the root lesion. There is no enamel around the roots, and the microorganisms appear to invade the cementum along Sharpey's fibers, or between bundles of fibers, in a manner comparable to invasion along dentinal tubules. The subsequent stages in the destruction of the root dentin probably parallel those of the coronal lesions.

As the defensive response of the odontoblasts is overwhelmed, an acute inflammatory reaction develops within the pulp *(pulpitis).* Acute pulp infection may result in a localized abscess or total pulp necrosis. Both conditions are very painful, and extirpation of the pulp (with root canal filling) or extraction of the tooth is required. If the condition is allowed to persist without therapy, the infection spreads through the periapical periodontium and the alveolar bone to other surrounding structures. The severity of the resultant infection varies according to the type and virulence of the offending microorganism or microorganisms, the immune state (resistance) of the host, the strategic location of the infected tooth, and the timing and effectiveness of therapy (such as antibiotics, incision and drainage).

The resultant infection may be limited to a painful periapical abscess that, in time, will drain through the gingiva. Frequently, chronic mild periapical infection results in the formation of a *periapical granuloma,* a well-circumscribed radiolucency surrounding the end of the decayed tooth. This focus of granulation tissue within the resorbed bone contains lymphocytes, plasma cells, histiocytes, and odontogenic epithelium. The epithelium in the rests of Malassez can be stimulated to proliferate by the inflammation and a cyst lined by squamous epithelium forms. This periapical, or *radicular,* cyst is discussed in the next section of this chapter.

Uncontrolled infection may spread along fascial planes in the floor of the mouth or face to cause localized cellulitis. Rarely, the infection extends to the orbit, cranial cavity, neck, or mediastinum and causes death (Fig. 50-16).

Fortunately, it is unnecessary to prepare sections of teeth to diagnose dental caries because gross and radiologic diagnosis suffices.

Gingivitis and periodontal disease

There are numerous varieties of inflammatory gingival and periodontal disease, and only the most important types are briefly discussed here.

Inflammation restricted to the gingival margin that is characterized by painless swelling, redness, and gingival bleeding is a common condition known as *chronic marginal gingivitis.* A survey by the National Institute of Dental Research indicates that 44% of employed adults in the United States have some degree of gingivitis. In most individuals the lesion is nonprogressive, especially if therapy is instituted.[233]

In 5% to 15% of the adult population, there is progressive inflammation associated with destruction of the periodontal ligament, variable loss of alveolar bone support around the teeth, and the formation of "pockets" (see below). This is a more serious condition known as *chronic adult periodontitis.*

As just described with dental caries, marginal gingivitis and adult periodontitis are initiated by microorganisms and accumulation of dental plaque. The microorganisms associated with the plaque in these lesions differ from those implicated in caries. The location of the plaque also differs; with periodontal disease, the supragingival plaque extends down the gingival sulcus and into the developing periodontal pocket.

The microbial flora change as the periodontal plaque becomes established, and there is no evidence that one organism alone is the specific cause of any of the clinically distinct forms of gingivitis and periodontal disease. Generally, in the initial stages, significant numbers of gram-negative anaerobic cocci *(Veillonella* species*)* and facultative and obligate anaerobic bacilli (such as *Actinomyces* species) are present. In time, the flora changes with increased numbers of gram-positive bacilli (especially *Actinomyces israelii)* and gram-negative rods (such as *Bacteroides* species). In plaque associated with chronic marginal gingivitis, the following organisms are reportedly present in equal proportions: streptococci, *Actinomyces* species, gram-negative bacilli such as *Bacteroides* species, and *Fusobacterium* species. In the periodontal pockets of advanced periodontal disease, the plaque microflora is composed overwhelmingly of anaerobes. Gram-negative bacilli and spirochetes (such as *Treponema* species) are present in large number, whereas the number of gram-positive bacilli (such as *Actinomyces* species) are proportionately reduced.

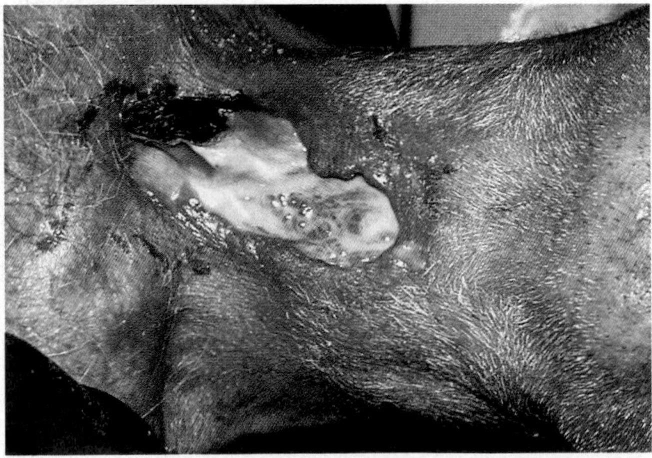

Fig. 50-16 Severe infection of dental origin (Ludwig angina) that descended to the neck. There is a large area of tissue necrosis with suppuration in the neck. The patient died a few days later because of a ruptured carotid artery.

The histopathology of marginal gingivitis and periodontal disease is well characterized. A few days after the accumulation of dental plaque, an acute inflammatory response (with neutrophils and edema) is found in the marginal gingiva (Fig. 50-17, *B*). Swelling of the gingiva can deepen the gingival sulcus to form a "pseudopocket." If the plaque persists, the inflammatory response becomes chronic, with stromal fibrosis and variable numbers of lymphocytes and plasma cells (Fig. 50-17, *C*). The intensity of the inflammatory response increases with time and reactive squamous epithelial proliferation occurs. Erosions of gingival epithelium and destruction of underlying stroma can occur. Immunoglobulin deposition has been demonstrated in the stroma in areas of gingivitis.

If marginal gingivitis progresses to involve the periodontal ligament and alveolar bone destructively, it is termed "periodontitis." As the periodontal ligament is destroyed and alveolar bone is resorbed, the alveolar sulcus deepens to form a fissure or "pocket." A *periodontal pocket* is defined as a crypt more than 3 mm in depth below the neck of the tooth, formed within the periodontal tissue by the burrowing action of lytic microbial and inflammatory products (Fig. 50-17, *D*). The gingival epithelial attachment ("junctional epithelium") migrates apically onto the exposed root surface or may ulcerate. Exposure of the root to the plaque permits root caries to develop.

Typically, areas of periodontitis undergo variable periods of quiescence and exacerbation, and the degree of inflammation differs in different periodontal pockets. After the inflammation subsides, bone deposition can replace some of the resorbed bone but not at the crest of the alveolar bone. Therefore, vertical bone loss is irreversible and can eventually lead to loss of the tooth.

Although the histologic picture is well defined, the mechanisms by which the microorganisms cause the destruction remain controversial. Microorganisms in the plaque produce a variety of factors that damage the periodontium either directly or indirectly by initiating the inflammatory response. Among these factors are exotoxins, endotoxins, enzymes (such as collagenase, hyaluronidase, proteases), lipoteichoic acid, and peptidoglycan. Immunologic mediators that have been implicated include prostaglandins (especially PGE_2), interleukin-1, and tumor necrosis factor.

Therapy of periodontal disease involves several modalities:

1. Removal of the plaque mechanically or chemically by introduction of antibiotics and anti-inflammatory agents into the pocket

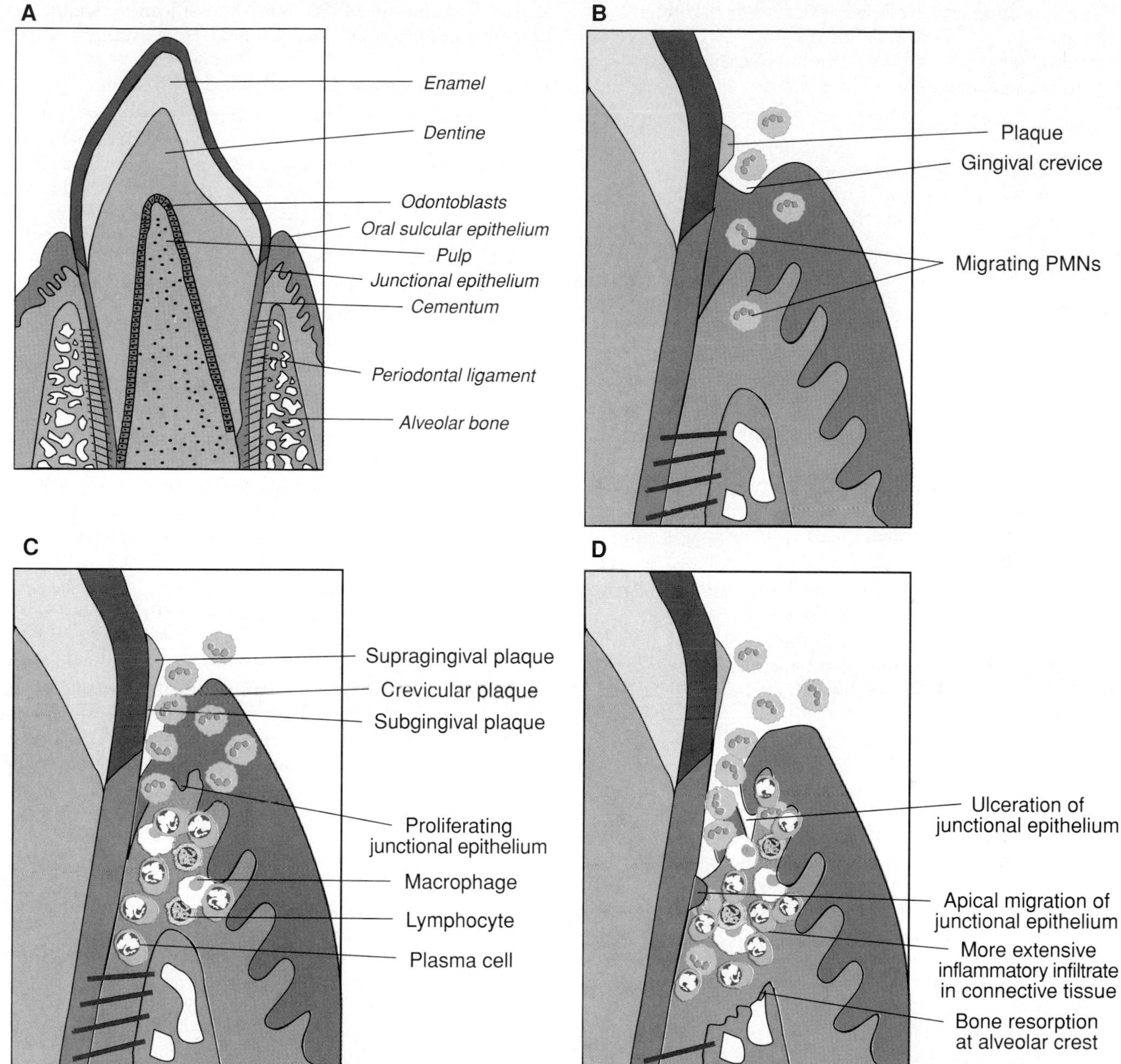

Fig. 50-17 **A,** Overview of normal tooth and periodontal structures. A healthy tooth is maintained in its socket by the periodontal ligament, a highly specialized collagenous connective tissue connecting the cementum covering the root surface to the alveolar bone. A shallow sulcus (gingival crevice) lies between the tooth and the gingiva that, under ideal conditions, is less than 1 mm deep. **B,** Initial changes in the gingival crevice after accumulation of dental plaque. Within 2 to 4 days there is an increase in the flow of gingival crevicular fluid, accompanied by the emigration of polymorphonuclear neutrophils (PMN) through the oral sulcular epithelium into the crevice. **C,** Gingival infiltrate in chronic marginal gingivitis. Rete peg proliferation is evident in the lateral part of the junctional epithelium. Emigration of PMN into the crevice continues, accompanied by a chronic inflammatory infiltrate in the underlying connective tissue. This infiltrate contains macrophages and T-lymphocytes, but plasma cells predominate. **D,** Changes seen in chronic adult periodontitis. The inflammatory infiltrate is more extensive than that in chronic marginal gingivitis. Pronounced apical migration of junctional epithelium has been accompanied by loss of the connective tissue attachment, leading to pocket formation. The most striking feature of the lesion, however, is resorption of alveolar bone, with loss of vertical bone height at the alveolar crest. (From Williams DW: Gingivitis and periodontal disease. In McGee JO'D, Isaacson PG, Wright NA, editors: *Oxford textbook of pathology,* vol 2, *Pathology of systems,* Oxford, 1992, Oxford University Press.)

2. Surgical elimination of deep pockets in the gingiva or bone
3. Faithful attention to brushing and flossing to reduce plaque reaccumulation.

Localized juvenile periodontitis occurs most often in teenagers and young adults. It is characterized by pocket formation, connective tissue attachment loss, and alveolar bone loss, mainly affecting the first molars and incisors. This entity has a familial tendency, and 70% of patients have reduced migration of neutrophils to chemotactic agents. The youngsters with this form of periodontitis rarely show calculus or plaque formation and often exhibit little or no preceding gingivitis.

Acute necrotizing ulcerative gingivitis begins as an infection of the interdental papillae, with pain and necrosis. It and a similar but more chronic form of ulcerative gingivitis has been reported in patients infected with HIV.[234]

CYSTS OF THE JAWS (LINED BY EPITHELIUM)

A true cyst is a cavity lined by epithelium that contains fluid or semisolid material. The term *cyst* is also used for sharply defined, radiolucent bone lesions even when they do not have the structure of a true cyst, such as an aneurysmal bone cyst. This section deals with true cysts. In the oral cavity and jawbones, cysts can arise from epithelial remnants of either dental or nondental origin and are therefore divided into odontogenic and nonodontogenic cysts.

There are several classifications of oral and jaw cysts.[235-237] Table 50-12 shows the 1985 World Health Organization (WHO) classification of these cysts, and Table 50-13 shows the revised, concise 1992 WHO classification. Figure 50-18 demonstrates the basic sites of the different cysts.[238]

Odontogenic cysts

Odontogenic cysts are true cysts lined by epithelium of dental origin and are divided into two categories: developmental or inflammatory cysts. *Developmental cysts* arise from spontaneous proliferation of odontogenic epithelial rests. In *inflammatory cysts* the epithelial proliferation is secondary to inflammatory stimulation caused by advanced caries with tooth pulp infection and necrosis. The cysts are further subtyped according to the stage of odontogenesis when they occur and their relationship to a tooth. Most odontogenic cysts are intraosseous, but they sometimes occur in the gingiva.

Clinical and radiographic information is needed, in addition to histologic examination, to assign a specific subtype to an odontogenic cyst.[239] In general, these cysts should be completely submitted for histologic examination to exclude the possibility of odontogenic keratocyst.

Dentigerous (follicular) cyst. The dentigerous cyst is the most common developmental odontogenic cyst. It is associated with the crown of an impacted or unerupted tooth, usually the mandibular and maxillary third molars, cuspids, and bicuspids. It arises from fluid accumulation, either between the crown of a tooth and the tooth follicle or between the layers of the reduced enamel epithelium.[240]

The dentigerous cyst is a lesion of children and young adults and occurs more frequently in males. They are usually discovered on routine dental x-ray films, but sometimes a slowly enlarging mass is observed. Radiographs usually show a unilocular radiolucency (sometimes with a sclerotic margin) surrounding the crown of an unerupted tooth. When the cyst

Table 50-12 1985 WHO classification of cysts of the jaws

Classification	Site	Suggested origin
1. Developmental		
a. Odontogenic		
Odontogenic keratocyst	Usually mandibular angle or ramus	Dental lamina or tooth germ
Follicular cyst	Around crown of unerupted tooth	Follicle and reduced enamel epithelium
Eruption cyst	Around crown of unerupted tooth	Follicle and reduced enamel epithelium
Lateral periodontal	Periodontal ligament	Dental lamina rests or reduced enamel epithelium
Gingival cyst of adults	Gingiva	Dental lamina rests or reduced enamel epithelium
Alveolar cyst of infants	Gum pads	Dental lamina
b. Non-odontogenic		
Nasopalatine duct cyst	Incisive canal and foramen	Oronasal duct epithelium
Nasolabial cyst	Soft tissues of buccal sulcus adjacent to upper canines	Nasolacrimal duct epithelium
Mid-palatal cyst of infants	Midline palate	Palatal process epithelium
2. Inflammatory		
Radicular cyst	Root apex	Rests of Malassez
Residual cyst	Edentulous alveolus	Rests of Malassez
Inflammatory lateral periodontal cyst	Periodontal ligament	Rests of Malassez
Paradontal cyst	Adjacent to partially erupted tooth involved by pericoronitis	Rests of Malassez or reduced enamel epithelium
Inflammatory	Follicle of unerupted permanent tooth below an infected deciduous tooth	Follicle and reduced enamel epithelium

Modified from Tinkler S: The jaws. In McGee JO'D, Isaacson PG, Wright NA, editors: *Oxford textbook of pathology: pathology of systems*, vol 2a, Oxford, 1992, Oxford University Press.
Based on Main DMG: Epithelial jaw cysts: 10 years of the WHO classification, *J Oral Pathol* 14:1, 1985.

Table 50-13 1992 WHO classification of cysts of the jaws

Developmental
Odontogenic
Gingival cysts of infants (Epstein pearls)
Odontogenic keratocyst (primordial cyst)
Dentigerous (follicular) cyst
Eruption cyst
Lateral periodontal cyst
Gingival cyst of adults
Glandular odontogenic cyst; sialo-odontogenic cyst
Non-odontogenic
Nasopalatine duct (incisive canal) cyst
Nasolabial (nasoalveolar) cyst
Inflammatory
Radicular cyst
Apical and lateral cysts
Residual cyst
Paradental (inflammatory collateral, mandibular infected buccal) cyst

From Kramer IRH, Pindborg JJ, Shear M: *Histological typing of odontogenic tumors*, ed 2, Berlin, 1992, Springer-Verlag.

lies in the bone adjacent to the unerupted crown, it is called a *lateral dentigerous cyst.* Uncommonly, the cyst is present in the soft tissue over an erupting tooth (usually a deciduous tooth and is referred to as an *eruption cyst).*

Histologically, the cyst lining is not specific, and clinical information helps distinguish it from other odontogenic cysts or an enlarged (hypertrophic) dental follicle. The lining is usually a thin, nonkeratinizing, stratified, squamous epithelium, two to three layers thick, resembling the reduced enamel epithelium. Mucus-secreting or ciliated cells are sometimes present, reflecting the pluripotential properties of the cyst epithelium[241,242] (Fig. 50-19, *A*). The cyst epithelium lies on a thin fibrous capsule. Sometimes islands of inactive odontogenic epithelium are present in the cyst wall. When inflamed, the cyst epithelium may become hyperplastic. When the epithelium is parakeratotic or orthokeratotic, the cyst should be classified as an odontogenic keratocyst (see below).

If left untreated, the dentigerous cyst can become large and cause extensive destruction of the jawbone. Enucleation of these cysts is usually curative. Between 15% and 33% of ameloblastomas arise in association with a dentigerous cyst, either from the epithelium lining the cyst lumen or the epithelial rests in the cyst wall[243] (Fig. 50-19, *B*). These *unicystic ameloblastomas* occur more often in teenagers, are often treated with simple enucleation, and have a lower recurrence rate than ameloblastomas unassociated with a cyst. Squamous and mucoepidermoid carcinomas have rarely been reported to arise in dentigerous cysts.[244,245]

Lateral periodontal cyst and gingival cyst of adults. Lateral periodontal cysts and gingival cysts of adults are uncommon odontogenic cysts found, respectively, in the bone lateral to a vital tooth and in the gingiva. These noninflammatory developmental cysts are lined by stratified nonkeratinized squamous epithelium, cuboidal cells, and occasionally fusiform or water-clear cells. The gingival cyst of adults is discussed earlier in this chapter, with other cysts of the gingiva.

Odontogenic keratocyst. Odontogenic keratocysts account for 5% to 10% of all jaw cysts. Its diagnosis is based on specific histologic criteria and not on the stage of odontogenesis or relationship to a tooth. The term *odontogenic keratocyst (OKC)* was introduced by Philipsen in 1956 to describe keratin-filled jaw cysts.[246] In 1981 Wright distinguished two types based on differences in histology and behavior: the more common *parakeratotic odontogenic keratocyst* (P-OKC) and the less common *orthokeratotic odontogenic keratocyst* (O-OKC).[247] Some authors consider odontogenic keratocyst to be synonymous with *primordial cyst,*

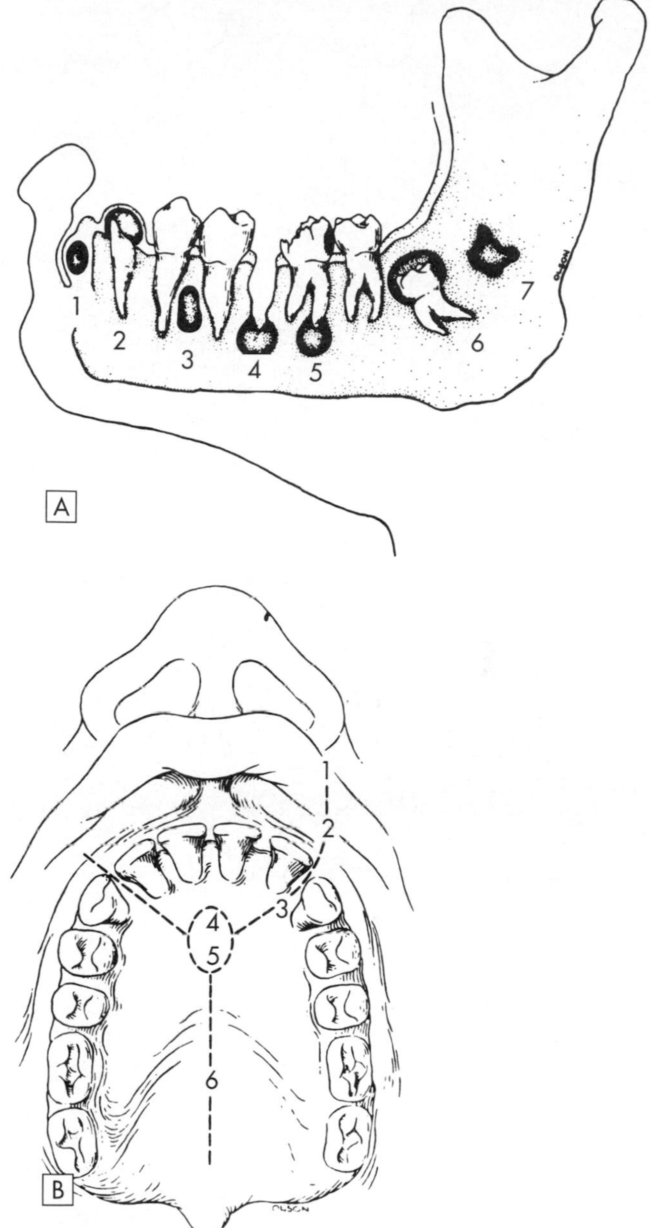

Fig. 50-18 Diagrams of the site of odontogenic, **A,** and fissural (nonodontogenic) cysts, **B,** in the mandible and maxilla respectively. **A:** *1,* gingival; *2,* eruption; *3,* lateral periodontal; *4,* residual; *5,* periapical (radicular); *6,* dentigerous; *7,* primordial. **B:** *1,* nasolabial cyst; *2,* nasoalveolar cyst, *3,* globulomaxillary cyst; *4,* nasopalatine cyst; *5,* cyst of palatine papilla; *6,* median palatal cyst. (From Batsakis JG: *Tumors of the head and neck: clinical and pathological considerations,* ed 2, Baltimore, 1979, Williams & Wilkins.)

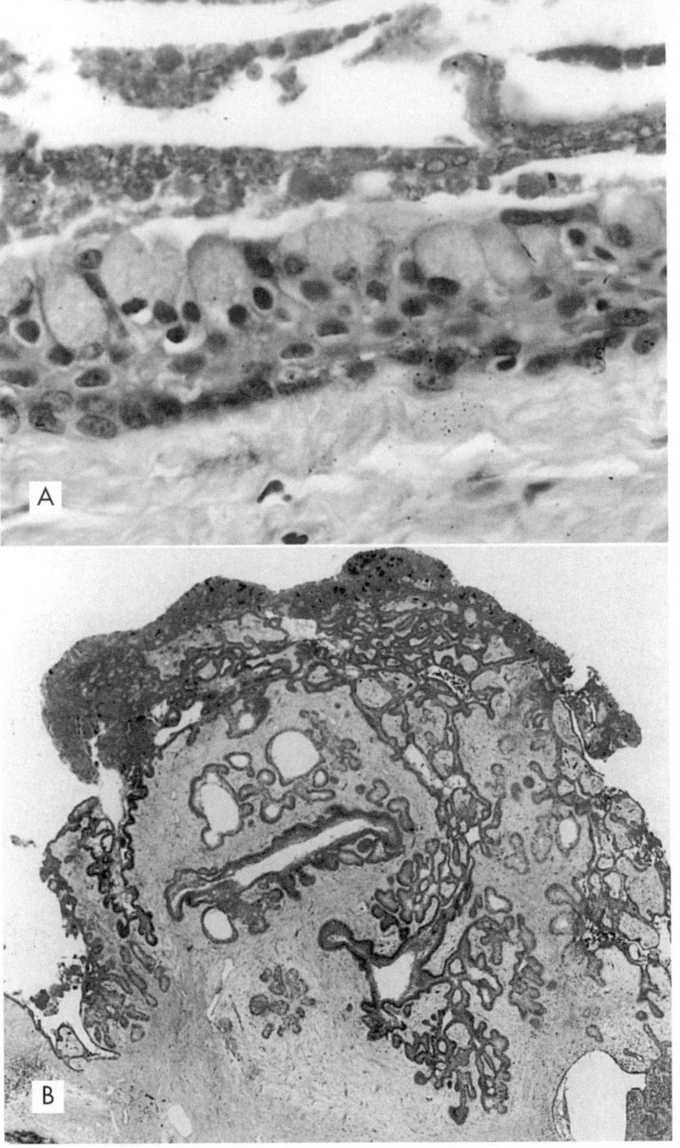

Fig. 50-19 Dentigerous cyst. **A,** The lining epithelium is stratified squamous with considerable mucus metaplasia. **B,** Dentigerous cyst with an intraluminal ameloblastoma. Notice the abrupt intraluminal ameloblastic proliferation and its deep penetration into the connective tissue wall.

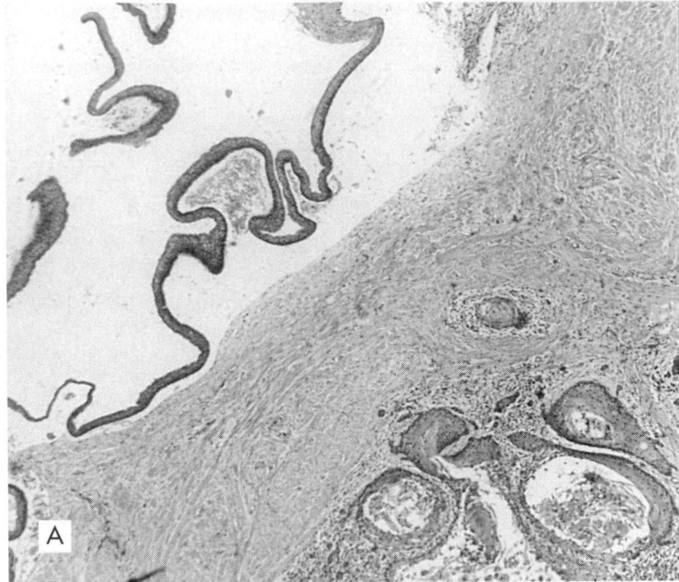

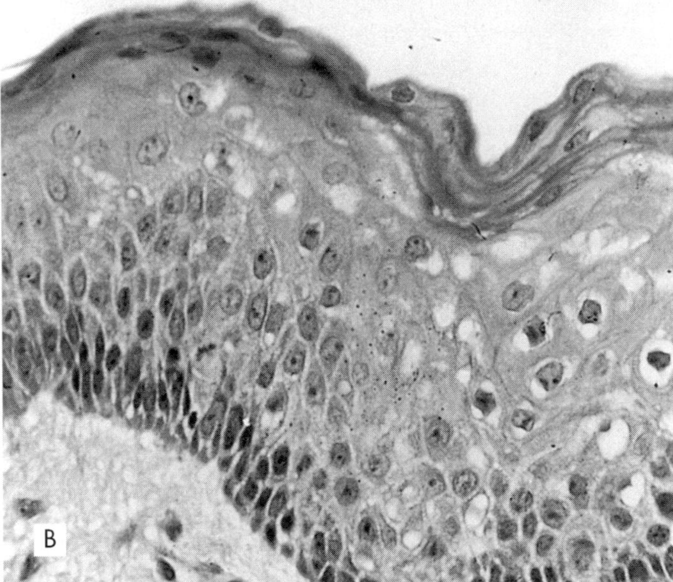

Fig. 50-20 Parakeratotic cyst. **A,** The cyst is lined by partially detached, corrugated, squamous epithelium. Daughter cysts are present deep in the capsule. **B,** The squamons epithelium at higher magnification shows basal cell hyperplasia and surface parakeratosis.

whereas others restrict the term *primordial cyst* to odontogenic cysts that form in place of a tooth and do not necessarily exhibit the characteristic histology of the OKC.

The P-OKC should be recognized for two reasons. First, the P-OKC has more aggressive growth potential and a higher recurrence rate than the O-OKC and other odontogenic cysts.[248-252] Second, in a minority of patients (particularly young patients with multiple cysts), the P-OKC is part of the nevoid basal cell carcinoma syndrome (described below).

The histogenesis of P-OKC is uncertain, but origin from the dental lamina or oral epithelium has been inferred. The diagnosis of P-OKC is based on characteristic histologic features (Fig. 50-20):

1. There is a thin and uniform squamous epithelial lining, five to eight cells thick, with a fairly flat base.
2. The epithelium has a well-developed basal layer of palisaded cuboidal or columnar cells with polarized, hyperchromatic nuclei.
3. The squamous cells progressively flatten toward the lumen.
4. The luminal surface is corrugated and at least partially lined by parakeratotic cells.
5. The lumen has an irregular, folded contour and may contain keratin.
6. The epithelial lining rests on a fibrous capsule, which is generally thin and uninflamed.

Of course, portions of the cyst may exhibit other histologic features. The epithelium may become detached from the capsule during processing. Focally the surface of the epithelium may be flattened or orthokeratotic. Occasionally, cholesterol or hyaline bodies are found in the capsule. If the cyst is inflamed, the epithelium may show squamous hyperplasia, loss of keratinization, erosions, and so forth, and the capsule may become thickened. Sometimes, buds of basal epithelium project into the surrounding stroma. Microcysts (also known as *daughter cysts* or *satellite cysts*) may occasionally be found in the wall. A few mitoses may be present. Epithelial atypia or dysplasia is infrequently seen in the cyst lining and basilar buds.

The P-OKC has a peak incidence in the second and third decades of life and is more common in males. It usually occurs in the mandibular angle and molar and ramus regions. Sometimes, it is associated with an unerupted tooth. Clinically the P-OKC can mimic a dentigerous, primordial, residual, lateral periodontal or even a radicular cyst. Radiographically, it may be unilocular or multilocular, with the latter encountered less frequently and in larger lesions.[253]

Although benign, the recurrence rate of P-OKC is high, ranging from 12% to 62.5%, and multiple recurrences are not unusual.[254] Because of this, the surgical management varies in aggressiveness from simple enucleation or curettage to ostectomy with curettage of the adjacent bone. Some large, destructive cases require segmental resection of the involved jawbone with immediate or delayed reconstruction. In any case, periodic clinical and radiologic follow-up examinations are recommended for early diagnosis of recurrences.

On the basis of experimental work, the aggressive clinical behavior of the P-OKC has been ascribed to several biologic properties including high mitotic activity,[255] high turnover rate of the epithelium,[256,257] and active collagenase in the lining tissues.[258,259] Some investigators have suggested that the P-OKC should be regarded as a benign neoplasm rather than a nonneoplastic cyst.[260]

Rare examples of ameloblastoma and carcinoma have been reported in association with OKC.[261]

Multiple odontogenic keratocysts of the jaws are a major component of the *nevoid basal cell carcinoma syndrome,* which is referred to by several names, including "Gorlin's syndrome."[262] In 1960, Gorlin and Goltz welded together the main features of this syndrome.[263,264] This autosomal dominant syndrome has almost 100% penetrance but very variable expressivity. Multiple basal cell carcinomas (usually on the face, beginning early in life) and multiple P-OKCs (also beginning early in life, occurring anywhere in the jaws, with frequent recurrences) are the hallmarks of this syndrome, but there are numerous other manifestations. These manifestations are grouped into five categories: cutaneous, skeletal, ophthalmologic, neurologic, and sexual. Other skin lesions include milia and palmar-plantar keratotic pitting. Common skeletal anomalies include frontal and temporoparietal bossing, kyphoscoliosis, bifurcated ribs, and spina bifida. Neurologic problems include medulloblastoma, dysgenesis of the corpus callosum, and calcification of the falx cerebri. Male hypogonadism and ovarian fibrosarcoma have infrequently been found.

Less than 10% of patients with multiple P-OKCs have other manifestations of the nevoid basal cell carcinoma syndrome, but it has been suggested that multiple P-OKCs alone may be a *forme fruste* of the syndrome. However, when the pathologist finds more than one P-OKC in a patient, particularly when the patient is young or has lesions in unusual locations, the clinician should be apprised of the possibility of this syndrome.

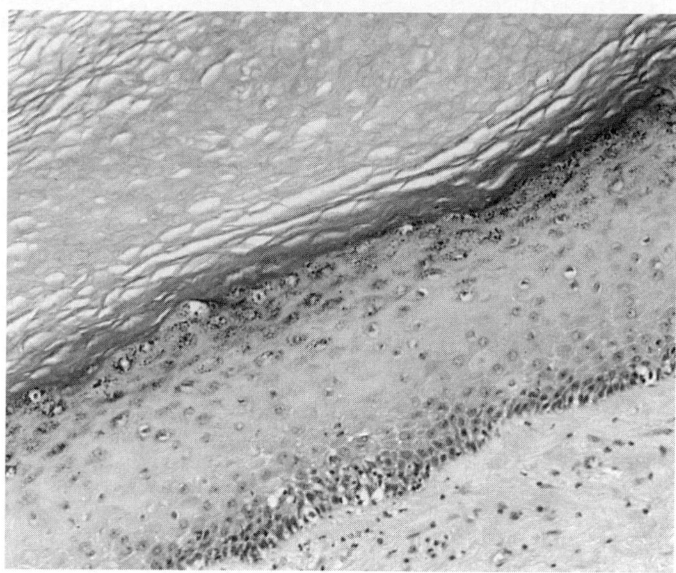

Fig. 50-21 Orthokeratotic odontogenic keratocyst. The cyst is lined by keratinizing epithelium covered with orthokeratin that fills its lumen.

The *orthokeratotic odontogenic keratocyst* (O-OKC) is histologically and clinically distinct from the P-OKC (Fig. 50-21). The distinguishing histologic features include the following:

1. The basal cell layer of the epithelium is flattened or cuboidal, without palisading and without polarized, hyperchromatic nuclei.
2. The surface of the epithelium is thin and uniformly orthokeratinized, with a prominent subjacent granular cell layer and without surface corrugations.
3. A substantial amount of fibrillar orthokeratin usually fills the cyst lumen.

O-OKCs are virtually always unilocular, are less aggressive than P-OKCs with very low or no recurrence rate, and there has been no association with the nevoid basal cell carcinoma syndrome. Some OKCs have a combination of the histologic features of both variants and, based on their behavior, should be classified as the parakeratotic subtype.

Radicular cyst. Radicular cysts are the most common cysts of the jaws. They develop from the odontogenic epithelial residues present in the periodontal ligament, the rests of Malassez and are related to chronic inflammation of the dental pulp. The inflammatory by-products from the pulp gain access to the periapical bone and form a localized focus of inflamed granulation tissue. This lesion, called a *periapical granuloma,* may also contain cholesterol clefts, histiocytes, macrophages, foreign body type of giant cells, and varying numbers of nests of odontogenic epithelium. Persistent inflammation stimulates these epithelial rests, which become hyperplastic, and eventually a microcyst lined by stratified squamous epithelium will form. As the inflammatory focus and cyst enlarge within the alveolar bone and the lesion becomes more defined, it gradually transforms into a radicular cyst. Sometimes during these intermediate stages, it is difficult to distinguish between granuloma and cyst, on either radiologic or histologic grounds.

There are several subtypes of radicular cysts, based on location. The most common is the *periapical cyst,* which forms in the alveolar bone around the tip (apex) of the root. The *lateral radicular cyst* forms in the bone beside the root. The *residual radicular cyst* is retained in the jaw after removal of the associated carious nonviable tooth.

The radicular cyst lining is usually nonkeratinized stratified squamous epithelium with considerable proliferation of the rete processes when there is ongoing inflammation. (If the epithelium exhibits significant keratinization, it should be classified as an odontogenic keratocyst.) Neutrophils may infiltrate the epithelium, and plasma cells (often with prominent Russell bodies) are often prominent in the stroma beneath the cyst epithelium. After the inflammation subsides, the cyst epithelium often becomes flat and attenuated, and the cyst capsule may become hyalinized.

Rushton, or hyaline, bodies are striking but rarely observed in the epithelium of radicular cysts. These are curving, eosinophilic laminated bodies with occasional foci of basophilic mineralization. These bodies are also rarely seen in the epithelium of dentigerous cysts but are almost unique to odontogenic cysts. Their nature is controversial, and they have been proposed as being keratinous, odontogenic, or hematogenous in origin.

If untreated, the radicular cyst can enlarge and cause destruction and weakening of the jaw. There are several methods to ablate the cyst, including extracting the associated tooth and curetting the lesion. Recurrences are unexpected but, with incomplete removal of the cyst epithelium, a residual radicular cyst may develop.

Nonodontogenic cysts

The second major category of true cysts within the jawbones, nonodontogenic cysts, includes a group of uncommon lesions, the epithelial lining of which is not of dental origin. Formerly these cysts were divided into fissural and developmental subtypes, but the concept that the fissural cysts arose from tissue entrapped during fusion of the embryonic processes is now widely discredited. The nasopalatine duct cyst is often lined, at least in part, by columnar epithelium resembling that lining the respiratory passages. It should be remembered, however, that many odontogenic cysts can be focally lined by cuboidal-columnar, mucous, or ciliated cells.

Nasopalatine duct (incisive canal) cyst. The nasopalative duct cyst arises from proliferation and cystic enlargement of epithelial residues of the nasopalatine duct (incisive canal) within the midline of the maxillary bone in the anterior palate. The nasopalatine duct cyst is the most common nonodontogenic cyst.[265] Rarely the cyst is entirely within the soft tissue of the palatine papilla and is then usually referred to as a *cyst of the palatine papilla.* Also rare is the formation of the cyst more posteriorly in the palate; this was previously distinguished as a *median palatine cyst* but is now often included as a nasopalatine duct cyst.

Clinically this cyst can appear as a painless swelling in the midline of the anterior palate. Middle-aged males are most often affected. Radiographically the nasopalatine duct cyst is a sharply defined radiolucency in the midline of the maxilla, usually just posterior to the central incisors, best seen on occlusal views. Occasionally it lies to one side of the midline. Its shape is oval, round, or, most characteristically, heart shaped. When large, the cyst may cause anterior maxillary and palatal bony expansion. The associated incisors are vital and not associated with the development of this cyst.

Reflecting its origin between the oral and nasal cavities, the cyst epithelium can be stratified squamous, cuboidal-columnar, or both types. The columnar type is often pseudostratified and can have ciliated or goblet cells, or both types. The stroma around the cyst contains mucous glands, nerves, blood vessels, adipose tissue, and varying numbers of inflammatory cells. An occasional island of hyaline cartilage may be present.

Other nonodontogenic cysts. Several other cysts that were believed to be fissural cysts, including the globulomaxillary cyst and the median mandibular cyst, have been described. Reexamination of these cysts indicates that many examples are actually odontogenic cysts (such as radicular cysts, lateral periodontal cysts, and OKC).

ODONTOGENIC TUMORS

Odontogenic tumors, arising from tooth-forming tissues, form a complex group of lesions of diverse histologic patterns and clinical behavior. They are uncommon lesions and, even in the specialized oral pathology laboratory, they constitute only about 1% to 2% of accessioned cases.[266] Odontogenesis is a complex process involving interaction of epithelium and mesenchyme, with the eventual formation of mature calcified dental tissues. Neoplastic and hamartomatous aberrations can occur at any stage, resulting in lesions with varying proportions of proliferating odontogenic epithelium or odontogenic mesenchyme, with or without calcified structures. A simplified classification of odontogenic tumors is presented in Table 50-14; this does not include some of the rare and transitional types, and more extensive works on the subject should be referred to for additional information.[267-269]

Table 50-14 Odontogenic tumors

Benign
Epithelial origin
Ameloblastoma
Odontogenic adenomatoid tumor
Calcifying epithelial odontogenic tumor
Mesenchymal origin
Myxoma
Odontogenic fibroma
Cemental tumors
Mixed epithelial and mesenchymal origin
Ameloblastic fibroma
Ameloblastic fibro-odontoma
Complex and compound odontomas
Malignant
Epithelial origin
Malignant ameloblastoma
Ameloblastic carcinoma
Mesenchymal origin
Ameloblastic fibrosarcoma

Benign odontogenic tumors of epithelial origin

Ameloblastoma. Ameloblastoma is the most common of the clinically significant odontogenic tumors. Its incidence is nearly equal to the combined incidence of all other odontogenic tumors, excluding odontomas (because odontomas are more common in the general population but are easily diagnosed and are seldom clinically significant). Ameloblastomas appear to originate from cell rests of enamel organ epithelium, from the epithelial lining of odontogenic cysts (chiefly dentigerous cysts), or occasionally from the basal layer of the oral mucosa.

Ameloblastomas appear most commonly in the third to fifth decades of life.[270,271] Although they may occur at younger ages, the diagnosis of ameloblastoma should be made in a youth only after exclusion of the benign ameloblastic fibroma and odontogenic adenomatoid tumor, to avoid overtreatment.

No sex or racial predilection is noted. Over 80% occur in the mandible, and 70% of these arise in the molar-ramus area. Rarely, an extraosseous (peripheral) example is discovered, usually in the gingiva.[272,273] Ameloblastomas may cause facial asymmetry by expanding the jaw. Radiographs show a multilocular (less commonly unilocular) radiolucency in the bone, sometimes with an embedded tooth (Fig. 50-22, *A*). The multilocular radiolucencies within the jaw, separated by delicate bony septa, has been described as resembling "soap bubbles." Although suggestive, this x-ray appearance is not specific for ameloblastoma and may be seen with central giant cell granuloma, myxoma, odontogenic keratocyst, and so forth.

Many histologic subtypes or patterns, including follicular, plexiform, acanthomatous, granular cell, and basal cell varieties, have been described. However, two or more patterns may occur within the same tumor, and there is no evidence that any histologic subtype is more aggressive than any other. Nearly all ameloblastomas demonstrate some microcystic degeneration, within either the epithelial component or the stroma.

Most ameloblastomas show one of the two predominant patterns, follicular or plexiform, the former being the more common. In the follicular type, islands (follicles) of cells, mimicking the dental organ epithelium, are separated by hypocellular, loose connective tissue. The outermost cells of the islands resemble those of the inner enamel epithelium of the developing tooth follicle, the ameloblastic layer. These cells are tall and columnar, with polarization of their nuclei away from the basement membrane.[274] The central portion of the epithelial islands is composed of a loose network of cells resembling stellate reticulum. Microcystic degeneration in the epithelial islands is common.

The plexiform pattern demonstrates irregular masses and interdigitating cords of epithelial cells, generally with a less developed stellate reticulum than that found in the follicular pattern (Fig. 50-22, *B*). There is also less stroma, and microcystic degeneration often occurs in the stromal component.

Prominent squamous metaplasia, particularly within the islands of the follicular pattern, gives rise to the acanthomatous variant. Occasionally, the tumor cells enlarge because of the excessive accumulation of eosinophilic granular particles (lysosomes) within the cytoplasm; when extensive, this gives rise to the granular cell variant. In the basal cell variant, most of the tumor cells are small and basaloid.

A distinct histologic variant of ameloblastoma with a pronounced stromal desmoplasia is now recognized and is termed "desmoplastic ameloblastoma"[275]; this constitutes about 12% of all ameloblastomas. This variant shares with the classical ameloblastoma a similar age of incidence and sex distribution; however, the desmoplastic variant occurs more frequently in the maxilla and more commonly in the anterior portion of the jaws.

The *unicystic ameloblastoma* is an odontogenic cyst with ameloblastic cell lining (Fig. 50-19, *B*). The ameloblastic cells project into the cyst cavity or infiltrate into the wall of the cyst but do not involve surrounding bone.

Ameloblastomas are generally benign but are locally invasive. Peripheral (extraosseous) and unicystic ameloblastomas have the best prognosis and are treated more conservatively. Other types of ameloblastoma tend to infiltrate the marrow spaces of the adjacent cancellous bone, and treatment by curettage alone is accompanied by a 55% to 90% incidence of recurrence.[276] Ameloblastomas may cause death by progressive infiltration into vital structures; posterior maxillary tumors are particularly notable in this respect.[277] Therefore ameloblastomas are often treated by block excision or segmental resection.

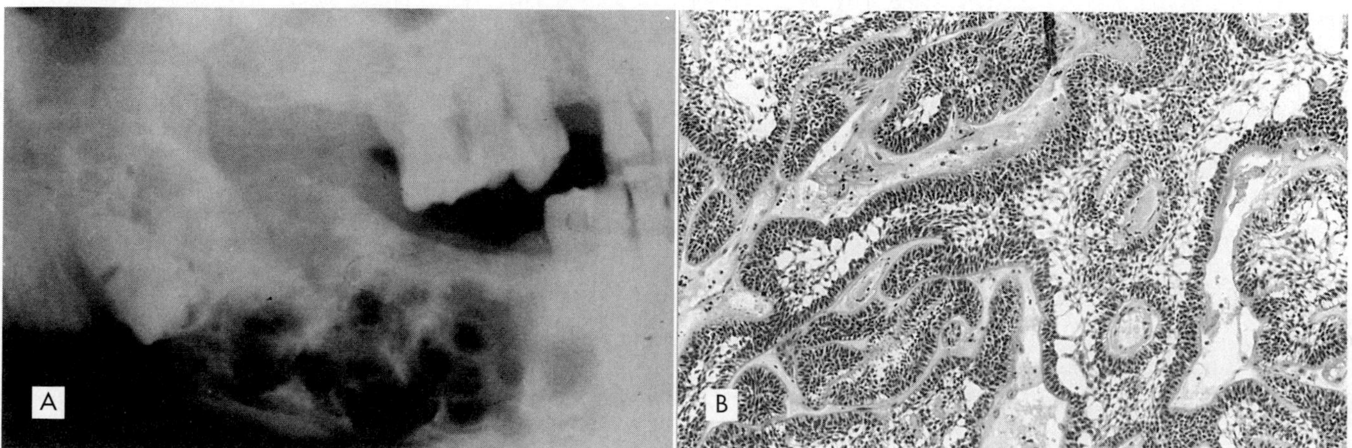

Fig. 50-22 Ameloblastoma in the right angle of the mandible. **A,** Radiograph shows a multilocular lesion. **B,** Plexiform pattern of ameloblastic proliferation.

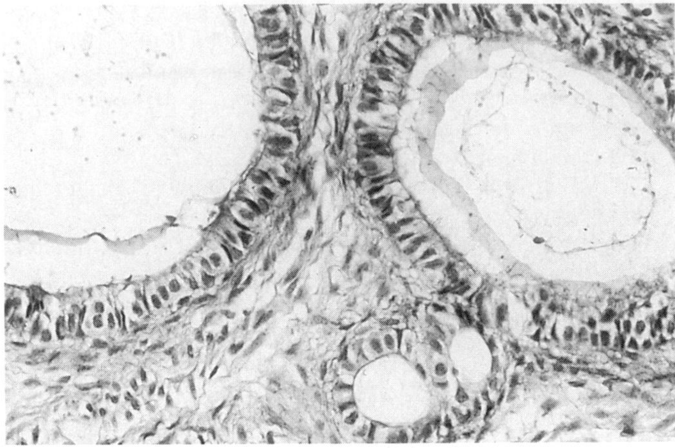

Fig. 50-23 Odontogenic adenomatoid tumor. The tumor is composed of ductlike structures that are lined by cuboidal or columnar cells.

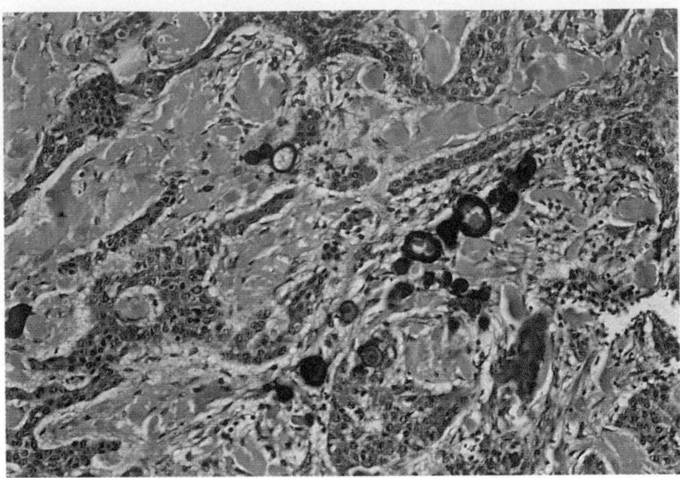

Fig. 50-24 Calcifying epithelial odontogenic tumor showing islands of polyhedral epithelial cells with nuclear pleomorphism and extracellular eosinophilic material.

Metastases are rare and usually occur in tumors of long duration (malignant ameloblastomas are discussed later).

Odontogenic adenomatoid tumor (adenomatoid odontogenic tumor). The odontogenic adenomatoid tumor (OAT) is a benign neoplasm that appears more commonly in females, arises more often in the anterior region of the upper jaw, and occurs most frequently in the second decade of life. Frequently, it is associated with an unerupted canine tooth. On x-ray film it resembles a dentigerous cyst.

Microscopically, the OAT consists of congeries of small nests and ductlike structures lined by cuboidal to tall columnar epithelium and swirling strands of spindle-shaped cells (Fig. 50-23). Eosinophilic material and small calcified foci are often scattered throughout the epithelial tissue. There is very scant fibrous stroma, and the lesion is encapsulated.

Although the tumor expands the jawbone, it is not invasive, and it does not recur even after extremely conservative surgical therapy.[278,279]

Calcifying epithelial odontogenic tumor (Pindborg tumor). The calcifying epithelial odontogenic tumor (CEOT) is a relatively rare lesion. It occurs most commonly in the fourth and fifth decades of life. There is no sex predilection. About 65% of reported cases have arisen in the mandibular premolar-molar area in association with an embedded tooth.[280-282] It usually presents as a slowly enlarging, painless mass. Radiographs show a mixed radiolucent-radiopaque lesion, often near the crown of an unerupted tooth.

Microscopically, the CEOT is composed of nests of closely packed, polyhedral epithelial cells that frequently demonstrate nuclear pleomorphism. Mitoses are rare. An extracellular eosinophilic homogeneous material staining like amyloid is characteristic of this tumor (Fig. 50-24). Concentric calcified deposits, resembling psammoma bodies but called "Liesegang rings," are formed in the amyloid material; these structures can become large and dense. The nature of the amyloid-like material is unknown, but the material appears to derive from the epithelial cells.

This slow-growing neoplasm may be invasive and recur locally, behaving like an ameloblastoma. There is a 10% to 15% recurrence rate.

Benign odontogenic tumors of mesenchymal origin

Myxoma (odontogenic myxoma, myxofibroma). The myxoma is one of the more common odontogenic tumors. Since most investigators believe that myxomas do not occur in the extragnathic skeleton, all myxomas of the jaws represent odontogenic tumors. The myxoma presumably arises from primitive odontogenic mesenchyme and bears a close histologic resemblance to the mesodermal portion of a developing tooth, the dental papilla.

The myxoma is encountered most often in young adults and occurs in the mandible and maxilla with about equal frequency. In some instances, tumor growth is fairly rapid and may result in noticeable bone expansion. Myxomas may thin the cortex and extend into the soft tissue. The radiologic appearance varies from an ill-defined radiolucency within a jaw to multiple small radiolucencies separated by delicate bony septa ("soap bubbles"). These x-ray appearances may also be seen with ameloblastomas.

Microscopy reveals sparsely cellular, loosely arranged spindle and stellate cells separated by abundant myxoid stroma (Fig. 50-25). The stromal mucin is hyaluronic acid. There is no capsule, and the margin is often ill defined. The nuclei of the myxoma cells may be hyperchromatic but do not exhibit significant atypia. Mitoses are exceedingly rare (the occasionally rapid tumor growth is presumably attributable to mucin production). Some tumors contain small rests of odontogenic epithelium, but their presence is not required for the diagnosis. Since the myxoma is histologically identical to the dental papilla of a developing tooth, the latter may occasionally be misdiagnosed as a myxoma if the clinical and radiologic findings are not appreciated.

There is generally little fibrous tissue within myxomas, but some myxomas have increased collagen fibers; these are designated as *myxofibromas* (or *fibromyxomas*).[283,284] Very rarely, a myxoma is hypercellular and has significant cytologic atypia and locally aggressive behavior; this is designated a *myxosarcoma.*[285]

Myxomas may exhibit infiltrative growth, and recurrence rates of up to 25% have been reported after curettage.

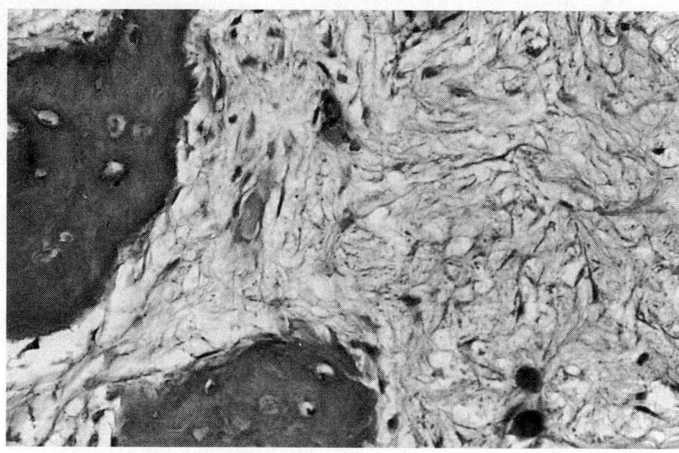

Fig. 50-25 Odontogenic myxoma. The bone has been replaced by spindle-shaped cells in a myxomatous background.

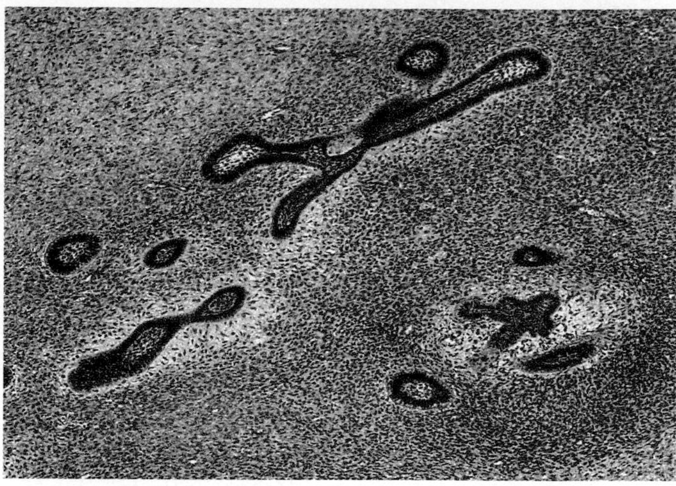

Fig. 50-26 Ameloblastic fibroma. Odontogenic epithelial islands and strands are surrounded by a very cellular connective tissue stroma.

Odontogenic fibroma. Odontogenic fibroma is an uncommon, ill-defined, and controversial lesion. Cases have been reported in patients over a wide age range, and the mandible is involved more often than the maxilla.

The lesion designated in the WHO classification as *odontogenic fibroma* is composed of plump fibroblasts and collagen fibers arranged in an interlacing pattern. Strands and nests of odontogenic epithelium are scattered through the lesion and may be prominent. Calcified cementum like structures and osteoid or dysplastic dentin may be present.[286-288] The histologically identical lesion occurring in the gingival mucosa is designated as the *peripheral* (extraosseous) *odontogenic fibroma.*[289]

Another form of odontogenic fibroma is composed of plump stellate fibroblasts with fine collagen fibers and considerable ground substance.[290] Occasionally, small rests of odontogenic epithelium may be observed. This variant merges with the histologic appearance of the myxofibroma.

The relationship between the two lesions, both referred to as odontogenic fibroma, is as yet unresolved. Both types are benign and respond well to conservative treatment.

Cemental tumors. Three main types of cemental lesions are recognized in the WHO classification of odontogenic tumors: benign cementoblastoma, cemento-ossifying fibroma, and cemento-osseous dysplasia. These are histologically similar lesions that combine neoplastic as well as nonneoplastic processes and are logically discussed in the next section, Fibro-osseus-cemental lesions of jaws.

Benign odontogenic tumors of mixed epithelial-mesenchymal origin

Ameloblastic fibroma. The benign tumor ameloblastic fibroma is characterized by proliferation of both epithelial and mesenchymal elements in the absence of hard tooth structures.[291] In contrast to ameloblastoma, the tumor for which it is most commonly mistaken, the ameloblastic fibroma usually occurs in a young age group, rarely being seen in persons over 21 years of age. It usually involves the molar region of the mandible and is often associated with an unerupted tooth.

Microscopy shows strands and buds of epithelial cells in a very cellular connective tissue stroma (Fig. 50-26). The presence of this mesenchymal portion differentiates this lesion from ameloblastoma. For the most part, the cells composing the strands of epithelium are cuboid and are two cell layers thick. Occasionally, a stellate reticulum is present. The lesion may be encapsulated.

In contrast to ameloblastoma, simple curettage of the ameloblastic fibroma is usually adequate treatment, though a comprehensive review showed an 18% incidence of local recurrences after curettage.[292]

Ameloblastic fibroodontoma. The benign tumor ameloblastic fibroodontoma shows the features of ameloblastic fibroma but also contains a variably sized component of dentin and enamel. Some lesions diagnosed as "ameloblastic fibroodontoma" probably represent only a stage in the development of an odontoma. However, other lesions grow to considerable size, cause bone destruction, and clearly represent neoplasms. The ameloblastic fibroodontoma is a well-circumscribed lesion that responds readily to conservative enucleation.[293]

Odontoma. An odontoma is the most common odontogenic tumor. Odontomas are considered to be hamartomatous lesions that, when fully developed, consist of enamel, dentin, and cementum. Odontomas are divided into complex and compound types. *Complex odontomas* consist of a haphazard mass of dentin, enamel, and cementum. The more common *compound odontoma* is composed of numerous small, misshapen toothlike structures separated by fibrous tissue.[294] Some odontomas have features of both.

These hamartomas are somewhat more common in the maxilla than in the mandible, and most patients are under 15 years of age. Compound odontomas are more often located in the anterior maxilla, whereas complex odontomas favor the posterior mandible. Most odontomas are small lesions that do not exceed the size of a tooth in the area in which they are located. Rarely, however, an odontoma may exceed 6 cm in diameter and cause expansion of the jaw.

Odontomas may interfere with tooth eruption or be found in place of a tooth. The majority of odontomas are asymptomatic and are detected during the course of routine dental radiographic examination. The radiologic appearance of the compound odontoma is characteristic, with numerous small toothlike structures, but the complex odontoma appears as a nonspecific amorphous radiodensity. These benign lesions are cured by simple excision.[295]

A very rare lesion, the *ameloblastic odontoma,* probably represents the simultaneous occurrence of an ameloblastoma and an odontoma;[296] these may be locally aggressive and behave in a manner similar to that of the ameloblastoma.

Malignant odontogenic tumors

Malignant behavior of odontogenic tumors is rare but well documented.

Malignant ameloblastoma. The term *malignant ameloblastoma* is currently applied to the rare examples of a histologically typical ameloblastoma that metastasize. Metastases of ameloblastoma have been demonstrated in regional lymph nodes, lungs, pleura, other bones, and occasionally other viscera. Both the primary tumor and metastatic deposits are histologically similar to most ameloblastomas that do not metastasize.

Ameloblastic carcinoma. The term *ameloblastic carcinoma* is applied to a tumor that has the general microscopic features of an ameloblastoma but shows cytologic evidence of malignancy in the primary tumor, in a recurrent tumor, or in a metastasis. These lesions are characterized by aggressive local behavior, frequent recurrences, and occasional metastases.[297,298]

Ameloblastic fibrosarcoma. The rare cancer ameloblastic fibrosarcoma is the malignant counterpart of the ameloblastic fibroma. Some tumors are malignant *ab initio* whereas others develop as a recurrence of a previously benign ameloblastic fibroma. Pain, ulceration, and extensive bone destruction are usually present. Microscopy demonstrates islands or strands of benign odontogenic epithelium similar to those seen in an ameloblastic fibroma, together with a cell-rich mesenchymal component exhibiting histologic features of fibrosarcoma. Mitoses and bizarre tumor cells are found. This tumor invades into adjacent tissues and is clinically aggressive. Metastasis of an ameloblastic fibrosarcoma, however, has not been convincingly documented.[299]

FIBROOSSEOUSCEMENTAL LESIONS OF JAWS

The umbrella term *benign fibroosseous lesions* is widely applied to diverse lesions involving the craniofacial skeleton that are all characterized by a fibrous stroma containing various combinations of bone and cementumlike material. A wide variety of developmental, dysplastic, and neoplastic lesions are included under this general designation. More specific diagnosis requires histologic correlation with history, clinical, and radiographic findings. In the absence of this information, the pathologist can seldom be more specific than to report that the lesion in question represents a benign fibroosseous lesion. The more important types of fibroosseous lesions are discussed in this section.

Fibrous dysplasia

The jaws may be involved in both monostotic and polyostotic forms of fibrous dysplasia. The monostotic form is more common and is most often seen in children and young adults. Maxillary lesions are most common and may not be strictly monostotic, involving contiguous bones (sphenoid, occiput, and zygoma). Polyostotic fibrous dysplasia, in addition to occurring in several or many bones, may be accompanied by melanotic pigmentation of the skin and various endocrine disturbances (McCune-Albright syndrome).

Fibrous dysplasia is manifest by painless swelling of the affected bone. Radiographically the lesion has a characteristic "ground-glass" appearance and ill-defined borders that blend imperceptibly with surrounding bone. Microscopically the jaw lesions of fibrous dysplasia tend to be more ossified than their counterparts in the extragnathic skeleton. The bone trabeculae are immature and form irregular shapes, likened to Chinese characters, that are separated by cellular fibrous tissue (Fig. 50-27).[300,301] Over time, the metaplastic bone in this self-limited condition tends to be replaced by lamellar bone.

Ossifying fibroma (cementifying fibroma, cemento-ossifying fibroma)

Ossifying fibromas of the jaws and craniofacial skeleton are generally considered to be benign neoplasms. Young adult women are most often affected. They occur most often in the molar area of the mandible and present as circumscribed, expansile tumors that on occasion may grow to massive size. Large lesions can cause pain or paresthesias. Radiologically they are well-circumscribed lesions that may be radiolucent or radiopaque.

Grossly the tumor is well circumscribed and may be encapsulated. Microscopically the ossifying fibroma is composed of a cellular fibrous connective tissue containing varying combinations of trabecular, woven, or lamellar bone, or relatively acellular calcifications resembling cementum. Lesions with the latter component predominating have been considered by the WHO[302] and others to be cementifying fibromas and classified as a separate type of odontogenic tumor. This appears to be an arbitrary and unnecessary division, and there is a growing tendency to include all these variations under the rubric of "ossifying fibroma."[303]

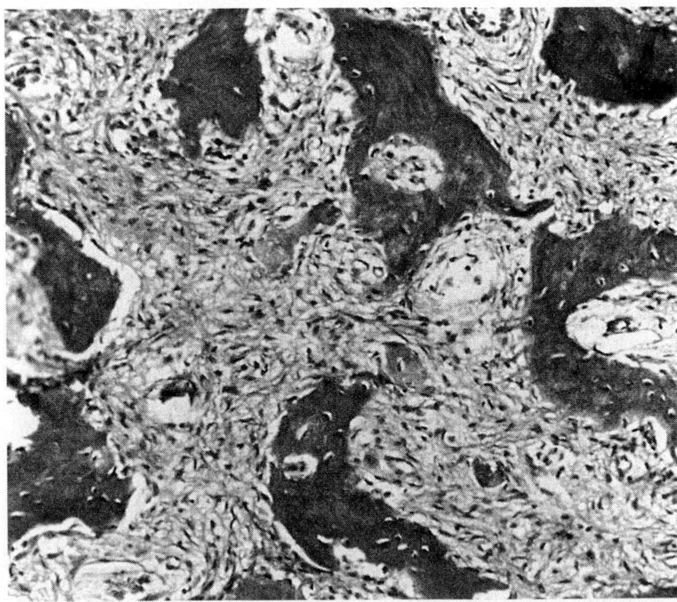

Fig. 50-27 Fibrous dysplasia of the maxilla. Notice the dysplastic bone trabeculae (likened to Chinese characters) separated by cellular fibrous tissue.

Most ossifying fibromas of the jaws respond well to simple enucleation, with a low incidence of recurrence. Large lesions, however, may require block resection and bone grafting.

Ossifying fibromas also occur in the extragnathic craniofacial skeleton, particularly in the ethmoid and frontal bones; these tend to be larger, more radiographically diffuse, and often more histologically cellular than those in the mandible or maxilla.[304] These lesions have been variously designated as aggressive, active, juvenile, or psammomatoid ossifying fibroma[305-307] and aggressive fibrous dysplasia.[308] The relationship of craniofacial ossifying fibromas to ossifying fibromas of the jaws or the long bones is uncertain.[309] Ossifying fibromas should be distinguished from the peripheral (extraosseous) ossifying fibroma that occurs on the gingiva (discussed earlier in this chapter); although both lesions are called ossifying fibroma, they are not histologically identical.

Benign cementoblastoma

The cementoblastoma is a rare benign neoplasm most often involving the roots of the mandibular first molar in young adult patients. The lesion causes pain, especially with mastication, and swelling. It radiographically presents as a sharply defined, densely calcified mass intimately associated with and resorbing the roots of the involved tooth. Histologically the tumor is composed of sheets of mineralized material (bone and cementum) bordered by large blastlike cells. The histologic features are very similar to those of osteoblastoma, and some investigators believe that cementoblastoma of the jaws is best classified as a form of osteoblastoma.[310-312]

Periapical cemental dysplasia (periapical cementoma)

Periapical cemental dysplasia is a frequent lesion, particularly in middle-aged black women. It is a nonneoplastic, presumably dysplastic condition. The anterior mandibular teeth are most often involved by asymptomatic periapical radiolucencies that, in older lesions, become increasingly calcified. In the early stages, the lesion may be confused with periapical inflammatory disease. This condition is self-limited, and treatment is not required.

Florid cementoosseous dysplasia

Florid cementoosseous dysplasia is less common and has been reported under various designations. This condition is usually seen in middle-aged or elderly black women. Radiographs show extensive sclerotic areas, often symmetrically involving the posterior quadrants of the mandible and the maxilla.[313] The microscopic appearance is indistinguishable from that of periapical cemental dysplasia, and both are similar to the ossifying fibroma.

GIANT CELL LESIONS OF JAWS

Central giant cell granuloma

Central giant cell granuloma is an uncommon, benign osseous lesion, occurring almost exclusively in the jawbones (it has been infrequently reported in other facial bones and elsewhere). A more common but histologically identical gingival lesion, the peripheral giant cell granuloma, was discussed earlier. It is generally believed that these lesions represent reactive or reparative processes, possibly in response to bone hemorrhage, trauma, or inflammation.

It typically presents with painless enlargement, usually in the second and third decades of life. Radiographs usually show a well-defined, multilocular radiolucency within the jaw (resembling ameloblastomas), though some lesions are unilocular or poorly defined.

Microscopy shows spindled fibroblasts in a well-vascularized fibrous stroma. Multinucleate giant cells are scattered through the lesion, sometimes evenly but usually in aggregates around vessels. Hemorrhages, hemosiderophages, inflammatory cells, dystrophic calcifications, and osteoid are variably present. It can resemble the other giant cell lesions discussed in the section below. Aggressive curettage of the lesion is usually curative.[314,315]

Brown tumor of hyperparathyroidism

Brown tumors are nonneoplastic bone lesions of hyperparathyroidism (sometimes referred to as *von Recklinghausen's disease of bone*, or *osteitis fibrosa cystica*) and have become infrequent, since the diagnosis is now often made on the basis of elevated serum calcium levels in asymptomatic adults.[316,317] Radiographically, brown tumors resemble bone cysts but may be multilocular or multiple (x-ray films may also show other osseous manifestations of hyperparathyroidism).

Histologically, the brown tumor consists of groups of multinucleated giant cells in a well-vascularized, cellular fibrous stroma. Hemosiderin from hemorrhages imparts the color for which the lesion is named. Clinical and radiologic information, particularly the serum calcium, distinguishes this lesion from the other giant cell lesions.

Aneurysmal bone cyst

Aneurysmal bone cyst is a very rare lesion in the jaws, occurring more often in the mandible than in the maxilla.[318-320] It histologically overlaps with some very vascular examples of central giant cell granuloma and other giant cell lesions. Separation is made on the basis of the cavernous spaces filled with blood and of clinical features. Aneurysmal bone cysts may be present with other bone lesions (such as fibrous dysplasia, hemangioma).

Cherubism (familial multilocular cystic disease of the jaws)

Cherubism, a benign but destructive condition, affects the jaws and usually presents in early childhood.[321] It can be sporadic or familial with autosomal dominant inheritance. The mandible is always involved, but it also usually involves the maxilla. The mandible is symmetrically enlarged, most commonly at the angles. Maxillary expansion causes fullness of the cheeks and downward retraction of the lower eyelids (exposing the lower sclera, so it appears that one is gazing heavenward) to give afflicted children a cherubic appearance. Dental development is disrupted, and teeth may be absent, displaced, or prematurely shed.

X-ray films show numerous multilocular radiolucencies and bone expansion. There can be such extensive osteolysis that the teeth lose their bony support and appear to "float in space" on radiographs. The diagnosis can be difficult in early lesions, which may be asymmetric or primarily involve the maxilla.

The histologic appearance varies. Active lesions consist of well-vascularized, cellular fibrous tissue with variable numbers of multinucleated giant cells, often in groups around hemorrhages, and spindle cells. Distinctive perivascular collagen deposits forming eosinophilic cuffs around small blood vessels are occasionally found. With regression, the lesion is gradually replaced by fibrous tissue and new bone, and the giant cells disappear. The histologic differential diagnosis includes the fibro-osseous and other giant cell lesions, but these can usually be excluded on clinical and radiologic grounds.

There is often regression after puberty. Some investigators advocate treatment of lesions with curettage.

Giant cell tumor

The neoplasms called *giant cell tumors* rarely occur in the jaws where they are likely to be associated with Paget's disease of bone. Clinically they may grow slowly and expand the bone, like the more common central giant cell granuloma, or they may grow more rapidly, causing pain and paresthesia. Radiographically they resemble the central giant cell granuloma.

Histologically they also resemble cellular examples of central giant cell granuloma, with numerous multinucleated giant cells evenly dispersed among mononuclear stromal cells. Differentiation can be difficult; the giant cells may be more evenly dispersed, be larger, and have more nuclei in the giant cell tumor, but there is overlap.[322]

NONODONTOGENIC NEOPLASMS INVOLVING THE JAWS

This section describes two bone neoplasms with a special affinity for the maxilla and mandible, and several neoplasms where jaw involvement has characteristics differing from involvement of bones elsewhere.[323]

Osteoma

The osteoma is an uncommon benign tumor of bone with a predilection for the jaws and other facial bones. The cause is unknown. Osteomas are usually single, but multiple osteomas can occur with Gardner's syndrome (discussed earlier). They occur at any age, but usually between 20 and 60 years of age. They are often small, asymptomatic, and incidentally discovered on x-ray films performed for unrelated reasons. An osteoma may present as a slowly enlarging, painless mass. Occasionally, lesions in the paranasal sinuses cause headaches, recurrent sinusitis, and ocular problems. Osteomas may be subperiosteal (peripheral) or endosteal (central).[324,325] Radiographs show a well-circumscribed, radiopaque mass. A peripheral lesion may radiologically resemble an exostosis or the rare parosteal osteosarcoma; a central lesion may resemble an odontoma, focal sclerosing osteomyelitis, cementoma, or heavily calcified fibro-osseous lesion.

Osteomas consist of mature bone, which may be compact, lamellar bone without marrow spaces, spongy (trabecular) bone with marrow spaces, or a combination of the two patterns. Although benign, they are usually excised to establish the diagnosis or because of symptoms.

Melanotic neuroectodermal tumor of infancy

The very rare tumor melanotic neuroectodermal tumor of infancy is probably of neural crest origin. It almost always occurs in infants less than 1 year old. This tumor most often occurs in the anterior maxilla, generally presenting as an osteolytic, rapidly enlarging swelling. The tumors are firm, usually with grossly visible pigmented areas. Microscopy reveals tubular or alveolar nests of cells separated by a vascular fibrous stroma. The peripheral cells in the nests are larger, cuboidal, or flattened, and some contain melanin. The neuroblastic cells in the centers of the nests are small and round with hyperchromatic nuclei. This tumor is incompletely or not encapsulated. Treatment is conservative excision with a good prognosis, but there are occasional recurrences.[326]

This tumor has a distinctive immunophenotypic profile. In one small series, the larger pigmented epithelioid cells stained with cytokeratin and the melanoma-associated antigen HMB-45, whereas the small cells (in two of three tumors) reacted with neuron-specific enolase and synaptophysin.[327] Both cell types reacted with vimentin antibody. Fairly similar results were obtained in another study.[328]

Osteoblastoma

Osteoblastoma is an uncommon, benign lesion of bone that occasionally occurs in the jaws. Osteoblastomas occur most often in the vertebrae and long bones, but the mandible is the most frequent site in the head and neck region. Clinically, radiologically, and histologically, osteoblastomas of the jaws resemble their extrafacial counterparts. However, in the jaws, the histologic differential diagnosis is complicated by its resemblance to fibro-osseous lesions, particularly the cementoblastoma (discussed previously).[329]

Osteosarcoma

About 5% of osteosarcomas occur in the jaws.[330-333] The mandible and maxilla are involved with about equal frequency. The average age at diagnosis is 34 years, about a decade older than for extragnathic osteosarcomas. Symptoms include pain, swelling, paresthesia, and loosening of teeth. Maxillary tumors may also present with epistaxis, nasal obstruction, or ocular symptoms.

Radiographs show variable radiopacity and radiolucency, depending on the degree of calcification and bone destruction. The tumor margins are ill defined, and the roots of involved teeth may be resorbed. The periodontal ligament normally forms a narrow radiolucent line around teeth, and osteosarcoma within the alveolar bone may cause widening of this line.[334] The "sunburst" pattern of radiating radiodense lines, caused by the bony periosteal reaction, is occasionally seen but is not diagnostic.

All the histologic varieties of osteosarcoma occur in the jaws, but the chondrosarcomatous, fibrosarcomatous, and fibrohistiocytomatous patterns occur relatively more commonly than in the long bones (in which the osteoblastic pattern predominates). Osteosarcomas in the jaws are also often of lower grade than extrafacial osteosarcomas.

Radical mandibulectomy or maxillectomy is usually combined with adjuvant chemotherapy because of the high incidence of recurrences. Radiation therapy is often used for incompletely excised or recurrent cancers, though it is also used as adjuvant therapy. The 5-year survival is approximately 40%, and is better in patients less than 21 years of age and with mandibular lesions (maxillary lesions sometimes spread extensively through the sinuses before detection and are closer to vital structures).

Chondrosarcoma

Chondrosarcomas of the jaws are very rare; only about 1% of chondrosarcomas occur in this site. Benign chondroid tumors in the jaws are even more rare. The anterior maxilla is the most common location. The average age at presentation has been variously reported but is older than that for extrafacial chondrosarcomas. Painless swelling is the most common presenting symptom. Radiographic findings are variable and can resemble those of osteosarcomas. Speckled radiodensities, attributable to foci of tumoral calcification, are suggestive.

Chondrosarcomas of the jaws histologically resemble their extrafacial counterparts.[335] In the jaws, osteosarcomas are more common and often have chondroid areas; therefore, the diagnosis of a cartilaginous tumor should be made only after careful consideration of the possibility of chondroblastic osteosarcoma. Benign chondroid neoplasms may be difficult to distinguish from low-grade chondrosarcomas.[336] Chondrosarcomas with prominent myxoid areas can resemble myxoma/myxofibroma and chondromyxoid fibroma in the bone and chondroid metaplasia in the mandibular joint space.

The prognosis for chondrosarcomas of the jaws is worse than that for those occurring in other sites. The best results are obtained when the tumor is excised with a wide margin, which requires surgery ranging from en bloc resection to radical mandibulectomy or maxillectomy.

Metastatic carcinoma

It is estimated than 1% of malignant neoplasms with bone metastases involve the jaws. Metastatic disease in the jawbones originates most commonly from primary carcinoma of the breast, kidney, lung, colon, prostate, and thyroid, in descending order.[337-341] The route of metastasis is generally hematogenous, either directly from the primary tumor or indirectly from a lung metastasis.[342]

Patients developing jaw metastases are usually elderly. The body and angle of the mandible are the most common sites for jaw metastases. Jaw metastases can present by swelling, pain, loosening of teeth, lip paresthesia, and pathologic fracture. Radiographically the lesion is usually an irregular, "moth-eaten," expansile radiolucency. Occasionally, the metastatic lesion is osteoblastic, producing irregular radiopacities; most notable for this are prostate and breast carcinomas.

Microscopically, metastatic carcinomas vary considerably, reflecting the type and grade of the tumor. Immunohistochemical stains are occasionally helpful in determining the origin of the cancer when the primary site is unknown. In roughly 20% to 30% of cases, the jaw metastasis is the first indication of the cancer.

REFERENCES

General reviews

1. Arnold WJ, Laissue JA, Friedmann I, Naumann HH, editors: *Diseases of the head and neck: an atlas of histopathology,* New York, 1987, Thieme Medical Publishers.
2. Barnes L, editor: *Surgical pathology of the head and neck,* New York, 1985, Marcel Dekker.
3. Bhaskar SN: *Synopsis of oral pathology,* ed 7, St. Louis, 1986, Mosby.
4. Cawson RA, Eveson JW: *Oral pathology and diagnosis: color atlas with integrated text,* Philadelphia, 1987, Saunders.
5. Cawson RA, Lucas RB: The mouth. In Symmers WS, editor: *Systemic pathology,* vol 3, Edinburgh, 1987, Churchill Livingstone.
6. Cawson RA, Lucas RB: The teeth and supporting tissues; tumours of the mouth and jaws. In Symmers WS, editor: *Systemic pathology,* vol 3, Edinburgh, 1987, Churchill Livingstone.
7. Schuller DE, Schleuning AJ II: *DeWeese and Saunders' otolaryngology–head and neck surgery,* ed 8, St. Louis, 1994, Mosby.
8. Jones JH, Mason DK, editors: *Oral manifestations of systemic disease,* London, 1980, Saunders.
9. McClatchey KD, Zarbo RJ: The jaws and oral cavity. In Sternberg SS, editor: *Diagnostic surgical pathology,* ed 2, New York, 1994, Raven Press.
10. Pindborg JJ: *Atlas of diseases of the oral mucosa,* ed 5, Copenhagen, 1992, Munksgaard.
11. Regezi JA, Sciubba J: *Oral pathology: clinical-pathologic correlations,* ed 2, Philadelphia, 1993, Saunders.
12. Scully C, Welbury R: *Color atlas of oral diseases in children and adolescents,* London, 1994, Wolfe Publishing (Mosby–Year Book Europe Limited).
13. Wenig BM: *Atlas of head and neck pathology,* Philadelphia, 1993, Saunders.

Normal development and structure

14. Avery JK: *Essentials of oral histology and embryology,* St. Louis, 1992, Mosby.
15. Beck F, Moffat DB, Davies DP: *Human embryology,* ed 2, Oxford, 1985, Blackwell Scientific Publications.
16. Gartner LP: *Essentials of oral histology and embryology,* Baltimore, 1986, Jen House Publishing.
17. Davis WL: *Oral histology: cell structure and function,* Philadelphia, 1986, Saunders.
18. Berkovitz BKB, Holland GR, Moxham BJ: *Color atlas and textbook of oral anatomy, histology and embryology,* ed 2, St. Louis, 1992, Mosby.
19. McClatchey, KD: Periodontium, minor salivary glands, and maxillary sinus. In Sternberg SS, editor: *Histology for pathologists,* New York, 1992, Raven Press.
20. Fechner RE, Mills SE: Larynx and pharynx. In Sternberg SS, editor: *Histology for pathologists,* New York, 1992, Raven Press.

Developmental anomalies

21. Gorlin RJ, Pindborg JJ, Cohen MM: *Syndromes of the head and neck,* ed 2, New York, 1976, McGraw-Hill.
22. Scully C: Down's syndrome: aspects of dental care, *J Dent* 4:167, 1976.
23. Buckley RH: Assessing inheritance of agammaglobulinemia, *N Engl J Med* 330:1526, 1994.
24. Jones JH, Mason DK, editors: *Oral manifestations of systemic disease,* Philadelphia, 1980, Saunders.

Infectious diseases

25. Winkler JR, Grassi M, Murray PA: Clinical description and etiology of HIV-associated periodontal diseases. In Robertson PB, Greenspan JS, editors: *Perspectives on oral manifestations of AIDS,* Littleton, Mass, 1988, PSG Publishing.
26. Rao MS, Kameswari VR, Ramula C, Reddy CRRM: Oral lesions in granuloma inguinale, *J Oral Surg* 34:1112, 1976.
27. Maher A, Bassiouny A, Bucci TJ et al: Tonsillomycosis: a mycohistopathological study, *J Laryngol Otol* 96:229, 1982.
28. Miller CS, Redding SW: Diagnosis and management of orofacial herpes simplex virus infections, *Dent Clin North Am* 36:879, 1992.
29. Topazian RG: Osteomyelitis of the jaws. In Topazian RG, Goldberg MH, editors: *Oral and maxillofacial infections,* ed 2, Philadelphia, 1987, Saunders.
30. Lichty G, Langlais R, Aufdemorte T: Garré's osteomyelitis: literature review and case report, *Oral Surg Oral Med Oral Pathol* 50:309, 1980.

Inflammatory diseases of skin and oral mucosa

31. DePanfilis G, Manara G, Ferraric et al: Imbalance in phenotype expression of T-cell subpopulations during different evolutional stages of lichen planus, *Acta Derm Venereol* 63:369, 1984.
32. Lacy MF, Reade PC, Hay KD: Lichen planus: a theory of pathogenesis, *Oral Surg Oral Med Oral Pathol* 56:521, 1983.

33. Vincent SD, Fotos PG, Baker KA, Williams TP: Oral lichen planus: the clinical, historical, and therapeutic features of 100 cases, *Oral Surg Oral Med Oral Pathol* 70:165, 1990.
34. Olsen RG, DuPlessis D, Barron G et al: Lichen planus specific epidermal antigen in affected patients, *J Clin Lab Immunol* 10:103, 1983.
35. Valsecchi R, Bontempelli M, Rossi A et al: HLA-DR3 and DQ antigens in lichen planus, *Acta Derm Venereol* 68:77, 1988.
36. Porter K, Scully C, Bidwell J, Porter S: Class I and II HLA antigens in British patients with oral lichen planus, *Oral Surg Oral Med Oral Pathol* 75:176, 1993.
37. Saurat JH, Gluckman E, Bussel A et al: The lichen planus–like eruption after bone marrow transplantation, *Br J Dermatol* 92:675, 1975.
38. Eisenberg E, Krutchkoff DJ: Lichenoid lesions of oral mucosa: diagnostic criteria and their importance in the alleged relationship to oral cancer, *Oral Surg Oral Med Oral Pathol* 73:699, 1992.
39. Krutchkoff DJ, Eisenberg E: Lichenoid dysplasia: a distinct histopathologic entity, *Oral Surg Oral Med Oral Pathol* 60:308, 1985.
40. Holmstrup P, Pindborg JJ: Erythroplakic lesions in relation to oral lichen planus, *Acta Derm Venereol 59(suppl 85):77, 1979.*
41. Holmstrup P: The controversy of premalignant potential of oral lichen planus is over, *Oral Surg Oral Med Oral Pathol* 73:704, 1992.
42. Silverman S Jr, Gorsky M, Lozada-Nur F: A prospective follow-up study of 570 patients with oral lichen planus: persistence, remission, and malignant association, *Oral Surg Oral Med Oral Pathol* 60:30, 1985.
43. Fulling HJ: Cancer development in oral lichen planus: a follow-up study of 327 patients, *Arch Dermatol* 108:667, 1973.

Systemic diseases involving the mouth

44. Grossman ME, Stevens AW, Cohen PR: Brief report: herpetic geometric glossitis, *N Engl J Med* 329:1859, 1993.
45. Greenspan J, Greenspan D, Lenette ET et al: Replication of Epstein-Barr virus within the epithelial cells of oral "hairy" leukoplakia, an AIDS-associated lesion, *N Engl J Med* 313:1465, 1986.
46. Jones JH, Mason DK, editors: *Oral manifestations of systemic disease,* Philadelphia, 1980, Saunders.
47. Snyder MB, Cawson RA: Oral changes in Crohn's disease, *J Oral Surg* 34:594, 1976.
48. Sánchez MA, Zali MR, Khalil AA et al: Be aware of Gardner's syndrome: a review of the literature, *Am J Gastroenterol* 71:68, 1979.
49. Cawson RA: Gingival changes in Wegener's granulomatosis, *Br Dent J* 118:30, 1965.
50. Patten SF, Tomecki KJ: Wegener's granulomatosis: cutaneous and oral mucosal disease, *J Am Acad Dermatol* 28:710, 1993.
51. Willman CL, Busque L, Griffith BB et al: Langerhans'-cell histiocytosis (histiocytosis X)—a clonal proliferative disease, *N Engl J Med* 331:154, 1994.
52. Zuendel MT, Bowers DF, Kramer RN: Recurrent histiocytosis X with mandibular lesions, Oral Surg *Oral Med Oral Pathol* 58:420, 1984.

Other inflammatory, reactive, or ulcerative conditions of the mouth

53. Axell T, Henricsson V: Association between recurrent aphthous ulcers and tobacco habits, *Scand J Dent Res* 93:239, 1985.
54. Scully C, Porter SR: Recurrent aphthous stomatitis: current concepts of etiology, pathogenesis, and management, *J Oral Pathol Med* 18:300, 1989.
55. Antoon JW, Miller RL: Aphthous ulcers: a review of literature on etiology, pathogenesis, diagnosis and treatment, *J Am Dent Assoc* 101:803, 1980.
56. Landesberg R, Fallon M, Insel R: Alterations of T-helper/inducer and T suppressor/inducer cells in patients with recurrent aphthous ulcers, *Oral Surg Oral Med Oral Pathol* 69:205, 1990.
57. Pedersen A, Klausen B, Hougen HP, Ryder LP: Peripheral lymphocyte subpopulations in recurrent aphthous ulcerations, *Acta Odontol Scand* 49:203, 1991.
58. MacPhail LA, Greenspan D, Greenspan JS: Recurrent aphthous ulcers in association with HIV infection, *Oral Surg Oral Med Oral Pathol* 73:283, 1992.
59. Shafer WG, Hine MK, Levy BM: *Text book of oral pathology,* ed 4, Philadelphia, 1983, Saunders.
60. Regezi JA, Sciubba J: *Oral pathology: clinical-pathologic correlations,* ed 2, Philadelphia, 1993, Saunders.
61. Grattan CE, Gentle TA, Basa MK: Oral papillary plasmocytosis resembling candidiasis without demonstrated fungus in the lesions, *Clin Exp Dermatol* 17:112, 1992.
62. Elzay RP: Traumatic ulcerative granuloma with stromal eosinophilia (Riga-Fede's disease and traumatic eosinophilic granuloma), *Oral Surg Oral Med Oral Pathol* 55:497, 1983.
63. Bhaskar SN, Hilly GZ: Traumatic granuloma of the tongue (human and experimental), *Oral Surg Oral Med Oral Pathol* 18:206, 1964.
64. El-Mofty SK, Swanson PE, Wick MR, Miller AS: Eosinophilic ulcer of the oral mucosa: report of 38 new cases with immunohistochemical observations, *Oral Surg Oral Med Oral Pathol* 75:716, 1993.
65. Doyle IL, Geary W, Baden E: Eosinophilic ulcer, *J Oral Maxillofac Surg* 47:349, 1989.
66. Brannon RB, Fowler CB, Hartman KS: Necrotizing sialometaplasia: a clinicopathologic study of sixty-nine cases and review of the literature, *Oral Surg Oral Med Oral Pathol* 71:317, 1991.

Disorders of mucosal pigmentation

67. Buchner A, Hansen LS: Pigmented nevi of the oral mucosa: a clinicopathologic study of 36 new cases and review of 155 cases from the literature, *Oral Surg Oral Med Oral Pathol* 63:676, 1987.
68. Jones JH, Mason DK, editors: *Oral manifestations of systemic disease,* Philadelphia, 1980, Saunders.
69. Cawson RA, Eveson JW: *Oral pathology and diagnosis,* Philadelphia, 1987, Saunders.
70. Buchner A, Hansen LS: Amalgam pigmentation (amalgam tattoo) of the oral mucosa: a clinicopathologic study of 268 cases, *Oral Surg Oral Med Oral Pathol* 49:139, 1980.

Benign epithelial proliferations

71. Abbey LM, Page DG, Sawyer DR: The clinical and histopathologic features of a series of 464 oral squamous cell papillomas, *Oral Surg Oral Med Oral Pathol* 49:419, 1980.
72. Harrist TJ, Murphy GF, Mihm MC: Oral warty dyskeratoma, *Arch Dermatol* 116:929, 1980.
73. Wechsler HL, Fisher ER: Oral florid papillomatosis: clinical, pathological, and electron microscopic observations, *Arch Dermatol* 86:480, 1962.
74. Van Wyck CW, Staz J, Farman AG: Focal epithelial hyperplasia in a group of South Africans: its ultrastructural features, *J Oral Pathol* 6:14, 1977.

Premalignant lesions and conditions

75. Morgan PR: Neoplasms and precancerous conditions of the oral mucosa. In McGee JO, Isaacson PG, Wright NA, editors: *Oxford textbook of pathology: pathology of systems,* vol 2a, Oxford, 1992, Oxford University Press.
76. WHO Collaborating Centre for Oral Precancerous Lesions: Definition of leukoplakia and related lesions: an aid to studies of oral precancer, *Oral Surg Oral Med Oral Pathol* 46:518, 1978.
77. Pindborg JJ: Oral precancer. In Barnes L, editor: *Surgical pathology of the head and neck,* vol 1, New York, 1985, Marcel Dekker.
78. Shafer WG, Hine MH, Levy BM: Benign and malignant tumors of the oral cavity. In *A textbook of oral pathology,* ed 4, Philadelphia, 1983, Saunders.
79. Pindborg JJ, Renstrup G, Pousen H, Silverman S: Studies in oral leukoplakia: V. Clinical and histologic signs of malignancy, *Acta Odontol Scand* 21:407, 1963.
80. Silverman S Jr, Shilliote EJ: Etiology and predisposing factors. In Silverman S Jr, editor: *Oral cancer,* ed 3, Atlanta, 1990, The American Cancer Society.
81. Waldron CA, Shafer WG: Leukoplakia revisited: a clinicopathologic study of 3256 oral leukoplakias, *Cancer* 36:1386, 1975.
82. Silverman S, Bhargave K, Mani NJ et al: Malignant transformation and natural history of oral leukoplakia in 57,518 industrial workers of Gujarat, India, *Cancer* 38:1790, 1976.
83. Pindborg JJ, Renstrup G, Joist O et al: Studies in oral leukoplakia: a preliminary report on the period prevalence of malignant transformation in

leukoplakia based on a follow-up study of 248 patients, *J Am Dent Assoc* 76:767, 1968.

84. Bánóczy J, Csiba A: Comparative study of clinical picture and histopathologic structure of oral leukoplakia, *Cancer* 29:1230, 1972.
85. Richtsmeier WJ: Biologic modifiers and chemoprevention of cancer of the oral cavity, *N Engl J Med* 328:58, 1993.
86. Queyrat L: Erythroplasie de gland, *Bull Soc Fr Dermatol Syphilique* 22:378, 1911.
87. Shear M: Erythroplasia of the mouth, *Int Dent J* 22:460, 1972.
88. Mashberg A, Meyers H: Anatomical site and size of 222 early asymptomatic squamous cell carcinomas: a continuing prospective study of oral cancer, *Cancer* 37:2149, 1976.
89. Shafer WG, Waldron CA: Erythroplasia of the oral cavity, *Cancer* 36:1021, 1975.
90. Mashberg A, Morrissey JB, Garfinkel L: A study of the appearance of early asymptomatic oral squamous cell carcinoma, *Cancer* 32:1436, 1973.
91. Mashberg A: Erythroplasia: the earliest sign of asymptomatic oral cancer, *J Am Dent Assoc* 96:615, 1978.
92. Pindborg JJ, Mehta FS, Gupta PC et al: Reverse smoking in Andhra Pradesh, India: a study of palatal lesions among 10,169 villagers, *Br J Cancer* 25:10, 1971.
93. Gupta PC, Mehta FS, Daftary DK et al: Incidence rates of oral cancer and natural history of oral precancerous lesions in a 10-year follow-up study of Indian villagers, *Comm Dent Oral Epidemiol* 8:287, 1980.
94. Ahlbom HE: Simple achlorhydric anemia, Plummer-Vinson syndrome, and carcinoma of the mouth, pharynx and oesophagus in women, *Br Med J* 2:231, 1936.
95. Vinson PP: Hysterical dysphagia, *Minn Med* 5:107, 1922.
96. Paymaster JC: Cancer of the buccal mucosa: a clinical study of 650 cases in Indian patients, *Cancer* 9:431, 1956.
97. Pindborg JJ: Is submucous fibrosis a precancerous condition in the oral cavity? *Int Dent J* 22:474, 1972.

Primary epithelial cancers

98. Silverman S Jr, editor: *Oral cancer,* ed 3, Atlanta, 1990, The American Cancer Society.
99. Vokes EE, Weichselbaum RR, Lippman SM, Hong WK: Head and neck cancer, *N Engl J Med* 328:184, 1993.
100. Gaham S, Dayal H, Rohrer J et al: Dentition, diet, tobacco and alcohol in epidemiology of oral cancer, *J Natl Cancer Inst* 59:1611, 1977.
101. Mashberg A, Garfinkel L, Harris S: Alcohol as a primary risk factor in oral squamous carcinoma, *CA* 31:146, 1981.
102. Ernster VL: Trends in smoking, cancer risks, and cigarette promotion: current priorities for reducing tobacco exposure, *Cancer* 62:1702, 1988.
103. Spitz Mr, Fueger JJ, Geopfert H et al: Squamous cell carcinoma of the upper aerodigestive tract: a case comparison analysis, *Cancer* 61:203, 1988.
104. Alston R, Jacoway J: Verrucous carcinoma of the oral mucosa in North Carolina (abstract 158), *J Dent Res* 59(special issue A):307, 1980.
105. Talamini R, Franceschi S, Barra S, La Vecchia C: The role of alcohol in oral and pharyngeal cancer in non-smokers, and of tobacco in non-drinkers, *Int J Cancer* 46:391, 1990.
106. Centers for Disease Control and Prevention: Mortality trends for selected smoking-related cancers and breast cancer—United States, 1950-1990, *MMWR* 42:857, 1993.
107. Public Health Service: *The health consequences of using smokeless tobacco: a report of the Advisory Committee to the Surgeon General* (DHHS # PHS 86-2874) Bethesda, Md, 1986, US Department of Health and Human Services.
108. Wynder L, Bross IJ, Feldman RM: A study of the etiological factors in cancer of the mouth, *Cancer* 10:1300, 1957.
109. McCoy GD, Wynder EL: Etiological and preventive implications in alcohol carcinogenesis, *Cancer Res* 39:2844, 1979.
110. Schmidt W, Popham RE: The role of drinking and smoking in mortality from cancer and other causes in male alcoholics, *Cancer* 47:1031, 1981.
111. Blot WJ, McLaughlin JK, Winn DM et al: Smoking and drinking in relation to oral and pharyngeal cancer, *Cancer Res* 48:3282, 1988.
112. Walton L, Masouredis C: The epidemiology of maxillofacial malignancy, *Oral Maxillofac Clin North Am* 5:207, 1993.
113. Blot WJ, Winn DM, Fraumeni JF: Oral cancer and mouthwash, *J Natl Cancer Inst* 70:251, 1983.
114. Winn DM, Blot WJ, McLaughlin JK et al: Mouthwash use and oral conditions in the risk of oral and pharyngeal cancer, *Cancer Res* 51:3044, 1991.
115. Wynder EL, Kabat C, Rosenthal S et al: Oral cancer and mouthwash use, *J Natl Cancer Inst* 70:255, 1983.
116. Kabat GC, Herbert JP, Wynder EL: Risk factors for oral cancer in women, *Cancer Res* 49:2803, 1989.
117. Mashberg A, Barsa P, Grossman ML: A study of the relationship between mouthwash use and oral and pharyngeal cancer, *J Am Dent Assoc* 110:731, 1989.
118. Pearson GR, Weiland LH, Neel HB III et al: Application of Epstein-Barr Virus (EBV) serology to diagnosis of North American nasopharyngeal carcinoma, *Cancer* 51:260, 1983.
119. Giller RH, Grose C: Epstein-Barr virus: the hematologic and oncologic consequences of virus-host interaction, *CRC Crit Rev Oncol Hematol* 9:149, 1989.
120. Abaza NA, Iczkovitz ML, Henefer EP: American Burkitt's lymphoma manifested in a solitary submandibular lymph node, *Oral Surg Oral Med Oral Pathol* 51:121, 1981.
121. Newland JR, Adler-Storthz K: Cytomegalovirus in intraoral Kaposi's sarcoma, *Oral Surg Oral Med Oral Pathol* 67:296, 1989.
122. Milde K, Loning T: Detection of papillomavirus DNA in oral papillomas and carcinomas: application of *in situ* hybridization with biotinylated HPV 16 probes, *J Oral Pathol* 15:292, 1986.
123. Matland NJ, Cox MF, Lynas C et al: Detection of human papillomavirus DNA in biopsies of oral tissue, *Br J Cancer* 56:245, 1987.
124. Adler-Storthz K, Newland JR, Tessin BA et al: Human papillomavirus type 2 DNA in oral verrucous carcinoma, *J Oral Pathol* 15:472, 1986.
125. Hirsh JM, Johansson SL, Vahlne A: Effect of snuff and herpes simplex virus I on rat oral mucosa: possible association with development of squamous cell carcinoma, *J Oral Pathol* 13:52, 1984.
126. Wingo PA, Tong T, Bolden S: Cancer Statistics, 1995, *CA* 45:8, 1995.
127. Public Health Service: *Cancers of the oral cavity and pharynx: a statistics review monograph 1973-1987* (DHHS #PHS 91-50212), Bethesda, Md, 1991, US Department of Health and Human Services.
128. Ries LAB, Edwards BK, editors: *Cancer statistic review, 1973-1987* (DHHS #NIH 90-2789), Bethesda, Md, 1990, US Department of Health and Human Services.
129. Silverman S Jr, Dillon WP: Diagnosis. In Silverman S Jr, editor: *Oral cancer,* ed 3, Atlanta, 1990, The American Cancer Society.
130. Maksem JA, Fu YS: Electron microscopy: the application of ultrastructural analysis to tumors of the head and neck region. In Barnes L, editor: *Surgical pathology of the head and neck,* New York, 1985, Marcel Dekker.
131. Rosai J: Special techniques in surgical pathology. In Rosai J, editor: *Ackerman's surgical pathology,* ed 7, St. Louis, 1989, Mosby.
132. Moll R, Franke WW, Schiller DL et al: The catalog of human cytokeratins: patterns of expression in normal epithelia, tumours and cultured cells, *Cell* 31:11, 1982.
133. Moll R, Krepler R, Franke WW: Complex cytokeratin polypeptide patterns observed in certain human carcinomas, *Differentiation* 23:256, 1983.
134. Cooper D, Schermer A, Sun TT: Biology of disease: classification of human epithelia and their neoplasms using monoclonal antibodies to keratins: strategies, applications, and limitations, *Lab Invest* 52:243, 1985.
135. Ranken R, Kaplan MJ, Gottfried TG et al: A monoclonal antibody to squamous cell carcinoma, *Laryngoscope* 97:657, 1987.
136. Morgan PR: Neoplasms and precancerous conditions of the oral mucosa. In McGee JO, Isaacson PG, Wright NA, editors: *Oxford textbook of pathology: pathology of systems,* vol 2a, Oxford, 1992, Oxford University Press.
137. Silverman S: Clinical diagnosis and early detection of oral cancer, *Oral Maxillofac Clin North Am* 5:199, 1993.
138. Shklar G, Cataldo E, Meyer I: Reliability of cytologic smear in diagnosis of oral cancer: a controlled study, *Arch Otolaryngol* 91:158, 1970.
139. Abaza NA, Miloro M: Fine-needle aspiration in oral and maxillofacial diagnosis, *Oral Maxillofac Clin North Am* 6:401, 1994.
140. Fu K, Silverman S Jr: Prognosis. In Silverman S Jr, editor: *Oral cancer,* ed 3, Atlanta, 1990, The American Cancer Society.

141. Dreyfuss AI, Clark JR: Analysis of prognostic factors in squamous cell carcinomas of the head and neck, *Hematol Oncol Clin North Am* 5:701, 1991.
142. Hermanek P, Sobin LH, editors: *TNM classification of malignant tumours,* ed 4, Berlin, 1987, Springer-Verlag.
143. McClatchey KD, Zarbo J: The jaws and oral cavity. In Sternberg SS, editor: *Diagnostic surgical pathology,* ed 2, New York, 1994, Raven Press.
144. Heppt H, Issing W: The role of flexible endosonography in diagnostic imaging of carcinomas of the oral cavity and oropharynx, *J Craniomaxillofac Surg* 20:34, 1992.
145. Westesson PL: Diagnostic imaging of oral malignancies, *Oral Maxillofac Surg Clin North Am* 5:207, 1993.
146. Stern WBR, Silva CE, Sipher BA et al: Computed tomography of the clinical and negative neck, *Head Neck* 12:109, 1990.
147. Heissler E, Steinkamp HJ, Heim T et al: Value of magnetic resonance imaging in staging carcinomas of the oral cavity and oropharynx, *Int J Oral Maxillofac Surg* 23:22, 1994.
148. Lindberg R: Distribution of cervical lymph node metastases from squamous cell carcinoma of the upper respiratory and digestive tracts, *Cancer* 29:1446, 1972.
149. Moore C, Flynn MB, Greenberg RA: Evaluation of size in prognosis of oral cancer, *Cancer* 58:158, 1986.
150. De Braud F, Heilburn LK, Ahmed K et al: Metastatic squamous cell carcinoma of an unknown primary localized to the neck: advantages of aggressive treatment, *Cancer* 64:510, 1989.
151. Merino OR, Lindberg RD, Fletcher GH: An analysis of distant metastases from squamous cell carcinoma of the upper respiratory and digestive tract, *Cancer* 40:145, 1977.
152. Papac RJ: Distant metastases from head and neck cancer, *Cancer* 53:342, 1984.
153. Galante M, Phillips TL, Silverberg IJ et al: Treatment. In Silverman S Jr, editor: *Oral cancer,* ed 3, Atlanta, 1990, The American Cancer Society.
154. De Conti RC: Perspective on chemotherapy of head and neck cancer, *Cancer Control J Moffitt Cancer Center* 1:24, 1994.
155. Endicott J, Trotti A: Organ preservation in patients with head and neck cancer, *Cancer Control J Moffit Cancer Center* 1:13, 1994.
156. Meyskens FL Jr: Coming of age—the chemoprevention of cancer, *N Engl J Med* 323, 1990.
157. Smith MA, Parkinson DR, Cheson BD et al: Retinoids in cancer therapy, *J Clin Oncol* 10:839, 1994.
158. Tepperman BS, Fitzpatrick PJ: Second respiratory and upper digestive tract cancers after oral cancer, *Lancet* 2:547, 1981.
159. Cooper JS, Pajak TJ, Rubin P et al: Second malignancies in patients who have head and neck cancer: incidence, effect on survival and implications based on the RTOG experience, *Int J Radiat Oncol Biol Phys* 17:449, 1989.
160. Banks ER, Frierson HF Jr, Mills SE et al: Basaloid squamous cell carcinoma of the head and neck: a clinicopathologic and immunohistochemical study of 40 cases, *Am J Surg Pathol* 16:939, 1992.
161. Leventon GS, Evans HL: Sarcomatoid squamous cell carcinoma of the mucous membranes of the head and neck: a clinicopathologic study of 20 cases, *Cancer* 48:994, 1981.
162. Gerughty RM, Hennigar GR, Brown RM: Adenosquamous carcinoma of the nasal, oral and laryngeal cavities: a clinicopathologic survey of ten cases, *Cancer* 22:1140, 1968.
163. Crissman JD, Kessis T, Shah KV et al: Squamous papillary neoplasia of the adult upper aerodigestive tract, *Hum Pathol* 19:1387, 1988.
164. Kraus FT, Pérez-Mesac: Verrucous carcinoma: clinical and pathologic study of 105 cases involving the oral cavity, larynx and genitalia, *Cancer* 19:26, 1966.
165. McCoy JM, Waldron CA: Verrucous carcinoma of the oral cavity: a review of forty-nine cases, *Oral Surg Oral Med Oral Pathol* 52:623, 1981.
166. Sundström B, Mörinstad H, Axéll T: Oral carcinomas associated with snuff dipping: some clinical and histological characteristics of 23 tumours in Swedish males, *J Oral Pathol* 11:245, 1982.
167. Ackerman LV: Verrucous carcinoma of the oral cavity, *Surgery* 23:670, 1948.
168. Fedder M, González MF: Nasopharyngeal carcinoma: a brief review, *Am J Med* 79:365, 1985.
169. Neel HB III: Nasopharyngeal carcinoma: clinical presentation, diagnosis, treatment, and prognosis, *Otolaryngol Clin North Am* 18:479, 1985.
170. Eneroth CM: Malignant melanoma of the oral cavity, *Int J Oral Surg* 4:191, 1975.
171. Kenichi O, Tsutomu K, Nobuyuki T et al: Malignant melanomas of the oral cavity: heterogeneity of pathological and clinical features, *Virchow's Arch [A] Pathol Anat* 420:43, 1992.
172. Silverman S Jr, Boles R, Dedo H et al: Other head and neck cancers. In Silverman S Jr, editor: *Oral cancer,* ed 3, Atlanta, 1990, The American Cancer Society.
173. Maghadam BK, Gier R: Melanin pigmentation disorders of the skin and oral mucosa, *Compend Contin Educ Dent* 12:14, 1991.
174. Rapini RP, Golitz LE, Greer Ro Jr et al: Primary malignant melanoma of the oral cavity: a review of 177 cases, *Cancer* 55:1543, 1985.
175. Pliskin ME: Malignant melanoma of the oral cavity. In Clark WH Jr, Goldman LI, Mastrangelo MJ, editors: *Human malignant melanoma,* New York, 1979, Grune & Stratton.
176. Eisen D, Voorhees JJ: Oral melanoma and other pigmented lesions of the oral cavity, *J Am Acad Dermatol* 24:577, 1991.

Cysts of the mucous membranes and soft tissues

177. Kreshover SJ: The incidence and pathogenesis of gingival cysts, *J Dent Res* 35:19, 1957.
178. Monteleone L, McLellan MS: Epstein's pearls (Bohn's nodules) of the palate, *J Oral Surg* 22:301, 1964.
179. Wysocki GP, Brannon RB, Gardner DG, Sapp P: Histogenesis of the lateral periodontal cyst and the gingival cyst of the adult, *Oral Surg Oral Med Oral Pathol* 50:327, 1980.
180. Regezi JA, Sciubba J: *Oral pathology: clinical-pathologic correlations,* ed 2, Philadelphia, 1993, Saunders.
181. Buchner A, Hansen LS: Lymphoepithelial cysts of the oral cavity: a clinicopathologic study of thirty-eight cases, *Oral Surg Oral Med Oral Pathol* 50:441, 1980.

Nonepithelial tumors and tumorlike lesions of mucous membranes and soft tissues

182. Shaffer WG, Hine MK, Levy RM: *Text book of oral pathology,* Philadelphia, 1983, Saunders.
183. Farman AG: The peripheral odontogenic fibroma, *Oral Surg Oral Med Oral Pathol* 40:82, 1975.
184. Kerr DA: Granuloma pyogenicum, *Oral Surg Oral Med Oral Pathol* 4:188, 1951.
185. McDonald RH: Granuloma gravidarum, *Am J Obstet Gynecol* 72:1132, 1956.
186. Bhasker SN, Jacoway JR: Pyogenic granuloma—clinical features, incidence, histology, and results of treatment: report of 242 cases, *J Oral Surg* 24:391, 1966.
187. Eversole LR, Rovin S: Reactive lesions of the gingiva, *J Oral Pathol* 1:30, 1972.
188. Giansanti JS, Waldron CA: Peripheral giant cell granuloma: review of 720 cases, *J Oral Surg* 27:787, 1969.
189. Anderson L, Fejerskon O, Philipsen HP: Oral giant cell granuloma: a clinical and histological study of 129 new cases, *Acta Pathol Microbiol Scand [A]* 81:606, 1973.
190. Dayan D, Buchner A, David R: Myofibroblasts in peripheral giant cell granuloma: light and electron microscopic study, *Int J Oral Maxillofac Surg* 18:258, 1989.
191. El-Mofty SK, Osdoby P: Growth behavior and lineage of isolated and cultured cells derived from giant cell granuloma of the mandible, *J Oral Pathol* 14:539, 1985.
192. Burkes EJ Jr, White JR: A peripheral giant cell granuloma manifestation of primary hyperparathyroidism: report of a case, *JAMA* 118:62, 1989.
193. Shafer WG: Verruciform xanthoma, *Oral Surg Oral Med Oral Pathol* 31:784, 1971.
194. Helm KF, Hopf RM, Kreider JW, Lookingbill DP: Verruciform xanthoma in an immunocompromised patient: a case report and immunohistochemical study, *J Cutan Pathol* 20:84, 1993.
195. Jensen JL, Liao SY, Jeffes, EW: Verruciform xanthoma of the ear with coexisting epidermal dysplasia, *Am J Dermatol* 14:426, 1992.

196. Travis WD, Davis GE, Tsokos M et al: Multifocal verruciform xanthoma of the upper aerodigestive tract in a child with a systemic lipid storage disease, *Am J Surg Pathol* 13:309, 1989.
197. Meyers DC, Woosley JT, Reddick RL: Verruciform xanthoma in association with discoid lupus erythematosis, *J Cutan Pathol* 19:36, 1992.
198. Wright BA, Jackson D: Neural tumors of the oral cavity, *Oral Surg Oral Med Oral Pathol* 49:509, 1980.
199. Sist TC, Greene GW: Traumatic neuromas of the oral cavity, *Oral Surg Oral Med Oral Pathol* 51:394, 1981.
200. Carney JA, Sigemore GW, Lovestadt SA: Mucosal ganglioneuromatosis, medullary thyroid carcinoma and pheochromocytoma: multiple endocrine neoplasia type 2b, *Oral Surg Oral Med Oral Pathol* 41:739, 1976.
201. Khari MRA, Dexter RN, Burzinski NJ, Johnston CC: Mucosal neuroma, pheochromocytoma and medullary thyroid carcinoma: multiple endocrine neoplasia syndrome type 3, *Medicine* 54:89, 1975.
202. Muzur MT, Shultz JJ, Myers JL: Granular cell tumor: immunohistochemical analysis of 21 benign tumors and one malignant tumor, *Arch Pathol Lab Med* 114:692, 1990.
203. Okada H, Yamamoto H, Kawanga T et al: Granular cell tumor of the tongue: an electron microscopical and immunohistochemical study, *J Nihon Univ School of Dentistry* 32:35, 1990.
204. Mittal KR, True LD: Origin of granules in granular cell tumor: intracellular myelin formation with autodigestion, *Arch Pathol Lab Med* 112:302, 1988.
205. Blair AE: Congenital epulis of the newborn, *Oral Surg Oral Med Oral Pathol* 43:687, 1977.
206. Tucker MC, Rusnock EJ, Azumi N et al: Gingival granular cell tumors of the newborn: an ultrastructural and immunohistochemical study, *Arch Pathol Lab Med* 114:895, 1990.
207. Laek EE, Worsham GF, Callihan MD et al: Gingival granular cell tumors of the newborn (congenital "epulis"): a clinical and pathologic study of 21 patients, *Am J Surg Pathol* 5:37, 1981.
208. Enzinger FM, Weiss SW: *Soft tissue tumors,* ed 3, St. Louis, 1995, Mosby, p 616.
209. Renshaw AA, Rosai J: Benign atypical vascular lesions of the lip, *Am J Surg Pathol* 17:557, 1993.
210. Kwon HJ, Browne GA, Posalaky LP, Warte DE: Hemangiopericytoma of the tongue: report of a case, *J Am Dent Assoc* 109:583, 1984.
211. Tajima Y, Weathers DR, Neville BW et al: Glomus tumor (glomangioma) of the tongue: a light and electron microscope study, *Oral Surg Oral Med Oral Pathol* 52:288, 1981.
212. Gorlin RJ, Pindborg JJ, Cohen MM: *Syndromes of the head and neck,* ed 3, New York, 1990, Oxford University Press.
213. McDaniel RK, Adcock JE: Bilateral symmetrical lymphangiomas of the gingiva, *Oral Surg Oral Med Oral Pathol* 63:224, 1987.
214. Hatziotis JC: Lipoma of the oral cavity, *Oral Surg Oral Med Oral Pathol* 31:511, 1971.
215. Vindenes H: Lipomas of the oral cavity, *Int J Oral Surg Oral Med Oral Pathol* 7:162, 1975.
216. Damm DD, Neville BW: Oral leiomyomas, *Oral Surg Oral Med Oral Pathol* 47:343, 1979.
217. Hagy DM, Halprin V, Wood C: Leiomyoma of the oral cavity, *Oral Surg Oral Med Oral Pathol* 17:748, 1964.
218. Corio RL, Lewis DM: Intraoral rhabdomyoma, *Oral Surg Oral Med Oral Pathol* 48:525, 1979.
219. Kroll SO, Jacoway JR, Alexander WN: Osseous choristoma of intraoral soft tissues, *Oral Surg Oral Med Oral Pathol* 32:588, 1971.
220. Eisenbud L, Sciubba J, Mir R et al: Oral presentation of non-Hodgkin's lymphoma: a review of thirty-one cases, *Oral Surg Oral Med Oral Pathol* 56:151, 1983.
221. Handlers JP, Howell RE, Abrams AM et al: Extranodal oral lymphoma; part I: a morphologic and immunoperoxidase study of 34 cases, *Oral Surg Oral Med Oral Pathol* 61:362, 1986.
222. Howell RE, Handlers JP, Abrams AM et al: Extranodal oral lymphoma; part II: relationships between clinical features and the Lukes-Collins classification of 34 cases, *Oral Surg Oral Med Oral Pathol* 64:597, 1987.
223. Abaza NA, Iczkovitz ML, Henefer EP: American Burkitts's lymphoma manifested in a solitary lymph node, *Oral Surg Oral Med Oral Pathol* 51:121, 1981.
224. Baden E, Al Saati T, Caverivier P et al: Hodgkin's lymphoma of the oropharyngeal region: report of four cases and diagnostic value of monoclonal antibodies in detecting antigens associated with Reed-Sternberg cells, *Oral Surg Oral Med Oral Pathol* 64:881, 1987.
225. Barnes L: Tumors and tumorlike lesions of the soft tissues. In Barnes L, editor: *Surgical pathology of the head and neck,* New York, 1985, Marcel Dekker.
226. Bras J, Batsakis JG, Luna MA: Malignant fibrous histiocytoma of the oral tissues, *Oral Surg Oral Med Oral Pathol* 64:57, 1987.
227. Bras J, Batsakis JG, Luna MA: Rhabdomyosarcoma of the oral soft tissues, *Oral Surg Oral Med Oral Pathol* 64:585, 1987.

Diseases of teeth and their supporting structures

228. Nikiforuk, G: *Understanding dental caries—etiology and mechanisms—basic and clinical aspects,* Basel, 1985, Karger.
229. Genco RJ, Goldman HM, Cohen DW: *Contemporary periodontics,* St. Louis, 1990, Mosby.
230. Shafer WG, Hine MH, Levy BM: *A textbook of oral pathology,* ed 4, Philadelphia, 1983, Saunders.
231. Williams DW: Dental caries. In McGee JOD, Isaacson PG, Wright NA, editors: *Oxford textbook of pathology: pathology of systems,* vol 2a, Oxford, 1992, Oxford University Press.
232. Chandrasoma P, Taylor CR: *Concise pathology,* Norwalk, 1991, Appleton & Lang.
233. Williams DW: Gingivitis and periodontal disease. In McGee JOD, Isaacson PG, Wright NA, editors: *Oxford textbook of pathology: pathology of systems,* vol 2a, Oxford, 1992, Oxford University Press.
234. Winkler JR, Murray PA, Grassi M, Hammerle C: Diagnosis and management of HIV-associated periodontal lesions, *J Am Dent Assoc* 225(suppl), 1989.

Cysts of the jaws (lined by epithelium)

235. Pindborg JJ, Kramer IRH, Torlini H: *Histological typing of odontogenic tumours, jaw cysts, and allied lesions,* Geneva, 1971, World Health Organization.
236. Kramer IRH, Pindborg JJ, Shear M: *Histological typing of odontogenic tumours,* ed 2, Berlin, 1992, Springer-Verlag.
237. Verbin RS, Barnes L: Cysts and cystlike lesions of the oral cavity, jaws and neck. In Barnes L, editor: *Surgical pathology of the head and neck,* New York, 1985, Marcel Dekker.
238. Tinkler S: The jaws. In McGee JO'D, Isaacson PG, Wright NA, editors: *Oxford textbook of pathology: pathology of systems,* vol 2a, Oxford, 1992, Oxford University Press.
239. Main DMG: Epithelial jaw cysts: 10 years of the WHO classification, *J Oral Pathol* 14:1, 1985.
240. Shaffer WG, Hine MK, Levy RM: *Text book of oral pathology,* Philadelphia, 1983, Saunders.
241. Gorlin RJ: Potentialities of oral epithelium manifest by mandibular dentigerous cysts, *Oral Surg Oral Med Oral Pathol* 10:271, 1957.
242. Shear M: Secretory epithelium in the linings of dental cysts, *J Dent Assoc S Afr* 15:117, 1960.
243. Stanley HR, Diehl DK: Ameloblastoma potential of follicular cysts, *Oral Surg Oral Med Oral Pathol* 20:260, 1965.
244. Gardner AF: The odontogenic cyst as a potential carcinoma: a clinicopathologic appraisal, *J Am Dent Assoc* 78:746, 1969.
245. Browand BC, Waldron CA: Central mucoepidermoid tumors of the jaws, *Oral Surg Oral Med Oral Pathol* 40:631, 1975.
246. Philipsen HP: Om keratocyster (kolesteatomer) i kaeberne, *Tandlaegebladet* 60:963, 1956.
247. Wright JM: The odontogenic keratocyst: orthokeratinized variant, *Oral Surg Oral Med Oral Pathol* 51:609, 1981.
248. Brannon RB: The odontogenic keratocyst: a clinicopathologic study of 312 cases, part I: clinical features, *Oral Surg Oral Med Oral Pathol* 42:54, 1976.

249. Brannon RB: The odontogenic keratocyst: a clinicopathologic study of 312 cases, part II: histologic features, *Oral Surg Oral Med Oral Pathol* 43:233, 1977.
250. Willias TP: Surgical treatment of odontogenic keratocysts, *Oral Maxillofac Clin North Am* 3:137, 1991.
251. Woolgar JA, Rippin JW, Browne RM: Comparative study of the clinical and histological features of recurrent and non-recurrent odontogenic keratocysts, *J Oral Pathol* 16:124, 1987.
252. Browne RM: The odontogenic keratocyst: histological features and their correlations with clinical behavior, *Br Dent J* 131:249, 1971.
253. Haring JI, Van Dis ML: Odontogenic keratocysts: a clinical, radiographic and histopathologic study, *Oral Surg Oral Med Oral Pathol* 66:145, 1988.
254. Browne RM: The odontogenic keratocyst, *Br Dent J* 128:225, 1970.
255. Main DMG: Epithelial jaw cysts: a clinicopathological reappraisal, *Br J Oral Surg* 8:114, 1970.
256. Scharffetter K, Balz-Herrmann C, Lagrange W et al: Proliferation kinetic study of the growth of keratocysts, *J Craniomaxillofac Surg* 1:226, 1989.
257. Toller PA: Autoradiography of explants from odontogenic cysts, *Br Dent J* 131:57, 1971.
258. Donoff RB, Harper E, Guralnick C: Collagenolytic activity in keratocysts, *J Oral Surg* 30:879, 1972.
259. Vitto VJ, Ylipäävälniemi P: Alterations in collagenolytic activity caused by jaw cyst fluids, *Proc Finn Dent Soc* 73:197, 1977.
260. Ahlfors E, Larsson A, Sjögren S: The odontogenic keratocyst: a benign cystic tumor? *J Oral Maxillofac Surg* 42:10, 1984.
261. Herbener GH, Gould AR, Neal DC, Farman AG: An electron and optical microscopic study of juxtaposed odontogenic keratocyst and carcinoma, *Oral Surg Oral Med Oral Pathol* 71:322, 1991.
262. Gorlin RJ: Nevoid basal-cell carcinoma syndrome, *Medicine* 66:98, 1987.
263. Gorlin RJ, Goltz WR: Multiple nevoid basal-cell epitheliomas, jaw cysts and bifid rib, *N Engl J Med* 262:908, 1960.
264. Rogerson KC: Gorlin's syndrome: an update on diagnosis and management, *Oral Maxillofac Surg Clin North Am* 3:155, 1991.
265. Cabrini RL, Barros RE, Albano H: Cysts of the jaws: a statistical analysis, *J Oral Surg* 28:485, 1970.

Odontogenic tumors

266. Regezi JA, Kerr DA, Courtney RM: Odontogenic tumors: analysis of 706 cases, *J Oral Surg* 36:771, 1978.
267. Kramer IRH, Pindborg JJ, Shear M: *Histological typing of odontogenic tumors,* ed 2, Geneva, 1992, Springer-Verlag.
268. Waldron CA: Odontogenic tumors and selected jaw cysts. In Gnepp DR, editor: *Pathology of the head and neck,* New York, 1988, Churchill Livingstone.
269. Regezi JA, Sciubba J: *Oral pathology: clinical-pathologic correlations,* ed 2, Philadelphia, 1993, Saunders.
270. Melisch DR, Dahklin DC, Masson JK: Ameloblastoma: a clinicopathologic report, *J Oral Surg* 30:9, 1972.
271. Waldon CA, El-Mofty SK: A histopathologic study of 116 cases of ameloblastomas with special reference to the desmoplastic variant, *Oral Surg Oral Med Oral Pathol* 63:441, 1987.
272. Buchner A, Sciubba JJ: Peripheral epithelial odontogenic tumors: a review, *Oral Surg Oral Med Oral Pathol* 63:432, 1987.
273. El-Mofty SK, Gerard NO, Farish SE, Rader B: Peripheral ameloblastoma: a clinical and histologic study of 11 cases, *J Oral Maxillofac Surg* 49:970, 1991.
274. Vickers RA, Gorlin RJ: Ameloblastoma: delineation of early histopathologic features of neoplasia, *Cancer* 26:699, 1970.
275. Yoshimura Y, Saito H: Desmoplastic variant of ameloblastoma: report of a case and review of the literature, *J Oral Maxillofac Surg* 84:1231, 1990.
276. Müller H, Slootweg PJ: The ameloblastoma: the controversial approach to therapy, *J Maxillofac Surg* 13:79, 1984.
277. Tsankis PJ, Nelson JF: The maxillary ameloblastoma: an analysis of 24 cases, *J Oral Surg* 38:336, 1980.
278. Courtney RM, Kerr DA: The odontogenic adenomatoid tumor: a comprehensive review of twenty-one cases, *Oral Surg Oral Med Oral Pathol* 39:424, 1975.
279. Toida M, Hyodo I, Okuda T et al: Adenomatoid odontogenic tumor: report of 2 cases and survey of 126 cases in Japan, *Oral Maxillofac Surg* 48:404, 1990.
280. Franklin CD, Martin MV, Clark A et al: An investigation into the origin and nature of the "amyloid" in calcifying epithelial odontogenic tumor, *J Oral Pathol* 10:417, 1981.
281. Franklin CD, Pindborg JJ: The calcifying epithelial odontogenic tumor, *Oral Surg Oral Med Oral Pathol* 42:753, 1976.
282. Krolls SO, Pindborg JJ: Calcifying epithelial odontogenic tumor: a survey of 23 cases and discussion of histomorphologic variations, *Arch Pathol* 98:139, 1974.
283. Barros RE, Domínguez Fu, Cabrini RL: Myxoma of the jaws, *Oral Surg Oral Med Oral Pathol* 27:225, 1969.
284. White DK, Chin S, Mohnoc AM: Odontogenic myxoma: a clinical and ultrastructural study, *Oral Surg Oral Med Oral Pathol* 39:901, 1975.
285. Lamberg MA, Colonius B, Menkinen JE et al: A case of malignant myxoma (myxosarcoma) of the maxilla, *Scand J Dent Res* 92:352, 1984.
286. Lers JP, Abrams AM, Melrose RJ et al: Central odontogenic fibroma: clinicopathologic features of 19 cases and review of the literature, *J Oral Maxillofac Surg* 49:46, 1991.
287. Dunlap CL, Barker BF: Central odontogenic fibroma of the WHO type, *Oral Surg Oral Med Oral Pathol* 57:390, 1984.
288. Gardner DG: The central odontogenic fibroma: an attempt at clarification, *Oral Surg Oral Med Oral Pathol* 50:425, 1980.
289. Buchner A, Ficarra G, Hansen LS: Peripheral odontogenic fibroma, *Oral Surg Oral Med Oral Pathol* 64:432, 1987.
290. Wesley RK, Wysocki GP, Miatz SM: The central odontogenic fibroma, *Oral Surg Oral Med Oral Pathol* 40:235, 1975.
291. Gardner DG: The mixed odontogenic tumors, *Oral Surg Oral Med Oral Pathol* 58:166, 1984.
292. Trodahl JN: Ameloblastic fibroma: a survey of cases from the Armed Forces Institute of Pathology, *Oral Surg Oral Med Oral Pathol* 33:547, 1972.
293. Miller AS, López CF, Pullon PA, et al: Ameloblastic fibro-odontoma, *Oral Surg Oral Med Oral Pathol* 41:354, 1975.
294. Budnick SN: Compound and complex odontomas, *Oral Surg Oral Med Oral Pathol* 42:501, 1975.
295. Kaugars GE, Miller ME, Abbey LM: Odontomas, *Oral Surg Oral Med Oral Pathol* 67:172, 1989.
296. La Briola JD, Steiner M, Bernstein M: Odontoameloblastoma, *J Oral Surg* 38:139, 1980.
297. Corio RL, Goldblatt LI, Edwards PA et al: Ameloblastic carcinoma: a clinicopathologic study and assessment of eight cases, *Oral Surg Oral Med Oral Pathol* 64:570, 1987.
298. Slootweg PJ, Müller H: Malignant ameloblastoma or ameloblastic carcinoma, *Oral Surg Oral Med Oral Pathol* 57:168, 1984.
299. Leider AS, Nelson JP, Trodahl JN: Ameloblastic fibrosarcoma, *Oral Surg Oral Med Oral Pathol* 33:559, 1972.

Fibroosseouscemental lesions of jaws

300. Waldron CA: Fibro-osseous lesions of the jaws, *J Oral Maxillofac Surg* 43:249, 1985.
301. Eversole LR, Sabes WR, Rouvin S: Fibrous dysplasia: a nosologic problem in the diagnosis of fibro-osseous lesions of the jaws, *J Oral Pathol* 1:189, 1972.
302. Kramer IRH, Pindborg JJ, Shear M: *Histologic typing of odontogenic tumors,* ed 2, Geneva, 1992, Springer-Verlag.
303. Eversole LR, Leider AS, Nelson K: Ossifying fibroma: a clinicopathologic study of sixty-four cases, *Oral Surg Oral Med Oral Pathol* 60:505, 1985.
304. Fu YS, Perzia KH: Non-epithelial tumors of the nasal cavity, paranasal sinuses and nasopharynx: a clinicopathologic study: II. Osseous and fibro-osseous lesions, *Cancer* 33:1289, 1974.
305. Damjanov I, Maenza RM, Snyder GG et al: Juvenile ossifying fibroma, *Cancer* 42:2668, 1978.
306. Makek M: *Clinical pathology of fibro-osseous-cemental lesions in the craniofacial and jaw bones,* Basel, 1983, Karger.
307. Margo CE, Ragsdale BD, Perman KI et al: Psammomatoid (juvenile) ossifying fibroma of the orbit, *Ophthalmology* 92:150, 1983.
308. Shapiro LG, Vanel D, Ackerman LV: Aggressive fibrous dysplasia of the maxillary sinus, *Skeletal Radiol* 22:563, 1993.

309. Schoenecker PJ, Swanson K, Sheridan JJ: Ossifying fibroma of the tibia, *J Bone Joint Surg* 63A:483, 1981.
310. Abrams AM, Kirby JW, Melrose RJ: Cementoblastoma: a clinicopathologic study of seven new cases, *Oral Surg Oral Med Oral Pathol* 38:394, 1974.
311. Monks FT, Bradley JC, Turner EP: Central osteoblastoma or cementoblastoma?—a case report and 12-year review, *Br J Oral Surg* 19:29, 1981.
312. Zachariades N, Skordalaki A, Papanicolaou S et al: Cementoblastoma: review of literature and report of a case in a seven-year-old girl, *Br J Oral Maxillofac Surg* 23:456, 1985.
313. Melrose RJ, Abrams AM, Mills BG: Florid osseous dysplasia, *Oral Surg Oral Med Oral Pathol* 41:62, 1976.

Giant cell lesions of jaws

314. Chuong R, Kaban LB, Kozakewich H, Pérez-Atayde A: Central giant cell lesions of the jaws: a clinicopathologic study, *J Oral Maxillofac Surg* 44:708, 1986.
315. Eisenbud L, Stern M, Rothberg M, Sachs SA: Central giant cell granuloma of the jaws: experiences in the management of 37 cases, *J Oral Maxillofac Surg* 46:376, 1988.
316. Petti GH: Hyperparathyroidism, *Otolaryngol Clin North Am* 23:339, 1990.
317. Parisien M, Silverberg SJ, Shane E, et al: Bone disease in primary hyperparathyroidism, *Endocrinol Metabol Clin North Am* 19:19, 1990.
318. Eisenbud L, Attie J, Garlick J, Platt N: Aneurysmal bone cyst of the mandible, *Oral Surg Oral Med Oral Pathol* 64:202, 1987.
319. Struthers PJ, Shear M: Aneurysmal bone cyst of the jaws: I. Clinicopathologic features, *Int J Oral Surg* 13:85, 1984.
320. Struthers PJ, Shear M: Aneurysmal bone cyst of the jaws: II. Pathogenesis, *Int J Oral Surg* 13:92, 1984.
321. Peters WJN: Cherubism: a study of twenty cases from one family, *Oral Surg Oral Med Oral Pathol* 47:307, 1979.
322. Auclair PL, Cuenin P, Kratochvil FJ et al: A clinical and histomorphologic comparison of the central giant cell granuloma and the giant cell tumor, *Oral Surg Oral Med Oral Pathol* 66:197, 1988.

Nonodontogenic neoplasms involving the jaws

323. Hoffman S, Jacoway JR, Krolls SO: *Intraosseous and parosteal tumors of the jaws,* Washington, DC, 1987, Armed Forces Institute of Pathology.
324. Schneider LC, Dolinsky HB, Gradjesk JE: Solitary peripheral osteoma of the jaws: report of case and review of the literature, *J Oral Surg* 38:452, 1980.
325. Rajayogeswaran V, Eveson JW: Endosteal (central) osteoma of the maxilla, *Br Dent J* 150:162, 1981.
326. Johnson RE, Scheithauer BW, Dahlin DC: Melanotic neuroectodermal tumor of infancy, *Cancer* 52:661, 1983.
327. Raju U, Zarbo RJ, Regezi JA et al: Melanotic neuroectodermal tumors of infancy: intermediate filament-, neuroendocrine-, and melanoma-associated antigen profiles, *Appl Immunohistochem* 1:69, 1993.
328. Kapadia SB, Frisman DM, Hitchcock CL, Popek EJ: Melanotic neuroectodermal tumor of infancy: clinicopathological, immunohistochemical, and flow cytometric study, *Am J Surg Pathol* 17:566, 1993.
329. Greer RO, Berman DN: Osteoblastoma of the jaws: current concepts and differential diagnosis, *J Oral Maxillofac Surg* 36:304, 1978.
330. Clark JL, Unni KK, Dahlin DC et al: Osteosarcoma of the jaw, *Cancer* 51:2311, 1983.
331. Foltz J, Jackson D: Osteogenic sarcoma of the mandible: a 24-year follow-up study, *J Oral Maxillofac Surg* 40:48, 1982.
332. Frierson HF, Mills SE: Osteosarcoma of the mandible, *Arch Otolaryngol* 110:416, 1984.
333. Slootweg PJ, Müller H: Osteosarcoma of the jaw bones: analysis of 18 cases, *J Maxillofac Surg* 13:158, 1985.
334. Gardner D, Mills D: The widened periodontal ligament of osteosarcoma of the jaws, *Oral Surg Oral Med Oral Pathol* 41:652, 1976.
335. Hackney FL, Aragon SP, Aufdemorte TB et al: Chondrosarcoma of the jaws: clinical findings, histopathology, and treatment, *Oral Surg Oral Med Oral Pathol* 71:139, 1991.
336. Chandhry AP, Robinovitch MR, Mitchell DF, Vickers RA: Chondrogenic tumors of the jaws, *Am J Surg* 102:403, 1961.
337. Regezi JA, Sciubba JJ: *Oral pathology, clinical-pathologic correlations,* ed 2, Philadelphia, 1993, Saunders.
338. Castigliano SG, Rominger CJ: Metastatic malignancy of the jaws, *Am J Surg* 87:496, 1954.
339. MacAffee KA II, Quinn PD, Abaza NA: Adenocarcinoma of the colon metastatic to the temporomandibular joint: a case report, *J Oral Maxillofac Surg* 51:793, 1993.
340. Stypulkowska J, Bartokowski S, Panas M et al: Metastatic tumors to the jaws and oral cavity, *J Oral Surg* 37:805, 1979.
341. Meyer I, Shklar G: Malignant tumors metastatic to the mouth and jaws, *Oral Surg Oral Med Oral Pathol* 20:350, 1965.
342. Cash CD, Royer RD, Dahlin DC: Metastatic tumors of the jaws, *Oral Surg Oral Med Oral Pathol* 14:897, 1961.

51 Salivary Glands

Douglas R. Gnepp
Samir K. El-Mofty

NORMAL SALIVARY GLAND

Development. All salivary glands arise from the ectoderm of the oral cavity. The glandular anlage first appears in the form of solid epithelial buds in the sixth embryonal week. The first to develop are the submandibular glands, and the last are the minor salivary glands, the development of which is initiated by the tenth week.

There are three stages in the development of salivary glands.[1] In the first stage, branching dichotomous ducts develop from the salivary anlagen. In the second stage the ducts acquire lumens and gland lobules form, and this continues through the seventh embryonal month. The third stage begins in the fifth embryonal month with the differentiation of acini and further maturation of the gland, together with a considerable reduction in the initially abundant connective tissue. The interstitium in which the parotid glands develop is rich in lymphoid tissue; this explains why intragranular lymph nodes are relatively abundant and why epithelial glandular tissue inclusions are frequently seen within some of the parotid lymph nodes. This feature is almost totally absent in the submandibular and sublingual glands.[1]

Early in the development of the salivary glands, the primitive duct buds are composed of an inner lining of duct cells and an outer myoepithelial cell layer. At later stages of development, as the branching duct system acquires spherical glandular acini as functional end units, the number of myoepithelial cells decreases until they eventually are located only at the distal segments of ducts and in the primitive acini.

Anatomy. All salivary glands consist of acinar and duct systems. Acini that are composed of serous or mucinous cells produce saliva. Serous cells contain periodic acid–Schiff (PAS)–positive granules, a large basal nucleus, and a rich rough endoplasmic reticulum. The mucous cells have a small, round basal nucleus surrounded by cytoplasm filled with vacuoles that contain acid and neutral sialomucins. The endoplasmic reticulum is limited to a narrow basal layer.

Fig. 51-1 is a diagram showing how the acini and ducts of salivary glands are organized. Contractile myoepithelial cells are enclosed within the basement membrane of the acinar cells and the intercalated and striated duct cells.[2] They are basket shaped, and their cytoplasm contains actin and myosin. The intercalated ducts are relatively short and are lined with cuboidal cells. Striated ducts succeed the intercalated duct system and are lined with tall columnar cells that are rich in mitochondria and exhibit numerous basal cytoplasmic invaginations that are arranged in a parallel fashion. The striated ducts are followed by the interlobular duct system. This system shows multiple layers of duct epithelium, but the number of layers varies with the caliber of the duct. The portions of the ducts closest to the striated ducts are lined with pseudostratified columnar epithelium with occasional goblet cells. The lining changes into stratified columnar epithelium

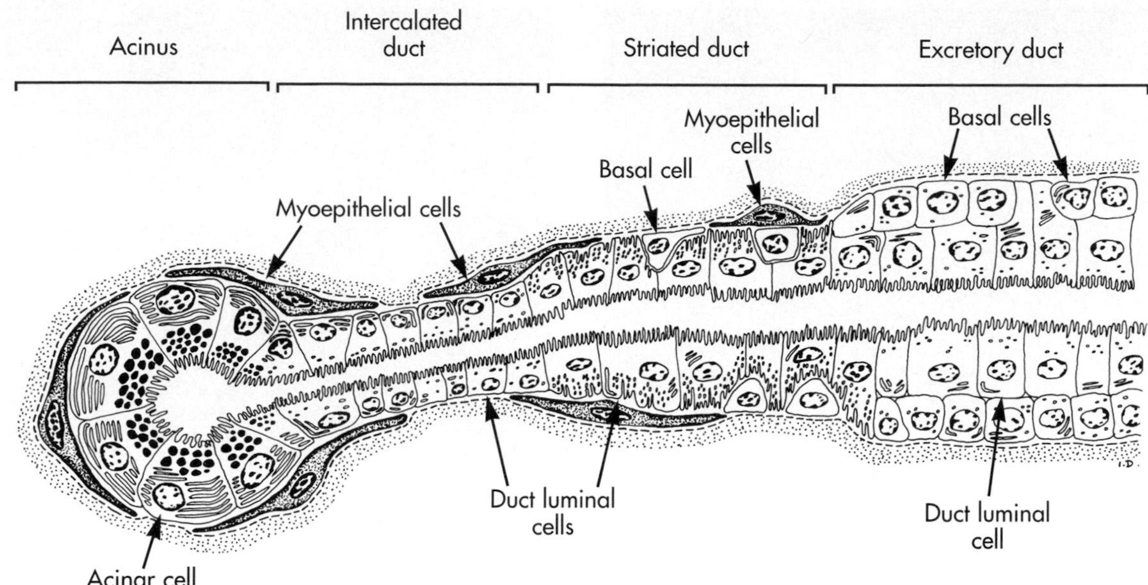

Fig. 51-1 The cellular organization of the acinus and ducts of a normal salivary gland. (From Burns BR, Dardick I, Parks WR: *Virchows Archiv [A] Pathol Anat Histopathol* 418:103, 1988.

and then to stratified squamous epithelium as the ducts approach the oral epithelium. Both the parotid and the submandibular glands are well encapsulated, but the sublingual gland is not.

DEVELOPMENTAL DISORDERS

The major salivary glands can be the site of many developmental anomalies. One or more lobules and rarely the entire gland may be congenitally absent or aplastic. A total absence of all major glands also has been reported;[1] this results in xerostomia and its complications such as rampant caries and periodontal disease. Rarely a major salivary duct may be congenitally atretic, imperforate, or duplicated. Salivary gland ectopia has been noted at different sites,[3] including lymph nodes of the head and neck, as well as in the mandible, tonsils, and neck. Inflammatory, obstructive, and neoplastic salivary diseases can develop in the ectopic tissue.[4]

Two developmental anomalies are of particular interest because they can easily be misdiagnosed as neoplastic disease. These are adenomatoid hyperplasia of the mucous glands and polycystic (dysgenetic) disease of the parotid gland.

Adenomatoid hyperplasia of mucous glands

Adenomatoid hyperplasia of the mucous glands affects the palate. It is believed to represent a hamartomatous proliferation of the minor salivary glands.[5] Clinically, adenomatoid hyperplasia is usually manifested as a painless, firm palatal mass that is covered with normal or bluish mucosa but shows no ulceration. Microscopically the mucosal connective tissue contains numerous, usually crowded and enlarged lobules of normal mucous acini and ducts. It is important to identify this anomaly to prevent overtreatment. The condition is usually harmless, though a case was reported in which a palatal mucoepidermoid carcinoma developed 12 years after adenomatoid hyperplasia of mucous glands was diagnosed.[5]

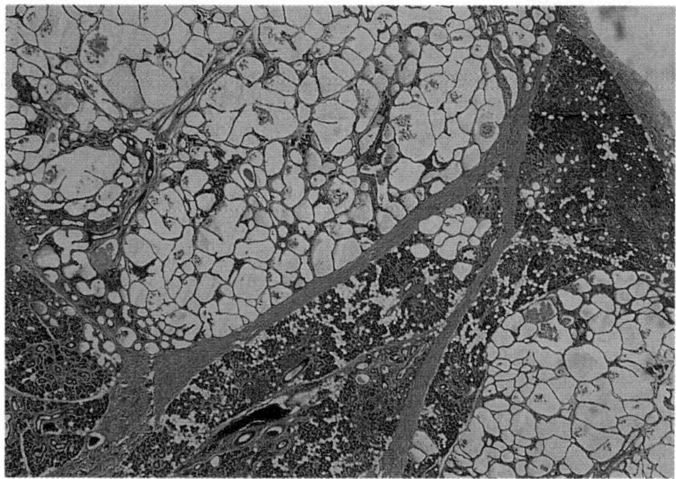

Fig. 51-2 Polycystic (dysgenetic) disease of the parotid glands. Parotid gland lobules are replaced with epithelium-lined cystic spaces. The overall architecture is preserved.

Polycystic (dysgenetic) disease of the parotid glands

Polycystic (dysgenetic) disease of the parotid glands is very rare. It may affect one but usually affects both salivary glands. It resembles polycystic disorders that involve other organs such as the kidney, pancreas, or lung. It is believed to be a developmental malformation of the duct system.[6] The condition more commonly affects female offspring. It is usually manifested during childhood but occasionally may become evident during adulthood. Typically a recurrent, painless swelling of the affected gland is the presenting symptom, but there is no abnormality of salivary flow.

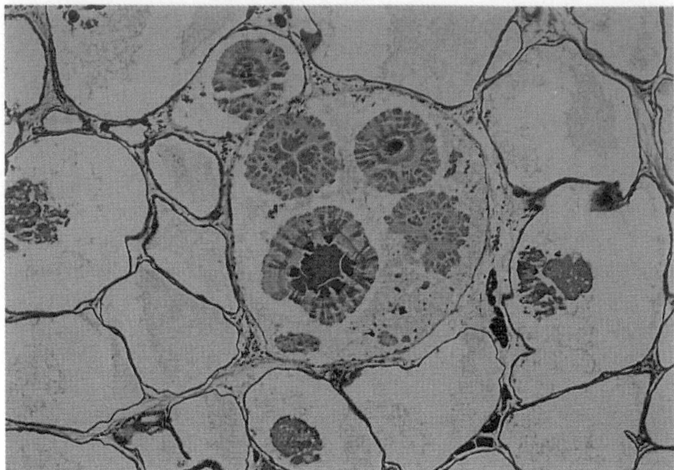

Fig. 51-3 Polycystic (dysgenetic) disease of the parotid gland. Eosinophilic bodies with concentric radial patterns within the lumens of the cysts in a polycystic parotid gland.

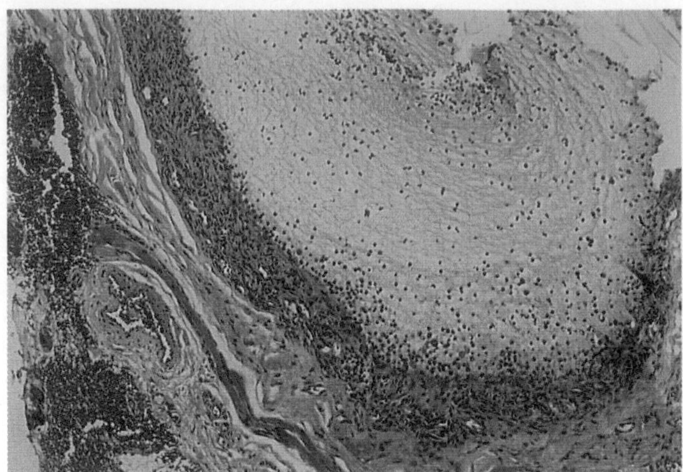

Fig. 51-4 A band of granulation tissue surrounds extravasated mucus in a mucocele of the lower lip.

Microscopically the overall architecture of the gland is preserved; the lobules appear distended and are replaced with epithelium-lined cystic spaces that may show short septal projections (Fig. 51-2). The epithelial cells of the lining vary from flat to cuboidal to columnar; occasionally columnar cells possess a round, snoutlike luminal border similar to the appearance of apocrine cells.[5] Cytoplasmic vacuolization is common, and these vacuoles may stain positively with fat stains.[7] Remnants of glandular acini may be found between the cysts. Occasional ducts communicate directly with the cystic cavities. The lumens of the cysts contain secretions and occasionally eosinophilic bodies with concentric radial patterns similar to those of the spheroliths and microliths (Fig. 51-3). There may also be a few scattered macrophages.

OBSTRUCTIVE DISORDERS

Lesions resulting from obstruction of ducts of the major and minor salivary glands are common. They can result either from severance or blockage in the duct system. Three common primary obstruction conditions are recognized: *mucocele, mucous retention cyst,* and *sialolithiasis.*

Mucocele

Mucocele is the most common of the obstructions and results from physically induced injury to minor salivary gland ducts and the subsequent extravasation and pooling of mucus in the surrounding tissues. It usually affects young persons during the first to third decades of life. The lower lip is the most frequent site, but they can arise almost anywhere in the mouth except where there are no salivary glands, such as those in the gingiva. Mucoceles are usually small, averaging about 1 cm in diameter. They are manifested clinically as raised, soft, fluctuant masses and may be bluish or translucent. Superficial lesions commonly appear vesicular, but deeper-seated mucoceles are usually covered with normal mucosa. Mucoceles may rupture, but they usually reform, which is responsible for causing the fluctuation in size typically seen.

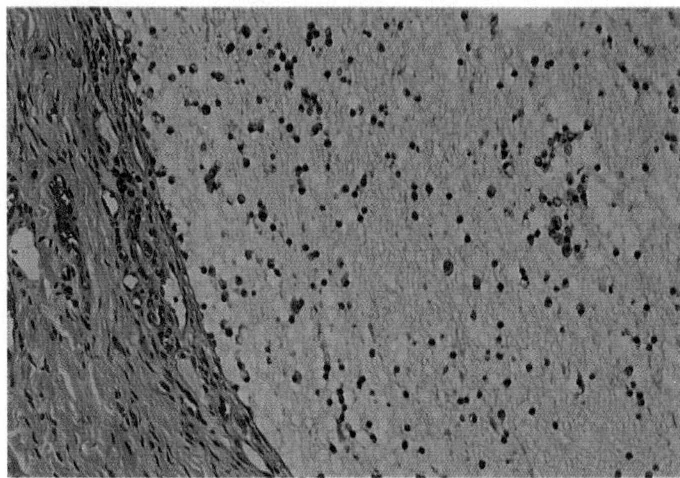

Fig. 51-5 Higher-magnification view of Fig. 51-4 showing inflammatory cells, including mucus-laden macrophages.

Large mucoceles of the floor of the mouth are called *ranulas*; when they extend through the myelohyoid muscle into the submandibular space and the soft tissue of the neck, they are termed *plunging,* or *cervical, ranulas.*[8]

Microscopically, mucoceles show extravasated, pooled mucus that appears as a circumscribed area of eosinophilic hyaline material. A band of granulation tissue is commonly seen at the periphery of the extravasated mucus (Fig. 51-4). Inflammatory cells, particularly mucus-laden macrophages with vacuolated cytoplasm, are often present in the granulation tissue and within the pooled mucus (Fig. 51-5).

Treatment is by excision of both the mucocele and the surrounding minor salivary glands. The mucocele may recur if the glands are not completely removed.

Mucus retention cyst

Mucus retention cysts are far less common than mucoceles. They develop as a result of the cystic dilatation of an obstructed salivary gland duct, more commonly in the major glands than the minor ones. The patients are usually older

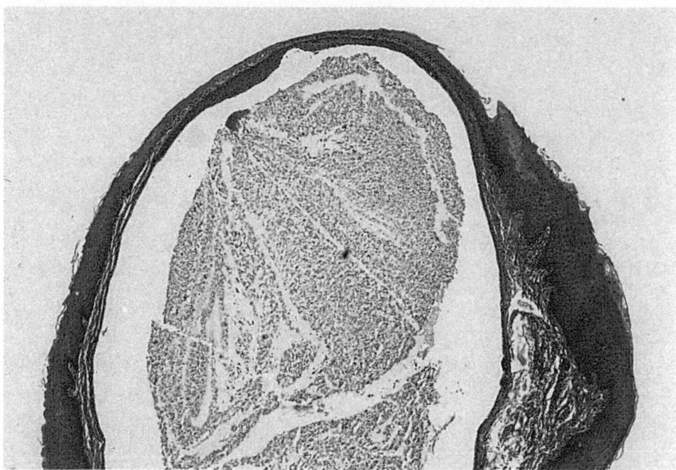

Fig. 51-6 Mucus retention cyst in a minor salivary gland of the oral cavity. The epithelial lining shows focal stratified squamous epithelium.

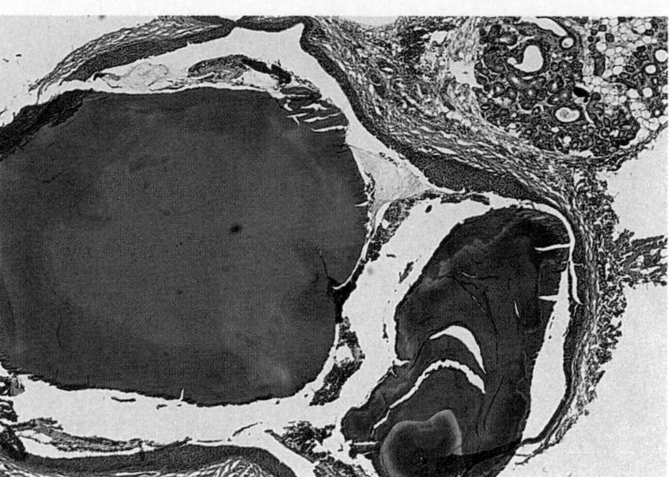

Fig. 51-7 Two salivary stones within a dilated duct. One sialolith shows concentric laminations.

than those affected by mucocele, with an average age of 50 years at the time of presentation. Microscopically these are true cysts with an epithelial lining composed of a single layer of uniform cuboidal or low columnar cells or more likely stratified squamous epithelium[9] (Fig. 51-6). Mucous cells may be scattered throughout the epithelial lining. The cyst lumen is filled with mucus. Inflammation is usually not a prominent feature, but rarely these cysts become secondarily infected.

The cause of the obstruction is not easily detectable, but it can be caused by a microlith, an inspissated secretion, or external compression or bending of the duct system.

SIALOLITHIASIS

Sialolithiasis denotes various calcified masses that form in the ducts of salivary glands. They stem from the calcification of an intraluminal organic nidus such as a dried secretion, bacterial colonies, or cellular debris. The formation of salivary stones is not related to metabolic disorders of calcium or phosphate. Their exact cause is not known, but inflammation of the salivary duct and the viscosity and stasis of saliva have been suggested as predisposing factors.[9,10]

The submandibular duct is the most common site of sialolithiasis, and in the mouth the upper lip glands are more likely to be involved than other locations. Its incidence peaks in the fourth and fifth decades.

Patients suffer episodic swelling and pain, particularly around mealtime, as the presenting symptoms, but their severity depends on the extent of obstruction. Sialolithiasis affecting minor glands is usually asymptomatic; it is manifested as a small, firm nodule that may be yellowish. Salivary stones, particularly larger ones in the submandibular duct, are easily demonstrated radiographically. The stones are predominantly composed of calcium phosphate in the form of hydroxyapatite.[11]

Grossly, sialoliths vary in size. They can be round or oval, their surface texture can be smooth or rough, and their color varies from white to yellowish. In cross section they show concentric laminations (Fig. 51-7). Microscopically the duct epithelium is usually compressed and may show squamous, oncocytic, or mucous cell metaplasia. Recurrent retrograde infection of the gland is common. This in combination with the long-term retention of secretions eventually leads to parenchymal atrophy and scarring of the affected gland.[9]

SIALADENITIS AND RELATED CONDITIONS

Inflammation of salivary glands is caused by a variety of mechanical, physical, microbial, and immunologic factors.

Mechanical obstruction of salivary ducts can be either partial or complete and may be intraluminal or extraductal. It leads to chronic and recurrent sialadenitis that can result in the partial or total destruction of the affected gland.

Radiation is an important physical cause of sialadenitis. Inadvertent exposure of the salivary glands to high doses of radiation is a common complication of the radiotherapy used in the management of head and neck cancer. Serous acini of the parotid gland are particularly radiosensitive.[12] An initial acute inflammatory response is later followed by a chronic sclerosing sialadenitis and resultant xerostomia.[12,13]

Infectious sialadenitis

Acute suppurative sialadenitis

Acute suppurative sialadenitis is usually caused by *Staphylococcus aureus* and group A streptococci that ascend through the salivary ducts from the oral cavity. Reduced or absent salivation is an important factor in its genesis, and the infection typically accompanies dehydration states. In recent years it has become a less frequent postoperative complication of major abdominal surgery. Clinically the presenting symptom of acute suppurative parotitis is a tender, diffuse, or localized swelling that may be fluctuant. Fistula-draining purulent material may form.[12] Microscopically there is edema, hyperemia, and acute inflammation. A periductal and intraductal accumulation of neutrophils is associated with destruction of the ductal epithelium. Acini are lost and parenchymal microabscesses form as the inflammatory process progresses.

Tuberculosis

Tuberculous lymphadenitis of the parotid gland is the most common form of tuberculosis (TB) to affect the salivary glands. Parenchymal TB is rare. The intraparotid and paraparotid lymph nodes become infected either as the result of lymphatic drainage of the glandular duct system, with the infection originating from a tuberculous focus in the mouth and pharynx, or as a result of the dissemination of pulmonary TB.[14]

Unlike pulmonary TB, tuberculous lymphadenitis may go unrecognized for a longer time because no constitutional symptoms are manifested. The disease usually is manifested clinically as a painless, discrete, solid nodule that is commonly mistaken for a tumor.[12] There may be multiple masses. The overlying skin is usually smooth and not erythematous, though scrofula occurs occasionally; the symptoms may exist for weeks to years. Submandibular and sublingual salivary glands are much less frequently involved. Multiple necrotizing granulomas, often confluent, are typical microscopic features. The caseating center is surrounded by epithelioid macrophages, foreign-body and Langhans' giant cells, and lymphocytes. Acid-fast bacilli are difficult to demonstrate in the sections, and bacterial cultures are usually required to demonstrate the pathogen.

Viral sialadenitis

Several viruses are known to be etiologic agents of sialadenitis; these include coxsackieviruses A and B, echovirus, Epstein-Barr virus, influenza A virus types I and III, parainfluenza virus, cytomegalovirus (CMV), and mumps virus.[12] Of these, paramyxovirus (the mumps virus) is the best known of the sialadenotropic viruses.

Mumps. Mumps is a self-limiting disease that predominantly affects children. It is caused by droplet infection of the upper respiratory tract. Viremia develops during an incubation period lasting 16 to 18 days, after which one or both of the parotid glands become painful and swollen. Stimulation of salivation intensifies the pain. Diagnosis is usually made on clinical grounds and is supported by the serologic findings. The glands are very rarely examined microscopically. When reported,[12,15] dense interstitial lymphoplasmacytic infiltrates, acinar cell vacuolization, and ductal dilatation are the microscopic features. The changes are reversible, and treatment is predominantly symptomatic. Orchitis, meningoencephalitis, pancreatitis, and arthritis are extremely rare complications that usually affect adults and can lead to serious consequences such as sterility and deafness.

Cytomegalovirus. Cytomegalovirus (CMV) is a DNA virus of the herpes group. Most of the adult population in the United States is seropositive for the virus. Like other herpesviruses, it can cause primary, latent, or persistent generalized infection. Numerous infections occur congenitally and perinatally, and it is the most common congenital infection. However, only 10% of congenitally infected infants suffer acute cytomegalic inclusion disease. The virus in these congenitally infected infants can be isolated from most body fluids.[16] Most immunocompetent adults and children with antibodies to CMV remain asymptomatic, or they may rarely experience an infectious mononucleosis-like disease.

In the settings of the acquired immunodeficiency disease (AIDS) and other immunocompromising states, CMV infection is often symptomatic, presenting in the form of retinitis, colitis, pneumonitis, encephalitis, or kidney and liver disease.[17] However, pronounced CMV salivary gland disease is rare, even though many patients with AIDS excrete CMV in their saliva.[18-20] The chronic parotid swelling observed in some infants with AIDS is believed to be acute CMV parotitis. Microscopically, CMV-infected cells are large and have large basophilic nuclear inclusions as well as smaller cytoplasmic inclusions. A chronic inflammatory cell infiltrate is usually detected.

Sjögren's syndrome and myoepithelial sialadenitis

Sjögren's syndrome is an autoimmune disease characterized by the progressive lymphocytic infiltration and destruction of exocrine glands, particularly the salivary and lacrimal glands. The clinical hallmarks of Sjögren's syndrome are keratoconjunctivitis sicca, xerostomia, and rheumatoid arthritis or some other connective tissue disease, such as systemic lupus erythematosus, dermatomyositis, systemic sclerosis, or mixed connective tissue disease.[21] When xerostomia and xerophthalmia occur in the absence of connective tissue disease, this is termed *primary Sjögren's syndrome*[22]; it is called the *sicca syndrome* in the older literature.[21] The other form of the disease, this one associated with connective tissue disease, is called *secondary Sjögren's syndrome.* The lymphocytic infiltrate that appears in the salivary glands commonly occurs in association with changes in the salivary ducts, producing a characteristic histologic appearance known as *myoepithelial sialadenitis*, or *benign lymphepithelial lesion.* Myoepithelial sialadenitis may occur unrelated to Sjögren's syndrome,[23,24] but the pathogenetic mechanism responsible for the development of these lesions is not known.

Clinical features. As much as 90% of the patients with Sjögren's syndrome are female. The average age at diagnosis is 50 years, and it is very rare for the disease to affect persons under 20 years of age. However, it may rarely occur in children.[25] The principal clinical symptoms are dryness of the eye and mouth, resulting in keratoconjunctivitis[26] and in difficulty speaking and swallowing food. Occasionally patients experience a burning sensation in the oral mucosa as well as recurrent and rapidly progressive dental caries and periodontal disease.[27]

Firm, diffuse enlargement of the salivary glands, which is usually but not always bilateral, is present in many patients. Induration of the glands without enlargement may be evident early in the disease.[23] These changes are usually painless, or there can be slight tenderness.

A typical sialographic feature of the affected parotid is the formation of punctate cavitary defects filled with radiopaque contrast media that look like a "fruit-laden, branchless tree." This characteristic appearance is believed to result from the leakage of contrast material through the weakened salivary gland ducts.[28]

Pathology. Biopsies are commonly performed on parotid tail or labial salivary glands are commonly biopsied as part of the diagnostic workup in patients with suspected Sjögren's syndrome. The histopathologic changes are similar in both sites.[29,30] The microscopic hallmark is a lymphocytic sialadenitis. In the early stages of the disease focal aggregates of lymphocytic infiltrates are seen in the parenchyma of the gland lobules (Fig. 51-8) and there is acinar involution at the site of the infiltrate. A focus score of greater than one focus per 4 mm^2 is considered a diagnostic sign of the disease,[31] with a focus consisting of 50 lymphocytes or more. As the inflammation pro-

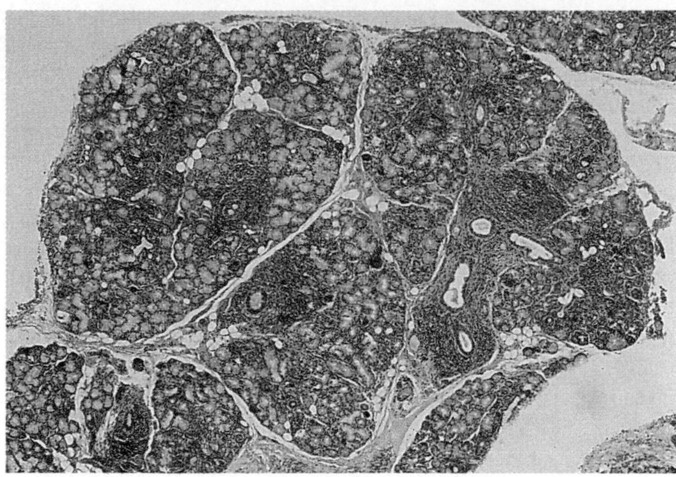

Fig. 51-8 Focal lymphocytic aggregates in the parenchyma of the lobules of lip salivary glands in a patient with Sjögren's syndrome.

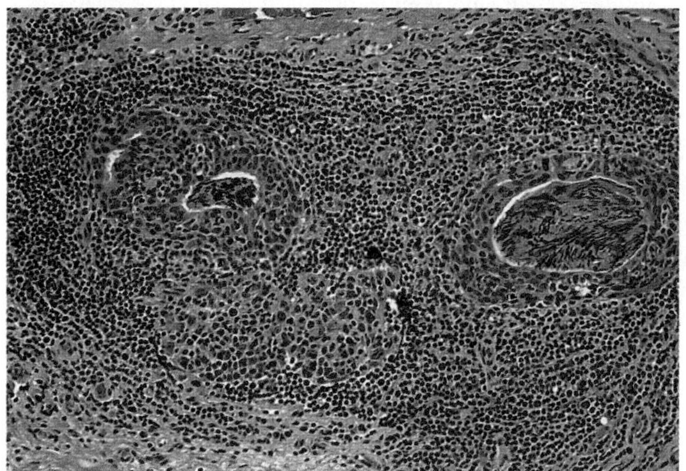

Fig. 51-9 Myoepithelial sialadinitis in a biopsy specimen of the parotid gland from a patient with Sjögren's syndrome.

gresses, partial and then total parenchymal loss become evident and the lymphocytic infiltrate dominates. Lymphoid follicles with germinal centers may be present, but plasma cells are not conspicuous. In later stages epithelial and myoepithelial duct cells proliferate and show the metaplastic changes responsible for producing the epimyoepithelial islands characteristic of myoepithelial sialadenitis[32] (Fig. 51-9).

The risk for non-Hodgkins lymphoma is 43.8 times greater in patients with Sjögren's syndrome than in age-matched controls.[33] The lymphoma is commonly nodal. It may arise in sites other than the head and neck, but the salivary glands, especially the parotid gland, may be the primary sites. A progressive unilateral swelling in an enlarged parotid gland in a patient with Sjögren's syndrome, particularly in an older woman, is suggestive of such an outcome. In these cases the lymphocytic infiltrate is monotypical and usually monoclonal and extends beyond the glandular lobules and capsule, with effacement of the glandular architecture.[34] The developing malignant lesion is usually a low-grade, monocytoid B-cell lymphoma.[35] In its early stage a primary B-cell lymphoma may be difficult to diagnose on the basis of light microscopy

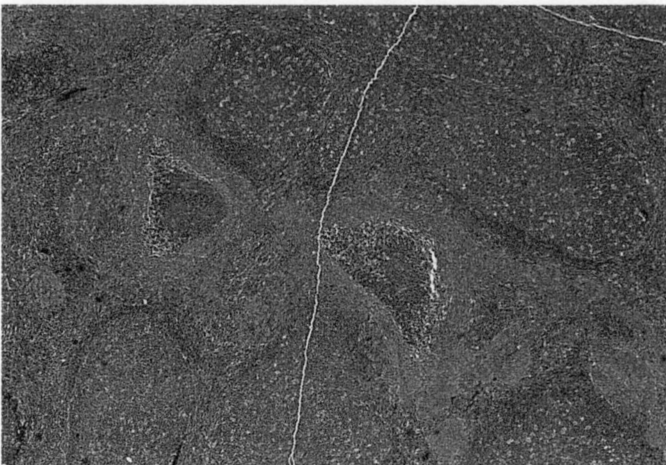

Fig. 51-10 Keratin-filled lymphoepithelial cysts and epimyoepithelial islands in the parotid gland of an HIV-positive patient. Also seen is the follicular hyperplasia of the lymphoid tissue.

findings alone, and immunohistochemical or molecular biology techniques, or both, may be needed to demonstrate the monoclonality typical of lymphoma.

HIV infection–associated lymphoepithelial cysts of the parotid

The lymphoepithelial cysts of the parotid that form in the setting of the human immunodeficiency virus (HIV) infection are keratin-filled cysts that are derived from metaplastic ductal epithelium of the parotid gland. The condition usually occurs as a component of persistent generalized lymphadenopathy[36,37] and presents as a unilateral or bilateral enlargement of the parotid. It persists for several months or longer. The pathologic changes are limited to the intraglandular lymphoid tissue and the paraparotid lymph nodes. Microscopic examination reveals the existence of a florid follicular hyperplasia. The follicles are irregularly shaped, enlarged, and increased in number. Follicular lysis and sinus histiocytosis are common. Both squamous epithelium–lined cysts containing keratin and epimyoepithelial islands are seen throughout the lesion[36-38] (Fig. 51-10).

The lymphoepithelial cysts forming in the absence of HIV infection are seen in the parotid gland and have been termed *branchial cleft cysts*.[39,40] They are usually small, averaging 2.5 cm in diameter. The pathogenetic events responsible for the formation of these cysts is not known. They are believed to arise either from salivary epithelium entrapped within lymphoid tissue or from the branchial apparatus.[40]

NECROTIZING SIALOMETAPLASIA

Necrotizing sialometaplasia (NSM) is a benign lesion of unknown cause that affects the minor salivary glands. It may be clinically and histologically misdiagnosed as a malignant neoplasm, particularly a mucoepidermoid carcinoma or squamous cell carcinoma. The lesion shows a combination of acinar necrosis and ductal squamous metaplasia that is believed to stem from local ischemia. Before its identification in 1973,[41] some patients with NSM were overtreated with aggressive surgery.

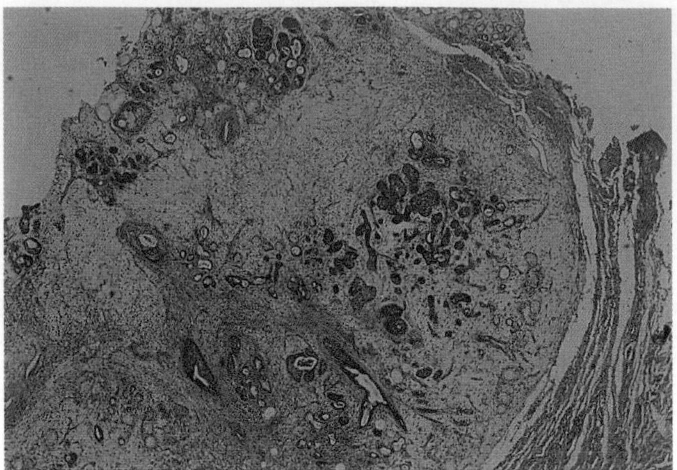

Fig. 51-11 Necrotizing sialometaplasia. Islands of stratified squamous epithelium are surrounded by necrotic mucous acini. The lobular architecture is maintained.

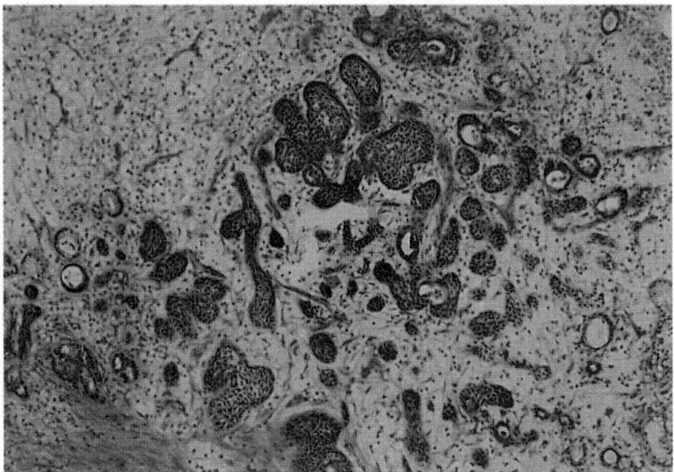

Fig. 51-12 Higher-magnification view of Fig. 51-11 showing residual ductal luminal spaces in some of the metaplastic squamous islands.

Clinical features. NSM most commonly affects the minor salivary glands of the palate but has also been found in other sites in the mouth, in extraoral locations in the upper aerodigestive tract,[42,43] and in the major salivary glands.[44] In the palate it is usually manifested as a deep, craterlike ulcer, but it occasionally starts as a submucosal nonulcerating nodule.[41] The ulcer is usually small, measuring 1 to 3 cm in its maximum diameter. Bilateral lesions also occur. Most cases are asymptomatic, though a few patients complain of numbness or a burning sensation. The symptoms typically last only for a few days or a few weeks; NSM remits spontaneously. The average age of patients at the time of its occurrence is 45.5 years. The male-to-female ratio is 1.8:1.[45] Ischemia is the most accepted cause of NSM; this is supported by the inability to isolate or culture specific microorganisms from the lesions, by their development in association with surgical procedures, and by experimental evidence.[46-48]

Pathology. The salivary gland lobules show either complete or partial necrosis of their mucous acini that is intermixed with squamous metaplasia of the ducts, thereby producing scattered squamous epithelial islands. Pools of mucin occasionally form within the necrotic lobules. The interlobular septa commonly show degenerative changes, acute inflammatory cell infiltrates, and foam cell macrophages (Fig. 51-11). Granulation tissue is usually present near the surface,[46] at the base of the ulcer. The metaplastic squamous cells may show reactive atypia, but they are patterned after the lobular architecture of the salivary gland lobule and occasionally contain luminal spaces (Fig. 51-12). Mucous cells might be present within the squamous epithelial islands, and this finding may cause the lesion to be mistaken for mucoepidermoid carcinoma. Necrosis of mucous acini and preservation of the lobular architecture are the most important features of NSM that distinguish it from squamous and mucoepidermoid carcinomas.

BENIGN NEOPLASMS

Pleomorphic adenoma

Pleomorphic adenoma, or benign mixed tumor, is the most common benign salivary gland tumor. It is characterized by a widely diverse morphologic appearance, consisting of epithelial and mesenchymal components that vary considerably in their relative amount and in their histologic growth pattern. Benign mixed tumors account for 60% to 70% of tumors of the parotid gland, 40% to 60% of those of the submandibular gland, and 40% to 70% of those of all minor salivary glands.[49-51]

Clinical features. Pleomorphic adenoma can occur at any age; however, it peaks in incidence in patients between 30 and 50 years of age (mean age, 41.2 years).[52] Women are more commonly affected, and the female-to-male ratio ranges from 3:1 to 4:1.[52] Tumors are manifested as slowly growing, painless, firm masses that can become very large if not treated. In the parotid gland most tumors arise in the superficial lobe near the angle of the mandible. Ten percent of parotid mixed tumors occur in the deep lobe and present as a parapharyngeal mass. Intraorally the palate is more commonly involved than other sites, and these tumors usually present as a firm submucosal mass that rarely ulcerates. When ulcers occur, trauma to the surface mucosa is usually the cause and not the tumor itself.

Pathology. Grossly the tumor appears as a sharply demarcated nodular mass. Mixed tumors in major glands are usually encapsulated or very well defined, though rarely a true capsule is not present. Tumors in the minor glands are usually well circumscribed, and there is not always a true capsule. Morphologic diversity is evident among different tumors and within the same lesion. The epithelial component in pleomorphic adenoma might form into ducts, cell nests, solid sheets, or interlacing cords. The mesenchymal stroma might be myxoid, chondroid, or fibrous. Ossification takes place in some tumors (Figs. 51-13 and 51-14). Squamous metaplasia, mucus-containing goblet cells, oncocytic cells, plasmacytoid myoepithelial cells, and sebaceous cells may be present, and occasionally adenoid cyst–like areas and clear cell foci are noted. Crystalloid structures, which are most commonly composed of tyrosine or collagen, are seen in some cases.[53,54] Mixed tumors have been classified into five categories on the basis of the ratio of the number of cells to the volume of the stroma, ranging from poorly cellular to extremely cellular.[55] The hypocellular tumors are more common in the parotid gland than are

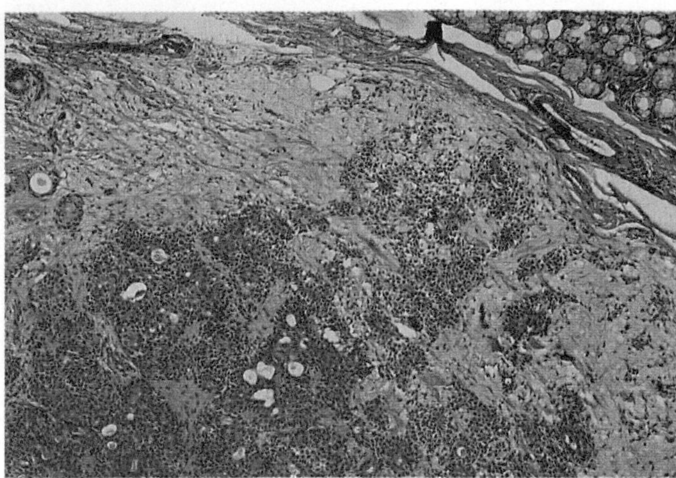

Fig. 51-13 Pleomorphic adenoma. The epithelial components are dispersed in myxoid stroma. The margin of the tumor is well defined; a fibrous capsule separates the tumor from the normal glandular parenchyma.

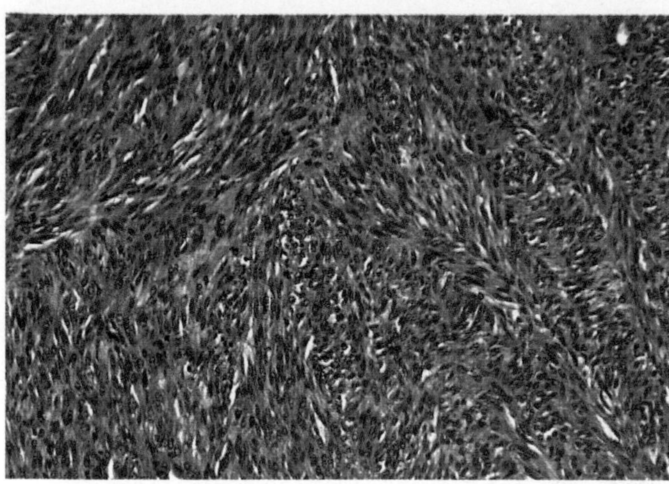

Fig. 51-15 Myoepithelioma composed of short fascicles of spindle-shaped myoepithelial cells.

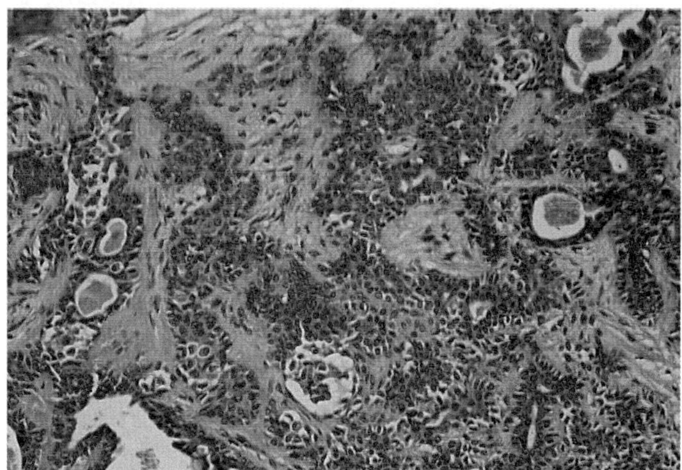

Fig. 51-14 Pleomorphic adenoma showing epithelial structures in a fibrous stroma.

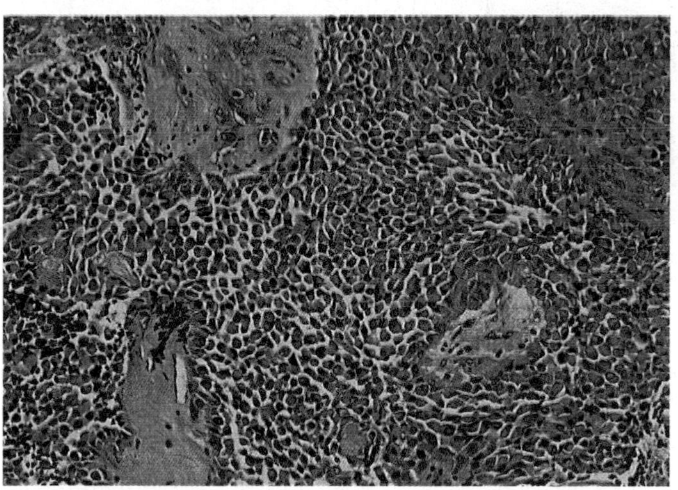

Fig. 51-16 Myoepithelioma. Plasmacytoid cells with eccentric nuclei and hyaline eosinophilic cytoplasm form solid sheets.

the more cellular ones, and in general minor salivary gland tumors tend to be more cellular than those of the major salivary glands.

Immunohistochemically the tumor cells show signs of epithelial or myoepithelial cell differentiation, or they may show a mixture of both. Myoepithelial cells stain with antibodies to cytokeratin, muscle-specific actin, smooth muscle actin, and vimentin. S-100 protein and glial fibrillary acidic protein are also found. The cells that form ducts and solid nests are immunoreactive with antibodies to cytokeratin, epithelial membrane antigen, and carcinoembryonic antigen.[52]

Therapy and prognosis. Pleomorphic adenoma is treated by surgical excision, and recurrence is negligible if the tumor is adequately removed.[56] When the tumor is in the parotid glands, superficial parotidectomy with nerve preservation is the method of choice in most cases. Intraoral tumors are excised with adequate surgical margins. The high recurrence rates that were reported in the past were most likely the consequence of undertreatment with enucleation.[57] Inadequate excision is often associated with multifocal, local recurrence.[58]

Myoepithelioma

Myoepithelioma of the salivary glands is composed entirely or predominantly of myoepithelial cells.[60-61] It represents one extreme in the histologic continuum of pleomorphic adenoma.[59,62]

Clinical features. Myoepitheliomas occur with equal frequency in the major and minor salivary glands. The age and sex distribution and clinical presentation of myoepithelioma are similar to those of mixed tumors.

Pathology. Myoepithelioma is a well-circumscribed or encapsulated tumor composed of several cells that can be classified as spindle shaped, plasmacytoid, polygonal epithelioid, and rarely clear[62,63] (Figs. 51-15 or 51-16). There may be combinations of these patterns within the same tumor. The spindle cell pattern, in which usually the cells are arranged in diffuse sheets or short fascicles, is the most common.[62,63] The plasmacytoid cells have eccentric nuclei and an eosinophilic, often hyaline cytoplasm. The polygonal cells can be arranged in clusters or sheets and exhibit some variations in size and form. Some epithelioid cells may have clear cytoplasm. The stroma in most myoepitheliomas is fibrous and scanty; there may be areas of myxoid change in some tumors. Positive staining for cytokeratin and muscle-specific actin, smooth muscle actin, or S-100 protein confirms the myoepithelial nature of the tumor.[52,62,64]

Therapy. The treatment of myoepithelioma is similar to that used for pleomorphic adenoma and is by total excision. Most myoepitheliomas behave in a benign fashion, with a minimal tendency to recur. A few cases of malignant myoepithelioma in the parotid as well as in the minor salivary glands have been reported; these are characterized histologically by cellular atypia and an infiltrative growth pattern and are capable of metastasizing.[62-65]

Papillary cystadenoma lymphomatosum (Warthin's tumor)

Papillary cystadenoma lymphomatosum is a slow-growing, benign tumor that arises almost exclusively in the parotid gland, commonly in its lower portion over the angle of the mandible. It constitutes about 5% to 6% of all parotid tumors.[66,67] Its peak incidence is in persons ranging from 40 to 70 years of age, and it is five times more common in men than in women. Tumors arise bilaterally in 7% of the patients.[67]

Pathology. Most tumors measure 2 to 3 cm at the time of diagnosis. The histologic appearance of papillary cystadenoma lymphomatosum is distinctive and pathognomonic. The tumor is composed of a lymphoid matrix containing epithelium-lined cystic spaces showing numerous papillary projections (Fig. 51-17). The epithelial lining of the cystic spaces and of the papillae is composed of two rows of oncocytic cells. The inner layer is made up of tall columnar cells, and the cells in the outer row are cuboidal and polygonal. The cytoplasm in both cells is granular and intensely eosinophilic. Rarely mucin-secreting cells and foci with squamous differentiation may be seen. The lumens of the cystic spaces are often filled with homogeneous eosinophilic, granular material. The lymphoid stroma is reactive. Cells are often arranged in follicles and may contain germinal centers.

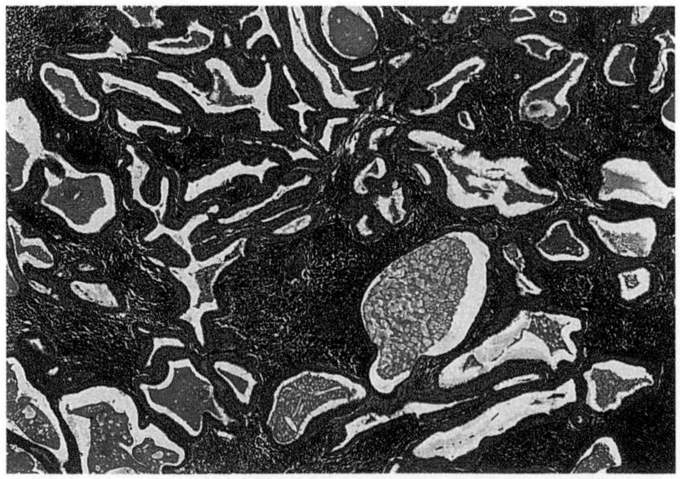

Fig. 51-17 Papillary cystadenoma lymphomatosum. Cystic spaces and papillary projections are lined with two rows of oncocytic cells in a lymphoid stroma.

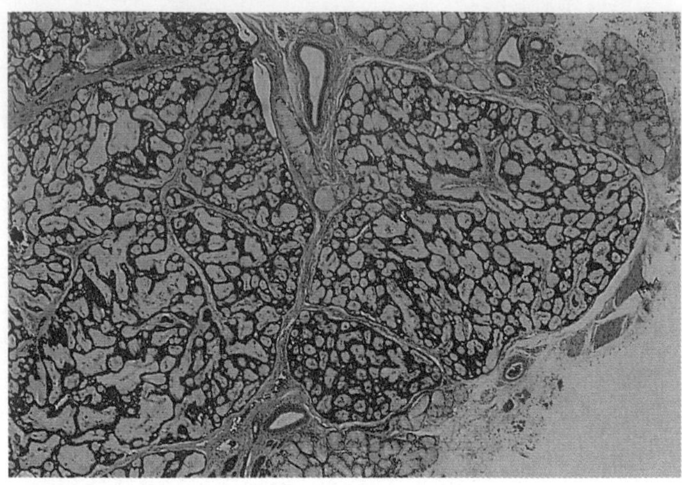

Fig. 51-18 Canalicular adenoma. Cuboidal cells are arranged in cords of single cells that form parallel columns.

Several theories on the pathogenesis of Warthin's tumor have been advanced. The most accepted one is that the tumor develops from parotid ductal epithelium present in lymph nodes in the immediate vicinity of or within the parotid gland.[67,68]

Therapy. Superficial parotidectomy with preservation of the facial nerve is the established method of treatment, particularly because some tumors tend to be multicentric.[67,69] Indeed, recurrence after a conservative excision is more likely to be a consequence of incomplete removal of multicentric lesions rather than a true recurrence.

Canalicular adenoma and basal cell adenoma

Because of similarities between canalicular adenoma and basal cell adenoma of the salivary glands, they have both been classified as *monomorphic adenoma.* There are, however, enough clinicopathologic differences between the two to warrant their identification as separate and distinct entities.

Canalicular adenoma

Canalicular adenoma arises exclusively from the minor salivary glands of the oral cavity. It commonly affects older patients, with a peak incidence in the eighth decade. The average age of patients ranges from 60 to 67 years.[70,71] Women are more commonly affected than men, and the female-to-male ratio revealed by different studies ranges from 1.2 to 1.8 : 1.[70-72] Clinically, canalicular adenoma presents as a slow-growing asymptomatic nodule, most commonly in the upper lip. In different series it has been found in this location in 73% to 100% of the cases.[51,71,72] These tumors arise in the buccal mucosa in a minority of cases.

Pathology. The mass is usually small at the time of diagnosis, with a mean diameter of 1.7 cm.[71] The covering mucosa is usually intact and normal in appearance; occasionally it might be slightly bluish. The microscopic appearance of canalicular adenoma is characteristic (Fig. 51-18). The cells are uniformly cuboidal or columnar; they usually have scanty eosinophilic cytoplasm and indistinct borders; and the nuclear chromatin is diffuse and granular. The cells are arranged in cords of single cells that form parallel columns producing long "canals." Typically the rows are separated periodically, producing ductal structures. The stroma of canalicular adenoma is delicate, richly vascular, and sparsely cellular (Fig. 51-19). The lesions are well circumscribed and are often surrounded by a thin fibrous capsule.[72] It is not uncommon for canalicular adenoma to be multifocal; in these cases the main tumor commonly is encapsulated but the smaller foci often are not.[71] It is rare for the tumor to recur after surgical removal, and if it does, this probably is the result of multifocality.

Basal cell adenoma

More than 80% of basal cell adenomas arise in the major salivary glands, most often the parotid. Basal cell adenoma of the parotid gland is commonly misdiagnosed on the basis of clinical findings as mixed tumor.

Pathology. Basal cell adenomas tend to occur in the superficial lobe and are freely movable. Unlike pleomorphic adenoma, they usually do not exceed 3 cm in diameter.[71,74] Microscopically, basal cell adenoma is composed of basaloid cells that form solid sheets, nests, cords, and ducts that are dispersed in a scanty fibrous stroma (Fig. 51-20). The tumors are composed of two types of cells. The first type are small cells that are cuboidal or columnar and contain round, deeply staining nuclei. These cells are usually congregated at the periphery of the cell masses and commonly show nuclear palisading. The second type of cells are larger and have a paler-staining oval nucleus; these cells predominate and form most of the central portions of the tumor nests, sheets, and trabeculae (Fig. 51-21).

There are several subtypes of basal cell adenoma classified according to the cellular growth pattern: solid, trabecular, and tubular.[73] A fourth type is membranous basal cell adenoma, also known as "dermal analog tumor" because of its histologic similarity to cutaneous cylindroma.[71,74]

The most common type of basal cell adenoma is the solid variant.[71,75] The cells in these tumors form solid sheets and islands. Eddies of squamous cells are occasionally formed by the larger, paler-staining central cells. The trabecular type resembles the solid type, except that the cells form trabeculas and cords, but ductal structures are the main feature in the tubular type. Basal cell adenomas have well-defined borders and are often encapsulated. However, only 50% of the membranous basal cell adenoma is encapsulated. They tend to be multilobular and multicentric.

The membranous basal cell adenoma characteristically is composed of solid nests of cells that are surrounded by a thick eosinophilic hyaline material (membrane) (Fig. 51-22). Similar material is often present within the islands in the form of interepithelial droplets. In contrast to other basal cell adenomas, the membranous variant is associated with a higher recurrence rate after surgical removal. Recurrence rates of 25% to 37%, similar to those associated with dermal cylindroma, have been reported.[74,76] Occasional membranous basal cell adenomas are a component of skin and salivary gland diathesis; in addition to the salivary gland adenoma, the patients also suffer multiple dermal cylindromas (turban tumor), trichoepithelioma, and eccrine spiradenoma.[76-78]

Malignant transformation of basal cell adenoma is exceedingly rare and may produce a hybrid basal cell adenoma–

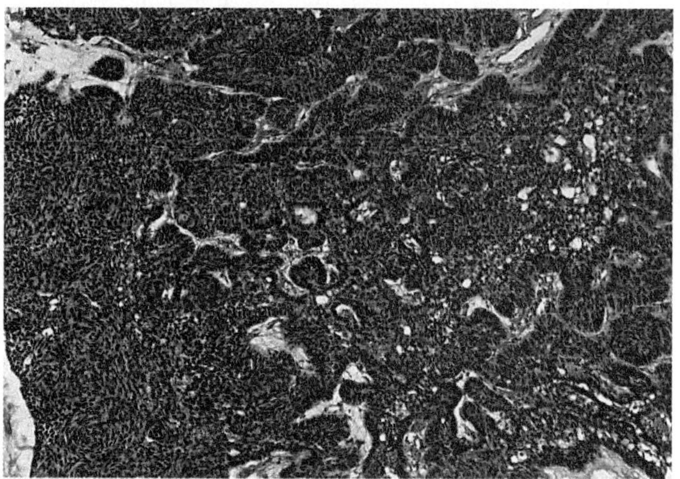

Fig. 51-20 Basal cell adenoma, with basaloid cells forming solid sheets.

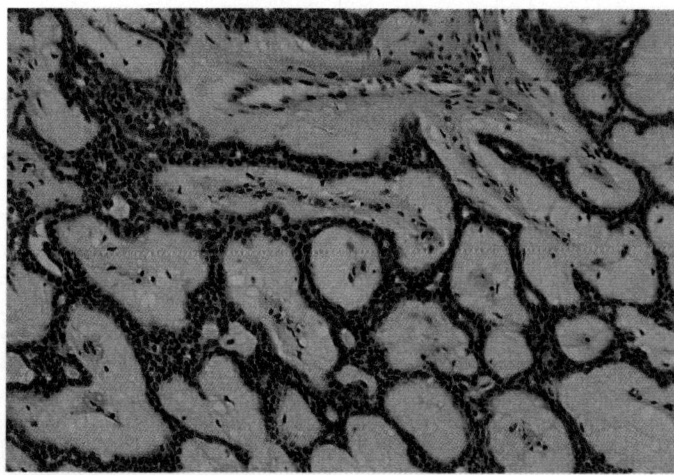

Fig. 51-19 Higher-magnification view of Fig. 51-18 showing canalicular structures in a delicate, richly vascular hypocellular stroma.

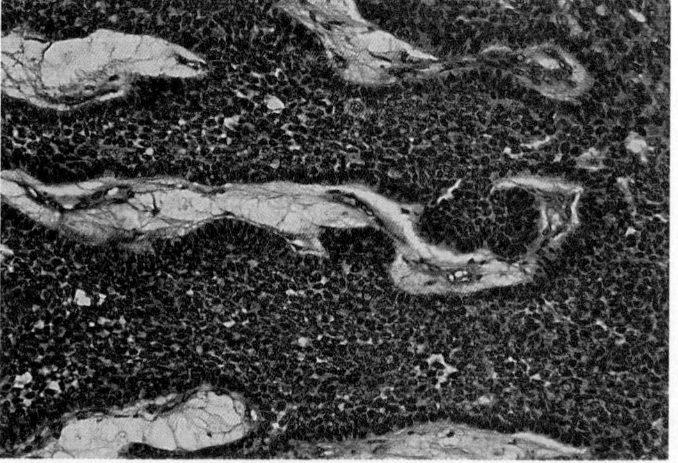

Fig. 51-21 Trabeculae of basal cell adenoma with palisaded columnar and cuboidal cells in the periphery and larger cells in the center.

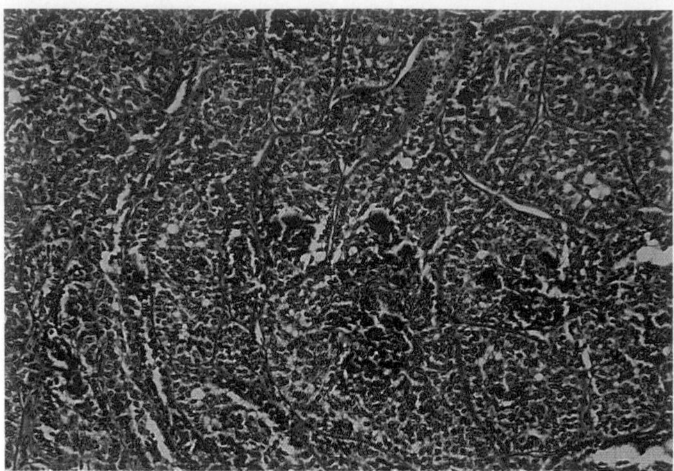

Fig. 51-22 Membranous basal cell adenoma. Basaloid cell nests surrounded with eosinophilic hyaline material form a membrane. Similar material exists in interepithelial droplets within the cell nests.

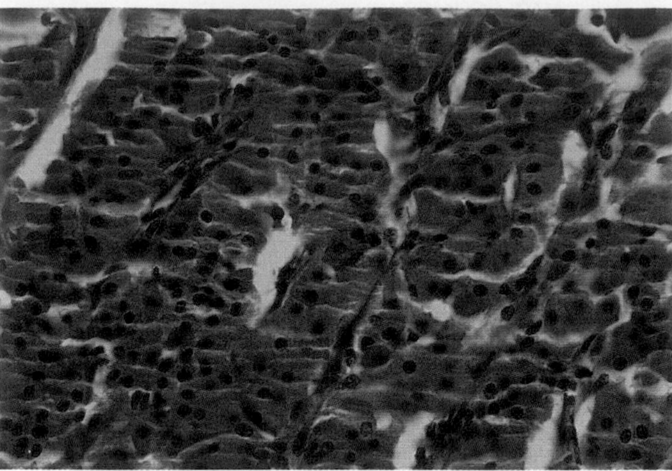

Fig. 51-23 Oncocytoma. Cords of oncocytic cells with bright eosinophilic and with granular cytoplasm and centrally placed nuclei.

adenoid cystic carcinoma.[79] There are rare reports of basal cell adenocarcinomas developing from membranous basal cell adenoma.[80,81]

Oncocytoma

Oncocytoma is an uncommon benign salivary gland tumor composed of mitochondria-rich oxyphilic cells called "oncocytes." In most studies it accounts for less than 1% of all salivary tumors.[82] Oncocytomas involve the parotid gland in most patients. The minor glands are much less frequently affected.

Clinical features. Oncocytoma has been reported to affect patients of all ages from the first to the tenth decade; however, its peak incidence is in the seventh and eight decades. It affects women more commonly than men and usually at a younger age. The average age of men at the time of diagnosis is 64 years, the average age of women is 59 years.[83] Its presenting clinical characteristics are similar to those of other benign adenomas of salivary glands. Patients are initially found to have slow-growing, asymptomatic, firm nodules commonly in the superficial lobe of the parotid. The tumor does not usually exceed 4 cm in diameter, and the masses are freely movable.[82] Occasionally they are multifocal.

Pathology. Microscopically, oncocytoma is usually well circumscribed to encapsulated, though rare tumors may have areas with irregular margins. The oncocytes are large and contain an intensely eosinophilic granular cytoplasm and a centrally located nucleus (Fig. 51-23). Nuclei may be large and vesicular with prominent nucleoli, or they may be small and darkly staining. The cells form solid sheets, cords, and alveolar or organoid patterns that occasionally have a central lumen.[82,83] There may be scattered groups of cells with clear cytoplasm, or they may form focal masses (Fig. 51-24). Tumors with a prominent clear cell component are referred to as "clear cell oncocytoma."[84] Fibrous connective tissue septa are rarely present within the tumor. Occasional oncocytomas show cellular pleomorphism and atypia, but in contrast to oncocytic carcinoma, they do not infiltrate into the glandular parenchyma or adjacent tissues.

Oncocytes contain numerous mitochondria that are best demonstrated by electron microscopy.[85] Phosphotunystic acid–hematoxylin staining can also be used to the same end.[82]

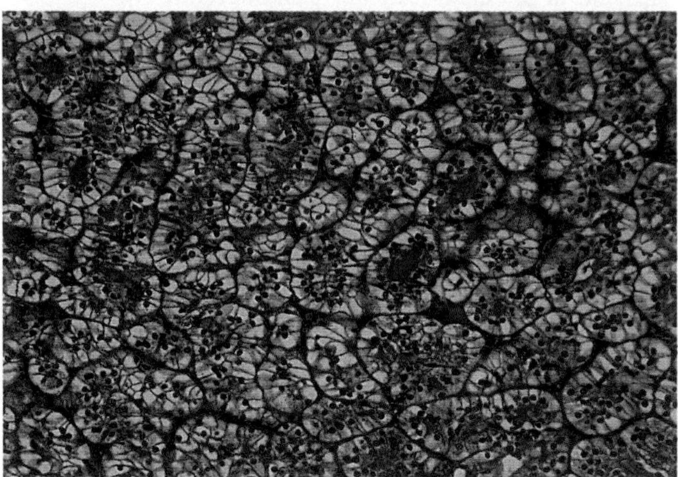

Fig. 51-24 Oncocytoma. Clear oncocytic cells are arranged in an alveolar pattern.

A true oncocytoma should be differentiated from *oncocytosis*. This latter process also commonly involves the parotid gland in patients over 50 years of age. Histologically, oncocytosis is often multifocal but usually retains a lobular pattern of arrangement and appears to be associated with aging. Oncocytosis is believed to be a metaplastic or hyperplastic process characterized by the replacement of normal acini or ducts with oncocytes. Rarely an oncocytoma arises in a background of oncocytosis.

Therapy and prognosis. Surgical removal is the treatment of choice for oncocytoma.[82,86,87] A superficial parotidectomy with preservation of the facial nerve is commonly employed for tumors in the parotid gland. Recurrence is rare. However, locally aggressive and frankly malignant changes in oncocytomas have been reported.[88]

Ductal papillomas

Papillomatous lesions of the salivary gland ducts are classified as (1) intraductal papilloma; (2) sialadenoma papilliferum, which is analogous to syringocystadenoma papilliferum of the sweat glands; and (3) inverted ductal papilloma.

Intraductal papilloma

Intraductal papilloma is a rare tumor that is more likely to arise in the ducts of minor salivary glands of the lip.[89] Clinically it presents as a small, asymptomatic submucosal mass and commonly occurs in patients in the fifth or sixth decade. Microscopically the papilloma is seen to arise from the surface of the salivary duct, which shows cystic dilatation. It is usually located away from the orifice. The papilloma is unicystic and is composed of papillary fronds that extend into the cystic lumen. The projections have delicate fibrovascular cores and are covered by bland cuboidal or columnar and occasional mucinous epithelium similar to that lining the cystically dilated salivary duct.[89] The proliferating fronds do not extend out of the salivary duct. If the process involves more than one duct, it is best classified as a cyst adenoma.

Sialadenoma papilliferum

The frequency of sialadenoma papilliferum cited in the literature varies; they are reported to constitute from 0.6% to 2% of benign salivary gland tumors.[51,89-91] Although the tumor can be found in the major salivary gland ducts, it is much more common in the minor glands of the mouth, particularly the palate. This lesion forms near or at the orifice of the salivary duct and presents as a papillary surface lesion, which is usually small. Clinically it is commonly misdiagnosed as a squamous papilloma. Most of the patients are adults whose average age is 56 years. It is more frequent in men.[89]

Pathology. Microscopically the tumor has exophytic and endophytic components (Fig. 51-25). The outer portion is a typical papilloma with fingerlike projections supported by delicate fibrous connective tissue cores that extend above the level of the adjacent mucosa. The covering epithelium of the fronds is stratified squamous, and it can be hyperkeratotic or parakeratotic. A mixed inflammatory cell infiltrate composed of lymphocytes, plasma cells, and neutrophils is usually present in this aspect of the lesion. The deeper endophytic component is unencapsulated and composed of branching ducts that are continuous with the interpapillary clefts of the surface component. Some of the ducts may be dilated and have intraluminal papillary projections. The epithelial lining of the ducts and cysts is usually composed of a double layer of cells—a tall columnar luminal cell layer and a cuboidal basal cell layer (Fig. 51-26). Both cell types are brightly eosinophilic and exhibit oncocytic features.[92] Inflammatory cells are present in the stroma.

Inverted ductal papilloma

Inverted ductal papilloma is the rarest of the ductal papillomas.[89,91,93] A review of the limited number of cases reported in the literature reveals that they occur in the minor salivary glands of adults at a mean age of 50 years. The lower lip and the buccal mucosa are more frequently affected than other oral sites are. Clinically this tumor presents as a firm nodule located below a normal-appearing mucosa. Like sialadenoma papilliferum, it forms near the orifice of salivary ducts and does not usually exceed 1.5 cm in diameter.

Pathology. Histologically, inverted ductal papilloma is a well-circumscribed outgrowth of basaloid and squamous cells that extend in a thick papillary configuration from a luminal surface into the lamina propria of the oral mucosa. The ductal lumen from which the inverted papilloma arises may communicate with the surface with an opening. It is covered with cuboidal duct cells and occasional scattered mucous cells.

Therapy. The treatment of ductal papillomas is surgical excision, which is curative.

Cystadenoma

Cystadenoma is a benign cystic neoplasm of salivary glands, representing 2% to 8.1% of all benign salivary tumors.[51,94] It affects both the major and minor salivary glands. The mean age of patients at the time of diagnosis is 53.5 years, and the highest incidence has been noted in patients who are in the sixth to eighth decades of life.[94] Of the major glands, the parotid is the most common site of the tumor. Cystadenoma of minor salivary glands occurs more frequently in the lip and buccal mucosa than in the palate.[51] The tumor is asymptomatic and presents as a small nodule that usually does not exceed 1 cm in its greatest dimension.[51]

Pathology. The diagnostic histologic criteria of cystadenoma are debated. The tumor is multicystic and well defined

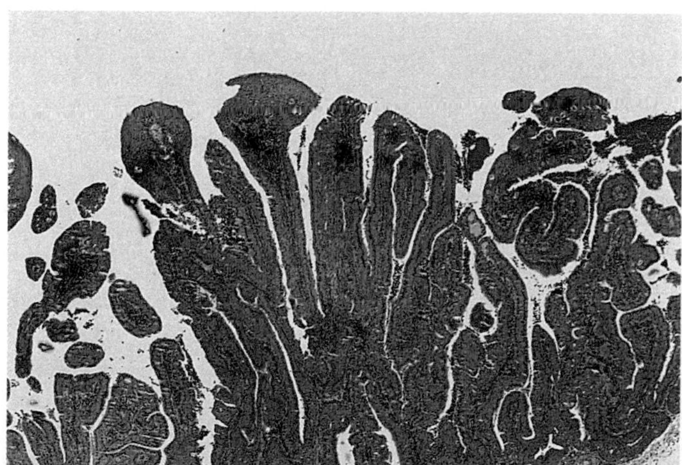

Fig. 51-25 Sialadenoma papilliferum. A papillary exophytic component is covered with stratified squamous epithelium, and a deeper endophytic component is composed of oncocytic cells.

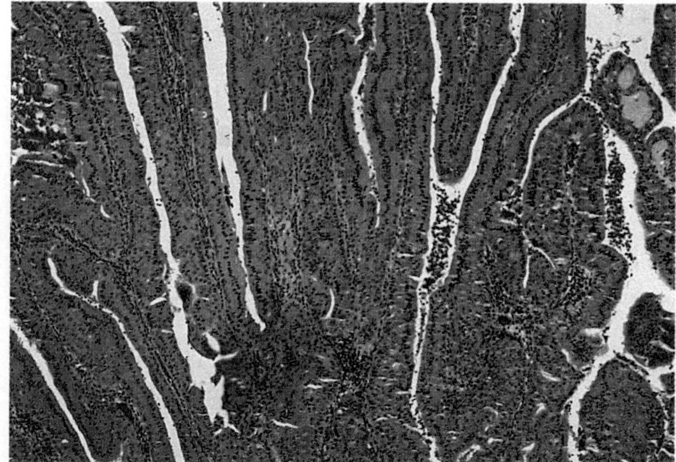

Fig. 51-26 Higher-magnification view of the endophytic component of sialadenoma papilliferum seen in Fig. 51-25 showing papillae lined with a double layer of oncocytic cells.

and may be encapsulated. The number and size of the cystic structures vary among tumors. The epithelial lining of the cysts can be cuboidal, flat, or columnar. Cellular atypia is not usually a fixture of this neoplasm. Oncocytic as well as mucous changes of the lining may exist and occasionally are dominant. The thickness of the cell lining varies, and a focal thickening that produces papillary projections is not uncommon (Fig. 51-27). It is because of these variations in the histologic features of cystadenoma that some lesions have been variably called *duct ectasia, salivary duct cyst, oncocytic papillary cystadenoma, papillary mucous cystadenoma,* and *papillary hyperplasia.*[94]

Therapy. The lesion is treated by conservative surgical excision, which is usually curative.

Sebaceous neoplasms

Sebaceous gland rests are commonly found in the submandibular and parotid glands but are rare in the sublingual gland. In the buccal mucosa they are known as *Fordyce's granules* and are found in up to 80% of persons.[94] Although sebaceous differentiation is common, primary sebaceous neoplasms are rare. Unlike sebaceous tumors of the skin, those arising in the salivary glands are not known to be associated with an increased risk for the development of colonic carcinoma or any other visceral malignancies.[94,95]

Two benign sebaceous tumors of salivary glands are known: *sebaceous adenoma* and *sebaceous lymphadenoma.* Sebaceous lesions can also occur in association with other salivary gland neoplasms.

Sebaceous adenoma

Sebaceous adenoma is a very rare salivary neoplasm, and most have been found in the parotid gland.[94-96] The tumors are generally small, not exceeding 3 cm in diameter. Men are more commonly affected than women.

Pathology. Microscopically the lesion is well circumscribed or encapsulated and is composed of sebaceous cell nests. The neoplastic cells show minimal atypia and are not invasive. Oncocytic metaplasia, histiocytic infiltration, and foreign body giant cells have been observed in some cases. Recurrence after surgical excision has not been reported.

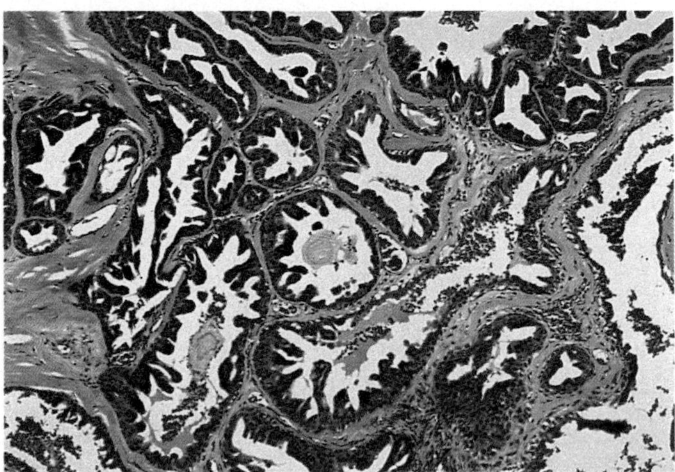

Fig. 51-27 Cystadenoma. Multiple cystic structures are seen, and their lining forms intraluminal papillary projections.

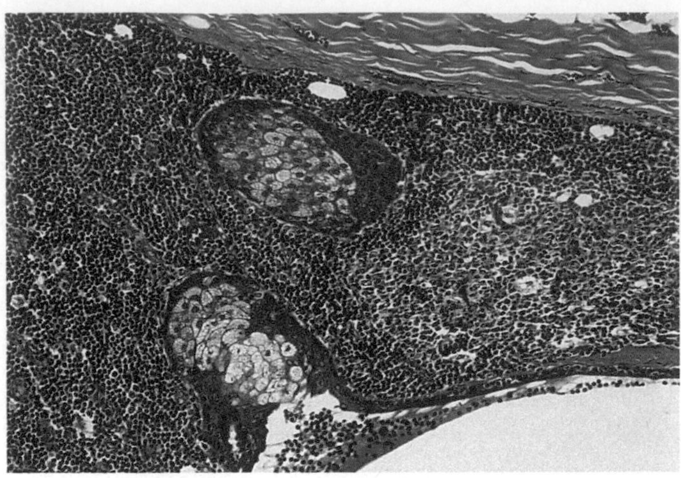

Fig. 51-28 Sebaceous lymphadenoma showing sebaceous glands and salivary ducts in a lymphoid stroma. There is a thick fibrous capsule at the periphery of the tumor.

Sebaceous lymphadenoma

Sebaceous lymphadenoma is also a very rare salivary tumor. It is believed to arise from intranodal sebaceous rests within salivary glands. The tumor occurs in older adults and shows a slight female bias. The majority arise from the parotid gland, and they range from 1.3 to 6 cm in diameter.[94,95]

Pathology. Microscopically most sebaceous lymphadenomas are encapsulated and composed of sebaceous glands admixed with salivary ducts in a background of lymphocytes and lymphoid follicles (Fig. 51-28). Histiocytes and giant cell nests surrounding areas of spilled sebum are commonly seen. Cytologic atypia is minimal, and the tumor does not invade surrounding structures. Adequate surgical excision is the recommended treatment.

Sebaceous differentiation in other salivary neoplasms

Several salivary gland tumors, including both benign and malignant neoplasms, have been noted to have associated areas showing sebaceous differentiation.[94-96] These include pleomorphic adenoma, oncocytoma, Warthin's tumor, carcinoma ex pleomorphic adenoma, mucoepidermoid carcinoma, adenoid cystic carcinoma, and acinic cell carcinoma.

MALIGNANT NEOPLASMS

Malignant salivary gland epithelial tumors are less common than their benign counterparts; the ratios of benign to malignant neoplasms noted in most series range between 3 to 4:1. This ratio is greatest for tumors of the parotid gland (4:1), lower for those of the submandibular gland (2:1), and lowest for those of the sublingual, minor salivary, and seromucinous glands (1:1). These neoplasms may be malignant from their onset or can develop in a preexisting benign tumor, most often a pleomorphic adenoma. Little is known about environmental causes of salivary gland tumors other than radiation exposure, for which there is good evidence of an increased incidence in exposed populations.

Mucoepidermoid carcinoma

Mucoepidermoid carcinoma is the most common malignant tumor of the salivary gland. It constitutes 2% to 10% of the tumors of the major salivary glands and 10% to 41% of the tumors of the minor salivary glands, representing the most common type of malignant minor salivary gland tumor.[49,51,97,98] Ninety percent of the tumors that affect the major glands occur in the parotid gland. Those that affect the minor salivary glands most commonly arise on the palate, but a significant number may also be found in the retromolar area, the floor of the mouth, the buccal mucosa, the lip, and the tongue.[49,51] These tumors may also arise within the body of the mandible or in the maxilla.[99] This tumor is most common in the 35- to 65-year age group; but no age group is exempt. Mucoepidermoid carcinoma is also the most common malignant salivary gland tumor to affect children and adolescents under 20 years of age.[97,100-102]

The most common etiologic factor that has been implicated in the development of mucoepidermoid carcinomas is therapeutic irradiation.[97,103] Mucoepidermoid carcinomas usually present as slowly growing, firm masses that are clinically indistinguishable from the more common pleomorphic adenoma. Pain is unusual and more often associated with high-grade tumors. High-grade tumors have poorly defined margins and may be fixed to the adjacent skin and soft tissue. In one large series high-grade mucoepidermoid carcinoma was the carcinoma most often associated with facial nerve palsy.[104]

Pathology. On gross examination the tumor may appear circumscribed, but it is seldom encapsulated. Cystic features are common and may be prominent. The tumors usually range from 1 to 4 cm in their greatest dimension; however, occasionally larger tumors are encountered. Microscopically, mucoepidermoid carcinomas are composed of epidermoid cells, mucus-secreting cells, and cells with an intermediate differentiation between these two cell types. Clear cells, many of which contain glycogen or mucin, or both, are present in many mucoepidermoid carcinomas and often are a prominent feature. These tumors show varying proportions of cell types in a given tumor (Fig. 51-29). These tumors are classified histologically as low, intermediate, and high grade. Suggested grading criteria have included the relative proportions of the cell types, the degree of tumor invasiveness, the pattern of invasion, the degree of maturation of the various cellular components, and the relative proportions of cystic spaces to areas of solid growth. In a recent review of 143 intraoral mucoepidermoid carcinomas, Auclair and coworkers[105] documented the histopathologic features that indicated aggressive behavior. These included an intracystic component of less than 20%, four or more mitotic figures per 10 high-power fields, nerve invasion, tumor necrosis, and cellular anaplasia.

Low-grade tumors commonly exhibit a nesting pattern consisting of numerous well-circumscribed squamous nests that contain numerous clear cells, some of which contain intracytoplasmic mucin. Many low-grade tumors, especially those in the minor salivary glands, contain a prominent mucin-secreting component composed of columnar cells lining cystic spaces. Nuclear atypia, mitotic activity, and an infiltrative growth pattern are not features of low-grade tumors. *Intermediate-grade tumors* tend to manifest as larger, more irregular nests of squamous cells containing more basilar or intermediate cells that less frequently display a cystic component. Minor nuclear atypia and mitotic activity may be present, and there is usually a small infiltrative component. *High-grade tumors* are predominantly solid and are very similar to the infiltrating epidermoid carcinomas that arise in other anatomic regions. These are infiltrative tumors that produce scanty mucin, and a careful search and special staining may be needed to identify intracellular mucin.

Therapy and prognosis. The histologic grade is directly related to the prognosis and clinical staging of these tumors. The survival rate in patients with low-grade tumors ranges from 90% to 100%. Complete surgical excision is the treatment of choice. An adequate excision is important; the recurrence rates are higher in those patients whose surgical margins show residual disease. Survival is better in younger patients and women and is worse in patients older than 60 years.[106] Intermediate- and high-grade tumors have a greater tendency to infiltrate, recur, and metastasize, with reported survival rates in such patients varying from 40% to 60%. Palliative radiation therapy should also be considered in patients with high-grade tumors and in those with residual microscopic disease at the surgical margins.

Acinic cell carcinoma

Acinic cell carcinoma is a relatively rare tumor with a histologic appearance similar to that of normal acinar serous cells. These tumors account for 2% to 3% of salivary gland tumors; they most often arise in the parotid gland but occasionally may involve the submandibular, minor salivary, or seromucinous glands.[107] These tumors commonly arise in patients in the fifth decade, but they may present from early childhood to old age. Acinic cell carcinoma is the second most common malignant

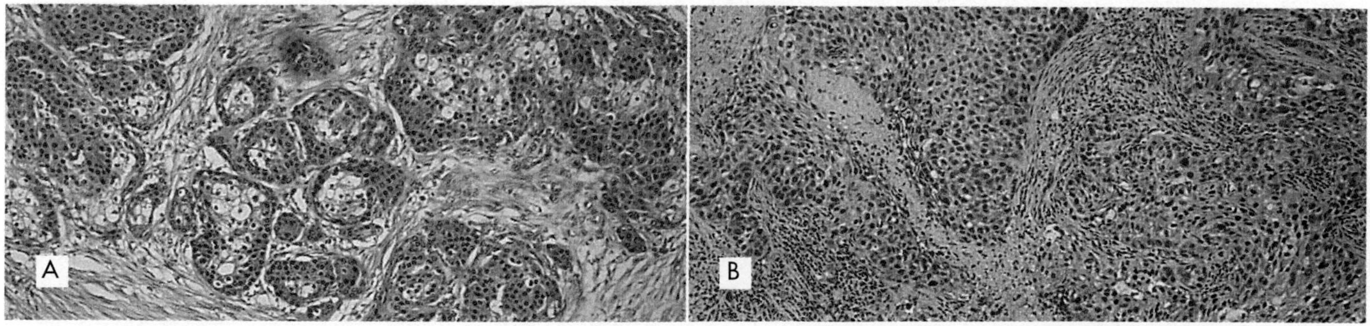

Fig. 51-29 Mucoepidermoid carcinoma. **A,** Low-grade tumor. Notice the bland squamous nests with central larger cells containing clear cytoplasm. **B,** High-grade tumor composed of pleomorphic, atypical squamous cells.

tumor in the pediatric population,[100-107] and there is a slight female preponderance. Acinic cell carcinoma is the most common malignant tumor involving more than one salivary gland. (3% to 4.8% of tumors).[108]

Pathology. On gross examination the tumor appears as a well-circumscribed mass with a diameter in the 2 to 4 cm range; however, they may also be multinodular and are rarely completely encapsulated. These tumors are usually grayish white to reddish gray, and most are solid, though occasional tumors may contain variably sized cystic spaces. Histologically, the tumor may be composed of several types of cells, including serous acinar cells, and intercalated ductlike cells, as well as vacuolated, clear, and nonspecific glandular cells.[107,109] These tumors can be grouped into four patterns: classic solid, microcystic, papillary cystic, and follicular[107] (Fig. 51-30). The *solid* pattern is the most typical one and is more commonly seen in tumors of the parotid gland. It is easily recognized because of the numerous well-differentiated serous acinar cells that closely resemble the cells of normal parotid parenchyma but without striated ducts. In this pattern there are sheets of tumor cells that contain abundant grayish blue, slightly granular cytoplasm. In the *microcystic* pattern, which is slightly more common than the solid pattern, there are numerous small cystic spaces that are usually 5 to 15 times the size of acinar cells and may be filled with mucinous or proteinaceous material. Collections of well-differentiated acinic cells are usually easy to find between the cystic spaces, though they may be very scarce in occasional tumors. Tumor cells in this pattern may be arranged in trabeculae; intercalated duct-like cells also may be prominent. The *papillary cystic* type is characterized by one or more variably sized cystic structures with papillary fronds containing proliferating epithelium that is similar to that found in the normal intercalated ducts. The thickness of the epithelium lining the cysts and projecting into their lumens is quite variable, ranging from a single layer to multiple layers. Cells composing this portion of the tumor are usually uniform; they are cuboidal and contain a moderate amount of cytoplasm. Mucicarmine staining often yields a markedly positive reaction in the cystic spaces. The *follicular* pattern of acinic cell carcinoma is the least frequently encountered one and has a thyroidlike appearance manifesting as variably-sized follicles lined by cuboidal to columnar epithelial cells. Approximately 75% of all acinic cell carcinomas exhibit multiple cell types and growth patterns. In our experience, PAS is the most helpful histologic stain, with and without diastase to stain the zymogen granules, which are PAS positive and diastase resistant. In the classic pattern there are numerous areas of positivity; in the other three patterns there may be only scattered single cells or small foci containing demonstrable zymogen granules. One of the more unusual features of this tumor is the dense lymphoid aggregate that is often intermingled with the tumor cells. This dense infiltrate may cause a false-negative diagnosis to be rendered on frozen section examination.[110]

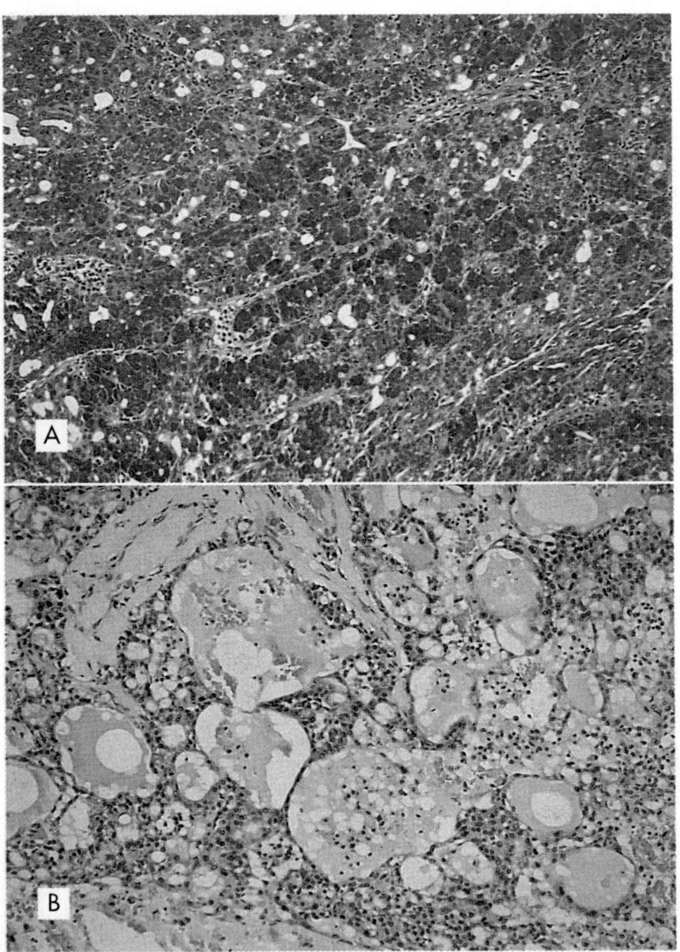

Fig. 51-30 Acinic cell adenocarcinoma. **A,** Classic solid pattern with sheets of well-differentiated serous acinar cells. **B,** Follicular pattern with many variably sized follicular structures.

Therapy and prognosis. Acinic cell carcinomas are regarded as low-grade malignant tumors. The prognosis in affected patients does not appear to correlate at all with the previously described histologic subtypes. An infiltrative growth pattern, multinodularity, and stromal hyalinization appear to be associated with more aggressive clinical behavior. However, the clinical stage of the disease seems to be the most important prognostic factor.[111,112] Acinic cell carcinomas are one of the lowest-grade salivary gland carcinomas, in that the prognosis in patients with this disease is better than that in patients with many mucoepidermoid carcinomas, as well as adenoid cystic carcinoma, and malignant mixed tumors. In a review, Hickman and colleagues[113] found the 5- and 10-year survival rates in patients with acinic carcinomas to be 82% and 68%, respectively. The 20-year survivals are only slightly lower. Patients die as the result of local recurrence; regional metastasis may occur in approximately 5% to 10% of patients, usually late in the disease, and rarely tumors may metastasize to distant sites, especially the lung. Wide local excision is the treatment of choice; radiotherapy may be added to the regimen when local disease is extensive and cannot be removed surgically. Rarely, acinic cell carcinomas occur in association with poorly differentiated carcinomas in the same tumor.[111] Whether these are examples of collision tumors or of dedifferentiation of the original tumor requires further clarification. However, the nature of the therapy in patients with these tumors should be decided on the basis of the poorly differentiated carcinoma component.[107,114]

Adenoid cystic carcinoma

Adenoid cystic carcinomas account for 3% to 10% of all salivary gland tumors.[115,116] They arise more commonly in the minor salivary glands and in the seromucinous glands of the upper respiratory tract than in all the major glands combined.[117-121] Twenty-five percent to 30% of adenoid cystic carcinomas occur in the major salivary glands, and they are much more common in the submandibular and sublingual glands than they are in the parotid; it is the most common malignant tumor to affect the submandibular gland.[122,123] Histologically similar tumors may also be found in the lacrimal glands, ear canal, tracheobronchial tree, breast, and other body sites. There is a considerable variation in the frequency of adenoid cystic carcinoma in relationship to mucoepidermoid carcinoma reported for the populations of different countries. Most reports from the United States indicate that mucoepidermoid carcinoma is the more frequently encountered tumor. In England and Western Europe adenoid cystic carcinoma appears to be the more common of the two.[49]

Adenoid cystic carcinomas occur most frequently in persons in the fourth to sixth decades of life; however, they may arise at any age, ranging from 4 days to 86 years.[124-126] Patients with tumors in the major glands commonly present with a painful mass; those with tumors in the minor or seromucinous glands commonly complain of respiratory obstruction, pain, epistaxis, or nasal discharge, or a combination of these symptoms. If the lower portion of the maxillary sinus is involved, ulceration and necrosis of the palate may be seen.

Pathology. Grossly, adenoid cystic carcinoma usually appears as a well-defined to locally invasive solid, firm mass that on microscopic examination is found to infiltrate into surrounding tissues. It is white or whitish gray and microscopically is composed of a rather uniform population of dark-staining, basaloid tumor cells containing a minimal amount of cytoplasm and arranged in three growth patterns: cribriform, solid, and tubular (Fig. 51-31). The *cribriform* pattern is the most characteristic and recognizable form. It manifests as a punched-out, or "Swiss cheese," arrangement of the tumors cells, usually surrounding acellular spaces that may contain mucoid or hyaline material. The hyaline material is actually reduplicated basement membrane. The tumor cells are composed of dense basophilic nuclei containing very inconspicuous or nonexistent nucleoli. Mitotic figures are rarely found. As the amount of basement membrane material increases, slender strands of tumor cells may form in an extensive hyaline background. The *tubular* type of adenoid cystic carcinoma contains tumor cells identical to those observed in the cribriform pattern; however, they form single tubular or ductal structures that are constructed of layers of isomorphic cells surrounded by hyalinized stroma. The lumens of the tubular structures often contain a mucinous, faintly eosinophilic material. Transitional areas between cribriform and tubular regions are common. The *solid* type of adenoid cystic carcinoma is characterized by large masses or nests of somewhat uniform basaloid tumor cells containing occasional intercalated duct-like structures and few if any of the circular punched-out spaces that characterize the cribriform pattern. Occasionally, areas of necrosis may be prominent within the central portion of these solid nests. Cellular pleomorphism is usually minimal, but mitotic activity may be prominent.

Therapy and prognosis. Wide surgical excision is the treatment of choice, possibly combined with aggressive radiotherapy to achieve better local control, especially if there is microscopic evidence of disease at or near the surgical margins. Chemotherapy is usually not included in the early treatment of these tumors, though recently positive responses to chemotherapeutic agents have been documented.[49] The various histologic patterns are often intermixed, and numerous studies have attempted to correlate the extent of the various patterns with prognosis. Much of the data are contradictory, though there is consensus that the outcome appears to be more favorable in patients with the cribriform and tubular patterns and worse in patients with a prominent solid pattern. Adenoid cystic carcinomas grow in an infiltrative and invasive fashion; perineural invasion is characteristic of this neoplasm and is often very conspicuous within the tumor and in nerves adjacent to and occasionally some distance from the primary tumor mass. This feature seems to account for the poor long-term outcome in patients with this tumor.

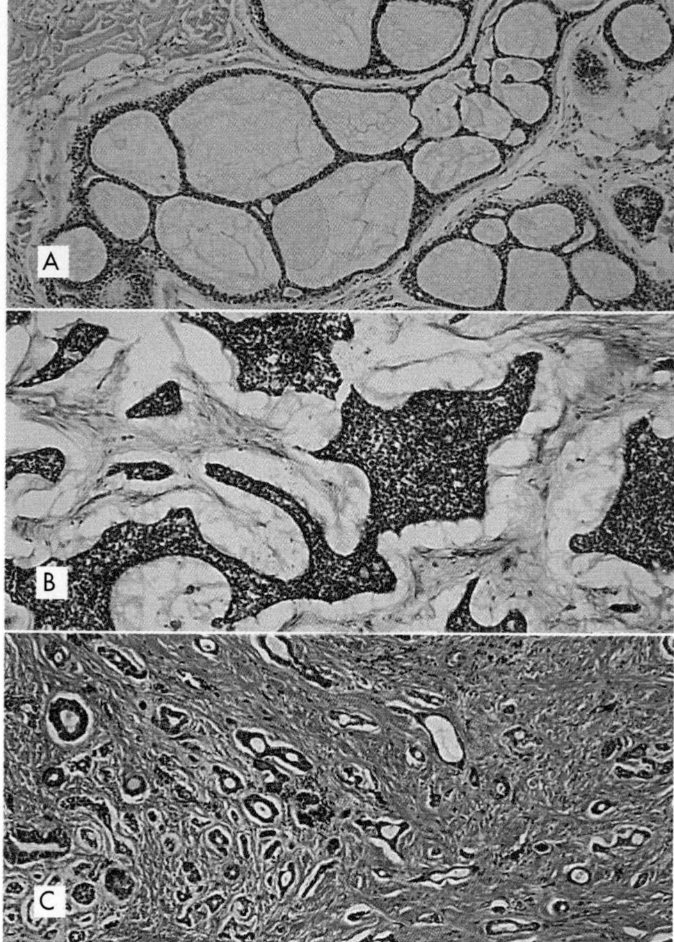

Fig. 51-31 Adenoid cystic carcinoma. **A,** Cribriform pattern. **B,** Solid pattern. **C,** Tubular pattern.

Despite its slow growth and often deceptively benign clinical features, the long-term survival in patients with this tumor is poor. Adenoid cystic carcinomas commonly recur locally and may spread to the central nervous system by way of the cranial nerves. Metastasis to the cervical lymph nodes occurs in approximately 15% of the patients; 28% to 58% of the tumors metastasize hematogenously to the lung, skeleton, liver, or brain.[117,121,127,128] Rarely adenoid cystic carcinomas metastasize before the primary tumor is detected.[129] Although 5-year survival rates of as much as 70% have been reported for patients with parotid adenoid cystic carcinomas, the rate in those with adenoid cystic carcinoma declines to 5% to 15% at 20 years, with the worst prognosis in patients who have tumors of the minor salivary, seromucinous, and submandibular glands. Because more than 20% of patients with metastatic adenoid cystic carcinoma may live 5 years or more after metastasis occurs, aggressive therapy is indicated.[121,130]

Malignant mixed tumor

Malignant mixed tumor comprises three different clinical pathologic entities: carcinoma arising in a benign mixed tumor (carcinoma ex pleomorphic adenoma), carcinosarcoma, and metastasizing mixed tumor. The first accounts for most of the malignant mixed tumors, and the second and third are extremely rare and account for only a small percentage of the tumors in this group. Many large series of cases of carcinoma ex mixed tumors have been collected and their findings have been summarized in a recent report.[136] Malignant mixed tumors constitute approximately 12% of malignant salivary gland tumors (range, 2.8% to 42.4%), 6.2% of all mixed tumors (range, 1.9% to 23.3%), and 3.6% of all salivary gland neoplasms (range, 0.9% to 14%).

Carcinoma ex pleomorphic adenoma

Carcinoma ex mixed tumor, also known as carcinoma ex pleomorphic adenoma or carcinoma arising in a benign mixed tumor, is a mixed tumor in which a second neoplasm, a carcinoma, arises. This tumor accounts for well over 95% of all so-called malignant mixed tumors.[131-133] Carcinoma ex pleomorphic adenoma most frequently arises in the parotid gland, but it may also involve the submandibular, minor salivary, or seromucinous glands. Tumors may present at any age in adults, but usually in the sixth or seventh decade and at an average age that is approximately one decade later than that in patients with pleomorphic adenomas; they are extremely rare in patients under 20 years of age. In the most typical history, patients have a long-standing mass that grows rapidly over the course of 3 to 6 months; however, a significant proportion of patients may present with a clinical history of less than 3 years.[106,134] Patients frequently complain of a painless mass, but pain with facial nerve palsy and skin fixation may also be noted.

Pathology. On average carcinoma ex pleomorphic adenoma is more than twice the size of its benign counterpart, ranging up to 25 cm in its greatest diameter.[133,135] Grossly, tumors are usually poorly circumscribed and many are extensively infiltrative. Occasional tumors, however, may be well circumscribed or completely encapsulated. Tumors are usually hard and white to tan-gray. The relative proportions of the benign and malignant components can be quite variable, and extensive sampling may be necessary to demonstrate the benign component. The malignant component is most commonly a poorly differentiated adenocarcinoma or undifferentiated carcinoma; however, virtually any form of carcinoma that can arise in the salivary glands can be the carcinoma component[131] (Fig. 51-32). The infiltrative, destructive growth pattern is the most reliable criterion establishing the diagnosis of carcinoma ex mixed tumor.

Therapy and prognosis. Carcinoma ex pleomorphic adenoma is an extremely aggressive malignant tumor. Approximately 40% to 50% of the patients develop one or more recurrences.[132,134,135] The metastatic rate varies from series to series, with as many as 70% of the patients developing local or distant metastasis.[136] Sites of distant metastases, in order of frequency, are the lungs, bone (especially the spine), abdominal area, and central nervous system.[133,137] The prognosis is excellent in patients whose carcinoma component is contained within the tumor capsule, similar to the prognosis in those with typical benign mixed tumor. However, patients with tumors penetrating the capsule have a poor prognosis, with 5-year survival rates of 25% to 65%, 10-year survival rates of 24% to 50%, 15-year survival rates of 10% to 35%, and 20-year survival rates of nil to 38%.[131,138] Therefore it is important to designate carcinoma ex pleomorphic adenoma confined within the capsule as opposed to those penetrating the capsule as noninvasive and invasive, respectively. Tortoledo and associates[135] reviewed their experience in 37 patients and found that none whose tumor extended less than 8 mm beyond the capsule died of tumor-related causes, whereas all patients whose tumor extended more than 9 mm beyond the capsule died of tumor-related causes. They also found the local recurrence rates were 70.5% when the malignant component extended 6 mm beyond the capsule and only 16.6% when it extended less than 6 mm beyond the capsule. They also correlated 5-year survival rates with the histologic subtype of carcinomas and found that 30% of those with undifferentiated carcinomas, 50% of those with myoepithelial carcinomas, 62% of

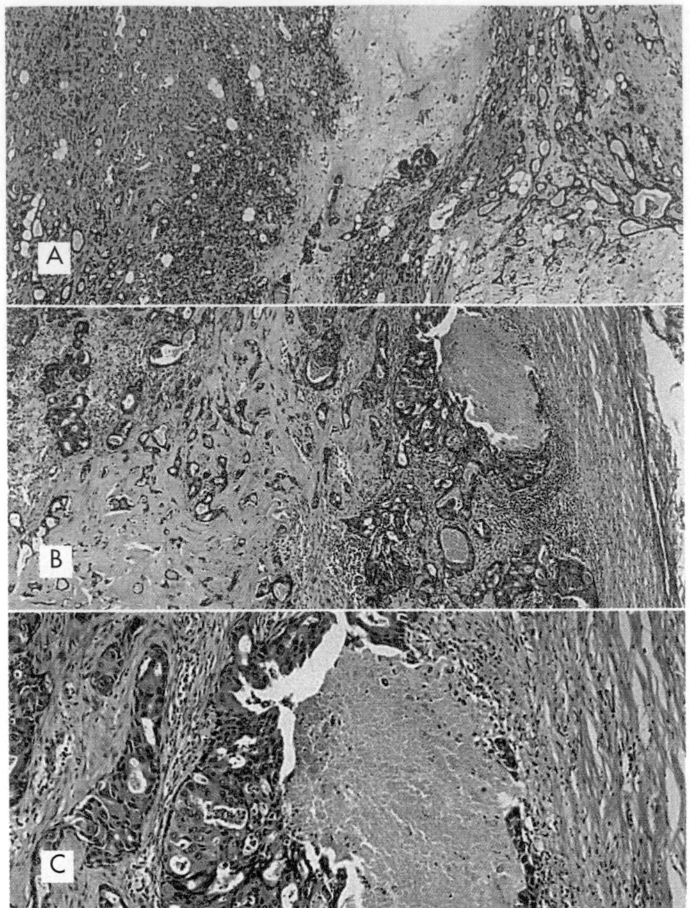

Fig. 51-32 Carcinoma ex pleomorphic adenoma. **A,** Benign mixed tumor portion with ductal and myxoid elements. **B,** An adjacent region with adenocarcinoma. **C,** Detail of carcinoma.

those with ductal carcinomas, and 96% of those with terminal duct carcinomas were still alive at 5 years. The best form of therapy for these aggressive tumors appears to be wide surgical excision together with contiguous lymph node dissection and adjuvant radiation therapy.

Carcinosarcoma

Carcinosarcoma is composed of both carcinomatous and sarcomatous elements. Unlike carcinoma ex mixed tumor, in which only the malignant component may metastasize, in carcinosarcoma, both the carcinoma and sarcomatous elements are capable of metastases. The carcinosarcoma variant of malignant mixed tumor is extremely rare, with slightly more than 40 cases reported so far.[131] Two thirds have arisen in the parotid glands, approximately 19% in the submandibular glands, and 14% in the palate. The mean age of these patients at presentation was 58 years and ranged from 14 to 87 years. Chondrosarcoma and osteosarcoma elements are the most common sarcomatous elements, and moderately or poorly differentiated ductal carcinoma and an undifferentiated carcinoma are the most common carcinoma component (Fig. 51-33). Local tissue infiltration and destruction are characteristic of this neoplasm, with almost 60% of the patients dying of locally recurrent or metastatic disease, usually within 30 months of the time of diagnosis.

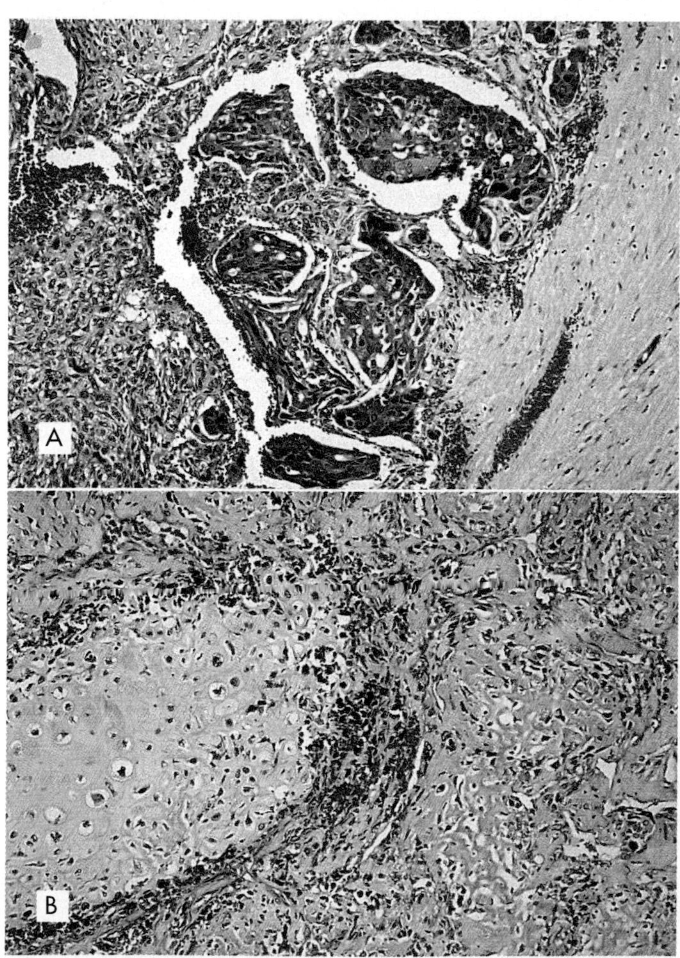

Fig. 51-33 Carcinosarcoma. **A,** An area with nests of poorly differentiated carcinoma. **B,** Poorly differentiated chondrosarcoma *(left)* with adjacent osteosarcoma *(right).*

Metastasizing mixed tumor

The metastasizing mixed tumor, the least common of the three types of malignant mixed tumor, is a neoplasm in which both the primary salivary gland tumor and its metastatic lesions are composed of typical benign-appearing mixed tumor (Fig. 51-34). Up to now, just over 25 cases have been described in the literature; more than three fourths of the tumors arose in the parotid gland, 13% in the submandibular gland, and 9% in the palate.[131,138] These tumors are characterized by local recurrences and there is typically a long interval between the initial development of the original mixed tumor and the appearance of the metastatic lesion. This interval has varied from 1.5 to 51 years. Half of the tumors in these patients metastasized to bone, 30% to the lung, and 30% to the lymph nodes; rarely tumors metastasized to other body sites. The treatment of choice is surgical excision with aggressive treatment of distant metastatic tumors. Forty percent of the patients have died of the disease, usually from distant metastases; 47% were alive and well, and 13% were alive with disease at the time of the review.

Clear cell carcinoma

Clear cell carcinoma of salivary gland origin is a group of uncommon neoplasms that contain a large proportion of tumor cells with clear cytoplasm that do not fit into other categories of carcinoma. Evidence accumulating over the past decade indicates that the clear cell carcinomas are really a heterogeneous group of neoplasms, most of which fall within the range of epithelial-myoepithelial carcinoma. However, as more information accumulates, it appears that other subtypes of primary clear cell carcinoma distinct from the epithelial-myoepithelial carcinoma are being encountered. One newly described tumor is the hyalinizing clear cell carcinoma.[139] This is a very low grade carcinoma that is characterized by nests of clear cells in a densely hyalinized stroma (Fig. 51-35). As evidence accumulates, it is one of the author's belief (D.R.G.) that additional subtypes of clear cell carcinoma, distinct from these carcinomas, will be identified.

In 1972 Donath and associates[140] described eight cases of a previously unrecognized clear cell tumor of salivary gland ori-

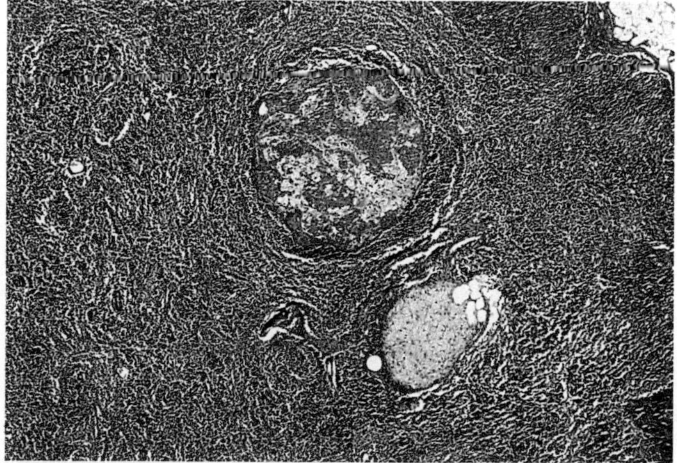

Fig. 51-34 Metastasizing mixed tumor in a lymph node. Notice two nests of benign-appearing mixed tumor surrounded by lymphoid stroma.

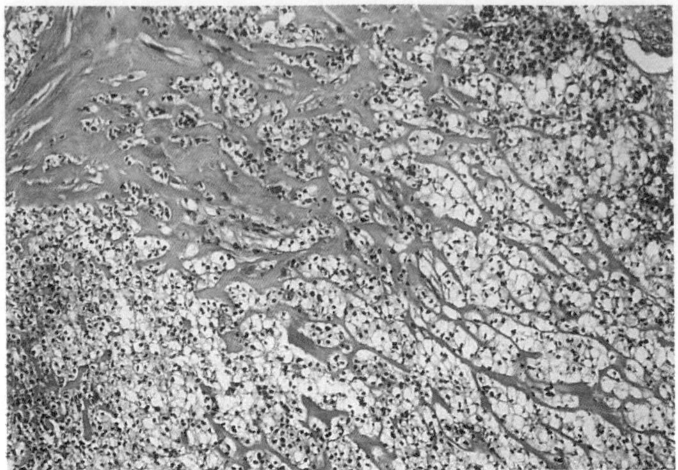

Fig. 51-35 Hyalinizing clear cell carcinoma with thin cords of clear cells in a densely hyalinized stroma.

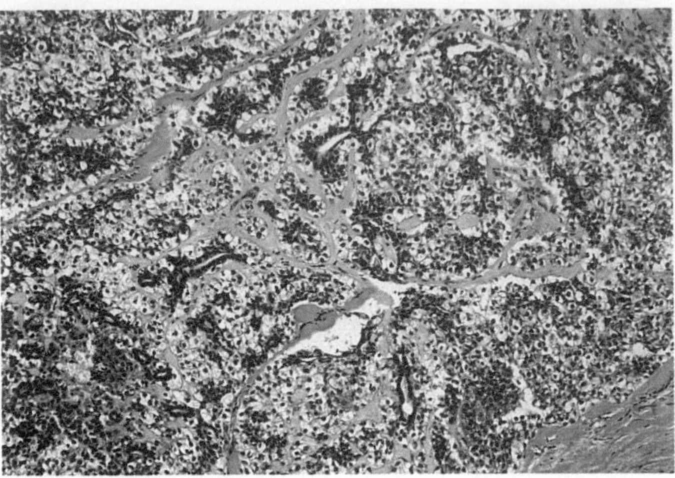

Fig. 51-36 Epithelial-myoepithelial carcinoma. There are numerous ductal structures rimmed with clear myoepithelial cells.

gin that they termed *epithelial-myoepithelial carcinoma.* However, it was not until 1982, when Corio and colleagues[141] published their report, that this neoplasm was described in the English language literature. Epithelial-myoepithelial carcinoma is one of the more uncommon carcinomas, accounting for less than 0.5% of the salivary gland neoplasms.[140,142] It most often afflicts older persons, usually in the sixth or seventh decade of life. Female patients have outnumbered male patients by a ratio of 2 : 1. Eighty-four percent of the tumors have occurred in the parotid gland, and 11% and 5% have occurred in the submandibular and minor salivary glands respectively. Patients typically initially have slowly enlarging masses, usually without other symptoms, but pain or facial nerve weakness has been noted in approximately 25%.

Pathology. Grossly, these neoplasms are well delineated and firm and may show areas where the tumor has infiltrated into adjacent tissue. They range up to 8 cm in their greatest dimension.[142,143] Histologically these tumors typically are well circumscribed; they may exhibit a single or multinodular growth pattern and are usually surrounded, at least partially, by a thick fibrous capsule. Upon close scrutiny, tumor nests are usually found to have penetrated the capsule and invaded adjacent parenchyma. Histologically these are biphasic tumors with islands of tumor cells composed of an inner layer of small ducts, lined by cuboidal epithelium similar to that in normal intercalated ducts, that are surrounded by varying numbers of clear cells; in turn these are often surrounded by dense, hyalinized basement membrane material (Fig. 51-36). Rarely, columnar cells and small foci of early squamous metaplasia are seen proliferating within ductal structures. The clear cell component may also be arranged in solid nests or sheets. The percentage and arrangement of the nodular aggregates of the biphasic component and the sheets of clear cells vary greatly from tumor to tumor. The clear cell component predominates in occasional tumors, and the more typical biphasic portions of the neoplasm may not be readily apparent. Areas of necrosis may also be seen; however, mitotic figures are usually not prominent. The clear cell component contains abundant glycogen and ultrastructurally and immunohistochemically has characteristics of myoepithelial differentiation. The lumens of the ductal structures occasionally contain mucinous material, but intracellular mucin is not found in the clear cell component or in the ductal epithelial cells. Perineural and intravascular growth are also occasionally found.

The *differential diagnosis* consists of other salivary gland tumors that may have clear cell foci, including benign mixed tumor, clear cell oncocytoma, the rare clear cell myoepithelioma, sebaceous adenoma and carcinoma, acinic cell carcinoma, mucoepidermoid carcinoma, and polymorphous low-grade adenocarcinoma. Finally, metastatic renal cell carcinoma should be considered in the differential diagnosis of all clear cell tumors of salivary origin. However, the finding of ductal differentiation characteristic of the epithelial-myoepithelial carcinoma eliminates renal cell carcinoma from the differential diagnosis.

Therapy and prognosis. Wide surgical excision is the treatment of choice for this neoplasm; however, even with complete excision, recurrence and distal metastasis can rarely occur.[144] Thirteen of the 37 patients in the reported series have experienced tumor recurrence, with one patient suffering as many as six episodes of recurrence; two patients have suffered metastasis and died of their disease. The metastases have involved regional lymph nodes, lung, and kidney.[140,141,143] To date the data are insufficient to determine the efficacy of adjuvant postoperative radiotherapy.

Polymorphous low-grade adenocarcinoma

Polymorphous low-grade adenocarcinoma is a recently described form of adenocarcinoma of salivary gland origin. It was first described in 1983 and is referred to in the literature also as "terminal duct carcinoma" or "lobular carcinoma."[145,146] Up to now, well over 200 cases have been reported, with most of the tumors arising in minor salivary glands.[145-155] Approximately 60% of the tumors have involved the palate, and most of the others arose in various other intraoral sites. Fourteen have involved major salivary glands, two arose in the nasal cavity, and one occurred in the nasopharynx. Approximately two thirds of the patients are women and most are in the fifth through eighth decades of life; however, as with many salivary gland tumors, there is a wide range in the age of patients with the tumor (21 to 94 years). Up to now, these tumors have not been encountered in the pediatric population.

Polymorphous low-grade adenocarcinoma is the second most common intraoral malignant neoplasm after mucoepidermoid carcinoma, accounting for 26% of carcinomas.[156] The tumors are firm, elevated, usually painless, and nonulcerated and range from 1 to 6 cm in their maximum dimension.[147] These masses are usually present for varying periods, ranging from 2 weeks to 30 years, before the patients come to medical attention.

Pathology. Histologically, polymorphous low-grade adenocarcinomas are characterized by an infiltrative growth pattern, histologic blandness, cytologic uniformity, and diversity in the cellular organization. Tumor cells are usually small and uniform; they contain bland, minimally hyperchromatic nuclei and scant to moderately abundant, clear to eosinophilic cytoplasm. Mitoses may be present but are usually sparse. These tumors are unencapsulated and may be well circumscribed; however, foci of peripheral infiltrative growth into normal tissue are seen in all cases. Occasionally, multiple sections must be sampled before small foci of tumor invasion are found. Tumors commonly invade adjacent soft tissue and salivary gland lobules and may infiltrate into adjacent bone. Perineural growth is common. The tumors cells are arranged in varied patterns, including sheets, interconnecting cords, islands, small tubules, ducts, and cystic and cribriform areas; other foci exhibit a single-file or "Indian-file" pattern (Fig. 51-37). The differential diagnosis includes a cellular mixed tumor and adenoid cystic carcinoma. The former tumors are not invasive, and the latter are usually composed of cells that are slightly more hyperchromatic and usually more infiltrative than polymorphous low-grade adenocarcinomas; they also lack the varied growth patterns typical of polymorphous low-grade adenocarcinoma.

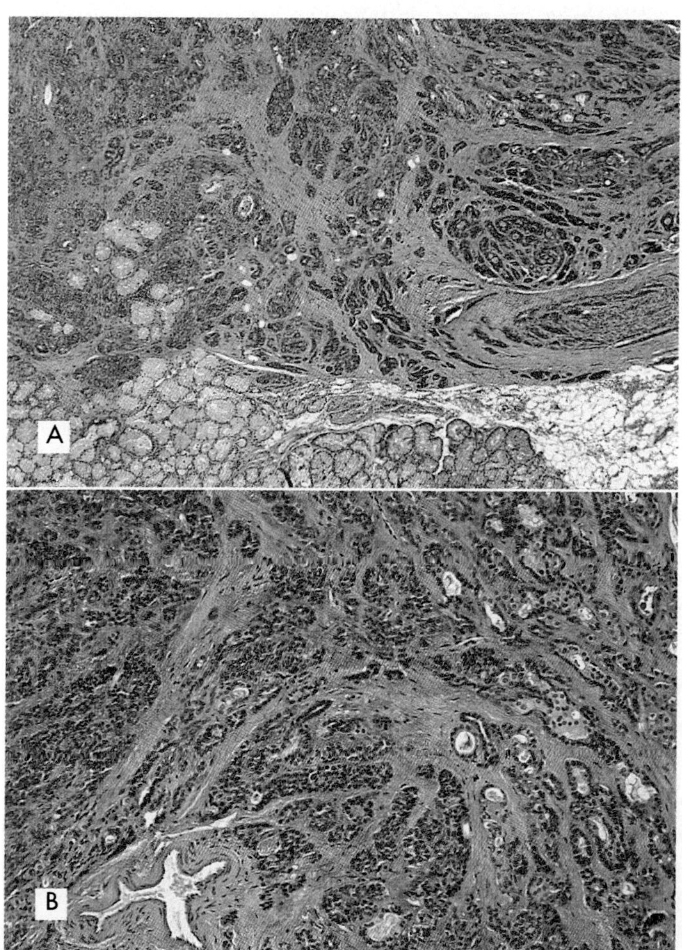

Fig. 51-37 Polymorphous low-grade adenocarcinoma. Notice the infiltrating margin of tumor, **A,** composed of irregular collections of uniform, bland basaloid tumor cells, **B.**

Therapy and prognosis. The treatment of choice is wide local surgical excision with the possible addition of radiation therapy in the event of recurrences. Polymorphous low-grade adenocarcinoma has a recurrence rate of 24%; cervical lymph node metastasis may rarely occur (6% of patients). Distant metastatic lesions have not been documented up to now. Only one patient has died of disease, and this was the result of extensive local recurrence with invasion of vital contiguous structures.[147]

Some authors consider low-grade papillary adenocarcinomas arising in the palate as a subtype of polymorphous low-grade adenocarcinoma.[157] These tumors are histologically different and distinct from polymorphous low-grade adenocarcinoma and are more aggressive biologically; therefore we believe they should be classified as papillary cystadenocarcinoma or papillary adenocarcinoma.

Malignant sebaceous neoplasms

Primary sebaceous neoplasms of salivary gland origin are extremely uncommon; fewer than 40 cases have been reported in the world literature to date.[95,158-163] Malignant neoplasms with sebaceous differentiation can be classified into three separate categories: sebaceous carcinoma, sebaceous lymphadenocarcinoma, and malignant salivary gland tumors with sebaceous differentiation.

Sebaceous carcinoma

Sebaceous carcinoma is the most common of the three types and is composed of variably sized nests or sheets of sebaceous cells showing different degrees of maturity, pleomorphism, nuclear atypia, and invasiveness (Fig. 51-38). The age distribution of this tumor is a biphasic, with a peak incidence in both

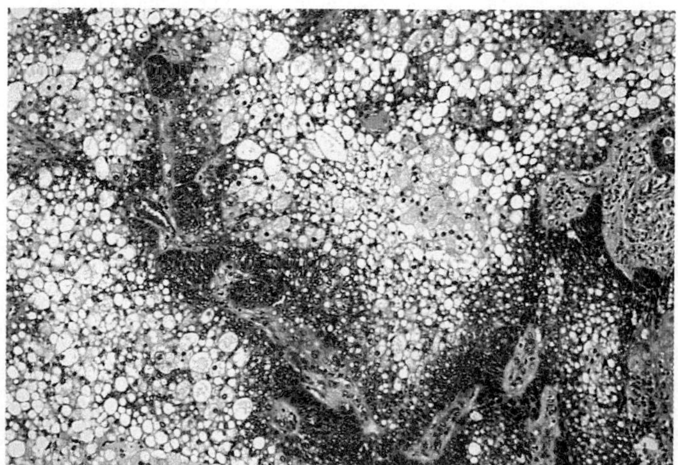

Fig. 51-38 Sebaceous carcinoma composed of atypical basaloid cells with minimal cytoplasm that mature into cells with abundant clear cytoplasm.

the third and in the seventh and eighth decades.[95,158] Patients commonly present with painful masses and often have facial paralysis.

Pathology. Tumors have ranged up to 6 cm in their maximum diameter and were described either as encapsulated or locally invasive. Cellular pleomorphism and cytologic atypia are uniformly present; tumor cells are hyperchromatic and contain abundant clear to slightly eosinophilic cytoplasm. Foci of necrosis and fibrosis are common; perineural invasion may be observed.

Treatment and prognosis. Wide surgical excision together with adjunctive radiation therapy is the treatment of choice for higher-stage tumors. The 5-year survival rate of 62% is slightly less than that in patients with similar tumors arising in the skin and orbit.[95] The longest recorded survival, 13 years, occurred in a patient who was 22 years old at the time of diagnosis; however, because of insufficient data, it is not yet possible to predict whether the survival rates differ between younger and older patients.

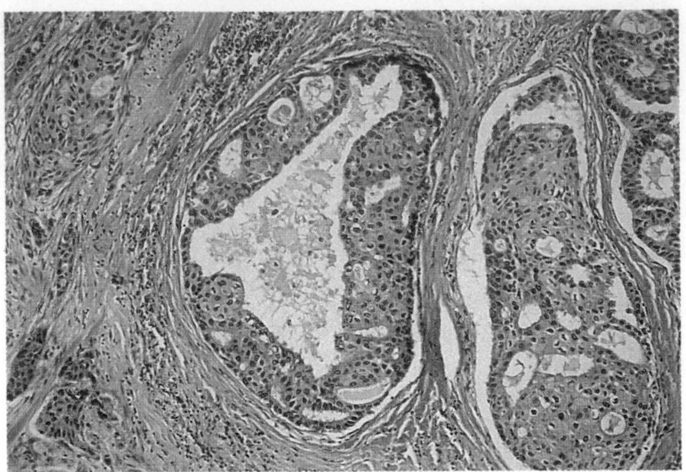

Fig. 51-39 Salivary duct carcinoma. Notice the tumor nests with back-to-back glands and areas of cribriform growth resembling ductal carcinoma of the breast.

Sebaceous lymphadenocarcinoma

Sebaceous lymphadenocarcinoma, the rarest primary sebaceous tumor, with only three reported cases,[95,158,163] is a carcinoma arising in an otherwise benign sebaceous lymphadenoma. All three patients were in their sixties, and their tumors arose in the parotid gland or in a periparotid lymph node. Appropriate therapy consists of wide local excision with the possible addition of adjunctive radiation therapy when tumors are clinically aggressive. Available follow-up information is minimal, but pulmonary metastasis did occur in one patient.

Rarely other malignant salivary gland tumors exhibit focal sebaceous differentiation. This is most common in carcinoma ex pleomorphic adenoma, but it has also been noted in mucoepidermoid and adenoid cystic carcinoma.[95,164]

Salivary duct carcinoma

Salivary duct carcinoma was initially described by Kleinsasser and associates in 1968.[165] Since its initial description, many have used this term in a more generic sense to refer to any primary adenocarcinoma that demonstrates focal ductal differentiation. Although many tumors originate from the salivary duct system, we believe this term should be reserved *only* for tumors that histologically resemble ductal carcinomas of the breast.

Salivary duct carcinoma is uncommon, but its incidence in our experience is greater than the incidences cited in the literature. Up to now, more than 100 cases have been described.[166] These tumors usually arise in men older than 50 years of age; more than 80% involve the parotid gland, with occasional tumors arising in the submandibular gland or in minor salivary glands.[162] Typically the tumor is of relatively recent onset and has shown rapid growth, but occasionally the clinical histories are longer.

Pathology. These tumors are usually infiltrative and poorly circumscribed and may range up to 7 cm in their greatest dimension. Histologically the tumor is arranged in nests or cords composed of atypical cells, usually containing abundant eosinophilic cytoplasm, that form back-to-back glands and often exhibit cribriform, papillary, or solid patterns (Fig. 51-39). Cellular pleomorphism may vary from mild to severe. Rarely an apocrine-like change may be seen. The comedo type of necrosis is common and often abundant but is occasionally absent. An associated intraductal component is usually present, which helps identify this neoplasm as a primary one. Rare tumors are found to have only an intraductal component. A desmoplastic reaction may be prominent in invasive tumors, and vascular or perineural growth, or both, is a frequent finding. Intracytoplasmic and intraductal mucin material is also found occasionally.

Therapy and prognosis. Salivary duct carcinoma is an aggressive, high-grade malignant tumor that should be treated with wide surgical excision combined with irradiation. In addition, because of the high incidence (59%) of cervical nodal metastasis, the neck should be treated with lymph node dissection or irradiation. Approximately 33% of patients have suffered local recurrence and 46% have developed distant metastases; more than 60% of patients have died of their disease, usually within 4 years of diagnosis.[166]

Basal cell adenocarcinoma

Basal cell adenocarcinoma is the malignant counterpart of basal cell adenoma. To date more than 43 cases have been reported, amounting to approximately 1% to 2% of all malignant epithelial salivary gland tumors in the Armed Forces Institute of Pathology (AFIP) Registry.[167] Ninety-one percent of the tumors have involved the parotid gland, and the remaining 9% have arisen in the submandibular gland. This tumor appears to occur in adults, 80% of the patients are more than 50 years of age, and they range in age from 27 to 92 years. Swelling is the principal presenting symptom, but pain or tenderness are also occasionally noted.

Pathology. The tumors average 2 cm in their maximum diameter but can be as large as 4 cm. Microscopically the tumor is composed of variably sized nests or cords of cells with a histological appearance similar to that of basal cell adenoma (Fig. 51-40); however, unlike basal cell adenoma, the tumor grows in an infiltrative, destructive fashion, and necrosis and an active mitotic rate have also been noted in a few cases. Cellular and nuclear pleomorphism are minimal. Approximately a third of the tumors have exhibited perineural invasion and almost a fourth intravascular growth.[167] In addition, approximately 10% of patients have had associated der-

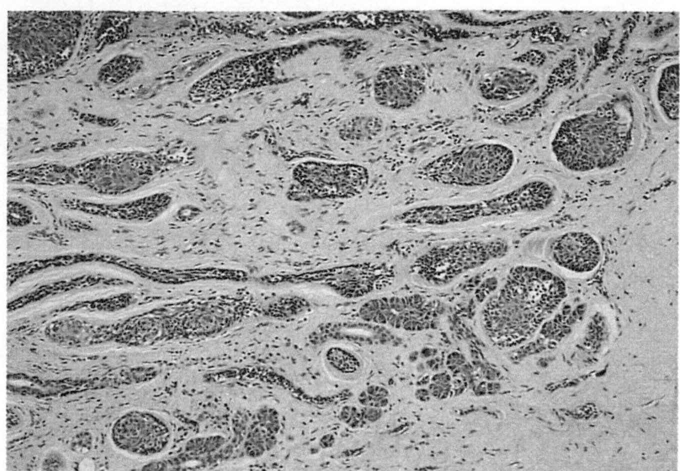

Fig. 51-40 Basal cell adenocarcinoma with numerous nests of tumor resembling the appearance of basal cell adenoma but growing in an infiltrative, destructive fashion.

mal cylindromas of the scalp, a finding similar to that noted in patients with basal cell adenoma.

Therapy and prognosis. The treatment of these neoplasms is similar to that adopted for other low-grade carcinomas of salivary gland origin and is by complete surgical excision with a neck dissection performed only in patients who have evidence of metastatic disease. Slightly more than 25% of the patients have suffered recurrence, and 12% have developed metastasis to cervical lymph nodes; one of the patients in the latter group also had metastatic spread to the lung. One patient died as a result of local spread of the disease.[168]

Undifferentiated carcinoma

Undifferentiated carcinomas of salivary gland origin are unusual and most commonly involve the parotid gland, though rarely they have been reported to arise in the submandibular or minor salivary glands. Undifferentiated carcinomas account for approximately 0.4% to 1% of the epithelial tumors arising in the salivary glands.[169,170] Three subtypes are described here: *lymphoepithelial carcinoma,* also known as *malignant lymphoepithelial lesion; undifferentiated large cell carcinoma;* and *undifferentiated small cell carcinoma.*

Lymphoepithelial carcinoma

Lymphoepithelial carcinomas occur mostly in North American and Greenland Eskimos and in Asians.[171] More than 100 cases have been reported. The parotid gland is involved in more than 90% of the tumors arising in the Eskimo and white population and a third to a half of the tumors in the Oriental population arise in the submandibular gland. Patients complain of an indurated mass, and this is often associated with pain or discomfort. The lymphoepithelial carcinoma that occurs in the white population may be associated with benign lymphoepithelial lesion, but in those patients living in the Arctic region, there is no association with either benign lymphoepithelial lesion or Sjögren's syndrome. Although the histologic appearance of this lesion is identical to that of similar tumors in the nasopharynx, the association of Epstein-Barr virus with the salivary gland lesions is much less than that observed for similar tumors in the nasopharynx.[171] Because of the histologic similarity of salivary gland tumors to nasopharyngeal primary tumors, a nasopharynx primary tumor must be ruled out before a tumor can be considered a primary.

Pathology. Lymphoepitheliomas present as solid masses averaging 2 to 3 cm in diameter. Microscopically they are composed of sheets or irregular nests, or both, that may interconnect and are surrounded by a benign dense lymphoid stroma. Tumor cells are large and have somewhat vesicular nuclei and abundant cytoplasm but show no evidence of keratinization or glandular differentiation (Fig. 51-41). Perineural invasion is frequent, and mitotic activity is easy to find. Tumors that arise in Eskimos seem to behave more aggressively, with higher rates of regional metastasis (30% to 50%) and distant metastasis (30% to 40%) than those noted for Oriental patients with similar tumors.[171]

Treatment and prognosis. Several observers have classified the tumors as high and low grade on the basis of the presence or absence of circumscription, the cytologic features, and the amount of the lymphoid component. Patients with low-grade tumors have fared extremely well with only a minimal mortality. By contrast, the prognosis in patients with high-grade tumors is very poor, with a high incidence of local recurrence and of regional and distant metastases. Most have died within 2 years of the diagnosis. Treatment should be by a complete surgical excision, possibly in combination with radiotherapy. Unfortunately, a rapid downhill course is almost always inevitable in patients with high-grade tumors regardless of the therapy used.

Large cell undifferentiated carcinoma

There are only scant data on large cell undifferentiated carcinomas because in most studies the data on the large or small cell variants are not segregated. In one Japanese study two thirds of these tumors were found to present in the fourth to fifth decades, but in a study from the AFIP, most of the tumors presented in the sixth, seventh, and ninth decades.[171,172]

Pathology. Large cell undifferentiated carcinomas are usually poorly encapsulated and markedly infiltrative, and they commonly invade adjacent skin and soft tissues. They are

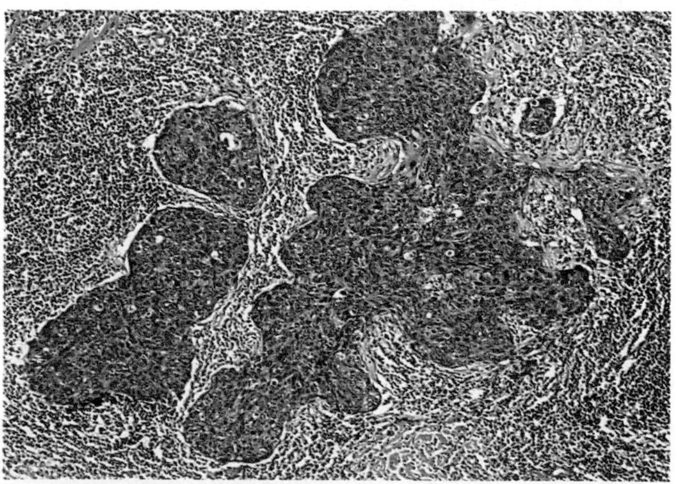

Fig. 51-41 Undifferentiated carcinoma of the lymphoepithelial type composed of collections of poorly differentiated carcinoma cells surrounded by lymphocytes.

solid and grayish white, and areas of necrosis may be prominent. These tumors are defined as a malignant epithelial neoplasm that is too poorly differentiated to be placed in any of the other better-recognized groups of carcinomas. A few authors include very minor foci of more recognizable forms of carcinoma with them.[173,174] The tumor cells are usually polygonal or spindle shaped and form sheets, trabeculae, or thin cords that may be separated by a fibrovascular stroma. Mitotic activity is usually brisk, and hemorrhage and necrosis may be noted. Occasional tumors also have a small cell component. The differential diagnosis consists of lymphoma, amelanotic melanoma, metastatic carcinoma (especially from a nasopharyngeal primary), primary lymphoepithelial carcinoma, olfactory neuroblastoma, and various sarcomas.

Therapy and prognosis. Wide local excision and aggressive radiotherapy are the treatments of choice. Follow-up data are minimal, but these tumors are typically aggressive, with local recurrences, regional nodal metastasis and distant metastasis occurring in more than half of the patients; more than 60% of the patients died of tumor-related causes.[175] Tumor size seems to predict behavior; patients with tumors exceeding 4 cm have survived a mean of 7.7 months and all have died of their disease; those with tumors less than 4 cm have survived a mean of 46 months, and 50% have died of their disease.[175]

Small cell carcinoma

Small cell carcinoma of salivary gland origin is histologically identical to small cell carcinomas of the lung. These are rare primary salivary gland tumors; less than 65 have been reported to arise in the major salivary glands.[171,176-182] However, there may be a higher incidence of occurrence in the minor salivary glands where small cell carcinoma accounted for 2.8% of 492 minor salivary gland tumors.[51] Small cell carcinomas most often occur during the fifth to seventh decades, but tumors have been found in patients ranging from 5 to 84 years of age. These tumors are slightly more common in men than in women, and on gross examination are found to be poorly circumscribed and infiltrative.

Pathology. Histologically, small cell carcinomas are composed of sheets, ribbons, or nests of anaplastic round to oval cells with hyperchromatic nuclei and minimal (small cell subtype) (Fig. 51-42) to moderate (intermediate subtype) amounts of cytoplasm. Nucleoli, if present, are inconspicuous. Mitoses are frequent, and tumor necrosis is usually prominent. Vascular and perineural tumor invasion is often noted, and true rosette formation may be found. Focal areas of ductal differentiation may also be observed, and occasionally areas of the small cell carcinoma seem to arise from basilar and ductal epithelium. Current immunohistochemical evidence indicates that all small cell salivary gland carcinomas may have neuroendocrine characteristics, though only 30% are found to actually contain neuroendocrine granules on ultrastructural examination.[183]

Treatment and prognosis. The treatment of choice is wide local excision. Lymphadenectomy is performed only when disease is palpable because this tumor commonly metastasizes hematogenously, a behavior similar to that of small cell carcinoma elsewhere in the body. Small cell carcinomas arising in the salivary glands may metastasize to cervical lymph nodes and other body sites; however, they do not metastasize as frequently as small cell carcinomas of the lung or larynx do. Their prognosis also is better. The 2- and 5-year survival rates for patients with small cell carcinomas arising in the major

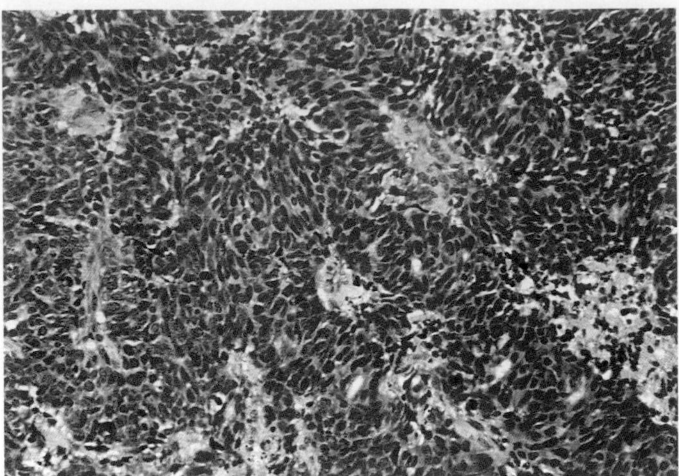

Fig. 51-42 Small cell carcinoma composed of interconnecting ribbons of oval, hyperchromatic tumor cells with minimal cytoplasm.

salivary glands are 70% and 46%, respectively[176]; the rates for those with tumors arising in the larynx are only 16% and 5% respectively.[184] Survival figures for small cell carcinoma of the lung are similar to those of the larynx. The survival rates in patients with small cell carcinomas arising primarily in the minor salivary glands appear to be better than those in patients with tumors arising in the lung.[185]

Oncocytic carcinoma

Oncocytic carcinoma is the malignant counterpart of benign oncocytoma. It is an uncommon salivary gland neoplasm that accounts for approximately 5% of the oncocytic salivary gland tumors.[186] To date approximately 50 cases predominantly involving the parotid gland (more than 75% of patients) have been reported, with occasional tumors documented in the submandibular gland, oral cavity, nasal cavity, and neck.[162] These tumors usually arise in the elderly, with an average age at occurrence of approximately 60 years. Rarely, tumors occur in middle-aged persons.

Pathology. Histologically, tumors are composed of large polygonal, round, or oval cells with abundant eosinophilic, finely granular cytoplasm that may be arranged in sheets or cords; occasionally they assume an alveolar pattern. There is a much greater degree of nuclear and cellular pleomorphism, and the number of mitotic figures is greater than that found in benign oncocytoma (Fig. 51-43). These tumors are usually unencapsulated and infiltrate into adjacent glandular or soft tissues. Vascular or neural invasion, or both, may be noted. It can occasionally be difficult to differentiate it from benign oncocytoma because the benign neoplasm may be multifocal and unencapsulated; often multiple foci of benign oncocytosis are accompanying features. These foci should not be construed as malignant. The finding of a destructive, infiltrating growth pattern, usually associated with cellular pleomorphism and atypia, vascular or neural invasion, or evidence of metastatic spread, or combinations of these findings, is necessary to establish the diagnosis of malignancy.

Therapy and prognosis. The treatment of choice is predominantly surgical and is by wide local excision and preservation of the facial nerve if possible. Adjunctive radiation therapy and possibly lymph node dissection should be consid-

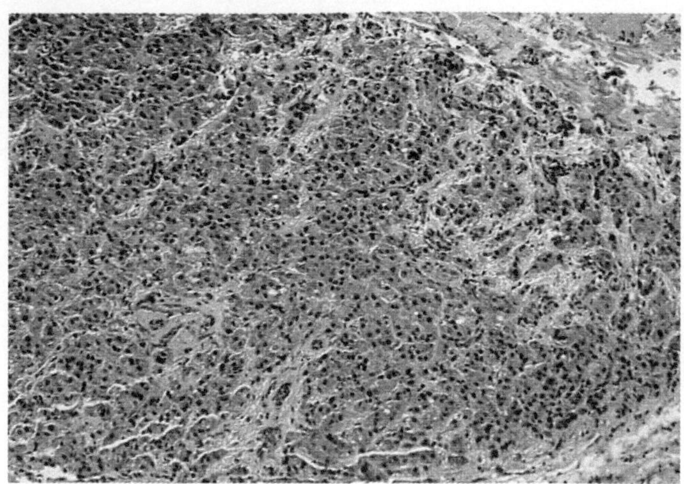

Fig. 51-43 Oncocytic carcinoma composed of an infiltrating sheet of moderately atypical tumor cells with abundant eosinophilic cytoplasm.

ered in patients with higher-stage disease. Follow-up information in the literature is scant; however, the tumor has recurred in approximately a third of the reported cases; 60% of the patients have suffered regional lymph node or distant metastasis and approximately 30% have died of their disease.[162]

Epidermoid carcinoma

Primary epidermoid carcinoma, also known as *squamous cell carcinoma,* is rare in salivary glands. It should be distinguished from squamous cell carcinoma of the mucosa or skin invading the salivary glands and from metastatic lesions originating from other organs. In our experience most epidermoid carcinomas involving the salivary glands represent metastatic lesions from other sites. However, according to the literature, primary epidermoid carcinomas constitute 1.6% to 3.6% of all benign and malignant salivary gland tumors from all sites and 6% to 13.9% of all malignant tumors arising in the major salivary glands.[187] In addition, several investigators have noted an increased incidence of epidermoid carcinoma in patients who have undergone radiotherapy in the head and neck regions.[103,199] Epidermoid carcinomas usually arise in the parotid glands (75% to 88% of tumors) of elderly men in the sixth or seventh decade.[103,187-189] These are clinically aggressive tumors; in one series almost 60% of the patients had facial nerve paralysis at the time of presentation.[189]

Pathology. Grossly, tumors are unencapsulated, poorly demarcated, white, and hard. Histologically these tumors are similar to epidermoid carcinomas at other sites, ranging from low-grade highly keratinized neoplasms to poorly differentiated sheets of tumors cells with minimal keratinization. Adjacent soft tissue invasion and regional metastasis are common.

The differential diagnosis includes metastatic squamous cell carcinoma and high-grade mucoepidermoid carcinoma. The former is identified by careful clinical evaluation; the finding of intracellular mucin-containing cells in the neoplasm is necessary to establish a diagnosis of the latter. Although slight keratin production may be found in mucoepidermoid carcinomas, extensive keratinization is exceedingly unusual and much more common in primary or metastatic epidermoid carcinoma.

Treatment and prognosis. Treatment is by radical parotidectomy or submandibulectomy, usually combined with radical neck dissection and adjunct postoperative radiotherapy. Biologically these are aggressive tumors; treatment fails in more than 60% of patients during the first year.[188] Cervical lymph node metastasis occurs in almost 50%, and approximately a third of patients develop metastasis. Cure rates at 5, 10, 15, and 20 years are 24%, 18%, 17%, and 17% respectively.[188] The fact that there is no significant change in these survival rates highlights the importance of 5-year follow-up in patients with these neoplasms; this is in contrast to the gradually declining rates observed in patients with most other forms of malignant salivary gland neoplasia.

Adenocarcinoma, not otherwise specified

Many of the previously described malignant salivary gland tumors are adenocarcinomas, but their histomorphologic features are specific enough to allow them to be meaningfully classified into a defined group. *Adenocarcinoma, not otherwise specified,* is a term that should be reserved for those salivary gland neoplasms exhibiting histologic characteristics typical of adenocarcinoma but not displaying histomorphologic features that allow them to be classified as one of the more typically recognized variants. If classified in this way, these neoplasms would rank as the third to fifth most common malignant neoplasms arising in the salivary glands. Approximately two thirds involve the minor salivary glands or seromucinous glands of the upper respiratory tract and a third involve the major salivary glands.[190] The parotid gland is the most common site of those tumors arising in the major glands and oral cavity.[191] Patients usually have asymptomatic solitary masses, but occasionally patients complain of pain. The histologic appearance is quite variable, and the diagnosis of adenocarcinoma, not otherwise specified, depends on the exclusion of more characteristic variants of salivary gland carcinoma. Tumors may range from low to high grade and should be classified on the basis of their grade because there is good correlation with survival rates in patients with grade I and grade III tumors. These are associated with 69% and 8% 5-year survival rates and 54% and 3% 15-year rates respectively.[190] The most accurate predictor of outcome appears to be clinical stage: stage I, II, and III tumors are associated with 15-year cure rates of 67%, 35%, and 8% respectively. Treatment for low-grade and low-stage tumors should be wide local excision, but tumors of a higher grade and stage should be treated more aggressively with adjunctive radiotherapy and treatment to the neck requiring irradiation or lymph node dissection, or both.

Cystadenocarcinoma

Cystadenocarcinomas are dominated by large cystic structures lined by epithelium that often may exhibit a papillary growth pattern.[162] These tumors do not display the histologic features characteristic of recognizable forms of salivary gland carcinomas that may form cystic structures, such as acinic cell carcinoma, mucoepidermoid carcinoma, or polymorphous low-grade adenocarcinoma. We would classify the low-grade papillary adenocarcinoma reported by Mills and coworkers[192] as cystadenocarcinomas. We do not believe these represent a special subtype of polymorphous low-grade adenocarcinoma. Cystadenocarcinomas are rare in our experience, and many contain mucicarmine-positive intracellular or extracellular material. The cells lining the cystic spaces vary from tall

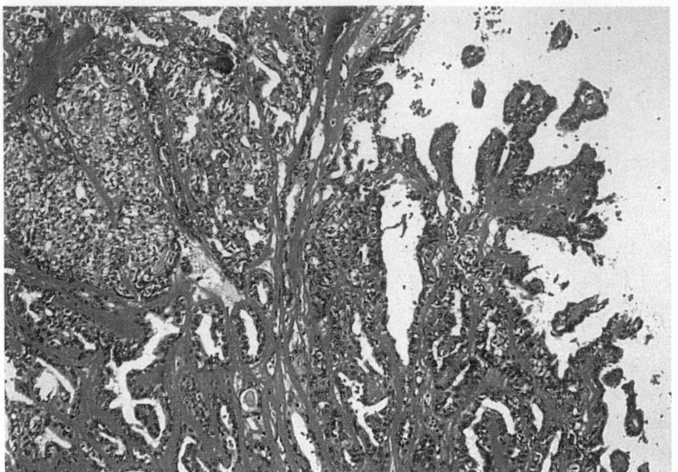

Fig. 51-44 Low-grade papillary cystadenocarcinoma. Notice the solid growth *(upper left)* and papillary cystic growth *(right)*.

columnar to cuboidal to simple squamous and may be mucus secreting or have areas of clear, oncocytic, or basaloid features (Fig. 51-44). Papillary features are common. Solid areas, usually located between cystic spaces, may be found.

These tumors are usually unencapsulated but may range from being encapsulated to being markedly invasive. Many of the tumors are of low to moderate grade, but occasional tumors are of high grade. Because of the rarity of this neoplasm and differences in the classification criteria used in various series, specific survival data are not available. The prognosis varies depending on the grade and clinical stage of the tumor, with the survival rate and prognosis in patients with lower-grade and lower clinical stage neoplasms being much better than those in patients with higher-stage and higher-grade neoplasms. Treatment should therefore be determined by the grade and stage of the tumor.

Malignant myoepithelioma

Malignant myoepithelioma or myoepithelial carcinoma is one of the rarest salivary gland neoplasms. Fewer than 10 cases have been reported in the world literature.[162] These tumors are similar histologically to benign myoepithelioma in that they have plasmacytoid and spindle cell features; however, they are invasive and grow in a more aggressive, destructive fashion than their benign counterpart, showing greater cellular pleomorphism, atypia, and increased mitotic activity. The proper treatment is wide surgical excision and possibly also irradiation in patients with higher-stage and higher-grade neoplasms.

Mucinous adenocarcinoma

Mucinous adenocarcinoma is a poorly characterized and defined neoplasm, not fitting into any of the previously described groups of neoplasms that have the common histologic feature of very prominent mucin-secreting tumor cells. Many of the mucin-secreting neoplasms described in the literature have characteristics more common to the cystadenocarcinoma group, and therefore are included in this category. Primary mucinous carcinomas of salivary gland origin are extremely unusual and histologically are similar to the mucin-secreting neoplasms that arise in the skin and breast. Because of their rarity, their clinical behavior is difficult to predict. Additional studies that isolate this tumor and better characterize their clinical behavior are necessary.

Metastasis to major salivary glands

Metastatic involvement of the major salivary glands or of the lymph nodes adjacent to the major salivary glands is common. The parotid glands contain from 3 to 32 (average, 20) intraglandular lymph nodes that are interconnected by a plexus of lymph vessels that drain the skin from the side of the head above the parotid gland and in the eye areas, as well as the nose, upper lip, external auditory canal, eustachian tube, and tympanic membrane.[193,194] In comparison, the submandibular gland proper does not contain any intraparenchymal lymph nodes.

Metastasis to the parotid region and submandibular gland is fairly common, and such lesions constitute 1% to 42% of salivary gland neoplasms in various series.[194] Approximately 90% of the metastatic tumors involve the parotid region, with the remainder involving the submandibular gland. Metastasis to the sublingual gland has not been reported. Epidermoid carcinoma and melanoma are the most common neoplasms metastasizing to the major salivary gland area, accounting for 60% and 14.5% of the metastatic tumors, respectively. Eighty-four percent of the tumors that metastasized to the parotid or parotid area originated in the head and neck region, with 85% arising from skin sites in the head and neck region. Only 14% of the metastatic tumors originated from sites other than the head or neck, most commonly the lung, kidney, and breast.[194] The opposite was true of the lesions in the submandibular gland, with 85% arising from sites other than the head or neck, most commonly also the breast, kidney, and lung.[194]

Mesenchymal neoplasms

Nonepithelial tumors, excluding lymphoid neoplasms, account for 1.9% to 4.5% of salivary gland tumors,[169,195,196] with benign neoplasms being more common than sarcomas. The ratio of benign to malignant mesenchymal neoplasms varies from series to series and ranges from 18:1 to 2.4:1.[169,196] More than 85% of soft-tissue neoplasms involve the parotid gland, more than 10% arise in the submandibular gland, and only rarely does a tumor involve the sublingual gland.

Vascular tumors are the most common benign mesenchymal neoplasm, representing almost 40% of the benign tumors. Seventy-five percent to 80% of vascular neoplasms are hemangiomas, and they occur most frequently in children in the first decade. Most of the other vascular tumors are lymphangiomas. Other types of benign soft-tissue neoplasms arising in the major salivary glands include neural tumors, fibrous tumors, lipomas, and miscellaneous other tumors (Table 51-1).

Patients with salivary gland *sarcomas* are older than those with the benign counterpart of this tumor. Virtually any type of sarcoma can arise primarily in the salivary gland (Table 51-2). In the largest published series,[197] hemangiopericytoma, malignant schwannoma, fibrosarcoma, and malignant fibrous histiocytoma were the most common neoplasms, accounting for 16%, 15%, 14%, and 11% of the sarcomas, respectively. These are aggressive neoplasms, with 40% to 64% of patients suffering recurrence, 38% to 64% developing metastasis (usually hematogenous), and 36% to 64% dying of their disease, most often within 3 years of diagnosis.[197,198] The most successful treatment has been wide surgical excision or surgery combined with irradiation.

Table 51-1 Benign mesenchymal salivary gland tumors

Type of tumor	AFIP Registry[169]	University of Hamburg Registry[196]	Total	%
Vascular/lymphatic				
Hemangioma	67	39	106	32
Lymphangioma	16	14	30	9
Mixed hemangioma and lymphangioma	—	7	7	2
Hemangiopericytoma	—	3	3	1
Neural tumors				
Schwannoma	36	9	45	14
Neurofibroma	31	9	40	12
Neurofibromatosis	—	3	3	1
Meningioma	1	—	1	0.3
Adipose tissue				
Lipoma	19	22	41	12
Fibrous tissue				
Nodular fasciitis	17	—	17	5
Fibrous histiocytoma	11	—	11	3
Fibromatosis	8	—	8	2
Myxoma	3	—	3	1
Myofibromatosis	1	—	1	0.3
Fibroma	—	1	1	0.3
Smooth muscle				
Angiomyoma	3	—	3	1
Other				
Granular cell tumor	3	2	5	1.5
Giant cell tumor	3	—	3	1
Glomangioma	1	—	1	0.3
Osteochondroma	—	2	2	0.6
TOTAL	220	111	331	

AFIP, Armed Forces Institute of Pathology.

Table 51-2 Nonlymphoid salivary gland sarcomas

Tumor type	AFIP Registry[169]	Luna et al[198]	University of Hamburg Registry[196]
Hemangiopericytoma	14	—	—
Malignant schwannoma	13	2	2
Fibrosarcoma	12	2	—
Malignant fibrous histiocytoma	9	3	4
Rhabdomyosarcoma	7	2	2
Angiosarcoma	5	—	—
Synovial sarcoma	4	—	—
Kaposi's sarcoma	3	3*	—
Leiomyosarcoma	3	—	—
Liposarcoma	2	—	—
Alveolar soft part sarcoma	2	—	—
Epithelioid sarcoma	1	—	—
Extraosseous chondrosarcoma	1	—	—
Osteosarcoma	—	2	—
Malignant hemangioendothelioma	—	—	1
Sarcoma, poorly differentiated	9	—	—
TOTAL	85	14	9

AFIP, Armed Forces Institute of Pathology.
*Arose in intraparotid lymph nodes.

Malignant lymphoma

Malignant lymphomas originating in salivary glands are unusual, accounting for 2.5% to 4.5% of salivary gland tumors and 7.5% to 16% of all malignant salivary gland tumors.[169,199-201] More than 90% are non-Hodgkin's lymphoma. The parotid is the salivary gland most commonly involved by lymphoma, but the submandibular gland may be involved in 15% to 23% of patients.[199] Involvement of the sublingual gland is rare.

Salivary gland lymphomas may be divided into those that develop in association with a benign lymphoepithelial lesion or Sjögren's syndrome and those that do not. Most primary lymphomas fall into the latter category. Lymphomas not associated with Sjögren's syndrome are usually B-cell or follicular center cell tumors, but may be of other types as well. A follicular pattern is found in most tumors and appears to account for the favorable clinical outcome in many of the patients with these tumors. Approximately 60% of lymphomas are of low grade; high-grade tumors are unusual.

REFERENCES

General reviews and developmental disorders

1. Seifert G, Miehlke A, Haubrich J et al, editors: *Diseases of salivary glands,* Stuttgart, 1986, Georg Thieme Verlag.
2. Dardick I: Histogenesis and morphogenesis of salivary gland tumors. In Ellis GL, Auclair PL, Gnepp DR, editors: *Surgical pathology of the salivary glands,* Philadelphia, 1991, Saunders.
3. Warnock GR, Jensen JL, Kratochvil FJ: Developmental diseases. In Ellis GL, Auclair PL, Gnepp DR, editors: *Surgical pathology of the salivary glands,* Philadelphia, 1991, Saunders.
4. Zajtchuk JT, Patow CA, Hyams V: Cervical heterotopic salivary gland neoplasms: a diagnostic dilemma, *Otolaryngol Head Neck Surg* 90:178, 1981.
5. Arafat A, Brannon RB, Ellis GL: Adenomatoid hyperplasia of mucous salivary glands, *Oral Surg Oral Med Oral Pathol* 52:51, 1981.
6. Seifert G, Thomsen ST, Donath K: Bilateral dysgenetic parotid glands: morphological analysis and differential diagnosis of a rare disease of the salivary glands, *Virchows Arch [A] (Pathol Anat Histopathol)* 390:273, 1981.
7. Dobson CM, Ellis HA: Polycystic disease of the parotid glands: case report of a new entity and review of the literature, *Histopathology* 11:953, 1987.

Obstructive disorders

8. Zafarulla MYM: Cervical mucocele (plunging ranula): an unusual case of mucous extravasation cyst, *Oral Surg Oral Med Oral Pathol* 62:63, 1986.
9. Koudelka BM: Obstruction disorders. In Ellis GL, Auclair PL, Gnepp DR, editors: *Surgical pathology of the salivary glands,* Philadelphia, 1991, Saunders.
10. Shafer WG, Hine MK, Levy BM: A textbook of oral pathology, ed 4, Philadelphia, 1983, Saunders.
11. Anneroth G, Eneroth CM, Isacsson G: Morphology of salivary calculi: the distribution of the inorganic component, *J Oral Pathol* 4:257, 1975.

Sialadenitis and related conditions

12. Seifert G, Miehlke A, Haubrich J et al, editors: *Diseases of salivary glands,* Stuttgart, 1986, Georg Thieme Verlag.
13. Fajardo FE, Berthrong LF: Radiation injury in surgical pathology: Part III. Salivary glands, pancreas, and skin, *Am J Surg Pathol* 5:279, 1981.
14. Werning J: Infections and systemic diseases. In Ellis GL, Auclair RL, Gnepp DR, editors: *Surgical pathology of the salivary glands,* Philadelphia, 1991, Saunders.
15. Hanson D, St. Siegel Strano AJ, Primack A et al: Mumps virus sialadenitis: an autopsy report, *Arch Pathol* 92:469, 1971.
16. Drew WL: Diagnosis of cytomegalovirus infection, *Rev Infect Dis* 10:S468, 1988.
17. Jacobsen MA, Mills J: Serious cytomegalovirus disease in the acquired immunodeficiency syndrome (AIDS), *Ann Intern Med* 108:585, 1988.
18. Marder MZ, Barr CE, Mandel ID: Cytomegalovirus presence and salivary composition in acquired immunodeficiency syndrome, *Oral Surg Oral Med Oral Pathol* 60:372, 1985.
19. Pialoux G, Ravisse P, Trotot P et al: Cytomegalovirus infection of the submandibular gland in a patient with AIDS, *Rev Infect Dis* 13:338, 1991.
20. Scott GB, Buck BE, Leterman JG et al: Acquired immunodeficiency syndrome in infants, *N Engl J Med* 310:76, 1984.

Sjögren's syndrome

21. Bloch KS, Buchanan WW, Whol MJ et al: Sjögren's syndrome: a clinical, pathological, and serological study of sixty-two cases, *Medicine* 44:187, 1965.
22. Moutsopoulos HM, Mann DL, Johnson AH et al: Genetic differences between primary and secondary sicca syndrome, *N Engl J Med* 301:761, 1979.
23. Daniels TE: Benign lymphoepithelial lesions and Sjögren's syndrome. In Ellis GL, Auclair PL, Gnepp DR, editors: *Surgical pathology of the salivary glands* Philadelphia, 1992, Saunders.
24. Ostberg Y: The clinical picture of benign lymphoepithelial lesions, *Clin Otolaryngol* 8:381, 1983.
25. Chudwin DS, Daniels TE, Wara DW et al: Spectrum of Sjögren syndrome in children, *J Pediatr* 98:213, 1981.
26. Whitcher JP: Clinical diagnosis of dry eye, *Int Ophthalmol Clin* 27:7, 1987.
27. Daniels TE, Silverman S, Michalski JP et al: The oral components of Sjögren's syndrome, *Oral Surg Oral Med Oral Pathol* 39:875, 1975.
28. Sam PM, Shugar JM, Train JS, Biller HF: Manifestations of parotid gland enlargement: radiographic, pathologic, and clinical correlations. Part I. The autoimmune pseudosialectasis, *Radiology* 141:415, 1981.
29. Chisholm DM, Waterhouse JP, Mason DK: Lymphocytic sialadenitis in the major and minor glands: a correlation in postmortem subjects, *J Clin Pathol* 23:690, 1970.
30. Botram V, Hjorting-Hansen E: Punch biopsy of minor salivary glands in the diagnosis of Sjögren's syndrome, *Scand J Dent Res* 78:295, 1970.
31. Chisholm DM, Mason DK: Labial salivary gland biopsy in Sjögren's syndrome, *J Clin Pathol* 21:636, 1968.
32. Batsakis JG: Lymphoepithelial lesion and Sjögren's syndrome, *Ann Otol Rhinol Laryngol* 96:354, 1987.
33. Kassan S, Thomas T, Moutsopoulos HM et al: Increased risk of lymphoma in sicca syndrome, *Ann Intern Med* 89:888, 1978.
34. Sciubba JJ, Auclair PL, Ellis GL: Malignant lymphoma. In Ellis GL, Auclair RL, Gnepp DR, editors: *Surgical pathology of the salivary glands,* Philadelphia, 1992, Saunders.
35. Shin SS, Sheibani K, Fishleder A et al: Monocytoid B-cell lymphoma in patients with Sjögren's syndrome: a clinicopathologic study of 13 patients, *Hum Pathol* 22:422, 1991.

HIV-infection–associated lymphepithelial cysts

36. Ryan JR, Ioachim HL, Marmer J et al: Acquired immune deficiency syndrome–related lymphoadenopathies presenting in the salivary gland and lymph nodes, *Arch Otolaryngol* 111:554, 1985.
37. Holliday RA, Cohen WA, Schinella RA et al: Benign lymphoepithelial parotid cysts and hyperplastic cervical adenopathy in AID-risk patients: a new CT appearance, *Radiology* 168:439, 1988.
38. Smith FB, Rajdeo H, Panesar N et al: Benign lymphoepithelial lesion of the parotid gland in intravenous drug users, *Arch Pathol Lab Med* 112:742, 1988.
39. Wyman A, Dunn LK, Talati VK et al: Lymphoepithelial "branchial" cysts within the parotid gland, *Br J Surg* 75:818, 1988.
40. Jensen JL: Idiopathic disease. In Ellis G, Auclair P, Gnepp DR, editors: *Surgical pathology of salivary glands,* Philadelphia, 1992, Saunders.

Necrotizing sialometaplasia

41. Abrams AM, Melrose RJ, Howell FV: Necrotizing sialometaplasia: a disease simulating malignancy, *Cancer* 32:130, 1973.
42. Maisel RH, Johnston WH, Anderson HA et al: Necrotizing sialometaplasia involving the nasal cavity, *Laryngoscope* 87:429, 1977.
43. Walker GK, Fechner RE, Johnes ME et al: Necrotizing sialometaplasia of the larynx secondary to atheroscleromatous embolization, *Am J Clin Pathol* 77:221, 1982.

44. Batsakis JG, Manning JT: Necrotizing sialometaplasia of major salivary glands, *J Laryngol Otol* 101:962, 1987.
45. Anneroth G, Hansen LS: Necrotizing sialometaplasia: the relationship of its pathogenesis to its clinical characteristics, *Int J Oral Surg* 11:283, 1982.
46. Brannon RB, Fowler CB, Hartman KS: Necrotizing sialometaplasia: a clinicopathologic study of sixty-nine cases and review of the literature, *Oral Surg Oral Med Oral Pathol* 72:317, 1991.
47. Sneige N, Batsakis JG: Necrotizing sialometaplasia, *Ann Otol Rhynol* 101:282, 1992.
48. Standish SM, Shafer WG: Several histologic effects of rat submandibular and sublingual salivary gland duct and blood vessel ligation, *J Dent Res* 36:866, 1957.

Benign neoplasms

Pleomorphic adenoma

49. Eveson JW, Cawson RA: Salivary gland tumors: a review of 2410 cases with particular reference to histologic types, site, age and sex distribution, *J Pathol* 146:51, 1985.
50. Spiro RH: Salivary neoplasms: overview of 35 year experience with 2807 patients, *Head Neck Surg* 8:177, 1986.
51. Waldron CA, El-Mofty SK, Gnepp DR: Tumors of the intraoral minor salivary glands: a demographic and histopathologic study of 426 cases, *Oral Surg Oral Med Oral Pathol* 66:323, 1988.
52. Waldron CA: Mixed tumor (pleomorphic adenoma) and myoepithelioma. In Ellis GL, Auclair PL, Gnepp DR, editors: *Surgical pathology of the salivary glands,* Philadelphia, 1991, Saunders.
53. Thomas K, Hatt MS: Tyrosine crystals in salivary gland tumors, *J Clin Pathol* 34:1003, 1981.
54. Campbell WGJ, Priest RC, Weathers DR: Characterization of two types of crystalloids in pleomorphic adenomas of minor salivary glands: a light microscopic, electron microscopic and histochemical study, *Am J Pathol* 118:194, 1985.
55. Foot FW Jr, Frazell EL: Tumors of the major salivary glands. In *Atlas of tumor pathology,* section 4, fascicle 2, series 1. Washington, D.C., 1954, Armed Forces Institute of Pathology.
56. Seifert G, Miehlke A, Haubrich J et al: *Diseases of the salivary glands: diagnosis, pathology, treatment, facial nerve surgery,* Stuttgart, 1980, Georg Thieme Verlag.
57. Kroll SO, Boyers RC: Mixed tumors of salivary glands: long term follow up, *Cancer* 30:276, 1972.
58. Woods JE: Parotidectomy versus limited resection for benign parotid masses, *Am J Surg* 149:749, 1985.

Myoepithelioma

59. Sciubba JJ, Brannon R: Myoepithelioma of salivary glands: report of 23 cases, *Cancer* 47:562, 1982.
60. Batsakis JG: Myoepithelioma, *Ann Otol Rhinol Laryngol* 94:523, 1985.
61. Barnes L, Appel BN, Perez H et al: Myoepithelioma of the head and neck: case report and review, *J Surg Oncol* 28:21, 1985.
62. Dardick I, Cavell S, Vorvin M et al: Salivary gland myoepithelioma variants: histological, ultrastructural and immunocytological features, *Virchows Arch [A] (Pathol Anat)* 416:25, 1989.
63. Dardick I, Van Nostrand AWF: Myoepithelial cells in salivary gland tumors—revisited, *Head Neck Surg* 7:395, 1985.
64. Dardick I, Thomas MJ, Van Nostrand AWP: Myoepithelioma: new concepts of histology and classification: a light and electron microscopic study, *Ultrastruct Pathol* 13:187, 1989.
65. El-Mofty SK, O'Leary TR, Swanson PE: Malignant myoepithelioma of salivary glands: clinicopathologic and immunophenotypic features: review of literature and report of 2 new cases, *Int J Surg Pathol 2:133, 1994.*

Papillary cystadenoma lymphomatosum (Warthin's tumor)

66. Chaudry AD, Gorlin RJ: Papillary cystadenoma lymphomatosum, *Am J Surg* 95:923, 1958.
67. Warnock GR: Papillary cystadenoma lymphomatosum (Warthin's tumor). In Ellis GL, Auclair PL, Gnepp DR, editors: *Surgical pathology of the salivary glands,* Philadelphia, 1991, Saunders.
68. Azzopardi JG, Hou LT: The genesis of adenolymphoma, *J Pathol* 88:213, 1964.
69. Shugar JM, Som PM, Biller HF: Warthin's tumor: a multifocal disease, *Ann Otol Rhinol Laryngol* 91:246, 1982.

Canalicular adenoma and basal cell adenoma

70. Mintz GA, Abrams AM, Melrose RJ: Monomorphic adenoma of the major and minor salivary glands: report of 21 cases and review of the literature, *Oral Surg Oral Med Oral Pathol* 53:375, 1982.
71. Kratochvil FJ: Canalicular adenoma and basal cell adenoma. In Ellis GL, Auclair PL, Gnepp DR, editors: *Surgical pathology of the salivary gland,* Philadelphia, 1991, Saunders.
72. Daley TD, Gardner DG, Smout MS: Canalicular adenoma: not a basal cell adenoma, *Oral Surg Oral Med Oral Pathol* 57:181, 1984.
73. Levine J, Krutchkoff DJ, Eisenberg E: Monomorphic adenoma of minor salivary glands: a reappraisal and report of nine new cases, *J Oral Surg* 39:101, 1981.
74. Batsakis JG, Brannon RB, Sciubba JJ: Monomorphic adenoma of major salivary glands: a histologic study of 69 tumours, *Clin Otolaryngol* 6:129, 1981.
75. Ellis GL, Gnepp DR: Unusual salivary gland tumors. In Gnepp DR, editor: *Pathology of the head and neck,* New York, 1988, Churchill Livingstone.
76. Batsakis JG, Brannon RB: Dermal analogue tumors of major salivary glands, *J Laryngol Otol* 95:155, 1981.
77. Ferrandiz C, Campo E, Baumann E: Dermal cylindromas (turban tumor) and eccrine spiradenoma in a patient with membranous basal cell adenoma of the parotid gland, *J Cutan Pathol* 12:72, 1985.
78. Headington JT, Batsakis JG, Beals TF et al: Membranous basal cell adenoma of the parotid gland, dermal cylindroma and trichoepithelioma, *Cancer* 39:2460, 1977.
79. Bernacki EG, Batsakis JG, Johns ME: Basal cell adenoma: distinctive tumor of salivary glands, *Arch Otolaryngol* 99:84, 1974.
80. Hyams BA, Scheithauer BW, Weiland LH et al: Membranous basal cell adenoma of the parotid gland: malignant transformation in a patient with multiple dermal cylindroma, *Arch Pathol Lab Med* 112:209, 1988.
81. Luna MA, Batsakis JG, Tortaledo ME, Del Junco GW: Carcinoma ex-pleomorphic adenoma of salivary glands, *J Laryngol Otol* 103:756, 1989.

Oncocytoma

82. Good RK: Oncocytoma. In Ellis GL, Auclair PL, Gnepp DR, editors: *Surgical pathology of salivary gland tumors,* Philadelphia, 1991, Saunders.
83. Hastrup N, Bretlau P, Kroudahl A et al: Oncocytoma of the salivary glands, *J Laryngol Otol* 96:1027, 1982.
84. Ellis GL: Clear cell oncocytoma of salivary glands, *Hum Pathol* 19:862, 1988.
85. Sun CN, White HJ, Thompson BW: Oncocytoma (mitochondrioma) of the parotid gland: an electron microscopical study, *Arch Pathol Lab Med* 99:208, 1975.
86. Porgel MA: Tumours of the salivary glands: a histological and clinical review, *Br J Oral Surg* 17:47, 1979.
87. Damm DD, White DK, Geissler RH et al: Benign solid oncocytoma of intraoral minor salivary glands, *Oral Surg Oral Med Oral Pathol* 67:84, 1989.
88. Goode RK, Cario RL: Oncocytic adenocarcinoma of salivary glands, *Oral Surg Oral Med Oral Pathol* 65:61, 1988.

Ductal papillomas

89. Ellis GL, Auclair PA: Ductal papillomas. In Ellis GL, Auclair PL, Gnepp DR, editors: *Surgical pathology of the salivary glands,* Philadelphia, 1991, Saunders.
90. Mitre BK: Sialadenoma papilliferum: report of a case and review of literature, *J Oral Maxillofac Surg* 44:469, 1986.
91. Regezi JA, Lloyd RV, Zarbo RJ, McClatchey KD: Minor salivary glands tumors: a histologic and immunohistochemical study, *Cancer* 55:108, 1985.
92. Fantasia JE, Nocco CE, Lally ET: Ultrastructure of sialadenoma papilliferum, *Arch Pathol Lab Med* 110:523, 1986.
93. White DK, Miller AS, McDaniel RK et al: Inverted duct papilloma: a distinctive lesion of minor salivary glands, *Cancer* 49:519, 1982.
94. Auclair PL, Ellis GL, Gnepp DR: Other benign epithelial neoplasms. In Ellis GL, Auclair PL, Gnepp DR, editors: *Surgical pathology of the salivary glands,* Philadelphia, 1991, Saunders.

Sebaceous neoplasms

95. Gnepp DR: Sebaceous neoplasms of salivary gland origin: a review, *Pathol Annu* 18(pt I):71, 1983.
96. Seifert G, Miehlke A, Haubrich J, Chilla R: *Diseases of the salivary glands: Pathology, diagnosis, treatment, facial nerve surgery,* Stuttgart, 1986, Thieme Verlag.

Malignant neoplasms

Mucoepidermoid carcinoma

97. Auclair PL, Ellis GL: Mucoepidermoid carcinoma. In Ellis GL, Auclair PL, Gnepp DR, editors: *Surgical pathology of the salivary glands,* Philadelphia, 1991, Saunders.
98. Eveson JW, Cawson RA: Tumours of the minor (oropharyngeal) salivary glands: a demographic study of 336 cases, *J Oral Pathol* 14:500, 1985.
99. Browand BC, Waldron CA: Central mucoepidermoid tumors of the jaws: report of 9 cases and review of the literature, *Oral Surg Oral Med Oral Pathol* 40:631, 1975.
100. Krolls SO, Trodahl JN, Boyers RC: Salivary gland lesions in children: a survey of 430 cases, *Cancer* 30:459, 1972.
101. Castro EB, Huvos AG, Strong EW, Foote FW Jr: Tumors of the major salivary glands in children, *Cancer* 29:312, 1972.
102. Seifert G, Okabe H, Caselitz J: Epithelial salivary gland tumors in children and adolescents: analysis of 80 cases (Salivary Gland Registry 1965-1984), *ORL J Otorhinolaryngol Relat Spec* 48:137, 1986.
103. Spitz MR, Batsakis JG: Major salivary gland carcinoma: descriptive epidemiology and survival of 498 patients, *Arch Otolaryngol* 110:45, 1984.
104. Spiro RH, Huvos AG, Strong EW: Cancer of the parotid gland: a clinicopathologic study of 288 primary cases, *Am J Surg* 130:452, 1975.
105. Auclair PL, Goode RK, Ellis GL: Mucoepidermoid carcinoma of intraoral salivary glands: evaluation and application of grading criteria in 143 cases, *Cancer* 69:2021, 1992.
106. O'Brien CJ, Soong SJ, Herrera GA et al: Malignant salivary tumors—analysis of prognostic factors and survival, *Head Neck Surg* 9:82, 1986.

Acinic cell carcinoma

107. Ellis GL, Auclair PL: Acinic cell adenocarcinoma. In Ellis GL, Auclair PL, Gnepp DR, editors: *Surgical pathology of the salivary glands.* Philadelphia, 1991, Saunders.
108. Gnepp DR, Schroeder W, Heffner D: Synchronous tumors arising in a single major salivary gland, *Cancer* 63:1219, 1989.
109. Ellis GL, Corio RL: Acinic cell adenocarcinoma: a clinicopathologic analysis of 294 cases, *Cancer* 52:542, 1983.
110. Gnepp DR, Rader WR, Cramer SF et al: Accuracy of frozen section diagnosis of the salivary gland, *Otolaryngol Head Neck Surg* 96:325, 1987.
111. Levitt SH, McHugh RB, Gomez-Marin O et al: Clinical staging system for cancer of the salivary gland: a retrospective study, *Cancer* 47:2712, 1981.
112. Spiro RH, Huvos AG, Strong EW: Acinic cell carcinoma of salivary origin: a clinicopathologic study of 67 cases, *Cancer* 41:924, 1978.
113. Hickman RE, Cawson RA, Duffy SW: The prognosis of specific types of salivary gland tumors, *Cancer,* 54:1620, 1984.
114. Stanley RJ, Weiland LH, Olsen KD, Pearson BW: Dedifferentiated acinic cell (acinous) carcinoma of the parotid gland, *Otolaryngol Head Neck Surg* 98:155, 1988.

Adenoid cystic carcinoma

115. Spiro RH, Huvos AG, Strong EW: Adenoid cystic carcinoma of salivary gland origin—a clinicopathologic study of 242 cases, *Am J Surg* 128:512, 1974.
116. Seifert G, Miehlke A, Haubrich J, Chilla R: *Diseases of the salivary glands: pathology, diagnosis, treatment facial nerve surgery,* New York, 1986, Georg Thieme Verlag.
117. Eby LS, Johnson DS, Baker HW: Adenoid cystic carcinoma of the head and neck, *Cancer* 29:1160, 1972.
118. Leafstedt SW, Gaeta JF, Sako K et al: Adenoid cystic carcinoma of major and minor salivary glands, *Am J Surg* 122:756, 1971.
119. Perzin KH, Gullane P, Clairmont AC: Adenoid cystic carcinomas arising in salivary glands: a correlation of histologic features and clinical course, *Cancer* 42:265, 1978.
120. Smith LC, Lane N, Rankow RM: Cylindroma (adenoid cystic carcinoma): a report of fifty-eight cases, *Am J Surg* 110:519, 1965.
121. Thackray AC, Lucas RB: Tumors of the major salivary glands, Philadelphia, 1970, Saunders. In *Atlas of tumor pathology,* series 2, fasc 10, Washington, D.C., 1974, Armed Forces Institute of Pathology.
122. Evans RW, Cruickshank AH: *Epithelial tumours of the salivary glands,* Philadelphia, 1970, Saunders.
123. Spiro RH, Huvos AG, Strong EW: Adenoid cystic carcinoma: factors influencing survival, *Am J Surg* 138:579, 1979.
124. Oppenheim H, Landau GH, Dorman DW et al: Cylindroma involving the paranasal sinuses, *Eye Ear Nose Throat Monogr* 47:86, 1968.
125. Tomich CE: Adenoid cystic carcinoma. In Ellis GL, Auclair PL, Gnepp DR, editors: *Surgical pathology of the salivary glands,* Philadelphia, 1991, Saunders.
126. Barnes L, Verbin O, Gnepp DR: Diseases of the nose, paranasal sinuses and nasopharynx. In Barnes L, editor: *Surgical pathology of the head and neck,* New York, 1986, Marcel Dekker.
127. Conley J, Dingman DL: Adenoid cystic carcinoma in the head and neck (cylindroma), *Arch Otolaryngol* 100:81, 1974.
128. Marsh WL, Allen MS Jr: Adenoid cystic carcinoma: biologic behavior in 38 patients, *Cancer* 43:1463, 1979.
129. Warren CJ, Gnepp DR, Rosenblum BN: Adenoid cystic carcinoma metastasizing before detection of the primary lesion, *South Med J* 82;1277, 1989.
130. Spiro RH, Koss LG, Hajdu SI, Strong EW: Tumors of minor salivary origin: a clinicopathologic study of 492 cases, *Cancer* 31:117, 1973.

Malignant mixed tumor

131. Gnepp DR: Malignant mixed tumors of the salivary glands: a review, *Pathol Annu* 28(Pt 1):279, 1993.
132. Spiro RH, Huvos AG, Strong EW: Malignant mixed tumor of salivary origin: a clinicopathologic study of 146 cases, *Cancer* 39:388, 1977.
133. Foote FW Jr, Frazell EL: Tumors of the major salivary glands, *Cancer* 6:1065, 1953.
134. LiVolsi VA, Perzin KH: Malignant mixed tumors arising in salivary glands: I. Carcinomas arising in benign mixed tumors: a clinicopathologic study, *Cancer* 39:2209, 1977.
135. Tortoledo ME, Luna MA, Batsakis JG: Carcinomas ex pleomorphic adenoma and malignant mixed tumors, *Arch Otolaryngol* 110:172, 1984.
136. Gerughty RM, Scofield HH, Brown FM, Hennigar GR: Malignant mixed tumors of salivary gland origin, *Cancer* 24:471, 1969.
137. Thomas WH, Coppola ED: Distant metastases from mixed tumors of the salivary glands, *Am J Surg* 109:724, 1965.
138. Gnepp DR, Wenig GM: Malignant mixed tumors. In Ellis GL, Auclair PL, Gnepp DR, editors: *Surgical pathology of the salivary glands,* Philadelphia, 1991, Saunders.

Clear cell carcinoma

139. Milchgrub S, Gnepp DR, Vuitch FM et al: Hyalinizing clear cell carcinoma of the salivary gland, *Am J Surg Pathol* 18:74, 1994.
140. Donath K, Seifert G, Schmitz R: Zur Diagnose and Ultrastruktur des tubularen Speichelgangcarcinoms: epithelial-myoepitheliales Schaltstückcarcinom, *Virchows Arch [A] Pathol Anat* 356:16, 1972.
141. Corio RL, Sciubba JJ, Brannon RB, Batsakis JG: Epithelial-myoepithelial carcinoma of intercalated duct origin: a clinicopathologic and ultrastructural assessment of sixteen cases, *Oral Surg Oral Med Oral Pathol* 53:280, 1982.
142. Daley TD, Wysocki GP, Smout MS, Slinger RP: Epithelial-myoepithelial carcinoma of salivary glands, *Oral Surg Oral Med Oral Pathol* 57:512, 1984.
143. Luna MA, Ordóñez NG, Mackay B et al: Salivary epithelial-myoepithelial carcinomas of intercalated ducts: a clinical, electron microscopic, and immunohistochemical study, *Oral Surg Oral Med Oral Pathol* 59:482, 1985.
144. Stiernberg CM, Batsakis JG, Bailey BJ, Clark WD: Epithelial-myoepithelial carcinoma of the parotid gland, *Otolaryngol Head Neck Surg* 94:240, 1986.

Polymorphous low-grade adenocarcinoma

145. Freedman PD, Lumerman H: Lobular carcinoma of intraoral minor salivary gland origin: report of twelve cases, *Oral Surg Oral Med Oral Pathol* 56:157, 1983.

146. Batsakis JG, Pinkston GR, Luna MA et al: Adenocarcinomas of the oral cavity: a clinicopathologic study of terminal duct carcinomas, *J Laryngol Otol* 97:825, 1983.
147. Wenig BM, Gnepp DR: Polymorphous low-grade adenocarcinoma of minor salivary glands, In Ellis GL, Auclair PL, Gnepp DR, editors: *Surgical pathology of the salivary glands,* Philadelphia, 1991, Saunders.
148. Evans HL, Batsakis JG: Polymorphous low-grade adenocarcinomas of minor salivary glands: a study of 14 cases of a distinctive neoplasm, *Cancer* 53:935, 1984.
149. Frierson HF, Mills SE, Garland TA: Terminal duct carcinoma of minor salivary glands: a nonpapillary subtype of polymorphous low-grade adenocarcinoma, *Am J Clin Pathol* 84:8, 1985.
150. Aberle AM, Abrams AM, Bowe R et al: Lobular (polymorphous low-grade) carcinoma of minor salivary glands: a clinicopathologic study of twenty cases, *Oral Surg Oral Med Oral Pathol* 60:387, 1985.
151. Luna MA, Batsakis JG, Ordóñez NG et al: Salivary gland adenocarcinomas: a clinicopathologic analysis of three distinctive types, *Semin Diagn Pathol* 4:117, 1987.
152. Gnepp DR, Chen JC, Warren C: Polymorphous low-grade adenocarcinoma of minor salivary gland: an immunohistochemical and clinicopathologic study, *Am J Surg Pathol* 12:461, 1988.
153. Dardick I, van Nostrand AWP: Polymorphous low-grade adenocarcinoma: a case report with ultrastructural findings, *Oral Surg Oral Med Oral Pathol* 66:459, 1988.
154. Ritland F, Lubensky I, LiVolsi VA: Polymorphous low-grade adenocarcinoma of the parotid salivary gland, *Arch Pathol Lab Med* 117:1261, 1993.
155. Kotliar S, Kemp B, Luna MA et al: Terminal duct adenocarcinoma of the parotid gland: a report of twelve cases and review of the literature, *Mod Pathol* 7:100A, 1994.
156. Waldron CA, El-Mofty SK, Gnepp DR: Tumors of the intraoral minor salivary glands: a demographic and histologic study of 426 cases, *Oral Surg Oral Med Oral Pathol* 66:323, 1988.
157. Mills SE, Garland TA, Allen MS: Low-grade papillary adenocarcinoma of palatal salivary gland origin, *Am J Surg Pathol* 8:367, 1984.

Malignant sebaceous neoplasms

158. Gnepp DR, Brannon R: Sebaceous neoplasms of salivary gland origin: report of 21 cases, *Cancer* 53:2155, 1984.
159. Takashi T, Ogawa I, Nikai H: Sebaceous carcinoma of the parotid gland, an immunohistochemical and ultrastructural study, *Virchows Arch [A] (Pathol Anat Histopathol)* 414:459, 1989.
160. Granstrom G, Aldenborg F, Jeppsson P-H: Sebaceous carcinoma of the parotid gland: report of a case and review of the literature, *J Oral Maxillofac Surg* 45:731, 1987.
161. Miyamoto K, Yanagawa T, Azuma M et al: Establishment of a transformed human epithelial cell line with a sebaceous cell phenotype and effect of epidermal growth factor and dibutyryl cyclic adenosine 3′:5′-monophosphate on the cellular phenotype, *Cancer J* 3:414, 1989.
162. Ellis GL, Auclair PL, Gnepp DR, Goode RK: Other malignant epithelial neoplasms. In Ellis GL, Auclair PL, Gnepp DR, editors: *Surgical pathology of the salivary glands,* Philadelphia, 1991, Saunders.
163. Linhartova A: Sebaceous glands in salivary gland tissue, *Arch Pathol* 98:320, 1974.
164. Cramer S, Gnepp DR: Sebaceous differentiation in an adenoid cystic carcinoma of the parotid gland, *Cancer* 46:1405, 1980.

Salivary duct carcinoma

165. Kleinsasser O, Klein HJ, Hübner G: Speichelgangcarcinom: eine der Milchgangcarcinomen der Brustdrüse analoge Gruppe von Speicheldrüsentumoren, *Arch Klin Exp Ohren Nasen Kehlkopfheilkd* 192:100, 1968.
166. Barnes L, Rao U, Krause J, et al: Salivary duct carcinoma. Part 1: A clinicopathologic evaluation and DNA image analysis of 13 cases with review of the literature, *Oral Surg Oral Med Oral Pathol* 78:64, 1994.

Basal cell adenocarcinoma

167. Ellis GL, Auclair PL: Basal cell adenocarcinoma. In Ellis GL, Auclair PL, Gnepp DR, editors: *Surgical pathology of the salivary glands,* Philadelphia, 1991, Saunders.
168. Ellis GL, Wiscovitch JG: Basal cell adenocarcinomas of the major salivary glands, *Oral Surg Oral Med Oral Pathol* 69:461, 1990.

Undifferentiated carcinoma

169. Auclair PL, Ellis GL, Gnepp DR et al: Salivary gland neoplasms: general considerations, In Ellis GL, Auclair PL, Gnepp DR, editors: *Surgical pathology of the salivary glands,* Philadelphia, 1991, Saunders.
170. Seifert G, Miehlke A, Haubrich J, Chilla R: *Diseases of the salivary glands: pathology, diagnosis, treatment facial nerve surgery.* New York, 1986, Thieme Verlag.
171. Eversole LR, Gnepp DR, Eversole GM: Undifferentiated carcinoma, In Ellis GL, Auclair PL, Gnepp DR, editors: *Surgical pathology of the salivary glands,* Philadelphia, 1991, Saunders.
172. Nagao K, Matsuzak O, Saiga H et al: Histopathologic studies of undifferentiated carcinoma of the parotid gland, *Cancer* 50:1572, 1982.
173. Blanck C, Bäckström A, Eneroth C-M, Jakobsson PA: Poorly differentiated solid parotid carcinoma, *Acta Radiol* 13:17, 1974.
174. Donath K, Seifert G, Sunder-Plassmann E: Ultrastrukturelle Subklassifikation undifferenzierter Parotiscarcinome: Analyse von 11 Fällen, *J Cancer Res Clin Oncol* 103:75, 1982.
175. Hui KK, Luna MA, Batsakis JG et al: Undifferentiated carcinomas of the major salivary glands, *Oral Surg Oral Med Oral Pathol* 69:76, 1990.
176. Gnepp DR, Corio RL, Brannon RB: Small cell carcinoma of the major salivary glands, *Cancer* 58:705, 1986.
177. Patterson SD: Oat-cell carcinoma, primary in parotid gland, *Ultrastruct Pathol* 9:77, 1985.
178. Wirman JA, Battifora HA: Small cell undifferentiated carcinoma of salivary gland origin: an ultrastructural study, *Cancer* 37:1840, 1976.
179. Leipzig B, Gonzales-Vitale JC: Small cell epidermoid carcinoma of salivary glands, *Arch Otolaryngol* 108:511, 1982.
180. Kraemer BB, Mackay B, Batsakis JG: Small cell carcinomas of the parotid gland: a clinicopathologic study of three cases, *Cancer* 52:2115, 1983.
181. Yaku Y, Kanda T, Yoshihara T et al: Undifferentiated carcinoma of the parotid gland, *Virchows Arch [A] Pathol Anat* 401:89, 1983.
182. Dubois PJ, Orr DP, Meyers EN, Barnes LE: Undifferentiated parotid carcinoma with osteoblastic metastases, *Am J Roentgenol* 129:744, 1977.
183. Gnepp DR, Wick MR: Small cell carcinoma of the major salivary glands: an immunohistochemical study, *Cancer* 66:185, 1990.
184. Gnepp DR, Ferlito A, Hyams V: Primary anaplastic small cell (oat cell) carcinoma of the larynx: review of the literature and report of 18 cases, *Cancer* 51:1731, 1983.
185. Koss LC, Spiro RH, Hajdu S: Small cell (oat cell) carcinoma of minor salivary gland origin, *Cancer* 30:737, 1972.

Oncocytic carcinoma

186. Goode RK, Corio RL: Oncocytic adenocarcinoma of salivary glands, *Oral Surg Oral Med Oral Pathol* 65:61, 1988.

Epidermoid carcinoma

187. Auclair PL, Ellis GL: Primary squamous cell carcinoma, In Ellis GL, Auclair PL, Gnepp DR, editors: *Surgical pathology of the salivary glands,* Philadelphia, 1991, Saunders.
188. Shemen LJ, Huvos AG, Spiro RH: Squamous cell carcinoma of salivary gland origin, *Head Neck Surg* 9:235, 1987.
189. Seifert G, Miehlke A, Haubrich J, Chilla R: *Diseases of the salivary glands; pathology, diagnosis, treatment, facial nerve surgery,* New York, 1986, Thieme Verlag.

Adenocarcinoma, not otherwise specified

190. Spiro RH, Huvos AG, Strong EW: Adenocarcinoma of salivary origin: clinicopathologic study of 204 patients, *Am J Surg* 144:423, 1982.
191. Auclair PL, Ellis GL: Adenocarcinoma, not otherwise specified. In Ellis GL, Auclair PL, Gnepp DR, editors: *Surgical pathology of the salivary glands,* Philadelphia, 1991, Saunders.

Cystadenocarcinoma

192. Mills SE, Garland TA, Allen MS: Low-grade papillary adenocarcinoma of palatal salivary gland origin, *Am J Surg Pathol* 8:367, 1984.

Metastasis to major salivary glands

193. Feind CR: The head and neck. In Haagensen CD, Feind CR, Herter FP et al, editors: *The lymphatics in cancer,* Philadelphia, 1972, Saunders.
194. Gnepp DR: Metastatic disease to the major salivary glands, In Ellis GL, Auclair PL, Gnepp DR, editors: *Surgical pathology of the salivary glands,* Philadelphia, 1991, Saunders.

or altered esophageal motility. Incompetence of the LES is usually idiopathic, but it may also be attributable to alcohol ingestion, cigarette smoking, or the use of therapeutic drugs (such as estrogens). The LES tone is also lowered during pregnancy and nasogastric intubation.

Symptoms of reflux esophagitis include heartburn, chest pain, regurgitation, and dysphagia. Complications such as aspiration into the lungs and esophageal strictures may develop in long-standing cases. Gastroesophageal reflux may be a factor in bronchial asthma.[27]

Pathology. Microscopically, reflux esophagitis is characterized by basal cell hyperplasia, elongation of papillae beyond the normal 50% extension into the epithelium (Ismail-Beigi criteria),[28] capillary proliferation within the papillae, and congestion (Kobayashi criteria)[29] (Fig. 52-7). Eosinophils in the epithelium have been described as markers for reflux esophagitis but are seldom observed in adults.[30,31] Ulceration is accompanied by infiltrates of neutrophiles; lymphocytes and macrophages are usually present in variable numbers. Reactive fibrosis of the submucosa may cause esophageal stricture, usually close to the LES. The long-term consequence of reflux esophagitis is the replacement of the squamous epithelium by columnar–cell lined mucosa (Barrett's esophagus).

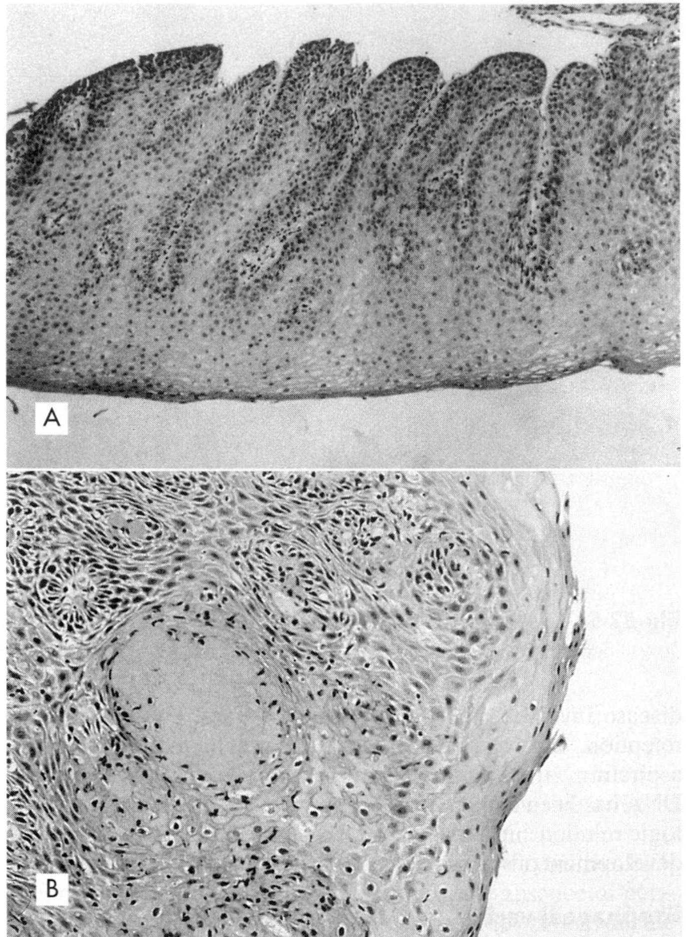

Fig. 52-7 Reflux esophagitis **A,** Ismail-Beigi criteria. Microscopic section showing basal cell hyperplasia and elongated papillae. **B,** Kobayashi criteria. Pronounced capillary proliferation with congestion within the papillae.

Infectious esophagitis

Viruses and fungi are the most common pathogens. Among the viruses, herpes simplex infections occur in patients with leukemias and lymphomas[32,33] and in immunocompetent patients.[34] Chickenpox also may affect the esophagus. Cytomegalovirus (CMV) esophagitis is observed in AIDS and transplant patients. Human papillomavirus (HPV) may infect the esophagus, but the prevalence of this form of infection is unknown. The infection is associated with focal epithelial hyperplasia or papilloma formation. Histologic signs of HPV infection include koilocytosis, anisonucleosis, giant cell formation, and disturbance of maturation and keratinization of squamous epithelium.[35,36] Viral infections cause painful plaques and ulcerations, which tend toward coalescence.

Human immunodeficiency virus (HIV) infection causes symptomatic esophagitis in a significant number of patients, complicated by superimposed infections with *Mycobacterium tuberculosis, Mycobacterium avium, and Cryptosporidium.*[37] Pseudomembranes may cover the ulcerations. Microscopically intranuclear inclusions in epithelial cells and giant cell formation are features of herpes infection (Fig. 52-8), whereas

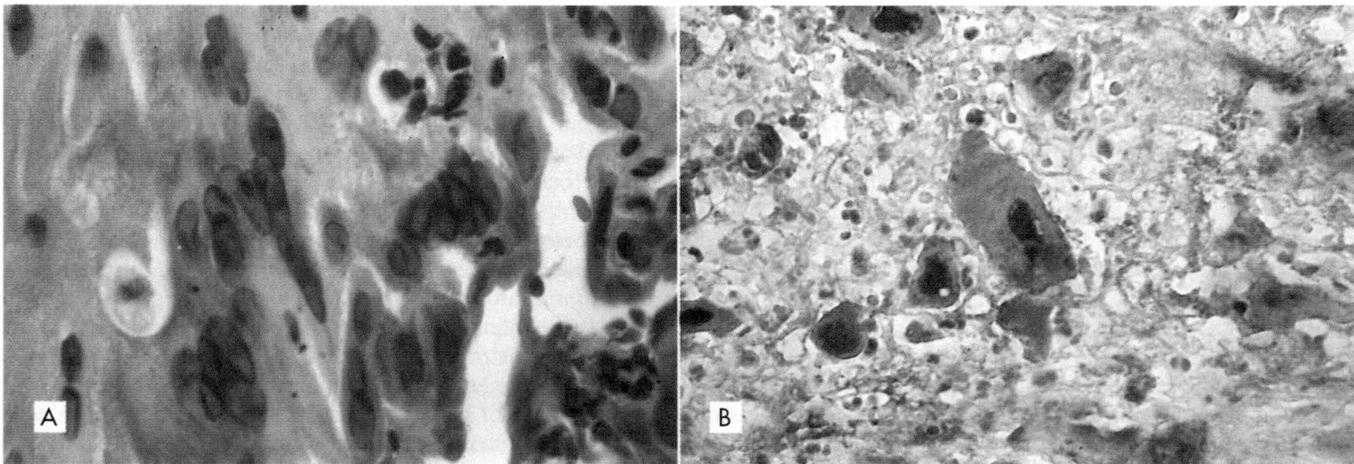

Fig. 52-8 Herpes esophagitis. **A,** Microscopic section showing giant cell formation and necrosis. **B,** Immunoperoxidase method demonstrating the intranuclear viral inclusions.

enlarged epithelial cells with intranuclear and intracytoplasmic inclusions are observed in CMV infection (Fig. 52-9).

Fungi are found in approximately 5% of endoscopic esophageal biopsy specimens but are most common in debilitated and immunocompromised patients, or in patients receiving chemotherapy for malignancies. Diabetes mellitus also predisposes to fungal esophagitis. Fungal infection is often superimposed on other esophageal diseases such as cancer, reflux esophagitis, or stricture.

Candida albicans is the most common pathogen, but other fungi such as *Mucor* or *Aspergillus* may be found as well. Areas of ulceration, usually in the lower third of the esophagus, may be covered by pseudomembranes, which contain fungal hyphae, fibrin, and necrotic cells (Fig. 52-10). White mucosal plaques are typically found in 50% of infected patients.

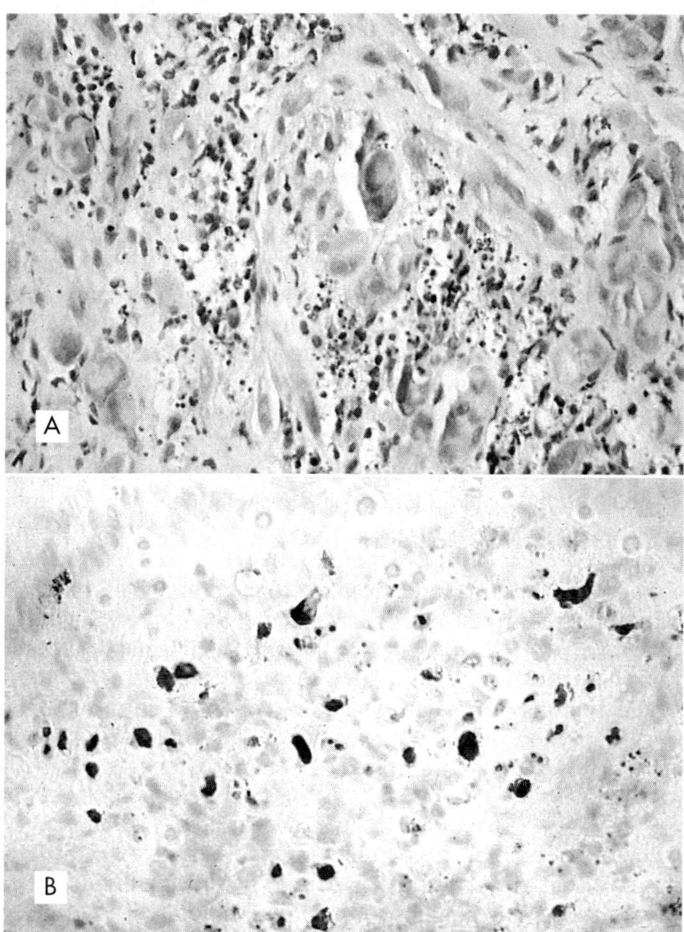

Fig. 52-9 Cytomegalovirus esophagitis. **A,** Microscopic section showing large cells with bizarre nuclei. **B,** Immunoperoxidase method demonstrating intranuclear and cytoplasmic viral inclusions.

Esophagitis caused by chemical or physical agents

Esophagitis may be caused by ingestion of strong acids and alkali, industrial chemicals, or agricultural poisons. The most severe corrosive esophagitis occurs after lye ingestion, either in attempted suicides in adults or accidental poisoning in children. This alkaline agent causes liquefaction and necrosis of the esophageal and gastric wall, associated with severe inflammation and perforation (Fig. 52-11). Lye ingestion is followed by significant mortality; recently the mortality has been decreased by early aggressive surgical resection of the affected portions of esophagus and stomach. The ingestion of substances containing sulfuric or hydrochloric acid (such as cleaning agents), either accidental or suicidal, causes coagulation necrosis of the esophageal wall. Physical agents capable of producing esophageal damage include external radiation for the treatment of thoracic malignancies. Chemical or physical injury of esophagus is often complicated by fibrous strictures. Cytotoxic drugs may cause esophagitis and ulcerations, often complicated by fungal infections.

Esophagitis in systemic illness

Esophagitis may be present in systemic illnesses, especially skin diseases characterized by blister formation such as epidermolysis bullosa and bullous pemphigoid. Esophageal blisters containing fluid usually rupture, leaving weeping ulcerations. Strictures may develop in protracted bullous diseases.

Bone marrow transplant patients may develop esophageal ulcerations, usually in the upper esophagus, as a consequence of graft-versus-host disease. Uremia also causes esophagitis. Functional disturbances caused by scleroderma or diabetes mellitus also predispose to esophagitis.

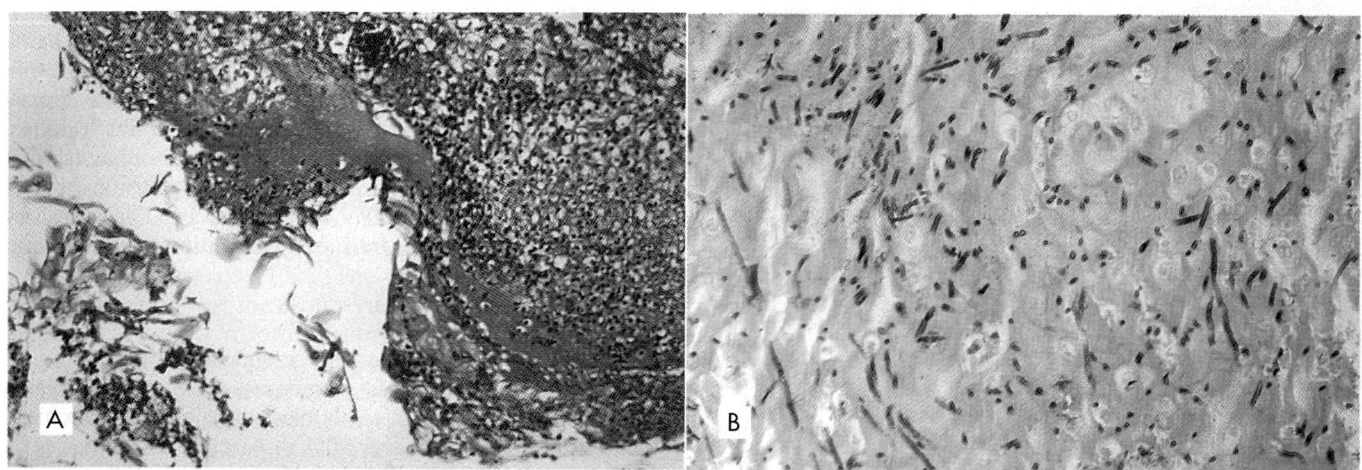

Fig. 52-10 Candida albicans esophagitis. **A,** Multiple hyphae are seen in a fibrinous exudate. **B,** Silver stain demonstrating long, pseudoseptate hyphae.

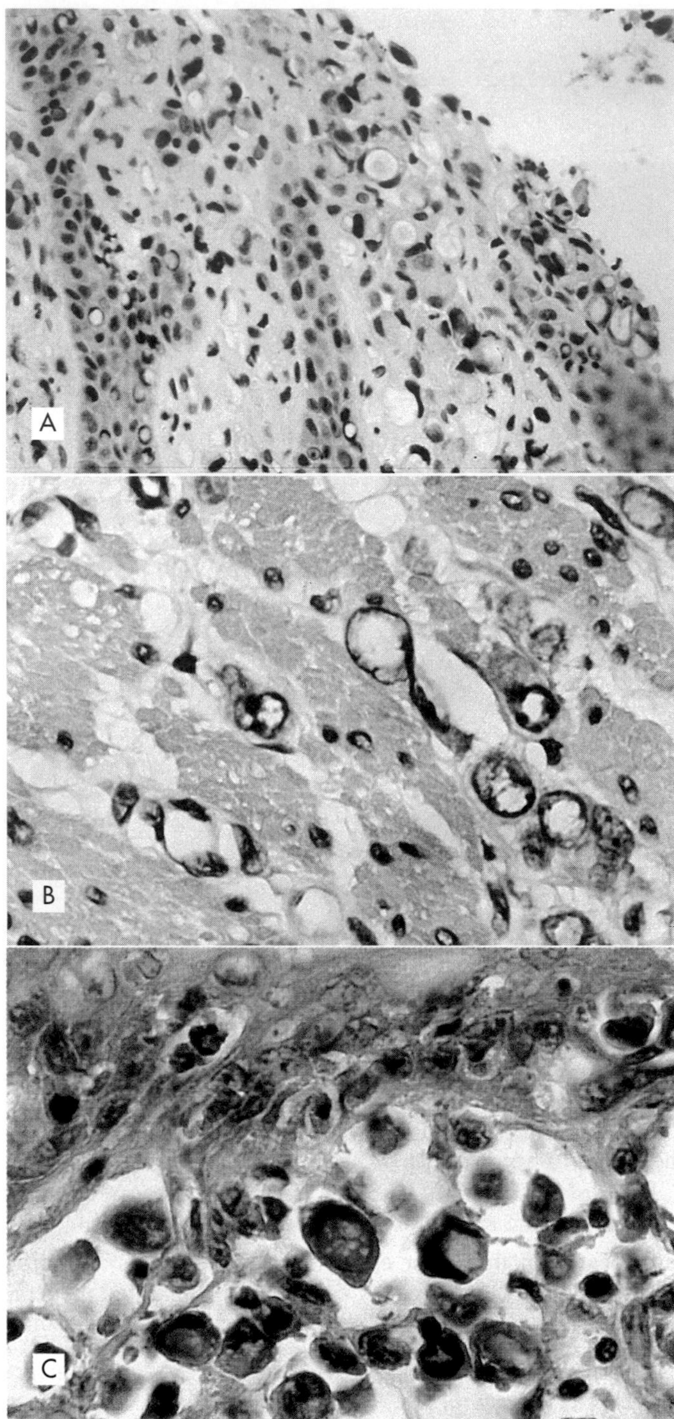

Fig. 52-17 Linitis plastica carcinoma of esophagus. **A,** Microscopic section showing an area of ulceration undermined by signet-ring cells. **B,** Infiltration of the muscularis layer by signet-ring cells. **C,** Mucicarmine stain showing the presence of mucin in the cytoplasm of signet-ring cells *(red).*

poid tumors containing epithelioid or spindle-shaped cells (Fig. 52-18). The degree of melanin pigmentation is quite variable. The prognosis is poor; the mean survival is 2 months.[58,59]

Sarcoma

Esophageal sarcomas represent less than 2% of all malignant tumors of the esophagus. Leiomyosarcomas are the most

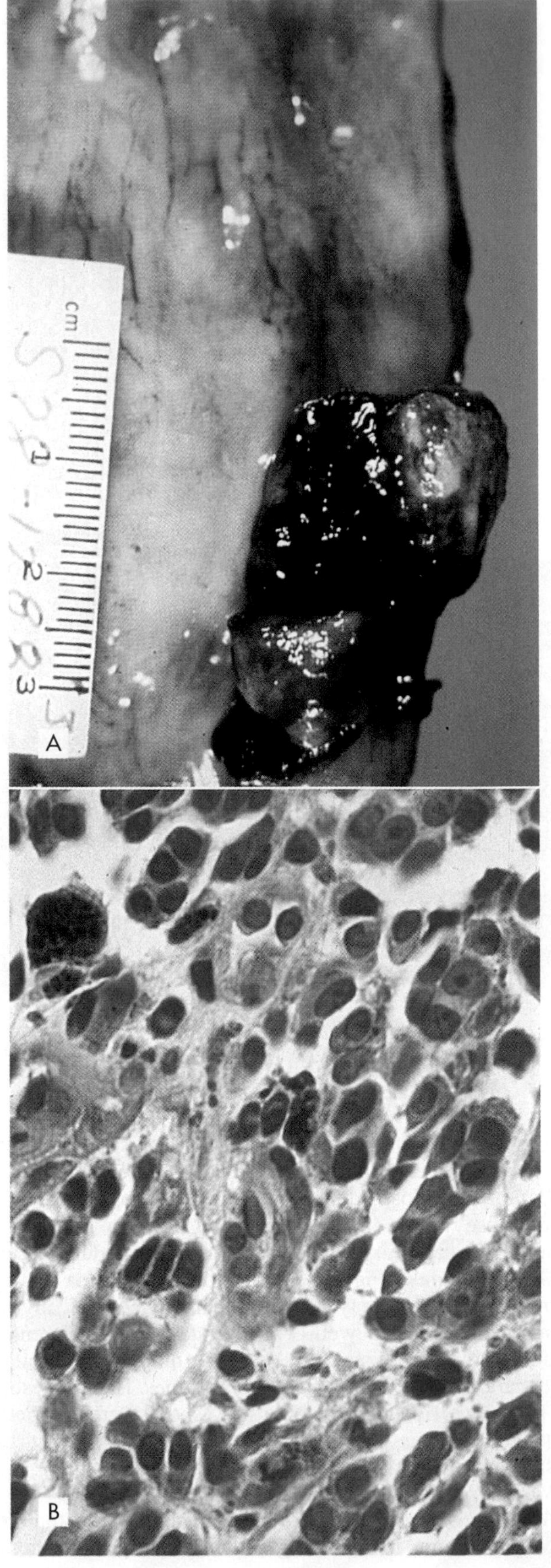

Fig. 52-18 Malignant melanoma. **A,** Gross specimen showing a dark, intraluminal nodular mass. **B,** Microscopic section showing tumor cells containing melanin.

common, formed by neoplastic smooth muscle cells.[60] Primary rhabdomyosarcomas, composed of striated muscle cells, have also been reported.[61] Patients infected with HIV may develop Kaposi's sarcoma.

Metastases

Secondary tumors invading the esophagus usually originate from the adjacent structures, that is, stomach, lungs, and breast, but may also reach the esophagus from distant sites by blood-borne metastases.

REFERENCES

Normal esophagus

1. Eroschenko VP: *diFiore's Atlas of histology,* Philadelphia 1993, Lea & Febiger.
2. Enterline H, Thompson J: *Pathology of the esophagus,* New York, 1984, Springer-Verlag.
3. Sadler TW: *Langman's medical embryology,* ed 6, Baltimore, 1990, Williams & Wilkins.
4. Bogomoletz WV, Geboes K, Feydy P et al: Mucin histochemistry of heterotopic gastric mucosa of the upper esophagus in adults, *Hum Pathol* 19:1301, 1988.
5. West JB: *Best and Taylor's physiological basis of medical practice,* ed 12, Baltimore, 1991, Williams & Wilkins.

Diseases affecting the lumen and motor functions of the esophagus

6. Chittmittrapap S, Spitz L, Kiely EM, Brereton RJ: Oesophageal atresia and associated anomalies, *Arch Dis Child* 64:364, 1989.
7. Stern Z, Sharon P, Ligumsky M et al: Glycogenic acanthosis of the esophagus, *Am J Gastroenterol* 74:261, 1980.
8. Okamura H, Tsutsumi S, Inak S, Mori T: Esophageal web in Plummer-Vinson syndrome, *Laryngoscope,* 98:994, 1988.
9. Sehgal VN, Jain VK, Bhattacharya SN et al: Esophageal web in generalized epidermolysis bullosa, *Int J Dermatol* 30:51, 1991.
10. Schatzki R, Gary JE: Dysphagia due to diaphragm-like localized narrowing in lower esophagus ("lower esophageal ring"), *Am J Roentenol* 70:911, 1953.
11. Eastridge CE, Pate JW, Mann JA: Loser esophageal ring: experiences in treatment of 88 patients, *Ann Thorac Surg* 37:103, 1984.
12. Bousvaros A, Antoioli DA, Winter HS: Ringed esophagus: an association with esophagitis, *Am J Gastroenterol,* 87:1187, 1992.

Diverticula and hernias

13. Duda M, Sery Z, Vojacek K et al: Etiopathogenesis and classification of esophageal diverticula, *Int Surg* 70:291, 1985.
14. Medeiros LJ, Doos WG, Balogh K: Esophageal intramural pseudodiverticulosis, *Hum Pathol* 19:928, 1988.
15. Bowdler DA, Stell PM: Carcinoma arising in posterior pharyngeal pulsion diverticulum (Zenker's diverticulum), *Br J Surg* 74:561, 1987.
16. Texter EC, Van Dersteppen G, Chejfec G et al: Criteria for the diagnosis of hiatal hernia, *Arch Intern Med,* 110:827, 1962.
17. Cohen S: Motor disorders of the esophagus, *N Engl J Med* 301:184, 1979.
18. Csendes A, Smook G, Braghetto I et al: Histological studies of Auerbach's plexuses of the esophagus, stomach and colon in patients with achalasia of the esophagus, *Gut* 33:150, 1992.
19. Goldblum JR, Whyte RI, Orringer MB et al: Achalasia: a morpliologic study of 42 resected specimens, *Am T Surg Pathol* 18:327, 1996.

Inflammation

20. Robertson SC, Martin BAB, Atkinson M: Varicella-zoster virus DNA in the esophageal myenteric plexus in achalasia, *Gut* 34: 299, 1993.
21. Meijssen MAC, Tilanus HW, Van Blankenstein M et al: Achalasia complicated by esophageal squamous cell carcinoma: a prospective study in 195 patients, *Gut,* 33:155, 1992.
22. Hirata M, Kawasaki S, Sanjo K, Idezuki Y: Histopathological study of oesophageal mucosa in patients with varices: a comparison between bleeders and non-bleeders, *Br J Surg* 78:1352, 1991.
23. Saltzman JR, Arora S: Complications of esophageal variceal band ligation: *Gastrointest Endosc,* 39:185, 1993.
24. Sugawa C, Benishek D, Walt AJ: Mallory-Weiss syndrome: a study of 224 patients, *Am J Surg* 145:30, 1983.
25. Boerhaave H, cited by Fitz RH: Rupture of healthy esophagus, *Am J Med* 73:17, 1877.
26. Michel L, Grillo HC, Malt RA: Operative and non-operative management of esophageal perforations, *Ann Surg* 194:57, 1981.
27. Sontag S, O'Connell S, Chejfec G et al: Is gastroesophageal reflux a factor in some asthmatics, *Am J Gastroenterol* 82:119, 1987.
28. Ismail-Beigi F, Horton PF, Pope CE: Histological consequences of gastroesophageal reflux in man, *Gastroenterology* 58:163, 1970.
29. Kobayashi S, Kasugai T: Endoscopic and biopsy criteria for the diagnosis of esophagitis with a fiberoptic esophagoscopy, *Dig Dis Sci* 19:345, 1974.
30. Winter HS, Madara JL, Stafford RJ et al: Intraepithelial eosinophils: a new diagnostic criterion for reflux esophagitis, *Gastroenterology* 83:818, 1982.
31. Frierson JF Jr: Histology in the diagnosis of reflux esophagitis, *Gastroenterol Clin North Am* 19:631, 1990.
32. Matsumoto J, Sumiyoshi A: Herpes simplex esophagitis, *Am J Clin Pathol* 84:96, 1985.
33. Greenson JK, Beschorner WE, Boitnott JK, Yardley JH: Prominent mononuclear cell infiltrate is characteristic of herpes esophagitis, *Hum Pathol* 22:541, 1991.
34. Galbraith JC, Shafran SD: Herpes simplex esophagitis in the immunocompetent patient: report of four cases and review, *Clin Infect Dis* 14:894, 1992.
35. Goldman H, Antonioli DA: Mucosal biopsy of the esophagus, stomach and proximal duodenum, *Hum Pathol* 13:423, 1982.
36. Winkler B, Capo V, Reumann W et al: Human papilloma-virus infection of the esophagus, *Cancer* 55:149, 1985.
37. Wilcox CM: Esophageal disease in the acquired immunodeficiency syndrome: etiology, diagnosis and management, *Am J Med* 92:412, 1992.

Tumors of the esophagus

38. Chejfec G, Schnell T, Sontag S: Editorial: Barrett's esophagus: a preneoplastic disorder, *Am J Clin Pathol* 98:5, 1992.
39. Polepalle SC, McCallum RW: Barrett's esophagus, *Gastroenterol Clin North Am* 19:733, 1990.
40. Cantero D, Tada M, Okita K: Esophageal leiomyoblastoma: the role of endoscopic procedures in the pre-operative diagnosis, *Gastrointest Endosc* 39:568, 1993.
41. Moses FM: Squamous cell carcinoma of the esophagus: natural history, incidence, etiology and complications, *Gastroenterol Clin North Am* 20:703, 1991.
42. Mimic Y, Garabrant DH, Peters JM et al: Tobacco, alcohol, diet, occupation and cancer of the esophagus, *Cancer Res 48:3843, 1988.*
43. Hille JJ, Markowitz S, Margolinsk A et al: Human papillomavirus and carcinoma of the esophagus, *N Eng J Med* 213:1707, 1985.
44. Marger RS, Marger D: Carcinoma of the esophagus and tylosis, *Cancer* 72:17, 1993.
45. Patil P, Redkar A, Patel SG et al: Prognosis of operable squamous cell carcinoma of the esophagus, *Cancer* 72:20, 1993.
46. Gschmossmann JM, Bonner JA, Foote RL et al: Malignant tracheoesophageal fistula in patients with esophageal cancer, *Cancer* 72:1513, 1993.
47. Ellis FH Jr: Treatment of carcinoma of the esophagus or cardia, *Mayo Clin Proc* 64:945, 1989.
48. Linder J, Stein RB, Roggli VL et al: Polypoid tumor of the esophagus, *Hum Pathol* 18:692, 1987.
49. Takubo K, Tsuchiya S, Nakagawa H et al: Pseudosarcoma of the esophagus, *Hum Pathol* 13:503, 1982.
50. Sotus PC, Majmudar B, Symbas PN: Carcinoma in situ of the esophagus, *JAMA* 239:335, 1978.
51. Chejfec G: Atypias, dysplasias and neoplasias of the esophagus and stomach, *Semin Diagn Pathol* 2:31, 1985.

peritoneal cavity. The gastric serosa is a continuum with the major and lesser omenta.

Duodenum

The duodenum is the first portion of the small intestine, extending between the stomach, through the pylorus, and the jejunum, with which it establishes a transition at the ligament of Treitz.[2,3] The duodenum, which measures between 25 and 35 cm in length, is divided into four portions: (1) first, superior, or bulb, (2) second, or descending; (3) third, or horizontal; and (4) fourth, or ascending. It forms a C-shaped loop that surrounds the head of the pancreas and is located anterior to the abdominal aorta at the level of the L1-L2 vertebrae. Fig. 53-2 includes a diagram of the gross anatomy of the duodenum. In the second portion is the ampulla of Vater, a small mucosal protrusion provided with the muscular sphincter of Oddi, in which open the common bile duct and the main pancreatic duct, sometimes separately, at times jointly. The arterial supply originates from the hepatic, right gastric, and superior pancreaticoduodenal branches of the celiac trunk and from the inferior pancreaticoduodenal artery, arising from the superior mesenteric artery. The venous return is directed into the superior mesenteric vein, one of tributaries of the portal system. Most of the innervation arises from the celiac plexus, with a sympathetic component accompanying the arterial vessels.

Histology. The duodenal wall is composed of four layers: mucosa, submucosa, muscularis propria, and serosa.[3,6] The *mucosa* is arranged in broad folds, which in the more distal portions describe the valves of Kerckring, and consists of villi and glands. The villi are thin, fingerlike projections that are covered by enterocytes; these cells are tall and columnar and form a single layer that rests on a basal lamina. The enterocytes are characterized by an apical surface composed of tightly packed microvilli, described by light microscopy as "brush border," which provides a greatly increased membrane surface highly suited for absorption of nutrients, and a well-defined system of tight intercellular junctions, which prevent passive passage of contents from the lumen into the lamina propria. Interspersed among the enterocytes are goblet cells, characterized by a flattened basal nucleus and the presence of a large apical mucus vacuole, and a few finely granulated endocrine cells. The glands contain a mixture of mucous cells, among which are the actively reproducing uncommitted stem cells, endocrine cells, and Paneth's cells. The endocrine cells are characterized by the presence of small secretory granules with a characteristic ultrastructural appearance and containing a variety of products such as gastrin, somatostatin, serotonin, secretin, cholecystokinin, and others. The Paneth's cells are characterized by the presence of coarse apical eosinophilic granules that contain lysozyme. The muscularis mucosae of the duodenum, unlike that of other areas of the gut, is not continuous because it is split widely by the *Brunner's glands*. These racemose structures, composed of branching and coiling glands, occupy a significant portion of the submucosa and sometimes are noted in the deeper reaches of the mucosa. Their cells are tall and cuboidal and have a clear cytoplasm that contains mucus and pepsinogen II in humans. Brunner's glands communicate with the surface by ductal structures that open at the base of the villi and contain scattered endocrine cells. The remainder of the submucosa consists of loose fibroconnective tissue containing blood and lymphatic vessels and a robust neural plexus of Meissner. Because of the presence of the Brunner's glands, as well as that of frequent lymphoid follicles in the submucosa, sometimes the duodenal villi appear somewhat short and blunted under normal circumstances.

The *muscularis propria* consists of two layers: the internal or circular layer, composed of tightly coiled smooth muscle fascicles, and the external or longitudinal, composed of very loosely coiled smooth muscle. Between these two layers of muscle there is the myenteric plexus of Auerbach, essentially identical to the same structure in the stomach. The *serosa* is represented by a thin layer of subserosal tissue covered by a continuous single lining mesothelial cells. The morphology of the small intestine is covered in greater detail in Chapter 54.

Examination and tissue sampling

Gross examination and sampling

Since the advent of efficacious therapy for most peptic ulcers with the introduction of histamine (H_2)-receptor blockers and proton pump inhibitors, most gastrectomy specimens are the result of surgery for neoplasia. Therefore this is the protocol given here. Fig. 53-4 is a diagram of the gross examination and sampling of a gastrectomy specimen.

Before opening the gastrectomy specimen, note whether it is a total or a subtotal resection and describe the length of both lesser and greater curvature as well as that of the attached duodenal cuff, if it is a distal excision, or of the esophageal segment, if it is a proximal resection. Describe also any lesions visible on inspection of the outer aspect of the specimen. Then proceed to open it along the greater curvature, unless the lesion is located there; in this case, open along the lesser cur-

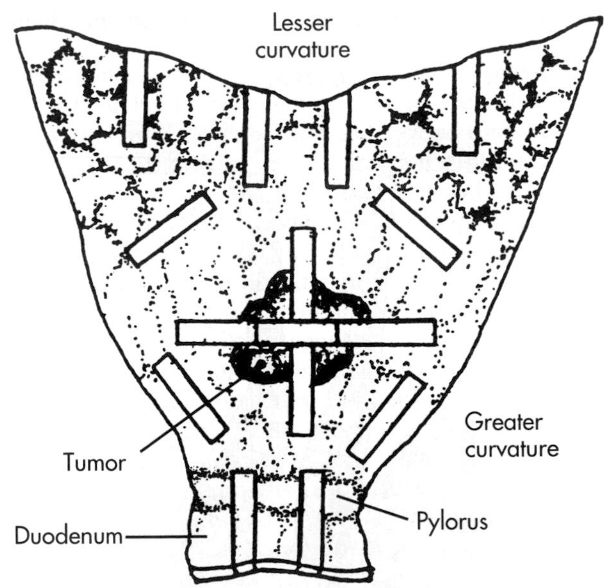

Fig. 53-4 Schema of the gross examination and sampling of distal stomach removed because of a tumor, present in the antrum at the lesser curvature. Samples should be taken from both proximal (gastric) and distal (duodenal) resection margins; it is important, when one is sampling the tumor, to take areas of transition between tumor and nonneoplastic mucosa, as well as a section from the most central part of the tumor; this is usually the site of deepest penetration, information essential for the staging of the tumor. Additional samples of surrounding nonneoplastic mucosa should also be taken to assess aspects such as gastritis, submucosal lymphatic spread, and others.

vature. Describe the neoplasm in terms of location, size (two or three dimensions), shape, consistency, form (ulcerated, excavated, flat, polypoid, exophytic), depth of invasion assessed grossly, and serosal involvement. Describe also other mucosal lesions and the appearance of the surrounding gastric mucosa (disposition and prominence of folds, vascularity, erosions, hemorrhages, and so on). After taking gross pictures, pin the specimen and fix in 10% buffered formalin for 6 to 18 hours. Then paint with India ink all resection margins and sample the specimen as follows: tumor (through the center, or the deepest penetration into the wall by gross inspection, and four quadrants of transition between the lesion and the surrounding mucosa), any other mucosal lesions, representative sections of the surrounding mucosa (antral, oxyntic, other), proximal and distal resection margins, taking care to include all the layers (not just the mucosa), and lymph nodes. For the last, note their presence, divide them into three groups (pyloric, greater curvature, and lesser curvature), and fix separately for better results. If omentum or spleen is included, omental or perisplenic lymph nodes are also sampled. All recovered nodes need to be submitted and examined for metastatic spread.

Endoscopic examination and biopsy sampling

The availability of modern flexible gastroduodenoscopes has provided an enormous boost to the diagnostic capabilities of gastroenterologists, thus affording a thorough exploration of the stomach.[7] In addition, their biopsy and therapeutic channels allow the retrieval of pedunculated lesions,[8] of substantial biopsy samples, and of brush cytology specimens.[9] Endoscopic visualization of the gastric mucosa not only permits the recognition of lesions such as ulcers, erosions, mucosal irregularities, and polyps, but also provides additional information such as color, texture, and degree of vascularity of the mucosa. An additional method, little used in Western countries but popular in Japan, is the application of intravital dyes such as toluidine blue or Congo red to the gastric mucosa. Whereas normal and metaplastic mucosa take up the dye readily, foci of severe dysplasia and early carcinoma do not and thus stand as gray-white areas next to the colored mucosa. This affords the opportunity to search the mucosa for lesions perhaps too subtle to be detected by routine endoscopic inspection.

It is essential that endoscopist and pathologist function as a team when a biopsy is obtained in order to provide the maximum benefit to the patient. The pathologist depends on the endoscopist to (1) obtain the appropriate samples based on his or her observation, (2) handle, label, and deliver the delicate tissue samples adequately and in a timely fashion, and (3) provide the pertinent information regarding the patient and the nature and location of the biopsy samples. The ideal number of biopsy samples procured during endoscopy varies with the type of lesion. If an ulcer is being investigated, samples must be obtained from the bed, four quadrants of the edges, and the surrounding mucosa. If it is an exophytic lesion, this must be sampled thoroughly from the top, the base or pedicle, and the surrounding mucosa to rule out in situ malignancy. In the case of possible dysplasia or endocrine cell hyperplasia and dysplasia, it is important to sample generously antrum, corpus, and fundus, paying special attention to the lesser curvature mucosa and to other features such as areas of granularity, thickening of the mucosal folds, or discoloration. Whereas advanced carcinoma of the stomach is relatively easy to see and sample, subtler early lesions including early carcinoma may require a minimum of eight biopsy samples for a 95% to 99% of positive results to be obtained. Finally, in the evaluation of the gastric mucosa for most types of gastritis, a minimum of two samples from antrum and two from corpus, one each from lesser and greater curvature respectively, are regarded as advisable for optimal results.

Endoscopically directed brush cytologic sampling is also an important diagnostic tool in the detection of malignant and premalignant lesions of the gastric mucosa. This approach alone provides a positivity rate of 80% to 85% of cases of gastric carcinoma. When applied with biopsy sampling, it yields a positive result in virtually all cases and reduces the number of directed biopsies necessary to attain such result.[10] Another cytologic approach used to explore submucosal biopsy specimens not accessible to brush cytology involves the use of needle aspiration carried with a sclerotherapy cannula passed through the therapeutic port of the endoscope.[11]

Microscopic examination

Most of the aspects of microscopic examination pertaining to biopsy samples also apply, albeit to a variable degree, to surgical resection specimens. The ideal orientation of a gastrointestinal specimen is one that provides a view perpendicular to the plane of the wall and will include the surface epithelium, full length of the glands, and full cross sections of submucosa, muscularis propria, and serosa, when present. In the case of biopsies, there are differences of opinion regarding orientation. Some authors like to orient the samples flat, with the mucosal side up, on a base of synthetic material before fixing; in this manner, the sample can later be embedded properly and perpendicular sections as described above can be obtained from mucosa and, when present, submucosa.[12] This approach is preferable in the case of large biopsy specimens, obtained with "jumbo" forceps, which have to be evaluated carefully for parameters such as atrophy, villus blunting, and others. When samples are small, or if very skilled operators capable of extracting, orienting, and fixing the samples gently and in a few seconds are not available, it is best to simply drop the biopsy samples in the fixative. Appropriate orientation of a significant portion of the specimen is generally achieved by cutting several levels for each block and examining the sections in search of the perpendicularly oriented mucosal portions. The pathologist has little use for a sample, no matter how well oriented, if it shows mechanical or dehydration artifacts that interfere significantly with the diagnosis.

The ideal fixative for gastrointestinal tissues would be one that is inexpensive, penetrates tissue structures rapidly, is capable of preserving cytologic detail, allows the application of all necessary histologic, histochemical, and immunohistochemical procedures, has a long shelf life in a ready-for-use form, and is not excessively toxic or poses disposal problems. Whereas such a paragon does not exist, 10% buffered formalin at pH 7.2-7.4 fulfills a significant number of these criteria and, with few exceptions, is used universally. Since this fixative does not provide ideal nuclear detail and may result in considerable fibrous tissue retraction, some workers are partial to other media, such as B5, Bouin's, or Hollande's fixative. All of these, however, contain heavy metals, which are toxic and must be specially disposed of, are more expensive, and must often be prepared in the laboratory shortly before use. Processing of small biopsy samples must take into account their size and avoid long dehydration and infiltration protocols in automated processors, which may result in brittle and hard-to-section tissues. Before processing, it is advisable to stain the tissue samples with eosin or methylene blue (not Mercurochrome!) for their better and complete visualization and to wrap them in tissue paper to prevent dispersion and actual loss of tissue. Embedding must be attempted with all samples together as much as possible and on edge for ideal visualization. Three or four slides containing two ribbons with multiple levels each should be stained, and, if there is a possibility that special or immunocytochemical stains may be needed, extra slides containing unstained tissues must be picked up the first time around; having to section a small tissue block for the second time may result in significant loss of valuable tissue.

Routine hematoxylin and eosin (H&E)–staining is regarded as adequate for most needs in gastrointestinal pathology. Some centers advocate the use of variants such as hematoxylin-phloxin-saffron or the combination of hematoxylin, phloxin, Alcian blue, and saffron because these allow easier recognition of collagen and mucin than the others. Such techniques, however, are more complicated and expensive and are not available to all laboratories. Special circumstances may dictate the need to execute more sophisticated techniques to demonstrate the presence of certain structures, organisms, or chemical substances. For example, Giemsa's technique is quite effective in highlighting mast cells, *Giardia, Cryptosporidium,* or *Helicobacter pylori*. The last is also well demonstrated by the silver techniques of Warthin-Starry or the Steiner modification. Fungal organisms are well demonstrated with either periodic acid–Schiff (PAS) stain after diastase application, or with the methenamine silver technique. All mucins, including neutral ones, are better demonstrated also with PAS with diastase, whereas acid sialomucins are evidenced with Meyer's mucicarmine and with Alcian blue pH 2.5, and sulfated mucins are shown with high-iron diamine (HID) stain or with Alcian blue pH 1.0. Endocrine cells can be demonstrated with Fontana-Masson silver technique, if they are argentaffin, or with the variants of Grimelius, Churukian-Schenk, or Sevier-Munger if they are only argyrophilic. Immunohistochemical techniques are widely used with increasing frequency, but their individual application is extensive and beyond the scope of this chapter.

Interpretation of the biopsy requires, as commented above, close collaboration and free communication between endoscopist and pathologist. Endoscopic photographs providing a clear idea of both appearance and size of the lesion biopsy specimens are invaluable to the pathologist. When one is exploring for malignancy or premalignancy, which may not be endoscopically obvious, it is very advisable to place samples from different areas in different, clearly identified, containers. It is important to be able to pinpoint exactly the place from which a sample showing early invasion or significant dysplasia was obtained in order to guide subsequent attempts for further evaluation or for surgical therapy.

Finally, some artifacts are often encountered in endoscopic biopsy specimens of the upper gastrointestinal tract: their existence and sometimes their inevitability must be known and expected to avoid catastrophic pitfalls in interpretation. The most common artifact is compression caused by the biopsy forceps: distortion of glands may be suggestive of the existence of adenocarcinoma, compression of nuclei may provide a spurious hyperchromasia interpreted as dysplasia, compression of lymphocytes in the lamina propria may raise the possibility of nonexistent significant inflammation, and compression of collagen may cause the pathologist to diagnose fibrosis in normal tissues. The presence of small mucosal hemorrhages may present a dilemma as to whether such a phenomenon is real or represents the effects of instrumentation during the procedure. In cases in which such ambiguity may not be resolvable, it is prudent to make a notation of its presence but to introduce at the same time the caveat that it may represent the result of iatrogenic trauma.

DEVELOPMENTAL ABNORMALITIES

Duplications, diverticula, and cysts

Congenital duplications, diverticula, and cysts of the alimentary tract are most frequent in the ileum but may occur in other parts as well.[13] Cysts and duplications usually present as rounded masses encased in the mesentery of the organ from which they arise. They are hollow and lined by a mucosa that may be identical to that of the neighboring intestinal segment or may be different, sometimes heterotopic. Diverticula are outpouchings separated by a passage of variable dimensions from the main lumen of the gut. Duplications and cysts of the stomach are generally located along the greater curvature,[14,15] whereas those of the duodenum are rare lesions often located in the submucosa that bulge into the lumen and may cause obstruction.[16] Congenital diverticula of the stomach and the duodenum are very rare.[13,17] Congenital duodenal diverticula are outpouchings from the posterior wall of the intestine that may traverse the diaphragm and make contact with defective vertebral bodies.[18]

Pyloric and duodenal atresia

Membranous atresia of the pylorus is an infrequent malformation, incompatible with postnatal life; usually, it has no known association with other conditions.[13] Duodenal atresia is comparatively more common and is believed to be the result of a failure of recanalization of the embryonal gut early in its development.[19,20] Stenosis of the duodenum, also resulting from defective recanalization, is less common than atresia.[13] Duodenal stenosis and atresia have a membranous configuration and are often associated with other congenital malformations such as congenital heart disease, annular pancreas, and intestinal malrotations. Between 25% and 30% of infants with duodenal stenosis or atresia have trisomy 21.[20]

Congenital pyloric stenosis

The relatively common condition congenital pyloric stenosis generally affects between 0.3% and 0.4% of all live-born infants. It is more frequently found in males than females and in white than black children, and firstborns are affected more often than subsequent children.[21]

Clinically, congenital pyloric stenosis presents with "projectile" vomiting between the second and the fourth postnatal week. The vomitus may be streaked with blood but, understandably, contains no bile. As vomiting persists, there is severe dehydration, alkalosis, and malnutrition with weight loss and failure to thrive. In many of these thin infants, it is possible to observe strong gastric peristaltic waves and the presence of a mass, which can also be readily palpated, upon visual inspection of the abdomen. In severe cases, death may ensue.[22]

The pathogenesis of congenital pyloric stenosis is not known. Because this condition presents a definite familial clustering, a recessive genetic origin has been suggested but not proved. The muscular hypertrophy that characterizes this lesion is believed to originate in utero, though the functional consequences may not be apparent for a couple of weeks. It is not clear whether changes in the myenteric plexus, on the other hand, may be the cause or the effect of the disease.[23]

Grossly, there is an elongated and narrowed pyloric canal resulting from a pyloric ring muscle, which is both elongated up to twice the normal length and thickened up to three or four times the normal adult thickness. This thickened pyloric ring merges with the muscle of the stomach but ceases abruptly in its transition into the duodenum.[13,24] The hypertrophic muscle forms a mass that projects into the lumen of the duodenum, resembling the protrusion of the cervix uteri into the vagina. Microscopically, the typical change manifests as both hypertrophy and hyperplasia of the pyloric sphincter smooth muscle, without increase in the collagenous tissue. The thickened circular muscle is made up of interlacing fascicles of smooth muscle fibers, running in different directions, and reminiscent of the structure of a leiomyoma. Ill-defined degenerative changes have been observed in the myenteric neural plexus within the pylorus, and loss of neuronal bodies has been reported.[25] These changes have not been clearly defined, particularly regarding the neurotransmitters that may be involved. In severe cases resulting in protracted and frequent vomiting, the submucosa may show thickening by edema and congestion, further contributing to the narrowing of the pyloric canal. Pyloromyotomy, a relatively simple surgical operation not requiring entry into the gastric cavity, results in quick and complete relief of the obstruction, though the pyloric hypertrophy itself may persist for quite some time.[26]

Heterotopias

Heterotopic structures are not rare in the stomach, particularly in the antral region and along the pyloric canal. Two types have been described.

Heterotopic pancreatic tissue is composed of ducts and acini and rarely contains discrete endocrine islets. These lesions appear as small mounds located in the submucosa and abutting into the lumen, measuring between 0.5 and 3.0 cm in maximum diameter. The overlying mucosa may show a central umbilication or even ulceration.[27]

Myoepithelial hamartomas or *adenomyomas* are also found in the submucosa and are composed of a combination of ducts, interlacing smooth muscle fascicles and Brunner's glands.[28] Because occasional nests of pancreatic tissue are often found in these hamartomas, many authors do not make a clear distinction between heterotopic pancreas and adenomyomas in the stomach.[13,28]

The duodenum is also a relatively common site of heterotopias. Whereas superficial gastric heterotopia is known to be a metaplastic process associated with gastric acid hypersecretion, the presence of areas of full-thickness gastric oxyntic mucosa, containing prominent parietal cells, is regarded as a true malformation.[29] Another common malformation is the presence of ectopic pancreatic tissue. This presents as a nodule in the submucosal compartment in the vicinity of the ampulla of Vater and usually contains both endocrine and exocrine cells.[30] Another location of aberrant pancreatic tissue is the pyloric ring; these lesions consist of acinar and endocrine elements, embedded within the pyloric muscle, and sometimes causing pyloric stenosis with obstruction similar to that encountered in congenital pyloric stenosis.[31]

Congenital diaphragmatic hernias

Most congenital diaphragmatic hernias are known as *pleuroperitoneal hernias* and are the result of a persistent pleuroperitoneal canal or foramen of Bochdalek.[32,33] The defect is located in a posterolateral position, and the left side is involved several times more often than the right side. There is a good deal of variation in the size of these hernias and hence of the symptoms associated with their existence. Small defects may not be diagnosed for years until signs of obstruction appear. In contrast, large defects may allow the passage of massive quantities of abdominal viscera resulting in displacement and compression of the thoracic organs. These in turn lead to displacement of the normal heartbeat, cyanosis and dyspnea, vomiting, and, in the most serious cases, death. Other, less frequent, types of diaphragmatic hernia are the *retrosternal hernia,* resulting from patency of one or both foramens of Morgagni,[34] and the *pericardiodiaphragmatic hernia,* as a consequence of the defective formation of the septum transversum. The latter condition is generally accompanied by a series of other congenital defects including those in the heart, abdominal wall, sternum, and so forth sometimes associated with trisomy 18.[35]

CIRCULATORY DISTURBANCES

Ischemia

The richly anastomotic arterial blood supply from multiple sources that supplies the stomach makes vascular narrowing or occlusion extremely rare causes of ischemic damage. The gastric mucosa, however, is vulnerable to the ischemia resulting from reduced blood supply to the splanchnic circulation that accompanies the severe hypotension occurring during the course of certain systemic conditions, particularly shock.[36-38] This is the underlying pathogenetic mechanism of stress ulcers and acute erosions (see later).

Congestive gastropathy

The stomach of patients with cirrhosis is often affected by various mucosal changes collectively known as *congestive gastropathy*.[39] The cardinal alteration is a mucosal vasculopathy characterized by vascular ectasia; inflammation is infrequent and, if present, apparently unrelated to the underlying venous hypertension. Endoscopically, the gastric mucosa has been compared to "snake skin," "scarlatina rash," and "measles rash." These and other colorful terms describe the types of congested or hemorrhagic appearance of the mucosa, which may also show petechiae, hemorrhagic erosions, and multiple bleeding spots. Microscopically, congestion of capillaries, dilatation of superficial vessels, edema, and hyperplasia of the muscularis mucosae have been observed. The presence of congestive gastropathy is a significant risk indicator of both chronic and overt bleeding, but it does not appear to affect survival independently.[40] It is important to differentiate between portal hypertensive gastropathy and gastric antral vascular ectasia (see below), since their treatment and outlook are quite different.[41]

Because the lower portion of the esophagus and the cardiac region of the stomach share the same venous drainage, patients with portal hypertension and esophageal varices frequently have also varices around the cardiac orifice and in the most proximal portion of the lesser curvature. The presence of dilated gastric veins in the absence of esophageal varices is extremely rare.

Gastric antral vascular ectasia

Gastric antral vascular ectasia ("watermelon stomach") is a rare cause of occult gastrointestinal bleeding and iron deficiency anemia characterized by a distinctive endoscopic appearance of the gastric antrum. Although less than 100 patients have been reported up to now, there appears to be a prevalence of elderly women and a weak association with atrophic gastritis and systemic sclerosis. The main findings are prominent flat or raised erythematous "watermelon stripes" radiating in spokelike fashion from the pylorus[42] (Fig. 53-5). Microscopically the characteristic features are dilated capillaries with focal thrombosis, dilated tortuous submucosal veins, and fibromuscular hyperplasia in the lamina propria of the antral mucosa[43] (Fig. 53-6); the corpus is usually normal. The pathogenesis of this lesion is unknown, but some authors have proposed mucosal trauma as a possible initial mechanism.[44] Antrectomy is usually the treatment of choice, but, because many patients are elderly and have associated conditions, endoscopic laser coagulation appears to be a safe and efficacious therapeutic alternative.[45]

Vasculitis

Gastrointestinal manifestations occur in 30% to 70% of patients with polyarteritis nodosa and systemic lupus erythem-atosus and more rarely in patients with rheumatoid arthritis, hypersensitivity angiitis, and Wegener's granulomatosis. The lesions in the gastrointestinal tract are related to the ischemic injury caused by occlusion of the affected vessels, which results in focal or diffuse mucosal necrosis and the formation of erosions or ulcers. Although the small intestine and the colon are affected more commonly, gastric lesions have been described in association with virtually all the above diseases.[46-49]

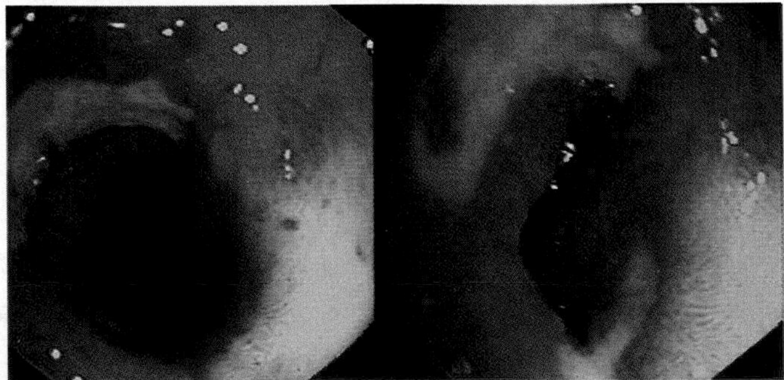

Fig. 53-5 Endoscopic photographs illustrating the typical appearance of the so-called watermelon stomach, which is characterized by alternating pink and deep red streaks as a result of focal vascular ectasia.

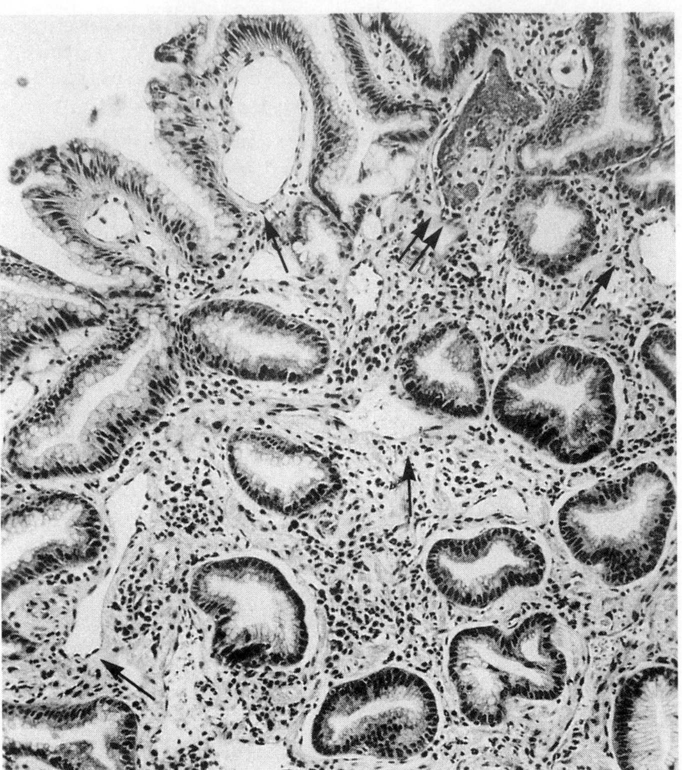

Fig. 53-6 Medium-power microphotograph of the gastric mucosa in "watermelon stomach." The lamina propria is expanded by fibrosis, increased numbers of smooth muscle fibers, scattered chronic inflammatory cells, and numerous thin-walled, dilated blood vessels *(arrows);* one of the latter contains a fibrin thrombus in its lumen *(double arrows).*

GASTRITIS

Gastritis is a term that conveys different meanings to different people. Pathologists view gastritis as an inflammatory process involving the gastric mucosa. Endoscopists often associate the term with a reddened, edematous, or eroded lining of the stomach. To many clinicians and lay persons the term *gastritis* evokes a wide range of poorly defined upper abdominal signs and symptoms. Despite or perhaps because of the many classifications of gastritis proposed in the last two decades, today's pathologists confronted with a gastric biopsy specimen have many good reasons to remain confused, and many sidestep the issue by releasing broadly descriptive but imprecise diagnoses. Before proceeding to illustrate the most important types of gastritides, this section briefly recapitulates the history of the modern classification of gastritis, highlighting the difficulties associated with the attempt to link cause, pathogenesis, and morphology in a single system.

Early classifications

Soon after it became possible to visualize the living stomach through the endoscope and examine histologically samples of gastric mucosa obtained through the biopsy forceps, researchers were baffled by the lack of correlation between a patient's symptoms, the endoscopic appearance of the stomach, and the degree of inflammation seen microscopically. As more patients of all ages were being endoscoped, it became apparent that the histologic markers of gastritis were detected in large segments of the asymptomatic population and that the prevalence of histologic gastritis increased steadily with age. Was chronic gastritis a disease or merely part of the normal process of aging? Later, interesting epidemiologic and geographic differences emerged: in the industrialized Western world, about 50% of subjects over 60 years of age have chronic gastritis; in some developing countries virtually everybody has gastritis by 50 years of age. Because of the extraordinary difficulties of correlating clinical, epidemiologic, and endoscopic findings with the histologic features of the mucosa, several pathologists went on to classify gastritis on strictly morphologic criteria. Among these classifications, the one put forward by Whitehead and his colleagues in 1972 became the most widely accepted.[50] These authors essentially ignored the issue of acute gastritis, an entity very rarely seen under the microscope, and, following earlier concepts espoused by Motteram[51] more than two decades earlier, divided chronic gastritis in superficial, atrophic, and gastric atrophy. They also introduced the terms *type A*, for the rare autoimmune atrophy seen in patients with pernicious anemia, and *type B*, for the more common chronic gastritis of unknown cause. This division was reinforced and clarified by Strickland and MacKay shortly thereafter.[52]

These early classifications, often slightly modified by subsequent investigators, were used for several years until it became generally accepted that many forms of gastritis are caused by or at least associated with *Helicobacter pylori*. This bacterium, briefly known as *Campylobacter pyloridis* and then *Campylobacter pylori*, acquired its current name in 1989,[53] only 6 years after its first description as "unidentified curved bacilli on gastric epithelium" by Warren and Marshall.[54,55] *H. pylori* is a gram-negative bacterium with a distinctive spiral shape, which is easily identified in histologic specimens. The bacterium measures between 2.5 and 4.0 μm in length and between 0.5 and 1.0 μm in diameter; its extremities are rounded, and it has two or more polar flagella.[56,57] One of the most distinctive biochemical features of *H. pylori* is its ability to produce large amounts of urease, an activity to which it devotes a tremendous amount of its metabolic resources.[58] Urease may have a number of important functions, including enabling the initial colonization of the gastric mucosa and allowing its survival in an acid environment.[59,60] Predictably, the discovery that *H. pylori* was associated with and perhaps responsible for the overwhelming majority of cases of the previously "idiopathic" chronic active gastritis made possible new classifications that would take into account etiology. New modifications of the existing schemes emerged, including the Sydney system.

The Sydney system

Aware of the inconsistencies among classifications and of the schism separating users from the conceivers, a group of gastroenterologists and pathologists formed a working party at the ninth World Congress of Gastroenterology in Sydney, Australia, in 1990, and generated a new comprehensive classification of gastritis.[61] The aims of the Sydney system, as it was called, were to create a flexible matrix of rules that respond to the changing demands of the subject and to produce a simple, easy-to-apply, comprehensive, and comprehensible classification, which is flexible and capable of correlation with preexisting ideas. This classification was divided in two parts. The endoscopic division is a system for reporting the endoscopic appearance of the stomach, so that a database can be created for the correlation with the microscopic aspects. The histological division incorporates "a logical combination of etiology, topography, and morphology." More of a recording/reporting system than a truly innovative classification, the Sydney system diagnosis of a typical set of biopsies from the antrum and the corpus from a patient with chronic active gastritis would read: *"Helicobacter pylori*–associated chronic pangastritis, with moderate activity, no atrophy, and no intestinal metaplasia." Now almost 6 years old, the Sydney system has been largely ignored by pathologists outside Europe. At the time of this writing, new panels of pathologists from various parts of the world are forming to reappraise the Sydney system and make it more usable.

For the purposes of this chapter, we consider the conditions of the stomach generally known as *gastritides* into two major categories, acute and chronic. The classification of acute gastritis, for which there is a good etiologic and clinical correlation, is largely free of debate. The chronic gastritides, on the other hand, are divided into categories, roughly corresponding to nosologic entities, as follows: (1) *chemical gastritis,* (2) *autoimmune* gastritis, (3) *chronic nonatrophic H. pylori* gastritis, and (4) *environmental* gastritis, also referred to as *multifocal atrophic gastritis* (MAG). The main characteristics of these four entities are compared in Table 53-1. A fifth group, referred to as *miscellaneous* chronic gastritis, is composed of a variety of conditions and is dealt with separately.

Acute infectious gastritis

Primary infections of the stomach used to be considered extremely uncommon and limited to rare circumstances in which a patient's pH remained elevated for a period of time sufficient to allow bacterial overgrowth. Two sets of circumstances that have required a radical revision of this concept occurred in the last decade. One is the discovery that *H. pylori* is responsible for chronic active gastritis and that chronic infection with this bacterium is one of the most prevalent infections of humankind. The other is the pandemic of the acquired immunodeficiency syndrome (AIDS), which has made a large segment of the population susceptible to infectious agents previously found only in the unusual immunosuppressed patient; these agents include viral, fungal, bacterial, and parasitic organisms capable of infecting the stomach. Infection with *H. pylori* is extensively discussed with chronic gastritis; therefore, in this section we limit our discussion to the other causes of infectious gastritis.

Viral gastritis

Although many common enteroviruses are believed to infect the gastric mucosa, so few patients with acute gastroenteritis undergo gastric biopsy that no information is available on the morphologic features of these infections. The only viral infections of the stomach with a distinct pathologic appearance are those caused by cytomegalovirus (CMV). CMV gastritis is seen only in patients with AIDS[62,63] or those receiving immunosuppressive doses of corticosteroids[64,65] and is usually associated with concurrent CMV infection of other sites of the digestive tract. Endoscopically the gastric mucosa may appear

Table 53-1 Main types of chronic gastritis

	Chemical	Autoimmune	Chronic active	Environmental
Synonyms	Reflux	Type A	Type B	Type AB
Etiology	D-G reflux or NSAID administration	Antibodies to proton pump and to pepsinogens	*H. pylori* infection	*H. pylori* infection Low vitamin C and high salt intake Nitrosamination
Location	Antrum + + Corpus +	Corpus + + + Antrum –	Antrum + + + Corpus +	Antrum + + + Corpus + +
Atrophy	+ +	+ + + +	±	+ + +
Associations	Erosive gastritis	Pernicious anemia	Peptic ulcer disease	Multifocal atrophic gastritis
Complications	Hemorrhage	Carcinoids	Ulceration, MALToma	Adenocarcinoma, MALToma

D-G, Duodenal-gastric; *NSAID,* nonsteroidal anti-inflammatory drugs.

completely normal or show erosions or shallow ulcers. The histopathologic appearance varies depending on the patient's ability to mount an immune response.[66] In some patients, particularly those with very low CD4 counts, numerous CMV inclusions may be seen in mucosal and endothelial cells as well as in macrophages, with little of no inflammatory response in the adjacent tissues. In other patients one may see a florid mixed inflammatory reaction with abundant granulation tissue, and typical CMV inclusions may be difficult to detect without the use of immunohistochemistry or in situ hybridization techniques. Herpesvirus may rarely infect the gastric mucosa of AIDS patients.[67,68]

Bacterial gastritis

Acute suppurative gastritis, caused by pyogenic bacteria, is an extremely rare condition also known as *phlegmonous gastritis*.[69,70] This life-threatening condition, sometimes present in pediatric patients, is characterized by the presence of large areas of purulent necrosis involving the full thickness of the gastric wall. When caused by gas-forming organisms, the term *emphysematous gastritis* has been used.[71] Infiltration of the gastric wall by gas has also been described in association with disseminated strongyloidiasis[72] and with the ingestion of lye.[73]

Bacterial overgrowth is believed to occur in the achlorhydric stomach, secondary to gastric atrophy associated with pernicious anemia, after complete antrectomy or vagotomy, or with the continuous use of H_2-receptor antagonists and acid pump inhibitors. The bacterial colonization of the achlorhydric stomach rarely results in symptomatic or histologically detectable gastritis. In patients with disseminated tuberculosis, mycobacteria may rarely involve the stomach, where they may elicit the formation of mucosal necrotizing granulomas identical to those found in other locations.[74,75] Another mycobacterium that has gained prominence with the spread of AIDS is *Mycobacterium avium–intracellulare.* When the stomach is involved, the typical lesions manifest as accumulations of foamy histiocytes in the lamina propria of the mucosa, sometimes with formation of ill-defined granulomas, but without necrosis. Staining for acid-fast bacilli reveals large numbers of positive microorganisms both within the histiocytes and extracellularly, in the stroma.[76]

Like tuberculous gastritis, gastric syphilis was a medical curiosity in the years preceding the AIDS pandemic. Recently, however, an increasing number of cases has been reported in HIV-infected patients.[77] When associated with secondary syphilis, syphilitic gastritis is characterized by a prominent mixed inflammatory infiltrate consisting predominantly of plasma cells and by mucosal ulcerations. Spirochetes may be seen in sections stained with appropriate silver stains (Dieterle, Steiner's, or Warthin-Starry).[78] The infiltrate may be dense enough to cause the swelling of gastric folds, which may also undergo erosion and ulceration, sometimes mimicking the endoscopic appearance of lymphoma or infiltrating carcinoma.[79]

Fungal gastritis

Candida species, *Histoplasma capsulatum,* and Mucoraceae have been found in the stomach of immunocompromised individuals, particularly AIDS patients, with disseminated infections. Endoscopically, gastric candidiasis appears as whitish patches scattered on the mucosa; microscopically, yeast forms are seen lying on and sometimes invading the eroded gastric mucosa. Hyphae of *Candida* spp. may be found at the base of a large portion of gastric ulcers, but they are believed to represent the secondary colonization of preexisting peptic ulcers.[80-82] Histoplasmosis is diagnosed when the typical intracellular organisms are found within macrophages of the mucosa, which may be grossly intact, eroded, or ulcerated.[83,84] Gastric invasion by mucormycosis agents, belonging to the Phycomycetes class, is rarely encountered and only in severely debilitated, immunocompromised patients. The typical lesions consist of extensive hemorrhage and necrosis accompanied by abundant inflammatory infiltrate but without granuloma formation. Although the lesions are primarily mucosal, they can extend deeply into the wall and cause perforation.[85,86]

Parasitic gastritis

The stomach is not a preferred site for human parasitic infections. Both *Cryptosporidum* spp.[87] and *Strongyloides sterco-*

ralis[88] have been found in the stomach of patients with disseminated infections. *Anisakis* larvae ingested by eating raw fish may penetrate and even perforate the gastric wall. In the few surgically resected specimens available for examination during this event, large numbers of eosinophils have been observed at the site of penetration,[89] whereas a granulomatous reaction usually surrounds the parasitic organisms in chronic cases.[90]

Chemical gastritis

The expression *chemical gastritis* was first utilized by O'Connor and coworkers in reference to the changes that appear in the gastric mucosa after exposure to bile reflux.[91] However, this term has later been applied to similar morphologic changes resulting from exposure to other chemical injury, most prominently the group of drugs collectively referred to as *nonsteroidal anti-inflammatory drugs (NSAIDs)*.

Indeed, some of the most common lesions of the stomach in developed countries are caused by the ingestion of NSAIDs. All these drugs, which include aspirin, ibuprofen, naproxen, and a variety of other products, are prostaglandin inhibitors and interfere with the cytoprotective action of the gastric mucus, thus exposing the mucosa to the corrosive effects of acid. Because the effect of these drugs is systemic, direct contact of the pill with the mucosa is not necessary, and similar lesions may be observed in both oral and parenteral users of NSAIDs. Typically the acute, early NSAID-induced lesions are small hemorrhagic mucosal erosions.[92] Endoscopically, they appear as isolated or multiple shallow mucosal lesions, located most often in the antrum. The remainder of the mucosa is usually normal. Earlier injuries, particularly those associated with the ingestion of large amounts of alcohol or drugs, such as aspirin, that affect the coagulation system, may show only superficial vascular dilatation and congestion, with fresh hemorrhage in the lamina propria without significant epithelial damage and with no polymorphonuclear infiltration.[93,94] In more advanced lesions the mucosa shows loss of the superficial layers, often limited to the surface epithelium; a deposit of fibrin, mixed with blood and neutrophils fills the mucosal gap and often extrudes above the level of the surface epithelium. The epithelium adjacent to the damaged area may be infiltrated by low numbers of inflammatory cells and shows regenerative changes. These erosions are limited to the mucosa and are repaired without the formation of granulation tissue. When a biopsy is done during the healing phase, one may observe prominent foveolar cell hyperplasia. The amount of inflammation is scanty and strictly limited to the area involved. In addition to a moderate degree of glandular atrophy and distortion, variable amounts of fibrosis and abundant smooth muscle can be appreciated in the intervening lamina propria (Fig. 53-7).

The relationship between NSAID ingestion and chronic peptic ulcer is still being evaluated. As is to be expected, a significant number of patients who are affected with NSAID-induced gastritis are, at the same time, infected with *pylori*. In such cases, it is difficult to sort out the pathogenesis of the range of lesions present.[95] It is clear that the prevalence of gastric ulcers is significantly increased in individuals who ingest NSAIDs on a regular basis.[91,94] These lesions are more often located in the distal portion of the antrum, on the greater curvature.[96] In addition, although it does not appear that NSAID exposure results in an increased prevalence of duodenal ulcers, these tend to bleed more often in patients who take NSAIDs.[97]

Bile reflux causes a type of chronic gastritis similar in location and in histopathologic appearance to that seen in the healing phases of NSAID-related gastritis.[98,99] The damage induced by the bile appears to be compounded by the presence of pancreatic juice, which causes the formation of lysolecithin.[100] The degree of damage induced in nonoperated patients by reflux of bile from duodenum to stomach through an incompetent pylorus tends to be limited and is restricted in great measure to the antral mucosa.[98] Mucosal erosion and ulceration are rare and, when present, minimal. Again the effects of a concomitant infection with *H. pylori* may represent a poorly defined confounding factor in a substantial number of patients.[101,102] Furthermore, because it is not uncommon to find combinations of what appears to be bile reflux and NSAID intake, some workers believe that pure bile reflux gastritis in nonoperated patients may be a rare occurrence.[103,104]

By contrast, in the diminishing cohort of patients subjected to antrectomy, the effects of bile and pancreatic juice reflux into the stomach may be a good deal more dramatic.[99,105,106] It is important to remember that in such patients elimination of the mucosal trophic effects by gastrin and vagal innervation leads to significant atrophy of the glandular component of the oxyntic mucosa.[107] Intestinal metaplasia does not appear to be a significant feature in this type of gastritis and, when present, has been related to the presence of concomitant *H. pylori* infection.[108] In antrectomized patients, particularly those subjected to a Billroth II procedure, the glandular atrophy and foveolar hyperplasia are particularly prominent; the latter acquires a tortuous configuration, sometimes conferring the mucosal surface a pseudovilliform pattern. In severe, long-standing cases, this hyperplasia leads to the formation of visi-

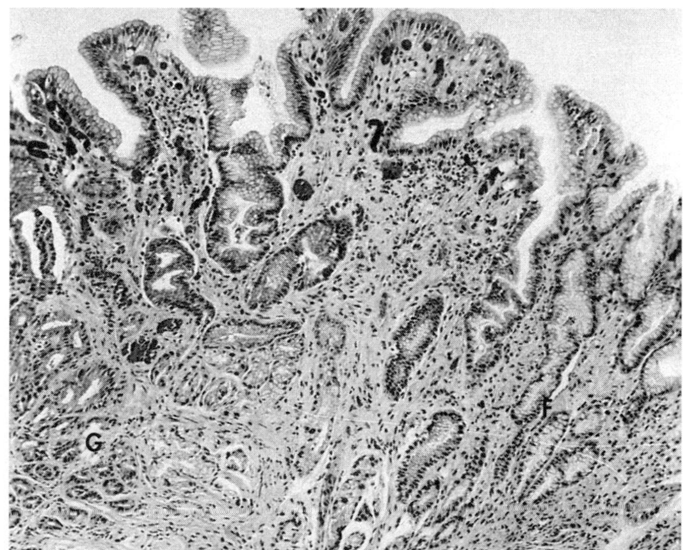

Fig. 53-7 Low-power microphotograph of the gastric mucosa in the so-called chemical gastritis. The antral glands *(G)* are somewhat atrophic, whereas the foveolar compartment *(F)* is significantly enlarged and reactive. The intervening lamina propria is considerably expanded by fibrosis and the presence of smooth muscle fibers and contains numerous congested capillaries, particularly toward the surface. Of note is the paucity of inflammatory cells in the lamina propria in this condition.

ble lesions in the proximity of the stoma. These are characterized either as *gastritis cystica polyposa,*[109,110] or, when the cystically dilated glands are seen under the muscularis mucosae, they are called *gastritis cystica profunda.*[111-113] The latter must be distinguished, on the basis of the cytologic features of the epithelial cells, from a well-differentiated adenocarcinoma of the stomach.

Autoimmune gastritis

Autoimmune gastritis, also known as *type A,* or *diffuse corporal atrophic, gastritis,* is a distinctive clinicopathological entity generally seen in association with the pernicious anemia syndrome.[114,115] This progressive lesion, commonly inherited as an autosomal dominant trait with incomplete penetrance[116] commonly affects patients with a northern European ethnic background.[115] These patients show the presence of circulating autoantibodies against the alpha and beta subunits of the parietal cell proton pump and the chief cell pepsinogens.[117,118] The gastritic process, resulting in almost total loss of oxyntic mucosa through atrophy, also leads to loss of intrinsic factor and failure of vitamin B_{12} absorption, ultimately resulting in pernicious anemia.[115]

Autoimmune, or type A, gastritis is restricted to the oxyntic corpus and fundus mucosa of the stomach and is characterized by a progressive replacement of the normal mucosa by patches of antral, pseudoantral, and later intestinal metaplasia. As a rule, small patches of oxyntic mucosa remain intact, even in advanced disease.[119-121] True antral metaplasia differs from the pseudoantral variety by the presence of gastrin-immunoreactive cells, absent from the latter. Pseudoantral metaplasia, on the other hand, exhibits the presence of enterochromaffin-like (ECL) cells and of pepsinogen I when investigated by immunocytochemistry.[121] The intestinal metaplasia is generally of the so-called complete or small intestinal type. This is characterized by the presence of enterocytes and goblet cells at the surface and by the presence of crypt, Paneth's, and endocrine cells in the basal portions of the metaplastic mucosa.[122,123] Figs. 53-8 and 53-9 illustrate the histologic appearance of the gastric mucosa in autoimmune gastritis. The mucins stored are nonsulfated sialomucins, and as a rule there is no significant atypia or dysplasia associated with this metaplastic change.[123] Variable degrees of chronic inflammation are observed in the lamina propria of both fundus and, with a superficial location, of the antral mucosa. Superficial antral gastritis has been reported in younger subjects with autoimmune fundal gastritis;[124] however, with advancing age, the fundal gastritis progresses, with generalized atrophy as the end

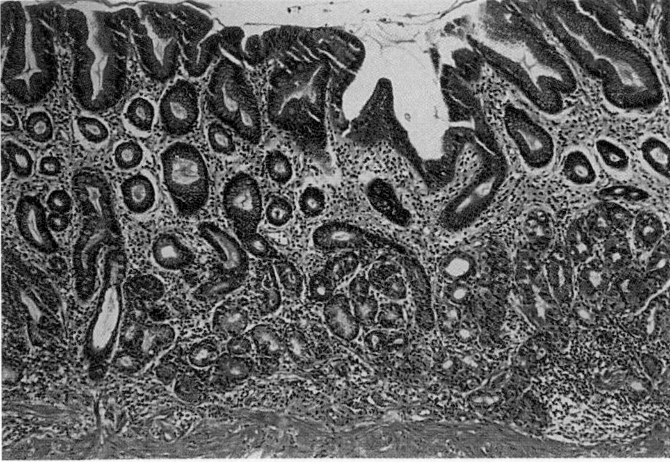

Fig. 53-8 Low-power microphotograph of the gastric oxyntic mucosa exhibiting autoimmune diffuse atrophic gastritis associated with pernicious anemia. A small island of recognizable oxyntic mucosa persists on the right hand side, whereas most of the rest is replaced by pseudoantral metaplasia. The intervening lamina propria shows mild edema and the presence of a few scattered inflammatory cells.

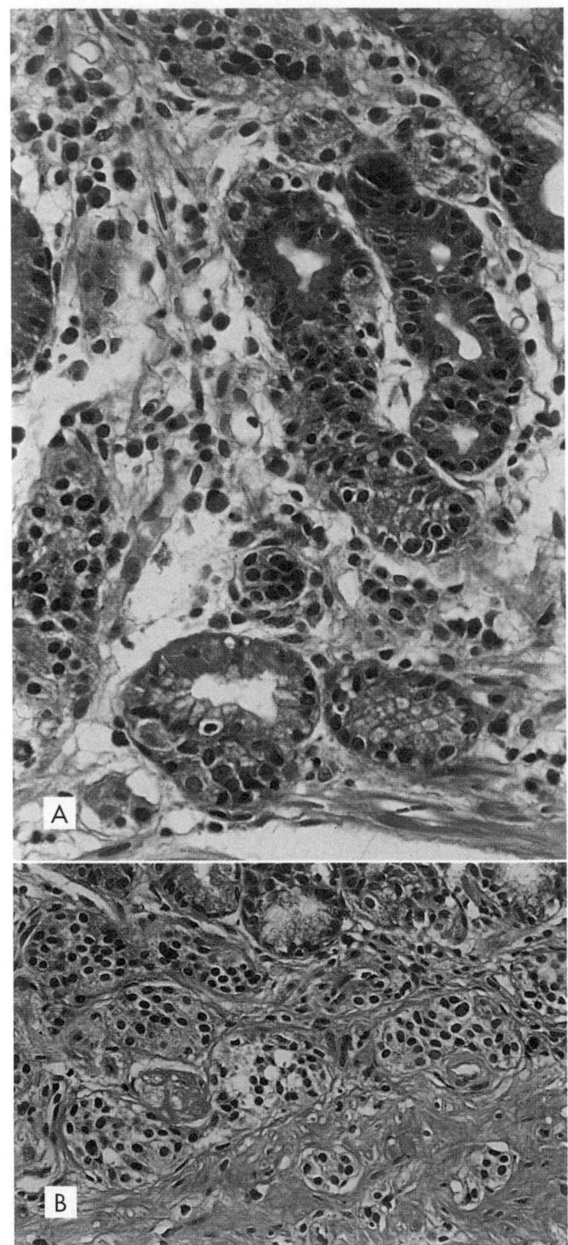

Fig. 53-9 Autoimmune atrophic gastritis. **A,** Medium-power photomicrograph atrophic pseudoantral glands. Some of these show clusters of polygonal clear cells, representing hyperplastic endocrine cells. Notice that the intervening lamina propria contains only moderate numbers of inflammatory cells. **B,** Close-up view of the bottom of the mucosa, including the muscularis mucosae at the bottom, showing numerous clusters of endocrine cells with light cytoplasm. These not only are present independent of the glands in the lamina propria, but also are found embedded in the muscularis mucosae.

point, whereas the antral gastritis decreases.[125,126] Loss of gastric acid production, the normal negative-feedback mechanism for the release of antral gastrin, results in stimulation of gastrin-producing (G) cells, with occurrence of G-cell hyperplasia and hypergastrinemia.[121,127] The latter, in turn, serves as a powerful trophic factor for the ECL-cells of the oxyntic mucosa, which exhibit variable degrees of hyperplasia.[128,129] In several cases, ECL, hyperplasia evolves into dysplasia, microcarcinoid formation, and the appearance of invasive gastric carcinoid tumors.[130]

Chronic nonatrophic gastritis

Chronic gastritis caused by infection with *H. pylori* is one of the most common chronic conditions of humankind, affecting an estimated two thirds of the world population.[131] The histopathological and clinical manifestations of *H. pylori* infection ranges from a mild indolent inflammatory infiltrate localized to the superficial layers of the antral mucosa (chronic antral gastritis) to a severe active inflammation affecting the entire stomach from antrum to cardia (pangastritis).[132] Depending on the multifactorial influence of yet unidentified bacterial virulence factors, individual host responses, and environmental determinants, chronic *H. pylori* gastritis may remain essentially unchanged for years, may cause the development of duodenal ulcer, or may evolve into atrophic gastritis, a condition that creates the background for the development of gastric ulcer and gastric carcinoma.[131] In a smaller subset of patients *H. pylori* gastritis may create a milieu favorable to the development of primary gastric lymphomas of the MALT type.[133] Fig. 53-10 depicts the multiple possible pathways resulting from *H. pylori* infection of the gastric mucosa.

Helicobacter pylori *Gastritis*

In a fashion similar to other bacterial infections, one of two possible occurrences follows the entrance of *H. pylori* into the host: either the organism is eliminated because of insufficient size of the inoculum, low virulence, or effective host responses, or it may initiate an infection. When it does so, *H. pylori* initially induces an inflammatory reaction that is predominantly polymorphonuclear and may be accompanied by the clinical features of acute gastritis, with epigastric pain, malaise, vomiting, and transient hypochlorhydria.[134,135] When this response subsides, the inflammatory infiltrate becomes mixed and includes polymorphonuclear leukocytes along with lymphoplasmacytic infiltrates with development of lymphoid follicles. At this stage, the clinical manifestations usually disappear. Although often intense and virtually always associated with local and systemic humoral responses, this combined reaction appears ineffective in eradicating the organism. A balance apparently develops between host and bacterium, which allows *H. pylori* to attain a certain biomass and survive, presumably unharmed, as long as appropriate conditions exist within the gastric ecosystem.

The typical histopathologic features of *H. pylori* chronic antral gastritis have been abundantly described[120,132] and are depicted in Fig. 53-11. The architecture of the mucosa is well preserved, with often only minor disarray of the pits caused by the lymphoplasmacytic infiltrate occupying the lamina propria. Neutrophils and variable numbers of eosinophils are mixed with the mononuclear infiltrate, but they are most prominent within the foveolar epithelium, where they are seen individually or in minute clusters. Small aggregates of neutrophils can often be seen on the surface epithelium and within the pits, forming the so-called pit abscesses. The antral glands may be separated by the infiltrate in the lamina propria. *H. pylori* organisms are located singly or in clusters along the surface and foveolar epithelium, entrapped within mucus strands, freely floating in the foveolar spaces, adherent to the columnar cells, or inserted between mucus cells (Fig. 53-12). Only exceptionally are rare isolated organisms seen in the lumen of mucus glands or within the lumen of oxyntic glands. Surface epithelial damage in various degrees of intensity almost invariably accompanies *H. pylori* infection and may occur in both antrum and corpus.[132,136] These cellular alterations manifest as flattening of the surface cells, formation of hyperplas-

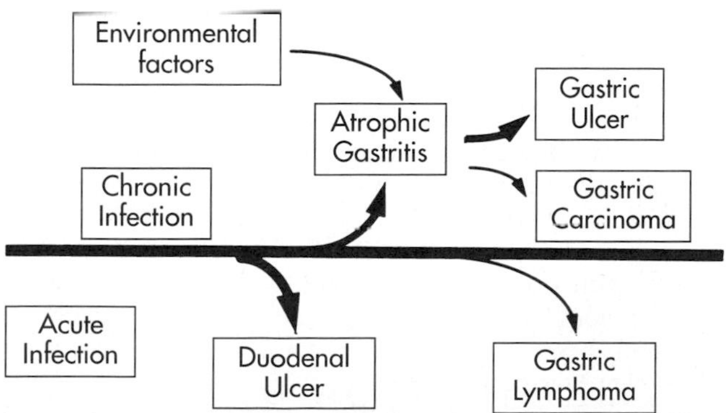

Fig. 53-10 Different pathways that may result from chronic infection with *Helicobacter pylori* and possible outcomes related to additional factors.

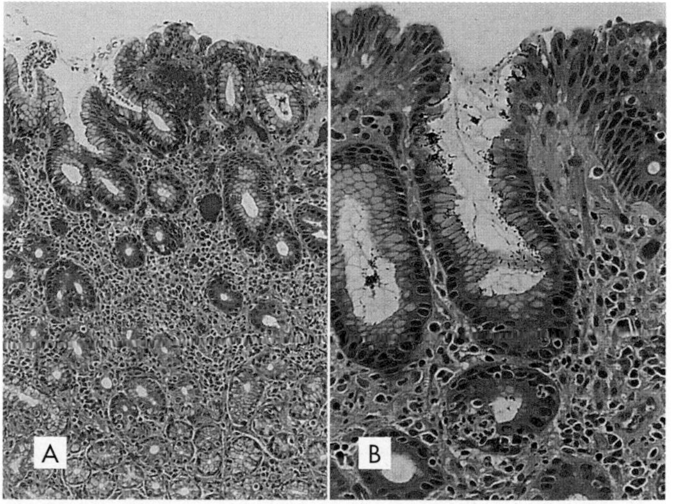

Fig. 53-11 Gastric antral mucosa exhibiting chronic active gastritis associated with *Helicobacter pylori*. **A,** Low-power photomicrograph. The lamina propria is expanded and contains increased numbers of inflammatory cells. The foveolae show mild reactive changes. **B,** High power photomicrograph. The intervening lamina propria contains increased numbers of chronic as well as scattered acute inflammatory cells. Several polymorphonuclear leukocytes are seen penetrating into and distorting a cross section of a gastric pit. Numerous *H. pylori* organisms are seen stained in black on the surface of the foveolar epithelium. (Steiner silver stain counterstained with hematoxylin and eosin.).

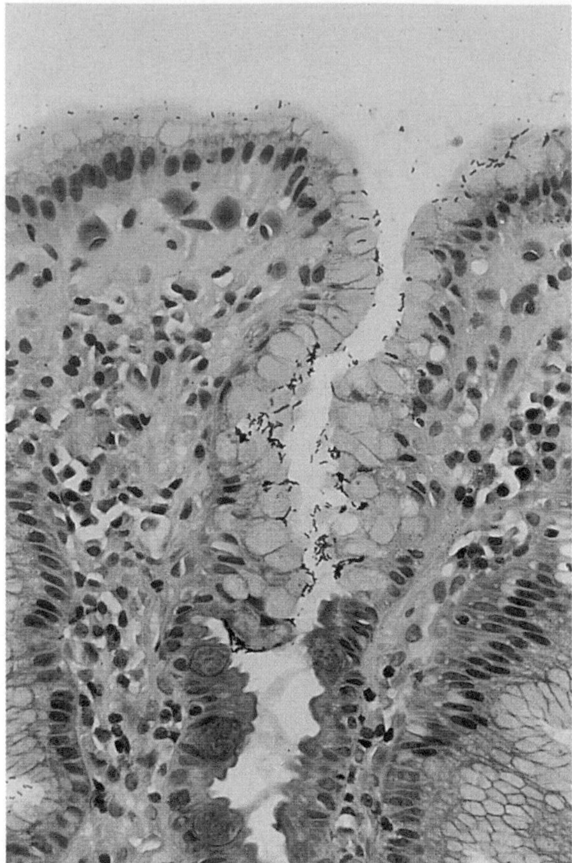

Fig. 53-12 *Helicobacter pylori* organisms are found in significant numbers lying over the surface mucous cells of the gastric mucosa and over the foveolar mucous cells. Notice, however, that they are absent from the lower aspect of the central foveola, which has undergone intestinal metaplasia. (Genta's modification of Steiner silver stain.)

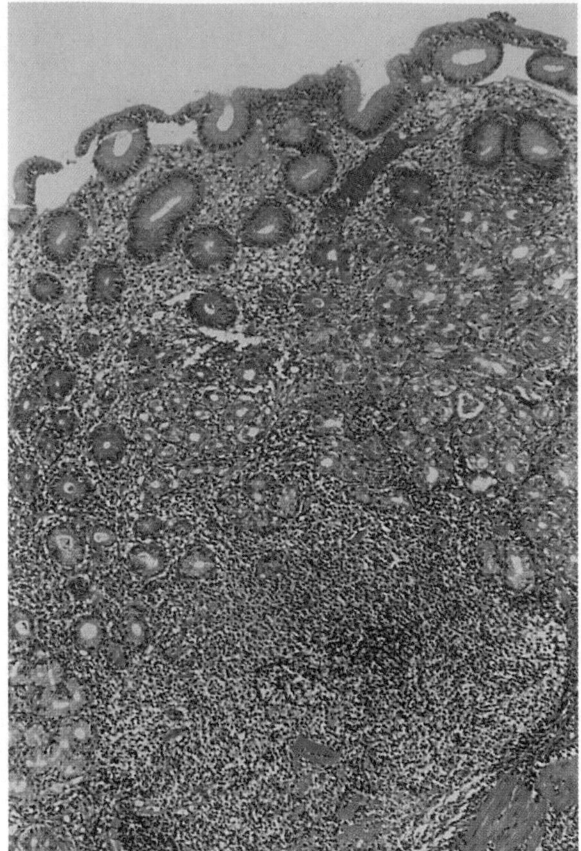

Fig. 53-13 Low-power microphotograph of gastric antral mucosa with chronic active gastritis associated with *Helicobacter pylori* infection. Notice the presence of a prominent lymphoid follicle in addition to the diffuse infiltration of the lamina propria. This type of lesion is highly characteristic of *H. pylori* infection.

tic-looking cellular tufts, and other subtler changes. This typical appearance can vary considerably depending on the size and relative proportions of the different components of the inflammatory infiltrate. Intraepithelial neutrophils may be so rare that they are difficult to find, even in the presence of large numbers of organisms. On the other hand, gross destruction of heavily infiltrated and dilated pits may be seen, and large numbers of polymorphonuclear cells may be mixed with the background mononuclear infiltrate. Lymphoid follicles, absent from the normal gastric mucosa, are being increasingly recognized as typical, if not pathognomonic, of *H. pylori* infection.[137,138] Fig. 53-13 illustrates the microscopic appearance of typical chronic active gastritis associated with *H. pylori* infection.

Although the density of organisms in the corpus of *H. pylori*–infected stomachs is slightly lower than that of the antrum, the prevalence of infection is essentially the same. In general, but not always, the overall inflammatory response is less intense in the corpus than in the antrum. When inflammation is present, it often has the appearance of what used to be known as superficial gastritis. A bandlike infiltrate of mononuclear cells separates the slightly elongated pits from the subjacent oxyntic mucosa, and usually very small numbers of neutrophils populate the columnar epithelium. Lymphoid follicles, though less prevalent than in the antrum, are frequently found in the corporal mucosa, even in cases when this area shows no other evidence of infection.[138]

Environmental gastritis

Our understanding of the natural evolution of the histopathologic features of *H. pylori*–associated gastritis is limited by the dearth of prospective long-term cohort studies. Data obtained from cross-sectional studies in populations with a high prevalence of *H. pylori* infection indicate that in a considerable percentage of patients the inflammation may eventually become exclusively mononuclear and slowly vanish over a period of years whereas at the same time the gastric glands decrease in number and the surface and foveolar epithelium undergoes intestinal metaplasia. The sequence of these changes represents the hypothetical pathway from *H. pylori*–associated chronic active gastritis to atrophic gastritis and eventually to gastric metaplasia and atrophy.[131,139] This manifestation of chronic gastritis was first called "multifocal" by Lambert[140] in 1977: *multifocal atrophic gastritis* seems the most appropriate name for this entity.

Chronic multifocal atrophic gastritis (MAG) is a variant of chronic atrophic gastritis, which is relatively uncommon in the United States but quite common and easily diagnosed in places with high incidence of gastric adenocarcinoma, such as many areas of Latin America, Japan, and China and less well recognized in Scandinavian and other European countries.[139,141-143] Since this entity is also found in the United States, particularly among socioeconomically disadvantaged populations,[139,144] it is important that it be recognized and diagnosed on a timely basis. This type of gastritis is generally associated with a high incidence of gastric adenocarcinoma[144-147] and one can recognize a variety of environmental factors, such as deficient intake of fresh fruits and vegetables,[148,149] high levels of $NaCl_2$ consumption,[150,151] and high rate of intragastric nitrosamine formation,[144,152,153] in addition to *H. pylori* infection, in its etiopathogenesis.

Chronic MAG is a process that starts at the antrofundic junction in the lesser curvature of the stomach and which extends, both distally and proximally, involving in a patchy fashion antral and oxyntic mucosae (Fig. 53-14). The characteristic lesion consists of patchy areas of atrophy and disappearance of either antral or oxyntic glands, which are replaced by intestinal metaplasia.[139,154,155] The intervening mucosa may be virtually normal in appearance, particularly in the oxyntic area, or it may show the presence of *H. pylori*–associated gastritis, characterized by increased numbers of chronic inflammatory cells in the lamina propria, foci of acute inflammation present in lamina propria and in glandular structures, and reactive features of the foveolar epithelium. Superficial erosions may also be present, accompanied by focal acute inflammation. Variable numbers of *Helicobacter*-like organisms may be seen in both foveolae and the mucus overlying the surface epithelium; these microorganisms generally can be seen in tissues stained with H&E, but when they are very scanty, it may be necessary to use special stains. Areas of intestinal metaplasia or of dysplasia as a rule do not contain *Helicobacter*-like organisms.[156] With the passage of time, these areas of atrophy and metaplasia tend to coalesce, the complete intestinal metaplasia becomes incomplete, also called "colonic" or "Type III," with appearance of sulfated mucins in intermediate as well as goblet cells.[157,158] This type of intestinal metaplasia is regarded as a reliable marker for malignant potential,[158-160] and some workers consider it as part of a continuum leading to neoplastic transformation.[161,162] Fig. 53-15 illustrates different aspects of MAG, or environmental gastritis.

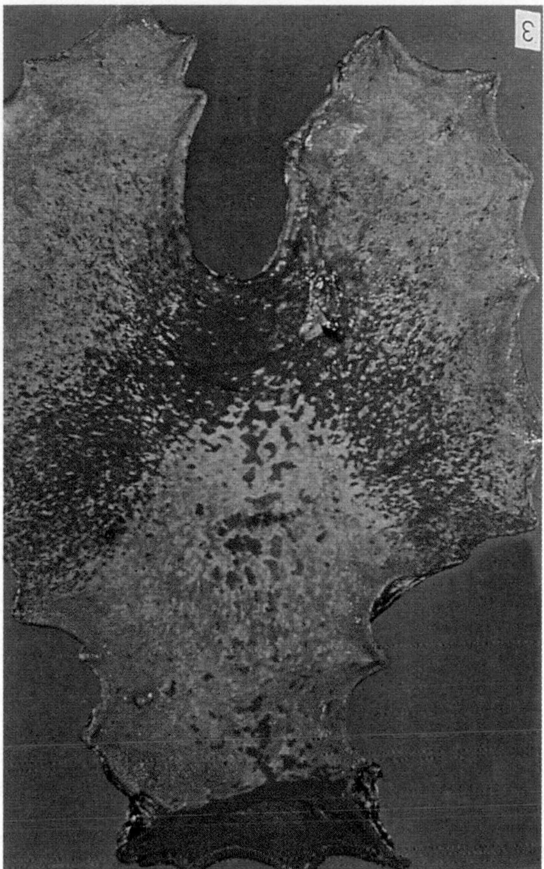

Fig. 53-14 Gross photograph of a subtotal gastrectomy specimen stained for acid phosphatase. Notice that the duodenum mucosa, at the bottom, stains brightly red. The antral-oxyntic boundary, describing an inverted V-shape with the apex at the lesser curvature, is also brightly stained in red, an indication of the degree of intestinal metaplasia experienced by the mucosa. In addition, multiple small foci of intestinal metaplasia surround the main lesion, all of which are characteristic of multifocal atrophic gastritis (MAG). This type of gastritis recognizes an environmental, multifactorial pathogenesis. (From Stemmerman GN, Hayashi T: *J Natl Cancer Inst* 41:627, 1968.)

Miscellaneous forms of gastritis

Eosinophilic gastritis

Eosinophilic gastritis is often part of the so-called eosinophilic gastroenteritis, an ill-defined group of conditions with the presence of infiltrates of eosinophile granulocytes as the common denominator.[163] This generic group of conditions, which affects pediatric patients more often than adults,[164] has been divided into a serosal type and a mural type, both of which are of unknown cause, and a mucosal type, generally the result of an allergic process.[165] In the mucosal form, the antrum is affected most frequently, and the intensity and extent of the process may vary widely.[166] Minor degrees of food allergy may acquire the form of scattered foci of eosinophilic infiltrates that involve individual glands and cause focal destruction; multiple biopsies may be necessary to arrive at the correct diagnosis in such instances. On the other hand, severe cases of allergic gastroenteritis will result in florid lesions consisting of widespread eosinophilic infiltration of the lamina propria of the mucosa, with extension to the submucosa and the superficial muscularis propria, and involvement of both glandular structures and surface epithelium, which may be eroded. This type of gastritis does not have a tendency to become chronic and must be separated from other conditions, such as parasitic diseases and Crohn's disease of the stomach, which may also present with eosinophilic infiltrates. The essential distinguishing feature of eosinophilic gastritis is the *destruction of glands* by the eosinophilic infiltrate. The mural variant, in contrast, is characterized by infiltration of the muscular wall with inflammatory infiltrate in which histiocytes and mature eosinophils are particularly prominent. This inflammation often forms an ill-defined mass, which may cause pyloric obstruction when it is located in the distal antrum. The overlying mucosa may show ulceration.[167,168]

Granulomatous gastritis

Granulomatous gastritis is a generic descriptor term that encompasses a variety of conditions, some idiopathic and some with a known cause. The granulomatous disorders of the stomach include infectious diseases, foreign-body reactions, Crohn's disease, sarcoidosis, and isolated granulomatous gas-

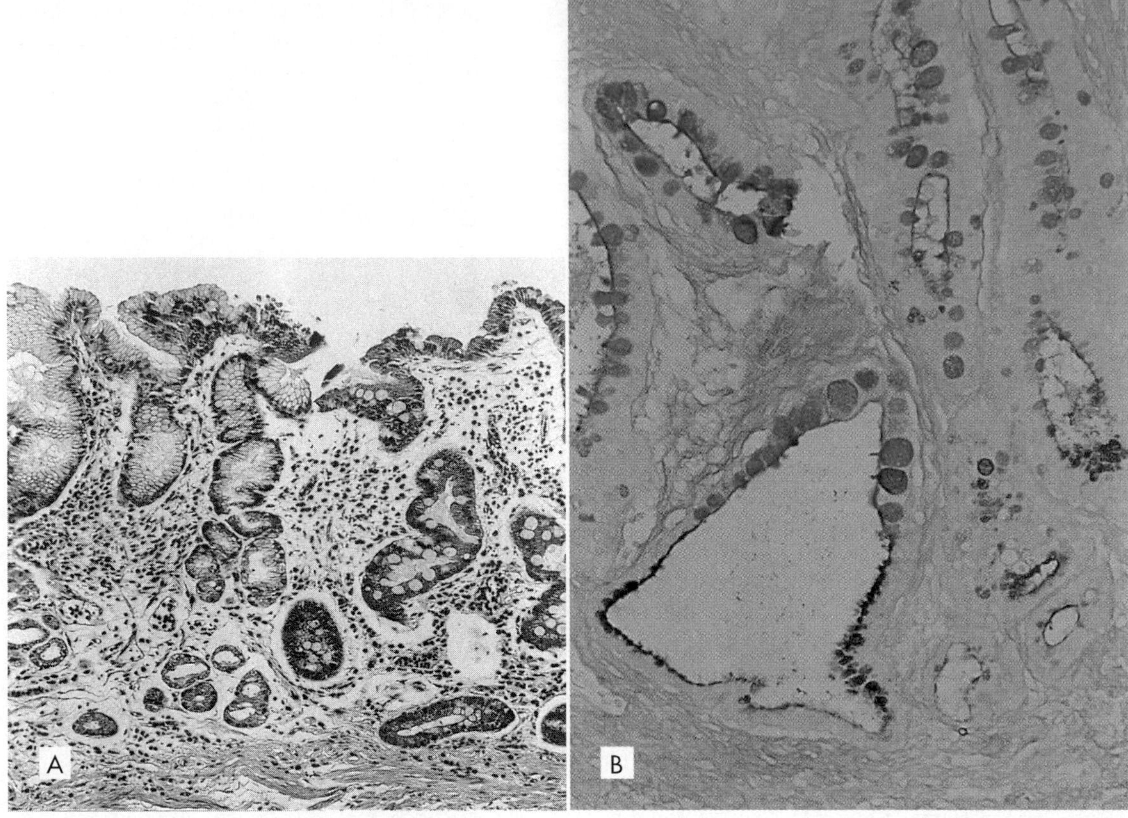

Fig. 53-15 **A,** Medium-low magnification photomicrograph of gastric antral mucosa exhibiting multifocal atrophic gastritis (MAG). The antral mucosa on the right side is replaced by intestinal metaplasia, whereas on the left side it exhibits considerable atrophy of the glands and reactive hyperplasia of the foveolar compartment. The lamina propria is expanded by fibrosis and contains moderate numbers of chronic inflammatory cells. **B,** Photomicrograph of type III intestinal metaplasia characterized by the presence of dark-staining sulfomucins in both columnar intermediate cells and occasional goblet cells. (Steiner's high-iron diamine [HID] stain, counterstained with Alcian blue pH 2.5.)

tritis.[120,169] The infectious variants may be attributable to tuberculosis[74,75] and histoplasmosis[83,84] and, with mounting frequency since the advent of AIDS, also to *Mycobacterium avium–intracellulare*.[76,120,169] In patients with Crohn's disease, the gastric manifestation takes the form of patchy acute lesions with glandular destruction and the appearance of occasional, sometimes ill-formed, small histiocytic granulomas.[170,171] Since Crohn's disease affecting exclusively the stomach is exceptional, the diagnosis of this disease can be made with confidence only in the presence of coexisting Crohn's disease lesions elsewhere. Likewise, because sarcoidosis only rarely affects the digestive system, it should be diagnosed in the stomach only when typical lesions of sarcoidosis are present in other organs such as lung or skin.[172] Fig. 53-16 presents the histologic appearance of granulomatous gastritis.

Isolated granulomatous gastritis, a term coined by Fahimi and coworkers,[173] is used to refer to an unusual form of unknown cause that affects generally the antral mucosa of older patients who present with symptoms of gastritis or, on occasion, of gastric outlet obstruction.[173,174] The diagnosis of this particular disorder can be made only by exclusion of other known causes, as discussed above, and in the face of negative investigation with special stains and culture for microorganisms. This disease tends to be self-limiting, and its symptoms disappear in a few weeks to months, whether or not corticosteroid treatment is carried out.[169]

Lymphocytic gastritis

The term *lymphocytic gastritis* has been applied to a situation where large numbers of small T-cell lymphocytes are seen to populate both glandular and superficial gastric epithelium, causing variable degrees of disruption.[175] This infiltration is typically found, on a patchy basis, as part of the so-called *varioliform gastritis,* also referred to as "chronic erosive gastritis."[176,177] This condition involves the oxyntic mucosa more consistently than that of the antrum and is characterized by its endoscopic appearance in which small multiple erosions alternate with small polypoid mucosal lesions. Histologically the erosions show focal disappearance of the superficial epithelium, surrounded by areas of reactive epithelial hyperplasia, cystically dilated glands and foveolae, and acute inflammatory infiltration of both lamina propria and glandular structures (Fig. 53-17). The latter, however, tend to be reasonably well preserved.

An infiltration similar to that described in varioliform gastritis is found in patients with celiac sprue, but in this case the

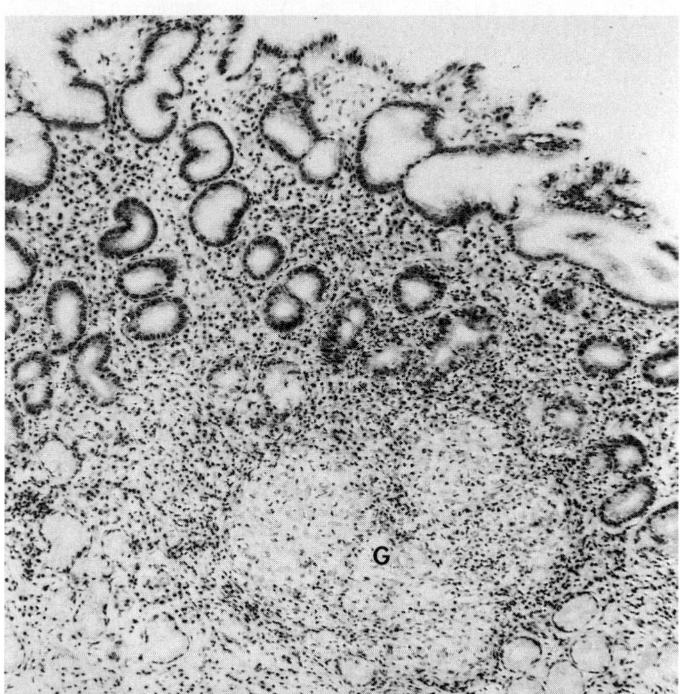

Fig. 53-16 Low-magnification photomicrograph showing several confluent small granulomas in the lamina propria of the gastric antral mucosa *(G)*. The lesions are composed of epithelioid histiocytes surrounded by a halo of lymphocytes and occasional plasma cells. The remainder of the lamina propria exhibits moderate chronic inflammation.

typical lesions of chronic erosive gastritis are not present.[178] Some cases of chronic atrophic gastritis reported from Latin America, which recognize a complex etiopathogenesis combining *H. pylori* infection and environmental factors, often show focal areas of intense lymphocytic infiltration of glandular and foveolar epithelium. In this case, however, the lymphocytic lesion is found in the antrum with a frequency similar or even higher than in the body of the stomach.

Xanthomatous gastritis

The name *xanthomatous gastritis* is applied to discrete raised yellow lesions that are found more frequently in the antro-oxyntic mucosa and measure a few millimeters each in maximum diameter[179] (Fig. 53-18). Under the microscope, the lesions are characterized by the presence of clusters and accumulations of large histiocytes with a clear vacuolated cytoplasm caused by the presence of lipids (Fig. 53-19). These cells are present in the lamina propria of the mucosa and are covered by normal or sometimes hyperplastic gastric epithelium. Xanthomas are often encountered in chronic gastritis, in particular postgastrectomy reflux gastritis; however, they may be found in the absence of significant inflammation, in which case the denomination *gastritis* would be somewhat of a misnomer. It is thought that xanthomas are formed as a consequence of prior hemorrhage into the mucosa.[180] The lipids stored in the histiocytes would be derived from destroyed red blood cells. This condition, which is usually discovered fortuitously at endoscopy, does not appear to be associated with any particular clinical manifestation, and it is believed to regress spontaneously. However it may be confused with muciphages, very rare in the stomach, or with a mucin-producing diffuse adenocarcinoma. In both instances, the cells contain mucins, which stain positively with PAS stain with diastase. Foamy histiocytes in *Mycobacterium avium–intracellulare* infection may also pose a differential diagnostic problem. However, these are usually clustered in small groups and are positive with stains that demonstrate acid-fast bacilli. The histiocytes in the gastric xanthoma are negative for both mucin and acid-fast special stains.

GASTRIC AND DUODENAL ULCERS

Acute gastric ulcers

From a histologic point of view, discontinuities in the mucosal lining have been divided into *erosions* and *ulcers*. An erosion is defined as a circumscribed superficial loss of substance that does not go beyond the muscularis mucosae. An ulcer, in contrast, consists of a circumscribed loss of substance that transcends the mucosa and may involve submucosa and beyond. These histologic definitions, however, cannot be directly translated into nosologic entities, since, within one such entity, erosions may evolve into ulcerations. Furthermore, endoscopic observation, a fundamental component in the description of many conditions, is not capable of discriminating between an erosion and a shallow ulceration. Gastric erosions are acute lesions that may be associated with a wide variety of etiopathogenetic mechanisms including stress, burns, trauma, sepsis, NSAID administration, and excessive alcohol intake, or be part of the so-called varioliform gastritis, already discussed above.

Stress ulcers

In cases of massive stress, gastric or duodenal erosions may fail to heal, and loss of mucosa occurs beyond the muscularis mucosae.[181-183] Acute stress ulcers tend to be multiple and exhibit well-delineated craters of variable depth but generally below the muscularis mucosae. These ulcers tend to bleed profusely because they are associated with congestion of the submucosal blood vessels.[184] Acute inflammatory exudate and necrotic debris may be found in the bed of the ulcer, but at this early stage there is only limited reparative activity. When they are associated with extensive burns or massive trauma, these are called "Curling's ulcers": these tend to be multiple, are of a more superficial nature, and are located preferentially in the body and fundus of the stomach, though they were originally described in the duodenum.[185] Fig. 53-20 illustrates the gross appearance of a gastric stress ulcer. Another type of acute gastroduodenal ulceration is found in patients with severe head trauma or with growing intracranial masses, and these are called "Cushing's ulcers." These tend to be deeper than Curling's ulcers and are distributed with comparable frequency in the esophagus, body of the stomach, the pyloric antrum, or the duodenum.[186] These Cushing's ulcers are distinctive in that they are accompanied by gastric hyperacidity, probably of vagal origin because it can be suppressed by anticholinergic agents. Both Curling's and Cushing's ulcers appear to be associated with reduced mucosal blood flow, a phenomenon that in the presence of gastric acid, whether normal or exaggerated, results in damage to the superficial epithelium followed by destruction of the underlying mucosa.[187,188]

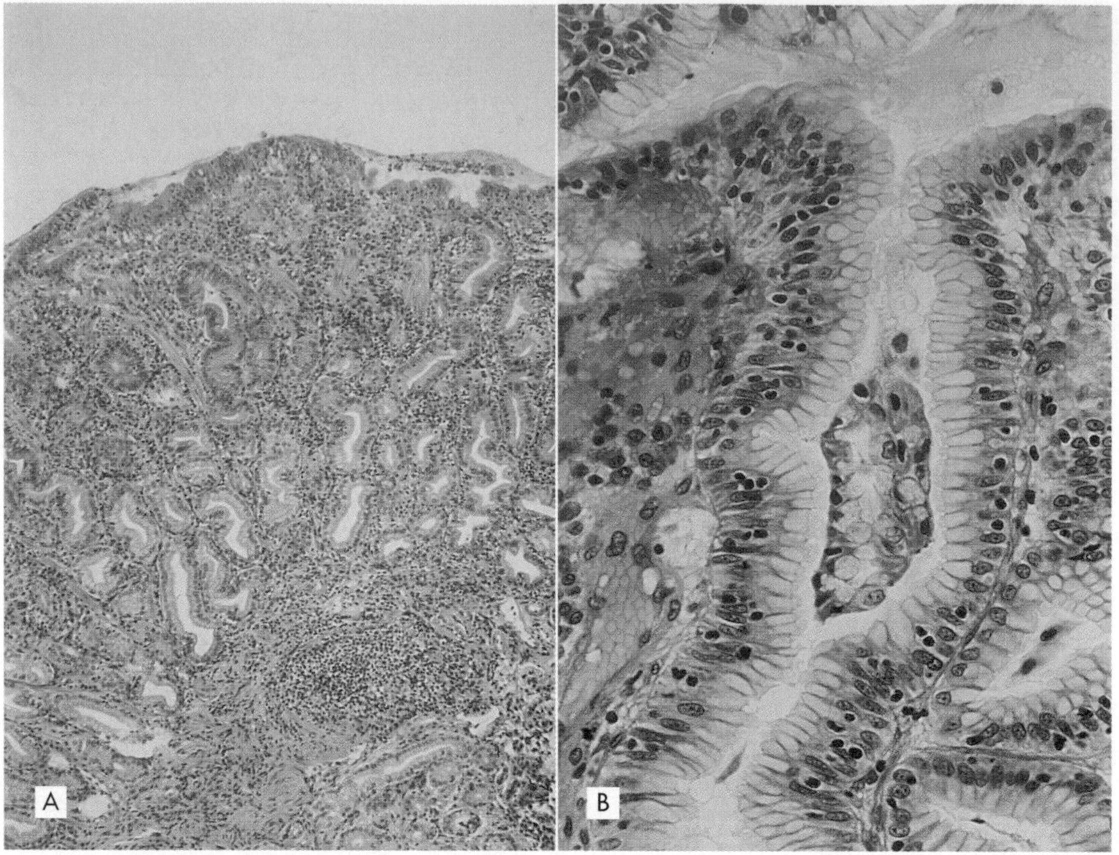

Fig. 53-17 Gastric antral mucosa with lymphocytic gastritis. **A,** Low-power microphotograph shows relative atrophy of the glandular compartment and hyperplasia of the foveolar compartment. In addition, the intervening mucosa contains large numbers of chronic inflammatory cells, which, at the bottom, are seen to form a small lymphoid aggregate. **B,** Close-up view of **A,** illustrating large numbers of small lymphocytes in the lamina propria, as well as traversing the foveolar and surface epithelium.

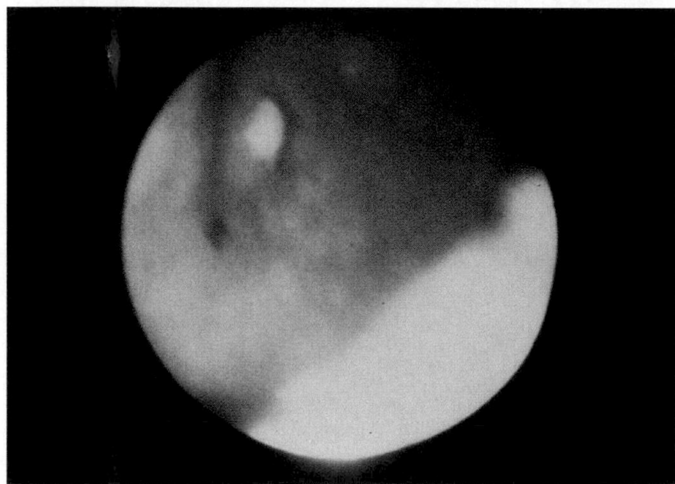

Fig. 53-18 Endoscopic photograph showing the appearance of a gastric xanthoma. This appears at the upper left as a small protuberance that is pale yellow and contrasts with the surrounding pink-reddish mucosa.

Peptic ulcer disease

Peptic ulcers are chronic, most often solitary lesions that occur at any level of the gastrointestinal tract exposed to the action of acid and peptic juices.[189] The basic pathologic characteristics of all ulcers are similar, irrespective of the site, and are therefore described together. Differences peculiar to a specific anatomic site are delineated. In descending order of frequency, ulcers occur in the duodenum, the stomach, the distal esophageal mucosa, the margins of a gastrectomy, and heterotopic gastric mucosa in Meckel's diverticulum. Approximately 98% of peptic ulcers occur in the stomach and duodenum, with a ratio of about 1:4. Ulcers may occur at virtually any age and affect both sexes; however, duodenal ulcers are more common in men between 20 and 50 years of age, whereas gastric ulcers affect almost equally men and women, most commonly in their fifth and sixth decade.

Epidemiology

The epidemiology of gastric and duodenal ulcer is intimately related to that of *H. pylori* infection, gastritis, and gastric cancer.[126] Studies carried out in various parts of the world have shown that the prevalence of *H. pylori* is essentially identical to the prevalence of gastritis reported in previous studies. The association of chronic gastritis with low socioeconomic status,

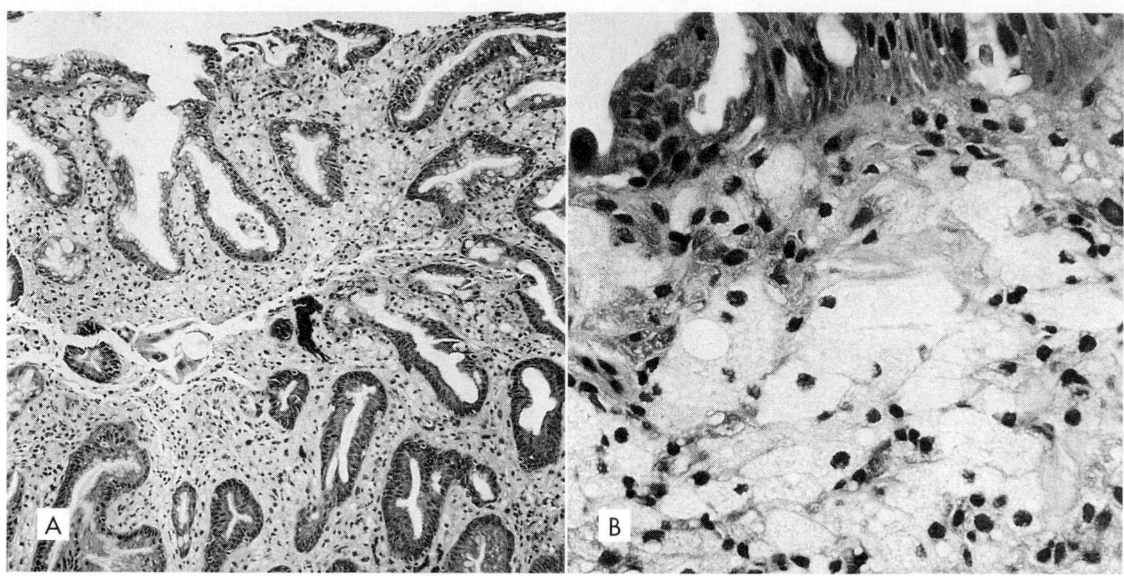

Fig. 53-19 **A,** Low-power microphotograph of gastric antral mucosa containing a xanthomatous lesion. **B,** High-power magnification of the gastric xanthoma showing the lamina propria entirely replaced by large histiocytes with clear foamy cytoplasm and slightly eccentric, small, bland-appearing nuclei.

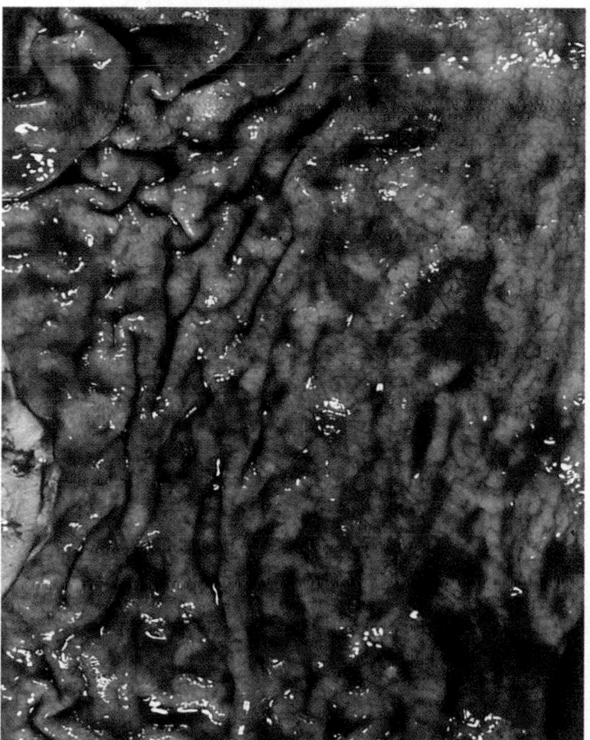

Fig. 53-20 Gross photograph of the gastric mucosa in a patient with superficial bleeding gastric ulcers, Curling type. These are shown as hemorrhagic patches over a mucosa that is congested and edematous.

age, peptic ulcer disease, and gastric carcinoma, demonstrated in such diverse areas of the world as Central and South America, Finland, and China, remain valid for *H. pylori* infection.[141,143,145,190-192] The prevalence of *H. pylori* in adults approximates 100% in many developing tropical countries; cross-sectional studies in these regions have shown that the percentage of infected children is very high, an indication that exposure to the bacteria occurs early in life. In the established industrialized parts of the world (Western Europe, United States and Canada, and Australia) exposure occurs later, resulting in a lower percentage of infected adults (around 50% by 50 years of age). In the emerging economies of Eastern Asia (such as Japan and Korea), where widespread sanitation has been introduced more recently, a clear trend in the epidemiology of *H. pylori* shows the change from a "third-world" to a "first-world" pattern.[193-196]

Pathogenesis

The pathogenesis of peptic ulcer is not known but is believed to involve an imbalance between aggressive and defensive factors.[197] In numerous gastric ulcers (perhaps as many as 30% in industrialized nations) and in a few duodenal ulcers (less than 2%), this imbalance appears to be the result of prostaglandin inhibition caused by the chronic ingestion of NSAIDs.[198] Prostaglandins PGE_2 and PGI_2 have a pivotal role in the normal protective mechanisms of the gastric and small intestinal mucosa.[199,200]

Helicobacter pylori infection is the major cause of peptic ulcer not associated with the use of NSAIDs.[201] This organism has been detected in the stomach of virtually all the patients with duodenal ulcer and in more than 90% of gastric ulcer patients who were not NSAID users.[202] Cure of *H. pylori* in these patients (achieved with complex courses of antibiotics or, more recently, with combinations of antibiotics and proton-pump inhibitors) facilitates the cure of peptic ulcer and essentially prevents its recurrence, an event that occurs within 1 year in more than 80% of patients treated with acid-inhibiting therapy alone.[203, 204]

Whereas the evidence linking *H. pylori* to peptic ulcer is incontrovertible, the pathogenetic mechanism or mechanisms whereby the organism predisposes to or causes ulcer remain uncertain. Possibilities include (1) disruption of the mucus barrier by production of ammonia, cytotoxin, or phospholipase, or the combination of all three; (2) enhancement of aggressive factors, such as acid, platelet activating factor, and pepsin; (3) activation of monocytes and macrophages, with release of tumor necrosis factor, interleukin-1, and reactive oxygen metabolites; (4) production of autoantibodies directed against the organism that cross-react with gastric tissue; and (5) enhanced release of gastrin. This last effect of *H. pylori* is receiving considerable attention, and an intriguing possible mechanism recently proposed would involve the inhibition of somatostatin secretion.[205]

Pathology

In the stomach, almost all peptic ulcers occur on the lesser curvature in the antrum, in an area close to the incisura angularis.[206] Gastric ulcers occurring on the greater curvature and in other parts of the stomach, such as the fundus, are much more likely to be associated with chronic use of NSAIDs than with *H. pylori* gastritis. In the duodenum, peptic ulcers most commonly occur in the first part, either on the anterior or posterior walls. When ulcers occur at both the anterior and posterior wall of the prepyloric area simultaneously, they are known as "kissing ulcers."

Peptic ulcers are usually sharply demarcated from the surrounding mucosa, which is generally slightly reddened, edematous, and elevated around the margins of the lesion. They tend to be relatively small, measuring between 0.5 and 2 cm in diameter. Some patients have very large ulcers, measuring more than 2 to 3 cm in diameter. Such ulcers have been defined as giant ulcers; the distinction is relevant because they may be misdiagnosed endoscopically as malignant.[207] The ulcer walls are perpendicular and limit a crater of variable depth, which may perforate the wall and penetrate into the adjacent structures, most commonly the pancreas. The base of the crater is grayish and may contain necrotic debris mixed with blood or appear clean, showing a whitish rim of fibrous tissue. The mucosa surrounding ulcers not complicated by extensive fibrosis appears grossly normal. In the stomach, particularly in the antrum, rugal folds may appear to radiate from long-standing chronic ulcers in an orderly fashion, like beams from a light source (Fig. 53-21). This feature, considered useful to differentiate benign ulcers from malignant ulcerating tumors, which lack this mucosal arrangement, is either missing or greatly attenuated in benign gastric ulcer arising in an atrophic stomach.[208]

Microscopically an area of necrosis with inflammatory cells, fibrin, debris, and sometimes microorganisms represents the active ulcer, the area of gastric or duodenal wall that is actually being destroyed. Fibrosis, the result of healing of the ulcer at its edges, forms a rim extending from around the crater to beneath the epithelium into the surrounding connective and muscular tissues (Fig. 53-22). Depending on the age of the ulcer and the number of previous recurrences, the fibrous component may be small enough to escape detection in the examination of an endoscopic biopsy specimen, or large and hard enough to mimic the gross appearance and the consistency of a malignant tumor. A lymphoid infiltrate, often arranged in lymphoid follicles, is usually found around the ulcer edges; rarely, the infiltrate may be so severe as to mimic malignant lymphoma of the stomach. Below the necrotic base of an ulcer, vessels show prominent inflammation, and some degree of arteritis obliterans is often found. When disrupted by the ulcerative process, these arteries bleed into the ulcer, and the magnitude of the hemorrhage depends on the size of the damaged vessels.[208-210] The mucosa immediately surrounding the ulcer shows chronic active inflammation, which becomes progressively more intense in the immediate vicinity of the ulcer crater. There, regenerative changes with large cells exhibiting bizarre nuclei and frequent mitoses are so widespread that when small samples of such areas are examined in biopsy specimens, the histologic diagnosis of dysplasia or even cancer is occasionally entertained.[208-210] However, in regeneration there is usually evidence of surface maturation, mitotic activity is confined to the deeper foveolar regions, and nuclei are blander and more uniform in appearance. In contrast, the appearance of dysplasia is essentially that of an adenoma, with pronounced cytologic abnormalities, atypia, loss of surface maturation, and cytoplasmic basophilia attributable to mucin depletion. These distinctions, however, can be treacherous, and quite appropriately an old pathologists' adage

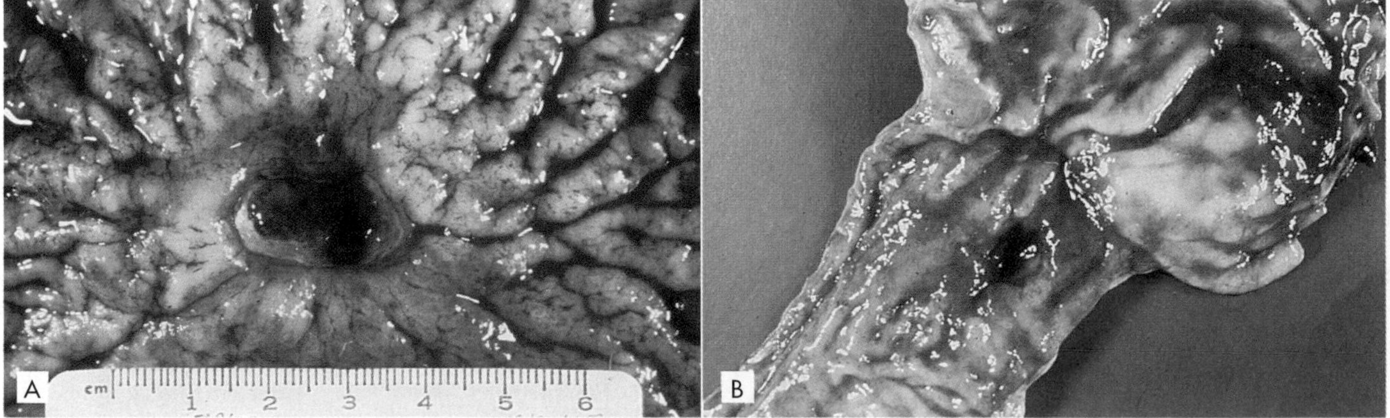

Fig. 53-21 **A,** Gross photograph of a chronic peptic ulcer located in the lesser curvature, straddling the antrum and corpus of the stomach. The ulcer is approximately 2 cm in maximum diameter and has a regular shape and a hemorrhagic but relatively clean fundus; its edges are slightly edematous; and the gastric folds radiate in all directions from the lesion, **B,** Gross photograph of a chronic peptic ulcer located in the first portion of the duodenum. This ulcer is smaller and also shows a hemorrhagic fundus.

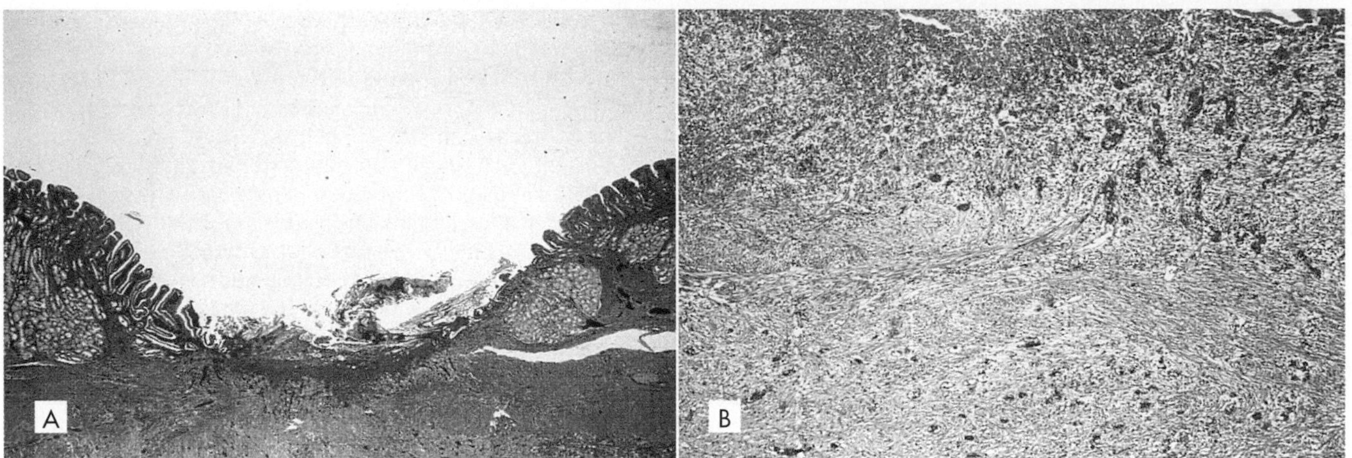

Fig. 53-22 **A,** Low-power photomicrograph of a peptic ulcer in the duodenum. The lesion consists of a mucosal defect located in the central portion that erases mucosa as well as muscularis mucosa and deeply penetrates the submucosa. Inflammatory reaction permeates the subjacent muscle. **B,** High-power photomicrograph illustrating the four layers that characterize the bed of a peptic ulcer. From top to bottom, these are necrotic debris, granulation tissue, inflammation (not particularly developed in this example), and fibrosis.

warns "Never diagnose cancer within three glands from an ulcer."

Complications

The most common complications of peptic ulcer disease in order of frequency are hemorrhage, penetration with or without perforation, and obstruction.[211] Approximately a third of the patients experience one of these complications at some point during the course of their disease; ulcers most commonly associated with complications are those located in the pyloric channel and in the postbulbar duodenum.

Bleeding occurs when an ulcer erodes into a vessel. The erosion of small vessels is rarely associated with distinctive upper gastrointestinal signs or symptoms; such patients usually present with iron deficiency anemia as a result of the chronic blood loss. Of the major arteries, those most commonly eroded are the gastroduodenal artery in duodenal ulcers, and the left gastric artery in gastric ulcers. Rupture of one of these vessels constitutes a medical emergency, which accounts for approximately 50% of all acute upper gastrointestinal bleeding events. Patients present with hematemesis, melena, and other signs of acute blood loss, such as hypotension, tachycardia, and shock. Interestingly, during bleeding events, many patients report a relief of their ulcer pain, a fact probably related to the neutralization of the gastric acid by blood. Regular use of NSAIDs greatly increase the risk of peptic ulcer bleeding, particularly in elderly patients.[212]

Perforation results when the ulcer erodes through the serosa of the viscus.[213] The acute free perforation of an ulcer into the abdominal cavity is accompanied by a dramatic intensification of the patient's symptoms; it is often accompanied by pneumoperitoneum and peritonitis and is an indication for immediate surgery. The search for perforation in a resected stomach or duodenum often requires careful handling and examination of the ulcer. The actual perforation may be barely visible and is often obscured by the presence of coagulated blood, fibrin, and other debris. Examination of the serosa in the vicinity of the ulcer will invariably reveal severe acute inflammation.

An ulcer may burrow in an area where the stomach or the duodenum are in intimate contact with a solid organ such as the pancreas or liver. In such cases, the ulcer continues its penetration beyond the wall of the viscus and invades the parenchyma of the organ, where it usually elicits a dramatic inflammatory response, followed by fibrous buildup, which clinically and radiographically may mimic a tumor.[214] The examination of such specimens is often complicated because it is rarely possible to separate the portion of gastrointestinal tract from the penetrated organ, to which it becomes fused into a hard fibrous mass. Rarely, the perforation occurs in the vicinity of another hollow structure, like a small intestinal loop, the transverse colon, or the gallbladder, followed by formation of a fistula.

Gastric outlet obstruction is the clinical syndrome resulting from the distortion and narrowing of the pyloric area caused by fibrosis, edema, or smooth muscle spasm. It occurs almost exclusively in patients with a long-standing peptic ulcer of the pyloric channel or the duodenum. Surgical repair is often necessary after medical management of the obstruction is carried out.

Zollinger-Ellison syndrome

In 1955, Zollinger and Ellison reported the existence of a syndrome characterized by massive gastric hyperacidity and intractable peptic ulcerations involving stomach and upper small intestine, associated with islet cell tumors of the pancreas.[215] It was later determined that the substance produced by such tumors was gastrin, and therefore the neoplasms were called *gastrinomas*.[216] It is currently accepted that approximately 75% of gastrinomas arise in the pancreas, 20% in the duodenum, and 5% are found in peripancreatic or gastroduodenal lymph nodes without a primary ever being identified. As many as 50% of gastrinomas, and particularly those arising in the duodenum, are part of the multiple endocrine neoplasia (MEN) syndrome, type 1.[217-219] The pathogenesis of the peptic ulcerations found in these patients is predicated upon the production of massive quantities of very low pH gastric juice that overwhelms both the ability of the gastric mucus to protect the mucosa and the buffering capacity of the bicarbonate-rich pancreatic juice secreted into the second portion of the duodenum. As a consequence of the latter, large amounts of very acidic chyme find their way into the upper small intestinal mucosa, normally suited for a neutral pH, and cause peptic ulcerations as well as diarrhea.

The gastric antral mucosa in the Zollinger-Ellison syndrome, in addition to one or more peptic ulcerations, shows variable degrees of chronic inflammation containing foci of acute inflammatory activity.[208] It is not clear whether the latter may result from the presence of *H. pylori,* which may also be encountered in these patients. Peptic ulceration, however, may occur in the stomach of patients with the Zollinger-Ellison syndrome in the absence of *H. pylori.*[220] The oxyntic mucosa lining gastric corpus and fundus, in contrast, tends to be free of inflammation and shows variable, sometimes considerable, degrees of hyperplasia of both the foveolar and the glandular compartment because of the trophic effect of circulating gastrin.[221] This same trophic effect causes proliferation of the argyrophilic ECL cells of the oxyntic mucosa, which may present diffuse, linear, micronodular, or adenomatoid patterns.[222,223] This hyperplasia may progress with formation of argyrophilic carcinoids of low malignancy, only in those cases where the gastrinoma is part of the MEN 1 grouping of endocrine neoplasms.[223,224]

DUODENITIS

Nonspecific duodenitis

The pylorus is an anatomic and physiologic valve that regulates the emptying of gastric contents into the duodenum, rendering the duodenal environment intimately associated with the physiologic events occurring in the stomach. Thus it is hardly surprising that alterations of the normal gastric physiology result in alterations of the mucosa of the first part of the duodenum.[225-227] The quintessential example of this is a duodenal ulcer, a condition associated with predominantly antral *H. pylori* gastritis, gastric hyperacidity, hypergastrinemia, and the development of gastric metaplasia in the duodenal mucosa. The events leading to the formation of peptic duodenal ulcer are discussed on p. 1687. Even in the absence of a duodenal ulcer, however, the duodenum may show inflammatory changes in patients both with and without *H. pylori* gastritis. Particularly common is the duodenitis associated with uremia and chronic renal dialysis. The degree of duodenal inflammation has been graded as mild, moderate, or severe, whereas Whitehead has proposed a division into three grades.[228] In grade I only the mononuclear cell population of the lamina propria is increased; in grade II there are also neutrophils in the lamina propria and the epithelium; in grade III duodenitis the changes of grade II are associated with erosions or ulcerations. Endoscopically there is very little correlation between grade I and II duodenitis with the appearance of the mucosa, which may be normal or show various degrees of edema and erythema. The correlation is better in erosive duodenitis (grade III), in which erosions are seen both endoscopically and histologically. Changes in the villous architecture generally parallel the density of the inflammatory infiltrate: in grade I the villi are virtually always normal, whereas in grade III severe villous flattening or complete atrophy are common.

A very common finding in the duodenitis that accompanies gastric hypersecretory states is the so-called gastric metaplasia of the duodenal surface epithelium. There is replacement of the normal enterocytes and goblet cells by tall columnar cells containing apical mucin, which is of the gastric (neutral) type. These patches of metaplastic epithelium, the extent of which appears to be directly proportional to the degree of hyperacidity, are often colonized by *H. pylori* and exhibit the same type of surface cell disruption seen in the stomach. It has been postulated that this damage to the metaplastic duodenal epithelium is the mechanism that initiates the appearance of a peptic ulcer in the duodenum.[229,230]

Nodular duodenum and Brunner gland hyperplasia

Frequently described as nodular duodenitis, the nodular duodenum is a condition of uncertain clinical significance characterized endoscopically by multiple erythematous nodules in the proximal duodenum. In a recent study,[231] duodenitis grade I was found in more than half of 83 patients examined, Brunner's gland hyperplasia was found in 10% of the patients, and gastric heterotopia in another 10%. The remainder of the patients had a histologically normal duodenum.

NONNEOPLASTIC POLYPS

Inflammatory polyps

Elevated lesions consisting mostly of granulation tissue are often called *inflammatory polyps,* though they are not epithelial proliferations and therefore should not be classified as polyps.[232] A special form of inflammatory polypoid lesion is the inflammatory fibroid polyp, also known as *Vanek's polyp.*[233] Grossly, this lesion consists of solitary or multiple polypoid masses ranging from 1 to 10 cm in diameter. The stroma is compact and reminiscent of that of leiomyomas. These tumors are composed of fibroblasts arranged in whirls around blood vessels; inflammatory cells, particularly eosinophils, are prominent. Inflammatory polyps are not known to be associated with carcinoma.[234-237]

Hyperplastic polyps

Hyperplastic polyps, also known as *regenerative polyps,* are composed of elongated, grossly distorted, branching and dilated hyperplastic foveolae laying in an edematous stroma with varying degrees of chronic and active inflammation and small, haphazardly distributed smooth muscle bundles[232,234] (Fig. 53-23). Hyperplastic polyps are usually small, measuring 0.5 to 1.5 cm in diameter, and are often multiple. Frequently, areas of the surface epithelium are eroded; this may result in chronic blood loss and iron-deficiency anemia, one of the most common clinical manifestations of hyperplastic polyps of the stomach. Although most authors agree that neither cellular atypia nor malignant transformation are common features of hyperplastic polyps, well-documented sporadic reports of adenocarcinoma arising within hyperplastic polyps have been published.[234-237]

Fundic gland polyps

Fundic gland polyps, originally described in the stomach of patients with familial polyposis, have later been seen in a large

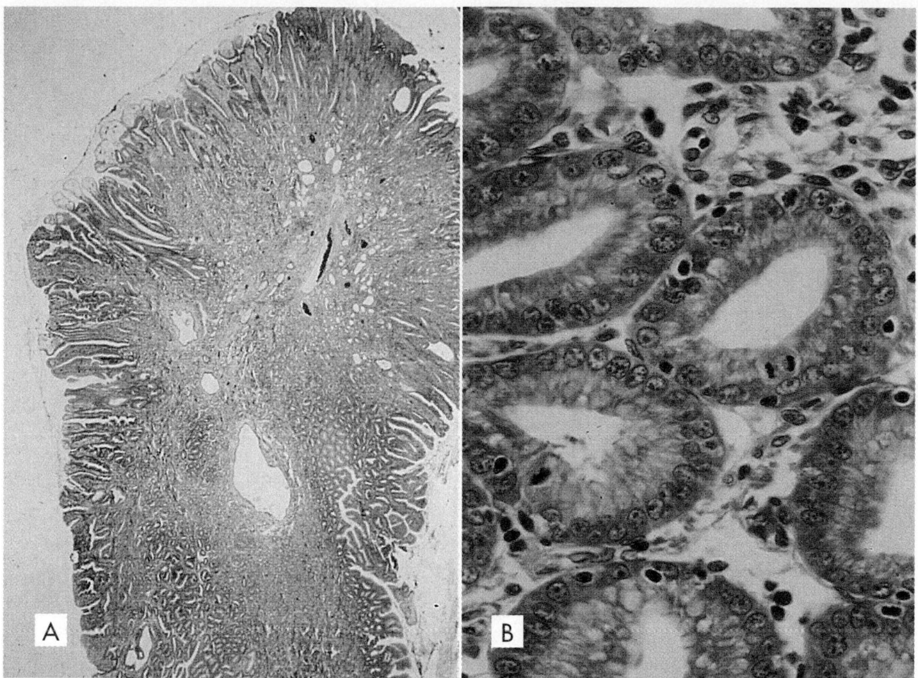

Fig. 53-23 **A,** Low-power photomicrograph of a large hyperplastic polyp arising in the gastric antral mucosa. This lesion is composed of well-vascularized fronds of fibrovascular tissue. The overlying mucosa is thickened by the excessive growth of the foveolar compartment, acquiring a villiform texture; **B,** Close-up view of the same lesion showing it to be formed by foveola-like structures lined by a single layer of tall columnar mucous cells with a bland cytologic appearance. Although several mitoses can be discerned, no significant cellular atypia is seen. The intervening mucosa contains occasional lymphocytes.

variety of individuals with gastritis, gastroenteric anastomosis, treated with proton-pump inhibitors, or in seemingly normal stomachs.[238,239] These lesions tend to be small (1 to 5 mm in diameter), often multiple, sessile, smooth nodules localized in the proximal gastric mucosa. Generally regarded as malformations, these polyps are composed of normal-appearing oxyntic mucosa exhibiting a normal or shortened foveolar compartment and the presence of small cystic dilatations in the upper portion of individual glands. Although their natural history is unclear, there is no evidence that these lesions may possess a malignant potential.[240,241]

Hamartomatous and heterotopic polyps

Hamartomatous polyps are nodules composed of tissue normally present in the stomach but arranged in a disorganized fashion.[242] These polyps are most commonly found in several hereditary gastrointestinal polyposis syndromes, such as Peutz-Jeghers syndrome, Gardner's syndrome, familial polyposis, and juvenile polyposis. These are described in Chapter 55.

Heterotopic polyps are composed of normal tissues not normally occurring in the stomach. The most common heterotopia in the stomach manifests as foci of heterotopic pancreas. These are usually submucosal lesions located in the prepyloric region. They may be eroded or ulcerated, and they frequently present with either occult or overt bleeding.

Peutz-Jeghers syndrome

Peutz-Jeghers syndrome is the result of a hereditary autosomal dominant trait characterized by the presence of hamartomatous polyps in stomach, small bowel, and large bowel, associated with a characteristic mucocutaneous pigmentation.[243] Pigmented melanotic spots measuring between 1 and 5 mm in diameter, generally present in the lips and oral mucosa, are observed in 95% of the patients. Clinical manifestations generally become apparent in the third decade of life and consist in abdominal pain caused by obstruction and intestinal bleeding, in turn the consequence of ulceration and infarction of large polyps.[244,245] The typical lesions are quite distinctive and consist of pedunculated polyps formed by fronds of lamina propria containing smooth muscle derived from the muscularis mucosae. Such fronds are covered by benign epithelial elements, normally found in the mucosa from which the polyp originates, that give rise to multiple villoglandular structures. Although the lesions of the Peutz-Jeghers syndrome are histologically benign, some studies have shown that this entity is associated with a significant increase in the incidence of malignancy, both systemically as well as in the stomach and duodenum within the digestive tract.[246]

Cronkhite-Canada syndrome

The Cronkhite-Canada syndrome is a multiple polyposis of unknown cause that lacks hereditary transmission and presents with hamartomatous polyps, similar to juvenile polyps, in the stomach, small bowel, and large bowel.[247] The syndrome, which usually becomes clinically manifest between 50 and 60 years of age, includes diarrhea, steatorrhea, alterations in the equilibrium of water and circulating electrolytes, malnutrition, anemia, hypoalbuminemia resulting from protein-losing enter-opathy, alternating hyperpigmentation and vitiligo, alopecia, and trophic alterations in fingernails. Histologic examination of the typical lesions reveals the presence of polypoid lesions composed of deformed glands with a benign appearance exhibiting remarkable tortuosity and, often, cystic dilatation of their lumen. The intervening lamina propria contains edema and a variable chronic inflammatory infiltrate. Histologic traits similar to those found in the polyps may be appreciated in the flat mucosa separating individual polyps. Because the disease does not have a specific treatment, approximately 50% of the cases have a fatal outcome.[248] Treatment with antibiotics, periods of parenteral nutrition, and a lactose-free diet reduce the symptoms and, in some instances, have resulted in remission.

Ménétrier's disease

Ménétrier's disease is an uncommon condition manifesting as diffuse and generalized hyperplasia of foveolar and surface mucous gastric cells, leading to hypertrophy of the rugal folds mostly in the proximal stomach, and associated with hypochlorhydria and protein-losing enteropathy[249] (Fig. 53-24). Most cases of Ménétrier's disease occur in men between 30 and 60 years of age. The glands show normal or only slightly reduced numbers of parietal and chief cells, and the hypoacidity in these patients is believed to be attributable to dilution of normal amounts of acid by exaggerated amounts of mucus and fluid secreted by the hyperplastic foveolar cells. This foveolar cell hypersecretion, in turn, is the substrate for the protein-losing enteropathy that is found almost invariably. A characteristic of Ménétrier's mucosal lesion is the lack of significant inflammatory infiltrate in the lamina propria, as well as of epithelial lesions such as erosions, intestinal metaplasia, or cellular atypia.[250-252] It is not clear whether there is a link between Ménétrier's disease and the development of gastric adenocarcinoma, despite a few reports that have described such association.[253,254] The lesions characteristic of Ménétrier's disease, of course, must be differentiated from the hypertrophic gastropathy associated with the Zollinger-Ellison syndrome, described above.

A somewhat different subset of Ménétrier's disease is a group of pediatric patients in whom there is often a concomitant history of respiratory infection and peripheral eosinophilia.[255] The pathogenetic link between the gastric lesions and the seemingly allergic reaction has not been established. Unlike in adults, these pediatric cases seem to be self-limiting and regress within weeks to months without specific therapy. These cases must be distinguished from severe manifestations of allergic gastroenteritis, a condition in which substantial inflammation of the gastric mucosa with widespread eosinophilic infiltration may cause the appearance of thickened mucosal folds. However, in the latter, the lesion is located preferentially in the antrum rather than in the corpus, and the eosinophilic infiltrate seen upon microscopic examination is virtually diagnostic.

NEOPLASMS

Adenomas

Neoplastic polyps of the stomach may be adenomas or adenocarcinomas. The prevalence of gastric adenomas parallels the incidence of gastric adenocarcinomas and therefore varies considerably in different populations. Adenomas increase in prevalence with age and affect men twice as often as women. Their most common location is the antrum, and they are usually solitary.[232,234,235]

The World Health Organization (WHO) has classified gastric adenomas into tubular, tubulovillous, and villous (or papillary).[256] Tubular adenomas are generally flat or slightly depressed lesions (flat adenomas). Their size varies between a few millimeters and several centimeters. The epithelium is formed by proliferating glands lined by rows of cells with hyperchromatic picket-fenced nuclei, in which as a rule neither mitoses nor pleomorphism are prominent (Fig. 53-25). These lesions, however, have clear malignant potential, and foci of carcinoma are found in at least 10% of flat adenomas. Villous adenomas are polypoid elevated lesions with a velvety papillary appearance. They are usually larger than flat adenomas, with an average size of about 4 cm. In contrast to tubular adenomas, the epithelium commonly shows severe dysplasia with mitoses, nuclear pleomorphism, and crowding (Fig. 53-26). These changes reflect their greater malignant potential: between 5% and 75% of gastric villous adenomas have been

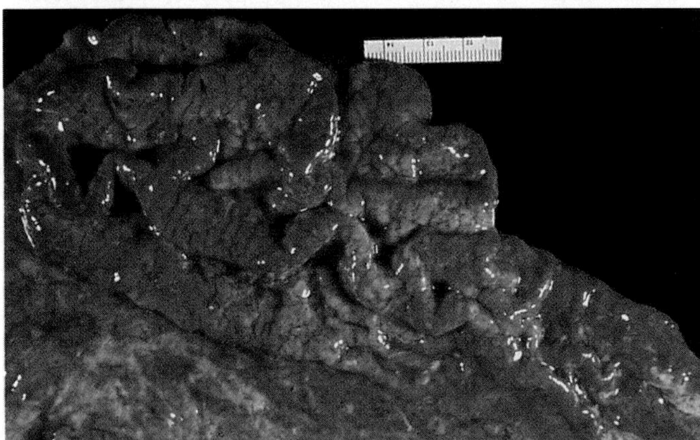

Fig. 53-24 Gross photograph illustrating the mucosa of the gastric corpus in Ménétrier's disease. The rugal folds are greatly enlarged and show congestion and edema. The mucosa is covered by glistening mucus.

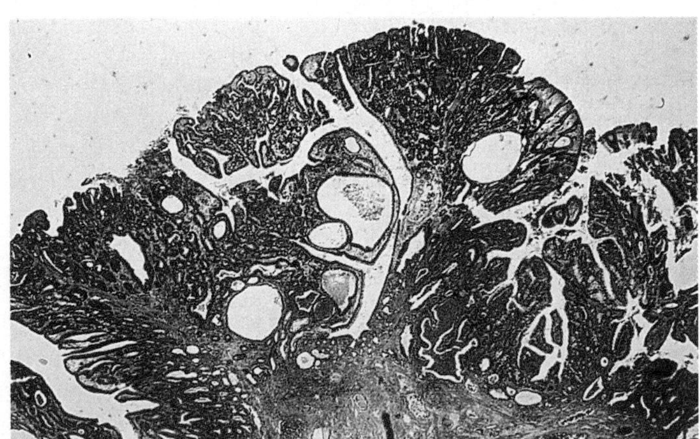

Fig. 53-25 Low-power photomicrograph of a tubulovillous tumor of the gastric mucosa. Unlike its hyperplastic counterpart, this lesion shows a good deal of hyperchromasia and intense proliferation of both glandular and villous structures. The underlying fibrovascular stroma contains focal aggregates of chronic inflammatory cells.

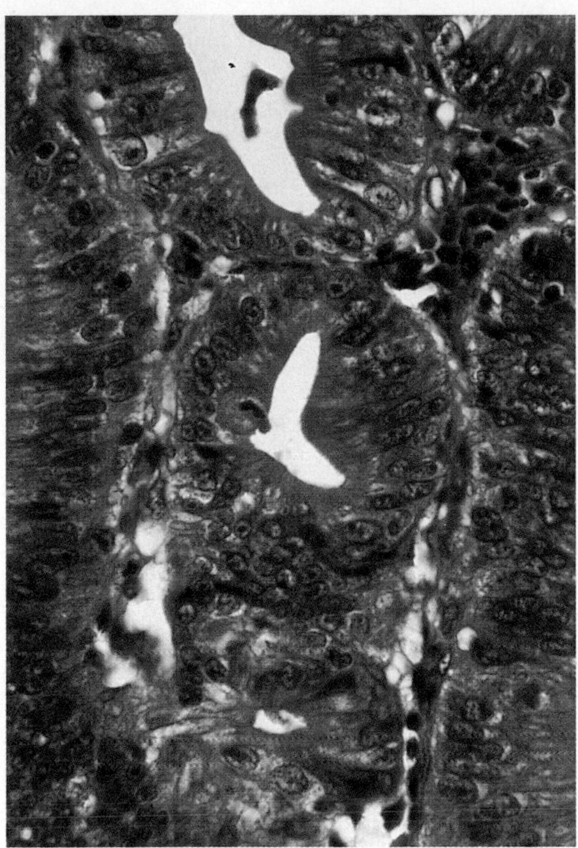

Fig. 53-26 Close-up view of an area within a tubulovillous adenoma of the stomach showing significant atypical atypia. The glandlike structures are closely apposed to each other, back to back, and are lined by stratified nuclei that show mild pleomorphism. Occasional mitotic figures are also seen.

reported to contain foci of invasive carcinoma. Furthermore, independent synchronous (occurring at the same time) or metachronous (occurring at another time, usually later) carcinoma has been found in up to 40% of the patients with a benign villous adenoma. This percentage clearly indicates that a common factor may be involved in the genesis of gastric adenomas and adenocarcinomas.[257]

Adenocarcinomas of stomach

Epidemiology

Although the death rate from gastric cancer has been steadily declining in Europe and North America and, to a lesser extent, in many developing countries for the past six decades, it still remains the second most common cancer in the world.[258] The development of better diagnostic and therapeutic measures may account for a small part of the declining death rate, but this is mostly attributable to a real reduced incidence of adenocarcinoma of the gastric antrum and corpus. In contrast, during the last two decades there has been a considerable increase in the incidence of adenocarcinoma of the cardia, particularly in countries such as the United States, the United Kingdom, and Sweden.[259,260]

The incidence of gastric adenocarcinoma has a wide geographic variation among different countries and even within different regions of the same country. The highest incidence is found in Costa Rica, Japan, and Chile; the lowest in Australia, Canada, and the United States.[261] The epidemiology of gastric adenocarcinoma parallels that of chronic gastritis, which, in turn, is intimately connected with the prevalence of *Helicobacter pylori* infection. A growing body of knowledge provides compelling evidence in favor of a strong causal link between *H. pylori* infection, chronic atrophic gastritis, and gastric carcinoma.[141-162,190-192] All these findings point to a powerful association between early infection with *H. pylori* and the presence of precancerous lesions of the stomach, that is, chronic atrophic gastritis involving antrum and body and the accompanying intestinal metaplasia. In his dissertation on human gastric carcinogenesis, Correa acknowledged the crucial role of *H. pylori* in initiating the chain of events leading to gastritis and to the eventual appearance of gastric carcinoma.[151] However, he also sounded a note of caution against regarding *H. pylori* infection as the main determining factor in such chain of events. He stated that *H. pylori* infection is a contributory but not sufficient factor in gastric carcinogenesis. Many pieces of evidence, originating from different areas of the world, point to the fact that, whereas *H. pylori* infection is a well-defined and early event in the process leading to the appearance of chronic atrophic gastritis, other factors must enter the picture for such outcome to take place.[148-153]

Premalignant lesions

Whereas diffuse adenocarcinomas generally do not recognize a precursor lesion and appear de novo, the intestinal type has been associated with several precursor conditions including *chronic multifocal atrophic gastritis* associated with *gastric dysplasia, gastric adenomas,* postgastrectomy *gastric remnant,* and, arguably, *Ménétrier's disease.*[143,144-147,154,155,262-266] In contrast, *chronic gastric ulcer,* once it has been proved benign, is no longer regarded as a significant premalignant condition.[267]

In advanced stages of multifocal atrophic (environmental) gastritis, foci of type III intestinal metaplasia, also called *incomplete* or *colonic,* characterized by the presence of significant amounts of sulfated mucins and of cellular atypia, may appear.[146,147,157-162] This type of metaplasia constitutes a significant marker for the development of gastric adenocarcinoma and probably represents a precursor lesions for such malignancy.

A further step in the malignant progression of MAG is the appearance of gastric epithelial dysplasia (GED),[268] an incompletely defined change that represents a common denominator with other conditions such as adenomas, gastric remnants, and, rarely, Ménétrier's disease. Under the microscope, GED shows the presence of distorted, often budding glands lined by stratified cells that exhibit variable pleomorphism, nuclear hyperchromasia, increased nuclear/cytoplasmic (N/C) ratio, and increased mitotic rate (Fig. 53-27). GED has been divided into mild, moderate, and severe, or, in more modern classifications, into a *low grade* and a *high grade.* Although low-grade GED was considered to be a relatively banal lesion, with a reported a regression rate of 66%, a recent study indicates that all grades of GED represent potentially premalignant lesions.[269] High-grade GED, by contrast, rarely regresses, and progression to carcinoma has been shown to between 57% and 75% during an 18-month follow-up period.[269,270] It has been reported recently that GED is the most reliable predictor for malignant transformation of the gastric mucosa.[271] The term "dysplasia" is utilized when the changes described above appear against a background of inflammation and multifocal

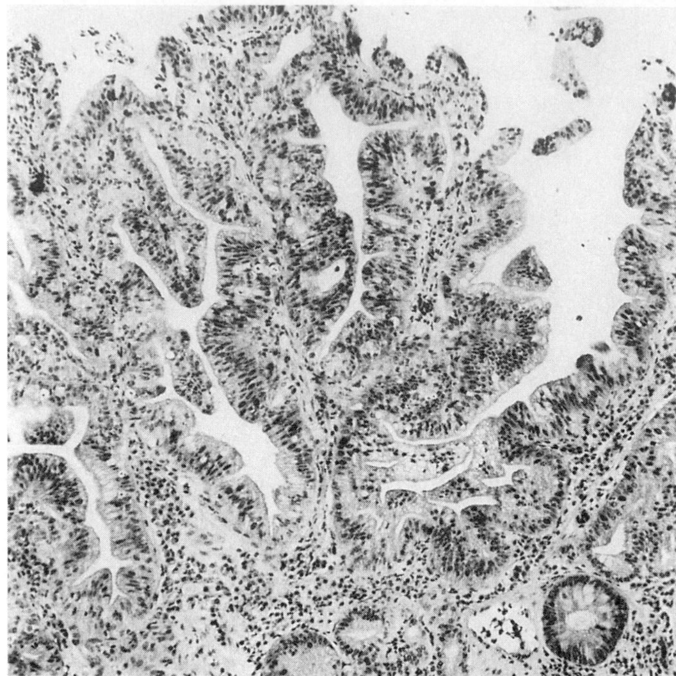

Fig. 53-27 Low-magnification photomicrograph showing high-grade dysplasia of the gastric mucosa in a patient with multifocal atrophic gastritis. The foveolar and surface epithelium has adopted a villiform configuration and is composed of stratified cells exhibiting hyperchromasia, moderate nuclear pleomorphism, increased mitotic rate, and partial loss of mucin. Next to this lesion, an invasive adenocarcinoma was found.

proliferative changes. Although adenomas, by definition, connote the existence of dysplasia, many authors prefer to restrict the term *adenoma* to describe solitary, grossly identifiable lesions devoid of inflammation.

Adenomas of the gastric mucosa are lesions of variable size, ranging from 0.5 up to 5 cm in diameter when left untreated, composed of proliferating glandular structures that exhibit variable degrees of atypia. The malignant potential of these lesions has been reported to range between 10% and 75%, depending largely on the size of the lesions being studied in individual series.[232,234,235] With the advent of flexible endoscopy, many adenomas are currently diagnosed when they are 2 cm or less in diameter, and therefore most are benign.[272] On the other hand, cancers tend to occur in adenomas measuring 2 cm or more in diameter;[273] therefore, such lesions must be either removed upon discovery or, failing this, very thoroughly sampled to rule out malignant transformation. After resection, a 6.1% local recurrence rate has been recorded within 1 year of the original polypectomy. The appearance of new polyps, sometimes hyperplastic and often adenomatous, has been noted in as many as a third of the cases, and occurrence of malignancy has been encountered in 3% to 25% of patients with gastric adenomas.[271-274]

Several studies have shown that adenocarcinomas may arise in the gastric remnant after partial gastrectomy.[275,276] However, it is less clear whether the incidence of such neoplasias is higher than that of an unoperated comparable population. This may become a moot point in the future since modern treatment of peptic ulcer disease with H_2-receptor antagonists, proton-pump inhibitors, and antibiotic therapy against *H. pylori* has drastically reduced the need for surgical intervention and particularly for antrectomy. It is important to distinguish between gastrectomy carried out for early gastric cancer, where recurrence usually takes place within 5 years, and that done for the treatment of benign peptic ulcer, with a 15- to 25-year lag period. Therefore, for a cancer to be considered as arising de novo in a gastric remnant it must be diagnosed 5 years or longer after gastrectomy to rule out the possibility that the malignancy was already present at a very early stage at the time of surgery.[277] Although statistics as to the true prevalence of adenocarcinoma in gastric remnants are quite disparate, it is accepted that the highest degree of risk is present in patients in whom surgery takes place at or before 40 years of age and who have been operated on for at least 15 to 20 years.[271]

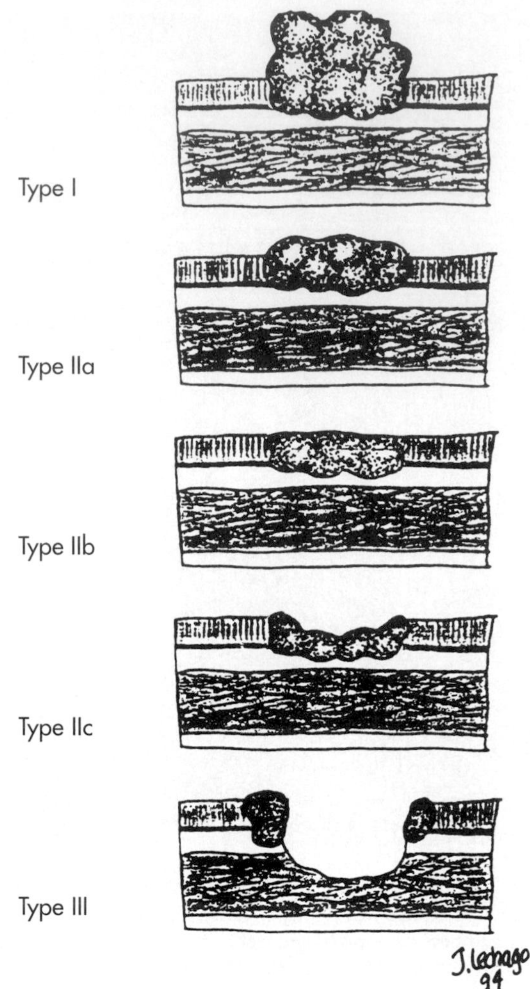

Fig. 53-28 Schema of the main types of early gastric carcinoma. *Type I,* protruded; *type IIa,* superficial elevated, *type IIb,* superficial flat; *type IIc,* superficial depressed; *type III,* excavated.

Early gastric cancer

Another significant development in this area is the characterization of the *early gastric cancer,* first described by Japanese workers.[278] This entity is defined as the presence of adenocarcinoma confined to mucosa and submucosa, regardless of whether there is metastatic involvement of the regional lymph nodes. Fig. 53-28 depicts the different types of early gastric

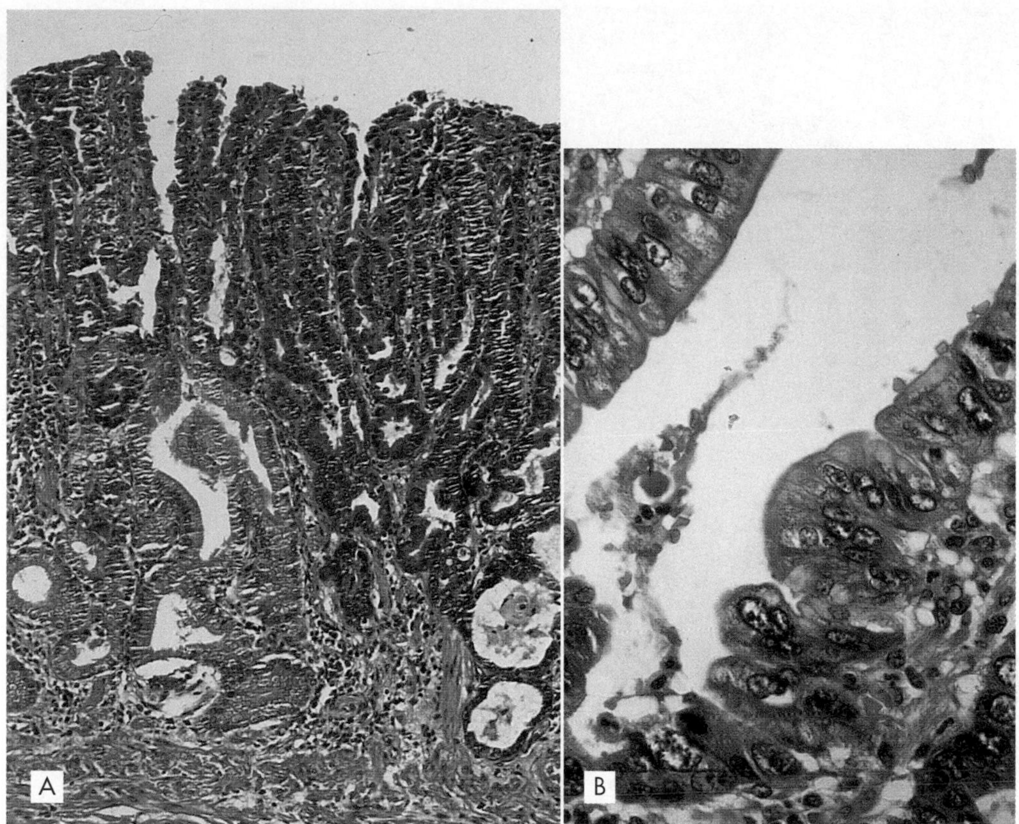

Fig. 53-29 **A,** Low-power photomicrograph of an intramucosal gastric carcinoma arising in a gastric mucosa with multifocal atrophic gastritis. The lesion involves the superficial half toward the left and the full thickness of the mucosa toward the right and consists of numerous glands and pitlike structures lined by cells that are stratified and contain hyperchromatic nuclei. The neoplastic tissue is contained within the muscularis mucosae, seen at the bottom of the picture. **B,** Close-up photomicrograph of the intramucosal carcinoma showing the high nuclear pleomorphism and hyperchromasia of the cells that cover the involved pits.

carcinoma of the stomach. When diagnosed and treated at this early stage, these carcinomas have a 90% to 95% 5-year survival rate.[279] Even though the frequency of early gastric cancer is relatively low in the United States, increasing awareness of its existence and of the radiologic and endoscopic parameters leading to its recognition have resulted in their representing 13% to 27% of all gastric cancers being diagnosed.[280] Grossly, these tumors have been classified as superficial, polypoid, fungating, ulcerated, or diffusely infiltrative.[281] Although it is largely descriptive, this classification has some clinical value: the superficial carcinoma corresponds to the histologic stage of early carcinoma, a Japanese usage defined as *"a primary carcinoma of the stomach with carcinomatous infiltration limited to the mucosa and submucosal layer, irrespective of the presence or absence of lymph node metastases."*[278] Fig. 53-29 depicts the histologic appearance of an intramucosal gastric carcinoma with a poorly differentiated pattern. Patients in whom gastric cancer is detected at this stage have a 5-year survival rate higher than 90%.[278-280] However, recurrences have been reported, particularly in a subset of patients demonstrating features such as expansile submucosal spread, cancer cell aneuploidy, and lymph node metastases.[271,282,283]

Invasive carcinoma

Approximately one half of gastric adenocarcinomas arise in the antrum, one fourth arise in the corpus, and the remaining fourth extend in both antrum and corpus, making it impossible to determine the site of origin.[281] Many carcinomas of the cardiac region are believed to originate from Barrett's columnar metaplasia in the distal portion of the esophagus and, as such, are not regarded as true gastric carcinomas. The size of gastric carcinoma at the time of diagnosis depends on the diligence with which such carcinomas are searched for in various compartments. Therefore, in series from Japan, where endoscopic screening and follow-up programs are widespread, early gastric carcinomas as small as 2 cm in diameter are represented much more often than in series from areas where the incidence of gastric cancer is lower and the degree of suspicion among physicians tends to be blunted.[271,282]

Grossly, adenocarcinomas of the stomach may show a variety of patterns. In addition to the early or superficial carcinoma, already discussed above, the more advanced carcinomas of the stomach have been divided into four groups by Borrmann:[281] (1) *polypoid,* consisting of a nodular tumor, often showing malignant transformation of an adenomatous polyp, presenting a broad base and no mucosal ulceration; (2) *fungating,* also a protruding lesion, larger and more frondous than the polypoid variety and often showing extensive ulceration of the top (Fig. 53-30); (3) *ulcerated,* an excavated lesion with an ulcer base below the surface of the mucosa and slightly elevated borders (Fig. 53-30). Although no single gross parameter is pathognomonic for the distinction of benign

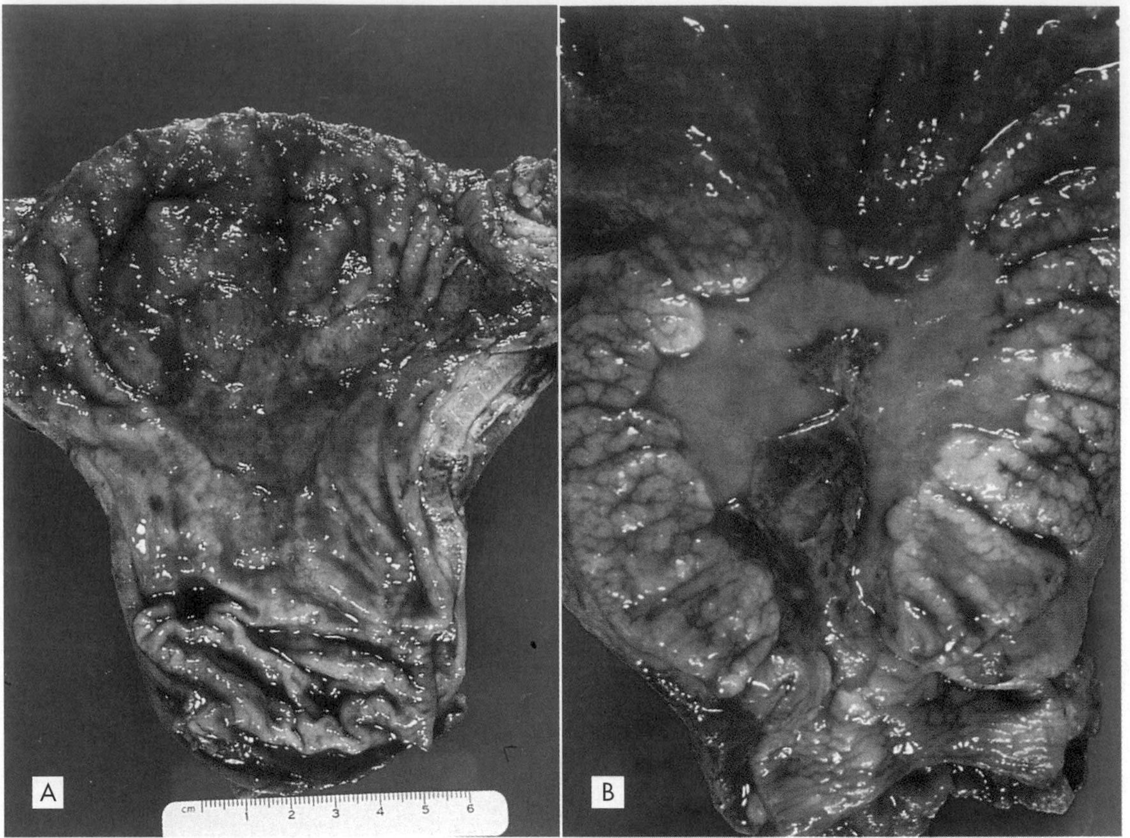

Fig. 53-30 **A,** Gross photograph of a gastric adenocarcinoma, fungating type. The lesion has a cauliflower-like appearance and is located over the lesser curvature, straddling the distal corpus and the proximal antrum. **B,** Gross photograph of a gastric adenocarcinoma, ulcerated type. The lesion is large, has an irregular profile, shows necrosis in its fundus, and interrupts the gastric mucosal folds.

Table 53-2 **Gross features of benign and malignant gastric ulcers**

	Benign	Malignant
Size	Smaller	Larger
Shape	Regular	Irregular
Borders	Edematous	Heaped up
Mucosal folds	Radiating	Interrupted
Ulcer bed	Clean (hemorrhagic)	Necrotic

from malignant gastric ulcers, observation of several features often permits such differentiation with a moderate degree of confidence. Table 53-2 is a comparison of the main gross features of benign and malignant ulcers of the stomach. The final group (4) is *diffusely infiltrative,* which gives the stomach, wall the thickened, rigid appearance classically described as the "leather-bottle" stomach or "linitis plastica."

Several classifications have been proposed for the histologic types of gastric adenocarcinomas. The WHO has divided carcinomas in four types: (1) papillary, (2) tubular, (3) mucinous, and (4) signet ring.[256] Because this classification has neither epidemiologic nor prognostic value, it has not been widely employed. In 1965, the Finnish pathologist Laurén, proposed a simple division in two types:[284] (1) *intestinal,* with features resembling those of a colonic adenocarcinoma as it forms recognizable glandular structures and adopts an expansive or exophytic pattern (Fig. 53-31); and (2) *diffuse,* composed originally of dispersed cells that do not form recognizable glandular structures, tends to grow with an infiltrative pattern, and may show variable degrees of signet-ring cell formation, partly corresponding to the WHO's signet-ring cell type (Fig. 53-31). This classification has the advantage that it is simple and highly reproducible and has considerable prognostic value: the survival rates of patients with the infiltrative type are less than one half of those with the intestinal type. Furthermore, the epidemiology of the intestinal type correlates well with the distribution of chronic atrophic gastritis and, today, with the prevalence of *H. pylori* infection. The drawback of Laurén's system is that between 10% and 20% of the gastric carcinomas do not fit in either category and have to be left out as "unclassified." This is attributable, in part, to the fact that once gastric adenocarcinomas become widely invasive, the intestinal type of tumors may show extensive areas with the infiltrating pattern and, conversely, originally infiltrating tumors may later show glandular formations. In 1977 Ming proposed a new classification dividing gastric carcinomas into *expanding* and *infiltrative* lesions;[281] most expanding carcinomas correspond to Laurén's intestinal type and virtually all infiltrative carcinomas are Laurén's diffuse type. According to Ming, most of the tumors that remained unclassified according to Laurén's system are expanding carcinomas in his classification.

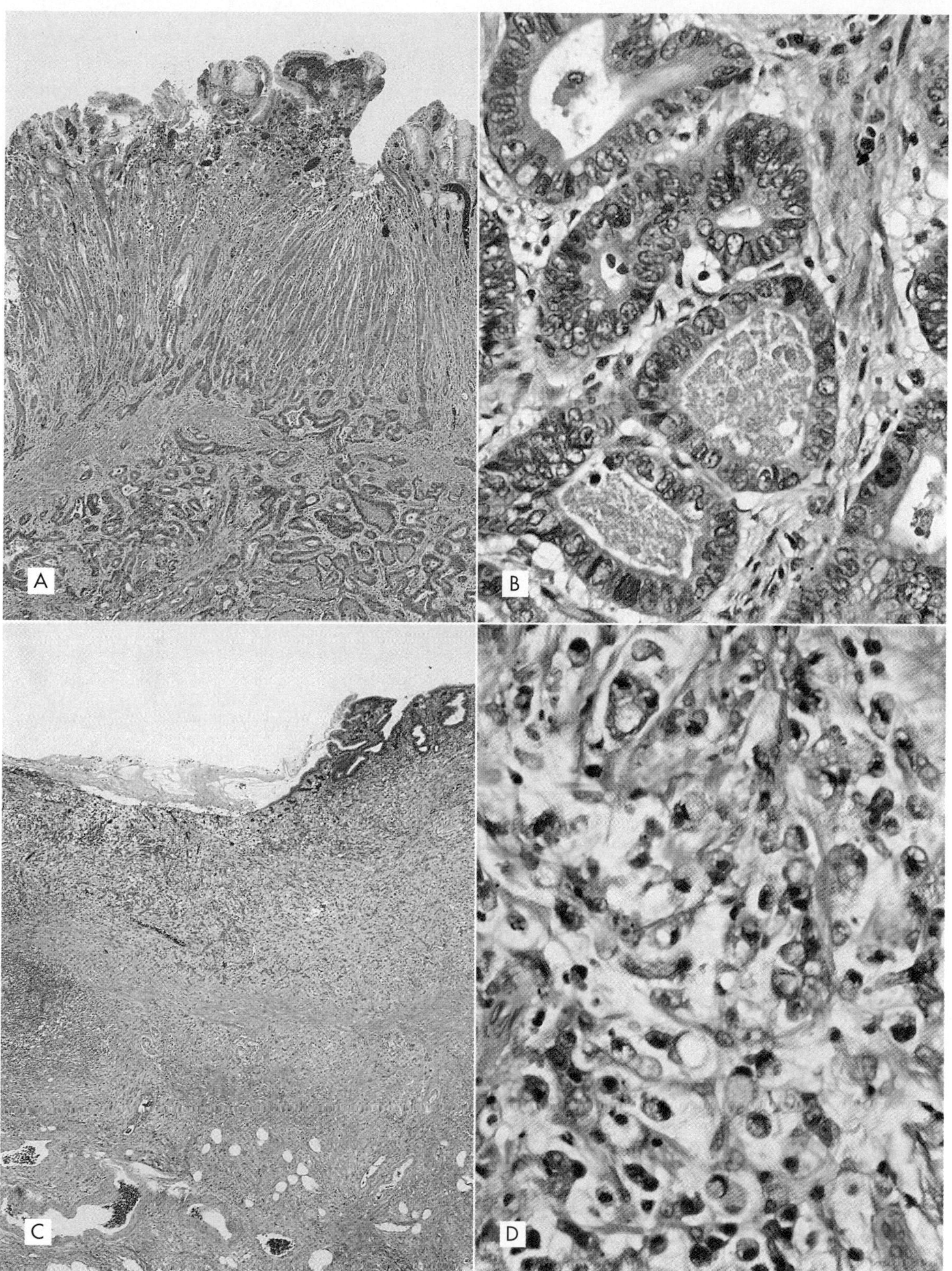

Fig. 53-31 **A,** Low-power photomicrograph of a gastric adenocarcinoma, intestinal or tubular type. The lesion arises from a mucosa that shows gastritis and invades submucosa and muscular layers, at the bottom of the picture. Glandlike structures are the main component of this neoplasia. **B,** Close-up view of the intestinal type of adenocarcinoma depicted in **A.** The individual glands are composed of stratified, highly pleomorphic cells, one of which shows an atypical tripolar mitosis. **C,** Low-power photomicrograph of a diffuse type adenocarcinoma. In this lesion, the malignancy is present, albeit unrecognizable at this low magnification, at the bottom of a mucosal ulceration seen at left. There is infiltration of the muscle, which appears disrupted on the left as well. **D,** Close-up view of the diffuse adenocarcinoma depicted in **C.** The neoplasm is composed of scattered individual cells that have clear, sometimes foamy cytoplasm and hyperchromatic nuclei. These cells infiltrate deeply into all layers but fail to form a discernible mass.

When one is evaluating gastric adenocarcinomas microscopically, it is convenient to consider three levels of differentiation. *Well-differentiated* tumors (corresponding to Laurén's intestinal type) are characterized by an abundance of glandular or tubular formation. Adenocarcinomas of this type are usually composed of tall columnar epithelial cells, sometimes containing goblet and Paneth's cells, and their elongated or oval nuclei show various degrees of atypia, ranging from a relatively monotonous shape with regular arrangement to a more pleomorphic and piled-up distribution. Their stroma is generally sparse but rich in capillaries, especially when the tumor has a polypoid pattern. In most cases, mucus production is entirely lost in the neoplastic epithelial cells. However, in some cases, the mucin production may be abundant, giving the tumor the appearance of a mucinous, gelatinous, or mucoid adenocarcinoma. These well-differentiated adenocarcinomas tend to grow both within and out of the gastric wall without losing the tight connections of the epithelial cells. In the largest, more advanced tumors, lymphatic invasion and metastasis to regional lymph nodes are frequently seen. Direct invasion of the cancer cells into intramural and extramural venules, causing liver metastasis through the portal circulation, is also not uncommon in this type.

In *moderately differentiated* carcinomas the nests of neoplastic tissue are relatively small and the cells forming the glands are mostly cuboidal or flat and lack a brush border, goblet cells, or Paneth's cells. In some of these tumors the nests are arranged in various glandular patterns (cribriform, acinar, solid, reticular) somewhat reminiscent of those of lobular carcinoma of the breast. The amount of stroma is moderate in most cases, but sometimes the abundance of stroma confers to these tumors a scirrhous appearance. The border of the cancerous lesion with the surrounding tissue is neither expanding nor infiltrating, but ragged or zigzagged. These features are best seen in low-power views of the histologic specimens. Whereas some of these tumors can still be classified as "intestinal type" according to the Laurén classification, most correspond to that portion of gastric adenocarcinoma considered of "unclassified" type.

When little or no glandular formation is detectable and the tumor cells are arranged mostly in minute solid clusters, anastomosing or trabecular patterns of non–mucin producing small cells, or isolated infiltrating tumor cells detached from cell clusters or cords, the tumor is considered *poorly differentiated*. In these cases, which almost invariably correspond to Laurén's infiltrating tumors, the histologic diagnosis of adenocarcinoma is often reached only on the basis of glandular arrangements faintly seen in some parts of the lesion. In some cases, immunocytochemical stains are necessary to distinguish these tumors from lymphomas. These tumors often invade the lymphatics, especially in the submucosa, but direct invasion of blood vessels is hardly ever seen.

Most "signet-ring" cell carcinomas have the pattern of these undifferentiated carcinomas, with large numbers of signet-ring cells mixed with other tumor cells widely infiltrating into the gastric wall. If the gastric resection specimen is carefully sectioned, even in these very poorly differentiated tumors it is often possible to detect areas of transition between the nonneoplastic and the neoplastic gastric mucosa.

In general, gastric adenocarcinomas tend to traverse the muscularis mucosae relatively early and invade the muscular wall. They may spread to neighboring structures, particularly to the lower esophagus, permeate lymphatics, and involve regional lymph nodes or, particularly the diffuse type, may spread along the serosa and cause the appearance of peritoneal implants and mucinous tumors in the ovaries, known as *Krukenberg's* tumors.[285] It is important to determine the extent of spread, as prognosis and subsequent treatment modalities are predicated upon the stage of the tumor at the time it is diagnosed. The American Joint Committee on Cancer (AJCC) has developed a staging system, called *TNM staging*, based on tumor invasion (T), lymph node involvement (N), and distant metastasis (M)[286] (Table 53-3). The presence of residual tumor (R) at curative surgery was also taken into account to further stratify these patients with a better predictive power.[287] Taking the TNM plus R into account, it has been found that stage I has a 5-year survival of 90%, stage II 50%, stage III 10%, and stage IV virtually nonexistent. A study from the United Kingdom attributes the improvement in the 5-year survival rates after curative surgery noted between 1970 and 1990 to a better patient selection, in turn the result of improved staging.[288]

Table 53-3 AJCC staging of gastric cancer

Stage	Primary tumor	Lymph node	Distant metastasis
0	Tis	N0	M0
IA	T1	N0	M0
IB	T2	N0	M0
IIA	T3	N0	M0
IIB	T4	N0	M0
IIIA	T_{any}	N1	M0
IIIB	T_{any}	N2	M0
IV	T_{any}	N_{any}	M1

This table represents a modification of the original American Joint Committee on Cancer (AJCC) staging and incorporates parameters from the UICC staging table, as well as the interpretation contained in G.R. Davis's chapter in Sleisinger MH, Fordtran JS, editors: *Gastrointestinal disease: pathophysiology/diagnosis/treatment,* ed 5, Philadelphia, 1993, Saunders.

Tis, Intraepithelial tumor; *T1,* invasive to submucosa; *T2,* invasive into muscularis; *T3,* invasive thru muscularis into subserosa; *T4,* invasive thru serosa into adjacent tissue; *N0,* no lymph node metastasis; *N1,* <3 metastatic nodes; *N2,* >3 metastatic nodes; *M0,* no distant metastasis; *M1,* distant metastasis present.

Ampullary carcinoma

Ampullary carcinoma is defined as an epithelial malignant neoplasm centered in and presumably arising from the ampulla of Vater.[289] The features that characterize this type of tumor are not merely topographic but also histogenetic: ampullary carcinomas are considered to arise from the epithelium that lines the ampulla of Vater or the immediate surrounding duodenal mucosa.[290,291] This assumption is based on the common presence of a preexisting villous or villolandular lesion in the area from which the malignancy arises.[290-293] The distinction between an ampullary and a pancreatic duct carcinoma is of more than academic interest inasmuch as the former connotes a definitely rosier prognosis.[294-296] In advanced cases, however, such distinction may not be possible because the tumor has overrun all structures in the vicinity. As a result, terms such *ampulla-head-of-pancreas,*[296] *periampullary,*[293-294] or *pancreatoduodenal*[295] carcinoma have been proposed. It is not clear whether the better prognosis of the

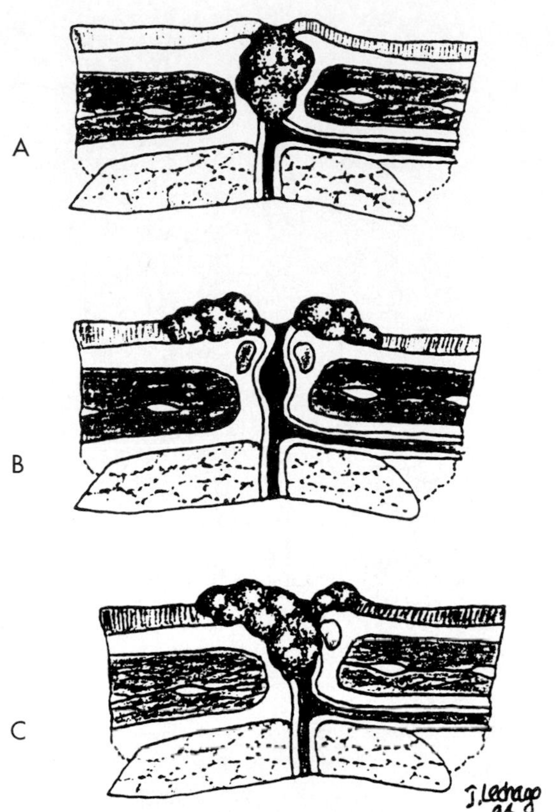

Fig. 53-32 Schema of the main variants of ampullary carbinoma. **A,** Intra-ampullary. **B,** Extra-ampullary. **C,** Mixed type.

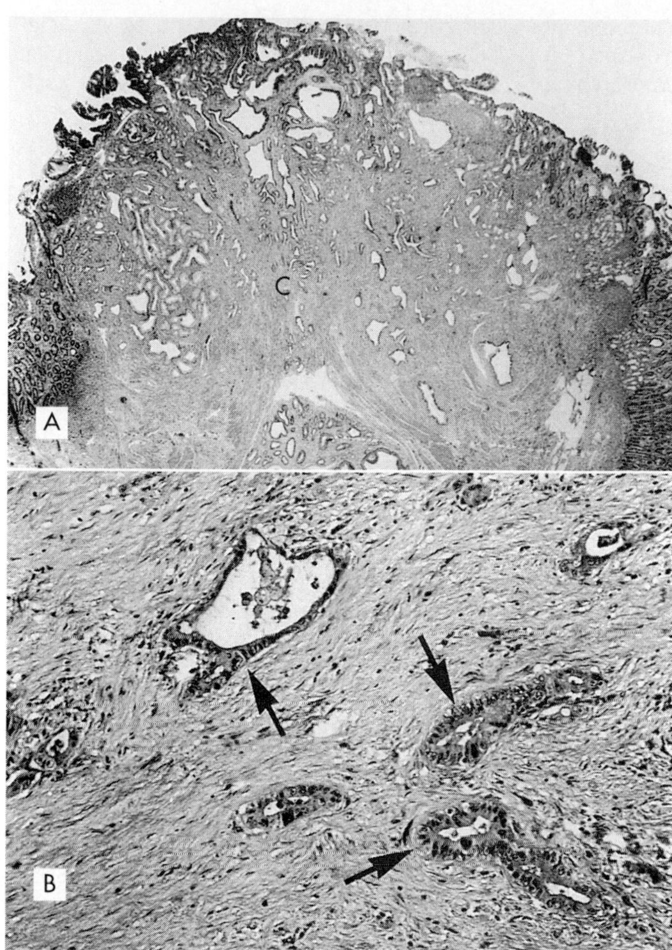

Fig. 53-33 **A,** Photomicrograph providing a panoramic view of the ampulla of Vater containing an intra-ampullary adenocarcinoma *(C)*. **B,** High-power photomicrograph showing the moderately differentiated adenocarcinoma. This is composed of scattered misshapen glands exhibiting moderate pleomorphism *(arrows)* and separated by abundant desmoplastic reaction.

ampullary neoplasms is the result of an intrinsic quality of their tumor cells, or of its generally early symptoms resulting in diagnosis and treatment at a preinvasive or early invasive stage in many instances.

There is overwhelming evidence that a significant number of periampullary and intra-ampullary carcinomas originate from preexisting benign villoglandular lesions.[290,292] These tumors are composed of intestinal type of cells, sometimes containing apical mucin and sometimes possessing a brush border. Goblet, endocrine, and Paneth's cells are very commonly found intermingled with the main cell type.[296] Variable degrees of atypia, from mild to carcinoma in situ, are found when these tumors are thoroughly sampled and investigated.[290,292,297] The presence of carcinoma in situ in adenomas and of residual adenoma in many ampullary carcinomas reinforce the theoretical concept of adenoma-carcinoma sequence in this location. The carcinomas have been classified on the basis of their location into (1) intra-ampullary, (2) periampullary, and (3) mixed type[296] (Fig. 53-32). This classification is useful because the survival rates of the three types differ considerably, with the intra-ampullary lesions having the better prognosis.[296] Irrespective of their location, many lesions consist of adenocarcinomas exhibiting poor differentiation at the deeper invasive front while showing a relatively benign villous or villoglandular pattern at the surface[298] (Fig. 53-33). This common finding must be kept in mind when one is assessing the tumor preoperatively using superficial endoscopic biopsy, ERCP-obtained tissue, or cytologic specimens.[298]

Malignancies arising in the ampulla of Vater or surrounding duodenal mucosa, as they grow, tend to infiltrate the wall of the duodenum, invade subjacent pancreatic parenchyma, give out metastases to the regional lymph nodes, and later metastasize to the liver or other organs.[296] Whereas unresected malignancies are invariably fatal within 5 years, radical pancreatoduodenectomy (Whipple's procedure) provides an overall 5-year survival of 50 to 55%.[299,300] The most important prognostic factor appears to be the stage of the neoplasm at the time of radical surgery.[301] Five-year survival rates are stage I (limited to the ampulla of Vater), 98 to 100%; stage II (invading duodenal wall or 2 cm or less into the pancreas, without metastases), 60% to 64%; stage III (positive regional lymph nodes, whether intraampullary or invading into the pancreas up to 2 cm), 12% to 15%; and stage IV (invading more than 2 cm into the pancreas, or with distant metastases irrespective of other parameters), <1%. The presence of regional lymph node metastases, histologic grade, and particularly the presence of perineural invasion constitute significant independent prognostic factors.[293,299,302,303]

Other malignant epithelial tumors

Tumors containing elements of adenocarcinoma together with squamous cells, occasionally producing keratin, are rarely found in the stomach and are called adenosquamous carcinomas or adenoacanthomas.[304] Their biologic behavior is similar to that of adenocarcinomas without squamous differentiation.

Pure squamous cell carcinomas of the stomach exist but are extremely rare.[305] Teratomas,[306] choriocarcinomas,[307] and carcinosarcomas[308] all have been reported to occur in the stomach.

Neuroendocrine hyperplasias and tumors

Endocrine cell hyperplasias

Hyperplasias of the gastrin-producing cells, generally referred to as *G-cell hyperplasias,* have been demonstrated in a variety of conditions and have been classified as *secondary* hyperplasias, when they are associated with a known cause, and *primary* hyperplasias, when such cause has not been identified.[127,309] Secondary G-cell hyperplasias have been associated with several pathogenic mechanisms such as hypochlorhydria, antropyloric distention, hypercalcemia, and less common entities such as acromegaly and chronic uremia.[127,310] Conditions associated with hypochlorhydria include chronic atrophic gastritis, particularly when it is associated with pernicious anemia, iatrogenic exclusion of the antrum, post–truncal vagotomy syndrome, and protracted treatment with H_2-receptor blockers or with proton-pump inhibitors. Primary G-cell hyperplasias have been associated with hypergastrinemia, gastric hyperacidity, and so-called intractable peptic ulcer disease, often requiring surgery. This type of hyperplasia is rather infrequent, and only a limited number of instances has been published and convincingly documented so far.[311] In such cases, antrectomy was followed by a return of circulating gastrin and gastric acid secretion values to normal levels. There is still a measure of controversy regarding whether common peptic ulcer disease is found in association with G-cell hyperplasia. Although some believe that this association does exist,[127] others maintain that such hyperplasia, if it exists at all, is probably secondary to vagotomy.[312]

G-cell hyperplasias, whether primary or secondary, have been described in the gastric antropyloric mucosa and have been characterized morphologically by the following parameters: (1) increase in the numbers of gastrin-immunoreactive cells in the antral mucosa (192 to 259 G-cells per linear millimeter; normal: 41 to 93 G-cells per linear millimeter),[121] (2) expansion of the compartment occupied by such cells within the antral glands, both toward the surface and toward the basal portion, and (3) appearance of characteristic clusters or "clones" of G-cells in the antral mucosa.[313] Fig. 53-34 is an example of G-cell hyperplasia as demonstrated by immunocytochemistry.

ECL-cell hyperplasias are characterized by the presence of increased numbers of argyrophil cells with a characteristic ultrastructure in the glands of the gastric oxyntic mucosa. This change has been recorded in association with *pernicious anemia*[128,314] and with the *Zollinger-Ellison syndrome.*[223,315] Although these two entities would appear to be totally opposed in terms of their functional manifestations, both share as a common denominator the presence of hypergastrinemia. Experimental and clinical evidence indicates that gastrin acts as a powerful trophic factor for the ECL cells, both in rats and in humans; sustained and significant elevations in circulating gastrin have been shown to result in ECL-cell hyperplasia.[129,316] On the basis of the morphologic pattern, the ECL-cell hyperplasias have been divided into simple, linear, micronodular, and adenomatoid[317] (Fig. 53-35). In patients with long-standing pernicious anemia, this hyperplasia may evolve into dysplasia and eventually into neoplasia with formation of microcarcinoids and intramucosal carcinoids and finally into invasive carcinoids.[128,314,317,318] In the Zollinger-Ellison syndrome, the ECL-cell hyperplasia does not cause the appearance of carcinoid tumors, except in such cases where the syndrome is part of the MEN I picture.[217] In patients with extensive ECL-cell hyperplasia secondary to pernicious anemia, antrectomy has resulted in regression of both hyperplasia and some of the ensuing carcinoid tumors, thus confirming the postulate that gastrin is a determinant factor in their pathogenesis.[319,320]

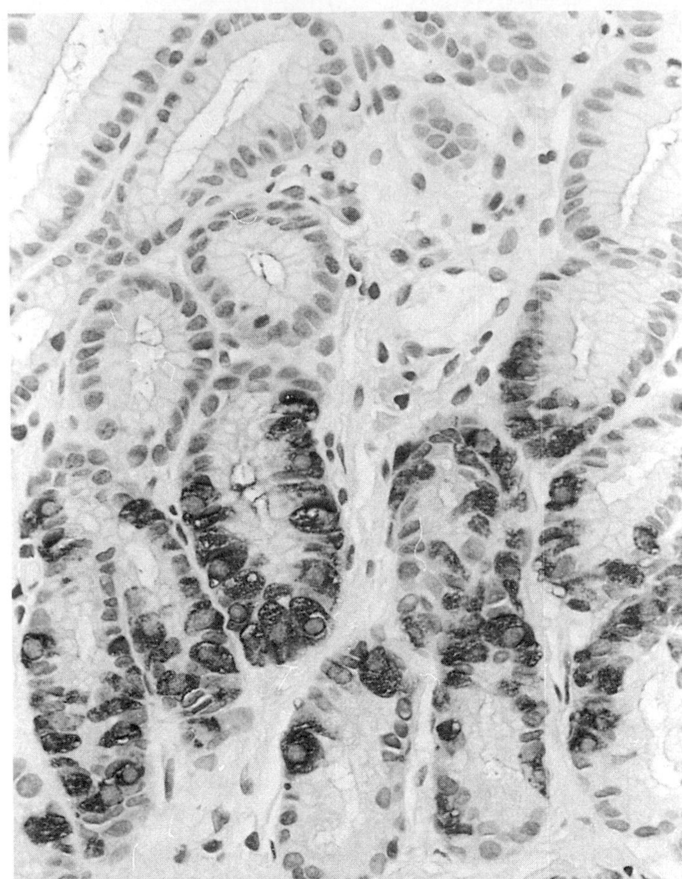

Fig. 53-34 High-power view of the gastric antral mucosa of a patient with fundal chronic atrophic gastritis associated with pernicious anemia. This picture illustrates the characteristic clustering of the G-cells, which not only are increased in number, but also form "clonal" aggregates. (ABC immunoperoxidase against gastrin.)

Hyperplasia of the enterochromaffin (EC) cells has been described in biopsy specimens of the small intestinal mucosa of patients with untreated celiac sprue.[321] This seems to be directly related to the severity of the concomitant disease and has been interpreted as a nonspecific response to the chronic inflammation and subsequent reparative activity, as it regresses when a gluten-free diet is instituted. Similar increases in EC-cell numbers have been observed in chronic gastritis, in appendicitis, and in the vicinity of intestinal constrictions.[127] No instances have been published documenting progression of EC-cell hyperplasias into carcinoid tumors in the small intestine.

Carcinoid tumors

Carcinoid tumors were classified by Williams and Sandler on the basis of their embryogenesis into three groups: foregut, midgut, and hindgut.[322] Although this classification represents

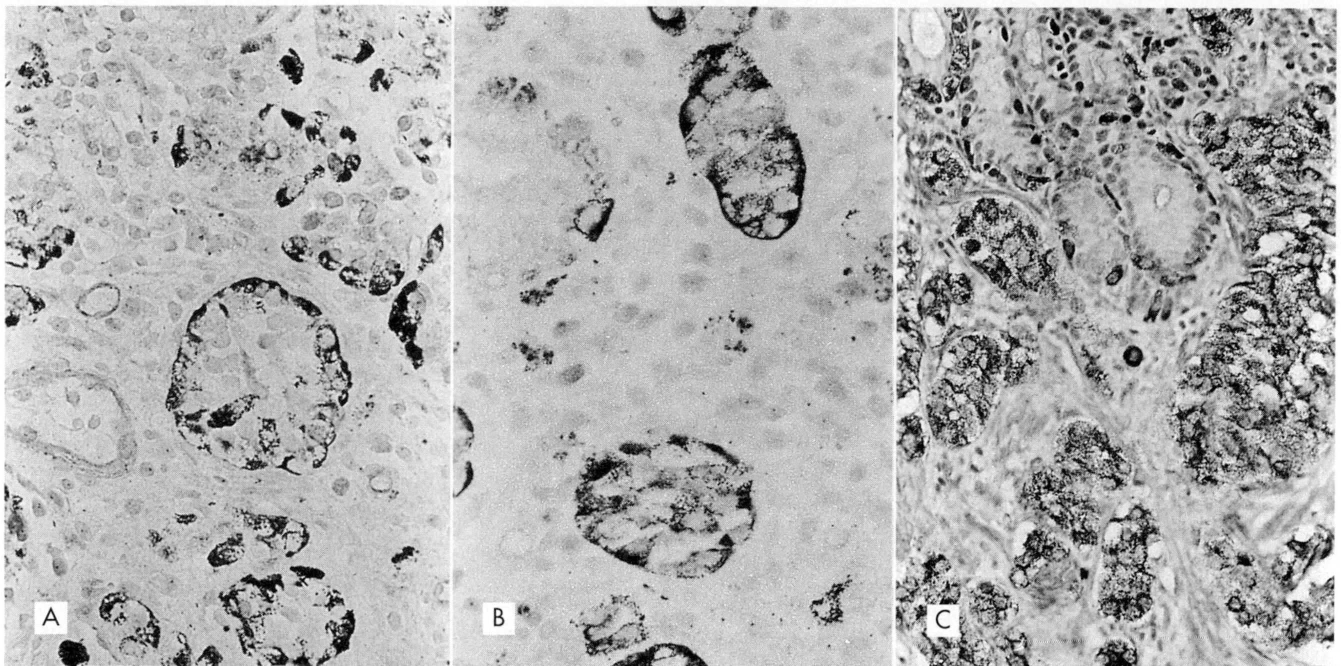

Fig. 53-35 Gastric oxyntic mucosa of a patient with fundic chronic atrophic gastritis associated with pernicious anemia. **A,** High-power photomicrograph depicts the linear pattern of ECL-cell proliferation. **B,** High-power photomicrograph of a different area from the same patient illustrating the ECL cells, this time arranged in micronodular pattern. **C,** High-power photomicrograph, also from the same patient, this time illustrating adenomatoid hyperplasia of the ECL cells. These are seen not only within glands, but also in the lamina propria forming extensive aggregates. Notice that these adenomatoid, dysplastic ECL cells are much less heavily granulated than their purely hyperplastic counterparts depicted in **A** and **B.** (Grimelius silver stain.)

an oversimplification and contains many exceptions, it nonetheless provides a useful functional basis for the categorization and investigation of such neoplasms. Although originally it was believed that the carcinoid tumors were benign, it has been seen that they are quite capable of invading adjacent organs and of metastasizing to distant sites. With few exceptions, histologic and cytologic parameters are not reliable indices of malignancy: most of these tumors, whether primary or metastatic, display a low mitotic rate and little cellular atypia. The only reliable marker for malignancy is the existence of distant metastases, invasion of neighboring structures, or the permeation of vascular structures. One of the most reliable prognostic parameters would appear to be the size of the tumor at the time of diagnosis. Whereas tumors measuring less than 1 cm in diameter only exceptionally exhibit metastatic activity, lesions measuring more than 2 cm in diameter often follow a malignant course.[323,324]

Foregut carcinoids are generally similar among themselves and to carcinoids from other parts of the digestive tube from the viewpoint of conventional morphology. However, silver stains, ultrastructural studies, and immunocytochemical investigations have revealed a remarkable variability within this group of tumors.[322] Indeed, diagnostically these lesions do not constitute a well-defined nosologic entity but rather represent a general category integrated by a variety of individual entities.[311] Gastric carcinoids may be *sporadic*[325] or *secondary* to ECL-cell hyperplasia resulting from pernicious anemia and long-standing gastric atrophy[314,318,325] (Fig. 53-36). These tumors are generally argyrophilic but not argentaffin, and electron microscopic examination reveals the secretory granules each with a small, electron-dense, eccentric core typical of the ECL cells.[314,318,325] Sporadic gastric carcinoids tend to behave more aggressively than those associated with pernicious anemia; the latter seldom metastasize and have not been reported as a direct cause of death so far.[325]

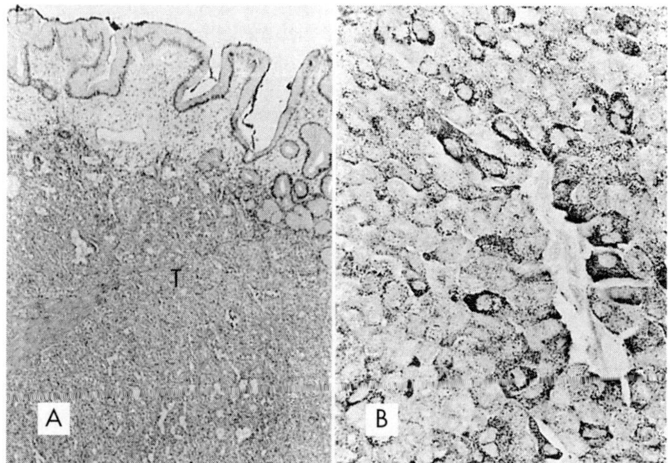

Fig. 53-36 **A,** Low-power photomicrograph of a gastric carcinoid tumor in a patient with fundal atrophic gastritis associated with pernicious anemia. The tumor *(T)* is present in the lower mucosa, replacing the glandular elements. **B,** High-power photomicrograph of the same tumor, stained with Grimelius silver stain. Some cells are densely granulated, whereas others are virtually agrandular. (From Lechago J: *Hum Pathol* 25:1114, 1994.)

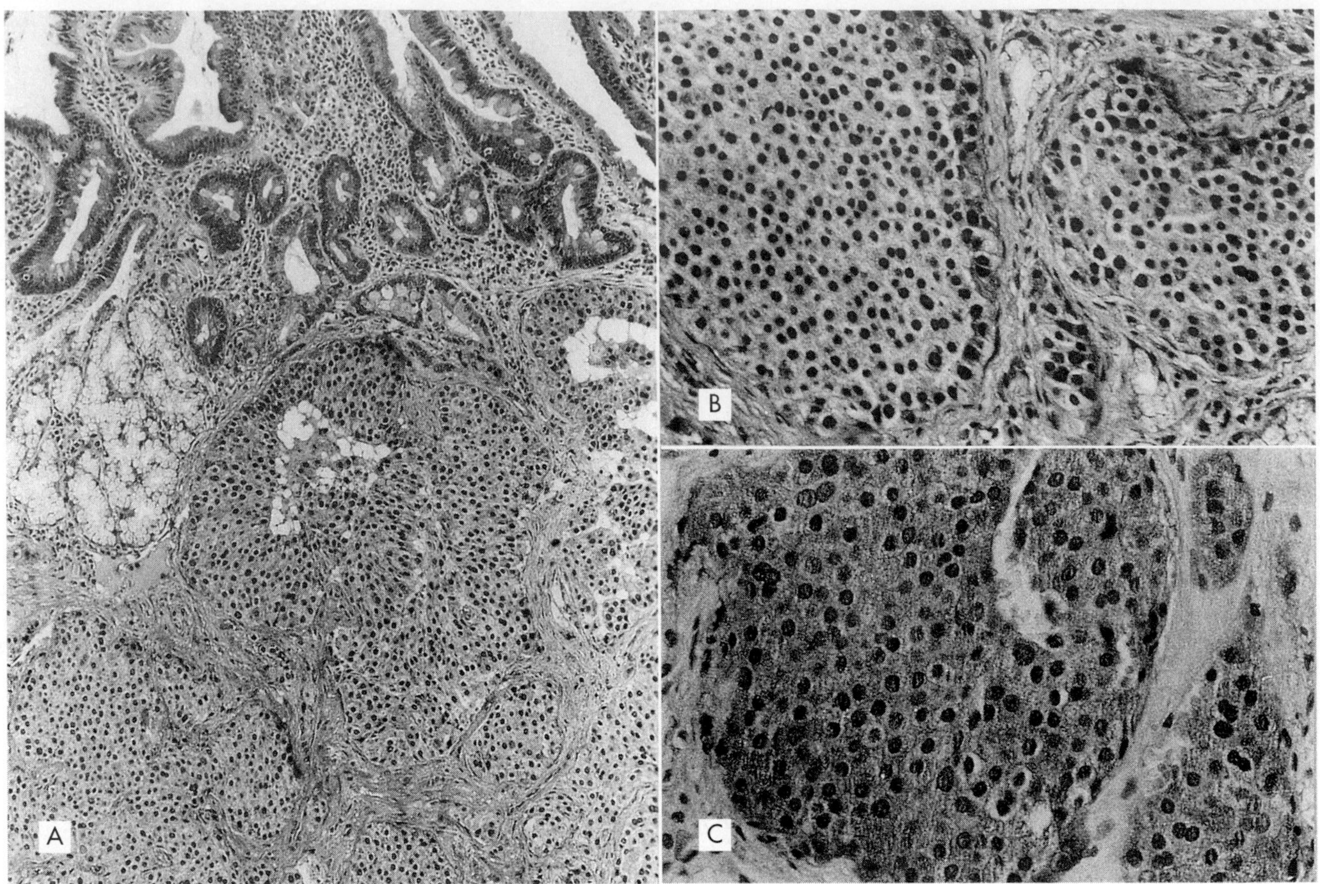

Fig. 53-37 Duodenal gastrinoma **A,** Low-power photomicrograph. The tumor is present in the lower region of the mucosa and submucosa and does not appear to arise from the mucosa itself. **B,** Close-up view of the tumor, illustrating its organoid pattern. The tumor cells are arranged in clusters of variable size separated by thin fibrovascular strands. The tumor cells are uniform and do not show significant pleomorphism or mitotic rate. **C,** High-power photomicrograph of same tumor immunostained for gastrin. Virtually all tumor cells show moderate granular staining of their cytoplasm.

A variety of endocrine tumors have been described in the duodenum: among the most common are *gastrinomas,* generally associated with the Zollinger-Ellison syndrome[326,327] (Fig. 53-37), and *somatostatinomas,* which sometimes coexist with neurofibromatosis and often contain characteristic psammoma bodies[328] (Fig. 53-38).

Poorly differentiated neuroendocrine carcinomas

Small cell undifferentiated carcinomas, originating from endocrine precursors, have been found in all segments of the digestive tube, from esophagus to colon.[313] These tumors are relatively more common in the esophagus and in the colon, whereas only rare examples have been reported in the stomach and proximal small intestine,[329,330] including the ampulla of Vater.[331] They are characterized by the presence of sheets of small cells with scanty cytoplasm and hyperchromatic elongated nuclei, exhibiting focal necrosis and a brisk mitotic rate. These lesions are positive with antibodies against neuron-specific enolase, but poorly positive or negative with antibodies to chromogranin and silver stains, since, as a rule, they are very scantily granulated. By electron microscopy, the few scattered cytoplasmic granules identified are round, small (100 to 120 nm in diameter), and electron dense. These tumors, like those of the lung, tend to respond readily to chemotherapy, but death ensues, nonetheless, within 6 to 9 months after diagnosis.[332]

Gangliocytic paragangliomas

Gangliocytic paragangliomas are rare lesions encountered almost exclusively in the second portion of the duodenum composed of a mixture of neuroectodermal cells morphologically similar to those of paragangliomas or carcinoid tumors, mature neurons, and scattered Schwann cells[333] (Fig. 53-39). Immunocytochemical analysis reveals the presence of multiple peptides both in the endocrine cells and the neurons, including somatostatin, serotonin, and pancreatic polypeptide.[333,334] These tumors, more frequent in males than in females with an age range between midtwenties and mideighties, are almost invariably benign and tend to present as polypoid lesions that may bleed into, or partially obstruct, the intestinal lumen. Rare instances of malignant behavior, including metastatic spread, have been reported.[335] Although quite diagnostic because of the presence of mature neurons, sometimes these lesions may pose a differential diagnostic problem with the more potentially malignant carcinoid tumors, when the pathologist is presented with a small mucosal biopsy that does not include such

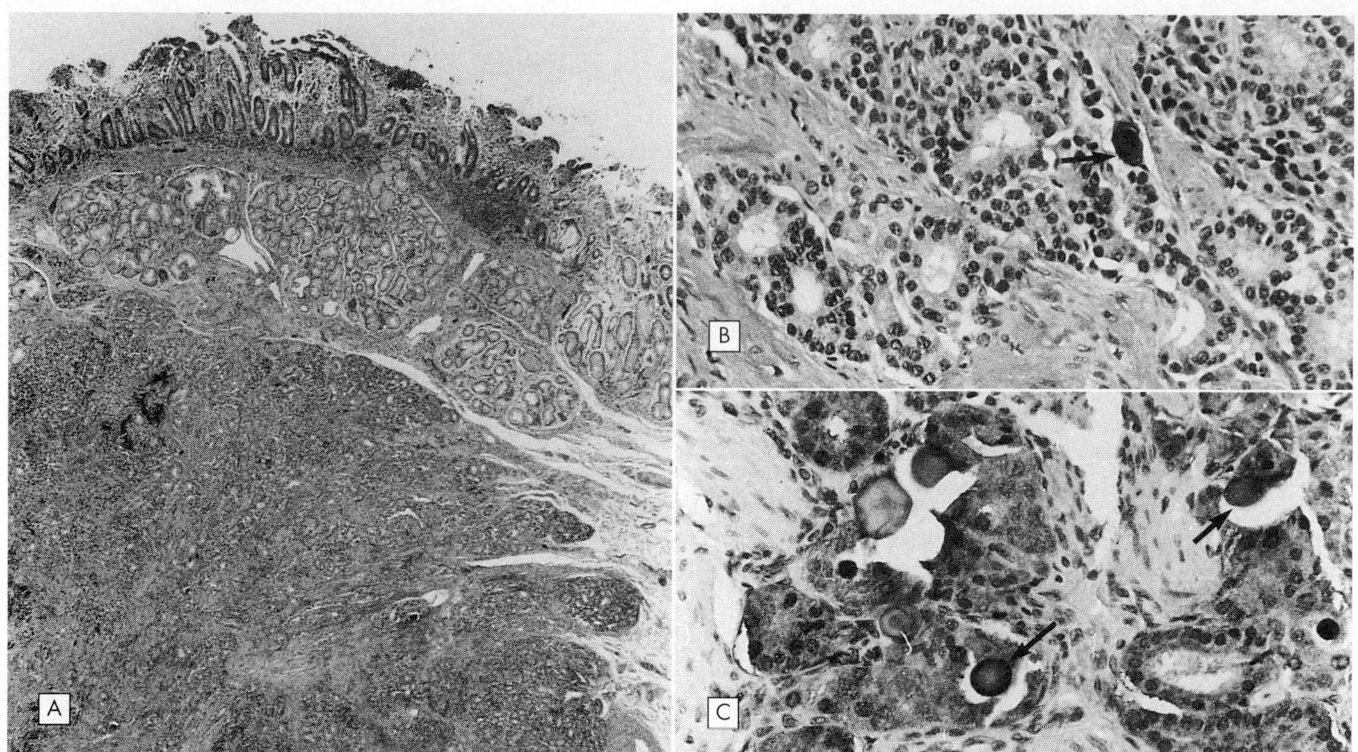

Fig. 53-38 Histologic appearance of a duodenal somatostatinoma. **A,** Low-power photomicrograph. The tumor is present in the submucosa and penetrates into the muscular layer. There is only focal mucosal involvement. **B,** Close-up photomicrograph illustrating the rosette and trabecular arrangement of the neoplastic cells in this duodenal somatostatinoma. The intervening lamina propria shows dense fibrosis. A psammoma body, characteristic of this type of tumor, is found in the stroma *(arrow)*. **C,** Close-up photomicrograph of same tumor immunostained with antibodies against somatostatin. The tumor cells are moderately positive and several psammoma bodies are also noted *(arrows)*.

neurons and shows only the carcinoid-like pattern. Immunocytochemical investigation for S-100 protein is useful in solving this problem, since it is positive in the Schwann cells that are part of the gangliocytic paraganglioma (Fig. 53-39) but negative in carcinoid tumors.[334]

Lymphomas

Gastric lymphomas constitute over 50% of all digestive lymphomas;[336] their prevalence has increased notably in the last few years.[337] This is an intriguing statistic considering that the normal gastric mucosa does not contain a lymphoid population comparable to that of the small and the large intestine, generally referred to as *gut-associated lymphoid tissue* (GALT), or *mucosa-associated lymphoid tissue* (MALT).[338]

A majority of gastric lymphomas present as high-grade, large-cell immunoblastic lymphomas.[339] These lesions tend to present as visible lesions with thickening of the rugal folds and frequent ulceration (Fig. 53-40). Under the microscope, these high-grade lymphomas may be relatively monomorphic, composed of large cells with abundant cytoplasm and vesicular nuclei endowed with prominent nucleoli[338] (Fig. 53-41). Variants of this type include mixtures of large cells, immunoblasts, and small lymphocytes, or a peculiar sclerosing type with interstitial collagen deposition.[340]

Other lymphomas of the stomach present as low-grade, small lymphocytic well-differentiated B-cell lymphomas, categorized as MALTomas by Isaacson and coworkers[338,341] (Fig. 53-42). These lymphomas are characterized by proliferation of monocytoid cells and by the presence of lymphoepithelial lesions;[341] the latter can be best demonstrated with keratin immunostains (Fig. 53-42). Whereas most MALTomas tend to be of low grade and indolent in nature, some would appear to evolve in later stages into a high-grade type.[338,342] Grade and stage are of prognostic significance among MALTomas.[337] It has been proposed that such MALTomas arise from the lymphoid follicles that appear in *chronic nonatrophic gastritis,*[138] often associated with peptic ulcer disease and with *H. pylori* infection.[133]

An interesting entity, sometimes referred to as *pseudolymphoma,* is currently under scrutiny: whereas some regard it merely as a benign nodular lymphoid proliferation, often associated with mucosal ulceration, others believe it to be an early or noninvasive stage of MALToma.[343] Indeed, numerous examples of lymphoma have been reported seemingly arising from a pseudolymphoma.[344] Whether this entity represents or not an early malignancy, consensus is progressively emerging in that the term *pseudolymphoma* lends itself to confusion and should probably be discarded.

Stromal tumors

The stomach is the site of origin of about 50% of all gastrointestinal stromal tumors.[345] These present grossly as masses of

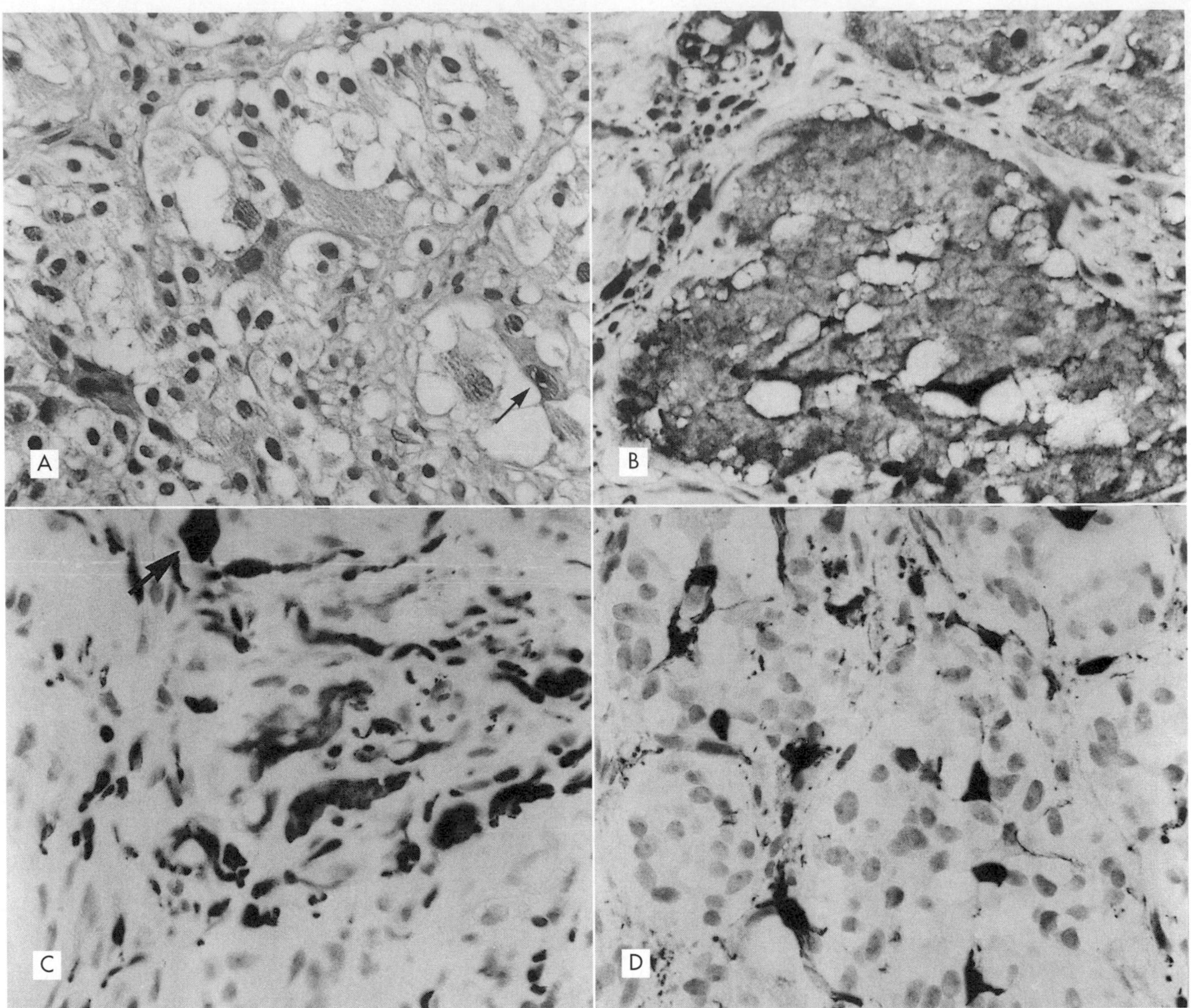

Fig. 53-39 Duodenal gangliocytic paraganglioma. **A,** High-power photomicrograph. The lesion is composed of nests and clusters of cells with abundant clear, faintly granular cytoplasm possessing small bland-appearing nuclei. Occasional neurons can be seen *(arrow)* and are characterized by abundant irregular cytoplasm and vesicular nuclei with prominent nucleoli. **B,** Immunostaining with antibodies against neuron-specific enolase *(NSE);* all component cells, as well as nerve structures, are moderately to strongly positive. **C,** Immunostaining with antibodies against neurofilaments; nerve bundles of variable thickness are strongly positive, along with a neuronal body *(arrow).* **D,** Immunostaining with S-100 protein antibodies. Small sustentacular cells with multiple thin processes are strongly immunostained. By contrast, the neuroendocrine and neuronal elements are negative.

variable size, generally well delimited, arising in the wall of the stomach and sometimes abutting the lumen or the serosa. Their cut surface tends to be homogeneous and have a whorled appearance (Fig. 53-43). When these lesions become obviously malignant, necrosis, hemorrhage, and degeneration may become grossly apparent. Of these lesions, the most common variety, generally present in body and fundus, is the *epithelioid cell leiomyoma,*[345,346] also named *leiomyoblastoma* in earlier descriptions when the true malignant potential of these lesions was not known.[347] The epithelioid leiomyomas are usually multilobulated or multinodular tumors composed of rounded or polygonal cells with abundant pale cytoplasm (Fig. 53-44). This typical pattern often alternates with another composed of plump spindle cells or with the presence of giant multinucleated tumor cells, varying from one area or nodule to another.[345,348] Its malignant counterpart, the epithelioid leiomyosarcoma, appears much more commonly in fundus and cardia than in the antrum and is characterized by the presence of smaller, more uniform cells endowed with a significant mitotic rate and variable pleomorphism. These tumors are more frequent in older patients and women exhibit a slight predominance. Some of these epithelioid leiomyosarcomas appear in the context of a familiar condition, generally in young women and accompanied by pulmonary chondromas

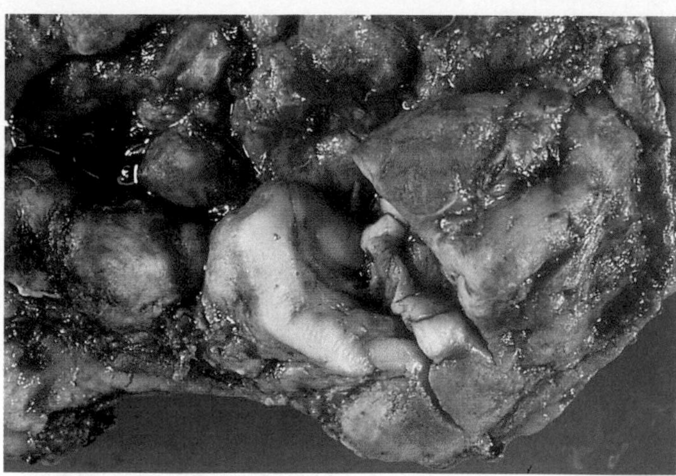

Fig. 53-40 Gross photograph of a high-grade lymphoma infiltrating the gastric mucosa. The gastric mucosal folds are greatly thickened and exhibit areas of hemorrhage. Where the mucosa has been cut it is greatly thickened, and the cut section has a "fish-flesh" appearance.

and extra-adrenal functioning paragangliomas, known as *Carney's triad.*[349]

Another group of tumors, generally referred to as *cellular leiomyomas,* consist of interlacing sheets, palisades, and fascicles of uniform spindle cells with elongated nuclei[346] (Fig. 53-45). In benign tumors, many cells contain small cytoplasmic vacuoles that indent one of the poles of the nucleus. Whereas these vacuoles are clearly artifactual, their presence appears to be a reliable marker for benignity because they are not found in leiomyosarcomas.[348] In a minority of cases, these tumors exhibit the ultrastructural (cytoplasmic filaments, pinocytotic vesicles, and basement membrane) and immunocytochemical (desmin and alpha-actin) markers of smooth muscle cells and are readily classified as leiomyomas, or leiomyosarcomas when they are malignant. Most, however, lack such ultrastructural or immunocytochemical markers, or exhibit other phenotypic traits, such as positivity for S-100 protein, which raises the possibility of their originating from a Schwann cell precursor. Because of this ambiguity, many prefer to call these tumors *stromal cell tumors,* thus sidestepping the relatively inconsequential issues of their origin, or even of their phenotypic differentiation.[350]

Whether these are stromal cell tumors, leiomyoblastomas, or smooth muscle tumors, all may present variable potentials

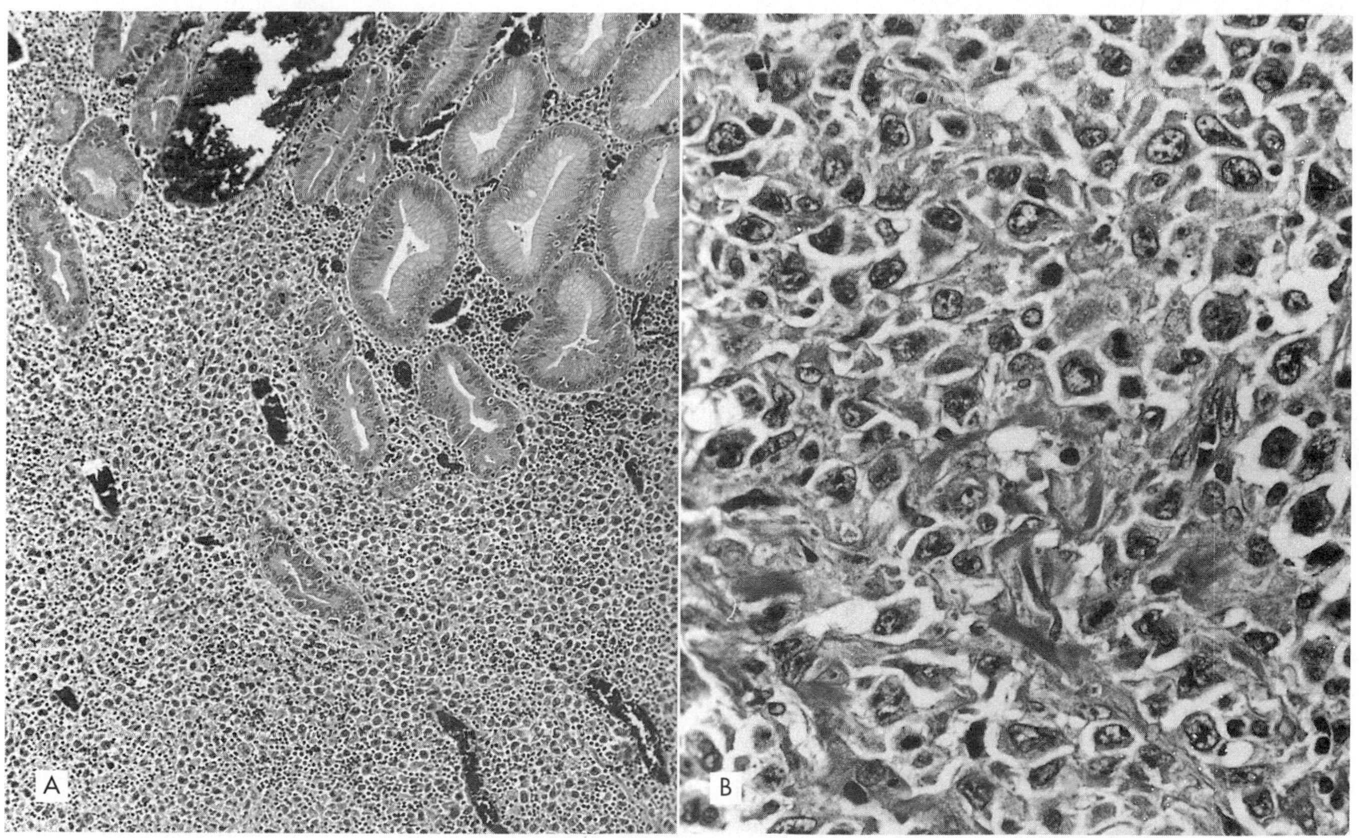

Fig. 53-41 **A,** Low-power photomicrograph of a high-grade lymphoma in the gastric mucosa. The lamina propria is greatly expanded and filled with large lymphoid cells with a moderately homogenous appearance. **B,** High-power view of the malignant lymphoid infiltrate illustrated in **A.** The cells are moderately discohesive and characterized by moderately abundant cytoplasm and vesicular nuclei containing prominent nucleoli. Occasional mitotic figures can be seen.

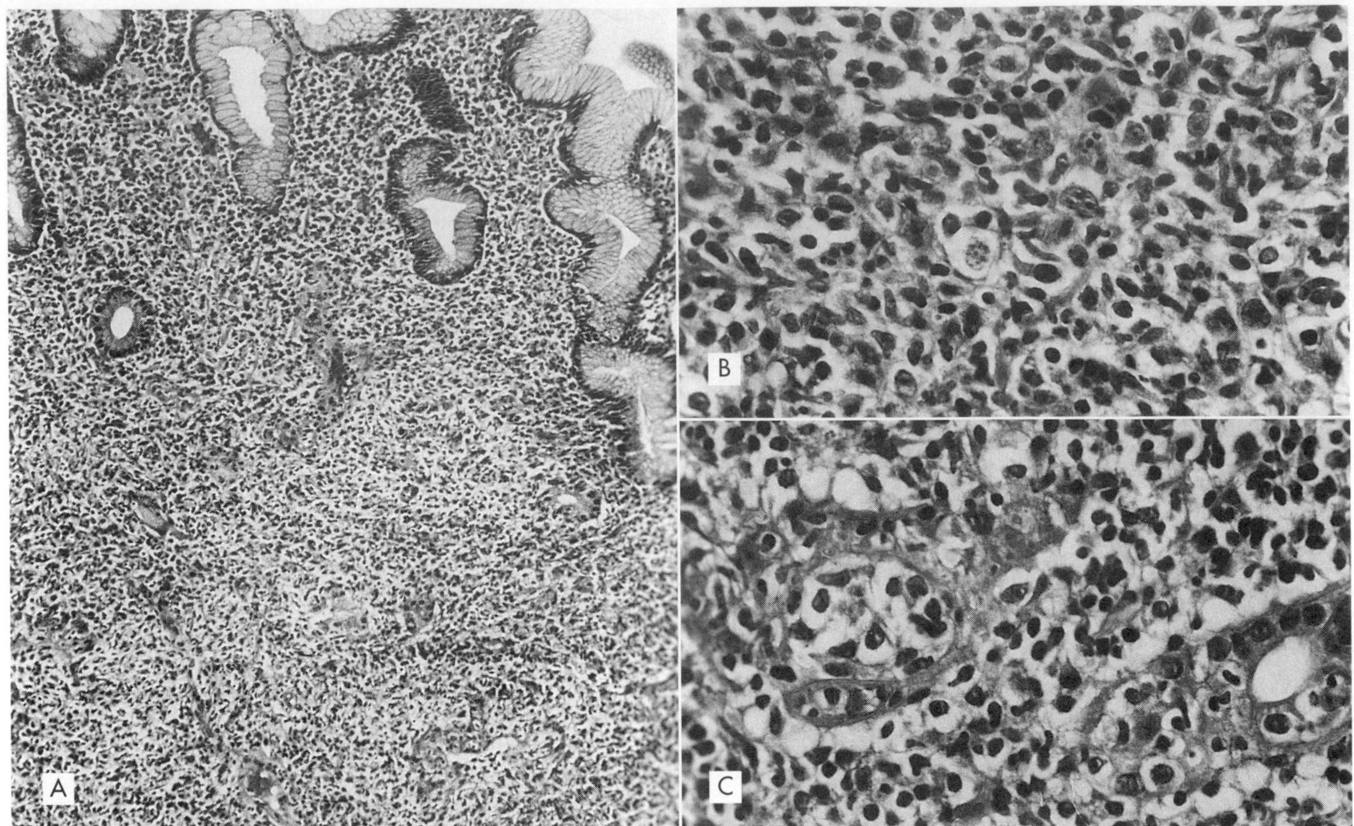

Fig. 53-42 **A,** Histologic appearance of a low-grade lymphoma (MALToma) in the antral gastric mucosa. In this low-power photomicrograph the glandular compartment has been almost entirely replaced by a homogenous infiltrate of small lymphoid cells. **B,** High-power photomicrograph of the infiltrating malignant cells. With exceptions, these contain a small amount of cytoplasm and nuclei exhibiting no significant atypia. Occasional larger cells with a blastic appearance can be found. Mitotic rate is low, and cellular atypia is rare. **C,** High-power photomicrograph illustrating the presence of lymphoepithelial lesions *(arrows),* characteristic of this low-grade lymphoma. The glands are greatly distorted and show infiltration by clusters of small lymphoid cells (*L*).

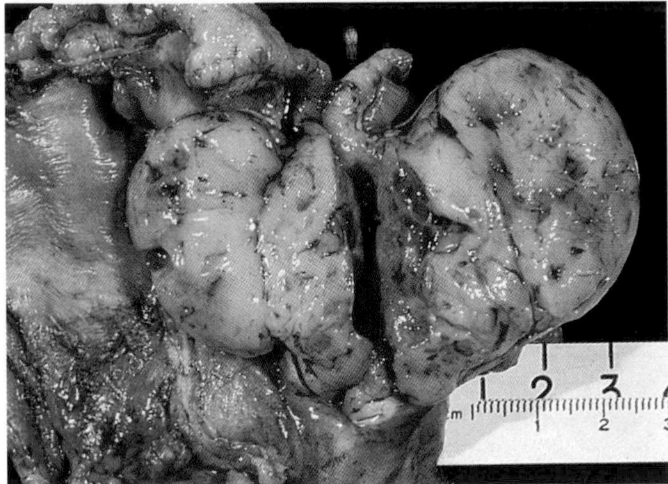

Fig. 53-43 Gross photograph of a gastric stromal tumor situated on the serosal aspect of the corpus of the stomach. The cut section of the tumor, which has been bisected, shows a glistening, slightly bulging, "meaty" appearance and contains scattered focal hemorrhages. No significant gross necrosis is observed.

for malignant behavior. After examining numerous possible factors, it is generally accepted that size of the tumor, cellularity, and mitotic rate are the most reliable indicators for malignancy, with significant differences existing between different segments of the digestive tract.[348,350] In the stomach, tumors that are less than 6 cm in diameter almost never metastasize, whereas those that measure 6 to 10 cm have an undetermined malignant potential, and those measuring more than 10 cm in diameter have a better than 50% chance of being metastatic. Cellularity is also a reliable indicator because most malignant tumors are highly cellular whereas poorly cellular tumors only exceptionally metastasize. Finally, mitotic rate is also significant, inasmuch as tumors with more than 1 mitosis per 10 high-power fields have a high probability of behaving in a malignant fashion. Necrosis and pleomorphism, though generally present in overtly malignant, invasive, or metastatic lesions (Fig. 53-46), have not been found to be reliable prognostic indicators in early lesions. Ploidy studies have disclosed that aneuploidy is a significant marker toward malignant behavior, but it is not clear whether it constitutes a reliable independent marker.[351] The cell type, however, seems to be

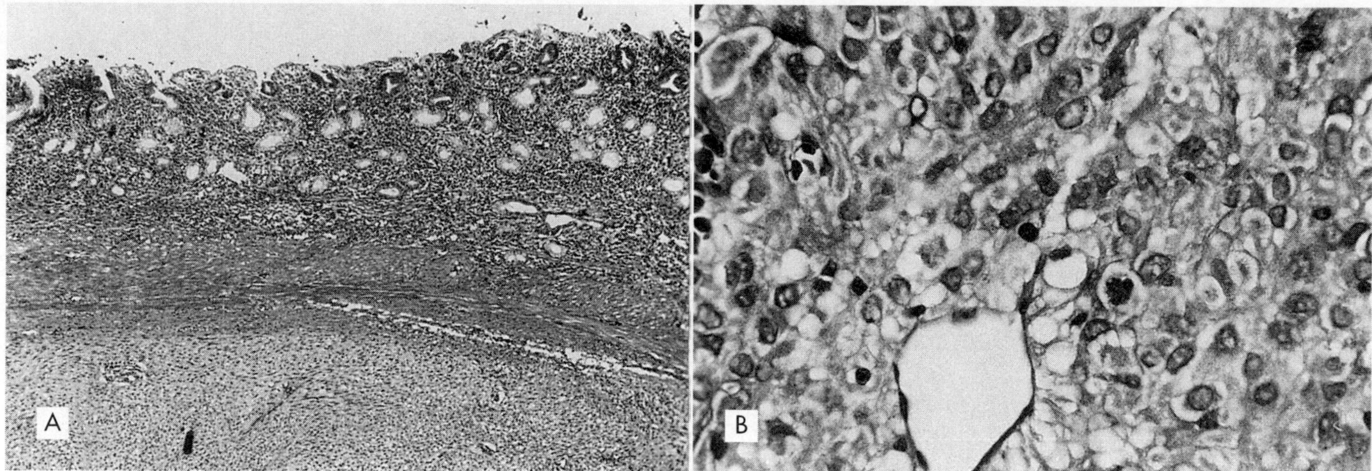

Fig. 53-44 Gastric epithelial leiomyoma in the submucosa of the gastric antrum. **A,** Low-power photomicrograph. The tumor shows several patterns, with predominance of epithelioid plump cells. The mucosa covering the lesion shows moderate inflammation. **B,** High-power photomicrograph of the same tumor, which is composed of large sheets of epithelioid cells with abundant cytoplasm exhibiting only mild pleomorphism. Occasional mitotic figures are seen.

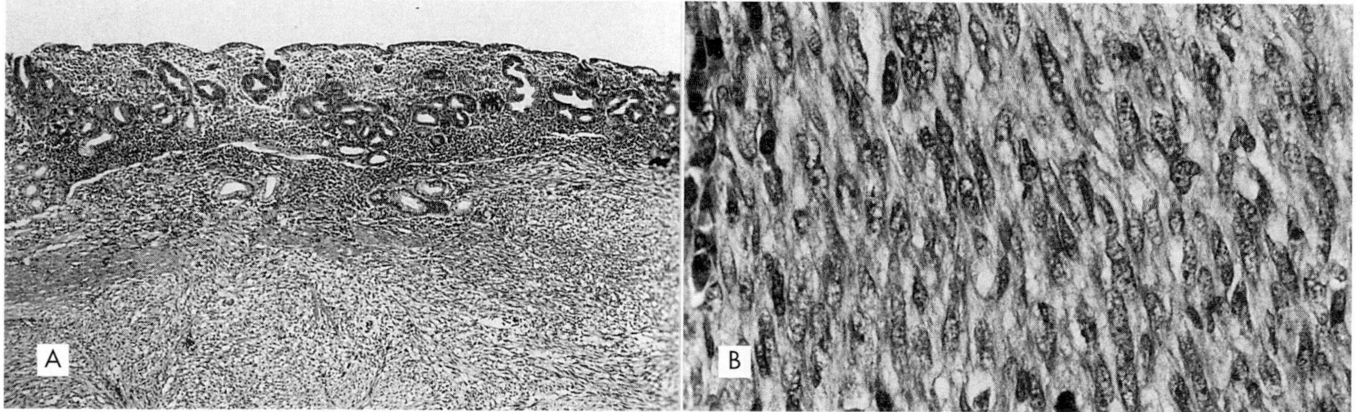

Fig. 53-45 Spindle cell leiomyoma arising in the gastric antrum. **A,** Low-power photomicrograph. The tumor, which occupies mostly the wall, penetrates at right into the mucosal compartment. The predominating pattern is that of interlacing fascicles of spindle cells. **B,** High-magnification photomicrograph of the same tumor, which is composed of homogenous fascicles of cells that are spindled in shape and are characterized by elongated nuclei with rounded tips. Occasional microvacuolar change is noted at the tips of some of the nuclei. Rare mitotic figures are sometimes seen.

important within the group of stromal sarcomas, in terms of survival. Whereas spindle cell sarcomas measure their survival time in terms of months (6 to 10) from the date of diagnosis, the mean survival time of the epithelioid cell sarcomas is slightly in excess of 5 years.[348]

Glomus tumors, neoplasms closely related to leiomyomas and leiomyoblastomas, have been described in the stomach.[352] These tumors consist of epithelioid cells with a clear cytoplasm arranged around small blood vessels, which sometimes show dilatation.[353] All cases so far reported have been benign.

Metastatic tumors

Metastases to the stomach from distant sites are uncommon, constituting 0.2% of all autopsy subjects in one series[354] and, when present, are generally found in the submucosa. Upon endoscopic examination, they may appear as polypoid protrusions lined by mucosa, and, in some instances, they may show a central umbilication or be ulcerated. The most common primary sites are lung, skin melanoma, and, in women, breast cancer. Other sites, such as esophagus, pancreas, and colon have been occasionally reported.[355]

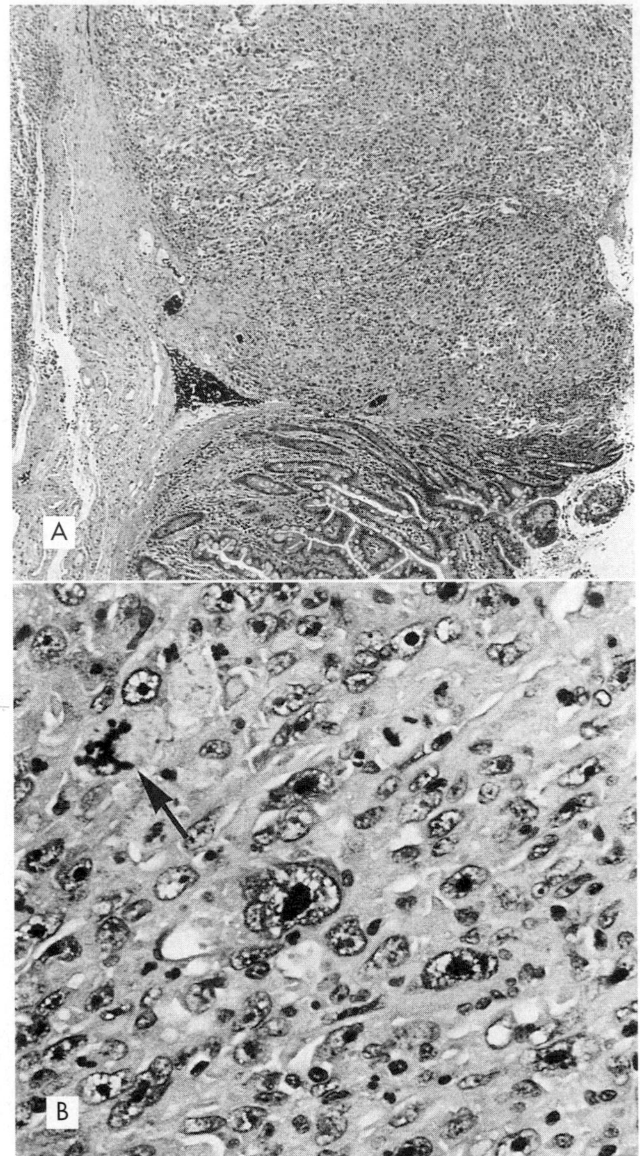

Fig. 53-46 Malignant stromal tumor arising in the pylorus. **A,** Low-power photomicrograph. The tumor arises from and replaces the muscular propria and also obliterates part of the mucosal compartment. A portion of the duodenal mucosa is also seen. **B,** High-magnification photomicrograph of the same tumor, which is composed of large sheets of cells endowed with abundant faintly eosinophilic cytoplasm and nuclei that show moderate to severe pleomorphism. Frequent mitotic figures, some of them atypical *(arrow),* are found.

REFERENCES

Normal stomach and duodenum

1. Moore KL, Persaud TVN: *The developing human: clinically oriented embryology,* ed 5, Philadelphia, 1993, Saunders.
2. Griffith CA: Anatomy. In Nyhus LM, Wastell C, editors: *Surgery of the stomach and duodenum,* Boston, 1977, Little, Brown.
3. Antonioli DA, Madara JL: Functional anatomy of the gastrointestinal tract. In Ming SC, Goldman H, editors: *Pathology of the gastrointestinal tract,* Philadelphia, 1992, Saunders.
4. Owen DA: Normal histology of the stomach, *Am J Surg Pathol* 10:48, 1986.
5. Helander HF: Fine structure of gastric glands. In Motta PM, Fujita H, editors: *Ultrastructure of the digestive tract,* Boston, 1988, Martinus-Nijhoff.
6. Madara JL, Trier JS: Functional morphology of the mucosa of the small intestine. In Johnson LR, editor: *Physiology of the gastrointestinal tract,* New York, 1987, Raven Press.
7. Morrissey JF: The 1982 A.S.G.E. Distinguished Lecture: Gastrointestinal endoscopy—20 years of progress, *Gastrointest Endosc* 29:53, 1983.
8. Williams CB: Diathermy-biopsy: a technique for the endoscopic management of small polyps, *Endoscopy* 5:215, 1973.
9. Witte S: Cytologic techniques and diagnosis. In Ming SC, Goldman H, editors: *Pathology of the gastrointestinal tract,* Philadelphia, 1992, Saunders.
10. Graham DY, Schwartz JT, Cain GD, Gyorkey F: Prospective evaluation of biopsy number in the diagnosis of esophageal and gastric carcinoma, *Gastroenterology* 82:228, 1982
11. Iishi H, Yamamoto R, Tatsuta M, Okuda S: Evaluation of fine-needle aspiration biopsy under direct vision gastrofiberscopy in diagnosis of diffusely infiltrative carcinoma of the stomach, *Cancer* 57:1365, 1986.
12. Haggitt RC, Rubin CE: Endoscopy and endoscopic biopsy. In Ming SC, Goldman H, editors: *Pathology of the gastrointestinal tract,* Philadelphia, 1992, Saunders.

Developmental abnormalities

13. Arey JB, Valdes-Dapena M: Embryology and developmental disorders. In Ming SC, Goldman H, editors: *Pathology of the gastrointestinal tract,* Philadelphia, 1992, Saunders.
14. Parker BC, Guthrie J, France NE, Atwell JD: Gastric duplications in infancy, *J Pediatr Surg* 7:294, 1972.
15. Dresler CM, Patterson GA, Taylor BR, Moote DJ: Complete foregut duplication, *Ann Thorac Surg* 50:306, 1990.
16. Bergman KS, Jacir NN: Cystic duodenal duplication: staged management in a premature infant, *J Pediatr Surg* 28:1584, 1993.
17. Eells RW, Simril WA: Gastric diverticula: report of thirty-one cases, *Am J Roentgenol Radium Ther Nucl Med* 68:8, 1952.
18. Colborn GL, Gray SW, Pemberton LB et al: The duodenum. Part 3: Pathology, *Ann Surg* 55:469, 1989.
19. Feggetter S: Congenital intestinal atresia, *Br J Surg* 42:378, 1955.
20. Grosfeld JL, Rescorla FJ: Duodenal atresia and stenosis: reassessment of treatment and outcome based on antenatal diagnosis, pathologic variance, and long-term follow up, *World J Surg* 17:301, 1993.
21. Benson DC: Infantile pyloric stenosis, *Prog Pediatr Surg* 1:63, 1970.
22. Scharli A, Sieber WK, Kiesewetter WB: Hypertrophic pyloric stenosis at the Children's Hospital of Pittsburgh from 1912 to 1967, *J Pediatr Surg* 4:108, 1969.
23. Ling LL, Ma AC: The pathology and pathogenesis of congenital hypertrophic pyloric stenosis, *Chin Med J* 78:228, 1959.
24. Lane-Roberts PA: Pathology of infantile hypertrophic pyloric stenosis, *Proc R Soc Med* 52:1022, 1959.
25. Friesen SR, Boley JO, Miller DR: The myenteric plexus of the pylorus: its early normal development and its changes in hypertrophic pyloric stenosis, *Surgery* 39:21, 1956.
26. Wollstein M: Healing of hypertrophic pyloric stenosis after the Fredet-Rammstedt operation, *Am J Dis Child* 23:511, 1922.
27. Martínez NS, Morlock CG, Dockerty MB et al: Heterotopic pancreatic tissue involving the stomach, *Ann Surg* 147:1, 1958.
28. Clarke BE: Myoepithelial hamartoma of the gastrointestinal tract: a report of eight cases with comment concerning genesis and nomenclature, *Arch Pathol* 30:143, 1940.
29. Lessels AM, Martin DF: Heterotopic gastric mucosa in the duodenum, *J Clin Pathol* 35:591, 1982.
30. de Castro Barbosa JJ, Dockerty MB, Waugh JM: Pancreatic heterotopia, *Surg Gynecol Obstet* 82:527, 1946.
31. MacKinnon D, Nash FW: Pyloric obstruction due to pancreatic heterotopia in a child, *Br Med J* 1:87, 1957.
32. Ahrend T, Thompson B: Hernia of the foramen of Bochdalek in the adult, *Am J Surg* 122:612, 1971.
33. Stokes KB: Unusual varieties of diaphragmatic herniae, *Prog Pediatr Surg* 27:127, 1991.
34. Comer T, Clagett O: Surgical treatment of hernia of the foramen of Morgagni, *J Thorac Cardiovasc Surg* 52:461, 1966.

35. Soper SP, Roe LR, Hoyme HE, Clemmons JJ: Trisomy 18 with ectopia cordis, omphalocele, and ventricular septal defect, *Pediatr Pathol* 5:481, 1986.

Circulatory disturbances

36. Sarfeh IJ, Rypins EB: Physiology and pathophysiology of the digestive organs in critical illness, *Crit Care Clin* 3:395, 1987.
37. Fiddian Green RG, Stanley JC, Nostrant T, Phillips D: Chronic gastric ischemia: a cause of abdominal pain or bleeding identified from the presence of gastric mucosal acidosis, *J Cardiovasc Surg* 30:852, 1989.
38. Casey KM, Quigley TM, Kozarek RA, Raker EJ: Lethal nature of ischemic gastropathy, *Am J Surg* 165:646, 1993.
39. Quintero E, Pique JM, Bombi JA et al: Gastric mucosal vascular ectasias causing bleeding in cirrhosis, *Gastroenterology* 93:1054, 1987.
40. D'Amico G, Montalbano L, Traina M et al: Natural history of congestive gastropathy in cirrhosis, *Gastroenterology* 99:1558, 1990.
41. Ligenfelser T, Krige JE: The stomach in cirrhosis: the legend of Proteus retold, *J Clin Gastroenterol* 17:92, 1993.
42. Gostout CJ, Viggiano TR, Ahlquist DA et al: The clinical and endoscopic spectrum of the watermelon stomach, *J Clin Gastroenterol* 15:256, 1992.
43. Gilliam JH III, Geisinger KR, Wu WC et al: Endoscopic biopsy is diagnostic in gastric antral vascular ectasia: the "watermelon stomach," *Dig Dis Sci* 34:885, 1989.
44. Fraser AG, Koelmeyer T, White AC, Nicholson GI: Antral vascular ectasia: the watermelon stomach, *NZ Med J* 105:338, 1992.
45. Labenz J, Borsch G: Bleeding watermelon stomach treated by Nd-YAG laser photocoagulation, *Endoscopy* 25:240, 1993.
46. Hoffman BI, Katz WA: The gastrointestinal manifestations of systemic lupus erythematosus: a review of the literature, *Semin Arthritis Rheum* 9:237, 1980.
47. Weber TR, Grosfeld JL, Bergstein J, Fitzgerald J: Massive gastric hemorrhage: an unusual complication of Henoch-Schönlein purpura, *J Pediatr Surg* 18:576, 1983.
48. Hashikata Y, Nishioka K: Multiple gastric ulcers in Wegener's granulomatosis: a follow-up report, *Dermatologia* 166:325, 1983.
49. Norris TH: Vascular disorders. In Ming SC, Goldman H, editors: *Pathology of the gastrointestinal tract,* Philadelphia, 1992, Saunders.

Gastritis

Classification

50. Whitehead R, Truelove SC, Gear MWL: The histological diagnosis of chronic gastritis in fiberoptic gastroscope biopsy specimens, *J Clin Pathol* 25:1, 1972.
51. Motteram RA: A biopsy study of chronic gastritis and gastric atrophy, *J Pathol Bacteriol* 63:389, 1951.
52. Strickland RG, MacKay IR: A reappraisal of the nature and significance of chronic atrophic gastritis, *Am J Dig Dis* 18:426, 1973.
53. Goodwin CS, Armstrong JA, Chilvers T et al: Transfer of *Campylobacter pylori* and *Campylobacter mustelae* to *Helicobacter* gen. nov. as *Helicobacter pylori* comb. nov. and *Helicobacter mustelae* comb. nov. respectively, *Int J Syst Bacteriol* 39:397, 1989.
54. Warren JR, Marshall BJ: Unidentified curved bacilli on gastric epithelium in active chronic gastritis, *Lancet* 1:1273, 1983.
55. Marshall BJ, Warren JR: Unidentified curved bacilli in the stomach of patients with gastritis and peptic ulceration, *Lancet* 1:1311, 1984.
56. Rollason TP, Stone J, Rhodes JM: Spiral organisms in endoscopic biopsies of the human stomach, *J Clin Pathol* 37:23, 1984.
57. Price AB, Levi J, Dolby JM et al: *Campylobacter pyloridis* in peptic ulcer disease: microbiology, pathology, and scanning electron microscopy, *Gut* 26:1183, 1985.
58. Mobley HLT, Foxall PA: *H. pylori* urease. In Hunt RH, Tytgat GNJ, editors: *Helicobacter pylori: basic mechanisms to clinical cure,* London, 1994, Kluwer Academic Publishers.
59. Marshall BJ, Barrett LJ, Prakash C et al: Urea protects *Helicobacter pylori* from the bactericidal effect of acid, *Gastroenterology* 99:697, 1990.
60. Eaton KA, Brooks CL, Morgan DR, Krakowka S: Essential role of urease in pathogenesis of gastritis induced by *Helicobacter pylori* in gnotobiotic piglets, *Infect Immun* 59:2470, 1991.
61. Price AB: The Sydney System: histological division, *J Gastroenterol Hepatol* 6:209, 1991.

Acute infectious gastritis

62. Freeman HJ, Schnitka TK, Piercey JRA, Weinstein WM: Cytomegalovirus infection of the gastrointestinal tract in a patient with late onset immunodeficiency syndrome, *Gastroenterology* 73:1397, 1977.
63. Knapp AB, Horst DA, Eliopoulos G et al: Widespread cytomegalovirus gastroenterocolitis in a patient with acquired immunodeficiency syndrome, *Gastroenterology* 85:1399, 1983.
64. Franzin G, Muolo A, Criminelli T: Cytomegalovirus inclusions in the gastroduodenal mucosa of patients after renal transplantation, *Gut* 22:698, 1981.
65. Strayer DS, Phillips GB, Barker KH et al: Gastric cytomegalovirus infections in bone marrow transplant patients, *Cancer* 48:1478, 1981.
66. Hinnant KL, Rotterdam HZ, Bell ET et al: Cytomegalovirus infection of the alimentary tract: a clinicopathological correlation, *Am J Gastroenterol* 81:944, 1986.
67. Howiler W, Goldberg HI: Gastroesophageal involvement in herpex simplex, *Gastroenterology* 70:775, 1976.
68. Sperling HV, Reed WG: Herpetic gastritis, *Am J Dig Dis* 22:1034, 1977.
69. González-Crussi F, Hackett RL: Phlegmonous gastritis, *Arch Surg* 93:990, 1966.
70. Miller AI, Smith M, Rogers AI: Phlegmonous gastritis, *Gastroenterology* 68:231, 1975.
71. Gonzalez L, Schowengerdt C, Skinner H, Lynch P: Emphysematous gastritis, *Surg Gynecol Obstet* 116:79, 1963.
72. Williford ME, Foster WL, Halvorsen RA, Thompson WM: Emphysematous gastritis secondary to disseminated strongyloidiasis, *Gastrointest Radiol* 7:123, 1982.
73. Clearfield HR, Shin H, Shriebman BK: Emphysematous gastritis secondary to lye ingestion, *Am J Dig Dis* 14:195, 1969.
74. Chazan B, Aitchinson J: Gastric tuberculosis, *Br Med J* 2:1288, 1960.
75. Subei I, Attar B, Schmitt G, Levendoglu H: Primary gastric tuberculosis: a case report and literature review, *Am J Gastroenterol* 82:769, 1983.
76. Roth RI, Owen RZ, Keren DF, Volberding PA: Intestinal infection with *Mycobacterium avium* in acquired immune deficiency syndrome (AIDS): histological and clinical comparison with Whipple's disease, *Dig Dis Sci* 30:497, 1985.
77. Fyfe B, Poppiti RJ Jr, Lubin J, Robinson MJ: Gastric syphilis: primary diagnosis by gastric biopsy: report of four cases, *Arch Pathol Lab Med* 117:820, 1993.
78. Besses C, Sans-Sabrofen J, Badia X et al: Ulceroinfiltrative syphilitic gastropathy: silver stain diagnosis from biopsy specimen, *Am J Gastroenterol* 82:773, 1987.
79. Morin ME, Tan A: Diffuse enlargement of gastric folds as a manifestation of secondary syphilis, *Am J Gastroenterol* 74:170, 1980.
80. Katzenstein ALA, Maksen J: Candidal infection of gastric ulcers: histology, incidence and clinical significance, *Am J Clin Pathol* 71:137, 1979.
81. Gotlieb-Jensen K, Andersen J: Occurrence of *Candida* in gastric ulcers: significance for the healing process, *Gastroenterology* 85:535, 1983.
82. Loffeld RJ, Loffeld BC, Arends JW et al: Fungal colonization of gastric ulcers, *Am J Gastroenterol* 83:730, 1988.
83. Fisher JR, Sanowski RA: Disseminated histoplasmosis producing hypertrophic gastric folds, *Dig Dis Sci* 23:282, 1978.
84. Miller DP, Everett ED: Gastrointestinal histoplasmosis, *J Clin Gastroenterol* 1:233, 1979.
85. Lawson H, Schmaman A: Gastric phycomycosis, *Br J Surg* 61:743, 1974.
86. Lyon DT, Schubert TT, Mantia AG, Kaplan MH: Phycomycosis of the gastrointestinal tract, *Am J Gastroenterol* 72:379, 1979.
87. Garone MA, Winston BJ, Lewin JH: Cryptosporidiosis of the stomach, *Am J Gastroenterol* 81:465, 1986.
88. Genta RM, Caymmi-Gomes A: Pathology of strongyloidiasis. In Grove DI, editor: *Strongyloidiasis: an important roundworm infection of man,* London, 1989, Taylor & Francis.
89. Watt IA, McLean NR, Girdwood RWA et al: Eosinophilic gastroenteritis associated with a larval anisakine nematode, *Lancet* 2:893, 1979.
90. Asami K, Watanuki T, Sakai H et al: Two cases of stomach granuloma caused by *Anisakis*-like larval nematodes in Japan, *Am J Trop Med Hyg* 14:119, 1965.

Chemical gastritis

91. O'Connor HJ, Wyatt JI, Dixon MF, Axon ATR: *Campylobacter*-like organisms and reflux gastritis, *J Clin Pathol* 39:531, 1986.
92. Roth SH, Bennet RE: Nonsteroidal anti-inflammatory drug gastropathy: recognition and response, *Arch Intern Med* 147:2093, 1987.
93. Silvoso GR, Ivey KJ, Butt JH et al: Incidence of gastric lesions in patients with rheumatic disease in chronic aspirin therapy, *Ann Intern Med* 91:517, 1979.
94. Larkai EN, Smith JL, Lidsky MD, Graham DY: Gastroduodenal mucosa and dyspeptic symptoms in arthritic patients during chronic nonsteroidal anti-inflammatory drug use, *Am J Gastroenterol* 82:1153, 1987.
95. Upadhyay R, Howatson A, McKinlay A et al: *Campylobacter pylori* associated gastritis in patients with rheumatoid arthritis taking nonsteroidal anti-inflammatory drugs, *Br J Rheumatol* 27:113, 1988.
96. MacDonald WC: Correlation of mucosal histology and aspirin intake in chronic gastric ulcer, *Gastroenterology* 65:381, 1973.
97. McIntosh JH, Byth K, Piper DW: Environmental factors in aetiology of chronic gastric ulcer: a case control study of exposure variables before the first symptoms, *Gut* 26:789, 1985.
98. Niemela A: Duodenogastric reflux in patients with upper abdominal complaints or gastric ulcer with particular reference to reflux-associated gastritis, *Scand J Gastroenterol* 115:1, 1985.
99. Dixon MF, O'Connor HJ, Axon ATR et al: Reflux gastritis: distinct histopathological entity? *J Clin Pathol* 39:524, 1986.
100. Ivey KJ, DenBesten L, Clifton JA: Effect of bile salts on ionic movement across the human gastric mucosa, *Gastroenterology* 59:683, 1970.
101. Stein HJ, Smyrk TC, DeMeester TR et al: Clinical value of endoscopy and histology in the diagnosis of duodenogastric reflux disease, *Surgery* 112:796, 1992.
102. Karttunen T, Niemelä S: *Campylobacter pylori* and duodenogastric reflux in peptic ulcer disease and gastritis, *Lancet* 1:118, 1988.
103. Müller-Lissner SA: Ist duodenogastraler Reflux pathogen? *Z Gastroenterol* 26:637, 1988.
104. Sobala GM, King RF, Axon AT, Dixon MF: Reflux gastritis in the intact stomach, *J Clin Pathol* 43:303, 1990.
105. Weinstein WM, Buch KL, Elashoff J et al: The histology of the stomach in symptomatic patients after gastric surgery: a model to assess selective patterns of gastric mucosal injury, *Scand J Gastroenterol* 20(suppl 109):77, 1985.
106. Bechi P, Amorosi A, Mazzanti R et al: Gastric histology and fasting bile reflux after partial gastrectomy, *Gastroenterology* 93:335, 1987.
107. Karttunen T, Niemelä S, Lehtola J et al: *Campylobacter*-like organisms and gastritis: histopathology, bile reflux, and gastric fluid composition, *Scand J Gastroenterol* 22:478, 1987.
108. Sobala GM, O'Connor HJ, Dewar EP et al: Bile reflux and intestinal metaplasia in gastric mucosa, *J Clin Pathol* 46:235, 1993.
109. Koch HK, Lesch R, Cremer M, Oehlert W: Polyps and polypoid foveolar hyperplasia in gastric biopsy specimens and their precancerous prevalence, *Front Gastrointest Res* 4:183, 1979.
110. Koga S, Watanabe H, Enjoji M: Stomal polypoid hypertrophic gastritis: a polypoid gastric lesion at gastroenterostomy site, *Cancer* 43:647, 1979.
111. Honore LH, Lewis AS, Ohara KE: Gastritis glandularis et cystica profunda: report of 3 cases with discussion of etiology and pathogenesis, *Dig Dis Sci* 24:48, 1979.
112. Franzen G, Novelli P: Gastritis cystica profunda, *Histopathology* 5:535, 1981.
113. Fonde EC, Rodning CB: Gastritis cystica profunda, *Am J Gastroenterol* 81:459, 1986.

Autoimmune gastritis

114. Fenwick S: On atrophy of the stomach, *Lancet* 2:78, 1870.
115. Strickland RG, Mackay IR: A reappraisal of the nature and significance of chronic atrophic gastritis, *Am J Dig Dis* 18:426, 1973.
116. Kekki M, Siurala M, Varis K et al: Classification principles and genetics of chronic gastritis, *Scand J Gastroenterol* 22(suppl 141):1, 1987.
117. Mardh S, Song YH: Characterization of antigenic structures in autoimmune atrophic gastritis with pernicious anaemia: the parietal cell H,K-ATPase and the chief cell pepsinogen are the two major antigens, *Acta Physiol Scand* 136:581, 1989.
118. Burman P, Mardh S, Norberg L, Karlsson FA: Parietal cell antibodies in pernicious anemia inhibit H+,K+-adenosine triphosphatase, the proton pump of the stomach, *Gastroenterology* 96:1434, 1989.
119. Correa P: Chronic gastritis (non-specific). In Whitehead R, editor: *Gastrointestinal and oesophageal pathology*, Edinburgh, 1989, Churchill-Livingstone.
120. Yardley JH: Pathology of chronic gastritis and duodenitis. In Goldman H, Appelman HD, Kaufman N, editors: *Gastrointestinal pathology*, Baltimore, 1990, Williams & Wilkins.
121. Solcia E, Capella C, Fiocca R et al: Exocrine and endocrine epithelial changes in types A and B chronic gastritis. In Malfertheiner P, Ditschuneit H, editors: *Helicobacter pylori, gastritis, and peptic ulcer*, Heidelberg, 1990, Springer-Verlag.
122. Teglbjaerg PS, Nielsen HO: 'Small intestinal type' and 'colonic type' intestinal metaplasia of the human stomach, *Acta Pathol Microbiol Scand* 77:187, 1969.
123. Silva S, Filipe MI: Intestinal metaplasia and its variants in the gastric mucosa of Portuguese subjects: a comparative analysis of biopsy and gastrectomy material, *Hum Pathol* 17:988, 1986.
124. Lewin KJ, Dowling F, Wright JP, Taylor KB: Gastric morphology and serum gastrin levels in pernicious anaemia, *Gut* 17:551, 1976.
125. Kekki M, Varis K, Pohjanpalo H: Course of antrum and body gastritis in pernicious anemia families, *Dig Dis Sci* 28:698, 1983.
126. Sipponen P, Kekki M, Siurala M: Age-related trends of gastritis and intestinal metaplasia in gastric carcinoma patients and controls representing the population at large, *Br J Cancer* 49:521, 1984.
127. Dayal Y, DeLellis RA, Wolfe HJ: Hyperplastic lesions of the gastrointestinal endocrine cells, *Am J Surg Pathol* 11(suppl 1):87, 1987.
128. Hodges JR, Isaacson P, Wright R: Diffuse enterochromaffin-like (ECL) cell hyperplasia and multiple gastric carcinoids: a complication of pernicious anaemia, *Gut* 22:237, 1981.
129. Creutzfeldt W: The achlorhydria-carcinoid sequence: role of gastrin, *Digestion* 39:61, 1988.
130. Solcia E, Fiocca R, Villani L et al: Morphology and pathogenesis of endocrine hyperplasias, precarcinoid lesions, and carcinoids arising in chronic atrophic gastritis, *Scand J Gastroenterol* 26(suppl 180):146, 1991.

Chronic nonatrophic gastritis

131. Lambert JR, Lin SK: Prevalence/disease correlates of *H. pylori*. In Hunt RH, Tytgat GNJ, editors: *Helicobacter pylori: basic mechanisms to clinical cure*, London, 1994, Kluwer Academic Publishers.
132. Dixon MF: Spectrum and implications of inflammation with *H. pylori*. In Hunt RH, Tytgat GNJ, editors: *Helicobacter pylori: basic mechanisms to clinical cure*, London, 1994, Kluwer Academic Publishers.
133. Wotherspoon AC, Ortiz-Hidalgo C, Falzon MR, Isaacson PG: *Helicobacter pylori*–associated gastritis and primary B-cell gastric lymphoma, *Lancet* 338:1175, 1991.
134. Rocha GA, Queiroz DM, Mendes EN et al: *Helicobacter pylori* acute gastritis: histological, endoscopical, clinical, and therapeutic features, *Am J Gastroenterol* 86:1592, 1991.
135. Axon ATR: Acute infection with *H. pylori*. In Hunt RH, Tytgat GNJ, editors: *Helicobacter pylori: basic mechanisms to clinical cure*, London, 1994, Kluwer Academic Publishers.
136. Chan WY, Hui PK, Leung KM, Thomas TMM: Modes of *Helicobacter* colonization and gastric epithelial damage, *Histopathology* 21:521, 1992.
137. Eidt S, Stolte M: Prevalence of lymphoid follicles and aggregates in *Helicobacter pylori* gastritis in antral and body mucosa, *J Clin Pathol* 46:832, 1993.
138. Genta RM, Hamner HW, Graham DY: Gastric lymphoid follicles in *Helicobacter pylori* infection: frequency, distribution, and response to triple therapy, *Hum Pathol* 24:577, 1993.

Environmental gastritis

139. Correa P: Chronic gastritis: a clinico-pathological classification, *Am J Gastroenterol* 83:504, 1988.
140. Lambert R: Chronic gastritis, *Digestion* 7:83, 1972.
141. Correa P, Haenszel W, Cuello C et al: Gastric precancerous process in a high risk population: cohort follow-up, *Cancer Res* 50:4737, 1990.
142. Kato I, Tominaga S, Ito Y et al: A prospective study of atrophic gastritis and stomach cancer risk, *Jpn J Cancer Res* 83:1137, 1992.

143. You WC, Blot WJ, Li JY, et al: Precancerous gastric lesions in a population at high risk of stomach cancer, *Cancer Res* 53:1317, 1993.
144. Correa P, Zavala D, Fontham E et al: Determinants of gastritis phenotype in *H. pylori* infection. In Hunt RH, Tytgat GNJ, editors: *Helicobacter pylori: basic mechanisms to clinical cure,* London, 1994, Kluwer Academic Publishers.
145. Fox J, Correa P, Taylor N et al: *Campylobacter pylori*–associated gastritis and immune response in a population at increased risk of gastric carcinoma, *Am J Gastroenterol* 84:775, 1989.
146. Craanen ME, Blok P, Dekker W et al: Subtypes of intestinal metaplasia and *Helicobacter pylori, Gut* 33:597, 1992.
147. Guarner J, Mohar A, Parsonnet J, Halperin D: The association of *Helicobacter pylori* with gastric cancer and preneoplastic gastric lesions in Chiapas, Mexico, *Cancer* 71:297, 1993.
148. Block G: Vitamin C and cancer prevention: the epidemiologic evidence, *Am J Clin Nutr* 53:2705, 1991.
149. Caygill CPJ: UK subgroup of ECP-EURONUT-IM study group: plasma vitamin concentration in patients with intestinal metaplasia and in controls, *Eur J Cancer Prev* 1:177, 1992.
150. Sato T, Fukuyama S, Susuki T, Takanagi J: The relationship between gastric cancer mortality and salted food intake in several places in Japan, *Bull Inst Public Health* 8:187, 1959.
151. Correa P: A human model of gastric carcinogenesis, *Cancer Res* 48:3854, 1988.
152. Stillwell WG, Glogowski S, Xu HX et al: Urinary excretion of nitrate, *N*-nitrosoproline, 3-methyladenine and 7-methylguanine in a Colombian population at high risk for gastric cancer, *Cancer Res* 51:190, 1991.
153. Xu GP, So PJ, Reed PI: Hypothesis on the relationship between gastric cancer and intragastric nitrosation: *N*-nitrosamines in gastric juice of subjects from a high risk area for gastric cancer and the inhibition of *N*-nitrosamine formation by fruit juices, *Eur J Cancer Prev* 2:25, 1993.
154. Stemmerman GN, Hayashi T: Intestinal metaplasia of the gastric mucosa: a gross and microscopic study of its distribution in various disease states, *J Natl Cancer Inst* 41:627, 1968.
155. Recavarren Arce S, Leon Barua R, Cok J et al: *Helicobacter pylori* and progressive gastric pathology that predisposes to gastric cancer, *Scand J Gastroenterol* 181:51, 1991.
156. Steer HW: Surface morphology of the gastroduodenal mucosa in duodenal ulceration, *Gut* 25:1203, 1984.
157. Jass JR, Filipe MI: A variant of intestinal metaplasia associated with gastric carcinoma: a histochemical study, *Histopathology* 3:191, 1979.
158. Filipe MI, Potet F, Bogomoletz W et al: Incomplete sulphomucin-secreting intestinal metaplasia for gastric cancer: preliminary data from a prospective study from three centres, *Gut* 26:1319, 1985.
159. Sipponen P, Seppälä K, Varis K et al: Intestinal metaplasia with colonic-type sulphomucins in the gastric mucosa; its association with gastric carcinoma, *Acta Pathol Microbiol Scand A* 88:217, 1980.
160. Turani H, Lurie B, Chaimoff C, Kessler E: The diagnostic significance of sufated acid mucin content in gastric intestinal metaplasia with early gastric cancer, *Am J Gastroenterol* 81:343, 1986.
161. Rokkas T, Filipe MI, Sladen GE: Detection of an increased incidence of early gastric cancer in patients with intestinal metaplasia type III who are closely followed up, *Gut* 32:1110, 1991.
162. Tosi P, Filipe MI, Luzi P et al: Gastric intestinal metaplasia type III cases are classified as low-grade dysplasia on the basis of morphometry, *J Pathol* 169:73, 1993.

Miscellaneous gastritis

163. Klein NC, Hargrove RL, Sleisenger MH, Jeffries GH: Eosinophilic gastroenteritis, *Medicine* (Baltimore) 49:299, 1970.
164. Goldman H, Proujansky R: Allergic proctitis and gastroenteritis in children: clinical and mucosal biopsy features in children, *Am J Surg Pathol* 10:75, 1986.
165. Talley NJ, Shorter RG, Zinsmeister AR: Eosinophilic gastroenteritis: a clinicopathological study of patients with disease of the mucosa, muscle layer, and subserosal tissues, *Gut* 31:54, 1990.
166. Katz AJ, Goldman H, Grand RJ: Gastric mucosal biopsy in eosinophilic (allergic) gastroenteritis, *Gastroenterology* 73:705, 1977.
167. Ureles AL, Alschibaja T, Lodico D, Stabins SJ: Idiopathic eosinophilic infiltration of the gastrointestinal tract, diffuse and circumscribed: a proposed classification and review of the literature, with two additional cases, *Am J Med* 30:899, 1961.
168. Johnstone JM, Morson BC: Eosinophilic gastroenteritis, *Histopathology* 2:335, 1978.
169. Goldman H: Gastritis. In Goldman H, Appelman HD, Kaufman N, editors: *Gastrointestinal pathology,* Baltimore, 1990, Williams & Wilkins.
170. Haggitt RC, Meissner WA: Crohn's disease of the upper gastrointestinal tract, *Am J Clin Pathol* 59:613, 1973.
171. Korelitz BI, Waye JD, Kreuning J et al: Crohn's disease in endoscopic biopsies of the gastric antrum and duodenum, *Am J Gastroenterol* 76:103, 1981.
172. Chinitz MA, Brandt LJ, Frank MS et al: Symptomatic sarcoidosis of the stomach, *Dig Dis Sci* 30:682, 1985.
173. Fahimi HD, Deren JJ, Gottlieb LS, Zamcheck N: Isolated granulomatous gastritis: its relationship to disseminated sarcoidosis and regional enteritis, *Gastroenterology* 45:161, 1963.
174. Grimaste VV, Janowitz HD, Waye JD: Granulomatous gastritis: a case report and review of the literature, *Am J Gastroenterol* 84:1315, 1989.
175. Haot J, Hamichi L, Wallez L, Mainguet P: Lymphocytic gastritis: a newly described entity: a retrospective endoscopic and histologic study, *Gut* 29:1258, 1988.
176. Lambert R, André C, Moulinier B, Bugnon B: Diffuse varioliform gastritis, *Digestion* 17:159, 1978.
177. Haot J, Jouret A, Willette M et al: Lymphocytic gastritis—prospective study of its relationship with varioliform gastritis, *Gut* 31:282, 1990.
178. De Giacomo C, Gianatty A, Negrini R et al: Lymphocytic gastritis: a positive relationship with celiac disease, *J Pediatr* 124:57, 1994.
179. Kimura K, Hiramoto T, Buncher CR: Gastric xanthelasma, *Arch Pathol Lab Med* 87:110, 1969.
180. Domellof L, Ericksson S, Helander HF et al: Lipid islands in the gastric mucosa after resection for benign ulcer disease, *Gastroenterology* 72:14, 1977.

Gastric and duodenal ulcers

181. Szabo S, Glavin GB: Hans Selye and the concept of biologic stress: ulcer pathogenesis as a historical paradigm, *Ann N Y Acad Sci* 597:14, 1990.
182. Gonzalez ER: Pathophysiologic changes in the critically ill patient: risk factors for ulceration and altered drug metabolism, *Drug Intell Clin Pharm* 24:5, 1990.
183. Kleiman RL, Adair CG, Ephgrave KS: Stress ulcers: current understanding of pathogenesis and prophylaxis, *Drug Intell Clin Pharm* 22:452, 1988.
184. Geus WP, Lamers CB: Prevention of stress ulcer bleeding: a review, *Scand J Gastroenterol* 178:32, 1990.
185. Curling TB: On acute ulceration of the duodenum in cases of burns, *Med Surg Trans* (London) 25:260, 1842.
186. Cushing H: Peptic ulcers and the interbrain, *Surg Gynecol Obstet* 55:1, 1932.
187. Flynn R, Stuart RC, Gorey TF et al: Stress ulceration and gastric mucosal cell kinetics: the influence of prophylaxis against acute stress ulceration, *J Surg Res* 55:188, 1993.
188. Schuster DP: Stress ulcer prophylaxis: in whom? With what? *Crit Care Med* 21:4, 1993.
189. Soll AH: Gastric, duodenal and stress ulcer. In Sleisenger MH, Fordtran JS, editors: *Gastrointestinal disease—pathophysiology/diagnosis/treatment,* ed 5, Philadelphia, 1993, Saunders.
190. Nomura A, Stemmermann GN, Chyou PH et al: *Helicobacter pylori* infection and gastric carcinoma among Japanese Americans in Hawaii, *N Engl J Med* 325:1132, 1991.
191. Parsonnet J, Friedman GD, Vandersteen DP et al: *Helicobacter pylori* infection and the risk of gastric carcinoma, *N Engl J Med* 325:1127, 1991.
192. Sipponen P, Hyvärinen H: Role of *Helicobacter pylori* in the pathogenesis of gastritis, peptic ulcer and gastric cancer, *Scand J Gastroenterol* 196:3, 1993.
193. Grossman MI: Peptic ulcer: definition and epidemiology. In Rotter J, Samloff IM, Rimoin DL, editors: *The genetics and heterogeneity of common gastrointestinal disorders,* New York, 1980, Academic Press.

194. Kurata HJ: Ulcer epidemiology: an overview and proposed research framework, *Gastroenterology* 96:569, 1989.
195. Sonnenberg A: The US temporal and geographic variations of diseases related to *Helicobacter pylori, Am J Public Health* 83:1006, 1993.
196. Graham DY: *Helicobacter pylori* in human populations: the present and predictions of the future based on the epidemiology of polio. In Menge H, Gregor M, Tytgat GNJ et al, editors: *Helicobacter pylori 1990: Proceedings of the Second International Symposium on Helicobacter pylori,* Berlin, 1991, Springer-Verlag.
197. Silen W: Gastric mucosal defense and repair. In Johnson LR, editor: *Physiology of the gastrointestinal tract,* ed 2 New York, 1987, Raven Press.
198. Borody T J, Brandl S, Andrews P et al: *Helicobacter pylori*–negative gastric ulcer, *Am J Gastroenterol* 87:1403, 1992.
199. Miller TA: Protective effects of prostaglandins against gastric mucosal damage: current knowledge and proposed mechanisms, *Am J Physiol* 245:G601, 1983.
200. Kimmey MB: NSAID, ulcers, and prostaglandins, *J Rheumatol* 19(suppl 36):68, 1992.
201. Dixon M: Acid, ulcers, and *H. pylori, Lancet* 342:384, 1993.
202. Labenz J, Borsch G: Evidence for the essential role of *Helicobacter pylori* in gastric ulcer disease, *Gut* 35:19, 1994.
203. Graham DY: Treatment of peptic ulcers caused by *Helicobacter pylori, N Engl J Med* 328:349, 1993.
204. Hunt RH: pH and Hp—gastric acid secretion and *Helicobacter pylori:* implications for ulcer healing and eradication of the organism, *Am J Gastroenterol* 88:481, 1993.
205. McHenry L Jr, Vuyyuru L, Schubert ML: *Helicobacter pylori* and duodenal ulcer disease: the somatostatin link? *Gastroenterology* 104:1573, 1993.
206. Oi M, Oshida K, Sugimura S: The location of gastric ulcer, *Gastroenterology* 36:45, 1959.
207. Lumsden K, MacLarnon JC, Dawson J: Giant duodenal ulcer, *Gut* 1:592, 1970.
208. Goldman H: Stress ulcer and chronic peptic ulcer disease. In Ming SC, Goldman H, editors: *Pathology of the gastrointestinal tract,* Philadelphia, 1992, Saunders.
209. Trier JS: Morphology of the gastric mucosa in patients with ulcer disease, *Am J Dig Dis* 21:138, 1976.
210. Lechago J: Histopathology of peptic ulcer. In Brooks FP, Cohen S, Soloway RD, editors: *Peptic ulcer disease,* New York, 1985, Churchill Livingstone.
211. Graham DY: Ulcer complications and their nonoperative treatment. In Sleisenger MH, Fordtran JS, editors: *Gastrointestinal disease: pathophysiology/diagnosis/treatment,* ed 5, Philadelphia, 1993, Saunders.
212. Bartle WR, Gupta AK, Lazor J: Non-steroidal anti-inflammatory drugs and gastrointestinal bleeding: a case control study, *Arch Intern Med* 146:2365, 1986.
213. Kozoll DD, Meyer KA: Symptoms and signs in the prognosis of gastroduodenal ulcers: an analysis of 1,904 cases of acute perforated gastroduodenal ulcers, *Arch Surg* 82:528, 1961.
214. Norris JR, Hubrich WS: The incidence and clinical features of penetration in peptic ulceration, *JAMA* 178:386, 1961.

Zollinger-Ellison syndrome

215. Zollinger RM, Ellison EH: Primary peptic ulcerations of the jejunum associated with islet tumors of the pancreas, *Ann Surg* 142:709, 1955.
216. Waldum HL, Mignon M, Sandvik AK et al: Biologic and immunologic gastrin activity in serum of patients with gastrinoma, bioassay of gastrin activity in serum, *Scand J Gastroenterol* 27:1039, 1992.
217. Solcia E, Capella C, Fiocca R et al: Gastric argyrophil carcinoidosis in patients with Zollinger-Ellison syndrome due to type I multiple endocrine neoplasia: a newly recognized association, *Am J Surg Pathol* 14:503, 1990.
218. Lehy T, Cadiot G, Mignon M et al: Influence of multiple endocrine neoplasia type I on gastric endocrine cells in patients with the Zollinger-Ellison syndrome, *Gut* 33:1275, 1992.
219. Cadiot G, Laurent Puig P, Thuille B et al: Is the multiple endocrine neoplasia type I gene a suppressor for fundic argyrophil tumors in the Zollinger-Ellison syndrome? *Gastroenterology* 105:579, 1993.
220. McColl KE, el Nujumi AM, Chittajallu RS et al: A study of the pathogenesis of *Helicobacter pylori* negative chronic duodenal ulceration, *Gut* 34:762, 1993.
221. Solcia E, Capella C, Buffa R et al: Pathology of the Zollinger-Ellison syndrome. In Fenoglio CM, Wolff M, editors: *Progress in surgical pathology,* vol 1, New York, 1980, Masson.
222. Solcia E, Rindi G, Silini E et al: Enterochromaffin-like (ECL) cells and their growths: relationships to gastrin, reduced acid secretion and gastritis, *Baillieres Clin Gastroenterol* 7:149, 1993.
223. Cadiot G, Lehy T, Mignon M: Gastric endocrine cell proliferation and fundic argyrophil carcinoid tumors in patients with the Zollinger-Ellison syndrome, *Acta Oncol* 32:135, 1993.
224. Goldfain D, le Bodic MF, Lavergne A et al: Gastric carcinoid tumours in patients with Zollinger-Ellison syndrome on long-term omeprazole, *Lancet* 1:776, 1989.

Duodenitis

225. Lawson HH: The duodenal mucosa in health and disease: a clinical and experimental study, *Surg Annu* 21:157, 1989.
226. Jonsson KA, Gotthard R, Bodemar G, Brodin U: The clinical relevance of endoscopic and histologic inflammation of gastroduodenal mucosa in dyspepsia of unknown origin, *Scand J Gastroenterol* 24:385, 1989.
227. Maratka Z: Endoscopic gastritis and duodenitis, *Gastrointest Endosc* 39:868, 1993.
228. Whitehead R, Roca M, Meikle DD et al: The histological classification of duodenitis in fibreoptic biopsy specimens, *Digestion* 13:129, 1975.
229. Madsen JE, Vetvik K, Aase S: *Helicobacter*-associated duodenitis and gastric metaplasia in duodenal ulcer patients, *APMIS* 99:997, 1991.
230. Wyatt JI, Rathbone BJ, Sobala GM et al: Gastric epithelium in the duodenum: its association with *Helicobacter pylori* and inflammation, *J Clin Pathol* 43:981, 1990.
231. Triadafilopoulos G: Clinical and pathologic features of the nodular duodenum, *Am J Gastroenterol* 88:1058, 1993.

Nonneoplastic polyps

232. Goldman DS, Appleman HS: Gastric mucosal polyps, *Am J Clin Pathol* 58:434, 1972.
233. Vanek J: Gastric submucosal granuloma with eosinophilic infiltration, *Am J Pathol* 25:397, 1941.
234. Ming SC, Goldman H: Gastric polyps: a histogenetic classification and its relation to carcinoma, *Cancer* 18:721, 1965.
235. Tomasulo J: Gastric polyps: histologic types and their relationship to gastric carcinoma, *Cancer* 27:1346, 1971.
236. Laxén F: Gastric polyps and gastric carcinoma, *Ann Clin Res* 13:154, 1981.
237. Laxén F, Sipponen P, Ihamäki L et al: Gastric polyps: their morphological and endoscopical characteristics and relation to gastric carcinoma, *Acta Pathol Microbiol Immunol Scand* 90:221, 1982.
238. Watanabe H, Enjoji M, Yao T et al: Gastric lesions in familial adenomatosis coli, *Hum Pathol* 9:269, 1978.
239. Tatsuta M, Okuda S, Tamura H et al: Gastric hamartomatous polyps in the absence of familial polyposis coli, *Cancer* 45:818, 1980.
240. Stolte M: Fundic gland polyps: a rare, innocuous, and reversible disturbance, *Gastroenterology* 105:1590, 1993.
241. Hizawa K, Iida M, Matsumoto T et al: Natural history of fundic gland polyposis without familial adenomatosis coli: follow-up observations in 31 patients, *Radiology* 189:429, 1993.
242. Iishi H, Tatsuta M, Okuda S: Clinicopathological features and natural history of gastric hamartomatous polyps, *Dig Dis Sci* 34:890, 1989.
243. Burdick D, Prior JT: Peutz-Jeghers syndrome: a clinicopathologic study of a large family with a 27-year follow-up, *Cancer* 50:2139, 1982.
244. Finan MC, Ray MK: Gastrointestinal polyposis syndromes, *Dermatol Clin* 7:419, 1989.
245. Buck JL, Harned RK, Lichtenstein JE et al: Peutz-Jeghers syndrome, *Radiographics* 12:365, 1992.
246. Hizawa K, Iida M, Matsumoto T et al: Neoplastic transformation arising in Peutz-Jeghers polyposis, *Dis Colon Rectum* 36:953, 1993.
247. Cronkhite LW, Canada WJ: Generalized gastrointestinal polyposis: an unusual syndrome of polyposis, pigmentation, alopecia and onychotrophia, *N Engl J Med* 299:49, 1955.
248. Daniel ES, Ludwig SL, Lewin KJ et al: The Cronkhite-Canada syndrome: an analysis of the pathologic features and therapy in 55 patients, *Medicine* 61:293, 1982.

249. Appelman HD: Localized and extensive expansions of the gastric mucosa: mucosal polyps and giant folds. In Appelman HD, editor: *Pathology of the esophagus, stomach and duodenum: contemporary issues in surgical pathology,* New York, 1984, Churchill Livingstone.
250. Meuwissen SG, Ridwan BU, Hasper HJ et al: Hypertrophic protein-losing gastropathy: a retrospective analysis of 40 cases in the Netherlands: the Dutch Ménétrier Study Group, *Scand J Gastroenterol* 194:1, 1992.
251. Komorowski RA, Caya JG: Hyperplastic gastropathy: clinicopathologic correlation, *Am J Surg Pathol* 15:577, 1991.
252. Wolfsen HC, Carpenter HA, Talley NJ: Ménétrier's disease: a form of hypertrophic gastropathy or gastritis? *Gastroenterology* 104:1310, 1993.
253. Mosnier JF, Flejou JF, Amouyal G et al: Hypertrophic gastropathy with gastric adenocarcinoma: Ménétrier's disease and lymphocytic gastritis? *Gut* 32:1565, 1991.
254. Hsu CT, Ito M, Kawase Y et al: Early gastric cancer arising from localized Ménétrier's disease, *Gastroenterol Jpn* 26:213, 1991.
255. Kraut JR, Powell R, Hruby MA, Lloyd-Still JD: Ménétrier's disease in childhood: report of two cases and a review of the literature, *J Pediatr Surg* 16:707, 1981.

Neoplasms

256. Watanabe H, Jass JR, Sobin LH: *Histological typing of oesophageal and gastric tumours: World Health Organization international histological classification of tumours,* Berlin, 1990, Springer-Verlag.
257. Ming SC: Epithelial polyps of the stomach. In Ming SC, Goldman H, editors: *Pathology of the gastrointestinal tract,* Philadelphia, 1992, Saunders.

Adenocarcinoma

258. Parkin DM, Pisani P, Fearly J: Estimates of worldwide incidence of eighteen major cancers in 1985, *Int J Cancer* 54:594, 1993.
259. Hansson LE, Sparen P, Nyren O: Increasing incidence of carcinoma of the gastric cardia in Sweden from 1970 to 1985, *Br J Surg* 80:374, 1993.
260. Blot WJ, Devesa SS, Kneller RW, Fraumeni JF Jr: Rising incidence of adenocarcinoma of the esophagus and gastric cardia, *JAMA* 265:1287, 1991.
261. World Health Organization Statistics 1986: *Age standardized death rates for selected causes by sex, latest available year,* Geneva, 1986, World Health Organization.
262. Wee A, Kang JY, Teh M: *Helicobacter pylori* and gastric cancer: correlation with gastritis, intestinal metaplasia, and tumour histology, *Gut* 33:1029, 1992.
263. Bearzi I, Ranaldi R, Santinelli A et al: Epithelial dysplasia of the gastric mucosa, a morphometric and ploidy pattern study, *Pathol Res Pract* 188:550, 1992.
264. Kushima R, Hattori T: Histogenesis and characteristics of gastric-type adenocarcinomas in the stomach, *J Cancer Res Clin Oncol* 120:103, 1993.
265. Kushima R, Jancic S, Hattori T: Association between expression of sialosyl-Tn antigen and intestinalization of gastric carcinomas, *Int J Cancer* 55:904, 1993.
266. Wood MG, Bates C, Brown RC, Losowsky MS: Intramucosal carcinoma of the gastric antrum complicating Ménétrier's disease, *J Clin Pathol* 36:1071, 1983.
267. Hole DJ, Quigley EM, Gillis CR, Watkinson G: Peptic ulcer and cancer: an examination of the relationship between chronic peptic ulcer and gastric carcinoma, *Scand J Gastroenterol* 22:17, 1987.
268. Ming SC, Bajtai A, Correa P et al: Gastric dysplasia: significance and pathologic criteria, *Cancer* 54:1794, 1984.
269. Rugge M, Farinati F, Baffa R et al: Gastric epithelial dysplasia in the natural history of gastric cancer: a multicenter prospective follow-up study, *Gastroenterology* 107:1288, 1994.
270. Rugge M, Farinati F, Di Mario F et al: Gastric epithelial dysplasia: a prospective follow-up study from the interdisciplinary group on gastric epithelial dysplasia, *Hum Pathol* 22:1002, 1991.
271. Antonioli DA: Precursors of gastric carcinoma: a critical review with a brief description of early (curable) gastric cancer, *Hum Pathol* 25:995, 1994.
272. Kamiya T, Morishita T, Asakura H et al: Long-term follow-up study on gastric adenoma and its relation to gastric protruded carcinoma, *Cancer* 50:2946, 1982.
273. Ming SC: Malignant potential of epithelial polyps of the stomach. In Ming SC, editor: *Precursors of gastric cancer,* New York, 1984, Praeger.
274. Laxén F, Sipponen P, Ihamäki T et al: Gastric polyps: their morphological and endoscopical characteristics and relation to gastric carcinoma, *Acta Pathol Microbiol Immunol Scand A* 90:221, 1982.
275. Lundegårdh G, Adami HO, Helmrick C et al: Stomach cancer after partial gastrectomy for benign ulcer disease, *N Engl J Med* 319:195, 1988.
276. Offerhaus GJA, Tersmette AC, Huibregtse K et al: Mortality caused by stomach cancer after remote partial gastrectomy for benign conditions: 40 years of follow up of an Amsterdam cohort of 2633 postgastrectomy patients, *Gut* 29:1588, 1988.
277. Gad A: Carcinoma of the resected stomach. In Ming SC, editor: *Precursors of gastric cancer,* New York, 1984, Praeger.
278. Japanese Research Society for Gastric Cancer: The general rules for the gastric cancer study in surgery and pathology, *Jpn J Surg* 11:127, 1981.
279. Bogomoletz WV: Early gastric cancer, *Am J Surg Pathol* 8:38, 1984.
280. Green PHR, O'Toole KM, Slonim D et al: Increasing incidence and excellent survival of patients with early gastric cancer: experience in a United States medical center, *Am J Med* 85:658, 1988.
281. Ming SC: Gastric carcinoma: a pathobiological classification, *Cancer* 39:2475, 1977.
282. Hirota T, Ming SC: Early gastric carcinoma. In Ming SC, Goldman H, editors: *Pathology of the gastrointestinal tract,* Philadelphia, 1992, Saunders.
283. Sano T, Sasako M, Kinoshita T et al: Recurrence of early gastric cancer: follow-up of 1475 patients end review of the Japanese literature, *Cancer* 72:3174, 1993.
284. Laurén P: The two histological main types of gastric carcinoma: diffuse and so-called intestinal type carcinoma: an attempt at histoclinical classification, *Acta Pathol Microbiol Immunol Scand* 64:31, 1965.
285. Yakushiji M, Tazaki T, Nishimura H, Kato T: Krukenberg tumors of the ovary: a clinicopathologic analysis of 112 cases, *Nippon Sanka Fujinka Gakkai Zasshi (Acta Obstet Gynaecol Jpn)* 39:479, 1987.
286. American Joint Committee for Cancer Staging and End-Results Reporting: *Manual for Staging of Cancer,* Chicago, 1977, American Joint Committee.
287. Davis GR: Neoplasms of the stomach. Sleisenger MH, Fordtran JS, editors. *Gastrointestinal disease: pathophysiology/diagnosis/treatment,* ed 5, Philadelphia, 1993, Saunders.
288. Akoh JA, Macintyre IM: Improving survival in gastric cancer: review of 5-year survival rates in English language publications from 1970, *Br J Surg* 79:293, 1992.

Ampullary carcinoma

289. Yamaguchi K, Enjoji M: Carcinoma of the ampulla of Vater: a clinicopathologic study and pathologic staging of 109 cases of carcinoma and 5 cases of adenoma, *Cancer* 59:506, 1987.
290. Yamaguchi K, Enjoji M: Adenoma of the ampulla of Vater: putative precancerous lesion, *Gut* 32:1558, 1991.
291. Seifert E, Schulte F, Stolte M: Adenoma and carcinoma of the duodenum and papilla of Vater: a clinicopathologic study, *Am J Gastroenterol* 87:37, 1992.
292. Baczako K, Büchler M, Beger HG et al: Morphogenesis and possible precursor lesions of invasive carcinoma of the papilla of Vater: epithelial dysplasia and adenoma, *Hum Pathol* 16:305, 1985.
293. Wise L, Pizzimbono C, Dehner LP: Periampullary cancer: a clinicopathologic study of sixty-two patients, *Am J Surg* 131:141, 1976.
294. Nakase A, Matsumoto Y, Uchida K, Honjo I: Surgical treatment of cancer of the pancreas and the periampullary region: cumulative results in 57 institutions in Japan, *Ann Surg* 185:52, 1977.
295. Yamaguchi K, Enjoji M, Tsuneyoshi M: Pancreatoduodenal carcinoma: a clinicopathologic study of 304 patients and immunohistochemical observation for CEA and CA 19-9, *J Surg Oncol* 47:148, 1991.
296. Cubilla AL, Fitzgerald PJ: Surgical pathology aspects of cancer of the ampulla-head-of-pancreas region. In Fitzgerald PJ, Morrison AB, editors: *The pancreas,* Baltimore, 1980, Williams & Wilkins.
297. Rosenberg J, Welch JP, Pyrtek LJ et al: Benign villous adenomas of the ampulla of Vater, *Cancer* 58:1563, 1986.
298. Yamaguchi K, Enjoji M, Kitamura K: Endoscopic biopsy has limited accuracy in diagnosis of ampullary tumors, *Gastrointest Endosc* 36:588, 1990.

299. Shutze WP, Sack J, Aldrete JS: Long-term follow-up of 24 patients undergoing radical resection for ampullar carcinoma, 1953 to 1988, *Cancer* 66:1717, 1990.
300. Nakao A, Harada A, Nonami T et al: The results and problems of surgical treatment of cancer of the duodenal papilla of Vater, *Nippon Geka Gakkai Zasshi* 93:805, 1992.
301. Mori K, Ikei S, Yamane T et al: Pathological factors influencing survival of carcinoma of the ampulla of Vater, *Eur J Surg Oncol* 16:183, 1990.
302. Neoptolemos JP, Talbot IC, Shaw DC, Carr-Locke DL: Long-term survival after resection of ampullary carcinoma is associated independently with tumor grade and a new staging classification that assesses local invasiveness, *Cancer* 61:1403, 1988.
303. Yamaguchi K, Nishihara K: Long- and short-term survivors after pancreatoduodenectomy for ampullary carcinoma, *J Surg Oncol* 50:195, 1992.

Miscellaneous epithelial tumors

304. Mori M, Iwashita A, Enjoji M: Adenosquamous carcinoma of the stomach: a clinicopathologic analysis of 28 cases, *Cancer* 57:333, 1986.
305. Callery CD, Sanders MM, Pratt S, Turnbull AD: Squamous cell carcinoma of the stomach: a study of four patients with comments on histogenesis, *J Surg Oncol* 29:166, 1985.
306. Haley T, Dimler M, Hollier P: Gastric teratoma with gastrointestinal bleeding, *J Pediatr Surg* 21:949, 1986.
307. Saigo PE, Brigati DJ, Sternberg SS et al: Primary gastric choriocarcinoma: an immunohistological study, *Am J Surg Pathol* 5:333, 1981.
308. Tanimura H, Furuta M: Carcinosarcoma of the stomach, *Am J Surg* 113:702, 1967.

Neuroendocrine hyperplasias and tumors

309. Lechago J: Endocrine cells of the gut and their disorders. In Goldman H, Appelman HR, editors: *Gastrointestinal pathology,* Baltimore, 1989, Williams & Wilkins.
310. Russo A, Buffa R, Grasso G et al: Gastric gastrinoma and diffuse G-cell hyperplasia associated with chronic atrophic gastritis, *Digestion* 20:416, 1980.
311. Lewin KJ, Yang K, Ulich T et al: Primary gastrin cell hyperplasia: report of five cases with a review of the literature, *Am J Surg Pathol* 8:821, 1984.
312. Creutzfeldt W, Arnold R: Endocrinology of duodenal ulcer, *World J Surg* 3:605, 1979.
313. Lechago J: Gastrointestinal neuroendocrine cell proliferations, *Hum Pathol* 25:1114, 1994.
314. Borch K, Renvall H, Kullman E et al: Gastric carcinoid associated with the syndrome of hypergastrinemic atrophic gastritis: a prospective analysis of 11 cases, *Am J Surg Pathol* 11:435, 1987.
315. Bordi C, Cocconi G, Togni R et al: Gastric endocrine cell proliferation: association with Zollinger-Ellison syndrome, *Arch Pathol* 98:274, 1974.
316. Larsson H, Carlsson E, Mattson H et al: Plasma gastrin and gastric entero-chromaffin-like cell activation and proliferation: studies with omeprazole and ranitidine and in intact and antrectomized rats, *Gastroenterology* 90:391, 1986.
317. Solcia E, Bordi C, Creutzfeldt W et al: Histopathologic classification of nonantral gastric endocrine growths in man, *Digestion* 41:185, 1988.
318. Creutzfeldt W, Stockman F: Carcinoids and carcinoid syndrome, *Am J Med* 82(suppl 5B):4, 1987.
319. Kern SE, Yardley JH, Lazenby AJ et al: Reversal by antrectomy of endocrine cell hyperplasia in the gastric body of pernicious anemia: a morphometric study, *Mod Pathol* 3:561, 1990.
320. D'Adda T, Pilato F, Sivelli R et al: Gastric carcinoid tumor and its precursor lesions: ultrastructural study of a case before and after antrectomy, *Arch Pathol Lab Med* 118:658, 1994.
321. Sjölund K, Alumets J, Berg NO et al: Enteropathy of celiac disease in adults: increased numbers of enterochromaffin cells in the duodenal mucosa, *Gut* 23:42, 1982.
322. Williams ED, Sandler M: The classification of carcinoid tumours, *Lancet* 1:238, 1963.
323. Godwin JD, II: Carcinoid tumors: an analysis of 2837 cases, *Cancer* 36:560, 1975.
324. Zakariai YM, Quan SH, Hajdu S: Carcinoid tumors of the gastrointestinal tract, *Cancer* 35:588, 1975.
325. Rindi G, Luinetti O, Cornaggia M et al: Three subtypes of gastric argyrophil carcinoid and the gastric neuroendocrine carcinoma: a clinicopathologic study, *Gastroenterology* 104:994, 1993.
326. DeLellis RA, Gagel RF, Kaplan MM, Curtis LE: Gastrinoma of duodenal G-cell origin, *Cancer* 38:201, 1976.
327. Vesoulis Z, Petras RE: Duodenal microgastrinoma producing the Zollinger-Ellison syndrome, *Arch Pathol Lab Med* 109:40, 1985.
328. Dayal Y, Doos WG, O'Brien MJ et al: Psammomatous somatostatinomas of the duodenum, *Am J Surg Pathol* 7:653, 1983.
329. Matsusaka T, Watanabe H, Enjoji M: Oat cell carcinoma of the stomach, *Fukuoka Acta Med* 67:65, 1976.
330. Swanson E, Dykoski D, Wick MR et al: Primary duodenal small-cell neuroendocrine carcinoma with production of vasoactive intestinal polypeptide, *Arch Pathol Lab Med* 110:317, 1986.
331. Lee CS, Machet D, Rode J: Small cell carcinoma of the ampulla of Vater, *Cancer* 70:1502, 1992.
332. Kelsen DP, Weston E, Kurtz R et al: Small cell carcinoma of the esophagus: treatment by chemotherapy alone, *Cancer* 45:1558, 1980.
333. Perrone T, Sibley RK, Rosai J: Duodenal gangliocytic paraganglioma: an immunohistochemical and ultrastructural study and a hypothesis concerning its origin, *Am J Surg Pathol* 9:31, 1985.
334. Scheithauer BW, Nora FE, Lechago J et al: Duodenal gangliocytic paraganglioma: clinicopathologic and immunocytochemical study of 11 cases, *Am J Clin Pathol* 86:559, 1986.
335. Dookhan DB, Miettinen M, Finkel G, Gibas Z: Recurrent duodenal gangliocytic paraganglioma with lymph node metastases, *Histopathology* 22:399, 1993.

Lymphomas

336. Brooks JJ, Enterline HT: Primary gastric lymphomas: a clinicopathologic study of 58 cases with long-term follow-up and literature review, *Cancer* 51:701, 1983.
337. Cogliatti SB, Schmid U, Schumacher U et al: Primary B-cell gastric lymphoma: a clinicopathological study of 145 patients, *Gastroenterology* 101:1159, 1991.
338. Isaacson PG: Gastrointestinal lymphoma, *Hum Pathol* 25:1020, 1994.
339. Vimadalal SD, Said JW, Voyles H III: Gastric lymphoreticular neoplasms: an immunological study of 36 cases, *Am J Clin Pathol* 80:792, 1983.
340. Lewin KJ: Disorders of the lymphoid system. In Ming SC, Goldman H, editors: *Pathology of the gastrointestinal tract,* Philadelphia, 1992, Saunders.
341. Isaacson PG, Wright DH: Malignant lymphoma of mucosa-associated lymphoid tissue: a distinctive type of B-cell lymphoma, *Cancer* 52:2515, 1983.
342. Chan JKC, Ng CS, Isaacson PG: Relationship between high-grade lymphoma and low-grade B-cell mucosa-associated lymphoid tissue lymphoma (MALToma) of the stomach, *Am J Pathol* 136:1153, 1990.
343. Saraga P, Hurlimann J, Ozzello L: Lymphomas and pseudolymphomas of the alimentary tract: an immunohistochemical study with clinicopathological correlations, *Hum Pathol* 12:713, 1981.
344. Wolf JA Jr, Spjut HJ: Focal lymphoid hyperplasia of the stomach preceding gastric lymphoma: case report and review of the literature, *Cancer* 48:2518, 1981.

Stromal tumors

345. Appelman HD: Stromal tumors of the esophagus, stomach, and duodenum. In Appelman HD, editor: *Pathology of the esophagus, stomach, and duodenum,* New York, 1984, Churchill Livingstone.
346. Appelman HD, Helwig EB: Cellular leiomyomas of the stomach in 49 patients, *Arch Pathol Lab Med* 101:373, 1977.
347. Stout AP: Bizarre smooth muscle tumors of the stomach, *Cancer* 15:400, 1962.
348. Appelman HD: Mesenchymal tumors of the gastrointestinal tract. In Ming SC, Goldman H, editors: *Pathology of the gastrointestinal tract,* Philadelphia, 1992, Saunders.

349. Carney JA: The triad of gastric epithelioid leiomyosarcoma, pulmonary chondroma, and functioning extra-adrenal paraganglioma: a five-year review, *Medicine* (Baltimore) 62:159, 1983.
350. Appelman HD: Mesenchymal tumors of the gut: historical perspectives, new approaches, new results, and does it make any difference? In Goldman H, Appelman HD, Kaufman N, editors: *Gastrointestinal pathology,* Baltimore, 1990, Williams & Wilkins.
351. Federspiel BH, Sobin LH, Helwig EB et al: Morphometry and cytophotometric assessment of DNA in smooth-muscle tumors (leiomyomas and leiomyosarcomas) of the gastrointestinal tract, *Analyt Quant Cytol* 9:105, 1987.
352. Appelman HD, Helwig FB: Glomus tumors of the stomach, *Cancer* 23:203, 1969.
353. Osamura RY, Watanabe K, Yoneyama K, Hayashi T: Glomus tumor of the stomach: light and electron microscopic study with literature review of related tumors, *Acta Pathol Jpn* 27:533, 1977.

Metastatic tumors

354. Ming SC: Tumors of the esophagus and stomach. In *Atlas of tumor pathology,* series 2, fasc 7, Washington, D.C., 1973, Armed Forces Institute of Pathology.
355. Green LK: Hematogenous metastases to the stomach: a review of 67 cases, *Cancer* 65:1596, 1990.

54 Small Intestine

Ivan Damjanov

NORMAL ANATOMY AND FUNCTION

The small intestine is a 4- to 5-meter-long portion of the alimentary tract that extends from the pylorus to the ileocecal valve. It consists of three parts: the *duodenum, jejunum,* and *ileum.*[1-5] The duodenum, which is relatively short, is located mostly in the retroperitoneal space and is fixed to the abdominal wall. The jejunum and ileum consist of freely movable loops located in the peritoneal cavity and attached to the posterior abdominal wall with a long mesentery. The jejunum accounts for the first three fifths of the intestinal loops, whereas the jejunum constitutes the remaining distal portion. The duodenum derives its name from the fact that it measures approximately 12 inches long (Latin *duodecim* 'twelve'). The jejunum was so named by the ancient anatomists because in the cadaver it is typically devoid of chyme and contains only air (Latin *jejunum* 'empty,'). The loops of the ileum appeared twisted to the prosectors of yore, and this part was named accordingly (Greek *eilein* 'to roll up').

Histology. Histologically the small intestine is composed of four layers: the mucosa, submucosa, muscularis propria, and serosa. The mucosa of the proximal, middle, and distal small intestine has the same general features but shows some distinct differences.[1-3] The main function of the small intestinal mucosa is absorption of the food, and thus it must have a large absorptive surface. To this end the mucosa forms large folds, called *plicae circulares of Kerkring,* which can be seen by the naked eye. The mucosa also forms elongated villi, visible with a dissecting microscope, and further increases the absorptive surface. The absorptive surface is further augmented by slender microvilli that extend into the lumen of the intestine from the apical cell membrane. They can be seen with the electron microscope. There are two kinds of villi: leaf-shaped broad and finger-shaped narrow. The leaf-shaped villi predominate in the duodenum and proximal jejunum, whereas the ileum contains only finger-shaped villi (Fig. 54-1). The spaces between the villi contain tubular glands, called the *crypts of Lieberkühn,* which extend through the lamina propria mucosae almost into the muscularis mucosae.

The villi and the crypts are lined by five types of epithelial cells. Four of these types are differentiated, but the fifth represents their common precursor—the undifferentiated intestinal stem cell (Fig. 54-1). The differentiated cells include *absorptive cells, goblet cells, neuroendocrine cells,* and *Paneth's cells.* The absorptive cells (also known as *enterocytes* or *villus columnar cells*) are tall columnar cells and predominate along the surface of the villi. They have a basally located nucleus, a well-developed cytoplasm, and an apical brush border that under the light microscope appears as a refractile surface lining. Goblet cells, which are scattered between the absorptive cells, appear plump because their supranuclear cytoplasm is distended by mucin. The neuroendocrine cells have a less developed cytoplasm and are intercalated between the other cells in the crypts. They have round nuclei and a clear perinuclear halo that contains neuroendocrine granules visible only by electron microscopy. These cells synthesize polypeptide hormones. It has been shown by immunohistochemical analysis that the neuroendocrine cells are a heterogeneous population and contain some 10 to 20 different hormones.

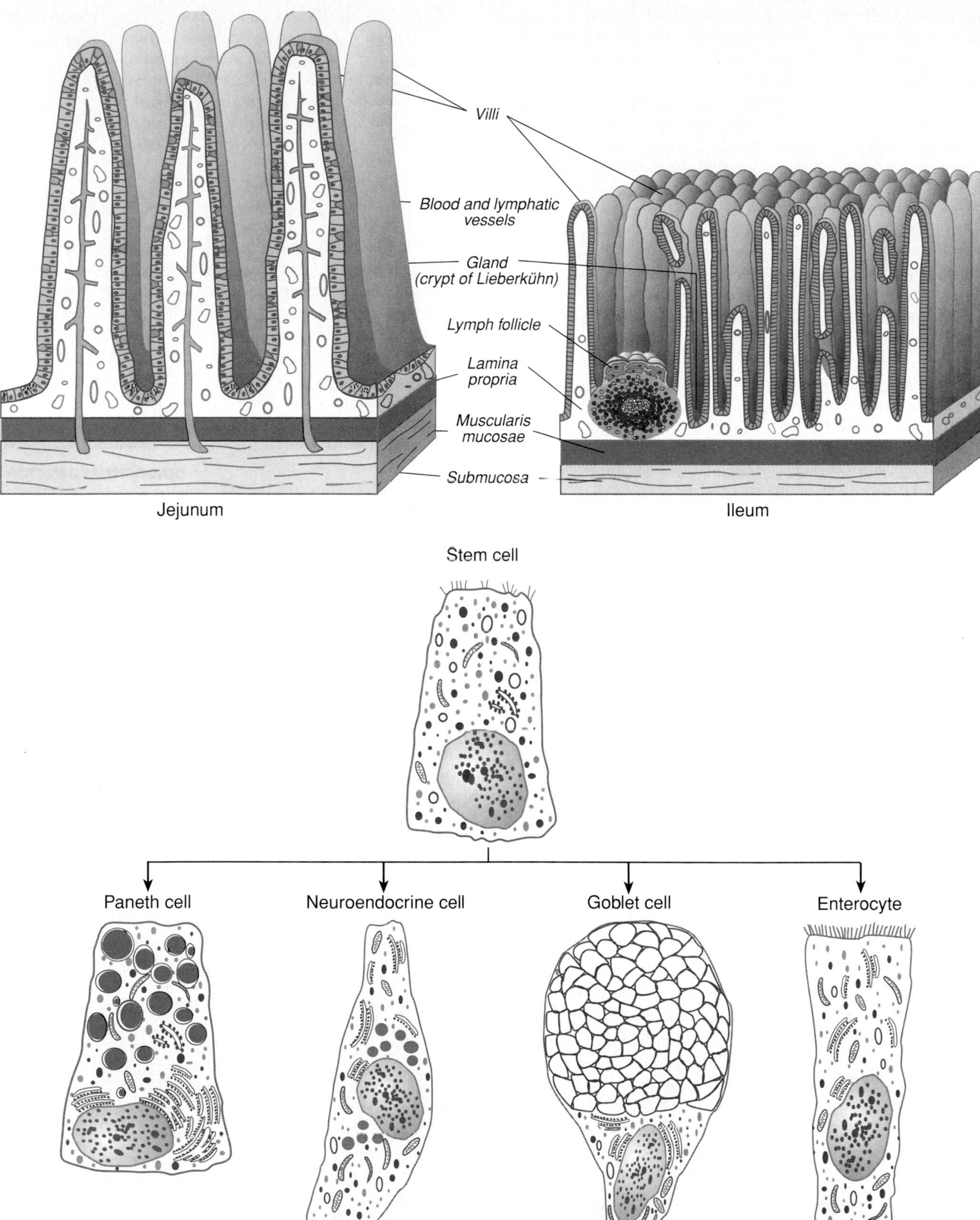

Fig. 54-1 Diagram of the mucosa and submucosa of the jejunum and ileum, and the main epithelial cells of the small intestine. (Modified from the original concepts developed by Dr. C. P. Leblond, Montreal, P.Q., Canada.)

The Paneth cells are large pyramid-shaped cells located at the base of the crypts. They have basally placed nuclei and a well-developed cytoplasm filled with large eosinophilic granules. Their function is unknown.

The lamina propria mucosae is composed of loose, highly vascularized connective tissue richly infiltrated with lymphocytes, plasma cells, and macrophages. It forms the core of the villi and surrounds the crypts occupying the space between the base of the crypts and the muscularis mucosae. Inside the villi the lamina propria contains centrally located blood vessels and lymphatics (lacteals), which are essential for absorption of food. The basal portion of the lamina propria is especially rich in lymphocytes, which may be arranged into follicles. In the ileum such lymphoid follicles are more prominent and often aggregate into *Peyer's patches,* which can be recognized as nodules by the naked eye.

The muscularis mucosae consists of thin bundles of smooth muscle cells arranged into an inner circular and an outer longitudinal layer. The outer muscle layer merges with the loose connective tissue of the submucosa, which contains large blood vessels and lymphatics, nerves, and ganglion cells of the *Meissner plexus.*

The muscle coat of the intestine (*lamina muscularis propria* or *lamina muscularis externa*) is the thickest layer of the intestine. It consists of an inner circular and an outer longitudinal layer of smooth muscles. It also contains nerves and the ganglion cells of the *myenteric plexus of Auerbach* located in the loose connective tissue that separates the two muscle layers.

External to the lamina muscularis the intestine is covered with a layer of loose connective tissue *(subserosa)* and a continuous layer of mesothelium, which forms the *peritoneal serosal surface.* The serosa also covers the mesentery, which represents the root of the intestine. The mesentery keeps the intestines attached to the posterior abdominal wall. It also holds the major blood vessels destined for the jejunum and ileum, all of which are derived from the *superior mesenteric artery,* one of the main branches of the aorta. The *superior mesenteric vein* drains the venous blood into the portal vein.

Function. The small intestine has the pivotal role in the uptake of nutrients. Its functions can be summarized as follows:

1. *Mixing of the food and digestive juices.* This mixing is accomplished by contractions of the circular layer of the muscularis.
2. *Propulsion of food.* The food is moved by continuous peristaltic contractions of the circular and longitudinal muscle fibers, which occurs in a coordinated, wavelike manner. This movement is integrated by intestinal nerves and is regulated by a series of reflexes and neurohormonal stimuli.
3. *Secretory function.* The intestinal cells secrete numerous enzymes essential for digestion. They also secrete fluids, electrolytes, and mucins, as well as biologically active substances such as lysozyme, immunoglobulins, transport proteins, and activators of pancreatic enzymes.
4. *Neuroendocrine function.* The neuroendocrine cells secrete a variety of bioactive substances (such as serotonin) and polypeptide hormones (such as cholecystokinin, enteroglucagon, and bombesin) that have paracrine and endocrine functions.
5. *Absorption of nutrients.* Carbohydrates, proteins, lipids, minerals, and many other essential nutrients are absorbed in the intestine. The enterocytes do not distinguish between the useful and the noxious substances. Hence, xenobiotics, toxic substances, and drugs are absorbed equally as well as nutrients.

DEVELOPMENTAL AND GENETIC DISEASES

Normal development. The small intestine develops from the fetal midgut.[6,7] The primitive gut, which is initially straight, becomes folded, forming the intestinal loops that are attached to the posterior abdominal wall by the fetal mesentery. The elongation and folding of the tube are associated with a counterclockwise rotation that brings the future large intestine anterior to the small intestine. The mesentery that follows the coiling of the intestinal loops fuses with the peritoneal lining of the abdominal cavity over the distal duodenum, which thus becomes retroperitoneal. The jejunal and ileal mesentery remains elongated but is fixed at its root, which extends transversely from the left superior to the right inferior portion of the posterior abdominal wall. This final intestinal positioning is completed by the sixth gestational week. The primitive intestinal epithelium begins proliferating during the latter part of this developmental period. By the sixth and seventh weeks of gestation the lumen of the intestines is completely obliterated. Thereafter the epithelium begins forming villi and crypts, which occurs at the same time as the cytodifferentiation specific to each portion of the intestine. By the end of the second trimester the intestines are lined by all the types of cells normally found in the adult intestine. However, these cells retain a fetal phenotype and lack many enzymes and functions of the adult intestines. The intestines mature fully only after birth.

Anomalies of positioning

The initial formation of the intestines occurs in the fetal abdominal cavity, which is too small to accommodate all the loops. The intestines protrude and are thus normally outside of the body boundaries up to the tenth week of pregnancy. Thereafter, as the abdominal cavity enlarges, the intestines are internalized and become covered with the anterior abdominal wall. If the intestines do not recede into the fetal abdominal cavity and the anterior abdominal wall is not completely formed, a congenital herniation known as *omphalocele* results (Fig. 54-2). The loops protrude from the abdominal cavity and are covered with a thin transparent layer composed of peritoneum on the inside and the amnion on the outside. Omphaloceles occur in 1 in 3500 births. More than 50% of these infants are stillborn, and many also have other congenital malformations.

Congenital umbilical hernia manifests as an abnormally large umbilical ring through which the fetal intestine protrudes. This hernia is closely related to omphalocelle and represents another, less severe, defect resulting from abnormal closure of the anterior abdominal wall.

Abnormal rotation of the fetal small intestines may assume several forms.[6,7] It may be isolated or combined with malpositioning of the colon. The variants include nonrotation or reversed rotation of the small intestine, mobile cecum, subhepatic cecum, or a complete *situs inversus viscerum.* Situs inversus viscerum may be part of *Kartagener's syndrome,* which is

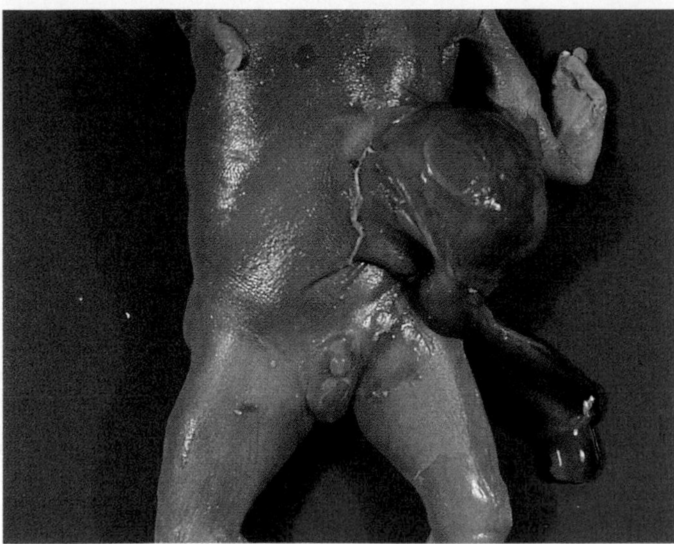

Fig. 54-2 Omphalocele.

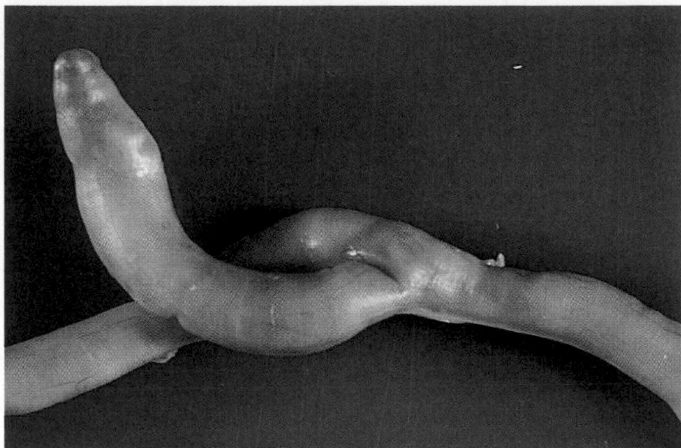

Fig. 54-3 Meckel's diverticulum in an infant.

characterized by immotile cilia, bronchiectasis, and immotile sperm. The malpositioning of the intestines may be mild and asymptomatic, but this malformation may also predispose to the development of volvulus and intestinal loop strangulation. These abnormalities can be diagnosed by use of modern radiologic and sonographic techniques.[8]

Vitelline duct remnants

During early development the midgut is linked to the yolk sac by a stalk that serves as the reference point for the initial intestinal rotations. As the yolk sac involutes and disappears by the sixteenth week of pregnancy, the enterovitelline duct undergoes atresia and disappears. The most common remnant of the vitelline duct is the *Meckel's diverticulum,* a blind pouch of the ileum[9] (Fig. 54-3). According to the *rule of 2s,* which is a mnemonic device, Meckel's diverticulum is found in 2% of the population at 2 feet from the cecum, is 2 inches long, and causes clinical symptoms in 2% of cases.[5] Meckel's diverticulitis may cause symptoms similar to those of appendicitis, except that the point of maximal tenderness is in the left lower abdominal quadrant. Meckel's diverticulum may contain ectopic pancreatic cells or gastric mucosa that can undergo peptic ulceration. It may be attached to the anterior abdominal wall by fibrous strand remnants of the vitelline duct. If the duct does not undergo complete atresia but remains patent, a vitelline (umbilicoileal) fistula connecting the ileal lumen with the umbilicus may form. Volvulus around the vitelline duct remnant is yet another rare complication.

Abnormalities of intestinal wall

Complete obliteration of the intestinal lumen, *atresia,* or pronounced narrowing of the lumen, *stenosis,* are rare. These malformations occur most often in the duodenum and less commonly in the jejunum and ileum. Intestinal atresia and stenosis are the consequences of intestinal recanalization in the third month of pregnancy. Absent recanalization and the resulting morphogenetic abnormalities may also cause intestinal *reduplication,* which assumes several forms: connected enteric duplication, disconnected enteric duplication, and bilateral duplication of false diverticula.[7]

The muscle layer of the intestine may also be focally defective and missing. Such sites may predispose to the formation of *diverticula.* Although diverticula develop at the sites of presumably congenital intestinal weakness, they are rarely found in persons before 40 years of age.[4] The muscularis may also contain inclusions and cysts of heterotopic mucosa or peritoneum and choristomas composed of gastric or pancreatic tissue.

The small intestine in 10% of children with Hirschsprung's disease may show agangliosis.[10] The ileal lesions are similar to those of the large intestine. The affected segment is typically devoid of ganglion cells but contains normal nerves. These nerves can be best visualized with antibodies to neurofilaments or acetylcholinesterase, which is typically increased in content in the aganglionic intestinal segment.

Cystic fibrosis

The abnormalities in intestinal and pancreatic secretion typical of cystic fibrosis may affect the intestines during prenatal development. In the most severe cases the viscid intestinal contents cause an obstruction known as *meconium ileus.*[11] The meconium is dark green or black, thick, and adherent to the mucosa, most prominently in the terminal ileum. The consequent obstruction of the ileum with meconium is associated with violent peristaltic movements that ultimately cause the intestine to rupture and meconium to dissipate throughout the abdominal cavity *(meconium peritonitis).* The affected ileum shows typical histologic features that include the accumulation of mucus in the crypts and between the villi. The crypts appear to be dilated with inspissated mucus. The villi appear flattened and are covered with chyme intermixed with mucus streaming out from the intervillous spaces.[12]

Abetalipoproteinemia

Abetaliproproteinemia is a rare autosomal recessive disorder characterized by a defect in the assembly of chylomicrons.[13] The defect involves the gene encoding the large subunit of the microsomal triglyceride transfer protein, which is essential for the synthesis of apolipoprotein B. Apolipoprotein B cannot be produced without this protein, and accordingly the intestines cannot form the chylomicrons essential for the transport of lipids into the liver. Lipids absorbed from the food remain in the enterocytes of the small intestine, imparting to those cells a vacuolated appearance. Chylomicron retention disease *(Andersen's disease)* is a related chylomicron-formation defect.[14] Such defects typically cause malabsorption and steatorrhea.

Carbohydrate absorption defects

Congenital deficiencies of lactase, sucrase, isomaltase, trehalase, and galactase result in the malabsorption of carbohydrates.[15] The most common of these disorders is lactase deficiency. It occurs in several forms,[16] some of which become apparent only in adulthood. Congenital sucrase-isomaltase deficiency is especially common in Eskimos, 10% of whom are affected.[17] These congenital enzyme deficiencies produce no histologic changes in the intestine, and the diagnosis is made only after the defect has been demonstrated functionally.

Intestinal lymphangiectasia

Intestinal lymphangiectasia is a rare congenital defect typically associated with protein-losing enteropathy.[18] The disease may be limited to the bowel, or it may be part of generalized familial lymphedema *(Milroy's disease)*. The dilated lymphatics can be seen by the naked eye as cystic spaces that distort segments of the intestine (Fig. 54-4). Histologically it presents with dilatation of the lacteals in the intestinal villi. The villi appear distended and edematous, and the lamina propria may contain lipid-laden foamy macrophages. Morphologically congenital lymphangiectasia cannot be distinguished from secondary obstructive lymphangiectasia caused by tumors, infections, or radiation.

Vascular malformations

Vascular malformations of the intestine, which may be congenital or acquired, are known by several names, such as *angiodysplasia, vascular ectasia, arteriovenous malformation,* and *telangiectasia.*[19-21] These defects may involve any part of the intestine and are an important cause of bleeding.[19] Although most often found in the cecum of the elderly, vascular lesions can occur in the small intestine as well.[20] The lesions are typically identified by angiography and are evident as bleeding nodules at operation. Histologically the abnormal vessels have thick walls and appear to be anastomosing with one another in the submucosa. True arteriovenous malformations appear as nodules or cysts.[21] However, angiodysplastic mucosal vascular spaces usually collapse and may not be evident in resected intestinal segments unless the blood vessels were injected with a dye that would allow the histologic identification of abnormal vascular spaces.[4]

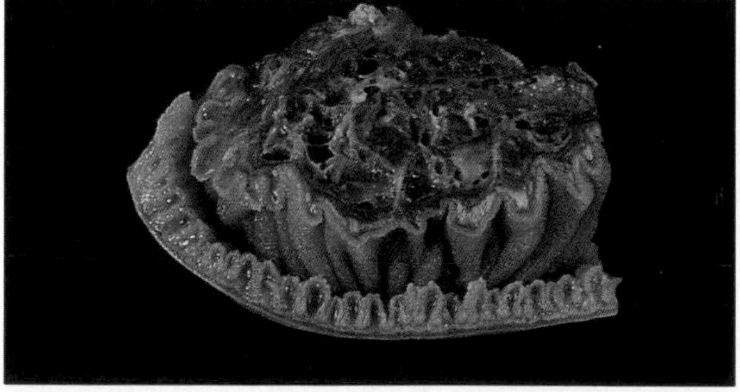

Fig. 54-4 Lymphangiectasia of the small intestine. Cystic spaces distorting the resected intestinal loop represent dilated lymphatics. (Courtesy Dr. W.V. Harrer, Camden, N.J.)

Congenital multifocal telangiectasia of the intestines occurs in the *Osler-Weber-Rendu disease.*[22] The intestinal lesions of this syndrome, which are associated with the skin and mucosal lesions, consist of dilated small blood vessels in the submucosa and the lamina propria mucosae. Multiple hemangiomas are found also in patients with *Maffucci's syndrome* in conjunction with multiple enchondromas and in patients with the *Kasabach-Merritt syndrome,* characterized by the triad of hemorrhagic diathesis, thrombocytopenia, and multiple hemangiomas.[4]

Visceral myopathy

Disorders of smooth muscle that cause motility problems may be congenital or acquired. The congenital disorders may occur in the context of systemic myopathic disorders such as myotonic dystrophy or Duchenne's muscular dystrophy. Motility problems also occur in an isolated form known as *familial autonomic visceral myopathy.*[23] Histologically the intestines show atrophy of the smooth muscle cells in the mucosa and the muscularis propria. The degenerating muscle cells appear vacuolated. These cells have indistinct margins and are ultimately replaced by fibrous tissue.[5] Extensive fibrosis imparts a honeycomb appearance to the muscle layer that is histologically indistinguishable from the changes caused by systemic sclerosis.

Visceral neuropathy

Several forms of familial visceral neuropathies involving the intestines are on record. These diseases, inherited as autosomal recessive or autosomal dominant traits, all present with intestinal pseudoobstruction caused by impaired motility.[24] Histologically the intestines contain a decreased number of neurons. Neuronal intranuclear inclusions may be seen in submucosal ganglion cells and the myentric plexus in some forms of familial visceral neuropathy.[5] Such neuronal changes must be distinguished from those of Chagas' disease, cytomegalovirus infection, and the paraneoplastic neuropathy. The last disease is usually associated with infiltrates of lymphocytes and plasma cells, which are not a feature of familial visceral neuropathy.

DILATATIONS AND OBSTRUCTIONS OF THE INTESTINAL LUMEN

Diverticulosis

Diverticula and pseudodiverticula may develop in any part of the small intestine but are most common in the jejunum. The pathogenesis of these jejunal outpouchings is not known. The diverticula are typically located along the mesenteric insertion line and are multiple. Histologically the wall of the diverticula is composed of mucosa and submucosa. Many of the congenital outpouchings are, however, *pseudodiverticula,* the walls of which consist of all four layers of the intestine. The mucosal epithelium often shows signs of atrophy brought on by distention. The muscle layer of pseudodiverticula usually shows fibrosis.

Intestinal obstruction

Obstruction of the intestine may arise as the result of intraluminal objects, intestinal disease, or external pressure.

Intraluminal objects that can obstruct the intestines include foreign bodies that have been swallowed accidentally or intentionally, gallstones, trichobezoars, and phytobezoars.[25]

Intramural causes of intestinal obstruction include various benign and malignant tumors, Crohn's disease, and radiation enteritis.

External causes of intestinal obstruction include peritoneal fibrous bands, adhesions, and tumors. Such adhesions may be sequelae of infectious peritonitis, surgical operations, chronic intestinal diseases characterized by serosal inflammation, and fistula formation (such as that stemming from Crohn's disease).

Intussusception is the invagination of one segment of the intestine into another. Typically it occurs in infants and is most common in the 3- to 6-month age group.[26] Most of the infantile cases of intussusception are idiopathic and probably result from irregularities in the contractions of intestines. The ileocecal area is most often affected.

Intussusception occurs less commonly in adults and it is usually secondary to tumors or some other readily identifiable abnormality of the intestinal wall (such as Meckel's diverticulum and an enterostomy site) or of the intestinal contents (such as a foreign body). In adults the intussusception may occur at any site, and unlike in infants, it does not show a predilection for occurring in the ileocecal area.[27]

Volvulus occurs when the intestinal loops rotate around their stalk. Intestinal obstruction typically ensues. Mesenteric twisting may also interrupt the blood flow and cause intestinal infarction. Volvulus most often occurs in the small intestine, which is affected in about 70% of cases. If the obstruction is not recognized, the intestinal loop affected by volvulus will necrotize, resulting in peritonitis. Chronic volvulus is typically caused by repeated attacks of intestinal ischemia.

Herniation of the intestinal loops into an extra-abdominal space may cause obstruction. This is especially common in the setting of hernias accompanied by inflammation and fibrosis, which may cause adhesions to form between the intestine and the wall of the hernia. Intestinal loops that are normally retractile may become incarcerated or strangulated, which ultimately leads to ischemic necrosis of the intestinal wall, rupture of the intestine, and peritonitis.

Pneumatosis cystoides intestinalis

Pneumatosis cystoides intestinalis is a rare condition in which air accumulates in the wall of the intestine. Its pathogenesis is obscure. Some of these cysts probably represent dilated lymphatics, but this cannot be proved even under the best of circumstances. Pneumatosis most often affects the colon, but it may involve the small intestine as well.[4] Histologically the lesions consist of thin-walled cysts lined by endothelial cells. The cysts are separated by connective tissue that may contain inflammatory cells. The lumens of the cysts may contain proteinaceous fluid and occasionally even bacteria. The mucosa overlying the cysts may show abnormal glandular architecture, and the condition can be confused with Crohn's disease or ulcerative colitis. The air spaces may also extend into the subserosal space and even into the mesentery.

CIRCULATORY DISORDERS

In the normal intestinal circulation the small intestine receives the arterial blood through the superior mesenteric artery. The main arterial trunk gives rise to several branches forming arcades that interanastomose in the mesentery of intestinal loops. The arteries originating at a right angle from the arches do not anastomose but enter the wall of the intestine. These branches form a major subserosal meshwork and also extend into penetrating arteries that cross through the muscularis toward the mucosa. The submucosal arterial branches give rise to arterioles that supply blood to the villi. The intestinal veins follow the arteries and ultimately form the superior mesenteric vein, which is a tributary of the portal vein.

Circulatory disorders in adults

The intestinal circulatory disturbances that occur in adults can be divided into four major groups[28]: (1) sudden complete occlusion of the superior mesentric artery or its major branches; (2) hypoperfusion of the intestines stemming from circulatory (pump) failure; (3) chronic ischemia stemming from a narrowing of the superior mesenteric artery or its major branches; and (4) mesenteric vein thrombosis.

Arterial thrombosis and embolism

Sudden arterial occlusion is most often a complication of atherosclerosis.[28] Atheromas typically develop at the orifice of the superior mesenteric artery, but ischemia occurs only after 70% of the original lumen has been obstructed. Complete occlusion is typically caused by thrombi, and this accounts for half of the cases of sudden intestinal ischemia. Emboli are the cause in a third of the cases, and other less common events such as arteritis, a dissecting aneurysm of the aorta, a retroperitoneal tumor, or surgical mishaps are the cause in the few remaining cases.

Grossly such intestines are suffused with blood and are edematous (Fig. 54-5). Histologically the entire intestinal wall is necrotic. Within hours bacteria invade the necrotic wall, and this invasion leads to gangrene and peritonitis. Intestinal infarcts are associated with a high mortality.

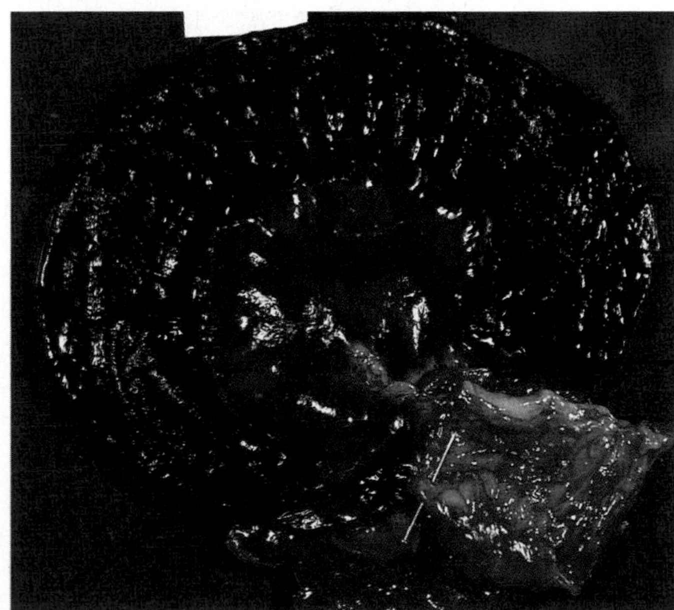

Fig. 54-5 Hemorrhagic infarction of the intestine.

Acute hypotensive hypoperfusion

Acute hypoperfusion of the intestine is a common feature of acute heart failure and shock. Under normal circumstances the splanchnic circulation constitutes 20% of the cardiac output. However, the intestinal blood supply can be dramatically reduced in the event of shock, and this is brought about either by catecholamine-induced constriction of the arteriolar sphincters or a general drop in blood pressure stemming from central pump failure (Fig. 54-6). Sudden hypoperfusion without arterial occlusion is the cause in a third of the patients with acute intestinal infarctions. The pathologic changes in the intestine are, however, the same regardless of the mechanism responsible for the acute ischemia.

Although the extent of necrosis varies from one patient to another, the early changes brought about by hypoperfusion are most prominent at the tip of villi, because these structures are the last to receive arterial blood. Additional ischemia affects the entire mucosa and submucosa. Histologically the mucosa and submucosa are necrotic. When the small mucosal vessels rupture, typically blood then extravasates into the interstitial spaces and into the lumen of the intestine. Bacterial invasion of the necrotic intestine is a common complication. Such hypotensive episodes are often lethal, but some patients recover. The intestines in these patients show widespread foci of mucosal ulceration and scarring.

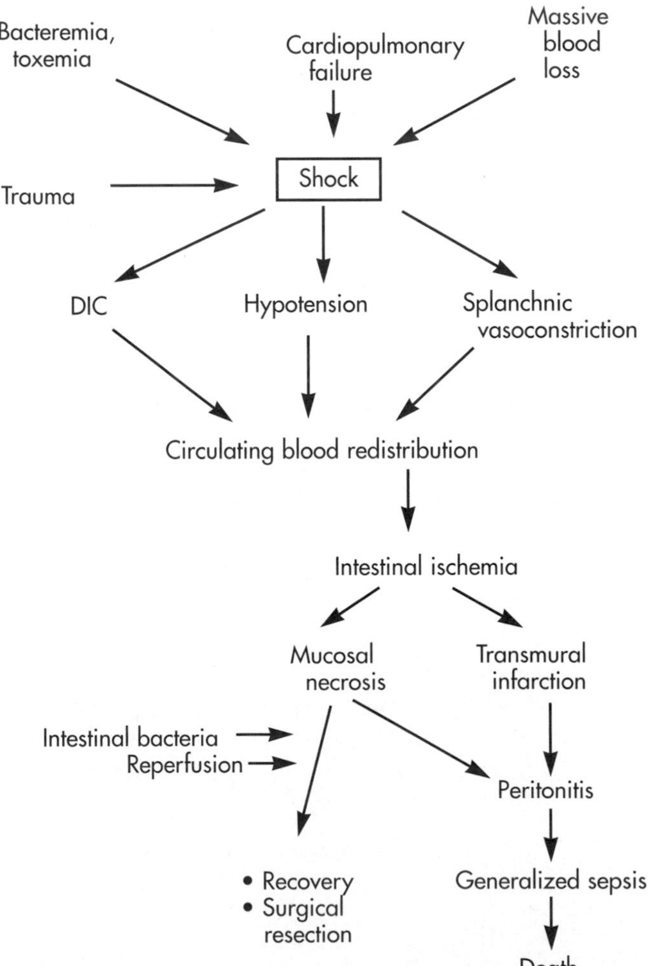

Fig. 54-6 Pathogenesis of intestinal infarcts caused by hypotensive hypoperfusion.

Chronic intestinal ischemia

Chronic intestinal ischemia often occurs in the setting of generalized atherosclerosis. However, the symptoms are highly variable, and therefore it is controversial whether it should be considered a distinct clinicopathologic entity. Low-grade ischemia, which may present with pain accentuated by food intake, is referred to as *postprandial angina*.[4] More pronounced chronic ischemia eventuates in focal intestinal necrosis. Mucosal ulcers are usually shallow and heal by scarring, imparting a cobblestone appearance to the intestine. Such lesions may mimic those of Crohn's disease.[29]

Mesenteric vein thrombosis

Mesenteric vein thrombosis leads to intestinal congestion, mucosal hemorrhages, and ischemia, which typically develop over several days.[30] Focal hemorrhagic necrosis of the intestines presents with hematochezia and diarrhea. Extensive transmural necrosis results in peritonitis.[30]

Neonatal necrotizing enterocolitis

Neonatal necrotizing enterocolitis is a disease that affects premature infants, typically occurring during the first 10 days of life. It is a multifactorial disease related to feeding the infant with baby formula and infection with gram-negative bacteria.[31] The disease has a dramatic course characterized by profuse vomiting, abdominal distention, and rectal bleeding. Radiologically the intestines appear dilated and show pneumatosis. Necrosis of the intestinal loops leads to rupture and peritonitis, events associated with a high mortality.

On gross examination the affected intestinal loops appear hemorrhagic and friable. Small bubbles of gas can be palpated in the distended intestinal wall and may be seen even underneath the serosa. Histologically there is necrosis, which may be transmural or patchy in the form of mucosal ulcers. Intestinal contents may be found in the abdominal cavity after the necrotic loops rupture. Most children who survive have no residual problems, but intestinal strictures may develop in some.[32]

Mesenteric vasculitis

Vasculitis of the intestines may occur in the setting of systemic vasculitis or in association with Crohn's disease.[33] Mesenteric inflammatory venoocclusive disease, a recently described entity, is yet another form of intestinal ischemia.[34] This vasculitis of unknown cause is limited to the mesenteric veins. Mesenteric vein thrombosis and intestinal infarction are the presenting events.

INFECTIONS

Infectious gastroenteritis is a major health problem worldwide. These infections are most prevalent in underdeveloped countries but are also of considerable significance in the United States, especially in day care centers, hospitals, and extended care facilities. Epidemics caused by contaminated water or food are still widespread in many parts of Asia and Africa. Undernourished children, debilitated patients with chronic disease, and those suffering from immunodeficiency are at greatest risk. Travelers to the tropics are also commonly affected.

Gastroenteritis may be caused by bacteria, viruses, fungi, and protozoa, the most important of which are discussed briefly.

Bacterial infections

The pathogenicity of bacteria depends on their own virulence and the capacity of the host to mount an efficient defense. Under normal circumstances the duodenum, jejunum, and upper ileum contain commensals, primarily diphtheroids, streptococci, and lactobacilli that have been swallowed with food. In the ileum the bacterial flora changes and *Escherichia coli* and anaerobic *Bacteroides* predominate. All these bacteria are normally present in small numbers. In the proximal bowel, bacterial counts do not exceed 10^4 to 10^5 per milliliter. Bacterial numbers increase temporarily after meals. In the ileum the number of bacteria ranges from 10^9 to 10^{11} per milliliter.

Bacterial gastroenteritis develops when the number of normal commensals increases and this causes them to become noxious or when the intestines are invaded by pathogens that are not normally part of the intestinal flora. Infection with *Vibrio cholerae* or *E. coli* requires an intake of 10^5 to 10^8 microbes. On the other hand, the ingestion of as few as 10 to 10^3 *Campylobacter jejuni* or *Giardia lamblia* may cause disease.

Bacterial overgrowth syndromes

Normal peristalsis is the primary equilibrator of the bacterial flora in the intestines. There are, however, other defense mechanisms that prevent excessive growth of commensals and the entry of potential pathogens. These mechanisms include the hydrochloric acid and proteolytic enzymes of the gastric juices, bile and pancreatic secretion, intestinal immunoglobulins, and bactericidal proteins (such as lysozyme). Bacterial overgrowth occurs if these protective mechanisms fail.

Various causes of bacterial overgrowth and the pathogenesis of the ensuing malabsorption syndrome are depicted in Fig. 54-7. Typically the intestinal volume is increased and contains an increased number of bacteria. Broad-spectrum antibiotic therapy is usually effective, with the steatorrhea and concomitant nutritional deficiency alleviated as a result. The histologic changes in the small intestine are nonspecific, however, and include minor mucosal changes such as edema of the villi and mild villous atrophy.

Bacterial diarrhea

Diarrhea is the main clinical consequence of bacterial enteritis. Three types of bacterial diarrheas are recognized: noninflammatory (toxin caused), inflammatory, and enteric fever. The most common are *the noninflammatory diarrheas* caused by enterotoxicogenic pathogens such as *E. coli* or *V. cholerae*. These microbes do not invade the mucosa and do not cause inflammation. Instead they reside in the upper intestines and produce diarrhea by secreting toxins that interfere with the absorptive or secretory function of intestinal cells. Enteropathogenic strains of *E. coli* produce a similar effect, even though these bacteria do not secrete distinct enteric toxins.

Inflammatory diarrhea is usually caused by invasive pathogens. Although the primary infection is in the large intestine, in most cases the small intestine may be involved as well. Among the pathogens that produce hemorrhagic stools and

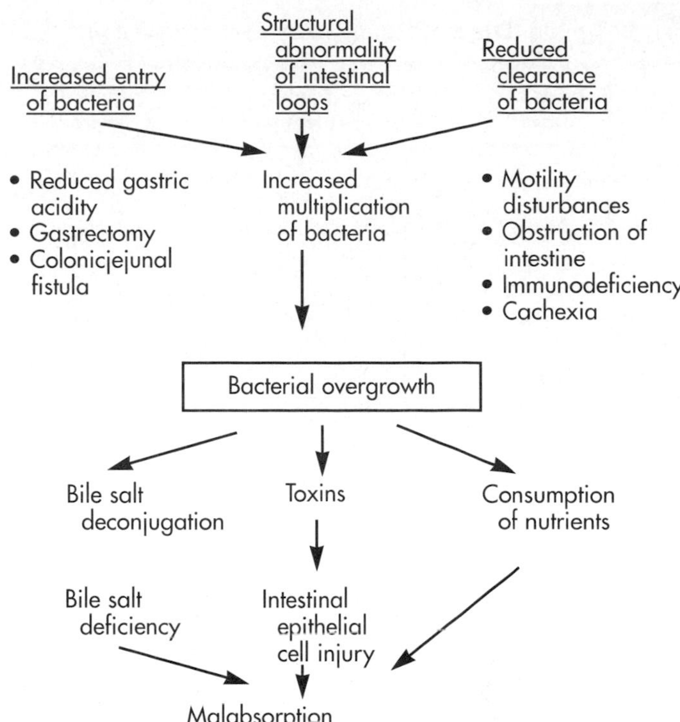

Fig. 54-7 Pathogenesis of malabsorption because of bacterial overgrowth.

rich inflammatory exudate are *Shigella, Salmonella, Campylobacter, Clostridium* species. Affected intestines show ulceration, mucosal inflammation, and even pseudomembrane formation.

The third type of intestinal infection, the so-called *enteric fever,* is typically caused by pathogens such as *Salmonella typhi, Campylobacter fetus,* or *Yersinia enterocolitica.* These pathogens invade the wall of the intestine overlying Peyer's patches and enter the lymphoid tissue, from which they gain access to local lymphatics and ultimately the systemic circulation. *Salmonella* reaches the biliary tract and is introduced into the intestine in bile. Other pathogens that cause enteric fever probably enter the intestine by a similar enterohepatic route. Histologically, these pathogens cause intestinal ulcers that typically overlie the enlarged Peyer's patches. The lymphoid tissue in Peyer's patches shows follicular hyperplasia and sinus histiocytosis. Mesenteric lymph nodes are also enlarged and show similar histologic features. Bacteria can be identified in macrophages. The spleen and liver also enlarge and show increased phagocytic cell activity or foci of inflammation.

Escherichia coli infection. *E. coli* is normally found in the human ileum and colon, where several species live as commensals. Infection with a pathogenic strain could, however, cause diarrhea. These strains are divided into four categories (Table 54-1).

Enteropathogenic strains of *E. coli* were originally isolated from the feces of infants and young children with diarrhea. These strains do not produce toxins, and the mechanism of their action is unknown. The affected intestines show only minimal mucosal inflammation.

Enterotoxicogenic strains of *E. coli* are capable of binding to the surface of small intestinal epithelial cells. In the intestine these organisms adhere to the surface of small intestinal

Table 54-1 Diarrhea caused by *Escherichia coli*

Types of *E. coli*	Clinical presentation	Type of diarrhea
Enteropathogenic	Endemic and epidemic diarrhea in infants	Watery
Enterotoxicogenic	Infantile diarrhea in developing countries and "traveler's diarrhea"	Watery
Enteroinvasive	Diarrhea with fever	Bloody
Enterohemorrhagic	Hemorrhagic colitis and hemolytic uremic syndrome	Bloody

epithelial cells and produce two types of toxins: heat labile and heat stable.[35] Heat-labile enterotoxins have the same biologic effects as cholera toxin. These *E. coli* species are an important cause of diarrhea in small children and undernourished infants. Heat-stable toxins activate guanylate cyclase, which triggers an increase in the transport of fluid into the lumen of the intestine. These species of *E. coli* are usually ingested with contaminated food or water and are the most common cause of traveler's diarrhea. The affected intestines do not show any significant histologic changes.

Enteroinvasive strains of *E. coli* primarily affect the large intestine, where they produce necrosis of the mucosa and severe inflammation. *Enterohemorrhagic strains* of *E. coli* also affect the large intestine. These *E. coli* produce a potent toxin that can be tested on vero cells and are therefore called *vero cytoxin–producing* E. coli. These organisms cause hemorrhagic colitis and hemolytic uremic syndrome, which usually occur sporadically after the ingestion of contaminated food or raw milk.

Salmonella infection. Various species of *Salmonella* are pathogenic in both human beings and animals and are thus an important cause of zoonoses. The infection is most often acquired by eating contaminated food. Water-borne infection and person-to-person transmission are less common. *S. typhi* and *S. paratyphi* are the most common isolates, and these microbes cause enteric fever and diarrhea. The bacteria invade the ileal mucosa overlying Peyer's patches, causing local ulceration and inflammation. The villi adjacent to the ulcerated mucosa show edematous widening and congestion. The submucosa is congested and contains neutrophils, plasma cells, and prominent macrophages that have eosinophilic cytoplasm. The cytoplasm of the macrophages appears granular because it contains phagocytosed bacteria, red blood cells, and tissue debris. The adjacent lymph nodes, like the lymphoid follicles in Peyer's patches, appear hyperplastic and show sinus histiocytosis. *Salmonella* spp. cause systemic symptoms, and the hematogenous dissemination of pathogens is accompanied by nonspecific inflammation in the liver, spleen, and other organs.

Campylobacter infection. *Campylobacter* spp. are gram-negative rods that appear slightly curved and are pathogenic both for human beings and animals. Human infection occurs after the ingestion of contaminated meat and poultry or milk and water. *C. jejuni* is the most common isolate. It produces ulceration and intestinal bleeding, most prominently in the jejunum but also in the ileum and colon. The pathogenesis of these lesions is not known, but it appears that the ulcerations result from toxins produced by the *Campylobacter* organisms. Invasion of tissue has been demonstrated in children and undernourished persons.[35]

Yersinia infection. *Yersinia enterocolitica* and *Y. pseudotuberculosis* are gram-negative rods that cause food-borne gastroenteritis. Preschool children are most often affected. The disease presents with diarrhea, abdominal colic, and fever. The infection of the intestines is often associated with mesenteric lymphadenitis, and it may mimic acute appendicitis. In adults *Y. enterocolitica* infection is self-limited, but it may also cause protracted diarrhea. The most prominent histologic changes are found in the terminal ileum and cecum. These lesions may resemble those of Crohn's disease, in that the inflammation is typically transmural and may contain epithelioid granulomas.[36] Nevertheless, most granulomas also contain neutrophils and often show central abscess formation. Mucosal ulcers, serosal inflammation, and involvement of the intramural blood vessels are also found.[36] Mesenteric lymph nodes are enlarged and show follicular hyperplasia with a "starry-sky" appearance resulting from an abundance of macrophages. Necrotizing granulomas reminiscent of those seen in cat-scratch disease[37] are also seen.

Cholera. *Vibrio cholerae* is a short, curved gram-negative rod. It is responsible for causing water-borne epidemics that are still prevalent in Southeast Asia, Africa, and South America. Outside the endemic areas, asymptomatic carriers appear to be the main source of infection, which is usually transmitted by contaminated food. *V. cholerae* produces massive watery diarrhea. The bacterium resides in the small intestine and is noninvasive. However, it secretes a potent enterotoxin that activates the adenocyclase in the enterocytes, stimulating them to secrete water into the lumen. The high mortality in victims of cholera (50% if untreated) stems from dehydration and loss of essential minerals, which leads to hypovolemic shock. The mortality is less than 1% when patients undergo adequate fluid replacement therapy.[35] Histologically the intestines show no significant pathologic changes.

Shigellosis. Several species of *Shigella* are known to cause diarrheal disease in human beings, the most important of which are *Sh. sonnei,* which causes mild disease; *Sh. flexneri* and *Sh. boydii,* which cause severe diarrhea; and *Sh. dysenteriae,* which causes the most profound disease. Like *V. cholerae, Shigella* species have no animal reservoir. In contrast to *V. cholerae,* which may survive in the environment and is thus transmitted by contaminated food and water, *Shigella* spp. are transmitted only by the fecal-oral route.

Shigellae are highly pathogenic, and an infection can arise from the ingestion of less than 100 microbes. The pathogens attach to the mucosal surface in the ileum and colon, causing intestinal cell necrosis. Mucosal ulceration and inflammation develop fast but heal spontaneously. The prognosis in patients with infection is usually good, except in malnourished children in whom it may aggravate the general symptoms of protein-calorie deficiency *(kwashiorkor).*

Tuberculosis. *Mycobacterium tuberculosis* and *M. bovis* were important intestinal pathogens before the antibiotic era.[38] Today, intestinal tuberculosis is uncommon in the United States, but it is still prevalent in underdeveloped countries. The intestinal infection is a feature of secondary tuberculosis and is typically acquired by swallowing the bacteria expectorated from the lungs, or it is acquired hematogenously from a primary pulmonary focus. The ileocecal region is involved in most cases, but the disease may involve other parts of the gastrointestinal tract as well.[4]

M. tuberculosis invades the intestine, causing intestinal ulceration and fibrosis *(ulcerohypertrophic form)*. In a minority of cases the ulceration is not evident; instead the intestine shows confluent nodules and fibrosis extending into the mesentery *(hypertrophic form)*. It has been stated that the mucosal ulcers of tuberculosis tend to be circumferential and perpendicular to the long axis of the intestine,[4] but scarring may deform the intestine and obscure the original ulcer. Histologically the lesions contain caseating granulomas surrounded by prominent fibrosis.

Mycobacterium avium–intracellulare (MAI), a ubiquitous acid-fast microbe, has become an important cause of intestinal tuberculosis in patients with the acquired immunodeficiency syndrome (AIDS).[39] MAI typically involves the small intestine, causing diarrhea and malabsorption. Histologically the intestine shows focal superficial ulceration and contains mucosal infiltrates of periodic acid–Schiff (PAS)–positive macrophages (Fig. 54-8) similar to those seen in Whipple's disease. These macrophages contain numerous acid-fast MAI bacilli.

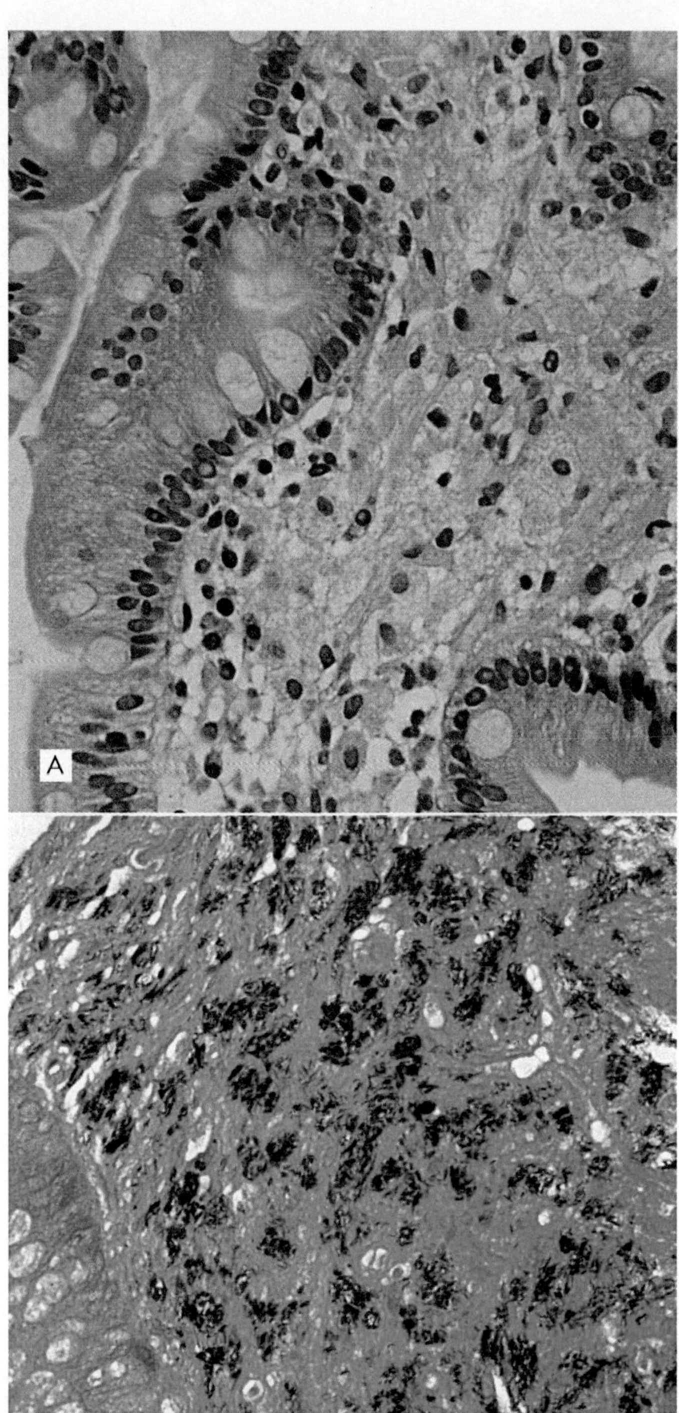

Fig. 54-8 Intestinal infection with *Mycobacterium avium–intracellulare* (MAI). **A,** The lamina propria contains numerous foamy macrophages. **B,** Microphages are filled with MAI, which are acid fast (Ziehl-Neelsen Stain).

Whipple's disease

In 1907 George H. Whipple described a disease that has since been known by his name, or as *intestinal lipodystrophy*.[39] This rare disease that typically presents with diarrhea and malabsorption is accompanied by systemic symptoms such as fever, arthralgia, hyperpigmentation of the skin, and anemia. The bacillus causing the disease, *Tropheryma whippelii*,[40] can be demonstrated by electron microscopy in the intestinal macrophages.

The most prominent changes are seen in the jejunum and ileum. Histologically the villi of the intestine are distorted and show dilated lacteals. The villi contain prominent infiltrates composed of PAS-positive macrophages and an increased number of lymphocytes (Fig. 54-9). Deposits of fat are found in the mucosa and the mesenteric lymph nodes. Like the dilatation of the lacteals, these changes probably stem from lymphatic obstruction. The macrophages appear to be impaired functionally. The lymphocytes in the mucosa are of the CD8 type. There is a reduced number of CD4 lymphocytes and IgA-secreting plasma cells. There is an increased number of IgM-positive cells.[39]

Viral enteritis

Viruses are an important cause of gastroenteritis[41] and are estimated to account for 30% to 40% of all the cases of infectious diarrhea in the United States. Rotavirus is currently the most common cause of diarrhea in infants and young children. The most important viral pathogens are listed in Table 54-2. In most instances the upper small intestine is the primary site of entry, whereas the stomach and colon are spared.[4]

The histologic findings in the small intestine may be prominent but are nonspecific. These changes include shortening of the villi and hyperplasia of the crypts, which usually contain an increased number of mitotic figures and appear dilated. The diagnosis can be facilitated by the electron microscopic finding of viruses in stool or mucosal biopsy specimens.

Fungal enteritis

Fungal infections occur predominantly in immunosuppressed persons.[42] Overall the incidence of mycotic infections revealed

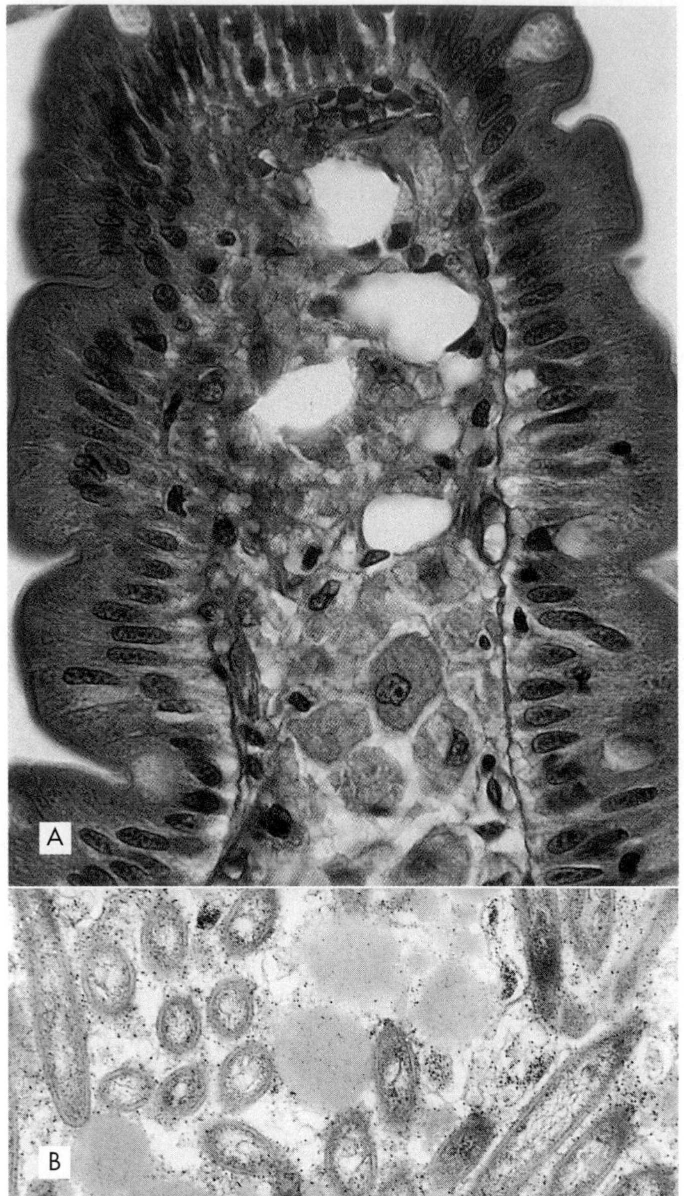

Fig. 54-9 Whipple's disease. **A,** Light microscopy study showing prominent macrophages in the lamina propria and dilated lacteals. **B,** Electron microscopy study of the pathogenic bacteria in the cytoplasm of intestinal macrophages. (Courtesy Dr. N. Ectors, Louvain, Belgium.)

by autopsy studies has been reported to range from 1% to 2%, but the incidence in immunosuppressed persons is about 20%. Infection of the intestines is found in 40% patients who have systemic mycoses.[42] The most common pathogens are *Aspergillus fumigatus* and *Candida albicans,* and the infections are most often limited to the mucosa and submucosa.

Parasitic infections

Parasitic infections caused by protozoa and worms are important causes of gastrointestinal disturbances. In the small intestine the most important protozoal pathogens are *Giardia lamblia* and *Cryptosporidium parvum.* Among the worms the most important are *Ascaris lumbricoides, Trichuris trichiura,* the hookworms *Ancylostoma duodenale* and *Necator americanus,* and *Strongyloides stercoralis.*[35]

Giardia lamblia was originally described by Anthony van Leeuwenhoek, the discoverer of the microscope, who examined his own feces. It is the most common intestinal parasite in the United States and Western Europe. In most instances it does not produce any symptoms, but it may cause diarrhea and malabsorption. Histologically the intestinal villi show either normal morphologic characteristics or some atrophy and nonspecific inflammation.[43] The parasites adhere to the surface of the villi and are readily identifiable in small intestinal biopsy specimens.

Cryptosporidium parvum is a coccidial protozoan that produces diarrhea in children in day care centers and in immunosuppressed persons, especially those suffering from AIDS.[43] Occasional water-borne infections are reported.[44,45] The infected small bowel contains parasites that adhere to the surface of the enterocytes. The parasite in its various stages of development, such as schizonts, merozoites, and macrogametocytes, can be visualized best by electron microscopy (Fig. 54-10).

Isospora belli is yet another parasite that can be found in the small intestinal biopsy specimens of patients with AIDS. Microsporida such as *Enterocytozoon bieneusi* and *Septata intestinalis* are obligate, intracellular, spore-forming protozoa.[46] These pathogens have also been noted with increasing frequency in patients with AIDS.

Worm infections are acquired by swallowing the infective eggs, as in ascariasis, or by transdermal infection with larvae, as occurs in *Ancylostoma duodenale* or *Strongyloides stercoralis* infection. Adult worms, larvae, or eggs can be detected in the intestinal contents or the crypts of the intestine in biopsy specimens.

Sarcoidosis

Sarcoidosis of the intestines is a rare disease of unknown cause. The disease is multisystemic and the intestines are typically involved, together with other organs. Sarcoidosis of the intestines can occasionally precede the symptoms of other organ involvement.[47]

MALABSORPTION SYNDROMES

The malabsorption of nutrients results from the ineffective uptake of substances from the intestinal lumen. Malabsorption may be the result of several pathogenetic mechanisms that impair the normal digestion and absorption of nutrients, and the resulting abnormalities can be classified as

1. Diseases affecting the intraluminal stage of digestion
2. Diseases affecting the intestinal stage of digestion and the absorption of nutrients
3. Diseases impairing the transport of absorbed nutrients
4. Endocrine and metabolic diseases affecting the functions of the intestines (Table 54-3).

Small intestinal biopsy specimens may be needed for the diagnosis of malabsorption syndromes to be established. The morphologic findings may be pathognomonic, or they may be significant but not diagnostic. Intestinal biopsy findings may also help identify the pathogens causing malabsorption. In

Table 54-2 Viral enteritis

Virus	Characteristics of virion (nm)	Epidemiologic characteristics
Rotavirus		
Group A	RNA (70-75)	Severe diarrhea in infants and young children
Group B	RNA (70-75)	Epidemics of diarrhea in adults and children (China)
Group C	RNA (70-75)	Sporadic cases of diarrhea in young children
Enteric adenovirus	DNA (70-80)	Diarrhea in infants and young children
Norwalk virus	RNA (27-32)	Epidemics of vomiting and diarrhea in older children and adults, often associated with consumption of shellfish, other food, or water
Calicivirus	RNA (27-38)	Diarrhea in children; in adults associated with consumption of food or shellfish
Astrovirus	RNA (27-32)	Pediatric diarrhea; reported in residents of nursing homes

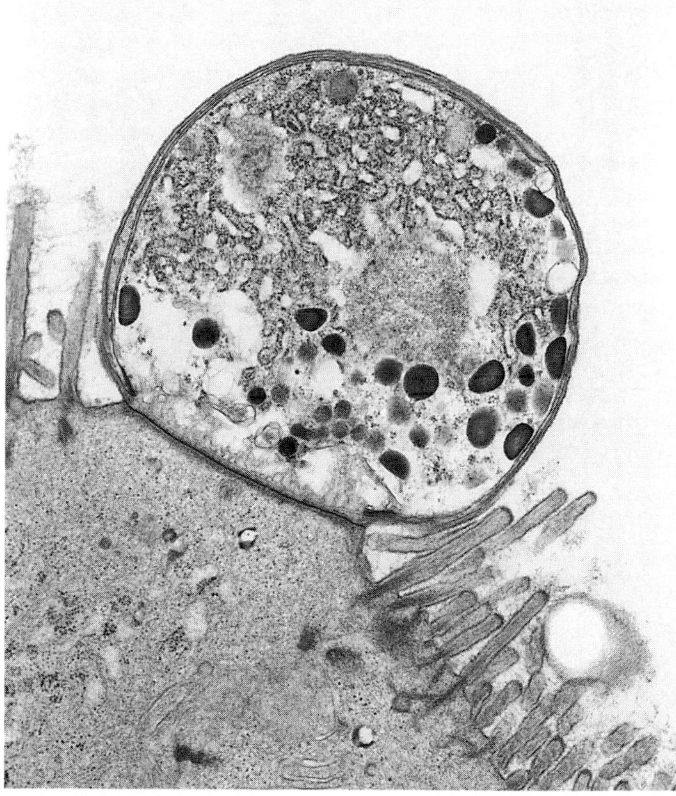

Fig. 54-10 *Cryptosporidium* attached to intestinal cell photographed by an electron microscope.

many instances the mucosal changes are mild or negligible, but even so, they may help in establishing the diagnosis through the process of exclusion (Table 54-4).

Celiac disease

Celiac disease, also known as *celiac sprue, nontropical sprue,* and *gluten-sensitive enteropathy,* is a multifactorial disease of uncertain pathogenesis.[48,49] It involves the formation of typical, though not pathognomonic, intestinal mucosal lesions, which are aggravated by the gluten in food and can be eliminated by a gluten-free diet.

The pathogenesis of celiac disease is not fully known, but it seems that genetic, nutritional, and immunologic factors play an important role. The disease usually commences in childhood and begins upon exposure to food containing grains. The most important precipitating factor is wheat gluten, which consists of a mixture of glutamine-rich and prolamin-rich gliadin polypeptides. Although gliadin is not intrinsically toxic to the intestinal mucosal cells, it causes the formation of typical mucosal lesions in susceptible persons. These abnormalities are eliminated once gluten is removed from the patient's diet, which indicates that diet has a critical pathogenetic role. Gluten-induced lesions occur only in genetically predisposed persons who have certain class II human lymphocyte antigens (HLAs). Celiac disease has been associated with HLA-DR3 and HLA-DQ2. These haplotypes have been found in 70% to 90% of all patients, irrespective of their ethnic origin and domicile. However, it is not known how having these particular HLA haplotypes predisposes these persons to the development of celiac disease, and it has been postulated that additional factors must play a role because most people who have these HLA markers are healthy. Immunologic factors have been implicated, and indeed most patients with celiac disease have IgA and IgM antibodies to gliadin. These antibodies are useful in establishing the diagnosis of celiac diseases. However, not all patients have antibodies to gliadin, and there is no direct proof that the antibodies detected in the serum or secreted *in vitro* from explants of mucosa are the cause of mucosal lesions or malabsorption.

The incidence of celiac disease is different in different countries and has been reported to be as high as 3 to 4 per 1000 in Ireland and Scandinavian countries.[50] It has been proposed that these differences may in part stem from the diet of the residents of these countries, but may also stem from differences in the fact that many mild cases are not diagnosed until adulthood or never at all. Set diagnostic criteria have been proposed by the European Society for Paediatric Gastroenterology and Nutrition[51] so that more cases will be diagnosed.

Celiac disease is diagnosed on the basis of the clinical and immunologic data in combination with the typical biopsy findings. Antigliadin tests can be used for screening asymptomatic pediatric populations, and results are typically positive in 60% of symptomatic patients. Most patients have diarrhea, but many patients do not. Anemia resulting from iron or folate deficiency, weight loss, weakness and depression, and amenorrhea may be the presenting symptoms in these latter patients. Children may show growth retardation and an increased sus-

Table 54-3 Classification of malabsorption syndromes

Disorders of intraluminal digestion
Gastric causes
Postgastrectomy syndromes
Pancreatic causes
Cystic fibrosis
Chronic pancreatitis
Pancreatic neoplasia
Hepatobilary causes
Cirrhosis
Cholestasis
Intestinal bacterial overgrowth
Hypomotility status (such as diabetes and scleroderma)
Anatomic abnormalities (such as diverticula, strictures, fistulas, and blind loop)
Parasites (such as *Giardia lamblia* and *Strongyloides stercoralis*)
Drugs (such as neomycin and cholestyramine)
Intestinal mucosal disorders
Genetic enzymatic defects (such as abetalipoproteinemia and disaccharide deficiency)
Celiac sprue
Inflammatory disorders
Viral or bacterial enteritis
Whipple's disease
Crohn's disease
Tropical sprue
AIDS-related disorders
Infiltrative disorders
Collagenous sprue
Amyloidosis
Scleroderma
Postradiation fibrosis
Neoplasia
Lymphoma
Carcinoids
Mastocytosis
Intestinal resection or bypass
Vascular and lymphatic disorders
Congestive heart failure
Mesenteric atherosclerosis
Vasculitis
Intestinal lymphangiectasia
Mesenteric fibrosis
Endocrine and metabolic disorders
Diabetes mellitus
Insufficiency of endocrine glands (thyroid, parathyroid, and adrenals)
Hyperfunctioning neuroendocrine tumors (carcinoid, gastrinoma, vasoactive intestinal polypeptide secreting tumor (VIPoma), and medullary carcinoma of thyroid)

Table 54-4 Small intestinal biopsy in malabsorption syndromes

Diseases associated with normal mucosal histologic features
Postgastrectomy syndromes
Inborn disaccharidase deficiencies
Short bowel syndrome
Hepatobiliary diseases
Pancreatic insufficiency
Drug-induced enteropathies
Alcoholism
Diseases associated with nonspecific changes
Celiac sprue
Tropical sprue
Dermatitis herpetiformis
Collagenous sprue
Microvillus inclusion enteropathy
Eosinophilic enteritis
Intraluminal bacterial overgrowth
Disturbances of intestinal motility
Zollinger-Ellison syndrome
Graft-versus-host disease
Radiation enteritis
Protein-calorie malnutrition
Mucosal lesions with identifiable pathogens
Viral infections
Cytomegalovirus infections
Bacterial infections
Mycobacterium avium–intracellulare
Whipple's disease
Fungal infections
Candidiasis
Histoplasmosis
Protozoan parasitic infections
Giardiasis
Cryptosporidiosis
Microsporidiosis
Coccidiosis
Metazoan parasitic infections
Ancylostomiasis
Strongyloidiasis
Capillariasis
Schistosomiasis
Diseases associated with diagnostic tissue changes
Abetalipoproteinemia
Amyloidosis
X-linked immunodeficiency
Lipid storage diseases
Chronic granulomatous disease
Lymphangiectasia
Mastocytosis
Waldenström's macroglobulinemia
Lipoid proteinosis

ceptibility to infections. The ultimate diagnosis, however, is made on the basis of the histologic appearance of intestinal biopsy specimens. Histologically the intestinal mucosa shows atrophy of the villi and lengthening of the crypts (Fig. 54-11). The number of mitotic cells in the crypts has been noted to be increased.[52] The intestinal cells lining the crypts appear cuboidal and have a more basophilic cytoplasm than normal cells do. The epithelium may show signs of hyperplasia and a loss of polarity, in that their nuclei are not in the basal part of the cytoplasm. The lamina propria appears hypercellular and contains an increased number of plasma cells, lymphocytes, macrophages, and eosinophils. The lymphocytes may be seen infiltrating the epithelial layer ("transepithelial migration of lymphocytes"). These intestinal changes are reversible, however, and disappear upon withdrawal of gluten from the diet.

The major pitfalls in diagnosing celiac disease on the basis of histologic findings occur because of poor sampling of tissue and tangential sectioning.[53] The most important intestinal complica-

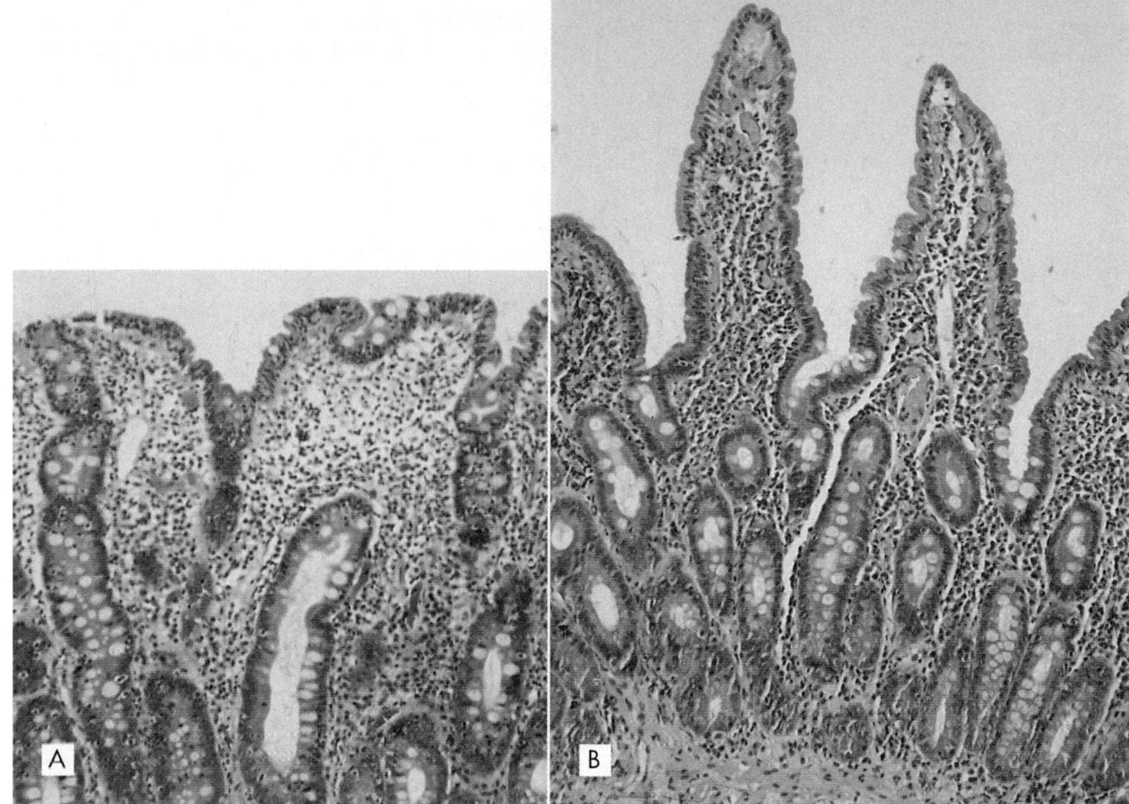

Fig. 54-11 Celiac disease. **A,** Intestinal biopsy specimen shows atrophy of the villi and lengthening of the crypts. **B,** After the patient was on a gluten-free diet for six months, the intestine shows almost normal features.

tion of celiac disease is lymphoma, which occurs in approximately 8% to 10% of the patients. Lymphomas usually develop in patients older than 50 years and are of the T-cell type.[48]

Tropical sprue

Tropical sprue is an imprecise term that is applied to a variety of diseases, presumably of infectious origin, that occur in residents of the tropics, with diarrhea being the presenting symptom. The pathogenesis is not known. The histologic findings in such patients are indistinguishable from those with celiac disease. In contrast to celiac disease, which predominantly affects the duodenum and ileum, tropical sprue uniformly involves the entire small intestine.[54] Broad-spectrum antibiotics are effective treatment.

Eosinophilic gastroenteritis

Eosinophilic gastroenteritis is a rare and poorly defined disorder.[55] The diagnosis, which is one of exclusion, should be rendered only in clinically symptomatic patients who do not have systemic eosinophilia or intestinal parasites. Isolated small intestinal disease is uncommon, and in most cases the intestinal involvement is associated with gastric lesions, which are more prominent. Because the predominant infiltrates are in the muscle layer and the subserosa, a mucosal intestinal biopsy specimen may be inadequate for arriving at a final diagnosis.

Microvillus inclusion disease

Microvillus inclusion disease is a congenital, rare malabsorption disease that presents with watery diarrhea in infants shortly after birth.[56] The intestines have a thin wall and flattened mucosa. There are no inflammatory cells, and the crypts do not show increased mitotic activity as they do in celiac disease. Ultimately the diagnosis is made on the basis of the electron microscopy finding of the inclusion of microvilli in the apical cytoplasm of enterocytes. Patients with the disease have a poor prognosis.

Intestinal microvillous dystrophy is another recently described entity that presents in infancy as an intractable diarrhea.[57] The diagnosis is made on the basis of electron microscopy findings.

Intestinal infiltrative disorders

Malabsorption can develop as a result of the excessive deposition of various substances in the wall of the intestine. Such material can be readily identified in intestinal biopsy specimens. Specific entities include *amyloidosis,*[58] *macroglobulinemia of Waldenström,*[59] which is occasionally associated with lymphangiectasia,[59] and *lipoid proteinosis*[60] (Fig. 54-12).

Deposits of collagen are seen in the settings of scleroderma and radiation enteritis, but also in the setting of *collagenous enterocolitis,* which is considered a rare variant of celiac disease.[61]

Small intestinal ulcerations

Ulceration can occur in the context of many intestinal diseases, including celiac disease.[62] Ulcers beyond the distal duodenum are rare, however. Causes of isolated jejunal ulcers include infectious diseases, foci of heterotopic gastric mucosa, ischemia, radiation enteritis, vasculitis, and tumors. Enteric-coated potassium tablets were the cause of small bowel ulcera-

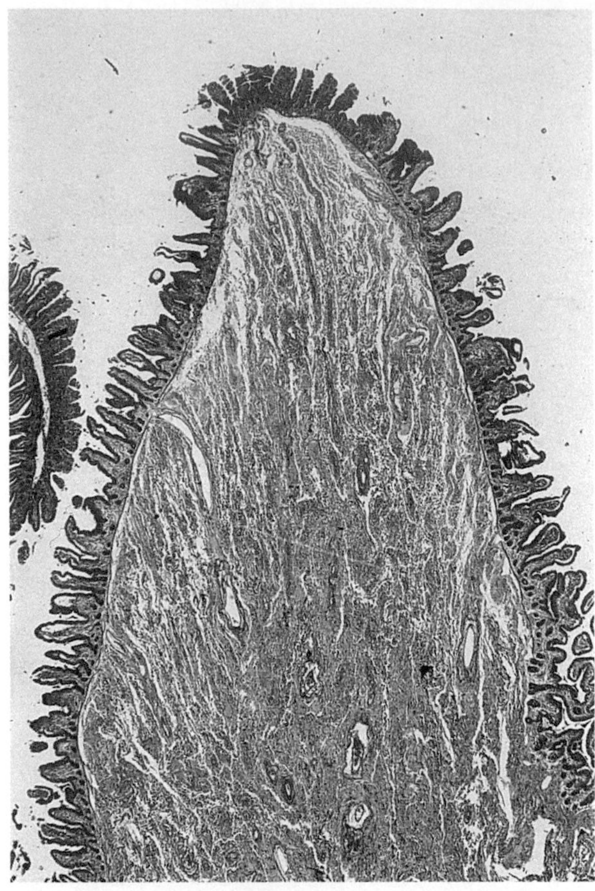

Fig. 54-12 Lipoid proteinosis. (Courtesy Dr. D. Caccamo, Detroit, Mich.)

tions in the 1960s, but these tablets are not used anymore.[63] Since the mid-1980s, the long-term use of nonsteroidal anti-inflammatory agents has been the most common cause of small bowel ulcerations. Such ulcerations may persist for a long time or recur and can rarely even lead to the development of perforations or strictures.[64]

Ulcers that cannot be related to specific causes are considered idiopathic. The term *ulcerative jejunitis* has been used for multiple ulcers of the small intestine found in some patients with malabsorption unrelated to gluten sensitivity.[65] Crohn's disease, which typically involves terminal ileus, is discussed in Chapter 56.

NEOPLASMS

Epidemiology and pathogenesis. Neoplasms of the small intestine are rare in comparison with those of the stomach or the large intestine; fewer than 2% of all alimentary tract tumors occur in the duodenum, jejunum, and ileum, even though these part of the intestines constitutes 75% of the total intestinal length and 90% of the surface area of the gastrointestinal tract.[66] Small intestinal cancer represents 0.5% of all malignant tumors of internal organs. The age-adjusted incidence per 100,000 is 1.4.[67]

Most malignant tumors of the small intestine can be classified as adenocarcinomas, carcinoids, lymphomas, or sarcomas. Ashley and Wells[66] surveyed 11 reviews of small intestinal cancer and found that carcinoids account for 35%, adenocarcinomas for 32%, and lymphomas for 21% of all malignant tumors. Di Sario and coworkers[68] reviewed the Utah Cancer Registry data and found that 41% of the tumors were carcinoids, 24% were adenocarcinomas, 22% were lymphomas, and 11% were sarcomas.

Weiss and Yang[67] calculated that the annual incidences of small intestinal malignant tumors, expressed as the number of cases per million, were as follows: carcinoids, 3.9; adenocarcinomas, 2.9; lymphomas, 1.6; and sarcomas, 1.2. Other studies have shown that adenocarcinoma is the most common malignant tumor of the small intestine.[68-70] From these studies it appears that adenocarcinoma accounts for approximately 40% of small intestinal cancer; carcinoids are the second most common neoplasm, accounting for 25% to 35% of cases; and sarcomas and lymphomas make up the remainder. The reported incidence of lymphomas is highly variable because it is often difficult to determine whether the tumor is a primary intestinal lesion or the intestine is involved secondarily by a systemic disease that presented only with intestinal symptoms but actually began in the abdominal lymph nodes.[71]

Studies that have investigated the etiology of small intestinal neoplasms have implicated several preexisting conditions in the pathogenesis of these tumors. Tuberculosis, Crohn's disease, and other chronic infections could all presumably predispose to the development of adenocarcinoma.[72] It has been generally accepted that celiac disease predisposes to the development of intestinal lymphoma.[73] An increased incidence of adenocarcinomas has also been observed in patients with celiac disease,[74,75] but a causal relationship between the intestinal disease and epithelial neoplasia has not been established.

Small intestinal epithelial polyps, like those in the large intestine, have a capacity to become malignant, and an adenoma-carcinoma sequence has been shown.[76] Familial adenomatous polyposis may involve the small intestine, and small intestinal cancer may develop in these polyps.[77] The bile may be an intestinal carcinogen,[78] but such a hypothesis needs additional corroboration.

Benign tumors

The exact prevalence of benign small intestinal tumors cannot be assessed precisely because many of these tumors are asymptomatic. Furthermore, the small intestines are often inadequately examined during routine autopsies and small lesions may remain unnoticed or go unrecorded. Nevertheless, Boyle and Lack[79] estimate that 60% to 75% of all small intestinal tumors are benign.

Adenoma

Small intestinal adenomas have the same features as the more common adenomas of the colon. Perzin and Bridge[80] noticed that most of these adenomas have a malignant component and most are located in the duodenum. Familial adenomatous polyposis is almost invariably associated with adenomas of the duodenum,[78] but other parts of the small intestine are not spared. Other familial polyposis syndromes such as Gardner's syndrome, Turcot's syndrome, Peutz-Jeghers syndrome, Cowden's disease, Canada-Cronkhite syndrome, and the Devon family syndrome are also characterized by small intestinal adenomatous polyps, which are often multiple.

Mesenchymal tumors

Mesenchymal tumors of the intestines include leiomyomas, schwannomas, lipomas, fibromas, lipomas, and hemangiomas.

Table 54-5 Immunohistochemical characteristics of gastrointestinal stromal tumors

Feature	Leiomyoma	Schwannoma	Gastrointestinal stromal tumors
Histologic appearance	Spindle cell neoplasm often with palisading	Spindle cell neoplasm often with palisading	Spindle cell neoplasm without palisading
Nuclei	Cigar shaped, perinuclear halo	Comma shaped	Fusiform
Electron microscopy	Fusiform dense bodies, filament bundles, pinocytotic vesicles, cell junctions usually absent, indistinct pericellular basal membrane partially present	Nondescript cytoplasm, rare cell junctions, pericellular basal membrane	Nondescript cytoplasm, no filament bundles, no pinocytotic, vesicles, no cell junctions, rare basal membrane
Vimentin	+	+	+
Desmin	+	–	+/–
Alpha smooth muscle cell actin	+	–	+/–
CD31 antigen	–	–	–
CD34 antigen	–	–	+
S-100 protein	–	+	–

Based on data from Pike AM et al: *Hum Pathol* 19:830, 1988; van de Rijn M et al: *Hum Pathol* 25:766, 1994; Miettinen M et al: *Am J Surg Pathol* 19:207, 1995.

The term *gastrointestinal stromal tumors* (GIST) has been proposed as an all-encompassing term[81,82] for spindle cell neoplasms. However, if histochemical analysis is done carefully, some tumors turn out to be leiomyomas and schwannomas (Table 54-5) and the term *GIST* should be reserved only for lesions that cannot be readily classified.[83] Hemangiomas of the small intestines may cause bleeding.[79] Lipomas are probably more common than the statistics show, but most are asymptomatic. Lipomas are most often found in the area of the ileocecal valve (Fig. 54-13).

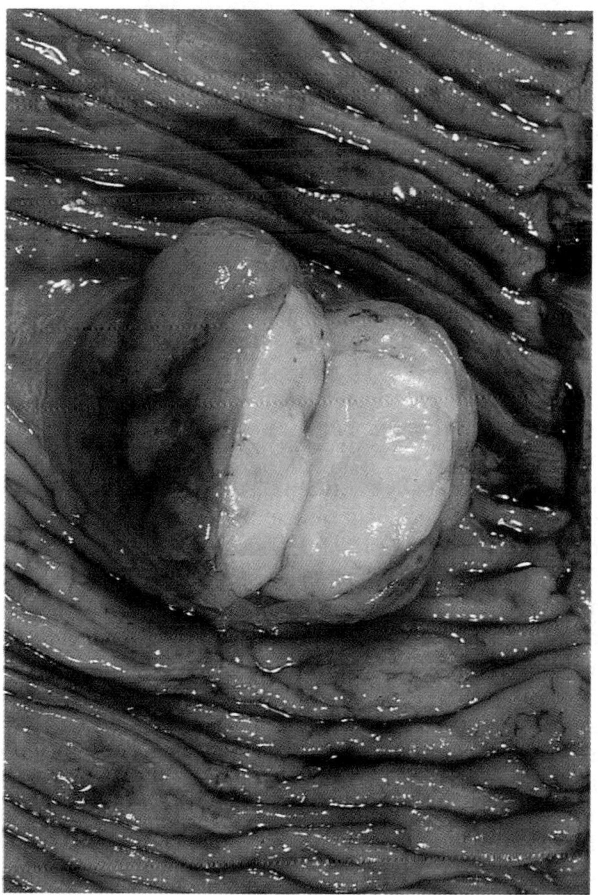

Fig. 54-13 Lipoma of the small intestine. (Courtesy Dr. W. V. Harrer, Camden, N.J.)

Malignant tumors

Most malignant tumors of the small intestine belong to one of four categories: adenocarcinomas, carcinoids, lymphomas, and sarcomas.

Adenocarcinoma

Most adenocarcinomas of the small intestine are found in the duodenum (40%) and jejunum (35%). Those that affect the distal ileum are rare but important complications of Crohn's disease. Overall, adenocarcinomas are more common in the elderly and show no sex predominance. Clinically they present with obstruction in 90% of the patients, whereas perforation, volvulus, and massive bleeding are less common presenting symptoms. Low-grade bleeding and anemia are common. On gross examination the tumors may be polypoid, ulcerated, or diffusely infiltrating. Metastatic lesions are typically found in local lymph nodes and the liver but are also found in other distant sites. Peritoneal seeding is also common. The prognosis is generally unfavorable, mostly because the tumors are detected late.

Carcinoids

Carcinoids occur in the small intestine approximately as often as they do in the appendix and the bronchi.[84-94] The ileum is the part most often affected (Table 54-6).

The age of patients varies, but most tumors arise in patients ranging from 50 to 70 years of age. Approximately 60% of patients have no systemic symptoms; the carcinoid syndrome, manifesting as diarrhea and flushing, occurs in 25%, whereas the remaining 20% of the patients have either diarrhea or flushing. Treatment may alleviate some symptoms and retard tumor growth,[84] but complete cure can be achieved only exceptionally once the tumor has metastasized.

Carcinoids are composed of neuroendocrine cells that structurally and functionally correspond to normal neuroendocrine cells of the gastrointestinal tract. The neuroen-

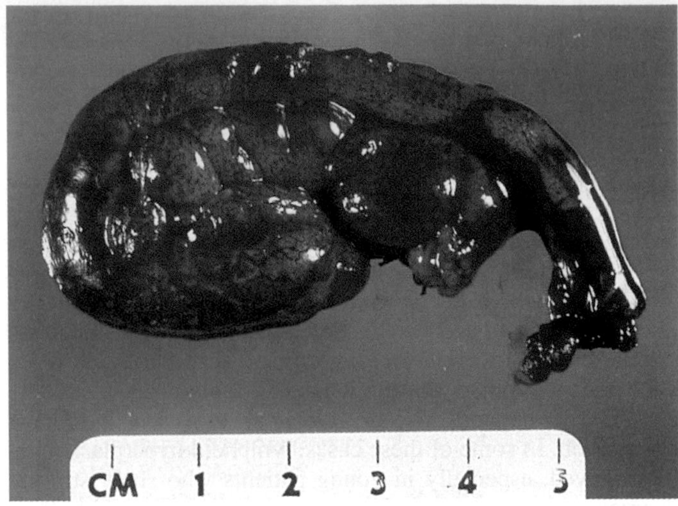

Fig. 55-1 Acute appendicitis with congestion of subserosal blood vessels.

may show marginating neutrophils in the lamina propria, as well as small collections of intraluminal neutrophils. Some authors believe that mucosal ulceration is required to accompany these changes to differentiate early acute appendicitis from artifacts of surgical manipulation,[34] whereas others believe that ulceration is not required.[35]

As the inflammation becomes more extensive, increased numbers of neutrophils can be found in the mucosa, causing cryptitis and crypt abscesses. The submucosa and muscularis propria are also inflamed, and extensive suppuration may result in gangrene and the development of focal defects in the appendiceal wall with subsequent perforation, resulting in periappendiceal abscess and peritonitis. Other complications include inflammation of the blood vessels draining the appendix and subsequent pylephlebitis, which can lead to the formation of liver abscesses or portal-vein thrombosis.

The existence of chronic appendicitis as a distinct clinicopathologic condition has been debated. Certainly, an organizing phase of acute appendicitis occurs, with the histologic findings of granulation tissue, a mixture of acute and chronic inflammatory cells and young connective tissue. However, true chronic appendicitis, with lymphocytes and plasma cells in the muscularis propria and serosa without significant acute inflammation, is rare.

Other specific bacterial infections

Typical acute appendicitis is usually caused by mixed coliform flora. Less often, appendicitis is caused by other bacteria, including *Escherichia coli*, *Enterococcus* spp., and other enteric bacteria.[36]

Actinomycosis

Actinomyces israelii is a normal constituent of the anaerobic flora of the mouth. On occasion, this organism may reach the appendix and cause mucosal injury, resulting in a suppurative appendicitis that may be complicated by a chronic periappendiceal abscess, or the formation of sinus tracts or fistulas.[37] This organism should be considered in any patient who develops a sinus tract or fistula after appendectomy. Histologically, neutrophils can be seen surrounding characteristic "sulfur granules," which represent masses of filamentous organisms.

Campylobacter infection

Campylobacter fetus subspecies *jejuni* usually causes a self-limited acute gastroenteritis but may cause a clinical presentation identical to acute appendicitis. In these cases, the mesenteric lymph nodes are often enlarged, and the appendix is grossly normal. Histologically, the changes in the appendix are similar to those described in *Campylobacter*-associated colitis.[38] Neutrophils, eosinophils, or both, are found in the lamina propria and in the surface and crypt epithelium, sometimes forming ulcers or crypt abscesses.[39] The histologic changes are limited to the mucosa and may resemble primary inflammatory bowel disease, but usually there are no indicators of chronic mucosal injury that are typical of primary inflammatory bowel disease. When stained with a Warthin-Starry stain, *Campylobacter* organisms can sometimes be seen as curved rods. Sometimes other techniques, such as immunoperoxidase or indirect immunofluorescence, can lead to a more specific identification.

Tuberculosis

On rare occasion, tuberculosis may be isolated to the appendix,[40,41] but it is usually associated with pulmonary or gastrointestinal disease. The presentation of tuberculous appendicitis may be similar to that of acute appendicitis and is characterized by the presence of necrotizing granulomas. The diagnosis may be confirmed by finding acid-fast bacilli with special stains or by culture.

Yersiniosis

Infection by *Yersinia pseudotuberculosis* or *Yersinia enterocolitica*, may cause a fatal systemic illness or a self-limited enteritis. Both organisms are small, gram-negative pleomorphic coccobacilli and may cause mesenteric adenitis with or without involvement of the terminal ileum, appendix, or cecum. Most patients are young and present with fever and colicky abdominal pain.[42,43]

Histologically, mesenteric lymph nodes show lymphofollicular hyperplasia with prominent germinal center formation and suppurative granulomas, often in the germinal centers.[42] Palisading histiocytes are found around a necrotic center, often with microabscesses. Similar changes are found in the appendix when it is involved[43] (Fig. 55-2). The differential diagnosis includes Crohn's disease, tuberculosis, sarcoidosis, tularemia, amebiasis, schistosomiasis, and actinomycosis. Careful histologic examination, serologic tests, and microbial cultures aid in this distinction.

Spirochetosis

Spirochetosis of the appendix has been found in patients with histologically proved acute appendicitis, but it is more common in patients who present with the clinical signs and symptoms of acute appendicitis with histologically noninflamed appendices ("pseudoappendicitis").[44] These organisms can be seen on hematoxylin and eosin–stained sections as a thickening or accentuation of the absorptive cell brush border, but identification is enhanced by use of special stains, such as Warthin-Starry or by electron microscopy. Epithelial damage is usually not seen. The significance of spirochetosis as a cause of appendicitis is debated.[35]

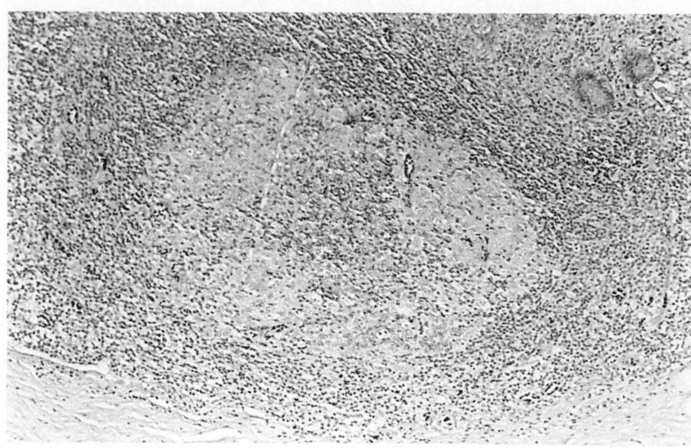

Fig. 55-2 Yersiniosis of the appendix, which shows lymphofollicular hyperplasia as well as a central microabscess surrounded by palisading histiocytes.

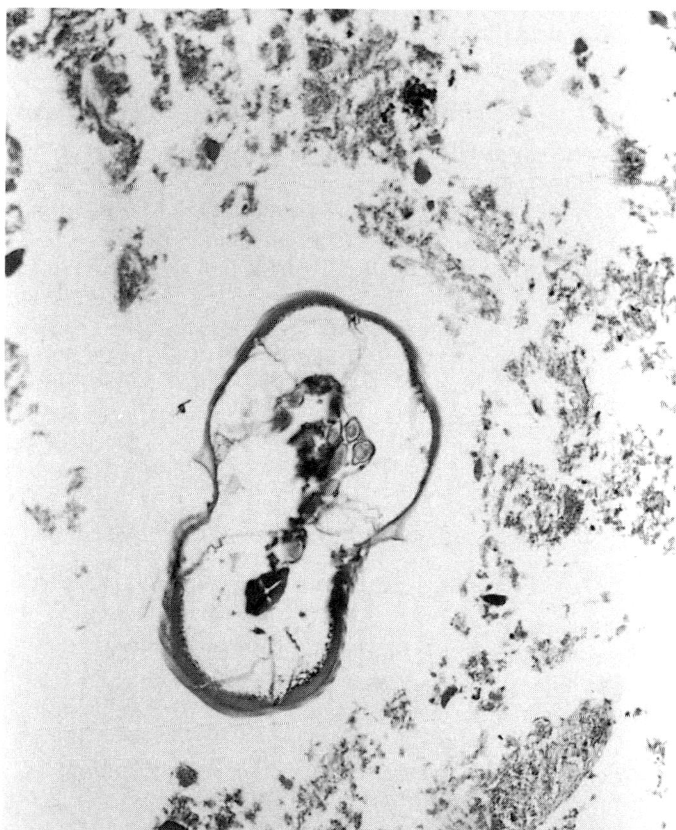

Fig. 55-3 Appendiceal enterobiasis. The mature female nematode is found in the appendiceal lumen and is characterized by its lateral cuticular alae.

Parasitic infections

Enterobiasis (pinworms)

Enterobius vermicularis is the most common nematode infection in humans. It is found in up to 3% of appendices in the United States.[45] The mature female nematode lives in the terminal ileum, cecum, appendix, and proximal ascending colon and migrates to the anal canal to deposit eggs in the perianal skin.[46] The role of this parasite in causing acute appendicitis is controversial. The adult worm is usually identified in the appendiceal lumen by recognition of its lateral cuticular alae[47-49] (Fig. 55-3).

Schistosomiasis

Schistosomiasis of the appendix is rare in the United States.[50,51] Although adult worms do not elicit an inflammatory response, a severe tissue reaction accompanies deposition of ova in the appendiceal wall. The organism may cause granulomatous schistosomal appendicitis, or the fibrosis induced by the ova may result in luminal obstruction, bacterial overgrowth, and the development of obstructive acute appendicitis.[52]

Strongyloides stercoralis infection (eosinophilic appendicitis)

Eosinophilic appendicitis is characterized by granulomas, often with central necrosis, and by associated tissue infiltration by eosinophilic leukocytes. Signs and symptoms vary, but only severe infection presents with clinical acute appendicitis.[53] Intact *Strongyloides* larvae have been identified in these granulomas only rarely.[54] Nevertheless, this parasite is believed to be the causative agent.

Viral infections

Measles

Characteristic histologic changes, similar to those found in the tonsils and adenoids, occur in the appendix during the prodromal stage of measles. These changes include lymphofollicular hyperplasia and the presence of Warthin-Finkeldey giant cells.[55] Patients may present with a clinical picture similar to that of acute appendicitis.[56] Measles virus ribonucleic acid has been detected in appendiceal lymphoid tissue by in situ hybridization in a patient infected by the measles virus, before the onset of subacute sclerosing panencephalitis.[57]

Adenovirus infection

The presence of adenovirus in the appendix has been strongly implicated in the pathogenesis of ileocecal intussusception.[58] It has been postulated that the virus may alter intestinal motility or cause lymphofollicular hyperplasia, predisposing to intussusception.[59] Histologically, smudgy, dark epithelial nuclei ("smudge cells") or eosinophilic intranuclear inclusions surrounded by a halo in epithelial cells are suggestive of adenovirus infection.[27] Infection can be confirmed by immunohistochemistry, in situ hybridization, or electron microscopy.

Cytomegalovirus infection

Gastrointestinal cytomegalovirus infection, most commonly of the esophagus or colon, is not uncommon in immunocompromised patients, particularly those with acquired immunodeficiency syndrome.[60] Appendiceal cytomegalovirus infection may occur, but it is rare.[61,62] Typical intranuclear and intracytoplasmic inclusions are identified in fibroblasts, in endothelial cells, and less commonly in epithelial cells. Ulcers with a neutrophilic infiltrate and even perforation have occasionally been seen in appendiceal cytomegalovirus infection.[63]

Infectious mononucleosis

Epstein-Barr infection and acute infectious mononucleosis rarely present with abdominal pain. However, those patients who undergo appendectomy often have histologic changes virtually identical to those seen in the lymph nodes of these patients. There is typically pronounced lymphofollicular hyperplasia with an expansion of the interfollicular zone by a polymorphous infiltrate of lymphoid cells, including immunoblasts, some of which bear a striking resemblance to Reed-Sternberg cells.[64]

Inflammatory bowel disease

Crohn's disease

The appendix is involved in over 25% of all cases of Crohn's disease coming to operation. However, reported examples of Crohn's disease first diagnosed and limited to the appendix number less than 100. These patients may present with signs and symptoms of acute appendicitis, or they may present with a mass in the right lower quadrant. Although some investigators believe that primary appendiceal Crohn's disease is a harbinger of disease that will appear later in other portions of the gastrointestinal tract,[65,66] others dispute this finding. Several studies have found that only about 7% to 10% of these patients eventually developed Crohn's disease at other sites,[67,68] and a fistula after appendectomy virtually never occurred. These authors believe that these cases are best classified as chronic (idiopathic) granulomatous appendicitis, a condition not nosologically related to Crohn's disease in the majority of cases.[67,69]

Histologic changes resemble those of Crohn's disease at other sites and are characterized by transmural inflammation with prominent lymphoid aggregates, patchy mucosal distortion, ulceration and fissures, and loose epithelioid granulomas. Differentiating this lesion from sarcoidosis, yersiniosis, tuberculosis, or parasitic infections may be difficult and often requires additional clinical information and special stains.

Ulcerative colitis

The appendix is involved in up to 50% of cases of resected ulcerative colitis.[70] The histologic changes in the appendix are similar to those in the colon, with mucosal distortion, expansion of the lamina propria by plasma cells, and variable epithelial damage. Although some authors have found that appendiceal ulcerative colitis may occur as a skip lesion, that is, appendiceal inflammation in the absence of cecal inflammation,[71,72] others have found appendiceal involvement to occur always in continuity with adjacent involved cecum, though disease activity may differ between the two sites[73,74]

Mucosal hyperplasia

Hyperplasia of the appendiceal mucosa may occur in response to mucosal injury and has been reported as a localized polyp or a diffuse process.[75-77] Most cases are found incidentally. There are reports of cases of nonneoplastic mucosal hyperplasia producing enough mucus to cause the gross appearance of a mucocele, but we believe that probably all these cases represent neoplastic cystadenomas. Females are affected more frequently, probably reflecting the increased frequency of incidental appendectomy in females. Most patients are older than 40 years.[75] Histologically, localized polyps closely resemble the more common hyperplastic polyps of the large intestine. There is elongation of tubules with serration of the luminal outlines and a proliferation of columnar and goblet cells, with occasional endocrine and Paneth cells. Although some investigators report subtle differences between these appendiceal hyperplastic polyps and typical colonic hyperplastic polyps, such as an increase in the goblet cell population relative to the number of columnar cells, and a lack of a thickened subsurface basement membrane,[78] we have not encountered these differences.

NEOPLASMS

The neoplasms of the appendix are rarely recognized clinically, and many are found incidentally in appendices removed for other reasons. The classification of epithelial neoplasms in this location is fraught with confusing terms, including *mucocele* and *pseudomyxoma peritonei*. These lesions have been classified by Appelman as follows:[78]

1. Colonic-type, noncystic, localized adenoma
2. Circumferential adenoma or cystadenoma
3. Adenocarcinoma
   a. colonic type
   b. mucinous
   c. signet-ring type

Mucocele

Few terms in appendiceal pathology have caused as much confusion as *mucocele*. It is probably best to consider mucocele as nothing more than a term used to describe a grossly dilated appendix filled with mucus. Mucocele cannot be used as a specific diagnostic term because its use in the literature embraces a morphologically and pathogenetically diverse group of conditions, both neoplastic and nonneoplastic. The neoplastic conditions, mucinous cystadenoma and cystadenocarcinoma, account for most of the appendices with a gross appearance of a mucocele.

Myxoglobulinosis is a rare variant of mucocele characterized by intraluminal mucinous and pearl-like globules, which occasionally calcify.[79] Histologically, the globules consist of faintly eosinophilic laminations of mucin around an amorphous granular and mucinous core. Myxoglobulinosis, like mucocele, is merely a descriptive term and does not imply any specific cause.

As stated above, we think it unlikely that other nonneoplastic conditions can ever result in the gross appearance of a mucocele, though several authors have advocated mucosal hyperplasia and retention (simple) cysts as causes of this condition. The term *retention cyst* was introduced by Aho in 1973 and refers to an appendix with a sterile outflow obstruction with resultant intraluminal mucus accumulation and luminal dilatation.[80] By definition, the mucosa is normal or flattened and lacks the features of hyperplasia or dysplasia. Obstruction may be caused by a variety of conditions, including fecaliths, endometriosis, carcinoid tumor, or a cecal tumor. It is possible that many of the cases reported as "retention cyst" actually represent cystadenomas in which the neoplastic epithelium was not sampled or was overlooked.

Adenoma

Colonic-type, noncystic localized adenoma

Localized adenomas, identical to those seen in the colon, occur in the appendix, but they are extremely rare.[81] Architecturally, they may be tubular, tubulovillous, or villous. Most are sessile, but, rarely, a small stalk can be seen. The epithelium has all the features of dysplastic colonic epithelium, with mucus depletion, cellular crowding and stratification, nuclear elongation, hyperchromatism, pleomorphism, and increased numbers of mitotic figures. Adenomas of the appendix may be isolated, associated with colonic adenomas, or can be seen in the setting of familial adenomatous polyposis.[82]

Circumferential adenoma or cystadenoma

Diffuse, circumferential adenomas or cystadenomas of the appendix are much more common than the colonic-type, localized adenomas. The distinction between these conditions is somewhat arbitrary, in that as localized or diffuse adenomas increase in size, they likely cause intraluminal accumulation of mucus with resultant luminal dilatation (cystadenoma).

Diffuse adenomas or cystadenomas occur in patients in the second through ninth decades of life, with a peak incidence in the seventh decade. Although a substantial percentage of cases are discovered incidentally, some patients present with signs and symptoms identical to those of acute appendicitis. Others have a palpable abdominal mass, usually in the presence of rupture with extravasation of mucus into the peri-appendiceal soft tissues, or pseudomyxoma peritonei (see the following page).

Cystadenomas may only be appreciable on microscopic examination of an incidentally removed, grossly normal appendix. Most patients with cystadenoma who present with acute right lower quadrant pain also have gross and microscopic evidence of acute appendicitis.[78]

Cystadenomas show variable cystic luminal dilatation and are filled with viscid mucus. The appendiceal wall often becomes thin and fibrotic as a result of the effects of pressure. Some show evidence of rupture and fibrosis of the surrounding soft tissues caused by a localized reaction to extravasated mucus (Fig. 55-4).

Most circumferential adenomas are composed of crowded columnar cells with basally oriented, elongated, hyperchromatic nuclei with large blobs of apical mucin. Epithelial ulceration may occur, and the mucin can elicit a stromal response of foreign-body reaction, granulation tissue, chronic inflammation, and occasionally calcification.[83] The luminal contour may be flat, slightly undulating, or villous (Fig. 55-5). Less commonly, circumferential adenomas may closely resemble ovarian mucinous tumors of borderline malignancy, with a villous luminal contour, serration of crypts, and stratification of mucus cells.[78] Either type may become highly dysplastic and may be found adjacent to an invasive carcinoma, suggestive of an adenoma (dysplasia)-carcinoma sequence similar to that proposed in the colon.[84,85]

When significant amounts of mucus accumulate in the lumen, the resultant increased intraluminal pressure may cause the adenomatous epithelium to herniate through points of weakness in the muscularis mucosae, resulting in epithelium that lies deep in the appendiceal wall.[86] This herniation may be difficult to distinguish from true invasion, which typically elicits a desmoplastic reaction in the surrounding stroma.[87] Pools of mucus may also dissect into and through the appendiceal wall and spill into the peri-appendiceal soft tissues, eliciting a fibrotic response (localized pseudomyxoma peritonei).[88] On rare occasions, large amounts of mucus may be found extruded into the peritoneal cavity (diffuse pseudomyxoma peritonei).

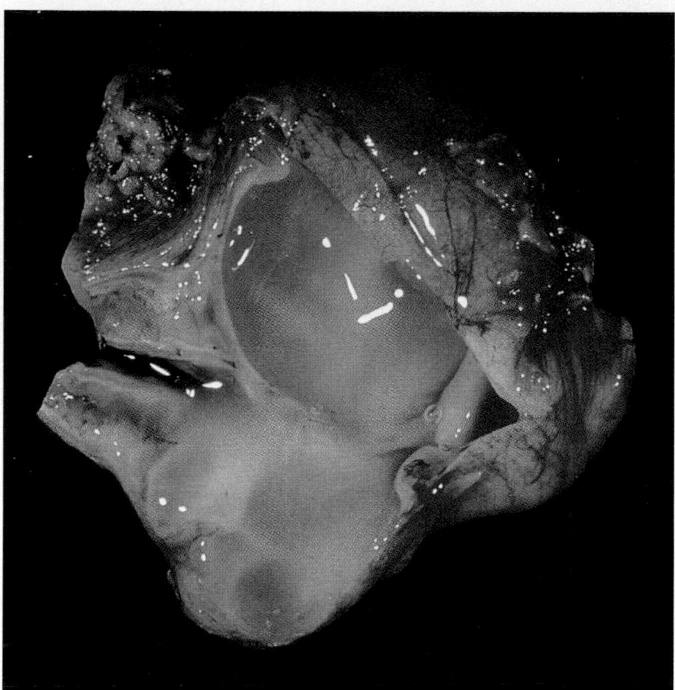

Fig. 55-4 Mucinous cystadenoma of the appendix with rupture and extravasation of mucus into the periappendiceal soft tissue.

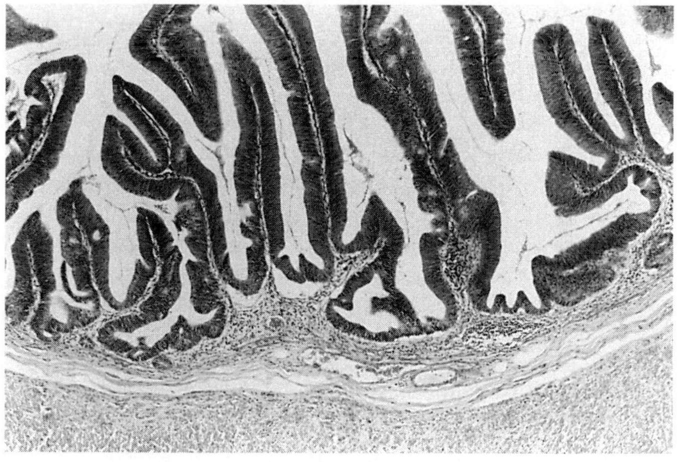

Fig. 55-5 Appendiceal cystadenoma with high grade dysplasia. The luminal contour has a villous configuration and severe cytologic atypia. However, invasive carcinoma is not present.

Adenocarcinoma

Invasive adenocarcinoma of the appendix

Invasive adenocarcinomas of the appendix are rare, and are less common than adenomas. They present as a solid, noncystic mass or as a cystic mucinous tumor (mucinous cystadenocarcinoma). Histologically, they can be classified as colonic-type, mucinous, or signet-ring adenocarcinomas.[78]

The peak age of incidence is similar to that of colonic adenocarcinoma, being found most often in the fifth to seventh decades.[89] There is a slight male predominance.[90] About 25% of cases are discovered incidentally. Seventy-five percent of patients are symptomatic and may present with signs and

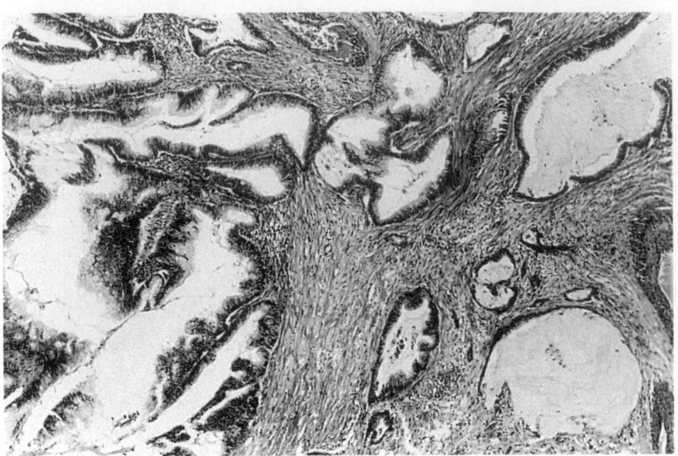

Fig. 55-6 Invasive adenocarcinoma of the appendix. Mucus-filled tubules are infiltrating the appendiceal wall and are associated with a desmoplastic stromal response.

symptoms of acute appendicitis, a palpable abdominal mass, or complications of pseudomyxoma peritonei (intestinal obstruction).

Mucinous cystadenocarcinomas may be indistinguishable from cystadenomas on gross examination and presentation.[81] If rupture occurs, a localized or diffuse form of pseudomyxoma peritonei may be found. In some cases, a firm nodule that infiltrates the appendiceal wall is seen.

In many cases of cystadenocarcinoma, the remnants of an adenoma with high-grade dysplasia can be seen at the edges of the neoplasm, supporting the existence of an adenoma (dysplasia)-carcinoma sequence.[84] When these tumors invade, mucus-filled tubules often become dilated, forming small intramural cysts (Fig. 55-6). There is a desmoplastic stromal response, which is useful in differentiating true from pseudoinvasion.[87]

The colonic type of adenocarcinomas, with the formation of small infiltrating glands, are rare. Signet-ring carcinomas, which closely resemble those found in the stomach, are even rarer and have a poor prognosis.[91] These lesions should be distinguished from adenocarcinoids (see below), which characteristically arise from the basoglandular portion of the mucosa, spare the luminal mucosa, show evidence of neuroendocrine differentiation, and have a generally better prognosis than that of signet-ring adenocarcinoma.

Although there is some disagreement, most studies advocate a right hemicolectomy (rather than simple appendectomy) for any invasive adenocarcinoma of the appendix.[81,92-95] This surgery is sometimes a two-step procedure, given that these neoplasms may be discovered in an incidentally removed appendix or in an appendix removed for clinically benign disease. If pseudomyxoma peritonei is present, meticulous removal of the mucus and peritoneal implants should be attempted ("bailing-out procedure").[96-98] Repeat laparotomy with aggressive debulking procedures to relieve bowel obstruction and recurrent disease increases survival.[92,96,98,99]

Pseudomyxoma peritonei

There is a great deal of confusion in the literature regarding the term *pseudomyxoma peritonei*. Some have used the term to refer to an accumulation of gelatinous ascites in the peritoneal cavity, regardless of whether epithelium is present.[83,100] This is the definition we ascribe to.[101] Others reserve this term for diffuse peritoneal involvement by a malignant, mucin-producing tumor.[81,96,97,102] Regardless of the definition, rupture of either a mucinous cystadenoma or cystadenocarcinoma can lead to pseudomyxoma peritonei. We agree with those authors who believe that adenomatous epithelium can be found in peritoneal mucus from a noninvasive appendiceal cystadenoma[84,100,101] and disagree with those who diagnose an appendiceal cystadenocarcinoma if any epithelium (even epithelium with low-grade dysplasia) is found in peritoneal mucus, regardless of whether actual invasion of the appendiceal wall is found.[81,96] However, regardless of what the primary appendiceal lesion is considered, it is generally agreed that the finding of epithelium in peritoneal mucus portends a worse prognosis, with recurrence of disease and increased complications, such as bowel obstruction.[96,101]

Patients with circumferential adenomas or cystadenomas with localized pseudomyxoma peritonei or no peritoneal mucus at all have an excellent prognosis after simple appendectomy. Patients with diffuse peritoneal mucus do somewhat worse, and the finding of epithelial cells in the extravasated mucus generally imparts a worse prognosis (regardless of whether they are considered cystadenomas or cystadenocarcinomas).[101] Finally, those patients with pseudomyxoma peritonei associated with a frankly invasive mucinous cystadenocarcinoma have a grave prognosis.

Coexistent appendiceal and ovarian neoplasms

The relationship, if any, between appendiceal and ovarian mucinous tumors remains controversial. Generally, spread of ovarian neoplasms to the appendix is relatively common, but it is typically limited to the outer appendiceal wall and is associated with disease in other sites.[103,104] In those female patients with concurrent appendiceal and ovarian mucinous tumors, some authors believe that in most cases, the lesions are independent and arise as part of a multifocal neoplastic process.[105,106] We believe that invariably the ovarian tumors represent metastases or implantation from a primary appendiceal mucinous neoplasm. This argument is supported by the increased frequency of bilateral ovarian tumors in the presence of an appendiceal tumor, as compared with ovarian tumors alone[103,107] as well as a preponderance of right-sided ovarian tumors in these cases, an indication that this predilection may be the result of the proximity of the appendix to the right ovary.[103]

Carcinoid

Carcinoids are neuroendocrine neoplasms that most likely originate from the mucosal neuroendocrine complex. This complex is located in the lamina propria of the appendix and contains a well-developed mucosal nervous plexus composed of collections of neuroendocrine cells, Schwann cells, neural processes, and occasional neurons. The complex can be accentuated using immunohistochemical stains (S-100, neuron-specific enolase, chromogranin).[108] The mucosal neuroendocrine complex is located just beneath the crypts, the area in which carcinoid tumors of the appendix are typically located.

Carcinoid tumors are the most common appendiceal neoplasm and have been found in up to 0.32% of surgically resected appendices.[109] Most are found incidentally in appendices removed for other reasons, but some patients do present with signs and symptoms of acute appendicitis. Patients rarely develop the carcinoid syndrome, which is almost always associated with a serotonin-producing tumor that has metastasized to the liver.[110] Even more rare is the development of an ACTH-producing tumor resulting in Cushing's syndrome.[111] The peak age of incidence for carcinoid tumor is between the third and fifth decades, and females are affected slightly more often than males, again probably reflecting the increased frequency of incidental appendectomy in females.

Pathology. Most carcinoids arise in the appendiceal tip, and measure less than 1 cm.[109] Although some tumors are appreciable only on a microscopic level, most form a well-circumscribed, homogeneous, white-to-yellow mass that infiltrates the appendiceal wall.

Appendiceal carcinoid tumors resemble other midgut carcinoids and are composed of a uniform population of small tumor cells that are arranged in sheets, nests, and cords, with occasional rosette or acinar formation[112] (Fig. 55-7). The nuclear chromatin pattern has a "salt-and-pepper" stippled appearance that is typical of neuroendocrine neoplasms in general. The cytoplasm is scanty and eosinophilic. Mitotic figures are difficult to identify. Some mucin may be seen in carcinoid tumors but not to the extent seen in goblet-cell carcinoids (see below). Invasion of lymphatic spaces is not uncommon.

Silver stains reveal the cells to be both argentaffin and argyrophil. Immunohistochemically, carcinoid tumors are typically positive for cytokeratin, neuron-specific enolase, chromogranin, and serotonin, though rare S-100–positive cells are also found, lending additional evidence that these tumors are derived from the mucosal neuroendocrine complex.[113] A variety of other peptide hormones, such as substance P, glucagon, and somatostatin, may also be found.[114] Ultrastructurally, membrane-bound neurosecretory granules are seen.

The prognosis of appendiceal carcinoids is excellent as a group. Lymph node metastases are rare and, when present, are usually found in tumors over 2 cm, though rare cases of carcinoids less than 1 cm have metastasized.[115,116] Invasion of the mesoappendix[116] and young age[115] may be indicators of aggressive behavior in tumors less than 2 cm. Simple appendectomy is adequate therapy for most cases, except for those tumors greater than 2 cm, those with evidence of metastatic disease, and cases with a tumor at the appendiceal margin. In these cases, right hemicolectomy has been recommended.[117,118]

Goblet-cell carcinoid

Since the late 1960s, over 100 cases of an appendiceal tumor that is distinct from carcinoid and adenocarcinoma but that has features of both have been described. Within this short period, several names have been given to this fascinating neoplasm including *crypt-cell carcinoma, mucinous carcinoid, adenocarcinoid, microglandular carcinoma,* and *composite carcinoma,* reflecting the controversy over its histogenesis.

Patients with this tumor are typically older than those with typical carcinoids, with most patients presenting in the sixth decade. Males and females are equally affected. Over 75% present with acute appendicitis, but occasionally this tumor is found incidentally.[78] Bilateral ovarian metastases are present at the time of presentation in a small number of patients.[119,120]

Pathology. The neoplasm may be found in any part of the appendix but is most common in the distal part of the appendix near the tip. These tumors usually do not produce a distinct mass but rather cause a thickening or induration of the appendiceal wall as a result of diffuse infiltration.[78]

Goblet-cell carcinoids arise from the basoglandular portion of the mucosa, typically sparing the luminal mucosal surface. No mucosal precursor lesion has been identified. The cells are arranged in tubular or glandular structures with occasional lumen formation and are composed of a mixture of intestinal cells that resemble those found in the normal intestinal crypt epithelium (hence the designation of *crypt-cell carcinoma*).[121] There are variable numbers of signet-ring and goblet cells that are filled with acid mucin (as shown with an Alcian blue stain), scattered Paneth cells, and occasional endocrine cells (which stain with chromogranin). Individual or groups of cells may be suspended in pools of extracellular mucus (hence the term *mucinous carcinoid*).[122] Most of the nuclei lay peripherally, and there is little nuclear pleomorphism or mitotic activity. As the tumor infiltrates the appendiceal wall, groups of cells lay widely scattered, often in a parallel array, with little stromal reaction[78] (Fig. 55-8). Perineural and lymphatic invasion are commonly seen.

The criteria for diagnosing goblet cell carcinoids vary. Burke and colleagues have distinguished between tubular carcinoids, goblet-cell carcinoids, and mixed carcinoid-adenocarcinoma.[123] Tubular carcinoids are nonargentaffin and express glucagon, unlike typical carcinoids. Intraluminal acid

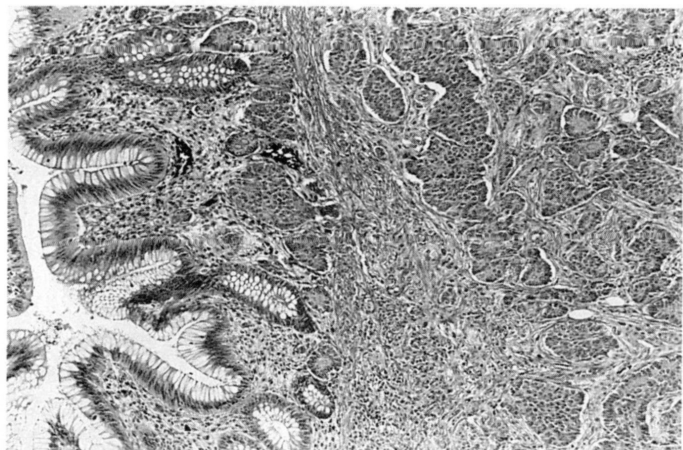

Fig. 55-7 Appendiceal carcinoid with nests of small uniform cells infiltrating the appendiceal wall.

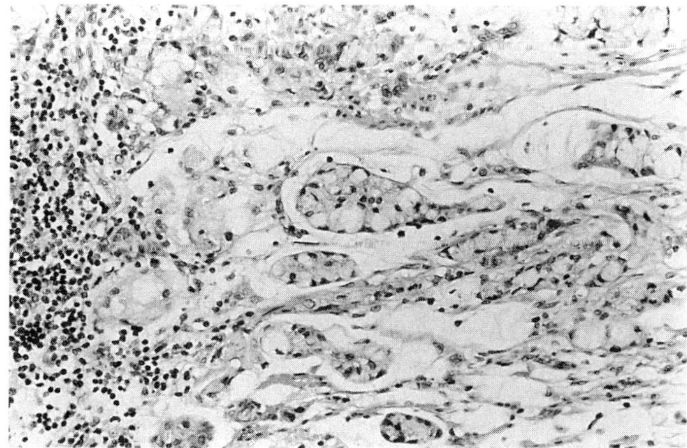

Fig. 55-8 Goblet cell carcinoid of the appendix with infiltration of nests, which resemble crypts containing goblet cells. These nests are suspended in pools of extracellular mucus.

mucin can be found, but the intracellular mucin that is characteristic of goblet-cell carcinoids is not prominent. Because all of their tubular carcinoids behaved in a clinically benign fashion, they classified these tumors as carcinoids. On the other hand, they reported on a subgroup of cases previously reported as goblet-cell carcinoids in which more than 50% of the tumor was composed of areas with typical invasive adenocarcinoma of the intestinal type. These tumors were clinically aggressive and had evidence of endocrine differentiation; some had foci identical to typical goblet-cell carcinoid. Because of the predominant carcinomatous growth pattern and the more aggressive behavior, these lesions were classified as mixed carcinoid-adenocarcinomas. Their typical goblet-cell carcinoids (described above) were associated with a prognosis worse than typical carcinoid and tubular carcinoid but better than mixed carcinoid-adenocarcinoma and typical invasive adenocarcinoma.

Ultrastructurally, both cytoplasmic mucin droplets and neurosecretory granules have been identified; however, there are conflicting data as to whether these are found in the same cell.[124,125] These tumors stain diffusely for cytokeratin, as well as for carcinoembryonic antigen and chromogranin in portions of the tumor showing adenocarcinomatous and neuroendocrine differentiation, respectively.

The prognosis of goblet-cell carcinoids has been considered to be intermediate between that of appendiceal carcinoid and adenocarcinoma. However, it is unclear what percentage of the cases in the literature are truly goblet-cell carcinoids (as opposed to typical carcinoids, tubular carcinoids, or mixed carcinoid-adenocarcinomas). Metastases were found in 20% of cases in one series,[126] but some of these cases were reclassified in another study as mixed carcinoid-adenocarcinoma, which the authors believed to be a separate condition with a worse prognosis.[123] Thus the true incidence of metastasis of these tumors is unclear. Several studies have documented bilateral ovarian metastases that resemble Krukenberg tumors and that may be mistaken for a metastasis from a gastric carcinoma.[119,120] Although some have identified a neuroendocrine component in the ovarian metastases,[127] others have not.[120] However, some of these cases may be metastases from mixed carcinoid-adenocarcinomas.

The optimal method of treatment of these tumors is also controversial, primarily because it has been difficult to obtain enough data. Although some advocate right hemicolectomy in virtually all cases,[128,129] others have found that appendectomy is all that is required if the surgical margin is tumor free.[123] Several studies have found that right hemicolectomy should be done in those cases with one or more of the following features: (1) spread beyond the appendix, (2) moderate-to-severe nuclear anaplasia, or (3) two or more mitoses per 10 high-power fields.[126,130]

Other tumors

Neurofibroma

Neurofibromas may be found anywhere in the gastrointestinal tract, but they are most common in the stomach and small intestines. Rare cases of appendiceal neurofibroma have been described, several of which have been manifestations of von Recklinghausen's disease.[131,132] However, solitary appendiceal neurofibromas have also been described.[133] These tumors resemble neurofibromas elsewhere, with wavy cells found in a mast cell–rich, loose myxoid matrix. The majority of cells showed the presence of S-100 protein. Neuromatous hyperplasia, which may resemble neurofibroma, is a common change typically found in the distal part of the appendix, particularly in elderly individuals.

Granular cell tumor

The gastrointestinal tract is a rare site for this tumor. In a study of gastrointestinal granular cell tumors, 4 of 75 cases were found in the appendix.[134] All four patients presented with signs and symptoms of acute appendicitis. The tumors are composed of polygonal cells with bland nuclei and granular cytoplasm. Immunohistochemically, they are strongly S-100 protein positive, and the membrane-bound lysosomal type of granules can be seen by electron microscopy. Granular cell transformation of the appendiceal smooth muscle cells does occur[135] and may give the appearance of granular cell tumor, but these cells are S-100 protein negative and ultrastructurally have actin-like filaments, indicative of their smooth muscle origin.

Paraganglioma

A paraganglioma is extremely rare in the gastrointestinal tract, being most common in the duodenum.[136] However, a mesoappendiceal paraganglioma with the typical nesting of cells *(Zellballen)* has been described.[137]

Lymphoma

The gastrointestinal tract is the most common site of extranodal lymphoma. Although the appendix may be involved by direct extension of an intestinal lymphoma, primary appendiceal lymphomas are exceedingly rare.[138] However, if the lymphoma is localized to the appendix, appendectomy may be curative.[139,140] Any type of non-Hodgkin's lymphoma may involve the appendix, but a preponderant number of cases are Burkitt's lymphoma.[141] Patients may present with a right lower quadrant mass, or with the clinical signs and symptoms of acute appendicitis.

MISCELLANEOUS LESIONS

Heterotopias

Heterotopic tissues may rarely be found in the appendix, including pancreatic,[6] esophageal, and gastric tissues.[142]

Hirschsprung's disease (aganglionosis)

In some cases, the loss of colonic ganglion cells may extend as far as the appendix, typically presenting as intestinal obstruction in a neonate.[143] Early surgical treatment is required for survival. As a result of the increased intraluminal pressure, appendiceal dilatation and perforation may result.[144]

Sarcoidosis

Sarcoidosis is a multisystem granulomatous disease that may affect the gastrointestinal tract and rarely the appendix. Most of the case reports describe noncaseating epithelioid granulomas in patients with histologic evidence of acute appendicitis.[145,146] However, sarcoidosis of the appendix may produce signs and symptoms in the absence of acute inflammation.[147] Evidence of systemic sarcoidosis is useful in distinguishing this condition from Crohn's disease.[148]

Endometriosis

Endometriosis of the appendix has been found in up to 3% of patients with documented pelvic endometriosis.[149] On occasion, the appendix may be the only site of involvement. Patients are often asymptomatic, and endometriosis is usually found incidentally. However, patients may present with signs and symptoms of acute appendicitis,[150] and preoperative differentiation of these two conditions may be difficult. Appendiceal endometriosis may be complicated by appendiceal rupture or intussusception.[151] Histologically, endometrial glands and stroma with associated hemosiderin are found, typically in the seromuscular layers, and often associated with hypertrophy of the muscularis propria.

Cystic fibrosis

The appendix is often involved in cystic fibrosis. Typically, the appendix is dilated or occluded with inspissated mucus. Histologically there is hyperplasia and hypersecretion by goblet cells, distention of crypts by eosinophilic secretions, and thick luminal mucus adherent to the mucosal surface.[152]

Patients may present with a right lower quadrant mass caused by fecal impaction, intestinal obstruction, or intussusception.[153] Patients may also have recurrent abdominal pain, prompting laparotomy and appendectomy before the diagnosis of cystic fibrosis.[154] Although acute appendicitis actually occurs less frequently in patients with cystic fibrosis than in the general population, possibly as a result of the distention of the appendiceal lumen by mucus,[155] the diagnosis of acute appendicitis in these patients may be difficult and is often delayed, frequently resulting in the development of periappendiceal abscesses.[156]

Intussusception

Appendiceal intussusception is very rare, being found in only 0.01% of appendices.[6] Patients may be of any age group and may be asymptomatic or present with acute or chronic episodic right lower quadrant pain. On endoscopy, the intussuscepted appendix may be mistaken for a cecal mass and biopsied, with the risk of a resultant peritonitis.[157]

Organic lesions, such as appendiceal endometriosis,[151] cystadenoma,[158] adenocarcinoma,[159] or a carcinoid tumor,[160] may cause intussusception. Other, more common appendiceal conditions, such as lymphofollicular hyperplasia or a fecalith, may rarely cause this condition.[161] The classification of the type of intussusception depends on the extent and portion of the appendix involved.[159] The extent of surgical therapy depends on the underlying cause.[162]

Fibrous obliteration (appendiceal neuroma)

Partial or complete obliteration of the appendiceal lumen is relatively common and has been reported in up to 35% of surgical specimens. This process typically affects the tip or distal aspect of the appendix, but occasionally the entire lumen is obliterated. Histologically the lumen is replaced by a collection of spindled cells in a loose fibromyxoid background, mixed with variable numbers of chronic inflammatory cells, fat, and collagen. Usually, there is a loss of mucosa, crypts, and lymphoid follicles.

Recent studies have suggested that most of these cases represent a neurogenic proliferation and have been termed *appendiceal neuromas*, or *neurogenic appendiculopathy*.[163,164] Immunohistochemically, most of the spindled cells are S-100 positive and ultrastructurally have the features of Schwann cells. There are also cells that stain with neuron-specific enolase and chromogranin, an indication that neuroendocrine cells may be an integral part of this proliferation.[163]

Intramucosal neuromas that resemble the central obliterative form may also occur and expand the lamina propria and separate the crypts.[163] These neuromas are typically found incidentally in appendectomy specimens. They are composed of cells that stain with S-100, neuron-specific enolase, and chromogranin. Ganglioneuromas do occur but are extremely rare.[165] They have been associated with von Recklinghausen's disease.[166]

The pathogenesis of the process remains unclear. Most investigators doubt that it is a sequela of appendicitis, and many believe that fibrous obliteration–neuroma may be the result of hyperplasia of neuroendocrine cells.[163] Interestingly, "appendiceal carcinoids" are often reported in association with fibrous obliteration–neuroma. Perhaps the excellent prognosis of appendiceal carcinoids relative to other gut carcinoid tumors is the result of the fact that many reported cases may be exaggerated endocrine-cell hyperplasia seen in otherwise typical fibrous obliteration. Therefore, we have strict criteria for the diagnosis of appendiceal carcinoid: (1) there must be neoplastic cells with a definite insular pattern and extension of cells into or through the muscularis propria, and (2) these cells must be associated with a gross nodular thickening of the appendiceal wall.[35]

REFERENCES

Normal appendix

1. Buschard K, Kjaeldgaard A: Investigation and analysis of the position, fixation, length, and embryology of the vermiform appendix, *Acta Chir Scand* 139:293, 1973.
2. Gray GF Jr, Wackym PA: Surgical pathology of the vermiform appendix, *Path Annu* 21(pt 2):111, 1986.
3. Segal GH, Petras RE: Vermiform appendix. In Sternberg SS, editor: *Histology for pathologists*, New York, 1992, Raven Press.
4. Gershon MD, Erde SM: The nervous system of the gut, *Gastroenterology* 80:1571, 1981.
5. Krishnamurthy S, Schuffler MD: Pathology of neuromuscular disorders of the small intestine and colon, *Gastroenterology* 93:610, 1970.

Developmental abnormalities

Duplications

6. Collins DC: 71,000 human appendix specimens: a final report summarizing 40 years' study, *Am J Proctol* 14:365, 1963.
7. Waugh TR: Appendix vermiformis duplex, *Arch Surg* 42:311, 1941.
8. Wallbridge PH: Double appendix, *Br J Surg* 50:346, 1963.
9. Bluett MK, Halter SA, Salhany KE, O'Leary JP: Duplication of the appendix mimicking adenocarcinoma of the colon, *Arch Surg* 122:817, 1987.
10. Ravitch MM: Hindgut duplication: doubling of colon and genital-urinary tracts, *Ann Surg* 137:588, 1953.

Agenesis and hypoplasia

11. Shand JE, Bremner DN: Agenesis of the appendix in a thalidomide child, *Br J Surg* 64:203, 1977.
12. Bremner DN, Mooney G: Agenesis of the appendix: a further thalidomide anomaly (Letter), *Lancet* 1:826, 1978.

Malposition

13. Moore KL, Persaud TVN: *The developing human: clinically oriented embryology*, ed 5, Philadelphia, 1993, Saunders.

Diverticulosis

14. Collins DC: Diverticula of the vermiform appendix, *Ann Surg* 104:1001, 1936.
15. George DH: Diverticulosis of the vermiform appendix in patients with cystic fibrosis, *Hum Pathol* 18:75, 1987.

16. Srouji MN, Chatten J, David C: Pseudodiverticulosis of the appendix with neonatal Hirschsprung's disease, *J Pediatr* 93:988, 1978.
17. Favara BE: Multiple congenital diverticula of the vermiform appendix, *Am J Clin Pathol* 49:60, 1968.
18. Deschenes L, Couture J, Garneau R: Diverticulitis of the appendix, *Am J Surg* 121:706, 1971.
19. Gardham AJ, Choyce CC, Randall M: Diverticulosis of the appendix in pseudomyxoma peritonei, *Br J Surg* 16:62, 1928.
20. Trollope ML, Lindenauer M: Diverticulosis of the appendix: a collective review, *Dis Col Rect* 17:200, 1974.

Inflammatory disorders

Acute appendicitis

21. Basta M, Morton NE, Mulvihill JJ et al: Inheritance of acute appendicitis: familial aggregation and evidence of polygenic transmission, *Am J Hum Genet* 46:377, 1990.
22. Addiss DG, Shaffer N, Fowler BS, Tauxe RV: The epidemiology of appendicitis and appendectomy in the United States, *Am J Epidemiol* 132:910, 1990.
23. Wangensteen OH, Bowers WF: Significance of the obstructive factor in the genesis of acute appendicitis, *Arch Surg* 34: 496, 1937.
24. Pieper R, Kager L, Tidefeldt U: Obstruction of appendix vermiformis causing acute appendicitis: an experimental study in the rabbit, *Acta Chir Scand* 148:63, 1982.
25. Chang AR: An analysis of 3,003 appendices, *Aust NZ J Surg* 51:169, 1981.
26. Nathans AA, Merenstein H, Brown S: Lymphoid hyperplasia of the appendix, *Pediatrics* 12:516, 1955.
27. Reif RM: Viral appendicitis, *Hum Pathol* 12:193, 1981.
28. Packard GB, McLauthlin CH: Acute appendicitis in children, *J Pediatr* 39:708, 1951.
29. Williams JS, Hale HW Jr: Acute appendicitis in the elderly: review of 83 cases, *Ann Surg* 162:208, 1965.
30. Blind J, Dahlgren S: The continuing challenge of the negative appendix, *Acta Chir Scand* 152:623, 1986.
31. Blair NP, Brigis SP, Turner LJ, MacCleod MM: Review of the pathologic diagnoses of 2,216 appendectomy specimens, *Am J Surg* 165:618, 1993.
32. Schirmer BD, Schmieg RE, Dix J et al: Laparoscopic versus traditional appendectomy for suspected appendicitis, *Am J Surg* 165:670, 1993.
33. Therkelson F: On histologic diagnosis of appendicitis, *Acta Chir Scand* 94(suppl 108):1, 1948.
34. Butler C: Surgical pathology of acute appendicitis, *Hum Pathol* 12:870, 1981.
35. Petras RE: Non-neoplastic intestinal diseases. In Sternberg SS, editor: *Diagnostic surgical pathology*, New York, 1994, Raven Press.

Bacterial infections

36. Bennion RS, Baron EJ, Thompson JE et al: The bacteriology of gangrenous and perforated appendicitis—revisited, *Ann Surg* 211:165, 1990.
37. Goner S, Allard M, Boileau GR: Appendicovesicle fistula caused by ileocecal actinomycosis, *Can J Surg* 25:23, 1982.
38. Van Spreeuwal JP, Duursma GC, Meijer CJLM et al: *Campylobacter* colitis: histologic, immunohistochemical, and ultrastructural findings, *Gut* 26:945, 1985.
39. Van Spreeuwal JP, Lindeman J, Bax R et al: *Campylobacter*-associated appendicitis: prevalence and clinicopathologic features, *Pathol Annu* 22(PT1):55, 1987.
40. Mittal VK, Kahnna SK, Gupta NM, Aikat M: Isolated tuberculosis of the appendix, *Am Surg* 41:172, 1975.
41. Morrison H, Mixter CG, Schlessinger MJ, Ober WB: Tuberculosis localized in the vermiform appendix, *N Engl J Med* 246:329, 1978.
42. El-Miraghi NRH, Mair NS: The histopathology of enteric infection with *Yersinia pseudotuberculosis*, *Am J Clin Pathol* 71:631, 1979.
43. Bennion RS, Thompson JE Jr, Gil J, Schmit PJ: The role of *Yersinia enterocolitica* in appendicitis in the southwestern United States, *Am Surg* 57:766, 1991.
44. Henrik-Nielsen R, Lundbeck FA, Teglbjaerg PS et al: Intestinal spirochetosis of the vermiform appendix, *Gastroenterology* 88:971, 1985.

Parasitic infections

45. Ashburn LL: Appendiceal oxyuriasis: its incidence and relationship to appendicitis, *Am J Pathol* 17:841, 1941.
46. Symmers WSC: Pathology of oxyuriasis, *Arch Pathol* 50:475, 1950.
47. Aschoff L: Appendicopathia oxyurica (pseudoappendicitis exoxyure), *Med Klin* 9:249, 1913.
48. Eastwood EH: The relation between appendicitis, *Oxyuris vermicularis* and local eosinophilia in the appendix wall, *J Pathol Bacteriol* 26:69, 1923.
49. Mogensen K, Pahle E, Kowalski K: *Enterobius vermicularis* and acute appendicitis, *Acta Chir Scand* 151:705, 1985.
50. Adebamowo CA, Akang EEU, Ladipo JK, Ajao OG: Schistosomiasis of the appendix, *Br J Surg* 78:1219, 1991.
51. Onuigbo WIB: Appendiceal schistosomiasis: method of classifying oviposition and inflammation, *Dis Col Rect* 28:397, 1985.
52. Satti MB, Tamimi DM, Sohaibani MO, Quorain AAL: Appendicular schistosomiasis: a cause of clinical acute appendicitis? *J Clin Pathol* 40:424, 1987.
53. Stemmerman GN: Eosinophilic granuloma of the appendix: a study of its relation to *Strongyloides* infestation, *Am J Clin Pathol* 36:524, 1961.
54. Noodleman JS: Eosinophilic appendicitis: demonstration of *Strongyloides stercoralis* as a causative agent, *Arch Pathol Lab Med* 105:148, 1981.

Viral infections

55. Herzberg M: Giant cells in the lymphoid tissue of the appendix in the prodromal stage of measles, *JAMA* 98:1139, 1932.
56. Elek E, Pinter A: Histologic changes in the appendix in the prodromal stage of measles, *Morphol Igazsagugyi Orv Sz* 30:230, 1990.
57. Fournier JG, Lebon P, Bouteille M et al: Subacute sclerosing panencephalitis: detection of measles virus RNA in appendix lymphoid tissue before clinical signs, *Br Med J* 293:523, 1986.
58. Porter HJ, Padfield CJH, Peres LC et al: Adenovirus and intranuclear inclusions in appendices in intussusception, *J Clin Pathol* 46:154, 1993.
59. Yunis EJ, Atchison RW, Michaels RH, DeCicco FA: Adenovirus and ileocecal intussusception, *Lab Invest* 33:347, 1975.
60. Knapp AB, Horst DA, Eliopoulos G et al: Widespread cytomegalovirus gastroenterocolitis in a patient with acquired immunodeficiency syndrome, *Gastroenterology* 85:1399, 1983.
61. Tucker RM, Swanson S, Wenzel RP: Cytomegalovirus and appendiceal perforation in a patient with AIDS, *South Med J* 82:1056, 1989.
62. Valerdiz-Casasola S, Pardo-Mindán FJ: Cytomegalovirus infection of the appendix in a patient with the acquired immunodeficiency syndrome, *Gastroenterology* 101:247, 1991.
63. Neumayer LA, Makai R, Ampel NM, Zukoski CF: Cytomegalovirus appendicitis in a patient with human immunodeficiency virus infection, *Arch Surg* 128:467, 1993.
64. O'Brien A, O'Briain DS: Appendiceal lymphoid tissue involvement parallels characteristic lymph node changes, *Arch Pathol Lab Med* 109:680, 1985.

Crohn's disease

65. Ewen SWB, Anderson J, Galloway JMD et al: Crohn's disease initially confined to the appendix, *Gastroenterology* 60:853, 1971.
66. Nugent FW: Crohn's disease of the appendix (Editorial), *Am J Gastroenterol* 65:83, 1976.
67. Ariel I, Vinograd I, Hershlag A et al: Crohn's disease isolated to the appendix: truths and fallacies, *Hum Pathol* 17:1116, 1986.
68. Timmcke AE: Granulomatous appendicitis: Is it Crohn's disease? Report of a case and review of the literature, *Am J Gastroenterol* 81:283, 1986.
69. Dudley TH, Dean PJ: Idiopathic granulomatous appendicitis, or Crohn's disease of the appendix revisited, *Hum Pathol* 24:595, 1993.

Ulcerative colitis

70. Lumb G, Protheroe RHB: Ulcerative colitis: a pathologic study of 152 surgical specimens, *Gastroenterology* 34:381, 1958.
71. Cohen T, Pfeffer RB, Valensi O: "Ulcerative appendicitis" occurring as a skip lesion in ulcerative colitis: report of a case, *Am J Gastroenterol* 62:151, 1974.

72. Davison AM, Dixon MF: The appendix as a "skip lesion" in ulcerative colitis, *Histopathology* 16:93, 1990.
73. Goldblum JR, Appelman HD: Appendiceal involvement in ulcerative colitis, *Mod Pathol* 5:607, 1992.
74. Jahadi MR, Shaw ML: The pathology of the appendix in ulcerative colitis, *Dis Col Rect* 19:345, 1976.

Mucosal hyperplasia

75. Qizilbash AH: Hyperplastic (metaplastic) polyps of the appendix, *Arch Pathol* 97:385, 1974.
76. MacGillivray JB: Mucosal metaplasia in the appendix, *J Clin Pathol* 25:809, 1972.
77. Pagnozzi JA, Mueller SC, Cioroiu MG: Mucosal hyperplasia (mucocele) of the vermiform appendix, *Dis Col Rect* 31:735, 1988.
78. Appelman HD: Epithelial neoplasia of the appendix. In: Norris HT, editor: *Pathology of the colon, small intestine, and anus,* New York, 1991, Churchill Livingstone.

Neoplasms

Mucocele

79. González JE, Hann SE, Trujillo YP: Myxoglobulosis of the appendix, *Am J Surg Pathol* 12:962, 1988.
80. Aho AJ, Heinonen R, Lauren P: Benign and malignant mucocele of the appendix, *Acta Chir Scand* 139:192, 1973.

Adenomas and adenocarcinomas

81. Higa E, Rosai J, Pizzimbono CA, Wise L: Mucosal hyperplasia, mucinous cystadenoma, and mucinous cystadenocarcinoma of the appendix: a re-evaluation of appendiceal "mucocele," *Cancer* 37:1525, 1973.
82. Mibu R, Itoh H, Iwashita A et al: Carcinoma in situ of the vermiform appendix associated with adenomatosis of the colon, *Dis Col Rect* 24:482, 1981.
83. Qizilbash AH: Mucoceles of the appendix: their relationship to hyperplastic polyps, mucinous cystadenomas, and cystadenocarcinomas, *Arch Pathol* 99:548, 1975.
84. Wolff M, Ahmed N: Epithelial neoplasms of the vermiform appendix (exclusive of carcinoid): I. Adenocarcinoma of the appendix, *Cancer* 37:2493, 1976.
85. Williams GR, Du Boulay CEH, Roche WR: Benign epithelial neoplasms of the appendix: classification and clinical associations, *Histopathology* 21:447, 1992.
86. Wolff M, Ahmed N: Epithelial neoplasms of the vermiform appendix (exclusive of carcinoid): II. Cystadenomas, papillary adenomas, and adenomatous polyps of the appendix, *Cancer* 37:2511, 1976.
87. Muto T, Bussey HJR, Morson BC: Pseudocarcinomatous invasion in adenomatous polyps of the colon and rectum, *J Clin Pathol* 26:25, 1973.
88. Jurgeleit HC: Pseudomyxoma peritonei: a localized, benign variant of appendiceal origin, *Dis Col Rect* 29:469, 1986.
89. Cohen SE, Wolfman EF: Primary adenocarcinoma of the vermiform appendix, *Am J Surg* 127:704, 1974.
90. Edmonson HT Jr, Hobbs ML: Primary adenocarcinoma of the appendix, *Am Surg* 33:717, 1967.
91. Qizilbash AH: Primary adenocarcinoma of the appendix: a clinicopathologic study of 11 cases, *Arch Pathol* 99:556, 1975.
92. Aranha GV, Reyes CV: Primary epithelial tumors of the appendix and a reappraisal of the appendiceal mucocele, *Dis Col Rect* 22:472, 1979.
93. Chang P, Attiyeh FF: Adenocarcinoma of the appendix, *Dis Col Rect* 24:176, 1981.
94. Lenriot JP, Huguier M: Adenocarcinoma of the appendix, *Am J Surg* 155:470, 1988.
95. Rutledge RH, Alexander JW: Primary appendiceal malignancies: rare but important, *Surgery* 11:244, 1992.
96. Smith JW, Kemeny N, Caldwell C et al: Pseudomyxoma peritonei of appendiceal origin, *Cancer* 70:396, 1992.
97. Fernández RN, Daly JM: Pseudomyxoma peritonei, *Arch Surg* 115:409, 1980.
98. Mann WJ, Wagner J, Chumas J et al: The management of pseudomyxoma peritonei, *Cancer* 66:1636, 1990.
99. Ghosh BC, Huvos AG, Whitely HW: Pseudomyxoma peritonei, *Dis Col Rect* 15:420, 1972.
100. Gibbs NM: Mucinous cystadenoma and cystadenocarcinoma of the vermiform appendix with particular reference to mucocele and pseudomyxoma peritonei, *J Clin Pathol* 26:413, 1973.
101. Prayson RA, Hart WR, Petras RE: Pseudomyxoma peritonei: a clinicopathologic study of 19 cases with emphasis on site of origin and nature of associated ovarian tumors, *Am J Surg Pathol* 18:591, 1994.
102. Landen S, Bertrand C, Maddern GJ et al: Appendiceal mucoceles and pseudomyxoma peritonei, *Surg Gynecol Obstet* 175:401, 1992.
103. Young RH, Gilks CB, Scully RE: Mucinous tumors of the appendix associated with mucinous tumors of the ovary and pseudomyxoma peritonei: a clinicopathologic analysis of 22 cases supporting an origin in the appendix, *Am J Surg Pathol* 15:415, 1991.
104. Malfetano JH: The appendix and its metastatic potential in epithelial ovarian cancer, *Obstet Gynecol* 69:396, 1987.
105. Seidman JD, Elsayed AM, Sobin LH et al: Association of mucinous tumors of the ovary and appendix: a clinicopathologic study of 25 cases, *Am J Surg Pathol* 17:22, 1993.
106. Sumithran E, Susil BJ: Concommitant mucinous tumors of appendix and ovary: result of a neoplastic field change? *Cancer* 70:2980, 1992.
107. Hart WR: Ovarian epithelial tumors of borderline malignancy (carcinomas of low malignant potential), *Hum Pathol* 8:841, 1977.
108. Papadaki L, Rode J, Dhillon AP, Dische FE: Fine structure of a neuroendocrine complex in the mucosa of the appendix, *Gastroenterology* 84:490, 1983.

Carcinoid tumor

109. Moertel CG, Dockerty MB, Judd ES: Carcinoid tumors of the vermiform appendix, *Cancer* 21:270, 1968.
110. Markgraf WH, Dunn TM: Appendiceal carcinoid with carcinoid syndrome, *Am J Surg* 107:730, 1964.
111. Johnston WH, Waisman J: Carcinoid tumor of the vermiform appendix with Cushing's syndrome, *Cancer* 27:681, 1971.
112. Soga J, Tazawa K: Pathologic analysis of carcinoids: histologic re-evaluation of 62 cases, *Cancer* 28:990, 1971.
113. Lundqvist M, Wilander E: Subepithelial neuroendocrine cells and carcinoid tumors of the human small intestine and appendix: a comparative immunohistochemical study with regard to serotonin, neuron-specific enolase and S-100 protein reactivity, *J Pathol* 148:141, 1986.
114. Iwafuchi M, Watanabe H, Kijima H et al: Argyrophil, nonargentaffin carcinoids of the appendix vermiformis: immunohistochemical and ultrastructural studies, *Acta Pathol Jpn* 37:1237, 1987.
115. Moertel CG, Weiland LH, Nagorney DM, Dockerty MB: Carcinoid tumor of the appendix: treatment and prognosis, *N Engl J Med* 317:1699, 1987.
116. MacGillivray DC, Heaton RB, Rushin JM, Cruess DF: Distant metastasis from a carcinoid tumor of the appendix less than one centimeter in size, *Surgery* 111:466, 1992.
117. Bowman GA, Rosenthal D: Carcinoid tumors of the appendix, *Am J Surg* 146:700, 1983.
118. Parkes SE, Muir KR, Sheyyab MA et al: Carcinoid tumours of the appendix in children 1957-1986: incidence, treatment and outcome, *Br J Surg* 80:502, 1993.

Goblet-cell carcinoid

119. Hood IC, Jones BA, Watts JC: Mucinous tumor of the appendix presenting as bilateral ovarian tumors, *Arch Pathol Lab Med* 110:336, 1986.
120. Hirschfield LS, Kahn LB, Winkler B et al: Adenocarcinoid of the appendix presenting as bilateral Krukenberg's tumors of the ovaries: immunohistochemical and ultrastructural study and literature review, *Arch Pathol Lab Med* 109:930, 1985.
121. Isaacson P: Crypt cell carcinoma of the appendix (so-called adenocarcinoid tumor), *Am J Surg Pathol* 5:213, 1981.
122. Klein HZ: Mucinous carcinoid of the vermiform appendix, *Cancer* 33:770, 1974.
123. Burke AP, Sobin LH, Federspiel BH et al: Goblet cell carcinoids and related tumors of the vermiform appendix, *Am J Clin Pathol* 94:27, 1990.
124. Abt AB, Carter SL: Goblet cell carcinoid of the appendix: an ultrastructural and histochemical study, *Arch Pathol Lab Med* 100:301, 1990.
125. Cooper PH, Warkel RL: Ultrastructure of the goblet cell type of adenocarcinoid of the appendix, *Cancer* 42:2687, 1978.

126. Warkel RL, Cooper PHP, Helwig EB: Adenocarcinoid, a mucin-producing carcinoid tumor of the appendix, *Cancer* 42:2781, 1978.
127. Ikeda E, Tsutsumi Y, Yoshida H, Yanagi K: Goblet cell carcinoid of the vermiform appendix with ovarian metastasis mimicking mucinous cystadenocarcinoma, *Acta Pathol Jpn* 41:455, 1991.
128. Edmonds P, Merino MJ, LiVolsi VA, Duray PH: Adenocarcinoid (mucinous carcinoid) of the appendix, *Gastroenterology* 86:302, 1984.
129. Park K, Blessing K, Kerr K et al: Goblet cell carcinoid of the appendix, *Gut* 31:322, 1990.
130. Bak M, Asschenfeldt P: Adenocarcinoid of the vermiform appendix: a clinicopathologic study of 20 cases, *Dis Col Rect* 51:605, 1987.

Other tumors

Neurofibroma

131. Hochberg FH, Dasilva AB, Galdabini J, Richardson EP: Gastrointestinal involvement in von Recklinghausen's neurofibromatosis, *Neurology* 24:1144, 1974.
132. Merck C, Kindblom LG: Neurofibromatosis of the appendix in von Recklinghausen's disease: a report of a case, *Acta Pathol Microbiol Scand (A)* 83:623, 1975.
133. Olsen BS: Giant appendicular neurofibroma: a light and immunohistochemical study, *Histopathology* 11:851, 1987.

Granular cell tumor

134. Johnston J, Helwig EB: Granular cell tumors of the gastrointestinal tract and perianal region: a study of 74 cases, *Dig Dis Sci* 26:807, 1981.
135. Sobel HJ, Marquet E, Schwarz R: Granular degeneration of appendiceal smooth muscle, *Arch Pathol* 92:427, 1971.

Paraganglioma

136. Cohen T, Zweig SJ, Tallis A: Paraganglioneuroma of the duodenum, *Am J Gastroenterol* 75:197, 1981.
137. Clark DE, Stocks JF, Wilkis JL: Mesoappendiceal paraganglioma, *Am J Gastroenterol* 80:340, 1985.

Lymphoma

138. Lewin KJ, Ranchod M, Dorfman RF: Lymphomas of the gastrointestinal tract, *Cancer* 42:693, 1978.
139. Loehr WJ, Mujahed Z, Zahn D et al: Primary lymphoma of the gastrointestinal tract: a review of 100 cases, *Ann Surg* 170:232, 1969.
140. Rao SK, Aydinalp N: Appendiceal lymphoma: a case report, *J Clin Gastroenterol* 13(5):588, 1991.
141. Sin IC, Ling E-T, Prentice RS: Burkitt's lymphoma of the appendix: report of two cases, *Hum Pathol* 11:465, 1980.

Miscellaneous lesions

Heterotopias

142. Droga BW, Levine S, Baber JJ: Heterotopic gastric and esophageal tissue in the vermiform appendix, *Am J Clin Pathol* 40:190, 1963.

Hirschsprung's disease

143. Adams BE, Adams RM: Hirschsprung's disease with extensive aganglionic segments, *Am J Surg* 98:248, 1959.
144. Martin LW, Perrin EV: Neonatal perforation of the appendix in association with Hirschsprung's disease, *Ann Surg* 166:799, 1967.

Sarcoidosis

145. Tinker MA, Viswanathan B, Laufer H, Margolis IB: Acute appendicitis and pernicious anemia as complications of gastrointestinal sarcoidosis, *Am J Gastroenterol* 79:868, 1984.
146. Munt PW: Sarcoidosis of appendix presenting as appendiceal perforation and abscess, *Chest* 66:295, 1974.
147. Clarke H, Pollett W, Chittal S, Ra M: Sarcoidosis with involvement of the appendix, *Arch Intern Med* 143:1603, 1983.
148. Byström J: Localized sarcoidosis of the appendix simulating MB Crohn, *Acta Chir Scand* 134:163, 1968.

Endometriosis

149. Lane RE: Endometriosis of the vermiform appendix, *Am J Obstet Gynecol* 79:372, 1960.
150. Uohara JK, Kovara TY: Endometriosis of the appendix: report of twelve cases and review of the literature, *Am J Obstet Gynecol* 121:423, 1975.
151. Mann WJ, Fromowitz F, Saychek T et al: Endometriosis asssociated with appendiceal intussusception: a report of two cases, *J Reprod Med* 29:625, 1984.

Cystic fibrosis

152. Jeffrey I, Durrans D, Wells M, Fox H: The pathology of meconium ileus equivalent, *J Clin Pathol* 36:1292, 1983.
153. Dolan TF, Meyers A: Mild cystic fibrosis presenting as an asymptomatic distended appendiceal mass: a case report, *Clin Pediatr* 14:862, 1975.
154. McIntosh JC, Mroczek EC, Baldwin C, Mestre J: Intussusception of the appendix in a patient with cystic fibrosis, *J Pediatr Gastroenterol Nutr* 110:542, 1990.
155. Shields MD, Levison H, Reisman JJ et al: Appendicitis in cystic fibrosis, *Arch Dis Child* 66: 307-310, 1991.
156. McCarthy VP, Mischler EH, Hubbard VS et al: Appendiceal abscess in cystic fibrosis, *Gastroenterology* 86:564, 1984.

Intussusception

157. Fazio RA, Wickremesinghe PC, Arsura EL, Rando J: Endoscopic removal of an intussuscepted appendix mimicking a polyp: an endoscopic hazard, *Am J Gastroenterol* 77:556, 1982.
158. Holck S, Wolff M: Intussusception with incarceration of a cystadenoma of the appendix: case report and review of the complications of appendiceal adenomas, *Dis Col Rect* 22:133, 1979.
159. Langsam LB, Raj PK, Galang CG: Intussusception of the appendix, *Dis Col Rect* 27:387, 1984.
160. Skaane P, Eide TJ: Malignant appendiceal carcinoid with intussusception of the base manifesting as a cecal tumor: report of a case, *Dis Col Rect* 20:511, 1977.
161. Itoh J, Soeno T, Koizumi R: Intussusception of the appendix with a calcified fecalith, *Jpn J Surg* 17:195, 1987.
162. Jevon GP, Dya D, Qizilbash AH: Intussusception of the appendix: a report of four cases and review of the literature, *Arch Pathol Lab Med* 116:960, 1992.

Fibrous obliteration

163. Stanley MW, Cherwitz D, Hagen K, Snover DC: Neuromas of the appendix: a light microscopic, immunohistochemical and electron-microscopic study of 20 cases, *Am J Surg Pathol* 10:801, 1986.
164. Aubock L, Ratzenhofer M: "Extraepithelial enterochromaffin cell-nerve-fibre complexes" in the normal human appendix and in neurogenic appendiculopathy, *J Pathol* 136:217, 1982.
165. Zarabi M, LaBach JP: Ganglioneuroma causing acute appendicitis, *Hum Pathol* 13:1143, 1982.
166. Lie KA, Lindboe CF, Kolmannskog SV et al: Giant appendix with diffuse ganglioneuromatosis: an unusual presentation of von Recklinghausen's disease, *Eur J Surg* 158:127, 1992.

56 Large Intestine and Anus

David A. Owen
James K. Kelly

LARGE INTESTINE

NORMAL STRUCTURE AND FUNCTION

Anatomically the large bowel may be divided into several segments: cecum, ascending colon, transverse colon, descending colon, sigmoid colon, and rectum. Clinically it is convenient to divide it simply into the right colon, left colon, and rectum. The colon receives its blood supply from a fan-like distribution of vessels within the mesentery. From the cecum to the splenic flexure, these are derived from the superior mesenteric artery, and from the splenic flexure distally they are derived from branches of the inferior mesenteric artery. A portion of the lower rectum is supplied by branches of the internal iliac vessels. Venous blood drains to the portal vein, except in the lower rectum, where there are portosystemic anastomoses. Lymphatics start in the basal third of the mucosa and drain initially to nodes located adjacent to the outer aspect of the bowel wall. From here, they pass via mesenteric nodes to the ileocolic group of retroperitoneal nodes. In the lower rectum there may be drainage to the internal iliac or inguinal nodes.

The histologic appearances are similar at all sites. The mucosa consists of surface epithelium, crypts, lamina propria, and lamina muscularis mucosae (Fig. 56-1). Beneath this are the submucosa, muscularis propria, and subserosa. The large bowel mucosa has a unique appearance, but other layers are similar to the rest of the gastrointestinal tract. The surface epithelium consists of absorptive cells and mucin-containing goblet cells. T-lymphoctyes are present between epithelial cells, with the normal number being approximately 5 lymphocytes per 100 epithelial cells. Small numbers of apoptotic surface epithelial cells are normally encountered. These may be recognized as globular bodies containing nuclear fragments. The crypt epithelium also contains absorptive and goblet cells. Mature cells populate the upper half of the crypts, and immature cells are present in the lower half. Immature goblet cells contain smaller amounts of mucus.[1]

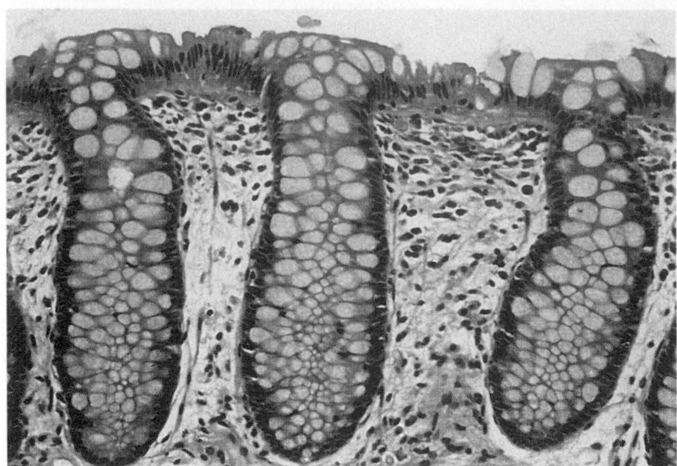

Fig. 56-1 Normal colonic mucosa. Notice the predominance of goblet cells in the epithelium and the light infiltrate of inflammatory cells in the lamina propria.

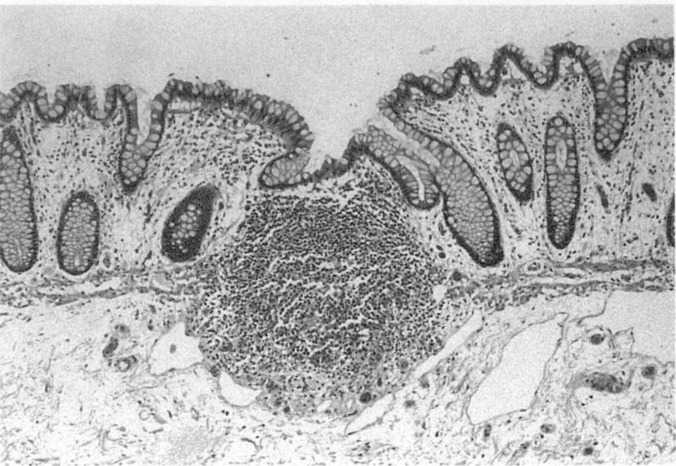

Fig. 56-2 Normal mucosal crypts displaced laterally by a lymphoid follicle.

Endocrine cells are present at the base of the crypts. They are triangular in shape and contain subnuclear eosinophilic granules. Most endocrine cells are argyrophilic, but only a few are argentaffinic. They show positive results with immunostains for chromogranin, vasoactive intestinal polypeptide (VIP), glucagon, substance P, somatostatin, and motilin.[2] Small numbers of Paneth cells are normally found at the base of crypts in the cecum and ascending colon but not in other parts of the large bowel. They have large pink granules located in the cytoplasm on the luminal side of the nucleus.

Large bowel crypts are regular structures with a smooth outline and are oriented perpendicularly to the mucosal surface. They are not branched unless the mucosa has been subject to chronic inflammation. The base of the crypts extends to a position immediately superficial to the muscularis mucosae. The surface of the mucosa is flat except at the site of the innominate grooves. On histologic cross section, the grooves appear as shallow V-shaped depressions. Crypts may empty into the base of these grooves, giving an appearance of branching. Mucosal irregularity may also occur adjacent to lymphoid follicles, where the follicle may displace the crypts sidewards, producing a splayed appearance (Fig. 56-2).

The lamina propria contains a loose collection of fibroblasts, vessels, nerves, smooth muscle, and inflammatory cells. The vessels are predominantly capillaries. Lymphatics are confined to the lower third of the lamina propria. Muscle fibers in the lamina propria are oriented perpendicularly to the surface. Normally, they are exceedingly slender but become more prominent if mucosal prolapse has occurred. Inflammatory cells normally present include lymphocytes, plasma cells, mast cells, eosinophils, and histiocytes. Most lymphocytes are helper/suppressor T-cells. Killer cells and B-cells are also present but in smaller numbers. They may be diffusely distributed throughout the lamina propria, or organized into lymphoid follicles. Typically the follicles span the entire thickness of the muscularis mucosae, with a portion present in the lamina propria and a portion in the submucosa. Plasma cells are chiefly IgA secreting and tend to be located in the upper half of the mucosa, below the superficial epithelium. Eosinophils are commonly present in small numbers, though there is considerable individual variation. Sheets of eosinophils, however, are considered abnormal. Macrophages and mast cells are found occasionally, though usually in lesser numbers than eosinophils. Macrophages often contain small quantities of mucus within their cytoplasm.

Fibroblasts may be found as isolated cells throughout the lamina propria, or as pericryptal fibroblasts, adjacent to the basement membrane of the superficial portion of the crypt. The basement membrane beneath the surface epithelium usually measures 1 to 2 μm but may be thickened up to 7 μm in adults and up to 4 μm in children.

The nerve supply to the colon generally follows the vessels. Sympathetic nerves originate from the paravertebral ganglia, and parasympathetic nerves originate from the celiac branch of the posterior vagus. There are three nerve plexuses in the bowel wall: an unnamed mucosal plexus, the submucosal plexus of Meissner, and the myenteric plexus of Auerbach. Ganglion cells are generally confined to Meissner's and Auerbach's plexuses, though occasionally they may be encountered within the lamina propria.

Biopsy artifacts

Biopsy specimens of the large bowel mucosa, obtained during endoscopy, frequently show stretching or compression artifact. Stretching of a biopsy specimen may simulate edema. Compression may produce a spurious hypercellularity, which should not be diagnosed as mild chronic inflammation unless accompanied by cryptitis or epithelial changes, such as nuclear enlargement, presence of prominent nucleoli, and cytoplasmic mucin depletion. Loss of surface epithelium without a vital response is usually an artifact of the biopsy. Crushed lymphoid follicles are usually identifiable by their position and surroundings.

An artifact termed *pseudolipomatosis*[3] (Fig. 56-3) may be caused by the endoscopist filling the colon with air under too much pressure. Some air escapes into the lamina propria through a small defect in the surface epithelium, producing changes that may be recognized on biopsy as multiple clear spaces giving a lacy, bubbly appearance.

Before a colonoscopy is performed, it is usually necessary to empty the colon of feces by enema preparation. Enemas

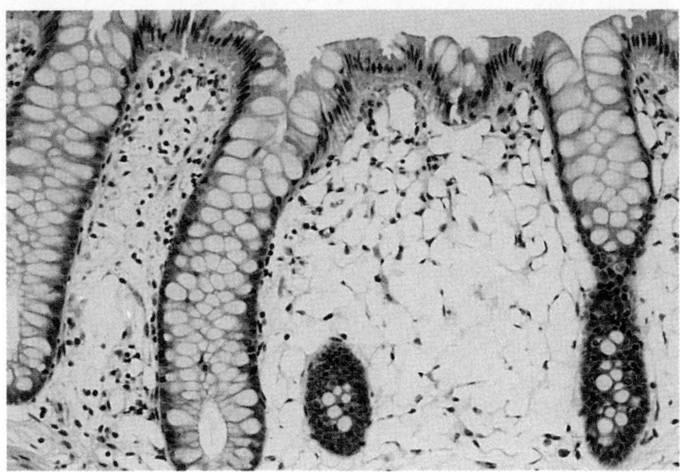

Fig. 56-3 Pseudolipomatosis, an artifact created by air entering the lamina propria.

using polyethylene glycol produce no histologic changes. However, bisacodyl enemas can cause mucin depletion, sloughing of superficial epithelial cells, and a scanty neutrophil infiltrate in the superficial lamina propria and epithelium.[4] Soap suds enemas can produce a low-grade colitis that can last for several months.[5]

HEREDITARY AND DEVELOPMENTAL DISORDERS

Hereditary and developmental disorders of the large intestine are rare but may be important causes of bowel obstruction in the neonatal period and infancy. They include the various forms of malrotation, atresias, webs, and strictures.

Malrotation

Malrotation is defined as a failure or abnormality of the usual bowel rotation that occurs in fetal life as the extruded bowel returns to the abdominal cavity. The bowel itself is usually normal, except that it is malpositioned.

Malrotation may occur in several forms. The most common and least significant form of malrotation occurs when the cecum does not become attached to the posterior wall of the abdominal cavity but retains its mesentery. This is referred to as a mobile cecum.[6] The most severe but least common abnormality is a nonrotation, where the small bowel is present in the right side of the abdominal cavity and the large bowel on the left side. Less often, rotation does occur but is incomplete (mixed rotation), with the cecum present in the epigastrium or just below the liver.

The cause of malrotation is unknown. An increased incidence has been reported in association with chromosomal abnormalities, such as trisomy 21, 13, or 18, and congenital metabolic disorders, such as Zellweger's syndrome.

Malrotation is usually asymptomatic but may result in some complications, the most important of which is volvulus. This involves twisting of the bowel around a fixed point, often the superior mesenteric artery. This occurs because the bowel is not tethered in its usual position.

Volvulus presents initially as intestinal obstruction. Later, if the volvulus persists, there may be ischemia with perforation. Volvulus occurring secondarily to malrotation must be distinguished from an acquired type of volvulus, occurring in adults and usually affecting the sigmoid colon.[7]

Congenital atresia and stenosis

Atresia may be defined as a discontinuity of the bowel lumen and stenosis as luminal narrowing. Most congenital atresias and stenosis presumably result from fetal intestinal anoxia during pregnancy or from an episode of neonatal necrotizing enterocolitis. Atresia and stenosis are increased in incidence in patients with chromosomal abnormalities, particularly Down's syndrome.

Atresias[8] of the gastrointestinal tract occur in one of every 1500 to 2000 births, however, only 10% involve the large bowel. Two major types are recognized. In the first, the affected segment is transformed into a fibrous band. In the second type, the muscularis propria is intact, but the mucosa is absent and the lumen is obliterated by loose fibrous tissue. Very short atretic segments are called "webs," or "diaphragms." Incomplete atresia leads to stenosis.

Cystic fibrosis

Cystic fibrosis[9] may present with intestinal obstruction caused by tenacious meconium (meconium ileus). The meconium plug may cause colonic rupture, resulting in meconium peritonitis. In about 10% of cases, the colon is hypoplastic (microcolon). Microscopic changes manifest as a mild dilatation of crypts, which contain inspissated pink-staining mucus.

Hirschsprung's disease

Hirschsprung's disease[10] is a congenital disorder that results from an absence of ganglion cells in the plexuses of Meissner and Auerbach. This is accompanied by hypertrophy of nerve trunks. The condition results from a failure of intrauterine ganglion cell development, possibly on an ischemic basis. It affects 1 in 5000 neonates and has a male-to-female predominance of 4:1. The condition is commoner in infants with Down syndrome and other congenital anomalies. There is also a strong familial tendency. If one child is affected, the risk for other siblings is 10% for long segment disease and 1% to 5% for short segment disease.

Hirschsprung's disease involves the distal sigmoid colon and rectum in about 90% of cases (short segment Hirschsprung's). In 10% of cases the whole colon, or even a portion of the terminal ileum, are devoid of ganglion cells. Rarer variants include *ultrashort segment disease* (anal region only), *zonal aganglionosis* (skip areas affected), *hypoganglionosis* (reduced numbers of ganglion cells), and *gangliocytic dysplasia* (enlarged coarse nerve fibers with an excess of immature ganglion cells).

On gross examination of the large bowel, the affected segment is contracted because of the unopposed action of the parasympathetic nerves. The unaffected segment, which lies proximal to the aganglionic colon, is typically dilated (megacolon). The intervening area is a cone-shaped zone, where ganglion cells are present in reduced numbers.

Microscopically,[11] the affected bowel contains hypertrophic nerves but no ganglion cells. The muscularis propria is normal. The diagnosis is made by a biopsy, which must include not only mucosa but the deeper layers of the submucosa as

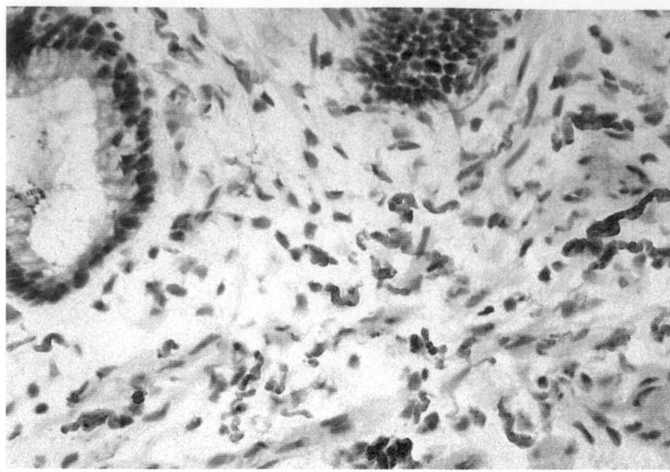

Fig. 56-4 Hirschsprung's disease, showing a proliferation of fine nerve fibres within the lamina propria (immunostain for acetyl cholinesterase). (Courtesy Dr. James Dimmick, British Columbia Children's Hospital, Vancouver, Canada.)

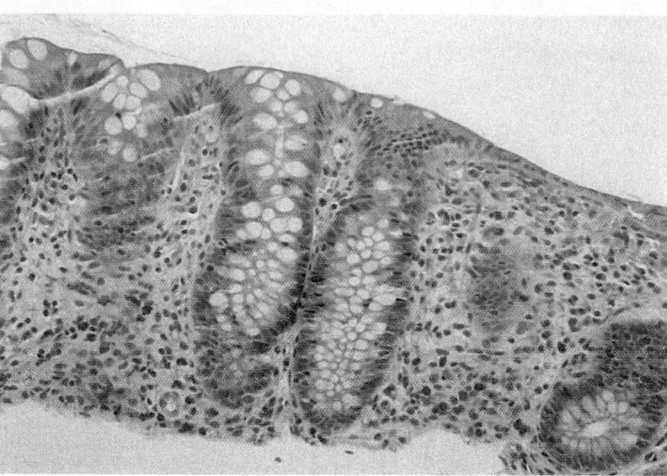

Fig. 56-5 Eosinophilic proctitis in a child with milk allergy. Notice the diffuse infiltrate of eosinophils in the lamina propria. (Courtesy Dr. James Dimmick, British Columbia Children's Hospital, Vancouver, Canada.)

well. Since submucosal ganglion cells are normally sparse, it is usually necessary to examine 20 to 50 serial sections to conclude that they are absent. Immunoperoxidase stains for neuron-specific enolase (NSE) may be helpful in identifying ganglion cells, particularly in premature infants, where they may be poorly developed and resemble lymphocytes. Additional diagnostic assistance may also be obtained by examination of frozen sections stained for acetylcholinesterase. This stain highlights the proliferation of cholinergic nerve fibers within the mucosa and muscularis mucosae (Fig. 56-4).

Hirschsprung's disease is a congenital disorder that typically presents in the neonatal period with severe constipation and failure to pass meconium. If untreated, perforation of the proximal bowel may occur. Surgical resection of the aganglionic segment of the colon with end-to-end anastomosis gives excellent clinical results.

DISEASES CAUSED BY INJURY FROM EXOGENOUS FACTORS

Allergic (eosinophilic) proctitis and colitis

The topic of allergy and eosinophilic infiltrates in the gastrointestinal tract is confusing and replete with overlapping terminology. Three major "entities" are described: eosinophilic gastroenteritis,[12] allergic gastroenteritis,[13] and allergic proctitis and colitis.[14] Before making a diagnosis of any of these conditions, one needs to exclude other more specific diseases. Crohn's disease and ulcerative colitis may on occasion exhibit large numbers of eosinophils in the lamina propria. Eosinophils are particularly prominent when the disease is declining in intensity, as it enters a phase of remission. Eosinophil infiltration is also seen in parasitic disease,[15] drug reactions,[16] and collagen vascular disease.[17]

The canine hookworm, *Ancylostoma caninum,* is a major cause of eosinophilic gastroenteritis in Queensland, Australia, but the parasite is rarely identified in resected bowel.[15] This organism may account for many more cases of eosinophilic gastroenteritis among residents of the tropics and subtropics than has yet been recognized. The nematode *Anisakis* is also associated with a localized eosinophilic response. This can be acquired in North America by ingestion of uncooked salmon and codfish.

Eosinophilic gastroenteritis[12] may be defined as a symptomatic condition characterized by histologic evidence of infiltration of one or more segments of the gastrointestinal tract by large numbers of eosinophil polymorphs. There is no obvious cause, such as parasites or systemic disease. This condition is commonest in the gastric antrum and rarely involves the large bowel. It has been described as having three forms, with the preponderance of eosinophil infiltration localized either to the mucosa, the bowel wall (submucosa and muscularis propria), or the subserosa. The last form may present with ascites and chronic peritonitis. Typically, patients with eosinophilic gastroenteritis are adults. A history of food allergy is uncommon, though a peripheral eosinophilia may be present. Disease involving the bowel wall can give rise to symptoms of obstruction.

The term *allergic gastroenteritis*[13] has been used to describe mucosal eosinophilic infiltrates in patients with documented food allergy. *Allergic proctitis and colitis*[13,14] (Fig. 56-5) is a localized form of eosinophilic gastroenteritis where the eosinophilic infiltrates are confined to the large bowel. Most cases are infants between 6 months and 2 years of age who are sensitive to cow's milk. Less commonly, soy protein is the provoking factor. Histologically, the changes manifest as a diffuse infiltrate of eosinophils in the lamina propria (Fig. 56-5). In severe cases, this may be accompanied by extension of eosinophil infiltration into the epithelium or submucosa. Unlike inflammatory bowel disease, the crypts do not become distorted or atrophic. As a general guide, up to 6 eosinophils per high-power field are considered normal in children. Numbers in excess of this are considered to constitute presumptive evidence of food allergy. The clinical symptoms of allergic proctitis and colitis include rectal bleeding, diarrhea, and vomiting. There may also be weight loss and abdominal pain. A mild blood eosinophilia is usually present. In most cases, the child "outgrows" the allergy and by adulthood is able to tolerate milk protein.

Drug-induced diseases

A wide variety of prescription and nonprescription drugs may affect the large bowel. The most important of these are antibiotics, which, by suppressing normal flora, allow proliferation of potentially pathogenic organisms. The best example of this situation is *Clostridium difficile,* producing pseudomembranous colitis. This is discussed in the section on colonic infections.

The next most common group of drugs producing large bowel disease are the nonsteroidal anti-inflammatory agents (NSAIDs), which appear to reduce the mucosal content of prostaglandins and allow accumulation of neutrophils in the lamina propria in response to substances within the bowel lumen. There is some evidence that NSAIDS produce an acute colitis[18] and may rarely cause colonic diaphragm disease.[19] These diaphragms consist of an expanded, fibrotic, submucosal core covered by normal mucosa, except at the orifice, where ulceration may be present. Diaphragms are considered to represent extremely short segment strictures. A suggestion has been made that NSAIDS may also produce nonspecific chronic ulcers.[20] The nature of the acute colitis caused by NSAIDS is controversial. The changes are said to be similar to those of microscopic colitis consisting mainly of increased numbers of chronic inflammatory cells in the lamina propria without cryptitis or crypt distortion.[18] Endoscopically, the changes are described as mucosal erythema without ulceration.

In some instances, nonspecific ulcers and strictures of the large bowel (sometimes called "solitary ulcer of the cecum") have been linked to ingestion of NSAIDS. However, the etiologic description of these ulcers is complex, and additional possible causes include localized ischemia and other ulcerogenic drugs, such as potassium chloride. They tend to occur in the right side of the colon and may be single or multiple. The ulcers are "punched out" and extend into the muscularis propria, where considerable fibrosis may be present. They may be circumferential. Typically, the adjacent mucosa and even the base of the ulcer is only minimally inflamed. The histologic findings are nonspecific and do not provide clues about the causes of ulceration.

Other drug-related large bowel diseases include submucosal hemorrhage related to anticoagulants,[21] ischemia secondary to vasospasm from vasopressin or ergot compounds,[22] and allergic enterocolitis[16] attributable to gold compounds or penicillamine. Anticancer chemotherapeutic drugs[23] cause a focal colitis characterized by preserved mucosal architecture, attenuated crypt lining cells, and a scanty cryptitis and lamina propria inflammatory infiltrate. The regenerating crypt cells may show cytologic atypia.

Melanosis coli[24] results from abuse of the anthraquinone type of purgatives. Only the mucosa is affected. Grossly, it may appear deep brown. Microscopically the lamina propria contains pigment-laden macrophages (Fig. 56-6). The pigment stains positively with Schmorl's or Fontana-Masson but is more closely related to lipofuscin than to melanin. Melanosis coli itself is asymptomatic, though the associated purgative abuse may result in diarrhea.

Barium granulomas[25] may occur if there is an escape of radiologic contrast media into the bowel wall. The tissue reaction is rich in histiocytes, with smaller numbers of foreign-body giant cells. Barium crystals may readily be identified on routine sections and are doubly refractile under polarized light.

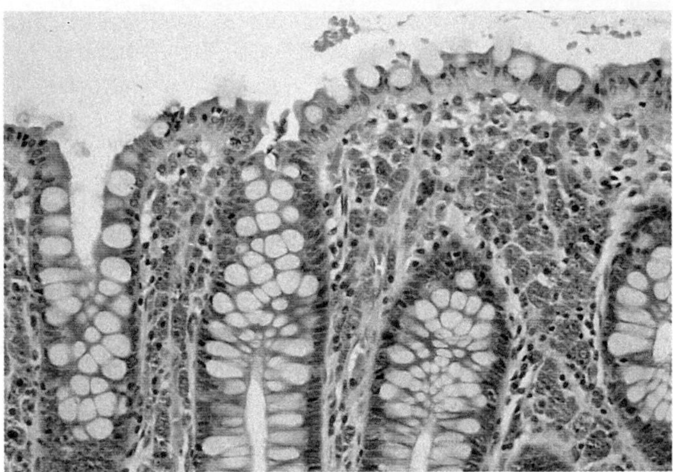

Fig. 56-6 Melanosis coli. Notice the golden brown pigment within lamina propria macrophages.

Stercoral ulcers

Stercoral ulcers are relatively common lesions occurring in the distal area of the colon and the rectum, particularly of older people.[26] They are the result of fecal impaction and pressure necrosis of the mucosa. Grossly the ulcers tend to be shallow, with well-circumscribed rounded or oval contours. The histologic features are nonspecific, though mucosa from the edge can show features of ischemic injury.

Radiation colitis

Radiation injury[27] of the large bowel may follow treatment of gynecologic, prostatic, or urinary bladder tumors. Damage is particularly likely in the rectum and rectosigmoid. Changes are dose dependent, but there are also variations in individual susceptibility.

Acute changes include mucosal edema and deposition of fibrinoid material in the walls of vessels. Epithelial cells show mucin depletion and bizarre nuclear forms. Mitoses, however, are usually absent. In more severe damage, degenerating cells are present within dilated crypts. These may be identified as apoptotic bodies by the karyorrhexis of nuclei. Ultimately, with very high doses of radiation, total mucosal sloughing occurs, and there is acute ulceration.

Chronic changes may first become manifest long after radiation therapy. They are characterized by mucosal atrophy and submucosal fibrosis. The crypts are short and irregular in outline, and the lamina propria contains increased amounts of collagen but with reduced numbers of inflammatory cells. In the fibrotic areas, atypical "radiation fibroblasts" are occasionally seen. These have enlarged nuclei with prominent nucleoli and abundant basophilic cytoplasm. Larger submucosal vessels show an obliterative endarteritis with thickened sclerotic walls. Capillaries, particularly within the mucosa, are telangiectatic and can contain fibrin thrombi.

NONINFECTIOUS DISEASES OF UNCERTAIN CAUSE

Diverticular disease

Diverticula are outpouchings of the mucosa through defects in the weakened muscularis propria of the colon.

Diverticulosis may be right sided or left sided in distribution. From the etiologic and epidemiologic point of view, these are entirely separate conditions, though the pathologic conditions are similar at both locations.

Left-sided diverticulosis is exceedingly common in North America and Europe but rare in Asia, Africa, and South America. About 50% of the elderly population of the Western world is affected, though it is uncommon in individuals under 40 years of age. The condition shows no predilection for either sex. The pathogenesis is unknown, though there is circumstantial evidence linking it to a diet low in fiber.[28] It is postulated that a low-residue diet results in abnormal peristaltic activity producing increased intraluminal pressure. Diverticular outpouchings occur through points of weakness in the wall of the colon. The tendency to produce diverticula may be accentuated by degenerative changes in connective tissue. For example, individuals with Marfan's syndrome or the Ehlers-Danlos[29] syndrome may develop diverticula at a young age.

Diverticular disease should be regarded as a range of changes, which includes hypertrophy of the muscularis propria,[30] formation of uncomplicated diverticula,[31] and secondary diverticulitis.[32] It is probable that the muscular abnormality is the most significant factor in the genesis of symptoms, since many of these appear to be related to a reduction in diameter of the bowel lumen. When diverticula form, they occur as two rows of either side of the colon between the antimesenteric teniae, at the site of perforation of the muscularis propria by medium-sized arteries, where they represent a point of weakness. Most diverticula measure up to 1.0 cm in diameter, and in many instances fecaliths are impacted within the diverticular sacs (Fig. 56-7). In fully developed disease, the mucosa develops a series of transverse ridges, between which are the mouths of the diverticula. Left-sided diverticula occur predominantly in the sigmoid colon, a part of the colon in which the feces become solid and elicit maximal resistance to the peristaltic activity. The intraluminal pressure generated in this way may be important in the pathogenesis of disease. Rarely, the disease spreads proximally to involve the transverse colon or even the ascending colon. This proximal disease probably has the same pathogenesis as sigmoid diverticulosis and is different from isolated right-sided diverticular disease.

Histologically, the diverticula are lined by mucosa and submucosa only (Fig. 56-8). The mucosa is often attenuated but is otherwise unremarkable. Low-grade inflammation may be present, usually in the form of cryptitis or isolated crypt abscesses. In diverticulitis, the mucosa is ulcerated, and the lumen of the diverticulum contains pus. The wall of the diverticulum now consists of inflammatory slough, granulation tissue, and surrounding fibrosis.

Approximately 10% of patients with diverticulosis develop symptoms, usually crampy left-sided abdominal pain with alternating episodes of diarrhea and constipation. Diverticulitis or intestinal hemorrhage are the usual complications and occur in 20% to 25% of patients. Diverticulitis may produce severe abdominal pain with fever. Intramural and pericolic abscesses

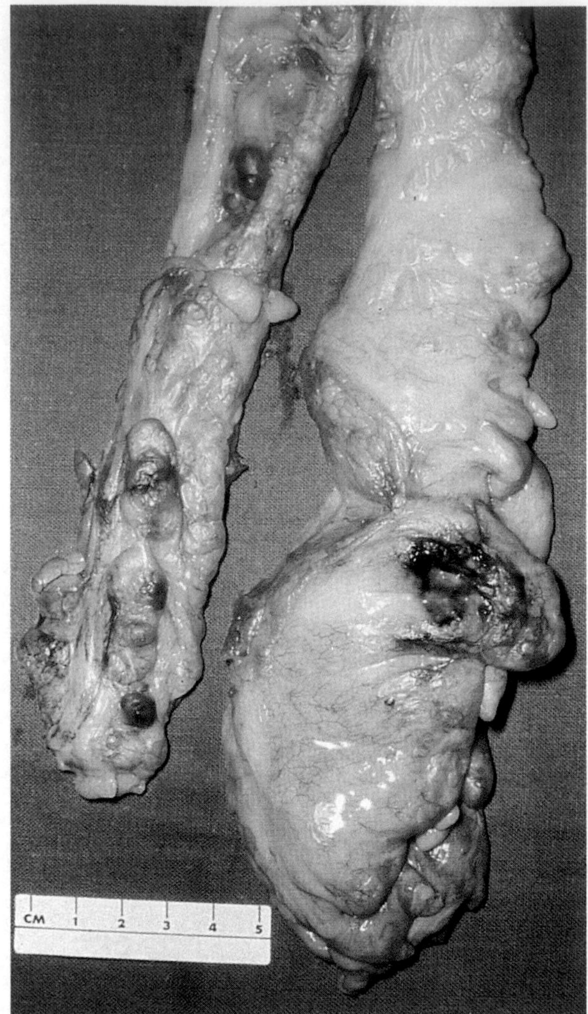

Fig. 56-7 Diverticulosis of the colon with fecaliths present in diverticular sacs.

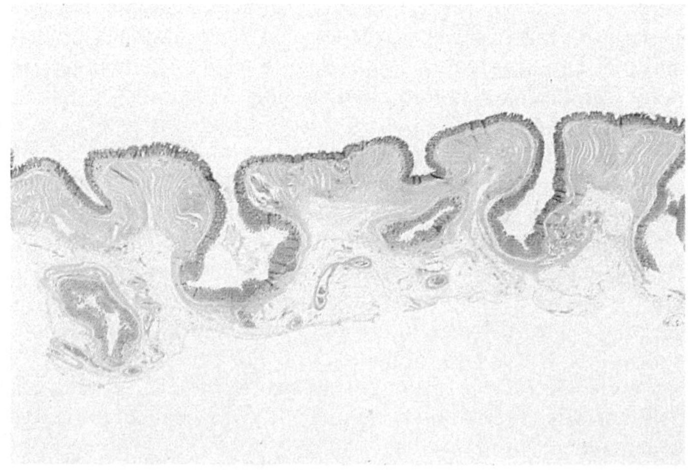

Fig. 56-8 Diverticula protruding through the muscularis propria into the subserosal fat.

may form, and the resulting fibrosis and distortion can result in narrowing of the bowel mimicking a carcinoma. Bleeding, usually massive painless hemorrhage, occurs after erosion of one of the colonic arteries as it passes adjacent to the neck of a diverticulum. An unusual but interesting complication is the development of mucosal polyps within the affected segment of colon.[33] These arise from the transverse mucosal ridges and histologically show features of mucosal prolapse, similar to those seen in the solitary rectal ulcer syndrome.

Right-sided diverticular disease[34] is most common in Asian populations, particularly the Japanese. The pathogenesis is unknown. The diverticula appear at a younger age and the male-to-female sex ratio is 3:1. Lesions are solitary in 20% of cases, and in an additional 60% there are less than 10 lesions. Histologically, they are similar to left-sided diverticula, except that some of them have attenuated muscularis propria in their wall.

Volvulus

Volvulus involving the sigmoid colon is a distinct clinicopathologic entity.[7] Typically, it is not the result of a congenital anomaly but is the consequence of an acquired lengthening of the sigmoid loop. It is particularly common in sub-Saharan Africa, Asia, and South America, where sigmoid enlargement may be secondary to a diet rich in fiber. In North America and western Europe, sigmoid volvulus occurs in elderly patients with a long history of chronic constipation, often associated with and possibly secondary to long-standing general medical or psychiatric problems.

Intestinal pseudo-obstruction

As the name implies, the term *pseudo-obstruction* refers to cases that manifest clinically with the symptoms of large bowel obstruction but have no gross lesion to account for it. Pseudo-obstruction may be acute or chronic. Acute pseudo-obstruction, also called Ogilvie's syndrome,[35] occurs in a variety of clinical situations but especially in patients who are seriously ill from other causes. Its cause is unknown, but the pathogenesis is presumably related to an acquired functional abnormality of visceral nervous function. Patients are generally elderly and men predominate. Apart from colonic dilatation, there are no morphologic abnormalities in the bowel.

Chronic pseudo-obstruction may result from visceral myopathies or neuropathies. Visceral myopathies[36] are the more common cause. There are several forms, such as autosomal dominant, autosomal recessive, and sporadic types. The large bowel pathologic condition is similar in the various forms, though extracolonic manifestations are different. The bowel can be affected diffusely or segmentally. Depending on the stage of the disease, the bowel wall may be thickened or thinned, or there may be diverticula present. Commonly, in the late stages, there is considerable dilatation with the formation of wide-mouthed diverticula. Histologically, there is vacuolar degeneration of the fibers of the muscularis propria, particularly the outer longitudinal layer. Gradually, the muscle is replaced by fibrous tissue. Inflammation is not seen, and the degeneration does not affect the muscularis mucosae, or the vascular smooth muscle. Visceral myopathy must be distinguished from systemic sclerosis, which tends to affect the inner circular muscle and is characterized by fibrosis without preceding vacuolar degeneration.

Visceral neuropathy[37] also occurs in autosomal dominant, autosomal recessive, and sporadic forms. Some of the sporadic types may be secondary to an underlying carcinoma. The pathologic description of all forms is exceedingly subtle and complex. Basically, there is a patchy degeneration of ganglion cells and nerves within the myenteric plexuses. Reduced numbers of nerve fibers are present and abnormally shaped ganglion cells are encountered. In the familial forms of the disease, some ganglion cells may have eosinophilic intranuclear inclusions resembling those of cytomegalovirus. In sporadic cases, there may be a chronic ganglionitis manifesting as infiltration by lymphocytes and plasma cells.

Brown bowel syndrome

The condition brown bowel syndrome may affect any part of the gastrointestinal tract. It is the result of an accumulation of lipofuscin pigment within the cytoplasm of muscle cells of the muscularis propria and muscularis mucosae.[38] There is a variety of causes, all of which have in common a malabsorption of fat and vitamin E. These include chronic pancreatitis, Whipple's disease, and cholestatic jaundice. Lack of vitamin E may also result from dietary deficiencies occurring in vegans.

Amyloidosis

Gastrointestinal involvement occurs in over 50% of cases with systemic amyloidosis.[39] In most cases, the distribution is diffuse, but rare examples of amyloid tumors are described. All types of amyloidosis result in deposition of amyloid material within the walls of submucosal vessels. In AL (primary) amyloidosis associated with myeloma, deposition typically also occurs in the muscularis propria and muscularis mucosae. In AA (secondary) amyloidosis secondary to long-standing inflammatory conditions, deposition also occurs in the lamina propria. The pattern of amyloid distribution shows some overlap, however, so that in an individual case it may not be possible to predict the underlying cause.

Amyloid of the gut is rarely symptomatic. Occasionally, it may result in malabsorption, secondary to mucosal infiltration. Gastrointestinal bleeding may occur secondary to vascular friability and coagulation defects. Heavy vascular involvement can cause ischemic ulceration. Muscle and nerve infiltration can produce pseudo-obstruction. If amyloid is suspected clinically, a rectal biopsy that includes submucosal vessels should be performed.[39]

CIRCULATORY DISORDERS

Colonic ischemia

Clinical syndromes of colonic ischemia[40] (Table 56-1) include ileocolic infarction, segmental colonic infarction, ischemic stricture, transient colonic ischemia, multifocal ischemia, venous ischemia,[41,42] and ischemia after pancreatitis.[42-46] The arterial factors responsible for colonic ischemia include atherosclerosis, thrombosis, embolism, vasculitis[42-50], thromboangiitis obliterans, systemic hypotension,[51] and spasm,[52,53] These etiologic factors may operate alone or in combination. For example, emboli may result from thrombi or atheromatous plaques and develop either spontaneously, after trauma, or after arterial catheterization.[54] Larger emboli occlude major vessels, whereas smaller emboli occlude the ileocolic, right colic, or middle colic arteries, or their branches. Superior mesenteric artery occlusion may cause infarction of small bowel and large bowel in continuity. The inferior mesenteric artery is routinely sacrificed during aortofemoral bypass operations, and approximately 7% of patients develop ischemia in its territory thereafter.[55] Nonocclusive ischemia is attributable to prolonged hypotension, combined hypotension and arterial stenosis, or arterial spasm. Intravenous, or crack cocaine causes acute, nonocclusive bowel ischemia in young adults because of arterial spasm.[52,53] Venous causes of ischemia (Table 56-1) include mechanical occlusion of major veins, venulitis, infection, or thrombosis caused by thrombophilias.

Recently described causes of colonic ischemia include idiopathic myointimal hyperplasia of mesenteric veins,[41] immunotherapy with interleukin-2 and interferon-alpha,[56] amyloid deposition in patients receiving long-term hemodialysis,[57] and segmental ischemic colitis in renal transplant recipients.[58]

Colonic injury from deprivation of blood supply ranges from minor degrees of mucosal injury to complete infarction. The pathologic features are variable, depending on cause, duration, and severity. Involvement is usually segmental within the colon. The region of the splenic flexure, at the junction of the territories supplied by the superior and inferior mesenteric arteries, is most commonly involved. Early ischemia produces a red, edematous mucosa (Fig. 56-9). Later, ulceration occurs secondary to mucosal necrosis. Scarring and contraction of the muscle coat leads to thickening of the bowel wall and symptoms of pain and obstruction in chronic lesions. Full-thickness infarction produces a green or black, soft, thin, friable bowel wall with eventual perforation and peritonitis. Extreme congestion and hemorrhage of mucosa and submucosa typifies venous obstruction, but this appearance can also occur after reperfusion after arterial occlusion. Multisegmental disease is typical of arteritis, embolism, or hypoperfusion injury. Between the patches of disease, the mucosa is normal.

The mucosal epithelium is most sensitive to ischemia. Initial injury causes rapid epithelial turnover. The crypts are lined by an immature epithelium without differentiation. The mucosa is thinned, and the surface cells are flattened. Once ulceration occurs, an inflammatory exudate forms a pseudomembrane on the surface. Grossly, ischemic pseudomembranes are diffuse, unlike the plaques of infectious pseudomembranous colitis. Inflammatory cell infiltration in ischemic bowel disease is often light. The mucosal capillaries become congested, and there is extravasation of blood. In more severe ischemia, the mucosa and sometimes the entire bowel wall undergo infarction (Fig. 56-10). Necrotic tissue

Table 56-1 Causes of large bowel ischemia

Arterial
- Vascular stenosis or occlusion
  - Atherosclerosis
  - Emboli, thrombotic or atherosclerotic
  - Aortofemoral bypass surgery
- Hypotension
- Vasculitis
  - Polyarteritis nodosa
- Spasm
  - Cocaine abuse
- Radiation
- Carcinoid tumor
- Mechanical factors
  - Twisting of vascular pedicle

Venous
- Mechanical factors
  - Torsion, volvulus
  - Intussusception
  - Adhesion bands
  - Hernias
- Thrombophilias (hereditary hypercoagulable states)
  - Antithrombin III deficiency
  - Deficiency of protein S or heparin cofactor II
  - Defects of plasminogen and plasminogen activators
- Acquired hypercoagulable states
  - Myeloproliferative disorders
  - Hyperviscosity states
  - Estrogen therapy
  - Recent surgery
  - Acute pancreatitis
  - Carcinomatosis
  - Paroxysmal nocturnal hemoglobinuria
  - Lupus anticoagulants

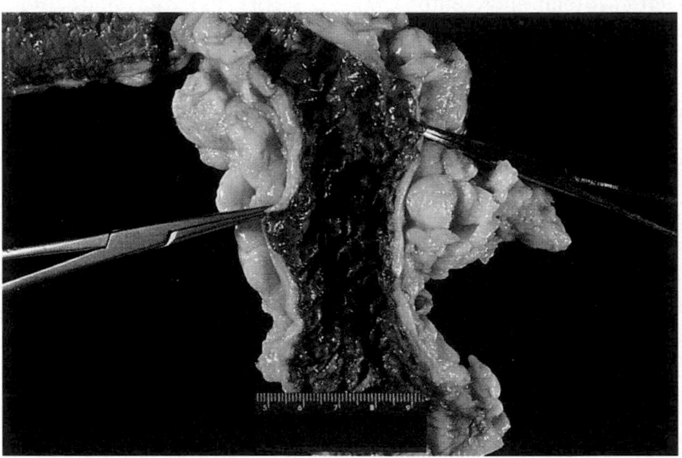

Fig. 56-9 Acute large bowel ischemia. Notice the hemorrhagic mucosal discoloration.

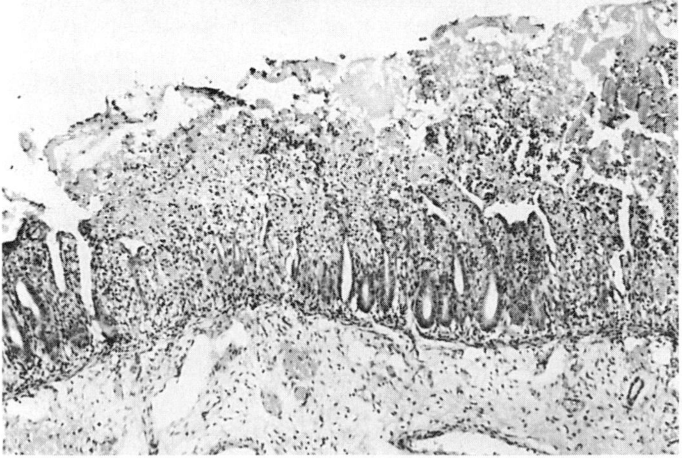

Fig. 56-10 Mucosal infarction from a case of ischemic bowel disease. A poorly organized membrane is present on the surface.

initially retains the ghosted cell outlines but is rapidly degraded by the bowel flora to amorphous debris.

Segmental ischemia that causes mucosal infarction and ulceration can be associated with transmural inflammation and a thickened bowel wall, simulating Crohn's disease. Extensive ulceration may heal with fibrosis rich in hemosiderin. Strictures and inflammatory pseudopolyps develop weeks or months after the initial insult. Very large ulcers persist indefinitely. Ischemic colonic muscle shows vacuolization and degeneration of fibers, especially in the circular coat.[59] Organizing occlusive arterial thrombi, cholesterol emboli, or vasculitis establishes the diagnosis of ischemia conclusively. A thrombus should be searched for on gross examination by serially sectioning of the vessels, but often the diagnosis of ischemic stricture is presumptive, since a vascular disorder cannot be documented.

Endoscopic biopsy specimens aid in the diagnosis of ischemia but are rarely if ever pathognomonic. Ischemic ulcers show nonspecific features, such as granulation tissue and exudate. The mucosa at the margin of the ulcers is thinned and shows mucin depletion, hyalinization of the lamina propria, and decreased numbers of inflammatory cells. The features of colonic infection by enterohemorrhagic *Escherichia coli* may be indistinguishable from ischemia, and this organism probably accounts for earlier reports of spontaneously resolving ischemia in young people.[60] Endoscopic biopsy reports usually have to be couched in terms of diagnostic possibilities, rather than a definitive diagnosis.

Pain is a major symptom of ischemic bowel disease. It is typically colicky and periumbilical at the onset but soon becomes continuous, severe, and poorly localized. A second symptom, bleeding, may range in severity from staining of stool to voluminous blood loss capable of producing shock. Barium examination may demonstrate thumbprinting indicating submucosal edema or, in more advanced cases, superficial ulcers, and ultimately strictures. Extreme narrowing of the mesenteric arteries without actual occlusion may cause intestinal angina, a syndrome of cramping abdominal pain, which begins within minutes of eating. Transient ischemia may be attributable to vascular occlusion, cardiac disease, or atherosclerosis, especially if complicated by hypotension or dehydration, in elderly patients.

Hemangiomas and vascular anomalies

Hemangiomas and vascular anomalies are classified (on the basis of histologic type, vessel size, and clinical associations Table 56-2).[61] The precise nature and pathogenesis of some of the lesions is obscure, and the terminology is often confusing, since acquired vascular abnormalities are sometimes called *malformations,* a term that usually implies a lesion that is formed during development.

Angiodysplasia[62,63] is a telangiectasia that causes acute or recurrent colonic hemorrhage. They are common in the elderly but rare in children and adolescents. The mean age at diagnosis is 65 years. A leash of dilated, thin-walled capillaries and venules arises from a feeding arteriole and appears as a cherry-red spot, less than 10 mm in diameter, in the mucosa. Biopsies may be done with little risk and are treated by fulguration.[64] There is an increased risk of angiodysplasia in patients with von Willebrand's disease,[65] calcific aortic stenosis, cirrhosis, occlusive vascular disease,[66] chronic renal failure,[67] and myelofibrosis.[68] The pathogenesis is obscure, but it is hypothesized that submucosal veins are obstructed as they traverse the muscle coat, resulting in increased pressure and dilatation. Lesions tend to be clustered in specific areas of the bowel,[69] and two thirds of these lesions are located in the cecum or ascending colon.[66] They may be delineated by angiography, but colectomy may occasionally have to be performed for acute hemorrhage when no lesion has been demonstrated.

Angiodysplasias have been most convincingly demonstrated by injection of the vessels and preparation of corrosion casts, but these methods are too time consuming for routine practice. Angiodysplasias collapse once the specimen is cut open, and so lesions are rarely found in resected segments of colon. One can demonstrate them by filling the bowel with formalin, stripping the mucosa, and examining it under a hand lens.[63] Histologically, they consist of a group of dilated capillaries in the lamina propria and submucosa (Fig. 56-11).

Table 56-2 Vascular abnormalities of the gut

Vascular abnormalities of the gut
Arteriovenous anomalies and telangiectasias
Angiodysplasia
Hereditary hemorrhagic telangiectasia
Turner's syndrome
Systemic sclerosis and CREST syndrome
Multiple varicosities and phlebectasias
Hemangiomas
Capillary
Cavernous
Mixed capillary-cavernous
Blue rubber bleb nevus syndrome
Klippel-Trénaunay-Weber syndrome
Peutz-Jeghers syndrome
Disorders of connective tissue affecting blood vessels
Pseudoxanthoma elasticum
Ehlers-Danlos syndromes
Dieulafoy lesion

CREST, Calcinosis, Raynaud's phenomenon, esophageal dysmotility, sclerodactyly, telangiectasia syndrome.

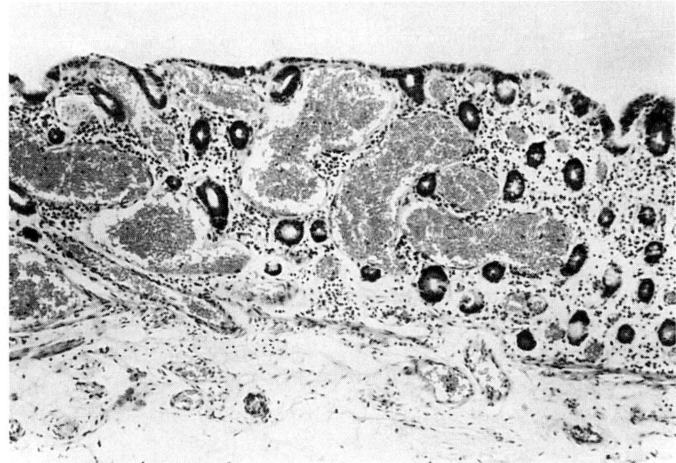

Fig. 56-11 Angiodysplasia of the colon. Notice the dilated, thin-walled vessels.

Hereditary hemorrhagic telangiectasia (Osler-Weber-Rendu syndrome) may affect the colon. The patients are young and have other features of the syndrome, such as telangiectasias of the lips and mouth, nosebleeds, and a positive family history. These telangiectasias may have a sclerotic stromal component and involve the muscularis propria and serosa, as well as the mucosa. Telangiectasias may occur in any part of the gastrointestinal tract in Turner's syndrome. These telangiectasias regress spontaneously with time.[61] Telangiectasias in systemic sclerosis[70] and CREST syndrome may also cause gastrointestinal bleeding. There is no consistent gross or microscopic appearance that permits a distinction between the various types of vascular ectasia. Reliance has to be placed on clinical findings.

Severe congestion of the colon occurs in patients with portal hypertension who may present with hematochezia or anemia and show cherry-red spots, angiodysplasia-like lesions, or nonspecific erythema.[71] *Varices* of the colorectum can occur in four situations—in the context of portal hypertension, as a familial syndrome (without portal hypertension), as an isolated varix, and as multiple varices localized to one part of the colon or affecting the whole colon. Anorectal and pararectal varices are found in 90% of patients with portal hypertension if they are sought by transvaginal ultrasonography. They infrequently cause bleeding. Isolated rectal or colonic varices and familial varices,[72] occurring in the absence of portal hypertension, are rare causes of massive recurrent bleeding.

Hemangiomas of the colon are rare and include capillary hemangiomas, cavernous hemangiomas, and mixed types. They are more often cavernous than capillary and usually single, diffusely infiltrative, circumferential, or segmental. Capillary hemangiomas are proliferations of small, closely packed capillaries with prominent endothelium, whereas cavernous hemangiomas consist of sinusoidal vessels, which may thrombose and calcify. Diffuse cavernous hemangiomas present in childhood with intermittent rectal bleeding but may go undiagnosed for many years. The angiomas affect a segment of colon or rectum and may involve adjacent viscera or the retroperitoneum and they may be associated with lymphangiomatosis or protein-losing enteropathy. Hemangiomas of the intestine have also been described in Peutz-Jeghers syndrome, blue rubber bleb nevus syndrome, and the Klippel-Trénaunay-Weber syndrome.

INFECTIOUS DISEASES

The most important infectious diseases of the colon are listed in Table 56-3.

Table 56-3 Infectious diseases of the large bowel

Bacteria
Acute self-limited colitis
Nontyphoid *Salmonella*
Shigella sp.
Campylobacter jejuni
Yersinia enterocolitica
Pseudomembranous colitis
Clostridium difficile
Escherichia coli
Neutropenic enterocolitis
Clostridium septicum
Gonococcal proctitis
Syphilis
Chlamydial proctitis
Granuloma inguinale
Malakoplakia
Viruses
Herpes proctitis
Cytomegalovirus
Parasites
Entamoeba histolytica
Balantidium coli
Enterobiasis
Trichuriasis
Schistosomiasis

Bacterial diseases

Diarrhea caused by Escherichia coli

Escherichia coli is the most numerous aerobe of the normal human colonic flora but also may cause several distinct forms of diarrheal disease and dysentery.[73] *E. coli* is serotyped by three major antigens: the lipopolysaccharide O antigen, the heat-labile flagellar H antigen, and the capsular (K) antigens. One hundred sixty-nine O serogroups and more than 60 H antigens are recognized. Each distinct class of pathogenic *E. coli* includes a restricted set of O serogroups and O:H serotypes, bears distinct K (capsular) antigens, and possesses distinctive virulence attributes.[73]

E. coli is transmitted by the fecal-oral route, by contaminated water or food, or by direct contact. In underdeveloped and tropical countries that lack sanitation or water treatment, *E. coli* diarrhea is a major cause of infantile and childhood diarrhea and contributes significantly to malnutrition, growth retardation, and death. Gastric acid is an important barrier to *E. coli,* and achlorhydria increases the risk of infection. Normal mucus, bowel flora, and motility are also significant barriers.[74]

E. coli that cause diarrhea are currently classified into five groups: enteropathogenic (EPEC), enterohemorrhagic (EHEC), enterotoxigenic (ETEC), enteroaggregative (EAggEC), and enteroinvasive (EIEC).[75] Specific serotypes are associated with production of specific toxins and with other virulence mechanisms confirming the value of serotyping.[73] Most pathogenic *E. coli* colonize the intestine by elaborating surface proteins that bind complementary receptors on host epithelial cells. They also form one or more toxins that cause fluid secretion, cell injury, or cell death.

Enteropathogenic *E. coli* (EPEC) are strains isolated from outbreaks of infantile diarrhea or summer diarrhea that do not elaborate heat-labile (LT) or heat-stable (ST) enterotoxins, do not invade the mucosa, or cause disseminated sepsis and belong to certain classic strains.[76] Duodenal biopsy specimens show a flat mucosa with crypt hyperplasia and a row of bacteria attached along the brush border diffusely or in patches. Rectal biopsy specimens may show similar features. Infants present with watery diarrhea without blood or mucus, accompanied by vomiting, low-grade fever, and, in severe cases, dehydration and electrolyte imbalance. The average total duration of diarrhea is about 9 days, though the duration tends to be longer than 14 days in younger children.[77]

Outbreaks of hemorrhagic colitis caused by EHEC infection have been reported worldwide. Miniepidemics, limited to nursing homes or day-care centers, have also been reported.[78,79] The incidence is highest in the elderly and in children. Infection may be complicated by the hemolytic-uremic syndrome. In patients over 65 years of age, the death rate may be as high as 26%. The source of infection most often implicated is improperly cooked ground beef, both in sporadic cases and in outbreaks.[78] EHEC possess both a plasmid-encoded adherence protein that mediates early mucosal interaction and a chromosomally encoded protein that mediates attachment and effacement. In addition, EHEC produce phage-encoded Shiga-like toxins I or II (SLT-I, SLT-II), or both.[80] These toxins were initially identified as being toxic to the Vero cell line and are also known as *verotoxins*. The pathogenesis of the hemolytic uremic syndrome, and thrombotic-thrombocytopenic purpura, may be related to combined effects of absorbed Shigatoxin and endotoxin on human vascular endothelial cells. This may account for the swelling of glomerular endothelial cells, fibrin deposition, and inflammatory cell infiltrates seen in the kidneys.[81]

Biopsy specimens of the rectosigmoid may show normal mucosa or mild acute inflammation indistinguishable from other infectious colitides. The main pathologic lesions are usually in the ascending and transverse colon. Biopsy specimens at these sites show a range of change including normal areas, edema and neutrophil infiltration characteristic of infectious colitis, and superficial mucosal necrosis and exudation resembling ischemic colitis.[82] The latter lesions may be associated with fibrin/platelet thrombi within mucosal capillaries. Pseudomembranous lesions may occur and may be indistinguishable from those caused by *Clostridium difficile*.

Infection with *E. coli* O157:H7 produces a range of illness from asymptomatic infection through mild diarrhea to hemorrhagic colitis with hemolytic uremia syndrome and death. Typically there is crampy abdominal pain, followed soon by watery diarrhea, and, within 48 hours the diarrhea becomes grossly bloody.

Enterotoxigenic *E. coli* (ETEC) produce heat-labile (LT) or heat-stable (ST) enterotoxins, which promote fluid secretion by the gut and cause secretory diarrhea.[83] Classical LT resembles cholera toxin and activates adenyl cyclase promoting intraluminal chloride secretion.[83] ETEC is a major cause of diarrhea in both children and adults in developing countries, in travelers to developing countries, and in outbreaks in the developed world.[83,84] Contaminated food and water are the main vehicles of transmission. Light microscopic examination of small bowel and large bowel biopsies is within normal limits. Ultrastructural examination reveals widening of intracellular spaces and junctional complexes. On the epithelial surface, there are disrupted microvilli and cytoplasmic processes projecting into the lumen.

Enteroaggregative *E. coli* (EAggEC) produce a toxin named EAST (enteroaggregative *E. coli* heat-stable enterotoxin). EAggEC has been incriminated as a cause of childhood diarrhea in Mexico and India. As the name implies, the presumed mechanism of disease is adherence to small and large bowel enterocytes. Biopsy specimens may reveal organisms adhering to the mucosal surface, but the tissue is otherwise unremarkable.

Enteroinvasive *E. coli* (EIEC) cause a dysenteric illness similar to shigellosis.[85] Most EIEC share antigenic and physiologic similarities with *Shigella* and are closely related genera, which cannot be distinguished by DNA/DNA hybridization. The morphology of the colonic mucosa in EIEC infection is not documented but is presumed to be that of an acute self-limited colitis.

Acute self-limited infectious colitis

Acute infectious or self-limited colitis (ASLC) may be caused by nontyphoid *Salmonella*,[86,87] *Shigella*,[88] *Campylobacter jejuni*,[89] *E. coli*, *Clostridium difficile*, or rarely *Yersinia enterocolitica*[90] However, these pathogens are cultured in only 50% to 60% of cases. It is not possible to identify by biopsy appearances in which infectious agent is present.

Nontyphoid *salmonella* is usually acquired from domestic animals, particularly via poultry, eggs, or from shellfish. The organisms remain localized in the small and large bowel mucosa. Diarrhea develops 8 to 36 hours after ingestion of food and is usually watery, only rarely bloody. Fluid and electrolyte replacement is the mainstay of treatment. Patients with ulcerative colitis appear to have an increased susceptibility to *Salmonella* infection, and the possibility of dual pathologic conditions should always be considered.

Four species of *Shigella* produce human disease: *Sh. dysenteriae*, *Sh. flexneri*, *Sh. boydii*, and *Sh. sonnei*. The disease is spread by fecally contaminated water. Only a small number of organisms are required to produce infection and children are particularly vulnerable. Shigellas are phagocytosed by epithelial cells, digest the membranous vacuoles that initially surround them, and escape into the lamina propria. Damage is mediated by a potent cytotoxin Shiga toxin, which has the ability to kill macrophages. *Sh. dysenteriae* serotype 1 is the most virulent species, being responsible for pandemic dysentery in Central America and the Indian subcontinent. A patient presents with severe abdominal pain, low-volume bloody diarrhea, tenesmus, and high fever, which may be complicated by the hemolytic-uremic syndrome. The colon and rectum show widespread ulceration, perforation, or pseudomembrane formation. Like most other bacterial diarrheas, shigellosis is usually a pancolitis that is most severe distally. The other shigellas produce milder disease, indistinguishable from acute self-limited colitis.

Campylobacter jejuni is part of the normal bowel flora in many domestic and wild animals. It is transmitted to humans by the ingestion of undercooked poultry, unpasteurized milk, or contaminated water. Very small numbers of organisms can transmit the disease. Most cases are sporadic, but large outbreaks have been reported. The organism produces a heat-labile toxin resembling cholera toxin that also produces a self-limited enterocolitis.

Yersinia enterocolitica typically causes an ileocecitis,[91] but it also accounts for up to 10% of cases of acute self-limited colitis[92] and some cases of segmental colitis. Disease is characterized grossly by aphthoid ulcers, erythema, and friability. Occasionally, larger ulcers are present. Microscopically, the inflammation may be localized to lymphoid follicles, or the areas of ulceration may be characterized by diffuse mucosal changes resembling ulcerative colitis.

Diarrhea, abdominal pain, vomiting, fever, and malaise are the main symptoms of ASLC, irrespective of the causative organism. Histologically[93] the crypt architecture is normal. There is neutrophil infiltration, edema, capillary congestion, and mucin depletion. The number of basally located plasma cells is not increased. Typically, the inflammation involves the luminal half of the mucosa and spares the base. Cryptitis is common, but crypt abscesses are rare. Plasma cells increase late in the course of infection and may make distinction from idiopathic inflammatory bowel disease difficult.[93,94]

Pseudomembranous colitis

Pseudomembranous colitis is a descriptive term for a particular form of large bowel disease that has characteristic appearances but multiple causes. In most cases it is caused by *Clostridium difficile*. Rarer causes include ischemia, verocytotoxin-producing *E. coli,* and *Shigella dysenteriae* type I infection. However, not all infections with *C. difficile* produce a pseudomembranous picture, and many may give the picture of nonspecific acute self-limited colitis. Pseudomembranous colitis generally occurs after antibiotic therapy that allows the selective proliferation of the organism within the bowel. In most instances, the disease is confined to the large bowel. However, it may rarely involve the small bowel, especially in children.[95]

C. difficile elaborates two major toxins.[96] Toxin A, a classical enterotoxin that in experimental animals causes fluid secretion from isolated loops of bowel, is also a cytotoxin and is responsible for pseudomembrane formation. Toxin B is a cytotoxin, the role of which in pathogenesis of lesions is presently unclear.

Grossly pseudomembranes are elevated flat-topped plaques. The intervening mucosa is normal. The plaques are cream colored or greenish in appearance. Initially, they are pinpoint in size, but as the disease advances, they may spread to cover several centimeters. Characteristically they are firmly attached to the mucosa and do not easily rub off. Microscopically,[97] the earliest lesions consist of a small volcano-like eruption of fibrin, mucin, and neutrophils from the intercryptal surface epithelium (Fig. 56-12). Later, the superficial portions of the crypts dilate and become incorporated in the membrane. In advanced lesions, the mucosa is totally destroyed. Pseudomembranes associated with *C. difficile* are typically lamellated with a characteristic streaming of incorporated neutrophils. Pseudomembranes occurring secondarily to ischemia often lack this streaming appearance and contain more fibrin than mucin.

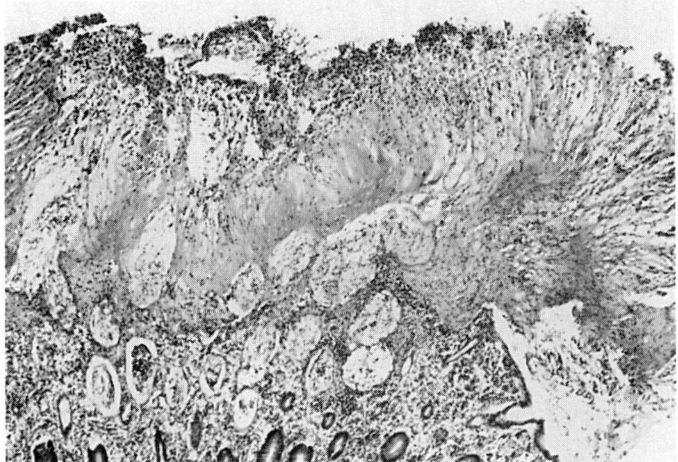

Fig. 56-12 Pseudomembranous colitis caused by *Clostridium difficile.*

Most patients present with watery diarrhea. Severe cases may be complicated by hypoalbuminemia, hypokalemia, and, rarely, bloody diarrhea, fever and shock, toxic megacolon, or perforation.[98]

Neutropenic enterocolitis

Neutropenic enterocolitis, which is also called *necrotizing cecitis* or *typhlitis,* is seen in patients who are profoundly neutropenic from anticancer chemotherapy, or cyclic neutropenia. The clinical syndrome manifests as fever, right lower quadrant abdominal pain, and rectal hemorrhage. The main organism causing neutropenic enterocolitis is *Clostridium septicum,*[99,100] but a variety of other clostridia have been implicated. Most patients have received antibiotics, which may disturb the balance of the bowel flora.

The disease involves chiefly the right side of the colon and the cecum. Grossly the cecum shows edema, hemorrhage, mucosal or transmural necrosis, patchy ulceration, and pseudomembrane formation with mucosal discoloration and friability. Microscopically, the surviving mucosa shows hemorrhage and congestion and may contain an increased number of dilated capillaries with fibrin thrombi. The submucosa is edematous and paradoxically may be infiltrated by neutrophils. The ulcers are nonspecific, and the pseudomembranes resemble those seen in ischemia. Cytomegalovirus inclusions are commonly identified and are assumed to represent a coinfection. Gram stain displays bacteria, usually a mixed flora, in the wall.

Sexually transmitted diseases

Rectal syphilis

Rectal syphilis[101] occurs after anal intercourse and occurs typically in promiscuous homosexual men. It presents as an ulcer or proctitis, which may be concurrent with chancres in the anal canal or at the anal margin. The duration from intercourse to presentation may be up to eight weeks. The biopsy specimen[102] shows intense inflammation, mainly plasma cells and lymphocytes, but sometimes granulomas or nonspecific proctitis is present. Serologic tests may be negative early in the course of the disease. Rectal syphilis may grossly mimic solitary ulcer syndrome, or a neoplasm,[103] particularly lymphoma, because of the associated adenopathy. Clinically, it may be asymptomatic or associated with pain, constipation, or rectal bleeding.

Gonococcal proctitis

Gonococcal proctitis is transmitted by anal intercourse. Endoscopically, a variety of changes may be encountered, ranging from normal to severe erythema, edema, and even ulceration.

The microscopic appearances[103,104] are highly variable and nonspecific, usually being similar to acute self-limited colitis, though in about one third of cases there is a prominent lymphocytosis and plasmacytosis. Rare instances when *Neisseria meningitidis* has been cultured from rectal swabs have been described.[104] These are assumed to have arisen after oral or anal intercourse.

Chlamydial proctitis

Both (lymphogranuloma venereum) (LGV) and non-LGV strains of chlamydia may cause proctitis after anal intercourse.[105,106]

LGV generally causes the most severe disease with pain and rectal discharge. Mucosal edema, erythema, and ulceration are present in the early stages. Later, the disease may produce inflammatory masses and heal by fibrosis with stricture formation. Biopsy specimens of these may show nonspecific acute and chronic inflammation with eosinophils, or there may be isolated giant cells and necrotizing granulomas.[105] In about 50% of patients, the disease spreads to involve the remainder of the colon or even the terminal ileum, and the late stages of this extensive disease may grossly and microscopically mimic Crohn's disease.

Non-LGV chlamydial infection results in less severe disease, which grossly and microscopically is only mildly abnormal. Clinically it is often asymptomatic.

Spirochetosis

Spirochetes are identified on the surface of colorectal mucosa in about 2% of unselected biopsy specimens[107] but are considerably more frequent (28% to 36%) in male homosexuals.[105] They are generally considered to be nonpathogenic, though some cases with diarrhea do respond to antibiotic therapy.[108] A variety of organisms have been identified, one of the commonest being *Brachyspira aalborgi*. Histologically the mucosa is completely normal, apart from a fuzzy blue band on the mucosal surface (Fig. 56-13). On closer inspection, slender curved organisms may be identified. Optimum recognition may be achieved by use of a silver stain, such as Warthin-Starry.[105]

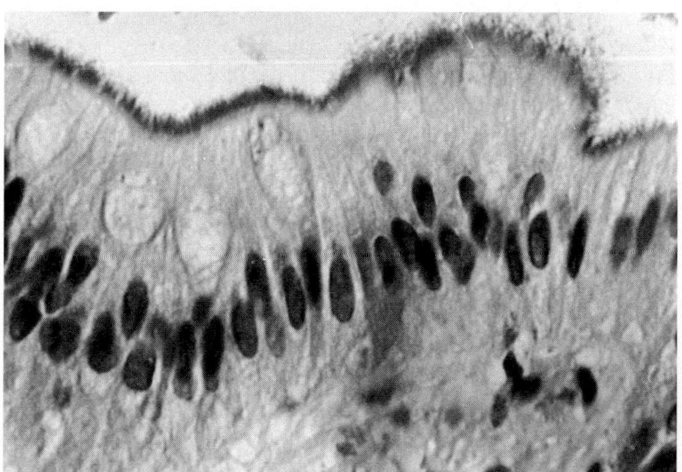

Fig. 56-13 Spirochetosis. Notice the fuzzy zone of organisms on the mucosal surface.

Viral infections

Herpes colitis and proctitis

Herpes simplex virus (HSV) proctitis is a relatively common venereally acquired infection that may affect immunocompetent and immunodeficient individuals.[109] Between 80% and 90% of cases are attributable to HSV type II infection. Herpes involving the more proximal colon appears to be extremely rare, with only one documented case that occurred in an immunosuppressed individual.

Clinically, HSV presents with perianal vesicles or small ulcers. On endoscopic examination, the mucosa is friable with superficial ulcers and vesicles. In severely immunosuppressed persons, the ulcers may be deeper and undermined. Histologically the rectal biopsy changes may be difficult to distinguish from other causes of infectious colitis. The crypt architecture is preserved and there is a predominance of acute inflammatory cells within the lamina propria. Generally the superficial ulcers are nonspecific, but, in some cases, typical HSV multinucleated giant cells with intranuclear inclusions may be encountered. Biopsy specimens from the submucosa may show a perivenular lymphocytic infiltrate.

Symptomatically, patients complain of intense anorectal pain, tenesmus, and constipation. Radicular pain and parasthesia can be referred to the skin overlying the buttocks and upper thigh.

Cytomegalovirus colitis

There are three clinical situations where cytomegalovirus (CMV) may involve the large bowel. The first of these is a self-limited, venereally acquired proctitis in immunocompetent patients.[110] These individuals develop rectal pain with hematochezia. Endoscopic examination reveals friable mucosa with serpiginous ulceration. Biopsy of this mucosa shows nonspecific acute and chronic inflammation, in which there may be small numbers of CMV inclusions.

The second pattern of CMV colitis occurs rarely in patients with fulminant ulcerative colitis who are taking corticosteroids.[111] Resection specimens from these cases generally show small numbers of CMV inclusions, and it is not clear to what degree the virus is contributing to tissue damage. Superinfection by CMV may provoke fulminant disease, or, alternatively, steroid therapy given for preexisting severe disease may reactivate the latent virus.

In immunosuppressed patients, CMV may cause a primary enteritis or colitis, characterized by friable hemorrhagic mucosa with ulcers that are typically serpiginous and punched out. Rarely, deep ulcers may perforate. Histologic changes vary in severity from nonspecific inflammation to acute ulceration. The inflammatory infiltrates are usually neutrophilic. Endothelial cells contain the typical owl-eyed nuclear or granular cytoplasmic inclusions. Because of this vascular involvement, it has been postulated that ischemia, secondary to capillary occlusion, may play a contributory role in the pathogenesis of ulceration. Epithelial cells may also contain inclusions.

Parasitic diseases

Amebiasis

Entamoeba histolytica[112,113] is the most common human pathogenic protozoon. Amebiasis affects the colon and terminal ileum. It occurs worldwide but is particularly prevalent in the tropics and subtropics, where spread occurs as a result of poor hygiene and sanitation. The amebas cause damage by a combination of processes, including contact-dependent cytolytic cell death and the production of proteolytic enzymes and cytotoxins.[112] Only specific enzyme-producing types of *E. histolytica* are pathogenic; they are recognized by their enzyme patterns, or zymodemes ('enzyme-populations').

The clinical severity of amebic colitis varies. At one extreme are asymptomatic carriers and at the other are cases of life-threatening fulminant colitis. The reasons for this difference in patterns of disease are variations in the zymodeme patterns and virulence attributes of the organisms. However, host factors, including genetic predisposition, nutritional status, immunologic competence, and the presence of cofactors, such as altered colonic bacterial flora, also play a role.

The life cycle of *E. histolytica* is very simple. In the human large bowel, the vegetative form is the trophozoite; it is distinguished from other amebas by the presence of ingested red blood cells within the cytoplasm. The trophozoites undergo binary fission or form cysts, which are excreted in the feces. There is no intermediate animal host. Cysts are ingested when fecal contamination of food or water occurs. The cysts survive gastric acid and small bowel digestion and release up to eight new trophozoites when they excyst in the large intestine.

On gross examination,[113] the changes include edema, mucosal friability, and ulcers covered by exudate and necrosis. In some instances, there is diffuse involvement similar to ulcerative colitis, but in others the ulceration is segmental and may heal with stricture formation. Early ulcers are pinpoint erosions, but as they enlarge, they become flask-shaped "collar stud ulcers" because of undermining. In advanced disease, the ulcers may be serpiginous and irregularly shaped. Occasionally, inflammatory masses resembling neoplasms may occur as localized lesions in the bowel or even in the perianal region. These masses are termed "amebomas," or amebic granulomas.

Initial microscopic changes[113] include edema, neutrophilic infiltration, mucin depletion, and microulceration. Later, there is deep ulceration with granulation tissue at the base and overlying necrotic debris (so-called dirty necrosis) containing trophozoites. Between ulcers, the mucosa may show active inflammation with cryptitis and crypt abscesses or may be relatively uninflamed. Amebas are located within slough at the surface of ulcers, in flecks of mucus on the intact mucosa, or on the luminal side of dirty necrosis (Fig. 56-14). The trophozoites are approximately 25 μm in diameter and resemble large histiocytes. Their cytoplasm is granular and bluish gray and may contain ingested red blood cells. The nucleus is inconspicuous, centrally located, or eccentric, with a single central karyosome that is often difficult to identify on hematoxylin and eosin–stained sections. The cytoplasm is PAS positive, which can be extremely helpful in identifying small numbers of organisms in large inflammatory masses. Complications of amebiasis can include dissemination to other organs, especially liver and brain, perforation, fulminant colitis, toxic megacolon, strictures, and inflammatory polyposis.

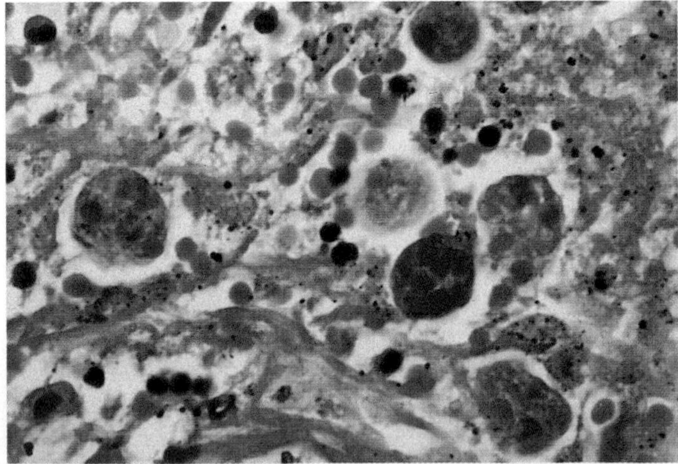

Fig. 56-14 Trophozoites of *Entamoeba histolytica* present in a zone of "dirty necrosis."

Other amebic diseases

Other rarely encountered potentially pathogenic amebas are *Balantidium coli*[114] and *Blastocystis hominis.*[115] Balantidiasis is rarely encountered outside of the tropics, where it infects domestic and wild animals. The clinical symptoms and method of transmission are similar to *E. histolytica*. Morphologically, *Balantidia* are oval-shaped organisms 50 to 100 μm in length, with a macronucleus and abundant cilia. Most infections are asymptomatic; others are similar to amebic dysentery.

Blastocystis hominis is probably nonpathogenic when it occurs in small numbers. Significant disease is considered to be present when at least 5 organisms are present in each high-power (objective × 40) field of wet mount fecal smears.[116] It is not uncommonly encountered in traveler's diarrhea in the company of *Dientamoeba fragilis*.

Enterobiasis

The nematode *Enterobius vermicularis* is also known as pinworm, threadworm, or *Oxyuris*[117] It is spread by the fecal-oral route from person to person. There is no intermediate host and no animal reservoir. Eggs hatch in the large bowel, producing male and female adults. The male dies soon after copulation, but the gravid female migrates to the perianal zone, where eggs are deposited.

Adult females are approximately 1.0 cm in length and up to 0.5 mm in cross section. They may be recognized by the presence of ovaries in the internal organs. The males are smaller, measuring 0.2 to 0.5 cm in length and up to 0.2 cm in cross section. Externally, both sexes have a thick cuticle and lateral alae. Adult worms and eggs may be encountered in the appendix or segments of large bowel removed for other reasons. Generally they do not penetrate the bowel mucosa or cause intestinal disease, other than pruritus ani. Some authorities believe that a heavy infestation may cause acute appendicitis by obstructing the lumen, but they are more often an incidental finding. Rarely, adult female worms migrate into unusual locations, such as the peritoneal cavity and the female genital tract.

Trichuriasis

Trichuris trichiura, or whipworm, has a worldwide distribution but is particularly prevalent in tropical and subtropical areas.[118,119] The adult nematode worms embed in the right side of the colon and shed eggs into the feces. Reinfection may occur by the fecal-oral route. There is no intermediate host. Adult worms measure up to 5 cm in length and are attached to the mucosal surface. In histologic cross section, they have a thick cuticle but no lateral alae. They may elicit a light mucosal infiltrate of lymphocytes and eosinophils, but often the mucosa is normal. They rarely cause symptoms, though severe infections result in diarrhea and abdominal pain and may stunt the growth of children.

Schistosomiasis

Three major forms of schistosomiasis are recognized, and all may affect the large bowel.[120] *Schistosoma mansoni* mainly affects the left side of the colon and may be identified by the presence of eggs with a lateral spine. *Schistosoma japonicum* also has eggs with a lateral spine, but these tend to be smaller sized than those of *S. mansoni*. It predominantly affects the right side of the colon and small bowel. *Schistosoma hematobium* is largely confined to the rectum and has a terminal spine on its eggs.

Infection is acquired by skin contact with freshwater contaminated by human feces. The schistosome eggs hatch and release miracidia, which infect a species of snail. The cercarial form of the organism emerges from the snail and penetrates intact human skin to reach the venous system. Mature adult worms live in veins in the bowel wall. After copulation, the adult females produce large quantities of eggs, many of which ultimately pass through the wall of the bowel into the gut lumen to complete the life cycle.

Light infections are usually asymptomatic. Heavy infections result in a large egg burden, many of which are retained in the submucosa, where they may die and create an intense inflammatory reaction in which eosinophils can be prominent.[120] Strictures may ultimately result, but more commonly the bowel mucosa may show ulceration or inflammatory polyps.

Malakoplakia

The colon is the commonest site of malakoplakia outside the urogenital tract.[121] Colonic malakoplakia has a bimodal age incidence, with one peak in children under 13 years of age and a second in middle-aged adults.[122] There is a slight excess in males over females. Some colonic malakoplakias are incidental foci adjacent to a carcinoma. Other cases are primary and may be associated with immunodeficiency or opportunistic infections. Primary large bowel malakoplakia presents with abdominal pain, mass, fever, anemia, diarrhea, or colitis and may show ulcerated or umbilicated yellowish mucosal nodules or polyps endoscopically.[123] At laparotomy, tumorlike masses may be found, or it may simulate Crohn's disease with ulcers and fistulas. The bladder is rarely involved concomitantly with large bowel.[124]

Histologically, malakoplakia consists predominantly of histiocytes, with smaller numbers of plasma cells and lymphocytes. The histiocytes contain Michaelis-Gutmann bodies, which are rounded, concentrically laminated, hematoxyphilic inclusions 5 to 8 μm in diameter. These stain positively for phosphorus, calcium, and iron. Ultrastructurally, the histiocytes in 50% of cases may contain phagolysosomes, in which there are degenerating bacteria. *E. coli* or *Klebsiella* are the organisms most often cultured from malakoplakia.

IDIOPATHIC INFLAMMATORY BOWEL DISEASE

Idiopathic inflammatory bowel disease (IIBD) includes two major conditions: ulcerative colitis (UC) and Crohn's disease (CD). They have many common epidemiologic, clinical, and morphologic features, though there are also some characteristic differences.

Ulcerative colitis

Ulcerative colitis is a chronic idiopathic inflammation of the rectal and colonic mucosa that affects a variable length of the large bowel in continuity from the anus. The incidence rate varies from country to country with a range from 2.2 per 100,000 per year in Baltimore to 15.1 per 100,000 in North Tees, England. Reported prevalence rates vary from 39 per 100,000 in Rochester, Minnesota, to 99 per 100,000 in North Tees, England. In many countries, the incidence rates have stabilized after showing steady increases for several years.[125] Mortality from IIBD is low; 0.05% of all United States deaths are attributable to IIBD.[125] IIBD may present at any time between infancy and old age, but the primary mode for clinical onset is between 15 and 25 years of age for both sexes. A second rise in incidence in the seventh decade has been described in some countries. Female incidence rates are about 30% higher for both ulcerative colitis and Crohn's disease in several populations of northern European origin. Nonwhite Americans of both sexes are one third as likely to develop ulcerative colitis and one fifth as likely to have Crohn's disease as the white population, but the difference between the races is closing with time.[125] Jews are at higher risk of developing IIBD than other ethnic groups. A strong hereditary influence is documented for both forms of IIBD, and between 10% and 40% of cases of ulcerative colitis have first-degree relatives with inflammatory bowel disease. In Denmark, the rate of ulcerative colitis among first-degree relatives of probands was increased by a factor of 9.5 over the general population. Twin studies show that as a cause the genetic factor is weaker in ulcerative colitis than that in Crohn's disease. There is a pronounced geographic variation in the occurrence of inflammatory bowel disease, and both Crohn's disease and ulcerative colitis are considerably more frequent in northern latitudes and in urban areas.[126] There is a positive association with the HLA-DR2 allele and a negative association with DR4 and DRW6.

The pathogenesis of IIBD is unknown. The prevailing view is that ulcerative colitis and Crohn's disease are separate conditions, though there are overlapping clinical, morphologic, and immunologic features. It seems likely that for the diseases to develop, there must be a provoking agent in the bowel lumen (infective or chemical), with an inappropriate host immune response that perpetuates the inflammatory reaction.

Ulcerative colitis[127] varies in extent from a distal proctitis affecting a few centimeters of bowel to total colonic involvement with extension into the terminal ileum (backwash ileitis). The gross, microscopic, and clinical features vary considerably with the degree and duration of disease activity. For descriptive purposes, the terms *active colitis, resolving colitis, chronically active colitis, quiescent colitis,* and *fulminant colitis* have been used for disease activity. Endoscopic and gross features of active disease are mucosal hyperemia, friability, granularity, ulcers, and erosions with blood in the lumen (Fig. 56-15). The junction between inflamed and uninflamed mucosa is usually gradual but may be sharp. Fulminant colitis exhibits extensive ulceration and may be associated with toxic dilatation (diameter greater than 5.5 cm on plain film), perforation, and peritonitis. In chronic quiescent colitis, the colon is shortened and the mucosa is flat and featureless (Fig. 56-16), except where inflammatory polyps or focal ulceration break the monotony (Fig. 56-17).

Inflammatory polyps are found endoscopically in about 20% of cases. They occur after episodes of severe disease, in which ulcers undermine the mucosa and when epithelium regenerates over the floors of the ulcers the islands remain elevated and become inflammatory polyps.

The rectal mucosa may grossly appear less diseased than the remainder of the colon, especially after treatment with steroid enemas. This rectal sparing should not be interpreted as representing a segmental colitis or misdiagnosed as Crohn's disease.

Histologic examination in an active phase reveals a diffuse increase in inflammatory cells within the lamina propria,

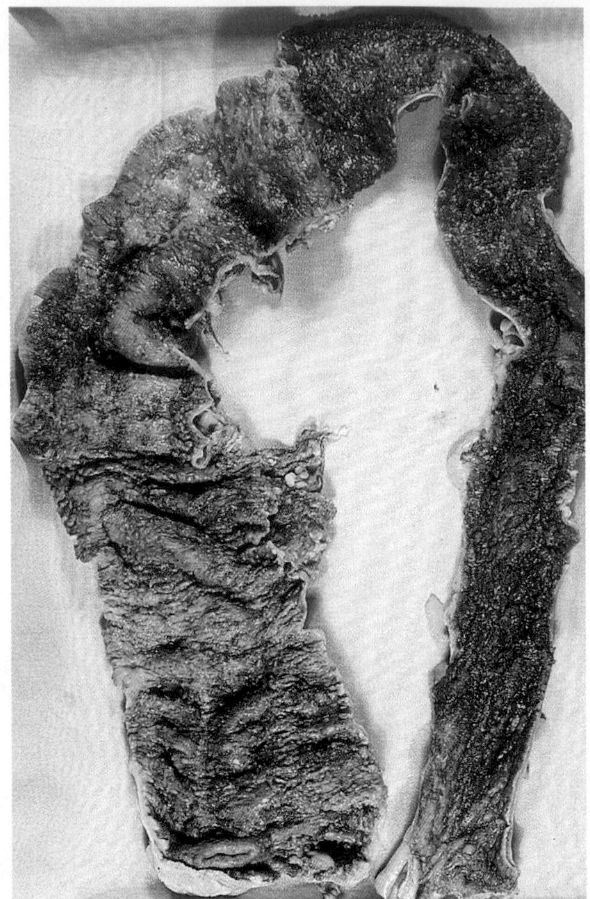

Fig. 56-15 Acute ulcerative colitis with extensive mucosal ulceration involving the entire colon.

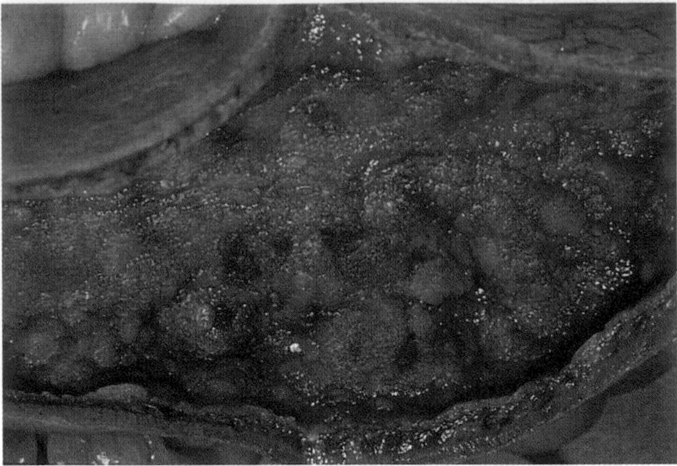

Fig. 56-16 Flat featureless mucosa from a case of chronic ulcerative colitis.

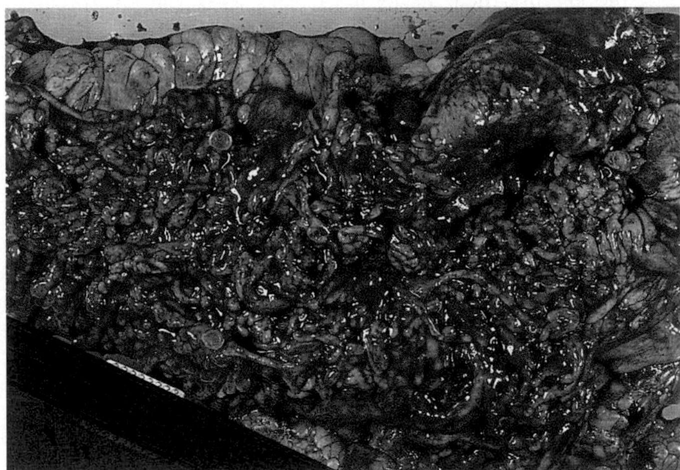

Fig. 56-17 Ulcerative colitis with inflammatory polyposis (pseudopolyps).

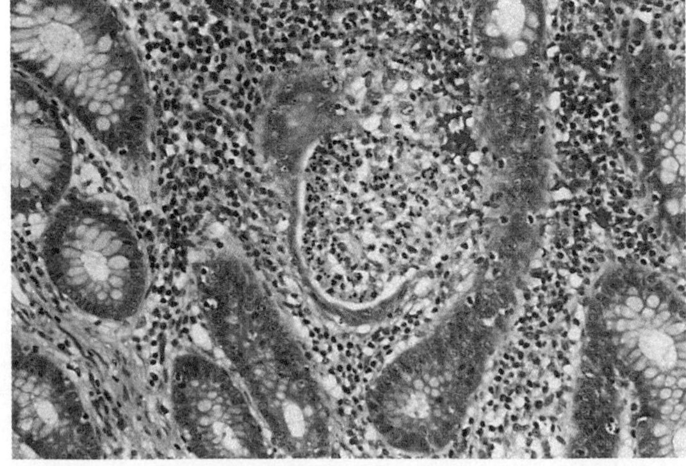

Fig. 56-18 Acute ulcerative colitis with crypt abscess formation.

including plasma cells, eosinophils, lymphocytes, macrophages, and neutrophils. The normal superficial predominance of the infiltrate is lost, and there is basal plasmacytosis. The capillaries are congested and dilated. The crypts show evidence of regeneration: branching (fission), shortening, irregularity, dilatation, and villiform change. Neutrophils infiltrate the surface and crypt epithelium and accumulate in crypt lumens to form abscesses (Fig. 56-18). Traditionally, neutrophil infiltration is regarded as the prime indicator of disease activity. Crypts that contain abscesses invariably show small foci of ulceration if serially sectioned. Macroscopic ulcers originate when crypt abscesses expand into the lamina propria and destroy the mucosa. If the muscularis mucosae is breached, the inflammation spreads laterally, undermining the mucosa, which sloughs and increases the area of ulceration. Such ulcers are extensive only in fulminant cases. As the disease undergoes resolution, neutrophils disappear from the epithelium and lamina propria. Later, chronic inflammatory cells diminish. This process may not occur uniformly but may be patchy, giving rise to local differences in intensity of inflammation. This must not be confused with Crohn's disease, where *normal* mucosa may be present immediately adjacent to heavily inflamed mucosa.

The mucosa of inactive colitis (Fig. 56-19) may show minimal or no inflammation and may have a villiform appearance because of crypt dilatation. It may be thinned and atrophic with short crypts that fail to reach the muscularis mucosae, branching crypts, and crypt dropout. Paneth cell metaplasia and increased numbers of enterochromaffin cells are present. The muscularis mucosae may be thickened, and this thickening accounts for cases of ulcerative colitis that have strictures of the sigmoid.[128] Lymphoid follicular hyperplasia may be prominent in quiescent or active disease, particularly in the rectum *(follicular proctitis).*

Ninety percent of patients have asymptomatic periods and relapses, whereas only 10% have continuous symptoms without remission. The symptoms vary with the extent of colonic involvement and severity of inflammation. Hematochezia, mild diarrhea, crampy abdominal pain, low-grade fever, iron-deficiency anemia, fatigue, and tenesmus are the main symptoms. Up to 20% of patients suffer from constipation and use laxatives. More than half of all patients have mild symptoms. Most cases have disease confined to the rectum (proctitis) or rectosigmoid, but disease that is initially confined to the distal area of the colon may subsequently spread proximally. Patients with moderate symptoms have several loose, blood-stained bowel movements per day. Severe or fulminant colitis may interrupt the course of mild or moderate disease or occur during the first bout of disease. It is characterized by profuse and bloody diarrhea, abdominal pain, and tenesmus. There may be severe and progressive anorexia, weight loss, fever, anemia, weakness, leukocytosis, hypokalemia, and hypoalbuminemia. The colon may become hypotonic and distended with gas, a condition called *toxic dilatation.*[129] Endoscopically the mucosa is friable, granular, and extremely congested and may be extensively ulcerated. Other local complications include ischiorectal and pararectal abscess formation. Extraintestinal manifestations of IIBD[130] include arthritis, uveitis, iritis, pyoderma gangrenosum, and erythema nodosum. Eighty percent of all cases of primary sclerosing cholangitis occur in young men with idiopathic ulcerative colitis.

The *differential diagnosis* of ulcerative colitis includes Crohn's disease, infectious colitis, diversion proctitis, and indeterminate colitis. Gross and microscopic features of practical value in the distinction of UC and CD are listed in Table 56-4. *Crohn's colitis* is distinguished[131] by patchy or discontinuous disease, ulcers separated by normal mucosa, strictures, sinuses or fistulas, anal fistulas and tags, granulomas, and an absence of diffuse continuous mucosal inflammation and hemorrhage. Terminal ileal disease may occur in both ulcerative colitis and Crohn's disease. However, in ulcerative colitis it is always in continuity with cecal inflammation. In some instances, ulcerative colitis may involve the appendix, even though the cecum and ascending colon are not affected.[132] Prolonged *shigellosis, gonorrhea,* or *syphilis* of the rectum may histologically resemble chronic inflammatory bowel disease. Stool cultures help to establish the diagnosis. Infectious or pseudomembranous colitis may complicate and exacerbate inflammatory bowel disease.

The term *indeterminate colitis*[133,134] may be used for cases of inflammatory bowel disease in which there is diagnostic uncertainty, with mixed features of Crohn's disease and ulcerative colitis. Indeterminate colitis is usually a severe pancolitis with an unremitting course from initial presentation to colectomy and may be complicated by toxic megacolon. Slit-shaped ulcers, transmural inflammation, and maintained goblet cells may be found. Acute fissures are accompanied by myocytolysis and capillary engorgement. The transmural inflammation is diffuse and is not composed of lymphoid aggregates. If biopsy specimens from a preceding phase of low-grade illness are available, they may help in establishing a specific diagnosis. The majority of cases with indeterminate colitis behave like ulcerative colitis.

Crohn's disease

Crohn's disease (CD) is an idiopathic, chronic, relapsing ulceroinflammatory disease of the gastrointestinal tract that most often affects the terminal ileum. The colon may be affected, either in association with small bowel disease, or as an isolated finding (20%).[127,133]

Crohn's colitis shows discontinuous segments of disease and large and small ulcers separated by normal (noncongested) mucosa. The earliest gross manifestations of CD are aphthoid ulcers.[135,136] These consist of small mucosal erosions 1 to 2 mm in diameter with a hemorrhagic edge and gray-white base. Commonly they are located on top of lymphoid follicles. As the disease progresses, the aphthoid ulcers enlarge to form discrete, confluent, serpiginous, or linear ulcers. Linear longitudinal (railroad track) ulcers often overlie teniae coli and with

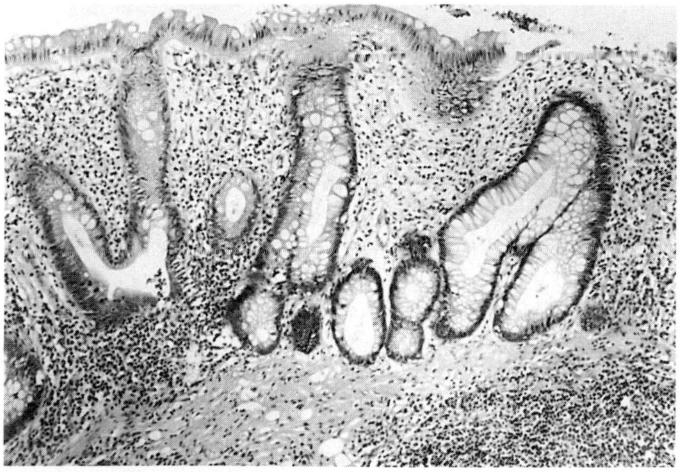

Fig. 56-19 Chronic ulcerative colitis with considerable crypt distortion. No active cryptitis is seen.

Table 56-4 Morphologic features useful in the distinction of ulcerative colitis and Crohn's disease*

Features suggestive of Crohn's disease
Focal mucosal inflammation
Terminal ileal involvement
Linear ulcers or "cobblestone" mucosa (gross feature)
Predominance of right-sided inflammation
Features highly suggestive of Crohn's disease
Discontinuous segments of inflammation (skip zones)
Aphthoid ulcers
Features virtually pathognomonic of Crohn's disease
Noncaseating granulomas
Transmural inflammation with subserosal lymphoid aggregates
Fistulas (at sites other than the anus)

*These features are most valuable when other causes of large bowel inflammation have been excluded.

transverse ulcers may dissect the mucosa into a cobblestone pattern (Fig. 56-20). Strictures (secondary to ulcers), sinuses, fistulas, and inflammatory polyps are often present. Fistulas may develop between the colon and the duodenum, small bowel, bladder, or vagina. Transmural inflammation consisting of lymphoid follicles is seen beneath chronic ulcers (Fig. 56-21). Granulomas may be found in any layer of the bowel wall but are not necessary for a positive diagnosis (Fig. 56-22). If the edematous skin tag at the apex of an anal fissure is examined histologically, it often shows follicular lymphoid inflammation or granulomas.

The differential diagnosis of colonic Crohn's disease includes idiopathic ulcerative colitis, segmental colitis, infectious colitis, and ischemic colitis (Table 56-4). *Ulcerative colitis* is distinguished by the presence of diffuse mucosal inflammation in continuity from the anus. There is mucosal congestion and hemorrhage, absence of granulomas, and absence of transmural inflammation (except under deep ulcers). *Segmental colitis* occurs in persons with *diverticular disease.* The inflammation is confined to the area of affected bowel. It is important not to confuse diverticulitis with fistula formation in Crohn's disease fistula formation. Chronic ischemic stricture is usually solitary and is associated with pronounced fibrosis, hemosiderin deposition, and vascular occlusion. *Irradiation injury* is suggested as a result of the history, and the resulting damage is ischemic in cause.

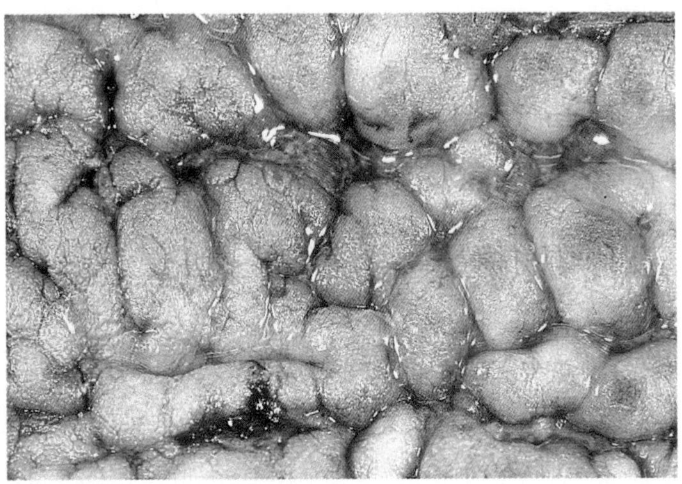

Fig. 56-20 Crohn's disease, showing a "cobblestone" pattern of the mucosa.

The clinical features of colonic CD depend on the extent and severity of involvement. Extensive colitis causes chronic diarrhea, abdominal pain, weight loss, and debility, but blood loss and anemia are usually less prominent than in ulcerative colitis. Anal disease encompasses fissures, mucosal tags, sinuses, fistulas, and perianal abscesses. Anal fistulas are usually associated with ulcers of the low rectum, above the anal sphincter, and are refractory to treatment while the rectal ulceration persists. Low ulcers tend to cause anal stenosis. Complications include internal fistulas, toxic dilatation, amyloidosis (rarely), dysplasia, carcinoma, and, occasionally, acute massive hemorrhage. Associated diseases include ankylosing spondylitis (5%), anterior uveitis (2%), and rarely sclerosing cholangitis.

Dysplasia and malignancy in inflammatory bowel disease

Dysplasia is a premalignant change that precedes the majority of colorectal cancers complicating IIBD.[137-139] Patients with chronic ulcerative colitis have a tenfold increase in the risk of colorectal carcinoma, and carcinoma complicating ulcerative colitis accounts for about 1% of all large bowel cancers. The risk of colonic and ileal adenocarcinoma is also increased in Crohn's disease and is preceded by dysplasia.[139] The severity of disease has no statistically demonstrable effect, and many carcinomas arise in patients with quiescent colitis. The principal risk factors for colorectal carcinoma are the extent and duration of colitis. The risk of dysplasia begins after 10 years of disease and increases progressively thereafter. Patients with inflammation confined to the rectum are at no greater risk for carcinoma than the general population is. Patients with total colitis are at highest risk, and patients with an intermediate extent of disease have a corresponding increase in risk. The cumulative risk of developing carcinoma varies, depending on the patient population studied. In studies from England,[140,141]

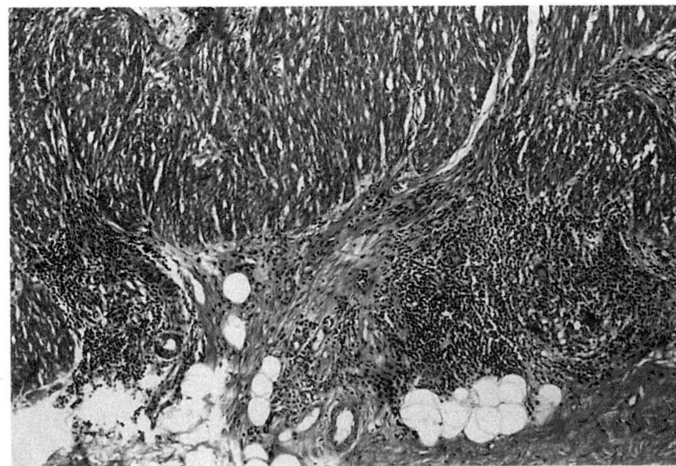

Fig. 56-21 Transmural chronic inflammation in Crohn's disease affecting the colon.

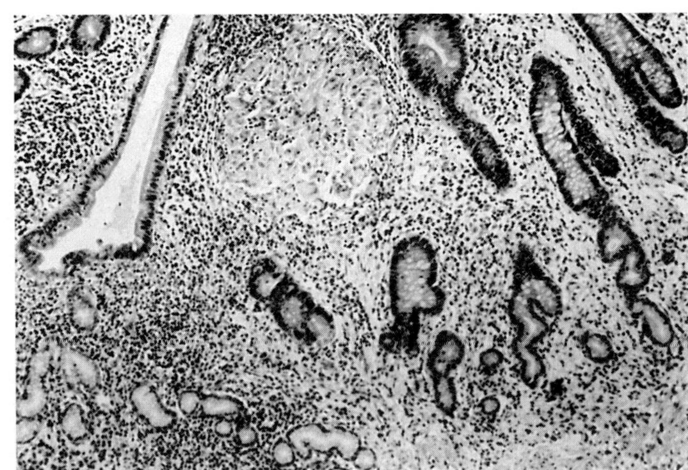

Fig. 56-22 Crohn's disease of the colon, showing a noncaseating granuloma *(center)* and gastric metaplasia (lower left).

8% to 13% of ulcerative colitis patients developed cancer 25 years after the initial diagnosis. A study from Sweden[142] found a 34% incidence after 25 years, but this is counterbalanced by a recent Danish report[143] claiming no excess morbidity from cancer. It might be speculated that, since 35% of the Danish patients with total colitis received a colectomy within the first 5 years of diagnosis, this low incidence may be attributable to the effects of treatment. In a series of private practice patients in the United States,[144] there was an 11.5% cancer incidence at 26 years.

Grossly, dysplasia often appears as an elevated poorly circumscribed plaque or nodule, which may have a velvety appearance. In some instances, however, it is indistinguishable from the adjacent mucosa on endoscopic or gross inspection. Carcinoma in ulcerative colitis is often flat, ill-defined, deeply infiltrating, and stricturing. In 25% of cases, there is more than one primary tumor.

Histologically, biopsy specimens from surveillance colonoscopies are classified either as negative, indefinite, or positive for dysplasia.[145] The last category is divided into low-grade and high-grade dysplasia. Dysplasia often resembles a villous adenoma. Dysplastic epithelium shows nuclear stratification and hyperchromatism, mitoses high in the crypts, and lack of maturation with diminished mucin confined to the apical portions of the cells (Fig. 56-23). In low-grade dysplasia, the atypical nuclei are confined to the lower half of the epithelium and are elongated, hyperchromatic, and mildly pleomorphic. Rarely, large numbers of endocrine cells or Paneth cells are present. The nuclei of high-grade dysplasia extend into the upper half of the epithelium and may reach the surface. They are stratified, pleomorphic, and hyperchromatic and may show clearing of the nucleoplasm and nucleoli (Fig. 56-23). Variants of dysplasia include cases that show incomplete maturation with a single cell layer containing nuclei that are large and hyperchromatic, nonmucin clear cell change, and dystrophic goblet cells. Dystrophic goblet cells are inverted, and so the nucleus is on the luminal aspect of the goblet, and the cell border may not reach the lumen.

Desmoplasia of the stroma, accompanied by high-grade dysplasia, establishes a diagnosis of invasive carcinoma, but invasion can occasionally occur without desmoplasia. The presence of mucin lakes also makes carcinoma more likely. Carcinomas arising in colitis are more frequently high-grade or colloid carcinomas than sporadic large bowel cancers. The prognosis for cancer in colitis is similar to sporadic colonic cancer, stage for stage.

Biopsy specimens are classified indefinite for dysplasia if the pattern of morphologic changes is not diagnostic but dysplasia cannot be excluded. Such cases may include inflammatory atypia and regenerative change. Regenerative or inflamed mucosa may show nuclei occupying half of the cell height with stratification or a single layer of large, open nuclei. Usually, some degree of surface maturation is retained (Fig. 56-24). The glands are not crowded, the mucosal thickness is normal or decreased, and the surface is not villiform.

Pedunculated dysplastic lesions in patients with ulcerative colitis are best regarded as adenomas arising coincidentally with colitis. This is obvious when a pedunculated adenoma arises in the right side of a colon with left-sided colitis. Dysplasia may arise in an inflammatory polyp but no more frequently than in flat mucosa.

DNA aneuploidy, detected by flow cytometry on endoscopic biopsy specimens, precedes histologic dysplasia and may identify a subset of IIBD patients without dysplasia who are more likely to develop dysplasia and who might benefit from increased frequency of colonoscopy.[146] However, histologic examination remains the standard for diagnosis of dysplasia. The histologic diagnosis of dysplasia is frequently very difficult and the described changes may be hard to distinguish from regeneration. In these cases, repeat biopsy should be performed. A diagnosis of high-grade dysplasia should be confirmed by a second pathologist before colectomy is performed.

Dysplasia is an asymptomatic condition. Surveillance colonoscopy aims to reduce the incidence of cancer by detecting and treating premalignant dysplasia. It is highly successful, except for patients who opt out (about 15% of patients). Compliance with surveillance diminishes when IIBD is in remission and patients become asymptomatic.

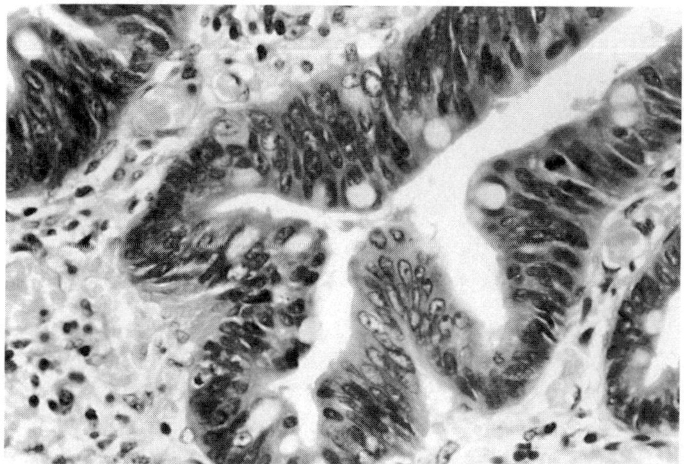

Fig. 56-23 High-grade dysplasia from a case of chronic ulcerative colitis.

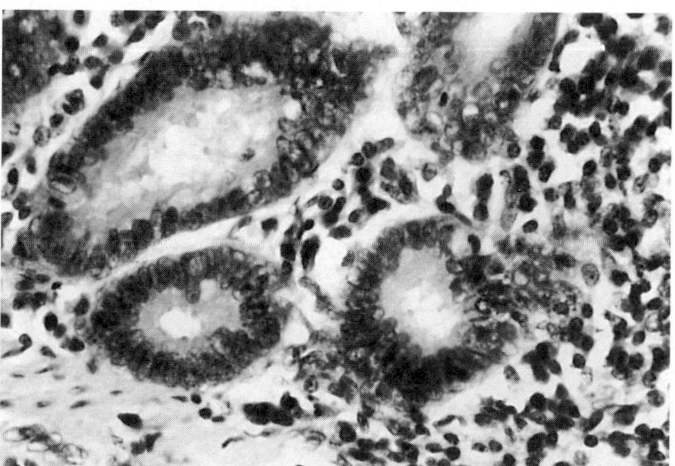

Fig. 56-24 Reactive (nondysplastic) changes in a case of chronic ulcerative colitis.

NONINFECTIOUS INFLAMMATORY CONDITIONS

Collagenous colitis

Biopsy specimens from patients with collagenous colitis show low-grade nonspecific mucosal inflammation, with a thickened subepithelial collagen band.[147] In adults the normal subepithelial collagen band measures up to 7 μm in thickness. Collagenous colitis is considered to be present when it exceeds 10 μm. The cause of increased collagen deposition by pericryptal fibroblasts,[148] the main pathologic process in this disease, is unknown. In some patients, there is a history of long-standing ingestion of aspirin or other nonsteroidal anti-inflammatory agents.[149] In others, there is a history of rheumatoid arthritis, thyroid disease, or celiac disease.[150] No microbial pathogens have ever been identified in the stool or colonic mucosa.

Women account for 80% of cases of collagenous colitis. The disease affects all parts of the large bowel, though involvement is patchy. Rectal sparing may occur in 25% of cases. A single rectal biopsy may therefore be inadequate to exclude the diagnosis.

By endoscopic examination, the bowel appears normal. Histologically[147] the subepithelial collagen band is confined to the surface of the mucosa and does not extend alongside crypts (Fig. 56-25). The thickening may be patchy and irregular. The crypt architecture is preserved with no atrophy or branching. The lamina propria contains an increased number of inflammatory cells, diffusely throughout the mucosa but most prominently in the superficial one third. The cells are mainly lymphocytes. Epithelial cells on the surface may become cuboidal, and there are increased numbers of intraepithelial lymphocytes. This epithelium has increased friability and can easily become stripped off the basement membrane by the biopsy procedure.

Patients present with watery intermittent diarrhea, usually lasting several months to several years.[151] This is never bloody. There may also be mild colicky abdominal pain. Collagenous colitis does not appear to be related in any way to ulcerative colitis or Crohn's disease but shares many similarities with lymphocytic colitis.

Lymphocytic (microscopic) colitis

As the name suggests, lymphocytic colitis is characterized by a colonic mucosal lymphocytosis. The cause is unknown, though some patients have celiac disease, which indicates that it may represent a nonspecific response to a variety of luminal antigens.[152] The mechanism of diarrhea has been shown to be a decrease in the absorption of water and sodium chloride.[153]

Lymphocytic colitis may occur at any age but is particularly common in middle-aged women. On endoscopic examination, the mucosa appears normal. Histologically,[154] lymphocytosis affects both lamina propria and epithelium. The changes are maximal in the surface epithelium, where there are typically 30 lymphocytes per 100 epithelial cells (normally 5 per 100 epithelial cells),[152] but also involve the superficial portion of the crypts (Fig. 56-26). The lymphocytes are almost exclusively suppressor T-cells. The epithelial cells show a loss of cytoplasmic mucin, nuclear enlargement, and prominent nucleoli. The lamina propria also contains excess lymphocytes, particularly in the superficial one third. When compared with cases of collagenous colitis, the lamina propria infiltrates in lymphocytic colitis are generally less intense.

Patients present with watery diarrhea that is not blood stained. Although there are many clinical and morphologic similarities between collagenous colitis and lymphocytic colitis, it is rare for one disease to evolve into the other. At the present time, they are best regarded as part of the same disease continuum with separate but occasionally overlapping features.[154,155]

Mucosal prolapse syndrome

The pathogenesis of mucosal prolapse syndrome (solitary rectal ulcer syndrome, or SRUS) is unclear.[156-159] It has been postulated that there is a failure of the normal relaxation by the puborectalis muscle during the act of defecation. This necessitates an increase in intra-abdominal pressure to achieve expulsion of stool. The pressure then forces a rectal mucosal fold to prolapse into the anal canal. Localized ischemia of the prolapsed mucosa as a result of local vascular compromise then produces the characteristic histologic changes of SRUS.

SRUS affects both sexes, over a wide age range, but is most common in women 20 to 40 years of age. Most lesions

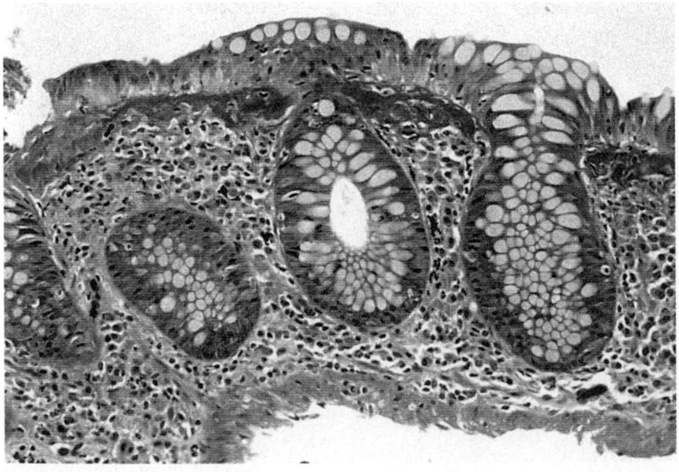

Fig. 56-25 Collagenous colitis, showing considerable subepithelial collagen deposition. (Trichrome stain.)

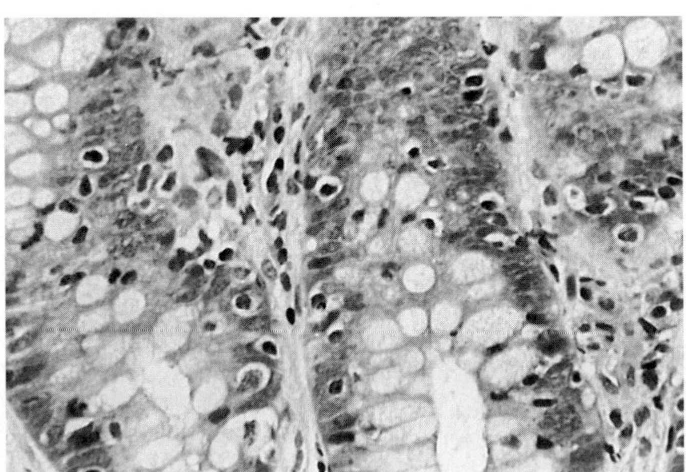

Fig. 56-26 Lymphocytic colitis. Notice the large number of intraepithelial lymphocytes.

occur on the anterior rectal wall, but SRUS may involve the bowel anywhere from the sigmoid to the anorectal junction. Despite the designation *solitary ulcer,* in 10% to 15% of cases multiple ulcers may be present within the single patch of diseased mucosa. Endoscopically only about half the patients with SRUS have an actual ulcer (Fig. 56-27). This is generally sharply demarcated, sometimes with a nodular edge. The remaining patients have an area of mucosal erythema, mucosal nodules, or frank polyps, which may or may not have surface ulceration.[159] Microscopically[160] (Fig. 56-28) SRUS shows mucosal thickening with capillary congestion and irregular proliferation and branching of crypts. The cells show enlarged, hyperchromatic nuclei, excess mitotic activity, and mucin-depleted goblet cells. Crypt dilatation may impart a villiform appearance to the rectal mucosa. Regeneration can be so pronounced that a spurious appearance of dysplasia may be noted. The lamina propria is hypocellular and tongues of muscle extend upward from the muscularis mucos to the surface epithelium. Surface ulceration is accompanied by capillary dilatation. The ulcers themselves may have no special features but can have a thin pseudomembrane on the surface.

Patients with SRUS present with a mucus rectal discharge and rectal bleeding. They may give a history of straining at stool, or a feeling of rectal obstruction. Since no specific treatment is available, the disorder tends to persist for prolonged periods of time.

Proctitis cystica profunda is a complication of SRUS.[161] It occurs after full-thickness mucosal ulceration, when surface epithelium grows down into the submucosa and becomes trapped there during the healing period. Histologically it is characterized by the presence of mucosa-lined cysts in the submucosa. The lining of the cysts is similar to the regenerative epithelium encountered in the surface mucosa.

Colitis cystica profunda is a morphologically similar condition that occurs outside the anorectal region. It is also a consequence of ulceration and is often secondary to various types of inflammatory bowel disease. In most instances, it is an incidental finding at colectomy, though occasionally raised patches of mucosa or sessile polyps may be identified endoscopically.

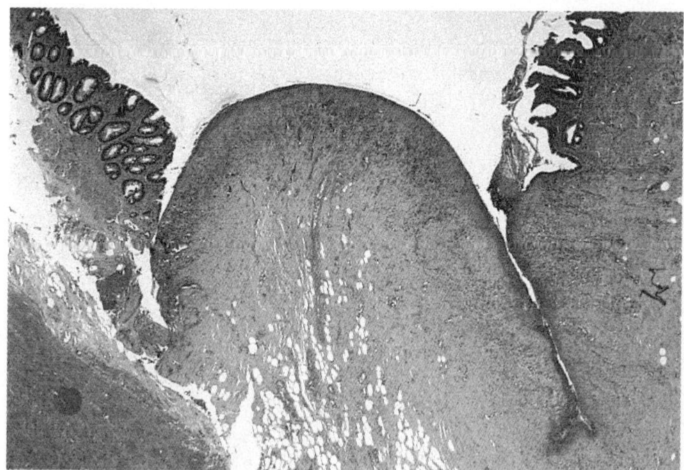

Fig. 56-27 Solitary rectal ulcer syndrome, showing extensive fibrosis involving the mucosa and submucosa.

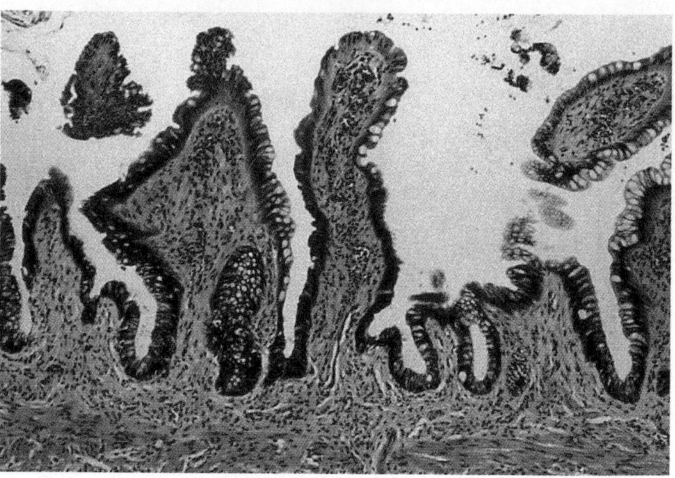

Fig. 56-28 Solitary rectal ulcer syndrome, showing pronounced crypt irregularity, mucosal fibrosis, and congestion. There is relative absence of inflammatory cells.

The term *inflammatory cloacogenic polyp*[162] refers to the presence of polypoid mucosal prolapse at the anorectal junction. The polyp consists of a mixture of rectal columnar epithelium and squamous transitional zone mucosa. Both show regenerative features. The stroma often shows more chronic inflammation than is usual for SRUS but contains the usual proliferating smooth muscle bundles.

The term *rectal prolapse* refers to a prolapse of the whole thickness of the proximal bowel wall through the anal sphincter. This is really a short-segment intussusception and is not etiologically related to the SRUS, though a biopsy specimen of a chronically prolapsed segment shows similar mucosal histologic features. Acute rectal prolapse may occur in dysentery, or in any massive diarrheal disorder, particularly in childhood. Nodular lymphoid hyperplasia may present as rectal prolapse. Rectal prolapse is also seen in old age.

Pneumatosis cystoides intestinalis

Pneumatosis cystoides intestinalis is defined as the presence of gas-filled cysts in the wall of the small or large bowel. It comprises two separate conditions with different causes, clinical features, and morphology. The first of these,[163] which is most common in children, often accompanies necrotizing enterocolitis, ischemia, or obstruction, and is attributable to a gas-producing anaerobic bacterial infection. This condition is better termed *emphysematous enterocolitis* to distinguish it from the adult form of pneumatosis.

Most adult cases of pneumatosis are associated with some other gastrointestinal disease or chronic obstructive pulmonary disease.[164] Of particular importance are bowel diseases that produce a breach in the mucosa, such as peptic ulcer, inflammatory bowel disease, or surgical anastomoses. Emphysema and asthma are the commonest associated pulmonary diseases. The gas is derived from the bowel lumen and is forced into the wall during coughing. This theory is supported by the fact that the gas in the cysts is identical in composition to flatus.[164] Any breach in the mucosa allows gas to enter the wall and spread via lymphatics or through the interstitium.

Pneumatosis may involve any part of the bowel and may present as noncommunicating cysts in the mucosa, submucosa, or subserosa. The cyst size may vary from a few millimeters to several centimeters (Fig. 56-29). On the mucosal surface, the endoscopic appearance is one of broad-based, smooth-surfaced polyps. Larger cysts have a thin, fibrous wall often lined by attenuated, multinucleated giant cells. These are considered to be a foreign-body reaction to extravasated lymph.[165,166]

In adult pneumatosis, symptoms are generally uncommon though, rarely, there may be subacute intestinal obstruction, requiring treatment. In the case of localized disease, this may be accomplished by surgical resection. Widespread disease is usually responsive to therapy with hyperbaric oxygen. Resolution of the cysts occurs slowly, as the relatively insoluble nitrogen is absorbed.

Diversion colitis

As the name implies, this condition develops in segments of colon or rectum that have been surgically disconnected from the fecal stream and persists indefinitely unless reanastomosis is performed.[167] Its cause is unknown, but recently it has been postulated that it is attributable to an absence of luminal short-chain fatty acids, which are the preferred metabolic substrates of intestinal epithelium. The colitis disappears when these nutrients are artificially instilled into the excluded segment.[168] Grossly, diversion colitis displays mucosal friability, erythema, and superficial ulceration. Microscopically (Fig. 56-30) there is a mucosal lymphoid hyperplasia,[169] patchy cryptitis, and crypt abscess formation.

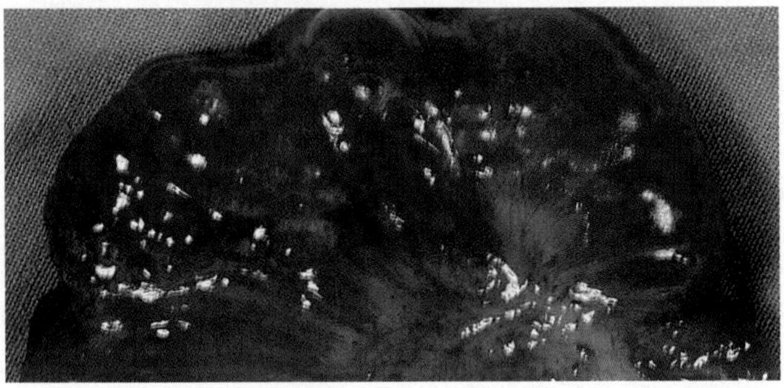

Fig. 56-29 Pneumatosis coli with extensive subserosal cyst formation.

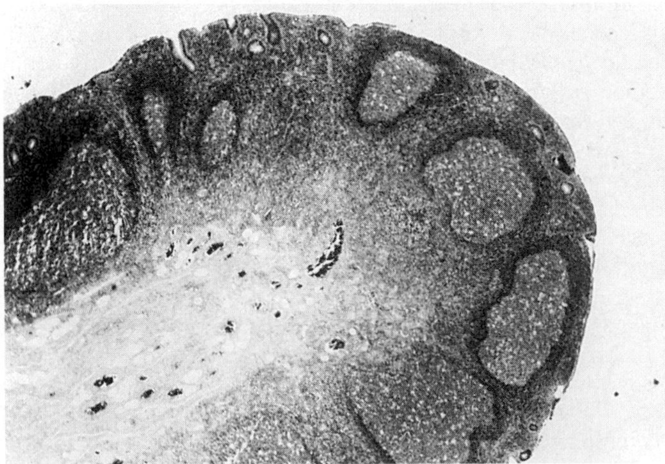

Fig. 56-30 Diversion colitis. Notice the extreme degree of lymphoid hyperplasia.

Behçet's syndrome

Behçet's syndrome includes iritis, with oral or genital ulcers and associated abnormalities, such as arthritis, erythema nodosum, and thrombophlebitis. Gastrointestinal symptoms are present in 50% of cases and most often relate to a colitis resembling Crohn's disease. Typical lesions include aphthoid ulcers,[170,171] patchy mucosal inflammation, and a cobblestone appearance of the mucosa. Granulomas are present occasionally, and some patients may demonstrate a lymphocytic venulitis.[171] Rarely, there are deep ulcers that can perforate.[172] All these findings are nonspecific, and the diagnosis on rectal biopsy can be made only if the clinical history is known. The cause of Behçet's syndrome is unknown, and the outcome, after corticosteroid treatment, is unpredictable.

TUMORS

Polyps

The term *polyp* is used as a gross description for any lesion that projects into the bowel lumen. A large polyp or any nonpolypoid mass may be referred to as a *tumor*. However, only by microscopic examination is it possible to determine the underlying nature of these lesions and whether they are neoplastic or nonneoplastic.

A classification of polyps is given in Table 56-5.

Hyperplastic polyps

Hyperplastic polyps are unique to the large bowel and do not occur in any other part of the gastrointestinal tract. Hyperplastic polyps of the stomach, which are probably secondary to inflammation and regeneration, are unrelated to colonic lesions that carry the same name.

The cause of hyperplastic polyps of the large bowel is unknown. They are believed to arise from a failure of the normal sloughing of cells that occurs at the epithelial surface. At

Table 56-5 Classification of large bowel polyps

Nonneoplastic polyps
Metaplastic
Hamartomatous
Juvenile polyp
Peutz-Jeghers syndrome
Cowden's syndrome
Ganglioneuromatosis
Cronkhite-Canada syndrome
Inflammatory
Inflammatory bowel disease
Inflammatory fibroid polyps
Lymphoid hyperplasia
Mucosal prolapse
Solitary rectal ulcer syndrome
Diverticular disease
Pneumatosis cystoides intestinalis
Neoplastic polyps
Adenoma
Villous, tubular, flat
Carcinoma
Carcinoid
Mesenchymal tumors

the base of the crypts, they contain hyperplastic cells that migrate superficially in a spiral fashion resulting in a serrated appearance on longitudinal section. At midcrypt level, the cells are fully mature; as they reach the surface, they fail to exfoliate and are thus referred to as being *hypermature*.

Hyperplastic polyps are a common finding in patients living in parts of the world where colorectal cancer is common, such as North America and Europe. In the third world where colorectal cancer is rare, hyperplastic polyps are less common.[173] This has given rise to speculation that hyperplastic polyps are a precursor of adenomas and carcinomas. At the present time, however, the evidence indicates that this transformation may occur infrequently and that the clinical finding of hyperplastic polyps does not place an individual patient at risk of having synchronous cancer or developing cancer at a later time.

Approximately 85% of persons living in North America and Europe will develop at least one hyperplastic polyp by 65 years of age.[173] Frequently the polyps are multiple. If more than 10 polyps are present, the designation "hyperplastic polyposis" may be used. Autopsy studies indicate that in a majority of cases the polyps may be evenly distributed throughout the colon, though in clinical practice most are removed from the rectosigmoid region. Occasionally, excised segments of bowel containing carcinomas may have hyperplastic polyps grouped around the tumor.[174]

Most hyperplastic polyps measure less than 5 mm in diameter, though rarely they may reach 2 cm.[175] Small lesions are sessile, but larger polyps may be pedunculated. They are brownish yellow in color, similar to normal mucosa, but are usually paler, resembling dewdrops. Microscopically they consist of serrated or saw-toothed crypts (Fig. 56-31). In the surface and midportions of the crypts, the number of goblet cells is diminished and the absorptive cells undergo metaplasia and resemble gastric surface epithelium. Absorptive cells are generally inconspicuous. At the base of the crypts, the features of hyperplasia are evident, with crowded stratified nuclei and increased mitotic activity. Occasionally, this hyperplasia is so pronounced that it may resemble a well-differentiated adenoma.

Hyperplastic polyps are asymptomatic and are usually discovered incidentally. They require no specific treatment but are usually excised to make a histologic diagnosis. Occasionally, *combined hyperplastic-adenomatous polyps* are encountered.[176] These are generally larger than 1 cm in diameter. Microscopically, they show serrated glands with dysplasia, either low grade or high grade. They should be regarded as an adenoma and treated as such.

Hyperplastic polyposis is an ill-defined condition that occurs sporadically. The colon may contain 10 to 30 polyps. Some of these may be larger than usual, and some may be combined hyperplastic-adenomatous lesions.[177] At the time of colonoscopy, the larger polyps should be excised, since there appears to be a low but definite risk of malignancy developing.

Inverted hyperplastic polyps[178] grow downward into the superficial submucosa, have a growth pattern that is more complex than usual, and may create the false impression of an infiltrating neoplasm.

Juvenile polyps

Juvenile polyps are hamartomatous lesions that are usually solitary and occur mostly in the large bowel, particularly the rectum.[179] As the name indicates, they are commonest in the first 5 years of life. Grossly they appear as rounded smooth-surfaced polyps 1 to 2 cm in diameter, with a short stalk. The color varies from bright red to deep brown. Histologically, they consist of excess lamina propria containing cystically dilated crypts lined by normal large bowel epithelium, or by epithelium that shows regenerative features (Fig. 56-32). Surface ulceration is common, leading to inflammation of the lamina propria and its replacement by granulation tissue.

Juvenile polyps readily undergo torsion and present with rectal bleeding and anemia. They may autoamputate and pass per rectum. There have been rare instances when solitary juvenile polyps have undergone neoplastic change, with the development first of dysplasia and later invasive carcinoma.

Juvenile polyposis[180] occurs when more than 10 polyps are present. There are familial (25%) and nonfamilial (75%) forms of the disease. Familial juvenile polyposis is inherited as an autosomal dominant trait. It is not known if nonfamilial juvenile polyposis is the result of a new gene mutation or is secondary to the action of environmental factors. Both forms present in the first or second decade of life. Most polyps occur in

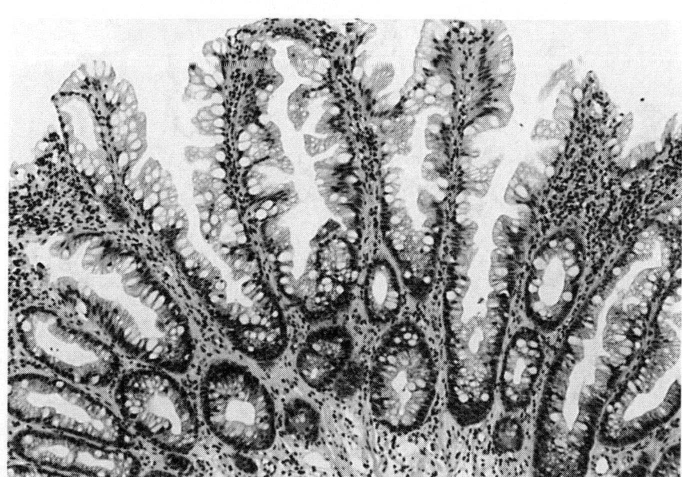

Fig. 56-31 Hyperplastic polyp. Notice the serrated appearance of the crypts.

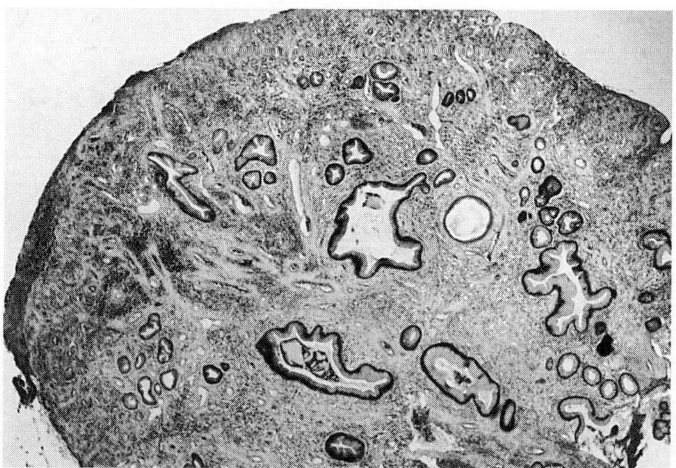

Fig. 56-32 Juvenile polyp, showing surface ulceration and cystically dilated crypts.

the large bowel, but occasionally other parts of the gastrointestinal tract, especially the stomach, may be involved. In most instances, the lesions are similar to solitary polyps, except that they tend to be larger. In approximately 10% of polyposis patients, the polyps become malignant. Most of these patients have the familial form of the disease.

The *Ruvalcaba-Myhre-Smith syndrome*[180] is probably a variant of juvenile polyposis in which the patients may also develop macrocephaly, mental deficiency, pigmented macules on the penis, and fibrous nodules of the tongue.

Other hamartomatous polyps

Peutz-Jeghers polyps, typically more common in the small bowel and stomach, may be found within the colon and rectum.[180] Histologically they are sessile arborizing lesions with a core of smooth muscle that is covered by normal mucosa. Typically, endocrine cells are also present at the base of the crypts. In those rare instances where the syndrome is complicated by development of an adenocarcinoma, the malignancies occur most frequently in the stomach and duodenum, not in the large intestine.

Cowden's syndrome[180,181] is inherited as an autosomal dominant condition. It manifests as oral mucosal papillomas and multiple cutaneous lesions, predominantly facial trichilemmomas and acral hyperkeratosis. There is a 50% risk in females of developing breast cancer. Thirty-five percent of patients have intestinal polyposis. The polyps may occur at any site and consist of sessile lesions showing cystic gland formation, overgrowth of the muscularis mucosae, and fibrosis of the lamina propria. In the large bowel, lymphoid hyperplasia, and adipose tissue within the lamina propria have also been described.

The *Cronkhite-Canada syndrome*[182] is characterized by the presence of numerous polyps throughout the gastrointestinal tract with dystrophic changes in the nails (onychodystrophy). There is no evidence that this syndrome is hereditary. Because of the large number of polyps, a protein-losing enteropathy may be present. The polyps are similar to juvenile polyps with the presence of excess lamina propria and epithelial cysts and are considered by some to represent diffuse hamartomas. The affected patients are older than those with juvenile polyposis and in the series of Burke and Sobin[182] ranged in age from 34 to 83 years.

Neoplasms

Adenoma

Adenomas are benign neoplasms arising from the crypt-forming epithelium. By convention, the term *adenoma* is restricted to localized lesions (polyps), and the term *dysplasia* is applied to diffuse noninvasive neoplastic changes, which may occur in inflammatory bowel disease. However, the morphology of these lesions is similar, and they are both precursors of invasive adenocarcinoma.

Sporadically occurring adenomas are rare before 40 years of age, but thereafter are progressively more common. By 70 years of age, 25% to 50% of the population in North America and western Europe have solitary or multiple adenomas in their large bowel.[183,184] There is a slight male predominance. Adenomas may develop at any site within the large bowel, though approximately one third are located in the rectum and sigmoid region. Recent evidence is suggestive that distal adenomas develop at a younger age and that more proximal tumors occur in older patients.[185] The natural history of adenomas is unknown, but there is evidence to suggest[186] that the majority remain the same size. Some adenomas will grow slowly, and about 15% will regress. It is, however, well recognized that adenomas tend to cluster within particular segments of bowel.[187] The larger an adenoma and the higher the degree of dysplasia, the more likely it is to be accompanied by additional polyps.

Grossly, three major types of adenoma may be identified: pedunculated (Fig. 56-33), sessile, and flat (depressed)[188] (Fig. 56-34). Intermediate forms may also be recognized. Pedunculated adenomas are the most common (90%) type. These tend to be small, with most of them measuring less than 1.0 cm in diameter. They may be reddish purple in color and have a surface that is coarsely lobulated. The stalk, which is covered by nonneoplastic mucosa, is generally longer with larger polyps. Lesions larger than 2 cm tend to be sessile (broad based) and have a surface villous appearance. Flat adenomas[189] are usually less than 1.0 cm in diameter and have the appearance of a slightly raised plaque, with a central depressed area (Fig. 56-34).

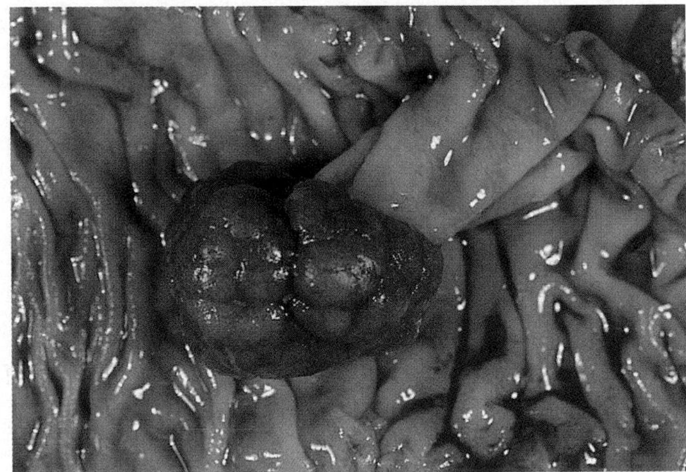

Fig. 56-33 Pedunculated adenoma of the colon.

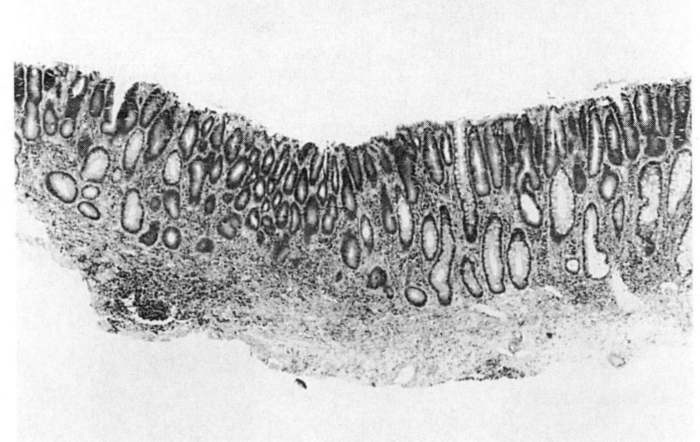

Fig. 56-34 Flat adenoma of the colon (also called "depressed adenoma").

By definition, all adenomas contain dysplastic epithelium. For descriptive purposes, it is best to restrict the grading of dysplasia to low grade and high grade (incorporating carcinoma in situ). In low-grade dysplasia, the nuclei are cigar shaped, crowded, and hyperchromatic. They are limited to the lower half of the epithelium, the remainder of which contains enterocyte cytoplasm and a mucus vacuole. In high-grade dysplasia, virtually the entire epithelium is composed of cells that have very scant cytoplasm. No mucus filled vacuoles are seen around the nuclei, which show crowding and loss of cell polarity. Polyps are rarely homogeneous with regard to dysplasia, and foci of high-grade dysplasia are commonly found in lesions that are otherwise low grade. This is not a practical diagnostic problem, however, since all adenomas should normally be excised irrespective of the grade of dysplasia.

On the basis of microscopic architecture, adenomas are classified as tubular (Fig. 56-35), villous (Fig. 56-36), or tubulovillous. The designation tubulovillous polyp is used only when both components exceed 25%. There is an approximate correspondence between the gross form of a polyp and its microscopic appearance; small pedunculated polyps and flat adenomas are almost always tubular; most large pedunculated polyps or sessile polyps are tubulovillous; and only rare sessile polyps are purely villous.

In addition to columnar epithelium, a minority of adenomas contain squamous cell, Paneth cell, or endocrine cell differentiation. This does not carry prognostic implications.

Pedunculated polyps may undergo torsion, resulting in intramucosal and submucosal hemorrhage, hemosiderin deposition and displacement of dysplastic epithelium into the submucosa, resulting in a phenomenon variously termed *pseudoinvasion*,[190] or adenoma cystica profunda. The misplaced glands may be dilated, ruptured, or associated with pools of extravasated mucus (Fig. 56-37). Correctly diagnosing pseudoinvasion and distinguishing it from early invasive adenocarcinoma is not always straightforward. Invasive carcinoma is generally accompanied by a focus of intramucosal carcinoma, which demonstrates high-grade dysplasia and a back-to-back tubular configuration. There is also a desmoplastic stroma. Misplaced glands in an adenoma have the same grade of dysplasia as the remainder of the polyp. They are surrounded by typical lamina propria.

Invasive adenocarcinoma in endoscopically resected polyps occurs with increasing frequency, proportionate to the size of the polyp, its villous component, and the degree of dysplasia. For example, 1% of tubular adenomas under 1 cm in diameter contain invasive carcinoma, but 53% of villous adenomas over 2 cm will demonstrate an invasive component.[191] A polyp consisting entirely of invasive carcinoma is termed a *polypoid carcinoma*. The criterion for adenocarcinoma is high-grade dysplasia with desmoplasia or invasion. When an adenocarcinoma has arisen in an adenoma but the invasive component is confined to the lamina propria, there is virtually no metastatic

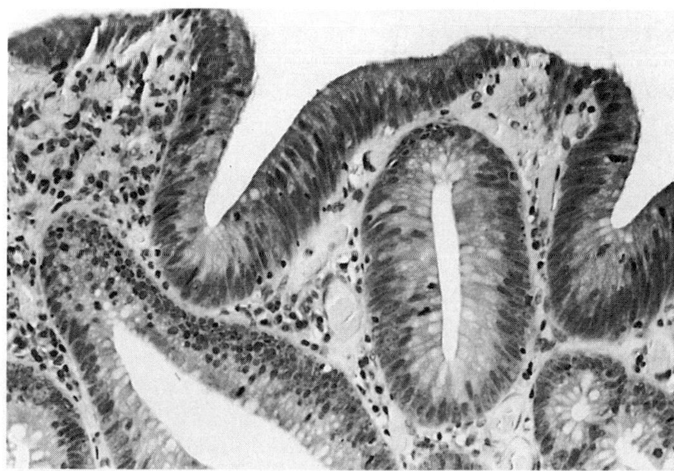

Fig. 56-35 Tubular adenoma of the colon. (There is low-grade dysplasia only).

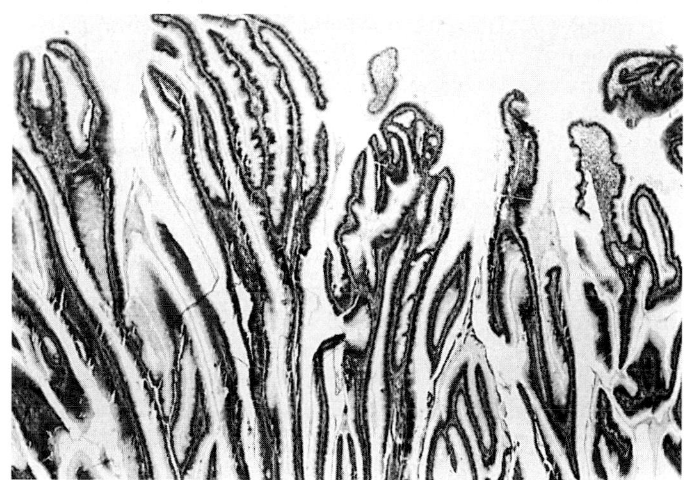

Fig. 56-36 Villous adenoma of the colon.

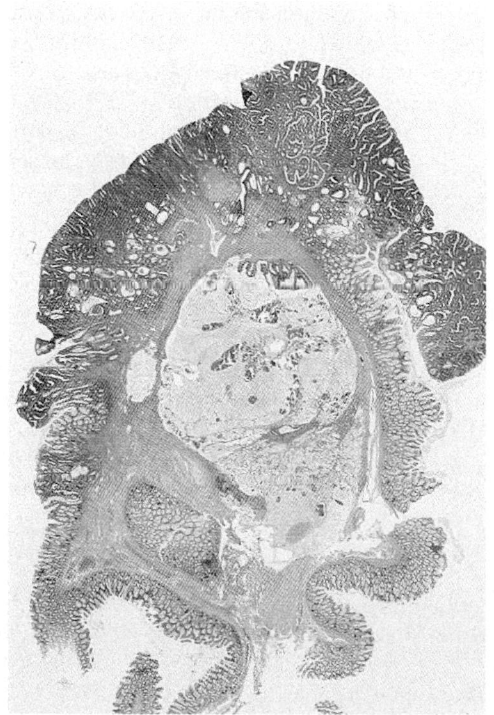

Fig. 56-37 Misplaced epithelium within the stalk of an adenoma (pseudoinvasion).

potential because of the paucity of intramucosal lymphatics.[192] However, once carcinoma has penetrated the muscularis mucosae, the chance of metastatic spread increases. The risk of metastasis in an early invasive carcinoma is closely related to its degree of differentiation, its depth of spread, and the presence of lymphatic involvement.[192,193] Tumors that are well or moderately differentiated with no lymphatic or vascular invasion and where the invasion involves only the head or stalk of the polyp have an exceedingly low risk of metastasis and are adequately treated by local excision. In this latter circumstance, a radical abdominal excision probably carries a greater risk of operative mortality than any theoretical benefit that might accrue from excision of an early lymph node metastasis.[193] Radical treatment should be reserved for those polyps that have any of the following features: poorly differentiated carcinoma, vascular invasion, tumor at the resection margin, or tumor that has invaded to a depth equivalent to the level of the submucosa in adjacent nonneoplastic mucosa (Fig. 56-38). The last situation is most likely to occur in sessile polyps.

Adenoma-carcinoma sequence

There is strong evidence to suggest that virtually all colonic adenocarcinomas arise within preexistent adenomas, or areas of dysplasia.[194] The risk of malignancy increases as an adenoma becomes larger, has a greater villous component, or has more high-grade dysplasia. However, exceptions exist, and some carcinomas probably develop in small and highly dysplastic flat adenomas. Carcinomas, arising anew from normal mucosa, have never been convincingly documented. Removal of adenomas endoscopically prevents colorectal cancer developing.[195]

Recent advances in molecular genetics have now begun to unravel events responsible for the adenoma-carcinoma sequence.[196] The earliest change may involve the acquired mutation of a suppressor gene at the APC (adenomatous polyposis coli) region of chromosome 5, or an adjacent region termed MCC (mutated in colon cancer). Subsequent events include point mutation of *ras* oncogenes and the deletion of suppressor genes on chromosome 18 (DCC, or deleted in colon cancer) and p53 on chromosome 17. In particular, the p53 gene has attracted considerable attention, since it appears to play a key role in the conversion of an adenoma to a carcinoma. p53 is involved in the normal regulation of transcription and arrests progress through the cell cycle in G_1 when DNA damage is present. Mutations of p53 and specific site mutations of K-*ras* correlate with short survival in carcinoma of the large bowel.[197]

Adenocarcinoma

The incidence of colorectal adenocarcinoma worldwide is highly variable. In North America and western Europe, it is 30 to 55 per 100,000 and only slightly less frequent than breast or lung cancer. In about 45% of cases, it proves fatal. By contrast, in Africa the incidence is only 5 per 100,000, even when the incidence is age corrected.[198] This difference appears to be lifestyle and diet related, since migrants from low-risk to high-risk geographic areas rapidly assume the higher risk. The exact dietary factors and carcinogenic mechanism have yet to be elucidated; however there is compelling evidence that excess fat (particularly animal fat)[198] and a lack of fiber and fresh vegetables may be responsible. One hypothesis indicates that excessive dietary fats may result in increased production of bile acids, which may themselves be carcinogenic, or may be converted to carcinogens by the action of bacteria within the bowel lumen. Fiber may protect by decreasing bowel transit time. Vegetables may protect by providing vitamins B, C, and E.

The gross appearances of colorectal carcinomas are variable. Small tumors may be indistinguishable from adenomas, and portions of the lesion may in fact consist of a precursor adenoma. Larger carcinomas usually have a central area of ulceration with a rolled (everted) edge (Fig. 56-39). Circumferential growth round the bowel wall results in stricture formation. Rarer gross forms include bulky exophytic lesions, bulky tumors with a mucinous component, and sclerotic linitis plastica lesions.

Histologically, most tumors are well or moderately differentiated and composed of irregularly shaped glands and branching cords of tumor cells. A papillary component may be present but is usually minor. The glands and papillae are lined by tall columnar to cuboidal epithelium corresponding to the degree of differentiation (Fig. 56-40).

In mucinous (colloid) tumors,[199] there are large quantities of extracellular mucin secreted, and the tumors distend and

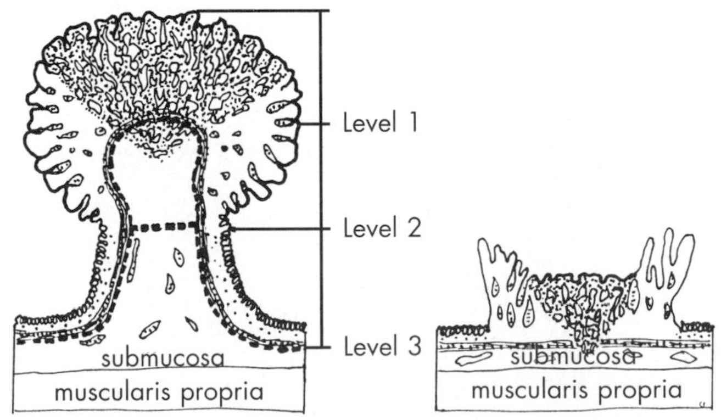

Fig. 56-38 Adenocarcinoma arising in large bowel adenomas. The risk of metastasis increases dramatically when carcinoma reaches the level of the normal lamina muscularis mucosae (level 3). (Modified from Haggitt RC, Glotzback RE, Soffer EE et al: *Gastroenterology* 89:328, 1985.)

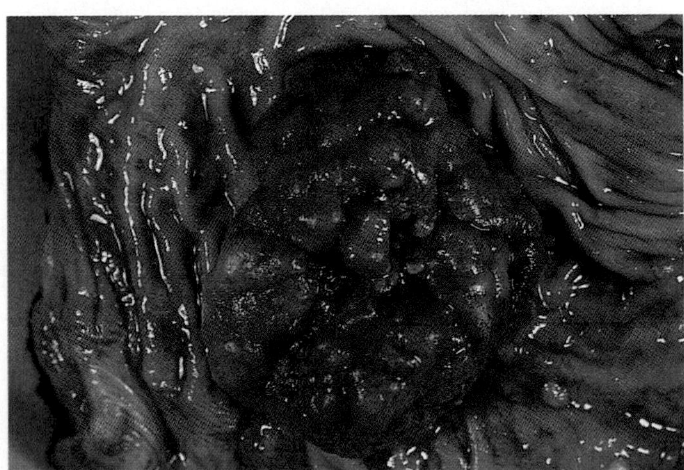

Fig. 56-39 Adenocarcinoma of the colon with a central area of ulceration.

form pools in the stroma (Fig. 56-41). Many colorectal adenocarcinomas have a minor mucinous component, but the designation *mucinous carcinoma* should be reserved for those neoplasms with at least 60% mucinous component. In 10% to 15% of mucinous tumors, a prominent signet-ring cell component may be identified.[200] When defined rigorously, as above, mucinous carcinomas have a poorer prognosis than nonmucinous adenocarcinomas have. At least part of the explanation for this is that mucinous tumors present at a more advanced stage than nonmucinous tumors do and are more likely to have a poorly differentiated component. The majority of mucinous carcinomas occur in the right side of the colon.

Rarely, adenocarcinomas that straddle the anorectal junction become colonized by melanocytes, which transfer pigment to the carcinoma cells. This phenomenon has been called *melanotic adenocarcinoma*.[201]

Malakoplakia or cytomegalovirus infection is occasionally found as localized responses adjacent to large bowel adenocarcinomas.[202]

The most important factor influencing survival in colorectal carcinoma is the stage of the disease (Table 56-6). Tumors that have not penetrated through the muscularis propria have a 95% 5-year survival; those that have penetrated through the muscularis propria but have not spread to lymph nodes have an 80% 5-year survival; those that have metastasized to nodes have a 20% to 40% 5-year survival, depending on how many nodes are affected. The original staging system was devised by Dukes[203] (Table 56-6). This has subsequently undergone several modifications, of which the one most widely used is the scheme developed by Astler and Coller.[204] The TNM[205] system (primary tumor, regional nodes, metastasis) may also be used. The weakness of all these systems is that they do not allow prediction of which patients without nodal disease have a poor prognosis and which patients with nodal disease have a good prognosis and will survive. This is important if chemotherapy is to be instituted. Conventional histopathologic analysis has shown that tumor grade, infiltrating border, lack of inflammatory reaction, and fibroblastic response allow prediction of a poor prognosis at each Dukes stage.[206] Flow cytometric analysis of tumors for DNA content has also shown that aneuploidy is correlated with a poor prognosis.[207] More recent work has indicated that, for Dukes B and C tumors, prognosis is closely linked to the presence of specific K-*ras* and p53 mutations.[197,208] K-*ras* mutations are present in 25% of cases with a good prognosis and 71% of cases that develop recurrent disease.

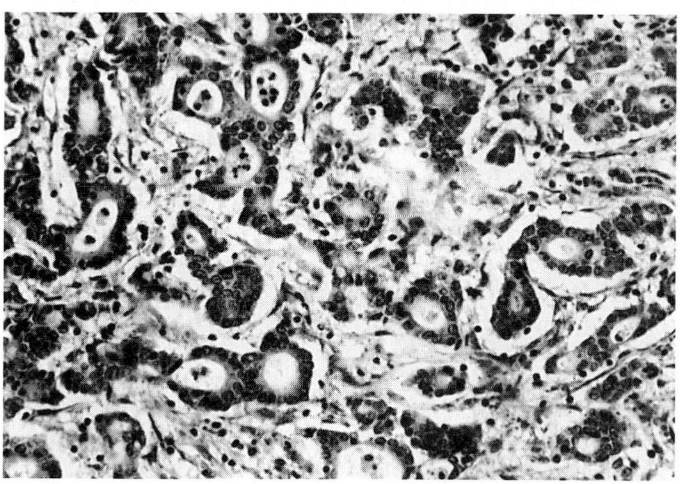

Fig. 56-40 Moderately well-differentiated adenocarcinoma of the large bowel.

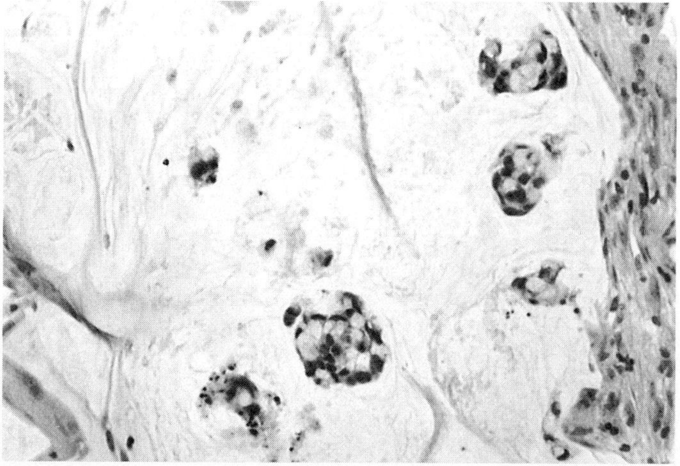

Fig. 56-41 Mucinous carcinoma of the colon. It contains pools of mucin with tumor cells floating in it.

The majority of patients with colorectal carcinoma present with diarrhea or constipation, or symptoms of early obstruction. Hemorrhage resulting in rectal bleeding is also common, and occult bleeding may lead to iron-deficiency anemia. A minority of patients present with perforation or advanced metastatic disease in the liver or peritoneal cavity. Lymph-borne metastasis occurs first to nodes in the pericolic fat immediately adjacent to the tumor. The tumor then spreads to nodes within the mesentery. Ultimately the retroperitoneal and porta hepatis nodes are affected.

Familial adenomatous polyposis (FAP)

Adenomatous polyposis is considered to be present when the large bowel contains over 100 adenomas.[180] In most instances, however, many thousands of polyps occur (Fig. 56-42). The disease is inherited through a mutated autosomal dominant gene (APC gene), located on the long arm of chromosome 5 (5q21).[209] The mutations are mostly changes in single base

Table 56-6 Schemes for the staging of colorectal carcinoma

Involved tissues	Dukes	Astler-Coller	TNM
Mucosa	—	A	Tis
Submucosa	A	B_1	T_1
Muscularis propria	A	B_1	T_2
Subserosa	B	B_2	T_3
Adjacent organs			T_4
Nodes beneath tumor	C_1	C_1 or C_2*	
Apical mesenteric node	C_2	C_1 or C_2*	
1 to 3 nodes			N_1
4+ nodes			N_2
Distant metastases			M_1

*In the Astler-Coller system, a B_1 tumor with nodal metastases is staged C_1 and a B_2 tumor with nodal metastasis is C_2.
TNM, Primary tumor, regional nodes, and metastasis.

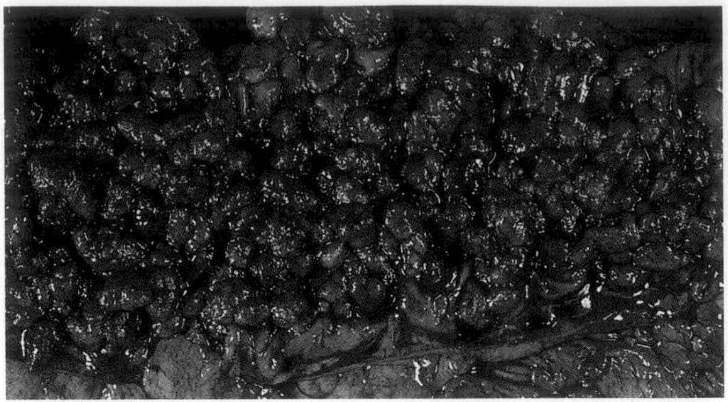

Fig. 56-42 Adenomatous polyposis coli in which the large bowel mucosa is carpeted with polyps.

pairs, insertions, or deletions and result in truncated gene products and protein. FAP with extraintestinal manifestations is called "Gardner's syndrome."

In FAP, the adenomas develop shortly after puberty. By 17 years of age carcinomas may arise within the larger lesions. By 25 years of age over 80% of individuals have cancer. By age 40, virtually 100% of individuals have cancer, unless a prior colectomy has been carried out.

Patients with FAP may develop gastric fundic gland polyposis (50% of cases), duodenal adenomas, and gastric, pancreatic, biliary, or distal small bowel neoplasms.[180] In Gardner's syndrome there are abdominal desmoid tumors, osteomas particularly of the jaw, and epidermal cysts, manifestations that appear to be a pleiotropic effect of the gene.[180] Turcot's syndrome[210] manifests as malignant brain tumors occurring in patients with FAP. At the present time, it is not clear whether this is a variant of Gardner's syndrome, or a separate entity.

On gross and microscopic examination, the lesions of FAP are similar to those seen in sporadic adenomas, with pedunculated, sessile, and flat lesions, which may have a tubular or villous architecture. Grossly, many thousands of polyps are usually present, and on microscopic examination many additional monocryptal adenomas can be detected.

Other inherited forms of colorectal cancer

Other inherited forms of colorectal cancer involve at least four related conditions that have also been referred to as the "cancer family syndrome." These patients presenting with this syndrome do not have adenomatous polyposis (that is, more than 100 polyps), though they may have multiple adenomas, from which the cancers are assumed to arise.

The hereditary flat adenoma syndrome (HFAS) was first described by Muto and colleagues.[191] These patients have multiple flat adenomas predominantly located in the right side of the colon. This syndrome is inherited as an autosomal dominant trait. The gene is also located on chromosome 5, giving rise to the suggestion that HFAS is an attenuated form of FAP.[211] Patients develop cancers at a age later than they do in classical FAP or in the Lynch syndrome.

Two separate but related variants of the Lynch syndrome (hereditary nonpolyposis colorectal cancer, or HNPCC) have been described.[212,213] In the Lynch 1 syndrome, patients develop colon cancer at an average age of 44 years predominantly (70%) in the right colon. Patients with the Lynch II syndrome develop extracolonic malignancies in addition. These include endometrial cancer, transitional carcinoma of ureter and renal pelvis, and adenocarcinomas of stomach, small bowel, ovary, pancreas, and biliary tract.

For diagnosis of the Lynch syndrome, the following criteria must be satisfied:[214] (1) There must be three affected relatives, one of whom is a first-degree relative of the other two; (2) colorectal cancer must be present in at least two generations; (3) one or more of the cancers must have developed before 50 years of age. The Lynch syndrome is inherited as an autosomal dominant trait encoded by a gene on chromosome 2.[215] This produces widespread alterations in short repeated DNA sequences on chromosomes 5q, 15q, 17q, and 18q.[216] Thus, numerous replication errors occur during tumor development. It is postulated that up to 13% of all colon cancer patients have the Lynch syndrome (type I and type II). The Muir-Torre syndrome[217] is characterized by multiple intestinal carcinomas associated with genitourinary and skin tumors, particularly sebaceous neoplasms. It is very rare. It may be a variant of Lynch syndrome type II.

Lastly, it is known that colon cancer occurs more frequently in the relatives of affected individuals than one would expect by chance.[212] At least by the current definitions, these patients do not have FAP, HFAS, or the Lynch syndrome, though the mode of inheritance is also believed to be an autosomal dominant gene. These cancers do not develop at an early age, but two or more metachronous or nonmetachronous tumors may occur.

Rare types of primary large bowel carcinoma

Unusual histologic types of colonic and rectal carcinoma include adenosquamous carcinoma,[218] pure squamous carcinoma,[219] spindle cell carcinoma,[220] choriocarcinoma,[221] and clear cell carcinoma.[222]

Adenosquamous carcinomas[218] may occur in patients with ulcerative colitis, familial adenomatous polyposis, and schistosomiasis; however, most affected patients have no known risk factor. These tumors constitute less than 0.5% of all colorectal cancers and occur equally frequently in both sexes. The median age at presentation is 55 years, but they can occur in adults of any age. A majority of adenosquamous carcinomas arise in the right side of the colon, particularly cecum, where they appear grossly similar to pure adenocarcinomas. Histologically, they consist of an intimate mixture of variably differentiated squamous and glandular elements. *Adenoacanthomas*[223] are a variant of adenosquamous carcinoma, in which the squamous component is present as benign-appearing squamous pearls. Nevertheless, both components are regarded as malignant, and both may be present in metastases. In occasional cases, these carcinomas produce a parathormone-like substance and present with hypercalcemia.[224] The clinical behavior of adenosquamous carcinomas is more aggressive than that of pure adenocarcinomas. Eighty percent have nodal or hepatic metastases at the time of presentation, and only 30% of patients survive longer than 5 years.

Pure squamous carcinomas occur in the large intestine sporadically or under special conditions. Risk factors include sinuses, fistulas, previous irradiation, and squamous metaplasia. The tumors occur predominantly in young adult males and are also mainly located in the right side of the colon. Histologically, most squamous carcinomas are poorly differentiated keratinizing lesions.[219] These should not be confused with small-cell undifferentiated carcinomas, which can show small foci of squamous differentiation. Rare examples of basaloid tumors, resembling anal carcinomas, have been described.[225] Generally the prognosis is poor.

Spindle cell carcinomas[220] are exceedingly rare in the large bowel. They may occur in a pure form or combined with squamous carcinoma or adenocarcinoma (carcinosarcoma). The spindle cells can differentiate to form metaplastic bone, cartilage, or striated muscle.

Choriocarcinomatous differentiation within poorly differentiated adenocarcinomas[221] usually takes the form of isolated syncytiotrophoblast-like cells that are immunopositive for human chorionic gonadotrophin. This type of neoplasm tends to affect young adults and involves the right side of the colon. The prognosis is poor.

Clear cell carcinomas[222] are another rare type of primary colonic neoplasm that may occur in a pure form or combined with an adenocarcinoma. The clear cells resemble those of a renal carcinoma and may contain glycogen or lipid. However, unlike renal carcinomas, these primary large bowel tumors are generally immunopositive for carcinoembryonic antigen.

Neuroendocrine cell tumors

Neuroendocrine cell tumors include hind-gut carcinoids,[226] goblet cell carcinoids,[227] combined adenocarcinoma/carcinoid,[228] and endocrine cell carcinomas.[229,230]

Hind gut carcinoids constitute approximately 25% of all gastrointestinal neuroendocrine tumors. The rectum is the most commonly involved site, and most tumors are solitary. Approximately 80% of rectal carcinoids are less than 1.0 cm in diameter and are discovered incidentally as dome-shaped lesions covered by intact mucosa. Histologically, they have a trabecular or alveolar growth pattern of monotonous polygonal cells with indistinct cell borders and regular nuclei containing small nucleoli (Fig. 56-43). Histochemically they may contain small amounts of mucus, and a minority are argyrophilic. Multiple hormones may be secreted and can be demonstrated by immunohistochemistry. Pancreatic polypeptide and glucagon are especially common.[231] They almost never give rise to the carcinoid syndrome. The prognosis of colorectal carcinoids is related to their size. Tumors under 1 cm in diameter are benign. Tumors over 2 cm in diameter are likely to be malignant. Invasion of the muscularis propria is the only consistently reliable criterion of malignancy.[232]

Goblet cell carcinoids[227] may rarely occur in the large bowel but have been described in the ascending colon and rectum. Histologically they are similar to goblet cell carcinoids of the appendix with small nests of widely infiltrating tumor cells. The nuclei are eccentric and compressed by the globule of cytoplasmic mucus resulting in a signet-ring appearance. They are weakly argyrophilic. These are very aggressive tumors with wide local spread and considerable metastatic potential.

The term *composite adenocarcinoma/carcinoid*[228] is applied to tumors consisting of discrete areas of adenocarcinoma, alternating with areas of carcinoid. Either tumor may be well or poorly differentiated. When metastases occur, these may also have a composite appearance. It is very common for large bowel carcinomas to have occasional endocrine cells scattered through them. These are not regarded as composite tumors and behave as typical adenocarcinomas. The term *amphicrine tumor*[233] is applied to a neoplasm in which single cells may show both endocrine and exocrine differentiation. Goblet cell carcinoid is an example of an amphicrine tumor.

Neuroendocrine cell carcinomas (Fig. 56-44) are of two types: large cell (atypical or malignant carcinoid),[230] or small cell (oat cell carcinoma).[229] Large cell tumors may be hard to distinguish from poorly differentiated adenocarcinomas or large cell lymphomas on light microscopy. They have a sheet-like growth pattern and are composed of polygonal cells with prominent nucleoli, abundant mitotic figures, and areas of necrosis. Small cell carcinoma of the colon is histologically indistinguishable from small cell carcinoma of the lung. Both large-cell and small-cell endocrine cell carcinomas of the colorectum have a poor prognosis and both may form part of a composite adenocarcinoma/carcinoid neoplasm.

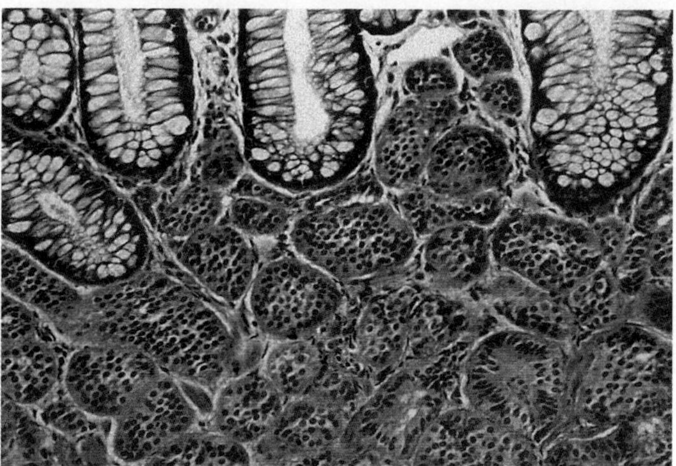

Fig. 56-43 Rectal carcinoid tumor having an alveolar growth pattern.

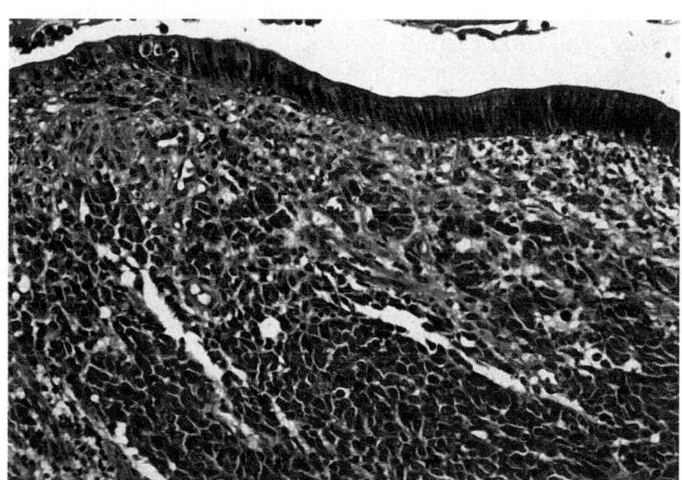

Fig. 56-44 Small cell type of colonic neuroendocrine carcinoma.

Endocrine cell tumors may rarely complicate long-standing inflammatory bowel disease, particularly ulcerative colitis.[230,234] A wide range of tumor types have been described, and in some instances the neoplasms have arisen in foci of endocrine cell hyperplasia. Multiple large bowel carcinoids have been described in patients with and without inflammatory bowel disease.[234]

Lymphoid hyperplasia and lymphoma

Lymphoid hyperplasia in the large bowel is a benign lesion that may be focal or diffuse. Focal hyperplasia (Fig. 56-45) occurs almost exclusively in the rectum (rectal tonsil),[235] where it may be present in association with hemorrhoids, a fissure, or a carcinoma. Secondary diffuse lymphoid hyper-

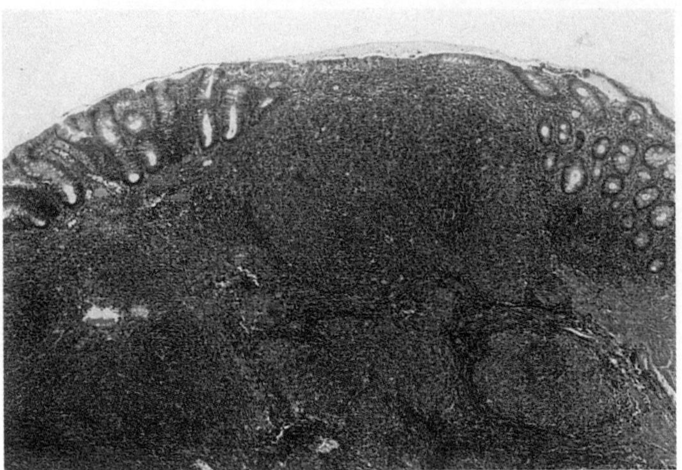

Fig. 56-45 Focal rectal lymphoid hyperplasia.

plasia may occur in a variety of conditions, such as ulcerative colitis (follicular colitis), diversion colitis, and pouchitis (postsurgical ileal pouch inflammation). In most instances, however, there is no known predisposing factor. In two thirds of cases, the hyperplasia is present as a single polyp commonly 1 to 2 cm in diameter but occasionally measuring up to 5 cm. Less commonly, there are several polyps, or even rectal polyposis. On histologic examination, the lesion occupies the submucosa and mucosa. It consists of multiple large follicles with germinal centers. Surface ulceration is generally not present.

Primary diffuse lymphoid hyperplasia of the bowel may be associated with hypogammaglobulinemia, and in these instances the hyperplasia is most obvious in the small bowel, and the colon is affected to a lesser extent, or not at all.[236] When lymphoid hyperplasia occurs without hypogammaglobulinemia,[237] it is most prominent in the colon and probably represents overgrowth of the normal colonic lymphoid follicles. It may cause hematochezia in children, but most cases are asymptomatic. It may also be a feature of HIV infection in the stage of generalized lymphadenopathy. Grossly, diffuse lymphoid hyperplasia presents as multiple mucosal nodules, measuring up to 4 mm in diameter. Histologically, these are similar to the enlarged follicles seen in focal hyperplasia.

Primary malignant lymphoma of the colon and rectum is an unusual tumor accounting for only 0.2% of large bowel malignancies.[238] It may occur sporadically or in association with AIDS,[239] organ transplantation,[240] and inflammatory bowel disease.[241] Histologically, the majority (64%) originate from mucosa-associated lymphoid tissue (MALT): 35% are low grade, and 29% are high grade. Most remaining cases are examples of mantle zone lymphoma presenting with lymphomatous polyposis (24%). Most have immunohistochemical features of B-lymphoctyes.

Benign and malignant stromal tumors

Leiomyomas[242] are the most common stromal lesion in the large bowel. They generally measure less than 1 cm in diameter and arise from the muscularis mucosae. Usually, they are discovered incidentally and have no malignant potential. Histologically, they are composed of regular spindle cells and often show extensive fibrosis. Malignant smooth muscle tumors[243] are large, fleshy, lobulated tumors that show zones of necrosis and resemble adenocarcinomas in their gross appearance and clinical presentation. They have a poor prognosis. Histologically they consist of pleomorphic cells with a sheetlike growth pattern and abundant mitotic activity. Between these two extremes of morphologic appearance and clinical behavior, there are rare examples of cellular spindle cell stromal tumors greater than 1.0 cm in diameter arising in the muscularis propria. They tend to occur particularly in the anorectal region. Despite a bland histologic appearance, they tend to recur and metastasize.[242]

Neurogenic tumors of the large bowel, such as schwannomas, neurofibromas, and ganglioneuromatosis, are rare. Schwannomas and neurofibromas are difficult to distinguish from other stromal tumors on routine sections but demonstrate positive immunostaining for neuron-specific enolase (NSE) and S-100 protein. Schwannomas are encapsulated and show characteristic nuclear palisading (Verocay bodies). Neurofibromas are circumscribed but unencapsulated. They may occur sporadically but are most frequent in patients with von Recklinghausen's disease. Ganglioneuromatosis[244] manifests as a mucosal and submucosal proliferation of mature nerves and ganglion cells. It tends to affect the bowel in a diffuse fashion. Patients with this condition may have von Recklinghausen's disease, multiple endocrine adenomatosis type 2b, Cowden's disease, or familial adenomatous polyposis.

Lipomas[245] may be found at any site within the large bowel but seem to be most common on the right side. They appear as well-circumscribed intramural masses that are yellow on the cut surface. The overlying mucosa may be attenuated or ulcerated. Rarely they can become pedunculated. Histologically they consist of mature adipose tissue. Small lipomas tend to present as incidental findings, but larger tumors may produce abdominal pain, rectal bleeding, or obstruction.

The term *lipomatous hypertrophy of the ileocecal valve*[246] refers to the tendency of this structure to undergo fatty infiltration. Most patients with the abnormality are middle-aged women. In most instances, it is of no clinical significance. Varying degrees of this abnormality occur, and in more fully developed cases dramatic enlargement may resemble a neoplasm on barium enema examination. Histologically the submucosa of the valve is expanded by mature adipose tissue dissected by broad and narrow fibrous trabeculas. The lesion is nonencapsulated.

Other rare soft-tissue lesions encountered in the large bowel include inflammatory fibroid polyps[247] and malignant fibrous histiocytoma.[248]

ANUS

NORMAL STRUCTURE AND FUNCTION

The anal canal extends from the lower margin of the rectum to the anal verge and is approximately 5 cm in length (Fig. 56-46). The upper and lower borders correspond approximately to the margins of the external sphincter. The only grossly identifiable landmark is the dentate (pectinate) line, which runs circumferentially in a wavy fashion.[249]

The zone below the dentate line is termed the *anal margin*. This is covered by squamous epithelium. Close to the dentate line, the epithelium is nonkeratinizing, but toward its lower margin, where it merges with hair-bearing skin, it becomes keratinizing.

Above the dentate line is the transitional zone, which is covered either by nonkeratinizing squamous epithelium, or by transitional epithelium (resembling urothelium) (Fig. 56-47). At its upper margin, this merges with rectal mucosa. This junction is very irregular and is not grossly identifiable. The columns of Morgani consist of 6 to 10 longitudinal mucosal folds, joined at their bases by semilunar valves. These lie immediately superior to the dentate line.

Mucus-secreting glands are present in the lamina propria of the transitional zone. The ducts, which are lined by transitional epithelium, open immediately above the anal valves.

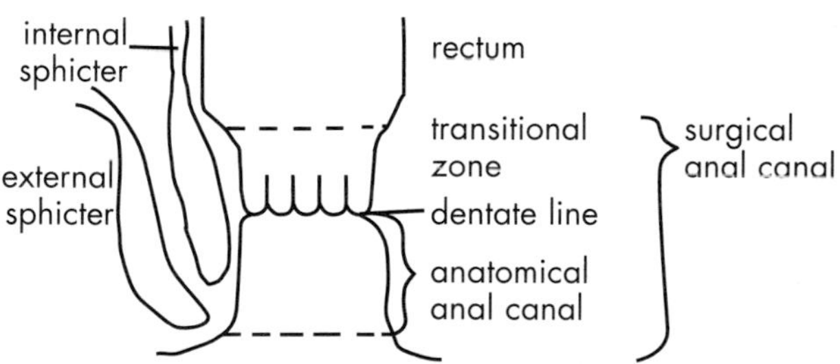

Fig. 56-46 Normal anatomy of the anal canal.

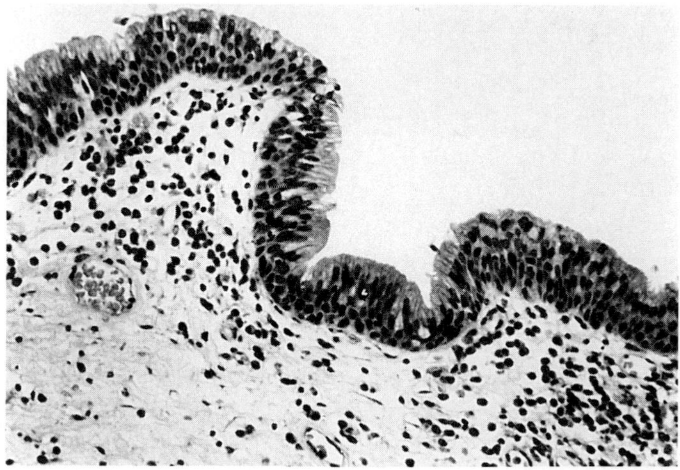

Fig. 56-47 Normal transitional mucosa of the anal canal.

NONNEOPLASTIC CONDITIONS

Hemorrhoids

Hemorrhoids are formed by a dilatation of veins in the external and internal hemorrhoidal plexuses.[250] Although it has been suggested that some cases are the result of straining at stool, or the result of pelvic congestion in pregnancy, their cause is unknown in most cases. Low-fiber diets that are common in Westernized societies can result in small quantities of compact stool that are hard to expel. In some individuals, there may be a genetic predisposition, evidenced by loosening of connective tissue of the vein wall and varicose veins of the lower extremities.

Hemorrhoids occurring above the dentate line are called *internal hemorrhoids;* below the dentate line they are termed *external hemorrhoids*. Clinically, hemorrhoids are classified into four grades. Nonprolapsing hemorrhoids are considered first-degree hemorrhoids. Prolapsing hemorrhoids that spontaneously reduce themselves are considered second degree. Hemorrhoids that require digital manipulation for reduction are considered third degree. Nonreducable hemorrhoids are considered fourth degree.

Histologically, hemorrhoids consist of dilated veins in the mucosa and submucosa. There may be evidence of thrombosis or hemosiderin deposition from a previous episode of bleeding. Depending on whether the hemorrhoids arise above or below the dentate line, they may be covered by columnar, transitional, or nonkeratinizing squamous mucosa.

Fistulas and sinuses

Sinuses are blind-ended tracts, extending from the mucosal surface into the deeper tissues. Fistulas are tracts that communicate between two epithelial surfaces.[251] In the anal region, both lesions may arise spontaneously or develop as a complication of inflammatory bowel disease,[252] tuberculosis, lymphogranuloma venereum, or actinomycosis. Sinuses and fistulas arise after a primary infection of the anal glands. This results in an intersphincteric abscess, which may rupture and drain in various directions. The most common type of fistula is purely intersphincteric and joins the surface epithelium to the intersphincteric space. A transsphincteric fistula connects the intersphincteric plane with the ischiorectal fossa by perforating the external sphincter. A suprasphincteric fistula connects the bowel superior to the external sphincter with the ischiorectal space by perforating the levator ani. An extrasphincteric fistula passes from the rectum outside the sphincters to the perianal skin.

Fistulas and sinuses are lined by inflammatory granulation tissue in which large numbers of foreign-body giant cells are present. In Crohn's disease, the typical noncaseating sarcoid type of granulomas may be encountered.

Anal fissure

Anal fissures are[253] longitudinal defects in the anal mucosa extending downward from the dentate line. At the lower margin, there is often a fibroepithelial polyp (so-called sentinal pile). Most fissures are caused by the trauma associated with passing a large firm stool through an area scarred by previous surgery.

Fissures are most common in young and middle-aged adults. More than 90% occur in the posterior midline. The remainder are in the midline anteriorly. The microscopic changes are nonspecific and manifest as chronic inflammation with granulation tissue formation.

Infectious diseases

Condyloma acuminatum

The term *condyloma* implies the presence of a wart occurring on a mucosal surface. In the case of anal condylomas, the cause is human papillomavirus (HPV), usually types 6 and 11;[254] however, a variety of other types have also been detected. The wart virus is spread venereally; consequently condylomas are most common in young sexually active adults. They are frequently multiple and grossly appear as papillary (cauliflower) lesions measuring up to several centimeters in diameter, generally located in the anal marginal zone.

Microscopically, condylomas consist of hyperplastic squamous epithelium, covering fibrovascular cores (Fig. 56-48). There may be koilocytic changes in which some intermediate and superficial squamous cells have a clear cytoplasm and pyknotic nuclei. Immunologic techniques or in situ hybridization will show evidence of intracellular papillomavirus. Cytogenetic analysis reveals many tetraploid and octaploid cells.

Most condylomas are completely benign. Condylomas with cytologic atypia are considered to carry a risk of malignant change and may give rise to verrucous carcinomas and squamous carcinomas. An association between anal condyloma, genital condyloma, and carcinoma of the cervix and vagina has also been shown, an indication of spread or transmission of viruses from one site to another.

Actinomycosis

Actinomycosis is a chronic infection caused by the filamentous, gram-positive anaerobic bacterium *Actinomyces israeli.* Occasionally, this may involve the anus and perianal regions, producing an inflammatory mass containing fistulas and pockets of pus.[255] Grossly the colonies appear as "sulfur granules."[256] Microscopically, these have a characteristic filamentous form with radiating eosinophilic material at the edge. If the lesion heals, there may be dense fibrosis with rectal stricturing.

Granuloma inguinale

Granuloma inguinale is a venereal disease caused by *Calymmatobacterium granulomatis,* which occurs predominantly in tropical and subtropical areas of the world. Grossly it is characterized by multiple anal and genital ulcers that are painless, red, and elevated. There may be inguinal lymphadenopathy. Histologically the ulcers contain mixed infiltrates of plasma cells, neutrophils, and large, pale-staining histiocytes that contain rod-shaped bacilli (Donovan bodies). These are best demonstrated with silver stains, such as Warthin-Starry.

ANAL NEOPLASMS

Anal intraepithelial neoplasia (AIN)

The term *anal intraepithelial neoplasia* incorporates squamous carcinoma in situ, Bowen's disease, and squamous dysplasia.[257] For simplicity, it is best to recognize only two grades of AIN: low grade and high grade. In almost all cases, it is the result of a venereally acquired infection by human papillomavirus types 16 and 18.[258] AIN is most common in young adults, particularly homosexual males.

The diagnosis of AIN is mainly histologic, since there are no distinct gross lesions. Any part of the anal canal may be involved, along with the circumanal skin. It may occur within condylomas or in patches of flat hyperkeratotic reddened mucosa or skin. In approximately 10% of hemorrhoidectomy specimens, AIN is present as an incidental finding.

The key histologic feature in the diagnosis is the presence of epithelial dysplasia (Fig. 56-49). In low-grade AIN, the changes involve the lower third to half of the mucosa. In high-grade AIN, the changes are full thickness, or virtually full thickness. Dysplasia may be recognized by the presence of nuclear crowding, enlargement, and pleomorphism. Mitotic activity may occur in a suprabasal location, and there may be atypical mitoses. Individual cell keratinization may be present. Koilocytic changes may be found, but these should be regarded only as evidence of HPV infection. They do not affect the grade of AIN or its biologic behavior. AIN is a precursor of invasive squamous carcinoma.

Squamous carcinoma

Anal squamous carcinoma[259-261] may arise above or below the dentate line. Tumors arising in the transitional zone account

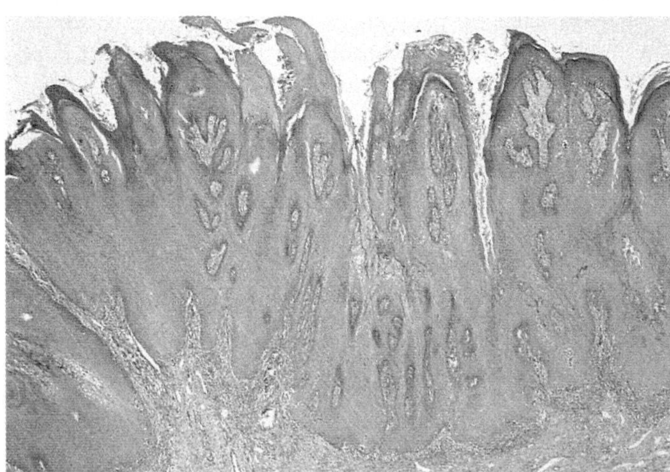

Fig. 56-48 Anal condyloma.

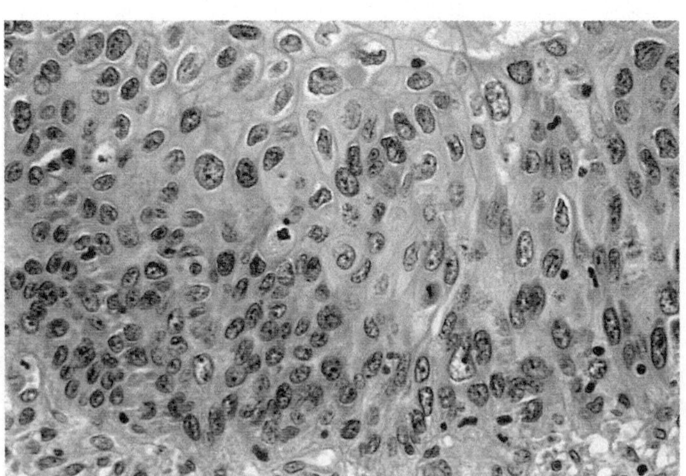

Fig. 56-49 Anal intraepithelial neoplasia.

for 75% of all anal carcinomas. They behave aggressively and are twice as common in women as they are in men. Carcinomas arising in the anal margin account for the remaining neoplasms. These are relatively less aggressive and are four times commoner in men than in women. Anal margin tumors occur more frequently in third world countries. Tumors at either site may occur in association with AIN, condylomas, and Crohn's disease.

The macroscopic features of anal carcinomas are identical to those of rectal adenocarcinomas. Most are ulcerated, with a rolled edge, though some may be polypoid. Microscopically the tumors arising in the anal margin zone are moderately to well differentiated and keratinizing. Two thirds of transitional zone tumors are keratinizing but are generally moderately to poorly differentiated. The remaining one third of cases are cloacogenic (basaloid) in appearance (Fig. 56-50). These consist of basal cells with small quantities of cytoplasm. They grow in islands with central necrosis and peripheral palisading. The mitotic rate is high, and they behave as poorly differentiated carcinomas.

Verrucous carcinoma

Verrucous carcinoma tumors, which have also been called the "giant condyloma of Bushke and Loewenstein," occur mainly in the anal margin mucosa.[262] Generally, they are large lesions with an exophytic growth pattern. Although they may spread laterally and invade underlying tissues, they very rarely metastasize. In some instances, these tumors contain koilocytic cells, indicating HPV infection. However, it is not clear whether all verrucous carcinomas have a viral origin and develop from preexistent condylomas.

Histologically, verrucous carcinomas are exceedingly well differentiated, and so on a small biopsy they may be impossible to distinguish from a condyloma (Fig. 56-51). A high index of suspicion should be present for all verrucous lesions over 2.0 cm in diameter. Biopsy specimens of the base of the lesion show superficial invasion, which may be recognized by the presence of tongues of squamous epithelium in the reticular dermis.

Anal gland carcinoma

Anal gland carcinoma tumors are unusual and arise from the ducts of anal glands. Three histologic subtypes are recognized:

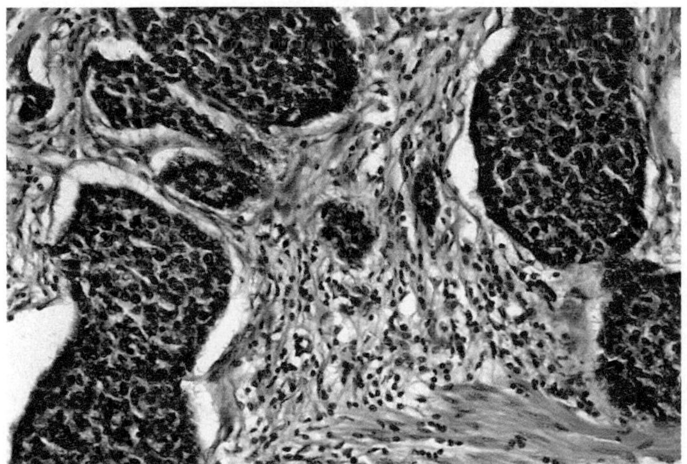

Fig. 56-50 Basaloid anal squamous carcinoma. Notice the peripheral palisading.

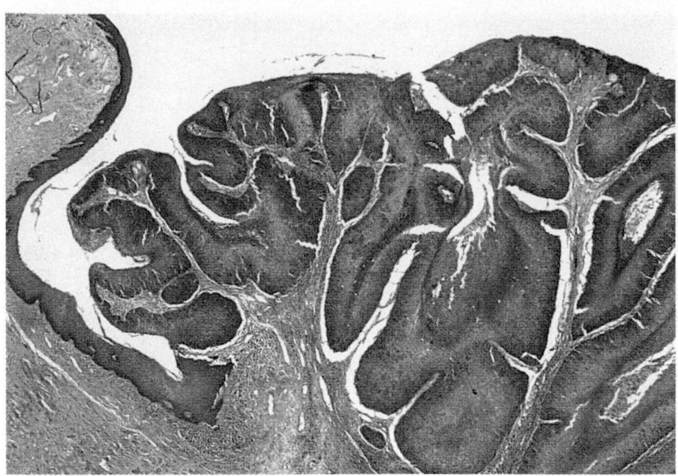

Fig. 56-51 Verrucous carcinoma of the anal region.

well-differentiated carcinoma,[263] mucinous carcinoma,[264] and mucoepidermoid carcinoma.[265] The well-differentiated carcinomas consist of well-formed ductlike structures lined by a bland columnar epithelium similar to a large bowel adenoma. They have a good prognosis. Mucinous tumors are histologically similar to colloid carcinomas of the large bowel. They have a poor prognosis and are difficult to excise locally because of extensive infiltration. Mucoepidermoid carcinomas appear like a mixture of cloacogenic squamous carcinoma and colloid carcinoma.

Malignant melanoma

Anal melanomas[266] arise in the transitional zone from melanocytes normally present at that site. They occur in adults of all age groups and present clinically as a bleeding mass that is grossly indistinguishable from other malignancies. Two thirds of cases show variable degrees of pigmentation. Microscopically they resemble cutaneous melanomas and consist predominantly of plump epithelioid cells with smaller numbers of spindle cells. At the edge of the main neoplasm there may be junctional melanocytic activity. Anal melanomas may show positive results with histochemical stains for melanin (Schmorl's or Masson-Fontana) and with immunohistochemical stains for S-100 protein and HMB45.

They are treated by local or radical excision. About 40% are confined to the anorectum, 40% have regional spread, and 20% have distal spread, at the time of diagnosis. The 1-year survival is 50%, and the 5-year survival is 15%.[267]

Perianal and anal Paget's disease

Paget's disease[268] in this region mainly affects the circumanal skin but may also extend into the anal margin. A substantial number of cases are associated with an underlying carcinoma. The primary may be located in the ducts of anal glands or in the rectal mucosa, just above the transitional zone. Smaller numbers of cases arise anew from the surface epithelium. There are no sufficiently large or well-controlled series to permit a precise determination of the relative frequency of each possibility. Histologically, anal Paget's disease is similar to Paget's disease of the breast. Solitary tumor cells or tumor cells in groups are present within the squamous epithelium. Paget cells have a clear cytoplasm and irregularly hyperchro-

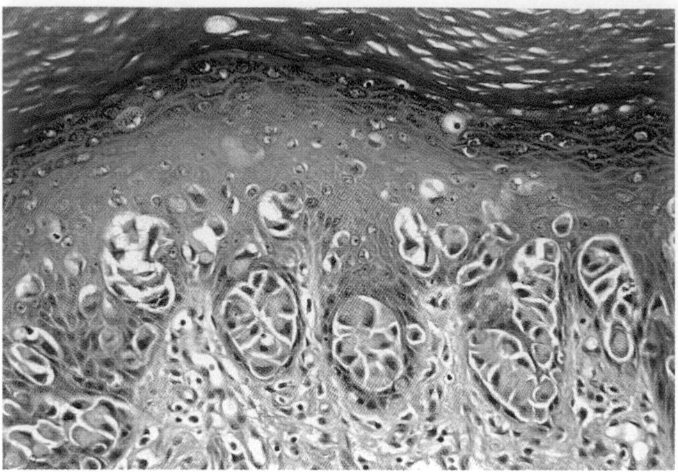

Fig. 56-52 Paget's disease of the anus. Notice the clear cells, which contain mucus.

matic nuclei. Their cytoplasm may contain mucin that stains with PAS (Fig. 56-52) or alcian blue and is immunoreactive with antibodies to CEA or cytokeratin. These features serve to distinguish Paget's disease from melanoma or AIN.

REFERENCES

The large intestine

Normal structure and function

1. Levine DS, Haggitt RC: Colon. In Sternberg SS, editor: *Histology for pathologists,* New York, 1992, Raven Press.
2. Cristina ML, Lehy T, Zeitoun P et al: Fine structural classification and comparative distribution of endocrine cells in normal human large intestine, *Gastroenterology* 75:20, 1978.
3. Snover DC, Sandstad J, Hutton S: Mucosal pseudolipomatosis of the colon, *Am J Clin Pathol* 84:575, 1985.
4. Meisel JL, Bergman D, Graney D et al: Human rectal mucosa: proctoscopic and morphological changes caused by laxatives, *Gastroenterology* 72:1274, 1977.
5. Pike BF, Phillippi PJ, Lawson EH: Soap colitis, *N Engl J Med* 285:217, 1971.

Hereditary and developmental disorders

6. Rogers RL, Hardford FJ: Mobile cecum syndrome, *Dis Colon Rectum* 27:399, 1984.
7. Habr Gama A, Haddad J, Simonsen O et al: Volvulus of the sigmoid colon in Brazil: a report of 230 cases, *Dis Colon Rectum* 19:314, 1976.
8. Grosfeld JL, Ballantine TV, Shoemaker R: Operative management of intestinal atresia and stenosis based on pathologic findings, *J Pediatr Surg* 14:368, 1979.
9. Oppenheimer EH, Esterly JR: Pathology of cystic fibrosis: review of the literature and comparison with 146 autopsied cases, *Perspect Pediatr Pathol* 2:241, 1975.
10. Blisard KS, Kleinman R: Hirschsprung's disease: a clinical and pathologic overview, *Hum Pathol* 17:1189, 1986.
11. Heitz PU, Komminoth P: Biopsy diagnosis of Hirschsprung's disease and related disorders, *Curr Top Pathol* 81:257, 1990.

Diseases caused by injury from exogenous factors

ALLERGIC DISORDERS

12. Talley NJ, Shorter RG, Zinsmeister AR: Eosinophilic gastroenteritis: a clinicopathological study of patients with disease of the mucosa, muscle layer and subserosal tissues, *Gut* 31:54, 1990.
13. Goldman H, Proujansky R: Allergic proctitis and allergic gastroenteritis in children: clinical and mucosal biopsy features in 53 cases, *Am J Surg Pathol* 10:75, 1986.
14. Jenkins HR, Pincott JR, Soothill JF et al: Food allergy: the major cause of infantile colitis, *Arch Dis Child* 59:326, 1984.
15. Croese J, Loukas A, Opdebeeck J, Drocir P: Occult enteric infection by *Ancylostoma caninum*: a previously unrecognized zoonosis, *Gastroenterology* 106:3, 1994.
16. Martin DM, Goldman JA, Gillam J et al: Gold induced eosinophilic enterocolitis: response to oral cromolyn sodium, *Gastroenterology* 80:1567, 1981.
17. De Schryver-Kecskemeti K, Clouse RE: A previously unrecognized subgroup of "eosinophilic gastroenteritis": association with connective tissue diseases, *Am J Surg Pathol* 8:171, 1984.

DRUG-INDUCED DISEASES

18. Lee FD: Importance of apoptosis in the histopathology of drug related lesions in the large intestine, *J Clin Pathol* 46:118, 1993.
19. Huber T, Ruchti C, Halter F: Non-steroidal anti-inflammatory drug-induced colonic strictures: a case report, *Gastroenterology* 100:1119, 1991.
20. Fortson WC, Tedesco FJ: Drug-induced colitis: a review, *Am J Gastroenterol* 79:878, 1984.
21. Herbert DC: Anticoagulant therapy and the acute abdomen, *Br J Surg* 55:353, 1968.
22. Stillman AE, Weinberg M, Mast WC et al: Ischemic bowel disease attributable to ergot, *Gastroenterology* 72:1336, 1977.
23. Weston JT, Guin GH: Epithelial atypias with chemotherapy in 100 acute childhood leukemias, *Cancer* 8:179, 1955.
24. Koskela E, Kulju T, Collan Y: Melanosis coli: prevalence, distribution and histologic features in 200 consecutive autopsies at Kuopio University Central Hospital, *Dis Colon Rectum* 32:235, 1989.
25. Lewis JW, Kerstein MD, Koss N: Barium granuloma of the rectum: an uncommon complication of barium enema, *Ann Surg* 181:418, 1975.

STERCORAL ULCERS

26. Grinvalsky HT, Bowerman CI: Stercoraceous ulcers of the colon, *JAMA* 171:1941, 1959.

RADIATION COLITIS

27. Berthrong M, Fajardo LF: Radiation injury in surgical pathology. II. Alimentary tract, *Am J Surg Pathol* 5:153, 1981.

Noninfections diseases of uncertain cause

DIVERTICULAR DISEASE

28. Painter NS, Burkitt DP: Diverticular disease of the colon, a 20th century problem, *Clin Gastroenterol* 4:3, 1975.
29. Beighton PH, Murdoch JL, Votteler T: Gastrointestinal complications of the Ehlers-Danlos syndrome, *Gut* 10:1004, 1969.
30. Hughes LE: Post-mortem survey of diverticular disease of the colon. Part II. The muscular abnormality in the sigmoid colon, *Gut* 10:344, 1969.
31. Morson BC: Pathology of diverticular disease of the colon, *Clin Gastroenterol* 4:37, 1975.
32. Ming SC, Fleischner FG: Diverticulitis of the sigmoid colon: re-appraisal of the pathology and pathogenesis, *Surgery* 58:627, 1965.
33. Kelly JK: Polypoid prolapsing mucosal folds in diverticular disease, *Am J Surg Pathol* 15:871, 1991.
34. Segal I, Leibowitz B: The distributional pattern of diverticular disease. *Dis Colon Rectum* 32:227, 1989.

INTESTINAL PSEUDO-OBSTRUCTION

35. Freilich HS, Chopra S, Gillam JI: Acute colonic pseudo-obstruction or Ogilvie's syndrome, *J Clin Gastroenterol* 8:457, 1986.
36. Schuffler MD, Lowe MC, Bill AH: Studies of idiopathic intestinal pseudo-obstruction. I. Hereditary hollow visceral myopathy: clinical and pathological studies, *Gastroenterology* 73:327, 1977.
37. Krishnamurthy S, Schuffler MD: Pathology of neuromuscular disorders of the small intestine and colon, *Gastroenterology* 93:610, 1987.

LIPOFUSCINOSIS AND AMYLOIDOSIS

38. Fox B: Lipofuscinosis of the gastrointestinal tract in man, *J Clin Pathol* 20:806, 1967.
39. Cohen AS: Amyloidosis, *N Engl J Med* 277:522, 574, 628, 1967.

Circulatory disorders

COLONIC ISCHEMIA

40. Whitehead R: The pathology of ischemia of the intestine. In Sommers SC, editor: *Pathology Annual,* New York, 1976, Appleton-Century-Crofts.

41. Genta RM, Haggitt RC: Idiopathic myointimal hyperplasia of mesenteric veins, *Gastroenterology* 101:533, 1991.
42. Sarago EP, Costa J: Idiopathic enterocolic lymphocytic phlebitis, *Am J Surg Pathol* 13:303, 1989.
43. Schein M, Saadia R, Decker G: Colonic necrosis in acute pancreatitis: a complication of massive retroperitoneal suppuration, *Dis Colon Rectum* 28:948, 1985.
44. Lindahl F, Vejlsted H, Backer OG: Lesions of the colon following acute pancreatitis, *Scand J Gastroenterol* 7:375, 1972.
45. Hunt DR, Mildenhall P: Etiology of strictures of the colon associated with pancreatitis, *Dig Dis Sci* 20:941, 1975.
46. Mohiuddin S, Sakiylak P, Gullick HD et al: Stenosing lesions of the colon secondary to pancreatitis, *Arch Surg* 102:229, 1971.
47. Gladman DD, Ross T, Richardson B et al: Bowel involvement in systemic lupus erythematosus: Crohn's disease or lupus vasculitis? *Arthritis Rheum* 28:466, 1985.
48. Bienenstock H, Menick R, Rogoff B: Mesenteric arteritis and intestinal infarction in rheumatoid arthritis, *Arch Intern Med* 119:359, 1967.
49. Adler RH, Norcross BM, Lockie LM: Arteritis and infarction of the intestine in rheumatoid arthritis, *JAMA* 180:922, 1962.
50. Weiser MM, Andres GA, Brenjens JR et al: Systemic lupus erythematosus and intestinal venulitis, *Gastroenterology* 81:570, 1981.
51. Bailey RW, Hamilton SR, Morris JB et al: Pathogenesis of nonocclusive ischemic colitis, *Ann Surg* 203:590, 1986.
52. Nalbandian H, Sheth N, Dietrich R, Georgiou J: Intestinal ischemia caused by cocaine ingestion: report of two cases, *Surgery* 97:374, 1985.
53. Mustard R, Gray R, Maziak D et al: Visceral infarction caused by cocaine abuse: a case report, *Surgery* 112:951, 1992.
54. Romano TJ, Graham SM, Chuong J et al: Bleeding colonic ulcers secondary to atheromatous microemboli after left heart catheterization, *J Clin Gastroenterol* 10:693, 1988.
55. Welling RE, Roedersheimer R, Arbaugh JJ, et al: Ischemic colitis following repair of ruptured aortic aneurysm, *Arch Surg* 120:1368, 1985.
56. Sparano JA, Dutcher JP, Kaleya R et al: Colonic ischemia complicating immunotherapy with intraleukin-II and interferon-alpha, *Cancer* 68:1538, 1991.
57. Choi H-S H, Heller D, Picken MM et al: Infarction of intestine with massive amyloid deposition in two patients on long-term hemodialysis, *Gastroenterology* 90:230, 1989.
58. Komorowski RA, Cohen EB, Kauffman HM et al: Gastrointestinal complications in renal transplant recipients, *Am J Clin Pathol* 86:161, 1986.
59. Salinas-Madrigal L, Bruk A, DeMello DE: Myofibrillar degeneration and necrosis of the visceral smooth musculature, *Hum Pathol* 18:815, 1987.
60. Duffy TJ: Reversible ischemic colitis in young adults, *Br J Surg* 68:34, 1981.

HEMANGIOMAS AND VASCULAR ANOMALIES

61. Camilleri M, Chadwick VS, Hodgson HJF: Vascular anomalies of the gastrointestinal tract, *Hepatogastroenterology* 31:149, 1984.
62. Pounder DJ, Roland R, Pieterse AS et al: Angiodysplasias of the colon, *J Clin Pathol* 35:824, 1982.
63. Thelmo WL, Vetrano JA, Wibowo A et al: Angiodysplasia of colon revisited: pathologic demonstration without the use of intravascular injection technique, *Hum Pathol* 23:37, 1992.
64. Stamm B, Heer M, Buhler H et al: Mucosal biopsy of vascular ectasia (angiodysplasia) of the large bowel detected during routine colonoscopic examination, *Histopathology* 9:639, 1985.
65. Duray PH, Marcal JM, LiVolsi VA et al: Gastrointestinal angiodysplasia: a possible component of von Willebrand's disease, *Hum Pathol* 15:539, 1984.
66. Heer M, Sulser H, Haney A: Angiodysplasia of the colon: an expression of occlusive vascular disease, *Hepatogastroenterology* 34:127:1987.
67. Marcuard SP, Weinstack JV: Gastrointestinal angiodysplasia in renal failure, *J Clin Gastroenterol* 10:482, 1988.
68. Freedman SD, Drews RE, Glotzer DJ et al: Recurrent gastrointestinal bleeding associated with myelofibrosis and diffuse intestinal telangiectasias, *Gastroenterology* 101:1432, 1991.
69. Cappell MS: Spatial clustering of simultaneous nonhereditary gastrointestinal angiodysplasia, *Dig Dis Sci* 37:1072, 1992.
70. Marshall JB, Moore GF, Settles RH: Colonic telangiectasis in scleroderma, *Arch Intern Med* 140:1121, 1980.
71. Viggiano TR, Gostout CJ: Portal hypertensive intestinal vasculopathy: a review of the clinical, endoscopic and histopathologic features, *Am J Gastroenterol* 87:944, 1992.
72. Iredale JP, Ridings P, McGinn FP et al: Familial and idiopathic colonic varices: an unusual cause of lower gastrointestinal hemorrhage, *Gut* 33:1285, 1992.

Infectious diseases

BACTERIAL DISEASES

73. Levine MM: *Escherichia coli* infections, *N Engl J Med* 313:445, 1985.
74. Boedeker EC: Enteroadherent (enteropathogenic) *Escherichia coli*. In Farthing MJG, Keusch GT, editors: *Enteric infection: mechanisms, manifestations and management,* London, 1989, Chapman & Hall.
75. Levine MM: *Escherichia coli* that cause diarrhea: enterotoxigenic, enteropathogenic, enteroinvasive, enterohemorrhagic and enteroadherent, *J Infect Dis* 155:377, 1987.
76. Neter E: Enteritis due to enteropathogenic *Escherichia coli, Am J Dig Dis* 10:883, 1965.
77. Rothbaum R, McAdams AJ, Giannella R et al: A clinicopathologic study of enterocyte-adherent *Escherichia coli:* a cause of protracted diarrhea in infants, *Gastroenterology* 83:441, 1982.
78. Riley LW, Remis RS, Helgerson SD et al: Outbreaks of hemorrhagic colitis associated with a rare *E. coli* serotype, *N Engl J Med* 308:681, 1983.
79. Carter AO, Borczyk AA, Carlson JAK et al: A severe outbreak of *Escherichia coli* O157:H7-associated hemorrhagic colitis in a nursing home, *N Engl J Med* 317:1496, 1987.
80. Bobak DA, Guerrant RL: New developments in enteric bacterial toxins, *Adv Pharmacol* 23:85, 1992.
81. Richardson SE, Karmali MA, Becker LE et al: The histopathology of the hemolytic uremic syndrome associated with verocytotoxin-producing *Escherichia coli* infections, *Hum Pathol* 19:1102, 1988.
82. Kelly JK, Oryshak A, Wenetsek M et al: The colonic pathology of *Escherichia coli* O157:H7 infection, *Am J Surg Pathol* 14:87, 1990.
83. Guerrant RL, Moore RA, Kirschenfeld PM et al: Roles of toxigenic and invasive bacteria in acute diarrhea in childhood, *N Engl J Med* 293:567, 1975.
84. Echeverria P, Blacklow NR, Sanford LB et al: Traveller's diarrhea among peace corps volunteers in Thailand, *J Infect Dis* 143:767, 1981.
85. Dupont HL, Formal SB, Hornick RB et al: Pathogenesis of *Escherichia coli* diarrhea, *N Engl J Med* 285:1, 1971.
86. Day DW, Mandal BK, Morson BC: The rectal biopsy appearance of *Salmonella* colitis, *Histopathology* 2:117, 1978.
87. McGovern VJ, Slavutin LJ: Pathology of *Salmonella* colitis, *Am J Surg Pathol* 3:483, 1979.
88. Butler T, Dunn D, Dahms B et al: Causes of death and the histopathologic findings in fatal shigellosis, *Pediatr Infect Dis J* 8:767, 1989.
89. Price AB, Jewkes J, Sanderson PJ: Acute diarrhea: *Campylobacter* colitis and the role or rectal biopsy, *J Clin Pathol* 32:990, 1979.
90. Gleason TH, Patterson SD: The pathology of *Yersinia enterocolitica* enterocolitis, *Am J Surg Pathol* 6:347, 1982.
91. Simmonds SD, Noble MA, Freeman HJ: Gastrointestinal features of culture positive *Yersinia enterocolitica* infection, *Gastroenterology* 92:112, 1987.
92. Kumar NB, Nostrant TT, Appelman HD: The histopathologic spectrum of acute self-limited colitis (acute infectious-type colitis), *Am J Surg Pathol* 6:523, 1982.
93. Nostrant TT, Kumar NB, Appelman HD: Histopathology differentiates acute self-limited colitis from ulcerative colitis, *Gastroenterology* 92:318, 1987.
94. Surawicz CM, Belie L: Rectal biopsy helps to distinguish acute self-limited colitis from idiopathic inflammatory bowel disease, *Gastroenterology* 86:104, 1984.
95. Buts J-P, Weber Am, Morin CL: Pseudomembranous enterocolitis in children, *Gastroenterology* 73:823, 1977.
96. Trnka YM, LaMont JT: *Clostridium difficile* colitis, *Adv Intern Med* 29:85, 1984.
97. Price AB, Davis DR: Pseudomembranous colitis, *J Clin Pathol* 30:1, 1977.
98. Cone JB, Wetzel W: Toxic megacolon secondary to pseudomembranous colitis, *Dis Colon Rectum* 25:478, 1982.

99. King A, Rampling A, Wright DG et al: Neutropenic enterocolitis due to *Clostridium septicum* infection, *J Clin Pathol* 37:335, 1984.
100. Ahsar N, Sun C-C, Di John D: Acute ileotyphlitis as presenting manifestation of acute myelogenous leukemia, *Am J Clin Pathol* 89:407, 1988.
101. Bassi O, Cosa G, Colavolpe A et al: Primary syphilis of the rectum—endoscopic and clinical features: report of a case, *Dis Colon Rectum* 34:1024, 1991.
102. Quinn TC, Lukehart SA, Goodell S et al: Rectal mass caused by *Treponema pallidum:* confirmation by immunofluorescent staining, *Gastroenterology* 82:135, 1982.
103. McMillan A, Lee FD: Sigmoidoscopic and microscopic appearance of the rectal mucosa in homosexual men, *Gut* 22:1035, 1981.
104. McMillan A, McNeillage G, Gilmour HM et al: Histology of rectal gonorrhea in men, with a note on anorectal infection with *Neisseria meningitidis, J Clin Pathol* 36:511, 1983.
105. Surawicz CM, Goodell SE, Quinn TC et al: Spectrum of rectal biopsy abnormalities in homosexual men with intestinal symptoms, *Gastroenterology* 91:651, 1986.
106. Quinn TC, Goodell SE, Mkrtichian E et al: *Chlamydia trachomatis* proctitis, *N Engl J Med* 305:195, 1981.
107. Tompkins DS, Foulkes SJ, Goodwin PG: Isolation and characterization of intestinal spirochetes, *J Clin Pathol* 39:535, 1986.
108. Henrik-Nielsen R, Orholm M, Pederson JO et al: Colorectal spirochetosis: clinical significance of the infestation, *Gastroenterology* 85:62, 1983.

VIRAL INFECTIONS

109. Goodell SE, Quinn TC, Mkrtichian E et al: Herpes simplex virus proctitis in homosexual men, *N Engl J Med* 308:868, 1983.
110. Surawicz CA, Myerson D: Self-limited cytomegalovirus colitis in immunocompetent individuals, *Gastroenterology* 94:194, 1988.
111. Cooper H, Raffensburger EC, Joknas L et al: Cytomegalovirus inclusions in patients with ulcerative colitis and toxic dilatation requiring colonic resection, *Gastroenterology* 72:1253, 1977.

PARASITIC DISEASES

112. Ravdin J: Pathogenesis of disease caused by *Entameba histolytica:* studies of adherence, secreted toxin and contact dependent cytolysis, *Rev Infect Dis* 8:247, 1986.
113. Brandt H, Tamayo P: Pathology of human amebiasis, *Hum Pathol* 1:351, 1970.
114. Castro J, Vázques-Inglesias JL, Arnal-Montréal: Dysentery caused by *Balantidium coli:* report of two cases, *Endoscopy* 15:272, 1983.
115. Vanatta HB, Adamson D, Mullican K: *Blastocystis hominis* infection presenting as recurrent diarrhea, *Ann Intern Med* 102:495, 1985.
116. Pikula ZP: *Blastocystis hominis* and human disease, *J Clin Microbiol* 24:1581, 1986.
117. Symmers W StC: Pathology of oxyuriasis, *Arch Pathol* 50:475, 1950.
118. Neafie RC, Connor DH: Trichuriasis. In Binford CH, Connor DH, editors: *Pathology of tropical and unusual diseases,* vol 2, Washington, DC, 1976, Armed Forces Institute of Pathology.
119. Gilman RH, Chong TH, David C et al: The adverse consequences of heavy *Trichuris* infection, *Trans R Soc Trop Med Hyg* 77:432, 1983.
120. Cheever AW, Kamel IA, Elwi AM et al: *Schistosoma mansoni* and *S. hematobium* infections in Egypt. III. Extra-hepatic pathology, *Am J Trop Med Hyg* 27:939, 1978.

MALAKOPLAKIA

121. McClure J: Malakoplakia of the gastrointestinal tract, *Postgrad Med J* 57:95, 1981.
122. McClure J: Malakoplakia, *J Pathol* 140:275, 1983.
123. Ghosh S, Pattniak S, Jalan R et al: Malakoplakia simulating rectal carcinoma, *Am J Gastroenterol* 85:910, 1990.
124. Lewin KJ, Harell GS, Lee AS et al: Malakoplakia: an electron-microscope study: demonstration of bacilliform organisms in malakoplakic macrophages, *Gastroenterology* 66:28, 1974.

Idiopathic inflammatory bowel disease

125. Calkins BM, Lilienfeld AM, Garland CF et al: Trends in incidence rates of ulcerative colitis and Crohn's disease, *Dig Dis Sci* 29:913, 1984.
126. Sonnenberg A: Geographic variation in the incidence of and mortality from inflammatory bowel disease, *Dis Colon Rectum* 29:854, 1986.
127. Price AB, Morson BC: Inflammatory bowel disease: the surgical pathology of Crohn's disease and ulcerative colitis, *Hum Pathol* 6:7, 1975.
128. Goulston SJ, McGovern VJ: The nature of benign strictures in ulcerative colitis, *N Engl J Med* 281:290, 1969.
129. Greenstein AJ, Sachar DB, Fibas A et al: Outcome of toxic dilatation in ulcerative colitis and Crohn's disease, *J Clin Gastroenterol* 7:137, 1985.
130. Danzi JT: Extraintestinal manifestations of idiopathic inflammatory bowel disease, *Arch Intern Med* 148:297, 1988.
131. Lockhart-Mummery HE, Morson BC: Crohn's disease (regional enteritis) of the large intestine and its distinction from ulcerative colitis, *Gut* 1:87, 1960.
132. Davidson AM, Dixon MF: The appendix as a skip organ in ulcerative colitis, *Histopathology* 16:93, 1990.
133. Price AB: Overlap in the spectrum of non-specific inflammatory bowel disease—"colitis indeterminate." *J Clin Pathol* 31:567, 1978.
134. Lee KS, Medline A, Shockey S: Indeterminate colitis in the spectrum of inflammatory bowel disease, *Arch Pathol Lab Med* 103:173, 1979.
135. Poulsen SS, Tinggaard-Pedersen N, Jarnum S: "Microerosions" in rectal biopsies in Crohn's disease, *Scand J Gastroenterol* 19:609, 1984.
136. Kelly JK, Sutherland LR: The chronological sequence in the pathology of Crohn's disease, *J Clin Gastroenterol* 10:28, 1988.
137. Collins RH, Feldman M, Fordtran JS: Colon cancer, dysplasia and surveillance in patients with ulcerative colitis, *N Engl J Med* 316:1654, 1987.
138. Yardley JH, Bayless TM, Diamond MP: Cancer in ulcerative colitis, *Gastroenterology* 76:221, 1979.
139. Hamilton SR: Colorectal carcinoma in patients with Crohn's disease, *Gastroenterology* 89:398, 1985.
140. Prior P, Gyde SN, Macartney JC et al: Cancer morbidity in ulcerative colitis, *Gut* 23:490, 1982.
141. Lennard-Jones JE, Melville DM, Morson BC et al: Pre-cancer and cancer in extensive ulcerative colitis: findings among 407 patients over 22 years, *Gut* 31:800, 1990.
142. Kewenter J, Ahlman H, Hulten I: Cancer risk in extensive ulcerative colitis, *Ann Surg* 188:824, 1978.
143. Langholz E, Munkholm P, Davidsen M et al: Colorectal cancer risk and mortality in patients with ulcerative colitis, *Gastroenterology* 103:1444, 1992.
144. Katzka I, Brody RS, Morris E et al: Assessment of colo-rectal cancer risk in patients with ulcerative colitis: experience from private practice, *Gastroenterology* 85:22, 1983.
145. Riddell RH, Goldman H, Ranshoff DF et al: Dysplasia in inflammatory bowel disease: standard classification with provisional clinical applications, *Hum Pathol* 14:931, 1983.
146. Rubin CE, Haggitt RC, Burmer GC et al: DNA aneuploidy in colonic biopsies predicts future development of dysplasia in ulcerative colitis, *Gastroenterology* 103:1611, 1992.

Noninfectious inflammatory conditions

147. Jesserun J, Yardley JH, Giardiello FM et al: Chronic colitis with thickening of the subepithelial collagen layer (collagenous colitis): histopathologic findings in 15 patients, *Hum Pathol* 18:839, 1987.
148. Hwang WS, Kelly JK, Shaffer EA et al: Collagenous colitis: a disease of pericryptal fibroblast sheath, *J Pathol* 149:33, 1986.
149. Riddell RH, Tanaka M, Mazzoleni G: Non-steroidal anti-inflammatory drugs as a possible cause of collagenous colitis: a case control study, *Gut* 33:683, 1992.
150. Hamilton I, Sanders S, Hopwood D et al: Collagenous colitis associated with small intestinal villous atrophy, *Gut* 27:1394, 1986.
151. Palmer KR, Berry H, Wheeler PJ et al: Collagenous colitis: a relapsing and remitting disease, *Gut* 27:578, 1986.
152. Wolber R, Owen D, Freeman H: Colonic lymphocytosis in patients with celiac sprue, *Hum Pathol* 21:1092, 1990.
153. Read NW, Krejs GJ, Read MG et al: Chronic diarrhea of unknown origin, *Gastroenterology* 78:264, 1980.
154. Lazenby AJ, Yardley JH, Giardello FM et al: Lymphocytic ("microscopic") colitis: a comparative histologic study with particular reference to collagenous colitis, *Hum Pathol* 20:18, 1989.
155. Yardley JH, Lazenby AJ, Giardello FM et al: Collagenous, "microscopic," lymphocytic and other gentler and more subtle forms of colitis, *Hum Pathol* 21:1089, 1990.

156. Rutter KP, Riddell RH: The solitary ulcer syndrome of the rectum, *Clin Gastroenterol* 4:505, 1975.
157. Womack NR, Williams NS, Holmfield JH et al: Pressure and prolapse, the cause of the solitary rectal ulcer syndrome, *Gut* 28:1228, 1987.
158. duBoulay CE, Fairbrother J, Isaacson PG: Mucosal prolapse syndrome: a unifying concept for solitary ulcer syndrome and related disorders, *J Clin Pathol* 36:1264, 1983.
159. Ford MJ, Anderson JR, Gilmour HM et al: Clinical spectrum of "solitary ulcer" of the rectum, *Gastroenterology* 84:1533, 1983.
160. Saul SH, Sollenberger LC: Solitary rectal ulcer syndrome: its clinical and pathological underdiagnosis, *Am J Surg Pathol* 9:411, 1985.
161. Levine DS: Solitary rectal ulcer syndrome. Are "solitary" rectal ulcer syndrome and "localized" colitis cystica profunda analogous syndromes caused by rectal prolapse? *Gastroenterology* 92:243, 1987.
162. Saul SH: Inflammatory cloacogenic polyp: Relationship to solitary rectal ulcer syndrome/mucosal prolapse and other bowel disorders, *Hum Pathol* 18:1120, 1987.
163. Thomas DF: Neonatal necrotizing enterocolitis. In Marston A, editor: *Vascular disease of the gastrointestinal tract: pathophysiology, recognition and management,* Baltimore, 1986, Williams & Wilkins.
164. Galandiuk S, Fazio VW: Pneumatosis cystoides intestinalis, *Dis Colon Rectum* 29:358, 1986.
165. Pieterse AS, Leong AS, Rowland R: The mucosal changes and pathogenesis of pneumatosis cystoides intestinalis, *Hum Pathol* 16:683, 1985.
166. Habouri NY, Honan RP, Hasleton PS et al: Pneumatosis coli: a case report with ultrastructural study, *Histopathology* 8:145, 1984.
167. Glotzer DJ, Glick ME, Goldman A: Proctitis and colitis following diversion of the fecal stream, *Gastroenterology* 80:438, 1981.
168. Harig JM, Soergel KH, Komorowski RA et al: Treatment of diversion colitis with short chain fatty acids, *N Engl J Med* 320:23, 1989.
169. Murray FE, O'Brien MJ, Birkett DH et al: Diversion colitis: pathologic findings in a resected sigmoid colon and rectum, *Gastroenterology* 93:1404, 1987.
170. Lakhanpal S, Tani K, Lie JT et al: Pathologic features of Behçet's syndrome: a review of Japanese autopsy registry data, *Hum Pathol* 16:790, 1985.
171. Lee RG: The colitis of Behçet's syndrome, *Am J Surg Pathol* 10:888, 1986.
172. Kasahara Y, Tanaka S, Nishino M et al: Intestinal involvement in Behçet's syndrome: review of 136 surgical cases from the Japanese literature, *Dis Colon Rectum* 24:103, 1981.

Large bowel polyps

173. Correa P: Epidemiology of polyps and cancer. In: Morson BC, editor: *Pathogenesis of colorectal cancer,* Philadelphia: 1978, Saunders.
174. Cappell MS, Forde KA: Spatial clustering of multiple hyperplastic, adenomatous and malignant colonic polyps in individual patients, *Dis Colon Rectum* 32:641, 1989.
175. Franzin G, Zamboni G, Scarpa A et al: Hyperplastic (metaplastic) polyps of the colon: a histologic and histochemical study, *Am J Surg Pathol* 8:687, 1981.
176. Longacre TA, Fenoglio-Preiser CM: Mixed hyperplastic adenomatous polyps/serrated adenomas: a distinct form of colo-rectal neoplasia, *Am J Surg Pathol* 14:524, 1990.
177. Williams GT, Arthur JF, Bussey HJ et al: Metaplastic polyps and polyposis of the colo-rectum, *Histopathology* 4:155, 1980.
178. Sobin LH: Inverted hyperplastic polyps of the colon, *Am J Surg Pathol* 9:265, 1985.
179. Dajani YF, Kamal MF: Colorectal juvenile polyps: an epidemiological and histopathological study of 144 cases in Jordanians, *Histopathology* 8:765, 1984.
180. Haggitt RC, Reid BJ: Hereditary gastrointestinal polyposis syndromes, *Am J Surg Pathol* 10:871, 1986.
181. Carlson GJ, Nitavongs S, Snover DC: Colorectal polyps in Cowden's disease (multiple hamartoma syndrome), *Am J Surg Pathol* 8:763, 1984.
182. Burke AP, Sobin LH: The pathology of Cronkhite-Canada polyps: a comparison to juvenile polyposis, *Am J Surg Pathol* 13:940, 1989.

Large bowel neoplasms

183. Rickert RR, Auerbach O, Garfinkel L et al: Adenomatous lesions of the large bowel: an autopsy study, *Cancer* 43:1847, 1979.
184. Williams AR, Balasooriya BA, Day DW: Polyps and cancer of the large bowel: a necropsy study in Liverpool, *Gut* 23:835, 1982.
185. Granqvist S: Distribution of polyps of the large bowel in relation to age, *Scand J Gastroenterol* 16:1025, 1981.
186. Hoff G, Foerster A, Vatn MH et al: Epidemiology of polyps in the rectum and colon: recovery and evaluation of unresected polyps two years after detection, *Scand J Gastroenterol* 21:852, 1986.
187. Eide TJ, Schweder T: Clustering of adenomas in the large intestine, *Gut* 25:1262, 1984.
188. Thompson JJ, Enterline HT: The macroscopic appearance of colorectal polyps, *Cancer* 48:151, 1981.
189. Muto T, Kamiya J, Sawada T et al: Small "flat adenoma" of the large bowel with special reference to its clinico-pathologic features, *Dis Colon Rectum* 28:847, 1985.
190. Muto T, Bussey HJ, Morson BC: Pseudo-carcinomatous invasion in adenomatous polyps of the colon and rectum, *J Clin Pathol* 26:25, 1973.
191. Muto T, Bussey HJ, Morson BC: The evolution of cancer of the colon and rectum, *Cancer* 36:2251, 1975.
192. Morson BC, Whiteway JE, Jones EA et al: Histopathology and prognosis of malignant colorectal polyps treated by endoscopic polypectomy, *Gut* 25:437, 1984.
193. Haggitt RC, Glotzback RE, Soffer EE et al: Prognostic factors in colorectal carcinomas arising in adenomas: implications for lesions removed by polypectomy, *Gastroenterology* 89:328, 1985.
194. Morson BC: The polyp-cancer sequence of the large bowel, *Proc R Soc Med* 67:451, 1974.
195. Winawer SJ, Zauber AG, Ho MH et al: Prevention of colorectal cancer by colonoscopic polypectomy, *N Engl J Med* 329:1977, 1993.
196. Hamilton SR: The molecular genetics of colorectal neoplasia, *Gastroenterology* 105:3, 1993.
197. Hamelin R, Laurent-Puig P, Olschwang S et al: Association of p53 mutations with short survival in colorectal cancer, Gastroenterology 106:42, 1994.
198. Alabaster O: Colorectal cancer: Epidemiology, risks and prevention. In: Ahlgren JD, MacDonald JS, editors: *Gastrointestinal oncology,* Philadelphia, 1992, Lippincott.
199. Connelly JH, Robey-Cafferty SS, Cleary KR: Mucinous carcinomas of the colon and rectum, *Arch Pathol Lab Med* 115:1022, 1991.
200. Sasaki O, Atkin WS, Jass JR: Mucinous carcinoma of the rectum, *Histopathology* 22:259, 1987.
201. Coma del Corral MJ, Pérez-Serrano L, Razquin-Lizarraga S: Melanotic adenocarcinoma of the ano-rectum, *J Clin Gastroenterol* 12:114, 1990.
202. Sandmeier D, Guillou L: Malakoplakia and adenocarcinoma of the caecum: a rare association, *J Clin Pathol* 46:959, 1993.
203. Dukes CE: The classification of cancer of the rectum, *J Pathol Bacteriol* 35:323, 1932.
204. Astler VA, Coller FA: The prognostic significance of direct extension of carcinoma of the colon and rectum, *Ann Surg* 139:846, 1954.
205. Spierse B, Beahrs OH, Hermanek P et al: *TNM atlas,* ed 3, Berlin, 1992, Springer-Verlag.
206. Halvorsen TB, Seim E: Association between invasiveness, inflammatory reaction, desmoplasia and survival in colorectal cancer, *J Clin Pathol* 42:162, 1989.
207. Visscher DW, Zarbo RJ, Ma CK et al: Flow cytometric DNA and clinicopathologic analysis of Dukes' A & B colonic adenocarcinomas: a retrospective study, *Mod Pathol* 3:709, 1990.
208. Benhattar J, Losi L, Chaubert P et al: Prognostic significance of K-*ras* mutations in colorectal carcinoma, *Gastroenterology* 104:1044, 1993.

INHERITED FORMS OF COLORECTAL CANCER

209. Burt RW, Bishop DT, Cannon-Albright L et al: Hereditary aspects of colo-rectal adenomas, *Cancer* 70:1296, 1992.
210. Turcot J, Depres JP, St Pierre F: Malignant tumors of the central nervous system associated with familial polyposis of the colon, *Dis Colon Rectum* 2:465, 1959.
211. Lynch HT, Smyrk TC, Watson P et al: Hereditary flat adenoma syndrome: a variant of familial adenomatous polyposis? *Dis Colon Rectum* 35:411, 1992.
212. Lynch HT, Watson P, Smyrk TC et al: Colon cancer genetics, *Cancer* 70:1300, 1992.

213. Lynch HT, Smyrk TC, Watson P et al: Genetics, natural history, tumor spectrum, and pathology of hereditary non-polyposis colo-rectal cancer: an updated review, *Gastroenterology* 104:1535, 1993.
214. Vasen HF, Mecklin J-P, Meera Khan P et al: The international collaborative group on hereditary non-polyposis colorectal cancer, *Dis Colon Rectum* 34:424, 1991.
215. Aaltonen LA, Peltomäki P, Leach FS et al: Clues to the pathogenesis of familial colorectal cancer, *Science* 260:812, 1993.
216. Thibodeau SN, Bren G, Schaid D: Microsatellite instability in cancer of the proximal colon, *Science* 260:816, 1993.
217. Alessi E, Brambilla L, Luporini G et al: Multiple sebaceous tumors and carcinomas of the colon: Torre syndrome, *Cancer* 55:2566, 1985.

RARE TYPES OF PRIMARY LARGE BOWEL CARCINOMA

218. Cerezo L, Alvarez M, Edwards O et al: Adenosquamous carcinoma of the colon, *Dis Colon Rectum* 28:597, 1985.
219. Williams GT, Blackshaw AJ, Morson BC: Squamous carcinoma of the colon and its genesis, *J Pathol* 129:139, 1979.
220. Weidner N, Zekan P: Carcinosarcoma of the colon: report of a unique case, with light and immunohistochemical studies, *Cancer* 58:1126, 1986.
221. Ordóñez NG, Luna MA: Choriocarcinoma of the colon, *Am J Gastroenterol* 79:39, 1984.
222. Jewell LD, Barr R, McCaughey WTE et al: Clear-cell epithelial neoplasms of the large bowel, *Arch Pathol Lab Med* 112:197, 1988.
223. Comer TP, Bears OH, Dockerty MB: Primary squamous cell carcinoma and adenocanthoma of the colon, *Cancer* 28:1111, 1971.
224. Mill UE, Ilardl CF, Zuna R et al: A biologically active parathyroid hormone-like substance secreted by an adenosquamous carcinoma of the transverse colon, *Hum Pathol* 18:1287, 1987.
225. Strate RW, Richardson JD, Bannayan GA: Basosquamous (transitional cloacogenic) carcinoma of the sigmoid colon, *Hum Pathol* 13:497, 1982.

NEUROENDOCRINE CELL TUMORS

226. O'Briain DS, Dayal Y, DeLellis RA et al: Rectal carcinoids as tumors of hindgut endocrine cells: a morphological and immunohistochemical analysis, *Am J Surg Pathol* 6:131, 1982.
227. Watson PH, Alguacil-García A: Mixed crypt cell carcinoma: a clinicopathologic study of the so-called goblet cell carcinoid, *Virchows Arch A* 412:175, 1987.
228. Moyana TN, Qizilbash AH, Murphy F: Composite glandular-carcinoid tumor of the colon, *Am J Surg Pathol* 12:607, 1988.
229. Wick MR, Weatherby RP, Weiland L: Small cell neuroendocrine carcinoma of the colon and rectum, *Hum Pathol* 18:9, 1987.
230. Owen DA, Hwang WS, Thorlakson RH et al: Malignant carcinoid tumor complicating chronic ulcerative colitis, *Am J Clin Pathol* 76:333, 1981.
231. Yang K, Ulich T, Cheng L et al: The neuroendocrine products of intestinal carcinoids: an immunoperoxidase study of 35 carcinoid tumors stained for serotonin and eight polypeptide hormones, *Cancer* 51:1918, 1983.
232. Burke M, Shepherd N, Mann CV: Carcinoid tumors of the rectum and anus, *Br J Surg* 74:358, 1987.
233. Chejfec G, Capella C, Solcia E et al: Amphicrine cells, dysplasias and neoplasias, *Cancer* 56:2683-2690, 1985.
234. Gledhill A, Hall PA, Cruse JP et al: Enteroendocrine cell hyperplasia, carcinoid tumors and adenocarcinoma in long-standing ulcerative colitis, *Histopathology* 10:501, 1986.

LYMPHOID HYPERPLASIA AND LYMPHOMA

235. Cornes JS, Wallace H, Morson BC: Benign lymphomas of the rectum and anal canal, *J Pathol Bacteriol* 82:371, 1961.
236. Ajdukiewicz AB, Youngs GR, Bouchier IA: Nodular lymphoid hyperplasia with hypogammaglobulinemia, *Gut* 13:589, 1972.
237. Robinson MJ, Padron S, Rywlin AM: Enterocolitis lymphofollicularis; morphologic, pathologic and serum immunoglobulin patterns, *Arch Pathol* 96:311, 1973.
238. Shepherd NA, Hall PA, Coates PJ et al: Primary malignant lymphoma of the colon and rectum: a histopathological and immunohistochemical analysis of 45 cases with clinicopathological correlations, *Histopathology* 12:235, 1988.
239. Levine AM, Gill PS, Muggia F: Malignancies in the acquired immunodeficiency syndrome, *Curr Probl Cancer* 11:209, 1987.
240. Hanto DW, Frizzera G, Purtillo DT et al: Clinical spectrum of lymphoproliferative disorders in renal transplant recipients and evidence for the role of Epstein-Barr virus, *Cancer Res* 41:4253, 1981.
241. Greenstein AJ, Mullin GE, Strauchen JA et al: Lymphoma in inflammatory bowel disease, *Cancer* 69:1119, 1992.

BENIGN AND MALIGNANT STROMAL TUMORS

242. Walsh TH, Mann CV: Smooth muscle neoplasms of the rectum and anal canal, *Br J Surg* 71:597, 1984.
243. Akwari DE, Dozois RR, Weiland LH et al: Leiomyosarcoma of the small and large bowel, *Cancer* 42:1375, 1978.
244. Carney JA, Go VL, Sizemore GW et al: Alimentary tract ganglioneuromatosis, *N Engl J Med* 295:1287, 1976.
245. Michowitz M, Lazebnik N, Noy S et al: Lipoma of the colon: a report of 22 cases, *Am Surg* 51:449, 1985.
246. Boquist L, Bargdahl L, Andersson A: Lipomatosis of the ileocecal valve, *Cancer* 29:136, 1972.
247. Johnstone JM, Morson BC: Inflammatory fibroid polyp of the gastrointestinal tract, *Histopathology* 2:349, 1978.
248. Baratz M, Ostrzega N, Michowitz M et al: Primary inflammatory malignant fibrous histiocytoma of the colon, *Dis Colon Rectum* 29:462, 1986.

Anus

249. Fenger C: Anal canal. In Sternberg SS, editor: *Histology for pathologists*, New York, 1992, Raven Press.
250. Thomson WH: The nature of hemorrhoids, *Br J Surg* 62:542, 1975.
251. Parks AG, Gordon PH, Hardcastle JD: A classification of fistula-in-ano, *Br J Surg* 63:1, 1976.
252. Lockhart-Mummery HE: Anal lesions in Crohn's disease, *Br J Surg* 72:595, 1985.
253. Lieberman D: Common anorectal disorders, *Ann Intern Med* 101:837, 1984.
254. Ferenczy A, Mitae M, Nagai N et al: Latent papilloma virus and recurring genital warts, *N Engl J Med* 313:784, 1985.
255. Cowgill R, Quan S: Colonic actinomycosis mimicking carcinoma, *Dis Colon Rectum* 12:45, 1979.
256. Udagawa SM, Portin BA, Bernhoft WH: Actinomycosis of the colon and rectum: report of two cases, *Dis Colon Rectum* 17:687, 1974.
257. Marfing TE, Abel ME, Gallagher DM: Perianal Bowen's disease and associated malignancies: results of a survey, *Dis Colon Rectum* 30:782, 1987.
258. Frazer IH, Medley G, Crapper RM et al: Association between ano-rectal dysplasia, human papilloma virus and human immunodeficiency virus in homosexual men, *Lancet* 2:657, 1986.
259. Greenall MJ, Quan SH, Stearns MW et al: Epidermoid cancer of the anal margin: pathologic features, treatment and clinical results, *Am J Surg* 149:95, 1985.
260. Boman B, Moertel CG, O'Connell MJ, et al: Carcinoma of the anal canal: a clinical and pathological study of 188 cases, *Cancer* 54:114, 1984.
261. Papillon J, Montbaron JT: Epidermoid carcinoma of the anal canal: a series of 276 cases, *Dis Colon Rectum* 30:324, 1987.
262. Bogomoletz WV, Potet F, Molas G: Condylomata acuminata, giant condyloma acuminatum (Bushke-Loewenstein tumour) and verrucous squamous carcinoma of the perianal and anorectal region: a continuous precancerous spectrum? *Histopathology* 9:155, 1985.
263. Jensen SL, Shokouh-Amiri MH, Hagen K et al: Adenocarcinoma of the anal ducts: a series of 21 cases, *Dis Colon Rectum* 31:268, 1988.
264. Prioleau PG, Allen MS, Roberts T: Perianal mucinous adenocarcinoma, *Cancer* 39:1295, 1977.
265. Berg JW, Love F, Stearns MW: Mucoepidermoid anal cancer, *Cancer* 13:914, 1960.
266. Cooper PH, Mills SE, Allen MS: Malignant melanoma of the anus: report of 12 patients and analysis of 255 additional cases, *Dis Colon Rectum* 25:693, 1982.
267. Weinstock MA: Epidemiology and prognosis of anorectal melanoma, *Gastroenterology* 104:174, 1993.
268. Beck DE, Fazio VW: Perianal Paget's disease, *Dis Colon Rectum* 30:263, 1987.

57 Liver

Kamal G. Ishak
Rodney S. Markin

NORMAL LIVER

Embryology

During the third to fourth week of gestation, the liver arises as a hepatic diverticulum from the endodermal lining of the foregut.[1] The hepatic diverticulum differentiates in a cranial direction, proliferating into hepatic cords. Proliferation in a caudal direction forms the gallbladder and extrahepatic biliary tree. The cords of hepatic epithelial cells then grow into the mesenchyme of the septum transversum. During development of the hepatic cords, they become intertwined with the growing capillary plexus arising from the vitelline veins that form the primitive hepatic sinusoids.

Mesenchymal cells from the septum transversum also become interposed between the sinusoids and the hepatic cords and form the connective tissue elements and capsule. Rudimentary bile canaliculi are apparent at 5 to 7 weeks of gestation (10 mm in length).

The intrahepatic bile ducts arise from the proximal segment of the primitive hepatic cords. This process is linked to the matching of the portal vein and its surrounding mesenchyme. The first layer of epithelial cells that come into contact with the portal vein are transformed into cells that become the epithelial cells of the bile ducts. The differentiation of the intrahepatic ducts is recognized in embryos at 8 to 10 weeks of gestational age (23 to 30 mm in length). Although the hepatocytes and bile duct epithelium arise from the same cell lineage, they are both structurally and functionally distinct without any detectable intermediate forms.

Anatomy

The adult liver weighs approximately 1500 g and represents approximately 1/50 of the adult human body weight. In the newborn, the liver has a much greater percentage of the total body weight (approximately 5%) that is related to its function, including extramedullary hematopoiesis,[2,3] than that of the adult.

The liver is located in the right upper quadrant and is partially protected by the rib cage. It is wedge shaped with the adult organ measuring approximately 10 by 15 by 20 cm in greatest dimensions.

The topography of the liver is commonly used to describe its gross features. The relationship between topography and the functional subsegments is not linear. The liver is divided into two large lobes—the right and the left—and two smaller lobes—the caudate and the quadrate. The superior, anterior, and lateral surfaces of the liver are covered by peritoneum except for a small area on the dome of the liver called the "bare area." This bare area represents the attachment of the liver to the diaphragm. The posterior surface of the liver also contains a "bare area" through which the inferior vena cava passes. The gallbladder fossa is located below the right lobe separating the quadrate lobe from the left and right lobes.

The functional topology of the liver is described by segments and subsegments. Specimens received from resections will be divided not along the topologic landmarks of the liver, but along the segmental or subsegmental landmarks based upon arterial and portal blood supply and bile drainage.

Histology

The hexagonal lobule has served as the microscopic unit of the liver for many decades. The classical lobule has an efferent (central) vein from which the hepatic plates radiate outward toward the portal areas; some three to six of these portal areas are located at the periphery of the lobule. The central veins vary in size and are lined by endothelial cells surrounded by a ring of collagen fibers. The large veins and sublobular veins contain some smooth muscles and thin wavy elastic fibers. The hepatocytes (liver cells) form plates ("cellae murales") one cell thick (except in young children in whom two–cell thick plates may be seen), which are surrounded on two sides by sinusoids. The layer of liver cells abutting the portal area is known as the *limiting plate*. It is separated from the portal area by a tissue space, the *space of Mall,* that probably serves as a lymphatic channel linking the spaces of Disse to the portal area lymphatics.

Hepatocytes are polygonal and have well-defined borders and an eosinophilic, finely granular cytoplasm. Prominent granularity is associated with an increase in the number of mitochondria. When present, ill-defined basophilic granules usually represent focal proliferation of the endoplasmic reticulum with ribosomes attached. Considerable amounts of glycogen and occasional fat vacuoles are present in the cytoplasm. A finely granular pigment, lipofuscin, with a golden brown color, is normally present in liver cells around the efferent veins, but little or no pigment is seen in the livers of children. Hepatocytic nuclei account for less than 7.3% of the liver cell volume.[4] Most liver cells contain one nucleus, but cells with two nuclei are not infrequently seen. Mitoses are exceptionally rare. The nuclei are round, have a fine chromatin pattern and one or more clearly defined amphophilic nucleoli. Glycogenated ("hydropic") nuclei may be a normal finding in periportal cells, particularly in children.

The normal liver should not contain any iron or copper demonstrable by special stains except during the first few weeks of life.[5] The newborn liver contains six to eight times the copper concentration of the adult liver. Concentrations fall to the adult value of about 30 μg/g of dry tissue within 6 months of birth.[6] Sinusoids are lined by endothelial and Kupffer cells, both of which have inconspicuous flattened nuclei and ill-defined cytoplasmic margins. The two cells cannot be distinguished by light microscopy unless the latter cell has phagocytosed pigment or other materials. An enormous body of literature has accumulated about the structure and function of Kupffer cells and other endothelial lining cells of the liver, including a monograph devoted to the topic and the published proceedings of several international symposia.[7-10]

The sinusoids contain blood cells and, in the neonate, hematopoietic elements. A space, the *space of Disse,* separates the surface of the hepatocyte facing the sinusoid from the endothelial lining cells. This space, which is not usually visualized in biopsy material, contains reticulin fibers, which can be stained as a continuous network by silver impregnation techniques. It also contains the perisinusoidal lipocytes or *Ito cells,* which are recognized only with difficulty in paraffin sections but are readily identified in thick sections of Epon-embedded material. Ito cells are elongated (5 to 10 μm in length), have relatively large nuclei, and generally contain fewer than six fat globules per cell. The fat globules store vitamin A, which is autofluorescent when sections are examined by ultraviolet microscopy. In addition to storing vitamin A, these cells play a pivotal role in hepatic fibrogenesis.[11] The Ito cells can be immunostained with antibodies to α-smooth muscle actin.[12] A recent review of the perisinusoidal lining cells is recommended for further reading.[13]

Bile canaliculi are located between adjacent hepatocytes and form a continuous network that drains bile into canals of Hering and then into the bile ducts in the portal areas. They are not easily seen in the normal liver but may appear as a tiny hole in the membranes separating two (or, less often, three) liver cells, or as short lengths of fine tubing. Bile canaliculi can be specifically stained by special stains,[14] by enzyme histochemical methods, such as those for alkaline phosphatase, adenosine diphosphatase, or adenosine triphosphatase,[15] or by an immunostain for polyclonal carcinoembryonic antigen (CEA).

The *canals of Hering* are difficult to identify in the normal liver. Several bile canaliculi generally drain into one canal, which traverses the space of Mall to empty into the intra-acinar (interlobular) bile ducts. Each canal of Hering is lined by low cuboidal to flattened cells, which, for part of its length, may alternate with small liver cells. The term "cholangiole," or "ductule" refers to the pathologic proliferation of small ducts around portal areas. They are probably of hepatocellular origin, since they are connected to the liver plates but end blindly at the other end.[16] The significance of ductular proliferation in diseases of the liver is reviewed recently by Burt and MacSween.[17]

The small bile ducts in portal areas have been referred to as "interlobular (intra-acinar) bile ducts," whereas large ones with an internal diameter greater than 100 μm have been termed "septal bile ducts."[18] They are lined by a single layer of cuboidal or mucin-secreting columnar cells respectively that rest on a basement membrane and some concentrically arranged collagenous fibers. The wall of the septal ducts may also contain smooth muscle and delicate elastic fibers.

The bile ducts in portal areas generally accompany an artery of approximately equal diameter. They are supplied by a rich arterial plexus of vessels, which can be demonstrated by the use of immunostains for laminin and collagen IV.

The portal areas are composed of collagenous connective tissue that surrounds the bile ducts described above, as well as arteries, branches of the portal vein, lymphatics, and autonomic nerve fibers. A few lymphocytes, macrophages, and mast cells may be normally present in portal areas.[19]

In histopathologic descriptions the classical lobule has for the most part been replaced by the hepatic *acinus*, or the functional liver unit related to the terminal branches of the afferent microcirculation.[2] The simple acinus is an irregular mass of parenchyma arranged around an axis consisting of a terminal hepatic arteriole, terminal portal venule, and bile duct. The simple liver acinus has three circulatory zones; the one nearest the portal area is called "zone 1." Cells in zone 1 receive blood with the highest amount of oxygen, insulin, glucagon, and various nutrients. The cells in zone 3 are the most vulnerable to damage from ischemia, anoxia, and nutritional deficiency because of their location.[2] The enzymatic specificity and metabolic heterogeneity of these zones also has implications for toxic liver injury. The complex acinus consists of at least three simple acini and a sleeve of parenchyma around the preterminal vessels and biliary branches. The largest microscopic acinar unit, the acinar agglomerate, consists of at least three complex acini.

For further information on the microanatomy of the liver, refer to the reviews of Rappaport and Wanless[2] and MacSween and Scothorne.[20] The normal ultrastructure of the liver, as revealed by transmission electron microscopy (TEM), is described in detail and illustrated lavishly in the atlas of Phillips and colleagues,[21] and the appearance of the liver by scanning electron microscopy (SEM) is covered in the monographs of Motta and colleagues[22] and Vonnahme.[23] A considerable body of information has accumulated regarding the cytoskeleton of the liver cell, stimulated largely by efforts to determine the pathogenesis and nature of Mallory bodies. Several recent reviews provide a wealth of information about the normal and abnormal cytoskeleton of the hepatocyte,[24-28] a subject that cannot be covered in this chapter because of the limitations of space.

EVALUATION OF LIVER DISEASES

Clinical manifestations

The liver supports many essential physiologic processes including the production of albumin and plasma proteins, regulation of postabsorptive glucose concentrations, low glucose concentrations, lipid synthesis, endogenous and exogenous detoxification, and other regulatory functions. In addition, the liver serves to buffer and detoxify components absorbed through the digestive tract, providing both regulatory and protective functions. The clinical manifestations of liver disease are highly variable. Clues that alert the clinician may be very subtle. A careful history and clinical evaluation may reveal changes of early hepatic encephalopathy such as increased fatigue, reversal of sleep pattern, or personality changes. The presence of prominent breast tissue and small testes in a male may represent undiagnosed cirrhosis. The identification of underlying liver disease may first be suspected by clinical laboratory values obtained during routine physical checkups, that is, elevated serum aminotransferases or alkaline phosphatase.

Specific symptoms such as fatigue, malaise, changes in sleep patterns or behavior, anorexia, fever, weight loss, and diminished libido may or may not be useful when attempting to evaluate the patient but may provide a starting point. Pruritus is an important symptom of cholestasis and is usually coupled with jaundice and skin excoriations. Jaundice, characterized by scleral icterus and yellow discolorization of the skin, is usually the first feature noticed by patients or their families. Right upper quadrant pain or discomfort could result from a rapidly enlarging liver with distention of the capsule; a variety of different diseases and disorders may cause this change. Other major presentations include ascites (gradual if the result of cirrhosis or sudden if related to the Budd-Chiari syndrome), upper or lower gastrointestinal bleeding (suggestive of portal hypertension from a variety of causes), or an upper abdominal mass caused by diffuse hepatomegaly or a mass lesion such as a benign or malignant tumor.

Important historical considerations include etiologic or predisposing factors. A working diagnosis of viral hepatitis should be considered when the patient had been exposed to persons known to have hepatitis, had received blood products or blood transfusions, or is an intravenous abuser of drugs. A large number of therapeutic drugs can also lead to a hepatitic or cholestatic liver injury. Populations of employees such as health professionals are subject to a variety of disorders that may be transmitted from the patient. Foreign travel and employment with livestock or other similar working conditions may be suggestive of a parasitic disease or Q fever. A family history of jaundice or liver disease may be suggestive of an inherited disorder such as α_1-antitrypsin deficiency, genetic hemochromatosis, or Wilson's disease.

Liver biopsy

The liver biopsy is an essential tool in the investigation of diseases of the liver. In experienced hands it is a safe procedure and can be performed on outpatients.[29-32] It is usually performed percutaneously, but a transjugular approach has also been employed successfully in patients with impaired coagulation or ascites.[33] The indications for liver biopsy are listed in Table 57-1.[31,32]

In addition to evaluating needle biopsy specimens, the surgical pathologist must render opinions on wedge biopsy specimens, lobectomy specimens obtained at laparotomy, and total hepatectomy specimens. For the study of medical diseases of the liver it is essential that the pathologist be informed of the patient's clinical condition, the results of laboratory tests, and radiographic studies. The correct diagnosis is likely to be arrived at when the pathologist and clinician work as a team. Adequate pathologic interpretation of liver diseases requires experience; however, the diagnosis of disease is partly dependent on the size of the biopsy specimen.

Clinical laboratory analyses

A variety of nonspecific and specific laboratory tests are used to evaluate the liver, its function, and tissue damage.[34] The metabolism of bilirubin and its conversion from indirect to direct by means of conjugation with sugar represents the liver's ability to conjugate bilirubin. Elevated bilirubin without an elevation of serum aminotransferases may be found in disorders such as Dubin-Johnson or Gilbert's disease. The decreased secretion of bilirubin through the biliary tract is usually associated with dysfunction of the liver. The term *cholestasis* is used to represent the impairment of secretion of bile and may occur at the cellular level. Cholestasis may be a harbinger of mechanical obstruction, hemolytic disease, or metabolic, drug, or viral disorders.

Serum aminotransferases, including aspartate aminotransferase (AST) and alanine aminotransferase (ALT), catalyze specific reactions to transfer amino groups. These enzymes are increased in liver injury and represent the leaking of injured or

Table 57-1 Indications for liver biopsy

Primary liver disease
Acute cholestasis (such as neonatal cholestasis, intrahepatic versus extrahepatic obstruction)
Chronic cholestasis (such as paucity of intraphepatic bile ducts, primary biliary cirrhosis, primary sclerosing cholangitis)
Disorders of bilirubin metabolism (such as Dubin-Johnson syndrome)
Developmental abnormalities (such as congenital hepatic fibrosis, polycystic disease)
Vascular disorders (such as venocclusive disease, hepatic vein thrombosis, hepatoportal sclerosis)
Inherited metabolic diseases (such as α_1-antitrypsin deficiency, Wilson's disease, genetic hemochromatosis, glycogenoses, hepatic porphyrias, tyrosinemia)
Chronic hepatitis
Drug-induced liver disease
Alcoholic liver disease
Cirrhosis (for presence or absence, degree of activity, cause)
Benign and malignant tumors and pseudotumors

Involvement of liver in diseases of other organs
Infectious diseases (such as viral infections, Q fever, tuberculosis, atypical mycobacterioses, brucellosis, leptospirosis, systemic mycoses, schistosomiasis, and other parasitic diseases)
Sarcoidosis
Investigation of fever of unknown origin
Diabetes mellitus
Differential diagnosis of liver disease in pregnancy (such as benign recurrent cholestasis, acute fatty liver of pregnancy, toxemia of pregnancy)
Nature of liver disease in inflammatory bowel diseases
Type of liver disease in rheumatoid and connective tissue disorders
Amyloidosis
Liver disease in hematopoietic disorders and staging of lymphomas
Metastases
Type of liver disease in patients after liver or bone marrow transplantation, especially development of acute rejection (and its grading) and chronic rejection

Patient management
Before initiation of medical or surgical therapy or before treatment of chronic hepatitis
For assessment of medical or surgical therapy
Assessment of long-term effects of severe hepatocellular injury, such as viral or drug-induced hepatitis
Baseline histopathologic description of transplanted liver for comparison with subsequent biopsy material for possible transplant rejection or other complications

lysed cells. Increases in AST and ALT usually reflect diseases primarily affecting the hepatocytes. ALT is much more specific for hepatobiliary disease when compared to AST. Aminotransferases are very valuable for monitoring the course of either acute or chronic parenchymal disease over time.

Alkaline phosphatase and gamma-glutamyl transpeptidase (GGT) are two enzymes that are associated with biliary tract disease. Serum levels of these enzymes are usually increased in cholestasis or bile duct obstruction. They may also be increased in parenchymal disease or infiltrative or mass lesions of the liver. Elevations of alkaline phosphatase, however, may represent disease from another organ system.

Albumin is synthesized exclusively in the liver. Its production is influenced by a variety of different conditions including systemic diseases, liver diseases, and suboptimal nutritional state. Hypoalbuminemia may be an important sign of liver disease. It may also be a useful indicator for monitoring hepatic function over a longer time (months to years).

Prothrombin time is one of the true liver function tests. It is dependent on the production of functional clotting factors from the liver. The synthesis is dependent on an adequate supply of vitamin K and should therefore be evaluated in that context. Prothrombin time measurements are utilized extensively in the early posttransplantation period for evaluating the function of the allograft.

A variety of assays for the detection of virally produced proteins, RNA and DNA, are currently available. The presence of virally produced proteins, RNA or DNA, may be suggestive of the underlying cause of a liver disease. The correlation between clinical laboratory values and the histologic findings are very important. A positive hepatitis C antibody test result, for example, does not indicate the presence of current hepatitis C viral (HCV) infection and should be carefully correlated with the biopsy results.

Gross appearance

A hand lens can be quite helpful during gross examination. A green color denotes cholestasis but does not help in distinguishing intrahepatic from extrahepatic cholestasis unless the specimen is large enough to reveal bile plugs in intra-acinar bile ducts, a feature favoring extrahepatic obstruction. Prominent portal areas or a white network of tissue usually denotes fibrosis. Dilated bile ducts may be seen in Caroli's disease, recurrent pyogenic cholangitis, and intrahepatic lithiasis and may contain biliary sludge or bilirubin calculi. Their wall may be thickened by chronic inflammation and fibrosis. The small (1 or 2 mm) or large nodules of a cirrhotic liver, surrounded by fibrous tissue septa, are usually readily recognized grossly. Large cirrhotic nodules (greater than 10 mm in diameter) are termed *macroregenerative nodules*. Nodular lesions with ill-defined or infiltrative margins are suggestive of carcinoma, as are large tumor masses. Invasion of portal vein branches or bile ducts may be visible grossly. Nodular regenerative hyperplasia (nodular transformation) differs from cirrhosis by the absence of fibrous septa between the nodules. Steatosis, whether in an architecturally normal or in a cirrhotic liver, gives the specimen a yellow color and imparts a greasy sensation to the examining fingers; when this change is extensive, a section may float in the fixative. Excessive iron accumulation, as in genetic hemochromatosis, imparts a rusty brown color to the liver. A diffuse slate gray color is seen in malaria or the Dubin-Johnson syndrome, whereas a patchy black color might be evident in metastases of malignant melanoma. Light tan to white foci or nodules can indicate involvement by lymphoma or carcinoma.

Solitary cysts are usually unilocular; multilocular cysts with a smooth lining are biliary cystadenomas. Roughened areas or papillary growths within the locules should raise the suspicion of malignancy. Multiple cysts of varied size that contain clear fluid are suggestive of autosomal dominant polycystic kidney disease. Echinococcal cysts are thick walled and can be calcified. They may contain brood capsules and translucent daughter cysts, or semisolid grumous material. Amebic abscesses have a shaggy lining and contain chocolate-colored material, unless there is secondary bacterial infection when the contents may be purulent. Pyogenic abscesses typically contain yellow or greenish pus, which can be odorless or foul smelling, depending on the causative organism.

Varying sized cavities containing liquid or clotted blood may be seen in peliosis hepatis and angiosarcoma; in the latter tumor, however, there is often firm, gray-white tumor tissue between the cavities. Thrombi, recent or old, may be noted grossly in intrahepatic veins in hepatic vein thrombosis. A nutmeg pattern of severe congestion may be seen in that condition, in venocclusive disease, and in congestive heart failure.

The benign and malignant tumors often have characteristic gross morphologic features, which are discussed in the section on tumors.

Methodology for histopathologic evaluation

Surgical material from the liver includes needle biopsy specimens (usually obtained percutaneously but sometimes at laparoscopy, by a transjugular approach, or during laparotomy), wedge biopsy specimens, lobectomy specimens, or, in centers where transplantation is performed, total hepatectomy specimens. The methodology for evaluation of autopsy material is similar to that for surgical specimens.

Frozen sections are rarely used for rapid histologic diagnosis except when open wedge biopsy specimens are available and then only to allow one to diagnose the nature of a tumor or other space-occupying lesion or to determine the suitability of a donor organ before transplantation. Frozen sections of formalin-fixed biopsy material stained with oil red O are useful for demonstration of neutral lipid in liver cells in a variety of conditions or in cells of benign or malignant tumors, fat globules of Ito cells, cholesterol crystals (which are also birefringent when examined under polarized light), and lipofuscin in liver or Kupffer cells. Cholesterol can be specifically stained in frozen sections by the Schultz modification of the Liebermann-Burchardt reaction, a stain useful for the diagnosis of Wolman's disease or cholesteryl ester storage disease. Baker's acid hematin with pyridine extraction is useful in identifying phospholipid in frozen sections, as in Niemann-Pick disease. Metachromatic granules in macrophage cells and bile duct epithelium in metachromatic leukodystrophy are best demonstrated in frozen sections by the use of stains such as cresyl violet or toluidine blue.

Some immunohistochemical stains can only be performed or are best evaluated in cryostat sections fixed in acetone.

Fixation and sectioning. The preferred fixative for routine processing for light microscopy is 10% neutral formalin. The preferred fixative for electron microscopy is 2.5% glutaraldehyde. Special fixatives are required in the evaluation of certain metabolic diseases in which the "storage" product is water soluble. Tissue from patients with mucopolysaccharidoses should be fixed in Lindsay's dioxane picrate solution[35] whereas that from patients with cystinosis is best fixed in alcohol. After routine processing, several sections should be cut at 4 to 5 μm and stained with hematoxylin and eosin (H&E). Serial sections are rarely necessary, but focal lesions such as granulomas, parasitic eggs, or larvae can be searched for in such sections if the clinical findings are strongly suggestive of their presence.

Most pathologists continue to evaluate sections of paraffin-embedded material. There has been increasing use of "thick" sections (actually thin sections 1 to 2 μm in thickness) made from biopsy material embedded in water-soluble resins.[36,37] These provide excellent cytologic detail and can be used for special stains and for immunohistochemistry.

Histochemistry. For the methodology of most of the stains cited, refer to the book *Laboratory Methods in Histotechnology* of the Armed Forces Institute of Pathology.[38] A preparation stained for iron (such as Mallory's stain for iron) is useful not only for demonstrating that metal but also for enhancing the green color of bile and the golden brown color of lipofuscin, both of which can be masked by overstaining with either eosin or hematoxylin. A reticulin stain (such as Wilder's or Manuel's stain) is useful for outlining areas of focal or zonal necrosis, thick liver cell plates, nodules of regeneration, septa linking portal areas to one another or to terminal hepatic venules, or septa partly or completely surrounding cirrhotic nodules. The Masson trichrome stain is very useful for demonstrating the location and extent of fibrosis and in assessment of changes involving veins or arteries, such as the lesions of venocclusive disease and hepatic vein thrombosis. The Movat or Musto pentachrome stains are particularly useful for vascular lesions, since they stain elastica and acid mucopolysaccharide, in addition to collagen and smooth muscle. Elastic tissue can also be demonstrated clearly by orcein, Victoria blue, or aldehyde fuchsin; any of the three stains can be used for identification of the hepatitis B surface antigen (HBsAg) in liver cells.[39] These stains also identify copper-binding protein (metallothionein),[40,41] but copper is best demonstrated specifically by the rubeanic or rhodanine stains.[42,43]

A periodic acid–Schiff (PAS) stain demonstrates glycogen; a much more useful stain that should be employed routinely is the PAS stain after pretreatment with diastase (PAS-D). The PAS-D stain strikingly demonstrates the presence of lipofuscin (and cell debris) in Kupffer cells and portal macrophages in acute hepatocellular injury. Dubin-Johnson pigment in liver cells stains variably with PAS-D. In both type IV glycogenosis and Lafora's disease (myoclonus epilepsy), liver cells contain PAS-positive inclusions that resist diastase digestion but can be digested by pectinase.[44] This appearance is also mimicked by cyanamide-induced hepatotoxicity. The globules of α_1-antitrypsin are strongly PAS positive and diastase resistant; they are of variable size (1 to 40 μm) and, in the precirrhotic liver, are located largely in periportal hepatocytes. Their identity should, however, be confirmed by an immunohistochemical method. The PAS stain is also useful for staining the basement membrane of intraacinar bile ducts. Basement membrane changes include destruction in primary biliary cirrhosis (PBC) or thickening in primary sclerosing cholangitis (PSC). Other uses for the PAS stain include the demonstration of fibrin (as in eclampsia or disseminated intravascular coagulopathy), amyloid, starch, amebas, and pathogenic fungi, though the last are more readily identified by the Gomori methenamine silver stain. The small cytoplasmic inclusions of cytomegalovirus infection are well demonstrated by the PAS-D stain.

Other stains that find occasional use in the study of hepatic biopsy material include the osmium tetroxide method for fat droplets;[45] the Hall stain for bile; the Fontana stain for lipofuscin and Dubin-Johnson pigment; the phosphotungstic acid–hematoxylin stain for fibrin or mitochondria; the ferric ferricyanide stain for uroporphyrin crystals;[46] an acid-fast stain for tubercle bacilli, schistosome eggs, or the hooklets in the scoleces of echinococcal cysts; a Warthin-Starry stain for spirochetes, leptospira, *Rochalimaea henselae* (the organism responsible for cat-scratch disease and bacillary peliosis in patients with AIDS); a Giemsa stain for *Toxoplasma* or *Leishmania* or for staining eosinophils and mast cells; and a Brown-Hopps stain for bacteria. An acid-phosphatase stain is useful for staining Gaucher cells and cells of hairy cell leukemia. Amyloid can be stained with Congo red and Sirius red, revealing green birefringence. Amyloid AA positivity is abolished by pretreatment with potassium permanganate in contrast to amyloid AL, which is permanganate resistant.[47] Amyloid, regardless of type, is metachromatic when stained with crystal violet or methyl violet.

Argyrophilic nucleolar organizer regions have been studied in a variety of neoplastic and medical diseases of the liver.[48,49] In one study, adenomatous hyperplasia could be distinguished from adenomatous hyperplasia with atypia or focal malignancy.[49] In another study, the quantitation of nucleolar organizer regions was found helpful in grading hepatocellular carcinoma.[48]

Immunohistochemistry (Table 57-2). Immunostains are now routinely utilized in the diagnosis of hepatic neoplasms; however, fewer applications have emerged in the study of medical diseases of the liver. With reference to the normal liver, antibodies to polyclonal cytokeratin, epithelial membrane antigen, and CEA stain bile ductal and ductular cells but not hepatocytes. Bile canaliculi are also stained by antibodies to polyclonal CEA. Bile ductal cells are reactive with monoclonal anticytokeratins 7, 8, 18, and 19, whereas liver cells are reactive with monoclonal antibodies to cytokeratins 8 and 18.[50]

Two pooled monoclonal antibodies to cytokeratins, have been used by Ray[51] to immunostain Mallory bodies. In our experience, a more reliable method is immunostaining for ubiquitin, a heat-shock protein that binds to Mallory bodies.[52] Continuous deposits of IgA along hepatic sinusoids have been regarded as a distinctive feature of alcoholic liver disease by some investigators but have been deemed nonspecific by others.[53] Several immunostains can identify the mesenchymal components of the normal liver, but few (nonneoplastic) diagnostic applications have emerged. Thus, factor VIII–related antigen can be identified in endothelial cells of arteries and veins but not these lining sinusoids. Cells of epithelioid hemangioendothelioma produce large quantities of factor VIII–related antigen.[54-57] Recently reported monoclonal antibodies to CD34 antigen (QB-END/10) of endothelium has been found useful in diagnosis of benign and malignant vascular tumors.[55-57] Lysozyme expression is characteristic of Kupffer cells. Desmin is demonstrable in perisinusoidal lipocytes (Ito cells), at least in the rat liver.[58,59] Burt and MacSween[60] have identified desmin-containing (stellate) cells in portal areas and have concluded that this intermediate filament protein is a useful stain for myofibroblasts within acini and in portal areas. Ito cells also synthesize and secrete fibronectin.[61] In our experience, an immunohistochemical stain for smooth muscle actin is superior for demonstrating myofibroblasts. Increased amounts of fibronectin have been identified in the livers of chronic alcoholics.[62] The deposition of fibronectin does not appear to be related to steatosis or steatonecrosis but is considered to be of significance in the early development of hepatic fibrosis in the alcoholic.[62]

Smooth muscle cells in portal area arteries and veins react with antibodies to muscle-specific actin. Laminin and type IV collagen are present in the basement membrane of bile ducts and vessels in portal areas. Collagen types I and V are found in the connective tissue of portal area and around terminal hepatic venules, and type III collagen (*reticulin* fibers) is present in spaces of Disse. Nerve fibers in the portal area can be immunostained with antibodies to S-100 and neurofibrillary protein. Different types of amyloid can now be characterized by commercially available antisera.[63,64] Looi and Sumithran[64] showed that AA ("secondary") amyloid was limited to the walls of vessels in the portal areas, whereas AL ("primary") amyloid characteristically had a sinusoidal pattern, though it was also found in vessel walls. The rare globular form of amyloid[65,66] consists of AA amyloid.[67] Nonamyloid light chain deposits resembling amyloid (but not staining with Congo red) in spaces of Disse have been reported by Lindner and associates.[68] These investigators identified kappa light chain immunoglobulin in the deposits by an immunofluorescent technique. Amyloid-like deposits of β_2-microglobulin are also Congo red positive but are not birefringent, as reported recently in a patient with end-stage renal disease who had been receiving hemodialysis for 2 years.[69]

The aberrant expression of class I and class II HLA has been studied in viral hepatitis, PBC, hepatic neoplasms, and allograft rejection. Space does not permit discussion of this important topic; refer to other sources for additional information.[70-74]

Immunostaining for viral antigens in the different types of viral hepatitis has been used for investigational purposes and, to a lesser extent, for diagnosis. Antisera to hepatitis A are currently not commercially available for immunohistochemistry. Delta virus antigen has been identified in nuclei of liver cells in both acute and chronic infections by several investigators.[75-78] Its tissue identification has proved especially useful in retrospective studies of endemic and epidemic delta virus infections[77] where sera were not available for testing for antibodies to the virus.

Antisera to HBsAg and hepatitis B core antigen (HBcAg) are commercially available; false-positive staining has been reported with some antisera.[79] Staining for these two antigens

Table 57-2 Immunohistochemistry: hepatic applications (excluding hematopoietic malignancies)

Tissue antigen	Application
Blood group antigen	Hemangioendothelioma; angiosarcoma, cholangiocarcinoma
Factor VIII–related antigen	Hemangioma; epithelioid hemangioendothelioma; angiosarcoma
Ulex europeus	Benign vascular tumors; angiosarcoma
CD34	Hemangioma; epithelioid hemangioendothelioma
Myoglobin	Embryonal rhabdomyosarcoma of bile ducts
Desmin	Rhabdomyosarcoma; leiomyosarcoma; Ito cells
Vimentin	Tumors of mesenchymal origin, such as fibrosarcoma; endothelial cells
Smooth muscle cell actin	Myofibroblasts; smooth muscle cells; smooth muscle tumors
S-100 protein	Malignant melanoma, metastatic; neurogenic tumors; granular cell tumors of extrahepatic bile ducts
HMB 45	Malignant melanoma; angiomyolipoma
Lysozyme	Kupffer cells; ductal cells
Carcinoembryonic antigen, polyclonal	Cholangiocarcinoma; metastatic adenocarcinoma; normal and neoplastic bile canaliculi; ductal/ductular cells
Alpha-fetoprotein	Hepatocellular carcinoma; hepatoblastoma
α_1-antitrypsin	α_1-antitrypsin deficiency
Transferrin receptor	Hepatocellular carcinoma
Ferritin	Hepatocellular carcinoma; hepatoblastoma
Cytokeratin "cocktails"(such as AE1/AE3)	Cholangiocarcinoma; metastatic adenocarcinoma; ductal/ductular cells; ductular metaplasia
Ubiquitin	Mallory bodies
Epithelial membrane antigen	Cholangiocarcinoma; metastatic adenocarcinoma
Amyloid A	Secondary amyloidosis
Hepatitis C virus*	Chronic hepatitis C
HBsAg	Chronic hepatitis B infection
HBcAg	Chronic hepatitis B infection
Delta agent*	Chronic delta agent infection
Herpesvirus	Herpesvirus types 1 and 2
Cytomegalovirus (CMV)	CMV antigen in infected liver and ductal cells
Adenovirus	Adenovirus antigen in nuclei of infected hepatocytes

*Not commercially available in the United States.

is used mainly for the carrier state, chronic hepatitis, and cirrhosis associated with that virus infection. The immunostain for HBcAg is particularly useful, since that antigen (unlike HBsAg) cannot be stained histochemically. Only if the antigen is present in excess does it impart a "sanded" appearance to the affected liver cell nucleus in an H&E preparation.[80] Several patterns of expression of HBsAg and HBcAg have been recognized.[81,82] The expression of preS1 and preS2 closely follows that of HBsAg.[83-85] The preS1 proteins have not been found useful as markers of viral replication. There are several recent reports of the immunohistochemical detection of HCV antigens, both in fresh-frozen and formalin-fixed tissue, as discussed later.

Several viral antigens, other than those of viral hepatitis, can be detected in the liver by the use of commercially available antisera. They include HIV,[86,87] adenovirus, herpes simplex virus,[88] and cytomegalovirus (CMV). In the case of CMV in situ hybridization was found to be more sensitive than immunohistochemical staining in one study[89,90] but not in another.[91] The polymerase chain reaction (PCR) appears to be the most sensitive method for detection of CMV.[92]

Antigens of nonviral microorganisms are also increasingly being detected by immunohistochemical methods. Examples include leptospiral antigen[93] and the antigen of *Pneumocystis carinii*.[94]

Immunohistochemical studies have been performed in a variety of liver diseases in an attempt to characterize the inflammatory cell types. Several investigators have focused their attention on PBC.[95-97] In the study of Krams and colleagues[95] the predominant cell type in the mononuclear infiltrate in that disease was the $CD3^+$, $CD4^+$ T-lymphocyte bearing the T-cell receptor xB. Additionally, $CD20^+$ B-cells and Ig^+ cells were found in the lymphoid infiltrate, and immunoglobulin was detected on the surface of biliary epithelium. These investigators concluded that the mechanisms involved in the pathophysiology of PBC may include both T-cells and antibody mechanisms. Another immunohistochemical study of liver tissues of patients with PSC likewise found T-cells to be the major component (78%) of the mononuclear cells in portal areas.[98] In a comparative study of lymphocytes in PBC, autoimmune chronic hepatitis, and PSC, Hashimoto and colleagues[97] found that the infiltrates were similar in the first two diseases. However, natural killer cells were twice as common in PSC as in PBC. A study of acute viral hepatitis B or non-A, non-B revealed that the majority of inflammatory cells were cytotoxic/suppressor cells.[99] Cytotoxic T-cells were also identified in a liver biopsy specimen from an adult patient with rubella hepatitis.[100] Other studies of chronic hepatitis have demonstrated an increase of cytotoxic/suppressor over helper/inducer cells.[97,100-104] Overall, the aforementioned lymphocyte subpopulation studies have proven helpful in unraveling pathogenetic mechanisms in necroinflammatory and chronic cholestatic disorders but have had few diagnostic applications.

Special light microscopy techniques. Polarizing microscopy is useful in identifying talc in portal macrophages or Kupffer cells in abusers of intravenous drugs,[105] or talc, starch, or suture material on the surface of the liver from previous surgery. Silica particles in the liver are birefringent.[106,107] Both malarial and schistosomal pigments, which are brown to black, are birefringent under polarized light. Formalin pigment (which is also black and birefringent) is often needle shaped and generally seen in vascular lumens in relation to erythrocytes, in contrast to parasitic pigment, which is finely granular and accumulates in reticuloendothelial cells. Anthracotic pigment is black but not birefringent. It is, however, often associated with needle-shaped particles of silica, which are birefringent. Usually, both of these particulate materials are found in macrophages. Two metals that can accumulate in the liver, titanium and gold, appear as black granules, and have a pink to orange birefringence. Titanium is present in reticuloendothelial cells in the liver of intravenous drug abusers and may be admixed with talc particles.[108] Gold salts accumulate in lipogranulomas[109] or in reticuloendothelial cells of the liver of patients with rheumatoid arthritis. In frozen sections cholesterol crystals (in the livers of patients with Wolman's disease and cholesterol ester storage disease) are birefringent, as cystine crystals are in cystinosis. Acicular uroporphyrin crystals in liver cells can be visualized by polarizing microscopy of unstained frozen or paraffin sections in porphyria cutanea tarda.[110] Red birefringent Maltese crosses and amorphous material are characteristic of protoporphyrin accumulation in canaliculi or Kupffer cells in erythropoietic protoporphyria.[111] Collagen (type I collagen), as opposed to reticulin fibers (type III collagen), has a silvery birefringence under polarized light. Amyloid has a characteristic apple green birefringence when sections stained with Congo red are examined by polarizing microscopy.

Ultraviolet (UV) microscopy is useful in studying the hepatic porphyrias. Unfixed, air-dried frozen sections of the liver in porphyria cutanea tarda and erythropoietic protophorphyria reveal red autofluorescence when examined by UV microscopy. Vitamin A that is stored in perisinusoidal lipocytes has a green and rapidly fading autofluorescence in UV radiation.

A granular yellow-green autofluorescence is characteristic of lipofuscin examined by UV microscopy. UV microscopy has been used in identifying various antigens in the liver such as α_1-antitrypsin, HBsAg and HBcAg, HCV antigens, and several oncofetal proteins in primary benign and malignant tumors.

Phase contrast microscopy is of limited value in studying medical diseases of the liver. It has been utilized in visualizing Thorotrast in Kupffer cells[112] and silicone particles in portal macrophages of hemodialysis patients.[113]

Scanning electron microscopy. Scanning electron microscopy (SEM) has many investigational but only a limited number of diagnostic applications. This is related to the cost of the equipment that is generally not available except in large academic centers and to lack of experience. Several atlases have dealt with the normal structure of the liver.[22,23] Reviews dealing with the normal or diseased liver have also appeared.[114,115] The diagnostic applications of this technique are largely limited to particulate material. This is especially so when energy-dispersive x-ray microanalysis is combined with SEM.[115] Examples include the identification of Thorotrast, silicone, silica, talc, titanium, gold, and barium sulfate.

Transmission electron microscopy. Several atlases of transmission electron microscopy (TEM) are available.[21,116,117] The most recent and by far the most comprehensive is that of Phillips and colleagues.[21] These investigators and others[117,118] have clearly demonstrated the value of electron microscopy in the interpretation of biopsy specimens from patients with known or suspected metabolic disorders, as well as drug-induced and cholestatic diseases. Among the metabolic diseases, distinctive or pathognomonic ultrastructural findings are present in hereditary fructose intolerance, α_1-antitrypsin deficiency, erythropoietic protoporphyria, Farber's disease, glycogenoses types II and IV, Gaucher's disease, metachromatic leukodystrophy, Dubin-Johnson syndrome, Wilson's disease, Zellweger's syndrome, and many others.

Drug-induced injury causes changes in many organelles of the liver depending on the type of drug, duration of use, and other factors. Many drugs (such as phenytoin, phenobarbital) and toxins (such as DDT and other pesticides) lead to proliferation of the smooth endoplasmic reticulum of liver cells ("induced" hepatocytes), which results in a characteristic ground-glass appearance by light microscopy. Megamitochondria, sometimes assuming monstrous forms, are considered typical of drug reactions.[21] Lysosomal phospholipidosis is highly typical of several drugs. The drugs amiodarone, perhexilene maleate, and $4,4^1$-diethylaminoethoxyhexestrol have been implicated in this change.[119-123] By light microscopy, phospholipidosis results in a foamy transformation of Kupffer cells and hepatocytes that resembles the changes in Niemann-Pick disease. Ultrastructurally the affected cells contain electron-dense, laminated lysosomal inclusions.

Viral particles are often readily identified ultrastructurally in liver cell nuclei and cytoplasm, even in autolyzed postmortem specimens. Examples include herpes simplex viruses, adenovirus, HBcAg, HBsAg, and even the complete hepatitis B virion (Dane particle).

Morphometry and flow cytometry have only limited diagnostic applications in diseases of the liver.

Molecular biology techniques. In situ DNA hybridization has been utilized successfully in detection of many infectious agents such as viruses, bacteria, and parasites. Applications of in situ hybridization in viral hepatitis have been reviewed recently by Negro and colleagues,[124] whereas applications of PCR in the study of viral infections of the liver were reviewed by Brechot.[125] Most of the molecular biologic studies have involved hepatitis B virus (HBV) DNA, but several recent reports have used PCR for detection of HCV DNA in liver tissue from patients with chronic hepatitis, cirrhosis, or hepatocellular carcinoma associated with HCV.[126-128]

The general diagnostic and prognostic applications of oncogenes in surgical pathology have been reviewed by Bartow.[129] Oncogene expression in liver regeneration and hepatocarcinogenesis has been reviewed by Fausto and Shank[130,131] and Gulbis.[132] The expression of eight cellular oncogenes in various liver diseases and in normal subjects was studied by Himeno and colleagues.[133] No significant differences in mRNA levels of c-*fos*, N-*myc*, N-*ras*, Ha-*ras*, c-*erb*-B, and c-*abl* were found among patients with hepatocellular carcinoma, cirrhosis, chronic hepatitis, or normal subjects. Increased c-*myc* expression was noted in patients with cirrhosis and hepatocellular carcinoma. The sustained activation of the c-*myc* genes in cirrhotic hepatocytes is believed to contribute to the development of hepatocellular carcinoma.[133] In a recent study Boix and colleagues[134] found overexpression of c-*met* mRNA in almost half of the hepatocellular carcinoma they studied, but the biologic relevance of that finding is not known.

Systematic histopathologic evaluation

Evaluation of diseases affecting the liver, whether intrinsic or secondary, requires a careful and methodical approach.[135-137] At the light microscopic level, sections stained with H&E are evaluated first, followed by the study of appropriate special stains. All fragments of a needle-biopsy specimen should be scanned at low-power magnification so that focal lesions, which may be present only in one fragment, are not missed. At low-power magnification, architectural distortion (as by fibrosis, cirrhosis, nodular transformation) or various "space-occupying" lesions may be readily identified. If none are visualized, the medium-power and high-power magnifications are then used. Since many (particularly acute) lesions involve zone 3, it is better to identify terminal hepatic venules (THVs) and then to proceed "centrifugally" to the portal areas. The THVs themselves should first be scrutinized for lesions (such as endotheliitis, phlebosclerosis, venoocclusive changes, thrombi), after which the various "systems" should be carefully and methodically evaluated in zone 3, followed by zones 2 and 1. The evaluation should include hepatocytes (such as ballooning with or without necrosis with dropping-out of cells, acidophilic bodies, coagulative degeneration, Mallory bodies, megamitochondria, steatosis), bile canaliculi (manifested by presence of deposits of protoporphyrin, bile plugs, dilatation with pseudogland formation), sinusoidal contents and lining cells, Kupffer cells, perisinusoidal lipocytes, and abnormalities in the spaces of Disse (such as fibrosis, amyloid deposits).

After examination of the various systems within the acinus, the morphologist should turn his or her attention to the limiting plates and the portal areas. The periportal region should be carefully inspected for hemosiderin accumulation, glycogenated nuclei, storage material (such as eosinophilic globules of α_1-antitrypsin, elongated megamitochondria, Lafora bodies) and for evidence of acute necrosis (such as hepatitis A, eclampsia, or toxic injury by phosphorus) or lymphocytic piecemeal necrosis (as in chronic hepatitis). Periportal fibrosis may accompany chronic necroinflammatory disease, chronic diseases of the biliary tract (whether extrahepatic or intrahepatic), and a variety of other conditions, and the portal areas may be linked together or to THVs, depending on the cause. Chronic cholestasis (as in PBC, PSC, prolonged extrahepatic biliary obstruction) leads to several changes involving periportal liver cells; these include bile pigmentation, pseudoxanthomatous transformation, copper storage, and Mallory body formation. Regeneration is characterized by two-cell-thick liver plates around portal areas. Ductular (cholangiolar) proliferation (with or without neutrophilic infiltration and bile plugging) can occur in a variety of circumstances and must be assessed in light of all other changes affecting that particular liver.

Changes in the portal area connective tissue (such as edema, focal scars) should be evaluated next, together with the types and distribution of inflammatory cells; the relative frequency of the various cell types should be noted. Lymphomas typically infiltrate portal areas and their contents (such as vessels, bile ducts) but often extend beyond them to destroy adjacent parenchyma. Granulomas are frequently located in portal or periportal areas. Hypertrophied portal macrophages should be searched for and their contents identified; such cells may contain pigments (such as hemosiderin, anthracotic pigment, malarial or schistosomal pigment, lipofuscin), extraneous particulate matter (such as talc, silica, Thorotrast, silicone, gold, titanium), mineral oil (with or without formation of lipogranulomas), and metabolites in several of the inherited metabolic diseases.

A variety of lesions may affect intra-acinar bile ducts; they may be acute (such as suppurative cholangitis, dilatation, presence of bile plugs in the lumen) or chronic (such as nonsuppurative destructive cholangitis or periductal sclerosis). Acute changes may be superimposed on chronic lesions. On the other hand, recognizing the absence of bile ducts (ductopenia) in portal areas of crucial importance in the diagnosis of chronic cholestatic disorders (as in arteriohepatic dysplasia, PSC, or PBC in adults).

The vessels in portal areas always need careful assessment. Thus, portal vein branches may reveal phlebosclerosis, pylephlebitis, or pylethrombosis (recent or old) or may contain tumor emboli. They are also frequently infiltrated by malignant cells of primary vascular tumors of the liver, such as angiosarcoma and epithelioid hemangioendothelioma. Cases of hepatoportal sclerosis are characterized by paucity of small portal vein branches; elastic stains are useful in identifying the sclerosed vessels. Hepatic artery branches may be involved by an arteritis (periarteritis, giant cell arteritis, rejection arteriopathy), endothelial hyperplasia (as in cystathioninuria or in women taking oral contraceptives), amyloidosis, or atherosclerotic changes.

After systematic appraisal of all the various systems in sections stained with H&E, the special stains should be evaluated. Minimally, these should include a connective tissue stain (such as Masson trichrome), a PAS stain after diastase digestion, a stain for iron, and one of the "Shikata" stains (such as orcein). A stain for reticulin fibers is useful for confirming the presence of nodules in suspected nodular transformation, particularly in needle biopsy specimens. Additional special stains and techniques, including immunohistochemical stains and special microscopy, are utilized as needed. Needless to say, after all the histopathologic changes are evaluated, the morphologist should correlate them with the clinical, biochemical, and radiographic findings to arrive at the correct diagnosis.

ACUTE HEPATOCELLULAR INJURY

The expression of acute hepatocellular injury can vary from spotty to massive necrosis, and the underlying type of degeneration can also differ depending on the etiology, as shown in Table 57-3 and discussed in the succeeding paragraphs.

Ischemic necrosis (ischemic hepatitis)

Coagulative necrosis of zone 3 (which can extend to zone 2) may occur after shock,[138-141] left-sided heart failure,[142] or right-sided failure associated with hypotension.[143-145] Clinically the presentation may mimic viral hepatitis.[142,143] A recent study has shown that an early massive rise in lactate dehydrogenase, rapid fall in aminotransferase values, and early mild to moderate renal failure should be strongly suggestive of ischemic hepatitis.[145] Liver cells that have undergone coagulative necrosis are shrunken, have an intensely eosinophilic cytoplasm, and show nuclear pyknosis or lysis (Fig. 57-1). When an inflammatory response is present, it is invariably neutrophilic. Clearing of the dead hepatocytes leads to condensation of reticulin fibers and fibrosis in some cases. Kupffer cells are hypertrophied and contain lipofuscin in adult patients. Although the changes in ischemic hepatitis are highly characteristic, they are not pathognomonic, since they can be mimicked by acute acetaminophen hepatotoxicity.

Table 57-3 Acute necroinflammatory disease

Pattern of injury	Morphology of lesions	Etiologic examples
Spotty necrosis	Apoptosis with or without ballooning	Viral hepatitis B, C, A, rubella, rubeola, drug induced
	Apoptosis with or without ballooning with or without cholestasis and granulomas	Drug induced (such as phenylbutazone, phenytoin)
Spotty necrosis and sinusoidal lymphocytosis	Apoptosis with or without ballooning	Infectious mononucleosis, CMV mononucleosis, drug induced (such as phenytoin, dapsone)
Spotty/patchy necrosis	Coagulative necrosis	Hepatitis due to Rift Valley, Lassa, Ebola, Coxsackie, dengue viruses
Patchy and confluent necrosis	Coagulative necrosis	Herpes virus hepatitis, varicella-zoster hepatitis, adenovirus hepatitis
Submassive (zonal) necrosis		
Zone 3	Ballooning	Viral hepatitis B, drug induced (such as halothane, methyldopa, isoniazid), toxic (such as CCl_4 and steatosis)
	Ballooning and Mallory bodies with or without steatosis	Alcoholic hepatitis; pseudoalcoholic hepatitis
	Coagulative necrosis	Ischemic necrosis, drug induced (such as acetaminophen), toxic (such as mushroom toxicity)
Zone 2	Coagulative necrosis	Yellow fever hepatitis
Zone 1	Ballooning	Viral hepatitis A, infectious mononuclesis, drug induced (such as halothane), toxic (such as phosphorus poisoning)
	Ballooning and Mallory bodies	Amiodarone injury
	Coagulative necrosis	Toxic injury (such as $FeSO_4$ toxicity in children), adenovirus hepatitis
Massive necrosis	Ballooning	Viral hepatitis (B with or without D coinfection, hepatitis A, hepatitis C), drug induced (such as halothane, phenytoin)
	Coagulative necrosis	Ischemic necrosis, viral infections (such as echovirus hepatitis), drug induced (acetaminophen), toxic injury (such as mushroom toxicity)
Microvesicular steatosis, panacinar	Spotty necrosis	Alcohol, drug induced (such as tetracycline, valproate), toxic (such as Jamaican vomiting sickness), fatty liver of pregnancy

Acute viral hepatitis

Although "hepatitis" may be caused by several viruses, the term *viral hepatitis* is reserved for inflammation of the liver caused by the viruses of hepatitis A, hepatitis B, hepatitis D (delta), hepatitis C, and hepatitis E. Characteristics of these five hepatotropic viruses are listed in Table 57-4.

Hepatitis A virus (HAV) is an RNA virus belonging to the picornaviruses (enteroviruses). It is transmitted by the fecal-oral route and causes an acute self-limited disease. Fulminant hepatitis is a rare complication; the death rate in one series was 0.14%.[146] Although a protracted or relapsing course can occur, there is no chronic liver disease or carrier state.[147-149] Acute hepatitis A is diagnosed readily by serologic testing for IgM anti-HAV, an antibody that appears at the onset of the illness and persists for 6 to 12 months. IgG anti-HAV is a serologic marker for past infection with HAV.

HBV is a member of the hepadnaviruses. In the serum of infected patients three types of particles may be seen: *spheres* (20 nm in diameter) and *tubules* (20 nm in diameter and 100 nm in length), that represent excess surface antigen (HBsAg), and 42 nm *Dane particles,* which are the complete HBV virion. The Dane particle has a shell of surface antigen (HBsAg) and a core that consists of DNA, DNA polymerase, core antigen (HBcAg), and e antigen (HBeAg); HBeAg is probably part of the core. The HBV genome is a small, circular, partly double-stranded DNA molecule composed of about 3200 nucleotides; in infected hepatocytes it can exist in a freely replicating form or integrated into the host genome.[150] Mutations of HBV (precore, core, and surface mutants) have been reported.[151] The clinically relevant mutations are the precore ones; they are involved in the pathogenesis of fulminant hepatitis B, as well as in severe exacerbations of chronic hepatitis B.[152-155]

The diagnosis of hepatitis B is made when one finds HBsAg in the serum; it appears in the blood about 6 weeks after infection and usually disappears in 3 months. The carrier state is characterized by persistence of HBsAg for more than 6 months. There is considerable variation in the incidence of the carrier rate worldwide, as from 0.1% to 0.2% in the United States or United Kingdom to 10% to 15% in Africa and the Far East. The presence of IgM antibody to HBcAg (IgM anti-HBc) indicates acute infection with HBV. The serologic markers of acute and chronic hepatitis B are listed in Table 57-4. For additional information the review of Hoofnagle and Schaefer is recommended.[156]

Hepatitis B is mainly transmitted by whole blood or its products; it is acquired parenterally or by intimate (often sexual) contact. It leads to both acute and chronic liver disease; some 5% to 10% of adults and 30% to 100% of neonates and children infected with HBV develop hepatitis. In about 25% to 30% of patients chronic hepatitis B progresses to cirrhosis, and some of the patients eventually develop hepatocellular carcinoma.[157-161] Patients with chronic hepatitis B usually have high serum levels of HBsAg and HBV DNA. HBcAg

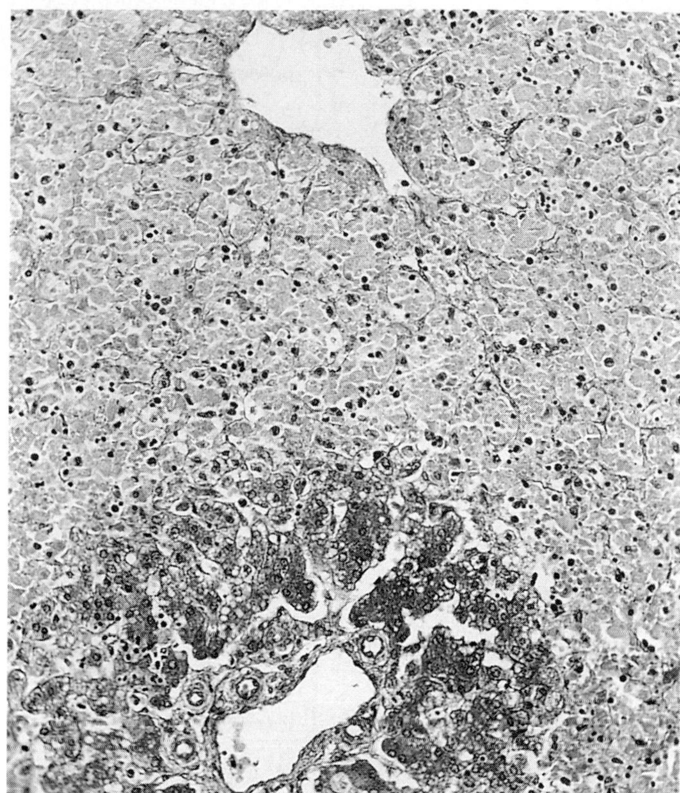

Fig. 57-1 Ischemic necrosis. Notice the collar of surviving hepatocytes (darkly stained) around a portal area.

and HBsAg are detectable in the liver by immunohistochemical methods. Hepatitis B can now be prevented by vaccination.

Hepatitis delta virus (HDV) is a defective RNA pathogen that is dependent for its replication on HBV. The virion (36 nm) is composed of the RNA genome and delta antigen enclosed in an HBsAg coat.[162] Since its discovery in 1977, HDV and the diseases it causes have generated a large body of literature, including the proceedings of two international symposia.[163-165] Infection with the virus is worldwide; the high prevalence areas include the Mediterranean basin, the Middle East, Africa, and the Amazon basin. In Western countries, including the United States,[163,166-170] the disease mainly affects persons with frequent blood contact (drug addicts, hemophiliacs, hemodialysis patients). Infections may be acute or chronic, the diagnosis being established by serologic tests for the presence or absence of anti-delta antibodies (IgG and IgM) and delta antigen.

HCV is a single-stranded RNA virus with a lipid envelope; it measures 50 to 60 nm in diameter. The diagnosis of hepatitis C is based on the detection of anti-HCV antibodies or the presence of HCV RNA in the serum. The epidemiology of parenterally transmitted HCV hepatitis is similar to that of hepatitis B. At present, 75% to 95% of posttransfusion hepatitis in the United States and other countries is caused by HCV.[171-174] A long-term follow-up study of posttransfusion non-A, non-B (NANB) hepatitis has failed to reveal an increased mortality, though there was a small but statistically significant increase in the number of deaths related to liver disease.[175]

Other than transfused patients, persons with coagulation disorders receiving factor VIII and other blood products, patients and staff of hemodialysis units, recipients of organ transplants, and drug addicts, are at risk for infection. There are four phenotypes of HCV in different countries.[176] About 20% to 40% of cases of sporadic hepatitis are attributable to HCV; the mode of transmission in these cases is not established but may be nonparenteral. Patients with "community-acquired" hepatitis C in the United States have a high rate of chronic hepatitis.[177] Similarly, several long-term follow-up studies of posttransfusion hepatitis C from the United States,[178] the United Kingdom,[179] Italy,[180] and Japan[181] have all shown a high rate of progression to chronic liver disease (greater than 60%) . There is also considerable evidence implicating hepatitis C in the development of hepatocellular carcinoma.[161,182-184]

Hepatitis E virus (HEV) is enterically transmitted by fecal contamination of drinking water.[185-190] Hepatitis E has been confirmed as the cause of epidemics of acute (usually cholestatic) hepatitis in India, Pakistan, Central Asia, North Africa, and Mexico. The highest attack rates are in young adults, but infection has been associated with a high death rate (up to 10%) in pregnant women.[188] No chronic hepatitis has been attributed to that disease.

Histopathology of acute viral hepatitis (Table 57-5). The appearance of the liver under the scanning objective of the light microscope is one of acinar disarray caused by the sum total of the changes to be described (Fig. 57-2). Two morphologic changes predominantly affect hepatocytes in viral hepatitis, namely, ballooning and apoptosis. These are seen throughout the acinus in various combinations, and not all hepatocytes in a given acinus are affected. In some cases of hepatitis B, however, ballooning tends to be more severe in zone 3.

Apoptosis is a type of cell death that leads to elimination of dead cells; it results in fragmentation of the injured hepatocyte.[191] Recent studies have shown that it is induced by transforming growth factor-β1.[192] In ultrastructural studies of apoptosis the nuclear outline becomes convoluted and the chromatin aggregates in dense, sharply circumscribed masses that abut on the nuclear membrane.[191] At the same time the condensed cytoplasm of the liver cell develops protuberances that separate and are released into spaces of Disse and sinusoids while the nucleus breaks up into discrete masses. Microscopically, the larger cell fragments, which may contain parts of the nucleus, are generally referred to as "acidophilic" or "hyaline" bodies (Fig. 57-3). The apoptotic bodies are quickly phagocytosed by Kupffer cells or adjoining liver cells.

Ballooning degeneration refers to the swelling of hepatocytes, often to several times the normal size. Affected cells have an indistinct cell membrane, and sometimes the membranes between adjacent hepatocytes disintegrate (Fig. 57-4). The cytoplasm is rarefied, often with perinuclear condensation of a small quantity of cytoplasmic remnants. There may be bile retention in some ballooned hepatocytes. Karyolysis is the typical nuclear degenerative change. The fate of ballooned hepatocytes is lysis, with disappearance, or "dropping out." The remnants of these cells attract lymphocytes and, less often, other types of inflammatory cells (focal necrosis) (Fig. 57-5) as well as hypertrophied and focally hyperplastic Kupffer cells.

Regenerative activity, both amitotic and mitotic, may be seen shortly after the onset of viral hepatitis. The number of regenerating cells gradually increases as the patient recovers.

Cholestasis is not a significant component of the histopathologic characteristics of acute viral hepatitis, except for the cholestatic variety. When present, it is usually seen as an occasional, haphazardly distributed canalicular bile plug.

Table 57-4 Viral characteristics and serologic and clinical aspects of five types of viral hepatitis

Type of hepatitis	Virus	Virus family	Transmission (predominant)	Acute mortality (%)	Carrier state (%)	Chronic hepatitis (%)	Cirrhosis (%)	Hepato-cellular carcinoma	Serologic markers
A	HAV 27 nm, single-stranded RNA	Picornaviridae	Enteral	0.2	No	No	No	No	IgM anti-HAV
E	HEV 32 nm, single-stranded RNA	Calciviridae	Enteral	<1.0 (10.0 in pregnant women)	No	No	No	No	Anti-HEV
B	HBV 42 nm, double-stranded DNA	*Hepadnavirus*	Parenteral	1.0	Yes <1.0-20.0 (0.3-1.5 in North America)	Yes 1.0-10.0	Yes <5	Yes	•HBsAg, IgM anti-HBc (acute) •IgM anti-HBc (acute) •HBsAg (early acute or chronic) •HBsAg, HBcAg, HBV DNA (chronic with continuing infection and high infectivity, or early acute)
D (coinfection with HBV)	HDV 37 nm, single-stranded RNA	Viroid	Parenteral	<1.0	Yes 5.0	Yes	1-5	?	IgM anti-HDV
C	HCV 50 nm, single-stranded RNA	Flaviviridae	Parenteral	<1.0 <1.0	Yes 50.0	50.0	10-20	Yes	•Anti-HCV •HCV RNA

Table 57-5 **Comparison of histopathology of different types of acute viral hepatitis**

Histopathologic change	Types of hepatitis				
	A	B	D	C	E
Spotty necrosis*	+	+	+	+	+
Zone 3 ballooning	−	±	+	±	−
Zone 1 ballooning	+	−	−	−	−
Panacinar ballooning	−	+	−	−	−
Massive necrosis	+	+	+	+	?
Steatosis†	±	+	+	−	±
Pronounced cholestasis with or without pseudogland formation	±	−	−	−	+
Kupffer cell hypertrophy and iron or lipofuscin, or both	+	+	+	+	−
Kuppfer cell hypertrophy and bile accumulation	±	−	−	−	+
Portal inflammation	+	+	+	+	+
Types of inflammatory cells‡	P, L, E, N	L, P	L, P	L, P	N, L
Ductular proliferation	±	±	±	±	±
Bile duct degeneration	−	−	−	±	−
Fibrosis	−	+	−	−	−

*Includes apoptosis, unicellular acidophilic and ballooning degeneration, and focal necrosis.
†Microvesicular steatosis; seen only in posttransplantation "reinfection."
‡*E,* Eosinophils; *L,* lymphocytes; *N,* neutrophils; *P,* plasma cells.

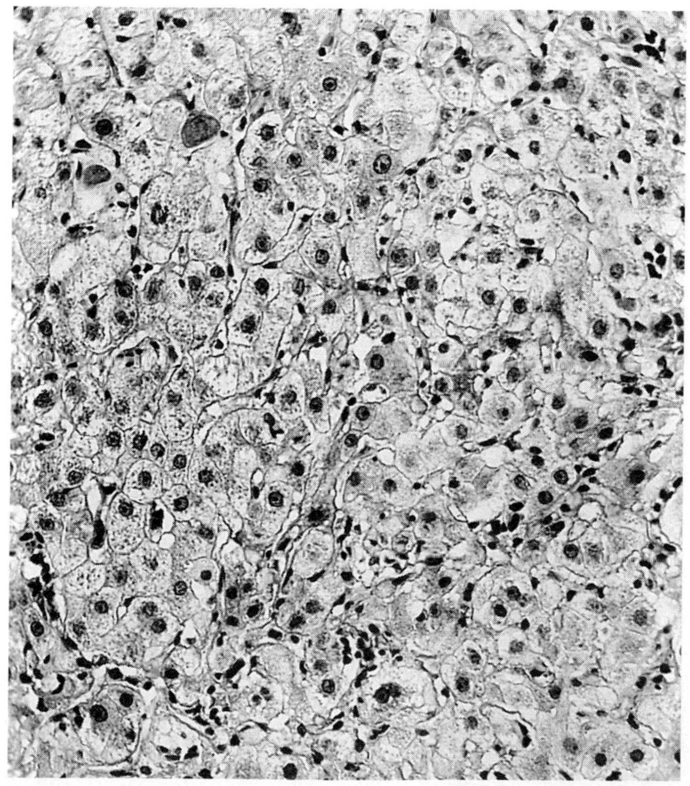

Fig. 57-2 Acute viral hepatitis. Acinar "disarray" with variable ballooning, focal necrosis, apoptotic body formation, and activation of Kupffer cells.

In addition to hepatocellular degeneration and regeneration, the acute phase of viral hepatitis is characterized by pronounced hypertrophy and hyperplasia of Kupffer cells. These cells also contain a light brown, finely granular pigment presumed to be phagocytosed from necrotic hepatocytes, in addition to apoptotic bodies of various sizes. The portal areas in viral hepatitis are usually heavily infiltrated with inflammatory cells (Fig. 57-6); lymphocytes predominate, but a small number of plasma cells, eosinophilic leukocytes, and neutrophils may be present. The inflammatory response often extends beyond the confines of the portal areas, leading to some blurring of outline of the limiting plate. Vessels in the portal areas show no noticeable changes in acute viral hepatitis. Occasional cases may reveal abnormalities of the bile ductal epithelium, such as swelling, necrosis, and infiltration by lymphocytes.

There is still controversy about histopathologic differences between the various types of viral hepatitis. Some investigators believe that there are no significant differences between acute viral hepatitis A, B, or C.[193,194] Other investigators believe that hepatitis A differs from hepatitis B and hepatitis C in the periportal predominance of the injury.[195-199] In one recent study, bile duct degenerative changes were considered diagnostic of acute viral hepatitis C.[199] Hepatitis E and some cases of hepatitis A are associated with a cholestatic type of acute hepatitis. It is characterized by pronounced cholestasis, pseudoglands, and only mild necroinflammatory changes. The comparative histopathologic characteristics of acute hepatitis caused by HAV, HBV, HDV, HCV, and HEV are listed in Table 57-5.

The subsiding phase of viral hepatitis is characterized by diminution of degenerative changes and increased regeneration. The differences between this and the active phase are, however, mainly quantitative. Acinar disarray diminishes or disappears, and the hepatic parenchyma gradually reverts to a

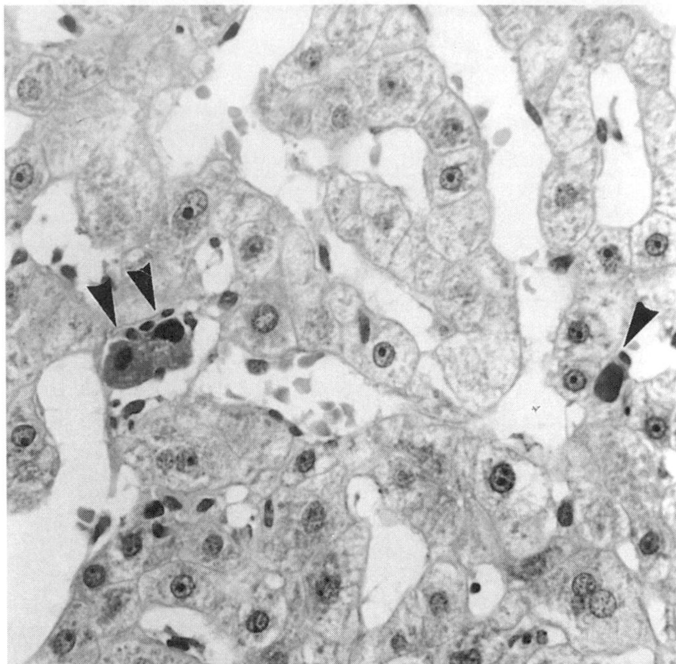

Fig. 57-3 Acute viral hepatitis: apoptotic bodies *(arrowheads)*.

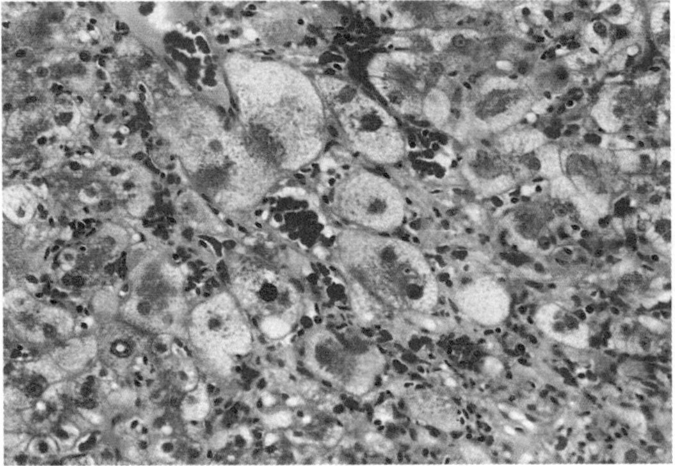

Fig. 57-4 Acute viral hepatitis. Darkly stained apoptotic body in a sinusoid contains a nucleus.

normal appearance, though varying degrees of unrest are still evident. The liver cell plates display some irregularity of alignment, and any slight damage that may have affected the reticulin network has been repaired. Only occasional degenerating cells and small foci of necrosis are evident. A minimal degree of cholestasis in zone 3 is often noted in subsiding hepatitis. One of the striking features is the continuing hypertrophy and focal hyperplasia of Kupffer cells and portal macrophages. They become relatively more conspicuous because the hepatocytes are less swollen. These cells now contain hemosiderin in addition to lipofuscin, and characteristically these two pigments are admixed in varying proportions in sections from the same biopsy specimen. The portal area inflammatory response gradually diminishes and becomes spotty. Uncomplicated viral hepatitis is not followed by any significant periportal or intra-acinar fibrosis.

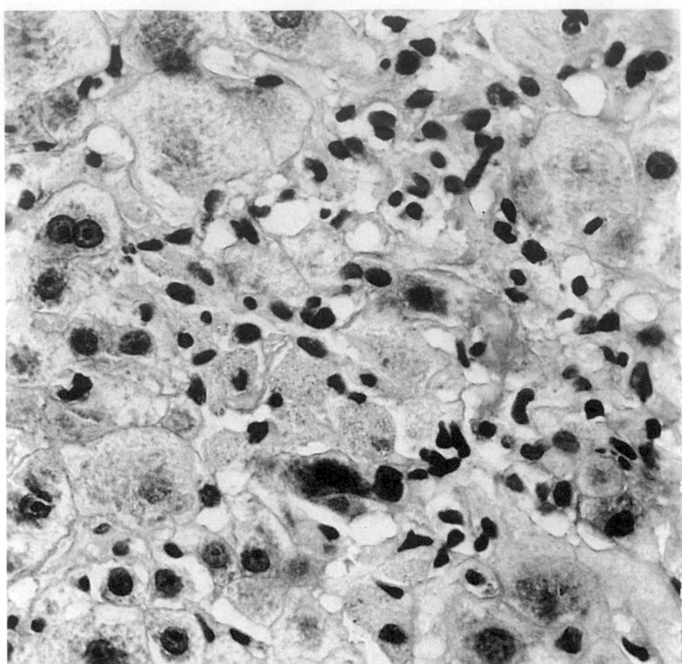

Fig. 57-5 Acute viral hepatitis. Ballooned hepatocytes *(left)* and focal necrosis.

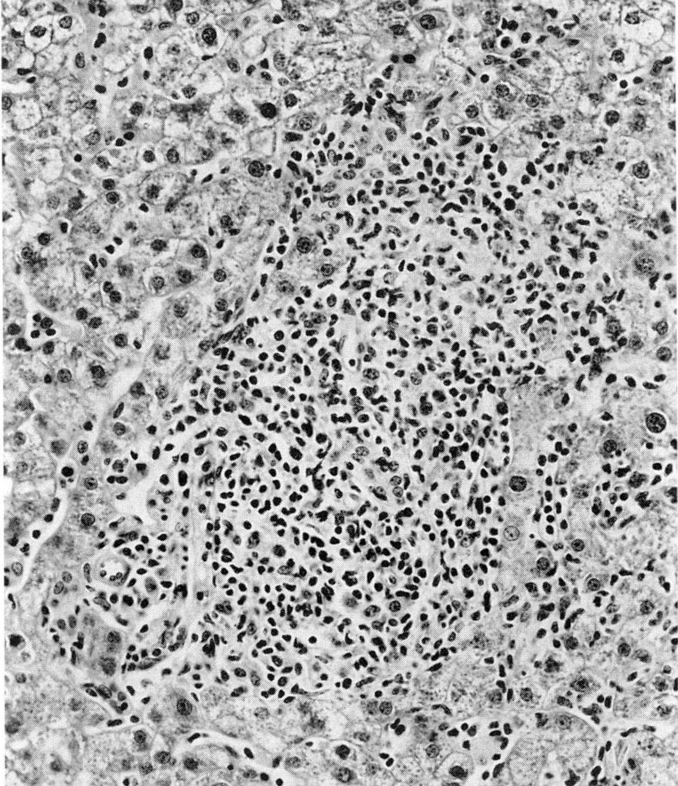

Fig. 57-6 Acute viral hepatitis. Foci of necrosis and reactive inflammatory changes.

Rarely the features of acute hepatitis may persist for many months or even years, and the histologic changes may not differ on light or electron microscopy from those of acute hepatitis. The term *chronic lobular hepatitis* has been used for this entity, which is characterized clinically by relapses and remissions. There is no fibrosis, and recovery eventually occurs, with or without therapy.

Severe acute viral hepatitis is associated with submassive necrosis. When necrosis occurs in hepatitis B it involves zone 3, sometimes with extension into zone 2 of the hepatic acini, but cases of severe viral hepatitis A are characterized by necrosis predominantly involving zone 1.[198] The zones of necrosis with the collapsed reticulin framework may be linked together ("bridging necrosis"). Boyer and Klatskin[200] found that bridging necrosis indicated a severe form of the disease that could lead to hepatic failure or the development of cirrhosis in a significant number of patients. In patients with a subacute course who subsequently die, regenerative nodules, often having a tumorlike appearance, may be seen grossly. These have an irregular alignment of reticulin fibers, plates of hepatocytes that are two cells thick, and varying degrees of cholestasis. The surrounding reticulin framework of the necrotic parenchyma is progressively compressed as the nodules enlarge and may eventually become collagenized.

The most severe cases of acute viral hepatitis are associated with massive necrosis. Sections from the liver show uniform disappearance (dropping out) of hepatocytes, but occasionally, haphazardly distributed cells survive, forming a cuff of cells around portal areas (Fig. 57-7). The reticulin framework is usually intact but frequently collapsed because of loss of liver cells, with resultant approximation of portal areas. The sinusoids can be empty or engorged with blood.

Variable numbers of inflammatory cells are present in spaces of Disse and sinusoids. They include lymphocytes and plasma cells as well as a lesser number of eosinophilic leukocytes and neutrophils. Central vein endophlebitis may be present. Kupffer cells reveal considerable hypertrophy and hyperplasia, and their cytoplasm is packed with lipofuscin. Zone 1 of the hepatic acinus shows a characteristic neocholangiolar proliferation with neutrophilic infiltration. The portal areas are variably infiltrated with inflammatory cells similar to those in the acini as well as pigment-laden macrophages; the inflammatory cells may infiltrate the periportal areas. This "spillover" can be distinguished from piecemeal necrosis of chronic hepatitis by the lack of separation of liver cells from the limiting plate and by the absence of periportal fibrosis. Several reviews of the histopathology of viral hepatitis are recommended for further reading.[201-205]

Drug-induced and toxic injury

Acute drug-induced and toxic liver injury can lead to a variety of lesions that range from mild spotty necrosis to massive necrosis. The types of injury and examples of causative drugs or toxins are listed in Table 57-6. In general, the morphologic expressions of drug-induced hepatocellular injury parallel those of viral hepatitis, though differences are apparent in

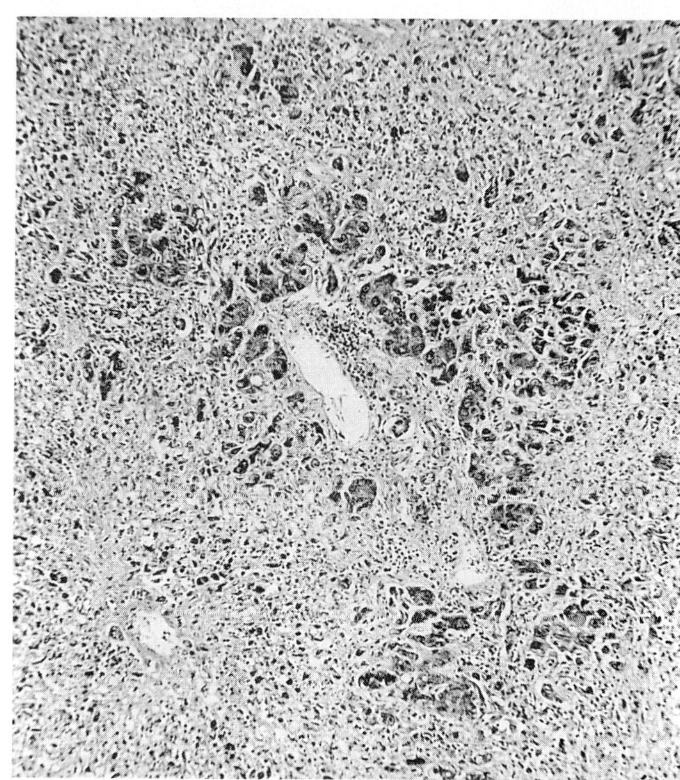

Fig. 57-7 Acute viral hepatitis B. Massive necrosis; only a few clusters of liver cells *(darkly stained)* have survived.

Table 57-6 Acute drug-induced and toxic hepatocellular injury

Type of injury	Examples
Panacinar spotty necrosis	
Resembling classic viral hepatitis	Drugs: isoniazid, paraminosalicylic acid, sulfonamides, antidepressants, propylthiouracil, methyldopa, diphenylhydantoin, papaverine
Submassive necrosis	
Acinar zone 3	Drugs: isoniazid, halothane, methoxyflurane, isoflurane, acetaminophen, allopurinol, dantrolene, ticrynafen, diclofenac Toxins: copper sulfate, carbon tetrachloride,* trichloroethylene,* chlorinated naphthalenes,* diethylene glycol, tannic acid,* toxic mushrooms,* pennyroyal oil
Acinar zone 1	Drugs: paraaminosalicylic acid, halothane, cocaine Toxins: phosphorus,* ferrous sulfate, mushrooms,* pennyroyal oil
Massive necrosis	Drugs: isoniazid, halothane, methyldopa, propylthiouracil, diphenylhydantoin, phenelzine, ticrynafen Toxins: carbon tetrachloride,* tetrachloroethane,* trinitrotoluene,* chloroethane, chlorinated naphthalenes

*Hepatocellular degeneration and necrosis may be or often are accompanied by steatosis.

some cases. For example, the inflammatory response may be mild or totally lacking, as may be the case with halothane-associated hepatic injury. On the other hand, the intra-acinar and portal and periportal inflammation may be prominent, but the cells may be predominantly neutrophils and eosinophils, unlike the lymphoplasmacytic response in viral hepatitis. Such a response has been observed by the authors in acute hepatocellular injury associated with propylthiouracil or ticrynafen. In hypersensitivity drug reactions associated with peripheral blood eosinophilia, the portal and intra-acinar cellular infiltrate is often rich in eosinophils, and these cells are also present in sinusoidal spaces.

Regardless of specific morphologic features that can be appreciated in a given case, the distinction between drug-induced injury and viral hepatitis must rely heavily on clinicopathologic correlations. These include establishing temporal eligibility of the drug, knowledge of previously reported adverse reactions of the suspect drug, and ruling out other possible causes by the biochemical, serologic, and morphologic findings. The interested reader is referred to several sources for further reading.[206-212] Other than morphologic differences, drug-induced injury may have a prognosis different from that of viral hepatitis. Thus Spitz and collegues [213] found that drug-induced bridging necrosis does not appear to be associated with an increased risk of development of active chronic liver disease.

With reference to direct hepatotoxins, the zonality of the injury in many cases (see Table 57-6), together with the type of hepatocellular degeneration and associated steatosis, will often be sufficient to distinguish it from viral hepatitis (Fig. 57-8 and 57-9).

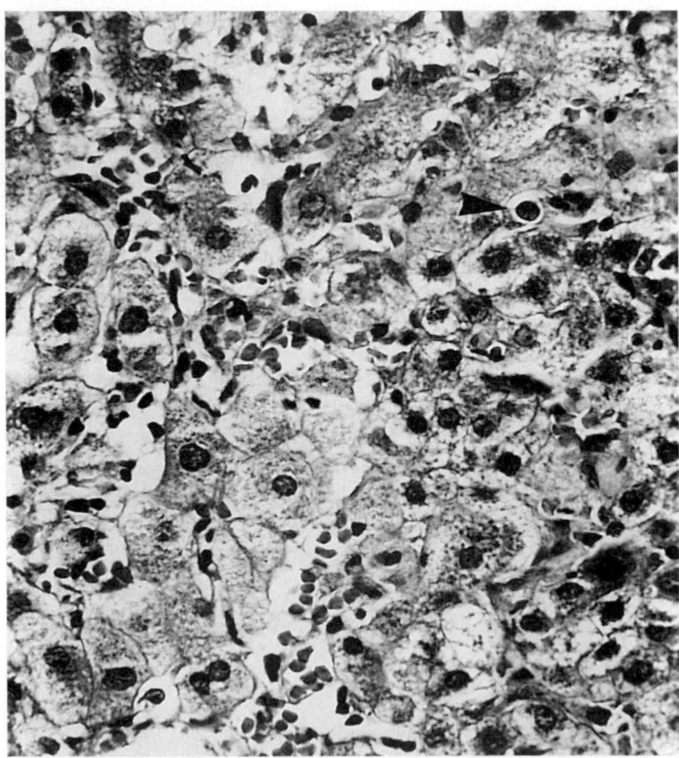

Fig. 57-8 Acute hepatocellular injury with spotty necrosis (hepatitis-like) as a result of isoniazid therapy. Notice disarray, ballooning, focal necrosis, and an apoptotic body *(arrowhead).*

Acute hepatocellular injury associated with infectious diseases other than viral hepatitis

Acute hepatocellular injury can be caused by viruses, rickettsiae, spirochetes, and bacteria. Because of the limitations of space, only the relatively more common diseases are described briefly.

Herpesvirus hepatitis

Lesions in the liver in adults in disseminated herpesvirus infection consist of variably sized and haphazardly distributed foci of coagulative degeneration and necrosis[214,215] (Fig. 57-10). An inflammatory response is usually lacking but, when present, is neutrophilic. Cowdry type A intranuclear inclusions are almost invariably found, particularly in partially degenerated liver cells at the periphery of the foci of necrosis (Fig. 57-11). The presence of herpes simplex antigen in infected liver cells can be definitively established by immunohistochemical methods. The viral particles can also be visualized by electron microscopy, even in autopsy specimens.

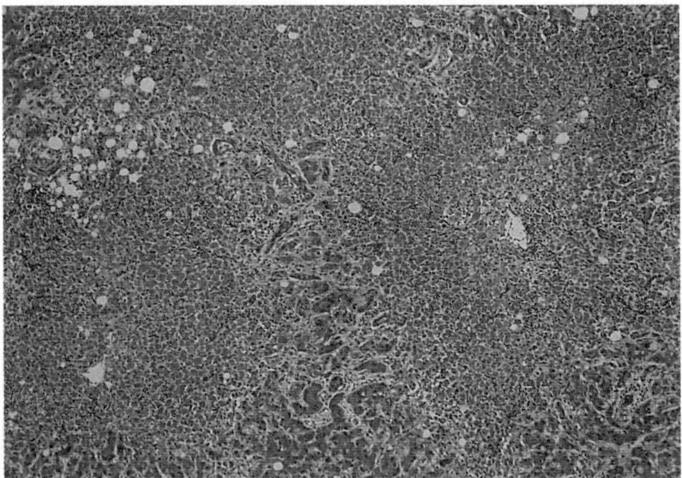

Fig. 57-9 Acetaminophen hepatotoxicity. Zone 3 necrosis with dropout of liver cells. Notice hypertrophied Kupffer cells *(darkly stained)* full of lipofuscin.

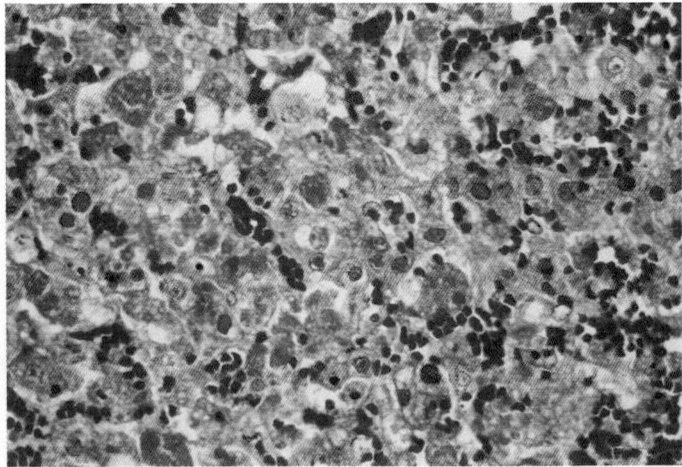

Fig. 57-10 Coagulative necrosis caused by herpesvirus hepatitis.

Adenovirus hepatitis

Adenovirus infection can lead to a severe hepatitis that resembles that of herpesvirus hepatitis. The intranuclear inclusions are, however, larger than that with herpesvirus and tend to be basophilic. Commercially available antisera can be used for immunohistochemical diagnosis in paraffin sections, and again the viral particles are readily identifiable in electron micrographs.

Infectious mononucleosis hepatitis

In comparison with viral hepatitis, the inflammatory response in this disease is more prominent whereas the hepatocellular injury is milder. Hepatocellular "unrest" is moderate to pronounced, and mitotic figures are often seen in hepatocytes, Kupffer cells, and portal mononuclear cells (Fig. 57-12). Apoptosis is present, but ballooning is absent or minimal. Small foci of necrosis can be present. Kupffer cells are usually greatly hypertrophied and hyperplastic and sometimes form tiny granulomatoid foci or, rarely, true granulomas. They may contain traces of hemosiderin but little if any lipofuscin. The hepatic sinusoids characteristically contain an increased number of lymphocytes, sometimes closely packed together in an "Indian-file" pattern. Portal areas are usually heavily infiltrated with inflammatory cells, which are preponderantly lymphocytes, though eosinophils and even neutrophils can be seen.

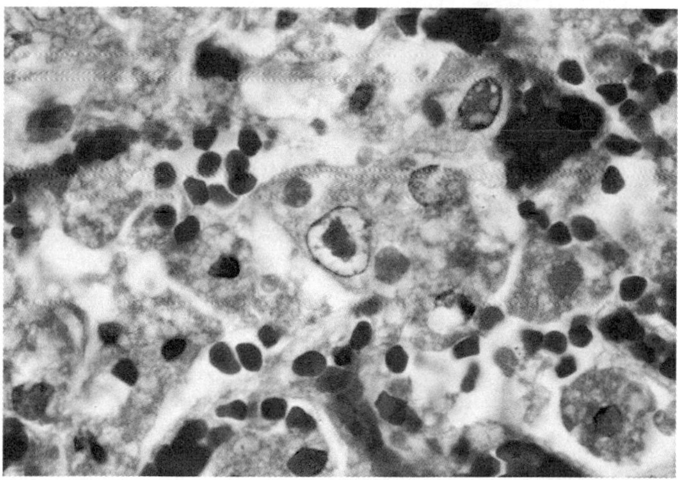

Fig. 57-11 Cowdry type A intranuclear inclusion in liver cell *(center)* in herpesvirus hepatitis.

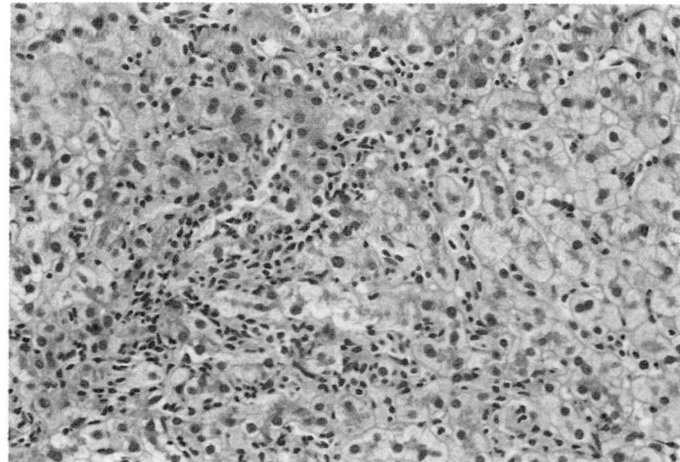

Fig. 57-12 Infectious mononucleosis hepatitis. Sinusoidal lymphocytosis and scattered focal necrosis.

The histologic differential diagnosis includes CMV mononucleosis,[216-219] toxoplasmic mononucleosis,[220] and drug-induced mononucleosis, such as that associated with phenytoin[221,222] or dapsone; the drug history is essential in the diagnosis of the latter. Serologic tests (the Monospot test and serologic tests for Epstein-Barr virus, CMV infection, and toxoplasmosis) are essential in the differentiation of CMV and toxoplasmic mononucleosis from infectious mononucleosis hepatitis inasmuch as diagnostic CMV inclusions and *Toxoplasma gondii* are not usually found in the hepatic lesions. Cytomegaly and characteristic intranuclear and cytoplasmic inclusions in bile duct (Fig. 57-13) and liver cells are seen only in CMV infections of the newborn and of adults who are immunocompromised.

Liver manifestations of Rocky Mountain spotted fever

The basic hepatic lesion in this disease is an inflammation of the portal triad in which large mononuclear cells and neutrophils predominate.[223] Other changes include portal vasculitis, erythrophagocytosis, cholestasis, and hepatocellular necrosis. Rickettsiae can be demonstrated in portal tract lesions in the majority of cases.[223]

Q-fever hepatitis

The typical lesion in Q-fever hepatitis is the noncaseating granuloma with a fibrin ring (often surrounding a fat vacuole) in its center (Fig 57-14), but focal necrosis, apoptosis, and

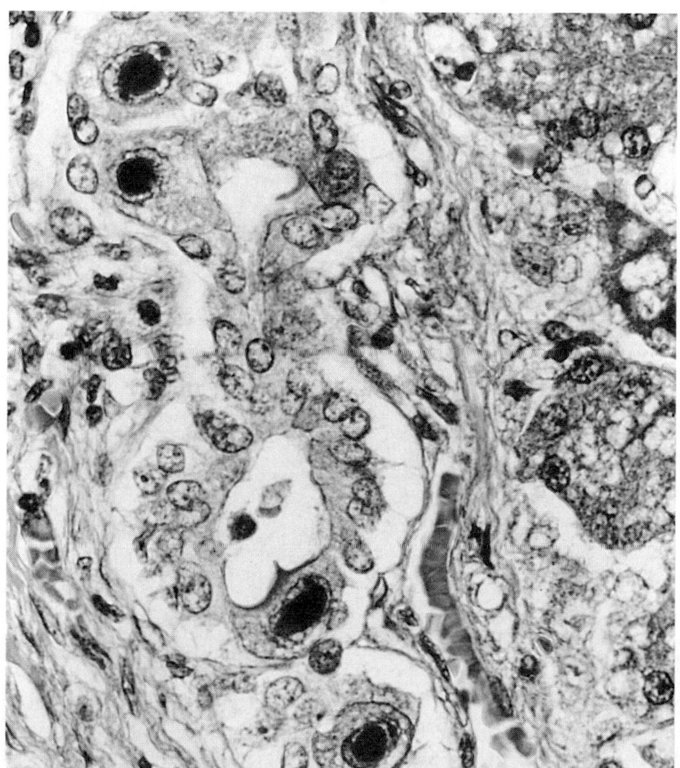

Fig. 57-13 Cytomegalovirus hepatitis. Infected bile ductal cells contain large, darkly stained intranuclear inclusions.

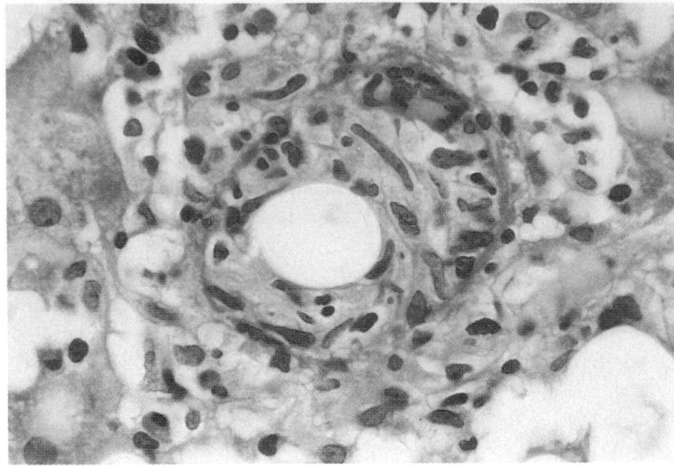

Fig. 57-14 Fibrin ring granuloma of Q-fever hepatitis.

lymphocytic portal infiltration are also seen.[224-229] The organism *Coxiella burnetii* is not identified in the lesions. Although fibrin ring ("doughnut") granulomas are typical of Q fever, they are by no means pathognomonic, since they have been reported in allopurinol hypersensitivity reactions,[230] infections with CMV[231] and Epstein-Barr virus (EBV),[232] bouttoneuse fever, and other conditions.[229]

Syphilis

A number of studies and reviews of hepatic changes in syphilis have been published.[233-244] The changes in early syphilis do not appear to be specific and include foci of necrosis, hypertrophy of Kupffer cells, portal inflammation, cholangitis, and rarely cholestatis.[233-240] Feher and colleagues [238] have proposed that the presence of foci of necrosis around efferent veins is characteristic of syphilitic hepatitis; they were able to demonstrate spirochetes in seven of 17 liver biopsy specimens.

Hepatic involvement in congenital syphilis has been reviewed by Oppenheimer and Hardy.[233] The early phase of congenital syphilis is characterized by a prominent portal and sinusoidal inflammatory infiltrate and foci of necrosis (Fig. 57-15). Lymphocytes, plasma cells, and hypertrophied Kupffer cells are particularly prominent. Spirochetes are more likely to be demonstrated by silver stains (such as Warthin-Starry) at this stage than in the healing phase. Progressive scarring in the sinusoids is accompanied by atrophy of hepatocytes. The pattern is that of "diffuse fibrosis" and lacks the nodularity and reorganization of cirrhosis.

The gummas of tertiary syphilis also heal by fibrosis. Broad-based scars eventually retract, giving rise to the deep clefts and a furrowed appearance of the hepatic surface, known as hepar lobatum.[234] It is worth noting at this juncture that hepar lobatum can also result from treatment of metastatic breast carcinoma with chemotherapy.[241]

Leptospirosis

In sections from hepatic biopsy material there are scattered sinusoidal acidophilic bodies, minimal to moderate hepatocellular unrest with increased mitotic activity, and minimal zone 3 cholestasis.[242] Kupffer cells are hypertrophied, and many reveal erythrophagocytosis. There is usually very little inflammatory response within the acinus or in portal areas. An additional change described in autopsy material is the dissociation of liver cell plates. Spirochetes are demonstrable in less than one fourth of the cases.

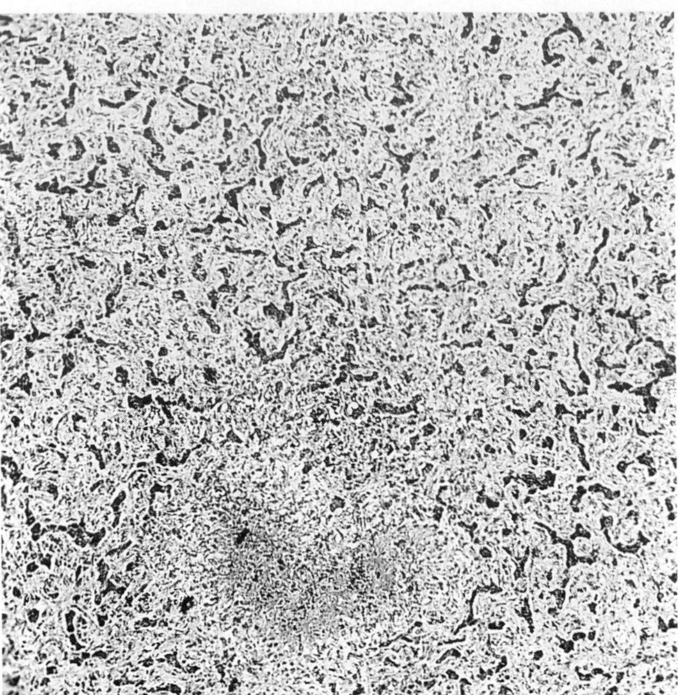

Fig. 57-15 Congenital syphilis.There is diffuse intra-acinar inflammation with disruption of liver cell plates. Notice the microgumma *(lower left)*.

Miscellaneous viral infections

Severe liver injury with confluent or massive necrosis can complicate many viral infections, which include echovirus, yellow fever, Lassa fever, Ebola fever, and several other hemorrhagic fevers. Several reviews of the clinicopathologic aspects of these diseases are recommended for further reading.[243-245]

CHRONIC HEPATOCELLULAR INJURY

Alcoholic liver disease and its differential diagnosis

Although some hepatic morphologic changes may appear after brief periods of alcohol ingestion, the characteristic lesions are believed to follow many years of heavy intake in susceptible individuals.[53,246-250] Steatosis can be demonstrated after a few days in healthy persons in whom alcohol has been substituted for some carbohydrate in the diet.[251] Lipogranulomas can be found but are rare in our experience. Ballooning degeneration can occasionally be present in early injury. We have observed such degeneration in association with zone 3 cholestasis, a combination that is difficult to distinguish from other forms of drug-induced injury.

The above changes are not considered specific for alcoholic liver disease and must be evaluated with the clinical history. When the disease is more active, a histologic pattern, usually referred to as "alcoholic hepatitis," can develop; it is diagnostic, though not pathognomonic. The most striking changes are found in zone 3. There is pronounced pleomorphism (unrest) of hepatocytes with focal necrosis. Many hepatocytes show cytoplasmic dissociation (clumping of part of the cytoplasm around the nucleus with rarefaction of the remainder). Some hepatocytes harbor Mallory bodies (alcoholic hyaline), a finding essential to the histologic diagnosis. Mallory bodies are irregular clumps or ropelike, eosinophilic structures occupying a portion of the cytoplasm of a liver cell (Fig. 57-16). They are PAS negative but are readily stained by monoclonal antibodies to ubiquitin (Fig. 57-17). Groups of neutrophils commonly infiltrate or surround degenerating hepatocytes harboring Mallory bodies (neutrophilic satellitosis). Steatosis (usually macrovesicular) of moderate or pronounced severity is usually present but can be mild or absent. Fibrosis tends to surround terminal hepatic venules, to extend in the spaces of Disse and sinusoids, and to envelop a single hepatocyte or groups of hepatocytes ("chicken-wire" fibrosis) (Fig. 57-18). The connective tissue can become a confluent mass, replacing zone 3 hepatocytes and obliterating the efferent veins. This stage of the disease is also known as *sclerosing hyaline necrosis*.[246] Venocclusive lesions have been described in terminal hepatic venules in both precirrhotic and cirrhotic stages of alcoholic hepatitis.[248] Periportal fibrosis may or may not be present. Ascites, believed to result from fibrous involvement of terminal and intercalated veins and possibly the hepatic sinusoids, can occur despite the absence of fully developed cirrhosis. The lesions appear to be reversible in some instances, though the exact determinants of prognosis are not clear.

Some biopsy specimens show fibrosis around terminal hepatic venules and pericellular fibrosis in zone 3 in the absence of any other prominent lesions (Fig. 57-19). This pattern is considered suggestive but not diagnostic of alcoholic liver disease. Lieber[251] maintains that such a pattern of injury identifies those at risk of developing cirrhosis and can progress to cirrhosis without an identifiable stage of "florid" necrosis and neutrophilic infiltration.

With progression of injury, fibrous bands begin to link zone 3 and portal areas, dissecting the acini into small segments that eventuate in a micronodular cirrhosis (Fig. 57-20). Ductular proliferation can be prominent near the portal areas. The presence of steatosis, neutrophilic infiltrates, and Mallory bodies provides clues to the diagnosis. However, these changes may be absent in some biopsy specimens, particularly those from patients who have ceased drinking for a considerable time. The clinical history might be the only means available to establish the diagnosis in the cirrhotic stage. The cirrhotic nod-

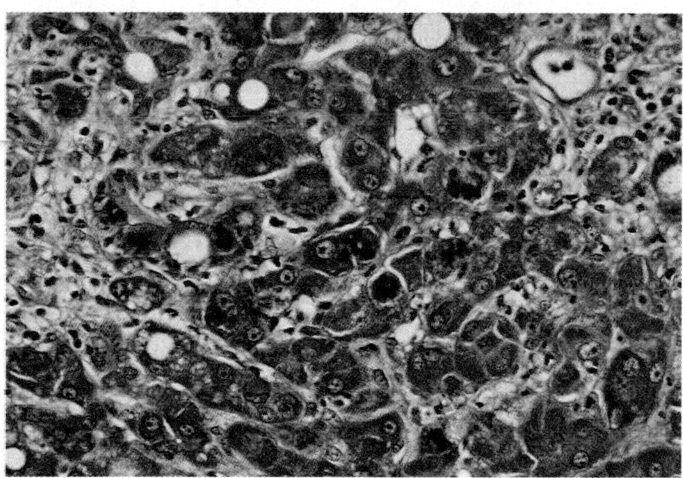

Fig. 57-16 Alcoholic hepatitis. Rope-like Mallory bodies in three hepatocytes.

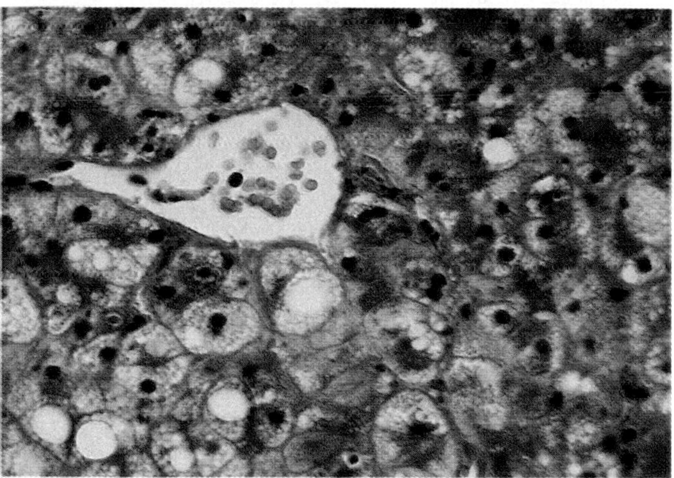

Fig. 57-18 Alcoholic hepatitis. Chicken-wire fibrosis in zone 3. (Mallory trichrome stain.)

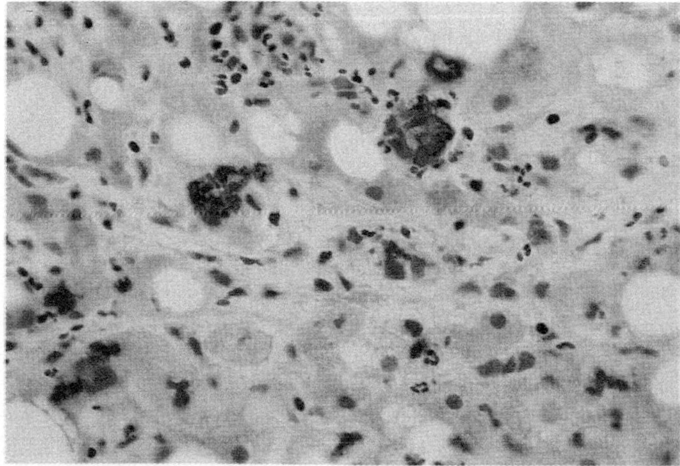

Fig. 57-17 Alcoholic hepatitis. Mallory bodies *(brown)* are immunostained with antibodies to ubiquitin.

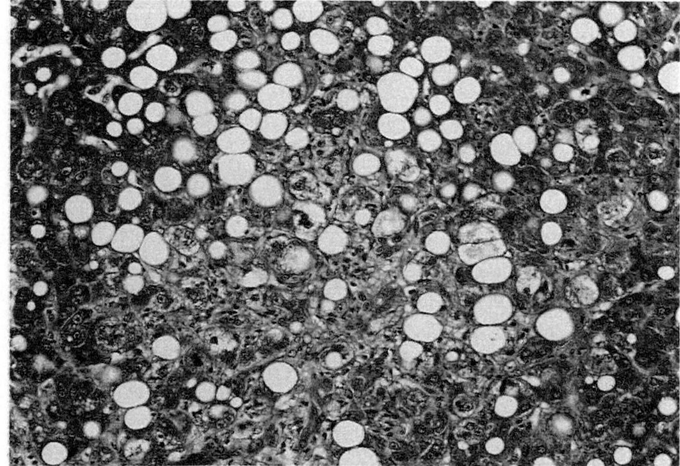

Fig. 57-19 Macrovesicular steatosis, alcoholic. Notice zone 3 fibrosis in center of field.

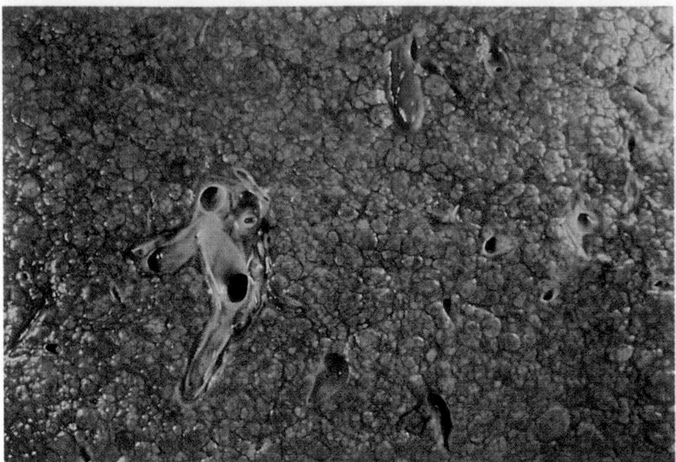

Fig. 57-20 Section of micronodular cirrhotic liver caused by alcohol abuse.

ules can undergo pronounced regeneration leading to development of a micronodular, a mixed, or rarely a macronodular cirrhosis.[252]

Although Mallory bodies are characteristic of the active phase of alcoholic hepatitis, they have been identified in other disorders and thus cannot be considered pathognomonic.[253,254] Changes resembling those of alcoholic hepatitis may occur in patients who are obese or have adult-onset diabetes mellitus. Several series of patients with this disease have now been published.[255-264] The term *nonalcoholic steatohepatitis* has been proposed for the entity,[259] but other terms, such as *fatty hepatitis, nonalcoholic steatonecrosis,* and *pseudoalcoholic hepatitis,* have been used. Mallory bodies have been observed in other conditions such as Wilson's disease, chronic cholestatic disorders such as PBC and PSC, Indian childhood cirrhosis, postjejunoileal bypass surgery,[255,265,266] hepatocellular carcinomas, and the condition after therapy with perhexiline maleate, amiodarone, or several other drugs. The location of the Mallory bodies, associated morphologic lesions, and the clinical and laboratory data should serve to distinguish these entities (see below).

Ultrastructurally, three types of Mallory bodies have been described: (1) type I consists of bundles of filaments (5 to 20 nm thick) arranged in parallel arrays, (2) type II is composed of randomly oriented fibrils (Fig. 57-21), and (3) type III consists of a granular or amorphous substance containing only scattered fibrils.[267] Simply stated, Mallory bodies are believed to result from derangement of the intermediate filament component of the cytoskeleton of liver cells. Extensive reviews of the pathogenesis of Mallory bodies have been published.[254,268-271]

Giant mitochondria are often found in hepatocytes of alcoholics.[272] Light microscopically, they are round, eosinophilic, sharply demarcated, and homogeneous and vary from about 1 to 7 μm in diameter. A second type of mitochondrion is needle or spindle shaped and is 7 μm or more in length and 1 μm in width. The rounded bodies can be confused with α_1-antitrypsin bodies but differ in that they are not periodic acid-Schiff positive and are more often found in zone 3. α_1-antitrypsin bodies are usually confined to zone 1 or the periphery of the cirrhotic nodule. Ultrastructurally, giant mitochondria often contain paracrystalline inclusions. Although giant mitochondria can be found with the electron microscope in a variety of conditions, it appears that with a light microscope they are seen mostly in alcoholics.[272]

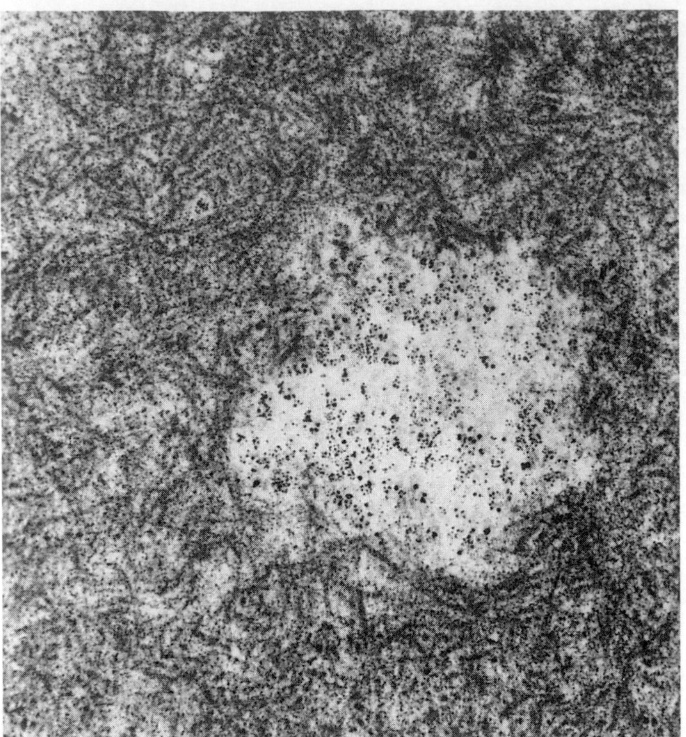

Fig. 57-21 Mallory body in a hepatocyte is composed of randomly oriented fibrils.

Hemosiderin can accumulate in hepatocytes in alcoholics and may at times lead to difficulties in differentiation of alcoholic liver disease from genetic hemochromatosis. The presence of Mallory bodies, neutrophilic satellitosis, and zone 3 sclerosis would, of course, provide evidence of alcoholic hepatitis. A very large amount of hemosiderin in hepatocytes and its presence in the epithelium of bile ducts would favor hemochromatosis, since iron accumulation is rarely pronounced in alcoholics.[273] The family history and the clinical and laboratory data are also helpful in distinguishing these two entities (see below). The iron overload in alcoholic liver disease might be attributable to increased iron absorption, to the iron content of alcoholic beverages, and to hemolytic episodes.

The relationship of hepatocellular carcinoma, which occurs in 10% to 15% of cirrhotic livers complicating alcoholic liver disease, is reviewed extensively by several investigators.[274-276]

Steatosis

Although the distinction is not always sharp, steatosis can be subclassified into two morphologic categories, macrovesicular and microvesicular. In routinely processed material, the lipid is dissolved by organic solvents, resulting in a vacuolated hepatocytic cytoplasm; in doubtful cases, frozen sections with special stains (such as oil red O) are necessary to confirm the presence of lipid.

Macrovesicular steatosis

Most affected hepatocytes contain a single, rounded vacuole that displaces the nucleus and cytoplasm to the periphery of the cell. The vacuoles are usually as large as or larger than a hepatocyte. A few hepatocytes can contain one or more smaller vacuoles. Associated conditions include alcoholism, malnutrition, diabetes mellitus, obesity, malabsorption, postjejunoileal bypass surgery, various debilitating disorders, some metabolic diseases, and exposure to various drugs and toxins.[277] The steatosis can be the only change, or it may be associated with other lesions, as after jejunoileal bypass surgery, in several metabolic diseases, and in drug-induced injury (see later section). The location of the fat is quite variable; it is most frequently diffuse but can be periportal or pericentral.

Periportal glycogenated nuclei (vacuolated or hydropic nuclei) are frequently associated with steatosis in diabetes mellitus, but the combination is not specific and can be found in the early stage of Wilson's disease (see later section). Glycogenated nuclei may be found in a variety of other disorders.

Steatosis can be induced by several drugs. Methotrexate can lead to macrovesicular steatosis as well as focal necrosis, nuclear pleomorphism, periportal fibrosis with piecemeal necrosis, and even cirrhosis.[278] Total parenteral nutrition in children can result in steatosis, but the dominant lesion is cholestasis. Fibrosis and, in occasional patients, cirrhosis can occur.[279]

Patients who have undergone jejunoileal bypass surgery for morbid obesity can develop hepatic disease of variable severity even though the liver may appear unremarkable at the time of operation. Steatosis can be the only change, but some patients develop prominent fibrosis.[255] The lesions frequently resemble those of alcoholic hepatitis.[265] Perivenular fibrosis can identify patients at risk to develop this hepatic injury and cirrhosis; the lesions occur in older patients who have greater weight loss after bypass surgery.[266] Hepatic fibrosis, hepatic failure, and other complications have led some to reverse the bypass in an attempt to reduce morbidity or mortality.[266] Severe hepatic injury resembling alcoholic hepatitis has also been reported after intestinal resection,[280] and it may progress to cirrhosis.

Glucocorticoids can produce a variable degree of steatosis depending on dosage. Steatosis caused by some hepatotoxins is usually accompanied by hepatocellular necrosis. In poisoning with carbon tetrachloride, chloroform, tetrachloroethane, tannic acid, or toxic mushrooms, the necrosis affects zone 3. With phosphorus poisoning, necrosis is periportal and can be less prominent than steatosis.

Microvesicular steatosis

Affected hepatocytes show a central nucleus surrounded by sharply defined small vacuoles. In autolyzed autopsy specimens, the cytoplasm can have a clear appearance, and the vacuoles might not be readily discernible. Reye's syndrome,[281] acute fatty liver of pregnancy[282,283] (Fig. 57-22), alcoholic liver injury ("alcoholic foamy degeneration"),[284] drug-induced injury (such as that caused by salicylates or valproic acid),[285,286] and several inherited metabolic diseases (such as acyl-CoA dehydrogenase deficiency)[281] are all manifested histopathologically by microvesicular steatosis. Epidemic delta virus superinfection of chronic hepatitis B is dominated histopathologically by microvesicular steatosis.[287] Other causes and pathogenetic mechanisms have been reviewed by Sherlock.[283]

Chronic Hepatitis

Histopathology

The histopathologic features of chronic hepatitis, regardless of causes, are characterized by several lesions, the most important of which is piecemeal necrosis.[288-290] Other changes, such as bile duct lesions, portal inflammation, intra-acinar degeneration and necrosis, and periportal and bridging fibrosis, are present to a variable extent. Additional specific features may be present, depending on the cause (such as ground-glass cells of the HBV carrier state).

Piecemeal necrosis. The necroinflammatory change sometimes referred to as "lymphocytic" piecemeal necrosis[289] initially destroys the limiting plate of liver cells (that is, is periportal). In the untreated patient there is continuous erosion of the hepatic parenchyma with closer and closer approximation of expanded portal areas. The necroinflammatory changes are succeeded by fibrosis. Piecemeal necrosis may not involve all portal areas equally in a given case and can affect either a segment or the entire perimeter of a portal area. It can continue unabated in the cirrhotic liver complicating chronic hepatitis, thus contributing to the "activity" of the cirrhotic process.

Degenerative changes affecting liver cells in piecemeal necrosis include cytoplasmic dissociation (a change characterized by swelling of liver cells with cytoplasmic rarefaction and coarse clumping of cytoplasmic organelles and eventually by lysis of nuclei and cell membranes)[201] and apoptosis.[290-292] The latter change results in the formation of variably sized, often rounded, fragments of liver cells that are located in the liver plates or sinusoids (Fig. 57-23). The larger apoptotic bodies, sometimes containing nuclear fragments, are often referred to as "acidophilic bodies." Within the sinusoids, the apoptotic bodies are hardly ever "free" but are usually phagocytosed and ultimately digested by Kupffer cells. The ultra-

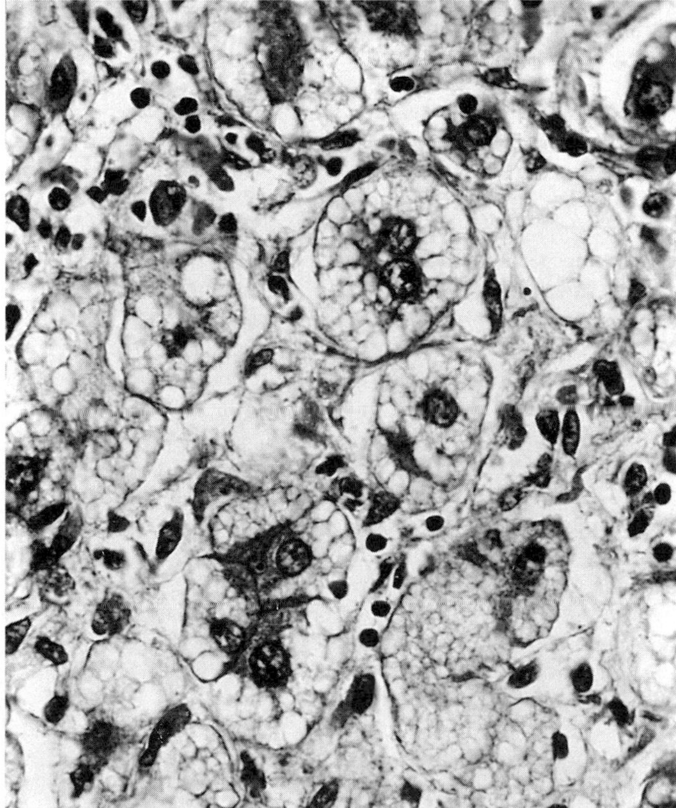

Fig. 57-22 Microvesicular steatosis in fatty liver of pregnancy. The hepatocytes are enlarged, and their cytoplasm is occupied by multiple small vacuoles. Notice central location of the nuclei.

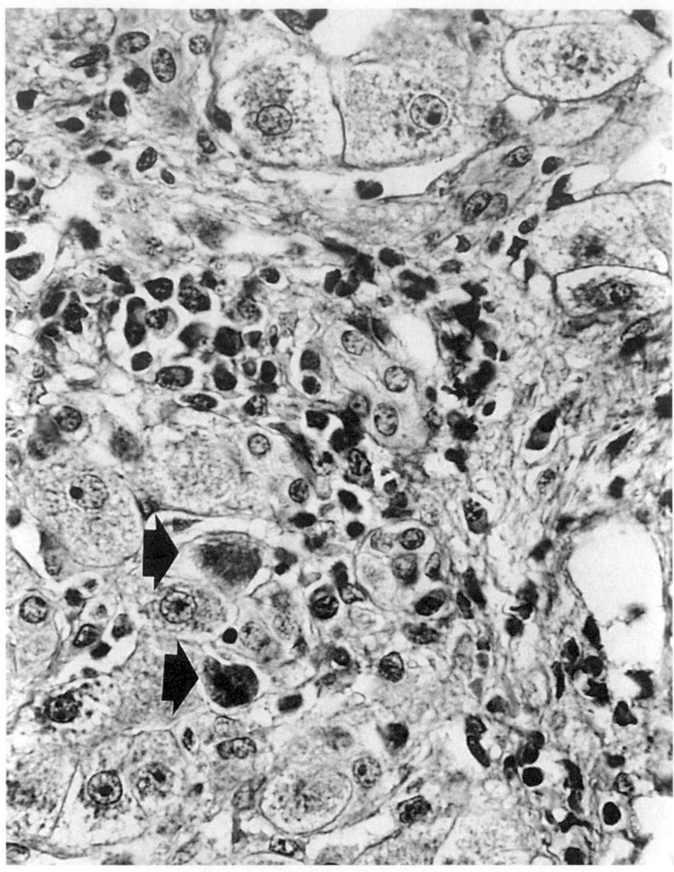

Fig. 57-23 Chronic hepatitis. Periportal liver cells reveals cytoplasmic dissociation, and there is infiltration by plasma cells. Notice acidophilic bodies *(arrows)*.

structural features of apoptosis in the liver are described in detail by Searle and colleagues.[191]

There is a very intimate relationship between lymphocytes and liver cells in chronic hepatitis[293,294] that is apparent even on cursory examination. The degenerating hepatocytes and inflammatory cells are closely apposed, with the lymphocytes often being located in spaces of Disse, with indentation of the cytoplasm of liver cells (polesis). Sometimes the hepatocyte completely encircles a lymphocyte or plasma cell (emperipolesis).[295] There is loss of microvilli of the plasma membrane of the liver cell facing the lymphocyte.[294] It should be noted that the processes of polesis and emperipolesis can be seen in chronic hepatitis and are seen not only in the areas of "periportal" piecemeal necrosis, but also throughout the hepatic acini, at varying distances from the leading edge of the piecemeal necrosis. In a semiquantitative study of emperipolesis in chronic hepatitis, Bechtelsheimer and colleagues[295] were of the opinion that change was much more pronounced in severe (chronic aggressive hepatitis) than in less severe forms (chronic persistent hepatitis) of the disease. The complex interactions between effector cells (T-lymphocytes) and liver cells (target cells) in the immune response in chronic autoimmune hepatitis are reviewed by Dienes and colleagues.[294] In the case of chronic hepatitis C, specific cytotoxic T-lymphocytes recognize epitopes in the highly conserved core protein and the more variable E2 envelope protein.[296] Koziel and colleagues[296] believe that identification of these epitopes recognized by HCV-specific cytotoxic T-lymphocytes will facilitate exploration of their role in disease pathogenesis as well as provide information useful for development of therapeutic intervention and vaccines.

A recent study of apoptosis has shown that it is mediated by Fas antigen, a cell surface antigen that belongs to the receptor family that includes tumor necrosis factor receptor, nerve growth factor receptor, B-cell CD40 antigen, and T-cell OX40 antigen.[297] Hiramatsu and colleagues[298] studied the immunohistochemical expression of Fas antigen and hepatitis C core antigen in chronic hepatitis C. Fas antigen was expressed in the cytoplasm of liver cells among infiltrating lymphocytes at the advancing edge of piecemeal necrosis; more expression was observed in areas of active inflammation than in areas with no inflammation. The prevalence of Fas antigen was higher in the cases expressing HCV core antigen than in those that were not. These investigators suggested that Fas expression could be triggered directly by HCV infection, or indirectly through the immune system, with resultant cytotoxic T-lymphocyte-induced DNA fragmentation. Regardless of the mechanism, these observations have demonstrated an important role for Fas antigen expression in the inflammatory response and piecemeal necrosis in chronic hepatitis C and probably in other types of chronic hepatitis.

Portal area lesions. In chronic hepatitis the portal connective tissue is variably infiltrated by lymphocytes and plasma cells. Lymphoid aggregates or follicles with reactive centers may be present. They are now considered typical though not pathognomonic of chronic hepatitis C. Immunohistochemical studies of these aggregates have been performed by two groups of investigators;[299,300] they are regarded as true functional lymphoid follicles. Mosnier and colleagues[300] found that they contained activated B-cells in germinal centers surrounded by a follicular dendritic cell network. A mantle zone of B-cells surrounds the activated B-cells. The B-cell follicle in turn is surrounded by a T-cell zone. In chronic hepatitis B some of the plasma cells may contain anti-HBs and anti-HBc.[301] Portal macrophages are often hypertrophied and contain PAS-positive, diastase-resistant, granular material.

A histopathologic feature that is highly characteristic, if not pathognomonic of chronic hepatitis, is the isolation and entrapment of single liver cells or groups of liver cells in the expanded portal areas.[135,201,302] Bile duct lesions have been reviewed by Vyberg.[303] He recognized three types of hepatitis-associated bile duct lesions. The type 2 lesion is the one most frequently seen in chronic hepatitis. It involves bile ducts with an outer diameter of 15 to 40 μm. The abnormal ducts are frequently surrounded by a lymphoid aggregate or follicle and often are not accompanied by a duct. Some represent preexisting ducts undergoing degeneration with swelling, cytoplasmic vacuolization, nuclear pyknosis or karyorrhexis, and infiltration by mononuclear inflammatory cells (Fig. 57-24). The basement membrane is usually not destroyed, and actual destruction of ducts is rare. Some of the abnormal "ducts" are actually composed of cells with an abundant eosinophilic cytoplasm suggestive of metaplasia of duct cells to hepatocytes.[303] Such metaplasia of bile duct cells to hepatocytes has been documented ultrastructurally and immunohistochemically by Nomoto and colleagues.[304]

Periportal fibrosis and associated changes. The usually progressive necroinflammation of piecemeal necrosis in chronic hepatitis is associated with collagenization of spaces of Disse and deposition of basement membrane material, a

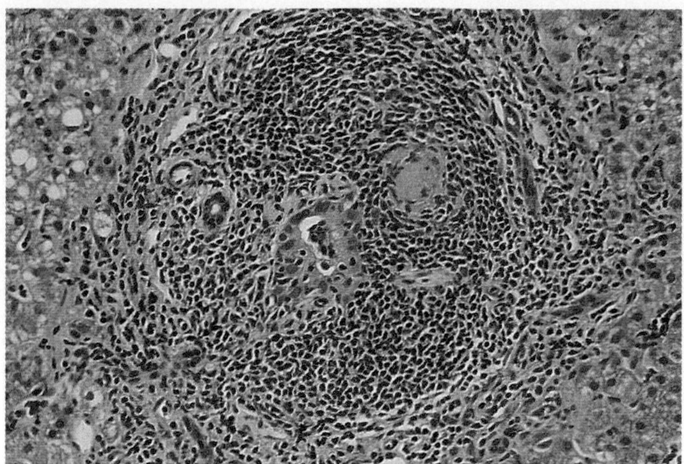

Fig. 57-24 Chronic hepatitis C. Degenerating bile duct is surrounded by a dense infiltrate of lymphocytes.

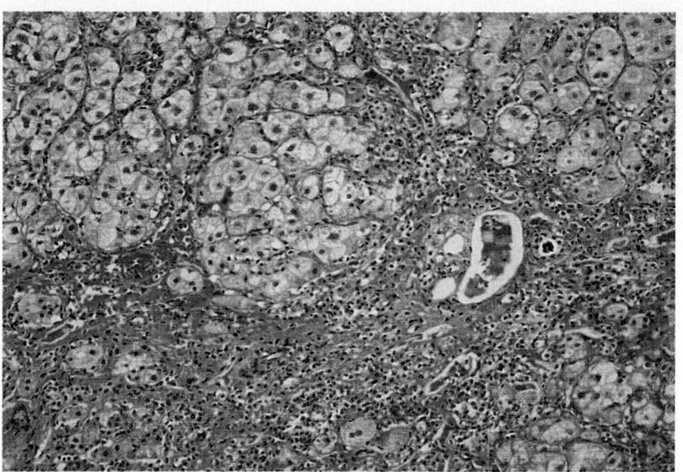

Fig. 57-25 Chronic hepatitis B. Pronounced fibrous expansion of portal areas with bridging. There is considerable portal inflammation and piecemeal necrosis.

process of "capillarization" that was described many years ago by Schaffner and Popper.[305] Central to this process is the extracellular matrix (interstitial and basement membrane collagens, glycoproteins, and proteoglycans) that is greatly increased as a result of synthesis by fat storing (Ito) cells and transitional cells.[306] Initially the fibrosis has a characteristic "stellate" or "arachnoidal" appearance. Capillarization of sinusoids around regenerated, two-cell-thick plates of liver cells leads to "rosette" formation. One group of investigators believes that "hepatic" rosettes are a form of liver cell regeneration.[307] A typical rosette consists of four to six hepatocytes, resting on a basement membrane and fibrous tissue, that surround a small, centrally located canaliculus. Rosetting is believed to be more characteristic of autoimmune than viral chronic hepatitis.[302,308]

As the fibrosis progresses, portal-to-portal fibrous bridges are formed (Fig. 57-25). Central-to-portal (and even central-to-central) fibrous bridges can develop from superimposed episodes of necrosis involving zone 3, as described later. Broad areas of fibrosis can result from the healing in bouts of multiacinar necrosis. Elastic fibers are deposited during healing, in addition to collagen fibers;[309] their presence can be demonstrated by the same stains used for identification of HBsAg in tissue sections, namely, orcein, aldehyde fuchsin, and Victoria blue. The result is the development of cirrhosis, in which the necroinflammatory changes of piecemeal necrosis (now periseptal) can continue unabated.

Intra-acinar lesions. Most instances of chronic hepatitis reveal intra-acinar necroinflammatory changes of variable severity, in addition to periportal piecemeal necrosis. In the typical case they are focal ("spotty") and consist mainly of apoptosis. Scattered apoptotic bodies of varied size are observed, as well as focal necrosis with aggregates of lymphocytes and plasma cells and polesis and emperipolesis. Hypertrophied Kupffer cells that have scavenged the apoptotic bodies and other granular debris are also present in the foci of necrosis. Steatosis, mild to moderate and generally macrovesicular, is now considered typical of chronic hepatitis C, as is noted later. It is an infrequent finding in chronic hepatitis B or in autoimmune chronic hepatitis (unless the patient had been treated with corticosteroids).

Hepatocellular injury in exacerbations and relapses. More severe intra-acinar injury is generally seen in exacerbations and relapses of chronic hepatitis. In chronic hepatitis B these may be spontaneous,[310-317] secondary to withdrawal of cytotoxic or immunosuppressive therapy,[318-320] or associated with delta virus[313,321] or HIV infection.[322,323] In addition to spontaneous exacerbations and relapses after interferon therapy, there is a recent report of reactivation of chronic hepatitis C after withdrawal of immunosuppressive therapy.[324]

Spontaneous flare-ups of chronic hepatitis C may be related to sequence variations of the hypervariable region of HCV.[325] In addition to the clinical and biochemical findings, acute exacerbations of chronic hepatitis B are characterized by increases in serum HBV DNA and IgM anti-HBc titers.[326-328] Villari and colleagues[329] analyzed the histologic features of seven patients with an acute exacerbation of chronic hepatitis B. In all cases, changes typical of acute hepatitis were superimposed on those of chronic hepatitis. In our experience, one or more of the following additional changes can be observed in exacerbations or relapses: (1) an increase in the degree of spotty necrosis, (2) ballooning degeneration, often most severe in zone 3, with dropout of hepatocytes and central-to-central and central-to-portal bridging necrosis that is subsequently followed by fibrosis. Ballooning degeneration may be associated with variable cholestasis; in such cases there is significant periportal cholangiolar proliferation, with infiltration of the cholangioles by neutrophils (acute cholangiolitis), (3) multiacinar necrosis, followed eventually by the formation of irregularly shaped, multiacinar scars.

Until recently, the pathogenesis of the exacerbations in chronic hepatitis has remained unclear. Maruyama and colleagues[330] studied 19 patients with chronic hepatitis B for alterations in HBV DNA, HBsAg, anti-HBc, and HBsAg-specific immune complex formation before, during, and after spontaneous acute exacerbations of liver injury. They found significant correlations between increasing levels of these serum markers and liver injury and suggested that the cyclic injury may reflect increases in HBV replication followed by an increase in the immune responses that mediate the liver injury.

Regeneration. Regeneration is typically seen in the form of two-cell-thick plates (periportal and periseptal) and an increased number of binucleated and trinucleated cells. Mitoses may be present in cases with recent exacerbations or relapses. A high proliferative rate of liver cells was demonstrated by immunohistochemistry for proliferating cell nuclear antigen in chronic viral hepatitis (both B and C) by Nakamura and colleagues.[331]

Cirrhosis. The continuous piecemeal necrosis with resultant periportal fibrosis, and the bridging and multiacinar necrosis with healing by fibrous bridges and irregular scars eventually lead to cirrhosis. Variable degrees of continuing necroinflammatory changes are usually present, and their extent should be noted by the histopathologist. Episodes of gastrointestinal hemorrhage can result in anoxic (coagulative) necrosis. Delta virus superinfection of HBV cirrhosis can lead to extensive necrosis with decompensation and liver failure.[332,333]

The cirrhosis occurring after chronic hepatitis is either macronodular, or mixed macronodular and micronodular in type. Liver cell dysplasia (large or small cell type), adenomatoid hyperplasia, and macroregenerative nodules, when present, should be noted in the histopathologic diagnosis because of their putative preneoplastic significance.[334-341]

Etiologic subtypes of hepatitis

The various etiologic subtypes of chronic hepatitis are compared in Table 57-7.

Chronic Hepatitis B (with or without delta virus). The specific markers of HBV infection, demonstrable by light or electron microscopy or immunohistochemically,[81-82] are of paramount importance in differential diagnosis. Ground-glass cells (Fig. 57-26) that contain HBsAg can be positively identified by special stains (orcein, Victoria blue, or aldehyde fuchsin). The differential diagnosis of ground-glass cells is listed in Table 57-8. Sanded liver cell nuclei caused by excess HBcAg accumulation[80] are difficult to recognize histopathologically. Furthermore, similar nuclei have been seen in HDV.[342] Both HBsAg and HBcAg are readily demonstrable immunohistochemically in liver cells in paraffin sections by commercially available antibodies, as well as in ductular cells[343] (Fig. 57-27).

The expression of pre-S1 and pre-S2 was studied in 44 patients with chronic hepatitis B by Chu and Liaw.[85] All had synthesis and display of the two antigens. Their distribution and quantitative expression were closely related to the status of HBV replication but not to the histologic activity. Concurrent HDV superinfection did not appear to modulate the synthesis and expression of the pre-S peptides in the liver.

Delta antigen can be demonstrated in tissue sections immunohistochemically. The antigen is located mainly in nuclei of liver cells, but there may be occasional cytoplasmic expression. In situ hybridization studies for HBV and HDV have been reviewed recently by Negro and colleagues,[124] as previously noted. Routine assays for serum HBV DNA or liver HBcAg are more sensitive and reliable and less time consuming than in situ hybridization of tissue HBV nucleic acids.[124]

Several viruses have been implicated in superinfections of patients with chronic hepatitis B. They include HAV,[344,345] HDV,[332,346-352] HCV,[353-357] CMV,[358,359] and HIV.[360-364]

Superimposed hepatitis A appears to have no adverse effect on the course of chronic hepatitis B. Superinfection with HDV, on the other hand, is associated with acute exacerbations,[313,321] with a sudden worsening and a fatal outcome,[321] or with more severe and progressive chronic liver disease.[332,348,351,352] However, in one study of 30 patients with chronic B hepatitis from Taiwan, HDV superinfection was not particularly different from spontaneous acute exacerbations, and the progression of the disease was slow.[365] In general, most experts agree that the degree of degeneration and necrosis is greater in delta-positive than in delta-negative chronic hepatitis B. The prognosis appears to depend to some extent on the individual immune response;[350] it is much poorer in drug addicts than in nonad-

Table 57-7 Etiology and histologic features of chronic hepatitis

Etiology	Distinctive histologic features
Viral hepatitis	
Hepatitis B virus	Ground-glass cells: "sanded" nuclei: positive immunohistochemical stains for HBsAg and HBcAg; core and surface antigen particles in liver cell nuclei and cytoplasm respectively (electron microscopy)
Hepatitis C virus	Bile duct degeneration; lymphoid aggregates and follicles; steatosis
Drug injury	
Isoniazid, methyldopa, oxyphenisatin, nitrofurantoin, dantrolene, diclofenac, and others	None
Inherited metabolic disease	
Wilson's disease	Copper accumulation in liver cells; Mallory bodies (zone 1); steatosis; glycogenated nuclei; heterogeneity of mitochondria with separation of inner and outer membranes of cristae (electron microscopy)
α_1-antitrypsin deficiency	Eosinophilic PAS-positive globules in liver cells: positive immunocytochemical stains for α_1-antitrypsin; amorphous inclusions in endoplasmic reticulum (electron microscopy)
Autoimmune	Rosettes; many plasma cells; giant hepatocytes
Idiopathic	None

dicts.[346] Occasionally, some patients may clear both hepatitis B and delta infections after delta virus superinfection.[347]

Double infections with HBV and HCV have been reported by several groups of investigators.[353-357] The chronic infections with the two viruses can be acquired simultaneously or at different times. Coinfection with both viruses has been documented in at least one study of posttransfusion hepatitis[357] An inverse relation between HBV and HCV replication was found in a study of 55 patients with double infections by Pontisso and colleagues.[355] Liver disease activity was generally milder in patients with an active HCV infection and inactive HBV status, an indication that HBV replication might be more harmful than HCV replication in that particular subgroup of patients.

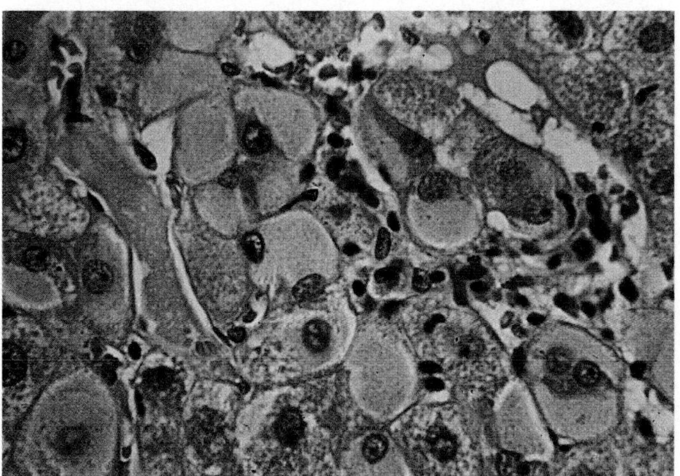

Fig. 57-26 Ground-glass cells in liver of HBsAg carrier.

CMV infection superimposed on HBsAg-positive chronic hepatitis can lead to a fatal outcome.[358,359]

As already noted, HIV infection can result in reactivation of hepatitis B. In HIV and HBV coinfection the liver disease (biochemically and histologically) tends to be less severe with less fibrosis than in HIV-negative HBV carriers. HIV superinfection of an HBV carrier is also associated with less liver inflammation and decreased aminotransferase values, though viral replication is increased.[360,361] Immunohistochemically, many more HBe-positive and HBc-positive hepatocytic nuclei are seen, resembling the findings in patients on immunosuppressive drugs; there is a negative correlation with histopathologic disease activity.[360]

Chronic hepatitis C. The histopathologic features of chronic hepatitis C have been delineated in a recent flurry of publications from several countries.[366-370] The studies leading to these publications were made possible by the commercial availability of serologic tests for diagnosis of HCV infection. Earlier reports of detailed studies of NANB hepatitis in hemophiliacs and other patients had, however, accurately described most of the changes now considered characteristic of chronic hepatitis C.[371,372] In 1987 Bianchi and colleagues[371] found that steatosis, sinusoidal inflammatory infiltrates, prominence of Kupffer cells, lymphoid follicle formation, and bile duct epithelial changes were histologic features favoring chronic NANB hepatitis. Similar observations were made by Lefkowitch and Apfelbaum[372] in 1989. Varying degrees of all these features were described in the recently reported studies of chronic hepatitis C (Table 57-9). Bile duct loss was reported in only one study,[367] and the presence of Mallory body-like material in another.[369] Of all the lesions in chronic hepatitis C, the most characteristic (but not always present or pathognomonic) are the lymphoid aggregates and follicles, bile duct damage, and the steatosis (Figs. 57-24 and 57-28). It must be emphasized at

Table 57-8 Ground-glass cells in viral hepatitis and other conditions

Location	PAS	Orcein, Aldehyde Fuchsin, Victoria Blue	Ultrastructure	Diagnosis
			Nonneoplastic liver	
Haphazard	–	+	SER* proliferation and tubular or round HBsAg particles	HBsAg carrier without clinical disease or with chronic hepatitis, or cirrhosis
Acinar zone 3 or panacinar	–	–	SER proliferation	Drug-induced change (such as phenobarbital, diphenylhydantoin, chlorpromazine)
Acinar zone 1	+	–	Non-membrane bound secondary lysosomes, degenerating organelles, glycogen and lipid droplets	Drug-induced injury from cyanamide
	+	–	Fibrillar non-membrane bound material and glycogen	Type IV glycogenosis
	+	–	Large aggregates of SER and glycogen	Lafora's disease
			Neoplastic liver	
Haphazard	–	–	Amorphous cytoplasmic material (fibrinogen)	Hepatocellular carcinoma, fibrolamellar type
	–	+	SER proliferation and tubular or round HBsAg particles	Hepatocellular carcinoma

**SER*, Smooth endoplasmic reticulum.

this point that the fundamental lesions of chronic hepatitis, as described in an earlier section, that is, the diffuse portal inflammation, piecemeal necrosis, spotty necrosis and apoptosis, and the sequelae of the necroinflammation (periportal fibrosis, bridging fibrosis, and cirrhosis), are all an integral part of the morphologic continuum of chronic hepatitis C. Indeed, it is these latter features that must be relied on for the diagnosis of chronic hepatitis C, since bile duct lesions and lymphoid aggregates have been described in acute hepatitis C.[199] A recent study has shown an interesting correlation between the mode of transmission of HCV and severity of the chronic hepatitis.[373] Thus, transfusion-acquired hepatitis C was found to be associated with more aggressive histologic inflammatory activity than hepatitis resulting from intravenous drug use. In this context it is worth noting that in another recent study the prevalence of hepatitis C in injecting drug abusers was 86%.[374]

Immunohistochemical studies of the lymphoid aggregates and follicles in chronic hepatitis C have been noted in an earlier section. HLA-DR expression in bile ducts undergoing damage was studied by Danque and colleagues.[375] In that study, HLA-DR was not detected in any of 30 liver biopsy specimens from patients with chronic hepatitis C, 90% of whom had histologic evidence of bile duct damage. It was concluded that the mechanism of bile duct injury in chronic hepatitis C must be different from that of other liver diseases with bile duct damage that do express HLA-DR antigen, such as PBC, PSC, graft-versus-host disease and allograft rejection. Similar conclusions were arrived at in another study by Broome and colleagues,[376] who found HLA-DR expression on biliary epithelium in PBC and PSC but not in those with chronic hepatitis C or alcoholic cirrhosis or normal controls. In a recent study by Chu and colleagues,[377] the genomic and replicative HCV RNA sequences were correlated with the histologic activity of chronic hepatitis C. It was concluded that a direct viropathic effect is less important than other mechanisms (such as the host immune response) in the pathogenesis of hepatocyte and bile duct injury in chronic hepatitis C.[377]

PCR has been used to detect HCV RNA in sera or liver tissue (fresh or paraffin embedded) by several groups of investigators.[378-380] Immunohistochemistry has been successfully utilized to detect HCV antigens in fresh frozen,[381-383] or paraffin-embedded tissue.[384] HCV RNA has been demonstrated in liver tissue by in situ hybridization[385-387] and more recently by in situ PCR.[388,389] In all cases the HCV antigens have been located in the cytoplasm of liver cells. Immunoelectron microscopy in one study revealed HCV-N35 antigen along the endoplasmic reticulum.[383]

Autoimmune chronic hepatitis. A new classification of autoimmune hepatitis was recently proposed by Stechemesser and colleagues.[390] It includes three different subgroups: *type 1a,* lupoid hepatitis (antinuclear antibody positive, with or without actin antibody); *type 1b,* only actin antibody positive; *type 2,* liver-kidney microsomal antibody positive; *type 3,* liver-pancreas antibody positive (with or without other autoantibodies). There are no histologic features that reliably distinguish autoimmune chronic hepatitis from chronic hepatitis B, other than the specific markers of HBV infection in the latter (such as ground-glass cells and the demonstration of surface or core antigen by various techniques). Dienes[391,392] believes that hypocellular areas of collapse and microacinus formation (rosettes) are suggestive of autoimmune chronic hepatitis. A predominance of plasma cells in portal areas is characteristic of autoimmune chronic hepatitis, being most helpful in distinguishing it from chronic hepatitis C in which the predominant cell is the lymphocyte. However, an abundance of plasma cells can be found in chronic hepatitis B and some cases of drug-induced chronic hepatitis. Bach and colleagues[367] recently compared autoimmune chronic hepatitis with chronic hepatitis

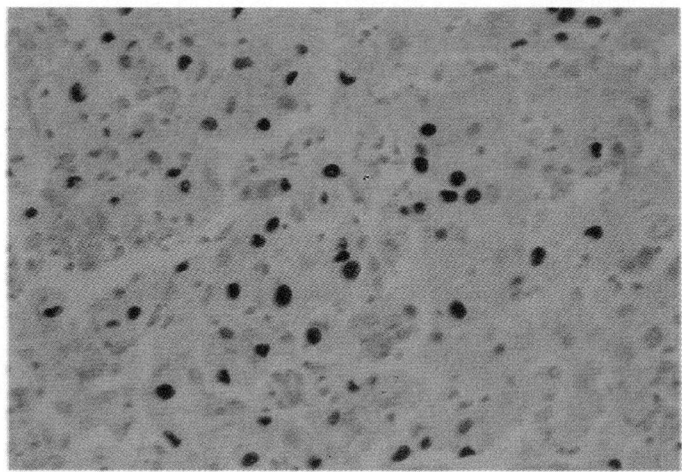

Fig. 57-27 Expression of HBcAg in nuclei of liver cells *(brown)* is demonstrated by anti-HBcAg immunostain.

Table 57-9 Histopathology of chronic hepatitis C

Lesion	Authors (% change)				
	Scheuer[366]	Bach et al[367]	Gerber et al[368]	Lefkowitch et al[369]	Roberts et al[370]
Bile duct damage	22.2	91.0	76.0	31.2	25.4
Bile duct loss	0	91.0	0	0	0
Lymphoid aggregates and follicles	78.0	49.0	45.0	49.4	68.2
Steatosis	53.7	72.0	31.0	68.9	42.9
Mallory bodies	0	0	0	17.6	0

Data from Scheuer PJ, Ashrafzadeh P, Sherlock S et al: *Hepatology* 15: 567, 1992; Bach N, Thung SN, Schaffner F: *Hepatology* 15: 572, 1992; Gerber MA, Krawczynski K, Alter MJ et al: *Mod Pathol* 5: 483, 1992; Lefkowitch JH, Schiff ER, Davis GL et al: *Gastroenterology* 104: 595, 1993; Roberts JM, Searle JW, Coolesley WGE: *Gastroenterol Jpn* 28: 901, 1993.

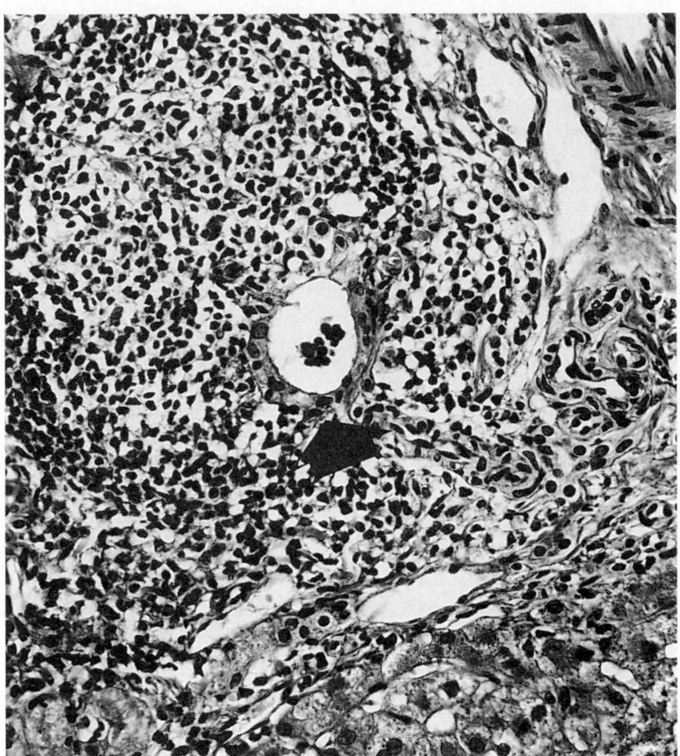

Fig. 57-28 Bile duct damage in viral hepatitis C.

C. They found that severe intra-acinar necrosis and inflammation, piecemeal necrosis, multinucleated hepatocytes, and broad areas of parenchymal collapse were seen more often in autoimmune chronic hepatitis than in chronic hepatitis C (in which bile duct damage, steatosis, and lymphoid aggregates were more common).

It is important to mention briefly that anti-HCV has been detected in one subtype of autoimmune chronic hepatitis, type 2, which is characterized by liver-kidney microsomal (LKM-1) antibodies.[393-398] Autoantibodies to cytosol antigen type 1 appear to be a more specific marker for autoimmune chronic hepatitis type 2 than anti-LKM-1 autoantibodies are.[399] Several groups of investigators have concluded that HCV might be directly responsible for the development of type 2 (anti-LKM-1 positive) autoimmune chronic hepatitis in genetically predisposed persons.[394,396,397] Up to now, no histopathologic differences between the various subtypes of autoimmune chronic hepatitis have emerged.

Multinucleated giant cells have been reported in some cases of autoimmune chronic hepatitis, other disorders with autoimmune features, and numerous hepatotropic viral infections.[400-410] The terms *postinfantile giant cell hepatitis*,[403] *syncytial giant cell hepatitis*,[405] and *postinfantile giant cell transformation in hepatitis*[406] have been used to identify such cases. Phillips and colleagues[405] reported 10 patients, four with subacute hepatic failure and six with severe chronic hepatitis. Electron microscopy revealed structures resembling *Paramyxovirus* nucleocapsids, and it was suggested that the virus could be the cause of the liver disease. Two subsequent series[406,407] have questioned the conclusions of Phillips and colleagues[405] that postinfantile liver disease with giant cell transformation is a single entity or that it always carries an ominous prognosis. In the series of Devaney and colleagues[406] the most frequently identified association was with autoimmune disease. A recently reported case associated with anti-M2 mitochondrial antibodies supports that association.[410] Corticosteroid therapy has led to clinical, biochemical, and histologic improvement in some cases.[409]

Cryptogenic chronic hepatitis. The label *cryptogenic chronic hepatitis* (as well as its end-stage, *cryptogenic cirrhosis*) has been used in the past as a catch-all term for chronic necroinflammatory disease of unknown cause. Many such cases now have been shown to be related to hepatitis C. Thus 18% of cases of cryptogenic chronic hepatitis studied at the Mayo Clinic were found to be anti-HCV positive.[411] In another study from the United Kingdom, 67% of cases of cryptogenic chronic liver disease had hepatitis C nucleocapsid antibodies.[412] In a third study from Spain, 82% of cases of cryptogenic chronic hepatitis were anti-HCV positive.[413] Cases not attributable to hepatitis C are infrequently associated with autoantibodies, an indication that cryptogenic cirrhosis may be distinct from autoimmune liver disease.[414] However, in a recent comparative study of 12 patients with cryptogenic hepatitis and 94 patients with autoimmune hepatitis, Czaja and colleagues[415] found no differences in clinical expression, genetic phenotype, and corticosteroid responsiveness between the two groups. They concluded that cryptogenic hepatitis may be an autoimmune disorder that has escaped detection by conventional immunoserologic markers.[415] Histopathologically, there are no characteristic features of "true" cryptogenic hepatitis or cirrhosis; the cirrhosis is generally inactive with little inflammation.[414]

Chronic hepatitis and alcohol. The combined effects of alcoholism and infection with either HBV or HCV have interested clinical investigators for many years.[416,417] Space does not permit more than a few comments about this important topic. The morphologic changes of chronic alcoholic hepatitis are characteristic and not likely to be confused with chronic hepatitis.[53,249,250] Changes that should implicate a viral cause for chronic hepatitis in the alcoholic who shows the presence of HBsAg[418] or anti-HCV[419-421] include piecemeal necrosis and lymphoplasmacytic portal and parenchymal inflammation. In cases with HCV infection, Freni and colleagues[422] found that there is close contact of cytotoxic T-cells to hepatocytes expressing class I HLA in areas of periportal and intra-acinar necrosis. Needless to say, the serologic tests for hepatitis B and C markers and the biochemical findings (in particular the GGT and the AST/ALT ratio) are critical in differential diagnosis.

Drug-induced chronic hepatitis. Many drugs have been incriminated in the causation of chronic hepatitis.[423-427] They have included acetaminophen, aspirin, amineptine, clometacine, dantrolene, diclofenac, fenofibrate, glafenine, isoniazid, isoxonine, methyldopa, nitrofurantoin, oxyphenisatin, papaverine, pemoline, perhexilene maleate, propylthiouracil, sulfonamides, ticrynafen, and tolazamide. Although this list appears lengthy, only one or two instances were reported with some of the drugs. Furthermore, many of the older reports antedated the discovery of HCV, making at least some suspect. Histopathologic differences between drug-induced and other types of chronic hepatitis (other than the specific or distinctive features of chronic hepatitis B or C) have not been forthcoming. In the case of some drugs, such as nitrofurantoin, serologic "autoimmune" markers may be demonstrable,[427] thus raising the possibility that the drugs could have triggered an autoimmune chronic hepatitis.

Chronic hepatitis associated with the inherited metabolic diseases. Chronic hepatitis is a recognized stage in the evolution of the liver disease in Wilson's disease.[428-430] It should always be considered in differential diagnosis of chronic hepatitis in a young person. Helpful histopathologic clues include steatosis, glycogenated nuclei in zone 1, cytochemically demonstrable copper accumulation, presence of Mallory's bodies in periportal liver cells (in the absence of other features of cholestasis), and clusters of oxyphil hepatocytes; these changes are in addition to the other features that are found in all cases of chronic hepatitis (piecemeal necrosis, portal inflammation, and so forth) regardless of cause. The ultrastructural changes, particularly the pleomorphism of mitochondria and widening of their intercristal spaces, are pathognomonic of Wilson's disease.

Chronic hepatitis was reported in heterozygotes (MZ phenotype) with α_1-antitrypsin deficiency by Hodges and colleagues,[431] in 1981. Recently, Propst and colleagues[432] found that most instances of chronic hepatitis in adults with homozygous and heterozygous α_1-antitrypsin deficiency that they studied were related to hepatotropic viruses (80% had HCV infection) or other risk factors (such as autoimmune hepatitis).

Nomenclature of chronic hepatitis

Several recent editorials and reviews have called for abandoning the widely used division of chronic hepatitis into CPH, CAH, and CLH; using one designation for chronic necroinflammatory disease—*chronic hepatitis,* with varying degrees of *activity,* and emphasizing the *cause.*[433-439] The need for reassessment of the existing classification is the extensive experience gained from morphologic studies of all types of chronic hepatitis, in particular hepatitis C, the availability of new drugs (such as interferon) for treatment of chronic viral hepatitis, and the long-term follow-up studies that have shown a discordance between the prognosis and the histologic subtype of chronic necroinflammatory disease of the liver. The histopathologic state at any given time in the course of a patient's illness is no more than a "snapshot" that can change from CPH to CLH to CAH, depending on the natural course of the disease (quiescent phase versus reactivations or relapses), therapy, superinfection with other viral agents, underlying genetic diseases (such as α_1-antitrypsin deficiency and hepatitis C), or modifying disorders (such as alcoholism). Sampling error may also lead to an erroneous subcategorization of the chronic liver disease in different biopsy specimens, even when they are obtained at the same time or within close intervals of time. Scheuer[433] has commented that, from the point of view of treatment, the separation of CPH from mild CAH is fundamentally unsound and ethically unacceptable; it betrays misunderstanding of the evolution of chronic hepatitis and may deprive patients of effective treatment. Scoring systems for the degree of activity of chronic hepatitis, and the stage of the disease (resulting from fibrosis and cirrhosis) are listed in Tables 57-10 and 57-11.

Table 57-10 Degree of activity in chronic hepatitis

	Lesions and degree of injury			
Category	**Portal area inflammation**	**Piecemeal necrosis**	**Spotty necrosis**	**Bridging or multiacinar necrosis, or both**
Mild	Mild, patchy	Absent or mild	Mild	Absent
Moderate	Moderate	Moderate	Moderate	Absent
Pronounced	Pronounced	Pronounced	Pronounced	Absent
Severe	Severe	Severe	Severe	Present

Table 57-11 Degree of fibrosis in chronic hepatitis

	Component lesions		
Category	**Fibrous expansion of portal areas**	**Bridging fibrosis***	**Bridging with nodules (cirrhosis)**
Mild	Absent of mild	Absent	Absent
Moderate	Moderate	Absent†	Absent
Pronounced	Pronounced	Pronounced	Absent‡
Severe	Severe	Severe	Present

*Bridging fibrosis can be portal, portal to zone 3 (central), or zone 3 to zone 3.
†Occasional bridging may be present.
‡Occasional nodule may be present ("incomplete cirrhosis").

CHOLESTASIS

Extrahepatic biliary obstruction

Lesions that can cause mechanical obstruction of bile flow include choledocholithiasis, neoplasms (benign and malignant), strictures (neoplastic, inflammatory, postoperative), sclerosing cholangitis, pancreatitis, choledochal cysts, pancreatic pseudocysts, biliary atresia, and several parasitic diseases (such as ascariasis, fascioliasis). Extrinsic pressure by enlarged lymph nodes, tumors, aneurysms, and so forth can also lead to obstruction of bile flow.

The occurrence of cholestasis depends on the degree of obstruction; it is not usually found in the absence of obvious or complete obstruction. Acinar zone 3 and sometimes zone 2 are the first to be affected by cholestasis (Fig. 57-29). Zone 3 hepatocytes can show slight pleomorphism (unrest). Cholangiolar proliferation and acute cholangiolitis are common though not specific findings. There can be edema and neutrophilic infiltration of the portal tracts. The epithelium of the intra-acinar bile ducts can show irregularity, hyperplasia, or edema, or all three. Bile plugs are sometimes present in bile duct lumens. Severe acute cholangitis occasionally is complicated by rupture with development of abscesses in the region of the affected bile ducts (cholangitic abscesses) (Fig. 57-30). Remnants of the disrupted biliary epithelium, bile, and mucin are often located within the abscesses. Xanthomatous cells and foreign-body giant cells with phagocytosed bile may also be present. Bile lakes (bile extravasates) (Fig. 57-31) and bile infarcts are of limited diagnostic significance, since they are seen only in advanced cases.

Any combination of the above findings can be suggestive of biliary obstruction, but the most reliable diagnostic findings are the presence of acute cholangitis, plugs of bile in the ducts, or bile staining of ductal epithelium.[440] Choledocholithiasis is more likely to produce cholangitis; the degree of cholestasis is highly variable. Acute suppurative cholangitis has also been reported with choledochal sludge.[441] Pronounced cholestasis with minimal or no cholangitis is likely to be associated with neoplastic obstruction of the biliary tree.

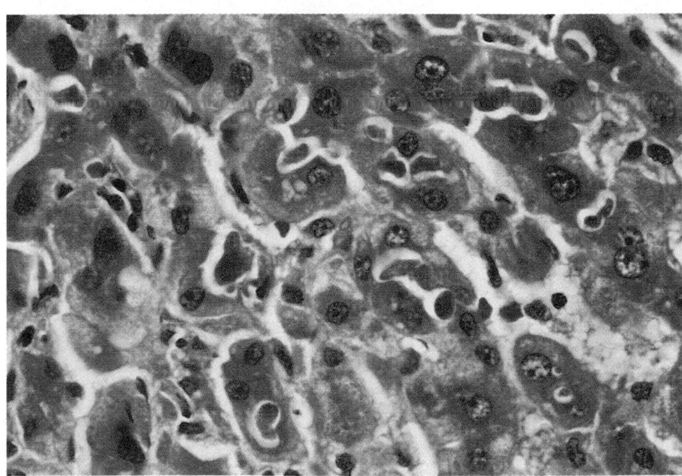

Fig. 57-29 Canalicular cholestasis in zone 3.

Although an acute cholangitis most often denotes extrahepatic biliary tract disease with an ascending infection, rare nonobstructive causes should be mentioned. They include heatstroke,[442] toxic shock syndrome[443] (Fig. 57-32), Kawasaki disease,[444] several toxins (paraquat, methylene diamine, and the toxin of toxic oil syndrome), and numerous drugs, such as chlorpropamide, chlorpromazine, and allopurinol.

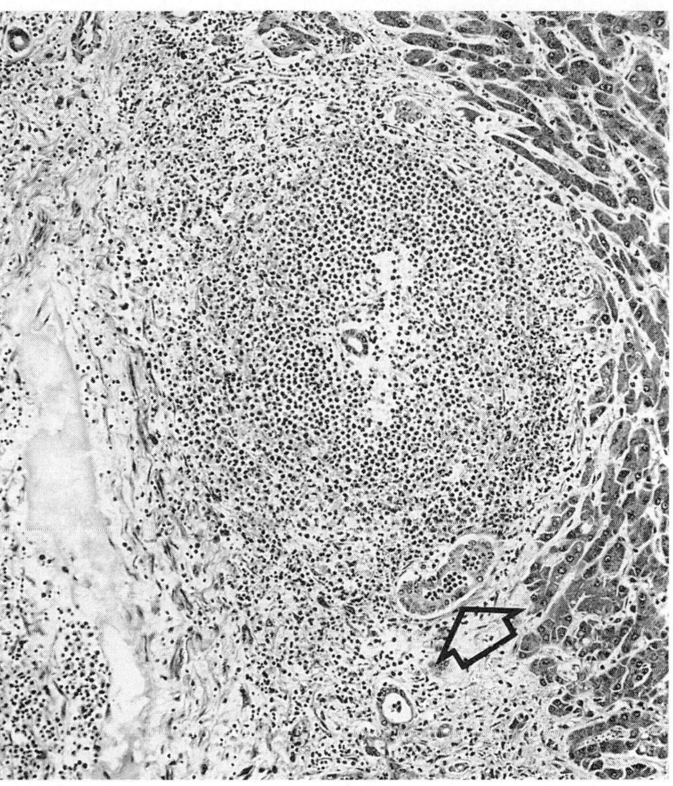

Fig. 57-30 Cholangitic abscess in portal area in patient with choledocholithiasis. Notice suppurative cholangitis in adjacent bile duct *(arrow)*.

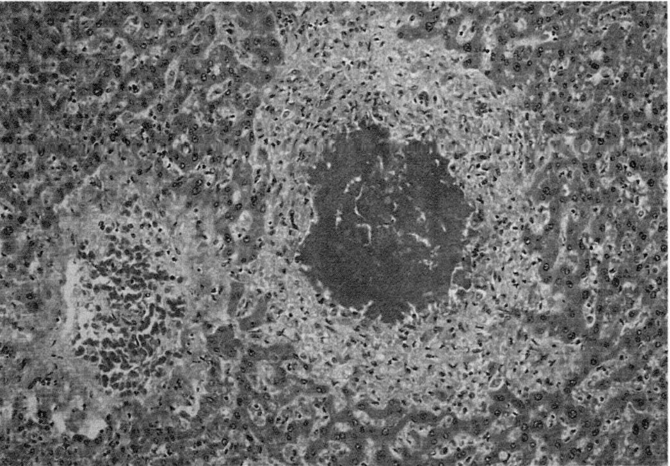

Fig. 57-31 Bile lake in patient with extrahepatic biliary obstruction from carcinoma of the head of the pancreas. Darkly stained bile is surrounded by xanthomatous cells.

Acute intrahepatic cholestasis

Many disorders, including alcoholic liver disease, drug-induced hepatotoxicity, viral hepatitis (see later section), and various developmental and metabolic diseases can be associated with intrahepatic cholestasis. Their clinical and morphologic features are usually distinct from those of biliary obstruction.

Bacterial sepsis can lead to intrahepatic cholestasis.[445,446] The tissue hallmark of sepsis is the presence of bile plugs in dilated cholangioles (ductular cholestasis). The cholangioles can also be surrounded and infiltrated by neutrophils. Intra-acinar cholestasis is present, but the bile ducts appear histologically normal.

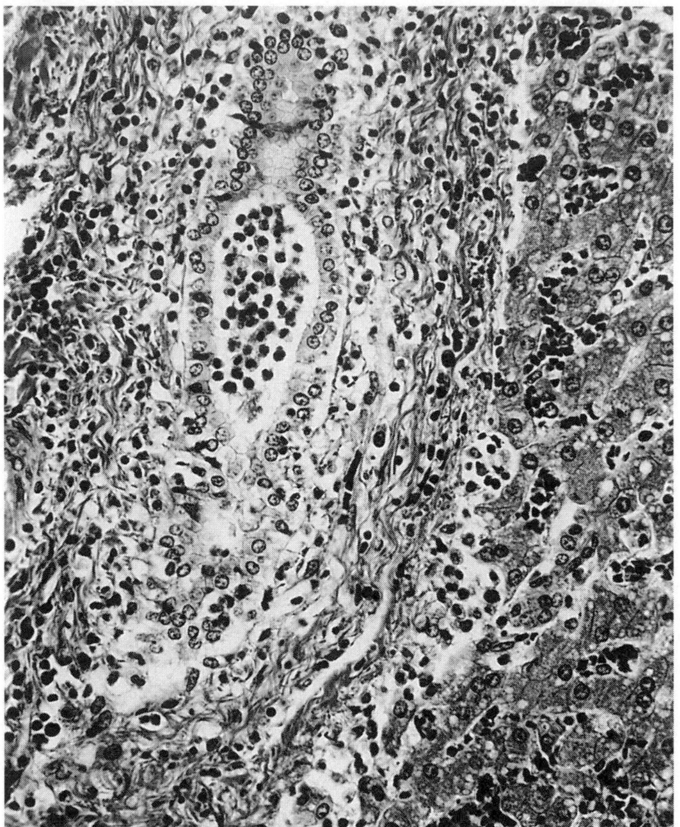

Fig. 57-32 Acute cholangitis in patient with toxic shock syndrome.

Many drugs can be complicated by intrahepatic cholestasis[447-450] (Table 57-12). An associated hepatocellular injury helps to differentiate the drug-induced changes from biliary obstruction. The cholestasis of anabolic and contraceptive steroids, however, is unaccompanied by hepatocellular injury of more than minimal degree.[451]

Certain drugs can produce a cholestatic syndrome that resembles obstructive jaundice. Example of such drugs are chlorpromazine and its derivatives, erythromycin, allopurinol, phenylbutazone, and chlorpropamide. Other than the clinical setting, the histologic findings that help to rule out biliary obstruction include one or more of the following: (1) the frequent finding of mild hepatocellular injury; (2) the absence of bile in ducts; (3) modestly elevated transaminase values; (4) morphologic features of hepatocellular injury; (5) tissue eosinophilia; (6) noncaseating granulomas. However, it should be remembered that some drugs, in addition to causing a cholestatic or combined cholestatic and hepatocellular injury, can also lead to an associated acute cholangitis; examples include chlorpromazine, chlorpropamide, allopurinol, and trimethoprim-sulfamethoxazole.

Benign recurrent cholestasis is a familial disorder characterized by recurrent bouts of cholestasis, usually starting before 30 years of age, that are self-limited and not followed by fibrosis or cirrhosis.[452-455] Studies by Minuk and Shaffer[454] suggest that the condition is secondary to an intrinsic abnormality in hepatocyte bile salt secretion. Biopsy specimens show moderate to pronounced cholestasis and little or no hepatocellular injury. Similar findings are noted in the syndrome of recurrent jaundice of pregnancy.[456]

Chronic cholestasis

Bile that is chronically retained in the lumen of canaliculi, cholangioles, and intra-acinar bile ducts undergoes inspissation and lamination, presumably as a result of absorption of water. In chronic cholestatic conditions, bile stasis tends to be mainly

Table 57-12 Drugs associated with acute cholestasis

Drug category	Examples
Anabolic and androgenic steroids	Methyltestosterone, fluoxymesterone
Contraceptive steroids	Estradiol, mestranol
Tranquilizers	Chlorpromazine, fluophenazine, mepazine, perphenazine, prochlorpenazine, thioridazine, trifluoperazine, chlordiazepoxide, diazepam
Antidepressants	Amitriptyline, imipramine, iprindole
Analgesics and drugs used in musculoskeletal diseases	Naproxen, propoxyphene hydrochloride, gold salts
Drugs used in cardiovascular diseases	Methyldopa, ajmaline, disopyramide
Diuretics	Furosemide, chlorothiazide, hydrochlorothiazide
Antimicrobials	Erythromycin estolate or succinate, penicillins, oleandomycin, trimethoprim-sulfamethoxazole, sulfones, nitrofurantoin
Oral hypoglycemics	Acetohexamide, tolbutamide, chlorpropamide
Antithyroid drugs	Methimazole, carbimazole
Immunosuppressive and antineoplastic drugs	6-Mercaptopurine, azathioprine
Miscellaneous	Warfarin, D-penicillamine, nicotinic acid, total parenteral nutrition

periportal. The lipid component of bile accumulates in the cytoplasm of liver cells (often around dilated canaliculi) and Kupffer cells, leading to pseudoxanthomatous and xanthomatous transformation respectively. Affected cells display a foamy, bile-tinged cytoplasm and pyknotic nuclei. Accumulation of copper in periportal liver cells, as well as the formation of Mallory bodies, is characteristic of chronic cholestasis. Bile lakes are a late manifestation of extrahepatic biliary obstruction. Other changes seen in chronic cholestasis include variable cholangiolar proliferation, periportal fibrosis with portal to portal linkage, and eventually a micronodular biliary cirrhosis.

Many of the diseases leading to chronic cholestasis are associated with a loss of bile ducts. In extrahepatic biliary atresia, the destruction of bile ducts can continue despite satisfactory bile drainage after hepatoportoenterostomy.[457,458] A sharp reduction of bile ducts is the hallmark of paucity of the intrahepatic bile ducts, which may be syndromic (arteriohepatic dysplasia; Alagille's syndrome) or nonsyndromic.[459-463] Cholangiodestructive lesions have been observed in early childhood in patients with arteriohepatic dysplasia, and the loss of bile ducts appears to be progressive.[460,461,463] Distinctive ultrastructural changes involving the Golgi apparatus of liver cells have been reported.[462] Nonsyndromic paucity of bile ducts can occur in adults and has been referred to as "idiopathic adulthood ductopenia."[464,465]

Reduction in the number of intrahepatic bile ducts has also been reported after intrauterine CMV infection[466,467] and in α_1-antitrypsin deficiency,[468] coprostanic acidemia,[469,470] and several other rare developmental syndromes.

Progressive familial cholestatic disorders, not specifically associated with reduction of bile ducts, include some that are well characterized, such as Byler's disease[471-475] and the familial cholestasis of North American Indians[476,477] and Greenland Eskimo children,[478] and others that are not.[479,480] These disorders usually culminate in cirrhosis; Byler's syndrome has also been complicated rarely by hepatocellular carcinoma.[472,474]

The two major chronic cholestatic disorders of adults are primary biliary cholangitis and primary sclerosing cholangitis.

Primary biliary cirrhosis

The characteristic clinical and laboratory features of and disorders associated with PBC are discussed in several reviews.[481-483] Fatigue and pruritus are the most frequent initial presentations. Approximately 80% of patients are women, usually 40 years of age or older. About half the patients are asymptomatic and are discovered incidentally because of cholestatic liver chemical analysis. Increased values of the serum alkaline phosphatase and gamma-glutamyltransferase (GGT) are characteristic. An increased titer of antimitochondrial antibody (AMA) that is greater than 1:40 is seen in more than 90% of patients. When symptoms are present, they include easy fatigability and pruritus. Hepatosplenomegaly, hyperbilirubinemia, signs of portal hypertension, and stigmas of chronic liver disease are later manifestations. The mean survival is about 12 years. Many patients with end-stage disease have now undergone successful liver transplantation.

Histopathologic features of PBC are described by many investigators.[484-487] As with biliary obstruction, particular attention to the condition of the intra-acinar bile ducts is critical in histologic evaluation. Affected ducts show variable chronic inflammation and destruction (chronic nonsuppurative destructive cholangitis) (Fig. 57-33). Histometric and serial-section observations have shown that the small ducts with a lumen diameter less than 70 to 80 μm are the ones destroyed in this disease.[488] Lymphocytes and plasma cells penetrate the basement membrane and wedge themselves between the epithelial cells, and there is destruction of epithelial cells. Segments of the basement membrane are simultaneously destroyed, a change best demonstrated with a PAS-stained section. Lymphoid follicles can be found around or adjacent to the degenerating bile ducts. Epithelioid granulomas are located in the portal areas, or less often in the parenchyma, in about one fourth of the cases.

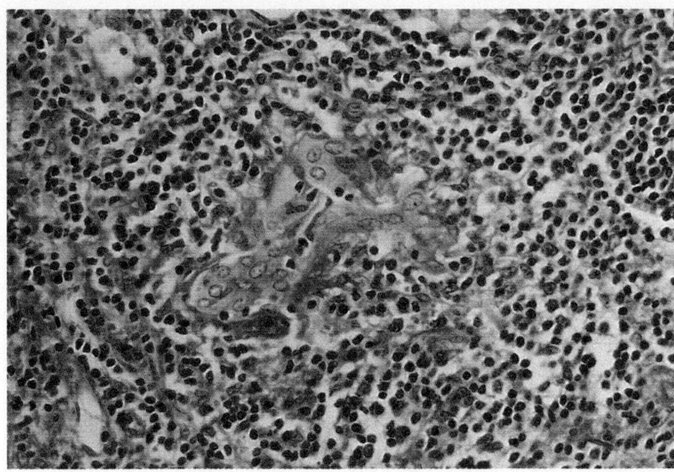

Fig. 57-33 Primary biliary cirrhosis. Distorted and degenerated bile duct is surrounded by many inflammatory cells.

Chronic nonsuppurative destructive cholangitis is considered pathognomonic of PBC. The degree of cholangitis varies greatly from one portal tract to another; some ducts can appear completely normal, whereas others exhibit striking inflammation or even complete destruction. Thus the active diagnostic lesion can be absent in small biopsy samples, and the pathologist is then compelled to apply other criteria and clinical data to the evaluation.

In most patients with PBC, more than half the portal tracts lack bile ducts (Fig. 57-34), in contrast to persons without PBC who have one or more bile ducts in 87% or more of portal tracts.[484] Also helpful is the frequent presence of periportal cholestasis and foci of pseudoxanthomatous change (Fig. 57-35). Small to moderate amounts of copper-binding protein (stainable with Victoria blue or orcein) and copper (specifically stained with rhodanine) (Fig. 57-36) are detected frequently in hepatocytes in the periportal area. Cholangiolar proliferation can be prominent in PBC, particularly in portal areas that lack bile ducts. Hepatocytes are relatively spared in PBC, though in advanced cases periportal "biliary" piecemeal necrosis, followed by fibrosis and nodular regeneration, can develop. Periportal Mallory bodies are found in about a fourth of the cases.[485] Fibrous linkage of portal tracts can result in a micronodular biliary cirrhosis.

As mentioned in an earlier section, some cases of chronic hepatitis, particularly chronic hepatitis C, show degenerative changes of the intra-acinar bile ducts. The changes can at times be suggestive of the diagnosis of PBC; in chronic hepatitis, however, lymphocytic piecemeal necrosis is typi-

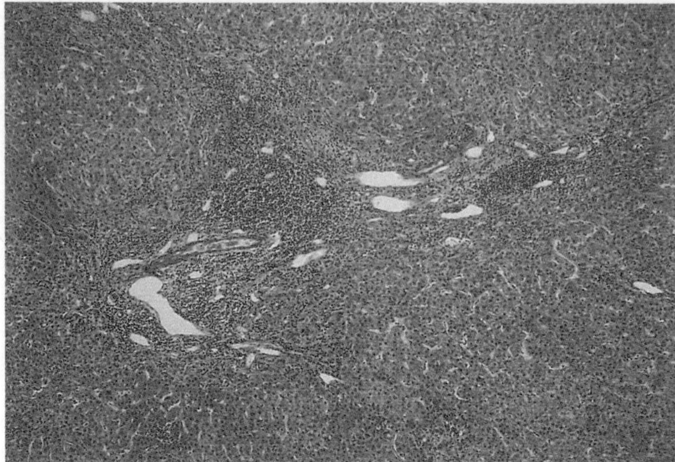

Fig. 57-34 Primary biliary cirrhosis. Late stage of the disease is characterized by pronounced ductopenia. Two fibrotically expanded portal areas are bridged by fibrous tissue and show moderate inflammation.

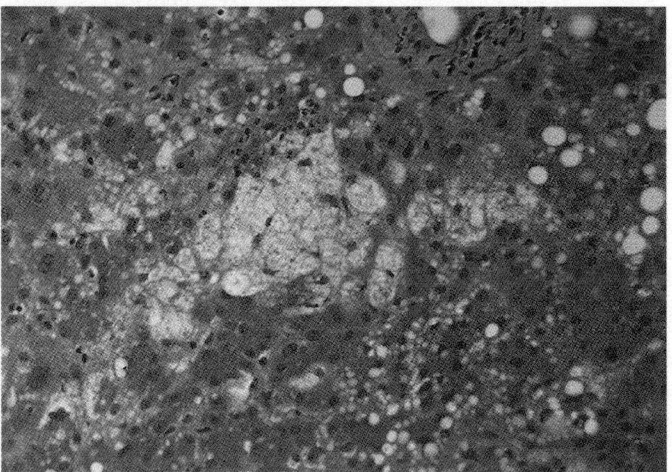

Fig. 57-35 Primary biliary cirrhosis. Clusters of xanthomatous cells in dilated sinusoids.

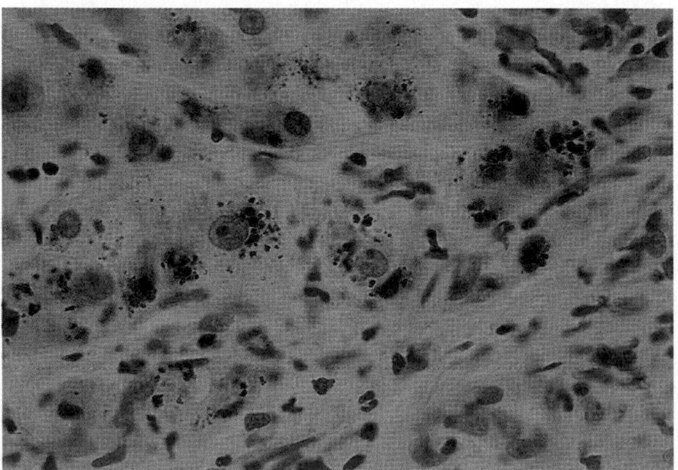

Fig. 57-36 Primary biliary cirrhosis. Copper accumulation *(red granules)* in periportal hepatocytes. (Rhodanine stain.)

cally more prominent, and chronic cholestasis does not develop. There is no ductopenia. Although the two diseases can usually be distinguished, occasional "mixed forms" may show features of both;[489] differentiation of the mixed forms by the use of different types of AMA is discussed by Berg and colleagues.[490] Another entity, referred to as *immunocholangitis,* or *autoimmune cholangitis,* has similar histologic features to those of PBC, but the AMA test results are negative.[491-496] Instead, antinuclear antibodies are present, often in high titer.

It is important to correlate the biochemical and serologic data with the histopathologic features for the diagnosis of PBC. Information of value would include a positive AMA test, greatly increased serum alkaline phosphatase activity, and elevated serum cholesterol and IgM values. The AMAs recognize the central, E2 components of the 2-oxo-acid dehydrogenase complexes. The major antigen is the core enzyme of the mitochondrial inner membrane pyruvate dehydrogenase complex, dihydrolipoamide acetyltransferase.[497,498]

As discussed above, the process of destructive cholangitis varies in degree from one portal tract to another; this variability makes any histologic staging system of very limited value.

An increased prevalence of hepatocellular carcinoma and breast cancer has been reported in PBC.[499]

Primary sclerosing cholangitis

The clinical aspects of PSC are discussed in several reviews and studies of large series from several centers worldwide.[483,500-505] The disease may be idiopathic or associated with other diseases, such as ulcerative colitis or retroperitoneal fibrosis. The onset may be in childhood,[506] but the usual presentation is between 25 and 40 years of age, and the male-to-female ratio is 2:1. Median survival is about 12 years. The incidence of bile duct carcinoma complicating PSC has varied from 4% to 19%.[505] As is the case with PBC a cholestatic biochemical profile is present in all patients. The AMA test results are negative. Recently, perinuclear antineutrophil cytoplasmic antibodies (p-ANCA) have been found to be present in a high percentage of patients with PSC, as well as in patients with ulcerative colitis, but not in PBC.[507,508] In one series p-ANCA were found in 82% of patients with PSC and in 25% of their relatives.[508] Radiographic studies, particularly ERCP (endoscopic retrograde cholangiography) are diagnostic in over 80% of the cases of PSC; they show a characteristic pattern of alternating strictures and dilatations of the bile ducts ("beading"). Laparotomy should be reserved for the minority of patients with complete obstruction of the common bile duct in order to exclude bile duct carcinoma. The disease usually involves the entire biliary tract, but there are occasional cases that affect only extrahepatic or intrahepatic ducts. The extrahepatic ducts are thick and cordlike and have a narrowed lumen.

Detailed histopathologic observations of PSC have been reported by many investigators.[509-512] Changes in the acini resemble those of chronic extrahepatic biliary obstruction of other causes; cholestasis is sometimes minimal or absent, since obstruction is rarely complete. Clues to the diagnosis can be observed in the portal areas. Some intra-acinar bile ducts can show much periductal fibrosis with prominent compression and distortion of the epithelium; the epithelium can be almost unidentifiable or even completely atrophic while a small nodule (cross section of a cord) of fibrous tissue remains in its place (Figs. 57-37 and 57-38). The basement membrane is intact and often thickened but eventually disappears when the duct is completely fibrosed. The bile ducts are reduced in number or are totally absent, depending on the stage of the disease. The degree of ductular proliferation is variable; cytokeratin stain often discloses many more ductules that are visible in H&E preparations. Dilated segments of the intrahepatic bile ducts may be seen histopathologically and have been referred to as *cholangiectases*.[512] Chronic cholestatic features, with pseudoxanthomatous transformation and accumulation of copper-binding protein and copper, are always present. Granulomas are, in our opinion, exceptionally rare, though reported in 10% of cases in one series.[500]

Differential diagnosis

Both PBC and PSC are chronic cholestatic disorders and may require differentiation from chronic active hepatitis, whereas that of PSC may mimic extrahepatic biliary tract obstruction (chronic or recurrent). The three diseases are compared and contrasted in Table 57-13. Other diseases that, on occasion, require differentiation from PSC include idiopathic adulthood ductopenia,[464,465] AIDS-related cholangiopathy that may be secondary to infection with CMV, *Cryptococcus neoformans, Cryptosporidium,* or *Trichosporon,*[513-515] ischemic cholangiopathy associated with intra-arterial infusion of floxuridine for treatment of liver metastases,[516-519] or cholangiopathy resulting from the injection of formalin into echinococcal cysts.[520] Conditions that must be differentiated from PBC include sarcoidosis with protracted jaundice,[521-523] a syndrome with features overlapping those of PBC and sarcoidosis,[524] and chronic drug-induced or toxic cholestatic injury.[448,449,] Examples of drugs and toxins leading to chronic cholestasis include

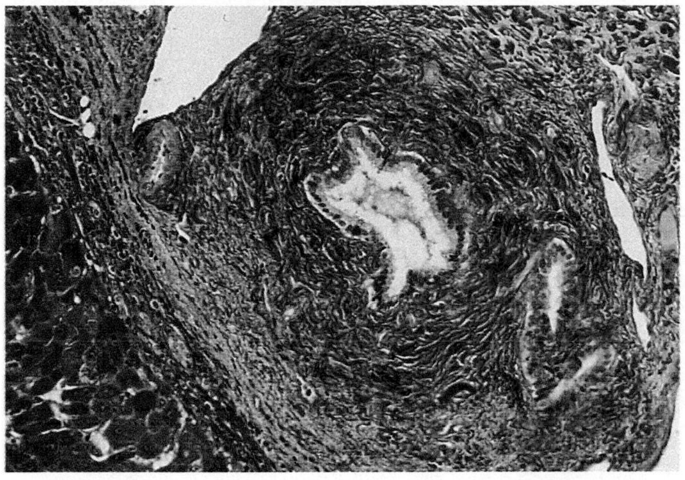

Fig. 57-37 Primary sclerosing cholangitis. Pronounced periductal sclerosis.

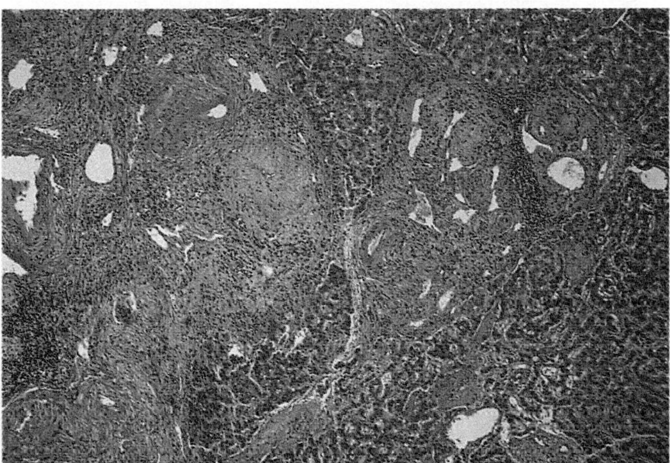

Fig. 57-38 Primary sclerosing cholangitis. No bile ducts are noted in fibrotic portal areas. Sclerosed ducts are replaced by round scars. Notice residual portal inflammation.

Table 57-13 Histologic differentiation of chronic hepatitis from primary biliary cirrhosis (PBC) and primary scerosing cholangitis (PSC)

Change	Chronic hepatitis*	PBC	PSC
Lymphocytic piecemeal necrosis	1+ to 3+	0 to 1+	0 to 1+
Acidophilic (apoptotic) bodies	1+ to 3+	0 to 1+	0
Focal necrosis	1+ to 3+	0 to 1+	0
Panacinar hepatitis–like injury	0 to 3+	0	0
Zone 3 necrosis (with or without bridging)	0 to 3+	0	0
Multiacinar necrosis	0 to 3+	0	0
Ground-glass cells	In HBV+ cases	0	0
Sanded nuclei	In HBV+ or HDV+ cases	0	0
Chronic nonsuppurative cholangitis†	0	2+ to 3+	0
Periductal sclerosis	0	0 to 1+	2+ to 3+
Ductopenia	0	1+ to 3+	1+ to 3+
Zone 1 cholestasis	0	1+ to 3+	1+ to 3+
Zone 1 pseudoxanthomatous change	0	1+ to 3+	1+ to 3+
Copper-binding protein and copper storage in zone 1	0 to 2+ (Wilson's disease)	1+ to 3+	1+ to 3+
Mallory bodies in zone 1	0 to 1+ (Wilson's disease)	0 to 3+	0+ to 3+
Granulomas (portal, intra-acinar)	0	0 to 2+	0
Portal inflammation	1+ to 3+	1+ to 3+	1 to 3+
Lymphoid aggregates and follicles	1+ to 3+ (especially hepatitis C)	0 to 2+	0 to 2+

**HBV,* Hepatitis B virus; *HCV,* hepatitis C virus; *HDV,* hepatitis delta virus; *0,* absent; *1+,* minimal; *2+,* moderate; *3+,* pronounced.
†Ducts in chronic hepatitis may show degenerative changes.

haloperidol,[525] ketoconazole,[526] oral contraceptives,[527] ampicillin,[528] flucloxacillin,[529] and Spanish toxic oil.[530] The most frequently reported association has been with the phenothiazines and ajmaline derivatives.[531-533] Acute cholangitis progressing to ductopenia is believed to be the underlying mechanism.[531] It is important at this point to emphasize that bile duct lesions resembling or indistinguishable from those of PBC, which may or may not culminate in chronic cholestasis, have been identified in several diseases. They include sarcoidosis,[534] chronic (as well as acute) graft-versus-host disease (discussed later), acute and chronic rejection of human liver allografts, Hodgkin's disease,[535] and, as already noted, chronic hepatitis, particularly that caused by HCV.

Before leaving this section we should mention several important chronic disorders of the intrahepatic bile duct. They include recurrent pyogenic cholangitis,[536] the closely related intrahepatic lithiasis (hepatolithiasis),[537] and parasitic infestations such as clonorchiasis and opisthorchiasis.[538] These diseases are characterized by dilatation of the bile ducts, which also may have thickened walls. Thickening of the wall is attributable to chronic cholangitis, mucus gland hyperplasia, and fibrosis; there may be a superimposed acute cholangitis. The epithelium may be ulcerated or hyperplastic, and the lumen often contains adult parasites (in the case of clonorchiasis and opisthorchiasis) or bilirubin calculi (in hepatolithiasis and recurrent pyogenic cholangitis). Caroli's disease (segmental intrahepatic dilatation of the bile ducts) is also associated with dilatation and chronic and acute inflammation of the ducts; it too may be complicated by intrahepatic lithiasis. Caroli's disease may be associated with congenital hepatic fibrosis. Patients with Caroli's and the other aforementioned diseases are at risk for development of intrahepatic cholangiocarcinoma.

HEPATOCELLULAR PIGMENT STORAGE

Lipofuscin and lipofuscin-like pigments

The two inherited conjugated hyperbilirubinemias, the Dubin-Johnson syndrome and Rotor's syndrome, have been reviewed recently by Zimniak[539] and Berk and Noyer[540] and are discussed briefly in the succeeding paragraphs.

Dubin-Johnson syndrome

Grossly, the liver is gray-black to black in color. Liver biopsy specimens do not reveal cholestasis. Instead, hepatocytes in zones 3 and 2 contain abundant, coarse granules of a dark, golden-brown pigment that resemble lipofuscin; it is most abundant in the pericanalicular region (Fig. 57-39). The pigment stains variably with oil red 0, D-PAS, Fontana-Masson, and acid-fast stains and shows yellow autofluorescence; thus it has some histochemical similarity to lipofuscin and melanin. Electron microscopy demonstrates that the lysosomal pigment differs from lipofuscin in being more pleomorphic and of variable electron density.[21] The pigment is the result of deposition of products of amino acid catabolism that cannot be excreted into bile.[541]

The Dubin-Johnson syndrome is inherited as an autosomal recessive trait. The typical clinical features include intermittent jaundice (often precipitated by intercurrent infections or oral contraceptives), cramping right upper quadrant pain, and possibly epigastric distress, fatigue, or dark urine. The total and direct bilirubin levels are elevated (approximately 1.5 to 6.0 mg/dl), with the direct fraction constituting more than 50% of the total. A very characteristic feature is a high sulfobromophthalein value at 90 and 120 minutes that is frequently higher than the 45-minute value, but this test is no longer used in diagnosis. Almost all patients have a nonvisualizing gallbladder by oral cholecystography. New diagnostic approaches to the Dubin-Johnson syndrome are the results of the 24-hour urine coproporphyrin determination and Tc-Disofenin scintigraphy.[542] Patients with the syndrome have an inversion of the normal ratio of the isomers of coproporphyrin recovered from the urine, though the total 24-urine coproporphyrin levels are normal.

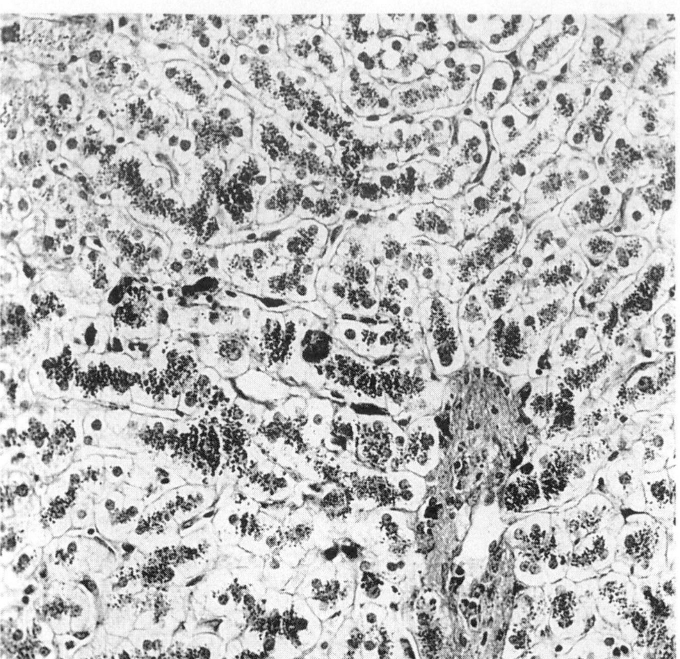

Fig. 57-39 Dubin-Johnson syndrome. Large accumulation of coarsely granular pigment in zone 3 liver cells. (PAS after diastase digestion.)

The Dubin-Johnson syndrome, as well as the related conjugated hyperbilirubinemia conditions found in sheep and rats, are most likely caused by a congenital impairment of an ATP-dependent transport system specific for a variety of multivalent organic anions, including bilirubin diglucuronide.[539] Bilirubin is thus conjugated but inefficiently excreted into bile.

Rotor's syndrome

Rotor's syndrome is characterized by chronic hyperbilirubinemia, predominantly conjugated; it appears to be a variant of the Dubin-Johnson syndrome. Several features serve to distinguish Rotor's syndrome, however. Oral cholecystograms are normal, and sulfobromophthalein tests do not show a rise at 90 and 120 minutes.[543] Differences in excretion of urinary coproporphyrins have also been established.[544] The liver is usually normal histologically.

Gilbert's syndrome

Gilbert's syndrome is characterized by a mild, chronic unconjugated hyperbilirubinemia. Patients are usually asymptomatic, and positive physical findings are limited to the possible presence of icterus, usually recognized in the late teens or early twenties.[545] Patients have a deficiency of glucuronyl transferase.

The diagnosis is partly one of exclusion. Other causes of unconjugated hyperbilirubinemia to be ruled out include shunt hyperbilirubinemia, exposure to some drugs (rifampicin and novobiocin) and cholecystographic agents, portacaval shunt, a wide variety of acquired diseases, and hemolysis.[545-548]

The histologic appearance of the liver may be virtually normal, though many cases show an excess of lipofuscin pigment, predominantly in zones 3 and 2.[549] The pigment is less in quantity and not so coarse as that of the Dubin-Johnson syndrome. A small amount of hemosiderin can accumulate in Kupffer cells and even in hepatocytes, possibly as a result of the mild hemolysis that can occur in some patients. The ultrastructural findings are not uniform.[24] In some biopsy specimens there are alterations in the sinusoidal membrane of hepatocytes (flattening and loss of microvilli and an increase in collagen fibers in the space of Disse). In other biopsy specimens giant mitochondria with paracrystalline inclusions are frequently observed, whereas in still others there is great proliferation of the smooth endoplasmic reticulum with dilatation of the rough endoplasmic reticulum.[549] An increase in lipofusin granules is a common finding.

The presence of hemolysis can greatly complicate the diagnosis, but a method using radioactive chromium is of great value in distinguishing patients with hemolysis and Gilbert's syndrome from those with hemolysis alone.[550]

Crigler-Najjar syndrome

The Crigler-Najjar syndrome, an autosomal recessive disease, is also associated with unconjugated hyperbilirubinemia, but it is more severe than in Gilbert's syndrome.[546,548,551] The biochemical defect is complete absence of bilirubin glucuronyl transferase. Patients with the disorder develop kernicterus and die, usually in childhood. Cholestasis, particularly in the form of canalicular bile plugs, can be identified in biopsy specimens. The variant described by Arias and colleagues[552] is less severe and can respond to treatment with phenobarbital. Hepatic transplantation has been reported and is advocated for patients whose serum bilirubin levels cannot be maintained at a safe level by phototherapy.[553]

Drug-induced lipofuscinosis

Therapy with certain drugs, including the phenothiazines, *Cascara sagrada,* aminopyrine, and phenacetin, can be followed by the cytoplasmic accumulation of lipofuscin in liver cells.[209] This phenomenon has little clinical significance save for possible resemblance to the Dubin-Johnson syndrome. The latter usually shows more prominent pigment and is readily differentiated by the characteristic laboratory and roentgenographic features.

Iron storage disease

Genetic hemochromatosis

In the earliest stages of genetic hemochromatosis, also known as hereditary or idiopathic hemochromatosis, there is accumulation of hemosiderin in hepatocytes in the periportal area (Fig. 57-40). As the quantity of iron increases, the cells of zones 2 and 3 become affected. Pigment also begins to accumulate in bile duct cells (Fig. 57-41). Scattered apoptotic bodies and foci of necrosis are found infrequently. Steatosis is absent or minimal unless other factors that account for it are present. Fibrous septa eventually creep from the portal areas into the surrounding parenchyma. The septa can show variable (usually mild) ductular proliferation, but inflammation is scanty. It is important to remember that patients with genetic hemochromatosis who have features of chronic hepatitis are likely to have HBV or HCV infection.[554] It is believed that hepatitis viral infections can act synergistically with iron in accelerating the development of liver damage in genetic hemochromatosis.[554]

As the liver damage progresses in genetic hemochromatosis, fibrous bands from adjacent portal tracts join and dissect the parenchyma into irregular micronodules. The overall pattern resembles that of biliary cirrhosis. In addition to its location in hepatocytes and duct cells, some hemosiderin accumulates in Kupffer cells and, late in the disease, in the wall of blood vessels and extracellularly in the fibrous septa.

Regeneration is not usually prominent, but regenerative nodules offer striking contrast to the remaining parenchyma by their lack of stainable iron.[555] A recent study has demonstrated that iron-free foci are preneoplastic and can develop into hepatocellular carcinoma.[555] Hepatocellular carcinomas in hemochromatotic livers are also devoid of iron. Hepatocellular

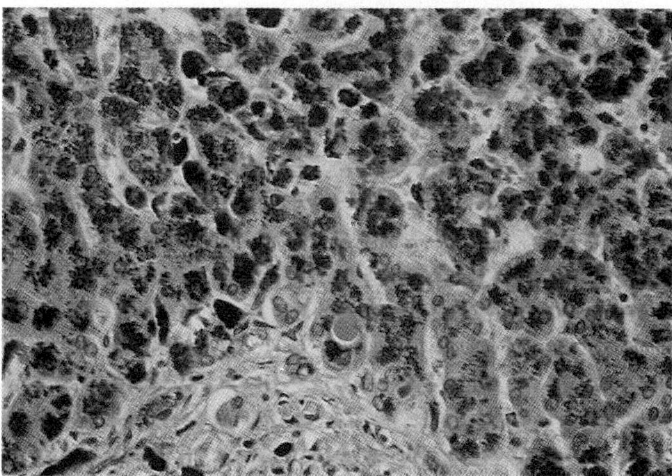

Fig. 57-40 Genetic hemochromatosis. Hemosiderin accumulation is most prominent in zone 1 hepatocytes. (Mallory stain for iron.)

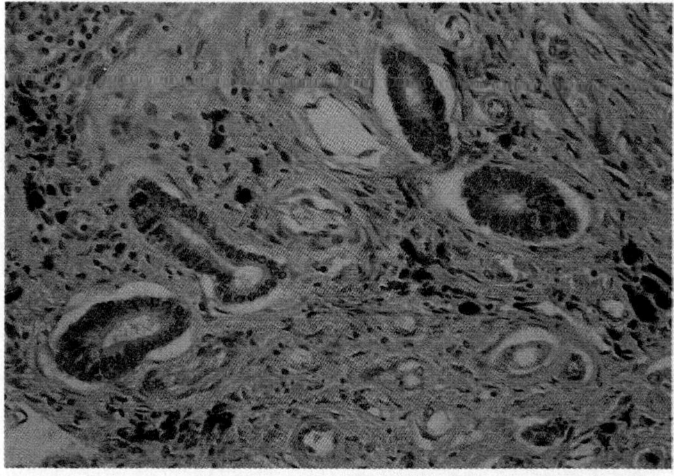

Fig. 57-41 Genetic hemochromatosis. Large hemosiderin accumulation in bile ducts, as well as in periportal liver cells. (Mallory stain for iron.)

carcinoma is 219 times more frequent in patients with hemochromatosis than in the normal population.[556]

It must be emphasized that the histologic findings in genetic hemochromatosis are not pathognomonic. Usually it is possible to differentiate it from other types of cirrhosis or alcoholic liver disease. Genetic hemochromatosis is more likely to be associated with significant cardiac or endocrine involvement, and the degree of hemosiderosis is usually considerably more than in such conditions. Other types of iron overload (such as beta-thalassemia) are less easily distinguished from genetic hemochromatosis.

Ultimately the diagnosis of genetic hemochromatosis is established by correlation of clinical, laboratory, and histologic findings.[556-561] The classical clinical triad includes cirrhosis, diabetes mellitus, and pigmentation of the skin. Patients with early disease may not necessarily show any of the three findings. Cardiac abnormalities, various endocrine deficiencies, and arthropathy can also develop. The serum iron is high, as it can be in other hepatic diseases, but the iron-binding capacity is low and saturated in hemochromatosis. Various means of quantitating the degree of iron excess have been devised, but not all are practical. A histologic grading method has been proposed by Brissot and associates.[562] They found a good correlation between their histologic grading system and the liver iron concentration. A determination of the hepatic iron concentration, usually by atomic absorption, is of diagnostic value.[563] The concentration is often greater than 10,000 µg/g dry weight in untreated hemochromatosis. The *hepatic iron index* is the most useful aid in diagnosis. It is derived from the hepatic iron concentration in micromoles per gram of dry weight (derived by dividing the concentration in mg/g dry weight by 56) divided by the age of the patient. Patients with hemochromatosis have an iron index greater than 2.[563]

The serum ferritin is usually elevated in genetic hemochromatosis but has limited diagnostic value. The test can be used with the percentage transferrin saturation to detect preclinical hemochromatosis in relatives of patients.[561] HLA typing can be used to predict the risk of hemochromatosis in family studies.

Perinatal hemochromatosis

Perinatal hemochromatosis is characterized by massive accumulation of iron in hepatocytes, pancreatic islet cells, and other organs and tissues.[564-568] The normal hepatic architecture is replaced by pseudoacini, fibrosis, and multinucleated giant cells (Fig. 57-42). Survival beyond 4 months of age is rare. The condition is clinically and pathologically distinct from Zellweger's cerebrohepatorenal syndrome and tyrosinemia, neonatal diseases in which large stores of iron are present in hepatocytes. A possible genetic defect has not been established. Recently, it has been shown that iron per se does not have a direct etiologic role in hemochromatosis.[568] Rather, it has been suggested that putative environmental agents (hypoxia, viruses, drugs) may interact with a factor or factors intrinsic to the developing fetal liver to initiate perinatal hemochromatosis.[568]

Hematologic disorders

Patients with various types of hemolytic and nonhemolytic refractory anemias can develop excessive hepatic iron storage and, infrequently, a clinicopathologic picture identical to that of genetic hemochromatosis. Etiologic factors include excessive iron absorption induced by erythroid hyperplasia, iron release after breakdown of hemoglobin, and exogenous iron from transfusions or oral compounds.[569,570] With early or slight hemolysis, hemosiderin is localized primarily in Kupffer cells. More advanced cases can have a histologic picture resembling genetic hemochromatosis, but clinical and laboratory findings, of course, point to the underlying hematologic disturbance.

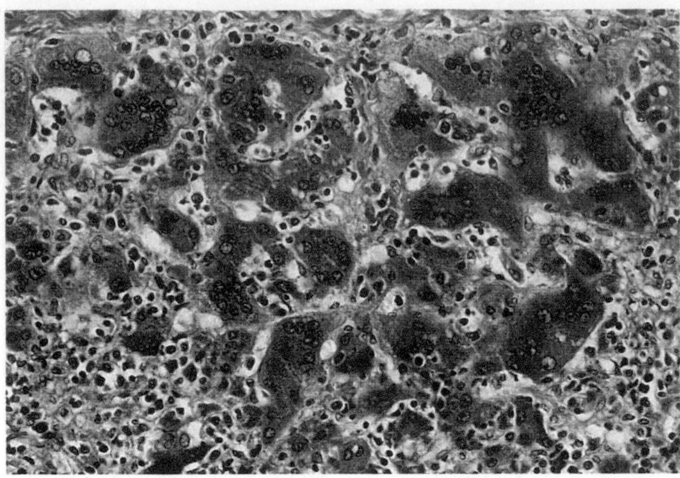

Fig. 57-42 Neonatal hemochromatosis. Many of the disrupted liver cells are multinucleated, and there is intra-acinar fibrosis and inflammation.

Dietary iron overload

The development of massive iron overload and pathologic changes resembling genetic hemochromatosis in the South African Bantu, who cook with iron utensils and drink a beer high in iron content, had indicated in the past that dietary overload alone can be responsible for iron storage disease. However, recent genetic studies have shown that an unidentified heritable trait may account for a substantial portion of the variability in transferrin saturation in these patients. The defect may occur in over 30% of the population and appears to be distinct from the genetic factor controlling hemochromatosis in white populations.[571] Although dietary iron overload is decreasing in the urban black population of South Africa, it persists in rural sub-Saharan Africa, specifically in Zimbabwe.[571] The phenomenon of dietary iron storage disease is less well established outside of Africa. The development of hepatic disease in some individuals who have ingested large quantities of iron for prolonged periods and who are otherwise normal[569] indicates that a careful dietary and drug history (including reference to nonprescription drugs) may be essential in the evaluation of an iron storage disorder.

Transfusional iron overload

Hemosiderin can be found in Kupffer cells after transfusions of blood. With many transfusions administered chronically, histologic changes resembling those of genetic hemochromatosis may develop.[570]

Undoubtedly most patients receiving multiple transfusions have an underlying hematologic disorder and fall into the category of hematologic disorders discussed above. Iron storage disease in such patients is usually multifactorial.

Other conditions such as congenital atransferrinemia, iron overload associated with porphyria cutanea tarda, and iron overload associated with chronic renal failure and portacaval shunt are discussed by Searle and associates.[559]

Other storage diseases

Wilson's disease

The metabolic defect in Wilson's disease (hepatolenticular degeneration) has not been elucidated, but the defective gene is on chromosone 13, closely linked to the esterase D locus. Tissue damage is related to accumulation of an excess of copper. The liver is the earliest site of progressive copper accumulation; copper is then released into the bloodstream to accumulate in other organs.[572] A diagnosis of Wilson's disease in the early or precirrhotic stage is imperative, since it is one of the few hepatic diseases for which specific therapy (that is, penicillamine) is available. The most helpful determinations include decreased serum ceruloplasmin, elevated hepatic copper content, increased urinary excretion of copper, and presence of Kayser-Fleischer rings by slit-lamp ocular examination. These findings are variably present in different stages of the disease and must be assessed accordingly.[572-575]

The earliest microscopic lesions in Wilson's disease include steatosis, periportal glycogenated nuclei (Fig. 57-43), and rare foci of necrosis or apoptotic bodies.[576] Although the hepatic copper content is elevated, copper is often not identifiable histochemically. Ultrastructural changes believed to be characteristic, if not pathognomonic, involve the mitochondria; these include pleomorphism, separation of the inner and outer membranes, enlarged intercristal spaces, and various types of inclusions.[21,573,575]

More advanced cases show lesions that resemble those of chronic hepatitis of other causation.[428-430] Piecemeal necrosis with variable periportal fibrosis is present. Periportal glycogenated nuclei are frequently present. The portal inflammatory infiltrate is predominantly lymphoplasmacytic, and Mallory

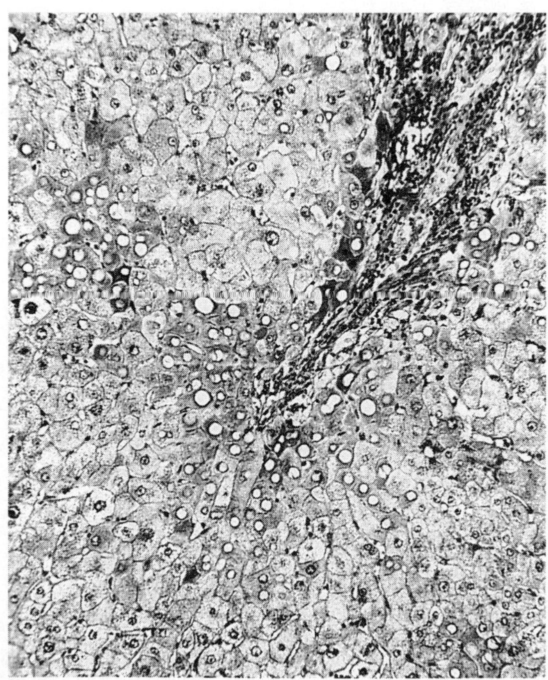

Fig. 57-43 Wilson's disease. Periportal fibrosis and numerous glycogenated nuclei in liver cells in zone 1.

bodies, with their characteristic neutrophilic response, may be present in liver cells in zone 1. Copper is commonly demonstrable in the periportal areas with special stains.[576] In contrast, copper is usually absent in other types of chronic hepatitis.

A variety of patterns of cirrhosis can develop in the later stages, but a macronodular type is the most common.[576] In general, areas of prominent copper deposition are accompanied by hepatocellular degeneration, classic Mallory bodies, and sometimes cholestasis. Regenerative foci lack identifiable copper. Thus the absence of stainable copper in a cirrhotic biopsy, particularly if the sample is small, would not rule out Wilson's disease. On the other hand, a large amount of copper in a cirrhotic liver is strongly suggestive of Wilson's disease. Hepatocellular carcinoma is an infrequent complication of Wilson's disease.[577]

Buffered formalin is recommended as the fixative of choice for the histochemical demonstration of copper. The rhodanine method has the best correlation with hepatic copper content, but the rubeanic acid technique is acceptable.[42,43] Copper-binding protein can be stained by orcein, Victoria blue, or aldehyde fuchsin. If the diagnosis is suspected before biopsy, a small portion of the sample can be saved for quantitation of copper by atomic absorption spectrophotometry or neutron activation analysis.

Indian childhood cirrhosis

Indian childhood cirrhosis is a rapidly progressive disorder usually presenting before 5 years of age. Three clinical stages have been delineated.[578,579] Many of the histopathologic changes resemble those of alcoholic liver disease, but steatosis is minimal or absent, and regeneration seems to be greatly impaired.[578-581] Although little is known of the early changes, a precirrhotic stage has been recognized; Mallory bodies and prominent inflammatory infiltrates can be identified even at this stage. The cirrhosis is usually micronodular, small groups or nodules of hepatocytes are surrounded by fibrous bands, and there is diffuse fibrosis within the nodules isolating individual hepatocytes. The considerable copper accumulation demonstrated by histochemical and quantitative methods[582,583] in Indian childhood cirrhosis may be of pathogenetic significance. The source of the copper may be dietary inasmuch as a high copper content has been found in milk stored in brass containers and ingested by infants in India.[584] Corroborative evidence comes from descriptions of a liver disease resembling Indian childhood cirrhosis (reported from Germany) in infants who had chronically ingested well water with a high content of copper.[585]

α_1-antitrypsin deficiency

Individuals with α_1-antitrypsin deficiency can develop hepatic or pulmonary disease of variable severity.[586-591] Many different phenotypes have been identified by electrophoresis in an acid-starch medium followed by antigen-antibody crossed electrophoresis. A system of codominant alleles, each controlling the production of a single type of α_1-antitrypsin molecule, appears to be operative; more than 70 allelic variants have been described. The occurrence of severe hepatic or pulmonary disease is well documented only with phenotypes associated with severe deficiency, namely, PiZZ, PiSZ, PiMZ, PiFZ, and Pi-null (that is, associated with minimal of no α_1-antitrypsin production).

Jaundice affects approximately 11% of PiZZ infants. Other PiZZ infants may show variable clinical or biochemical signs suggestive of liver disease. Jaundice usually occurs within the first 3 or 4 months of life and clears by the sixth to eighth month. Biopsy specimens from affected infants show intrahepatic cholestasis, sometimes associated with acute hepatocellular injury in the form of acidophilic bodies or ballooning and with no or mild giant cell transformation. Variable degrees of periportal fibrosis and ductular proliferation can be observed. PAS-positive globules are usually not detectable in infants under 3 months of age. Histologic changes in those with neonatal cholestasis have not always provided clues to the subsequent clinical course, but about 55% of affected infants later develop cirrhosis. Occasional cases are associated with paucity of the intrahepatic bile ducts, and these appear to have the worst prognosis.

α_1-antitrypsin deficiency (both homozygous and heterozygous) is characterized by the presence of characteristic globules. In the noncirrhotic liver they are located in periportal hepatocytes. They are round, homogeneous, and eosinophilic and vary from 1 to 40 μm in diameter. Usually, they are separated from the remainder of the cytoplasm by a halo that is probably artifactual. They are intensely PAS-positive (Fig. 57-44), unlike Mallory bodies and giant mitochondria. Diastase digestion does not affect the staining with PAS. The bodies are antigenically identical to α_1-antitrypsin by immunohistochemical techniques. Ultrastructurally, they are amorphous, moderately electron-dense deposits located in the endoplasmic reticulum.[21]

Liver biopsy specimens from adults with the deficiency may reveal only the characteristic globules in periportal regions. Other cases show erosion of the limiting plate associated with chronic inflammation and periportal fibrosis. Such cases appear similar to chronic hepatitis of other causes. A recent study by Propst and colleagues[432] has shown that a high prevalence of chronic viral infection (hepatitis C or B) and other risk factors such as alcoholism, rather that the α_1-antitrypsin deficiency per se, may be the cause of chronic liver disease in adult patients.

The cirrhotic stage has a very variable morphologic appearance; most cases reveal a macronodular or mixed pattern, but an occasional micronodular pattern may be found. Mild cholestasis can be present, and mild to moderate steatosis is not uncommon. Prominent cholestasis can occur in cases associated with paucity of bile ducts. The globules are usually more heavily concentrated at the periphery of the cirrhotic nodules.

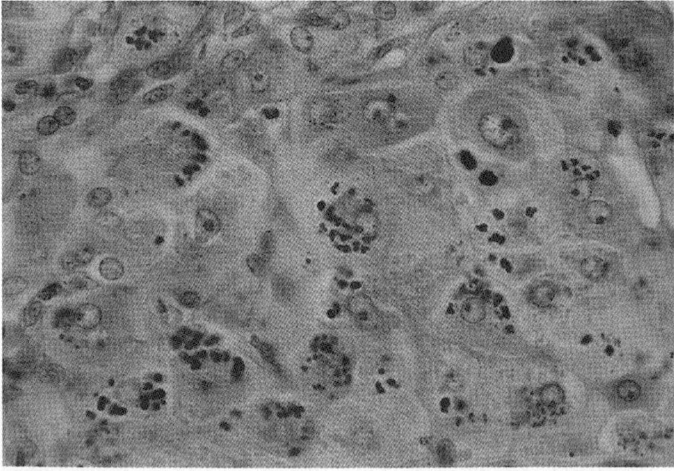

Fig. 57-44 α_1-antitrypsin globules are periodic acid-Schiff positive. (PAS after diastase digestion.)

The differential diagnosis of α_1-antitrypsin globules includes fibrinogen globules in fibrinogen storage disease[592,593] and plasma inclusions (also referred to as *congestion globules*)[594] that are seen in congestive failure or a variety of other conditions. The former are weakly PAS-positive, whereas the latter are PAS-negative. Fibrinogen globules are immunoreactive to antifibrinogen antibodies, whereas congestion globules contain a variety of plasma proteins (since they are plasma inclusions in the cytoplasm of liver cells).

Several reports have documented the occurrence of hepatocellular carcinoma in some patients with α_1-antitrypsin deficiency; all had an underlying cirrhosis.[595-597]

Glycogen storage diseases (glycogenoses)

A disorder of glycogen storage should be suspected in any child with unexplained hepatomegaly, cardiomegaly, hypoglycemia, muscular weakness, central nervous system deterioration, or growth failure. Morphologic findings in biopsy specimens from the liver and other organs are not specific but are of value in suggesting or confirming a diagnosis of glycogenosis and distinguishing the various types.[598] Definitive diagnosis depends on the demonstration of the specific enzymatic defect.

Alcohol is the most suitable fixative for the histochemical demonstration of glycogen. Tissues destined for enzymatic analysis are usually frozen and must be handled with care because of lability of enzymes and potential contamination from such sources as starch in surgical gloves.

Liver biopsy specimens in types I, III, and IV show enlarged hepatocytes with a clear or finely vesiculated cytoplasm (Fig. 57-45). The plate architectural pattern is not

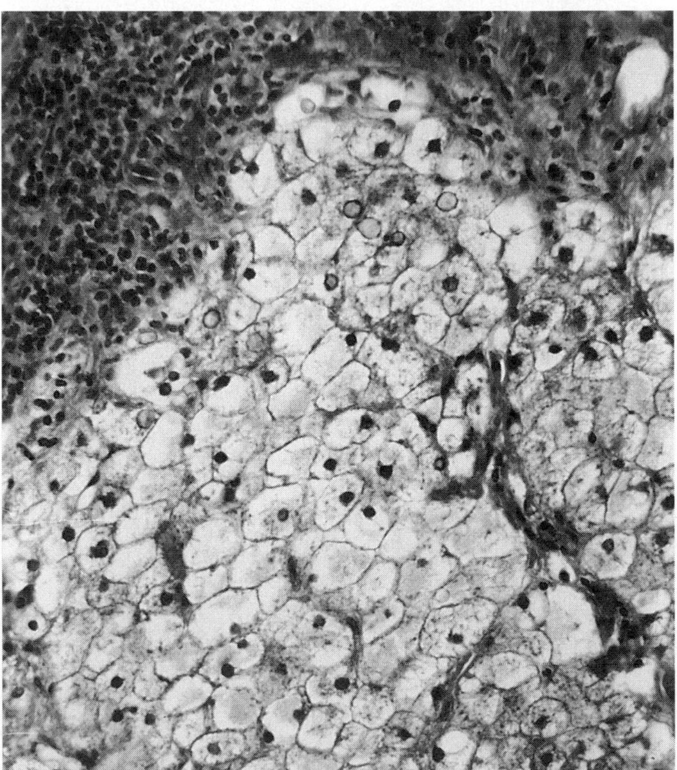

Fig. 57-45 Glycogenesis type III. Liver cells are greatly swollen and have a rarefied cytoplasm and pyknotic nuclei. Notice fibrous septum to the left and glycogenated nuclei.

apparent; instead, the greatly enlarged hepatocytes are arranged in a sheetlike or mosaic pattern, obscuring the compressed sinusoidal spaces.[598]

Several morphologic differences can be cited. Steatosis is more prominent in types I and III and infrequent in type VI. Periportal fibrosis is limited to types III and VI, but a fully developed cirrhosis is rare, except in type IV. Ultrastructurally, large uniform accumulations of glycogen displace intracellular organelles.

Hepatocytes in type II show only mild hypertrophy with a finely vacuolated cytoplasm. The vacuoles correspond to lysosomes packed with glycogen, as one can demonstrate by electron microscopy.

Type IV is associated with the accumulation of an abnormal glycogen molecule, an amylopectin-like material, in hepatocytes. This distinctive material is homogeneous and colorless or lightly eosinophilic. It typically appears as a circumscribed inclusion displacing the remainder of the cytoplasm and the nucleus to the periphery and stains intensely with PAS, Best's carmine, colloidal iron, and Lugol's iodine. The inclusions resist digestion with diastase or amylase but can be digested with pectinase.[599] Ultrastructurally, the material consists of randomly oriented fibrils, glycogen rosettes, and fine granules.[21] The abnormal glycogen accumulates mainly in zone 1 hepatocytes. Periportal fibrosis, usually present, is progressive and eventuates in cirrhosis of a micronodular or mixed type.

Hepatocellular adenomas and even carcinomas have been reported in some cases of type I glycogen storage disease.[600,601]

The reader is referred to the review of McAdams[598] for discussion of the rarer types of glycogen storage disease and of those types that do not involve the liver.

Hereditary tyrosinemia

Heredity tyrosinemia, a disorder of amino acid metabolism, is transmitted as an autosomal recessive trait. Acute and chronic forms are recognized. The onset of the acute form is within weeks or months of birth. There is failure to thrive, anemia, vomiting, diarrhea, hepatosplenomegaly, a bleeding diathesis, and rickets. Death results from liver failure, associated with bleeding or infections, within the first year of life. The chronic form is manifested in the first year of life by growth retardation, gastrointestinal symptoms, multiple renal tubular defects with secondary rachitic changes, and hepatic failure. Hereditary tyrosinemia is characterized by a deficiency of fumarylacetoacetate, the last enzyme in the degradation of tyrosine. The defect results in the accumulation of fumarylacetoacetate and maleylacetoacetate, which lead to cellular damage.

The livers of fatal cases are enlarged, yellow, fibrotic, and nodular. Histopathologically there is steatosis, cholestasis, pseudogland formation, intra-acinar and periportal fibrosis, and nodular regeneration, including macroregenerative nodules.[602-604] Liver cell dysplasia and multifocal hepatocellular carcinoma may be present. Hepatocellular carcinoma occurs in 37% of patients who survive beyond 2 years of age.

Readers interested in additional information on the hepatic pathology of inherited metabolic diseases not covered in this section are referred to other sources.[605,606]

RETICULOENDOTHELIAL REACTIONS

For convenience reticuloendothelial (RE) reactions can be subclassified into nongranulomatous and granulomatous types with the full realization that the cells involved in both lesions are derived from the mononuclear-phagocyte system that, in the liver, comprises Kupffer cells and portal macrophages.

Nongranulomatous disorders

Careful examination of Kupffer cells and portal macrophages is an essential part of the morphologic study of the liver. These cells respond to infections and a variety of other noxious stimuli by undergoing hypertrophy and hyperplasia, and this activation leads to enhanced phagocytic and other functions. They often phagocytose pigments (such as lipofuscin or bile) and cell debris derived from the host's liver cells or from damaged circulating cells (such as hemosiderin released from lysed erythrocytes). Erythrophagocytosis by Kupffer cells occurs in leptospirosis, relapsing fever, malaria, and the reactive hemophagocytic syndrome associated with viral or other infections and occurs with extramedullary hematopoiesis. It is a frequent finding in the liver of patients with the acquired immunodeficiency syndrome, but its pathogenesis in that disease is unclear. Sickled erythrocytes can be avidly phagocytosed by Kupffer cells.

Many of the inherited errors of metabolism are manifested by the excessive accumulation of a metabolite in Kupffer cells. The most important of these, together with the appearance of the stored material by H&E, special stains, and special microscopy, are listed in Table 57-14. For further details, refer to other sources.[605,606] The ultrastructural appearance of these stored metabolites is comprehensively covered in the monograph by Phillips and associates.[21]

Cells of the RE system in the liver can phagocytose a variety of infectious agents including bacteria, mycobacteria, fungi, and protozoa. Tubercle bacilli are generally not found within granulomas in the immunocompetent host. Patients with the acquired immunodeficiency syndrome (AIDS) are highly susceptible to infection with *Mycobacterium avium-intracellulare*.[607,608] The liver is frequently involved with "macrophagic" granulomas composed of hypertrophied, gray-blue macrophages (Fig. 57-46) containing hundreds of acid-fast bacilli. The bacilli are also phagocytosed by Kupffer cells and portal macrophages. Giant cells and inflammatory cells are generally absent, as is caseation necrosis. In lepromatous leprosy, lepra bacilli accumulate in enlarged RE cells that have a foamy cytoplasm (lepra cells) and are clustered in granuloma-like formations; in the untreated patient numerous acid-fast bacilli can be demonstrated in these cells. Of the pathogenic fungi, *Histoplasma capsulatum* and, less often, *Cryptococcus neoformans* are typically found in RE cells of the liver. Affected cells have a foamy cytoplasm, but the fungi are difficult to identify in H&E-stained sections. They are readily stained with Gomori's methenamine silver stain and, in the case of *C. neoformans,* with Alcian blue or mucicarmine (because of the capsular mucopolysaccharide). Lytic foci of varied size that contain numerous fungi may be seen in cryptococcosis; they are generally not associated with an inflammatory response.

Hepatic involvement is well recognized in toxoplasmosis and visceral leishmaniasis (kala-azar). Organisms are rarely found in the liver in the former disease but have been identified by immunofluorescence in one study.[609] In visceral leishmaniasis Kupffer cells and portal macrophages are hypertrophied and filled with Leishman-Donovan bodies, which can be demonstrated with a reticulin or Giemsa stain. The Kupffer cells may form granulomatoid nodules or true granulomas.[610,611]

Other than the actual presence of infectious agents there can be accumulation of parasitic pigment in the RE cells of the

Table 57-14 Hepatic reticuloendothelial (RE) storage in inherited metabolic diseases

Disease	Stored material	Histology (H&E)	Other results
Erythropoietic protoporphyria	Protoporphyrin	Brown, round to amorphous crystals) (canaliculi, liver, and RE cells	Birefringent red crosses and granular crystals; red autofluorescence
Mucopolysaccharidoses (Hurler's and Hunter's disease)	Acid mucopolysaccharide	Colorless material (liver and RE cells)	Colloidal iron +
Cystinosis	Cystine	Colorless, amorphous, refractile crystals (RE cells)	Silvery birefringence
Fabry's disease*	Ceramide trihexoside (with cholesterol)	Light tan, finely granular cytoplasm (RE and liver cells)	PAS+*; ORO +; Schultz stain +†
Metachromatic leukodystrophy	Sulfatide	Light tan, finely granular, cytoplasm (RE and ductal cells)	PAS+; metachromatic with cresyl violet and toluidine blue; red color with Masson's trichrome
Gaucher's disease	Glycosyl ceramide	Striated cytoplasm (Kupffer cells), iron stain +	PAS+; acid phosphatase stain+; lysozyme immunostain+
Niemann-Pick disease	Sphingomyelin (and cholesterol)	Foamy cytoplasm (liver and RE cells)	PAS+; ORO+; Baker's acid hematin + but negative after pyridine extraction
Wolman's disease and cholesteryl ester storage disease	Neutral lipid and cholesterol	Foamy cytoplasm; occasional cells have cleftlike spaces (liver and RE cells)	ORO and Schultz+; silvery birefringence
Chronic granulomatous disease	Lipofuscin	Light tan, granular pigment (RE cells)	ORO +; PAS+; argentaphilic
Hermansky-Pudlak syndrome	Ceroid	Tan, granular pigment (RE cells)	Yellow autofluorescence
Atransferrinemia; genetic hemochromatosis; porphyria cutanea tarda; Zellweger syndrome; hereditary tyrosinemia	Hemosiderin	Brown, coarsely granular, refractile pigment (liver, ductal, or RE cells)	Iron stains +

+, Presence of (or positive); *H&E,* hematoxylin and eosin; *ORO,* oil red O; *PAS,* periodic acid-Schiff stain; *RE,* reticuloendothelial.
*Positive stain caused by storage of cholesterol or lipofuscin (in addition to metabolite).

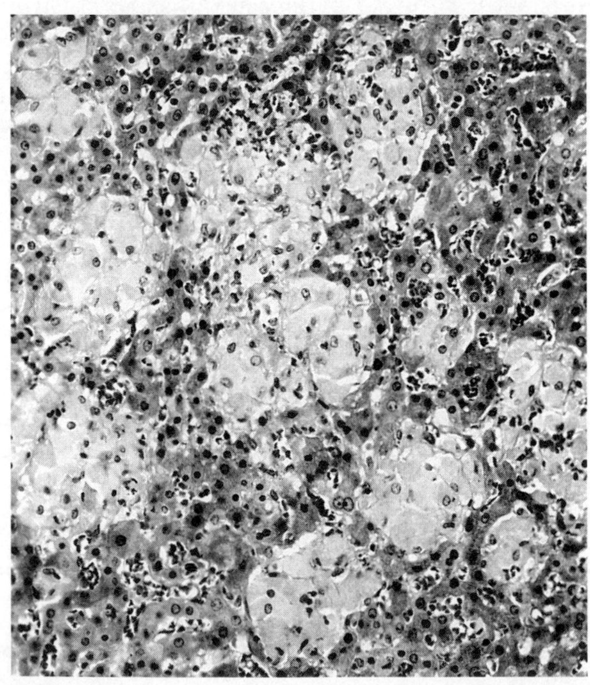

Fig. 57-46 *Mycobacterium avium-intracellulare* infection in patient with AIDS. Granulomas are composed of hypertrophied macrophage cells. Giant cells and inflammatory cells are absent.

liver. A brown to black and finely granular pigment (hemozoin) is phagocytosed by Kupffer cells and portal macrophages in malaria[612] (Fig. 57-47) and schistosomiasis;[613] in the latter disease it can also be identified in macrophages within egg-incited granulomas. The pigment is birefringent and, after microincineration, can be shown to contain traces of iron.

A variety of foreign materials can accumulate in RE cells of the liver.[115,613,614] Intravenous lipid emulsions may lead to accumulation of a lipofuscin-like pigment in RE cells in children.[615,616] Polyvinylpyrrolidone (at one time used as a plasma expander and later as a binder or retarding agent in some subcutaneously injected drugs) accumulates in RE cells of the liver;[617] it is blue gray, amorphous, and Congo red positive. However, unlike amyloid, which also stains positively with Congo red, it does not display apple green birefringence. Silicone rubber can be released from cracked prosthetic devices[618,619] or from silicone elastomer (Silastic) tubing in hemodialysis equipment;[115] it is refractile and colorless in sections stained with H&E and special stains and is best demonstrated by phase-contrast microscopy. The silicone may be engulfed by multinucleated giant cells that line hepatic sinusoids or are located in portal areas. It can be visualized by scanning electron microscopy, and the element silicon can be identified by x-ray microanalysis.[115]

Talc and sometimes other materials (such as titanium) may be present in RE cells of the liver of abusers of intravenously

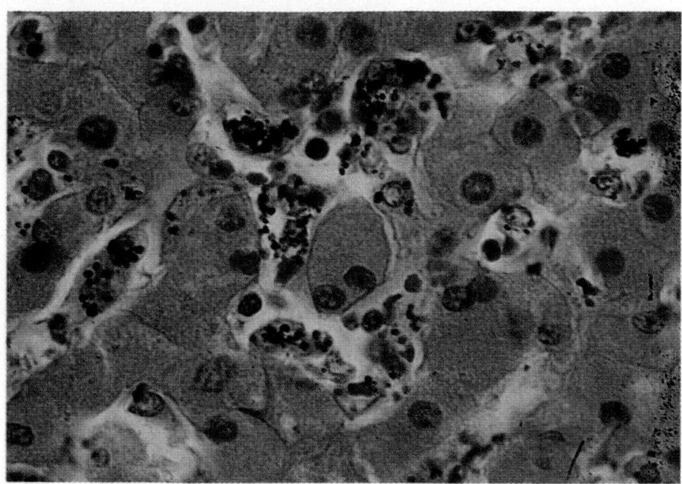

Fig. 57-47 Black, granular hemozoin pigment in Kupffer cells in patient with falciparum malaria.

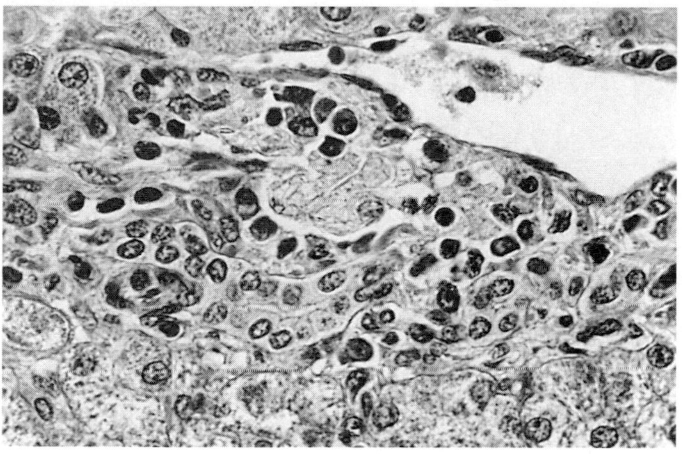

Fig. 57-48 Clusters of hypertrophied perivenular Kupffer cells (above) contain talc crystals that are birefringent (below). Patient was an intravenous abuser of heroin.

administered drugs,[105] as noted previously (Fig. 57-48). Silica, silicates, and anthracotic pigment can accumulate in RE cells of the liver (with or without a granulomatous response), usually in persons occupationally exposed to dusts containing these substances.[620] The silica and silicates are needle shaped or amorphous, colorless, and birefringent. Anthracotic pigment is black and disappears after microincineration.

A formerly used radiographic contrast material, Thorotrast (a colloidal suspension containing thorium dioxide) may be found in RE cells of the liver. It rarely excites a granulomatous reaction; more frequently, it is extracellular and lies trapped in portal or periportal fibrous tissue. It has a pink-brown color in H&E sections and is refractile and coarsely granular but not birefringent. Thorotrast has a characteristic appearance by SEM, and the element thorium can be positively identified in the deposits by energy-dispersive x-ray analysis.[115] The material remains in the RE system for the life of the patient and, after a latency of many years, can incite various primary hepatic malignancies, such as cholangiocarcinoma and angiosarcoma.

Granulomatous disorders

A granuloma is defined as a focal aggregate of epithelioid cells derived from mononuclear phagocytes. Conceptually, granulomas evolve in three stages: the development of an infiltrate of young mononuclear phagocytes, the maturation and aggregation of these cells into a mature granuloma, and the potential further maturation of these cells into an epithelioid granuloma.[621]

Hepatic granulomas, including drug-induced and toxic ones, have been reviewed previously.[613,614] The study of hepatic granulomas must take into account the history (including the occupational and drug history), the laboratory data, the results of imaging studies, skin and serologic tests, and results of cultures of hepatic biopsy material for aerobic and anaerobic bacteria, mycobacteria, and fungi. Microscopic study should include examination of all fragments from a biopsy specimen, the use of special stains (for acid-fast bacilli, fungi, bacteria, and other organisms), special microscopy (such as polarizing microscopy or phase contrast), SEM or TEM, and immunohistochemistry, in selected cases. Other specialized techniques, including microradiography, x-ray diffraction, and energy dispersive x-ray microanalysis, are useful in some cases.[614]

Noncaseating granulomas having no specific identifying features are characteristic of PBC, sarcoidosis, chronic beryl-liosis, brucellosis, drug-induced injury and most of the conditions listed in the "miscellaneous" category in Table 57-15. Some of the diseases, however, are characterized by lesions, other than the granulomas, that are suggestive of the diagnosis. For example, the liver in PBC also reveals chronic cholestasis and cholangiodestructive lesions in portal areas. Drug-induced granulomas can be accompanied by hepatocellular injury or combined hepatocellular and cholestatic injury, as is typical of the liver injury associated with phenylbutazone and a few other drugs.[613,622] Also there may be an associated tissue eosinophilia.

Granulomatoid foci or granulomas found in the liver in viral infections (such as infectious mononucleosis and CMV mononucleosis) and rickettsial infections, such as Q fever, have already been discussed. Granulomas in tuberculosis may or may not reveal central necrosis ("caseation") or acid-fast bacilli. Lepra bacilli are difficult to find in granulomas in tuberculoid leprosy but can be demonstrated in large numbers with special stains in untreated lepromatous leprosy.[623,624] The granulomas associated with bacille Calmette-Guérin (BCG) (used either for vaccination or immunotherapy for malignant melanoma) may or may not contain acid-fast bacilli.[625,626] Granulomas caused by the systemic mycoses often contain the fungal spores or hyphae, which are best demonstrated with the Gomori methenamine silver stain.

Several parasitic diseases can involve the liver with a granulomatous response. By far the most important of these is *schistosomiasis,* caused by either *Schistosoma mansoni* or *S. japonicum.*[613] The granulomas in this disease usually contain intact eggs or their chitinous remnants (Fig. 57-49); the latter are colorless and can be better identified by their acid-fastness. The granulomas in the same biopsy specimen can be of differing ages, from "active" granulomas with many epithelioid cells and eosinophils to round scars containing fragments of egg chitin. Calcified eggs are characteristic of *S. japonicum* but not *S. mansoni* infection. Schistosomal pigment is usually readily identified in the RE cells in livers harboring active granulomas. Healing of the granulomas can lead to oblitera-

Table 57-15 Hepatic granulomas

Causes	Examples
Viral infections	Infections mononucleosis, cytomegalovirus infection
Rickettsial infections	Q-fever, boutonneuse fever
Bacterial infections	Brucellosis, melioidosis, cat-scratch disease, salmonellosis, Whipple's disease, yersiniosis
Mycobacterial infections	Tuberculosis, atypical mycobacterioses, leprosy, bacille Calmette-Guérin (BCG) therapy
Spirochetal infections	Syphilis
Protozoal infections	Visceral leishmaniasis, toxoplasmosis
Mycotic infections	Histoplasmosis, coccidioidomycosis
Parasitic disease	Visceral larva migrans, schistosomiasis, capillariasis
Metallic injury	Berylliosis, chronic copper toxicity, aluminum toxicity
Drug-induced injury	Sulfonamides, hydralazine, quinidine, methyldopa, phenylbutazone, diphenylhydantoin, carbamazepine
Foreign nonviable material	Talc, starch, silica, silicone, anthracotic pigment, mineral oil
Extruded cell components	Lipogranuloma, bile granuloma
Inherited matabolic diseases	Chronic granulomatous disease
Hepatic neoplasms	Hepatocellular adenoma, focal nodular hyperplasia, hepatoblastoma
Miscellaneous	Sarcoidoisis, primary biliary cirrhosis, chronic ulcerative colitis, regional enteritis, polymyalgia rheumatica (arteritica)

tion of intrahepatic portal vein branches with resultant portal hypertension, or extensive scarring.[627] Grossly the thickened fibrotic portal areas resemble pipestems, hence the term *pipestem cirrhosis*. Rarely, coarse lobulation may lead to hepar lobatum.[628] It is worth noting at this point that the usual (albeit rare) cause of hepar lobatum is the healing of syphilitic gummas.[628a] Another recently reported cause is the chemotherapeutic regression of metastases to the liver.[241,629] It is important to remember that patients with schistosomiasis may have changes of chronic hepatitis or cirrhosis that are secondary to infection with either HBV or HCV.[630,631] The clinical features of schistosomiasis were reviewed recently by Nompleggi and colleagues.[632]

Other parasitic diseases in which eggs can be found in association with a granulomatous response include hepatic capillariasis, fascioliasis, paragonimiasis, clonorchiasis, and ascariasis. *Visceral larva migrans,* usually ascribable to the larvae of *Toxocara canis* or *I. cati,* can affect the livers of young children. The infection in infants and young children is typically acquired by ingestion of earth contaminated with the feces of dogs or cats. Irregular, often confluent granulomatous lesions are associated with a massive outpouring of eosinophils and often reveal areas of central necrosis resulting from degeneration and degranulation of eosinophils; there can be Charcot-Leyden crystals in the necrotic foci, but larvae are only rarely identified. The areas of necrosis are surrounded by palisaded epithelioid cells and scattered giant cells, which are intimately intermingled with eosinophils.

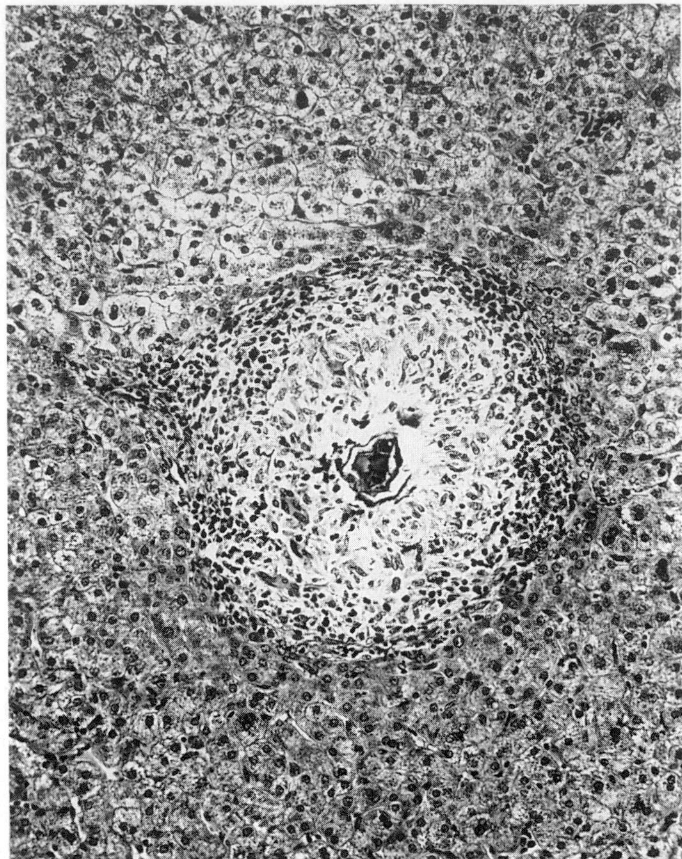

Fig. 57-49 Schistosomiasis. Liver granuloma caused by *S. mansoni* contains a cross-sectioned schistosome egg.

Hepatic granulomas can be associated with occupational exposure to metals, such as beryllium or copper. The actual metal has been identified within the granulomas and RE cells of the livers of vineyard sprayers exposed to copper.[633]

Lipogranulomas can result from rupture of fat-laden hepatocytes (fat "cyst")[634] but are more often the result of accumulation of mineral oil in the liver[635-638] (Fig. 57-50). They consist of variable numbers of fat vacuoles, histiocytes, and lymphocytes; there can be some associated focal fibrosis. Typically, mineral oil granulomas are located in portal areas or in the vicinity of terminal hepatic venules.

The extravasation of bile from bile ducts, usually in cases of prolonged extrahepatic biliary obstruction, may be associated with granuloma formation, with or without giant cells.[613]

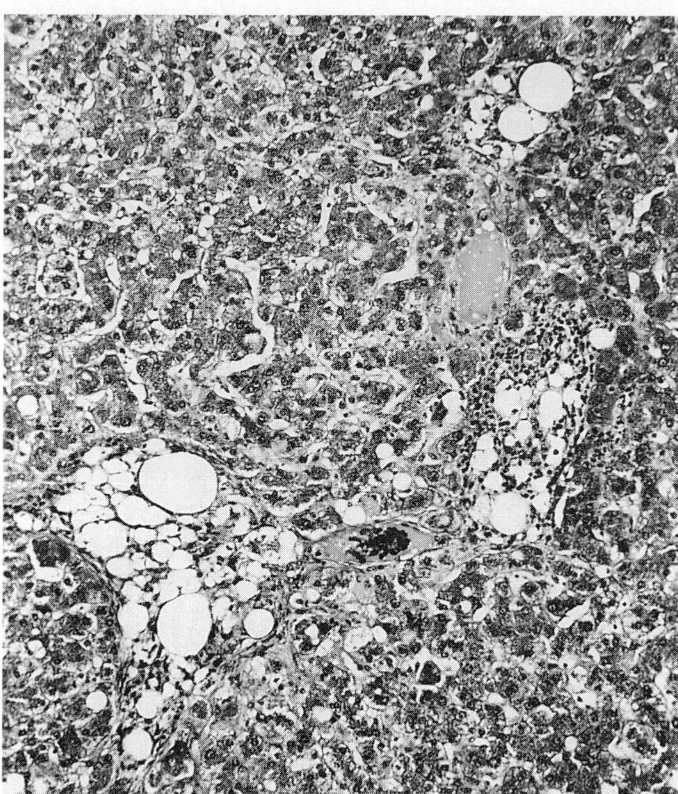

Fig. 57-50 Two lipogranulomas near a central vein are composed of lipophages.

VASCULAR DISORDERS

Portal vein disorders

Thrombosis of the portal vein, with or without intrahepatic extension, is usually secondary to other processes, such as myeloproliferative disorders, cirrhosis, pylephlebitis, neoplastic invasion (hepatocellular carcinoma, hepatoblastoma, and other intra-abdominal neoplasms, such as pancreatic carcinoma), shunt procedures for portal hypertension, nodular regenerative hyperplasia, and, rarely, hepatic venous outflow obstruction. Protein C deficiency has emerged as an important cause of portal vein thrombosis.[639] It is a particularly troublesome complication in children after liver transplantation.[640] The deficiency in reported cases of portal vein thrombosis has been an acquired disorder,[639,640] but a congenital deficiency of protein C is also recognized.[641] Rarely, oral contraceptive therapy can lead to thrombosis of the portal vein.[642,643]

Thrombosis or obstruction of portal veins can be associated with no additional hepatic lesions or can lead to *infarcts of Zahn*. The latter are not true infarcts but, rather, foci of hepatocellular atrophy and sinusoidal congestion.[644] Grossly, they appear as irregular areas of hyperemia and are sometimes located near neoplasms. They can undergo fibrosis and may mimic hepatocellular carcinoma in imaging studies. In a recent histopathologic and postmortem angiologic study, Saegusa and colleagues[645] have suggested that portal vein thrombosis is a more important cause of hepatic infarction than either hepatic vein thrombosis or hepatic arterial damage.

Portal pylephlebitis may complicate intra-abdominal suppurative processes (such as diverticulitis, appendicitis) or acute omphalitis of the newborn. Thrombosis or pylephlebitis can complicate umbilical vein catheterization in children[646-648] but is no longer of clinical significance.

Cavernomatous transformation of the portal vein is a condition in which the vessel is replaced by a spongy venous lake with extension into the gastroduodenal ligament. It is one of the causes of portal hypertension in children and can result from thrombosis of the portal vein after omphalitis or umbilical vein catheterization.[648]

An *endothelialitis* (endotheliitis) of terminal hepatic venules or portal vein branches is one of the major histopathologic changes of acute liver transplant rejection; it is characterized by attachment of lymphocytes to the endothelium of terminal hepatic venules or portal vein branches.

Hepatoportal sclerosis (noncirrhotic portal fibrosis) is characterized by sclerosis and obliteration of small portal venules and dilatation of the larger branches of the portal vein. Intimal fibrosis and varying stages of thrombosis and organization are commonly present.[649-652] There is portal and periportal fibrosis. This disorder is notable for its common association with portal hypertension in the absence of fully developed cirrhosis. It is a recognized complication of chronic exposure to arsenic.[653-655] Most of the idiopathic cases have been reported from India and Japan.[650-652]

Hepatic artery disorders

Thrombosis can follow trauma, ligation, invasion by malignant neoplasms, or perfusion with antineoplastic agents. Hyaline thrombi (composed of fibrin) in hepatic arterioles are typical of idiopathic thrombocytopenic purpura.[656]

Various types of *arteritis* can involve not only the hepatic artery but also its smaller branches and thus can be seen in liver biopsy material. Included are polyarteritis nodosa, syphilitic arteritis, arteritis caused by rickettsial diseases, and hypersensitivity arteritis, such as that secondary to drugs. An arteritis may be seen in acute rejection of transplanted livers and portends a poor outcome. It is characterized by thickening of the arterial wall and infiltration by lymphocytes. The accumulation of foam cells in the intima of arteries *(rejection arteriopathy)* is one of the highly characteristic lesions of chronic transplant rejection.

Infarcts are usually the result of occlusion of the hepatic artery, particularly if distal to the origin of the gastroduodenal branch. Multiple causes including ligation, thrombosis, aneurysms, arteriosclerosis, and polyarteritis nodosa are recognized.[657-660] The diagnosis is being made more frequently during life as a result of the use of computerized tomography.[658,659] Occlusion of the portal vein and even shock have been incriminated in hepatic infarction.[645,660] An infarct is characterized by an irregular area of coagulative necrosis involving many contiguous acini. In contrast to confluent necrosis, such as that associated with shock or congestive heart failure, portal tracts with their contents are also infarcted. If the patient survives, the infarct is infiltrated by neutrophils and can undergo organization and ultimately fibrosis.

Hepatic involvement is freqently in *amyloidosis,* and liver biopsy has been advocated as a means of establishing the diagnosis.[661] Amyloid deposition can be limited to the arteries but can also be found in the parenchyma (Fig. 57-51). The eosinophilic material gradually accumulates in the space of Disse, eventually leading to atrophy of the hepatic plates. A

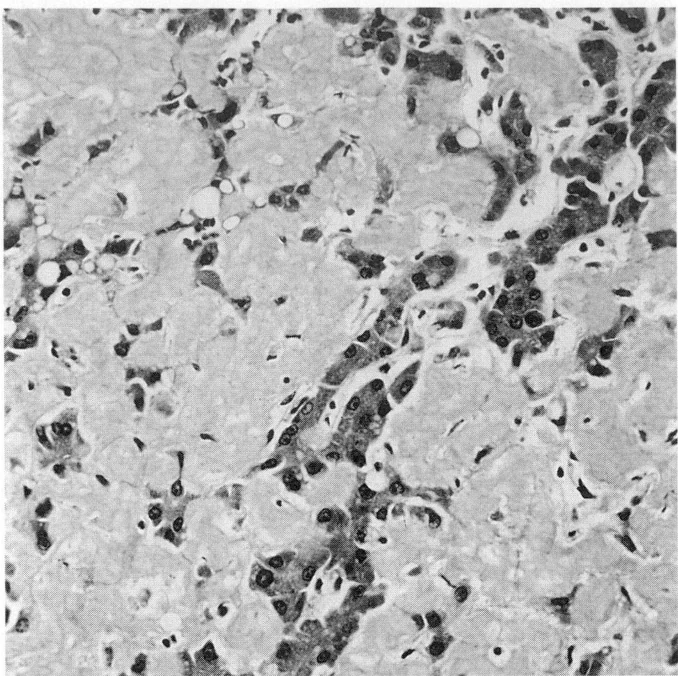

Fig. 57-51 Hepatic amyloidosis. Considerable intra-acinar amyloid deposition has caused atrophy and disruption of the hepatic plates.

special type of hepatic amyloidosis with globular deposits has already been mentioned. The globules are present in spaces of Disse and rarely in sinusoids where they are engulfed by Kupffer cells, as well as in portal areas and terminal hepatic venules. They have a characteristic hillock or "sombrero" shape by SEM.[115] The histochemical and immunohistochemical staining reactions of amyloid have already been alluded to in a previous section.

Sinusoidal disorders

Dilatation

Chronic congestive heart failure leads to the gradual development of dilatation and congestion of sinusoids and, subsequently, to atrophy of hepatocytes.[662,663] Zone 3 is predominantly affected. Grossly the alternating congested and noncongested parenchyma give sections of the liver a nutmeg-like pattern. Fibrosis can develop in zone 3, and ultimately, fibrous linkage of adjacent efferent veins results in the pattern of "cardiac," or congestive, cirrhosis. Thick liver plates (periportal) and nodular regenerative hyperplasia can be seen in advanced cases.

Cases complicated by severe *acute congestive heart failure* or by shock can develop anoxic necrosis in zone 3. The hepatocytes are particularly susceptible to oxygen deprivation and show coagulative necrosis (see Fig. 57-1). The affected cells are shrunken and display intense cytoplasmic eosinophilia, and nuclear pyknosis, karyorrhexis, and karyolysis. A neutrophilic response is typical if the patient lives for a few days. Later, as cell debris is cleared, empty areas of cell dropout punctuated by lipofuscin-laden macrophages are all that remain. The appearance can then be indistinguishable from that resulting from other types of necrosis (such as ballooning). Anoxic necrosis of zone 3 can occur in patients who have congestive heart failure and have developed prolonged shock, usually lasting longer than 24 hours.

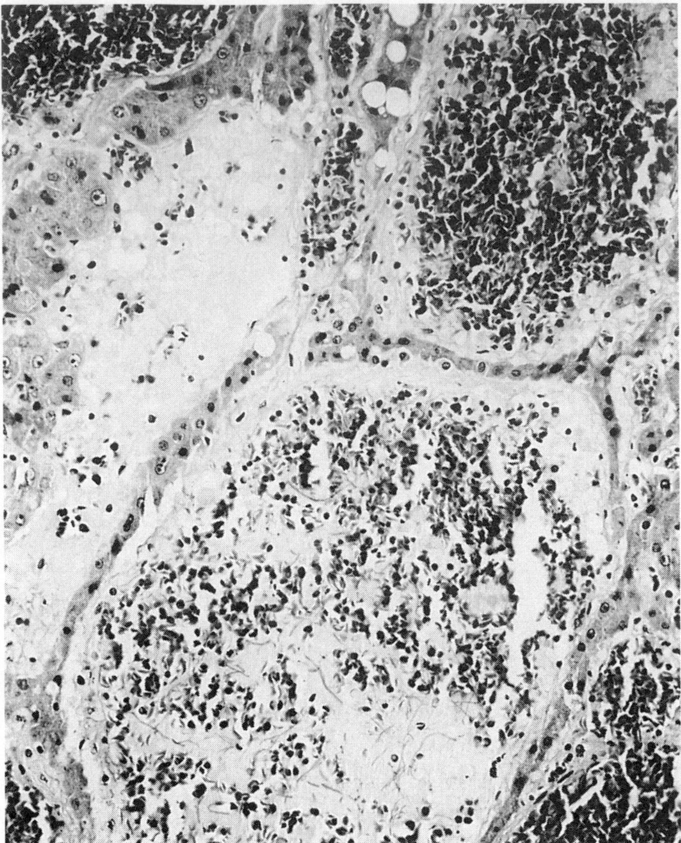

Fig. 57-52 Peliosis hepatis in patient treated with anabolic steroids. Blood filled cavities are separated by atrophic liver cells and do not have an endothelial lining.

A characteristic type of sinusoidal dilatation sometimes occurs after the use of oral contraceptives.[664-666] The periportal zones and sometimes the midzones are affected. Liver plates show variable degrees of atrophy. The change affects all acini, unlike the focal sinusoidal dilatation seen sometimes near hepatic masses. We have seen one case in which the surgeon described the involved liver as dark red, distended, and pulsating. Ultrastructurally, striking perisinusoidal fibrosis has been observed, and there is proliferation and enhanced activity of endothelial and perisinusoidal cells.[666] There is no current evidence to indicate a relationship between this condition and peliosis hepatis. Rupture of the liver would seem to be a plausible complication of the dilatation but has not been reported.

Peliosis hepatis is characterized by scattered cavities of varied size that are filled with blood (Fig. 57-52). The process is now considered to be the result of endothelial injury that allows blood to accumulate in spaces of Disse with resultant formation of the cavities. In the past, peliosis hepatis was recognized as a complication of debilitating disorders, such as tuberculosis and malignancies, and was discovered at autopsy as an incidental finding. At the present time its most frequent cause is therapy with androgenic or anabolic steroids.[667,668] Other causes include therapy with tamoxifen[669] or danazol,[670] hypervitaminosis A,[671] and prior use of Thorotrast.[672] Some cases of *bacillary peliosis hepatis* (bacillary angiomatosis) complicating AIDS have been reported.[673-677] As already noted, this condition is caused by a newly described organism, *Rochalimaea henselae,* which is also the etiologic agent of cat-scratch disease. Peliosis hepatis can be diagnosed by radiologic imaging techniques thereby avoiding the potentially disastrous complications such as hepatic rupture or hepatic failure.[678]

An endothelial lining is usually lacking in peliotic cavities. Inflammation is not a feature, but older lesions can show organization of the contents. Varying degrees of sinusoidal dilatation can be present near some of the lesions. In bacillary peliosis hepatis numerous bacillary organisms are present in the lesions; they are best demonstrated by the Warthin-Starry stain.

Irregular dilatation of sinusoids and hemorrhages are phenomena that occur within various hepatocellular neoplasms, whether associated with use of steroids or not; such hemorrhages should not be referred to as "peliosis hepatis."

Panacinar sinusoidal dilatation can be found in sickle cell disease; the dilated sinusoids are packed with masses of sickled erythrocytes[679] (Fig. 57-53). Variable dilatation, lacking any particular zonal localization, can be associated with other disorders, notably neoplasms and granulomatous diseases and rheumatoid arthritis.[680,681] Sinusoidal dilatation of the liver is one of the systemic manifestations of Hodgkin's disease.[682] A characteristic triad of histologic changes, that is focal sinusoidal dilatation, proliferation of ductules, and infiltration of edematous portal areas by neutrophils, has been observed in the vicinity of space-occupying lesions.[683]

Fibrin thrombosis

Patients with *toxemia of pregnancy* may have no evidence of liver disease. Those who do frequently have deposits of fibrin in sinusoids.[684] Occasionally the deposits are associated with hepatocellular necrosis of variable severity. The necrosis is of the coagulative type and often is located in the periportal area, though foci of necrosis in other zones can be present. By the time a sample is obtained, active necrosis is not usually observed. Instead, areas of hepatocellular dropout are infiltrated by a few inflammatory cells. The phosphotungstic acid hematoxylin (PTAH) and PAS stains are frequently helpful in delineating the fibrin deposits; the fibrin has also been demonstrated by immunohistochemical methods.[685]

Disseminated intravascular coagulation can be associated with a similar pattern of injury, but the sinusoidal fibrin deposition need not be restricted to the periportal areas[685] (Fig. 57-54).

Cellular infiltrates

Many types of cellular infiltrates may be observed in the sinusoids.[135] If sufficiently prominent, they can lead to mild sinusoidal dilatation. Sepsis and other extrahepatic suppurative processes (associated with peripheral leukocytosis with a shift to the left) can be manifested by prominent sinusoidal neutrophilic infiltrates. Numerous lymphocytes in sinusoids are characteristic of mononucleosis and mononucleosis-like syndromes and the tropical splenomegaly syndrome ("big spleen" disease).

Neoplastic infiltrates from metastatic carcinoma, leukemias, primary or secondary lymphomas, systemic mastocytosis, and multiple myeloma can be observed in sinusoids. In hairy cell leukemia the sinusoidal lining cells are destroyed and replaced by the leukemic cells.[686,687] Some primary lymphomas of the liver, in particular, T-cell lymphomas, have a characteristic pattern of sinusoidal infiltration.[688,689] In systemic mastocytosis, mast cells are present also in inflammatory cellular infiltrates in the parenchyma and portal areas.[690-692]

Sinusoidal extramedullary hematopoiesis in the adult is an abnormal finding and is suggestive of a hematologic disturbance. Portal hypertension may be a complication of agnogenic myeloid metaplasia; the pathogenesis is multifactorial, being related to the presence of hematopoietic cells, transformation of Ito cells into fibroblasts or myofibroblasts, and deposition of basement membrane-like material.[693] Extramedullary hematopoiesis is a normal finding in the neonate but is seen to

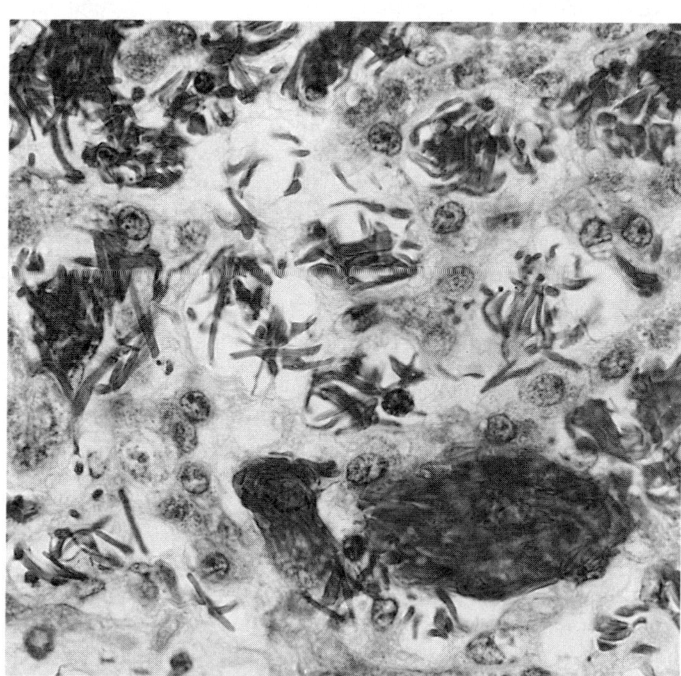

Fig. 57-53 Numerous sickled erythrocytes are present in sinusoids of liver of patient with sickle cell disease.

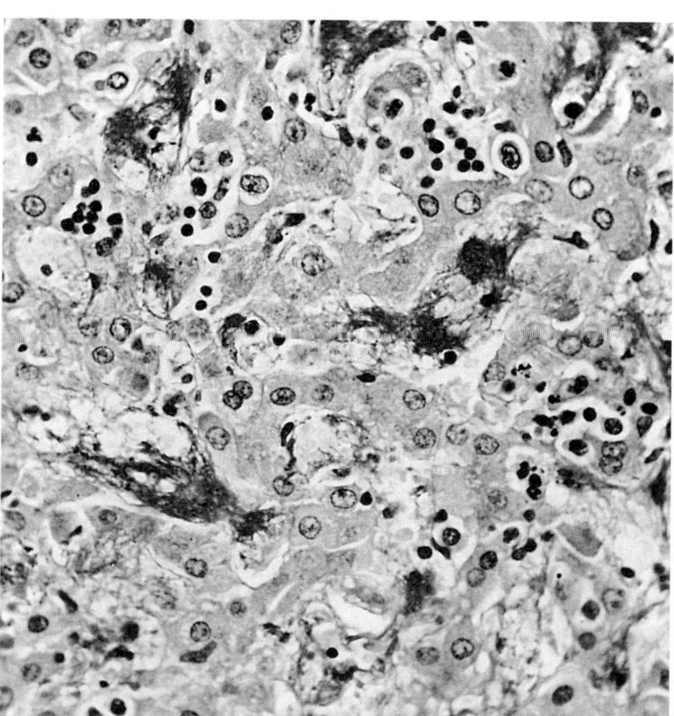

Fig. 57-54 Fibrin deposits in sinusoids of liver of patient with neonatal listeriosis and disseminated intravascular coagulopathy. (PAS after diastase digestion.)

excess in newborns who have various infections, or hematologic and metabolic disorders, or who are premature.

Parasites (such as malaria, microfilariae) are occasionally identified in the sinusoids as well as in other vessels. Larvae of *Strongyloides stercoralis* can be seen in sinusoids in disseminated strongyloidiasis in immunosuppressed patients[694-696] and can lead to formation of granulomas.[697]

Venous outflow tract

The terminal hepatic venules (THV), intercalated (sublobular) veins, hepatic veins, and inferior vena cava are included in this anatomic grouping. In biopsy specimens, only the THV and intercalated veins are commonly sampled. Obstruction of any portion of the outflow tract can be followed by changes in other vessels, such as sinusoidal dilatation and, rarely, thrombosis of portal venules.

Outflow obstruction is subclassified into that type associated with thrombotic involvement of the hepatic veins or vena cava primarily (Budd-Chiari syndrome) and that characterized by occlusion of the THV and intercalated veins (venoocclusive disease). In practice, it is not always possible to distinguish the two in the liver biopsy specimens, since the usual samples do not include the larger veins. Additionally, some cases show overlap in that both large and small vessels are affected. Nevertheless, the subclassification has value in serving to delineate various etiologic categories.

Hepatic vein thrombosis (Budd-Chiari syndrome)

Nearly half of all cases are idiopathic; others are associated with hypercoagulable states (such as lupus anticoagulant, protein C and antithrombin III deficiency, oral contraceptives, pregnancy, myeloproliferative disorders, and paroxysmal nocturnal hemoglobinuria), neoplastic involvement of veins, hepatic abscesses or cysts, and fibrous webs or diaphragms occluding the inferior vena cava.[698-704] The latter occur most frequently in the Orient, but cases have been reported from the United States.[704]

The clinical findings of abdominal pain, hepatomegaly, and ascites can be suggestive of the correct diagnosis but frequently are ascribed to cirrhosis. Imaging techniques (computerized tomography, ultrasound and hepatic venography, magnetic resonance imaging) and biopsy of the liver play an important role in the diagnosis.

The histologic findings are commonly confused with congestive heart failure or drug-induced injury and must be interpreted with care. Many of the changes do resemble those of congestive heart failure but differ by showing variability of involvement among acini, particularly well visualized with open (wedge) biopsy specimens. Those acini with acute changes show severe sinusoidal dilatation and congestion, most pronounced in zone 3, but sometimes extending to the portal tracts.[705] Coagulative necrosis is frequently in the acute stage.[705] Progressive sinusoidal dilatation is accompanied by atrophy of hepatocytes. Zone 3 fibrosis can follow either type of injury and can link adjacent THV. The caudate lobe is typically uninvolved because of its separate venous drainage and often undergoes compensatory hypertrophy.

Other histologic features are distinctive. Erythrocytes in the congested areas are packed into the spaces of Disse and crowd the degenerating hepatocytes. The THV and intercalated veins can show thrombosis, recanalized thrombi, or fibrous mural thickening (Fig. 57-55). The thrombotic changes are not observed in congestive heart failure. Also, although erythrocytes can replace necrotic hepatocytes in congestive heart failure[706] and other disorders, the extravasation into the space of Disse near viable hepatocytes appears to be unique to venous outflow obstruction.

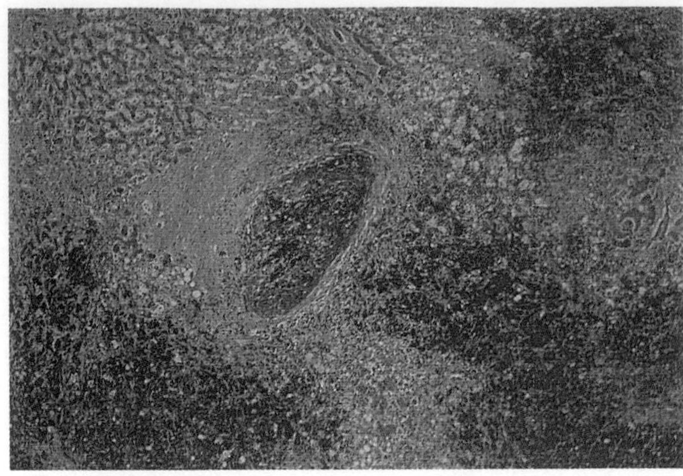

Fig. 57-55 Budd-Chiari syndrome in patient who had used oral contraceptives for many months. There is organized thrombus in vein *(center)* and necrosis involving zone 3.

Venoocclusive disease

The most notable cause of venoocclusive disease is the ingestion of pyrrolizidine alkaloids, which are components of many plants, such as *Senecio* and *Crotolaria* species. First reported in South Africa, the disorder was later discovered in Jamaican children and has since been recognized in many developing countries and occasionally in the United States.[633] Herbal decoctions brewed from plants containing the alkaloids and contamination of grain by the alkaloids have been implicated in human cases.

Excessive radiation and the administration of urethane, 6-thioguanine, azathioprine, dacarbazine, combination cancer chemotherapy, and hypervitaminosis A are also capable of causing venoocclusive disease.[707] Venoocclusive disease occurring after bone marrow transplantation appears to be related to chemoradiotherapy given for pretransplantation conditioning.[708,709] Hepatic venular stenosis resembling venocclusive disease has been reported after orthotopic liver transplanation, it may be related to rejection or to recurrent viral hepatitis.[710]

The range of morphologic parenchymal changes resembles that of the Budd-Chiari syndrome, but in the early stages, lesions of the THV and intercalated veins are distinctive. Changes are limited to the intrahepatic veins. Intimal edema is followed by the subendothelial deposition of reticulin and collagen fibers and progressive narrowing of the lumen (Fig. 57-56). Extravasated erythrocytes are frequently situated between the fibers. Inflammation is sparse or absent, and superimposed thrombi are not seen. Cases with severe acute injury may show necrosis of venous walls. With progressive fibrosis of the walls, the veins become difficult to identify, appearing as small hyalinized cylinders.

Although a poor prognosis accompanies venous outflow obstruction, early diagnosis is important. Some types might be amenable to therapeutic measures, such as membranotomy for vena cava webs, various shunt procedures, discontinuation of the offending drug or toxin, or liver transplantation.

FIBROSIS AND CIRRHOSIS

Fibrosis

Hepatic fibrosis is the increase in the collagen content of the liver. It results from a variety of injuries but can occur in the absence of any identifiable morphologic alterations.

Hepatic fibrosis in the nonneoplastic liver has been classified as follows:[135](1) capsular and subcapsular fibrosis, as may occur after peritonitis or exposure to vinyl chloride; (2) focal fibrosis that results from healing of granulomas, gummas, abscesses, or infarcts, and, when extensive, can result in hepar lobatum; (3) segmental or lobar fibrosis secondary to occlusion of a bile duct or vessels supplying a segment or lobe; (4) diffuse intra-acinar fibrosis that can be panacinar or zonal, as in zone 3 after alcoholic injury ("chicken-wire" fibrosis), or in zone 1 after chronic cholestatic conditions or chronic hepatitis; diffuse fibrosis with nodule formation by definition is cirrhosis; (5) "system fibrosis" that involves bile ducts (such as periductal fibrosis in primary sclerosing cholangitis) or vessels (such as phlebosclerosis, venocclusive disease, or healed thrombosis).

Some diseases associated with hepatic fibrosis can lead to portal hypertension in the absence of cirrhosis.[711] Among the most frequent is alcoholic liver disease.

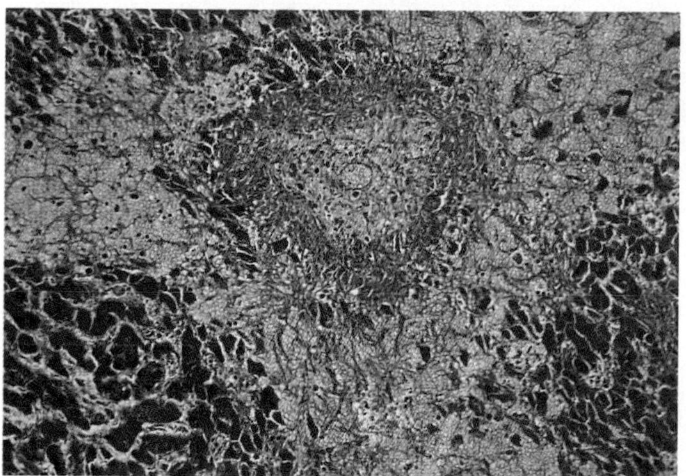

Fig. 57-56 Venoocclusive disease caused by *Senecio* toxicity. Terminal hepatic venule *(top)* is almost completely occluded by intimal edema. There is perivenular congestion and necrosis.

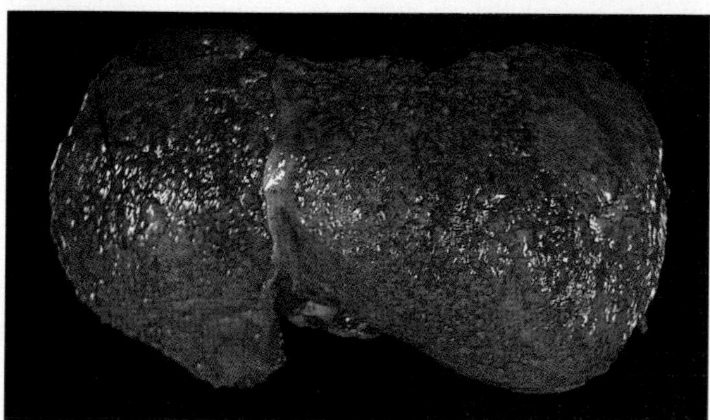

Fig. 57-57 Micronodular cirrhosis.

Cirrhosis

Cirrhosis is a diffuse process characterized by fibrosis and conversion of the normal liver architecture into structurally abnormal nodules. Three basic morphologic categories are recognized:[712] (1) a micronodular type, which includes cases in which the nodules are less than 3 mm in diameter; (2) a macronodular type, in which most nodules are greater than 3 mm in diameter and usually show striking variation in size; (3) a mixed type characterized by approximately equal numbers of micronodules and macronodules (Figs. 57-57 and 57-58). Regenerative nodules are not essential for the diagnosis of cirrhosis; in both biliary cirrhosis and hemochromatosis, for example, regeneration may be minimal or absent.

The diagnosis of cirrhosis is difficult to establish by percutaneous needle biopsy, particularly if the pattern is macronodular. In part, the difficulty is attributable to the preferential sampling of parenchyma as the biopsy needle rebounds from the fibrous septa. Microscopic clues to the diagnosis are alluded to in other publications.[135,713] Biopsy specimens are commonly fragmented, and the fragments have rounded edges (Fig. 57-59). Fibrous septa can course through the fragments but sometimes are represented by thin septa hugging margins of the fragments. Stains for collagen are frequently necessary to detect them. Such stains are also valuable for distinguishing collapsed reticulin that follows extensive necrosis ("passive septa") from fibrosis, and for demonstrating thick liver plates in regenerative nodules of the cirrhotic liver.

In macronodular cirrhosis, silver stains usually demonstrate a very irregular reticulin pattern because of alterations in the growth of hepatocytes. Nodules within nodules (adenomatous hyperplasia) may be seen. Many cell plates are greater than one cell in thickness, and the compressed sinusoidal spaces may be nearly invisible. Hepatocytes are pleomorphic, unless the process is entirely inactive. An alteration of the spatial relationship between the portal vessels and THV is typical. Micronodular cirrhosis is less difficult to diagnose by needle biopsy than macronodular cirrhosis, since the diameter of the biopsy needle usually exceeds that of the small cirrhotic nodules.

The capsule of the liver in some noncirrhotic patients may be thickened by an increase in fibrous tissue, vessels, and ductules. A small biopsy specimen from such an area (particularly a superficial wedge biopsy) should be interpreted with caution and not diagnosed as cirrhosis.

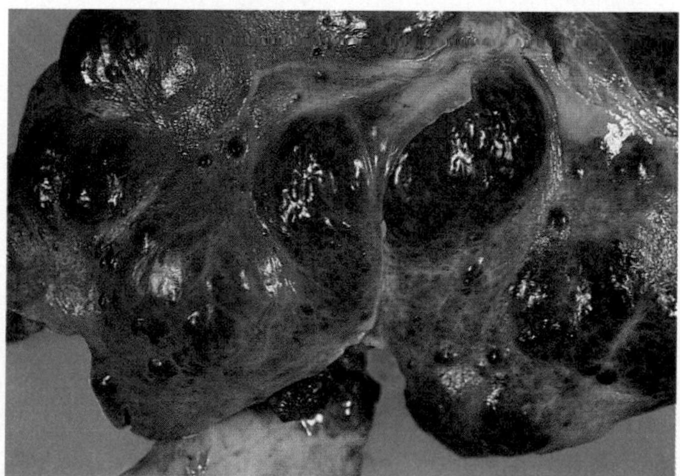

Fig. 57-58 Macronodular cirrhosis.

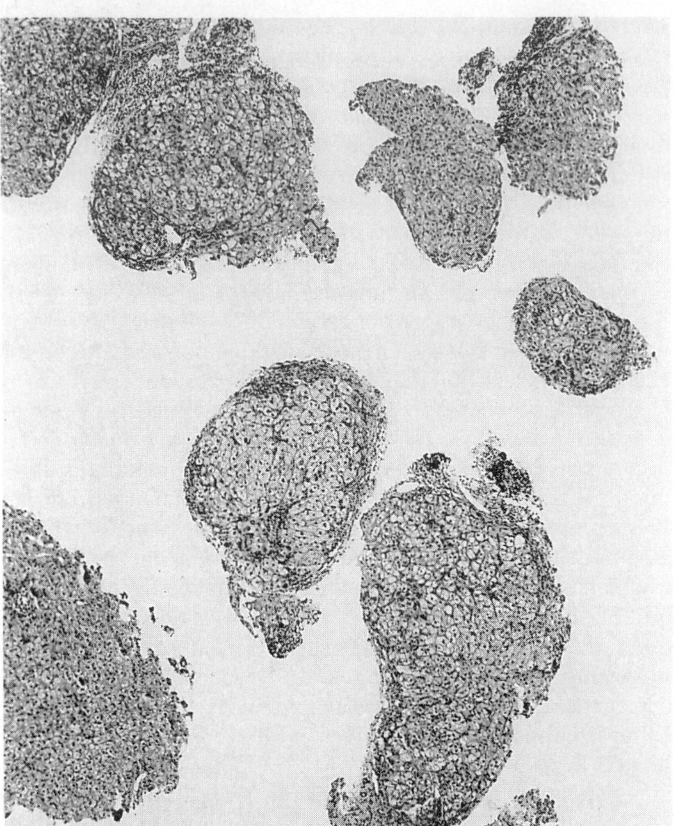

Fig. 57-59 Fragmented needle biopsy specimen from a cirrhotic liver; some of the fragments are invested by delicate septa.

The morphologic approach in cirrhosis should include an assessment of whether cirrhosis is fully developed or incomplete, the basic morphologic type (micronodular, macronodular, or mixed), the degree of activity, and the presumptive cause, if possible. Biopsy specimens showing occasional nodules and incomplete septa can be designated as incomplete cirrhosis, but the term *cirrhosis* should be reserved for those with diffuse nodules surrounded by septa. The activity of the cirrhosis is based on the degree of hepatocellular degeneration and necrosis and the amount of inflammation in the nodules and in the fibrous septa. Periseptal piecemeal necrosis should also be considered when one is assessing the degree of activity.

Every effort should be made to establish the underlying cause, though this is not always possible. Refer to accounts in the preceding sections for the histologic appearances in individual disorders. An etiologic diagnosis can sometimes be established by changes observed in hematoxylin and eosin-stained sections alone (such as absence of bile ducts and chronic cholestasis, an indication of a biliary cirrhosis secondary to PBC or PSC). Special stains are often helpful in establishing an etiologic diagnosis. Particularly useful are stains for copper or copper-binding protein in Wilson's disease and chronic cholestatic diseases, the PAS stain for α_1-antitrypsin deficiency, aldehyde fuchsin, orcein, or Victoria blue stains for viral hepatitis type B, and an iron stain for hemochromatosis. Immunocytochemical techniques may also be used in α_1-antitrypsin deficiency and viral hepatitis (such as those for HBsAg, HBcAg, HCV, and HDV antigens).

Conditions associated with the micronodular pattern of cirrhosis include alcoholic liver disease, nonalcoholic steatohepatitis, biliary cirrhosis (primary and secondary), glycogenosis type IV, genetic hemochromatosis, postjejunoileal bypass disease, Indian childhood cirrhosis, galactosemia, and congestive (cardiac) cirrhosis.

Macronodular cirrhosis is more likely to be seen in cases of viral hepatitis, Wilson's disease, hereditary tyrosinemia, α_1-antitrypsin deficiency, and drug-induced injury. These disorders, as well as alcoholism, can also lead to a mixed micronodular-macronodular pattern.

Complicating lesions may be found. *Liver cell dysplasia* is apparently more frequent in posthepatitis cirrhosis than in other types. It is characterized by nuclear and cytoplasmic enlargement, nuclear hyperchromasia, prominent nucleoli, and occasionally multinucleation.[714] *Adenomatous hyperplasia* (including *macroregenerative nodules,* which have a diameter greater than 8 to 10 mm) is a nodular lesion that occurs in cirrhosis and is believed to progress to hepatocellular carcinoma through an "intermediate" lesion.[715-719] Adenomatoid hyperplasia occurs as an ill-defined nodule within a cirrhotic nodule ("nodule-in-nodule" formation) that is best recognized by compression of surrounding reticulin fibers and different orientation of the liver plates. It is considered likely that this lesion, rather than liver cell dysplasia, is the precusor of hepatocellular carcinoma in the cirrhotic liver.

Cirrhotic livers are particularly susceptible to anoxia because of their altered vascular relationships. Shock, resulting from bleeding esophageal varices or other causes, produces irregular circumscribed areas of coagulative necrosis termed *anoxic pseudolobular necrosis,* or *ischemic hepatitis in cirrhosis.*[720] Henrion and colleagues[720] found ischemic hepatitis in 1.5% of 130 consecutive cases of cirrhosis admitted to their intensive care unit for gastrointestinal hemorrhage.

Hemosiderosis is not uncommon, particularly in the cirrhosis of the alcoholic. It also complicates portacaval shunts. The amount of iron that accumulates in these patients, however, is far less than that in genetic hemochromatosis and is unlikely to lead to tissue injury.[721] Cholestasis of varied cause can be present. Pathognomonic changes in intra-acinar bile ducts should be observed before a diagnosis of superimposed biliary obstruction is rendered.

SPACE-OCCUPYING LESIONS

Cysts and cystic dilatations

Developmental cysts

Caroli's disease. Although Caroli's disease generally involves the entire liver, it may be segmental or lobar. The inheritance is autosomal recessive. Clinically, patients suffer from bouts of recurrent fever and pain. Jaundice occurs only when a stone blocks the common bile duct.[722,723] Leukocytosis is observed typically when acute cholangitis develops. Liver tests are generally normal except during episodes of obstructive jaundice. The diagnosis is established by cholangiography (intravenous, transhepatic), endoscopic retrograde cholangiopancreatography, ultrasonography, and computerized tomography. The complications include recurrent cholangitis, abscess formation, septicemia or pyemia, intrahepatic lithiasis, and amyloidosis. Adenocarcinomas, including some arising in cases with a lobar distribution, have also been reported.[724,725] Surgical treatment is by internal or external drainage procedures. Segmental or lobar forms of Caroli's disease can be treated by partial hepatectomy.

Macroscopically the intrahepatic cystic dilatations are round or lanceolate, are 1 to 4.5 cm in diameter, and may be separated by stretches of essentially normal duct. Inspissated bile or soft and friable bilirubin calculi may be noted in the lumen. Microscopically the dilated ducts usually show severe chronic inflammation, with or without superimposed acute inflammation, and varying degrees of fibrosis. The epithelium may appear normal (cuboidal to tall columnar), may be partly or completely ulcerated, or may be focally hyperplastic; all these changes can be found in different ducts in the same case. Mucous glands (sometimes in abundance) may be present in the fibrotic and inflamed wall. Areas of severe epithelial dysplasia or carcinoma in situ are seen rarely.[726,727] The lumen contains admixtures of inspissated mucin and bile, calcareous material, or frank pus during the bouts of acute cholangitis. Caroli's disease can be associated with congenital hepatic fibrosis.

According to Desmet[728] the pathogenesis of Caroli's disease seems to involve total or partial arrest of remodeling of the ductal plate of the larger intrahepatic bile ducts. In Caroli's "syndrome" (Caroli's disease with congenital hepatic fibrosis) the hereditary factor causing the arrest of remodeling seems to exert its influence not only during the early period of bile duct embryogenesis, but also later during development of the more peripheral biliary ramifications (the interlobular bile ducts).

Autosomal recessive polycystic kidney disease (ARPKD)

Infantile presentation. Autosomal recessive polycystic kidney disease (ARPKD) is inherited in an autosomal recessive manner. The prevalence is estimated to be between 1:10,000 to 1:60,000.[729] The gene for this disorder has not been mapped. There is an equal sex incidence. Depending on the age of presentation and the degree of renal involvement, ARPKD has been divided into four types by Blyth and Ockenden[730]—perinatal, neonatal, infantile, and juvenile. ARPKD has been reviewed by several authors.[731-734]

The *perinatal* type is the most severe form of this condition. Some affected patients are stillborn. In the series of Blyth and Ockenden[730] no infant survived beyond 6 weeks of age. Most patients were admitted with signs of respiratory distress (from various forms of pulmonary insufficiency) and had obvious abdominal distension because of huge symmetrical renal masses. Liver test abnormalities were uncommon. Surviving patients with the *neonatal* type of the disease develop gradually increasing renal insufficiency and hypertension. Pyelonephritis is common. Portal fibrosis and cystic dilatation of bile ducts are more pronounced, and cholangitis is a frequent complication. In the *infantile* group the clinical picture is either of chronic renal failure or of increasing portal hypertension. Portal fibrosis is moderate. The *juvenile* group typically includes children (1 to 5 years old) who present with portal hypertension. Liver pathologic changes are noticeable. It is likely that this group represents cases of congenital hepatic fibrosis, as suggested by Landing and colleagues.[733] Gang and Herrin[735] have found that ARPKD has a continuum of phenotype expression with prognostic implications but believe that all cases do not fit into the sharply defined subgroups of Blyth and Ockenden.[730] In their study of 11 patients, four had 90% or more renal cystic change; these patients did not survive beyond 20 days of birth. In contrast, five of the seven less severely diseased patients with a 20% to 75% range of cystic changes in the kidneys were all alive at 6 to 21 years of age.

The liver in ARPKD does not appear abnormal macroscopically, though it may be enlarged and firm. Histologically, there is a striking increase in the number of biliary channels that arise in portal areas and extend irregularly and deeply into the lobules. They appear to branch or "anastomose" and often show polypoid projections. A circular (often interrupted) appearance (ductal plate malformation) is believed to represent arrested development of the bile ducts[736] (Fig. 57-60). Normal interlobular ducts are not seen. According to Witzleben[734] the biliary channels are in continuity with the rest of the biliary system ("communicating" cystic disease), in contrast to the noncommunicating autosomal dominant polycystic kidney disease. The supporting connective tissue is very scanty, and in the intralobular extensions the basement membrane of the epithelium appears to be in direct contact with the liver cell plates. The epithelial lining consists of a single layer of low columnar to cuboidal cells. The dilated channels may contain a small quantity of a pink or orange material or, rarely, pus.

Juvenile and adult presentation—congenital hepatic fibrosis (CHF). Congenital hepatic fibrosis occurs predominantly in children and adolescents. Patients typically come to medical attention because of hepatosplenomegaly or bleeding from esophageal varices secondary to portal hypertension that is usually presinusoidal, but asymptomatic cases have been reported.[737,738] Cholangitis as a manifestation of CHF has been emphasized by Fauvert and Benhamou.[739] These investigators recognize four clinical forms—portal hypertensive, cholangitic, mixed portal hypertensive-cholangitic, and latent forms. The pure cholangitic form is rare. In the mixed form patients suffer from recurrent bouts of cholangitis, with or without jaundice, in addition to the manifestations of portal hypertension.

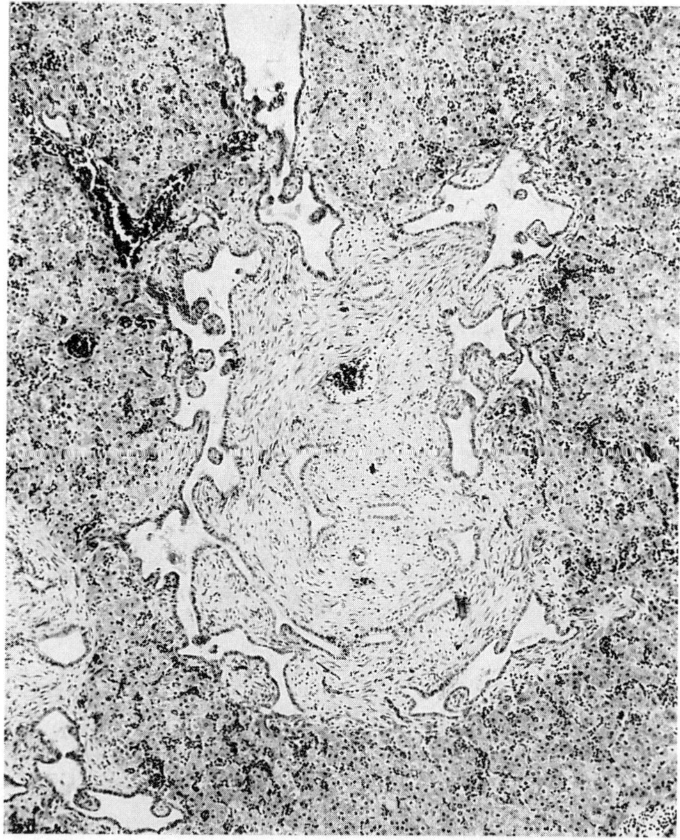

Fig. 57-60 Neonatal liver from patient with autosomal recessive polycystic disease of the kidneys and liver showing the ductal plate malformation.

The usual kidney disease, when present, is medullary tubular ectasia, a fusiform or cystic dilatation of tubules (particularly the collecting ducts), detected by intravenous pyelography and renal angiography, but some patients may have cystic kidneys resembling those of polycystic disease, and others may have nephronophthisis.[737,740,741] The organ most affected, be it kidney or liver, may vary within the same family. Routine liver function tests are usually normal, but the serum alkaline phosphatase activity may be increased.

The combination of a patent portal vein and well-preserved liver function makes patients with CHF ideal candidates for portosystemic shunt surgery. Of 75 published cases reviewed by Sommerschild and colleagues,[737] 50% had died; the major causes of death were renal failure and uncontrollable hemorrhage. One complication that should be noted is the rare development of cholangiocarcinoma.[742]

Grossly the liver in CHF is enlarged, has a firm to hard consistency, and shows a fine reticular pattern of fibrosis; no cysts are visible to the naked eye. Microscopically, there is diffuse periportal fibrosis, with the bands of fibrous tissue varying in thickness (Fig. 57-61). Irregularly shaped islands of hepatic tissue, some incorporating several acini, may be seen. When the bands of fibrous tissue are thick, THVs may be encroached upon and become incorporated within the fibrous tissue. Numerous uniform and generally small bile ducts are scattered in the fibrous tissue. An interrupted circular arrangement of the ducts (ductal plate malformation) may be recognizable. The ducts are lined by cuboidal to low columnar epithelium and may contain bile or traces of mucin. They may be slightly dilated and irregular in outline. Paucity of portal vein branches has been noted in some studies[737] and has usually been invoked as the cause of the portal hypertension. There is generally little inflammation in CHF except in cases associated with cholangitis, when numerous neutrophils infiltrate the ducts and surrounding connective tissue; rupture of the ducts can result in microabscess formation. Histopathologically the latter cases may be difficult to differentiate from extrahepatic biliary obstruction with ascending infection, particularly since there may be an associated tissue cholestasis. The correct diagnosis must be based on the history, clinical findings, and the results of radiographic studies. It is important to reiterate at this point that CHF may be associated with Caroli's disease or, rarely, with choledochal cyst.

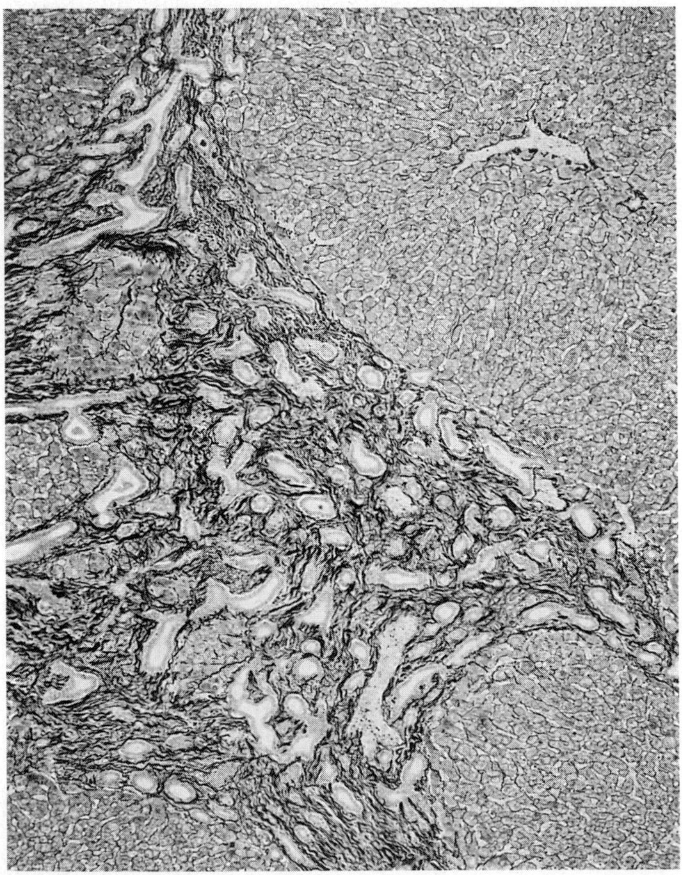

Fig. 57-61 Congenital hepatic fibrosis. Septum contains numerous small ducts. (Manuel's reticulin stain.)

Many malformation syndromes, characterized by hepatic morphologic changes that resemble those of CHF can be differentiated by the associated findings (Table 57-16).[733,743]

Autosomal dominant polycystic kidney disease (ADPKD). The abnormal gene of ADPKD-1 is on the short arm of chromosome 16, closely linked to the α-hemoglobin and phosphoglycolate phosphatase genes, and can be identified by a DNA probe 16S4 when there are two other affected family members.[744-747] The incidence of this mutant gene is one in 1000 and constitutes 90% of cases. In adults, the other (non-ADPKD-1) 10% of patients present with a milder form of polycystic disease. In one series of 173 autopsies of individuals with polycystic kidneys, one to several liver cysts were found in 16%, and numerous cysts were present in 21%.[748] The renal disease can be present at birth, but hepatic manifestations are rare before 16 years of age.[749]

The incidence of liver involvement and its complications have been reviewed in a large series of ADPKD, including 132 patients receiving hemodialysis and 120 patients not receiving hemodialysis.[750] Liver cysts were found by noninvasive radiologic procedures in 85 of 124 patients receiving dialysis; sex

Table 57-16 Differential diagnosis of malformation syndromes resembling congenital hepatic fibrosis (CHF)

Syndrome	Associated findings
Meckel's syndrome	Encephalocele Polydactyly Cystic kidneys
Ivemark's syndrome	Dysplasia of the pancreas, liver, and kidneys Cysts in pancreas and liver (in some cases)
Ellis–van Creveld syndrome (chondroectodermal dysplasia)	
Nephronophthisis-CHF syndrome	Retinal lesions Mental retardation Cerebellar hypoplasia Osseous abnormalities
Jeune syndrome	Skeletal dysplasia Pulmonary hypoplasia Retinal lesions
Vaginal atresia syndrome	
Tuberous sclerosis	
Medullary cystic disease	

distribution was equal. In contrast, the nondialyzed population demonstrated a 75% incidence of liver cysts in females and 44% incidence in males, with the peak incidence occurring 10 years sooner in females. The cysts were larger and greater in number in that population, and there was a correlation with the number of pregnancies. There were reported nineteen autopsies in which 5 deaths were liver related. Risk factors for the development of hepatic cysts in ADPKD were also examined in a large series (39 patients and 189 unaffected family members) by Gabow and colleagues.[747] The hepatic expression of the disease was found to be modulated by age, female sex, pregnancy, severity of the renal lesion, and kidney function.

The leading complication in ADPKD is infected liver cysts, with cholangiocarcinoma the second most common complicaton. A recent study examining hepatic cyst infection indicates that the incidence increases from 1% to 3% during end-stage renal failure.[751] In that study Enterobacteriaceae were cultured from the infected cysts in 9 out of 12 patients.[751] Conditions associated with ADPKD include colon diverticula (70%), cardiac valve complications (25%), ovarian cysts (40%), inguinal hernia (15%), and intracranial aneurysms (10%), suggestive of a diffusely abnormal matrix.

Grossly the liver in ADPKD is enlarged and diffusely cystic, with the cysts varying from less than 1 mm to 12 cm or more in diameter. Occasionally one lobe, usually the left, is affected. Diffuse dilatation of the intrahepatic and extrahepatic bile ducts has been reported in some cases of ADPKD.[752] The cysts contain a clear, colorless, or light yellow fluid.

Microscopically the cysts are lined by columnar or cuboidal epithelium, but the larger cysts have a flat epithelium. Collapsed cysts resemble corpora atretica of the ovary. The supporting connective tissue is scanty except in relation to von Meyenburg's complexes, a frequently associated lesion, where it may be dense and hyalinized. A small number of inflammatory cells, usually lymphocytes, may infiltrate the supporting stroma. Infected cysts contain pus and may rupture. Calcification of the wall of hepatic (and renal) cysts in ADPKD has been reported.[753]

Von Meyenburg's complexes are considered part of the continuum of adult polycystic disease. A histomorphometric and clinicopathologic study of 28 cases of ADPKD by Ramos and colleagues[754] supports the view that the cysts of ADPKD arise by progressive dilatation of the abnormal ducts in von Meyenburg's complexes. The complexes are small (less than 0.5 cm in diameter) and usually scattered in both lobes. Their color is grayish white or green. They are occasionally associated with cavernous hemangiomas. Microscopically the lesions are discrete, round to irregular in shape, and periportal in location. The constituent ducts are embedded in a collagenous stroma and are often round (but may be irregular in shape) and have slightly dilated lumens (Fig. 57-62). They are lined by low columnar or cuboidal epithelium and contain pink amorphous material, which may be bile stained, or actual bile. Cholangiocarcinomas have been reported in association with von Meyenburg's complexes, as well as with multiple hepatic cysts considered a type of ADPKD.[755-758]

Solitary (nonparasitic) cyst. A solitary cyst is usually subdivided into unilocular (95%) and multilocular (biliary cystadenoma) (5%) varieties; the latter is discussed in the section on tumors. Solitary cysts occur at all ages, though the majority present in the fourth to sixth decades of life. The female-to-male ratio in two reviews was 4:1[759] and 5.25:1.[760] Cysts less than 8 to 10 cm rarely cause symptoms and may be found incidentally at laparotomy for some other disease. Symptoms, when present, include an upper abdominal mass with fullness, nausea, and occasional vomiting. Rapid enlargement has been reported in infancy.[761] An acute abdominal crisis may result from torsion, strangulation, and hemorrhage into the cyst or rupture.[762,763] Jaundice is an infrequent complication.[764,765] Diagnosis is established by ultrasonography or computerized tomography. In the past the treatment of choice was excision, but aspiration and injection of sclerosing solutions have now obviated the need for surgery in many cases.

Solitary cysts involve the right lobe twice as often as the left. Very rarely, they can arise in the falciform ligament.[766] The cysts are round to oval and well encapsulated, and they may be pedunculated. They can contain up to 17 liters of fluid and fill the abdominal cavity. The fluid is usually clear.

The lining of the cysts usually consists of a single layer of flat, cuboidal, or columnar epithelium, but it may be squamous in type. The cells rest on a basement membrane and are supported by a fibrous stroma. The wall may contain lipofuscin-laden macrophages, cholesterol crystals with an associated foreign-body giant cell reaction, and varying numbers of inflammatory cells. Malignant tumors may arise in unilocular cysts and are usually adenocarcinomas, but occasional squamous cell carcinomas and even a carcinoid tumor have been reported.[767-769]

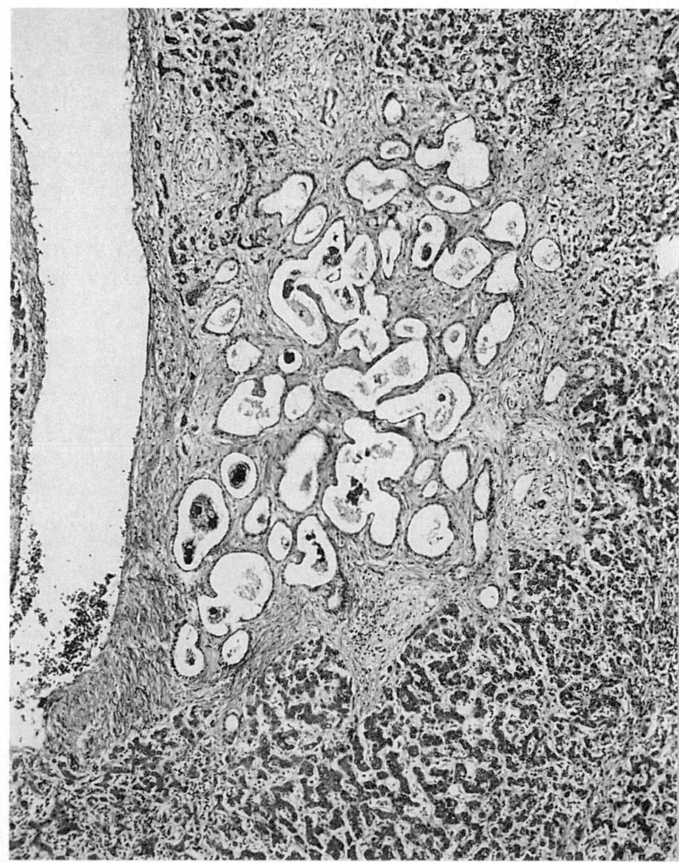

Fig. 57-62 Von Meyenburg's complex composed of small, somewhat irregular bile ducts set in a fibrous stroma. Some of the ducts contain bile.

Acquired

Hydatid cyst (echinococcosis). The disease hydatid cyst, or echinococcosis, is a worldwide health problem, being especially endemic in countries where sheep raising is common (such as Greece, Spain, Turkey, Argentina, Uruguay, Australia, New Zealand, and South Africa). It is caused by the larval stages of various cestode (tapeworm) species of the genus *Echinococcus*. *Echinococcus granulosus* causes cystic hydatid disease and has a worldwide distribution. *E. multilocularis* causes alveolar hydatid disease and occurs only in the northern hemisphere (Alaska and Canada in North America). *E. vogeli,* which causes polycystic echinococcosis, is very rare in humans, and has been reported in Central and South America. Major definitive hosts are the dog (for *E. granulosus*), fox, dog, and cat (for *E. multilocularis*). The intermediate hosts are sheep, cattle, pigs, horses, and camels (for *E. granulosus*), rodents (for *E. multilocularis*) and pacas, a type of wild rodent (for *E. vogeli*). Hydatid disease occurs when man becomes an accidental intermediate host by swallowing the eggs of the parasite. The larvae (or oncospheres) are freed in the duodenum, burrow their way through the intestinal mucosa, and enter the lumen of blood vessels. The liver is the major organ affected in all three species; in the case of *E. granulosus* primary cysts are found in the liver in 60% of cases, in the lungs in 20% of cases, and in other organs in the remainder.

Clinical findings in a series of 226 cases included right upper quadrant pain (66%), hepatomegaly (44%), a palpable mass (39%), and anorexia and weight loss (25%).[770] Complications include obstructive jaundice, rupture into the common bile duct or peritoneum, infection of the cyst, and inferior vena cava thrombosis.[770-776] Alveolar echinococcosis (caused by *E. multilocularis*) invades not only hepatic and biliary tissue, but also vessels of the liver, the inferior vena cava, and the diaphragm. The diagnosis of echinococcosis of the liver is established by imaging studies, beginning with ultrasound examination; in one series the cysts were demonstrated with 94% accuracy by that technique.[770]

Most hydatid cysts are located in the right lobe of the liver. Their size varies with their age. Cysts of *E. granulosus* grow approximately by 1 cm per year; clinical symptoms do not usually develop until the cyst is 10 cm in diameter.[777] The hydatid cyst has an inner germinal layer (supported by a semipermeable laminated cuticle) from which many brood capsules develop (Fig. 57-63). The brood capsules contain the scolices representing the future head of the adult tapeworm; they contain a double row of scimitar-shaped hooklets, which are acid fast. Calcification of the wall occurs in old cysts. An outer adventitial layer, formed by the host, separates the cyst from the liver (Fig. 57-63). The cyst of *E. multilocularis* (alveolar echinococcosis) consists of a spongy pale tissue in which are scattered multiple small cysts. Microscopically a laminated membrane lines the cysts, but scoleces are found in less than 10% of cysts.[778] A granulomatous inflammatory response is frequently seen in the wall.[778] *E. vogeli* leads to polycystic hydatid cysts that histopathologically resemble those of alveolar echinococcosis.[779]

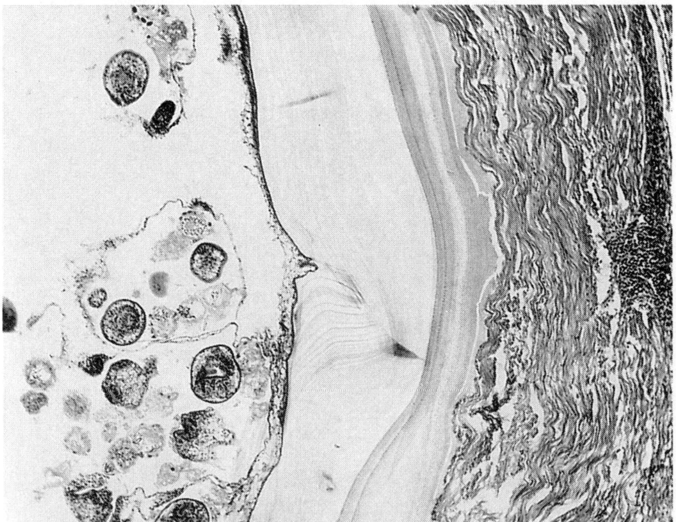

Fig. 57-63 Echinococcal cyst consists of an adventitial fibrous wall *(right),* a laminated membrane, and detached brood capsules and scoleces *(left).*

Medical and surgical treatment of hepatic echinococcosis, including orthotopic liver transplantation for incurable alveolar echinococcosis, are discussed in several publications.[780-781]

Pseudocysts. Two cases of pancreatic pseudocyst have been reported in the left lobe of the liver; one occurred after trauma to the liver, and the other was a complication of alcoholic pancreatitis.[782] Cystic degeneration of hepatic malignancies, both primary (such as hepatocellular carcinoma, cholangiocarcinoma) and metastastic (such as neuroendocrine tumors), may pose difficulties in imaging studies but are unlikely to cause problems in histopathologic interpretation.[783-785]

Abscess

Pyogenic abscess

About one fifth of all pyogenic abscesses are cryptogenic.[786] The remainder are secondary to diseases of the biliary tract (cholangitic abscesses), intra-abdominal sepsis with spread of the infection by means of the portal venous system (pylephlebitic abscesses), extra-abdominal foci of suppuration with bacteria reaching the liver by way of its arterial supply, spread from contiguous infections in adjacent viscera or organs, and spread from penetrating or blunt trauma. Examples of recently reported associations of hepatic abscess have included chronic pancreatitis,[787] hemorrhoidectomy,[788] and Crohn's disease.[789] Currently, biliary tract disease is the leading cause of pyogenic hepatic abscess[786,790] (Fig. 57-64). *Escherichia coli* is the most frequently isolated organism; other organisms include *Klebsiella, Proteus, Pseudomonas,* and enterococci. Earlier diagnosis and more refined therapeutic methods have radically reduced the high mortalities seen a decade or more ago.[786] The mortality is higher with multiple (41%) than with single abscesses (15%).[791] The diagnostic approach to liver abscess is discussed by De Cock and Reynolds.[790] The roles of percutaneous drainage (which is replacing open drainage) and medical management have been discussed by several authors.[790-792]

Pyogenic abscesses are either single or multiple. The contents may be yellow or green and are frequently foul smelling. Microscopically, acute abscesses contain pus; bacteria may or may not be identified with tissue Gram stains. The wall of subacute or chronic abscesses is replaced by granulation and fibrous tissue. In some abscesses the source of infection may be identified in tissue sections by the presences of an associated suppurative cholangitis (cholangitic abscess) or portal pylephlebitis (pylephlebitic abscess).

Amebic abscess

The mortality from uncomplicated amebic abscess is now less than 3%, but rupture can raise that figure to 7% to 15%.[790,793-796] The significant reduction in mortality in recent years has been achieved by early diagnosis (aspiration, serologic tests), accurate localization by radiologic methods (nuclear scanning, ultrasound, computerized tomography), drug therapy, and ultrasound-guided percutaneous drainage when indicated.[790] Surgery is now reserved for drainage of a ruptured abscess or treatment of a coexistent surgical condition.[56,288]

Amebic abscesses are more often single (70%) than multiple and measure from 10 to 15 cm in diameter. The lining is ragged. The contents are typically chocolate brown or like anchovy paste, but they may be purulent if secondary bacterial infection had occurred. They are odorless; a foul smell indicates secondary bacterial infection. Wet preparation made from material aspirated from an amebic abscess should be searched for trophozoites. Fixed preparation can be studied by routine stains or after staining with PAS, Heidenhain's iron hematoxylin stain, or the Gomori methenamine silver stain. Microscopically the abscess wall consists of necrotic, amorphous, eosinophilic, material and may contain trophozoites with ingested erythrocytes (Fig. 57-65). The amebas are PAS positive and argentophilic, but nuclear details are best demonstrated by the Heidenhain stain. Indirect immunofluorescence has also been utilized for detection of *Entamoeba histolytica* in tissue sections.[797] In healing amebic abscesses the necrotic tissue is replaced by granulation tissue, and eventually the entire abscess is replaced by a fibrous scar. Readers interested in additional information regarding the pathology of amebiasis should consult the excellent review of Brandt and Tamayo.[798]

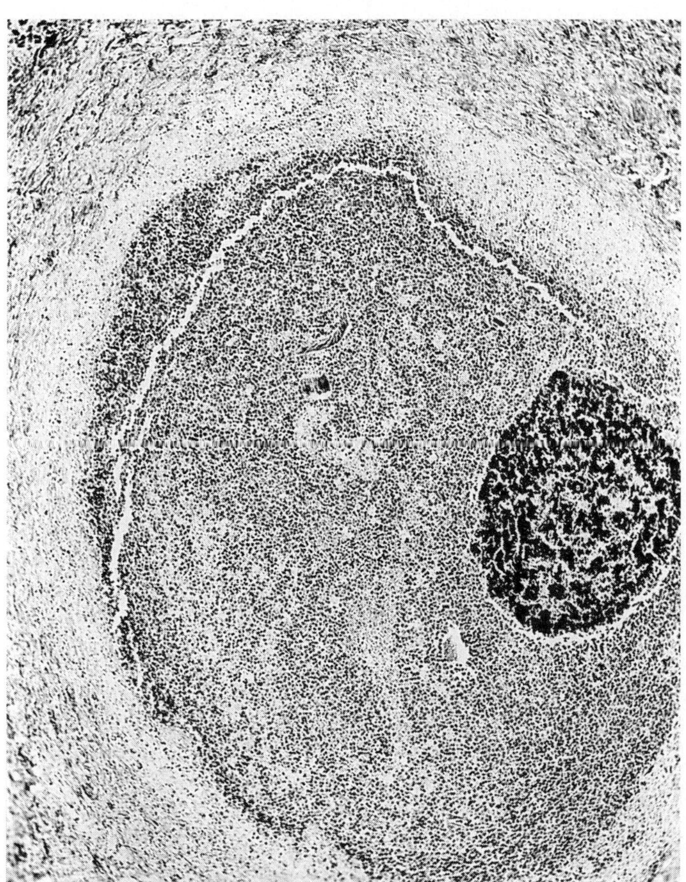

Fig. 57-64 Cholangitic abscess contains a darkly stained bolus of bile *(right)*.

Tumorlike conditions

Mesenchymal hamartoma

Mesenchymal hamartoma[799,800] occurs almost exclusively in young children. The average age is approximately 15 months, with the lesion occurring twice as often in males as in females. A primary clinical presentation is that of progressive abdominal enlargement. The tumor may weigh as much as 1 kg because of fluid accumulation.

Mesenchymal hamartoma consists of a loose, myxoid connective tissue in which are scattered branched, tortuous bile ducts; a ductal plate–like arrangement of ducts may be present. Fluid accumulation in the connective tissue leads to cyst formation. Numerous blood vessels and even lymphatics are seen. Hematopoiesis is also a frequent feature. Hepatocytes are scattered throughout the fibrous tissue in small clusters or sheets. Partial or total excision results in a cure. The recent findings of translocation involving 19q13.4 and aneuploidy in some cases indicate that mesenchymal hamartoma may be a true neoplasm and not a developmental anomaly.[801,802] A case of a possible transition of a mesenchymal hamartoma to an undifferentiated sarcoma was reported recently.[803]

Focal nodular hyperplasia

Focal nodular hyperplasia may be single or multiple; it occurs in noncirrhotic livers. It has been described in patients varying in age from children through late adulthood.[804-807] Most of these lesions are identified in the third to fifth decade of life, with the female-to-male ratio being approximately 2:1. Most of these lesions are discovered accidentally. Patients rarely present with pain or abdominal discomfort because of the mass. Hemorrhage or rupture is very rare. In one study focal

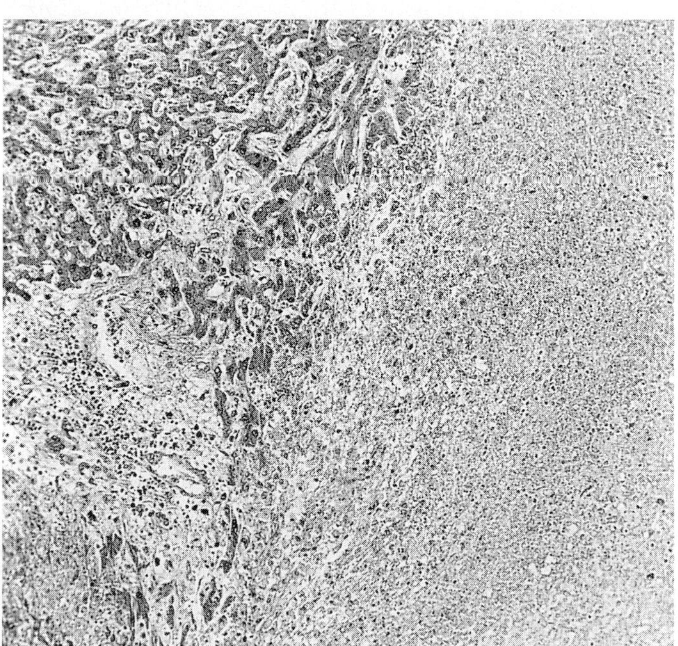

Fig. 57-65 Amebic abscess contains amorphous material.

nodular hyperplasia was associated with hepatic hemangioma in 23% of cases.[808] A syndrome of multiple focal nodular hyperplasia associated with widespread vascular malformations and malignant brain tumors was reported by Wanless and colleagues.[809]

Focal nodular hyperplasia occurs in a normal liver and appears as a spherical mass, approximately 5 cm in diameter. Larger masses up to 15 cm in diameter have been described. The largest masses tend to distort the liver surface and may be pedunculated. When sectioned, the lesion bulges from the surrounding liver. There is a characteristic central stellate scar with fibrous septa radiating peripherally in a wagon-wheel pattern (Figs. 57-66 and 57-67). Histopathologically, focal nodular hyperplasia is composed of normal-appearing hepatocytes arranged in two-cell-thick plates between septa of fibrous tissue. Eccentrically or concentrically thickened arteries are usually present in the fibrous core and septa. Variable numbers of ducts, formed by a process of ductular metaplasia, are present at the interface of the septa with the hepatocytes.[810] Copper storage, usually in periseptal liver cells, is a frequent finding. An underlying spiderlike arterial malformation is believed to be the cause of the lesion.[811]

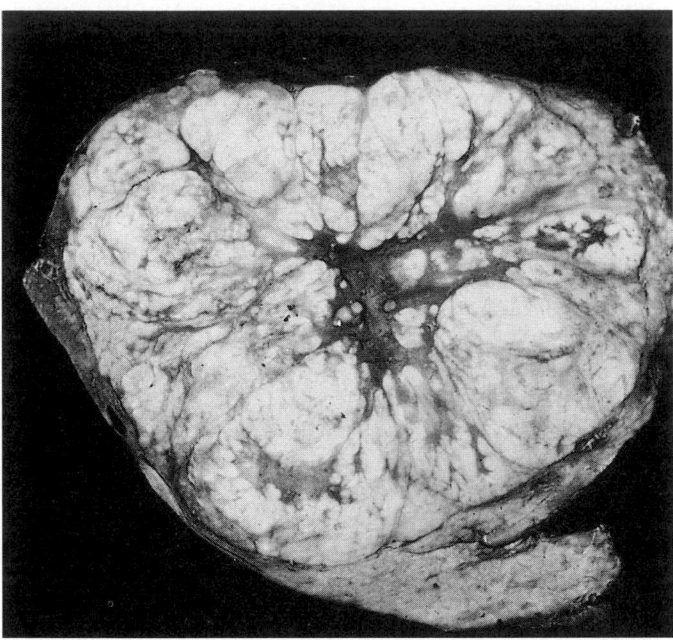

Fig. 57-66 Section of focal nodular hyperplasia showing central sear and radiating septa.

Nodular transformation (nodular regenerative hyperplasia)

Nodular transformation is characterized by diffuse hepatic nodularity without fibrosis or cirrhosis. It has been associated with rheumatoid arthritis, CREST (calcinosis, Raynaud's phenomenon, esophagitis, sclerodactyly, telangiectasia) syndrome, myeloproliferative disorders, autoimmune diseases, polyarteritis nodosa, subacute bacterial endocarditis, diabetes mellitus, lymphomas, chronic inflammatory bowel disease, and contraceptive or anabolic steroid use.[812-817]

Nodular transformation is more frequent in adults than in children. Symptoms and signs are usually attributable to the associated disease; however, some patients may develop portal hypertension or hepatic failure. Rupture of the liver is very rare. Clinically and histologically the condition may be confused with cirrhosis. Histopathologic diagnosis is more easily made using a wedge biopsy than a needle biopsy. Nodules of hyperplastic hepatocytes are arranged in two-cell-thick plates (Fig. 57-68). No fibrous septa are present, and thin rims of compressed atrophic parenchyma are present at the pushing margins. The features of nodular transformation are best appreciated in reticulin-stained slides (Fig. 57-69). There is typically an associated acinar atrophy of the intervening hepatic parenchyma. Occlusive vascular lesions, particularly of the small intrahepatic portal vein branches, may be seen. The pathogenesis has been attributed to a portal venopathy (leading to atrophy and compensatory hyperplasia)[813,814] or to long-term drug therapy.[812]

Inflammatory pseudotumor of the liver

The rare inflammatory pseudotumor of the liver occurs more frequently in the lung, skin, breast, kidney, stomach, spleen, and other organs.[818,819] Its pathogenesis is obscure. It is usually intrahepatic; rarely, when located near the hilum, it may

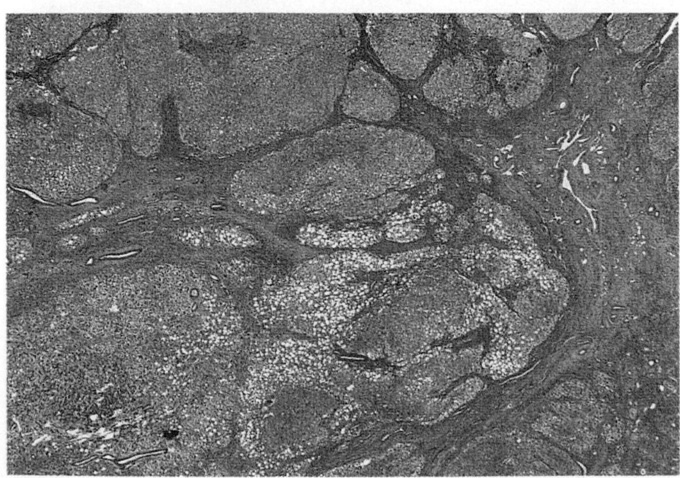

Fig. 57-67 Histologically the central scar of nodular hyperplasia extends into thinner septa.

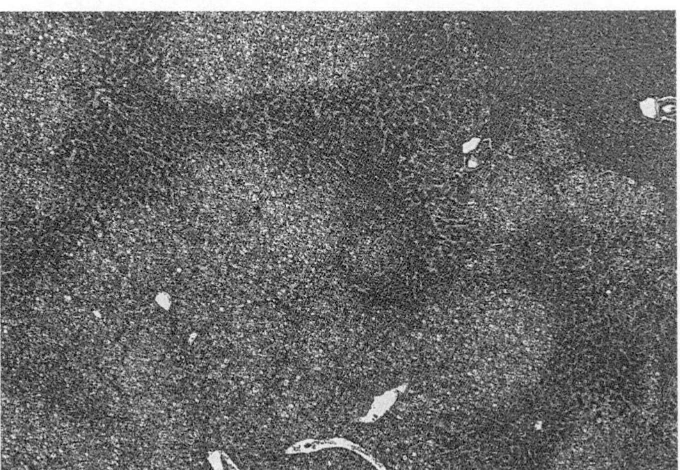

Fig. 57-68 Nodular transformation. Nodules are sharply defined, and the constituent cells are larger and paler than the normal hepatocytes. Some of the cells in the nodules contain fat vacuoles.

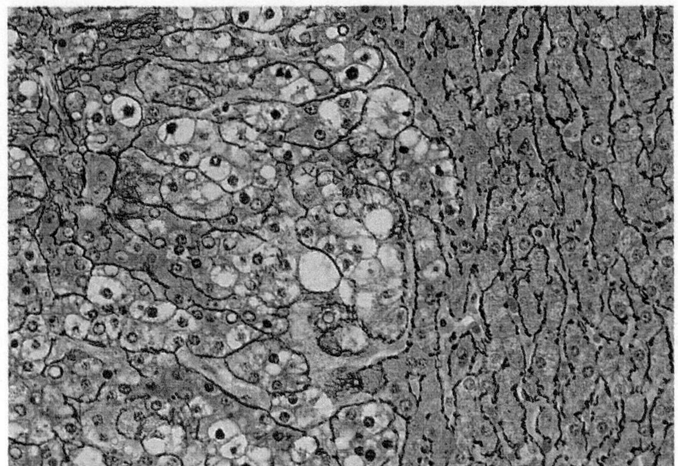

Fig. 57-69 Nodular transformation. Nodule *(top)* with thick liver cell plates is surrounded by an atrophic parenchyma with compressed reticulin fibers. (Manuel's reticulin stain.)

cause obstructive jaundice or portal hypertension. Histopathologically, there is an admixture of polyclonal plasma cells, macrophages, and fibroblasts, with variable collagen deposition. Xanthomatous cells, noncaseating granulomas, and a phlebitis may be seen in some cases. Microorganisms are usually not demonstrable by special stains.

NEOPLASMS

Benign epithelial tumors

There are several benign epithelial tumors, all of which are fairly uncommon, except for hepatocellular adenoma.

Bile duct adenoma

Bile duct adenomas are rare and usually an incidental finding at surgery or autopsy in adults.[820,821] Grossly, they are often mistaken for metastases. Bile duct adenomas are usually single and typically measure less than 1 cm in maximum dimension.

Microscopically, bile duct adenomas are composed of small ducts embedded in fibrous tissue. The stroma may be dense and hyalinized. The tumors are sharply defined but nonencapsulated. Often, normal portal areas are embedded within the adenoma; they are best seen in Masson-stained sections.

The differential diagnosis includes metastatic adenocarcinoma, intrahepatic cholangiocarcinoma, and von Meyenburg's complex. Cholangiocarcinomas are usually larger; both they and metastatic adenocarcinomas show histologic features of an invasive malignant neoplasm. Von Meyenburg's complexes are often multiple and may be associated with cysts. The constituent bile ducts may have an irregular pattern with polypoid intraluminal projections. Bile or, in infected cases, pus may be found in the lumen.

Biliary papillomatosis

Biliary papillomatosis is an underreported condition.[822-824] Multiple tumors are present within intrahepatic and extrahepatic bile ducts and occasionally within the gallbladder. They may produce obstruction that can be aggravated by hemobilia or infection. Although these tumors do have malignant potential, the patients usually die of other complications before malignancy is diagnosed. Curettage is one proposed form of therapy, but orthotopic liver transplantation is probably the treatment of choice. Histopathologically, dilated intrahepatic and extrahepatic bile ducts are filled with papillary excrescences composed of tall columnar cells supported by fibrovascular stalks.

Bile duct cystadenoma

Bile duct cystadenomas occur in the fourth or fifth decades, predominantly in women.[825-828] The main symptoms are abdominal discomfort or pain caused by the large size of the tumors, which are found primarily in the right lobe. Elevated serum levels of the tumor-associated antigen CA 19-9 have been reported in several cases, a finding helpful in differential diagnosis from other cystic conditions, such as hydatid cyst.[829] The tumors are multilocular and contain mucoid or clear fluid. Histologically the locules are lined by cuboidal to columnar epithelium that is mucin secreting. Secondary infection is uncommon. The surrounding stroma is usually compact and cellular, resembling ovarian stroma. Cholesterol clefts and macrophages containing hemosiderin and lipofuscin may be deposited around the cystic spaces, usually with ulceration of the epithelium. These tumors tend to recur if inadequately excised and have malignant potential. A rare variant, serous cystadenoma, is composed of small locules lined by glycogen-rich cuboidal cells; it lacks the mesenchymal stroma of the mucinous variety.[828]

Hepatocellular adenoma

The hepatocellular adenoma is the most important benign hepatocellular tumor. Its association with oral contraceptives has been well documented by case control studies.[830,831] Rooks and colleagues[831] demonstrated a direct relationship between the duration of use of oral contraceptives and the development of hepatocellular adenoma. They estimated annual incidence of hepatocellular adenoma in the United States to be 3.4 out of 100,000 oral contraceptive users.[831] Androgenic and anabolic steroids have also been shown to be associated with hepatocellular adenoma; most of these have developed in patients with Fanconi's anemia.[832] All the drugs that have been associated with hepatocellular adenoma up to now have been synthetic hormones derived from 7-alpha-ethinyl-substituted and not natural 17-alkyl derivatives. There is no evidence that any progesterone components of current formulations of oral contraceptives play a role in the increased risk of hepatocellular adenoma.

The pathologic features of hepatocellular adenoma are characteristic. It usually occurs in a normal liver and is a single, large lesion that can measure up to 15 cm in diameter. Occasionally, multiple tumors of varied size may be seen. Grossly the tumors are well defined; however, a capsule is usually not present. The cut surface is tan to yellow and may be focally hemorrhagic or infarcted.

Histopathologically, liver cell adenoma is composed of a sheetlike growth of cells resembling normal liver cells. Focal areas of recent or old hemorrhage and irregular scarring may be present. The plates of liver cells are two cells thick with slitlike compression of the sinusoids. The tumor cells are usually larger than normal and have a low nuclear to cytoplasmic ratio. The cytoplasm is often clear or rarefied because of the presence of glycogen or fat. Canalicular bile plugs may be present. Extramedullary hematopoesis is seen rarely. The presence of a reticulin framework and the lack of a trabecular pattern are helpful in differentiating hepatocellular adenoma from hepatocellular carcinoma. Intravascular invasion, when present, is diagnostic of carcinoma. Liver cell dysplasia may be seen; however, the relationship between that change and the development of hepatocellular carcinoma is not clear. That complication is well documented but rare.[833,834]

Hepatocellular adenomas may also occur with high frequency in patients with type I glycogen storage disease[835,836] and have been reported in cases of familial diabetes mellitus.[837]

Benign mesenchymal tumors

Hemangioma

Hemangioma is the most common benign tumor of the liver; it occurs at all ages and in both sexes. Many hemangiomas are found, incidentally, at autopsy. Only tumors with a diameter greater than 10 cm (giant hemangioma) are likely to cause symptoms. Hemangiomas occasionally enlarge rapidly during pregnancy. Patients who are symptomatic usually present with a palpable mass in the upper abdomen and vague discomfort. Episodes of pain are believed to be associated with thrombosis and infarction. Thrombocytopenia and hypofibrinogenemia may complicate giant hemangiomas.

Macroscopically, hemangiomas are usually solitary and less than 5 cm in diameter. They frequently present as flat surfaced or bulging, subcapsular lesions that are reddish blue and well delineated. Large tumors may become pedunculated. Microscopically they are composed of cavernous vascular channels and may contain thrombi or rarely phleboliths; calcification or prominent scarring with hyalinization may occur (sclerosed hemangioma). Malignant transformation is unknown.

Infantile hemangioendothelioma

Although rare, infantile hemangioendothelioma is the most common mesenchymal tumor arising in the liver in infancy.[838,839] Most present during the first few months of life. Hepatomegaly and cardiac failure caused by arteriovenous shunts within the tumor are common manifestations. Complications include microangiopathic hemolytic anemia, thrombocytopenia, and hypofibrinogenemia.

The tumors may be single or multiple with ill-defined margins, and they can be locally aggressive. Macroscopically they are red-brown and spongy, with a fibrous, focally calcified center. Microscopically they are composed of multiple communicating vascular channels and spaces lined by plump endothelial cells. In some areas tufts of epithelial cells may project into the vascular lumens. The amount of supporting stroma present is variable and usually contains small bile ducts. As with other tumors of childhood, extramedullary hematopoiesis is often present. Rare tumors undergo malignant transformation with histologic features resembling angiosarcoma in the adult.[840]

Some pediatricians advocate no treatment for infantile hemangioendothelioma, but when the tumor is single, it is usually excised. Other modalities of therapy include hepatic artery ligation and arterial embolization.

Angiomyolipoma

The majority of angiomyolipomas have been reported in adults and are usually asymptomatic.[841] Many more of these tumors are being diagnosed as a result of modern radiologic imaging techniques. Only rarely are they associated with tuberous sclerosis.

The tumors are usually single and vary in size. They are composed of admixtures of mature adipose tissue; tortuous, thick-walled, and often hyalinized vessels; and smooth muscle. They often express muscle specific actin, as well as S-100 protein and HMB-45.[842,843] Melanin pigment may be present in the epithelioid cells and can be demonstrated by a Fontana stain or a Warthin-Starry stain at pH 3.2 (one that is specific for melanin).[844] The proportions of adipose tissue and smooth muscle are quite variable, and occasional tumors are composed largely of one or the other component. Hematopoietic foci are frequently found in angiomyolipomas; when this is a prominent finding, the terms *myelolipoma* and *angiomyomyelolipoma* have been used.

Malignant epithelial tumors

Bile duct cystadenocarcinoma

Bile duct cystadenocarcinoma is the malignant counterpart of the benign bile duct cystadenoma.[825-828] Most patients present with an abdominal mass. The features of invasion, cellular pleomorphism, and a papillary growth pattern are indicative of malignancy. These tumors may invade adjacent organs and can metastasize to distant sites.

Intrahepatic cholangiocarcinoma

Cholangiocarcinoma (peripheral cholangiocarcinoma)[845-847] is one of the two major carcinomas arising within the liver in the adult. Its incidence is lower than that of hepatocellular carcinoma. Cholangiocarcinoma has been associated with liver fluke infestations of the liver, such as clonorchiasis and opisthorchiasis in Southeast Asia.[848,849] Other etiologic factors associated with the development of bile duct carcinoma include intrahepatic lithiasis.[850,851] Chronic ulcerative colitis and PSC have been causally related to hilar cholangiocarcinoma.[852,853] Developmental anomalies of the biliary tract, including Caroli's disease, CHF, choledochal cysts, von Meyenburg's complexes, and solitary and multiple liver cysts, are all known to be complicated by the development of cholangiocarcinoma.[854-861] Cholangiocarcinoma is the most common malignant hepatic tumor in patients who had received Thorotrast, a discontinued radiologic contrast medium.[862,863] Occasional cases have been reported in women taking oral contraceptives[864] or in patients using anabolic or androgenic steroids.[865]

Two thirds of intrahepatic cholangiocarcinomas are solitary, and one third are multifocal; they are found more frequently in the right lobe. The peak incidence is in the sixth decade, and there is an equal sex distribution. Patients most commonly present with malaise and abdominal pain. Jaundice is present in approximately one third of the patients but is rare as an initial presentation. There are no diagnostic laboratory features, and alpha-fetoprotein levels in the peripheral blood are not elevated.

Intrahepatic cholangiocarcinomas arise in noncirrhotic livers. They may be single or multicentric, are firm to hard, and are gray-white; some are focally calcified. Histopathologically they have a large component of fibrous tissue and have a tubular or papillary pattern[844] (Fig. 57-70). Squamous differentiation may occur in tumors that have arisen in congenitally dilated ducts. Cholangiocarcinomas stain positively for mucin, cytokeratin, epithelial membrane antigen, and CEA.

The prognosis of patients with cholangiocarcinoma is poor. The survival rate is approximately 6 months from the time of diagnosis. Metastases are usually present at autopsy and are mainly in regional lymph nodes; however, lung metastases may also be present. Seeding of the peritoneal cavity may occur.

Hepatocellular carcinoma

Hepatocellular carcinoma (HCC) is one of the most common cancers in man. There are wide variations in the geographic incidence of HCC.[866] The populations with the highest number of cases per year reside in Africa and Southeast Asia (more than 30 cases per 100,000 persons per year). Japan, the Middle East, and south central Europe represent a population with an intermediate incidence (5 to 20 cases per 100,000 persons per year). The populations with the lowest relative incidence of HCC reside in northwest and central Europe, North, Central, and South America, India, Pakistan, Australia, and the white population of South Africa (<5 cases per 100,000 persons per year).

Several different causes have been associated with HCC. The role of HBV in the development of HCC continues to increase in importance.[157-161,867-870] Age also is related to the development of HCC depending on the geography and its incidence. In high-incidence areas, there has been a strong tendency toward development of HCC in younger age groups. In parts of Africa and Southeast Asia, 50% of the patients developing HCC are less than 30 years old. The male-to-female ratio ranges from 4:1 to 8:1, depending on the geographic area.

Hepatitis C virus has emerged as an important risk factor for HCC in the past few years.[182-184] There are considerable geographic variations, with high prevalence rates in Japan and Italy. In the United States the relative risk of HCC in patients with chronic HCV infection increased fivefold to sevenfold. It is estimated that in the United States about 7% and 11% of HCC cases are related to HBV and HCV infection respectively.

In areas where the incidence of HBV infection is uncommon, HCC is often associated with alcohol induced cirrhosis. The relative risk in different studies has varied from 1.3 to 12.0.[871,872] The incidence of HCC arising in a background of cirrhosis is approximately 15%.

Many naturally occurring carcinogens in foodstuffs, including pyrrolizidine alkaloids, phytanic acid, nitrosamines, and mycotoxins, have been implicated in the cause of HCC. Hepatitis B and aflatoxin appear to be synergistic risk factors in China.[873,874] Other risk factors include tobacco smoking and long-term use of oral contraceptives; the relative risk for oral contraceptive use is 3.8 to 13.5.[875] HCC has been reported in patients with a great variety of inherited metabolic diseases,[876] in particular genetic hemochromatosis.[877]

Frequently, patients present with hepatomegaly and ascites and complain of abdominal pain and weight loss. By the time the diagnosis is made, the potential for cure is poor. There is usually no antecedent history of liver disease even though the majority of patients have developed cirrhosis.

A variety of paraneoplastic syndromes, both endocrine and hematologic, have been reported in association with HCC.[878] Hypoglycemia is frequently seen in Southeast Asia but is less common in other locations. Hypercalcemia may occur in both HCC and cholangiocarcinoma. Ectopic parathyroid hormone, prostaglandin E, vitamin D, and osteoclastic activating substances may also be present.

Alpha-fetoprotein (AFP) is present in the serum of about half the patients with HCC.[879-881] Serum AFP levels in healthy adults range from 0.1 to 5.8 ng/ml. The concentrations of AFP in the serum in HCC are in excess of 500 ng/ml; values greater than 10,000 ng/ml are found in 50% to 70% of patients. The continuous increase of serum AFP using serial determinations is consistent with the presence of HCC. Metastases to the liver, particularly from gastric carcinoma, may be associated with elevated serum concentrations, but the concentrations are usually less than 150 ng/ml. It is also worth noting that elevated serum levels of AFP may be detected in patients with hepatitis and cirrhosis, but the levels are usually below 1000 ng/ml.

HCC forms a soft, hemorrhagic and sometimes bile stained mass with a tendency toward central necrosis. The tumors may be multinodular, solitary, massive, or diffuse with replacement of almost the entire liver (Figs. 57-71 and 57-72). The tumors show no fibrosis except for the fibrolamellar variant, which often reveals fibrous septa mimicking the appearance of focal nodular hyperplasia (Fig. 57-73). A collaborative study of autopsy material from Japan, the United States, and South Africa determined three major growth patterns of tumor growth: expanding, spreading, and multifocal.[882] Tumor extension may be found within the portal vein, major hepatic veins, the inferior vena cava, and intrahepatic and extrahepatic bile ducts. Widespread obstruction of vessels in the liver is a major factor in the development of portal hypertension.

HCC occurs in several histologic patterns:[844]

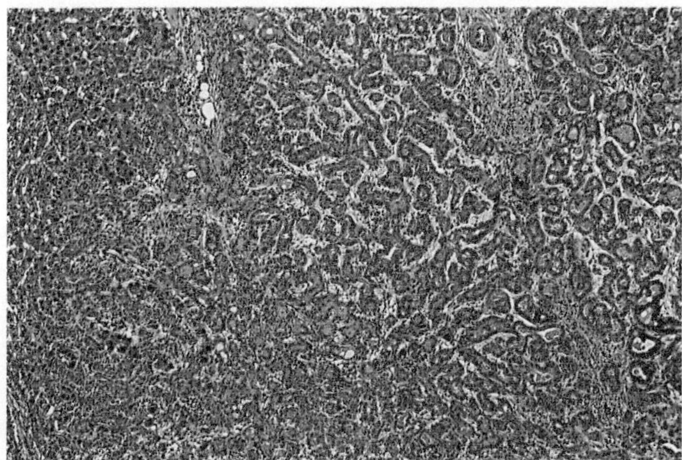

Fig. 57-70 Intrahepatic cholangiocarcinoma with a tubular pattern.

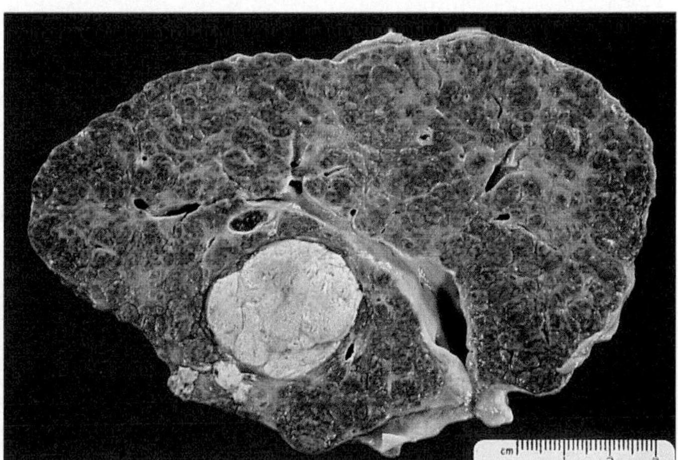

Fig. 57-71 Section of cirrhotic liver with a solitary nodule of hepatocellular carcinoma. (Courtesy Dr. James Fishback, Kansas City, Kans.)

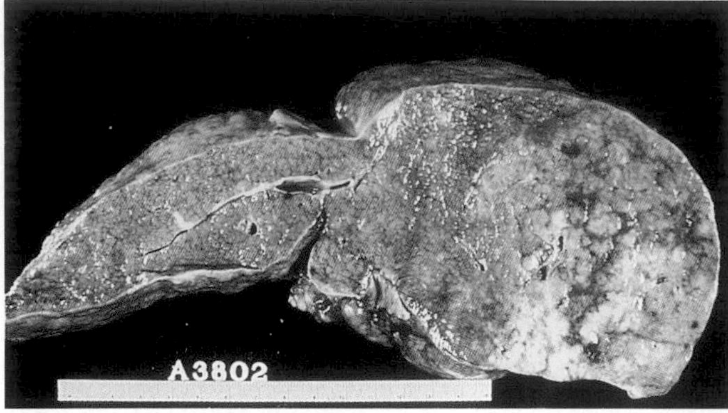

Fig. 57-72 Massive hepatocellular carcinoma is poorly demarcated from the remaining liver.

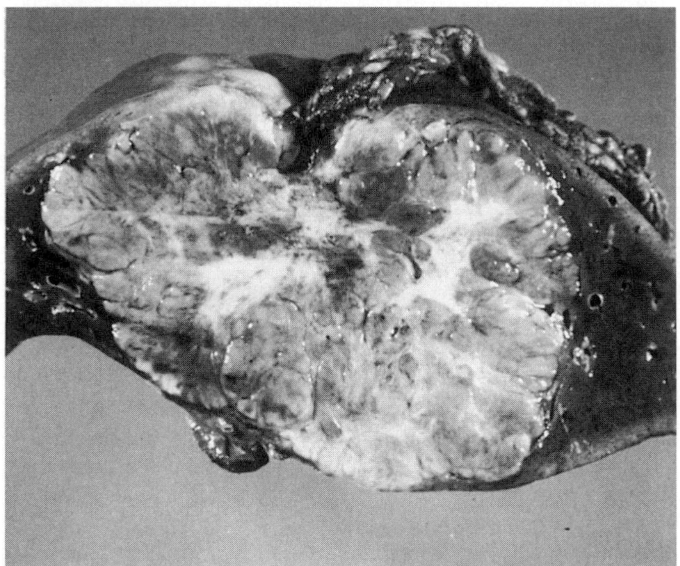

Fig. 57-73 Section of fibrolamellar variant of hepatocellular carcinoma showing nodularity and several white fibrous scars.

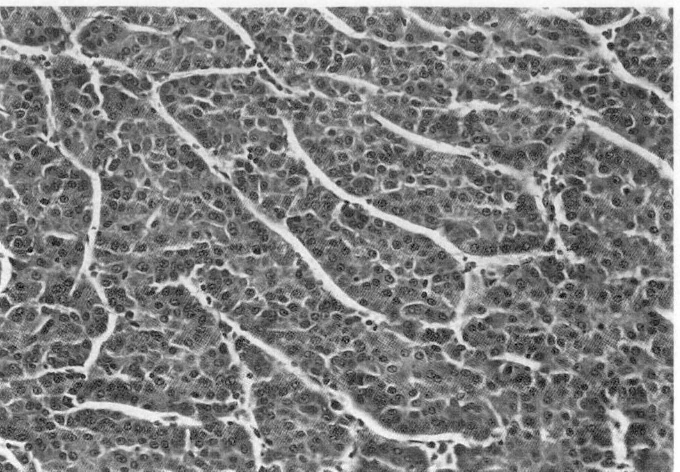

Fig. 57-74 Hepatocellular carcinoma with a trabecular pattern.

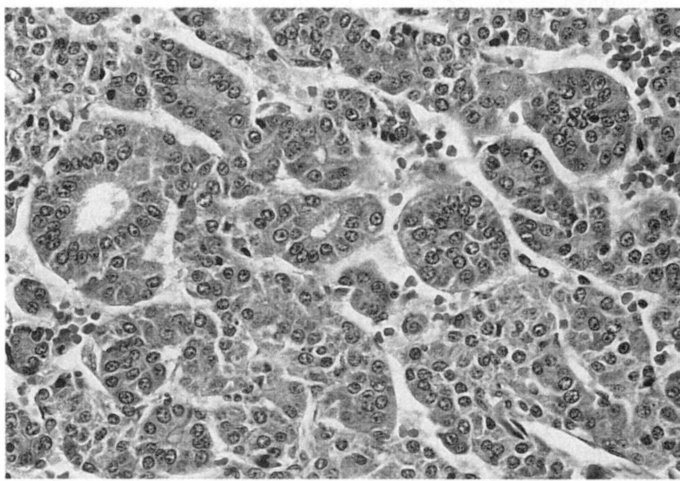

Fig. 57-75 Hepatocellular carcinoma. The tumor has a pseudoglandular pattern.

1. *Trabecular.* This is the most common form of HCC (Fig. 57-74). The tumor forms trabeculae or plates of varying cell thicknesses. There is no stroma between the cells; however, the sinusoids are lined by endothelial cells. Kupffer cells have been demonstrated in some cases. Canaliculi may be clearly visible between tumor cells in H&E preparations and may contain bile.
2. *Compact.* The compact pattern results from compression of the sinusoids, thus resulting in a solid appearance to the tumor.
3. *Pseudoglandular (acinar).* Large dilated canaliculi in the trabeculae, with or without bile, lead to this pattern (Fig. 57-75). Sometimes, cystic spaces containing colloid-like, PAS-positive material may also be present. This material is fibrin and should not be mistaken for mucus.
4. *Scirrhous.* The scirrhous pattern is usually attributable to secondary scarring within the tumor.
5. *Fibrolamellar.* The fibrolamellar pattern consists of dense fibrous lamellae separating tumor cells arranged in compact sheets, small trabeculas, or pseudoglands (Fig. 57-76). The tumor cells are polygonal and have an intensely eosinophilic cytoplasm that appears coarsely granular because of the presence of many mitochondria. Globular, PAS-positive inclusions, as well as pale bodies, are seen in the cytoplasm in this variant.

Morphologically, HCCs have cells that are polygonal with vesicular nuclei, prominent nucleoli, and a finely granular cytoplasm. The degree of differentiation is variable. In general, the larger the tumor cell, the more well differentiated it is and the more it resembles an hepatocyte. The poorly differentiated tumor cells are smaller with more variable nuclei and a scanty basophilic cytoplasm. Clear cells are commonly seen; however, the tumor is rarely composed entirely of them. The clear cell variant may be confused with clear cell carcinoma of the kidney. The clear cytoplasm is usually attributable to large amounts of glycogen. A foamy or vacuolated cytoplasm may be attributable to the presence of fat. A pleomorphic cytologic variant is characterized by considerable variation in cell size, nuclear size, shape, and staining and the presence of bizarre multinucleated cells. At this juncture it is worth reiterating that the most important diagnostic features of HCC are a trabecular pattern, the presence of canaliculi between tumor cells, and the

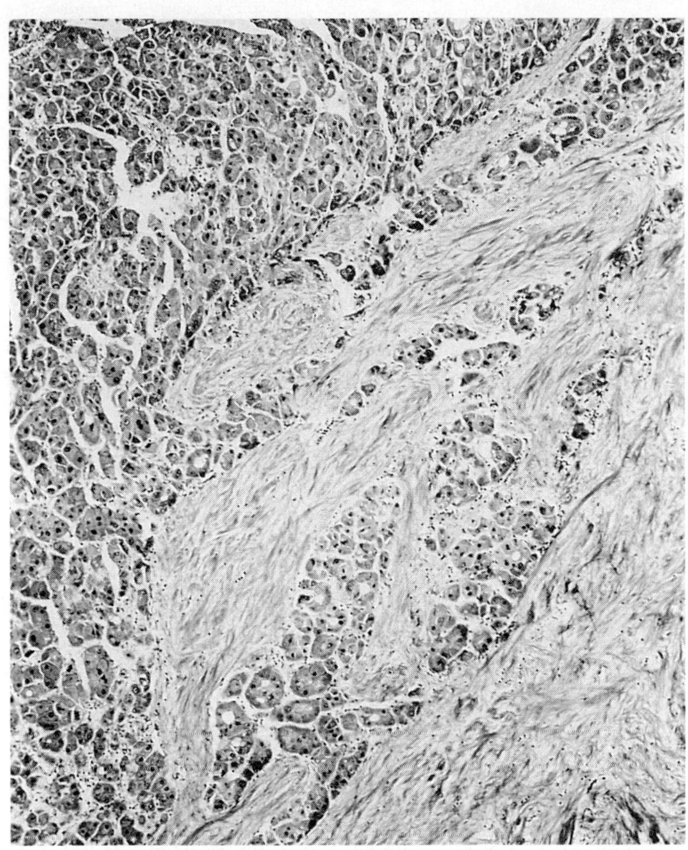

Fig. 57-76 Fibrolamellar variant of hepatocellular carcinoma with lamellae of dense fibrous tissue intersecting the tumor, which displays both microtrabecular and pseudoglandular patterns.

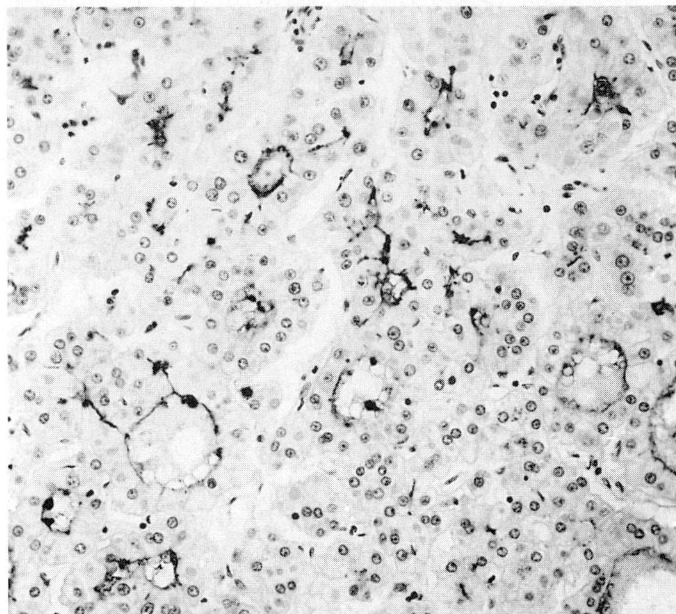

Fig. 57-77 Canaliculi in hepatocellular carcinoma are outlined by an immunostain for polyclonal carcinoembryonic antigen.

identification of bile in canaliculi or in the cytoplasm of tumor cells. A particularly useful immunostain for demonstration of canaliculi is the polyclonal CEA (Fig. 57-77).

Intracytoplasmic inclusions are found in a large number of HCC. They consist primarily of globular hyaline bodies, which may be intracellular or extracellular and are acidophilic. They are usually PAS positive; immunohistochemical methods have shown them to be composed of AFP, α_1-antitrypsin, fibrinogen, ferritin, and albumin. Pale bodies are composed mainly of fibrinogen. Classical Mallory bodies may also be present in the cytoplasm, and they can be immunostained with antibodies to ubiquitin. It is worth nothing that Mallory bodies also can be found in benign tumors such as hepatocellular adenoma and focal nodular hyperplasia.

HCC differentiation is related to prognosis. Poorly differentiated HCCs are more likely to stain positive with AFP, and they are also more likely to metastasize than the well-differentiated HCCs. In Hong Kong, the clear cell variant of HCC appears to have a better prognosis than other histologic or cytologic variants.[883] Fibrolamellar carcinoma occurs in adolescents and young adults of either sex.[884-886] It is not associated with HBV or alcoholism, and there is no underlying cirrhosis. AFP levels are not significantly elevated. The tumor is usually single and large and more frequently found in the left lobe. It is slow growing and amenable to surgical resection. The mean survival time is approximately 68 months, with 5-year survival rates of 82% and 63% respectively in some series.

Hepatoblastoma

Hepatoblastoma is a childhood tumor that accounts for approximately 0.2% to 5% of childhood malignancies.[887-891] It occurs early in life and is associated with a variety of congenital anomalies including hemihypertrophy, congenital absence of the portal vein, Beckwith-Wiedemann syndrome and familial adenomatosis coli. Hepatoblastoma occurs twice as frequently in males as in females, with the majority presenting in the first 2 years of life. The patients usually have progressive enlargement of the abdomen because of a hepatomegaly, with or without a palpable mass. Other signs include failure to thrive, fever, vomiting, diarrhea, and weight loss. Serum AFP levels are invariably elevated.

Grossly, hepatoblastoma is most commonly found in the right lobe and varies in size from 5 to 25 cm in diameter. It is usually well circumscribed, with focal areas of cystic degeneration, necrosis, and hemorrhage.

Microscopically, hepatoblastoma consists of cells in a range of maturation stages embedded within a variable mesenchymal matrix. The epithelial component is prominent and always present. It consists of (1) *embryonal type cells,* which are small, fusiform, and darkly staining with uniform hyperchromatic nuclei, and (2) *fetal cells,* which are large with more cytoplasm; some are filled with glycogen or fat. Over 90% of the tumors synthesize AFP, which can be demonstrated in tumor cells immunohistochemically. Squamous epithelium with or without keratinization may be present. The mesenchymal component consists of a primitive mesenchyme and osteoid (Figs. 57-78 and 57-79). Extramedullary hematopoiesis is a constant feature. A variant, teratoid hepatoblastoma may also contain melanin, cartilage, and muscle.[892,893]

Hepatoblastoma is a rapidly progressing tumor. Patients usually succumbs to a rupture of the tumor, liver failure, or metastasis to lymph nodes, lung, brain, heart, and bone. Chemotherapy combined with early surgical resection has improved the prognosis.

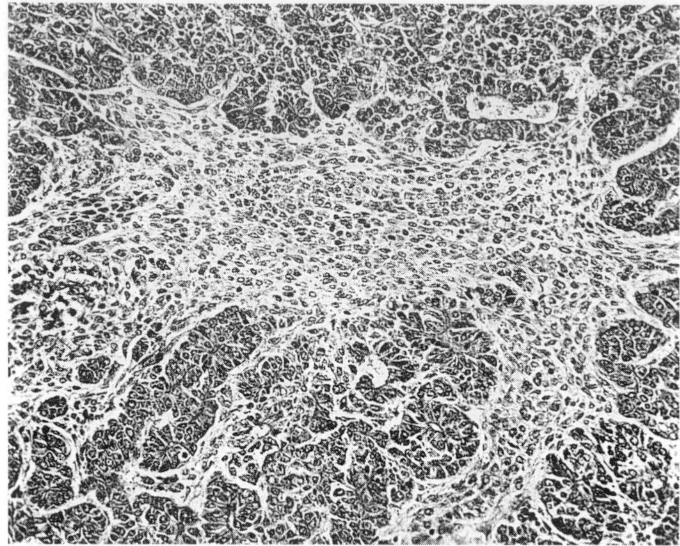

Fig. 57-78 Hepatoblastoma. Primitive mesenchyme is surrounded by embryonal cells forming cords and acini.

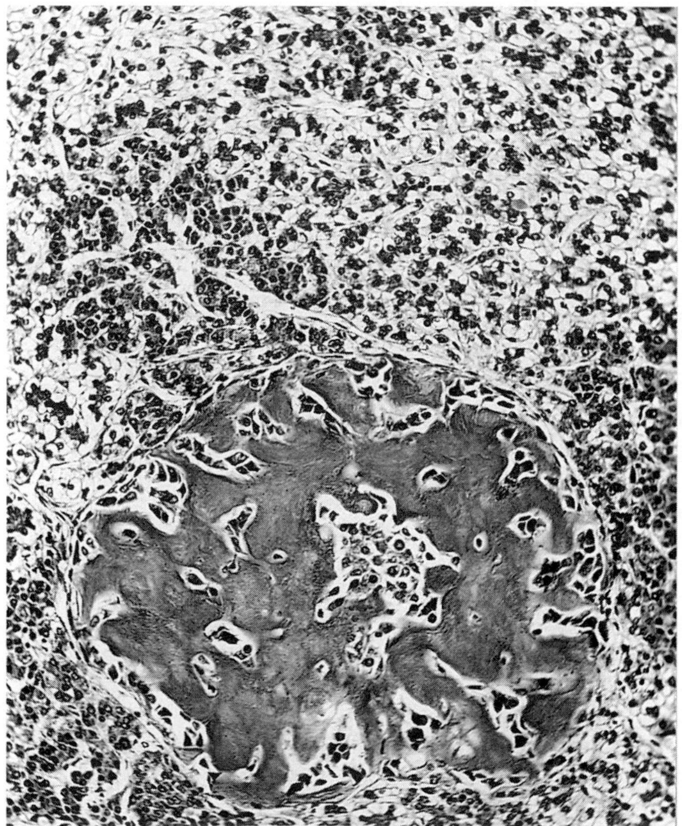

Fig. 57-79 Hepatoblastoma. Fetal type cells ("light and dark") have a compact pattern without distinct trabeculas. Notice osteoid focus *(bottom)*.

Combined hepatocellular and cholangiocarcinoma

Goodman and colleagues[894] described 24 cases of this tumor. The gross appearance is similar to that of HCC. Four of these cases were considered collision tumors, 12 were transitional tumors (with an intimate intermingling of hepatocellular and cholangiocellular components), and eight were fibrolamellar carcinomas with mucin-producing pseudoglands.

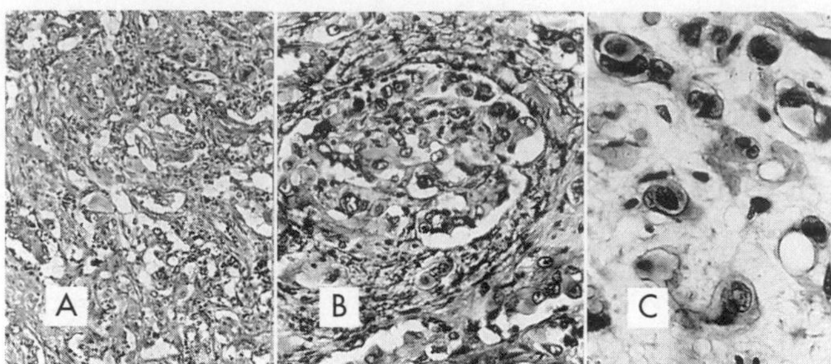

Fig. 57-80 Epithelioid hemangioendothelioma. **A,** Tumor cells growing in sinusoidal spaces are supported by a scanty fibrous stroma. **B,** Tumor is growing in lumen of a portal vein branch. **C,** Epithelioid tumor cells are surrounded by a loose fibrous stroma. Vacuoles represent intracellular vascular lumens.

Malignant mesenchymal tumors

Epithelioid hemangioendothelioma

Epithelioid hemangioendothelioma was described by Weiss and Enzinger.[895] Before their description, this tumor was regarded as a sclerotic form of cholangiocarcinoma. A study of 32 cases of hepatic epithelioid hemangioendothelioma by Ishak and colleagues[54] showed that this tumor arises more frequently in females with an average age of approximately 50 years. The patient presentation is nonspecific with weight loss, abdominal discomfort, and occasionally jaundice. Rare initial presentations include the Budd-Chiari syndrome or liver failure.

Epithelioid hemangioendothelioma is usually multicentric and involves both lobes.[54,896] Grossly the tumors are white and firm. Microscopically, tumor cells are spindled or epithelioid in appearance, with an abundant cytoplasm and vesicular nuclei. They grow in the sinusoids and intrahepatic veins but also form their own intracellular vascular lumens[54,896] (Fig. 57-80). With time the tumor becomes progressively more sclerotic and focally calcified. von Willebrand factor (factor VIII) and CD34 (QB-END/10) are usually positive in the cytoplasm of tumor cells and vascular lumens.[55] Growth is slow, and the 5-year survival rate is 33%. Many of these tumors have now been successfully treated by orthotopic liver transplantation with long-term survival.[897,898]

Angiosarcoma

The rare tumor angiosarcoma occurs most frequently in specific occupations and after exposure to Thorotrast.[899] An increased incidence of angiosarcoma has been reported in workers exposed to vinyl chloride monomer, the substrate for the production of polyvinyl chloride (PVC).[900] Thorotrast, a colloidal suspension of thorium dioxide used in the past as a radiologic contrast medium, has also been associated with development of angiosarcoma, with a latent period of 15 to 20 years.[901,902] Thorium is a radioactive element with a half-life of approximately 400 years. Seventy percent of an injected dose is taken up by the liver, 20% by the spleen, and 10% by the bone marrow; there is no significant elimination of the material. Thorotrast particles are coarse, pink-brown, and refractile; they are often extracellular but may be engulfed by reticuloendothelial cells. They are readily seen by scanning electron microscopy in paraffin sections, and the element thorium can be positively identified by x-ray microanalysis.

The clinical features of angiosarcoma are discussed by Locker and colleagues.[903] Grossly, angiosarcoma is usually multicentric and appears as ill-defined, spongy, hemorrhagic nodules scattered throughout the liver. It frequently metastasizes to the spleen, lungs, bone, lymph nodes, and adrenals. Histopathologically, large, cavernous, blood-filled spaces may contain papillary projections. Solid cellular masses resembling fibrosarcoma may be seen. The tumor cells also grow along preexisting sinusoids. They are elongated, spindled, or pleomorphic, with hyperchromatic nuclei. Multiple nuclei and mitotic activity are variable. Extramedullary hematopoiesis is usually present. Extension of the tumor into portal and hepatic vein branches is a frequent finding.

Undifferentiated sarcoma

Undifferentiated (embryonal) sarcomas are found primarily in children between 6 and 10 years of age.[904,905] Occasionally they are reported in older patients. Patients usually present with a rapidly growing abdominal mass. Jaundice is rare. AFP levels are characteristically low. The tumors are large, soft, and grey-white with gelatinous and hemorrhagic areas. Microscopically they resemble embryonic mesenchyme and contain spindle and stellate cells, and occasionally, bizarre multinucleated cells. The stroma is loose and myxoid. Rhabdomyoblastic or leiomyosarcomatous differentiation is rare. Tumor cells often contain round, eosinophilic globules that are PAS positive and express α_1-antitrypsin. Poorly formed bile ducts are usually present at the periphery of the tumor and are believed to represent entrapped nonneoplastic liver. In the past, the prognosis was poor with most patients succumbing to their disease within a year; however, survival has improved after combination chemotherapy, radiation, and surgical excision.[906]

Metastatic tumors

The liver is the most common site for metastases from lung, breast, and gastrointestinal tract.[744,907] The most frequent diagnosis is that of adenocarcinoma; the exact primary site often cannot be determined histopathologically, even with the use of immunohistochemical analysis.[908] However, a list of possibilities should be enumerated for consideration by the clinician. Metastatic liver disease may mimic other diseases of the liver. Occasionally, patients present with fulminant hepatic failure[909,910] or with jaundice.[911] Diagnosis is largely based on imaging studies and fine-needle aspiration biopsy.

Tumors with distinct histopathologic features may be identified with a high degree of accuracy in biopsy material. Among these are carcinoid and islet cell tumors, melanoma, Hodgkin's and non-Hodgkin's lymphoma, small cell carcinomas, squamous carcinomas, and clear cell carcinoma of the kidney. Immunohistochemical analysis may be helpful in identifying carcinoma of the prostate (presence of prostate-specific antigen), follicular carcinoma of the thyroid (thyroglobulin), yolk sac tumor (alpha-fetoprotein), and beta-human chorionic gonadotropin. Metastatic sarcomas bear a striking resemblance to the primary; their source may be clinically evident in most cases.

LIVER DISEASE AFTER BONE MARROW TRANSPLANTATION

Graft-versus-host disease

Bone marrow transplantation (BMT) is currently an accepted therapy for a variety of conditions, including immunodeficiency syndromes, aplastic anemia, hematologic malignancies, and some genetic disorders. It is also an experimental therapy for some nonhematologic malignancies, including breast cancer.

The complications associated with BMT include an increased immunodeficiency (beyond that associated with the disease being treated) and graft-versus-host disease (GVHD). GVHD may present with a variety of clinical signs and symptoms, including rash, diarrhea, and jaundice. Involvement of the liver is usually associated with GVHD in other organ systems, in particular, the skin.

There are two recognized forms of disease: acute and chronic GVHD. These two subgroups differ in their pathogenetic mechanism, the time of onset of symptoms, and the organs involved. GVHD develops in approximately one half of all allogeneic bone marrow recipients and is a contributing factor in the death of up to 40% of the cases.[912,913]

Acute graft-versus-host disease

Acute GVHD usually occurs within the first 6 weeks after transplantation. Three organ systems are primarily involved—skin, gastrointestinal tract, and liver. Liver involvement is manifested clinically by hepatomegaly with associated increases in serum bilirubin and serum alkaline phosphatase levels. These findings, though nonspecific, are usually sufficient to implicate GVHD of the liver when either skin or gastrointestinal involvement, or both, are also present. Liver biopsy is usually performed when either the clinical features are atypical or when the only manifestations of the disease are abnormal liver tests.

The major histologic feature associated with acute GVHD is damage to the interlobular bile ducts.[914-921] The affected ducts show irregular epithelial cells with focal nuclear pleomorphism, cytoplasmic vacuolation, and intracellular lymphocytes (Fig. 57-81). Occasionally, individual epithelial cell necrosis and mitoses are also present. The portal tracts may contain a mild lymphocytic infiltrate that varies significantly, depending on the patient's peripheral white blood cell count. In some cases, endotheliitis may be present.[917,918]

Biopsy specimens obtained early in the course of the GVHD show mild nonspecific changes, including hepatocellular ballooning, focal hepatocytic necrosis, and some acidophilic bodies. As the disorder progresses, the acinus may become more involved with pronounced canalicular cholestasis and more prominent hepatocyte injury (ballooning and numerous acidophilic bodies). In some cases, prominent periportal fibrosis may be present.

The histologic findings in posttransplantation biopsy material may be very nonspecific. In such cases, it is important to determine the ratio of portal to acinar abnormalities. A false-positive diagnosis of GVHD may be found in up to 15% of the cases evaluated.

Chronic graft-versus-host disease

Chronic GVHD develops between 80 and 400 days after transplantation. It is usually preceded by acute GVHD but may

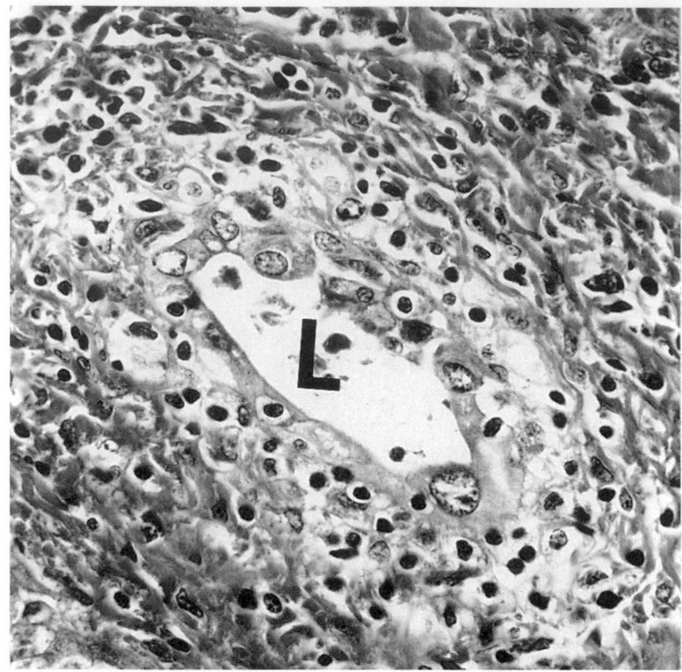

Fig. 57-81 Graft-versus-host disease. Bile duct in portal area is extensively damaged and is infiltrated by lymphocytes. *L*, Lumen.

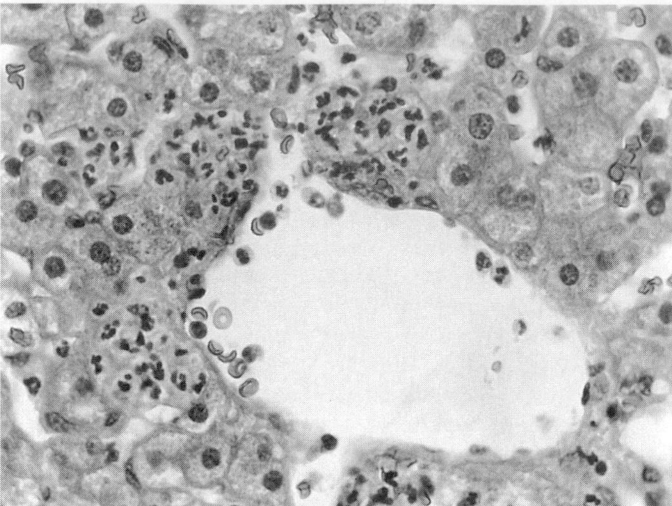

Fig. 57-82 Open surgical biopsy artifact. Multiple foci of necrosis, with infiltration by neutrophils, surround a terminal hepatic venule.

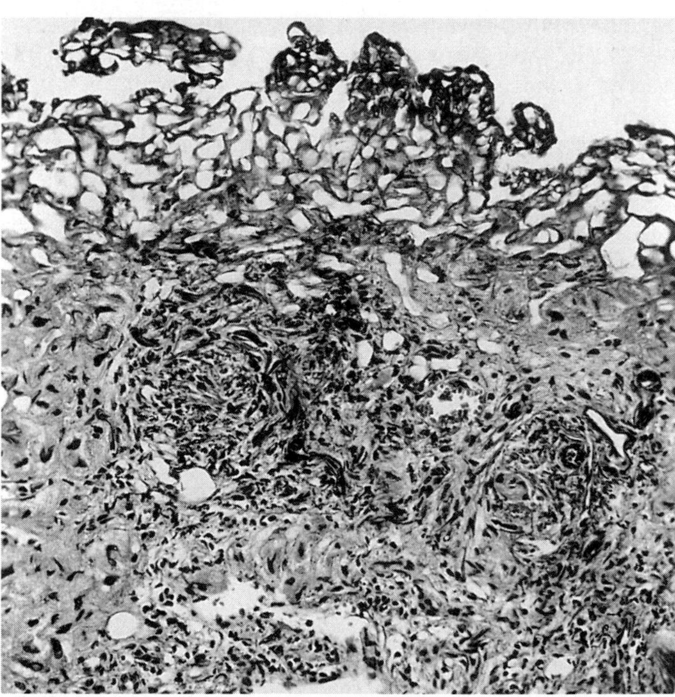

Fig. 57-83 Electrocautery artifact. Surface of open biopsy specimen *(top)* has been destroyed by heat.

occur in the absence of acute GVHD in approximately 25% of the cases. In addition to the skin, gastrointestinal tract, and liver, chronic GVHD may involve the minor salivary glands, lymph nodes, mouth, eyes, lungs, and the musculoskeletal system. Hepatic involvement, present in approximately 90% of the cases, is characterized by variable increases in serum bilirubin and aminotransferase values and by prominent increases in serum alkaline phosphatase values.[920,921]

Histologically the changes of chronic GVHD are similar to those of acute GVHD but differ in degree and extent. The changes in the bile ducts are more prominent that those in acute GVHD, and there may be ductopenia. There is prominent portal inflammation, consisting primarily of lymphocytes and plasma cells, with some associated periportal fibrosis. Piecemeal necrosis may also be present.

Intra-acinar changes include prominent canalicular cholestasis and acidophilic bodies. As the original interlobular ducts are destroyed, chronic cholestasis, progressive periportal fibrosis, and eventual cirrhosis may develop.[922-924]

Differentiating between chronic GVHD and chronic hepatitis (particularly that caused by HCV) may be difficult. Both disorders share features of portal inflammation, periportal fibrosis, bile duct injury, and individual cell necrosis.[925] Liver biopsy specimens obtained from BMT patients should always be interpreted in light of the clinical findings.

NONSPECIFIC CHANGES AND ARTIFACTS

Histopathologic changes that cannot be correlated with the clinical or biochemical data should be labeled "nonspecific." The term *nonspecific reactive hepatitis* should be avoided because the grouping of changes is not a histologic entity. The nonspecific changes include focal necrosis, mild steatosis, patchy portal inflammation, sinusoidal dilatation, and activation of Kupffer cells.

Other nonspecific changes may be seen in the vicinity of space-occupying lesions. Such changes include compression atrophy of liver cell plates, periportal ductular proliferation, edema of portal area connective tissue with infiltration by neutrophils, and focal sinusoidal dilatation.

Open-wedge biopsy specimens may show changes that can be misleading and even be suggestive of cirrhosis.[926] They include focal subcapsular fibrosis, periportal fibrosis with portal-to-portal or portal-to-capsular bridging, and acinar atrophy. A normal acinar architecture should alert the hepatic morphologist to the facility and nonspecificity of these surface alterations.

Many artifacts seen in biopsy material from the liver are also seen in other tissues.[927] One artifact that should be kept in mind occurs in wedge biopsy specimens obtained at laparotomy.[928-930] The changes are proportionately more severe the longer the duration of the abdominal surgery. They include foci of necrosis infiltrated by neutrophils, usually in the vicinity of THV (Fig. 57-82). Extravasation of neutrophils and erythrocytes is also evident beneath Glisson's capsule. The perivenular foci of necrosis progressively diminish in severity from the surface to the depths of the biopsy specimen. The changes are generally believed to be anoxic rather than traumatic in cause.

A recently described "sponge artifact" manifests as angulated, often triangular holes in the tissue sections.[931,932]

Wedge biopsy specimens obtained with the electric cautery show burn effects at the periphery (Fig. 57-83). They include charring and discoloration, destruction of cytologic features, and the formation of spaces (from accumulation of steam) in the interstices of the biopsy tissue.

REFERENCES

Normal liver

Embryology

1. Clearfield HR: Embryology, malformations, and malposition of the liver. In Berk JE, Haubrich WS, Kalser MH et al, editors: *Bockus gastroenterology,* ed 4, Philadelphia and London, 1985, Saunders.

Gross anatomy

2. Rappaport AM, Wanless IR: Physioanatomic considerations. In Schiff L, Schiff ER, editors: *Diseases of the liver,* ed 7, Philadelphia, 1993, Lippincott.
3. Schaffner F, Popper H: Structure of the liver. In Berk JE, Haubrich WS, Kalser MH et al, editors: *Bockus gastroenterology,* ed 4, Philadelphia, 1985, Saunders.

Microscopic anatomy

4. Rohr HP, Luthy J, Gudat F et al: Stereology: a new supplement to the study of human liver biopsy specimens, *Prog Liver Dis* 5:25, 1976.
5. Reed GR, Butt EM, Landing BH: Copper in childhood liver disease, *Arch Pathol* 93:249, 1972.
6. Sternlieb I: Copper and the liver, *Gastroenterology* 78:1615, 1980.
7. Wisse E, Knook DL, editors: *Kupffer cells and other liver sinusoidal cells,* Amsterdam, 1977, Elsevier/North Holland Biomedical Press.
8. Liehr H, Grün M: *The reticuloendothelial system and the pathogenesis of liver disease,* Amsterdam, 1980, Elsevier/North Holland Biomedical Press.
9. Kirn A, Knook DL, Wisse E, editors: *Cells of the hepatic sinusoid,* vol 1, Rijswijk, the Netherlands, 1986, Kupffer Cell Foundation.
10. Bioulac-Sage, Balabaud C: *Sinusoids in human liver: health and disease,* Rijswijk, the Netherlands, 1988, Kupffer Cell Foundation.
11. Kuiper J, Brouwer A, Knook DL, Van Berkel TJC: Kupffer and sinusoidal endothelial cells. In Arias IM, Boyer JL, Fausto N et al, editors: *The liver: biology and pathobiology,* ed 3, New York, 1994, Raven Press.
12. Enzan H, Himeno H, Iwamura S et al: Immunohistochemical identification of Ito cells and their myofibroblastic transformation in adult human liver, *Virchows Arch* 424:249, 1994.
13. Geerts A, Bleser PD, Hautekeete ML et al: Fat-storing (Ito) cell biology. In Arias IM, Boyer JL, Fausto N et al, editors: *The liver: biology and pathobiology,* ed 3, New York, 1944, Raven Press.
14. Badaruddin RH, Waldrop FW, Puchtler H: Alterations of the myoid pericanalicular layer in the liver, *Arch Pathol Lab Med* 100:616, 1976.
15. Wachstein M: Cyto- and histochemistry of the liver. In Rouiller C, editor: *The liver,* vol 1, New York, 1963, Academic Press.
16. Tanaka M, Shimoda T, Takaki K et al: Hepatic fibrosis: the relation between proliferating bile ductules and alpha 1-antitrypsin, *Acta Pathol Jpn* 30:695, 1980.
17. Burt AD, MacSween RNM: Bile duct proliferation—its true significance, *Histopathology* 23:599, 1993.
18. Masuko K, Rubin E, Popper H: Proliferation of bile ducts in cirrhosis, *Arch Pathol* 78:421, 1964.
19. Murata K, Okudaira M, Akashio K: Mast cells in human liver tissue: increased mast cell number in relation to the component of connective tissue in the cirrhotic process. *Acta Derm Venereol* Suppl (Stockh) 73:157, 1973.
20. MacSween RNM, Scothorne RJ: Developmental anatomy and normal structure. In MacSween RNM, Anthony PP, Scheuer PJ, editors: *Pathology of the liver,* ed 2, Edinburgh, 1987, Churchill Livingstone.
21. Phillips MJ, Poucell S, Patterson J, Valencia P: *The liver: an atlas and text of ultrastructural pathology,* New York, 1987, Raven Press.
22. Motta PM: Scanning electron microscopy of the liver, *Prog Liver Dis* 7:1, 1982.
23. Vonnahme F-J: *The human liver: a scanning electron microscopic atlas,* Basel, 1993, Karger.
24. Denk H, Franke WW: Cytoskeletal filaments. In Arias I, Popper H, Schachter D, Shafritz DA, editors: *The liver: biology and pathobiology,* New York, 1982, Raven Press.
25. French SW: Present understanding of the development of Mallory's body, *Arch Pathol Lab Med* 107:445, 1983.
26. Denk H, Lackinger E, Vennigerholz F: Pathology of the cytoskeleton of hepatocytes, *Prog Liver Dis* 8:237, 1986.
27. Phillips MJ, Satir P: The cytoskeleton of the hepatocyte: organization, relationships, and pathology. In Arias, IM, Jakoby WB, Popper H et al, editors: *The liver: biology and pathobiology,* ed 2, New York, 1988, Raven Press.
28. French SW: Cytoskeleton: intermediate filaments. In Arias IM, Boyer JL, Fausto N et al: *The liver: biology and pathobiology,* ed 3, New York, 1994, Raven Press.

Evaluation of liver diseases

Liver biopsy

29. Krauer CM: Percutaneous biopsy of the liver as a procedure for outpatients, *Gastroenterology* 74:101, 1978.
30. Perrault J, McGill DB, Ott BJ et al: Liver biopsy: complications in 1000 inpatients and outpatients, *Gastroenterology* 74:103, 1978.
31. Ishak KG, Schiff ER, Schiff L: Needle biopsy of the liver. In Schiff L, Schiff ER, editors: *Diseases of the liver,* ed 6, Philadelphia, 1987, Lippincott.
32. Schiff ER, Schiff L: Needle biopsy of the liver. In Schiff L, Schiff ER, editors: *Diseases of the liver,* vol 1, ed 7, Philadelphia, 1993, Lippincott.
33. Rosch J, Lakin PC, Antonovic R et al: Transjugular approach to liver biopsy and transhepatic cholangiography, *N Engl J Med* 289:227, 1973.

Clinical laboratory analysis

34. Kaplan MM: Laboratory tests. In Schiff L, Schiff ER: *Diseases of the liver,* vol 1, ed 7, Philadelphia, 1993, Lippincott.

Fixation and sectioning

35. Lindsay S, Reilly WA, Gotham IJ et al: Gargoylism: study of pathologic lesions and clinical review of 12 cases, *Am J Dis Child* 76:239, 1948.
36. Chi EY, Smuckler EA: A rapid method for processing liver biopsy specimens for 2m sectioning, *Arch Pathol Lab Med* 100:457, 1976.
37. Zerpa H, Malik NJ, Arborgh BA, Scheuer PJ: Application of routine and immunohistochemical staining methods to liver tissue embedded in a water-soluble resin, *Liver* 1:62, 1981.

Histochemistry

38. Prophet EB, Mills B, Arrington JB, Sobin LH: *Laboratory methods in histotechnology,* Washington, D.C., 1992, American Registry of Pathology, Armed Forces Institute of Pathology.
39. Shikata T, Uzawa T, Yoshiwara N et al: Staining methods of Australia antigen in paraffin section: detection of cytoplasmic inclusion bodies, *Jpn J Exp Med* 44:25, 1974.
40. Sipponen P: Orcein positive hepatocellular material in long standing biliary diseases. I. Histochemical characteristics, *Scand J Gastroenterol* 11:545, 1976.
41. Jain S, Scheuer PJ, Archer B et al: Histologic demonstration of copper and copper-associated protein in chronic liver disease, *J Clin Pathol* 31:784, 1978.

42. Lindquist RR: Studies on the pathogenesis of hepatolenticular degeneration: II. Cytochemical methods for the localization of copper, *Arch Pathol* 87:370, 1969.
43. Irons RD, Schenk EA, Lee JCK: Cytochemical methods for copper, *Arch Pathol Lab Med* 101:298, 1977.
44. Nishimura R, Ishak KG, Reddick R et al: Lafora's disease: diagnosis by liver biopsy, *Ann Neurol* 8:409, 1980.
45. Hall P, Gormley BM, Jarvis LR, Smith RD: A staining method for the detection and measurement of fat droplets in hepatic tissue, *Pathology* 12:605, 1980.
46. Fakan F, Chlumska A: Demonstration of needle-shaped hepatic inclusions in porphyria cutanea tarda using the ferric ferricyanide reduction test, *Virchows Arch [A]* 411:365, 1987.
47. Wright JR, Calkins E, Humplirey RL: Potassium permanganate reaction in amyloidosis, *Lab Invest* 36:274, 1977.
48. Nonomura A, Mizukami Y, Matsubara F, Nakanuma Y: Identification of nucleolar organizer regions in non neoplastic and neoplastic hepatocytes by the silver-staining technique, *Liver* 10:229, 1990.
49. Terasaki S, Terada T, Nakanuma Y et al: Argyrophilic nucleolar organizer regions and alpha-fetoprotein in adenomatous hyperplasia in human cirrhotic livers, *Am J Clin Pathol* 95:850, 1991.

Immunohistochemistry

50. Osborn M, van Lessen G, Weber K et al: Methods of laboratory investigation: differential diagnosis of gastrointestinal carcinomas by using monoclonal antibodies specific for individual keratin polypeptides, *Lab Invest* 55:497, 1986.
51. Ray MB: Distribution patterns of cytokeratin antigen determinants in alcoholic and non-alcoholic liver diseases, *Hum Pathol* 18:61, 1987.
52. Vyberg M, Leth P: Ubiquitin: an immunohistochemical marker of Mallory bodies and alcoholic liver disease, *APMIS Suppl* 23:46, 1991.
53. Ishak KG, Zimmerman HJ, Ray MB: Alcoholic liver disease: pathologic, pathogenetic and clinical aspects, *Alcohol Clin Exp Res* 15:45, 1991.
54. Ishak KG, Sesterhenn IA, Goodman ZD et al: Epithelioid hemangioendothelioma of the liver: a clinicopathologic and follow-up study of 32 cases, *Hum Pathol* 15:839, 1984.
55. Anthony PP, Ramani P: Endothelial markers in malignant vascular tumors of the liver: superiority of QB-END/10 over von Willebrand and *Ulex europaeus* agglutinin 1, *J Clin Pathol* 44:29, 1991.
56. Ramani P, Bradley NJ, Fletcher CDM: QBEND/10, a new monoclonal antibody to endothelium: assessment of its diagnostic utility in paraffin sections, *Histopathology* 17:237, 1990.
57. Traweek ST: The human hematopoietic progenitor cell antigen (CD34) in vascular neoplasia, *Am J Clin Pathol* 96:25, 1991.
58. Tsutsumi M, Takada A, Takese S: Characterization of desmin-positive rat liver sinusoidal cells, *Hepatology* 7:277, 1987.
59. Yokoi Y, Namihisa T, Kuroda H et al: Immunocytochemical detection of desmin in fat-storing cells (Ito cells), *Hepatology* 4:709, 1986.
60. Burt AD, MacSween RNM: Immunolocalization of desmin in fixed rat and human liver. In Kern A, Knook DL, Wisse E, editors: *Cells of the hepatic sinusoid,* vol 1, Rijswijk, 1986, Kupffer Cell Foundation.
61. Ramadori G, Rieder H, Knittel T et al: Fat storing cells (FSC) of rat liver synthesize and secrete fibronectin, *J Hepatol* 4:190, 1987.
62. Junge J, Horn T, Christoffersen P: The occurrence and significance of fibronectin in livers from chronic alcoholics, *Acta Pathol Microbiol Scand (A)* 98:56, 1988.
63. Chastonay P, Hurlimann J: Characterization of different amyloids with immunological techniques, *Pathol Res Pract* 181:657, 1986.
64. Looi L-M, Sumithran E: Morphologic differences in the pattern of liver infiltration between systemic AL and AA amyloidosis, *Hum Pathol* 19:732, 1988.
65. French SW, Schloss GT, Stillman AE: Unusual amyloid bodies in human liver, *Am J Clin Pathol* 75:400, 1981.
66. Kanel GC, Uchida T, Peters RL: Globular hepatic amyloid: an unusual morphologic presentation, *Hepatology* 1:647, 1981.
67. Osick LA, Lee T-P, Pedemonte MB et al: Hepatic amyloidosis in intravenous drug abusers and AIDS patients, *J Hepatol* 19:79, 1993.
68. Lindner J, Wollmer RT, Croker BP et al: Systemic kappa light-chain deposition: an ultrastructural and immunohistochemical study, *Am J Surg Pathol* 7:85, 1983.
69. Terreros DA, Knight JA, Peric-Golia L, Cheung AK: Generalized β_2-microglobulin deposition: a preamyloidosis disorder? *Arch Pathol Lab Med* 113:31, 1989.
70. Demetris AJ: The pathology of liver transplantation, *Prog Liver Dis* 9:687, 1990.
71. Franco A, Barnaba V, Natali P et al: Expression of class I and class II major histocompatibility complex antigens on human hepatocytes, *Hepatology* 8:449, 1988.
72. Gouw ASH, Huitema S, Grond J et al: Early induction of MHC antigens in human liver grafts: an immunohistologic study, *Am J Pathol* 133:82, 1988.
73. Senaldi G, Lobo-Yeo A, Mowat AP et al: Class I and class II major histocompatibility complex antigens on hepatocytes: importance of the method of detection and expression in histologically normal and diseased livers, *J Clin Pathol* 44:107, 1991.
74. van den Oord JJ, de Vos R, Desmet VJ: HLA expression in liver disease, *Prog Liver Dis* 9:73, 1990.
75. Govindarajan S, De Cock KM, Peters RL: Morphologic and immunohistochemical features of fulminant delta hepatitis, *Hum Pathol* 16:262, 1985.
76. Govindarajan S, Lim B, Peters RL: Immunohistochemical localization of delta antigen associated with hepatitis B virus in liver biopsy sections embedded in Araldite, *Histopathology* 8:63, 1984.
77. Popper H, Thung SN, Gerber MA et al: Histologic studies of severe delta agent infection in Venzuelan Indians, *Hepatology* 3:906, 1983.
78. Stocklin E, Gudat F, Krey G et al: Delta antigen in hepatitis B: immunohistology of frozen and paraffin-embedded liver biopsies and relation to HBV infection, *Hepatology* 1:238, 1981.
79. Goodman ZD, Langloss JM, Bratthauer GL et al: Immunohistochemical localization of hepatitis B surface antigen and hepatitis B core antigen in tissue sections: a source of false positive staining, *Am J Clin Pathol* 89:533, 1988.
80. Bianchi L, Gudat F: Sanded nuclei in hepatitis B, *Lab Invest* 35:1, 1976.
81. Bianchi L, Spichtin HP, Gudat F: Chronic hepatitis. In MacSween RNM, Anthony PP, Scheuer PJ, editors: *Pathology of the liver,* Edinburgh, 1987, Churchill Livingstone.
82. Gerber MA, Thung SN: The diagnostic value of immunohistochemical demonstration of hepatitis viral antigens in the liver, *Hum Pathol* 18:771, 1987.
83. Fraiese A, Pontisso P, Cavalletto D et al: Expression of preS1 and preS2 in the liver of chronic hepatitis B virus carriers, *J Hepatol* 7:157, 1988.
84. Yuki N, Hayashi N, Katayama K et al: Quantitative analysis of pre-S1 and pre-S2 in relation to HBsAg expression, *Hepatology* 11:38, 1990.
85. Chu CM, Liaw YF: Intrahepatic expression of pre-S1 and pre-S2 antigens in chronic hepatitis B: virus infection in relation to hepatitis B virus replication and hepatitis delta virus superinfection, *Gut* 33:1544, 1992.
86. Housset C, Boucher O, Girard PM et al: Immunohistochemical evidence for human immunodeficiency virus-1 infection of liver Kupffer cells, *Hum Pathol* 21:404, 1990.
87. Hoda SA, White JE, Gerber MA: Immunohistochemical studies of human immunodeficiency virus-1 in liver tissue of patients with AIDS, *Mod Pathol* 4:578, 1992.
88. Goodman ZD, Ishak KG, Sesterhenn IA: Herpes simplex in apparently immunocompetent adults, *Am J Clin Pathol* 85:694, 1986.
89. Keh WC, Gerber MA: In situ hybridization for cytomegalovirus DNA in AIDS patients, *Am J Pathol* 131:490, 1988.
90. Masih AS, Linder J, Shaw BW Jr et al: Rapid identification of cytomegalovirus in liver allograft biopsies by in situ hybridization, *Am J Surg Pathol* 12:362, 1988.
91. Paya CV, Hermans PE, Wiesner RH et al: Cytomegalovirus hepatitis in liver transplantation: prospectve analysis of 93 consecutive liver transplantations, *J Infect Dis* 160:752, 1989.
92. Persons DL, Moore JA, Fishback JL: Comparison of polymerase chain reaction, DNA hybridization, and histology with viral culture to detect cytomegalovirus in immunosuppressed patients, *Mod Pathol* 4:149, 1991.
93. Alves VAF et al: Detection of leptospiral antigen in the human liver and kidney using an immunoperoxidase staining procedure, *J Pathol* 151:125, 1987.

94. Lachman MF, Cartun RW, Pedersen CA, Cole SR: Immunocytochemical identification of *Pneumocystis carinii* in formalin-fixed, paraffin-embedded tissues, *Lab Med* 11:808, 1990.
95. Krams SM, Van de Water J, Coppel RL et al: Analysis of hepatic T-lymphocytes and immunoglobulin deposits in patients with primary biliary cirrhosis, *Hepatology* 12:306, 1990.
96. Yamada G, Hyodo L, Nishihara T et al: Light and electron microscopic observations of lymphocyte subsets in liver of patients with primary biliary cirrhosis by immunoperoxidase method using monoclonal antibodies, *Acta Hepatol Jpn* 26:645, 1985.
97. Hashimoto E, Lindor KD, Homburger HA et al: Immunohistochemical characterization of hepatic lymphocytes in primary biliary cirrhosis in comparison with primary sclerosing cholangitis and autoimmune chronic active hepatitis, *Mayo Clin Proc* 68:1049, 1993.
98. Whiteside TL, Lasky S, Si L et al: Immunologic analysis of mononuclear cells in liver tissue and blood of patients with primary sclerosing cholangitis, *Hepatology* 5:468, 1985.
99. Govindarajan S, Uchida T, Peters RL: Identification of T-lymphocytes and subsets in liver biopsy cases of acute viral hepatitis, *Liver* 3:13, 1983.
100. Onji M, Kumon I, Kanaoka M et al: Intrahepatic lymphocyte subpopulations in acute hepatitis in an adult with rubella, *Am J Gastroenterol* 83:320, 1988.
101. Colucci G, Colombo N, Del Ninno E et al: In situ characterization by monoclonal antibodies of the mononuclear cell infiltrate in chronic active hepatitis, *Gastroenterology* 85:1138, 1983.
102. Eggink HF, Houthoff HJ, Huitema S et al: Cellular and humoral immune reactions in chronic active liver disease. I. Lymphocyte subsets in liver biopsies of patients with untreated idiopathic autoimmune hepatitis, chronic active hepatitis B and primary biliary cirrhosis, *Clin Exp Immunol* 50:17, 1982.
103. Husby G, Blomhoff JP, Elgjo K et al: Immunohistochemical characterization of hepatic tissue lymphocyte subpopulations in liver disease, *Scand J Gastroenterol* 17:855, 1982.
104. Si L, Whiteside TL, Van Thiel DH et al: Lymphocyte subpopulations at the site of "piecemeal" necrosis in end-stage chronic liver diseases and rejecting liver allografts in cyclosporine-treated patients, *Lab Invest* 50:341, 1984.

Special light microscopy techniques

105. Allaire GS, Goodman ZD, Ishak KG, Rabin L: Talc in liver tissue of intravenous drug abusers with chronic hepatitis: a comparative study, *Am J Clin Pathol* 92:583, 1989.
106. Pimentel JC, Menezes AP: Pulmonary and hepatic granulomatous disorders due to the inhalation of cement and mica dusts, *Thorax* 33:219, 1978.
107. Carmicheal GP, Targoff C, Pintar K et al: Hepatic silicosis, *Am J Clin Pathol* 73:720, 1980.
108. Coelho Filho, JC, Moreira RA, Crocker PR et al: Identification of titanium pigment in drug addict's tissues, *Histopathology* 19:190, 1991.
109. Landas SK, Mitros FA, Furst DE, LaBrecque DR: Lipogranulomas and gold in the liver in rheumatoid arthritis, *Am J Surg Pathol* 16:171, 1992.
110. Cortes JM, Iliva H, Paradinas FJ et al: The pathology of the liver in porphyria cutanea tarda, *Histopathology* 4:471, 1980.
111. Klatskin G, Bloomer JR: Birefringence of hepatic pigment deposits in erythropoietic protoporphyria, *Gastroenterology* 67:294, 1974.
112. Terzakis JA, Sommers SC, Synder RW et al: X-ray microanalysis of hepatic thorium deposits, *Arch Pathol* 98:241, 1974.
113. Leong ADY, Disney APS, Gove DW: Refractile particles in liver of haemodialysis patients, *Lancet* 1:889, 1981.

Scanning electron microscopy

114. Grisham JW, Nopanitanya W, Compagno J: Scanning electron microscopy, *Prog Liver Dis* 5:1, 1976.
115. Ishak KG: Applications of scanning electron microscopy to the study of liver disease, *Prog Liver Dis* 8:1, 1986.

Transmission microscopy

116. Johannessen JV, editor: Electron microscopy in human medicine, vol 8, *The liver,* New York, 1979, McGraw-Hill.
117. Tanikawa K: *Ultrastructural aspects of the liver and its disorders,* Tokyo, 1979, Igaku-Shoin.
118. Spycher MA: Electron microscopy: a method for the diagnosis of inherited metabolic storage diseases, *Pathol Res Pract* 167:118, 1980.
119. Guigui B, Perrot S, Barry JP et al: Amiodarone hepatic phospholipidosis: a morphological alteration independent of pseudoalcoholic liver disease, *Hepatology* 8:1063, 1988.
120. Pessayre O, Bichara M, Feldmann G et al: Perhexilene maleate induced cirrhosis, *Gastroenterology* 76:170, 1979.
121. Poucell S, Ireton J, Valencia-Mayoral P et al: Amiodarone-associated phospholipidosis and fibrosis of the liver: light, immunohistochemical and electron microscopic studies, *Gastroenterology* 86:926, 1984.
122. Poupon R, Rosensztajn L, Prudhomme de Saint-Maur P et al: Perhexilene maleate–associated hepatic injury: prevalence and characteristics, *Digestion* 20:145, 1980.
123. Shikata T, Kanetaka T, Endo Y et al: Drug-induced generalized phospholipidosis, *Acta Pathol Jpn* 22:517, 1972.

Molecular biology techniques

124. Negro F, Pacchioni D, Mondardini A et al: In situ hybridization in viral hepatitis, *Liver* (spec. issue) 12:217, 1992.
125. Brechot C: Polymerase chain reaction: a new tool for the study of viral infections in hepatology, *J Hepatol* 11:124, 1990.
126. Ohkoshi S, Kato N, Kinoshita T et al: Detection of hepatitis C virus RNA in sera and liver tissues of non-A, non-B hepatitis patients using the polymerase chain reaction, *Jpn J Cancer Res* 81:862, 1990.
127. Akyol G, Dash S, Shieh YSC et al: Detection of hepatitis C virus RNA sequences by polymerase chain reaction in fixed liver tissue, *Mod Pathol* 5:501, 1992.
128. Nuovo GJ, Lidonnici K, MacConnell P, Lane B: Intracellular localization of polymerase chain reaction (PCR)—amplified hepatitis C cDNA, *Am J Surg Pathol* 17:683, 1993.
129. Bartow SA: Diagnostic and prognostic applications of oncogenes in surgical pathology, *Am J Surg Pathol* 14(suppl 1):5, 1990.
130. Fausto N, Shank PR: Oncogene expression in liver regeneration and hepatocarcinogenesis, *Hepatology* 3:1016, 1983.
131. Fausto N, Shank PR: Analysis of proto-oncogene expression during liver regeneration and hepatocarcinogenesis. In Okuda K, Ishak KG, editors: *Neoplasms of the liver,* Tokyo, 1987, Springer-Verlag.
132. Gulbis B, Galand P: Immunodetection of the p21-*ras* products on human normal and preneoplastic tissues and solid tumors: a review, *Hum Pathol* 24:1271, 1993.
133. Himeno Y, Fukuda Y, Hatanaka M, Imura H: Expression of oncogenes in human liver disease, *Liver* 8:208, 1988.
134. Boix L, Rosa JL, Ventura F et al: C-*met* mRNA overexpression in human hepatocellular carcinoma, *Hepatology* 19:88, 1994.

Systematic histopathologic evaluation

135. Ishak KG: New developments in diagnostic liver pathology. In Farber E, Phillips MJ, Kaufman N, editors: *Pathogenesis of liver diseases,* Baltimore, 1987, Williams & Wilkins.
136. Ishak KG, Stromeyer FW: Medical diseases of the liver. In Silverberg SG, editor: *Principles and practice of surgical pathology,* vol 2, ed 3, New York, 1990, Churchill Livingstone.
137. Ishak KG: Hepatic histopathology. In Schiff L, Schiff ER, editors: *Diseases of the liver,* vol 1, ed 7, Philadelphia, 1993, Lippincott.

Hepatocellular injury

Ischemic necrosis (ischemic hepatitis)

138. Clarke WTW: Centrilobular hepatic necrosis following cardiac infarction, *Am J Pathol* 26:249, 1949.
139. Ellenberg M, Osserman KE: The role of shock in the production of liver cell necrosis, *Am J Med* 2:170, 1951.
140. Monte SM, Arcidi JM, Moore GW, Hutchins GM: Midzonal necrosis of hepatocellular injury after shock, *Gastroenterology* 86:627, 1984.
141. Nunes G, Blaisdell FW, Margaretten W: Mechanism of hepatic dysfunction following shock and trauma, *Arch Surg* 100:546, 1970.
142. Cohen JA, Kaplan MM: Left-sided heart failure presenting as hepatitis, *Gastroenterology* 74:583, 1978,
143. Bynum TE, Boitnott JH, Maddrey WC: Ischemic hepatitis, *Dig Dis Sci* 24:129, 1979.
144. Arcidi JM, Moore GW, Hutchins GM: Hepatic morphology in cardiac dysfunction: a clinicopathologic study of 1000 subjects at autopsy, *Am J Pathol* 104:159, 1981.

145. Gitlin N, Serio KM: Ischemic hepatitis: widening horizons, *Am J Gastroenterol* 87:831, 1992.

Viral hepatitis

146. Gust ID, Feinstone SM; *Hepatitis A,* Boca Raton, Fla., 1988, CRC Press.
147. Lemon SM: Type A hepatitis: new developments in an old disease, *N Engl J Med* 313:1059, 1985.
148. Fienstone SM: Hepatitis A, *Prog Liver Dis* 8:299, 1986.
149. Glikson M, Galun E, Oren R et al: Relapsing hepatitis A: review of 14 cases and literature survey, *Medicine* 71:14, 1992.
150. Tiollais P, Dejean A, Brechot C et al: Structure of hepatitis B virus DNA. In Vyas GN, Dienstag JL, Hoofnagle JH, editors: *Viral hepatitis and liver disease,* Orlando, Fla., 1984, Grune & Stratton.
151. Carman W, Thomas H, Domingo E: Viral genetic variation: hepatitis B as a clinical example, *Lancet* 341:349, 1993.
152. Omata M, Ehata T, Yokosuka O et al: Mutations in the precore region of hepatitis B virus DNA in patients with fulminant and severe hepatitis, *N Engl J Med* 324:1699, 1991.
153. Liang TJ, Hasegawa K, Rimon N et al: A hepatitis B virus mutant associated with an epidemic of fulminant hepatitis, *N Engl J Med* 324:1705, 1991.
154. Carman WF, Fagan EA, Hadziyannis S et al: Association of a precore genomic variant of hepatitis B virus with fulminant hepatitis, *Hepatology* 14:219, 1991.
155. Yotsumoto S, Kojima M, Shoji I et al: Fulminant hepatitis related to transmission of hepatitis B variants with precore mutations between spouses, *Hepatology* 16:31, 1992.
156. Hoofnagle JH, Schafer DF: Serologic markers of hepatitis B infection, *Semin Liver Dis* 6:1, 1986.
157. Popper H, Shafritz DA, Hoofnagle JH: Relation of hepatitis B carrier state to hepatocellular carcinoma, *Hepatology* 7:764, 1987.
158. Brechot C: Hepatitis B virus (HBV) and hepatocellular carcinoma: HBV DNA status and its implications, *J Hepatol* 4:269, 1987.
159. DiBisceglie AM, Rustgi VK, Hoofnagle JH et al: Hepatocellular carcinoma, *Ann Intern Med* 108:390, 1988.
160. Colombo M: Hepatocellular carcinoma, *J Hepatol* 15:225, 1992.
161. Sherlock S: Viruses and hepatocellular carcinoma, *Gut* 35:828, 1994
162. Rizzetto M: The delta agent, *Hepatology* 3:729, 1983.
163. Rizzetto M, Hadziyarenis S, Hansson BG et al: Hepatitis delta virus infection in the world: epidemiological patterns and clinical expression, *Gastroenterol Int* 3:18,1992.
164. Rizzetto M, Gerin JL, Purcell RH, editors: *The hepatitis delta virus and its infection,* New York, 1987, Alan R Liss.
165. Verme G, Bonino F, Rizzetto M, editors: *Viral hepatitis and delta infection,* New York, 1983, Alan R Liss.
166. Shiels MT, Czaja AJ, Taswell HF et al: Frequency and significance of delta antibody in acute and chronic hepatitis B: a United States experience, *Gastroenterology* 89:1230, 1985.
167. Jacobson IM, Dienstag JL, Werner BG et al: Epidemiology and clinical impact of hepatitis D virus (delta) infection, *Hepatology* 5:188, 1985.
168. De Cock KM, Govindarajan S, Chin KP et al: Delta hepatitis in the Los Angeles area: a report of 126 cases, *Ann Intern Med* 105:108, 1986.
169. Kunches LM, Craven DE, Werner BG: Seroprevalence of hepatitis B and delta agent in parenteral drug abusers, *Am J Med* 81:591, 1986.
170. Rizzetto M, Verme G: Delta hepatitis—present status, *J Hepatol* 1:187, 1985.
171. Esteban R: Epidemiology of hepatitis C virus infection, *J Hepatol* 17(suppl. 3):567, 1993.
172. Alter HJ, Hoofnagle JH: Non-A, non-B hepatitis. I. Recognition, epidemiology and clinical features. II. Experimented transmission, putative virus agents, markers and prevention, *Gastroenterology* 85:439, 462, and 743, 1983.
173. Dienstag JL, Alter HJ: Non-A, non-B hepatitis: evolving epidemiologic and clinical perspective, *Semin Liver Dis* 6:67, 1986.
174. Thomas HC: Non-A, non-B hepatitis, *Q J Med* 65:793, 1987.
175. Seeff LB, Buskell-Bales Z, Wright EC et al: Long-term mortality after transfusion-associated non-A, non-B hepatitis, *N Engl J Med* 327:1906, 1992.
176. Takada N, Takase S, Takada A, Date T: Differences in the hepatitis C virus genotypes in different countries, *J Hepatol* 17:277.
177. Alter MJ, Margolis HS, Krawczynski K et al: The natural history of community-acquired hepatitis C in the United States, *N Engl J Med* 327:1899, 1992.
178. DiBisceglie AM, Goodman ZD, Ishak KG et al: Long-term clinical and histopathological follow-up of chronic post transfusion hepatitis, *Hepatology* 14:969, 1991.
179. Patel A, Sherlock S, Dusheiko G et al: Clinical course and histological correlations in post-transfusion hepatitis C: the Royal Free Hospital experience, *Eur J Gastroenterol Hepatol* 3:491, 1991.
180. Tremolada F, Casarin C, Alberti A et al: Long-term follow-up of non-A, non-B (type C) post-transfusion hepatitis, *J Hepatol* 16:273, 1992.
181. Takahashi M, Yamada G, Miyamoto R et al: Natural course of chronic hepatitis C, *Am J Gastroenterol* 88:240, 1993.
182. Simonetti RG, Camm C, Fiorello F et al: Hepatitis C virus infection as a risk factor for hepatocellular carcinoma in patients with cirrhosis, *Ann Intern Med* 116:97, 1992.
183. Resnick RH, Koff R: Hepatitis C–related hepatocellular carcinoma, *Arch Intern Med* 153:1672, 1993.
184. Lee H-S, Han CJ, Kim CY: Predominant etiologic association of hepatitis C virus with hepatocellular carcinoma compared with hepatitis B virus in elderly patients in a hepatitis B–endemic area, *Cancer* 72:2564, 1993.
185. Maynard JE: Epidemic non-A, non-B hepatitis, *Semin Liver Dis* 4:336, 1984.
186. Bradley DW, Maynard JE: Etiology and natural history of post-transfusion and enterically-transmitted non-A, non-B hepatitis, *Semin Liver Dis* 6:56, 1986.
187. Ramalingaswami V, Purcell RH: Waterborne non-A, non-B hepatitis, *Lancet* 1:571, 1988.
188. Bradley DW: Enterically transmitted non-A, non-B hepatitis, *Br Med Bull* 46:442, 1990.
189. Reyes GR: Hepatitis E virus (HEV): molecular biology and emerging epidemiology, *Prog Liver Dis* 11:203, 1993.
190. Krawczynski K: Hepatitis E, *Hepatology* 17:932, 1993.
191. Searle J, Harmon BV, Bishop CJ et al: The significance of cell death by apoptosis in hepatobiliary disease, *J Gastroenterol Pathol* 2:77, 1987.
192. Oberhammer F, Bursch W, Tiefenbacher R et al: Apoptosis is induced by transforming growth factor-β1 within hours in regressing liver without significant fragmentation of the DNA, *Hepatology* 18:1238, 1993.
193. Kryger P, Christoffersen P: Liver histopathology of the hepatitis A virus infection: a comparison with hepatitis type B and non-A, non-B, *J Clin Pathol* 36:650, 1983.
194. Okuno T, Sano A, Deguchi T et al: Pathology of acute hepatitis A in humans: comparison with acute hepatitis B, *Am J Clin Pathol* 81:162, 1984.
195. Abe H, Ikejiri N, Sata M et al: Histological findings of the liver in viral hepatitis type A: a comparison with hepatitis type B, *Acta Hepatol Jpn* 22:22, 1981.
196. Abe H, Beninger PR, Ikejiri N et al: Light microscopic findings of liver biopsy specimens from patients with hepatitis A and comparison with type B, *Gastroenterology* 82:938, 1982.
197. Teixeira MR Jr, Weller IVD, Murray A et al: The pathology of hepatitis A in man, *Liver* 2:53, 1982.
198. Ishak KG: Hepatitis A infection: pathology. In Seeff LB, Lewis JH, editors: *Current perspectives in hepatology,* Festschift for Hyman J. Zimmerman, M.D., New York, 1989, Plenum Medical.
199. Kobayashi K, Hashimoto E, Ludwig J et al: Liver biopsy features of acute hepatitis C compared with hepatitis A, B, and non-A, non-B, non-C, *Liver* 13:69, 1993.
200. Boyer JK, Klatskin G: Pattern of necrosis in acute active viral hepatitis: prognostic value of bridging (subacute hepatic necrosis), *N Engl J Med* 283:1063, 1970.
201. Ishak KG: Light microscopic morphology of viral hepatitis, *Am J Clin Pathol* 65:787, 1976.
202. Ishak KG: Viral hepatitis. In Binford CH, Connor DH, editors: *Pathology of tropical and extraordinary diseases,* vol 1, Washington, D.C., 1976, Armed Forces Institute of Pathology.
203. MacSween RNM: Pathology of viral hepatitis and its sequelae, *Clin Gastroenterol* 9:23, 1980.

204. Phillips MJ, Purcell S: Modern aspects of the morphology of viral hepatitis, *Hum Pathol* 12:1060, 1981.
205. Scheuer PJ: Viral hepatitis. In MacSween RNM, Scheuer PJ, Anthony PP, editors: *Pathology of the liver,* Edinburgh, 1987, Churchill Livingstone.
206. Review by International Group: Guidelines for diagnosis of therapeutic drug-induced liver injury in liver biopsies, *Lancet* 1:854, 1974.

Drug-induced and toxic injury

207. Davidson CS, Leevy CM, Chamberlayne EC: *Guidelines for detection of hepatotoxicity due to drugs and chemicals,* Washington, D.C., 1978, U.S. Government Printing Office.
208. Zimmerman HJ: *Hepatotoxicity,* New York, 1978, Appleton-Century-Crofts.
209. Ishak KG: The liver. In Riddell RH, editor: *Pathology of drug-induced and toxic diseases,* New York, 1982, Churchill Livingstone.
210. Ishak KG, Mullick FG: Drug-induced and toxic liver injury. In Peters RL, Craig JR, editors: *Liver pathology,* New York, 1986, Churchill Livingstone.
211. Stricker BHC: *Drug-induced hepatic injury,* ed 2, Amsterdam, 1992, Elsevier.
212. Zimmerman HJ, Maddrey WC: Toxic and drug-induced hepatitis. In Schiff L, Schiff ER, editors: *Diseases of the liver,* ed 7, Philadelphia, 1993, Lippincott.
213. Spitz RD, Keren DF, Boitnott JK et al: Bridging hepatic necrosis: etiology and prognosis, *Am J Dig Dis* 23:1076, 1978.

Herpes simplex hepatitis

214. Singer DB: Pathology of neonatal herpes virus infection, *Perspect Pediatr Pathol* 6:243, 1981.
215. Goodman ZD, Ishak KG, Sesterhenn IA: Herpes simplex in apparently immunocompetent adults, *Am J Clin Pathol* 85:694, 1986.

Infectious mononucleosis hepatitis

216. Bonkowsky HL, Lee LV, Klatskin G: Acute granulomatous hepatitis: occurrence in cytomegalovirus mononucleosis, *JAMA* 233:1284, 1975.
217. Snover DC, Horwitz CA: Liver disease in cytomegalovirus mononucleosis: a light microscopical and immunoperoxidase study of six cases, *Hepatology* 4:408, 1984.
218. Ten Napel CHH, Houthoff HJ: Cytomegalovirus hepatitis in normal and immune compromised hosts, *Liver* 4:184, 1984.
219. Griffiths PD: Cytomegalovirus and the liver, *Semin Liver Dis* 4:307, 1984.
220. Remington JS, Barnett CH, Meikel M et al: Toxoplasmosis and infectious mononucleosis, *Arch Intern Med* 110:744, 1962.
221. Mullick FG, Ishak KG: Hepatic injury associated with diphenylhydantoin therapy: a clinicopathologic study of 20 cases, *Am J Clin Pathol* 74:442, 1980.
222. Cook LF, Shilkin KB, Reed WD: Phenytoin induced granulomatous hepatitis, *Aust NZ J Med* 11:539, 1981.

Liver manifestations of Rocky Mountain spotted fever

223. Adams JS, Walker DH: The liver in Rocky Mountain spotted fever, *Am J Clin Pathol* 75:156, 1981.

Q-fever hepatitis

224. Pellegrin M, Delsol G, Auvergnat JC et al: Granulomatous hepatitis in Q-fever, *Hum Pathol* 11:51, 1980.
225. Dupont HL, Hornick RB, Levin HS et al: Q-fever hepatitis, *Ann Intern Med* 74:198, 1871.
226. Hofmann CE, Heaton JW Jr: Q-fever hepatitis: clinical manifestations and pathological findings, *Gastroenterology* 83:474, 1982.
227. Qizilbash AH: The pathology of Q-fever as seen in liver biopsy, *Arch Pathol Lab Med* 107:364, 1983.
228. Srigley JR, Geddie WR, Vellend H et al: Q-fever: the liver and bone marrow pathology, *Am J Surg Pathol* 9:752, 1985.
229. Marazuela M, Moreno A, Yebra M et al: Hepatic fibrin-ring granulomas: a clinico-pathologic study of 23 patients, *Hum Pathol* 22:607, 1991.
230. Vanderstigel M, Zafrani ES, Legone JL et al: Allopurinol hypersensitivity as a cause of hepatic fibrin-ring granulomas, *Gastroenterology* 90:188, 1986.
231. Lobdell DH: "Ring" granulomas in cytomegalovirus hepatitis, *Arch Pathol Lab Med* 111:881, 1987.
232. Nenert M, Mavier P, Dubuc N et al: Epstein-Barr virus infection and hepatic fibrin-ring granulomas, *Hum Pathol* 19:608, 1988.

Syphilis

233. Oppenheimer EH, Hardy JB: Congenital syphilis in the newborn infant: clinical and pathological observations in recent cases, *Johns Hopkins Med J* 129:63, 1971.
234. Islam N, Wadud A: Tertiary syphilis of the liver: case report, *J Trop Med Hyg* 75:183, 1972.
235. Baker AL, Kaplan MM, Wolfe HJ et al: Liver disease associated with early syphilis, *N Engl J Med* 282:1422, 1971.
236 Lee RV, Thornton GF, Conn HO: Liver disease associated with secondary syphilis, *N Engl J Med* 284:1423, 1971.
237. Sobel HJ, Wolfe EH: Liver involvement in early syphilis, *Arch Pathol* 93:565, 1972.
238. Feher J, Somogyi T, Timmer M et al: Early syphilitic hepatitis, *Lancet* 2:896, 1975.
239. Tiliakos N, Shammaa JM, Nasrallah SM: Syphilitic hepatitis, *Am J Gastroenterol* 73:60, 1980.
240. Veeravahn M: Diagnosis of liver involvement in early syphilis: a critical review, *Arch Intern Med* 145:132, 1984.
241. Qizilbash A, Kontozoglou T, Sianos J et al: Hepar lobatum associated with chemotherapy and metastatic breast cancer, *Arch Pathol Lab Med* 111:58, 1987.

Leptospirosis

242. Dooley JR, Ishak KG: Leptospirosis. In Binford CH, Connor DH, editors: *Pathology of tropical and extraordinary diseases,* Washington, D.C., 1976, Armed Forces Institute of Pathology.

Miscellaneous viral infections

243. Zuckerman AJ, Simpson DIH: Exotic virus infections of the liver, *Prog Liver Dis* 6:425, 1979.
244. Ishak KG, Walker DH, Coetzer JAW et al: Viral hemorrhagic fevers with hepatic involvement: pathologic aspects with clinical correlations, *Prog Liver Dis* 7:495, 1982.
245. Howard CR, Ellis DS, Simpson DIH: Exotic viruses and the liver, *Semin Liver Dis* 4:361, 1984.

Alcoholic liver disease

246. Edmondson HA, Peters RL, Reynolds TB et al: Sclerosing hyaline necrosis of the liver in the chronic alcoholic: a recognizable clinical syndrome, *Ann Intern Med* 59:646, 1963.
247. Review by an International Group: Alcoholic liver disease: morphologic manifestations, *Lancet* 3:707, 1981.
248. Goodman ZD, Ishak KG: Occlusive venous lesions in alcoholic liver disease: a study of 200 cases, *Gastroenterology* 83:786, 1982.
249. French SW, Nash J, Shitabata P et al: Pathology of alcoholic liver disease, *Semin Liver Dis* 13:154, 1993.
250. Harrison DJ, Burt AD: Pathology of alcoholic liver disease, *Bailliere's Clin Gastroenterol* 7:641, 1993.
251. Rubin E, Lieber CS: Alcohol-induced hepatic injury in non-alcoholic volunteers, *N Engl J Med* 278:869, 1968.
251a. Lieber CS: Pathogenesis and early diagnosis of alcoholic liver injury, *N Engl J Med* 298:888, 1978.
252. Rubin E, Krus S, Popper H: Pathogenesis of postnecrotic cirrhosis in alcoholics, *Arch Pathol* 73:40, 1962.
253. Gerber MA, Orr W, Denk H et al: Hepatocellular hyaline in cholestasis and cirrhosis: its diagnostic significance, *Gastroenterology* 64:89, 1973.
254. French SW: The Mallory body: structure, composition and pathogenesis. *Hepatology* 1:76, 1981.
255. Marubbio AT, Buchwald H, Schwartz et al: Hepatic lesions of central pericellular fibrosis in morbid obesity, and after jejunoileal bypass, *Am J Clin Pathol* 66:684, 1976.
256. Holzbach RT: Nonalcoholic fatty liver, *Cleve Clin J Med* 55:136, 1988.
257. Adler M, Schaffner F: Fatty liver hepatitis cirrhosis in obese patients, *Am J Med* 67:811, 1979.
258. Falchuk KR, Fiske SC, Haggitt RC et al: Pericentral hepatic fibrosis and intracellular hyalin in diabetes mellitus, *Gastroenterology* 78:535, 1980.
259. Ludwig J, Viggiano TR, McGill DB et al: Nonalcoholic steatohepatitis: Mayo Clinic experience with a hitherto unnamed disease, *Mayo Clin Proc* 55:434, 1980.

260. Bacon BR, Farahvash M, Janney CG, Neuschwander-Tetri BA: Nonalcoholic steatohepatitis: an expanded clinical entity, *Gastroenterology* 107:1103, 1994.
261. Itoh S, Yougel T, Kawagoe K: Comparison between nonalcoholic steatohepatitis and alcoholic hepatitis, *Am J Gastroenterol* 82:650, 1987.
262. Diehl AM, Goodman ZD, Ishak KG: Alcohol-like liver disease in nonalcoholics, *Gastroenterology* 95:1056, 1988.
263. French SW, Eidus LB, Freeman J: Nonalcoholic fatty hepatitis: an important clinical condition, *Can J Gastroenterol* 3:109, 1989.
264. Powell EE, Cooksley WGE, Hanson R et al: The natural history of nonalcoholic steatohepatitis: a follow-up study of forty-two patients for up to 21 years, *Hepatology* 11:74, 1990.
265. Peters RL, Gay T, Reynolds TB: Post-jejunoileal bypass hepatic disease: its similarity to alcoholic hepatic disease, *Am J Clin Pathol* 63:318, 1975.
266. Haines NW, Baker AL, Boyer JL et al: Prognostic indicator of hepatic injury following jejunoileal bypass performed for refractory obesity: a prospective study, *Hepatology* 1:161, 1981.
267. Yokoo H, Minick OT, Batti F et al: Morphologic variants of alcoholic hyalin, *Am J Pathol* 69:25, 1972.
268. Denk H, Krepler R, Lackinger E et al: Immunological and biochemical characterization of the keratin-related component of Mallory bodies: a pathological pattern of hepatocytic cytokeratins, *Liver* 2:165, 1982.
269. French SW: Present understanding of the development of Mallory's body, *Arch Pathol Lab Med* 107:445, 1983.
270. Denk H, Lackinger E: Cytoskeleton in liver diseases, *Semin Liv Dis* 6:199, 1986.
271. French SW, Okanone T, Swierenga SHH et al: The cytoskeleton of hepatocytes in health and disease. In Farber E, Phillips MJ, Kaufman N, editors: *Pathogenesis of liver diseases,* Baltimore, 1987, Williams & Wilkins.
272. Yokoo H, Singh SK, Hawasli AH: Giant mitochondria in alcoholic liver disease, *Arch Pathol Lab Med* 102:213, 1978.
273. Jakobovits AW, Morgan MY, Sherlock S: Hepatic siderosis in alcoholics, *Dig Dis Sci* 24:305, 1979.
274. MacSween RNM: Alcohol and cancer, *Br Med Bull* 38:31, 1982.
275. Leevy CM, Sameshima Y, McNeil G et al: Hepatocellular carcinoma in the alcoholic, *IARC Sci Publ* 63:143, 1984.
276. Lieber CS, Garro A, Leo MA et al: Alcohol and cancer, *Hepatology* 6:1005, 1986.

Steatosis

277. Zimmerman HJ, Ishak KG: Nonalcoholic steatohepatitis and other forms of pseudoalcoholic liver disease. In Hall P, editor: *Alcoholic liver disease,* ed 2, Kent, UK, 1994, Edward Arnold.
278. Dahl MGC, Gregory MM, Scheuer PJ: Liver damage due to methotrexate in patients with psoriasis, *Br Med J* 1:625, 1971.
279. Mullick FG, Moran CA, Ishak KG: Total parenteral nutrition: a histopathologic analysis of the liver changes in 20 children, *Mod Pathol* 7:190, 1994.
280. Peura DA, Stromeyer FW, Johnson LF: Liver injury with alcoholic hyaline after intestinal resection, *Gastroenterology* 79:128, 1980.
281. Balistreri WF: Idiopathic Reye's syndrome and its metabolic-mimickers. In Balistreri WF, Stocker JT, editors: *Pediatric hepatology,* New York, 1990, Hemisphere Publishing Corp.
282. Rolfes DB, Ishak KG: Acute fatty liver in pregnancy: a clinicopathologic study of 35 cases, *Hepatology* 5:1149, 1985.
283. Sherlock S: Acute fatty liver of pregnancy and the microvesicular fat diseases, *Gut* 24:265, 1983.
284. Uchida T, Kao H, Quispe-Sjögren M et al: Alcoholic foamy degeneration: a pattern of acute alcoholic injury of the liver, *Gastroenterology* 84:683, 1983.
285. Starko KM, Mullick FG: Hepatic and cerebral pathology findings in children with fatal salicylate intoxication: further evidence of a causal relationship between salicylate and Reye's syndrome, *Lancet* 1:326, 1983.
286. Zimmerman HJ, Ishak KG: Valproate induced hepatic injury: analyses of 23 fatal cases, *Hepatology* 2:591, 1982.
287. Popper H, Thung SN, Gerber MA et al: Histologic studies of severe delta agent infection in Venezuelan Indians, *Hepatology* 3:906, 1983.

Chronic hepatitis

288. Review by an International Group: Acute and chronic hepatitis revisited, *Lancet* 2:914, 1977.
289. Baptista A, Bianchi L, DeGroote J et al: The diagnostic significance of periportal hepatic necrosis and inflammation, *Histopathology* 12:569, 1988.
290. Kerr JFR, Cooksley WGE, Searle J et al: The nature of piecemeal necrosis in chronic active hepatitis, *Lancet* 2:827, 1979.
291. Carson DA, Ribeiro JM: Apoptosis and disease, *Lancet* 341:1251, 1993.
292. Alison MR, Sarraf CE: Liver cell death: patterns and mechanisms, *Gut* 35:577, 1994.
293. Kawanishi H: Morphological association of lymphocytes with hepatocytes in chronic liver disease, *Arch Pathol Lab Med* 101:286, 1977.
294. Dienes HP, Autschbach F, Gerber MA: Ultrastructural lesion in autoimmune hepatitis and some of the immune response in liver tissue, *Semin Liver Dis* 11:197, 1991.
295. Bechtelsheimer H, Gedigk P, Miller R, Klein H: Aggressive Emperipolesis bei chronischen Hepatitiden, *Klin Wochenschr* 54:137, 1976.
296. Koziel MJ, Dudley D, Afdhal N et al: Hepatitis C virus (HCV)-specific cytotoxic T-lymphocytes recognize epitopes in the case and envelope proteins of HCV, *J Virol* 67:7522, 1993.
297. Itoh N, Yonehara S, Ishii A et al: The polypeptide encoded by the DNA for human cell surface antigen Fas can mediate apoptosis, *Cell* 66:233, 1991.
298. Hiramatsu N, Hayashi N, Katayama K et al: Immunohistochemical detection of Fas antigen in liver tissue of patients with chronic hepatitis C, *Hepatology* 19:1354, 1994.
299. Hino K, Okuda M, Konishi T et al: Analysis of lymphoid follicles in liver of patients with chronic hepatitis C, *Liver* 12:387, 1992.
300. Mosnier J-F, Degott C, Marcellin P et al: The intraportal lymphoid nodule and its environment in chronic active hepatitis C: an immunohistochemical study, *Hepatology* 17:366, 1993.
301. Petrovic IM, Scheuer PJ: Anti-HBs- and anti-HBc-containing plasma cells in livers of patients with type B hepatitis, *J Hepatol* 7:7, 1988.
302. Bianchi L, Spichtin HP, Gudat F: Chronic hepatitis. In MacSween RNM, Anthony PP, Scheuer PJ, editors: *Pathology of the liver,* Edinburgh, 1987, Churchill Livingstone.
303. Vyberg M: The hepatitis-associated bile duct lesion, *Liver* 13:289, 1993.
304. Nomoto M, Uchikosi Y, Kajikazawa N et al: Appearance of hepatocytelike cells in the interlobular bile ducts of human liver in various disease states, *Hepatology* 16:1199, 1992.
305. Schaffner F, Popper H: Capillarization of hepatic sinusoids in man, *Gastroenterology* 44: 239, 1963.
306. Takahara T, Nakayama Y, Ito H et al: Extracellular matrix formation in piecemeal necrosis: immunoelectron microscopic study, *Liver* 12:368, 1992.
307. Nagore N, Howe S, Boxer L, Scheuer PJ: Liver cell rosettes: structural differences in cholestasis and hepatitis, *Liver* 9:43, 1989.
308. Dienes HP, Hutteroth T, Hes G, Meuer SC: Immunoelectron microscopic observations on the inflammatory infiltrates and HLA antigens in hepatitis B and non-A, non-B, *Hepatology* 7:1317, 1987.
309. Bedossa P, Lemaigre G, Paraf F, Martin E: Deposition and remodelling of elastic fibres in chronic hepatitis, *Virchows Arch [A] (Pathol Anat)* 417:159, 1990.
310. Davis GL, Hoofnagle JH, Waggoner JG: Spontaneous reactivation of chronic type B hepatitis, *Gastroenterology* 84:1370, 1982.
311. Liaw Y-F, Tai D-I, Chu C-M et al: Acute exacerbation in chronic type B hepatitis: comparison between HBeAg and antibody-positive patients, *Hepatology* 7:20, 1987.
312. Koike K, Iino S, Kurai K et al: IgM anti-HBc in anti-HBe positive chronic type B hepatitis with acute exacerbations, *Hepatology* 7:573, 1987.
313. Chu C-M, Liaw Y-F, Pao C-C, Huang M-J: The etiology of acute hepatitis superimposed upon previously unrecognized asymptomatic HBsAg carrier, *Hepatology* 9:452, 1989.
314. Fattovich G, Brollo L, Alberti A et al: Spontaneous reactivation of hepatitis B virus infection in patients with chronic type B hepatitis, *Liver* 10:141, 1990.
315. Levy P, Mancellin P, Martenol-Peignoux M et al: Clinical course of spontaneous reactivation of hepatitis B virus infection in patients with chronic hepatitis B, *Hepatology* 12:570, 1990.
316. Lok ASF, Lai C-L: Acute exacerbations in Chinese patients with chronic hepatitis B virus (HBV) infection, *J Hepatol* 10:29, 1990.

317. Meyer RA, Duffy MC: Spontaneous reactivation of chronic hepatitis B infection leading to fulminant hepatic failure: report of two cases and review of the literature, *J Clin Gastroenterol* 17:231, 1993.
318. Bird GLA, Smith H, Portmann B et al: Acute liver decompensation on withdrawal of cytotoxic chemotherapy and immunosuppressive therapy in hepatitis B carriers, *Q J Med* 73:895, 1989.
319. Hoofnagle JH, Dusheiko GM, Schafer DF et al: Reactivation of chronic hepatitis B virus infection by cancer chemotherapy, *Ann Intern Med* 96:447, 1982.
320. Lau JYN, Lai CL, Lin HJ, Lok ASF et al: Fatal reactivation of chronic hepatitis B virus infection following withdrawal of chemotherapy in lymphoma patient, *Q J Med* 73:911, 1989.
321. Chu C-M, Farci P, Liaw Y-F et al: The role of delta superinfection in acute exacerbations of chronic type B hepatitis, *Liver* 6:26, 1986.
322. Waite J, Gilson RJC, Weller IVD et al: Hepatitis B virus reactivation or reinfection associated with HIV infection, *AIDS* 2:443, 1988.
323. Lazizi Y, Grangeot-Keros L, Delfraissy J-F: Reappearance of hepatitis B virus in immune patients infected with the human immunodeficiency virus type 1, *J Infect Dis* 158:666, 1988.
324. Gruber A, Lundberg L-G, Bjorkholm M: Reactivation of chronic hepatitis C after withdrawal of immunosuppressive therapy, *J Intern Med* 234:223, 1993.
325. Kurosaki M, Enomoto N, Marumo F, Sato C: Rapid sequence variation of the hypervariable region of hepatitis C virus during the course of chronic infection, *Hepatology* 17:1293, 1993.
326. Liaw Y-F, Pao C-C, Chu C-M: Changes in serum HBV-DNA in relation to serum transaminase during acute exacerbation in patients with chronic type B hepatitis, *Liver* 8:231, 1988.
327. Krogsgaard K, Aldershvile J, Kryger P et al: Reactivation of viral replication in anti-HBe positive chronic HBsAg carriers, *Liver* 10:54, 1990.
328. Raimondo G, Rodino G, Smedile V et al: Hepatitis B virus (HBV) markers and HBV-DNA in serum and liver tissue of patients with acute exacerbation of chronic type B hepatitis, *J Hepatol* 10:271, 1990.
329. Villari D, Raimondo G, Brancatelli S et al: Histological features in liver biopsy specimens of patients with acute reactivation of chronic type B hepatitis, *Histopathology* 18:73, 1991.
330. Murayama T, Iino S, Koike K et al: Serology of acute exacerbation in chronic hepatitis B virus infection, *Gastroenterology* 105:1141, 1993.
331. Nakamura T, Hayama M, Sakai T et al: Proliferative activity of hepatocytes in chronic viral hepatitis as revealed by immunohistochemistry for proliferating cell nuclear antigen, *Hum Pathol* 24:750, 1993.
332. Sagnelli E, Felaco FM, Filippini P et al: Influence of HDV infection on clinical, biochemical and histological presentation of HBsAg positive chronic hepatitis, *Liver* 9:229, 1989.
333. Liaw Y-F, Chen T-J, Chu C-M, Lin H-H: Acute hepatitis delta virus superinfection in patients with liver cirrhosis, *J Hepatol* 10:41, 1990.
334. Watanabe S, Okita K, Harada T et al: Morphologic studies of the liver cell dysplasia, *Cancer* 51:2197, 1983.
335. Anthony PB: Liver cell dysplasia. What is its significance? *Hepatology* 7:394, 1987.
336. Lefkowitch JH, Apfelbaum TF: Liver cell dysplasia in non-A, non-B hepatitis, *Arch Pathol Lab Med* 111:170, 1987.
337. Nakanuma Y, Terada T, Terasaki S et al: Atypical adenomatous hyperplasia in liver cirrhosis: low-grade hepatocellular carcinoma or borderline lesion? *Histopathology* 17:27, 1990.
338. Kondo F, Ebara M, Suriura N et al: Histological features and clinical course of large regenerative nodules: evaluation of their precancerous potentiality, *Hepatology* 12:592, 1990.
339. Theise ND, Schwartz M, Miller C, Thung SN: Macroregenerative nodules and hepatocellular carcinoma in forty-four sequential adult liver explants with cirrhosis, *Hepatology* 16:949, 1992.
340. Ferrell L, Wright T, Roberts J, Ascher N: Incidence and diagnostic features of macroregenerative nodules vs. small hepatocellular carcinoma in cirrhotic livers, *Hepatology* 16:1372, 1992.
341. Nakanuma Y, Terada T, Ueda K et al: Adenomatous hyperplasia of the liver as a precancerous lesion, *Liver* 13:1, 1993.
342. Moreno A, Ramon Y, Cajal S et al: Sanded nuclei in delta patients, *Liver* 9:367, 1989.
343. Deleadetsima JK, Vafiadis I, Tassopoulos NC et al: HBcAg and HBsAg expression in ductular cells in chronic hepatitis B, *Liver* 14:71, 1994.
344. Conteas C, Kao H, Rakela J: Acute type A hepatitis in three patients with chronic HBV infection, *Dig Dis Sci* 28:684, 1983.
345. Zachoval R, Roggendorf M, Deinhardt F: Hepatitis A infection in chronic carriers of hepatitis B virus, *Hepatology* 3:528, 1983.
346. Butti M, Mas A, Sanchez, Tapias JM: Chronic hepatitis D in intravenous drug addicts and non-addicts, *J Hepatol* 7:169, 1988.
347. Chin KP, Govindarajan S, Redeker AG: Permanent HBsAg clearance in chronic hepatitis B viral infection following acute delta superinfection, *Dig Dis Sci* 33:851, 1988.
348. Craxi A, Raimondo G, Longo G et al: Delta agent infection in acute hepatitis and chronic HBsAg carriers with and without liver disease, *Gut* 25:1288, 1984.
349. Kanel GC, Govindarajan S, Peters RL: Chronic delta infection and liver biopsy changes in chronic active hepatitis B, *Ann Intern Med* 101:286, 1984.
350. Negro F, Baldi M, Bonino F et al: Chronic HDV (hepatitis delta virus) hepatitis: intrahepatic expression of delta antigen, histologic activity and outcome of liver disease, *J Hepatol* 6:8, 1988.
351. Rizzeto M, Verme G, Recchia S: Chronic hepatitis in carriers of hepatitis B surface antigen with intrahepatic expression of the delta infection, *Ann Intern Med* 98:437, 1983.
352. Lok A, Lindsay A, Scheuer PJ, Thomas HC: Clinical and histological features of delta infection in chronic hepatitis B carriers, *J Clin Pathol* 38:530, 1985.
353. Fattovich G, Tagger A, Brollo L et al: Hepatitis C infection in chronic hepatitis B virus carriers, *J Infect Dis* 163:400, 1991.
354. Fong T-L, DiBisceglie AM, Waggoner JG et al: The significance of antibody to hepatitis C in patients with chronic hepatitis B, *Hepatology* 14:64, 1991.
355. Pontisso P, Ruvoletto MG, Fattovich G et al: Clinical and virological profiles in patients with multiple hepatitis C infections, *Gastroenterology* 105:1529, 1993.
356. Hanley JP, Dolan G, Day S et al: Interaction of hepatitis B and hepatitis C infection in haemophilia, *Br J Haematol* 85:611, 1991.
357. Mimms LT, Moseley JW, Hollinger FB et al: Effect of concurrent acute infection with hepatitis C virus on acute hepatitis B infection, *Br Med J* 307:1095, 1993.
358. Vandelli C, Zannini A, Piaggi V et al: What is the effect of a cytomegalovirus infection when superimposed on HBsAg-positive chronic hepatitis? *J Hepatol* 4:343, 1987.
359. Marinelli RMA, Monache MD, Gerardi R et al: Liver pathology in cytomegalovirus infection associated with hepatitis B virus, *J Intern Med Res* 21:154, 1993.
360. McDonald JA, Harris S, Waters JA, Thomas HC: Effect of human immunodeficiency virus (HIV) infection on chronic hepatitis B hepatic viral antigen display, *J Hepatol* 4:337, 1987.
361. Perrillo RP, Regenstein PG, Roodman ST: Chronic hepatitis B in asymptomatic homosexual men with antibody to human immunodeficiency virus, *Ann Intern Med* 105:382, 1986.
362. Krogsgaard K, Lindhardt BO, Nielsen JO et al: The influence of HTLV III infection on the natural history of hepatitis B virus infection in male homosexual HBsAg carriers, *Hepatology* 7:37, 1987.
363. Goldin RD, Fish DE, Hay A et al: Histological and immunohistochemical study of hepatitis B virus in human immunodeficiency virus infection, *J Clin Pathol* 43:203, 1990.
364. McNair ANB, Main J, Thomas HC: Interactions of the human immunodeficiency virus and the hepatotropic viruses, *Semin Liver Dis* 12:188, 1992.
365. Lin H-H, Liaw Y-F, Chen T-J et al: Natural course of patients with chronic type B hepatitis following acute delta virus superinfection, *Liver* 9:129, 1989.
366. Scheuer PJ, Ashrafzadeh P, Sherlock S et al: The pathology of hepatitis C, *Hepatology* 15:567, 1992.
367. Bach N, Thung SN, Schaffner F: The histological features of chronic hepatitis C and autoimmune chronic hepatitis, *Hepatology* 15:572, 1992.
368. Gerber MA, Krawczynski K, Alter MJ et al: Histopathology of community acquired chronic hepatitis C, *Mod Pathol* 5:483, 1992.

369. Lefkowitch JH, Schiff ER, Davis GL et al: Pathological diagnosis of chronic hepatitis C: a multicenter comparative study with chronic hepatitis B, *Gastroenterology* 104:595, 1993.
370. Roberts JM, Searle JW, Coolesley WGE: Histological patterns of prolonged hepatitis C infection, *Gastroenterol Jpn* 28:901, 1993.
371. Bianchi L, Desmet VJ, Popper H et al: Histologic patterns of liver disease in hemophiliacs with special reference to morphologic characteristics of non-A, non-B hepatitis, *Semin Liver Dis* 7:203, 1987.
372. Lefkowitch JH, Apfelbaum TF: Non-A, non-B hepatitis: characterization of liver biopsy pathology, *J Clin Gastroenterol* 11:225, 1989.
373. Gordon SC, Elloway RS, Long JC, Dmuchowsky CF: The pathology of hepatitis C as a function of transmission: blood transfusion vs. intravenous drug use, *Hepatology* 18:1338, 1993.
374. Fingerhood MI, Jasinski DR, Sullivan JT: Prevalence of hepatitis C in a chemically dependent population, *Arch Intern Med* 153:2025, 1993.
375. Danque POV, Bach N, Schaffner F et al: HLA-DR expression in bile duct damage in hepatitis C, *Mod Pathol* 6:327, 1993.
376. Broom U, Scheynius A, Hultcrantz R: Induced expression of heat-shock protein on biliary epithelium in patients with primary sclerosing cholangitis and primary biliary cirrhosis, *Hepatology* 18:298, 1993.
377. Chu H-W, Dash S, Gerber MA: Genomic and replicative hepatitis C virus RNA sequences and histologic activity in chronic hepatitis C, *Hum Pathol* 25:160, 1994.
378. Ohkoshi S, Kato N, Kinoshita T et al: Detection of hepatitis C virus RNA in sera and liver tissues of non-A, non-B hepatitis patients using the polymerase chain reaction, *Jpn J Cancer Res* 81:862, 1990.
379. Shieh YSC, Shim K-S, Lampertico P et al: Detection of hepatitis C virus sequences in liver tissue by the polymerase chain reaction, *Lab Invest* 66:408, 1991.
380. Bresters D, Cuypers HTM, Recsnik HW et al: Detection of hepatitis C viral RNA sequences in fresh and paraffin-embedded liver biopsy specimens of non-A, non-B hepatitis patients, *J Hepatol* 15:391, 1992.
381. Krawczynski K, Beach MJ, Brandley DW et al: Hepatitis C antigen in hepatocytes: immunomorphologic detection and identification, *Gastroenterology* 103:622, 1992.
382. Sansonno D, Dammacco F: Hepatitis C virus c100 antigen in liver tissue from patients with acute and chronic infection, *Hepatology* 18:240, 1993.
383. Tsutsumi M, Urashima S, Takada A et al: Delection of antigens of hepatitis C virus RNA encoding the NS5 region in the livers of patients with chronic type C hepatitis, *Hepatology* 19:265, 1994.
384. Infantolino D, Bonino F, Zanetti AR et al: Localization of hepatitis C virus (HCV) antigen by immunohistochemistry on fixed-embedded liver tissue, *Ital J Gastroenterol* 22:198, 1990.
385. Blight K, Trowbridge R, Rowland R, Gowans E: Detection of hepatitis C virus RNA by in situ hybridization, *Liver* (spec. issue) 12:286, 1992.
386. Yamada G, Nishimoto H, Endou H et al: Localization of hepatitis C viral RNA and capsid protein in human liver, *Dig Dis Sci* 38:882, 1993.
387. Tanaka Y, Enomoto N, Kojima S et al: Detection of hepatitis C virus RNA in the liver by in situ hybridization, *Liver* 13:203, 1993.
388. Akyol G, Dash S, Shieh C et al: Detection of hepatitis C virus RNA sequences by polymerase chain reaction in fixed liver tissue, *Mod Pathol* 5:501, 1992.
389. Nuovo GJ, Lidonnici K, MacConnell P, Lane B: Intracellular localization of polymerase chain reaction (PCR)—amplified hepatitis C cDNA, *Am J Surg Pathol* 17:683, 1993.
390. Stechemesser E, Klein R, Berg PA: Characterization and clinical relevance of liver-pancreas antibodies in autoimmune hepatitis, *Hepatology* 18:1, 1983.
391. Dienes HP: *Viral and autoimmune hepatitis: morphologic and pathogenetic aspects of cell damage in hepatitis with potential chronicity,* Stuttgart, 1989, Gustav Fischer Verlag.
392. Dienes HP, Popper H, Manns M et al: Histologic features in autoimmune hepatitis, *Gastroenterology* 27:325, 1989.
393. Fasconi M, Lenzi M, Ballardini G et al: Anti-HCV in autoimmune hepatitis and primary biliary cirrhosis, *Lancet* 336:823, 1990.
394. Garson JA, Lenzi M, Ring C et al: Hepatitis C viraemia in adults with type 2 autoimmune hepatitis, *J Med Virol* 34:223, 1991.
395. Lenzi M, Johnson PJ, McFarlane IG et al: Antibodies to hepatitis C virus in autoimmune liver disease: evidence for geographical heterogeneity, *Lancet* 338:277, 1991.
396. Todros L, Touscoz G, D'Urso N et al: Hepatitis C virus-related chronic liver disease with autoantibodies to liver-kidney microsomes (LKM), *J Hepatol* 13:128, 1991.
397. Bianchi FB, Lenzi M, Cassani F et al: Immunology and autoimmunity in hepatitis C. In Meyer zum Buschenfelde K-H, Hoofnagle JH, Manns M, editors: *Immunology and liver,* Dordrecht, 1993, Kluwer Academic Publishers.
398. Pawlotsky J-M, Ben Yahia M, Andre C et al: Immunological disorders in C virus chronic active hepatitis: a prospective case-control study, *Hepatology* 19:841, 1994.
399. Abuaf N, Johenet C, Chretien P et al: Characterization of the liver cytosol antigen type 1 reacting with autoantibodies in chronic active hepatitis, *Hepatology* 16:892, 1992.
400. Richey J, Rogers S, Van Thiel DH, Leser R: Giant multinucleated hepatocytes in an adult with chronic active hepatitis, *Gastroenterology* 73:570, 1977.
401. Bernard O, Hadchouel M, Scotto J et al: Severe giant cell hepatitis with autoimmune hemolytic anemia in early childhood, *J Pediatr* 99:704, 1981.
402. Shinozaki T, Saito K, Shiraki K: HBsAg-positive giant-cell hepatitis with cirrhosis in a 10-month-old infant, *Arch Dis Child* 56:64, 1981.
403. Thaler H: Post-infantile giant cell hepatitis, *Liver* 2:293, 1982.
404. Thijs JC, Bosna KA, Henzen-Longmans SC, Meuwissen SGM: Post-infantile giant cell hepatitis in a patient with multiple autoimmune features, *Am J Gastroenterol* 80:294, 1985.
405. Phillips MJ, Blendis LM, Poucell S et al: Syncytial giant cell hepatitis: sporadic hepatitis with distinctive pathological features, a severe clinical course, and paramyxoviral features, *N Engl J Med* 324:455, 1991.
406. Devaney K, Goodman ZD, Ishak KG: Post-infantile giant-cell transformation in hepatitis, *Hepatology* 16:327, 1992.
407. Lau JYN, Koukoulis G, Mieli-Vergani G et al: Syncytial giant-cell hepatitis—a specific disease entity? *J Hepatol* 15:216, 1992.
408. Sanna G, Faa G, Forresu S et al: Syncytial giant cell hepatitis: a new form of chronic liver disease, *Eur J Intern Med* 4:155, 1993.
409. Weinstein U, Valderrama E, Pettei M, Livine J: Early steroid therapy for the treatment of giant cell hepatitis with autoimmune hemolytic anemia, *J. Pediatr Gastroenterol Nutr* 17:313, 1993.
410. Rabinovitz M, Demetris AJ: Post infantile giant cell hepatitis associated with anti-M2 mitochondrial antibodies, *Gastroenterology* 107:1162, 1994.
411. Czaja AJ, Hay JE, Rakela J: Clinical features and prognostic implications of severe corticosteroid cryptogenic chronic active hepatitis, *Mayo Clin Proc* 65:23, 1990; comment: 65:119, 1990.
412. Brown J, Dourakis S, Karayainnis P et al: Seroprevalence of hepatitis C virus nucleocapsid antibodies in patients with cryptogenic chronic liver disease, *Hepatology* 15:175, 1992; comment: 15:350, 1992.
413. Sanchez-Tapias JM, Barrera JM, Costa J et al: Hepatitis C virus infection in patients with nonalcoholic chronic liver disease, *Ann Intern Med* 112:921, 1990.
414. Greeve M, Ferrell L, Kim M et al: Cirrhosis of undefined pathogenesis: absence of evidence for unknown viruses or autoimmune processes, *Hepatology* 17:593, 1993.
415. Czaja AJ, Carpenter HA, Santrach PJ et al: The nature and prognosis of severe cryptogenic chronic active hepatitis, *Gastroenterology* 104:1755, 1993.
416. MacFarlane IG: Hepatitis C and alcoholic liver disease, *Am J Gastroenterol* 88:982, 1993.
417. Villa E, Baldini G, DiStabile S et al: Alcohol and hepatitis B virus infection, *Acta Med Scand Suppl* 703:97, 1986.
418. Murata T, Takanari H, Watanabe S et al: Enhancement of chronic viral hepatic changes by alcohol intake in patients with persistent HBs-antigenemia, *Am J Clin Pathol* 94:270, 1990.
419. Noguchi O, Yamaoka K, Ikeda T et al: Clinicopathologic analysis of alcoholic liver disease complicating chronic type C hepatitis, *Liver* 11:225, 1991.
420. Rosman AS, Paronetto F, Galvin K et al: Hepatitis C virus antibody in alcoholic patients: association with the presence of portal and/or lobular hepatitis, *Arch Intern Med* 153:965, 1993.

421. Fong T-L, Kanel GC, Conrad A et al: Clinical significance of concomitant hepatitis C infection in patients with alcoholic liver disease, *Hepatology* 19:554, 1994.
422. Freni MA, Ajello A, Resta ML et al: HCV infection, hepatic HLA display and composition of the mononuclear cell inflammatory infiltrate in chronic alcoholic liver disease, *Eur J Clin Invest* 21:586, 1991.
423. Goldstein GB, Lam KC, Mistilis SP: Drug-induced active chronic hepatitis, *Am J Dig Dis* 18:177, 1973.
424. Wright R: Drug-induced chronic hepatitis, *Scand J Gastroenterol* 9:93, 1974.
425. Zimmerman HJ: Drug-induced chronic liver disease. In Farber E, Fisher MM, editors: *Toxic injury of the liver,* Part B, New York, 1980, Marcel Dekker.
426. Pessayre D, Larrey D: Acute and chronic drug-induced hepatitis, *Balliere's Clin Gastroenterol* 2:385, 1988.
427. Sharp JR, Ishak KG, Zimmerman HJ: Chronic active hepatitis and severe hepatic necrosis associated with nitrofurantoin, *Ann Intern Med* 92:14, 1980.
428. Sternlieb I, Scheinberg IH: Chronic hepatitis as a first manifestation of Wilson's disease, *Ann Intern Med* 76:59, 1972.
429. Archer GJ, Morrie RD: Wilson's disease and chronic active hepatitis, *Lancet* 1:486, 1977.
430. Scott J, Gollan JL, Samourian S, Sherlock S: Wilson's disease presenting as chronic active hepatitis, *Gastroenterology* 74:645, 1978.
431. Hodges JR, Millward-Sadler GH, Barbatis C, Wright R: Heterozygous MZ $alpha_1$ - antitrypsin deficiency in adults with chronic hepatitis and cryptogenic cirrhosis, *N Engl J Med* 304:557, 1981.
432. Propst T, Propst A, Dietzeo et al: High prevalence of viral infection in adults with homozygous and heterozygous $alpha_1$-antitrypsin deficiency and chronic liver disease, *Ann Intern Med* 117:641, 1992.
433. Scheuer PJ: Classification of chronic viral hepatitis: a need for reassessment, *J Hepatol* 13:372, 1991.
434. Zetterman RK: Chronic hepatitis: is it persistent, active, or just chronic? *Am J Gastroenterol* 88:1, 1993.
435. Gerber MA: Chronic hepatitis C: the beginning of the end of a time-honored nomenclature? *Hepatology* 15:733, 1992.
436. Ludwig J: The nomenclature of chronic active hepatitis: an obituary, *Gastroenterology* 105:274, 1993.
437. Czaja AJ: Chronic active hepatitis: the challenge for a new nomenclature, *Ann Intern Med* 119:510, 1993.
438. Desmet VJ, Gerber M, Hoofnagle JH et al: Classification of chronic hepatitis: diagnosis, grading and staging, *Hepatology* 19:1513, 1994.
439. Ishak KG: Chronic hepatitis: morphology and nomenclature, *Mod Pathol* 7:690, 1994.

Cholestasis

Extrahepatic biliary obstruction

440. Gall EA, Dobrogorski O: Hepatic alterations in obstructive jaundice, *Am J Clin Pathol* 41:126, 1964.
441. Grier JF, Cohen SW, Grafton WD et al: Acute suppurative cholangitis associated with choledochal sludge, *Am J Gastroenterol* 89:617, 1994.
442. Rubel LR, Ishak KG: The liver in exertional heatstroke, *Liver* 3:249, 1983.
443. Ishak KG, Rogers WA: Cryptogenic acute cholangitis: association with toxic shock syndrome, *Am J Clin Pathol* 76:619, 1981.
444. Gear JHS, Meyers KEC, Steele M: Kawasaki disease manifesting with acute cholangitis: a case report, *S Afr Med J* 81:31, 1992.

Intrahepatic cholestasis

445. Banks JG, Foulis AK, Ledingham IM et al: Liver function in septic shock, *J Clin Pathol* 35:1249, 1982.
446. Lefkowitch JH: Bile ductular cholestasis: an ominous histopathologic sign related to sepsis and "cholangitis lenta," *Hum Pathol* 13:19, 1982.
447. Zimmerman HJ: Intrahepatic cholestasis, *Arch Intern Med* 139:1038, 1979.
448. Zimmerman HJ, Lewis JH: Drug-induced cholestasis, *Med Technol* 2:112, 1987.
449. Larrey D, Erlinger S: Drug-induced cholestasis, *Bailliere's Clin Gastroenterol* 2:423, 1988.
450. Ishak KG: Hepatic lesions caused by anabolic and contraceptive steroids, *Semin Liver Dis* 1:116, 1981.
451. Stricker BHC: *Drug-induced hepatic injury,* ed 2, Amsterdam, 1992, Elsevier.
452. de Pegter AGF, van Berge Henegouwen GP, ten Bokkel Huinink JA, Brandt KH: Familial benign recurrent cholestasis, *Gastroenterology* 71:202, 1976.
453. Summerfield JA, Scott J, Berman M et al: Benign recurrent intrahepatic cholestasis: studies of bilirubin kinetics, bile acids, and cholangiography, *Gut* 21:154, 1980.
454. Minuk GY, Shaffer EA: Benign recurrent intrahepatic cholestasis: evidence for an intrinsic abnormality in hepatocyte secretion, *Gastroenterology* 93:1187, 1987.
455. Brenard R, Geubel AP, Benhamou JP: Benign recurrent intrahepatic cholestasis: a report of 26 cases, *J Clin Gastroenterol* 11:546, 1989.
456. Reyes H: The spectrum of liver and gastrointestinal disease seen in cholestasis of pregnancy, *Gastroenterol Clin North Am* 21:905, 1992.

Chronic cholestatic injury

457. Alagille D: Extrahepatic biliary atresia, *Hepatology* 4:75, 1984.
458. Gautier M, Valayer J, Odievre M, Alagille D: Histological liver evaluation 5 years after surgery for extrahepatic biliary atresia: a study of 20 cases, *J Pediatr Surg* 19:263, 1984.
459. Alagille D, Estrade A, Hadchouel M et al: Syndromatic paucity of interlobular bile ducts (Alagille's syndrome) or arteriohepatic dysplasia: review of 80 cases, *J Pediatr* 110:195, 1987.
460. Dahms BB, Petrelli M, Wyllie R et al: Arteriohepatic dysplasia in infancy and childhood: a longitudinal study of six patients, *Hepatology* 2:350, 1982.
461. Kahn EL, Daum F, Markowitz J et al: Arteriohepatic dysplasia. II. Hepatobiliary morphology, *Hepatology* 3:77, 1983.
462. Valencia-Mayoral P, Weber J, Cutz E et al: Possible defect in the bile secretory apparatus in arteriohepatic dysplasia (Alagille's syndrome): a review with observations on the ultrastructure of the liver, *Hepatology* 4:691, 1984.
463. Kahn C: Paucity of interlobular bile ducts: arteriohepatic dysplasia and nonsyndromatic duct paucity, *Perspect Pediatr Pathol* 14:168, 1991.
464. Ludwig J, Wiesner RH, LaRusso NF et al: Idiopathic adulthood ductopenia: a cause of chronic cholestatic liver disease and biliary cirrhosis, *J Hepatol* 7:193, 1988.
465. Zafrani ES, Metreau J-M, Douvin C et al: Idiopathic biliary ductopenia in adults: a report of five cases, *Gastroenterology* 99:1823, 1990.
466. Finegold MJ, Carpenter RJ: Obliterative cholangitis due to cytomegalovirus: a possible precursor of paucity of intrahepatic bile ducts, *Hum Pathol* 13:662, 1982.
467. Kage M, Kosai K-I, Kojiro M et al: Infantile cholestasis due to cytomegalovirus infection of the liver, *Arch Pathol Lab Med* 117:942, 1993.
468. Hadchouel M, Gautier M: Histopathological study of the liver in the early cholestatic phase of alpha-1 antitrypsin deficiency, *J Pediatr* 89:211, 1976.
469. Eyssen H, Parmentier G, Compernolle F et al: Trihydroxycoprostanic acid in the duodenal fluid of two children with intrahepatic bile duct anomalies, *Biochim Biophys Acta* 273:212, 1972.
470. Hanson RF, Isenberg JN, Williams GC et al: The metabolism of 3α, 7α, 12α-trihydroxy-5β-cholestan-26-oic acid in two siblings with cholestasis due to intrahepatic bile duct anomalies: an apparent inborn error of cholic acid synthesis, *J Clin Invest* 56:577, 1975.
471. Clayton RJ, Iber FL, Ruebner BH et al: Byler disease, *Am J Dis Child* 117:112, 1969.
472. Dahms BB: Hepatoma in familial cholestatic cirrhosis of childhood: its occurrence in twin brothers, *Arch Pathol Lab Med* 103:30, 1979.
473. De Vos R, de Wolf-Peeters C, Desmet V et al: Progressive intrahepatic cholestasis (Byler's disease): case report, *Gut* 16:943, 1975.
474. Ugarte N, Gonzalez-Crussi F: Hepatoma in siblings with progressive familial cholestatic cirrhosis of childhood, *Am J Clin Pathol* 76:172, 1981.
475. Riely C: Familial intrahepatic cholestatic syndromes, *Semin Liver Dis* 89:202, 1987.
476. Weber AM, Tuchweber B, Yousef I et al: Severe familial cholestasis in North American Indian children: a clinical model of microfilament dysfunction? *Gastroenterology* 81:653, 1981.

477. Weber AM et al: Cholestasis induced by microfilament dysfunction. In Daum F, editor: *Extrahepatic biliary atresia,* New York, 1983, Marcel Dekker.

478. Ornvold K, Nielsen I-M, Poulsen H. Fatal familial cholestatic syndrome in Greenland Eskimo children, *Virchows Arch [A] (Pathol Anat)* 415:275, 1989.

479. Jones EA, Rabin L, Buckley CH et al: Progressive intrahepatic cholestasis of infancy and childhood: a clinicopathological study of a patient surviving to the age of 18 years, *Gastroenterology* 71:675, 1976.

480. Kaplinsky C, Sternlieb I, Javitt N, Rotem Y: Familial cholestatic cirrhosis associated with Kayser-Fleischer rings, *Pediatrics* 65:782, 1980.

Primary biliary cirrhosis

481. Sherlock C, Scheuer PJ: The presentation and diagnosis of 100 patients with primary biliary cirrhosis, *N Engl J Med* 289:674, 1983.

482. Kaplan MM: Primary biliary cirrhosis, *N Engl J Med* 316:521, 1987.

483. Weisner RH, LaRusso NF, Ludwig J et al: Comparison of the clinicopathologic features of primary sclerosing cholangitis and primary biliary cirrhosis, *Gastroenterology* 88:108, 1985.

484. Baggenstoss AH, Foulk, WT, Butt HR et al: The pathology of primary biliary cirrhosis with emphasis on histogenesis, *Am J Clin Pathol* 42:259, 1965.

485. Goudie RB, MacSween RNM, Goldberg DM: Serological and histological diagnosis of primary biliary cirrhosis, *J Clin Pathol* 19:527, 1966.

486. MacSween RNM: Primary biliary cirrhosis. In Peters RL, Craig JR, editors: *Liver pathology,* New York, 1986, Churchill Livingstone.

487. Portmann B, MacSween RNM: Diseases of the intrahepatic bile ducts. In MacSween RNM, Anthony PP, Scheuer PJ, editors: *Diseases of the liver,* ed 2, Edinburgh, 1987, Churchill Livingstone.

488. Nakanuma Y, Ohta G: Histometric and serial section observations of intrahepatic bile ducts in primary biliary cirrhosis, *Gastroenterology* 76:1325, 1979.

489. Klöppel G, Seifert G, Lindner H et al: Histopathological features in mixed types of chronic aggressive hepatitis and primary biliary cirrhosis, *Virchows Arch [A] (Pathol Anat)* 373:143, 1977.

490. Berg PA, Wiedmann KH, Sayers T et al: Serological classification of chronic cholestatic liver disease by the use of two different types of antimitochondrial antibodies, *Lancet* 2:1329, 1980.

491. Brunner G, Klinge O: A cholangitis with antinuclear antibodies (immunocholangitis) resembling chronic nonsuppurative destructive cholangitis, *Dtsch Med Wochenschr* 112: 1454, 1987.

492. Williamson JMS, Chalmers DM, Clayden AD et al: Primary biliary cirrhosis and chronic active hepatitis: an examination of clinical, biochemical, and histopathological features in differential diagnosis, *J Clin Pathol* 38:1007, 1985.

493. Lindor KD, Wiesner RH, LaRusso NF, Dickson ER: Chronic active hepatitis. overlap with primary biliary cirrhosis and primary sclerosing cholangitis. In Czaja AJ, Dickson ER, editors: *Chronic active hepatitis, the Mayo Clinic experience,* New York, 1986, Marcel Dekker.

494. Carrougher JG, Shaffer RT, Canales LI, Goodman ZD: A 33-year-old woman with an autoimmune syndrome, *Semin Liver Dis* 11:256, 1991.

495. Ben-Ari Z, Dhillon AP, Sherlock S: Autoimmune cholangiopathy: part of the spectrum of autoimmune chronic active hepatitis, *Hepatology* 18:10, 1993.

496. Taylor S, Dean P, Riely C: Primary autoimmune cholangitis: an alternative to antimitrochondrial antibody-negative primary biliary cirrhosis, *Am J Surg Pathol* 18:91, 1994.

497. Fussey SPM, Guest JR, James OFW et al: Identification and analysis of the major M2 autoantigens in PBC, *Proc Natl Acad Sci USA* 85:8654, 1988.

498. Coppel RL, McNeilage J, Surh CD et al: Primary structure of the human M2 mitochondrial autoantigen of PBC: dihydrolipoamide acetyl transferase, *Proc Natl Acad Sci USA* 86:7317, 1988.

499. Krasner N, Johnson PJ, Portmann B et al: Hepatocellular carcinoma in primary biliary cirrhosis: report of four cases, *Gut* 20:255, 1979.

Primary sclerosing cholangitis

500. Chapman RWG, Arborgh BA, Rhodes JM et al: Primary sclerosing cholangitis: a review of its clinical features, cholangiography, and hepatic histology, *Gut* 21:870, 1980.

501. LaRusso NF, Wiesner RH, Ludwig J: Primary sclerosing cholangitis, *N Engl J Med* 310:899, 1984.

502. Wiesner RH, Ludwig J, LaRusso NF et al: Diagnosis and treatment of primary sclerosing cholangitis, *Semin Liver Dis* 5:241, 1985.

503. Chapman RW: Primary sclerosing cholangitis, *J Hepatol* 1:179, 1985.

504. Wiesner PH, Grambsch PM, Dickson ER et al: Primary sclerosing cholangitis: natural history, prognostic factors and survival analysis, *Hepatology* 10:430, 1989.

505. Porayko MK, LaRusso NF, Wiesner RH: Primary sclerosing cholangitis: a progressive disease, *Semin Liver Dis* 11:18, 1991.

506. Amédée-Manesme O, Bernard O, Brunelle F et al: Sclerosing cholangitis with neonatal onset, *J Pediatr* 111:225, 1987.

507. Hardarson S, LaBrecque DR, Mitros FA et al: Antineutrophil antibody in inflammatory bowel and hepatobiliary diseases, *Am J Clin Pathol* 99:277, 1993.

508. Seibold F, Slametschka D, Gregor M, Weber P: Neutrophil autoantibodies: a genetic marker in primary sclerosing cholangitis and ulcerative colitis, *Gastroenterology* 107:532, 1994.

509. Lefkowitch JH: Primary sclerosing cholangitis, *Arch Intern Med* 142:1157, 1982.

510. Ludwig J, LaRusso NF, Wiesner RH: Primary sclerosing cholangitis. In Peters RL, Craig JR, editors: *Liver pathology,* New York, 1986, Churchill Livingstone.

511. Ludwig J, MacCarty RL, Larusso NF et al: Intrahepatic cholangiectases and large-duct obliteration in primary sclerosing cholangitis, *Hepatology* 6:500, 1986.

512. Harrison RF, Hubscher SG: The spectrum of bile duct lesions in end-stage primary sclerosing cholangitis, *Histopathology* 19:321, 1991.

513. Cello JP: Acquired immunodeficiency syndrome cholangiopathy: spectrum of disease, *Am J Med* 86:539, 1989.

514. Dowsett JF: Sclerosing cholangitis in acquired immunodeficiency syndrome, *Scand J Gastroenterol* 23:1267, 1988.

515. Patel SA et al: Borges MC, Batt MD, Rosenblate HJ: *Trichosporon* cholangitis associated with hyperbilirubinemia and findings suggesting primary sclerosing cholangitis on endoscopic retrograde cholangiopancreatography, *Am J Gastroenterol* 85:84, 1990.

516. Bolton JE, Bowen JC: Biliary sclerosis associated with hepatic artery infusion of floxuridine, *Surgery* 99:119, 1986.

517. Doria MI, Shepard KV, Levin B et al: Liver pathology following hepatic arterial infusion chemotherapy: hepatic toxicity with FUDR, *Cancer* 58:855, 1986.

518. Hohn DC, Rayner AA, Economou JS et al: Toxicities and complications of implanted pump hepatic arterial and intravenous floxuridine infusion, *Cancer* 57:465, 1986.

519. Ludwig J, Kim CH, Wiesner RH, Krom RAF: Floxuridine-induced sclerosing cholangitis: an ischemic cholangiopathy, *Hepatology* 9:215, 1989.

520. Belghiti J, Benhamou J-P, Houry S et al: Caustic sclerosing cholangitis: a complication of the surgical treatment of hydatid disease of the liver, *Arch Surg* 121:1162, 1986.

521. Rudzki C, Ishak KG, Zimmerman HJ: Chronic intrahepatic cholestasis of sarcoidosis, *Am J Med* 59:573, 1975.

522. Valla D, Pessegueiro-Miranda H, Degott C et al: Hepatic sarcoidosis with portal hypertension: a report of seven cases with a review of the literature, *Q J Med* 242:531, 1987.

Differential diagnosis of PSC and PBC

523. Devaney K, Goodman ZD, Epstein MS et al: Hepatic sarcoidosis: clinicopathologic features in 100 patients, *Am J Surg Pathol* 17:1272, 1993.

524. Fagan EA, Moore-Gillon JC, Turner-Warwick M.: Multiorgan granulomas and mitochondrial antibodies, *N Engl J Med* 308:572, 1983.

525. Dincsoy HP, Saelinger DC: Haloperidol-induced chronic cholestatic liver disease, *Gastroenterology* 83:694, 1982.

526. Benson GD, Anderson PK, Combes B, Ishak KG. Prolonged jaundice following ketoconazole-induced hepatic injury, *Dig Dis Sci* 33:240, 1988.

527. Lieberman J, Keeffe EB, Stenzel P: Severe and prolonged oral contraceptive jaundice, *J Clin Gastroenterol* 6:145, 1984.

528. Cavanzo FJ, Garcia CP, Botero RC: Chronic cholestasis, paucity of bile ducts, red cell aplasia and the Stevens-Johnson syndrome: an ampicillin-associated case, *Gastroenterology* 99:854, 1990.

529. Olsson R, Wiholm B-E, Sand C et al: Liver damage from flucloxacillin, cloxacillin and dicloxacillin, *J Hepatol* 15:154, 1992.

530. Díaz de Rojas FD, García MC, Borda IA et al: Hepatic injury in the toxic oil syndrome, *Hepatology* 5:166, 1985.
531. Degott C, Feldmann G, Larrey D et al: Drug-induced prolonged cholestasis in adults: a histological semiquantitative study demonstrating progressive ductopenia, *Hepatology* 15:244, 1992.
532. Larrey D, Pessayre D, Duhamel G et al: Prolonged cholestasis after ajmaline-induced hepatitis, *J Hepatol* 2:81, 1986.
533. Ishak KG, Irey NS: Hepatic injury associated with the phenothiazines: a clinicopathologic and follow-up study of 36 cases, *Arch Pathol* 93:283, 1972.
534. Nakanuma Y, Ohta G, Yamazaki Y, Doishita K: Intrahepatic bile duct destruction in a patient with sarcoidosis and chronic intrahepatic cholestasis, *Acta Pathol Jpn* 29:211, 1979.
535. Cavalli G, Casali AM, Lambertini F, Busachi C: Changes in the small biliary passages in the hepatic localization of Hodgkin's disease, *Virchows Arch [A] (Pathol Anat)* 384:295, 1979.
536. Craig JR: Recurrent pyogenic cholangitis. In Peters RL, Craig JR, editors: *Liver pathology,* New York, 1986, Churchill-Livingstone.
537. Nakanuma Y, Yamaguchi K, Ohta G, Terada T: Pathologic features of hepatolithiasis in Japan, *Hum Pathol* 19:1181, 1988.
538. Marcial MA, Marcial-Rojas RA: Parasitic diseases of the liver. In Schiff L, Schiff ER, editors: *Diseases of the liver,* ed 6, Philadelphia, 1987, Lippincott.

Hepatocellular pigment storage

539. Zimniak P: Dubin-Johnson and Rotor syndromes: molecular basis and pathogenesis, *Semin Liver Dis* 13:248, 1993.
540. Berk PD, Noyer C: The familial conjugated hyperbilirubinemias, *Semin Liver Dis* 14:386, 1994.

Dubin-Johnson syndrome

541. Swartz HM, Sarna T, Varma RR: On the nature and excretion of the hepatic pigment in the Dubin-Johnson syndrome, *Gastroenterology* 76:958, 1979.
542. Pinos T, Constansa JM, Palacin A, Figueras C: A new diagnostic approach to the Dubin-Johnson syndrome, *Am J Gastroenterol* 85:91, 1990.

Rotor's syndrome

543. Wolpert E, Pascasio FM, Wolkoff AW et al: Abnormal sulfobromophthalein metabolism in Rotor's syndrome and obligate heterozygotes, *N Engl J Med* 296:1099, 1977.
544. Wolkoff AW, Wolpert E, Pascasio FN et al: Rotor's syndrome: a distinct inheritable pathophysiologic entity, *Am J Med* 60:173, 1976.

Gilbert's syndrome

545. Powell LW, Hemingway E, Billing B et al: Idiopathic unconjugated hyperbilirubinemia (Gilbert's syndrome), *N Engl J Med* 277:1108, 1967.
546. Reichen J: Familial unconjugated hyperbirubinemia syndromes, *Semin Liver Dis* 3:24, 1983.
547. Berk PD: Bilirubin metabolism and the hereditary hyperbilirubinemias. In Berk JE, editor: *Bockus gastroenterology,* vol 5, Philadelphia, 1985, Saunders.
548. Berk PD, Noyer C. The familial unconjugated hyperbilirubinemias, *Semin Liver Dis* 14:356, 1994.
549. Barth RF, Grimley PM, Berk PD et al: Excess lipofuscin accumulation in constitutional hepatic dysfunction (Gilbert's syndrome): light and electron microscopic observations, *Arch Pathol* 91:41, 1971.
550. Berk PD, Baschke TF: Detection of Gilbert's syndrome in patients with hemolysis: a method using radioactive chromium, *Ann Intern Med* 77:527, 1972.

Crigler-Najjar syndrome

551. Crigler JF, Najjar VA: Congenital familial nonhemolytic jaundice with kernicterus, *Pediatrics* 10:169, 1952.
552. Arias IM, Gartner LM, Cohen M et al: Chronic nonhemolytic unconjugated hyperbilirubinemia with glucuronyl transferase deficiency: clinical, biochemical, pharmacologic, and genetic evidence for heterogeneity, *Am J Med* 47:395, 1969.
553. Kaufman SS, Wood RP, Shaw BW et al: Orthotopic liver transplantation for type I Crigler-Najjar syndrome, *Hepatology* 6:1259, 1986.

Genetic hemochromatosis

554. Piperno A, Fargion S, D'Alba R et al: Liver damage in Italian patients with hereditary hemochromatosis is highly influenced by hepatitis B and C virus infection, *J Hepatol* 16:364, 1992.
555. Deugnier YM, Charalambous P, Le Quilleuc D et al: Preneoplastic significance of hepatic iron-free foci in genetic hemochromatosis: a study of 185 patients, *Hepatology* 18: 1363, 1993.
556. Niederau C, Fischer R, Sonnenberg A et al: Survival and causes of death in cirrhotic and in noncirrhotic patients with primary hemochromatosis, *N Engl J Med* 313:1256, 1985.
557. Bassett ML, Holliday JW, Powell LW: Genetic hemochromatosis, *Semin Liver Dis* 4:217, 1984.
558. Powell LW, Holliday JW: Hemochromatosis. In Berk JE, editor: *Bockus gastroenterology,* vol 5, *Liver,* Philadelphia, 1985, Saunders.
559. Searle JW, Kerr JFR, Holliday JW et al: Iron storage disease. In MacSween RNM, Anthony PP, Scheuer PJ, editors: *Pathology of the liver,* ed 2, Edinburgh, 1987, Churchill Livingstone.
560. Chapman RW, Laulicht M, Hoffbrand AV et al: Hepatic iron stores and markers of iron overload in alcoholics and patients with idiopathic hemochromatosis, *Dig Dis Sci* 27:909, 1982.
561. Powell LW, Halliday JW: The detection of early hemochromatosis, *Am J Dig Dis* 23:377, 1978.
562. Brissot P, Bourel M, Herry D et al: Assessment of liver iron content in 271 patients: a reevaluation of direct and indirect methods, *Gastroenterology* 80:557, 1981.

Perinatal hemochromatosis

563. Summers KM, Halliday JW, Powell LW: Identification of homozygous hemochromatosis by measurement of hepatic iron index, *Hepatology* 12:20, 1990.
564. Goldfisher S, Gritsky NW, Change CH et al: Idiopathic neonatal iron storage involving the liver, pancreas, heart, and endocrine and exocrine glands, *Hepatology* 1:58, 1981.
565. Knisely AS, Magid MS, Dische R et al: Neonatal hemochromatosis. In *Birth defects: original article series,* vol 23, New York, 1987, March of Dimes Birth Defects Foundation.
566. Adams PC, Searle J: Neonatal hemochromatosis: a case and review of the literature, *Am J Gastroenterol* 83:422, 1988.
567. Colletti, RB, Clemmons JJW: Familial neonatal hemochromatosis with survival, *J Pediatr Gastroenterol Nutr* 7:39, 1988.
568. Silver MM, Valberg LS, Cutz E et al: Hepatic morphology and iron quantitation in perinatal hemochromatosis: comparison with a large perinatal control population, including cases with chronic liver disease, *Am J Pathol* 143:1312, 1993.

Hematologic disorders

569. Turnberg LA: Excessive oral iron therapy causing hemochromatosis, *Br Med J* 1:1360, 1965.
570. Schafer AI, Cheron RG, Dluhy R et al: Clinical consequences of acquired transfusional iron overload in adults, *N Engl J Med* 304:319, 1981.

Dietary iron overload

571. Gordeuk VR, Boyd RD, Brittenham GM: Dietary iron overload persists in rural sub-Saharan Africa, *Lancet* 1:1310, 1986.

Wilson's disease

572. Diess A, Lynch RE, Lee GR et al: Long-term therapy of Wilson's disease, *Ann Intern Med* 75:57, 1971.
573. Sternlieb I: Evolution of the hepatic lesion in Wilson's disease (hepatolenticular degeneration), *Prog Liver Dis* 4:11, 1972.
574. Sternlieb I: The development of cirrhosis in Wilson's disease, *Clin Gastroenterol* 4:367, 1975.
575. Scheinberg IH, Sternlieb I: *Wilson's disease*, Philadelphia, 1984, Saunders.
576. Stromeyer FW, Ishak KG: The histopathology of the liver in Wilson's disease: a study of 34 cases, *Am J Clin Pathol* 73:12, 1980.
577. Cheng WSC, Govindarajan S, Redeker AG: Hepatocellular carcinoma in a case of Wilson's disease, *Liver* 12:42, 1992.

Indian childhood cirrhosis

578. Bhagwat AG, Walia BN, Koshy A, Banerji CK: Will the real Indian childhood cirrhosis please stand up? *Cleve Clin Q* 50:323, 1983.
579. Nayak NC: Indian childhood cirrhosis. In MacSween RNM, Anthony PP, Scheuer PJ, editors: *Pathology of the liver*, Edinburgh, 1987, Churchill Livingstone.
580. Smetana HF, Hadley GG, Sirsat SM: Infantile cirrhosis: an analytic review of the literature and a report of 50 cases, *Pediatrics* 28:107, 1961.
581. Joshi VV: Indian childhood cirrhosis, *Perspect Pediatr Pathol* 11:175, 1987.

582. Tanner MS, Portmann B, Mowatt AP et al: Increased hepatic copper concentration in Indian childhood cirrhosis, *Lancet* 1:1203, 1979.

583. Popper H, Goldfischer S, Sternlieb I et al: Cytoplasmic copper and its toxic effects: studies in Indian childhood cirrhosis, *Lancet* 1:1205, 1979.

584. Tanner MS, Kantarjian AH, Bhave SA, Pandit AN: Early introduction of copper-contaminated animal milk feed as a possible cause of Indian childhood cirrhosis, *Lancet* 2:992, 1983.

585. Müller-Höcker J, Meyer U, Wiebecke B et al: Copper storage disease of the liver and chronic dietary copper intoxication in two further German infants mimicking Indian childhood cirrhosis, *Pathol Res Pract* 183:39, 1985.

α_1-antitrypsin deficiency

586. Sharp HL: The current status of α_1-antitrypsin, a protease inhibitor, in gastrointestinal disease, *Gastroenterology* 70:611, 1976.

587. Morse JO: α_1-antitrypsin deficiency, *N Engl J Med* 299:1045 and 1099, 1978.

588. Sveger T: α_1-antitrypsin defficiency in early childhood, *Pediatrics* 62:22, 1978.

589. Sharp HL: α_1-antitrypsin: an ignored protein in understanding liver disease, *Semin Liver Dis* 2:314, 1982.

590. Alagille D: α_1-antitrypsin deficiency, *Hepatology* 4:11S, 1984.

591. Perlmutter DH: Liver disease associated with α_1-antitrypsin deficiency, *Prog Liver Dis* 11:139, 1993.

592. Pfeifer U, Ormanns W, Klinge O: Hepatocellular fibrinogen storage in familial hypofibrinogenemia, *Virchows Arch* 36:247, 1981.

593. Callea F, De Vos R, Togni R et al: Fibrinogen inclusions in liver cells: a new type of ground-glass hepatocyte: immune, light and electron microscopic characterization, *Histopathology* 10:65, 1986.

594. Klatt EC, Koss MN, Young TS et al: Hepatic hyaline globules associated with passive congestion, *Arch Pathol Lab Med* 112:510, 1988.

595. Eriksson S, Carlson J, Velez R: Risk of cirrhosis and primary liver cancer in α_1-antitrypsin deficiency, *N Engl J Med* 314:736, 1986.

596. Eriksson S: α_1-antitrypsin deficiency and liver cirrhosis in adults: an analysis of 35 Swedish autopsied cases, *Acta Med Scand* 221:461, 1987.

597. Rakela J, Goldschmiedt M, Ludwig J: Late manifestation of chronic liver disease in adults with α_1-antitrypsin, *Dig Dis Sci* 32:1358, 1987.

Glycogen storage diseases (glycogenoses)

598. McAdams AJ, Hug G, Bove KE: Glycogen storage disease, types I to X: criteria for morphologic diagnosis, *Hum Pathol* 5:463, 1974.

599. Reed G-B Jr, Dixon JF, Neustein JB et al: Type IV glycogenosis, *Lab Invest* 19:546, 1968.

600. Fink AS, Appelman HD, Thompson NW: Hemorrhage into a hepatic adenoma and type Ia glycogen storage disease: a case report and review of the literature, *Surgery* 97:117, 1985.

601. Coire CI, Qizilbash AH, Castelli MF: Hepatic adenomata in type Ia glycogen storage disease, *Arch Pathol Lab Med* 111:166, 1987.

Hereditary tyrosinemia

602. Dehner LP, Snover DC, Sharp HL et al: Hereditary tyrosinemia type I (chronic form): pathologic findings in the liver, *Hum Pathol* 20:149, 1989.

603. Mieles LA, Esquival CO, van Thiel DH et al: Liver transplantation for tyrosinemia: a review of 10 cases from the University of Pittsburgh, *Dig Dis Sci* 35:153, 1990.

604. Weinberg AG, Mize CE, Worthen HE: The occurrence of hepatoma in the chronic form of hereditary tyrosinemia, *J Pediatr* 88:434, 1976.

605. Ishak KG: Pathology of inherited metabolic disorders. In Balistreri WF, Stocker JT, editors: *Pediatric hepatology,* Washington, D.C., 1990, Hemisphere Publishing Corp.

606. Ishak KG, Sharp HL: Metabolic errors and liver disease. In MacSween RNM, Anthony PP, Scheuer PJ et al, editors: *Pathology of the liver,* Edinburgh, 1994, Churchill Livingstone.

Reticuloendothelial reactions

Nongranulomatous disorders

607. Hawkins CC, Gold JWM, Whimbey E et al: *Mycobacterium avium* complex infections in patients with the acquired immunodeficiency syndrome, *Ann Intern Med* 105:804, 1986.

608. Farhi DC, Mason UG III, Horsburgh CR: Pathologic findings in disseminated *Mycobacterium avium-intracellulare* infection: a report of two cases, *Am J Clin Pathol* 85:67, 1986.

609. Vischer TL, Bernheim C, Engelbrecht E: Two cases of hepatitis due to *Toxoplasma gondii, Lancet* 2:919, 1967.

610. Gupta S, Chakravarty NK, Ray HN et al: The liver in kala-azar, *Ann Trop Med Parasitol* 50:252, 1956.

611. Danneshbod K: Visceral leishmaniasis (kala-azar) in Iran: a pathologic and electron microscopic study, *Am J Clin Pathol* 57:156, 1972.

612. Lawrence C, Olson JA: Birefringent hemozoin identifies malaria, *Am J Clin Pathol* 80:300, 1986.

613. Ishak KG: Granulomas of the liver. In Ioachim HL, editor: *Pathology of granulomas,* New York, 1983, Raven Press.

614. Ishak KG, Zimmerman HJ: Drug-induced and toxic granulomatous hepatitis, *Clin Gastroenterol* 2:463, 1988.

615. Jacobson S, Ericsson JL, Obel AL: Histopathological and ultrastructural changes in the human liver during intravenous nutrition for seven months, *Acta Clin Scand* 138:335, 1971.

616. Passwell JH, David R, Katznelson D et al: Pigment disposition in the reticuloendothelial system after fat emulsion infusion, *Arch Dis Child* 51:366, 1976.

617. Reske-Nielsen E, Bojsen-Moller M, Vetner M et al: Polyvinylpyrrolidone-storage disease, *Acta Pathol Microbiol Scand[A]* 84:397, 1976.

618. Hameed K, Ashfaq S, Waugh DOW et al: Ball fracture and extrusion in Starr-Edwards aortic valve prosthesis with dissemination of ball material, *Arch Pathol* 86:520, 1968.

619. Ridolfi RL, Hutchins GM: Detection of ball variance in prosthetic heart valves by liver biopsy, *Johns Hopkins Med J* 134:131, 1974.

620. Le Fevre MF, Green FHY, Joel DD et al: Frequency of black pigment in livers and spleens of coal workers, *Hum Pathol* 13:1121, 1982.

Granulomatous disorders

621. Adams DO: The granulomatous inflammatory response: a review, *Am J Pathol* 84:164, 1976.

622. Benjamin SB, Ishak KG, Zimmerman HJ et al: Phenylbutazone liver injury: a clinical-pathologic survey of 23 cases and review of the literature, *Hepatology* 1:255, 1981.

623. Karat ABA, Job CK, Pao PSS: Liver in leprosy: histological and biochemical findings, *Br M J* 1:307, 1971.

624. Chen TSN, Drutz DJ, Whelan GE: Hepatic granulomas in leprosy: their relation to bacteremia, *Arch Pathol Lab Med* 100:182, 1976.

625. Bodurtha A, Kim YH, Laucius JF et al: Hepatic granulomas and other hepatic lesions associated with BCG immunotherapy for cancer, *Am J Clin Pathol* 61:747, 1974.

626. Grant RM, Mackie R, Cochran AJ et al: Results of administering BCG to patients with melanoma, *Lancet* 2:1096, 1974.

627. Andrade ZA, Cheever AW: Alterations of the intrahepatic vasculature in hepatosplenic schistosomiasis mansoni, *Am J Trop Hyg* 20:425, 1971.

628. Tsui WMS, Choro LTC: Advanced schistosomiasis as a cause of hepar lobatum, *Histopathology* 23:495, 1993.

628a. Symmers D, Spain D: Hepar lobatum, *Arch Pathol* 42:64, 1946.

629. Chin NW, Chapman I, Jiménez FA: Complete chemotherapeutic regression of hepatic metastases with resultant hepar lobatum, *Am J Gastroenterol* 82:149, 1986.

630. Bassily S, Dunn MA, Farid S et al: Chronic hepatitis B in patients with schistosomiasis mansoni, *J Trop Med Hyg* 86:67, 1983.

631. Koshy A, Al-Nakib B, Al-Mufti S et al: Anti-HCV-positive cirrhosis associated with schistosomiasis, *Am J Gastroenterol* 88:1428, 1993.

632. Nompleggi DJ, Farraye FA, Singer A et al: Hepatic schistosomiasis: report of two cases and literature review, *Am J Gastroenterol* 86:1658, 1991.

633. Pimentel JC, Menezes AP: Liver disease in vineyard sprayers, *Gastroenterology* 72:275, 1977.

634. Christoffersen P, Braendstrup O, Juhl E et al: Lipogranulomas in human liver biopsies with fatty change: a morphological, biochemical and clinical investigation, *Acta Pathol Microbiol Scand[A]* 79:150, 1971.

635. Boitnott JK, Margolis S: Saturated hydrocarbons in human tissues. III. Oil droplets in the liver and spleen, *Johns Hopkins Med J* 127:65, 1970.

636. Dincsoy HP, Weesner RE, MacGee J: Lipogranulomas in non-fatty human livers: a mineral oil induced environmental disease, *Am J Clin Pathol* 78:35, 1982.
637. Cruickshank B, Thomas MJ: Mineral oil (follicular) lipidosis. II. Histologic studies of spleen, liver, lymph nodes and bone marrow, *Hum Pathol* 15:731, 1984.
638. Wanless IR, Geddie IR: Mineral oil lipogranulomata in liver and spleen, *Arch Pathol Lab Med* 109:283, 1985.

Vascular disorders

Portal vein disorders

639. Mitchell CA, Rowell JA, Hau L et al: A fatal thrombotic disorder associated with an acquired inhibitor of protein C, *N Engl J Med* 317:1638, 1987.
640. Harper PL, Edgar PF, Luddington RJ et al: Protein C deficiency and portal thrombosis in liver transplantation in children, *Lancet* 2:924, 1988.
641. Matsuda M, Sugo T, Sakata T et al: A thrombotic state due to an abnormal protein C, *N Engl J Med* 319:1265, 1988.
642. Ishak KG: Morphologic hepatic lesions associated with oral contraceptive (O.C.) and anabolic steroids (A.S.). In Oliver G, editor: *Advances in pharmacology and therapeutics,* vol 8, Oxford, 1979, Pergamon Press.
643. Ishak KG: Hepatic lesions caused by anabolic and contraceptive steroids, *Semin Liver Dis* 1:116, 1981.
644. Matsumoto T, Kuwabara N, Abe H et al: Zahn infarct of the liver resulting from occlusive phlebitis in portal vein radicles, *Am J Gastroenterol* 87:365, 1992.
645. Saegusa M, Takano Y, Okudaira M: Hepatic infarction: histopathological and postmortem angiological studies, *Liver* 11:239, 1993.
646. Scott JM: Iatrogenic lesions in babies following umbilical vein catheterization, *Arch Dis Child* 40:426, 1965.
647. Wigger HJ, Bransilver BR, Blanc WA: Thromboses due to catheterization in infants and children, *J Pediatr* 76:1, 1970.
648. Larroche JL: Umbilical catheterization: its complications, *Biol Neonate* 16:101, 1970.
649. Aikat BK, Bhusnurmaath SR, Chhuttani PN et al: The pathology of noncirrhotic portal fibrosis: a review of 32 autopsy cases, *Hum Pathol* 10:405, 1979.
650. Nayak NC: Pathology of noncirrhotic portal fibrosis in India. In Okuda K, Omata M, editors: *Idiopathic portal hypertension,* Tokyo, 1983, University of Tokyo Press.
651. Kage M, Arakawa K, Fukuda T et al: Histopathological study of surgical liver biopsies in IPH. In Okuda K, Omata M, editors: *Idiopathic portal hypertension,* Tokyo, 1983, University of Tokyo Press.
652. Aida Y, Okudaira M, Ohbu M et al: Pathological features of the liver in idiopathic portal hypertension in Japan: a study on typical autopsy cases. In Okuda K, Omata M, editors: *Idiopathic portal hypertension,* Tokyo, 1983, Tokyo University Press.
653. Morris JS, Schmid M, Newman S et al: Chronic arsenical poisoning and noncirrhotic portal hypertension, *Gastroenterology* 64:86, 1974.
654. Huet PM, Guillaume E, Cote et al: Noncirrhotic perisinusoidal portal hypertension associated with chronic arsenical intoxication, *Gastroenterology* 68:1270, 1975.
655. Datta DV, Mita SK, Chuttani PN et al: Chronic arsenic intoxication as a possible aetiological factor in idiopathic portal hypertension (noncirrhotic portal fibrosis) in India, *Gut* 20:378, 1979.

Hepatic artery disorders

656. Craig JM, Gitlin D: The nature of the hyaline thrombi in thrombotic thrombocytopenic purpura, *Am J Pathol* 33:251, 1957.
657. Chen V, Hamilton J, Qizilbash A: Hepatic infarction, *Arch Pathol Lab Med* 100:32, 1976.
658. Dammann HG, Hagemann J, Runge M et al: *In vivo* diagnosis of massive hepatic infarction by computed tomography, *Dig Dis Sci* 27:73, 1982.
659. Adler DD, Glazer GM, Silver TM: Computed tomography of liver infarction, *Am J Roentgenol* 142:315, 1984.
660. Seeley TT, Blumenfeld TM, Ikeda R et al: Hepatic infarction, *Hum Pathol* 3:265, 1972.
661. Stauffer MH, Gross JB, Fould WT et al: Amyloidosis: diagnosis with needle biopsy of the liver in eighteen patients, *Gastroenterology* 41:92, 1961.

Sinusoidal disorders

662. Dunn GD, Hayes P, Breen KJ et al: The liver in congestive heart failure: a review, *Am J Med Sci* 265:174, 1973.
663. Bras G, Brandt KH: Vascular disorders. In MacSween RNM, Anthony PP, Scheuer PJ, editors: *Pathology of the liver,* Edinburgh, 1987, Churchill Livingstone.
664. Winkler K, Poulsen H: Liver diseases with periportal sinusoidal dilatation: a possible complication to contraceptive steroids, *Scand J Gastroenterol* 10:699, 1975.
665. Spellberg MA, Mirro J, Chowdhurry L: Sinusoidal dilatation related to oral contraceptives, *Am J Gastroenterol* 72:248, 1979.
666. Balázs M: Sinusoidal dilatation of the liver in patients on oral contraceptives: electron microscopical study of 14 cases, *Exp Pathol* 35:231, 1988.
667. Boyer JL: Androgenic-anabolic steroid associated peliosis hepatitis in man: a review of 38 reported cases. In Oliver G, editor: *Advances in pharmacology and therapeutics,* vol 8, 1979, Pergamon Press.
668. Ishak KG, Zimmerman HJ: Hepatotoxic effects of the anabolic/androgenic steroids, *Semin Liver Dis* 7:230, 1987.
669. Loomus GN, Anija P, Botta RA: A case of peliosis hepatis in association with tamoxifen therapy, *Am J Clin Pathol* 80:881, 1983.
670. Nesher G, Dollberg L, Zimran A et al: Hepatosplenic peliosis after danazol and glucocorticoids for ITP, *Lancet* 1:242, 1986.
671. Zafrani ES, Bernuau D, Feldmann G: Peliosis-like ultrastructural changes of the hepatic sinusoids in human chronic hypervitaminosis A: report of three cases, *Hum Pathol* 15:1166, 1984.
672. Dejgaard A, Krogsgaard K, Jacobsen M: Veno-occlusive disease and peliosis of the liver after Thorotrast administration, *Virchows Arch [A] (Pathol Anat)* 403:87, 1984.
673. Czapar CA: Peliosis hepatis in the acquired immunodeficiency syndrome, *Arch Pathol Lab Med* 110:611, 1986.
674. Scoazec J-Y, Marche C, Girard P-M et al: Peliosis hepatis and sinusoidal dilatation during infection by the human immunodeficiency virus (HIV), *Am J Pathol* 131:38, 1988.
675. Perkocha LA, Geaghan SM, Yen TSB et al: Clinical and pathological features of bacillary peliosis hepatis in association with human immunodeficiency virus infection, *N Engl J Med* 323:1581, 1990.
676. Leong SS, Cazen RA, Yu GSM et al: Abdominal visceral peliosis associated with bacillary angiomatosis, *Arch Pathol Lab Med* 116:866, 1992.
677. Granter SR, Barnhill RL: Bacillary angiomatosis, *Adv Pathol Lab Med* 6:491, 1993.
678. Tsukamoto Y, Nakata H, Kimoto T et al: CT and angiography in peliosis hepatitis, *Am J Roentgenol* 142:539, 1984.
679. Bauer TW, Moore GW, Hutchins GM: The liver in sickle cell disease: a clinicopathologic study of 70 patients, *Am J Med* 69:833, 1980.
680. Bruguera M, Aranguibel F, Ros E et al: Incidence and clinical significance of sinusoidal dilatation in liver biopsies, *Gastroenterology* 75:474, 1978.
681. Laffón A, Moreno A, Gutierrez-Bucero A et al: Hepatic sinusoidal dilatation in rheumatoid arthritis, *J Clin Gastroenterol* 11:653, 1989.
682. Bruguera M, Caballero T, Carreras E et al: Hepatic sinusoidal dilatation in Hodgkin's disease, *Liver* 7:76, 1987.
683. Gerber MA, Thung SN, Bodenheimer HC Jr et al: Characteristic histologic triad in liver adjacent to metastatic neoplasm, *Liver* 6:85, 1986.
684. Rolfes DB, Ishak KG: Liver disease in toxemia of pregnancy, *Am J Gastroenterol* 81:1138, 1986.
685. Isaki Y, Hirokawa K, Fukozawa T et al: Immunohistochemical study on the liver in autopsy cases with disseminated intravascular coagulation (DIC) with reference to clinicopathologic analysis, *Virchows Arch [A] (Pathol Anat)* 404:229, 1984.
686. Nanba K, Soban EJ, Bowling MC et al: Splenic pseudosinuses and hepatic angiomatous lesions: distinctive features of hairy cell leukemia, *Am J Clin Pathol* 67:415, 1977.
687. Roquet M-L, Zafrani E-L, Farcet J-P et al: Histopathological lesions of the liver in hairy cell leukemia: a report of 14 cases, *Hepatology* 5:496, 1985.
688. Anthony PP, Sarsfield P, Clarke T: Primary lymphoma of the liver: clinical and pathological features of 10 patients, *J Clin Pathol* 43:1007, 1990.
689. Zafrani ES, Gaulard P: Primary lymphoma of the liver, *Liver* 13:57, 1993.
690. Yam LT, Chan C, Li CY: Hepatic involvement in systemic mast cell disease, *Am J Med* 80:819, 1986.

691. Travis WD, Li C-Y, Bergstrath EJ et al: Systemic mast cell disease: analysis of 58 cases and literature review, *Medicine* 67:345.

692. Horny H-P, Kaiserling E, Campbell M et al: Liver findings in generalized mastocytosis: a clinicopathologic study, *Cancer* 63:532, 1989.

693. Roux D, Merlio JP, Quinton A et al: Agnogenic myeloid metaplasia, portal hypertension and sinusoidal abnormalities, *Gastroenterology* 92:1067, 1987.

694. Masur H, Jones TC: Protozoal and helminthic infections. In Greico MH, editor: *Infections in the abnormal host,* New York, 1980, Yorke Medical Books.

695. Hennequin C, Pialoux G, Taillet-Bellemere C et al: Hyperinfestation anguillules chez un patient sous corticothérapie: révélation hépatobiliaire. *Gastroenterol Clin Biol* 15:87, 1991.

696. Haque AK, Schnadig V, Rubin SA, Smith JH: Pathogenesis of human strongyloidiasis: autopsy and quantitative parasitological analysis, *Mod Pathol* 7:276, 1994.

697. Palterra AA, Katsimbura: Granulomatous hepatitis due to *Strongyloides stercoralis*, *J Pathol* 113: 241, 1974.

Hepatic veins

THROMBOSIS (BUDD-CHIARI SYNDROME)

698. Maddrey WC: Hepatic vein thrombosis (Budd-Chiari syndrome), *Hepatology* 4:445, 1984.

699. Gupta S, Blumgart LH, Hodgson HJF: Budd-Chiari syndrome: long term survival and factors affecting mortality, *J Med* 60: 781, 1986.

700. Dilawari JB, Bamberg P, Chawla Y et al: Hepatic outflow obstruction (Budd-Chiari syndrome): experience with 177 patients and a review of the literature, *Medicine* 73: 21, 1994.

701. Lewis JH, Tice HL, Zimmerman HJ: Budd-Chiari syndrome associated with oral contraceptive steroids: review and treatment of 47 cases, *Dig Dis Sci* 28:673, 1985.

702. Levy VG, Ruskone A, Baillou C et al: Polycythemia and the Budd-Chiari syndrome: study of the serum erythropoietin and bone marrow erythroid progenitors, *Hepatology* 5:858, 1985.

703. Maddrey WC: Hepatic vein thrombosis (Budd-Chiari syndrome): possible association with the use of oral contraceptives, *Semin Liver Dis* 7:32, 1987.

704. Rector WG, Yu Y, Goldstein L et al: Membranous obstruction of the inferior vena cava in the United States, *Medicine* 64:134, 1985.

705. Ishak KG: The Budd-Chiari syndrome. Pathologic aspects with clinical correlations. In Seeff LB, Lewis J, editors: *Current perspectives in hepatology: a Festschrift for Hyman J. Zimmerman,* New York, 1989, Plenum Press.

706. Chen JA, Kaplan MM: Left-sided heart failure presenting as hepatitis, *Gastroenterology* 74:583, 1978.

VENOOCCLUSIVE DISEASE

707. Zimmerman HJ, Ishak KG: Do estrogens cause venocclusive disease of the liver? *Gastroenterology* 93:384, 1987.

708. McDonald GB, Sharma P, Mathews DE et al: Venocclusive disease of the liver after bone marrow transplantation: diagnosis, incidence, and predisposing factors, *Hepatology* 4:116, 1984.

709. McDonald GB, Hinds MS, Fisher LD et al: Veno-occlusive disease of the liver and multiorgan failure after bone marrow transplantation: a cohort study of 355 patients, *Ann Intern Med* 118:255, 1993.

710. Dhillon AP, Burroughs AK, Hudson M et al: Hepatic venular stenosis after orthotopic liver transplantation, *Hepatology* 19:106, 1994.

Fibrosis and cirrhosis

711. Ishak KG: Nodular regenerative hyperplasia, blood disorders and other uncommon diseases associated with intrahepatic portal hypertension. In Okuda K, Benhamou J-P, editors: *Portal hypertension,* Tokyo, 1991, Springer-Verlag.

712. Anthony PP, Ishak KG, Nayak NC et al: The morphology of cirrhosis, *J Clin Pathol* 31:395, 1978.

713. Scheuer PJ: *Liver biopsy interpretation*, London, 1988, Bailliere-Tindall.

714. Anthony PP, Vogel CL, Barker LF: *Liver cell dysplasia*: a premalignant condition, *J Clin Pathol* 26:217, 1973.

715. Theise ND, Schwartz M, Miller C, Thung SN: Macroregenerative nodules and hepatocellular carcinoma in forty-four requential adult liver explants with cirrhosis, *Hepatology* 16:949, 1992.

716. Ferrell L. Wright T, Lake J et al: Incidence and diagnostic features of macroregenerative nodules vs. small hepatocellular carcinoma in cirrhotic liver, *Hepatology* 16:1372, 1992.

717. Terada T, Terasaki S, Nakanuma Y: A clinicopathologic study of adenomatous hyperplasia of the liver in 209 consecutive cirrhotic livers examined by autopsy, *Cancer* 72:1551, 1993.

718. Nakanuma Y, Terada T, Ueda K et al: Adenomatous hyperplasia of the liver as a precancerous lesion, *Liver* 13:1, 1993.

719. Ferrell LD, Crawford JM, Dhillon AP et al: Proposal for standardized criteria for the diagnosis of benign, borderline, and malignant lesions arising in chronic advanced liver disease, *Am J Surg Pathol* 17:1113, 1993.

720. Henrion J, Colin L, Schmitz A et al: Ischemic hepatitis in cirrhosis: rare but lethal, *J Clin Gastroenterol* 16:35, 1993.

721. Adams PC, Bradley C, Frei JV: Hepatic iron and zinc concentrations after portacaval shunting for nonalcoholic cirrhosis, *Hepatology* 19:101, 1994.

Space-occupying lesions

Cysts

722. Caroli J: Diseases of the intrahepatic biliary tree, *Clin Gastroenterol* 2:147, 1973.

723. Mercadier M, Chigot JP, Clot JP, Langlois P, Lansieux P: Caroli's disease, *World J Surg* 8:22, 1984.

724. Phinney PR, Austin GE, Kadell BM: Cholangiocarcinoma arising in Caroli's disease, *Arch Pathol Lab Med* 105:194, 1981.

725. Chen KTK: Adenocarcinoma of the liver: association with congenital hepatic fibrosis and Caroli's disease, *Arch Pathol Lab Med* 105:294, 1981.

726. Fozard JBJ, Wyatt JI, Hall RI: Epithelial dysplasia in Caroli's disease, *Gut* 30:1150, 1989.

727. Joly I, Choux R, Baroni JL et al: Carcinome in situ sur maladie de Caroli localisée, *Gastroenterol Clin Biol* 14:90, 1990.

728. Desmet VJ: Congenital diseases of intrahepatic bile ducts: variations on the theme "ductal plate malformation," *Hepatology* 16:1069, 1992.

729. McDonald RA, Avner EA: Inherited polycystic kidney disease in childhood, *Semin Nephrol* 11:632, 1991

730. Blyth H, Ockenden BG: Polycystic disease of kidneys and liver presenting in childhood, *J Med Genet* 81:257, 1971.

731. Bradford WD, Bradford JW, Porter FS, Sidbury JB Jr: Cystic disease of liver and kidney with portal hypertension: a cause of sudden unexpected hematemesis, *Clin Pediatr* 7:249, 1968.

732. Lieberman E, Salinas-Madrigal L, Gwinn JL et al: Infantile polycystic disease of the kidneys and liver, *Medicine* 50:227, 1971.

733. Landing BH, Walls TR, Claireaux AE: Morphometric analysis of liver lesions in cystic diseases of childhood, *Hum Pathol* 11:549, 1980.

734. Witzleben CL: Cystic diseases of the liver. In Zakim D, Boyer TD, editors: *Hepatology: a textbook of liver disease,* ed 2, Philadelphia, 1990, Saunders.

735. Gang DL, Herrin JT: Infantile polycystic disease of the liver and kidneys, *Clin Nephrol* 25:28, 1986.

736. Jørgensen MJ: The ductal plate malformation, *APMIS* 257(suppl):1, 1977.

737. Sommerschild HC, Langmark F, Maurseth K: Congenital hepatic fibrosis: report of two new cases and review of the literature, *Surgery* 73:53, 1973.

738. Averback P: Congenital hepatic fibrosis: asymptomatic adults without renal anomaly, *Arch Pathol Lab Med* 101:260, 1977.

739. Fauvert R, Benhamou JP: Congenital hepatic fibrosis. In Schaffner F, Sherlock SJ, Leevy CM, editors: *The liver and its diseases,* New York, 1974, Intercontinental Medical Book.

740. Boichis H, Passwell J, David R, Miller H: Congenital hepatic fibrosis and nephronophthisis, *J Med* 42:221, 1973.

741. Kerr DNS, Harrison CV, Sherlock S, Walker RM: Congenital hepatic fibrosis, *Q J Med* 30:91, 1960.

742. Scott J, Shousha S, Thomas HC, Sherlock S: Bile duct carcinoma: a late complication of congenital hepatic fibrosis, *Am J Gastroenterol* 73:113, 1980.

743. Bernstein J: Hepatic and renal involvement in malformation syndromes, *Mt Sinai J Med* 53:421, 1986.

744. Reeders ST, Breuning MH, Davies KE et al: A highly polymorphic DNA marker linked to adult polycystic kidney disease on chromosome 16, *Nature* 317:542, 1985.

745. Parfrey PS, Bear JC, Morgan J et al: The diagnosis and prognosis of autosomal dominant polycystic kidney disease, *N Engl J Med* 323:1085, 1990.
746. Kimberling WJ, Pieke-Dahl SA, Kumar S: The genetics of cystic diseases of the kidney, *Semin Nephrol* 11:596, 1991.
747. Gabow PA: Autosomal dominant polycystic kidney disease: more than a renal disease, *Am J Kidney Dis* 16:403, 1990.
748. Melnick PJ: Polycystic liver, *Arch Pathol* 59:162, 1955.
749. Dalgaard OZ: Bilateral polycystic disease of the kidneys: a follow-up of 284 patients and their families, *Acta Med Scand* 328 (suppl):13, 1957.
750. Fick GM, Johnson AM, Strain JD et al: Characteristics of very early onset autosomal dominant polycystic kidney disease, *J Am Soc Nephrol* 3:1863, 1993.
751. Telenti A, Torres VE, Gross JB Jr et al: Hepatic cyst infection in autosomal dominant polycystic kidney disease, *Mayo Clin Proc* 65:933, 1990.
752. Terada T, Nakanuma Y: Congenital biliary dilatation in autosomal dominant adult polycystic disease of the liver and kidneys, *Arch Pathol Lab Med* 112:1113, 1988.
753. Coffin B, Hadengue A, Degos F, Benhamou J-P: Calcified hepatic and renal cysts in adult dominant polycystic kidney disease, *Dig Dis Sci* 35:1172, 1990.
754. Ramos A, Torres VE, Holley KE et al: The liver in autosomal dominant polycystic kidney disease, *Arch Pathol Lab Med* 114:180, 1990.
755. Homer LW, White HJ, Reed RC: Neoplastic transformation of von Meyenburg complexes of the liver, *J Pathol Bacteriol* 96:499, 1968.
756. Bonfors M: The development of cholangiocarcinoma from multiple bile-duct adenomas, *Acta Pathol Microbiol Immunol Scand Sect A* 92:285, 1984.
757. Honda N, Cobb C, Lechago J: Bile duct carcinoma associated with multiple Von Meyenburg complexes in the liver, *Hum Pathol* 17:1287, 1986.
758. Bruns CD, Kuhms JG, Wieman J: Cholangiocarcinoma in association with multiple biliary microhamartomas, *Arch Pathol Lab Med* 114:1287, 1990.
759. Geist DC: Solitary nonparasitic cyst of the liver, *Arch Surg* 71:867, 1955.
760. Flagg RS, Robinson DW: Solitary nonparasitic hepatic cysts, *Arch Surg* 95:964, 1967.
761. Byrne WJ, Fonkalsrud EW: Congenital solitary nonparasitic cyst of the liver: a rare cause of a rapidly enlarging abdominal mass in infancy, *J Pediatr Surg* 17:316, 1982.
762. Ayyash K, Haddad J: Spontaneous rupture of a solitary nonparasitic cyst of the liver, *Acta Chir Scand* 154:241, 1988.
763. Shipley P, Bayles B, Hershfield N et al: Spontaneous rupture of a nonparasitic hepatic cyst associated with peritonitis, *Can J Gastroenterol* 5:171, 1991.
764. Clinkscales NB, Trigg LP, Poklepovic J: Obstructive jaundice secondary to benign hepatic cyst, *Radiology* 154:643, 1985.
765. Cappell MS: Obstructive jaundice from benign nonparasitic hepatic cysts: identification of risk factors and percutaneous aspiration for diagnosis and treatment, *Am J Gastroenterol* 83:93, 1988.
766. Enterline DS, Rauch RE, Silverman PM et al: Cyst of the falciform ligament of the liver, *Am J Roentgenol* 142:327, 1984.
767. Greenwood N, Orr W McN: Primary squamous-cell carcinoma arising in a solitary nonparasitic cyst of the liver, *J Pathol* 107:145, 1972.
768. Bloustein PA, Silverberg SG: Squamous cell carcinoma originating in a hepatic cyst: case report with a review of the hepatic cyst–carcinoma association, *Cancer* 38: 2002, 1976.
769. Pliskin A, Cualing H, Stenger RJ: Primary squamous cell carcinoma originating in congenital cysts of the liver, *Arch Pathol Lab Med* 116:105, 1992.
770. Bilge A, Sozuer EM: Diagnosis and surgical treatment of hepatic hydatid disease, *HPB Surg* 6:57, 1992.
771. McCorkell SJ: Echinococcal cysts in the common bile duct: an uncommon cause of obstruction, *Gastrointest Radiol* 10:390, 1985.
772. Stuive PC, Overbosch D, Jongsma CK et al: Jaundice caused by hydatid disease of the liver, *Neth J Med* 35:241, 1989.
773. Dadoukis J, Gamvros O, Aletras H: Intrabiliary rupture of the hydatid cyst of the liver, *World J Surg* 8:786, 1984
774. Van Steenbergen W, Fevery J, Broeckaert L et al: Hepatic echinococcosis ruptured into the biliary tract, *J Hepatol* 4:133, 1987.
775. Lewall DB, McCorkell SJ: Rupture of echinococcal cysts: diagnosis, classification and clinical implications, *AmJRoentgenol* 146:391, 1986.
776. Koçak ES, Bumim C, Erden E et al: Unusual complication of hydatid cysts: acute inferior vena caval thrombosis, *Dig Surg* 10:114, 1993.
777. Marcial MA, Marcial-Rojas RA: Parasitic diseases of the liver. In Schiff L, Schiff ER, editors: *Diseases of the liver,* ed 6, Philadelphia, 1987, Lippincott.
778. Miguel JP, Bresson-Hadni S, Vuitton D: Echinococcosis of the liver. In McIntyre N, Benhamou J-P Bircher J et al editors: *Oxford textbook of clinical hepatology,* Oxford, 1991, Oxford University Press.
779. Menegelli UG, Martinelli ALC, Llorach Velludo MAS et al: Polycystic hydatid disease *(Echinococcus vogeli):* clinical, laboratory and morphological findings in nine Brazilian patients, *J Hepatol* 14: 203, 1992.
780. Behrns KE, van Heerden JA: Surgical management of hepatic hydatid disease, *Mayo Clin Proc* 66:1193, 1991.
781. Bresson-Hadni S, Franza A, Miguet JP et al: Orthotopic liver transplantation for incurable alveolar echinococcosis of the liver: report of 17 cases, *Hepatology* 13:1061, 1991.
782. Okuda K, Sugita S, Tsukada E et al: Pancreatic pseudocyst in the left hepatic lobe: a report of two cases, *Hepatology* 13:359, 1991.
783. Kumada T, Nakano S, Kitamura K et al: Cystic degeneration of liver malignancies: study by US and CT, *Jpn J Gastroenterol* 30:837, 1983.
784. Thompson NW, Eckhauser FE, Vinik AI et al: Cystic neuroendocrine neoplasms of the pancreas and liver, *Ann Surg* 199:158, 1984.
785. Dent GA, Feldman JM: Pseudocystic liver metastases in patients with carcinoid tumors: report of three cases, *Am J Clin Pathol* 82:275, 1994.

Abscess

786. Greenstein AJ, Lowenthal D Hammer GS et al: Continuing changing patterns of disease in pyogenic liver abscess: a study of 36 patients, *Am J Gastroenterol* 79:217, 1994.
787. Ammann R, Münch R, Largiader F et al: Pancreatic and hepatic abscesses: a late complication in 10 patients with chronic pancreatitis, *Gastroenterology* 103:560, 1994.
788. Parikh SR, Molinelli B, Dailey T H: Liver abscess after hemorrhoidectomy: report of two cases, *Dis Colon Rectum* 37:185, 1994.
789. Vakil N, Hayne G, Sharma A et al: Liver abscess in Crohn's disease, *Am J Gastroenterol* 89:1090, 1994.
790. De Cock KM, Reynolds TB: Amebic and pyogenic liver abscess. In Schiff L, Schiff ER, editors: *Diseases of the liver,* ed 7, Philadelphia, 1993, Lippincott.
791. McDonald MI, Corey GR, Gallis HA, Durack ST: Single and multiple pyogenic liver abscesses: natural history, diagnosis and treatment, with emphasis on percutaneous drainage, *Medicine* 63:291, 1994.
792. McCorkell SJ, Niles NL: Pyogenic liver abscess: another look at medical management, *Lancet* 1:803, 1985.
793. Greaney GC, Reynolds TB, Donovan AJ: Ruptured amebic liver abscess, *Arch Surg* 120:555, 1985.
794. Katzenstein D, Rickerson V, Porande A: New concepts of amebic liver abscess derived from hepatic imaging, serodiagnosis, and hepatic enzymes in 67 consecutive cases in San Diego, *Medicine* 61:337, 1982.
795. Knight R: Hepatic amebiasis, *Semin Liver Dis* 4:277, 1984.
796. Greenstein AJ, Barth J, Sicker A et al: Amebic liver abscess: a study of 11 cases compared with a series of 38 patients with pyogenic liver abscess, *Am J Gastroenterol* 80:472, 1985.
797. Parelkar SN, Stamm WP, Hill KR: Indirect immunofluorescent staining of *E. histolytica* in tissues, *Lancet* 1:212, 1971.
798. Brandt H, Tamayo RP: Pathology of human amebiasis, *Hum Pathol* 1:351, 1970.

Mesenchymal hamartoma

799. Stocker JT, Ishak KG: Mesenchymal hamartoma of the liver: report of 30 cases and review of the literature, *Pediatr Pathol* 1:245, 1983.
800. Lack EE: Mesenchymal hamartoma of the liver: a clinical and pathologic study of nine cases, *Am J Pediatr Hematol Oncol* 8:91, 1986.
801. Mascavello JT, Krous HF: Second report of a translocation involving 19q13.4 in mesenchymal hamartoma of the liver, *Cancer Genet Cytogenet* 58:141, 1992.
802. Otal TM, Hendricks JB, Pharis P, Donnelly WH: Mesenchymal hamartoma of the liver: DNA flow cytometric analyisis of eight cases, *Cancer* 74:1237, 1994.
803. de Chadarevian J-P, Pawel BR, Faerber EN, Weintraub WH: Undifferentiated (embryonal) sarcoma arising in conjunction with mesenchymal hamartoma of the liver, *Mod Pathol* 7:490, 1994.

Focal nodular hyperplasia

804. Ishak KG, Rabin L: Benign tumors of the liver, *Med Clin North Am* 59:995, 1987.
805. Knowles DM, Wolff M: Focal nodular hyperplasia of the liver: a clinicopathologic study and review of the literature, *Hum Pathol* 7:533, 1976.
806. Stocker JT, Ishak KG: Focal nodular hyperplasia of the liver: a study of 21 pediatric cases, *Cancer* 48:336, 1981.
807. Ishak KG: Benign tumors and pseudotumors of the liver, *Appl Pathol* 6:82, 1988.
808. Mathieu D, Zafrani ES, Anglode M-C, Dhumeaux D: Association of focal nodular hyperplasia and hepatic hemangioma, *Gastroenterology* 97:154, 1989.
809. Wanless IR, Albrecht S, Bilbao J et al: Multiple focal nodular hyperplasia of the liver associated with vascular malformations of various organs and neoplasia of the brain: a new syndrome, *Mod Pathol* 2:456, 1989.
810. van Eyken P, Sciot R, Callea F, Desmet VJ: A cytokeratin-immunohistochemical study of focal nodular hyperplasia: further evidence that ductular metaplasia of hepatocytes contributes to ductular "proliferation," *Liver* 9:372, 1989.
811. Wanless IR, Mawdsley C, Adams R: On the pathogenesis of focal nodular hyperplasia of the liver, *Hepatology* 5:1194, 1985.
812. Stromeyer FW, Ishak KG: Nodular transformation (nodular regenerative hyperplasia) of the liver: a clinicopathologic study of 30 cases, *Hum Pathol* 12:60, 1981.
813. Wanless IR, Godwin TA, Allen F, Feder A: Nodular regenerative hyperplasia in hematologic disorders: a possible response to obliterative portal venopathy: a morphometric study of nine cases with an hypothesis on the pathogenesis, *Medicine* 59:387, 1980.
814. Wanless IR: Micronodular transformation (nodular regenerative hyperplasia) of the liver: a report of 64 cases among 2500 autopsies and a new classification of benign hepatocellular nodules, *Hepatology* 11:787, 1990.
815. Moran CA, Mullick FG, Ishak KG: Nodular regenerative hyperplasia of the liver in children, *Am J Surg Pathol* 15:449, 1991.
816. Washington K, Lane KL: Nodular regenerating hyperplasia in partial hepatectomy specimens, *Am J Surg Pathol* 17:1151, 1993.
817. Buffet C, Altman C: Hyperplasia nodulaire régénérative, *Gastroenterol Clin Biol* 18:123, 1994.

Inflammatory pseudotumor

818. Anthony PP: Inflammatory pseudotumour (plasma cell granuloma) of lung, liver and other organs, *Histopathology* 23:501, 1993.
819. Shek TWH, Ng IOH, Chan KW: Inflammatory pseudotumor of the liver: report of four cases and review of the literature, *Am J Surg Pathol* 17:231, 1993.

Bile duct adenoma

820. Govindarajan S, Peters RL: The bile duct adenoma, *Arch Pathol Lab Med* 108:922, 1994.
821. Allaire GS, Rabin L, Ishak KG, Sesterhenn IA: Bile duct adenoma: a study of 152 cases, *Am J Surg Pathol* 12:708, 1988.

Biliary papillomatosis

822. Mercadier M, Bodard M, Fingerhut A, Chigot JP: Papillomatosis of the intrahepatic bile ducts, *World J Surg* 8:30, 1984.
823. Padfield CJH, Ansell ID, Furness PN: Mucinous biliary papillomatosis: a tumour in need of wider recognition, *Histopathology* 13:687, 1988.
824. Bottger T, Sorger K, Jenny E, Junginger T: Progressive papillomatosis of the intrahepatic and extrahepatic bile ducts, *Acta Chir Scand* 155:125, 1989.

Bile duct cystadenoma

825. Ishak KG, Willis GW, Cummins SD et al: Biliary cystadenoma and cystadenocarcinoma: report of 14 cases and review of the literature, *Cancer* 39:322, 1977.
826. Wheeler DA, Edmondson HA: Cystadenoma with mesenchymal stroma (CMS) in the liver and bile ducts: a clinicopathologic study of 17 cases, 4 with malignant change, *Cancer* 56:1434, 1985.
827. Akwari OE, Tucker A, Siegler HF, Itani KMF: Hepatobiliary cystadenoma with mesenchymal stroma, *Ann Surg* 211:18, 1990.
828. Devaney K, Goodman ZD, Ishak KG: Hepatobiliary cystadenoma and cystadenocarcinoma: a light microscopic and immunohistochemical study of 70 patients, *Am J Surg Pathol* 18:1078, 1994.
829. Thomas JA, Scriven MW, Puntis MCA et al: Elevated serum CA 19-9 levels in hepatobiliary cystadenoma with mesenchymal stroma, *Cancer* 70:1841, 1992.

Hepatocellular adenoma

830. Edmondson HA, Henderson B, Benton B: Liver-cell adenomas associated with the use of oral contraceptives, *N Engl J Med* 294:470, 1976.
831. Rooks JB, Ory HW, Ishak KG et al: Epidemiology of hepatocellular adenoma: the role of contraceptive use, *JAMA* 242:644, 1979.
832. Touraine RL, Bertrand Y, Foray P et al: Hepatic tumours during androgen therapy in Fanconi anaemia, *Eur J Pediatr* 152:692, 1993.
833. Ferrell LD: Hepatocellular carcinoma arising in a focus of multilobular adenoma: a case report, *Am J Surg Pathol* 17:525, 1993.
834. Foster JH, Berman MM: The malignant transformation of liver cell adenomas, *Arch Surg* 129:712, 1994.
835. Fink AS, Appelman HD, Thompson NW: Hemorrhage into a hepatic adenoma and type Ia glycogen storage disease: a case report and review of the literature, *Surgery* 97:117, 1985.
836. Poe R, Snover DC: Adenomas in glycogen storage disease type I: two cases with unusual histologic features, *Am J Surg Pathol* 12:477, 1988.
837. Foster JH, Donohue TA, Berman MM: Familial liver-cell adenomas and diabetes mellitus, *N Engl J Med* 299:238, 1978.

Infantile hemangioendothelioma

838. Dehner LP, Ishak KG: Vascular tumors of the liver in infants and children: a study of 30 cases and review of the literature, *Arch Pathol* 92:101, 1971.
839. Selby DM, Stocker JT, Maclawin MA et al: Infantile hemangioendothelioma of the liver, *Hepatology* 20:39, 1994.
840. Selby DM, Stocker JT, Ishak, KG: Angiosarcoma of the liver in childhood: a clinicopathologic and follow-up study of 10 cases, *Pediatr Pathol* 12:485, 1992.

Angiomyolipoma

841. Goodman ZD, Ishak KG: Angiomyolipomas of the liver, *Am J Surg Pathol* 8:745, 1984.
842. Weeks DA, Arneson M, Zuppan C et al: Hepatic angiomyolipoma with striated granules and positivity with melanoma-specific antibody (HMB-45): a report of two cases, *Ultrastruct Pathol* 15:563, 1991.
843. Tsui WMS, Yuen AKT, Ma KF, Tse CCH: Hepatic angiomyolipomas with a deceptive trabecular pattern and HMB-45 positivity, *Histopathology* 21:569, 1992.
844. Ishak KG, Anthony PP, Sobin LH: *Histological typing of tumours of the liver,* Berlin, 1994, Springer-Verlag.

Intrahepatic cholangiocarcinoma

845. Mori W, Nagasako K: Cholangiocarcinoma and related lesions. In Okuda K, Peters RL, editors: *Hepatocellular carcinoma,* New York, 1976, Wiley & Sons.
846. Sugihara S, Kojiro M: Pathology of cholangiocarcinoma. In Okuda K, Ishak KG, editors: *Neoplasms of the liver,* Tokyo, 1987, Springer-Verlag.
847. Nakajima T, Kondo Y, Miyazaki M, Okui K: A histopathologic study of 102 cases of intrahepatic cholangiocarcinoma: histologic classification and modes of spreading, *Hum Pathol* 19:1228, 1988.
848. Choi BI, Park JH, Kim YI et al: Peripheral cholangiocarcinoma and clonorchiasis: CT findings, *Radiology* 169:149, 1988.
849. Kurathong S, Lerdveresirikul P, Wongpaitoon V et al: *Opisthorchis viverrini* infection and cholangiocarcinoma: a prospective, case-controlled study, *Gastroenterology* 89:151, 1985.
850. Nakanuma Y, Terada T, Tanaka Y, Ohta G: Are hepatolithiasis and cholangiocarcinoma etiologically related? A morphological study of 12 cases of hepatolithiasis associated with cholangiocarcinoma, *Virchows Arch [A](Pathol Anat)* 406:45, 1985.
851. Koga A, Ichimiya H, Yamaguchi K et al: Hepatolithiasis associated with cholangiocarcinoma: possible etiologic significance, *Cancer* 55:2826, 1985.
852. Ritchie JK, Allan RN, Macartney J et al: Biliary tract carcinoma associated with ulcerative colitis, *Q J Med* 43:263, 1974.
853. Wee A, Ludwig L, Coffey RJ et al: Hepatobiliary carcinoma associated with primary sclerosing cholangitis and chronic ulcerative colitis, *Hum Pathol* 16:719, 1985.

854. Phinney PR, Austin GE, Kadell BM: Cholangiocarcinoma arising in Caroli's disease, *Arch Pathol Lab Med* 105:194, 1981.
855. Kchir N, Haouet S, Boubaker S et al: Maladie du Caroli associée a un hépatocarcinome: à propos d'une observation et revue de la littérature, *Sem Hôp Paris* 66:1962, 1990.
856. Daroca PJ, Tuthill R, Reed RJ: Cholangiocarcinoma arising in congenital hepatic fibrosis, *Arch Pathol* 99:592, 1975.
857. Kagawa Y, Kashihara S, Kuramoto S, Maetani S: Carcinoma arising in a congenitally dilated biliary tree, *Gastroenterology* 72:1286, 1978.
858. Voyles CR, Smadja C, Shanda C, Blumgart LH: Carcinoma in choledochal cysts: age-related incidence, *Arch Surg* 118:986, 1983.
859. Burns CD, Kuhns JG, Wieman TJ: Cholangiocarcinoma in association with multiple biliary microhamartomas, *Arch Pathol Lab Med* 114:1287, 1990.
860. Imamura M, Miyashita T, Tani T et al: Cholangiocellular carcinoma associated with multiple liver cysts, *Am J Gastroenterol* 79:790, 1984.
861. Rossi RL, Silverman ML, Braasch JW et al: Carcinomas arising in cystic conditions of the bile ducts: a clinical and pathologic study, *Ann Surg* 205:377, 1987.
862. Rubel LR, Ishak KG: Thorotrast-associated cholangiocarcinoma: an epidemiologic and clinicopathologic study, *Cancer* 50:1408, 1982.
863. Ito Y, Kojiro M, Nakashima T et al: Pathomorphologic characteristics of 102 cases of Thorotrast-related hepatocellular carcinoma, cholangiocarcinoma, and hepatic angiosarcoma, *Cancer* 62:1153, 1988.
864. Littlewood ER, Barrison IG, Murray-Lyon IM, Paradinas FJ: Cholangiocarcinoma and oral contraceptives, *Lancet* 1:310, 1980.
865. Stromeyer FW, Smith DH, Ishak KG: Anabolic steroid therapy and intrahepatic cholangiocarcinoma, *Cancer* 43:440, 1979.

Hepatocellular carcinoma

866. Parkin DM, Stjernward J, Muir CS: Estimates of the worldwide frequency of twelve major cancers, *Bull WHO* 62:163, 1984.
867. Muñoz N, Bosch X: Epidemiology of hepatocellular carcinoma. In Okuda K, Ishak KG, editors: *Neoplasms of the liver,* Tokyo, 1987, Springer-Verlag.
868. Bosch FX, Muñoz N: Hepatocellular carcinoma in the world: epidemiologic questions. In Tabor E, DiBisceglie AM, Purcell RH, editors: *Etiology, pathology, and treatment of hepatocellular carcinoma in North America,* Houston, 1991, Gulf Publishing.
869. Beasley RP: Hepatitis B virus: the major etiology of hepatocellular carcinoma, *Cancer* 61:1842, 1987.
870. Lieberman HM, Tur-Kaspa R, Shafritz DA: Hepatitis B virus infection and hepatocellular carcinoma. In Okuda K, Ishak KG, editors: *Neoplasms of the liver.* Tokyo, 1987, Springer-Verlag.
871. Tabor E: Hepatocellular carcinoma: possible etiologies in patients without serologic evidence of hepatitis B infection, *J Med Virol* 27:1, 1989.
872. Austin H: The role of tobacco use and alcohol consumption in the etiology of hepatocellular carcinoma. In Tabor E, DiBisceglie AM, Purcell RH, editors: *Etiology, pathology, and treatment of hepatocellular carcinoma in North America,* Houston, 1991, Gulf Publishing.
873. Zhang Y-J, Chen C-J, Lee CS et al: Aflatoxin B_1-DNA adducts and hepatitis B virus antigens in hepatocellular carcinoma and non-tumorous liver tissue, *Carcinogenesis* 12:2247, 1991.
874. Li D, Cao Y, He L et al: Aberrations of p53 gene in human hepatocellular carcinoma from China, *Carcinogenesis* 14:169, 1993.
875. Thomas DB: Exogenous steroid hormones and hepatocellular carcinoma. In Tabor E, DiBisceglie AM, Purcell RH, editors: *Etiology, pathology, and treatment of hepatocellular carcinoma in North America,* Houston, 1991, Gulf Publishing.
876. Ishak KG: Hepatocellular carcinoma associated with the inherited metabolic diseases. In Tabor E, DiBisceglie AM, Purcell RH, editors: *Etiology, pathology and treatment of hepatocellular carcinoma in North America,* Houston, 1991, Gulf Publishing.
877. Bradbear RA, Halliday JW, Bassett ML, Cooksley WG: Hepatocellular carcinoma in hemochromatosis. In Okuda K, Ishak KG, editors: *Neoplasms of the liver,* Tokyo, 1987, Springer-Verlag.
878. Kew MC: Clinical manifestations and paraneoplastic syndromes of hepatocellular carcinoma. In Okuda K, Ishak KG, editors: *Neoplasms of the liver,* Tokyo, 1987, Springer-Verlag.
879. Wepsic HT, Kirkpatrick A: Alpha-fetoprotein and its relevance to human disease, *Gastroenterology* 77:787, 1979.
880. Sawabu N, Hattori N: Serological tumor markers in hepatocellular carcinoma. In Okuda K, Ishak KG, editors: *Neoplasms of the liver,* Tokyo, 1987, Springer-Verlag.
881. Takeda K: α-Fetoprotein: reevaluation in hepatology, *Hepatology* 12:1420, 1990.
882. Okuda K, Peters RL, Simson IW: Gross anatomic features of hepatocellular carcinoma from three disparate geographic areas, *Cancer* 54:2165, 1984.
883. Lai CL, Wu PC, Lam KC, Todd D: Histologic prognostic indicators in hepatocellular carcinoma, *Cancer* 44:1677, 1979.
884. Craig JR, Peters RL, Edmondson HA, Omata M: Fibrolamellar carcinoma of the liver: a tumor of adolescents and young adults with distinctive clinicopathologic features, *Cancer* 46:372, 1980.
885. Berman MM, Libbey NP, Foster JH: Hepatocellular carcinoma of polygonal cell type with fibrous stroma—an atypical variant with a favorable prognosis, *Cancer* 46:1448, 1980.
886. Rolfes DB: Fibrolamellar carcinoma of the liver. In Okuda K, Ishak KG, editors: *Neoplasms of the liver,* Tokyo, 1987, Springer-Verlag.

Hepatoblastoma

887. Ishak KG, Glunz PR: Hepatoblastoma and hepatocarcinoma in infancy and childhood: report of 47 cases, *Cancer* 20:396, 1967.
888. Lack EE, Neave C, Vauster GF: Hepatoblastoma: a clinical and pathologic study of 54 cases, *Am J Surg Pathol* 6:693, 1982.
889. Abenoza P, Manivel JC, Wick MR et al: Hepatoblastoma: an immunohistochemical and ultrastructural study, *Hum Pathol* 18:1025, 1987.
890. Haas E, Muczynski KA, Krailo M et al: Histopathology and prognosis in childhood hepatoblastoma and hepatocarcinoma, *Cancer* 64:1082, 1989.
891. Conran RM, Hitchcock CL, Maclawin MA et al: Hepatoblastoma: the prognostic significance of histologic types, *Pediatr Pathol* 12:167, 1992.
892. Manivel C, Wick MR, Abenoza P et al: Teratoid hepatoblastoma: the nosologic dilemma of solid embryonic neoplasms of childhood, *Cancer* 57:2168, 1986.
893. Ruck P, Kaiserling E: Melanin-containing hepatoblastoma with endocrine differentiation: an immunohistochemical and ultrastructural study, *Cancer* 72:361, 1993.

Combined hepatocellular and cholangiocarcinoma

894. Goodman ZD, Ishak KG, Langloss JM et al: Combined hepatocellular-cholangiocarcinoma: report of 14 cases and review of the literature, *Cancer* 39:322, 1977.

Epithelioid hemangioendothelioma

895. Weiss SW, Enzinger F: Epithelioid hemangioendothelioma: a vascular tumor often mistaken for a carcinoma, *Cancer* 50:970, 1982.
896. Weiss SW, Ishak KG, Dail DH et al: Epithelioid hemangioendothelioma and related lesions, *Diagn Histopathol* 3:259, 1986.
897. Marino IR, Todo S, Tzakis AG et al: Treatment of hepatic epithelioid hemangioendothelioma with liver transplantation, *Cancer* 62:2079, 1988.
898. Kelleher MB, Iwatsuki S, Sheahen DG. Epithelioid hemangioendothelioma of liver: clinicopathological correlation of 10 cases treated by orthotopic liver transplantation, *Am J Surg Pathol* 13:999, 1989.

Angiosarcoma

899. Ishak KG: Mesenchymal tumors of the liver. In Okuda K, Peters RL, editors: *Hepatocellular carcinoma,* New York, 1976, Wiley & Sons.
900. Popper H, Thomas LB, Teller NC et al: Development of hepatic angiosarcoma induced by vinyl chloride, Thorotrast and arsenic: comparison with cases of unknown etiology, *Am J Pathol* 92:349, 1978.
901. Falk H, Telles NC, Ishak KG et al: Epidemiology of Thorotrast-induced hepatic angiosarcoma in the United States, *Environ Res* 18:65, 1979.
902. Telles NC, Thomas LB, Popper H et al: Evolution of Thorotrast-induced hepatic angiosarcomas, *Environ Res* 18:74, 1979.
903. Locker GY, Doroshow JH, Zwelling LA, Chabner BA. The clinical features of hepatic angiosarcoma: a report of four cases and a review of the English literature, *Medicine* 58:48, 1979.

Undifferentiated sarcoma

904. Stocker JT, Ishak KG: Undifferentiated embryonal sarcoma of the liver, *Cancer* H2:336, 1978.
905. Lack EE, Schloo BL, Azami N et al: Undifferentiated (embryonal) sarcoma of the liver: clinical and pathologic study of 16 cases with emphasis on immunohistochemical features, *Am J Surg Pathol* 15:1, 1991.

906. Urban CE, Mache CL, Schwinger W et al: Undifferentiated (embryonal) sarcoma of the liver in childhood: successful combined-modality therapy in four patients, *Cancer* 72:2511, 1993.

Metastatic tumors

907. Craig JR, Peters RL, Edmondson HA: *Tumors of the liver and intrahepatic bile ducts,* Washington, D.C., 1988, Armed Forces Institute of Pathology.
908. Mack, Zarbo RJ, Trierson HF, Lee MW: Comparative immunohistochemical study of primary and metastatic carcinomas of the liver, *Am J Clin Pathol* 99:551, 1993.
909. Harrison HB, Middleton HM, Crosby JH, Dasher MN: Fulminant hepatic failure: an unusual presentation of metastatic liver disease, *Gastroenterology* 80:820, 1981.
910. Trimble MS, Ghent CN, Grant DR, McLeen CA: Metastatic breast cancer presenting as fulminant hepatic failure: a case report and literature review, *Can J Gastroenterol* 3:149, 1989.
911. McArthur MS, Teergarden DK: Metastatic melanoma presenting as obstructive jaundice with hemobilia, *Am J Surg* 145:830, 1983.

Liver disease after bone marrow transplantation

Graft-versus-host disease

912. Ferrara JLM, Deeg HJ: Graft-versus-host disease. *N Engl J Med* 324:667, 1991.
913. Gale RP: Graft-versus-host disease, *Immunol Rev* 88:193, 1985.
914. Bernuau D, Gisselbrecht C, Devergie A et al: Histologic and ultrastructural appearance of the liver during graft-versus-host disease complicating bone marrow transplantations, *Transplantation* 29:236, 1980.
915. Beschorner WE, Pino J, Boitnott JK et al: Pathology of the liver with bone marrow transplantation: effects of busulfan, carmustine, acute graft-versus-host disease and cytomegalovirus infection, *Am J Pathol* 99:369, 1980.
916. Sloane JP, Farthing MJG, Powles RL: Histopathological changes in the liver after allogeneic bone marrow transplantation, *J Clin Pathol* 33:344, 1980.
917. Snover DC, Weisdorf SA, Ramsay NK et al: Hepatic graft versus host disease: a study of the predictive value of liver biopsy in diagnosis, *Hepatology* 4:123, 1984.
918. Shulman HM, Sharma P, Amos D et al: A coded histologic study of hepatic graft-versus-host disease after human bone marrow transplantation, *Hepatology* 8:463, 1988.
919. McDonald GB, Shulman HW, Sullivan KM et al: Intestinal and hepatic complications of human bone marrow transplantation. Part I. *Gastroenterology* 90:460, 1986.
920. Shulman HM, McDonald GB: Liver disease after marrow transplantation. In Sale GE, Shulman HM, editors: *The pathology of bone marrow transplantation,* New York, 1984, Masson Publishing.
921. McDonald GB, Shulman HW, Sullivan KM et al: Intestinal and hepatic complications of human bone marrow transplantation. Part II. *Gastroenterology* 90:770, 1986.
922. Knapp AB, Crawford JM, Rappeport JM et al: Cirrhosis as a consequence of graft-versus-host disease, *Gastroenterology* 92:513, 1987.
923. Stechschulte DJ Jr, Fishback JL, Emani A et al: Secondary biliary cirrhosis as a consequence of graft-versus-host disease, *Gastroenterology* 98:223, 1990.
924. Geubel AP, Cnudde A, Ferrant AM et al: Diffuse biliary tract involvement mimicking primary sclerosing cholangitis after bone marrow transplantation, *J Hepatol* 10:23, 1990.
925. Snover DC: Biopsy interpretation in bone marrow transplantation, *Pathol Annu* 24(Pt 2):63, 1989.

Nonspecific changes and artifacts

926. Petrelli M, Scheuer PJ: Variation in subcapsular liver structure and its significance in the interpretation of wedge biopsies, *J Clin Pathol* 20:743, 1987.
927. Thompson SW, Luna LG: *An atlas of artifacts encountered in preparation of microscopic tissue sections,* Springfield, Ill., 1978, Charles C Thomas.
928. Keller TC, Smetana HF: Artifact in liver biopsies, *Am J Clin Pathol* 20:728, 1950.
929. Sunzel H, Zettergren L: Histological liver lesions developing during abdominal operations, *Gastroenterology* 105:45, 1966.
930. Christoffersen P, Poulsen H, Skeie E: Focal liver cell necrosis accompanied by infiltration by granulocytes during operation, *Acta Hepato-Splenol* 17:240, 1970.
931. Landas SK, Bromley CM: Sponge artifact in biopsy specimens, *Arch Pathol Lab Med* 114:1285, 1990.
932. Kepes JL, Oswald HT: Tissue artifact caused by sponge in imbedding cassettes, *Am J Surg Pathol* 15:810, 1991.

58 Gallbladder and Extrahepatic Biliary Ducts

José Jessurun
Jorge Albores-Saavedra

THE NORMAL GALLBLADDER AND EXTRAHEPATIC DUCT

Gross anatomy. The gallbladder is located in a depression on the inferior surface of the right and quadrate lobes of the liver known as the *gallbladder bed*. Although its normal dimensions in adults vary and are dependent on the volume of bile contained within, the gallbladder may be up to 10 cm long, 3 to 5 cm wide, and have a wall thickness of 0.1 to 0.2 cm. The blind end that projects beyond the anterior liver margin is known as the *fundus*. Most of the organ is formed by the central body, or corpus, a portion of which bulges toward the upper margin of the first portion of the duodenum forming the infundibulum, or Hartmann's pouch. The neck is a short and narrow segment located between the body and the cystic duct.

The organ is attached to the liver by loose connective tissue that contains blood vessels, lymphatics, and occasionally bile ducts. A peritoneal fold known as the "cholecystoduodenal ligament" attaches the infundibulum to the first portion of the duodenum.

The vascular supply of the gallbladder is the cystic artery, which usually originates from the right hepatic artery.[1] Venous blood is carried through small veins that traverse the gallbladder bed and drains into the liver. Lymph drains to several distant groups of lymph nodes: the retropancreatic, the celiac, and the superior mesenteric. The cystic node primarily drains the anterior surface of the gallbladder. The gallbladder and extrahepatic bile ducts receive sympathetic and parasympathetic nerve fibers from the anterior and posterior hepatic plexuses.[2]

The cystic duct is a 3 cm long structure located in the right free edge of the lesser omentum. At the junction with the gallbladder neck several mucosal folds project into the lumen. These enfoldings, called the *spiral valve of Heister*, contain thin groups of smooth muscle fibers that regulate the filling and emptying of the gallbladder according to the pressure in the biliary system.

After emerging from the liver, the right and left hepatic ducts fuse into a 2 to 3 cm long common hepatic duct, which continues as the common bile duct after combining with the cystic duct. Except for the latter, these ducts are covered by the serous layers of the lesser omentum. The common hepatic duct is about 5 cm long and 0.1 cm in diameter. Based on its relation to the duodenum and pancreas, it is divided into four segments: supraduodenal, retroduodenal, pancreatic, and intraduodenal.

Most of their blood supply is provided by branches from the right, left, and common hepatic arteries and the retroduodenal, cystic, gastroduodenal, and retroportal arteries. Venous blood drains directly into the liver or portal vein. Lymphatic channels drain into lymph nodes near the porta hepatis or into deep pancreatic nodes. The nerve supply is provided by the hepatic plexus.[3]

Histology. The wall of the gallbladder has three layers: mucosa, muscularis, and adventitia.

The mucosa, composed of surface epithelium and lamina propria, projects into the lumen as branching folds that increase in height as the gallbladder contracts and are less prominent in the distended organ. Three types of epithelial cells are normally found in the mucosa: columnar, "pencil-like," and basal. A single layer of columnar cells, with basally oriented nuclei, forms the surface epithelium. This cell has a lightly eosinophilic cytoplasm and few small apical vacuoles. Ultrastructural examination shows short microvilli projecting into the lumen. Invaginations of the apical portions of the luminal cell membrane give rise to pinocytotic vesicles. These cells are tightly joined together by apical junctional complexes. The lateral membranes of neighboring cells interdigitate and surround an extracellular space, the width of which varies according to the content of water and electrolytes actively transported into it.[4]

The "pencil-like" cell, occasionally seen in the surface epithelium, is a narrow columnar cell with dark eosinophilic cytoplasm. This cell is not a squeezed or compressed columnar cell, since ultrastructurally it contains more organelles and shows basal cytoplasmic extensions that penetrate the basement membrane.[5]

The basal cell is a rarely observed type of epithelial cell found in contact with and parallel to the basement membrane.

In addition to the epithelial cells, a few T-lymphocytes are normally present between the surface columnar cells. Endocrine cells and melanocytes are normally absent.

Several tubuloalveolar glands are present in the neck of the normal gallbladder. These mucous glands are composed of low columnar or cuboidal cells with clear cytoplasm and basally located nuclei. It is important to remember their exclusive location in the neck, since when glands with a similar appearance are seen elsewhere they usually represent pyloric gland metaplasia.

Rokitansky-Aschoff sinuses describe the pathologic herniations of the mucosa into or through the muscularis (Fig. 58-1). In this sense, they are analogous to colonic diverticuli. Enfoldings of the mucosa in the lamina propria are common in the contracted gallbladder and should not be regarded as abnormal.

The lamina propria is composed of loose connective tissue, nerve fibers, blood vessels, and lymphatics. Small numbers of lymphocytes, IgA-containing plasma cells, mast cells, and macrophages may be present.

The muscular layer is a slightly thickened version of the muscularis mucosa of the intestine composed of bundles of loosely arranged smooth muscle separated by fibrovascular connective tissue.

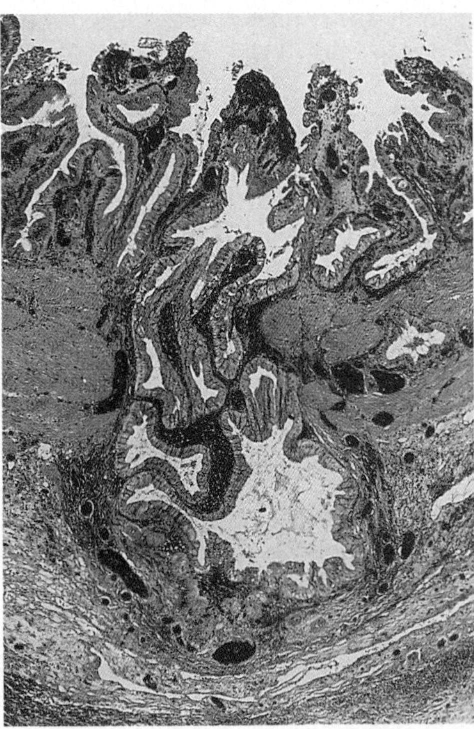

Fig. 58-1 Rokitansky-Aschoff sinuses are abnormal mucosal outpouchings into or through the muscularis caused by increased intraluminal pressure.

The adventitia is composed of loose connective tissue, blood vessels, lymphatics, nerves, and fatty tissue. Its abdominal side is covered by serosa. Rare paraganglia may be seen adjacent to the vessels.[4] On the hepatic side, Luschka ducts may be seen in the adventitia. These small, usually microscopic, bile ducts may be solitary or multiple and are lined by cells similar to those of the intrahepatic bile ducts. Larger accessory biliary ducts may occasionally be present in the adventitia. Leakage of bile into the peritoneum may occur if these ducts are left patent after a cholecystectomy.[6]

The extrahepatic bile ducts are lined by a single layer of tall columnar cells that, except for containing less mucin, are otherwise similar to the those present in the gallbladder. The epithelium invaginates into the stroma, forming pockets or pits called "sacculi of Beale." On tangential sections, they may deceivingly appear as deep glands unconnected with the surface epithelium. It is through these saccules that the secretions produced by the biliary glands drain. These unevenly distributed glands have a lobular arrangement and are surrounded by dense stroma. They are lined by mucin-producing low-columnar to cuboidal cells.[4]

The stroma beneath the surface epithelium is dense and contains very few inflammatory cells. In most instances, no smooth muscle fibers are found in the common bile duct except for the intrapancreatic and intraduodenal segments where prominent muscle fibers form the sphincter choledochus.

Embryology. The gallbladder, bile ducts, liver, and primitive ventral pancreas originate from a diverticulum that appears on the ventral surface of the primitive foregut near the yolk stalk. At 4 weeks of gestation, three separate buds can be recognized: the cranial penetrates into the splanchnic mesenchyme of the septum transversum and develops into the liver, the caudal becomes the gallbladder, and a smaller basal bud gives rise to the ventral pancreas. Their centrifugal migration causes elongation of those segments originally attached to the foregut, which become the hepatic, cystic, and common bile ducts. Proliferation of epithelial cells transform these hollow structures into solid cords that acquire a lumen by vacuolization of the cells around the seventh week of gestation.[3]

Physiology. The continuous secretion of bile by the liver totals approximately 1000 ml each day. The direction in which bile flows is a consequence of the reciprocal activity of the smooth muscle in the gallbladder and sphincter of Oddi. When food is ingested, the gallbladder contracts and the sphincter of Oddi relaxes causing the release of bile into the duodenum. Fatty meals and to a lesser degree proteins stimulate the gallbladder smooth muscle to contract mainly through the action of cholecystokinin, a polypeptide hormone secreted by the proximal small intestine.[4] Contraction of the gallbladder during the interdigestive period is most probably mediated by motilin, another polypeptide hormone found in the epithelium of the duodenum and jejunum. By contrast somatostatin, a hormone secreted from the intestine and pancreas after the ingestion of a fatty meal, inhibits gallbladder contraction. Even though cholecystokinin and somatostatin are released by the same meal stimuli, their opposing actions indicate that these hormones probably "balance" each other.[7]

During fasting, contraction of the sphincter of Oddi causes the progressive accumulation of bile in the common bile duct. When the pressure in this system exceeds the resting pressure of the gallbladder (approximately 10 mm Hg), bile flows into the latter. Although the capacity of the gallbladder is small (40 to 70 ml), a larger quantity of bile constituents are effectively stored through concentration. Water is absorbed by the epithelial cells through a osmotic gradient generated by a NaK-ATPase-mediated sodium-coupled transport of chloride.[8]

An additional function of the gallbladder is the secretion of mucin by the surface epithelial cells and neck mucous glands. Recently, these mucosubstances have been extensively investigated, since, as will be explained subsequently, they may be important in the formation of gallstones.

CONGENITAL AND DEVELOPMENTAL ABNORMALITIES

Abnormalities of the gallbladder

Even though congenital anomalies of the gallbladder are rare, they may represent a challenge for the diagnostic radiologist and for the surgeon while performing a cholecystectomy. Congenital malformations include anomalies in *shape, number,* and *position.*

Abnormalities of shape

The most common abnormality in shape is an angulation of the fundus called *Phrygian cap* because of its resemblance to the folded hats worn in an ancient country of Asia Minor called Phrygia. Microscopic examination shows a mucosal fold with some disorientation of the underlying muscle bundles. Although clinically unimportant, it may be mistaken on radiologic examination for a stone or a pathologic septum.[9] *Congenital diverticula* are very rare. They consist of saccular outpouchings of the gallbladder wall. Although multiple diverticula may occur, they are usually single and may be located anywhere. Congenital diverticula may be clinically inapparent or may contain stones and become infected.

Septation of the gallbladder is characterized by the presence of one or multiple septa that divide the gallbladder lumen into several chambers.[10] (Fig. 58-2). This anomaly probably results from incomplete fusion of the vacuoles that give rise to the lumen after the solid stage. In some cases the septa contain muscle fibers that are continuous with those of the outer wall. This finding has been used as an argument to support a developmental cause.[11] However, smooth muscle may be absent. It should be noted that inflammatory diseases of the gallbladder can produce internal compartmentalization. The inflammatory septa are usually thicker than the congenital septa and are composed of inflamed fibrous tissue. In some cases, particularly those associated with gallstones, the distinction between inflamed congenital septa and acquired compartmentalization is impossible. Septation of the gallbladder has been associated with intermittent abdominal pain in young adults. Rare cases in children have also been reported.[12] Stones are usually but not invariably absent.

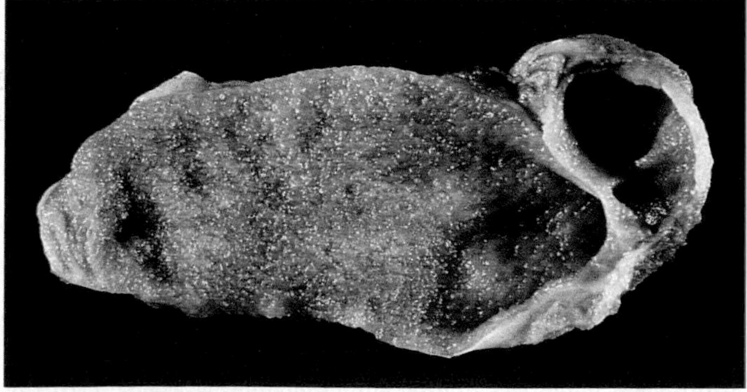

Fig. 58-2 Septated gallbladder. This congenital malformation may be associated with abdominal pain in children and young adults.

The term *hourglass gallbladder* has been used to describe those cases with a transverse septum that divides the lumen into a proximal and distal cavity. Inflammatory changes and stone formation tend to occur more frequently in the distal cavity.

Cystic malformations of the gallbladder may be analogous to the more common choledochal cysts or may arise by occlusion of the neck of a diverticulum.[13] In addition, dilatation of Luschka's ducts may give rise to multilocular cysts around the gallbladder.

Failure of development of the caudal foregut diverticulum results in *agenesis* of the gallbladder. It can either occur as an isolated phenomenon or be associated with other anomalies, the most common one being choledocholithiasis. Other abnormalities associated with gallbladder agenesis include absence of ascending colon, polycystic kidneys, tracheoesophageal fistulas, cardiac defects, imperforate anus, annular pancreas, the Klippel-Feil syndrome, and horseshoe kidney combined with malrotation of the gut.[14]

A *hypoplastic* gallbladder may result as a consequence of incomplete development of the caudal bud or failure of recanalization of the solid stage. It may be found in association with congenital biliary atresia and in cystic fibrosis. This condition should be differentiated from acquired post-inflammatory fibrotic retraction of the gallbladder.[14]

Numerical abnormalities

In contrast, excessive budding of the caudal diverticulum gives rise to gallbladder *duplication* or even *triplication.* Most commonly, the cystic ducts enter the common bile duct separately (H type) or unite to form a common cystic duct (Y type). Less frequently, they drain independently into the hepatic ducts. Stones, inflammatory conditions, and tumors may preferentially involve one of the gallbladders.[14]

Abnormalities of position

The gallbladder may be located in *abnormal sites.* It may be found on the left side as the only malpositioned organ or, more commonly, as part of situs inversus. In other instances, the gallbladder is retroplaced, within the falciform ligament or abdominal wall, or totally surrounded by liver parenchyma *(intrahepatic gallbladder).* Another abnormality that may be clinically relevant is the so-called wandering, or floating, gallbladder. In this instance, the gallbladder is completely surrounded by peritoneum without a firm attachment to the liver. Its extreme mobility predisposes to kinking of the cystic duct that compromises bile flow, or twisting of the nutrient vessels, which may result in hemorrhagic infarction.[15,16]

Abnormalities of bile ducts

Abnormalities of the bile ducts may occur as isolated phenomena or in association with gallbladder malformations. Absence of the cystic duct is usually associated with agenesis of the gallbladder. Duplication generally parallels duplication of the

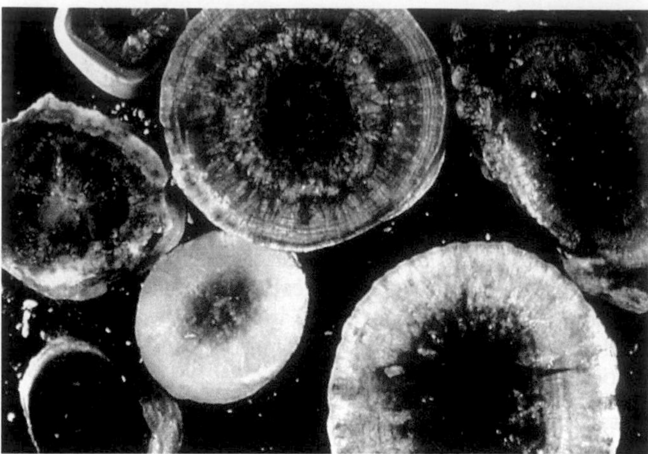

Fig. 58-5 The center of a cholesterol gallstone is frequently pigmented because of a concentration of calcium bilirubinate salts in this area higher than that in the outer portions.

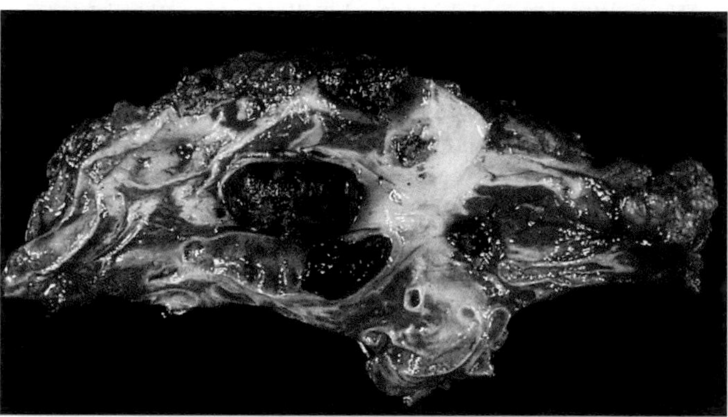

Fig. 58-6 The bile ducts have been opened to reveal numerous pigmented (brown) stones.

Bile acids are secreted by the liver cells through a different transport mechanism. Although they are soluble in water, beyond a certain concentration they aggregate into simple micelles. The chemical properties of bile acids render an extremely water-soluble structure because of the orientation of the hydrophobic portions away from water and the exposure of the hydrophilic surfaces to the aqueous environment. As detergents, bile acids can dissolve portions of vesicles and incorporate them as mixed micelles. These structures are disks composed of cholesterol and phospholipids surrounded by bile acids.[25-27]

As the concentration of cholesterol increases, more of it is carried in vesicles. In addition, during micellation, more phospholipid than cholesterol is transferred from vesicles to mixed micelles. The resulting cholesterol-enriched unilamellar vesicles are unstable and fuse into large multilamellar vesicles. When the cholesterol-to-phospholipid ratio exceeds 1, cholesterol crystallizes at their surface. Enhancement of crystallization is influenced by the concentration of solutes in bile, since aggregation occurs more efficiently when cholesterol carriers are close to each other.[25,26,28]

Cholesterol is most soluble in a mixture of lipids containing at least 50% bile acids and a smaller amounts of phospholipids. Supersaturation occurs when a solution contains more cholesterol molecules than can be incorporated into mixed micelles. Bile supersaturation may be attributable to hypersecretion of cholesterol, hyposecretion of bile acids, or a combination of both. An increase in biliary cholesterol output is the most common cause of supersaturation that is the result of increased synthesis or uptake of endogenous (transported by low-density lipoproteins) or exogenous (by chylomicrons) cholesterol by the hepatocytes. The secretion of cholesterol increases and that of bile acids decreases when the activity of a microsomal rate-limiting enzyme, called 7α-hydroxylase, that converts cholesterol to bile acids is low. Adequate bile acid secretion depends of the integrity of the enterohepatic circulation. This circulation occurs 3 to 12 times per day and consists of the active absorption of more than 90% of bile acids in the terminal ileum and their return to the liver via the portal system where active and passive uptake by the hepatocyte makes them again available for secretion. Any interference with this mechanism will contribute to bile acid hyposecretion and cholesterol supersaturation.[25-27]

Supersaturation of cholesterol is a necessary but not sufficient condition for the formation of cholesterol gallstones. For a given degree of cholesterol saturation, patients with gallstones form cholesterol crystals more rapidly than individuals without gallstones. That a nucleation defect is also required was demonstrated when it was shown that equally saturated biles from stone patients and controls nucleate cholesterol at different rates: the former did so rapidly and the latter slowly. It has become apparent that the tendency of bile to nucleate its cholesterol depends on the balance between substances that promote and prevent nucleation. Pronucleating substances include mucous glycoproteins, immunoglobulins, aminopeptidase N, phospholipase C, fibronectin, and orsomucoid. Antinucleating substances comprise apolipoproteins A-1 and A-2 and biliary glycoproteins belonging to the cytokeratin family of proteins.[29-32] (Fig. 58-7).

Alterations in one or several of the mechanisms may be correlated with some clinical conditions known to be associated with gallstone formation.

Epidemiology. The prevalence of cholesterol gallstones varies greatly with age, sex, country, and ethnic group. Geographic differences are most probably related to the interaction of genetic and environmental factors. In the United States at least 10% of adults have gallstones.[24] When segregated by ethnic groups, Native Americans[33] and Mexican-Americans[34,35] have the highest prevalence rates, and African-Americans the lowest. In other parts of the world, gallstones are extremely common in Chile and the Scandinavian countries whereas their incidence in most of Asia and Africa is very low. Ultrasound surveys and autopsy studies have consistently shown that women develop stones more than twice as often as men and that their prevalence increases with age.[36,37]

An increased risk for gallstones is associated with number of pregnancies, estrogen-replacement therapy, oral-contraceptive use, obesity, and rapid weight loss but not with diabetes mellitus.[26]

Pigment gallstones

Pathogenesis. There are two types of pigment stones: black and brown.[38] The distinction is important because they differ in their cause, associated clinical conditions, morphology, and chemical composition. Black stones are composed of

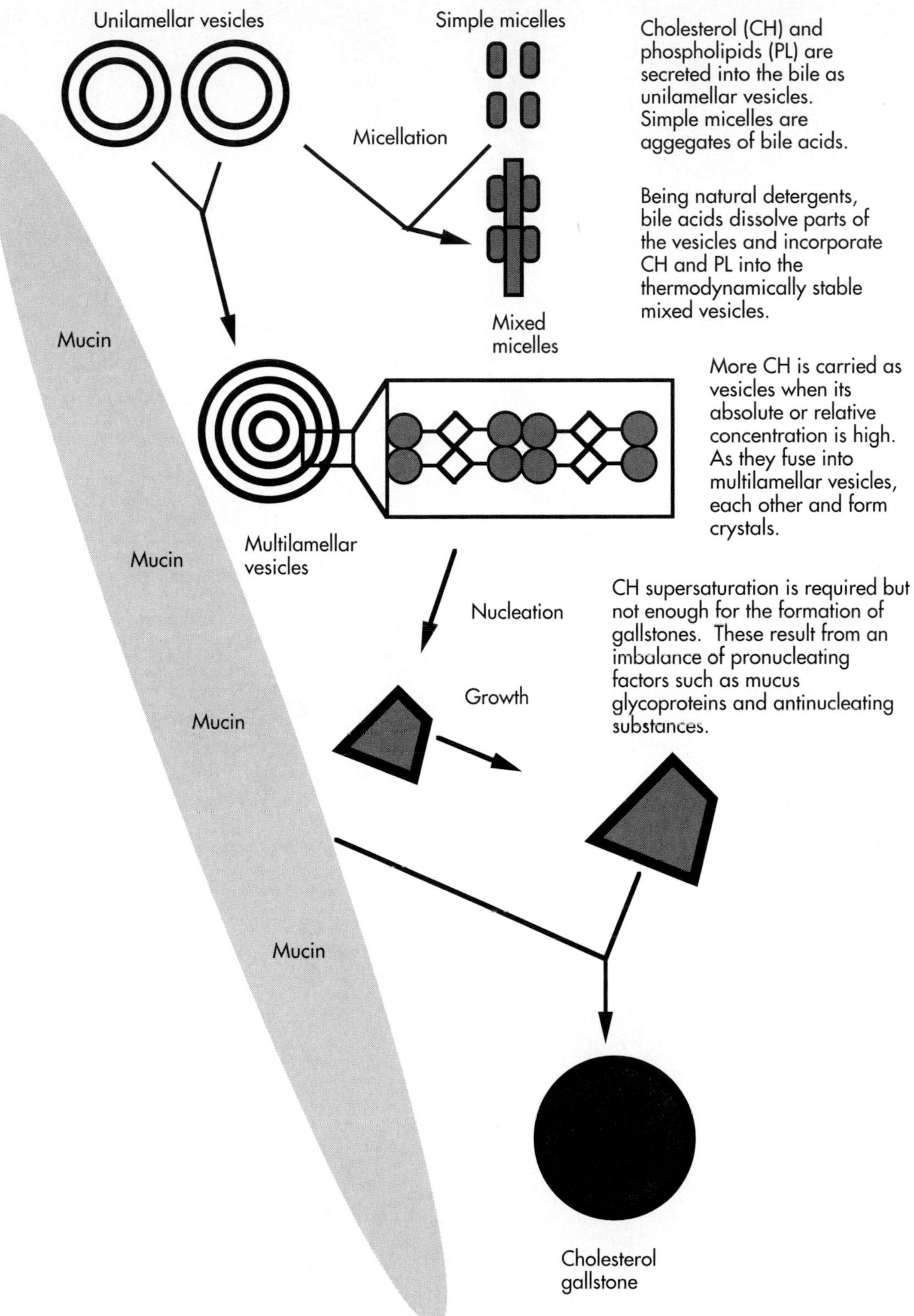
Unilamellar vesicles
Simple micelles
Cholesterol (CH) and phospholipids (PL) are secreted into the bile as unilamellar vesicles. Simple micelles are aggegates of bile acids.
Micellation
Being natural detergents, bile acids dissolve parts of the vesicles and incorporate CH and PL into the thermodynamically stable mixed vesicles.
Mixed micelles
Mucin
More CH is carried as vesicles when its absolute or relative concentration is high. As they fuse into multilamellar vesicles, each other and form crystals.
Multilamellar vesicles
Mucin
Nucleation
CH supersaturation is required but not enough for the formation of gallstones. These result from an imbalance of pronucleating factors such as mucus glycoproteins and antinucleating substances.
Growth
Mucin
Mucin
Cholesterol gallstone

Fig. 58-7 Pathogenesis of cholesterol gallstones.

calcium bilirubinate, phosphate, and carbonate embedded in a glycoprotein matrix; the cholesterol concentration is very low. Brown stones contain calcium salts of bilirubin and fatty acids, mainly palmitate, and cholesterol in a glycoprotein matrix. Calcium carbonate and phosphate are usually not present.[28,38]

Unconjugated bilirubin plays a central role in the formation of both types of stones. In normal bile, 1% to 2% of the total bilirubin is unconjugated bilirubin, most of which is solubilized by mixed micelles. Free unconjugated bilirubin combines with calcium to produce calcium bilirubinate. An increase in unconjugated bilirubin results from nonenzymatic

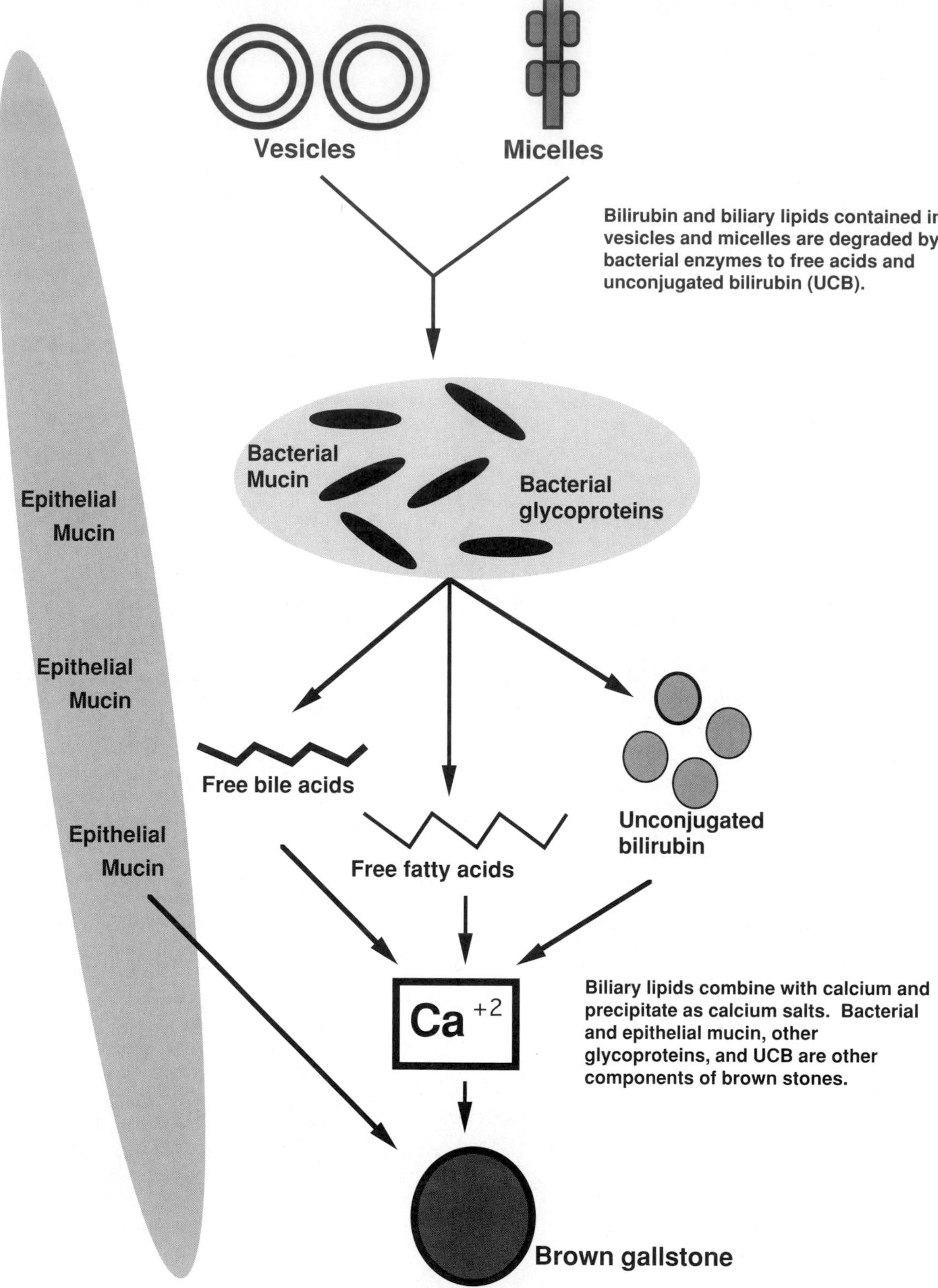
Vesicles
Micelles
Bilirubin and biliary lipids contained in vesicles and micelles are degraded by bacterial enzymes to free acids and unconjugated bilirubin (UCB).
Epithelial Mucin
Bacterial Mucin
Bacterial glycoproteins
Epithelial Mucin
Free bile acids
Free fatty acids
Unconjugated bilirubin
Epithelial Mucin
Ca +2
Biliary lipids combine with calcium and precipitate as calcium salts. Bacterial and epithelial mucin, other glycoproteins, and UCB are other components of brown stones.
Brown gallstone

Fig. 58-8 Pathogenesis of brown gallstones.

or enzymatic hydrolysis of bilirubin conjugates by bacterial or endogenous β-glucuronidase activity.

Brown pigment stone disease results from bile infection, which is usually secondary to stasis. Production of enzymes by bacteria play a central role in stone formation. In addition to β-glucuronidase, bacteria elaborate phospholipase A, which cleaves phospholipids to form lysolecithin and free fatty acids, and hydrolases, which generate free bile acids from conjugated bile salts. The resulting insoluble unconjugated bilirubin and free fatty acids (mainly palmitic and stearic) precipitate as calcium salts. Furthermore, depletion of bile acids from micelles enhances cholesterol supersaturation and promotes its precipitation. Bacteria are present within the matrix of most brown stones.[24,38] (Fig. 58-8).

Black pigment stone disease is not associated with bacterial infection. An increased concentration of unconjugated bilirubin originates from an increment in the secretion of bilirubin conjugates as occurs in hemolysis and chronic alcoholism, followed by nonbacterial enzymatic or nonenzymatic hydrolysis. An analogous effect may occur if there is a decrease in the secretion of bile salts, as occurs in cirrhotics, since these compounds are required to solubilize unconjugated bilirubin and buffer ionized calcium.[28] Gallstone growth is enhanced by the structural framework provided by gallbladder mucin (Fig. 58-9).

Epidemiology. Pigment gallstones occur in all countries. Although they account for only 20% to 25% of stones in the United States, they are the most common type worldwide. Like cholesterol gallstones, pigment stones develop more frequently in females and their incidence increases with age; however, at variance with the former, race does not appear to be a factor.

The clinical conditions associated with black gallstones include hemolytic anemia, cirrhosis, alcoholism, malaria, pancreatitis, total parenteral nutrition, and advanced age. Brown stones are associated with consumption of a low protein diet and juxtapapillary duodenal diverticula. Most importantly, brown stones can develop throughout the intrahepatic and extrahepatic ducts in addition to the gallbladder; for this reason, they constitute most of the common bile duct stones formed de novo. Another important difference is their association with polymicrobial bacterial infection; *Escherichia coli* is frequently cultured.[28,38]

CHOLECYSTITIS

Inflammatory diseases of the gallbladder are a frequent cause of morbidity in Western countries. For their diagnosis and treatment, more than $5 billion were spent in direct cost in 1990 in the United States. This heterogeneous group of diseases is discussed according to the clinicopathologic classification outlined in Table 58-2.

Acute cholecystitis

Acute cholecystitis is clinically defined as an episode of acute biliary pain accompanied by fever and right hypochondrial tenderness and guarding, with persistence of the symptoms beyond 24 hours.[39] Most of the cases (90%) are associated with gallstones. Because of their unique clinical or pathologic characteristics, the three types of acute cholecystitis that warrant separate discussion are acute calculous cholecystitis, acute acalculous cholecystitis, and emphysematous cholecystitis.

Acute calculous cholecystitis

The precipitating event for the development of acute calculous cholecystitis appears to be occlusion of the neck of the gallbladder or cystic duct by a stone. The increased intraluminal pressure causes dilatation of the gallbladder and edema of its wall. However, outflow obstruction does not always cause acute cholecystitis. Shrinkage of the gallbladder is the sole consequence of cystic duct ligation or obliteration in animal models.[40] Other contributing factors for acute cholecystitis may be mucosal ischemia secondary to visceral distention or external compression of the nearby cystic artery by the impacted stone, formation of inflammatory mediators such as lysolecithin and prostaglandins, and mucosal injury by bile acids.[41] It has been postulated that trauma to the mucosa caused by stones releases phospholipase from lysosomes residing in mucosal epithelial cells. This enzyme converts lecithin to lysolecithin, which is an active detergent known to be toxic to the mucosa.[42]

When bile cultures are obtained early enough (within 48 hours of onset), bacteria can be identified in 81% of the cases.[39] The predominant organisms are intestinal: *Escherichia coli,* other gram-negative aerobic rods, enterococci, and in 20% of the cases anaerobes.[42,43] Most authorities agree that bacterial invasion is most probably a secondary event.

Pathology. The gallbladder is usually enlarged and its wall is considerably thickened by edema, vascular congestion, and hemorrhage (Fig. 58-10). The serosa is dull and covered with patches of fibrinopurulent exudate. As mentioned previously, a gallstone is frequently found obstructing the outflow pathway. Thick, cloudy bile admixed with blood and pus fills the lumen. Depending on the severity of the inflammatory response, the mucosal changes range from edema and congestion to widespread ulcers and necrosis. Histologically, an acute inflammatory reaction characterized by edema, vascular congestion, hemorrhage, scant to abundant neutrophilic infiltration, and necrosis predominates in specimens obtained early in the course of the disease. Intramural microabscesses and secondary vasculitis may be present.

As the disease evolves, lymphocytes, plasma cells, macrophages, and variable number of eosinophils appear. Granulation tissue and collagen deposition replace previously ulcerated or necrotic tissue.

Complications of acute calculous cholecystitis include empyema, gangrene, and perforation. The latter complication is usually sealed off by the omentum, leading to the formation of pericholecystic adhesions or abscess; however, life-threatening septic and biliary peritonitis may ensue.[39]

Clinical Features. Most patients are women with a peak age incidence of 50 to 70 years. The typical symptoms are right upper quadrant pain of recent onset accompanied by abdominal guarding and local tenderness. These symptoms may be deceptively mild or even absent in the elderly. Sometimes, the enlarged gallbladder may be palpated, or pain may be elicited while one is palpating the right upper quadrant when the patient inhales deeply (Murphy's sign). Some patients are febrile and jaundiced and most show leukocytosis. Documentation of the diagnosis is achieved by imaging techniques, mainly ultrasonography and CT scan, which show an enlarged and thickened gallbladder containing stones.[44]

Acute acalculous cholecystitis

The infrequent but clinically serious disease called "acute acalculous cholecystitis" is found in approximately 5% of all patients undergoing cholecystectomy.[45] It predominantly affects individuals with other clinicopathologic conditions including trauma, nonbiliary surgical procedures, sepsis, burns, parenteral nutrition, mechanical ventilation, numerous blood transfusions, and use of narcotics or antibiotics. Its exact pathogenesis is not fully understood though it appears to be multifactorial.[46] Increased bile viscosity from stasis with obstruction of the cystic duct has been suggested as a con-

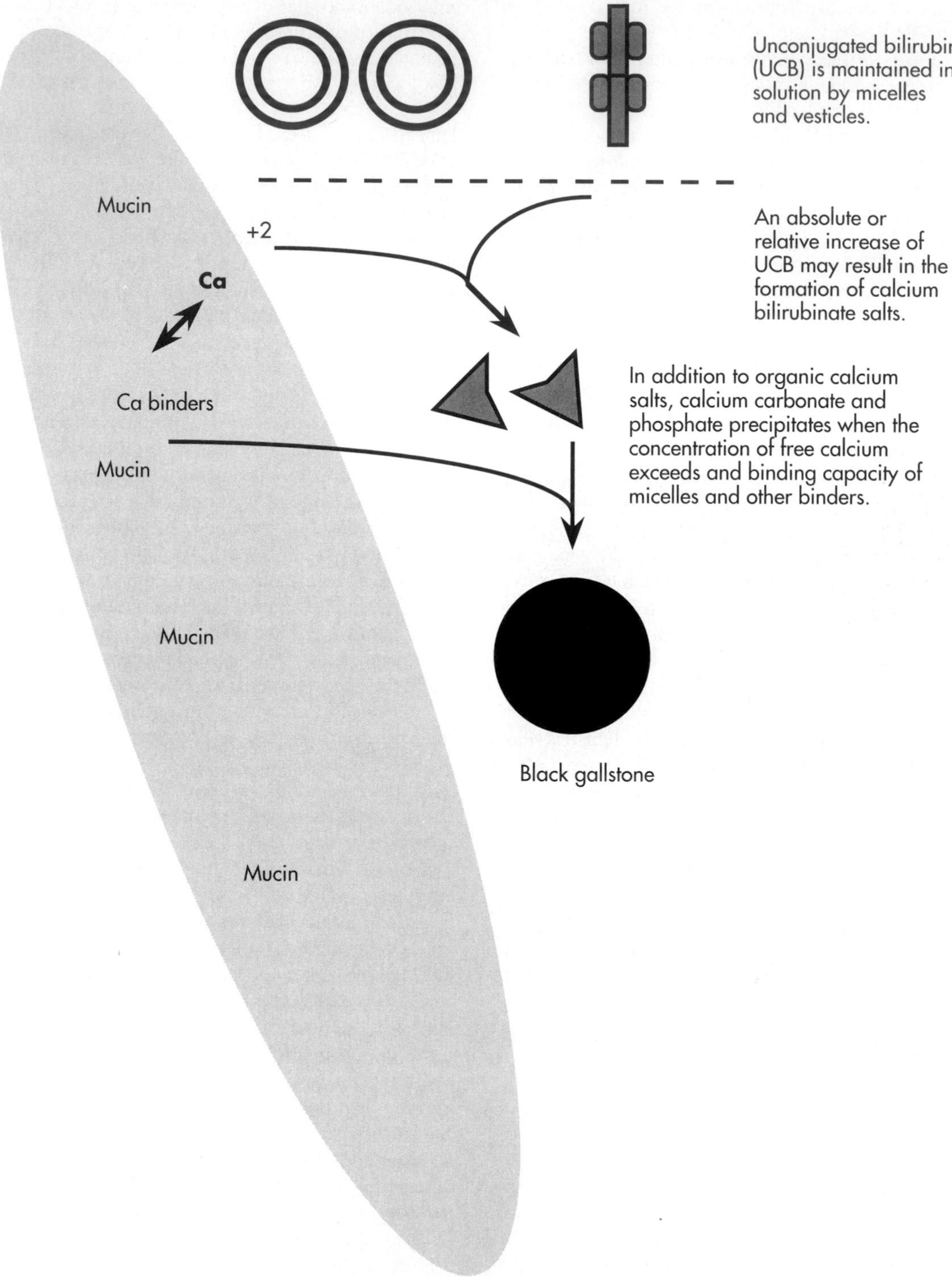
Unconjugated bilirubin (UCB) is maintained in solution by micelles and vesicles.
Mucin
+2
Ca
An absolute or relative increase of UCB may result in the formation of calcium bilirubinate salts.
Ca binders
In addition to organic calcium salts, calcium carbonate and phosphate precipitates when the concentration of free calcium exceeds and binding capacity of micelles and other binders.
Mucin
Mucin
Black gallstone
Mucin

Fig. 58-9 Pathogenesis of black gallstones.

tributing factor. This hypothesis is supported by the association of acute acalculous cholecystitis with clinical conditions that have in common gallbladder stasis such as fasting, use of narcotics, dehydration, and anesthesia. Undoubtedly, mucosal ischemia is a major culprit in elderly patients with underlying cardiovascular diseases or those that develop acute acalculous cholecystitis after trauma, sepsis, or surgical procedures. Bile cultures are generally negative; however, secondary bacterial infections by enteric organisms may supervene.

There are no specific clinical or histologic differences between acute calculous and acalculous cholecystitis except for a higher proportion of men and an increased rate of complications and overall mortality for the latter condition.[45,46]

Acute emphysematous cholecystitis

Acute emphysematous cholecystitis is an uncommon variant of acute cholecystitis characterized by the production of gas by the infecting bacterial organism. On plain roentgenograms

Table 58-2 Classification of cholecystitis

Acute
Calculous
Acalculous
Emphysematous
Chronic
Calculous
Acalculous
Xanthogranulomatous
Other

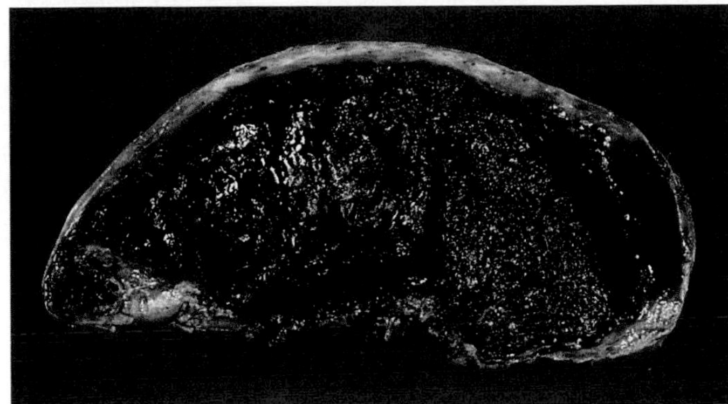

Fig. 58-10 Acute cholecystitis. This opened specimen shows a hemorrhagic and friable mucosa. Microscopic examination of the thickened wall showed edema, hemorrhage, and a predominantly neutrophilic infiltrate.

of the abdomen, a characteristic pattern of air is seen in the gallbladder lumen, its wall, and in the pericholecystic area. It occurs most frequently in men between 50 and 60 years of age and in persons with diabetes mellitus. As a result of frequent complications such as gangrene and perforation, the overall mortality is high (15% versus 4.1% for acute calculous cholecystitis). About half of bile cultures are positive for clostridial organisms, the most common being *C. welchii.* Vascular occlusion of the cystic artery or its branches by atherosclerosis and small vessel disease (both frequent complications of diabetes mellitus) is the major contributory factor of emphysematous cholecystitis.[47,48]

Pathology. During cholecystectomy, the gallbladder is found to be distended, tense, and encased by the omentum, fibrous adhesions, or an abscess. A necrotic, friable wall frequently leads to fragmentation of the gallbladder during removal. Upon opening, gas and foul-smelling purulent exudate escape from the lumen. Gallstones, frequently of the pigment type, are found in 70% of the cases. The mucosa appears necrotic, congested, and hemorrhagic. On microscopic examination colonies of gram-positive bacilli are often found within a necrotic and acutely inflamed mucosa. Gas bubbles are occasionally present within the wall or in the subserosal connective tissue.

Chronic cholecystitis

Chronic cholecystitis is almost always associated with gallstones. The pathogenesis of this common disorder is poorly understood. It has been suggested that chronic cholecystitis develops as a result of recurrent attacks of mild acute cholecystitis. However, a clinical history supportive of this hypothesis is provided by only a minority of patients. The inflammatory and reparative changes may be in part explained by repetitive mucosal trauma produce by gallstones. However, it is doubtful that gallstones are solely responsible, since there is a poor correlation between the severity of the inflammatory response and the number of stones or their volume. A more likely explanation for this association is that both cholelithiasis and chronic cholecystitis are a consequence of bile with an abnormal composition leading to stone formation and chemical injury to the mucosa. At variance with the high percentage of positive bile cultures in patients with acute cholecystitis, bacteria, mostly *E. coli* and enterococci, are cultured in less than a third of the cases of chronic cholecystitis.[19]

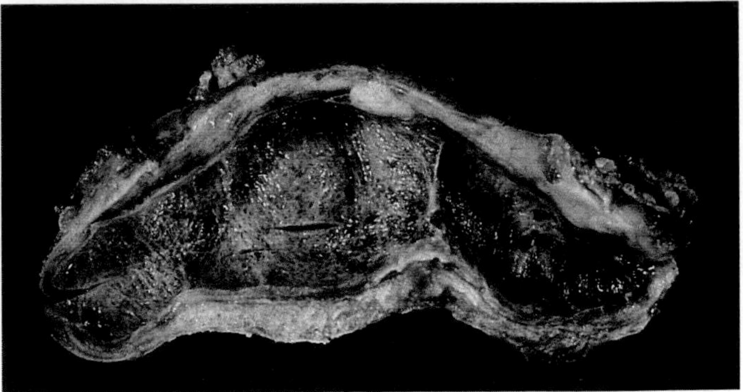

Fig. 58-11 Chronic cholecystitis. The gallbladder wall is thickened and the mucosa appears fibrotic and trabeculated. Several large cholesterol gallstones were removed from the lumen.

Pathology. The variable appearance of the gallbladder in chronic cholecystitis is a reflection of differences in the degree of inflammation and fibrosis. The gallbladder may be distended or shrunken. Fibrous serosal adhesions are suggestive of previous episodes of acute cholecystitis. On section, the wall is usually thickened, but it may be thin. The mucosa may be intact with preservation or accentuation of its folds or, in cases with outflow obstruction, flattened. Mucosal erosions or ulcers are frequently found in association with impacted stones (Fig. 58-11). The presence of gallstones is not sufficient or necessary for the diagnosis of chronic cholecystitis. This diagnosis is based on the demonstration of any of the following microscopic features: (1) a predominantly mononuclear inflammatory infiltrate, (2) fibrosis, or (3) metaplastic changes.

The degree of the inflammatory reaction is variable. In some cases, the infiltrate is exclusively located in the mucosa, whereas in others it extends into the muscularis and serosa. The distribution of the infiltrate varies from focal to patchy to diffuse. Most of the cells are mononuclear; lymphocytes usually predominate over plasma cells and histiocytes. Occasionally, follicular lymphoid hyperplasia with formation of lymphoid polyps occur. Although the lymphoid hyperplasia is usually focal and confined to the lamina propria, it may infiltrate the full thickness of the gallbladder wall. When extensive, the term *follicular cholecystitis* is used to describe this condition[50] (Fig. 58-12). A minor component of eosinophils and neutrophils may be present. When neutrophils are predominantly found within the epithelium in a setting of chronic cholecystitis, it is prefer-

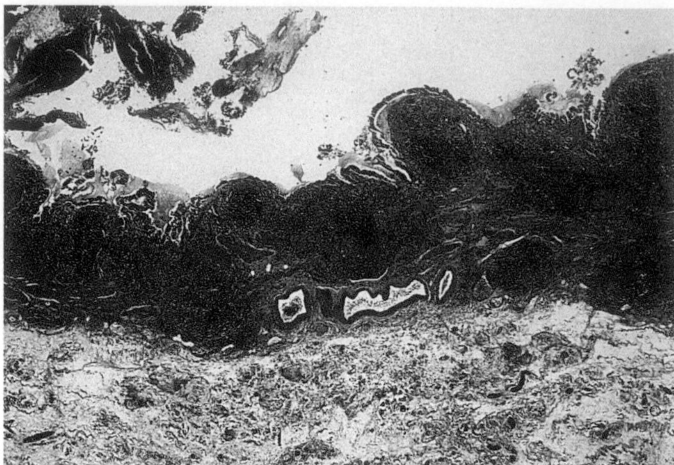

Fig. 58-12 Chronic cholecystitis. Transmural lymphocytic infiltrates are apparent. The term *follicular cholecystitis* is used when numerous lymphoid follicles expand the lamina propria, as in this case.

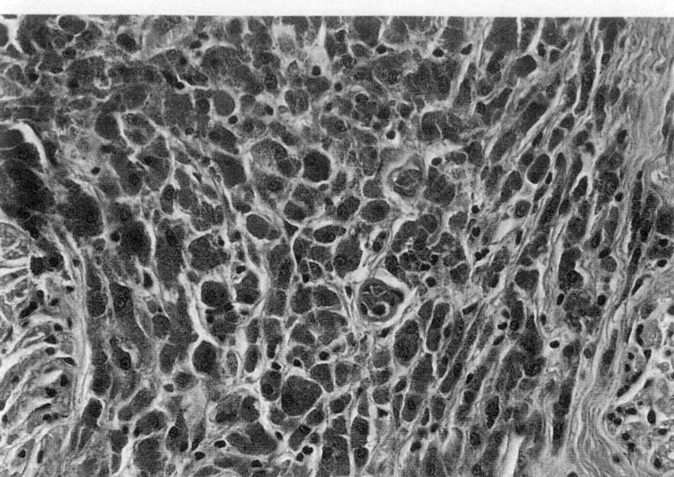

Fig. 58-14 Ceroid granulomas. These lesions are formed by aggregates of histiocytes containing intracytoplasmic dark golden brown pigment.

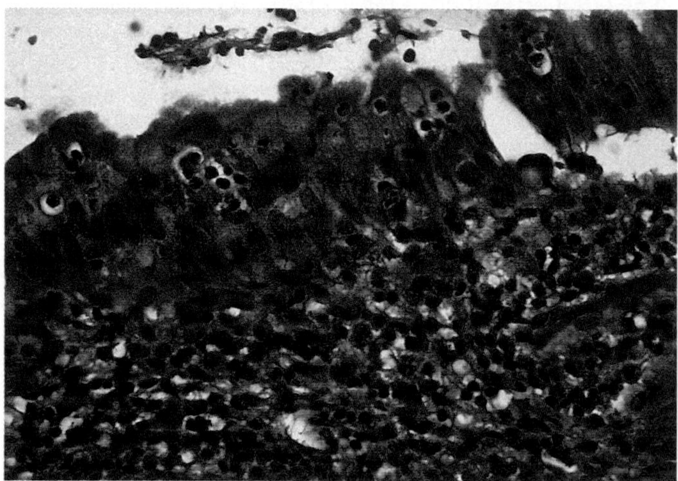

Fig. 58-13 Chronic active cholecystitis. In the setting of chronic cholecystitis, an "active" lesion is identified by neutrophilic infiltration of the biliary epithelium.

able to view them as evidence of "activity" of the inflammatory process rather than as a mixed acute and chronic or subacute condition. The term *chronic active cholecystitis* may better define these cases (Fig. 58-13).

When bile penetrates into the subepithelial layers through mucosal ulcers or fissures, it frequently elicits an inflammatory reaction composed of closely packed histiocytes with pale cytoplasm containing abundant brown pigmented granules. In addition to its color, this pigment, referred to as *ceroid*, is characterized histochemically by its acid-fastness and periodic acid-schiff (PAS) positivity, which is diastase resistant (Fig. 58-14). A sparse lymphocytic reaction usually accompanies the histiocytes.[51,52] Most importantly, ceroid granulomas trigger a reparative response leading to the deposition of dense collagen that eventually replaces those areas previously involved by the inflammatory process or even the whole gallbladder. Dystrophic calcifications within this fibrous tissue may diffusely involve the gallbladder giving rise to the so-called porcelain gallbladder[53,54] (Fig. 58-15). For unknown

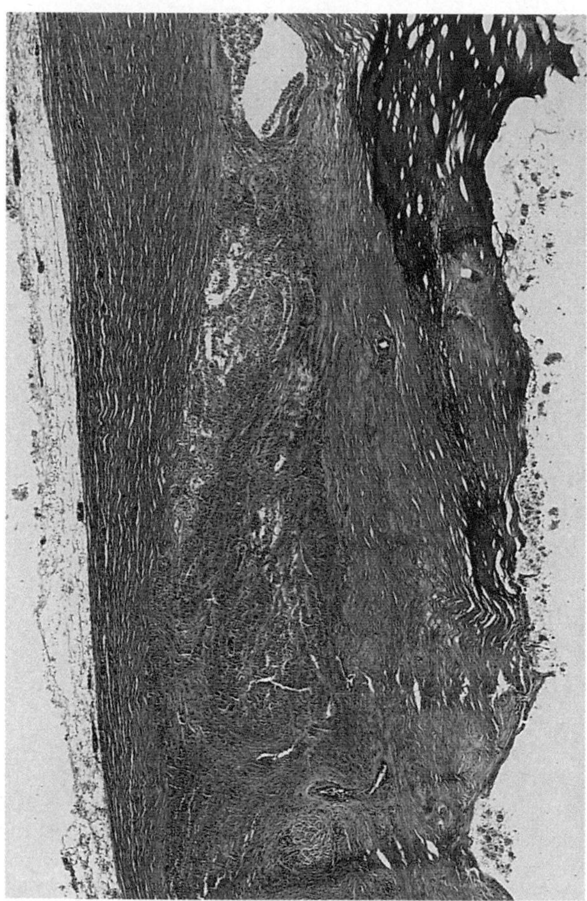

Fig. 58-15 "Porcelain" gallbladder. The mucosa and muscularis have been replaced by dense fibrous tissue with dystrophic calcifications. A ceroid granuloma is seen in the center of the lesion.

reasons, carcinoma of the gallbladder is more frequently associated with this condition than with other forms of chronic cholecystitis.[55,56] In addition to ceroid granulomas, foreign-body granulomas characterized by aggregates of multinucleated giant cells and foamy histiocytes may be seen around

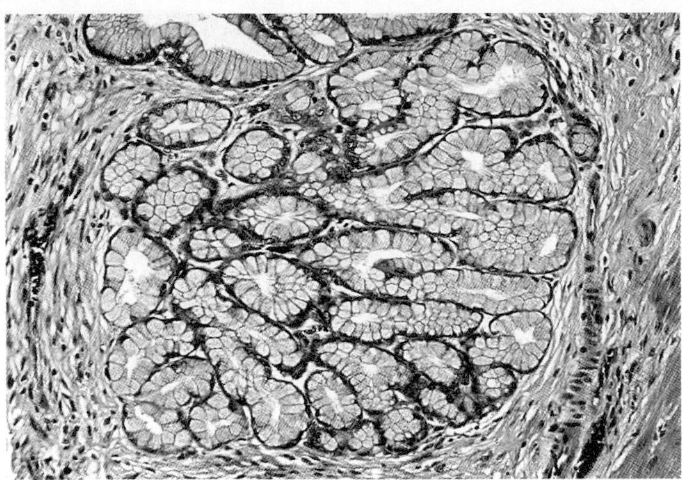

Fig. 58-16 Chronic cholecystitis with antral metaplasia. A nodule of the metaplastic pyloric type of glands is seen in the lamina propria of the gallbladder.

clefts containing cholesterol crystals or concretions of bile. Foamy histiocytes are also the predominant cells in xanthogranulomas, usually in association with plasma cells and occasional giant cells or ceroid-containing histiocytes. These cells may form tumorlike aggregates that are sometimes confused with neoplasms.[57-60]

As a result of chronic injury, metaplastic changes can result.[61,62] The most common type of metaplasia is of the antral (or pyloric) type (Fig. 58-16). It is characterized by tubular glands in the lamina propria formed by clear cells with abundant mucin vacuoles identical to those found in the gastric antrum. The surface epithelium frequently undergoes metaplasia of superficial gastric type. This change is characterized by focal or diffuse replacement of the columnar epithelium of the gallbladder by taller, mucin-rich, PAS-positive, columnar cells. Less frequently, intestinal metaplasia may occur and is identified by the appearance of cells with intestinal phenotypes, such as goblet cells, absorptive columnar cells, Paneth cells, and gut endocrine cells. Very infrequently, squamous metaplasia may be found.

Clinical features. Uncertainty still prevails as to the precise symptom complex associated with gallstone disease and chronic cholecystitis. It is probable that most persons with gallstones never experience biliary colic. The only symptom that has been proved to be related to gallstones is episodic upper abdominal pain.[63] Dyspeptic symptoms, belching, bloating, abdominal discomfort, heartburn, and food intolerances are frequently attributed both by the patients and their physicians to cholelithiasis and chronic cholecystitis. However, most of these symptoms are probably unrelated to these conditions and frequently persist after cholecystectomy. From this discussion it is apparent that it is easier to define chronic cholecystitis by its pathologic features than by clinical characteristics.

In the United States, laparoscopic cholecystectomy has become the preferred treatment for patients with cholelithiasis.[63a] This minimally invasive surgical procedure offers the advantages of shorter hospitalization, limited postoperative pain, diminished disability, and improved cosmesis.[63a,63b] In most instances, the gallbladder is easily removed through the umbilical puncture wound. Difficulties may be encountered when the gallbladder is distended by bile or gallstones and when inflammation and fibrosis give rise to a thick, noncollapsible wall. This problem is usually solved by extension of the umbilical incision or by removal of the bile and stones after the neck of the gallbladder has been pulled through the skin and amputated. Large stones can be pulverized by mechanical devises, ultrasound, or laser energy.[63c] When examining a gallbladder, the pathologist should differentiate the numerous artifacts produced by these procedures from the pathologic changes caused by the disease process.

Chronic acalculous cholecystitis

About 12% to 13% of patients with chronic cholecystitis do not have gallstones.[64] It has been suggested that postinflammatory stenosis or anatomic abnormalities of the cystic duct might impede normal emptying of the gallbladder. Such patients may pose diagnostic difficulties, since ultrasound scans and oral cholecystograms are often normal. Patients that may benefit from cholecystectomy might be identified by a cholecystokinin (CCK) provocative test. A positive test result is obtained when pain is induced 5 to 10 minutes after an intravenous injection of cholecystokinin.[65] Furthermore, incomplete emptying of the gallbladder and poor concentration can be documented when this test is performed at the same time as oral cholecystography.[66]

Histopathologic analysis of the excised gallbladders of some patients with acalculous cholecystitis show abundant eosinophils. This condition has been referred to as *lymphoeosinophilic cholecystitis* when eosinophils compose 50% to 75% of the total number of inflammatory cells and *eosinophilic cholecystitis* when the infiltrate is composed almost exclusively of eosinophils. It has been hypothesized that abnormal biliary contents or certain hepatic metabolites may evoke a hypersensitivity reaction recruiting a large number of eosinophils that cause mucosal damage and gallbladder dysmotility.[67]

A form of chronic cholecystitis has been recently identified characterized by a diffuse lymphoplasmacytic infiltrate confined to the lamina propria. Intraepithelial neutrophils (active lesions) may be seen. In the absence of gallstones, this form of chronic cholecystitis is found almost exclusively in patients with sclerosing cholangitis.

Xanthogranulomatous cholecystitis

Xanthogranulomatous cholecystitis is an uncommon form of chronic cholecystitis characterized by a focal or diffuse inflammatory process frequently accompanied by fibrosis. Its incidence is approximately 1.8% of excised gallbladders. The pathogenesis of this condition is uncertain; it has been proposed that a xanthogranulomatous reaction results from the penetration of bile into the gallbladder wall from mucosal ulcers or ruptured Rokitansky-Aschoff sinuses in conjunction with outflow obstruction by calculi and infection.[57-60] Positive bile cultures, mostly for enterobacteria, are found in about 50% of the patients.

Pathology. As mentioned before, the areas involved by the xanthogranulomatous process may appear as poorly demarcated, firm, yellow masses that resemble a carcinoma clinically and macroscopically.[58] Histologic examination shows rounded to spindle-shaped lipid-laden macrophages, plasma cells, and fibrosis. Cholesterol clefts, foreign-body giant cells, the Touton type giant cells, and other inflammatory cells (lymphocytes, eosinophils, and neutrophils) are commonly found. Quite frequently, the xanthogranulomatous reaction occupies a limited area of the gallbladder and the remainder shows "conventional" chronic cholecystitis, often with lymphoid follicles (Fig. 58-17).

Xanthogranulomatous inflammation should be differentiated from malakoplakia, which has been reported in the gallbladder.[68] The characteristic microscopic findings of malakoplakia are a diffuse proliferation of histiocytes with abundant eosinophilic granular cytoplasm, some of which contain spherules positive by PAS and von Kossa's (calcium) stains.

Clinical features. The diagnosis of xanthogranulomatous cholecystitis cannot be established on clinical grounds alone. It may be suspected when a history of at least one previous episode of acute cholecystitis is obtained. Imaging studies demonstrate, in almost all patients, a thickened wall and gallstones. Recovery after surgery is usually uneventful.

Cholecystitis in patients with AIDS

Acalculous cholecystitis has been cited in several reports as a complication of HIV infection.[69-71] Pathologic examination of the excised gallbladders has shown infection with CMV or *Cryptosporidium*. CMV infection is usually associated with mucosal ulceration and a mixed inflammatory reaction. Both nuclear and cytoplasmic inclusions are typically present in endothelial cells, mononuclear cells in the lamina propria, and occasionally epithelial cells. The cryptosporidia colonize the biliary cells and elicit an inflammatory response of variable intensity, being mild in most cases. Rare instances of infection by *Mycobacterium avium* have been reported. The diffuse histiocytic proliferation induced by this organism may mimic xanthogranulomatous cholecystitis or malakoplakia.

Cholesterolosis

Cholesterolosis is defined as the presence of aggregates of lipid-containing macrophages in the lamina propria of the gallbladder. Autopsy and surgical studies have shown a prevalence of 12% and 9% to 26% respectively.[72-74] Its etiology and pathogenesis are poorly understood. The accumulation of cholesterol esters and triglycerides may reflect an increased hepatic synthesis of these lipids or increased absorption and esterification by the gallbladder. Recall that the normal gallbladder can absorb small amounts of cholesterol from the bile. Patients with cholesterolosis, as those with cholesterol stones, have supersaturated bile; as expected, the two conditions frequently coexist. It is therefore probable that cholesterolosis results from an increased cholesterol uptake from bile containing a high concentration of this lipid. Another theory postulates the existence of a defect in macrophages that fail to metabolize or excrete the cholesterol absorbed from the bile.[74]

Pathology. On gross examination, the lipid deposits appear as yellow flecks against a dark green background, an appearance that has been called *strawberry gallbladder* because of its alleged resemblance to that fruit (though our experience with strawberries and cholesterolosis does not support this allegation) (Fig. 58-18). When extensive, these deposits may form polypoid excrescences that project into the lumen. Commonly referred to as *cholesterol polyps* but more properly called *cholesterolosis polyps*, these lesions are generally small but may be large enough to be detected by imaging techniques. Cholesterol gallstones are present in half of the surgical cholesterolosis cases and in 10% of autopsy series.

Microscopically the diagnostic feature is the accumulation of foamy macrophages within an expanded lamina propria that forms the core of a thickened fold or polyp. The adjacent mucosa is either normal or inflamed; the latter situation occurs almost exclusively in patients with coexistent stones (Fig. 58-19).

Clinical features. More than a century after its identification, uncertainty still prevails as to whether cholesterolosis is a clinically relevant condition. Some investigators have shown that cholecystectomy alleviates severe symptoms in some patients, whereas others have suggested that cholesterolosis is an inconsequential finding in patients with unexplained abdominal pain. If the prevalence of cholesterolosis derived from autopsy studies reflects the actual frequency in the general population, it is obvious that most individuals with cholesterolosis do not develop symptoms. Some studies have suggested that cholesterolosis is associated with symptoms in patients having acalculous biliary disease. Colicky abdominal pain and selective food intolerance are the most common. Most symptomatic patients that have their pain reproduced by an intravenous injection of cholecystokinin appear to normalize after cholecystectomy.[75] Recent evidence indicates a possi-

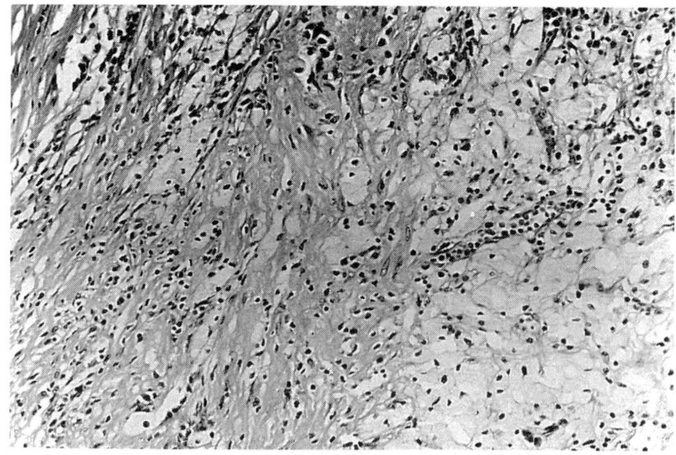

Fig. 58-17 Xanthogranulomatous cholecystitis. The characteristic inflammatory infiltrate consists of a mixture of foamy histiocytes and other inflammatory cells, mostly plasma cells and lymphocytes.

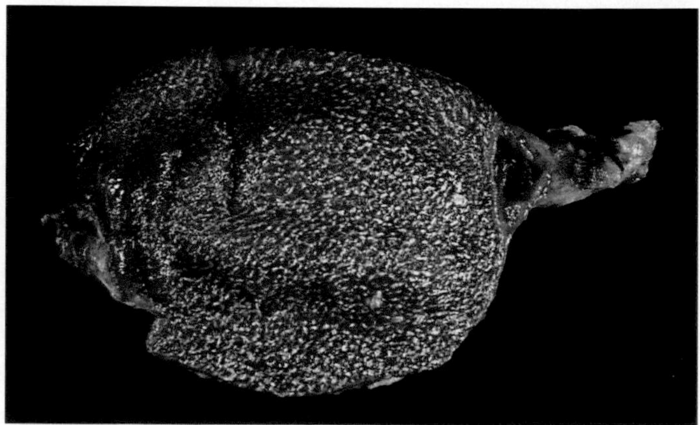

Fig. 58-18 Cholesterolosis.

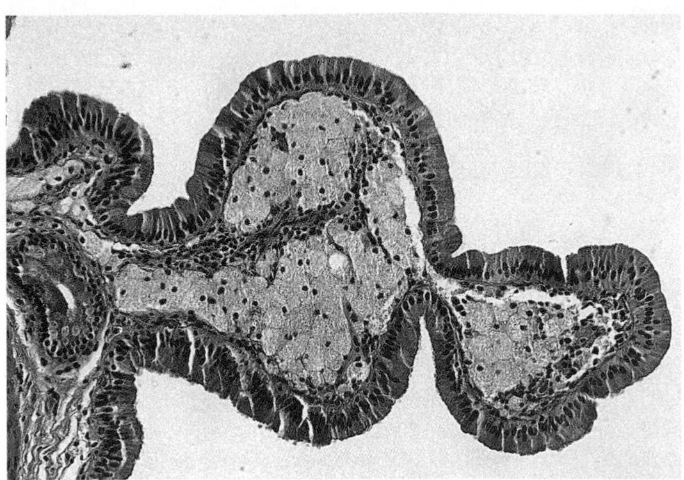

Fig. 58-19 Cholesterolosis. The lamina propria is expanded by foamy histiocytes. Other inflammatory cells are usually absent. The accumulation of this type of histiocytes does not elicit tissue damage or fibrosis.

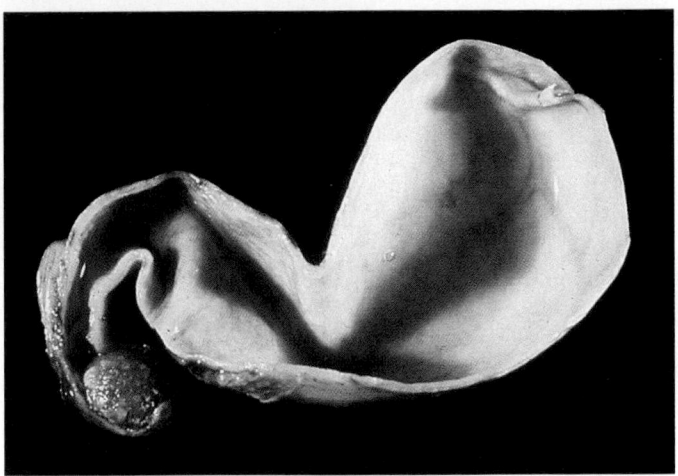

Fig. 58-20 Hydrops of the gallbladder. The dilated lumen was filled with a watery fluid. Obstructing the cystic duct is a cholesterol gallstone.

ble relationship between cholesterolosis and acute pancreatitis.[76] Temporary impaction of cholesterolosis polyps at the sphincter of Oddi producing recurrent attacks of acute pancreatitis has been postulated as the most likely event.

Other conditions affecting the gallbladder

Hydrops and mucocele

Distention of the gallbladder by a clear and watery or mucoid material has been called *hydrops* or *mucocele,* respectively, and accounts for 3% of the pathologic gallbladders in adults.[14] In this age group, the most common cause is an impacted stone in the neck of the gallbladder or cystic duct. Less frequent causes include tumors, fibrosis, or kinking of the cystic duct or external compression by inflammatory or neoplastic masses. In children it is usually an acute process associated with infectious diseases or other inflammatory disorders such as streptococcal infections, mesenteric adenitis, typhoid, leptospirosis, viral hepatitis, familial Mediterranean fever, or Kawasaki syndrome. These cases may resolve with conservative treatment.[14,76]

Pathology. The gallbladder is considerably distended and may contain over 1500 ml of fluid. When associated with numerous stones, the wall is usually thickened. By contrast, a thin wall is the rule when a single stone obstructs the cystic duct or in acute cases of childhood (Fig. 58-20). Microscopic examination usually reveals a flattened mucosa lined by low columnar or cuboidal cells. As a result of increased intraluminal pressure, Rokitansky-Aschoff sinuses may be plentiful. The amount of inflammatory cells varies from sparse to abundant. An acute cholecystitis with edema of the lamina propria and abundant neutrophils occurs in some patients with Kawasaki syndrome.[76]

Diverticula

Congenital and traction diverticula are the two types of "true" diverticula that occur in the gallbladder. The congenital lesions have been discussed previously. They are differentiated from the more common acquired pseudodiverticula by the constituents of their wall: the former have all the elements of the normal wall while the latter usually have little or no smooth muscle. The walls of traction diverticula are also composed of all the elements. These diverticula are caused by the pulling action of postinflammatory fibrous adhesions anchoring the serosa of the gallbladder to adjacent structures. Erosion by stones, healing fistulas, widespread peritonitis of any cause, or previous intra-abdominal surgery precede their formation. Traction diverticula are distinguished from congenital outpouchings mainly by their relationship with intra-abdominal lesions in the vicinity of the gallbladder and by the predominance of the inflammatory and fibrosing changes in the external layers rather than in the mucosa. In some cases, this distinction may be impossible.

Acquired pseudodiverticula are mucosal herniations between the smooth muscle bundles of the wall and should be regarded as prominent Rokitansky-Aschoff sinuses. Almost invariably, these pulsion diverticula are associated with stones and chronic cholecystitis or with outflow obstruction. Similar to diverticular disease of the colon, the intervening smooth muscle is usually hypertrophied. The mucosal outpouchings and the prominent muscle may form a localized tumorlike lesion that has been referred to as *adenomyoma* or may diffusely thicken the gallbladder, a condition known as *adenomyomatosis,* or *cholecystitis glandularis proliferans.*[77,78]

Ischemic diseases

Deprivation of arterial blood flow or obstruction to venous drainage may result in infarction of the gallbladder. As mentioned previously, the gallbladder is supplied by the cystic artery, which in most cases originates from the right hepatic artery. The latter is a branch of the celiac artery. Venous blood is carried though small veins that drain into the liver. Atherosclerosis and its common complication, thrombosis, is the usual cause of obliteration of the arterial blood flow. Embolic occlusion may occur as a complication of valvular heart disease or bacterial endocarditis. Another cause may be a dissecting aneurysm extending into the celiac artery with occlusion of the site of origin of the hepatic artery. External compression of the arteries or interference with venous drainage may result from impingement on these vessels by stones, tumors, or occlusion by iatrogenic ligation.[79-80]

As a consequence of abnormal mobility, the gallbladder may twist on its pedicle, a condition known as *torsion*, or *volvulus*. As mentioned previously (see the discussion of congenital abnormalities), this condition may result when the gallbladder is completely surrounded by peritoneum without a firm attachment to the liver. Torsion may also result from loosening of the connective tissue with aging or shrinkage of a cirrhotic liver leading to detachment of the gallbladder from its bed and visceroptosis.[14]

Uncommonly, ischemic lesions result from vasculitis. Among the primary vascular diseases that may involve the gallbladder, polyarteritis nodosa appears to be the most frequent.[81] Other forms of vasculitis that affect this organ include allergic granulomatosis (Churg and Strauss), rheumatoid vasculitis, and a form of small-vessel vasculitis restricted to the gallbladder known as *localized or focal visceral angiitis*. Lymphocytic venulitis and acalculous chronic cholecystitis may be seen in patients with sarcoidosis. Secondary vasculitis frequently occurs in patients with calculous cholecystitis.

Pathology. The gallbladder wall is thickened, and the mucosa is congested or hemorrhagic. Microscopic examination reveals partial or complete loss of the epithelium, edema, or hemorrhage in the lamina propria. When occlusion to venous outflow predominates, there is extensive, often transmural, hemorrhagic infarction. Ischemic lesions associated with primary vasculitis are often focal and confined to the mucosa. In patients with calculous cholecystitis, superimposed ischemic damage caused by secondary vasculitis or small vessel thrombosis is frequently found. Healed ischemic lesions are at least partially responsible for the deposition of fibrous tissue in so-called sclerosing cholecystitis.

Clinical features. Most of the cases occur in patients older than 60 years. The preoperative clinical diagnosis is rarely made, since the symptoms mimic those of acute cholecystitis.

Trauma

The gallbladder is seldom damaged from abdominal trauma, since it is partially protected by the ribs and liver. Blunt abdominal trauma can disrupt a distended gallbladder causing contusion, laceration, avulsion, or intraluminal hemorrhage.[82] Penetrating wounds may damage the gallbladder, usually in association with injury to the adjacent organs. Iatrogenic injury can result from needles used for liver biopsy or percutaneous transhepatic cholangiography. An acute cholecystitis with mucosal necrosis followed by fibrosis may occur as a result of repeated infusion of chemotherapeutic agents through a catheter placed in the hepatic artery for the treatment of liver metastasis.[83]

Biliary fistulas

In most cases, fistulas between the biliary tract and adjacent hollow organs are a consequence of gallstone-associated necrosis and inflammation of the gallbladder or bile ducts. Inflammatory adhesions precede their formation; these lesions may form masses that could be confused with a fixed inoperable tumor. A classical cholecystectomy in the presence of fistulas carries a high risk of injury to the bile ducts. The most common fistulas are cholecystoduodenal, followed by cholecystocolic and choledochoduodenal fistulas.[14] Biliobiliary fistulas form between the gallbladder and the common bile duct. This complication should be suspected in patients with cholelithiasis and jaundice.[84]

NONNEOPLASTIC DISEASES OF EXTRAHEPATIC BILE DUCTS

Cholangitis

The inflammatory diseases of the bile ducts are collectively referred to as cholangitis. A clinically relevant classification groups these disorders as simple obstructive cholangitis, recurrent cholangitis syndromes, and primary sclerosing cholangitis.

Simple obstructive cholangitis

In Western countries obstructive cholangitis is the most common type.[85] The conditions that may cause biliary obstruction include choledocholithiasis, bile-duct cysts and diverticula, tumors, fistulas, extrinsic processes such as pancreatic tumors, chronic pancreatitis, ampullary lesions, cystic duct gallstones (Mirizzi's syndrome), and scarring from previous surgical procedures.[86]

Choledocholithiasis is the most frequent cause of obstruction. In Western countries, most of the stones are cholesterol calculi that originate in the gallbladder and migrate into the bile ducts. Approximately 15% of patients with cholelithiasis have stones within the bile ducts. As previously discussed, those that form primarily within the bile ducts are pigment stones.

It seems that obstruction alone does not produce cholangitis. In addition, it has been shown in animal models that bacterial colonization does not necessary result in cholangitis. In humans, colonization of the biliary tract by enteric bacteria has been demonstrated even in patients without biliary disease. Inflammatory lesions of bile ducts are most probably produced by the concerted action of partial or complete obstruction, biliary stasis, and bacterial proliferation. The organisms most commonly found are enteric bacteria such as *Escherichia coli, Streptococcus faecalis, Clostridium, Klebsiella, Enterobacter, Pseudomonas, and Proteus*.[87] The route by which bacteria colonize the biliary system remains unknown. Contamination from an infected gallbladder, duodenal reflux, and lymphatic, hepatic arterial, or portal venous bacteremia have been proposed. Strong support for portal bacteremia has been obtain from animal experiments and could account for the predominance of enteric bacteria. However, portal bacteremia in humans appears to be very rare.

Pathology. In acute cholangitis the extrahepatic bile ducts show edema and a predominantly neutrophilic infiltrate in the lamina propria that focally infiltrates the epithelium. Degenerative and regenerative epithelial changes, ulcers, and erosions are also seen. Involvement of the intrahepatic biliary system, referred to as ascending cholangitis, occurs in the majority of the cases.

Clinical features. The classic clinical symptoms associated with acute obstructive cholangitis are known as *Charcot's triad* and consist of intermittent abdominal pain, fever, and jaundice. Its complete form is manifested in 20% to 70% of the cases. Most patients have leukocytosis and abnormal liver function tests, mainly hyperbilirubinemia with elevated alkaline phosphatase and aminotransferases not exceeding 500 IU/L. Serum amylase is increased in 40% of the patients and does not necessarily indicate concomitant pancreatitis. Blood cultures positive for multiple enteric organism should be suggestive of biliary sepsis.

A few unfortunate patients develop a severe form of illness with a high mortality known as *acute suppurative* or *toxic cholangitis*. The typical symptoms associated with this condition constitute Reynolds' pentad and manifest as abdominal pain, fever, jaundice, shock, and delirium. The risk for progression to toxic cholangitis is apparently increased in patients who failed to respond to initial antibiotic management and in those with congenital or malignant obstructions.

Acute renal failure and intrahepatic abscesses are the two most common complications of acute cholangitis. Renal failure is believed to be attributable to hypoperfusion from sepsis, endotoxemia, and tubular injury from bile pigments.[88-92]

Recurrent pyogenic cholangitis

The syndrome recurrent pyogenic cholangitis, also known as *oriental cholangiohepatitis*, *intrahepatic pigment-stone disease*, and *biliary obstruction syndrome of the Chinese* is characterized by recurrent abdominal pain, fever, chills, and jaundice.[93] The bile ducts show dilated and stenotic segments, fibrosis, inflammatory cells, and pigment stones. First described in the Chinese population in Hong Kong, it is now recognized as a serious health problem in China, Taiwan, Japan, Korea, Singapore, Vietnam, Malaysia, and the Philippines.[94] Sporadic cases have been reported in Europe and South Africa. In the United States and Canada, the disease is largely limited to Asian immigrants.[95]

The cause of this disease is unknown. The two most popular theories attribute the cause to parasites and malnutrition. The former postulates that the inflammatory and fibrosing changes are secondary to chronic infestation of the biliary tree with endemic parasites such as *Clonorchis sinensis*, now known as *Opisthorchis sinensis*, and *Ascaris lumbricoides*. Initially, bile flow is hampered by adult flukes or eggs. Stagnation leads to secondary bacterial infection, pigment stone formation, and pyogenic cholangitis.[96] In support of this theory is the observation that the stones frequently contain ova or fragments of parasites. However, patients with recurrent cholangitis have only a slightly higher rate of infestation by *O. sinensis* than the general population in endemic areas. In these countries, numerous individuals are infected with liver flukes without ever developing cholangitis. In other areas where the parasitic infection is less common, such as Japan, no conclusive association has been demonstrated.[97]

The second theory postulates that recurrent infectious gastroenteritis in malnourished people causes frequent episodes of portal bacteremia. As discussed before, the synergistic action of obstruction plus infection are required for the development of cholangitis. This theory would explain the much higher incidence of the disease in patients from a low socioeconomic class.[98]

Pathology. The main pathologic changes are located in the intrahepatic and extrahepatic bile ducts. An enlarged, irregularly scarred liver with capsular adhesions is the usual appearance, but after multiple attacks it may become shrunken, especially the lateral segment of the left lobe. The intrahepatic bile ducts show alternating areas of stricture and dilatation. An unusual feature is the abrupt tapering toward the periphery of the dilated segments; this contrasts with the diffuse dilatation seen in patients with other causes of obstruction. Within the lumen, pigment stones and secretions are usually found. In most cases, the extrahepatic ducts are not stenotic except for the most distal segment where repeated passage of stones through the sphincter of Oddi may cause postinflammatory strictures. The dilated segments are not strictly related to the location of the stones.[93] Bile duct stones are present in 75% to 80% of cases and gallstones in about 50% to 70%.

Histologically the portal tracts show the characteristic cluster of changes of bile duct obstruction: proliferation of bile ducts, inflammatory cells, mainly neutrophils, and variable edema. Periductal fibrosis is frequently present. Histologic changes in the extrahepatic ducts include a predominantly neutrophilic infiltrate and fibrosis, with epithelial changes ranging from loss of cells to adenomatous hyperplasia.

Cholangiocarcinoma develops in 2.4% to 4.9% of patients with recurrent pyogenic cholangitis.[99,100] It has been suggested that continuous epithelial injury caused by chronic infection and inflammation, or resulting from mechanical irritation by stones, may lead to the sequence of adenomatous hyperplasia to dysplasia to cholangiocarcinoma.[101]

Clinical features. Most of the cases occur in persons 20 to 40 years of age; there is no sex predilection. As mentioned before, there is a strong association with lower socioeconomic class. A history of recurrent attacks is frequent. These are characterized by abdominal pain, nausea, vomiting, fever, shaking chills, and jaundice. The findings on physical examination include epigastric tenderness and rigidity, enlargement of the liver, and a palpable gallbladder. Laboratory findings include leukocytosis and an elevated alkaline phosphatase. Most of the patients have positive bile cultures for enteric bacteria. Various imaging studies have been used to demonstrate the presence of stones and dilated biliary ducts.[93]

Primary sclerosing cholangitis

Primary sclerosing cholangitis (PSC) is an idiopathic, rare disorder characterized by chronic, fibrosing inflammation of the intrahepatic and extrahepatic bile ducts.[102] This disorder occurs primarily in young men and is clinically characterized by gradual onset of progressive fatigue and pruritus followed by jaundice with slow progression to cirrhosis. A cholestatic biochemical profile is usually present. Between 50% to 70% of the cases are associated with inflammatory bowel disease, mainly ulcerative colitis.[102,103] Recent evidence that indicates the probable participation of immune mechanisms in its pathogenesis include an increased prevalence of HLA-B8, HLA-DR3, and HLA-DRw52a haplotypes, an aberrant expression of HLA-DR antigen in intrahepatic bile ducts, an increased CD4/CD8 ratio of circulating and portal tract T-lymphocytes, a defective suppressor T-cell function, peripheral blood lymphocytes sensitized to bile antigens, and the recent demonstration of cytoplasmic and nuclear antineutrophil antibodies. Whether some of these findings have direct pathogenic importance remains to be determined.[104-107]

Pathology. The extrahepatic ducts may appear as "fibrous cords." Strictures involving segments of bile ducts of variable length are distributed throughout the intrahepatic and extrahepatic bile ducts. A feature that is better demonstrated by cholangiograms than by gross examination is the presence of alternating areas of stricture and normal or slightly dilated ducts, producing a characteristic "beaded" appearance. About one fourth of the cases show diverticulum-like outpouchings. Microscopic examination of the extrahepatic bile ducts reveals a diffuse and dense inflammatory infiltrate composed predominantly of lymphocytes and plasma cells with ulceration of the epithelium and disruption of the muscular wall.

Neutrophils may be found in the lumen and infiltrating the epithelial cells but usually not within the wall, a differentiating feature from suppurative cholangitis. In more advanced lesions, dense fibrosis may predominate with entrapment of the periluminal glands. The architectural distortion of these glands coupled with the reactive cytologic atypia of the lining cells may closely simulate an infiltrating adenocarcinoma[108-110] (Fig. 58-21).

The gallbladder is almost always inflamed.[109-113] A form of cholecystitis frequently associated with PSC is characterized by a diffuse subepithelial infiltrate composed predominantly of plasma cells and lymphocytes. The muscularis is usually spared. In the absence of gallstones, these histologic features are almost exclusively seen in PSC.[113] Involvement of pancreatic ducts with associated acinar pancreatitis may occur.

Clinical Features. As mentioned before, most patients are male and under 45 years of age. More than half have a history of inflammatory bowel disease, usually ulcerative colitis and much less commonly Crohn's disease. Less commonly associated diseases include thyroiditis, pancreatitis, the sicca syndrome, retroperitoneal and mediastinal fibrosis, pseudotumor of the orbit, sarcoidosis, histiocytosis X, Peyronie's disease, angioblastic lymphadenopathy, Weber-Christian disease, rheumatoid arthritis, autoimmune hemolytic anemia, and immunodeficiency syndromes. Patients with PSC have a variable clinical course: some evolve rapidly to liver failure, whereas others are asymptomatic for many years. Typically the symptoms appear insidiously, the most frequent being fatigue, pruritus, and jaundice. Right upper quadrant pain and fever are also common. Liver-function tests reveal a cholestatic profile. The alkaline phosphatase is always elevated, but the levels can fluctuate. Serum aminotransferase and bilirubin levels are elevated. There are no consistent serologic markers useful in the diagnosis of this disorder. Cholangiographic examination demonstrates multifocal strictures involving the intrahepatic and extrahepatic ducts. As mentioned before, the strictures are typically short and annular, alternating with normal or dilated segments producing the characteristic "beaded" appearance. The strictures may be associated with outpouchings resembling diverticula.

The natural history of PSC has not been clearly defined. It appears to be a progressive disease with considerable morbidity and mortality, with an average survival of 6 years after symptoms develop. At present no effective medical treatment is available. Liver transplantation is currently offered to patients with end-stage disease.[110,114,115]

Long-standing PSC is a risk factor for cholangiocarcinoma. The development of this tumor is analogous to the increased frequency of colonic adenocarcinomas in patients with ulcerative colitis and is possibly related to the chronic inflammatory process with continuous damage and regeneration of the biliary epithelium. PSC may also be a risk factor for hepatocellular carcinoma just as other forms of cirrhosis constitute a risk factor.[116]

Parasitic infections

Opisthorchis sinensis (Clonorchis sinensis)

It is estimated that 19,000,000 persons worldwide are infected with *Opisthorchis sinensis (Clonorchis sinensis),* mainly those living in the Far East.[117] Routine stool screening of Chinese immigrants to the United States has demonstrated active infection in 25%.[118] The infection is acquired by eating raw fresh-

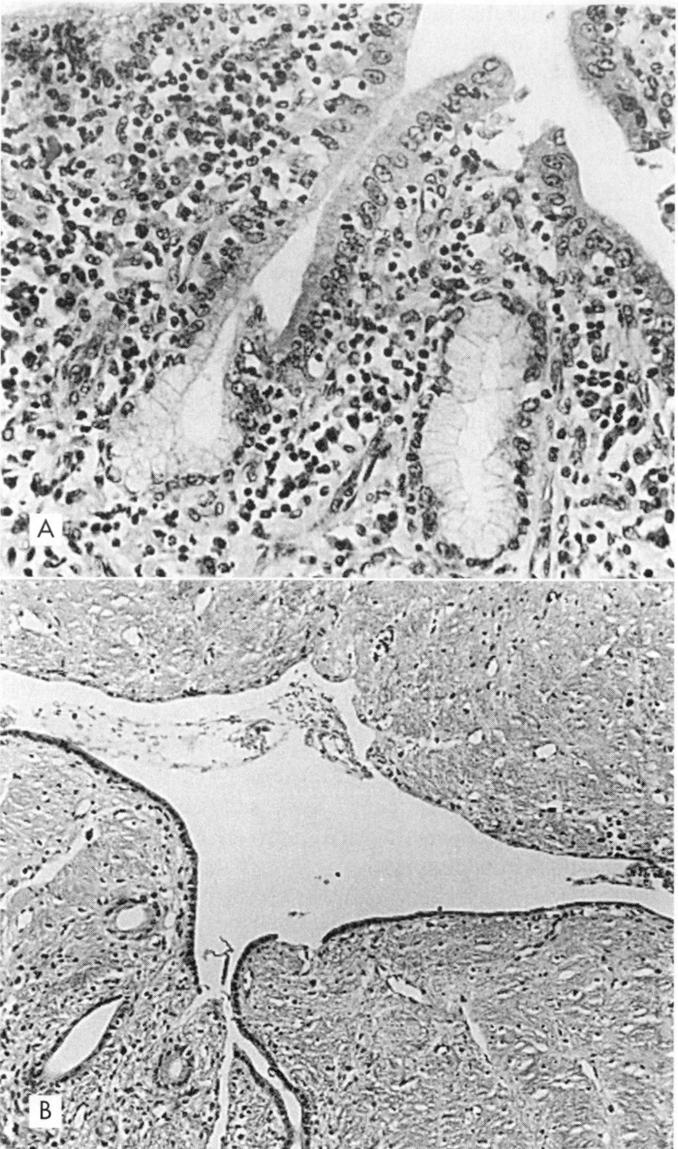

Fig. 58-21 Primary sclerosing cholangitis. Luminal obstruction is secondary to ductal inflammation, **A,** or fibrosis, **B.**

water fish infected with the metacercariae of this parasite. In humans it leads to the formation of immature flukes that ascend from the duodenum into the biliary tree where they mature. Since the flukes have a long life-span, infected persons can harbor them for decades.

Symptoms are related to the fluke burden. Persons with fewer than 100 flukes are usually asymptomatic, whereas those with 100 to 1000 flukes have anorexia, nausea, epigastric pain, and diarrhea. A higher fluke load is accompanied by biliary colic and right upper quadrant tenderness.[117] On cholangiographic studies, the presence of wavy, filamentous filling defects in the bile ducts is pathognomonic for clonorchiasis.[119]

The pathologic findings in patients with *O. sinensis* infection vary. Since the parasite does not invade the bile ducts, little inflammatory response is elicited. Initially the biliary mucosa is edematous with intact or desquamating epithelium. With persistent infection, the epithelium undergoes mucinous metaplasia and becomes hyperplastic. Periductal fibrosis is the hallmark of long-standing infections. At this stage, it is common for organisms to be absent and for mucinous metaplasia to decrease. Uncomplicated lesions contain few or no inflammatory cells. When complicated by pyogenic cholangitis, a heavy neutrophilic response is always present and is suggestive of bacterial superinfection. The most common bacterium in this setting is *E. coli*. As a result of disruption of the eggs by the inflammatory cells, granulomas rich in eosinophils may form.

Ascaris lumbricoides

Adult worms of *Ascaris lumbricoides* may migrate from the intestine into the biliary tree producing biliary obstruction. As with *O. sinensis*, bacterial superinfection may lead to recurrent pyogenic cholangitis. The worms are easily visualized by imaging techniques such as cholangiograms and ultrasound studies.[120]

Fasciola hepatica

Fasciola hepatica is another parasite that can produce biliary obstruction, cholangitis, and rarely cholecystitis. The infection occurs more frequently in Europe, Asia, Africa, and South America and is acquired by the ingestion of water plants containing encysted metacercariae. In the duodenum, the metacercariae excyst, migrate through the wall of the intestine, penetrate Glisson's capsule, burrow through the parenchyma of the liver, and invade the bile ducts and occasionally the gallbladder. In the acute phase an inflammatory infiltrate rich in eosinophils may be seen, followed by regenerative hyperplasia of the bile duct epithelium, and fibrosis.[102]

AIDS-related lesions

Several bile duct lesions unrelated to gallstones, malignant disease, or previous surgery, collectively called HIV-associated cholangiopathy, have been recognized in patients with HIV infection. These include papillary stenosis, a sclerosing cholangitis-like disorder, a combination of both, and long extrahepatic bile duct strictures.[121-125]

Pathology. The extrahepatic bile ducts in most cases show mixed inflammatory infiltrates, fibrosis, and usually no identifiable organisms. When present, they usually are CMV or *Cryptosporidium,* the microsporidia species *Enterocytozoon bieneusi,* and rarely *Mycobacterium avium.* In the liver, the portal tracts show increased fibrous tissue and sparse lymphocytic inflammation. The interlobular bile ducts are either absent or show degenerative epithelial changes. Inflammatory cells are characteristically sparse.

Clinical features. Patients with HIV-associated cholangiopathy present with right upper quadrant or epigastric pain and fever. Most have an elevated serum alkaline phosphatase, but only 15% have elevated bilirubin levels. Endoscopic retrograde cholangiopancreatography frequently demonstrates ductal irregularities and a "beaded" appearance. In patients with papillary stenosis, endoscopic sphincterotomy is followed by a great relief of pain. However, because of ongoing intrahepatic duct disease, serum alkaline phosphatase levels continue to increase.

The cause of HIV-associated cholangiopathy remains to be determined. Some of the cases may be related to either CMV or *Cryptosporidium* infection. However, by itself, *Cryptosporidium* is an unlikely candidate, since it usually elicits a very mild inflammatory response (Fig. 58-22). The histologic changes associated with CMV infection vary from mild to severe. Interestingly, in the neonate this organism may infect bile duct epithelium and cause obliterative cholangitis and paucity of bile ducts. In addition, its propensity to infect endothelial cells may induce vasculitis and ischemic damage.[126] Recently, it has been demonstrated that infection of the biliary tract with *Enterocytozoon bieneusi* is associated with and may be a cause of AIDS-related cholangitis.[125] The altered immune status of HIV-infected patients may well contribute to the pathogenesis of bile duct damage as happens in some patients with congenital immunodeficiencies. In addition, it has been proposed that persistent portal bacteremia in HIV-infected patients with enteric infections may invoke an ulcerative colitis-like ductal sclerosis.

Nonneoplastic biliary strictures

Nonneoplastic biliary strictures most frequently result from either iatrogenic injury or a blunt or penetrating abdominal trauma. More than 80% of bile duct strictures occur after cholecystectomy. The incidence of this complication is roughly 2 per 1000 operations. Inadvertent damage of the bile ducts may occur as a result of failure to recognize unexpected anatomic variations or poor visualization because of encasement of the ducts by an abscess or fibrous tissue. Attempts to gain hemostasis when bleeding from the cystic or hepatic arteries occurs may lead to bile duct injury. Even in expert hands, extreme friability of acutely inflamed tissues makes dissection of the Calot's triangle a formidable task. A classical cholecystectomy in the presence of a biliobiliary fistula carries

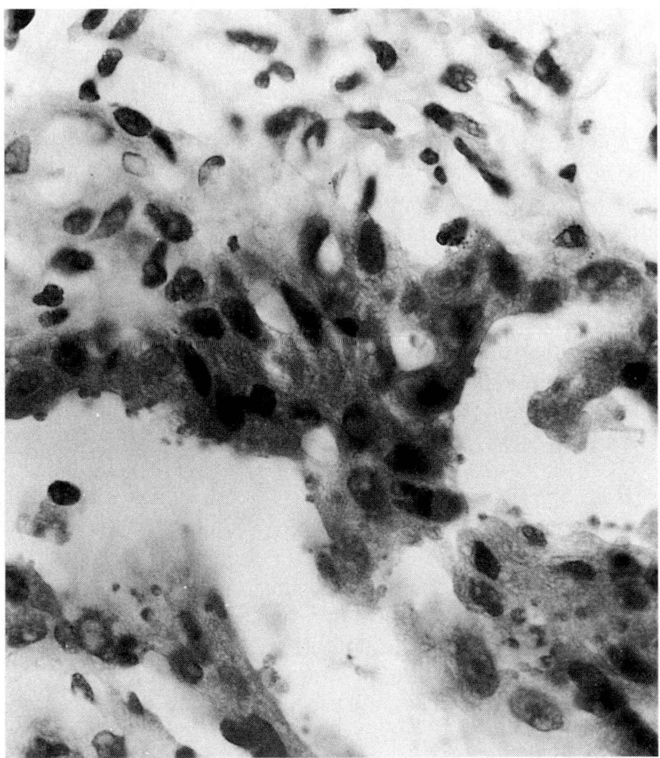

Fig. 58-22 Cryptosporidiosis. An endoscopic biopsy specimen of the distal common bile duct in a 27-year-old HIV-positive male patient revealed numerous extracellular round organisms consistent with *Cryptosporidium.*

Table 58-3 Bile duct strictures

Type	Location of stricture	Incidence (%)	Successful outcome after surgical repair (%)
1	Low CHD or CBD (CHD > 2 cm)	18 - 26	100
2	Mid CHD (CHD < 2 cm)	27 - 38	59
3	Hilar	20 - 33	87
4	Destruction of hilar	14 - 16	71
5	Right hepatic branch alone or with CHD	0 - 7	33

Modified from Lillemoe KD, Pitt HA, Cameron JL: *Surg Clin North Am* 70:1355, 1990.
CHD, Common hepatic duct; *CBD,* common bile duct

a high risk of injury to the right or the common hepatic duct. The importance of ischemia in the formation of postoperative strictures has been recently emphasized. Damage to the vessels that nourish the bile ducts may result in ischemic necrosis and fibrous occlusion of the ducts.

Other conditions that affect the biliopancreatoduodenal area that may give rise to postinflammatory bile duct strictures include subhepatic abscesses, chronic duodenal ulcers, chronic pancreatitis, and granulomatous lymphadenitis.

The location of the stricture is essential in planning the type of surgical repair and predicting the outcome. This information is summarized in Table 58-3.[127,128]

NEOPLASMS

Although the gallbladder and extrahepatic bile ducts have a simple histologic structure, they give rise to a wide variety of neoplasms. In fact the morphologic spectrum of both benign and malignant epithelial tumors of the extrahepatic biliary tract is as broad as that of tumors of the intestine. The histologic classification of tumors of the gallbladder and extrahepatic bile ducts we endorse is that proposed by the World Health Organization,[129] which appears in Table 58-4. This classification is based primarily on the microscopic characteristics and histologic patterns of the tumors as seen by conventional light microscopy and not on histogenesis.

Benign tumors

Adenoma of the gallbladder

Adenomas of the gallbladder are uncommon benign neoplasms of glandular epithelium that are typically polypoid and well demarcated. They are found in 0.3% to 0.5% of gallbladders removed for cholelithiasis or chronic cholecystitis.[130] Some investigators have reported an incidence of 10% to 12% in cholecystectomy specimens but have included some other tumorlike lesions such as adenomas. The malignant potential of adenomas has been the source of controversy. Some authors believe that most carcinomas of the gallbladder and extrahepatic bile ducts arise from preexisting adenomas because they have identified presumed remnants of adenomas in nearly all carcinomas.[131] In our experience, however, adenocarcinomas of the gallbladder often show a

Table 58-4 Histologic classification of tumors of the gallbladder and extrahepatic bile ducts

Epithelial tumors
Benign
Adenoma
Tubular
Papillary
Tubulopapillary
Cystadenoma
Papillomatosis (adenomatosis)
Dysplasia
Malignant
Carcinoma in situ
Adenocarcinoma
Papillary adenocarcinoma
Adenocarcinoma, intestinal type
Mucinous adenocarcinoma
Clear cell adenocarcinoma
Signet-ring cell carcinoma
Adenosquamous carcinoma
Squamous cell carcinoma
Small cell carcinoma (oat cell carcinoma)
Undifferentiated carcinoma
Endocrine tumors
Carcinoid tumor
Mixed carcinoid-adenocarcinoma
Paraganglioma
Nonepithelial tumors
Benign
Granular cell tumor
Leiomyoma
Lipoma
Hemangioma
Lymphangioma
Neurofibroma
Ganglioneurofibromatosis
Neurofibromatosis
Malignant
Rhabdomyosarcoma
Kaposi's sarcoma
Leiomyosarcoma
Malignant fibrous histiocytoma
Angiosarcoma
Miscellaneous tumors
Carcinosarcoma
Malignant melanoma
Malignant lymphomas
Unclassified tumors
Secondary tumors
Tumorlike lesions
Regenerative epithelial atypia
Papillary hyperplasia
Adenomyomatous hyperplasia
Intestinal metaplasia
Pyloric gland metaplasia
Squamous metaplasia
Heterotopias
Xanthogranulomatous cholecystitis
Cholecystitis with lymphoid hyperplasia
Inflammatory polyp
Cholesterol polyp
Malakoplakia
Congenital cyst
Amputation neuroma
Primary sclerosing cholangitis

broad spectrum of cytologic abnormalities that range from minimal nuclear atypia to overt malignant changes. The areas with minimal atypia may be interpreted as remnants of an adenoma. Likewise, hyperplasia of the pyloric type of glands often found in the vicinity of carcinomas can be confused with adenomas.[130] In a series of 32 adenomas only 2 progressed to invasive adenocarcinoma.[132] Studies of in situ and small invasive carcinomas of the gallbladder have shown that only few contain remnants of preexisting adenomas (5% in one series, 13% in another).[132,133] Moreover, the prevalence of adenoma is not high in geographic areas where cholelithiasis is endemic, as has been documented with carcinoma. In fact, adenomas are much less common than carcinomas, making unlikely the assertion that the adenoma-carcinoma sequence is the usual route for the development of invasive carcinoma.

Clinical features. Adenomas of the gallbladder are more common in women than in men. In our series of 37 patients, 26 were females (70%). The age of the patients range from 17 to 79 years with a mean of 58 years. Only rarely gallbladder adenomas occur in children.[134] These benign tumors are often small, asymptomatic, and usually discovered incidentally during cholecystectomy. However, when they arise in the neck and are able to block the flow of bile, producing gallbladder distention, when larger than 2 cm, or when multiple and filling the gallbladder lumen, they can produce symptoms similar to those of chronic cholecystitis. Some can be seen as fixed radiolucent defects on cholecystograms; the majority are now recognized by ultrasound or CT scan. Occasionally adenomas of the gallbladder occur in association with Gardner's syndrome[135] or with Peutz-Jeghers syndrome.[136,137] Adenomas of the gallbladder have also been reported in patients with an anomalous pancreatobiliary duct union.[138] Whether this association is coincidental or has a casual relationship is not yet known. The suggestion has been made that regurgitation of pancreatic juice leads to inflammation, metaplasia, and adenoma formation. If this hypothesis is correct, one would expect to find adenomas in the extrahepatic bile ducts in addition to the gallbladder, an association that to our knowledge has not been documented.

Pathology. Adenomas of the gallbladder are usually solitary, either pedunculated or sessile, and as a rule measure less than 2 cm in diameter.[139,140] They are most commonly located in the body, followed in frequency by the fundus and neck. Approximately 10% are multiple.[141] When multiple they may fill the entire gallbladder lumen.[132] According to different series from 50% to 65% of adenomas are associated with cholelithiasis.

A tubular adenoma initially appears as a soft, nodular pink elevation on the mucosa. As the lesion enlarges, it projects into the lumen. At this stage the adenoma resembles a lobulated berrylike nodule similar to the tubular adenomas of the large intestine. Papillary adenomas exhibit the typical cauliflower-like appearance with a fine granular surface.

According to their growth pattern, adenomas of the extrahepatic biliary tree are divided into three types: tubular, papillary, and tubulopapillary. Cytologically they are classified into pyloric gland type, intestinal type, and biliary type.

Tubular adenoma, pyloric gland type

Pathology. The tubular adenoma of the pyloric gland type is a benign tumor composed of closely packed short tubular glands, similar to pyloric glands lined by dysplastic epithelium. In its early phase of development the pyloric gland type of tubular adenomas appears as well-demarcated nodules embedded in the lamina propria and covered by normal biliary epithelium. (Fig. 58-23). They are composed of closely packed pyloric type glands, some of which appear cystically dilated (Fig. 58-24). The glands, which form lobules, are lined by columnar or cuboidal cells with vesicular or hyperchromatic nuclei and small nucleoli. A variable amount of cytoplasmic mucin is present. Dysplastic changes are more pronounced in larger adenomas. Foci of carcinoma in situ are present in approximately 9% of the adenomas and invasive adenocarcinoma in 7%. Nodular aggregates of cytologically bland spindle cells with eosinophilic cytoplasm but without keratinization or intercellular bridges known as squamoid morules are present in about 10% of the cases, whereas frank squamous metaplasia is exceedingly rare.[132,142] Approximately 20% of the tumors contain Paneth cells as well as a population of endocrine cells. By immunohistochemistry serotonin and a variety of peptide hormones, including somatostatin, pancre-

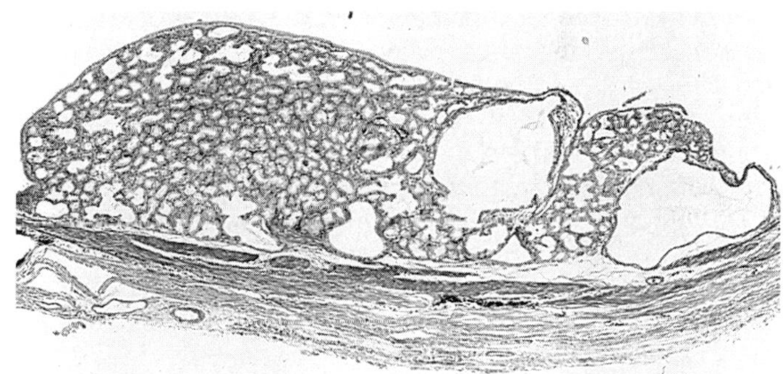

Fig. 58-23 Tubular adenoma of the pyloric gland type. Well-demarcated nodule composed of tubular glands, some of which appear cystically dilated, is embedded in the lamina propria and covered by normal gallbladder epithelium.

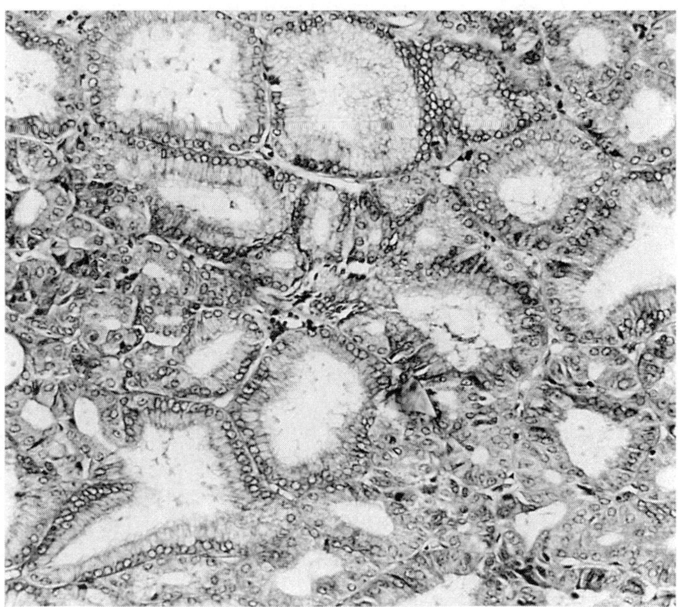

Fig. 58-24 Tubular adenoma of the pyloric gland type. Closely packed tubular glands lined by cuboidal epithelial cells with vesicular nuclei and cytoplasm containing variable amounts of mucin.

atic polypeptide and gastrin, have been demonstrated in the cytoplasm of these cells. As they enlarge, most adenomas develop a pedicle and project toward the lumen. Rarely, they extend into or can arise from Rokitansky-Aschoff sinuses, a finding that should not be confused with carcinoma. The connective tissue stroma is usually minimal but can become edematous or partially hyalinized and may contain lymphocytes. It is continuous with the connective tissue in the lamina propria. When the connective tissue stroma is abundant and edematous and there are only scattered glands, the microscopic picture is reminiscent of a fibroadenoma of the breast.

Tubular adenoma, intestinal type

Pathology. The tubular adenoma of the intestinal type is a benign tumor composed of tubular glands lined by cells with intestinal phenotype showing variable degrees of dysplastic changes (Fig. 58-25). This type of adenoma closely resembles colonic adenomas. It consists of tubular glands lined by pseudostratified columnar epithelium that is usually more atypical than that of pyloric gland adenomas. Clusters of goblet, Paneth, and endocrine cells are usually admixed with the columnar cells. Serotonin and less frequently peptide hormones have been identified in the endocrine cells by immunohistochemistry. The adenomatous epithelium may extend into the Rokitansky-Aschoff sinuses and should not be confused with stromal invasion. Hyperplasia of the pyloric type of glands is often seen at the base of the adenomas.

Papillary adenoma, intestinal type

Pathology. The papillary adenoma of the intestinal type is a benign tumor composed predominantly of papillary structures lined by dysplastic cells with intestinal phenotype. The predominant cell is columnar with elongated hyperchromatic nuclei and little or no cytoplasmic mucin (Fig. 58-26). The cells are pseudostratified and mitotically active and are indistinguishable from those of papillary adenomas of the large intestine. Tubular glands lined by the same type of epithelium but representing less than 20% of the tumor may also be found. Dysplastic changes are more severe than in the pyloric-gland type of adenomas. Admixed with the columnar cells are goblet, Paneth, and serotonin-containing cells. Some of these endocrine cells are immunoreactive for peptide hormones. These adenomas usually arise in a background of pyloric gland hyperplasia. In our series, one of five papillary adenomas, intestinal type, progressed to invasive adenocarcinoma.

Papillary adenoma, biliary type. The biliary type of papillary adenoma consists of well-defined papillary structures lined by columnar cells, which except for the presence of more cytoplasmic mucin, show minimal variation from normal gallbladder epithelium. So far, no endocrine cells or Paneth cells have been found in these adenomas. Only mild dysplastic changes are noted, and in situ or invasive adenocarcinoma has not been reported in association with these adenomas.

Tubulopapillary adenoma. When tubular glands and papillary structures each constitute more than 20% of the tumor, the term *tubulopapillary adenoma* is applied. Two types are recognized. One manifest as tubular glands and papillary structures similar to those of mixed intestinal adenomas. The other type manifests as tubular glands similar to pyloric glands and papillary structures often lined by foveolar type of epithelium. Paneth and endocrine cells are seen in either type. Dysplastic changes are present in both types.

Adenomas of the extrahepatic bile ducts

Adenomas of the extrahepatic bile ducts are much less common than those that arise in the gallbladder. They usually arise from the common bile duct, cause biliary obstruction, and clinically mimic malignant tumors. Adenomas are classified as tubular, papillary, and mixed and have a cell composition similar to those in the gallbladder.

Cystadenoma. Cystadenoma, a rare but distinctive neoplasm, belongs to a family of mucinous cystic tumors that can

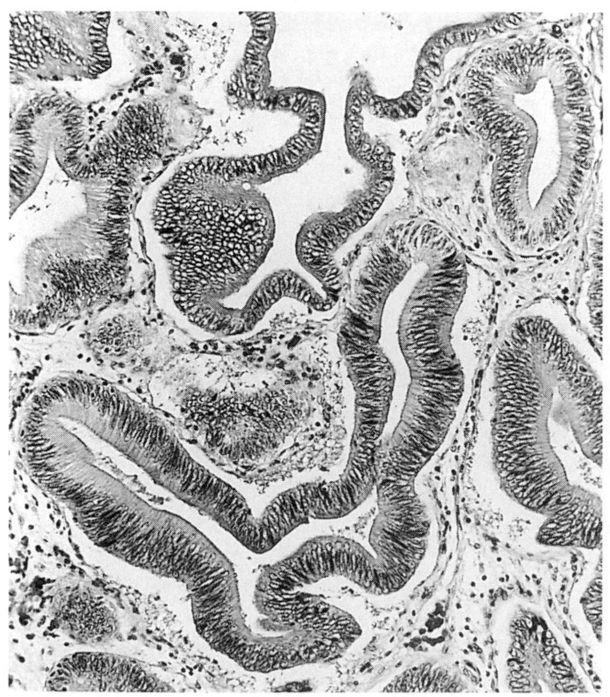

Fig. 58-25 Intestinal type of adenoma of the gallbladder. Adenoma composed of tubular glands resembling colonic glands.

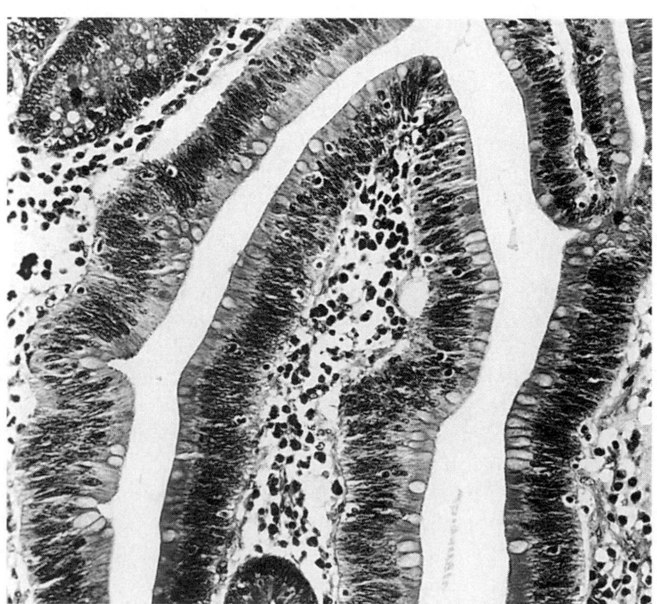

Fig. 58-26 Papillary adenoma. Papillary structures lined by pseudostratified columnar cells having hyperchromatic elongated nuclei. Goblet cells are admixed with the columnar cells.

arise in the pancreas, within the liver, in the extrahepatic biliary tree, and even in the retroperitoneum unattached to any organ.[130,143-146]

Cystadenomas are more common in the extrahepatic bile ducts than in the gallbladder.[130,132] They are larger than noncystic adenomas and are almost invariably symptomatic. Some of these tumors may be as large as 20 cm in diameter, leading to obstructive jaundice or chronic cholecystitis-like symptoms.

Pathology. Grossly the tumors are cystic and multiloculated. The thickness of the cyst wall varies from 0.3 to 3 cm. The locules contain mucinous fluid, and the inner surface is finely granular or trabeculated. Small polypoid structures project into the lumen.

Microscopically, the cyst wall is characterized by an inner layer of cuboidal or columnar biliary type of epithelium that contains mucin, a cellular mesenchymal stroma, and an outer layer of hyalinized fibrous tissue. In some tumors an occasional serotonin-containing (EC) cell is seen among the columnar or cuboidal epithelial cells. The cellular mesenchymal stroma closely resembles ovarian stroma (Fig. 58-27). This impression is further substantiated by the close similarity of the well-demarcated hyalinized areas to corpus albicans. However, ectopic ovarian tissue has never been reported in cystadenomas of the extrahepatic biliary tree. Chronic inflammatory cells, edema, hemorrhage, and extensive fibrosis may distort or even efface the three-layer architecture.

Recently estrogen and progesterone receptors have been detected in the spindle-shaped cells of the mesenchymal stroma by immunohistochemistry.[147] The biliary epithelium, on the other hand, does not have steroid receptors. The clinical significance of this finding, if any, is unknown. The demonstration of estrogen and progesterone receptors in the mesenchymal stroma of mucinous cystic neoplasms of the liver and pancreas further substantiates that these tumors belong to the same family.

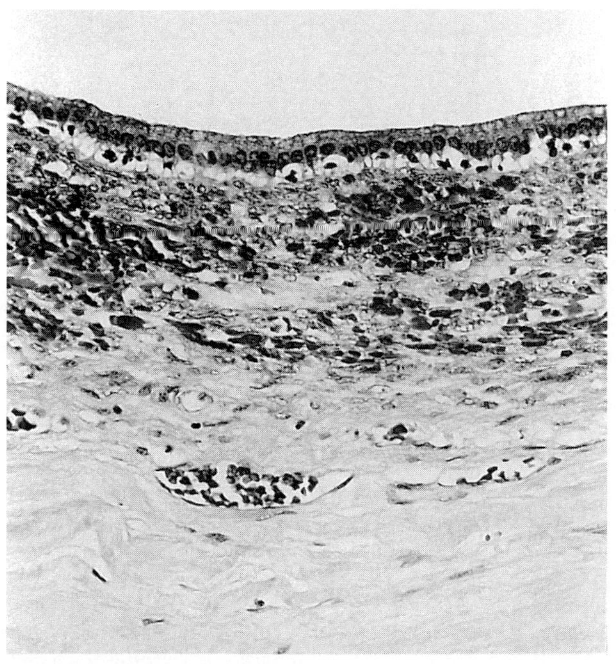

Fig. 58-27 The three characteristic layers of biliary cystadenoma are clearly seen: columnar epithelium, primitive mesenchymal stroma, and dense fibrous tissue.

Biliary cystadenomas may recur after incomplete excision.

Papillomatosis. Papillomatosis, a rare clinicopathologic condition, is characterized by multifocal papillary tumors prone to local recurrence.[148-150] It usually occurs in adult patients between 40 and 50 years of age. The papillary structures are lined by columnar cells with bland nuclei. Focal carcinomatous changes are seen in some cases. The lesion involves extensive areas of the extrahepatic bile ducts and may even extend into the gallbladder, intrahepatic bile ducts, and main pancreatic duct. For many years papillomatosis of the biliary tree was considered to be a benign papillary epithelial proliferation that could become malignant. However, recent studies indicate that on rare occasions even the benign-appearing cells may invade the wall of the ducts or metastasize to lymph nodes and liver. Because of this, the term *low-grade multicentric intraductal papillary carcinoma* has been proposed for this neoplasm, which has been compared with a similar tumor involving the main pancreatic duct.[132]

Other benign tumors

Benign mesenchymal tumors. Benign mesenchymal tumors are exceedingly rare and their morphologic features are similar to those seen in other organs. Leiomyomas, hemangiomas, lipomas, lymphangiomas and osteomas have been reported.

Granular cell tumor is the most common nonepithelial neoplasm of the extrahepatic bile ducts.[151-153] It usually causes biliary obstruction and microscopically may simulate a malignant neoplasm because it may extend to the periductal fibroadipose tissue and even to lymph nodes. Reactive hyperplasia of the overlying epithelium occurs in a few cases. Some granular cell tumors of the biliary tree are multicentric. Granular cell tumors of the gallbladder are often asymptomatic and are less common than those that arise in the bile ducts.

Ganglioneuromatosis of the gallbladder is a component of the type IIb multiple endocrine neoplasia syndrome.[154] Neurofibromatosis of the gallbladder can occur in association with neurofibromatosis types I and II.[155]

Paragangliomas and carcinoid tumors. Paragangliomas are small (less than 1 cm) and exceedingly rare tumors that usually represent an incidental finding in cholecystectomy specimens.[156] In the bile ducts, however, these tumors may cause obstructive jaundice.[157]

Carcinoid tumors of the gallbladder and extrahepatic bile ducts represent less than 1% of all digestive tract carcinoids.[158,159] Grossly these tumors appear as yellow to gray nodules. The neoplastic cells are arranged in cords, trabeculae or nests. (Figs. 58-28). In some tumors tubular structures predominate (so-called tubular carcinoid). Most carcinoid tumors of the extrahepatic biliary tree synthesize serotonin. With liver metastases, they can give rise to the carcinoid syndrome. Some carcinoids produce peptide hormones such as somatostatin and gastrin. Somatostatinomas are most commonly seen in the region of the ampulla. Characteristically these tumors contain psammoma bodies and usually do not produce the somatostatinoma syndrome.[160] Occasionally somatostatinomas of the ampulla are associated with MEN 1 syndrome or neurofibromatosis.[161]

Tumors showing a mixture of carcinoid and adenocarcinoma have been documented in the biliary tree.[162]

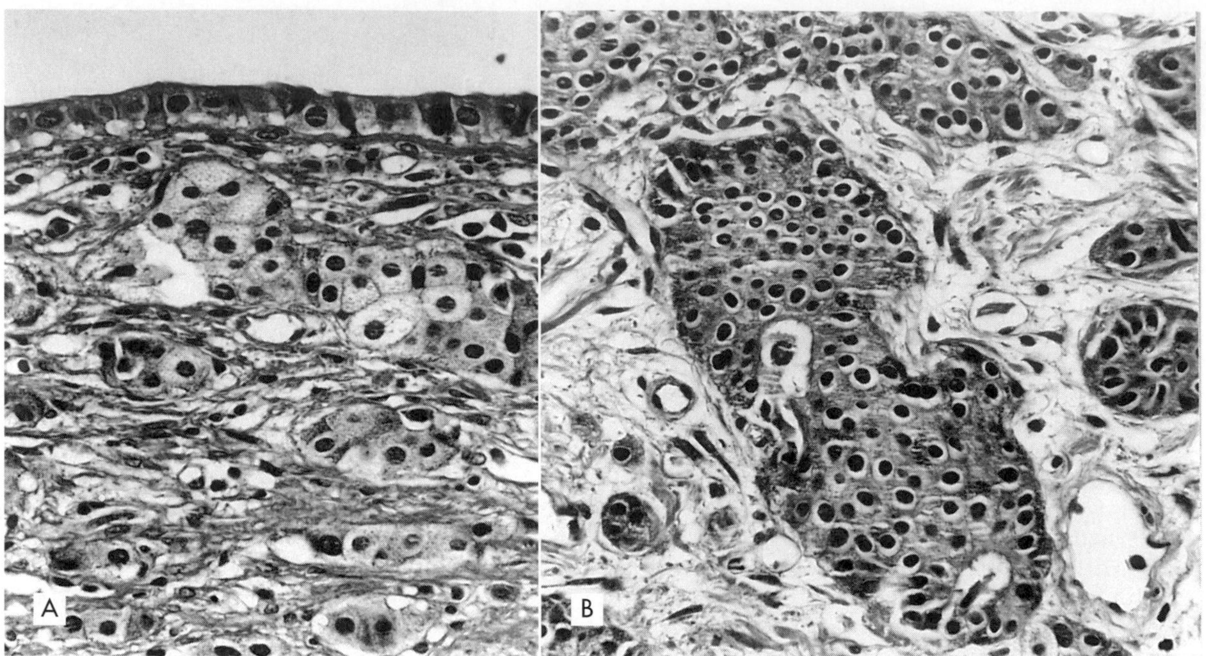

Fig. 58-28 Carcinoid tumor of common bile duct. **A,** Cords of small regular cells with round hyperchromatic nuclei and clear or granular cytoplasm infiltrate the fibrous stroma. The overlying biliary epithelium is normal. **B,** Insular growth pattern of the same tumor.

Malignant tumors

Dysplasia and carcinoma in situ

It is now accepted that most invasive carcinomas of the gallbladder and extrahepatic bile ducts are preceded by dysplasia and carcinoma in situ. Only a small proportion of invasive tumors arise from preexisting adenomas. It is therefore believed that the dysplasia-carcinoma in situ sequence is the usual route for the development of invasive carcinoma.[163-172] The following facts have been offered in support of this hypothesis: dysplasia and carcinoma in situ are found in the mucosa adjacent to most carcinomas of the gallbladder and extrahepatic bile ducts;[163-173] multiple sections of gallbladders removed for cholelithiasis have shown dysplasia and carcinoma in situ in 13.5% and 3.5% of the cases respectively;[163] the anatomic distribution of these lesions is similar to that of invasive carcinoma.[164]

Since dysplasia and carcinoma in situ are often seen in association with cholelithiasis, they usually arise in an abnormal mucosa showing pyloric gland or intestinal metaplasia. Dysplasia and carcinoma in situ usually begin on the surface epithelium and extend laterally and downward into Rokitansky-Aschoff sinuses and metaplastic glands.[171] Rarely dysplasia and carcinoma in situ may arise in metaplastic glands, in Rokitansky-Aschoff sinuses, or in adenomyomatous hyperplasia.

Dysplasia is characterized by columnar or cuboidal cells with or without stratification, nuclear enlargement and hyperchromatism, prominent nucleoli, loss of polarity, and mitotic figures (Fig. 58-29). Flat and papillary growth patterns have been recognized. In carcinoma in situ the above-mentioned changes are more pronounced than in dysplasia and a cribriform architecture may be present (Fig. 58-30). Other histologic forms of dysplasia and carcinoma in situ include squamous and intestinal types. It is important to emphasize that distinction between severe dysplasia and carcinoma in situ is often subjective and sometimes impossible. Recently it has been suggested that morphometric analysis is useful in differentiating dysplasia from carcinoma.[174]

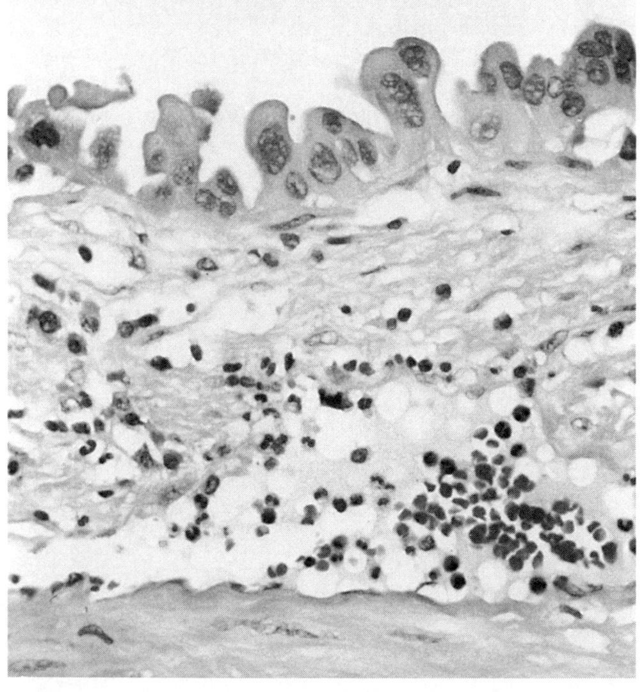

Fig. 58-29 Severe dysplasia. Cells of the surface gallbladder epithelium show loss of polarity and contain large hyperchromatic nuclei located in the apical, central, or basal portions of the cells.

Carcinoma of the gallbladder and extrahepatic bile ducts

Because of histologic similarities, malignant epithelial tumors of the gallbladder and extrahepatic bile ducts are usually discussed under the same heading in many pathology text books. However, these neoplasms show more differences than similarities (Table 58-5).

The incidence of carcinoma of the gallbladder varies in different parts of the world. Considerable variation is also found in different ethnic groups within the same country. In the United States, for example, carcinoma of the gallbladder is more common in American Indians than in whites or in blacks.[175] The rate for female American Indians is 21 per 100,000 compared with 1.4 per 100,000 among white females. The rate for Hispanic-American females is intermediate between female American Indians and white females (10 per 100,000).[176] In Latin American countries the highest rates are found in Chile, Mexico, and Bolivia. There is no geographic variation in the incidence of extrahepatic bile duct carcinoma. The incidence of carcinoma of the gallbladder correlates with the incidence of cholelithiasis. No such correlation exists for extrahepatic bile duct carcinoma, which is seen more often in patients with ulcerative colitis and primary sclerosing cholangitis.[177,178] Carcinomas of the gallbladder show a strong female predominance and are recognized late in their course, usually after they have spread to the liver or regional lymph nodes, whereas extrahepatic bile duct carcinomas are slightly more common among males and produce early biliary obstruction. The dominant and initial sign of extrahepatic bile duct cancer is jaundice occurring in more than 90% of patients, whereas the symptoms of gallbladder carcinoma often are those of preexisting cholecystitis with cholelithiasis.[171] Cholangiography is essential for the diagnosis of extrahepatic bile duct carcinomas, and ultrasound and CT scan are useful tools for the preoperative diagnosis and staging of gallbladder carcinoma.[179] Patients with carcinoma of the gallbladder or extrahepatic bile ducts have high levels of serum carcinoembryonic antigen (CEA) and the carbohydrate antigen CA-19-9, a tumor-associated antigen.[180] However, these tumor markers lack specificity, and their usefulness is limited to the follow-up study of the patients.

Malignant epithelial tumors of the gallbladder are more common than carcinomas of the extrahepatic bile ducts. In the Surveillance, Epidemiology, and End Results Program of the National Cancer Institute, which covers 9.6% of the population of the United States, 3038 cases of gallbladder carcinoma and 1766 cases of extrahepatic bile duct cancer were recorded during a 10-year period (1977-1986).[181,182]

Sex and age distribution. Carcinoma of the gallbladder predominates in females. According to different series the female-male ratio varies from 2:1 to 5:1. In contrast, carcinoma of the extrahepatic bile ducts is slightly more common in males.

Carcinoma of the biliary tract is a disease of older age groups. For extrahepatic bile duct cancer the peak age is in the range 65 to 69 years and for gallbladder carcinoma 70 to 79 years. Approximately 10% of patients 65 years or older undergoing surgery for biliary tract disease can be expected to have carcinoma of the gallbladder or bile ducts.

Etiologic factors. Many epidemiologic studies have suggested a genetic susceptibility for carcinoma of the gallbladder among American Indians.[175,176] Familial aggregations of gallbladder carcinoma have been reported in the United States and in other countries. The high incidence of carcinoma of the gallbladder in Hispanic Americans appears to be the result of racial intermixture, since the Iberian Spaniards do not have high rates of gallbladder cancer. Most likely the high rates observed in most Latin American countries is also the result of racial intermixture by the Spanish immigrants and native American Indians.

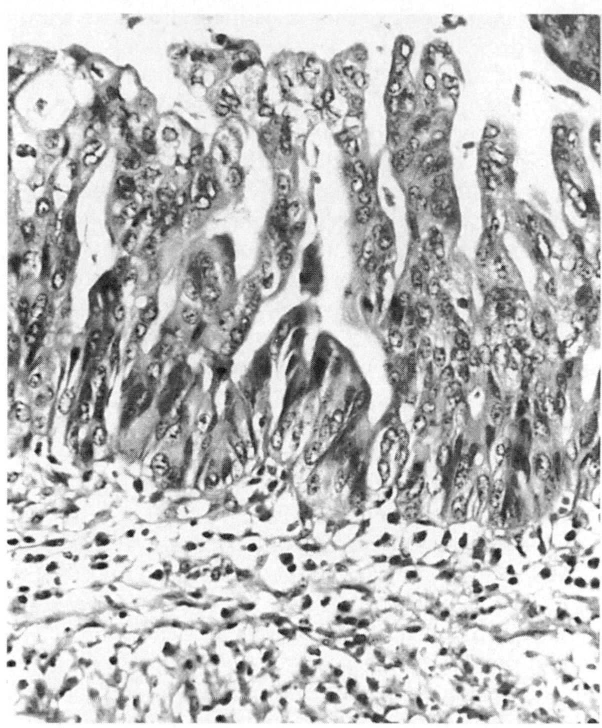

Fig. 58-30 Carcinoma in situ. The gallbladder epithelium is stratified and shows cytologic features of malignancy.

Table 58-5 Comparison of gallbladder and extrahepatic bile duct carcinomas

	Gallbladder	Extrahepatic bile ducts
Geographic variation in incidence	Yes	No
More common in certain ethnic groups	Yes	No
Female predominance	Yes	No
Associated with gallstones	Yes	No
Increased incidence with ulcerative colitis and primary sclerosing cholangitis	No	Yes
Biliary obstruction is usually the initial sign	No	Yes
Cholangiography essential for diagnosis	No	Yes
Adenocarcinoma, the most common histologic type	Yes	Yes
Elevated serum carcinoembryonic antigen	Yes	Yes
Poor prognosis	Yes	Yes

The association of carcinoma of the gallbladder with gallstones has been known for over 100 years. In our series of 386 patients with gallbladder carcinoma 78% had stones. Multivariate analysis has shown that the presence of gallstones is a risk factor independent of age or sex. The association of gallbladder cancer and stones has been interpreted by many as indicating a causal relationship. Some investigators believe that irritation caused by stones promotes neoplastic transformation. Others believe that a carcinogen present in the bile or the stones is responsible for the development of carcinomas. None of these hypothesis have been proved. Most carcinomas of the gallbladder are associated with the cholesterol type of stones. Biochemical studies have shown that stones from gallbladder cancer patients are formed through standard mechanisms for cholesterol precipitation and are not secondary to stasis or infection.

Diffuse calcification of the gallbladder, so-called porcelain gallbladder, carries a high risk for malignant transformation, estimated between 12% and 21%.[183] Because of this, prophylactic cholecystectomy has been recommended in patients with porcelain gallbladders.

Extrahepatic bile duct carcinoma. Patients with ulcerative colitis and primary sclerosing cholangitis often develop carcinoma of the extrahepatic bile ducts. The relative risk for individuals with ulcerative colitis is about 31.3 times greater than that in the general population.[178] In fact, nearly half of the patients with both ulcerative colitis and primary sclerosing cholangitis eventually develop extrahepatic bile duct cancer.[177] However, the mechanism by which these two diseases induce carcinomas of the bile ducts is unknown.

Choledochal cysts also predispose to extrahepatic bile duct carcinoma. The incidence of carcinoma in choledochal cysts has been estimated to be 20 times greater than the incidence in the general population. A mixture of bile and gastroduodenal contents may promote the development of carcinoma, since half of the reported cases developed carcinoma after a mean interval of 4 years after internal drainage of the cyst. Adenocarcinoma is the most common tumor found in the cyst wall, but other neoplasms, including rhabdomyosarcoma and carcinoid tumors, have been reported.

In the Orient, *Opisthorchis viverrini* and *Opisthorchis sinensis* infestations have been associated with carcinoma of the intrahepatic bile ducts[184] and occasionally with carcinoma of the extrahepatic bile ducts.[185] The parasites cause a chronic inflammatory reaction with considerable epithelial proliferation of bile ducts followed by metaplastic changes and neoplastic transformation. However, the fact that humans may harbor *O. viverrini* and *O. sinensis* in their bile ducts for long periods and only some patients develop malignant tumors indicates that the carcinogenic stimulus is multifactorial.

Pathology of gallbladder carcinoma. Approximately 10% to 15% of invasive gallbladder carcinomas cannot be recognized with certainty on gross examination. The microscopic findings in these cases are similar to those of chronic cholecystitis. However, most tumors appear as a focal thickening of the gallbladder wall, a raised mucosal plaque, a bulging submucosal nodule, a polypoid structure protruding into the lumen, an infiltrating gray-white mass, or a diffuse thickening and induration of the entire wall. Papillary carcinomas show a polypoid or cauliflower-like appearance. Mucinous carcinomas have mucoid or gelatinous cut surfaces. Most carcinomas (60%) originate in the fundus, 30% in the body, and 10% in the neck.

Gross features of carcinoma of extrahepatic bile ducts. Grossly these tumors can be classified into three types: nodular, polypoid, or diffusely infiltrating. A combination of these features is sometimes seen. Not infrequently there is only a focal thickening or induration of the wall, with partial obstruction of the bile duct showing a roughened or granular mucosa. This type

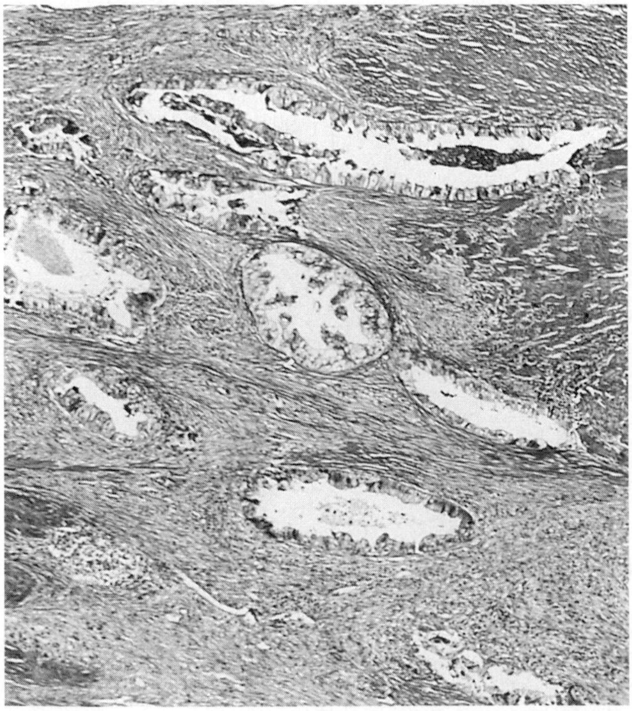

Fig. 58-31 Well-differentiated adenocarcinoma. The tumor is composed of glands of different sizes that are infiltrating the fibrotic gallbladder wall.

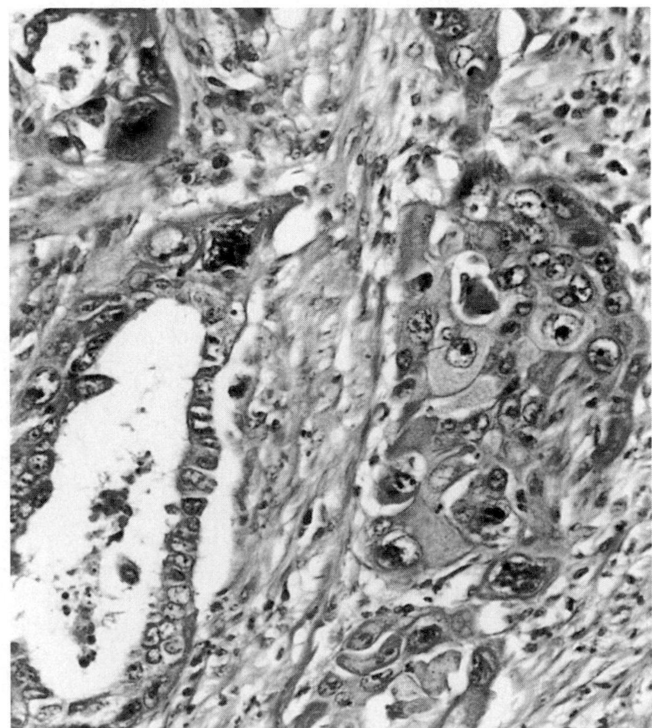

Fig. 58-32 Adenosquamous carcinoma of common bile duct. The tumor consists of both glands and squamous elements.

of carcinoma can easily be overlooked by both surgeons and pathologists. It has been reported that carcinoma of the bile ducts has been missed in as many as 20% of patients at the time of the initial surgical exploration for obstructive jaundice. Even obtaining biopsy specimens of high proximal carcinomas may be extremely difficult. Approximately 50% of all carcinomas are located in the upper third, 25% in the middle third, and 19% in the lower third. In 7%, it is not possible to specify the site of origin because of diffuse involvement of the bile ducts.

Microscopic features. Most malignant epithelial tumors of the biliary tree are well to moderately differentiated adenocarcinomas (Fig. 58-31). Some of these are papillary and grow predominantly into the lumen of the gallbladder or bile ducts. Others are composed of cells with intestinal phenotype.[186] Clear cell adenocarcinomas closely mimic renal cell carcinoma.[187] Mucinous adenocarcinomas are those in which more than 50% of the tumor contains extracellular mucin. Some adenocarcinomas may be composed predominantly of signet-ring cells. Rarely adenocarcinomas contain trophoblastic elements.[188] Adenosquamous carcinomas show in addition to glands a squamous component (Fig. 58-32). Small cell carcinomas are similar to those that occur in the lung[189-191] (Fig. 58-33). These tumors may be pure or contain foci of adenocarcinoma or squamous cell carcinoma. Endocrine differentiation can be demonstrated by immunohistochemistry or electron microscopy in most of these small cell tumors. Undifferentiated carcinomas consist predominantly of spindle and giant cells and resemble sarcomas[188,192] (Figs. 58-34 and 58-35). Although glandular structures are typically absent, foci of adenocarcinoma can be identified in some of these undifferentiated carcinomas after extensive sampling. Approximately 70% of them, however, express cytokeratin, the presence of which supports their epithelial derivation. Some undifferentiated car-

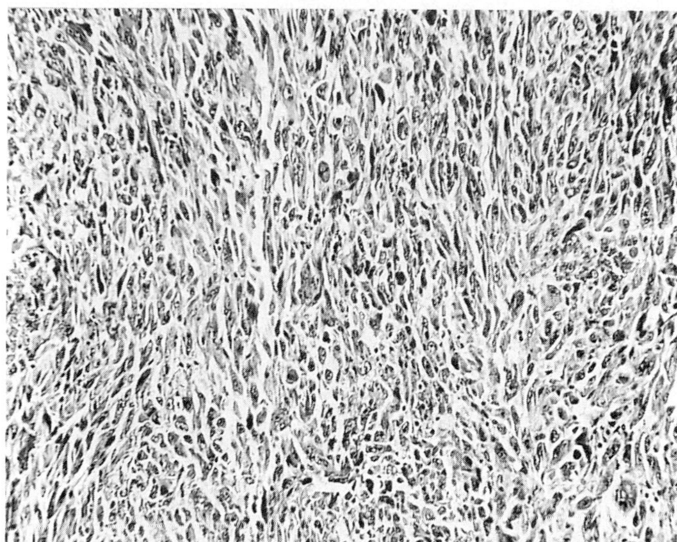

Fig. 58-34 Undifferentiated carcinoma, spindle cell type, of the gallbladder. The predominant cell is spindle shaped and is arranged in fascicles. A few multinucleated giant cells are seen.

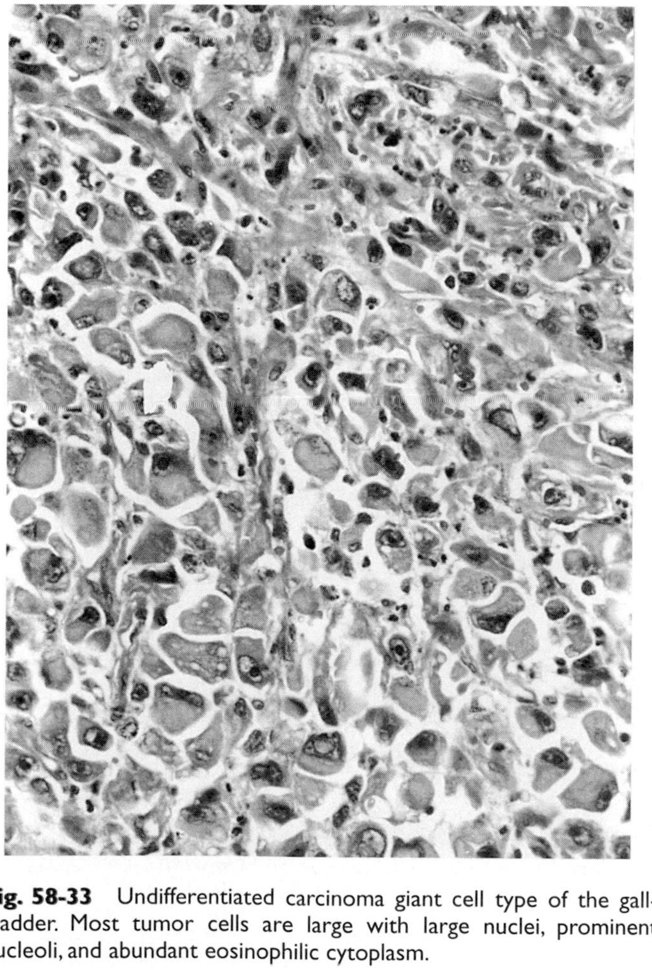

Fig. 58-33 Undifferentiated carcinoma giant cell type of the gallbladder. Most tumor cells are large with large nuclei, prominent nucleoli, and abundant eosinophilic cytoplasm.

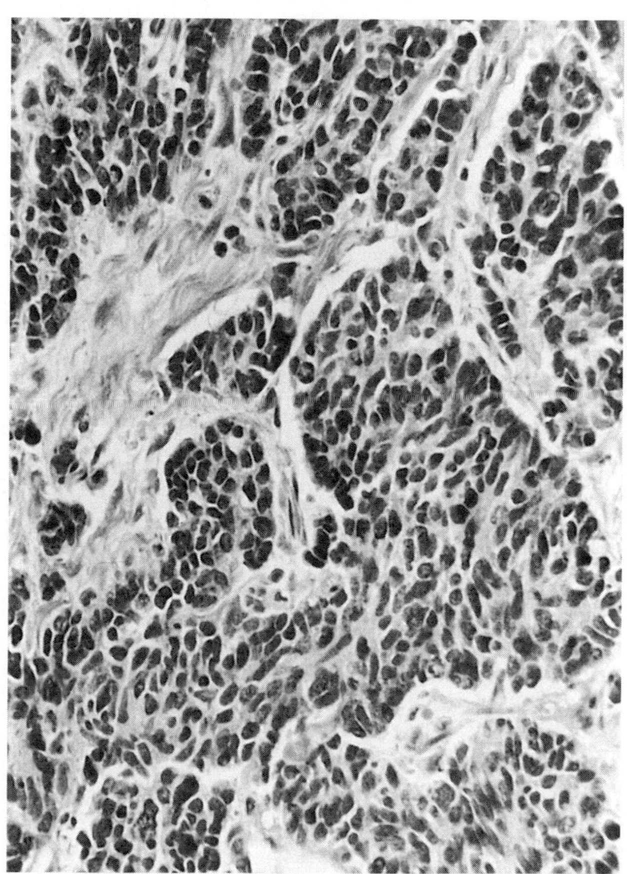

Fig. 58-35 Small cell carcinoma of gallbladder. Small round cells with hyperchromatic nuclei and finely dispersed chromatin are arranged in cords and nests.

cinomas consist of small cells without endocrine differentiation.

Many well to moderately differentiated adenocarcinomas of the gallbladder and extrahepatic bile ducts contain a population of endocrine cells, which can be identified by silver stains or by immunohistochemistry.[193,194] Regardless of the number of endocrine cells present, a diagnosis of carcinoid or adenocarcinoid is not warranted. The clinical significance of these endocrine cells is unknown.

Most adenocarcinomas of the gallbladder and extrahepatic bile ducts are immunoreactive for CEA and the carbohydrate tumor-associated antigen CA-19-9.[180,195,196] Rarely undifferentiated carcinomas as well as adenocarcinomas with trophoblastic differentiation are reactive for human chorionic gonadotropin.[197,198] Alpha-fetoprotein has occasionally been demonstrated by immunohistochemistry in clear cell adenocarcinomas of the gallbladder.[187,199] Most small cell carcinomas of the gallbladder express cytokeratin and show the presence of neuron-specific enolase.[190] A small number of these tumors are immunoreactive for chromogranin. Rarely serotonin and peptide hormones have been identified in neoplastic cells. Recently, genetic analysis has shown a variety of molecular abnormalities in gallbladder carcinomas, including p53 mutations and loss of heterozygosity at chromosome locations 9p and 8p and at the DCE gene.[200b]

The expression of p53 and C-*erb* B-2 proteins has recently been demonstrated by immunohistochemistry in dysplasia and invasive adenocarcinomas of the gallbladder.[200] The suggestion has been made that p53 mutations might be an early event in the evolution of some gallbladder carcinomas.

Prognosis. Prognosis of gallbladder and extrahepatic bile duct carcinoma is poor. The two most important factors having the greatest effect on survival are pathologic stage of disease and histologic grade of the tumor. Patients with in situ carcinoma are cured by cholecystectomy. For patients with carcinoma limited to the gallbladder wall the 5-year survival rate is 32%.[181] Patients with known liver metastases or direct extension to adjacent organs die soon after diagnosis. Patients with papillary adenocarcinoma are associated with the best survival, whereas patients with undifferentiated carcinomas, spindle and giant cell types, and small cell carcinomas have the worse prognosis. Although carcinomas of the extrahepatic bile ducts are better differentiated than carcinomas of the gallbladder, they have a worse prognosis. The 5-year survival rate for patients with stage I disease was 11% in the largest series recorded so far.[182] However, patients with tumors in the distal third of the common bile duct have a better prognosis than those with tumors in the middle or proximal portion of the ductal system.[179]

Carcinosarcoma, malignant lymphoma, and malignant melanoma

Carcinosarcomas occur predominantly in females over 50 years of age with cholelithiasis. These tumors consist of a mixture of two components: carcinomatous and sarcomatous. The epithelial elements usually form glands but may be arranged in cords or sheets. The mesenchymal component in addition to spindle cells may include heterologous elements such as cartilage, osteoid, and rhabdomyoblasts.[201] Cytokeratin and CEA are absent from the mesenchymal component. This helps to distinguish carcinosarcomas from undifferentiated carcinomas composed predominantly of spindle and giant cells.

Malignant lymphoma of the gallbladder is usually the manifestation of systemic disease. Primary malignant lymphomas of the gallbladder are exceedingly rare.[202] Small lymphocytic, large cell, and immunoblastic types have been described. Most of these tumors have a B-cell phenotype.

Primary malignant melanoma of the gallbladder is basically a diagnosis of exclusion. The absence of a primary tumor elsewhere and the presence of junctional activity favors a primary in the gallbladder.[203]

Malignant mesenchymal tumors. Because of the AIDS epidemics, Kaposi's sarcoma is now the most common soft-tissue sarcoma of the gallbladder and extrahepatic bile ducts. However, this tumor has little clinical significance, since it is usually an incidental autopsy finding. Only rarely is Kaposi's sarcoma of the gallbladder symptomatic. The hemorrhagic lesions involve the serosa, subserosa, or muscular wall of the gallbladder or the periductal connective tissue of the bile ducts.

Embryonal rhabdomyosarcoma (sarcoma botryoides, botryoid sarcoma) is the most common malignant neoplasm of the biliary tree in childhood. The usual clinical presentation is biliary obstruction and jaundice. The tumor, which is more common in the bile ducts than in the gallbladder, forms soft polypoid structures with a characteristic grapelike appearance.[204] Microscopically the polypoid structures are covered with normal biliary epithelium (Fig. 58-36). Beneath the epithelium is a concentration of primitive mesenchymal cells, some with abundant eosinophilic cytoplasm. Cross striations are found in 20% to 30% of the tumors. Muscle-specific actin, desmin, and myoglobin can be demonstrated in tumor cells by immunocytochemistry. With the use of multimodality therapy the prognosis of this tumor has improved.[205]

Other malignant mesenchymal tumors of the biliary tree, such as leiomyosarcomas, angiosarcomas, and malignant fibrous histiocytomas, are so rare that they constitute medical curiosities.

Tumorlike lesions. A wide variety of tumorlike lesions have been described in the biliary tree. Some of these are metaplastic mucosal changes associated with cholelithiasis,

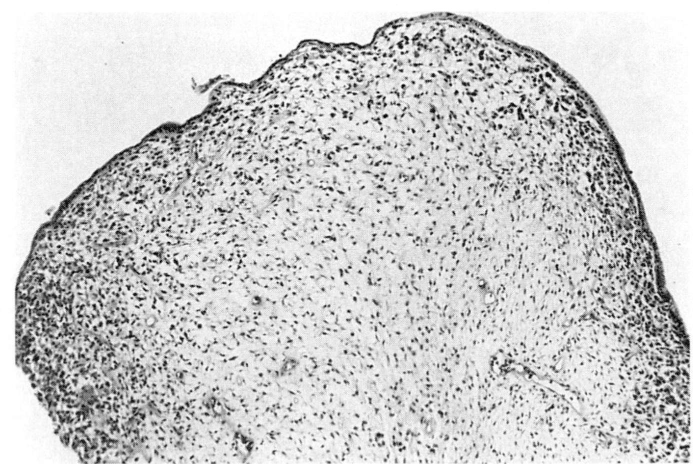

Fig. 58-36 Embryonal (botryoid) rhabdomyosarcoma of common bile duct. The polypoid mass is covered by normal biliary epithelium and is composed of primitive malignant mesenchymal cells. Extensive myxoid areas are present.

such as pyloric gland hyperplasia and squamous and intestinal metaplasia, which may play a role as cancer precursors. Epithelial atypia secondary to repair is a reactive lesion associated with acute and chronic cholecystitis that is often confused with in situ carcinoma. Similar reactive changes are also seen in the mucosa of the bile ducts with acute and chronic inflammation. Ectopic gastric mucosa and pancreatic tissue occur more frequently in the gallbladder than in the bile ducts and are often symptomatic in both sites. Ectopic adrenal cortex, thyroid, and liver have been reported in the gallbladder and usually constitute surgical or autopsy findings. Amputation neuroma may occur shortly or many years after cholecystectomy. Rarely a neuroma may grow into the lumen of the extrahepatic bile ducts, causing obstructive jaundice and clinically mimicking a malignant neoplasm.

REFERENCES

The normal gallbladder

1. Moosman DA, Coller FA: Prevention of traumatic injury to the bile ducts: a study of the structures of the cystohepatic angle encountered in cholecystectomy and supraduodenal choledochostomy, *Am J Surg* 82:132, 1951.
2. Frierson HF: The gross anatomy and histology of the gallbladder, extrahepatic bile ducts, vaterian system, and minor papilla, *Am J Surg Pathol* 13:146, 1989.
3. Lindner HH: Embryology and anatomy of the biliary tree. In Way LW, Pellegrini CA, editors: *Surgery of the gallbladder and bile ducts,* Philadelphia, 1987, Saunders.
4. Frierson HF: Gallbladder and extrahepatic biliary system. In Sternberg SS, editor: *Histology for pathologists,* New York, 1992, Raven Press.
5. Albores-Saavedra J, Henson DE: Tumors of the gallbladder and extrahepatic bile ducts, Washington, DC, 1986, Armed Forces Institute of Pathology.
6. Moosman DA: Accessory bile ducts: their significance during cholecystectomy, *Mich Med* 63:355, 1964.
7. Fisher RS, Rock E, Levin G et al: Effects of somatostatin on gallbladder emptying, *Gastroenterology* 92:885, 1987.
8. Frizzell RA, Heintze K: Transport functions of the gallbladder. In Javitt NB, editor: *Liver and biliary tract physiology I. International Review of Physiology,* vol 21, Baltimore, 1980, University Park Press.

Congenital and developmental abnormalities

9. Williams I, Slavin G, Cox A et al: Diverticular disease (adenomyomatosis) of the gallbladder: a radiological-pathological survey, *Br J Radiol* 59:29, 1986.
10. Esper E, Kaufman DB, Crary GS et al: Septate gallbladder with cholelithiasis: a cause of chronic abdominal pain in a 6-year-old child, *J Pediatr Surg* 27:1560, 1992.
11. Bhagavan BS, Amin PB, Land AS et al: Multiseptate gallbladder: embryogenetic hypotheses, *Arch Pathol* 89:382, 1970.
12. Haslam RH, Gayler BW, Ebert PA: Multiseptate gallbladder: a cause of recurrent abdominal pain in childhood, *Am J Dis Child* 112:600, 1966.
13. Lobe TE, Hayden CK, Merkel M: Giant congenital cystic malformation of the gallbladder, *J Pediatr Surg* 21:447, 1986.
14. Weedon D: *Pathology of the gallbladder,* New York, 1984, Masson.
15. Chiavarini RL, Chang SF, Westerfield JD: The wandering gallbladder, *Radiology* 115:37, 1975.
16. Ashby BS: Acute and recurrent torsion of the gall-bladder, *Br J Surg* 52:182, 1965.
17. Todani T, Watanabe Y, Narusue M et al: Congenital bile duct cysts: classification, operative procedures, and review of thirty-seven cases including cancer arising from choledochal cyst, *Am J Surg* 134:263, 1977.
18. Flanigan PD: Biliary carcinoma associated with biliary cysts, *Cancer* 40:880, 1977.
19. Tan KC, Howard ER: Biliary atresia, *Bailliere's Clin Gastroenterol* 3:211, 1989.
20. Nietgen GW, Vacanti JP, Pérez-Atayde AR: Intrahepatic bile duct loss in biliary atresia despite portoenterostomy: a consequence of ongoing obstruction? *Gastroenterology* 102:2126, 1992.
21. Dussaix E, Hadchouel M, Tardieu M et al: Biliary atresia and Reo virus type 3 infection, *N Engl J Med* 311:658, 1984.
22. Carmi R, Magee CA, Neill CA et al: Extrahepatic biliary atresia and associated anomalies: etiologic heterogeneity suggested by distinctive patterns of associations, *Am J Med Genet* 45:683, 1993.
23. Lawrence D, Howard ER, Tzannatos C et al: Hepatic portoenterostomy for biliary atresia, *Arch Dis Child* 56:460, 1981.

Gallstones

24. Moser AJ, Abedin MZ, Roslyn JJ: The pathogenesis of gallstone formation, *Adv Surg* 26:357, 1993.
25. Bowen JC, Benner HI, Ferrante WA et al: Gallstone disease: pathophysiology, epidemiology, natural history, and treatment options, *Med Clin North Am* 76:1143, 1992.
26. Everson GT: Gallbladder function in gallstone disease, *Gastroenterol Clinb North Am* 20:85, 1991.
27. Paumgartner G, Sauerbruch T: Gallstones: pathogenesis, *Lancet* 338:1117, 1991, comment, 339:241, 1992.
28. Donovan JM, Carey MC: Physical-chemical basis of gallstone formation, *Gastroenterol Clin North Am* 20:47, 1991.
29. Holan KR, Holzbach RT, Hermann RE et al: Nucleation time: a key factor in the pathogenesis of cholesterol gallstone disease, *Gastroenterology* 77:611, 1979.
30. Harvey PRC, Strasberg SM: Will the real cholesterol-nucleating and -antinucleating proteins please stand up? *Gastroenterology* 104:646, 1993.
31. Ohya T, Schwarzendrube J, Busch N et al: Isolation of a human biliary glycoprotein inhibitor of cholesterol crystallization, *Gastroenterology* 104:527, 1993.
32. Abei M, Kawczak P, Nuutinen H et al: Isolation and characterization of a cholesterol crystallization promoter from human bile, *Gastroenterology*104:539, 1993.
33. Weiss KM, Ferrell RE, Hanis CL et al: Genetics and epidemiology of gallbladder disease in New World native peoples, *Am J Hum Genet* 36:1259, 1984.
34. Maurer KR, Everhart JE, Ezzati TM et al: Prevalence of gallstone disease in Hispanic populations in the United States, *Gastroenterology* 96:487, 1989.
35. Maurer KR, Everhart JE, Knowler WC et al: Risk factors for gallstone disease in the Hispanic population of the United States, *Am J Epidemiol* 131:836, 1990.
36. Méndez-Sánchez N, Jessurun J, Ponciano-Rodríguez G et al: Prevalence of gallstone disease in Mexico: a necropsy study, *Dig Dis Sci* 38:680, 1993.
37. Simonovis NJ, Wells CK, Feinstein AR: *In-vivo* and postmortem gallstones: support for validity of the "epidemiologic necropsy" screening technique, *Am J Epidemiol* 133:922, 1991.
38. Trotman BW: Pigment gallstone disease, *Gastroenterol Clin North Am* 20:111, 1991.

Cholecystitis

39. Sen M, Williamson RCN: Acute cholecystitis: surgical management, *Bailliere's Clin Gastroenterol* 5:817, 1991.
40. Salomonowitz E, Frick MP, Simmons RL et al: Obliteration of the gallbladder without formal cholecystectomy, *Arch Surg* 119:725, 1984.
41. Sjödahl R, Wetterfors J: Lysolecithin and lecithin in the gallbladder wall and bile; their possible roles in the pathogenesis of acute cholecystitis, *Scand J Gastroenterol* 9:519, 1974.
42. Pellegrini CA, Way LW: Acute cholecystitis. In Way LW, Pelllegrini CA, editors: *Surgery of the gallbladder and bile ducts,* Philadelphia, 1987, Saunders.
43. Claesson BEB, Holmlund DEW, Matzsch TW: Microflora of the gallbladder related to duration of acute cholecystitis, *Surg Gynecol Obstet* 162:531, 1986.
44. Adams A, Roddie ME: Acute cholecystitis: radiological management, *Bailliere's Clin Gastroenterol* 5:787, 1991.
45. Babb RR: Acute acalculous cholecystitis: a review, *J Clin Gastroenterol* 15:238, 1992.

46. Frazee RC, Nagorney DM, Mucha P: Acute acalculous cholecystitis, *Mayo Clin Proc* 64:163, 1989.
47. Mentzer RM, Golden GT, Chandler JG et al: A comparative appraisal of emphysematous cholecystitis, *Am J Surg* 129:10, 1975.
48. Lee BY, Morilla CV: Acute emphysematous cholecystitis: a case report and review of the literature, *NY State J Med* 92:406, 1992.
49. Bergan T, Dobloug I, Liavag I: Bacterial isolates in cholecystitis and cholelithiasis, *Scand J Gastroenterol* 14:625, 1979.
50. Albores-Saavedra J, Gould E, Manivel-Rodríguez C et al: Chronic cholecystitis with lymphoid hyperplasia, *Rev Invest Clin (Mex)* 41:159, 1989.
51. Hanada M, Tujimura T, Kimura M: Cholecystic granulomas in gallstone disease, *Acta Pathol Jpn* 31:221, 1981.
52. Amazon K, Rywlin AM: Ceroid granulomas of the gallbladder, *Am J Clin Pathol* 73:123, 1980.
53. Ashur H, Siegal B, Oland Y et al: Calcified gallbladder (porcelain gallbladder), *Arch Surg* 113:594, 1978.
54. Weiner PL, Lawson TL: Porcelain gallbladder, *Am J Gastroenterol* 64:224, 1975.
55. Berk RN, Armbuster TG, Saltzstein SL: Carcinoma in the porcelain gallbladder, *Radiology* 106:29, 1973.
56. Polk HC: Carcinoma and the calcified gallbladder, *Gastroenterology* 50:582, 1966.
57. Roberts KM, Parson MA: Xanthogranulomatous cholecystitis: clinicopathological study of 13 cases, *J Clin Pathol* 40:412, 1987.
58. Howard TJ, Bennion RS, Thompson JE: Xanthogranulomatous cholecystitis: a chronic inflammatory pseudotumor of the gallbladder, *Am Surg* 57:821, 1991.
59. Goodman ZD, Ishak KG: Xanthogranulomatous cholecystitis, *Am J Surg Pathol* 5:653, 1981.
60. Dao AH, Wong SW, Adkins RB: Xanthogranulomatous cholecystitis: a clinical and pathologic study of twelve cases, *Am J Surg* 55:32, 1989.
61. Kozuka S, Hachisuka K: Incidence by age and sex of intestinal metaplasia in the gallbladder, *Hum Pathol* 15:779, 1984.
62. Albores-Saavedra J, Nadji M, Henson DE et al: Intestinal metaplasia of the gallbladder: a morphologic and immunocytochemical study, *Hum Pathol* 17:614, 1986.
63. Diehl AK: Symptoms of gallstone disease, *Bailliere's Clin Gastroenterol* 6:635, 1992.
63a. Soper NJ, Flye MW, Brunt LM et al: Diagnosis and management of biliary complications of complications of laparoscopic cholecystectomy, *Am J Surg* 165:663, 1993.
63b. Deziel DJ, Millikan KW, Economou SG et al: Complications of laparoscopic cholecystectomy: a national survey of 4,293 hospitals and an analysis of 77,604 cases, *Am J Surg* 165:9, 1993.
63c. Fitzgibbons RJ, Annibali R, Litke BS: Gallbladder and gallstone removal, open versus closed laparoscopy, and pneumoperitoneum, *Am J Surg* 165:497, 1993.
64. Raptopoulos V, Compton CC, Doherty P et al: Chronic acalculous gallbladder disease: multiimaging evaluation with clinical-pathologic correlation, *Am J Roetgenol* 147:721, 1986.
65. Sykes D: The use of cholecystokinin in diagnosing biliary pain, *Ann R Coll Surg Engl* 64:114, 1982.
66. Giffen WO, Bivins BA, Rogers EL et al: Cholecystokinin cholecystography in the diagnosis of gallbladder disease, *Ann Surg* 191:636, 1980.
67. Dabbs DJ: Eosinophilic and lymphoeosinophilic cholecystitis, *Am J Surg Pathol* 17:497, 1993.
68. Charpentier P, Prade M, Bognel C et al: Malacoplakia of the gallbladder, *Hum Pathol* 14:827, 1983.
69. Kavin N, Jonas RB, Chowdhury L et al: Acalculous cholecystitis and cytomegalovirus infection in the acquired immunodeficiency syndrome, *Ann Intern Med* 104:53, 1986.
70. Blumberg RS, Kelsey P, Perrone T et al: Cytomegalovirus and *Cryptosporidium*-associated acalculous gangrenous cholecystitis, *Am J Med* 76:1118, 1984.
71. Lebovics E, Dworkin BM, Heir SK et al: The hepatobiliary manifestations of human immunodeficiency virus infection, *Am J Gastroenterol* 83:1, 1988.

Cholesterolosis

72. Feldman M, Feldman M Jr: Cholesterosis of the gallbladder: an autopsy study of 165 cases, *Gastroenterology* 27:641, 1954.
73. Salmenkivi K: Cholesterosis of the gallbladder: a clinical study based on 269 cholecystectomies, *Acta Chir Scand* 324(suppl):1, 1964.
74. Jacyna MR, Bouchier IAD: Cholesterolosis: a physical cause of "functional" disorder, *Br Med J* 295:619, 1987.
75. Parrilla-Paricio P, García-Olmo D, Pellicer-Franco E et al: Gallbladder cholesterolosis: an etiological factor in acute pancreatitis of uncertain origin, *Br J Surg* 77:735, 1990.

Other conditions

76. Suddleson EA, Reid B, Woolley MM et al: Hydrops of the gallbladder associated with Kawasaki syndrome, *J Pediatr Surg* 22:956, 1987.
77. Williams I, Slavin G, Cox A et al: Diverticular disease (adenomyomatosis) of the gallbladder: a radiological-pathological survey, *Br J Radiol* 59:29, 1986.
78. Berk RN, van-der-Vegt JH, Lichtenstein JE: The hyperplastic cholecystoses: cholesterolosis and adenomyomatosis, *Radiology* 146:593, 1983.
79. Matz LR, Lawrence-Brown MMD: Ischaemic cholecystitis and infarction of the gallbladder, *Aust NZ J Surg* 52:466, 1982.
80. Hallendorf LC, Dockerty MB, Waugh JM: Gangrenous cholecystitis: a clinical and pathologic study of 100 cases, *Surg Clin North Am* 28:979, 1948.
81. Dillard BM, Black WC: Polyarteritis nodosa of the gallbladder, *Surgery* 67:427, 1970.
82. Penn I: Injuries of the gallbladder, *Br J Surg* 49:636, 1962.
83. Corrasco CH, Freeny PC, Chuang VP et al: Chemical cholecystitis associated with hepatic artery infusion chemotherapy, *Am J Roentgenol* 141:703, 1983.
84. Venkatesh-Rao PS, Tandon RK, Kapur BML: Biliobiliary fistula: review of nine cases, *Am J Gastroenterol* 83:652, 1988.ä

Acquired conditions of the bile ducts

85. Thompson JE Jr, Tompkins RK, Longmire WP Jr: Factors in management of acute cholangitis, *Ann Surg* 195:137, 1982.
86. Koehler RE, Melson GL, Lee JK et al: Common hepatic duct obstruction by cystic duct stone: Mirizzi syndrome, *AJR* 132:1007, 1979.
87. Warren KW, Williams CI, Tan EGC: Diseases of the gallbladder and bile ducts. In Schiff L, Schiff ER, editors: *Diseases of the liver*, Philadelphia, 1987, Lippincott.
88. Dineen P: The importance of the route of infection in experimental biliary tract obstruction, *Surg Gynecol Obstet* 119:1001, 1964.
89. O'Connor MJ, Schwartz ML, McQuarrie DG et al: Acute bacterial cholangitis: an analysis of clinical manifestation, *Arch Surg* 117:437, 1982.
90. Boey JH, Way LW: Acute cholangitis, *Ann Surg* 191:264, 1980.
91. Sinanan MN: Acute cholangitis, *Infect Dis Clin North Am* 6:571, 1992.
92. Lipsett PA, Pitt HA: Acute cholangitis, *Surg Clin North Am* 70:1297, 1990.
93. Lim JH: Oriental cholangiohepatitis: pathologic, clinical, and radiologic features, *AJR* 157:1, 1991.
94. Nakayama F, Koga A: Hepatolithiasis: present status, *World J Surg* 8:9, 1984.
95. Ho CS, Wesson DE: Recurrent pyogenic cholangitis in Chinese immigrants, *Am J Roentgenol Radium Ther Nucl Med* 122:368, 1974.
96. Seel DJ, Park YK: Oriental infestational cholangitis, *Am J Surg* 146:188, 1983.
97. Nakanuma Y, Yamaguchi K, Ohta G et al: Pathologic features of hepatolithiasis in Japan, *Hum Pathol* 19:1181, 1988.
98. Ong GB: A study of recurrent pyogenic cholangitis, *Arch Surg* 84:199, 1962.
99. Koge A, Ichimiya H, Yamaguchi K et al: Hepatolithiasis associated with cholangiocarcinoma: possible etiologic significance, *Cancer* 55:2826, 1985.
100. Chen MF, Jan Y-Y, Wang C-S et al: Intrahepatic stones associated with cholangiocarcinoma, *Am J Gastroenterol* 84:391, 1989.
101. Nakanuma Y, Terada T, Tanaka Y et al: Are hepatolithiasis and cholangiocarcinoma aetiologically related? *Virchows Arch* [A] 406:48, 1985.
102. LaRusso NF, Wiesner RH, Ludwig J et al: Primary sclerosing cholangitis, *N Eng J Med* 310:899, 1984.
103. Pokorny CS, McCaughan GW, Gallagher ND et al: Sclerosing cholangitis and biliary tract calculi-primary or secondary? *Gut* 33:1376, 1992.
104. Snook JA, Chapman RW, Fleming KA et al: Peripheral blood and portal tract lymphocytes populations in primary sclerosing cholangitis, *J Hepatol* 9:36, 1989.
105. Chapman RW, Varghese Z, Gaul R et al: Association of primary sclerosing cholangitis with HLA-B8, *Gut* 24:38, 1983.

106. Chapman RW, Kelly P, Heryet A et al: Expression of HLA-DR antigens on bile duct epithelium in primary sclerosing cholangitis, *Gut* 29:422, 1988.
107. Lo SK, Fleming KA, Chapman RW: Prevalence of anti-neutrophil antibody in primary sclerosing cholangitis and ulcerative colitis using an alkaline phosphatase technique, *Gut* 33:1570, 1992.
108. Ludwig J: Surgical pathology of the syndrome of primary sclerosing cholangitis, *Am J Surg Pathol* 13(suppl 1):43, 1989.
109. Jeffrey GP, Reed WD, Carrello S et al: Histological and immunohistochemical study of the gall bladder lesion in primary sclerosing cholangitis, *Gut* 32:424, 1991.
110. Harrison RF, Hubscher SG: The spectrum of bile duct lesions in end-stage primary sclerosing cholangitis, *Histopathology* 19:321, 1991.
111. Lefkowitch JH: Primary sclerosing cholangitis, *Arch Intern Med* 142:1157,1982.
112. Brandt DJ, MacCarty TL, Charboneau JW et al: Gallbladder disease in patients with primary sclerosing cholangitis, *AJR* 150:571, 1988.
113. Jessurun J, Bolio-Solis A, Manivel JC: Diffuse plasmalymphocytic acalculous cholecystitis: a distinctive form of chronic cholecystitis associated with primary sclerosing cholangitis (PSC), *Mod Pathol* 6:51A, 1993.
114. Wiesner RH, Grambsch PM, Dikson R et al: Primary sclerosing cholangitis: natural history, prognostic factors and survival analysis, *Hepatology* 10:430, 1989.
115. Dikson ER, Murtaugh PA, Wiesner RH et al: Primary sclerosing cholangitis: refinement and validation of survival models, *Gastroenterology,* 103:1893, 1992.
116. Wee A, Ludwig J, Coffey RJ et al: Hepatobiliary carcinoma associated with primary sclerosing cholangitis and chronic ulcerative colitis, *Hum Pathol* 16:719, 1985.
117. Lin AC, Chapman SW, Turner HR et al: Clonorchiasis: an update, *South Med J* 80:919, 1987.
118. Schwartz DA: Cholangiocarcinoma associated with liver fluke infection: a preventable source of morbidity in Asian immigrants, *Am J Gastroenterol* 81:76, 1986.
119. Viranuvatti V, Stitnimankarn T: Liver fluke infection and infestation in Southeast Asia, *Prog Liver Dis* 4:537, 1972.
120. Schulman A, Loxton AJ, Heydenrych JJ et al: Sonographic diagnosis of biliary ascariasis, *AJR* 139:485, 1982.
121. Margulis SJ, Jacobson IM: Hepatobiliary and pancreatic manifestations of AIDS, *Semin Gastrointest Dis* 2:49, 1991.
122. Cello JP: Human immunodeficiency virus-associated biliary tract disease, *Semin Liver Dis* 12:213, 1992.
123. Viteri AL, Greene JF Jr: Bile duct abnormalities in the acquired immune deficiency syndrome, *Gastroenterology* 92:2014, 1987.
124. Bonacini M: Hepatobiliary complication in patients with human immunodeficiency virus infection, *Am J Med* 92:404, 1992.
125. Pol S, Romana CA, Richard S et al: Microsporidia infection in patients with the human immunodeficiency virus and unexplained cholangitis, *N Eng J Med* 328:95, 1993.
126. Finegold MJ, Carpenter RJ: Obliterative cholangitis due to cytomegalovirus: a possible precursor of paucity of intrahepatic bile ducts, *Hum Pathol* 13:662, 1982.
127. Standfield NJ, Salisbury JR, Howard ER: Benign non-traumatic inflammatory strictures of the extrahepatic biliary system, *Br J Surg* 76:849, 1989.
128. Lillemoe KD, Pitt HA, Cameron JL: Postoperative bile duct strictures, *Surg Clin North Am* 70:1355, 1990.

Neoplasms

Benign tumors

ADENOMAS

129. Albores-Saavedra J, Henson DE, Sobin LE: *Histological typing of tumours of the gallbladder and extrahepatic bile ducts,* World Health Organization, Berlin, 1991, Springer-Verlag.
130. Albores-Saavedra J, Henson DE: Tumors of the gallbladder and extrahepatic bile ducts, *Atlas of Tumor Pathology,* second series, Fasc 22, Washington, DC, 1986, Armed Forces Institute of Pathology.
131. Kosuka S, Tsubone M, Yasui A, Hachisuka K: Relation of adenoma to carcinoma in the gallbladder, *Cancer* 50:2226, 1982.
132. Albores-Saavedra J, Vardaman C, Vuitch F: Non-neoplastic polypoid lesions and adenomas of the gallbladder, *Pathol Annu* (Pt 1) 28:145, 1993.
133. Kijima H, Watanabe H, Iwafuchi M, Ishihara N: Histogenesis of gallbladder carcinoma from investigation of early carcinoma and microcarcinoma, *Acta Pathol Jpn* 39:235, 1989.
134. Mogilner JG, Dharan M, Siplovich L: Adenoma of the gallbladder in childhood, *J Pediatr Surg* 26:223, 1991.
135. Tantachamrun T, Borvonsombat S, Theetranont C: Gardner's syndrome associated with adenomatous polyp of the gallbladder, *J Med Assoc Thai* 62:441, 1979.
136. Foster DR, Foster DBE: Gallbladder polyps in Peutz-Jeghers syndrome, *Postgrad Med J* 56:373, 1980.
137. Wada K, Tanaka M, Yamaguchi K, Wada K: Carcinoma and polyps of the gallbladder associated with Peutz-Jeghers syndrome, *Dig Dis Sci* 32:943, 1987.
138. Yamaguchi K, Maeda S, Kitamura K: Papillary adenoma of the gallbladder associated with regurgitation of pancreatic juice through abnormally shaped union, *Acta Chir Scand* 155:549, 1989.
139. Christensen AH, Ishak KG: Benign tumors and pseudotumors of the gallbladder: report of 180 cases, *Arch Pathol* 90:423, 1970.
140. Yamaguchi K, Enjoji M: Gallbladder polyps: inflammatory, hyperplastic and neoplastic types, *Surg Pathol* 1:203, 1988.
141. Lin G, Hägerstrand I: Multiple adenomas of the gallbladder, *Acta Pathol Microbiol Immunol Scand, Sect. A,* 91:475, 1983.
142. Nishihara K, Yamaguchi K, Hashimoto H, Enjoji M: Tubular adenoma of the gallbladder with squamoid spindle cell metaplasia, *Acta Pathol Jpn* 41:41, 1991.

CYSTADENOMA

143. Ishak KG, Willis GW, Cummins SD, Bullock AA: Biliary cystadenoma and cystadenocarcinoma, *Cancer* 39:322, 1977.
144. Albores-Saavedra J, Gould EW, Angeles-Angeles A, Henson DE: Cystic tumors of the pancreas, *Pathol Annu* 25(pt 1):19, 1990.
145. Simmons T, Miller C, Pesigan A, Lewin K: Cystadenoma of the gallbladder, *Am J Gastroenterol* 84:1427, 1989.
146. Wheeler DA, Edmondson HA: Cystadenoma with mesenchymal stroma (CMS) in the liver and bile ducts: a clinicopathologic study of 17 cases, 4 with malignant change, *Cancer* 56:1434, 1985.
147. Vuitch F, Battifora H, Albores-Saavedra J: Demonstration of steroid hormone receptors in pancreato-biliary mucinous cystic neoplasms, *Lab Invest* 68:114A, 1993.

PAPILLOMATOSIS

148. Madden JJ Jr, Smith GW: Multiple biliary papillomatosis, *Cancer* 34:1316-20, 1974.
149. Neumann RD, LiVolsi VA, Rosenthal NS et al: Adenocarcinoma in biliary papillomatosis, *Gastroenterology* 70:779, 1976.
150. Böttger ThK, Sorger E, Junzinger Th: Progressive papillomatosis of the intrahepatic and extrahepatic bile ducts, *Acta Chir Scand* 155:125, 1989.

GRANULAR CELL TUMORS

151. Jain KM, Hastings OM, Rickert RR et al: Granular cell tumors of the common bile duct, *Am J Gastroenterol* 71:401, 1979.
152. Aisner SC, Khaneja S, Ramïrez O: Multiple granular cell tumors of the gallbladder and biliary tree, *Arch Pathol Lab Med* 106:470, 1982.
153. Eisen RN, Kirby WM, O'Quinn JL: Granular cell tumor of the biliary tree, *Am J Surg Pathol* 15:460, 1991.

GANGLIONEUROFIBROMATOSIS

154. Carney JA, Sizemore GW, Hayles AM: Multiple endocrine neoplasia, type 2b, *Pathobiol Annu* 8:105, 1978.
155. Rutgeents P, Hendrickx H, Geboes K et al: Involvement of the upper digestive tract by systemic neurofibromatosis, *Gastrointest Endosc* 1:22, 1981.

PARAGANGLIOMA

156. Miller TA, Weber TR, Appelman HD: Paraganglioma of the gallbladder, *Arch Surg* 105:637, 1972.
157. Sarma DP, Rodríguez FH, Hoffman EO: Paraganglioma of the hepatic duct, *South Med J* 73:1677, 1980.

CARCINOID TUMORS

158. Vitaux J, Salmon RJ, Languille O et al: Carcinoid tumor of the common bile duct, *Am J Gastroenterol* 76:360, 1981.
159. Angeles-Angeles A, Quintanilla L, Larriva J: Primary carcinoid of the common bile duct: immunohistochemical characterization of a case and review of the literature, *Am J Clin Pathol* 96:341, 1991.

160. Tanaka K, Iida Y, Tsutsumi Y: Pancreatic polypeptide-immunoreactive gallbladder carcinoid tumor, *Acta Pathol Jpn* 115:118, 1992.
161. Barrón-Rodríguez P, Manivel C, Méndez-Sánchez N et al: Carcinoid tumor of the common bile duct: evidence for its origin in metaplastic endocrine cells, *Am J Gastroenterol* 86:1073, 1991.
162. Goodman ZD, Albores-Saavedra J, Lundblad D: Somatostatinoma of the cystic duct, *Cancer* 53:498, 1984.
163. Burke AP, Sobin LH, Federspiel BH et al: Carcinoid tumors of the duodenum: a clinicopathologic study of 99 cases, *Arch Pathol Lab Med* 114:700, 1990.
164. Burke AP, Sobin LH, Shekitkas KM et al: Somatostatin-producing duodenal carcinoids in patients with von Recklinghausen's neurofibromatosis: a predilection for black patients, *Cancer* 65:1591, 1990.
165. Wisniewski M, Toker C: Composite tumor of the gallbladder exhibiting both carcinomatous and carcinoidal patterns, *Am J Gastroenterol* 58:633, 1972.
166. Wada A, Ishiguro S, Tateishi R et al: Carcinoid tumor of the gallbladder associated with adenocarcinoma, *Cancer* 51:1911, 1983.

Malignant tumors

DYSPLASIA AND CARCINOMA IN SITU

167. Albores-Saavedra J, Alcántara-Vázquez A, Cruz-Ortis H, Herrera-Geopfert H: The precursor lesions of invasive gallbladder carcinoma, *Cancer* 45:919-27, 1980.
168. Albores-Saavedra J, Manrique JJ, Angeles-Angeles A, Henson DE: Carcinoma in situ of the gallbladder: a clinicopathologic study of 18 cases, *Am J Surg Pathol* 8:323, 1984.
169. Laitio M: Histogenesis of epithelial neoplasms of human gallbladder. I. Dysplasia, *Pathol Res Pract* 178:51, 1983.
170. Duarte I, Llanos O, Domke H et al: Metaplasia and precursor lesions of gallbladder carcinoma, *Cancer* 72:1878, 1993.
171. Yamaguchi A, Hachisuka K, Isogai M, Tsubone M: Carcinoma in situ of the gallbladder with superficial extension into the Rokitansky-Aschoff sinuses and mucous glands, *Gastroenterol Jpn* 27:765, 1992.
172. Suzuki M, Takahashi T, Ouchi K, Matsuno S: The development and extension of hepatohilar bile duct carcinoma: a three-dimensional tumor mapping in the intrahepatic biliary tree visualized with the aid of a graphics computer system, *Cancer* 64:658, 1989.
173. Harvath AC, Manley PN, Groll A et al: Bile duct carcinoma and biliary tract dysplasia in chronic ulcerative colitis, *Arch Pathol Lab Med* 113:434, 1989.

CARCINOMA OF THE GALLBLADDER AND EXTRAHEPATIC BILE DUCTS

174. Nakajo S, Yamamoto M, Tahara E: Morphometric analysis of gallbladder adenocarcinoma: discrimination between carcinoma and dysplasia, *Virchows Arch [A] Pathol Anat]* 416:133, 1989.
175. Rudolph R, Cohen JJ, Gascoigne RH: Biliary cancer among Southwestern American Indians, *Ariz Med* 27:14, 1970.
176. Morris DL, Buechley RW, Key CR et al: Gallbladder disease and gallbladder cancer among American Indians in tricultural New Mexico, *Cancer* 42: 2472, 1978.
177. Wiesner RH, Ludwig J, LaRusso NF et al: Diagnosis and treatment of primary sclerosing cholangitis, *Semin Liver Dis* 5:241, 1985.
178. Mir-Madjlessi SH, Farmer RG, Sivak MV: Bile duct carcinoma in patients with ulcerative colitis, *Dig Dis Sci* 32:145, 1987.
179. Rossi RL, Heiss FW, Beckmann CF et al. Management of cancer of the bile duct, *Surg Clin North Am* 65:59, 1985.
180. Yamaguchi K, Enjoji M: Carcinoma of the gallbladder: a clinicopathology of 103 patients with a newly proposed staging, *Cancer* 62:1425, 1988.
181. Henson DE, Albores-Saavedra J, Corle D: Carcinoma of the gallbladder: histologic types, stage of disease, grade and survival rates, *Cancer* 70:1493, 1992.
182. Henson DE, Albores-Saavedra J, Corle D: Carcinoma of the extrahepatic bile ducts: histologic types, stage of disease, grade, and survival rates, *Cancer* 70: 1498, 1992.
183. Ashner H, Siegal B, Oland Y et al: Calcified gallbladder (porcelain gallbladder), *Arch Surg* 113:594, 1978.
184. Belamaric J: Intrahepatic bile duct carcinoma and *C. sinensis* infection in Hong Kong, *Cancer* 31:468, 1973.
185. Flavell DJ: Liver-fluke infection as an aetiological factor in bile duct carcinoma of man, *Trans R Soc Trop Med Hyg* 75:814, 1981.
186. Albores-Saavedra J, Nadji M, Henson DE: Intestinal type adenocarcinoma of the gallbladder: a clinicopathologic and immunocytochemical study of seven cases, *Am J Surg Pathol* 10:19, 1986.
187. Vardaman C, Albores-Saavedra J: Clear cell carcinomas of the gallbladder and extrahepatic biliary ducts, *Am J Surg Pathol* 19:91, 1995.
188. Albores-Saavedra J, Cruz-Ortíz H, Alcántara-Vázquez A et al. Unusual types of gallbladder carcinoma: a report of 16 cases, *Arch Pathol Lab Med* 105:287, 1981.
189. Albores-Saavedra J, Soriano J, Larraza-Hernández O et al: Oat cell carcinoma of the gallbladder, *Hum Pathol* 15:639, 1984.
190. Cavazzana AO, Fassina AS, Tallot M, Ninfo V: Small cell carcinoma of the gallbladder: an immunocytochemical and ultrastructural study, *Pathol Res Pract* 187:472, 1991.
191. Johnstone A, Zuch RH, Anders KH: Oat cell carcinoma of the gallbladder: a rare and highly lethal neoplasm, *Arch Pathol Lab Med* 117:1009, 1993.
192. Ke-Jian G, Yamaguchi K, Enjoji M: Undifferentiated carcinoma of the gallbladder: a clinico-pathologic, histochemical and immunohistochemical study of 21 patients with a poor prognosis, *Cancer* 61:1872, 1988.
193. Albores-Saavedra J, Nadji M, Henson DE, Angeles-Angeles A: Enteroendocrine cell differentiation in carcinomas of the gallbladder and mucinous cystadenocarcinomas of the pancreas, *Path Res Pract* 183:169, 1988.
194. Yamamoto M, Takahashi I, Iwamoto T et al: Endocrine cells in extrahepatic bile duct carcinomas, *J Cancer Res Clin Oncol* 108:331, 1984.
195. Albores-Saavedra J, Nadji M, Morales AR, Henson DE: Carcinoembryonic antigen in normal preneoplastic and neoplastic gallbladder epithelium, *Cancer* 52:1069, 1983.
196. Maxwell P, Davis RI, Sloan JM: Carcinoembryonic antigen (CEA) in benign and malignant epithelium of the gallbladder, extrahepatic bile ducts and ampulla of Vater, *J Pathol* 170:73, 1993.
197. Fukuda T, Ohnishi Y: Gallbladder carcinoma producing human chorionic gonadotropin, *Am J Gastroenterol* 85:1403, 1990.
198. Abu-Farsakh H, Fraire AE: Adenocarcinoma and (extragonadal) choriocarcinoma of the gallbladder in a young woman, *Hum Pathol* 22:614, 1991.
199. Ikeda M, Okada S, Morozumi A et al: Alpha-feto-protein producing carcinoma of the gallbladder associated with anomalous arrangement of the pancreaticobiliary ductal system: early detection through an attack of acute pancreatitis, *Gastroenterol Jpn* 27:668, 1992.
200. Kamel D, Paakko P, Nerorva K et al: p53 and c-*erb* B-2 protein expression in adenocarcinomas and epithelial dysplasias of the gallbladder, *J Pathol* 170:67, 1993.
200b. Wistuba II, Sugio K, Hung J et al: Allele specific mutations involved in the pathogenesis of endemic gallbladder carcinoma in Chile, *Cancer Res*, 55:2511, 1995.

CARCINOSARCOMA, MALIGNANT LYMPHOMA, AND MALIGNANT MELANOMA

201. Albores-Saavedra J, Henson DE, Sobin L: The World Health Organization histologic classification of tumors of the gallbladder and extrahepatic bile ducts: a commentary on the second edition, *Cancer* 70:410, 1992.
202. Albores-Saavedra J, Gould E, Manivel C et al: Chronic cholecystitis with lymphoid hyperplasia, *Rev Invest Clin* (Mex) 41:159, 1989.
203. Peison B, Rabin L: Malignant melanoma of the gallbladder, *Cancer* 37:2448, 1976.

RHABDOMYOSARCOMA

204. Lack EE, Pérez-Atayde AR, Schuster SR: Botryoid rhabdomyosarcoma of the biliary tract, *Am J Surg Pathol* 5:643, 1981.
205. Ruymann FB, Raney B, Crist WM et al: Rhabdomyosarcoma of biliary tree in childhood: a report from the intergroup rhabdomyosarcoma study, *Cancer* 56:575, 1985.

59 Pancreas

Daniel S. Longnecker

NORMAL PANCREAS

The pancreas is a combined exocrine and endocrine gland that is highly specialized in its ability to synthesize and secrete a wide variety of specific proteins. This chapter focuses on diseases of the exocrine pancreas but begins with a brief review of the normal structure, function, and development of the pancreas to provide an immediate context for understanding the nature of the diseases that affect it, the most prevalent of which are acute and chronic pancreatitis, cystic fibrosis, and carcinoma.

Anatomy. The pancreas weighs 70 to 140 g in adults. The gross appearance of the normal pancreas varies with the person's state of nutrition and vascular perfusion. The normal pancreas is tan to yellow, it is pale relative to the liver, and it is less translucent than adipose tissue. The pancreas is compact and elongate, extending from the duodenum to the hilum of the spleen (Fig. 59-1). Its configuration varies from one person to another. In one series, the length of most pancreases in young adults was found to vary from 16 to 21 cm, and the weight averaged approximately 100 g.[1] The duodenal portion is called the *head*, the splenic portion the *tail*, and the middle portion the *body*. This topographic subdivision is arbitrary but is useful for the purpose of description. In human beings the pancreas is narrow in the axis of the aorta and the superior mesenteric vessels. This segment is sometimes designated as the *neck* and marks the boundary between the head and body. The body and tail are not demarcated by any distinct anatomic landmarks. The pancreas is retroperitoneal in location and is surrounded by fat except where the head abuts on the duodenum; the ventral surface lies close to the peritoneum.

Pancreatic ducts are classified according to their size and location as the main duct, interlobular ducts, intralobular ducts, and ductules. The pancreatic duct system originates in the lobules as ductules that join to form intralobular ducts that then join interlobular ducts. The latter drain into the main pancreatic duct that extends from the tail to its entry point into the duodenum through the ampulla of Vater. The main pancreatic duct (called the *duct of Wirsung*) ranges from 1 to 2 mm in diameter and may either open into the bile duct in the head of the pancreas (called the *common channel*), or open directly into the duodenum at the ampulla. An accessory duct in the head (termed the *duct of Santorini*) may open separately into the duodenum proximal to the ampulla through a minor papilla. A lobule is defined as that portion of the pancreas served by one intralobular duct and its branches. Lobules of acinar tissue and the major ducts are visible grossly. Islets and intralobular ductules are not visible to the naked eye.

Histologically the exocrine pancreas is composed of two basic cell types, acinar cells and ductal cells. More than 80% of the gland consists of pancreatic acinar cells, and the duct system constitutes 2% to 4%. Cells of the terminal ductules that abut on or are interspersed among acinar cells are commonly designated as *centroacinar cells*. Islets are interspersed in the exocrine tissue but have no constant relationship to the lobular or duct system. Ductules may extend into the islets, and a variable fraction of normal islets contain a few acinar cells.

Acinar cells are pyramid-shaped cells arranged to form a tubuloacinar network that convolutes on itself within the lobules.[2] The acinar tubules and acini are surrounded by a basement membrane and have a small central lumen. The paranuclear basal portion of the acinar cell is basophilic, reflecting its high content of rough endoplasmic reticulum (RER), and the apical cytoplasm (near the acinar lumen) is granular and eosinophilic, reflecting the presence of zymogen granules. These secretory granules contain the digestive enzymes. More than half of the acinar cells in adults have two nuclei.

The typical ultrastructural features of acinar cells, that is abundant RER and zymogen granules, reflect their secretory activity. The cells also contain elongate mitochondria and have well-developed Golgi complexes at the interface between the RER and zymogen granules. The cells are linked to adjacent cells by junctional complexes located along the lateral cell membranes, and these tight junctions are in the apical region near the acinar lumen. Apical microvilli protrude from the cell membrane into the lumen.

Ductal cells are smaller than acinar cells and have a single nucleus. Main and interlobular ducts are normally lined by a

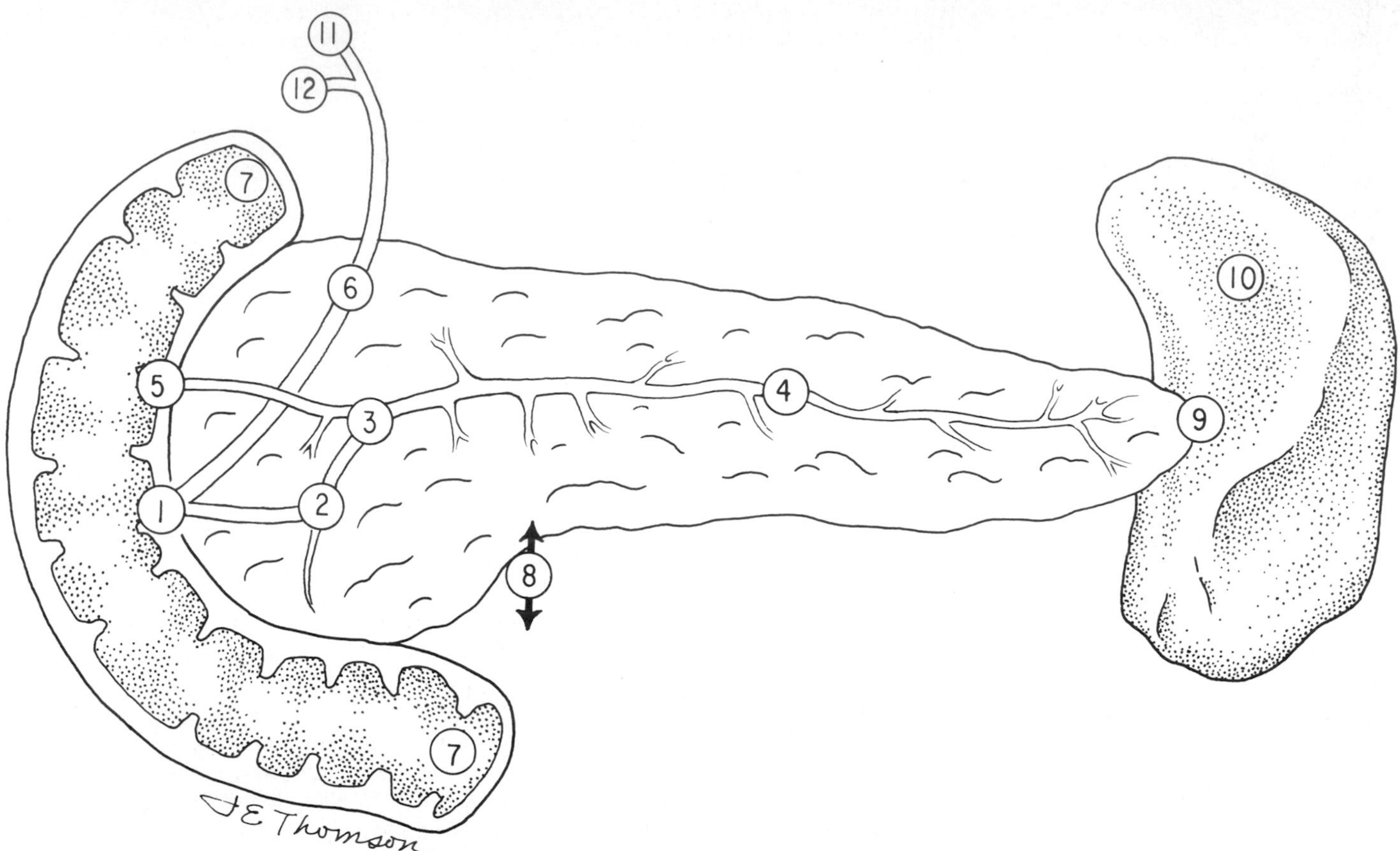

Fig. 59-1 Gross anatomic relationships of the pancreas depicting aspects of development and variation in the duct system.

1 Major papilla (ampulla of Vater) where the common bile duct and the main pancreatic duct enter the duodenum. The ducts may join proximal to the ampulla to form a common channel, join in the ampulla, or open separately into the duodenum.
2 Main pancreatic duct (duct of Wirsung) in the head of the pancreas. This portion of the duct and the pancreatic parenchyma are derived from the ventral anlage of the pancreas.
3 Junction of the ducts of Wirsung and Santorini in the head of the pancreas. Failure of the ducts to join at this point during development causes pancreas divisum.
4 Main pancreatic duct in the body of the pancreas. This portion of the duct and the parenchyma are derived from the dorsal anlage of the pancreas.
5 Minor papilla where the accessory pancreatic duct (duct of Santorini) enters the duodenum if the papilla has remained patent during development. In pancreas divisum this is the entry point for the main pancreatic duct.
6 Common bile duct passes behind the duodenum and courses through the posterior aspect of the head of the pancreas to the ampulla.
7 Duodenum bordering the head of the pancreas. The stomach lies anterior to the pancreas.
8 Axis of the superior mesenteric artery and portal vein marks the junction of the pancreatic body and head.
9 The tail of the pancreas extends to the hilum of the spleen and lies ventral to the left kidney.
10 Spleen.
11 The common hepatic duct extends to the liver.
12 The cystic duct extends to the gallbladder.

single layer of cuboidal or low columnar cells. The lumen of the main pancreatic duct is surrounded by a thick collagenous layer that is five to 10 times thicker than the epithelium. Numerous small branch ducts extend peripherally through the wall. Interlobular ducts also have a thick collagenous wall that thins as the ducts become intralobular. The smallest branches of the duct system, the intralobular ductules, are lined by cuboidal or slightly flattened ductal cells. The smallest intralobular ductules are surrounded by a basement membrane but lack a collagenous sheath. The cytoplasm of ductal cells is pale and eosinophilic. Ultrastructurally the cytoplasm contains relatively small amounts of RER and smooth endoplasmic reticulum as well as prominent mitochondria. Mucoprotein secretory granules may be present in the apical cytoplasm. The lateral cell membranes form tight junctions, and the luminal surface forms microvilli. The basilar cell membrane abuts on a basement membrane.

Embryonic development. Both exocrine cell types and islets are derived from a common pool of precursor cells derived from the dorsal and ventral portions of the embryonic midgut. The dorsal and ventral primordia fuse during normal development. The ventral anlage forms the inferior and posterior parts of the head of the pancreas (see Fig. 59-1), and the dorsal anlage gives rise to the remainder of the head, body, and tail of the pancreas.

Physiology. Acinar cells secrete digestive enzymes through the exocytosis of zymogen granules into the acinar lumen, either in response to cholinergic vagal nerve stimuli, the dominant control mechanism in human beings, or in response to specific circulating peptide hormones for which the cells have receptors. Cholecystokinin and bombesin are two peptides that stimulate pancreatic secretion. Several of the digestive enzymes are synthesized as inactive proenzymes that are activated by proteolytic cleavage in the intestinal lumen. Trypsinogen is normally activated by enterokinase, a protease secreted by the duodenal mucosa, but it can also be activated by active trypsin or certain lysosomal enzymes. Trypsin activates the other proenzymes secreted by the pancreas. Pancreatic enzymes are required for the normal digestion and absorption of food in the gastrointestinal tract, especially for the hydrolysis of lipids.

Duct cells secrete water, chloride, and bicarbonate, which buffers the pancreatic juice, maintaining it at a pH of approximately 6.5, and stabilizes the proenzymes. Duct secretion is stimulated by vagal nerves and by secretin, which reaches the cells through the circulation. Ductal secretions transport the proenzymes into the duodenum.

Xenobiotics may reach the pancreas through the bloodstream after absorption and systemic distribution. Thus exposure to toxic chemicals could result from skin contact, inhalation, injection, or ingestion. The possibility also exists that ingested xenobiotics in the duodenum may enter the pancreatic duct by reflux and thus reach the ductal cells. Such reflux has been documented in experimental animals when the duodenal luminal pressure is increased, but this probably does not occur often in human beings.

The pancreas contains both phase I and phase II drug-metabolizing enzymes. However, such enzymatic activity represents only about 1% of that which takes place in liver cells. Both acinar and ductal cells contain such enzymes but in different amounts. The induction of cytochrome p-450 enzymes by xenobiotics, such as betanaphthalflavone, has been demonstrated in hamsters and rats. The pancreas may metabolize and activate indirectly acting toxins and procarcinogens, as has been shown in experimental animals. There are significant species differences with regard to the effect of xenobiotics, and the data obtained in animals cannot be extrapolated directly to human beings.

DEVELOPMENTAL ABNORMALITIES

Abnormalities of the pancreas include gross anomalies of development, minor structural changes of little clinical significance, and biochemical abnormalities.

Malformations

Annular pancreas

Annular pancreas is a malformation in which the pancreas encircles the duodenum and results from the abnormal fusion of the two pancreatic anlagen. Annular pancreas is a rare cause of duodenal obstruction.

Pancreas divisum

Pancreas divisum is the division of the pancreas into two parts, either functionally or in a gross configuration that involves the duct of the ventral pancreas emptying through the major ampulla with the common bile duct and the duct of the dorsal pancreas emptying through a minor papilla proximal to the ampulla of Vater in the duodenum. These duct systems normally fuse during development to form the main pancreatic duct (Wirsung) that extends from the tail to the ampulla and a minor or accessory duct (Santorini) that extends from the major duct in the head of the pancreas toward the minor papilla, which may or may not remain patent (see Fig. 59-1). Failure of the two duct systems to fuse causes a major duct to form that is dependent on drainage through the minor papilla, with a portion of the head of the pancreas draining through the ampulla. Its prevalence is estimated to be in the range of 5%.[3]

Ectopic pancreas

Ectopic pancreas (heterotopic pancreas) is the presence of pancreatic tissue in the wall of the stomach, duodenum, or jejunum. Primitive cells in the gut wall are related developmentally to the cells that give rise to the pancreas. Occasionally such cells proliferate and differentiate into pancreatic tissue. An ectopic pancreas may develop as part of Meckel's diverticulum in the ileum.

Pancreatic hamartoma

Pancreatic hamartoma is an apparent tumor consisting of an abnormally arranged mixture of mature acinar, islet, and duct cells surrounded by fibrous tissue. The ductal elements are dilated, and in one case the islet cells were found to be dispersed among acinar cells rather than aggregated as islets.[4] The mixture of mature cell types that do not show atypical changes indicates that this may be a malformation rather than a neoplasm.

Ectopic splenic tissue

Ectopic splenic tissue may be found within the tail of the pancreas.[5]

Duplication of the duodenum

Duplication of the duodenum such that an intrapancreatic cyst forms in the head of the pancreas has been described. Such duplications may retain a connection with the bowel lumen and therefore functionally be a diverticulum rather than a cyst.

Aplasia

Rarely the exocrine pancreas fails to develop or one of the two anlagen fails to develop so that most of the pancreas is then derived from either the dorsal or ventral portion. Partial agenesis with origin primarily from the ventral lobe results in a "short pancreas".[6] In some patients a congenital short pancreas is associated with polysplenia.[7]

Genetic diseases

Cystic fibrosis

Cystic fibrosis is the major genetically determined disease affecting the exocrine pancreas. *Fibrocystic disease* of the pancreas and *mucoviscidosis* are alternate names. Cystic fibrosis is an inherited systemic disease in which the mucinous secretions are abnormally viscous. The genetic abnormalities and the mode of inheritance are discussed in Chapter 14.

The pancreas is invariably affected, but the extent of pathologic changes and the time of their onset vary from person to person. All pancreatic changes can be explained by the hyperviscosity of mucus. Obstruction of the pancreatic duct by abnormal secretions in patients with cystic fibrosis causes pancreatitis. Malabsorption stemming from deficient enzyme secretion by the exocrine pancreas becomes an important part of the clinical picture in 85% of patients with cystic fibrosis, but 15% have a functioning pancreas. This is a consistent feature among affected siblings, implying the existence of a genetically mediated influence on the severity of the pancreatic disease. The discovery of the common cystic fibrosis mutation enabled Kerem and others[8] to test this hypothesis and demonstrate that pancreatic insufficiency was present in 99% of the patients homozygous for the ΔF508 mutation, 72% of the patients heterozygous for the ΔF508 mutation, and only 36% of the patients with other mutations. Pancreatic enzyme, fluid, and electrolyte secretion was severely impaired in the patients who were homozygous for the ΔF508 mutation. The pancreatic pathologic characteristics of cystic fibrosis are discussed in the section Pancreatitis.

Familial pancreatitis

Familial pancreatitis has been described as an autosomal dominant, non–sex-linked disease with limited penetrance[9-11] and is much less prevalent than cystic fibrosis. The clinical course is characterized by episodes of acute pancreatitis of mild to moderate severity that begin in childhood, with subsequent progression to chronic pancreatitis. Pancreatic lithiasis is typical late in the course when chronic pancreatitis has developed.[9] Ductal strictures have been noted in some cases. Aminoaciduria accompanies the disease in some kinships. The pathogenesis of the pancreatitis is not clear and may differ in various kinships. The risk of pancreatic carcinoma is increased in these patients.[10]

Shwachman-Diamond syndrome

The Shwachman-Diamond syndrome, with an incidence about one tenth that of cystic fibrosis, and the even less common Johanson-Blizzard syndrome are associated with pancreatic insufficiency.[12] In the former, the pancreas shows diminished acinar tissue and replacement by fat, whereas the findings are variable in the latter syndrome.

Single enzyme deficiencies, that is, failure of the acinar cells to produce one of the pancreatic digestive enzymes, have been described, but a hereditary basis has not been established for all variants.[11] A defect in the gene that codes for duodenal enterokinase, which is essential for the activation of pancreatic zymogens, has also been described. This defect results in malabsorption.

MINOR PATHOLOGIC CHANGES

Several adaptive and focal developmental, necrotic, and proliferative changes in the pancreas, including lesions of minor importance or rare occurrence, may be encountered as incidental findings at autopsy or in pancreases surgically resected for the treatment of pancreatitis or neoplasms.

Changes affecting the pancreas diffusely

Adiposity

Adiposity of the pancreas has been defined by Stamm[1] as replacement of more than 25% of the parenchyma by adipose tissue. The fat cells are both intralobular and perilobular. The change has also been called "adipose atrophy" and "stromal fatty ingrowth." Such adiposity is associated with aging, diabetes, and systemic atherosclerosis.[1] It is commonly noted that the acinar cell mass decreases and the pancreas contains increasing numbers of fat cells as persons age.

Focal necrosis

A 30% incidence of focal necrosis of parenchymal or fat cells in foci measuring 1 to 3 mm in diameter was noted in one autopsy series.[1] Systemic bacterial disease was implicated as a cause. Ischemic injury to the pancreas causes a transient coagulative necrosis to occur that quickly becomes liquefactive because of the activation of endogenous pancreatic lysosomal and digestive enzymes. The leakage of pancreatic lipases causes the necrosis of adipose tissue and the characteristic fat necrosis of peripancreatic and mesenteric fat.

Regeneration

Both acinar and ductal cells have the ability to divide, and the exocrine pancreas can regenerate lost cells as long as the stromal framework is preserved. Thus mitoses may be seen in these cell types in adults. When portions of the pancreas have been resected in experimental animals, the remaining pancreas has been observed to enlarge to compensate partially for the loss. This might be regarded as a physiologic hyperplasia.

Changes in acinar cells

A physiologic hypertrophy occurs cyclically in well-nourished persons, who store a considerable amount of protein in zymogen granules during the fasting state. On the other hand, malnourished, protein-deficient, or starved persons store comparatively small amounts of zymogens in acinar cells, which therefore appear atrophic.

Acinar cells may swell or accumulate fat in the cytoplasm as a result of toxic injury. At the ultrastructural level, cell swelling has been accompanied by vesiculation of the RER and dilatation of cisternae. Iron is deposited in acinar cells in hemochromatosis, but to a lesser degree than it is in hepatocytes.

Autophagy

Autophagy is a conspicuous change in acinar cells that have been subjected to cytotoxic injury (Fig. 59-2). It has been demonstrated experimentally that acinar cells can extrude autophagic vacuoles and residual bodies either into the duct lumen or into the interstitium such that residual bodies (lipochrome pigment) do not accumulate in acinar cells.[13] The pancreas of rodents can reduce its mass through the apoptosis of acinar cells, and it seems likely that a similar mechanism is at work in the human pancreas during the pancreatic atrophy that occurs in kwashiorkor.[14] Fragments of deleted acinar cells may be phagocytosed by adjacent acinar or ductal cells, and this process may be difficult to differentiate morphologically from autophagy (Fig. 59-2).

Acinar dilatation

Acinar dilatation occurs without a known cause in patients with bacterial disease or uremia.[1] The change may be focal or

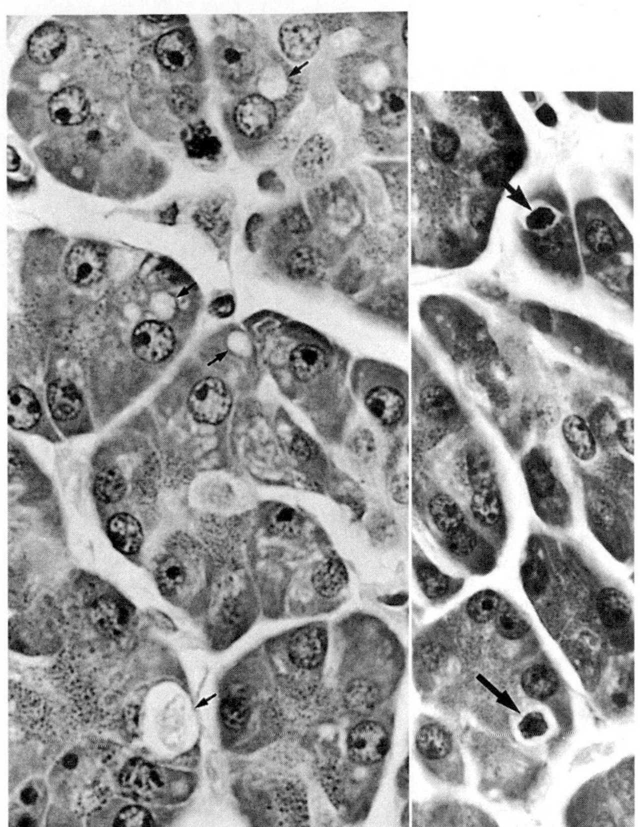

Fig. 59-2 Autophagy. This collage from a single microscopic field contains several acinar cells with vacuoles. Most vacuoles appear empty *(small arrows)*, and a few contain dense residual bodies *(large arrow)*. The largest of these dense bodies may reflect the presence of apoptosis.

diffuse. Diffuse dilatation was found in 7% and focal dilatation in 15% of the autopsies analyzed by Stamm.[1]

Focal acinar cell change

Focal acinar cell change represents a group of lesions characterized by irregular but sharply outlined groups of acinar cells, ranging from islet size to 3 mm in their greatest dimension. The foci have characteristics of a clonal population of cells, in that the cells all show similar changes. In one variant designated as *eosinophilic degeneration*, the cytoplasm of the acinar cells often shows a homogeneous eosinophilia (loss of basophilia).[1] In such foci the cells and their nuclei are often similar in size to the surrounding acinar cells. In other variants the cytoplasm may be vacuolated or the zymogen content of the cells may be decreased. The nuclei may be normal in size and contain dense chromatin or they may be enlarged (Fig. 59-3). Mitoses are infrequent, and inflammatory infiltrates are absent. Variants of focal acinar cell change have been given various names, including *acinar adenomatous hyperplasia*,[15] *focal acinar cell dysplasia*,[16,17] "acinar cell adenoma,"[18] and "hyperplastic acinar cell nodule."[19] The reported incidence of focal acinar cell changes increases during the first two decades of life[20] and has been reported to range from 1.2% to 43.5% in various series.[1,16,17,19] The lesions in this category have been noted to resemble those induced in rodents by pancreatic carcinogens.[16,18]

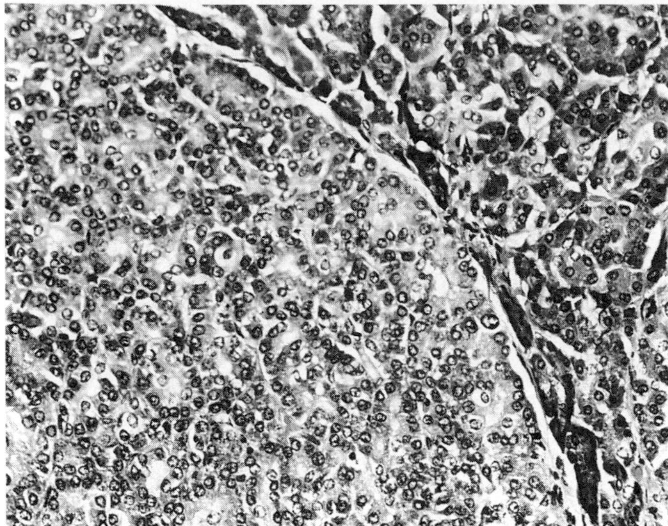

Fig. 59-3 Focal acinar cell change. The lefthand portion of the field contains cells of a nodule composed of small acinar cells with slightly enlarged nuclei. Normal acinar cells lie on the right. This is one of several variants of focal acinar cell change.

This is a heterogeneous group of lesions in human beings. Because their biologic and clinical significance is unknown, it seems appropriate to group them together and to note distinctive features descriptively. Few of these lesions seem to merit a diagnosis of acinar cell adenoma in human beings, and this diagnosis should be reserved for large, presumably neoplastic lesions.

Ductal metaplasia

Pancreatic acinar cells can undergo metaplasia and assume a ductal phenotype. Loss of apical cytoplasm appears to be the initial step in this process. Ductal metaplasia of acinar cells may contribute to the formation of tubular complexes (see later discussion).

Changes in ductal epithelium

Ductal epithelial lesions consist of ulceration, squamous metaplasia, and a continuum of hyperplastic changes that includes lesions regarded as preneoplastic.

Cysts

Small nonneoplastic cysts that lack an apparent communication with the duct system measure up to 1 cm in diameter (Fig. 59-4). These cysts have fibrous walls that vary in thickness and are lined by columnar, cuboidal, or flattened ductal cells. Multiple contiguous small cysts have been called cystic ductal complexes (Fig. 59-5). Their lumens may contain proteinaceous secretions that are sometimes condensed into laminated concretions. Similar condensed proteins may form "plugs" in intralobular and interlobular ducts.

Calculi

Larger ducts may contain calculi that are composed of calcium carbonate and a protein matrix. Calculi are often elongated and may be several centimeters long and up to 1 to 2 cm in diameter.

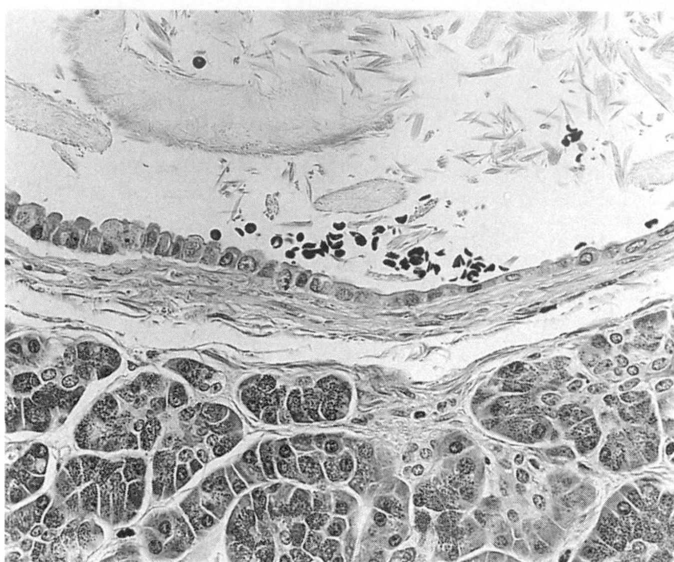

Fig. 59-4 Nonneoplastic cyst with a thin fibrous wall lying in normal acinar tissue. The cells lining the cyst appear to be of the ductal type and are cuboidal or slightly flattened. The cyst contains proteinaceous concretions and a few erythrocytes.

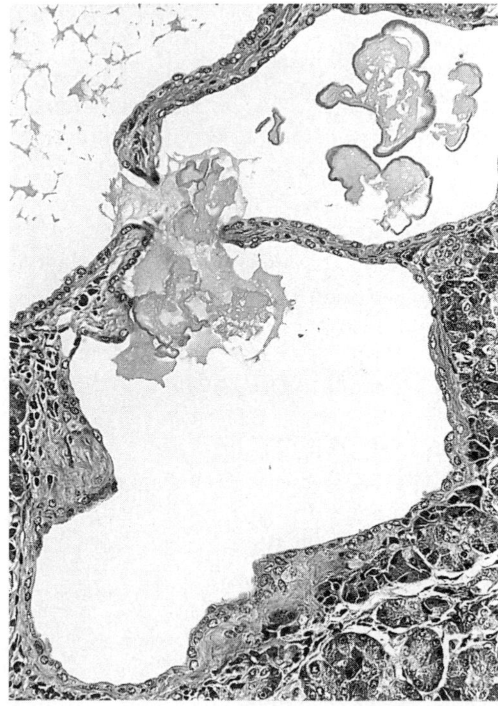

Fig. 59-5 Cystic ductal complex. These adjacent small cysts are lined by flattened epithelium and have a thin fibrous wall. The three lumens communicate. The cyst in the upper left corner was the largest of the three. Proteinaceous precipitate forms concretions in the cystic spaces.

Squamous metaplasia

Squamous metaplasia can occur in ductal epithelium. This is typically found in the setting of chronic pancreatitis with intraductal calculi. Frequently only a portion of the main duct or a ductule is involved. This lesion is found in 8% to 47% of the nontumorous pancreases as well as in chronically inflamed pancreases.[21] Extensive squamous metaplasia may occur in the main pancreatic duct after prolonged stenting or secondary to infection with *Clonorchis sinensis*.[22] Focal epithelial hyperplasia, which is a condition involving an increase in the number of epithelial layers in conjunction with slight squamous metaplasia,[21,23] can be regarded as the immature variant of squamous metaplasia (Fig. 59-6). The surface layer in the immature variant may retain mucous cells. Although the incidence of squamous metaplasia increases with age,[19] no association with pancreatic cancer has been noted.

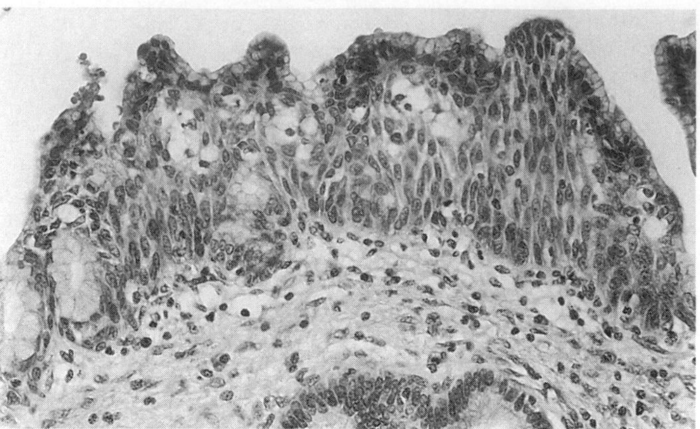

Fig. 59-6 Incomplete squamous metaplasia in a duct showing ductal hyperplasia. Most of the stratified area is still capped by low columnar cells.

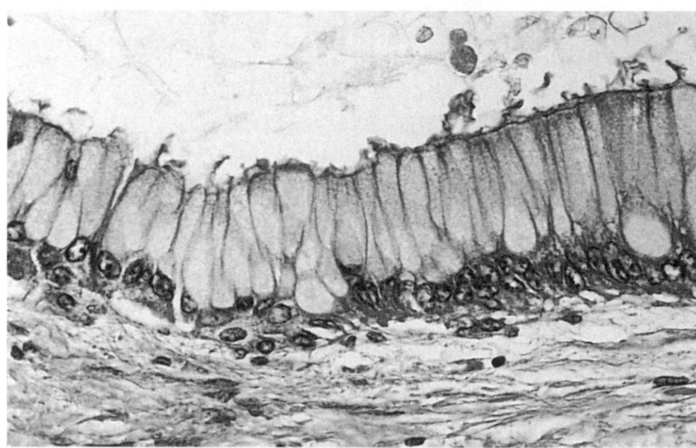

Fig. 59-7 Nonpapillary ductal hyperplasia in an intralobular duct lined by tall columnar, mucin-containing cells.

Nonpapillary ductal hyperplasia

Nonpapillary ductal hyperplasia is characterized by the replacement of normal epithelium of the ducts by tall columnar cells containing elongated basal nuclei and considerable supranuclear mucin (Fig. 59-7). These cells appear crowded, and their elongated nuclei are arranged perpendicularly to the basement membrane. Thus the term *hyperplasia* seems appropriate even though mitoses are seldom seen. This is the most frequent epithelial change affecting the pancreatic ducts and is found in up to 90% of nontumorous pancreases at autopsy. Changes of this type were noted in 55% of of the pancreases in Stamm's series.[1] Ductal hyper-

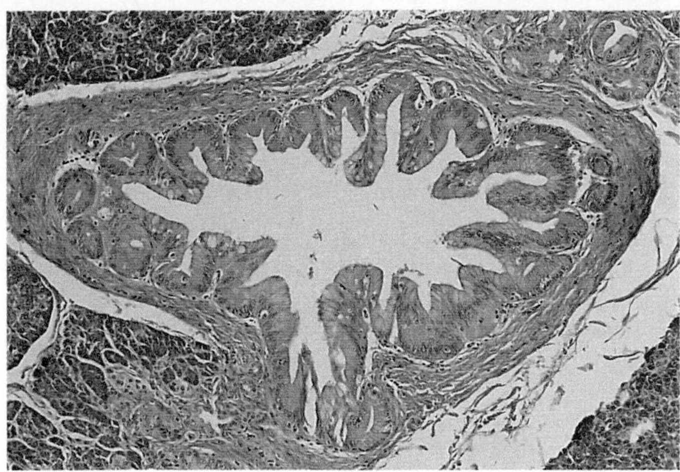

Fig. 59-8 Papillary ductal hyperplasia in an interlobular duct. The duct is lined by tall columnar, mucin-containing cells that form papillary folds. The stromal core can be seen in several of the papillary folds.

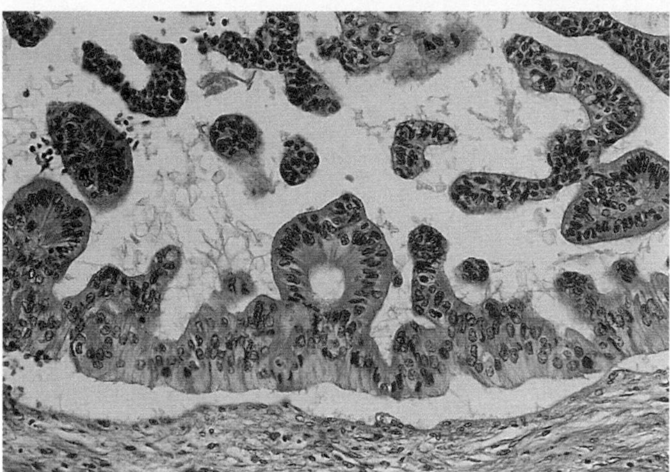

Fig. 59-9 Papillary ductal hyperplasia with severe atypia. Some of the papillary projections lack stromal cores. The nuclear/cytoplasmic ratio is high in some cells.

plasia is particularly prevalent in association with moderate obstruction and chronic pancreatitis, and its incidence in patients with pancreatic cancer has been observed to be about the same as that in a matched control group of patients with other types of nonpancreatic cancer.[21,24] "Mucinous cell hypertrophy," "mucous metaplasia," "mucoid transformation," "goblet cell metaplasia," "nonpapillary epithelial hypertrophy," and "ductal hyperplasia (grade 1)" are alternative names. Neutral mucin and sialomucin are found in these cells, but the amount of sulfated mucin that is normally produced in the ducts is markedly reduced. Ultrastructurally the appearance of the mucin granules in these cells is altered compared with their appearance in the cells of normal large ducts.[25] Occasionally there are also metaplastic pyloric-type gland cells that stain intensely with periodic acid–Schiff reagent (PAS).[25] Pure metaplastic pyloric-type glands are found mainly in the connective tissue surrounding main or interlobular ducts that show hyperplasia.

Papillary ductal hyperplasia

Papillary ductal hyperplasia is characterized by the intraductal papillary proliferation of duct cells showing mucinous hypertrophy. The papillary epithelial folds typically contain a vascular tissue stalk (Fig. 59-8). The lesion has also been called *ductal hyperplasia (grades 2 and 3)*.[19,26] The incidence of ductal papillary hyperplasia increases with age, and it has been observed to be higher in patients with pancreatic cancer than in control autopsy patients without pancreatic cancer (50% versus 12%).[21,24] Papillary hyperplasia in secondary ducts may cause duct obstruction in elderly patients.

Papillary ductal hyperplasia with severe atypia

Papillary ductal hyperplasia with severe atypia is discussed with ductal carcinoma in the section Carcinoma in Situ (Fig. 59-9). Such lesions are rare compared with papillary hyperplasia without atypia.

Focal adenomatous ductal hyperplasia

Focal adenomatous ductal hyperplasia is an aggregation of small ducts lined by epithelium with mucinous hypertrophy and often with pyloric gland metaplasia (Fig. 59-10). Occasionally, hyperplasia may lead to formation of small adenomalike nodules,[27] but such lesions are not considered neoplasms. Ductular cystic hyperplasia[18] may be a variant. Papillary ductal hyper-

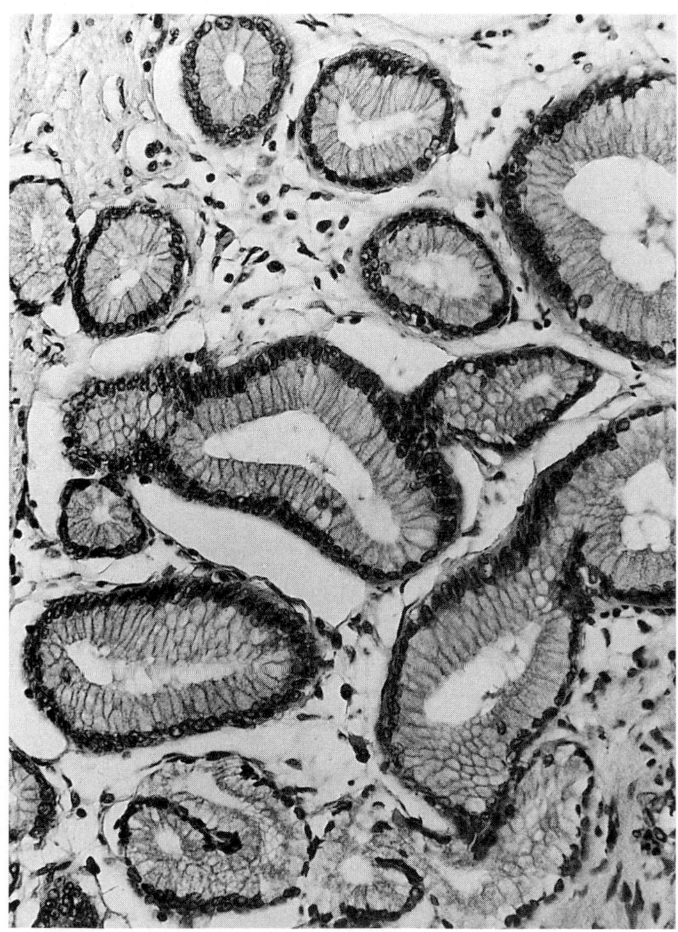

Fig. 59-10 Focal adenomatous ductal hyperplasia. Several adjacent ductules are lined by hyperplastic mucinous, columnar cells, a few of which have flattened basilar nuclei characteristic of pyloric glands.

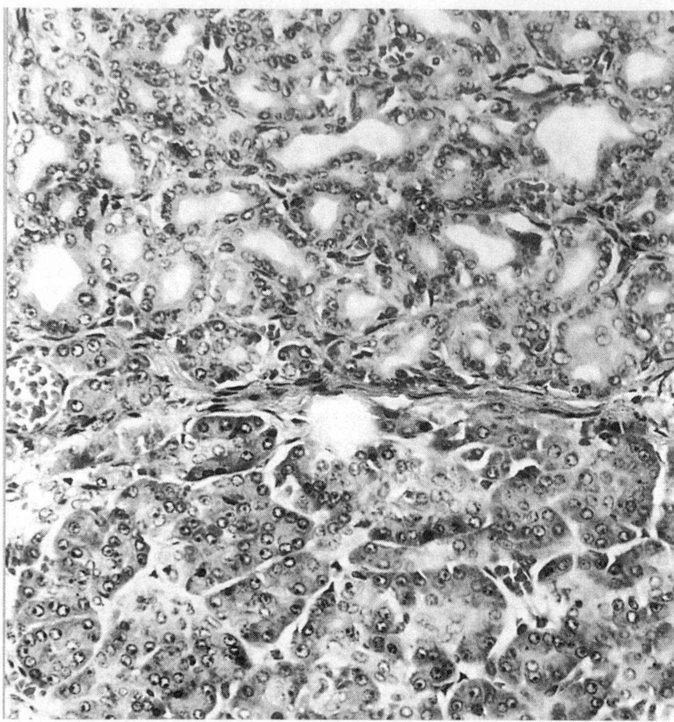

Fig. 59-11 Tubular complex. Acinar tissue occupies the lower half of the field and is replaced in the upper half by ductules with wide lumens and lacking any substantial fibrous wall. This tubular change is focal and blends in with the appearance of surrounding acinar tissue.

plasia may occur in conjunction with focal adenomatous duct hyperplasia.[28]

Tubular complex

Tubular or ductular structures may focally replace acinar tissue in the lobules. This lesion has been called a *tubular complex*[29] and *focal acinar dilatation.*[1] The cells lining these structures most often have characteristics of centroacinar cells, but acinar cells may be interspersed. They are seen in the settings of chronic pancreatitis,[29] uremia,[1] and cachexia. In the context of chronic pancreatitis they seem to reflect the presence of atrophic or regressive changes.

Another type of tubular complex may replace acinar tissue in apparently normal pancreases (Fig. 59-11). These lesions have also been called *ductular hyperplasia*[19] and "ductal metaplasia,"[30] reflecting the uncertainty as to whether they arise as a result of the proliferation of ductular cells or of the metaplasia of acinar cells. The cells lining these structures do not appear atrophic and may contain or lack mucin. Some lesions show no fibrosis but some show considerable fibrosis around the ductules, though inflammation is invariably absent. Lesions with a high mucus content may represent a variant of adenomatous duct hyperplasia.

PANCREATITIS

Pancreatitis constitutes a group of diseases in which the basic pathologic processes are injury to the exocrine cells and inflammation in the pancreas. The severity and duration

Table 59-1 Relationships of the varying degrees and duration of pancreatitis to the final pathologic outcome

Process	Clinical course	Outcome
Interstitial pancreatitis	Transient →	Resolution and recovery
	Persistent →	Chronic pancreatitis
Focal acute pancreatitis	Single or sporadic episodes →	Focal scarring
	Recurrent episodes →	Chronic pancreatitis
Severe acute pancreatitis	Survival →	Pseudocyst formation or scarring
	Fulminant →	Death

of pancreatitis vary, and thus pancreatitis gives rise to a range of clinical diseases and pathologic changes (Table 59-1).

Classification

A mild form of acute pancreatitis that is attended by complete recovery after a short illness is designated as interstitial pancreatitis. At the opposite end of the range of acute disease is the potentially lethal and severe acute pancreatitis; this is characterized by abdominal pain and shock and may be complicated by the development of pulmonary edema, hypoxemia, renal failure, and other systemic manifestations (multisystem organ failure).[31] Mild or moderate pancreatitis may persist or recur over the course of months or years in some patients, resulting in the progressive destruction of the pancreas. This is designated as chronic pancreatitis, and its major clinical feature may be pain that may be accompanied by signs of malabsorption as pancreatic exocrine function is lost.

Etiology and pathogenesis. The causes of interstitial, acute, and chronic pancreatitis overlap, as do the pathogenetic mechanisms that operate during its evolution (Table 59-2). Acinar cell injury and duct obstruction are the two key processes, and the activation and release of pancreatic enzymes within the pancreas play a crucial role in the initiation of pancreatitis (Fig. 59-12, *A*). However, the severity of the inflammation and necrosis, the duration of the disease, and the amount of pancreas involved vary depending on the causes.

Pancreatic digestive enzymes are similar to lysosomal enzymes in terms of their substrate specificity and are active at the intracellular pH. The acinar cell is normally protected from the action of its own enzymes (for example, proteinases, deoxy ribonuclease, ribo nuclease, lipase, phospholipase A, and amylase) through the elaborate intracellular compartmentalization of enzymes within the cytocavitary network of endoplasmic reticulum, Golgi complex, and zymogen granules; through the synthesis of several of the enzymes in inactive forms, (such as trypsinogen); and through the presence of trypsin inhibitors in the cells, pancreatic juice, interstitial fluid, and plasma. Acinar cells live in a delicate balance because the activation of these enzymes within the cell can result in damage to cell organelles, leading to autophagy or cell death and necrosis. Trypsin is a key enzyme in this balance because it activates other proenzymes, such as chymotrypsinogen, procarboxypeptidase, proelastase, and prophospholipase (Fig. 59-12, *B*). Trypsin also activates mediators of inflammation in the kallikrein-kinin system. Lysosomal cathepsin B can activate trypsinogen,[32] providing a possible intracellular mechanism for the initiation of an enzyme activation cascade. Minor episodes of acinar cell injury appear to be common because autophagic vacuoles are found in scattered acinar cells in "normal" pancreases. The number of autophagic vacuoles and necrotic cells increases in proportion to the severity of injury.

Necrosis of acinar cells causes the release of the enzymes into the interstitium. These activated enzymes injure the adjacent cells and amplify the damage. Fat cells are damaged and their lipids are hydrolyzed by phospholipase A and pancreatic lipase (fat necrosis). Vessels are damaged, especially by elastase and proteases, and this results in hemorrhage.

The causes of pancreatic acinar cell injury include toxic chemicals or drugs, viruses (such as mumps and cytomegalovirus), ischemia, and interstitially activated pancreatic enzymes. Acute pancreatitis can be induced in animals by the administration of chemicals that are cytotoxic to acinar cells. Numerous chemical agents, including some drugs, are known or suspected to induce acinar cell damage or necrosis. There are sporadic reports of acute pancreatitis associated with the use of specific therapeutic agents such as thiazide diuretics, and the list of implicated drugs is now quite long.[35] The evidence implicating a drug as a cause of pancreatitis is often circumstantial, however. Rigid criteria for a causal relationship have been proposed.[33]

The pancreatic involvement in patients with mumps is variable and is usually mild, that is, interstitial pancreatitis. Cytomegalovirus infection has been observed to induce pancreatitis in immunosuppressed patients.[36] Injury inflicted by free radicals generated in an antioxidant-depleted pancreas has also been implicated as a cause of acinar cell damage. Pancreatic ischemia is apparently expressed clinically as acute pancreatitis, and pancreatitis has been encountered in patients with several forms of arteritis.

Trauma to the upper abdomen can precipitate acute pancreatitis. Contusion of acinar tissue and disruption of the duct system with the subsequent interstitial leakage of enzymes are possible mechanisms.

The presence of hyperlipidemia, including certain hereditary types, seems to predispose to the development of acute pancreatitis.[37] One mechanism proposed to explain this is the hydrolysis of triglycerides (TGs) in the interstitial fluid of the

Table 59-2 Causes of pancreatitis grouped according to probable mechanism

Causes of acinar cell injury
Ischemia
Mumps
Cytomegalovirus
Hepatitis virus
Toxic chemicals
Drugs*
Asparaginase
Azathioprine
Sulfonamides
Thiazide diuretics
Furosemide
Estrogens
Tetracycline
Causes of ductal obstruction
Gallstones
Neoplasms (primary or secondary)
Pancreas divisum
Parasites (*Ascaris lumbricoides, Clonorchis sinensis*)
Increased ductal pressure and leakage
Endoscopic retrograde cholangiopancreatography
Miscellaneous mechanisms
Abdominal trauma
Hypertriglyceridemia
Hyperparathyroidism
Tuberculosis
Penetrating duodenal ulcer
Mechanism unknown
Alcohol abuse (acute and chronic)

*Drugs exhibiting the strongest association with acute pancreatitis are listed.[33] Additional drugs have a probable association.[33,34]

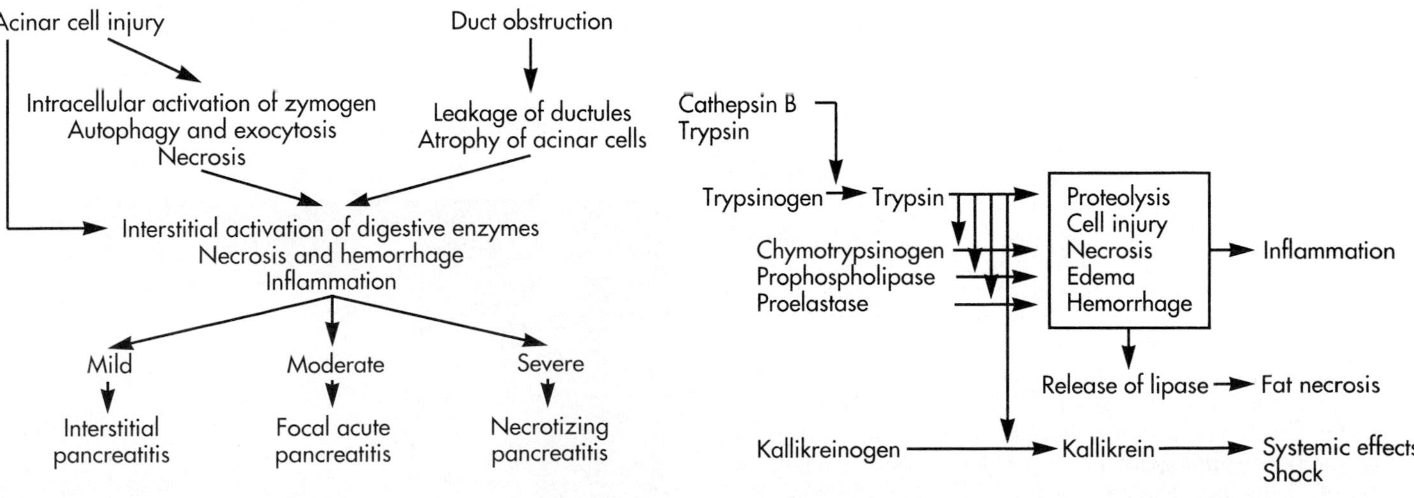

Fig. 59-12 **A,** Pathogenetic relationships of acinar cell injury and duct obstruction to pancreatitis. **B,** Intrapancreatic mechanisms of enyzme activation in pancreatitis.

pancreas by "leaked" pancreatic lipase–releasing free fatty acids, which are cytotoxic and can initiate acinar cell injury.[38] Acute pancreatitis is sometimes associated with familial hyperlipoproteinemia (types I and V), chronic renal failure, and estrogen therapy, including birth control pills. Each of these is associated with elevated serum levels of TGs, implicating the pathogenic mechanism just described.

Pancreatitis is an inconstant complication of hyperparathyroidism when there is moderate or severe hypercalcemia. Hyperparathyroidism may stem from a functioning parathyroid neoplasm or hyperplasia, and a hereditary form is transmitted as an autosomal dominant trait. Ca^{2+} is a cofactor for the "autocatalytic activation" of trypsinogen by trypsin, and this provides a possible, but unproved, mechanism.

The second major mechanism in the pathogenesis of pancreatitis is duct obstruction. In experimental animals it has been observed that small ducts leak when intraductal pressure is elevated as a result of pancreatic duct obstruction. This causes the release of pancreatic enzymes into interstitial tissue, where they can initiate tissue damage and inflammation. Duct obstruction affects the pancreas of various animal species in several ways: it induces acute pancreatitis, interstitial pancreatitis, and atrophy and fibrosis of the pancreas.[32]

Pancreatitis has been noted to occur in a variety of clinical conditions in which pancreatic duct obstruction can be demonstrated or its existence assumed. Causes of pancreatic duct obstruction include gallstones, precipitated protein and glycoprotein secretions in intrapancreatic ducts, ductal anomalies such as pancreas divisum, and neoplasms.

A third to half of the cases of acute pancreatitis are associated with biliary tract disease. Gallstones can cause pancreatic duct obstruction when there is a common channel. The impaction of gallstones in the ampulla of Vater seems to predispose to the development of acute pancreatitis. Recently the presence of multiple small biliary stones ("sludge") in the bile has been found to be associated with episodes of acute pancreatitis; this presumably also arises as the result of obstruction.[35] The mixing of bile and pancreatic juice in the duct system with reflux into the pancreas may play a role in the pathogenesis of pancreatitis in such patients. The pancreatic enzyme phospholipase A can hydrolyze lecithin (in bile) to form lysolecithin, which is cytotoxic by virtue of its ability to interact with cell membranes.

The incidence of pancreas divisum is higher among patients who suffer recurrent bouts of pancreatitis than among those who have no history of pancreatitis,[3] pointing toward an association with partial obstruction. Less common causes of obstruction of the distal pancreatic duct or common channel are tumors of the ampulla of Vater or pancreatic duct such as villous adenomas or submucosal carcinoids. Persistent intrapancreatic duct obstruction predisposes to the development of chronic pancreatitis. The pancreatic lesion of cystic fibrosis serves as an example.

In the United States most cases of chronic pancreatitis of known cause are associated with chronic alcoholism, but chronic pancreatitis is a clinical problem in only a small fraction of alcoholics. The concentration of protein in pancreatic juice is increased in chronic alcoholics, and it is common for protein to precipitate within ducts to form plugs. These protein plugs sometimes calcify to form intraductal "stones." The importance of these plugs as a cause of intrapancreatic duct obstruction has been questioned, however, and it appears that other mechanisms such as direct damage to the ductal epithelium play a more important role in the pathogenesis of alcohol-associated pancreatitis.[39] Alcohol has been reported to cause fat to accumulate in acinar cells, but it is not severely cytotoxic.

In some cases of acute pancreatitis, inflammation of the ducts with destruction of the epithelium is severe (Fig. 59-13). When large plugs or calculi are present (Fig. 59-14), duct epithelium may become eroded and the underlying duct wall inflamed.[13] Destruction of the duct epithelium may contribute to the leakage and activation of exocrine enzymes.

It is usually accepted that some cases of chronic pancreatitis represent the end stage of damage that has accumulated during multiple recurrent episodes of nonfatal pancreatitis stemming from alcoholism or other causes. Hereditary pancreatitis, which has also been called "chronic recurrent pancreatitis" because of its clinical course, is a rare but documented cause of chronic pancreatitis.[9]

Acinar cell injury and pancreatic duct obstruction are key factors in the etiology and pathogenesis of pancreatitis. Both lead to the intrapancreatic release and activation of the digestive enzymes, followed by cell injury, necrosis, hemorrhage, and inflammation. Acute pancreatitis is attributed to either gallstone disease or alcoholism in about 70% of cases, but a small percentage of the cases are attributed to other specific causes (see Table 59-2). The remainder are regarded as idio-

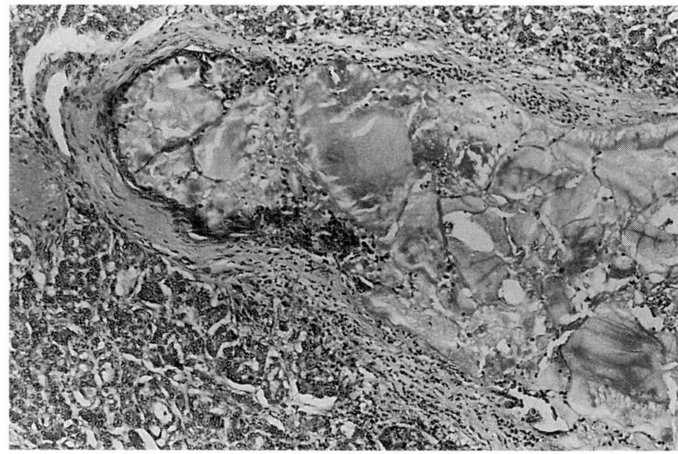

Fig. 59-13 Inflamed duct. The collagenous tissue of the duct wall surrounds a mass of dense protein secretions in the lumen. The duct epithelium has been destroyed, and the wall is acutely inflamed.

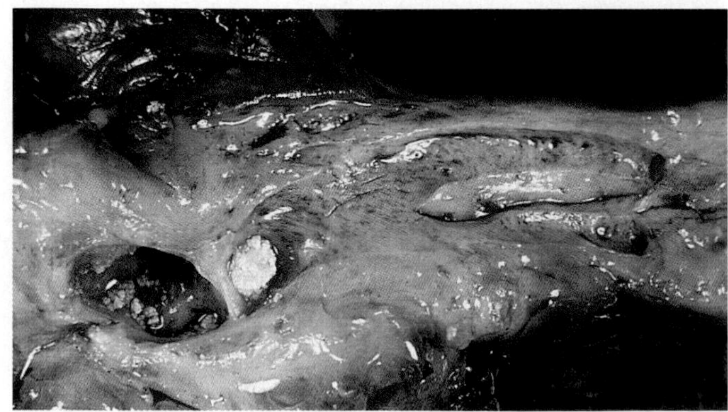

Fig. 59-14 Chronic pancreatitis with pancreatic calculi. The main pancreatic duct in the head and body of the pancreas is greatly dilated. Acinar lobules appear to be replaced by fat and fibrous tissue.

pathic. The cause of chronic pancreatitis is also often unknown (idiopathic). The clinical and pathologic outcomes depend on the severity and duration of the pancreatitis, as well as on the number of recurrent episodes.

Interstitial (edematous) pancreatitis

The major changes of mild acute pancreatitis are acute inflammation and edema in the stroma (Fig. 59-15). The gross characteristics of increased firmness and swelling are the result of edema. Infiltrating leukocytes initially include a high fraction of neutrophils. There is no necrosis of the acinar tissue and stroma, but there may be limited fat necrosis that is predominantly peripancreatic.

Acute pancreatitis

Severe acute pancreatitis has also been called *acute hemorrhagic pancreatitis* and *necrotizing pancreatitis*—portraying two key pathologic features of the disease. The major changes are necrosis of the acinar tissue, stroma, and adjacent fat (Fig. 59-16). Because of the necrosis of vessels, which is typical but varies in degree, extravasated blood permeates the necrotic tissue. On gross examination the pancreas exhibits a variegated appearance, with areas of hemorrhage, liquefactive necrosis, and fat necrosis resembling muddy oil. The process is typically multifocal or patchy rather than involving the whole pancreas uniformly. Isolated areas where fat necrosis constitutes the major change are opaque white or yellow-white, reflecting the hydrolysis of lipids and the deposition of calcium salts of fatty acids ("soaps"). In the setting of severe acute pancreatitis focal fat necrosis may take place in mesenteric and retroperitoneal fat and other intra-abdominal sites remote from the pancreas. Subcutaneous fat necrosis has been observed in severe cases.

Histologically there is acute inflammation at the interface between necrotic areas and viable tissue early in the process, although edema may be a more conspicuous feature than infiltration by leukocytes. Nonviable acinar tissue rapidly undergoes complete liquefactive necrosis because of the high content of digestive enzymes. Therefore it may be impossible to recognize acinar tissue if the process is more than a few hours old. Peripancreatic fat is destroyed more slowly. Fat necrosis is recognized by the altered staining of the cell membranes and nuclei and by the deposition of calcium salts in the cytoplasm of the fat cells (blue in hematoxylin and eosin–stained sections). Foci of fat necrosis may be recognizable for days to weeks after the initial injury.

In patients who survive acute pancreatitis, the acute inflammation gradually abates and the necrotic and hemorrhagic lesions are gradually replaced by fibrous tissue. This process may take weeks. Pancreatic acinar and ductal cells are able to divide and replenish cell losses unless the lobular stroma has been totally destroyed. When inflammation subsides completely, the amount of fibrous tissue diminishes.

The change characteristic of acute pancreatitis, that is necrosis with inflammation, may involve only small amounts of pancreatic tissue in single or multiple sites. It is probably best to render a diagnosis of focal necrosis in those patients with small lesions who show no clinical evidence of pancreatic disease and to reserve a diagnosis of acute pancreatitis for those patients with lesions that appear to be extensive enough to have potential clinical significance.

Complications of acute pancreatitis

The most important complications of acute pancreatitis are infection and the formation of pseudocysts and abscesses. Necrotic pancreatic tissue may become infected (infected necrosis) with bacteria, most often enteric organisms, and progress to form an abscess. Abscesses may occur early or late in the course of pancreatitis. Infection is said to arise in 40% of the patients with pancreatic necrosis and is associated with

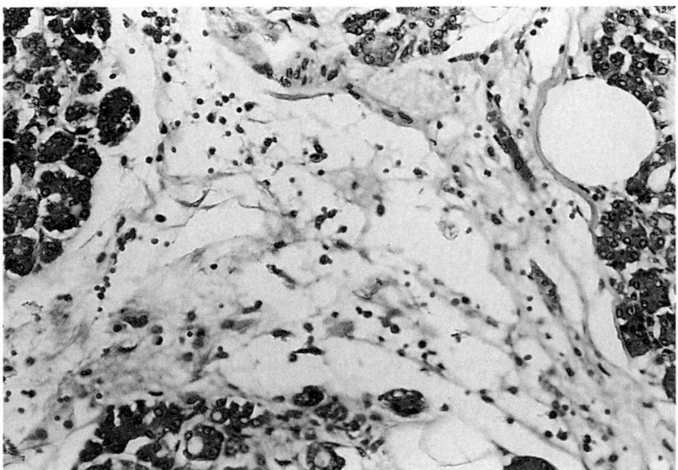

Fig. 59-15 Interstitial pancreatitis. The interlobular space is widened as the result of edema and contains leukocytes. Notice the absence of necrosis of the acinar cells in the lobules.

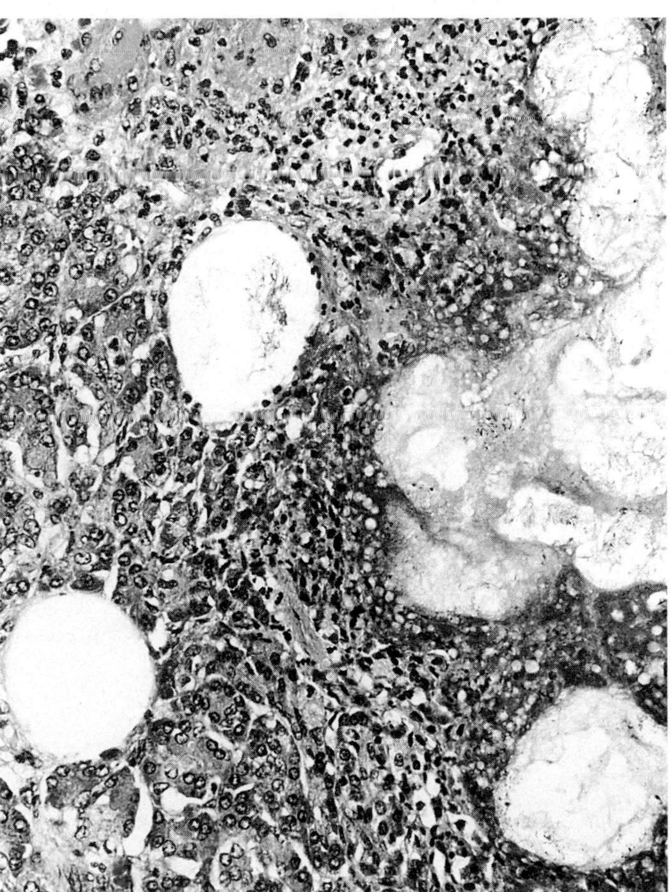

Fig. 59-16 Acute necrotizing pancreatitis. Acinar cell necrosis, fat necrosis, and a sparse leukocytic infiltrate can be seen. Acinar cells at the left of the field appear to be viable.

an increased mortality.[40] Peripancreatic fluid collections commonly develop during the early phase of acute pancreatitis and may become infected.[31]

Pseudocyst formation is a complication of acute pancreatitis that takes 4 or more weeks to occur.[31] A pseudocyst forms when the mass of necrotic tissue becomes too large to be absorbed and is walled off by scarring to form a fibrous-walled cavity filled with semisolid or liquid debris (Fig. 59-17). The pseudocyst may be intrapancreatic or peripancreatic in location. Because the pancreatic duct system in the adjacent viable pancreas may drain into a pseudocyst, the cyst typically contains a high concentration of pancreatic enzymes. Pseudocysts range from 1 to 30 cm in diameter. The larger cysts extend into the peripancreatic tissue and may involve adjacent organs such as the spleen, stomach, or colon.

Large pseudocysts may rupture into the peritoneal cavity, causing chemical peritonitis, or they may compress and obstruct the duodenum or the common bile duct, or both. Uncommonly a pseudocyst erodes into a major vessel, causing fatal hemorrhage, or extends through the diaphragm into the mediastinum or pleural space. Its contents are typically sterile. If a pseudocyst becomes infected by bacteria, the lesion is transformed into an abscess and sepsis becomes a major concern.

Chronic pancreatitis

In chronic pancreatitis the pancreas becomes small and hard as the result of the scarring and atrophy of acinar tissue (Fig. 59-18). The changes typical of chronic pancreatitis may be diffuse in that form resulting from duct obstruction, or they may be multifocal and patchy. In the latter setting, which is typical of the chronic pancreatitis that occurs in alcoholic patients, the duct system is distorted. During active phases of chronic pancreatitis, there is an infiltration of lymphocytes, and the frank changes typical of acute pancreatitis, including the formation of pseudocysts, may be superimposed upon those characteristics of chronic pancreatitis; alcoholics are an example of the victims of this process. Later, however, the inflammation may subside, and the major changes then become atrophy and fibrosis. Fibrosis develops both around lobules (perilobular) and within them (intralobular). In advanced stages of chronic pancreatitis, acinar tissue may become completely atrophic and may be replaced by dense fibrous tissue, with variable persistence of ducts. Islets persist longer than the exocrine elements. Plugs formed from secreted proteins and glycoproteins may arise in the smaller ducts. The duct system may be dilated and contain calculi.[41] These are often found in patients with hereditary pancreatitis and less commonly in those with alcoholic pancreatitis. There is also an increased incidence of intraductal epithelial hyperplasia, which may be rather extensive.

In patients with chronic pancreatitis, it appears that malabsorption does not occur until atrophy and scarring cause enzyme secretion to be reduced to less than 10% of the normal levels.[42]

Cystic fibrosis

The pancreases of patients with cystic fibrosis show varying degrees of obstructive pancreatitis. This may begin in utero or in childhood. At the time of death there are usually macroscopic and microscopic signs of chronic pancreatitis. Interlobular and intralobular ducts are characteristically filled with solid mucinous or proteinaceous secretions. The ducts are focally or diffusely dilated. Early in the disease there is diffuse interstitial pancreatitis that may persist and progress to chronic

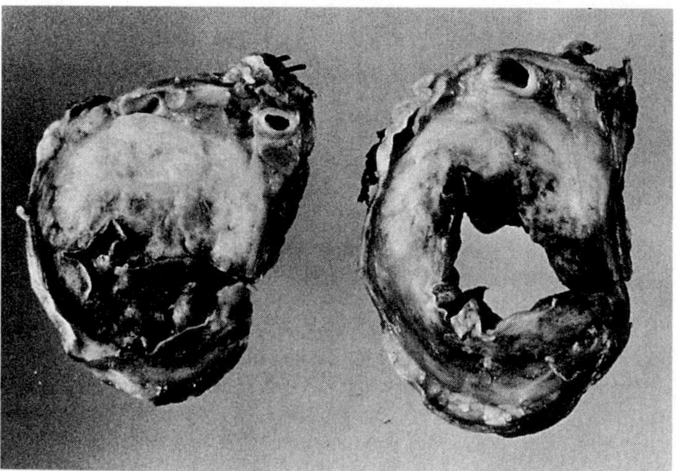

Fig. 59-17 Pseudocyst. The pancreas was resected because of a persistent pseudocyst that was located centrally in the pancreas and did not extend into surrounding tissues. The splenic artery is at the top of the transections. The necrotic cavity is 2 to 3 cm in diameter.

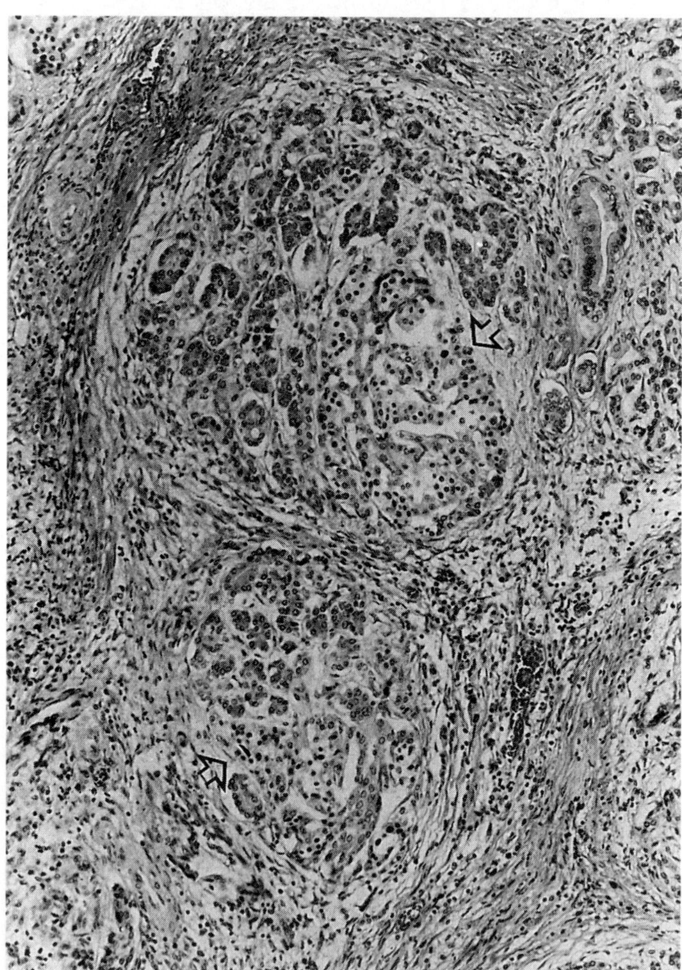

Fig. 59-18 Chronic pancreatitis. Two atrophic lobules are separated by fibrous tissue and infiltrating lymphocytes and macrophages. Each lobule contains surviving islet tissue *(arrows)*. The small duct appears normal except for the presence of mild epithelial hyperplasia *(upper right)*. This represents an active phase of chronic pancreatitis.

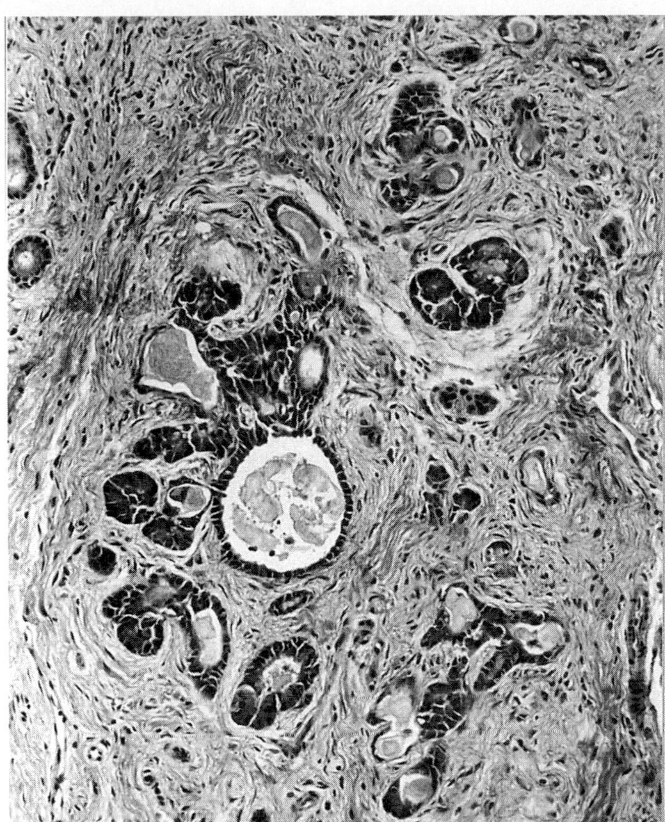

Fig. 59-19 Cystic fibrosis. A duct and intralobular ductules are dilated and contain dense secretions. Acinar tissue is largely atrophic, and the lobule is infiltrated and surrounded by dense scar tissue. Only a few leukocytes persist.

pancreatitis. Later, when acinar tissue is largely atrophic, the inflammation subsides and the pancreas consists of ducts and islets embedded in fibrous or adipose tissue, or a mixture of both (Fig. 59-19).

NEOPLASMS

Neoplasms of the pancreas arise from ductal, acinar, stromal, or islet cells. The term *carcinoma of the pancreas* is customarily used only in reference to exocrine tumors and rare mixed exocrine-endocrine carcinomas. Neoplasms, including carcinomas composed primarily of endocrine cells, are collectively termed *islet cell tumors* (see Chapter 64). Carcinoma of the pancreas is responsible for causing approximately 25,000 deaths annually in the United States.[43] It is usually diagnosed after there has been local invasion or metastasis; as a result, treatment is seldom effective. The average survival is less than 1 year after diagnosis; the 5-year survival is less than 5%. A large composite series spanning several decades of experience has provided data regarding survival in patients who undergo resection (Table 59-3).

Most pancreatic neoplasms are malignant,[44] but benign tumors and tumors with a variable malignant potential also occur. Thus the classification has both a clinical and prognostic significance. Several classification schemes are used, and this has created a need for standardization of terms. A classification scheme proposed by the World Health Organization (WHO) groups neoplasms according to clinical behavior (Table 59-4).

Table 59-3 **Rate of resectability and 5-year survival in patients undergoing resection in a composite series of patients with carcinoma of the pancreas**

Total cases	22,319
Resected cases	2,398
Percentage resected	10.7
Percentage of 5-year survivals	3.7

From Gudjonsson B: *Cancer* 60:2284, 1987.

Table 59-4 **Histologic classification of tumors of the exocrine pancreas proposed by the World Health Organization**

1.1 Benign tumors
1.1.1 Serous cystadenoma
1.1.2 Mucinous cystadenoma
1.1.3 Intraductal papillary-mucinous adenoma
1.1.4 Mature teratoma
1.2 Borderline tumors (uncertain malignant potential)
1.2.1 Mucinous cystic tumor with moderate dysplasia
1.2.2 Intraductal papillary-mucinous tumor with moderate dysplasia
1.2.3 Solid-pseudopapillary tumor
1.3 Malignant tumors
1.3.1 Severe ductal dysplasia-circinoma in situ
1.3.2 Ductal adenocarcinoma
1.3.2.1 Mucinous noncystic carcinoma
1.3.2.2 Signet ring cell carcinoma
1.3.2.3 Adenosquamous carcinoma
1.3.2.4 Undifferentiated (anaplastic) carcinoma
1.3.2.5 Mixed ductal-endocrine carcinoma
1.3.3 Osteoclastlike giant cell tumor
1.3.4 Serous cystadenocarcinoma
1.3.5 Mucinous cystadenocarcinoma
1.3.5.1 noninvasive
1.3.5.2 invasive
1.3.6 Intraductal papillary-mucinous carcinoma
1.3.6.1 noninvasive
1.3.6.2 invasive
1.3.7 Acinar cell carcinoma
1.3.7.1 Acinar cell cystadenocarcinoma
1.3.7.2 Mixed acinar-endocrine carcinoma
1.3.8 Pancreatoblastoma
1.3.9 Solid-pseudopapillary carcinoma
1.3.10 Miscellaneous carcinomas

Overall survival is excellent in patients who undergo excision of benign tumors; it is longer for patients with tumors in the "uncertain" category than for those with malignant tumors. Less than 10% of the exocrine pancreatic tumors are deemed benign or uncertain. The uncertain tumors include those that may be cured by excision, that is, those that are apparently benign, but also include tumors that will ultimately exhibit overt malignant behavior if they are not resected completely.

Etiology and pathenogenens

Demographic data. The demographic data regarding pancreatic cancer are dominated by ductal adenocarcinomas and its variants, which together constitute approximately 90% of the cases.[45] The special demographic characteristics of less common carcinomas are given with their descriptions. The incidence of

Table 59-5 Incidence of pancreatic neoplasms in two large series

Common (80-85% of pancreatic neoplasms)
Ductal adenocarcinoma
Uncommon (2-5% of pancreatic neoplasms)
Undifferentiated carcinoma
Intraductal papillary-mucinous adenomas and tumors with moderate dysplasia
Mucinous noncystic carcinoma
Adenosquamous carcinoma
Serous cystadenoma
Rare (in the range of 1% or less)
Mucinous cystadenocarcinoma
Acinar cell carcinoma
Mucinous cystic adenoma and tumors with moderate dysplasia
Intraductal papillary-mucinous carcinoma
Solid pseudopapillary tumor
Pancreatoblastoma
Serous cystadenocarcinoma
Small cell carcinoma
Mature cystic teratoma

From Cubilla AL, Fitzgerald PJ: Tumors of the exocrine pancreas. In *Atlas of tumor pathology*, series 2, fasc 19, Washington, D.C., 1984, Armed Forces Institute of Pathology; Gold EB, Cameron JL: *N Engl J Med* 328:1485, 1993.

pancreatic carcinoma appeared to increase in the United States from 1930 to 1970 but has essentially leveled off in the meantime. The incidence is higher among men than among women (ratio, 1.6:1) and increases with age until the ninth decade. The incidence among African-Americans is consistently higher than that among whites living in the United States.

Cigarette smoking is the only clearly established exogenous risk factor to which there is widespread exposure among victims of the cancer. The incidence of pancreatic cancer in smokers is double that in nonsmokers. The incidence of carcinomas of the pancreas and bladder has been observed to be higher in a small cohort of workers exposed to beta-naphthylamine and benzidine than that in the control population,[46] but exposure to these chemicals or to others that have been implicated as causes of carcinoma of the pancreas accounts for only a small fraction of the total number of cases. The risk of carcinoma of the pancreas has been reported to be increased in patients with chronic pancreatitis,[47] but the fraction of cases that can be attributed to this cause is less than 1%.[48] Epidemiologic studies have provided few other clues regarding possible causes of pancreatic cancer in human beings, and in most cases the cause is really unknown. In the past, when the incidence of carcinoma of the pancreas in Japan was low compared with that in the United States, its incidence among Japanese who immigrated to the United States became similar to that in the native United States white population. Thus lifestyle and dietary factors appear to play a major role in the etiology of carcinoma of the pancreas, but the detailed basis of such influences remains uncertain.

Experimental data. Several animal models for the induction of pancreatic carcinoma by chemicals have furnished examples of carcinomas that arise in both acinar cells and ductal cells and exhibit spectra of histologic types; these carcinomas provide a match for the major types of carcinomas encountered in human beings. Several nitrosamines and closely related compounds have been effective in inducing such pancreatic cancers in animals.[49] This raises the question whether nitrosamines generated endogenously in the stomach might also reach and affect the pancreas. Findings from experimental studies involving the use of chemical carcinogens also support the possibility that environmental chemical agents might reach and affect the pancreas. Avenues for the histogenesis of pancreatic carcinoma have been outlined using as their basis data yielded by several animal models (see the following section).

The development of the carcinomas in the animal models is promoted by feeding the animals a high-fat diet. In rats testosterone seems to foster and estrogen to suppress the development of the carcinomas, and the incidences of both carcinomas and preneoplastic changes are higher in male rats than in female rats. The administration of several peptide hormones such as cholecystokinin has also been found to modify carcinogenesis in the rat. Thus carcinogenesis in the pancreas appears to be a complex process that can be influenced by exposure to chemical carcinogens, dietary factors, and endogenous hormonal factors.[49]

Histogenesis. The origin of pancreatic neoplasms has been studied extensively in animal models. Proliferative lesions of the ductal cells seem to be the source of most ductal carcinomas in hamsters. Proliferative lesions of the acinar cells seem to become acinar cell carcinomas in rats and mice. Carcinomas with a ductal phenotype appear to develop from acinar cells in rats and guinea pig models, indicating that malignant transformation and ductal metaplasia may occur simultaneously in acinar cells. It is unclear whether this pathway operates in the human form of the cancer.

The rare association of ductal carcinomas with intraductal papillary-mucinous tumors in human subjects has been noted, but the low incidence of the latter lesions indicates that they may not be the major precursor to the former. Intraductal hyperplasia with severe atypia (carcinoma in situ) also arises in the absence of an intraductal papillary tumor. Such lesions are the most widely acknowleged precursors to ductal carcinomas. They appear to be analogous to the intraductal preneoplastic lesions identified in nitrosamine-treated hamsters.

Molecular changes. Results of recent studies indicate that approximately 75% of human pancreatic carcinomas have an activated c-K-*ras* oncogene, usually possessing a mutation in codon 12.[50] Other studies have revealed that the normal p53 protein is lost in approximately half of the pancreatic carcinomas.[27] Expression of transforming growth factor–alpha in concert with overexpression of the receptors for epidermal growth factor, forming an autocrine growth-stimulating mechanism, also appears to be prevalent in pancreatic cancer cells.[51] Expression of other growth factors, such as the basic fibroblast growth factor, and their receptors by pancreatic carcinomas is also reported.[52] These and other changes in oncogenes and tumor suppressor genes may someday be used in establishing the diagnosis or predicting the prognosis of carcinomas in the pancreas. Too little information has accrued to form a sound basis for such application of molecular markers at present.

Pathology. The gross characteristics of exocrine neoplasms overlap among the various histologic types. Features of importance for classification and staging include the size and consistency of the tumor, and whether the tumor is solid or cystic. Typical ductal adenocarcinomas are desmoplastic and they are hard. A soft consistency in a solid tumor indicates that the tumor is one of the less common types. Cystic tumors are often large, measuring up to 20 cm in diameter. Most carcinomas are found in the head of the pancreas. Some tumors involve two regions or extend diffusely throughout the entire pancreas. Small cystic tumors may be intraductal. Thus the relationship of a cystic tumor to the duct system should be noted carefully.

At the histologic level, variation in the differentiation and cell type within a neoplasm is common, especially in larger tumors. Tumors exhibiting varied patterns should be classified according to the dominant pattern, usually the one constituting 80% or more of the tumor.[18] With the advent of immunostaining, it became possible to detect minor cell populations with greater sensitivity than was possible in the past. It is now known that a high fraction of ductal adenocarcinomas contain the islet type of endocrine cells that can be identified using markers such as chromogranin or specific islet hormones. On the other hand, a few ducts may be present in islet cell tumors. A mixture of cells with exocrine and endocrine differentiation is common in certain special types of neoplasms (papillary cystic tumors and pancreatoblastoma) that are assumed to arise from a primitive cell type. Rarely there appear to be equivalent exocrine and islet cell components in a neoplasm, and such tumors have been designated as duct-islet, or acinar-islet carcinoma.[18] These are included under miscellaneous carcinomas in the WHO classification.

Benign tumors

Serous cystadenoma

The serous cystadenoma is composed of multiple small cysts (1 mm to 2 cm in diameter) lined by cuboidal epithelium with a clear, glycogen-containing cytoplasm within a fibrous capsule (Fig. 59-20, *A* and *B*). The cysts contain serous fluid. Most of these neoplasms appear to be benign, but a few tumors with a similar histologic appearance have been reported to be malignant.[53] These are classified as microcystic serous cystadenocarcinoma (Fig. 59-20 *C*). These tumors are malignant, as evi-

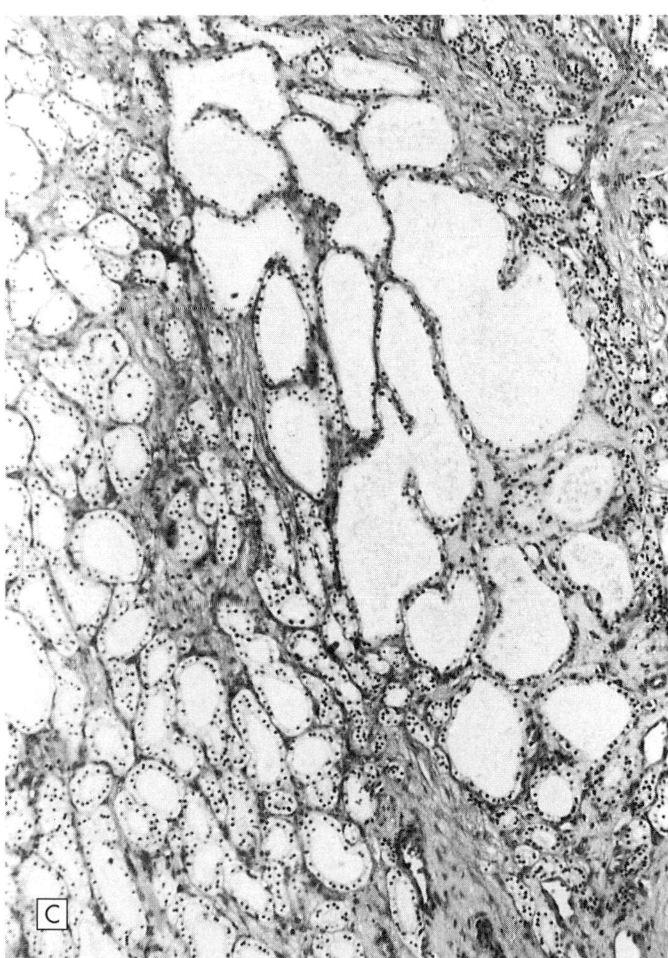

Fig. 59-20 A, Serous cystadenoma. The tumor is oval and encapsulated. Portions of the pancreas are attached *(top* and *lower right).* **B,** Serous cystadenoma. Cysts of varying sizes are lined by cuboidal or slightly flattened epithelial cells containing pale cytoplasm and are separated by moderately dense fibrous tissue. **C,** Serous cystadenocarcinoma. (Photomicrograph by Dr. G. Klöppel, Brussels, from specimen supplied by George HD, Murphy F, Michalski et al: *Am J Surg Pathol* 13:61, 1989.)

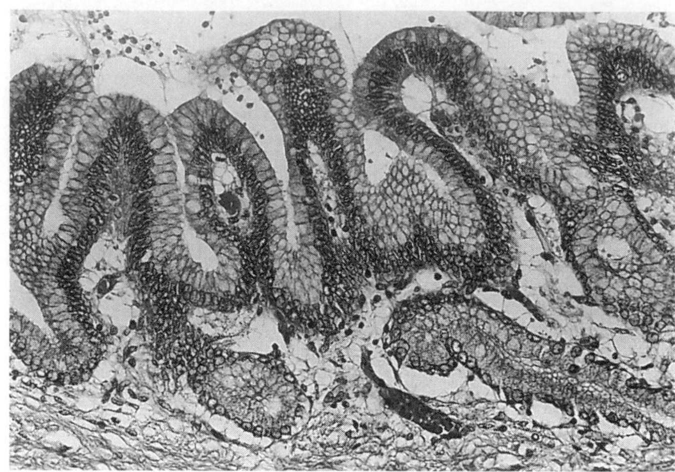

Fig. 59-21 Intraductal papillary-mucinous adenoma. The duct is lined by a highly differentiated mucinous epithelium that has formed a complex papillary, intraductal mass. This tumor was an incidental finding at autopsy.

denced by the fact that they invade local tissue, in one case the stomach and spleen,[54] and metastasize to the liver.

Mature teratoma

The mature cystic teratoma (termed *dermoid cyst*) is composed of a mixture of mature cell and tissue types with a cystic component that is usually lined by squamous epithelium.[18] Less complex cysts lined by keratinizing squamous epithelium and surrounded by lymphoid tissue with germinal centers have been classified as lymphoepithelial cysts and may represent a distinct category of benign cystic lesion.[55]

Intraductal papillary-mucinous neoplasms

Intraductal papillary-mucinous neoplasms appear to represent a closely related group of neoplasms that range from benign to malignant. Overall they appear to grow and progress slowly. Men and women are equally affected, and most are older than 50 years of age.

The neoplasms develop in the main pancreatic duct or in major side branches. Most of the intraductal papillary tumors secrete large amounts of mucin, which causes the main pancreatic duct to dilate; this is the reason why they are called *ductectatic mucin-hypersecreting tumors*. Grossly they are cystic neoplasms that communicate with the duct system. The tumors are usually multiloculated, measuring up to 4 cm and averaging 2 cm in diameter.

The benign counterpart of this group, called intraductal papillary-mucinous adenoma, lacks the usual histologic or cytologic signs of malignancy, exhibiting no more than a mild dysplastic change (Fig. 59-21). The columnar epithelium is highly differentiated, and there is no evidence of invasion. Papillary projections have well-developed stromal cores and form an intraductal mass. These lesions have also been called *intraductal papilloma*, *papillary adenoma*, and *villous adenoma of the pancreatic duct*.

Intraductal papillary-mucinous tumors of borderline malignant potential have a complex papillary growth pattern with epithelium that shows moderate dysplasia but lacks severe dysplasia, invasion, and metastasis (Fig. 59-22). The epithe-

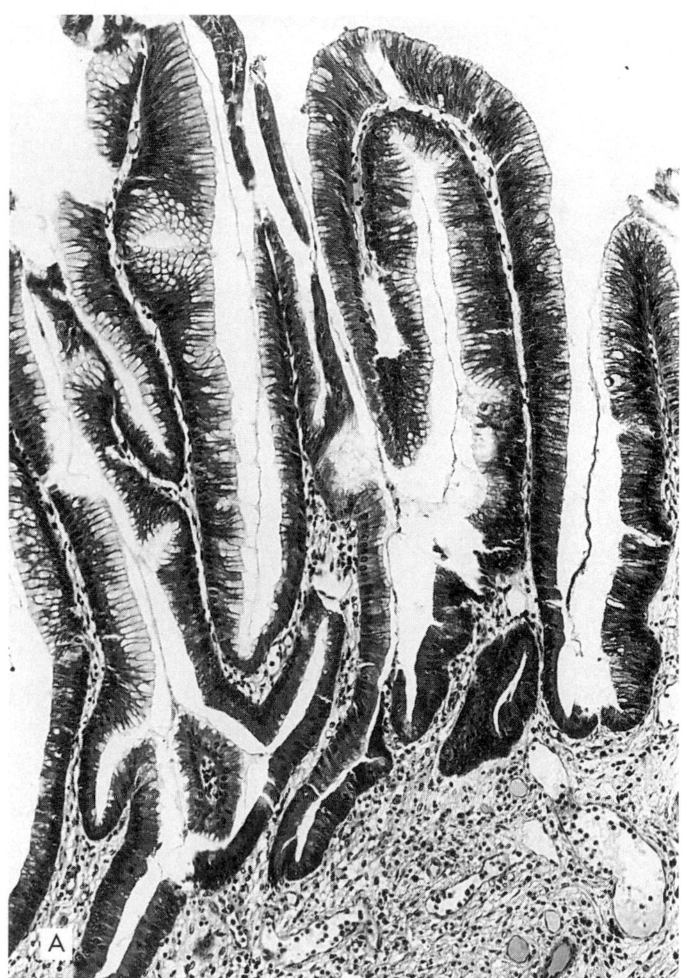

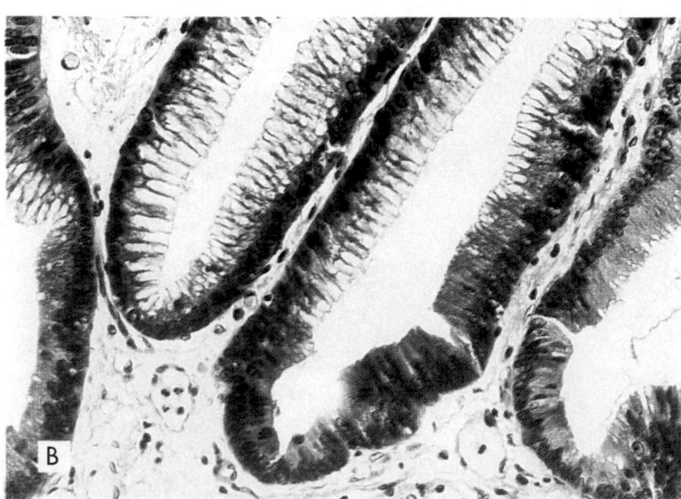

Fig. 59-22 Intraductal papillary-mucinous tumor with borderline malignant potential. **A,** The long papillary folds are covered by columnar, mucinous epithelium; the epithelium at the base of the folds (**A** and **B**) shows dysplastic changes with nuclei lying near the surface.

lium may or may not secrete mucus, and many of these tumors fall into the ductectatic mucin-hypersecreting group.

Intraductal papillary-mucinous carcinoma (Fig. 59-23) may be purely intraductal and show severe dysplasia of carcinoma in situ grade, or it may show evidence of invasion or metastasis. The invasive component may show a papillary cystic, ductal, or noncystic mucinous pattern.

The overall survival for patients with adenomas and borderline tumors after resection is clearly longer than that for patients with variants that exhibit clear evidence of invasion or metastasis. Intraductal papillary neoplasms are assumed to represent an adenoma-carcinoma sequence that progresses relatively slowly, with delayed spread to lymph nodes, liver, and the peritoneum. Thus they may be identified before invasion becomes evident and be cured by resection. A few examples of the close association of intraductal papillary-mucinous neoplasms with a component of ductal or mucinous noncystic adenocarcinoma are suggestive that some of the intraductal tumors become more aggressive carcinomas.

Borderline tumors

Mucinous cystic neoplasms

Mucinous cystic adenoma is a cystic tumor with a dense fibrous wall lined by highly differentiated, columnar, mucin-secreting epithelium, typically arranged in papillary projections (Fig. 59-24). The tumors usually range from 2 to 20 cm in diameter and may be multilocular. They are typically located in the tail or body of the pancreas, away from the main pancreatic duct, though peripheral tumors in the head have also been reported. Some authorities believe that these tumors arise in interlobular or intralobular ducts that subsequently cease to communicate with the duct system because of scarring. The benign form is regarded as part of a range that includes *mucinous cystic tumor of borderline malignant potential* and *mucinous cystadenocarcinoma.* The histologic features of the *mucinous cystic neoplasms* generally parallel those exhibited by intraductal-papillary mucinous neoplasms. The mucinous cystic tumors usually occur in women, and the patients are typically younger than those with intraductal papillary-mucinous tumors or ductal adenocarcinomas.

Mucinous cystadenocarcinoma is a predominantly cystic neoplasm filled with mucin and cellular debris. The epithelium lining the cysts typically is papillary, columnar, and mucin secreting (Fig. 59-25, *A*). Varying degrees of atypia are present. Invasion or metastasis provides evidence of malignancy (Fig. 59-25, *B*). The cystadenocarcinomas probably arise from preexisting intraductal papillary-mucinous tumors or mucinous cystic tumors.

The average survival in patients with mucinous cystadenocarcinoma is longer than that in those with ductal carcinomas.

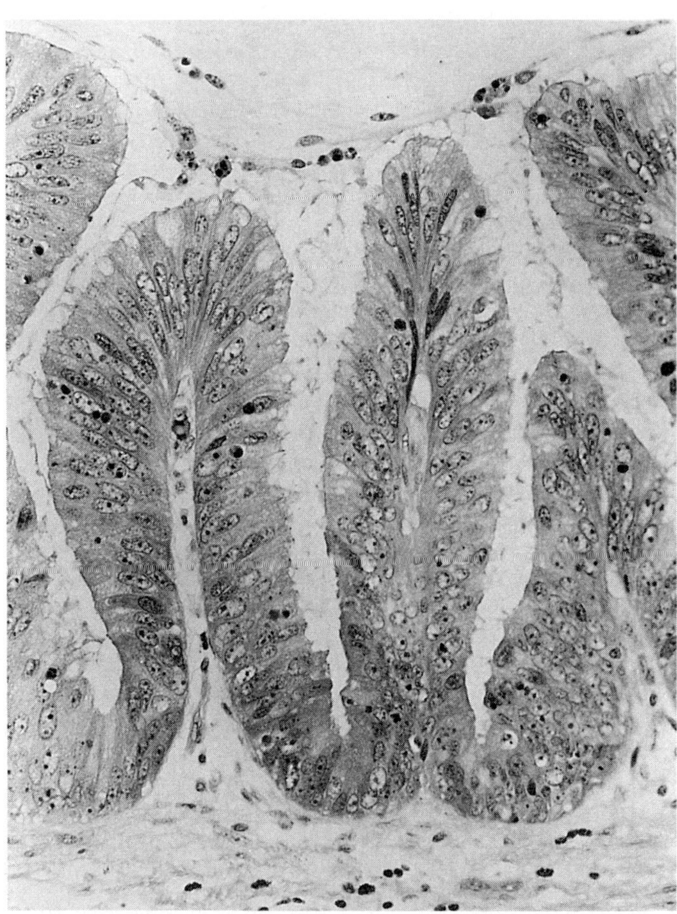

Fig. 59-23 Intraductal papillary-mucinous carcinoma. The surface epithelium lining a cystic space is columnar and retains evidence of mucus secretion. The pancreatic duct was dilated to 1 cm in diameter and was filled with mucus. The tumor in the head of the pancreas was 2.1 cm in diameter. Invasion was noted elsewhere in the specimen.

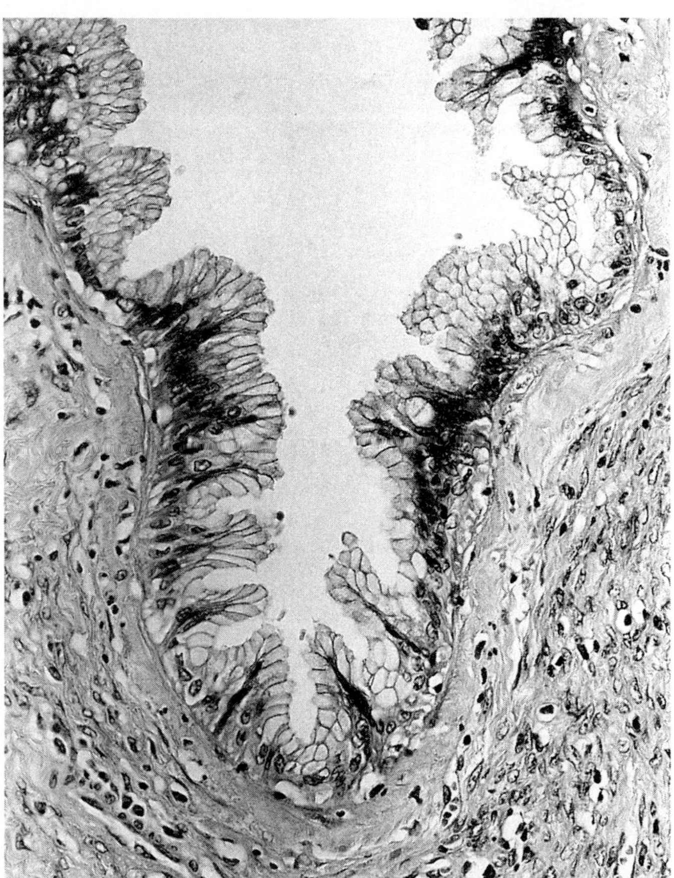

Fig. 59-24 Mucinous cystadenoma. The epithelium lining the cystic spaces is columnar and mucinous; it is highly differentiated and forms a few abortive papillary folds.

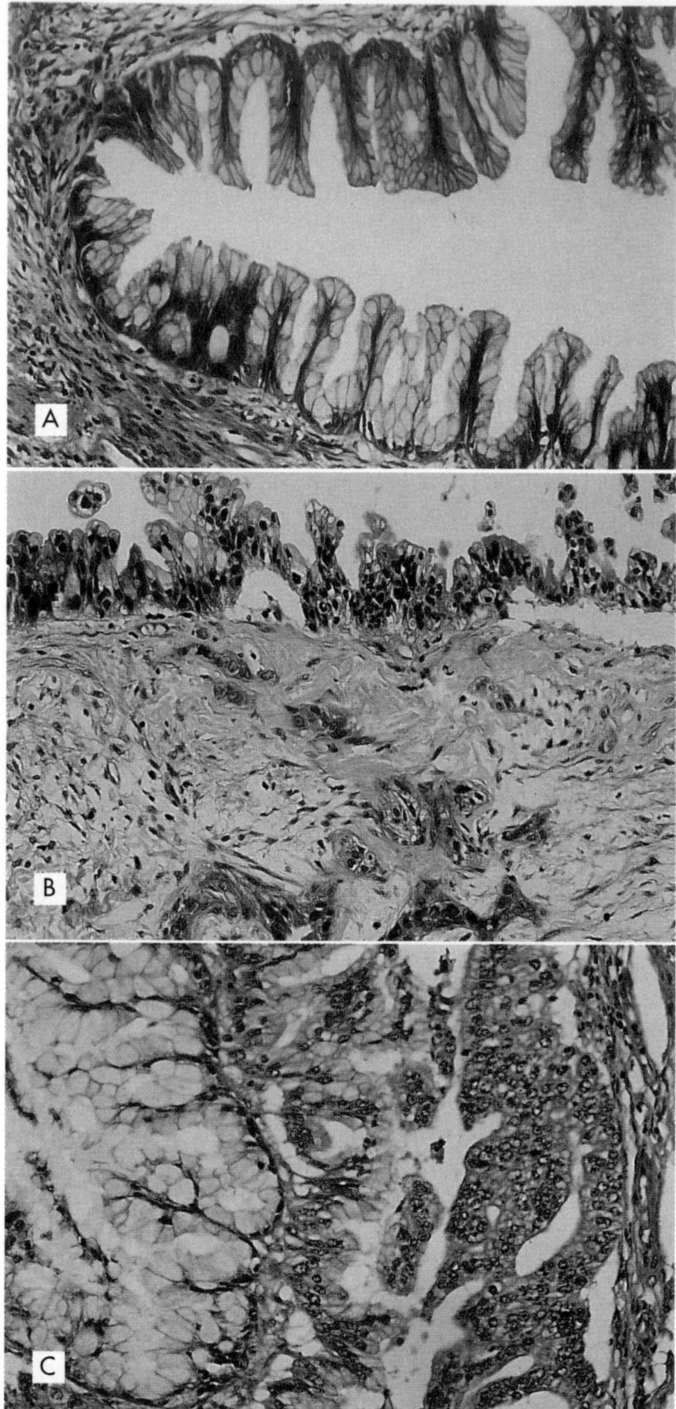

Fig. 59-25 Mucinous cystadenocarcinoma. In **A**, well-differentiated papillary-mucinous epithelium lines a cyst. In **B** (from the same specimen), the cyst lining is dysplastic and there is stromal invasion. **C**, Intraductal papillary-mucinous carcinoma (same tumor as Fig. 59-23).

An adenoma-carcinoma sequence with slow progression is assumed, and a close relationship to the intraductal papillary-mucinous neoplasms is implied, though it has been questioned.[27]

Differential diagnosis. It may be difficult to assign neoplasms to the interrelated categories of intraductal papillary-mucinous and mucinous cystic neoplasms. Whether a neoplasm is deemed an adenoma rather than placed in the next higher category (that "with uncertain malignant potential") depends on how severe the dysplasia, if present, is judged to be. If there is moderate dysplasia that is free of invasion or metastasis, then the "uncertain" category is most appropriate. Large tumors that lack clear evidence of malignancy should be sampled liberally because the histologic features may vary regionally and invasion can be focal. A neoplasm that is apparently entirely intraductal and shows severe atypical cellular changes is deemed an intraductal papillary-mucinous carcinoma, though the lesion may be regarded as a carcinoma in situ.

Neoplasms of the intraductal papillary-mucinous and mucinous cystic groups have been encountered more frequently in the population of Japan than in that of the United States and Europe.[45,56,57] However, it is not yet clear whether this reflects a true difference in incidence or inconsistencies in classification and nomenclature. This emerging group of tumors has received a variety of names, including *intraductal papillary neoplasm*, *ductectatic mucinous cystadenoma*, *mucin-hypersecreting carcinoma*, and *mucinous ductal ectasia*. This inconsistent nomenclature complicates comparison of the incidences in various series. The terminology and classification guidelines for these tumors are still evolving.

Solid pseudopapillary tumor

Solid pseudopapillary tumor constitutes a group of tumors that includes both apparently benign and overtly malignant variants. *Solid-cystic tumor* is a common alternative name. These tumors characteristically occur in young women, beginning in adolescence, though they also arise in older patients and in men (10% to 15%). Macroscopically they are either solid or cystic, range from 2 to 18 cm in diameter (averages 9 cm),[58] and have a fibrous capsule. In their basic pattern they consist of a solid growth of small polygonal cells with round or oval nuclei and either eosinophilic or clear cytoplasm (Fig. 59-26). The tumor is traversed by fibrovascular septa. Necrosis occurs in more than half of the tumors, and it has been suggested that the papillary pattern results from the preservation of tumor cells near the fibrovascular cores, with degeneration or necrosis of the cells distant from the blood supply. This has been termed a *pseudopapillary* pattern. There may be hemorrhage into the tumor. Immunohistochemical studies have demonstrated the existence of both exocrine and endocrine markers, and electron microscopy has shown the tumors contain both zymogen and neurosecretory granules. This implies that the neoplasm originates from a primitive epithelial cell that can differentiate along either exocrine or endocrine pathways. Ten percent to 20% of the neoplasms are malignant, which is manifested initially by venous invasion and later by metastasis to regional nodes or liver. In one study the presence of venous invasion, high-grade nuclear atypia or aneuploidy, and conspicuous necrotic foci showed a positive correlation with malignant behavior.[58]

Malignant tumors of ductal origin

Ductal adenocarcinoma

Ductal adenocarcinoma is the most common histologic type of human pancreatic cancer, accounting for 80% to 85% of the cases in large series. These carcinomas vary in their differentiation, often secrete mucin, and typically are accompanied by the proliferation of stromal fibrous tissue. Macroscopically they are solid, pale, and hard, commonly ranging from 2 to 10

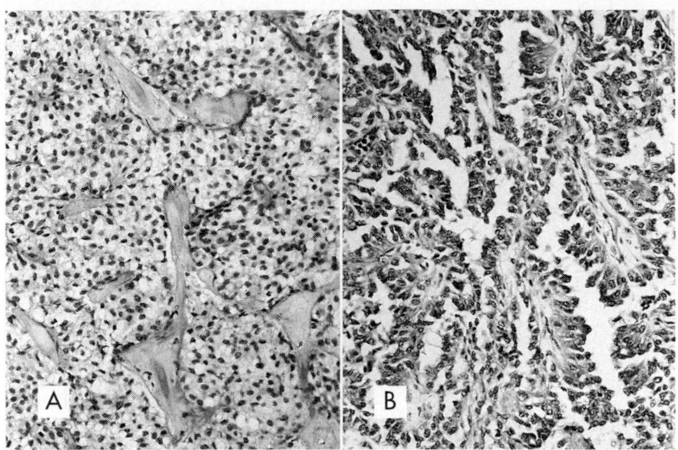

Fig. 59-26 Papillary cystic (solid-cystic) tumor. **A,** Solid pattern. The tumor is composed of small polygonal cells. **B,** Pseudopapillary pattern. The tumor is composed of polygonal cells surrounding stromal cores that provide a blood supply. This pattern is typically seen at the margin of cystic areas of the tumor.

cm in diameter. A few small carcinomas with a diameter in the range of 1 cm have been reported, but most are larger than 2 cm. In one large series the average size (largest diameter) of ductal adenocarcinomas found in the head of the pancreas was 5 cm, whereas those in the body or tail averaged 10 cm in diameter.[18] This size difference is believed to reflect the fact that carcinomas arising in the head of the pancreas are diagnosed earlier because in this site even a small cancer can cause bile or pancreatic duct obstruction that is manifested clinically by jaundice or pancreatitis. The tumor size noted in recently compiled series tends to be smaller. This is probably the result of earlier diagnosis made possible by the improved resolution of imaging methods and by the use of pancreatography after endoscopy with cannulation of the pancreatic duct.

Histologically, typical ductal adenocarcinomas of the pancreas are composed of ductlike structures surrounded by abundant fibrous stroma. The carcinomas are graded according to their cytologic appearance as well differentiated, moderately differentiated, or poorly differentiated (grades 1, 2, and 3, respectively).[59] The cells in well-differentiated carcinomas surround lumens of moderate size, whereas the cells in poorly differentiated variants grow in small cords that form abortive or incomplete lumens (Fig. 59-27). Epithelial cells are columnar or cuboidal. Mucin secretion serves as an index of differentiation. It is prominent in grade 1 carcinomas and absent or negligible in grade 3 carcinomas. When grading is done carefully, survival has been found to correlate (inversely) with the grade.[59] Perineural invasion in peripancreatic nerves is common, even when the primary carcinoma is small and well differentiated (Fig. 59-28), and invasion into the nerve trunks is sometimes noted. Extension along nerves into the retroperitoneal region has been reported.[60]

Immunohistochemistry testing is of limited diagnostic value. Immunostaining for markers such as carcinoembryonic antigen and CA19-9 may yield positive results. Tumor cells express several cytokeratins (types 7, 8, 18, and 19) that are also found in normal ductal epithelium.[27] None of these markers can be used to distinguish between primary pancreatic carcinomas and adenocarcinomas originating from other sites.

The differential diagnosis between adenocarcinoma of the pancreas and chronic pancreatitis can be difficult at the gross level because both exhibit a hard and fibrotic appearance and at the histologic level because of superficial similarities in appearance. Differential points include the preservation of lobular architecture in chronic pancreatitis even when there is extensive fibrosis, whereas the lobular pattern is violated by invasive carcinomas. The cells that compose the ducts and ductules derived from acinar tissue in chronic pancreatitis have small or normal nuclei, whereas the nuclei of malignant cells are commonly enlarged. The number of mitoses in well-differentiated carcinomas is low, and mitoses are to be anticipated in pancreatic epithelium attempting regeneration. Thus the number of mitoses is not a helpful distinguishing feature when the epithelium is well differentiated. More mitoses are seen in grades 2 and 3 ductal adenocarcinomas,[59] whereas the number of mitoses in atrophic pancreatic epithelium in the late stages of chronic pancreatitis is low. Perineural invasion is a useful criterion for pancreatic malignancy. Sympathetic ganglia occur in the pancreas, and the finding of ganglia cells in nerve trunks should be distinguished from invasion by malignant cells.

Carcinoma in situ

Severe atypia of the duct epithelium with or without papillary projections may be found in the vicinity of ductal adenocarcinomas and has been termed *carcinoma in situ.* When this change is found in the presence of an overt ductal adenocarcinoma, the intraductal component may represent invasion rather than an independent, in situ, lesion. Lesions of ductal epithelium with atypia of carcinoma in situ grade in patients who do not have invasive pancreatic carcinoma have been described but are rare.[19,61] Important criteria for severe ductal atypia include loss of cell polarity, nuclear pleomorphism and enlargement, and a cribriform papillary growth pattern (see Fig. 59-9). Severe atypia of carcinoma in situ grade has also been noted in ductular epithelium.[19]

Undifferentiated carcinoma

Undifferentiated carcinoma includes solid anaplastic carcinomas either dominated by tumor giant cells or with a dominant spindle cell pattern (Fig. 59-29). Alternate terms for the tumor are *anaplastic carcinoma, pleomorphic carcinoma, giant cell carcinoma*, and *sarcomatoid carcinoma*. The clinical behavior of the *giant cell carcinomas* observed in the series reported on by Cubilla and Fitzgerald[18] seems comparable to that of grade 3 ductal adenocarcinomas because the prognosis in these patients was worse than the average one in patients with ductal carcinomas, except that a rare variant with osteoclastlike cells seems to carry a better prognosis.

Adenosquamous carcinoma

Adenosquamous carcinoma is regarded as a variant of ductal carcinoma that includes both glandular and squamous elements (Fig. 59-30). The glandular element is like that of a typical ductal adenocarcinoma, and the squamous element may contain highly keratinized foci. *Squamous cell carcinomas* of the pancreas have been noted in some series, and this is apparently an alternative designation for adenosquamous carcinoma. Other designations for this group of tumors include *mucoepidermoid* and *adenoacanthoma*. Pure squamous cell carcinomas of the pancreas are rare, and their existence has

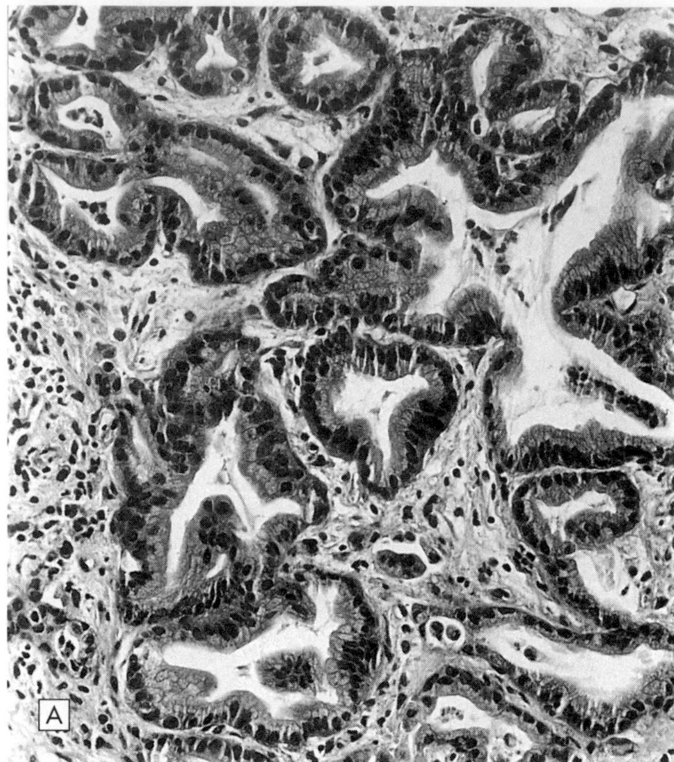

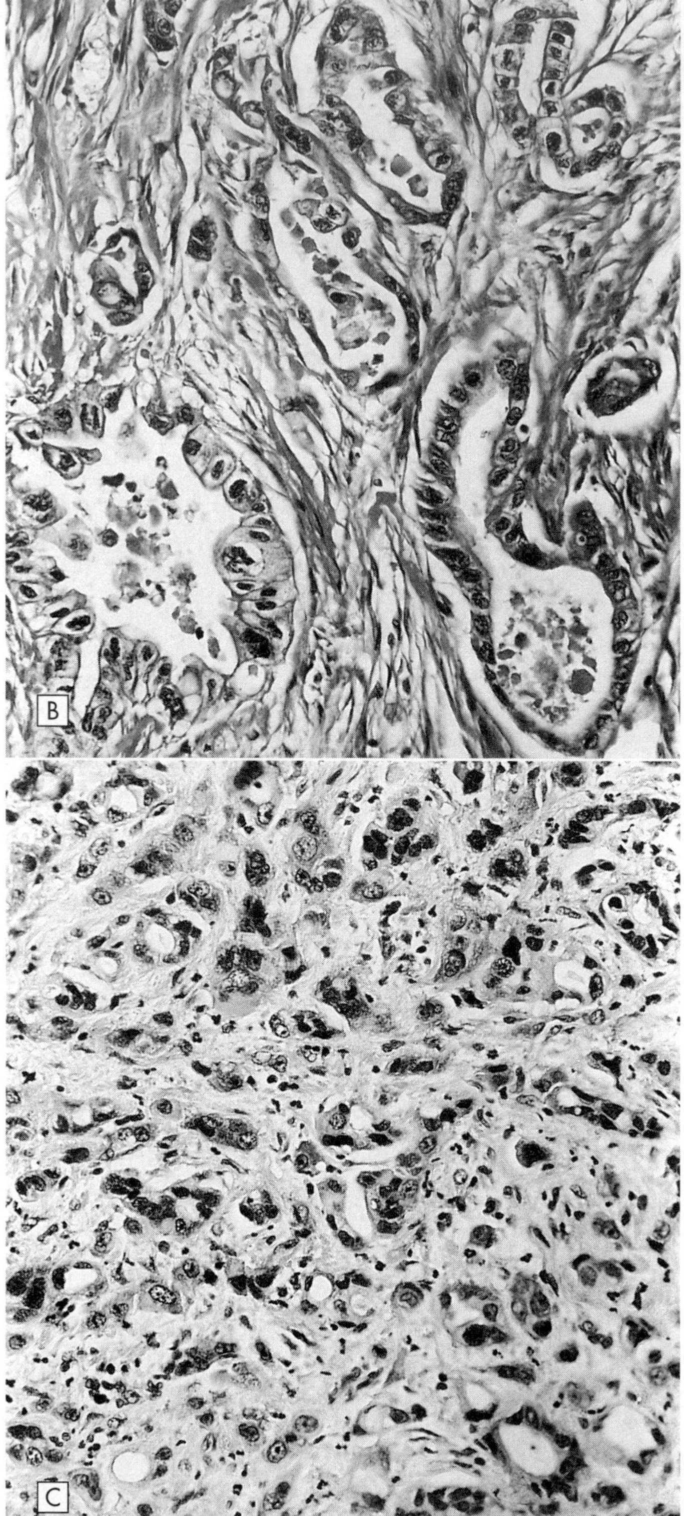

Fig. 59-27 Ductal adenocarcinomas. **A,** Well-differentiated form (grade 1). Columnar cells line ductlike structures. **B,** Moderately differentiated form (grade 2). Ductlike spaces are lined by cuboidal cells. **C,** Poorly differentiated form (grade 3). Several poorly formed ducts, a few signet-ring cells, cellular pleomorphism, and moderate desmoplasia are present.

been questioned. In some cases deemed pure squamous cell carcinoma, only a small portion of a large tumor has been examined histologically, leaving open the possibility that a glandular component has been missed.[62] The prognosis for adenosquamous carcinomas is similar to that for ductal carcinomas.

Mucinous noncystic carcinoma

Mucinous noncystic adenocarcinoma is a solid neoplasm with a high content of mucin that is distributed in the interstitium surrounding malignant glandular epithelium as well as within glandular lumens, as is characteristic of mucinous carcinomas in other tissues (Fig. 59-31). Alternative terms for the tumor are *colloid carcinomas*, *mucinous adenocarcinoma*, and *gelatinous carcinoma*. These neoplasms are regarded as a variant of ductal adenocarcinoma and have a similar prognosis. "Signet-ring cell carcinoma" is the name for a solid carcinoma composed of mucin-containing (signet-ring) cells that do not form glandular or cystic structures. The signet ring cells may "float" in mucin. This has been regarded as a variant of mucinous noncystic carcinoma.[18]

Acinar cell carcinoma

Acinar cell carcinoma is a rare solid neoplasm composed of differentiated acinar cells that either form acini or tubules or form solid sheets of polygonal cells with markers of acinar cell differentiation. Either the acinar pattern or the solid pattern may predominate (Fig. 59-32). Antibodies to trypsinogen, lipase, or amylase may be used in immunohistochemical stains to elicit evidence that the cells retain markers of acinar cell differentiation.[63,64] A small fraction of acinar cell carcinomas are cystic. The survival in a group of 28 patients with the tumors was clearly longer than the average survival in patients with ductal adenocarcinomas.[64]

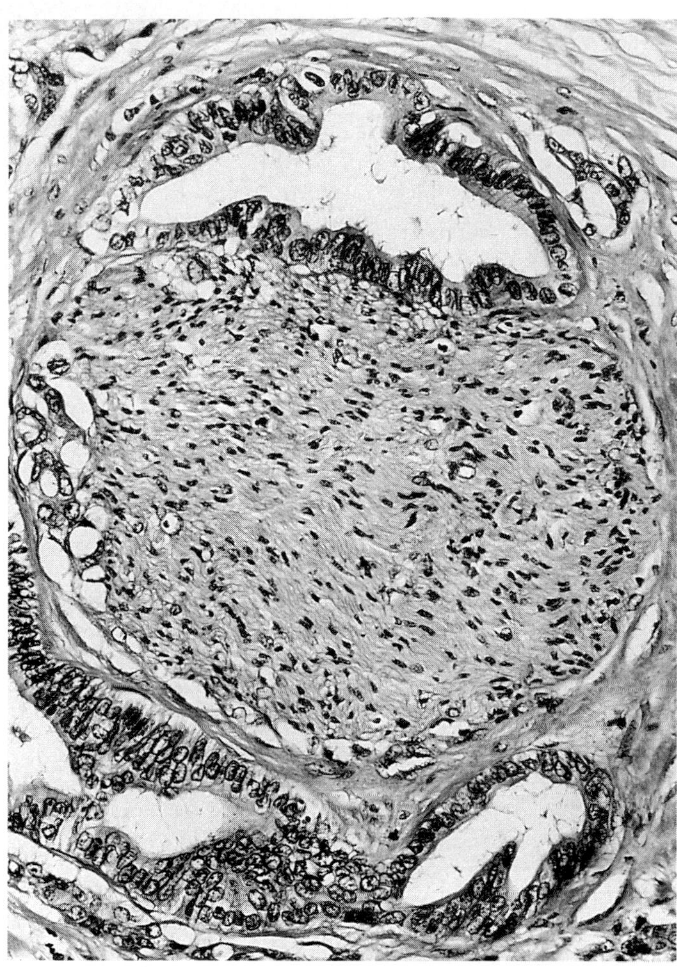

Fig. 59-28 Ductal adenocarcinoma invading the perineural space. A few cells have invaded the nerve trunk. The carcinoma is well differentiated.

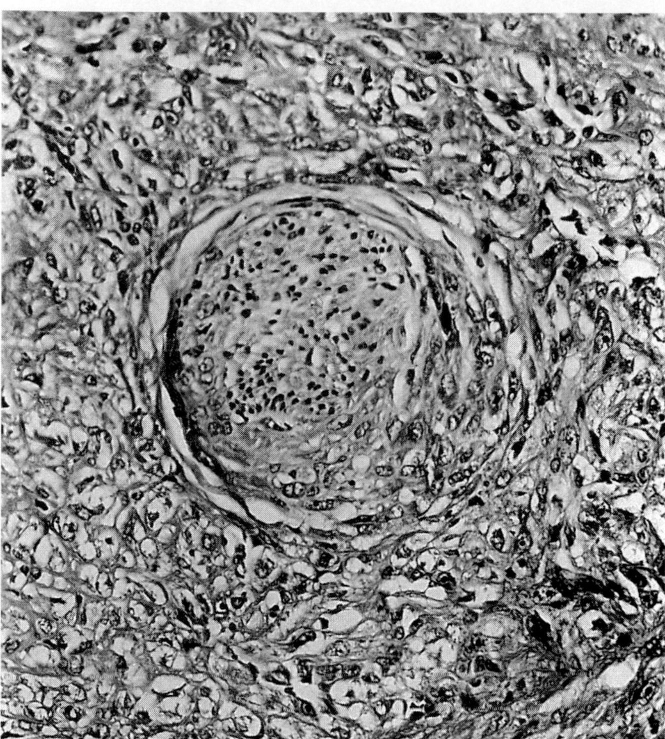

Fig. 59-29 Undifferentiated carcinoma. This field contains pleomorphic, spindle-shaped cells surrounding a nerve *(center)*. A few of the cells near the nerve are polygonal and appear epithelial.

Other tumors

Pancreatoblastoma

Pancreatoblastoma is a rare tumor that is usually found in infants and children between 1 and 17 years of age,[65] but it is also encountered in adults. These are usually solid encapsulated tumors, but a portion of the tumor may be cystic. Primitive cell types may predominate, and these appear as small, undifferentiated epithelial cells, as polygonal cells of intermediate size, or as spindle-shaped cells with scant cytoplasm (Fig. 59-33). Horie and others[65] noted an organoid pattern in small masses of cells, indicating the possible formation of primitive lobules with glandular structures in the periphery enclosing undifferentiated cells and with a core of squamoid cells. These elements are sometimes present in a less-ordered fashion. Both endocrine and exocrine differentiation have been identified in component cells, such that ductal, acinar, and islet cells may be seen at the histologic (Fig. 59-34) or ultrastructural level. Stromal elements may be present and occasionally display aberrant differentiation into bone or cartilage. The name *pancreatoblastoma, mixed type*, has been proposed for the tumors that have both epithelial and mesenchymal components. Individual tumors differ in their histologic appearance, and the key to diagnosis is the finding of mixed patterns of differentiation in a background of primitive cells. Both pure epithelial and mixed pancreatoblastomas may be cured by complete resection, but these tumors have a malignant potential. Pancreatoblastoma appears to be the counterpart of childhood tumors such as Wilms' tumor and hepatoblastoma that arise from stem cells in other organs.

Miscellaneous carcinomas

Variants of pancreatic carcinoma have been given a variety of names in earlier classifications.[18,27] Mixed exocrine-endocrine carcinomas include tumors with nearly equal differentiated ductal and endocrine components. Immunohistochemical markers may be used to document the endocrine component.

Other rare patterns include ciliated cell carcinoma, oncocytic carcinoma, and clear cell carcinoma.[27] One variant, termed *microadenocarcinoma*, is a solid glandular tumor with multiple small lumens and no desmoplasia.[18] This pattern occurs in some acinar cell carcinomas, indicating that the microglandular pattern may sometimes be a variant of this group rather than a distinct type. Special stains can demonstrate the mucin content in clear cell carcinomas.

The miscellaneous pancreatic tumors are rare, and so far their prognoses and therapeutic implications are not clear. This may stem from the fact that data are available for only a few cases. In general these tumors occur in adults. Perhaps the greatest significance of the rare patterns is the difficulty in recognizing the pancreatic origin in a biopsy specimen from a metastatic site.

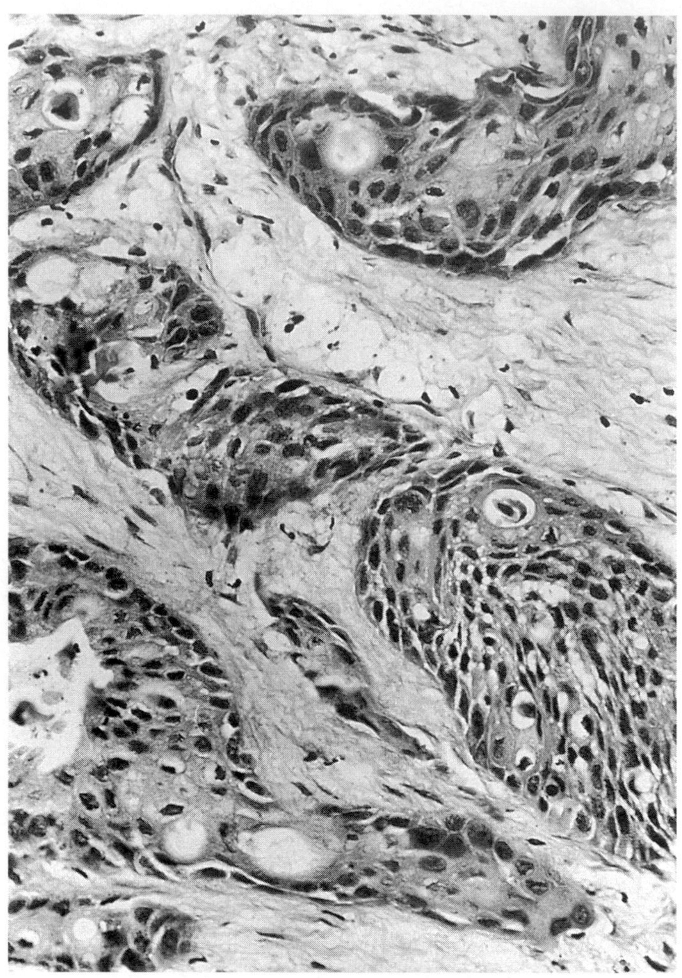

Fig. 59-30 Adenosquamous carcinoma. Most cells show squamous differentiation. The tumor was highly invasive and desmoplastic.

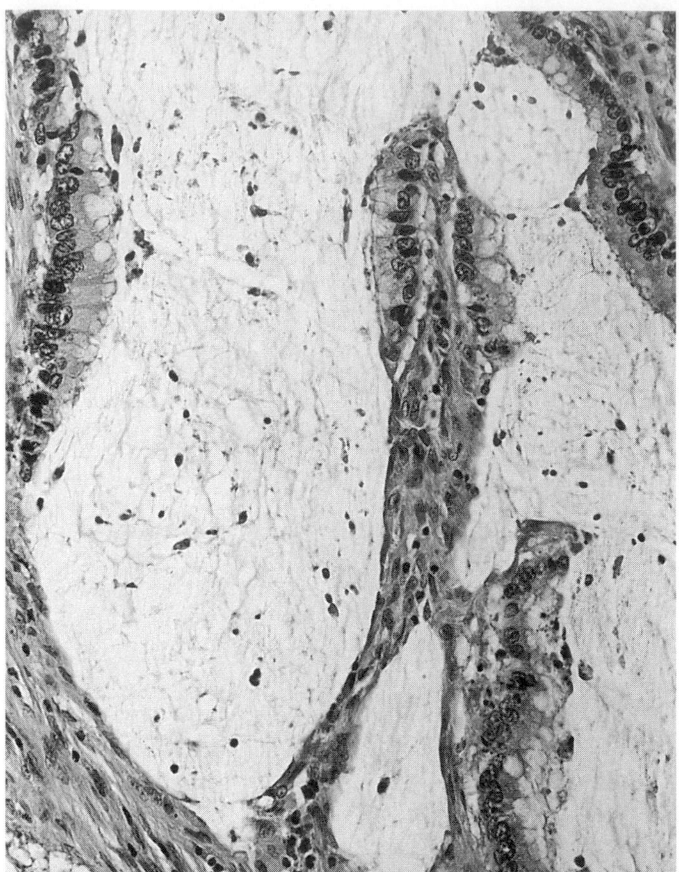

Fig. 59-31 Mucinous noncystic carcinoma. Mucin-filled spaces are partially lined by columnar, mucin-secreting epithelium and are partially bounded by connective tissue. This is a recurrent pattern.

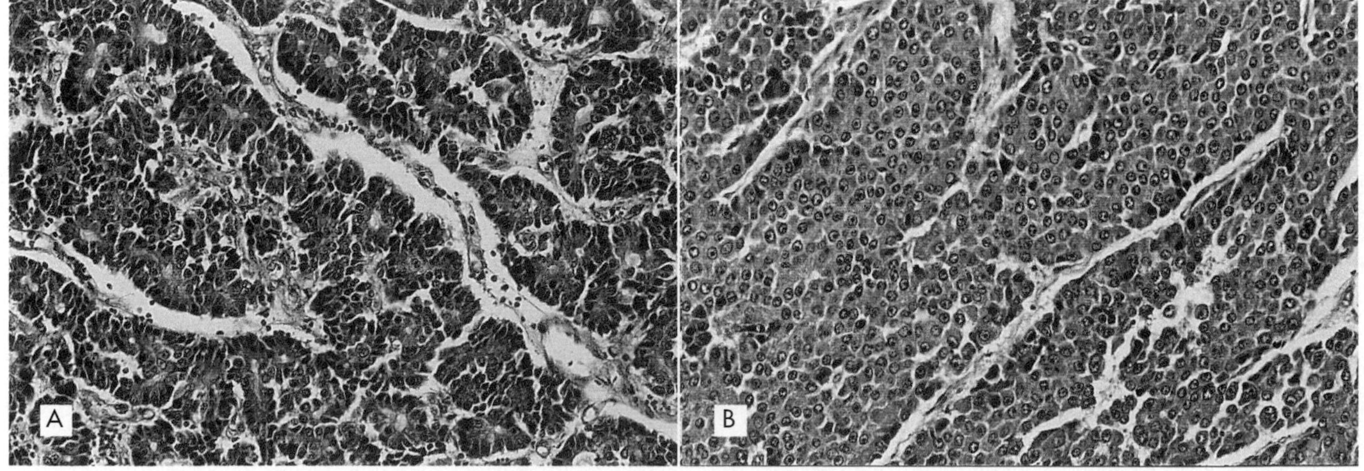

Fig. 59-32 Acinar cell carcinoma. Two different types of tumors are illustrated. **A,** Well-differentiated acinar pattern. The neoplastic cells are smaller than normal acinar cells but have larger nuclei. They form acini or acinar tubules. There is virtually no fibrous stroma. **B,** Solid pattern. The tumor is composed of monomorphic cells of moderate size that do not form glands or acini.

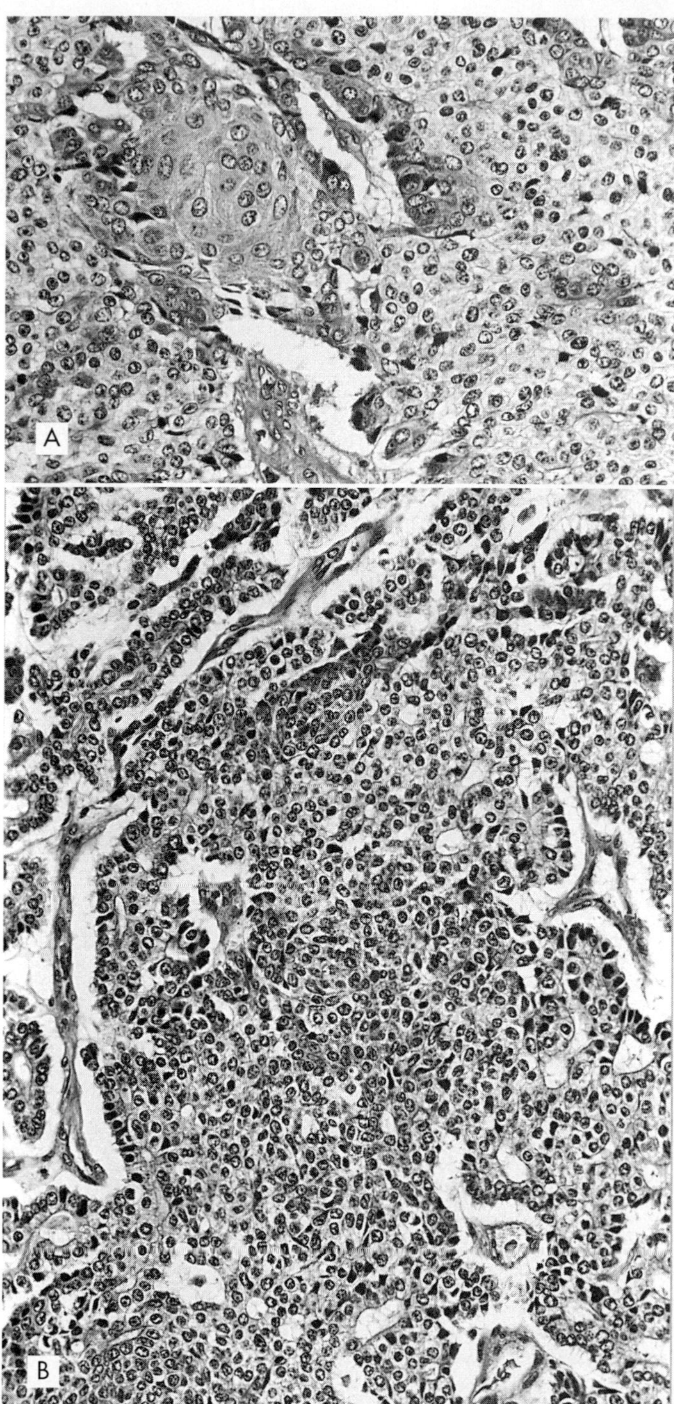

Fig. 59-33 Pancreatoblastoma. Two different tumors are shown. **A,** The dominant cell type is polygonal and moderate in size and contains a light cytoplasm. These grow in solid masses. Cells at the edge of these masses contain darker cytoplasm and form groups suggestive of acini. A nest of squamoid cells can be seen *(upper left)*. **B,** As in **A,** the dominant cell type is polygonal and contains clear cytoplasm. The cells grow in a solid pattern with occasional glandlike spaces. In a few areas cuboidal cells with a darker cytoplasm form a single layer on stromal cores.

Small cell carcinoma

Small cell carcinoma is the term used for rare solid tumors composed of small monomorphic cells that contain scant cytoplasm with a size in the range of lymphocytes and that are similar in appearance to small cell carcinoma of the lung (Fig. 59-35). The fact that they possess neuroendocrine markers, demonstrable immunohistochemically,[66] and neurosecretory granules, demonstrable ultrastructurally, indicates that these tumors may be variants of islet cell carcinoma, though they are commonly grouped with exocrine carcinomas. A primary small cell carcinoma of the pancreas is diagnosed only when other primary tumors, including a primary lung tumor, have been excluded. These carcinomas are highly malignant, but some have shown a response to chemotherapy.

Metastatic spread

Pancreatic carcinomas metastasize to regional nodes, peritoneum, liver, lungs, and pleura. Lymphatic spread usually precedes hematogenous spread. The groups of lymph nodes most frequently involved by metastatic pancreatic carcinoma are located around, and especially dorsal to, the head of the pancreas. Lymphatic involvement extends retroperitoneally to nodes around the superior mesenteric artery and adjacent aorta and to nodes around the celiac artery and its branches.

Pancreatic carcinoma is staged according to the tumor size, the status of local extension and lymph node involvement, and the presence or absence of distant metastasis. Systems proposed by the American Joint Committee on Cancer (Table 59-6) and the Union Internationale Contre Cancer[67] differ slightly. There is greater emphasis on tumor size in the latter system. Precise assignment to stages I to III in either system requires careful evaluation of resected specimens, but operative findings or the results of imaging studies are used as the basis for a stage IV classification.

Unfortunately, the remote internal location of the pancreas makes early detection on the basis of cytologic or biopsy findings very difficult. Cytologic study involves either collecting specimens through a fiberoptic duodenoscope possessing a special cannula that allows the pancreatic duct to be entered through the ampulla of Vater or aspirating material through a percutaneous "skinny needle" guided by ultrasound imaging. Biopsy specimens of ductal mucosa can be obtained by the endoscopic route.

New complex therapeutic protocols based on biologic approaches (gene therapy and immunotherapy) may take several months for completion. Thus it is important to identify variants of pancreatic carcinoma that are associated with survivals that might allow such treatment. The current prognostic indicators include the tumor phenotype, the grade of the ductal adenocarcinomas, and the stage. In the future, molecular markers may assume importance in this evaluation.

Nonepithelial tumors

Nonepithelial tumors that may involve the pancreas include benign soft tissue tumors, sarcomas, and lymphomas.[27] All but secondary cases of involvement by lymphoma are rare.

Secondary neoplasms

The pancreas is uncommonly the site of metastasis from primary carcinomas in other organs such as the breast, colon, and lung. In some cases this appears to result from extension from paraaortic lymph nodes rather than from direct metastasis to the pancreas.

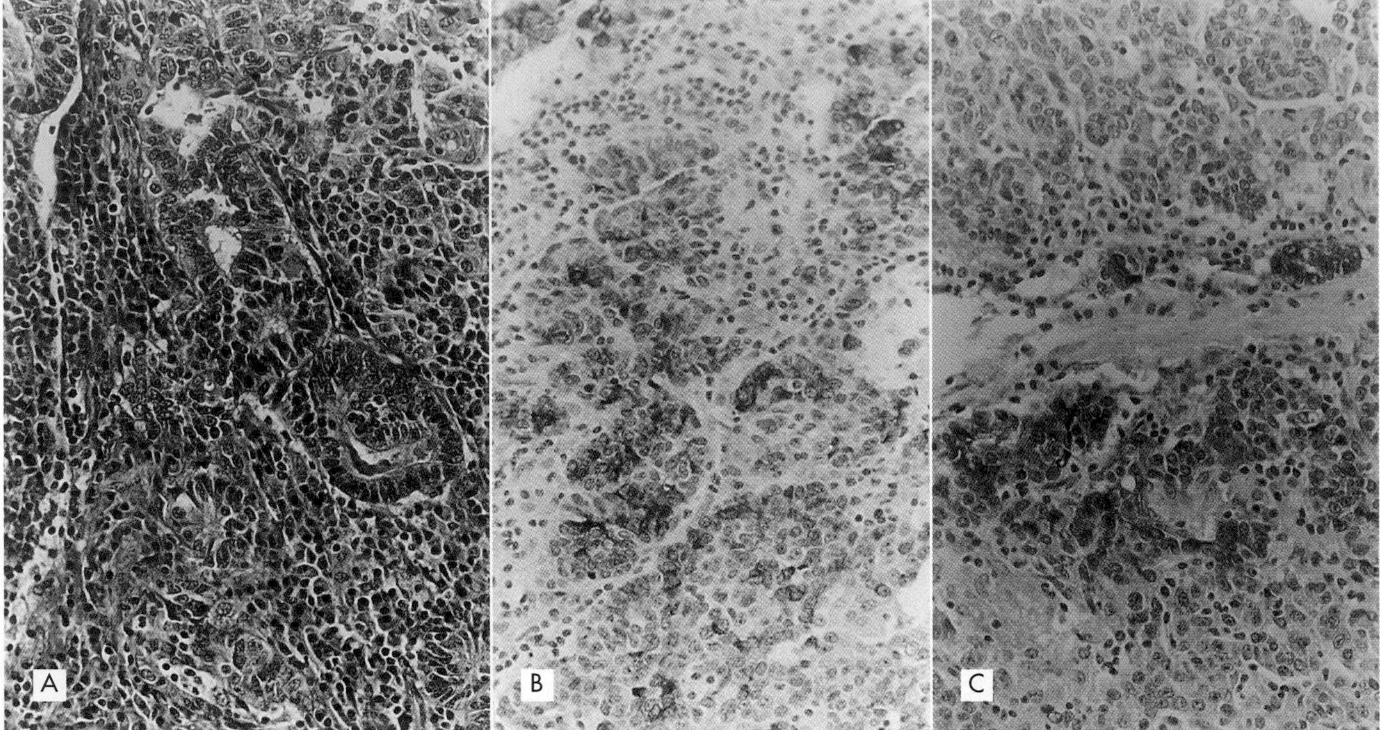

Fig. 59-34 Pancreatoblastoma with a mixture of exocrine and endocrine cell types. **A,** Ductlike structures are intermixed with solid masses of "bland"-appearing cells indicative of an islet cell tumor. **B,** Scattered cells are stained using antibody to chromogranin. (Hematoxylin and immunoperoxidase.) **C,** Cells in acinar groups are stained using antibody to trypsin. (Hematoxylin and immunoperoxidase.)

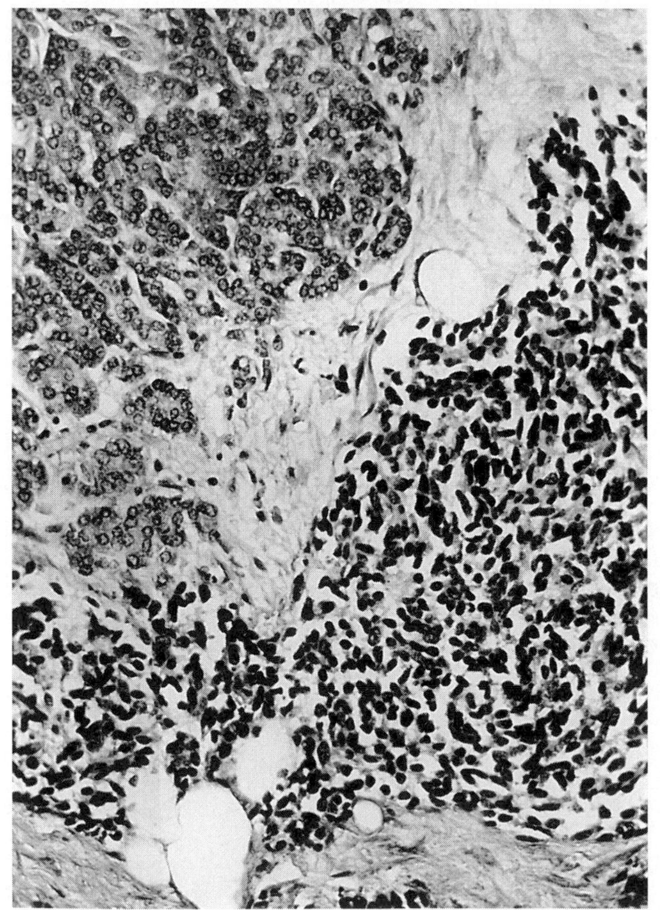

Fig. 59-35 Small cell carcinoma. Normal acinar tissue is present *(upper right).* (Courtesy Dr. G. Klöppel, Brussels.)

Table 59-6 American Joint Committee for Cancer Staging and End Results reporting guidelines for carcinoma of the pancreas

TNM classification criteria	
T1	No direct extension of the primary beyond the pancreas
T2	Limited direct extension to the duodenum, bile duct, or stomach
T3	Advanced direct extension incompatible with surgical resection
TX	Direct extension not assessed
N0	Regional nodes not involved
N1	Regional nodes involved
NX	Regional lymph nodes not assessed
M0	No distant metastasis
M1	Distant metastasis present
MX	Distant metastasis not assessed
TNM stages	
Stage I	T1-2, N0, M0
Stage II	T3, N0, M0
Stage III	T1-3, N1, M0
Stage IV	Any T or N, M1

FURTHER READING

Multiauthored reference works provide a wealth of detail regarding the normal pancreas, its function, and its diseases.[68-70] The clinically oriented volume edited by Bradley[70] provides reviews on all aspects of acute pancreatitis, including a chapter on pathology prepared by Klöppel. Prior reviews,[13,71] monographs,[72] and the Armed Forces Institute of Pathology's *Atlas of Tumor Pathology*[18] provide additional relevant photomicrographs that supplement those included here.

ACKNOWLEDGMENTS

Photomicrographs of acinar cell carcinoma, pancreaticoblastoma, and papillary cystic tumors were made from slides provided by Dr. Clara Heffess, Armed Forces Institute of Pathology, Washington, D.C. Photomicrographs are also derived from slides provided by Drs. Yo Kato, Tokyo, Japan; Mark Silverman, Boston, MA; and Günther Klöppel, Brussels, Belgium.

REFERENCES

1. Stamm BH: Incidence and diagnostic significance of minor pathologic changes in the adult pancreas at autopsy: a systematic study of 112 autopsies in patients without known pancreatic disease. *Hum Pathol* 15:677, 1984.
2. Bockman DE: Anatomy of the pancreas. In Go VLW, DeMagno EP, Gardner JD, et al, editors. *The pancreas: biology, pathobiology and disease,* New York, Raven Press, 1993.
3. Cotton PB: Congenital anomaly of pancreas division as cause of obstructive pain and pancreatitis, *Gut* 21:105, 1980.
4. Flaherty MJ, Benjamin DR: Multicystic pancreatic hamartoma: a distinctive lesion with immunohistochemical and ultrastructural study, *Hum Pathol* 23:1309, 1992.
5. Hayward I, Mindelzun RE, Jeffrey RB: Intrapancreatic accessory spleen mimicking pancreatic mass on CT, *J Comput Assist Tomogr* 16:984, 1992.
6. Gilinsky NH, del Favero G, Cotton PB et al: Congenital short pancreas: a report of two cases, *Gut* 26:304, 1985.
7. Soler R, Rodríguez E, Comesana ML et al: Agenesis of the dorsal pancreas with polysplenia syndrome: CT features, *J Comput Assist Tomogr* 16:921, 1992.
8. Kerem E, Corey M, Kerem BS et al: The relation between genotype and phenotype in cystic fibrosis—analysis of the most common mutation (ΔF508). *N Engl J Med* 323:1517, 1990.
9. Comfort MW, Steinberg AG: Pedigree of a family with hereditary chronic relapsing pancreatitis, *Gastroenterology* 21:54, 1952.
10. Girard RM, Dube S, Archambault AP: Hereditary pancreatitis: report of an affected Canadian kindred and review of the disease. *Can Med Assoc J* 125:576, 1981.
11. Roberts IM: Disorders of the pancreas in children, *Gastroenterology* 19:963, 1990.
12. Lerner A, Lebenthal E: Hereditary diseases of the pancreas. In Go VLW, DeMagno EP, Gardner JD, et al, editors: *The pancreas: biology, pathobiology and disease,* New York, 1993, Raven Press.
13. Longnecker DS: Pathology of pancreatitis. In Braganza JM, editor: *The pathogenesis of pancreatitis,* Manchester, England, 1991, Manchester University Press.
14. Brooks SE, Golden MH: The exocrine pancreas in kwashiorkor and marasmus: light and electron microscopy, *West Indian Med J* 41:56, 1992.
15. Glenner G, Mallory GK: The cystadenoma and related nonfunctional tumors of the pancreas. Pathogenesis, classification, and significance, *Cancer* 9:980, 1956.
16. Longnecker DS, Shinozuka H, Dekker A: Focal acinar cell dysplasia in human pancreas, *Cancer* 45:534, 1980.
17. Kishi K, Nakamura K, Yoshimori M et al: Morphology and pathological significance of focal acinar cell dysplasia of the human pancreas, *Pancreas* 7:177, 1992.
18. Cubilla AL, Fitzgerald PJ: Tumors of the exocrine pancreas. In *Atlas of Tumor Pathology,* series 2, fasc 19, Washington, DC, 1984, Armed Forces Institute of Pathology.
19. Pour PM, Sayed S, Sayed G: Hyperplastic, preneoplastic and neoplastic lesions found in 83 human pancreases, *Am J Clin Pathol* 77:137, 1982.
20. Longnecker DS, Hashida Y, Shinozuka H: Relationship of age to prevalence of focal acinar cell dysplasia in the human pancreas, *J Natl Cancer Inst* 65:63, 1980.
21. Cubilla AL, Fitzgerald PJ: Morphological lesions associated with human primary invasive nonendocrine pancreas cancer, *Cancer Res* 36:2690, 1976.
22. Chan P, Teoh TB: The pathology of *Clonorchis sinensis* infestation of the pancreas, *J Pathol* 93:185, 1967.
23. Oertel JE: The pancreas: non-neoplastic alterations, *Am J Surg Pathol* 13:50, 1989.
24. Klöppel G, Bommer G, Rückert K et al: Intraductal proliferation in the pancreas and its relationship to human and experimental carcinogenesis, *Virchows Arch [A] Pathol Arat Histol* 387:221, 1980.
25. Sessa F, Bonato M, Frigerio B et al: Ductal cancers of the pancreas frequently express markers of gastrointestinal epithelial cells, *Gastroenterology* 98:1655, 1990.
26. Kozuka S, Sassa R, Taki T et al: Relation of pancreatic duct hyperplasia to carcinoma, *Cancer* 43:1418, 1979.
27. Klöppel G: Pathology of nonendocrine pancreatic tumors, *Pancreas* 871, 1993.
28. Sommers SC, Murphy SA, Warren S: Pancreatic duct hyperplasia and cancer, *Gastroenterology* 27:629, 1954.
29. Bockman DE: Cells of origin of pancreatic cancer: experimental animal tumors related to human pancreas, *Cancer* 47:1528, 1981.
30. Parsa I, Longnecker DS, Scarpelli DG et al: Ductal metaplasia of human exocrine pancreas and its association with carcinoma, *Cancer Res* 45:1285, 1985.
31. Bradley EL III: The necessity for a clinical classification of acute pancreatitis: the Atlanta system. In Bradley EL III, editor: *Acute pancreatitis: diagnosis and therapy,* New York, 1994, Raven Press.
32. Steer ML: How and where does acute pancreatitis begin?, *Arch Surg* 127:1350, 1992.
33. Mallory A, Kern F Jr: Drug-induced pancreatitis: a critical review, *Gastroenterology* 78:813, 1980.
34. Marshall JB: Acute pancreatitis, *Arch Intern Med* 153:1185, 1993.
35. Marshall JB, Kretschmar JM, Gerhardt DC: Gastrointestinal manifestations of mixed connective tissue disease, *Gastroenterology* 98:1232, 1990.
36. Wilcox CM, Forsmark CE, Grendell JH et al: Cytomegalovirus-associated acute pancreatic disease in patients with acquired immunodeficiency syndrome: report of two patients, *Gastroenterology* 99:263, 1990.
37. Toskes PP: Hyperlipidemic pancreatitis, *Gasterenterol Clin North Am* 19:783, 1990.
38. Saharia P, Margolis S, Zuidema GD et al: Acute pancreatitis with hyperlipidemia: studies with an isolated perfused canine pancreas, *Surgery* 82:60, 1977.
39. Singh M, Simsek H: Ethanol and the pancreas. Current status, *Gastroenterology* 98:1051, 1990.
40. Traverso LW: Infections complicating severe pancreatitis, *Infect Dis Clin North Am* 6:601, 1992.
41. Pitchumoni CS, Mohan AT: Pancreatic stones, *Gastroenterol Clin North Am* 19:873, 1990.
42. DiMagno EP, Malagelada JR, Go VLW: Relationship between alcoholism and pancreatic insufficiency, *Ann NY Acad Sci* 252:200, 1975.
43. Boring CC, Squires TS, Tong T: Cancer statistics, *CA Cancer J Clin* 43:7, 1993.
44. Gudjonsson B: Cancer of the pancreas: 50 years of surgery, *Cancer* 60:2284, 1987.
45. Longnecker DS, Kato Y, Konishi Y et al: Comparison of histologic type and stage of exocrine pancreatic neoplasms from surgical series in Europe, Japan and the United States. In Beger H, Büchler M, editors: *Cancer of the pancreas: molecular biology, progress in diagnosis and treatment* Heidelberg, in press, Springer-Verlag.
46. Manusco TF, El Attar AA: Cohort study of workers exposed to naphthylamine and benzidine, *J Occup Med* 9:227, 1967.
47. Lowenfels AB, Maisonneuve P, Cavallini G et al: Pancreatitis and the risk of pancreatic cancer, *N Engl J Med* 328:1433, 1993.

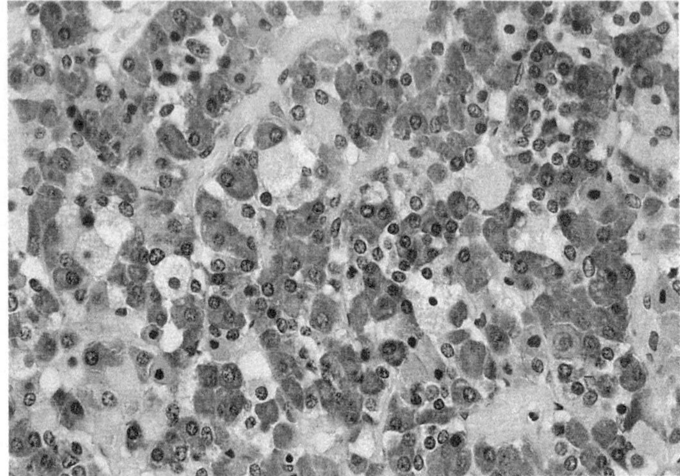

Fig. 60-6 Growth hormone cells in the anterior pituitary are the most numerous cell type (Immunoperoxidase).

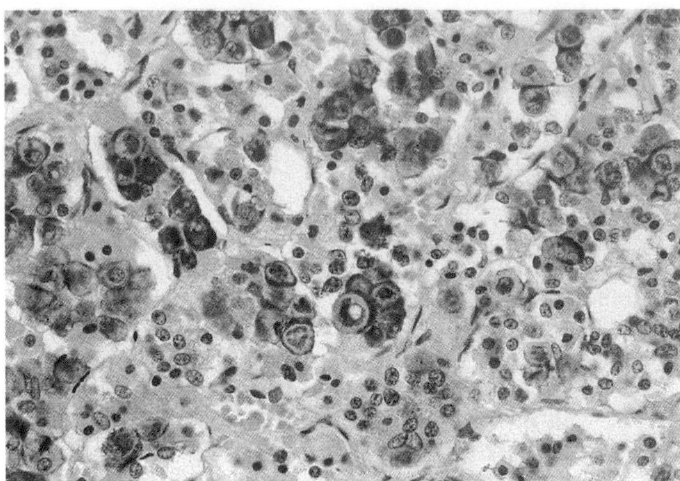

Fig. 60-8 Nests of corticotrophs staining positively for adrenocorticotropin (Immunoperoxidase).

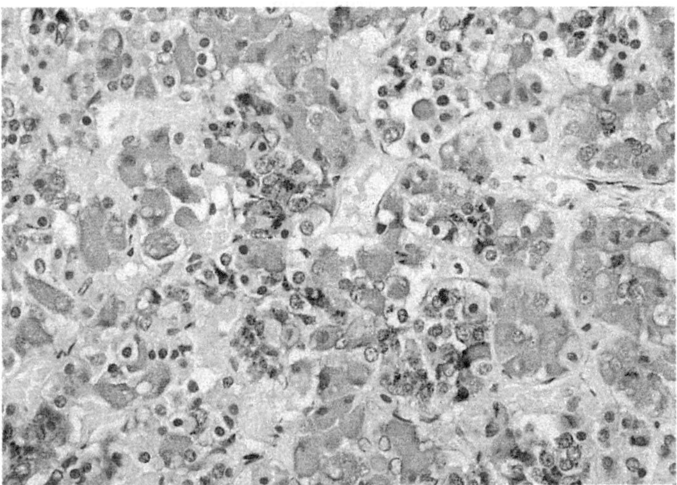

Fig. 60-7 Prolactin cells in the anterior pituitary showing a distinct juxtanuclear immunoreactive prolactin hormone in many cells (Immunoperoxidase).

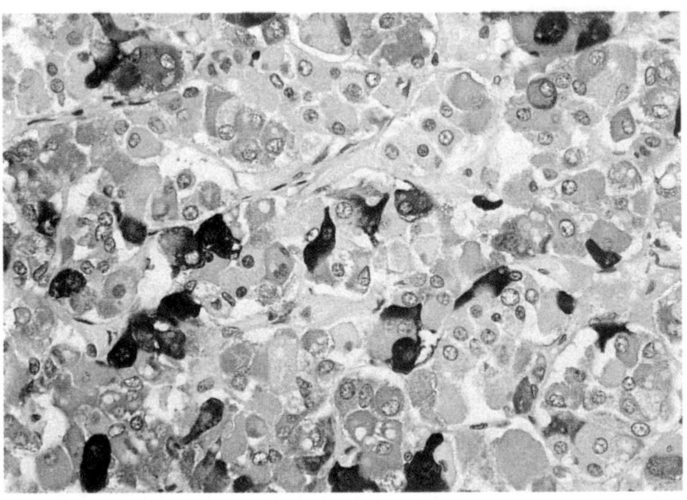

Fig. 60-9 Thyrotrophs have a distinctly angular shape and constitute about 5% of anterior pituitary cells (Immunoperoxidase).

dopamine agonists, are small cells with heterochromatic nuclei, smaller secretory granules, scanty rough endoplasmic reticulum (RER), and inconspicuous Golgi apparatuses.[16]

Mammosomatotrophs (GH/PRL cells). Bihormonal cells that produce both GH and PRL are present in the normal pituitary.[21] They increase in number during pregnancy, indicating a contribution of mammosomatotrophs to PRL production.[22]

Corticotrophs (ACTH cells). Corticotrophs are basophilic cells that are numerous in the central mucoid wedge (Fig. 60-8). They stain positively with periodic acid–Schiff (PAS) and are easily identified because of the presence of large perinuclear vacuoles called *enigmatic bodies* that ultrastructurally correspond to phagolysosomes. Some corticotrophs extend into the posterior lobe. This process, referred to as *basophil invasion*, may become prominent with increasing age.[7] The proopiomelanocortin (POMC) gene is located on chromosome 2 and consists of three exons. Corticotrophs produce ACTH, a 39–amino acid, single-chain peptide derived from the precursor POMC molecule. POMC is a 31kD glycoprotein processed into different biologically active peptides by the proprotein convertases present in the pituitary.[23] The POMC-derived peptides are stored in round, drop-shaped, or heart-shaped secretory granules measuring 300 to 500 nm. The ultrastructural markers of corticotrophs are perinuclear bundles of type 1 keratin filaments.

ACTH stimulates the adrenal cortex to secrete glucocorticoids, mineralocorticoids, and sex steroids. Corticotrophs are stimulated by corticotropin-releasing hormone. Glucocorticoids have a rapid inhibitory effect on ACTH secretion, and the inhibited corticotrophs are easily identified at the light microscopic level by the progressive perinuclear accumulation of type 1 filaments, a process known as "Crooke's hyalinization."

Thyrotrophs (TSH cells). Thyrotrophs account for approximately 5% of the anterior lobe cells and are located mainly in the anteromedian area of the mucoid wedge (Fig. 60-9). The angular thyrotroph cells contain PAS-positive droplets in their cytoplasm. The TSH beta-gene is located on chromosome 1 and consists of three exons. TSH is formed by the association of an alpha- and beta-subunit and is stored in small secretory granules (100 to 300 nm). It stimulates the thyroid to acceler-

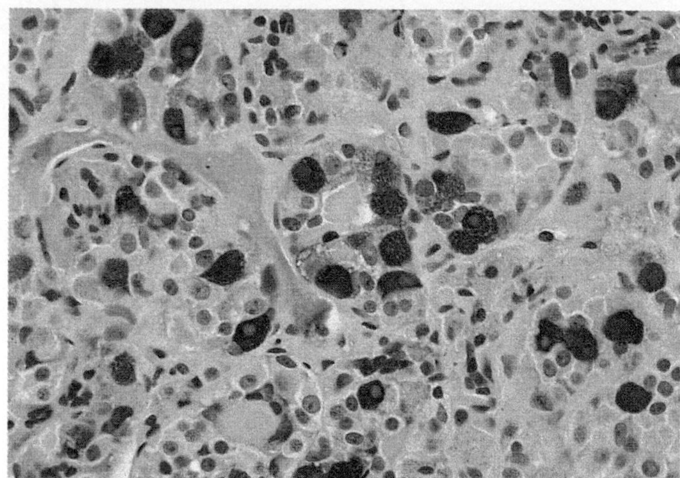

Fig. 60-10 Gonadotrophs in the anterior pituitary staining for luteinizing hormone (LH)–beta. These cells commonly express both follicle-stimulating and LH glycoproteins (Immunoperoxidase).

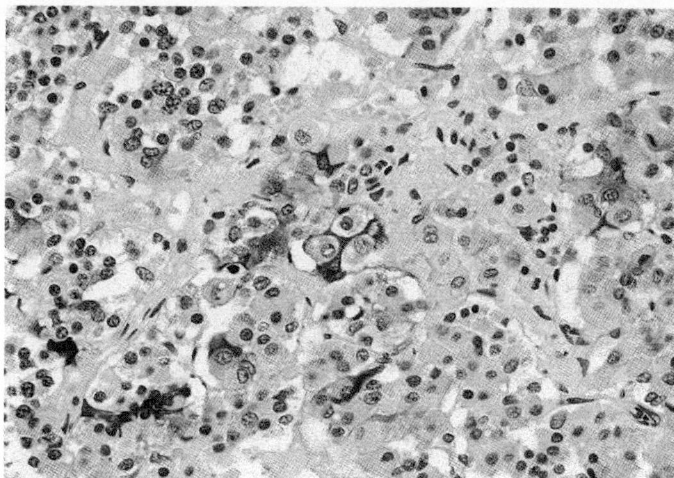

Fig. 60-11 Folliculostellate cells have cytoplasmic projections that extend between hormone-producing cells and are strongly positive for S-100 protein (Immunoperoxidase).

ate thyroid hormone production. TRH stimulates the thyrotrophs, and SRIF blocks TRH-induced secretion. TSH secretion is inhibited by thyroid hormones and by glucocorticoids as well. In the setting chronic hypothyroidism an increased number of stimulated thyrotrophs called *thyroidectomy cells* are present in the pituitary.[16,24]

Gonadotrophs (FSH/LH cells). Gonadotrophs are basophilic cells that are evenly distributed throughout the pars distalis. Most are bihormonal cells, in that they are immunoreactive for both FSH and LH (Fig. 60-10). The two glycoprotein hormones are composed of alpha- and beta-subunits and are located in large (300 to 600 nm) and small (approximately 200 nm) spherical secretory granules. The FSH beta-gene is located on chromosome 11 and consists of three exons. FSH stimulates spermatogenesis and the growth of ovarian follicles. The LH beta-gene is located on chromosome 19 and consists of three exons. LH induces the ovulation and luteinization of the ovarian follicle and ovarian steroidogenesis and it stimulates Leydig's cells to produce testosterone and the ovary to elaborate luteal phase hormones. Primary hypogonadism or surgical gonadectomy results in the formation of *gonadectomy cells*, which represent stimulated gonadotrophs.[16,24]

Folliculostellate cells. Folliculostellate cells are nongranulated cells and are shaped like stars because of their long, thin cytoplasmic processes that extend between hormone-producing cells (Fig. 60-11). Folliculostellate cells can be identified by immunocytochemical staining for S-100 protein.[25] They have a phagocytic function and produce growth factors and other cytokines in some species.[26] However, their exact role in the human pituitary is still uncertain.[27]

Neurohypophysis

The posterior lobe is composed of pituicytes—glial cells that contain a yellow-brown pigment that accumulates with age, as well as nerve fibers and capillaries. The nerve fibers originate in the hypothalamic magnacellular neurons that produce vasopressin and oxytocin. The hormones are transported to the posterior lobe as dense-core secretory granules along the axoplasm of unmyelinated nerve processes. Focal axonal dilatations called *Herring bodies* are filled with hormone-containing secretory granules.[28]

REACTIVE CHANGES

Pregnancy

Hyperplasia of PRL cells in the pituitary gland takes place during pregnancy[20,22] (Fig. 60-12). Bihormonal mammosomatotrophs producing PRL and GH increase in number as the pregnancy progresses. Immunohistochemical analyses and in situ hybridization of the pituitary in pregnancy have shown a decrease in the GH level and number of gonadotrophs along with an increase in the PRL content and the number of bihormonal cells.[20,22] Because of the increased size of the pituitary during pregnancy, there is an increased risk of infarction occurring during delivery secondary to hypotension stemming from massive blood loss or other causes (Sheehan's syndrome). The gland decreases in weight after delivery but remains larger in multiparous women.

Distinct morphologic changes in the anterior pituitary cells are associated with the increased or decreased function of other endocrine tissues. Although some of these morphologic changes, such as Crooke's hyaline change, are almost pathognomonic, a variety of physiologic or pharmacologic alterations may lead to the same or related morphologic changes.

Hormonal syndromes

Hypothyroidism

Primary hypothyroidism is commonly associated with hypertrophy and hyperplasia of the pituitary gland[29-31] (Fig. 60-13). In experimental animals, treatment with radioactive iodine, specific drugs that inhibit thyroid hormone synthesis such as propylthiouracil, or surgical extirpation of the thyroid has been observed to lead to TSH cell hyperplasia or the formation of TSH-producing pituitary adenomas.[32] Immunohistochemical studies in human beings have shown nodular hyperplasia of TSH-secreting cells and adenomas associated with primary hypothyroidism.[35] Hyperplasia of PRL cells may be associated with hypothyroidism,[33] which can be explained by the depletion of hypothalamic dopamine stores. The enlargement of the sella turcica in some patients with hypothyroidism and associated hyperprolactinemia may result from reversible thyrotroph and lactotroph hyperplasia, rather than from true adenomas.[34]

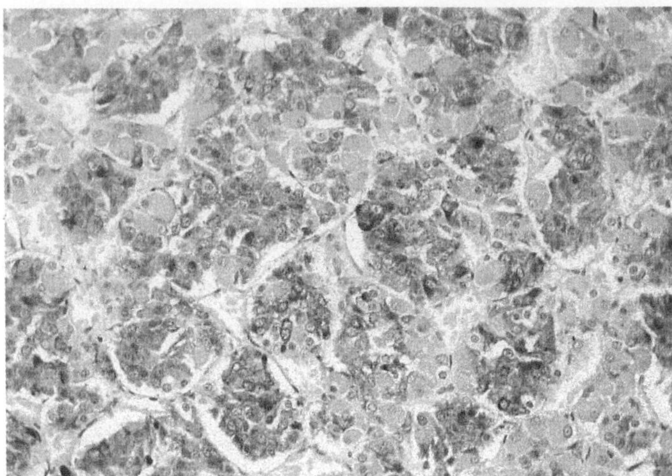

Fig. 60-12 This pituitary gland from a pregnant woman shows prominent prolactin cell hyperplasia (Immunoperoxidase).

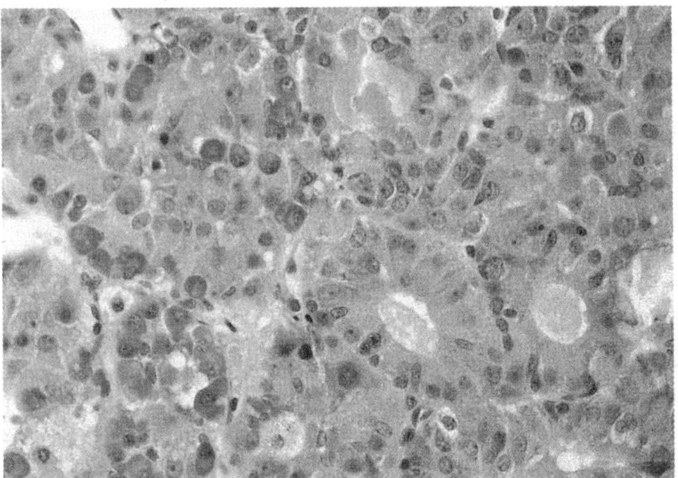

Fig. 60-13 Thyrotroph hyperplasia in the setting of hypothyroidism. There are enlarged acini with hypertrophied thyroid-stimulating hormone cells and an intermingling of other cell types.

Hyperthyroidism

The pituitary glands of patients with hyperthyroidism may exhibit regression of TSH cells.[35,36] In a study of 33 patients who died as the result of thyrotoxicosis, immunohistochemical studies revealed that there were decreased numbers of TSH-containing cells. This loss of immunoreactivity appears to be reversible in patients treated for hyperthyroidism.[37]

Addison's disease

The pituitary gland enlarges in patients with Addison's disease.[38] Histochemical stains often show the presence of degranulated basophil cells. Immunohistochemical studies of the pituitary performed in 18 patients with untreated Addison's disease revealed the existence of diffuse and nodular hyperplasia of the ACTH cells, the extent of which corresponded to the duration of the disease.[39] ACTH-producing adenomas may develop in these patients. An increased number of TSH cells as been noted in patients with Addison's disease, and this may be indirectly related to the association of immune destruction

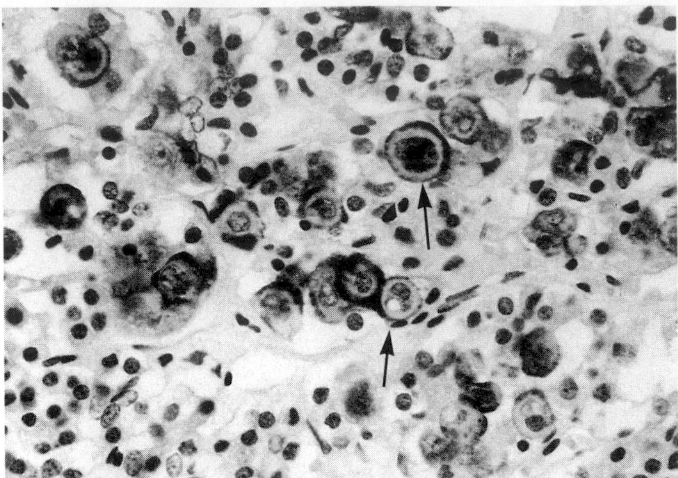

Fig. 60-14 Crooke's hyaline change in adrenocorticotropin cells in the setting of hyperadrenocorticism. The granules are pushed to the cell periphery by the accumulating intermediate filaments *(arrows).*

of the adrenal glands with atrophy of the thyroid (Schmidt's syndrome).[40,41]

Hyperadrenocorticism

The excessive production of glucocorticoids precipitates specific morphologic changes in the anterior pituitary (Crooke's hyaline change) and these result from the accumulation of cytokeratin filaments[42-46] (Fig. 60-14). This condition can be caused by the administration of glucocorticoids, by the excessive production of glucocorticoids by adrenocortical hyperplasia or neoplasms, and by the ectopic production of ACTH by neoplasms such as small cell, undifferentiated carcinoma of the lung. Crooke's hyaline change is reversible once the excess glucocorticoid stimulus is eliminated.[44] Crooke's hyaline can be seen in adenomatous as well as non neoplastic pituitary cells associated with ACTH production.

Hypogonadism

Gonadectomy in rodents leads to hypertrophy of the gonadotrophs. These cells have an increased cytoplasmic volume ("castration cells") and ultrastructurally are characterized by a cystically dilated RER. Prominent "castration cells" are less conspicuous in human subjects who have undergone gonadectomy.[47,48] Ultrastructural abnormalities of gonadotrophs may be seen in the settings of some gonadal deficiency syndromes or in menopause.[47]

Effects of drugs

Specific types of cells of the anterior pituitary and pituitary adenomas show functional and morphologic alterations after drug treatment[24,49] (Table 60-3). Most of these drugs are used in the medical therapy of pituitary adenomas, as an alternative to surgical treatment. Dopamine agonists such as bromocriptine interact with the D_2–receptor and inhibit PRL secretion. The use of dopamine agonists in the treatment of prolactinomas brings about a dramatic reduction in tumor size in most patients.[50] There is usually only minimal tumor cell necrosis. In most cases the effects on tumor size are reversible after discontinuation of the drug.[50] During bromocriptine treatment the prolactinoma cells contain less cytoplasm and the endoplasmic reticulum and Golgi complexes in the cells are reduced in

Table 60-3 Effects of specific drugs on anterior pituitary cells and tumors

Drug	Specific effect
Dopamine agonists (bromocriptine)	Inhibit prolactin secretion and reduce size of prolactinomas
Somatostatin analogs (octreotide)	Inhibit GH secretion and cause variable reduction in GH adenoma size
Estrogens	Stimulate PRL secretion and produce PRL cell hyperplasia
GnRH analogs	Stimulate and subsequently inhibit LH and FSH secretion from pituitary High doses suppress gonadal function

GH, growth hormone; *PRL*, prolactin; *GnRH*, FSH- and LH-releasing hormone; *LH*, luteinizing hormone; *FSH*, follicle-stimulating hormone.

extent. With protracted treatment there is fibrosis of the tumor. In situ hybridization studies have shown decreased PRL mRNA in the pituitary of patients who have undergone bromocriptine treatment.[51] SRIF analogs such as octreotide primarily affect GH cells, with the result that GH secretion and plasma GH levels are decreased. The effect on tumor size is variable and not as striking as the effect of dopamine agonists on prolactinoma cells.[52] GH adenoma cells treated with SRIF analogs may show a variable decrease in cytoplasmic volume.[52]

Estrogens are known to induce PRL cell hyperplasia and tumor development in rodents.[32] The effects of estrogens in human beings are less pronounced, but high dosages are associated with the development of hyperprolactinemia and PRL cell hyperplasia.[53] Pituitary adenomas secondary to high-dose estrogen therapy have been observed rarely, but estrogens can accelerate the growth of prolactinomas.[53,54] Many drugs alter the secretory function and morphologic appearance of the human pituitary gland,[24] but few of these are used in the treatment of pituitary adenomas.

Hereditary and developmental diseases

Many hereditary diseases are associated with abnormal pituitary function. These range from classic syndromes such as multiple endocrine neoplasias to newly observed entities resulting from mutations of specific regulatory transcription factors.

Multiple endocrine neoplasia, type I (MEN I), is associated with the development of hyperplasias and tumors of the pituitary, pancreas, and parathyroids and with the development of gastric and duodenal ulcers secondary to gastrinomas.[55,56] The gene defect responsible in MEN I has been localized to chromosome 11.[57] The syndrome is inherited as an autosomal dominant trait. Pituitary adenomas develop in patients with MEN I, but it is not known whether these patients also have anterior pituitary cell hyperplasia. The pituitary adenomas associated with MEN I are more often endocrinologically functional and more frequently produce GH or PRL compared with the behavior of sporadically developing pituitary adenomas.[58]

Kallmann's syndrome, or isolated gonadotropin deficiency, results from a defect in the formation and migration of FSH- and LH-releasing hormone (GnRH) neurons to the hypothalamus and is associated with agenesis of the olfactory bulb.[59,60] The syndrome may be inherited as an X-linked, autosomal dominant or as an autosomal recessive trait. An X-linked inheritance is most common. This syndrome is more common in male offspring and is associated with anosmia, color blindness, hypogonadism, and midline defects such as cleft lip and palate.[60] Affected women are eunuchoid and have low gonadotropin levels stemming from defects in the release of GnRH. The size of the pituitary is normal and histologically it appears unremarkable. However, the gonadotrophs are often devoid of immunoreactive gonadotropin hormones.

The Pit-1/GHF-1 transcription factor is important for the development of GH and PRL cells, and it also regulates TSH cell secretion.[61,62] This transcription factor binds to the promoter regions of GH, PRL, and TSH–beta genes. Various types of mutations, including both missense and nonsense mutations, have resulted in "transcription factor"–related diseases such as familial dwarfism and cretinism.[61-65] If diagnosed early, these conditions can be ameliorated with appropriate replacement therapy.

Isolated hormone deficiencies

Rare cases of isolated pituitary hormone deficiencies have an inherited basis. For example, a few reported cases of isolated GH deficiency may have been secondary to deletion of the GH gene (type 1A).[66] Molecular analyses have revealed the existence of variable genotypes, with one copy of the GH gene in some patients and another copy of the variant GH gene in others. Morphologic and immunohistochemical analyses carried out in a patient with isolated GH deficiency revealed the presence of abundant immunoreactive GH cells and exocytosis of secretory granules.[67] Deficiencies of other hormones such as gonadotropins result from the hypothalamic defects that occur in Kallmann's syndrome in conjunction with hypogonadism and anosmia.[59,60]

Agenesis and hypoplasia of pituitary

Congenital absence of the pituitary gland is a rare condition that is usually associated with hypoplasia of the adrenals, thyroid, and gonads.[68-75] It probably stems from failed fusion of Rathke's pouch with the infundibular process, a step that appears to be critical to normal pituitary development. Posterior pituitary gland tissue may be identified in many cases of congenital absence of the anterior pituitary.

Hypoplasia of the pituitary gland is a rare condition that usually occurs with anencephaly, although in a few cases patients have not had anencephaly.[72,73,76] In anencephaly the sella turcica is flattened and filled with spongy vascular tissue. The number of ACTH cells in the hypoplastic anterior pituitary are decreased, but the numbers of other anterior pituitary gland cells are normal. The ACTH cells show ultrastructural changes such as poorly developed organelles. The adrenal glands are usually hypoplastic. The weight of the thyroid and gonads of anencephalic neonates is within the normal range.

Empty sella syndrome

The empty sella syndrome results from a reduction in the volume of the sellar contents.[7,9] This syndrome may be primary or secondary, in origin. The primary empty sella syndrome is characterized by an incomplete or absent sellar diaphragm. The resulting increased cerebrospinal fluid pressure leads to

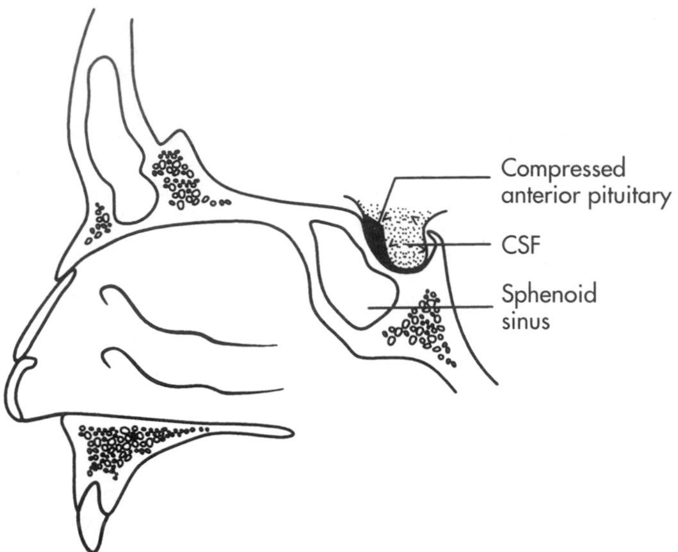

Fig. 60-15 Primary empty sella syndrome. The pituitary is compressed as the result of the increased cerebrospinal fluid pressure. *CSF,* Cerebrospinal fluid.

compression of the sellar contents (Fig. 60-15), such that the hypophyseal fossa enlarges and the pituitary is compressed and flattened. All adenohypophyseal cells can be identified by immunohistochemical studies. The secondary empty sella syndrome results from infarction, necrosis, or hypophysectomy, and the hypophyseal fossa in affected patients contains a small pituitary or no pituitary tissue at all.

Circulatory disorders

Pituitary apoplexy is usually secondary to hemorrhage in the pituitary gland.[77,79] Infarcts that involve more than 25% of the pituitary are noted in as much as 8% of unselected autopsies. Apoplexy was found in 7% of 560 patients who had undergone surgery for pituitary tumors.[79] The pituitary function has a considerable functional reserve, such that a loss of 50% or less of the anterior lobe cells is usually asymptomatic. Moderate symptoms of hypopituitarism occur when there is a 60% to 75% loss of anterior pituitary tissue, and severe hypophyseal deficiency becomes apparent when 90% of the hormone producing cells are destroyed.[7]

Sheehan's syndrome, postpartum necrosis of the pituitary (Fig. 60-16), is usually secondary to the hypotension caused by excessive blood loss during delivery.[77] Vasospasm may trigger the ischemia that leads to infarction in patients with Sheehan's syndrome. The necrosis may be focal or involve more than 90% of the adenohypophysis. Because the posterior

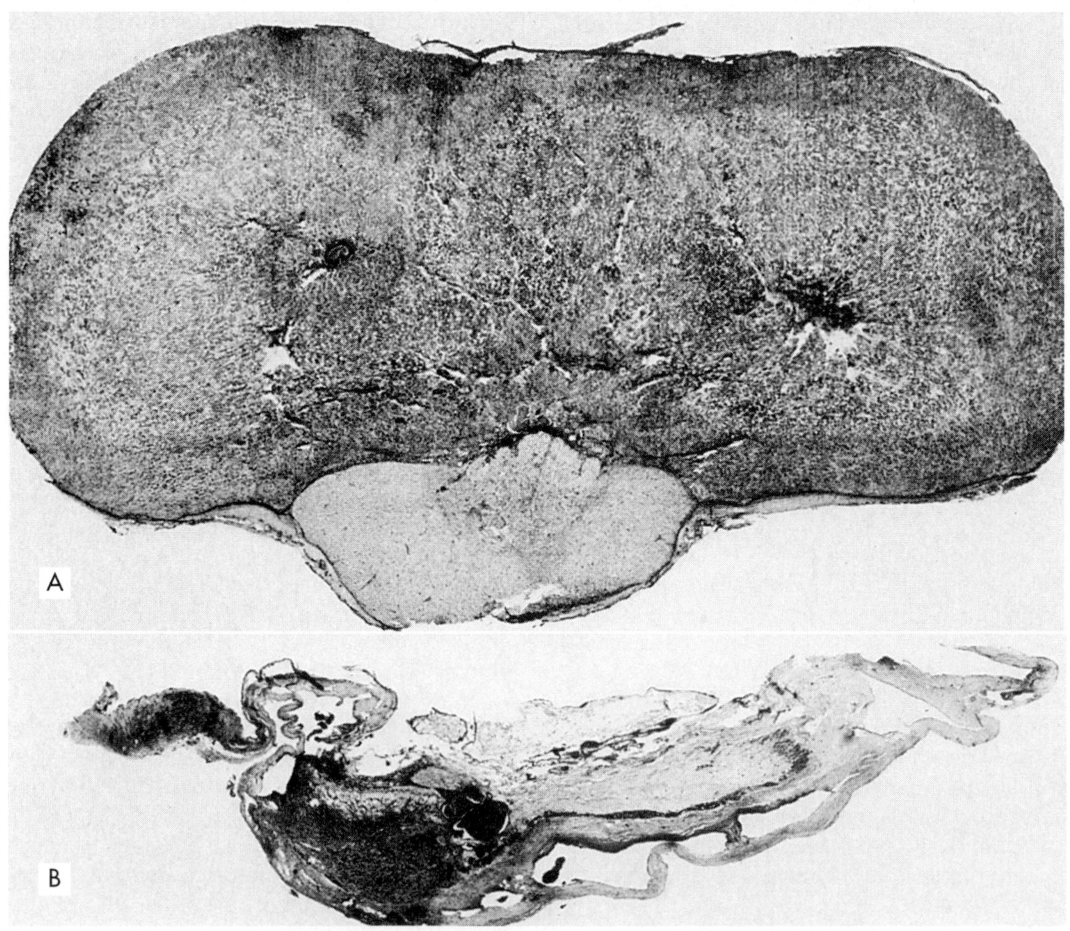

Fig. 60-16 Postpartum necrosis of pituitary gland. **A,** Most of the anterior lobe is affected. **B,** Shrunken and deformed gland. This patient survived for many years. (Courtesy Prof. H.L. Sheehan and Dr. A. R. Currie.)

pituitary has a rich arterial blood supply, which is independent of the portal vasculature, it is usually not affected. With healing, fibrosis and scar formation may be extensive, leading to a further loss of hormone-producing cells.

Various other conditions can cause infarction of the pituitary. These include physically induced head injury, massive cerebrovascular accidents, disseminated intravascular coagulation, and severe thrombocytopenia. Hemorrhagic infarcts may be associated with pituitary macroadenomas and are most common in patients with large adenomas.

EXOGENOUS INJURY

Physically induced injury to the head or surgical trauma can precipitate hypopituitarism. Disruption of the pituitary stalk secondary to surgery or head injury produces a characteristic pattern of anterior and posterior pituitary dysfunction.[80] This develops as the result of a loss of specific neural and vascular connections to the hypothalamus, and also in part results from variable degrees of pituitary infarction.[80] Diabetes insipidus is a common consequence and is found in approximately 80% of cases. Menses cease after transection of the stalk,[82] though gonadotropins may still be detectable in the urine. There may be a dramatic increase in adrenocortical secretion secondary to the release of preformed ACTH stores.[80] TSH and GH secretion decreases greatly, and PRL levels increase after stalk section. Some patients may experience galactorrhea, which is normally under dopaminergic inhibition.

Radiation-induced injury to the pituitary or hypothalamus can result in hypopituitarism.[82-84] GH deficiency usually develops in children with leukemia or brain tumors treated with irradiation,[83,84] but adults with pituitary tumors treated with irradiation suffer multiple endocrine deficiencies that worsen with higher doses of radiation.[84] In a recent study of adults and children treated with 39.6 to 70.2 Gy of radiation for brain tumors, 28% had symptoms of thyroid deficiency and 62% had low serum total or free thyroxine or triiodothyronine concentrations.[83] Of the postpubertal patients, 61% had evidence of hypogonadism and 50% had hyperprolactinemia.[83] The mechanism of injury may be related to direct injury to the pituitary or the hypothalamic neurons that produce releasing and inhibitory hormones, or the stroma or microvasculature, or both, may be injured. It is generally thought that cranial irradiation is a more common cause of hypothalamic dysfunction than is pituitary dysfunction.[83]

METABOLIC DISORDERS

Many metabolic abnormalities lead to the deposition or accumulation of specific substances in the pituitary.[7,85] Amyloid deposition has been observed to occur in the settings of systemic diseases and pituitary adenomas.[86,87] The amyloid is usually found in blood vessels or it may also be found in interstitial connective tissue, especially when multiple myeloma is the cause. Prolactinomas are the most common pituitary neoplasm associated with interstitial deposits of amyloid. Iron deposits in the pituitary may be found in the settings of hemosiderosis or hemochromatosis. The gonadotrophs usually contain more iron than do the other cells.[88,89] The fibrosis developing secondary to iron deposition may cause pituitary insufficiency.

Inborn errors of metabolism, including several lysosomal storage diseases, may affect the pituitary. For example, Hurler's syndrome, or gargoylism, is associated with the abnormal storage of mucopolysaccharides in many tissues, including the anterior pituitary. The cytoplasm of pituitary cells is vacuolated, and ultrastructural studies typically show the existence of many membrane-bound vesicles possessing concentric osmiophilic lamellae known as *Zebra bodies.*[90]

INFECTIOUS DISEASES

Patients with sepsis may suffer purulent hypophysitis or pituitary abscess, but this is more likely in patients with pituitary cysts.[91] Purulent meningitis may cause acute hypophysitis by direct spread into the subarachnoid space around the pituitary. Other conditions such as otitis media, sinusitis, and thrombophlebitis of the cavernous sinus may also be associated with acute hypophysitis.

Granulomatous inflammation can involve the entire pituitary, and a variety of granulomatous processes, including tuberculosis and fungal infections,[92] may also involve the pituitary. The histologic appearance of the pituitary, consisting of multinucleated giant cells, is similar to the changes seen in the lung and other tissues (Fig. 60-17). There may be extensive destruction of the adenohypophysis followed by the development of hypopituitarism. Sarcoidosis can involve the anterior or posterior pituitary but primarily involves the hypothalamus, leading to the destruction of cells in the hypothalamus that produce pituitary regulatory peptides. Syphilis can also lead to extensive destruction of the pituitary.[93]

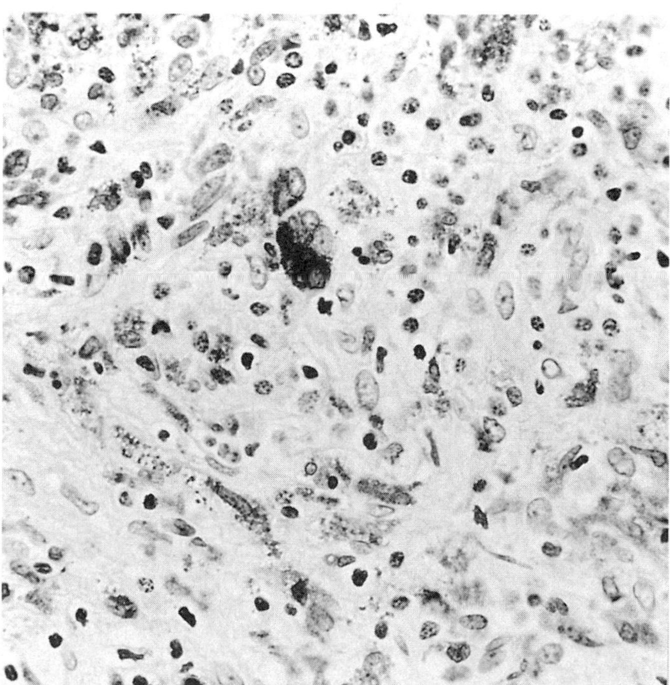

Fig. 60-17 Granulomatous inflammation of the pituitary. Staining for acid-fast organisms and fungi was negative. Immunohistochemical staining with monoclonal antibody CD68, which recognizes macrophages, has produced a positive reaction in the multinucleated cells (Immunoperoxidase).

The pituitary gland in patients with the acquired immunodeficiency syndrome may show acute necrotic foci and is frequently involved with infections.[94] Infections are caused by a variety of pathogens, including cytomegalovirus, *Pneumocystis carinii,* and *Toxoplasma gondii.* In all cases, there has been a systemic infection with these pathogens.[94]

AUTOIMMUNE DISEASES

Autoimmune diseases of the pituitary have not been completely delineated. Some may be restricted to the pituitary, and others may be part of systemic autoimmune diseases.

Lymphocytic hypophysitis is probably an autoimmune disease of the pituitary gland.[95-97] Most cases arise in women during pregnancy or in the postpartum period. Patients in one series were noted to range from 22 to 74 years of age. Most patients presented within 1 year postpartum, except for the 59- and 74-year-old patients whose disease was diagnosed at autopsy. The histologic features include cellular infiltrates composed mainly of lymphocytes and some plasma cells (Fig. 60-18), and prominent oncocytes are found in the anterior pituitary on electron microscopy. Lymphoid follicles with germinal centers may also be present. Some patients may have inflammatory disorders involving the thyroid, adrenals, and other endocrine tissues.[96,97] Treatment is with glucocorticoids, which may suppress the inflammatory response in these patients.[98]

Central diabetes insipidus can be caused by various conditions. Patients with this disorder have polyuria and polydipsia stemming from the vasopressin deficiency. In addition to familial diabetes insipidus, which is characterized by autosomal dominant inheritance, and secondary diabetes insipidus, which is caused by tumors, infections, trauma, and other lesions, a third form, designated as *idiopathic diabetes insipidus*, has recently been characterized as an autoimmune disease (infundibuloneurohypophysitis).[99] In patients with this form of diabetes insipidus, the pituitary stalk becomes thickened or the neurohypophysis can be enlarged, both of which can be recognized by magnetic resonance imaging in many patients who have had the disorder for less than 2 years. Histologic examinations may show an infiltration of T-cells and plasma cells.[99] In addition to diabetes insipidus, patients may have mild hyperprolactinemia.

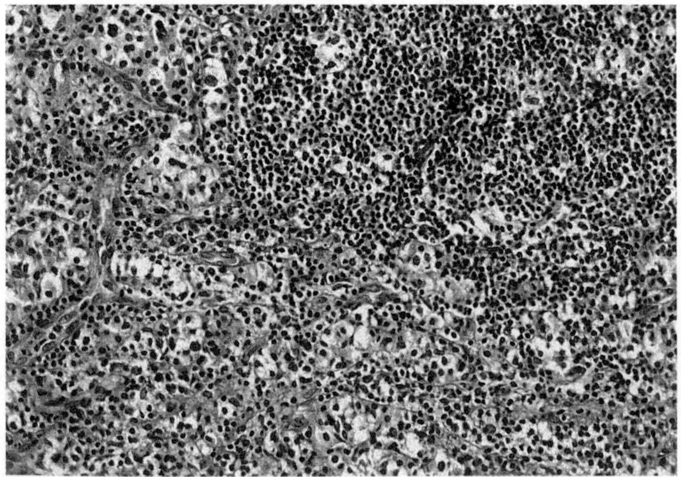

Fig. 60-18 Lymphocytic hypophysitis showing infiltration of the pituitary by a predominantly lymphocytic infiltrate.

Autoantibodies to pituitary cells have been detected in the setting of many disorders, including the empty sella syndrome, specific hormone deficiencies, and hypopituitarism.[100,101] Antibodies against specific pituitary cell lines have been detected in more than half the patients with the primary empty sella syndrome.[100]

Autoimmune polyglandular syndromes are a group of poorly understood autoimmune diseases associated with the hypofunction of various endocrine tissues. There are two types: type I, comprising adrenal insufficiency, mucocutaneous candidiasis, and hypoparathyroidism; and the more common type II, comprising adrenal insufficiency, hyperthyroidism or primary hypothyroidism, insulin-dependent diabetes mellitus, primary hypogonadism, myasthenia gravis, and celiac disease. Patients with the type II syndrome typically have two or more of these diseases.[102]

IDIOPATHIC AND POORLY UNDERSTOOD DISEASES

Giant cell granuloma

Giant cell granuloma of the pituitary is a rare idiopathic inflammatory disorder.[103] Similar findings may be encountered in the adrenal cortex, gonads, or thyroid gland. Sarcoidosis, a disease of unknown cause with many features implying an immune cause, may involve the pituitary.[104] Giant cell granuloma differs from sarcoidosis by the fact that the process is limited to the adenohypophysis and does not involve the hypothalamus or neurohypophysis. Like sarcoidosis, the granulomas are usually noncaseating. Giant cell granulomas may lead to the progressive destruction of the adenohypophysis with resultant hypopituitarism. Sarcoidosis of the pituitary and hypothalamus remains an enigmatic disease.[105] Because it is a diagnosis of exclusion, special staining for organisms should routinely be performed before this diagnosis is rendered.

Anterior pituitary hyperplasia

Hyperplasia of the anterior pituitary is an uncommon disorder and may be caused by a hypothalamic dysfunction associated with an excess of hypothalamic hormones. These hormones may also be of ectopic origin and come from neoplasms of the lungs, pancreas, and other sites.[106,107] Gangliocytic hamartomas of the hypothalamus and other sites are yet another possible site of origin. However, in most cases of pituitary hyperplasia, a specific cause cannot be identified.[108,109]

GH and ACTH cell hyperplasias are the most common patterns and can be diffuse or nodular. The nodular pattern is more easily recognized histologically. Reticulin and immunohistochemical staining is helpful in arriving at a diagnosis of pituitary hyperplasia because it can demonstrate the expansion and preservation of acini as well as the hypertrophy and hyperplasia of anterior pituitary cells.[7] GH cell hyperplasia is frequently associated with ectopic growth hormone–releasing hormone production.[106,107] ACTH cell hyperplasia may be nodular or diffuse. Nodular hyperplasia is associated with enlargement of the acini and hypertrophy of individual ACTH cells.[104] Diffuse hyperplasia is characterized by an increase in the number of ACTH cells, especially in the mucoid wedge area, with very little distortion of the acinar pattern.

NEOPLASMS

Pituitary adenomas

Pituitary tumors are common lesions that are typically found in the anterior part of the gland. Almost all are benign adenomas, and only a few cases of primary malignant neoplasms of the pituitary have been reported.[7] Small pituitary adenomas, which are not grossly apparent, are found at 5% to 20% of routine autopsies. Hormonally active, clinically symptomatic tumors account for approximately 10% to 15% of the surgically resected intracranial tumors.[7]

The unique features of pituitary tumors are dictated by the heterogeneous cellular composition of the gland and, its anatomic location and relationship to the hypothalamus and other endocrine glands. Anatomically the pituitary is composed of two parts, each of which can give rise to tumors. However, most of the tumors arise from the anterior pituitary and the posterior pituitary tumors account for less than 1% of all neoplasms.

Histologically the pituitary is composed of several cell types. All of these cells can give rise to tumors, and there are several types of pituitary tumors as a result (Table 60-4).

The relationship of the pituitary to the hypothalamus, which contains releasing factors, and the peripheral endocrine glands, which are controlled by the pituitary, determines the nature of the clinical symptoms of endocrine lesions. It may also be important in determining the pathogenesis of some lesions.

The anatomic location of the pituitary is critical to the understanding of the symptoms caused by these tumors and the surgical treatment used for the neoplasms. Because of their intrasellar location, pituitary adenomas can compress the optic nerves at the chiasm and produce specific patterns of visual loss. The unique location of the pituitary enables the surgeon to resect these tumors transsphenoidally, and most pituitary microadenomas are currently resected in this way.

Table 60-4 Frequency of pituitary adenomas*

Adenoma type	Percentage
GH cell adenoma, densely granulated	7.2
GH cell adenoma, sparsely granulated	6.4
PRL cell adenoma, densely granulated	0.4
PRL cell adenoma, sparsely granulated	26.5
Mixed (GH cell–PRL cell) adenoma	3.7
Mammosomatotroph adenoma	1.3
Acidophil stem cell adenoma	1.7
Corticotroph adenoma	9.9
Silent "corticotroph" adenoma, subtype 1	1.5
Silent "corticotroph" adenoma, subtype 2	2.1
Silent adenoma, subtype 3	1.4
Thyrotroph adenoma	1.0
Gonadotroph adenoma	9.3
Null cell adenoma	12.7
Oncocytoma	13.1
Unclassified adenoma	1.8

GH, Growth hormone; *PRL*, prolactin.
*Based on unselected surgical material involving 1910 cases.

The pathogenesis of pituitary adenomas is unclear. Most if not all GH cell, PRL cell, gonadotroph, and clinically nonfunctioning adenomas arise as autonomous, solitary tumors.[7] Results of clonality studies also support the monoclonal origin of various adenoma types.[110] Hypothalamic factors may be operative in a small number (10% to 15%) of patients with Cushing's disease whose pathologic lesion is not an adenoma but hyperplasia or a combination of hyperplastic and neoplastic changes. With the notable exception of some thyrotroph adenomas, target organ failure does not seem to play an important role in the induction of pituitary tumors.

Classification of the pituitary tumors on the basis of the tinctorial properties of tumor cells or the histologic pattern seen in routine hematoxylin and eosin–stained preparations is only of historic interest. In the past it was customary to classify adenomas of the pituitary into three types: those composed of acidophilic, basophilic, or chromophobe cells. Using this imprecise classification the derivation of tumors and their function could be predicted in less than 25% of all cases.[111] The subdivision of tumors on the basis of growth pattern into diffuse, sinusoidal, and papillary neoplasms has not been informative either. Most of the GH- and PRL-producing adenomas, clinically nonfunctional null cell adenomas, and oncocytomas show a diffuse pattern of growth. The sinusoidal pattern predominates in ACTH- and LH/FSH-producing tumors. The papillary pattern is seen in some PRL- and LH/FSH-producing tumors. Pituitary tumors are currently classified on the basis of their immunohistochemical and electron microscopy features (see Table 60-4). Using this approach, one can classify pituitary tumors into several categories: hormone-secreting tumors that correspond to the five cell types of the normal pituitary, hormonally plurifunctional tumors, hormonally inactive tumors, and so on.

Pituitary adenomas less than 10 mm in diameter are considered microadenomas, and tumors 10 mm or greater are considered macroadenomas (Fig. 60-19). Every type of pituitary cell gives rise to one or more morphologic type of adenoma. The occurrence of three ultrastructurally distinct tumors that are not related to the known cell types implies the existence of as yet uncharacterized cell types.[112-115] The relative incidences of the various types of adenoma are noted in autopsy material different from those noted in surgical material. In adult autopsy material there is an almost equal percentage of PRL-producing and clinically nonfunctioning (null cell and, oncocytoma) adenomas, leaving only a small percentage of cases representing the other types. The prominence of these two groups is much more subdued in surgical material (see Table 60-4).

Immunohistochemical analysis is the most widely used technique to obtain information on the cell derivation and hormone content of various types of adenomas. However, the results must be assessed with caution. Plurihormonality, that is, the production of more than one hormone by a cell, is widespread in the pituitary; thus the immunohistochemical profiles of several type of tumors overlap.[116-119] In nearly all dubious cases, the electron microscopy findings can decide the diagnosis if well-preserved tissue is available for analysis.

GH-producing adenomas

Approximately 20% of surgically removed pituitary adenomas are associated with a clinically elevated GH level (see Table 60-4). When these tumors arise in childhood or adolescence,

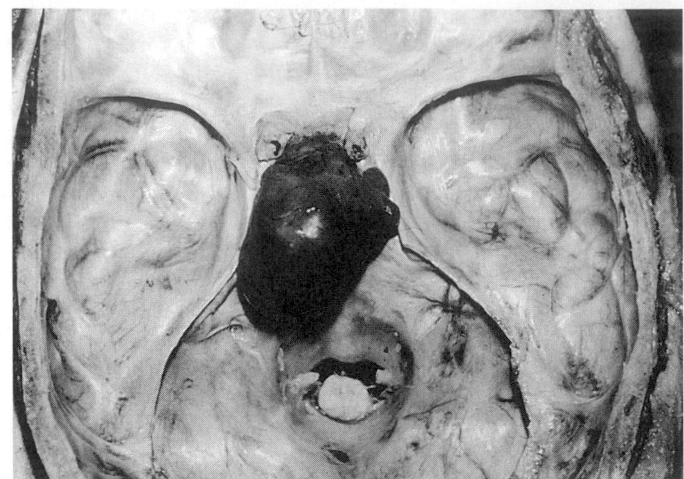

Fig. 60-19 Pituitary macroadenoma in a postmortem case. The tumor is very vascular and hemorrhagic.

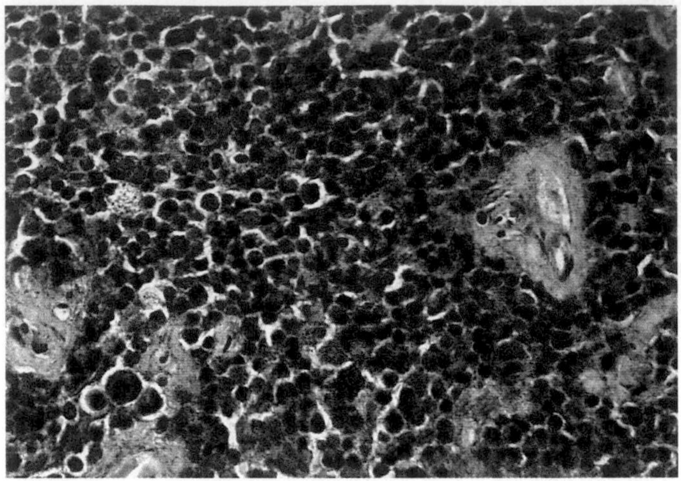

Fig. 60-20 In situ hybridization detection of growth hormone messenger RNA in a growth hormone adenoma.

gigantism is the result. Gigantism is uncommon because most GH-secreting tumors develop in adults, resulting in the enlargement of acral parts (jaw, nose, and phalanges), the accumulation of soft tissue, and the development of visceromegaly. Among the various severe metabolic consequences of GH overproduction, the cardiovascular diseases account the most for the shortened life-span of acromegalic patients.

Many tumor cell types cause acromegaly.[7,112-114,120] The *densely granulated GH cell adenoma* corresponds to the typical acidophil adenoma, which usually shows slow, expansive growth resulting in the well-known "ballooning" of the sella turcica. These tumors are composed of acidophilic cells arranged in a diffuse or, less frequently, a trabecular growth pattern. Cytoplasmic GH can be shown by immunohistochemical,[21,64] and most tumors are plurihormonal, containing the alpha-subunit of PRL and other glycoprotein hormones.[112,121] The significance of this phenomenon is still unclear. In situ hybridization studies show a diffuse expression of GH mRNA (Fig. 60-20). On electron micrographs the cells that make up these tumors resemble normal somatotrophs; typical features include a centrally placed nucleus, parallel cisternae of RER usually located at the cell periphery, a prominent Golgi apparatus, and numerous, mostly spherical, evenly electron-dense secretory granules with a diameter chiefly in the range of 400 to 600 nm (Fig. 60-21).

The *sparsely granulated* GH cell adenomas are more aggressive, often invasive tumors and are likely to have reached the macroadenoma stage by the time of surgery. They are composed of chromophobic cells that contain immunoreactive perinuclear GH mainly within the Golgi sacculi (Fig. 60-22). The immunoreactive, small, scanty secretory granules of GH may not be perceptible on light microscopy studies. Plurihormonality is uncommon, and if present, there is usually only a weak positivity for PRL the alpha-subunit or both. On electron microscopy studies the cells of sparsely granulated GH cell tumors are not found to resemble any cell type of the normal pituitary. The irregular or rounded cells have eccentric, often flattened or crescent-shaped nuclei, variable quantities of RER, and a fairly prominent Golgi apparatus. The Golgi apparatus, however, is often displaced to the cell periphery by the so-

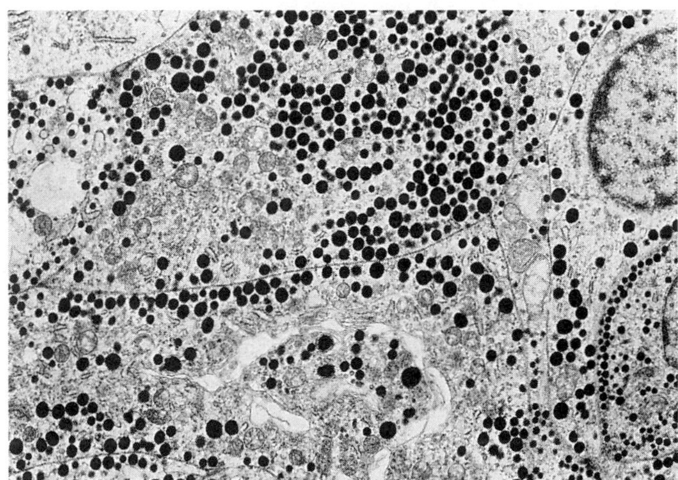

Fig. 60-21 Densely granulated growth hormone cell adenoma with large electron-dense secretory granules.

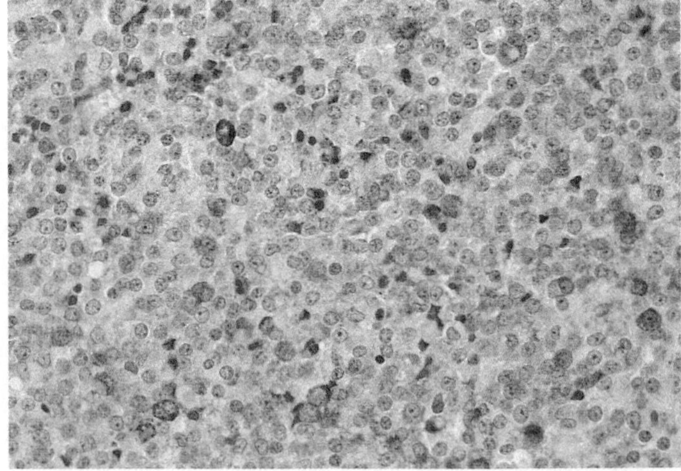

Fig. 60-22 Growth hormone cell adenoma showing positive, but variable, staining for growth hormone in a sparsely granulated tumor (Immunoperoxidase).

called fibrous body, which is consistently located within the Golgi region. This structure, a diagnostic feature of sparsely granulated GH adenomas, is composed of varying proportions of type 2 (cytokeratin) filaments and tubular smooth endoplasmic reticulum.[7,122] The secretory granules are sparse and very small, usually not exceeding 250 nm in diameter.

Acromegaly and gigantism may be caused by other uncommon bihormonal pituitary neoplasms capable of producing both GH and PRL.[112-114,117,118] The *bimorphous mixed adenoma,* consisting of densely granulated GH cells and sparsely granulated PRL cells, is the most common. This adenoma is associated with both elevated GH levels and hyperprolactinemia. The *mammosomatotroph adenoma* is accompanied by the signs and symptoms of GH overproduction, but hyperprolactinemia is rarely pronounced. This morphologic variant is similar to densely granulated GH cell adenoma. However, the cells also show exocytosis, a feature typical of PRL cells. The cells of the infrequently *acidophil stem cell adenoma* display the ultrastructural features of both sparsely granulated PRL cells and GH cells, but clinically the tumor is predominantly PRL producing and the clinical features of GH overproduction are not likely to be present.

Octreotide (Sandostatin), a somatostatin analog, is useful for the treatment of acromegaly.[123] Although it alleviates the severity of the clinical syndrome, the reduction in tumor size and alteration in the tumor morphologic appearance are minimal. The most frequent alterations are varying degrees of perivascular and interstitial fibrosis, an increase in the size and number of secretory granules, sometimes associated with a minor decrease in cell size, and the presence of large lysosomes and signs of crinophagy (uptake of secretory granules by lysosomes).

Table 60-5 Some causes of hyperprolactinemia

Drugs
Estrogen
Opiates
Phenothiazines
Reserpine
Tricyclic antidepressants
Hepatic disease
Hypothalamic disease
Irradiation
Tumors
Sarcoidosis
Hypothyroidism
Pituitary disease
Compression of pituitary stalk
Empty sella syndrome
Mixed prolactin–growth hormone adenomas
Prolactinoma
Stalk section

PRL-producing adenomas

PRL cell adenoma, accounting for approximately 27% of the cases of surgically removed adenomas, is the most common pituitary tumor.[7,112-114,124] Most of these tumors occur in women of reproductive age who present typically with amenorrhea, galactorrhea, and infertility. Diminished libido, impotence, and infertility are the common complaints in men. Microadenomas predominate in women, whereas postmenopausal women and men are more likely to have a macroadenoma at the time of pituitary surgery. Other conditions cause hyperprolactinemia (Table 60-5) and should be considered in the differential diagnosis of prolactinomas. There are considerable differences in the biologic behavior of PRL cell adenomas; some tumors progress slowly, whereas others are fast growing and invasive. They show variable responses to dopamine agonist treatment as well. Despite these differences, the morphology of these tumors is rather uniform.

Most PRL cell adenomas are composed of chromophobic or slightly acidophilic cells arranged in a diffuse, or less often, a papillary growth pattern. Some tumors show appreciable calcification.[7,125] Endocrine amyloid may form as well, though it is rarely discernible on light microscopy studies.[7,113,124] Immunoreactivity with anti-PRL is most evident in the Golgi apparatus, whereas the positivity of the small, sparse secretory granules may be negligible (Fig. 60-23). Elongate or irregular cells are noted on electron microscopy preparations. The nuclei contain large nucleoli. The RER is abundant, and the slender, parallel cisternae are often organized into concentric whorls. The prominent Golgi apparatus harbors numerous pleomorphic immature granules, and cytoplasmic secretory granules, which measure 150 to 300 nm in diameter, are sparse. Exocytosis, which is the extrusion of secretory granules either at the capillary side (orthotopic) or at the lateral cell membranes (misplaced), is present and is a reliable ultrastructural marker of PRL differentiation[7,113,124] (Fig. 60-24).

The treatment of PRL cell adenomas with dopamine agonists, introduced in the early 1970s, is an alternative to surgery in many cases. In patients with large macroadenomas, preoperative medical treatment reduces the size of the tumor, thus facilitating surgical removal. The injectable, long-acting form of bromocriptine is particularly effective.[51,50] Although most PRL cell adenomas are amenable to dopamine agonist therapy, patients may show unequal responses depending on the D_2-receptor content of the tumor cells. In tumors displaying significant suppression, a striking increase in cellularity and a considerable decrease in cell volume are noted, and these are largely a result of the involution of the RER and the Golgi complex. In such cells PRL immunoreactivity may be lost because of the suppressed transcription of the PRL gene.[51] The reduction in the tumor mass is often associated with varying degrees of fibrosis and sometimes with considerable calcification.

The acidophilic, densely granulated PRL cell adenoma is a rare morphologic variant.[7,124] PRL tumors with densely granulated areas are more likely to occur in patients with a remote history of dopamine agonist treatment.

ACTH-producing adenomas

The large majority of corticotroph adenomas are associated with Cushing's disease. The clinical signs and symptoms of hypercorticism are truncal obesity, plethoric face, buffalo hump, hirsutism, easy bruising, headache, hypertension, elevation of the serum cortisol levels with loss of diurnal variation, and an increased output of urinary free cortisol.[7,112] A minority of patients have Nelson's syndrome—a pituitary corticotroph adenoma that develops after removal of the adrenals to alleviate symptoms of preexisting hypercortisolism.

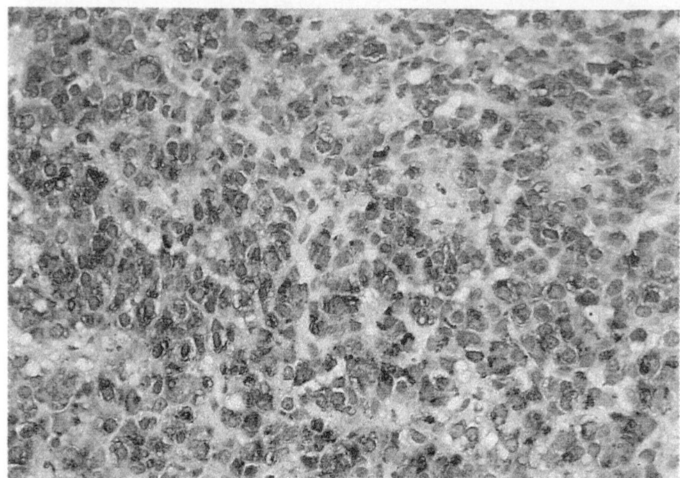

Fig. 60-23 Prolactin cell adenoma showing diffuse staining for immunoreactive prolactin. (Immunoperoxidase.)

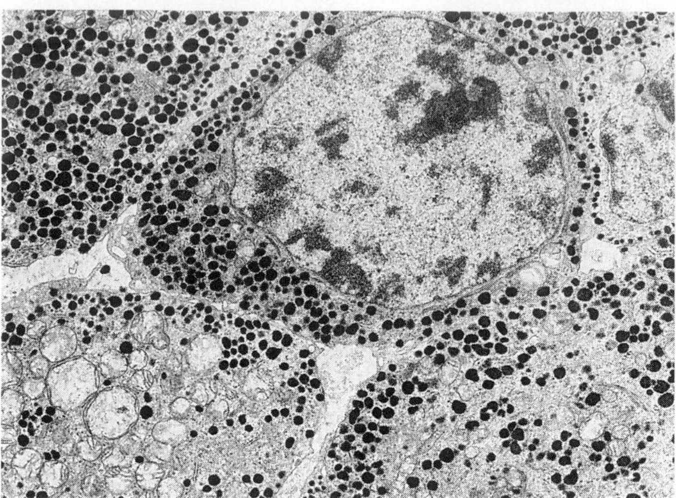

Fig. 60-25 Corticotroph adenoma. The tumor cells have large secretory granules that range from 250 to 450 nm in diameter.

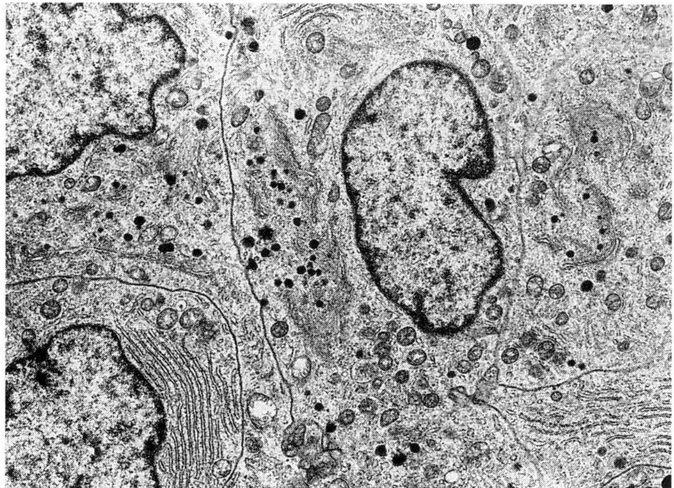

Fig. 60-24 Ultrastructure of a prolactin cell adenoma showing few secretory granules and misplaced exocytosis *(arrows)* or the extrusion of secretory granules at the lateral cell membranes.

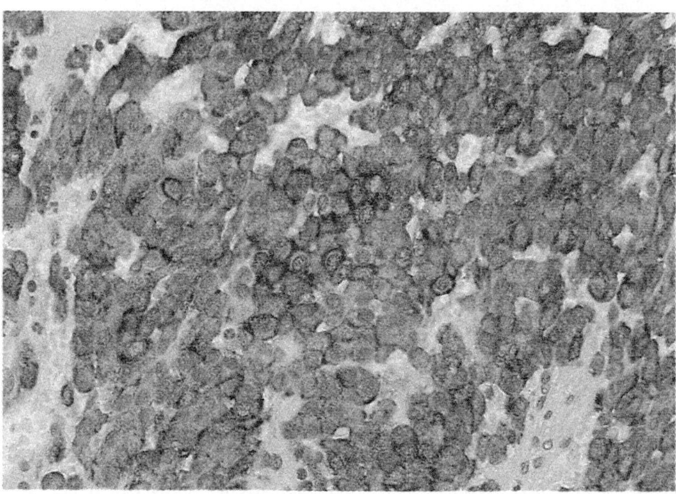

Fig. 60-26 Silent corticotroph adenoma containing cells with abundant immunoreactive adrenocorticotropin. (Immunoperoxidase.)

Because of the greatly improved accuracy in the diagnosis of pituitary-dependent Cushing's disease and advances in pituitary microsurgery, Nelson's syndrome is becoming a rarity. Most pituitary lesions causing Cushing's disease are microadenomas, whereas tumors causing Nelson's syndrome are large, and often invasive and difficult to treat. Unlike other pituitary hypersecretory syndromes caused by solitary adenomas, Cushing's disease may infrequently be induced by corticotroph hyperplasia, possibly stemming from hypothalamic regulatory disorders.[114,119,126]

Typical corticotroph microadenomas, as well as most tumors in patients with Nelson's syndrome, are composed of basophilic cells that are strongly PAS positive and are arranged in a sinusoidal growth pattern. The cells in macroadenomas are likely to have sparse granules and may appear chromophobic on routine histologic preparations. ACTH and other POMC peptides are abundant in corticotroph adenomas (Fig. 60-25). Ultrastructurally the cells of basophilic corticotroph adenomas are similar to normal corticotrophs (Fig. 60-25). The two important features are the numerous secretory granules with a diameter of 200 to 450 nm. These are usually spherical, but irregular, indented, and heart-shaped forms are found as well. Small bundles of cytokeratin filaments may surround the nucleus.[128] These type 1 filaments with a diameter of 7 to 10 nm are specific markers of the human ACTH cell. An excessive accumulation of keratin (Crooke's hyalinization) typically occurs in suppressed corticotrophs as the result of endogenous or exogenous hypercortisolism. Crooke's hyaline is found in a minority of the corticotroph adenomas associated with Cushing's disease.[112-114]

Not all pituitary adenomas that are immunoreactive with antibodies to ACTH are associated with Cushing's disease. Tumors with immunoreactive ACTH (Fig. 60-26) and rich in POMC mRNA, but not associated with Cushing's disease, are classified as silent corticotroph adenomas (see Table 60-4). The process whereby ACTH is released in these tumors may be defective, but the pathogenesis of this condition has not been elucidated.

TSH-producing adenoma

The TSH-producing adenoma is very rare.[7,112-114,129,130] Thyrotroph adenomas may be accompanied by hyperthyroidism and inappropriate TSH secretion or by long-standing hypothyroidism. Some adenomas with the histologic, immunohistochemical, and ultrastructural features of thyrotroph tumors occur in euthyroid patients. When diagnosed the tumor is often an invasive macroadenoma. Histologically they are composed of chromophobic cells arranged in a sinusoidal or diffuse growth pattern. Nuclear pleomorphism and focal fibrosis are common. Immunoreactive TSH and the alpha-subunit of glycoprotein hormones can be demonstrated (Fig. 60-27). Thyrotroph tumors may contain a few GH-positive cells. Ultrastructurally the cells of well-differentiated TSH adenomas appear moderately polar and angulated. The cytoplasm contains small (100 to 250 nm) secretory granules that often form a single layer underneath the plasmalemma (Fig. 60-28).

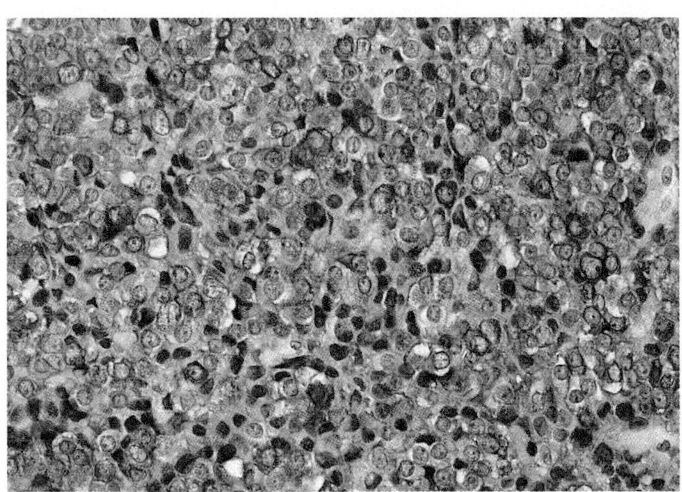

Fig. 60-27 Thyrotroph adenoma. The tumor cells are round to angular and contain abundant immunoreactive hormone (Immunoperoxidase).

FSH/LH-producing adenoma

Adenomas producing gonadotroph hormones are more frequent than previously thought,[7,114,115,125,131] but their prevalence is still not firmly established because of the lack of consensus on the diagnostic criteria. There are no distinct hypersecretory syndromes related to these tumors. The serum levels of FSH and LH may be elevated in men, but the levels in women are likely to be within the normal range for the patient's age.

Gonadotroph tumors are composed of chromophobic cells arranged in a diffuse or sinusoidal pattern with pseudorosette formation around vessels. The immunohistochemical findings are variable—FSH, LH, and the alpha-subunit of glycoprotein hormones can be demonstrated (Fig. 60-29). Ultrastructurally FSH/LH adenomas display a considerable variability, especially in men. Differentiation of glycoprotein hormones is suggested by the polarity of cells and uneven distribution of small secretory granules. The RER and Golgi complex are prominent in some cells but less so in others (Fig. 60-30). A characteristic vacuolar transformation of the Golgi apparatus (honeycomb Golgi complex) is found in most of the gonadotroph adenomas in women and is useful diagnostically (Fig. 60-31). An unusual morphologic variant in which the adenoma cells contain larger secretory granules (up to 450 nm) resembling those of normal gonadotrophs is found in both male and female patients.

Null cell adenoma, oncocytoma

Null cell adenoma and its oncocytic variant represent 25% of the surgically removed pituitary tumors[7,112-114,132,133]. These tumors are clinically nonfunctioning and occur mostly in older patients. Null cell adenomas have no immunohistochemical or ultrastructural markers indicative of their functional differentiation. Because of the absence of endocrine signs and symptoms, null cell adenoma and oncocytoma are usually diagnosed at the macroadenoma stage when mass effects become evident, such as compression of adjacent structures such as the optic chiasm. Because of the so-called stalk-section effect, mild or moderate hyperprolactinemia may be present and varying degrees of hypopituitarism may develop.

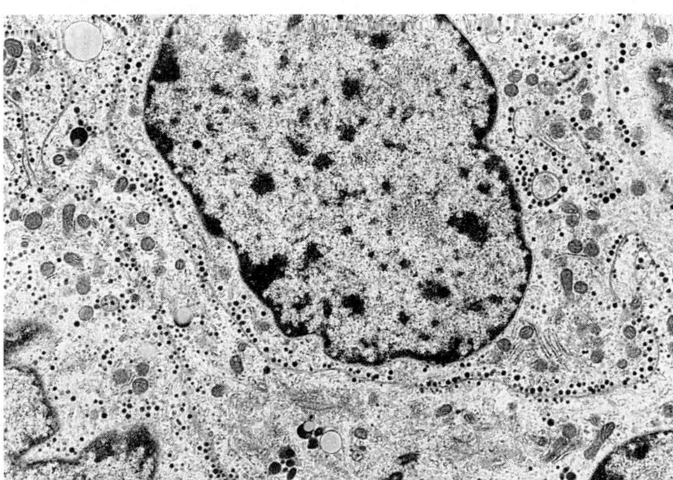

Fig. 60-28 Thyrotroph adenoma. The tumor cells have small secretory granules that range from 100 to 250 nm in diameter.

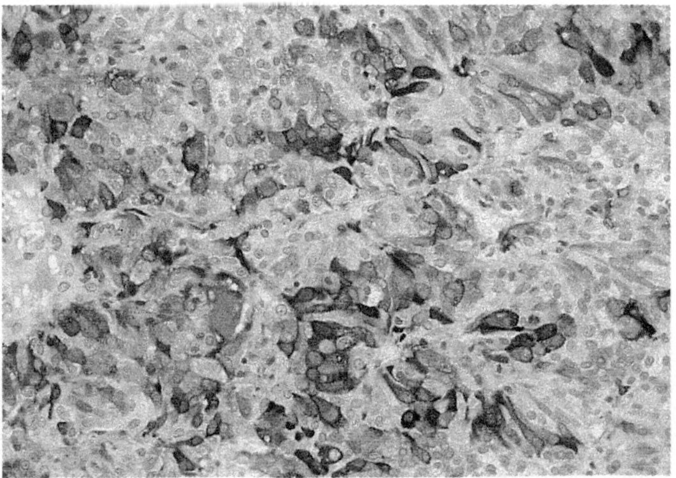

Fig. 60-29 Gonadotroph adenoma with a strong immunoreactivity for the alpha-subunit of glycoprotein hormone (Immunoperoxidase).

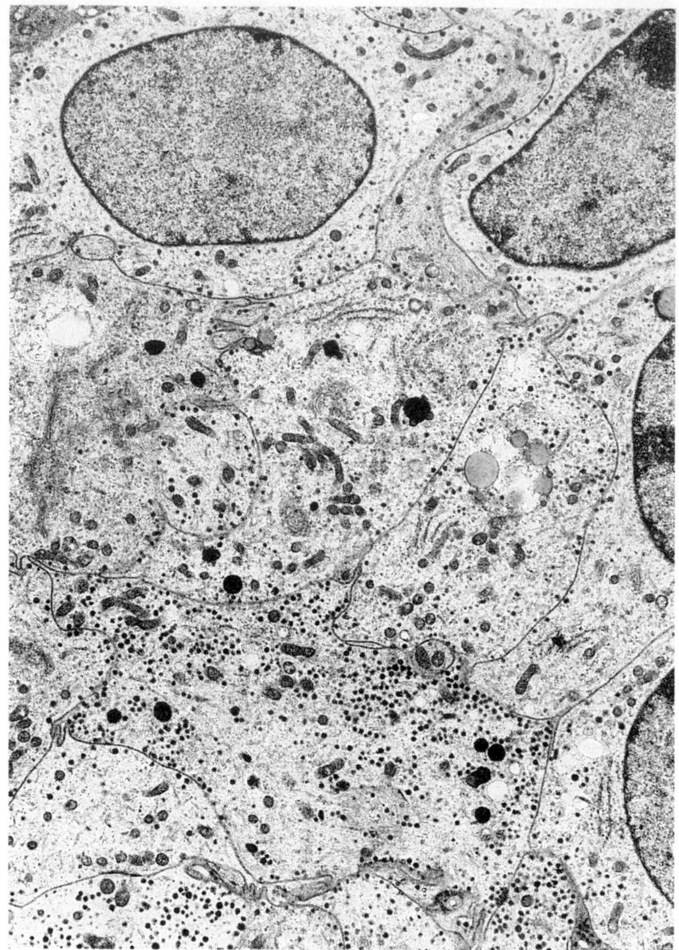

Fig. 60-30 Gonadotroph adenoma showing a male pattern of differentiation consisting of small secretory granules and an inconspicuous Golgi complex.

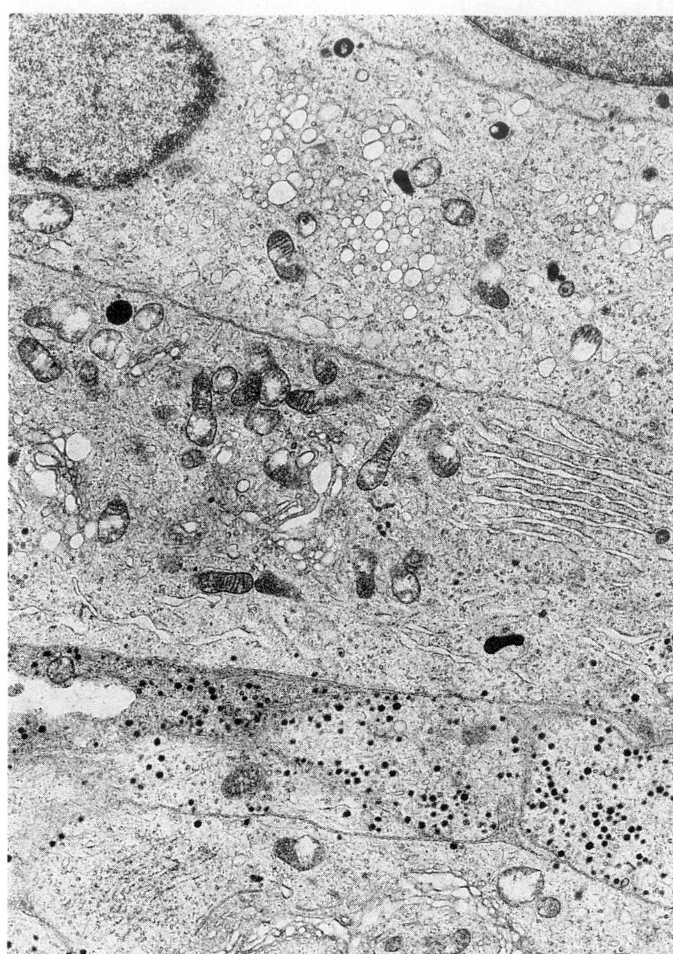

Fig. 60-31 Gonadotroph adenoma with a female pattern of differentiation. The Golgi complex shows vacuolar transformation exhibiting a distinct honeycomb pattern.

Null cell adenomas are composed of chromophobic cells. Oncocytomas are acidophilic because of the nonspecific uptake of acid dyes by mitochondria. Null cell adenomas exhibit a diffuse growth pattern, or pseudorosettes may form around vessels. Oncocytomas almost always grow in a diffuse pattern. Immunohistochemical studies may show nonreactivity or show scattered immunoreactivity with antibodies to FSH, LH, and the alpha-subunit. This, and the frequent expression of glycoprotein hormone genes in nonfunctioning adenomas, indicates a possible differentiation toward gonadotrophs.[115] Ultrastructurally null cell adenomas consist of rather small polyhedral cells possessing a poorly developed RER and Golgi complex and containing randomly scattered, sparse, and small (less than 250 nm) secretory granules (Fig. 60-32). The mitochondrial content is normal in most cells, though an oncocytic change may be evident in many null cell tumors. The cells that make up oncocytomas as a rule are larger than those in null cell tumors and harbor numerous mitochondria that often obscure other organelles (Fig. 60-33).

Invasive adenomas

Most pituitary adenomas are benign tumors that exhibit a slow rate of cell proliferation and expansive growth pattern. Although not encapsulated, they have a distinct border and are surrounded by condensed reticulin fibers and a few rows of compressed nontumorous adenohypophyseal cells.

Invasive adenomas grow across the normal anatomic barriers and infiltrate into adjacent structures.[134-136] These tumors may spread into the sphenoid sinus, the cavernous sinus, or the optic chiasm. They may damage the optic and other nerves and grow into the brain, disrupting the morphology and impairing the function of the hypothalamus.[137] Invading pituitary tumors may cause severe clinical symptoms such as headache, nausea, visual disturbances (even blindness), increased intracranial pressure and varying degrees of hypopituitarism; if untreated, they eventuate in death.

Invasion cannot be properly assessed using fragmented surgical material; for this, neighboring tissue must also be obtained. Imaging studies and the gross examination of a small surgically removed piece of the dura, during operation or histologic investigation are helpful in the evaluation of invasiveness. In earlier studies, the frequency of invasion was estimated to range from 10% to 20%. Recent evidence, however, indicates that invasion may occur in 30% to 50% of the patients with pituitary adenomas.[137]

All types of pituitary adenoma can be invasive. Overall, macroadenomas are more often invasive than are microadenomas. PRL- and GH-producing adenomas and silent corti-

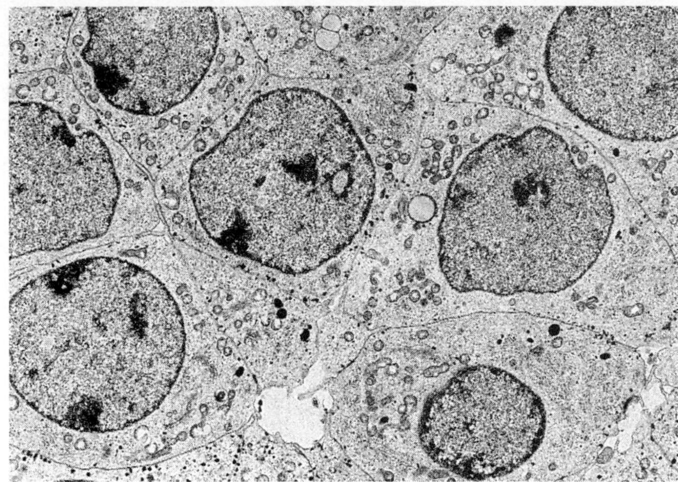

Fig. 60-32 Ultrastructural features of a null cell adenoma with small secretory granules (less than 250 nm) and a poorly developed rough endoplasmic reticulum and Golgi complex.

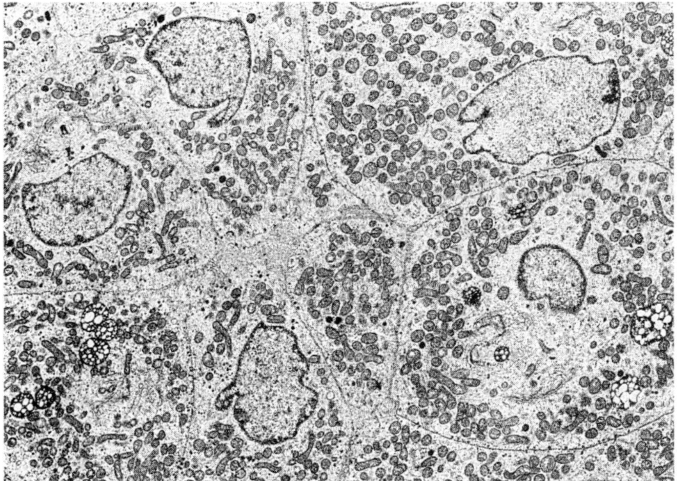

Fig. 60-33 Oncocytoma with many mitochondria and a few small secretory granules.

cotroph adenomas are the most common invasive tumors. The endocrinologically active corticotroph adenomas associated with Cushing's disease are least prone to invasion.[135] Because invading tumors lack a distinct border, complete surgical removal is difficult and recurrence is more common than in noninvasive adenomas.

Pituitary carcinoma

Carcinomas of adenohypophyseal cells are exceedingly rare, representing less than 0.001% of the tumors of the sella region.[138-144] They may produce GH, PRL, or ACTH, or they may be endocrinologically inactive. They can metastasize to the brain and spinal cord or to any organ outside the nervous system. There are no histologic differences between pituitary adenomas and pituitary carcinomas. Cellular and nuclear pleomorphism, the presence of mitotic figures, hemorrhage, necrosis, and even invasion are not regarded as proof of malignancy. The only reliable criterion for the diagnosis of pituitary carcinoma is the demonstration of distant metastatic lesions.[7]

Carcinomas producing PRL, GH, and ACTH are most common, and TSH carcinomas are rare.[142] Electron microscopic examination may fail to identify the cell type if the tumor is dedifferentiated. Exact classification can be important, because some tumors respond to medical treatment such as that consisting of dopamine agonists or somatostatin analogs. Surgical removal is often unsuccessful, though radiation treatment may be beneficial.

Flow cytometry data and other measures of cell proliferation such as nucleolar organizing regions, the Ki-67 antigen and proliferating cell nuclear antigen contents, and tumor expression of suppressor genes (such as p53) do not predict biologic behavior, growth rate, prognosis, or recurrence. Approximately 30% of histologically benign pituitary adenomas contain aneuploid nuclei. There is no correlation between the DNA content and tumor growth rate.

It is not clear why pituitary tumors, even invasive adenomas, rarely give rise to distant metastases. Whether this stems from peculiarities inherent in the vasculature, an inability of the tumor cells to penetrate into the vascular lumen, inherent cellular characteristics, or an inability to adapt to a new environment remains to be elucidated.

OTHER SELLAR LESIONS (Table 60-6)

Because of the pressure they exert on the pituitary, other tumors that arise in the sella turcica may cause endocrine symptoms, even though they do not secrete pituitary hormones. Diabetes insipidus becomes evident when the posterior lobe is destroyed or the pituitary stalk or hypothalamus is damaged. Vasopressin deficiency ensues, causing polyuria and polydipsia. Anterior hypopituitarism secondary to

Table 60-6 Intrasellar and parasellar lesions

Cysts
Epidermoid cyst
Rathke's cleft
Inflammatory lesions
Bacterial abscess
Granulomatous inflammation
Lymphocytic hypophysitis
Sarcoidosis
Tuberculosis
Miscellaneous lesions
Aneurysms
Empty sella syndrome
Hamartomas
Pituitary apoplexy
Neoplasms
Craniopharyngioma
Chordoma
Dermoid cyst
Germinoma
Granular cell tumor
Hypothalamic hamartoma
Langerhans' cell histiocytosis
Meningioma
Neuroma
Optic nerve glioma
Pituitary adenoma

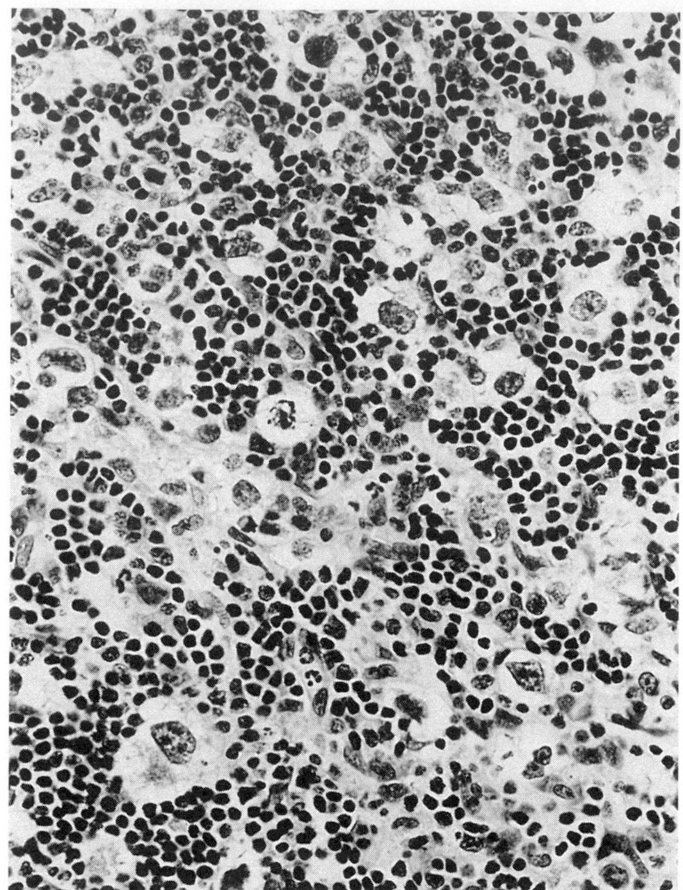

Fig. 60-34 Germinoma. The large tumor cells have clear cytoplasm and are surrounded by benign lymphocytes.

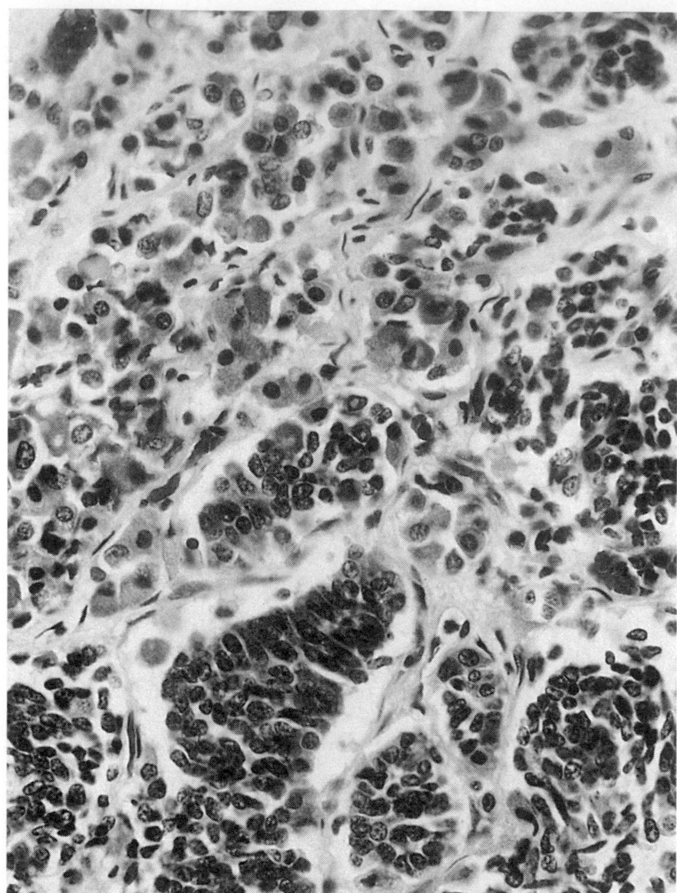

Fig. 60-35 Metastatic small cell (oat cell) carcinoma of lung to the anterior pituitary gland.

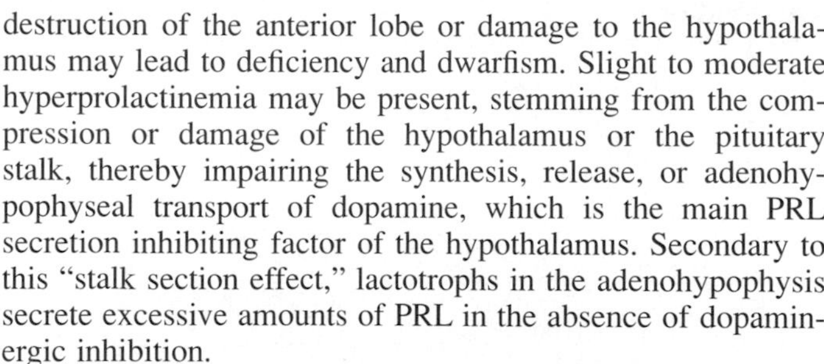

destruction of the anterior lobe or damage to the hypothalamus may lead to deficiency and dwarfism. Slight to moderate hyperprolactinemia may be present, stemming from the compression or damage of the hypothalamus or the pituitary stalk, thereby impairing the synthesis, release, or adenohypophyseal transport of dopamine, which is the main PRL secretion inhibiting factor of the hypothalamus. Secondary to this "stalk section effect," lactotrophs in the adenohypophysis secrete excessive amounts of PRL in the absence of dopaminergic inhibition.

The sella turcica may be invaded by metastatic carcinoma, craniopharyngioma, granular cell tumor, meningioma, chordoma, glioma, germinoma (Fig. 60-34), various mesenchymal tumors, sarcomas, lymphomas, and plasmacytomas.[145,146] Occasionally, fibrosarcoma or osteosarcoma develops in the sellar region of patients who have undergone radiation treatment many years earlier for a preexisting pituitary tumor.[7] The most common lesions are discussed in the following sections.

Metastatic carcinoma

Metastatic tumors in the pituitary occur in 1% to 6% of patients with disseminated carcinoma. Among women, breast carcinoma is the most frequent primary site.[147] Tumors of the lung, prostate, gastrointestinal tract, ovary, and other organs also metastasize to the pituitary[147-150] (Fig. 60-35). Metastatic tumors are more frequent in the posterior lobe than in the anterior lobe because the posterior lobe has a richer arterial blood supply.

Craniopharyngioma

Craniopharyngiomas account for 3% to 5% of intracranial tumors and, after pituitary adenomas, are the most common neoplasm in the sellar region[151-154] (Fig. 60-36). They most often arise in children or young adults and rarely occur in older patients.

Most craniopharyngiomas are suprasellar, but approximately 20% are located in the sella turcica. They are slow-growing, well-demarcated tumors and have the potential to invade by spreading into neighboring tissue, even to the hypothalamus.

The clinical symptoms include headache, visual disturbances, increased intracranial pressure, seizures, and cranial nerve palsies. Endocrinologically, various degrees of hypopituitarism, diabetes insipidus, and hyperprolactinemia may be apparent. If the tumor develops before puberty, dwarfism stemming from GH deficiency may be a leading symptom. The findings yielded by magnetic resonance imaging are valuable in establishing the diagnosis. Craniopharyngiomas often undergo massive calcification, which can be demonstrated by imaging techniques.

Histologically the tumors resemble ameloblastomas of the jaw (Fig. 60-37). They contain clusters of epithelial cells that are embedded in a connective tissue stroma, which may con-

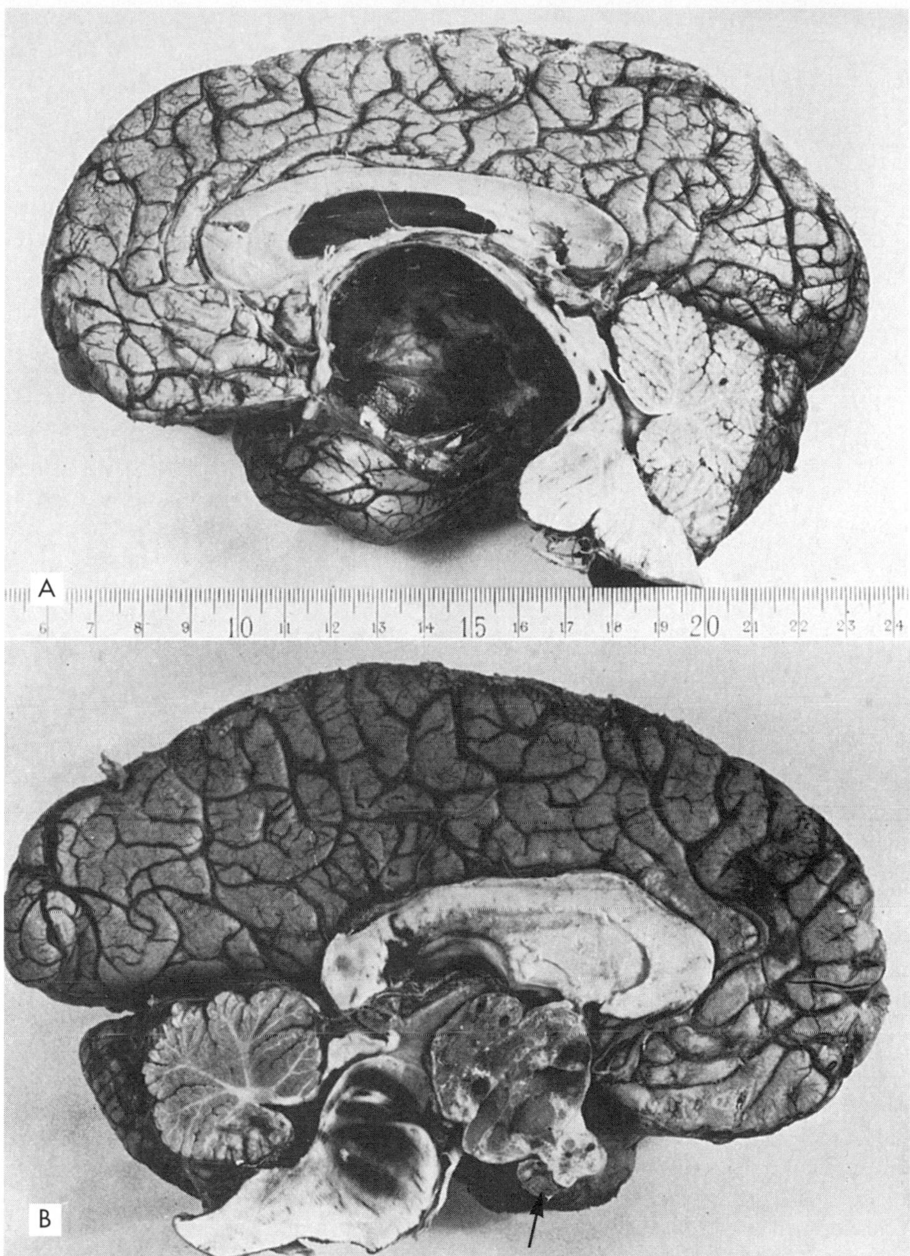

Fig. 60-36 **A,** Cystic suprasellar craniopharyngioma. **B,** Solid and cystic suprasellar tumor. *Arrow,* Pituitary gland. (Courtesy Dr. Dorothy S. Russell and A. R. Currie.)

tain numerous inflammatory cells. Calcification, cornification, and cyst formation are often seen, and cholesterol crystal clefts may be present. With a few exceptions, craniopharyngiomas are benign. They are endocrinologically inactive and contain no immunoreactive pituitary hormones. The findings noted on electron microscopy studies consist of epithelial cells attached by numerous desmosomes and bundles of cytoplasmic tonofilaments, but no secretory granules. There are no specific immunohistochemical markers for craniopharyngiomas, though epithelial cells mark with antikeratin and the stromal cells with vimentin.

The treatment of craniophyaryngiomas is surgical removal. If the tumor recurs, radiation therapy is an alterative treatment.

Granular cell tumor

In a substantial majority of cases granular cell tumors are small microscopic lesions.[155-159] They are typically found at incidentally autopsy in approximately 5% of adults. Granular cell tumors consist of small, well-demarcated, nonencapsulated nodules that form in the posterior lobe or in the distal part of the pituitary stalk. Histologically the nodules are composed of large, irregular cells with abundant granular, acidophilic cytoplasm. The granules are strongly PAS positive, are present in large numbers, and are randomly distributed in the cell cytoplasm (Fig. 60-38). Electron microscopy studies show that these granules correspond to large lysosomal bodies and not to mitochondria or secretory granules. The tumor cells are immunoreactive with anti–S-100 protein

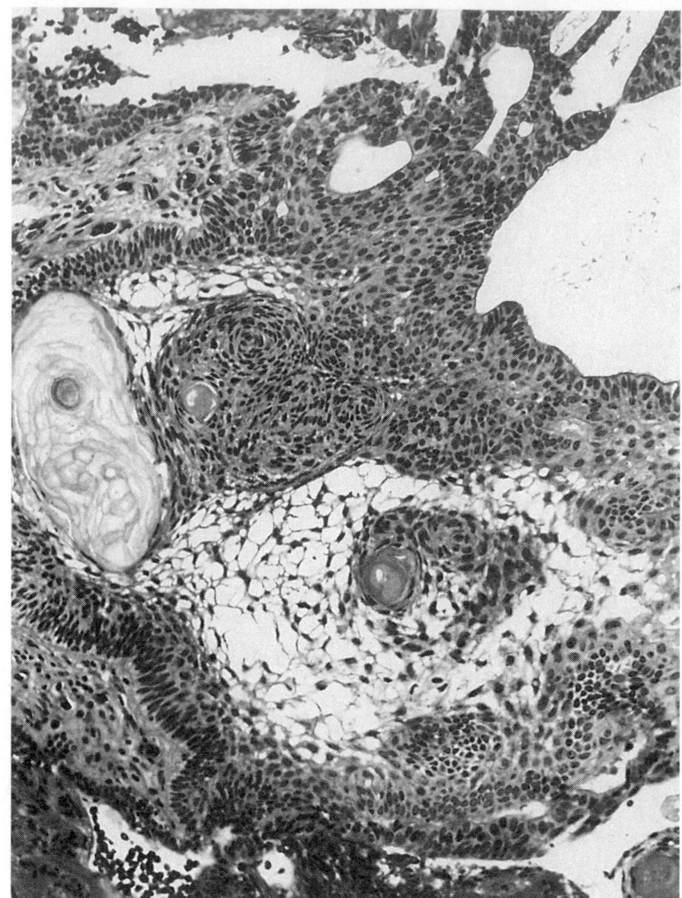

Fig. 60-37 Section of a craniopharyngioma showing cystic spaces, squamous differentiation, and a keratin pearl.

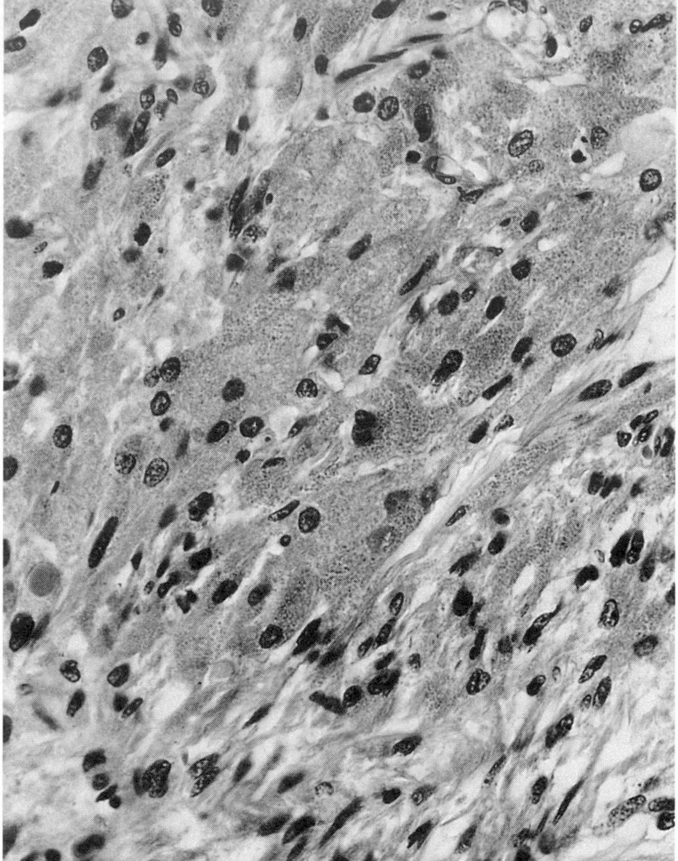

Fig. 60-38 Small granular cell tumor in the pars nervosa. The cells have abundant granular cytoplasm and small nuclei.

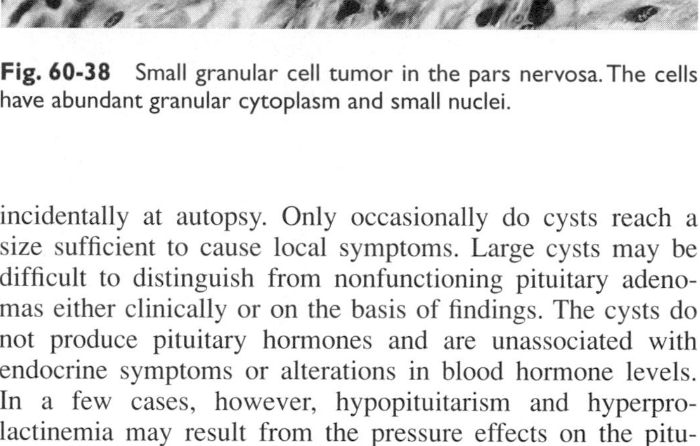

and lack all pituitary hormones. Results of immunohistochemical studies have indicated that granular cell tumors may arise from the "granular" pituicytes, as shown by the fact that they show a similar immunohistochemical profile.[158]

Rarely granular cell tumors grow faster than usual and become large space-occupying lesions that cause local symptoms and necessitate surgical removal.

Langerhans' cell histiocytosis

Histiocytosis X, that is, the neoplastic proliferation of cells that have features of Langerhans' cells, presents as Letterer-Siwe disease, Hand-Schüller-Christian (HSC) disease, or eosinophilic granuloma. The pituitary may be involved in all three syndromes but most often in HSC. Diabetes insipidus, calvarial bone defects and exophthalmus have been referred to as the "HSC triad." Typical histiocytic infiltrates are found in bone, orbital tissue, the posterior pituitary, infundibulum, and infundibular stem.[85] The ultrastructural identification of Birbeck granules is helpful in establishing a histologic diagnosis.

Cysts

Several types of cysts occur in the region of the sella turcica[160–164]; most produce no clinical symptoms and are found incidentally at autopsy. Only occasionally do cysts reach a size sufficient to cause local symptoms. Large cysts may be difficult to distinguish from nonfunctioning pituitary adenomas either clinically or on the basis of findings. The cysts do not produce pituitary hormones and are unassociated with endocrine symptoms or alterations in blood hormone levels. In a few cases, however, hypopituitarism and hyperprolactinemia may result from the pressure effects on the pituitary.

Cysts vary in size from small, clinically insignificant cavities to large space-occupying lesions. Rathke's cleft cysts that measure 1 to 10 cm in diameter are not uncommon at the pars anterior–pars intermedia interface. They are lined by a simple layer of flat, cuboidal, or columnar and often ciliated epithelium and are filled with an amorphous acidophilic material (Fig. 60-39). *Epidermoid cysts* are slow-growing, benign lesions lined by multiple layers of squamous epithelium. They may resemble cystic craniopharyngiomas. *Dermoid cysts* similar to those in the ovary are very rare in the sellar region. The wall of these teratoid tumors is lined by stratified squamous epithelium and contains connective tissue, sweat glands, sebaceous glands, hair follicles, and other tissues. Lymphocytes, macrophages, and occasional foreign-body giant cells may be seen in the wall of the cysts and adjacent normal structures.

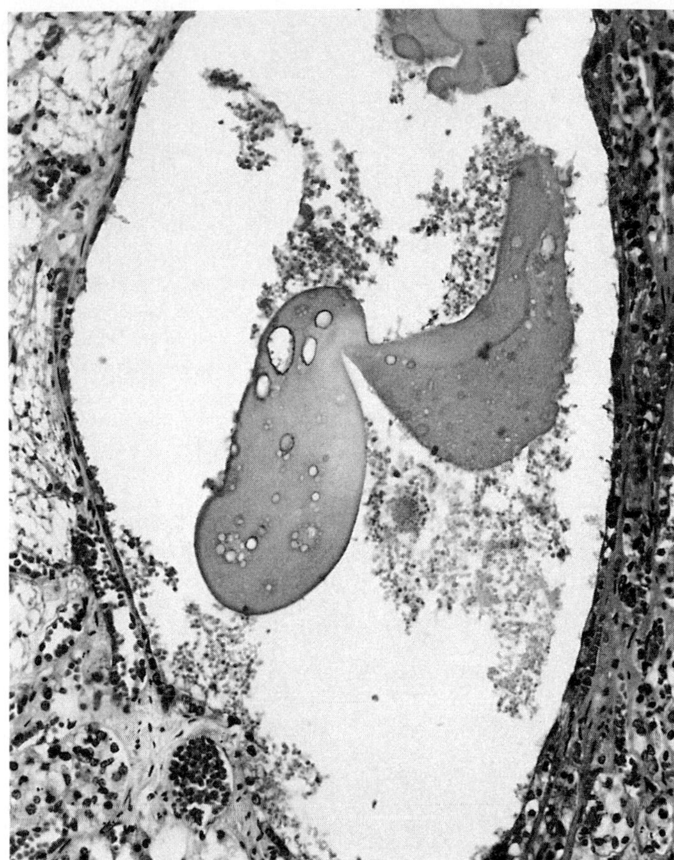

Fig. 60-39 Rathke's cyst lined by flattened ciliated epithelium. Proteinaceous material is present in the lumen. The cyst is compressing the adjacent anterior pituitary cells.

REFERENCES

Normal pituitary anatomy and physiology

Development

1. Goodyear CG, Guyda HJ, Giroud CJP: Development of the hypothalamic-pituitary axis in the human fetus. In Tolis G, Labrie F, Mortin JB, Nattolin F, editors: *Clinical neuroendocrinology: a pathophysiological approach,* New York, 1979, Raven Press.
2. Boyd JD: Observations on the human pharyngeal hypophysis, *J Endocrinol 14:66, 1956.*
3. Ciocca DR, Puy LA, Stati AO: Identification of seven hormone-producing cell types in the human pharyngeal hypophysis, *J Clin Endocrinol Metab* 60:212, 1985.
4. Lloyd RV, Chandler WF, Kovacs K, Ryan N: Ectopic pituitary adenomas with normal anterior pituitary gland, *Am J Surg Pathol* 10:546, 1986.
5. Baker BL, Jaffe RB: The genesis of cell types in the adenohypophysis of the human fetus as observed with immunocytochemistry, *Am J Anat* 143:137, 1975.
6. Osamura RY, Watanabe K: Histogenesis of the cells of the anterior and intermediate lobes of human pituitary glands: immunohistochemical studies, *Int Rev Cytol* 95:103, 1985.

Anatomy

7. Kovacs K, Horvath E: Tumors of the pituitary gland. In Atlas of tumor pathology, series 2, fasc 21, Washington, DC, 1986, Armed Forces Institute of Pathology.
8. Erdheim J, Stumme F: Über die Schwangerschaftsveränderung der Hypophyse, *Beitr Pathol Anat* 46:1, 1909.
9. Kaufman B, Chamberlin WB Jr: The ubiquitous "empty" sella turcica, *Acta Radiol* 13:413, 1972.
10. Goldberg GM, Eshbang DE: Squamous cell nests of the pituitary gland as related to the origin of craniopharyngiomas, *Arch Pathol* 70:293, 1960.
11. Bergland RM, Page RB: Pituitary-brain vascular relations: a new paradigm, *Science* 204:18, 1979.
12. Bergland RM, Page RB: Can the pituitary secrete directly to the brain? (affirmative anatomical evidence), *Endocrinology* 102:1325, 1978.
13. Gorczyca W, Hardy J: Arterial supply of the human anterior pituitary gland, *Neurosurgery* 20:369, 1987.
14. Sheehan HL, Kovacs K: Neurohypophysis and hypothalamus. In Bloodworth JMB Jr, editor: *Endocrine pathology,* ed 2, Baltimore, 1982, Williams & Wilkins.

Histology and physiology

15. Halmi NS: Current status of human pituitary cytophysiology, *NZ Med J* 80:551, 1974.
16. Horvath E, Kovacs K: Fine structural cytology of the adenohypophysis in rat and man, *J Electron Microsc* Tech 8:401, 1988.
17. Moriarty GC. Adenohypophysis: ultrastructural cytochemistry: a review, *J Histochem Cytochem* 21:855, 1973.
18. Pelletier G, Lechenc R, Lalerie F: Identification of gonadotropic cells in the human pituitary by immunoperoxidase technique, *Mol Cell Endocrinol* 6:123, 1976.
19. Asa SL, Penz G, Kovacs K, Ezrin C: Prolactin cells in the human pituitary: a quantitative immunocytochemical analysis, *Arch Pathol Lab Med* 106:360, 1982.
20. Scheithauer BW, Sano T, Kovacs K et al: The pituitary gland in pregnancy: a clinicopathologic and immunohistochemical study of 69 cases. *Mayo Clin Proc* 65:462, 1990.
21. Lloyd RV, Anagnostou D, Caw M et al: Analysis of mammosomatotrophic cells in normal and neoplastic human pituitary tissues by the reverse hemolytic plaque assay and immunocytochemistry, *J Clin Endocrinol Metab* 66:1103, 1988.
22. Stefaneanu L, Kovacs K, Lloyd RV et al: Pituitary lactotrophs and somatotrophs in pregnancy: a correlative in situ hybridization and immunocytochemical study, *Virchows Arch [B] (Cell Pathol)* 62:291, 1992.
23. Benjannet S, Rondeau N, Day R et al: PC1 and PC2 are proprotein convertases capable of cleaving proopiomelanocortin at distinct pairs of basic residues, *Proc Natl Acad Sci USA* 88:3564, 1991.
24. Saeger W: Effect of drugs on pituitary ultrastructure, *Microsc Res Tech* 15:162, 1976.
25. Girod C, Trouillas J, Dubois MP: Immunocytochemical localization of S-100 protein in stellate cells (folliculo-stellate cells) of the anterior lobe of the normal human pituitary, *Cell Tissue Res* 241:505, 1985.
26. Ferrara N, Schweigerer L, Neufeld G et al: Pituitary follicular cells produce basic fibroblast growth factor, *Proc Natl Acad Sci USA* 84:5773, 1989.
27. Marin F, Kovacs K, Stefaneanu L: S-100 protein immunopositivity in human nontumorous hypophyses and pituitary adenomas, *Endocr Pathol* 3:28, 1992.
28. Scheithauer BW, Horvath E, Kovacs K: Ultrastructure of the neurohypophsis, *Microsc Res Tech* 20:177, 1992.
29. Russfield AB: Hypophyseal changes in hypothyroidism induced by radioactive iodine in man, *Arch Pathol Lab Med 66*:79, 1958.
30. Vagenakis AG, Dole K, Braverman LE: Pituitary enlargement, pituitary failure, and primary hypothyroidism, *Ann Intern Med* 85:195, 1976.

Pituitary in disorders of other endocrine glands

31. Warner NE: Pituitary Gland. In Kissane JM, editor: *Pathology,* vol 2, Ed 9, St. Louis, 1981, Mosby.
32. Furth J, Clifton KH: Experimental pituitary tumors. In Harris GW, Donovan BT, editors: *The pituitary gland,* vol 2, Berkeley, 1966, University of California Press.
33. Scheithauer BW, Kovacs K, Randall RV, Ryan N: Pituitary gland in hypothyroidism: histologic and immunocytologic study, *Arch Pathol Lab Med* 109:499, 1985.
34. Pioro EP, Scheithauer BW, Laws ER Jr et al: Combined thyrotroph and lactotroph cell hyperplasia simulating prolactin-secreting pituitary adenoma in long-standing primary hypothyroidism, *Surg Neurol* 29:218, 1988.
35. Halmi NS: Current status of human pituitary cytophysiology, *NZ Med J* 80:551, 1974.

36. Murray S, Ezrin C: Effect of Graves' disease on the "thyrotroph" cell of the adenohypophysis, *J Clin Endocrinol* 26:287, 1966.
37. Scheithauer BW, Kovacs KT, Young WF Jr, Randall RV: The pituitary gland in hyperthyroidism, *Mayo Clinic Proc* 67:22, 1992.
38. Crooke AC, Russell DS: The pituitary gland in Addison's disease, *J Pathol Bacteriol* 40:255, 1935.
39. Scheithauer BW, Kovacs K, Randall RV: The pituitary gland in untreated Addison's disease: A histologic and immunocytologic study of 18 adenohypophyses, *Arch Pathol Lab Med* 107:484, 1983.
40. Bloodworth JMB Jr, Kirkendall WM, Carr TL: Addison's disease associated with thyroid insufficiency and atrophy (Schmidt syndrome), *J Clin Endocrinol* 14:540, 1954.
41. Carpenter CCJ, Solomon N, Silverberg SG et al: Schmidt's syndrome (thyroid and adrenal insufficiency): a review of the literature and a report of fifteen new cases including ten instances of coexistent diabetes mellitus, *Medicine* 43:153, 1964.
42. Crooke AC: A change in the basophil cells of the pituitary gland common to conditions which exhibit the syndrome attributed to basophil adenoma, *J Pathol Bacteriol* 41:339, 1935.
43. Halmi NS, McCormick WF: Effects of hyperadrenocorticism on pituitary thyrotropic cells in man, *Arch Pathol* 94:471, 1972.
44. Halmi NS, McCormick WF, Decker DA Jr: The natural history of hyalinization of ACTH/MSH cells in man, *Arch Pathol* 91:318, 1971.
45. Kilby RA, Bennett WA, Sprague RG: Anterior pituitary glands in patients treated with cortisone and corticotropin, *Am J Pathol* 33:155, 1955.
46. Saeger W: Surgical pathology of the pituitary in Cushing's disease, *Pathol Res Pract* 187:613, 1991.
47. Kovacs K, Horvath E: Gonadotrophs following removal of ovaries: a fine structural study of human pituitary glands, *Endocrinologie* 66:1, 1975.
48. Phifer RF, Midgley AR, Spicer SS: Immunohistologic and histologic evidence that follicle-stimulating hormone and luteinizing hormone are present in the same cell type in the human pars distalis, *J Clin Endocrinol Metab* 36:125, 1973.

Effects of drugs on the anterior pituitary

49. Müller EE, Nistico G: *Brain messengers and the pituitary,* San Diego, 1989, Academic Press.
50. Tindall GT, Kovacs K, Horvath E, Thorner MO: Human prolactin-producing adenomas and bromocriptine; a histological, immunocytochemical, ultrastructural and morphometric study, *J Clin Endocrinol Metab* 55:1178, 1982.
51. Kovacs K, Stefaneanu L, Horvath E et al: Effect of dopamine agonist medication on prolactin producing pituitary adenomas: a morphological study including immunocytochemistry, electron microscopy and in situ hybridization, *Virchows Arch [A] (Pathol Anat Histopathol)* 418:439, 1991.
52. Barkan AL, Lloyd RV, Chandler WF et al: Preoperative treatment of acromegaly with long-acting somatostatin analog SMS 201-995: shrinkage of invasive pituitary macroadenomas and improved surgical remission ratio, *J Clin Endocrinol Metab* 67:1040, 1988.
53. Scheithauer BW, Kovacs KT, Randall RV, Ryan N: Effects of estrogen on the human pituitary: a clinicopathologic study, *Mayo Clin Proc* 64:1077, 1989.
54. White MC, Anapliotou M, Rosenstock J et al: Heterogeneity of prolactin responses to ostradiol benzoate in women with prolactinomas, *Lancet* 1:1394, 1981.

Hereditary diseases

55. Underdahl LO, Woolner LB, Black BM: Multiple endocrine adenomas: report of 8 cases in which the parathyroids, pituitary and pancreatic islets were involved, *J Clin Endocrinol Metab* 13:20, 1953.
56. Wermer P: Genetic aspects of adenomatosis of endocrine glands, *Am J Med* 16:363, 1954.
57. Larsson C, Skogseid B, Oberg K et al: Multiple endocrine neoplasia type I gene maps to chromosome 11 and is lost in insulinomas, *Nature* 332:85, 1988.
58. Scheithauer BW, Laws ER Jr, Kovacs K et al: Pituitary adenomas in the multiple endocrine neoplasia type I syndrome. *Semin Diagn Pathol* 4:205, 1987.
59. Kallmann FJ, Schoenfeld WA, Barrera SE: The genetic aspects of primary eunuchoidism, *Am J Ment Defic* 48:203, 1944.
60. Petit C: Molecular basis of the X-chromosome linked Kallmann's syndrome, *Trends Endocrinol Metab* 4:8, 1993.
61. Li S, Crenshaw EB III, Rawson EJ et al: Dwarf locus mutants lacking three pituitary cell types result from mutations in the POU-domain gene Pit-1, *Nature* 347:528, 1990.
62. Voss JW, Rosenfeld MG: Anterior pituitary development: short tales from dwarf mice, *Cell* 70:527, 1992.
63. Pfaffle RW, Di Mattia GE, Parks JS et al: Mutation of the POU-specific domain of Pit-1 and hypopituitarism without pituitary hypoplasia, *Science* 257:1118, 1992.
64. Radovick S, Nations M, Du Y et al: A mutation in the POU-homeodomain of Pit-1 responsible for combined pituitary hormone deficiency, *Science* 257:1115, 1992.
65. Tatsumi K, Miyai K, Notomi T et al: Cretinism with combined hormone deficiency caused by a mutation in the Pit-1 gene, *Nature Genet* 1:56, 1992.

Isolated hormone deficiency

66. Vnencak-Jones CL, Phillips JA III, Chen EY, Seeburg PH: Molecular basis of human growth hormone gene deletions, *Proc Natl Acad Sci USA* 85:5615, 1988.
67. Schechter J, Kovacs K, Rimoin D: Isolated growth hormone deficiency: immunocytochemistry, *J Clin Endocrinol Metab* 59:798, 1984.

Developmental defects

68. Blizzard RM, Alberts M: Hypopituitarism, hypoadrenalism and hypogonadism in the newborn infant, *J Pediatr* 48:782, 1956.
69. Brewer D: Congenital absence of the pituitary gland and its consequences, *J Pathol Bacteriol* 73:59, 1957.
70. Kosaki K, Matsuo N, Tamai S et al: Isolated aplasia of the anterior pituitary as a cause of congenital panhypopituitarism: case report, *Horm Res* 35:226, 1991.
71. Moncrieff MW, Hill DS, Archer J, Arthur LJ: Congenital absence of pituitary gland and adrenal hypoplasia, *Arch Dis Child* 47:136, 1972.
72. Mosier HD: Hypoplasia of the pituitary and adrenal cortex, *J Pediatr* 48:633, 1956.
73. Osamura RY: Functional prenatal development of anencephalic and normal anterior pituitary glands. I. Human and experimental animals studied by peroxidase-labeled antibody method, *Acta Pathol Jpn* 27:495, 1977.
74. Reid JD: Congenital absence of the pituitary gland, *J Pediatr* 56:658, 1960.
75. Steiner MM, Boggs JD: Absence of pituitary gland, hypothyroidism, hypoadrenalism and hypogonadism in a 17-year-old dwarf, *J Clin Endocrinol Metab* 25:1591, 1965.
76. Ehrlich RM: Ectopic and hypoplastic pituitary with adrenal hypoplasia; case report, *J Pediatr* 51:377, 1957.

Circulatory disorders

77. Sheehan HL: Postpartum necrosis of the anterior pituitary, *J Pathol Bacteriol* 45:189, 1937.
78. Thorner MO, Vance ML, Horvath E, Kovacs K: The anterior pituitary. In Wilson JD, Foster DW, editors: *Williams textbook of endocrinology,* Philadelphia, 1992, Saunders.
79. Wakai S, Fukushima T, Teramoto A, Sano K: Pituitary apoplexy: its incidence and clinical significance, *J Neurosurg* 55:187, 1981.

Exogenous injury

80. Reichlin S: Neuroendocrinology. In Wilson JD, Foster DW, editors: *Williams textbook of endocrinology,* ed 8, Philadelphia, 1992, Saunders.
81. Dugger GS, Van Wyr JJ, Newsome JF: The effect of pituitary-stalk section on thyroid function and gonadotropic-hormone secretion in women with mammary carcinoma, *J Neurosurg* 19:589, 1962.
82. Clayton PE, Shalet SM: Dose dependency of time of onset of radiation-induced growth hormone deficiency, *J Pediatr* 118:226, 1991.
83. Constine LS, Woolf PD, Cann D et al: Hypothalamic-pituitaries dysfunction after radiation for brain tumors, *N Engl J Med* 328:87, 1993.
84. Littley MD, Shalet SM, Beardwell CG et al: Radiation-induced hypopituitarism is dose-dependent, *Clin Endocrinol* (Oxf) 31:363, 1989.

85. Sheehan HL, Kovacs K: Neurohypophysis and hypothalamus. In Bloodworth JMB Jr, editor: *Endocrine pathology*, ed 2, Baltimore, 1982, Williams & Wilkins.

Metabolic disorders

86. Bilbao J, Kovacs K, Horvath E: Pituitary melanocorticotrophinoma with amyloid deposition, *Can J Neurol Sci* 2:199, 1975.
87. Landolt AM, Kleihues P, Heitz PU: Amyloid deposits in pituitary adenomas: differentiation of two types, *Arch Pathol Lab Med* 111:453, 1987.
88. Bergeron C, Kovacs K: Pituitary siderosis: a histologic, immunocytologic and ultrastructural study, *Am J Pathol* 93:295, 1978.
89. Horvath E, Kovacs K: Pathology of the pituitary gland. In Ezrin C, Horvath E, Kaufman B, et al, editors: *Pituitary diseases*, Boca Raton, Fla, 1980, CRC Press.
90. Schochet SS Jr, McCormick WF, Halmi NS: Pituitary gland in patients with Hurler's syndrome: light and electron microscopic study, *Arch Pathol* 97:96, 1974.

Infectious diseases

91. Obenchain TG, Becker DP: Abscess formation in a Rathke's cleft cyst: case report, *J Neurosurg* 36:359, 1972.
92. Rickards AG, Harvey PW: "Giant cell granuloma" and the other pituitary granulomata, *Q J Med* 47:425, 1954.
93. Oelbaum MH: Hypopituitarism in male subjects due to syphilis, *Q J Med* 45:249, 1952.
94. Sano T, Kovacs K, Scheithauer BW et al: Pituitary pathology in acquired immunodeficiency syndrome, *Arch Pathol Lab Med* 113:1066, 1989.

Autoimmune diseases

95. Asa SL, Bilbao JM, Kovacs K et al: Lymphocytic hypophysitis of pregnancy resulting in hypopituitarism: a distinct clinicopathologic entity, *Ann Intern Med* 95:166, 1981.
96. Jensen MD, Handwerger BS, Scheithauer BW et al: Lymphocytic hypophysitis with isolated corticotropin deficiency, *Ann Intern Med* 105:200, 1986.
97. Meichner RH, Riggio S, Manz HJ, Earll JM: Lymphocytic hypophysitis causing pituitary mass, *Neurology* 37:158, 1987.
98. Feigenbaum SL, Martin MC, Wilson CB, Jaffe RB: Lymphocytic adenohypophysitis: a pituitary mass lesion occurring in pregnancy: proposal for medical treatment, *Am J Obstet Gynecol* 164:1549, 1991.
99. Imura H, Nakao K, Shimatsu A et al: Lymphocytic infundibuloneurohypophysitis as a cause of central diabetes insipidus, *N Engl J Med* 329:683, 1993.
100. Komatsu M, Kondo T, Yamauchi K et al: Antipituitary antibodies in patients with primary empty sella syndrome, *J Clin Endocrinol Metab* 67:633, 1988.
101. Pouplard A: Pituitary autoimmunity, *Horm Res* 16:289, 1982.
102. Eisenbarth GS, Jackson RA: The immunoendocrinopathy syndromes. In Wilson JD, Foster DW, editors: *Williams textbook of endocrinology*, ed 8, Philadelphia, 1992, Saunders.

Idiopathic and poorly understood diseases

103. Doniach I: Histopathology of the pituitary, *Clin Endocrinol Metab* 14:765, 1985.
104. McKeever PE, Koppelman MC, Metcalf D et al: Refractory Cushing's disease caused by multinodular, ACTH-cell hyperplasia, *J Neuropathol Exp Neurol* 41:490, 1982.
105. Plair CM, Perry S: Hypothalamic-pituitary sarcoidosis, *Arch Pathol* 74:527, 1962.
106. García-Luna PP, Leal-Cerro A, Montero C et al: A rare cause of acromegaly: ectopic production of growth hormone–releasing factor by a bronchial carcinoid tumor, *Surg Neurol* 27:563, 1987.
107. Thorner MO, Perryman RL, Cronin MJ et al: Somatotroph hyperplasia: successful treatment of acromegaly by removal of the pancreatic islet tumor secreting a growth hormone–releasing factor, *J Clin Invest* 70:965, 1982.
108. Kovacs K, Ilse G, Ryan N et al: Pituitary prolactin cell hyperplasia, *Horm Res* 12:87, 1980.
109. Saeger W, Ludecke DK: Pituitary hyperplasia: definition, light and electron microscopic structures and significance in surgical specimens, *Virchows Arch [A] Pathol Anat Histol* 399:277, 1983.

Neoplasms

Pituitary adenomas

110. Herman V, Fagin J, Gonsky R et al: Clonal origin of pituitary adenomas, *J Clin Endocrinol Metab* 71:1427, 1990.
111. Thapar K, Kovacs K, Laws ER Jr, Muller PJ: Pituitary adenomas; current concepts in classification, histopathology, and molecular biology, *Endocrinologist* 3:39, 1993.
112. Horvath E, Kovacs K: The adenohypophysis. In Kovacs K, Asa SL, editors: *Functional endocrine pathology*, Boston, 1991, Blackwell Scientific.
113. Horvath E, Kovacs K: Ultrastructural diagnosis of human pituitary adenomas, *Microsc Res Tech* 20:107, 1992.
114. Horvath E, Kovacs K: Ultrastructural diagnosis of pituitary adenomas and hyperplasias. In Lloyd RV, editor: *Surgical pathology of the pituitary gland (Major problems in pathology*, vol 27), Philadelphia, 1993, Saunders.
115. Jameson JL, Klibanski A, Black PM et al: Glycoprotein hormone genes are expressed in clinically nonfunctioning pituitary adenomas, *J Clin Invest* 80:1472, 1987.
116. Frawley LS, Bockfor FR: Mammosomatotropes: presence and functions in normal and neoplastic pituitary tissue, *Endocr Rev* 12:337, 1991.
117. Giannattasio G, Bassetti M: Human pituitary adenomas: recent advances in morphological studies, *J Endocrinol Invest* 13:435, 1990.
118. Lloyd RV, Gikas RVB, Chandler WF: Prolactin and growth hormone–producing pituitary adenomas: an immunohistochemical and ultrastructural study, *Am J Surg Pathol* 7:251, 1983.
119. McNicol AM: Patterns of corticotropic cells in the adult human pituitary in Cushing's disease, *Diagn Histopathol* 4:335, 1981.
120. Kovacs K, Horvath E: Pathology of growth hormone–producing tumors of the human pituitary, *Semin Diagn Pathol* 3:18, 1986.
121. Scheithauer BW, Horvath E, Kovacs K et al: Plurihormonal pituitary adenomas, *Semin Diagn Pathol* 3:69, 1986.
122. Neumann PE, Goldman JE, Horoupian DS, Hess MA: Fibrous bodies in growth hormone secreting adenomas contain cytokeratin filaments, *Arch Pathol Lab Med* 109:505, 1985.
123. Beckers A, Kovacs K, Horvath E et al: Effect of treatment with octreotide on the morphology of growth hormone–secreting pituitary adenomas: study of 24 cases, *Endocr Pathol* 2:123, 1991.
124. Horvath E, Kovacs K: Pathology of prolactin cell adenomas of the human pituitary, *Semin Diagn Pathol* 3:4, 1986.
125. Horvath E, Kovacs K: Gonadotroph adenomas of the human pituitary: sex-related fine structural dichotomy: a histologic, immunocytochemical, and electron microscopic study of 30 tumors, *Am J Pathol* 117:429, 1984.
126. Lloyd RV, Chandler WF, McKeever PF, Schteingart DE: The spectrum of ACTH-producing pituitary lesions, *Am J Surg Pathol* 10:618, 1986.
127. Robert F, Hardy J: Human corticotroph cell adenomas, *Semin Diagn Pathol* 3:34, 1986.
128. Neumann PE, Horoupian DS, Goldman JE, Hess MA: Cytoplasmic filaments of Crooke's hyaline change belong to the cytokeratin class: an immunocytochemical and ultrastructural study, *Am J Pathol* 116:214, 1984.
129. Beckers A, Abs R, Mahler C et al: Thyrotropin-secreting pituitary adenomas: report of seven cases, *J Clin Endocrinol Metab* 72:477, 1991.
130. Girod C, Trouillas J, Claustrat B: The human thyrotropic adenoma: pathologic diagnosis in five cases and critical review of the literature, *Semin Diagn Pathol* 3:58, 1986.
131. Trouillas J, Girod C, Sassolas G, Claustrat B: The human gonadotropic adenoma: pathologic diagnosis and hormonal correlations in 26 tumors, *Semin Diagn Pathol* 3:42, 1986.
132. Kovacs K, Asa SL, Horvath E et al: Null cell adenomas of the pituitary: attempts to resolve their cytogenesis. In Lechago J, Kameya T, editors: *Endocrine pathology update*, New York, 1990, Field & Wood.
133. Yamada S, Asa SL, Kovacs K: Oncocytomas and null cell adenomas of the human pituitary: morphometric and in vitro functional comparison, *Virchows Arch [A] (Pathol Anat Histol)* 413:333, 1988.

Invasive adenomas

134. Martins AN, Hayes GJ, Kempe LG: Invasive pituitary adenomas, *J Neurosurg* 22:268, 1965.
135. Pernicone PJ, Scheithauer BW: Invasive pituitary adenomas and pituitary carcinomas. In Lloyd RV, editor: *Surgical pathology of the pituitary gland.* (Major problems in pathology, vol 27), Philadelphia, 1993, Saunders.
136. Scheithauer BW, Kovacs KT, Laws ER Jr, Randall RV: Pathology of invasive pituitary tumors with special reference to functional classification, *J Neurosurg* 65:733, 1986.
137. Selman WR, Laws ER Jr, Scheithauer BW, Carpenter SM: The occurrence of dural invasion in pituitary adenomas, *J Neurosurg* 64:402, 1986.

Pituitary carcinomas

138. Atienza DM, Vigersky RJ, Lack EE et al: Prolactin-producing pituitary carcinoma with pulmonary metastases: a case report, *Cancer* 68:1605, 1991.
139. Graf CJ, Blinderman EE, Terplan KL: Pituitary carcinoma in a child with distant metastases, *J Neurosurg* 19:254, 1962.
140. Hashimoto N, Handa H, Nishi S: Intracranial and intraspinal dissemination from a growth hormone–secreting pituitary tumor, *J Neurosurg* 64:140, 1986.
141. Luzi P, Miracco C, Lio R et al: Endocrine inactive pituitary carcinoma metastasizing to cervical lymph nodes: a case report, *Hum Pathol* 18:90, 1987.
142. Mixson AJ, Friedman TC, Katz DA et al: Thyrotropin-secreting pituitary carcinoma, *J Clin Endocrinol Metab* 76:529, 1993.
143. Mountcastle RB, Roof BS, Mayfield RK et al: Case report: pituitary adenocarcinoma in an acromegalic patient: response to bromocriptine and pituitary testing: a review of the literature on 36 cases of pituitary carcinoma, *Am J Med Sci* 298:109, 1989.
144. Scheithauer BW, Randall RV, Laws ER Jr et al: Prolactin cell carcinoma of the pituitary: clinicopathologic, immunohistochemical and ultrastructural study of a case with cranial and extracranial metastases, *Cancer* 55:598, 1985.

Other sellar neoplasms

145. McKeever PE, Blaivas M, Sima AA: Neoplasms of the sellar region. In Lloyd RV, editor: *Surgical pathology of the pituitary gland.* (Major problems in pathology, vol 27), Philadelphia, 1993, Saunders.
146. Scheithauer BW: The hypothalamus and neurohypophysis. In Kovacs K, Asa SL, editors: *Functional endocrine pathology,* Boston, 1991, Blackwell Scientific.

Metastatic carcinomas

147. Hägerstrand I, Schonebeck J: Metastases to the pituitary gland, *Acta Pathol Microbiol Scand* 75:64, 1969.
148. Jin L, Lloyd RV: Metastatic neoplasms to the pituitary gland. In Lloyd RV, editor: *Surgical pathology of the pituitary gland.* (Major problems in Pathology, vol 27), Philadelphia, 1993, Saunders.
149. Max MB, Deck MD, Rottenberg DA: Pituitary metastasis: incidence in cancer patients and clinical differentiation from pituitary adenoma, *Neurology* 31:998, 1981.
150. Teears RJ, Silverman EM: Clinicopathologic review of 88 cases of carcinoma metastatic to the pituitary gland, *Cancer* 36:216, 1975.

Craniopharyngioma

151. Akimura T, Kameda H, Abiko S et al: Intrasellar craniopharyngioma, *Neuroradiology* 31:180, 1989.
152. Hoffman HJ: Craniopharyngiomas, *Prog Exp Tumor Res* 30:325, 1987.
153. Nelson GA, Bastian FO, Schlitt M, White RL: Malignant transformation in craniopharyngioma, *Neurosurgery* 22:427, 1988.
154. Petito CK, DeGirolami U, Earle KM: Craniopharyngiomas, *Cancer* 37:1944, 1976.

Granular cell tumor

155. Becker DH, Wilson CB: Symptomatic parasellar granular cell tumor, *Neurosurgery* 8:173, 1981.
156. Liwnicz BH, Liwnicz RG, Huff JS et al: Giant granular cell tumor of the suprasellar area: immunohistochemical and electron microscopic studies, *Neurosurgery* 15:246, 1984.
157. Luse SA, Kernohan JW: Granular cell tumors of the stalk and posterior lobe of the pituitary gland, *Cancer* 8:616, 1955.
158. Nashioka H: Immunohistochemical study of granular cell tumors and granular pituicytes of the neurohypophysis, *Endocr Pathol* 4:140, 1993.
159. Vaquero J, Leunda G, Gabezudo JM et al: Granular pituicytomas of the pituitary stalk, *Acta Neurochir* 59:209, 1981.

Cysts

160. Klonoff DC, Kahn DG, Rosenzweig W, Wilson CB: Hyperprolactinemia in a patient with a pituitary and an ovarian dermoid tumor: case report, *Neurosurgery* 26:335, 1990.
161. Kucharczyk W, Peck WW, Kelly WM et al: Rathke cleft cysts: CT, MR imaging, and pathologic features, *Radiology* 165:491, 1987.
162. Lee BCP, Deck MDF: Sellar and juxtasellar lesions detection with MR, *Radiology* 157:143, 1985.
163. Matsushima T, Fukui M, Fujii K: Epithelial cells in symptomatic Rathke's cleft cysts: a light- and electron-microscopic study, *Surg Neurol* 30:197, 1988.
164. Yoshida J, Kobayashi T, Kageyama N, Kanzaki M: Symptomatic Rathke's cleft cyst: morphological study with light and electron microscopy and tissue culture, *J Neurosurg* 47:451, 1977.

61 Thyroid Gland

Maria L. Carcangiu
Ronald A. DeLellis

THE NORMAL THYROID GLAND

The thyroid gland is unique among endocrine organs in many ways. It is the largest of all endocrine glands, and because of its superficial location, it is the only one that is amenable to direct physical examination and biopsy. Diseases of the thyroid, including a vast array of developmental, inflammatory, hyperplastic, and neoplastic disorders, are exceedingly common in clinical practice. The understanding of these diseases is greatly facilitated by an understanding of normal thyroid anatomy and physiology, which is briefly reviewed.

Embryology

The thyroid median anlage develops from the endoderm of the pharyngeal floor as a medial invagination that rapidly proliferates caudally, remaining connected with the oral cavity through a thin channel, the thyroglossal duct, which is later obliterated. Remnants of the thyroglossal duct are identifiable as the pyramidal lobe in approximately 40% of adults.[1-5] The thyroid precursor proliferates as a hollow vesicular structure, which later becomes solid, possessing two lateral protuberances that become the two lobes of the adult thyroid gland. Although most of the thyroid parenchyma originates from this medial pharyngeal precursor, the ultimobranchial body, which is derived from the fourth and fifth pharyngeal complex, partially contributes to the formation of the developing gland.[6] Parafollicular cells (C-cells) and solid cell nests originate from this structure, and the so-called lateral thyroids are also believed to be derived from it.[5,7-9] The C-cells, which are derived proximately from the neural crest, migrate to the ultimobranchial bodies before they are incorporated into the developing thyroid gland.[10,11]

As the fetal thyroid gland develops, the endodermal cells rapidly replicate, forming cords and trabeculas that later transform into follicular structures. A finely granular material collects within these primitive follicles and later acquires the features of colloid. The fetal thyroid gland develops rapidly until the fourth month (crown-rump length, 18 mm). Subsequently the thyroid growth rate parallels that of the body, reaching the normal adult weight (average, 15-35 g) at approximately 15 years of age.

Anatomy

The thyroid has a shape reminiscent of a butterfly, consisting of two bulky lateral lobes (average dimension, 4-5 × 2 cm) connected by a relatively thin isthmus. Occasionally the isthmus may be absent. A thin, delicate capsule invests the gland. From this capsule, numerous stromal septa of various thickness penetrate the thyroid parenchyma, irregularly dividing it into lobules. Each lobule consists of approximately twenty to forty individual follicles. The superior and inferior thyroid arteries, originating from the external carotid artery, provide the blood supply. The superior and middle thyroid veins collect the blood from the thyroid gland and transport it into the external jugular vein; the inferior thyroid vein drains into the brachiocephalic vein. The thyroid gland is richly supplied with lymphatic vessels. Those draining the superior portion of the thyroid and isthmus collect into the internal jugular lymph nodes; those draining the inferior portion of the thyroid collect into the pretracheal and paratracheal lymph nodes (the pretracheal lymph node situated close to the isthmus is also known as the *delphian node*).

Histology

The follicle represents the morphologic unit responsible for the endocrine function of the gland. It is spherical to ovoid and measures approximately 200 μm in diameter. It contains a proteinaceous material known as *colloid* and is lined by a single layer of epithelial cells resting on a well-defined basement

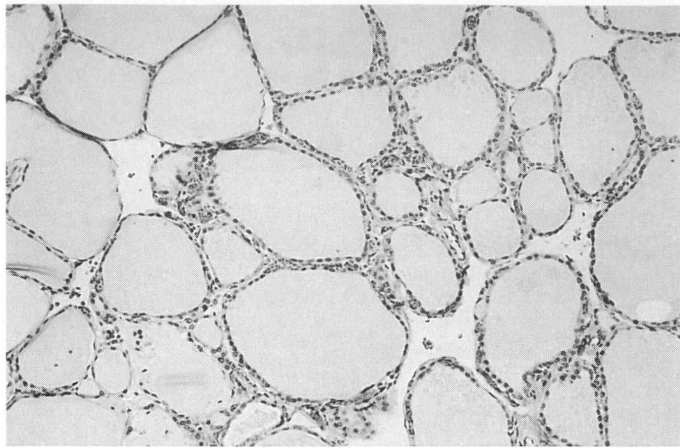

Fig. 61-1 Normal adult thyroid gland. Follicles of various size and shape are lined by a flattened epithelium. The lumen of the follicles contains colloid.

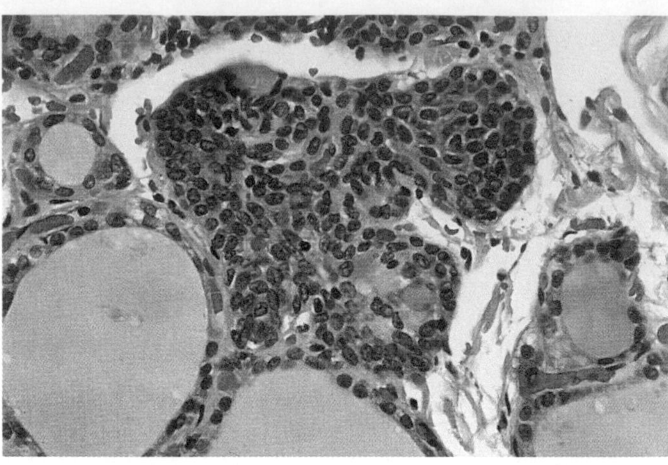

Fig. 61-2 Solid cell nest in normal adult thyroid gland. The nest is present in the interstitium of the gland and is composed of relatively small cells with round to ovoid nuclei.

membrane (Fig. 61-1). The size of the follicles, the morphologic features of the follicular epithelium, and the staining quality of the colloid change according to the functional activity of the gland. The epithelium is flattened in inactive thyroid glands, cuboidal in normally active glands, and tall and cylindrical in conditions associated with a high functional activity. The colloid is scanty in hyperfunction-ing glands, but it is dense, homogeneous, and intensely eosinophilic in hypoactivie glands. Calcium oxalate crystals seen in the colloid are more often associated with thyroid hypofunction, particularly in elderly persons.[12] Ultrastructurally the follicular cells show an abundant granular endoplasmic reticulum, a well-developed Golgi apparatus, numerous lysosomes (the number of which changes according to the functional activity of the cell), and numerous apical microvilli. Well-developed desmosomes are present, particularly on the sides of the cells near the luminal surface.[13]

Some thyroid conditions are characterized by the presence of large follicular cells with abundant eosinophilic granular cytoplasm and chromatin-rich nuclei. These cells are called *oncocytes,* or *Hürthle cells,* and represent modified forms of follicular cells that are particularly rich in mitochondria and oxidative enzymes.

Immunohistochemically both the colloid and the cytoplasm of follicular cells stain positively for thyroglobulin (with both monoclonal and polyclonal antibodies), triiodothyronine (T_3), and thyroxine (T_4), but oncocytes stain weakly for these products.[14-17] Follicular cells are also positive for keratin (low molecular weight), epithelial membrane antigen, and vimentin.[16-18] Estrogen and progesterone receptors are also detectable in some cells.[19]

The accumulation of melanin-like pigment in the cytoplasm of the follicular cells may result in a grossly *black thyroid;* this phenomenon is particularly common in patients who have been treated with tetracycline antibiotics[20,21] (such as minocycline).

Solid cell nests, which are most commonly found along the central axes of the middle and upper thirds of the lateral lobes, represent remnants of the ultimobranchial bodies. Most measure 0.1 mm in diameter, but occasional solid cell nests may measure up to 2 mm[22] (Fig. 61-2). They are composed of oval to polygonal cells with elongate nuclei containing finely granular chromatin. The cells contain low-molecular-weight cytokeratins, and occasional cells within the nests stain positively for thyroglobulin or calcitonin.[11] Solid cell nests are found in 3% of routinely examined thyroid glands and in 61% of glands that have been blocked serially at intervals of 2 to 3 mm.[22]

Thyroid follicular epithelium can undergo *squamous metaplasia.*[23] In addition, islands of *mature cartilage* (presumably derived from the branchial pouch), *skeletal muscle,* or *adipose tissue* can be identified within the thyroid parenchyma.[24] Occasionally, parathyroid glands can be located entirely within the substance of the thyroid.

C-cells. C-cells represent the second endocrine compartment of the thyroid. They are difficult to identify in hematoxylin and eosin–stained sections of normal adult thyroid gland. Although they can be stained selectively with some histochemical methods (for example, the Grimelius technique), immunohistochemical methods employing antibodies to calcitonin yield the most consistent and reproducible results[25,26] (Fig. 61-3). C-cells in the normal fetal and adult glands are concentrated in the middle to upper thirds of the lateral lobes, primarily along their central axes.[26] C-cells are considerably more numerous in the glands of neonates than in those of adults. Generally the thyroids of adults contain up to 50 C-cells per single low-power field.[27] Occasional normal adult glands, particularly in older persons, may also contain large C-cell nodules.[28] The presence of such nodules may reflect partial failure of embryonic C-cell migration and dispersion within the gland.

C-cells reside exclusively within thyroid follicles[26] (Fig. 61-3). The cells, which vary from being round to spindle shaped, are separated from the thyroid interstitium by the follicular basal lamina and from the luminal colloid by the overlying follicular cells. Occasional C-cells may have prominent cytoplasmic processes that extend beneath the adjacent follicular cells. Ultrastructurally, C-cells contain variable numbers of secretory granules that range from 60 to 550 nm in diameter.[29] The type I granules have an average diameter of 280 nm and moderately electron-dense, finely granular contents that are closely applied to the limiting membranes of the granules. Type II granules have an average diameter of 130 nm and

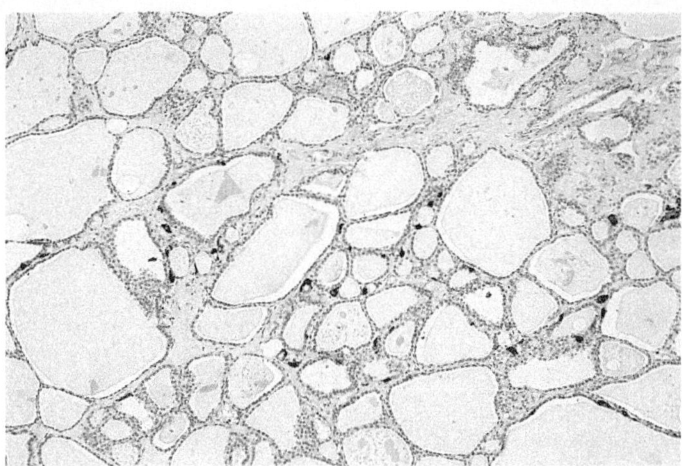

Fig. 61-3 C-cells in normal adult thyroid gland. This section was stained with antibodies to calcitonin combined with the peroxidase-antiperoxidase technique. C-cells are present exclusively within follicles.

more electron-dense contents that are separated from the limiting membranes by a narrow electron-lucent space.[29] Other granule types have also been identified ultrastructurally.

C-cells contain a variety of products that reflect their neuroendocrine phenotype, including neuron-specific enolase, chromogranin, and synaptophysin.[30] They show no neurofilament proteins but typically contain low-molecular-weight cytokeratins.

Physiology of follicular cells

The main function of the thyroid gland is the production of thyroid hormones, the most important of which are T_4 and T_3. The major functions of these hormones are to regulate the intermediate metabolism of carbohydrates and proteins and the consumption of oxygen.[31-33] The activity of the thyroid hormones is necessary for the normal development of the central nervous system: a reduction in or absence of these hormones in the first years of life results in irreversible mental retardation (cretinism). Body development and bone maturation also depend on the activity of thyroid hormones; however, after the first 2 years of life the body can compensate for a sharp reduction or absence of thyroid hormone levels by making complex hormonal readjustments. Steps in the biosynthesis of thyroid hormones include the ingestion of iodine present in water and food, the concentration of iodide within the thyroid, and the organification of iodide to iodine. This last step depends on the action of iodide peroxidase, which oxidates the iodide ion to a highly reactive form of iodine that in turn binds to tyrosine. The result is monoiodotyrosine (MIT) when one iodine molecule is attached or diiodotyrosine (DIT) when two iodine molecules are attached.[34] The iodotyrosine residues are condensed to form the biologically active thyroid hormones, T_4 and T_3. T_4 results from the coupling of two molecules of DIT and T_3 from the coupling of one molecule of MIT with a molecule of DIT.[35]

Thyroid hormones are stored as thyroglobulin, a large protein with numerous iodinated tyrosine residues, including the biologically active T_4 and T_3. Thyroglobulin is collected at the center of the thyroid follicles and is the main constituent of colloid. When the gland is activated by thyroid-stimulating hormone (TSH) to release thyroid hormones, the endocytosis of colloid and proteolysis of thyroglobulin by lysosomal enzymes occur.[35] T_3 and T_4 diffuse into the bloodstream, where they are transported primarily by the specific carrier protein T_4-binding globulin. This globulin normally transports more than 70% of T_3 and T_4. Approximately 20% of the circulating T_3 and T_4 is carried by transthyretin (prealbumin) and albumin.[36] Only a small proportion of circulating thyroid hormones (approximately 0.05% of T_3 and 0.015% of T_4) is unbound and therefore biologically active. Free, circulating, biologically active T_3 and T_4 are in equilibrium with the hormones bound to the carrier proteins. The amount of circulating T_4 is much greater than that of T_3; however, T_3 is about four times more active biologically, and as a result the final contribution of T_3 to the biologic activity of thyroid hormones equals that of T_4.[37]

Thyroid biosynthetic and secretory activities are controlled by TSH, a glycoprotein synthesized and secreted by the anterior pituitary gland. TSH binds to a specific receptor located on the external surface of follicular thyroid cells and regulates the complex mechanism responsible for T_3 and T_4 synthesis and release by activating the adenylate cyclase pathway.[38] TSH release is in turn regulated by a tripeptide secreted by the hypothalamus, thyrotropin-releasing hormone (TRH). TSH and TRH release are regulated by the circulating levels of free T_3 and T_4 by means of a negative-feedback on the pituitary and hypothalamus: low levels of free T_3 and T_4 stimulate the release of TSH and TRH. In contrast, TSH and TRH release are inhibited by high levels of circulating free T_3 and T_4[38-41] (Fig. 61-4).

Physiology of C-cells

Calcitonin is a 32–amino acid peptide that is released from the thyroid when the plasma calcium levels are increased.[42] When it is administered to experimental animals with a high bone turnover or to patients with Paget's disease, the plasma calcium levels decline. This effect is mediated by the inhibition of osteoclastic activity. Calcitonin also acts in the kidney to enhance the production of vitamin D. The major physiologic role of calcitonin is to protect the skeleton during periods of calcium stress such as during growth, pregnancy, and lactation.[42] The absence of calcitonin is not associated with hypercalcemia, but high levels of the hormone do not precipitate hypocalcemia. Calcium is a potent stimulator of calcitonin secretion. In addition, both gastrin and cholecystokinin act as calcitonin secretagogues, as does estrogen when administered long term.

The calcitonin gene is located on the short arm of chromosome 11 and consists of six exons that encode katacalcin (C-terminal flanking peptide) and the calcitonin gene–related peptide (CGRP).[42,43] The primary transcript of the calcitonin gene gives rise to two different messenger RNAs (mRNAS) by tissue-specific alternative splicing events, leading to the production of calcitonin and CGRP mRNAs. The calcitonin-CGRP gene is expressed both in thyroid and nervous tissues, but calcitonin is produced in large quantities only in the thyroid. Katacalcin is a 21–amino acid peptide that is cosecreted with calcitonin, but its function is unknown. CGRP is a 37–amino acid peptide that is a potent vasodilator and that also functions as a neuromodulator or neurotransmitter.[42]

Basal calcitonin levels in normal male adults range from 3 to 36 pg/ml (0.9 to 0.5 pmol/L), whereas levels in female adults range from 3 to 17 pg/ml (0.9 to 5.0 pmol/L). Stimu-

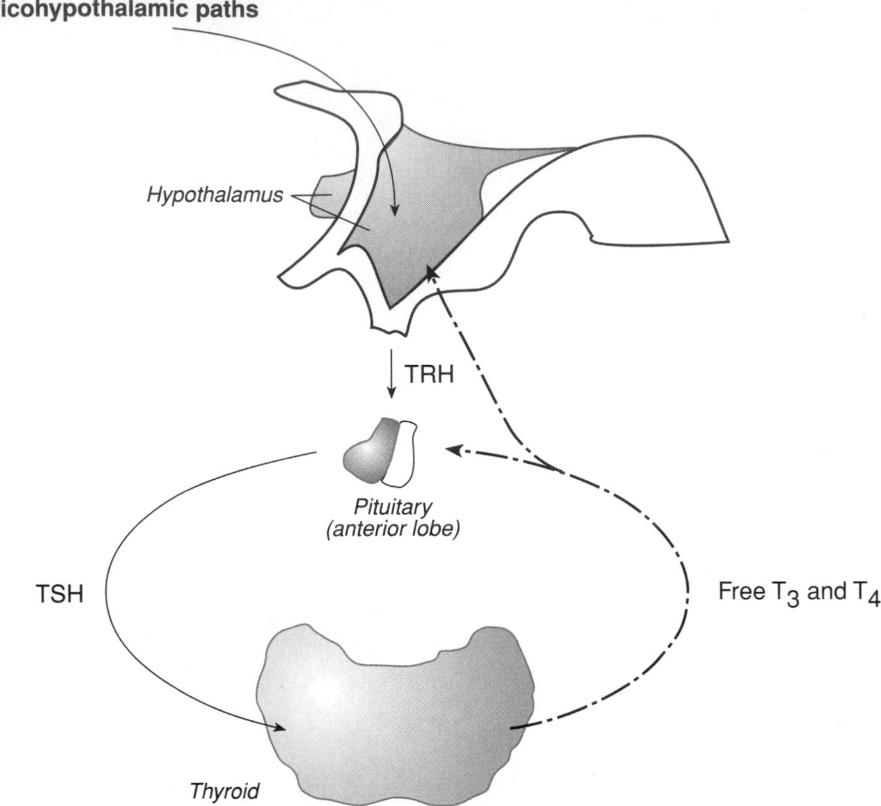

Fig. 61-4 Homeostatic regulation of thyroid function. Thyroid secretory activity is controlled by the level of thyroid-stimulating hormone *(TSH)*. TSH release is in turn regulated by the thyrotropin-releasing hormone *(TRH)*. Both TSH and TRH release are regulated by a negative-feedback mechanism acting on the pituitary and hypothalamus and the degree of release is inversely related to the amount of free triiodothyronine *(T_3)* and thyroxine *(T_4)* in the blood.

lated calcitonin levels (after the administration of pentagastrin) are less than 106 pg/ml (30.9 pmol/L) in men and less than 29 pg/ml (8.5 pmol/L) in women.[42]

In addition to calcitonin, the C-cells also contain a variety of other peptides, including somatostatin[44] and gastrin-releasing peptide.[45] C-cells also contain a variety of biologically active amines, including serotonin.[46] In some species C-cells also contain TRH.[47]

CONGENITAL ABNORMALITIES

The most serious congenital abnormality of the thyroid gland is total agenesis or aplasia of the thyroid.[48] This is a rare event and occurs in 1 in 4000 newborns. It represents the most frequent cause of cretinism in nongoitrogenous areas.[49] Of lesser clinical significance is *partial thyroid agenesis,* or simple hypoplasia, which generally results from absent or defective downward migration of the medial anlage from which the thyroid originates.[50-52] The persistence of residual thyroid tissue at the base of the tongue or along the thyroglossal duct is also a consequence of the faulty downward migration of the medial anlage.[53-55] *Lingual thyroid glands,* which are sometimes quite large, may be associated with a fully developed thyroid gland or with a complete absence of thyroid tissue in its normal anatomic location. Carcinomas in lingual thyroid glands have been encountered and are an exceptional occurrence.[56] *Accessory* or *aberrant thyroid glands* can also be found as small nodules in the neck region (in a median or lateral location), the submandibular region, larynx, trachea, mediastinum (more frequently in a retrosternal location and rarely in the pericardial region or in the heart), or in unusual locations (such as the porta hepatis and gallbladder).[57-62]

The rare occurrence of small islands of thyroid tissue within cervical lymph nodes can create differential diagnostic problems with the much more frequent lymph node metastases from clinically occult thyroid carcinomas.[63]

When the ultimobranchial body remnants fail to fuse to the median thyroid, nests of *solid- and cystic-squamous–appearing cells associated with lymphocytes* may also be found in the neck.[64-66]

Another important thyroid malformation is the *thyroglossal duct cyst.*[67,68] This cystic structure is mostly found in children but may be encountered in adults and the elderly as well. It arises from small segments of the thyroglossal ducts that failed to regress.[69] It is often small and is usually located medially in the neck, but sometimes it can become quite large when a large amount of fluid collects within its lumen or when inflammation occurs. Proximally located cysts are usually lined by squamous epithelium, whereas those located distally tend to be lined by columnar epithelium. The clinical relevance of these remnants depends on whether inflammation occurs, which can be acute (with abscess formation) or chronic. Chronic inflammation and scarring can result in the formation of sinus tracts. Infrequently, papillary carcinomas can develop from these remnants.[70-73]

Congenital abnormalities of the thyroid C-cells are rare. C-cells were reported as missing from the thyroid glands of patients with DiGeorge syndrome (thymic and parathyroid hypoplasia/aplasia, type B interrupted aortic arch, truncus arteriosus, and tetralogy of Fallot), as would be expected if these cells were derived exclusively from the cephalic neural crest. More recent studies, however, have indicated that the numbers of C-cells are reduced rather than absent even from patients with complete forms of the syndrome.[74,75] These observations imply that some thyroid C-cells may develop from sites other than the neural crest.

THYROIDITIS

Thyroiditis encompasses a group of disorders that include not only processes of clearcut inflammatory nature but also lesions of uncertain significance, in which sclerosis and lymphocytic infiltrates are the most relevant pathologic findings. An ideal classification of thyroiditides would require identification of either a distinctive morphologic appearance or a known cause. Because such criteria are often lacking, the commonly employed classification represents an odd combination of etiologic, clinical, morphologic, and even eponymic designations.

Acute thyroiditis

Acute thyroiditis is rare, probably because the thyroid gland is relatively resistant to the common bacterial or fungal infections.[76] The organisms most frequently responsible are *Staphylococcus aureus, Streptococcus pyogenes,* and *Streptococcus pneumoniae.* Thyroid involvement nearly always stems from the spread of an infectious process involving the oropharyngeal cavity or salivary glands. Rare cases of thyroiditis resulting from *Pneumocystis carinii,* cytomegalovirus, or fungi have been observed in immunodeficient patients.[77-79] Clinically, local inflammatory symptoms (pain, edema, enlargement of the gland, and abscess formation) may be associated with general symptoms and sepsis. Morphologically, acute thyroiditis is traditionally divided into suppurative and nonsuppurative forms. The suppurative form often follows inflammation and abscess formation in the piriform sinus tract.[80] Among the noninfectious acute thyroiditides of known cause are those resulting from radiation therapy. They present with a clinical picture similar to that of infectious thyroiditis, but the symptoms are usually milder and the disease is self-limited.[81]

Subacute (granulomatous) thyroiditis

"De Quervain's thyroiditis," "granulomatous thyroiditis," "pseudotuberculous thryroiditis," and "giant cell thyroiditis" are some of the synonyms used in the past for this form of thyroiditis. The available data, though inconclusive, point to a viral cause.[76] Subacute thyroiditis is often preceded by an inflammatory process involving the upper airways and is characterized clinically by fever and general symptoms of the type encountered in viral infections. In addition, its occurrence is often associated with outbreaks of viral diseases and increasing antibody titers against a variety of viral antigens (mumps, measles, rhinoviruses, and adenovirus) have been documented in approximately 50% of the patients.[82,83] The very clinical course of subacute thyroiditis, which is unresponsive to antibiotic treatment and which is characterized by spontaneous resolution of symptoms within several weeks or a few months, also seems to favor a viral cause. The immunologic findings are usually inconsequential, but circulating autoantibodies against the TSH receptor have been detected in a limited number of patients.[83] However, these do not correlate with clinical symptoms and tend to persist long after the process has resolved. There is no association between subacute thyroiditis and thyroid diseases in which autoimmune phenomena are known to play a major role, such as Hashimoto's thyroiditis and Graves' disease. It therefore appears likely that the presence of autoantibodies in patients with subacute thyroiditis simply reflects the presence of tissue damage to thyroid epithelium, a damage that probably stems from direct viral infection of the gland.[76] The association between subacute thyroiditis and HLA-Bw35 in a high percentage of patients supports a genetic predisposition to this disease.[84]

Clinical features. Subacute thyroiditis occurs most often in middle-aged women and is characterized by a sudden, often painful enlargement of the gland, up to two to three times its normal size. Local symptoms are accompanied by low-grade fever, malaise, weakness, and other general symptoms. Inflammation of the thyroid gland and damage to the follicular epithelium may trigger an increased release of thyroid hormones, resulting in moderate hyperthyroidism. Physical examination reveals fever, tachycardia, and an enlarged and more firm thyroid gland that is painful to palpation. Thyroid enlargement is characteristically asymmetric, even if the entire gland is involved.

Pathology. Grossly the thyroid is diffusely but irregularly enlarged; it is more nodular and adhers to the adjacent structures. The cut surface has a somewhat typical appearance: the most affected areas are yellow-white and raised against the red-brown background of the noninvolved thyroid parenchyma.

Histologically the intensity of the inflammatory process varies in different areas of the gland depending on the stage of the disease. Early on there is focal involvement with disruption of follicles, the infiltration of polymorphonuclear granulocytes in the follicular lumen, and microabscess formation. In later stages there are collections of macrophages, epithelioid cells, and Langhans type of giant cells that are actively phagocytosing colloid (Fig 61 5). With time these inflammatory cells replace the damaged follicles, resulting in granuloma for-

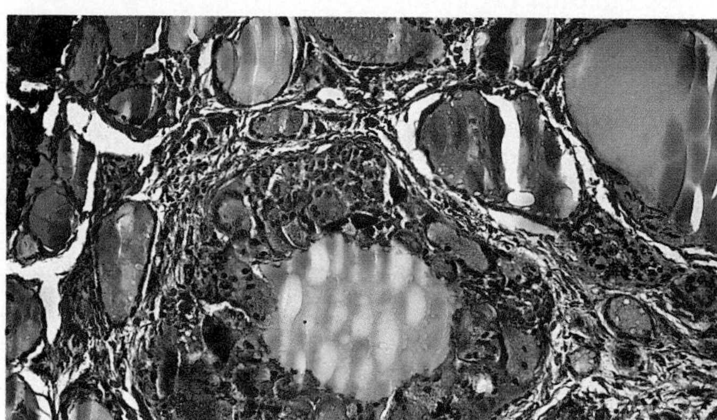

Fig. 61-5 Subacute (granulomatous) thyroiditis. Multinucleated giant cells surround residual colloid in a follicle.

mation with giant cells. The latter morphologic appearance has been emphasized in some of the older designations of subacute thyroiditis, that is, "giant cell thyroiditis" and "granulomatous thyroiditis." The final stages are characterized by the deposition of collagen, particularly in areas where there is more extensive tissue destruction. Areas in different stages of evolution often coexist in the same gland. Results of immunohistochemical studies support the view that the giant cells, at least in part, are derived from the follicular epithelium.

Other granulomatous inflammations

Palpation thyroiditis is the term coined by Carney and colleagues[85] to describe a peculiar histologic appearance of thyroid glands that have been excised for a variety of causes but which has no apparent clinical significance.[85] The findings consist of lymphocytes, histiocytes (some foamy), and a few multinucleated giant cells that have replaced the epithelium of small groups of scattered thyroid follicles, infiltrated into the adjacent parenchyma, and formed granulomatous lesions. This condition (also known as *multifocal granulomatous folliculitis*) is relatively common in surgically removed thyroids (40% of the cases in Carney's series) but less so in autopsy material, supporting the view that it is the result of vigorous palpation of the gland before surgical excision.[86]

Tuberculosis can involve the thyroid gland in the form of multiple granulomas. Although now rare, it is likely to occur with increased frequency because of the recent epidemics of tuberculosis refractory to conventional antibiotic treatment.[87] *Tertiary syphilis* is another extremely rare cause of granulomatous thyroiditis.[88] *Fungal infection* can involve the thyroid gland, particularly in immunocompromised patients, and cause the formation of granulomas.[89]

Autoimmune thyroiditis

Autoimmune thyroiditis, a term with pathogenetic implications, refers to Hashimoto's thyroiditis and its variants and to other closely related immunologically mediated disorders of the thyroid. Common features include goiter, a lymphocytic infiltrate in the gland, and the production of antibodies to a variety of thyroidal antigens. It is likely that most of the autoimmune processes involving the thyroid are interrelated and that their morphologic and clinical diversities are a function of the stage of the disorder or of the predominance of one feature over another.[90-92]

Hashimoto's thyroiditis

Hashimoto's thyroiditis, the most common form of autoimmune thyroiditis, was originally reported by the Japanese ophthalmologist Hashimoto in 1912 who coined the term *struma lymphomatosa* to incorporate its main features: enlargement of the gland ("struma") and prominent and widespread lymphocytic infiltrates.[93]

Clinical features. Classic Hashimoto's thyroiditis is considerably more common in women than in men, with a female-to-male ratio of 8-10: 1. The disease arises most commonly in patients between 30 and 50 years of age. The clinical picture is dominated by painless enlargement of the thyroid, which is sometimes accompanied by dysphagia and pressure symptoms resulting from goiter. There are generally no systemic symptoms. During the initial phases of the disease, most patients are euthyroid, but as the disease progresses, hypothyroidism of varying severity supervenes. As a matter of fact, Hashimoto's disease constitutes the most common cause of goitrous hypothyroidism in adults. Occasionally, hyperthyroidism, so-called *hashitoxicosis,* may develop. This association is more than coincidental because there are many similarities in the autoimmune phenomena that characterize both Hashimoto's thyroiditis and Graves' disease.

Pathogenesis. Hashimoto's thyroiditis is a prototypic autoimmune disorder, and both humoral and cell-mediated mechanisms have been implicated in its pathogenesis.[94] Autoimmune thyroiditis may develop as a result of a genetically determined dysfunction in antigen-specific suppressor T-cells. As a result there is an uncontrolled attack on follicular cells by cytotoxic T-cells. Concurrently, unregulated helper T-cell function results in the formation of autoantibodies by B-cells. Antibodies to thyroglobulin and thyroid peroxidase (antimicrosomal antibodies) have been identified in the serum of varying proportions of patients with Hashimoto's disease. There are several lines of evidence that suggest a possible role for complement-fixing antibodies against thyroid peroxidase in mediating cell injury of the follicular cells. Antibodies to thyroglobulin are capable of mediating antibody-dependent, cell-mediated cytotoxicity and could have a role in the development of the disease.[95] Antibodies to the TSH receptor have been detected in 10% to 15% of patients with Hashimoto's thyroiditis but are primarily TSH–receptor blocking antibodies.

The incidence of other autoimmune diseases, including Graves' disease, Sjögren's disease, lupus erythematosus, and rheumatoid arthritis, is increased in patients with Hashimoto's thyroiditis or members of their families. These data indicate genetic influence may also be involved in the development of this type of thyroiditis.[76] Involvement of the adrenal gland (lymphocytic adrenalitis) in the presence of Hashimoto's thyroiditis is referred to as *Schmidt's syndrome.*[96] The lymphocytic infiltration of other organs such as the lung has also been reported.[97]

Pathology. Grossly the thyroid may be three or four times its normal size and may reach a weight of 200 g or more. The enlargement is usually symmetrical, but in some instances it may have a nodular quality, with one lobe being substantially larger than the other. It is firm or rubbery but never stony hard as in Riedel's disease. The cut surface is smooth or vaguely lobulated, and uniformly gray or pale yellow, and it closely resembles that of a hyperplastic lymph node (Fig. 61-6, *A*). The capsule is thin and unaltered and does not adhere to the contiguous structures as in Riedel's thyroiditis.

Histologically the dominant feature is a massive lympho plasmacytic infiltration of the thyroid parenchyma. Lymphoid follicles with germinal centers are usually present. The number of thyroid follicles is decreased and the remaining ones are usually small and atrophic. The follicular epithelium shows a widespread oncocytic change (Fig. 61-6, *B* and *C*). This combination of numerous lymphocytes and oncocytes is important for the cytologic diagnosis of this disorder in fine-needle aspiration material. Rarely the follicular epithelium may undergo hyperplastic changes, sometimes of a nodular type, creating difficulties in differentiating the condition from papillary carcinoma. The follicular epithelium may also undergo squamous metaplasia. The follicular cells in patients with Hashimoto's thyroiditis, even in the absence of squamous metaplasia, show a stronger reactivity with antibodies to high-molecular-weight keratins than that displayed by normal follicular epithelium. The cells are also positive for thyroglobulin, S-100 protein, HLA-DR, and *N*-acetyl-α-D-galatosamine.[98]

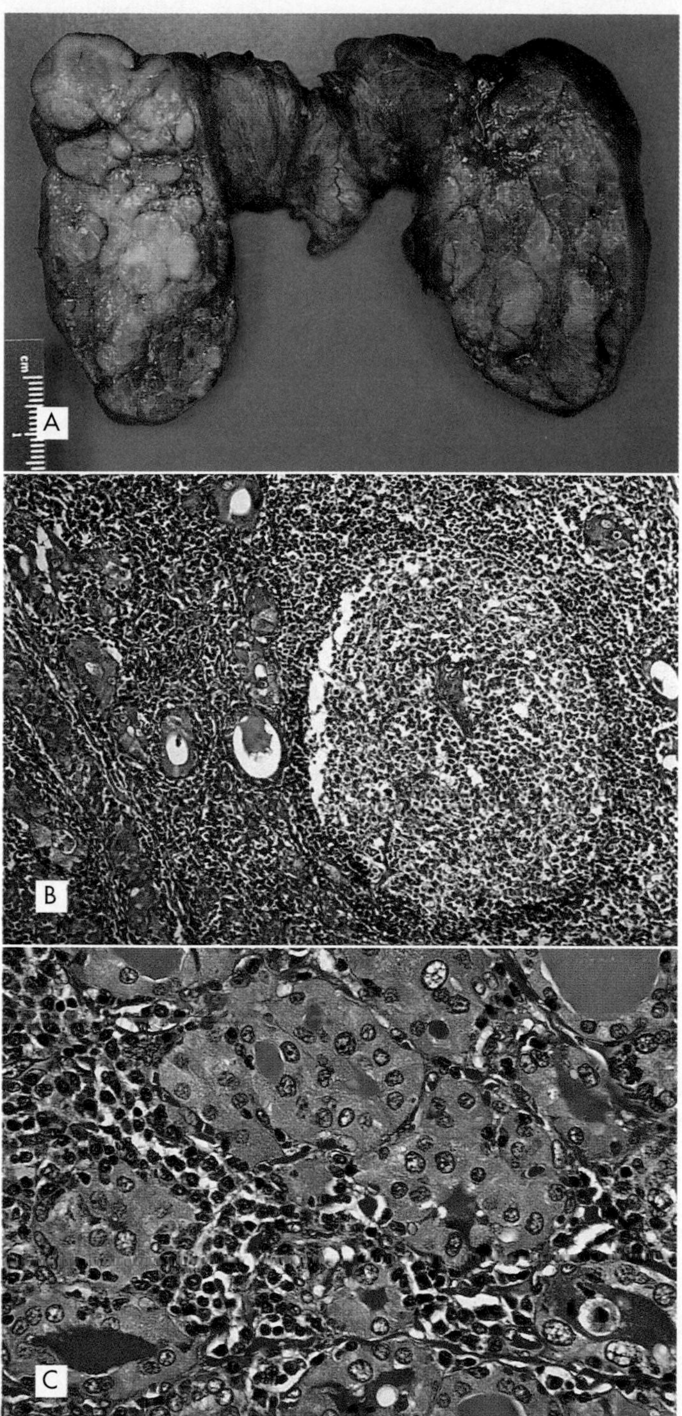

Fig. 61-6 Hashimoto's thyroiditis. **A,** Gross appearance. The thyroid is enlarged and on cut section shows a multinodular white appearance stemming from the replacement of the parenchyma by lymphocytes. **B** and **C,** Microscopic appearance. Pronounced lymphocytic infiltration with germinal center formation and oncocytic change of the follicular epithelium. At higher power the oncocytic cells show nuclei of various sizes with a vesicular appearance.

The risk of malignant neoplasms, particularly malignant lymphoma and leukemia, is increased in patients with Hashimoto's thyroiditis.[99,100]

Hashimoto's thyroiditis may spontaneously remit, particularly in children. The standard treatment includes the administration of synthetic thyroid hormone, with the dosage determined by the serum TSH levels. Surgical excision may become necessary if the goiter causes compression symptoms when the gland becomes unduly large or if a malignant tumor is suspected.[101]

Variants of Hashimoto's thyroiditis

The *fibrous variant* of Hashimoto's thyroiditis, which constitutes approximately 10% of the cases, is characterized by a prominent fibrosis that extensively replaces the thyroid parenchyma. Frequently there is also squamous metaplasia of the residual follicles and an inflammatory infiltrate predominantly made up of plasma cells. Grossly the thyroid is considerably enlarged and has a firm consistency. Clinically, compression symptoms, high titers of antithyroglobulin and antimicrosomal antibodies, and hypothyroidism are the rule.

It has been suggested that fibrous Hashimoto's thyroiditis bears some relation to the so-called *atrophic thyroiditis* (idiopathic myxedema).[102] Both conditions are more common in older persons, are associated with hypothyroidism, and involve elevated titers of antimicrosomal and antithyroglobulin antibodies. The main difference is that the fibrous variant of Hashimoto's thyroiditis is associated with goiter, as unlike the atrophy of the gland that occurs in atrophic thyroiditis. In the latter condition, thyroid growth-blocking antibodies may be responsible for the failure of the follicular epithelium to regenerate.[86,103-107]

Juvenile thyroiditis, which is more common in children and young women, is considered a variant of Hashimoto's thyroiditis.[108] The thyroid in this disorder is usually only slightly enlarged, and the patients are euthyroid with low titers of thyroid antibodies.[109] Histologically the main difference between this thyroiditis and typical Hashimoto's thyroiditis is the absence of prominent oncocytic changes of follicular cells. The epithelium may instead show focal hyperplasia.

Closely related to juvenile thyroiditis is the so-called *painless thyroiditis.* The different terms proposed for this form of thyroiditis reflect its clinical and morphologic features, and include *silent thyroiditis, indolent thyroiditis, lymphocytic thyroiditis, subacute thyroiditis, hyperthyroiditis,* and *self-resolving lymphocytic thyroiditis with hyperthyroidism.*[110-113] The cause is unknown, but the features of the lesion, laboratory data (high prevalence of autoantibodies in the serum), its association with other autoimmune diseases, and the familial clustering of the cases (increased frequency in association with HLA-DR3 and HLA-DR5) all point to an autoimmune pathogenesis.[114-117] At least two thirds of the reported cases occur in women, most commonly in the first months post partum. There is, however, a significant variability in the number of cases reported from different countries.[118-121] Clinically it differs from subacute thyroiditis in that there is no local pain, the symptoms are milder and there is a moderate, transient hyperthyroidism (less than 3 months' maximal duration). The thyroid may be normal or slightly enlarged. In approximately one third of the patients hyperthyroidism is followed by hypothyroidism, which is also transient. Overall the symptoms usually last less than 1 year.[76]

Histologically, painless thyroiditis shares several morphologic features with subacute (granulomatous) thyroiditis, including disruption of the follicular epithelium and fibrosis. However, it differs from it by the fact that there is an absence of giant cells, a more intense lymphocytic infiltrate, an oncocytic change of the thyroid epithelium, and a focal epithelial hyperplasia.[122] It is possible that some of the cases classified in the past as hashitoxicosis would be currently interpreted as painless thyroiditis.[86]

Nonspecific lymphocytic thyroiditis

Nonspecific lymphocytic thyroiditis, also known as *focal lymphocytic thyroiditis* and *simple chronic thyroiditis,* is the most common type of thyroiditis seen in pathologic material. It has been noted at autopsy in up to 40% of thyroids, but racial differences seem to exist.[123] It is more common in women, and because its incidence increases with age, it is believed to be an immunologic disorder associated with aging. Because affected patients have low titers of thyroid autoantibodies in the serum, it has been suggested that the incidence of nonspecific lymphocytic thyroiditis may parallel the presence of thyroid autoantibodies in the general population.[124] Thyroid function is usually not altered in patients with the disorder, and there are no clinical symptoms. Histologically there are focal aggregates of lymphocytes, frequently admixed with plasma cells, but the presence of germinal centers or oncocytic changes of the follicular epithelium are very rare.

Riedel's thyroiditis

Riedel's thyroiditis, a rare disorder described by Riedel in 1896, is characterized by extensive fibrosis replacing the thyroid tissue. *Invasive fibrous thyroiditis, ligneous thyroiditis,* and *struma fibromatosis* are other names for this disorder, which more frequently affects adults (average, 50 years) and shows a predilection for women.[125,126] In a large series from the Mayo Clinic, Riedel's thyroiditis was identified in 0.05% of all thyroidectomy specimens, confirming its extreme rarity.[126] The cause of Riedel's thyroiditis is unknown, but it may represent a manifestation of the group of idiopathic disorders of the connective tissue known as *multifocal idiopathic fibrosclerosis*, which also includes idiopathic retroperitoneal, mediastinal, and retroorbital fibrosis, as well as sclerosing cholangitis.[127,128]

Clinical features. The symptoms of Riedel's thyroiditis are nonspecific, and the diagnosis is suspected when a stone-hard goiter is noticed on palpation. The thyroid appears to be fixed and firmly adherent to adjacent structures in the neck. Compression symptoms may occur, and clinically the process may simulate carcinoma. Unlike subacute (granulomatous) thyroiditis, Riedel's thyroiditis is not preceded by an acute inflammatory process.

Pathology. Grossly, the process may involve the whole thyroid gland or a portion of it. In addition, contiguous structures, most often adjacent muscles, are also involved, in contrast to the behavior of subacute granulomatous thyroiditis and Hashimoto's thyroiditis and its fibrous variant. On cross section, the involved areas appear whitish and show no lobulation but the appearance of the spared areas is normal. Histologically, fibrous tissue, which is frequently extensively hyalinized, is found to replace normal thyroid structures and often invade the adjacent muscle tissue[129] (Fig. 61-7, *A*). The inflammatory infiltrate is focal and is composed predominantly of lymphocytes and plasma cells. Eosinophils may also be present. Characteristically, vasculitis and perivasculitis are present in the medium-sized veins in areas of fibro-

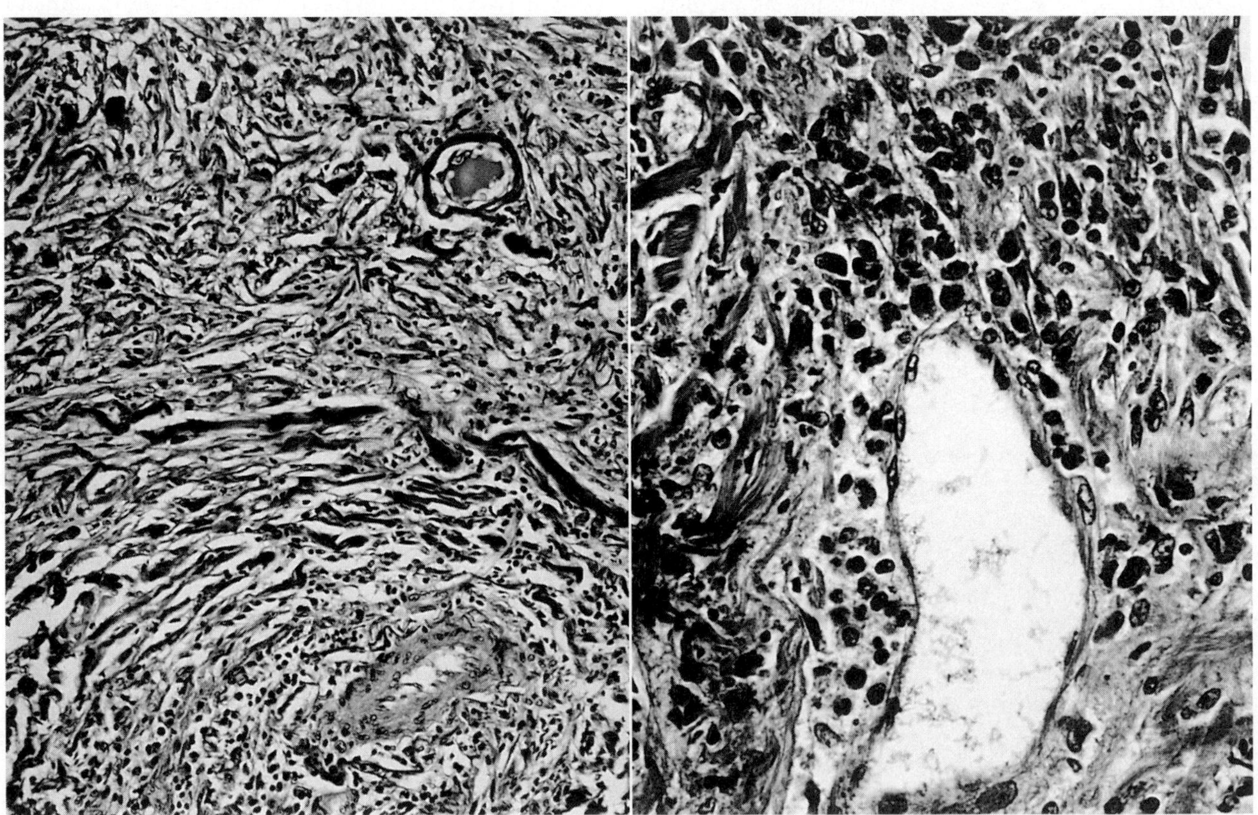

Fig. 61-7 Riedel's thyroiditis. **A,** Diffuse fibrosis and inflammatory cells replace the thyroid parenchyma. **B,** Medium-sized vein involved by vasculitis.

sis[130] (Fig. 61-7, *B*). Histologically, the other main disorder in the differential diagnosis is the fibrous variant of Hashimoto's thyroiditis. In the latter, the gland is firm but not stony hard. Furthermore, the process does not extend outside the thyroid gland; the noninvolved follicles show oncocytic changes and there is no vasculitis. Riedel's and Hashimoto's thyroiditides do not appear to be related despite the occasional coexistence of the two.[131]

GRAVES' DISEASE

Hyperthyroidism refers to any condition in which the body tissues are exposed to supraphysiological concentrations of thyroid hormones. Graves' disease and toxic nodular goiter are the most common causes of hyperthyroidism. Other less frequent causes are "toxic adenoma," inappropriate TSH secretion, trophoblastic tumors, thyroiditis associated with hormone leakage, struma ovarii iatrogenica (e.g., amiodarone-associated thyrotoxicosis). As already mentioned, Graves' disease is currently interpreted to be a manifestation of autoimmune thyroid disease, and as such it is closely related to Hashimoto's thyroiditis. An aggregation of Graves' disease and Hashimoto's thyroiditis in the same families has been found; furthermore, an association with the histocompatibility-type HLA-DR3 and high serum levels of autoantibodies against various thyroid antigens have been demonstrated in both diseases.[132-134] The cause of the autoimmune reaction in both diseases appears to be a genetically induced organ-specific defect in suppressor T-lymphocytes, which is responsible for the excessive production of thyroid antibodies.[135]

Almost all patients with Graves' disease exhibit high serum levels of the so-called thyroid-stimulating antibodies. There is strong evidence that these antibodies, which are IgGs, stimulate thyroid function, mimicking the effect of TSH, by binding to the TSH receptor of the follicular cell surface.[132,135] More specifically growth-stimulating antibodies, a specific class of thyroid-stimulating antibodies, are believed to be responsible for causing the thyroid enlargement in Graves' disease, and the thyroid-stimulating antibodies are believed to be the cause of hyperthyroidism (Fig. 61-8). The fact that antibodies have been detected that can block these thyroid autoantibodies indicates that the histologic and clinical differences between Graves' disease and Hashimoto's thyroiditis may be related to the different expression of these blocking antibodies.

The pathogenesis of Graves' ophthalmopathy and the role of ophthalmogenic immunoglobulins have not yet been defined, but it is likely that the damage to the orbital connective tissue is attributable to an autoimmune process.[132,136]

Clinical features. Graves' disease affects persons of all ages, most often during the third or fourth decade of life, and shows an approximately fivefold preponderance in women. Clinically, patients with the disorder exhibit the typical features of hyperthyroidism and diffuse goiter. In addition, eye symptoms occur in about half the patients. The mildest and

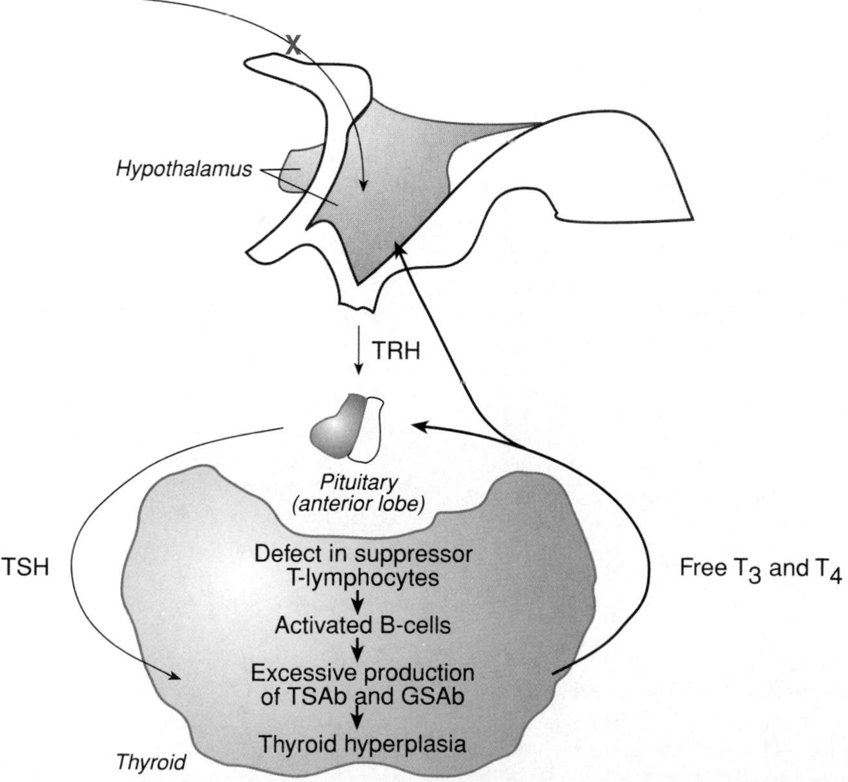

Fig. 61-8 Pathophysiologic mechanism of Graves' disease. A genetically induced organ-specific defect in suppressor T-lymphocytes is responsible for the excessive production of thyroid autoantibodies, that is, thyroid-stimulating antibodies *(TSAb)* and growth-stimulating antibodies *(GSAb),* with consequent enlargement of the thyroid gland and excessive production of triiodothyronine *(T_3)* and thyroxine *(T_4)*. The excess of T_3 and T_4 results in the suppression of thyrotropin-releasing hormone *(TRH)* and thyroid-stimulating hormone *(TSH)* production.

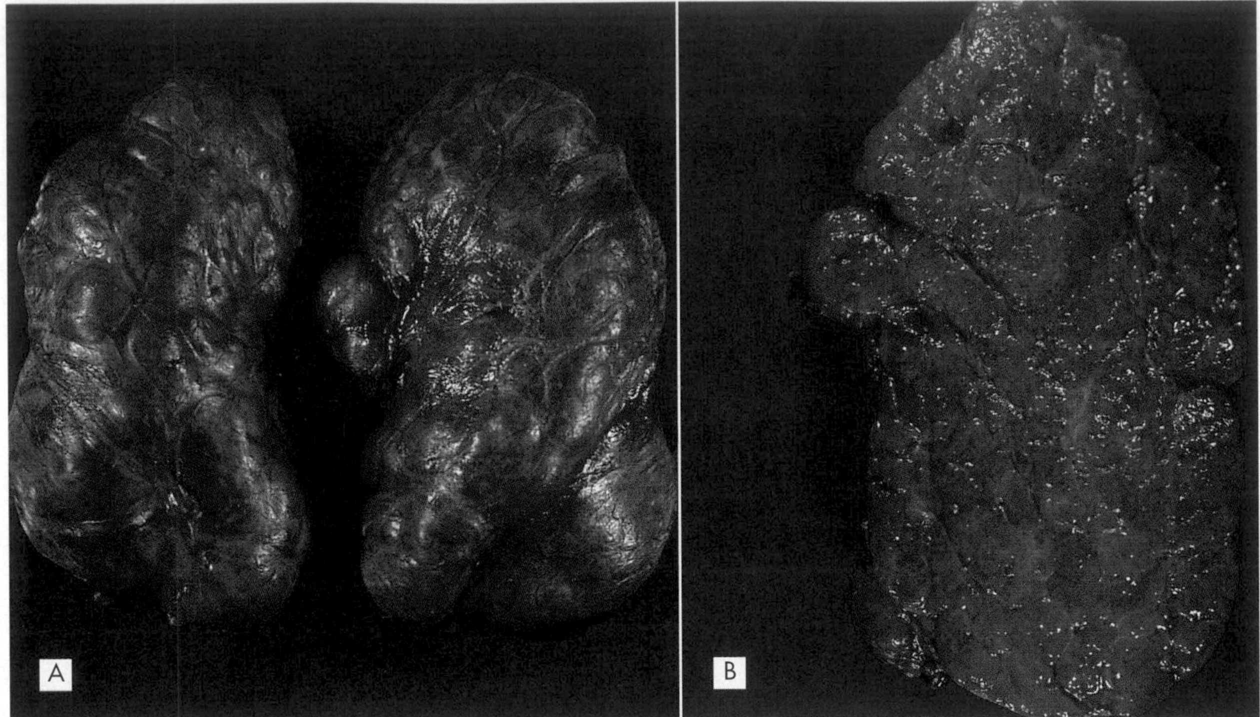

Fig. 61-9 Graves' disease. **A,** The thyroid is moderately and symmetrically enlarged. **B,** On a cut section the surface is homogeneous and hyperemic and the normal colloidal appearance is missing.

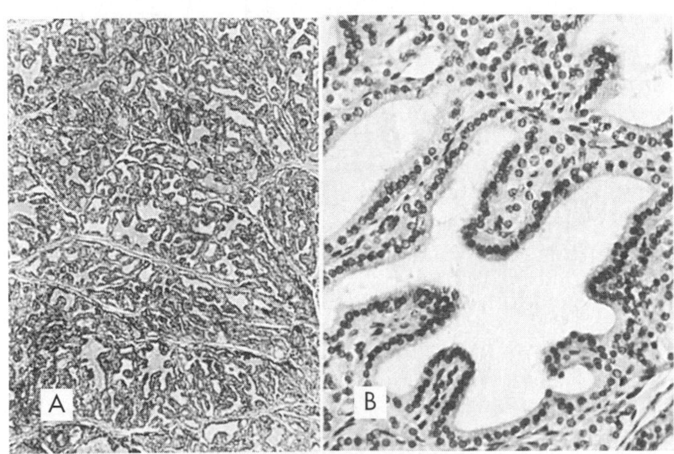

Fig. 61-10 Graves' disease. **A,** Epithelial hyperplasia in Graves' disease. The lobular architecture is preserved; the follicles are small and show papillary infoldings. **B,** Papillary infoldings projecting into the follicles are lined by a columnar epithelium with basally located nuclei and clear cytoplasm.

most common form is exophthalmos; in the most severe forms there is limitation of eye movements and optic nerve damage. Rarely patients may have pretibial myxedema or acropathy (peripheral soft tissue swelling and periosteal changes with clubbing of the fingers and toes).[137]

Pathology. Grossly the gland is moderately and symmetrically enlarged; in most cases it weighs less than 100 g (Fig. 61-9). On cut sections the surface is homogeneous and hyperemic and the normal colloidal appearance is lacking. Histologically the follicles are hyperplastic with papillary infoldings that may be difficult to distinguish from the appearance of papillary carcinoma[138] (Fig. 61-10). The cells are tall and columnar and contain a microvacuolated clear cytoplasm and basally located nuclei. Mitoses may be present. Oncocytic changes of the follicular cells may be seen, indicating a possible evolution toward Hashimoto's thyroiditis. The colloid is pale staining and finely vacuolated and shows prominent peripheral scalloping. The stroma is vascular and sometimes mildly fibrotic, and it frequently contains aggregates of lymphoid cells that form germinal centers. The hyperplastic process may involve follicles outside the thyroid, leading to a pseudoinvasive pattern of growth.

Surgical specimens often do not show the typical hyperplastic features of Graves' disease because nearly all patients have been treated with medications preoperatively. Iodine inhibits thyroid hormone synthesis and release, resulting in thyroid involution together with the accumulation of colloid in the follicles and a decrease in vascularity and follicular cell height.[139] Multiple adenomatous nodules with cystic changes, pronounced eosinophilia and nuclear atypia, and chronic thyroiditis make up the histologic picture of Graves' disease in patients who have undergone iodine therapy.[140] Antithyroid drugs inhibit thyroid hormone synthesis, causing an increase in the TSH level. As a result, the thyroid may become even more hyperplastic, though the patient is often clinically euthyroid.

Exophthalmos is caused by an increase in the volume of extraocular muscles and other orbital tissues. Histologically the extracellular spaces contain increased amounts of glycosaminoglycans, and there is edema and mononuclear inflammatory cells. These changes later progress to fibrosis.[136] In the setting of pretibial myxedema, metachromatic extracellular material is found in deeper layers of the dermis.[141]

A claim has been made that Graves' disease predisposes to the development of thyroid cancer. However, all the cases reported seem to be incidental carcinomas, usually of the papillary type. The 1% to 9% incidence of cancer noted in thyroids removed for Graves' disease[142] does not differ from that noted in glands not affected by thyroiditis.

Besides subtotal thyroidectomy, other treatments for Graves' disease comprise antithyroid drugs such as propylthiouracil, methimazole, and carbimazole as well as destruction of the thyroid with radioactive iodine.[143-146]

OTHER HYPERPLASTIC THYROID DISEASES

In addition to Graves' disease, in which the diffuse hyperplastic changes of the thyroid gland stem from an autoimmune process, there are three other well-defined thyroid diseases having as a common morphologic denominator the presence of either diffuse or (much more commonly) nodular thyroid hyperplasia leading to clinically detectable enlargement (goiter). These are best classified on the basis of their pathogenetic mechanism, which, alas, is unknown for the most common of these disorders (Table 61-1).

In *dyshormonogenetic goiter* the enlargement of the gland results from enzymatic defects in hormone biosynthesis.[147,148] Several types of this disorder have been described in terms of the enzyme involved (Table 61-2), but in some instances no biochemical abnormality is demonstrable. All appear to be inherited as Mendelian recessive traits.[148,149] This type of goiter is usually associated with cretinism, but the patient can be euthyroid if the enzymatic defect in hormone synthesis is only partial. *Cretinism* is the term given to congenital hypothyroidism when the lack of thyroid hormone is complete or almost complete and prolonged. In addition to hypothyroidism, patients with cretinism also suffer an intellectual defect and growth retardation that are caused by thyroid hormone deficiency during fetal life. Grossly, in dyshormonogenetic goiter the thyroid is usually large, asymmetric, and multinodular and exhibits frequent degenerative changes. Histologically, the formation of microfollicles and trabeculas, papillary proliferation, cellular pleomorphism in various degrees, and atypia characterize this type of goiter. Variations in the histologic composition of the goiters have been related to specific enzymatic defects.[150] Because the epithelial proliferation may be very cellular and include trabecular or papillary formations, increased mitotic activity, and pleomorphism, the differential diagnosis includes carcinoma, and it may be difficult to differentiate between the two[151] (Fig. 61-11). Furthermore, because of the TSH stimulus on the follicular epithelium, the hyperplastic process can be so florid as to simulate pseudoinvasion of the thyroid capsule or the thyroid vessels. Rare cases of carcinoma arising in patients with dyshormonogenetic goiter have been described, however.[152]

Iodine-deficient goiter (endemic goiter) is prevalent in several high mountainous areas or in areas far from the sea, such as the Alps, the Himalayas, and the Andes, where the iodine content in drinking water and food is low. Endemic goiter is a common disease: in 1960 it was estimated that 200 million people in the world were affected, but its prevalence is decreasing because of the prophylactic iodination of salt.[153,154] The endemic cretinism that occurs in the same areas where endemic goiter is prevalent is also becoming very rare.

Idiopathic nodular goiter (sporadic goiter) is the most common form of goiter seen in the population of the United States. Its clinical incidence in the general adult population is 3% to 5% and its autopsy incidence is approximately 50%.[155,156] Its pathogenesis remains obscure. A small subset is caused by inborn errors in the synthesis of thyroid hormone (see earlier discussion of dyshormonogenetic goiter). Goitrogens, substances that interfere with the production of thyroid hormone, like drugs used in the treatment of hyperthyroidism or like some foods (such as cabbage and cauliflower), are other rare causes of goiter. Suboptimal iodine intake, a slight impairment in hormone synthesis, an increased iodide clearance by the kidney, and autoimmune mechanisms leading to the production of thyroid-stimulating immunoglobulins have also been proposed as causes.[157,159] Growth-stimulating immunoglobulins or unknown locally arising growth factors have also been implicated.[160,161]

Whatever the cause, the sequence of events leading to nodular hyperplasia is the same. The long-term stimulation by TSH, because of the suboptimal production of thyroid hormone, results in epithelial hyperplasia that is often followed by involution. Both of these changes result in diffuse goiter. Nodular goiter is usually regarded as an end stage of diffuse goiter and is caused by the cyclic changes that take place during hyperplasia and involution.[162] This is supported by the fact that in endemic areas the goiter is hyperplastic in children, diffusely enlarged with colloid accumulation in adolescents, and nodular in adults.

The mechanisms responsible for the formation of thyroid nodules in this setting are largely unknown. Normal thyroid cells are heterogeneous from the standpoint of their iodinating capacity, peroxidase context, responsiveness to TSH, and replicative ability.[163] The development of nodules may therefore reflect the generation of new metabolically heterogeneous follicles derived from genetically distinct cells and cell clus-

Table 61-1 **Causes of thyroid hyperplasia**

Type of thyroid hyperplasia	Pathogenesis	Pathology	Functional status
Dyshormonogenetic goiter	Genetically determined enzymatic defects in hormone synthesis	Nodular	Hypothyroid
Iodine-deficient goiter	Iodine deficiency	Nodular	Usually euthyroid
Idiopathic nodular goiter	Unknown	Nodular	Usually euthyroid, sometimes hyperthyroid
Graves' disease	Autoimmune	Diffuse	Hyperthyroid

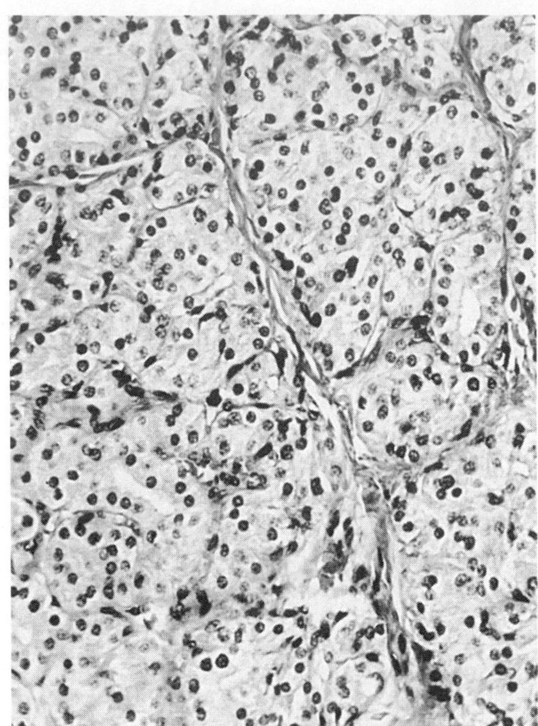

Fig. 61-11 Dyshormonogenetic goiter showing intense epithelial hyperplasia that may be difficult to differentiate from carcinoma.

Table 61-2 Genetic defects in thyroid hormone synthesis (dyshormonogenesis)

Iodide-transport defect (inability to concentrate iodide in the thyroid)
Organification defect (inability to bind iodide to thyroglobulin, caused by peroxidase deficiency)
Coupling defect (inability to couple monoiodotyrosine and diiodotyrosine to form triiodothyronine and thyroxine)
Dehalogenase defect (inability to deiodinate monoiodotyrosine and diiodotyrosine, caused by dehalogenase deficiency)
Defects in thyroglobulin synthesis

ters existing in the normal gland. With the development of new follicles and the uneven accumulation of colloid, tensions and stresses are produced within the thyroid that lead to rupture of adjacent follicles and vessels, followed by hemorrhage, scarring, and dystrophic calcification.[161]

Clinically, most adult patients present with a multinodular gland that may become very large and produce compression symptoms, which may be severe if the goiter extends substernally. Most patients are euthyroid, but hypothyroidism or hyperthyroidism may occur, the latter never accompanied by ocular symptoms.

Pathology. In *diffuse goiter* the thyroid is symmetrically and diffusely enlarged and may weigh several hundred grams. Histologically the hyperplastic stage is characterized by epithelial hyperplasia with small follicles, a tall epithelium showing papillary infoldings, and scanty colloid. In the involution stage, the stage usually seen in histologic specimens, large follicles distended by colloid and lined by flattened cells are the characteristic finding.

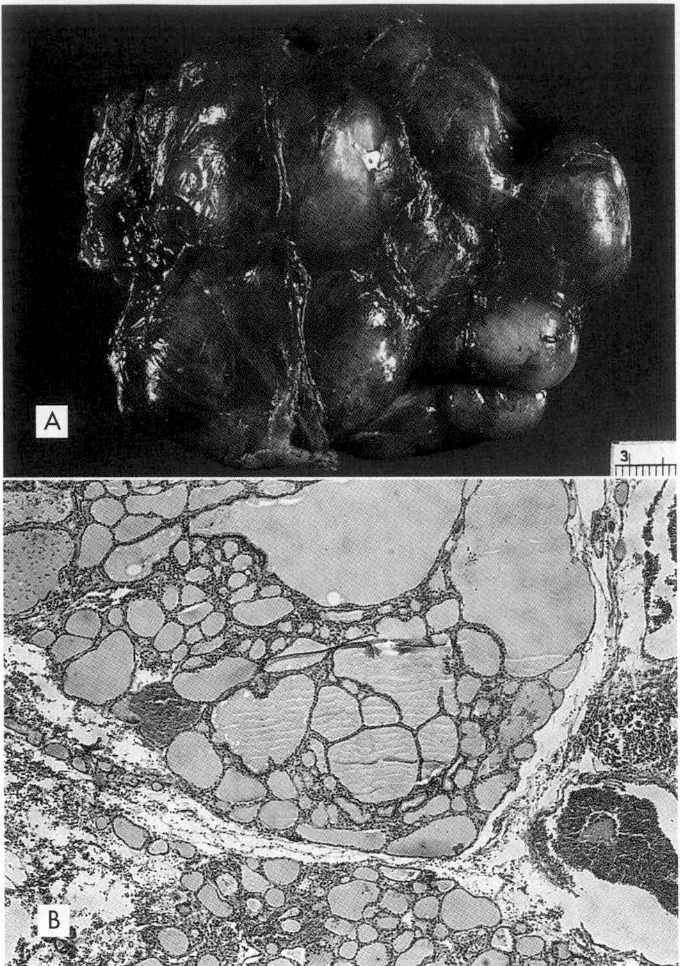

Fig. 61-12 Nodular goiter. **A,** Grossly the gland is asymmetric with nodules that vary considerably in size. **B,** Low-power appearance of a hyperplastic nodule composed of variously sized, but predominantly large, follicles. Hemorrhage and an inflammatory infiltrate are also seen.

In *nodular goiter* the thyroid usually weighs 50 to 100 g, but it can sometimes weigh more than 500 g. The gland is usually asymmetric, with nodules that vary considerably in size. Both grossly and histologically the thyroid shows considerable heterogeneity in its structure. Grossly the nodules may be colloidal or they may show degenerative features such as hemorrhage with hemosiderin deposits and cholesterol crystals, as well as calcifications, fibrous scarring, or cystic degeneration. The nodules may be totally or partially encapsulated (Fig. 61-12, *A*). Histologically the follicles may vary from small to large and the epithelium from flat to tall (Fig. 61-12, *B*). Some nodules may be composed of oncocytic cells, often arranged in cords, and some may exhibit micropapillary structures that may cause the condition to be diagnosed erroneously as papillary carcinoma. Within nodules, predominantly composed of large dilated follicles, it is common to find clusters of follicular cells exhibiting a solid or microfollicular pattern. These clusters have been interpreted to be the source of growth of the goiter. They are supposed to be able to replicate. As such they have have been referred as *foci of secondary proliferation,* and immunohistochemical studies have shown them to express p21 as the protooncogene product.[164]

It is not unusual for a nodule in multinodular goiter to become larger than the others and to acquire adenoma-like properties. Histologically the differential diagnosis between such a dominant nodule and a true adenoma is based on a series of criteria that are discussed in the section on follicular adenoma (see p. 1956).

Fine-needle aspiration of nodular goiter usually yields specimens that show abundant colloid, benign-appearing follicular cells, and histiocytes.

Nodular hyperplasia with mild enlargement of the thyroid usually does not necessitate any form of treatment. Subtotal thyroidectomy is performed when the large size of the gland causes symptoms.[165]

Toxic nodular goiter and *Plummer's disease* are names for nodular goiter with hyperthyroidism. Hyperthyroidism develops over many years, is more common in older women, and usually is not accompanied by ocular symptoms.[166] Scintigrams typically show hyperfunctioning areas in the thyroid.[167] Histologically, "hot" nodules do not differ from those that occur in nodular hyperplasia without hyperthyroidism, only in some instances showing a more active epithelial proliferation consisting of tall cells, papillary infolding, and scalloped colloid. Hyperplastic changes may also be seen in the thyroid tissue between the nodules. Sometimes only the intranodular thyroid tissue becomes hyperplastic.

Toxic adenoma is the name given a solitary thyroid nodule accompanied by usually mild hyperthyroidism that does not include ocular manifestations. The frequent absence of clinical manifestations and its nonneoplastic nature make the name "toxic adenoma" doubly inappropriate for this lesion. These lesions are better classified as autonomous *adenomatoid* nodules that are independent from TSH control and are able to produce thyroid hormone in large quantities. Histologically they may not differ from the nodules that occur in nodular hyperplasia or they may show signs of hyperactivity, such as tall epithelium and irregularly shaped follicles with papillary projections.[168]

Amyloid goiter is the enlargement of the thyroid that occurs in systemic amyloidosis. This rare manifestation of amyloidosis may be unilateral or bilateral and in severe cases may even cause symptoms of local compression. Rarely, medullary carcinomas contain so much amyloid that they simulate amyloid goiter.

THYROID TUMORS

The overwhelming majority (95%) of thyroid tumors are primary and epithelial in origin. The remainder include malignant lymphomas, rare mesenchymal neoplasms, and metastatic tumors.

Primary epithelial thyroid tumors can be divided into two major groups: those exhibiting evidence of follicular cell differentiation and those exhibiting features of C-cell differentiation, the former greatly predominating. Rare combined forms also exist. (Table 61-3). Classification of the tumors is based on the pattern of cell differentiation, that is, the phenotype of the tumor cells, rather than on the pattern of growth. Thus a tumor with follicular cell differentiation may exhibit a follicular, papillary, solid, or other type of growth, but a follicular (glandular, tubular) pattern of growth can rarely be seen in tumors of the C-cell type.

Most tumors (about 80%) of the follicular cells are benign, that is, adenomas. They are very common in adults and their frequency does not seem to be related to the level of iodine in the diet. Carcinomas represent the most common form of endocrine gland malignancy but constitute only about 1% of all the cases of cancer diagnosed in the United States. The annual incidence of thyroid cancer in the United States is 4 per 100,000, and the annual death rate is approximately 4 per 1,000,000. Thus, there are approximately 10,000 cancer cases reported every year and 1000 thyroid cancer–related deaths.

Table 61-3 Classification of thyroid tumors

Primary tumors
- ***Epithelial tumors***
  - A. Tumors of follicular cells
    - Benign: adenomas
      - Follicular adenoma (and variants)
      - Oncocytic (Hürthle cell) adenoma
    - Malignant: carcinomas
      - Well differentiated
        - Papillary carcinoma (and variants)
        - Follicular carcinoma
        - Oncocytic (Hürthle cell) carcinoma
      - Poorly differentiated
      - Undifferentiated (anaplastic)
  - B. Tumors of C-cells (medullary carcinoma)
  - C. Tumors of follicular and C-cells
- ***Malignant lymphomas***
- ***Mesenchymal tumors***
- ***Others (such as teratoma and paraganglioma)***

Metastatic tumors

As a group thyroid carcinomas have a strong predilection for women (from 60% to 70% of the cases) and can occur at any age. They also represent one of the most common forms of cancer in children and are often related to previous radiation exposure.[169-171] They run the gamut of behavior, from the extremely indolent and highly curable papillary carcinomas to the rapidly growing and inexorably fatal anaplastic carcinomas. There is a close correlation between the morphologic features and behavior, more so than that exhibited by carcinoma in many other sites. This requires that the pathologist carefully assess these features in order to predict the likelihood of recurrence, possible sites of metastatic deposits, the expected response to therapy, and outcome (Table 61-4). As a matter of fact, the thyroid is one of the organs for which the microscopic categorization of the tumor is as important as the staging of the disease. This is exemplified dramatically by the fact that undifferentiated carcinomas are regarded as stage IV even when limited to the thyroid gland.

Clinical features. Most thyroid tumors in general and carcinomas in particular present initially with a painless thyroid mass that is found to be "cold" on scintigrams. Because the large majority of clinically detectable thyroid nodules will prove to be benign and many not even neoplastic (that is, the appearance of a "dominant" nodule in the setting of nodular hyperplasia), it becomes important to select for surgical excision those patients in whom the likelihood of malignancy justifies the procedure. In this era of heightened concern about spiraling medical cost, and knowing that as much as 4% of the adult United States population has one or more palpable nodules, the magnitude of the problem becomes obvious.

Of all the techniques that have been used in the diagnosis of thyroid tumors, fine-needle aspiration biopsy clearly has

Table 61-4 Natural history of different types of thyroid carcinoma arising from follicular cells

Characteristic	Papillary carcinoma	Follicular carcinoma	Oncocytic (Hürthle cell) carcinoma	Poorly differentiated carcinoma	Undifferentiated carcinoma
Age	All ages (including children)	Middle and old age	Middle and old age	Middle and old age	Old age
Female-to-male ratio	About 2.5:1	About 2:1	About 2:1	About 1.5:1	About 1.5:1
Primary tumor	Usually intrathyroid	Usually intrathyroid	Usually intrathyroid	Often extrathyroid	Usually extrathyroid
Regional metastases	Common	Very rare	Rare	Common	Common
Distant organ metastases	Rare	Relatively common	Common	Common	Common
Ten-year survival	>90%	50% to 90%	60% to 70%	15% to 30%	<2%
Principal cause of death	Local invasion and distant metastases	Distant metastases	Distant metastases	Distant metastases	Local invasion and distant metastases

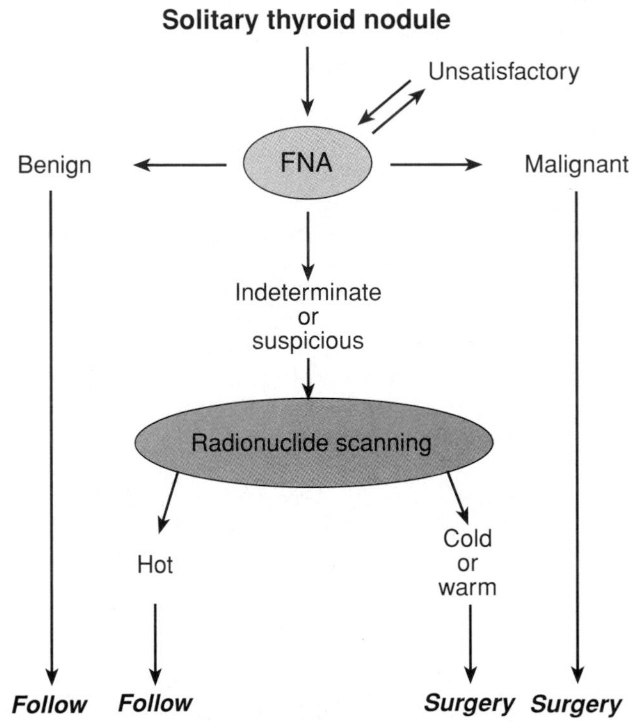

Fig. 61-13 Management of a solitary thyroid nodule.

proved the most useful, to the point that its use has dramatically altered the approach to this problem (Fig. 61-13). The number of patients undergoing unnecessary surgery has been drastically reduced, and the finding of carcinoma among the surgically resected glands has correspondingly increased in incidence.[172] In expert hands, the procedure has a very low complication rate and, the findings are sensitive and specific; it is also a rapid and relatively inexpensive procedure.[173] It is not possible to distinguish between a follicular adenoma and follicular carcinoma in the specimens obtained (although it is possible to identify the process as neoplastic and therefore deserving surgery), but most nonneoplastic (colloid) nodules, thyroiditides, and papillary carcinomas, plus the rare medullary and anaplastic carcinomas, can be identified.

Tumors of follicular cells

Follicular adenoma

Follicular adenoma is defined by the World Health Organization (WHO) committee as "a benign encapsulated tumor showing evidence of follicular cell differentiation."[174] Because it is frequently difficult to distinguish a true neoplastic process from a localized nodular manifestation of a hyperplastic process on the basis of histologic findings, some adjunctive criteria are necessary. Microscopically, adenoma should be diagnosed when the lesion is single and completely surrounded by a fibrous capsule and when its microscopic appearance substantially differs from that of the surrounding thyroid tissue. The clonal nature of lesions with such characteristics has been proved by analysis of the X chromosome.[175,176] However, adenomas may be multiple and a hyperplastic nodule may have a histologic appearance indistinguishable from that of an adenoma. Thus defined, follicular adenoma is a rather common neoplasm that occurs predominantly in young women, though it can occur in persons of both sexes and all ages.

Clinically it presents as a solitary thyroid nodule that frequently appears "cold" on isotopic scans. The largest lesions may cause symptoms related to compression.

Pathology. Follicular adenomas are round or oval and by definition are surrounded by a fibrous capsule that is usually thin (Fig. 61-14). Their size is highly variable, with the largest lesions reaching 10 cm or more in diameter. The cut surface is homogeneous and has a more fleshy appearance than that of the surrounding thyroid tissue. Secondary changes, including hemorrhage, calcification, or cystic degeneration, are seen but are less frequent than they are in hyperplastic nodules. Massive necrosis of the entire nodule can occur spontaneously or more frequently as a complication of a fine-needle aspiration procedure. The nodule varies from grayish white to red, depending on the cellular composition of the tumor, the amount of colloid, and the vascularity.

Microscopically the epithelial proliferation may exhibit a variety of architectural patterns, and this has led to the identification of numerous histologic variants, such as trabecular solid (embryonal), microfollicular (fetal), normofollicular (simple), and macrofollicular (colloid) adenoma (Fig. 61-15). These morphologic designations have no biologic or clinical

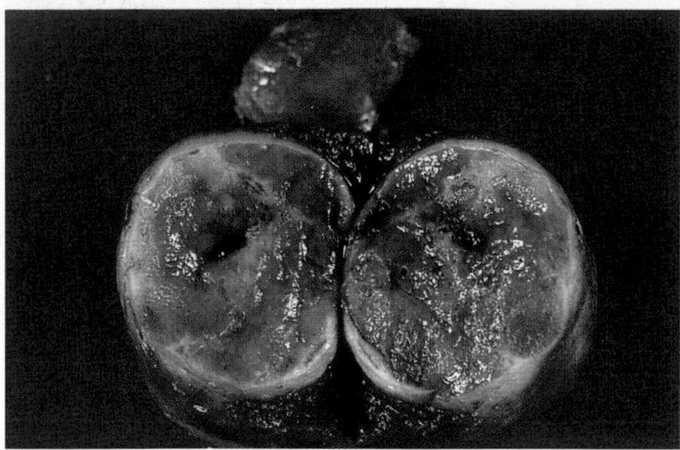

Fig. 61-14 Follicular adenoma. A well-circumscribed nodule surrounded by a fibrous capsule is seen. Cut section shows a homogeneous tan surface with focal hemorrhage.

implications. Hyperplastic changes in the form of papillary or pseudopapillary structures may be seen. Usually these papillae are short, have a poorly developed fibrovascular core, are devoid of the cytologic features typical of papillary carcinoma, and face the lumens of dilated follicles. Secondary degenerative changes such as hemorrhage, fibrosis, calcifications, and cyst formation are common.

We have already mentioned the need to distinguish a follicular adenoma from a hyperplastic nodule. Other important differential diagnoses include follicular carcinoma and the follicular variant of papillary carcinoma. Both follicular adenoma and follicular carcinoma can be very cellular. Mitoses are usually absent in follicular adenoma, but they usually are just as scanty in follicular carcinoma. The capsule of adenomas tends to be thinner than that of carcinomas and by definition uninvolved by tumor. The follicular variant of papillary carcinoma, which may also be encapsulated, must be considered when fibrous bands intersecting the neoplastic proliferation; scalloped, strongly eosinophilic colloid; and the nuclear changes typical of papillary carcinoma such as ground-glass nuclei and nuclear grooves are found.

Like normal follicles, the cells of follicular adenomas are immunohistochemically positive for thyroglobulin (less strongly than the surrounding parenchyma), low-molecular-weight keratins, and vimentin and are surrounded by a basement membrane containing laminin and type IV collagen.[177,178]

DNA aneuploidy has been detected by flow cytometry in about 25% of the follicular adenomas, particularly in cellular lesions, but this finding does not seem to add any important prognostic information to that yielded by the microscopic diagnosis.[179,180]

Fine-needle aspiration biopsy samples of follicular adenomas are usually cellular with only scanty colloid. These features, together with the absence of histiocytes, frequently allow it to be distinguished from a nodule in a goiter. However, in the differential diagnosis, it is impossible to distinguish between follicular adenoma and a well-differentiated follicular carcinoma. In such cases histologic examination of the nodule is mandatory to resolve the matter. Severe morphologic variants of follicular adenoma have been described.

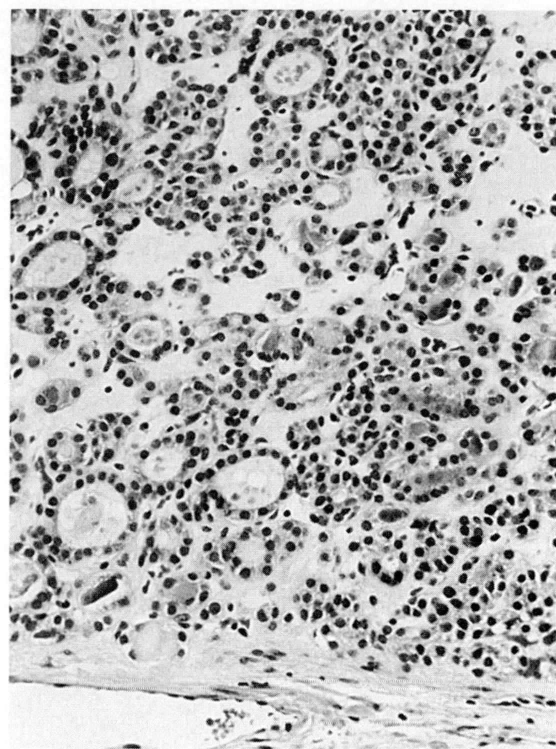

Fig. 61-15 Follicular adenoma. The neoplastic proliferation has a microfollicular pattern of growth and is sharply separated from the surrounding thyroid by a fibrous capsule.

Atypical follicular adenomas. Variants of follicular adenoma that deserve additional study have been described. As defined by the WHO committee, "the cellular proliferation [of these tumors] is more pronounced and the architecture and cytologic patterns are less regular."[174]

Hyalinized trabecular adenoma is a distinctive type of thyroid neoplasm characterized by a prominent hyaline appearance resulting from the perivascular deposition of collagen and the intracytoplasmic accumulation of intermediate filaments.[181] The cells are usually arranged in trabeculas or in solid nests reminiscent of the *Zellballen* of paraganglioma (Fig. 61-16, *A*). The nuclei may be round, oval, or, more frequently, elongated. Nuclear grooves, pseudoinclusions and perinuclear vacuoles are seen. The differential diagnosis includes medullary carcinoma and papillary carcinoma. The latter is particularly difficult to recognize on the basis of fine-needle aspiration findings. Immunohistochemically, hyalinizing trabecular adenoma stains positively for thyroglobulin; on some occasions, it has also shown a focal positivity for neuroendocrine markers such as neuron-specific enolase, chromogranin, and neurotensin.[182] This neoplasm is generally included among the adenomas. However, the possibility exists that it represents a special variant of papillary carcinoma with a very low grade of malignancy.

Adenoma with bizarre nuclei is a rare variant of follicular adenoma and is characterized by the presence of cells (usually arranged in clusters) containing gigantic hyperchromatic nuclei (Fig. 61-16, *B*).

Oncocytic (Hürthle cell) adenoma is be discussed with the closely related clear cell adenoma in the sections on thyroid tumors that exhibit oncocytic or clear features. The standard

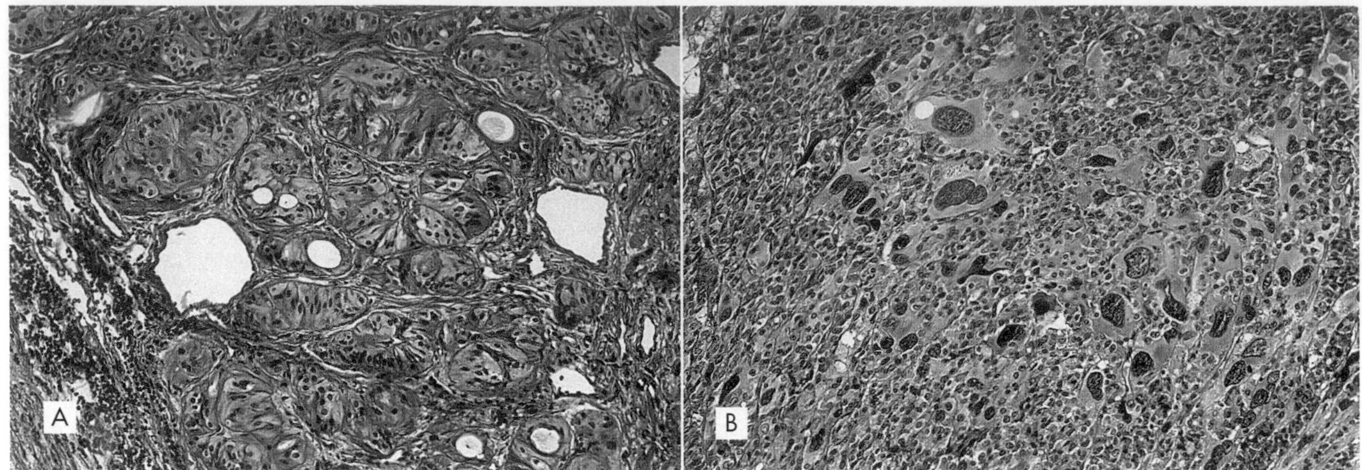

Fig. 61-16 Follicular adenoma variants. **A,** Hyalinizing trabecular adenoma. The cells are arranged in trabeculas and nests reminiscent of the *Zellballen* of paraganglioma. **B,** Adenoma with bizarre nuclei. Clusters of cells with huge, irregularly shaped nuclei are admixed with smaller monomorphic cells exhibiting a solid growth pattern.

treatment for follicular adenoma and its variants is lobectomy.

Papillary carcinoma

Papillary carcinoma is by far the most common type of thyroid malignancy. Its incidence appears to have increased in recent years, but this may be at least partially related to a change in the diagnostic criteria for this entity, particularly in connection with the recognition of the follicular variant.

Papillary carcinoma is more frequent in women than in men, with a male-to-female ratio of about 1:2.5. Peculiarly it can affect patients of any age, including children, but the mean age of onset ranges from approximately 35 to 40 years. There is a history of low-dose radiation exposure to the head or neck (for the treatment of acne) in 5% to 10% of the patients with this type of tumor. There appears to be a negative correlation between papillary carcinoma and endemic goiter, as shown by the fact that the incidence of the tumor is higher in iodine-rich areas and its relative frequency in Switzerland rose after the addition of iodine to the diet.[183-185] There have been indications of an increased incidence of papillary carcinoma in the settings of Graves' disease and Hashimoto's thyroiditis, but this has never been statistically proved.[186,187] In most cases papillary carcinoma presents as an indolent, slowly growing thyroid mass, with or without lymphadenopathy. Cervical lymphadenopathy is the initial manifestation of the disease in about 20% of the cases.[189] In most of these cases the primary thyroid tumor can be detected with isotopic scanning or by the fine-needle aspiration findings, but sometimes only after resection of the gland.

Pathology. The size of the primary tumor is extremely variable, ranging from microscopic to several centimeters (mean, 2.3 cm). The gross appearance of the nodule varies greatly. It may be either solid or cystic and either clearly invasive with an infiltrative or pushing pattern of growth or encapsulated (Fig. 61-17, *A*). Multicentric foci are seen grossly in about 20% of the cases, and extension to the perithyroidal soft tissues or muscle occurs on rare occasions. Microscopically the diagnosis of papillary carcinoma is made on the basis of certain architectural features (mainly papillae), but also on the basis of certain characteristic nuclear features, including optically clear nuclei (ground glass), nuclear pseudoinclusions, and nuclear grooves[189-192] (Fig. 61-17, *B* and *C*). The papillae vary greatly in size and shape. They can be long and slender with a central fibrovascular core, short and stubby, or very small and devoid of a central core (so-called abortive papillae) (Fig. 61-18). They can grow in a complex arborizing pattern or can be arranged in an orderly parallel fashion. The papillary stroma may be edematous or hyaline, and it may contain lymphocytes, foamy macrophages, hemosiderin, or psammoma bodies. The latter are calcific concretions with well-defined concentric laminations that are found in about 50% of papillary carcinomas, being more common in neoplasms with a papillary type of growth.[193] The nidus for the psammoma body formation is probably a necrotic cell around which the layers of calcium salt are deposited[194] (Fig. 61-19). Psammoma bodies in the thyroid are almost pathognomonic of papillary carcinoma; if they are found in benign-appearing thyroid parenchyma or in a cervical lymph node, this should always prompt a search for a nearby carcinoma.

The papillary proliferation is nearly always associated with areas exhibiting a follicular growth pattern. Areas in which the neoplastic proliferation has become solid or squamous are seen in 20% of the cases. Solid and squamous changes seem to be related events and are more common in certain variants of papillary carcinoma (Fig. 61-20). Squamous changes are seen more commonly at the advancing edge of the neoplastic growth where the tumor elicits a dense stromal proliferation. An abundant fibrous stroma is commonly present in papillary carcinoma. It sometimes becomes very cellular and dense and can rarely acquire a fasciitis-like quality that obscures the real nature of the neoplastic proliferation.[195] Lymphocytes are also seen, sometimes in large numbers.

Ultrastructurally the most characteristic feature of the cells that compose papillary carcinoma is the highly indented nuclear membrane. This may result in large invaginations within the nucleus, and these represent the counterpart at the electron microscopic level of the inclusion-like formations seen on light microscopy studies.

Immunohistochemically the cells of papillary carcinoma are positive for thyroglobulin, keratin, vimentin, S-100 pro-

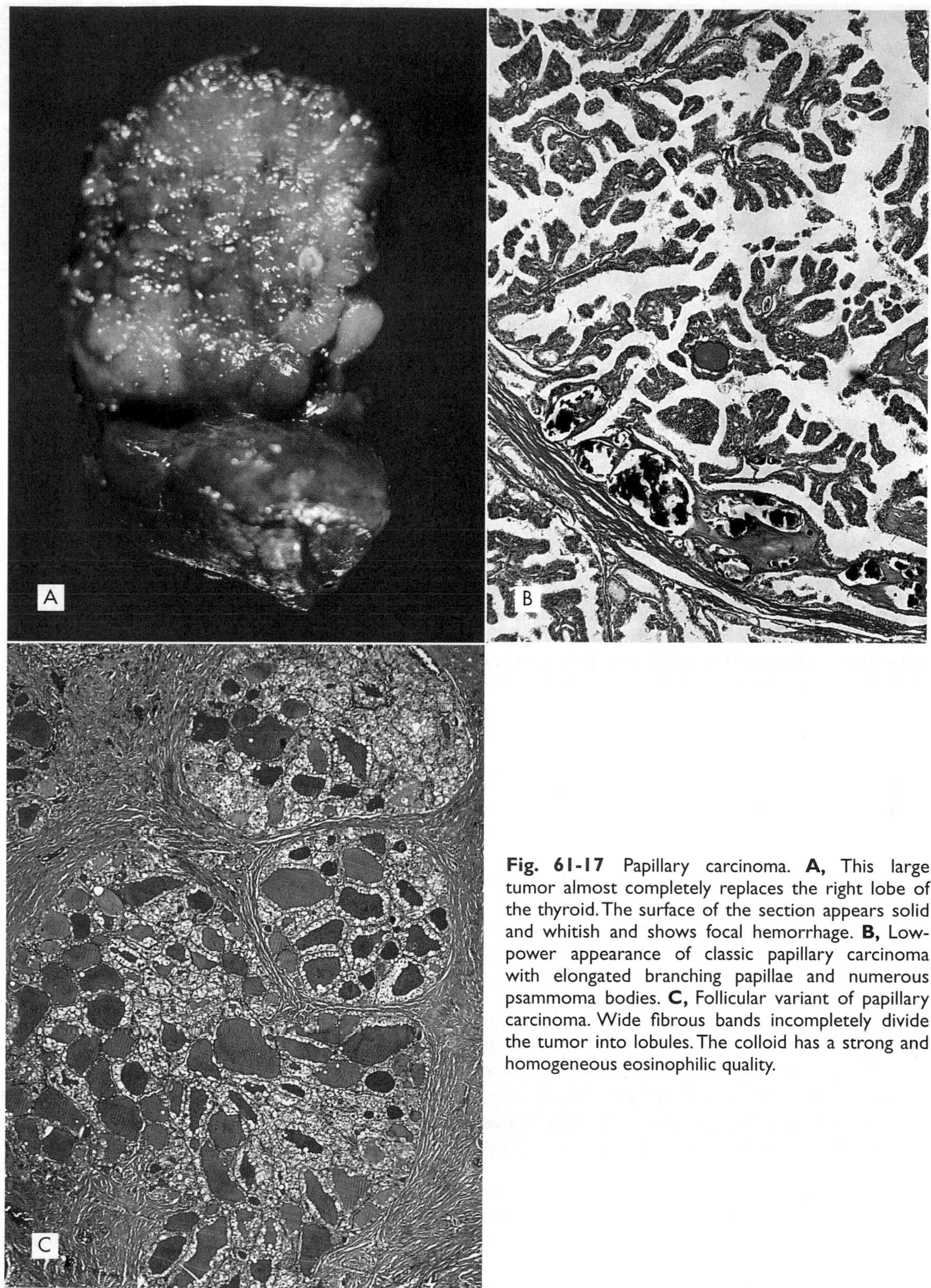

Fig. 61-17 Papillary carcinoma. **A,** This large tumor almost completely replaces the right lobe of the thyroid. The surface of the section appears solid and whitish and shows focal hemorrhage. **B,** Low-power appearance of classic papillary carcinoma with elongated branching papillae and numerous psammoma bodies. **C,** Follicular variant of papillary carcinoma. Wide fibrous bands incompletely divide the tumor into lobules. The colloid has a strong and homogeneous eosinophilic quality.

tein, and epithelial membrane antigen, and occasionally for carcinoembryonic antigen.[196,197] Both low- and high-molecular-weight keratins show positivity, the latter being more common when the tumor shows signs of squamous differentiation.[198] Estrogen receptor proteins have also been demonstrated.[199] Rearrangements of the *ret* and *trk* proto-oncogenes, located, respectively, on chromosomes 10 and 1, have been demonstrated but with some geographic differences in terms of their frequency.[200,201]

Fine-needle aspiration specimens from papillary carcinomas are usually very cellular and contain scanty colloid. Papillary formations and psammoma bodies can be found, but more

carcinomas. As a result of the exclusion of all these tumors from the category of follicular carcinoma, the number of thyroid tumors diagnosed as follicular carcinoma has notably decreased in the past 10 to 15 years. Although the supplementation of iodine in the water in iodine-deficient areas might be responsible for having led to a real diminution in the incidence of follicular tumors in these regions (with a corresponding increase in the incidence of papillary carcinoma), the changes in the diagnostic criteria for thyroid tumors most likely constitute the main source of this phenomenon.

Follicular carcinoma is more common in women than in men, and the average age of onset is 10 years older than that for papillary carcinoma. It rarely occurs in children. As already mentioned, an increased incidence of this tumor in iodine-deficient areas has been shown.

It typically presents as a solitary thyroid nodule, which is "cold" on scintigrams. Unlike papillary carcinoma, it is exceptional for it to metastasize to the cervical lymph nodes. Follicular carcinoma usually spreads through the hematogenous route. Symptoms related to distant metastases (such as a bone fracture) may be the first manifestation of the disease.

Follicular carcinoma is divided into two subtypes according to the degree of invasiveness: minimally invasive or encapsulated and widely invasive.

Minimally invasive follicular carcinoma appears grossly as a solitary round or ovoid nodule that is light tan or brown and surrounded by a thick capsule. The size is variable but usually exceeds 1 cm in diameter. Secondary degenerative changes may be present. The histologic and immunohistochemical features are similar to those of follicular adenoma, especially those of the embryonal, fetal, and atypical types. Less frequently there is increased mitotic activity (usually focal), nuclear atypia, and nucleolar prominence. Carcinoma should be suspected when these features are found, but should be diagnosed only when capsular invasion is discovered. Capsular invasion can be regarded as having occurred if the tumor is seen outside the capsule (Fig. 61-22). Clusters of follicular cells within the capsule or irregularities in the contour of the capsule are not diagnostic signs of invasion. Multiple sections are often needed so that the area of capsular rupture can be seen and the diagnosis made with certainty.[230] Vascular invasion, which is a more reliable criterion of malignancy than capsular invasion is, is identified by the presence of a compact tumor mass that is surrounded by vascular endothelium and located in a vessel situated within or outside the capsular wall. The mass should be attached at some point to the vessel wall; loose tumor cells in vascular lumens should not be accepted as evidence of vascular invasion because they might have resulted from manipulation of the tumor. The identification of vascular invasion poses considerable difficulty for the pathologist, and immunohistochemical or histochemical staining does not facilitate this process.[231-233]

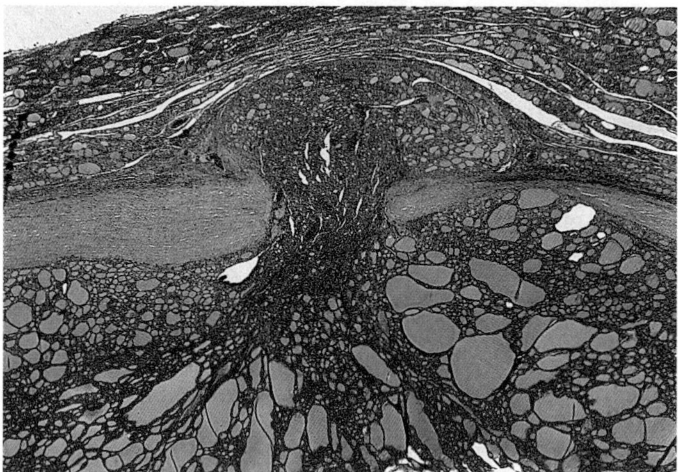

Fig. 61-22 Minimally invasive (encapsulated) follicular carcinoma. The neoplastic proliferation penetrates the entire thickness of the capsule.

Distinguishing follicular carcinoma from follicular adenoma (or from a dominant nodule of nodular hyperplasia) can be even more problematic after a fine-needle aspiration, because the tumor capsule may appear interrupted and distorted as a result of the reparative process secondary to the procedure.

As already mentioned, it is almost impossible to distinguish follicular adenoma from well-differentiated follicular carcinoma on the basis of the findings yielded by cytologic material. The less-differentiated tumors show hyperchromatic nuclei and prominent nucleoli, the cells are arranged in a microfollicular or solid pattern, and there is necrotic debris. The amount of colloid is scanty.

Widely invasive follicular carcinoma shows widespread infiltration of the thyroid parenchyma and blood vessels. Usually there is no capsule and microscopically the tumor shows architectural and cytologic features indicative of malignancy. A solid or trabecular pattern of growth is frequently seen, as is increased mitotic activity, nuclear hyperchromastism, and necrosis. Many of the histologic features of this type of follicular carcinoma overlap with those of the so-called poorly differentiated carcinoma.

In the encapsulated type of follicular carcinoma, the tumor by definition shows only minimal invasion of the thyroid parenchyma and never extrathyroid extension; this is instead a common finding in patients with widely invasive carcinomas.

Metastases are usually blood borne and are more common in lung and bone. The metastatic tumor may appear better differentiated than the primary thyroid tumor (the "metastasizing struma" or "metastasizing adenoma" described in the older literature). Metastases occur in less than 1% of the patients with the minimally invasive carcinomas with capsular invasion only, in less than 5% of those with vascular invasion, and in as many as 80% of those with the widely invasive tumors.[234-236]

Treatment and prognosis. Lobectomy or subtotal thyroidectomy with suppression of TSH secretion by T_4 is the most appropriate treatment for encapsulated, minimally invasive carcinoma. Total thyroidectomy followed by the administration of radioactive iodine is the treatment of choice for the widely invasive tumors. Metastatic disease is treated with radioactive iodine or externally administered radiation therapy, or both.

The prognosis also varies tremendously depending on the type of tumor.[237,238] Within one institution a 50% death rate was observed in those with a widely invasive tumor and a 3% rate in those with a minimally invasive tumor.[239,240] It is likely that this difference will become even greater with the use of the current diagnostic criteria.

Oncocytic (Hürthle cell) tumors

Oncocytic tumors consist of thyroid tumors that are composed exclusively or predominantly of oncocytic cells (see p. 1944). These modified follicular cells have been called by various names, including *Hürthle cells, Askanazy cells, oxyphilic cells,* and *oncocytes.* Askanazy was the first to describe human oncocytic cells. The designation *Hürthle cell neoplasm* is, however, the one most commonly encountered in the literature, even though the cells Hürthle found in the thyroid of dogs most likely would now be considered C-cells. The WHO committee has chosen to designate these cells as *oxyphilic,* and the term *oncocytic* (used to designate cells with similar characteristics in other organs) is frequently used as a synonym.[174]

Terminology is not the only controversial issue related to this type of tumor. Whether these lesions in fact constitute a distinct type of thyroid neoplasm has been questioned. Some authors (including the WHO committee) classify oncocytic tumors simply as follicular or papillary, depending on their architectural characteristics, implying that the oncocytic changes represent only an epiphenomenon devoid of any effect on the natural history of the tumor.[174] The body of evidence seems to favor the alternative point of view that neoplasms made up of oncocytes represent a separate category of thyroid tumors on the basis of their distinctive morphologic and clinical characteristics.[241,242] Hürthle cell tumors are more common in adults than children and predominate in female subjects, although the latter is a less prominent feature of carcinomas.

Pathology. Onocytic tumors appear as solitary, solid, tan and variously sized masses. Malignant tumors tend to be larger than adenomas; they can be well encapsulated or invade the thyroid parenchyma, usually in a multinodular fashion (Fig. 61-23). Microscopically the pattern of growth is follicular in most cases; less frequently it is solid and trabecular, and rarely it is papillary. The cells have the typical granular acidophilic cytoplasm, but it is not rare to see areas where the cytoplasm is clear. The nuclei are usually vesicular and uniform but may show pleomorphism with large hyperchromatic nuclei and prominent nucleoli (Fig. 61-24). In the setting of carcinoma the cells tend to be smaller and the pattern of growth is more frequently of the solid and trabecular type. The colloid tends to be very dense in the follicular tumors, and it is common to see inspissated colloid in the form of concentric laminations that simulate psammoma bodies. In contrast to those seen in papillary carcinoma, these formations are located in the follicular lumens. An infarct type of necrosis, which is sometimes massive, may be present as a consequence of the fine-needle aspiration procedure.

As in conventional follicular neoplasms, adenoma and carcinoma are distinguished by the presence or absence of clear-cut capsular or vascular invasion, or both. The same criteria used to diagnose malignancy in non-Hürthle follicular lesions should be applied in the diagnoses of oncocytic tumors.[243] The claim that all Hürthle cell tumors should be regarded as malignant or potentially malignant has been repeatedly disproved. Only tumors with the attributes of carcinoma have shown the ability to progress, spread, and metastasize.[241,242-246] Hürthle cell carcinoma spreads to the perithyroid soft tissue more frequently than does conventional follicular carcinoma. Distant metastasis (bone and lung) and metastasis to the regional lymph nodes are also more common.[247]

Rare tumors exhibit a papillary pattern of growth. True papillae have to be differentiated from pseudopapillae, frequently seen in follicular lesions, and represent a cutting artifact of the thin fibrous septa that divide enlarged follicles. Papillary Hürthle cell tumors, similar to their follicular counterparts, can be either encapsulated or invasive. Encapsulated tumors behave in a benign fashion, and the invasive ones are usually aggressive, probably more so than conventional papillary carcinoma.[248]

Ultrastructurally the cytoplasm of the cells is packed with mitochondria. Pronounced abnormalities in terms of the size, content, and shape of the mitochondria can be observed.[249] Some mitochondria may appear dilated, with the distortion and eventual disappearance of the cristae. When this process becomes prominent, the organelles acquire a round vesicular shape and may no longer be recognized as mitochondria. This is the ultrastructural equivalent of the clearing of the cytoplasm seen at the light microscopy level.

The material obtained by fine-needle aspiration is usually very cellular and is made up of polygonal cells with a relatively large eosinophilic and distinctly granular cytoplasm. Markedly atypical or binucleated nuclei are common features. The distinction between oncocytic carcinoma and oncocytic adenoma and between the latter and a hyperplastic nodule with oncocytic change may be almost impossible on cytologic grounds. Carcinoma cells, however, tend to be smaller with a high nucleocytoplasmic ratio and intranuclear cytoplasmic inclusions. On the other side, cells from an oncocytic adenoma

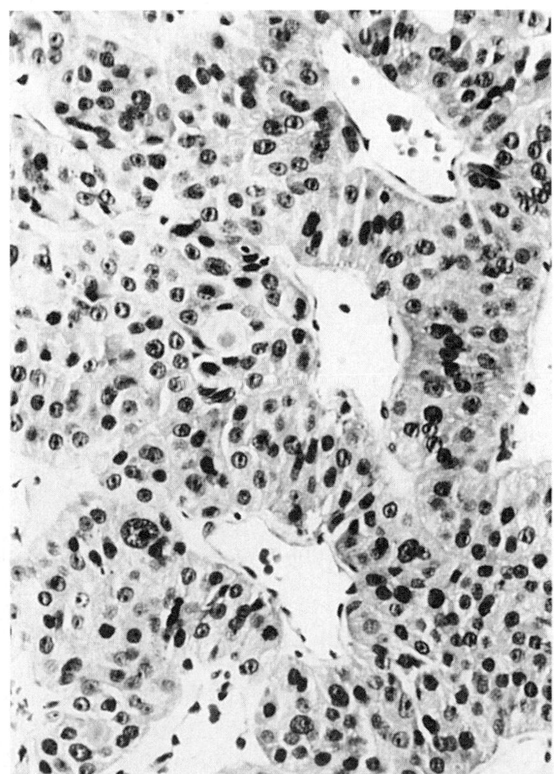

Fig. 61-23 Oncocytic (Hürthle cell) adenoma. The tumor has a predominantly trabecular growth pattern and is composed of large cells with abundant eosinophilic cytoplasm, large nuclei, and prominent nucleoli.

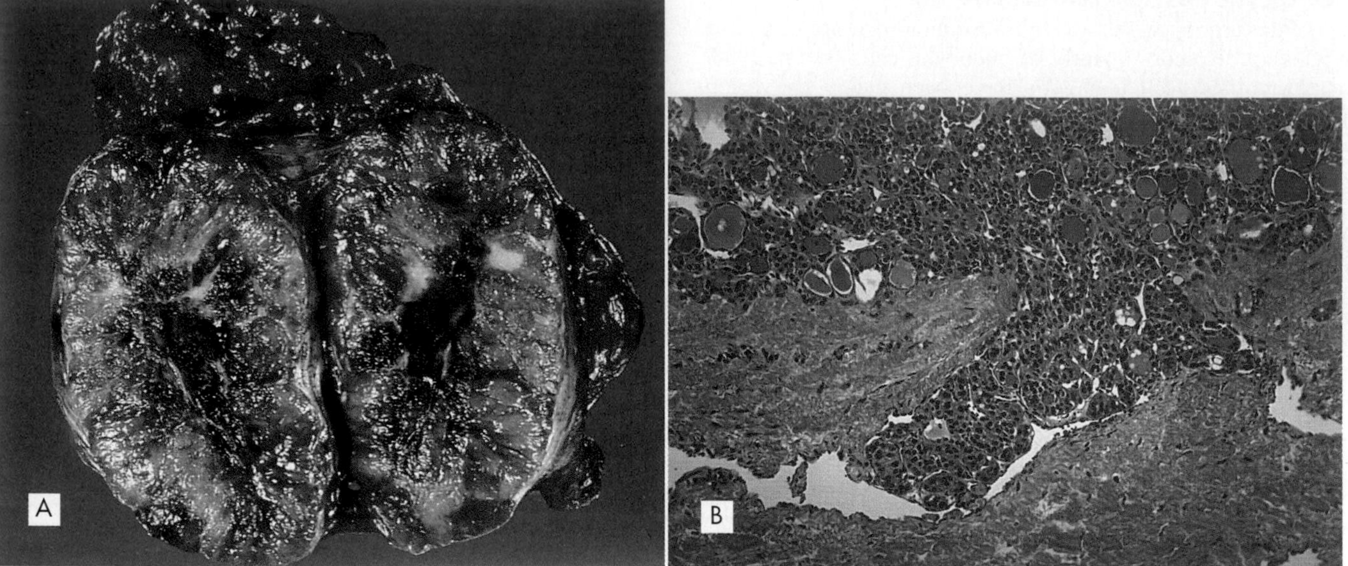

Fig. 61-24 Oncocytic (Hürthle cell) carcinoma. **A,** The cut section of this large oncocytic (Hürthle cell) carcinoma shows the typical tan color of this neoplasm. Necrosis and hemorrhage are also present, and the tumor grossly appears encapsulated. **B,** Tumor invades capsular vessels.

are less cohesive and their nuclei are smaller than those of a hyperplastic nodule.

Treatment and prognosis. Lobectomy is the treatment for Hürthle cell adenomas, and a total thyroidectomy is the therapy for the malignant lesions. Hürthle cell carcinoma is usually nonresponsive to radioactive iodine therapy, and consequently external radiation therapy is added.

Hürthle cell adenomas are always cured by excision. Carcinomas are aggressive neoplasms, more so than conventional follicular carcinoma, and the 5-year survival rate in these patients is approximately 60%.[250,251] No morphologic characteristic has proved to have prognostic significance.[241] DNA analysis has shown a higher incidence of invasive growth in aneuploid tumors, but it is unable to predict the final outcome of any individual tumor.[252]

Clear cell tumors

Clear cell changes can be seen in various histologic types of thyroid neoplasms. Most frequently they occur in Hürthle cell tumors as a result of the vesicular swelling of mitochondria.[253,254] Other mechanisms that cause clear cell changes in other types of tumors are the accumulation of glycogen, lipid, "mucin," and thyroglobulin.[253] The accumulation of thyroglobulin in the form of vacuoles confers the characteristic "signet-ring" appearance to some clear cell neoplasms, which are most frequently benign; these are the so-called signet-ring adenomas.[255]

Thus, clear cell tumors are not a specific type of tumor but represent follicular, papillary, or undifferentiated carcinomas that have superimposed clear changes[253,256] (Fig. 61-25).

In the differential diagnosis it is important to consider renal clear cell carcinoma, a tumor with a tendency to metastasize to the thyroid. Multiple nodules, clear (as opposed to finely granular) cytoplasm, sinusoidal blood vessels, and fresh hemorrhage are more in keeping with metastatic renal cell carcinoma. Immunohistochemical staining for thyroglobulin can be helpful, but caution should be used in interpreting the results because of the frequent artifacts stemming from diffusion of the thyroglobulin.

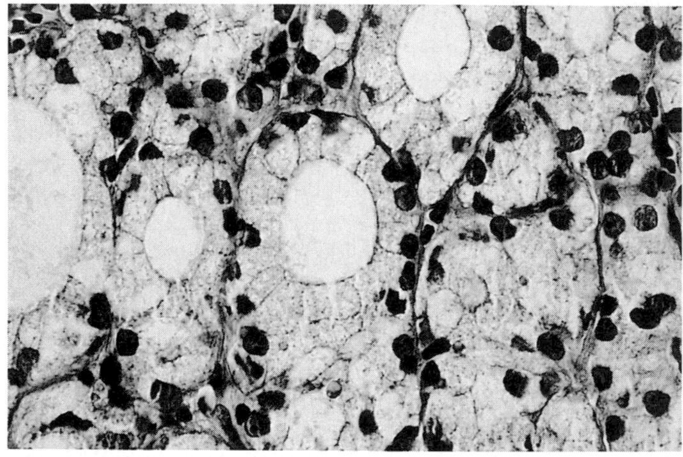

Fig. 61-25 Clear cell follicular adenoma. This tumor has a follicular growth pattern and is composed of follicular cells with a granular clear cytoplasm.

Poorly differentiated carcinoma

Poorly differentiated carcinoma is a recently described group of neoplasms that occupy an intermediate position between the well-differentiated carcinomas (follicular and papillary) and the undifferentiated (anaplastic) carcinomas, both in terms of their morphologic appearance and biologic behavior.[257]

Poorly differentiated carcinomas show a solid, trabecular, or microfollicular pattern of growth; high mitotic activity; and necrosis.[258,259] In the so-called insular carcinoma (the most common and better-illustrated variant), the cells are particularly small and contain round nuclei and scanty cytoplasm.[257] The predominant pattern of growth is solid, with an insular appearance accentuated by the artifactual retraction of the

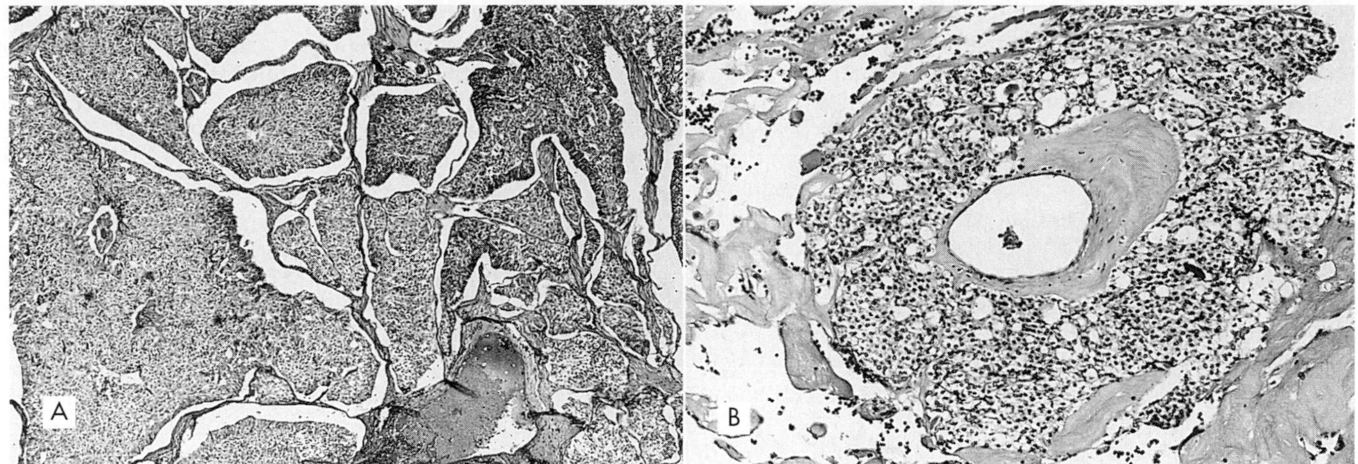

Fig. 61-26 Poorly differentiated carcinoma. **A,** Typical low-power appearance of poorly differentiated (insular) carcinoma. The neoplastic growth is solid and arranged in well-defined nests. **B,** Peritheliomatous pattern of poorly differentiated (insular) carcinoma. Necrosis has spared the neoplastic cells located around vessels.

tumor cells from the stroma (Fig. 61-26, *A*). The tumor can also form microfollicles containing dense colloid. Necrosis is common, resulting in a focal peritheliomatous appearance to the tumor growth (Fig. 61-26, *B*). Insular carcinoma in most instances represents a poorly differentiated follicular carcinoma, but its association with (or origin from) papillary carcinoma has also been demonstrated.[257]

The cells of insular carcinoma stain positively for thyroglobulin and keratin.[257] The positivity for thyroglobulin and negativity for calcitonin distinguishes this type of thyroid tumor from medullary carcinoma, with which it shares some morphologic features. Most likely some of the tumors diagnosed in the past as the compact subtype of small cell anaplastic carcinoma actually belong in this category.

Undifferentiated (anaplastic) carcinoma

According to the WHO classification undifferentiated carcinoma is a highly malignant tumor that appears partially or totally undifferentiated on standard light microscopy preparations, but there is some evidence of epithelial differentiation on morphologic, immunohistochemical, or ultrastructural grounds.[174] This type of thyroid carcinoma is rare, constituting 10% to 25% of all thyroid carcinomas. It is characteristically a tumor of old age, and it is slightly more common in women than in men.

Undifferentiated carcinoma usually presents as a rapidly enlarging neck mass that is associated with symptoms of compression such as dyspnea, dysphagia, and hoarseness.[260] Rarely distant metastases are the first sign of the disease.[261] The tumor appears "cold" on radioactive iodine scans.

Pathology. Undifferentiated carcinoma is usually manifested as a large and firm mass containing necrotic areas. It frequently replaces the entire thyroid gland and extends into the adjacent soft tissue, including the esophagus and trachea.

Histologically the tumor shows three distinct morphologic patterns, which frequently coexist. These are spindle cell, giant cell, and squamoid (Fig. 61-27). Tumors previously called "small cell undifferentiated carcinoma" have often been found instead to be malignant lymphoma, small cell medullary carcinomas, or poorly differentiated ("insular") carcinomas.[262]

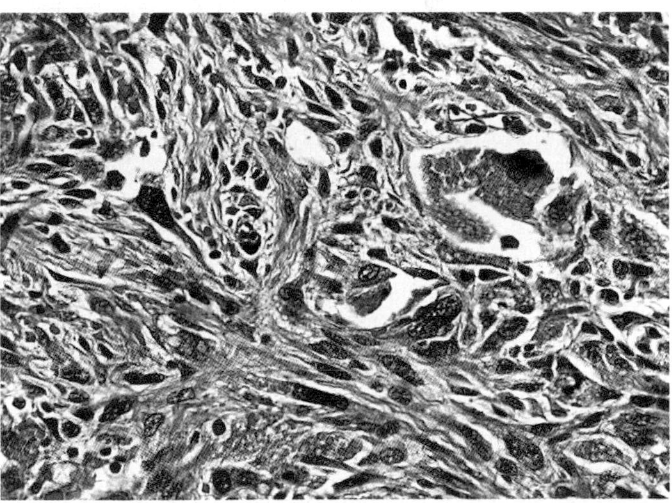

Fig. 61-27 Undifferentiated (anaplastic) carcinoma. This tumor is composed of a mixture of spindle and giant cells.

Cellular pleomorphism, high mitotic activity, necrosis, and pronounced invasiveness both in the gland and in the adjacent soft tissues are common to all types. Most tumors are composed of polygonal, spindle, and giant cells. Osteoclastlike, multinucleated giant cells, probably originating from circulating monocytes, may rarely be present.[263-265] The fasciculated or storiform pattern of growth frequently exhibited by spindle cell tumors may create diagnostic problems because of the resemblance to sarcomas. In the tumors displaying the squamoid pattern, which are the least common, the neoplastic growth resembles that of a nonkeratinizing squamous cell carcinoma of any other location.[260] Usually these tumors show other features typical of undifferentiated carcinoma, allowing them to be distinguished from the rarer squamous cell carcinoma of the thyroid or from esophageal or laryngeal squamous cell carcinoma involving the thyroid. Immunohistochemically most undifferentiated carcinomas stain positively for keratin, in keeping with their epithelial origin.[260,266,267] Thyroglobulin immunoreactivity is confined to areas showing papillary or follicular differentiation,[260] and carcino embryonic antigen immunoreactivity is demonstrable in the squamoid type. Ultrastructural examination is able to confirm the epithelial nature of the tumor in only half of the cases.[268,269]

A differentiated component, either papillary or follicular carcinoma, has been found to coexist with undifferentiated carcinoma in 8.5% to 80% of the cases, leading to the assumption that undifferentiated tumors arise from differentiated ones.[270-272] The presence of p53 gene mutations in a high percentage of the cases of undifferentiated carcinomas but not in the areas of residual papillary carcinoma suggests that these mutations play a role in the transformation of a well-differentiated tumor to an undifferentiated one.[273-275] An association between tall cell papillary carcinoma and spindle cell squamous carcinoma has been noted.[276]

Therapy and prognosis. The prognosis in patients with undifferentiated carcinoma is exceedingly poor. The 5-year survival rate is less than 10% and the mean survival is 6 months. Death is usually caused by local invasion of the tumor, though the tumor also metastasizes into both regional lymph nodes and distant organs, most often the lungs.[277,278] A combination of surgery, radiation therapy, and chemotherapy has only a palliative effect.[279,280]

Rare types of carcinoma

Mucoepidermoid carcinoma has been described as a distinct type of thyroid carcinoma that is characterized by a combination of squamous and mucin-producing features.[281] It has been suggested that it is probably derived from intrathyroidal "cell nests" that, as already discussed, are believed to be derived from ultimobranchial bodies. However, the multiple histologic and clinical similarities that this tumor shares with papillary carcinoma point toward a metaplastic follicular cell origin.[282] Of uncertain origin, but probably related to mucoepidermoid carcinoma, is the so-called *sclerosing mucoepidermoid carcinoma with eosinophilia* that usually arises in the thyroid glands of patients with Hashimoto's thyroiditis, often of the fibrous type.[283] Rare cases of *mucinous carcinoma* have also been described.[284,285] Primary *squamous cell carcinoma* of the thyroid is very rare and has to be differentiated from a primary laryngeal or esophageal carcinoma that extends to the gland and from the squamous type of undifferentiated thyroid carcinoma.[286] The differential diagnosis also includes tumors showing thymic or related branchial pouch differentiation. They can occur in the neck either close to or within the thyroid and exhibit squamous or mucinous differentiation. These tumors have been recently referred to by the acronyms SETTLE (*s*pindle *e*pithelial *t*umor with *t*hymuslike *d*ifferentiation) and CASTLE (*c*arcinoma *s*howing *t*hymuslike *d*ifferentiation).[287-293]

Tumors of C-cells

Medullary thyroid carcinoma

Medullary thyroid carcinoma (MTC) is a malignant tumor composed of cells showing evidence of C-cell differentiation.[294-296] These tumors account for up to 10% of all thyroid malignancies and occur sporadically or in familial forms that show autosomal dominant modes of inheritance. The sporadic tumors account for up to 70% of all cases in most large series, and they occur with equal frequencies in different parts of the world.[297] There is no apparent connection between irradiation to the head and neck area and the subsequent development of MTC. The sporadic form of MTC is primarily a tumor of middle-aged adults, with a female-to-male ratio of 1.3:1. Generally patients with sporadic tumors present with unilateral involvement of the gland with or without associated cervical lymph node metastases.[298]

Familial MTCs may rarely occur as isolated thyroid tumors but more commonly occur in association with hyperplastic or neoplastic lesions of the parathyroid glands and adrenal medulla (multiple endocrine neoplasia [MEN 2A]).[299] In a genetically distinct syndrome, MTC occurs in association with adrenal medullary hyperplasia or pheochromocytoma, together with gastrointestinal and ocular ganglioneuromas (MEN 2B)[300,301] (Table 61-5). In patients with MEN 2A, the mean age at the time of diagnosis of the thyroid tumors is approximately 20 years. With the advent of routine prospective screening studies in high-risk patients, however, the mean age at diagnosis has become progressively younger.[302] In patients with MEN 2B-associated MTCs, the mean age at diagnosis is now 15 years; this has an important bearing on survival because the prognosis in these patients is poorer than that in those with MEN 2A.[301]

The results of recent linkage analyses indicate that the putative gene responsible for MEN 2A and 2B maps to 10q 11.2, the site of the *ret* protooncogene that is consistently expressed in MTC and pheochromocytoma. Findings from the studies of Mulligan and coworkers[303] have in fact indicated that the

Table 61-5 Type 2 multiple endocrine neoplasia (MEN) syndromes*

Features	Syndromes: Type 2A†	Syndromes: Type 2B
Thyroid	C-cell hyperplasia–medullary thyroid carcinoma	C-cell hyperplasia–medullary thyroid carcinoma
Adrenal	Adrenal medullary hyperplasia–pheochromocytoma	Adrenal medullary hyperplasia–pheochromocytoma
Parathyroid	Hyperplasia–adenoma	—
Oral mucosa	—	Neuromatosis; megacolon
Skeletal system	—	Marfanoid habitus; pes cavus, talipes equinovarus, other skeletal abnormalities
Chromosomal localization	10q 11.2	10q 11.2

*Rarely, familial forms of medullary carcinoma may occur in the absence of other endocrine abnormalities.
†In a small number of families, type IIA MEN has occurred in association with hereditary cutaneous lichen amyloidosis.

ret oncogene is the MEN 2A gene.[303] Germline mutations of the *ret* oncogene have been identified in 20 of 23 families with MEN 2A but not in 23 normal controls subjects. Nineteen of the 20 mutations affected the same cysteine residue at the boundary of the *ret* extracellular and transmembrane domains. Patients with MEN 2B have mutations affecting the transmembrane domain of the ret proto-oncogene.[305a]

The laboratory diagnosis of sporadic and familial MTC depends on the demonstration of increased levels of calcitonin in the serum. The observation that calcitonin levels could be stimulated by the administration of calcitonin secretagogues (such as calcium and pentagastrin) has formed the basis for the implementation of large-scale screening studies directed toward the early diagnosis of familial MTC.[302] These studies have been effective in the detection of clinically occult MTCs as well as their precursor lesions, as discussed in the section on C-cell hyperplasia.

Pathology. MTCs range in size from those that are just visible to those that replace the entire thyroid.[295,304] The tumors are tan to pink and vary in consistency from soft to firm (Fig. 61-28). The larger lesions are sharply circumscribed but are not encapsulated. Sporadic tumors, even when quite large, generally are unilateral. Familial MTCs tend to be bilateral and multicentric, even when quite small (Fig. 61-28).

Typical MTCs may show solid, lobular, or insular patterns of growth[295,304] (Figs. 61-29 to 61-31). Individual tumor cells may be round, polygonal, or spindle shaped, and most tumors show admixtures of these patterns. The nuclei tend to be eccentric and are round to ovoid with coarsely clumped chromatin that often imparts a plasmacytoid appearance to the cells.[305] Areas of necrosis and hemorrhage tend to occur in larger tumors, particularly those measuring more than 1.5 cm in diameter. The cytoplasm of the tumor cells is finely granular and ranges from eosinophilic to amphophilic. The granularity of the cytoplasm can be enhanced by the use of argyrophil stains. Ultrastructurally the tumor cells contain variable numbers of dense-core secretory granules ranging from 60 to 550 nm in diameter.[306]

The familial tumors are indistinguishable histologically from those that occur sporadically. The familial tumors, however, are typically multicentric and bilateral. Moreover, examination of the nontumorous thyroid in C-cell–bearing areas typ-

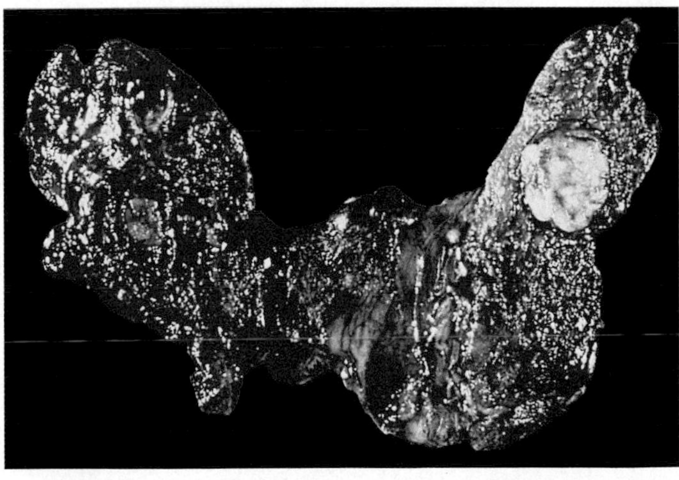

Fig. 61-28 Thyroidectomy specimen from a patient with type 2A multiple endocrine neoplasia. Tumor nodules are present bilaterally at the junctions of the upper and middle thirds of the lateral lobes.

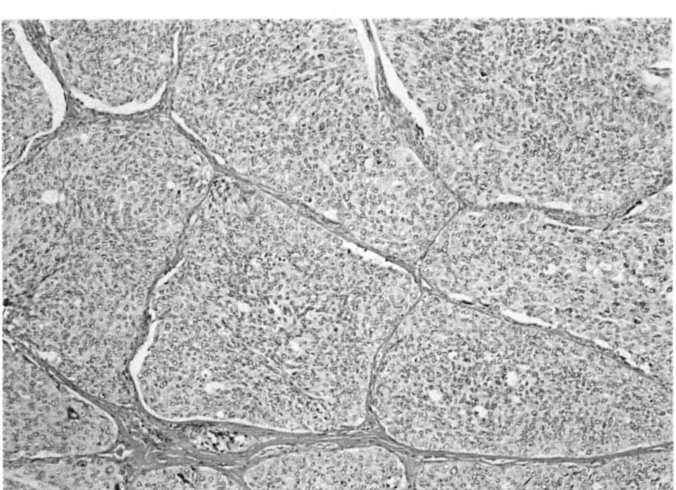

Fig. 61-30 Medullary thyroid carcinoma. This tumor shows a predominantly lobular pattern of growth.

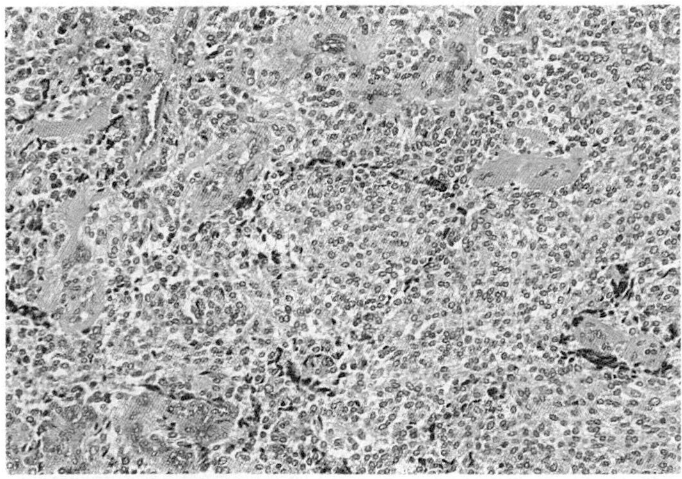

Fig. 61-29 Medullary thyroid carcinoma. This tumor shows a predominantly solid pattern of growth.

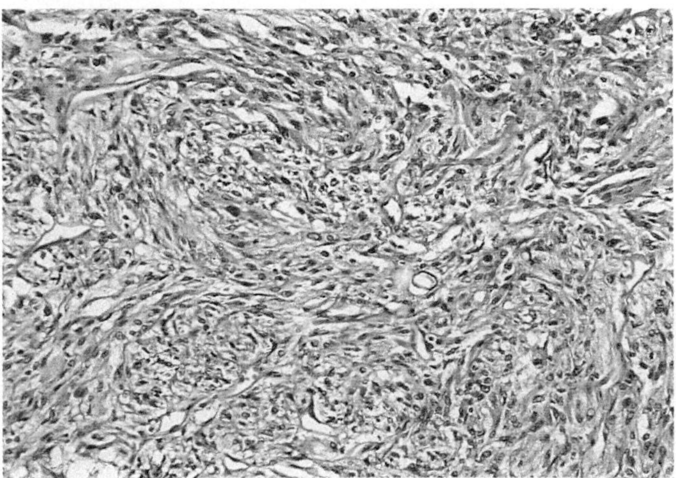

Fig. 61-31 Medullary thyroid carcinoma. This tumor shows a spindle cell pattern of growth.

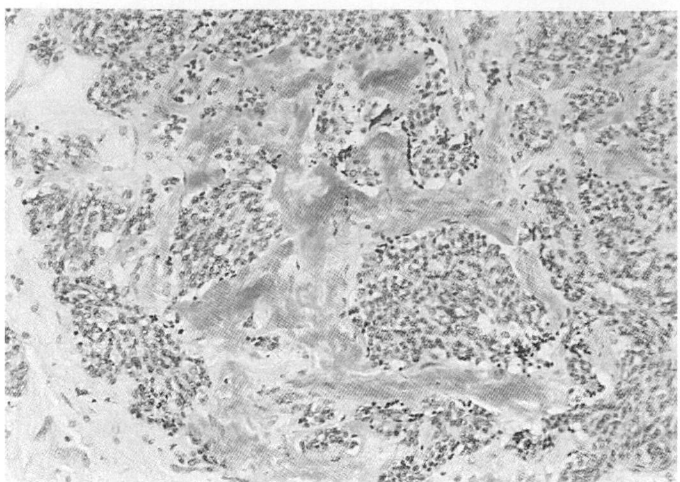

Fig. 61-32 Medullary thyroid carcinoma stained with Congo red. Amyloid deposits adjacent to the tumor cells are strongly congophilic.

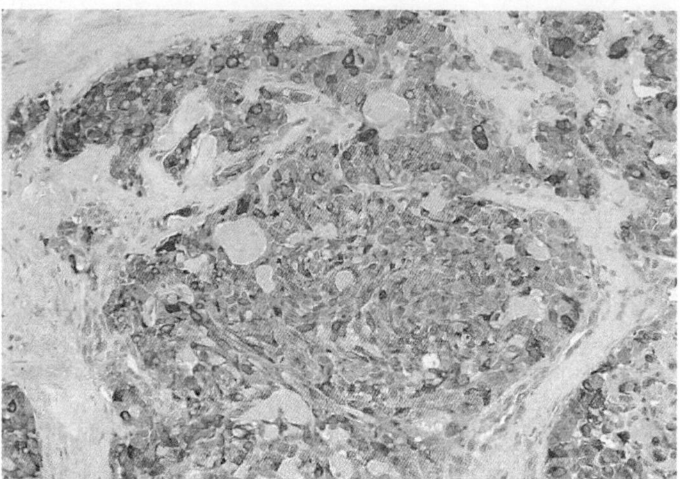

Fig. 61-33 Medullary thyroid carcinoma stained for calcitonin. This section was stained with a polyclonal antiserum to calcitonin using the peroxidase-antiperoxidase technique. Most of the tumor cells contain immunoreactive calcitonin.

ically reveals the presence of C-cell hyperplasia of both diffuse and nodular types (see p. 1970).

Amyloid deposits, which are evident in up to 80% of cases, can be demonstrated by Congo red staining (Fig. 61-32). Typically the amyloid deposits occur in the stromal compartment of the tumors, and in some instances they may be calcified. The amyloid deposits in cases of MTC are most likely derived from calcitonin or a calcitonin precursor.[307] The ultrastructural characteristics of MTC-associated amyloid are identical to those seen in the settings of AA or AL amyloidosis.

Immunoperoxidase studies have revealed the existence of calcitonin in approximately 80% of the cases of MTC (Figs. 61-33 and 61-34). Although many cases exhibit extensive calcitonin immunoreactivity, occasional cases may show only small foci of positive staining.[304] Tumors that show no calcitonin peptide may react positively with probes for calcitonin mRNA using in situ hybridization formats.[308] In addition to calcitonin, these tumors may contain a variety of other peptides, including somatostatin, gastrin-releasing peptide, adrenocorticotropin, beta-endorphin, leu-enkephalin, substance P, vasoactive intestinal peptide, glucagon, gastrin, and insulin.[309,310] Both serotonin and catecholamines are also present in some of these tumors.

MTCs contain low-molecular-weight cytokeratins and variable amounts of vimentin. Occasional tumor cells may also contain neurofilament proteins. The tumor cells react with antibodies for a variety of markers of neuroendocrine cells, including chromogranins, synaptophysin, histaminase, and neuron-specific enolase.[309,310] The specificity of the finding of neuron-specific enolase, however, is relatively low because this marker has also been identified in some tumors of follicular cell origin.

Carcinoembryonic antigen is present in most MTCs.[311] Indeed, some MTCs may lose their capacity to synthesize calcitonin while maintaining their ability to synthesize carcinoembryonic antigen. In patients with MTC, the finding of persistently elevated levels of carcinoembryonic antigen in the face of decreasing calcitonin levels has been a predictor of aggressive disease.[312]

Most often there are variable degrees of cellularity in fine-needle aspiration biopsy specimens of MTCs.[305] The tumor

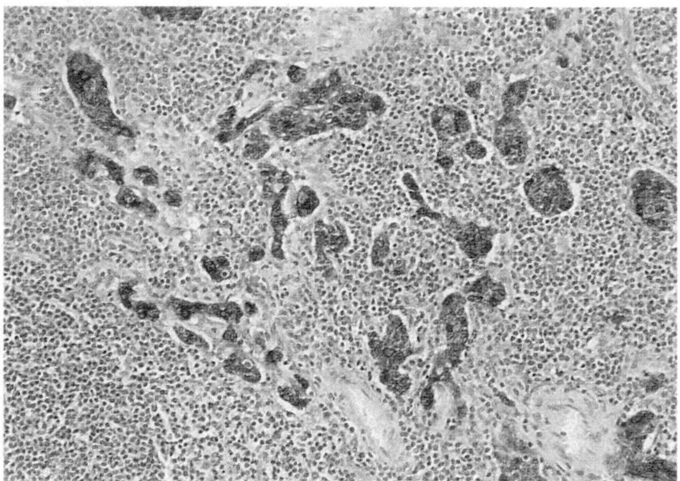

Fig. 61-34 Lymph node metastatic lesion of medullary thyroid carcinoma. The section was stained with a polyclonal antiserum to calcitonin using the peroxidase-antiperoxidase technique. The tumor cells contain immunoreactive calcitonin, and the surrounding lymphoid tissue shows a negative reaction.

cells are present singly or in small, loosely cohesive groups and often show considerable pleomorphism consisting of round, polygonal, and spindle shapes. Nuclei are often eccentrically placed; with coarsely clumped chromatin and generally inconspicuous nucleoli. The cytoplasm often has a fibrillary texture that is enhanced by Papanicolaou staining. In Wright-Giemsa–stained preparations the cytoplasm may exhibit a fine granularity. Amyloid deposits are often impossible to distinguish from colloid in Papanicolaou-stained preparations. However, the amyloid deposits will stain selectively with Congo red. MTCs tend to be overdiagnosed on the basis of cytologic findings; therefore, the diagnosis should be confirmed by immunoperoxidase staining for calcitonin.

Variants of medullary carcinoma. MTCs often exhibit a remarkable degree of diversity in their histologic patterns and may simulate a variety of other primary and metastatic tumors of the thyroid. Many MTCs contain isolated follicular structures. Occasional examples of these tumors may be composed wholly of tumor cells arranged in follicular patterns, and these tumors have been referred to as *follicular* or *tubular variants*[313] (Fig. 61-35). *Papillary variants* have also been described, but they are exceptionally uncommon.[314] A *pseudopapillary variant* is more common and results from degeneration or necrosis of tumor cells, such that viable cells appear to be attached to the stromal-vascular compartment of the neoplasm. The *small cell variant* resembles the intermediate type of bronchogenic carcinoma[315] (Fig. 61-36). These tumors may exhibit a compact, trabecular, or diffuse growth pattern with prominent mitotic activity and foci of necrosis. Although isolated tumor giant cells are found frequently in MTCs, the *giant cell variant* of this tumor is composed almost exclusively of giant cells.[316] Other variants of MTC include *oncocytic,*[317] *clear cell,*[318] *melanocytic,*[319] *squamous,*[317] and *amphicrine*[320] types of tumor. The amphicrine variant is composed of cells that contain both mucin and calcitonin. Occasional MTCs may show a *paraganglioma-like pattern.*[321] Although cases of C-cell adenoma have been reported,[322] most authors consider them to represent encapsulated MTCs.

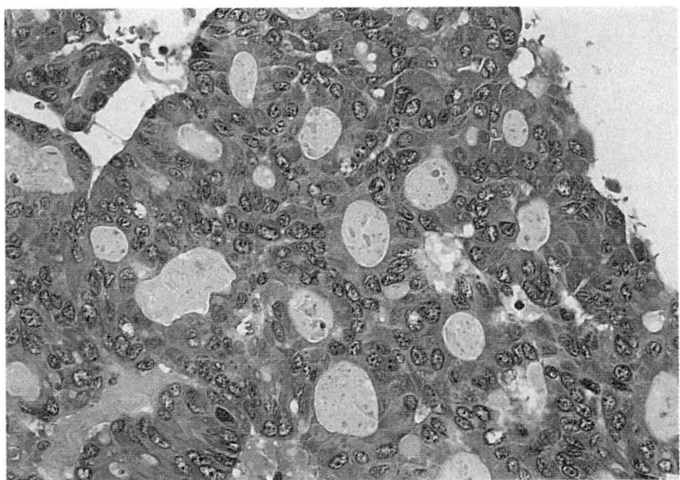

Fig. 61-35 Follicular variant of medullary thyroid carcinoma. This tumor is composed almost exclusively of tumor cells arranged in a follicular or tubular pattern.

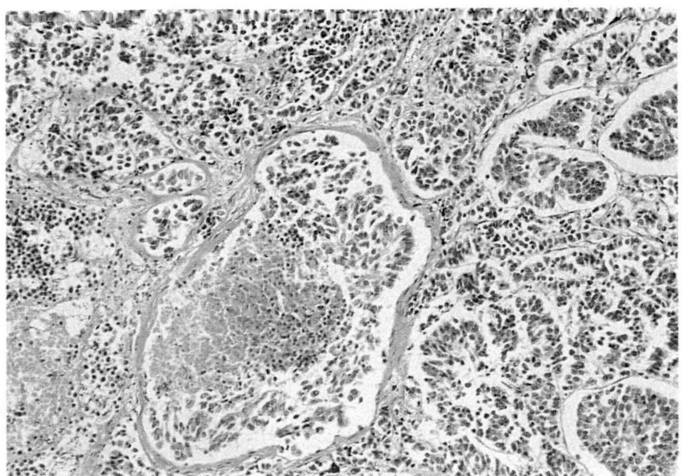

Fig. 61-36 Small cell variant of medullary thyroid carcinoma. Most of the tumor cells have a fusiform appearance. Areas of necrosis are evident.

Differential diagnosis. MTC must be distinguished from a wide variety of benign and malignant thyroid neoplasms, as well as from metastatic tumors to the thyroid.[304] Although true papillary variants are rare, the pseudopapillary pattern is quite common and tumors with these features should be distinguished from papillary carcinomas of follicular origin. The latter tumors typically have tumor cells aligned along fibrovascular cores, overlapping nuclei with finely dispersed chromatin, nuclear folds, and nuclear cytoplasmic invaginations. Follicular variants of MTC must also be distinguished from true follicular neoplasms and from MTCs with entrapped normal follicles. Although follicular carcinomas and entrapped normal follicles stain positively for thyroglobulin, follicular variants of MTC typically stain positively for calcitonin and negatively for thyroglobulin.[304]

Hyalinizing trabecular adenomas are characteristically encapsulated, as are occasional variants of MTC.[304] Both lesions may be focally hyalinized, but amyloid is a feature only of MTC. Moreover, MTCs stain positively for calcitonin but negatively for thyroglobulin, while the reverse is characteristic of hyalinizing trabecular adenomas.

MTCs must also be distinguished from poorly differentiated or insular carcinomas. The stroma of insular carcinomas typically is negative for amyloid and the tumor cells show at least a focal positivity for thyroglobulin but evidence of calcitonin immunoreactivity. MTCs must also be distinguished from anaplastic or undifferentiated carcinomas. This can be accomplished generally by the demonstration of calcitonin or amyloid, or both, in the spindle cell and giant cell variants of MTC. As noted previously, most diffuse, small cell malignant neoplasms of the thyroid represent malignant lymphomas. Immunohistochemical analysis typically reveals the presence of calcitonin peptide in small cell variants of MTC or in situ hybridization shows calcitonin mRNA. The so-called primary oat cell carcinoma of the thyroid typically stains negatively for calcitonin and calcitonin mRNA.[323] In some instances parathyroid adenomas may present as intrathyroidal masses simulating primary thyroid neoplasms.[304] The parathyroid adenomas are typically encapsulated and are composed of cords and nests of chief cells with small, centrally placed nuclei and pale cytoplasm. The chief cells stain negatively for calcitonin but may stain positively for chromogranin and parathyroid hormone.

Treatment and prognosis. MTCs are treated surgically by total thyroidectomy. The prognosis for patients with MTC is generally intermediate between that for patients with differentiated and those with undifferentiated thyroid carcinomas. In most large series the 5-year survival rates have ranged from 60% to 70% and the 10-year survival rates have ranged from 40% to 50%.[298] The prognosis in patients who are younger than 40 years of age at diagnosis is significantly better than that in older patients, while the prognosis in women is more favorable than that in men.

Tumors generally metastasize to cervical lymph nodes of the central and lateral neck, and the probability of nodal metastasis correlates positively with the size of the primary neoplasm. There are no apparent differences in survival among the patients with the different histologic patterns of MTC according to the results of most studies.[298] Calcitonin-poor MTCs are thought by some authors to pursue a more aggressive course than calcitonin-rich tumors.[324] The results of the studies conducted by Bigner and coworkers[325] indicate that tumors with high mitotic rates may be more aggressive than are tumors with low mitotic rates. There is also some indication that aneuploid tumors may be more likely to be associated with a more aggressive course. Generally the thyroid tumors in patients with MEN 2B tend to behave in a more malignant fashion than the tumors in patients with either MEN IIA or sporadic MTC do.

C-cell hyperplasia

C-cell hyperplasia is an uncommon entity characterized by multifocal proliferations of C-cells within the follicles of the thyroid. This entity was first recognized when increased secretion of calcitonin was noted after the administration of calcium gluconate or pentagastrin in persons at risk for the development of the familial form of MTC associated with MEN 2A.[326] Subsequently, C-cell hyperplasia was also identified in patients at risk for the development of MEN 2B–associated MTC. Results from a series of studies ultimately led to the concept that C-cell hyperplasia was a precursor of MTC in patients with familial forms of this tumor.[327]

Pathology. Thyroid glands from patients with C-cell hyperplasia associated with the MEN 2A or 2B syndromes show no apparent gross abnormalities. When C-cell hyperplasia is suspected on the basis of abnormal calcitonin secretory responses, each lobe of the gland should be blocked in its entirety for histologic examination.[328] Foci of C-cell hyperplasia are most likely to be found in the middle third of each lateral lobe. Because it is difficult to identify C-cell hyperplasia in hematoxylin and eosin–stained sections, immunoperoxidase procedures using polyclonal antisera or monoclonal antibodies to calcitonin should be used to identify them.

Diffuse C-cell hyperplasia is characterized by increased numbers of C-cells, as compared with the number in age- and sex-matched controls[327] (Fig. 61-37, 61-38, and 61-39). The process should involve both lobes, and there should be at least 50 C-cells per low-power microscopic field.[329] Occasional C-cells may appear enlarged and contain prominent nuclei. The C-cell proliferation is confined to the follicles. Generally the C-cells show strong positive staining for calcitonin (Fig. 61-38) and at the ultrastructural level contain abundant secretory granules. In some instances the C-cells within the follicle may surround the more centrally located follicular cells to form a complete circumferential collar.

Nodular C-cell hyperplasia is characterized by the complete obliteration of follicles by C-cells[329] (see Fig. 61-37). Because C-cell nodules may occasionally be found in normal glands, nodular hyperplasia should be diagnosed only when the process is extensive, bilateral, and multicentric.[330] A diagnosis of early MTC is made when C-cells extend through defects in the follicular basal lamina into the interstitium (Fig. 61-40). This phenomenon is often accompanied by fibrosis around the invading C-cells (Fig. 61-40).

In some instances it may be extremely difficult, if not impossible, to distinguish mild forms of diffuse C-cell hyperplasia from normal C-cell density. This diagnosis should therefore be made with extreme caution. In such equivocal cases, genetic analysis may be needed to determine whether the patient is a carrier of the abnormal gene.[305a,333]

Foci of nodular hyperplasia may be difficult to distinguish from a variety of other changes in hematoxylin and eosin–stained sections. These changes include squamous metaplasia, solid cell nests, tangential cuts of follicles, and intrathyroidal thymic or parathyroid rests. Immunoperoxidase staining for calcitonin is often necessary to resolve these differential diagnoses. Occasionally it may be difficult to distinguish intrathyroidal metastases of MTC from foci of C-cell hyperplasia. In such cases, however, the metastatic deposits are found within vascular or lymphatic channels. When tumor has penetrated the vascular wall, it may infiltrate into the adjacent thyroid parenchyma in a manner that is highly suggestive of a primary tumor site. The presence of C-cell hyperplasia adjacent to such foci is highly suggestive of a primary focus of MTC.

Treatment and prognosis. The treatment of choice for patients with C-cell hyperplasia is total thyroidectomy. In one large series of patients who were screened for calcitonin abnormalities by provocative testing with calcium gluconate

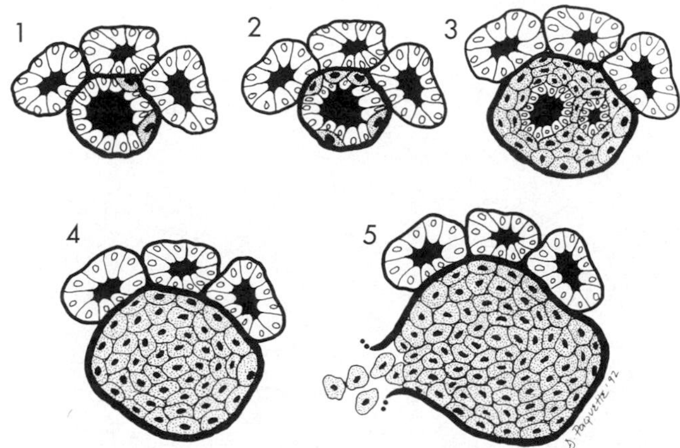

Fig. 61-37 Stages in the development of familial medullary thyroid carcinoma. C-cells are depicted with stippled cytoplasm. *1,* Normal C-cell topography; *2,* mild diffuse C-cell hyperplasia; *3* and *4,* nodular C-cell hyperplasia; *5,* medullary thyroid carcinoma. (From DeLellis RA: The pathology of medullary thyroid carcinoma and its precursors. In LiVolsi VA, DeLellis RA, editors: *Pathobiology of the parathyroid and thyroid glands,* Baltimore, 1993, Williams & Wilkins.)

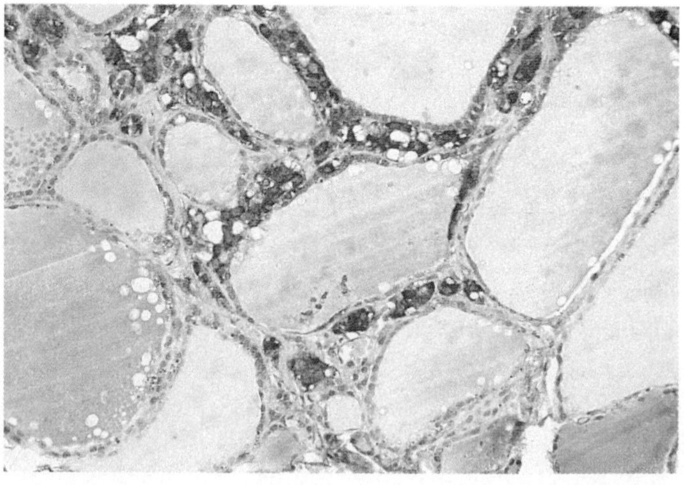

Fig. 61-38 C-cell hyperplasia stained for calcitonin with the peroxidase-antiperoxidase technique. Increased numbers of C-cells encircle the follicles.

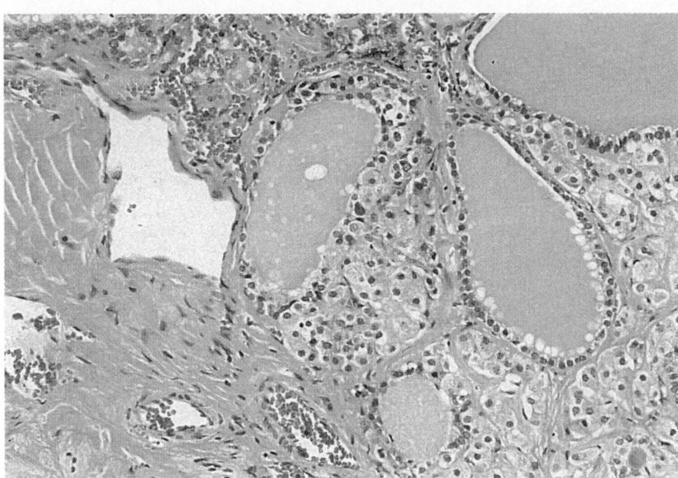

Fig. 61-39 C-cell hyperplasia from a patient with type 2A multiple endocrine neoplasia. The proliferation of C-cells involves this follicle in an eccentric fashion.

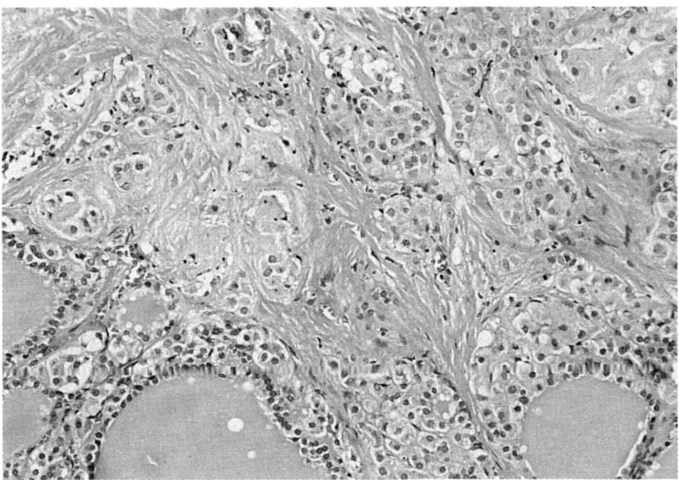

Fig. 61-40 C-cell hyperplasia with microscopic medullary thyroid carcinoma from a patient with type 2A multiple endocrine neoplasia (same case as shown in Fig. 61-39). C-cells have extended into the adjacent stroma.

or pentagastrin, 57% proved to have C-cell hyperplasia alone and 39.5% were found to have C-cell hyperplasia with microscopic foci of medullary carcinoma.[332] A single patient in this series was found to have no apparent C-cell abnormalities. None of the patients has exhibited evidence of nodal metastasis during more than 10 years of follow-up.

In addition to its presence in the type 2 MEN syndromes, C-cell hyperplasia has also been found in a variety of other conditions (Table 61-6). As might be expected in view of the secretagogue effects of calcium and gastrin on calcitonin secretion, C-cell hyperplasia may occur in patients with hypercalcemia of diverse causes and in patients with hypergastrinemia associated with the Zollinger-Ellison syndrome.[333] In addition, C-cell hyperplasia has been observed in occasional patients with Hashimoto's disease and hypothyroidism.[334-336] C-cell hyperplasia has also been reported to occur adjacent to papillary and follicular carcinomas of the thyroid.[337,338]

Table 61-6 C-cell hyperplasia

MEN 2 associated
Isolated (familial) medullary thyroid carcinoma
MEN 2A
MEN 2B
Non–MEN 2 associated
Hypercalcemia
Hypergastrinemia
Hashimoto's thyroiditis
Goitrous hypothyroidism
Peritumoral (adjacent to non–C-cell neoplasms)

MEN, multiple endocrine neoplasia.

Tumors of follicular and C-cells

Mixed medullary and follicular carcinoma

Tumors with combined features of medullary and follicular carcinoma are rare.[339] By definition these neoplasms, which have also been referred to as "intermediate carcinomas," should show morphologic evidence of follicular and C-cell differentiation and should contain thyroglobulin and calcitonin or other peptides.[340] The mixed medullary and follicular carcinomas should be distinguished from medullary carcinomas with entrapped normal thyroid follicles and the follicular variant of medullary carcinoma. Although the origin of mixed tumors is unknown, it has been suggested that they arise from uncommitted stem cells of the ultimobranchial body that have the capacity to differentiate into both C-cells and follicular cells.[341]

The mixed carcinomas most often have a fleshy appearance and may or may not be encapsulated. Microscopically they exhibit solid and follicular areas with or without cribriform areas[342] (Fig. 61-41). Follicular areas most often exhibit a microfollicular pattern. An important feature that distinguishes the mixed tumors from medullary carcinomas with entrapped follicles is the similarity of the nuclei in solid and follicular areas in the former. Entrapped normal follicles have normal-appearing nuclei.

Mixed medullary and follicular carcinomas stain positively for thyroglobulin. In the series of cases described by Ljungberg and coworkers,[342] 28% contained calcitonin, 57% contained somatostatin, and 71% contained neurotensin. In the cases reported by Holm and associates,[343] both calcitonin and thyroglobulin were present in the same tumor cells in both primary and metastatic lesions.

Mixed medullary and papillary carcinoma

Rare examples of mixed medullary and papillary carcinoma have been reported.[344] As expected, the medullary carcinoma cells stain positively for both calcitonin and carcinoembryonic antigen, but the papillary components stain positively only for thyroglobulin. Both components may also be evident in lymph node metastases (Fig. 61-42). Although mixed medullary and papillary neoplasms could arise from a common stem cell, the possibility that they represent collision tumors cannot be excluded.

Mesenchymal tumors

Benign mesenchymal tumors of the thyroid are very rare. Sarcomas such as fibrosarcoma[345] may occur in the thyroid, but a

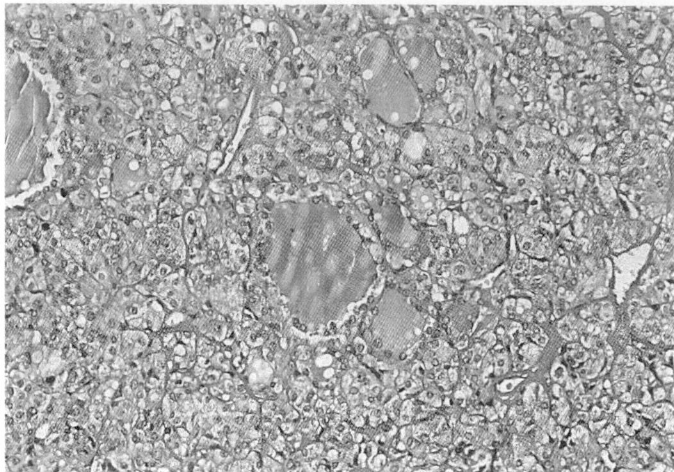

Fig. 61-41 Mixed follicular and medullary thyroid carcinoma. The tumor shows a predominantly solid pattern of growth.

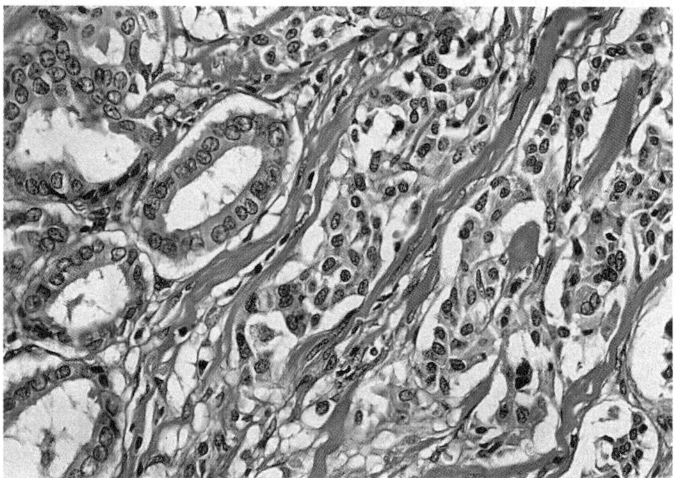

Fig. 61-42 Lymph node metastastic lesion of mixed papillary and medullary carcinoma. The papillary component shows a predominantly follicular growth pattern. Typical clear nuclei are present in the papillary component.

sarcoma can be diagnosed only after the alternative and more likely diagnosis of undifferentiated carcinoma has been ruled out. Several convincing cases of angiosarcoma of the thyroid have been reported.[346] Immunohistochemically the tumor cells show positivity for endothelial markers, including factor VIII and *Ulex europaeus,* and sometimes also for keratin.[347,348] Thyroid angiosarcomas are very aggressive tumors with a prognosis comparable to that of undifferentiated carcinoma.

Malignant lymphoma

The thyroid is involved in about 20% of the patients who die of generalized lymphoma. Primary thyroid lymphomas also occur; they constitute about 5% of all thyroid malignancies. They are more frequent in elderly women and present as a rapidly enlarging mass in the thyroid area, usually associated with compression symptoms such as dyspnea or dysphagia. Most thyroid lymphomas arise against a background of chronic lymphocytic thyroiditis (especially Hashimoto's thyroiditis). Grossly the thyroid is replaced by a whitish tan growth with a firm consistency. The adjacent lymph nodes are involved in a minority of cases, but extrathyroid extension is common.[349] Microscopically most thyroid lymphomas are of the diffuse large cell type[350] (Fig. 61-43). The second most common type is immunoblastic lymphoma; low-grade lymphomas composed of small or "intermediate" lymphocytes have also been described.[351] It has been suggested that low-grade thyroid lymphomas represent neoplasms of mucosa-associated lymphoid tissue.[352,353] The frequent recurrence of these lymphomas in the gastrointestinal tract seems to confirm this.[352]

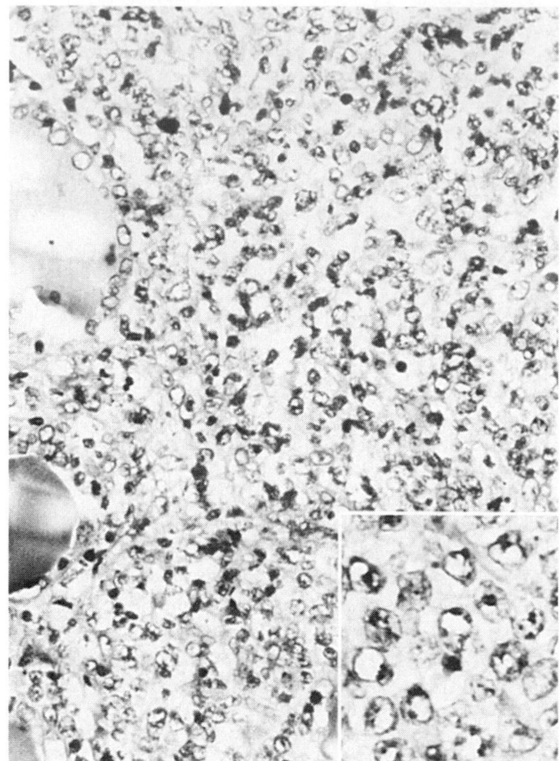

Fig. 61-43 Malignant lymphoma. Tumor cells invade between residual follicles with a diffuse pattern. *Inset,* Large vesicular nuclei and prominent nucleoli corresponding to large cell lymphoma.

Primary thyroid lymphomas stain positively for leukocyte common antigen and for markers indicative of B-cell derivation;[354-356] as such they are easily differentiated from other types of thyroid tumors, including poorly differentiated carcinoma and small cell medullary carcinoma.

The prognosis in patients with malignant lymphoma is better than that in patients with undifferentiated carcinoma, the 5-year survival being about 50%.[349]

The treatment for thyroid lymphoma consists of thyroidectomy followed by adjuvant therapy. *Plasmacytoma* may occur in the thyroid, and rare cases of *Hodgkin's disease* primarily involving the thyroid are on record.[357,358]

Metastatic tumors

Although clinically demonstrable metastastic lesions are uncommon in the thyroid, such lesions in the thyroid have been detected at autopsy in one fourth of the patients who have died of a metastasizing neoplasm.[359,360] The most common primary tumors are melanoma, breast carcinoma, and renal cell carcinoma. The latter may present as a thyroid nodule years after the removal of the kidney lesion.[361] Its differential diagnosis with primary clear cell thyroid tumors has been discussed in the section on clear cell tumors (see p. 1964)

REFERENCES

The normal thyroid gland

1. Arey LB: *Developmental anatomy,* Philadelphia, 1965, Saunders.
2. Gray H: *Anatomy of the human body,* Philadelphia, 1948, Lea & Febiger.
3. Hoyes AD, Kershaw DR: Anatomy and development of the thyroid gland, *Ear Nose Throat J* 64:318, 1985.
4. Norris EH: The early morphogenesis of the human thyroid gland, *Am J Anat* 24:443, 1918.
5. Sugiyama S: The embryology of the human thyroid gland including ultimobranchial body and others related, *Ergeb Anat Entwickl Gesch* 44:H2:6, 1971.
6. LiVolsi VA: Branchial and thymic remnants in the thyroid and cervical region: an explanation for unusual tumors and microscopic curiosities, *Endocr Pathol* 4:115, 1993.
7. Norris EH: The parathyroid glands and the lateral thyroid in man: their morphogenesis, histogenesis, topographic anatomy and prenatal growth, *Contrib Embryol Carneg Inst* 159:249, 1937.
8. Toran-Allerand CD: Normal development of the hypothalamic-pituitary-thyroid axis. In Ingbar SH, Braverman LE, editors: *Werner's The thyroid,* Philadelphia, 1986, Lippincott.
9. Weller GL: Development of the thyroid, parathyroid and thymus glands in man, *Contrib Gland Embryol Carneg Inst* 141:93, 1933.
10. LeDonavin N, Fontain J, LeLievre C: New studies on the neural crest origin of the avian ultimobranchial glandular cells—interspecific combinations and cytochemical characterization of C-cells based on the uptake of biogenic a immune precursors, *Histochemistry* 38:297, 1974.
11. Nadig J, Weber E, Hedinger C: C-cells in vestiges of the ultimobranchial body in human thyroid glands, *Virchows Arch* [B] 27:189, 1978.
12. Katoh R, Suzuki K, Hemmi A, Kawaoi A: Nature and significance of calcium oxalate crystals in normal human thyroid gland: a clinicopathological and immunohistochemical study, *Virchows Arch [A] (Pathol Anat Histopathol)* 422:301, 1993.
13. Klinck GH, Oertel JE, Winship T: Ulstrastructure of normal human thyroid, *Lab Invest* 22:2, 1970.
14. Kawaoi A, Okano T, Nemoto N, Shikata T: Production of thyroxine (T_4) and triiodothyronine (T_3) in nontoxic thyroid tumors: an immunohistochemical study, *Virchows Arch* [A] 390:249, 1981.
15. Kurata A, Ohta K, Mine M et al: Monoclonal antihuman thyroglobulin antibodies, *J Clin Endocrinol Metab* 59:573, 1984.
16. Permanetter W, Nathrath WBJ, Löhrs U: Immunohistochemical analysis of thyroglobulin and keratin in benign and malignant thyroid tumors, *Virchows Arch [A] (Pathol Anat Histopathol)* 398:221, 1982.
17. Stanta G, Carcangiu ML, Rosai J: The biochemical and immunohistochemical profile of thyroid neoplasia, *Pathol Annu* 23:129, 1988.
18. Bulley ID, Gatter KC, Hertet A, Mason DY: Expression of intermediate filament proteins in normal and diseased thyroid glands, *J Clin Pathol* 40:136, 1987.
19. Hiasa Y, Nishioka H, Kitahori Y et al: Immunohistochemical detection of estrogen receptors in paraffin sections of human thyroid tissues, *Oncology* 48:421, 1991.
20. Attwood HD, Dennett X: A black thyroid and minocycline treatment, *Br Med J* 2:1109, 1976.
21. Landas SK, Schelper RL, Tio FO et al: Black thyroid syndrome: exaggeration of a normal process?, *Am J Clin Pathol* 85:411, 1986.
22. Harach HR: Solid cell nests in the thyroid, *J Pathol* 155:191, 1988.
23. LiVolsi VA, Merino MJ: Squamous cells in the human thyroid gland, *Am J Surg Pathol* 2:113, 1978.
24. Finkle HI, Goldman RL: Heterotopic cartilage in the thyroid, *Arch Pathol* 95:48, 1973.
25. Braunstein H, Stephens CL: Parafollicular cells of the human thyroid, *Arch Pathol* 86:659, 1968.
26. DeLellis RA, Wolfe HJ: The pathobiology of the human calcitonin (C)-cell: a review, *Pathol Annu* 16:25, 1981.
27. O'Toole K, Fenoglio-Preiser C, Pushparaj N: Endocrine changes associated with the human aging process: III. Effects of age on the number of cal-citonin immunoreactive cells in the thyroid gland, *Hum Pathol* 16:991, 1985.
28. Gibson WC, Peng T-C, Croker BP: C-cell nodules in adult human thyroid: a common autopsy finding, *Am J Clin Pathol* 75:347, 1981.
29. DeLellis RA, May L, Tashjian AH Jr, Wolfe HJ: C-cell granule heterogeneity in man: an ultrastructural immunocytochemical study, *Lab Invest* 38:263, 1978.
30. DeLellis RA: Endocrine tumors. In Colvin RB, Bhan AR, McCluskey RT, editors: *Diagnostic immunopathology,* New York, 1988, Raven Press.
31. Müller MJ, Seitz HJ: Thyroid hormone action on intermediary metabolism. I. Respiration, thermogenesis and carbohydrate metabolism, *Klin Wochenschr* 62:11, 1984.
32. Müller MJ, Seitz HJ: Thyroid hormone action on intermediary metabolism. II. Lipid metabolism in hypo- and hyperthyroidism, *Klin Wochenschr* 62:49, 1984.
33. Müller MJ, Seitz HJ: Thyroid hormone action on intermediary metabolism. III. Protein metabolism in hyper- and hypothyroidism, *Klin Wochenschr* 62:97, 1984.
34. Green WL: Physiology of the thyroid gland and its hormones. In Green WL, editor: *The thyroid,* New York, 1987, Elsevier.
35. Ingbar S: The thyroid gland. In Wilson J, Foster D, editors: *William's textbook of endocrinology,* Philadelphia, 1985, Saunders.
36. Sterling K: Thyroid hormone action at the cell level, *N Engl J Med* 300:117, 1979.
37. Liddle GW, Liddle RA: Endocrinology. In Smith LH, Thier SO, editors: *Pathophysiology,* Philadelphia, 1981, Saunders.
38. Larsen R: Thyroid-pituitary interaction, *N Engl J Med* 306:23, 1982.
39. Pittman JA, Haigler ED et al: Hypothalamic hypothyroidism, *N Engl J Med* 285:844, 1971.
40. Pittmann JA: Thyrotropin-releasing hormone, *Adv Intern Med* 19:303, 1974.
41. Wilber JF: Thyrotropin releasing hormone: secretion and actions, *Annu Rev Med* 24:353, 1973.
42. MacIntyre I: Calcitonin: physiology, biosynthesis, secretion, metabolism and mode of action. In DeGroot LJ, editor: *Endocrinology,* Philadelphia, 1989, Saunders.
43. Amara SG, Jonas V, Rosenfeld MG et al: Alternative RNA processing in calcitonin gene expression generates mRNAs encoding different polypeptide products, *Nature* 298:240, 1982.
44. Scopsi L, Ferrari L, Pilotti S et al: Immunocytochemical localization and identification of prosomatostatin gene products in medullary carcinoma of human thyroid gland, *Hum Pathol* 21:820, 1990.
45. Sunday ME, Wolfe HJ, Roos BA et al: Gastrin releasing peptide gene expression in developing hyperplastic and neoplastic thyroid C-cells, *Endocrinology* 122:1551, 1988.
46. Nunez EA, Gershon MD: Thyrotropin induced thyroidal release of 5-hydroxytryptamine and accompanying ultrastructural changes in parafollicular cells, *Endocrinology* 113:309, 1983.
47. Gkonos PJ, Tavianini MA, Lui CC, Roos BA: Thyrotropin releasing hormone gene expression in normal thyroid parafollicular cells, *Mol Endocrinol* 3:2101, 1989.

Congenital abnormalities

48. Harada T, Nishikawa Y, Ito K: Aplasia of one thyroid lobe, *Am J Surg* 124:617, 1972.
49. Gaby M: The role of thyroid dysgenesis and maldescent in the etiology of sporadic cretinism, *J Pediatr* 60:830, 1962.
50. Burman KD, Adler RA, Wartofsky L: Hemiagenesis of the thyroid gland, *Am J Med* 58:143, 1975.
51. Melnick JC, Stemkowski PE: Thyroid hemiagenesis (hockey stick sign): a review of the world literature and a report of four cases, *J Clin Endocrinol Metab* 52:247, 1981.
52. Piera J, Garriga J, Calabuig R, Bargallo D: Thyroid hemiagenesis, *Am J Surg* 151:419, 1986.

53. Baughman RA: Lingual thyroid and lingual thyroglossal tract remnants, *Oral Surg* 34:781, 1972.
54. Neinas FW, Gorman CA, Devine KD, Woolner LB: Lingual thyroid: clinical characteristics of 15 cases, *Ann Intern Med* 79:205, 1973.
55. Reaume CE, Sofie VL: Lingual thyroid, *Oral Surg* 45:841, 1978.
56. Diaz-Arias AA, Bickel JT, Loy TS et al: Follicular carcinoma with clear cell change arising in lingual thyroid, *Oral Surg Oral Med Oral Pathol* 74:206, 1992.
57. Aguirre A, de la Piedra M, Ruiz R, Portilla J: Ectopic thyroid tissue in the submandibular region, *Oral Surg Oral Med Oral Pathol* 71:73, 1991.
58. Osammor JY, Bulman CH, Blewitt RW: Intralaryngotracheal thyroid, *J Laryngol Otol* 104:733, 1990.
59. Kantelip B, Lusson JR, DeRiberolles C et al: Intracardiac ectopic thyroid, *Hum Pathol* 17:1293, 1986.
60. Curtis LE, Sheahan DG: Heterotopic tissues in the gallbladder, *Arch Pathol* 88:677, 1969.
61. Johnson R , Hartman WH: The thyroid. In Silverberg S, editor: *Principles and practice of surgical pathology,* New York, 1983, Wiley Medical Publishers.
62. Rahn J: An unusual heterotopia of thyroid gland tissue, *Zentralbl Allg Pathol* 99:80, 1959.
63. Frantz VK, Forsythe R, Hanford JM, Rogers WM: Lateral aberrant thyroids, *Ann Surg* 115:161, 1942.
64. Janzer RC, Weber E, Hedinger C: The relation between solid cell nests and C-cells of the thyroid gland, *Cell Tissue Res* 197:295, 1979.
65. Sugiyama S: The embryology of the hyman thyroid gland including ultimobranchial body and others related, *Ergeb Anat Entwickl Gesch* 44:6, 1971.
66. Toran-Allerand CD: Normal development of the hypothalamic-pituitary-thyroid axis. In Ingbar SH, Braverman LE, editors, *Werner's the thyroid,* Philadelphia, 1986, Lippincott.
67. Allard RHB: The thyroglossal cyst, *Head Neck Surg* 5:134, 1982.
68. Dalgaard JB, Witteland P: Thyroglossal anomalies: a follow-up study of 58 cases, *Acta Chir Scand* 111:444, 1956.
69. Solomon JR, Rangecroft L: Thyroglossal-duct lesions in childhood, *J Pediatr Surg* 19:555, 1984.
70. Joseph TJ, Komorowski RA: Thyroglossal duct carcinoma, *Hum Pathol* 6:717, 1975.
71. Fernández JF, Ordóñez NG, Schultz PN et al: Thyroglossal duct carcinoma, *Surgery* 110:928, 1991.
72. LiVolsi VA, Perzin KH, Savetsky L: Carcinoma arising in median ectopic thyroid (including thyroglossal duct tissue), *Cancer* 34:1303, 1974.
73. Weiss SD, Orlich CC: Primary papillary carcinoma of a thyroglossal duct cyst: report of a case and literature review, *Br J Surg* 78:87, 1991.
74. Palacios J, Gamallo C, García M, Rodríguez JI: Decrease in thyrocalcitonin-containing cells and analysis of other congenital anomalies in 11 patients with DiGeorge syndrome, *Am J Med Genet* 46:641, 1993.
75. Pueblitz S, Weinberg AG, Albores-Saavedra J: Thyroid C-cells in the DiGeorge anomaly: a quantitative study, *Pediatr Pathol* 13:463, 1993.

Thyroiditis

76. Singer PA: Thyroiditis: acute, subacute and chronic, *Med Clin North Am* 75:61, 1991.
77. Frank TS, LiVolsi VA, Connor AM: Cytomegalovirus infection of the thyroid in immunocompromised adults, *Yale J Biol Med* 60:1, 1987.
78. Guttler R, Singer PA, Axline SG et al: *Pneumocystis carinii* thyroiditis: report of three cases and review of the literature, *Arch Intern Med* 153:393, 1993.
79. Ragni MV, Dekker A, DeRubertis FR et al: *Pneumocystis carinii* infection presenting as necrotizing thyroiditis and hypothyroidism, *Am J Clin Pathol* 95:489, 1991.
80. Miyauchi A, Matsuzuka F, Kuma K, Takai S: Piriform sinus fistula: an underlying abnormality common in patients with acute suppurative thyroiditis, *World J Surg* 14:400, 1990.
81. Holten I: Acute response of the thyroid to external radiation, *Acta Pathol Microbiol Scand* 91(suppl 283):9, 1983.
82. Eylan E, Zmucky R, Sheba C: Mumps virus and subacute thyroiditis: evidence of a causal association, *Lancet* 1:1062, 1967.
83. Volpé R, Row VV, Ezrin C: Circulating viral and thyroid antibodies in subacute thyroiditis, *J Clin Endocrinol Metab* 27:1275, 1967.
84. Nyulassy S, Hnilica P, Buc M et al: Subacute (de Quervain) thyroiditis: association with HLA-B35 antigen and abnormalities of the complement system immunoglobulins and other serum proteins, *J Clin Endocrinol Metab* 45:270, 1977.
85. Carney JA, Moore SB, Northcutt RC et al: Palpation thyroiditis (multifocal granulomatous folliculitis), *Am J Clin Pathol* 64:639, 1975.
86. LiVolsi VA: *Surgical pathology of the thyroid,* Philadelphia, 1990, Saunders.
87. Sachs MK, Dickinson G, Amazon K: Tuberculous adenitis of the thyroid mimicking subacute thyroiditis, *Am J Med* 85:573, 1988.
88. Harach MR, Williams ED: The pathology of granulomatous diseases of the thyroid gland, *Sarcoidosis* 7:19, 1990.
89. Kakudo K, Kanokogi M, Mitsunobu M et al: Acute mycotic thyroiditis, *Acta Pathol Jpn* 33:147, 1983.
90. Mizukami Y, Michigishi T, Kawato M et al: Chronic thyroiditis: thyroid function and histologic correlations in 601 cases, *Hum Pathol* 23:980, 1992.
91. Solomon DH, Beall GN, Tersaki PI et al: Autoimmune thyroid disease—Graves' and Hashimoto's, *Ann Intern Med* 88:379, 1978.
92. Volpé R, Farid NR, Von Westarp C, Row VV: The pathogenesis of Graves' disease and Hashimoto's thyroiditis, *Clin Endocrinol* 3:239, 1974.
93. Hashimoto H: Zur Kenntniss der lymphomatosen Veränderung der Schilddrüse (Struma lymphomatosa), *Arch Klin Chir* 97:219, 1912.
94. Davies TF, Kendler DL: Mechanisms of autoimmune thyroid disease. In LiVolsi VA, DeLellis RA, editors, *Pathobiology of the parathyroid and thyroid glands,* Baltimore, 1993, Williams & Wilkins.
95. Westman AP: Autoimmune thyroiditis: predisposition and pathogenesis, *Clin Endocrinol* 36:307, 1992.
96. Carpenter CCJ, Solomon N, Silverberg SG et al: Schmidt's syndrome (thyroid and adrenal insufficiency): a review of the literature and a report of fifteen new cases including ten instances of coexistent diabetes mellitus, *Medicine* (Baltimore) 43:153, 1964.
97. Khardori R, Eagleton LE, Soler NG, McConnachie PR: Lymphocytic interstitial pneumonitis in autoimmune thyroid disease, *Am J Med* 90:649, 1991.
98. Wick MR, Sawyer MD: Antigenic alteration in autoimmune thyroid diseases, *Arch Pathol Lab Med* 113:77, 1989.
99. Hamburger JI, Miller JM, Kini SR: Lymphoma of the thyroid, *Ann Intern Med* 99:685, 1983.
100. Holm L-E, Blomgren H, Löwhagen T: Cancer risks in patients with chronic lymphocytic thyroiditis, *N Engl J Med* 312:601, 1985.
101. Thomas CG Jr, Rutledge RG: Surgical intervention in chronic (Hashimoto's) thyroiditis, *Ann Surg* 193:769, 1981.
102. Katz SM, Vickery AL: The fibrous variant of Hashimoto's thyroiditis, *Hum Pathol* 5:161, 1974.
103. Drexhage HA, Bottazzo GF, Doniach D et al: Evidence for thyroid-growth stimulating immunoglobulins in some goitrous thyroid disease, *Lancet* 2:287, 1980.
104. Drexhage HA, Bottazzo GF, Bitensky L et al: Thyroid growth-blocking antibodies in primary myxoedema, *Nature* 289:594, 1981.
105. Konishi J, Iida Y, Kasagi K et al: Primary myxedema with thyrotropin-binding inhibitor immunoglobulins: clinical and laboratory findings in 15 patients, *Ann Intern Med* 103:26, 1985.
106. Valente WA, Yavin Z, Yavin E et al: Monoclonal antibodies to the thyrotropin receptor: the identification of blocking and stimulating antibodies, *J Endocrinol Invest* 5:293, 1982.
107. Valente WA, Vitti P, Rotella CM et al: Antibodies that promote thyroid growth, *N Engl J Med* 309:1028, 1983.
108. Greenberg AH, Czernichow P, Hung W et al: Juvenile chronic lymphocytic thyroiditis: clinical, laboratory and histological correlations, *J Clin Endocrinol Metab* 30:293, 1970.
109. Rallison ML, Dobyns BM, Keating FR et al: Occurrence and natural history of chronic lymphocytic thyroiditis in childhood, *J Pediatr* 86:675, 1975.
110. Gluck FB, Nusynowitz ML, Plymate S: Chronic lymphocytic thyroiditis, thyrotoxicosis, and low radioactive iodine uptake, *N Engl J Med* 293:624, 1975.
111. Nikolai TF, Brosseau J, Kettrick MA et al: Lymphocytic thyroiditis, *Arch Intern Med* 147:221, 1987.

112. Papapetrou PD, Jackson IMD: Thyrotoxicosis due to "silent" thyroiditis, *Lancet* 1:361, 1975.
113. Woolf PD: Transient painless thyroiditis with hyperthyroidism: a variant of lymphocytic thyroiditis? *Endocr Rev* 1:411, 1980.
114. Farid NR, Hawe BS, Walfish PG: Increased frequency of HLA-DR3 and 5 in the syndromes of painless thyroiditis with transient thyrotoxicosis: evidence for an autoimmune aetiology, *Clin Endocrinol* 19:699, 1983.
115. Mitani Y, Shigemasa C, Taniguchi S et al: Clinical course of silent thyroiditis in a patient with Sjögren's syndrome, *Arch Intern Med* 148:1974, 1988.
116. Singer PA, Gorsky JE: Familial postpartum transient hyperthyroidism, *Arch Intern Med* 145:240, 1985.
117. Volpé R: Is silent thyroiditis an autoimmune disease?, *Arch Intern Med* 148:1907, 1988.
118. Amino N, Mori H, Iwatani Y et al: High prevalence of transient postpartum thyrotoxicosis and hypothyroidism, *Med Intell* 306:849, 192.
119. Freeman R, Rosen H, Thysen B: Incidence of thyroid dysfunction in an unselected postpartum population, *Arch Intern Med* 146:1361, 1986.
120. Jansson R, Bernander S, Karlsson A et al: Autoimmune thyroid dysfunction in the postpartum period, *J Clin Endocrinol Metab* 58:681, 1984.
121. Nikolai TF, Brosseau J, Kettrick MA et al: Lymphocytic thyroiditis, *Arch Intern Med* 147:221, 1987.
122. Mizukami Y, Michigishi T et al: Silent thyroiditis: a histologic and immunohistochemical study, *Hum Pathol* 19:423, 1988.
123. Okayasu I, Hatakeyama S, Tanaka Y et al: Is focal chronic autoimmune thyroiditis an age-related disease? Differences in incidence and severity between Japanese and British, *J Pathol* 163:257, 1991.
124. Williams ED, Doniach I: The post-mortem incidence of focal thyroiditis, *J Pathol Bacteriol* 83:255, 1962.
125. Schwaegerle SM, Bauer TW, Esselstyn CB: Riedel's thyroiditis, *Am J Clin Pathol* 90:715, 1988.
126. Woolner LB, McConaher WM, Beahrs OH: Invasive fibrous thyroiditis (Riedel's struma), *J Clin Endocrinol Metab* 17:201, 1957.
127. Meyer S, Hausman R: Occlusive phlebitis in multifocal fibrosclerosis, *Am J Clin Pathol* 65:274, 1976.
128. Nielsen HK: Multifocal idiopathic fibrosclerosis: two cases with simultaneous occurrence of retroperitoneal fibrosis and Riedel's thyroiditis, *Acta Med Scand* 206:119, 1980.
129. Levine SN: Current concepts of thyroiditis, *Arch Intern Med* 143:1952, 1983.
130. Harach HR, Williams ED: Fibrous thyroiditis: an immunopathological study, *Histopathology* 7:739, 1983.
131. Taubenberger JK, Merino MJ, Medeiros LJ: A thyroid biopsy with histologic features of both Riedel's thyroiditis and the fibrosing variant of Hashimoto's thyroiditis, *Hum Pathol* 23:1072, 1991.

Graves' disease

132. Gossage AAR, Munro DS: The pathogenesis of Graves' disease, *Clin Endocrinol Metab* 14:299, 1985.
133. Jansson R, Karlsson A, Forsum U: Intrathyroidal HLA-DR expression and T-lymphocyte phenotypes in Graves' thyrotoxicosis, Hashimoto's thyroiditis and nodular colloid goitre, *Clin Exp Immunol* 58:264, 1984.
134. Hanafusa T, Pujol-Borrell R, Chiovato L et al: Aberrant expression of HLA-DR antigen of thyrocytes in Graves' disease: relevance for autoimmunity, *Lancet* 2:1111, 1983.
135. Volpe R: Autoimmune thyroid disease: a perspective, *Mol Biol Med* 3:25, 1986.
136. Bahn RS, Heufelder AE: Pathogenesis of Graves' ophthalmopathy, *N Engl J Med* 329:1468, 1993.
137. Nixon DW, Samols E: Acral changes associated with thyroid diseases, *JAMA* 212:1175, 1970.
138. Spjut HJ, Warren WD, Ackerman LV: A clinical pathologic study of 76 cases of recurrent Graves' disease, toxic (nonexophthalmic) goiter, and nontoxic goiter, *Am J Clin Pathol* 27:367, 1957.
139. Eggen PC, Seljelid R: The histological appearance of hyperfunctioning thyroids following various preoperative treatments, *Acta Pathol Microbiol Scand [A]* 81:16,1973.
140. Mizukami Y, Michigishi T, Nonomura A et al: Histologic changes in Graves' thyroid gland after 131I therapy for hyperthyroidism, *Acta Pathol Jpn* 42:419, 1992.
141. Johnson WC Hellwig EB: Cutaneous focal mucinosis: a clinicopathological and histochemical study, *Arch Dermatol* 93:13, 1966.
142. Farbota LM, Calandra DB, Lawrence AM, Paloyan E: Thyroid carcinoma in Graves' disease, *Surgery* 98:1148, 1985.
143. Caruso DR, Mazzaferri EL: Intervention in Graves' disease: choosing among imperfect but effective treatment options, *Postgrad Med* 92:117, 128, 133, 1992.
144. Falk SA: The management of hyperthyroidism: a surgeon's perspective, *Otolaryngol Clin North Am* 23:361, 1990.
145. Farrar JJ, Toft AD: Iodine-131 treatment of hyperthyroidism: current issues, *Clin Endocrinol* 35:207, 1991.
146. Sridama V, McCormick M, Kaplan EL et al: Long-term follow-up study of compensated low-dose 131I therapy for Graves' disease, *N Engl J Med* 311:426, 1984.

Hyperplasia

147. Lever EG, Medeiros-Neto GA, DeGroot LJ: Inherited disorders of thyroid metabolism, *Endocrinol Rev* 4:213, 1983.
148. Stanbury JB: Inborn errors of the thyroid, *Prog Med Genet* 10:55, 1974.
149. Barsano CP, DeGroot LJ: Dyshormonogenetic goitre, *Clin Endocrinol Metab* 8:145, 1979.
150. Kennedy JS: The pathology of dyshormonogenetic goiter, *J Pathol* 99:251, 1969.
151. Vickery AL: The diagnosis of malignancy in dyshormonogenetic goitre, *Clin Endocrinol Metab* 10:317, 1981.
152. Cooper DS, Axelrod L, DeGroot LJ et al: Congenital goiter and the development of metastatic follicular carcinoma with evidence for a leak of nonhormonal iodide: clinical, pathological, kinetic, and biochemical studies and a review of the literature, *J Clin Endocrinol Metab* 52:294, 1981.
153. Gaitan E, Nelson NC, Poole GV: Endemic goiter and endemic thyroid disorders, *World J Surg* 15:205, 1991.
154. Woeber KA: Iodine and thyroid disease, *Med Clin North Am* 75:169, 1991.
155. Mortensen JD, Woolner LB, Bennett WA: Gross and microscopic findings in clinically normal thyroid glands, *J Clin Endocrinol Metab* 15:1270, 1955.
156. Tunbridge WMG, Evered DC, Hall R et al: The spectrum of thyroid disease in a community: the Whickham survey, *Clin Endocrinol* 7:481, 1977.
157. Brown RS, Pohl SL, Jackson IMD, Reichlin S: Do thyroid-stimulating immunoglobulins cause non-toxic and toxic multinodular goitre? *Lancet* 1:904, 1978.
158. Hennemann G: Non-toxic goitre, *Clin Endocrinol Metab* 8:167, 1979.
159. Studer H, Ramelli F: Simple goiter and its variants: euthyroid and hyperthyroid multinodular goiters, *Endocr Rev* 3:40, 1982.
160. Doniach D, Chiovato L, Hanafusa T, Bottazzo GF: The implications of "thyroid-growth-immunoglobulins" (TGI) for the understanding of sporadic nontoxic nodular goitre, *Springer Semin Immunopathol* 5:433, 1982.
161. Ramelli F, Studer H, Bruggisser D: Pathogenesis of thyroid nodules in multinodular goiter, *Am J Pathol* 109:215, 1982.
162. Berghout A, Wiersinga WM, Smits NJ, Touber JL: Interrelationships between age, thyroid volume, thyroid nodularity, and thyroid function in patients with sporadic nontoxic goiter, *Am J Med* 89:602, 1990.
163. Peter HJ, Studer H, Forster R, Gerber H: The pathogenesis of hot and cold follicles in multinodular goiters, *J Clin Endocrin Metab* 55:941, 1982.
164. Studer H, Gerber H, Zbaeren J, Peter HJ: Histomorphological and immunohistochemical evidence that human nodular goiters grow by episodic replication of multiple clusters of thyroid follicular cells, *J Clin Endocrinol Metab* 75:1151, 1992.
165. Sugenoya A, Masuda H, Komatsu M et al: Adenomatous goitre: therapeutic strategy, postoperative outcome, and study of epidermal growth factor receptor, *Br J Surg* 79:404, 1992.
166. Davis PJ, Davis FB: Hyperthyroidism in patients over the age of 60 years, clinical features in 85 patients, *Medicine* 53:161, 1974.
167. Studer H, Peter HJ, Gerber H: Toxic nodular goitre, *Clin Endocrinol Metab* 14:351, 1985.

168. Hamburger JI: Solitary autonomously functioning thyroid lesions: diagnosis, clinical features and pathogenetic considerations, *Am J Med* 58:740, 1975.

Generalities and classification of thyroid tumors

169. Carr RF, LiVolsi VA: Morphologic changes in the thyroid after irradiation for Hodgkin's and non-Hodgkin's lymphoma, *Cancer* 64:825, 1989.
170. DeJong SA, Demeter JG, Jarosz H et al: Thyroid carcinoma and hyperparathyroidism after radiation therapy for adolescent acne vulgaris, *Surgery* 110:691, 1991.
171. Furmanchuk AW, Averkin JI, Egloff B et al: Pathomorphological findings in thyroid cancers of children from the Republic of Belarus: a study of 86 cases occurring between 1986 ("post-Chernobyl") and 1991, *Histopathology* 21:401, 1992.
172. Mazzaferri EL: Management of a solitary thyroid nodule, *N Engl J Med* 328:553, 1993.
173. Gharib H, Goellner JR: Fine-needle aspiration biopsy of thyroid: an appraisal, *Ann Intern Med* 118:282, 1993.

Tumors of follicular cells

174. Hedinger CE: *Histological typing of thyroid tumours,* Berlin, 1988, Springer-Verlag.
175. Hicks DG, LiVolsi VA, Neidich JA et al: Clonal analysis of solitary follicular nodules in the thyroid, *Am J Pathol* 137:553, 1990.
176. Namba H, Matsuo K, Fagin JA: Clonal composition of benign and malignant human thyroid tumors, *J Clin Invest* 86:120, 1990.
177. Dal Cin P, Sneyers W, Aly MS et al: Involvement of 19q13 in follicular thyroid adenoma, *Cancer Genet Cytogenet* 60:99, 1992.
178. Miettinen M, Virtanen I: Expresion of laminin in thyroid gland and thyroid tumors: an immunohistologic study, *Int J Cancer* 34:27, 1984.
179. Hostetter AL, Hrafnkelsson J, Wingren SO et al: A comparative study of DNA cytometry methods for benign and malignant thyroid tissue, *Am J Clin Pathol* 89:760, 1988.
180. Zedenius J, Auer G, Backdahl M et al: Follicular tumors of the thyroid gland: diagnosis, clinical aspects and nuclear DNA analysis, *World J Surg* 16:589, 1992.
181. Carney JA, Ryan J, Goellner JR: Hyalinizing trabecular adenoma of the thyroid gland, *Am J Surg Pathol* 11:583, 1987.
182. Katoh R, Jasani B, Williams ED: Hyalinizing trabecular adenoma of the thyroid: a report of three cases with immunohistochemical and ultrastructural studies, *Histopathology* 15:211, 1989.
183. Franssila K, Saxén E, Teppo L et al: Incidence of different morphological types of thyroid cancer in the Nordic countries, *Acta Pathol Microbiol Scand [A]* 89:49, 1981.
184. Williams ED, Doniach I, Bjarnason O et al: Thyroid cancer in an iodide-rich area, *Cancer* 39:215, 1977.
185. Hofstadter F: Frequency and morphology of malignant tumours of the thyroid before and after the introduction of iodine-prophylaxis, *Virchows Arch [A] (Pathol Anat Histol)* 385:263, 1980.
186. Farbota LM, Calandra DB, Lawrence AM, Paloyan E: Thyroid carcinoma in Graves' disease, *Surgery* 98:1148, 1985.
187. Ott RA, Calandra DB, McCall A et al: The incidence of thyroid carcinoma in patients with Hashimoto's thyroiditis and solitary cold nodules, *Surgery* 98:1202, 1985.
188. Carcangiu ML, Zampi G, Pupi A et al: Papillary carcinoma of the thyroid: a clinicopathologic study of 241 cases treated at the University of Florence, Italy, *Cancer* 55:805, 1985.
189. Carcangiu ML, Zampi G, Rosai J: Papillary thyroid carcinoma: a study of its many morphologic expressions and clinical correlates, *Pathol Annu* 20:1, 1985.
190. Tscholl-Ducommun J, Hedinger CE: Papillary thyroid carcinomas: morphology and prognosis, *Virchows Arch [A] (Pathol Anat Histol)* 396:19, 1982.
191. Vickery AL Jr: Thyroid papillary carcinoma, *Am J Surg Pathol* 7:797, 1983.
192. Scopa CD, Melachrinou M, Saradopoulou C, Merino MJ: The significance of the grooved nucleus in thyroid lesions, *Mod Pathol* 6:691, 1993.
193. Klinck GH, Winship T: Psammoma bodies and thyroid cancer, *Cancer* 12:656, 1959.
194. Johannessen JV, Sobrinho-Simões M: The origin and significance of thyroid psammoma bodies, *Lab Invest* 43:287, 1980.
195. Chan JK, Carcangiu ML, Rosai J: Papillary carcinoma of thyroid with exuberant nodular fasciitis-like stroma: report of three cases, *Am J Clin Pathol* 95:309, 1991.
196. Buley ID, Gatter KC, Heryet A, Mason DY: Expression of intermediate filament proteins in normal and diseased thyroid glands, *J Clin Pathol* 40:136, 1987.
197. Henzen-Logmans SC, Mullink H, Ramaekers FCS et al: Expression of cytokeratins and vimentin in epithelial cells of normal and pathologic thyroid tissue, *Virchows Arch [A]* 410:347, 1987.
198. Schelfhout LJ, Van Muijen GN, Fleuren GJ: Expression of keratin 19 distinguishes papillary thyroid carcinoma from follicular carcinomas and follicular thyroid adenoma, *Am J Clin Pathol* 92:654, 1989.
199. Diaz NM, Mazoujian G, Wick MR: Estrogen-receptor protein in thyroid neoplasms: an immunohistochemical analysis of papillary carcinoma, follicular carcinoma, and follicular adenoma, *Arch Pathol Lab Med* 115:1203, 1991.
200. Santoro M, Carlomagno F, Hay ID et al: *Ret* oncogene activation in human thyroid neoplasms is restricted to the papillary cancer subtype, *J Clin Invest* 89:1517, 1992.
201. Wajjwalku W, Nakamura S, Hasegawa Y et al: Low frequency of rearrangements of the *ret* and *trk* proto-oncogenes in Japanese thyroid papillary carcinomas, *Jpn J Cancer Res* 83:671, 1992.
202. Deligeorgi-Politi H: Nuclear crease as a cytodiagnostic feature of papillary thyroid carcinoma in fine-needle aspiration biopsies, *Diagn Cytopathol* 3:307, 1987.
203. Katoh R, Sasaki J, Kurihara H et al: Multiple thyroid involvement (intraglandular metastasis) in papillary thyroid carcinoma: a clinicopathologic study of 105 consecutive patients, *Cancer* 70:1585, 1992.
204. Russell WO, Ibañez ML, Clark RL, White EC: Thyroid carcinoma: classification, intraglandular dissemination and clinicopathological study based upon whole organ sections of 80 glands, *Cancer* 16:1425, 1963.
205. DeGroot LJ, Kaplan EL, McCormick M, Straus FH: Natural history, treatment, and course of papillary thyroid carcinoma, *J Clin Endocrinol Metab* 71:414, 1990.
206. McConahey WM, Hay ID, Wollner LB et al: Papillary thyroid cancer treated at the Mayo Clinic, 1946 through 1970: initial manifestations, pathologic findings, therapy, and outcome, *Mayo Clin Proc* 61:978, 1986.
207. Cady B: Papillary carcinoma of the thyroid, *Semin Surg Oncol* 7:81, 1991.
208. Cohn K, Bäckdahl M, Forsslund G et al: Prognostic value of nuclear DNA content in papillary thyroid carcinoma, *World J Surg* 8:474, 1984.
209. Joensuu H, Klemi P, Eerola E, Tuominen J: Influence of cellular DNA content on survival in differentiated thyroid cancer, *Cancer* 58:2462, 1986.
210. Bondeson L, Ljungberg O: Occult papillary thyroid carcinoma in the young and the aged, *Cancer* 53:1790, 1984.
211. Ha ID, Grant CS, van Heerden JA et al: Papillary thyroid microcarcinoma: a study of 535 cases observed in a 50-year period, *Surgery* 112:1139, 1992.
212. Klinck GH, Winship T: Occult sclerosing carcinoma of the thyroid, *Cancer* 8:701, 1955.
213. Evans HL: Encapsulated papillary neoplasms of the thyroid: a study of 14 cases followed for a minimum of 10 years, *Am J Surg Pathol* 11:592, 1987.
214. Schröder S, Böcker W, Dralle H et al: The encapsulated papillary carcinoma of the thyroid: a morphologic subtype of the papillary thyroid carcinoma, *Cancer* 54:90, 1984.
215. Lindsay A: *Carcinoma of the thyroid gland: a clinical and pathologic study of 293 patients at the University of California Hospital,* Springfield, Ill., 1960, Charles C Thomas.
216. Chen KTK, Rosai J: Follicular variant of thyroid papillary carcinoma: a clinicopathologic study of six cases, *Am J Surg Pathol* 1:123, 1977.
217. Rosai J, Zampi G, Carcangiu ML: Papillary carcinoma of the thyroid: a discussion of its several morphologic expressions, with particular emphasis on the follicular variant, *Am J Surg Pathol* 7:809, 1983.
218. Evans HL: Follicular neoplasms of the thyroid, *Cancer* 54:535, 1984.
219. Carcangiu ML, Bianchi S: Diffuse sclerosing variant of papillary thyroid carcinoma: clinicopathologic study of 15 cases, *Am J Surg Pathol* 13:1041, 1989.

220. Fujimoto Y, Obara T, Ito Y et al: Diffuse sclerosing variant of papillary carcinoma of the thyroid: clinical importance, surgical treatment, and follow-up study, *Cancer* 66:2306, 1990.
221. Mizukami Y Nonomura A, Michigishi T et al: Diffuse sclerosing variant of papillary carcinoma of the thyroid, *Acta Pathol Jpn* 40:676, 1990.
222. Soares J, Limbert E, Sobrinho-Simões M: Diffuse sclerosing variant of papillary thyroid carcinoma, *Pathol Res Pract* 185:200, 1989.
223. Flint A, Davenport RD, Lloyd RV: The tall cell variant of papillary carcinoma of the thyroid gland: comparison with the common form of papillary carcinoma by DNA and morphometric analysis, *Arch Pathol Lab Med* 115:169, 1991.
224. Johnson TL, Lloyd RV, Thompson NW et al: Prognostic implications of the tall cell variant of papillary thyroid carcinoma, *Am J Surg Pathol* 12:22, 1988.
225. Sobrinho-Simões M, Sambade C, Nesland JM, Johannessen JV: Tall cell papillary carcinoma, *Am J Surg Pathol* 13:79, 1989.
226. Berends D, Mouthaan PJ: Columnar-cell carcinoma of the thyroid, *Histopathology* 20:360, 1992.
227. Evans HL: Columnar-cell carcinoma of the thyroid: a report of two cases of an aggressive variant of thyroid carcinoma, *Am J Clin Pathol* 85:77, 1986.
228. Sobrinho-Simões M, Nesland JM, Johannessen JV: Columnar-cell carcinoma: another variant of poorly differentiated carcinoma of the thyroid, *Am J Clin Pathol* 89:264, 1988.
229. Meissner WA, Warren S: Tumors of the thyroid gland. In *Atlas of tumor pathology,* series 1, Washington, D.C., 1968, Armed Forces Institute of Pathology.
230. Yamashina M: Follicular neoplasms of the thyroid: total circumferential evaluation of the fibrous capsule, *Am J Surg Pathol* 16:392, 1992.
231. González Cámpora R, Montero C, Martin-Lacave I, Galera H: Demonstration of vascular endothelium in thyroid carcinomas using *Ulex europeaus* I agglutinin, *Histopathology* 10:261, 1986.
232. Harach HR, Jasani B, Williams ED: Factor VIII as a marker of endothelial cells in follicular carcinoma of the thyroid, *J Clin Pathol* 36:1050, 1983.
233. Stephenson TJ, Griffiths DWR, Mills PM: Comparison of *Ulex europaeus* I lectin binding and factor VIII–related antigen as markers of vascular endothelium in follicular carcinoma of the thyroid, *Histopathology* 10:251, 1986.
234. Cady B, Rossi R, Silverman M, Wool M: Further evidence of the validity of risk group definition in differentiated thyroid carcinoma, *Surgery* 98:1171, 1985.
235. Iida F: Surgical significance of capsule invasion of adenoma of the thyroid, *Surg Gynecol Obstet* 144:710, 1977.
236. Lang W, Choritz H, Hundeshagen H: Risk factors in follicular thyroid carcinomas: a retrospective follow-up study covering a 14-year period with emphasis on morphological findings, *Am J Surg Pathol* 10:246, 1986.
237. Brennan MD, Bergstralh EJ, van Heerden JA, McConahey WM: Follicular thyroid cancer treated at the Mayo Clinic, 1946 through 1970: initial manifestations, pathologic findings, therapy and outcome, *Mayo Clin Proc* 66:11, 1991.
238. van Heerden JA, Hay ID, Goellner JR et al: Follicular thyroid carcinoma with capsular invasion alone: a nonthreatening malignancy, *Surgery* 112:1130, 1992.
239. Woolner, LB, Beahrs OH, Black BM et al: Classification and prognosis of thyroid carcinoma, *Am J Surg* 102:354, 1961.
240. Woolner LB: Thyroid carcinoma: pathologic classification with data on prognosis, *Semin Nucl Med* 1:481, 1971.
241. Carcangiu ML, Bianchi S, Savino D et al: Follicular Hürthle cell tumors of the thyroid gland, *Cancer* 68:1944, 1991.
242. Tallini G, Carcangiu ML, Rosai J: Oncocytic neoplasms of the thyroid gland, *Acta Pathol Jpn* 42:305, 1992.
243. Rosai J, Carcangiu ML: Pathology of thyroid tumors: some recent and old questions, *Hum Pathol* 15:1008, 1984.
244. Bondeson L, Bondeson A-G, Ljungberg O, Tibblin S: Oxyphil tumors of the thyroid: follow-up of 42 surgical cases, *Ann Surg* 194:677, 1981.
245. Bronner MP, LiVolsi VA: Oxyphilic (Askanazy/Hürthle cell) tumors of the thyroid: microscopic features predict biologic behavior, *Surg Pathol* 1:137, 1988.
246. Horn RC Jr: Hürthle cell tumors of the thyroid, *Cancer* 7:234, 1954.
247. Watson RG, Brennan MD, Goellner JR et al: Invasive Hürthle cell carcinoma of the thyroid: natural history and management, *Mayo Clin Proc* 59:851, 1984.
248. Barbuto D, Carcangiu ML, Rosai J: Papillary Hürthle cell neoplasms of the thyroid gland: a study of 20 cases [abstract], *Mod Pathol* 3:7A, 1990.
249. Nesland JM, Sobrinho-Simões MA, Holm R et al: Hürthle-cell lesions of the thyroid: a combined study using transmission electron microscopy, scanning electron microscopy and immunocytochemistry, *Ultrastruct Pathol* 8:269, 1985.
250. Frazell EL, Duffy BJ Jr: Hürthle cell cancer of the thyroid: a review of forty cases, *Cancer* 4:952, 1951.
251. Gundry SR, Burney RE, Thompson NW, Lloyd R: Total thyroidectomy for Hürthle cell neoplasm of the thyroid, *Arch Surg* 118:529, 1983.
252. Schark C, Fulton N, Yashiro T et al: The value of measurement of *ras* oncogenes and nuclear DNA analysis in the diagnosis of Hürthle cell tumors of the thyroid, *World J Surg* 16:745, 1992.
253. Carcangiu ML, Sibley RK, Rosai J: Clear cell change in primary thyroid tumors: a study of 38 cases, *Am J Surg Pathol* 9:705, 1985.
254. Dickersin GR, Vickery AL Jr, Smith SB: Papillary carcinoma of the thyroid, oxyphil cell type, "clear cell" variant: a light- and electron-microscopic study, *Am J Surg Pathol* 4:501, 1980.
255. Schröder S, Böcker W: Signet-right cell thyroid tumors: follicle cell tumors with arrest of folliculogenesis, *Am J Surg Pathol* 9:619, 1985.
256. Schröder S, Böcker W: Clear cell carcinomas of thyroid gland: a clinicopathological study of 13 cases, *Histopathology* 10:75, 1986.
257. Carcangiu ML, Zampi G, Rosai J: Poorly differentiated ("insular") thyroid carcinoma: a reinterpretation of Langhans' *"wuchernde Struma." Am J Surg Pathol* 8:655, 1984.
258. Cabanne F, Gérard-Marchant R, Heimann R, Williams ED: Tumeurs malignes du corps thyroïde. Problèmes de diagnostic histopathologique: à propos de 692 lésions recueillies par le groupe coopérateur des cancers du corps thyroïde de l'OERTC, *Ann Anat Pathol* [Paris] 19:129, 1974.
259. Sakamoto A, Kasai N, Sugano H: Poorly differentiated carcinoma of the thyroid: a clinicopathologic entity for a high risk group of papillary and follicular carcinomas, *Cancer* 52:1849, 1983.
260. Carcangiu ML, Steeper T, Zampi G, Rosai J: Anaplastic thyroid carcinoma: a study of 70 cases, *Am J Clin Pathol* 83:135, 1985.
261. Barr R, Dann F: Anaplastic thyroid carcinoma metastatic to skin, *J Cutan Pathol* 1:201, 1974.
262. Schmid KW, Kroll M, Hofstadter F, Ladurner D: Small cell carcinoma of the thyroid. A reclassification of cases originally diagnosed as small cell carcinomas of the thyroid, *Pathol Res Pract* 181:540, 1986.
263. Gaffey MJ, Lack EE, Christ ML, Weiss LM: Anaplastic thyroid carcinoma with osteoclast-like giant cells: a clinicopathologic, immunohistochemical, and ultrastructural study, *Am J Surg Pathol* 15:160, 1991.
264. Hashimoto H, Koga S, Watanabe H, Enjoji M: Undifferentiated carcinoma of the thyroid gland with osteoclast-like giant cells, *Acta Pathol Jpn* 30:323, 1980.
265. Hutter RVP, Tollefsen HR, DeCosse JJ et al: Spindle and giant cell metaplasia in papillary carcinoma of the thyroid, *Am J Surg* 110:660, 1965.
266. LiVolsi VA, Brooks JJ, Arendash-Durand B: Anaplastic thyroid tumors: immunohistology, *Am J Clin Pathol* 87:434, 1987.
267. Miettinen M, Franssila K, Kehto V-P et al: Expression of intermediate filament proteins in thyroid gland and thyroid tumors, *Lab Invest* 50:262, 1984.
268. Johannessen JV, Gould VE, Jao W: The fine structure of human thyroid cancer, *Hum Pathol* 9:385, 1978.
269. Newland JR, Mackay B, Hills CS Jr, Hickey RC: Anaplastic thyroid carcinoma: an ultrastructural study of 10 cases, *Ultrastruct Pathol* 2:121, 1981.
270. Aldinger KA, Samaan NA, Ibañez M, Hills CS Jr: Anaplastic carcinoma of the thyroid: a review of 84 cases of spindle and giant cell carcinoma of the thyroid, *Cancer* 41:2267, 1978.

271. Fisher ER, Gregorio R, Shoemaker R et al: The derivation of so-called "giant-cell" and spindle-cell" undifferentiated thyroidal neoplasms, *Am J Clin Pathol* 61:680, 1974.

272. Harada T, Ito K, Shimaoka K et al: Fatal thyroid carcinoma: anaplastic transformation of adenocarcinoma, *Cancer* 39:2588, 1977.

273. Fagin JA, Matsuo K, Karmakar A, Chen DL et al: High prevalence of mutations of the p53 gene in poorly differentiated human thyroid carciomas, *J Clin Invest* 91:179, 1993.

274. Ito T, Seyama T, Mizuno T et al: Unique association of p53 mutations with undifferentiated but not with differentiated carcinomas of the thyroid gland, *Cancer Res* 52:1369, 1992.

275. Nakamura T, Yana I, Kobayashi T et al: p53 gene mutations associated with anaplastic transformation of human thyroid carcinomas, *Jpn J Cancer Res* 83:1293, 1992.

276. Bronner MP, LiVolsi VA: Spindle cell squamous carcinoma of the thyroid: an unusual anaplastic tumor associated with tall cell papillary cancer, *Mod Pathol* 4:637, 1991.

277. Nishiyama RH, Dunn EL, Thompson NW: Anaplastic spindle-cell and giant-cell tumors of the thyroid gland, *Cancer* 30:113, 1972.

278. Venkatesh YS, Ordóñez NG, Schultz PN et al: Anaplastic carcinoma of the thyroid: a clinopathologic study of 121 cases, *Cancer* 66:321, 1990.

279. Kim JH, Leeper RD: Treatment of anaplastic giant and spindle cell carcinoma of the thyroid gland with combination adriamycin and radiation therapy, *Cancer* 52:954, 1983.

280. Spanos GA, Wolk D, Desner MR et al: Preoperative chemotherapy for giant cell carcinoma of the thyroid, *Cancer* 50:2252, 1982.

281. Franssila KO, Harach HR, Wasenius V-M: Mucoepidermoid carcinoma of the thyroid, *Histopathology* 8:847, 1984.

282. Bondeson L, Bondeson AG, Thompson NW: Papillary carcinoma of the thyroid with mucoepidermoid features, *Am J Clin Pathol* 95:175, 1991.

283. Chan JK, Albores-Saavedra J, Battifora H et al: Sclerosing mucoepidermoid thyroid carcinoma with eosinophilia: a distinctive low-grade malignancy arising from the metaplastic follicles of Hashimoto's thyroiditis, *Am J Surg Pathol* 15:438, 1991.

284. Mizukami Y, Nakajima H, Annen Y et al: Mucin-producing poorly differentiated adenocarcinoma of the thyroid: a case report, *Pathol Res Pract* 189:608, 1993.

285. Sobrinho-Simõpes MA, Nesland JM, Johannessen JV: A mucin-producing tumor in the thyroid gland, *Ultrastruct Pathol* 9:277, 1985.

286. Huang T-Y, Assor D: Primary squamous cell carcinoma of the thyroid gland: a report of four cases, *Am J Clin Pathol* 55:93, 1971.

287. Chan JK, Rosai J: Tumors of the neck showing thymic or related branchial pouch differentiation: a unifying concept, *Hum Pathol* 22:349, 1991.

288. Damiani S, Filotico M, Eusebi V: Carcinoma of the thyroid showing thymoma-like features, *Virchows Arch [A] (Pathol Anat Histopathol* 418:463, 1991.

289. Harach HR, Saravia Day E, Franssila KO: Thyroid spindle cell tumor with mucous cysts: an intrathyroid thymoma? *Am J Surg Pathol* 9:525, 1985.

290. Kakudo K, Mori I, Tamaoki N, Watanabe K: Carcinoma of possible thymic origin presenting as a thyroid mass: a new subgroup of squamous cell carcinoma of the thyroid, *J Surg Oncol* 138:187, 1988.

291. Kingsley DP, Elton A, Bennett MH: Malignant teratoma of the thyroid, case report and a review of the literature, *Br J Cancer* 22:7, 1968.

292. Miyauchi A, Kuma K, Matsuzuka F et al: Intrathyroidal epithelial thymoma: an entity distinct from squamous cell carcinoma of the thyroid, *World J Surg* 9:128, 1985.

293. Murao T, Nakanishi M, Toda K, Konishi H: Malignant teratoma of the thyroid gland in an adolescent female, *Acta Pathol Jpn* 29:109, 1979.

Tumors of C cells

294. Hazard JB, Hawk WA, Crile G Jr: Medullary (solid) carcinoma of the thyroid: a clinicopathologic entity, *J Clin Endocrinol Metab* 19:152, 1959.

295. Williams ED, Brown CL, Doniach I: Pathological and clinical findings in a series of 67 cases of medullary carcinoma of the thyroid, *J Clin Pathol* 19:103, 1966.

296. Hedinger CE: *Histological typing of thyroid tumors,* Berlin, 1988, Springer-Verlag.

297. Saad MF, Ordóñez NG, Rashid RK et al: Medullary carcinoma of the thyroid: a study of the clinical features and prognostic factors in 161 patients, *Medicine* (Baltimore) 63:319, 1984.

298. Schroder S, Bocker W, Baisch H et al: Prognostic factors in medullary thyroid carcinoma: survival in relation to age, sex, stage, histology, immunocytochemistry and DNA content, *Cancer* 61:806, 1988.

299. Schimke RN, Hartman WH: Familial amyloid producing medullary thyroid carcinoma and pheochromocytoma: a distinct genetic entity, *Ann Intern Med* 63:1027, 1965.

300. Gorlin RJ, Sedano HO, Vickers RA, Cervenka J: Multiple mucosal neuromas, pheochromocytomas and medullary carcinoma of the thyroid—a syndrome, *Cancer* 22:293, 1968.

301. Carney JA, Sizemore GW, Hayles AB: Multiple endocrine neoplasia, type 2B, *Pathobiol Annu* 8:105, 1978.

302. Gagel RF, Tashjian AH Jr, Cummings T et al: The clinical outcome of prospective screening for multiple endocrine neoplasia, type 2a, *N Engl J Med* 318:478, 1988.

303. Mulligan LM, Kwok JBJ, Healey CS: Germ-line mutations of the RET protooncogene in multiple endocrine neoplasia type 2A, *Nature* 363:458, 1993.

303a. DeLellis RA: Multiple endocrine neoplasia syndromes revisited: clinical, morphological, and molecular features, *Lab Invest* 72:494, 1995.

304. Rosai J, Carcangiu ML, DeLellis RA: Tumors of the thyroid gland. In *Atlas of tumor pathology,* series 3, fasc 5, Washington, D.C., 1992, Armed Forces Institute of Pathology.

305. Kini SR: Thyroid. In Kline TS, editor: *Guides to clinical aspiration biopsy,* New York, 1987, Igaku-Shoin.

306. DeLellis RA, Wolfe HJ: The pathobiology of the human calcitonin (C)-cell, *Pathol Annu* 16:25, 1991.

307. Westermark P, Johnson KH: The polypeptide hormone–derived amyloid forms: nonspecific alterations or signs of abnormal peptide-processing, *Acta Pathol Microbiol Scand* 96:475, 1988.

308. Zajac JD, Penschow J, Mason T et al: Identification of calcitonin and calcitonin gene related peptide messenger RNA in medullary thyroid carcinoma by hybridization histochemistry, *J Clin Endocrinol Metab* 62:1037, 1986.

309. Uribe M, Fenoglio-Preiser CM, Grimes M et al: Medullary carcinoma of the thyroid gland: Clinical, pathological and immunohistochemical features with a review of the literature, *Am J Surg Pathol* 2:577, 1985.

310. Sikri KL, Varndell IM, Hamid QA et al: Medullary carcinoma of the thyroid: an immunocytochemical and histochemical study of 25 cases using 8 separate markers, *Cancer* 56:2481, 1988.

311. DeLellis RA, Rule AH, Spiler I et al: Calcitonin and carcinoembryonic antigen as tumor markers in medullary thyroid carcinoma, *Am J Clin Pathol* 70:587, 1978.

312. Mendelsohn G, Wells SA, Baylin SB: Relationship of tissue carcinoembryonic antigen and calcitonin to tumor virulence in medullary thyroid carcinoma: an immunohistochemical study in early, localized and virulent disseminated stages of disease, *Cancer* 54:657, 1984.

313. Harach HR, Williams ED: Glandular (tubular and follicular) variants of medullary carcinoma of the thyroid, *Histopathology* 7:83, 1983.

314. Kakudo K, Miyauchi A, Yakai SI et al: C-cell carcinoma of the thyroid, papillary type, *Acta Pathol Jpn* 29:633, 1979.

315. Mendelsohn G, Baylin SB, Bigner SH et al: Anaplastic variants of medullary thyroid carcinoma: a light microscopic and immunohistochemical study, *Am J Surg Pathol* 4:331, 1980.

316. Kakudo K, Miyauchi A, Ogihara T et al: Medullary carcinoma of the thyroid: giant cell type, *Arch Pathol Lab Med* 102:445, 1978.

317. Dominíquez-Malagon H, Delgado-Chávez R, Torres-Najera M et al: Oxyphil and squamous variants of medullary thyroid carcinoma, *Cancer* 63:1183, 1989.

318. Landon G, Ordóñez NG. Clear cell variant of medullary carcinoma of the thyroid, *Hum Pathol* 16:844 , 1985.

319. Marcus JN, Dise CA, LiVolsi VA: Melanin production in a medullary thyroid carcinoma, *Cancer* 49:2518, 1982.

320. Golough R, Us-Krasovec M, Auersperg M et al: Amphicrine composite calcitonin and mucin producing carcinoma of the thyroid, *Ultrastruct Pathol* 8:197, 1985.

321. Huss LJ, Mendelsohn G: Medullary carcinoma of the thyroid: an encapsulated variant resembling the hyalinizing trabecular (paraganglioma-like) adenoma of the thyroid, *Mod Pathol* 3:581, 1990.
322. Kodama T, Okamoto T, Fujimoto Y et al: C-cell adenoma of the thyroid: a rare but distinct clinical entity, *Surgery* 104:997, 1988
323. Eusebi V, Damiani S, Riva C et al: Calcitonin-free oat cell carcinoma of the thyroid gland, *Virchows Arch [A] (Pathol Anat Histopathol)* 417:267, 1990.
324. Lippman SM, Mendelsohn G, Trump DL et al: The prognostic and biological significance of cellular heterogeneity in medullary thyroid carcinoma, *J Clin Endocrinol Metab* 54:233, 1982.
325. Bigner SH, Cox EB, Mendelsohn G et al: Medullary carcinoma of the thyroid in the multiple endocrine neoplasia IIA syndrome, *Am J Surg Pathol* 5:459, 1981.
326. Wolfe HJ, Melvin KE, Cervi-Skinner SJ et al: C-cell hyperplasia preceding medullary thyroid carcinoma, *N Engl J Med* 289:437, 1973.
327. DeLellis RA, Nunnemacher G, Wolfe HJ: C cell hyperplasia: an ultrastructural analysis, *Lab Invest* 36:237, 1977.
328. DeLellis RA, Wolfe HJ: The pathobiology of the human calcitonin (C)-cell: a review, *Pathol Annu* 16:25, 1981.
329. DeLellis RA: The pathology of medullary thyroid carcinoma and its precursors. In LiVolsi VA, DeLellis RA, editors: *Pathobiology of the parathyroid and thyroid glands,* Baltimore, 1993, Williams & Wilkins.
330. Gibson WC, Peng T-C, Croker BP: C-cell nodules in adult human thyroid: a common autopsy finding, *Am J Clin Pathol* 75:347, 1981.
331. Ponder BAJ, Ponder MA, Coffey R et al: Risk estimation and screening in families of patients with medullary carcinoma, *Lancet* 1:397, 1988.
332. Gagel RF, Tashjian AH Jr, Cummings T et al: The clinical outcome of prospective screening for multiple endocrine neoplasia type 2A, *N Engl J Med* 318:478, 1988.
333. LiVolsi VA, Feind CR, LoGerfo P, Tashjian AH Jr: Demonstration by immunoperoxidase staining of hyperplasia of parafollicular cells in the parathyroid gland in hyperparathyroidism, *J Clin Endocrinol Metab* 37:550, 1973.
334. Albores-Saavedra J: C-cell hyperplasia, *Am J Surg Pathol* 13:987, 1988.
335. Biddinger PW, Brennan MF, Rosen PP: Symptomatic C-cell hyperplasia associated with chronic lymphocytic thyroiditis, *Am J Surg Pathol* 15:599, 1991.
336. Libbey NP, Nowakowski KJ, Tucci JR: C-cell hyperplasia of the thyroid in a patient with goitrous hypothyroidism and Hashimoto's disease, *Am J Surg Pathol* 13:71, 1989.
337. Albores-Saavedra J, Monforte H, Nadji M, Morales AR: C-cell hyperplasia in thyroid tissue adjacent to follicular cell tumors, *Hum Pathol* 19:795, 1988.
338. Scopsi L, DiPalma S, Ferrari C et al: C-cell hyperplasia accompanying thyroid diseases other than medullary thyroid carcinoma: an immunocytochemical study by means of antibodies to calcitonin and somatostatin, *Mod Pathol* 4:297, 1991.

Tumors of follicular and C-cells

339. Hales M, Rosenau W, Okerlund MD, Galante M: Carcinoma of the thyroid with a mixed medullary and follicular pattern: morphological, immunohistochemical and clinical laboratory studies, *Cancer* 50:1352, 1982.
340. Hedinger CHR, WIlliams ED, Sobin LH et al: Histological typing of thyroid tumors. In *WHO international classification of tumors,* ed, 2, Berlin, 1988, Springer-Verlag.
341. LiVolsi VA: Mixed thyroid carcinoma: a real entity? *Lab Invest* 57:237, 1987.
342. Ljungberg O, Bondeson L, Bondeson AG: Differentiated thyroid carcinoma, intermediate type: a new tumor entity with features of follicular and parafollicular carcinoma, *Hum Pathol* 15:218, 1984.
343. Holm R, Sobrino-Simões M, Nesland JM, Johannessen JV: Concurrent production of calcitonin and thyroglobulin by the same neoplastic cells, *Ultrastruct Pathol* 10:241, 1986.
344. Albores-Saavedra J, Gorráez de la Mora T, de la Torre-Rendón F, Gould E: Mixed medullary-papillary carcinoma of the thyroid: a previously unrecognized variant of thyroid carcinoma, *Hum Pathol* 21:1151, 1990.

Mesenchymal tumors

345. Hedinger CE: Sarcomas of the thyroid gland. In Hedinger CE, editor: *Thyroid cancer,* Berlin, 1969, Springer-Verlag.
346. Egloff B: The hemangioendothelioma. In Hedinger CE, editor: *Thyroid cancer,* Berlin, 1969, Springer-Verlag.
347. Eusebi V, Carcangiu ML, Dina R, Rosai J: Keratin-positive epithelioid angiosarcoma of thyroid: a report of four cases, *Am J Surg Pathol* 14:737, 1990.
348. van Haelst UJ, Pruszczynski M, ten Cate LN, Mravunac M: Ultrastructural and immunohistochemical study of epithelioid hemangioendothelioma of bone: coexpression of epithelial and endothelial markers, *Ultrastruct Pathol* 14:141,1990.

Malignant lymphoma

349. Compagno J, Oertel JE: Malignant lymphoma and other lymphoproliferative disorders of the thyroid gland: a clinicopathologic study of 245 cases, *Am J Clin Pathol* 74:1, 1980.
350. Burke JS, Butler JJ, Fuller LM: Malignant lymphomas of the thyroid: a clinical pathologic study of 35 patients including ultrastructural observations, *Cancer* 39:1587, 1977.
351. Aozasa K, Inoue A, Yoshimura H et al: Intermediate lymphocytic lymphoma of the thyroid: an immunologic and immunohistological study, *Cancer* 57:1762, 1986.
352. Anscombe AM, Wright DH: Primary malignant lymphoma of the thyroid—a tumour of mucosa-associated lymphoid tissue: review of seventy-six cases, *Histopathology* 9:81, 1985.
353. Isaacson PG, Androulakis-Papachristou A, Diss TC: Follicular colonization in thyroid lymphoma, *Am J Pathol* 141:43, 1992.
354. Fauré P, Chittal S, Woodman-Memeteau W et al: Diagnostic features of primary malignant lymphomas of the thyroid with monoclonal antibodies, *Cancer* 61:1852, 1988.
355. Maurer R, Taylor CR, Terry R, Lukes RJ: Non-Hodgkin lymphomas of the thyroid: a clinicopathological review of 29 cases applying the Lukes-Collins classification and an immunoperoxidase method, *Virchows Arch [A] (Pathol Anat Histol)* 383:293, 1979.
356. Mizukami Y, Michigishi T, Nonomura A et al: Primary lymphoma of the thyroid: a clinical, histological and immunohistochemical study of 20 cases, *Histopathology* 17:201, 1990.
357. Feigin GA, Buss DH, Paschal B et al: Hodgkin's disease manifested as a thyroid nodule, *Hum Pathol* 13:774, 1982.
358. Shimaoka K, Gailani S, Tsukada Y, Barcos M: Plasma cell neoplasm involving the thyroid, *Cancer* 41:1140, 1978.

Metastatic tumors

359. Ivy HK: Cancer metastatic to the thyroid: a diagnostic problem, *Mayo Clin Proc* 59:856, 1984.
360. Silverberg SG, Vidone RA: Metastatic tumors in the thyroid, *Pacif Med Surg* 74:175, 1966.
361. Carcangiu ML, Sibley RK, Rosai J: Clear cell change in primary thyroid tumors: a study of 38 cases, *Am J Surg Pathol* 9:705, 1985.

62 Parathyroid Glands

Sanford I. Roth

Metabolic aberrations of serum parathyroid hormone synthesis and secretion accompanied by alterations in the serum calcium concentration are the main result of diseases of the parathyroid glands. These alterations in serum calcium concentration produce significant signs and symptoms and even death if untreated. Nonfunctioning lesions of the parathyroid glands are rare, and it is even rarer for them to be clinically significant or to be discovered except as incidental autopsy findings. Hyperfunction (hyperparathyroidism) is a common disease and may require therapy.[1] Hypofunction (hypoparathyroidism) is much less frequent and most commonly is caused by iatrogenic loss attributable to thyroid or other surgery or cervical irradiation. Total absence of the glands because of congenital or developmental defects with or without adrenal and thymic agenesis, or idiopathic origins, or parathyroid involvement with systemic diseases,[2] or by end-organ defects (pseudohypoparathyroidism) also results in hypoparathyroidism.[3]

The most common disease of the parathyroid glands is *secondary hyperparathyroidism*. It is attributable to stimulation of parathyroid chief-cell proliferation and hypersynthesis and secretion of parathyroid hormone. The causes include hypocalcemia and hyperphosphatemia with or without vitamin D deficiency from renal, intestinal, or bone disease.[4] Hyperfunction of the parathyroid glands because of neoplasms or hyperplasias of the parathyroid glands is referred to as "primary hyperparathyroidism." *Tertiary hyperparathyroidism* is primary hyperparathyroidism in patients with preexisting secondary hyperparathyroidism.[5]

NORMAL PARATHYROIDS

Development

The parathyroid glands develop symmetrically and are first identifiable in 9 mm (crown-rump length) human embryos. They arise from the third and fourth branchial pouches during the fifth week of gestation.[6,7] The glands of the third pouch along with the thymus are referred to as parathyroid III (since the glands develop almost symmetrically, they are usually referred to in the singular) and become the inferior parathyroids. The glands of the fourth pouch become the superior glands, parathyroid IV. The first evidence of the glands is a proliferation of large, relatively clear well-demarcated, polygonal cells arising along the dorsolateral aspect of the dorsocephalic entoderm (endoderm) of the third pouch and from the dorsolateral entoderm with a narrow extension onto both the anterior and posterior surfaces of the fourth pouch before its union with the ectodermal cleft. One report[8] has suggested that the glands in the amphibian arise from the ectodermal portion of the branchial cleft. These researchers assumed that the parathyroids are therefore of ectodermal origin; however, Norris's study[6] clearly indicates that the human parathyroids originate from the endoderm and not from the ectoderm of the branchial cleft. In the case of parathyroid III, there is a concomitant proliferation of the cells of the thymic precursor, forming a bilobate mass.

Parathyroid IV is associated with a mass of cells that form medially in the fourth branchial pouch (the ultimobranchial or postbranchial body, which is combined with the cells from the adjacent neural crests to give rise to the calcitonin-secreting C-cells). As this bilobate complex separates from the branchial pouch, the ultimobranchial body is engulfed by the expanding lateral wings of the thyroid. Parathyroid IV separates and comes to lie near the middle of the thyroid gland, close to the crossing of the recurrent laryngeal nerve and the middle thyroid artery. Because there is little movement of parathyroid IV, its position is much more constant in the adult. It may, however, be engulfed by the lateral lobes of the thyroid and come to lie in the thyroid capsule or even within the thyroid gland. Anatomic evidence supports the concept that the glands are functioning in utero.[9,10]

Anatomy

The parathyroid glands begin as a few cells in the branchial endoderm. They grow exponentially from their first differentiation in the embryo until 25 years of age.[11] At 3 months the glands weigh a mean total of 5 to 9 mg. The glands are initially globular, but as the neck organs develop, they assume their adult shape as flattened ovulate disks with sharp edges. Initially the parathyroids are gray-tan, but as they develop, they assume a more yellow-to orange tan color. They reach an adult size of approximately 30 mg (6 by 4 by 2 mm) each (Fig. 62-1). With age the glands become a brighter yellow. The mean total weight of the glands in the adult male is 120 ±3.5 mg, whereas that of the female is 142 ±5.2 mg.[12-17] The lower glands are larger than the upper ones. In the adult the parenchymal cells average approximately 68.3% of the total gland weight in men and 62.6% in women. The mean parenchymal weight is 82.0 ±2.6 mg in men and 88.9 ±3.9 mg in women.[15] African-Americans have been reported to have a higher total gland weight than whites have.[16] The stroma consists of thin delicate strands of reticulum and collagen without significant stromal fat and does not show any significant alteration before puberty. Beginning at puberty there is an increase in the stroma, largely because of an increase in stromal fat (Fig. 62-2), which continues throughout life. The amount of stromal fat is difficult to measure and evaluate because of the extreme variability in the amount of stromal fat from patient to patient, gland to gland, and even region to region in the same gland. It is related not only to the functional state of the gland, but also to the nutritional state of the individual, his or her age and sex, and the cell types present in the stroma. The amount of stromal fat usually parallels the general body fat. It is affected by the degree of parenchymal cell proliferation.

Four parathyroid glands are present in 90% to 97% of individuals with a variation from two to 12 glands.[18-24] Two percent to 6.5% of patients have supernumerary glands, believed to be the result of embryonic division of one or more of the glands. These glands are typically located along the normal migratory tract of the glands. Hyperplasias or neoplasms forming in supernumerary glands have been reported.[15,25-29]

The location of the parathyroid glands is somewhat variable, though several studies have demonstrated that the upper glands are situated primarily along the posterior aspect of the middle third of the thyroid, and the lower glands have a more disparate distribution, with the most common site being near the lower pole of the thyroid[18-22] (Fig. 62-3). In addition to the usual ectopic locations—the anterior mediastinum,[18-22] the thymus,[18-22,30] the thyroid,[31,32] and the retroesophageal space[19]—glands have been reported in the vagus nerve,[33] the cervical ganglia,[34] the posterior pharyngeal wall,[35] and even in the vaginal wall.[36] This latter location most likely represents an incomplete teratoma, since it was associated with a nodule of thyroid. Interestingly, to the best of my knowledge (or that of Robert E. Scully, M.D., of the Massachusetts General Hospital), no parathyroid tissue has ever been reported in an ovarian or testicular teratoma.

In the absence of congenital developmental defects, it is rare for there to be less than four glands, and most cases with less than four glands are caused by failure of the autopsy prosector to identify one or more anomalously positioned glands.

Histology

The important features related to parathyroid pathology are the cell types and their relationships to the surrounding interstitium. The perivascular stroma shows an increase in collagen deposition with age.[16,37] Interstitial adipocytes are first seen late in the first decade and increase in number, reaching a peak in the third to fifth decade. Women manifest a sharp increase in stromal adipocytes at menarche. Despite the considerable variation in the amount of stromal fat, in adults adipocytes have been shown by morphometric studies to account for approximately 50% of the stromal volume.[7,14,38,39]

The glands have only one cell type, the *chief cell,* from their first appearance until puberty. In the adult the chief cells appear as cords, sheets, nests, and even as pseudofollicles containing eosinophilic proteinaceous material, which may stain for amyloid.[40-43] The chief cell cytoplasm contains abundant glycogen and, as a result of artifacts of fixation, may appear somewhat vacuolated. The adult chief cell is a spheroid measuring 8 to 12 μm in diameter. In children there is little intracytoplasmic fat.[44] As first recognized by Sandström,[45,46] 70% to 90% of normal adult chief cells have intracytoplasmic fat droplets.[15,32,44-48]

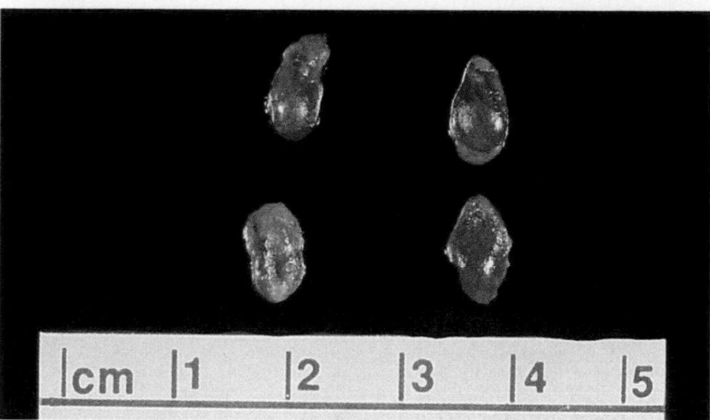

Fig. 62-1 Four normal adult parathyroid glands.

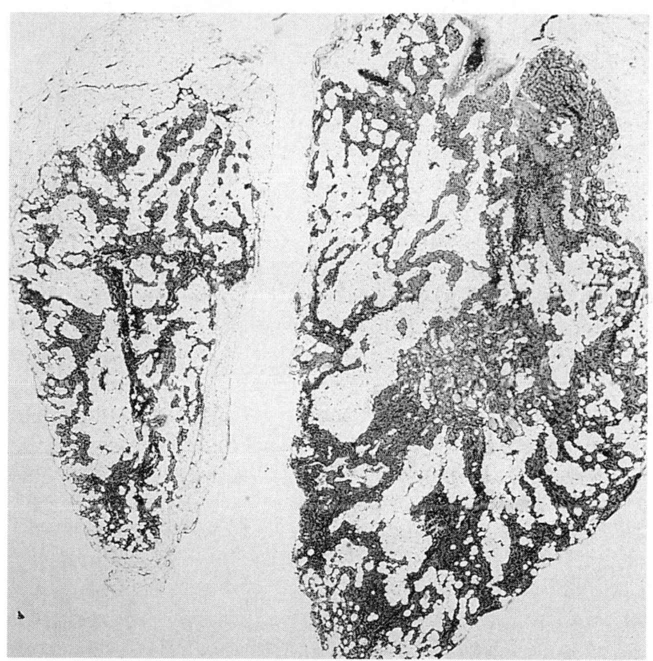

Fig. 62-2 Two normal adult parathyroid glands demonstrating abundant stromal fat. The parenchyma is composed of a mixture of chief cells and oxyphil cells. Notice the variability of the distribution of adipocytes and parenchymal cells.

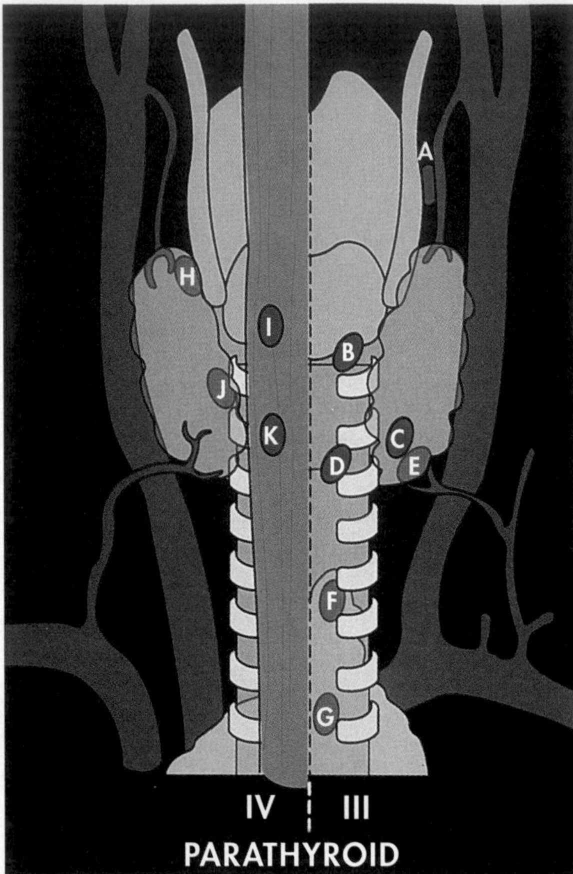

Fig. 62-3 The distribution of the normal parathyroid glands in man, derived from the studies of Wang, as seen from the dorsal surface of the trachea and thyroid.[15] The upper glands (IV) on the left, where the esophagus is also seen, whereas the lower glands (III) are on the right and much more variable in location. The most common location of the lower glands are *C* and *E*, whereas the upper glands are most commonly seen at location *J*.

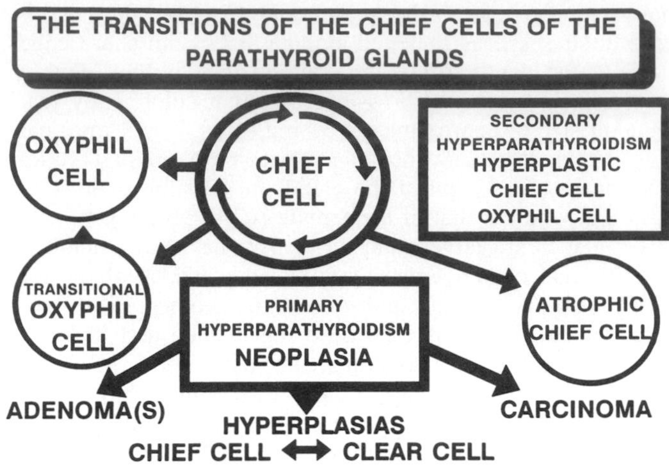

Fig. 62-4 The derivation of the cell types in the human parathyroid gland. The normal transitional oxyphil cells, the oxyphil cells of the normal glands, the atrophic chief cells of chronic suppression, and the chief and oxyphil (including transitional forms) cells of primary and secondary hyperplastic glands, and neoplastic glands (embracing adenomas and carcinomas) are derived from the chief cells. The oxyphil and chief cells of primary chief cell hyperplasias, and the vacuolated cells of clear cell hyperplasia originate from the chief cells.

The presence of stored parathyroid hormone (PTH) has been demonstrated in normal chief cells.[32,49-53] The amount of hormone per cell is variable, an indication of a difference in the quantity of stored hormone. Chromogranin is costored and cosecreted with PTH.[54-58] Chromogranin is largely limited to the chief cells, where the amount stored in each cell is also variable.[54-58] Products of chromogranin cleavage are smaller hormones that have been demonstrated to inhibit the secretion of PTH.[56,58-61] and other hormones.[62-67] The variation in the quantity of stored hormones is consistent with the theory that the chief cells are undergoing cyclical changes.[32,53,68-71] This cyclical theory is also supported by in situ localization by hybridization techniques that indicate a variable distribution of preproparathyroid hormone mRNA in the chief cells.[51-53,72,73]

Beginning around puberty, a second cell type, the *oxyphil cell,* appears in the parenchyma of the gland.[32,74-78] The oxyphil cells are 12 to 20 μm in diameter and have clearly demarcated cell membranes. The nuclei are small and somewhat pyknotic. The cytoplasm is homogeneous, granular, and brightly eosinophilic, resembling the Hürthle cells of the thyroid and the oncocytes of other endocrine organs.[75-78] The cytoplasm of oxyphil cells stains for mitochondria.[78a] There are transitional forms of the oxyphil cells with a variable lighter cytoplasm. The oxyphil and transitional oxyphil cells are believed to be derived from the chief cells[32] (Fig. 62-4). The number of oxyphil cells increases with age.[32,76,77] It is believed that the oxyphil cells are the result of a proliferation of mitochondria in the chief cells.[32,79,80] This can occur in individual chief cells, resulting in individual oxyphil cells among the chief cells.[76,77] The oxyphil cells are also believed to be capable of cell division with transmission of the oxyphil trait and ensuing formation of "oxyphil nodules." Intracellular fat is sparse in the oxyphil cell.[32,44,48] Balogh and Cohen,[79] Tremblay and Cartier,[80] and Fischer[81] demonstrated a high level of activity of a wide variety of oxidative enzymes in the oxyphil cells. These studies did not measure the level of activity per unit mitochondrial protein. Biochemical studies[82] of oxyphil cells of salivary gland tumors reveal a decreased level of mitochondrial enzymes per unit of mitochondrial protein. Munger and Roth[48] showed that the normal oxyphil cells lacked the organelles necessary for protein synthesis and secretion. Immunohistochemical localization of stored PTH[32,49] and chromogranin[50] and in situ hybridization of mRNA for preproparathyroid hormone show a low synthetic rate and low storage in the oxyphil cells.[51-53,72] Müller-Höcker[83] demonstrated a deficiency of cytochrome *c* oxidase in parathyroid oxyphil cells. These studies indicate a decreased function in the mitochondria and provide evidence that these cells are degenerating forms.

Ultrastructure and the secretory cycle

Ultrastructural studies on the chief cells of the human parathyroids first suggested a secretory cycle in the cells (Fig. 62-5). Munger and Roth[48] demonstrated that individual chief cells had disparate amounts of glycogen and secretory (dense-core) granules. The chief cell organelles associated with protein secretion were of different sizes and had a distinctive organization. On the basis of these findings they proposed that some

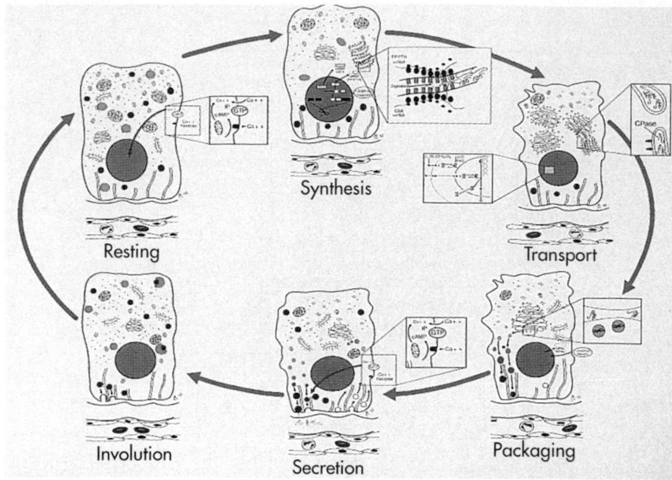

Fig. 62-5 The secretory cycle of the parathyroid chief cells. Although this is a continuum, typical stages have been recognized ultrastructurally. During the *resting phase* the cells are rich in glycogen and lipid bodies, with dispersion of the granular endoplasmic reticulum (GER) and free ribosomes. Dense core secretory granules are relatively uncommon and scattered throughout the cytoplasm. Rare lysosomes are seen. The Golgi apparatus is small and inconspicuous with few vesicles and vacuoles. The cell membranes are relatively straight with few interdigitations. At the end of the resting phase, presumably because of decreased cytoplasmic [Ca^{++}] and release of vitamin D metabolite from the upstream promotor site, the cell begins to synthesize parathyroid hormone (PTH).

As the *synthetic phase* begins, transcription of the gene for PTH begins with production of the complementary RNA for preproparathyroid hormone and presumably accompanied by a similar transcription of chromogranin. The mRNA, produced by removal of the introns and splicing of the exons, moves to the GER, which aggregates (the perinuclear body of Pappenheimer and Wilens[48]). This is accompanied by aggregation of the free ribosomes to polysomes. The preprohormone crosses into the lumen of the GER where the "pre-" portion of the molecule is removed by a ligase. Other alterations include depletion of the dense core granules, lysosomes, glycogen, and lipid bodies. The cell membrane increases in tortuosity probably because of the loss of cytoplasmic volume. The synthesis and secretion of hormone is halted, presumably by the action of 1α,25-dihydroxyvitamin D on the upstream promotor region of PTH and the cytosolic [Ca^{++}].

In the *transport phase,* the hormone, supposedly accompanied by chromogranin, is transported through the cisternae of the GER to the Golgi apparatus as the "pro-" segment is removed by a "clipase." The hormone is conveyed to the Golgi vesicles. Further depletion of lipid bodies, glycogen, and secretory granules occurs, and the cisternae of the GER disperse.

In the *packaging phase,* the hormone is bundled along with chromogranin into dense core granules, and the Golgi apparatus begins its involution.

Secretion occurs as the dense core granules containing PTH and chromogranin move along the microtubules, fuse with the cell membrane, and release the hormone into the pericapillary extracellular space. Depending on the ambient [Ca^{++}], the granules are rapidly passed along the microtubules and secreted (low [Ca^{++}]), or left free in the cytoplasm (high [Ca^{++}]) to be destroyed by lysosomes or to be secreted at a later time. The Golgi continues to decrease in size and complexity. The free ribosomes disaggregate.

The cells begin to involute toward the *resting phase* with gradual loss of secretory granules and further involution of the Golgi apparatus. The cells begin to accumulate glycogen and lipid bodies and approach the resting phase. Lysosomes, containing acid phosphatase, accumulate in the cells. These presumably serve to destroy excess hormone and unsecreted secretory granules.

cells were "active" and others were "resting." Experimental studies[68-71] led to the proposal that the chief cells underwent cyclical alteration and that each chief cell independently synthesized and secreted a "batch" of PTH. The control of this process in the parathyroid chief cells was proposed to be the method of the overall regulation of PTH synthesis and secretion. It was theorized that elevation of the ambient [Ca^{++}] increased the length of the resting phase and decreased overall PTH secretion. Lowering of the ambient [Ca^{++}] shortened the resting phase, thus increasing the synthesis and secretion of PTH. In an investigation using reverse hemolytic plaque assay, this hypothesis of cyclical PTH (and chromogranin) synthesis and secretion was confirmed in individual chief cells.[58,73] These studies have also proved that this cyclical secretion could be controlled by the ambient [Ca^{++}]. The two proteins, chromogranin and PTH, however, did not cosecrete in equivalent amounts.[73] This may be attributable to differential packaging of the two proteins in different states of the secretory cycle or it may be an artifact of the sensitivity of the antibodies used in the assay. It has been further confirmed that PTH secretion from a gland cannot be completely suppressed, and such incapacity indicates that the resting phase cannot be maintained by an individual chief cell indefinitely.[68,70,84]

The oxyphil cells have a cytoplasm filled with mitochondria. Although they have the typical interdigitating cristae, the mitochondria are often bizarre in size and shape.[48] The organelles associated with protein synthesis and secretion, Golgi, granular endoplasmic reticulum (GER), and secretory granules are sparse. Primary lysosomes are seen. Abundant glycogen is present between the mitochondria. In the absence of organelles associated with hormone synthesis and secretion and the absence of chromogranin and PTH in the oxyphil cells, it is believed that these cells in the normal gland do not synthesize PTH.

Transitional oxyphil cells have an ultrastructure intermediate between chief cells and oxyphil cells.[35,48] The mitochondria are increased in number compared with chief cells, but they also contain Golgi, GER, and secretory granules. It is not clear whether these cells retain the capacity to synthesize and secrete PTH and whether they respond normally to the ambient [Ca^{++}].

Physiology of calcium homeostasis

During the growth phase, humans are generally in positive calcium balance, whereas young adults have a calcium intake and thus bone formation that equals output[85-87] (Fig. 62-6). In later life almost all individuals are in negative calcium balance.[87] The main organs concerned with maintaining calcium balance are the parathyroid glands (control), gastrointestinal tract (intake), kidneys and sweat glands (excretion), and bones (storage).[85-87] In normal individuals the calcium balance is controlled by the parathyroid glands and vitamin D and its metabolites (Fig. 62-7). The role of calcitonin, the third hormone concerned with calcium metabolism, is still poorly understood in humans. It seems likely that it is involved in managing long-term stresses on calcium metabolism, such as those that occur during pregnancy, rather than on immediate control. Experimentally calcitonin generally opposes the action of PTH on bone resorption and renal calcium conservation (see Chapter 61).

The serum and extracellular calcium concentration is one of the most tightly regulated ions in mammals.[86] Although the ionized calcium is the biochemically significant form, the total serum calcium concentration (the sum of the ionized calcium

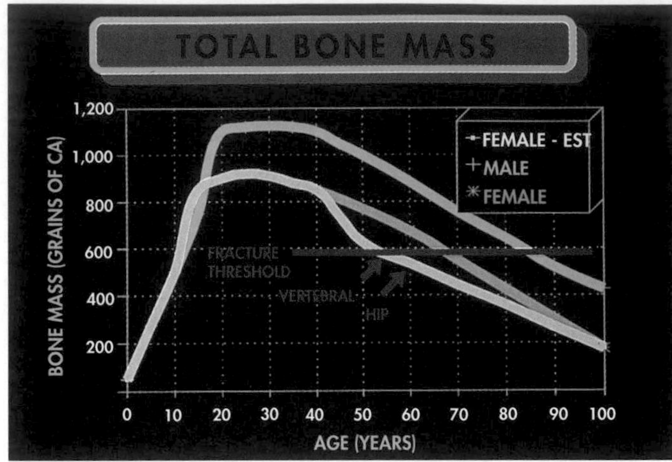

Fig. 62-6 The rate of bone formation and loss with age in men and women. Since the major storage site for calcium is the bone, bone formation exceeds bone resorption (bone growth) while individuals are in positive calcium balance, whereas bone loss occurs in individuals who are in negative calcium balance.

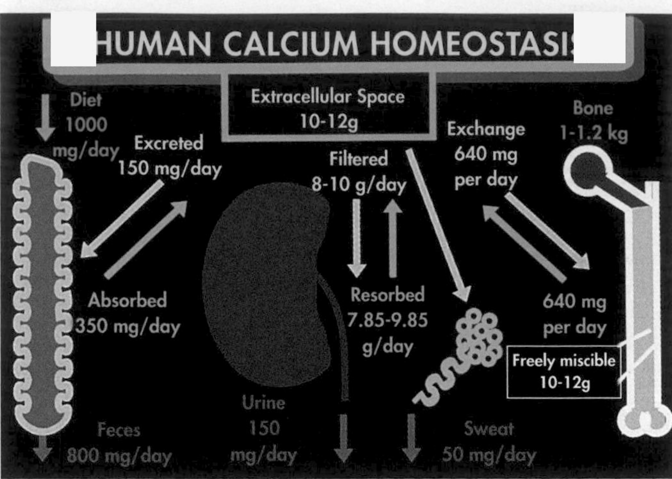

Fig. 62-8 Human calcium balance in a young adult in calcium balance. Of the total dietary calcium 200 mg/day is actually absorbed and excreted through the kidneys and sweat glands. The bone exchange is 640 mg/day.

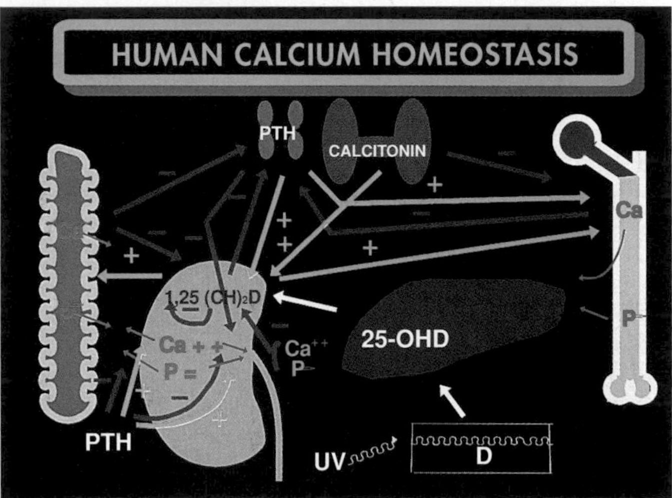

Fig. 62-7 Control of calcium metabolism. Parathyroid hormone (PTH) acts primarily on the bone and kidneys, whereas vitamin D (*D*) metabolites act on the intestines, bone, and parathyroid glands. Calcium-ion concentration acts on the parathyroid glands and the thyroid C-cells. In man calcitonin appears to play a relatively insignificant role in the rapid regulation of calcium metabolism. All effects of PTH and vitamin D (+) tend to elevate the ionic serum calcium, and such elevation results in a negative feedback on PTH. Calcitonin acts in opposition to PTH in most experimental conditions.

and the bound calcium) is the form most frequently measured and clinically evaluated.[86] The total calcium is easier to measure, and since in most patients it is directly proportional to the ionized calcium, this value is used in most clinical studies.[87] This relationship was first clearly stated by McLean and Hastings,[88] and their nomogram was used to estimate ionized calcium until technology permitted direct measurement of the ionized form.

The total body calcium in an adult is approximately 1000 to 1200 g, of which 99% is in the skeleton as crystalline hydroxyapatite. Of the skeletal calcium roughly 1% is readily exchangeable with the calcium of the extracellular fluid and serum. The extracellular (including serum) calcium and intracellular calcium are approximately 10 to 12 g respectively. These three compartments constitute the "miscible pool" of calcium. The concentration of extracellular and serum ionic calcium (1.18 mM) is approximately 10,000 times that of the intracellular calcium concentration (10^{-4} mM). The total serum calcium ranges from 9 to 11 mg/dl (2.2 to 2.7 mM), of which 48% is free ionized calcium. Another 46% is bound to serum proteins (largely albumin), and 3% is bound to diffusible ion complexes (citrate and phosphate), and the last 3% is bound to miscellaneous other substances.[85-87]

The most important factor in long-term control of calcium balance is intestinal calcium absorption from the diet.[89] The adult American diet consists of 200 to 2000 mg per day (Report of FAO/WHO Expert Group, WHO Technical Report Series 452 FAO/WHO, Geneva, 1970). The intestinal absorption of calcium varies with the dietary intake, from approximately 70% efficiency with deficient diets to 20% efficiency with high-calcium diets, resulting in a dietary absorption in the proximal small intestine of approximately 350 to 400 mg in an adult with an adequate diet (Fig. 62-8). In addition approximately 150 mg per day is excreted through the large intestine, resulting in a net dietary intake of approximately 200 to 250 mg (Fig. 62-8). This absorption is largely controlled by the level of $1\alpha,25(OH)_2$-dihydroxyvitamin D_3, or $1\alpha,25(OH)_2D_3$.[89] Elevation of $1\alpha,25(OH)_2D_3$ increases calcium absorption and depression of $1\alpha,25(OH)_2D_3$ decreases calcium absorption. In euparathyroid adults the urinary excretion of calcium amounts to 150 to 200 mg per day, and approximately 50 mg of calcium per day is secreted with the sweat.

Phosphate-ion concentration is less closely regulated than [Ca^{++}]. Large swings in phosphate occur with diet.[90] Increased bone resorption tends to raise the serum phosphate, whereas PTH decreases tubular reabsorption of phosphate. The net effect is a decrease in the serum phosphate under the influence of PTH.

Vitamin D_3, the form most effectively used by humans, is synthesized in the skin and obtained in the diet. Vitamin D_2 is obtained largely by supplemental addition to foods. In the skin the precursor of vitamin D_3, which is 7-dehydrocholesterol, is synthesized from squalene. Under the influence of ultraviolet B, 7-dehydrocholesterol is transformed to vitamin D_3, which enters the circulation. In the United States, milk and other products are fortified with vitamin D_2. Dietary vitamin D is absorbed with fat, enters the lymphatics with the chylomicrons, and enters the bloodstream through the thoracic duct. Still relatively ineffective as an antirachitic, vitamin D_2 or D_3, whether obtained from the skin or the diet, is transported to the liver where vitamin D 25-hydroxylase (from both the mitochondria and microsomes) converts it to 25-hydroxyvitamin D. Although there are probably other sites for this enzymatic conversion, the liver appears to be the principal site of conversion in humans. The vitamin D 25-hydroxylase is a regulated enzyme that is inhibited by a 1α,25-dihydroxyvitamin D, 25-hydroxyvitamin D, and vitamin D.[89]

25-Hydroxyvitamin D, a more effective antirachitic calcium mobilizer than vitamin D, requires further hydroxylation to the most active form, 1α,25-dihydroxyvitamin D. This hydroxylation occurs in the proximal convoluted tubules and the pars rectus of the kidneys, the principal locations of 1-α-hydroxylases. These mitochondrial enzymes are mixed-function, cytochrome P-450 oxidases that require NADPH and molecular oxygen. Both enzymes produce 1α,25-dihydroxyvitamin D or 1α,24,25-trihydroxyvitamin D from 25-hydroxy- or 24,25-dihydroxyvitamin D. These are the most active forms of vitamin D in antirachitic effects, increasing gastrointestinal calcium absorption and promoting bone resorption. The enzymatic activity of the proximal convoluted tubule is stimulated exclusively by PTH, whereas the enzyme of the pars rectus responds to calcitonin.[89]

Vitamin D and its metabolites are transported in the serum by a vitamin D–binding protein, which is believed to inhibit degradation, promote solubility, and act as a reservoir. Other metabolites of vitamin D have been reported to have a wide variety of miscellaneous functions.[89]

The main action of vitamin D is to promote calcium absorption from the proximal intestinal tract. This is believed to occur by means of a 1α,25-vitamin D receptor. The presence of this or similar receptors in other organs has opened up the possibility of a wide variety of other functions for vitamin D metabolites. The exact mechanisms of enhancement of intestinal calcium absorption by vitamin D remain under investigation. It is known to induce the synthesis of a calcium-binding protein, but this does not seem to explain all of the physiologic responses of vitamin D–deficient animals to 1α,25-dihydroxyvitamin D. Other actions of vitamin D include the enhancement of bone resorption, probably through activation of macrophages and osteoclast precursors, the inhibition of the transcription of the parathyroid gene, and possibly the increased proliferation of parathyroid cells responding to hypocalcemia.[89]

Parathyroid hormone

PTH is synthesized exclusively by the chief cells of the parathyroid glands.[32,50-53,72,91] The gene for PTH is located on the short arm of chromosome 11 (11p15.4).[91] Its location has been precisely identified with reference to several other genes on this chromosome. The gene order has been identified as centromere–catalase–calcitonin–FSHβ–PTH–β globin–Harvey ras–insulin. The gene for parathyroid hormones in several species thus far studied has a similar structure, exon I (a 5′ untranslated region), intron A (separates the untranslated region from the signal sequence), exon II (coding for the preproregion), intron B (separates exon III, which encodes for the hormone, and a 3′ untranslated region). Intron A varies in size in different species, being largest (about 3400 base pairs) in the human. Intron B is approximately 100 base pairs in all species studied. There is a termination codon immediately after the codon for glutamine at position 84. The gene is a single-copy gene, and there are no related duplicate or pseudogenes. The human gene contains two polymorphisms.[92] One is identified by the restriction endonuclease Pst I, which cleaves between the encoding sequence for residues 28 and 29 of the mature hormone, with the second site 2800 or 2200 base pairs downstream in the 3′ flanking region.[92] Seventy percent of the population have the longer fragment, 30% have the shorter one, and heterozygotes are common. The second polymorphism depends on the presence or absence of a Taq I cleavage site in intron B.[92] Both polymorphisms have been used in familial studies of disorders of calcium metabolism. Although studies on the promotor sequences are as yet incomplete, the upstream promoter sequences have been shown to be responsive to 1α,25-dihydroxyvitamin D, hypocalcemia, and cAMP.[92]

Parathyroid hormone–related protein (PTH-rP) is the hormone responsible for the hypercalcemia of malignancy.[92-96] It is located on chromosome 12, which is believed to be an ancient duplication of chromosome 11.[93-96] Apparently there are two messengers produced because of the presence of two functional TATA start sequences in the human gene. In contrast to PTH, PTH-rP undergoes differential splicing.[93-96]

Biosynthesis of PTH begins with transcription of the PTH gene to a precursor mRNA. The precursor mRNA is processed and spliced by removal of the introns to the mature mRNA for the preprohormone (a straight-chain polypeptide consisting of a 25–amino acid leader sequence (pre-), a 6–amino acid prosequence, and the 84–amino acid mature hormone.[91,92] The preproPTH is synthesized on the polyribosomes, which are bound to the endoplasmic reticulum by the leader sequence. The leader sequence and the C-terminal fragment are necessary for transfer of the hormone from the cytosol to the lumen of the endoplasmic reticulum. Here the leader sequence is removed by a signal peptidase. The prohormone is then transported to the Golgi region where it is packaged into secretory granules along with chromogranin (secretogranin I), and the presequence is removed[91-92] (Fig. 62-5). The C-terminal portion of the molecule is required for processing and secretion of the molecule.[97]

Mature PTH is a straight-chain polypeptide (relative molecular mass, approximately 9600) of 84 amino acids. The biologic activity is largely present in the N-terminal 34 amino acids.[91-92] There are three regions in the N-terminal portion, an activation domain (amino acids 1 to 6), an inhibitory domain (amino acids 7 to 24), and a principal binding domain (amino acids 25 to 34).[91-92] The C-terminal portion of the hormone is necessary for the binding of the polyribosomes to the endoplasmic reticulum and the transfer of the hormone to the lumen of the GER.[91-92]

Synthesis of PTH is controlled by 1α,25-dihydroxyvitamin D and $[Ca^{++}]$.[98] Alteration in the ambient $[Ca^{++}]$ results in a corresponding increase or decrease in the cytosolic $[Ca^{++}]$. This is accompanied by alterations in the cAMP and inositol pathways with a decrease in cytosolic $[Ca^{++}]$ increasing PTH secretion acutely and transcription and synthesis over the long run.[98] In addition a decrease in ambient and cytosolic $[Ca^{++}]$

eral human tumors, parathyroid adenomas, centrocytic lymphomas, and other B-cell tumors. The gene has been found to be the same as *bcl*-1 and encodes a novel protein, cyclin D1, an apparent regulator of the G_1/S phase transition. As with other housekeeping or growth-regulator genes, its promotor region has Sp1 binding sites and no TATA box.[138] In a parathyroid adenoma it was demonstrated that there was a clonal inversion around the centromere on one allele of chromosome 11,[137] such that the tissue-specific 5′-regulatory sequences of the PTH gene (from the short arm of chromosome 11) were brought into juxtaposition with the PRAD1 gene, causing overexpression. Since the other allele of chromosome 11 is normal, there is normal expression of PTH in the tumor cells. Although only approximately 5% of parathyroid tumors have had PRAD1/cyclin overexpression demonstrated, because the rearrangements may have different promoters or the promoters may be too far upstream to be detected by the methods used, the true incidence may be much higher.[139] The overexpressed cyclin is normal, and this normality indicates that its own promotor is being used. Furthermore, this promotor is apparently insulated from the 1α,25-dihydroxyvitamin D inhibitor. The identification of monoclonality in parathyroid adenomas adds further justification to the current recommended therapy for patients with adenomas and chief cell hyperplasia (see the discussion of therapy later). There is no evidence of mutations in the p53 gene in parathyroid adenomas.[139a]

Locations. Adenomas are found at all sites where normal parathyroid glands have been found. Parathyroid tumors have been reported near the carotid bifurcation cephalically, in the pericardial sac caudally, retroesophageally, in the anterolateral portion of the thyroid, and in the substernal mediastinum.[140-143] Encroachment on the esophagus, trachea, or thyroid and cervical or mediastinal lesions may be located by barium swallow, sequential cervical esophagrams, radiographs, computerized tomography (CT), magnetic resonance imaging, or differential cervical scintigrams, or as cold nodules on thyroid scans.

One percent to 3% of abnormal parathyroids are totally embedded within a normal thyroid, whereas capsular tumors may be engulfed within multinodular goiters.[15,141-143] Gravitational forces may pull a parathyroid tumor into the mediastinum, even one derived from a superior gland. Mediastinal adenomas may originate from aberrant glands or dystrophic fragments of glands. Although up to 21% of parathyroid tumors may be located beneath the thoracic inlet, less than 3% of these require mediastinotomy for removal.[25,143a]

Gross features. Adenomas in two glands were found along with one or two normal gland biopsy specimens in eight of our cases (0.9%). These patients were all apparently cured by removal of the two adenomas. Although so-called double adenomas were diagnosed more frequently in the past (6.8% to 39%),[144] most of these cases in fact represent primary chief cell hyperplasia. Since recurrences may require years, their absence is attributable to the shortness of follow-up study or to death of these elderly patients.

The average weight of parathyroid adenomas in patients with classic osteitis fibrosa cystica was approximately 10 g, with the largest weighing 53 g, whereas the average weight of adenomas in patients without radiographic bone disease was 1.3 g, with most being under 1 g and some under 0.5 g.[15] I have accepted an adenoma in a gland that weighed less than 35 mg total, since its removal cured the patient's hyperparathyroidism, but the diagnosis of any tumor weighing less than 100 mg must be confirmed by a surgical cure.[145-146] The correlation between tumor weight and the serum calcium and the PTH levels is probably not statistically significant.[15]

Even small adenomas usually involve the entire gland, though a small rim of normal parathyroid gland may be identified grossly or microscopically. The involved glands are ellipsoidal, with minimal swelling, and have more rounded edges and somewhat darker brown color than the normal glands have. Larger adenomas are ovate, spherical, or teardrop shaped (Fig. 62-9). They may be smooth or nodular, orange-tan to dark brown, soft and pliable. The capsule is usually thin, translucent, and gray with a fine capillary network. Rarely the capsule may be thick, tan, fibrous, and dense. Small tags of yellow adipose tissue, which may upon sectioning contain thymus or normal parathyroid, are occasionally identifiable attached to the capsule. The capsule may have a thin fibrous stalk, especially in mediastinal tumors. Less pliable dark red thyroid or gray-pink to black lymph nodes, lacking the surface capillary networks can be easily discriminated from parathyroid tumors. A darker, more chocolate color is observed if the tumor is largely constituted of oxyphil cells. Surgical manipulation often creates dark red hemorrhagic areas in the subcapsular and deep parenchyma.

The cross section of the parenchyma is orange-tan to red-tan, with areas of dark red hemorrhage, dark brown old hemorrhage, or gray-tan fibrosis. Clear, colorless to chocolate, watery fluid-filled, single or multiple cystic spaces, 0.1 to 1.0 cm in diameter, are occasionally seen. Large single functioning cysts may have originated as adenomas that have degenerated because of vascular insufficiency. Small gray-tan to brown remnants of the tumor in the fibrotic wall may be seen.

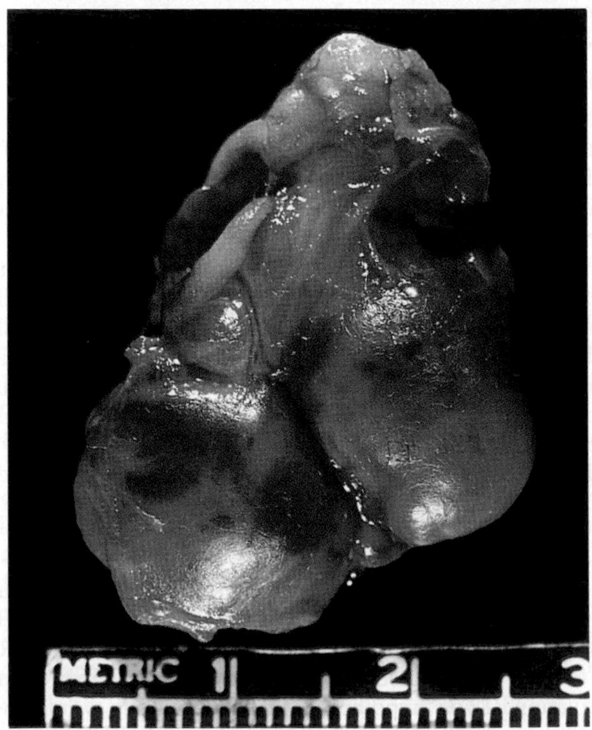

Fig. 62-9 A somewhat larger than typical parathyroid adenoma. The gland is teardrop shaped and somewhat nodular with a yellow-tan surface and a thin translucent capsule.

Microscopic features. The majority of adenomas are composed primarily of chief cells (Fig. 62-9). Oxyphil cells may be present, ranging from a few individual cells, to nests and nodules to involvement of the entire tumor.[15,37,47] The capsule is thin and composed of delicate collagen fibers. The intratumoral stroma is usually sparse with considerable vascularity, which can be easily identified as a histochemical reaction for endothelial alkaline phosphatase or an immunohistochemical reaction for factor VIIIa. Individual or small groups of adipocytes may focally be seen in the stroma. There are occasional areas of pseudogland formation around blood vessels, resembling Wright rosettes, or pseudoacini with a pink eosinophilic proteinaceous luminal substance[15,37,41,47] (Fig. 62-10). Rarely, an entire tumor has a pseudofollicular structure and may be difficult to differentiate from a thyroid tumor. Anoxic necrosis of the central cells in large spherical groups of tumor cells without central capillaries is believed to be the pathogenesis of the acinar formation. The luminal contents often show the presence of amyloid[41,43] and show a fibrillar structure reminiscent of amyloid on electron microscopic examination.[47] The acinar contents contain glycoproteins, giving a positive periodic acid–Schiff (PAS) reaction, whereas thyroid acinar fluid shows no PAS-positive material. Positive reactions for intracellular fat may be seen in the parathyroid acinar cells, but not in those of the thyroid. The lining cells vary from flattened to tall columnar cells with surface microvilli and basally located nuclei.

Classification of parathyroid adenomas on the basis of cell type and cell arrangement has not afforded worthwhile clinicopathologic correlations. All the cells of adenomas, hyperplasias, and normal glands originate from chief cells. It is worthwhile, however, for the surgical pathologist to appreciate the differences in histologic patterns present in tumors of parathyroid origin. The chief cells in adenomas are spherical and 9 to 14 μm in diameter. The cells are crowded, often with nuclear overlapping. The nuclei in adenomas are somewhat larger and more hyperchromatic and pleomorphic than those of the normal chief cells. Multinucleate cells with two to five small hyperchromatic nuclei are common, and giant nuclear forms up to 20 μm in diameter are seen in about 10% of adenomas (Fig. 62-11). Giant and highly pleomorphic nuclei with pronounced hyperchromatism are rarely seen (Fig. 62-12). Mitoses are uncommon, and small irregular pyknotic nuclei in adenomas should not be incorrectly called "mitotic figures." Since chief cell hyperplasia less frequently contains pleomorphic nuclei and multinucleated cells, this feature may assist one in distinguishing an adenoma from a chief cell hyperplasia.

The chief cell membranes are poorly demarcated. The cytoplasm is lightly eosinophilic, occasionally with granular or vacuolated cytoplasm in hematoxylin and eosin–stained paraffin-embedded sections. The chief cells of adenomas generally contain little intracellular fat, and what is present is usually in finely dispersed droplets.[44,147-151] In formalin-fixed tissue, a single large cytoplasmic vacuole may occur and may result in an apparent clearer separation of the cells. Care must be taken not to interpret this vacuolization of the chief cell cytoplasm as an involvement of the gland with the cells of a true water-clear cell hyperplasia (see later), which are rarely seen in adenomas.

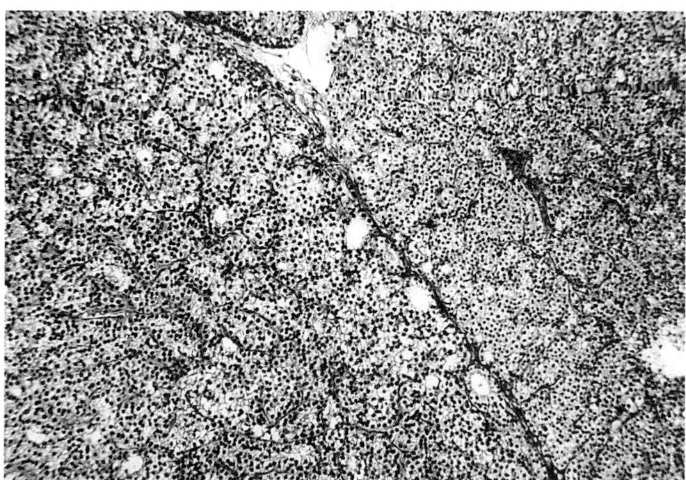

Fig. 62-10 A parathyroid adenoma composed almost purely of chief cells. In the right upper portion of the gland, the cells are arranged in uniform sheets and cords, whereas in the left lower portion of the micrograph the cells are arranged in sheets, cords, and pseudofollicles.

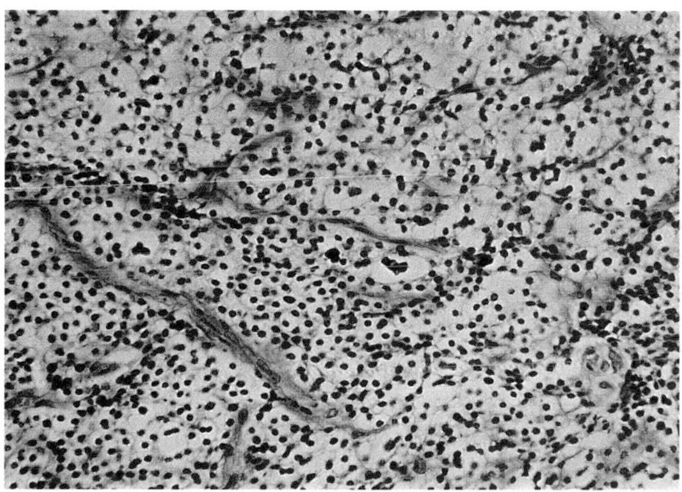

Fig. 62-11 Sheets of chief cells in an adenoma. Giant cells, both mononuclear and multinuclear, are seen in some cells.

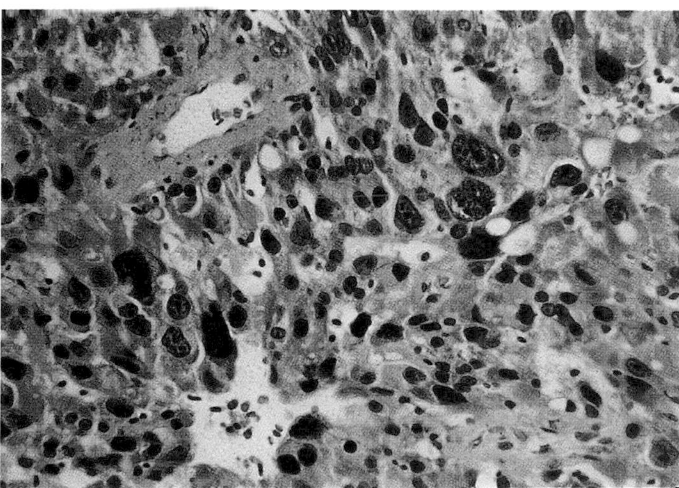

Fig. 62-12 An area of large atypical, highly pleomorphic chief cells in a parathyroid adenoma.

152. Arnold BM, Kovacs K, Horvath E et al: Functioning oxyphil cell adenoma of the parathyroid gland: evidence for parathyroid secretory activity of oxyphil cells, *J Clin Endocrinol Metab* 38:458, 1974.
153. McGregor DH, Lotuaco LG, Rao MS, Chu LL: Functioning oxyphil adenoma of parathyroid gland: an ultrastructural and biochemical study, *Am J Pathol* 92:691, 1978.
154. Ordóñez NG, Ibáñez MI, Mackay B et al: Functioning oxyphil cell adenomas of parathyroid gland: immunoperoxidase evidence of hormonal activity in oxyphil cells, *Am J Clin Pathol* 78:681, 1982.
155. Bedetti CD, Dekker A, Watson CG: Functioning oxyphil cell adenoma of the parathyroid gland: a clinicopathologic study of ten patients with hyperparathyroidism, *Hum Pathol* 15:1121, 1984.
156. Wolpert HR, Vickery AL Jr, Wang C-A: Functioning oxyphil cell adenomas of the parathyroid gland: a study of 15 cases, *Am J Surg Pathol* 13:500, 1989.
157. Shimada T, Higashi K, Kimura K et al: A case of primary hyperparathyroidism due to an oxyphil cell adenoma, *Endocrinol Jpn* 39:499, 1992.
158. Capps RB: Multiple parathyroid tumors with massive mediastinal and subcutaneous hemorrhage, *Am J Med Sci* 188:801, 1934.
159. Lee MC, McElhinney WT, Gall EA: Unusual manifestations of parathyroid adenoma, *Arch Surg* 71:475, 1955.
160. Lemann J, Donatelli AA: Calcium intoxication due to primary hyperparathyroidism, *Ann Intern Med* 60:447, 1964.
161. Chodack P, Attie NN, Groder MG: Hypercalcemic crisis coincidental with hemorrhage in parathyroid adenoma, *Arch Intern Med* 116:416, 1965.
162. Mannix H, Loehr WJ: Unusual aspects of hyperparathyroidism, *Surg Gynecol Obstet* 126:347, 1968.
163. DeGroote JW: Acute intermittent hyperparathyroidism with hemorrhage into a parathyroid adenoma, *JAMA* 208:2160, 1969.
164. Berry BE, Carpenter PC, Fultton RE, Danielson GK: Mediastinal hemorrhage from parathyroid adenoma simulating dissecting aneurysm, *Arch Surg* 108:740, 1974.
165. Santos GH, Tseng C-L, Frater RWM: Ruptured intrathoracic parathyroid adenoma, *Chest* 68:844, 1975.
166. Jordon FT, Harness JK, Thompson NW: Spontaneous cervical hematoma: a rare manifestation of parathyroid adenoma, *Surgery* 89:697, 1981.
167. Weiler R, Fircher-Colbrie R, Schmid KW et al: Immunological studies on the occurrence and properties of chromogranin A and B and secretogranin II in endocrine tumors, *Am J Surg Pathol* 12:877, 1988.
168. Dietel M, Lehmann E, Kaspar M, Heitz PH: Distribution pattern of PTH in human parathyroid adenomas: an immunohistochemical study, *Horm Metab Res* 12:640, 1980.
169. Berger G, Berger F, Billard F et al: Storage and degradation of secretory proteins in adenomatous and secondary hyperplastic parathyroid cells: an immunoelectron microscope study, *Virchows Arch [A] (Pathol Anat)* 415:305, 1989.
170. Weber CJ, Russell J, Costanzo K et al: Relationships of parathyroid hormone, parathyroid secretory protein, parathyroid hormone messenger RNA, parathyroid secretory protein mRNA, and replication in human parathyroid adenoma and secondary hyperplasia tissues and cultures, *Surgery* 112:1089, 1992.
171. Pesce C, Tobia F, Carli F, Antoniotti GV: The sites of hormone storage in normal and disease parathyroid glands: a silver impregnation and immunohistochemical study, *Histopathology* 15:157, 1989.
172. Schmid KW, Hittmair A, Ladurner D et al: Chromogranin A and B in parathyroid tissue of cases of primary hyperparathyroidism: an immunohistochemical study: *Virchows Arch [A] (Pathol Anat)* 418:295, 1991.
173. Danks JA, Ebeling PR, Hayman JA et al: Immunohistochemical localization of parathyroid hormone–related protein in parathyroid adenoma and hyperplasia, *J Pathol* 161:27, 1990.
174. Roth SI, Wang C-A, Potts JT Jr: The team approach to primary hyperparathyroidism, *Hum Pathol* 6:645, 1975.
175. de Menezes Y, Sesso A: Annulate lamellae as a precursor or a product of paired cisternae in human adenomatous parathyroid cells, *Acta Anat* 131:3, 1988.
176. Cinti S, Osculati F: Ribosome-lamellae complex in the adenoma cells of the human parathyroid gland, *J Submicrosc Cytol* 14:521, 1982.
177. Ober WB, Kaiser GA: Hamartoma of the parathyroid, *Cancer* 11:601, 1958.
178. Abul-Haj SK, Conklin H, Hewitt WC: Functioning lipoadenoma of the parathyroid gland: report of a unique case, *N Engl J Med* 266:121, 1962.
179. LeGolvan DP, Moore BP, Nishiyama RH: Parathyroid hamartoma: report of two cases and review of the literature, *Am J Clin Pathol* 67:31, 1977.
180. Weiland LH, Garrison RC, ReMine WH, et al: Lipoadenoma of the parathyroid gland, *Am J Surg Pathol* 2:3, 1978.
181. Geelhoed GW: Parathyroid lipoadenoma: clinical morphological features, *Surgery* 92:806, 1982.
182. Hargreaves HK, Wright TC Jr: A large functioning parathyroid lipoadenoma found in the posterior mediastinum, *Am J Clin Pathol* 76:89, 1980.
183. Gabbert H, Rothmund M, Hohn P: Myxoid lipoadenoma of the parathyroid gland, *Pathol Res Pract* 170:420, 1980.
184. DaRoca PJ Jr, Landau RL, Reed RJ et al: Functioning lipoadenoma of the parathyroid gland, *Arch Pathol Lab Med* 105:28, 1977.
185. Ducatman BS, Wilkerson SY, Brown JA: Functioning parathyroid lipoadenoma: report of a case diagnosed by intraoperative touch preparations, *Arch Pathol Lab Med* 110:645, 1986.
186. Rosai J, Levine JD: Tumors of the thymus. In *Atlas of tumor pathology,* series 2, fasc 13, Washington, D.C., 1976, Armed Forces Institute of Pathology.
187. van Hoeven KH, Brennan MF: Lipothymoadenoma of the parathyroid, *Arch Pathol Lab Med* 117:312, 1993.
188. Cope O, Keynes WM, Roth SI, Castleman B: Primary chief-cell hyperplasia of the parathyroid glands: a new entity in the surgery of hyperparathyroidism, *Ann Surg* 148:375, 1958.
189. Castleman B, Shantz A, Roth SI: Parathyroid hyperplasia in primary hyperparathyroidism: a review of 85 cases, *Cancer* 38:1668, 1976.
190. Frohner RN, Wolgamot JC: Primary hyperparathyroidism: five cases in one family, *Ann Intern Med* 40:765, 1954.
191. Williams ED: The parathyroid glands. In Symers VS, editor: *Systemic pathology,* vol 4, ed 2, Edinburgh, 1978, Churchill Livingstone.
192. Altenähr E, Seemann N, Seifert G: Pathologische Anatomie der Epithelkörperchen, *Prakt Chir* 82:1, 1969.
193. Tominaga Y, Grimelius L, Johansson H et al: Histological and clinical features of non-familial primary parathyroid hyperplasia, *Pathol Res Pract* 188:115, 1992.
194. Benson L, Ljunghall S, Åkerström G, Oberg K: Hyperparathyroidism presenting as the first lesion in multiple endocrine neoplasia type 1, *Am J Med* 82:731, 1987.
195. DeLellis RA, Dayal Y, Tischler AS et al: Multiple endocrine neoplasia (MEN) syndromes: cellular origins and interrelationships, *Int Rev Exp Pathol* 28:163, 1986.
196. Carney JA, Roth SI, Heath H III: The parathyroid glands in multiple endocrine neoplasia, type 2b, *Am J Pathol* 99:387, 1980.
197. Berg B, Biörklund A, Grimelius L et al: A new pattern of multiple endocrine adenomatosis: chemodectoma, bronchial carcinoid, G-H producing pituitary adenoma, and hyperplasia of the parathyroid glands, and antral and duodenal gastrin cells, *Acta Med Scand* 200:321, 1976.
198. Rode RL, Dhillon AP, Cotton PB et al: Carcinoid of the stomach and primary hyperparathyroidism—a new association, *J Clin Pathol* 40:546, 1987.
199. Wheeler MH, Curley IR, Williams ED: The association of neurofibromatosis, pheochromocytoma and somatostatin-rich duodenal carcinoid tumor, *Surgery* 100:1163, 1986.
200. Larraza-Hernández O, Albores-Saavedra J, Benavídes G et al: Multiple endocrine neoplasia, pituitary adenoma, multicentric papillary thyroid carcinoma, bilateral carotid body paraganglioma, parathyroid hyperplasia, gastric leiomyoma and systemic amyloidosis, *Am J Clin Pathol* 78:527, 1982.
201. Black WC III: Correlative light and electron microscopy in primary hyperparathyroidism, *Arch Pathol* 88:225, 1969.
202. Black WC III, Haff RC: The surgical pathology of parathyroid chief cell hyperplasia, *Am J Clin Pathol* 53:565, 1970.
203. Black WC III, Utely JR: The differential diagnosis of parathyroid adenoma and chief cell hyperplasia, *Am J Clin Pathol* 49:761, 1968.
204. King DT, Hirose FM: Chief cell intracytoplasmic fat used to evaluate parathyroid diseases by frozen section, *Arch Pathol Lab Med* 103:609, 1979.

205. Nilsson O: Studies on the ultrastructure of the human parathyroid glands in various pathological conditions, *Acta Pathol Microbiol Immunol Scand [A]* 263(suppl):1, 1977.
206. Wang C-A, Reider SV: A density test for the intraoperative differentiation of parathyroid hyperplasia from neoplasia, *Ann Surg* 187:63, 1978.
207. Åkerström G, Pertoft H, Grimelius L et al: Density determinations of hman parathyroid glands by density gradients, *Acta Pathol Microbiol Scand [A]* 87:91, 1979.
208. Fitko R, Roth SI, Hines JR et al: Parathyromatosis in hyperparathyroidism, *Hum Pathol* 21:234, 1990.
209. Straus FH II, Kaplan EL, Nishiyama RH, Bigos ST: Five cases of parathyroid lipohyperplasia, *Surgery* 94:901, 1983.
210. Clark OH: Hyperparathyroidism due to primary cystic parathyroid hyperplasia, *Arch Surg* 113:748, 1978.
211. Fallon MD, Haines JW, Teitelbaum SL: Cystic parathyroid gland hyperplasia—hyperparathyroidism presenting as a neck mass, *Am J Clin Pathol* 77:104, 1982.
212. Mallette LE, Malini S, Rappaport MP, Kirkland JL: Familial cystic parathyroid adenomatosis, *Ann Intern Med* 107:54, 1987.
213. Bradford WD, Wilson JW, Gaede JT: Primary neonatal hyperparathyroidism—an unusual case of failure to thrive, *Am J Clin Pathol* 59:265, 1973.
214. Rhone DP: Primary neonatal hyperparathyroidism: report of a case and review of the literature, *Am J Clin Pathol* 64:488, 1975.
215. Goldbloom RB, Gillis DA, Prasad M: Hereditary parathyroid hyperplasia: a surgical emergency of early infancy, *Pediatrics* 49:514, 1972.
216. García-Buñuel R, Kutchemeshgi A, Brandes D: Hereditary hyperparathyroidism: the fine structure of the parathyroid gland, *Arch Pathol* 97:399, 1974.
217. Albright F, Bloomberg E, Castleman B, Churchill ED: Hyperparathyroidism due to diffuse hyperplasia of all parathyroid glands rather than adenoma of one: clinical studies on three such cases, *Arch Intern Med* 54:315, 1934.
218. Castleman B, Cope O: Primary parathyroid hypertrophy and hyperplasia: a review of 11 cases at the Massachusetts General Hospital, *Bull Hosp Joint Dis* 12:368, 1951.
219. Roth SI: The ultrastructure of primary water-clear cell hyperplasia of the parathyroid glands, *Am J Pathol* 61:233, 1970.
220. Persson S, Hansson G, Hedman I et al: Primary parathyroid hyperplasia of water-clear cell type: transformation of water-clear cells into chief cells, *Acta Pathol Microbiol Immunol Scand [A]* 94:391, 1986.
221. Sandelin K, Auer G, Bondeson L et al: Prognostic factors in parathyroid cancer: a review of 95 cases, *World J Surg* 16:724, 1992.
222. Schantz A, Castleman B: Parathyroid carcinoma: a study of 70 cases, *Cancer* 31:600, 1973.
223. Smith JF, Coombs RRH: Histological diagnosis of carcinoma of the parathyroid gland, *J Clin Pathol* 37:1370, 1984.
224. Avramides A, Papamargaritis K, Antoniadis A, Gakis D: Large parathyroid functioning carcinoma (1,200 g) presenting as a substernal goiter, *J Endocrinol Invest* 15:39, 1992.
225. McCance DR, Kenny BD, Sloan JM et al: Parathyroid carcinoma: a review, *J R Soc Med* 80:505, 1987.
226. Hakaim AG, Esselstyn CB Jr: Parathyroid carcinoma: 50-year experience at the Cleveland Clinic Foundation, *Cleve Clin J Med* 60:331, 1993.
227. Shane E, Bilezikian JP: Parathyroid carcinoma: a review of 62 patients, *Endocr Rev* 3:218, 1982.
228. Wynne AG, van Heerden J, Carney JA, Fitzpatrick LA: Parathyroid carcinoma: clinical and pathologic features in 43 patients, *Medicine* 71:197, 1992.
229. Haghighi P, Astarita RW, Wepsic HT, Wolf PL: Concurrent primary parathyroid hyperplasia and parathyroid carcinoma, *Arch Pathol Lab Med* 107:349, 1983.
230. Frayha RA, Nassar VH, Dagher F et al: Familial parathyroid carcinoma, *Lab Med J* 25:299, 1972.
231. Mallette LE, Bilezikian JP, Ketcham AS, Aurbach GD: Parathyroid carcinoma in familial hyperparathyroidism, *Am J Med* 57:642, 1974.
232. Dinnen JS, Greenwood RH, Jones JH et al: Parathyroid carcinoma in familial hyperparathyroidism, *J Clin Pathol* 30:966, 1977.
233. Leborgne J, LeNeel J-C, Guzelin F, Malvy P: Cancer familial des parathyroïdes. Intérêt de l'angiographie dans le diagnostic des récidives locorégionales. Considérations à propos de deux cas, *J Chir* (Paris) 109:315, 1975.
234. Streeten EA, Weinstein LS, Norton JA et al: Studies in a kindred with parathyroid carcinoma, *J Clin Endocrinol Metab* 75:362, 1992.
235. Sieracki JC, Horn RC: Nonfunctioning carcinoma of the parathyroid, *Cancer* 13:502, 1960.
236. Yamashita H, Noguchi S, Murakami N et al: Immunohistological study of nonfunctional parathyroid carcinoma: report of a case, *Acta Pathol Jpn* 42: 279, 1992.
237. Ordóñez, NG, Samaan NA, Ibáñez ML, Hickey RC: Immunoperoxidase study of uncommon parathyroid tumors: report of two cases of nonfunctioning parathyroid carcinoma and one intrathyroid parathyroid tumor–producing amyloid, *Am J Surg Pathol* 7:535, 1983.
238. Merlano M, Conte P, Scarsi P: Non-functioning parathyroid carcinoma: a case report, *Tumori* 71:193, 1985.
239. Murphy MN, Glennon PG, Diocee MS: Nonsecretory parathyroid carcinoma of the mediastinum: light microscopic, immunocytochemical, and ultrastructural features of a case, and review of the literature, *Cancer* 58:2468, 1986.
240. Baba H, Kishihava M, Tohmon M et al: Identification of parathyroid hormone messenger ribonucleic acid in an apparently nonfunctioning parathyroid carcinoma transformed from a parathyroid carcinoma with hyperparathyroidism, *J Clin Endocrinol Metab* 62:247, 1986.
241. Barnicott NA: The local action of the parathyroid and other tissues on bone in intracerebral grafts, *J Anat* 82:233, 1948.
242. Chang H-Y: Grafts of parathyroid and other tissues to bone, *Anat Rec* 111:23, 1951.
243. Rapoport A, Sepp AH, Brown WH: Carcinoma of the parathyroid gland with pulmonary metastases and cardiac death, *Am J Med* 28:443, 1960.
244. Massachusetts General Hospital, Case Records: Case 50-1971, *N Engl J Med* 285:1422, 1971.
245. Wang C-A, Gaz RD: Natural history of parathyroid carcinoma: diagnosis, treatment and results, *Am J Surg* 148:522, 1985.
246. Shane E: Parathyroid carcinoma. In Bilezikian JP, Marcus R, Levine MA, editors: *The parathyroids: basic and clinical concepts,* New York, 1994, Raven Press.
247. Shane E, Bilezikian JP: Parathyroid carcinoma: a review of 62 patients, *Endocr Rev* 3:218, 1982.
248. Trigonis C, Cedermark B, Willems J et al: Parathyroid carcinoma—problems in diagnosis and treatment, *Clin Oncol* 10:11, 1984.
249. Sokol MS, Kavolius J, Schaaf M, D'Avis J: Recurrent hyperparathyroidism from benign neoplastic seed: a review with recommendations for management, *Surgery* 113:456, 1993.
250. Fraker DL, Travis WD, Merendino JJ Jr et al: Locally recurrent parathyroid neoplasms as a cause for recurrent and persistent primary hyperparathyroidism, *Ann Surg* 213:58, 1991.
251. Rattner DW, Marrone GC, Kasdon E, Silen W: Recurrent hyperparathyroidism due to implantation of parathyroid tissue, *Am J Surg* 149:745, 1985.
252. Snover DC, Foucar K: Mitotic activity in benign parathyroid disease, *Am J Clin Pathol* 75:345, 1981.
253. Chaitin BA, Goldman RL: Mitotic activity in benign parathyroid disease, *Am J Clin Pathol* 76:363, 1981.
254. Obara T, Fujimoto Y, Yamaguchi K et al: Parathyroid carcinoma of the oxyphil cell type: a report of two cases, light and electron microscopic study, *Cancer* 55:1482, 1985.
255. Edelson GW, Kleerekoper M, Talpos GB et al: Mucin-producing parathyroid carcinoma, *Bone* 13:7, 1992.
256. Sandelin K, Auer G, Bondeson L et al: Prognostic factors in parathyroid cancer: a review of 95 cases, *World J Surg* 16:724, 1992.
257. Bondeson L, Sandelin K, Grimelius L: Histopathological variables and DNA cytometry in parathyroid carcinoma, *Am J Surg Pathol* 17:820, 1993.
258. August DA, Flynn SD, Jones MA et al: Parathyroid carcinoma: the relationship of nuclear DNA content to clinical outcome, *Surgery* 113:290, 1993.

259. Obara T, Fujimoto Y, Hirayama A et al: Flow cytometric DNA analysis of parathyroid tumors with special reference to its diagnostic and prognostic value in parathyroid carcinoma, *Cancer* 65:1789, 1989.
260. Cryns VL, Thor A, Xu HJ et al: Loss of retinoblastoma tumor-suppressor gene in parathyroid carcinoma, *N Engl J Med* 330:757, 1994.
261. Åltenähr E, Saeger W: Light and electron microscopy of parathyroid carcinoma: report of 3 cases, *Virchows Arch [A] (Pathol Anat)* 360:107, 1973.
262. Bichel P, Thomsen OF, Askjaer SAA, Nielsen HE: Light and electron microscopic investigation of parathyroid carcinoma during dedifferentiation, *Virchows Arch [A] (Pathol Anat)* 386:363, 1980.
263. Irvin GL III, Taupier MA, Block NL, Reiss E: DNA patterns in parathyroid disease predict postoperative parathyroid hormone secretion, *Surgery* 104:1115, 1988.
264. Chahinian AP, Holland JF, Nieburgs, HE et al: Metastatic nonfunctioning parathyroid carcinoma: ultrastructural evidence of secretory granules and response to chemotherapy, *Am J Med Sci* 282:80, 1983.
265. Cinti S, Colussi G, Minola E, Dickersin GR: Parathyroid glands in primary hyperparathyroidism: an ultrastructural study of 50 cases, *Hum Pathol* 17:1036, 1986.
266. Boquist LLV: Nucleolar organizer regions in normal, hyperplastic and neoplastic parathyroid glands, *Virchows Archiv [A] (Pathol Anat)* 417:237, 1990.
267. Harlow S, Roth SI, Bauer K, Marshall RB: Flow cytometric DNA analysis of normal and pathologic parathyroid glands, *Mod Pathol* 4:310, 1991.
268. Bowlby LS, DeBault LE, Abraham SR: Flow cytometric DNA analysis of parathyroid glands: relationship between nuclear DNA and pathologic classifications, *Am J Pathol* 128:338, 1987.
269. Mallette LE: DNA quantitation in the study of parathyroid lesions: a review, *Am J Clin Pathol* 98:305, 1992.
270. Jacobi JM, Lloyd HM, Smith JF: Nuclear diameter in parathyroid carcinomas, *J Clin Pathol* 39:1353, 1987.
271. LiVolsi VA, Hamilton R: Intraoperative assessment of parathyroid gland pathology: a common view from the surgeon and the pathologist, *Am J Clin Pathol* 102:365, 1994.
272. Wang C-A: Surgery of the parathyroid glands. In Welch CE, Hardy JD, editors: *Advances in surgery,* vol 5, St. Louis, 1976, Mosby.
273. Wang C-A, Castleman B, Cope O: Surgical management of hyperparathyroidism due to primary hyperplasia: a clinical and pathologic study of 104 cases, *Ann Surg* 195:384, 1977.
274. Norton JA, Brennan MF, Wells SA Jr: Surgical management of hyperparathyroidism. In Bilezikian JP, Marcus R, Levine MA, editors: *The parathyroids: basic and clinical concepts,* New York, 1994, Raven Press.
275. Deftos LJ, Parthemore JC, Stabile BE: Management of primary hyperparathyroidism, *Annu Rev Med* 44:19, 1993.
276. Grimelius L, Åkerström G, Bondeson L et al: The role of the pathologist in diagnosis and decision making in hyperparathyroidism, *World J Surg* 15:698, 1991.
277. Worsey MJ, Carty SE, Watson CG: Success in unilateral neck exploration for sporadic primary hyperparathyroidism, *Surgery* 114:1024, 1994.
278. Silverberg SG: Imprints in the intraoperative evaluation of parathyroid disease, *Arch Pathol* 100:375, 1975.
279. Proye CAG, Goropoulos A, Franz C et al: Usefulness and limits of quick intraoperative measurements of intact (1-84) parathyroid hormone in the surgical management of hyperparathyroidism: sequential measurements in patients with multiglandular disease, *Surgery* 110:1035, 1991.
280. Kao PC, van Heerden JA, Taylor RL: Intraoperative monitoring of parathyroid procedures by a 15-minute parathyroid hormone immunochemiluminometric assay, *Mayo Clin Proc* 69:532, 1994.
281. Chapuis Y, Icard JD, Ferguson WR et al: Parathyroid adenomectomy under local anesthesia with intraoperative monitoring of UcAMP and/or 1-84 PTH, *World J Surg* 16:570, 1992.
282. Russell CF, Laird JD, Ferguson WR: Scan-directed unilateral cervical exploration for parathyroid adenoma: a legitimate approach? *World J Surg* 14:406, 1990.
283. Hosking SW, Jones H, du Boulay CE, McGinn PP: Surgery for parathyroid adenoma and hyperplasia: relationship of histology to outcome, *Head Neck* 15:24, 1993.
284. Kairaluoma MV, Mäkäräinen H, Kellosalo J et al: Results of surgery in primary hyperparathyroidism, *Ann Chir Gynaecol* 81:309, 1990.
285. Lucas R, Welsh RJ, Glover JL: Unilateral neck exploration for primary hyperparathyroidism, *Arch Surg* 125:982, 1990.
286. Duh QY, Uden P, Clark OH: Unilateral neck exploration for primary hyperparathyroidism: an analysis of a controversy using a mathematical model, *World J Surg* 16:654, 1992.
287. Mallette LE, Blevins T, Jordan PH, Noon GP: Autogenous parathyroid grafts for generalized primary parathyroid hyperplasia: contrasting outcome in sporadic hyperplasia versus multiple endocrine neoplasia type I, *Surgery* 101:738, 1987.
288. Vetto JT, Brennan MF, Woodruf J, Brut M: Parathyroid carcinoma: diagnosis and clinical history, *Surgery* 114:882, 1993.
289. Jansson S, Tisell L-E: Autotransplantation of diseased parathyroid glands into subcutaneous abdominal adipose tissue, *Surgery* 101:549, 1987.
290. Mozes MF, Soper WD, Jonasson O, Long GR: Total parathyroidectomy and autotransplantation in secondary hyperparathyroidism, *Arch Surg* 115:378, 1980.
291. Rothmund M, Wagner PK: Total parathyroidectomy and autotransplantation of parathyroid tissue for renal hyperparathyroidism: a one- to six-year follow-up, *Ann Surg* 197:7, 1983.
292. Wagner PK, Rothmund M: Replantation von autologem kältekonserviertem Nebenschilddrüsengewebe beim permanenten postoperativen Hypoparathyreoidismus, *Dtsch Med Wochenschr* 112:1160, 1987.
293. Niederle B, Roka R, Brennan MF: The transplantation of parathyroid tissue in man: development, indication, technique, and results, *Endocr Rev* 3:245, 1982.
294. Carty SE, Norton JA: Management of patients with persistent or recurrent primary hyperparathyroidism, *World J Surg* 15:716, 1991.
295. Wells SA Jr, Farndon JR, Dale JK et al: Long-term evaluation of patients with primary parathyroid hyperplasia managed by total parathyroidectomy and heterotopic autotransplantation, *Ann Surg* 192:451, 1980.
296. Klempa I, Steinau U, Frei U et al: Morphologische Aspekte der Parathyreoideatransplantation: Beitrag zur klinischen Relevanz des induzierten, invasiven Gewebswachstums, *Chirurgie* 49:704, 1982.
297. Brennan MF, Brown EM, Marx SJ et al: Recurrent hyperparathyroidism from an autotransplanted parathyroid adenoma, *N Engl J Med* 299:1057, 1978.
298. Frei U, Klempa I, Schneider M et al: Tumour-like growth of parathyroid autografts in uraemic patients, *Proc Eur Dial Transplant Assoc* 18:548, 1981.
299. Rattner DW, Marrone GC, Kasdon E et al: Recurrent hyperparathyroidism due to implantation of parathyroid tissue, *Am J Surg* 149:745, 1985.
300. Coulon G, Mantion G, Saint-Hillier Y et al: Récidive d'un hyperparathyroïdisme sur autogreffe parathyroïdienne, hyperplasie ou carcinome? *Ann Pathol* 6:340, 1986.
301. Posen S: Asymptomatic primary hyperparathyroidism: the case for conservative management, *Aust NZ J Med* 22:161, 1992.
302. Stock JL, Marcus R: Medical management of primary hyperparathyroidism. In Bilezikian JP, Marcus R, Levine MA, editors: *The parathyroids: basic and clinical concepts,* New York, 1994, Raven Press.
303. Mitlak BM, Daly M, Potts JT Jr et al: Asymptomatic primary hyperparathyroidism, *J Bone Miner Res* 6(suppl 2):S-100, 1991.
304. Gough I: Asymptomatic primary hyperparathyroidism: the case for surgical management, *Aust NZ J Med* 22:501, 1992.
305. Bilezikian JP: Guidelines for the medical or surgical management of primary hyperparathyroidism: to operate or not to operate. In Bilezikian JP, Marcus R, Levine MA, editors: *The parathyroids: basic and clinical concepts,* New York, 1994, Raven Press.
305a. Palnaes HC, Lau PM, Christensen L: Diagnosis, treatment and outcome of parathyroid cancer, *Eur J Surg* 157:517, 1991.
306. Haff RC, Ballinger WF: Causes of recurrent hypercalcemia after parathyroidectomy for primary hyperparathyroidism, *Ann Surg* 173:884, 1971.
307. Åkerström G, Rudberg C, Grimelius L et al: Causes of failed primary exploration and technical aspects of reoperation in primary hyperparathyroidism, *World J Surg* 16:562, 1992.

308. Levin KE, Clark OH: The reasons for failure in parathyroid operations, *Arch Surg* 124:911, 1989.
309. Wang C-A: Parathyroid reexploration, *Ann Surg* 186:140, 1977.
310. Nathaniels ED, Nathaniels AM, Wang C-A: Mediastinal parathyroid tumors: a clinical and pathological study of 84 cases, *Ann Surg* 171:165, 1970.
311. Potts JT Jr, Fradkin, JE, Aurbach GD et al, editors: Proceedings of NIH Consensus Development Conference on the diagnosis and management of asymptomatic primary hyperparathyroidism, *J Bone Miner Res* 6(suppl 2):S1, 1991.
312. Doppman JL, Miller DL: Localization of parathyroid tumors in patients with asymptomatic hyperthyroidism and no previous surgery, *J Bone Mineral Res* 6(suppl 2):S153, 1991.
312a. Heath ED, Heath EM: Conservative management of primary hyperparathyroidism, *J Bone Miner Res* 6(suppl 2):S117, 1991.
313. Wells SA Jr: Surgical therapy of patients with primary hyperparathyroidism: long-term benefits, *J Bone Miner Res* 6(suppl 2):S143, 1991.
314. Niederle B, Roka R, Kovarik J et al: Klinische Erfahrungen nach operative Therapie der Asymptomatischen und symptomatischen Nebenschilddrüsen über Funktion, *Klin Wochenschr* 64:917, 1986.
315. Augustin N, Wagner PK, Rothmund M: Asymptomatischer Hyperparathyreoidismus. Indikation zur Operation? *Dtsch Med Wochenschr* 112:636, 1987.
316. Cheung PS, Borgstrom A, Thompson NW: Strategy in reoperative surgery for hyperparathyroidism, *Arch Surg* 124:676, 1989.
317. Lafferty FW: Pseudohyperparathyroidism, *Medicine* 45:247, 1966.
318. Omenn GS, Roth SI, Baker WH: Hyperparathyroidism associated with malignant tumors of nonparathyroid origin, *Cancer* 24:1004, 1969.
319. Arnaud CD, Tenenhouse A: Parathyroid hormone. In Rasmussen H, editor: *International encyclopedia of pharmacology and therapeutics:* Pharmacology of the endocrine system and related drugs: parathyroid hormone, thyrocalcitonin and related drugs, sect 51, vol 1, New York, 1970, Pergamon Press, pp. 197.
320. Mohamed IA, Hubbard R, Ah-Sing E, Chakraborty J: Monoclonal antibodies to human parathyroid hormone (1-34) and their use in the immunochemical detection of parathyroid tumors, *Hybridoma* 6:381, 1987.
321. Nussbaum S, Gaz R, Arnold A: Hypercalcemia and ectopic secretion of parathyroid hormone by an ovarian carcinoma with rearrangement of the gene for parathyroid hormone, *N Engl J Med* 323:1324, 1990.
322. Strewler GJ, Budayr AA, Bruce RJ et al: Secretion of authentic parathyroid hormone by a malignant tumor, *Clin Res* 38:462A, 1990.
323. Yoshimoto K, Yamasaki R, Sakai H et al: Ectopic production of parathyroid hormone by small cell lung cancer in a patient with hypercalcemia, *J Clin Endocrinol Metab* 68:976, 1989.
324. Black KS, Mundy GR: Other causes of hypercalcemia. In Bilezikian JP, Marcus R, Levine MA, editors: *The parathyroids: basic and clinical concepts,* New York, 1994, Raven Press.

Secondary hyperparathyroidism

325. Coburn JW, Salusky IB: Hyperparathyroidism in renal failure: clinical features, diagnosis, and management. In Bilezikian JP, Marcus R, Levine MA, editors: *The parathyroids: basic and clinical concepts,* New York, 1994, Raven Press.
326. Castleman B, Mallory TB: Parathyroid hyperplasia in chronic renal insufficiency, *Am J Pathol* 13:553, 1937.
327. Roth SI, Marshall RB: Pathology and ultrastructure of the human parathyroid glands in chronic renal failure, *Arch Intern Med* 124:397, 1969.
328. Altenähr E, Seifert G: Ultrastruktueller Vergleich menschlicher Epithelköperchen bei sekundärem Hyperparathyreoidismus und primärem Adenom, *Virchows Arch [A]* 335:60, 1971.
329. Mallette LE: The functional and pathologic spectrum of parathyroid abnormalities in hyperparathyroidism. In Bilezikian JP, Marcus R, Levine MA, editors: *The parathyroids: basic and clinical concepts,* New York, 1994, Raven Press.

Familial hypocalciuric hypercalcemia

330. Law WM JR, Carney JA, Heath H III: Parathyroid gland in familial benign hypercalcemia (familial hypocalciuric hypercalcemia), *Am J Med* 76:1021, 1984.
331. Thorgeirsson V, Costa J, Marx SJ: The parathyroid glands in familial hypocalciuric hypercalcemia, *Hum Pathol* 12:229, 1984.
332. Law WM Jr, James EM, Charboneau JW et al: High-resolution parathyroid ultrasonography in familial benign hypercalcemia (familial hypocalciuric hypercalcemia), *Mayo Clin Proc* 59:153, 1984.

Hypoparathyroidism

333. Sherwood LM: Hypoparathyroidism. In Favus M, editor: *Primer on metabolic bone diseases and disorders of mineral metabolism,* ed 2, New York, 1993, Raven Press.
334. Thakker RV: Molecular genetics of hypoparathyroidism. In Bilezikian JP, Marcus R, Levine MA, editors: *The parathyroids: basic and clinical concepts,* New York, 1994, Raven Press.
335. Whyte MP: Autoimmune aspects of hypoparathyroidism. In Bilezikian JP, Marcus R, Levine MA, editors: *The parathyroids: basic and clinical concepts,* New York, 1994, Raven Press.

Pseudohypoparathyroidism

336. Albright F, Burnett CH, Smith PH: Pseudohypoparathyroidism: an example of "Seabright-Bantam syndrome," *Endocrinology* 30:922, 1942.
337. Horwitz CA, Meyers WPL, Foote FW Jr: Secondary malignant tumors of the parathyroid glands: report of two cases with associated hypoparathyroidism, *Am J Med* 52:797, 1972.
338. Keynes WM, Truscott BM: Large solitary cysts of the parathyroid gland, *Br J Surg* 44:23, 1956.
339. Wang C-A, Vickery AL Jr, Maloof F: Large parathyroid cysts mimicking thyroid nodules, *Ann Surg* 175:448, 1972.
340. Nylander PEA: Über parathyreoideale Halszysten, *Acta Chir Scand* 64:539, 1929.
341. Rogers LA, Fetter BF, Peete WPJ: Parathyroid cyst and cystic degeneration of parathyroid adenoma, *Arch Pathol* 88:476, 1969.
342. Simkin EP: Hyperparathyroidism associated with a parathyroid cyst: an unusual presentation, *Br J Surg* 63:927, 1976.
343. Troster M, Chie H-F, McLarty TD: Parathyroid cysts: report of a case with ultrastructural observations, *Surgery* 83:238, 1978.
344. Clark OH: Parathyroid cysts, *Am J Surg* 135:395, 1978.
345. Calandra DB, Shah KH, Prinz RA et al: Parathyroid cysts: a report of eleven cases including two associated with hyperparathyroid crisis, *Surgery* 94:887, 1983.
347. Albertson DA, Marshall RB, Jarman WT: Hypercalcemic crisis secondary to functioning parathyroid cyst, *Am J Surg* 141:175, 1981.
347. Silverman JF, Khazanie PG, Norris HT, Fore WW: Parathyroid hormone (PTH) assay of parathyroid cysts examined by fine-needle aspiration biopsy, *Am J Clin Pathol* 86:776, 1986.
348. Birnbaum J, Van Herle AJ: Immunoheterogeneity of parathyroid hormone in parathyroid cysts: diagnostic implications, *J Endocrinol Invest* 12:831, 1989.
349. Okamura K, Ikenoue H, Sato K et al: Sclerotherapy for benign parathyroid cysts, *Am J Surg* 163:344, 1992.
350. Turner A, Lampe HB, Cramer H: Parathyroid cysts, *J Otolaryngol* 18:311, 1989.
351. Cruse CW, Daouk AA: Mediastinal parathyroid cysts: report of a case and review of the literature, *Am J Surg* 135:714, 1978.
352. Buchanan G, Gregory MM: Giant functioning cervicomediastinal parathyroid cyst, *Ann Otol* 88:545, 1979.
353. Ramos Gabatin A, Mallette LE, Bringhurst FR, Draper MW: Functional mediastinal parathyroid cyst: dynamics of parathyroid hormone secretion during cyst aspirations and surgery, *Am J Med* 79:633, 1985.
354. Miyauchi A, Kakudo K, Fujimoto T et al: Parathyroid cyst: analysis of the cyst fluid and ultrastructural observations, *Arch Pathol Lab Med* 105:497, 1981.
355. Ortel YC, Wargotz ES: Diagnosis of parathyroid cysts, *Am J Clin Pathol* 88: 252, 1987.
356. Case Records of the Massachusetts General Hospital: Case 40-1969, *N Engl J Med* 281:783, 1969.

63 Adrenal Glands

Ernest E. Lack
John G. Gruhn

NORMAL ADRENALS

The adrenal glands are paired endocrine organs consisting of both cortex and medulla that differ in embryogenesis, structure, and function. The adrenal cortex is involved in synthesis and release of steroids that can be considered in three groups with different functional attributes: (1) *glucocorticoids* (principally cortisol), which are synthesized in the zona fasciculata and zona reticularis; (2) *mineralocorticoids,* the most important being aldosterone, which is synthesized in the zona glomerulosa; and (3) *sex steroids* (androgens and estrogens), which are synthesized largely in the zona reticularis and less so in the zona fasciculata. The adrenal medulla is composed of chromaffin cells, which synthesize and secrete catecholamines (mainly epinephrine), which mediate rapid adaptations to changes in the environment with responses that are dissipated quickly. There is no known deficiency syndrome attributable to the absence of the adrenal medullae, but by contrast the adrenal cortex is essential for life, as evidenced by the syndrome of insufficient cortical tissue described by Thomas Addison in 1855.[1]

Embryology

The adrenal glands are in essence bipartite endocrine structures, one within the other, of different embryogenesis; the cortex is derived from a specialized condensation of coelomic epithelium (mesodermal origin) in an area designated as the adrenal ridge, and the medulla is of neural crest origin. The adrenal primordium is evident at stage 14 (approximately 5 to 7 mm, 32 days) based on the embryologic studies of Crowder[2] and the Carnegie staging used by O'Rahilly.[3] A collection of proliferating cells becomes evident within the mesenchyme between the root of the dorsal mesentery and developing gonads at stage 15 (approximately 7 to 9 mm; 33 days). These cells are joined by a second wave of cells arising from coelomic epithelium with the adrenal primordium growing centrifugally through the addition of new cells in the subcapsular zone. Later in embryogenesis the developing cortex deep to the subcapsular zone is known as the "fetal or provisional cortex." The adrenal medulla is derived from primitive cells migrating from neural crest into the dorsal and medial aspect of the adrenal primordium. At stages 16 and 17 (approximately 11 to 14 mm; 41 days) the paraaortic neural plexus is a prominent structure with sympathetic nerve fibers and developing paravertebral paraganglia. It is remarkable that throughout fetal life the amount of adrenal chromaffin tissue is scanty compared with extraadrenal locations, particularly the collections of chromaffin cells described by Zuckerkandl.[4] These collections of extraadrenal chromaffin cells have been referred to as the "organs of Zuckerkandl," and following birth these cells undergo involution, with only microscopic collections occasionally found in adults. Many of the primitive cells of neural crest origin that migrate into the adrenal primordium are destined to mature into chromaffin cells and ultimately form the definitive adrenal medulla; other cells probably mature into ganglion cells, which can normally be found in adrenal medullae, some undergo spontaneous regression or involution, and others may linger as neuroblastic nodules until birth or early infancy. These neuroblastic nodules may enter into the differential diagnosis of in situ neuroblastoma.

Anatomy

The optimal way of examining adrenal glands in surgical specimens, or those obtained at autopsy, is to obtain the gland intact and then carefully remove all adherent connective tissue and fat. At times this may be laborious, particularly when there are projecting nodules or other irregularities of cortex and capsule, but this dissection affords the pathologist the opportunity to examine the external aspect of the gland in detail and permits proper orientation of the gland for transverse sectioning to inspect the cortical and medullary compartments. Transverse sections of about 3 mm thickness can be done with serial display of the sections side by side, thus allowing one to visualize the amount and distribution of medulla and cortex and appreciate any gross irregularity.

At birth the fetal cortex makes up approximately 80% of the adrenal gland, and within the first few weeks of life there is a near 50% reduction in weight caused by regression of cells of the fetal cortex. After this there is a gradual increase in combined weight of adrenal glands, as seen in Fig. 63-1. It is remarkable that the developing adrenal gland at about 4 months of gestational age is as large as the fetal kidney. The average combined weights of the adrenal glands of full-term infants studied at Children's Hospital, Boston, was about 6.5 g and decreased to about 2 g between 9 and 14 weeks of life.[4] In the study by Stoner and associates,[5] the average combined weight of adrenal glands was 10 g at birth (range of 2 to 17 g), 6 g at 7 days of age, and 5 g at 2 weeks of age. By necessity, data regarding the average weight and size of adrenal glands in younger individuals must be based on autopsy studies.[6] In adults there have been several studies of ostensibly healthy patients at autopsy who have died suddenly,[7] or in surgical series of adrenals removed from women with breast cancer.[8] In the autopsy study by Quinan and Berger,[7] the average weight of individual adrenal glands was 4.15 g without any

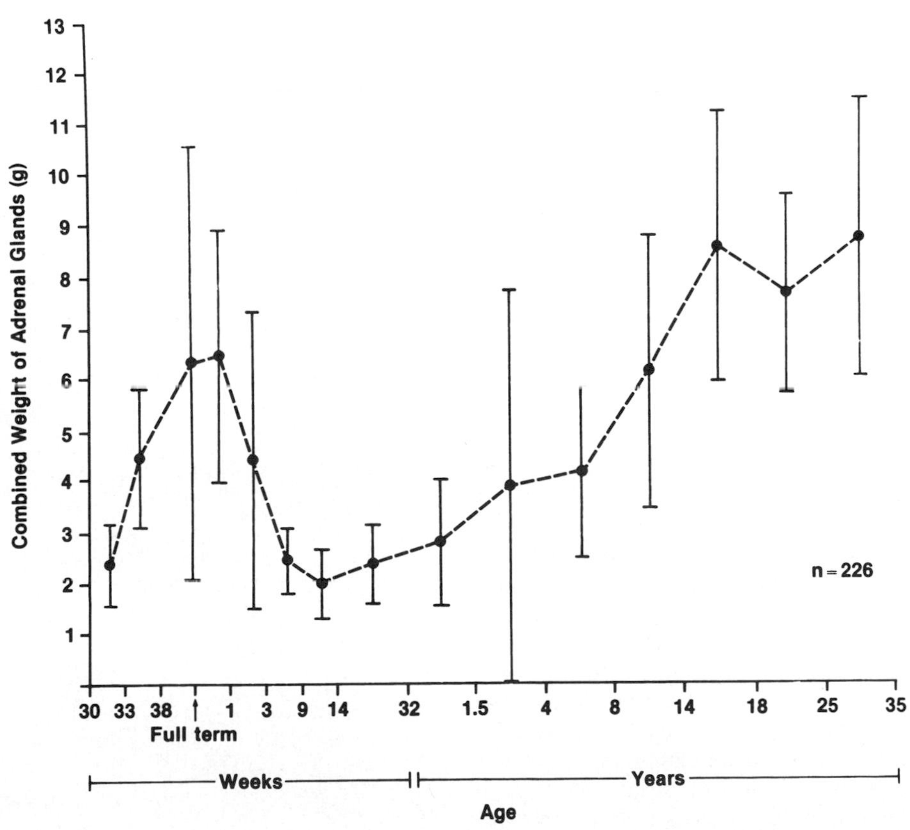

Fig. 63-1 Average combined weight of both adrenal glands from 226 patients at autopsy ranging in age from preterm to the fourth decade. Notice the almost 50% reduction in weight in the first few weeks of life caused by regression of the fetal cortex. (From Lack EE, Kozakewich HPW: Embryology, developmental anatomy, and selected aspects of non-neoplastic pathology. In Lack EE, editor: *Pathology of the adrenal glands,* New York, 1990, Churchill Livingstone.)

significant difference in weight from the right and left side.[7] In the study by Studzinski and associates[8] of adrenal glands obtained at surgery the average individual weight of adrenals was 4.0 g (1 standard deviation of 0.8 g); 99% of apparently normal adrenal glands weighed less than 6 g each, indicating that glands exceeding this weight should be viewed as potentially abnormal, provided of course that all connective tissue and fat is carefully removed. The adrenal glands obtained at autopsy from individuals with chronic or subacute health problems, or with prolonged debilitating illness, tend to be somewhat heavier, and this difference in weight is believed to be related to stress of the underlying illness and the effect of prolonged ACTH stimulation.

Gross morphology

On macroscopic inspection, the adrenal glands from newborns tend to have a smoother external surface than the glands of adults. On transverse section the fetal cortex is a pale grayish tan, but it may become quite dark because of a combination of regression of cortical cells and relative prominence of vascular sinusoids. This deep congestion and reddish-brown discoloration may give one the mistaken impression of adrenal hemorrhage or apoplexy. The adrenal glands in adult patients have a slightly different appearance. The right adrenal gland is roughly pyramidal in shape, and the left is more crescentic or elongate. The anterior surface of the gland as seen in situ is relatively flat, and this is where one may identify the central adrenal vein. The arterial supply to the glands is threefold: the superior adrenal artery arises from the inferior phrenic artery, the middle adrenal artery from the aorta, and the inferior adrenal artery from the renal artery on either side. The posterior surfaces of the adrenal glands are convex, with a prominent longitudinal ridge, or crista, that is flanked on either side by lateral extensions, or alae ('wings'). The glands can be roughly divided into three regions: the medial third, or head, of the gland, which is directly inferior and medial; the middle third, or body; and the lateral third, or tail.

In the adult gland the adrenal medulla is concentrated in the body and head, with relatively little extension into one or the other ala.[4] Medullary tissue makes up about 10% of the weight of the adrenal gland.[7] Using planimetry, the ratio of surface area occuppied by cortex to that of the medulla is approximately 10:1,[6] and under normal conditions there is little or no medullary tissue in the tail of the gland. Because of the concentration of chromaffin tissue in the head of the adrenal gland, lower cortical to medullary surface area ratios would be expected in this region of the gland compared with higher ratios in the body. Careful quantitation of surface areas may be informative when one is attempting to evaluate the adrenal gland for possible adrenal medullary hyperplasia. However, spuriously low cortical-to-medullary surface area may reflect adrenal cortical atrophy. In the normal adult the adrenal cortex measures 1 to 2 mm in thickness. Atrophy must be considered when the cortical thickness is less than 1 mm throughout. The cortical cells in the normal adult gland are usually well lipidized, giving a yellow hue macroscopically, which is often highlighted by a thin, darker inner zone representing the zona reticularis. The medullary compartment is typically gray-white. In the newborn adrenal gland, medullary tissue is usually not grossly discernible on transverse sections of the gland.

Histology

Developing adrenal cortex

In the newborn adrenal gland, the adult or definitive cortex forms a thin subcapsular band measuring 0.1 to 0.2 mm thick. Normally there is no zonation evident microscopically until near the end of the first month of life, when some differentiation of the zona glomerulosa and zona fasciculata can be detected. Cells of the definitive cortex are relatively small, with gradation into cells of the fetal or provisional zone. The latter cells are larger, with relatively abundant, compact, eosinophilic cytoplasm and larger vesicular nuclei containing a small nucleolus (Fig. 63-2). Occasionally, microcyst formation occurs within the definitive cortex,[9,10] particularly in premature infants.[9] Some investigators believe that these microcysts are merely a manifestation of normal developmental anatomy, whereas others consider it a stress-related phenomenon, related to fetal hypoxia or infection.

Adrenal cortex in adults

More distinct zonation is evident in the adrenal cortex of adults (Fig. 63-3). The zona glomerulosa consists of small ball-like aggregates of cells (hence the term *glomerulosa*) immediately beneath the capsule that have a modest amount of

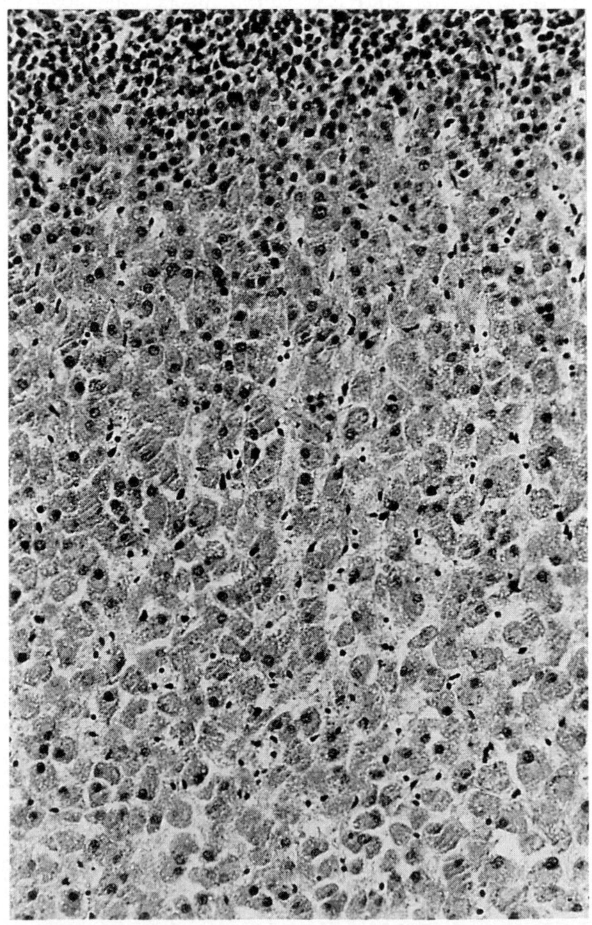

Fig. 63-2 Fetal adrenal cortex is composed of adult, or definitive, zone at the top of the field, with a gradual transition into larger cells of the fetal, or provisional, cortex. The fetal cortex makes up about 80% of the glands at this phase of development and undergoes pronounced regression soon after birth.

lipid-rich, pale-staining cytoplasm. This zone is poorly defined or discontinuous and is never prominent in the normal adrenal gland.[4] The zona fasciculata composes about 70% of the adrenal cortex in the normal adult gland and consists of radial cords of lipid-rich cells that merge with cells of the zona reticularis that have more lipid-depleted or compact, eosinophilic cytoplasm. Cells of the zona reticularis are arranged in small anastomosing cords (Fig. 63-3). Normally the junction between cortex and medulla is relatively smooth; however, there may be cortical-medullary intermingling, with small tonguelike extensions of cortical cells into adjacent medulla or discontinuous islets of cortical cells among chromaffin cells. On the other hand, there may be small nests of chromaffin cells within the cortex, even out near the capsule, but these are difficult to discern without special immunostains to highlight cells with neuroendocrine differentiation. The normal adult adrenal gland can have some degree of cortical nodularity, and this has been reported with increased frequency in elderly individuals[11] as well as those with hypertension[11,12] or diabetes mellitus.[12] It is not uncommon to see small extrusions of cortical tissue on the capsular surface of the adrenal glands, where they appear as small (usually less than 2 mm), spherical, or ovoid nodules. These nodules may have a complete fibrous capsule continuous with adjacent adrenal capsule, but careful sectioning may reveal continuity of the cortical cells with the underlying adrenal cortex. At times the nodules may be situated on the surface of the gland or reside free in periadrenal fat without any attachment to the gland.

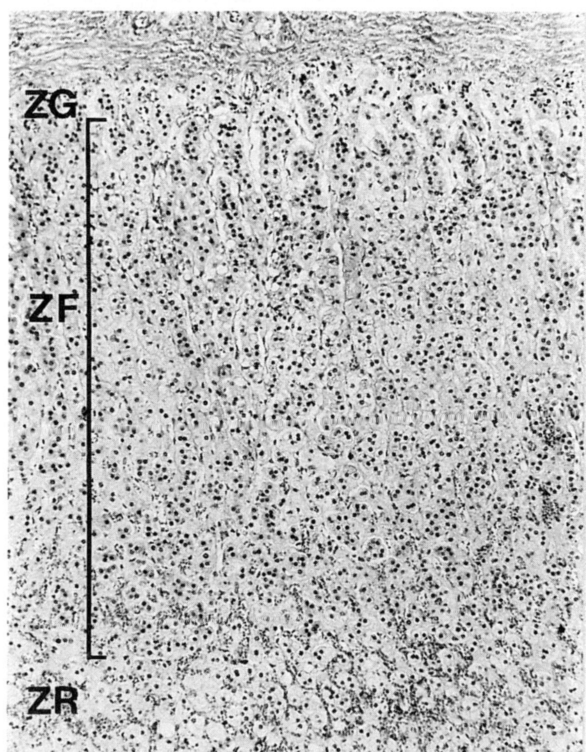

Fig. 63-3 Normal zonation of adrenal cortex in an adult. Zona glomerulosa *(ZG)* forms a thin, discontinuous layer beneath the adrenal capsule at top. Zona fasciculata *(ZF)* and zona reticularis *(ZR)* are indicated. Aldosterone is formed in ZG, and cortisol is synthesized primarily in the ZF with a small contribution from the ZR. The adrenal sex steroids (androgens and estrogens) are synthesized primarily in the ZR.

Adrenal medulla

Developing chromaffin cells of the adrenal medulla have relatively abundant pale-staining cytoplasm and vesicular, round to oval nuclei. The neuroblastic nodules are composed of cells that are considerably more immature, with scant cytoplasm and darkly stained nuclei, and that are most prominent in the fetus of 13 to 16 cm crown-rump length in terms of nodule size (average about 60 μm in diameter) and number (average 44 in serially embedded tissue).[13] During the first 6 months of postnatal life the adrenal medulla develops into a compact structure resembling adult chromaffin tissue, with well-developed clusters of cells with amphophilic to basophilic cytoplasm that is often finely granular. Later in life, with optimal fixation and processing, a myriad of pinpoint, intracytoplasmic granules can be identified by light microscopy. Most of these are the dense-core neurosecretory type of granules. Intracytoplasmic hyaline globules were identified by Dekker and Oehrle[14] in 79% of autopsies. These globules may be solitary but are more often multiple within individual cells, and are characteristically positive with the periodic acid–Schiff (PAS) stain and resistant to diastase predigestion. Intracytoplasmic globules of identical type have also been noted in pheochromocytomas.[15] Tributaries of the central adrenal vein can be readily seen in the medulla and are remarkable for the discontinuous, longitudinal bundles of smooth muscle. One may occasionally identify an intravascular protrusion of cortical or medullary cells through muscular deficiencies in the vein wall.[4]

Ultrastructure of adrenal cortex and medulla

As one might suspect from the normal histology of the adrenal cortex, the cells of the three zones differ in terms of intracytoplasmic lipid content. Cells of the zona fasciculata have relatively abundant intracytoplasmic lipid, with prominent mitochondria having tubular or vesicular cristae. Cells of the zona glomerulosa have a smaller cytoplasmic volume and lesser amounts of intracytoplasmic lipid. Mitochondria of these cells tend to be rounded or elongate, with lamellar cristae.[4] Cells of the zona reticularis contain fewer lipid droplets, thus accounting for the compact, eosinophilic appearance by routine light microscopy. Lipochrome pigment may be prominent within these cells. Smooth endoplasmic reticulum can be found within cells of all three zones, but it tends to be most prominent in zona fasciculata cells, where it may have vesicular or tubular array and occur in association with mitochondria and lipid material. It may be difficult to render a definitive description of "normal" ultrastructural morphology of adrenocortical cells, however, because they enter into a dynamic interaction with ACTH. The microvasculature of the cortex is lined by attenuated endothelial cells with cytoplasmic fenestrations, which are in turn usually limited by surrounding basement membrane.

The most characteristic ultrastructural feature of chromaffin cells are numerous cytoplasmic neurosecretory type granules limited by an investing membrane, with a core diameter usually ranging in size from 150 to 250 nm. Granules of the epinephrine type have a moderately electron-dense core with close, uniform apposition by a limiting membrane, thus imparting a symmetric appearance; granules of the norepinephrine type have a more asymmetric appearance, with an eccentric location of electron-dense core and wide halo of delimiting membrane. Epinephrine makes up approximately 85% of stored catecholamines in the normal adrenal medulla.[4] It has been estimated that almost 90% of circulating norepinephrine is derived from axonal terminals of sympathetic postganglionic neurons, with only a small portion from the adrenal medulla.[16] Catecholamine release is largely mediated by acetylcholine released from preganglionic sympathetic nerve endings terminating on chromaffin cells. The adrenal chromaffin cells can therefore be likened to postganglionic sympathetic neurons lacking dendritic or axonal extensions. There may be variation in overall electron density of chromaffin cell cytoplasm giving rise to populations of "light" and "dark" cells, but the functional significance of this feature is not known.

Anatomic variation

Accessory and heterotopic adrenal tissue

Accessory or heterotopic adrenal tissue can be found anywhere from the upper abdomen to sites along the lines of descent of the gonads. The close embryologic relationship between the developing adrenal primordia and gonadal structures helps to explain accessory or heterotopic adrenal tissue. Within the upper abdomen, the accessory or heterotopic adrenal tissue may consist of both cortex and medulla, but in sites further removed, the tissue almost always consists of cortical tissue alone, but without the distinctive zonation seen in the normal adult adrenal. One of the most frequent sites of heterotopic or accessory tissue is near the celiac artery (32%).[17] Other sites include the broad ligament near the ovary,[18] and, in males, almost anywhere along the line of gonadal descent, including connective tissue of the spermatic cord, region of epididymis, and testicular hilum. Accessory adrenocortical tissue has been noted in 7.5% of male infants under the age of 1 year,[19] and identical rests can be found in the connective tissue lining of hernia sacs. Accessory adrenal cortical tissue has also been noted in the kidney in a subcapsular location, particularly in the upper pole, where the accessory tissue usually appears as a bright yellow, flattened nodule usually less than 3 to 4 mm in diameter.[4] There are also some exotic locations of ectopic adrenal tissue that defy plausible embryologic explanation, including intracranial, pulmonary, and placental heterotopia.[4] Heterotopic adrenocortical tissue often appears as a round to ovoid encapsulated structure with a predominantly fascicular arrangement of lipid-rich cells. Rare examples of intratesticular and intraovarian adrenocortical rests have also been reported.[20,21]

Adrenal union, adhesion, and fusion

Adrenal union or adhesion with kidney or liver has been described. Adrenal gland union or adhesion is distinguished by whether a continuous connective tissue capsule separates the involved organs.[22] Another adrenal anomaly is fusion, which is sometimes associated with congenital midline defects or indeterminate visceral situs. In some cases of renal agenesis the adrenal glands may have an abnormal shape with an oval, smooth contour.

REACTIVE CHANGES

Morphologic changes associated with stress

Acute or prolonged physiologic stress may activate the hypothalamic-pituitary-adrenocortical axis, with increased action of ACTH and stimulation of glucocorticoid production. The individual or combined weights of the adrenal glands may increase within 2 to 4 days under the influence of ACTH with a near doubling in weight.[8] On transverse sections of the lipid-depleted gland, the cortex may appear homogeneous gray-tan, which microscopically represents conversion of the normal, pale-staining, lipid-rich cells of the zona fasciculata to cells with compact, eosinophilic cytoplasm relatively devoid of lipid (Fig. 63-4). This conversion to compact cells may simulate a widening of the zona reticularis with extension out to the zona glomerulosa or capsule. The lipid depletion observed in adults is often patchy or focal in distribution, whereas in young children, the pattern of lipid depletion and conversion to compact cells tends to be more diffuse. A pattern of focal lipid depletion has been described as lipid reversion in which the lipid is usually sparse to absent in the outer aspect of the cortex, scanty in the zona reticularis, and prominent in intervening zona fasciculata. This pattern overall might be mistaken for hyperplasia of zona glomerulosa. It suggests recovery from stress with gradual lipidization of cells of the inner zona fasciculata.

Lipid depletion may also be accompanied by foci of "tubular degeneration," changes that manifest as conversion of normally solid cords of cells in the outer cortex into tubular structures, sometimes with individual cell necrosis. The changes are most likely caused by excess hormonal stimulation by ACTH rather than bacterial toxins.[23] A peculiar vacuolization of fetal adrenocortical cells has been observed in infants with erythroblastosis fetalis,[24] and nearly identical changes have been detected in some patients with thalassemia.[4]

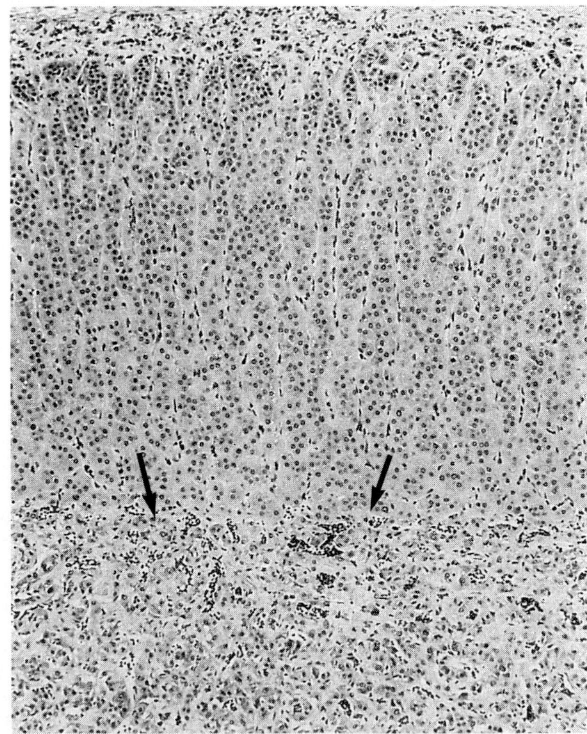

Fig. 63-4 Considerable depletion of lipid in cortical cells in an adrenal gland from a patient who died of acquired immunodeficiency syndrome (AIDS). Cortical cells have compact, eosinophilic cytoplasm. Notice junction with adrenal medulla in lower third of field *(arrows)*.

Iron overload

There may be considerable deposition of hemosiderin within cells of the outer adrenal cortex, particularly the zona glomerulosa, in iron overload conditions such as primary hemochromatosis and excess blood transfusions.[4] Hypothalamic and pituitary dysfunction has been reported in some patients with hemochromatosis and thalassemia major and is probably related to excess iron deposition. Hypothyroidism, adrenal insufficiency, and decreased production of gonadotrophins with loss of libido and testicular atrophy have also been reported. Hemosiderin is typically deposited within the cytoplasm of cells of the zona glomerulosa. This can easily be found on low-power microscopic examination with dark brown, granular material representing hemosiderin. Sometimes the hemosiderin deposition appears in cells deeper within the cortex than the usual zona glomerulosa type of cells. Prussian blue stain for iron will greatly highlight the accumulation of hemosiderin. The deposition may be so heavy that it appears as tan-brown discoloration on external examination of the intact gland, and it may be even more conspicuous in transverse sections.

Effects of drugs, cytotoxic agents, and radiation

Only a few drugs and cytotoxic agents have direct antiadrenal activity.[4] A selective cytotoxic effect on cells of the zona fasciculata was demonstrated with the insecticide DDT, and a derivative of this chemical agent, marketed as Mitotane (*o,p'*-DDD) has been used for the treatment (usually palliative) of patients with adrenocortical carcinoma. This drug appears to have a direct adrenolytic effect, with specificity for both normal and neoplastic adrenocortical cells. Aminoglutethimide, originally introduced as an anticonvulsant, was associated with secondary adrenal insufficiency and was withdrawn from general use. Metyrapone is a drug used in testing for pituitary reserve by selective inhibition of 11-beta-hydroxylation; with normal pituitary function ACTH is secreted in sufficient quantities to overcome the enzymatic block, resulting in near-normal secretion of cortisol. Some agents have antiadrenal activity without actually causing structural damage. Such an example is ketoconazole, a broad-spectrum antifungal drug that can block adrenal steroid synthesis; a rare side effect in patients receiving high doses is relative corticosteroid deficiency. A few steroidal agents have a direct inhibitory effect on steroidogenesis. Suramin, a potent competitive inhibitor of reverse transcriptase used in the treatment of acquired immunodeficiency syndrome (AIDS), has also been associated with adrenal insufficiency. Linear hyaline fibrosis has been reported in the zona reticularis after radiation, probably because of damage to the reticular vascular plexus.[25]

Adrenal cytomegaly

Adrenal cytomegaly is a focal or diffuse process restricted to cells of the fetal or provisional cortex and is evidenced by cellular and nuclear enlargement with hyperchromasia.[26] Sometimes the nucleomegaly may be striking. There may be intranuclear vacuoles, termed *pseudoinclusions*. Ultrastructural study has shown that these represent nuclear invaginations of cell cytoplasm.[27] Congenital adrenal cytomegaly is usually an incidental finding affecting about 3% of newborn infants and 6.5% of premature stillborns.[26] Even with considerable nuclear enlargement, mitotic figures are characteristically absent (Fig. 63-5).

Beckwith-Wiedemann syndrome

The Beckwith-Wiedemann syndrome[28,29] affects an estimated 1 in 13,000 newborns, with most cases cited in the literature (about 85%) occurring sporadically.[4] The disorder is also known as the "EMG syndrome" to emphasize the major triad of clinical findings: exomphalos, macroglossia, and gigantism. Familial cases have been reported and were suggestive of a pattern of mendelian inheritance; a recent segregation analysis of affected pedigrees suggested an autosomal-dominant inheritance with incomplete penetrance and variable expressivity.[30]

The adrenal glands are characteristically enlarged, with combined weights often ranging up to 16 g. Adrenal cytomegaly is a characteristic feature in this disorder and is typically bilateral. Adrenal chromaffin tissue has been characterized as being fully mature and in some instances hyperplastic.[31] Some of the affected infants have somatic gigantism, which may be asymmetric, giving rise to hemihypertrophy. Visceromegaly may involve the kidneys and pancreas; one of the important factors affecting prognosis in early life is neonatal hypoglycemia, which must be recognized and treated. In a review by Wiedemann, 7.5% of children developed a malignant intraabdominal tumor, usually nephroblastoma (Wilms' tumor) or adrenal cortical carcinoma.[32] Other neoplasms have been reported in this syndrome, such as neuroblastoma and pancreatoblastoma.[4]

CONGENITAL AND HEREDITARY ADRENOCORTICAL DISORDERS

Anencephaly

Anencephaly is a severe developmental disorder of anterior neural tube structures that is incompatible with life. There may be agenesis of much of the brain and cranial vault, with some distortion of the sella turcica. The pituitary is seldom identifiable on gross examination, but histologic sections usually demonstrate this tissue, though it may be reduced in amount. The adrenal glands are often extremely small. The average combined weight in one study was 1.8 g, and many weighed less than 1 g combined.[33] The fetal cortex is quite thin, though

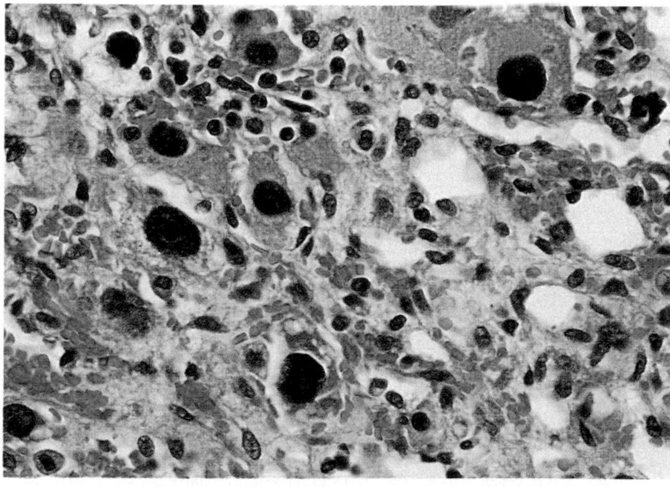

Fig. 63-5 Adrenal cytomegaly. Notice large cells of provisional, or fetal, cortex with enlarged hyperchromatic nuclei. Infant had the Beckwith-Wiedemann syndrome.

it may appear normal in size and structure until about week 20 of gestation. The average width of the adult or definitive cortex is about 0.3 mm, but this value may be high because of lack of fetal cortex. There appears to be about a 2% to 3% risk of central nervous system malformations in subsequent children after birth of an anencephalic infant.[34]

Adrenoleukodystrophy

Adrenoleukodystrophy (ALD) is a peroxisomal disorder, with the basic biochemical defect being a decreased capacity to oxidize unbranched, very long chain fatty acids of 24 to 30 carbon atoms.[35,36] Lipid material accumulates in tissue as cholesterol esters. ALD is a rare disease, with a complex clinical spectrum. A neonatal and childhood (juvenile) form of the disorder is recognized with a degenerating, demyelinating process, adrenal cortical atrophy, and variable adrenal hypofunction. In most patients with ALD, neurologic manifestations of the disease precede any clinical or laboratory evidence of adrenal involvement. In addition, an adult variant of ALD—adrenomyeloneuropathy (AMN)—usually begins in the second or third decade of life. The childhood form of ALD may have an X-linked pattern of inheritance, and neonatal ALD may have connatal presentation with an autosomal-recessive inheritance.

Typically, there is widespread central nervous system demyelination, especially the posterior cerebrum, cerebellum, and descending cortical spinal tracts. There may be either clinical evidence of adrenal insufficiency or decreased adrenocortical reserve on laboratory testing. The adrenocortical insufficiency is attributable to primary adrenal involvement. The glands are often small, with a normal-appearing medulla. A characteristic feature is the presence of enlarged cortical cells with a "striated" or "ballooned" appearance (Figure 63-6). This is particularly evident after routine processing because of extraction of intracytoplasmic lipids. Some investigators regard the lipid accumulation as having a cytotoxic effect, thus helping to explain the pathogenesis for adrenal and white-matter damage.

Congenital adrenal hypoplasia

There are two basic forms of congenital hereditary adrenal hypoplasia: a rare miniature type affecting both sexes, in which the adrenal glands are small but have relatively normal architecture, and a more common cytomegalic type with an X-linked pattern of inheritance.[37-39] The affected males in the latter disorder have small adrenal glands with abnormal architectural features and scattered cytomegalic cortical cells, which may show intranuclear "pseudoinclusions." Clinical presentation is usually in the newborn period with weight loss, dehydration, vomiting and severe salt-losing tendency. The onset of adrenocortical insufficiency in other cases is variable, depending on the adrenocortical reserve and the amount of functioning endocrine tissue. Males with the cytomegalic type of congenital adrenal hypoplasia usually have hypogonadotropic hypogonadism in the adolescent age group that is believed to be of hypothalamic origin.

Familial glucocorticoid deficiency

The rare disorder familial glucocorticoid deficiency affects both sexes and seems to be caused by a primary defect in the adrenal cortex resulting in deficient secretion of glucocorticoids and secondary increase in ACTH levels.[4,40-42] Synonyms include congenital adrenocortical unresponsiveness to ACTH or the ACTH insensitivity syndrome. Mineralocorticoid secretion is usually normal.[4] Although not yet identified, the primary defect may involve failure of attachment of ACTH to membrane receptor sites or absence of activation of adenyl cyclase by ACTH. Patients with this disorder usually become symptomatic in the first 2 years of life, with episodes of hypoglycemia, seizures, muscle weakness, and cutaneous hyperpigmentation.

Adrenal dysfunction in glycerol kinase deficiency

Adrenal insufficiency in this rare disorder is characterized by decreased production of both glucocorticoids and mineralocorticoids. The overwhelming predominance in males is suggestive of an X-linked mode of inheritance. Most children have symptoms of adrenal insufficiency; some may have other phenotypic abnormalities, such as moderate psychomotor retardation, spasticity, growth failure, Duchenne muscular dystrophy, and osteoporosis.[4] It has been proposed that the deficiency of glycerol kinase may inhibit conversion of cholesterol to pregnenolone (the early step in glucocorticoid biosynthesis).

Selective hypoaldosteronism

The rare disorder selective hypoaldosteronism was first described in 1957,[43] and has usually been attributed to decreased renin secretion in patients with chronic renal failure (hyporeninemic hypoaldosteronism). Recent reports suggest an isolated defect in function of the zona glomerulosa or endogenous abnormality in angiotensin II production.[4]

Congenital adrenal hyperplasia

Normal pathways of steroid biosynthesis. The biosynthetic pathway for steroidogenesis in the adrenal glands is

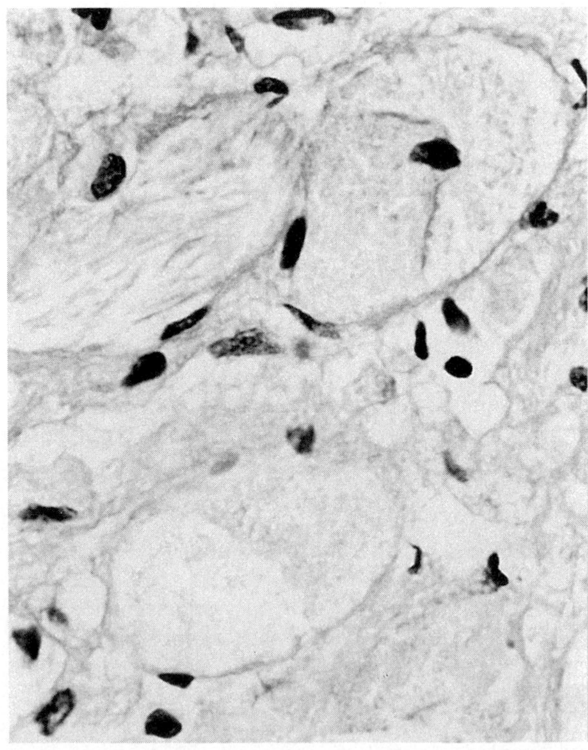

Fig. 63-6 Adrenoleukodystrophy. Large "ballooned" cortical cells have elongate cleftlike spaces within cytoplasm caused by extraction of lipid.

shown in Fig. 63-7. The three major classes of steroids are mineralocorticoids, glucocorticoids, and sex steroids. Congenital adrenal hyperplasia (CAH), also known as the "adrenogenital syndrome," results from a deficiency from any one of five different enzymes involved in steroid synthesis and has an autosomal-recessive pattern of inheritance. It is the most common cause of ambiguous genitalia in the newborn. The disorder may become manifest because of deficiency or absence of particular steroids such as cortisol. The enzymatic deficiency leads to accumulation of precursor steroids that "spill over" into alternate metabolic pathways, particularly those involving synthesis of androgens. The developing male infant is relatively unaffected by increased androgens in utero, such as testosterone, but in the female

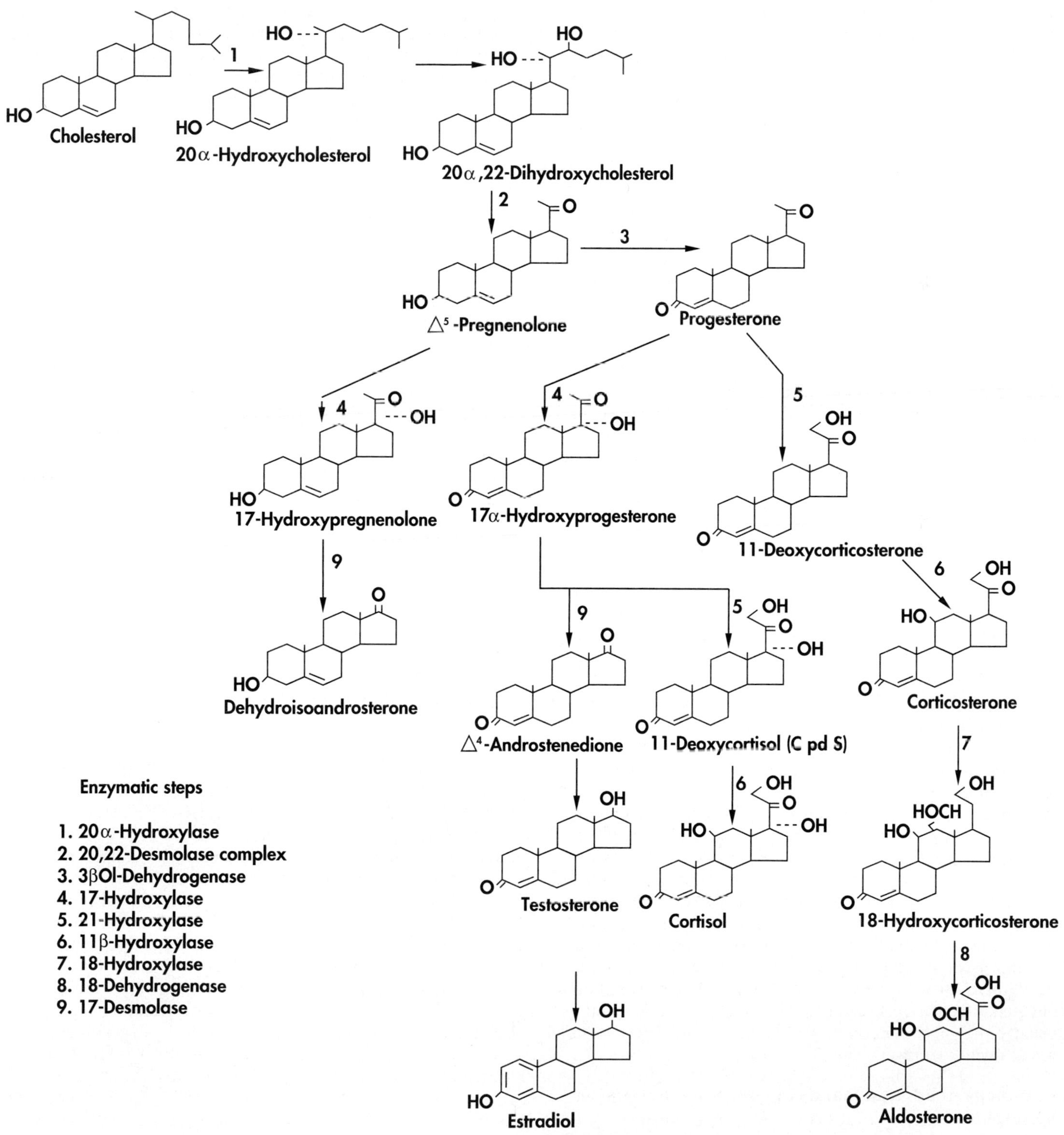

Fig. 63-7 Major biosynthetic pathways for adrenal steroids. The ezymatic steps are from *1* to 9.

the development of external genitalia may be severely affected.

21-Hydroxylase deficiency. 21-Hydroxylase deficiency accounts for 90% to 95% of all cases of CAH, with an incidence between 1 in 5000 and 1 in 15,000 live births in most populations.[44] A particularly high incidence has been observed in Yupik eskimos in Alaska. Three forms of the disorder have been recognized: *a classic* form, with the incidence noted; a *nonclassic* form, in which individuals are apparently normal at birth, but later develop signs and symptoms of androgen excess; and a *cryptic* form, in which there may be identical biochemical abnormalities, but patients are often entirely asymptomatic.[44] The genetic locus associated with 21-hydroxylase encoding is associated with the HLA major histocompatibility complex on the short arn of chromosome 6. In two thirds of the cases, the biosynthesis of aldosterone is deficient, with the resulting "salt-wasting" form of the disorder. If the biosynthetic block in aldosterone synthesis is severe, it may cause hypotension or death in the first few weeks of life. The ambiguous genitalia of female infants often alerts the physician to the correct diagnosis. In the remaining one third of cases, patients have a simple virilizing form of the disorder without aldosterone deficiency.

Affected males usually appear normal at birth because development of external genitalia is under the influence of androgens. Female infants, however, tend to display various degrees of ambiguous genitalia with clitoral enlargement and fusion of labial scrotal folds. The changes may be so extreme that the affected female infant is mistakenly assumed to be male at birth. If left untreated and the child survives, there may be rapid somatic growth with advanced bone age, though the early closure of epiphyseal growth plates may result in short stature. Skin hyperpigmentation can also be seen.

11-Beta-hydroxylase deficiency. 11-Beta-hydroxylase deficiency in its classic form accounts for about 5% to 8% of cases of CAH, and its incidence in the general white population is about 1 in 100,000 births.[44] Enzymatic block here results in accumulation of precursor steroids proximal to conversion of 11-deoxycortisol cortisol as well as a biosynthetic defect in the mineralocorticoid pathway. The disorder results in hypertension, hypokalemia, and effects of excess androgen secretion.

3-Beta-hydroxysteroid dehydrogenase deficiency. 3-Beta-hydroxysteroid dehydrogenase deficiency results in a defect affecting the synthesis of all three classes of steroids and is unique because there is intersexuality—both males and females are affected.[44] Females may show slight masculinization, and males may be incompletely masculinized with varying degrees of hypospadias.

17-Alpha-hydroxylase deficiency. As noted in Fig. 63-7 this enzymatic block interferes with synthesis of glucocorticoids and sex steroids, but synthesis of mineralocorticoids is not affected. Male patients are incompletely masculinized and females may have amenorrhea.

Cholesterol desmolase deficiency. Cholesterol desmolase deficiency is a rare enzymatic deficiency in which patients usually die in childhood from adrenal insufficiency despite replacement therapy.[44]

Pathology of adrenal glands in congenital adrenal hyperplasia

It is very uncommon today to see adrenal glands in cases of CAH that are unrecognized or untreated. The glands in this disorder are often 6 to 8 times larger than normal. Individual glands may weigh 10 to 15 g in children. In older individuals, the individual weights of adrenal glands may be 30 to 35 g.[4] Grossly, the adrenal glands often have a cerebriform external surface caused by redundant folding of cortex, and the gland may appear tan to dark brown because of prolonged and intense stimulation by ACTH. Microscopically, there is hyperplasia of the zona fasciculata with conversion of pale-staining, lipid-rich cells to cells that have compact, eosinophilic cytoplasm. This lipid depletion is attributable to trophic stimulation by ACTH. Heterotopic or accessory adrenocortical tissue in other sites may also become enlarged. In the rare deficiency of cholesterol desmolase there is accumulation of cholesterol and cholesterol esters, which gives the hyperplastic adrenal glands a bright yellow or whitish color on cross section. Cholesterol clefts can also be seen, with foreign-body giant cell reaction and some dystrophic calcification. The histologic picture of CAH may be modified somewhat by exogenous steroid administration or less severe forms of enzymatic deficiency. In some of these cases the expanded zona fasciculata may contain cells that are not so lipid depleted.

Association with adrenal and other neoplasms

There have been rare cases of adrenocortical neoplasms, both adenomas and carcinomas, reported in association with congenital adrenal hyperplasia.[4,45] This has been attributed to the persistent trophic stimulation by ACTH with neoplastic transformation of adrenocortical cells, but the precise mechanisms are not known. Rare cases of adrenal myelolipoma and a few nonadrenal tumors have also been reported.[46,47]

Testicular "tumors" of adrenocortical type

A rare complication of CAH in male patients, particularly those with the salt-losing form of 21-hydroxylase deficiency, is the development of testicular "tumors" in young adult life. The tumors are usually bilateral (83%), and patients typically have testicular pain and tenderness.[48] Some cases reported in the literature clearly indicate that the tumors are ACTH dependent.[49,50] Administration of dexamethasone may lead to reduction in testicular size and amelioration of symptoms such as pain because of suppression of ACTH levels.[50] About 65% of these testicular tumors present as palpable nodules, measuring 2 to 10 cm in diameter. Grossly, the tumor has a lobulated cut surface and is composed of light tan to dark brown nodules with intersecting bands of connective tissue. Individual tumor cells are polygonal with ample granular pink cytoplasm and relatively distinct cell borders, imparting a mosaic appearance. Microscopically, the neoplasms resemble Leydig (or interstital) cell tumors, but there are several important differences—ACTH dependency, bilaterality, the absence of crystalloids of Reinke, and benign biologic behavior.[48] These tumors may represent hyperplasia of multipotent testicular stromal cells capable of differentiation into either Leydig cells or ectopic adrenocortical cells, depending on the hormonal milieu or trophic stimulation by ACTH. Identical testicular tumors of adrenocortical type have been reported in male patients with Nelson's syndrome[51] (also characterized by increased ACTH), as well as in women with Nelson's syndrome with similar "adrenal rest" tumors in the region of the ovaries.[52]

ADRENOCORTICAL INSUFFICIENCY

Idiopathic Addison's disease

The seminal features of chronic adrenocortical insufficiency were originally described by Thomas Addison in 1855 and included wasting, weakness, and cutaneous pigmentation.[1] Recognition of this adrenoprival syndrome (Addison's disease) was an important landmark in the emerging discipline of endocrinology. Of the various causes of Addison's disease, the most common form today is the idiopathic, or autoimmune, type. Some investigators regard this as an organ-specific form of autoimmune adrenalitis. A proposed mechanism of autoimmune adrenalitis is the expression of class II major histocompatibility antigens by epithelial cells that then function as an adrenal-specific autoantigen, thus enabling helper T-lymphocytes to initiate an autoimmune response.[4] It is not known whether class II antigen expression is a primary event or one mediated by lymphokines related to the inflammatory infiltrate. Polyglandular autoimmune (PGA) syndromes involve organs, particularly thyroid and pancreas, in addition to the adrenal. There is a complex form known as PGA type I, or autoimmune polyendocrinopathy–candidiasis–ectodermal dysplasia (APECED), with Addison's disease, hypoparathyroidism, and mucocutaneous candidiasis, as well as dystrophic changes of dental enamel and nails.[53] There is also an association with chronic hepatitis, juvenile-onset diabetes mellitus, and primary hypogonadism. The type II PGA syndrome includes Addison's disease along with autoimmune thyroid disease or insulin-dependent diabetes mellitus.[54] The association between nontuberculous Addison's disease and primary hypothyroidism was reported in 1926 and is sometimes referred to as *Schmidt's syndrome*.[55]

The adrenal glands in idiopathic Addison's disease are typically small and waferlike, and on gross examination of the suprarenal area the glands may be difficult to identify. Sometimes liberal sampling of tissue from the suprarenal area may be necessary to uncover residual adrenal tissue. The adrenal cortex bilaterally has a remarkable endocrine reserve, and for functional impairment to occur, as much as 90% or more of cortical tissue must be ablated. Microscopically, the cortex is thin and may be discontinuous, with small islands of cells interspersed with lymphocytes and plasma cells (Fig. 63-8). There may be lymphoid follicles with reactive germinal centers. Residual cortical cells often appear enlarged, with ample, compact eosinophilic cytoplasm and occasional nuclear pseudoinclusions.

It should be noted that not infrequently in individuals without any signs of adrenal insufficiency one may see focal, nonspecific "adrenalitis" composed of mononuclear cells, mainly lymphocytes, particularly between cortical cells or around venules at the corticomedullary junction. A relation with abdominal inflammatory conditions such as chronic pyelonephritis has been suggested.

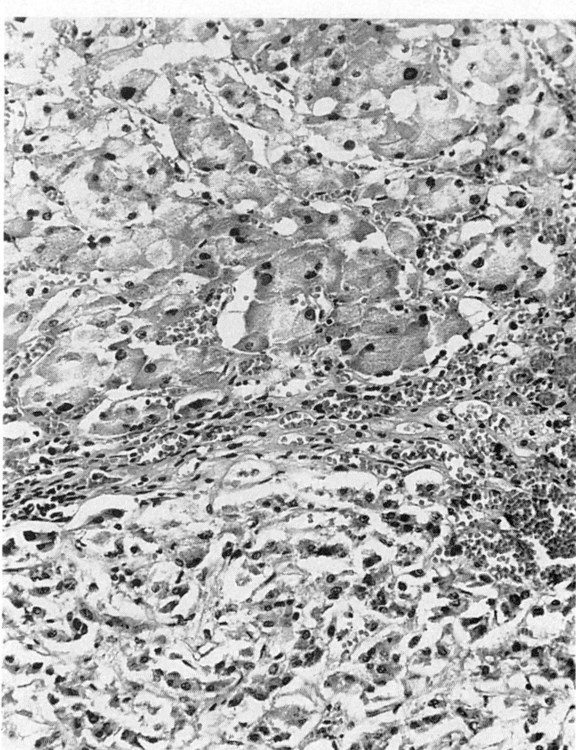

Fig. 63-8 Idiopathic (autoimmune) form of Addison's disease. Adrenal cortex was greatly reduced in volume with discontinuous islands of enlarged cells having compact, eosinophilic cytoplasm. Lymphoid aggregates with occasional germinal centers were present in other areas. Residual adrenal medulla was prominent (bottom third of field) relative to cortex.

Secondary Addison's disease

Adrenal tuberculosis

Historically, the most common cause of Addison's disease was adrenal tuberculosis with bilateral necrocaseous distruction of both glands. Over half of the cases of Addison's disease reported between 1900 and 1929 were secondary to tuberculosis, whereas only 19% were attributed to primary or idiopathic atrophy.[56,57] In recent decades, through appropriate public health measures and improvement in antituberculous therapy, Addison's disease attributable to tuberculosis has decreased. The adrenal glands involved by tuberculosis are bilaterally enlarged and show extensive caseation necrosis. There are usually few classic tuberculoid granulomas. The blunted granulomatous response within the adrenal glands has been attributed to locally high concentration of steroids. Adrenal calcification may also occur. It is interesting to note that in a recent study some patients with lepromatous leprosy were shown to have low adrenocortical reserve, but none had the clinical characteristics of Addison's disease.[58]

Adrenal histoplasmosis

In a review of 102 cases of disseminated histoplasmosis, the adrenal glands were involved in 82%, and 7% of patients had Addison's disease.[59] Similar to tuberculous infection, extensive caseous necrosis is a common feature. Three patterns of adrenal involvement have been described: (1) scattered macrophages containing *Histoplasma* organisms (Fig. 63-9) within sinusoids, (2) focal aggregates of more heavily parasitized macrophages, and (3) perivasculitis of extracapsular adrenal vessels, which may be associated with extensive necrosis. This third pattern of involvement was most often associated with sufficient parenchymal destruction to cause cortical insufficiency.

Other mycotic infections have also been reported to cause Addison's disease, including both North American and South

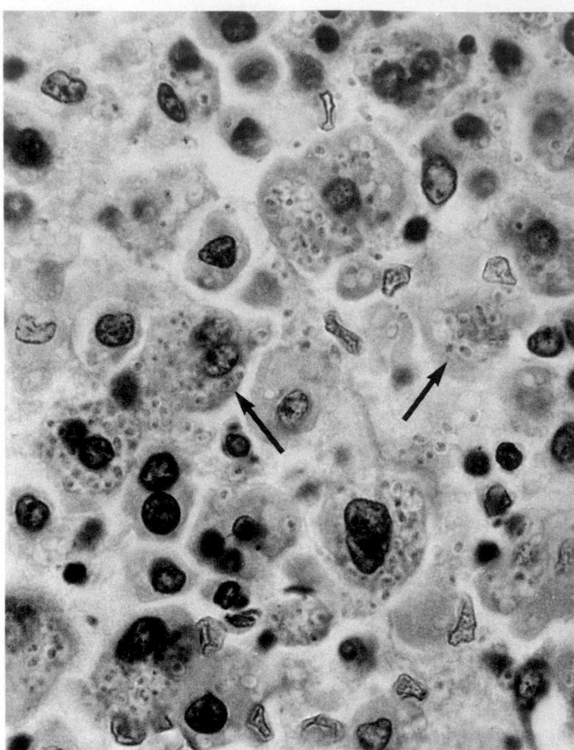

Fig. 63-9 Disseminated histoplasmosis. Histiocytes within adrenal cortex contain numerous round to oval organisms measuring 2 to 4 μm in diameter *(arrows)*.

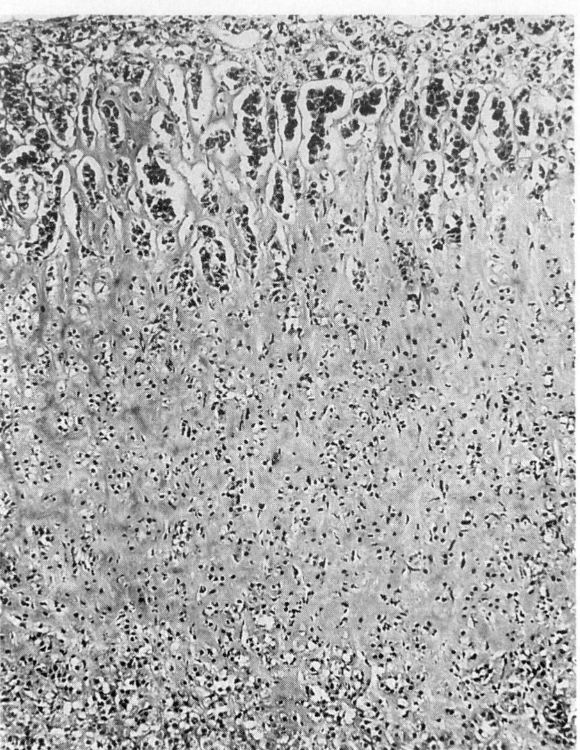

Fig. 63-10 Amyloidosis of adrenal gland. Much of zona fasciculata contains homogeneous eosinophilic material that was positive with Congo red stain and exhibited characteristic apple-green dichroism with polarized light.

American blastomycosis, coccidioidomycosis, and cryptococcosis.[4]

Amyloidosis

Amyloidosis is an unusual cause of Addison's disease. In the review by Guttman in 1930, involving 566 cases of Addison's disease, amyloidosis was the underlying cause in only 1.7% of cases.[56] The secondary form of amyloidosis (AA) is the one usually associated with extensive involvement of much of the cortex (Fig. 63-10). Homogeneous deposits of eosinophilic material occur between columns and cords of cortical cells, with secondary severe atrophy of cells of the zona fasciculata and the zona reticularis. There may be a small uninvolved rim of cortical cells in the immediate subcapsular zone. In primary amyloidosis, the deposition of amyloid is usually within walls of arterioles.

Metastatic malignant tumors

In patients with metastatic carcinoma, involvement of the adrenal glands is relatively common, particularly at autopsy.[60] Few, however, manifest Addison's disease during life.[61] In the large study by Guttman less than 1% of Addison's disease was attributable to metastatic carcinoma.[56] It is of interest to note in the original monograph by Addison in 1855 that several of his patients had metastatic carcinoma to both adrenal glands.[1] Other common primary sites associated with Addison's disease include lung, stomach, and colon. Addison's disease has also been reported on occasion in patients with malignant lymphoma,[62] of both Hodgkin's and non-Hodgkin's type, as well as a rare form of malignant lymphoma having distinct angiotropism, which was erroneously referred to as malignant "angioendotheliomatosis."[4]

Acquired immunodeficiency syndrome (AIDS)

Cytomegalovirus (CMV) has a distinct tropism for the adrenal glands and has been identified in up to one half of AIDS patients at autopsy.[63-67] The terminal course of some of these patients is punctuated as hypotension, hyponatremia, and hypovolemia, suggestive of underlying adrenocortical insufficiency. However, the maximum extent of adrenal necrosis (70%) may be less than that usually associated with chronic adrenocortical insufficiency. Another consideration in the AIDS pattern is concurrent adrenal tuberculosis, which causes extensive *parenchymal destruction*.[65] Infection of the adrenal glands by *Pneumocystis carinii* has been described, but adrenal insufficiency has not been documented.[68]

Herpetic adrenalitis

The adrenal glands can be infected by Herpesviridae, including cytomegalovirus (CMV), herpes simplex, and varicella-zoster virus (Fig. 63-11). Hepatoadrenal necrosis caused by herpes simplex infection in the newborn was described by Haas in 1935.[69] The involved glands usually show microscopic, sharply delineated, almost punched-out areas of the coagulation type of necrosis, with little or no inflammatory response.[70] At times the cortical necrosis can be extensive and confluent. Cellular effects of viral infection, such as multinucleation and intranuclear inclusions, are present in most cases.

Waterhouse-Friderichsen syndrome

Waterhouse-Friderichsen syndrome, classically associated with meningococcal sepsis, affects patients with bacterial sep-

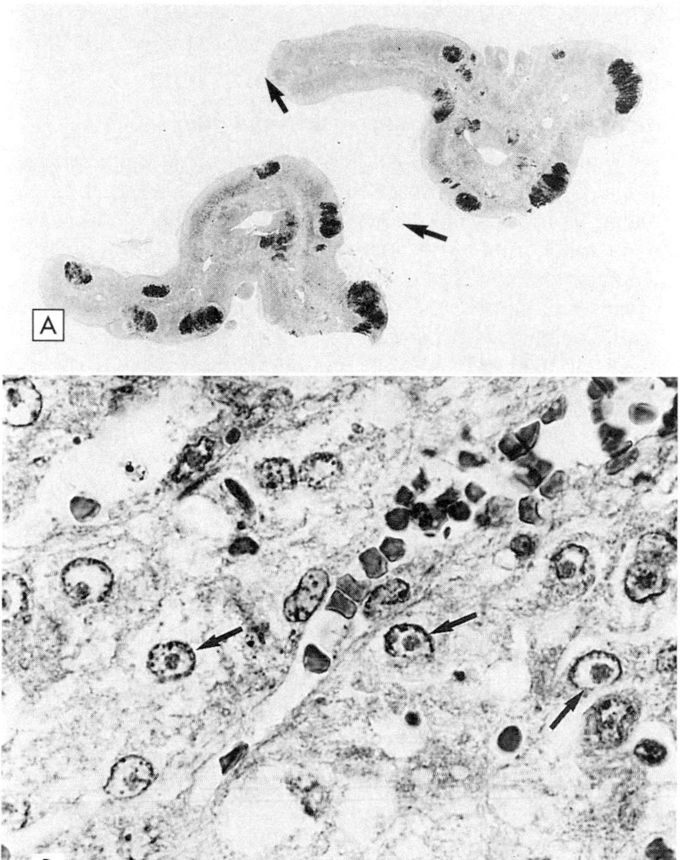

Fig. 63-11 **A,** Adrenal glands from an adult who died of disseminated varicella complicating treatment for an underlying malignancy. Notice sharply demarcated zones of necrosis with hemorrhage. **B,** Adrenal cortical cells of edge of necrotic zones have eosinophilic intranuclear inclusions with surrounding halo (Cowdry type A inclusions) *(arrows)*.

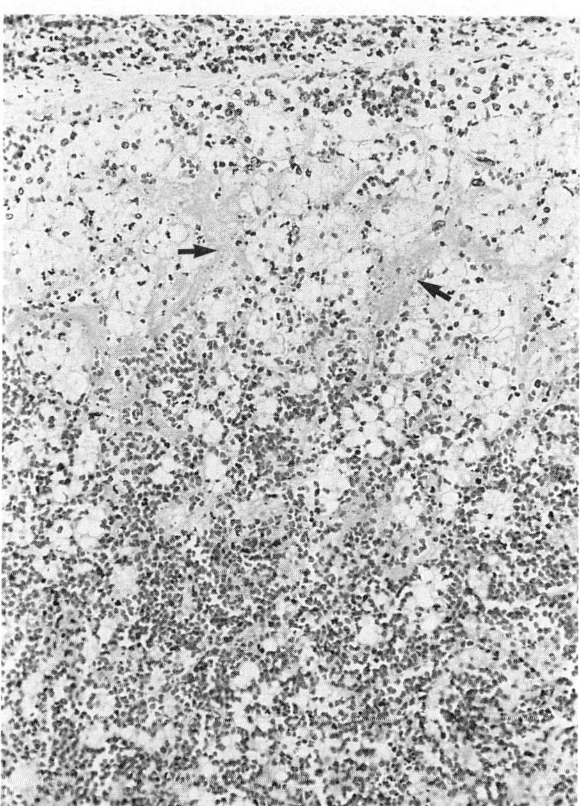

Fig. 63-12 Waterhouse-Friderichsen syndrome. There is hemorrhage and congestion of cortex with few fibrin thrombi in thin sinusoids *(arrows)*. Patient died of meningococcal sepsis.

sis caused by other organisms such as *Haemophilus influenzae* and *Streptococcus pneumoniae*. The clinical features are rapid onset of circulatory collapse and shock, along with a rash, which is usually a manifestation of disseminated intravascular coagulation. The syndrome may be rapidly fatal, often within 24 hours of onset.[4] Although the circulatory collapse has been attributed to acute adrenal failure, objective assessment of adrenocortical reserve is usually lacking. Endotoxemia may play a more important role. The adrenal glands at autopsy may not be particularly enlarged but show intense congestion and hemorrhage. At times the hemorrhage may be extensive with disruption of adrenal parenchyma and occasional extension into periadrenal connective tissue. Small fibrin thrombi are often found within sinusoids, along with extensive adrenal necrosis and hemorrhage (Fig. 63-12).

Adrenal hemorrhage, hematoma, and abscess formation

Adrenal hemorrhage can complicate anticoagulant therapy, adrenal or renal vein thrombosis, and other conditions. Many cases are associated with heparin administration with or without warfarin.[4] Consequences include vascular collapse and death from acute adrenal insufficiency, recovery with nonspecific symptoms or chronic adrenocortical insufficiency, which may necessitate steroid replacement therapy.[71] Neonatal adrenal hemorrhage has been associated with difficult labor or delivery, asphyxia, sepsis, brachycardia, and hemorrhagic disorders.[4] The adrenal hemorrhage in the neonatal period is often unilateral and is usually confined to the right adrenal gland. This fourfold predilection for the right adrenal gland has been explained by the potential compression of the right adrenal gland between the liver and spine and the venous drainage of the right adrenal, which flows directly into the inferior vena cava, increasing susceptibility to sudden changes in venous pressure. The affected neonate may have a smooth, immobile flank mass, or diffuse abdominal distention associated with retroperitoneal hemorrhage. The adrenal hematoma may resolve by shrinkage and calcification, undergo cyst formation, or develop into a secondary abscess. Neonatal adrenal abscess can also result from hematogenous bacterial seeding during the course of maternal infection or neonatal sepsis in the absence of gross adrenal hemorrhage.

Adrenal calcification

Adrenal calcification, which is usually patchy, can occur after traumatic delivery, neonatal sepsis, congenital toxoplasmosis, and possible viral infection.[4] Rarely, metaplastic bone formation may be present, presumably a remote consequence of hemorrhage or necrosis.

Lysosomal storage diseases

Adrenal abnormalities may accompany Wolman's disease, Niemann-Pick disease, and a few other storage diseases.[72,73] Wolman's disease is a rare autosomal-recessive abnormality of lipid metabolism with accumulation of cholesterol esters and triglycerides in multiple organs. The disease usually develops in the first few weeks of life, with persistent vomiting, feeding difficulties, and abdominal distention. Hepatosplenomegaly is a characteristic finding, along with anemia. There is bilaterally symmetric enlargement of adrenal glands in this disorder, with dystrophic calcifications, which may impart a gritty sensation to the glands on section. Microscopically, the inner zona fasciculata and entire zona reticularis are replaced by a broad expanse of cells having vacuolated cytoplasm and acicular spaces corresponding to cholesterol esters that have been extracted during routine processing (Fig. 63-13). The adrenal glands may also show some abnormalities in a related but milder disorder known as *cholesteryl ester storage disease*.

Ovarian thecal metaplasia

Ovarian thecal metaplasia, a peculiar lesion described initially as focal hyperplasia of the adrenocortical "blastema,"[74] derives its name from its resemblance to ovarian stroma.[75] It is a microscopic finding in about 4% of surgically resected adrenal glands.[76] Macroscopic tumefactive spindle cell lesions have also been described, with findings in one case suggestiive of origin from Schwann cells.[77] A case of granulosa cell tumor primary in the adrenal gland has also been reported.[78]

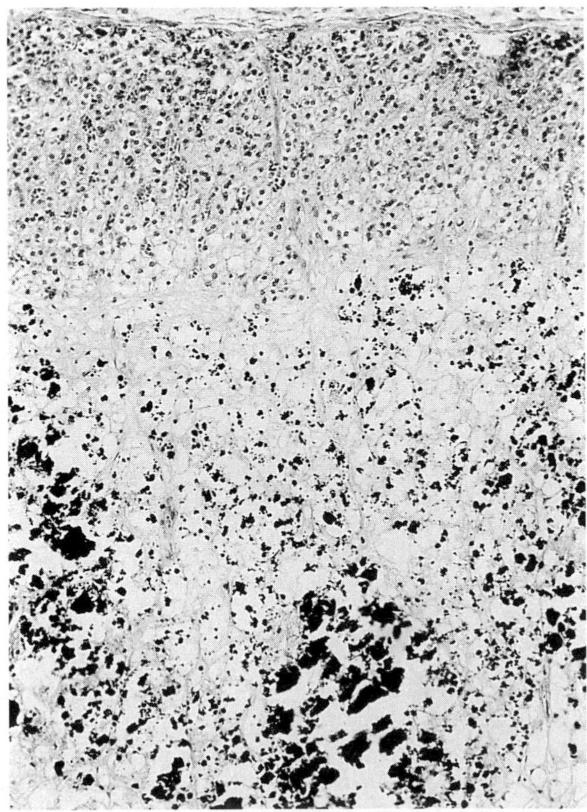

Fig. 63-13 Wolman's disease. Notice calcification within inner adrenal cortex and vacuolated spaces where lipid has been extracted during tissue processing.

CORTICAL HYPERPLASIA AND ADRENOCORTICAL HYPERFUNCTION

The nodular or hyperplastic adrenal gland

General considerations. Perhaps the most complex and confusing issue to confront the pathologist is evaluating the nodular or hyperplastic adrenal gland in which there is no obvious endocrine syndrome or biochemical abnormality on laboratory testing (Fig. 63-14). Hyperplasia usually indicates an increased number of cells in a tissue or organ, which is often associated with increase in size or weight; when hyperplasia is applied to the description of endocrine glands such as the adrenals, however, there is usually some implied or manifest endocrine hyperfunction with excess secretion of hormones. Hyperplasia of the adrenal cortex may be diffuse, nodular, or a mixture of both. The range of changes can be quite broad, ranging from a mild increase in amount of cortical tissue to large adrenal glands with thick cortex and numerous cortical macronodules.

The terms *micronocular hyperplasia* and *macronocular hyperplasia* frequently appear in the literature to subclassify hyperplastic adrenocortical nodules, but lack of uniform criteria hampers interpretation, and both may represent end points on a continuum of nodular cortical hyperplasia that can be found in the same gland. High-resolution radiologic imaging techniques have resulted in increased recognition of incidental nodular adrenocortical hyperplasia. Adrenocortical hyperplasia is almost always bilateral, though rare cases of unilateral adrenal hyperplasia have been noted.[4] The gross morphology of the nodular or diffusely hyperplastic adrenal gland may provide useful diagnostic information that can also be correlated with clinical and endocrinologic findings. The nodular adrenal gland with no evidence of hypercorticalism is probably the most common adrenal abnormality encountered by pathologists and radiologists.

Incidental cortical nodule or nodules—incidence and size at autopsy. The precise incidence of adrenocortical nodules is difficult to determine because there is no universally accepted morphologic definition of what constitutes a nodule, either a micronodule or macronodule. Early studies of adrenocortical nodules at autopsy considered any solitary nodule more than 3

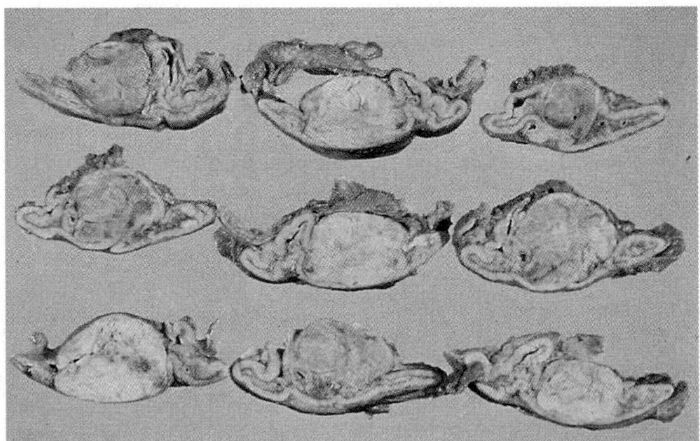

Fig. 63-14 Transverse sections of adrenal glands show multiple nodules within cortex, with several being over 1 cm in diameter.

to 5 mm in diameter to represent a "nonfunctional adenoma,"[79] whereas other autopsy series considered adrenocortical adenomas as being 1.5 cm or more in diameter.[80] Studies have identified cortical adenomas in 1.5% to 8.7% of autopsies.[12,81,82] The incidence appears increased in patients with hypertension (20%),[80] and those who are elderly (29%).[83]

The term *nodular adrenal* is preferable to hyperplasia to describe the increase in cortical tissue with aging and hypertension because there may be no evidence of adrenal hypercorticalism. It may also be inappropriate to use the term *adenoma,* which implies a true neoplasm. Adrenocortical nodularity is usually bilateral, and there may be significant disparity in the weight of glands from an individual patient.[84] Some of the cortical nodules may be 2 to 3 cm in diameter, but most are less than 1 cm in size. Close inspection may be necessary to appreciate more subtle intracortical nodules. The cortical nodules are composed of pale-staining, lipid-rich cells, similar to those seen in the zona fasciculata. There may be some variability in histologic appearance, even including a lipomatous or myelolipomatous component with or without osseous metaplasia. The incidental cortical nodules discovered at autopsy or in living patients do not appear to be "nonfunctional" but rather "nonhyperfunctional" without biochemical or clinical evidence of overproduction of adrenal steroids.

Incidence of cortical nodule or nodules in vivo. With the increase in sensitivity of CT scans, cortical nodules 0.5 cm or less in diameter may be detectable. Incidental adrenocortical nodules are seen in surgically resected adrenal glands (such a radical nephrectomy specimens), but only rarely does this result in a diagnosis of unsuspected adrenocortical hyperfunction. The frequency of incidental advenocortical nodules determined by CT scans of 5082 patients ranges from 0.6% to 1.3%,[85-87] with the average size from 2.4 to 2.8 cm.[87,88]

Incidental pigmented nodule or nodules. Small pigmented brown or black adrenocortical nodules, incidentally found at autopsy or in surgical specimens, range in size from 1 mm to 1.5 cm in diameter. These nodules are usually located in the zona reticularis adjacent to the medullary compartment. Retrospective autopsy studies have revealed pigmented adrenal nodules in 2.2% to 10.4% of cases,[89,90] but when adrenals are examined in a prospective fashion and sectioned at 3 mm intervals, the incidence of pigmented nodules was reported to be 37%, and in 11% of cases the lesions were bilateral.[89] Histologically, the cells resemble those of the zona reticularis with compact, eosinophilic cytoplasm and variable amount of intracytoplasmic amorphous pigment representing lipofuscin. These incidental pigmented adrenocortical nodules do not appear to be associated with any endocrine disturbance, electrolyte imbalance, or hypertension and should be distinguished from the rare "black adenoma" discussed subsequently. A recent study suggested that some of the pigment may represent neuromelanin.[90]

Management. The incidentally discovered adrenal nodule may present problems with differential diagnosis, particularly in a patient with known malignancy in which the stage of the neoplasm must be correctly assessed. In this situation fine-needle aspiration may provide valuable diagnostic information. Endocrinologic evaluation is important to rule out hypercorticalism (such as excess glucocorticoid or mineralocorticoid secretion) or evidence of a pheochromocytoma. Various investigators have used different sizes as being critical, including 3,[91] 4,[92] 5,[93] and 6 cm.[94,95] Magnetic resonance imaging (MRI) has been shown to be useful in the differentiation of adrenal masses; T_2-weighted imaging, for example, might allow separation of nonfunctioning adenomas (low signal intensity) from metastases and adrenocortical carcinoma (intermediate signal intensity) and from pheochromocytomas (very high intensity).[96] Although some initial reports of MRI indicate increased specificity related to lesion signal intensity, there appears to be sufficient overlap with tumors of various type that one must be cautious in trying to make a specific diagnosis.[97]

Adrenocortical hyperfunction with hypercortisolism

Pituitary-dependent hypercortisolism (Cushing's disease)

There are four basic causes of noniatrogenic Cushing's syndrome: (1) hypercortisolism caused by pituitary-dependent ACTH overproduction (Cushing's disease), which accounts for 60% to 70% of cases in adults[98,99] (Fig. 63-15); (2) autonomously secreting adrenocortical tumors, adenoma, or carcinoma (Fig. 63-16), which make up 17% to 25% of cases; (3) ectopic production of ACTH (15% to 16% of cases), or, rarely, the ectopic production of corticotropin-releasing factor (CRF) (Fig. 63-17); and (4) rare cases of adrenocortical hyperplasia caused by primary pigmented nodular adrenocortical disease or macronodular hyperplasia with marked adrenal enlargement. The incidence of these different forms of hypercortisolism depends on variables such as age group and sex. In early childhood, for example, autonomously secreting adreno-

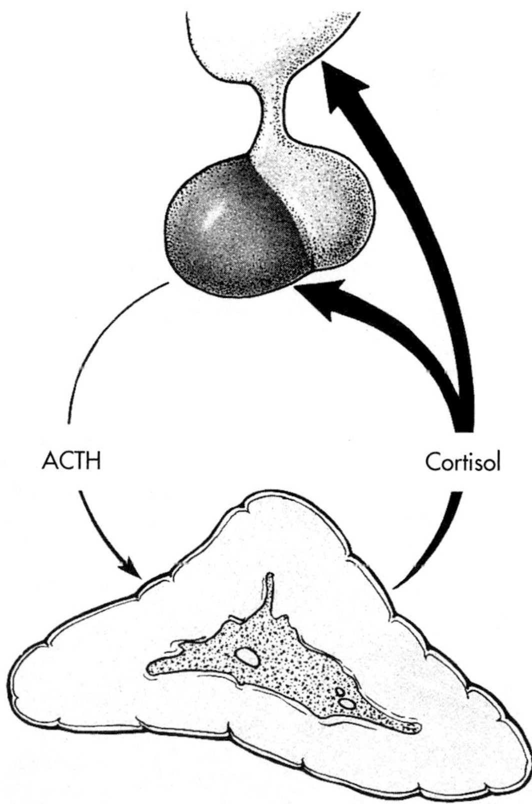

Fig. 63-15 Pituitary-dependent form of hypercortisolism (Cushing's disease) is usually caused by an ACTH-producing microadenoma of the pituitary. ACTH levels may be in the normal range or only mildly elevated.

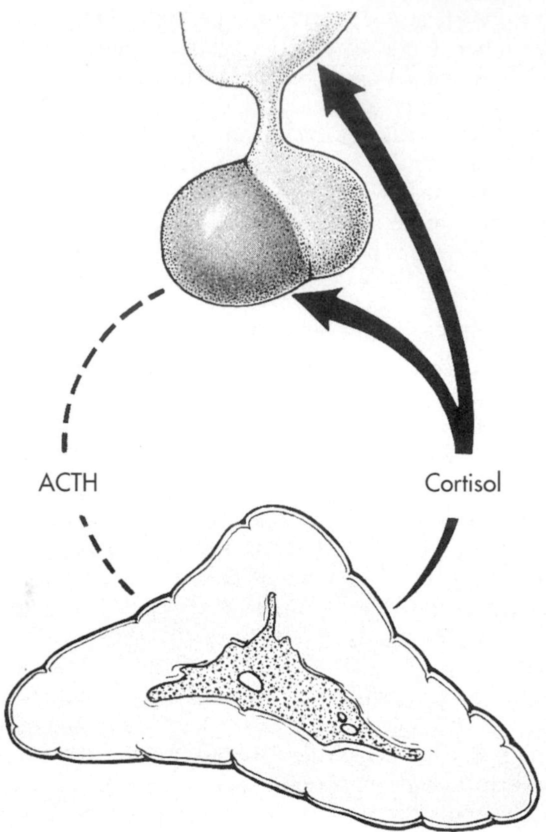

Fig. 63-16 Autonomous secretion of cortisol by an adrenocortical neoplasm. ACTH levels tend to be very low or undetectable.

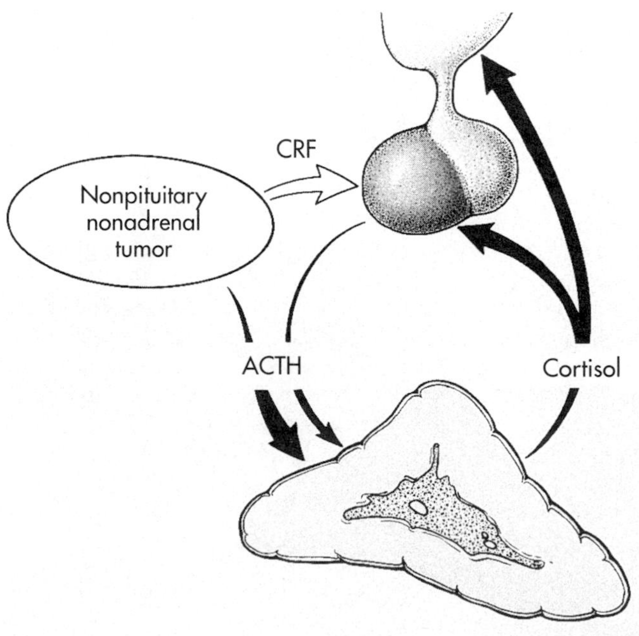

Fig. 63-17 With ectopic secretion of ACTH (or, rarely, corticotropin-releasing factor) levels of circulating ACTH are typically higher than that in Cushing's disease and are sometimes greatly elevated. Some tumors may secrete corticotropin releasing factor (CRF).

cortical tumors, either adenoma or carcinoma, cause over half of the cases of Cushing's syndrome under 8 years of age.[100] Cushing's syndrome caused by ectopic ACTH production in adults is largely a disease of men, whereas most examples of Cushing's disease occur in woman of reproductive age. The disease for which Cushing's name is applied (that is, Cushing's disease) specifically refers to the pituitary, ACTH-dependent form of hypercortisolism, which is attributable to either a microadenoma or a macroadenoma of ACTH-producing cells (corticotrophs), or, rarely, hyperplasia of ACTH-producing cells of the adenohypothesis.

Cushing, in his classic treatise published in 1932, presented detailed case histories of patients whose clinical findings could be ascribed to a basophil adenoma in the absence of any apparent alteration in the adrenal cortex, other than possible secondary hyperplasia, and he added that this will give pathologists reason in the future to scrutinize more carefully the anterior pituitary for lesions of similar composition.[101] Today the pathologist rarely has the opportunity to examine adrenalectomy specimens from patients with Cushing's disease because of the improved surgical technique for treatment of the disease at the level of the pituitary gland (such as a transsphenoidal pituitary adenomyectomy). In most cases the enlargement of the adrenal glands is only modest, with a near doubling in weight. The individual weight of most glands is between 6 and 12 g,[102] with the average weight being 8.2 g.[103] Infrequently, the adrenal glands may appear to be within the "normal" weight range but have subtle histologic abnormality. When sectioned in the transverse plane the adrenal glands may have a rounded contour, and some of the larger glands may show some cortical nodularity. The smaller nodules usually measure 1 to 3 mm in diameter and may appear as prominent capsular extrusions. Gross examination may show a faint irregular demarcation between the outer zona fasciculata, with its yellowish color, whereas the inner one third to one half of the cortex is dark tan to brown and reflects the conversion of pale, lipid-rich cells to cells that are lipid depleted with compact, eosinophilic cytoplasm. The gland thus simulates an expanded zona reticularis. Diffuse hyperplasia may be accompanied by a nodular component that is sometimes macronodular.

In most cases the thickness of the adrenal cortex is greater than 2 mm because of an increase in the thickness of the zona fasciculata. The broad inner zone of cortical cells with compact eosinophilic cytoplasm represents conversion of lipid-rich cells of the inner zona fasciculata (Fig. 63-18). Conversion of lipid-rich cortical cells may not be entirely uniform and may be influenced by physiologic factors. There may also be small micronodules of lipid-rich cells within the outer zona fasciculata. The zona glomerulosa, which is normally discontinuous and thin, may be even harder to identify because of the expanded zona fasciculata. Cells of the zona fasciculata may show irregular extensions into periadrenal fat or form prominent capsular extrusions with sharply demarcated or irregular borders, and cortical cells around tributaries of the central adrenal vein may become quite prominent. Correlation of histologic features with clinical and hormonal data may be crucial because some resected adrenal specimens may show only subtle alterations. Macronodular hyperplasia can be seen in Cushing's disease, and there is evidence indicating that it may represent a late stage of diffuse and micronodular hyperplasia in response to long-term trophic stimulation of the adrenal cortex.[103]

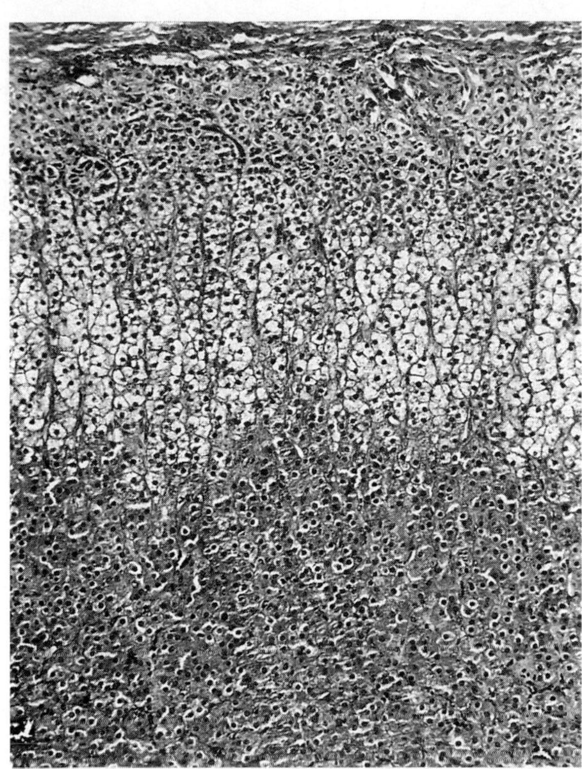

Fig. 63-18 Cushing's disease. Much of the zona fasciculata has been converted to cells with more compact, eosinophilic cytoplasm caused by lipid depletion.

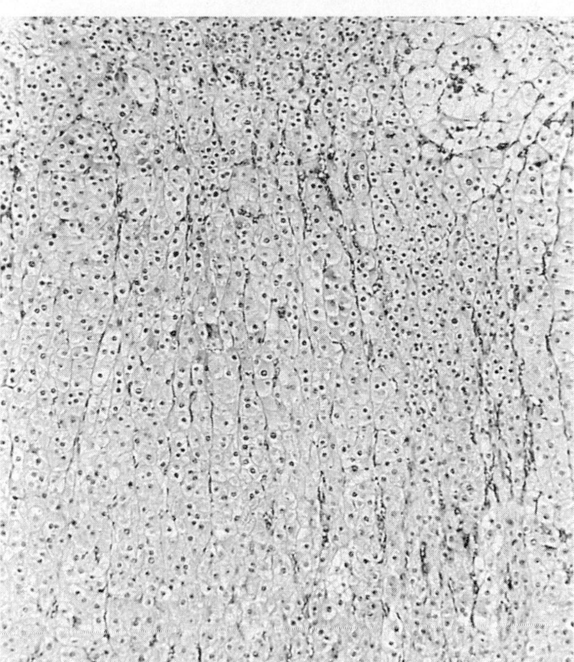

Fig. 63-19 Adrenal gland from a patient with ectopic ACTH syndrome caused by secretion of ACTH by an atypical bronchial carcinoid tumor. Notice pronounced hyperplasia of cortex with enlargement of many cells. Most cells have compact, eosinophilic cytoplasm.

Ectopic ACTH syndrome

ACTH is ectopically produced by a variety of extrapituitary tumors, including bronchial carcinoid tumors, pulmonary carcinomas, pancreatic islet cell carcinoma, medullary thyroid carcinoma, thymic carcinoid tumor, and ovarian adenocarcinoma.[79] Some, such as bronchial carcinoids, may be slow growing, and so the patient has florid Cushing's syndrome while the primary tumor remains undetectable; other, highly aggressive tumors, such as small cell undifferentiated carcinoma of the lung, may be associated with cachexia and electrolyte disturbances without a demonstrable Cushing's syndrome. The adrenal glands in the ectopic ACTH syndrome are usually symmetrically enlarged, frequently each 10 to 15 g, and, rarely, the weight may exceed 20 or 30 g.[79] The plasma ACTH levels are usually quite high. The cortical hyperplasia is diffuse, often with a brownish tint caused by conversion of pale-staining lipid-rich cells to cells with compact, eosinophilic cytoplasm. The widened columns and cords of zona fasciculata cells blend imperceptibly with cells of zona reticularis and may extend all the way out to the adrenal capsule (Fig. 63-19). Individual cortical cells are often enlarged, with abundant compact, pink cytoplasm, and nuclei may display a mild degree of pleomorphism. Occasional clusters of lipid-rich cortical cells may be scattered randomly within the outer zona fasciculata.

Primary pigmented nodular adrenocortical disease

Primary pigmented nodular adrenocortical disease (PPNAD) is a rare form of ACTH or pituitary-independent hypercortisolism. PPNAD is a descriptive designation without any particular reference to underlying pathogenesis. Biochemical findings supporting the autonomous nature of this disorder include (1) increased serum cortisol levels; (2) ACTH levels that are undetectable, low, or within the normal range; (3) lack of suppression of serum cortisol levels with low-dose or high-dose dexamethasone; and (4) no response to metyrapone or ACTH administration.[104] In general, the optimal treatment for patients with PPNAD is bilateral adrenalectomy, and in these cases the surgeon must be prepared to remove both adrenal glands even though they appear normal or even small in size. CT scan of the abdomen usually reveals normal or only slightly enlarged adrenal glands.[105] After bilateral adrenalectomy in cases of PPNAD, Nelson's syndrome has not been reported, which is a further factor supporting the primary autonomous nature of the hypercortisolism.

The average combined weight of resected adrenal glands in 29 cases of PPNAD was 9.5 g (range of 4 to 21 g), with a good correlation between size and weight of individual adrenal glands in each case.[79,106-110] Some of the glands on external examination may show pigmented nodules scattered on the surface, but the best way to see this gross morphology is in transverse sections of the glands (Fig. 63-20). The nodules are usually less than 5 mm in diameter and are often in the size range of 1 to 3 mm; the largest cortical nodules described in the study by Shenoy and associates[106] measured 1.8 cm in diameter. Usually the nodules are described as brown to dark brown or jet black, but other color combinations have been reported, even yellow or golden yellow.[107] In some cases the internodular cortex is atrophic, measuring less than 1 mm in thickness; however, some cases may not demonstrate cortical atrophy but instead appear hyperplastic. Many of the micronodules appear to reside within the zona reticularis and may encroach slightly on the medullary compartment (Fig. 63-21). Most of the cells in the micronodules have compact,

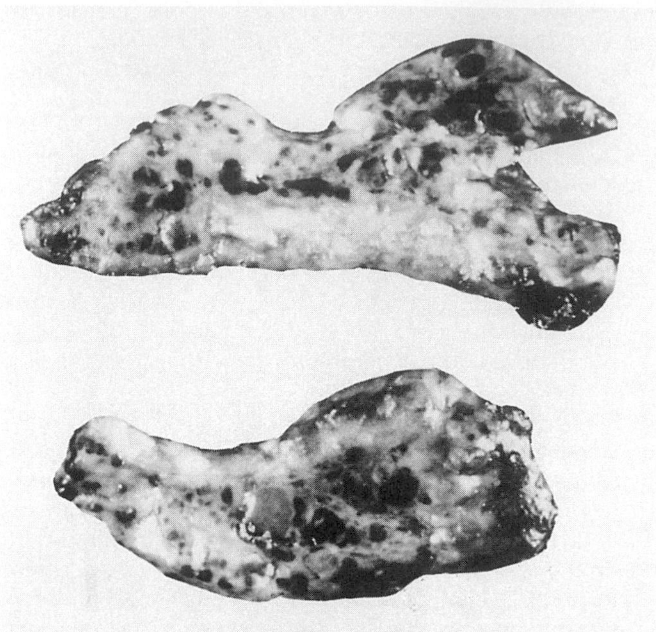

Fig. 63-20 Primary pigmented nodular adrenocortical disease (PPNAD). Sections of adrenal gland showed numerous darkly pigmented nodules studding all zones of the cortex. Patient underwent bilateral adrenalectomy.

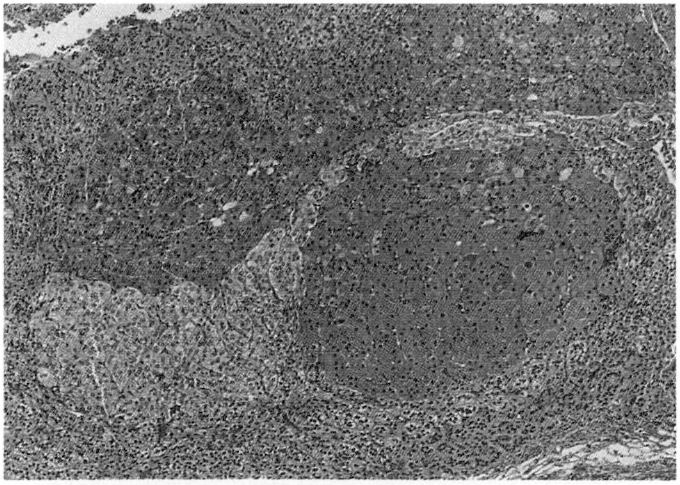

Fig. 63-21 Notice two nodules of cortical cells with compact, eosinophilic cytoplasm. One nodule contains cells with abundant cytoplasmic pigment representing lipofuscin. Intervening medulla is somewhat compressed.

eosinophilic cytoplasm with a variable amount of lipochrome pigment, which in some cells may be quite abundant. Nuclei are round to oval with vesicular appearance, and small, dotlike nucleoli. Occasionally there is significant nuclear enlargement compared with cells of the internodular cortex. An admixture of cells with pale-staining, lipid-rich cytoplasm may also be seen. Occasionally a lipomatous or myelolipomatous component is present within some of the micronodules. An unusual finding is protrusion of hyperplastic cortical cells into tributaries of the central adrenal vein.

The precise cause of PPNAD is unknown, but some have speculated that the cells within the micronodules may be overly sensitive to normal or subnormal levels of ACTH or become hyperactive for other reasons. Some have questioned the possibility of an organ-specific autoimmune disorder, and indeed familial cases were recently reported in which serum immunoglobulin stimulated growth of adrenocortical cells in vitro.[110,111] The study by Wulffraat and colleagues[110] provided evidence for an autoimmune receptor antibody disorder and suggested that the hypercortisolism in this condition is attributable to circulating immunoglobulins directed against ACTH receptors or domains of this receptor. On rare occasion, clinical Cushing's syndrome has been reported to regress spontaneously.[112]

A familial occurrence of PPNAD has been noted with involvement of more than one family member. The condition may also be associated with peculiar skin pigmentation, and a rare variant of testicular sex cord–stromal tumor, the large cell calcifying Sertoli cell tumor.[113] Carney and colleagues[114] identified an unusual complex in which two or more of the following features were present: Cushing's syndrome, cardiac myxoma, cutaneous myxoma, myxoid mammary fibroadenoma, and spotty cutaneous pigmentation.[114] Danoff and colleagues[109] noted the association of melanocytic schwannoma with PPNAD, and Carney[115] later reported several patients with psammomatous melanocytic schwannomas, some with the complex of myxomas, spotty pigmentation, and endocrine overactivity. The pigmented cutaneous lesions are of several types—lentigines or compound nevi and larger, darkly pigmented lesions consistent with blue nevi. Recently a study of several family pedigrees suggested a mendelian dominant inheritance pattern, either autosomal or X-linked,[116] but more studies may be needed to better define the familial aspects of this unusual complex. Echocardiography has been recommended in patients with spotty pigmentation of the type and distribution outlined, as well as patients with PPNAD, and those with bilateral or multifocal large cell calcifying Sertoli cell tumors of the testis to rule out an underlying or associated cardiac myxoma.[114]

Macronodular hyperplasia with marked adrenal enlargement

Macronodular hyperplasia with marked adrenal enlargement is a rare form of Cushing's syndrome in which the adrenal glands appear to function autonomously and show bilateral macronodular hyperplasia (Fig. 63-22). The glands in this disorder may be large enough to simulate a tumor with combined adrenal weights of 60 to 80 g or more.[79] In one recent study a combined weight of 176 g was reported.[117] There is an extraordinary degree of macronodular cortical hyperplasia, to the extent that the medullary compartment may be obscured. Some cases have occurred in patients with long-standing Cushing's disease, but there are instances in which there is no detectable abnormality of the sella even with prolonged careful follow-up study. The bilateral macronocular adrenocortical hyperplasia shown in Fig. 63-22 is from a 40-year-old woman who had long-standing Cushing's syndrome with combined adrenal weights of 94 g.[118] This patient was followed for nearly 30 years and at last examination had no evidence for a pituitary neoplasm.[119]

Macronodular hyperplasia with marked adrenal enlargement can have confusing biochemical aspects, and there is a recent report of a case that seemed to be a transition from a

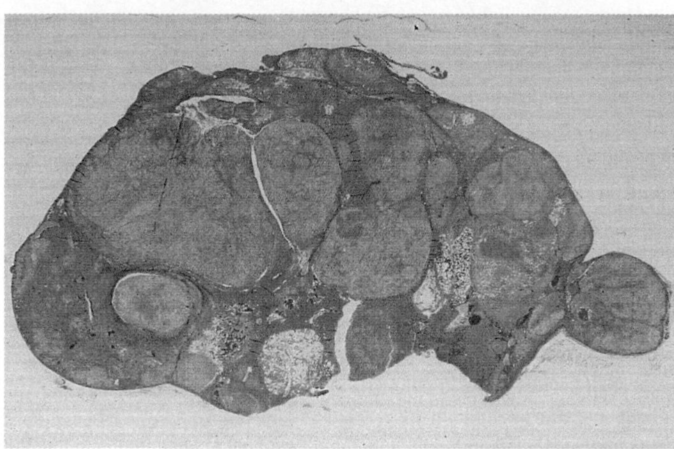

Fig. 63-22 Advanced macronodular hyperplasia with marked adrenal enlargement. Notice multiple macronodules composed of cells with pale-staining, lipid-rich cytoplasm. Foci of lipomatous metaplasia are also present.

pituitary- or ACTH-dependent (that is, Cushing's disease) to adrenal-dependent form of hypercortisolism.[120] Biochemical findings, such as low or undetectable ACTH levels and absence of suppression of serum cortisol with low or high levels of dexamethasone, coupled with tomographic evidence of an adrenal mass, are suggestive, in some cases, of an autonomously secreting adrenocortical tumor. It may be difficult to decide with confidence whether these large macronodules are truly neoplastic or represent autonomously hyperfunctioning, hyperplastic nodules that require either no ACTH or only very low levels to sustain hypercortisolism.[79]

Multiple endocrine neoplasia (MEN) syndrome type 1

In the review by Ballard and colleagues[121] of cases of MEN type 1, many endocrine glands were affected, including parathyroid (87%), pancreatic islets (81%), pituitary (65%), and adrenal glands (36%). The adrenal glands have been reported showing "adenomas," "miliary adenomas," and nodular hyperplasia, but relatively little clinical significance can be attached to the changes noted.[121] There are rare cases with clinical hypercorticalism. In a recent case report and literature review, Miyagawa and associates[122] could identify fewer than 10 cases of Cushing's disease occurring in MEN type 1. In a study at the Mayo Clinic, pituitary adenomas in MEN type 1 accounted for only 2.7% of the general population of 1500 patients with pituitary adenomas.[123] Only 3 of 41 pituitary adenomas from patients with a diagnosis of MEN type 1 were classified as being composed of ACTH-producing cells; two occurred in associated with Nelson's syndrome, and one probably was an example of a silent corticotrophic adenoma without evidence of clinical hyperfunction.[123]

Hyperaldosteronism

Primary hyperaldosteronism

Conn[124] described the clinical syndrome of primary hyperaldosteronism caused by an aldosterone-secreting adrenocortical adenoma.[124] At least five different settings for the syndrome of primary hyperaldosteronism have been recognized: (1) an aldosterone-producing adrenocortical adenoma (Conn's syndrome), (2) idiopathic hyperaldosteronism with bilateral hyperplasia of zona glomerulosa, (3) adrenocortical carcinoma, (4) glucocorticoid remediable hyperaldosteronism, and (5) an indeterminate category. Pathologists rarely have the opportunity today to study the nontumorous adrenal glands from patients with primary hyperaldosteronism because adrenalectomy is reserved mainly for patients with an aldosterone-producing cortical tumor who have a much more predictable response in terms of normalization of blood pressure after treatment. The glucocorticoid-remediable form of hyperaldosteronism has recently been shown to result from a genetic mutation (autosomal dominant) involving the aldosterone synthase gene and the 5′ regulatory region of the 11-β-hydroxylase gene, which allows illicit production of aldosterone by the zona fasciculata.[125]

From 15% to 35% of cases of primary hyperaldosteronism are idiopathic in nature with bilateral hyperplasia of zona glomerulosa.[79] The increasing complexity of primary hyperaldosteronism is reflected in some of these cases. Hyperplasia of zona glomerulosa can be divided into several groups: (1) hyperplasia of zona glomerulosa without nodules, (2) hyperplasia of zona glomerulosa with micronodules and macronodules, and (3) normal-appearing zona glomerulosa with micronodules.[126] The cause of this disorder without an identifiable tumor is obscure, though some have suggested an "aldosterone-stimulating factor" of anterior pituitary origin in the cause of idiopathic hyperaldosteronism.[127]

The gross examination the adrenal glands may be normal, or heavier than normal with visible micronodules or macronodules. One might question whether some of the cortical nodules are a result of hypertension rather than a cause of it. In the detailed study by Dobbie, capsular "arteriopathy" was implicated in pathogenesis of some cortical nodules in the aging population.[85] Hyperplasia of the zona glomerulosa may be evident as a continuous band of cells beneath the adrenal capsule or focal extension in an irregular fashion into adjacent cortex.[79] The hyperplasia of zona glomerulosa may be focal or diffuse, and the changes may vary in different parts of the gland, necessitating multiple sections to appreciate any significant abnormalities.

Secondary hyperaldosteronism

Activation of the renin-angiotensin system may cause secondary hyperaldosteronism as a normal physiologic response to changes in electrolytes and extracellular fluid volume. Secondary hyperaldosteronism or stimulation of aldosterone production occurs in patients with sodium depletion, severe dehydration, nephrotic syndrome, congestive heart failure, cirrhosis, and rare conditions such as a renin-secreting juxtaglomerular cell tumor. Hyperplasia of zona glomerulosa has been reported in the adrenal glands of patients with cystic fibrosis,[128] a disorder that may be complicated by substantial depletion of salt, particularly in hot weather, and of course some of these patients may develop hepatic cirrhosis.

ADRENOCORTICAL NEOPLASMS

Adrenocortical adenoma with Cushing's syndrome

Clinical features. Fully developed Cushing's syndrome has features dominated by fat deposition, centripetal obesity, moon facies, and formation of a "buffalo hump." Cutaneous striae, as well as systemic hypertension and a variety of other

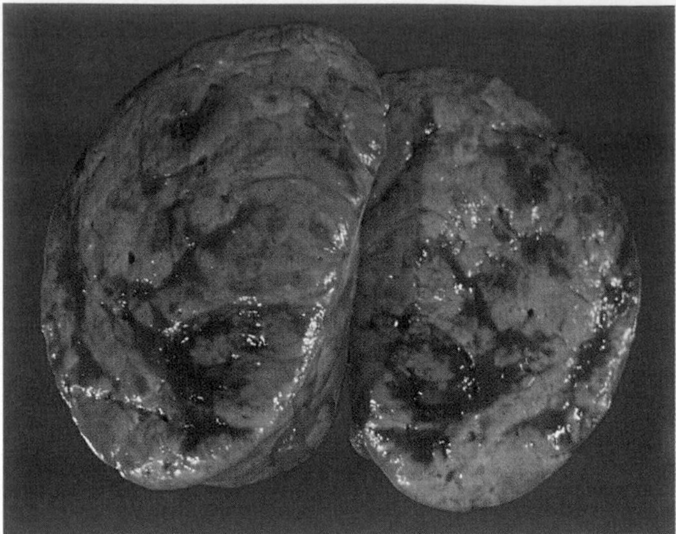

Fig. 63-23 Adrenocortical adenoma. Tumor on cross section is deep orange with tan-brown geographic areas. Darker zones correspond to areas of tumor in which cells are relatively depleted of lipid and have increased lipofuscin pigment.

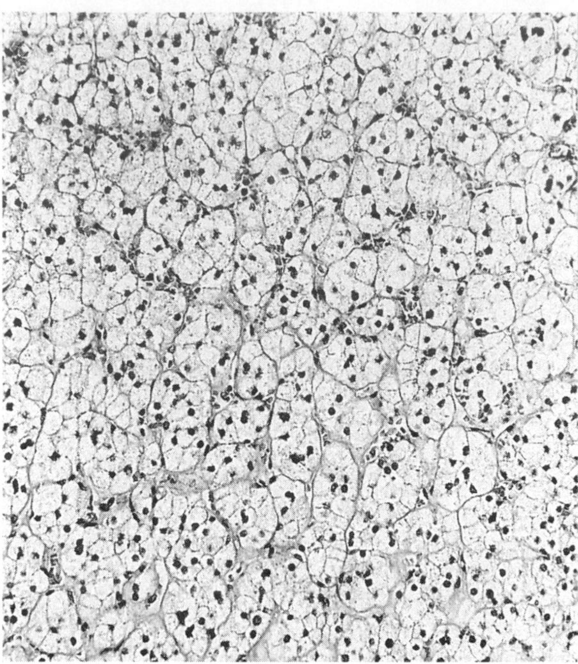

Fig. 63-24 Adrenocortical adenoma with hypercortisolism (Cushing's syndrome). Tumor cells are pale staining with abundant intracytoplasmic lipid, arranged in small nests or alveoli. Nuclei are relatively uniform in size and shape.

complaints, such as fatigue, backache, and abdominal pain, are present. Menstrual disturbances may occur in women, causing secondary amenorrhea.

Gross pathologic features. Adrenocortical adenomas characteristically synthesize and release steroids in a physiologically autonomous manner. Adenomas in the setting of Cushing's syndrome are usually less than 50 g in weight and measure 3 to 4 cm in diameter. Many of the tumors weigh 10 to 40 g, but occasionally tumors in excess of 100 g are seen.[129] Adrenocortical adenomas may have sharp circumscription or even appear encapsulated on cross section; however, on close microscopic examination this often appears to be pseudoencapsulation caused by compression of adjacent connective tissue, or the tumor may acquire its capsule from the adrenal gland itself. The tumors on cross section vary in color from yellow to golden yellow to tumors that are variegate in color, with dark brown or even black areas (Fig. 63-23). Some tumors can show focal degenerative change, but frank hemorrhage and confluent necrosis are unusual features that should cause one to suspect an underlying carcinoma, particularly if the tumor is large.

Microscopic pathologic features. Adenomas are composed of neoplastic cortical cells with pale, lipid-rich cytoplasm similar to cells of the zona fasciculata (Fig. 63-24). An admixture of cells with compact eosinophilic cytoplasm is not uncommon. The yellow color of cortical tumors is principally attributable to accumulation of intracellular lipid, which can be demonstrated in frozen sections with Oil red O or other lipid stains. Several architectural patterns may be seen, such as nesting or alveolar arrangement, and formation of trabeculae or short cords. Clusters of enlarged lipid-rich cells may appear ballooned. Nuclei are usually regular, are modestly enlarged with vesicular appearance, and have a small nucleolus; on occasion there may be considerable nuclear enlargement and pleomorphism, but this finding does not predict biologic behavior. As with functioning adrenocortical lesions including hyperplasia, adenoma, and carcinoma, there may be foci or lipomatous or myelolipomatous metaplasia.

Although the architectural pattern and cell composition may be typical for cortical adenomas associated with Cushing's syndrome, clinical correlation is required to distinguish the tumor from a nonhyperfunctioning macronodule or adenomas associated with an entirely different endocrine syndrome.[129] Atrophy of the attached (or contralateral) nonneoplastic cortex is a reliable indication of hypercortisolism.[130] A thickness of cortex of less than 1 mm throughout usually confirms cortical atrophy.

Adrenocortical adenoma with primary hyperaldosteronism (Conn's syndrome)

Gross pathologic features. Aldosterone-secreting adrenocortical adenomas are often referred to as *aldosteronomas*. In one study 92% were unilateral and solitary and 8% were multiple but still unilateral.[131] Most are small, less than 3 cm in diameter.[132] Grossly, the tumor usually projects from or distorts the surface of the gland; in other instances it is best seen on transverse sectioning of the adrenal gland, where it appears as a sharply demarcated, almost encapsulated mass. On cross section the tumor is often homogeneous with a yellow-orange or canary-yellow appearance (Fig. 63-25). Larger tumors may exhibit degenerative change.

Microscopic pathologic features. Although the tumor may appear encapsulated on gross examination, careful microscopic study often reveals a pushing, expansile border without true encapsulation. As with other cortical adenomas the tumor may compress adjacent connective tissue, thus acquiring a pseudocapsule, or with progressive expansion, the adrenal capsule itself may become part of the encapsulation. The tumor cells are arranged in nests or alveolar clusters, short

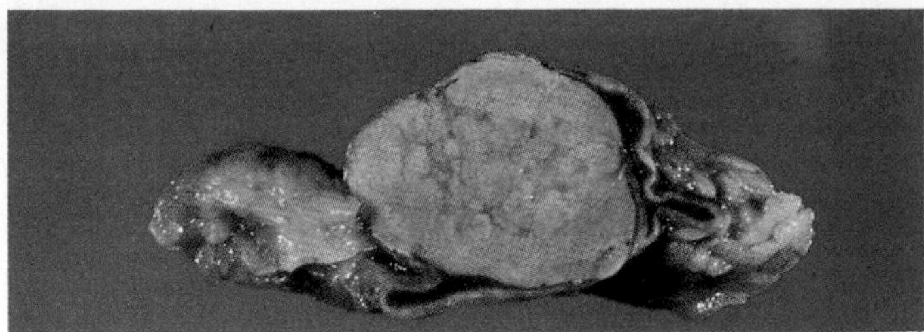

Fig. 63-25 Aldosterone-producing adrenocortical adenoma (aldosteronoma). Tumor is sharply circumscribed and yellow-orange on section.

cords, or short anastomosing trabeculae. Nuclei are relatively uniform and vesicular, often with a nucleolus. There may be nuclear irregularity. As with benign and malignant cortical neoplasms, there may be intranuclear pseudoinclusions representing invaginations of cell cytoplasm. The histologic appearance may substantially vary among microscoic fields.[126] Findings include cells that are large and rich in cytoplasmic lipid, analogous to cells of zona fasciculata, and cells with eosinophilic cytoplasm that resemble cells of zona reticularis. Smaller cells may be found with less abundant lipid-rich, pale cytoplasm, resembling cells of zona glomerulosa. A fourth cell type, intermediate in morphology between zona glomerulosa and zona fasciculata cells, is the hybrid cell. These cells have the unique capacity to elaborate hormones normally produced by either zona glomerulosa (aldosterone) or zona fasciculata.

Spironolactone bodies. Spironolactone bodies, originally described by Janigan in 1963,[133] are characteristic inclusions within the cytoplasm of zona glomerulosa cells that are associated with administration of the aldosterone antagonist spironolactone (Aldactone). The inclusions may appear as early as 10 days after treatment and may persist for 4 months after the last dose.[134,135] Subsequently, similar inclusions were seen in an aldosterone-producing adenoma. The structures are eosinophilic with scroll-like laminations and usually appear to reside within a clear zone or surrounded by a halo (Fig. 63-26, *A*). They are rich in lipid, and the inclusions usually stain medium blue with Luxol fast blue stain (Fig. 63-26, *B*). The inclusions are usually solitary, ranging in size from 2 to 12 μm, but are often nearly equal in size to the nucleus of the cortical cell in which they reside. In one study, the number of inclusions within aldosterone-producing adenomas correlated with the proportion of glomerulosa type of cells.[136] Aldosterone has been demonstrated within the cytoplasmic inclusions using immunohistochemistry.[137]

Functional "black" adenomas

Pigmented "black" adenomas are uncommon. Most have been associated with Cushing's syndrome, though a few have been reported with aldosterone hypersecretion. Pigmentation of adrenocortical adenomas, as seen in those with Cushing's syndrome, is not uncommon, but diffusely pigmented, black adenomas are very rare. Grossly the differential diagnosis of a black adenoma is adrenal hematoma or hemorrhage, hemorrhagic cortical neoplasm, or a malignant melanoma either metastatic to the adrenal glands or, rarely, primary. Most tumors are diagnosed in the third decade of life and appear to be more common in females. The tumors usually weigh less than 35 g with an average diameter of about 2.5 cm.[129]

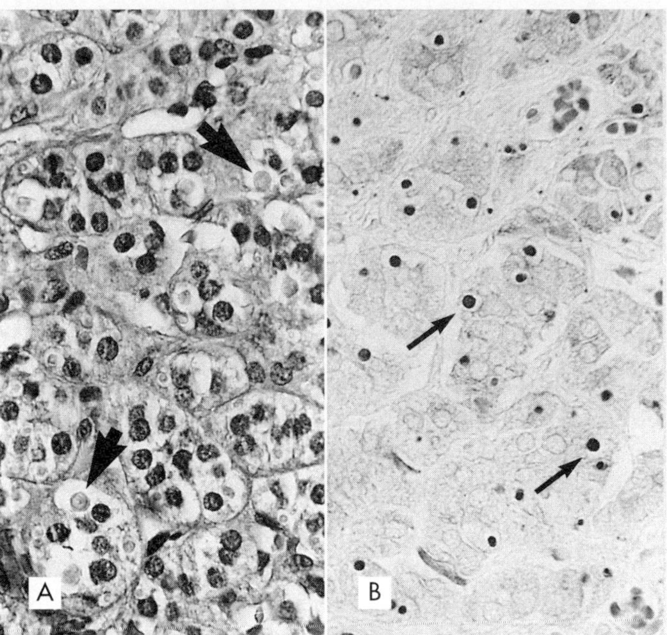

Fig. 63-26 **A,** Spironolactone bodies appear as eosinophilic structures with concentric laminations and surrounding clear space *(arrows).* **B,** Spironolactone bodies are highlighted by staining for phospholipid. Each inclusion appears blue-black *(arrows)* (Luxol fast blue stain).

Black adenomas are usually composed of cells with compact, eosinophilic cytoplasm with variable amount of brown or golden-brown pigment often showing some clearing of the cytoplasm immediately adjacent to the nucleus. The architectural arrangement of cells is similar to that in other adrenocortical adenomas, with short trabeculae or alveolar clusters. Special stains indicate that the pigment is lipofuscin. On ultrastructural examination, the tumor cells are relatively poor in lipid and contain a variable number of irregularly shaped electron-dense granules. Pigmented granules with ultrastructural features of typical melanosomes or premelanosomes are not evident.

Adrenocortical carcinoma

Incidence and epidemiology. Adrenocortical carcinoma (ACC) is a rare tumor with an estimated incidence in the population of about two cases per million population.[129] ACC occurs in all age groups, though some studies indicate a bimodal incidence peak in the fifth to seventh decades and in the first two decades of life. Pooling data from many series indicates a nearly equal sex distribution overall, but patients with Cushing's syndrome are more often females.[129] There are a few epidemiologic factors associated with ACC; some of them include the cancer family (Li-Fraumeni) syndrome,[138,139] Beckwith-Wiedemann syndrome,[32] and rare tumors seen in the setting of congenital adrenal hyperplasia.[4,45]

Clinical features. ACC may be functionally active. Steroids secretion can elicit a well-developed endocrine syndrome such as Cushing's syndrome, or more often, a mixed endocrine syndrome with Cushing's syndrome, virilization, or mineralocorticoid excess. The incidence of functionally active tumors ranges from 24% to 96%.[129] This variation may reflect differences in details of clinical evaluation or in assessment of biochemical data. The malignant potential of adrenocortical neoplasms cannot be predicted by their hormonal function. However, those causing feminization are cause for concern with regard to potential malignancy.[140] It should be noted that virilization has also been reported on rare occasions in adrenocortical adenomas containing crystalloids of Reinke, and some of these tumors have been reported as Leydig cell adenomas of the adrenal gland.[141,142]

ACC tend to be large neoplasms, and many tumors are over 12 cm in diameter with an average weight of about 1000 g.[143] They often elicit signs or symptoms of an abdominal mass with pain or a palpable tumor. Fatigue or weight loss may be a prominent feature. Low-grade intermittent fever has been seen in 10% to 20% of patients, and may be related to tumor necrosis. In some patients, however, weight loss is not a conspicuous feature and has been attributed to the anabolic effects of steroids. Metastases at the time of presentation occur in 25% or more of patients with ACC.[129]

Gross pathologic features. Data compiled from large clinical series show that 59% of tumors arose in the left adrenal gland and 41% in the right.[129] The average weight ranges from 705 to 1210 g, with some of the larger tumors weighing nearly 3 kg in weight. In the study by Tang and Gray[144] tumors weighing over 95 g proved to be clinically malignant whereas those under 50 g were benign. Weight alone, as a defining criterion for benign or malignant behavior, is too simplistic—some tumors weighing in excess of 1000 g may be clinically benign, whereas (rarely) those weighing less than 50 g may behave in a malignant fashion. Larger adrenocortical adenomas in the weight range of 100 to 400 g present the most significant diagnostic problems. ACC often presents as a bulky, resiliently firm tumor with coarse bosselations and, on cross section, may have an ominous macroscopic appearance with areas of necrosis, hemorrhage, and cystic degeneration (Fig. 63-27). Most of the larger tumors can be correctly assumed to be malignant on gross inspection alone.

Microscopic pathologic features. The architectural pattern of most ACC can be classified as trabecular, alveolar (or nesting), or diffuse. A broad anastomosing trabecular pattern is particularly characteristic, with interconnecting columns of cells separated by elongate to ectatic vascular spaces (Fig. 63-28). Many tumors have intersecting broad bands of fibrous tissue with a predominance of lipid-depleted cells with compact, eosinophilic cytoplasm, but other tumors may show an admixture of more lipid-rich, pale-staining cells. Nuclear pleomorphism can be a spectacular feature, but this feature alone does not permit correct typing of the tumor as malignant. Mitotic figures may be conspicuous in ACC and often provide important clues to the correct diagnosis, particularly if there are atypical mitotic figures. ACC may show vascular invasion, which often appears as loose discohesive plugs of tumor cells within vascular lumens. Capsular invasion or invasion of adjacent organs such as kidney may also be seen.

It may be extremely difficult to diagnose an ACC with absolute certainty using histologic or nonhistologic parameters. Using a statistical model, the following histologic features have the greatest predictive value: (1) broad fibrous bands, (2) diffuse growth pattern, and (3) vascular invasion.[145] Widespread tumor necrosis and increased numbers of mitoses were also found to have predictive value. In another review, the following features were found in clinically recurrent or metastatic tumors: (1) mitotic rate greater than 5 per 50 high-power fields (hpf), (2) atypical mitotic figures, and (3) venous invasion.[146] In another study, tumor weight as a nonhistologic parameter and mitotic activity had the highest discriminating value in diagnosing malignant tumors.[147] It is apparent from these and other studies that there is a small but significant number of adrenocortical neoplasms in which it is extremely difficult to predict biologic behavior.

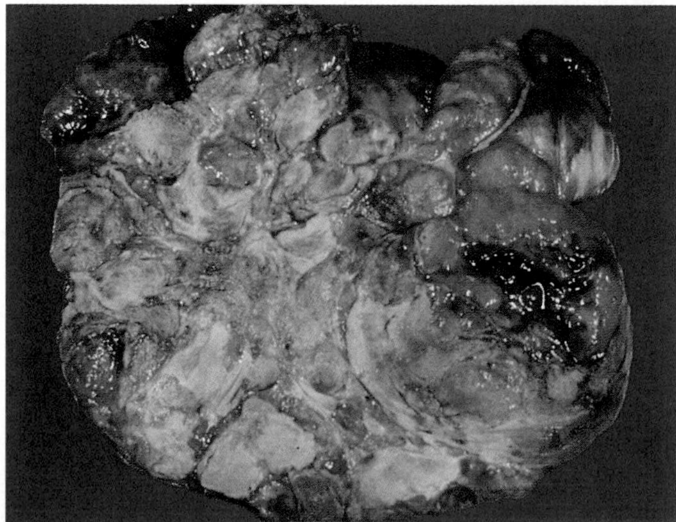

Fig. 63-27 Adrenocortical carcinoma resected from a teenage girl with virilization. Tumor weighed over 1000 g and on cross section is coarsely nodular with extensive areas of necrosis.

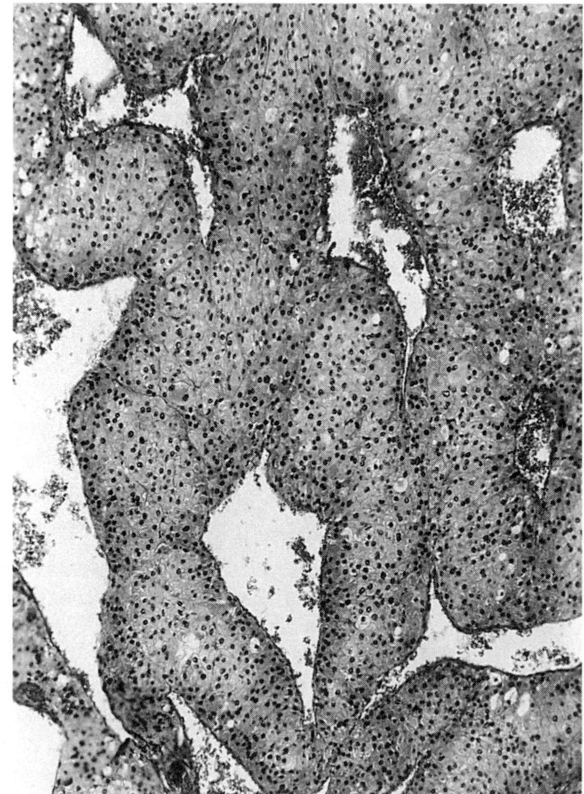

Fig. 63-28 Adrenocortical carcinoma. Tumor has broad anastomosing trabecular pattern with delicate sinusoids. Nuclei are relatively uniform, but some tumors can be greatly pleomorphic with enlarged hyperchromatic nuclei.

Prognostic factors and biologic behavior. ACC are often highly malignant tumors with advanced stage at diagnosis. The mortality varies from 70% to 92%.[129] Most cause death within 12 months of diagnosis, with sites of metastases reflecting both hematogenous and lymphatic dissemination. Liver and lung are the most common sites of distant spread, but a variety of other sites may be involved, such as retroperitoneum, inferior vena cava, lymph nodes (both intra-abdominal and thoracic), bone, and various other sites. In recent series using the TNM (tumor, node, metastasis) classification, 61.5% had stage 4 tumors, 7.3% stage 3, 30.3% stage 2, and only one was stage 1 at the time of initial diagnosis.[148,149] Some have attempted to grade ACC and correlate this with prognosis. Mitotic rate has been used in distinguishing low-grade ACC with a median survival of 58 months (≤20 mitoses per 50 hpf) from high-grade ACC with a median survival of only 14 months (>20 mitoses per 50 hpf).[150,151] Flow cytometric analysis of DNA content has been used in an attempt to predict biologic behavior, with conflicting results.[152-156] Analysis of DNA content complements conventional histologic methods in the diagnosis of ACC. The real value of DNA ploidy analysis appears to be restricted to patients who are undergoing curative surgical resection because in one study the prognosis of patients undergoing palliative surgery was dismal regardless of DNA ploidy patterns.[154] It must be remembered that aneuploid DNA peaks may be seen in adrenocortical and other endocrine neoplasms that prove to be clinically benign.[157]

Adrenocortical neoplasms in childhood

Most children with an adrenocortical neoplasm have endocrine symptoms or biochemical evidence of hypercorticalism.[129] Historical data are suggestive of a relatively poor prognosis for children with adrenocortical tumors, but because childhood tumors are so rare, it is difficult to fully characterize morphologic features that reliably indicate malignancy. There may be a greater tendency to diagnose these tumors as malignant in childhood.[156,158] A recent study revealed the following to be significant adverse findings in adrenocortical neoplasms: (1) large tumor size (average 11.9 cm) and weight (median 560 g), (2) older age at diagnosis (average 10 years), (3) high mitotic count (average 31 per 50 hpf), and (4) extensive tumor necrosis.[156,159]

Special studies

Fine-needle aspiration. Fine-needle aspiration under CT or ultrasound guidance can provide valuable information regarding the incidentally discovered adrenal mass, particularly in staging patients with primary extraadrenal malignancies. Careful correlation with clinical findings, endocrinologic data, and specifics about the mass on imaging studies such as size, location, and other factors will help enhance the sensitivity and specificity of cytologic interpretation. One must exercise extreme caution in trying to distinguish an ACC from a benign adrenocortical neoplasm on a cytologic basis alone (Fig. 63-29). Other benign adrenal neoplasms that can be diagnosed by FNA include myelolipoma. One must be aware of certain pitfalls in interpretation of FNA of adrenal masses; occasionally, metastatic carcinoma can mimic normal or neoplastic adrenocortical cells, and benign cortical nodules have been reported to mimic small round-cell malignancies, probably because of mechanical disruption of cell cytoplasm during the aspiration process.[129]

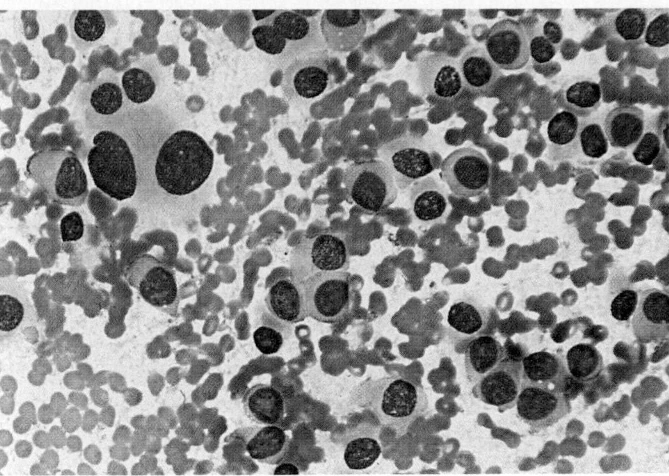

Fig. 63-29 Fine-needle aspiration of adrenocortical carcinoma. Tumor cells are greatly pleomorphic with considerable variation in nuclear size and shape (Diff Quik stain).

Immunohistochemistry. There are no immunohistochemical markers pathognomonic of adrenocortical neoplasms. Routinely processed, paraffin-embedded ACCs can contain vimentin and are usually not reactive with epithelial markers such as antikeratin and antiepithelial membrane antigen.[160-162] Some adrenocortical tumors, however, may mark with antikeratin after treatment of tissue with protease, or if fresh frozen tissue is examined. In contrast to pheochromocytoma, adrenocortical neoplasms are typically nonreactive with chromogranin. Some ACCs may demonstrate positive immunostaining for synaptophysin, which has been used as a neuroendocrine marker.[163]

ADRENAL MEDULLARY HYPERPLASIA

Adrenal medullary hyperplasia has been most convincingly demonstrated in the setting of MEN syndrome type 2, where it is regarded as a precursor for pheochromocytomas.[164-166] Adrenal medullary hyperplasia without features of MEN has been described in patients with signs and symptoms suggestive of pheochromocytoma, but at surgery there is no evidence of a discrete tumor.[16,167,168] Adrenal medullary hyperplasia has also been noted in the Beckwith-Wiedemann syndrome.[31] The criteria for adrenal medullary hyperplasia are (1) an increase in adrenal weight with diffuse or nodular expansion of the medullary compartment by chromaffin cells, often with extension into the tail or both alae of the gland, (2) a decrease in overall ratio of cortex to medulla, and (3) an increase in the calculated medullary weight or volume.

The distinction of diffuse or nodular adrenal medullary hyperplasia from early pheochromocytoma in MEN syndromes type 2A and 2B is arbitrary. Some have regarded nodules 1 cm or more in diameter as pheochromocytoma.[165] The histologic appearance of some of the nodules of adrenal medullary hyperplasia may vary with respect to architecture, cell size, and nuclear morphology. A frequent finding is the presence of intracytoplasmic hyaline globules and occasionally prominent vacuolated cells. Nuclear enlargement and hyperchromasia can be seen, often in a juxtacortical location.

PHEOCHROMOCYTOMA

Incidence. Fränkel[186] provided the first description of a patient with pheochromocytoma in 1886. The term *pheochromocytoma* (*phaios,* Greek for 'dusky' or 'dark'; *chromo-,* 'color'; *kytos,* 'cell') is based on the tinctorial staining of the tumor after exposure to chromium salts. Pheochromocytomas are relatively rare tumors in general practice; in a population-based study at the Mayo Clinic an average annual incidence rate of eight cases per million population was reported.[170] The incidence of clinically unsuspected or undiagnosed cases of pheochromocytoma detected at surgery or at autopsy ranges from 14% to as high as 53%.[16] The prevalence of undetected or undiagnosed pheochromocytoma appears to have declined with heightened clinical awareness, as well as availability of more sophisticated biochemical assays and high-resolution imaging procedures.

Clinical features. Pheochromocytomas are most commonly seen in the fourth and fifth decades of life, though the tumor can also occur in children. Familial tumors tend to be diagnosed at an earlier age than sporadic tumors. Over 90% of pheochromocytomas are sporadic, with the remainder having familial occurrence mainly in the MEN type 2A and 2B syndromes. In childhood there is an increased incidence of bilateral, multicentric, and extra-adrenal paragangliomas. It is important to note that the incidence of bilaterality in familial cases of pheochromocytomas is over 50%.

The most common signs and symptoms in patients with pheochromocytomas are severe headache, palpitations with or without tachycardia, diaphoresis, anxiety, and nervousness. These features are attributable to catecholamines, epinephrine, and norepinephrine. Hypertensive episodes are characteristic, and there may also be reflex bradycardia or possible hypotension.[171] In the presence of classic signs and symptoms it may be relatively easy to diagnose a pheochromocytoma, though the signs and symptoms may be mild and inconstant. Pheochromocytoma is a characteristic component of MEN type 2A (Sipple's syndrome) and MEN type 2B; tumors in these syndromes are usually multicentric and bilateral, and are often preceded by diffuse or nodular medullary hyperplasia. Only rarely are the tumors extra-adrenal in location.[16] In MEN type 2B the patients often have a characteristic phenotype that may draw attention to the disorder at an early stage. Gastrointestinal manifestations caused by ganglioneuromatosis and neuromatous nodules of the oral mucous membranes and other sites may be prominent features (Fig. 63-30). Medullary thyroid carcinoma can be a lethal component of this syndrome, thus making early detection essential.[16,168]

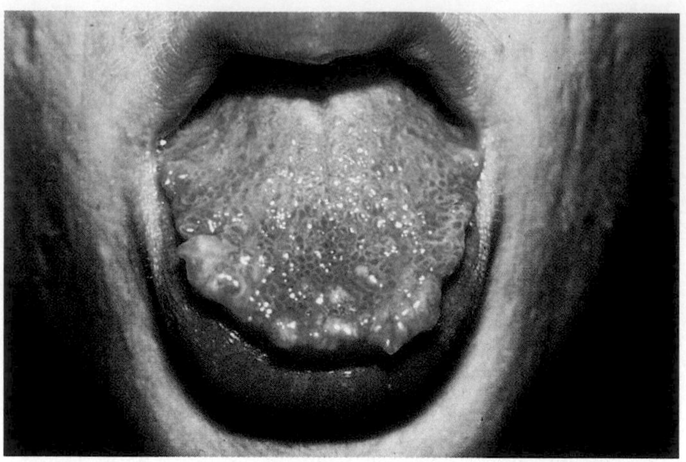

Fig. 63-30 Patient with multiple endocrine neoplasia (MEN) syndrome type 2B. Notice mucosal neuromatous nodules studding lateral borders and anterior aspect of tongue. Patient died of widely metastatic medullary thyroid carcinoma (the most lethal component of the syndrome).

Gross pathologic feratures. Sporadic pheochromocytomas are typically unilateral, solitary, and unicentric tumors that on gross inspection may be sharply circumscribed, almost encapsulated, similar to adrenocortical neoplasms. On close microscopic inspection this may represent pseudoencapsulation resulting from compression of adjacent connective tissue or expansion of the adrenal capsule itself. The average weight in several series is about 100 g, but the range in weight is quite variable.[16] Most tumors are 3 to 5 cm in diameter, and on cross section the tumors are usually resiliently firm and grayish or dusky red (Fig. 63-31). Degenerative changes can be seen with fibrosis, necrosis, and cystic alteration. Rarely, the tumor may undergo such pronounced cystic change that viable portions of tumor may be difficult to recognize on gross examination. Pheochromocytomas can invade the inferior vena cava or even extend into the right atrium on rare occasions.

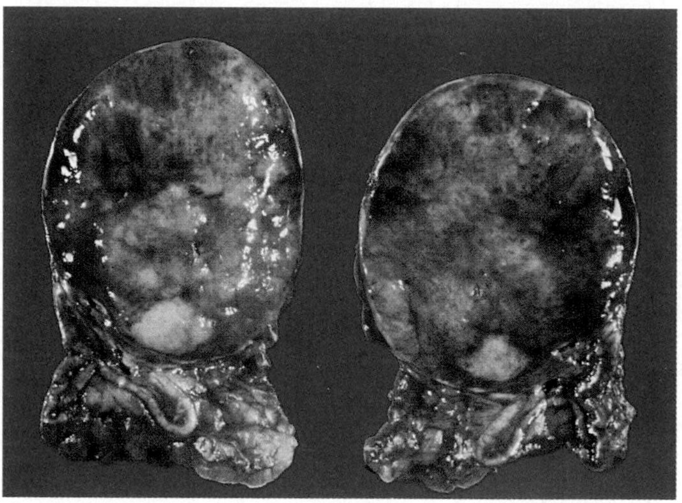

Fig. 63-31 Pheochromocytoma. Tumor has been bivalved and appears pale gray with mottled areas of congestion and hemorrhage. Residual adrenal and periadrenal fat are attached to lower portion of tumor.

Microscopic pathologic features. Three major histologic architectural patterns can be found in pheochromocytomas: an anastomosing cell cord or trabecular pattern (Fig. 63-32), alveolar pattern, and a diffuse or solid arrangement of cells. Occasionally a spindle cell pattern may be evident. These tumors have a prominent microvascular component that can be accentuated by staining for reticulum. Individual tumor cells are usually polygonal with a lightly eosinophilic cytoplasm having granular quality on close inspection; at times the cytoplasm may be basophilic or lavender in appearance and may resemble normal chromaffin cells. There may be some variation in nuclear shape, and on occasion nuclei can be pleomorphic, with enlarged hyperchromatic forms. This finding by itself does not indicate malignancy. Intracytoplasmic hyaline glob-

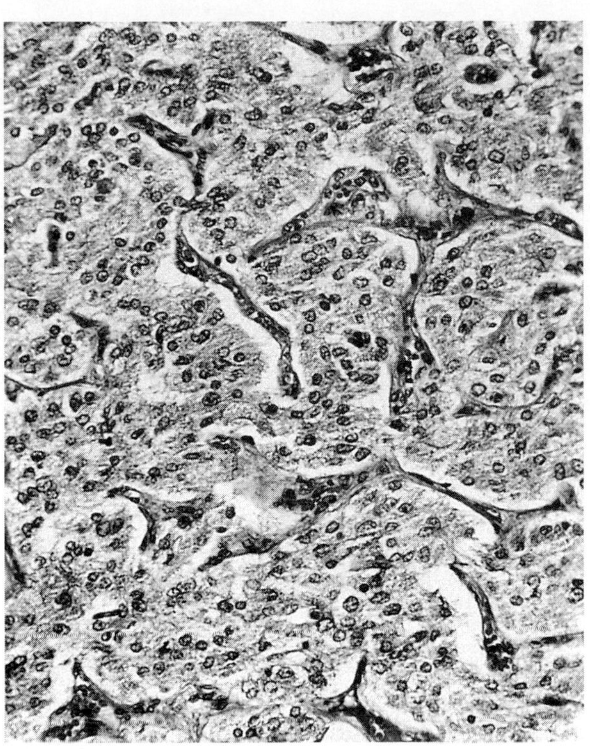

Fig. 63-32 Pheochromocytoma has anastomosing cell cord (or trabecular) pattern with prominent microvasculature. Cell borders are relatively indistinct, and nuclei are haphazardly arranged.

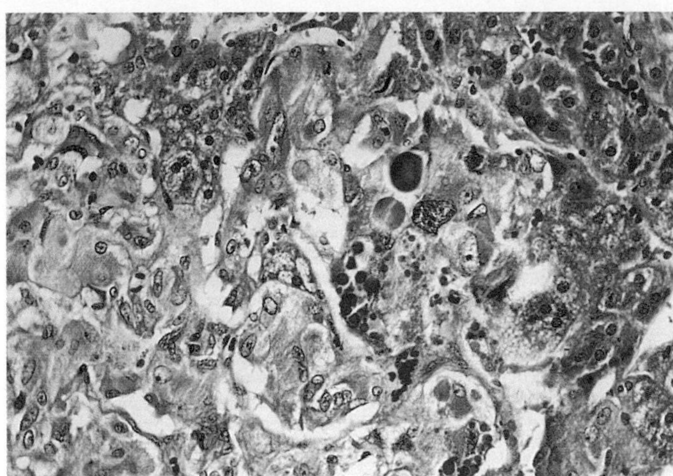

Fig. 63-33 Pheochromocytoma. Eosinophilic hyaline globules are numerous in this field and appear as round to oval intracytoplasmic structures.

ules have been observed in about 45% of pheochromocytomas;[16,168,172] in some tumors the globules are numerous, but in most cases they are difficult to find on casual inspection. These globules are eosinophilic, PAS positive, and resistant to diastase predigestion (Fig. 63-33). Nuclear pseudoinclusions have been seen in approximately one third of pheochromocytomas, and represent invaginations of cell cytoplasm into the nucleus. Periadrenal brown fat has also been noted in association with pheochromocytomas and has been related to catecholamine secretion by tumor with activation of depots of fetal (brown) fat. Some studies have cast doubt on the presence of this finding in pheochromocytomas.[173]

Pheochromocytomas may contain scattered neuronal cells or ganglion cells. Composite pheochromocytomas have morphologic features of both pheochromocytoma and other elements resembling neuroblastoma, ganglioneuroblastoma, or ganglioneuroma.[15,16,174,175] Composite pheochromocytomas accounted for less than 5% of all sympathoadrenal paragangliomas (including pheochromocytomas) seen at the National Cancer Institute.[15,16] These composite tumors with features of both neural and endocrine cells recall the phenotype of cells grown in vitro and the close relationship between the nervous system and the endocrine system. Rarely, these composite tumors have been associated with a watery diarrhea syndrome related to vasoactive intestinal peptide (VIP) secretion.[174] A rare example of composite pheochromocytoma and malignant peripheral nerve sheath tumor has also been reported.[168]

Ultrastructure. The hallmark of pheochromocytomas is the presence of dense-core neurosecretory granules, which usually range in diameter from 150 to 250 nm (Fig. 63-34, *A*). In contrast to normal chromaffin cells, which contain predominantly epinephrine, pheochromocytomas are rich in norepinephrine. These granules have a prominent eccentric membrane-bound space adjacent to the dense core (Fig. 63-34, *B*).[176] A more uniform ultrastructural morphology has been associated with biochemically "pure" epinephrine-secreting tumors in which granules lack the prominent electron-lucent halo.[176] The morphology of the dense-core granules may vary considerably, and given the broad array of regulatory peptides and hormones that can be localized within individual neoplastic cells, it becomes very difficult to associate one particular granule morphology with any particular secretory product.

Immunohistochemistry. Neoplastic cells of pheochromocytoma typically bind antibodies to neuroendocrine substances such as neuron-specific enolase, chromogranin (Fig. 63-35), and synaptophysin. They can also demonstrate positive immunostaining for a broad array of other regulatory peptides and hormones.[177] For the most part, these regulatory peptides and hormones have no known functional significance when expressed within neoplastic cells. There are important exceptions, however, such as the unusual pheochromocytoma associated with ectopic production of ACTH and development of Cushing's syndrome. Another rare occurrence is the pheochromocytoma that secretes VIP, causing a watery diarrhea syndrome, referred to as the Verner-Morrison syndrome, or WDHA (watery diarrhea, hypokalemia, achlorhydria), syndrome. Immunohistochemical demonstration of neuroendocrine markers, such as chromogranin A, can provide valuable diagnostic information, particularly when the tumor has unusual features, or morphologically simulates another type of neoplasm such as an adrenocortical tumor. As noted, hyaline globules are seen in a significant proportion of pheochromocytomas, though in about 10% of cases they may also be identified within adrenocortical neoplasms.[159] Another cell type that has been noted in pheochromocytoma is the sustentacular cell, which is apparent at the periphery of nests and cords of neoplastic chromaffin cells and is usually readily demonstrated in sections stained for S-100 protein.

Fine-needle aspiration. Although a variety of adrenal masses discovered incidentally during examination using abdominal imaging studies have been aspirated for diagnostic purposes, it is unusual, based on cases reported in the litera-

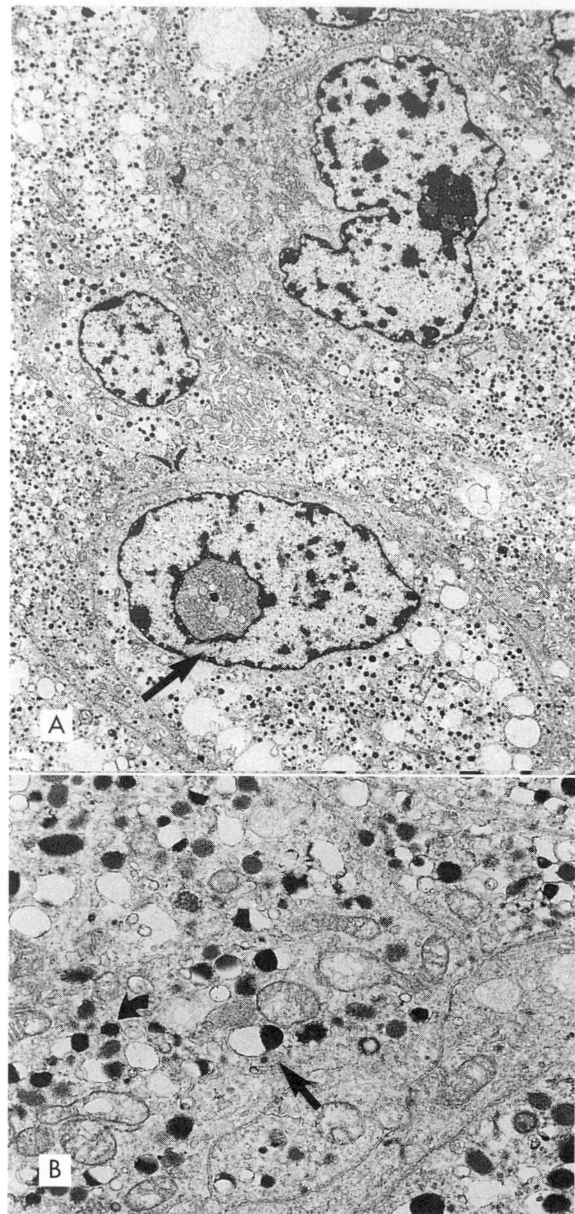

Fig. 63-34 **A,** Pheochromocytoma. Tumor cells contain abundant dense-core neurosecretory granules and show some interdigitation of cytoplasmic processes. Nucleus near bottom has irregular folding of membrane; nucleus of tumor cell near top of field has "pseudoinclusion" *(arrow)* caused by invagination of cell cytoplasm. **B,** Dense-core neurosecretory granules vary in size and shape; some have eccentric core and wide halo, which has been associated with norepinephrine storage *(straight arrow),* whereas others are more symmetric, with close investment by limiting membrane (epinephrine type, *curved arrow*).

ture, for pheochromocytomas. Several reports have underscored the potential danger for such a procedure because of the possibility of a catecholamine crisis or hemorrhagic complications with fatal outcome.[178,179] Interpretation of cytologic findings in a fine-needle aspiration of a pheochromocytoma may be a problem; the presence of irregular hyperchromatic nuclei may invite misinterpretation as a malignant tumor or a mistaken diagnosis of another neoplasm altogether.

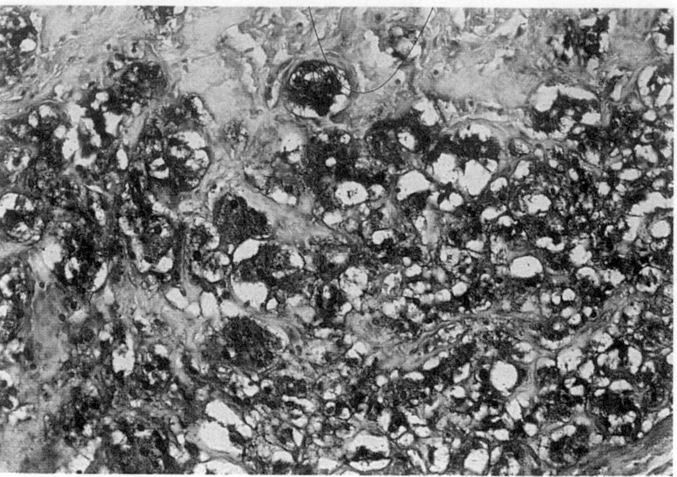

Fig. 63-35 Pheochromocytoma. Positive immunostain for chromogranin, a good neuroendocrine tumor marker, is evidenced by deep red reaction product within cytoplasm of tumor cells. Staining reaction accentuates the nesting and trabecular arrangement of tumor cells.

Prognostic factors and biologic behavior. The incidence of clinically malignant pheochromocytomas reported in the literature varies considerably. A large literature review reported a 2.8% malignancy rate in adults and 2.4% in children.[180] In more recent series, the reported rate of malignancy ranged from 7% to 14%.[16,181] The data can be skewed in series that include extra-adrenal paragangliomas because these tumors tend to have a clinically higher rate of malignancy.[16,168] Aside from documented metastases, it is notoriously difficult to render a reliable prediction of biologic behavior based on histopathologic features alone.[15] The most frequent sites of regional or distant metastases are liver, lymph nodes, lung, and bone; rarely, the initial manifestation may be that of an isolated lytic bone metastasis.[16] Quantitative determination of nuclear DNA content, either by flow cytometry or static image analysis, has permitted retrospective evaluation of pheochromocytomas for features that may be associated with malignancy, but the reported findings are not uniform.[16,168]

NEUROBLASTOMA AND GANGLIONEUROBLASTOMA

Incidence and location of tumors. Neuroblastoma is the most common malignancy in infants under the age of 1 year. In the pediatric age group it is second only to central nervous system malignancies in frequency of solid tumors.[168,182,183] The peak age at presentation is 2 years, and over half are diagnosed before 1 year of age. The incidence of neuroblastoma is 9.6 per million population per year, with about 500 new patients diagnosed yearly in the United States.[182] Neuroblastoma and ganglioneuroblastoma are basically tumors of the sympathetic nervous system. The distribution of primary sites of neuroblastoma based on 118 patients reported from the Dana Farber Institute is abdominal in 68% of cases (adrenal gland 38%, nonadrenal gland 30%), chest 20%, pelvis 3.4%, neck 3.4%, and unknown 5%.[184]

Clinical features. The child with adrenal neuroblastoma may have a firm abdominal mass or other nonspecific findings.

The staging system for neuroblastoma proposed by Evans and associates[185,186] continues to be used in many treatment centers, and recently an international staging system has been proposed.[187] Table 63-1 shows the current mortalities for patients with different-stage tumors.[188] Approximately two thirds of children with neuroblastoma have metastatic disease at presentation,[182] and features commonly noted are irritability, anorexia, fever, bone pain, and orbital metastases. The orbital involvement may be manifest by ecchymotic discoloration of soft tissues or proptosis, and it may be asymmetric in its presentation. On occasion a child may have widespread blue-gray, mobile nodules of cutaneous and subcutaneous metastatic neuroblastoma. Occasionally, children have severe watery diarrhea caused by VIP production by the tumor, and in other cases a paraneoplastic syndrome of opsoclonus with myoclonus may be present. Familial occurrence of neuroblastoma has also been noted and in some studies indicates a possible autosomal-dominant pattern of inheritance.[182] A subset of children with neuroblastoma have stage IVS disease,[189] which accounts for about 10% of childhood neuroblastoma and is usually diagnosed under 1 year of age. These children would ordinarily be stage I or stage II, but they have remote tumors confined to blood, skin, or bone marrow, without radiographic evidence of bone metastases. Despite this remarkable tumor burden, these patients have a very good prognosis (>80% survival[188] despite minimal or no treatment.[190,191]

Gross pathologic features. Adrenal neuroblastoma may appear as a discrete, small ovoid mass or a large multinodular tumor with apparent complete overgrowth of the underlying gland.[192] The tumor may invade surrounding tissue, despite the gross impression of encapsulation. On cross sections these tumors often have areas of hemorrhage and necrosis with coarse lobulations and bulging nodules of tumor (Fig. 63-36). The tumor may have a soft, encephaloid consistency. Those tumors showing a greater degree of differentiation or maturation may present foci that are more firm and homogeneous, tan yellow on section. Rarely, a neuroblastoma may become greatly cystic and simulate a simple adrenal cyst or hematoma.

Microscopic pathologic features. Neuroblastoma is the prototypical small, round, blue cell tumor of childhood. Varied morphologic patterns form a continuum from an undifferentiated neuroblastoma to ganglioneuroblastoma, which can show a high degree of differentiation. The tumor often has an ill-defined lobular pattern with thin fibrovascular septa, and individual cells may be separated by pale fibrillary material. This fibrillary material represents neuritic processes, which may be oriented around preformed vascular or connective tissue structures or may form the center of Homer Wright rosettes (Fig. 63-37). Homer Wright rosettes are the most characteristic features of neuroblastoma. Sometimes the matted fibrillar matrix may be more extensive and has been likened to neuropil of the central nervous system. Undifferentiated neuroblasts have ovoid to rounded nuclei with a stippled chromatin pattern; this is seen to best advantage in fresh touch imprints or smears of tumors (Fig. 63-38). As differentiation or maturation proceeds the neoplastic cells come to have neuronal or ganglion-like features, with more distinct cell borders, heightened eosinophilia of cell cytoplasm, and eccentric nuclei sometimes with a prominent nucleolus. In ganglioneuroblastoma there is clear cut ganglion cell differentiation. The age-linked classification system of Shimada and associates[193] is useful for establishing favorable and unfavorable histologic groups.[193,194] This classification system has the important feature of distinguish-

Table 63-1 International staging system for working party

Stage	Incidence (%)	Survival (%) at 5 years
I	5	≥90
IIa	10	70 to 80
IIb	10	
III	25	40 to 70 (depending on completeness of surgical resection)
IV	60	>60 (if <1 yr) 20 (if 1-2 yr) 10 (if >2 yr)
IVS	5	>80

Modified from Philip T: *Am J Pediatr Hematol/Oncol* 14:97, 1992.

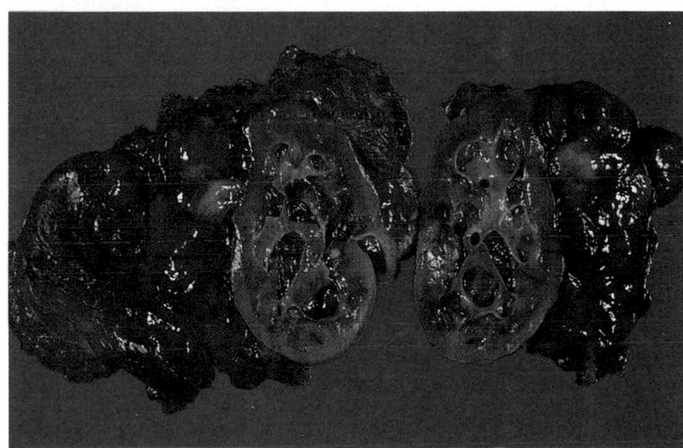

Fig. 63-36 Neuroblastoma involves adrenal and para-adrenal area. Tumor is lobulated and hemorrhagic and has a soft encephaloid consistency on gross examination. Kidney has been resected in continuity with tumor and has been bivalved in the coronal plane.

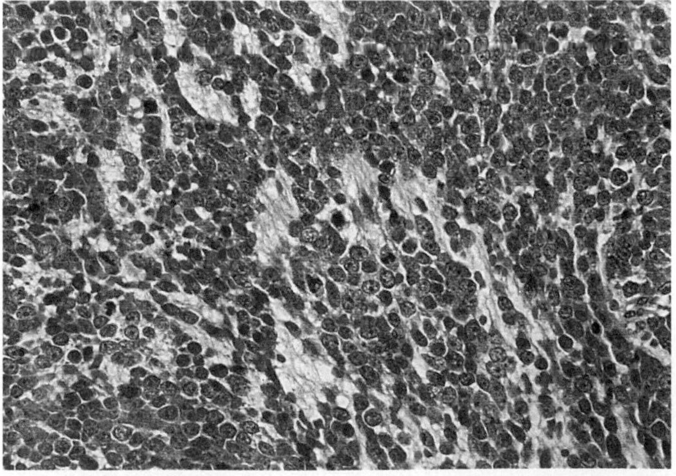

Fig. 63-37 Neuroblastoma. Tumor is composed of sheets of closely packed cells interrupted by irregular areas of pale fibrillar material representing Homer Wright rosettes.

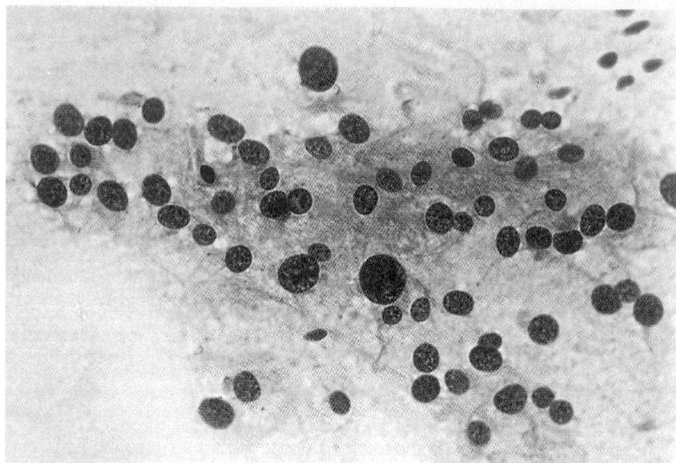

Fig. 63-38 Neuroblastoma. Imprint/smear shows cytologic detail. Nuclei have stippled, "salt-and-pepper" nuclear chromatin pattern. Nuclei are separated by pale fibrillar material representing poorly defined neuritic cell processes.

ing the character of the stromal component within the tumor. "Stroma-poor" tumors contain a variable proportion of fibrillar pink matrix (in some cases little to none can be found), and "stroma-rich" tumors contain an abundant spindle cell (or schwannian) matrix. In the stroma-rich group of tumors three subcategories are recognized: *well-differentiated* and *intermixed,* which fall into the favorable histologic subgroup and *nodular,* which corresponds to "composite ganglioneuroblastoma," a term introduced by Stout[195] in an early review of ganglioneuromas of the sympathetic nervous system. This latter group falls into the unfavorable histologic subgroup. Age enters as a distinguishing characteristic for the stroma-poor tumors, and in this category unfavorable histologic tumors can be separated out based on the combination of age at diagnosis, proportion of differentiating elements, and a derived morphologic finding in terms of the mitosis karyorrhexis index. Using this classification system, the good prognosis group of tumors include the favorable stroma-poor tumors and the well-differentiated and intermixed stroma-rich tumors (87% survival), and the poor prognosis group includes the unfavorable stroma-poor tumors and the nodular stroma-rich tumors (7% survival).[193] Newer classifications and terminology of childhood neuroblastoma have appeared.[196,197]

Ultrastructure. The fibrillary matrix of neuroblastomas and ganglioneuroblastomas consists of a tangled skein of neuritic cell processes that contain arrays of microtubules and intermediate filaments. An important diagnostic feature is the presence of small, dense-core neurosecretory granules, which may be very sparse (Fig. 63-39).

Immunohistochemistry. Four useful immunohistochemical markers for neuroblastomas are neuron-specific enolase, synaptophysin, chromogranin, and neurofilament proteins. These findings alone are not diagnostic of neuroblastoma but must be correlated with light microscopic morphology and clinical findings. Cells showing the presence of S-100 protein can often be identified near delicate fibrovascular septa, a location that is remarkably similar for sustentacular cells of pheochromocytomas. In a recent study of tumors designated as undifferentiated neuroblastoma, tumors with positive to intensely positive staining for S-100 protein seemed to have a better prognosis.[198] In cases of ganglioneuroblastoma associated with the watery diarrhea syndrome it is possible to identify cells that are immunoreactive for VIP, and increased levels of this neuropeptide (and also somatostatin) have been correlated with cellular differentiation.[199]

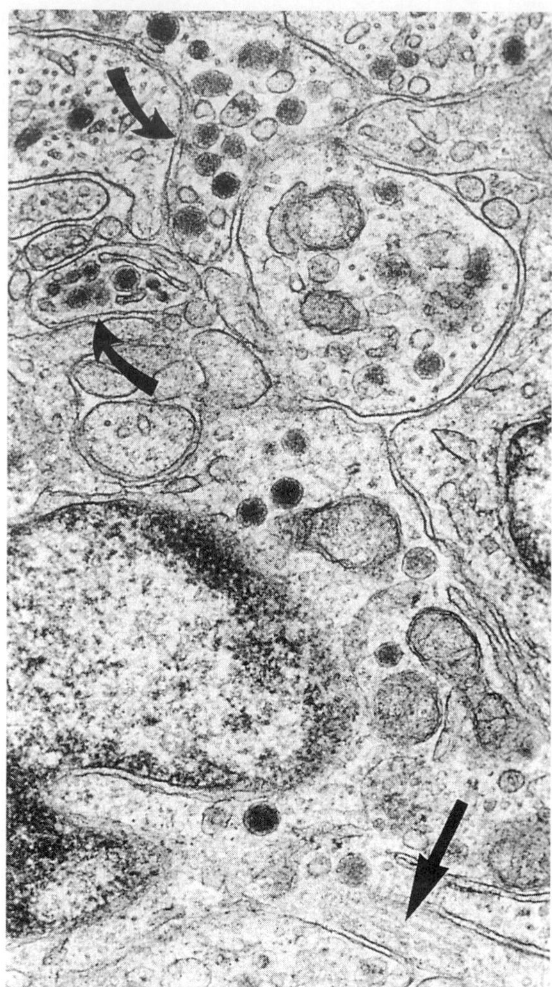

Fig. 63-39 Neuroblastoma shows complex intertwining of neuritic cell processes, which corresponds to the pale fibrillary matrix that forms the center of Homer Wright rosettes. Microtubules are present within cytoplasmic processes *(straight arrow)* along with neurosecretory type of granules *(curved arrows).*

Prognostic factors and biologic behavior. Metastases of neuroblastoma occur by both lymphatic and hematogenous routes, with the most frequent site being bone, especially the cortex of long bones and flat bones. Other sites of metastasis include lymph node, liver, skin, bone marrow, and skull. Metastases to skull and dura may be seen, but separate involvement of brain parenchyma is unusual.[200] Pepper[201] reported a group of infants in the first 6 weeks of life with a small primary tumor yet massive hepatic metastases, and these cases may well be the earliest reports of what is today regarded as stage IVS neuroblastoma. Many nonhistologic factors have an important correlation with prognosis; those that correlate with adverse outcome include older age at diagnosis, advanced stage (except for stage IVS), increased levels of neuron-specific enolase, and serum ferritin[182] and amplification of N-*myc* oncogene expression.[202]

In situ neuroblastoma. In situ neuroblastoma is defined as a distinct tumor nodule composed of immature cells, morphologically indistinguishable from classic childhood neuroblastoma, in which there is neither gross nor microscopic evidence of tumor elsewhere in the body.[203,204] Using these criteria, in situ neuroblastoma was identified in about 1 in every 200 autopsies on infants up to 3 months of age,[203] an incidence much greater than that of clinically overt neuroblastoma. The consensus is that if these lesions are truly neoplastic, most undergo spontaneous regression. The major controversy here is distinguishing incipient malignancy from the small developmental neuroblastic nodules that are an integral part of the normal developmental anatomy of the adrenal glands.[13] Knudson and Meadows[205] regard in situ and stage IVS neuroblastomas as representing hyperplastic lesions lacking a "second hit" or "event."

GANGLIONEUROMA

Anatomic location and clinical features. Ganglioneuroma is a fully differentiated, benign neoplasm that usually arises in the posterior mediastinum with only 10% to 15% of tumors originating primarily in the adrenal glands.[192] The age at diagnosis is usually older than that of children with neuroblastoma or ganglioneuroblastoma. In the study by Bove and McAdams[206] the average age of patients was 7 years (range of 2 to 15 years), and two thirds of the tumors arose in the posterior mediastinum.

Gross pathologic features. The tumors are rubbery, firm, and well circumscribed and on cross section are gray-white to yellowish, without areas of hemorrhage or necrosis. Calcification occurs in some of these tumors, evident on gross or radiographic examination.

Microscopic pathologic features. Ganglioneuroma is essentially an admixture of benign Schwann cells with a variable component of mature ganglion cells (Fig. 63-40). The distribution or density of ganglion cells varies tremendously in these tumors, and some sections may show only a spindle cell component suggestive of schwannoma or neurofibroma. Often the cells are arranged in broad fascicles that intersect in an irregular fashion. Ganglion cells are fully mature and may show conspicuous intracytoplasmic pigment or amorphous material at the periphery of the cell, resembling Nissl substance. Satellite cells can sometimes be observed adjacent to the ganglion cells. Some ganglioneuromas show blunt extensions into adjacent soft tissue. There may also be small clusters of lymphocytes that should not be mistaken for primitive neuroblasts. The identification of less-differentiated histologic features, however, has important prognostic implications. Rare ganglioneuromas have been reported to contain Leydig cells with typical Reinke crystalloids, and one has been associated with virilization.[207,208]

MISCELLANEOUS TUMORS AND TUMORLIKE LESIONS

Adrenal cysts

Adrenal cysts are rare tumefactive lesions common in the fifth to sixth decades of life, with less than 5% occurring in the pediatric age group (rarely congenital).[209] There is a 3:1 female-to-male ratio. Adrenal cysts may produce symptoms from compression of adjacent structures with abdominal pain, a palpable mass, or a variety of gastrointestinal symptoms; these lesions occur equally on either side and are reported to be bilateral in 5% to 8% of cases.

There are four types of adrenal cysts: (1) the common endothelial cysts (45%); (2) adrenal pseudocysts (39%), the most frequent to present clinically as a surgical lesion; (Fig. 63-41).[209] (3) epithelial cysts 9%; and (4) parasitic, which make up about 7% of all cases and are most commonly caused by echinococcal infection The endothelial type of adrenal cyst consists of lymphangiomatous and angiomatous variants. Many of these cysts are encountered incidentally at autopsy. The radiographic appearance of adrenal pseudocysts is characteristic enough that a correct diagnosis can be strongly suspected if the cystic mass has a peripheral rim of calcification. It may be impossible to distinguish this lesion from an adrenal neoplasm with secondary cystic change.

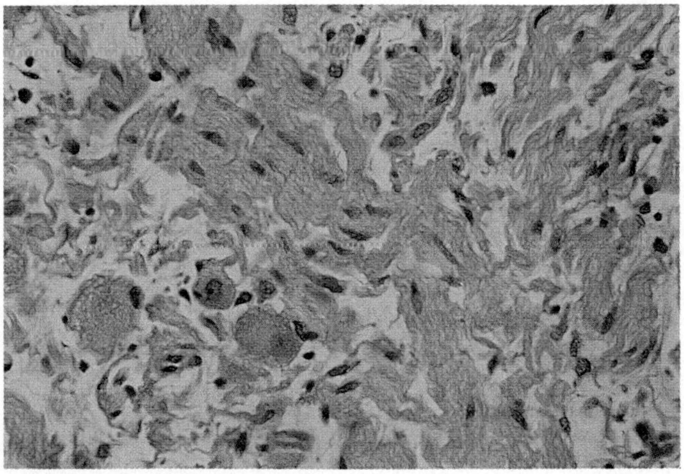

Fig. 63-40 Ganglioneuroma. Tumor has predominant spindle cell histologic features with randomly scattered relatively mature ganglion cells.

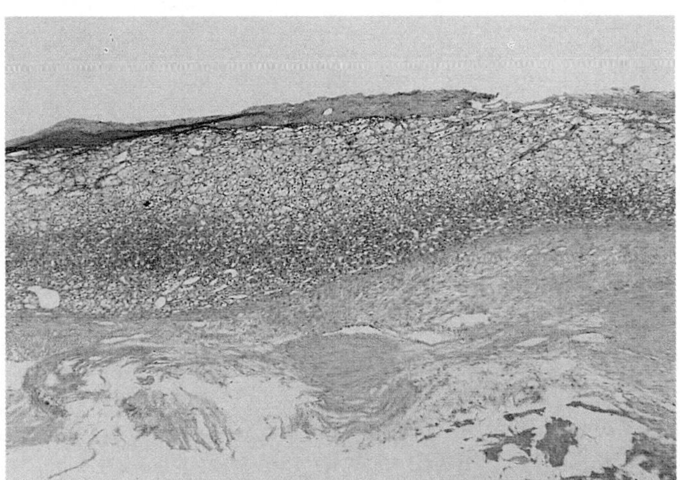

Fig. 63-41 Adrenal pseudocyst. Adrenal mass had an irregular fibrous wall with fibrin-rich material. No epithelial or endothelial lining could be identified.

Adrenal myelolipoma

Myelolipomas occur most commonly in the adrenal gland. Extra-adrenal sites include the mediastinum, perirenal, and presacral areas, as well as the liver and stomach.[209] Most common in the fifth to seventh decades of life, they are unusual under 30 years of age. There is a roughly equal sex predilection. In about half of patients with adrenal myelolipoma the lesion is an incidental finding. With the use of high-resolution CT and ultrasound, adrenal myelolipomas are discovered with increasing incidence. The most common symptoms are abdominal or flank pain followed by hematuria, palpable mass, hypertension, dysuria, or an associated hormonal disorder such as Cushing's syndrome.[209] Myelolipomas are grossly circumscribed. Microscopic sections show that the lesion is sharply demarcated but lacks a capsule. The lesions are usually solitary and unilateral, but this is not always the case. The gross appearance of the lesion on cross section depends on the amount of adipose tissue versus hematopoietic component. If the former predominates, the cut surface is frequently yellow, and the hematopoietic or myeloid constituent may appear red or purple. Adrenal myelolipomas can be large, measuring up to 34 cm in diameter, or the lesion may be discovered incidentally at autopsy and be quite small. Microscopically, myelolipomas consist of hematopoietic elements usually representing all three maturation sequences admixed with mature adipose tissue (Fig. 63-42). Occasionally one can see bony trabeculae.

Malignant lymphoma

Involvement of the adrenal glands by malignant lymphoma has been reported in 18% to 25% of autopsies of patients dying of this disease and is usually a manifestation of wide dissemination.[209] Primary malignant lymphoma of the adrenal gland is rare. In most cases with bilateral involvement of adrenal glands by malignant lymphoma, extra-adrenal disease is also present. Malignant lymphoma involving the adrenal glands may cause enlargement and hypofunction; patients rarely have Addison's disease because of lymphomatous infiltration of the adrenal glands.[62]

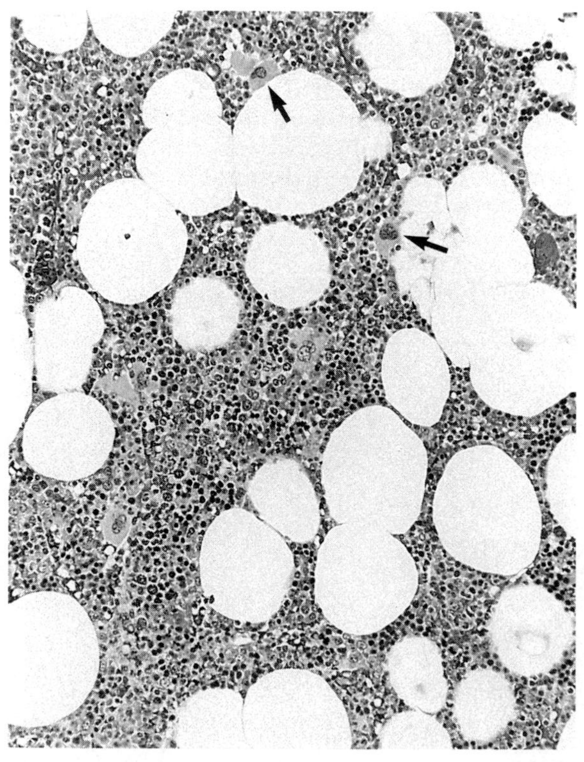

Fig. 63-42 Adrenal myelolipoma is composed of trilinear hematopoietic elements and admixed adipose tissue. Megakaryocytes are indicated by *arrows*.

Malignant melanoma

Adrenal malignant melanoma is usually a manifestation of disseminated disease from a primary cutaneous site. Few primary malignant melanomas of the adrenal gland have been adequately documented. A typical gross appearance of an adrenal malignant melanoma is a brown to jet-black mass, often with areas of hemorrhage and necrosis.[209,210] Tumor cells contain a variable amount of melanin pigment, which contributes to the dark coloration of the tumor grossly. The diagnosis can be supported by a combination of positive staining with the Fontana-Masson silver stain, immunoreactivity with S-100 protein and HMB-45, or ultrastructural identification of premelanosomes or melanosomes. Primary adrenal malignant melanoma enters into the differential diagnosis of pigmented adrenal tumors such as black adenomas.

Primary mesenchymal tumors

Primary mesenchymal tumors are rare. Some of them are vascular in type, including hemangioma and angiosarcoma. Kaposi's sarcoma has been observed secondarily involving the adrenal gland in the setting of AIDS. Adrenal smooth muscle tumors have also been reported, including leiomyoma and leiomyosarcoma.[211] Other rare mesenchymal tumors of the adrenal glands include adenomatoid tumor[212] and Leydig cell tumor.[141,142]

Schwannoma and neurofibroma have been reported arising in the adrenal gland, but they are extremely unusual. Malignant peripheral nerve sheath tumors (malignant schwannoma) can also arise in the adrenal gland, and several examples have been reported in adrenal ganglioneuroma occurring after radiation therapy for childhood neuroblastoma.[168]

METASTATIC TUMORS

The adrenal glands per unit weight are considered to be the organs most frequently involved by tumor metastases, with the most common primary sites being lung and breast.[60] The rich vascular supply of the adrenal glands and the sinusoidal vascularity have been considered to be factors conductive to metastases. Other types of tumor metastatic to the adrenal glands include malignant melanoma, gastric carcinoma, colorectal carcinoma, and renal cell carcinoma.[209] Rarely, metastatic tumor of the adrenal glands may cause clinical adrenal insufficiency with Addison's disease.[61] Bilateral adrenal involvement has been reported in 41% of autopsies of patients with metastatic malignancy involving the adrenal glands.[209] Occasionally, metastatic carcinoma may mimic a primary adrenal tumor. Metastatic large cell undifferentiated carcinoma of the lung and metastatic renal cell carcinoma are examples that can simulate a poorly differentiated adrenal cortical carcinoma, particularly if one is not aware of pertinent historical, clinical, or intraoperative findings.

REFERENCES

Normal adrenals

1. Addison T: *On the constitutional and local effects of disease of the supra-renal capsules,* London, 1855, S. Highley.
2. Crowder R: The development of the adrenal gland in man, with special reference to origin and ultimate location of cell types and evidence in favor of the "cell migration" theory, *Contrib Embryol Carnegie Inst* 36:193, 1957.
3. O'Rahilly R: The timing and sequence of events in the development of the human endocrine system during the embryonic period proper, *Anat Embryol* 166:439, 1983.
4. Lack EE, Kozakewich HPW: Embryology, developmental anatomy, and selected aspects of non-neoplastic pathology. In Lack EE, editor: *Pathology of the adrenal glands,* New York, 1990, Churchill Livingstone.
5. Stoner HB, Whiteley HJ, Emery JL: The effect of systemic disease on the adrenal cortex of the child, *J Pathol Bacteriol* 66:171, 1953.
6. Symington T: *Functional pathology of the human adrenal gland,* Baltimore, 1969, Williams & Wilkins.
7. Quinan C, Berger AA: Observations on human adrenals with especial reference to the relative weight of the normal medulla, *Ann Intern Med* 6:1180, 1933.
8. Studzinsky GP, Hay DCF, Symington T: Observations on the weight of the human adrenal gland and the effect of preparations of corticotropin with different purity on the weight and morphology of the human adrenal gland, *J Clin Endocrinol Metab* 23:248, 1963.
9. Oppenheimer E: Cyst formation in the outer adrenal cortex, *Arch Pathol* 87:653, 1969.
10. Rodin AE, Hsu FL, Whorton EB: Microcysts of the permanent adrenal cortex in perinates and infants, *Arch Pathol Lab Med* 100:499, 1976.
11. Dobbie JW: Adrenocortical nodular hyperplasia: the ageing adrenal, *J Pathol* 99:1, 1969.
12. Hedeland H, Ostberg G, Hokfelt B: On the prevalence of adrenocortical adenomas in an autopsy material in relation to hypertension and diabetes, *Acta Med Scand* 184:211, 1968.
13. Turkel SB, Itabashi HH: The natural history of neuroblastic cells in the fetal adrenal gland, *Am J Pathol* 76:225, 1974.
14. Dekker A, Oehrle JS: Hyaline globules of the adrenal medulla of man, *Arch Pathol* 91:353, 1971.
15. Linnoila RI, Keiser HR, Steinberg SM, Lack EE: Histopathology of benign versus malignant sympathoadrenal paragangliomas: clinicopathologic study of 120 cases including unusual histologic features, *Hum Pathol* 21:1168, 1990.
16. Lack EE: Adrenal medullary hyperplasia and pheochromocytoma. In Lack EE, editor: *Pathology of the adrenal glands,* New York 1990, Churchill Livingstone.
17. Graham LS: Celiac accessory adrenal glands. *Cancer* 6:149, 1953.
18. Falls JL: Accessory adrenal cortex in the broad ligament: Incidence and functional significance, *Cancer* 8:143, 1955.
19. Dahl EV, Bahn RC: Aberrant adrenal cortical tissue near the testis in human infants, *Am J Pathol* 40:587, 1962.
20. Roosen-Runge EC, Lund J: Abnormal sex cord formation and an intra-testicular adrenal cortical nodule in human fetus, *Anat Rec* 173:57, 1972.
21. Symonds DA, Driscoll SG: An adrenal rest within the fetal ovary: report of a case, *Am J Clin Pathol* 60:562, 1973.
22. Dolan MF, Janovski NA: Adreno-hepatic union (adrenal dystopia), *Arch Pathol* 86:22, 1968.

Reactive changes

23. Wilbur OM Jr, Rich AR: A study of the role of adrenocorticotropic hormone (ACTH) in the pathogenesis of tubular degeneration of the adrenals, *Bull Johns Hopkins Hosp* 93:321, 1954.
24. Bartman J, Driscoll SG: Fetal adrenal cortex in erythroblastosis fetalis, *Arch Pathol* 87:343, 1969.
25. Sommers SC, Carter ME: Adrenocortical postirradiation fibrosis, *Arch Pathol* 99:421, 1975.
26. Craig JM, Landing BH: Anaplastic cells of fetal adrenal cortex, *Am J Clin Pathol* 21:940, 1951.
27. Oppenheimer EH: Adrenal cytomegaly: studies by light and electron microscopy: comparison with the adrenal in Beckwith's and virilism syndromes, *Arch Pathol* 90:57, 1970.
28. Beckwith JB: Extreme cytomegaly of the adrenal fetal cortex, omphalocele, hyperplasia of kidneys and pancreas, and Leydig-cell hyperplasia—another syndrome? Paper presented at the annual meeting of the Western Society for Pediatric Research, Los Angeles, Calif., Nov. 11, 1963.
29. Wiedemann HR: Complexe malformatif familial avec hernie ombilicale et macroglossie, un "syndrome nouveau," *J Genet Hum* 13:223, 1964.
30. Pettenati MJ, Haines JL, Higgins RR et al: Wiedemann-Beckwith syndrome: presentation of clinical and cytogenetic data on 22 new cases and review of the literature, *Hum Genet* 74:143, 1986.
31. Beckwith JB: Macroglossia, omphalocele, adrenal cytomegaly, gigantism and hyperplastic visceromegaly, *Birth Defects* 5:188, 1969.
32. Wiedemann HR: Tumours and hemihypertrophy associated with Wiedemann-Beckwith syndrome, *Eur J Pediatr* 141:129, 1983.

Congenital and hereditary adrenocortical disorders

33. Benirschke K: Adrenals in anencephaly and hydrocelphaly, *Obstet Gynecol* 8:412, 1956.
34. Reed GB, Claireaux AE, Bain AD: *Diseases of the fetus and newborn; pathology, radiology, and genetics,* St. Louis, 1989, Mosby.
35. Jaffe R, Crumvine P, Hoshida Y et al: Neonatal adrenoleukodystrophy: clinical, pathologic and biochemical delineation of a syndrome affecting both males and females, *Am J Pathol* 108:100, 1982.
36. Powers JM, Moser HW, Moser, AB et al: Pathologic findings in adrenoleukodystrophy heterozygotes, *Arch Pathol Lab Med* 111:151, 1987.
37. Prader A, Zachmann M, Illig R: Luteinizing hormone deficiency in hereditary congenital adrenal hypoplasia, *J Pediatr* 86:421, 1975.
38. Hay ID, Smail PJ, Forsyth CC: Familial cytomegalic adrenocortical hypoplasia: an X-linked syndrome of pubertal failure, *Arch Dis Child* 56:715, 1981.
39. Martin MM, Martin ALA: The syndrome of congenital hereditary adrenal hypoplasia and hypogonadotropic hypogonadism, *Int J Adolesc Med Health* 1:119, 1985.
40. Shephard TH, Landing BH, Mason DC: Familial Addison's disease: case report of two sisters with corticoid deficiency unassociated with hypoaldosteronism, *Am J Dis Child* 97:154, 1959.
41. Lamberts SWJ, Koper JW, Biemond P et al: Cortisol receptor resistance: the variability of its clinical presentation and response to treatment. *J Clin Endocrinol Metab* 74:313, 1992.
42. Yamaoka T, Kudo T, Takuwa Y et al: Hereditary adrenocortical unresponsiveness to adrenocorticotropin with a postreceptor defect, *J Clin Endocrinol Metab* 75:270, 1992.
43. Hudson JB, Chobanian AV, Relman AS: Hypoaldosteronism: a clinical study of a patient with an isolated adrenal mineralocorticoid deficiency, resulting in hyperkalemia and Stokes-Adams attacks, *N Engl J Med* 257:529, 1957.
44. White PC, New MI, Dupont B: Congenital adrenal hyperplasia, *N Engl J Med* 316:1519, 1987.
45. Bauman A, Bauman CG: Virilizing adrenocortical carcinoma: development in a patient with salt-losing congenital adrenal hyperplasia, *JAMA* 248: 3140, 1982.
46. Boudreaux D, Waisman J, Skinner DG, Law R: Giant adrenal myelolipoma and testicular interstitial cell tumor in a man with congenital 21-hydroxylase deficiency, *Am J Surg Pathol* 3:109, 1979.
47. Condom E, Villabona CM, Gómez JM, Carrera M: Adrenal myelolipoma in a woman with congenital 17-hydroxylase deficiency, *Arch Pathol Lab Med* 109:1116, 1985.
48. Rutgers JL, Young RH, Scully RE: The testicular "tumor" of the adrenogenital syndrome: a report of six cases and review of the literature on testicular masses in patients with adrenocortical disorders, *Am J Surg Pathol* 12:503, 1988.
49. Kirkland RT, Kirkland JL, Keenan BS et al: Bilateral testicular tumors in congenital adrenal hyperplasia, *J Clin Endocrinol Metab* 44:369, 1977.
50. Radfar N, Bartter FC, Easley R et al: Evidence for endogenous LH suppression in a man with bilateral testicular tumors and congenital adrenal hyperplasia, *J Clin Endocrinol Metab* 45:1194, 1977.

51. Johnson RE, Scheithauer B: Massive hyperplasia of testicular adrenal rests in a patient with Nelson's syndrome, *Am J Clin Pathol* 77:501, 1982.
52. Verdonk C, Guerin C, Lufkin E, Hodgson SF: Activation of virilizing adrenal rest tissue by excessive ACTH production: an unusual presentation of Nelson's syndrome, *Am J Med* 73:455, 1982.

Adrenocortical insufficiency

53. Ahonen P, Myllarniemi S, Sipila I, Perheentupa J: Clinical variation of autoimmune polyendocrine-candidiasis-ectodermal dystrophy (APECED) in a series of 68 patients, *N Engl J Med* 322:1829, 1990.
54. Neufeld M, Maclaren NK, Blizzard RM: Two types of autoimmune Addison's disease associated with different polyglandular autoimmune (PGA) syndromes, *Medicine* 60:355, 1981.
55. Schmidt, MB: Eine biglanduläre Erkrankung (Nebennieren und Schilddrüse) bei morbus Addisonii, *Dtsch Pathol Ges* 21:212, 1926.
56. Guttman PH: Addison's disease: a statistical analysis of five hundred and sixty-six cases and a study of the pathology, *Arch Pathol* 10:742, 1930.
57. Dunlop D: Eighty-six cases of Addison's disease, *Br Med J* 5362:887, 1963.
58. Durairaj V, Radhabai K, Alagappan R et al: Adrenal cortical function and reserve in lepromatous leprosy, *Indian J Lepr* 56:828, 1984.
59. Goodwin RA Jr, Shapiro JL, Thurman GH et al: Disseminated histoplasmosis: clinical and pathologic correlations, *Medicine* 59:1, 1980.
60. Abrams HL, Spiro R, Goldstein N: Metastases in carcinoma: analysis of 1000 autopsied cases, *Cancer* 3:74, 1950.
61. Kung AWC, Pun KK, Lam K et al: Addisonian crises as presenting feature in malignancies. *Cancer* 65:177, 1990.
62. Serrano S, Tejedor L, García, B et al: Addisonian crises as the presenting feature of bilateral primary adrenal lymphoma, *Cancer* 71:4030, 1993.
63. Donovan DS Jr, Dluhy RG: AIDS and its effect on the adrenal gland, *Endocrinologist* 1:227, 1991.
64. Grinspoon SK, Bilezikian JP: HIV disease and the endocrine system, *N Engl J Med* 327:1360, 1992.
65. Rotterdam H, Dembitzer F: The adrenal glands in AIDS, *Endocr Pathol* 4:4, 1993.
66. Klatt EC, Shibata D: Cytomegalovirus infection in the acquired immunodeficiency syndrome: clinical and autopsy findings, *Arch Pathol Lab Med* 112:540, 1988.
67. Pulakhandam U, Dincsoy HP: Cytomegaloviral adrenalitis and adrenal insufficiency in AIDS, *Am J Clin Pathol* 93:651, 1990.
68. Cote RJ, Rosenblum M, Telzak EE et al: Disseminated *Pneumocystis carinii* infection causing extrapulmonary organ failure: clinical, pathologic, and immunohistochemical analysis, *Mod Pathol* 3:25, 1990.
69. Hass GM: Hepato-adrenal necrosis with intranuclear inclusion bodies: report of a case, *Am J Pathol* 11:127, 1935.
70. Singer DB: Pathology of neonatal herpes simplex virus infection, *Perspect Pediatr Pathol* 6:243, 1981.
71. Siu SCB, Kitzman DW, Sheedy PF II, Northcutt RC: Adrenal insufficiency from bilateral adrenal hemorrhage, *Mayo Clin Proc* 65:664, 1990.
72. Abramov A, Schorr S, Wolman M: Generalized xanthomatosis with calcified adrenals, *J Dis Child* 91:282, 1956.
73. Crocker AC, Vawter GF, Neuhauser EBD: Wolman's disease: three new patients with a recently described lipidosis, *Pediatrics* 36:627, 1963.
74. Reed RJ, Patrick JT: Nodular hyperplasia of the adrenal cortical blastema, *Bull Tulane Univ Med Fac* 26:151, 1967.
75. Wong TW, Warner NE: Ovarian thecal metaplasia in the adrenal gland, *Arch Pathol* 92:319, 1971.
76. Fidler WJ: Ovarian thecal metaplasia in adrenal glands, *Am J Clin Pathol* 67:318, 1977.
77. Carney JA: Unusual tumefactive spindle cell lesions in the adrenal glands, *Hum Pathol* 18:980, 1987.
78. Orselli RC, Bassler TJ: Theca granulosa cell tumor arising in adrenal, *Cancer* 31:474, 1973.

Cortical hyperplasia and adrenocortical hyperfunction

79. Lack EE, Travis WD, Oertel JE: Adrenal cortical nodules, hyperplasia, and hyperfunction. In Lack EE, editor: *Pathology of the adrenal glands,* New York, 1990, Churchill Livingstone.
80. Shamma AH, Goddard JW, Sommers SC: A study of the adrenal status in hypertension, *J Chronic Dis* 8:587, 1958.
81. Russi S, Blumenthal HT, Gray SH: Small adenomas of the adrenal cortex in hypertension and diabetes, *Arch Intern Med* 76:284, 1945.
82. Commons RR, Callaway CP: Adenomas of the adrenal cortex, *Arch Intern Med* 81:37, 1948.
83. Spain DM, Weinsaft P: Solitary adrenal cortical adenoma in elderly female: frequency, *Arch Pathol* 78:231, 1964.
84. Neville AM: The nodular adrenal, *Invest Cell Pathol* 1:99, 1978.
85. Dobbie JW: Adrenocortical nodular hyperplasia: the aging adrenal, *J Pathol* 99:1, 1969.
86. Glazer HS, Weyman PJ, Sagel SS et al: Non-functioning adrenal masses: incidental discovery on computed tomography, *AJR* 139:81, 1982.
87. Abecassis M, McLoughlin MJ, Langer B et al: Serendipitous adrenal masses: prevalence, significance and management, *Am J Surg* 149:783, 1985.
88. Francis IR, Smid A, Gross MD et al: Adrenal masses in oncologic patients: functional and morphologic evaluation, *Radiology* 166:353, 1988.
89. Robinson MJ, Pardo V, Rywlin AM: Pigmented nodules (black adenomas) of the adrenal: an autopsy study of incidence, morphology and function, *Hum Pathol* 3:317, 1972.
90. Damron TA, Schelper RL, Sorensen L: Cytochemical demonstration of neuromelanin in black pigmented adrenal nodules, *Am J Clin Pathol* 87:334, 1987.
91. Carpenter PC: Cushing's syndrome: update of diagnosis and management, *Mayo Clin Proc* 61:49, 1986.
92. Case Records of the Massachusetts General Hospital: Case 46-1988, *N Engl J Med* 319:1336, 1988.
93. Roubidoux M, Dunnick NR: Adrenal cortical tumors, *Bull NY Acad Med* 67:119, 1991.
94. Ross NS, Aron DC: Hormonal evaluation of the patient with an incidentally discovered adrenal mass, *N Engl J Med* 323:1401, 1990.
95. Bravo EL: Pheochromocytoma: new concepts and future trends, *Kidney Int* 40:544, 1991.
96. Doppman JL, Reinig JW, Dwyer AJ et al: Differentiation of adrenal masses by magnetic resonance imaging, *Surgery* 102:1018, 1987.
97. Case Records of the Massachusetts General Hospital: Case 6-1991, *N Engl J Med* 324:400, 1991.

Cushing's syndrome

98. Orth DN, Liddle GW: Results of treatment in 108 patients with Cushing's syndrome, *N Engl J Med* 285:243, 1971.
99. Gold EM: The Cushing syndrome: changing views of diagnosis and treatment, *Ann Intern Med* 90:829, 1979.
100. Thomas CG Jr, Smith AT, Griffith J et al: Hyperadrenalism in childhood and adolescence, *Ann Surg* 199:538, 1984.
101. Cushing H: The basophil adenomas of the pituitary body and their clinical manifestations (pituitary basophilism), *Bull Johns Hopkins Hosp* 50:137, 1932.
102. Neville AM, Symington T: The pathology of the adrenal gland in Cushing's syndrome, *J Pathol Bacteriol* 93:19, 1967.
103. Smals AGH, Pieters GFFM, van Haelst UJG et al: Macronodular adrenocortical hyperplasia in longstanding Cushing's disease, *J Clin Endocrinol Metab* 58:25, 1984.
104. Carney JA, Young WF Jr: Primary pigmented nodular adrenocortical disease and its associated conditions, *Endocrinologist* 2:6, 1992.
105. Doppman JL, Travis WD, Nieman L et al: Cushing syndrome due to primary pigmented nodular adrenocortical disease: findings at CT and MR imaging, *Radiology* 172:415, 1989.
106. Shenoy BV, Carpenter PC, Carney JA: Bilateral primary pigmented nodular adrenocortical disease: rare cause of the Cushing syndrome, *Am J Surg Pathol* 8:335, 1984.
107. Travis WD, Tsokos M, Doppman JL et al: Primary pigmented nodular adrenocortical disease: a light and electron microscopic study of eight cases, *Am J Surg Pathol* 13:921, 1989.
108. Larsen JL, Cathey WJ, Odell WD: Primary adrenocortical nodular dysplasia, a distinct subtype of Cushing's syndrome: case report and review of the literature, *Am J Med* 80:976, 1986.

109. Danoff A, Jormark S, Lorber D, Fleischer N: Adrenocortical micronodular dysplasia, cardiac myxomas, lentigines, and spindle cell tumors, *Arch Intern Med* 147:443, 1987.
110. Wulffraat NM, Drexhage HA, Wiersinga WM et al: Immunoglobulins of patients with Cushing's syndrome due to pigmented adrenocortical micronodular dysplasia stimulate *in vitro* steroidogenesis. *J Clin Endocrinol Metab* 66:301, 1988.
111. Van Berkhout FT, Croughs RJM, Wulffraat NM, Drexhage HA: Familial Cushing's syndrome due to nodular adrenocortical dysplasia is an inherited disease of immunoglobulin origin, *Clin Endocrinol* 31:185, 1989.
112. Young WF Jr, Carney JA, Musa BU et al: Familial Cushing's syndrome due to primary pigmented nodular adrenocortical disease: reinvestigation 50 years later, *N Engl J Med* 321:1659, 1989.
113. Proppe KH, Scully RE: Large-cell calcifying Sertoli cell tumor of the testis, *Am J Clin Pathol* 74:607, 1980.
114. Carney JA, Gordon H, Carpenter PC et al: The complex of myxomas, spotty pigmentation, and endocrine overactivity, *Medicine* 64:270, 1985.
115. Carney JA: Psammomatous melanotic schwannoma: a distinctive, heritable tumor with special associations, including cardiac myxoma and the Cushing syndrome, *Am J Surg Pathol* 14:206, 1990.
116. Carney JA, Hruska LS, Beauchamp GD, Gordon H: Dominant inheritance of the complex of myxomas, spotty pigmentation, and endocrine overactivity, *Mayo Clin Proc* 61:165, 1986.
117. Aiba M, Hirayama A, In H et al: Adrenocorticotropic hormone–independent bilateral adrenocortical macronodular hyperplasia as a distinct subtype of Cushing's syndrome: enzyme histochemical and ultrastructural study of four cases with a review of the literature, *Am J Clin Pathol* 96:334, 1991.
118. Kirschner MA, Powell RD Jr, Lipsett MB: Cushing's syndrome: nodular cortical hyperplasia of adrenal glands with clinical and pathological features suggesting adrenocrotical tumor, *J Clin Endocrinol* 24:947, 1964.
119. Doppman JL, Nieman LK, Travis WD et al: CT and MR imaging of massive macronodular adrenocortical disease: a rare cause of autonomous primary adrenal hypercortisolism, *J Comput Assist Tomogr* 15:773, 1991.
120. Hermus AR, Pieters GF, Smals AG et al: Transition from pituitary-dependent to adrenal-dependent Cushing's syndrome, *N Engl J Med* 318:966, 1988.

MEN type 1

121. Ballard HS, Frame B, Hartsock RJ: Familial multiple endocrine adenoma–peptic ulcer complex, *Medicine* 43:481, 1964.
122. Miyagawa K, Ishibashi M, Kasuga M et al: Multiple endocrine neoplasia type I with Cushing's disease, primary hyperparathyroidism and insulin-glucagonoma, *Cancer* 61:1232, 1988.
123. Scheithauer BW, Laws ER Jr, Kovacs K et al: Pituitary adenomas of the multiple endocrine neoplasia type I syndrome, *Semin Diagn Pathol* 4:205, 1987.

Hyperaldosteronism

124. Conn JW: Primary aldosteronism: a new clinical syndrome, *J Lab Clin Med* 45:6, 1955.
125. Lifton RP, Dluhy RG, Powers M et al: A chimaeric 11-beta-hydroxylase/aldosterone synthase gene causes glucocorticoid-remediable aldosteronism and human hypertension, *Nature* 355:262, 1992.
126. Neville AM, Symington T: Pathology of primary aldosteronism, *Cancer* 19:1854, 1966.
127. Carey RM, Sen S, Dolan LM et al: Idiopathic hyperaldosteronism: a possible role for aldosterone-stimulating factor, *N Engl J Med* 311:94, 1984.
128. Hawkins E, Singer DB: The adrenal cortex in cystic fibrosis of the pancreas, *Am J Clin Pathol* 66:710, 1976.

Adrenocortical neoplasms

129. Lack EE, Travis WD, Oertel JE: Adrenal cortical tumors. In Lack EE, editor: *Pathology of the adrenal glands,* New York, 1990, Churchill Livingstone.
130. Neville AM, Symington T: The pathology of the adrenal gland in Cushing's syndrome, *J Pathol Bacteriol* 93:19, 1967.
131. Neville AM, O'Hare MJ: Histopathology of the human adrenal cortex, *Clin Endocrinol Metab* 14:791, 1985.
132. Conn JW, Knopf RF, Nesbit RM: Clinical characteristics of primary aldosteronism from an analysis of 145 cases, *Am J Surg* 107:159, 1964.
133. Janigan DT: Cytoplasmic bodies in the adrenal cortex of patients treated with spironolactone, *Lancet* 1:850, 1963.
134. Jenis EH, Hertzog RW: Effect of spironolactone on the zona glomerulosa of the adrenal cortex: light and electron microscopy, *Arch Pathol* 88:530, 1969.
135. Davis DA, Medline NM: Spironolactone (aldactone) bodies: concentric lamellar formations in the adrenal cortices of patients treated with spironolactone, *Am J Clin Pathol* 54:22, 1970.
136. Cohn D, Jackson RV, Gordon RD: Factors affecting the frequency of occurrence of spironolactone bodies in aldosteronomas and non-tumorous cortex, *Pathology* 15:273, 1983.
137. Hsu SM, Raine L, Martin HF: Spirinolactone bodies: an immunoperoxidase study with biochemical correlation, *Am J Clin Pathol* 75:92, 1981.
138. Li FP, Fraumeni JF Jr, Mulvihill JJ et al: A cancer family syndrome in twenty-four kindreds, *Cancer Res* 48:5358, 1988.
139. Malkin D, Li FP, Strong LC et al: Germ line p53 mutations in a familial syndrome of breast cancer, sarcomas, and other neoplasms, *Science* 250:1233, 1990.
140. Gabrilove JL, Seman AT, Sabet R et al: Virilizing adrenal adenoma with studies on the steroid content of the adrenal venous effluent and a review of the literature, *Endocr Rev* 2:462, 1981.
141. Vasiloff J, Chideckel EW, Boyd CB, Foshag LJ: Testosterone-secreting adrenal adenoma containing crystalloids characteristic of Leydig cells, *Am J Med* 79:772, 1985.
142. Pollock WJ, McConnell CF, Hilton C, Lavine RL: Virilizing Leydig cell adenoma of adrenal gland, *Am J Surg Pathol* 10:816, 1986.
143. Gabrilove JL, Sharma DC, Wotiz HH, Dorfman RI: Feminizing adrenocortical tumors in the male: a review of 52 cases including a case report, *Medicine* 44:37, 1965
144. Tang CK, Gray GF: Adrenocortical neoplasms: prognosis and morphology, *Urology* 5:691, 1975.
145. Hough AJ, Hollifield JW, Page DL, Hartmann WH: Prognostic factors in adrenal cortical tumors: a mathematical analysis of clinical and morphologic data, *Am J Clin Pathol* 72:390, 1979.
146. Weiss LM: Comparative histologic study of 43 metastasizing and non-metastasizing adrenocortical tumors, *Am J Surg Pathol* 8:163, 1984.
147. van Slooten H, Schaberg A, Smeenk D, Moolenaar AJ: Morphologic characteristics of benign and malignant adrenocortical tumors, *Cancer* 55:766, 1985.
148. Henley DJ, van Heerden JA, Grant CS et al: Adrenal cortical carcinoma —a continuing challenge, *Surgery* 94:926, 1983.
149. Cohn K, Gottesman L, Brennan M: Adrenocortical carcinoma, *Surgery* 100:1170, 1986.
150. Weiss LM, Medeiros LJ, Vickery AL Jr: Pathologic features of prognostic significance in adrenal cortical carcinoma, *Am J Surg Pathol* 13:202, 1989.
151. Medeiros LJ, Weiss LM: New developments in the pathologic diagnosis of adrenal cortical neoplasms: a review, *Am J Clin Pathol* 97:73, 1992.
152. Bowlby LS, DeBault LE, Abraham SR: Flow cytometric analysis of adrenal cortical tumor DNA: relationship between cellular DNA and histopathologic classification, *Cancer* 58:1499, 1986.
153. Amberson JB, Vaughan ED Jr, Gray GF, Naus GJ: Flow cytometric analysis of nuclear DNA from adrenocortical neoplasms: a retrospective study using paraffin-embedded tissue, *Cancer* 59:2091, 1987.
154. Hosaka Y, Rainwater LM, Grant CS et al: Adrenocortical carcinoma: nuclear deoxyribonucleic acid ploidy studied by flow cytometry, *Surgery* 102:1027, 1987.
155. Cibas ES, Medeiros LJ, Weinberg DS et al: Cellular DNA profiles of benign and malignant adrenocortical tumors, *Am J Surg Pathol* 14:948, 1990.
156. Zerbini C, Kozakewich HPW, Weinberg DS et al: Adrenocortical neoplasms in childhood and adolescence: analysis of prognostic factors including DNA content, *Endocr Pathol* 3:116, 1992.
157. Joensuu H, Klemi PJ: DNA aneuploidy in adenomas of endocrine organs, *Am J Pathol* 132:145, 1988.
158. Cagle PT, Hough AJ, Pysher TJ et al: Comparison of adrenal cortical tumors in children and adults, *Cancer* 57:2235, 1986.

64 Diabetes and Endocrine Pancreas

Jürgen Roth
Paul Komminoth
Günter Klöppel
Philipp U. Heitz

Abbreviations

CGRP	Calcitonin gene–related peptide	PCR	Polymerase chain reaction
ECL cells	Enterochromaffin-like cells	PGP 9.5	Protein gene product 9.5
IAA	Insulin autoantibodies	PNHH	Persistent neonatal hyperinsulinemic hypoglycemia
IAPP	Islet amyloid polypeptide		
ICA	Islet cell antibodies	PP	Pancreatic polypeptide
ICSA	Islet cell surface antibodies	SSCP	Single-strand conformation polymorphism
IDDM	Insulin-dependent type I diabetes mellitus	VIP	Vasoactive intestinal polypeptide
MEN syndromes	Multiple endocrine neoplasia syndromes	WDHA syndrome	Watery diarrhea hypokalemia achlorhydria syndrome
NIDDM	Non–insulin-dependent type 2 diabetes mellitus		
NSE	Neuron-specific enolase	ZES	Zollinger-Ellison syndrome

NORMAL ENDOCRINE PANCREAS

Endocrine cells of the pancreas are arranged into anatomic units, called "islets of Langerhans," that are scattered throughout the entire organ and intermixed with the exocrine pancreas.

Embryology

The development of the endocrine pancreas is complex and interrelated with development of the exocrine portion of the organ. The course of the appearance of the various components is summarized in Table 64-1. It is now clear that both the exocrine and endocrine pancreas are of endodermal origin.[1,2] After the fusion of the ventral and dorsal pancreas anlage at around the seventh week of gestation, endocrine cells can be detected in 9- to 10-week-old human embryos.[3] Early on, four different endocrine cell types can be distinguished by immunocytochemistry.[4,5] Insulin (β)-, glucagon (α)-, somatostatin (δ)-, and pancreatic polypeptide (PP)-immunoreactive cells exist initially in the exocrine duct epithelium. Around the thirteenth week of gestation, formation of the islets of Langerhans commences with the appearance of duct-associated, nonvascularized buds that separate to form the mantle type of vascularized islets characterized by a central mass of insulin-producing cells surrounded by several layers of non-β cells.[6] Between the twenty-first and twenty-sixth weeks of gestation, non-β cells appear in peripheral and central parts of the islets, and the adult type of islets are formed. Islet formation persists during intrauterine life and can be seen at different phases of the neonatal period. Histologic sections of pancreas examined during this period show both the fetal and the adult type of islets.

Anatomy and histology

The islets of Langerhans are scattered throughout the adult human pancreas. The islets vary in size and shape. They are separated from the exocrine cells by a fine fibrous capsule that extends internally in the form of vascular and connective tissue bands subdividing the inside of the islets into subunits (Fig. 64-1). Two types of islets can be distinguished based on their particular composition of endocrine cells and anatomical locations.[7] The β cell–rich islets constitute sharply delineated, round to oval complexes present throughout the pancreas. In contrast, the PP cell–rich islets are trabecular, irregular in shape, and restricted to the posterior part of the pancreatic head. This region seems to be derived from the ventral pancreas anlage and forms a separate lobe. Single endocrine cells also may be found scattered through the exocrine pancreas and duct epithelium.

Table 64-1 Main stages of human pancreas development

Developmental key event	Embryo age (weeks)
Occurrence of dorsal anlage	3-4
Occurrence of ventral anlage	4
Fusion of the ventral and dorsal anlage	40
Endocrine cells in duct epithelium	9-10
Duct-associated, nonvascularized endocrine cell buds	13
Mantle type of vascularized islets	17
Adult type of islets	21-26

Electron microscopy

Various endocrine pancreatic cell types can be identified based on the morphology of their secretory granules. Unequivocal identification can be achieved only by immunoelectron microscopy using specific antibodies (Fig. 64-2). This approach is mandatory for the classification of endocrine pancreatic tumors, which often exhibit abnormal morphology of secretory granules. The β cells contain membrane-limited polymorphic secretory granules (200 to 300 nm in diameter) composed of a highly electron-dense, often paracrystalline core surrounded by a wide, electron-lucent halo; the α cell's secretory granules (250 to 400 nm in diameter) contain an eccentrically located, less electron-dense core surrounded by a narrow, electron-lucent halo. The material enclosed in the δ cell's secretory granules (150 to 400 nm in diameter) appears homogeneous and is of low electron density. The PP cells contain small, round to ovoid secretory granules (90 to 230 nm in diameter) filled with highly electron-dense material.

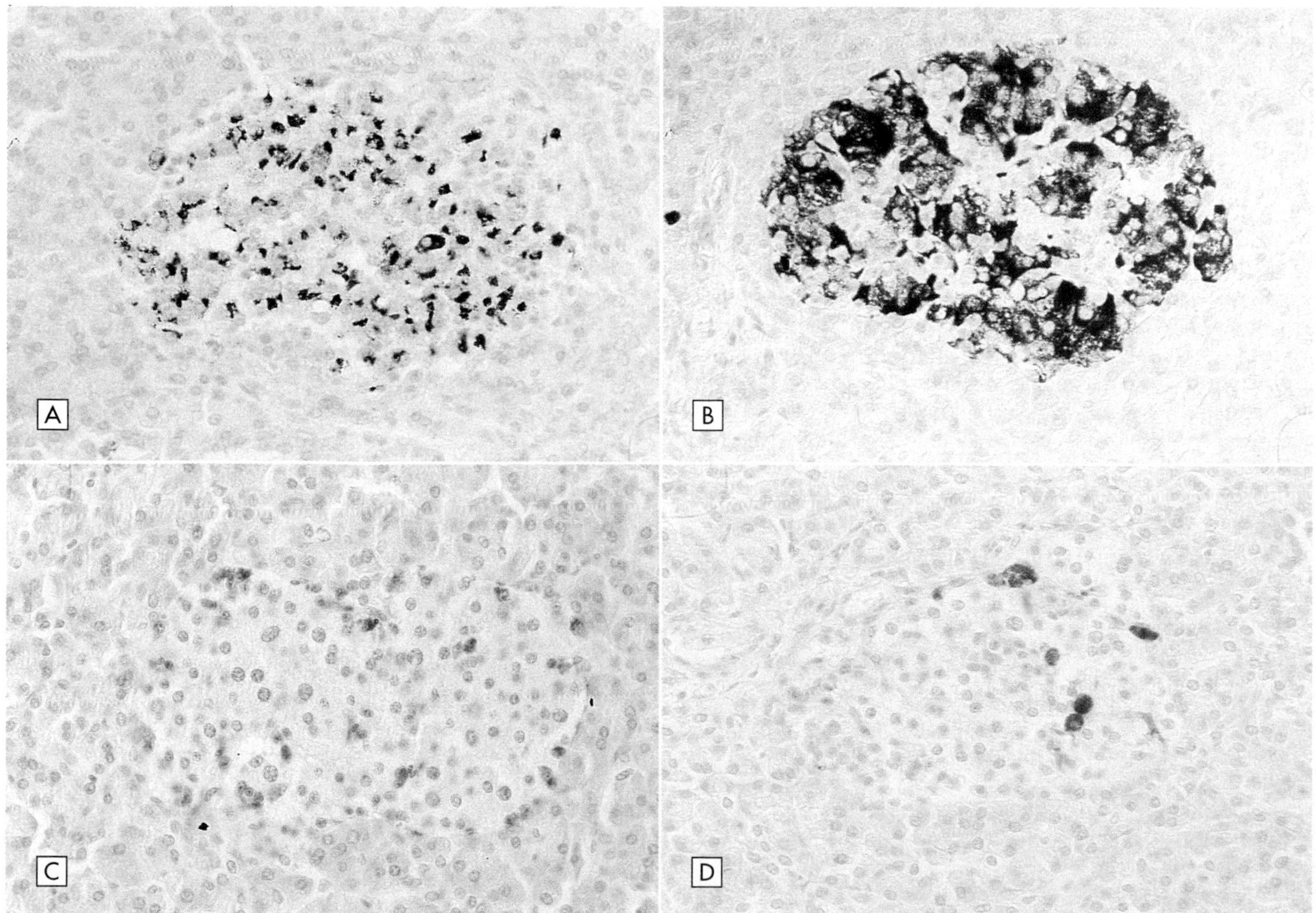

Fig. 64-1 Normal human pancreas. Immunohistochemical detection of proinsulin, **A,** and of insulin, **B,** Paraffin sections, monoclonal antibodies, immunogold-silver technique, nuclear fast red. Immunostaining for glucagon, **C,** and somatostatin, **D,** (Paraffin sections, polyclonal antibody, immunoperoxidase technique, hematoxylin.)

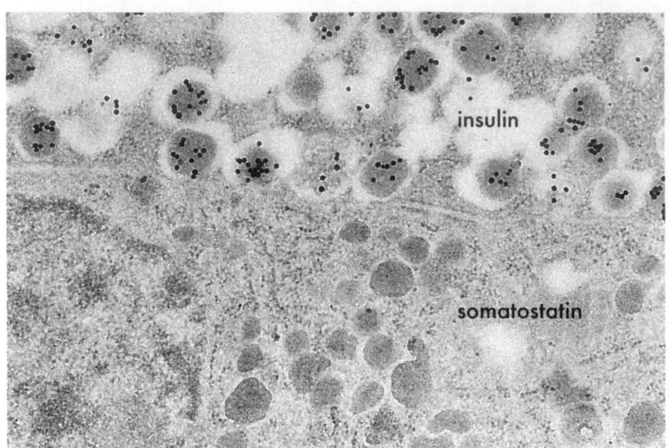

Fig. 64-2 Immunoelectron microscopic localization of insulin in secretory granules of a β cell; the adjacent D cell is unlabeled. (Ultrathin Epon section, protein A–gold technique.)

Most islet β cells are juxtaposed to other β cells, forming small groups with a polarized orientation to capillaries. Less often, β cells are juxtaposed to α cells and δ cells. Gap junctions between adjacent cells mediate communication, making possible the exchange of small molecules from β cells to other β cells and non-β cells of the islets. This process is influenced by glucose, calcium, and cyclic AMP levels.[8] The interactions between endocrine cells within the islets may also be mediated by paracrine secretion. In vitro and in vivo insulin release can be stimulated by glucagon, which binds to high-affinity receptors on β cells and exerts its effects at concentrations that seem to correspond to those present in the islet afferent arterioles.[9] The microvasculature of the islets[10] consists of one or two afferent arterioles that terminate into capillaries. The capillaries are lined by fenestrated endothelium and form a glomerulus-like network. Cholinergic fibers may regulate the blood flow through the afferent arterioles.[11] The efferent capillaries coalesce into collecting venules in the periphery of the islets. In the interstitium of the islets, neural endings with varying content of neurotransmitters exist that may exert a stimulatory[12] or inhibitory[12,13] effect on insulin secretion. Mononuclear phagocytes and dendritic cells, which express MHC class II surface antigens,[14] may function in the phagocytosis of damaged cells[15] or in the induction of a local immune reaction.[16]

Hormone synthesis

Like many other biologically active polypeptides, pancreatic hormones are synthesized as large preproproteins, which become converted by limited endoproteolysis into the smaller, mature proteins,[17,18] as illustrated for insulin by a sequence that leads to secretion.

The structure of the insulin gene, which is a member of a superfamily of structurally related peptides, is well known, and the regulation of its expression is highly complex.[19] The structure of insulin has been highly conserved phylogenetically. The mature hormone consists of an α-chain, composed of 21 amino acids, and a β-chain, composed of 30 amino acids, linked by two, interchain disulphide bonds (Fig. 64-3). The human preproinsulin consists of a signal peptide, the B-chain, a dibasic Arg-Arg pair, the connecting C-peptide, a dibasic Lys-Arg pair, and the A-chain (Fig. 64-3). The cotranslational removal of the signal peptide in the endoplasmic reticulum yields proinsulin. Proinsulin is converted into the mature hormone by the combined action of two endoproteases and a carboxypeptidase H (Fig. 64-3 and Table 64-2). The genes for both endoproteases have been cloned, and their substrate specificity is well established (Fig. 64-3).[17] One endoprotease, referred to as "PC 2," cleaves the dibasic pair, Arg_{31}-Arg_{32}, in the B-chain/C-peptide junction; the other, referred to as "PC 3," cleaves the dibasic pair Lys_{64}-Arg_{65} in the A-chain/C-peptide junction of proinsulin. The dibasic amino acids exposed by the endoproteases are removed by carboxypeptidase H. The different events yielding the mature insulin take place in various cellular compartments (Fig. 64-3). Proinsulin is transported to the Golgi apparatus. Immature secretory granules, which contain proinsulin, are formed in the *trans* Golgi network. The mechanism involved in the sorting of proinsulin and other prohormones into such dense-cored secretory granules is not yet clear. The immature, partially clathrin-coated, acidic secretory granules at the *trans* side of the Golgi apparatus seem to represent the major site of endoproteolytic prohormone conversion, as demonstrated by high resolution immunoelectron microscopy using monoclonal antibodies to proinsulin and insulin.[20] These monoclonal antibodies have also been applied to localize both proinsulin and insulin in sections of formaldehyde-fixed and paraffin-embedded human pancreas (Fig. 64-4).

Sample processing and investigation

The morphologic identification of endocrine cell types in normal or diseased pancreas can only be unequivocally achieved by immunocytochemistry or by in situ hybridization.[21-24] Histochemical techniques such as aldehyde-fuchsin staining, argyrophilic reactions, and others to identify neuroendocrine cell types are of limited value. At present, diagnosis can be fully achieved by immunohistochemistry, which has replaced conventional electron microscopic investigations, to detect and classify the endocrine type of secretory granules.

Polypeptide hormones, particularly insulin, are relatively resistant to various conditions of chemical fixation and embedding for subsequent immunohistochemical studies employing polyclonal and monoclonal antibodies.

Light microscopic immunolabeling. For light microscopic immunolabeling, fixation of thin tissue slices in buffered (pH 7.4) formaldehyde or Bouin's fluid, followed by standard paraffin embedding, is the procedure of choice. Various immunohistochemical techniques using gold-labeled secondary reagents and silver amplification[21] or traditional immunoenzyme protocols can be recommended, all of which produce acceptable results.

Electron microscopic immunolabeling. Fixation of 1 mm^3 tissue pieces in buffered, vacuum-distilled glutaraldehyde, with or without postfixation in osmium tetroxide, followed by resin embedding (Epon, Araldite, Durcupan, Lowicryl K4M, LR White or Gold), gives acceptable results. In our laboratory we routinely use, for each sample, Epon (with osmium tetroxide) and Lowicryl K4M (without osmium tetroxide) embedding for both fine structural analysis and immunolabeling. Before immunolabeling, thin sections of osmicated samples should be pretreated for antigen retrieval either with saturated aqueous sodium metaperiodate for about 1 hour or with 1% aqueous periodic acid for 4 minutes. Postembedding immunogold labeling[25,26] is, in our opinion,

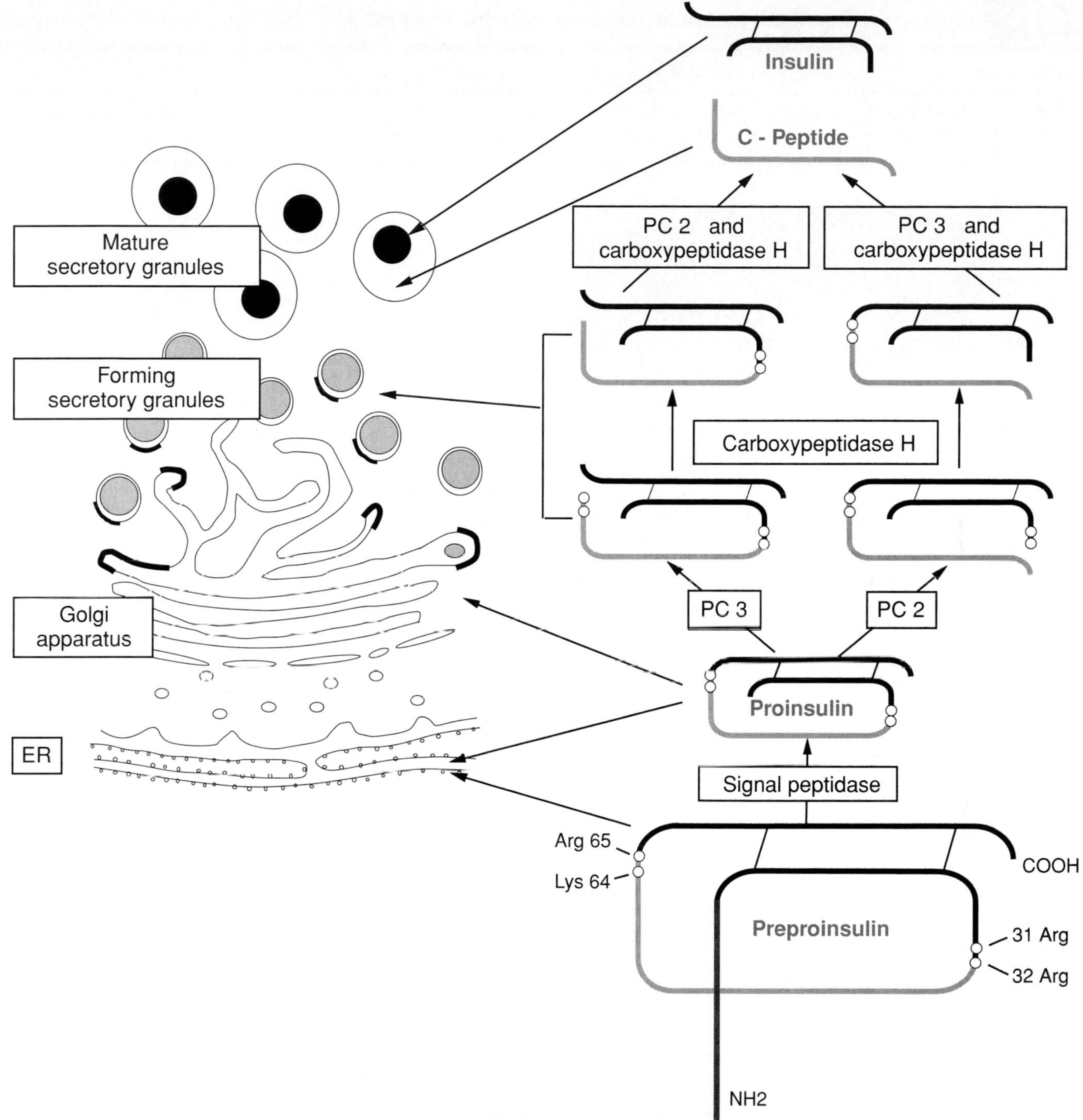

Fig. 64-3 Schema of the various processing steps yielding insulin in a normal β cell (for details, see text).

the method of choice and provides highest resolution and unequivocal identification of the labeled structures.

In situ hybridization. In situ hybridization for the detection of mRNA may be particularly helpful in identifying endocrine cells rapidly secreting their hormonal product or products without forming secretory granules.[23] For in situ hybridization, samples should be preferably fixed in 4% buffered (para)formaldehyde and frozen in a cryoprotectant (Fig. 64-5). Best results are obtained on frozen sections using cRNA or oligonucleotide probes.[22] However, successful mRNA detection has also been achieved on archival paraffin material.[24]

Molecular analysis. PCR, Southern and northern blotting, and SSCP, requiring purified DNA and RNA, are performed on freshly provided specimens, preferably freshly snap frozen.

DIABETES MELLITUS

Diabetes mellitus is not a single disease; it is a group of disorders characterized by hyperglycemia caused by either absolute or relative insulin deficiency. On the basis of clinical, genetic,

Table 64-2 Characteristics of the proinsulin endoproteases PC 2 and PC 3

Endoprotease	Substrate specificity	Optimum pH	Ion requirement
PC 2	-Arg_{31}-Arg_{32}-	5.5	millimolar Ca^{2+}
PC 3	-Lys_{64}-Arg_{65}-	5.5-7.5	micromolar Ca^{2+}

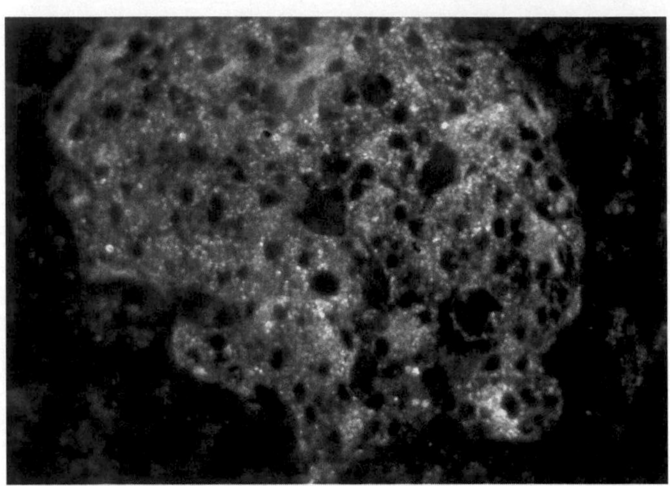

Fig. 64-4 Diffuse staining of human islet with FITC-labeled islet cell antibodies.

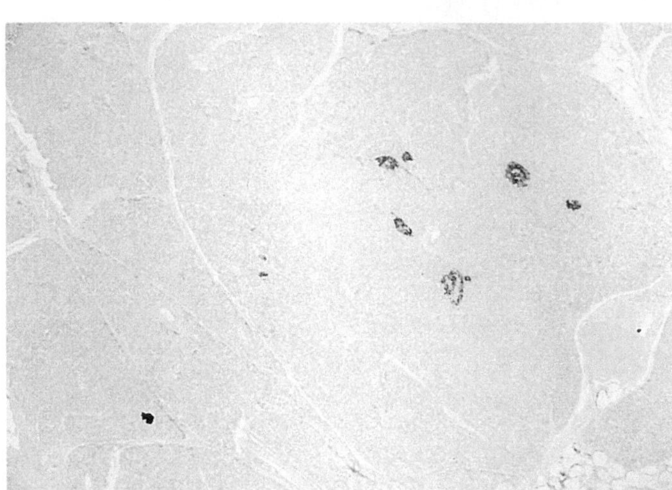

Fig. 64-5 Small group of insulin-positive islets in recent-onset type I diabetes, restricted to one lobule of the pancreas. (Immunostaining for insulin.)

and immunologic features, diabetes has been segregated into insulin-dependent type 1 diabetes (IDDM), non–insulin dependent type 2 diabetes (NIDDM), diabetes secondary to pancreatic diseases or hormone overproduction, and gestational diabetes (Table 64-3). From a morphologic point of view, the islet changes associated with the various types of diabetes can be divided into those with and those without severe (to absolute) β cell loss. Severe β cell loss is found in IDDM and in some uncommon forms of diabetes, such as virus-related diabetes and congenital diabetes. Islets without a severe loss of β cells are encountered in NIDDM and in the secondary forms of diabetes (Table 64-3).

Epidemiology. There are considerable racial and geographic differences in the incidences of IDDM and NIDDM. Thus IDDM diabetes is rare in some ethnic groups, such as Japanese, Indians, Chinese, and American Indians, whereas white populations in North America and Europe show a prevalence of 0.6 to 3.5 per 1000 and an incidence (subjects 0 to 14 years) of about 14 per 1,000,000. NIDDM is common in all populations of westernized countries and has dramatically increased in certain ethnic groups, in which it was originally low, with modernization of life. The highest prevalence rates are now seen in Pima Indians (35.0) and Micronesians (34.4) and the lowest in Eskimos and Alaska Indians (1.3 to 1.9). The incidence rate of Pima Indians is 19 times that of the white population in the United States.

In a number of tropical countries malnutrition appears to be associated with diabetes mellitus. This non–ketosis prone type of diabetes occurs in two forms: *J-type diabetes* (*J* for Jamaica) and *pancreatic fibrosis diabetes*. The latter type is most commonly encountered in India and South Africa and results from chronic calcifying pancreatitis, the cause and pathogenesis of which are obscure.

Insulin-dependent type I diabetes mellitus

Type 1 diabetes, or IDDM, is a disease of the endocrine pancreas that is characterized by an autoimmune-mediated destruction of the pancreatic insulin-producing β cells, resulting in insulin dependency (Table 64-3).

Etiology and pathogenesis. Insulitis and highly selective destruction of β cells are pathognomonic of IDDM[27] and have been demonstrated in early stages of the disease of many patients with IDDM. The lymphocytic nature of insulitis, its restriction to islets containing β cells, and association with acute β cell damage or clinical severity of the disease indicate that the insulin-producing cells may have been destroyed by an autoimmune process.

Other findings lending support to the autoimmune pathogenesis of β cell destruction are (1) demonstration of autoantibodies to islet cells (ICA, islet cell antibodies; ICSA, islet cell surface antibodies) (Fig. 64-4), insulin (IAA, insulin autoantibodies), and the GABA-synthesizing enzyme glutamic acid decarboxylase (GAD), of the islet cells, which can be present for several years before clinical onset of diabetes[28-30]; (2) association of IDDM with some well-known autoimmune diseases, such as Hashimoto's thyroiditis, idiopathic Addison's disease, and pernicious anemia[31]; (3) recurrence of insulitis in pancreatic isografts from HLA-identical donors in pancreas-transplanted patients with long-standing IDDM[32]; (4) experimental production of insulitis by active immunization of rabbits, cows, or sheep against homologous or heterologous insulin;[33] and (5) immune-related β cell destruction in BB rats[34] and NOD mice,[35] which serve as models for human IDDM.

The autoimmune destruction of the β cells may best be explained by the existence of a β cell–specific protein that, for

Table 64-3 **Features of the main types of diabetes mellitus**

Features	Type 1 (IDDM)	Type 2 (NIDDM)	Secondary diabetes
Incidence	>10%	>85%	1% to 2%
Age at onset	Predominantly before 20 years	Predominantly after 30-40 years	Depends on the primary disease
Clinical features	Sudden onset, thin, ketosis prone, insulin required	Gradual onset, obese, normally ketosis resistant, normally insulin not required	Similar to type 2 diabetes, except obesity
Family history	Increased prevalence (20%) of type 1 diabetes	Increased prevalence (60%) of type 2 diabetes	None
Monozygotic twins	<50% concordance	>90% concordance	None
HLA associations	Yes	No	None
Islet cell antibodies	Yes	No	None
Associated autoimmune endocrine disease	Yes	No	None
Islet changes	>80% loss of β cells	Amyloidosis, 10% to 50% β cell loss	Fibrosis 10% to 50% β cell loss
Insulin response to glucose	Flat or absent	Variable	Reduced

unknown reasons, acquires autoantigenic properties and eventually becomes the target for the autoimmune reaction. A recent working hypothesis focuses on the aberrant expression of class II HLA molecules on β cells, which thus would acquire the capability of class II–restricted antigen presentation of an autoantigen (or antigens) to helper T-lymphocytes. This assumption has been based on the observation of an exclusive class II HLA expression on insulin-containing cells in patients with recent-onset IDDM. However, class II HLA expression has also been detected on β cells of NIDDM patients whose disease is believed to be unrelated to autoimmunity.[36] We could not demonstrate class II HLA on β cells of two patients with recent-onset IDDM in another study (Lernmark and Klöppel, unpublished observation). It appears that other, as yet unknown immune mechanisms could be involved in the selective destruction of the β cells.

Although the exact immune recognition of the hypothetical β cell autoantigen is not known, accumulated evidence indicates that its expression is genetically predetermined. It is now well established that susceptibility to IDDM is increased in subjects expressing the HLA antigens DR3, DR4 or the heterozygous form, DR3/DR4. Recently, it was found that subjects who carry certain DR4 haplotypes in association with DQw8 have the highest risk of developing IDDM.[37] These data indicate that the gene or genes responsible for the development of IDDM may be located close to the HLA-DR and DQ cluster on chromosome 6. Because this region on chromosome 6 also contains immune response genes, it is conceivable that certain inherited HLA haplotypes may facilitate immune responses against autoantigens and thus contribute to the development of autoimmune diabetes.

Studies in monozygotic twins with IDDM revealed that the concordance in identical twins is less than 50%, indicating that environmental factors, such as toxins and viral agents, may have a pathogenic role as well. In support of viral pathogenesis are the temporal relationships between common childhood viral infections, such as mumps, rubella, cytomegalovirus, and coxsackievirus B, and the subsequent development of IDDM. Experimental production of β cell necrosis, insulitis, and diabetes in mice infected with encephalomyocarditis virus is yet another argument in favor of viral pathogenesis.[38] In addition, coxsackievirus B infections have been demonstrated in children dying in ketoacidotic coma and displaying insulitis[39] and typical changes of IDDM. These diabetics had an encephalitis and myocarditis as well, and so it appears that a coxsackievirus B infection was superimposed on a classical IDDM. If viruses or other environmental factors, therefore, play a role in the initiation of IDDM, it must be shown that they affected the β cells long before the clinical onset of the disease.

In summary, the classical IDDM appears to be an autoimmune-mediated process based on a genetic predisposition and possibly triggered by environmental factors, which are unknown so far. Gradual β cell loss becomes clinically manifest only when the β-cell mass is reduced to a critical point, after which metabolic compensation is not possible,[40] or the overstressed β cells, responding to incidental events (such as viral infection), cannot meet the demand functionally. The presence of ICA has been used to predict the onset of IDDM and to estimate its preclinical period.[41] However, as in long-term trials, ICAs were found to disappear from about 30% to 50% of subjects initially positive for these autoantibodies, and the role of these autoantibodies in the disease process and their relation to β cell destruction are not well understood. This holds also for the other autoantibodies so far recognized, including the GAD antigen.[42]

Pathology of the pancreas. Pancreases from patients who died shortly after onset of IDDM appear normal in size, shape, and weight.[43] Histologically, however, most islets are devoid of β cells.[43] The total β cell volume is therefore reduced by about 80%.[43] A minority of islets, which are unevenly distributed in the pancreas (Fig. 64-5), still contain β cells that are normal in number and distribution but may show nuclear hypertrophy and sparse granulation. The key finding of recent-onset IDDM is a lymphocytic infiltration around and within islets that still contain at least a few β cells (Fig. 64-6). Insulitis usually affects only single islets and can therefore be easily overlooked. The infiltrates consist primarily of T lymphocytes with only scarce β-lymphocytes and macrophages.[44] As a rule, insulitis is found only in diabetics younger than 15 years[45] and is particularly common in diabetic infants. These cellular infiltrates persist for a limited time, and most patients who die after a prolonged disease (1 to 2 years) usually show no residual infiltration of the islets.

Pancreases from patients with long-term IDDM with a duration of more than 1 year display a considerable reduction in weight and volume.[36] This volume reduction results from severe atrophy of the acinar cells, which is attributed to the deficiency of insulin, which usually has a trophic effect on acinar cells.[27] Histologically, islets are often difficult to recognize in hematoxylin and eosin–stained sections. This is attributable to their irregular outlines and the small size of the glucagon, somatostatin, and PP cells that remained. Quantitatively, these changes result in a relative hyperplasia of the non-β cells (Fig. 64-7). In some patients insulin cells do not disappear completely and may still be present even after 40 years of disease duration.[36]

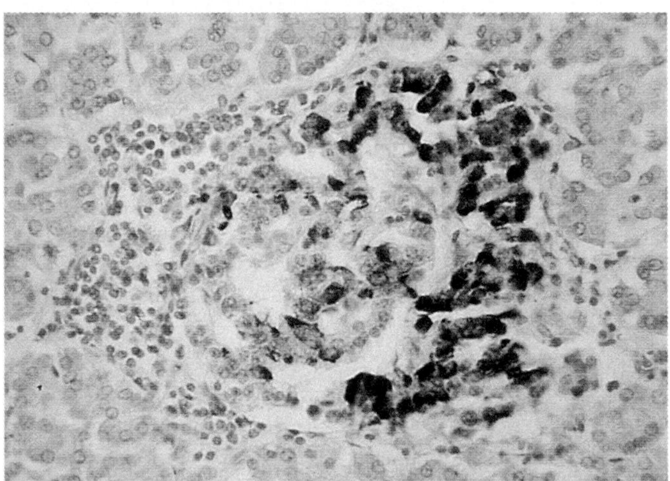

Fig. 64-6 Islet still containing β cells and showing infiltration by lymphocytes (insulitis). (Immunostaining for insulin.)

Islet amyloidosis is an exceptional finding in IDDM because the formation of islet amyloid requires insulin-producing cells (see NIDDM). Islet calcification and fibrosis are equally rare. Mitosis, as an unequivocal sign of cell replication and regeneration, has not been observed in surviving β cells of IDDM patients.

All acinar cells show considerable atrophy. The perilobular spaces and to some degree also the interacinar spaces are enlarged and contain loosely arranged connective tissue (Fig. 64-8). In some cases, fibrosis of the exocrine tissue is associated with a sparse and unevenly distributed lymphocytic infiltration.[45] The large arteries are often affected by arteriosclerosis, and the small vessels show diabetic microangiopathy.

Clinical presentation. IDDM can occur from the first months of life to the seventh decade, but most cases occur in the 4 to 14 years age group. First clinical symptoms, usually polydipsia, polyuria, and weight loss of a few weeks in duration, occur most often during autumn and winter months. Often the disease is recognized because of an exacerbation by a viral infection.

Older patients who develop IDDM in their fourth decade or later (late-onset IDDM) often exhibit a slowly progressive deterioration of β cell function, together with the immunologic and genetic characteristics of classical IDDM (ICA and HLA DR3/DR4).[41] Among these diabetics are those with polyglandular autoimmunity (autoimmune thyroiditis, adrenalitis, and pernicious anemia), which occurs primarily in middle-aged women, is strongly related to HLA-DR3 only, and has an insidious clinical onset and persisting islet cell antibodies. Histologically this diabetes type shows changes identical to those of classical IDDM.

Pancreatic islet grafts. Islets of Langerhans transplanted into patients with IDDM show various pathologic changes, the most common of which are cell necrosis and infarction. Inflammatory infiltration of the islets, mainly consisting of T8 ($CD8^+$) lymphocytes and macrophages, was noted in 25% of the grafts.[32] It is difficult to determine whether this form of insulitis is attributable to rejection or to recurrent IDDM. The most intense insulitis with evidence of selective β cell destruction was observed in the grafts of HLA-identical recipients.[32]

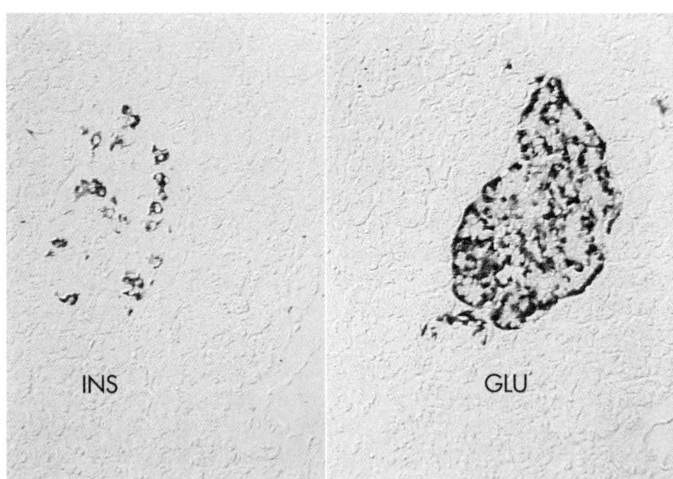

Fig. 64-7 Chronic type I diabetes of 21 years in duration: few surviving B (insulin) cells in an islet with relative hyperplasia of α cells. (Immunostaining for insulin, *INS,* and glucagon, *GLU.*)

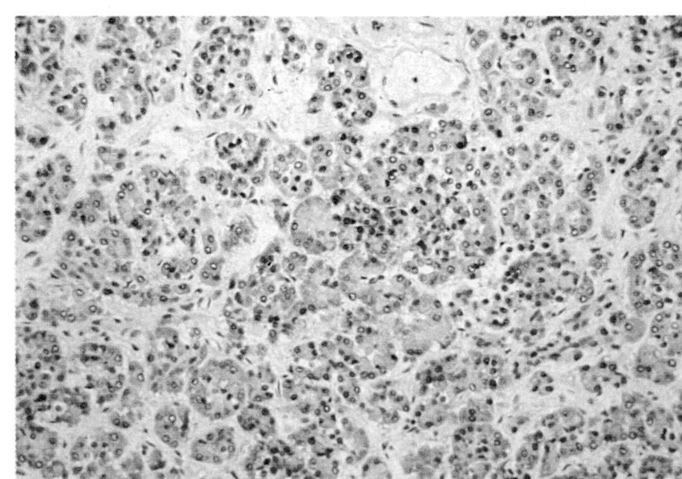

Fig. 64-8 Severe atrophy of the pancreatic acinar cells in long-lasting type I diabetes.

In these patients recurrent diabetes was therefore believed to be the consequence of the destruction of the β cells as a result of an anamnestic cytotoxic T-lymphocyte–mediated autoimmune response. However, graft dysfunction was also noted in patients without signs of acute rejection or islet damage. The pathophysiology of the recurrent diabetes in these patients remains to be explained. Cytomegalovirus infection has also been noticed in some grafts.

Non–insulin-dependent type 2 diabetes mellitus

Type 2 diabetes, or NIDDM, is a complex disease of the endocrine pancreas and the insulin-requiring tissues. It is characterized by a strong genetic susceptibility and by environmental influences, resulting in insulin resistance and impaired β cell function (Table 64-3).

Etiology and pathogenesis. In contrast to IDDM, there is no association with autoimmune phenomena or certain HLA antigens in NIDDM. Moreover, the β cells are present in the islets, though their number may be reduced to one half the norm. Consequently, these patients always have some endogenous insulin production and thus become not totally insulin dependent but develop a relative insulin deficiency.

Although these features are common to almost all patients with NIDDM, there is nevertheless evidence that they are not all affected by the same disease. Subsets are the maturity-onset diabetes of youth (MODY), with an apparent autosomal-dominant mode of inheritance of probably mutated glucokinase gene,[46,47] and diabetes caused by mutations of the insulin gene. For all the other patients who compose the majority of NIDDM patients, the most important factors relevant to the development of their disease are heredity, obesity, peripheral insulin resistance, and impaired β cell function.[48] The following pertinent questions are related to these factors: Which is the mode of inheritance, and what is the inherited defect? What is the role of obesity in the pathogenesis of NIDDM? What are the mechanisms of insulin resistance? How are the β cells damaged?

The major determinant of NIDDM appears to be genetic susceptibility. Monozygotic twins show close to 100% concordance, and families of NIDDM diabetics have a distinctly increased prevalence rate for this disease. However, despite strong evidence of inheritance, neither its mode nor its nature has so far been revealed.

Obesity and pregnancy appear to be the most important factors known to promote the appearance of NIDDM in genetically susceptible persons. Population-based studies have shown that obese subjects have a greater incidence of diabetes, and countries with the greatest prevalence of obesity have the highest incidence of the disease. NIDDM is therefore a disease of the "developed" countries and is rare in developing countries. This strong influence of obesity on the manifestation of diabetes is best explained by the fact that weight gain is associated with a considerable reduction in insulin sensitivity (reduced insulin-mediated glucose uptake by muscle and fat tissues and impaired suppression of hepatic glucose production) and a concomitant rise in serum insulin levels. A decline in insulin secretion caused by an exhaustion of the secretory capacity of the β cells then results in frank diabetes. However, not all obese subjects become diabetic; therefore, additional factors are required for the clinical disease to appear.

The pathogenesis of the assumed, late-onset β cell failure in NIDDM is obscure. It could be a primary, genetically predetermined reduction of the β cells or a functional and also genetically programmed abnormality of insulin secretion. A reduction of the β cell mass, usually in the order of 10% to 50%, can be found in most IDDM. However, because we still do not know exactly the critical mass of actively secreting β cells required to maintain normoglycemia, it remains unclear whether the modest decline in the number of β cells in diabetics fully explains their impaired function.[49] A functional damage to the β cells could therefore be more important for the development of NIDDM than a reduced β cell mass. Functional defects of the β cell response to glucose can be demonstrated by drugs and amino acid infusion, which typically elicit more rapid insulin responses than glucose in the affected persons. Morphologic signs of a functional insufficience, such as degranulation and compensatory cellular hypertrophy, are not apparent in most cases. If a decrease in the β cell mass adds to the functional abnormality (as has been suggested by experimental studies[49]), it may result from a reduced capacity for β cell replication and regeneration. This is then either the consequence of a second inherited defect, or hyperglycemia per se. Animal studies indicated that the genetic background is of importance for the growth response of β cells to hyperglycemia.[50] On the other hand, other studies have shown that sustained hyperglycemia per se exacerbates insulin deficiency.[49]

Another finding that also points to a functional abnormality of the β cells in NIDDM is the precipitation of islet amyloid polypeptide (IAPP)[51] or amylin[52] in the stroma surrounding the β cells. IAPP is a 37-amino-acid peptide with about 50% homology to human calcitonin gene-related peptide. It is a normal component of β cells in nondiabetic or diabetic humans and animals and is localized in the secretory granules and cosecreted with insulin.[51] Its metabolic function is unknown. In particular, there is yet no evidence that IAPP acts as a physiologically relevant modulator of insulin secretion or inducer of insulin resistance.[51] The gene for IAPP has been localized to the 12p chromosome, but no genetic defects in this protein have yet been recognized. In NIDDM subjects and, rarely, in obviously nondiabetic subjects, it forms amyloid fibrils, which are deposited between the β cells and the capillaries. The cause of amyloid formation is not known, but it indicates abnormalities within the cell. Considering the impaired insulin secretion in NIDDM, it is obvious to relate amyloid deposition to disturbances in the rate of synthesis, conversion, and secretion of IAPP and, perhaps, insulin in the diabetic pancreas. It is unclear whether islet amyloidosis affects the normal function of the β cell. The extent of islet amyloidosis in diabetics is variable[53] and therefore difficult to correlate to the severity and duration of the disease. However, it has been shown that in some NIDDM patients amyloid deposition may lead to 30% reduction in β cell population and that, in monkeys, the degree of amyloid formation and the number of islets affected increases with the progression of diabetes. This could indicate that progressive amyloid deposition around islet capillaries impairs islet function by creating a perivascular diffusion barrier that affects the glucose recognition and insulin secretion by the β cells.

In summary, it seems that two main defects are important for the pathogenesis of NIDDM: peripheral insulin resistance and a defective β cell function. How these defects relate to the known genetic susceptibility of NIDDM, and its influence by other factors, such as obesity, pregnancy, or the deposition of amyloid in the islets, remains speculative.

Pathology of the pancreas. No gross abnormalities of the pancreas, either qualitative or quantitative, are specific for NIDDM. Histologically, the islets may appear normal or show stromal amyloidosis (Fig. 64-9). Unlike the islets in IDDM, they always contain β cells in regular distribution and often in normal numbers (Fig. 64-10). There is no significant degranulation of β cells, except in patients dying in diabetic coma with sustained high glucose levels. In these patients, the β cells also display hydropic change of the cytoplasm caused by glycogen accumulation, a reversible lesion that can be experimentally produced by prolonged hyperglycemia.

Islet amyloidosis, which is found in up to 90% of the NIDDM subjects, occurs only in islets containing insulin-producing β cells. The amyloid is deposited between the capillaries and the endocrine cells. It stains brightly with thioflavin T, but weakly with Congo red. By electron microscopy, it consists of thin, branching fibrils with diameters of 7.5 to 10 nm that run into deep plasma membrane pockets of the β cells.[54] The major constituent of the amyloid fibrils is islet amyloid polypeptide (IAPP)[54] or amylin,[52] which can be immunocytochemically identified within the β cells as a normal component of the secretory granules. In islets with amyloid the storage of IAPP in the β cells is greatly reduced, though its mRNA can be detected in normal concentrations[53] (Fig. 64-11). The amyloid deposits form cords that appear to compress the islet cells. Amyloidosis affects the islets unevenly, and in only a small percentage of patients are all islets (except the PP islets in the head of the pancreas) involved. In these patients amyloidosis is associated with a reduced islet volume. Islet amyloidosis is, however, not specific for diabetes because it is occasionally also seen in subjects who had not suffered from overt diabetes.[53] In addition, there is a sharp correlation with age.[55] Amyloidosis is uncommon in patients younger than 50 years, but it affects about 50% of diabetics older than 70 years.

Quantitative data on the β cell mass and volume in NIDDM subjects range from normal to a distinct reduction by up to 50%.[56,57] This is probably caused by the apparent heterogeneity of the disease regarding age, disease duration, weight, and β cell function. In a study[58] that correlated quantitative data to five clinical parameters (obesity, age, sex, disease duration, and type of therapy), it was shown that the insulin-treated patients had a significantly lower endocrine cell volume (mean, 0.67 ml), and especially β cell volume (mean, 0.41 ml), than those treated with oral compounds and diet (mean endocrine cell volume, 0.81 g; mean β cell volume, 0.52 ml) or diet alone (mean endocrine cell volume, 1.26 ml; mean β cell volume, 0.8 ml). Sex, age, body weight, and disease duration had no significant effect on these variables. These data indicate that insulin deficiency in NIDDM is the consequence of the decreased β cell mass but that this reduction in β cells is not related to age or duration of the disease.

Clinical presentation. At the time of diagnosis most NIDDM subjects are between 30 and 60 years of age. Typical patients are obese and have a positive family history for diabetes. They may have polyuria and polydipsia or sometimes unexplained weakness or weight loss, but often patients are asymptomatic, and the diagnosis is made by blood or urine examinations. The onset of the disease may occur after an infection that may evoke symptoms in patients with previously latent diabetes.

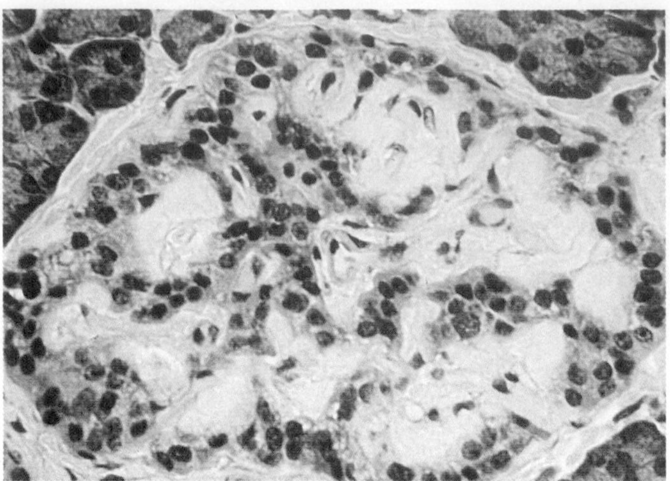

Fig. 64-9 Islet amyloidosis. Perisinusoidal deposits of amyloid replacing endocrine cells.

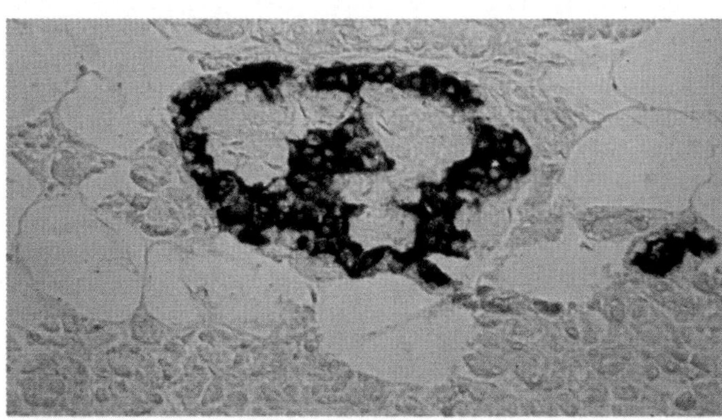

Fig. 64-10 Islet amyloidosis. B cells are normally distributed and well granulated. (Immunostaining for insulin.)

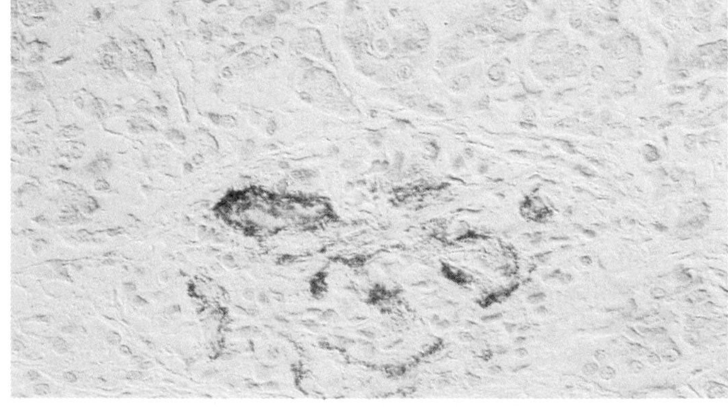

Fig. 64-11 Islet amyloid immunostained with antiserum to islet amyloid polypeptide. Notice that β cells are negative.

Uncommon forms of diabetes mellitus including viral diabetes and secondary diabetes

Permanent diabetes mellitus in newborns (congenital diabetes) is extremely rare. Except for aplasia of the pancreas, its pathologic basis has not been well established. In some cases congenital absence of the islets[59] or the β cells[29] has been suggested. In other cases the cause has remained entirely unclear.

Viral infections, such as mumps, herpes simplex, cytomegalovirus, and varicella, have been reported to affect the exocrine pancreas.[60] Acute islet cell damage (varying from clusters of cells with pyknotic nuclei to total islet necrosis), in addition to, or without, pancreatitis, has been observed in infants dying of culture-proved coxsackievirus encephalomyocarditis.[60]

Diabetes secondary to pancreatic diseases

This diabetes form includes all states of sustained hyperglycemia secondary to diseases that lead to disappearance, destruction, or severe alteration of the exocrine tissue of the pancreas and that are unrelated to genetic factors.

Aplasia. Congenital aplasia of the pancreas is extremely rare. Often it is combined with other malformations, such as gallbladder agenesis. The pancreatic parenchyma is replaced by soft tissue, mainly consisting of fatty tissue and nerve fibers. Because of the absence of exocrine and endocrine pancreatic tissue, malabsorption, diabetes, and growth retardation are the leading clinical symptoms.

Pancreatitis. Acute pancreatitis is only rarely followed by permanent diabetes. In chronic pancreatitis, diabetes mellitus occurs in increasing frequency with advancement of the disease, and, in end-stage chronic pancreatitis with distinct exocrine insufficiency and calcification, approximately 70% of the patients have overt diabetes mellitus. In India, as well as in other underdeveloped countries, chronic calcifying pancreatitis in adolescents is one of the most frequent causes of diabetes in this age group.[61] Indian pancreatic fibrosis is most likely a consequence of severe malnutrition.

Early forms of chronic pancreatitis, characterized by perilobular fibrosis, leave the distribution and architecture of the islets largely unchanged and are not associated with diabetes. In advanced chronic pancreatitis, when the acinar parenchyma is extensively replaced by connective tissue, the islets are qualitatively and probably also quantitatively changed. The disappearance of exocrine tissue causes the islets to aggregate in sclerosed tissue, where they may form adenoma-like complexes (Fig. 64-12) and eventually develop intrainsular fibrosis. Quantitatively these islets show a gradual loss of β cells (Fig. 64-13).[40] In advanced scarring of the pancreatic head there may also be a reduction of PP cells because in those cases only remnants of PP islets are encountered in the PP lobe. This finding correlates well with an impaired PP secretion observed in these cases. Although no data are available on the total endocrine cell volume in severe chronic pancreatitis, a reduction of the endocrine cell mass is likely to occur. Ultrastructurally, the remaining endocrine cells appear normal and show no evidence of cellular damage.[40] These morphologic features of chronic pancreatitis indicate that diabetes may result from fibrosis extending into the islets and thus reducing the total β cell mass.

Pancreatic carcinoma. Carcinomas, especially those localized in the head of the pancreas, are frequently associated with diabetes mellitus. This is probably caused by chronic obstructive pancreatitis. The islet system is affected in a way similar to chronic pancreatitis[40] and results in impaired insulin secretion. Malignancy-related insulin resistance may also play a role, but this relationship remains to be established more convincingly.[62]

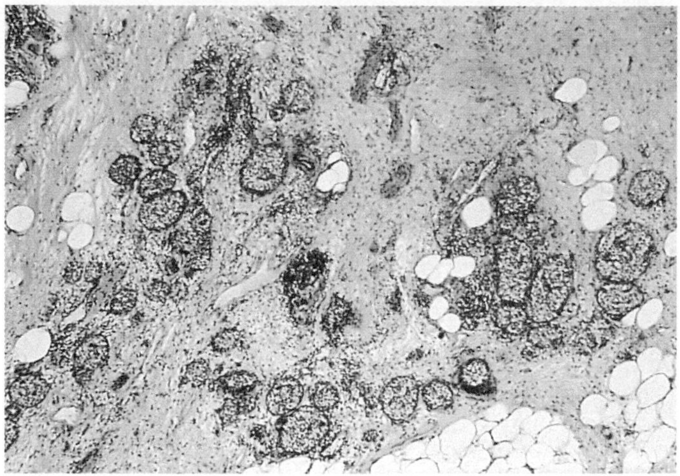

Fig. 64-12 Pancreas in advanced chronic pancreatitis with clustering and embedding of islets in fibrous tissue.

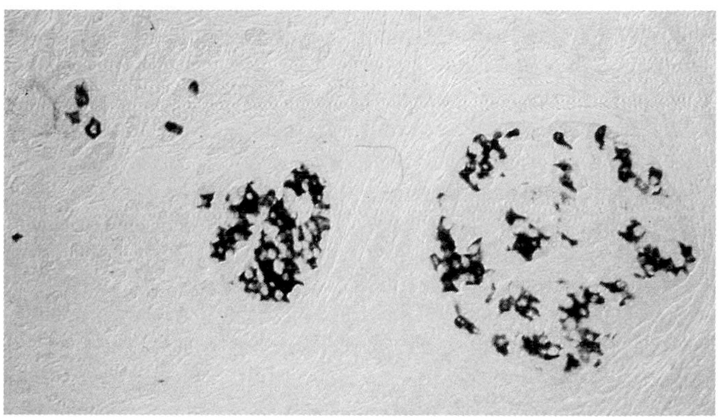

Fig. 64-13 Pancreas in advanced chronic pancreatitis. Islets with reduced β cell number. (Immunostaining for insulin.)

Cystic fibrosis. Diabetes mellitus occuring in association with cystic fibrosis used to be rare (1% to 2%). However, a rising incidence (8% to 13%) of overt diabetes has been reported in young adults with advanced cystic fibrosis, probably reflecting the increasing survival of these patients.[63] The clinical and functional features of this type of diabetes are essentially the same as in chronic pancreatitis. The long-standing duct occlusion, by inspissated secretion and subsequent acinar atrophy, focal fibrosis, and lipomatosis, leads to qualitative and quantitative islet changes similar to those in chronic pancreatitis.

Hemochromatosis. Diabetes is a well-known feature of primary hemochromatosis and secondary hemosiderosis. Initially, it can often be controlled by diet, but later it becomes insulin dependent because of impaired insulin secretion. Morphologically, it was found that, within the islets, iron is deposited in the β cells only (Fig. 64-14), which, in addition, are severely degranulated.[64] This indicates that iron overload of β cells may affect insulin biosynthesis and storage, thereby leading to diabetes. Because there is no β cell destruction, this type of diabetes is different from IDDM. It remains to be explained how iron interferes with β cell function and why non-β cells are not affected.

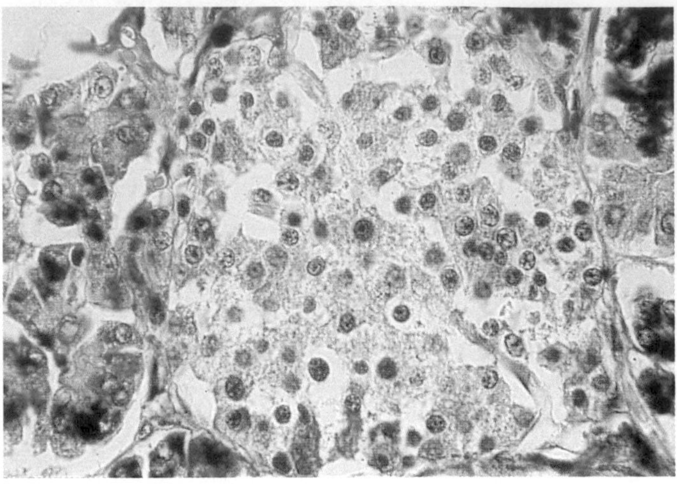

Fig. 64-14 Pancreas in hemochromatosis. Staining for iron shows positivity in most islet cells.

Diabetes secondary to endocrine diseases

Hormones with an insulin-antagonistic effect, such as growth hormone, glucocorticoids, catecholamines, thyroxine, and glucagon, cause impaired glucose tolerance or even overt diabetes, when produced in excess as a result of a tumor or hyperplasia of the respective gland of origin.[65] Endocrine syndromes frequently associated with carbohydrate abnormalities of variable intensity are acromegaly, Cushing's syndrome, pheochromocytoma syndrome, glucagonoma syndrome, hyperthyroidism, Conn's syndrome, and carcinoid syndrome. Although no changes of the islets can be observed in syndromes with mild glucose intolerance and those caused by hormones that inhibit insulin secretion, hypertrophic islets with signs of β cell stimulation may be found in syndromes that manifest diabetes caused by insulin resistance. This has been observed in some cases of Cushing's disease.

Rare causes of diabetes

Numerous rare genetic syndromes (lipoatrophic diabetes, leprechaunism, acanthosis nigricans types A and B, ataxia telangiectasia, stiff-man syndrome, Bardet-Biedl syndrome) may be associated with either glucose intolerance or overt diabetes.[47] The pathogenetic mechanisms of these diabetes forms vary, resulting either in absolute or relative insulin deficiency. Special islet lesions have not been described in any of the syndromes.

The high coincidence of cirrhosis and diabetes is long established (Naunyn's diabetes).[66] Possible causes of hepatogenic diabetes include reduced insulin degradation by the cirrhotic liver with subsequent hyperinsulinism, and insulin resistance.[67]

Chemically induced diabetes

Two groups of drugs causing permanent or transient hyperglycemia can be distinguished: (1) substances with a cytotoxic effect on β cells and (2) substances inhibiting insulin secretion without β cell destruction. The first group includes alloxan, glyoxal, streptozotocin, oxine, dithizone, and, recently, asparaginase, pentamidine isothionate, and *N*-3-pyridylmethyl *N'*-*p*-nitrophenyl urea (PNU).[68] Diazoxide, diphenylhydatoin, cyproheptadine, and mannoheptulose form the second group. The majority of these drugs have been used only experimentally in laboratory animals,[69] but some (streptozotocin for the treatment of malignant insulinomas; diazoxide for the treatment of hyperinsulinemic hypoglycemia) serve also as medications in clinical practice.

Complications of diabetes mellitus

The clinical range of the natural course of diabetes extends from acute metabolic complications, such as ketotic and hyperosmolar coma, to several other diseases that are now recognized as sequelae of chronic hyperglycemia (Fig. 64-15).

Before the introduction of insulin in the therapy of diabetes mellitus, coma was the major cause of death in diabetes. Since then, the life expectancy of treated diabetics is determined by the early occurrence of vascular complications. However, it must be emphasized that the susceptibility of the diabetic to angiopathy and also to other diseases, such as neuropathy, is highly variable.

Acute complications. Absolute or relative hypoinsulinemia results in inadequate glucose utilization. Glucose then appears in urine when the blood glucose level exceeds the renal threshold. Together with glucose, water leaves the body, causing severe dehydration if not compensated by polydipsia. Glucose can no longer be used as a fuel, and so the mobilization of energy reserves from fat and protein stores is accelerated. This in turn leads to considerable weight loss. Moreover, the breakdown of neutral fat results in an increase in free fatty acids, which are released into the circulation and oxidized by the liver to ketone bodies. Ketoacidosis occurs and eventually, together with the severe loss of water and electrolytes (particularly potassium) by the kidneys, causes ketoacedotic coma. In the so-called nonketotic hyperosmolar coma, which usually occurs in patients with NIDDM, ketosis is less severe, but hyperglycemia and dehydration (caused by extreme hyperosmolarity of the plasma) are more severe than in ketoacedotic coma.

Morphologic signs indicating or suggestive of severe, sustained hyperglycemia and diabetic coma are scarce. As a result of increased glycogen accumulation, glycogen nuclei may be found in the liver, Armanni-Ebstein cells in the kidneys, and hydropic degeneration of the β cells in the pancreas. The brain may show flattening of gyri and narrow sulci caused by edema. All other complications found in coma diabeticum are more likely related to the effects of circulatory failure and shock than to the diabetic situation itself.

Long-term complications. Vascular lesions of diabetes *(diabetic angiopathy)* are subdivided into *diabetic macroangiopathy,* the disease of the large and medium-sized muscular arteries, indistinguishable from atherosclerosis in nondiabetics, and *diabetic microangiopathy,* the disease of the arterioles and capillaries.

Macroangiopathy. In diabetics, atherosclerosis is more severe and starts earlier than in nondiabetics. Diabetics have, therefore, a greatly increased risk of myocardial infarction, cerebral stroke, and gangrene of the legs, and myocardial infarction is the major cause of death in diabetes.[70] It is not clear how diabetes contributes to the complex process of atherogenesis. Hypertension (one of every two adult diabetics is hypertensive), hyperlipidemia and hypercholesterolemia, sorbitol accumulation in cells of the vessel walls by the polyol pathway, and altered platelet aggregation undoubtedly play a role.

Microangiopathy. Degree and duration of hyperglycemia appear to be the main factors responsible for the development

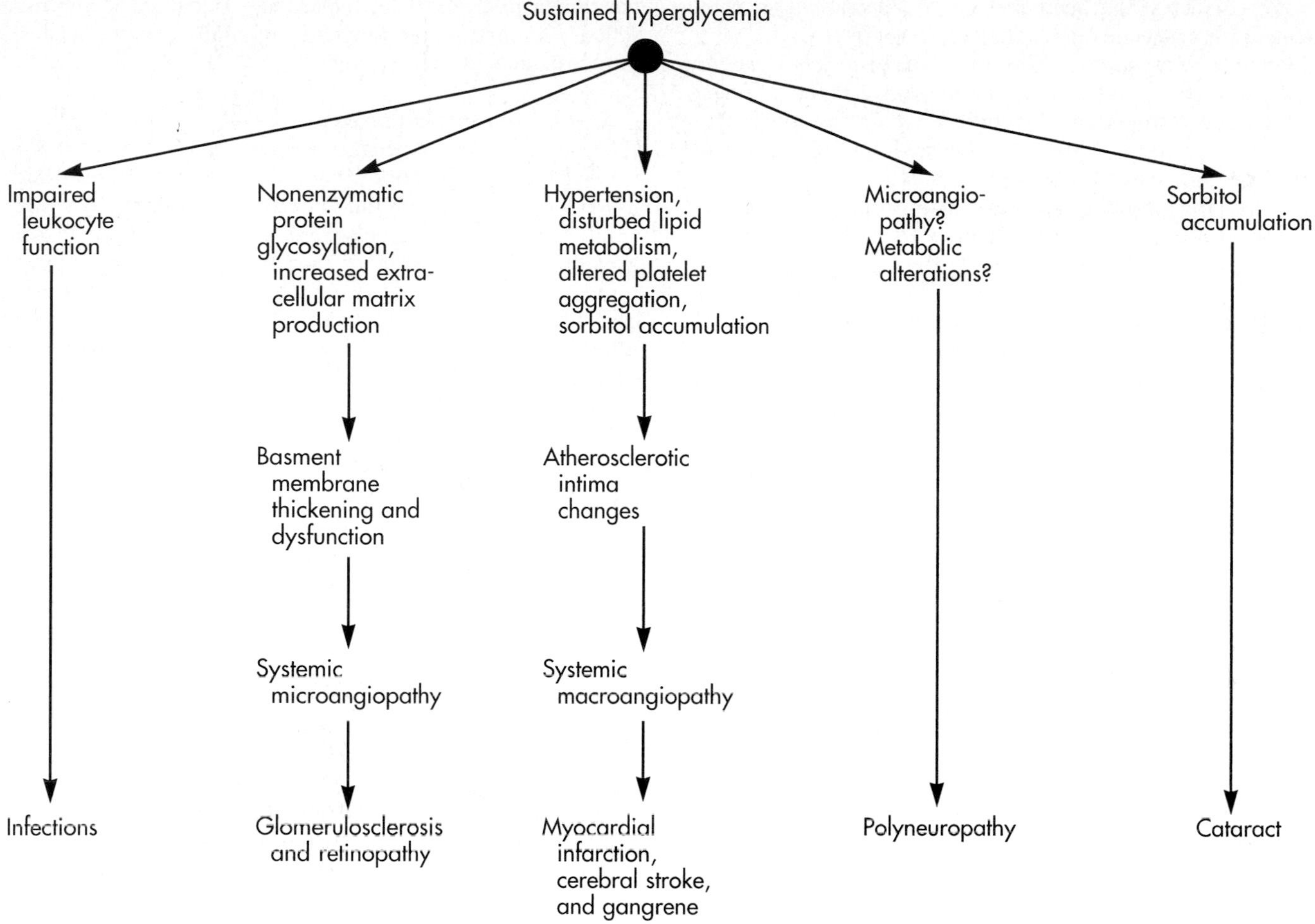

Fig. 64-15 Clinical consequences of sustained hyperglycemia in diabetes mellitus.

of microangiopathy because intensive therapy delays its onset and slows its progression.[71] Although the precise biochemical mechanisms linking sustained hyperglycemia, basement membrane thickening caused by increased accumulation of extracellular matrix proteins, and disturbed vascular function are not yet fully understood, there is evidence that glucose-induced increase in extracellular matrix protein synthesis, possibly in concert with nonenzymatic glycosylation of proteins, is involved.[72]

Diabetic microangiopathy occurs throughout the body, but clinically is most apparent in the kidneys and eyes, where it results in glomerular sclerosis and retinopathy respectively. About 90% of all adult diabetics show only minor signs of glomerular diseases (see Chapter 65). Diffuse or nodular glomerulosclerosis may develop in these patients.[73] Forty percent to 50% of IDDM patients with an onset of their disease before 15 years of age die of renal insufficiency. Among all diabetics nephropathy accounts for about 9% of the deaths[70] and is thus the second leading cause of death after myocardial infarction.

Diabetic retinopathy. Diabetic retinopathy starts with the development of microaneurysms, macular edema, PAS-positive lipid exudates (hard waxy exsudates), hemorrhages, and gray-white microinfarcts (cotton-wool spots). This nonproliferative stage is followed by proliferation of new small vessels and fibrous tissue, probably caused by retinal anoxia, within and on the inner surface of the retina. Adhesions between the newly developed fibrovascular tissue on the retina and the vitrous body finally lead to traction and retinal detachment and may result in blindness. A similar process may concomitantly affect the iris, resulting in glaucoma. Cataract formation, on the other hand, is directly related to the disturbed glucose metabolism and sorbitol accumulation in the lens.

Diabetic polyneuropathy. Diabetic polyneuropathy appears in different forms, the most common being the bilateral distal, sensorimotor syndrome (symmetrical peripheral polyneuropathy) symmetrically affecting the nerves of the lower extremities.[74] The nerves show sequential demyelinization and eventual irreversible injury to axons. Other forms of diabetic neuropathy include mononeuropathy, amyotrophy, and dysfunction of the autonomic nervous system.

Infections. Infections played a significant role in the preinsulin era in the natural course of diabetes but are nowadays of less importance. Infections most often affect the skin *(Candida albicans)* and the kidney (pyelonephritis with or without necrotizing renal papillitis).

Necrobiosis lipoidica. Necrobiosis lipoidica is a rare skin disease pathogenetically related to diabetes. It usually develops after diabetes has been present for years, but in some patients it may precede clinical diabetes.

Diabetic embryopathy. The term *diabetic embryopathy* includes all changes found in infants of diabetic mothers. Characteristic features are a significantly increased mortality caused by respiratory distress disease, high birth weight, macrosomia, increased amount of pancreatic endocrine tissue, and greater prevalence of congenital malformations. Incidence and severity of *embryopathia diabetica* depends on the control of diabetes during pregnancy.

Pathogenesis. The sustained effects of maternal hyperglycemia are the cause of the fetal changes. As glucose passively passes through the placenta, the elevated blood glucose levels of the mother stimulate fetal insulin production and secretion, thereby causing β cell hyperplasia and hypertrophy. The insulin released, on the other hand, cannot cross the placenta and thus promotes utilization of glucose in the fetus and, in addition, exerts growth-enhancing anabolic effects. This results in enlargement of the subcutaneous fat depots, glycogen storage, and eventually hypertrophy of visceral organs. For these reasons islet volume correlates with birth weight and maternal blood glucose levels.[75]

Pathology of the pancreas. Grossly, the pancreas is normal. Histologically the most conspicuous feature is the increased size of many islets (mean islet diameter 120 to 180 μm versus 60 to 100 μm in controls) caused by β cell hypertrophy and hyperplasia (Fig. 64-16).[75] This may lead to a doubling of the total islet volume. Occasionally there are infiltrates of lymphocytes and especially eosinophilic leukocytes surrounding large islets and in the interstitial septae. Infiltration of eosinophils is frequently associated with periinsular fibrosis and the deposition of Charcot-Leyden crystals. Its degree appears to be positively correlated with volume and size of the islets and the severity of maternal diabetes. The cause of these eosinophilic infiltrates has not been identified.

Hyperinsulinemic hypoglycemia

Three major lesions are known to cause persistent hyperinsulinemic hypoglycemia: (1) nesidioblastosis either in its diffuse or focal form; (2) islet hyperplasia, mainly caused by increased numbers of β cells; and (3) insulinoma. Whereas nesidioblastosis and islet hyperplasia occur in newborns and infants, insulinoma predominates in adults (see the discussion of tumors later in this chapter).

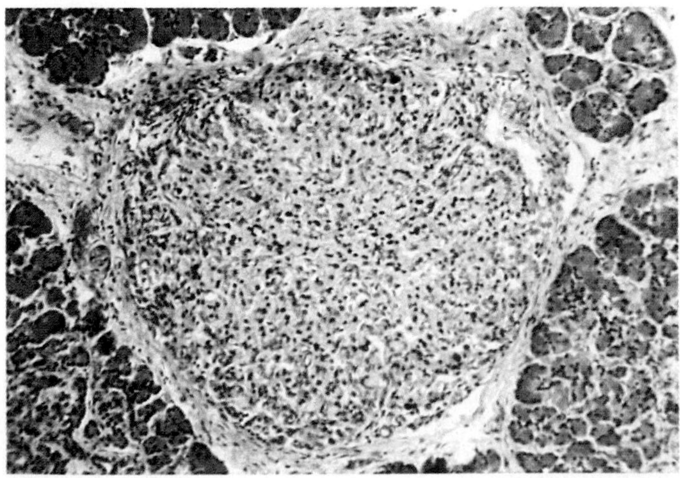

Fig. 64-16 Pancreas of newborn of diabetic mother. Islet with distinct hypertrophy.

Neonatal nesidioblastosis

Persistent neonatal hyperinsulinemic hypoglycemia (PNHH) is one of several pathophysiologic mechanisms resulting in hypoglycemia in the infant. Other causes of hypoglycemia are ketotic hypoglycemia, endocrine disorders (pituitary failure, growth hormone deficiency, adrenal insufficiency, hyperthyroidism), hepatic enzyme deficiency (glycogen storage diseases), and disorders of gluconeogenesis and immune-related diseases (antibodies to insulin receptor).[76,77] PNHH has been estimated to represent between 20% and 55% of all cases of persistent hypoglycemia in infancy.[78] All islet changes associated with PNHH are herein summarized under the term *nesidioblastosis*, though nesidioblastosis, strictly speaking, signifies only the physiologic process of budding off of endocrine cells from duct epithelium.

Pathogenesis. The etiology of PNHH and the pathogenesis of the inappropriate insulin secretion are obscure. Because both focal and diffuse nesidioblastosis have histologic characteristics in common, it is tempting to speculate that the two types of nesidioblastosis are various expressions or different stages of one basic defect rather than of different basic lesions.[79] In some patients the underlying defect appears to be genetically determined because familial cases with a suspected autosomal recessive trait of inheritance have been reported. Judging from the morphologic descriptions given in these reports, it seems that so far all familial cases had suffered from the diffuse type of nesidioblastosis whereas none had been affected by a focal lesion.

Distinct β cell hypertrophy, the morphologic hallmark of nesidioblastosis, may reflect an increase in secretory activity with continuing overproduction of insulin. It is not known whether this hyperactivity of the β cells (or a subset of β cells) is caused by a primary functional defect or is secondary to an abnormality of the mechanisms controlling the functional as well as structural differentiation of the endocrine pancreas. The latter hypothesis is largely based on the fact that some structural features of the fetal pancreas (scattering of small endocrine cell clusters throughout the acinar tissue, ductulo-insular complexes) are also present in the nesidioblastosis-involved pancreas.[79] The question as to whether the β cell defect is permanent or gradually improves with time can so far not be definitely answered because of a lack of long-term studies on the natural course of PNHH. However, no improvement has been noted in the disease on long-term follow-up study of a few patients.[80]

Morphology. The multitude of terms for the pancreatic disease underlying PNHH reflects the general lack of knowledge concerning this disease and the variability of its appearance. The following synonyms are currently used: nesidioblastosis, β cell nesidioblastosis, diffuse or generalized islet hyperplasia, focal or multifocal ductulo-insular proliferation, microadenomatosis, focal islet cell adenomatosis, endocrine cell dysplasia, and nesidiodysplasia.[80] Some authors did not find consistent abnormalities in the pancreas.

At present, it appears that basically two types of islet lesions (herein called *nesidioblastosis*) are associated with PNHH: a focal and a diffuse form of nesidioblastosis.[80]

In focal nesidioblastosis, a small, barely visible focus with increased consistency (diameter 5 to 8 mm) may be found in the pancreas at laparotomy. The lesions are usually unifocal, and most are found in the body and tail. Rarely, they are multifocal. Histologically the focal lesion is composed of huge, isletlike and partly confluent endocrine cell clusters, often encompassing small ducts (ductulo-insular complexes). The isletlike cell clusters push aside acinar tissue or are haphazardly dispersed between exocrine cells (Fig. 64-17). The endocrine cells vary in size, including large insulin-producing cells with prominent and giant nuclei. The diameter of these β cells was often one and a half times larger than normal. The histologic features of the well-demarcated nodules, which may macroscopically appear to be tumors, are in principle, comparable with those of the focal lesion. The only difference is the absence of acinar cells between the endocrine cell clusters, which are, instead, separated by fibrous stroma cords. Immunocytochemical analysis reveals the presence of insulin cells, glucagon cells, somatostatin cells, and PP cells in nearly normal spatial distribution. Insulin cells, however, are more numerous than normal. The islets outside the foci display endocrine cells that are normal in size, appearance, and distribution.

In diffuse nesidioblastosis there are no gross abnormalities. Histologically the main criteria for establishing the diagnosis are (1) distinct β cell hypertrophy with nuclear enlargement, often resulting in giant and bizarre nuclei (Figs. 64-18 and 64-19); (2) presence of islets of variable size, often with somewhat irregular outline; (3) irregularly sized and poorly defined endocrine cell clusters scattered in the acinar parenchyma; and (4) endocrine cell complexes, often intimately connected with small or larger ducts (ductulo-insular complexes) (Fig. 64-20).

Immunocytochemically, the islets, as well as the small endocrine cell aggregates and the ductulo-insular complexes, are composed of the four currently known endocrine cell types. Except for certain cases, there seems to be no increase in insulin cells. In some patients, a decrease of the volume density of D cells was reported,[81] but this could not be confirmed by others.[80] A decreased number of α cells, reported in a few patients, has not been observed in larger series.[80]

Clinical presentation. The leading symptoms are somnolence, ataxia, seizures, and loss of consciousness before meals. More than 75% of the patients have these symptoms during the

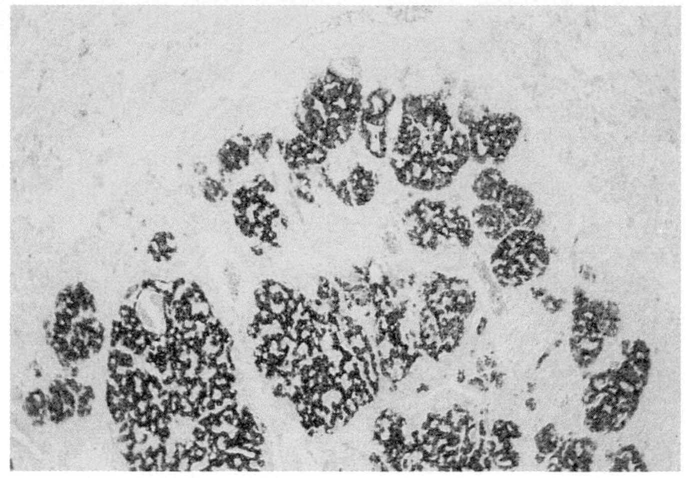

Fig. 64-18 Focal nesidioblastosis. Cluster of islets with β cells in normal spatial distribution. (Immunostaining for insulin.)

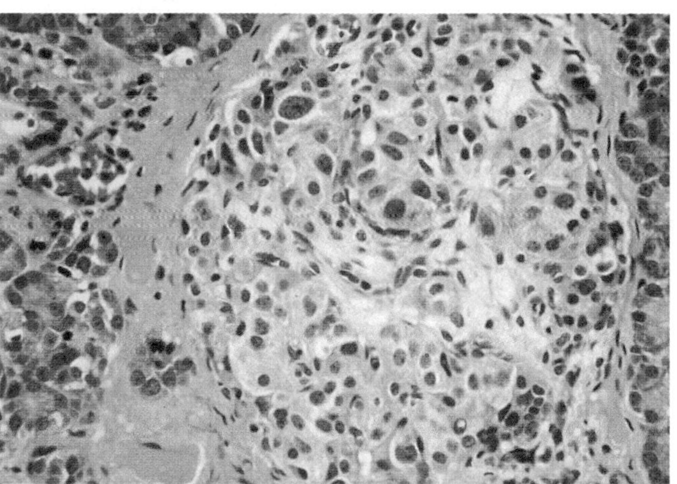

Fig. 64-19 Diffuse nesidioblastosis. Islet with distinct hypertrophy of nuclei.

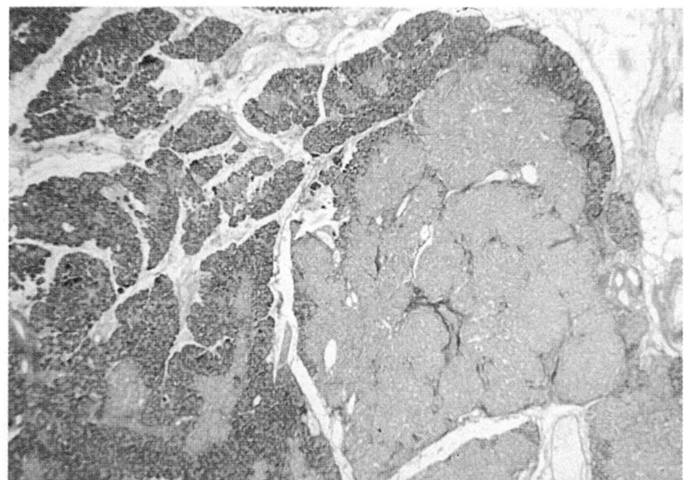

Fig. 64-17 Focal nesidioblastosis. Clustering of endocrine cell mass in the pancreas.

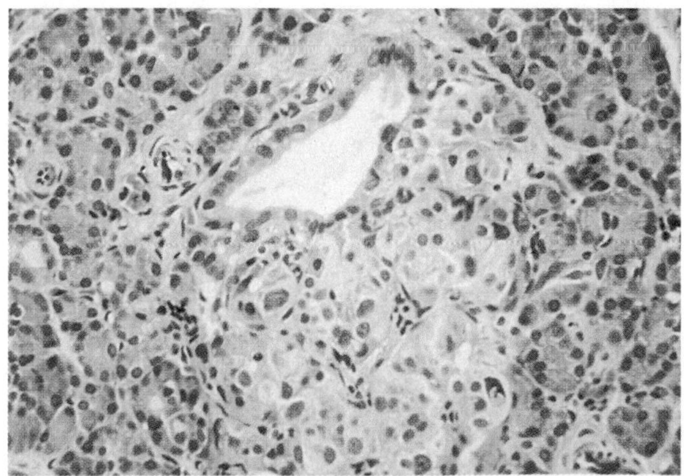

Fig. 64-20 Diffuse nesidioblastosis. Irregularly outlined islet associated with a small duct (ductulo-insular complex).

first 3 months of life, and more than 90% during the first year of life. Biochemically, a high insulin-to-glucose ratio in the blood is characteristic.[76] Moreover, many of the newborns with PNHH are large for gestational age and appear obese and plethoric. Early recognition and efficient prevention of hypoglycemia are essential for the prevention of permanent neurologic damage and severe mental retardation resulting from neuroglycopenia.[76] Prevention of recurrent hypoglycemic attacks may be achieved by frequent feeding and glucose infusions combined with adrenal steroids or glucagon administration, or substances inhibiting insulin secretion (such as diazoxide or protamine-zinc somatostatin). Despite recent advances in medical treatment, near-total pancreatectomy is often necessary.

Nesidioblastosis in adults

Persistent hyperinsulinemic hypoglycemia in adults, not caused by an insulinoma, is extremely rare. Up to now, some 22 patients have been reported.[82] Because the endocrine pancreas usually does not show the full range of the features seen in infants, diagnosis of nesidioblastosis in an adult should only be made after exclusion of an insulinoma by all clinical and morphologic means.

Islet hyperplasia caused by hyperglycemic stimulation

Islet hyperplasia as a consequence of sustained hyperglycemia is seen in infants of diabetic mothers (see the discussion of diabetic embryopathy earlier in this chapter).

Islet hyperplasia associated with genetic diseases

In addition to islet cell hyperplasia in infants of diabetic mothers, the same changes may occur in a number of congenital syndromes. The best known is the Beckwith-Wiedemann syndrome (omphalocele, macroglossia, gigantism, hyperplastic visceromegaly, renal dysplasia, Leydig cell hyperplasia, cytomegaly of the adrenal cortex, and increased incidence of tumors), which can be associated with hypoglycemia caused by hyperinsulinism.[32] The pancreas is increased in size and shows massive islet hyperplasia and hypertrophy (Fig. 64-21). The islets are abnormally large and occasionally confluent, but their distribution within the pancreas appears to be normal. The increase in endocrine tissue results from an increase in all endocrine cell types, particularly the insulin and glucagon cells. Qualitatively, a lack of segregation of glucagon and PP cells to distinct parts of the gland (PP cells to the dorsal part of the head of the pancreas and α cells to the remaining parts of the pancreas) has been observed.[32]

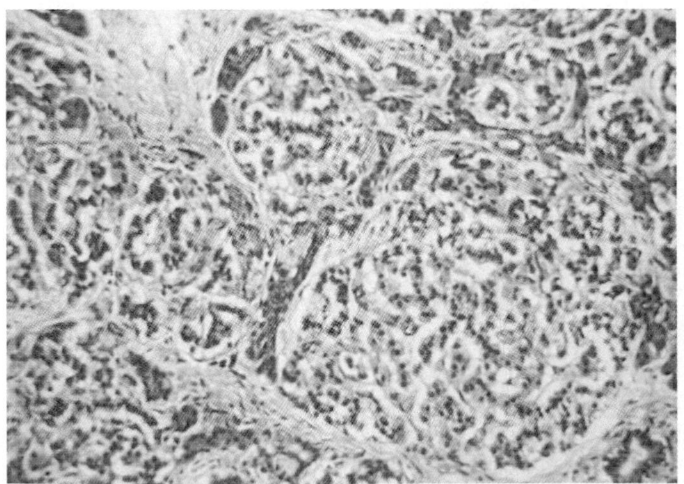

Fig. 64-21 Beckwith-Wiedemann syndrome. Pancreas shows islet hyperplasia and hypertrophy.

Hyperplasia and hypertrophy of islets have also been described in infants with congenital malformations of the heart and in patients with α-1-antitrypsin deficiency.[57] However, since these studies were not based an quantitative assessments, it remains to be established whether there is a true volume increase in islet tissue in these patients. Clinically, the observed islet changes were not associated with hyperinsulinemic hypoglycemia.

PANCREATIC NEUROENDOCRINE NEOPLASMS

Pancreatic neuroendocrine tumors are composed of cells that phenotypically may resemble those normally found in the islets of Langerhans but may also contain phenotypically identical but functionally "nonpancreatic" cells of the diffuse gastrointestinal neuroendocrine system. By electron microscopy these cells show neuroendocrine differentiation and, by immunohistochemical analysis, some common as well as cell type–specific markers. The precursors of these tumors are presumably developmentally multipotent in terms of their capacity to differentiate into various cell types producing various hormones and regulatory peptides. Whether these cells originate from the ductular epithelium or the islet cells is a matter of debate.[83]

Incidence and prevalence. Pancreatic neuroendocrine tumors are uncommon. Their prevalence has been estimated at less than 1 in 100,000. The incidence of insulinoma has recently been estimated at 4 cases per million per year.[84] In Northern Ireland, an incidence of 0.5 patients with gastrinoma per million per year was reported; in Denmark, an incidence of 1.5 patients with gastrinoma per million per year was reported. It seems that the incidence of gastrinoma has increased during recent years, probably because of improved diagnostic techniques.

Classification. Neuroendocrine tumors of the pancreas have been variously named, including islet cell tumors, insulinomas, nesidioblastomas, β-cell tumors, non–β cell tumors, carcinoid-islet cell tumors, and APUDomas. Because these names have created confusion and discussion, we prefer the term *neuroendocrine tumor of the pancreas*. If criteria of malignancy are present, the term *malignant* or *metastasizing* should be added. Tumors giving rise to well-defined hormonal syndromes are designated *functioning*. They are classified according to the hormone responsible for the clinical syndrome and detected by radioimmunoassay and immunocytochemistry. Consequently the tumors are called *insulinomas*, *gastrinomas*, and so on, even if they turn out to be multihormonal. Nonfunctioning (nonsecreting, inactive, hormonally silent) tumors may be named according to the major product detected by immunocytochemistry or radioimmunoassay, such as *pancreatic neuroendocrine tumor producing (synthesizing) insulin*.

In surgical series, functioning neuroendocrine tumors account for 60% to 85% of all pancreatic neuroendocrine neoplasms (Fig. 64-22). On the other hand, clinically insignificant or unrecognized and asymptomatic tumors, usually smaller

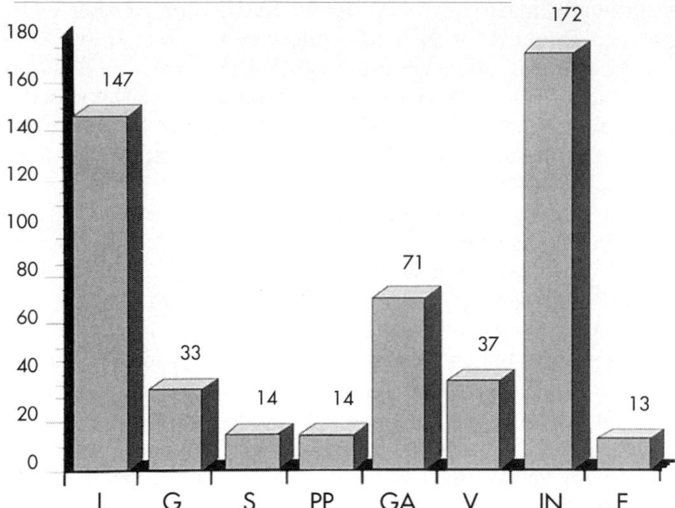

Fig. 64-22 Number of the various types of pancreatic neuroendocrine tumors in a series of 501 neoplasms. *E,* Ectopic hormone-producing tumors; *I,* insulinoma; *G,* glucagonoma; *S,* somatostatinoma; *PP,* PP-oma; *GA,* gastrinoma; *V,* vipoma, *IN,* nonfunctioning (inactive) tumors.

than 1 cm in diameter, have been found in 0.4% to 1.5% of unselected autopsies.[85]

Etiology and pathogenesis. No risk factors clearly associated with pancreatic neuroendocrine tumors are known. mRNA of the proto-oncogenes Ha-*ras,* Ki-*ras, fos,* c-*myc* was detectable as determined by in situ hybridization and quantitative northern blot analysis in neuroendocrine tumors of the pancreas and in nontumorous pancreatic tissues. N-*myc* and *sis* mRNA were not found. Ha-*ras* and Ki-*ras* mRNA was overexpressed up to 42 times in tumors as compared with nontumorous pancreatic tissue; metastasizing tumors revealed 2 to 6 times higher Ha-*ras* mRNA levels than benign neoplasias. Lower levels of *fos* m-RNA were found in all tumors as compared with normal pancreas. Significant differences of *fos* mRNA levels in malignant and benign pancreatic neuroendocrine tumors, however, were not found. High *fos* mRNA expression in a normal pancreas is in accordance with the recent evidence that the *fos* gene may be involved in the regulation of differentiation (and secretion) of neuronal and endocrine cells. These results indicate that Ha-*ras* and Ki-*ras* mRNA overexpression may be associated with progression of neuroendocrine pancreatic tumors and that the measurement of Ha-*ras* mRNA levels may contribute to the assessment of tumor prognosis.[86] Point mutation at codon 12 of the Ki-*ras* protooncogene, which is found in 75% to 90% of pancreatic ductal adenocarcinomas, was not detected in pancreatic neuroendocrine tumors. Together, these findings, many of which need to be confirmed, do not provide any definite clues about the pathogenesis of the neuroendocrine tumors of the pancreas.

Pathology. The majority of the tumors are well demarcated, solitary neoplasms with white-gray, yellow, or pinkish brown color and firm consistency. The size of the tumors is not related to the severity of hormonally induced symptoms. Usually their diameter ranges between 1 and 5 cm. Tumor nodules with a diameter below 0.5 cm are called "microadenomas." *Microadenomatosis* is a term signifying the occurrence of multiple microadenomas in the pancreas. However, as a rule, tumors associated with hormonally induced symptoms are larger than 0.5 cm in diameter. Among the functioning tumors, insulinomas are usually smaller (<2 cm) than gastrinomas, glucagonomas, vipomas, and other rare, functioning tumors. This indicates that the latter tumors may require a larger volume than insulinomas do to produce hormonally induced symptoms. Malignant tumors usually metastasize, but their spread is confined to regional lymph nodes and the liver. Extrahepatic metastases are rare.

Histology. Tumors may have a solid, trabecular, or glandular pattern. These patterns often differ considerably from one tumor to another and may vary within the same tumor. Most tumor cells are well differentiated. They have finely granular, eosinophilic cytoplasm and contain round-to-oval nuclei, often with distinct nucleoli. Pleomorphism of cells and nuclei is, in general, lacking, and mitotic figures are uncommon. The amount of vascular stroma and fibrosis vary. The histologic pattern of a tumor, in general, does not allow a conclusion as to its functional state or the type of hormone produced. There are two exceptions: amyloid deposits are indicative of insulinomas, and glandular structures containing psammoma bodies are commonly observed in somatostatinomas of the ampullary region. This endocrine amyloid is composed of the polypeptide islet amyloid polypeptide (IAPP), or amylin,[87-89] which is normally released by the pancreatic β cell together with insulin. It has been mapped to chromosome 12, and its amino acid sequence shows a strong homology with that of CGRP.

Electron microscopy. Electron-dense, membrane-bound secretory granules are the hallmark of neuroendocrine differentiation, which can be demonstrated by electron microscopy in many tumors. The tumors may be ultrastructurally classified as well differentiated or poorly differentiated. In well-differentiated tumors, including most insulinomas, secretory granule morphology is indicative of the hormone stored in the respective cell. However, in poorly differentiated tumor cells, morphology of the secretory granules is not diagnostic.

Precise classification of pancreatic neuroendocrine tumors requires analysis of the cell phenotype by immunocytochemistry. The tumor cells usually express markers (1) common to all neuroendocrine cells and (2) cell type–specific markers. Synaptophysin, chromogranins A and C, and protein gene product 9.5 (PGP 9.5) are markers common to many of the neuroendocrine cells. Synaptophysin is an integral membrane glycoprotein of synaptic vesicles. Chromogranins are components of the matrix of neuroendocrine secretory granules, and PGP 9.5 is a cytoplasmic protein. The expression of the markers is largely independent of that of the hormones. The staining pattern of chromogranins reflects the number and distribution of the secretory granules in the cell[90] because they are stored in the matrix of the secretory granules. In addition to the neuroendocrine markers, the tumors contain cytokeratins, 8, 18, and 19, and often neurofilaments. Cell type–specific products of the tumors are insulin, glucagon, somatostatin, and pancreatic polypeptide. In addition to these eutopic hormones, tumors may express hormones ectopic to the pancreas.

In the majority of functioning tumors, the hormone causing the syndrome can be detected by immunocytochemistry at the light and electron microscopic levels. Staining intensity or number of positive cells, however, are not related to the severity of symptoms. Using a battery of antibodies against pancreatic and ectopic hormones, many tumors turn out to be multihormonal. Pancreatic polypeptide is a frequent component of many types of pancreatic neuroendocrine tumors. Metastases may produce hormones not found in the primary.

The detection of mRNA at the cellular level can be accomplished by in situ hybridization, both on tissue sections and on single-cell preparations. The combination of immunocytochemistry and in situ hybridization on the same tissue sections revealed a high degree of heterogeneity regarding immunoreactive peptide hormone content and steady-state amounts of its mRNA in individual cells of pancreatic neuroendocrine tumors. These results indicate that hormone-secreting cells may not be positive by immunocytochemistry for a given peptide but may contain the related mRNA. The usual reason for this is nonregulated, constitutive hormone secretion.

Somatostatin receptors can be demonstrated in pancreatic neuroendocrine tumors. It was shown that the presence of somatostatin receptors on tumors correlated with the in vivo localization thereof by scanning and with the suppressive effect of the somatostatin analog octreotide on hormonal release by these tumors.[91,92]

Criteria of malignancy. In the majority of pancreatic neuroendocrine tumors, the biologic behavior cannot be predicted from the histologic data. Poorly differentiated and fast-growing neoplasms are the exception; they may resemble pulmonary small cell carcinoma or undifferentiated cancers, the neuroendocrine nature of which is barely recognizable by conventional histologic features. In all other slowly growing tumors, the only indisputable evidence of malignancy is angioinvasion, gross infiltration of adjacent organs, or metastasis to regional lymph nodes or the liver. To establish the benign nature of a tumor, a long clinical follow-up period is needed because metastases may become apparent only years after the removal of the primary. Nevertheless, well over 90% of insulinomas are benign. The majority (at least 60%) of all other types of pancreatic neuroendocrine tumors are malignant.

The α-chain of human chorionic gonadotropin (HCG-α) and, less frequently, HCG-β were repeatedly reported to be expressed by neuroendocrine tumors of the pancreas. Immunocytochemically, HCG-α was found to be produced by approximately 65% of malignant, functioning, pancreatic neuroendocrine tumors.[93,94] However, it is also produced by a small number of benign tumors. This marker is therefore of limited value in the differential diagnosis of benign and malignant tumors. In addition and in contrast to findings in nonneuroendocrine tumors, the histochemical detection of so-called β-1,6-branches of asparagine-linked oligosaccharides does not permit differentiation of metastasizing from nonmetastasizing insulinomas.[95]

Recent studies on the DNA content of pancreatic neuroendocrine tumors failed to establish a clear correlation between the ploidy status and clinical outcome.[96] Such DNA-ploidy analysis did not allow discrimination between benign and malignant pancreatic neuroendocrine neoplasms. It may, however, help to predict the prognosis because patients with malignant diploid pancreatic neuroendocrine tumors show a longer mean survival (5.7 years) than patients with aneuploid tumors (3.5 years) do. In line with these findings, it was found that all patients who lived longer than 10 years had diploid tumors.[97]

Differential diagnosis. Most neuroendocrine tumors of the pancreas are recognized without much difficulty. The morphology is typically monomorphic, and the number of mitotic figures is usually low. Problems may be encountered with functionally inactive or undifferentiated tumors. Using cytochemical markers for the neuroendocrine phenotype, the diagnosis can most often be established unequivocally. Caution must, however, be exerted in the detection of neuron-specific enolase (NSE) because many antibodies are not specific for NSE, and immunoreactivity for NSE is not restricted to neuroendocrine tumor cells.

One tumor that has been considered neuroendocrine for many years—the solid-cystic tumor of the pancreas—deserves further discussion. The tumor contains NSE, as visualized by immunocytochemistry and confirmed by western blotting, and its appearance resembles that of a neuroendocrine neoplasm. However, the tumor most often (1) does not produce systemic symptoms but only local effects; (2) is usually large (diameter >5 cm); (3) contains small cells and groups of larger cells with a clear cytoplasm; (4) shows broad, hyalinized septa with blood vessels; (5) displays hemorrhages and necrotic foci and cholesterol; (6) does not react with antibodies to neuroendocrine markers (except NSE); (7) does not produce hormones; (8) produces α-1-antitrypsin in large groups of cells; and (9) occurs predominantly in young women.

Clinical presentation. Pancreatic neuroendocrine tumors can produce life-threatening symptoms as a result of their inappropriate secretion of hormones. The clinical syndromes associated with or caused by inappropriate secretion of hormones by pancreatic neuroendocrine tumors are described under the headings of the various functioning tumors. Nonfunctioning tumors are not associated with a distinct clinical syndrome. They may become clinically apparent by their large size, by invasion of organs adjacent to the pancreas, or by the occurrence of metastases. Rarely, they present as obstructive pancreatitis.

The progression of the diseases is often remarkably slow, and survival of 5 to 10 years after appearance of liver metastases is common. It must be borne in mind, however, that functioning pancreatic neuroendocrine tumors are life threatening by their inappropriate secretion of hormones that cause hypoglycemia, gastric ulcers, and duodenal ulcers or watery diarrhea (vipomas). Surgery is the treatment of choice for small tumors. Increase in mass of metastasizing tumors can apparently be inhibited, or symptoms caused by inappropriate secretion of hormones may be relieved, at least temporarily, by somatostatin analogs if tumor cells possess functioning somatostatin receptors.

Insulinoma

Insulinoma is a neuroendocrine tumor that secretes insulin. The regulation of insulin secretion is impaired. This results in an inappropriate secretion of insulin; that is, it is not adequately suppressed upon the fall of the concentration of blood glucose. Insulinoma is the most common cause of persistent hyperinsulinemic hypoglycemia. The highest incidence is found between 30 and 60 years of age, with no predilection for either sex. Children below 15 years are rarely affected. Insulinomas are by far the most frequent of all functioning pancreatic neuroendocrine tumors (Fig. 64-22).

Pathology. Virtually all insulinomas are in or attached to the pancreas[98] (Fig. 64-23). Most tumors are small (less than 2 cm) and histologically indistinguishable from other neuroendocrine tumors. Histologic patterns of insulinoma can be solid, trabecular, glandlike, and mixed trabecular–solid (Fig. 64-24). By immunocytochemistry, insulin and proinsulin-producing

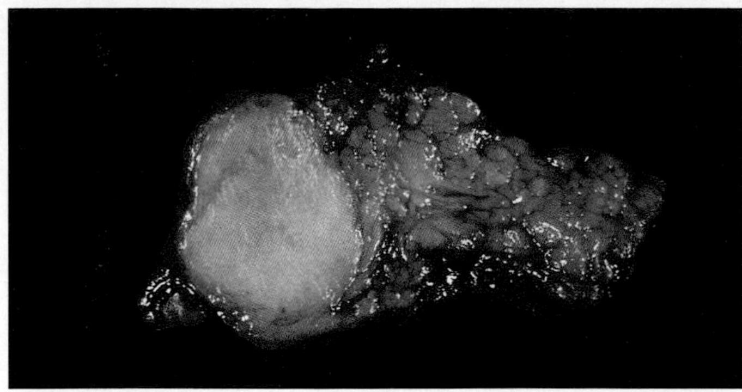

Fig. 64-23 Surgical specimen showing a well-circumscribed insulinoma.

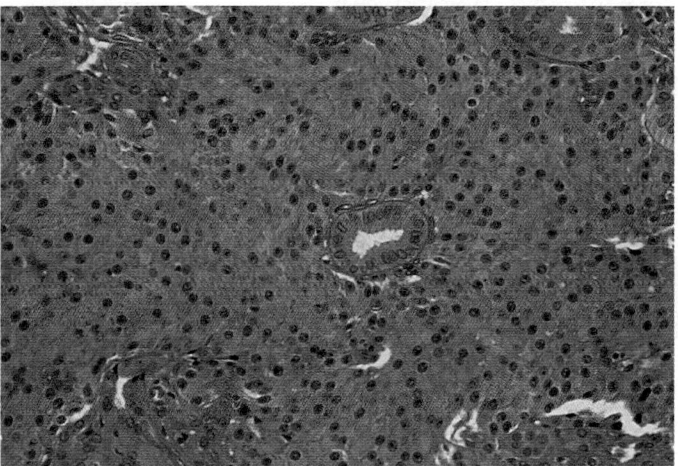

Fig. 64-24 Typical histologic pattern of a solid neuroendocrine tumor (insulinoma) of the pancreas.

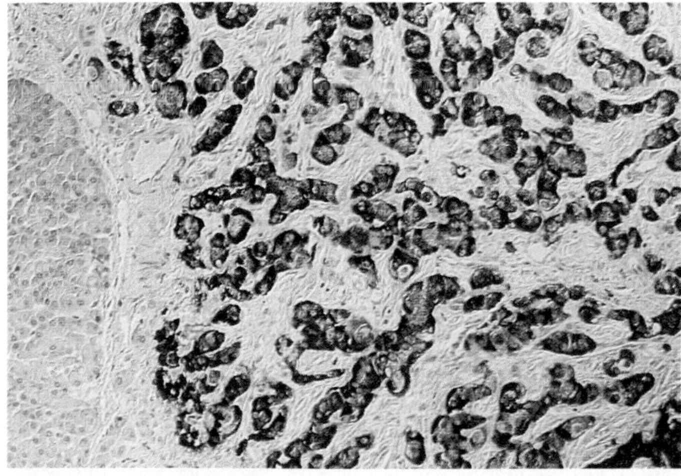

Fig. 64-25 Immunohistochemical demonstration of insulin with a polyclonal antiserum in a trabecular insulinoma. Adjacent to exocrine pancreatic parenchyma. (Paraffin section, immunoperoxidase technique, hematoxylin.)

cells can be identified in most insulinomas (Fig. 64-25). Typically, insulin-rich cells account for 60% to 80% of all tumor cells. Strong positivity for insulin at the secretory pole of the cells and proinsulin in the perinuclear region (the Golgi region) can be seen in some of the insulinomas irrespective of their histologic type (Fig. 64-26). However, more often, abnormal staining patterns for proinsulin and insulin are found, irrespective of the histologic type, the multihormonality, or the malignancy of the insulinoma[99] (Fig. 64-26). By immunoelectron microscopy, labeling for insulin is usually abundant over secretory granules in well-granulated tumor cells, irrespective of the secretory granule morphology (Fig. 64-27). Insulin mRNA can be detected by in situ hybridization (Fig. 64-28). About half of the insulinomas are multihormonal. In such tumors, insulin-rich cells are admixed with cells producing glucagon, somatostatin, or pancreatic polypeptide. Islet cell amyloid polypeptide (IAPP) is found in approximately 10% of the tumors.

Inappropriate proinsulin and insulin secretion is typical. The degree of differentiation of the tumors and the localization of proinsulin and insulin parallel the biochemical findings of their respective concentration in the tumor parenchyma and in the serum. The inadequately controlled insulin release apparently results from the constitutive secretion of newly synthesized prohormone. Recent immunocytochemical studies in insulinomas indicate a probable impaired proinsulin-insulin conversion, at least partly occurring within the Golgi apparatus of the tumor cells.[99]

By electron microscopy, well-granulated cells with typical β granules, cells with atypical, pleomorphic granules, and scarcely granulated cells have been described. In addition, cells with typical α and PP granules may be identified in multihormonal tumors.

Clinical presentation. The combination of fasting hypoglycemia (values less than 40 mg/dl glucose during an observed fast), neuroglycopenia, and the failure to suppress insulin secretion are diagnostic of an insulinoma. A gradual onset of sweating and palpitations (warning symptoms) is typical. Subsequently, tachycardia, anxiety and tremulousness appear (because of epinephrine release from the adrenal medulla), as well as symptoms of "neuroglycopenia" (confusion, headache, aberrant behavior, loss of consciousness, seizures, and blurred vision). These symptoms are relieved by food ingestion or glucose administration.

A high percentage of proinsulin in the total measured serum insulin concentration after an overnight fast and an elevated serum concentration of C peptide support the diagnosis of an insulinoma.

Gastrinoma

Gastrinoma is a neuroendocrine tumor with inappropriate secretion of gastrin. Gastrinoma is the second most frequent functioning neuroendocrine tumor of the pancreas (Fig. 64-22). In the United States, approximately 0.1% of the patients with duodenal ulcers may suffer from Zollinger-Ellison syndrome (ZES). ZES occurs more often in males than in females (3:2); the mean age at the onset of symptoms is approximately 38 years. Sixty percent to 75% of patients with ZES are found to suffer from sporadic ZES; in the remaining patients, ZES is part of a multiple endocrine neoplasia type 1 syndrome (see discussion of MEN type 1 later in this chapter). The large majority of gastrinomas are malignant.

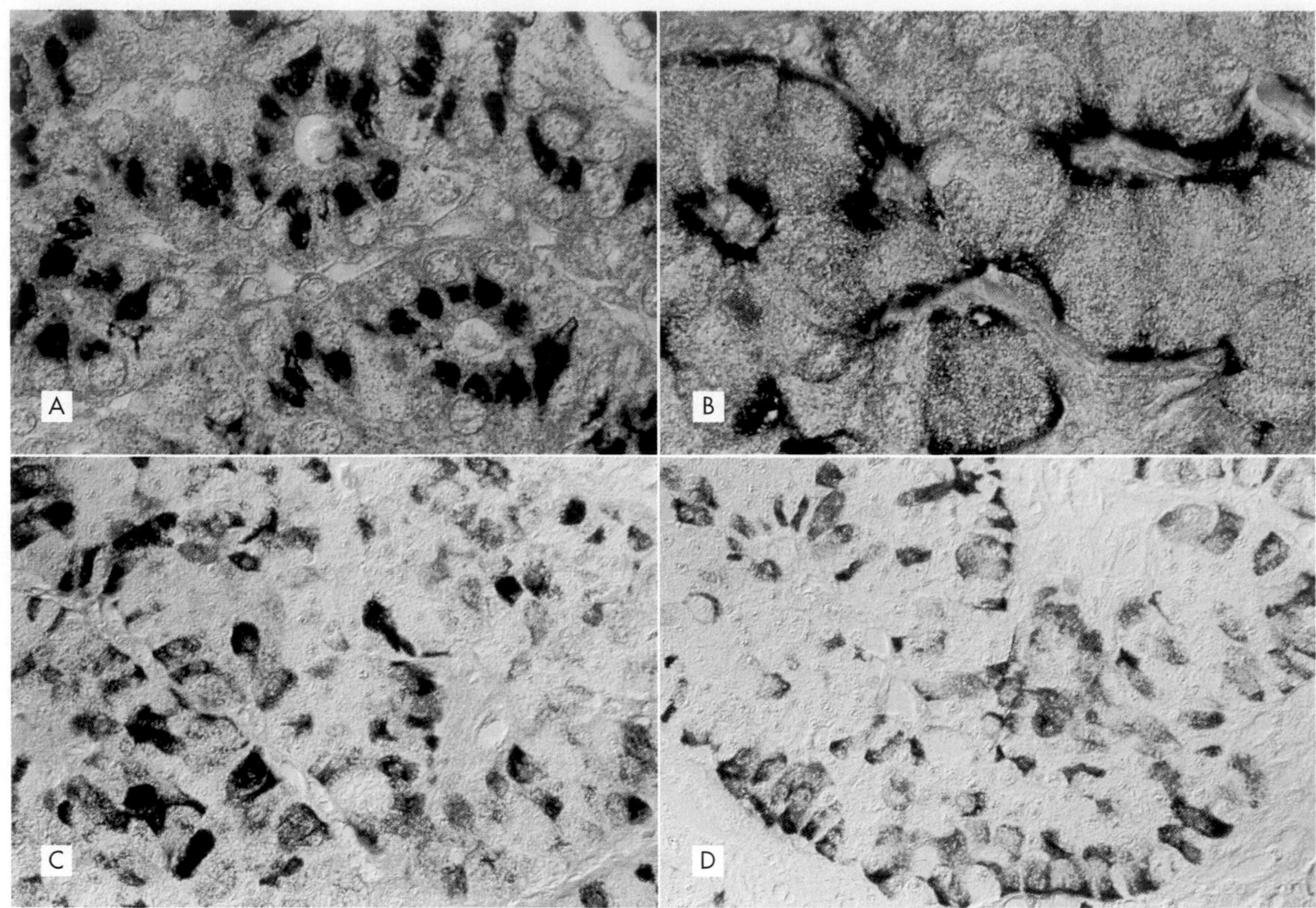

Fig. 64-26 Immunohistochemical localization of proinsulin and insulin with the respective monoclonal antibodies in insulinomas. Different patterns of immunostaining can be observed similar to the pattern found in normal B cells, **A** and **B** (compare with Fig. 64-1) or atypical with several positive cells and diffuse intracellular distribution of immunoreactivity, **C** and **D.** (Paraffin sections, immunogold-silver technique, nuclear fast red.)

Pathology. In sporadic ZES, 50% to 70% of the gastrinomas occur in the pancreas, particularly in its head, and the remainder are mainly found in the duodenum (Fig. 64-29). This anatomic area, comprising the head of the pancreas and the superior and descending portions of the duodenum, has been called the "gastrinoma triangle."[100] Unusual sites of primary gastrinomas are the stomach, jejunum, biliary tract, liver, kidney, and mesentery.

Some peripancreatic and periduodenal lymph node gastrinomas are believed to represent primary tumors rather than metastases from an occult primary in the duodenum. At present they are considered metastases of (generally small) duodenal gastrinomas.

Sporadic gastrinomas are usually solitary. In the pancreas their diameter generally exceeds 2 cm. In the duodenum most gastrinomas are less than 1 cm in diameter and are therefore easily overlooked.[101] Many duodenal gastrinomas are hormonally hyperactive and are detected at an early stage.

By immunocytochemistry, gastrin can be demonstrated in most gastrinomas (Fig. 64-30). Trabecular tumors often show a stronger gastrin positivity than tumors with a solid pattern. Some tumors may remain gastrin negative, probably because of the low content of gastrin in the tumor tissue. Approximately 50% of gastrinomas are multihormonal and secrete pancreatic polypeptide, glucagon, and insulin, in addition to gastrin.

Ultrastructural investigations of gastrinomas revealed that only about 15% of the tumors are composed of cells resembling antral type G cells. In general, two gastrin components, G17 and G34, are produced and secreted at different rates without obvious relationship to morphologic or clinical data. The tumors also contain neuroendocrine granules, but their morphology varies and is, therefore, not diagnostic of gastrinoma.

Metastases to regional lymph nodes are found in approximately 60% of patients with pancreatic gastrinomas. Metastases to the liver generally occur late and are seen only in a small percentage of patients at the time of surgery. Duodenal gastrinomas are less often malignant than are pancreatic gastrinomas, but this may be because of earlier detection. Nevertheless, they can metastasize while still very small and give rise to paraduodenal lymph node metastases that may be larger than the primary. It has, therefore, been suggested that the so-called lymph node gastrinomas are metastases of duodenal microgastrinomas that had been overlooked.

Pathology of the nontumorous pancreas and stomach. No definite effect of hypergastrinemia on the morphology of the exocrine pancreas in humans has been established so far. In the

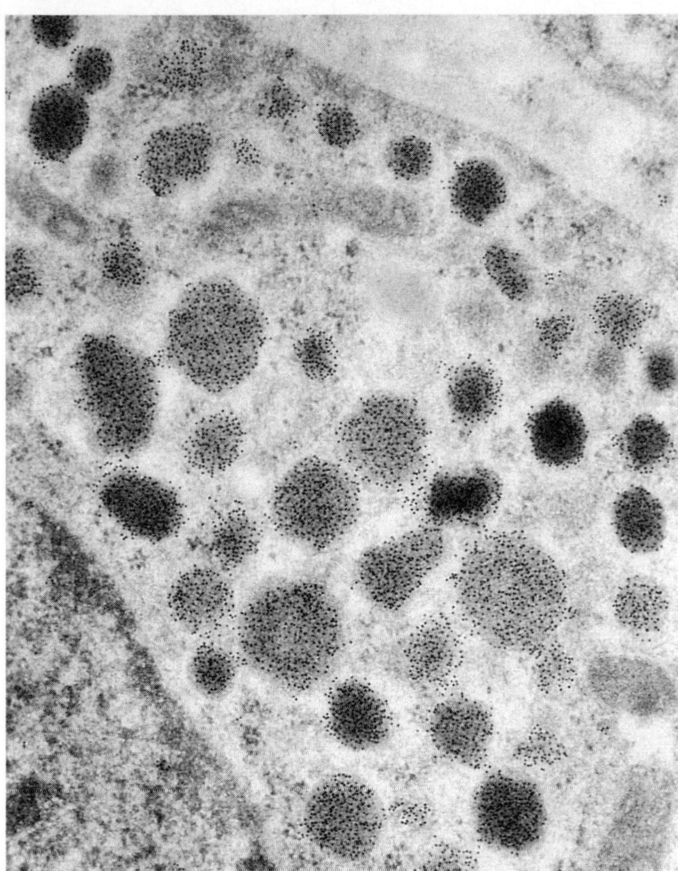

Fig. 64-27 Immunoelectron microscopic detection of insulin immunoreactivity with a monoclonal antibody in insulinoma. (Lowicryl K4M ultrathin section, protein A–gold technique.)

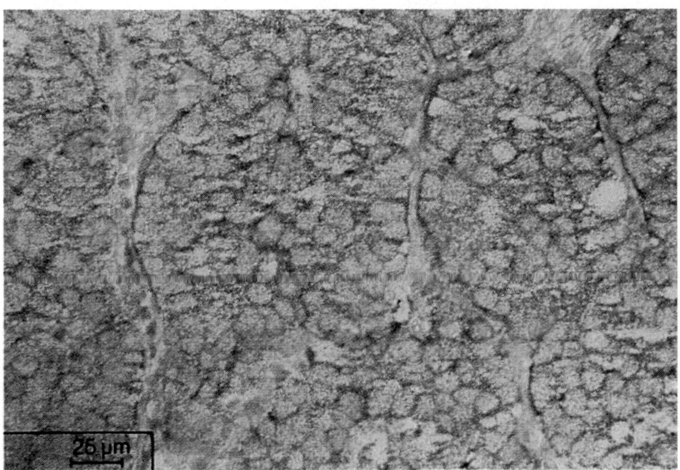

Fig. 64-28 Detection of insulin mRNA in an insulinoma by in situ hybridization. (Paraffin section, digoxigenin-labeled oligonucleotide antisense probes, immunogold-silver staining, nuclear fast red.)

stomach mucosa, sustained hypergastrinemia causes parietal cell hyperplasia, with thickening of the mucosal folds, and gastric acid hypersecretion. In addition, enterochromaffin-like cells (ECL cells), the specific product of which is unknown at present, are increased in number in the fundic mucosa.

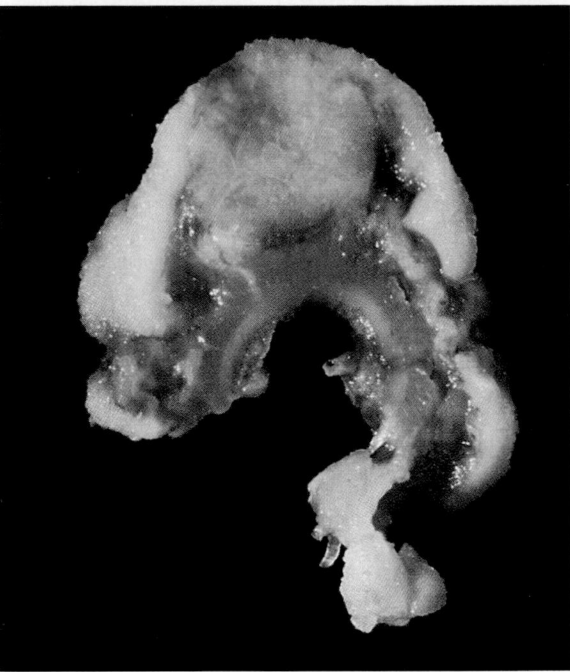

Fig. 64-29 Section through the duodenal wall showing a gastrinoma in typical submucosal localization (From Goossens A, Heitz P, Klöppel G: Pancreatic endocrine cells and their non-neoplastic proliferations. In Dayal Y, editor: *Endocrine pathology of the gut and pancreas,* Boca Raton, Fla, 1991, CRC Press.

Long-term treatment with omeprazol may induce ECL hyperplasia indirectly by inhibiting secretion of hydrochloric acid and thereby abolishing the inhibitory effect of gastric acid on the antral G cells. ECL cell carcinoids in the fundus of the stomach (probably caused by continuous stimulation of ECL cells by gastrin), which are well-known complications of patients suffering from pernicious anemia with chronic type A gastritis, appear to be very uncommon in patients with sporadic ZES.

Clinical presentation. Inappropriate gastrin secretion by gastrinomas causes ZES, characterized by gastric acid hypersecretion, intractable peptic ulceration, and occasional severe diarrhea. The term *pseudo-ZES* (also called ZES *type 1*, as opposed to ZES *type 2*, caused by a gastrinoma), was coined for a syndrome similar to ZES but caused by antral G cell hyperplasia.[102-104]

Vipoma

Vipoma is a neuroendocrine tumor with inappropriate secretion of vasoactive intestinal polypeptide (VIP). It may therefore produce the watery diarrhea, hypokalemia, and achlorhydria (WDHA) syndrome, also known as *Verner-Morrison's syndrome*. Vipomas occur more often in females than in males.

Most adult patients with WDHA have pancreatic vipomas. Rare VIP-producing pheochromocytomas and intestinal neuroendocrine tumors (carcinoids) can produce the same clinical symptoms. In children, WDHA syndrome has been reported in association with VIP-secreting ganglioneuromas and ganglioneuroblastomas.

Pathology. Pancreatic vipomas are usually solitary, large tumors. At least 80% of the tumors are malignant. By immunocytochemistry VIP can be visualized in most tumors.

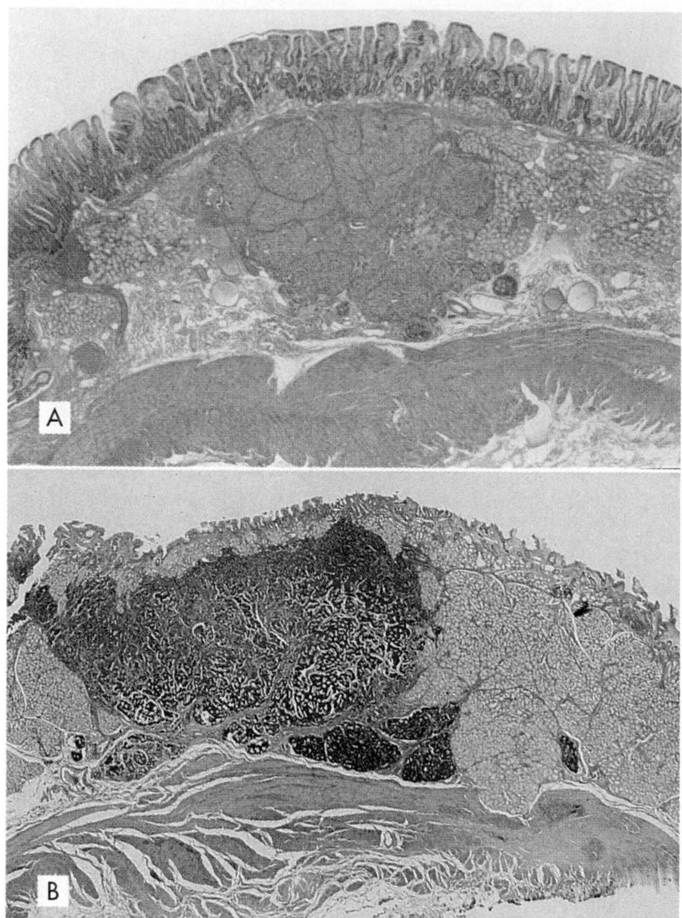

Fig. 64-30 Gastrinoma of the duodenum stained with hematoxylin and eosin, **A,** and for gastrin, **B.** Notice the adjacent, unlabeled Brunner's glands. (Paraffin section, immunoperoxidase technique, hematoxylin.)

In addition, it was shown that VIP and PP may be produced by the same tumor cell. This may explain the frequent occurrence of PP cells in vipomas. Other hormones commonly elaborated in vipomas are calcitonin and neurotensin.[105] By electron microscopy tumor cells contain noncharacteristic, small, neurosecretory granules.

Clinical presentation. Inappropriate secretion of VIP by vipomas causes WDHA. Although VIP is the most likely mediator of WDHA syndrome, other substances such as prostaglandins and neurotensin may also be involved.

Glucagonoma

Glucagonoma is a neuroendocrine tumor with inappropriate secretion of glucagon. It occurs most often between 40 and 70 years of age and is slightly more common in women than in men.

Pathology. The active tumors are generally rather large and occur in or are attached to the pancreas. For unknown reasons many immunocytochemically characterized, actively secreting glucagonomas do not cause symptoms of inappropriate glucagon secretion.[106]

Immunocytochemically, glucagon cells often stain weakly. In the tumors unreactive to glucagon, immunoreactivity to peptides derived from proglucagon (glicentin, glucagon-like peptides 1 and 2) can often be demonstrated. In addition, numerous PP cells can often be identified in glucagonomas.[107]

By electron microscopy, typical A cell granules can be recognized mainly in glucagonomas not causing the glucagonoma syndrome. Atypical secretory granules predominate in glucagonomas associated with the classical clinical syndrome.

Clinical presentation. The glucagonoma syndrome includes a skin rash (necrolytic migratory erythema), a mild glucose intolerance, normochromic normocytic anemia, weight loss, depression, and a tendency to develop deep vein thrombosis.[108] The syndrome reflects the catabolic action of highly elevated glucagon concentration in the serum.

Uncommon functioning tumors producing ectopic hormones

The aberrant production and secretion of ACTH (Cushing's syndrome), serotonin (atypical carcinoid syndrome), growth hormone–releasing hormone or growth hormone (acromegaly), and parathyroid hormone (PTH) or a PTH-like peptide (paraneoplastic hypercalcemia) by neuroendocrine tumors of the pancreas is uncommon. Many of these neoplasms are large and malignant. Histologically they do not differ from the more common tumors.

Tumors associated with combined hormonal syndromes

The systematic use of immunocytochemistry for analysis of the hormonal profile of pancreatic neuroendocrine tumors revealed that many of these tumors are multihormonal. Clinically, however, only a few of them give rise to a combination of syndromes or, more often, may switch from one syndrome to another. Known associations are ZES and hypercalcemia, ZES and Cushing's syndrome, hypoglycemia and Cushing's syndrome, and hypoglycemia with ZES or carcinoid syndrome. In a small number of tumors a glucagonoma syndrome switched to a hypoglycemic syndrome subsequent to cytostatic therapy.

It must be emphasized that some patients with combined clinical syndromes, in particular ZES and Cushing's syndrome, actually suffer from MEN 1.

Nonfunctioning tumors

Nonfunctioning neuroendocrine tumors of the pancreas include all neoplasms not associated with a distinct hormonal syndrome. Tumors containing a majority of cells elaborating PP (PPoma), neurotensin (neurotensinoma), calcitonin (calcitoninoma), or somatostatin (somatostatinoma) are also included in this group because they do not cause distinct clinical syndromes. The group represents approximately 30% of all pancreatic neuroendocrine tumors (Fig. 64-22).

The reasons for the lack of symptoms include the following: (1) the amount of hormone or hormones produced or released may be too low to cause symptoms; (2) the principal hormone elaborated and secreted by the tumor exerts no specific effects (PP and neurotensin); (3) the tumor secretes an inactive hormone precursor; and (4) the hormonal product of the tumor has yet to be identified.

Pathology. At least 64% of the surgically removed nonfunctioning tumors are malignant. The survival times of malignant nonfunctioning and functioning tumors, respectively, do not differ significantly. Many tumors measure more than 5 cm in diameter.

Immunocytochemically, only 10% of tumors have hormone-containing cells, which are usually sparse. Most lack neuroendocrine granules and do not react with antibodies to chromogranin. The reactions for synaptophysin and NSE are most often positive. Many of these cells nevertheless contain secretory granules, visible by electron microscopy.

PP is frequently found in nonfunctioning tumors. Because it is sometimes the only hormone present, these neoplasms have been called *PP-omas*. However, PP-omas produce no distinct clinical syndromes. Many of them occur in the setting of MEN 1. A small number of nonfunctioning tumors were found to produce serotonin.

Tumors rich in somatostatin cells (somatostatinomas) have been reported in association with diabetes, cholecystolithiasis, steatorrhea, indigestion, hypochlorhydria, and occasionally anemia. Additional features include weight loss, anemia, diarrhea, and abdominal pain.[109] Whether these symptoms can be ascribed to the inhibitory effect of somatostatin on secretory systems or are to be considered nonspecific is a matter of debate.[110]

Pancreatic somatostatinomas are often large, malignant, and preferentially located in the head of the gland. The tumors also occur in the second portion of the duodenum, often at the papilla of Vater. Some of these reveal psammoma bodies and are associated with neurofibromatosis type 1 and pheochromocytomas.[111]

Tumors described as *neurotensinomas* and *calcitoninomas* are either hormonally silent or are associated with syndromes that are difficult to relate to the effects of these hormones.

Mixed neuroendocrine-exocrine tumors

Truly mixed endocrine-exocrine tumors of the pancreas are extremely uncommon. The inclusion of apparently proliferating but otherwise normal ducts into neuroendocrine tumors, or the occurrence of endocrine cells attached to the neoplastic glands of ductal adenocarcinomas of the pancreas, cannot be considered evidence for a true amphicrine phenotype of tumor.

MULTIPLE ENDOCRINE NEOPLASIA (MEN) SYNDROMES

Multiple endocrine neoplasia (MEN) is a genetic predisposition to hyperplasia and tumors, or both, in two or more endocrine organs. The disease may appear simultaneously or sequentially in different organs. Distinct forms of MEN are MEN type 1, MEN type 2, MEN type 2A, and MEN type 2B.

MEN 1

MEN 1 (Wermer's syndrome) represents an autosomal-dominant inherited predisposition to tumors of parathyroid glands, anterior pituitary, the endocrine pancreas, and duodenum. In addition, endocrine tumors (carcinoids) of the stomach, ileum, lung, and thymus, adrenocortical hyperplasia or tumors, thyroid disease, lipomas, and pinealomas may occur.[112]

Etiology and pathogenesis. MEN 1 is inherited as an autosomal-dominant disorder with a high degree of penetrance (approximately 50% of children are affected) and variable expression. Sporadic cases of MEN 1 are related to spontaneous mutations. Tumorigenesis in MEN 1 involves the unmasking of a recessive mutation (rearrangement) at the MEN 1 locus, which has recently been mapped to the centromeric part of chromosomal region 11q (band 11q13) by genetic linkage analysis to restriction fragment length polymorphism (RFLP) markers.[113,114] The alterations of the MEN 1 locus may also involve the genes encoding insulin, calcitonin, and Ha-*ras,* all localized to chromosome 11, spanning from band p15 to q23. Rearrangement of this locus may lead to impaired regulation of the related genes.

Pathology. The neuroendocrine abnormalities occuring in MEN 1 are listed in Table 64-4. Parathyroid glands of MEN 1 patients show diffuse or nodular proliferation, composed predominantly of chief cells.[115] All parathyroid glands are usually involved, and recurrence after surgery is frequent. The outstanding feature of the pancreatic lesions is diffuse microadenomatosis (Fig. 64-31), possibly associated with one or several larger tumors (macrotumors) with diameters greater than 0.5 cm.[116] Histologically, most of the small tumors display a distinct trabecular pattern and may contain conspicuous connective tissue stroma. Immunohistochemically, these tumors consistently express multiple hormones, with one hormone usually prevailing. Most frequent are PPomas, followed by glucagonomas and insulinomas.[116] Despite the frequent occurrence of a ZES in MEN 1 patients, pancreatic gastrinomas are uncommon, though the pancreas of these patients may be studded with other neuroendocrine tumors of varying size. The gastrinomas in these patients most often reside in the proximal duodenum, where they commonly occur as multiple, very small (<1 cm) submucosal nodules.[117] Periduodenal lymph node metastases can be found in up to 60% of these patients. Pituitary lesions in MEN 1 tend to be multifocal. The majority of pituitary adenomas are clinically nonfunctional. Twenty-five percent express immunohistochemically and secrete prolactin or growth hormone. Basophilic ACTH-producing and other types of pituitary adenomas are rare.

Additional endocrine lesions may be encountered. These include thymic and gastrointestinal neuroendocrine tumors (carcinoids). Adrenocortical nodular hyperplasia or adenoma and thyroid follicular adenomas have also been observed. However, a recent study on such adrenocortical adenomas revealed no association with the genetic defect of MEN 1.[118]

Clinical presentation. The MEN 1 disease is uncommon (estimated prevalence between 0.02 and 0.2 per 1000). However, it has become apparent that incomplete forms of the syndrome exist. About 18% of unselected patients with primary hyperparathyroidism, 55% of patients with ZES, 4% with insulinomas, and 2.7% with pituitary tumors have evidence of MEN 1. No sex linkage has been shown, and both sexes are equally affected.

The clinical picture of MEN 1 may vary from case to case and depends largely on which glands are involved and whether the lesions secrete hormones. Clinical manifestations may reflect the interactions between simultaneously occurring endocrine lesions or may change according to proliferative lesions involving multiple endocrine glands. Although 45% of patients with MEN 1 may be clinically asymptomatic, hyperparathyroidism is the most frequent manifestation of this disease. The hyperparathyroidism is often mild and rarely leads to nephrocalcinosis. Symptoms related to pancreatic and duodenal lesions include, in 30% to 50% of patients, ZES (disseminated gastrointestinal ulcers caused by excessive gastrin secretion); in 10% to 30% of patients, hypoglycemia, caused by excessive insulin secretion; and in 2% to 10% of patients, WDHA (Verner-Morrison) syndrome, caused by excessive

Table 64-4 Multiple endocrine neoplasia syndrome 1 (MEN 1)

Organ/pathology	Incidence (approx.)	Hormones	Symptoms
Parathyroid glands	>90%	Parathyroid hormone	Hyperparathyroidism
Diffuse or nodular hyperplasia with adenomatosis			
Endocrine pancreas/duodenum	50% to 85%	Multihormonal	
Diffuse microadenomatosis of the pancreas with or without one or several macrotumors (>0.5 cm)			
PP-oma	Most frequent	Pancreatic polypeptide	
Insulinoma	10% to 30%	Insulin	Hypoglycemia
Vipoma	2% to 10%	VIP	Verner-Morrison syndrome (WDHA)
Glucagonoma	Rare	Glucagon	Glucagonoma syndrome
Somatostatinoma		Somatostatin	
Gastrinoma of the duodenum	30% to 50%		Hypergastrinemia, Zollinger-Ellison syndrome
Anterior pituitary	30% to 65%		
Inactive or GH adenoma	70%	Often inactive, growth hormone	Local symptoms, hypopituitarism, acromegaly
GH adenoma, prolactinoma	25%	Growth hormone, prolactin	Acromegaly, hyperprolactinemia
ACTH adenoma	Rare	ACTH	Cushing's disease
Gastrointestinal and thymic endocrine cells	5%		
Carcinoids			
Adrenal cortex	40%	Hypercorticism	
Nodular hyperplasia, adenoma			
Thyroid gland	20%	Hyperthyroidism, mild	
Follicular adenoma			

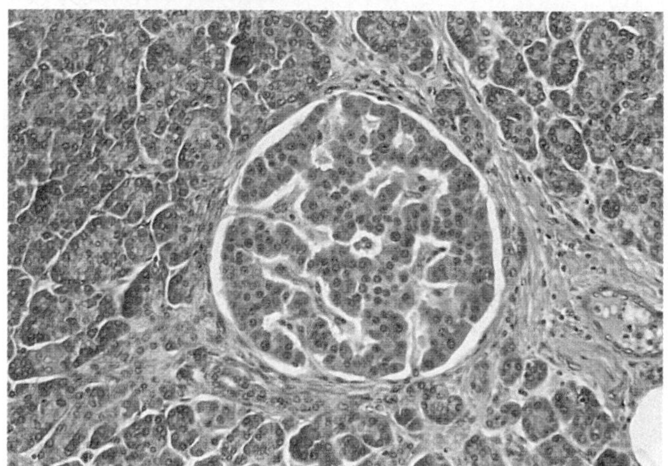

Fig. 64-31 Microadenoma of the pancreas in a patient with MEN 1.

VIP secretion. A glucagonoma syndrome or acromegaly, caused by excessive growth hormone secretion, are infrequently encountered. Amenorrhea is the most frequent manifestation of pituitary lesions in females affected with MEN 1. Local symptoms (such as visual disturbances), hypopituitarism, Cushing's disease, acromegaly, and hyperprolactinemia with impotence in males occur less frequently.

MEN 2

MEN 2 represents an autosomal-dominant genetic predisposition to neoplastic lesions of thyroid C-cells, adrenal medulla, and parathyroid glands. Some MEN 2 patients additionally show neurogenic tumors and a marfanoid habitus. Two types of MEN 2 can be distinguished: MEN type 2A (Sipple's syndrome) and MEN type 2B (Froboese's, or mucosal neuroma, syndrome).

MEN 2A

MEN 2A is characterized by the hyperplasia or neoplasia or thyroid C-cells, the adrenal medulla, and parathyroid glands.

Etiology and pathogenesis. MEN 2A is inherited as an autosomal-dominant disorder with a high degree of penetrance and variable expression. The MEN 2A gene has recently been localized to a 450 kilo–base pair region on chromosome 10q11.2.[119] This DNA segment encompasses the RET proto-oncogene, a receptor tyrosine kinase gene with a yet unknown ligand. It has been shown that germline missense mutations in the RET cysteine-rich domain may disrupt normal protein conformation, altering RET signal transduction and leading to the MEN 2A phenotype.[120,121]

Pathology. The neuroendocrine abnormalities encountered in MEN 2A are listed in Table 64-5. Proliferative thyroid C-cell lesions are present in more than 90% of MEN-2A patients. Medullary thyroid carcinomas are usually multifocal and bilateral (Fig. 64-32) and are typically preceded by diffuse and nodular C-cell hyperplasia[122] (Fig. 64-33). C-cell hyperplasia has been defined as the appearance of more than 50 C-cells per low-power field with clusters of 2 to 5 C-cells.[123] During progression of C-cell hyperplasia, C-cells begin to replace the follicular epithelium (diffuse C-cell hyperplasia), ultimately filling the follicles and producing small nodules of C-cells (nodular C-cell hyperplasia). Transition from nodular C-cell hyperplasia to microscopic medullary thyroid carcinoma is

Table 64-5 **Multiple endocrine neoplasia syndrome 2A (MEN 2A)**

Organ/pathology	Incidence (approximately)	Hormones	Symptoms
Thyroid	>90%		
Multifocal diffuse and nodular C-cell hyperplasia		Calcitonin, calcitonin gene–related peptide	
Medullary thyroid carcinoma (bilateral)			Diarrhea, tends to progress slowly
Adrenal medulla	20% to 40%		
Medullary hyperplasia	85% to 90%		
Pheochromocytoma	85% to 90%	Epinephrine, norepinephrine	Hypertension
Bilateral	70% to 80%		
Extraadrenal	10% to 15%		
Parathyroid glands	60%	Parathyroid hormone	Hyperparathyroidism, often asymptomatic
Chief-cell hyperplasia			

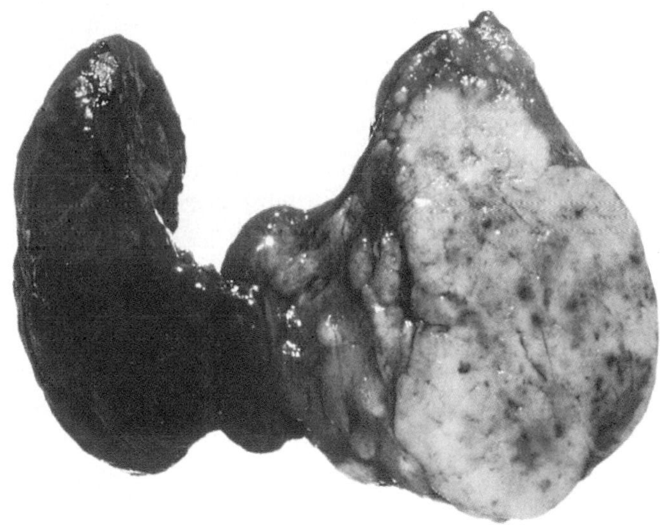

Fig. 64-32 Macroscopic appearance of a multicentric medullary thyroid carcinoma in a patient with MEN 2A.

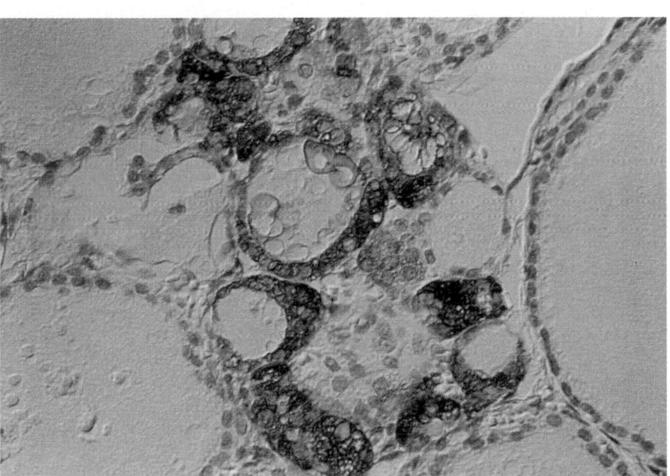

Fig. 64-33 Calcitonin immunostaining demonstrating diffuse thyroid C-cell hyperplasia in a patient with MEN 2A.

manifested by invasion of C-cells through the follicular basement membrane into the thyroid stroma,[124] leading to a stromal reaction. Medullary thyroid carcinoma is most often located in the middle and upper parts of the thyroid lobes, the major sites of C-cells also in unaffected thyroids. Familial and sporadic medullary thyroid carcinoma have the same histologic features, except that the familial form may show foci of hyperplastic C-cells in adjacent normal tissue.

Diffuse or nodular adrenal medullary hyperplasia occurs in the majority of patients with MEN 2A. Pheochromocytomas are mostly multicentric and bilateral and rarely show malignant behavior (Fig. 64-34). No specific histologic differences exist between sporadically occurring and familial pheochromocytoma.

Nodular hyperplasia of chief cells of the parathyroid glands occurs in up to 60% of MEN 2A patients.

Differential diagnosis. MEN 2A lesions must be distinguished from sporadic medullary thyroid carcinoma and

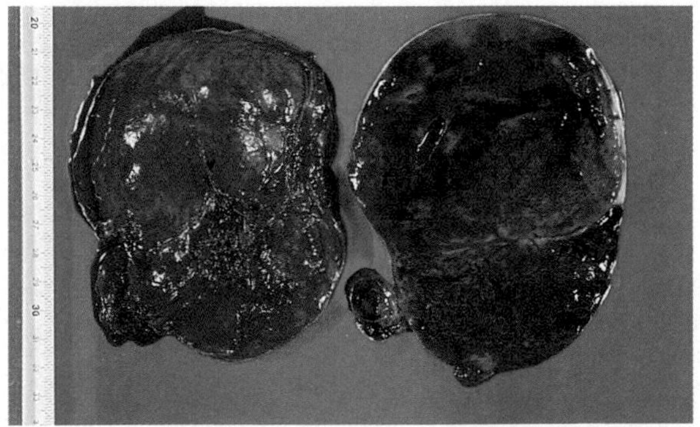

Fig. 64-34 Patient with MEN 2A suffering from bilateral pheochromocytoma. Encapsulated pheochromocytoma of the right adrenal. View of the capsule *(left)* and the cut surface *(right)*.

pheochromocytoma. Both are mostly solitary tumors and lack foci of C-cell hyperplasia or nodular medullary hyperplasia, respectively. Immunohistochemistry, such as that for polysialic acid (Fig. 64-35) or carinoembryonic antigen, can help distinguish primary from secondary (reactive) C-cell hyperplasia, occurring adjacent to follicular or papillary thyroid tumors, in chronic hypercalcemia and gastrinemia or in chronic lymphocytic (Hashimoto's) thyroiditis.[125]

Clinical presentation. Medullary thyroid carcinoma is the most frequent manifestation of MEN 2A. Mean age of presentation is approximately 30 years, in contrast to sporadic medullary thyroid carcinoma, which is usually diagnosed in the sixth or seventh decade. With biochemical screening tests (such as serum calcitonin levels), genetic linkage analysis, and single-strand conformation analysis to detect point mutation, affected members of kindreds with familial history of MEN 2A can be diagnosed at a younger age and tumors detected in early stages. Secretory diarrhea may be seen in MEN 2A patients, and associated pheochromocytoma can cause symptoms of excess catecholamine secretion. Hypercalcemia resulting from hyperparathyroidism is infrequent, and Cushing's syndrome is a rare manifestation.

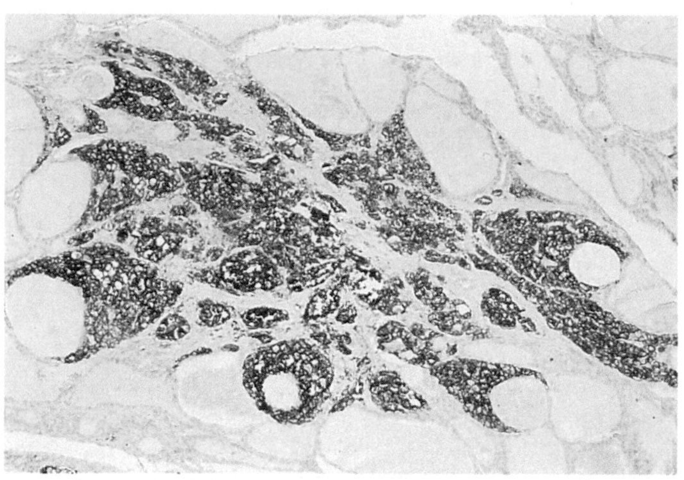

Fig. 64-35 Microscopic medullary thyroid carcinoma in a focus of C-cell hyperplasia exhibiting strong immunostaining for polysialic acid. (Immunogold-silver technique, nuclear fast red.)

MEN 2B

MEN type 2B is an uncommon variant of MEN 2 with earlier onset of tumors. Affected individuals show additional phenotypic features, including a marfanoid habitus, ganglioneuromatosis of the gastrointestinal wall, upper airways, oral cavity, and conjunctivae.

Etiology and pathogenesis. MEN 2B is inherited as an autosomal-dominant disorder. The MEN 2B gene has also been mapped to the chromosome 10q11.2 but to a larger region, as in MEN 2A. No mutations of the RET cysteine-rich domain have been detected,[119] but mutations of the tyrosine kinase domain in codon 918 have recently been found.[126]

Pathology. The neuroendocrine abnormalities encountered in MEN 2B are listed in Table 64-6. The thyroid and adrenal lesions in MEN 2B are identical to those occurring in MEN 2A. Mucosal neuromas involve the mucosae of the upper aerodigestive tract and conjunctivae and cause a typical facies of MEN 2B patients. The tumors histologically resemble amputation neuromas, showing nodular aggregates of irregularly arranged nerve bundles. Gastrointestinal ganglioneuromatosis is characterized by proliferations of nerves, ganglia, and Schwann cells in the submucosal and intramuscular plexus of the gastrointestinal wall (Fig. 64-36).

Clinical presentation. In addition to the clinical symptoms described in MEN 2A, patients affected with MEN 2B show a marfanoid habitus and a typical facies with thick lips, nodularity of the tongue, buccal mucosa, and conjunctivae, caused by the mucosal neuromas. Gastrointestinal ganglioneuromatosis may cause constipation or diarrhea, and a third of MEN 2B patients develop a megacolon. Medullary thyroid carcinoma in MEN 2B develops at a young age. It is usually highly aggressive, and few patients survive 5 years if not adequately treated.

Table 64-6 Multiple endocrine neoplasia syndrome 2B (MEN 2B)

Organ/pathology	Incidence (approximately)	Hormones	Symptoms
Thyroid	>90%		
Multifocal diffuse and nodular C-cell hyperplasia		Calcitonin, calcitonin gene–related peptide	
Medullary thyroid carcinoma (bilateral)			Diarrhea, tends to develop early and progress rapidly
Adrenal medulla	20% to 40%		
Medullary hyperplasia	85% to 90%		
Pheochromocytoma	85% to 90%	Epinephrine, norepinephrine	Hypertension
Bilateral	70% to 80%		
Extra-adrenal	10% to 15%		
Parathyroid glands	Rarely	Parathyroid hormone	No hyperparathyroidism detectable
Chief-cell hyperplasia			
Peripheral neural system	100%		
Marfanoid habitus	100%		
Mucosal neuromas	100%		
Intestinal ganglioneuromatosis	40% to 50%		Diarrhea or constipation, megacolon

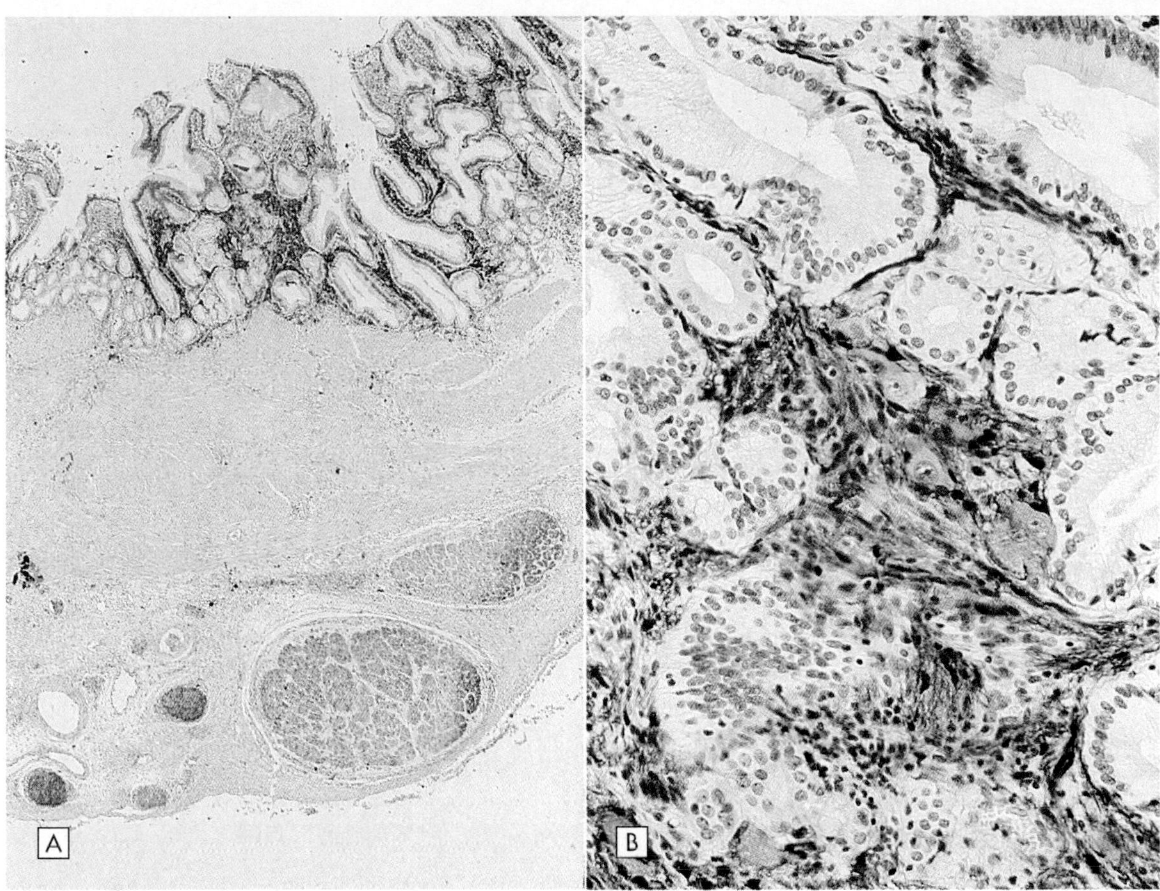

Fig. 64-36 Ganglioneuromatosis of the gall bladder in a patient with MEN 2B. **A,** There are prominent, S-100–positive nerve bundles in the wall. **B,** Numerous S-100–positive ganglion cells and nerves in the mucosa.

Mixed multiple endocrine neoplasia

Overlapping symptoms of MEN 1 and 2, as well as reports of multiple endocrine lesions associated with nonendocrine phenotypic abnormalities, are apparently very uncommon.[127,128]

The combination of parathyroid adenoma and papillary thyroid carcinoma has been termed MEN 3.[129] A familial pattern of occurrence has not yet been found, and the existence of this syndrome remains questionable.

REFERENCES

Embryology, anatomy, and physiology

1. Le Douarin N: *The neural crest. Developmental and cell biology series,* Cambridge, 1982, Cambridge University Press.
2. Le Douarin N: On the origin of pancreatic endocrine cells, *Cell* 53:169, 1988.
3. Pictet R, Rutter W: Development of the embryonic endocrine pancreas. In Greep R, Astwood E, Steiner D et al, editors: *Handbook of physiology,* Washington, DC, 1972, American Physiological Society.
4. Hahn von Dorsche H, Reiher H, Hahn H: Phases in the early development of the human islet organ, *Anat Anz* 166:69, 1987.
5. Like A, Orci L: Embryogenesis of the human pancreatic islets: a light and electron microscopic study, *Diabetes* 21:511, 1972.
6. Ferner H: *Das Inselsystem des Pankreas: Entwicklung, Histobiologie und Pathophysiologie mit besonderer Berücksichtigung des Diabetes mellitus,* Stuttgart, 1952, Thieme.
7. Orci L: Macro- and microdomains in the endocrine pancreas, *Diabetes* 31:538, 1982.
8. Meda P, Michaelis R, Halban P et al: In vivo modulation of gap junctions and dye coupling between B-cells of the intact pancreatic islet, *Diabetes* 32:858, 1983.
9. Samols E, Bonner-Weir S, Weir G: Intra-islet insulin-glucagon-somatostatin relationships, *Clin Endocr Metab* 15:33, 1986.
10. Bonner-Weir S: The microvasculature of the pancreas, with emphasis on that of the islets of Langerhans. In Go V, Dimagno E, Gardner J et al, editors: *The pancreas,* New York, 1993, Raven Press.
11. Jansson L, Hellerström C: Glucose-induced changes in pancreatic islet blood flow mediated by central nervous system, *Am J Physiol* 251:E664, 1986.
12. Ahrén B, Taborsky G, Porte D: Neuropeptidergic versus cholinergic and adrenergic regulation of islet hormone secretion, *Diabetologia* 29:827, 1986.
13. Schuit F, Pipeleers D: Differences in adrenergic recognition by pancreatic A and B cells, *Science* 232:875, 1986.
14. Farr A, Anderson S: In situ ultrastructural demonstration of cells bearing Ia antigens in the murine pancreas, *Diabetes* 34:987, 1985.
15. Pipeleers D, In't Veld P, Pipeleers-Marichal M et al: Presence of pancreatic hormones in islet cells with MHC-class II antigen expression, *Diabetes* 36:872, 1987.
16. In't Veld P, Pipeleers D: In situ analysis of pancreatic islets in rats developing pancreas: appearance of non-endocrine cells with surface MHC-II class antigens and cytoplasmic insulin immunoreactivity, *J Clin Invest* 82:1123, 1988.
17. Bailes E, Guest P, Hutton J: Insulin synthesis. In Ashcroft F, Ashcroft S, editors: *Insulin: molecular biology to pathology,* Oxford, 1992, IRL Press.
18. Loh Y, Beinfeld M, Birch N: Proteolytic processing of prohormones and proneuropeptides. In Loh Y, editor: *Mechanism of intracellular trafficking and processing of proproteins,* Boca Raton, Fla, 1993, CRC Press.
19. Clark A, Docherty K: The insulin gene. In Ashcroft F, Ashcroft S, editors: *Insulin: molecular biology to pathology,* Oxford, 1992, IRL Press.

20. Orci L, Ravazzola M, Storch M et al: Proteolytic maturation of insulin is a post-Golgi event which occurs in acidifying clathrin-coated secretory vesicles, *Cell* 49:865, 1987.
21. Roth J, Warhol MJ: Immunogold silver staining techniques for high resolution immunohistochemistry in clinical materials. In Bullock G, Van Velzen D, Warhol M J, editors: *Techniques in diagnostic pathology,* vol 3, London, 1992, Academic Press.
22. Komminoth P, Merk FB, Leav I et al: Comparison of ^{35}S- and digoxigenin-labeled RNA and oligonucleotide probes for in situ hybridization: expression of mRNA of the seminal vesicle secretion protein II and androgen receptor genes in the rat prostate, *Histochemistry* 98:217, 1992.
23. Lloyd R, Field K, Jin L et al: Analysis of endocrine active and clinically silent corticotropic adenomas by in situ hybridization, *Am J Pathol* 137:479, 1990.
24. Shorrock K, Roberts P, Pringle J et al: Demonstration of insulin and glucagon mRNA in routinely fixed and processed pancreatic tissue by in-situ hybridization, *J Pathol* 165:105, 1991.
25. Roth J: Postembedding labeling on Lowicryl K4M tissue sections: detection and modification of cellular components. In Tartakoff AM, editor: *Vesicular transport,* vol 31, San Diego, 1989, Academic Press.
26. Roth J, Heitz P: Immunolabeling with the protein A–gold technique: an overview, *Ultrastruct Pathol* 13:467, 1989.

Diabetes mellitus

27. Foulis AK, Stewart JA: The pancreas in recent-onset type I (insulin-dependent) diabetes mellitus: insulin content of islets, insulitis and associated changes in the exocrine acinar tissue, *Diabetologia* 26:456, 1984.
28. Baekkeskov S, Aanstoot HJ, Christgau S et al: Identification of the 64K autoantigen in insulin-dependent diabetes as the GABA-synthesizing enzyme glutamic acid decarboxylase, *Nature* 347:151, 1990.
29. Blum D, Dorchy H, Mouraux T et al: Congenital absence of insulin cells in a neonate with diabetes mellitus and mutase-deficient methylmalonic acidaemia, *Diabetologia* 36:352, 1993.
30. Wilkin TJ: Insulin autoantibodies as markers for type I diabetes, *Endocr Rev* 11:92, 1990.
31. Handwerger BS, Fernandes G, Brown DM: Immune and autoimmune aspects of diabetes mellitus, *Hum Pathol* 11:338, 1980.
32. Sibley RK, Sutherland DER: Pancreas transplantation: an immunohistologic and histopathologic examination of 100 grafts, *Am J Pathol* 128:151, 1987.
33. Klöppel G: Experimental insulitis. In Volk B, Arquilla E, Allen R, editors: *The diabetic pancreas,* ed 2, New York, 1985, Plenum.
34. Like AA, Weringer EJ: Autoimmune diabetes in the Bio Breeding/ Worcester rat. In Lefèbvre P, Pipeleers DG, editors: *The pathology of the endocrine pancreas in diabetes,* Berlin 1988, Springer.
35. Kolb H: Mouse models of insulin dependent diabetes: low-dose streptozocin-induced diabetes and nonobese diabetic (NOD) mice, *Diabetes Metab Rev* 3:751, 1987.
36. Löhr M, Bergstrome B, Maekawa R et al: Human cytomegalovirus in the pancreas of patients with type 2 diabetes: is there a relation to clinical features, mRNA and protein expression of insulin, somatostatin, and MHC class II? *Virchows Arch [A] (Pathol Anat)* 421:371, 1992.
37. Todd JA: Genetic control of autoimmunity in type I diabetes, *Immunol Today* 11:122, 1990.
38. Craighead JE, Steinke J: Diabetes mellitus–like syndrome in mice infected with encephalo-myocarditis virus, *Am J Pathol* 63:119, 1971.
39. Yoon JW, Austin M, Onodera T et al: Virus-induced diabetes mellitus: isolation of a virus from the pancreas of a child with diabetic ketoacidosis, *N Engl J Med* 300:1173, 1979.
40. Klöppel G, Bommer G, Commandeur G et al: The endocrine pancreas in chronic pancreatitis: immunocytochemical and ultrastructural studies, *Virchows Arch [A] (Pathol Anat)* 377:157, 1978.
41. Groop L, Miettinen A, Groop PH et al: Organ-specific autoimmunity and HLA-DR antigens as markers for beta-cell destruction in patients with type II diabetes, *Diabetes* 37:99, 1988.
42. Peterse JS, Russel ST, Marshall MO et al: Differential expression of glutamic acid decarboxylase in rat and human islets, *Diabetes* 42:484, 1993.
43. Klöppel G, Drenck CR, Oberholzer M et al: Morphometric evidence for a striking B-cell reduction at the clinical onset of type I diabetes, *Virchows Arch [A] Pathol Anat* 403:441, 1984.
44. Bottazzo GF, Pujol-Borrell R, Gale E: Etiology of diabetes: the role of autoimmune mechanisms. In Alberti KGMM, Krall LP, editors: *Diabetes annual I,* Amsterdam, 1985, Elsevier.
45. Foulis AK, Liddle CN, Farquharson MA et al: The histopathology of the pancreas in type I (insulin-dependent) diabetes mellitus: a 25-year review of deaths in patients under 20 years of age in the United Kingdom, *Diabetologia* 29:267, 1986.
46. Permutt MA, Chiu KC, Tanizawa Y: Glucokinase and NIDDM: a candidate gene that paid off, *Diabetes* 41:1367, 1992.
47. Vadheim CM, Rotter JI: Genetics of diabetes mellitus. In Alberti KGMM, De Fronzo RA, Keen H et al, editors: *International textbook of diabetes mellitus,* New York, 1992, John Wiley & Sons.
48. De Fronzo RA: Pathogenesis of type 2 (non-insulin dependent) diabetes mellitus: a balanced overview, *Diabetologia* 34:607, 1991.
49. Weir GC, Leahy JL, Bonner-Weir S: Experimental reduction of B-cell mass: implications for the pathogenesis of diabetes, *Diabetes Metab Rev* 2:125, 1986.
50. Andersson A: The influence of hyperglycaemia, hyperinsulinaemia and genetic background on the fate of intrasplenically implanted mouse islets, *Diabetologia* 25:269, 1983.
51. Johnson KH, O'Brien TD, Westermark P: Newly identified pancreatic protein islet amyloid polypeptide, *Diabetes* 40:310, 1991.
52. Cooper GJS, Willis AC, Clark A et al: Purification and characterization of a peptide from amyloid-rich pancreases of type 2 diabetic patients, *Proc Natl Acad Sci USA* 84:8628, 1987.
53. Westermark GT, Christmanson L, Terenghi G et al: Islet amyloid polypeptide: demonstration of mRNA in human pancreatic islets by in situ hybridization in islets with and without amyloid deposits, *Diabetologia* 36:323, 1993.
54. Westermark P: Fine structure of islets of Langerhans in insular amyloidosis, *Virchows Arch [A] (Pathol Anat)* 359:1, 1973.
55. Bell ET: Hyalinization of the islets of Langerhans in diabetes mellitus, *Diabetes* 1:341, 1952.
56. Klöppel G, Drenck CR: Immunzytochemische Morphometrie beim Typ-I und Typ-II-Diabetes mellitus, *Dtsch Med Wochenschr* 108:188, 1983.
57. Rahier J, Goebbels RM, Henquin JC: Cellular composition of the human diabetic pancreas, *Diabetologia* 24:366, 1983.
58. Klöppel G, Gepts W, In't Veld PA: Morphology of the pancreas in normal and diabetic states. In Alberti KGMM, De Fronzo RA, Keen H et al, editors: *International textbook of diabetes mellitus,* New York, 1992, John Wiley & Sons.
59. Dodge JA, Laurence KM: Congenital absence of islets of Langerhans, *Arch Dis Child* 52:411, 1977.
60. Ujevich MM, Jaffe R: Pancreatic islet cell damage: its occurence in neonatal coxsackievirus encephalomyocarditis, *Arch Pathol Lab Med* 104:438, 1980.
61. Harsha Rao R: Diabetes in the undernourished: coincidence or consequence? *Endocr Rev* 9:67, 1988.
62. Cersosimo E, Pisters PWT, Pesola G et al: Insulin secretion and action in patients with pancreatic cancer, *Cancer* 67:486, 1991.
63. Lebenthal E, Lerner A, Heitlinger L: The pancreas in cystic fibrosis. In Go VLW, Gardner JD, Brooks FP et al, editors: *The exocrine pancreas,* New York, 1986, Raven Press.
64. Rahier J, Loozen S, Goebbels RM et al: The haemochromatotic human pancreas: a quantitative immunohistochemical and ultrastructural study, *Diabetologia* 30:5, 1987.
65. Harrison LC, Flier JS: Diabetes associated with other endocrine diseases. In Podolsky S, Viswanathan M, editors: *Secondary diabetes: the spectrum of the diabetic syndromes,* London, 1980, Raven Press.
66. Creutzfeldt W, Sickinger K, Frerichs H: Diabetes und Lebererkrankungen. In Pfeiffer EF, editor: *Handbuch des Diabetes mellitus: Pathophysiologie und Klinik,* vol 2, München, 1971, Lehmanns.
67. Shankar TP, Solomon SS, Duckworth WC et al: Studies of glucose intolerance in cirrhosis of the liver, *J Lab Clin Med* 102:459, 1983.

68. Chang AY, Diani AR: Chemically and hormonally induced diabetes mellitus. In Volk BW, Arquilla ER, editors: *The diabetic pancreas,* ed 2, New York, 1985, Plenum Press.
69. Creutzfeldt W, Creutzfeldt C, Frerichs H et al: The morphological substrate of the inhibition of insulin secretion by diazoxide, *Horm Metab Res* 1:53-64, 1969.
70. Marble A: Late complications of diabetes: a continuing challenge, *Diabetologia* 44:193, 1976.
71. Diabetes Control and Complications Trial Research Group: The effect of intensive treatment of diabetes on the development and progression of long-term complications in insulin-dependent diabetes mellitus, *N Engl J Med* 329:977, 1993.
72. Kreisberg JI: Biology of disease: hyperglycemia and microangiopathy: direct regulation by glucose of microvascular cells, *Lab Invest* 67:416, 1992.
73. Bloodworth JMB Jr: A re-evaluation of diabetic glomerulosclerosis 50 years after the discovery of insulin, *Hum Pathol* 9:439, 1978.
74. Clements RS: Diabetic neuropathy—new concept of its etiology, *Diabetes* 28:606, 1979.
75. Hultquist GT, Olding LB: Endocrine pathology of infants of diabetic mothers, *Acta Endocrinol* 241(suppl):97, 1981.
76. Aynsley-Green A, Polak JM, Bloom SR et al: Nesidioblastosis of the pancreas: definition of the syndrome and the management of the severe neonatal hyperinsulinemic hypoglycemia, *Arch Dis Child* 56:496, 1981.
77. Elias D, Cohen IR, Schechter Y et al: Antibodies to insulin receptor followed by anti-idiotype: antibodies to insulin in child with hypoglycemia, *Diabetes* 36:348, 1987.
78. Pagliara AS, Karl IE, Haymond M et al: Hypoglycemia in infancy, *J Pediatr* 82(part 1):558-577, 82(part 2):365, 1973.
79. Klöppel G, Heitz PU: Nesidioblastosis: a clinical entity with heterogeneous lesions of the pancreas. In Falkmer S, Hakanson R, Sundler F, editors: *Evolution and tumour pathology of the neuroendocrine system,* Amsterdam, 1984, Elsevier.
80. Goossens A, Heitz PU, Klöppel G: Pancreatic endocrine cells and their non-neoplastic proliferations. In Dayal Y, editor: *Endocrine pathology of the gut and pancreas,* Boca Raton, Fla., 1991, CRC Press.
81. Bishop AE, Polak JM, Garin Chesa P et al: Decrease of pancreatic somatostatin in neonatal nesidioblastosis, *Diabetes* 30:122, 1981.
82. Albers N, Löhr M, Bogner U et al: Nesidioblastosis of the pancreas in an adult with persistent hyperinsulinemic hypoglycemia, *Am J Clin Pathol* 91:94, 1989.

Pancreatic neuroe.ndocrine neoplasms

83. Klöppel G, Heitz PU: Pancreatic endocrine tumors, *Pathol Res Pract* 183:155, 1988.
84. Service F, McMahon M, O'Brien P et al: Functioning insulinoma—incidence, recurrence, and long-term survival of patients: a 60-year study, *Mayo Clin Proc* 66:711, 1991.
85. Grimelius L, Hultquist G, Steinkvist B: Cytological differentiation of asymptomatic pancreatic islet cell tumors in autopsy material, *Virchows Arch [A] (Pathol Anat)* 365:275, 1975.
86. Höfler H, Ruhri C, Pütz B et al: Oncogene expression in endocrine pancreatic tumors, *Virchows Arch [B] (Cell Pathol)* 55:355, 1988.
87. Cooper G, Leighton B, Dimitriadis G et al: Amylin found in amyloid deposits in human type 2 diabetes mellitus may be a hormone that regulates glycogon metabolism in skeletal muscle, *Proc Natl Acad Sci USA* 85:7763, 1988.
88. Eissele R, Neuhaus C, Trautmann M et al: Immunoreactivity and expression of amylin in gastrenteropancreatic endocrine tumors, *Am J Pathol* 143:283, 1993.
89. Johnson K, O'Brien T, Betsholtz C et al: Islet amyloid, islet-amyloid polypeptide, and diabetes mellitus, *N Engl J Med* 321:513, 1989.
90. Bishop A, Power R, Polak J: Markers for neuroendocrine differentiation, *Pathol Res Pract* 183:119, 1988.
91. Reubi J, Hacki W, Lamberts S: Hormone-producing gastrointestinal tumors contain a high density of somatostatin receptors, *J Clin Endocrinol Metab* 65:1127, 1987.
92. Reubi J, Kvols L, Waser B et al: Detection of somatostatin receptors in surgical and percutaneous needle biopsy samples of carcinoids and islet cell carcinomas, *Cancer Res* 50:5969, 1990.
93. Graeme-Cook F, Nardi G, Compton C: Immunocytochemical staining for human chorionic gonadotropin subunits does not predict malignancy in isulinomas, *Am J Clin Pathol* 93:273, 1990.
94. Heitz PU, von Herbay G, Klöppel G et al: The expression of subunits of human gonadotropin (hCG) by non-trophoblastic, non-endocrine, and endocrine tumors, *Am J Clin Pathol* 88:467, 1987.
95. Li WP, Komminoth P, Heitz PU et al: Expression of β 1,6 branching of asparagine-linked oligosaccharides in malignant and benign insulinomas of the pancreas, *Pathol Res Pract* 189:740, 1993.
96. Alanen K, Joensuu H, Klemi P et al: DNA ploidy in pancreatic endocrine tumors, *Am J Clin Pathol* 93:784, 1990.
97. Donow C, Baisch H, Heitz PU et al: Nuclear DNA-content in 27 pancreatic endocrine tumors: correlation with malignancy, survival and expression of glycoprotein-hormone alpha-chain, *Virchows Arch [A] (Pathol Anat)* 419:463, 1991.
98. Stefanini P, Carboni M, Patrassi N et al: B-islet cell tumors of the pancreas: results of a study on 1,067 cases, *Surgery* 75:597, 1974.
99. Roth J, Klöppel G, Madsen O et al: Distribution pattern of proinsulin and insulin in human insulinomas: an immunocytochemical analysis in 76 tumors, *Virchows Arch [B] (Cell Pathol)* 63:51, 1992.
100. Donow C, Pipeleers-Marichal M, Schröder S et al: Surgical pathology of gastrinoma: site, size, multicentricity, association with multiple endocrine neoplasia type I and malignancy, *Cancer* 68:1329, 1991.
101. Pipeleers-Marichal M, Somers G, Willems G et al: Gastrinomas in the duodenums of patients with multiple endocrine neoplasia type I and the Zollinger-Ellison syndrome, *N Engl J Med* 322:723, 1990.
102. Friesen S, Tomita T: Pseudo–Zollinger-Ellison syndrome: hypergastrinemia, hyperchlorhydria without tumor, *Ann Surg* 194:481, 1981.
103. Jensen R, Doppman J, Gardner J: Gastrinoma. In Go VLW, Gardner J, Brooks JF et al, editors: *Biology, pathology, and disease,* New York, 1986, Raven Press.
104. Polak J, Stagg B, Pearse A: Two types of Zollinger-Ellison syndrome: immunofluorescent, cytochemical and ultrastructural studies of the antral and pancreatic gastrin cells in different clinical states, *Gut* 13:501, 1972.
105. Capella C, Polak J, Buffa R et al: Morphologic patterns and diagnostic criteria of VIP-producing endocrine tumors: a histologic, histochemical and biochemical study of 32 cases, *Cancer* 52:1860, 1983.
106. Ruttmann E, Klöppel G, Bommer G et al: Pancreatic glucagonoma with and without syndrome: immunocytochemical study of 5 tumor cases and review of the literature, *Virchows Arch [A] (Pathol Anat)* 388:51, 1980.
107. Bordi C, Ravazzola M, Baetens D et al: A study of glucagonomas by light end electron microscopy and immunofluorescence, *Diabetes* 28:925, 1979.
108. Mallinson C, Bloom S, Warin A et al: A glucagonoma syndrome, *Lancet* 2:1, 1974.
109. Krejs G, Orci L, Conlon J et al: Somatostatinoma syndrome, *N Engl J Med* 301:285, 1979.
110. Pipeleers D, Couturier E, Gepts W et al: Five cases of somatostatinoma: clinical heterogeneity and diagnostic usefulness of basal and tolbutamide-induced hypersomatostatinemia, *J Clin Endocrinol Metab* 56:1236, 1983.
111. Dayal Y, Kirsten K, Tallberg A et al: Duodenal carcinoids in patients with and without neurofibromatosis, *Am J Surg Pathol* 10:348, 1986.

Multiple endocrine neoplasia (MEN) syndromes

112. Brandi M, Marx S, Aurbach G et al: Familial multiple endocrine neoplasia type I: a new look at pathophysiology, *Endocr Rev* 8:391, 1987.
113. Larsson C, Nordenskjöld M: Multiple endocrine neoplasia, *Cancer Surv* 9:703-723, 1990.
114. Larsson C, Weber G, Kvanta E et al: Isolation and mapping of polymorphic cosmid clones used for sublocalization of the multiple endocrine neoplasia type 1 (MEN 1) locus, *Hum Genet* 89:187, 1992.
115. Castleman B, Schantz A, Roth S: Parathyroid hyperplasia in primary hyperparathyroidism: review of 85 cases, *Cancer* 38:1668, 1976.

116. Klöppel G, Willemer S, Stamm B et al: Pancreatic lesions and hormonal profile of pancreatic tumors in multiple endocrine neoplasia type I: an immunocytochemical study of nine patients, *Cancer* 57:1824, 1986.
117. Donow C, Pipeleers MM, Schröder S et al: Surgical pathology of gastrinoma: site, size, multicentricity, association with multiple endocrine neoplasia type 1, and malignancy, *Cancer* 68:1329, 1991.
118. Skogseid B, Larsson C, Lindgren PG et al: Clinical and genetic features of adrenocortical lesions in multiple endocrine neoplasia type 1, *J Clin Endocrinol Metab* 75:76, 1992.
119. Mole S, Mulligan L, Healey C et al: Localisation of the gene for multiple endocrine neoplasia type 2A to a 480 kb region in chromosome band 10q11.2, *Hum Molec Genet* 2:247, 1993.
120. Donis-Keller H, Dou S, Chi D et al: Mutations in the RET proto-oncogene are associated with MEN 2A and FMTC, *Hum Mol Genet* 2:851, 1993.
121. Mulligan L, Kwok J, Healey C et al: Germline mutations of the RET proto-oncogene in multiple endocrine neoplasia type 2A, *Nature* 363:458, 1993.
122. Wolfe H, Melvin K, Cervi-Skinner S et al: C-cell hyperplasia preceding medullary thyroid carcinoma, *N Engl J Med* 289:437, 1973.
123. LiVolsi V, Feind C, LoGerfo P et al: Demonstration by immunoperoxidase staining of hyperplasia of parafollicular cells in the thyroid gland in hyperparathyreoidism, *J Clin Endocrinol Metab* 37:550, 1973.
124. DeLellis R, Nunnemacher G, Wolfe H: C-cell hyperplasia: an ultrastructural analysis, *Lab Invest* 36:237, 1977.
125. Komminoth P, Roth J, Saremaslani P et al: Polysialic acid of the neural cell adhesion molecule in the human thyroid: a marker for medullary thyroid carcinoma and primary C-cell hyperplasia, *Am J Surg Pathol* 18:399, 1994.
126. Hofstra RMW, Landsvater RM, Ceccherine I et al: A mutation in the RET protooncogene associated with multiple endocrine neoplasia type 2B and sporadic medullary thyroid carcinoma, *Nature* 367:275, 1994.
127. Probst A, Lotz M, Heitz PU: Von Hippel-Lindau's disease, syringomyelia and multiple endocrine tumors: a complex neuroendocrinopathy, *Virchows Arch [A] (Pathol Anat)* 378:265, 1978.
128. Tateishi R, Wada A, Ishiguro S et al: Coexistence of bilateral pheochromocytoma and pancreatic islet cell tumor: report of a case and review of the literature, *Cancer* 42:2928, 1978.
129. Dralle H, Altenähr E: Pituitary adenoma, primary parathyroid hyperplasia and papillary (non-medullary) thyroid carcinoma, *Virchows Arch [A] (Pathol Anat)* 381:179, 1979.

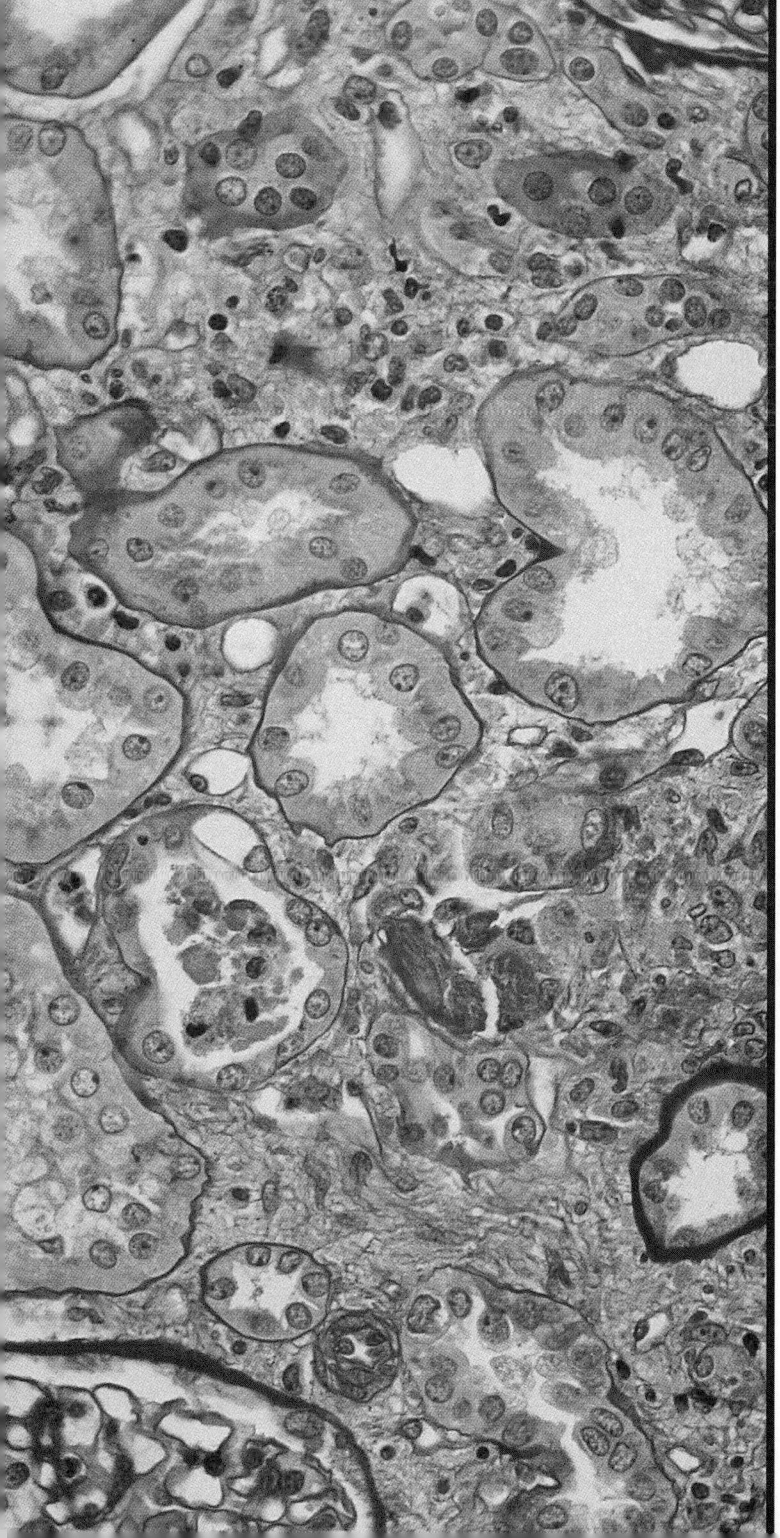

Part Seven

DISEASES OF THE UROGENITAL AND REPRODUCTIVE SYSTEMS

65 Kidney

A. NONNEOPLASTIC CONDITIONS

Arthur H. Cohen
Cynthia C. Nast

The kidneys are kidney bean–shaped paired organs in the retroperitoneum that have diverse physiologic functions, complex anatomy, and a wide range of pathologic processes and extremely interesting pathogenic mechanisms and microscopic morphologies, all leading to a wide variety of clinical and laboratory manifestations. This chapter covers some of the more important pathologic processes.

NORMAL ANATOMY AND PHYSIOLOGY

Each kidney in normal adults weighs approximately 150 g, with ranges of 125 to 175 g in men and 115 to 155 g in women. Both kidneys combined are 1/240 (0.4%) of the total body weight. Each kidney is supplied by a single renal artery originating from the abdominal aorta; the main renal artery branches to form anterior and posterior divisions at the hilum. Each artery divides further, and its branches penetrate the renal substance proper as interlobar arteries, which course between lobes. Interlobar arteries extend to the corticomedullary junction and give rise to arcuate arteries, which arch between cortex and medulla and course roughly perpendicular to interlobar arteries. Branches of the arcuate arteries, interlobular arteries, run perpendicularly to the arcuate arteries and extend through the cortex toward the capsular surface. Afferent arterioles are branches from the interlobular arteries and give rise to glomerular capillaries. The glomeruli represent a spherical bag of capillary loops arranged in several lobules; the capillaries merge to exit the glomerulus as efferent arterioles, which, in superficial nephrons, branch to form another capillary bed in the interstitium that surrounds cortical tubules. These capillaries are known as peritubular or interstitial capillaries. Efferent arterioles from juxtamedullary glomeruli extend into the medulla as vasa recta, or straight vessels, which supply the outer and inner medulla. The vasa recta and peritubular capillaries collect, forming into interlobular veins; the veins follow the arteries in distribution, size, and course, and leave the kidneys as renal veins, which empty into the inferior vena cava.

The kidneys have three major gross components: the cortex, the medulla, and the collecting system. On cut surface, the *cortex* is the pale outer region, approximately 1.5 cm in thickness; it has a granular appearance because of the presence of glomeruli and convoluted tubules. The *medulla,* a series of pyramidal structures with apical papillae, number normally 8 to 18, and have a striped or striated appearance because of the parallel arrangement of the tubular structures. The bases of the pyramids are at the corticomedullary junction and the apices extend into the collecting system. Cortical parenchyma extends into spaces between adjacent pyramids;

this portion of the cortex is known as *columns of Bertin*. A medullary pyramid with surrounding cortical parenchyma, which includes both columns of Bertin and the subcapsular cortex, constitutes a renal lobe. The *collecting system* consists of the pelvis, which represents the expanded upper portion of the ureter and is more or less funnel shaped. Each pelvis has two or three major branches known as the *major calyces*. Each calyx divides further into three or four smaller branches known as *minor calyces*. Each calyx usually receives one medullary papilla.

Each kidney contains approximately 1 million *nephrons*, which are the individual functioning units and are composed of glomeruli and tubules. Each *glomerulus* is a spherical collection of interconnected capillaries within a space (Bowman's space) lined by flattened parietal epithelial cells (Fig. 65-1 and 65-2). Bowman's space is continuous with the tubules, with the orifice of the proximal tubule generally at the pole opposite the glomerular hilus where the afferent and efferent arterioles enter and leave, respectively. The outer aspects of the glomerular capillaries are covered by a layer of visceral epithelial cells, or podocytes. Each visceral epithelial cell has a large body, which contains the nucleus, and cytoplasmic extensions, which divide, forming small fingerlike processes that interdigitate with similar structures from adjacent cells and cover the capillaries. These interdigitating processes, known as pedicels, are also called foot processes because of their appearance on transmission electron microscopy. The space between adjacent foot processes is known as the filtration slit; adjacent foot processes are joined together by a thin membrane known as the slit-pore diaphragm.

Epithelial cells cover the glomerular capillary basement membrane (GBM), a three-layered structure with a central thick layer that is slightly electron dense (lamina densa) and thinner electron-lucent layers beneath epithelial and endothelial cells (lamina rarae externa and lamina rarae interna, respectively). The GBM is composed predominantly of type IV collagen with small amounts of type V collagen, laminin, and proteoglycans, predominantly heparan sulfate. Entactin and fibronectin are also present. The GBM in adults measures approximately 340 to 360 nm in thickness and is significantly thicker in men than in women. The endothelial cells are thin and have multiple fenestrae, each measuring approximately 80 nm in diameter.

The capillary tufts are supported by the mesangium, which represents the intraglomerular continuation of the arteriolar walls. The mesangium has two components. The *extracellular matrix* has many structural, compositional, and, therefore, tinctorial properties similar to basement membrane. The *cells* of the mesangium, known as mesangial cells, of which there are two types, include modified smooth muscle cells, representing greater than 95% of the cellular population, and bone marrow–derived cells, representing the remainder. Mesangial cells have numerous functions, including contraction, production of extracellular matrix, secretion of inflammatory and other active mediators, phagocytosis, and migration from the central zone, where they are normally situated.

The proteoglycans of the GBM are negatively charged; similarly, the surfaces of both epithelial and endothelial cells are also anionically charged because of sialoglycoproteins in the cellular coats. Both of these negatively charged structures are responsible for the *charge selective barrier* to filtration of glomerular contents. The basement membrane, which along with the fenestrated endothelial cell allows for ready filtration of water and small substances, is known as the *size-selective barrier*. The visceral epithelial cell in the adult is responsible for the production and maintenance of basement membrane.[1-3]

The remaining portion of the nephron is divided into proximal tubules, which are often convoluted, the loop of Henle, with both descending and ascending limbs, and the distal tubule. The proximal tubular cells have well-developed, closely packed microvillous luminal surfaces known collectively as brush border. The cells are larger than those of the distal tubules, which have relatively few surface microvilli. The proximal tubular cells contain numerous mitochondria, resulting in granular cytoplasm. Each tubule is surrounded completely by a basement membrane. In tissue sections, adjacent tubular basement membranes are almost in direct contact with one another and are separated by a small amount of connective tissue, known as the interstitium, containing peritubular capillaries

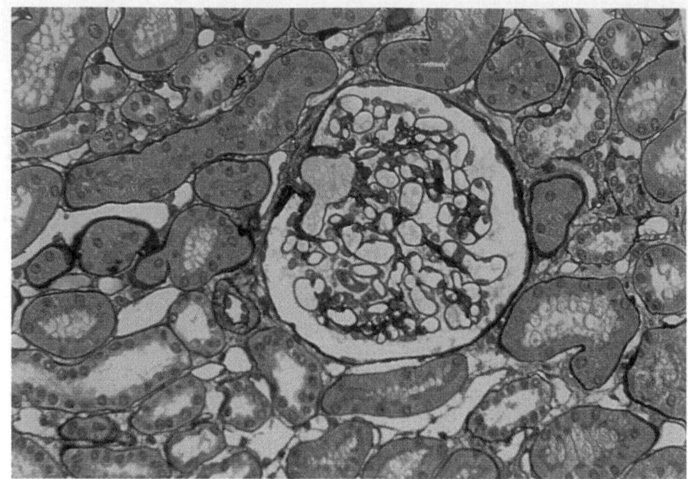

Fig. 65-1 Normal glomerulus; notice single-contoured walls, patent capillaries, inconspicuous mesangium, and degree of cellularity. (Periodic acid–methenamine silver.)

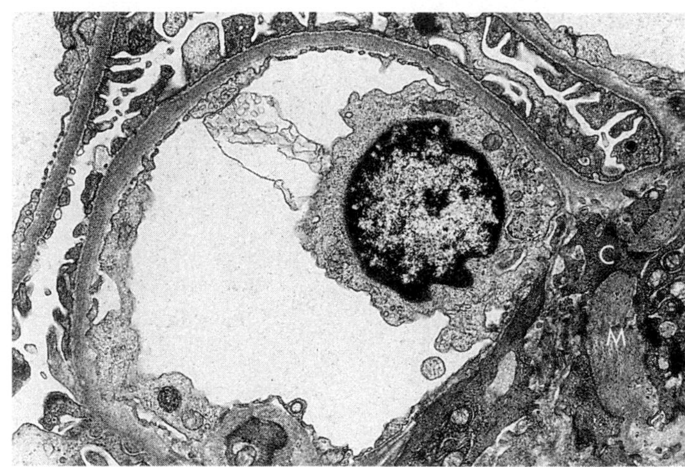

Fig. 65-2 Notice the intact epithelial foot processes, normal basement membrane, and attenuated cytoplasm of endothelial cell. The mesangium is of normal volume with matrix *(M)* and adjacent cell cytoplasm *(C)*.

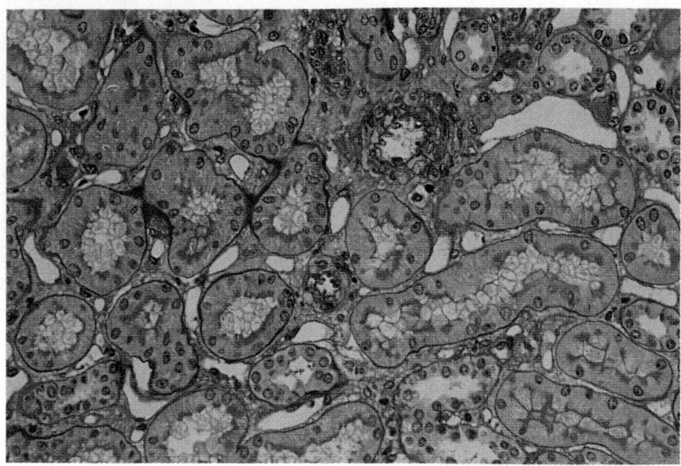

Fig. 65-3 Normal cortical tubules and interstitium. Notice brush border of proximal cells and close relationship of adjacent tubules to one another. (Periodic acid–Schiff.)

(Fig. 65-3). At the vascular pole of the glomerulus and the site of entrance of the afferent arteriole, the cells of the arteriolar wall are modified into secretory cells known as juxtaglomerular cells; these produce and secrete renin, contained in granules. The macula densa, a portion of the distal tubule at the glomerular hilum, is characterized by more crowded and smaller distal tubular cells, which are in contact with the juxtaglomerular cells. Surrounding the macula densa and afferent arteriole are lacis cells, mesenchymal cells similar to mesangial cells.[1]

The major function of the glomerulus is filtration of water and small solutes; the glomerular capillary wall provides an effective size and isoelectric charge–selective barrier to various substances, the most important of which are plasma proteins. Serum albumin, because of its anionic charge, is repelled by the negatively charged capillary wall and thus is not filtered. The other proteins are larger and are retained in the circulation because of their size. The major function of the tubules is resorption of water, bicarbonate, potassium, proteins, and glucose and chloride. The cells of the juxtaglomerular apparatus represent, in part, the endocrine component of the kidney, with secretion of renin.

EXAMINATION OF RENAL TISSUE

Because of the types of diseases and the components of the renal tissue that are abnormal in these diseases, the preparation of tissue specimens for examination is often different from that of most or all other tissues. In particular, the elucidation of lesions of glomeruli mandates that a variety of histochemical stains be used and that tissue sections be cut thinner than for other tissues. Furthermore, to take best advantage of the stains, many investigators and renal pathologists have found that formalin, Zenker's solution, and many of the more commonly used fixatives result in substandard preparations. Consequently, alcoholic Bouin's solution (Duboscq-Brasil) is the fixative of choice. For the elucidation of glomerular structure and pathologic condition, it is necessary that the extracellular matrix components (basement membrane, mesangial matrix) be preferentially stained. In paraffin-embedded sections, the hematoxylin and eosin stain does not ordinarily allow for distinction of extracellular matrix from cytoplasm in a clear or convincing manner. Periodic acid–Schiff (PAS), periodic acid–methenamine silver (Jones), and Masson's trichrome stains all provide excellent definition of extracellular material (Table 65-1). Each stain has its advantages and disadvantages, and as a rule, all are used in evaluating renal tissues, especially biopsy specimens. The PAS reagent stains GBM mesangial matrix, and tubular basement membranes red (positive), whereas the periodic acid–methenamine silver colors the same components black, providing clear contrast between positively and negatively staining structures. We prefer Masson's trichrome stain using aniline blue; with this method, extracellular glomerular matrix and tubular basement membranes stain blue and are clearly distinguished from the cells and abnormal material that accumulate in pathologic circumstances.[4] Congo red, elastic tissue, and other stains should be employed when indicated. The tissue sections in all but Congo red stains should be no greater than 2 to 3 μm in thickness because the definition of a glomerular pathologic condition, especially regarding cellularity, depends on sections of this thickness. Furthermore, the ability to detect subtle pathologic abnormalities is enhanced with thinner sections.

Especially for glomerular disease, *immunohistochemistry* is necessary for evaluation of renal tissues, especially for diagnosing glomerular diseases. Most laboratories utilize immunofluorescence for identifying and localizing immunoglobulins, complement, fibrin, and other immune substances within renal tissues. For renal biopsy studies and, when indicated on other renal specimens, we routinely employ the following fluorescein-labeled antibodies: IgG, IgA, IgM, C1q, C3, albumin, fibrin, and kappa and lambda immunoglobulin light chains. Fluorescence positivity in glomeruli is described as granular or linear. Regardless of the immunopathologic mechanisms responsible for the granular deposits, there is an electron microscopic counterpart to granular deposits; by electron microscopy, extracellular masses of electron-dense material correspond to the deposits[4] (Table 65-2). The granular deposits can be appreciated in tissue prepared for light microscopy; this is best demonstrated and documented with the use of Masson's trichrome stain, which makes granular deposits appear as bright fuchsinophilic (orange, red-orange) smooth homogeneous structures. It is for this reason that Masson's trichrome has achieved considerable popularity in the evaluation of renal specimens. There is no regular ultrastructural or light microscopic counterpart to linear staining.

Electron microscopy (EM) is routinely used in the study of renal tissues. For glomerular diseases this method helps localize deposits, detect extremely small deposits, and document alterations of cellular structure. In addition, immunofluorescence and EM are often necessary or helpful in diagnosing tubular, interstitial, and vascular lesions.[5]

These methods are in current use for all renal biopsy specimens in most institutions. The detection and diagnosis of many renal disorders observed in autopsy or nephrectomy specimens may also require a similar approach. Many important abnormalities can be still detected if a portion of the formalin-fixed surgical or autopsy tissue is processed for EM or if, should it be available, fresh tissue is evaluated by immunofluorescence.

Table 65-1 Staining characteristics of various renal structures

Structure	Stain: Hematoxylin and eosin	Periodic acid–Schiff	Periodic acid methenamine–silver (Jones)	Masson's trichrome
Glomerular and tubular basement membranes	Pink-red	Magenta	Black	Light blue
Mesangial matrix	Pink-red	Magenta	Black	Light blue
Interstitial type of collagen	Pink-red	Light pink	Gray	Dark blue
Cytoplasm endothelial, mesangial, smooth muscular	Pink granular	White-pink	Gray-pink	Rust colored, finely granular
Epithelial	Pink granular	White-pink	Gray-pink	Rust colored, coarsely granular
Proteinaceous material (deposits)	Pink or bright red	Homogeneous pale or bright pink (generally negative)	Homogeneous pink or red (counterstain negative)	Bright (or pale) orange, smooth
Fibrin	Pink or bright red	Slightly positive or negative	Pink or negative	Bright, brilliant red-orange fibrillar
Nuclei	Dark blue	Dark blue	Dark blue	Dark brown

Table 65-2 Glomerular granular immune deposits

Technique	Appearance
Immunofluorescence	Granular-mesangial or capillary wall
Electron microscopy	Dense (darkly staining) extracellular mass
Light microscopy with Masson's trichrome stain	Fuchsinophilic (bright, homogeneous)

Table 65-3 Distribution of glomerular lesions

Entire glomerular population

Focal—abnormality affects a portion (usually less than 50%) of the glomeruli

Diffuse—abnormality affects all or almost all glomeruli

Single glomerulus

Segmental—abnormality affects part of the capillary tuft

Global—abnormality affects the entire capillary tuft

GENERAL PATHOLOGY OF RENAL STRUCTURES

Before embarking on a description of the various renal diseases, we present first a discussion of basic abnormalities that characterize the renal structures.

Glomeruli

Increased cellularity. Hypercellularity may result from increase in intrinsic cells (mesangial or endothelial cells) or from accumulation of leukocytes in capillary lumens, beneath endothelial cells, or in the mesangium. Although this terminology is not entirely correct, glomerular lesions with increased cells in the tufts are often known as *proliferative glomerulonephritis.* Accumulation of cells within the urinary space is known as a *crescent.* Localization of abnormalities affecting portions of glomerular populations and glomeruli are indicated by specific terms (Table 65-3).

Increase in extracellular matrix. An increase in the extracellular matrix implies an increase in mesangial matrix or basement membrane material. In the former instance, this may be in a uniform and diffuse pattern in all lobules or may cause a nodular appearance to the mesangium. Increased basement membrane material most commonly takes the form of thickened basement membranes, an abnormality which is best appreciated by EM.

Sclerosis. Sclerosis refers to increased extracellular matrix and other material leading to obliteration of capillaries and solidification of all or part of the tufts. Sclerosis (glomerular scarring) may be associated with accumulation of collagen in and obliterating the urinary space along with increased extracellular matrix in the capillary tufts. When the entire glomerulus is involved, this is known as *complete sclerosis;* an older and less precise term is *glomerular hyalinization.* Segmental glomerulosclerosis implies a completely different pathologic process and often a disease. With segmental sclerosis, only portions of the capillary tufts are involved; capillaries are obliterated by increased extracellular matrix or large precipitates of plasma protein known as insudates.

Crescents. Crescents represent accumulation of cells and extracellular material in the urinary space. Crescents are the result of severe capillary wall damage with disruptions in continuity and spillage of fibrin from inside the damaged capillaries into the urinary spaces. This results in proliferation of visceral and perhaps parietal epithelial cells and accumulation of monocytes and other blood cells in the urinary space. The cellular composition of the crescent varies depending on the type of disease and associated damage to the basement membrane of Bowman's capsule. Crescents most commonly heal by organization. With an admixture of cells and collagen, the crescent is considered fibrocellular: with only collagen in the urinary space, the crescent is designated as fibrotic. With organization of the crescent, the capillary tuft is often collapsed and distorted.

Peripheral migration and interposition of mesangium. In certain diseases, the mesangial cells and often matrix extend from the central lobular portion of the tuft into the peripheral capillary wall, migrating between endothelial cell and basement membrane. In this location, with mesangial matrix between the interposed mesangial cell and endothelial cell, the capillary wall is thickened and has two layers of extracellular matrix. This two-layered or double-contoured appearance may involve a few or all capillaries depending on the disease process and the stimulus.

Alteration in visceral epithelial cell morphology. Detection of alteration in visceral epithelial cell morphology abnormality requires EM. In association with protein loss across the glomerular capillary wall, the epithelial cells change shape; the foot processes retract and swell, resulting in loss of individual foot processes and a near solid mass of cytoplasm covering the GBM. This loss, or *effacement of foot processes,* is also incorrectly known as fusion because it was believed that adjacent foot processes fused with one another. This is not the case because adjacent foot processes are from different cells and, as documented by scanning EM, the cells do not merge.[6,7]

Tubules

Atrophy. Atrophy results in irregular thickening and wrinkling of basement membranes even before diminution in size of tubules. Hence, under most circumstances, thickened or wrinkled basement membranes imply tubular atrophy.

Casts. Tubular casts are composed primarily of Tamm-Horsfall protein, a mucoprotein produced by cells of the thick ascending limb of Henle's loop. Under physiologic and pathologic circumstances, this protein may precipitate in the lumen and form internal casts of the distal nephron. It may be passed in the urine as hyaline casts. Tamm-Horsfall protein is best appreciated in PAS-stained sections because of its strong positivity. Tamm-Horsfall protein may be found in abnormal sites (proximal nephron, interstitium, vessels) in certain disorders.

Interstitium

Acute interstitial processes are defined by the presence of edema; this is best appreciated in PAS-stained or periodic acid methenamine silver–stained sections by separation of normal tubules from one another. Normal tubules are identified by normal basement membranes. Chronic interstitial processes are characterized by fibrosis; this is associated with tubular atrophy. The type of inflammatory cell (such as polymorphonuclear leukocyte or lymphocyte) does not determine the acute or chronic nature of the interstitial process.

Arteries and arterioles

With few exceptions (thrombotic microangiopathies, scleroderma) the changes in these structures are not unique to the kidney (see later in this chapter for further discussion).[7]

CLINICAL MANIFESTATIONS OF RENAL DISEASES

Our colleagues in nephrology have categorized the clinical and laboratory manifestations of renal disease in a variety of clinical syndromes.[6]

Nephrotic syndrome is characterized by loss of large amounts of albumin and other proteins (greater than 3.5 g per 24 hours) in the urine. This results in decreased serum albumin, peripheral edema, hyperlipidemia, and lipiduria. Some patients have heavy proteinuria alone without the other manifestations. Nephrotic syndrome is always a manifestation of glomerular injury.

Asymptomatic proteinuria or hematuria indicates less than nephrotic range proteinuria or microscopic hematuria detected in a patient without physical complaints. This category also includes patients who have gross hematuria. The findings are often of glomerular origin.

Acute nephritic syndrome manifests as a sudden onset of proteinuria, hematuria, diminished urine production with fluid retention, azotemia, hypertension, and often edema. This is attributable to abnormal glomeruli.

In *rapidly progressive glomerulonephritis* there is progressive and relentless loss of renal function over weeks to months associated with hematuria and variable proteinuria. This is also considered of glomerular origin.

Acute renal failure is acute loss of glomerular filtration with or without diminution in urine production. This may be of glomerular, tubular, interstitial, or vascular origin.

Tubular defects result in loss of amino acids, glucose, and other substances in the urine.

Hypertension may occur with or without any of the other mentioned renal syndromes.

Chronic renal failure is the appearance of azotemia or uremia often without other manifestations of renal disease.

Renal infection and urinary obstruction require no additional comments.

PATHOGENIC MECHANISMS IN RENAL DISEASES

Immunologic

Many glomerular and a small number of tubulointerstitial and vascular disorders are immunologically mediated[9] (Table 65-4). These may be the result of antibody-mediated or cell-mediated processes. In most instances in humans, the immediate cause or antigenic stimulus for the immune reaction is not known. There are ample numbers of animal models of immunologically mediated renal disease that correspond to human disorders and that have provided considerable insight into mechanisms of injury and clear understandings of the pathologic process. The detection of antibody-mediated damage in renal tissue depends on the use of immunofluorescence microscopy.

Most glomerulopathies are immunologically mediated and are the result of antibody-induced injury. This can occur as a consequence of antibody combining with an intrinsic antigen in the glomerulus or antibody combining either in situ or in the circulation with an extrinsic glomerular antigen, with immune complexes localizing or depositing in glomeruli. With *circulating immune complexes,* the antigens may be of endogenous or exogenous origin. Endogenous antigens occur in diseases such as systemic lupus erythematosus (SLE) and include components of nuclei such as DNA, histones, and so on. Exogenous antigens are usually of microorganism origin such as bacterial products, hepatitis B and C viral antigens, and malarial antigen. Circulating immune complexes are trapped or

Table 65-4 Types of immunologic renal injury

Humoral (antibody)-induced damage—glomerular, tubulointerstitial
- Circulating immune complex deposition
  - Endogenous antigens
  - Exogenous antigens
- In situ immune complex formation—glomerular, tubulointerstitial
  - Intrinsic antigen
    - Basement membrane (glomerular, tubular)
    - Glomerular visceral epithelial membrane
    - Others
  - Planted antigen
    - Endogenous antigens
    - Exogenous antigens

Cell-mediated damage—glomerular, tubulointerstitial, vascular

lodge in glomeruli in the mesangium and subendothelial aspects of capillary walls. Less commonly, they may be found in subepithelial locations. The electron microscope precisely localizes the deposits. Certain diseases are characterized by deposits in predominantly one site, whereas other diseases may be characterized by deposits in more than one location. Once immune complexes are deposited, complement is fixed and often leukocyte infiltration follows. The white blood cells accumulate in capillary lumens and infiltrate into the mesangium; in addition, intrinsic mesangial cells may divide and may also extend into peripheral capillary walls. The leukocytes, in part, may be responsible for removal of deposited immune complexes. The names of the many glomerular disorders, diagnostic criteria, and prognostic and therapeutic implications depend on the correct localization and identification of the immune complexes in the glomeruli.

The other mechanism of antibody-induced injury results from in situ immune complex formation. This can occur in two major situations. The antibody can be directed against an intrinsic component of the glomerulus such as a portion of the basement membrane or perhaps, as shown in experimental animals, a component glomerular cell such as visceral epithelial cell. Alternatively, antigen may arrive in the glomerulus from the circulation and be planted or trapped in a particular location. Antibody binds with the trapped antigen, forming an immune complex locally. The stimulus or stimuli for antibody production are often not known.

In humans, antibody directed against the basement membrane component is known as anti-GBM antibody. The pattern of florescence is of linear binding of the antibody to the basement membrane. Planted antigens in humans and epithelial cell antigen in experimental animals, when combined with antibody in situ, result in a pattern of granular fluorescence similar to glomeruli with deposition of circulating immune complexes. With planted antigens, the pattern of florescence is often of uniform granular deposits, most commonly in the capillary walls; EM often indicates that the resulting electron-dense deposits are in the subepithelial aspect of the capillary walls. Much less commonly, mesangial or subendothelial deposits may result from in situ immune complex formation.

Cell-mediated immune injury in human renal disease is evident in acute interstitial disorders such as drug-induced acute interstitial nephritis and certain forms of transplant rejection. On the other hand, cell-mediated immune mechanisms in glomerular disease are postulated with sound experimental and clinical reasoning, though at present there is no definitive evidence that such a mechanism is operative.[10]

It is not the purpose of this chapter to deal in detail with inflammatory mediators of injury; refer to Chapter 18 for a detailed discussion. In the kidneys, the main tissue components responsible for glomerular injury include leukocytes, which may be attracted because of complement activation and which release a large number of growth factors, oxygen free radicals, cytokines, and other substances.

Complement components, especially C5B-C9, may have a large role in producing structural and functional damage, especially in glomeruli. Recent and continuing evidence has documented important roles of cytokines, especially interleukin-1 and tumor necrosis factor, as well as platelet-derived growth factor and transforming growth factor–beta (TGF-β) in the genesis and progression of glomerular disease.

Nonimmunologic

Damage to glomerular visceral epithelial cells. Damage from a wide variety of influences causes swelling of glomerular visceral epithelial cells with disappearance or effacement of the individual foot processes. Further damage results in vacuolization, accumulation of protein in lysosomes (protein reabsorption droplets), and detachment of cell from the basement membrane.[11] Many investigators believe that the denuded basement membrane represents a site of major protein loss across the capillary wall.

Pronounced reduction in renal mass. With significant loss of functioning nephrons, the remnant nephrons undergo hypertrophy. This has been adequately documented in experimental animals and is believed to occur in human disease. Glomerular hypertrophy is associated with increased intracapillary and systemic blood pressures, with increase in blood flow and glomerular filtration. Although initially an adaptive process, these physiologic events are associated with the ultimate development of segmental glomerulosclerosis, diminution in glomerular filtration, and heavy proteinuria. It is likely that this mechanism is responsible for the progression of many forms of renal disease regardless of the primary site of injury.[12,13]

Mechanisms of tubular and interstitial injury. As noted, immunologic mechanisms may be responsible for certain forms of interstitial damage, but in contrast to the glomeruli, toxins, ischemia, and obstruction of urine outflow are important processes. Rather than discuss these mechanisms in general terms, they are dealt with in detail in the appropriate disorder.

DEVELOPMENTAL AND HEREDITARY DISORDERS

Autosomal recessive polycystic kidney disease

Autosomal recessive polycystic kidney disease (ARPKD) is an inherited form of renal disease, manifested predominantly in childhood, with constant hepatic abnormalities. Formerly known as infantile polycystic kidney disease, it is one of several forms of cystic disease of kidneys that may be apparent at birth or in early infancy. There are two forms of this disorder, one presenting in early infancy, and the other manifesting in older children and adults.

Etiology and pathogenesis. ARPKD is inherited in an autosomal recessive manner; however, the defective gene has not been identified. It is likely that the kidneys initially develop normally, but some as yet unidentified stimulus causes dilatation of collecting ducts. The hepatic abnormalities are probably caused by development arrest of bile duct formation, with fibrosis as a secondary process.[14,15]

Pathology. The kidneys are enlarged, are reniform in configuration, and are spongy. In newborns with severe involvement the kidneys may weight 300 g or more combined and result in pronounced abdominal distention. The cysts are small and elongated, extending from the corticomedullary junction radially toward the capsule (Fig. 65-4) These tubular channels usually measure 1 to 2 mm in diameter and 5 to 10 mm in length and represent dilated collecting tubules and ducts lined by uniform cuboidal epithelium (Fig. 65-5). The glomeruli and remainder of the nephron proximal to collecting tubules are normal or compressed by the cysts. In older children, there is less cystic involvement of the kidneys, though the cysts are irregularly distributed, larger, and more spherical. There is progressive scarring, with completely sclerotic glomeruli and tubular atrophy and interstitial fibrosis.[16]

The hepatic abnormalities also differ with the age of the patient. In neonates, there is an increase in the number of bile ducts that are tortuous, surround the portal tracts, and are dilated, extending into hepatic lobules. With age, there is increased portal fibrosis with ultimate bridging septa, regenerative nodules, and portal hypertension. When the early hepatic lesions of bile ductular increase and malformation occur as an isolated abnormality (no renal involvement), it is known as Caroli's disease. Similarly, the later hepatic lesions without concomitant renal changes are known as congenital hepatic fibrosis; the liver disease may be the dominant clinical manifestation in older children.[16,17]

Differential diagnosis. The gross and microscopic morphology of the kidneys in the neonatal period is distinctive, and confusion with other disorders usually does not occur. In older children with fewer but larger cysts, differentiation from autosomal dominant polycystic kidney disease is necessary.

Clinical presentation. ARPKD occurs most commonly in the newborn period and is manifested by oliguria and large kidneys with pronounced abdominal distention. Oligohydramnios and Potter facies (abnormal ears, beaked nose, small chin, and facial creases) are evident at birth. Because of small lungs, there is high mortality from pulmonary insufficiency. In older children, the presenting manifestations are more varied, with hepatic disease dominating—hepatomegaly, portal hypertension, splenomegaly, and esophageal varices. Renal enlargement and insufficiency are also variable. In most patients with ARPKD, death occurs in childhood, though some children survive into adulthood with renal insufficiency.[17]

Autosomal dominant polycystic kidney disease

Autosomal dominant polycystic kidney disease (ADPKD) is a common systemic genetic disorder characterized by the appearance of numerous cysts throughout the kidneys, often leading to end-stage renal failure and cysts in other organs, especially the liver. It is inherited as an autosomal dominant tract with nearly complete penetrance. Although other hereditary cystic diseases occur, this entity is quite specific in inheritance, pathology, and, often, clinical manifestations, and so it is not to be confused with the other disorders.[17]

Etiology and pathogenesis. A causative gene has been localized in most patients to the short arm of chromosome 16 and is known as ADPKD-1. Other genes may be operative in a small number of families, although a second gene has not yet been identified. The ADPKD-1 gene is considered responsible for the disease in greater than 90% of families in the white population. The disorder is world-wide in distribution and affects all races; there is no gender predilection.[18]

The pathogenesis is unknown, though several theories exist. One holds that epithelial cell proliferation, perhaps related to the effects of growth factors, is primary and results in papillary hyperplasia, which can lead to intranephron obstruction and proximal cystic dilatation.[19,20] Indeed, cellular papillae are not an uncommon feature of cyst walls. Another postulate is that the basic defect is in extracellular matrix pro-

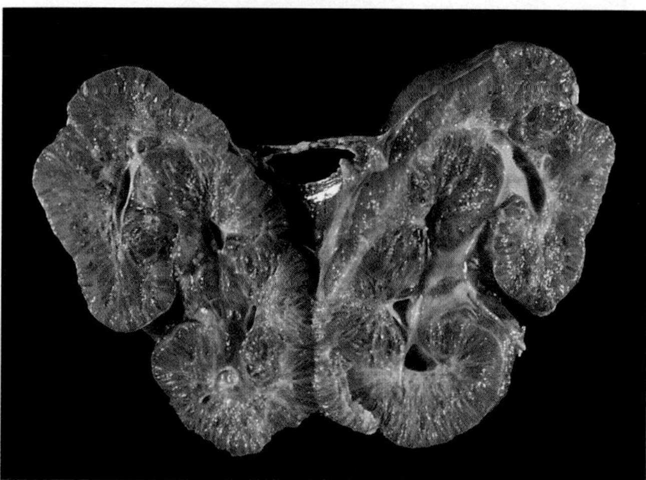

Fig. 65-4 Autosomal recessive polycystic kidney disease. The kidney is greatly enlarged, with prominent parallel elongated dilated channels.

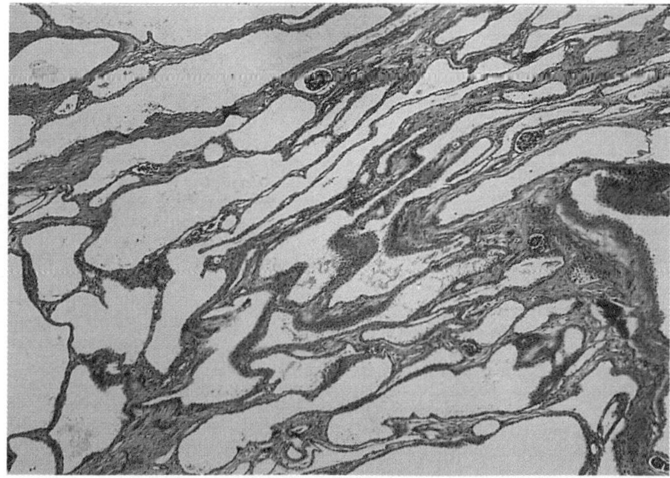

Fig. 65-5 Low-power photomicrograph demonstrating elongated cystically dilated collecting ducts in cortex of kidney illustrated in Fig. 65-4. (Periodic acid–Schiff.)

duction; altered basement membranes can result in tubular diverticula and cyst formation.[21] Abnormal vascular tissue associated with intracranial aneurysms and lesions of cardiac valves and hypertension are extrarenal manifestations of this disorder perhaps related to abnormal extracellular matrix. Cyst growth can be enhanced by altered sodium and water flux in the nephron; abnormal localization of Na^+, K^+-ATPase to the apical rather than basilar portion of epithelial cells has been documented and can cause sodium and fluid to move into rather than out of a cyst.[18] The pathogenic mechanisms responsible for hepatic bile cysts are also not known.

Pathology. The gross appearance of kidneys with fully established advanced ADPKD is striking and impressive. Both kidneys are involved, tend to be similar to one another, and maintain the reniform shape. They are greatly enlarged and can average in excess of 2000 g each and measure up to 40 cm in length (Fig. 65-6). The size, in part, depends on the severity of renal functional impairment, with the smallest kidneys occurring in patients without azotemia and the largest ones in patients with advanced azotemia or uremia. The cysts vary in size from a few millimeters to several centimeters and typically contain a clear fluid similar to urine in color and viscosity. Some cysts may contain blood (fresh or old), and a few may contain purulent material. In some series, neoplasms (carcinomas, adenomas) have been reported; most are several millimeters in diameter, though some may be several centimeters and easily visible on gross examination.[17,18]

The cysts are typically lined by thin and simplified epithelium (Fig. 65-7); the nephron segment from which the cyst arose cannot usually be ascertained by examination of the lining cells unless lectin binding or other methods are used. Cystically dilated Bowman's spaces or cysts of Bowman's capsules are often present. It is estimated that, in at least 80% of affected kidneys, hyperplastic lesions of lining epithelium will be present. These include flat hyperplasia with general increase in layers of lining cells, and polypoid hyperplasia with one or more polyps composed of a fibrovascular core covered by epithelium in each cyst. True intracystic papillary or solid adenomas may also be found.[22] The renal parenchyma between cysts may be normal; more often it displays compression, with tubular atrophy, interstitial fibrosis, and complete glomerular sclerosis. There may be variable interstitial lymphocyte accumulation. In addition, arterial and arteriolar changes of hypertension are often present.[17,18]

Clinical presentation. Most patients become symptomatic in the third or fourth decades with abdominal pain from the enlarged kidneys. Hematuria is common, probably from bleeding into one or more cysts. Approximately 50% of the patients develop hypertension. Early in the disorder, there is a decrease in renal concentrating ability. Bacterial infection of the cysts or renal parenchyma is common; cyst infection is difficult to treat because few antibiotics can effectively penetrate the cysts. Approximately 50% of the patients will develop end-stage renal failure by 60 years of age. Renal transplantation is the therapy of choice; most patients fare better than those with other forms of end-stage renal disease. Extrarenal manifestations include hepatic and other visceral cysts, often without major clinical significance. Mitral valve prolapse occurs in approximately 25% of the patients, and intracranial berry aneurysms are present in many patients; the exact frequency is unknown but is estimated to affect up to 40%.[18,23]

Differential diagnosis. The major lesions from which this disorder needs to be distinguished are acquired cystic disease and ARPKD. For both, a careful clinical history, including family history, is necessary. Faced with an enlarged multicystic kidney from an adult with advanced renal disease, one may find it difficult to distinguish acquired cystic disease from ADPKD; microscopic evaluation may be useful because in the former, the lining epithelium is more likely to be hyperplasic or papillary. The cysts in ARPKD are grossly more elongated

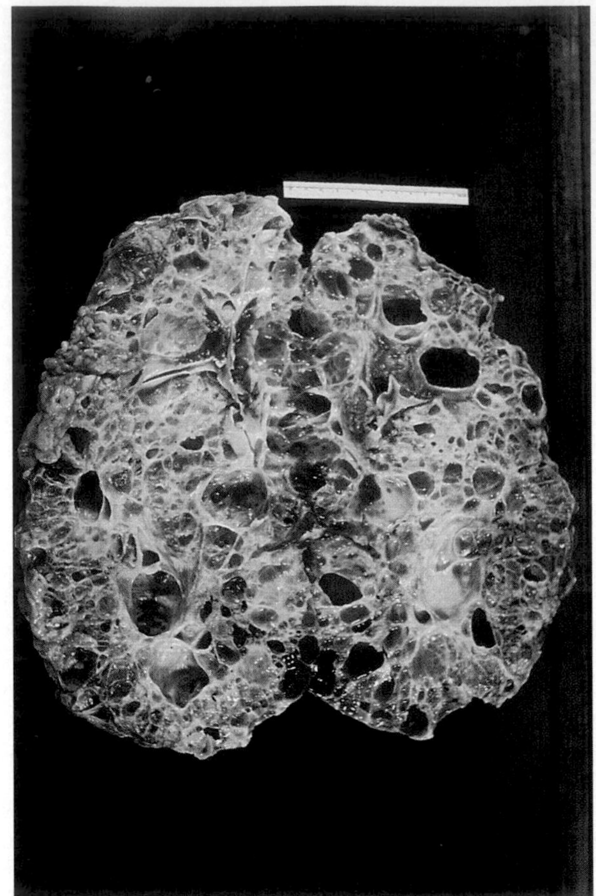

Fig. 65-6 Autosomal dominant polycystic kidney disease. The kidney is enormous, with multiple large cysts.

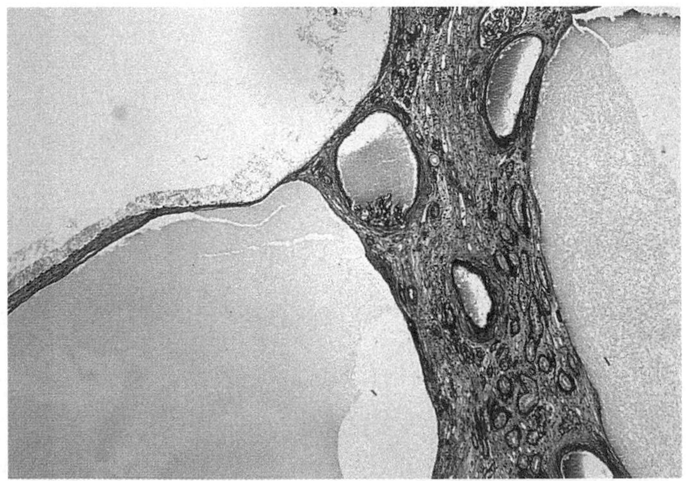

Fig. 65-7 Multiple large cysts and a cystically dilated Bowman's space are evident. The lining of all is flattened. (Periodic acid–Schiff.)

and occur perpendicularly to the capsular surface because they represent dilated collecting ducts. In ARPKD, as a rule, the kidneys are not as enlarged as those in ADPKD.

Familial juvenile nephronophthisis–medullary cystic disease complex

The disorder or group of disorders known as familial juvenile nephronophthsis–medullary cystic disease complex, usually hereditary in nature, is characterized initially by salt wasting, urine concentrating defect or other manifestations of tubular dysfunction, and, ultimately, small kidneys, often with medullary cysts. Extrarenal abnormalities are present in some patients. Familial juvenile nephronophthisis typically affects children, whereas medullary cystic disease, with a different pattern of inheritance, affects young adults. This form of renal disease is traditionally considered either one of the renal cystic diseases or, because of the major histologic findings, a form of chronic interstitial nephritis.[17]

Etiology and pathogenesis. Although there are sporadic cases of this complex, most are inherited. The autosomal recessive form, known as familial juvenile nephronophthisis, affects mainly children and accounts for approximately 67% of reported cases. Onset is usually during the first decade of life. The autosomal dominant form, medullary cystic disease, is an adult disorder, with onset occurring usually in the third decade. It is suggested that sporadic cases represent new dominant mutations. The precise gene or genes responsible for any component of this disease complex have not been identified.[17]

The basic defect responsible for the clinical and morphologic features has not been clearly defined; however, several studies have documented striking lesions of tubular basement membranes, suggesting that a primary abnormality of this structure may be responsible for the varied manifestations.

Pathology. As the name of the disorder implies the kidneys are characteristically small and shrunken especially with a long course of disease. There are cysts mainly at the corticomedullary junction, though deeper medullary cysts may occur. Approximately 25% of cases lack cysts.

Microscopic. The traditionally typical findings are of cortical interstitial fibrosis and tubular atrophy with prominently thickened tubular basement membranes. A variable infiltrate of lymphocytes is present in the fibrotic interstitium.[17] The cysts, considered to occur in the distal convoluted and collecting tubules, are lined by flattened epithelium and have thickened basement membranes. More recent work, however, has challenged this traditional consideration. Tubular basement membranes by both light and electron microscopy display pronounced alterations in apparently normal, as well as abnormal, tubules. The basement membranes range from extremely thin and attenuated to greatly thickened (Fig. 65-8). The thicker ones, as documented by EM, are often multilayered; both thick and thin portions often occur simultaneously in the same tubule, frequently with abrupt transitions.[24,26] In addition, interstitial masses of Tamm-Horsfall protein are evident in most kidneys.[24,27] It is suggested that the primary defect is abnormal tubular basement membrane production or formation; the very thin basement membranes are not compliant and may represent sufficient weakness in the tubular walls to allow cyst formation. These thin basement membranes are likely fragile and result in tubular rupture with spillage of contents into the surrounding interstitium.[24] Multilayered basement membranes may result from waves of thin basement membrane production and deposition. It is of note that the abnormal tubular basement membranes do not regularly bind with anti–tubular basement membrane serum, and such nonbinding indicates a lack of one or more normal basement membrane components.[24,26]

Differential diagnosis. There are few diseases from which the nephronophthisis-medullary cystic disease complex need to be distinguished by the pathologist. Grossly, because of medullary cysts, medullary sponge kidney, which is characterized by dilatation of collecting ducts of medullary pyramids in association with multiple papillary cysts, should be considered; this disorder, however, does not have any of the tubular basement membrane changes or cortical abnormalities microscopically. Other forms of cystic disease also lack both the gross and microscopic features. Perhaps most difficult, especially on renal biopsy in a patient without demonstrable cysts, is distinguishing nephronophthisis from chronic interstitial nephritis. The tubular basement membrane changes as documented by both light and electron microscopies, should allow appropriate diagnosis.

Clinical presentation. The clinical manifestations in children and adults are very similar; at presentation, polyuria, polydipsia, anemia, weakness, and azotemia are commonly documented. Urinary concentrating defects and sodium wasting are also evident. These features are manifestations of tubular dysfunction; glomerular abnormalities are not regularly encountered. Extrarenal abnormalities occur, with ocular, skeletal, hepatic, and cerebral involvement in variable combination. The best known of these rare syndromes, with renal disease and tapetoretinal degeneration, is known as renal-retinal dysplasia. Progression of the nephronophthisis–medullary cystic disease complex to end-stage renal failure averages approximately 5 years from presentation.[17]

Renal dysplasia

Renal dysplasia is a disorder in which abnormal metanephric development and differentiation result in a malformed kidney or kidneys. There is complete or partial absence of normal structures. The maldeveloped organ is composed of primitive ducts and metaplastic cartilage.

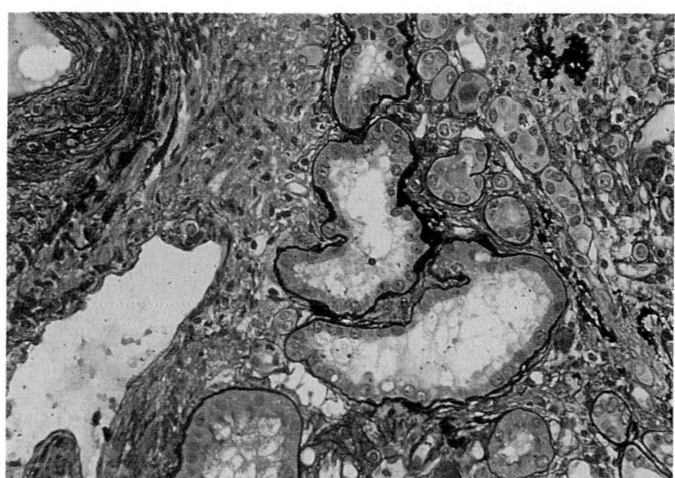

Fig. 65-8 Medullary cystic disease. There is considerable variation in thickness of tubular basement membranes, which range from very thick to quite thin. Interstitial fibrosis surrounds these three tubules, the central one of which best displays the basement membrane changes. (Periodic acid–methenamine silver.)

This disorder is a congenital malformation associated, with a high frequency, with other abnormalities of the urinary tract, most commonly some degree of obstruction. It is often but not always nonhereditary, though dysplasia may be a component of some hereditary syndromes.[28,29]

Etiology and pathogenesis. In most patients with renal dysplasia, urinary tract malformations invariably associated with urinary obstruction are also present.[30] This has led to the belief that, in the face of obstruction, an abnormal environment results in the kidneys during and after nephrogenesis and causes abnormal renal development.

Pathology. Renal dysplasia may be unilateral or bilateral and may be cystic or aplastic. Further, dysplasia may involve the entire kidney or a portion (usually the upper pole in duplicated kidneys with ectopic ureteroceles).

The typical but by no means constant gross appearance is of an enlarged multicystic structure that usually lacks reniform shape (multicystic dysplasia) (Fig. 65-9). The cysts are variable in size, ranging from a few millimeters to several centimeters, and are located peripherally around a more solid central core. There is invariably ureteral atresia and pyelocalyceal occlusion. The superior ureter is often absent. In aplastic dysplasia, the kidneys are very small irregular nubbins of solid tissue with atretic ureters.

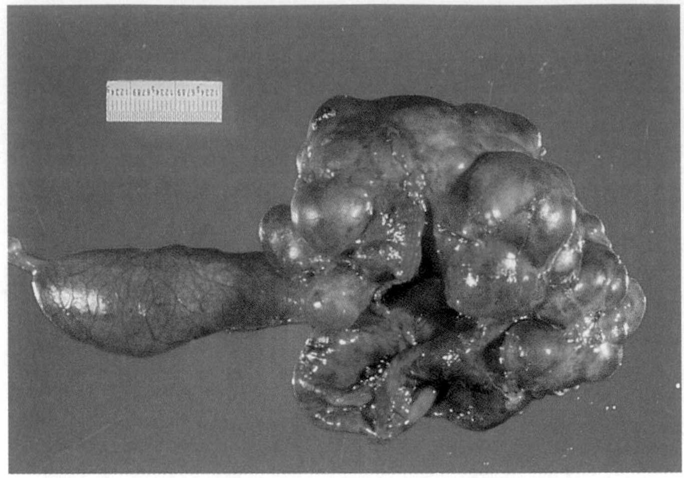

Fig. 65-9 Renal dysplasia. This kidney consists of several irregular cysts without identifiable normal renal parenchyma.

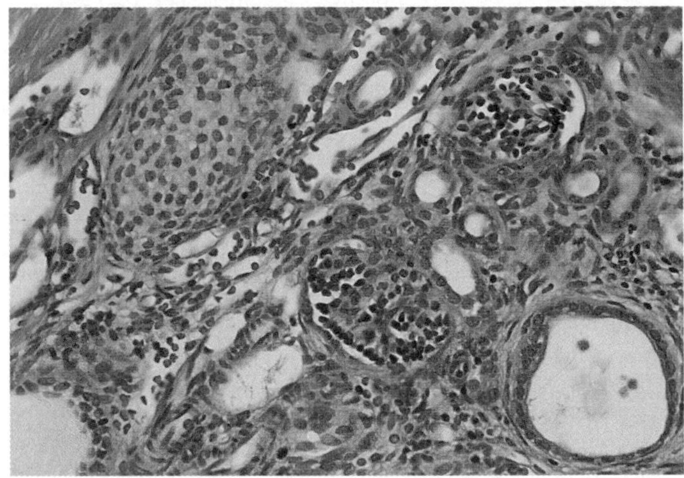

Fig. 65-10 Cartilage is adjacent to a glomerulus without normal surrounding parenchyma.

Microscopically the hallmarks are primitive ducts, which are often dilated and cystic in the multicystic variant, lined by undifferentiated columnar epithelium and surrounded by concentric layers of fibromuscular tissue. Small islands of metaplastic cartilage are common. Normal nephron structures are infrequent (Fig. 65-10).[28,29]

Differential diagnosis. The gross and, especially, microscopic features are distinctive.

Clinical presentation. Bilateral dysplastic kidneys are incompatible with life because they are nonfunctioning. Unilateral dysplasia may be asymptomatic, though an enlarged multicystic kidney may be detectable as a flank mass during a routine examination of an infant. As stated, most cases of dysplasia are sporadic, without a hereditary contribution. However, cystic dysplasia is a feature of many hereditary syndromes, including Meckel's syndrome (microcephaly and posterior encephalocele), Jeune's syndrome (asphyxiating thoracic dysplasia), and cerebrohepatorenal syndrome of Zellweger.[28] Rarely, various renal malignancies have been reported in dysplastic kidneys.[31]

Alport's syndrome

Alport's syndrome, also known as hereditary nephritis, was first described by Guthrie in 1902.[32] It is a familial disease characterized by a primary defect in type IV collagen within the GBM inducing hematuria. This biochemical defect is associated with the morphologic changes of basement membrane thinning, thickening, and layering. The syndrome also encompasses high-frequency hearing loss and, less commonly, ocular abnormalities, with males more severely affected.[33]

At present there is no subclassification of Alport's syndrome, though as the genetics and biochemistry become better understood classifications may arise based on the collagen abnormalities and modes of inheritance.

Etiology and pathogenesis. Most cases of Alport's syndrome are X-linked dominant traits resulting from deletion or point mutations of the COL4A5 gene in the Xq22 region of the long arm of the X chromosome.[34,35] Much less commonly, Alport's syndrome is inherited in an autosomal dominant or, rarely, an autosomal recessive manner. The X-linked form induces abnormalities of the alpha 5 chain of type IV collagen. Type IV collagen is a key constituent of glomerular basement membranes and contains two alpha 1 and one alpha 2 chains in a triple helix. Portions of GBM also contain type IV collagen triple helices composed of the alpha 3, alpha 4, and alpha 5 chains. When the COL4A5 gene is abnormal, the alpha 5 (IV) chain is not present or cannot form a helix with the other chains, leading to abnormal basement membranes lacking the alpha 3, 4, and 5 chains.[36,37] Over a period of years, the basement membrane changes lead to altered glomerular permselectivity and filtration with associated morphologic abnormalities. It is possible that there is accumulation of other collagens in abnormal amounts or locations as a consequence, with progression to advanced glomerular scarring. Of interest is the associated lack of the alpha 3 (IV) chain, which contains the Goodpasture antigen (see the discussion of anti-GBM disease).

Pathology. The light microscopic findings in Alport's syndrome are nonspecific and vary considerably depending on the severity of the disease. Early in the course of the disease the only glomerular lesion is the persistence of fetal glomeruli characterized by small rounded visceral epithelial cells with an immature appearance.[38] The tubules may contain red blood cells, and foam cells are often found within the interstitium (Fig. 65-11). Over time the glomeruli develop an increase in mesangial matrix material, occasionally with mild segmental increase in mesangial cellularity. Capillary walls become thickened and may have double contours. Ultimately there is focal and segmental glomerulosclerosis with capillary collapse, insudative lesions, and adherence to Bowman's capsule, as seen in the idiopathic form of focal sclerosis. Crescents occur rarely. The lesion progresses with an increased number of completely sclerotic glomeruli, ultimately leading to an end-stage kidney. The tubules and interstitium have variable degrees of atrophy and fibrosis, which worsens as the glomerular disease progresses, often with prominent interstitial foam cells. Late in the course nephrosclerosis is also observed.

Immunofluorescent findings are entirely nonspecific, with IgM and complement components in segments of sclerosis, scattered weak mesangial staining for IgM, and the same immunoglobulin in arteriolar walls. Of diagnostic significance is the lack of glomerular capillary wall staining in most cases when overlain with sera from patients with anti-GBM disease because the Goodpasture antigen is absent in Alport's syndrome.

EM is required for a diagnosis of Alport's syndrome. There is a range of abnormalities in the GBM, which may affect all or portions of variable numbers of capillary walls.[39] The basement membranes are usually thick and thin, measuring as little as 60 nm and becoming as wide as 1200 nm (normal GBM is 340 to 360 nm in adults). There is a great deal of variability in the range of basement membrane widths between cases. The thickened basement membranes have alternating electron-dense and electron-lucent irregular strata, giving a lamellated appearance (Fig. 65-12); electron-lucent areas may contain rounded 20 to 90 nm structures of variable electron density. The subepithelial aspect of capillary walls is scalloped and

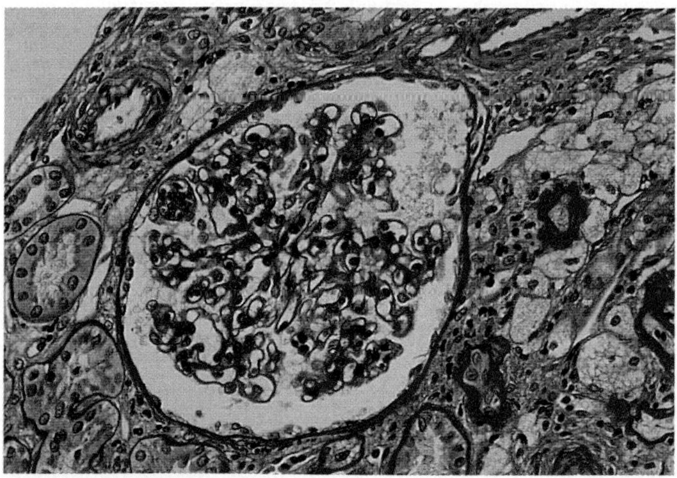

Fig. 65-11 Alport's syndrome. The glomerulus has single-contoured capillary walls and unremarkable or slightly expanded mesangial regions. There are foam cells in the interstitium, with focal tubular atrophy and interstitial fibrosis. (Periodic acid–Schiff.)

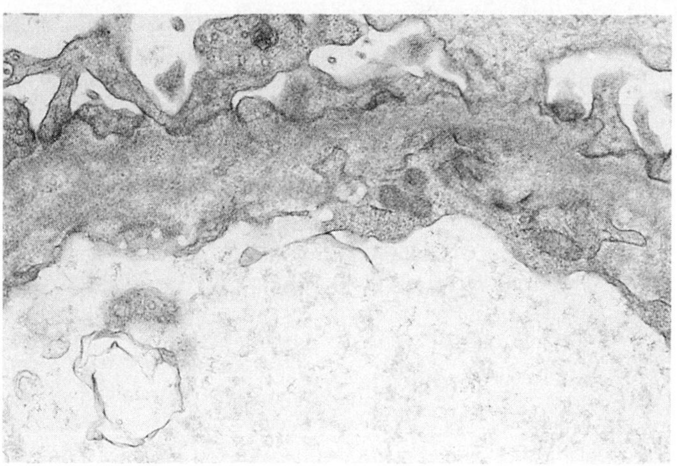

Fig. 65-12 Thickened capillary wall showing electron-dense and electron-lucent layering, subepithelial irregular surface (scalloping) and partial visceral epithelial cell foot process effacement.

irregular, with considerable effacement of visceral epithelial cell foot processes. Electron-dense immune complex deposits are not a feature of this disease. With progression there are increased mesangial matrix material and the changes of segmental glomerulosclerosis.

Differential diagnosis. A diagnosis of Alport's syndrome cannot be made by light or immunofluorescent microscopy, which may appear normal or mimic focal and segmental glomerulosclerosis. Early IgA nephropathy may appear normal by light microscopy but has characteristic immunofluorescent findings.

Ultrastructurally, advanced immune complex–mediated diseases such as IgA nephropathy may have basement membrane changes similar to those in Alport's syndrome but have the other features of the underlying disease. When Alport's syndrome contains only thin GBM without the layering and scalloping, it may be impossible to distinguish from thin basement membrane nephropathy; clinical correlation and a careful family history are required to classify the disease, and staining of the kidney with anti-GBM antiserum may prove helpful.

Clinical presentation. The disease is more severe and has an early onset in males, in whom the hallmark symptom is persistent microscopic hematuria, occasionally with episodes of gross hematuria. Heterozygous females may have intermittent hematuria. Proteinuria is related to the degree of basement membrane layering;[40] proteinuria and hypertension develop as the syndrome worsens, in association with the onset of segmental sclerosis. Chronic renal failure occurs in males as early as the third to fourth decade. Females fare much better and usually retain renal function. Other organ systems are affected by the type IV collagen abnormality in this syndrome. The most common is high-frequency hearing loss that develops in the second decade. Ocular defects, specifically anterior lenticonus, occur in 15% to 30% of individuals with Alport's syndrome.

There is no treatment for the renal disease in Alport's syndrome other than renal transplantation. Because this is a genetic abnormality of basement membranes, it cannot recur in the transplanted kidney. However, because the recipient's native kidney did not contain the Goodpasture antigen, these patients have a 5% risk of developing anti-GBM antibody glomerulonephritis in the donor graft, which contains the antigen.[41] Those at most risk have early onset chronic renal failure before 30 years of age, with the anti-GBM antibody nephritis occurring within the first posttransplantation year and often resulting in graft loss.

Thin basement membrane nephropathy

Thin basement membrane nephropathy is a renal lesion in which the only abnormality is thinning of the GBM. This is associated with hematuria or proteinuria and may or may not be a familial disorder. It is relatively common, occurring in 20% to 25% of patients with asymptomatic hematuria and 5% to 9% of the general population.[42]

This lesion may be classified according to the history, that is, whether this is a familial or sporadic abnormality.[43-45] The inherited disease has been termed *benign familial hematuria*. However, the same morphologic findings may occur in early Alport's syndrome, and it is not always possible to obtain a complete history. Therefore, all cases meeting this definition should be considered thin basement membrane nephropathy, and clinical correlation with careful follow-up study is necessary to determine the significance of the disease.

Etiology and pathogenesis. The familial form of thin basement membrane nephropathy is usually transmitted in an autosomal dominant fashion, though a few cases of apparent autosomal recessive inheritance have been reported.[43-45] The genetics of sporadic cases are not known because this entity has not been studied as completely as Alport's syndrome. The pathogenesis also is not understood. GBMs appear to contain all the normal components, though type IV collagen has been reported to occur in an abnormal location within the basement membrane.[46]

Pathology. The light microscopic appearance is usually normal, with scattered red cells in the tubular lumens. Rarely, glomeruli have mild mesangial widening without significant increased cellularity. There may be abnormalities related to other disease processes, such as ischemic change if nephrosclerosis occurs simultaneously. Immunofluorescence microscopy is negative, and overlaying of glomeruli with anti-GBM antiserum results in normal binding, in contrast to many cases of Alport's syndrome in which there is reduced or absent binding.

EM discloses thinning in some to all of the GBMs, ranging from the usual 340 to 360 nm width in adults to as thin as 60 to 80 nm (Fig. 65-13). An average width of less than 250 nm in adults and 200 nm in children is required for the diagnosis.[47,48] Thinning is primarily caused by the reduced width of the lamina densa.[49] The basement membranes have the usual medium–electron dense appearance without layering, lamellation, or subepithelial scalloping. Visceral epithelial foot processes are discrete, mesangial regions have no changes, and there are no electron-dense deposits.

Differential diagnosis. The light microscopic picture may be similar to Alport's syndrome and mild IgA nephropathy. Because these patients do not have nephrotic syndrome, minimal change disease is not in the differential diagnosis from a clinical standpoint. Immunofluorescence will identify those biopsy specimens with IgA nephropathy. EM examination is required to make the diagnosis; however, the findings may be identical to those in early Alport's syndrome. Family history, renal staining with anti-GBM anti-serum, and clinical follow-up study will aid in differentiating between these two entities, but clinical follow-up may be the only way to determine which is the real disorder.

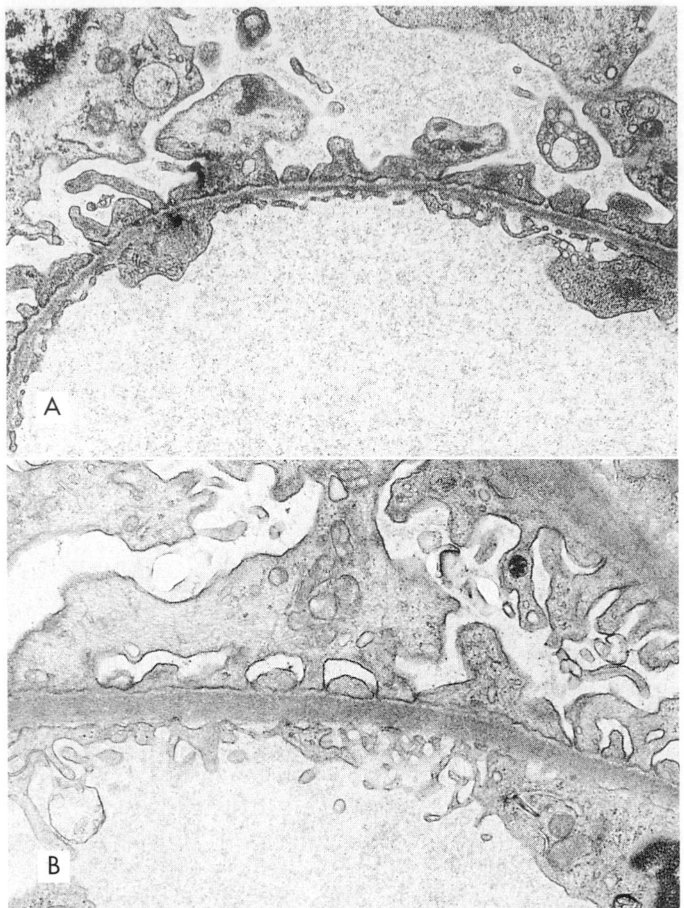

Fig. 65-13 Thin basement membrane nephropathy. **A,** The capillary wall is very thin, measuring 90 nm in width. The lamina densa has the usual homogeneous electron density, and overlying foot processes are discrete. **B,** Compare to a normal capillary wall, which is 360 nm in width.

Clinical presentation. Patients classically have persistent or intermittent microscopic hematuria, often in childhood but occasionally in adulthood. Proteinuria may be present, or, rarely, it may be the primary urinary abnormality; Alport's syndrome must be carefully sought in these patients.[42,50] The prognosis with true thin basement membrane nephropathy is excellent, with preservation of renal function. There is no therapy for this disorder.

Fabry's disease

Fabry's disease is an inherited disorder of α-galactosidase A deficiency with renal, neurologic, and cutaneous manifestations dominating. It is one of the sulfatidoses, one of many lysosomal storage diseases. It is in the same group of disorders that includes Gaucher's disease and Niemann-Pick disease.[51]

Etiology and pathogenesis. Fabry's disease is an X-linked disorder transmitted by a defective gene located on the long arm of the X-chromosome, Xq22>q24. Hemizygous males are affected predominantly; heterozygous females have variable clinical expression. The enzyme defect results in accumulation of the glycosphingolipid ceramide trihexoside in plasma and in tissues in epithelial, mesenchymal, and neural cells. The important affected organs include kidney, autonomic nervous system, skin, heart, and eyes.[51]

Pathology. In the kidney, ceramide trihexoside accumulates in epithelial cells of glomeruli (Fig. 65-14) most prominently, with lesser involvement of distal tubules and loop of Henle. In paraffin-embedded sections, the affected cells are enlarged and contain multiple uniform vacuoles.[51,52] As the disease progresses, glomeruli undergo segmental and then complete sclerosis.[53] Vacuolated cells are also in arteries and arterioles, and occasionally in the interstitium. The cellular inclusions have a distinctive ultrastructural appearance as multiple whorled or concentrically layered dense and pale "zebra bodies" or myelin figures (Fig. 65-15).

Differential diagnosis. The ultrastructural features are almost pathognomonic; similar but not as extensive inclusions have been described in glomerular visceral epithelium as a consequence of chloroquine therapy and, rarely, in patients with pulmonary silicosis. When faced with extensively involved renal tissue, the pathologist can make a very firm presumptive diagnosis with a recommendation for an α-galactosidase determination.

Clinical presentation. The renal manifestations of Fabry's disease are those of proteinuria usually begin in the third decade, with progression to end-stage renal disease with hypertension within 10 to 20 years. Males are more severely affected; female heterozygotes may be asymptomatic or have only proteinuria. No specific therapy exists; renal transplantation is effective. The cellular changes may recur in the transplanted organ, with little clinical significance.[51]

VASCULAR DISORDERS

Benign nephrosclerosis and atheromatous embolization

Nephrosclerosis is arteriosclerosis of arteries and arterioles in the kidney with associated ischemic injury of the tubules, interstitium, and glomeruli.[54] Atheromatous embolization is the lodging of embolized plaque in the renal vasculature.

Nephrosclerosis can be classified as having arterial and arteriolar components depending on the size of the affected vessels. This form of ischemic renal injury is different morphologically and pathogenetically from malignant nephrosclerosis, which is discussed separately. Atheromatous emboli can occur in any size vessel and may be fresh or remote.

Etiology and pathogenesis. Nephrosclerosis is usually intimately associated with hypertension, though blood pressure may be normal in many patients with nephrosclerosis. The mechanisms underlying nephrosclerosis encompass those involved in essential hypertension, which are discussed elsewhere. Genetic and environmental factors, aging, smooth muscle and endothelial cell responses to vasoactive factors, abnormal vascular responses, and structural changes to vessel walls may contribute to hypertension systemically and in the kidney.[55,56] There likely is much interaction among these elements of vascular damage, ultimately producing thickened vessel walls with hypertrophy or hyperplasia of medial smooth muscle cells, proliferation and migration of smooth muscle cells into the intima, and increased deposition of extracellular matrix material.[57] The smooth muscle cells may be reacting to the direct effect of wall stretch secondary to hypertension or to circulating or local mitogenic factors such as renin, angiotensin II, and endothelin. Paracrine or autocrine regulation by the smooth muscle cells may also occur through platelet-derived growth factor, TGF-β, and other cytokines. The level of hypertension correlates with deposition of extracellular matrix material, including elastin, collagens, and glycosaminoglycans. Experimental evidence indicates that these proteins may also influence maintenance of hypertension because blood pressure is reduced when collagen cross-linkage is blocked.

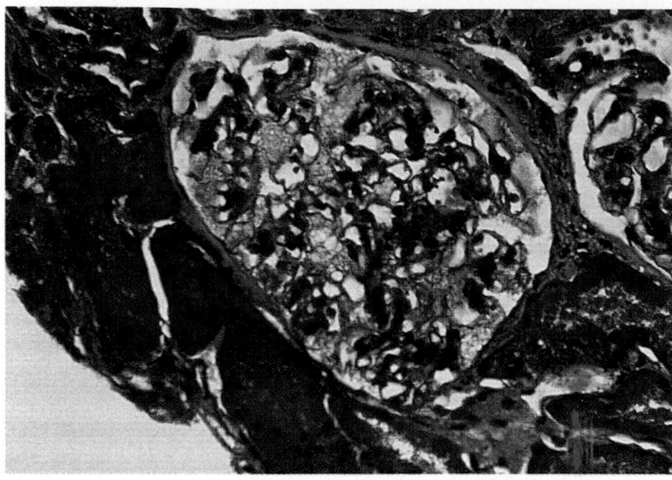

Fig. 65-14 Fabry's disease. In this glomerulus, the visceral epithelial cells are enlarged and finely vacuolated. (Masson's trichrome.)

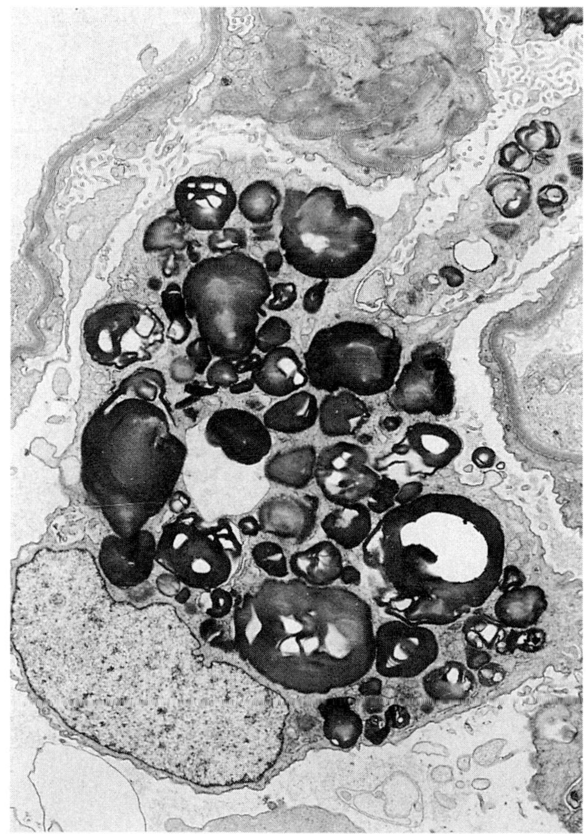

Fig. 65-15 Fabry's disease, electron microscopy. The visceral epithelial cell is filled with dense myelin figures representing stored sphingolipid.

Atheroemboli dislodge from plaques either spontaneously in patients with severe ulcerative artherosclerosis or secondary to minor trauma, surgery, or angiography.[58,59] They usually originate from the aorta or its major branches. The kidney is the most frequently affected organ with the interlobular (150 to 200µm) arteries involved to the greatest degree. After lodging in an artery or arteriole there is complement activation, leading to leukocyte recruitment and activation, with release of oxygen radicals and other lysosomal contents.[60] Endothelial damage results, further stimulating the myointimal proliferative response to embolization. Atheromatous material activates platelets in vitro, and this process may add to the vascular damage induced by complement and physical trauma.

Pathology. Kidneys from patients with nephrosclerosis are equally affected and appear small with an adherent capsule and finely granular surface (Fig. 65-16). On cut section the cortex is thin and there may be V-shaped subcapsular scars along the distribution of interlobular arteries. Arcuate arteries are prominent, and small cortical cysts (acquired cystic disease) may occur. Cortical infarcts may accompany atheromatous embolization.

Vessels of all calibers are variably involved, depending on the severity of the disease. The larger interlobar and arcuate arteries display thickened intimas with an increase in the extracellular matrix and narrowed lumens (Fig. 65-17). The internal elastic lamina is frayed and may be reduplicated. The smaller interlobular arteries have reduplication of the internal elastic lamina, smooth muscle proliferation, and variable fibrosis of the intima and may have accumulation of IgM and complement components (hyalinization) in the wall. Afferent arterioles display hypertrophy of the muscular wall, hyalinization, and, occasionally, degeneration of the basement membrane (Fig. 65-18). Efferent arterioles infrequently demonstrate these abnormalities. There is variable expansion of juxtaglomerular apparatus.[54]

The degree of renal ischemia is reflected in the tubular, interstitial, and glomerular changes.[61] There is focal tubular atrophy characterized by thickened tubular basement membranes and reduced tubular size; tubular dropout and hypertrophy of nonatrophic tubules occur focally in more severe cases. Tubular atrophy may take the form of "thyroidization," in which tubules are dilated with thinned epithelium and luminal casts. The tubular atrophy is accompanied by interstitial fibrosis with an associated mild mononuclear inflammatory infiltrate. Glomerular ischemia is characterized by thickened, wrinkled, and partially collapsed walls and an increase in mesangial matrix material, often with accumulation of collagen in Bowman's space adjacent to the arteriolar pole (Fig. 65-19). The number of completely sclerotic glomeruli may be increased.

Immunofluorescent microscopy reveals IgM and complement components in the walls of arterioles. EM reveals glomerular changes of ischemia, including thickened and

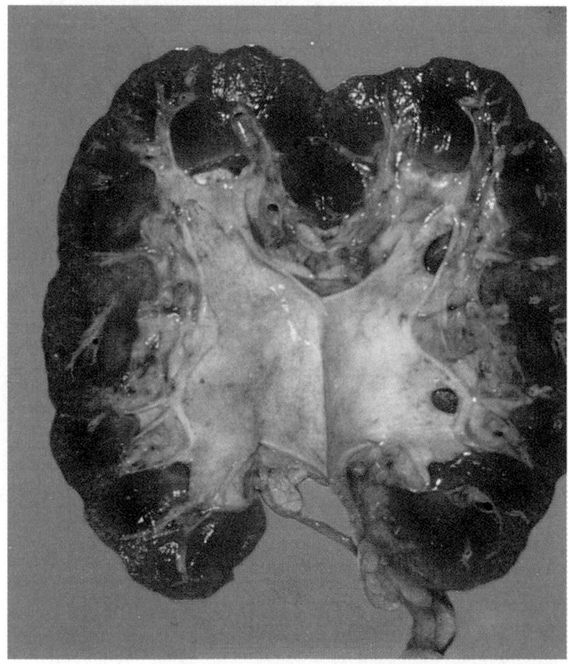

Fig. 65-16 Nephroclerosis. The cortex is irregularly thinned, with scattered, V-shaped indentations corresponding to areas of subcapsular scarring.

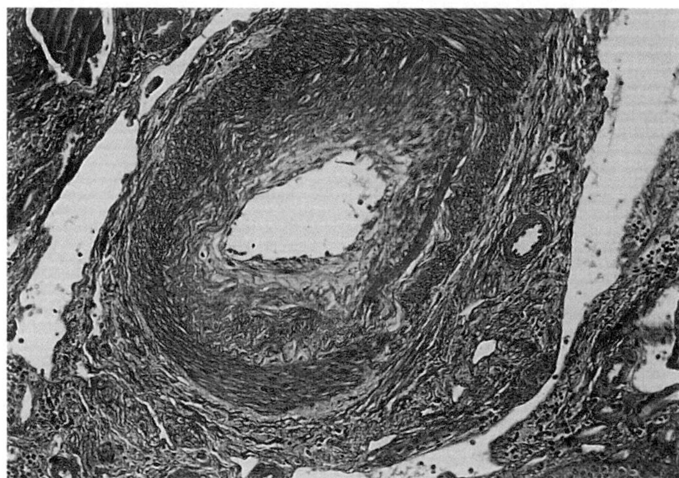

Fig. 65-17 Artery with intimal fibrosis and considerable narrowing of the lumen, with mild muscular hypertrophy. (Masson's trichrome.)

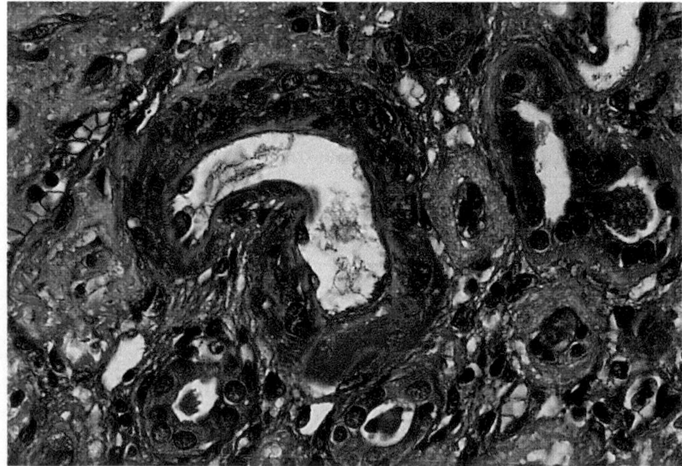

Fig. 65-18 Arteriole with muscular hypertrophy and plasma protein deposition (hyalinization) within the wall. (Masson's trichrome.)

wrinkled capillary basement membranes, partial effacement of visceral epithelial cell foot processes, subendothelial lucent zones in capillary walls, and a variable increase in mesangial matrix material.

Atheromatous emboli are superimposed on a background of significant nephrosclerosis. The emboli may be within vessels of any size and infrequently are in glomerular capillaries.[58,62,63] Any number of vessels may be involved by the emboli, which consist of acicular (needle-shaped) clear crystals (dissolved cholesterol) with or without adjacent proteinaceous material or lipid-laden macrophages (Fig. 65-20); smaller vessels often contain only the crystals. Acute lesions have fibrin and abundant plasma protein material in the lumens. As the emboli age they often become engulfed by activated macrophages with formation of foreign body giant cells, with associated fibroblast and endothelial cell proliferation and perivascular mononuclear cell infiltrates. Ultimately the emboli are incorporated in the thickened and fibrotic vascular wall. Crescents may occur when the crystals rupture glomerular capillary walls.

Differential diagnosis. The changes of nephrosclerosis are distinct and do not afford much diagnostic difficulty. This abnormality often accompanies other renal diseases and is a common finding in patients biopsied for other reasons; in this setting it is not possible to determine whether the nephrosclerosis is a primary or secondary process. Malignant hypertensive changes, including arterial and arteriolar mucoid intimal fibrosis, "onionskin" thickening of the muscularis, and fibrin deposition in vascular walls and lumens, may be superimposed on background features of nephrosclerosis. In some patients with severe hypovolemia secondary to nephrotic syndrome or other causes, there is glomerular ischemia without the attendant vascular changes. Similarly, in biopsy tissue from patients with arcuate or larger artery disease where the large artery is not sampled, glomerular and tubulointerstitial lesions are found without the accompanying vascular disease. Similarly, multiple sections and an adequate sample of arteries are often necessary for identification of athermomatous emboli.

Clinical presentation. Most patients with long-standing hypertension have some degree of renal involvement, which is initially asymptomatic. Additionally, systemic hypertension is absent in many people over 50 years of age who have nephrosclerosis. Over time, nephrosclerosis results in a gradual decline in renal function, accounting for up to 15% of all patients worldwide who develop end-stage renal disease (ESRD). Plasma renin levels are normal, and urinary findings include hyaline and granular casts and variable amounts of proteinuria infrequently reaching the nephrotic range.

Atheromatous emboli usually occur after 60 years of age in patients with severe atherosclerosis and hypertension. Symptoms include subacute and chronic renal failure, occasionally with accelerated hypertension. A history of recent vascular manipulation or radiographic procedures is often elicited.[58,59,62] If there is extensive embolization, there may be palpable purpura and other symptoms mimicking vasculitis. Five percent to 10% of patients exhibit elevated sedimentation rate, transient hypocomplementemia, or eosinophilia.[64-66] The urine analysis findings are similar to those observed in nephrosclerosis with scattered red and white blood cells. Systemic complications are referable to other involved organs.

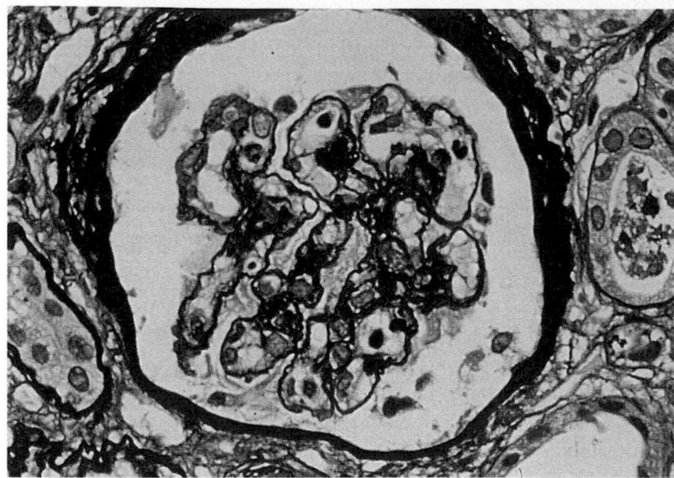

Fig. 65-19 Glomerulus demonstrating ischemic change. Capillary walls are thickened and wrinkled, with partial obliteration of lumans; mesangial regions have a mild increase in matrix material. Bowman's capsule is also thickened and wrinkled. (Periodic acid–methenamine silver.)

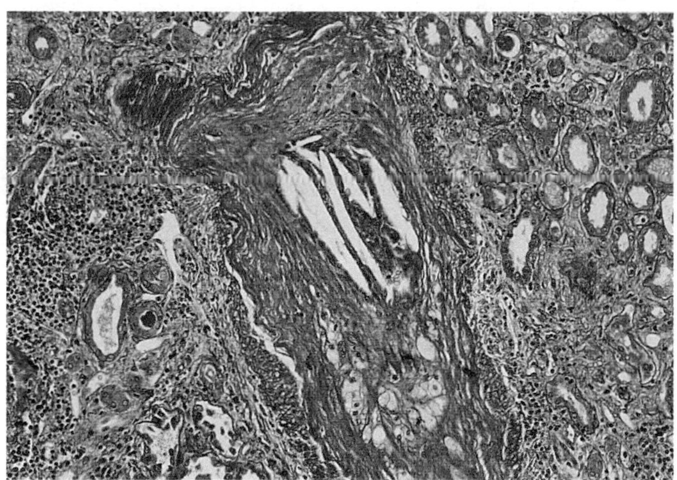

Fig. 65-20 Artery with intimal fibrosis and complete obliteration of the lumen caused by cholesterol crystals and foam cells (atheromatous embolus). Monocytes are surrounding the crystals. (Masson's trichrome.)

The kidneys in malignant hypertension, thrombotic microangiopathies, and progressive systemic sclerosis (scleroderma)

Renal structural involvement in malignant hypertension, thrombotic microangiopathies, and progressive systemic sclerosis (scleroderma) is virtually identical in all, with severe arterial, arteriolar, and glomerular damage and other acute ischemia with hemorrhage and infarction throughout the parenchyma. Furthermore, pathogenic mechanisms are very similar. Hence, they are discussed as a single entity.

Malignant hypertension, the clinical entity, is characterized by elevated diastolic blood pressure (in excess of 130 mm Hg), and the corresponding pathologic features in the kidney are known as malignant nephrosclerosis.[67] *Thrombotic microangiopathies* are a group of disorders characterized by microangiopathic hemolytic anemia, thrombocytopenia, and renal failure, though other organs may also be affected.[68] The major disorders are hemolytic uremic syndrome (HUS) and thrombotic thrombocytopenic purpura (TTP). *Scleroderma kidney* is the grouping of functional and structural renal abnormalities in patients with progressive systemic sclerosis.[69] All these entities are considered severe vascular disorders of the kidneys.

Etiology and pathogenesis. The pathogenesis of the vascular lesions in all these disorders is believed to be related to primary fibrin accumulation in the walls of the vessels. In all, luminal thrombi appear not to be the intitial event and may be a response to the endothelial damage induced by mural fibrin. The stimulus for fibrin deposits is not known and may well be different in the different disorders. In the thrombotic microangiopathies, primary endothelial injury is proposed; this may be related to mechanical injury, local immunologic reactions (anti–endothelial antibodies, immune complex deposition), direct toxic endothelial injury caused by infectious agents or drugs, or the effects of prostaglandins, especially prostacyclin. The pathogenesis of scleroderma may be related to abnormal coagulation, immune mechanisms, or other poorly defined considerations. In malignant hypertension, activation of the renin-angiotensin system, with pronounced vasoconstriction, sharp elevation of blood pressure, and consequent endothelial injury with increased vascular permeability, mural fibrin deposition and luminal thrombi, and mural necrosis have been suggested as a plausible mechanism. This may also be relevant to scleroderma kidney; however, it should be noted that the lesions of scleroderma kidney may be present in the absence of hypertension.[67-69]

Pathology. The basic lesions are in the arterial vasculature, involving interlobular arteries in scleroderma, microangiopathies and malignant hypertension, and arcurate arteries to a variable degree in thrombotic microangiopathies and malignant hypertension. Endothelial cells are swollen, and the subendothelial space is greatly widended by a combination of factors. There is accumulation of fibrin and perhaps other plasma proteins, erythrocytes (which are often deformed), concentrically arranged myointimal cells in a background of mucinous ground substance, and no changes to the underlying elastic lamina (Fig. 65-21).

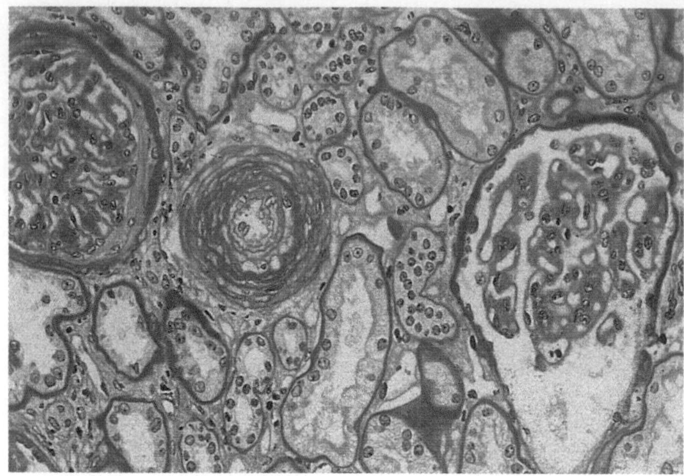

Fig. 65-21 Malignant hypertension. The interlobular artery wall is greatly thickened because of concentric intimal layering (onion skin lesion). One glomerulus displays considerable ischemia; the other has some thickened capillary walls with double contours and widened mesangial regions, features of fibrin-induced damage. (Periodic acid–Schiff.)

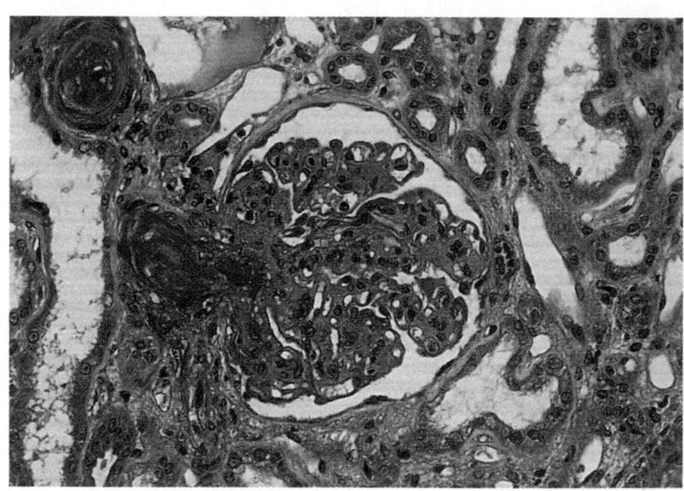

Fig. 65-22 The arteriole is thrombosed, with extension of the thrombotic lesion into the glomerulus. There is mesangial widening with mild increase in cellularity. (Masson's trichrome.)

Arterioles are consistently abnormal; the changes do not affect all arterioles simultaneously and, when present, involve the afferent vessels only. Endothelial cells are swollen, and fibrin and other plasma proteins accumulate in massive amounts between endothelium and muscularis. Although overt "fibrinoid necrosis" with luminal thrombosis (thrombonecrotic lesions) was once reasonably common in association with severe hypertension (Fig. 65-22), these abnormalities are rarely encountered currently, primarily because of effective antihypertensive therapy. Thrombosed arterioles may be aneurysmally dilated and have associated endothelial proliferation with organization of the thrombi; these infrequent lesions have the name *glomeruloid* structures because of their superficial resemblance to glomeruli. This finding is most often observed in HUS and TTP. There is enlargement of juxtaglomerular apparatus with increased granularity of juxtaglomerular cells; this is most common in malignant hypertension and scleroderma but is present in the thrombotic microangiopathies in association with hypertension.

The glomeruli are regularly abnormal, though the type and degree of involvement vary depending on severity and duration of the disease. Two types of changes are evident: those that result from fibrin deposition and those that result from ischemia. Capillary walls are thickened because of endothelial cell swelling and widening of the subendothelial space, sometimes associated with a double contour (Fig. 65-23). Capillary lumens may contain thrombi. Mesangial regions are widened, with increased cytoplasmic volume. Mesangiolysis (dissolution of matrix) is most common and prominent in the thrombotic microangiopathies; this is associated with the development of capillary microaneurysms. With healing of this process, increased mesangial matrix with subsequent sclerosis ensues, often with a lobular pattern. As a result, late stages of this process can at times be confused by light microscopy with membranoproliferative glomerulonephritis type I. With pronounced ischemia, glomerular wall collapse, alone or with the noted changes, occurs.

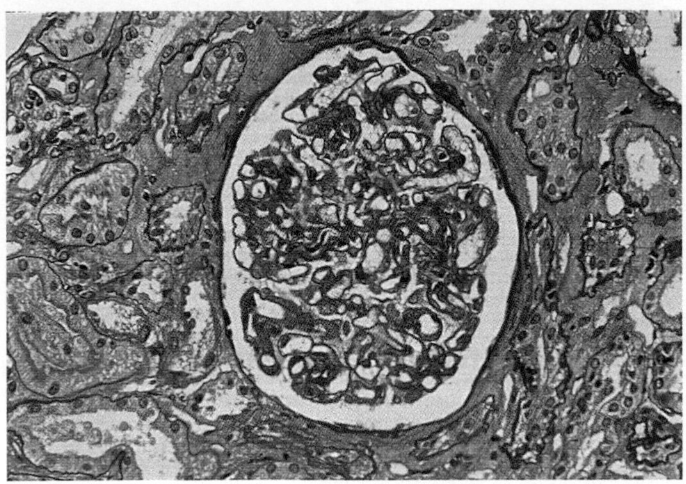

Fig. 65-23 Glomerulus with slight capillary wall wrinkling; some of the capillary walls are thickened, with double contours. Mesangial regions are minimally widened. (Periodic acid–Schiff.)

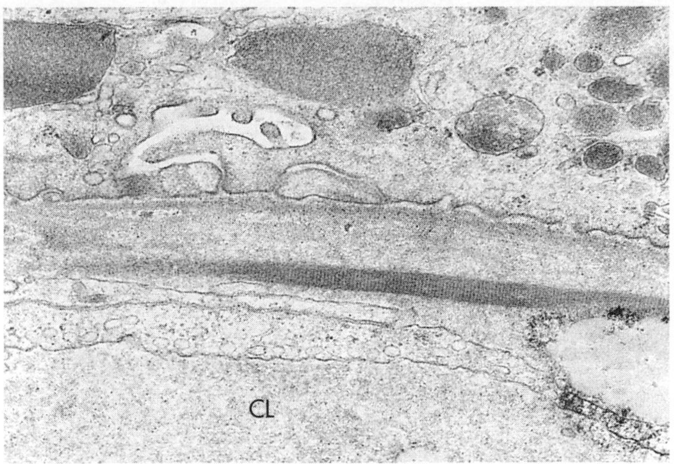

Fig. 65-24 Thrombotic microangiopathy. The subendothelial space is widened, with flocculent and lucent material and a single tactoid of fibrin. *CL*, Capillary lumen.

In all these disorders, vascular thrombi may ultimately result in infarction; when widespread, this leads to cortical necrosis.

The ultrastructural abnormalities of the arteries and arterioles are not unexpected given the light microscopic description. The glomerular lesions are better understood and documented. The subendothelial zones are greatly widened and filled with flocculent lucent material, rarely with well-defined tactoids of fibrin (Fig. 65-24). A thin subendothelial basement membrane is present; mesangial interposition may also be noted. Endothelial cells are prominently swollen.[67-72] The mesangial matrix may be permeated by flocculent lucent material as in the subendothelial spaces; this represents the early stages of mesangiolysis.[73]

Immunofluorescence in all disorders is similar. Fibrin is identified in glomerular capillary walls in a linear pattern and is in the walls of arteries and arterioles. In all these structures, fibrin corresponds to the subendothelial lucent and flocculent zones. IgM and C3 may be present in a similar pattern and distribution.[74]

Differential diagnosis. The morphologic abnormalities are so similar that the distinction of one from the other is often in the hands of the clinician. Sometimes it is not possible to be definitive because there are often overlapping clinical features.

Clinical presentation. The clinical renal manifestations of all of these disorders are similar, with different features more prominent in each. Thrombotic microangiopathies are characterized by diminished renal function with oliguria dominating, though anuria is not common. Moderate to pronounced proteinuria and hematuria are common. Hypertension is evident in approximately 50% of the patients; it may be quite severe. In scleroderma, oligoanuria, pronounced renal insufficiency, and severe hypertension are usual; rarely, the lesion may antedate the development of hypertension. The hematologic alterations (MAHA, thrombocytopenia) are not common. In malignant hypertension, decreased renal function, often with oliguria, hematuria, and proteinuria, and a microangiopathic peripheral blood with thrombocytopenia are common features.[76,77]

INFLAMMATORY DISORDERS

Immunologic glomerulopathies

Minimal change disease

Minimal change disease is a glomerular disorder characterized by mild morphologic abnormalities detected only by EM and responsible for the clinical picture of nephrotic syndrome. This disease is occasionally known by other names, including lipoid nephrosis, minimal change nephrotic syndrome, nil disease, foot process disease, and visceral epithelial cell disease; these largely reflect the types of structural abnormalities present.

Minimal change disease is one of the "primary" glomerulopathies responsible for the nephrotic syndrome[6,78] (Table 65-5). There is less than universal agreement as to the relationship of minimal change disease to focal and segmental glomerulosclerosis and to mesangial injury glomerulonephritis with IgM deposit (IgM nephropathy); some investigators consider these three lesions to be part of the same continuum of glomerular injury,[79] whereas others, including ourselves, consider each to be a separate entity.[80] If part of the same continuum, minimal change disease is on one end, with a favorable prognosis and corticosteroid responsiveness, and focal and segmental glomerulosclerosis is on the other end with a more ominous prognosis, including steroid resistance and progressive renal insufficiency often leading to ESRD.[78,79]

Etiology and pathogenesis. The cause of minimal change disease is not known, though much evidence indicates this to be an immunologically mediated disorder. Most investigators consider this disease to result from an abnormal lymphokine or other factor produced by abnormal T-cells. There is ample evidence supporting this concept,[81] though a factor or factors have not been isolated from lymphocytes or identified in the serum of affected patients. The frequent association of minimal change disease with atopy (allergen exposure) and its occurrence with lymphoreticular malignancies, including Hodgkin's disease, non-Hodgkin's lymphomas and chronic lymphocytic leukemia, and the disappearance of nephrotic syndrome with remission of the malignancy, are all suggestive of a link between T-lymphocytes and minimal change dis-

Table 65-5 "Primary" glomerulopathies responsible for nephrotic syndrome

Minimal change disease
Mesangial injury glomerulonephritis with IgM deposits
Focal and segmental glomerulosclerosis
Membranous glomerulonephritis
Membranoproliferative glomerulonephritis

ease. Other malignancies (such as mesothelioma, renal cell carcinoma) and medications including gold, nonsteroidal anti-inflammatory agents, and lithium carbonate are also associated with this glomerulopathy.[6,78]

Pathology. The description of the gross appearance of the kidneys is derived largely from reports in the precorticosteroid and preantibiotic eras, for there is little if any opportunity at present to examine grossly the kidneys of patients with uncomplicated minimal change disease. The typical features during nephrotic syndrome include mildly enlarged kidneys with pale to yellow cortices and smooth capsular surfaces.

By light microscopy, the glomeruli have a normal appearance; that is, they are not enlarged, there is no increased cellularity, and capillary walls and basement membranes are thin and single contoured (Fig. 65-25). Proximal and, occasionally, distal tubular cells contain lipid vacuoles, and proximal cells also contain protein reabsorption droplets in the form of multiple round bright globules with the tinctorial characteristics of plasma proteins. Both of these tubular cell abnormalities are not limited to minimal change disease; they are features of any glomerulopathy responsible for nephrotic syndrome. In this setting, hyperlipidemia and lipiduria are reflections of the metabolic disturbances that are integral features of the full-blown nephrotic syndrome. The cellular lipid has been identified as at least cholesterol and triglycerides; it represents filtered lipid that has been reabsorbed. Because this was the only morphologic abnormality identified in the original description of this entity by Munk in the early part of this century, it is not surprising that he thought that "lipid degeneration" of the tubules was pathogenetically important and that he termed the disorder *lipoid nephrosis*.[6,78]

Immunofluorescence microscopy typically discloses no immunoglobulin or complement deposits in glomeruli. Some reports have described IgM with or without C3 in mesangial regions in minimal change disease; the interpretation of whether the glomerulopathy is, indeed, minimal change disease with deposits or a separate entity is controversial. In addition, the prognostic significance of these deposits is also debated. (See description and the discussion of mesangial injury glomerulonephritis later in this chapter.) The protein reabsorption droplets in tubular epithelial cells stain for albumin.

EM demonstrates that the major glomerular abnormality is complete or near-complete effacement (or loss) of the foot processes of visceral epithelial cells (Fig. 65-26). There is frequent microvillous transformation of the free surfaces of these cells, thus increasing the surface area (presumably to allow for greater reabsorption of filtered protein). These epithelial cell changes are a reflection of glomerular proteinuria and as such are not specific for minimal change disease. However, these changes are the only structural lesions of a "primary" nature and are responsible for several of the terms used for this disease.[6]

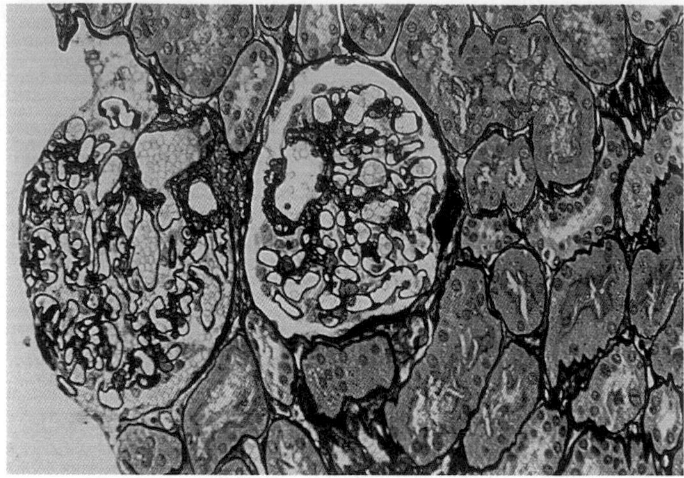

Fig. 65-25 Minimal change disease. The glomeruli are structurally normal. (Periodic acid–methenamine silver.)

Differential diagnosis. In the clinical setting of nephrotic syndrome, the structure of the glomeruli as evaluated by the three microscopic techniques is virtually pathognomonic for minimal change disease. However, perhaps the only lesions that may have this appearance are the "uninvolved" glomeruli in focal and segmental glomerulosclerosis. As described later in this chapter, glomeruli without sclerosis are enlarged,[82] which should permit distinction between these two disorders. On the other hand, should all three modalities of examination not be available, the differential diagnosis becomes a bit more broad; it should be kept in mind, however, that proper diagnosis mandates the use of all three methods. Nevertheless, if there is tissue only for light microscopy, in addition to minimal change disease, other entities to be considered include, once again, "uninvolved" glomeruli in focal and segmental glomerulosclerosis, mesangial injury glomerulonephritis with IgM deposits, and very early membranous glomerulonephritis. For the latter two, immunofluorescence easily distinguishes one from the other.[6,78]

Clinical presentation. As discussed, minimal change disease presents with the nephrotic syndrome and less commonly as heavy (nephrotic range) proteinuria without other features of the full-blown syndrome. Microscopic hematuria is infrequent. Unless otherwise complicated, renal insufficiency and hypertension are not present. In most patients, the proteinuria is steroid responsive, meaning that a course of prednisone will generally result in clearance of proteinuria, usually within a few weeks of initiation of treatment. Although relapses are not uncommon, the response to therapy is usually the same. On the other hand, untreated minimal change disease often undergoes spontaneous remissions, but it usually takes a considerably longer time than that induced by prednisone. Although the course in some patients may be of a steroid-dependent or steroid-resistant nature, it is sufficiently unusual to prompt a renal biopsy.

Mesangial injury glomerulonephritis with IgM deposits (IgM nephropathy, mesangial proliferative glomerulonephritis)

Mesangial injury glomerulonephritis is a glomerulopathy characterized by mesangial IgM deposits and responsible for

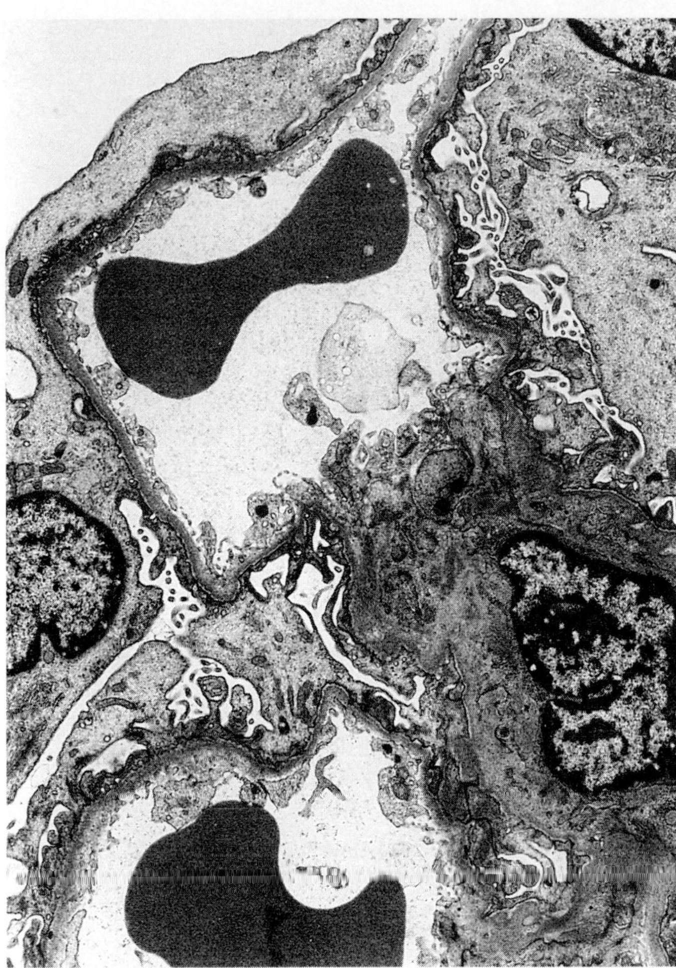

Fig. 65-26 There is complete effacement of the foot processes of visceral epithelial cells.

nephrotic syndrome.[80,83] Its classification is controversial; some investigators consider this to be a separate disease process, some consider it part of the minimal change disease spectrum, and some do not believe that such a lesion exists.[79,85]

Etiology and pathogenesis. The pathogenesis of this lesion is not known; IgM may not necessarily be part of an immune complex but may be trapped nonspecifically in an otherwise disordered mesangium.

Pathology. The glomeruli are normal to slightly abnormal, with diffuse widening and, usually, mild increase in cellularity of mesangial regions. By immunofluorescence, there is diffuse granular IgM deposition throughout all mesangial regions; this is occasionally accompanied by C3. By EM, in approximately 60% of the biopsy specimens, small, electron-dense deposits are in the mesangium; in the remainder, there are either ill-defined mesangial densities or no deposits. The foot processes of visceral epithelial cells are completely effaced.[78,80]

Differential diagnosis. When all three modalities of tissue examination are considered, there are no disorders from which this needs to be separated, if one assumes that the observer accepts this as an entity. In addition, because some "uninvolved" glomeruli in focal and segmental glomerulosclerosis may have mesangial IgM deposits, focal and segmental glomerulosclerosis need to be excluded.[85,86]

Clinical presentation. The most common manifestation is heavy proteinuria, often in the nephrotic range, sometimes with microscopic hematuria. This lesion does not regularly respond to corticosteroid therapy; most patients are steroid dependent. Follow-up study indicates that in some patients the nephrotic syndrome ultimately resolves whereas in others it persists and progressive renal insufficiency evolves. In some patients, the lesion has been found to recur in the transplant.[78,80,85,86]

Focal and segmental glomerulosclerosis

Focal and segmental glomerulosclerosis is, on the one hand, a glomerulopathy usually responsible for the nephrotic syndrome and, on the other hand, a description of morphologic glomerular abnormalities, which may occur in association with a large variety of lesions that affect the kidneys (Table 65-6). In both instances, by light microscopic evaluation of renal tissue, a portion of the glomerular population (focal) exhibits a complex abnormality with obliteration of some capillary lumens (segmental) by extracellular matrix, foam cells, or precipitates of plasma proteins ("insudative" lesion), all resulting in sclerosis. This seemingly convoluted definition and introduction will be clarified in the following.[6,78]

Focal and segmental glomerulosclerosis (as a disease) is one of the glomerulopathies responsible for the nephrotic syndrome. There is controversy as to whether it is a distinct entity or is part of the "minimal change disease spectrum." We believe that it is a specific disease and will discuss and describe it as such, and we will also explain this position.

Etiology and pathogenesis. The etiology and pathogenesis of this disorder are unknown, though evidence favors, in some instances, glomerular enlargement and increased intraglomerular capillary blood pressure as initiating factors. Note that, in segmental sclerosis as a complication to other forms of renal damage, evidence exists implicating, at least in experimental animals, intraglomerular capillary hypertension with resulting damage to visceral epithelium, endothelium, and mesangial cells. A serum factor has been recently described in humans and can be assayed.[87] Although the pathogenesis in both instances is not clear, the morphogenesis of the structural lesion in both is reasonably clear.

Pathology. In its classic appearance, focal and segmental glomerulosclerosis (the disease) has reasonably distinctive morphologic features. Microscopically, most of the glomeruli have a normal appearance, with patent capillary lumens, thin, single-contoured capillary walls, and no increase in cellularity; however, compared with age-matched controls, the glomeruli are increased in size. A portion of the population, characteristically in the deep cortex (juxtamedullary glomeruli), exhibits segmental sclerosis. The capillaries in a portion of the tuft are not patent. This may be the result of capillary wall collapse associated with increased mesangial matrix–basement membrane material or a nonimmunologic precipitate of plasma protein (IgM, C3) in lumens (Fig. 65-27). This latter abnormality is currently known as an "insudative" lesion and is also called "hyalinosis."[6,7,78] The precipitate stains brightly and often contains small or large vacuoles representing dissolved lipid (Fig. 65-28). The sclerotic segment is usually adherent to Bowman's capsule.

Although the above description is adequate for the fully developed lesion, it does not consider its development. Many investigators believe that the initial structural damage is to

Table 65-6 Focal and segmental glomerulosclerosis

"Primary"
Part of minimal change disease spectrum
Unique disease
Secondary
Heroin-associated nephropathy
HIV-associated nephropathy
Complicating other renal disorders
Reflux nephropathy and other sclerotic interstitial disorders
Glomerulonephritis (many types)
Nephrosclerosis
Familial-metabolic diseases
Chronic transplant rejection
Variants
Collapsing glomerulopathy
Tip lesion

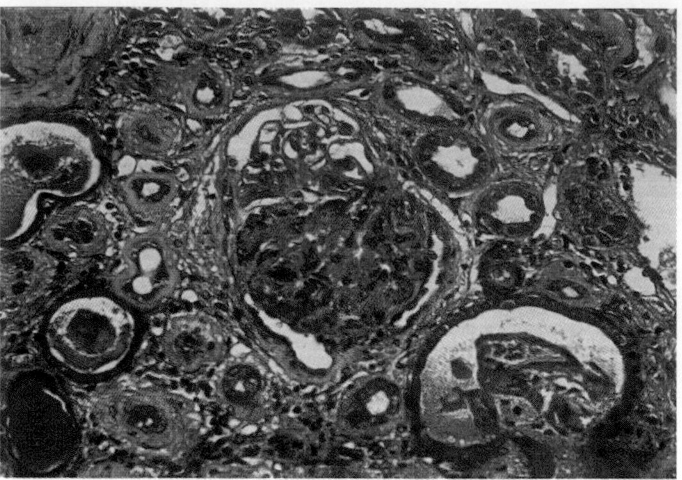

Fig. 65-27 Focal and segmental glomerulosclerosis. Glomerulus with extensive segmental sclerosis; many of the capillaries are obliterated by large insudative lesions. (Masson's trichrome.)

visceral epithelial cells;[6,88] initially, in the affected segment, these cells increase in size and number and develop coarse cytoplasmic vacuoles or blebs. Monocytes, most commonly with abundant cytoplasmic lipid (foam cells), accumulate in corresponding capillary lumens.[89] As the lesion progresses, endothelial cells and monocytes undergo degeneration, but at the same time precipitates of plasma protein form in these capillaries. The foam cells degenerate and liberate lipid, which becomes incorporated into the insudative lesion. The walls of some empty capillaries with overlying abnormal visceral epithelial cells become wrinkled and collapse; the epithelial cell cytoplasm is usually separated from the original basement membrane by a pale "halo" (Fig. 65-28). The various stages may be present in several glomeruli simultaneously, and both early and late stages may be evident in the same glomerulus.[6,78]

Typically, the tubules and interstitium are abnormal and likely represent lesions intrinsic to the glomerulopathy. In the early stages of the glomerular lesion, there may be tubular cell degeneration or necrosis, sometimes associated with interstitial edema. In the more advanced stages of the glomerulopathy, there is focal tubular atrophy with interstitial fibrosis. If hypertension is part of the clinical picture, as is often the case, concomitant arterial and arteriolar changes of nephrosclerosis will be present.[6,78]

Certain variations of focal and segmental glomerulosclerosis require further consideration. These include collapsing glomerulopathy and glomerular tip lesion. Each represents anatomic variations and clinical subgroups, which may have peculiar clinical courses and responses to therapy.

Collapsing glomerulopathy is an "entity" in which there are pronounced alterations of visceral epithelial cells (enlargement, increase in number, coarse cytoplasmic vacuolization, numerous protein reabsorption droplets) affecting virtually all cells of a single glomerulus, as well as affecting most glomeruli; this is associated with varying degrees of capillary wall wrinkling and collapse with ultimate luminal narrowing or obliteration.[90,91] Because these changes, at least qualitatively, are often similar to the early lesions of focal and segmental glomerulosclerosis, some investigators consider collapsing glomerulopathy to be a "virulent" form of

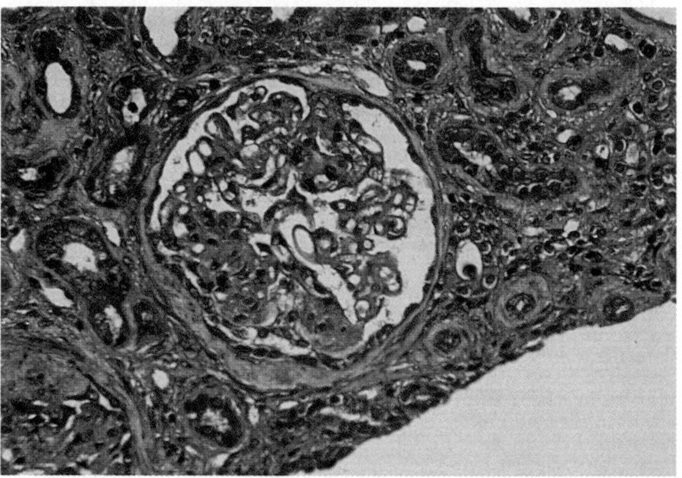

Fig. 65-28 In the sclerotic segments, the visceral epithelial cell cytoplasm is separated from the original basement membranes by a large, relatively clear zone, also known as a halo. (Masson's trichrome.)

focal and segmental glomerulosclerosis with the lesions all "shifted to the left." There are widespread tubulointerstitial changes with extensive tubular cell degeneration and necrosis and diffuse interstitial edema. Indeed, one form of this lesion occurs in patients infected with human immunodeficiency virus (HIV); the renal disease is known as HIV-associated nephropathy. In addition to the glomerular collapse and segmental sclerosis (Fig. 65-29), there are dramatic tubular changes. There is microcystic dilatation, with precipitates of plasma proteins in the lumens of many tubules (Fig. 65-30). Unlike other forms of focal and segmental glomerulosclerosis, there are numerous tubuloreticular structures in the cytoplasm of endothelial and other cells (Fig. 65-31), features indicative of HIV infection. As with other forms of segmental glomerulosclerosis, this lesion is more common in black patients.[91-93]

The *glomerular tip lesion* is so termed because the segment of sclerosis in all affected glomeruli is at the tubular pole (or

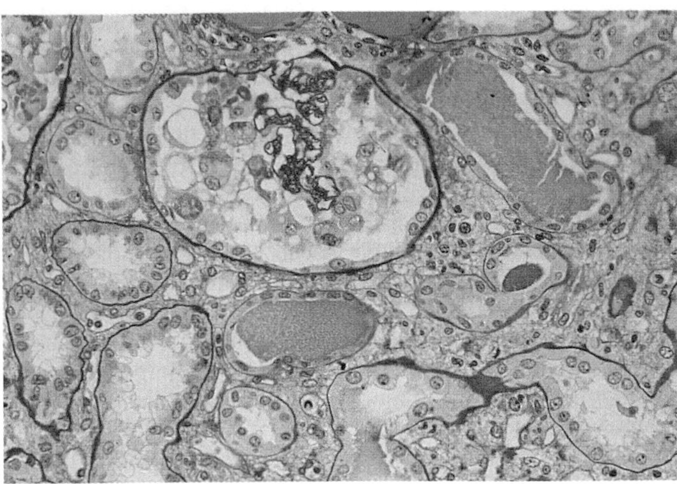

Fig. 65-29 HIV-associated nephropathy. The glomerular capillary walls are collapsing, and visceral epithelial cells are hyperplastic, hypertrophied, and vacuolated and contain protein droplets. Notice the loss of brush border staining for proximal tubular cells and the interstitial edema with mild infiltrate of mononuclear leukocytes. (Periodic acid–Schiff.)

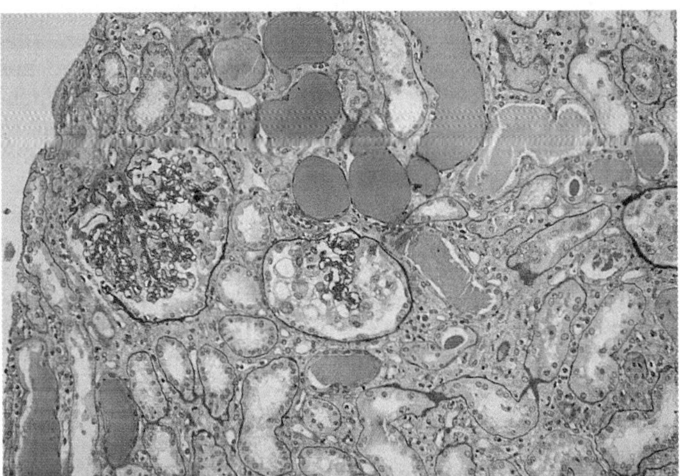

Fig. 65-30 Tubules are moderately dilated and contain a precipitate of plasma protein. The interstitium is edematous. The glomerular changes are well illustrated. (Periodic acid–Schiff.)

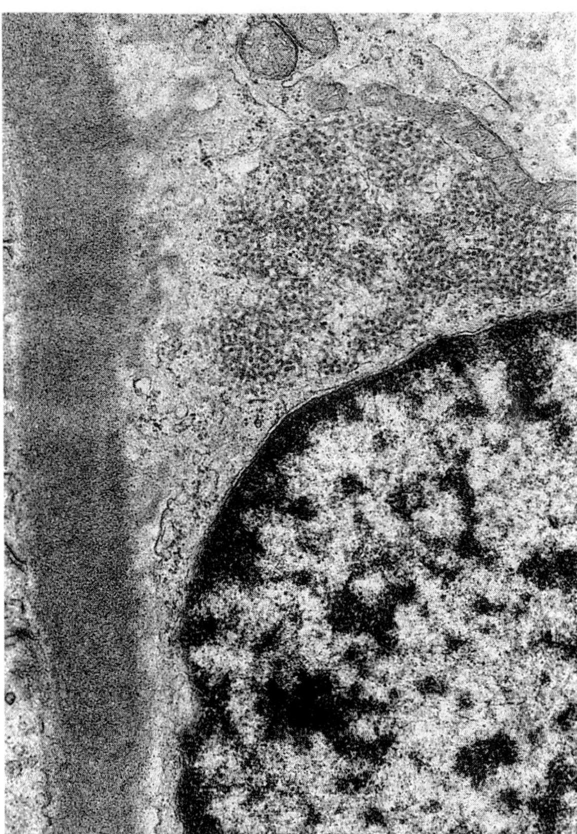

Fig. 65-31 Portion of glomerular endothelial cell with large tubuloreticular structure.

tip of the capillary tuft). Typically, the abnormal segment is in a relatively early stage of evolution, with slight increase in and other changes of visceral epithelium, and with foam cells alone or coexisting with small insudative lesions.[94] There is some debate as to whether this is a specific clinicopathologic entity or it is merely segmental sclerosis in an early to middle stage of evolution at the tubular pole.

Differential diagnosis. Because the pathologic evaluation of glomerular lesions requires immunofluorescence and EM examination, it is possible to exclude with certainty other lesions in which segmental glomerulosclerosis is a complicating factor. This task is easily accomplished if the following information is kept in mind: glomeruli without segmental sclerosis determine the diagnosis or nature of the disease process. Therefore, those glomeruli must be carefully evaluated. Evidence of immune-mediated diseases such as IgA nephropathy will, by definition, be found by immunofluorescence in the glomeruli without segmental sclerosis. Likewise, the characteristic GBM changes of Alport's syndrome will be found by EM. Similarly, segmental sclerosis occurring in a setting of reflux nephropathy–chronic interstitial nephritis immediately indicates the glomerular lesion to be a complication (or even an integral feature) of an advanced chronic tubulointerstitial process.[95] Thus, this is not the *disease* focal and segmental glomerulosclerosis but the lesion of segmental glomerulosclerosis.

Clinical presentation. The disease focal and segmental glomerulosclerosis most commonly presents with heavy proteinuria with or without the other features of the nephrotic syndrome; this is associated with some degree of renal insufficiency and hypertension. The disease and proteinuria are typically not responsive to corticosteroid therapy, and both may progress unabated to advanced renal failure over the course of many years; there are some instances in which ESRD may be reached in as little as 2 or 3 years from onset. Patients with this more rapid course are at risk for the development of recurrence of both morphologic and clinical manifestations in the transplanted kidney.[6]

Membranoproliferative glomerulonephritis

Membranoproliferative glomerulonephritis (MPGN) is a renal lesion with three distinct types, which may represent different disease entities and are grouped under the same heading for historical reasons; they require classification before they can be defined.[96,97] MPGN type I is an immune complex–mediated disease process with a specific morphologic pattern of injury

deposits may be found in mesangial and singly in subepithelial locations. In more advanced disease there is considerable capillary wall collapse, but the electron-dense character of the infiltrating material can still be identified. There is infrequent peripheral mesangial migration and interposition of capillary walls. Visceral epithelial cell foot processes are diffusely effaced.

MPGN type III encompasses variants of the other types of MPGN. Burkholder and colleagues[97] described a lesion having the basic features of MPGN type I with subepithelial deposits often with intervening projections of basement membrane material similar to membranous glomerulonephritis. The immunofluorescent features are those of MPGN with predominance of C3 staining. Others have independently reported glomerular changes of MPGN type I with layering of silver-negative material in the capillary basement membrane ultrastructurally and occasional clusters of subepithelial deposits.[106,112] The relationship of these uncommon lesions to MPGN types I and II is not known.

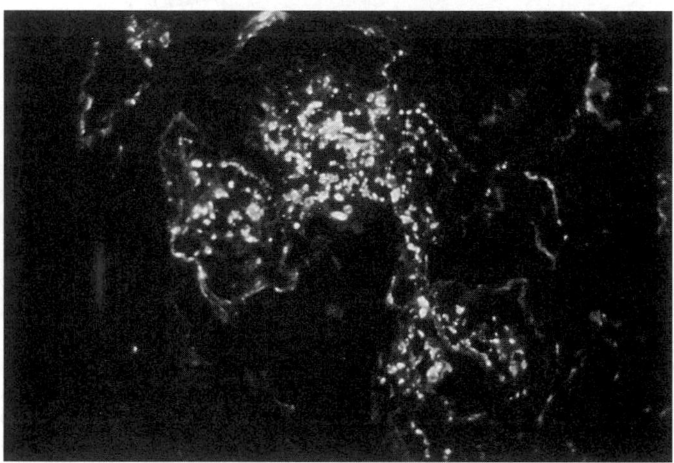

Fig. 65-36 Glomerulus showing coarse granular staining of mesangial regions, segmental capillary wall, and tubular basement membranes for C3.

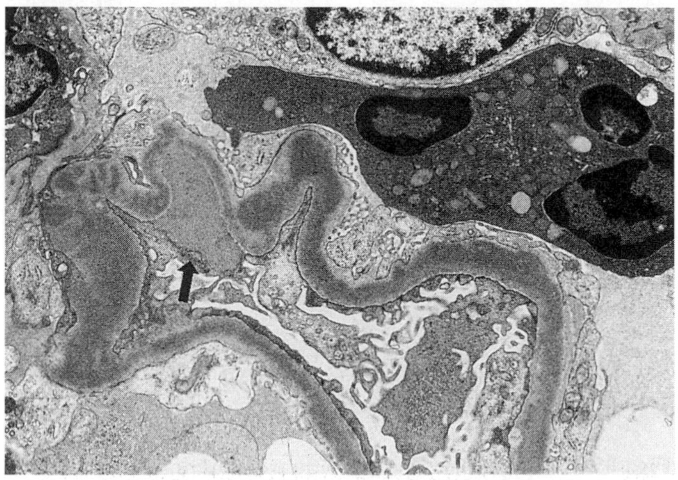

Fig. 65-37 Glomerular capillary walls with segmental replacement of the lamina densa by electron-dense, finely granular material. Notice the resorbing subepithelial hump-shaped deposit *(arrow)*.

Differential diagnosis. The light microscopic differential diagnosis of MPGN type I includes the other lobular glomerular lesions: diabetic nephropathy, light chain deposit disease, and amyloidosis. Lupus glomerulonephritis, cryoglobulins, fibrillary glomerulonephritis, and Henoch-Schönlein purpura, among others, may also have an MPGN type I pattern. Immunofluorescence and EM readily differentiate among these disease entities. It is more difficult to distinguish primary from secondary MPGN type I; clinical correlation is absolutely essential and testing for hepatitis C virus should be performed. It is not usually difficult to recognize MPGN type II, particularly ultrastructurally. MPGN type III is uncommon and must be differentiated from the previously noted diseases and from secondary forms of membranous glomerulonephritis; the predominant C3 on immunoflourescence allows this distinction to be made.

Clinical presentation. All types of primary MPGN occur in children and young adults. Type I most often presents with nephrotic syndrome and variable hematuria, frequently after a viral illness with hypocomplementemia.[96,107,108] Type II is less common; it constitutes 15% to 30% of all patients with MPGN and virtually never occurs after 30 years of age. This type more often presents with hematuria, acute nephritis, profound hypocomplementemia, and C3 nephritic factor; it is also associated with partial lipodystrophy.[113] These patients have a more rapid downhill course, can have hematuria or heavy proteinuria, and have a rate of progression similar to type I. Poor prognostic indicators include nephrotic syndrome, hypertension, renal insufficiency, and crescents on biopsy material. There is no effective treatment, and spontaneous remissions occur but are infrequent. All forms of MPGN tend to recur in renal allografts with the recurrence rate for type II approaching 100%.[114]

Membranous glomerulonephritis

Membranous glomerulonephritis is an immune complex–mediated form of glomerular injury associated with heavy proteinuria and the nephrotic syndrome. It is characterized by subepithelial immune deposits in the glomerular capillary walls, often with projections of basement membrane material adjacent to the deposits.

Membranous glomerulonephritis may be classified as a primary renal disease or as a secondary process in a variety of settings. The primary form occurs without relation to underlying diseases, use of drugs, or infections. Secondary forms are observed in association with illnesses such as SLE and carcinoma, with drugs such as gold and penicillamine, and with infections such as hepatitis[115] (Table 65-8). It is important to determine whether membranous glomerulonephritis is occurring as a primary or secondary lesion because this affects the therapy and prognosis of the disease.

Etiology and pathogenesis. Membranous glomerulonephritis is a disease in which immune complexes localize to the subepithelial region of the glomerular capillary walls.[116] There are two possible mechanisms for this distribution of antigen-antibody complexes. The most likely is immune complex formation in situ, with circulating antibodies binding to an intrinsic glomerular or an extrinsic "planted" antigen in the capillary walls.[117] Less likely, circulating immune complexes may deposit in the capillary walls.

In situ immune complex formation occurs in Heyman nephritis, an experimental form of membranous glomerulonephritis in which the antibody is directed against an intrinsic glomerular antigen (gp 330).[118,119] This antigen is similar to a proximal tubular antigen (Fx1A); however, few patients with membranous glomerulonephritis have antibodies against tubular antigens.[119,120] Other, unknown, intrinsic capillary wall antigens may be involved. Circulating antigens may localize to the subepithelial aspect of the capillary wall ("planted antigens").[121] Antigen charge and size are important factors in this process with direct binding of antigen to the capillary wall, autoimmune mechanisms, or biochemical factors also potentially involved.[122,123] Experimental membranous glomerulonephritis can be induced with cationic bovine serum albumin and ferritin, which "plant" in capillary walls, causing subepithelial immune deposition and proteinuria.[122]

The antigens responsible for primary membranous glomerulonephritis are not known. In some secondary forms of the disease, however, the antigen has been identified. Hepatitis e and less commonly B surface antigens and antibodies have been identified in the immune deposits in patients with hepatitis, and some patients with thyroiditis have thyroid antigens in the immune complexes.[124-126] Autoantibodies are found in those with SLE. Membranous glomerulonephritis associated with tumors may be related to unidentified tumor antigens.

Pathology. There are few opportunities to examine kidneys grossly from patients with membranous glomerulonephritis without other complicating lesions. Autopsy material has demonstrated large white kidneys with expanded renal cortices and smooth surface.

The light microscopic findings in membranous glomerulonephritis vary with the progression of the disease.[116] The very early lesion may have normal-appearing glomeruli. With progression, the capillary walls become thickened with patent capillary lumens, occasionally with a rounded appearance. Fuchsinophilic deposits are observed on the subepithelial aspect of capillary walls with the Masson's trichrome stain. Methenamine silver stain reveals subepithelial projections ("spikes") in subepithelial locations; these correspond to the deposition of new basement membrane material adjacent to the deposits (Fig. 65-38). The spikes and deposits may appear as small holes in tangentially sectioned capillary walls. In advanced disease, the deposits are completely surrounded by basement membrane material and are incorporated into the capillary walls; capillary walls may also have double contours. Crescents are rarely present; however, late stages of the disease may be associated with formation of anti-GBM antibodies and crescent formation.[127] Primary membranous has mesangial regions of the usual width and cellularity without deposits. Secondary forms have varying degrees of mesangial expansion, hypercellularity, and deposits, occasionally with crescents.[128]

Immunofluorescence microscopy discloses granular glomerular capillary wall staining for IgG, usually with C3 and light chains in primary membranous (Fig. 65-39). Secondary forms may have strong staining for other immunoglobulins in addition to IgG, and C1q is found in patients with SLE-associated membranous glomerulonephritis.

EM features have been used to subclassify membranous glomerulonephritis into four stages[116,129] (Fig. 65-40). Stage I is early disease with normal light microscopy. Ultrastructurally, there are small to medium subepithelial electron-dense deposits in the capillary walls, varying in number from few to many. All stages have extensive effacement of the overlying

Table 65-8 Common associations with secondary membranous glomerulonephritis

Infections
Hepatitis B
Syphilis
Autoimmune diseases
Systemic lupus erythematosus
Rheumatoid arthritis
Sjögren's syndrome
Thyroiditis
Drugs
Gold
Penicillamine
Mercury
Captopril
Malignancies
Diabetes mellitus
Renal transplantation

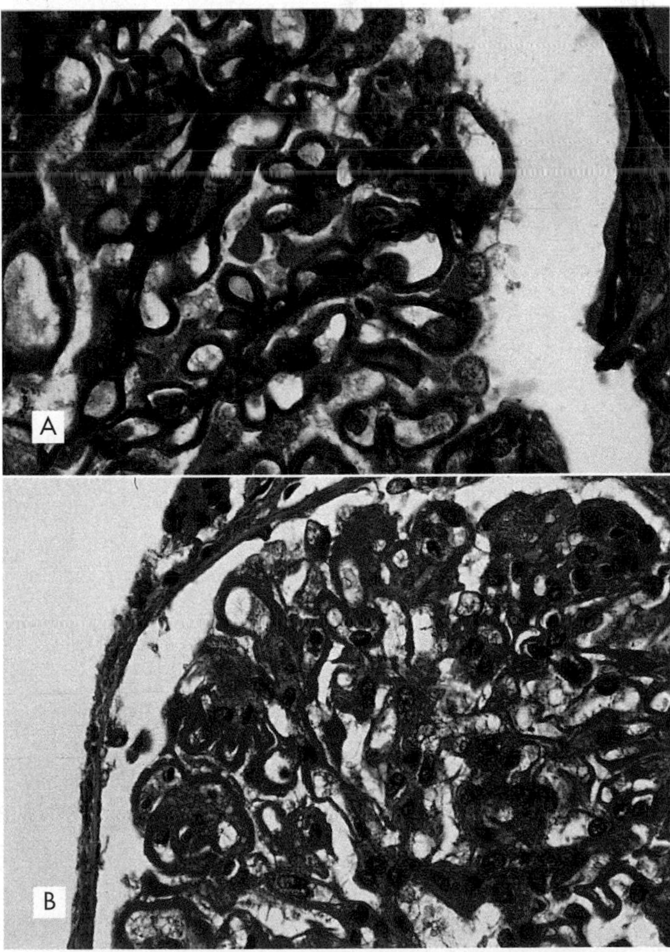

Fig. 65-38 Membranous glomerulonephritis. **A,** Glomerulus with projections ("spikes") of basement membrane material adjacent to deposits along the outer subepithelial aspect of capillary walls. Mesangial regions have no abnormalities. (Periodic acid–methenamine silver. **B,** Glomerulus with prominent subepithelial fuchsinophilic deposits along capillary walls. (Masson's trichrome.)

visceral epithelial cell foot processes. Stage II encompasses larger and more numerous deposits, with new basement membrane material laid down by visceral epithelial cells adjacent to the deposits (spikes). Stage III is characterized by incorporation of deposits into the capillary wall (intramembranous deposits) caused by completely surrounding new basement membrane material. In stage IV there are lucent areas in the deposits and thickened capillary walls, where resorption of deposits has occurred. The capillary walls are thickened, with layering of the basement membrane. Mesangial deposits are not found in the primary membranous form but are common in the secondary forms; tubuloreticular structures are within endothelial cell cytoplasm in SLE with membranous glomerulonephritis. Active disease is associated with homogeneous electron-dense deposits, and lucencies and fading of deposits are observed with resorption of deposits.[130] There are other changes associated with proteinuria, including microvillous transformation of visceral epithelial cell cytoplasm and cytofolds in endothelial cells.

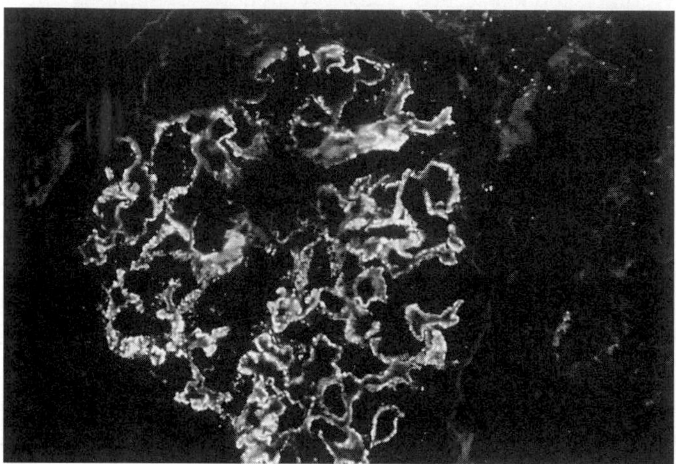

Fig. 65-39 Glomerulus showing diffuse granular capillary wall IgG.

Differential diagnosis. By light microscopy, early membranous glomerulonephritis may have normal morphology; thus in a nephrotic patient the differential diagnosis includes minimal change disease, IgM nephropathy or the uninvolved glomeruli in focal and segmental glomerulosclerosis. Immunofluorescence microscopy will readily distinguish these diseases from membranous, as will the EM features.

Clinical presentation. Nephrotic syndrome is the presenting manifestation, and membranous glomerulonephritis accounts for 20% of cases of adult onset nephrotic syndrome. Infrequently, it presents with asymptomatic proteinuria, and microscopic hematuria is found in a minority of patients. Males are more often affected, and most patients are over 30 years of age.[131] In secondary membranous glomerulonephritis, the age, sex, and systemic findings are related to the underlying disorder; lupus patients are often female and younger,

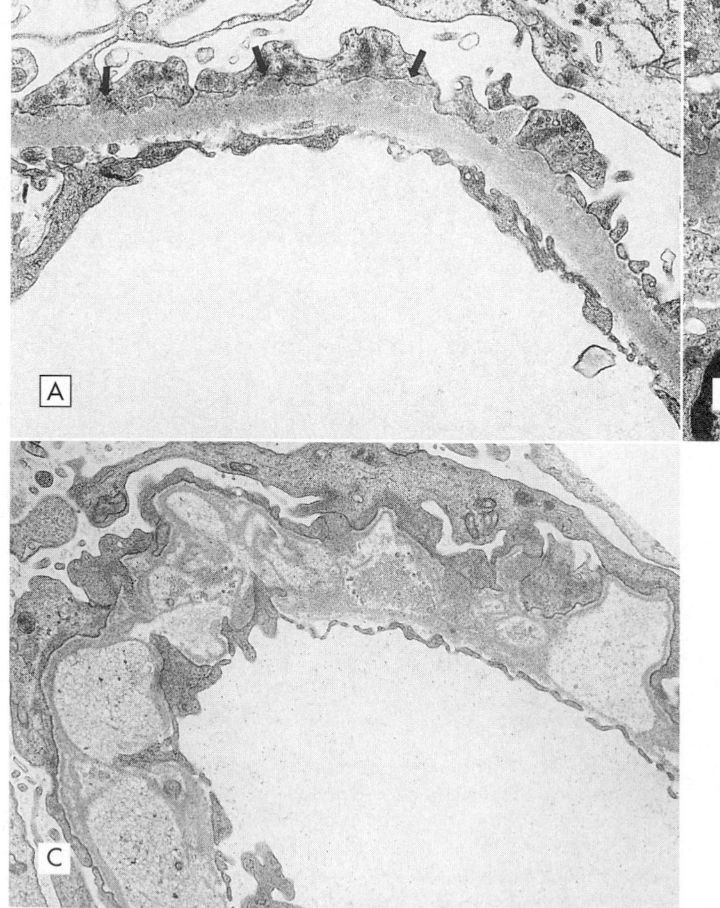

Fig. 65-40 Membranous glomerulonephritis **A,** Early (stage I) disease with small subepithelial electron-dense deposits *(arrows)* and effacement of visceral epithelial cell foot processes. **B,** Middle (stage II) lesion showing larger, more numerous deposits with intervening projections of new basement membrane material forming "spikes" *(arrows)*. The original basement membrane appears thinned, and foot processes are effaced **C,** Advanced (stage III to IV) membranous. Many deposits are completely covered by new basement membrane and have been partially resorbed, resulting in the irregular electron-lucent and electron-dense appearance. The capillary wall is thickened by intramembranous deposits.

those with associated malignancies tend to be older,[132] and those with underlying infections may have symptoms of the infectious disease. The course of the untreated primary disease is variable, with up to 50% having some degree of spontaneous remission. One quarter will have persistent nephrotic syndrome, and the rest will progress to renal failure; there is no satisfactory treatment, though various regimens using steroids and immunosuppressive agents have been used.[133,134] The secondary form may remit if the underlying disease is treated; therefore it is important to distinguish between the primary and secondary forms.

IgA nephropathy

IgA nephropathy (Berger's disease) is an immune complex–mediated glomerulonephritis with IgA as the sole or dominant antibody in the complexes, which localize preferentially in the mesangium. Although a similar immunopathologic picture may occur in association with hepatic or interstitial diseases and as part of the systemic disorder, Henoch-Schönlein purpura, IgA nephropathy is an idiopathic process.

IgA nephropathy is a "primary" glomerulonephritis and typically presents with the nephrologic syndrome of "asymptomatic hematuria or proteinuria," though during its course, many other renal manifestations may be evident. This disorder is the most common primary glomerulopathy in the world, with an exceptionally high incidence in Asia and Mediterranean countries.[135-137]

Etiology and pathogenesis. Many factors are believed to contribute to the development of IgA nephropathy. Among the more important are deposition of circulating IgA-containing immune complexes or macromolecular IgA, an intrinsic abnormality of IgA, altered regulation of the immune response (which is likely genetically determined), or immunologic reaction to a planted or intrinsic mesangial antigen. Although each of these is a distinctive mechanism, they may not be mutually exclusive and may contribute to this disorder's pathogenesis. Many but not all patients with IgA nephropathy will have elevated levels of serum IgA and IgA-fibronectin complexes.[135-139]

Pathology. The definition of this disorder and its diagnosis rest on immunofluorescence; there are mesangial deposits of IgA (Fig. 65-41) often with C3, and sometimes with IgG or IgM in lesser degrees of intensity. Granular deposits of IgA in some capillary walls are present in a small number of glomeruli. Mesangial deposits are associated with a variable light microscopic appearance of glomeruli. Most commonly, mesangial regions are widened, reflecting the presence of the deposits (Fig. 65-42); the deposits may be clearly identified with Masson's trichrome stain. There is usually increased mesangial cellularity, which ranges from mild to severe and which may affect different glomeruli and different lobules in each glomerulus to varying degrees resulting in a picture of a "focal and segmental proliferative" glomerulonephritis (Fig. 65-43). This picture may be complicated by crescents and by segments of sclerosis or capsular adhesions; segmental sclerosis usually reflects advanced disease and is associated with heavy proteinuria. Crescents may be observed during an episode of gross hematuria.[140] Most commonly, capillary walls are thin and single contoured, though double contours occasionally occur in a few capillaries of a small percentage of glomeruli.

Tubules are usually unremarkable; however, acute tubular necrosis has been noted in some patients with gross hematuria and acute renal failure. It is believed that release of large amounts of hemoglobin from intratubular lysed erythrocytes is directly tubulotoxic. In advanced IgA nephropathy, tubular atrophy and interstitial fibrosis are evident. Arteriolar walls are thickened, with plasma protein insudates ("hyalinization"), a feature correlated with hypertension and development of chronic renal insufficiency.[141,142]

By EM there are large, rounded, electron-dense deposits in paramesangial regions bordered by paramesangial basement membrane (Fig. 65-44). Capillary wall deposits in subendothelial or subepithelial sites are present in some glomeruli and are usually associated with basement membrane changes with thinning, decreased staining intensity, multiple layers, and disruptions. The capillary wall changes are likely the anatomic defect responsible for glomerular hematuria.[143] Depending upon the degree of proteinuria, there may be effacement of the foot processes of visceral epithelial cells.[135,136]

Differential diagnosis. The pathologic features, when considered as a whole, are indicative of an immune complex–

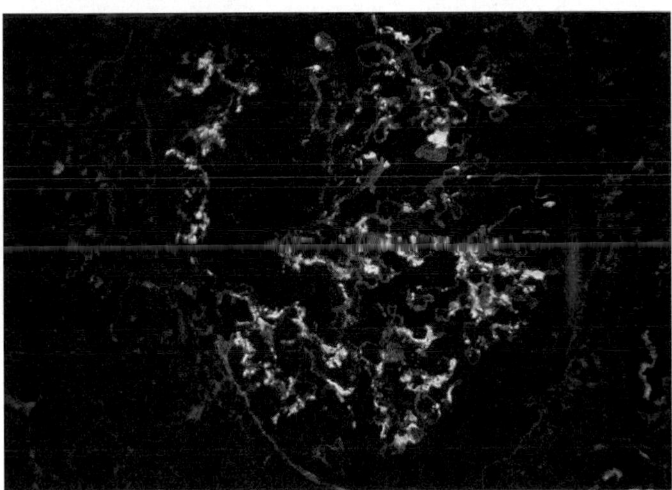

Fig. 65-41 IgA nephropathy. Diffuse granular mesangial deposits of IgA are present.

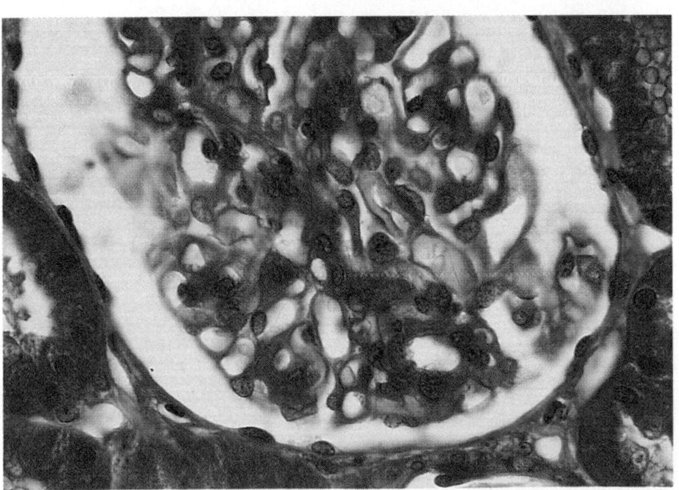

Fig. 65-42 IgA nephropathy. This glomerulus without mesangial hypercellularity contains large, rounded, fuchsinophilic paramesangial deposits in many lobules. (Masson's trichrome.)

mediated glomerulonephritis with dominant IgA deposits. There are several disorders with these findings; they include Henoch-Schönlein purpura nephritis, IgA nephropathy, and glomerular involvement in certain hepatic, intestinal, or cutaneous disorders. The most reliable manner to distinguish one from the other concerns a careful clinical history and evaluation of physical and laboratory features. From the viewpoint of the renal biopsy, some clues allow categorization of the glomerulopathy. Large rounded mesangial deposits as determined by light microscopy or EM are much more common in and clearly favor a diagnosis of IgA nephropathy (Berger's disease). Smaller and more numerous mesangial deposits by EM, more capillary wall deposits, and the presence of fibrin in mesangial deposits by immunofluorescence favors Henoch-Schölein purpura. Few and small deposits, very mild light microscopic glomerular abnormalities, and extracellular lipid accumulations in the mesangium point to hepatic disease. Although lupus glomerulonephritis may be characterized by IgA-containing deposits, IgA is not dominant and C1q is present; C1q is absent in IgA nephropathy and Henoch-Schölein purpura.

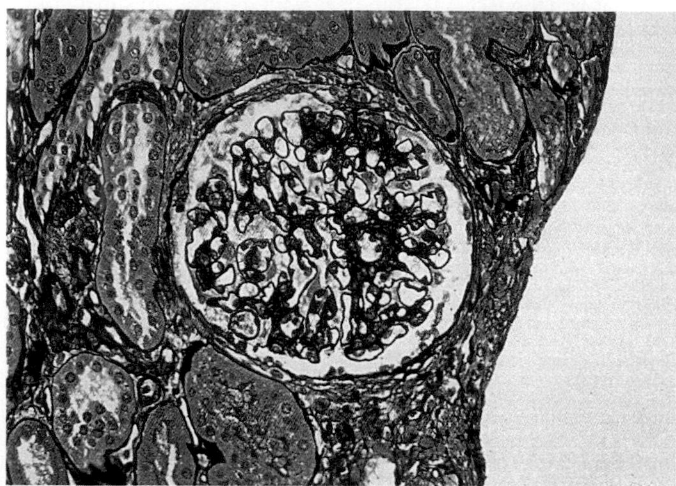

Fig. 65-43 IgA nephropathy. Glomerulus with mesangial widening and mild segmental increase in cellularity. A capsular adhesion along with a small segment of sclerosis is at 12 o'clock. (Periodic acid–methenamine silver.)

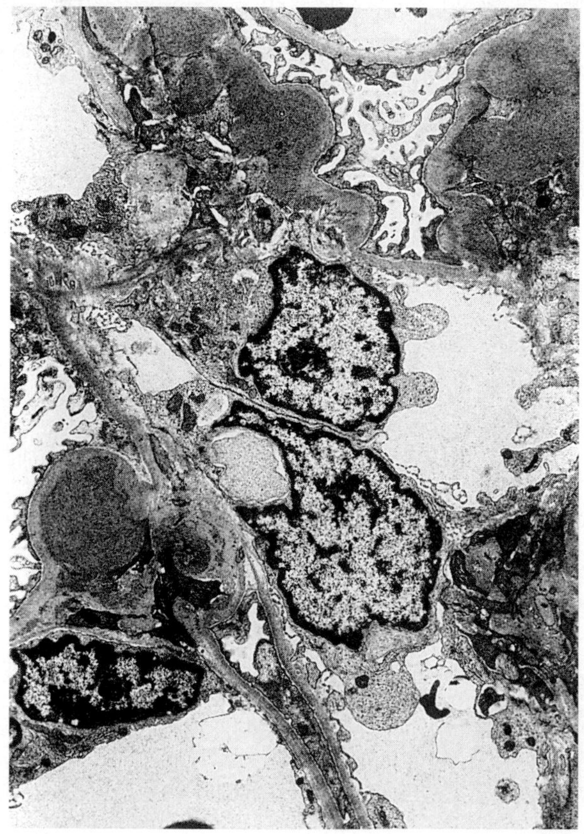

Fig. 65-44 IgA nephropathy. Large, round, electron-dense deposits in paramesangial locations. There are no capillary wall deposits.

Clinical presentation. As mentioned, this glomerulopathy is traditionally considered to be manifested as asymptomatic hematuria and proteinuria. However, virtually all of the nephrologic syndromes have been associated with IgA nephropathy and the clinical presentations are as varied as the light microscopic appearances of the glomeruli.[144] Gross hematuria, usually coincident with or within a few days after a sore throat (synpharyngitic), is most common; it is usually recurrent, with intervening urine demonstrating microscopic hematuria and low-grade or no proteinuria. However, microscopic hematuria, asymptomatic heavy proteinuria or nephrotic syndrome, rapidly progressive glomerulonephritis, acute renal failure, and varying degrees of hypertension may be initial manifestations of this disorder.

There is no effective therapy for IgA nephropathy; the secondary or complicating manifestations such as hypertension can be treated effectively, but the immunologic process and its glomerular damage are not modified by therapy. This glomerulopathy, once established, is chronic and not curable. It is estimated that up to 33% of patients followed for 20 years will develop ESRD.[135,136] IgA mesangial deposits recur in transplanted kidneys but are clinically insignificant and rarely lead to renal failure.[145]

Henoch-Schönlein purpura

Henoch-Schönlein purpura is a clinical syndrome incorporating renal, skin, joint and gastrointestinal symptoms.[146] The primary abnormality is a small vessel vasculitis with IgA deposits in the affected vessels; the renal lesion is a proliferative glomerulonephritis with predominantly mesangial IgA deposits.[147] This syndrome is also known as Schönlein-Henoch purpura, anaphylactoid purpura, and rheumatoid purpura.

Henoch-Schönlein purpura is characterized by mesangial IgA deposits and currently is believed to represent one end of the continuum of IgA-mediated renal diseases, with systemic involvement. There is a morphologic classification based on the degree of mesangial hypercellularity and crescent formation, including mesangiopathic, focal and segmental, diffuse proliferative, and endocapillary or extracapillary glomerulonephritides.[148] These are described in more detail below.

Etiology and pathogenesis. Much of the information available on the pathogenesis of IgA-mediated renal diseases has been obtained from studies of IgA nephropathy. Henoch-Schönlein purpura is an immune complex–mediated renal lesion with variable numbers of patients having circulating immune complexes containing IgA. The IgA antibody may emanate from the mucosal system of the gastrointestinal or respiratory tracts, or the bone marrow; there is little information about potential etiologic agents inducing the immune complexes found in Henoch-Schonlein purpura.[149-152] Defective clearance of IgA complexes, higher levels of circulating immune complexes, and large macromolecular IgA aggregates have been reported in patients with active disease. The degree of renal damage resulting from the IgA deposition is variable; complement activation and factors produced by mesangial cells in response to the deposits may mediate the glomerular injury.

Pathology. Little information is available regarding the gross appearance of the kidneys in Henoch-Schönlein purpura, but in most instances it likely is normal. If there is an active lesion with numerous crescents, the kidneys may be somewhat enlarged.

Light microscopy discloses a range of glomerular involvement, from minimal to severe. The basic abnormality is mesangial widening with increased cellularity, fuchsinophilic deposits, and a mild increase in matrix material (Fig. 65-45). Capillary walls may be involved in more severe cases, with scattered deposits and double contours. Crescents are variably present; with more active disease there may be disruptions in Bowman's capsule, with cells and fibrin extending from crescents into the surrounding interstitium. In more advanced lesions there may be glomeruli with fibrotic crescents, focal and segmental glomerulosclerosis, and complete sclerosis. The tubular cells may be necrotic with associated interstitial edema and mononuclear inflammatory cells in active disease, and tubular atrophy with interstitial fibrosis are associated with advanced changes (see the discussion of IgA nephropathy in this chapter).

There is a morphologic classification encompassing this variability, with mesangial hypercellularity and the number of crescents being the most important features.[148, 151] *Mesangiopathic glomerulonephritis* has mild mesangial hypercellularity and few fuchsinophilic deposits. *Focal and segmental glomerulonephritis* is characterized by segments of more pronounced mesangial hypercellularity, mild capillary wall involvement, and variable numbers of crescents or adhesions. *Diffuse proliferative (endocapillary) glomerulonephritis* has widespread, pronounced mesangial hypercellularity, more capillary wall deposits, and double contours, with capillary luminal leukocytes. Infrequently, there may be a lobular configuration to the glomeruli. *Endocapillary/extracapillary glomerulonephritis* encompasses the diffuse proliferative lesion with cellular crescents. This category is further divided into those with less than or greater than 50% crescents. Vasculitis is virtually never observed in renal tissues, though it is present in other organs such as skin and the gastrointestinal tract.

Immunofluorescence microscopy is required to make the diagnosis, which is defined as mesangial deposits of IgA in the appropriate clinical setting (Fig. 65-46). These are granular deposits of IgA, usually with C3, light chains, and, often, smaller amounts of IgG or IgM. The staining has greater intensity in more proliferative lesions and may involve capillary walls segmentally. When cellular crescents are present, glomeruli stain for fibrin in the urinary space.

EM reveals electron-dense deposits in mesangial regions, often underlying the paramesangial basement membrane but more diffuse than in typical IgA nephropathy (Fig. 65-47). The

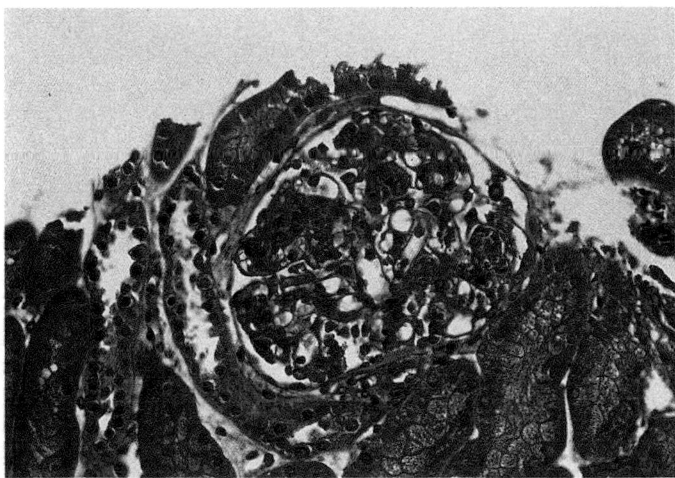

Fig. 65-45 Henoch-Schönlein purpura. The glomerulus displays variable mesangial expansion and hypercellularity. Capillary walls are single contoured, with few circulating leukocytes in capillary lumens. The appearance is similar to IgA nephropathy, though large paramesangial fuchsinophilic deposits are not so frequently observed. (Masson's trichrome.)

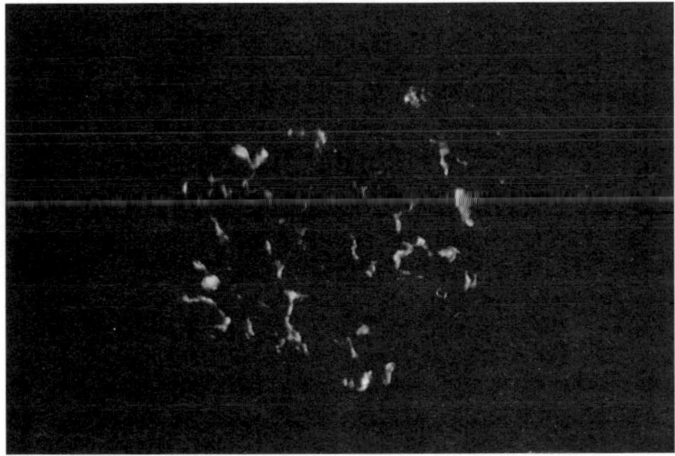

Fig. 65-46 Henoch-Schönlein purpura. Glomerulus with granular mesangial staining for IgA, similar to IgA nephropathy.

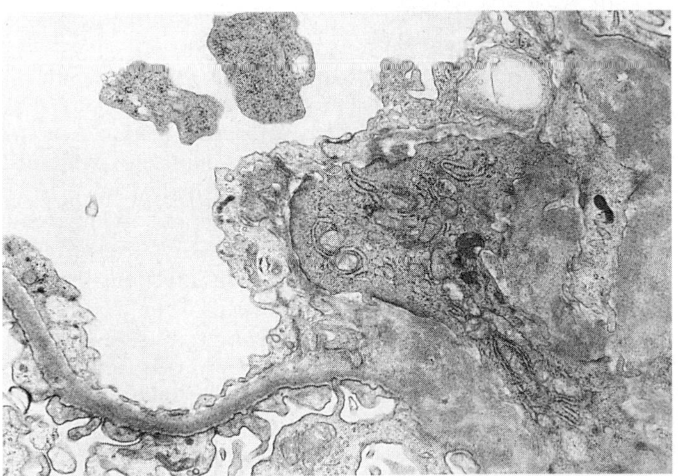

Fig. 65-47 Henoch-Schönlein purpura. Electron-dense deposits throughout a mesangial region. The capillary wall has no abnormalities.

deposits may be small but tend to be larger with more active disease. Occasionally there are scattered subepithelial deposits, at times hump shaped, and small subendothelial deposits associated with peripheral mesangial migration and interposition in capillary walls. Glomerular capillary basement membranes often demonstrate focal thinning or thickening and layering, changes also observed in IgA nephropathy. Visceral epithelial cell foot processes are variably effaced.

Differential diagnosis. The light microscopic findings in Henoch-Schönlein purpura can mimic IgA nephropathy or SLE. Infrequently, numerous crescents may be present, similar to pauci-immune crescentic glomerulonephritis, or subepithelial hump-shaped deposits simulate postinfectious glomerulonephritis. Immunofluorescence microscopy will easily distinguish among these (except IgA nephropathy). Although the electron dense deposits are a bit smaller and more diffusely located in Henoch-Schönlein purpura relative to IgA nephropathy, the clinical picture is the only sure means of differentiating these two entities.

Clinical presentation. This is primarily a disease of children and adolescents, rarely occurring in adults. Patients usually have extrarenal manifestations including palpable purpura of the lower extremities, arthralgias, and abdominal pain.[146,152,153] Clinical renal disease occurs in 10% to 25% of patients, manifesting as gross or microscopic hematuria, variable proteinuria up to the nephrotic range, and renal insufficiency in more severe cases. The morphologic classification correlates with clinical symptoms and outcome, which is worse in those with diffuse proliferative and crescentic lesions. There is no proved effective therapy for Henoch-Schonlein purpura, though steroids and immunosuppressive agents are occasionally used in patients with more severe symptoms.[154] This lesion infrequently recurs in renal transplants.

Postinfectious glomerulonephritides

Post-infectious glomerulonephritis is an immune complex–mediated form of glomerulonephritis occurring in association with certain infections and in which the antigen is thought to be directly or indirectly related to the infecting organism. Although infection with many microorganisms can be complicated by this form of glomerular injury, certain strains of group A streptococci are most commonly and characteristically involved, and poststreptococcal glomerulonephritis is considered to be the standard.

Postinfectious glomerulonephritis is an immune-mediated lesion that typically presents with the clinical manifestations of acute nephritis. This form of glomerulonephritis may be associated with deep-seated visceral abscesses, infected ventriculoatrial or other shunts, infective endocarditis, and so on.[6,155]

Etiology and pathogenesis. Postinfectious glomerulonephritis is the prototype of an immune complex–mediated disease. It follows or is associated with an infectious process, and soluble immune complexes are found in the serum. The disease is self-limited, and immune complexes are found in glomeruli. Although it was initially believed that the immune complexes from the circulation deposited in glomeruli, it is currently believed that an antigen of the microorganism is first planted in glomeruli and combined in situ with circulating antibody. Complement is found in glomeruli, and levels are depressed in serum. Accumulation of leukocytes such as neutrophils and monocytes ensues, resulting in glomerular damage and functional alterations such as hematuria, proteinuria, and decreased glomerular filtration. In some instances, antigen of microorganism can be identified in the glomerular deposits; in other patients or infectious agents, the antigen has not been identified and its existence is presumed.[6,155,156]

Pathology. The morphologic and immunomorphologic features vary somewhat depending on the chronicity of the infection and the time after the onset of glomerulonephritis that the tissue is examined.

Grossly, in the acute stage, the kidneys are enlarged, with pale capsular surface and cortex.

Microscopically, varied appearances are encountered. In poststreptococcal glomerulonephritis, all glomeruli are abnormal and appear reasonably similar to one another and are greatly hypercellular. This results from the accumulation of numerous monocytes in capillary lumens with varying numbers of neutrophils, eosinophils, and lymphocytes. Mesangial regions are widened, with infiltration by monocytes and, probably, replication of intrinsic mesangial cells. Capillary walls most often have single contours but are irregularly thickened because of subepithelial hump-shaped deposits, which vary considerably in quantity from one capillary to another (Fig. 65-48). Crescents occur but are not common. In glomerulonephritis associated with endocarditis, abscesses, and so on, the glomerular picture may be the same as just described or, more commonly, may be different, probably relating to duration of disease. The increased cellularity is more segmental in each tuft, and crescents are often smaller and fibrocellular or fibrotic. In long-standing infections, the morphology may assume a membranoproliferative glomerulonephritis type I pattern with lobular architecture, increased mesangial cellularity, and prominent, double-contoured capillary walls because of widespread peripheral migration and interposition of mesangium. In most instances, eradication of the underlying infection will result in clearing of or vast improvement in glomerular damage.

The interstitium is usually edematous, with variable but mild inflammation, mainly with mononuclear leukocytes.

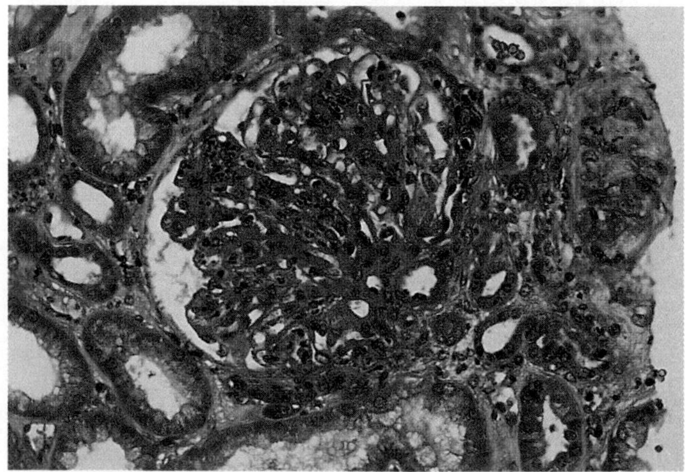

Fig. 65-48 Acute postinfectious glomerulonephritis. There is considerable increase in cellularity, mainly because of accumulation of numerous polymorphonuclear leukocytes in capillary lumens. Notice numerous subepithelial hump-shaped fuchsinophilic deposits in many capillary walls. There are protein precipitates ("hyalinization") in the arteriole. (Masson's trichrome.)

Tubules often contain leukocytes and erythrocytes of glomerular origin. Arteries and arterioles are usually normal unless hypertension coexists or there is concomitant necrotizing arteritis. The latter is exceedingly rare.

Immunofluorescence microscopy discloses granular deposits of C3 and IgG in glomerular capillary walls and mesangial regions (Fig. 65-49). The deposits are often irregularly distributed. In acute poststreptococcal glomerulonephritis, it is not unusual to find C3 without demonstrable IgG. IgM may also be present, though with considerably less intensity.

EM characteristically indicates electron-dense deposits in capillary walls and mesangial regions. The hallmark of this glomerulopathy is subepithelial, hump-shaped, often large deposits (Fig. 65-50); these may be in large or small numbers depending on the duration of the lesion. Electron-dense deposits are also not infrequently in subendothelial aspects of some capillary walls. Leukocytes are in capillary lumens and frequently in direct contact with capillary basement membrane. There is effacement of the foot processes of visceral epithelial cells.[6,158]

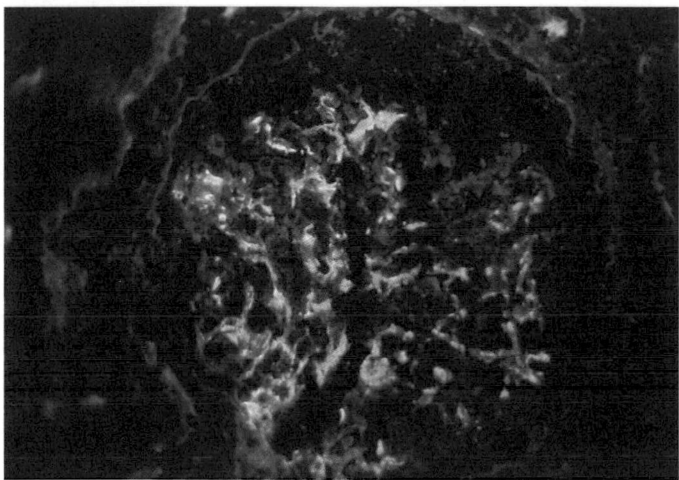

Fig. 65-49 Postinfectious glomerulonephritis. Irregular mesangial and capillary wall staining for C3.

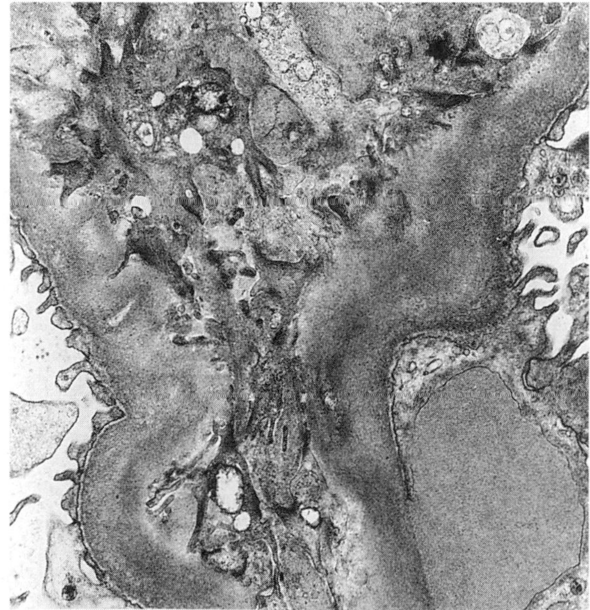

Fig. 65-50 Postinfectious glomerulonephritis. A large hump-shaped deposit is in a subepithelial location; deposits are often more dense than this one.

Differential diagnosis. Clinical, laboratory, and immunomorphologic findings are characteristic of postinfectious glomerulonephritis, though they are not always diagnostic. Furthermore, the morphology does not identify the type, source, or agent of infection. The pathologic features are those of an immune complex–mediated glomerulonephritis with hypercellularity; the hump-shaped deposits may rarely be observed also in Henoch-Schönlein purpura nephritis and complicating dense deposit disease (MPGN II), but immunofluorescence or EM should allow for distinguishing one entity from the other. Ultrastructurally, the three locations of deposits are not unlike SLE, but the appearance and size of the deposits, presence of tubuloreticular structures, and composition of deposits as determined by immunofluorescence should allow differentiation of postinfectious from lupus glomerulonephritis. Last, it should be pointed out that despite our pathologic sophistication and expertise, some renal specimens exhibit features that cannot be anything but a postinfectious glomerulonephritis but that are from patients without demonstrable infectious processes.

Clinical presentation. In the acute form, this glomerular lesion presents with the nephrologic syndrome of acute nephritis characterized by sudden onset of hematuria, proteinuria, hypertension, diminished glomerular filtration rate, and sodium and water retention. Serum complement (C3) is depresssed and, if associated with streptococcal infection, antistreptolysin O titer is elevated. The more chronic infections and glomerulonephritis present with heavy proteinuria and variable hematuria, variable renal insufficiency, and often hypocomplementemia. As mentioned, with identification and eradication of the infection (if possible), morphologic and clinical features improve.[6,155,158]

Hepatitis-associated glomerulonephritis and other renal lesions

There are numerous forms of renal disease secondary to hepatitis B and C infection. Linkage of a nephropathy to viral infection requires the presence of viral antigen or genome within the patient and the simultaneous occurrence of a renal lesion known to be induced by hepatitis; in hepatitis B cases, viral antigens have been detected in the renal immune complexes in all associated forms of renal disease.

Hepatitis B virus infection may induce a systemic vasculitis that mimics polyarteritis nodosa, which can involve the kidney.[159] The other associated lesions are immune complex–mediated glomerulonephritides, most often membranous glomerulonephritis, with fewer cases of MPGN types I and III, and cryoglobulinemia[160] (Table 65-9). Minimal change disease, focal and segmental glomerulosclerosis, and IgA nephropathy have been reported less often and their association is not certain; glomerular IgA deposition is related to chronic liver disease of any cause.[161] Hepatitis C virus may be a major cause of MPGN type I and cryoglobulinemia.[162,163] There are also scattered reports of membranous glomerulonephritis and polyarteritis nodosa linked to hepatitis C .[164,165]

Etiology and pathogenesis. The vascular and renal lesions induced by hepatitis B are immune complex–mediated abnor-

Table 65-9 Hepatitis-associated renal lesions

Well established
Mebranous glomerulonephritis
Membranoproliferative glomerulonephritis type I
Membranoproliferative glomerulonephritis type III
Cryoglobulinemia
Hepatic glomerulosclerosis
Polyarteritis nodosa
Poorly established
IgA nephropathy
Focal and segmental glomerulosclerosis

malities, resulting from deposition or in situ formation of hepatitis antigen-antibody complexes in patients with active infection.[159,166] The e antigen produces immune complexes of the appropriate size and charge to allow deposition primarily in glomerular capillary wall subepithelial locations, inducing a form of membranous glomerulonephritis. The surface antigen is found in larger cationic complexes, which tend to localize in the mesangium and peripheral capillary walls in association with an MPGN pattern of injury.[167] Hepatitis B core antibody infrequently has been identified in renal immune deposits.

Hepatitis C virus–infected patients remain viremic for life and are now recognized as having a high incidence of renal disease. This is also an immune complex–mediated disease in which a large number of patients with hepatitis C and cryoglobulinemia have anti-hepatitis C core antibody or hepatitis C RNA in the cryoprecipitate.[162] Frequently, IgM is also produced in these patients; this IgM has rheumatoid factor properties, binding to the IgG anti–hepatitis C antibody. Patients with membranous glomerulonephritis have been shown to contain hepatitis C RNA in renal tissue.[164]

Pathology. The pathologic features of the hepatitis-associated renal lesions are the same as those entities where hepatitis virus is not the etiologic agent, and they are described in the appropriate sections. Membranous glomerulonephritis secondary to infection usually has a mild mesangial proliferative component and may have immune complexes within mesangial regions in addition to the subepithelial deposits. MPGN type I, cryoglobulinemia, and vasculitis related to hepatitis infection cannot be distinguished morphologically from those diseases when they are idiopathic or linked to other etiologic factors. The vasculitis is usually not associated with crescentic glomerulonephritis, unlike many of the antineutrophil cytoplasmic antibody (ANCA)–associated vasculitides.

Differential diagnosis. The differential diagnosis for each entity is discussed in detail in the appropriate disease section.

Clinical presentation. Patients with the various renal abnormalities become symptomatic in the same manner as the primary renal disease with or without associated liver abnormalities. It is important to identify hepatitis as the cause of the renal lesion because this has significant therapeutic implications. Steroid therapy has been used in the past, but currently interferon-alpha is used with varying success in treating the underlying infection with subsequent resolution of the renal component.[168,169]

Anti–glomerular basement membrane disease

Anti-GBM disease is a form of immunologic glomerular injury induced by the binding of circulating autoantibodies to an epitope located in a homohexamer found within the globular noncollagenous domain of type IV collagen in GBMs. The resulting damage is most commonly in the form of a crescentic glomerulonephritis, often with coexisting renal tubular and pulmonary alveolar damage. Anti-GBM nephritis presents clinically with rapidly progressive glomerulonephritis. The clinical and pathologic manifestations may be limited to the kidneys (anti-GBM disease) or may be associated with pulmonary hemorrhage (Goodpasture's disease).[6,155,170]

Etiology and pathogenesis. As the name of the disease implies, anti–glomerular basement membrane disease is the result of the production of antibodies directed against an antigen in the GBM, binding of antibodies, and activation of inflammation with resultant severe damage to glomeruli. The antigen known as the Goodpasture antigen is normally hidden within the fully assembled globular domain of type IV collagen molecule and is a peptide on the alpha 3 chain. The antibody is almost always of IgG isotype, though, rarely, IgA antibodies have been documented. The cause of the disease is not known precisely, though clinical events such as the frequent occurrence of prodromal flulike symptoms is suggestive of a viral cause. In some patients, a history of volatile hydrocarbon exposure is elicited; both of these events are suggestive of pulmonary alveolar basement membrane damage as the initial event, exposing the basement membrane antigen and initiating antibody formation.[6,155,170-173] It is well known that the GBMs of some patients with Alport's syndrome lack the Goodpasture antigen.[41,155] Consequently, anti-GBM disease may occur in such patients who are transplanted with normal kidneys when their own kidneys fail.[41]

Pathology. The kidneys are grossly enlarged during the acute phase of the disease; this is largely because of interstitial edema and inflammation. There are often petechial hemorrhages on the capsular surface and throughout the cortex that represent hemorrhages in individual nephrons.

The major light microscopic features involve glomeruli; characteristically, there are crescents or fibrin in the urinary spaces of a variable percentage of the glomeruli (Fig. 65-51),

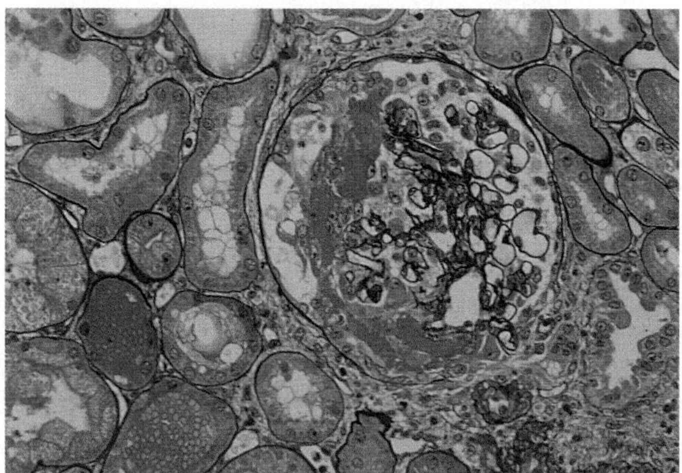

Fig. 65-51 Anti–glomerular basement membrane nephritis. Glomerulus with a fresh crescent consisting of fibrin and cells in the urinary space. There is disruption of the basement membrane of Bowman's capsule, with migration of cells from the interstitium into the urinary space. The capillary tufts are distorted and compressed because of the crescent. Notice the free erythrocytes in tubular lumens. The interstitium is mildly edematous. (Periodic acid–methenamine silver.)

though all glomeruli are the sites of bound anti-GBM antibody and complement fixation. Glomeruli without crescents have a variety of appearances, including segmental accumulation of leukocytes and fibrin in capillary lumens, breaks in capillary walls with spillage of fibrin (and cells) into the urinary spaces, and normal. Breaks in the basement membranes of Bowman's capsules, with cells and fibrin of the crescent extending into the surrounding interstitium, are common features. The interstitium is edematous and infiltrated with mononuclear leukocytes. Tubular cell degeneration and necrosis usually accompany the interstitial changes. Arteries and arterioles are normal except in those patients with coexisting ANCA; in this not infrequent circumstance, necrotizing lesions of these vessels may be observed.[174,175]

Immunofluorescence microscopy discloses linear staining of *all* GBMS for IgG (Fig. 65-52); isolated reports have described linear IgA or IgM. Complement (C3) may occur in a similar pattern or in an interrupted linear or globular pattern. Fibrin is in urinary spaces of glomeruli with crescents. Linear IgG is in tubular basement membranes (either focal or generalized) in approximately two thirds of the patients.

There are no characteristic or diagnostic features by EM; there is no ultrastructural counterpart of linear immune deposits. The luminal leukocytes and fibrin, capillary wall discontinuities, and fibrin and cells in the urinary spaces (crescents) reflect the light microscopic alterations as described previously.[6,7,170]

Differential diagnosis. Considering that the pathologic diagnosis of glomerular diseases requires the correlation of combined light microscopy, EM, and immunofluorescence with clinical and laboratory features, there is an exceedingly short list of entities to consider in the differential diagnosis. Without immunofluorescence, the pathologist is faced with a crescentic glomerulonephritis; if the glomeruli without crescents display prominent proliferative features (hypercellularity), this generally points away from anti-GBM disease. On the other hand, if the glomeruli without crescents are normal (or near normal), the other major lesion to consider is pauci-immune crescentic glomerulonephritis (either as part of a systemic vasculitis or limited to the kidneys). EM is of little assistance inasmuch as both anti-GBM disease and pauci-immune crescentic glomerulonephritis lack electron-dense deposits and the other abnormalities are common to both. Serologic tests (serum anti-GBM or ANCA) are necessary to distinguish one disorder from the other.[170]

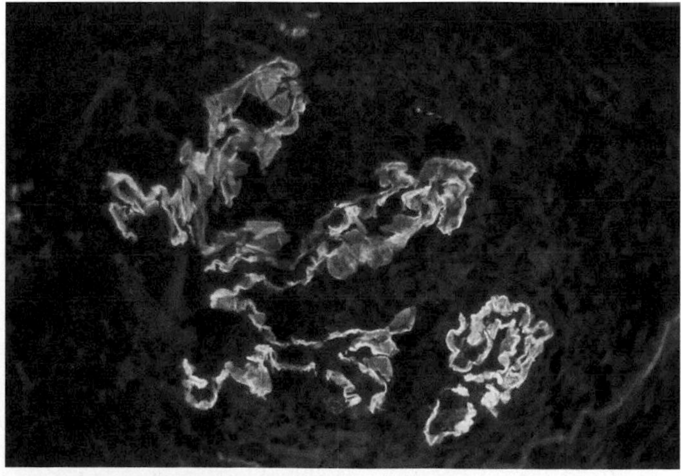

Fig. 65-52 Anti-glomerular basement membrane nephritis. Linear staining in all capillary walls for IgG.

Clinical presentation. The nephrologic syndrome most commonly associated with anti-GBM disease is rapidly progressive glomerulophritis, with relentless loss of renal function over weeks to months accompanied by hematuria and variable proteinuria.[176] If there are concomitant antibodies to pulmonary alveolar capillary basement membranes, which occurs in approximately 75% of patients, pulmonary infiltrates with hemoptysis are present and can be the major life-threatening manifestation.[155,170] Once believed to be a disorder of young males, anti-GBM disease may occur at any age; there are two peaks of age-dependent incidence, one in the third decade and the other in the sixth or seventh decade. By convention, the combination of circulating anti-GBM antibodies and tissue-bound glomerular and pulmonary antibodies with concomitant damage (crescentic glomerulonephritis, pulmonary hemorrhage) is known as Goodpasture's *disease*. Glomerulonephritis with pulmonary hemorrhage that is non–anti-GBM related is designated Goodpasture's *syndrome*.[170]

As alluded to previously, an important, indeed necessary, aspect of this disease is the demonstration of circulating anti-GBM antibodies by the clinical laboratory. By following the titer, it is possible to monitor the activity of the disease, including timing of renal transplantation when necessary. Therapy is aimed at suppressing the production of or removing circulating antibodies by immunosuppression and plasmapheresis respectively. This aggressive approach has been found to be effective in treating the renal component only if renal insufficiency is not advanced.[155,170]

Vasculitis and pauci-immune crescentic glomerulonephritis

The term *vasculitis* covers a wide range of abnormalities associated with inflammation of variously sized blood vessel walls in a range of clinical settings. In the kidney, vasculitis rarely presents as vascular inflammation but more commonly is manifested as pauci-immune crescentic glomerulonephritis (PICGN). This abnormality is characterized by glomerular crescents without significant immune deposits, glomerular hypercellularity, or involvement by anti-GBM antibody.[177] A diagnosis of vasculitis-associated renal injury requires correlation of the clinical, serologic, and morphologic data.

The classification of the vasculitides is a confusing area that has evolved over the past 130 years.[178] Classifications have been proposed based on the size and location of involved vessels, age of the lesions, proposed pathogenetic mechanisms, and clinical symptoms.[179] Currently, the availability of tests for ANCA has afforded a new rationale for the pathogenesis and overlap of symptoms in the vasculitides.[180] Neutrophils fixed in alcohol and overlain with labeled patient's serum containing ANCA give two staining patterns: a cytoplasmic (c-ANCA) pattern corresponding to anti–proteinase 3 antibody and a perinuclear (p-ANCA) pattern usually corresponding to anti–myeloperoxidase antibody.[180,181] An international consensus conference recently reviewed this topic and proposed a classification system for primary vasculitides based on vessel size and ANCA positivity.[182] The small vessel primary vasculitides emcompass most of those affecting the kidney and are the focus of this discussion.

Vasculitis also occurs as a secondary process in several systemic diseases that involve the kidney, such as SLE, rheumatoid arthritis, and cryoglobulinemia.[183,184] Vascular inflammation can also occur with some infections, drug reactions, and in association with tumors and radiation.[185-187]

Glomerulonephritis with crescents has been classified into three types by the World Health Organization. Type I is anti-GBM antibody nephritis; type II includes crescents, with an underlying immune complex–mediated glomerular disease such as lupus or postinfectious glomerulonephritis and type III PICGN, without immune deposits or anti-GBM antibodies. Type III is the form associated with vasculitis, and more recently the classification incorporates ANCA serologic studies. Therefore, both vasculitis and PICGN are grouped according to ANCA positivity.

Etiology and pathogenesis. The pathogenesis of the noninfectious vasculitides is not well known, as evidenced by the numerous classification systems that have been developed over the years. These lesions may eventually be understood in relation to those that are ANCA associated and those that are not; it is likely that the ANCA-associated vasculitides are pathogenetically related because there is considerable overlap in the clinical symptoms and response to therapy among this group of diseases. Primary and secondary vasculitides are initiated by humoral and cell-mediated mechanisms, accounting for the varied settings in which vasculitis occurs.[183,188,189]

Humoral (antibody-mediated) immunity with immune complex formation as observed in serum sickness models is one mechanism in the initiation and exacerbation of vasculitis, particularly secondary forms associated with systemic disease.[183,188,190] Antibodies can react with endothelial or vascular smooth muscle antigens, inducing complement activation and recruitment of leukocytes and resulting in inflammation and necrosis of vessel walls. Prior depletion of complement or neutrophils prevents the formation of antibody-mediated experimental vasculitis.[191] Immune complex deposits are infrequently observed in primary vasculitis not associated with immune complex–mediated systemic diseases; however, immune complexes are rapidly cleared, and it is possible that the initial deposition is not identified at the time biopsy is performed.

The discovery of ANCA has led to a new consideration of humoral factors in the development of primary vasculitis. Support for a pathogenetic role of ANCA includes the correlation between ANCA levels and disease activity, and the good specificity of ANCA for vasculitis.[192,193] These antibodies react with neutrophils in vitro inducing a respiratory burst with degranulation and formation of oxygen radicals, possibly inducing or worsening the vascular damage.[194] None of the studies up to now is conclusive, and the role of ANCA remains somewhat speculative.

A role for cell-mediated immunity is suggested by the mononuclear and granulomatous inflammatory components so often a part of vasculitis. Cytotoxic T-cells may respond to foreign antigens within vessel walls, inciting necrosis and a subsequent neutrophilic infiltrate. Endothelial cells have the capacity to express MHC class II antigens and adhesion molecules and may actively participate in this process. Wegener's granulomatosis is associated with vascular granulomas, and such an association is suggestive of a hypersensitivity T-cell–mediated reaction that can be mimicked by drug-induced or infection-induced vasculitides.

PICGN is the renal manifestation of primary vasculitides such as microscopic polyangiitis and Wegener's granulomatosis.[195] The same process that evokes vascular necrosis and inflammation elsewhere produces a glomerular capillary "vasculitis," resulting in capillary wall damage and disruption and allowing extrusion of cells and fibrin into the urinary space, forming crescents.[196] There may be breaks in Bowman's capsule with cells and fibrin extending into the interstitium and associated acute tubulointerstitial injury.

Pathology. The only large vessel vasculitis that commonly (Fig. 65-53) affects the kidney is macroscopic (classic) polyarteritis nodosa.[179] Grossly the kidneys are normal or reduced in size, with a coarse nodular appearance and foci of infarction. On a cut surface there are small aneurysms or thrombi in arcuate and interlobar arteries. In small vessel vasculitides with active PICGN kidneys are enlarged, often with areas of hemorrhage, and advanced disease produces small contracted kidneys.

Microscopically, macroscopic polyarteritis nodosa involves focal and segmental inflammation of medium-sized interlobar and arcuate arteries with lesions of varying age found simultaneously. Acute lesions have a circumferential or eccentric infiltrate composed of neutrophils, lymphocytes, monocytes, and, occasionally, eosinophils in the intima. There may be medial or adventitial involvement, often with adventitial plasma cells. Focal fibrin deposition with necrosis and cellular debris (fibrinoid necrosis) is in a limited or transmural pattern with disruption of the internal elastic lamina and swollen detached endothelial cells. Arteries may become thrombosed with ensuing focal cortical infarcts. There are tubular cell degeneration and regeneration, interstitial edema, and interstitial inflammation. Interstitial hemorrhage may be found, particularly in the medulla or adjacent to areas of infarction. Glomeruli have ischemic injury with capillary wall thickening and partial collapse. More advanced vascular lesions show healing, with a loose proliferation of myointimal cells, early collagen deposition, and mild tubular atrophy with interstitial fibrosis. Healed arteritis produces scars in areas of prior necrosis with narrowed arterial lumens and reduplicated elastic lamina; elastic stain discloses disruptions in the original internal elastic lamina.[197] The chronic tubular and interstitial changes are more severe, as is the glomerular ischemia.

Immunofluorescence and EM do not contribute to the diagnosis. It is unusual to find the changes of classic polyarteritis nodosa on biopsy material because the large arteries involved are not commonly sampled.

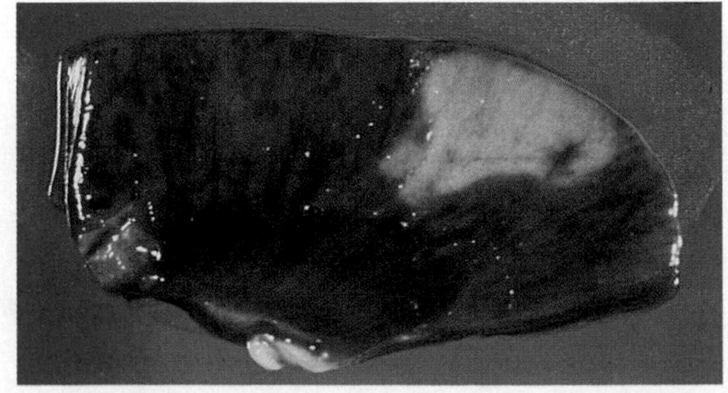

Fig. 65-53 Arteritis and pauci-immune crescentic glomerulonephritis. Section of kidney from a patient with macroscopic polyarteritis nodosa. There is a wedge-shaped cortical infarct caused by segmental involvement and occlusion of large and medium-sized arteries.

The small vessel primary vasculitides include Wegener's granulomatosis and microscopic polyangiitis and have similar morphologic appearances. The primary abnormality is PICGN, with focal necrotizing lesions and crescents ranging from cellular to fibrous depending on the duration of disease. In active disease, glomerular capillary walls have focal disruptions with mononuclear cells, occasional neutrophils, and fibrin in the urinary space in a segmental or circumferential fashion[198] (Fig. 65-54). There is often collapse or wrinkling of glomerular tufts in the portions underlying the crescents. The remaining glomerular tufts do not show hypercellularity or fuchsinophilic deposits. Capillary walls are single contoured, but lumens contain occasional circulating leukocytes. Disruptions in Bowman's capsule are not uncommon, with cells and fibrin extending into the interstitium. There are interstitial edema, mononuclear inflammation (occasionally with scattered eosinophils), and tubular necrosis. In advanced disease the crescents are fibrocellular to fibrous, with fibroblasts and collagen in the urinary space replacing the mononuclear cells and fibrin. Glomerular tufts are collapsed or sclerotic, and there is tubular atrophy with associated interstitial fibrosis. It is unusual to find vascular inflammation in the kidney, but when it occurs it involves the small interlobular arteries, arterioles, capillaries, and venules at the same stage simultaneously. Affected vessels have fibrinoid necrosis with neutrophil predominance in the intima with or without medial and adventitial damage (Fig. 65-55). Circumferential inflammation is more common; arterial aneurysms, thrombi, and infarcts are uncommon. Granulomas may be present with multinucleated giant cells but are infrequent even in Wegener's granulomatosis. There may be peritubular capillaritis with small fibrin thrombi as the only vessel involvement. Advanced vasculitis results in thickened fibrotic vessel walls.

Wegener's granulomatosis more often has granulomatous features with multinucleated giant cells in the crescents, but this is a nonspecific finding. Up to 20% of patients with Wegener's have papillary necrosis. Churg-Strauss syndrome has similar features to microscopic polyangiitis, but renal damage is usually mild.

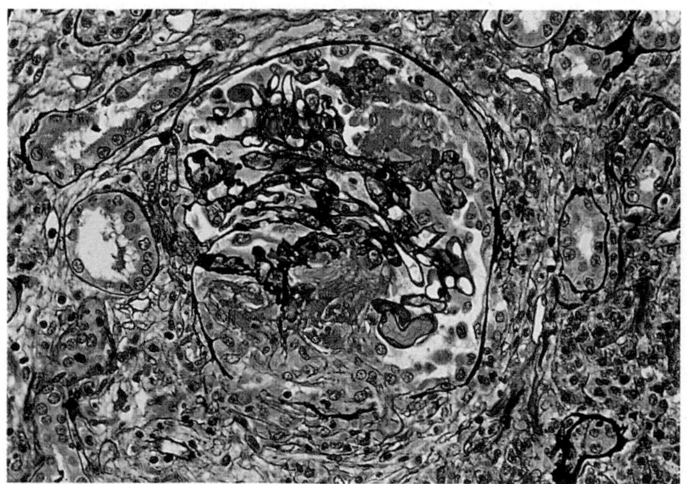

Fig. 65-54 Pauci-immune crescentic glomerulonephritis. Glomerulus with a cellular crescent containing fibrin and cells in the urinary space. There are disruptions of Bowman's capsule adjacent to the crescent. An uninvolved tuft has a normal appearance. (Periodic acid–methenamine silver.)

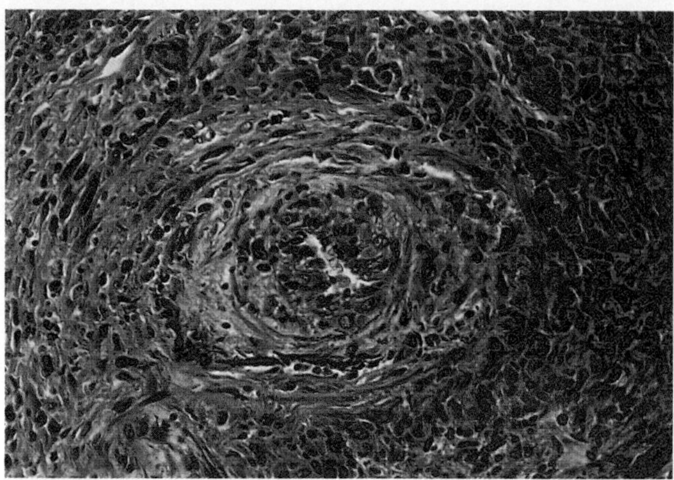

Fig. 65-55 Pauci-immune crescentic glomerulonephritis. Small interlobular artery with leukocytes throughout the focally edematous wall and fibrin deposition. (Masson's trichrome.)

Immunofluorescence is negative or weakly positive for immunoglobulins and complement components in glomerular mesangia or capillary walls with a granular pattern, hence the term *pauci-immune crescentic glomerulonephritis.* Fibrin is strongly positive in active crescents within Bowman's space and in damaged vessel walls (Fig. 65-56). EM usually fails to disclose electron-dense deposits; when present they are small and infrequent. Capillary basement membranes are normal, or thickened and wrinkled with small subendothelial lucent zones. When crescents occur there are focal disruptions in the capillary basement membranes; these structures may be darkened, and fibrin is evident within the urinary space.[198] Visceral epithelial cell foot processes are effaced or necrotic, and endothelial cell cytoplasm is swollen.

Differential diagnosis. When vasculitis is present in the kidney with normal glomeruli, large vessel size indicates macroscopic polyarteritis or temporal arteritis, and medium and small vessel inflammation is suggestive of the hypersensitivity or ANCA-associated diseases. When the primary lesion is crescentic glomerulonephritis, crescents may occur in a wide range of glomerulonephritides; careful examination of preserved glomeruli by light, immunofluorescent, and electron microscopies will allow a diagnosis of immune complex–mediated or anti-GBM antibody nephritis. Once the lesion is identified as pauci-immune crescentic glomerulonephritis, it may be difficult to distinguish the specific underlying form of vasculitis. Serologic tests may contribute in this regard; the majority of patients with Wegener's granulomatosis have anti–proteinase 3 antibody (c-ANCA), whereas those with microscopic polyangiitis tend to produce antimyeloperoxidase antibody (p-ANCA).[199] However, overlap syndromes often occur in which a specific diagnosis may never be reached.

Clinical presentation. Renal disease in patients with primary vasculitis has some common features.[195,200] Patients are usually male in the fifth to sixth decade, and 65% to 75% of those with Wegener's granulomatosis or microscopic polyangiitis demonstrate renal involvement. However, there are cases of Wegener's granulomatosis in the first 2 decades of life. Classical polyarteritis often induces hypertension without acute renal failure unless there is significant renal infarction; urine analysis shows granular and hyaline casts with mild proteinuria. The renal manifestations of Wegener's granulomatosis and microscopic polyangiitis include rapidly progressive glomerulonephritis with hematuria, red cell casts, and mild proteinuria. There may be anemia, arthralgias, fever, and other manifestations of systemic vasculitis, and pulmonary hemorrhage may occur in either (though it is more common in Wegener's). ANCA and anti-GBM antibody serologic tests are necessary to make the correct diagnosis; if ANCA is present, it is useful to follow the titers because they correlate with the clinical course. Treatment includes steroids and immunosuppressive agents such as cytoxan.[201,202] There is no clear role for plasma exchange in PICGN or vasculitis. Prognosis relates to the severity of renal failure at the time of diagnosis and the degree of pulmonary hemorrhage.

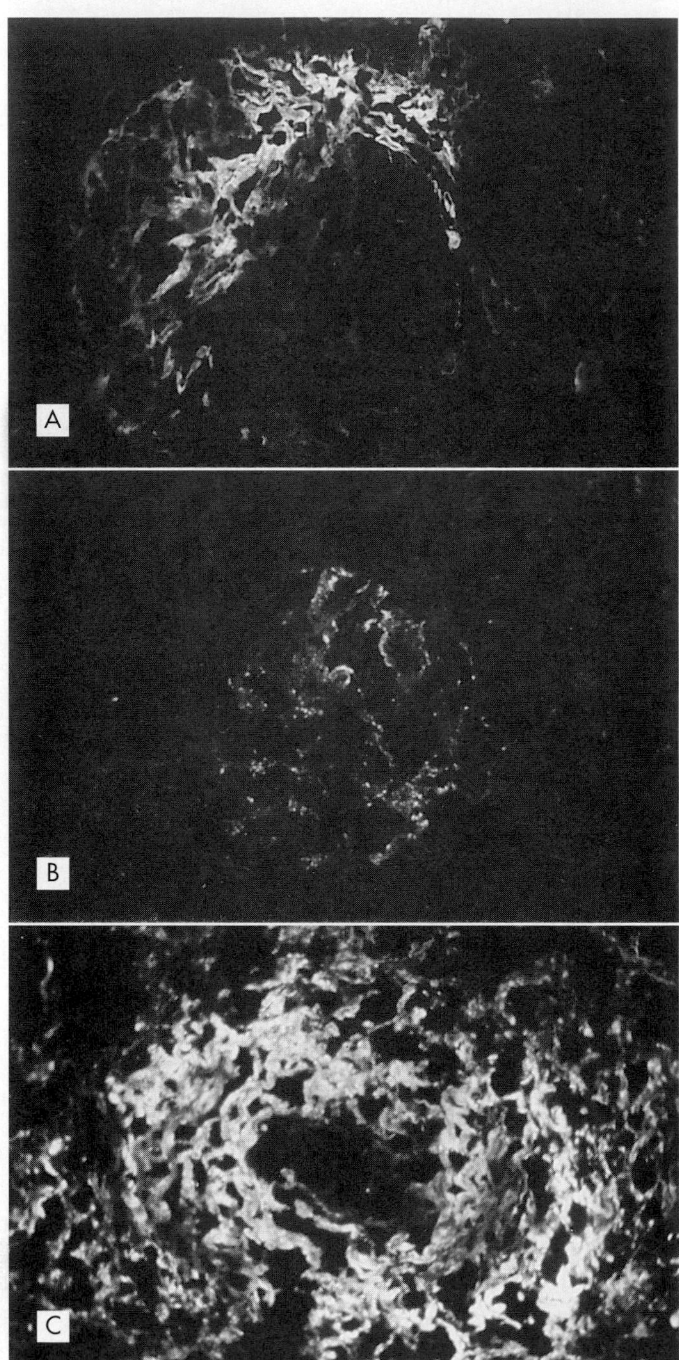

Fig. 65-56 Pauci-immune crescentic glomerulonephritis. **A,** Glomerulus with fresh crescent staining for fibrin within the urinary space; the glomerular tufts are negative. **B,** Glomerular mesangial regions with trace to 1+ staining for C3 in a granular pattern. **C,** Inflamed interlobular artery from patient with microscopic polyangiitis showing fibrin throughout the vascular wall.

Systemic lupus erythematosus nephritis

Lupus nephritis is renal involvement in SLE; this is in the form of immune complex–mediated injury primarily to glomeruli, with relatively minor effects on interstitium and vasculature.

Lupus nephritis is a disease process mediated by the deposition of immune complexes. The glomerular lesions are dominant and are traditionally classified into four different types based on morphology: mesangial (injury, proliferative) lupus glomerulonephritis, focal proliferative lupus glomerulonephritis, diffuse proliferative lupus glomerulonephritis and membranous lupus glomerulonephritis. The terminology is meant to be descriptive, but it is also very much outdated. The World Health Organization has assigned numbers to the various glomerular lesions[7,55,203] (Table 65-10).

Etiology and pathogenesis. The many known and postulated aspects of the cause and pathogenesis of SLE are considered in detail in Chapter 26. The specific pathogenic mechanisms responsible for lesions of the kidney are briefly discussed.

Most investigators agree that the immune complexes in glomeruli result from the deposition of circulating antibodies and antigens, especially DNA. However, the glomerular complexes may not always be the result of deposition of preformed circulating immune complexes; indeed, it is quite possible that there is also in situ immune complex formation, a process that is likely responsible for the subepithelial deposits in membranous lupus glomerulonephritis. As described later, the various glomerulopathies may result from both deposition of circulating complexes and in situ–formed complexes, with one mechanism dominating depending on the lesion.[155,204]

Pathology. Perhaps the best approach to considering the glomerular pathology is to note that virtually all patients with SLE have immune deposits in glomeruli; the basic location of the deposits is in mesangial regions. Stated somewhat differ-

Table 65-10 World Health Organization classification of lupus nephritis

Class	Lesion
I	No abnormalities by light, electron, and immunofluorescence microscopies
II	Mesangial (injury, proliferative) glomerulonephritis
A	No increased cellularity
B	Mild increase in mesangial cellularity
III	Focal and segmental proliferative glomerulonephritis
IV	Diffuse proliferative glomerulonephritis
V	Membranous glomerulonephritis
A	"Pure" membranous glomerulonephritis
B	With mesangial glomerulonephritis
C	With focal proliferative glomerulonephritis
D	With diffuse proliferative glomerulonephritis

ently, glomeruli of all patients with SLE at the very least harbor immune complex deposits in mesangia. Additional deposits and accumulation of cells in various locations are superimposed on the mesangial deposits and result in different morphologies and clinical manifestations. As a rule, in mesangial glomerulonephritis, IgG, C3, and, occasionally, C1q constitute the deposits, whereas in the other forms of glomerulonephritis, frequently all immunoglobulin classes (IgG, IgA, IgM) and complement components (C3, C1q) are deposited. This is known in renal pathology parlance as "full-house immunofluorescence."

Several ultrastructural peculiarities of lupus nephritis may be present in any of the lesions. These include tubuloreticular structures (cellular inclusions induced by interferon) in endothelial cells and occasionally monocytes and lymphocytes. The electron-dense deposits may have a crystalline organizational pattern with concentric curved lines having the appearance of fingerprints. The tubuloreticular structures are usually numerous and widespread; although they may be noted in other disorders, only HIV infection is also associated with similar large numbers of these inclusions as lupus. The fingerprint deposits appear to be unique to lupus.

In *mesangial lupus glomerulonephritis,* the glomeruli by light microscopy appear almost normal, with widening of mesangial regions; there may be normal cellularity or a mild, diffuse increase in mesangial cells (Fig. 65-57). By immunofluorescence, there are granular deposits in mesangial sites only. By EM, dense deposits are in the mesangium; they are usually small to medium in size (Fig. 65-58).

Focal proliferative lupus glomerulonephritis is characterized by segmental hypercellularity of the capillary tufts with segmental increase in mesangial cells and accumulation of leukocytes in capillary lumens (Fig. 65-59). These changes are superimposed on the "background" mesangial glomerulonephritis described previously. By convention, this form of glomerulonephritis affects no more than 50% of the glomerular population. Its designation is, by definition, a misnomer because it implies that some glomeruli are affected and others are not. In addition to increased cells, there may be segmental capillary wall necrosis, degenerating leukocytes with nuclear fragmentation, and crescent formation. Mesangial and subendothelial deposits are often seen with appropriate stains. Interstitial edema or inflammation are variable. Immunofluorescence microscopy reveals granular mesan-

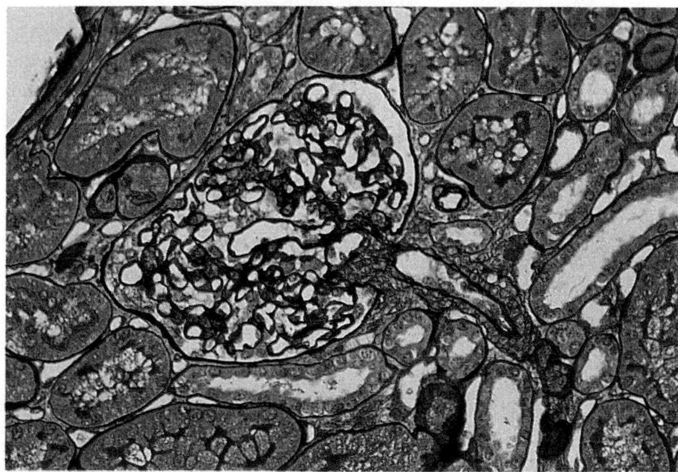

Fig. 65-57 Lupus nephritis. Mesangial proliferative (injury) lupus glomerulonephritis. There is mild widening and increase in cellularity of mesangial regions, the only structural alterations in this glomerulus. (Periodic acid–methenamine silver.)

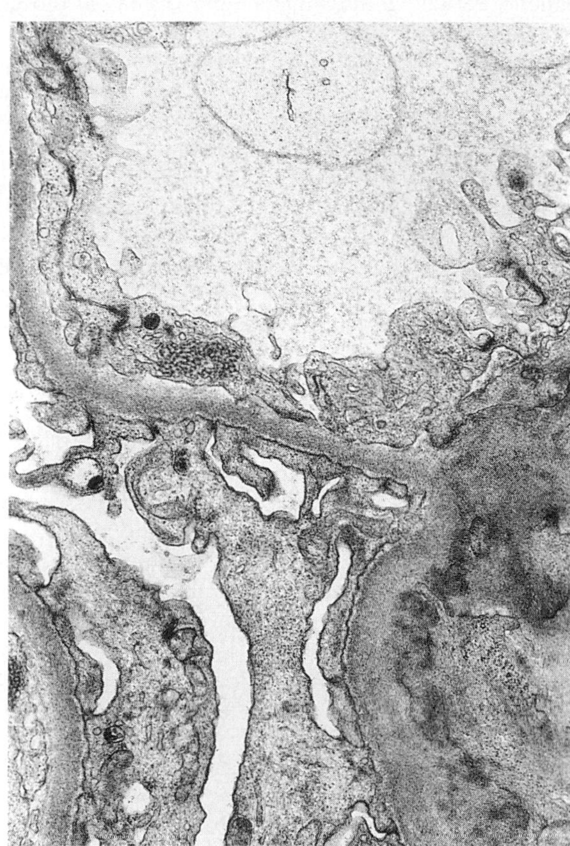

Fig. 65-58 Lupus nephritis. Electron-dense deposits are in the mesangium. Notice endothelial cell tubuloreticular structure.

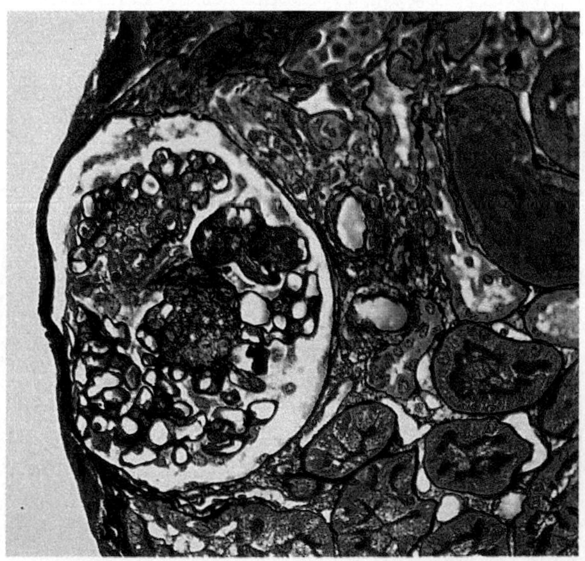

Fig. 65-59 Focal proliferative lupus glomerulonephritis. In this glomerulus, there is segmental increase in cellularity, primarily involving mesangial regions and with few leukocytes in the corresponding capillary lumens. Eosinophilic deposits are in mesangial regions. (Period acid–methenamine silver.)

gial deposits in all glomeruli and irregular granular capillary wall deposits in some. By EM, in addition to mesangial deposits, there are deposits in subendothelial aspects of some capillary walls, often associated with accumulation of leukocytes in capillary lumens. Peripheral mesangial migration may also occur in these capillary walls.

Diffuse proliferative lupus glomerulonephritis perhaps represents the more severe continuation of the focal proliferative lesion and the full-blown pathologic picture of immune complex–mediated glomerular damage. Typically, there is sharp increase in cellularity involving all or most of the capillary tufts in greater than 50% of the glomerular population; in most instances, most glomeruli exhibit these changes. There is considerable mesangial hypercellularity, sometimes imparting a lobular appearance to the tufts (Fig. 65-60). There are many leukocytes (monocytes and neutrophils most commonly) in capillary lumens; there may be degeneration of these cells, with resulting nuclear debris and hematoxylin bodies. These latter structures are infrequently encountered in current practice and likely represent degenerating nuclei with bound antibody; with hematoxylin and eosin stain, they are lilac colored and are usually clumped together.[206] Capillary walls are thickened, mainly because of large subendothelial deposits, which, when circumferential, are given the antiquated term *wire loops*. Capillary walls may have a double-contoured appearance that results from peripheral mesangial migration and interposition. Massive subendothelial deposits may protrude into the lumens and appear as brightly staining and homogeneous masses termed *hyaline thrombi*. These structures are neither hyaline (whatever that is) nor thrombi. However, true thrombi not related to these lesions have been described as a common finding in some biopsy series. Mesangial deposits are also present, often in large numbers. Local breaks in capillary walls with crescent formation are common. In addition, there is often interstitial edema with accumulation of mononuclear leukocytes. Arterial and arteriolar lesions are uncommon and variable. Accumulation of plasma proteins in the walls of arterioles with degeneration of smooth muscle cells and luminal narrowing (lupus arteriolopathy) and arteriolar thrombonecrotic lesions of thrombotic microangiopathies occur and usually correlate with severe hypertension. True necrotizing arteritis is exceedingly uncommon and may be associated with numerous crescents.

Immunofluorescence reveals mesangial granular and capillary wall granular and confluent granular deposits in virtually all glomeruli. In those with "hyaline thrombi," there are large luminal masses of immune material. Most kidneys with diffuse proliferative glomerulonephritis also are the sites of granular deposits along tubular basement membranes, in the walls of peritubular capillaries, and, rarely, in arterial and arteriolar walls. With crescents, fibrin is in the glomerular urinary spaces, in capillary lumens, and in walls in a linear pattern. As might be expected, EM discloses large and numerous deposits, primarily in mesangial and subendothelial locations (Fig. 65-61). A small number of subepithelial deposits are usually present. Deposits are also in tubular basement membranes, in peritubular capillary walls, and in the interstitium in those instances when extraglomerular deposits are documented by immunofluorescence (Fig. 65-62).

Membranous lupus glomerulonephritis has many of the features of idiopathic membranous glomerulonephritis; however, it should be kept in mind that they are superimposed on the basic lupus glomerular lesion of mesangial immune deposits. By light microscopy, virtually all capillary walls are uniformly thickened, with the degree correlating with the stage of the lesion. Therefore, there are uniform subepithelial deposits with intervening basement membrane projections or

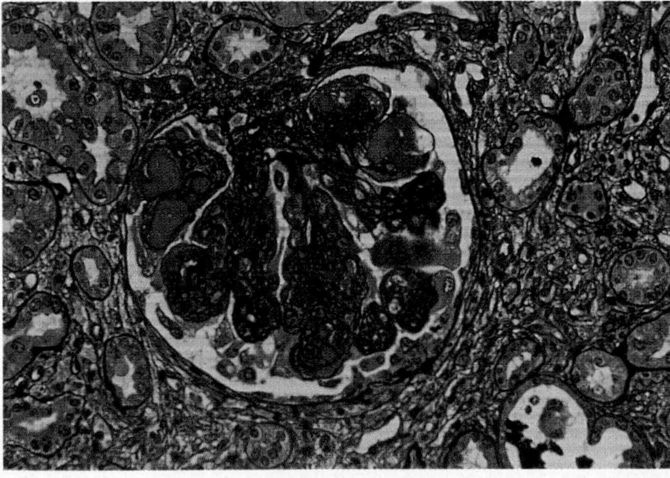

Fig. 65-60 Diffuse proliferative lupus glomerulonephritis with increase in mesangial cellularity, leukocytes in capillaries, and large subendothelial deposits in many capillary walls. There are also large "hyaline thrombi" in the lumens. (Periodic acid–methenamine silver.)

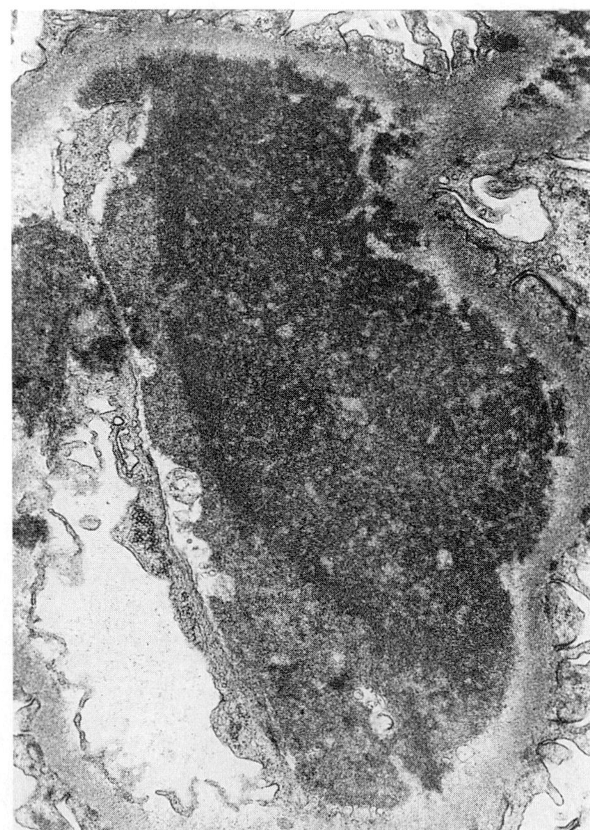

Fig. 65-61 Diffuse proliferative lupus glomerulonephritis with large subendothelial electron-dense deposit. Notice tubuloreticular structure in endothelial cell.

surrounding basement membrane material. Mesangial regions are slightly widened. There is little or no increased cellularity. Immunofluorescence reveals uniform granular capillary wall deposits. Electron microscopy indicates subepithelial electron-dense deposits and basement membrane material between or around deposits. In most instances, at least a few small deposits are found in mesangial regions (Fig. 65-63); they and the tubuloreticular structures distinguish this lupus lesion from idiopathic membranous glomerulonephritis. Rarely, small subendothelial deposits may also be present.

Membranous lupus glomerulonephritis may be combined with any of the other lupus glomerulopathies so that morphologically the glomeruli exhibit features of both simultaneously. For example, with mixed membranous and focal proliferative glomerulonephritis, all glomeruli have subepithelial uniform deposits (and spikes) and some also exhibit segmental increase in cellularity (mesangial and capillary lumens), even with crescents. The immunofluorescence and EM appearances are also merged. Similarly, mesangial proliferative and diffuse proliferative lesions coexist with membranous glomerulonephritis.[7,155,205,207,208]

A semiquantitative system for assessing the severity and potential reversibility of the tissue damage has been devised by investigators at the National Institutes of Health, largely by modifying work done in the 1960s and 1970s.[209] This activity and chronicity index, which has limitations because of lack of regular reproducibility, is used as a guide to therapy and prognosis. It divides the changes into active and chronic lesions and assigns values to each change to produce a numerical assessment (Table 65-11). These indices are currently in clinical use, though there is some skepticism concerning their value.[210]

Differential diagnosis. The pathologic evaluation of renal tissues is not limited to a consideration of the light microscopic abnormalities, and so the problem of distinguishing lupus from other forms of glomerulonephritis is not a particularly great one. Furthermore, although renal involvement may clearly be the initial manifestation of SLE, renal biopsies should be accompanied

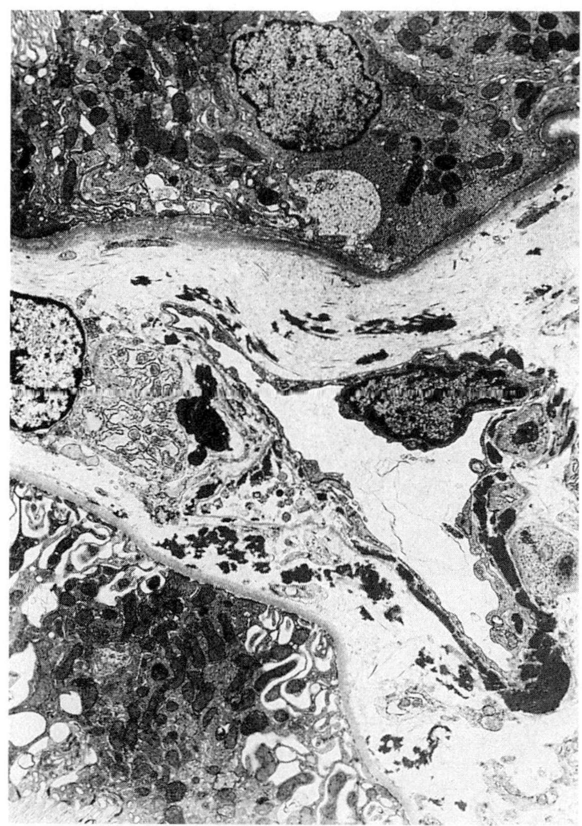

Fig. 65-62 Lupus nephritis with numerous interstitial and peritubular capillary electron-dense deposits.

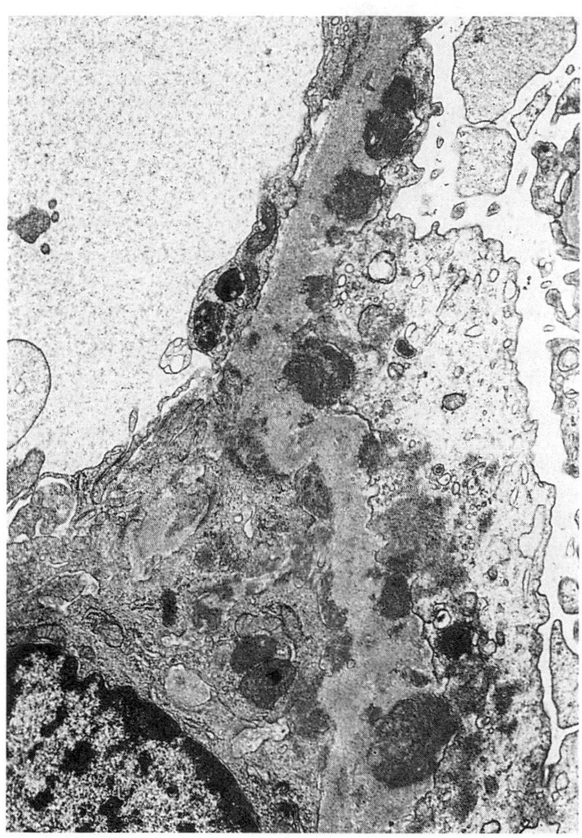

Fig. 65-63 Membranous lupus glomerulonephritis with subepithelial deposits and small mesangial deposits.

Table 65-11 Lupus nephritis scoring system of renal pathology

Active lesions	Chronic lesions
Glomerular	
Hypercellularity	Sclerosis
Leukocytic infiltration	Fibrous crescents
Necrosis, karyorrhexis*	
Crescents—cellular*	
"Wire loops"	
"Hyaline thrombi"	
Tubulointerstitial	
Mononuclear leukocyte infiltration	Interstitial fibrosis tubular atrophy

Each lesion is assigned a grade of 0, 1, 2, or 3; those with an asterisk are doubled. Add all active lesions for activity index (maximum number 27) and chronic lesions for chronicity index (maximum number 12).

by an appropriate clinical history and pertinent laboratory data, thereby providing information that the patient has lupus erythematosus. Hence, in most instances of tissue examination, it is a matter of determining the classification of the lesion and the extent of activity and chronicity. The concern about differentiating lupus from other glomerulonephritides is small. The immunofluorescence and EM features of focal proliferative and diffuse proliferative lupus glomerulonephritis, with full-house immunofluorescence and extraglomerular deposits along with the ultrastructurally defined tubuloreticular structures are so characteristic as to be diagnostic. However, the membranous variant, with no increased cellularity, may occur in a patient not known to have lupus either clinically or serologically; this variant requires careful consideration and differentiation from idiopathic membranous glomerulonephritis. Often, but not always, the deposits also contain C1q in lupus and not in the idiopathic or other forms of membranous glomerulonephritis. Ultrastructurally, in lupus small or larger mesangial deposits are present, small subendothelial deposits may be present, and endothelial cell tubuloreticular structures, especially if more than a small one or two, all point to lupus and away from virtually all other glomerulopathies, with two exceptions. These are the glomerulonephritis that occurs in mixed connective tissue disease (the renal lesions are identical to all forms of lupus glomerulonephritis) and membranous glomerulonephritis, perhaps related to hepatitis B or C infection, in an HIV-infected individual. The hepatitis component may be responsible for mesangial and subepithelial deposits, and HIV infection is associated with numerous tubuloreticular structures.[155,205]

Clinical presentation. Although one would intuitively expect each form of glomerulonephritis to have reasonably unique clinical and laboratory manifestations of renal disease, such is not the case in all patients.[203] At one extreme, there may be no evidence of renal involvement despite clear-cut and severe glomerular injury (as in the diffuse proliferative lesion); at the other extreme, nephrotic syndrome may be the presenting manifestation of focal proliferative glomerulonephritis, diffuse proliferative glomerulonephritis, and membranous glomerulonephritis.[155,211] Nevertheless, in many instances clinical features do reflect the changes. The mildest form of glomerular injury, mesangial glomerulonephritis, may be clinically silent or may be associated with mild hematuria or low-grade proteinuria. Focal proliferative glomerulonephritis usually presents with proteinuria, occasionally in the nephrotic range, hematuria, and some degree of renal insufficiency. Diffuse proliferative glomerulonephritis presents with considerable hematuria, heavy proteinuria, renal insufficiency (often severe and progressive), and hypertension. Last, membranous glomerulonephritis is associated with the nephrotic syndrome.[155,205]

Therapy for lesions that cause more significant clinical manifestations usually consists of corticosteroids, most often with cyclophosphamide. This is directed at patients with active (usually proliferative) lesions, especially in glomeruli; the use of the activity and chronicity indices has permitted some selection of patients who may benefit from this form of treatment. The prognosis for the different classes of glomerulonephritis differs, with mesangial proliferative the best, with little or no progression to advanced renal failure, and diffuse proliferative the worst, with a high percentage of untreated patients progressing to ESRD. Focal proliferative glomerulonephritis is intermediate. Membranous glomerulonephritis usually is a very slowly progressive disorder; however, combined with either focal proliferative or diffuse proliferative glomerulonephritis, the prognosis is poor in untreated patients and is about the same as diffuse proliferative glomerulonephritis.[155,205,212,213] Confusing the therapeutic and prognostic considerations is the well-known ability of the glomerular lesions to transform into a different type either spontaneously or under the influence of therapy. For example, focal proliferative may change to diffuse proliferative, and diffuse proliferative to membranous glomerulonephritis.[155,205] Most clinical manifestations and therapies consider glomerular involvement; tubulointerstitial involvement may be the dominant feature in some patients.[205]

Acute interstitial nephritis

Acute interstitial nephritis (AIN), also known as acute tubulointerstitial nephritis, is a form of renal interstitial injury characterized by infiltration of mononuclear leukocytes with or without eosinophils and a variable component of tubular inflammation with interstitial edema. Occasionally a granulomatous component may be present. This form of renal injury has an incidence of 1% in autopsy kidneys.

AIN may be classified by pathogenic mechanisms such as cell-mediated immunity, direct renal infection by viral and certain bacterial organisms, humoral immune responses, and hereditary and metabolic disorders[214,215] (Table 65-12). These forms cannot be distinguished morphologically and require clinicopathologic correlation.

Etiology and Pathogenesis. Various pathways lead to renal interstitial mononuclear inflammation[216] (Table 65-12). Cell-mediated immunity of the delayed hypersensitivity type is the likely mechanism for AIN secondary to drugs and as a renal reaction to systemic infection such as streptococcal disease, diphtheria, and measles.[217-219] Drugs, particularly antibiotics and nonsteroidal anti-inflammatory agents or their metabolites, may bind to tissue or altered tissue components, evoking a T-cell response[220] (Table 65-13). This response is idiosyncratic, not dose related, and may take up to 1 year of use to occur with nonsteroidal anti-inflammatory drugs (NSAIDs).[221]

Humoral immunity is a better understood but less frequent mechanism inducing AIN. Anti–tubular basement membrane

Table 65-12 Etiologies of acute interstitial nephritis

Etiology
Drug-induced
Allergic (hypersensitivity)
Toxic
Idiopathic
Immunologically mediated
Anti–tubular basement membrane disease
Immune complex deposition
T-cell mediated (sarcoid, idiopathic)
Infection associated
Reactive (viral, bacterial)
Direct (viral, leptospiral, rickettsial, mycobacterial)
Hereditary and metabolic
Crystal formation
Paraprotein mediated
Toxins
Hereditary
Radiation
Idiopathic

antibodies may occur as an idiopathic process or in renal transplant recipients with linear staining of tubular basement membranes for IgG and C3. However, in the setting of AIN, anti–tubular basement membrane antibody may be a secondary process when drugs interact with a portion of the basement membrane leading to macrophage digestion and presentation of new autoantigens in the 48 to 70 kD range.[222] In these cases, the antibody usually does not result in significant disease.

Other suggested mechanisms for the induction of AIN include augmented expression of MHC antigens and adhesion molecules on renal cells, possibly through upregulation of interferon-gamma and other proinflammatory cytokines.[223] Idiopathic forms of AIN also exist, including AIN associated with uveitis[224] and renal involvement in sarcoidosis.

Pathology. Grossly, kidneys with AIN are enlarged, with a district corticomedullary junction and pale cortex. Histologically there is diffuse interstitial edema with variable infiltrates of lymphocytes, plasma cells, and monocytes/macrophages in the cortex (Fig. 65-64). The inflammation may be prominent at the corticomedullary junction. Eosinophils compose from zero to 10% of the infiltrate, being more prevalent in the hypersensitivity forms of AIN.[225] When present, eosinophils often have a patchy distribution or may form scattered microabscesses. Neutrophils and basophils are infrequently observed; large numbers of neutrophils indicate acute infectious interstitial nephritis. Occasionally granulomas occur, particularly with sulfa-containing drugs, oxacillin, mycobacterial infection, and sarcoidosis[226] (Fig. 65-65 and Table 65-14). The lymphocytes and macrophages extend into the walls and lumens of tubules (tubulitis), with distal tubules affected most commonly.[227] There are scattered degenerating and regenerating tubular cells; desquamated tubular cells may be observed in tubular lumens. Proximal tubules often have focal loss of brush border staining. Immunofluorescent studies are usually negative but infrequently reveal granular deposits of complement in the tubular basement membranes and, rarely, fibrin in the interstitium. In cases of anti–tubular basement membrane antibody formation there is linear staining along these structures for IgG.

Direct renal infection may invoke a morphologic picture identical to AIN. Viral infections produce this form of interstitial inflammation, and if inclusions are not observed within cells in the kidney, a specific diagnosis may not be possible.[228] Certain

Table 65-13 Drugs that can induce acute interstitial nephritis

Diuretics	Nonsteroidal anti-inflammatory drugs
Chlorthalidone	Acetaminophen
Chlorothiazide	Aspirin
Hydrochlorothiazide	Clometacine
Furosemide	Diclofenac
Thienylic acid	Diflunical
Triamterene	Fenoprofen
Antibiotics	Ibuprofen
Acyclovir	Indomethicin
Amoxicillin	Ketoprofen
Ampicillin	Mefanamic acid
Carbenicillin	Naproxen
Cefaclor	Phenazone
Cefotaxime	Phenylbutazone
Cephalothin	Sulindac
Cephradine	Tolmetin
Cephalexin	Zomepirac
Chloramphenicol	**Other**
Ciprofloxacin	Aldomet
Erythromycin	Allopurinol
Ethambutol	Amphetamine
Foscarnet	Azathioprine
Gentamicin	Carbamazepine
Lincomycin	Captopril
Methicillin	Cimetidine
Minocycline	Clofibrate
Nafcillin	Contrast agents
Oxacillin	Glafenin
Penicillin G	Heroin
Polymyxin sulfate	Herbal medicines
Rifampin	Phenindione
Spiramycin	Interleukin-2
Sulfonamides	Phenobarbital
Tetracyclines	Phenylopropanolamine
Vancomycin	Phenytoin
	Recombinant interferon-α
	Sulfinpyrazone
	Warfarin

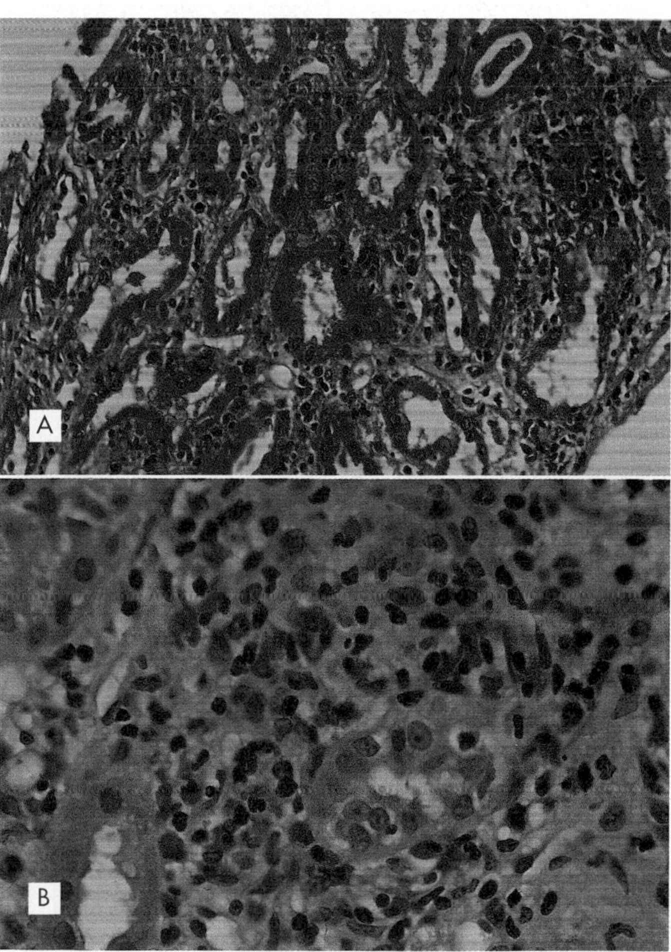

Fig. 65-64 A, Acute interstitial nephritis. There are interstitial edema, mononuclear inflammatory cells in the interstitium and tubular walls, and focal tubular cell degeneration. (Masson's trichrome.) **B,** The interstitium and tubules are similar to those in **A,** with the addition of eosinophils.

bacteria, including leptospirae, rickettsiae, and mycobacteria, also induce a cell-mediated response in the kidney.

EM studies do not contribute significantly to the diagnosis, though may be used to identify eosinophils.

Differential diagnosis. The differential diagnosis includes acute tubular necrosis with a mild inflammatory infiltrate; in fact, there may be no reason to distinguish between the two because there is considerable overlap in the initiating injuries resulting in these abnormalities. Differentiation from acute transplant rejection, which is a form of AIN, can be extremely difficult. A careful history, search for systemic illness, and clinicopathologic correlation are required to ascertain the underlying cause of AIN. Granulomatous AIN must be differentiated from sarcoidosis and infections such as tuberculosis.

Clinical presentation. Patients with AIN have varying degrees of acute renal failure.[229] There may be microscopic or macroscopic hematuria, low-grade proteinuria, and granular, hyaline, or white blood cell casts. When AIN is a hypersensitivity allergic response, there is often fever, rash, arthralgia, eosinophilia, and eosinophiluria. However, NSAIDs may not induce typical allergic symptoms and may be used for as long as a year before inducing symptoms. After withdrawal of the offending agent, most patients fully recover if the disease process is acute; those with NSAID-induced lesions may improve more slowly. Bad prognostic indicators for all patients with AIN include older age at onset, renal failure for more than 3 weeks, and more severe renal cortical inflammation. Steroids are occasionally used to improve renal function more rapidly.

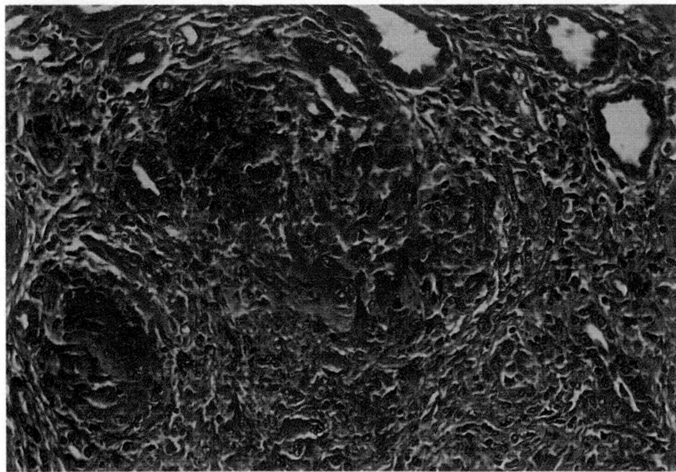

Fig. 65-65 Acute interstitial nephritis. The renal interstitium is edematous and contains confluent noncaseating granulomas with numerous multinucleated giant cells. (Masson's trichrome.)

Table 65-14 Causes of granulomatous interstitial nephritis

Causes
Drug hypersensitivity
Infection
Foreign bodies or particles
Sarcoidosis
Nephritis with uveitis syndrome
Wegener's granulomatosis
Idiopathic

Infectious diseases

Acute infectious interstitial nephritis

Acute infectious interstitial nephritis, also known as acute pyelonephritis, is a response to infection characterized primarily by neutrophil infiltrates in the kidney. It is classified by the route of infection, either ascending from the lower urinary tract or by hematogenous spread.[230] Ascending infection initially affects the medulla, with secondary cortical inflammation. Hematogenous spread begins in the cortex, often in association with microabscesses. Focal bacterial nephritis is infection limited to a single lobe of the kidney. Emphysematous pyelonephritis is characterized by the accumulation of gas in renal and perirenal tissues secondary to carbon dioxide production, primarily by gram-negative bacteria.

Etiology and pathogenesis. Bacterial and fungal organisms generally induce acute infectious interstitial nephritis; exceptions to this include the organisms that cause leptospirosis, toxoplasmosis, legionnaires' disease, and a few other organisms that evoke a mononuclear inflammatory response (Table 65-15). Viral infections do not induce neutrophilic infiltrates, and *Mycoplasma* organisms result in granulomatous inflammation. The more frequent pathway of renal infection is the ascending route from the lower urinary tract.[231,232] *Escherichia coli* is the most common offending organism initially infecting the urethra and bladder. The pathogen then travels up the ureter or ureters and periureteral lymphatics; this may or may not be associated with vesicoureteral reflux or obstruction. Bacterial attachment to the urothelium is facilitated by the P pili (fimbriae) found on some strains of *E. coli,* which are believed to play an important role in this pathway of infection.[233,234] The organisms gain access to the kidneys at the fornices and adhere to the renal epithelium in the collecting ducts and distal tubules, ultimately reaching the cortex through the medullary rays. Neutrophils accumulate in the peritubular capillaries in response to the infection and then migrate into the interstitium and tubules. The considerable parenchymal damage often observed in infectious interstitial nephritis is largely secondary to neutrophil activation with subsequent release of lytic enzymes and oxygen radicals. Tubular rupture occurs and bacteria gain access to the interstitium, inciting an additional inflammatory response.

Table 65-15 Organisms causing acute infectious interstitial nephritis

Ascending infection
Escherichia coli (most common)
Klebsiella
Proteus species
Pseudomonas
Streptococcus faecalis
Serratia
Alcaligenes species
Staphylococcus albus
Hematogenous spread
Staphylococcus aureus
Actinomyces species
Brucella species
Yeasts
Filamentous fungi
Mycobacterium tuberculosis

The hematogenous route of infection occurs in patients with bacteremia or sepsis. In experimental models, bacteria enter the peritubular capillaries with subsequent spread to the interstitium, initially infecting the cortex and then extending to other parts of the kidney. Multiple foci of cortical infection may be observed, and focal abscess formation is common.

Pathology. Grossly, the affected kidney is swollen, has a bulging surface, and may contain small abcesses (Fig. 65-66). On cut surface, infected papillae are blunted, congested, and have a purulent exudate. Foci of necrosis may be present, with zones of hyperemia alternating with white streaks extending between the cortex and medulla. Medullary abscesses are associated with ascending infection and those in the cortex with hematogenous seeding.

Microscopically, there is neutrophil infiltration in the interstitium, tubules, and peritubular capillaries (Fig. 65-67). In ascending infection, medullary and papillary inflammation is predominant, and neutrophils often collect in tubular lumens, forming microabscesses. Inflamed tubules may rupture, spilling Tamm-Horsfall protein and other tubular contents into the interstitium. When infection occurs hematogenously, there is cortical inflammation, with small abscesses and sparing of the papillae. Tubular cells are necrotic. Proximal cells show more vulnerability than cells of the distal tubules or collecting ducts though the latter more often have abscesses. The interstitium is edematous, and there may be areas of hemorrhage. If the infection has been present for a week or more, there is a concomitant mononuclear inflammatory infiltrate. The glomeruli and vasculature are not involved unless entrapped in an abscess or area of necrosis. Immunofluorescence and EM studies do not contribute to the diagnosis.

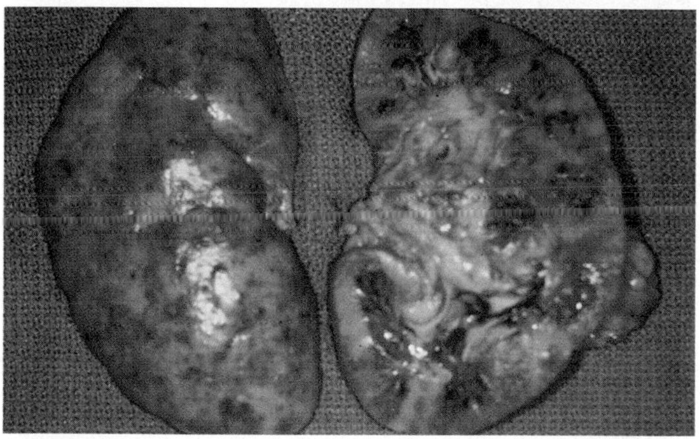

Fig. 65-66 Acute infectious interstitial nephritis. The kidney is from a patient with acute lymphocytic leukemia and systemic candidiasis. There is swelling with focal hemorrhage and small abscesses in the cortex.

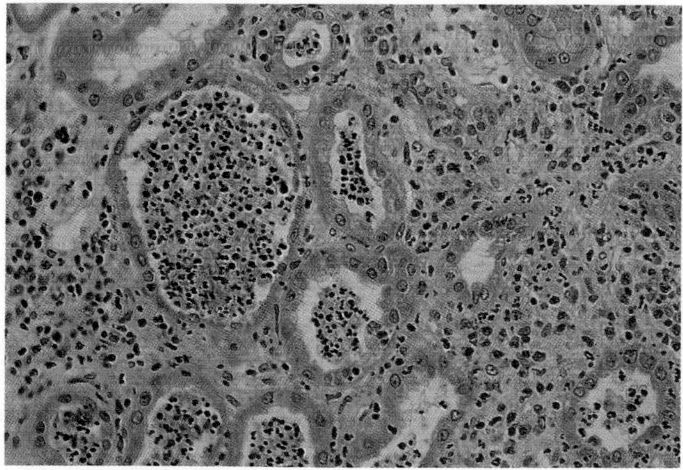

Fig. 65-67 Acute infectious interstitial nephritis. Neutrophils are within dilated tubular lumens and the edematous interstitium.

Differential diagnosis. Few other renal diseases mimic acute infectious interstitial nephritis. There is little difficulty in arriving at a diagnosis with nephrectomy or autopsy specimens. In renal biopsy tissue, areas adjacent to infarcted parenchyma display edema and neutrophils with or without hemorrhage and necrosis. However, the clinical setting allows for differentiation of these entities.

Clinical presentation. Patients with acute renal infection have fever, chills, and flank pain. There may be dysuria with urinary frequency, and with severe bilateral involvement there is renal functional impairment. Urine analysis reveals bacteria, pyuria with white blood cell casts, and variable hematuria. Urine culture should be performed and appropriate antibiotic therapy instituted as soon as possible.[235]

Chronic interstitial nephritis

Chronic interstitial nephritis is a renal lesion in which the primary abnormality is interstitial fibrosis with mononuclear leukocytic infiltrates and associated tubular atrophy. This chronic damage is unrelated to underlying vascular or glomerular injury, though changes of these renal elements may also occur in kidneys with chronic interstitial nephritis.

The disorder may be classified by cause. Obstruction and reflux induce chronic interstitial nephritis, usually with a component of infection. Other etiologic factors include drugs, radiation, uric acid, unusual miscellaneous diseases such as Balkan nephritis, Sjögren's syndrome and familial forms. These may all have a similar appearance, and classification requires clinicopathologic correlation. Unique morphologic forms of chronic interstitial nephritis, including xanthogranulomatous pyelonephritis, malakoplakia, and megalocytic interstitial nephritis, warrant separate classification.

Etiology and pathogenesis. The most common forms of chronic interstitial nephritis are those associated with reflux (reflux nephropathy) or obstruction (Table 65-16). *Reflux* entails the backflow of urine up the ureters to the kidney

Table 65-16 Causes of chronic interstitial nephritis

Obstruction*
Reflux*
Bacterial infection
Sjögren's syndrome
Drugs (lithium compounds, NSAIDs†)
Balkan nephropathy
Radiation
Juvenile nephronophthisis
Familial

*Usually with a component of infection.
†NSAID use more often causes papillary necrosis.

upon voiding. It results from abnormal positioning of the ureterovesical junction or inadequate length of the intravesical ureter.[236,237] This is found most commonly in children under 5 years of age when reflux tends to occur, with the abnormality subsiding after growth and lengthening of the ureter. A pig model has been used to demonstrate the role of the compound papillae at the renal poles during reflux; these papillae have large ducts of Bellini with broad openings, which allow refluxed urine greater access to the kidney than the smaller, more angulated openings of the simple papillae elsewhere in the kidney.[238-240] The urine enters the kidney, resulting in tubular rupture or forniceal tears with extension of the urinary contents into the renal parenchyma (intrarenal reflux). Renal infection usually follows and may be necessary for subsequent fibrosis and inflammation of the interstitium.[239]

Obstruction of urinary outflow is also associated with chronic interstitial nephritis, again likely requiring concomitant infection. Calculi, tumors, and prostatic enlargement are some of the more common causes of urinary obstruction. Urine remains in the ureters and kidney, with dilatation of the pelvises (hydronephrosis); ascending infection and chronic tubulointerstitial damage result.[241,242] Uric acid induces injury by initiating an inflammatory response,[243] and radiation directly damages renal tissue.[244] Drugs such as lithium and NSAIDs induce chronic interstitial injury through mechanisms that are not clear; chronic NSAID use more often induces papillary necrosis than chronic interstitial nephritis[245,246] (Table 65-17).

Xanthogranulomatous pyelonephritis is a specialized form of infection-associated chronic interstitial nephritis that may be related to poor urinary drainage or parenchymal hemorrhage in patients with *Escherichia coli* or *Proteus* species infections.[247,248] Malakoplakia and megalocytic interstitial nephritis occur in similar clinical settings to xanthogranulomatous pyelonephritis and are related to an abnormal host response. In patients with these diseases, macrophages are defective, with an inability to digest bacteria fully.[249,250]

Pathology. Grossly, reflux nephropathy has scarring at the renal poles with dilated calyces, overlying thinned parenchyma, and irregular broad scars with contraction (Fig. 65-68). The remainder of the kidney may be normal or have an ischemic appearance with a granular surface. Kidneys with obstruction as the underlying process have diffuse dilatation of the calyces with uniform parenchymal thinning; calculi may be present. The renal surface is smooth or finely granular with shallow scars.

Microscopically, kidneys with chronic interstitial nephritis of any cause have considerable areas of interstitial fibrosis with tubular atrophy and foci of tubular dropout in more severe cases (Fig. 65-69). Tubules may display "thyroidization," a form of tubular atrophy with thinned, dilated tubules containing casts. There is focal tubular rupture with extravasation of Tamm-Horsfall protein into the interstitium. Mononuclear leukocytes, including lymphocytes, monocyte/macrophages, and plasma cells, are in the interstitium, usually in large numbers and occasionally with lymphoid follicles.

If active infection is still present, there may be a component of neutrophils and few eosinophils. Cases of reflux or obstruction demonstrate mononuclear inflammation, fibrosis, and smooth muscle hypertrophy of the involved calyces; the transitional epithelium may be hyperplastic or may have undergone glandular or squamous metaplasia. In reflux nephropathy there is a sharp demarcation between the scarred and pre-

Table 65-17 Causes of papillary necrosis

Causes of papillary necrosis
Analgesic abuse
Acute infectious interstitial nephritis
Sickle cell disease
Nonsteroidal anti-inflammatory drugs
Diabetes mellitus
Obstruction

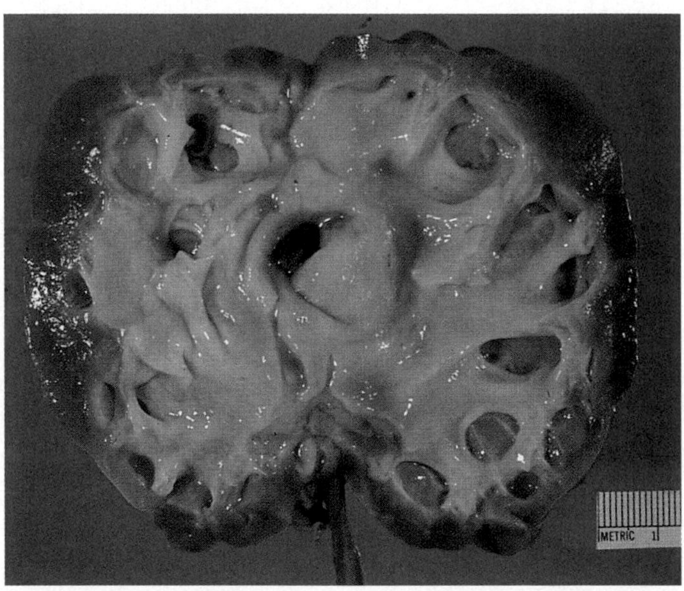

Fig. 65-68 Chronic interstitial nephritis. This kidney, from a patient with obstruction, shows diffuse calyceal dilatation with considerable thinning of the renal parenchyma.

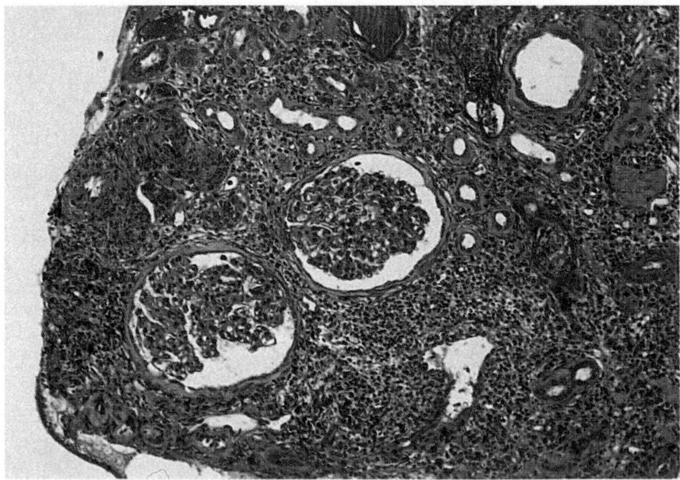

Fig. 65-69 Chronic interstitial nephritis. There is an extensive mononuclear leukocytic infiltrate within the interstitium in association with tubular atrophy, interstitial fibrosis, and considerable tubular dropout. The glomeruli are ischemic with thickened wrinkled capillary walls. (Masson's trichrome.)

served renal parenchyma, and in obstruction there is diffuse fibrosis and atrophy. Arteries and arterioles often have changes of nephrosclerosis, including intimal fibrosis, medial hypertrophy, and hyalinization of the walls of arterioles. Glomeruli have ischemic changes, with capillary wall wrinkling and collapse, periglomerular fibrosis, and often Tamm-Horsfall protein in the urinary space, particularly in obstruction. Preserved glomeruli undergo hypertrophy, and it is not uncommon to find focal and segmental glomerulosclerosis. Immunofluorescence and electron microscopies do not contribute significantly to the diagnosis.

Drug-induced chronic interstitial nephritis may have fewer numbers of leukocytes, particularly when lithium is the offending agent. Radiation nephritis may have an associated glomerular lesion with an appearance similar to thrombotic microangiopathy with prominent mesangiolysis.[251]

Xanthogranulomatous pyelonephritis grossly displays soft yellow nodules and cavities within the thinned parenchyma, particularly around the calyceal system and often with stone formation (Fig. 65-70). The calyces are dilated when obstruction is present. Microscopically there are sheets of foamy macrophages diffusely and in clusters, often with cholesterol crystals and granulomas. Plasma cells and lymphocytes are found in varying numbers with neutrophils when active infection is still present. Tissue destruction can be widespread, with necrosis of all renal elements and granulation tissue formation; this process may spread locally beyond the kidney.

Malakoplakia and megalocytic interstitial nephritis are more often bilateral lesions. Kidneys are enlarged, with yellow nodules in the cortex and medulla and fewer in the pelvis, though this process may be restricted to the pelvis. In malakoplakia the kidney is infiltrated with large histiocytes containing PAS-positive cytoplasm (von Hansemann cells) (Fig. 65-71) and lamellar calcified bodies containing iron and calcium (Michaelis-Gutmann bodies). Few foamy macrophages are observed. Megalocytic interstitial nephritis is similar, but there are no Michaelis-Gutmann bodies in the large histocytes, and glomeruli are more often spared.

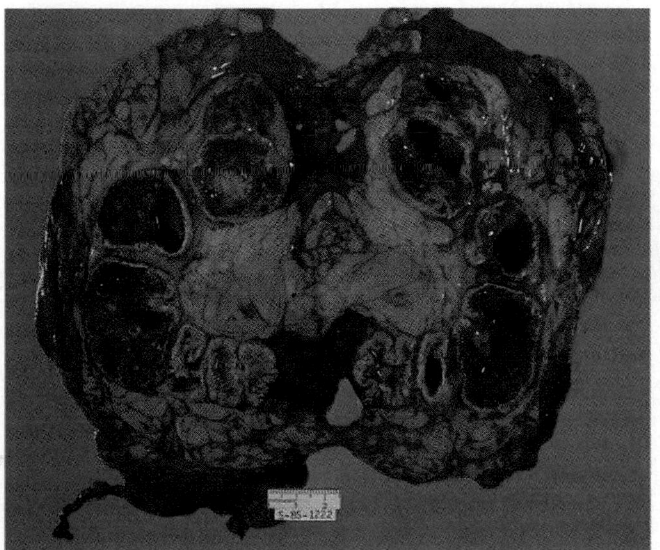

Fig. 65-70 Xanthogranulomatous pyelonephritis with calyceal dilatation and replacement of the attenuated parenchyma by large, yellow nodular tissue. Calyces contain calcified material.

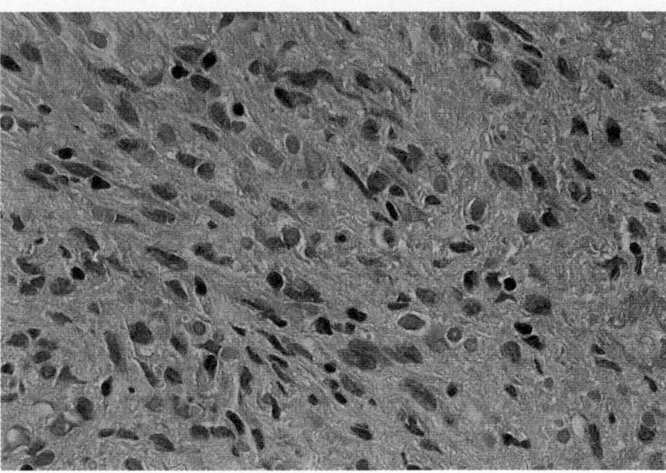

Fig. 65-71 Malakoplakia. The interstitium is replaced by infiltrating macrophages, which contain PAS-positive globules (von Hansemann histiocytes). (Periodic acid–Schiff.)

Differential diagnosis. The diagnosis of chronic interstitial nephritis is not difficult, but differentiating the causes of the disease is more challenging. The pelvicalyceal scarring and inflammation observed in nephrectomy or autopsy specimens with obstruction or reflux aid in determining the cause, as the degree of Tamm-Horsfall protein does in Bowman's space. Drug-induced or radiation nephritis may have less inflammation than chronic interstitial nephritis associated with infection. Xanthogranulomatous pyelonephritis and the other variants may grossly mimic carcinoma but are quite distinctive microscopically. The radiologic picture may be helpful, and, as with all renal lesions, correlation with the clinical findings is required.

Clinical presentation. Chronic interstitial nephritis usually presents with some degree of renal insufficiency when there is bilateral involvement. It is important to determine the cause because this affects therapy and prognosis. When obstruction or reflux are underlying causes, there may be a history of stones or childhood urinary tract infection. Reflux nephropathy is a disease of childhood, and the renal damage has likely occurred during the first 5 years of life; there is a familial component with links to MHC A9, B12, and W15 loci. If active infection is present, patients have flank pain, fever, malaise, and possibly renal failure. Hypertension and nephrotic range proteinuria occur when nephrosclerosis and focal and segmental glomerulosclerosis complicate the interstitial disease. Malakoplakia and to a lesser degree megalocytic interstitial nephritis present as acute renal failure. Treatment includes antibiotics for active infection, correction of reflux or obstruction if they are still present, or drug withdrawal if there is an offending agent. Xanthogranulomatous pyelonephritis and severe end-stage obstruction or reflux usually require nephrectomy.

METABOLIC, HORMONAL, AND TOXIC DISORDERS

Acute tubular necrosis

Acute tubular necrosis (ATN) is a reversible lesion that causes damage to tubular epithelial cells and that is associated with the clinical syndrome of acute renal failure. There are two forms of ATN—ischemic and toxic. The ischemic form is usually the result of peripheral circulatory collapse with reduced organ perfusion, and the toxic form can result from the direct effects of various drugs and chemicals (therapeutic, environmental, industrial) on tubular epithelium.[252]

Etiology and pathogenesis. The ischemic form of ATN results from acute and pronounced renal hypoperfusion as a consequence of circulatory collapse or hypovolemia. Common situations in which this occurs include sepsis, pronounced dehydration after severe diarrheal illnesses, trauma with excessive blood loss or decreased intravascular volume, physically induced muscle injury (crush) with rhabdomyolysis and myoglobinuria, pronounced hemolysis associated with incompatible blood transfusions, malaria, paroxysmal hemoglobinuria, and postsurgical shock (Table 65-18). Reduced renal perfusion especially affects medullary tubules and in particular cells of the thick ascending limb of the loop of Henle which are particularly vulnerable to ischemia/anoxia.[252-254]

A wide variety of substances are nephrotoxic; these include therapeutic agents (antibiotics such as aminoglycosides, cephalosporins, amphotericin B, sulfonamides), heavy metals (such as mercury, lead, platinum, and lithium), radiocontrast agents, organic solvents (such as ethylene glycol and carbon tetrachloride), some NSAIDs, and many other chemical and biologic compounds (Table 65-19). Tubular epithelium is especially susceptible to toxins because of several factors including the elaborate cellular/enzyme and transport systems for organic acids and ions, electrically charged cell surfaces for tubular resportion, and mechanisms for concentrating solutes.[255]

Tubular cell damage ensues; the exact mechanism or mechanisms responsible for acute renal failure are not known, though four sound hypotheses have been proposed. (It is not the intention of this chapter to dissect these in detail; refer to any standard work on renal pathophysiology for a more complete discussion.) The four hypotheses are (1) arteriolar vasoconstriction resulting from activation of renin-angiotensin system or release of endothelin, thromboxanes, renin, and other agents all consequent to glomerulotubular feedback; (2) intratubular obstruction because of casts, desquamated cells, and debris; (3) backleak of fluids from inside tubules through damaged cells into the interstitium; and (4) possible direct effect of uremic toxins on glomerular capillary wall ultrafiltration coefficient.[252-257]

Table 65-18 Causes of ischemic acute tubular necrosis

Causes
Shock
Trauma
Crush injuries
Burns
Transfusion reactions
Nontraumatic rhabdomyolysis
Sepsis
Hemorrhage
Postpartum
Operative, postoperative
Cardiogenic shock
Hepatorenal syndrome

Pathology. The microscopic lesions of ATN are best seen in renal biopsy material rather than autopsy specimens because the effects of autolysis on tubular epithelium make observation of subtle cellular changes difficult if not impossible to ascertain. Consequently, the diagnosis of ATN in postmortem material can be difficult.

Grossly the kidneys are usually moderately enlarged, with pale cortex and congested medulla.

In the ischemic form of ATN the important but by no means sole changes affect tubular epithelium. The major abnormality in tubular cells is loss of staining of brush border, a change best documented with PAS stain. The cells are flattened, with relatively dilated lumens resulting. With these two features, proximal tubules lose their morphologic distinction and become difficult to distinguish from distal tubules (Figs. 65-72 and 65-73). Distal tubular cells are also flattened and the lumens dilated. There is individual cell necrosis, with desqua-

Table 65-19 Causes of toxic acute tubular necrosis

Causes
Heavy metals
Mercury
Bismuth
Gold
Chromium
Uranium
Arsenic
Organic solvents
Carbon tetrachloride
Ethylene glycol
Insecticides
Antibiotics
Aminoglycosides, sulfonamides
Nonsteroidal anti-inflammatory drugs
Anesthetics
Cancer chemotherapeutic agents
Radio-contrast agents
Poisonous mushrooms
Poisonous fish, fish gallbladders

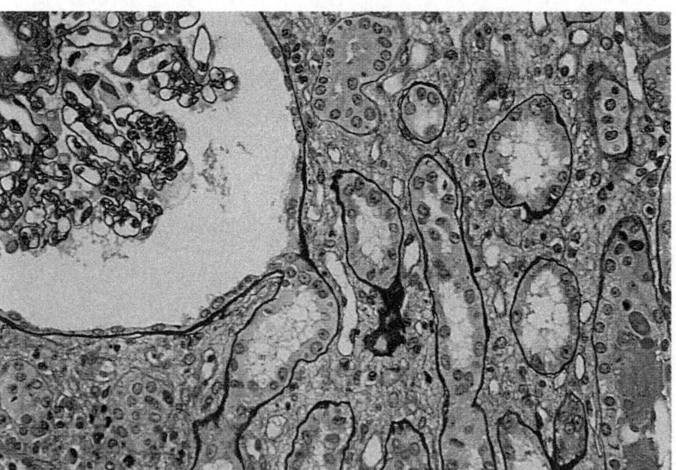

Fig. 65-72 Acute tubular necrosis. There is complete loss of brush border staining for proximal cells. In this particular slide, there is pronounced interstitial edema. Notice tubular metaplasia of the parietal epithelial cells. (Periodic acid–Schiff.)

mation of necrotic cells into the lumens; the site of cell loss appears as a localized defect in epithelial cells lining the tubular basement membrane (Fig. 65-74). This abnormality has been termed the *nonreplacement phenomenon*, though there is no convincing evidence that the missing cell or cells are not replaced. The medulla is especially vulnerable to ischemia because of its relatively small blood flow, especially in relation to the cortex, and so medullary and some cortical tubules may be prominently affected. The cells of the thick ascending limb of Henle are often involved; indeed, some investigators have postulated that acute injury to these cells could explain all the renal functional abnormalities in ATN.[252,256,258] In distal tubules desquamated cells and debris are incorporated into casts formed from precipitated Tamm-Horsfall protein. One of the less common abnormalities in ATN is disruption of the tubular wall, with spillage of contents into the adjacent interstitium. Masses of Tamm-Horsfall protein in the interstitium are occasionally associated with a localized mononuclear leukocytic infiltrate, forming ill-defined granulomas. With resolution of the process responsible for acute renal failure, basophilic cytoplasmic staining and mitotic figures become evident in tubular cells; tubular metaplasia[259] (tubularization) of parietal epithelial cells lining the basement membranes of Bowman's capsules may also occur at this time. There is also mild interstitial edema and mild inflammation with lymphocytes and monocytes. One of the more intriguing abnormalities is the accumulation of many nucleated cells in medullary vasa recta; these cells, which have been documented to be lymphocytes, monocytes, plasma cells, and granulocyte precursors, are in much larger numbers than in other vascular beds. Their presence in autopsy tissue in which the more subtle abnormalities described previously for tubular cells are obscured by autolysis may be interpreted as support for acute tubular necrosis in the appropriate clinical setting.[254,260]

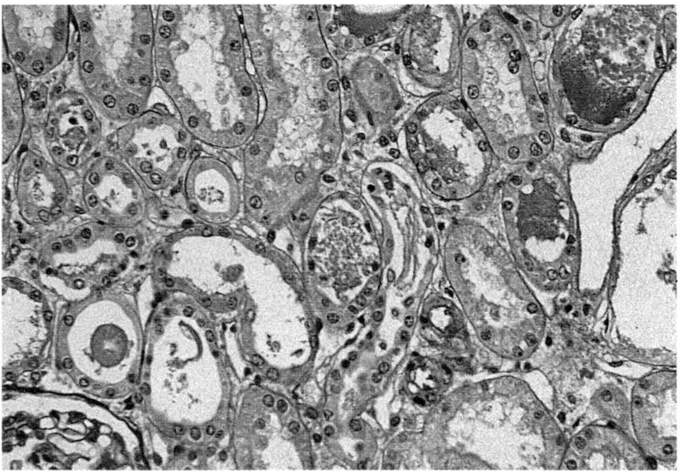

Fig. 65-73 Acute tubular nerosis. The tubule in the center contains granular debris in the lumen; the epithelial cells do not completely line the basement membrane because there are two foci lacking cells (nonreplacement phenomenon). (Periodic acid–Schiff.)

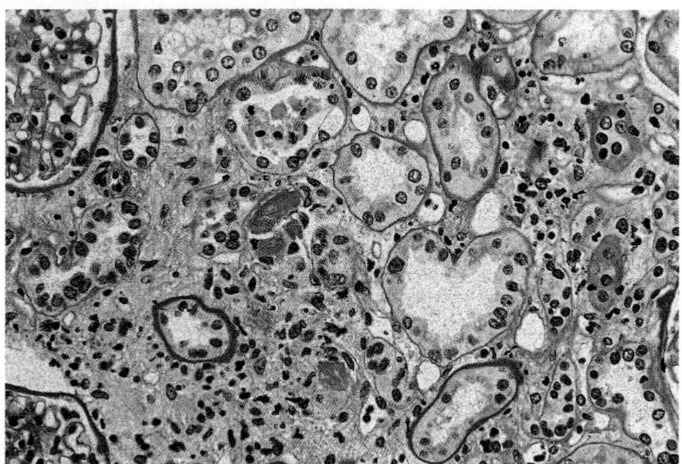

Fig. 65-74 Acute tubular necrosis. Small focus of interstitial Tamm-Horsfall protein. Notice adjacent tubule with abnormal cells and luminal debris. (Periodic acid–Schiff.)

In toxic ATN the morphologic features vary depending on the agent. With mercury ($HgCl_2$), for example, there is nearly complete necrosis of all proximal tubular cells, which resolves if the patient survives. On the other hand, acute renal failure with some agents such as lithium is associated with virtually no morphologic changes in tubular epithelium. Between these extremes are most of the toxins, which result in varying degrees of epithelial cell damage, which may or may not correlate with clinical features. In aminoglycoside-induced renal failure, proximal tubular cells often contain myeloid bodies (concentrically layered inclusions in lysosomes); these structures are indications of cell injury and do not correlate with renal function, though they may be a marker for aminoglycoside administration. Perhaps one of the more interesting situations occurs in patients with ethylene glycol (antifreeze) poisoning.[261] There is extensive tubular cell damage with features of ischemic ATN; in addition, there are numerous intratubular oxalate crystals. These are in far greater numbers than anticipated by the renal failure alone and represent a metabolite of ethylene glycol.[7]

Differential diagnosis. The microscopic lesions are distinctive whether as the sole structural abnormality or in association with or complicating another nephropathy. As described, interstitial edema with little inflammation is usual; with more extensive leukocytic infiltration, the distinction between acute interstitial nephritis (especially related to drug hypersensitivity) becomes blurred. Therefore it may not be possible to decide whether the lesion is primarily acute tubular necrosis or acute interstitial nephritis; in such instances, the term "acute tubulointerstitial nephritis" is used.

Clinical presentation. The nephrologic syndrome resulting from ATN is acute renal failure. There is initial diminution of excretion of nitrogenous wastes (elevated blood urea nitrogen and creatinine), sometimes associated with slight decrease in urine output (nonoliguric acute renal failure). The nonoliguric form accounts for approximately 30% of all cases and is usually associated with a drug-induced mechanism. Pronounced oliguria or anuria may develop during the maintenance stage, with considerable fluid and electrolyte imbalance and uremia. During this time, dialysis is often necessary. In the recovery phase, there is an increase in urine production, often to a considerable degree, with further electrolyte and acid-base instability and ultimate normalizing of serum creatinine.[252]

The ultimate prognosis of ATN depends primarily on the inciting event and the status of other vital organs. The renal status can return to or near base-line function; only rarely does significant permanent functional impairment occur.[252]

Diabetic nephropathy

Diabetic nephropathy encompasses the renal abnormalities associated with diabetes mellitus, including glomerular, vascular, and tubulointerstitial changes.[262] The hallmark lesions are those of glomerular diffuse or nodular increase in mesangial matrix material with thickened capillary basement membranes, plasma protein deposits in the walls of afferent and efferent arterioles, and varying degrees of tubular atrophy and interstitial fibrosis. Arterial nephrosclerosis is also usually present. Immune complex deposition is not a feature of diabetic nephropathy.

Diabetic glomerulosclerosis, the glomerular lesion of diabetic nephropathy, occurs in either diffuse or nodular patterns, which do not correlate with clinical symptoms. There is no other specific classification of diabetic renal disease.

Etiology and pathogenesis. The pathogenesis of diabetic glomerulosclerosis is incompletely understood; however, many of the contributory factors leading to glomerular hypertrophy, scarring, and reduced function have been identified. The diabetic milieu allows glycosylation of proteins, including those of the glomerular extracellular matrix.[263] Advanced glycosylated end products accumulate within glomeruli, and there is an increase in abnormal glomerular collagen synthesis with reduced degradation of extracellular matrix.[264–266] These factors result in matrix expansion, and glycosylated proteins additionally interact with leukocytes, inducing cytokine release and contributing to glomerular growth and hypertrophy.[267] Hemodynamic changes in diabetic patients include augmented glomerular filtration rate and renal plasma flow early in the disease, with subsequent increased glomerular intracapillary blood pressure further causing glomerular injury.[268,269] Ultimately, the final common pathway for scarring ensues, leading to glomerulosclerosis. Microvascular disease may also adversely affect the tubulointerstitium. Hypertension influences the accumulation of plasma proteins in arteriolar walls, with associated ischemic renal injury. These processes interact to induce renal damage, but their relative contributions are not known.

Pathology. Early in the course of the disease the kidneys grossly are enlarged with a smooth surface and are often large and swollen when patients have nephrotic syndrome. As the disease progresses and is complicated by hypertensive changes, the kidneys become progressively smaller and contracted, with a granular surface and irregular subcapsular scars. If infection is present, abscesses may be observed as described in the section on acute infectious interstitial nephritis, or there may be papillary necrosis.[270]

The light microscopic picture varies depending on the severity of renal involvement and the presence of complicating abnormalities. In early disease, glomerular capillary basement membranes are thickened, and there may be no appreciable increase in matrix material. As the lesion progresses, there is a diffuse increase in mesangial matrix material affecting all glomeruli, often with a mild degree of mesangial hypercellularity. Varying degrees of mesangiolysis may be seen. The diffuse lesion occurs alone or with accumulation of mesangial matrix in a nodular pattern (Kimmelstiel-Wilson disease)[271] (Fig. 65-75). When nodules are present, there is great variability in the numbers of glomeruli containing the nodules, as well as the number of nodules per glomerulus. As the lesion ages, matrix material may be replaced by collagen. Capillary microaneurysms often overlie the mesangial nodules, likely resulting from disruption of mesangial attachment of the basement membrane. There are "capsular drops" composed of plasma protein material located on the inner aspect of Bowman's capsule, but these are not specific for diabetic glomerulosclerosis. Segments of sclerosis not infrequently accompany the other glomerular changes and consist of capillary collapse, foam cells, adhesions to Bowman's capsule, and insudative lesions ("fibrin caps"). Glomeruli may also appear ischemic, with thickened and partially collapsed capillary walls and periglomerular fibrosis.

The hallmark vascular lesion is hyalinization (plasma protein deposition) in the walls of afferent and efferent arterioles. The ideal section demonstrates both arterioles simultaneously within one glomerulus. There is usually accompanying arteriolar and arterial muscular hypertrophy, with the arteries also containing intimal fibrosis, as in kidneys with nephrosclerosis.

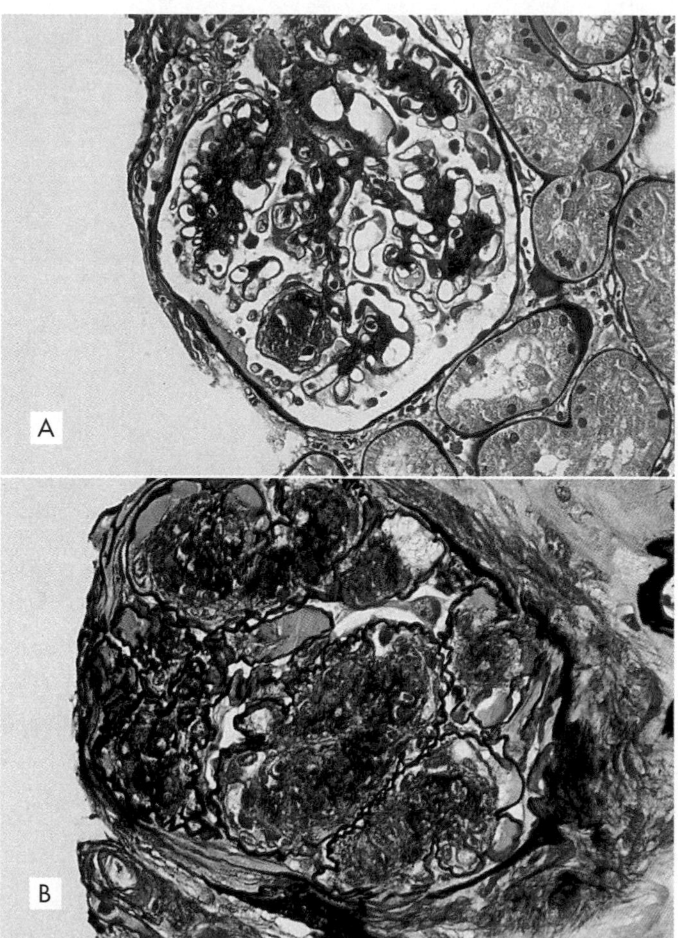

Fig. 65-75 **A,** Diabetic nephropathy. Glomerulus with diffuse expansion of mesangial regions caused by matrix accumulation with normal cellularity. One mesangial region has a nodular appearance. Capillary basement membranes are mildly thickened. **B,** Glomerulus showing considerable nodular expansion of mesangial matrix material with reduced cellularity. Capillary microaneurysms containing plasma protein insudates overlie the mesangial nodules. The capillary basement membranes are considerably thickened, with focal wrinkling. (Periodic acid–methenamine silver.)

There is tubular atrophy and interstitial fibrosis proportional to the severity of the glomerular and vascular injury. In patients with nephrotic syndrome, tubular epithelial cells contain protein reabsorption droplets and lipid vacuoles. The Armanni-Ebstein lesion is a tubular lesion unique to diabetes in which the proximal tubular epithelial cells are enlarged and contain glycogen droplets; because of improved therapy it is almost never encountered today.

Immunofluorescence microscopy reveals "pseudolinear" staining of glomerular capillary and tubular basement membranes for IgG and albumin (Fig. 65-76). Glomerular segments of sclerosis contain IgM and complement in an amorphous pattern segmentally along capillary walls. Arteriolar walls have prominent staining for IgM and complement corresponding to the plasma protein deposits.

EM examination discloses greatly thickened capillary basement membranes with a uniform electron density or accentuation of the fibrillary substructure[272] (Fig. 65-77). Visceral epithelial cell foot processes are effaced and are detached from the underlying basement membrane in areas of segmental sclerosis. Mesangial matrix material is expanded, and rarely there is mesangiolysis, the mechanism by which capillary walls detach and form microaneurysms. Electron-dense masses representing insudative lesions may be in subendothelial locations, but no typical electron-dense (immune complex) deposits are found.

Differential diagnosis. Diabetes must be distinguished from the other nodular or lobular glomerular lesions: amyloidosis, light-chain deposit disease, and MPGN type I (Table 65-11). Immunofluorescent and EM findings are distinctive in these diseases, allowing for differentiation. Patients with diabetes may also have secondary glomerular lesions such as membranous glomerulonephritis, which is found commonly in patients with diabetic nephropathy.[273] In these settings, immune complexes are superimposed on the typical changes of diabetic glomerulosclerosis.

Clinical presentation. Diabetes is usually present for greater than 10 years before renal manifestations become apparent. Low-grade albuminuria may occur for a period of time, followed by significant proteinuria and nephrotic syndrome with hypertension and variable degrees of renal insufficiency. The level of diabetic retinopathy mirrors the degree of renal injury in most cases.[274,275] Therapy includes control of hypertension and glucose levels; a recent study indicates that angiotensin-converting enzyme inhibition may be effective in slowing the onset of diabetic nephropathy.[276]

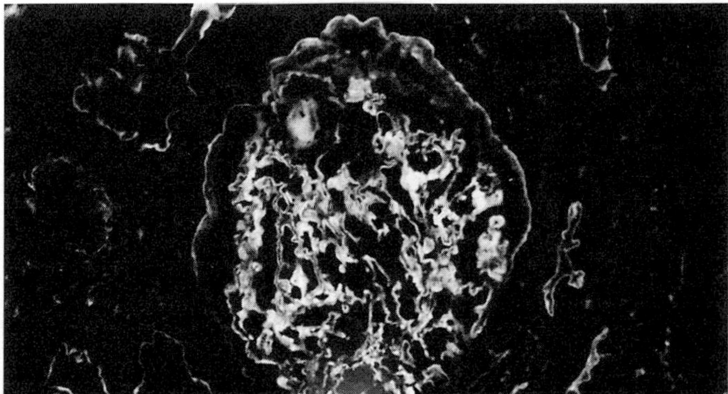

Fig. 65-76 Diabetic nephropathy. "Pseudolinear" staining for albumin along glomerular capillary walls, Bowman's capsule, and tubular basement membranes. There is some accentuation of mesangial regions with albumin as well.

Plasma cell dyscrasias (monoclonal immunoglobulin-induced renal damage)

In this section we discuss renal lesions that are direct consequence of the action or actions of monoclonal proteins (paraproteins) on renal parenchyma. Other lesions that indirectly result from plasma cell dysfunction or antineoplastic therapy, such as infection and tubular necrosis, may also occur. Although the paraprotein may be a complete immunoglobulin (heavy chain, light chain), heavy chain alone, or light chain alone, the major renal lesions are most commonly the result of the action or deposition of the abnormal light chain; infrequently, the entire immunoglobulin molecule or only the heavy chain may produce two of the lesions (Table 65-20). The three renal disorders are Bence Jones cast nephropathy, light-chain deposit disease, and amyloidosis.[277,278] Each lesion is considered separately, though the kidneys in a single patient may be affected by two or all three simultaneously. Amyloidosis is covered in considerably greater depth in Chapter 20. It is

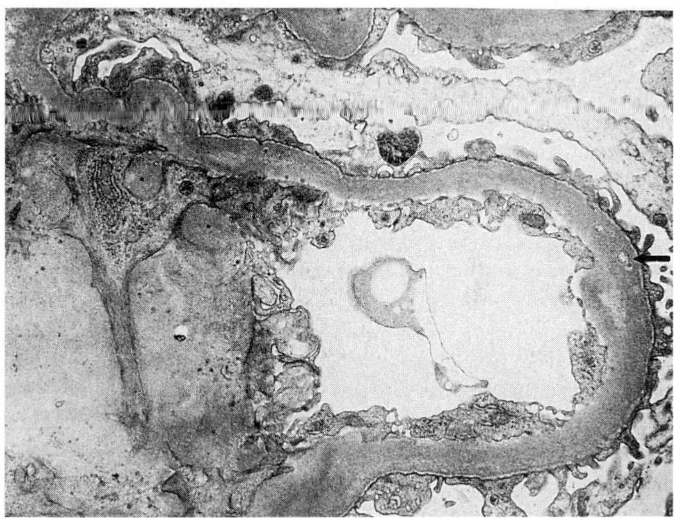

Fig. 65-77 Diabetic nephropathy. Glomerular capillary basement membranes are greatly thickened but retain the usual electron density with scattered striated membranous structures. Visceral epithelial cell foot processes are partially effaced. Mesangial matrix material is expanded, and the capillary lumen has a decreased caliber. There are no electron-dense deposits.

Table 65-20 Paraprotein-induced renal lesions

Kidney lesion	Paraprotein
Bence Jones cast nephropathy	Light chain (λ)
Light-chain deposit disease (systemic)	Light chain (κ) Light and heavy chain Heavy chain
Amyloidosis (systemic)	Light chain (λ VI) Heavy chain

a property of the abnormal light chain that determines the type of renal lesion.[279]

Bence Jones cast nephropathy

Bence Jones cast nephropathy is a tubular lesion occurring in patients with multiple myeloma characterized by the presence of structurally peculiar casts primarily composed of the abnormal light chain surrounded by multinucleated giant cells of the foreign body type.[280,281] It is one of the renal manifestations of multiple myeloma, usually associated with acute or chronic renal failure.

Etiology and pathogenesis. The casts and their consequences result from the action of abnormal light chains, which are freely filtered by the glomeruli; the light chains are partially reabsorbed by cells of proximal tubules and may cause tubular cell necrosis because they are tubulotoxic. The remaining free light chains pass down the rest of the nephron either because the resorptive capacity of intact proximal cells has been exceeded or because of tubular cell necrosis. The light chains precipitate in the tubular lumens; in the distal tubules, Bence Jones and Tamm-Horsfall proteins coprecipitate.[281] However, it appears that Bence Jones protein can precipitate alone because the abnormal casts can also be found in proximal tubules and even Bowman's spaces of glomeruli. It is likely that, as tubular cells are damaged because of the toxic actions of the light chain, defects in tubular wall integrity are produced, thus allowing free communication between interstitium and tubule lumens. It is through these defects that monocytes migrate into tubules, surround the casts, and merge to form multinucleated giant cells. The casts, which may be very large, and associated cellular reaction can and do obstruct individual nephrons. Acute renal failure is therefore multifactorial, with ATN, nephron obstruction, and AIN all contributing.[282]

Pathology. Kidneys with cast nephropathy alone are usually slightly enlarged grossly, primarily because of interstitial edema and inflammation. Microscopically the major abnormality is the presence of tubular casts. The casts have a variety of appearances. With hematoxylin and eosin, they are brightly eosinophilic and refractile; they are PAS negative and fuchsin positive with Masson's trichrome stain. They are not always uniformly stained; some contain elongated crystals, some have a multilayered appearance, and some display altered peripheral staining. This last feature may be the result of amyloid formation in the cast. In addition to these features, the casts characteristically contain "fracture lines" or are fragmented into multiple pieces, some of which have striking geometric shapes (rectangles, squares, parallelograms). As mentioned, a diagnostic feature is the presence of multinucleated foreign-body giant cells surrounding the casts or fragments. Tubular basement membranes are often discontinuous, and the surrounding interstitium is edematous with a small infiltrate of mononuclear leukocytes (Fig. 65-78). With time, tubules may undergo atrophy. The casts are most often located in distal tubules and collecting ducts, but they may also be found in proximal tubules and Bowman's capsules; indeed, myeloma cast nephropathy is the disorder with the longest casts and greatest distribution of them in the nephron.[280–282]

The composition of the casts has been delineated mainly by immunofluorescence. All investigators have documented the abnormal light chain to be present with the greatest degree of intensity. The other light chain and other plasma proteins (immunoglobulins, albumin, and so on) are also present, though usually with less staining intensity. As mentioned, Tamm-Horsfall protein is universally found in casts in the distal nephron. A characteristic feature of the immunofluorescence appearance of the casts is that their peripheries stain more intensely than the centers; this, however, does not necessarily correlate with the infrequently noted amyloid at the casts' periphery.[280,281]

The ultrastructural appearance of the casts is heterogeneous, though the basic structure is of deeply electron-dense material; the casts may be coarsely granular, finely granular, or homogeneous, and they incorporate cytoplasmic debris. Some casts may contain more pale-staining fibrils either admixed with the dense matrix or at the periphery; this material is likely Tamm-Horsfall protein, though amyloid may be similar in appearance. Congo-red staining on the paraffin-embedded tissue is necessary to document the latter protein.[281]

Differential diagnosis. The light microscopic appearance of the casts with fracture lines, and multiple fragments, crystals, and surrounding giant cells, is virtually pathognomonic of myeloma casts; indeed, it is not unusual for a renal pathologist to diagnose this lesion and, hence, multiple myeloma in the absence of clinical or laboratory evidence pointing to that disease. There are isolated single reports describing other disorders with similar renal tubular morphology; a single patient with pancreatic adenocarcinoma died with similar light microscopic tubular lesions and no evidence of a plasma cell dyscrasia at autopsy. A few patients with lymphoproliferative diseases have also been described to have similar renal lesions.[282]

Clinical presentation. Cast nephropathy is associated with renal failure; most patients have acute renal failure, though chronic renal failure may also be a manifestation. Proteinuria is usually evident; however, because light chains are not detected by the dipstick method, they must be sought specifically by urine immunoelectrophoresis, along with a 24-hour urine quantitation. Although at one time this was believed to be an irreversible lesion, reduction of circulating and filtered free light chain by chemotherapy and, in some instances, plasmapheresis has been associated with improvement of renal function and in clearing of casts.[277,283]

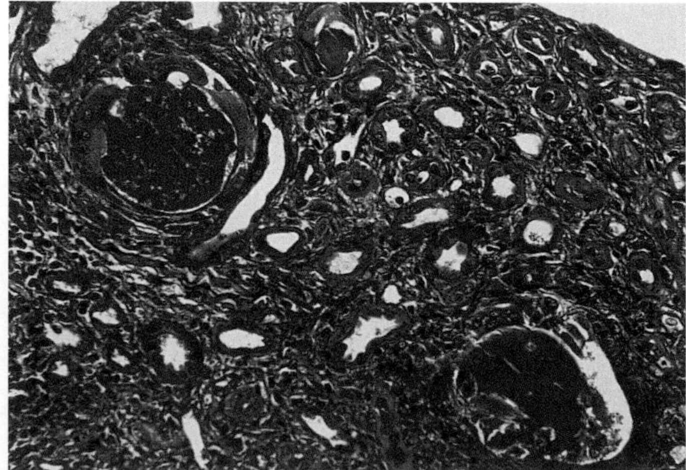

Fig. 65-78 Bence Jones cast nephropathy. Portion of renal medulla with three casts; all are fuchsinophilic, fragmented, and surrounded by multinucleated giant cells of the foreign-body type. (Masson's trichrome.)

Light-chain deposit disease

Light-chain deposit disease is a systemic disorder in which an abnormal monoclonal light chain is deposited in all basement membranes and other extracellular sites. In the kidneys, tubular and glomerular basement membranes and mesangial matrix are the major sites of deposition. In the majority of reported cases, the abnormal light chain is kappa.[277] In a few instances, an intact monoclonal immunoglobulin (light and heavy chain) molecule or an abnormal heavy chain alone are deposited. As a consequence, this disorder is incorrectly named and should probably be termed *monoclonal immunoglobulin deposition disease*.[284]

This systemic disease is considered a "metabolic" disorder and is conceptually and practically similar to AL amyloid.[277]

Etiology and pathogenesis. Light-chain deposit disease is the result of the nonimmune deposition of a monoclonal light chain. It is a disorder resulting from abnormally functioning plasma cells with the production of altered free light chains; multiple myeloma is not universally present. It is likely that more than 60% of the patients have overt myeloma; the rest have either plasmacytosis or numerically and structurally normal plasma cells. In this last instance, increased immunoglobulin synthesis with excess abnormal light chain production has been documented.[285] The property or properties of the abnormal light chain that promote tissue binding are not known, though many features have been investigated, including size (larger or smaller than normal), glycosylation, molecular weight, and isoelectric point. It has been determined, however, that it is an intrinsic feature of the light chain rather than an abnormality of extracellular matrix.[277,279,286,287,289]

Pathology. This disorder requires immunohistochemical analysis, most notably immunofluorescence on unfixed tissue, for diagnosis. Because there may be no light microscopic or ultrastructural lesions to be suggestive of this lesion, diagnosis on renal biopsy tissue mandates that the panel of reagents used for immunofluorescence include antisera to both light chains. By immunofluorescence, linear staining of all basement membranes for the abnormal light chain is evident; the tubular basement membranes are usually more intensely stained than GBM or mesangial matrix (Fig. 65-79). The light microscopic features are variable. Tubular basement membranes may be thickened, with two distinct layers, the outer one representing light-chain deposit. Glomeruli may appear normal or may display any of a variety of changes. Most characteristically, they have a nodular increase in the mesangial matrix without increased cellularity, features that are virtually indistinguishable from diabetic nodular glomerulosclerosis (Fig. 65-80). Capillary microaneurysms are common features in light-chain deposit disease, further emphasizing the similar morphologies.[289] Other patterns of glomerular injury include MPGN, focal and segmental glomerulosclerosis, and crescents.[283,290-292]

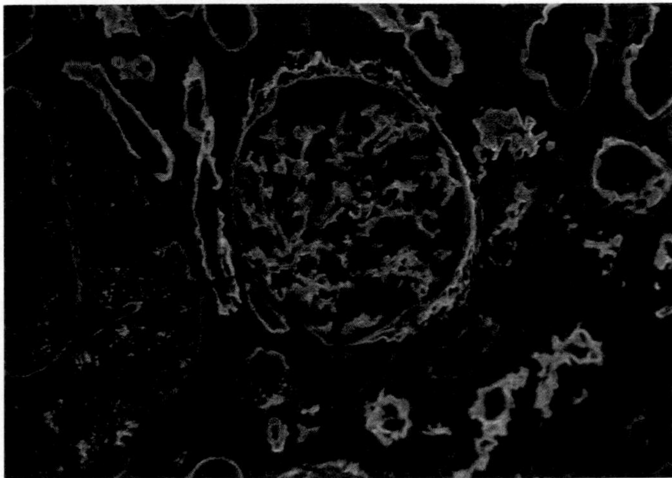

Fig. 65-79 Light-chain deposit disease with staining of all basement membranes for kappa light chain.

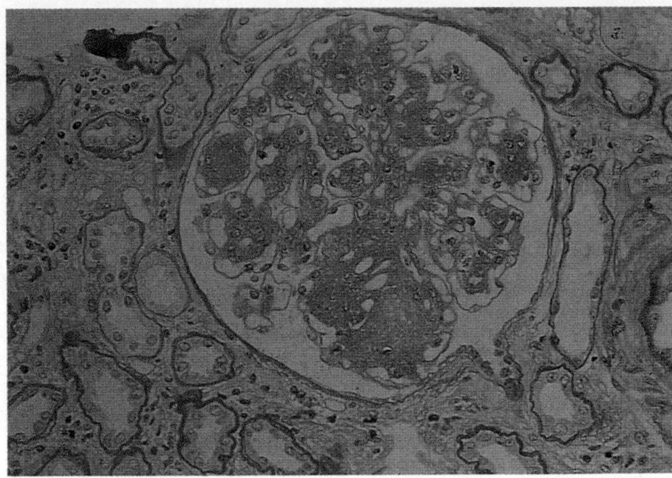

Fig. 65-80 Light-chain deposit disease. The mesangial regions are nodular and largely acellular, and the glomerulus has an appearance not unlike nodular diabetic glomerulosclerosis. (Periodic acid–Schiff.)

Ultrastructurally there are electron-dense granular "deposits" within GBM and in mesangial matrix and along outer aspects of tubular basement membranes (Fig. 65-81). In our experience, some specimens lack deposits in tubules and glomeruli. In glomeruli, there is usually effacement of epithelial foot processes. As mentioned, because there may be neither light microscopic nor EM abnormalities, the only manner of diagnosis rests with immunofluorescence microscopy. Because virtually all diagnostic laboratories use commercially prepared antisera for immunofluorescence, it is important to note that, on occasions, the tissue-bound light chain may be sufficiently abnormal, especially regarding antigenicity, that it may not bind with the antiserum. At times, another company's product may be directed against a conserved antigen, thus providing useful diagnostic information.

Differential diagnosis. Assuming preserved antigenicity of the abnormal light chain and assuming that the laboratory evaluating kidney specimens routinely uses antikappa and antilambda antisera, one can find virtually no differential diagnosis to consider. There are no disorders other than a plasma cell dyscrasia characterized by monotypic light-chain extracellular deposits. If, on the other hand, one approaches the specimen diagnostically by considering the light microscopic changes initially, several disorders need to be considered; these include, most prominently, diabetic glomerulosclerosis, though other glomerulopathies such as mesangial proliferative glomerulonephritis and MPGN need to be excluded (Table 65-21). In all of these, the key element is immunofluorescence.

Clinical presentation. The renal manifestations of light-chain deposit disease are heavy proteinuria (including but not limited to light chains) and renal insufficiency.[272,280] Although this is a systemic disease, the kidneys are most commonly and importantly affected. Other organs with clinically important involvement include the liver and heart.[292] As alluded to previously, not all patients have multiple myeloma when they become ill with renal disease. Most patients have demonstrable free light chains in urine or serum. Renal function deteriorates within a few years. Therapy is aimed at reducing light-chain production and tissue deposition; it includes chemotherapy and, in some instances, plasmapheresis. Unless abnormal light-chain production is abolished, the lesion will recur in a transplanted kidney.[277]

AL Amyloid

Refer to Chapter 20 for a detailed discussion. The pathologic aspects of AL amyloid are virtually indistinguishable from those of other forms of amyloid, especially AA, affecting the kidneys.

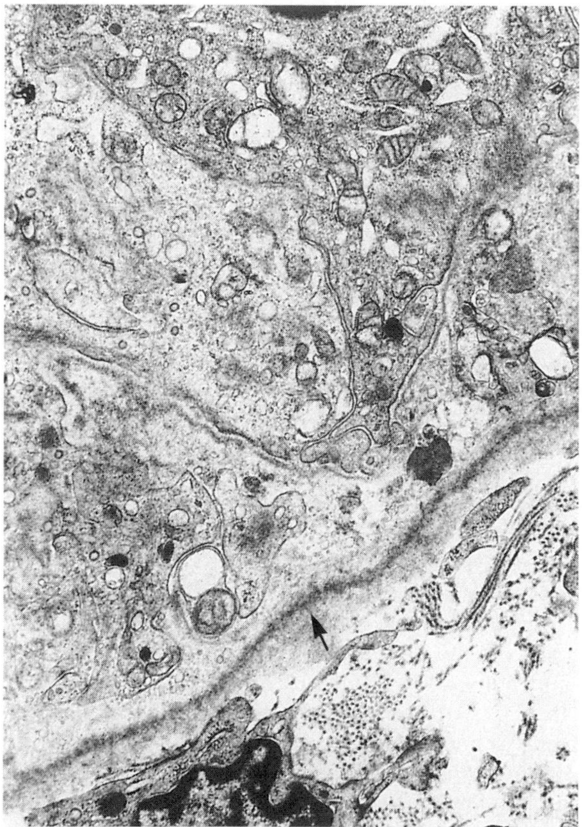

Fig. 65-81 Light-chain deposit disease. There is a thin, dense layer of finely granular "deposit" *(arrow)* of light chain in this tubular basement membrane.

Cryoglobulinemia

Cryoglobulins are plasma proteins that reversibly precipitate at low temperatures; cryoglobulinemic glomerulonephritis is the renal injury that occurs when cryoglobulins deposit in renal vessels, particularly the glomerular capillaries. This entity encompasses the glomerular response to the cryoglobulins, including inflammation, mesangial hypercellularity, and mesangial cell/monocyte interposition in capillary walls.

There are three forms of cryoglobulins, termed *types I, II, and III*[293] (Table 65-22). Type I is composed of a monoclonal immunoglobulin, occurs infrequently, and is associated with plasma cell dyscrasias such as multiple myeloma. Type II includes essential mixed cryoglobulins, the most common form and the type associated with renal disease. It is composed of a polyclonal IgG and secondary monoclonal IgM, usually with kappa light chain, exhibiting rheumatoid factor properties.[294] Infections, connective tissue diseases, and lymphomas may be underlying causes, though one third are classified as essential mixed cryoglobulinemia without a clear underlying cause.[295] Type III is composed of polyclonal IgG and anti-IgG antibody and is the least common form; it is associated with collagen-vascular diseases and chronic infections.

Etiology and pathogenesis. Almost all cryoglobulins affecting the kidney are the type II mixed variety. In 30% of the cases of mixed cryoglobulins there is no underlying cause found; these are termed *essential mixed cryoglobulinemia*. In the remainder, associations are found with B-cell lymphoproliferative disorders or infections, particularly hepatitis B and C. Hepatitis C is currently believed to induce perhaps the largest percentage of cryoglobulins of this type.[296] The IgG involved may be antigen bound or an anti-idiotypic antibody against IgM;[297] alternatively, the IgM may be reacting against the Fc or Fab portions of the IgG. Renal injury in cryoglobulinemia is believed to be secondary to glomerular deposition of serum cryoglobulins. The physicochemical properties inducing cryoprecipitation are not fully understood; however, increased concentration of cryoglobulins caused by glomerular filtration may enhance precipitation in the kidney. The cryoprecipitates activate complement and appear to act as immune complexes, inciting a leukocytic infiltrate in the glomeruli.[298] These cells, particularly monocytes, are activated and often contain cryoglobulins in secondary lysosomes. Further glomerular damage follows from release of lysosomal contents and oxygen radicals from the activated leukocytes.

Pathology. The glomeruli are the most affected part of the kidney, having an "MPGN" appearance by light microscopy (Fig. 65-82). There is a pronounced lobular pattern with mesangial hypercellularity. Capillary lumens are often

Table 65-21 Glomerulopathies with nodular or lobular appearance

Lesion	Nodule composition	Staining: PAS	Staining: Trichrome	Cellularity
Diabetic glomerulosclerosis	Mesangial matrix	Positive	Blue	Decreased
Light-chain deposit disease	Abnormal light chain	Positive	Blue	Normal to decreased
Amyloid	Amyloid	Negative	Pale blue	Decreased
Membranoproliferative glomerulonephritis	Mesangial cells, immune deposits	Mixture Positive and negative	Mixture of blue, rust, fuchsinophilic	Increased

occluded because of extensive infiltration by mononuclear leukocytes, particularly monocytes, which are present in glomeruli in higher numbers with this disease relative to any other glomerular lesion.[299] There are characteristic "plasma protein" thrombi in scattered capillary lumens, which are fuchsin and PAS positive and represent deposited cryoglobulins. Capillary walls have numerous double contours. There may be small numbers of crescents, and visceral epithelial cells contain protein reabsorption droplets. Approximately one third of the time cryoglobulins deposit in arterioles and arteries, where they incite a vasculitis; monocytes and neutrophils are in vessel walls in association with luminal thrombosis and vessel necrosis. The tubules exhibit variable necrosis, with interstitial edema and a mononuclear inflammatory infiltrate.

Immunofluorescence microscopy reveals capillary walls and the luminal plasma protein thrombi to stain for the immunoglobulins composing the cryoglobulin, usually IgG and IgM[300] (Fig. 65-83). There is accompanying C3 with variable light-chain staining. The capillary wall staining is granular, with peripheral accentuation, and thrombi have a globular appearance within capillary lumens. If vessels are involved with the cryoglobulin, the walls stain for the same immune reactants.

EM shows the cryoglobulins to stain as electron-dense material with a curved cylindrical or annular substructure measuring 2.5 to 3 nm in diameter[301] (Fig. 65-84). This mater-

Table 65-22 Types of cryoglobulins and associated abnormalities

Type I	Monoclonal immunoglobulin
	Plasma cell dyscrasias
Type II	Polyclonal IgG, monoclonal IgM
	Infection
	Autoimmune disorders
	Lymphomas
	Idiopathic (essential mixed)
Type III	Polyclonal IgG, polyclonal anti-IgG
	Autoimmune disorders
	Chronic infections

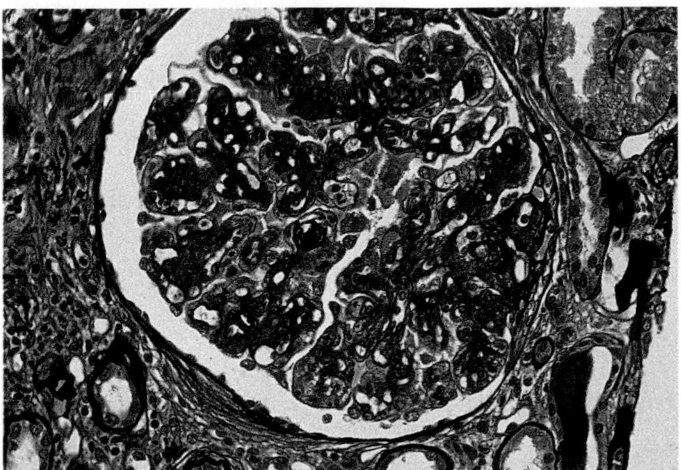

Fig. 65-82 Cryoglobulinemia. Glomerulus with somewhat lobular mesangial expansion and hypercellularity. There are capillary wall double contours, and monocytes are within capillary lumens. Two capillaries have plasma protein thrombi within the lumens. (Periodic acid–methenamine silver.)

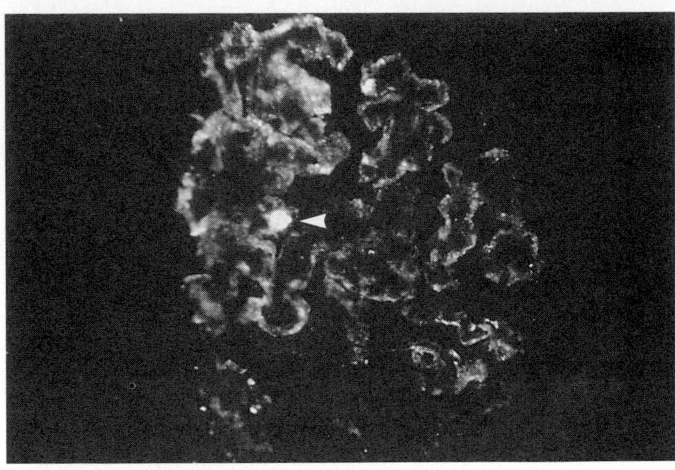

Fig. 65-83 Cryoglobulinemia. There is granular irregular capillary wall staining for IgM with a large intraluminal thrombus also containing IgM *(arrow)*.

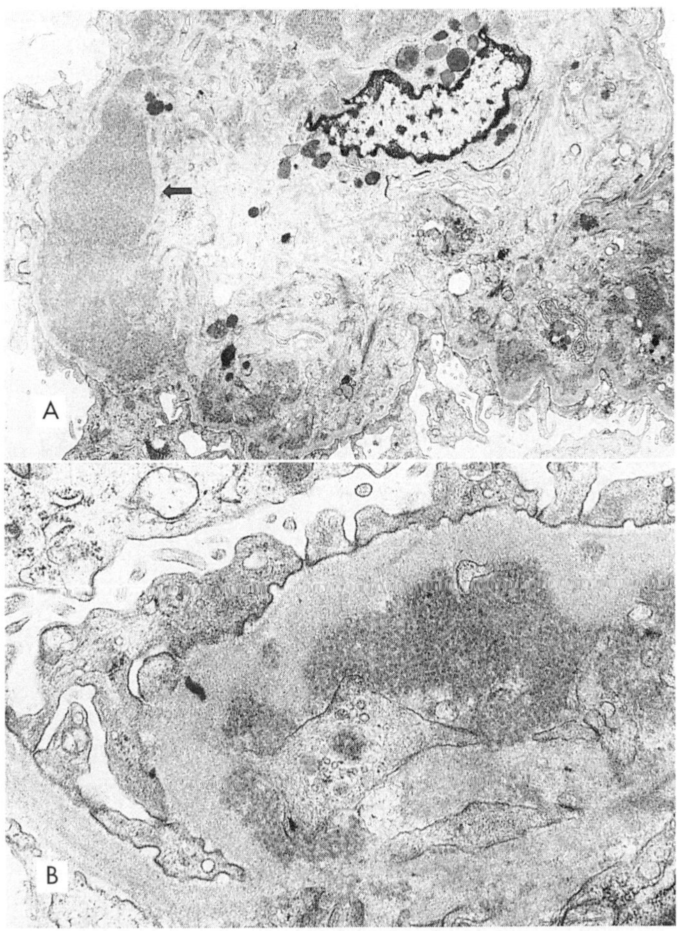

Fig. 65-84 Cryoglobulinemia. **A,** Glomerular capillary walls are thickened by subendothelial electron-dense masses of cryoglobulin *(arrow)* with extensive peripheral migration and interposition of cell cytoplasm. The almost occluded lumen contains a monocyte with numerous secondary lysosomes. Visceral epithelial cell foot processes are extensively effaced. **B,** The subendothelial electron-dense material has an annular to tubular appearance.

ial is located in subendothelial regions, thrombi, and involved vessels. Similar material is less commonly in mesangial regions adjacent to the capillary lumens and may be observed in secondary lysosomes of monocytes that have ingested the cryoglobulin. There is mesangial cell migration and interposition in capillary walls, and monocyte cytoplasm and nuclei are often interposed in capillary walls, with lying down of new subendothelial basement membrane material, forming double contours. Visceral epithelial cell foot process effacement is present, and protein reabsorption droplets are in the cytoplasm of these cells.

Differential diagnosis. The light microscopic pattern of glomerular injury mimics MPGN type I, and light-chain deposit disease and diffuse proliferative lupus glomerulonephritis may also have this appearance. Among these three, capillary luminal thrombi are observed only in the lupus lesion, and the thrombi are not PAS positive. Postinfectious glomerulonephritis has a comparable degree of capillary luminal hypercellularity; however, the leukocytes are more often neutrophils. Immunofluorescent microscopy of cryoglobulins lacks the Clq staining characteristic of lupus and the C3 predominance of postinfectious glomerulonephritis. The EM finding of the typical cylindrical substructure in primarily subendothelial deposits is virtually diagnostic of cryoglobulins.

Clinical presentation. Patients with mixed cryoglobulinemia usually have purpura associated with small vessel cryoglobulin deposition and often have arthralgias and hypertension. Renal involvement occurs in 20% to 60% of patients; it occurs as nephrotic syndrome in one fourth, acute nephritis or renal failure in one fourth, and variable proteinuria and hematuria in the remainder.[302] Complement levels are low, particularly C4; rheumatoid factor is elevated and a cryocrit can be obtained. Therapy is by use of plasmapheresis for removal of cryoglobulins and treatment of any underlying disease such as hepatitis C. In essential mixed cryoglobulinemia, treatment is by steroids, cytotoxic agents, and control of hypertension, with varying degrees of success. It is helpful to follow the cryocrit, which must be obtained with care to ensure an accurate result.

OTHER DISORDERS

Acquired cystic disease

Acquired cystic disease complicates many forms of moderate or advanced structural renal damage with varying degrees of scarring. It is characterized by cysts, tubular epithelial hyperplasia, and often neoplasms, some of which may behave in a biologically malignant fashion. This lesion is most pronounced in patients on long-term dialysis. Unlike many other forms of renal cystic disease with a congenital or hereditary basis, acquired cystic disease appears after many (or most) forms of chronic renal damage.[303]

Etiology and pathogenesis. The cause is unknown, though the appearance of cysts and tumors relates to the duration of renal disease and azotemia; the disorder becomes more prominent and clinically significant when the patient is treated with dialysis. It should be noted that initial reports of acquired cystic disease in the "modern era" stressed its relationship and linked its likely cause to hemodialysis; however, as mentioned, the onset of the changes occurs in relation to renal scarring.[304] One theory suggests that one or more factors produced in response to continued loss of functioning renal mass can result in tubular enlargement and cellular hyperplasia, cyst formation, and renal growth; the factors are not removed by dialysis, thereby explaining continued development and "flourishing" of the disease in that setting. The nature and identification of the factors are clearly not known.[305]

The cysts have been noted to occur in all segments of the nephron, and hyperplasia and tumors also appear to be of diverse origin.[306] Most but clearly not all of the neoplasms arise within cysts, though tumors can arise in solid parenchyma.[307]

Pathology. By definition, kidneys with acquired cystic disease are affected initially by some form of chronic damage; cystic disorders such as ADPKD are excluded in most reports of this entity, though these patients probably can develop superimposed acquired cystic disease.

In mild or early stages of the disease, the kidneys grossly display some degree of scarring, with a few or many cysts randomly throughout the parenchyma, including subcapsular, intracortical, and medullary in location.[308,309] Some investigators have suggested a minimum of 5 cysts to be considered diagnostic.[304] They vary in size from a few millimeters to several centimeters in diameter. With more advanced disease, more numerous cysts are evident, and kidney size may be increased. The cysts frequently contain clear fluid; they may also contain fresh or old blood.[294] Approximately 20% of kidneys with the more advanced lesion will harbor neoplasms (Fig. 65-85). These may be small, cortical, yellow or yellow-white masses, or they may be larger tumors arising either within cysts as polypoid masses or in solid parenchyma. It has been suggested that tumors greater than 1 cm in diameter be considered actually or potentially biologically malignant.[308-310]

Microscopically, the cysts are lined by low cuboidal epithelium. Some cysts may be lined by hyperplastic cells; in these, papillary hyperplasia is common (Fig. 65-86). Overt papillary tumors may arise in larger cysts and have the same microscopic characteristics as similar lesions not associated with acquired cystic disease (Fig. 65-87). Likewise, tumors in the noncystic parenchyma are morphologically similar to their counterparts in a noncystic setting.[307]

In the fully developed instance, the renal parenchymal changes are those of end-stage kidneys. These include complete and, occasionally, segmental sclerosis of glomeruli; extensive tubular atrophy, with interstitial fibrosis and variable interstitial lymphocyte accumulation; and pronounced thickening of artery

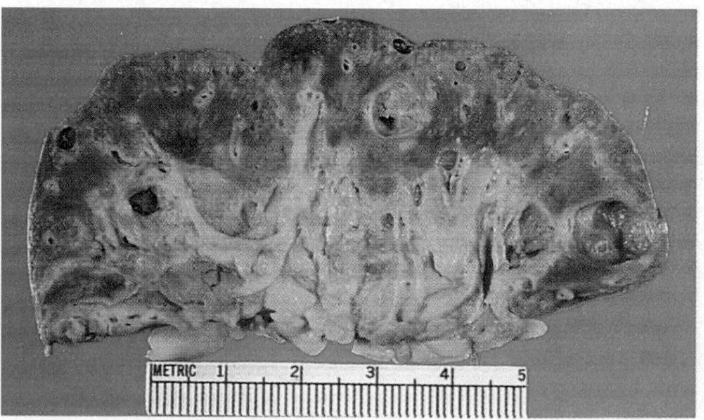

Fig. 65-85 Acquired cystic disease. Multiple cysts are in the cortex and medulla. An intracystic papillary neoplasm is also present.

walls, with luminal narrowing. Calcification may be extensive in tubules (cells and basement membranes) and glomeruli, and oxalate may be throughout tubules and interstitium.

Differential diagnosis. The major disorder from which acquired cystic disease needs to be differentiated is autosomal dominant (adult) polycystic kidney disease. Perhaps the most salient feature is the clinical history and the verification that a noncystic form of renal disease existed before the appearance of cysts. Furthermore, there is usually a family history. In general, the kidneys are larger in the genetic disorder and are far less likely to harbor neoplasms. Microscopically there is usually more epithelial hyperplasia and atypia of cyst epithelium in the acquired disorder. Moreover, there may be some residual evidence of the primary disease, such as various glomerulopathies, all of which are exceedingly uncommon in association with ADPKD.

Clinical presentation. Acquired cystic disease is usually clinically silent unless one of its two "complications" occur. These include metastases from a renal cell carcinoma and massive retroperitoneal or urinary tract bleeding from erosion of expanding cysts through a thick-walled artery. Both are more likely with advanced disease in a patient on dialysis. The most important clinical aspect is to identify the presence of acquired cystic disease, especially in patients entering chronic hemodialysis programs, and to monitor periodically by imaging procedures for the development of enlarging tumors.[310-314]

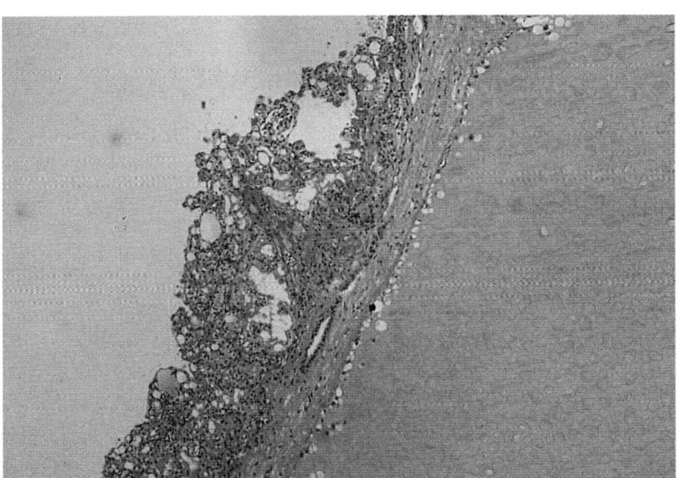

Fig. 65-86 Acquired cystic disease. There are two cysts, one with lumen filled with precipitate of pale-staining proteinaceous material and lined by a single layer of epithelium; the adjacent cyst is empty and lined by epithelium with pronounced hyperplasia, forming a large, flat papilla in the lumen. (Periodic acid–Schiff.)

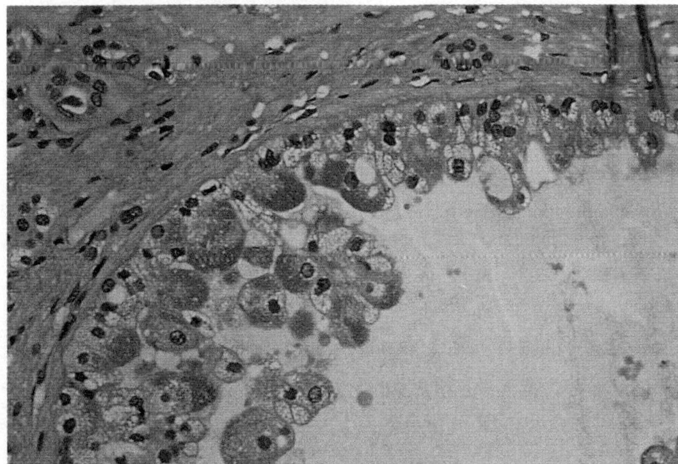

Fig. 65-87 Acquired cystic disease. A portion of cyst wall lined by hypertrophied cells forming hyperplastic papillae. (Periodic acid–Schiff.)

Renal transplant pathology

Renal transplants are usually assessed to determine the underlying cause of acute allograft failure, chronic allograft failure, or the presence of glomerular disease. The most common lesions inducing acute and chronic renal transplant failure are reviewed (Table 65-23).

Acute transplant failure

Acute allograft failure is an elevation in the serum creatinine level over a short time, usually days to weeks. This most often occurs within the first 3 to 6 months after engraftment but may happen at any time if, for example, the patient is noncompliant with antirejection medication.

Common causes of acute graft failure include acute transplant rejection, acute tubular necrosis, and acute cyclosporin A nephrotoxicity.[315] Less frequent abnormalities associated with graft insufficiency include viral infection, graft infarction, posttransplantation lymphoproliferative disorder,[316] obstruction, and surgical problems, such as lymphocele. All the causes of acute renal failure in native kidneys may also pertain to allografts, including drug-induced interstitial nephritis and acute infectious interstitial nephritis.

Etiology and pathogenesis. *Acute transplant rejection* is the result of recipient response to the foreign donor organ. In the more common cell-mediated rejection, recipient cytotoxic T-lymphocytes with lesser numbers of B-cells, NK cells, and macrophages infiltrate the graft and injure the organ parenchyma, resulting in graft failure.[317,318] This process is initiated by several cytokines from T-lymphocytes and macrophages, including interferon-gamma and interleukin-2, among many others.[319,320] These cytokines activate T-cells, which enter the parenchyma via the peritubular capillaries, inducing further clonal expansion and infiltration into the renal interstitium, tubular walls, and occasionally arteries. Vascular involvement

Table 65-23 **Causes of allograft dysfunction**

Acute
Rejection
Cyclosporin A toxicity
Acute tubular necrosis
Renal infection
Obstruction
Infarction
Acute interstitial nephritis (drug induced)
Chronic
Rejection
Cyclosporin A toxicity
Nephrosclerosis
Recurrent disease
De novo glomerulonephritis

generally implies a more severe rejection episode. In a small subset of patients there will be a component of humoral rejection caused by preformed or new antibodies directed against donor antigens.[321] This type of rejection involves arteries and is usually quite severe.

Acute tubular necrosis is the damage of tubular epithelium similar to that in the native kidney. It may be induced by renal ischemia in the preoperative or early postoperative period, or it may be related to factors in the donor kidney.[322] Drugs and hypoxia may further exacerbate tubular necrosis, as in the native kidney.

Acute cyclosporin A nephrotoxicity is a drug effect resulting in renal insufficiency. There is controversy regarding the pathogenesis of this form of renal injury. Cyclosporin A induces renal ischemia likely secondary to abnormalities in synthesis of eicosanoids, endothelin, and other paracrine factors.[323] The reduced blood flow, possibly combined with other effects of these cytokines and direct actions of cyclosporin A on renal cells, induces a decrement in renal function, which is readily reversible after cessation of the drug.[314]

Pathology. Grossly, kidneys with severe irreversible acute rejection are swollen and may have areas of hemorrhage or infarction. Microscopically, acute rejection has features similar to acute interstitial nephritis, with the abnormalities occurring primarily in the cortex. The interstitium is edematous, with a mononuclear leukocytic infiltrate primarily composed of lymphocytes and occasional monocyte/macrophages and eosinophils. Lymphocytes are also within the walls of tubules between the epithelial cells (tubulitis), a characteristic of acute rejection (Fig. 65-88). There is variable necrosis of tubular epithelial cells, usually in proportion to the degree of tubular inflammation, and peritubular capillaries may contain circulating leukocytes. When cell-mediated vascular rejection is present, the arteries or arterioles have swollen endothelial cells, which are detached from the elastic lamina and mononuclear leukocytes underneath the endothelium in the vascular wall (Fig. 65-89). There may be interstitial hemorrhage secondary to disruption of peritubular capillary walls. Glomeruli may have numerous lymphocytes and monocytes within capillary lumens (acute transplant glomerulopathy). Humoral rejection is characterized by a neutrophilic infiltrate within arterial walls with or without focal necrosis of arteries and thrombus formation.[325] In severe cell-mediated or humoral rejection there is vascular thrombosis with focal parenchymal infarction.

Acute tubular necrosis is characterized by necrosis of individual tubular cells and cytoplasmic debris in tubular lumens. Proximal tubular brush border staining is focally absent, and there is flattening of tubular epithelium with relative dilatation of tubular lumens. The interstitium is edematous and has a modest mononuclear inflammatory infiltrate; there is no significant tubular inflammation. Glomeruli and vessels are unremarkable.

Acute cyclosporin A nephrotoxicity may have characteristic morphologic abnormalities or may occur in kidneys with a normal appearance; therefore, occasionally it is a diagnosis of exclusion.[317,326,327] The characteristic lesion is proximal tubular cell small isometric cytoplasmic vacuoles, which correspond to dilated endoplasmic reticulum (Fig. 65-90). These are found in a small percentage of kidneys with acute cyclosporin A nephrotoxicity and occur in few tubular profiles, but they tend to involve most epithelial cells in the affected tubules. Other tubules may have flattened epithelium with dilated lumens without large numbers of necrotic tubular cells. In some cases the appearance is similar to tubular necrosis. The interstitium is edematous and may have foci of lymphocytic infiltrates without tubulitis. Arterioles have hyalinization of the walls, often affecting the outer aspect of the muscularis (Fig. 65-91), and muscular hypertrophy with associated expansion of juxtaglomerular apparatus. Arteries are usually normal, and glomeruli show only mild ischemia, with thickening and wrinkling of capillary walls. A form of acute cyclosporin A nephrotoxicity has all the features of a thrombotic microangiopathy in the native kidney.[328] Immunofluorescence and EM findings generally do not contribute significantly to the diagnosis but are necessary to evaluate kidneys for other possible abnormalities.

Differential diagnosis. Acute rejection must be differentiated from other forms of acute interstitial nephritis, including viral infection, particularly CMV and EBV, and drug-induced

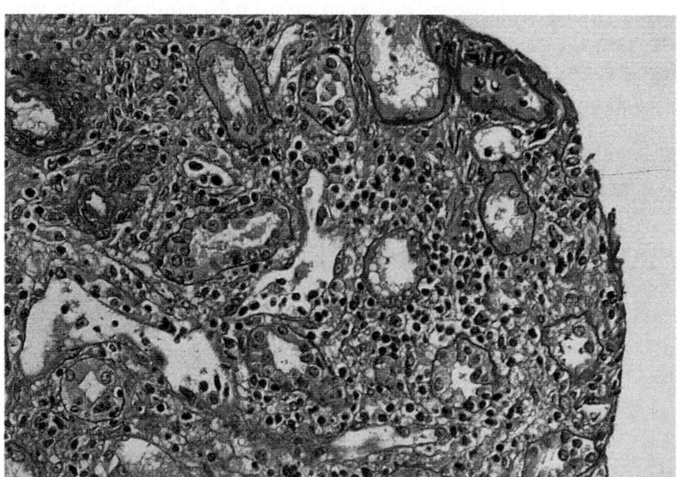

Fig. 65-88 Pathologic transplant characteristics. The interstitium is edematous and contains a lymphocytic infiltrate. Lymphocytes are also within the walls of tubules and the lumens of dilated peritubular capillaries. There is tubular injury characterized by loss of proximal cell brush border staining. (Periodic acid–Schiff.)

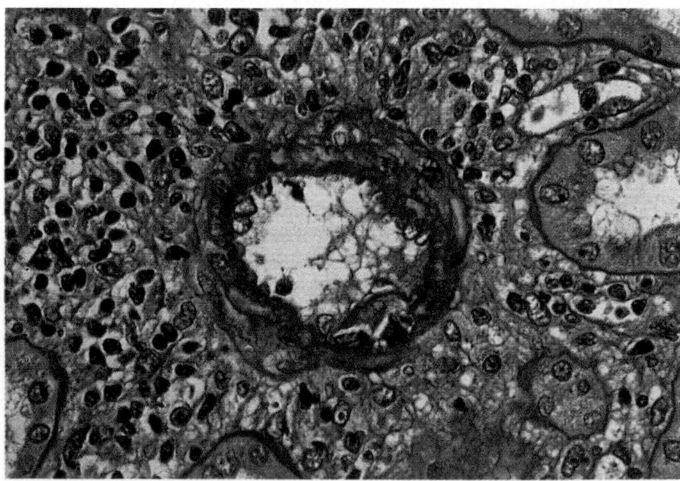

Fig. 65-89 Vascular transplant rejection. The artery has swollen endothelial cells focally detached from the basement membrane, with lymphocytes underneath the endothelium extending into the vascular wall. (Periodic acid–Schiff.)

lesions. Intracellular inclusions are diagnostic for CMV but often are not seen; immunochemical staining or in situ hybridization may be useful. A careful history is necessary for assessment of possible drug-induced lesions. Humoral rejection may simulate arteritis, but a careful history and appropriate serologic studies allow an accurate diagnosis. Acute cyclosporin A–associated renal insufficiency may be a functional abnormality without morphologic alterations of the kidney. The thrombotic microangiopathy associated with cyclosporin A must be differentiated from recurrent hemolytic uremic syndrome. Careful clinical correlation is required in these settings.

Clinical presentation. All three abnormalities usually develop within the first 3 to 6 months after transplantation as renal insufficiency. Acute rejection historically is associated with fever and graft tenderness, but this is less frequent in the cyclosporin A era.[329] Elevated cyclosporin A levels may be helpful in patients with acute cyclosporin A toxicity; however, the thrombotic microangiopathy is an idiosyncratic drug effect occurring with or without elevated levels. Renal biopsy is often required to differentiate among these causes of acute graft dysfunction. Acute rejection is treated with steroids or more aggressive therapy including anti–thymocyte globulin, OKT3 antibody, and FK506.[330] Cyclosporin A toxicity is corrected with reduction in the cyclosporin A dosage, and tubular necrosis requires supportive therapy.

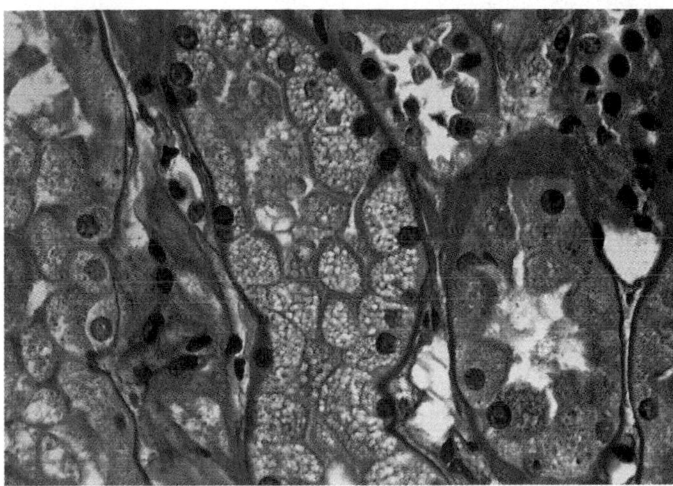

Fig. 65-90 Acute cyclosporin A nephrotoxicity. The large proximal tubule has small isometric cytoplasmic vacuoles in virtually all epithelial cells. Notice that the adjacent tubular profiles do not contain vacuoles. There is mild interstitial edema without an inflammatory infiltrate. (Periodic acid–Schiff.)

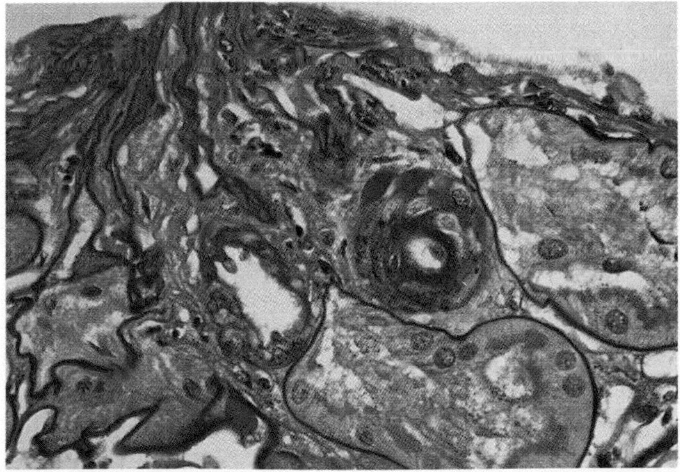

Fig. 65-91 Cyclosporin nephrotoxicity. Arteriole with muscular hypertrophy and plasma protein deposition (hyalinization) on the outer aspect of the muscular wall. (Periodic acid–Schiff.)

Chronic transplant failure

Chronic allograft dysfunction is characterized by a slow decline in renal function over months in a graft that has been in place for at least 6 months. The most common causes are chronic rejection, chronic cyclosporin A nephrotoxicity, and nephrosclerosis. It may be difficult to distinguish among these lesions, and they often occur together.

Etiology and pathogenesis. The pathogenesis of chronic rejection is not well understood.[331] The chronic renal changes are secondary to immunologic events in part; chronic rejection usually follows prior episodes of acute rejection.[332] The cell-mediated or humoral-mediated injury affects the renal vasculature and tubulointerstitium, resulting in renal scarring with added components of ischemia, further compounding the renal compromise. Chronic cyclosporin A nephrotoxicity is also an ischemic lesion, with cyclosporin A likely contributing by augmenting extracellular matrix–material production from renal cells directly and mediated by cytokines.[333] Nephrosclerosis occurs for the same reasons as in the native kidney, with immunologic factors possibly contributing.

Pathology. Chronic transplant rejection is primarily a cortical lesion, though the large arcuate arteries may be the first affected vessels. The characteristic abnormality is intimal fibrosis of arteries with mononuclear leukocytes and foam cells in the thickened arterial wall and disruption of the internal elastic lamina with luminal narrowing.[334] There is focal tubular atrophy with associated interstitial fibrosis and an infiltrate composed of lymphocytes and plasma cells (Fig. 65-92). White cells are within the walls of the atrophic tubules. Glomeruli are frequently involved, displaying capillary-wall double contours, mesangial expansion with mild hypercellularity, and an increase in matrix material, segmental sclerosis, and, rarely, mesangiolysis; these features constitute chronic transplant glomerulopathy[335] (Fig. 65-93). Immunofluorescence may show the presence of mesangial and capillary wall IgM, C1q, and C3. EM reveals subendothelial flocculent material similar to that observed in thrombotic microangiopathy, peripheral mesangial migration and interposition in capillary walls, and, infrequently, mesangial or subendothelial electron-dense deposits or insudative lesions (Fig. 65-94).

Chronic cyclosporin A nephrotoxicity has features similar to renal ischemia: "striped" tubular atrophy and interstitial fibrosis with a mild to absent associated inflammatory infiltrate[327] (Fig. 65-95). Arterioles have considerable hyalinization of the walls, and there is expansion of juxtaglomerular apparatus. The arteries are normal, and glomeruli show ischemic changes.

Nephrosclerosis has the same appearance as in the native kidney. Arteries have intimal fibrosis with luminal narrowing without leukocytes in the walls. There is hyalinization of arterioles and foci of tubular atrophy with interstitial fibrosis and variable inflammation. Glomeruli have the capillary wall thickening and wrinkling characteristic of ischemia.

Differential diagnosis. It may be difficult to distinguish among these abnormalities, and they often occur together (Table 65-24). Chronic rejection is present when there is arterial inflammation with fibrosis, and chronic transplant glomerulopathy is virtually diagnostic of chronic rejection but must be differentiated from recurrent or *de novo* glomerular lesions. Immunofluorescence and EM are necessary to make this distinction. Chronic cyclosporin A nephrotoxicity requires a lack of arterial fibrosis.

Clinical presentation. By definition these lesions present with slowly progressive renal failure in a patient with a transplant for at least 6 months. Hypertension is usually present, and there may be significant proteinuria with chronic transplant glomerulopathy.[336] The only therapy is control of hypertension with supportive therapy.

Glomerular disease in renal transplants is not uncommon. Recurrent glomerular lesions mimic the morphologic and often the clinical findings of the disease in the native kidney.[337] Focal and segmental glomerulosclerosis and MPGN type II (dense deposit disease) recur often and early and may cause graft loss.

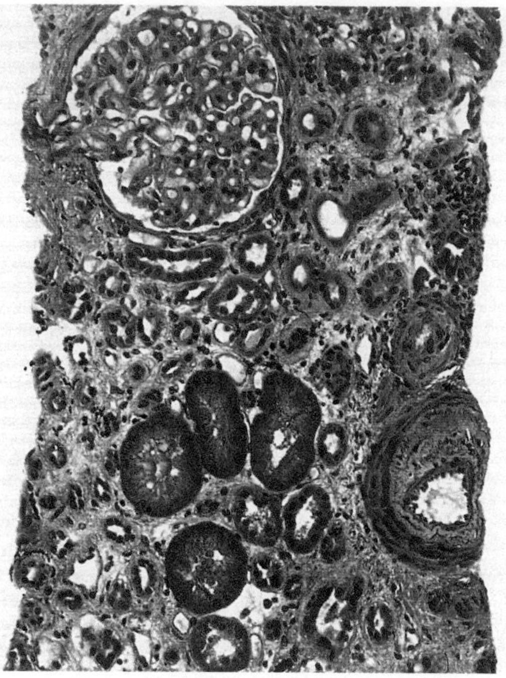

Fig. 65-92 Chronic transplant failure. The artery displays intimal fibrosis with entrapped mononuclear leukocytes and narrowing of the lumen. There is tubular atrophy with interstitial fibrosis and scattered interstitial lymphocytes. The glomerulus shows ischemic change characterized by capillary wall thickening and wrinkling. (Masson's trichrome.)

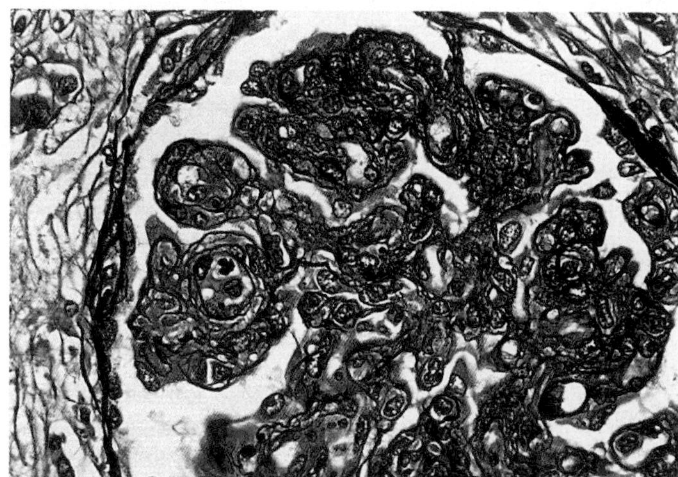

Fig. 65-93 Chronic transplant glomerulopathy. The glomerulus has many capillary wall double contours with mononuclear leukocytes in mesangial regions and some capillary lumens. There is mesangial matrix material widening, with hypercellularity. (Periodic acid–methenamine silver.)

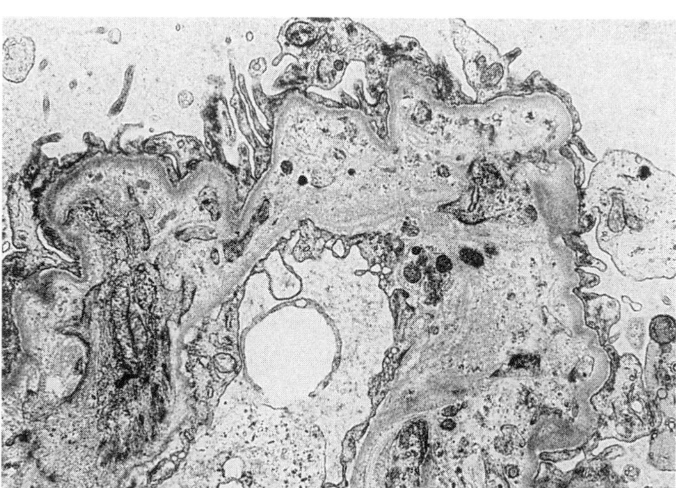

Fig. 65-94 Chronic transplant glomerulopathy. There is considerable thickening of the glomerular capillary wall from peripheral mesangial migration and interposition, with flocculent electron-lucent and electron-dense material in subendothelial regions. The lumen is narrowed, and there is partial effacement of visceral epithelial cell foot processes.

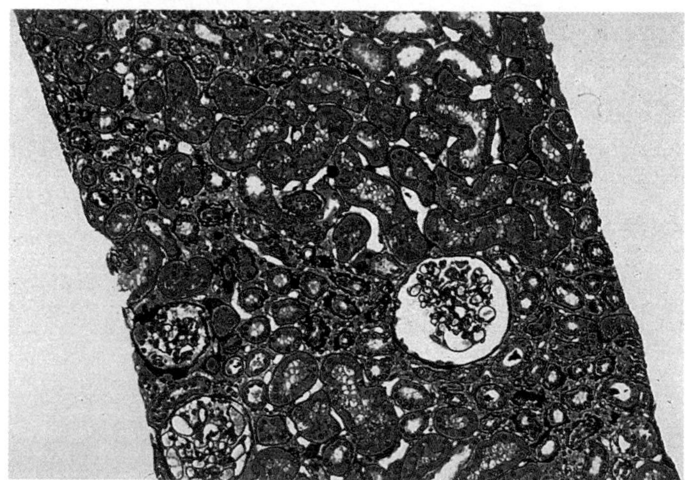

Fig. 65-95 Chronic cyclosporin A nephrotoxicity. There are zones of tubular atrophy and interstitial fibrosis (striped fibrosis) with a minimal inflammatory infiltrate. Intervening tubules have mild hypertrophy and the interstitium is unremarkable. Glomeruli are unremarkable or show slight thickening and wrinkling of capillary walls, representing ischemic change. (Periodic acid–methenamine silver.)

Table 65-24 Pathology of the major causes of allograft failure

Cause	Tubules	Interstitium	Vessels	Glomeruli
Acute cell-mediated rejection	Mural lymphocytes with or within necrosis	Lymphocytes Edema	Arterial mural lymphocytes, swollen endothelium	Capillary lymphocytes, monocytes
Acute tubular necrosis	Necrosis, mitotic figures	Edema	Normal	Normal
Acute cyclosporin A toxicity	Degeneration, flattened epithelium, isometric vacuoles	Edema	Arteriolar insudates	Normal or ischemic
Chronic rejection	Atrophy dropout	Fibrosis with or without mononuclear leukocytes	Arterial fibrosis, lymphocytes	Chronic transplant glomerulopathy
Chronic cyclosporine A toxicity	Atrophy	"Striped" fibrosis	Arteriolar insudates	Ischemic

In contrast, IgA nephropathy often recurs morphologically with mesangial IgA deposits but rarely is clinically significant. Systemic diseases also recur in the transplanted kidney, such as diabetic nephropathy, multiple myeloma, and amyloidosis.[338] New *(de novo)* glomerulopathies may arise in renal allografts, most often membranous glomerulonephritis and focal and segmental glomerulosclerosis.[339] All these abnormalities have the same clinical symptoms and morphologic features as in native kidneys.

REFERENCES

Normal anatomy and pathology

1. Clapp WL, Abrahamson DR: Development and gross anatomy of the kidney. In Tisher CC, Brenner BM, editors: *Renal pathology with clinical and functional correlations,* ed 2, Philadelphia, 1994, Lippincott.
2. Tisher CC, Brenner BM: Structure and function of the glomerulus. In Tisher CC, Brenner BM, editors: *Renal pathology with clinical and functional correlations,* ed 2, Philadelphia, 1994, Lippincott.
3. Jones DB: Mucosubstances of the glomerulus, *Lab Invest* 21:119, 1969.
4. Cohen AH: Masson's trichrome stain in the evaluation of renal biopsies: an appraisal, *Am J Clin Pathol* 65:631, 1976.
5. Pirani CL: Evaluation of kidney biopsy specimens. In Tischer CC, Brenner BM, editors: *Renal pathology with clinical and functional correlations* ed 2, Philadelphia, 1994, Lippincott.
6. Glassock RJ, Cohen AH, Adler SG et al: Primary glomerular disease. In Brenner BM, Rector FC Jr, editors: *The kidney,* ed 4, Philadelphia, 1991, Saunders.
7. Cohen AH, Nast CC: Atlas of renal pathology. In Massry SG, Glassock RJ, editors: *Textbook of nephrology,* ed 3, Baltimore, 1995, Williams & Wilkins.
8. Cohen AH: Morphology of renal tubular hyaline casts, *Lab Invest* 44:280, 1981.
9. Eddy AA, Michael AF: Immunopathogenic mechanisms of glomerular injury. In Tischer CC, Brenner BM, editors: *Renal pathology with clinical and functional correlations,* ed 2, Philadelphia, 1994, Lippincott .
10. Main IW, Nikolic-Paterson DJ, Atkins RC: T-cells and macrophages and their role in renal injury, *Semin Nephrol* 12:395, 1992.
11. Cohen AH, Mampaso F, Zamboni L: Glomerular podocyte degeneration in human renal disease: an ultrastructural study, *Lab Invest* 37:30, 1977.
12. Hostetter TH, Olson JL, Rennke HG et al: Hyperfiltration in remnant nephrons: a potentially adverse response to renal ablation, *Am J Physiol* 241:F85, 1981.
13. Rennke HG, Anderson S, Brenner BM: The progression of renal disease: structural and functional correlations. In Tisher CC, Brenner BM, editors: *Renal pathology with clinical and functional correlations,* ed 2, Philadelphia, 1994, Lippincott.

Developmental and hereditary disorders

14. Cole BR: Autosomal recessive polycystic kidney disease. In Gardner KD Jr, Bernstein J, editors: *The cystic kidney,* Boston, 1990, Kluwer Academic.
15. Gagnadoux MF, Habib R, Levy M et al: Cystic renal diseases in children, *Adv Nephrol* 18:33, 1989.
16. Rapola J, Kääriäinen H: Polycystic kidney disease: morphologic diagnosis of recessive and dominant polycystic kidney disease in infancy and childhood, *APMIS* 96:68, 1988.
17. Welling LW, Grantham JJ: Cystic disease of the kidney. In Tisher CC, Brenner BM, editors: *Renal pathology with clinical and functional correlations* ed 2, Philadelphia, 1990, Lippincott.
18. Gabow PA: Autosomal dominant polycystic kidney disease, *N Engl J Med* 329:332, 1993.
19. Evan AP, Gardner KD Jr, Bernstein J: Polypoid and papillary epithelial hyperplasia: a potential cause of ductal obstruction in adult polycystic disease, *Kidney Int* 6:743, 1979.
20. Grantham JJ, Geiser JL, Evan AP: Cyst formation and growth in autosomal dominant polycystic kidney disease, *Kidney Int* 31:1145, 1987.
21. Carone FA, Nakamura S, Punyarit P et al: Sequential tubular cell and basement membrane changes in polycystic kidney disease, *J Am Soc Nephrol* 3:244, 1992.
22. Gregoire JR, Torres VE, Holley KE et al: Renal epithelial hyperplastic and neoplastic proliferation in autosomal dominant polycystic kidney disease, *Am J Kidney Dis* 9:27, 1987.
23. Parfrey PS, Bear JC, Morgan J et al: The diagnosis and prognosis of autosomal dominant polycystic kidney disease, *N Engl J Med* 323:1085, 1990.
24. Cohen AH, Hoyer JR: Nephronophthisis: a primary tubular basement membrane defect, *Lab Invest* 55:564, 1986.
25. Zollinger HU, Mihatsch MJ, Edefonti A et al: Nephronophthisis (medullary cystic diseases of the kidney): a study using electron microscopy, immunofluorescence, and a review of the morphologic findings, *Helv Paediatr Acta* 35:509, 1990.
26. Gubler MC, Mounier F, Foidart JM et al: Ultrastructural and immunohistochemical study of RBM in familial juvenile nephronophthisis. In Price RG, Hudson BG, editors: *Renal basement membranes in health and disease,* London, 1987, Academic Press.
27. Zager RA, Cotran RS, Hoyer JR: Pathologic localization of Tamm-Horsfall protein interstitial deposits in renal disease, *Lab Invest* 38:52, 1978.
28. Bernstein J, Gilbert Barness E: Congenital malformations of the kidney. In Tisher CC, Brenner BM, editors: *Renal pathology with clinical and functional correlations,* ed 2, Philadelphia, 1994, Lippincott.
29. Bernstein J: Developmental abnormalities of the renal parenchyma: hypoplasia and dysplasia, *Pathol Annu* 3:213, 1968.

134. Pollak VE: Treatment of membranous glomerulonephropathy, *Am J Kidney Dis* 19:68, 1992.
135. Emancepator SN: Primary and secondary forms of IgA nephritis. In Heptinstall RH, editor: *Pathology of the kidney,* ed 4, Boston, 1992, Little, Brown.
136. Habib R, Niaudet P, Levy M: Schönlein-Henoch purpura nephritis and IgA nephropathy. In Tisher CC, Brenner BM, editors: *Renal pathology with clinical and functional correlations,* ed 2, Philadelphia, 1994, Lippincott.
137. Levy M, Berger J: Worldwide perspective of IgA nephropathy, *Am J Kidney Dis* 12:340, 1988.
138. van den Wall Bake AWL: Mechanisms of IgA deposition in the mesangium, *Contrib Nephrol* 104:138, 1993.
139. Endo Y, Kanbayashi H: Etiology of IgA nephropathy syndrome, *Pathol Int* 44:1, 1994.
140. Bennett WM, Kincaid-Smith P: Macroscopic hematuria in mesangial IgA nephropathy: correlation with glomerular crescents and renal dysfunction, *Kidney Int* 23:393, 1983.
141. Gallo GR, Katafuchi R, Neelakantappa K, Baldwin DS: Prognostic pathologic markers in IgA nephropathy, *Am J Kidney Dis* 12:362, 1988.
142. Katafuchi R, Vamvakas E, Neelakantappa K et al: Microvascular disease and the progression of IgA nephropathy, *Am J Kidney Dis* 15:72, 1990.
143. Lee HS, Choi Y, Lee JS et al: Ultrastructural changes in IgA nephropathy in relation to histologic and clinical data, *Kidney Int* 35:880, 1989.
144. Clarkson AR, Seymour AE, Thompson AJ et al: IgA nephropathy: a syndrome of uniform morphology, diverse clinical features and uncertain prognosis, *Clin Nephrol* 8:459, 1977.
145. Berger J: Recurrence of IgA nephropathy in renal allograft, *Am J Kidney Dis* 12:371, 1988.
146. Habib R, Murcia I, Beaufils H et al: Nephropathies in children, *Biomed Pharmacother* 44:159, 1992.
147. Tanizawa T, Okada T, Uenoyama F et al: Henoch-Schönlein's syndrome in childhood: renal histopathology. III. Immunofluorescent microscopic study, *Acta Med Biol* 31:153, 1984.
148. Levy M, Broyer M, Arsan A et al: Anaphylactoid purpura nephritis in childhood: natural history and immunopathology, *Adv Nephrol* 6:183, 1976.
149. Egido J, Sancho J, Mampaso F et al: A possible common pathogenesis of the mesangial IgA GN in patients with Berger's disease and Schönlein-Henoch syndrome, *Proc Eur Dial Transplant Assoc* 17:660, 1980.
150. Lanzkowsky S, Lanzkowsky L, Lanzkowsky P: Henoch-Schönlein purpura, *Pediatr Rev* 13:130, 1992.
151. Meadow SR, Glasgow EF, White RHR et al: Schönlein-Henoch nephritis, *Q J Med* 41:241, 1972.
152. Feldt R, Stickler GB: The gastrointestinal manifestations of anaphylactoid purpura in children, *Mayo Clin Proc* 37:465, 1962.
153. Case records of Massachusetts General Hospital: Case 12-1994, *N Engl J Med* 330:847, 1994.
154. Austin HA, Balow JE: Henoch-Schönlein nephritis: prognostic features and the challenge of therapy, *Am J Kidney Dis* 2:515, 1983.
155. Glassock RJ, Cohen AH, Adler SG et al: Secondary glomerular disease. In Brenner BM, Rector RC Jr, editors: *The kidney,* ed 4, Philadelphia, 1991, Saunders.
156. Paukewycz OG, Sturgill BC, Bolton WK: Proliferative glomerulonephritis: post-infectious, non-infectious, and crescentic forms. In Tisher CC, Brenner BM, editors: *Renal pathology with clinical and functional correlations,* ed 2, Philadelphia, 1994, Lippincott.
157. Gallo GR, Neugarten J, Baldwin DS: Glomerulonephritis associated with bacterial and viral infections. In Tisher CC, Brenner BM, editors: *Renal pathology with clinical and functional correlations,* ed 2, Philadelphia, 1994, Lippincott.
158. Adler SG, Cohen AH: Glomerulonephritis with bacterial endocarditis, ventriculovascular shunts, visceral infections. In Schrier RW, Gottschalk CW, editors: *Diseases of the kidney,* ed 5, Boston, 1993, Little, Brown.
159. Michalak T: Immune complex of hepatitis B surface antigen in the pathogenesis of periarteritis nodosa, *Am J Pathol* 90:619, 1978.
160. Takeda S, Kida H, Katagiri M et al: Characteristics of glomerular lesions in hepatitis B virus infection, *Am J Kidney Dis* 11:57, 198
161. Kawaguchi K, Koike M: Glomerular lesions associated with liver cirrhosis: an immunohistochemical and clinicopathologic analysis, *Hum Pathol* 17:1137, 1988.
162. Johnson RJ, Gretch DR, Yamabe H et al: Membranoproliferative glomerulonephritis associated with Hepatitis C virus infection, *N Engl J Med* 328:465, 1993.
163. Misiani R, Bellavita P, Fenili D et al: Hepatitis C virus infection in patients with essential mixed cryoglobulinemia, *Ann Intern Med* 117:573, 1992.
164. Davda R, Peterson J, Weiner R et al: Membranous glomerulonephritis in association with hepatitis C virus infection, *Am J Kidney Dis* 22:452, 1993.
165. Cacoub P, Lunel-Fabiani F, Huong Du LT: Polyarteritis nodosa and hepatitis C virus infection, *Ann Intern Med* 116:605, 1992.
166. Takekoshi Y, Tochimaru N, Nagata Y et al: Immunopathogenetic mechanisms of hepatitis B virus–related glomerulopathy, *Kidney Int* 35(suppl): 534, 1991.
167. Collins AB, Bhan AK, Dienstag JL et al: Hepatitis B immune complex glomerulonephritis: simultaneous glomerular deposition of hepatitis B surface and e antigens, *Clin Immunol Immunopathol* 26:137, 1983.
168. Lisker-Melman M, Webb D, Di Bisceglie AM et al: Glomerulonephritis caused by chronic hepatitis B virus infection: treatment with recombinant human alpha-interferon, *Ann Intern Med* 111:479, 1989.
169. Davis GL, Balart LA, Schiff ER: Treatment of chronic hepatitis C with recombinant interferon alpha: a multicenter randomized, controlled trial, *N Engl J Med* 321:1501, 1989.
170. Cohen AH, Glassock RJ: Anti-GBM glomerulonephritis, including Goodpasture's syndrome in renal pathology with clinical and functional correlations. In Tisher CC, Brenner BM, editors: *Renal pathology with clinical and functional correlations,* ed 2, Philadelphia, 1994, Lippincott.
171. Salant D: Immunopathogenesis of crescentic glomerulonephritis and lung purpura, *Kidney Int* 32:408, 1987.
172. Kelly PT, Haponik EP: Goodpasture syndrome: molecular and clinical advances, *Medicine* 73:171, 1994.
173. Hudson BG, Weislander J, Wisdom BJ Jr, Noelken ME: Goodpasture syndrome: molecular architecture and function of basement membrane antigen, *Lab Invest* 61:256, 1989.
174. Bonsib SM, Goeken J, Kemp J et al: Coexistent anti-neutrophil cytoplasmic antibody and antiglomerular basement antibody associated disease: report of six cases, *Mod Pathol* 6:526, 1993.
175. O'Donaghue DJ, Short CD, Brenchley PEC et al: Sequential development of systemic vasculitis with anti-neutrophil cytoplasmic antibodies complicating anti–glomerular basement membrane disease, *Clin Nephrol* 32:251, 1989.
176. Walker RG, Scheinkestel C, Becker GJ et al: Clinical and morphological aspects of the management of crescentic anti–glomerular basement membrane antibody (anti-GBM) nephritis/Goodpasture's syndrome, *Q J Med* 54:75, 1985.
177. Stilmant MM, Bolton WK, Sturgill BC et al: Crescentic glomerulonephritis without immune deposits: clinicopathologic features, *Kidney Int* 15:184, 1979.
178. Churg J: Nomenclature of vasculitic syndromes: a historical perspective, *Am J Kidney Dis* 18:148, 1991.
179. Rosen S, Falk RJ, Jennette JC: Polyarteritis nodosa including microscopic form and renal vasculitis. In Churg A, Churg J, editors: *Systemic vasculitis,* New York, 1991, Igaku-Shoin.
180. Jennette JC, Wilkman AS, Falk RJ: Anti-neutrophil cytoplasmic autoantibody–associated glomerulonephritis and vasculitis, *Am J Pathol* 135:921, 1989.
181. Jennette JC, Hoidal JR, Falk RJ: Specificity of anti-neutrophil cytoplasmic antoantibodies for proteinase 3, *Blood* 75:2263, 1990.
182. Jennette JC, Falk RJ, Andrassy K et al: Nomenclature of systemic vasculitides, *Arthritis Rheum* 37:187, 1994.
183. Breedveld FC, Heurkens AH, Lafeber GF et al: Immune complexes in sera from patients with rheumatoid vasculitis induce polymorphonuclear cell–mediated injury to endothelial cells, *Clin Immunol Immunopathol* 48:202, 1988.
184. McClusky RT, Fienberg R: Vasculitis in primary vasculitides, granulomatoses and connective tissue diseases, *Hum Pathol* 14:305, 1983.

185. Marcellin P, Calmus Y, Takahashi H: Latent hepatitis B virus infection in systemic necrotizing vasculitis, *Clin Exp Rheumatol* 9:23, 1991.
186. Sergent JS: Vasculitides associated with viral infections, *Clin Rheum Dis* 6:339, 1980.
187. Dubost JJ, Souteyrand P, Sauvezic B: Drug-induced vasculitides, *Baillieres Clin Rheumatol* 5:119, 1991.
188. Ronco P, Verroust P, Mignon F et al: Immunopathological studies of polyarteritis nodosa and Wegener's granulomatosis: a report of 43 patients with 51 renal biopsies, *Q J Med* 52:212, 1983.
189. Kallenberg CGM, Brouwer E, Weening JJ et al: cytoplasmic antibodies: current diagnostic and pathophysiological potential, *Kidney Int* 46:1, 1994.
190. Dixon FJ, Vasquez JJ, Weigle WO et al: Pathogenesis of serum sickness, *Arch Pathol* 65:18, 1958.
191. Mathieson PW, Peters DK: Deficiency and depletion of complement in the pathogenesis of nephritis and vasculitis, *Kidney Int* 42(suppl):513, 1993.
192. Jennette JC, Falk RJ: Anti-neutrophil cytoplasmic autoantibodies and associated disease: a review, *Am J Kidney Dis* 15:517, 1990.
193. Van der Woude RJ, Rasmussen N, Lobatto S et al: Autoantibodies against neutrophils and monocytes: tool for diagnosis and marker of disease activity in Wegener's granulomatosis, *Lancet* 1:425, 1985.
194. Falk RJ, Terrell RS, Charles LA et al: Anti-neutrophil cytoplasmic autoantibodies induce neutrophils to degranulate and produce oxygen radicals in vitro, *Proc Natl Acad Sci USA* 87:4115, 1990.
195. Serra A, Cameron JS, Turner DR et al: Vasculitis affecting the kidney: presentation, histopathology and long-term outcome, *Q J Med* 210:181, 1984.
196. Couser WG: Rapidly progressive glomerulonephritis: classification, pathogenetic mechanisms and therapy, *Am J Kidney Dis* 11:449, 1988.
197. Arkin A: A clinical and pathological study of periarteritisnodosa: a report of five cases, one histologically healed, *Am J Pathol* 6:401, 1930.
198. Min KW, Gyorkey F, Gyorkey P et al: The morphogenesis of glomerular crescents in rapidly progressive glomerulonephritis, *Kidney Int* 5:47, 1974.
199. Geffriaud-Ricouard C, Noel LH, Chauveau D et al: Clinical significance of ANCA in 98 patients, *Adv Exp Med Biol* 336:273, 1993.
200. Balow JE: Renal vasculitis, *Kidney Int* 27:954, 1985.
201. Bolton WK, Wilkowski MJ: Treatment and prognosis of renal and systemic vasculitis, *Contrib Nephrol* 94:72, 1991.
202. Hoffman GS, Kerr GS, Leavitt RY et al: Wegener granulomatosis: an analysis of 158 patients, *Ann Intern Med* 116:488, 1992.
203. Appel GB, Silva FG, Pirani CL et al: Renal involvement in systemic lupus erythematosus (SLE): a study of 56 patients emphasizing histologic classifications, *Medicine* 57:371, 1978.
204. Foster MH, Cizman B, Madaio MP: Nephritogenic autoantibodies in systemic lupus erythematosus: immunochemical properties, mechanisms of immune deposition, and genetic origins, *Lab Invest* 69:494, 1993.
205. Hill GS: Systemic lupus erythematosus and mixed connective tissue disease. In Heptinstall RH, editor: *Pathology of the kidney,* Boston, 1992, Little, Brown.
206. Cohen AH, Zamboni L: Ultrastructural appearance and morphogenesis of renal glomerular hematoxylin bodies, *Am J Pathol* 89:105, 1977.
207. Adler SG, Johnson K, Louie JS et al: Lupus membranous glomerulonephritis: different prognostic subgroups obscured by imprecise histologic classification, *Mod Pathol* 3:186, 1990.
208. Schwartz MM, Kawala K, Robert JL et al: Clinical and pathological features of membranous glomerulonephritis of systemic lupus erythematosus, *Am J Nephrol* 4:301, 1984.
209. Balow JE, Austin HA: Renal disease in systemic lupus erythematosus, *Rheum Dis Clin North Am* 14:117, 1988.
210. Schwartz MM, Bernstein J, Hall GS et al: Predictive value of renal pathology in diffuse proliferative lupus glomerulonephritis: lupus nephritis collaborative study group, *Kidney Int* 36:891, 1989.
211. Mahajan SK, Ordóñez NG, Feitelson PJ et al: lupus nephropathy without clinical renal involvement, *Medicine* 56:493, 1976.
212. Schwartz MM, Lan SP, Bonsib SM et al: Clinical outcome of three discrete histologic patterns of injury in severe lupus glomerulonephritis, *Am J Kidney Dis* 13:273, 1989.
213. Magil AB, Putterman ML, Ballon HS et al: Prognostic factors in diffuse proliferative lupus glomerulonephritis, *Kidney Int* 34:511, 1988.
214. Buysen JGM, Houthoff HJ, Krediet RT, Arisz L: Acute interstitial nephritis: a clinical and morphologic study in 27 patients, *Nephrol Dial Transplant* 5:94, 1990.
215. Cameron JS: Allergic interstitial nephritis: clinical features and pathogenesis, *Q J Med* 66:97, 1988.
216. Neilson EG: Pathogenesis and therapy of interstitial nephritis, *Kidney Int* 35:1257, 1989.
217. Baldwin DS, Levin BB, McCluskey RT, Gallo GR: Renal failure and interstitial nephritis due to penicillin and methicillin, *N Engl J Med* 279:1245, 1968.
218. Mallory GK, Keefer CS: Tissue reactions in fatal cases of *Streptococcus hemolyticus* infection, *Arch Pathol* 32:334, 1941.
219. Levy M, Gwesry P, Loirat C et al: Immunologically mediated tubulo-interstitial nephritis in children, *Contrib Nephrol* 16:132, 1978.
220. Sugisaki T, Yoshida T, McCluskey RT et al: Autoimmune cell-mediated tubulointerstitial nephritis induced in Lewis rats by renal antigens, *Clin Immunol Immunopathol* 15:33, 1980.
221. Brezin JH, Katz SM, Schwartz AB, Chinitz JL: Reversible renal failure and nephrotic syndrome associated with non-steroidal anti-inflammatory drugs, *N Engl J Med* 301:1271, 1979.
222. Steblay RW, Rudofsky U: Renal tubular disease and autoantibodies against tubular basement membrane induced in guinea pigs, *J Immunol* 107:589, 1971.
223. Mampaso F, Sánchez-Madrid F, Molina A et al: Expression of adhesion receptor and counterreceptors from the leukocyte-endothelial adhesion pathways LFA-1/ICAM-1 and VLA-4/VCAM-1 on drug-induced tubulointerstitial nephritis, *Am J Nephrol* 12:391, 1993.
224. Dobrin RS, Vernier RL, Fish AJ: Acute eosinophilic interstitial nephritis and acute renal failure with bone marrow–lymph node granulomas and anterior uveitis, *Am J Med* 59:325, 1975.
225. Ooi BS: Drug-induced interstitial nephritis. In Bertoni T, Remuzzi G, Garattini S, editors: *Drugs and the kidney,* vol 33, New York, 1986, Raven Press.
226. Magil AB: Drug-induced acute interstitial nephritis with granulomas, *Hum Pathol* 13:36, 1983.
227. Ivanyi B, Marcussen N, Kemp E, Olsen TS: The distal nephron is preferentially infiltrated by inflammatory cells in acute interstitial nephritis, *Virchows Arch [A]* 420:37, 1992.
228. Platt JL, Sibley RK, Michael AF: Interstitial nephritis associated with cytomegalovirus infection, *Kidney Int* 28:550, 1985.
229. Linton AL, Clark WF, Driedger AA et al: Acute interstitial nephritis due to drugs: review of the literature with a report of nine cases, *Ann Intern Med* 93:735, 1980.
230. Hill GS: Renal infection. In Hill GS, editor: *Uropathology,* New York, 1989, Churchill Livingtone.
231. Brumfilt W, Pereival A: Pathogenesis and laboratory diagnosis of non-tuberculous urinary tract infection: a review, *J Clin Pathol* 17:482, 1964.
232. Freedman LR: Natural history of urinary infection in adults, *Kidney Int* 4(suppl):S96, 1975.
233. Eden CS, Hansson HA: *Escherichia coli* pili as possible mediators of attachment to human urinary tract epithelial cells, *Infect Immun* 21:229, 1978.
234. Roberts JA: Etiology and pathophysiology of pyelonephritis, *Am J Kidney Dis* 17:1, 1991.
235. Heptinstall RH: Urinary tract infection, and clinical features of pyelonephritis. In Heptinstall RH, editor: *Pathology of the kidney,* Boston, 1992, Little, Brown.
236. King LR: Vesicoureteral reflux: history, etiology and conservative management. In Kelalis P, King LR, editors: *Clinical pediatric urology,* vol 1, Philadelphia, 1976, Saunders.
237. Ransley PG, Risdon RA, Godley ML: Effects of vesicoureteral reflux on renal growth and function as measured by GFR, plasma creatinine and urinary concentrating ability: an experimental study in the minipig, *Br J Urol* 60:193, 1987.
238. Hodson CJ, Maling TM, McManamon PJ, Lewis MG: The pathogenesis of reflux nephropathy (chronic atrophic pyelonephritis), *Br J Radiol* 13(suppl):1-26, 1975.
239. Bailey RR: The relationship of vesico-ureteric reflux to urinary tract infection and chronic pyelonephritis-reflux nephropathy, *Clin Nephrol* 1:132, 1973.

240. Ransley PG: Intrarenal reflux: anatomical, dynamic, and radiological studies—Part I, *Urol Res* 5:61, 1977.
241. Guze LB, Beeson PB: Experimental pyelonephritis. I. Effect of ureteral ligation on the course of bacterial infection in the kidney of the rat, *J Exp Med* 104:803, 1956.
242. Brumfitt W, Heptinstall RH: Experimental pyelonephritis: the influence of temporary and permanent ureteric obstruction on the localization of bacteria, *Br J Exp Pathol* 39:610, 1958.
243. Weismann G: The molecular basis of acute gout, *Hosp Pract* 6:43, 1971.
244. Madrazo A, Schwartz G, Churg J: Radiation nephritis: a review, *J Urol* 114:822, 1975.
245. Walker RG, Dowling JP, Alcorn D et al: Renal pathology associated with lithium therapy, *Pathology* 15:403, 1983.
246. Adams DH, Howie AJ, Mihatsch MJ et al: Nonsteroidal anti-inflammatory drugs and renal failure, *Lancet* 2:57, 1986.
247. McDonald GS: Xanthogranulomatous pyelonephritis, *J Pathol* 133:203, 1981.
248. Parsons MA, Harris SC, Longstaff AJ et al: Xanthogranulomatous pyelonephritis: a pathological, clinical and etiologic analysis of 87 cases, *Diagnost Histopathol* 6:203, 1983.
249. McClure J: Malakoplakia, *J Pathol* 140:275, 1983.
250. Garrett IR, McClure J: Renal malakoplakia: experimental production and evidence of a link with interstitial megalocytic nephritis, *J Pathol* 136:111, 1982.
251. Bergstein J, Andreoli SP, Provisor AK, Yum M: Radiation nephritis following total body irradiation and cyclophosphamide in preparation for bone marrow, *Transplantation* 41:63, 1986.

Metabolic, hormonal, and toxic disorders

252. Brezis M, Rosen S, Epstein FH: Acute renal failure. In Brenner BM, Rector FC Jr, editors: *The kidney,* ed 4, Philadelphia, 1991, Saunders.
253. Olsen S, Solez K: Acute tubular necrosis and toxic renal injury. In Tisher CC, Brenner BM, editors: *Renal pathology with clinical and functional correlations,* ed 2, Philadelphia, 1994, Lippincott.
254. Solez K: Acute renal failure (acute tubular necrosis, infarction, and cortical necrosis. In Heptinstall RH, editors: *Pathology of the kidneys,* ed 4, Boston, 1992, Little, Brown.
255. Bennett WM, Elzinga LW, Porter GA: Tubulointerstitial disease and toxic nephropathy. In Brenner BM, Rector FC Jr, editors: *The kidney,* ed 4, Philadelphia, 1991, Saunders.
256. Brezis M, Epstein FH: Cellular mechanisms of acute ischemic injury to the kidney, *Annu Rev Med* 44:27, 1993.
257. Bonventre J: Mechanisms of ischemic renal failure, *Kidney Int* 43:1160, 1993.
258. Brezis M, Rosen S, Silva P et al: Selective vulnerability of the medullary thick ascending limb to anoxia in the isolated perfused rat kidney, *J Clin Invest* 73:182, 1984.
259. Solez K, Morel-Maroger L, Sraer JD: The morphology of acute tubular necrosis in man: analysis of 57 renal biopsies and a comparison with the glycerol model, *Medicine* 58:362, 1979.
260. Bohle A, Jahnecke J, Meyer D et al: Morphology of acute renal failure: comparative data from biopsy and autopsy, *Kidney Int* 10(suppl):89, 1976.
261. Cohen AH: Two cases of acute renal failure of unknown etiology, *Am J Nephrol* 7:330, 1987.
262. Gellman DD, Pirani CL, Soothill JF et al: Diabetic nephropathy: a clinical and pathological study based on renal biopsies, *Medicine* 38:321, 1959.
263. Schober E, Pollak A, Coradello H et al: Glycosylation of glomerular basement membrane in type I (insulin-dependent) diabetic children, *Diabetologia* 23:485, 1982.
264. Brownlee M, Cerami A, Vlassara H: Advanced glycosylation end products in tissue and the biochemical basis of diabetic complications, *N Engl J Med* 318:1315, 1988.
265. Nerlich A, Schleicher E: Immunohistochemical localization of extracellular matrix components in human diabetic glomerular lesions, *Am J Pathol* 139:889, 1991.
266. Schleicher ED, Olgemöller B: Glomerular changes in diabetes mellitus, *Eur J Clin Chem Clin Biochem* 30:635, 1992.
267. Kirstein M, Brett J, Rodoff S et al: Advanced protein glycosylation induces transendothelial human monocyte chemotaxis and secretion of platelet-derived growth factor: role in vascular disease of diabetes and aging, *Proc Natl Acad Sci U S A* 87:9010, 1990.
268. Hostetter TH, Rennke HG, Brenner BM: The case for intrarenal hypertension in the initiation and progression of diabetic and other glomerulopathies, *Am J Med* 72:375, 1982.
269. Zatz R, Meyer TW, Rennke HG, Brenner BM: Predominance of hemodynamic rather than metabolic factors in the pathogenesis of diabetic glomerulopathy, *Proc Natl Acad Sci U S A* 82:5963, 1985.
270. Gupta KL, Sakhuja V, Khandelwal N et al: Renal papillary necrosis in diabetes mellitus, *J Assoc Phys India* 38:908, 1990.
271. Kimmelstiel P, Wilson C: Intercapillary lesions in glomeruli of kidney, *Am J Pathol* 12:83, 1936.
272. Lannigar R, Blainey JD, Brewer DB: Electron microscopy of the diffuse glomerular lesion in diabetes mellitus with special reference to early changes, *J Pathol Bacteriol* 88:255, 1964.
273. Yoshikawa Y, Truong LD, Mattioli CA et al: Membranous glomerulonephritis in diabetic patients: a study of 15 cases and review of the literature, *Mod Pathol* 3:36, 1990.
274. Parving HH, Gall MA, Skott P et al: Prevalence and causes of albuminuria in non–insulin dependent diabetic patients, *Kidney Int* 41:758, 1992.
275. Chahaz PS, Kohner EM: The relationship between diabetic retinopathy and diabetic nephropathy, *Diabetic Nephrop* 2:4, 1983.
276. Lewis EJ, Hunsicker LG, Bain RP, Rhode RD: The effect of angiotensin-converting-enzyme inhibition on diabetic nephropathy, *N Eng J Med* 329:1456, 1993.
277. Striker LJ MM, Preud'homme JS, D'Amico G et al: Monoclonal gammopathies, mixed cryoglobulinemias, and lymphomas. In Tisher CC, Brenner BM, editors: *Renal pathology with clinical and functional correlations,* ed 2, Philadelphia, 1994, Lippincott.
278. Solomon A, Weiss DT: Ominous consequences of immunoglobulin deposition, *N Engl J Med* 329:1422, 1993.
279. Solomon A, Weiss DT, Kattine AA: Nephrotoxic potentials of Bence Jones proteins, *N Engl J Med* 324:1845, 1991.
280. Silva FG, Pirani CL, Mesa-Tejeda R et al: The kidney in plasma cell dyscrasias: a review and a clinicopathologic study of 50 patients. In Fenoglio C, Wolff M, editors: *Progress in surgical pathology,* New York, 1984, Masson.
281. Border WA, Cohen AH: Renal biopsy diagnosis of clinically silent multiple myeloma, *Ann Intern Med* 93:43, 1980.
282. Cohen AH: The pathogenesis of cast nephropathy in the kidney in plasma cell dyscrasias. In Minetti L, D'Amico G, Ponticelli C, editors: The kidney in plasma cell dyscrasias, Dordrecht, 1988, Kluwer Academic.
283. Cohen AH: Pathology of light chain nephropathies. In Robinson RR, editor: *Nephrology,* New York, 1984, Springer-Verlag.
284. Buxbaum JN, Chuba JV, Hellman GC et al: Monoclonal immunoglobulin deposition disease: light chain and light and heavy chain deposition diseases and their relationship to light chain amyloidosis: clinical features, immunopathology, and molecular analysis, *Ann Intern Med* 112:455, 1990.
285. Gallo GR, Feiner HD, Katz LA et al: Nodular glomerulopathy associated with nonamyloidotic kappa light chain deposits and excess immunoglobulin light chain synthesis, *Am J Pathol* 99:621, 1980.
286. Cogne M, Preud'homme JL, Bauwens M et al: Structure of a monoclonal kappa chain of the V kappa IV subgroup in the kidney and plasma cells in light chain deposition disease, *J Clin Invest* 87:2186, 1991.
287. Sanders PW, Herrera GA: Monoclonal immunoglobulin light chain-related renal diseases, *Semin Nephrol* 13:324, 1993.
288. Gallo G: Renal complications of B-cell dyscrasia, *N Engl J Med* 324:1889, 1991 (editorial).
289. Sinniah R, Cohen AH: Glomerular capillary aneurysms in light chain nephropathy: an ultrastructural proposal of pathogenesis, *Am J Pathol* 118:298, 1985.
290. Hill GS, Morel-Maroger L, Mery JP: Renal lesions in multiple myeloma; their relationship to associated protein abnormalities, *Am J Kidney Dis* 2:243, 1983.

291. Noel LH, Droz D, Ganeval D et al: Renal granular monoclonal light chain deposits: morphological aspects in 11 cases, *Clin Nephrol* 21:263, 1984.
292. Peng SK, French WJ, Cohen AH et al: Light chain cardiomyopathy associated with small vessel disease, *Arch Pathol Lab Med* 112:844, 1988.
293. Brouet JC, Clauvel JP, Danon F et al: Biological and clinical significance of cryoglobulins: a report of 86 cases, *Am J Med* 57:775, 1974.
294. Meltzer M, Franklin EC, Elias K et al: Cryoglobulinemia: a clinical and laboratory study. II. Cryoglobulins with rheumatoid factor activity, *Am J Med* 40:837, 1966.
295. Zanussi C, Invernizzi F, Meroni PL: Classification of cryoglobulins. In Ponticelli C, Minetti L, D'Amico G, editors: *Antiglobulins, cryoglobulins and glomerulonephritis,* Boston, 1986, Martinus Nijhoff.
296. Agnello V, Chung RT, Kaplan LM: A role for hepatitis C virus infection in type II cryoglobulinemia, *N Engl J Med* 327:1490, 1992.
297. Geltner D, Franklin EC, Frangione B: Anti-idiotype activity in the IgM fractions of mixed cryoglobulins, *J Immunol* 125:1530, 1980.
298. Castiglione A, Bucci A, Fellin G et al: The relationship of infiltrating renal leukocytes to disease activity in lupus and cryoglobulinemic glomerulonephritis, *Nephron* 50:14, 1988.
299. Ferrario F, Castiglione A, Colasanti G et al: The detection of monocytes in human glomerulonephritis, *Kidney Int* 28:513, 1985.
300. Tarantino A, Devecchi A, Montagnino G et al: Renal disease in essential mixed cryoglobulinemia: long-term follow-up of 44 patients, *Q J Med* 50:1, 1981.
301. Monga G, Mazzuco G, Coppo R et al: Glomerular findings in mixed IgA-IgM cryoglobulinemia: light, electron microscopy, immunofluorescence and histochemical correlations, *Virchows Arch [B]* 20:185, 1986.
302. D'Amico G, Ferrario F, Colasanti G et al: Glomerulonephritis in essential mixed cryoglobulinemia. In Davison AM, Guillon PJ, editors: *Proceedings of the XXI Congress of the European Dialysis and Transplant Association,* London, 1985, Pitman.

Other disorders

303. Dunnill MS, Millard PR, Oliver D: Acquired cystic disease of the kidneys: a hazard of long-term intermittent maintenance hemodialysis, *J Clin Pathol* 30:868, 1979.
304. Grantham JJ, Levine E: Acquired cystic disease: replacing one kidney disease with another, *Kidney Int* 28:99, 1985.
305. Grantham JJ: Acquired cystic kidney disease, *Kidney Int* 40:143, 1991.
306. Deck MA, Verani R, Silva FG et al: Histogenesis of renal cysts in end-stage renal disease (acquired cystic kidney disease): an immunohistochemical and lectin study, *Surg Pathol* 1:391, 1988.
307. Chung WY, Nast CC, Ettenger RB et al: Acquired cystic disease in chronically rejected renal transplants, *J Am Soc Nephrol* 2:1298, 1992.
308. Hughson MD, Buchwald D, Fox M: Renal neoplasia and acquired cystic disease in patients receiving long-term dialysis, *Arch Pathol Lab Med* 110:592, 1986.
309. Hughson MD, Fox M, Garvin AJ: Pathology of the end-stage kidney after dialysis. In Damjanov I, Cohen AH, Mills SE, Young RH editors: *Progress in reproductive and urinary tract pathology,* New York, 1990, Field & Wood.
310. Ishikawa I: Uremic acquired cystic disease of the kidney, *Urology* 26:101, 1983.
311. Ishikawa I: Uremic acquired renal cystic disease: natural history and complications, *Nephron* 58:257, 1991.
312. MacDougall ML, Welling LW, Weigmann TB: Prediction of carcinoma in acquired cystic disease as a function of kidney weight, *J Am Soc Nephrol* 1:828, 1990.
313. Matson MA, Cohen EP: Acquired cystic kidney disease: occurrence, prevalence, and renal cancers, *Medicine* 69:217, 1990.
314. Bretan PN Jr, Busch MP, Hricak H: Chronic renal failure: a significant risk factor in the development of acquired renal cysts and renal cell carcinoma, *Cancer* 57:1871, 1986.
315. Colvin RB: Cellular and molecular mechanisms of allograft rejection, *Annu Rev Med* 41:361, 1990.
316. Ferry J, Jacobson J, Conti D et al: Lymphoproliferative disorders and hematologic malignancies following organ transplantation, *Mod Pathol* 2:583, 1989.
317. Hall BM: Cells mediating allograft rejection, *Transplantation* 51:1141, 1991.
318. Tötterman TH, Hanås E, Bergstrom R et al: Immunologic diagnosis of kidney rejection using FACS analysis of graft-infiltrating functional and activated T and NK cell subsets, *Transplantation* 47:817, 1989.
319. Dallman MJ: The cytokine network and regulation of the immune response to organ transplants, *Transplant Rev* 6:209, 1992.
320. Nast CC, Zuo XJ, Prehn J et al: Gamma-interferon gene expression in human renal allograft fine needle aspirates, *Transplantation* 57:498, 1994.
321. Cerilli J, Clarke J, Doolin T et al: The significance of a donor-specific vessel cross match in renal transplantation, *Transplantation* 46:359, 1988.
322. Finn WF: Prevention of ischemic injury in renal transplantation, *Kidney Int* 37:171, 1990.
323. Kopp JB, Klotman P: Cellular and molecular mechanisms of cyclosporine nephrotoxicity, *J Am Soc Nephrol* 1:162, 1990.
324. Myers BD: Cyclosporine nephrotoxicity, *Kidney Int* 30:964, 1986.
325. Sibley RK, Payne W: Morphologic findings in the renal allograft biopsy, *Semin Nephrol* 5:294, 1985.
326. Alexopoulos E, Leontsini M, Daniilidis M et al: Differentiation between renal allograft rejection and cyclosporine toxicity: a clinicopathologic study, *Am J Kidney Dis* 18:108, 1991.
327. Bergstrand A, Bohman O, Farnsworth A et al: Renal histopathology in kidney transplant recipients immunosuppressed with cyclosporin A: results of an international workshop, *Clin Nephrol* 24:107, 1985.
328. Shulman H, Striker G, Deeg HJ et al: Nephrotoxicity of cyclosporin A after allogeneic marrow transplantation, *N Engl J Med* 305:1392, 1981.
329. Morris PJ: The clinical and laboratory diagnosis of graft rejection. In Brent I, Sell RA, editors: *Organ transplantation: current clinical and immunologic concepts,* London, 1989, Bailliere Tindall.
330. Gruber SA, Chan GLC, Canafax DM: Immunosuppression in renal transplantation II: corticosteroids, antilymphocyte globulin and OKT3, *Clin Transplant* 5: 1725, 1989.
331. Hayry P, Mennander A, Ransanen-Sokolowski A et al: Pathophysiology of vascular wall changes in chronic allograft rejection, *Transplant Rev* 7:1, 1993.
332. Dennis MJ, Beckingham IJ, Blamey RW: Effect of acute damage from acute rejection and ischemia on long-term renal allograft histology, *Transplant Proc* 25:2101, 1993.
333. Rosen S, Greenfeld Z, Brezis M: chronic cyclosporine-induced nephropathy in the rat, *Transplantation* 49:445, 1990.
334. Kasiske BL, Kalil RSN, Lee HS et al: Histopathologic findings associated with a chronic progressive decline in renal allograft function, *Kidney Int* 40:514, 1991.
335. Maryniak RK, First MR, Weiss MA: Transplant glomerulopathy: evolution of morphologically distinct changes, *Kidney Int* 27:799, 1985.
336. Habib R, Zurowska A, Hinglais N et al: A specific glomerular lesion of the graft: allograft glomerulopathy. *Kidney Int* 42(suppl):S104, 1993.
337. Cameron JS: Recurrent primary disease and de novo nephritis following renal transplantation, *Pediatr Nephrol* 5:412, 1991.
338. Lim EC, Terasaki PI: Outcome of renal transplantation in different primary diseases, *Clin Transpl,* 293, 1991.
339. Neumayer HH, Kienbaum M, Graft S et al: Prevalence and long-term outcome of glomerulonephritis in renal allografts, *Am J Kidney Dis* 22:320, 1993.

B. NEOPLASMS

John N. Eble

BENIGN RENAL TUMORS	MALIGNANT RENAL TUMORS
Renal oncocytoma	Renal cell carcinoma
Mesenchymal neoplasms	Nephroblastoma (Wilms' tumor)
	Urothelial carcinoma of the renal pelvis and ureter

Renal neoplasms account for 1% to 2% of all cancers. The most important ones are nephroblastoma in children and renal cell carcinoma and carcinoma of the renal pelvic urothelium in adults. Overall, they are more common in males than in females. Symptoms of mass or hematuria are common. The cause is usually obscure, but genetic factors have been identified for renal cell carcinoma and nephroblastoma, and chemical carcinogens play a role in the development of renal pelvic carcinoma. The outlook for patients with nephroblastoma has improved steadily throughout this century; today almost all patients are cured. Renal cell carcinoma and renal pelvic carcinoma are resistant to radiation and chemotherapy, and the outlook for patients with these tumors is less favorable.

BENIGN RENAL TUMORS

Renal oncocytoma

Renal oncocytomas are uncommon benign neoplasms that arise from the distal tubules.[1] There is no consistent abnormality in nuclear DNA, but these tumors have consistent abnormalities in mitochondrial DNA.[2] The parenchyma is a distinctive mahogany brown, and large tumors often have central zones of gray edematous fibrous tissue. They consist of generally uniform cells growing in a compact pattern and have abundant, finely granular eosinophilic cytoplasm, which, at the ultrastructural level, is densely packed with mitochondria. The diagnosis of oncocytoma should not be made if the tumor contains mitotic figures, cells with clear cytoplasm, significant necrosis, or papillary architecture.[3]

Mesenchymal neoplasms

Angiomyolipomas are the most common mesenchymal tumors of the kidney and consist of variable mixtures of fat, smooth muscle, and thick-walled blood vessels (Fig. 65-96). The smooth muscle cells may be epithelioid and have noticeable nuclear pleomorphism; these are not indicators of malignancy. They occur in two distinct clinical settings: approximately half are associated with tuberous sclerosis and half occur sporadically. In patients with tuberous sclerosis, they usually are asymptomatic, multiple, bilateral, and small, whereas the sporadic ones usually are symptomatic, single, and large.[4,5] They are uncommon in the general population, but more than 50% of patients with tuberous sclerosis develop them. Although they are generally regarded as hamartomas, they may grow to great size and infiltrate surrounding structures, rarely growing into the renal vein and vena cava. A few patients have deposits of angiomyolipoma in regional lymph nodes;[6] these are regarded as multicentricity rather than metastasis. The only cases with metastasis and progression have been ones in which leiomyosarcoma has arisen in the angiomyolipoma.[7]

Mesoblastic nephromas are the most common renal tumors in the first three months of life but are quite rare after 6 months.[8] Their cut surface resembles that of a leiomyoma: firm, whorled, and light colored. Composed of spindle cells, polygonal cells, or mixtures of the two, they have infiltrative borders with the adjacent kidney and perirenal tissues.[9] An abdominal mass is the usual presenting finding. First recognized in 1966,[10] subsequent studies have shown this to be a morphologically distinct and prognostically favorable tumor. Almost all patients are cured by surgical resection; the few recurrences have been attributed to incomplete excision.

Renomedullary interstitial cell tumors are small, whitish nodules frequently found in the renal medullae at autopsy.[11] Composed of prostaglandin-containing renomedullary interstitial cells and spindle cells, it is uncertain whether these are neoplasms, hamartomas, or hyperplastic nodules. *Juxtaglomerular cell tumors,* also known as "reninomas," are

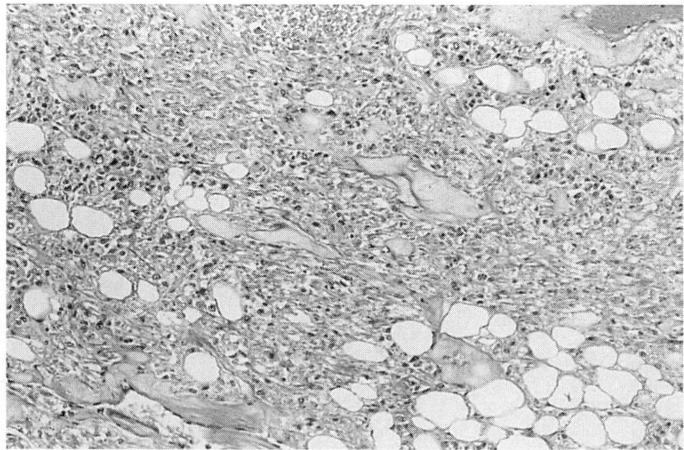

Fig. 65-96 Angiomyolipoma consists of a variable mixture of thick-walled blood vessels, smooth muscle, and fat.

benign tumors originating from the cells of the juxtaglomerular apparatus.[11] Often occurring in young adults and discovered in the course of clinical evaluations for hypertension, these tumors are solitary, and none has recurred or metastasized. Renal hemangiomas are uncommon and can cause hematuria.[12]

MALIGNANT RENAL TUMORS

Renal cell carcinoma

Renal cell carcinoma arises from the epithelium of the renal tubules and is the most important renal cancer in adults, with approximately 23,000 new cases annually in the United States.

Over the past two decades, the classification of renal cell neoplasms has grown more complex, and the schema shown in Table 65-25, based on that proposed by Thoenes and colleagues,[13] has gained acceptance. Whether the small neoplasms found at autopsy, usually resembling chromophil carcinomas but sometimes composed of clear cells, should be considered small carcinomas or adenomas has long been debated. The best candidates are lesions smaller than 10 mm, composed of cells with bland nuclei and small amounts of cytoplasm, usually arranged in a papillary architecture. Lesions composed of cells with clear cytoplasm should be regarded as small renal cell carcinomas, regardless of size.

Obesity, smoking, and exposure to industrial chemicals are risk factors for renal cell carcinoma.[14] Almost half of patients with von Hippel-Lindau disease develop renal cell carcinoma.[15] It also is associated with tuberous sclerosis and autosomal dominant polycystic kidney disease. Acquired renal cystic disease also is strongly associated with renal cell carcinoma.[16]

Table 65-25 Classification of renal cell neoplasia

Benign Neoplasms
Renal oncocytoma
Carcinomas
Renal cell carcinoma
Clear cell
Chromophil
Eosinophil
Basophil
Chromophobe
Typical
Eosinophil
Collecting duct carcinoma
Neuroendocrine tumors
Carcinoid
Small cell carcinoma

Losses of genetic material in the short arm of chromosome 3 are nearly constant findings in clear cell tumors, and many also have trisomy 7 and loss of the Y chromosome (Table 65-26). Chromophil tumors do not have the 3p deletion but instead frequently have loss of the Y chromosome and trisomy of 17, 7, or 16.[2]

Renal cell carcinomas range from tumors 1 to 2 cm in size found incidentally by radiologists to massive tumors weighing thousands of grams. They are usually well-circumscribed, solid, soft, lobulated masses (Fig. 65-97), but infiltration of the perinephric fat, renal parenchyma, or renal vein may be seen, especially in high-grade lesions. The yellow color typical of the clear cell type is the most common and distinctive, but most are variegated and some are tan or light brown. Multicentricity occurs within the same kidney in from 7% to 13% of cases, and tumors are present in both kidneys in approximately 1% of patients.

The histologic classification developed by Thoenes and colleagues[13] divides these tumors into clear cell, chromophil, and chromophobe types. Most are of the clear cell type, composed of cells with abundant clear cytoplasm, usually arranged in a diffuse or alveolar pattern (Fig. 65-98). The cytoplasm is clear because it contains much lipid and glycogen, which dissolve during tissue processing. The chromophil group encompasses two frequently seen types: *eosinophil,* with abundant cytoplasm, which is vividly eosinophilic; and those with small amounts of cytoplasm, which are called *basophil.* Both are usually arranged in a papillary architecture; these have also been called "papillary renal cell carcinoma." Chromophobe renal cell carcinoma is characterized by myriad minute intracytoplasmic vesicles that impart a pale, flocculent appearance to the cytoplasm.[17] In association with any of the cell types, approximately 5% of renal cell carcinomas contain areas resembling sarcoma.[18] The presence of sarcomatoid areas carries a poor prognosis. Rarely, carcinomas arise from the renal collecting ducts and are called "collecting duct carcinoma." Carcinoid tumors and small cell carcinomas rarely occur in the kidney.[11] The grading system for renal cell carcinoma consists of four grades based on the size and contour of nuclei and conspicuousness of nucleoli[19] (Table 65-27).

Clinically occult renal cell carcinomas that occur at distant sites with unknown primaries or that recur years after an apparently successful radical nephrectomy may pose special diagnostic problems. The coexpression of cytokeratin and vimentin, which occurs in a majority of renal cell carcino-

Table 65-26 Cytogenetic abnormalities in renal cell neoplasms

	Percentage of tumors with abnormality					
	−3p	+7	+17	+16	−Y	Mitochondrial
Clear cell	96	18	0	0	26	0
Chromophil	0	75	80	62	93	0
Chromophobe	Multiple losses					Yes
Oncocytoma	No consistent lesions					100

Nephrogenic metaplasia

Nephrogenic metaplasia, also known as *nephrogenic adenoma*, occurs particularly in the bladder and in rare cases occurs in the urethra, ureter, and renal pelvis. Approximately 75% of the lesions are seen in males and can occur at any age from infancy up to the ninth decade. Predisposing factors include chronic bladder infection, lithiasis, previous instrumentation, trauma, and catheterization and on rare occasions is seen in patients with organ transplants. The lesions are for the most part small. Thus 62% are 1 cm or less; 10% are larger than 4 cm. The lesions are single in 80% of the cases. The trigone is the most frequently affected site in the bladder, and the lesion cystoscopically appears polypoid, papillary, or sessile, or may simulate in situ carcinoma. Microscopically, the lesion may appear polypoid, papillary, or tubulocystic, and on rare occasions shows a diffuse pattern (Fig. 66-5). The tubules are usually small, round, and hollow (Fig. 66-6) and are delineated by a prominent periodic acid–Schiff (PAS)–positive basement membrane. Cystic dilatation of the tubules filled with eosinophilic material is not uncommon. The tubules and cysts are lined by cuboidal to low columnar epithelium with scanty cytoplasm. Larger cells with clear cytoplasm may be seen, and hobnail cells are present in one third of the cases. Mitosis and dysplastic features are almost nonexistent. Pronounced chronic inflammation is frequently seen. There is no evidence that nephrogenic metaplasia is a neoplastic lesion; the term "nephrogenic adenoma" should therefore be avoided. The main differential diagnosis is clear cell adenocarcinoma, but such tumors are rare, lack predisposing factors, are seen predominantly in middle-aged or older females, and are large with cellular atypia and mitoses.[1,3]

Preneoplastic lesions of the urothelium

Dysplasia

In dysplasia, the urothelium (either of normal thickness or hyperplastic) shows nuclear abnormalities. Nagy and colleagues[4] and Murphy and Soloway[5] listed 10 morphologic criteria to be used in the diagnosis of dysplasia. These include changes in the number of cell layers and polarity of cells, presence of mucosal denudations, cytoplasmic clearing, nuclear crowding, increased nuclear size, changes in chromatin pattern, nuclear irregularity, prominent nucleoli, and mitoses. All these criteria need not be present simultaneously. The authors applied the terms *mild*, *moderate*, and *severe dysplasia* in analogy with cervical dysplasia. Mostofi and Sesterhenn[6] have recommended the term "carcinoma in situ grades 1 and 2" for mild and moderate dysplasia respectively. We, however, agree with a panel of urologists and pathologists that use of the terms *carcinoma in situ grades 1 and 2* should be discouraged because such terminology may lead to unwarranted aggressive treatment.[7] Although dysplasia is frequently seen in bladders with papillary tumors, the biologic significance of dysplasia remains to be determined.

Carcinoma in situ

A diagnosis of carcinoma in situ (CIS) can be made when the entire thickness of the urothelium has been replaced by a population of malignant cells (Fig. 66-7). The lesion is flat (nonpap-

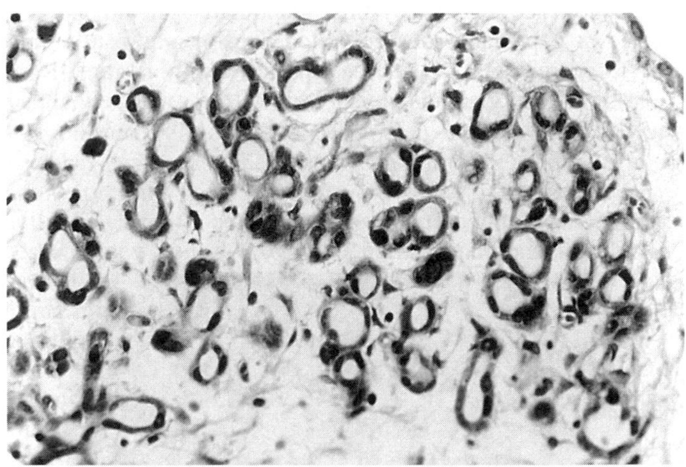

Fig. 66-6 Higher magnification of nephrogenic metaplasia. Notice the tubular structures resembling vascular spaces.

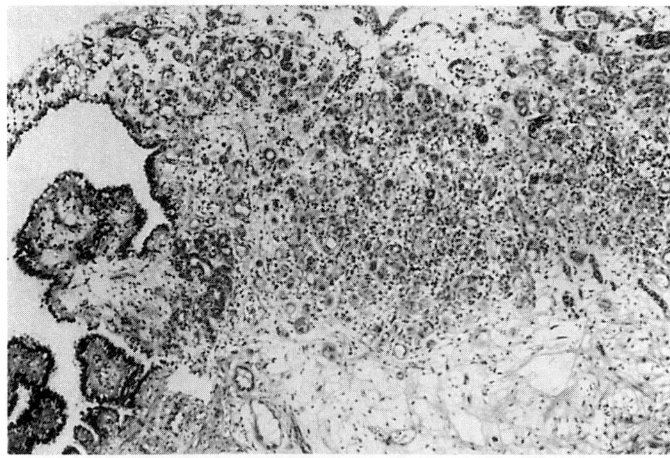

Fig. 66-5 Specimen from transurethral resection of the bladder showing nephrogenic metaplasia manifesting in abundant small tubular structures in an inflammatory edematous lamina propria. Notice the polypoid appearance.

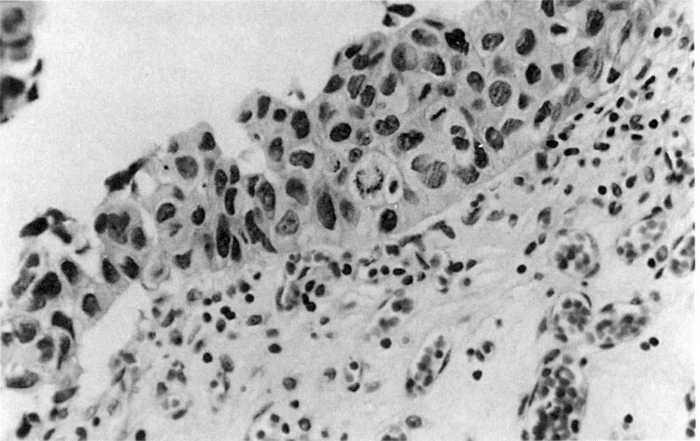

Fig. 66-7 Carcinoma in situ in bladder biopsy specimen. Patient had symptoms of urgency and frequency of urination. No tumors were detected by cystoscopy. Notice the malignant features of the cells as well as the disturbed polarity, mitosis, and absence of umbrella cells.

illary). CIS is most commonly seen in patients with high-grade papillary transitional cell carcinoma, and there is involvement of the distal ureters, urethra, and prostatic duct in 9% to 60% of the patients.[1,8] Primary CIS without associated urothelial tumors constitutes less than 10% of the cases. It is seen characteristically in males older than 50 years of age and is associated with irritative symptoms. In 70% of cases, multifocality is noted, and the majority of cases have cytologic features of malignancy. A majority of patients develop invasive carcinoma within 3 years of diagnosis if left untreated. By cystoscopy, the mucosa often shows a reddish, velvety appearance. The tumor cells have reduced cohesiveness, and it is common to receive biopsy specimens with denuded mucosa or with only a few malignant cells. Positive cytologic finding without obvious bladder lesions may represent CIS of the upper urinary tract or of the urethra, periurethral glands, or prostate.

BLADDER

Normal structure and function

The urinary bladder develops from the cloaca and the urogenital sinus; the latter is divided into the dorsal rectum and the ventral urogenital sinus. The urogenital sinus develops into the urinary bladder and the posterior urethra; the bladder and the proximal and middle urethral linings are of endodermal origin, whereas the distal urethral lining is of ectodermal origin. The stromal and muscular components of the ureters and bladder are of mesodermal origin.[9]

Normal anatomy and histology

The normal urinary bladder is a hollow organ located in the pelvis and connected to ureters on both sides and the urethra centrally. Anatomically, several distinct regions are recognized in it: the trigone, the lateral, posterior, and anterior walls, and the dome.

The urinary bladder has three histologic layers: the urothelium, the lamina propria, and the muscularis propria (detrusor muscle). In the bladder, the urothelium is up to seven cell layers thick. The number of layers depends on the distention of the bladder at the time of fixation. The urothelial lining is composed of superficial (or umbrella), intermediate, and basal cells, the last resting on a basal lamina. The suburothelial connective tissue is called the *lamina propria* and consists of loose connective tissue with blood and lymphatic vessels and thin nerves. The deep part of the lamina propria borders the detrusor muscle, consisting of interlacing bundles of smooth muscle fibers. At approximately one third of the distance from the basal lamina to the detrusor muscle, there are thin wisps of smooth muscle fibers forming the so-called muscularis mucosae (Fig. 66-8). Although muscularis mucosae was not described until 1983,[10] Ro and colleagues[11] systematically studied 100 consecutive bladder biopsy specimens and found it missing from only six. The muscularis mucosae, though discontinuous, is important for bladder cancer staging; the presence of relatively large vessels are helpful for its histologic identification.[12] The lamina propria is encased by the muscle layer that forms the detrusor muscle. Adipose tissue or peritoneum cover the detrusor muscle. Urachal rests are often present in the bladder, especially in the dome or anterior wall. The structure may be that of a narrow tube or microcyst or microcysts lined by flat urothelium-like cells.

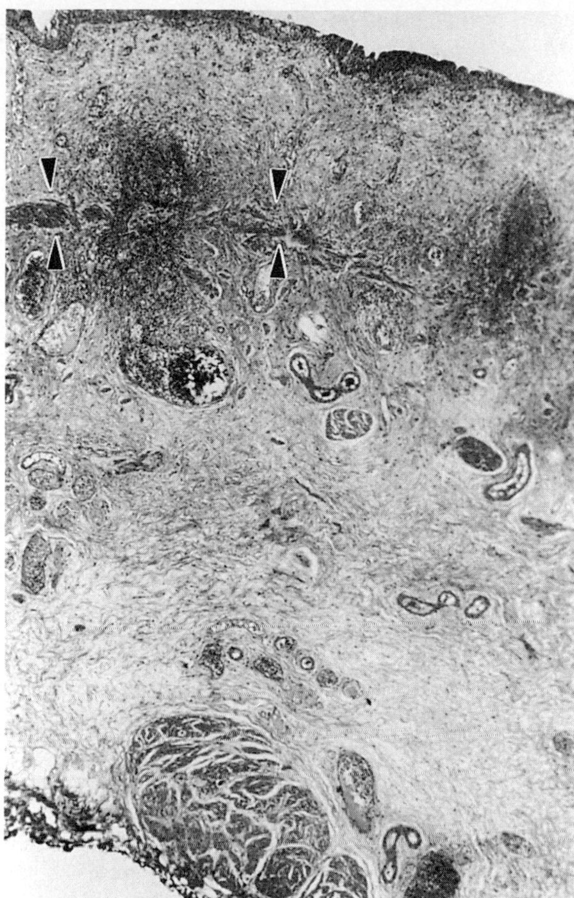

Fig. 66-8 Specimen from transurethral resection of the bladder showing normal structures of the bladder, urothelium, lamina propria, muscularis mucosae *(arrowheads)* and detrusor muscle *(bottom)*. Notice the distinct vasculature at the level of the muscularis mucosae.

Function. The lower urinary tract serves as a conduit for the transport and storage of urine and for the excretion (release) of urine and is partially permeable to urinary contents.[13] Storage of urine in the bladder is dependent primarily on the viscoelastic properties of the interlacing smooth muscle bundles of the detrusor muscle. Neurologic control of storage appears to be of secondary importance, with sympathetic fibers that arise from segments T10 to L2 of the spinal cord, being conducted along the pudendal and hypogastric nerves and possibly acting to relax the detrusor muscle and tighten the skeletal muscle outlet sphincter. Release is predominantly controlled by cholinergic parasympathetic nerves, which arise from the S2 to S4 segments and are carried through the pelvic nerve, as well as by somatic motor neurons that also arise from the sacral cord. These nerves produce increased smooth muscle contraction of the bladder and urethral relaxation. Supraspinal pathways control these neuronal responses. In addition, purine neurotransmitters appear to be involved with the later phases of bladder contraction, possibly to ensure complete emptying, and a variety of peptide neurotransmitters also are involved, though their specific role or roles are unclear. Afferent nerves are also important in providing a sense of fullness or urgency, signaling the need for release, but these nerves also carry signals for pain. These afferent nerves are carried in the pelvic nerve along with the parasympathetic neurons.

Abnormalities of bladder function are exceedingly common. *Incontinence* afflicts 12 to 15 million individuals in the United States yearly. It can be caused by suprasacral cord transection, trauma, peripheral nerve disorders, metabolic disorders, drugs, neurologic diseases, and other factors.[13] Cord transection actually leads to loss of micturition control; some function may return weeks to months later but with small volume and incomplete emptying. Peripheral nerve damage can result in either a flaccid, hypotonic, or hypertonic bladder. *Obstruction* of the bladder is also a common problem, which is often accompanied by pain, urinary dysfunction, and inflammation. Obstruction also produces detrusor hypertrophy and hyperactivity.

Examination of surgical specimens

Forceps or cold-cup biopsy specimens or material from transurethral resection of bladder (TURB) should be fixed properly and oriented for perpendicular sectioning. Material from bladder tumors obtained by TURB should be fractionated by the urologist, with the main part of the tumor and the deeper part including the detrusor muscle being placed in separate containers. TURB material almost invariably shows cautery damage, which sometimes makes interpretation and grading of tumors difficult or impossible.

Partial cystectomy specimens should be sent fresh to the pathology department or should be mounted on a cork plate and fixed in 10% neutral buffered formalin. The specimen and the tumor should be measured, and the tumor as well as the closest excision margins should be sampled. Nontumorous areas should also be sampled for dysplasia or for CIS. Nontumorous sections such as areas of ulceration and hemorrhages should be sampled randomly in addition to obvious lesions.

Total cystectomy specimens include small segments of the ureters, and those should be tied off. The bladder should be filled with approximately 100 to 200 ml of 10% neutral buffered formalin through a Foley catheter and submerged and fixed for 24 to 48 hours. The bladder should be opened through the dorsal urethra and the anterior wall dome. Sections should be taken from obvious tumors, previous TURB areas, and hemorrhagic areas. One to two random sections should also be taken from the bladder neck, the trigone, the left and right lateral walls, the posterior wall, the anterior wall, and the dome as well as from the proximal ureters, the proximal, middle, and distal parts of the urethra, and the prostate.

Congenital disorders

Exstrophy

Exstrophy is a congenital condition in which the entire anterior wall of the urinary bladder is missing or in which a vesicocutaneous fistula has developed as a result of incomplete closure of the anterior abdominal wall and the anterior bladder wall. The primary defect is not completely understood but is most likely associated with a lack of normal differentiation of the cloacal membrane. This structure occupies most of the lower anterior abdominal wall. Exstrophy is often associated with other anomalies such as lack of fusion of the symphysis pubis, and labia, and epispadias.[14] The condition is not hereditary and is somewhat more frequent in males than in females, with a frequency of 1 case in 50,000 births.[15] Because of contact with clothes and continuous drainage of urine, these individuals develop chronic urinary tract infection with squamous and glandular metaplasia (Fig. 66-4). Uncorrected exstrophy results in ascending urinary tract infection and impaired renal function. Surgical correction results in histologic improvement in only 25% of the cases. The affected patients are at a risk for bladder cancer; 80 such cases have been reported. The majority of these cancers are adenocarcinomas.[1]

Diverticulum

Diverticuli of the urinary bladder are relatively common, particularly in male patients over 50 years of age suffering from prostatic enlargement with partial obstruction. In contrast to these acquired diverticuli, those in younger individuals occur in the absence of obstruction and are congenital. In all ages, the majority of diverticuli are found around the ureteral orifices. Smaller diverticuli lack clinical significance, but larger ones predispose to infection and lithiasis, and in these cases surgical removal is indicated. Furthermore, 2% to 7% of patients with diverticuli develop tumors within the diverticuli.

Morphologically, the diverticulum has a narrow neck leading to a larger pouch (Fig. 66-9). It has been suggested that congenital diverticuli have smooth muscle fibers whereas acquired ones lack smooth muscle fibers. However, chronic inflammation results in fibrosis of the wall, and muscle fibers cannot be identified in either type of diverticulum after longstanding inflammation.[1]

Nonneoplastic conditions

Von Brunn's nests, cystitis cystica, cystitis glandularis, squamous metaplasia, and nephrogenic metaplasia occur in the urinary bladder very often. Histologically, these lesions have the same features as those already described in the calyces, pelves, and ureters.

Cystitis

Bacterial cystitis

Bacterial urinary tract infection (UTI) is most commonly caused by gram-negative organisms, especially *Escherichia coli.* Other organisms, such as *Klebsiella pneumoniae* and *Streptococcus fecalis,* are frequent causes of UTI, as are *Pro-*

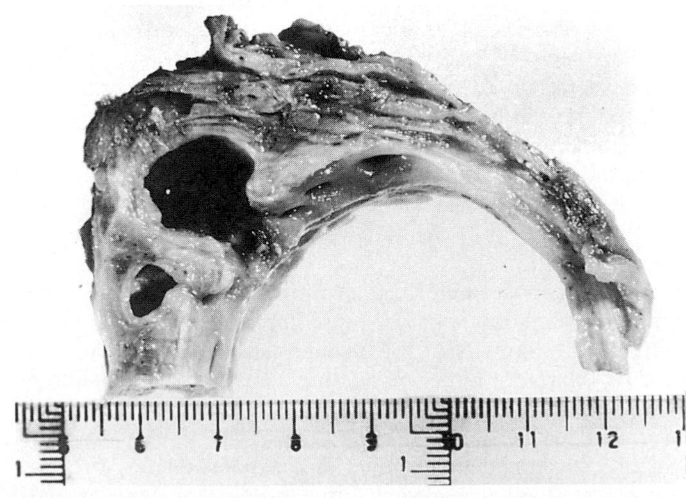

Fig. 66-9 Autopsy specimen of bladder from a male patient with benign prostatic hypertrophy showing multiple diverticuli.

teus vulgaris and *Pseudomonas aeruginosa. Chlamydia trachomatis, Mycoplasma hominis,* and *Ureaplasma urealyticum* can be cultured from bladder urine but are more important pathogens in the urethra, kidneys, and genital system. The mycoplasmas and ureaplasmas have been associated with an increased tendency to develop urinary tract stones but have not been implicated significantly in bladder infections. Normal urine is sterile, and the urinary bladder is resistant to an infection under normal circumstances. Bladder infections appear with two events, namely, colonization of the urine by organisms and impairment of host defenses. Adhesion of the bacteria to the urothelial surface has been suggested as a necessary step in the process. UTI is rare in young children without urinary tract malformation. The incidence increases in the sexually active female (the so-called honeymoon cystitis) and in the male suffering from benign prostatic hypertrophy caused by urinary retention. Predisposing factors also include a short female urethra, diverticula, foreign bodies such as stones or catheters, as well as agents causing mechanical destruction of the bladder mucosae.[1,16]

The diagnosis is based on clinical symptoms, urinalysis, and positive culture; biopsies should be avoided. Histologically, cystitis produces a typical acute inflammatory response, frequently with epithelial erosion and ulceration, which is associated with pyuria, hematuria, and bacteruria.

Tuberculosis

Infection with *Mycobacterium tuberculosis* results typically from downstream spread from the kidney and is very rare today. Identical lesions are commonly seen after intravesicular instillation of BCG (bacille Calmette-Guérin) for treatment of carcinoma in situ or superficial papillary bladder tumors. Histologically, the lesions are composed of epithelioid granulomas with or without central caseous necrosis (Fig. 66-10). They may be seen in the lamina propria and also in the detrusor muscle. Differentiation from vesical sarcoidosis requires special stains for acid-fast bacilli or culture.[16]

Schistosomal cystitis

Schistosoma hematobium, the main cause of schistosomal cystitis, is endemic in eastern Africa and the Middle East, but only occasional cases are found in the United States. The intermediate host is a snail from which the cercariae escape, swim to the human host, penetrate the skin, and, through the lymphatics, move to the liver, where maturation occurs. The worms mate in the mesenteric plexus and move to the bladder to deposit ova. The histologic appearance in the bladder varies depending on the stage, but generally a granulo-matous response is seen, with calcified eggs (Fig. 66-11), a variable degree of fibrosis, and squamous or glandular metaplasia.[17] Chronic infestation is associated with a greatly increased risk of bladder cancer, especially squamous cell carcinoma and adenocarcinoma. In addition to neoplasia, other serious complications include hydroureter, hydronephrosis, and pyelonephritis.

Fungal cystitis

The overwhelming majority of fungal infections of the urinary tract are caused by *Candida* species. Patients at risk include immunosuppressed individuals, such as AIDS patients and transplant recipients, patients with diabetes mellitus, patients undergoing antibiotic therapy, patients with indwelling catheters, and premature infants.[18] The histologic features include an inflammatory exudate with budding and nonbudding yeast cells and pseudohyphae.

Viral cystitis

Both RNA and DNA viruses may be identified in urine specimens. Immunosuppressed patients can develop cytomegalovirus infections, and cells characteristic of *Polyomavirus* infection are sometimes identified. These viruses usually are not associated with any significant symptoms.

Interstitial cystitis

The term *interstitial cystitis* (IC) was first used by Skene in the late 1800s but popularized later by Hunner who described the

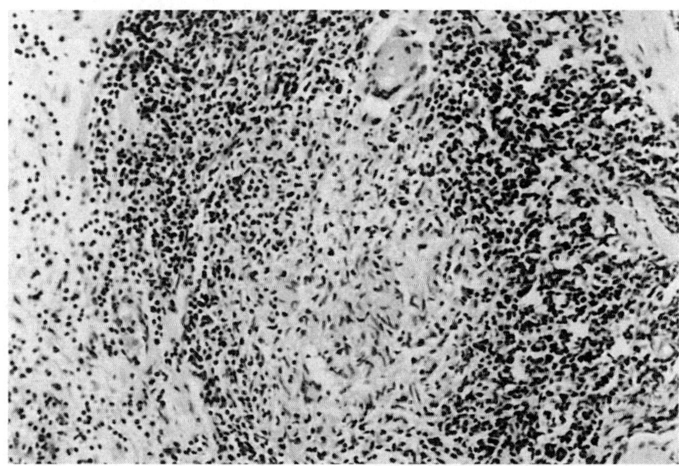

Fig. 66-10 Bladder biopsy from a patient with carcinoma in situ treated with BCG. Granuloma with a Langhans' giant cell can be seen.

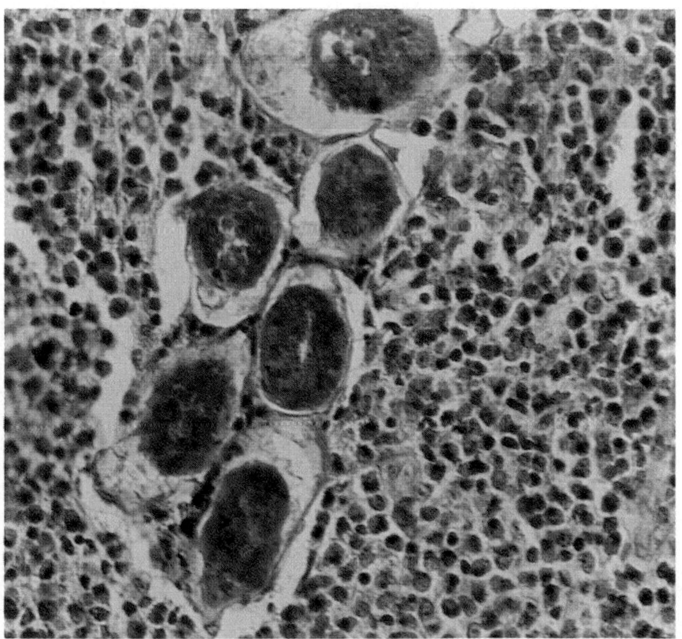

Fig. 66-11 Bladder biopsy showing schistosomal ova associated with considerable eosinophilia. (From Johansson SL: *Diseases of the urinary bladder,* video disc, Los Angeles, 1992, Intellipath.)

ulcer named after him. It is a condition of unknown cause and pathogenesis with a pronounced preponderance in females (approximately 90% of patients are females). The diagnosis is based on the clinical symptoms of urgency, frequency, and bladder pain. Cystoscopically, one group of patients shows pale areas with radiating vessels, and there are mucosal and vascular ruptures forming *Hunner's ulcer,* which can be seen when the bladder is distended to at least 70 cm of H_2O pressure (Fig. 66-12). In the second group of patients, there are no ulcers, only petechial, strawberry-like hemorrhages called *"glomerulations"* (Fig. 66-13). These appear on the second distention during cystoscopic evaluation. The diagnosis of IC is made clinically, but a biopsy must nevertheless be performed to exclude other forms of cystitis or CIS. The mean age of patients for nonulcer IC is 40 years and that for ulcer IC is 60 years, but there is no evidence that the former progresses to the latter. Histologically, IC with ulcers shows wedge-shaped ulcers covered with fibrin and erythrocytes (Fig. 66-14). The lamina propria displays pronounced edema, mucosal hemorrhage, and usually moderate to severe chronic inflammation dominated by lymphocytes, occasionally with germinal centers. The inflammation is generally limited to the lamina propria, but perineural inflammation is seen in 80% of the patients. Patients with identical symptoms, but who do not have ulcers show only suburothelial hemorrhage corresponding to the glomerulations and relatively often have mucosal ruptures (Fig. 66-15). The inflammatory response is usually mild or nonexistent. If appropriate fixation or staining methods are used, only the ulcer type of IC will show an increased number of mast cells in both the lamina propria and the muscularis.[19,20]

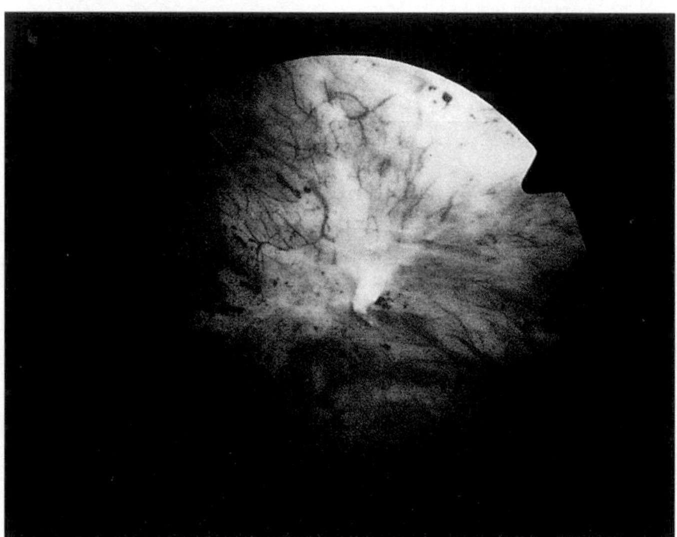

Fig. 66-12 Cystoscopic appearance of ulcer type of interstitial cystitis. Notice a central scar with a small fibrin deposit before distention. (From Johansson SL, Fall M: *J Urol* 143:1118, 1990.)

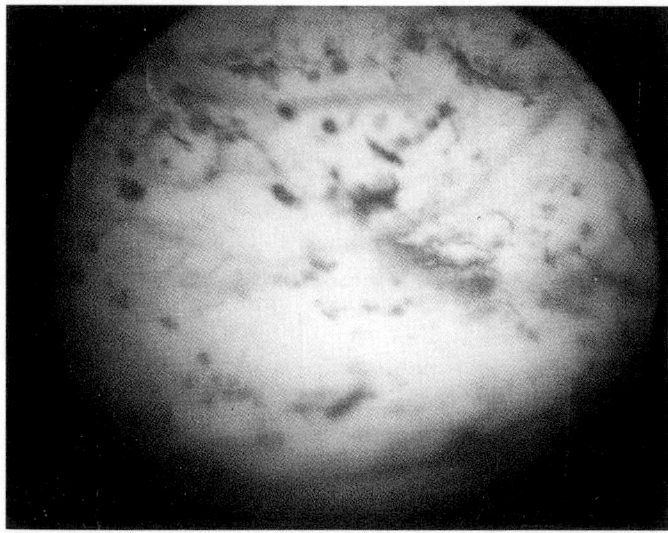

Fig. 66-13 Cystoscopic appearance showing postdistention glomerulations in a patient with nonulcer disease. (From Johansson SL, Fall M: *J Urol* 143:1118, 1990.)

Eosinophilic cystitis

The rare condition eosinophilic cystitis was first described in 1960. It affects males and females equally. Symptoms are similar to those of IC, but hematuria may also occur, and patients are often middle aged. Cystoscopically the mucosa is swollen, reddish, and sometimes tumorlike. Histologically, there is transmural inflammation with a strong preponderance of

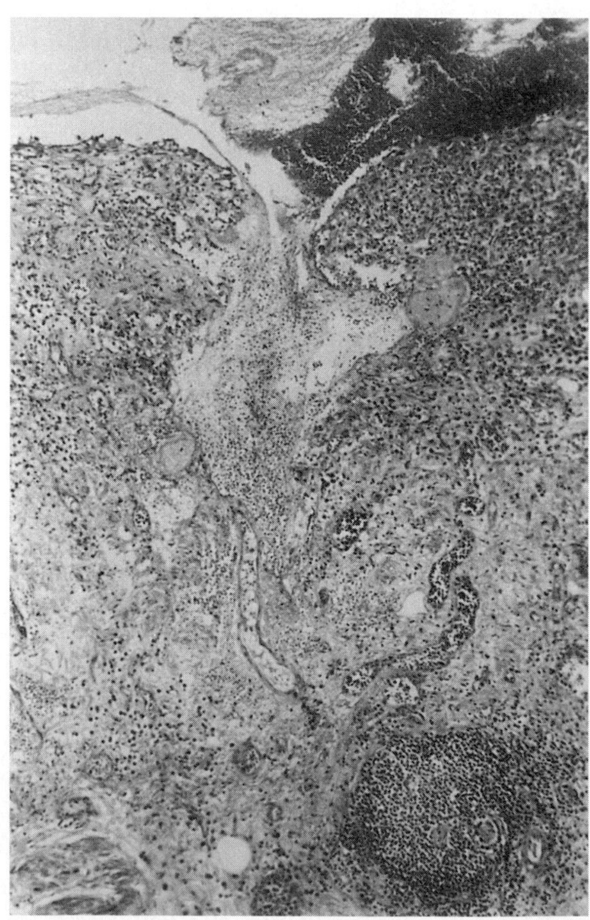

Fig. 66-14 Specimen from transurethral resection of the bladder showing ulcer type of interstitial cystitis. Notice the wedge-shaped Hunner's ulcer, blood and fibrin on the surface, granulation tissue, edema, and chronic inflammation.

eosinophils (Fig. 66-16). Inflammation and edema are more intense in the lamina propria. Focal muscle necrosis is also seen together with a variable degree of fibrosis. Involvement of the ureters with obstruction may occur. Some patients have predisposing allergic conditions, whereas others do not. Urine cultures are usually sterile. The characteristic morphologic features of eosinophilic cystitis are important for the differential diagnosis from other forms of cystitis, principally IC, which generally lacks eosinophils, muscle necrosis, and transmural inflammation.[21]

Emphysematous cystitis

Emphysematous cystitis is a rare condition occurring usually in elderly patients who have diabetes or are debilitated. Sometimes it may affect patients with bladder outlet obstruction, fistulas, and diverticula. In histologic sections, urothelial cysts appear as empty holes surrounded by slight inflammation, or occasionally by foreign-body giant cells (Fig. 66-17). The cysts contain gas produced by *E. coli* or *Aerobacter aerogenes* or sometimes *Clostridium perfringens.*[16]

Follicular cystitis

In follicular cystitis small, multiple, nodular lesions can be seen cystoscopically or in autopsy bladders. Histologically the diagnosis is confirmed by the presence, in the lamina propria, of lymphoid follicles with germinal centers, causing a slight elevation of the urothelium. Actually, the term is inadequate because the lesions are asymptomatic, no organism associated with follicular cystitis has been identified, and similar follicles may also be found in the upper urinary tract.[1]

Gangrenous cystitis

Gangrenous cystitis, in common with emphysematous cystitis, typically affects debilitated or elderly patients suffering from systemic infections or from compromised cardiovascular function. The lesions are not caused by a specific organism, and the bacteriologic findings are usually nonspecific. The urothelium over the entire bladder is often necrotic, and fibrinopurulent debris, mixed with red blood cells, forms a membrane on the urothelial surface. Inflammation and necrosis usually extend deeply and involve the detrusor muscle. Gangrenous cystitis is lethal in 60% of patients.[1]

Malakoplakia

Malakoplakia is a chronic inflammation that occurs as yellow plaques varying from a few millimeters to 2.5 cm in size. Although it has been reported in several extraurinary tract sites, at least one half of all cases originate in the urinary bladder. The cause of malakoplakia has not been determined, though there is a close association with *E. coli* infection and depressed immune status. A key factor in malakoplakia is an acquired defect in monocyte bactericidal activity, probably one of lysosomal degradation.[16] The clinical symptoms are those of infection or inflammation, frequency, urgency, dysuria, and hematuria. There is a pronounced preponderance of females. The condition has been described in all ages, but the peak incidence is in the fifth to seventh decades. Smith[22] described three histologic pictures related to time: (1) the early or prediagnostic phase showing stromal edema with lymphocytes and plasma cells and increasing numbers of histiocytes; (2) the classic phase dominated by abundant large von Hansemann histiocytes, and intracellular and extracellular pathogno-

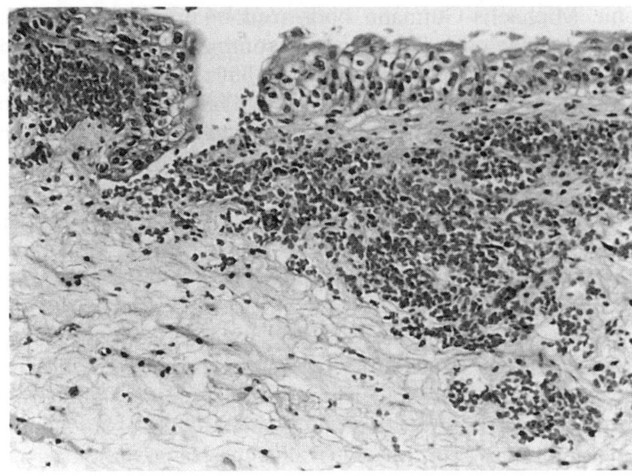

Fig. 66-15 Nonulcer type of interstitial cystitis showing mucosal rupture and suburothelial hemorrhage corresponding to glomerulation.

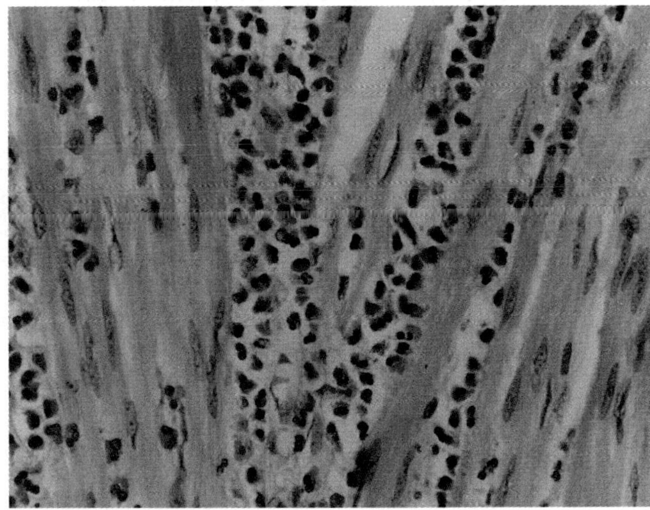

Fig. 66-16 Eosinophilic cystitis involving the detrusor muscle exhibiting a pronounced eosinophilic infiltrate.

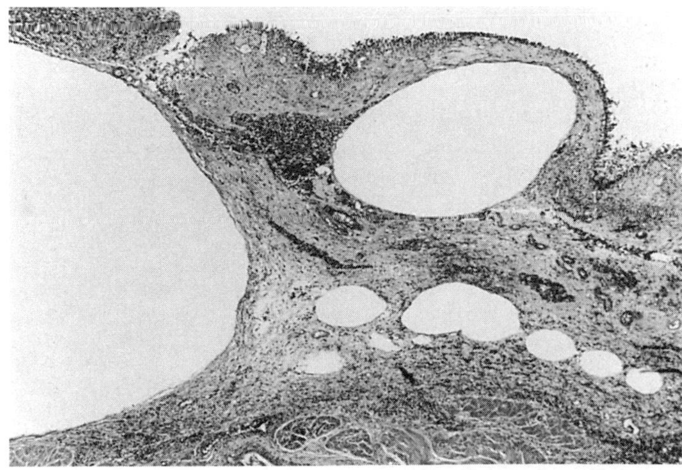

Fig. 66-17 Autopsy specimen from a patient with emphysematous cystitis. Notice the cystlike empty spaces in the lamina propria.

tus. In both the bladder and the urethra the appearance is identical to that of genital condylomas. In the urethra, the main differential diagnosis is squamous papilloma, which is exophytic with branching papillae.[16]

Amyloidosis

Amyloidosis of the urinary bladder is uncommon. The bladder may be involved by primary or secondary amyloidosis. Both sexes are equally affected, most of the cases being reported in the fifth to seventh decades, and men are affected at a slightly younger age than women. Painless gross hematuria is the main presenting symptom in 85% of the cases and is often massive in the secondary cases. The cystoscopic findings are not specific. The lesions are frequently localized and often indistinguishable from a bladder tumor before biopsy. Histologically, deposits of amyloid can be found in the arteries, arterioles, veins, the suburothelial stroma, and the inner layers of the muscularis propria. Foreign-body giant cell reaction and calcification may be present. Amyloid has also been described in the renal pelvis, ureter, and urethra.[1,3]

Endometriosis

Endometriosis of the bladder has been reported to occur in 1% of patients with this condition in the genital organs. Fifty percent of these patients have a history of pelvic surgery. It is diagnosed almost exclusively during the reproductive years.[3] Dysuria and hematuria are the two most common symptoms, and the lesions may be seen as bluish cysts by cystoscopy. IC-like symptoms in a patient with previous pelvic surgery may be caused by endometriosis. Histologically the lesion resembles endometriosis elsewhere in the body.

NEOPLASMS OF THE URINARY TRACT

Epidemiology

In the United States, bladder cancer accounts for about 7% of all cancer in males and 2% of all cancer in females, and the incidence is increasing, with approximately 50,000 new cases reported annually. The incidence of renal pelvic tumors is roughly one tenth that of bladder tumors, and the incidence of ureteral tumors is approximately one tenth that of tumors of the renal pelvis. The mean age at diagnosis is about 65 years, the majority of urothelial tumors being diagnosed between 50 and 80 years of age. Tumors in patients younger than 30 years of age are rare, with fewer than 100 cases reported. Tumors occur more commonly in males, with a ratio of three males to one female. More than 90% of lower urinary tract tumors are of transitional cell (urothelial) origin (Table 66-1).

Table 66-1 Classification of urinary bladder tumors (epithelial neoplasms)

Transitional cell (urothelial) neoplasms
- Papilloma
  - Inverted
  - Everted
- Carcinoma
  - Papillary
  - Nonpapillary (solid)
- Carcinoma in situ and possible precursor lesions
- Variants of transitional cell carcinoma
  - Transitional cell carcinoma with glandlike lumens
  - Transitional cell carcinoma, nested type
  - Lymphoepithelial carcinoma

Squamous cell carcinoma, conventional type

Verrucous squamous cell carcinoma

Villous adenoma

Adenocarcinoma
- Papillary, glandular, mucinous, signet-ring cell, and clear cell carcinoma

Small cell carcinoma (neuroendocrine carcinoma)

Mixed carcinoma

Other epithelial neoplasms
- Carcinosarcoma
- Carcinoid tumor

Table 66-2 Etiologic factors for cancer of the urinary tract

	Renal pelvis	Ureter	Bladder
Occupational			
Dyestuff industry	Yes	Yes	Yes
Leather industry			Yes
Rubber industry			Yes
Paint exposure			Yes
Organic chemical industry			Yes
Hair dressers			Yes
Cigarette smoking	Yes	Yes	Yes
Aromatic amines	Yes	Yes	Yes
Phenacetin-containing analgesics	Yes	Yes	Yes
Thorotrast	Yes	Yes	
Chlornaphazine			Yes
Radiation treatment			Yes
Cyclophosphamide	Yes		Yes
Balkan nephropathy	Yes	Yes	Yes
Arsenic (in Taiwan)?			Yes

Etiology

The cause of urinary tract tumors is generally unknown, though the epidemiologic data are suggestive of possible links with several environmental risk factors (Table 66-2). Chemicals implicated in the cause of urinary tract cancer and proved to be carcinogenic also in animals include the aromatic amines 2-naphthylamine, 4-aminobiphenyl, and benzidine, and the benzidine-derived azo dyes, which were widely used in the dyestuff and rubber industries. Other aromatic amines have also been implicated as causes of bladder cancer. It has been estimated that cigarette smoking accounts for 50% to 60% of all bladder cancer in the United States, whereas occupational exposure is responsible for 20% to 30% of bladder tumors. The 4-aminobiphenyl and other aromatic amines present in tobacco smoke may account for some of the associated bladder cancer. The antineoplastic agent chlornaphazine, used in the 1950s and 1960s to treat polycythemia, is a derivative of 2-naphthylamine and metabolically is converted to the amine.[28] An increasing number of cancers (usually high grade), especially in the bladder, have been reported after treatment (usually orally) with cyclophosphamide and related phosphamides.[3] Most likely the pathogenetic mechanism is related to the formation of acrolein, a cyclophosphamide metabolite, which is capable of DNA adduction. Sodium saccharin and related sodium and potassium salts, though capable of producing bladder tumors in the male rat at very high doses, do not appear to be human bladder carcinogens. Consumption of phenacetin-containing analgesics results particularly in the development of renal pelvic tumors, and relative risks of 10% and 4% have been reported for women and men, respectively.[29] An increased risk of ureteral and bladder tumors is also associated with phenacetin-related analgesic abuse. The majority of these patients also have renal papillary necrosis. The average induction time is 22 years, similar to that seen in occupational bladder cancer with aromatic amines.[30] Occupational exposure has been associated with increased risk of bladder cancer in the dye industry, chemical industry, textile manufacturing, and paper industry.[28] In Taiwan, arsenic in the drinking water has been linked to bladder cancer development, and in several Balkan countries there is an increased rate of bladder cancer in individuals with a nephropathy endemic to the area, but for which no cause has yet been defined. Chronic inflammation of the bladder, such as that attributable to neurogenic bladder, calculi, or diverticula, shows a weak association with bladder cancer development, with an increased proportion of these being squamous cell rather than transitional cell carcinomas.

Inverted papilloma

Inverted papilloma was originally described by Paschkis in 1927[31] and was rediscovered by Potts and Hirst in 1963.[32] Since then, more than 250 cases have been reported in the urinary tract, with the majority (75%) being in the bladder. It accounts for almost 2% of all bladder tumors. Thus, among 700 bladder tumors diagnosed in the southwestern part of Sweden during 1987-1988, 13 cases (1.8%) of inverted papilloma were found (unpublished observation), and Kunze found that, out of 1829 cases of tumors of the renal pelvis, ureter, bladder, and urethra, 2.2% were inverted papillomas.[33] There is a male preponderance; the male-to-female ratio is approximately 5:1, with a peak incidence in the fifth and sixth decades. Painless hematuria is the most common clinical presentation. Cystoscopically, the lesion, which in 80% of the cases is located in the trigone–bladder neck region, usually appears as a smooth, nodular, polypoid structure, though sessile and papillary tumors have been described. The bladder neck location helps explain the frequent occurrence of obstructive symptoms.

Most tumors measure 1 to 2 cm, though tumors measuring up to 7.5 cm have been described.[1,8] The light microscopic appearance is relatively characteristic. The smooth surface is lined by urothelium, which may be thinner than normal, of normal thickness, or even slightly hyperplastic, but without dysplasia and with preserved umbrella cell layer. The lesion is composed of anastomosing cords and columns of urothelial cells extending deep into the lamina propria (Fig. 66-23). The peripheral cells of the cords appear in palisades oriented perpendicularly to the basal lamina, giving the lesion a basal cell carcinoma–like appearance. Frequently, small cysts with proteinaceous or mucinous material are present, and foci of cells with a squamous appearance are common (Fig. 66-24). Kunze and colleagues recognized the above-mentioned variant of inverted papilloma and described a second one, the glandular type. The latter is best described as a hypertrophic tumorlike variant of cystitis glandularis with tall mucus-containing columnar cells.[33]

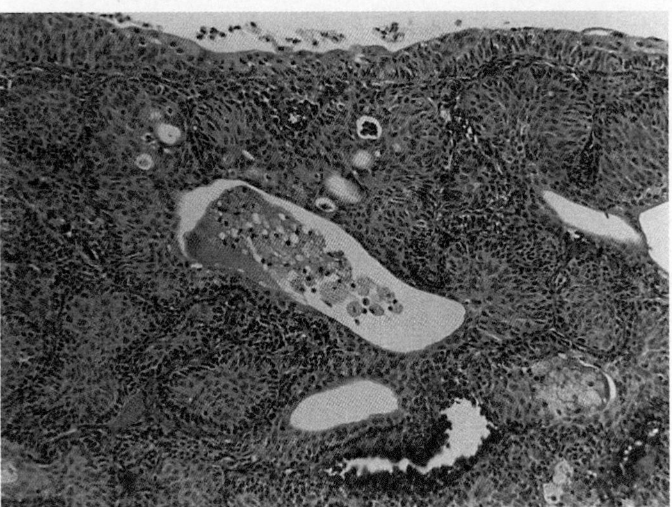

Fig. 66-23 Inverted papilloma showing a typical inverted pattern with anastomosing cords of blend urothelial cells with focal cystlike spaces. (From Johansson SL: *Diseases of the urinary bladder,* video disc, Los Angeles, 1992, Intellipath.)

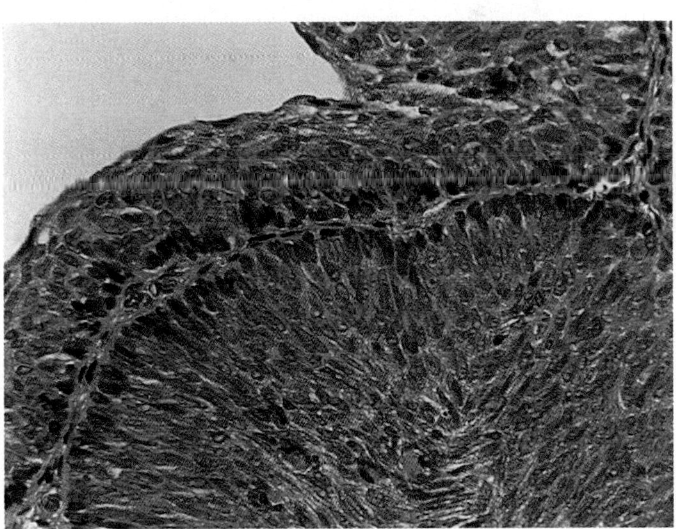

Fig. 66-24 Higher magnification of inverted papilloma showing peripheral palisading of bland urothelial cells. Notice the basal cell carcinoma–like appearance. (From Johansson SL: *Diseases of the urinary bladder,* video disc, Los Angeles, 1992, Intellipath.)

Inverted papilloma must be distinguished from carcinoma. Inverted papilloma usually has a bland cytologic appearance and lacks mitotic figures. If dysplasia and mitoses are identified, especially with squamous features and keratinization, the lesion represents a carcinoma with an inverted pattern. Some of these carcinomas may have deceptively benign features.[3]

Urothelial neoplasms

Gross appearance. Urothelial tumors may appear as single or as multiple (25% of tumors) lesions. Papillary tumors, which are the most common, cystoscopically have the appearance of "seaweed" protruding into the lumen of the bladder

(Fig. 66-25). Besides papillary tumors, sessile, nodular, and ulcerated masses may be identified (Fig. 66-26). Generally, papillary tumors are of low grade, whereas the others tend to be of high grade and invasive. Sixty percent of bladder tumors are located in the lateral and posterior walls and 20% in the trigone.

Histology. In the United States and Europe the majority of tumors in the renal pelvis, ureter, and bladder are urothelial (transitional cell) carcinomas. At least 90% are urothelial, 3% to 8% are squamous cell carcinomas, and less than 1% are adenocarcinomas (in the bladder). In the renal pelvis and ureter, adenocarcinomas are extremely rare. The configuration of the carcinomas may be papillary, papillary and solid, or solid. The majority of papillary carcinomas are noninvasive and usually of low grade, whereas almost all solid tumors are invasive. The most important factors for prognosis in urinary tract tumors are the grade and the stage of the tumor.

Several malignancy grading systems have been published; the two most widely used are the WHO system and the one presented by Bergkvist and associates.[34,35] The WHO grading system comprises three grades and undifferentiated carcinoma. Grade 1 is the least anaplastic, grade 3 the most anaplastic but still recognizable as urothelial carcinoma, and those tumors in between are grouped under grade 2 (Figs. 66-27 to 66-30). Although it is a simple system, it lacks specific histologic and cytologic criteria for the different grades. The original or modified Bergkvist's system[35] provides detailed criteria for

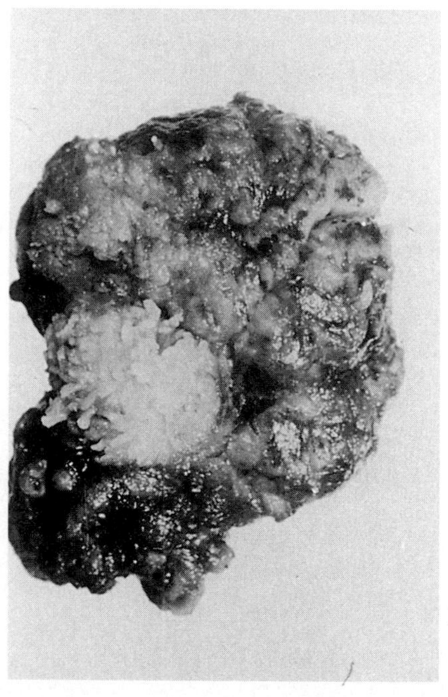

Fig. 66-25 Partial resection specimen of bladder showing a low-grade papillary transitional cell carcinoma.

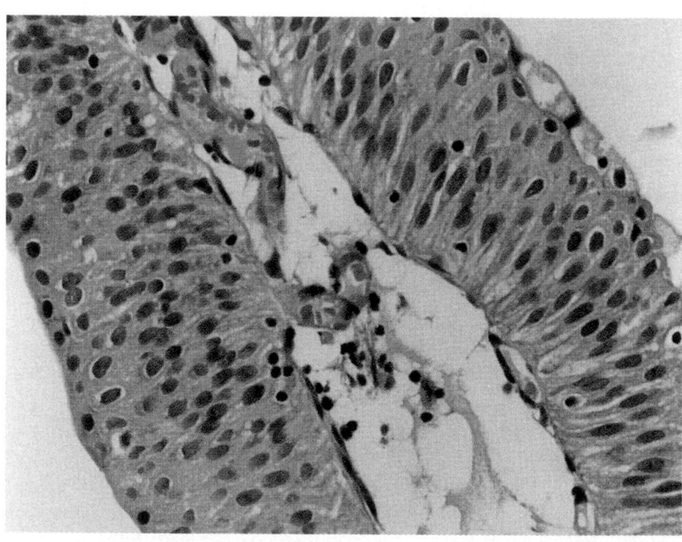

Fig. 66-27 Transitional cell papilloma, everted type. Notice the fibrovascular core lined by fewer than eight layers of normal-appearing urothelial cells with preserved umbrella cell layer.

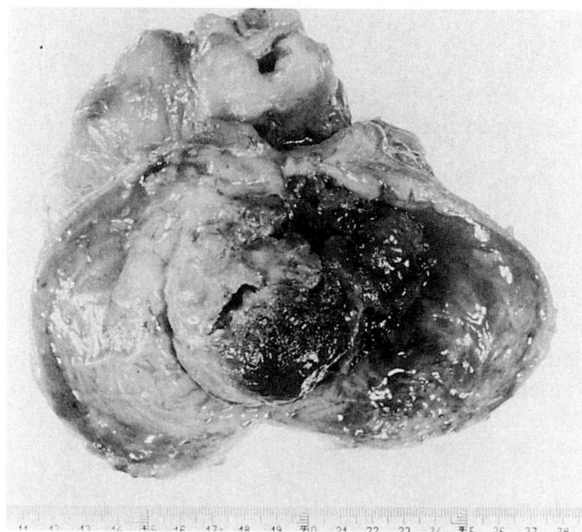

Fig. 66-26 Gross appearance of an autopsy specimen showing a large, solid, high-grade transitional cell carcinoma in a 56-year-old man refusing treatment for 3 years.

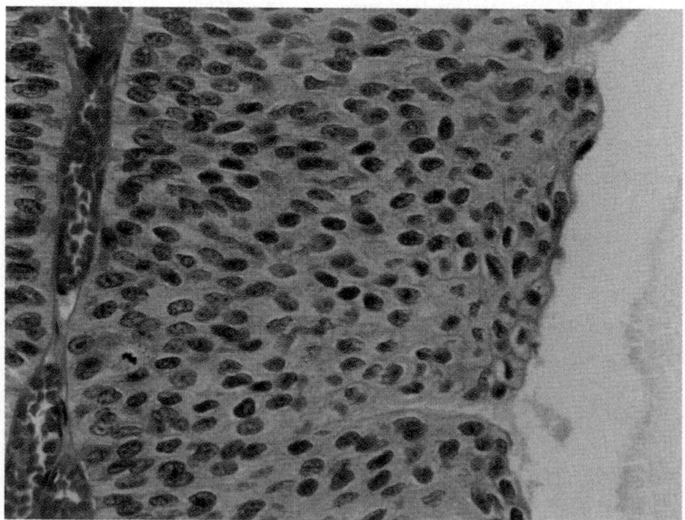

Fig. 66-28 Transitional cell carcinoma, grade 1, showing fewer than eight layers of urothelial cells with minimal nuclear abnormalities, well-preserved polarity of the cells, and umbrella cells.

malignancy grading, is based on deviation from the normal histologic appearance of the urothelium, and can easily be translated to the WHO system (Table 66-3). These grading systems are also applicable for urothelial tumors of the renal pelvis, ureter, and urethra.

Papilloma. In our opinion, everted or true papilloma as defined by Koss is a small papillary tumor composed of thin fibrovascular cores lined by up to seven layers of normal urothelium without significant dysplasia.[37] The umbrella cells are preserved, mitotic figures are absent, but degenerative changes with clearing of the cytoplasm can be seen (Fig. 66-27). The lesion is rare (constituting less than 1% of bladder tumors) and is usually seen in individuals 30 to 60 years of age. It is a single lesion, and recurrence of a true everted papilloma is unusual. It may be confused with polypoid cystitis, but in polypoid cystitis, which may have a papillary configuration, there is more edema instead of a distinct fibrovascular core, and microabscesses are frequently seen in the urothelium.

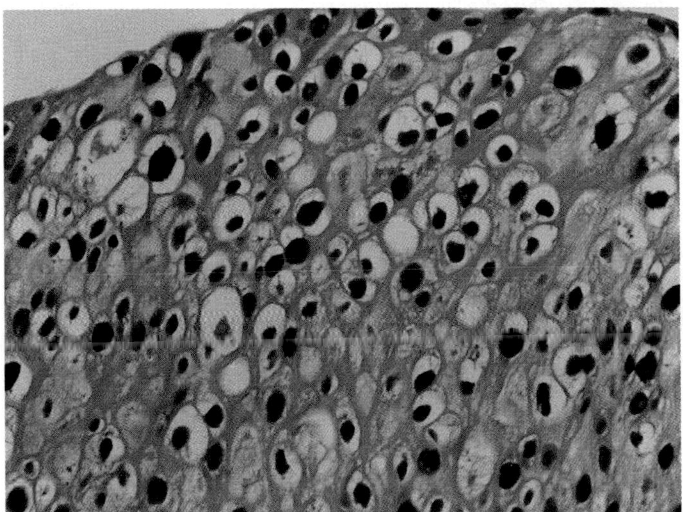

Fig. 66-29 Transitional cell carcinoma, grade 2, showing increase in numbers of cells and nuclear size, nuclear hyperchromasia, and disturbance in polarity.

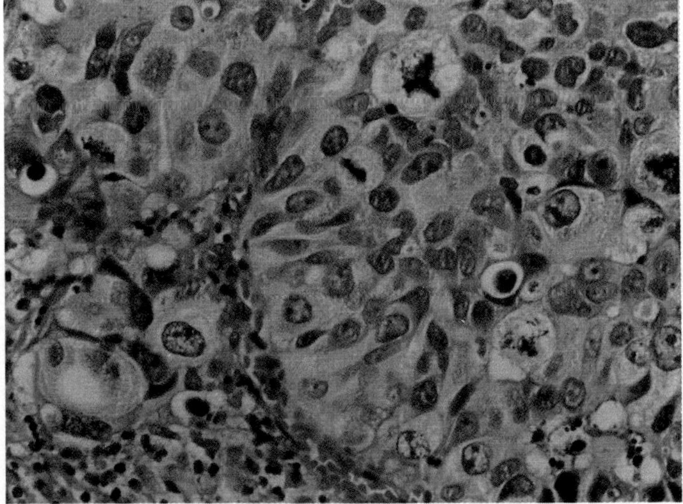

Fig. 66-30 Transitional cell carcinoma, grade 3, showing considerably disturbed polarity, increased cell and nuclear pleomorphism, enlarged nucleoli, hyperchromasia, and mitoses.

There has been some controversy about distinction of papilloma from papillary urothelial carcinoma, Bergkvist grades 1 and 2A (WHO grade 1), and some authors have included the latter lesions under the category of papilloma. The distinction is for the most part not of clinical significance because in our experience Bergkvist grade 1 tumors never infiltrate and less than 3% of grade 2A tumors invade. Both types, especially when present as single lesions, are treated conservatively with TURB. However, low-grade papillary carcinomas have a high propensity for recurrence, whereas true papillomas do not. We, therefore, favor retaining the distinction of papilloma from papillary carcinomas, grades 1 and 2A.[36]

Papillary carcinoma. The TNM system for staging of urinary bladder tumors is also used by the American Joint Committee on Cancer (AJCC).[38] The term *superficial bladder cancer* for stages Ta and T1 has previously been used but should be avoided, since there clearly is a difference in prognosis between stage Ta and T1.[39] In particular, tumors with deep lamina propria invasion, that is, invasion at or below the level of the muscularis mucosae, are associated with a worse prognosis.[12] The level of invasion should be accurately indicated in the pathology report. When present, the muscularis mucosae is easily identified in normal and nonneoplastic specimens, but in small, fragmented TURB or biopsy specimens of bladder tumors it may be difficult to differentiate muscularis mucosae from detrusor muscle. However, the presence of relatively large blood vessels at the level of the muscularis mucosae helps in the identification of this layer, should the question arise.[12] In the ureter and renal pelvis, no muscularis mucosae has been identified.[1]

Papillary urothelial tumors of stages Ta and T1 are generally treated with TURB. The natural history includes: (1) removal, no recurrence; (2) removal, recurrence usually of the same grade; (3) recurrence with progression to higher grade or stage. In cases with stages Ta and T1, 57% to 85% recur and between 4% to 30% develop progression with muscle invasion. Recent studies indicate that, in T1 tumors, patients with invasion to or beyond the muscularis mucosae have a worse prognosis than patients with invasion above the muscularis mucosae.

Important prognostic factors for recurrence or progression for papillary urothelial carcinomas have been identified:

High tumor grade
Interruption of basement membrane

Table 66-3 Comparison between the two main grading systems for bladder carcinoma

Malmström et al[36] (1987)	WHO[34] (1973)
Transitional cell carcinoma (TCC)	
Grade O (papilloma)	Papilloma
TCC—grade 1	TCC—grade 1
TCC—grade 2A	
TCC—grade 2B	TCC—grade 2
TCC—grade 3	TCC—grade 3

Invasion into or below the muscularis mucosae
Detrusor muscle involvement
Small vessel invasion (lymphatic or blood vessel)
Tentacular invasion
Associated carcinoma in situ
Tumor size and multiplicity

Five-year survival is 90% for patients with Ta tumors and 75% in patients with T1 tumors. Approximately 75% to 90% of bladder tumors are papillary tumors, whereas 20% are solid and invasive.

Solid, invasive tumors. Of the solid, invasive tumors, 80% to 91% are stage T2 to stage T3a tumors, displaying muscle invasion at the time of presentation, whereas the remaining 9% to 20% have a history of papillary transitional cell carcinoma (TCC), stages Ta or T1, which recurred and progressed to muscle invasion. The 5-year survival of patients with muscle invasive tumors usually has been reported to be between 20% to 50%, depending on whether invasion involves the superficial or the deep muscle layers. Metastases are encountered particularly in regional lymph nodes. Distant spread may involve bones, lungs, and liver.

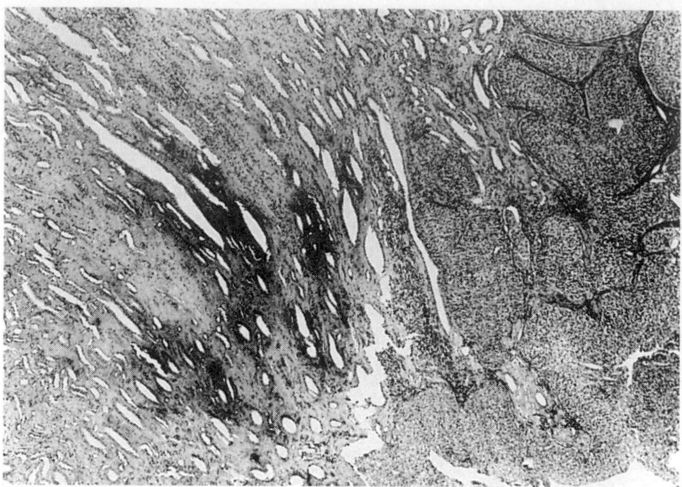

Fig. 66-31 Urothelial renal pelvic carcinoma invading a necrotic papilla. The patient was a 40-year-old abuser of phenacetin-containing analgesics.

Renal pelvic and ureteral tumors

The distribution of tumor grades in 170 Swedish patients with transitional cell carcinoma of the renal pelvis was 3%, 38%, 37%, and 22% for grades 1 to 4, respectively.[30,40,41] In the largest series from the United States, comprising 70 patients, the corresponding figures were 18%, 42%, 22%, and 15%.[42] The 5-year survival is related to grade and stage, and generally grade 3 and grade 4 tumors have poor prognosis. The AJCC TNM staging system for tumors of the renal pelvis and ureter has recently been published.[38] The overall 5-year survival of renal pelvic tumors has been reported to vary from 17% to 84%. In a series of 72 patients, the 5-year survival was 51% after simple nephrectomy with or without ureterectomy.[38] Sixty-six percent of the patients in that series who were dying from their tumor underwent an autopsy, and in 43%, the main finding was local recurrence. In a prospective study, 38 patients with renal pelvic carcinoma were treated with transabdominal perifascial nephrectomy with total ureterectomy, including a cuff of the bladder, which resulted in a 5-year survival of 84%.[41] However, in low-grade, noninvasive tumors located in the extrarenal pelvis, partial resection of the renal pelvis appears sufficient.[40,41,42] In patients with renal pelvic tumors induced by abuse of phenacetin-containing analgesics, the patients have renal papillary necrosis and interstitial nephritis with variable degree of renal insufficiency (Fig. 66-31). In these patients, parenchyma-saving resections of the kidney may be necessary to avoid renal insufficiency and hemodialysis. Regional and distant metastases involve regional lymph nodes, lungs, bones, and liver.

Renal pelvic tumors are relatively often associated with synchronous and metachronous tumors elsewhere in the urinary tract, particularly in the ipsilateral ureter and bladder (Fig. 66-32). Squamous cell carcinoma of the renal pelvis constitutes approximately 5% of renal pelvic tumors. Both in the renal pelvis and in the ureter (where it is even rarer), it is diagnosed as high-stage disease and is usually fatal.

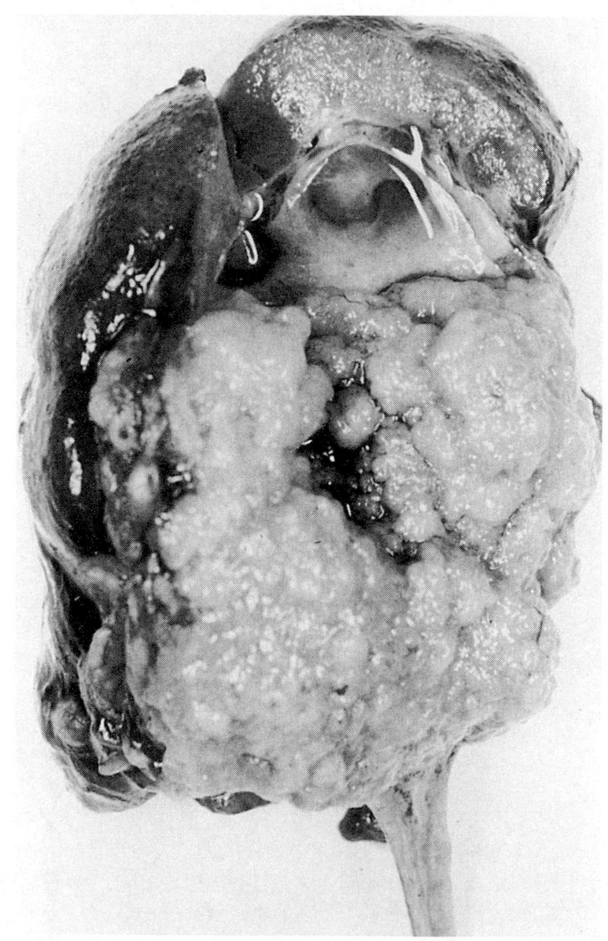

Fig. 66-32 Nephrectomy specimen with renal pelvic papillary transitional cell carcinoma.

Tumor grade and stage are closely correlated in tumors of the ureter and both parameters are important prognostic factors. The 5-year survival rate for noninvasive and lamina propria invasive tumors is 80% to 100%, whereas the mean survival is 47% for muscle invasive tumors.[1]

Tumor markers. Several tumor markers have been evaluated in attempts to determine potentially aggressive cases of stage Ta bladder cancer. The markers of particular interest are blood group ABH, Lewis, and T antigens. Blood group antigens (ABH) are normally present in many tissues including normal urothelium. Loss of ABH antigens from urothelial tumors correlates with a propensity for tumor progression. Generally, antigen expression is retained in low-grade, low-stage TCC, and deletion and discordant expression is seen in high-grade, high-stage carcinomas. The loss of these antigens preceded the decrease in histologic level of differentiation, and therefore immunohistochemical analysis was seen as a tool to predict the future behavior of low-grade, low-stage tumors. Technical and interpretative problems have, however, made it difficult to include ABH expression of bladder tumors into routine patient management schemes. A universally accepted standard for preparing and immunostaining human tissues has not been established. An additional drawback is the fact that a high percentage of patients (40% to 50% of whites in the United States) belong to the blood group O and do not possess the A or B determinants. Poor preservation of tissue, necrosis, hemorrhage, cautery effect, chemotherapy, and radiation therapy may also influence staining results.

Lewis antigens are closely related to the ABH structure, and more than 90% of the population possess the Lewis gene. Normal urothelium thus expresses one of the two Le determinants, Le^a and Le^b , and it is important to establish the normal distribution pattern for these antigens. Generally, high-grade tumors express a more irregular Le pattern.

The Thomsen-Friedenrich antigen (the T antigen) is another prognostic marker used in patients with bladder cancer. It is a precursor of the MN blood group substances and is present in normal urothelium. Detection requires enzymatic removal of the terminal sialic acid from the determinant. Once exposed by neuraminidase treatment the "cryptic" T antigen can be visualized by its affinity for peanut agglutinin or by specific monoclonal antibodies. Well-differentiated cancers in which the epithelium is similar to normal urothelium "hide" the antigen by means of terminal neuraminic acid moieties. If these moieties are lost from the MN blood group, direct detection of the T antigen without previous neuraminidase treatment is possible (the tumor is considered T antigen positive). If the T antigen cannot be detected despite neuraminidase treatment, it is likely to be a result of the decreased degree of differentiation of the tumor. Such a result is labeled "cryptic T-antigen negative." Both the loss of the T sequence and the spontaneous emergence of T antigen are considered to herald tumor recurrence and progression. Thus, Lange and Limas[43] reported that 37% of ABH-negative tumors progressed to being invasive, but 64% of the tumors that were simultaneously abnormal for T-antigen expression also progressed. Other reports, however, have failed to correlate tumor grade, T-antigen expression, and prognosis. It is, however, unusual to have ABH positivity in the presence of an abnormal T antigen because T-antigen abnormality occurs after ABH deletions. Overall, the ABH, Lewis, and T antigens have not proved to be reliable, independent indicators of tumor behavior and are generally not used routinely in clinicopathologic evaluation.[44]

Some 20 cytokeratins have been identified, and the urothelium expresses in particular cytokeratins 7, 8, 18, and 19. Expression is strongest in the umbrella cells; cytokeratin 18 is expressed only in the umbrella cells. However, in recent years, studies have shown that cytokeratins 8 and 18 are also expressed in high-grade bladder tumors. The importance of keratin expression in evaluation of bladder tumors has not been established.

In addition to the determination of tumor type, grade, and stage, many institutions also analyze chromosomal ploidy and cellular proliferation (the numbers of cells in S phase). Both flow cytometry and image analysis can successfully be performed on exfoliated cells from bladder washings, from fresh biopsy specimens, and from archival, formalin-fixed, paraffin-embedded material. Voided urine specimens are not well suited because of poor cellularity and degenerative cellular changes, which result in poor resolution of DNA by flow cytometry. Flow cytometry is more sensitive than cytologic testing, but it is valuable not so much in the diagnosis as in the follow-up study of patients with bladder tumors including the evaluation of conservatively treated Ta and T1 bladder carcinomas. Many institutions use the combination of DNA analysis and conventional urine cytologic testing. Chromosomal ploidy has, by a majority of investigations, been reported to be associated with an increased risk of recurrence and progression and with a poorer prognosis.[45,46] However, chromosomal ploidy has not been shown to be a prognostic factor in muscle-invasive bladder cancer.[47]

Cytogenetics and molecular biology. Beginning with the early observations of Falor and Ward, chromosomal abnormalities have been sought as prognostic markers of recurrence or progression and invasion.[48] They observed that abnormal chromosomes occurred in high-grade urothelial carcinomas and were predictive of eventual invasion by tumors that were still superficial. With improved techniques for determining karyotypes and with the development of more refined banding techniques, specific chromosomal alterations that are related to the biologic behavior of these tumors have been identified. Such studies have also provided strong support for the clonal origin of the malignancies. One or more defects in chromosome 9, as a monosome, or in the p or the q arms, are frequently detected in noninvasive, low-grade, papillary TCC. In contrast, high-grade, invasive TCC usually contains a defect on chromosome 17p, which represents an abnormality in the p53 gene.[49] Significantly, chromosome 9 abnormalities are relatively uncommon in papillary high-grade, stage Ta, or T1 TCC, or in CIS. In the few cases where low-grade papillary carcinoma and flat CIS were present together, an abnormal chromosome 9 was present in the papillary carcinoma, and a p53 abnormality was present in the CIS. These differences in p53 and chromosome 9 expression between low-grade and high-grade tumors provide additional evidence that they represent two different diseases. Spruck and colleagues[50] recently suggested two different pathways leading to the development of noninvasive bladder cancer. p53 gene inactivation seems to occur early in CIS, an observation supported by the fact that p53 mutations were found in patients with CIS without any previous history of bladder cancer, many of whom did not have detectable loss of either chromosome 9 or 17. In contrast, chromosome 9 alterations may be sufficient for superficial papillary tumors to develop. The progression of superficial papillary tumors and CIS may require subsequent acquisition of defects in p53 or additional defects in chromosome 9.[50] Other chromosomal alterations have been observed in bladder tumors, particularly in high-grade, invasive TCC, most frequently involving chromosomes 3, 5, 7, 8, 10, 11, and 13. Some of these most likely represent late, secondary changes related to the increasing genetic instability of DNA with progressing malignancy.[51,52]

Karyotypic abnormalities represent relatively gross changes in the DNA. Specific gene alterations that provide more specific molecular details about the mechanism and pathogenesis of bladder cancers have been identified. Mutations in the *ras* family of oncogenes were originally identified in human cancers by use of a cell line derived from a poorly differentiated bladder carcinoma. In subsequent studies, however, such mutations were observed only in 5% to 30% of TCC, and it became clear that a single genetic error was unlikely to be sufficient for development of malignancy. Mutations or altered expression of other oncogenes have also been observed, but none occurs in more than a relatively small minority of cases.

Abnormalities in tumor-suppressor genes have also been identified in bladder cancer. p53 mutations have been described in preceding paragraphs and are related to high-grade TCC, either in situ or invasive. In advanced, invasive TCC, abnormalities in the retinoblastoma gene (Rb) are frequently observed. Nevertheless, none of the alterations in oncogenes or suppressor genes have so far led to clinically useful markers for diagnosis, prognosis, or therapy.

Epidermal growth factor (EGF) is present in relatively large amounts in urine and acts as an endogenous enhancer of bladder tumor development. EGF receptors appear to increase with higher-grade urothelial tumors and recently a significant correlation between EGF receptor expression, high tumor stage, and poor patient outcome was reported, though EGF expression was not independent of stage.[53] Basic fibroblast growth factor (bFGF), originally described as urinary endothelial stimulating factor, also appears to increase with grade and stage. Although of scientific interest, these also have not become clinically applicable.[54]

Squamous cell carcinoma (SCC)

Squamous cell carcinoma accounts for 3% to 8% of all bladder tumors in the Western world with an age and sex distribution similar to TCC. Risk factors are urinary tract infection, lithiasis, chronic indwelling catheter, and schistosomiasis in areas where the parasite is endemic. The tumors are generally ulcerating and infiltrating rather than exophytic. Hematuria is a common symptom. Histologically they are identical to squamous cell carcinoma elsewhere. Most tumors are moderately to poorly differentiated, that is, grades 2 to 3. Associated keratinizing squamous metaplasia is present in 17% to 25% of the cases. The prognosis is unfavorable, with a 5-year survival of 7% to 20%. This is related to high stage at presentation and vascular invasion. The treatment of choice is total cystectomy. The therapeutic value of chemotherapy and radiation has not been determined.[1,3]

Verrucous squamous cell carcinoma, which was initially described by Ackerman in the oral cavity, has also been reported to occur rarely in the bladder.[3,55] It has a cauliflower-like appearance and is composed of well-differentiated squamous epithelium without significant dysplasia. It is well circumscribed with pushing borders and is locally aggressive but does not metastasize.

Undifferentiated carcinoma

Undifferentiated carcinoma includes sarcomatoid (spindle cell) carcinoma and small cell carcinoma. TCC, SCC, and adenocarcinoma can present as poorly differentiated spindle cell tumors with the appearance of sarcomatous elements (Fig. 66-33). The patients are usually over 60 years of age and present with hematuria. The tumors are usually polypoid, and the carcinomatous elements may be TCC, SCC, adenocarcinoma, small cell carcinoma, or a mixture of them. The spindle cells sometime blend with the malignant epithelial cells. Epithelial elements or in situ changes are often present, but if they are not identified morphologically, keratin and EMA stains are helpful in distinguishing these tumors from true sarcomas.[3]

Small cell undifferentiated carcinoma of the bladder is identical to its pulmonary counterpart and was first reported in 1981.[56] The incidence is between 0.5% to 1% of bladder tumors.[57,58] The tumors are generally diagnosed in the seventh and eighth decade, approximately 80% occurring in males. Fifty-six percent are pure small cell carcinoma at the time of biopsy, 20% are combinations of small cell carcinoma and TCC, and the remainder have various combinations of small cell carcinoma and TCC, SCC, or adenocarcinoma. (Fig. 66-34) Both oat cell and intermediate cell variants have been described. In the majority of cases, the tumor cells stain positive for neuron-specific enolase, keratin, and synaptophysin, and dense-core granules can be identified by EM. Prognosis is poor; only 10 of 115 reported patients survived 2 years.[59]

Adenocarcinoma

Adenocarcinoma constitutes approximately 1% of bladder tumors and is most often diagnosed in the fifth to the sixth decades, with a male preponderance. Risk factors include exstrophy, nonfunctional bladder, and schistosomiasis. Hematuria is the main symptom. About one third are urachal in ori-

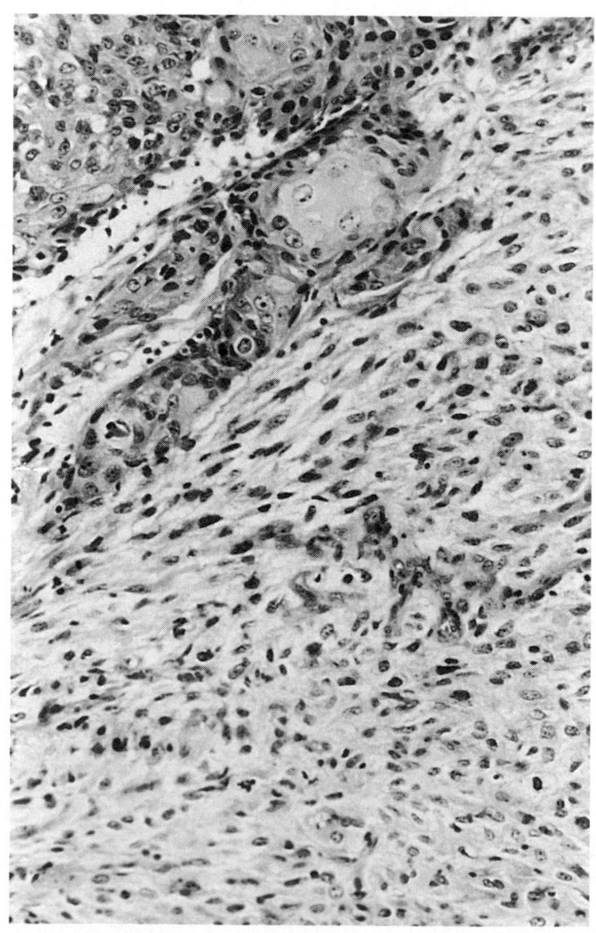

Fig. 66-33 Squamous cell carcinoma with spindle cell differentiation.

gin, the remainder originate elsewhere in the bladder. Tumors are usually solitary and in exceptional cases, multifocal. Histologically, most cases are glandular, mucinous, or papillary, but signet-ring cell carcinoma and clear cell carcinoma have also been reported[59,60] (Fig. 66-35). Different histologic patterns are often intermixed.

The differential diagnosis includes other extravesicular adenocarcinomas extending into the bladder, especially colorectal, gynecologic, or prostatic carcinoma. Adenocarcinomas of the prostate almost invariably show the presence of prostate-specific antigen (PSA) and prostatic acid phosphatase (PAP), whereas bladder adenocarcinomas do not. Clinical data may be critical in other cases. The prognosis is related to tumor size and type, and the 5-year survival rate varies between 6% and 33%. Recent studies have not found a difference in prognosis between urachal and nonurachal adenocarcinomas. The treatment of choice is partial bladder resection or cystectomy. The efficacy of chemotherapy or radiation treatment remains to be determined. Some 50 cases of adenocarcinoma of the renal pelvis and 16 of the ureter have been reported.[1,59]

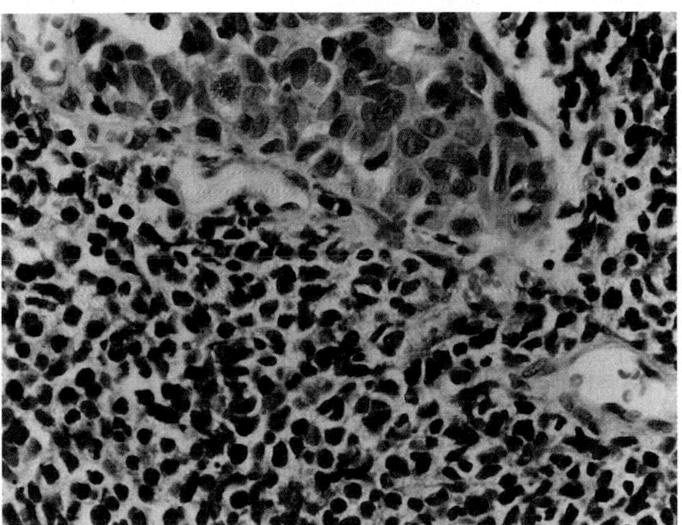

Fig. 66-34 Mixed tumor composed of high-grade transitional cell carcinoma, grade 3, and small cell carcinoma, oat cell type.

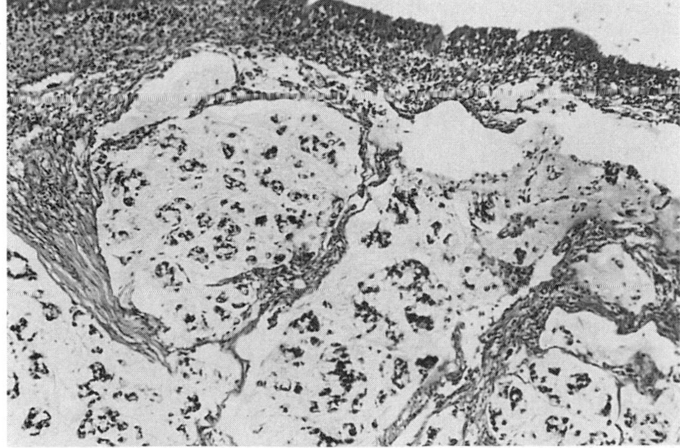

Fig. 66-35 Specimen from transurethral resection of the bladder from a patient with bladder tumor located at the dome showing features of mucinous adenocarcinoma. Notice the preserved, normal-appearing urothelium. This tumor fulfilled the criteria for urachal carcinoma.

Mixed tumors

Mixed differentiation in tumors of the renal pelvis, ureter, and bladder is common, and all possible combinations have been reported. The most common types are TCC and SCC. The predominating pattern, if any, is likely to determine the prognosis, with the possible exception of small cell or signet-ring cell carcinoma. When the components are present in approximately equal proportions, the tumor should be reported as a mixed tumor; patterns of differentiation present should be indicated.

Carcinosarcoma

Carcinosarcomas are malignant neoplasms consisting of carcinomatous and malignant mesenchymal elements. The tumors are large and ulcerating, and there is deep invasion of the wall. The sarcomatoid elements are usually chondroid or osteosarcomatous mixed with TCC and less frequently with SCC or adenocarcinoma. Prognosis is poor, and the patients usually succumb to local recurrence or distant metastases within 2 years. A few cases of carcinosarcomas of the renal pelvis and ureter have been reported.[61]

Mesenchymal neoplasms

Benign tumors

Leiomyoma. Fewer than 200 cases of vesical leiomyoma have been reported, occurring in all age groups. Approximately two thirds of the patients are women, which also is the case for leiomyoma of the renal pelvis, ureter, and urethra. The presenting symptoms include hematuria and dysuria. The tumor varies in size from a few millimeters to several centimeters. The morphologic appearance is identical to leiomyomas occurring in more common locations such as the uterus.[1]

Hemangioma. Hemangioma is uncommon in the bladder, with about 90 reported cases. It may occur at any age, but 60% of the patients are younger than 30 years of age. Clinical presentation is usually hematuria resulting from a nodular lesion on the lateral wall or dome. Biopsy is associated with a high risk of a major hemorrhage. The majority of tumors are of cavernous type. Hemangioma has also been reported in the renal pelvis and ureter. The treatment of choice is partial cystectomy.[61]

Other rare benign mesenchymal tumors include granular cell tumors, fibrous histiocytoma, neurilemoma, lymphangioma, lipoma, and adenofibroma. Neurofibroma of the bladder is usually seen in patients with von Recklinghausen's disease.

Malignant tumors

Leiomyosarcoma. Leiomyosarcoma is the most common mesenchymal malignancy in the adult bladder, though only about 100 cases have been reported. Because of the paucity of large study series of leiomyosarcoma of the bladder, the morphologic criteria for distinguishing leiomyoma from leiomyosarcoma in this location has not been established. Walker and colleagues[61] state that "it seems prudent to label as leiomyosarcoma any smooth muscle neoplasms demonstrating infiltrative, destructive invasion of the vesical musculature. The designation leiomyoma should be reserved for sharply circumscribed neoplasms demonstrating little or no mitotic activity and minimal cytologic atypia."

Grossly, leiomyosarcomas of the bladder are large masses, often with a polypoid, intraluminal component. The cut surface shows a "fish-flesh" or sometime gelatinous appearance. Histologically, they are virtually identical to leiomyosarcomas elsewhere in the body and are composed of spindle cells with cigar-shaped nuclei forming fascicles. Usually the cellularity is modest with mild to moderate nuclear pleomorphism and relatively few mitotic figures, though some tumors are highly pleomorphic with abundant mitoses. Myxoid changes are not uncommon. The cells stain positively for muscle-specific actin (MSA) and often for vimentin and desmin as well but are generally negative for EMA and keratin. Most are low-grade tumors with a tendency for local recurrence but seldom metastasize.

Rhabdomyosarcoma. Rhabdomyosarcoma is the main malignant pediatric bladder tumor with a peak incidence at 5 years of age. The presenting symptoms are bladder neck obstruction and hematuria. The tumor appears as multiple glistening, polypoid masses or as a large solitary mass bulging into the bladder or replacing the wall of the bladder. Usually the tumor shows features of embryonal rhabdomyosarcoma with a condensation of rhabdomyoblasts below the urothelium, the so-called cambium layer, and a more dispersed cell population in an edematous stroma. The large single mass shows a solid pattern often with focal alveolar features. Combination therapy is associated with a salvage rate of 54.5%.[62] Occasional cases of other mesenchymal tumors, such as malignant fibrous histiocytoma, fibrosarcoma, osteosarcoma, chondrosarcoma, liposarcoma, and extrarenal rhabdoid tumor, have been described in the bladder.[1,61]

Miscellaneous neoplasms

Pheochromocytoma. More than 100 cases of pheochromocytoma have been reported, with most patients being younger than 50 years of age. They present with hypertensive episodes during micturition as a result of catecholamine release during detrusor activity. Most patients have increased levels of catecholamines in the serum and urine. The tumor is composed of nests of tumor cells (Zellballen, 'cell balls') separated by a thin fibrovascular core. The lamina propria and detrusor muscle are frequently involved. The cells are uniform and polygonal with amphophilic, pale cytoplasm and fairly well-defined cell borders. Nuclear pleomorphism is common with some bizarre cells. Features of malignancy have been recorded in tumors from 19 of 128 patients.[1,61] There are, however, no reliable histologic criteria of malignancy.

Germ cell neoplasms. Germ cell tumors of the bladder are rare, and most pathologists will not encounter them; the majority of germ cell tumors are choriocarcinomas.

URETHRA

Normal anatomy

The male urethra can be divided into the proximal and distal segments. The proximal urethra commences at the internal urethral orifice and passes through the prostate as the membranous urethra. The two openings of the ejaculatory duct are present at the colliculus seminalis, and multiple urethral and prostatic ducts empty from the lateral walls. The distal urethra is divided into the bulbous and penile urethra. The latter widens to form the fossa navicularis, which is located immediately internal to the meatus (external urethral orifice). The proximal part of the urethra is lined by urothelium, which is continuous with that of the bladder. A gradual change to stratified columnar epithelium occurs in the distal parts of the membranous urethra and the distal urethra, and the fossa navicularis is lined by stratified squamous epithelium, which is continuous with that of the glans penis. The bulbourethral (Cowper's) glands are mucus secreting and empty into the distal urethra. The small mucus-secreting Littre's glands are present in the lateral wall of the distal urethra.

The female urethra is likewise lined by urothelium continuous with that of the bladder. In the proximal part, a transition from transitional epithelium to stratified columnar epithelium occurs, and near the external meatus there is a change to stratified squamous epithelium. The distal urethra contains the periurethral Skene's glands, which are similar to Littre's glands in the male.

Congenital disorders

Congenital disorders include epispadias, hypospadias, duplication, megalourethra, and posterior and anterior urethral valves.

Urethritis and related disorders

Urethritis may be caused by coliform bacteria or by sexually transmitted pathogens such as *Neisseria gonorrhoeae* and *Chlamydia* and *Mycoplasma* organisms. Gonorrhea has an incubation of 3 to 7 days, after which the patient experiences a thick, yellow discharge associated with voiding discomfort. If left untreated, the patient may develop urethral stricture or disseminated disease.

Urethral diverticulum is usually seen in females, and an incidence of 3% has been reported. The condition is mainly one of middle-aged individuals and characteristically is localized in the dorsolateral wall of the urethra. Symptoms include urgency, frequency, and postmicturition dripping. The diagnosis is made by physical examination and confirmed by ureterography. Because of infection and an increased risk of malignancy, the diverticulum should be resected. Histologically the mucosal surface frequently shows ulceration with acute and chronic inflammation and a variable degree of fibrosis.[1]

Polypoid urethritis is usually associated with the use of indwelling catheters and is a common disorder with features similar to those in polypoid cystitis.[63]

Urethral caruncle is diagnosed only in women, usually after menopause. The patients suffer from pain and bleeding. The lesions are located near the external meatus. Three morphologic variants are recognized: (1) papillary, (2) angiomatous, and (3) granulomatous. The consistent features are severe, acute and chronic inflammation of the epithelium and subepithelial tissue. The mucosa can be polypoid, papillary, or sometimes ulcerated and is lined by urothelium or squamous epithelium, which is occasionally hyperplastic and may be confused with carcinoma (Figs. 66-36 and 66-37). The subepithelial tissue may show abundant thin-walled vessels or granulation-like tissue with a variable degree of fibrosis. Separation into the three histologic types can be done on the basis of the predominant pattern. The cause and pathogenesis are unclear; prolapse of the mucosa may be a responsible factor. There is no increased risk of malignancy in urethral caruncles.[2]

Neoplastic disorders

Adenomatous polyp of the prostatic epithelium is a lesion of relatively young males (peak incidence is in the second to fourth decades). The patients suffer from hematuria, hemospermia, or both. Approximately 200 cases have been reported. The lesions are sessile, polypoid, or papillary and show a villoglandular pattern with prostatic type of epithelium (Fig. 66-38). PSA or PAP stains confirm the prostatic origin of the epithelium.[1]

Urethral carcinoma is uncommon, but in contrast to carcinoma of the renal pelvis, urethra, and bladder, almost three fourths of the cases are diagnosed in women.[64] In the female, squamous carcinomas constitute 48% of urethral carcinomas, whereas urothelial carcinomas and adenocarcinomas each constitute 15%. In the female, the mean age of the patients is approximately 60 years; the symptoms include bleeding, obstruction, and a palpable mass. The majority of tumors are of distal location and involve a large portion of the urethra. About one third of the patients have enlarged inguinal nodes at the time of presentation, and most of these contain metastatic tumor cells. The 5-year survival for patients with distal tumors is 14% to 40% as compared to 0% to 17% for proximal tumors.[1]

Carcinoma of the male urethra is less frequent than in females, and the majority of cases are *squamous cell carcinomas*. One third of the cases are associated with venereal disease and urethral stricture. The majority of patients are older than 60 years of age. The prognosis is related to location and stage.[1]

Clear cell adenocarcinoma is a rare malignancy of the urethra, almost exclusively involving middle-aged or older women. Approximately 30 cases have been reported, only two of which were in men.[60]

Cloacogenic carcinomas, originally described in the anorectal region, have also been reported in the urethra. *Malignant melanoma* has been reported in both the male and female urethra and may be pigmented or amelanotic. They are identical to cutaneous melanomas but often are epithelioid or spindle shaped. Immunoperoxidase staining with antibodies against S-100 protein or HMB-45 may help in diagnosing amelanotic cases. The prognosis is poor, with the majority of patients succumbing to metastatic disease within three years.[1]

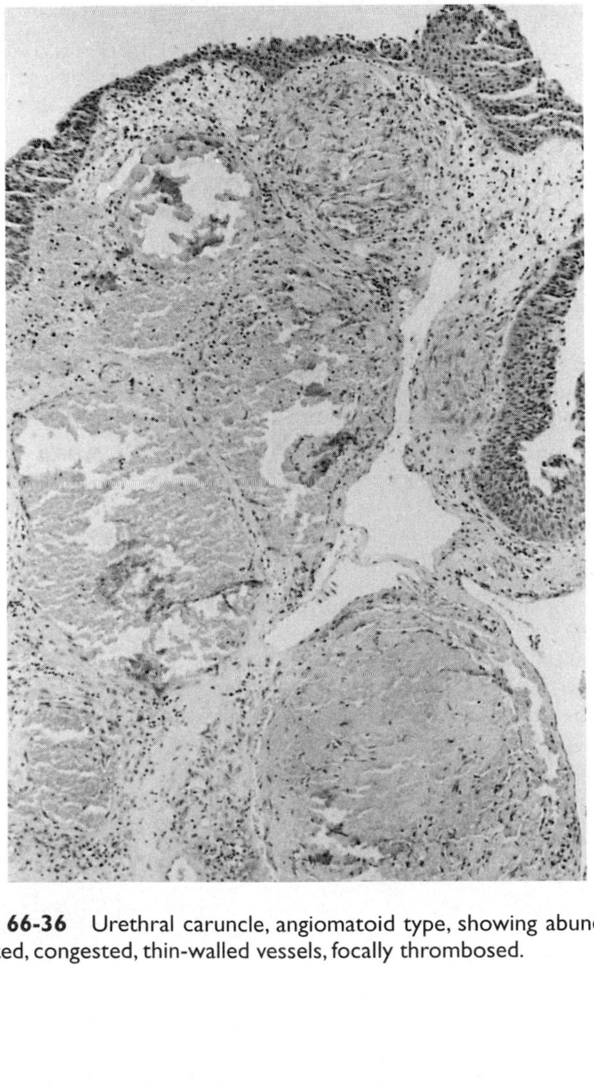

Fig. 66-36 Urethral caruncle, angiomatoid type, showing abundant dilated, congested, thin-walled vessels, focally thrombosed.

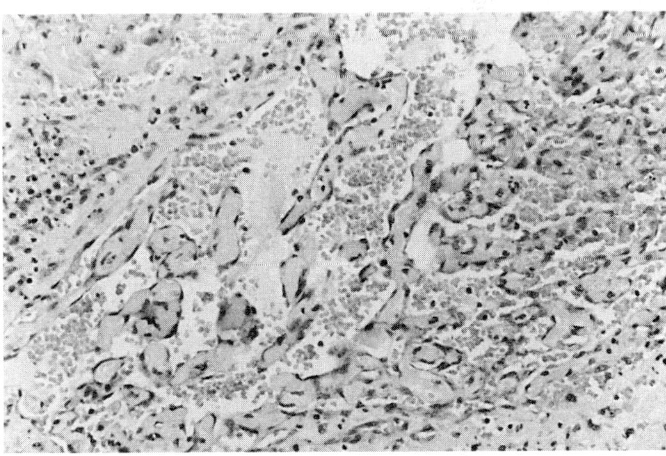

Fig. 66-37 Same case as in Fig. 66-36 showing another area with papillary endothelial hyperplasia in a dilated vessel.

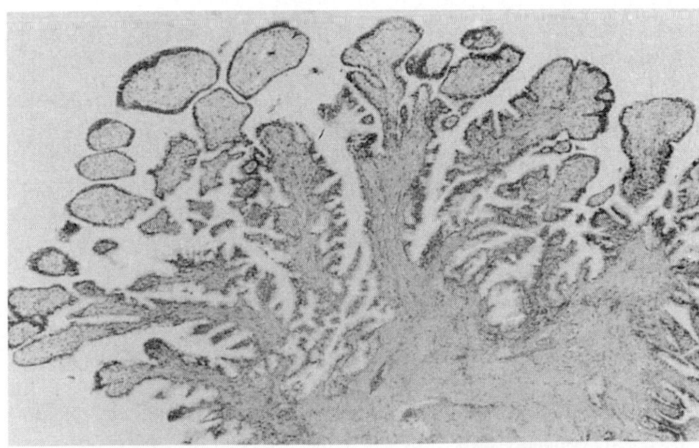

Fig. 66-38 Urethral polyp with prostatic epithelium from a 37-year-old man with hemospermia.

REFERENCES

General references

1. Peterson RO: *Urologic pathology,* ed 2, Philadelphia, 1992, Lippincott.
2. Murphy WM: Diseases of the urinary bladder, urethra, ureters and renal pelvis. In Murphy WM, editor: *Urological pathology,* Philadelphia, 1989, Saunders.
3. Young RH: Non-neoplastic epithelial abnormalities and tumor like lesions. In Young RH, editor: *Pathology of the urinary bladder.* New York, 1989, Churchill Livingstone.

Preneoplastic lesions

4. Nagy GK, Frable WJ, Murphy WM: Classification of premalignant urothelial abnormalities: a Delphi study of the National Bladder Cancer Collaborative Group A, *Pathol Annu* 17:219, 1982.
5. Murphy WM, Soloway MS: Developing carcinoma (dysplasia) of the urinary bladder, *Pathol Annu* 17:197, 1982.
6. Mostofi FK, Sesterhenn IA: Pathology of epithelial tumors and carcinoma in situ of bladder, *Prog Clin Biol Res* 162A:55, 1984.
7. Friedell GH, Soloway MS, Hilgar AG: Summary of workshop on carcinoma in situ of the bladder, *J Urol* 136:1047, 1986.
8. Ayala AG, Ro JY: Premalignant lesions of the urothelium and transitional cell tumors. In Young RH, editor: *Pathology of the urinary bladder,* New York, 1989, Churchill Livingstone.

Developmental anomalies

9. Moore KL: The urogenital system in the developing human. In *Clinically oriented embryology,* ed 3, Philadelphia, 1982, Saunders.
10. Dixon JS, Gosling JA: Histology and fine structure of the muscularis mucosae of the human urinary bladder, *J Anat* 136:265, 1983.
11. Ro JY, Ayala AG, El-Naggar A: Muscularis mucosae of urinary bladder: importance for staging and treatment, *Am J Surg Pathol* 11:668, 1987.
12. Younes M, Sussman J, True LD: The usefulness of the muscularis mucosae in the staging of invasive transitional cell carcinoma of the bladder, *Cancer* 66:543, 1990.
13. Steers WD: Physiology of the urinary bladder. In Walsh PC, Retik AB, Stamey TA, Vaughan ED Jr, editors: *Campbell's urology,* ed 6, Philadelphia, 1992, Saunders.
14. Muecke EC: Extrophy, epispadias, and other anomalies of the bladder. In Walsh PC, Gittes RF, Perlmutter AD, Stamey TA, editors: *Campbell's urology,* ed 5, Philadelphia, 1986, Saunders.
15. Engel RM, Wilkinson HA: Bladder exstrophy, *J Urol* 104:699, 1970.

Cystitis

16. McClure J, Young, RH: Infectious diseases of the urinary bladder including malakoplakia. In Young RH, editor: *Pathology of the urinary bladder,* New York, 1989, Churchill Livingstone.
17. Smith JH, Christie JD: Urinary schistosomiasis. In Young, RH, editor: *Pathology of the urinary bladder,* New York, 1989, Churchill Livingstone.
18. Roy JB, Geyer TR, Mohr JA: Urinary tract candidiasis, *Urology* 23:533, 1984.
19. Johansson SL, Fall M: Clinical features and spectrum of light microscopic changes in interstitial cystitis, *J Urol* 143:1118, 1990.
20. Johansson SL, Fall M: Pathology of interstitial cystitis, *Urol Clin North Am,* 21:55, 1994.
21. Johansson SL, Smout MS, Taylor RJ: Eosinophilic cystitis associated with symptomatic ureteral involvement, *J Urol Pathol* 1:69, 1993.
22. Smith BH: Malakoplakia of the urinary tract: a study of 24 cases, *Am J Clin Pathol* 43:409, 1965.
23. Spagnolo DV, Waring PM: Bladder granuloma after bladder surgery, *Am J Clin Pathol* 86:430, 1986.
24. Lundgren L, Aldenborg, F Angervall, L Kindblom, LG: Pseudosarcomatous spindle cell proliferations in the urinary bladder of adults, *Hum Pathol* 25:181, 1994.
25. Ekelund P, Johansson SL: Polypoid cystitis: a catheter associated lesion of the human bladder, *Acta Pathol Microbiol Scand[A]* 87:179, 1979.
26. Ekelund P, Anderström C, Johansson SL, Larsson P: The reversibility of catheter-associated polypoid cystitis, *J Urol* 130:456, 1983.
27. Stillwell TJ, Benson RC Jr: Cyclophosphamide-induced hemorrhagic cystitis: a review of 100 patients, *Cancer* 61:451, 1988.

Neoplasms of the urinary tract

28. Bryan GT: Etiology and pathogenesis of bladder cancer. In Bryan GT, Cohen SM, editors: *The pathology of bladder cancer,* vol 1, Boca Raton, Fla., 1993, CRC Press.
29. Mc Credie M, Ford JM, Taylor TS, Stewart JH: Analgesics and cancer of the renal pelvis in New South Wales, *Cancer* 49:2617, 1982.
30. Johansson SL, Angervall L, Bengtsson, U, Wahlqvist, L: Uroepithelial tumors of the renal pelvis associated with analgesic abuse, *Cancer* 33:743, 1974.
31. Paschkis R: Über Adenome der Harnblase, *Z Urol Chir* 21:315, 1927.
32. Potts IF, Hirst E: Inverted papilloma of the bladder, *J Urol* 90:175, 1963.
33. Kunze E, Schauer A, Schmitt M: Histology and histogenesis of two different types of inverted urothelial papillomas, *Cancer* 51:348, 1983.
34. Mostofi FK, Sobin LH, Torloni H: Histological typing of urinary bladder tumours. In *International histological classification of tumours,* no. 10, Geneva, 1973, World Health Organization.
35. Bergkvist A, Ljungqvist A, Moberger G: Classification of bladder tumors based on the cellular pattern, *Acta Chir Scand* 130:378, 1965.
36. Malmström P-U, Busch C, Norlén BJ: Recurrence, progression and survival in bladder cancer, *Scand J Urol Nephrol* 21:185, 1987.
37. Koss, LG: *Tumors of the urinary bladder. In Atlas of tumor pathology,* series 2, fasc 11, Washington, D.C., 1975, Armed Forces Institute of Pathology.
38. Beahrs OH, Henson DE, Hutter RVP, Kennedy BJ, editors: *Manual for staging of cancer,* ed 4, Philadelphia, 1992, Lippincott.
39. Anderström C, Johansson SL, Nilsson S: The significance of lamina propria invasion on the prognosis of patients with bladder tumors, *J Urol* 124:23, 1980.
40. Johansson SL, Angervall L, Bengtsson U, Wahlqvist L: A clinicopathologic and prognostic study of epithelial tumors of the renal pelvis, *Cancer* 37:1376, 1976.
41. Johansson, SL, Wahlqvist L: A prognostic study of urothelial renal pelvic tumors: a comparison between the prognosis of patients treated with intrafascial and perifascial nephrectomy, *Cancer* 43:2535, 1979.
42. Rubinstein MA, Walz BJ, Bucy JG: Transitional cell carcinoma of the kidney: a 25-year experience, *J Urol* 119:594, 1978.
43. Lange PH, Limas C: Molecular markers in the diagnosis and prognosis of bladder cancer. *Urology* 23(suppl):46, 1984.
44. Nochomowitz, LE: Epithelial neoplasms. In Nochomowitz, LE, editor: *Bladder biopsy interpretation,* New York, 1992, Raven Press.
45. Melamed MR: Flow cytometry for detection and evaluation of urinary bladder carcinoma, *Semin Surg Oncol* 8:300, 1992.
46. Al-AGadi H, Nagel R: Deoxyribonucleic acid content and survival rates of patients with transitional cell carcinoma of the bladder, *J Urol* 151:37, 1994.
47. Fosså SD, Berner AA, Jacobsen A-B et al: Clinical significance of DNA-ploidy and S-phase fraction and their relation to p-53 protein, c-*erb*-B-2 protein and HCG in operable muscle invasive bladder cancer, Br J Cancer 68:572, 1993.
48. Falor WH, Ward RM: Cytogenetic analysis: a potential index for recurrence of early carcinoma of the bladder, *J Urol* 115:49, 1976.
49. Olumi AF, Tsai YC, Nicholas PW et al: Allelic loss of chromosome 17p distinguishes high grade from low grade transitional cell carcinomas of the bladder, *Cancer Res* 50:7081, 1990.
50. Spruck CH, Ohneseit F, González-Zuleta M et al: Two molecular pathways to transitional cell carcinoma of the bladder, *Cancer Res* 54:784, 1994.
51. Miyao N, Tsai YC, Lerner SP et al: Role of chromosome 9 in human bladder cancer, *Cancer Res* 53:4066, 1993.
52. Knowles MA, Elder PA, Williamson M et al: Allelotype of human bladder cancer, *Cancer Res* 54:531, 1994.
53. Nguyen PL, Swanson PE, Jaszcz W et al: Expression of epidermal growth factor receptor in invasive transitional cell carcinoma of the urinary bladder, *Am J Clin Pathol* 101:166, 1994.

54. Perucca D, Szepetowski P, Simon, MP, Gaudray P: Molecular genetics of human bladder carcinomas, *Cancer Genet Cytogenet* 49:143, 1990.
55. Ackerman LV: Verrucous carcinoma of the oral cavity, *Surgery* 23:670, 1948.
56. Cramer SF, Aikawa M, Cebelin M: Neurosecretory granules in small cell invasive carcinoma of the urinary bladder, *Cancer* 47:724, 1981.
57. Murphy WM, Beckwith JB, Farrow GM: Tumors of the urinary bladder, urethra, ureters, renal pelvis and kidneys. In *Atlas of tumor pathology,* series 3, Washington, D.C., 1995, Armed Forces Institute of Pathology.
58. Holmäng S, Borghede G, Johansson SL: Primary small cell carcinoma of the urinary bladder: a report of 25 cases, *J Urol* 153:1820, 1995.
59. Johansson SL, Anderström CRK: Primary adenocarcinoma of the urinary bladder and urachus. In Williams CJ, Krikorian JG, Green MR, Raghavan D, editors: *Textbook of uncommon cancers,* Chichester, N.Y., 1988, John Wiley & Son.
60. Young RH, Scully RE: Clear cell adenocarcinoma of the bladder and urethra: a report of three cases and review of the literature, *Am J Surg* 9:816, 1985.
61. Walker AN, Mills SE, Young RH: Mesenchymal and miscellaneous other primary tumors of the urinary bladder. In Young RH, editor: *Pathology of the urinary bladder,* New York, 1989, Churchill Livingstone.
62. Broecker BH, Plowman N, Pritchard J, Ransley PG: Pelvic rhabdomyosarcoma in children, *Br J Urol* 61:427, 1988.
63. Norlen LJ, Ekelund P, Hedelin H, Johansson SL: Effects of indwelling catheters on the urethral mucosa (polypoid urethritis), *Scand J Urol Nephrol* 22:81, 1988.
64. Johansson SL: *Diseases of the urinary bladder,* Interactive video disc, Los Angeles, 1992, Intellipath.

67 Male Reproductive System

A. TESTIS, EPIDYDIMIS, AND PENIS

Ivan Damjanov

TESTIS, EPIDYDIMIS, AND VAS DEFERENS

Normal anatomy and physiology of testis

The testes are paired organs that have two principal functions: the production of sperm and the secretion of male sex hormones. Sperm is produced in the seminiferous tubules, whereas the sex hormones are produced by the interstitial Leydig cells. The hormonal and reproductive compartments of the testis are closely interrelated, and the cells of each compartment are in an endocrine-paracrine relationship to one another.[1] The testis is also part of the hypothalamic-pituitary—gonadal and adrenal hormonal axis, and its reproductive functions are centrally regulated.[2]

Normal development. The testes are derived developmentally from genital ridges, which develop in early embryos as pregonadal placodes on the mesonephros.[3] The genital ridge is populated by the primordial germ cells that migrate into them from their primary site of origin in the yolk sac. The germ cells interact with the stromal cells of the genital ridge—an interaction that finally determines whether the undifferentiated gonad develops into a fetal testis or an ovary. Fetal Sertoli cells secrete the antimüllerian hormone (AMH) which inhibits the meiosis of male germ cells. This is in contrast to the fetal ovary, which lacks AMH, allowing the meiosis of oocytes to start during fetal life. The AMH secreted by the fetal Sertoli cells promotes the involution of the müllerian ducts and inhibits the development of fallopian tubes, the uterus, and parts of the vagina in the male fetus. In the female fetus, whose ovaries do not produce AMH, these derivatives of the müllerian ducts develop normally and give rise to the internal female genital organs.

The fetal testis is originally located in the abdominal cavity, but it moves into the inguinal canal as the body develops and it has descended into the scrotum by the end of pregnancy. The inguinal canal subsequently obliterates, preventing the return of the testes into the abdominal cavity. In 4% to 6% of male infants the inguinal canal is not closed at the time of delivery and the testis is retractile. Approximately 25% of premature infants weighing less than 2500 g have undescended testes.[4] However, most of these testes eventually descend and are not retractable after the first 3 months of life. By the end of the first year, only 1% to 2% of all boys have clinically apparent cryptorchidism.[5]

The histologic maturation of the testes occurs in several stages, which are hormonally regulated, (Fig. 67-1). Within the seminiferous tubules the primordial germ cells differentiate into gonocytes, the progenitors of fetal spermatogonia, which at puberty mature into adult spermatogonia. The morphology of testes changes during infancy and childhood, and this is best illustrated by the changes in the ratio of Sertoli cells to germ cells that take place. During early childhood, Sertoli cells outnumber the germ cells, which are usually rather inconspicuous until prepuberty. These age-related dif-

Abbreviations

AFP	Alpha-fetoprotein
AMH	Antimüllerian hormone
CIS	Carcinoma in situ testis
EC	Embryonal carcinoma
FSH	Follicle-stimulating hormone
GnrH	Gonadotropin-releasing hormone
hCG	Human chorionic gonadotropin
HPV	Human papillomavirus
LH	Luteotropic hormone
NDFP	Nodular and diffuse fibrous proliferation
NSGCT	Nonseminomatous germ cell tumors
PLAP	Placental alkaline phosphatase

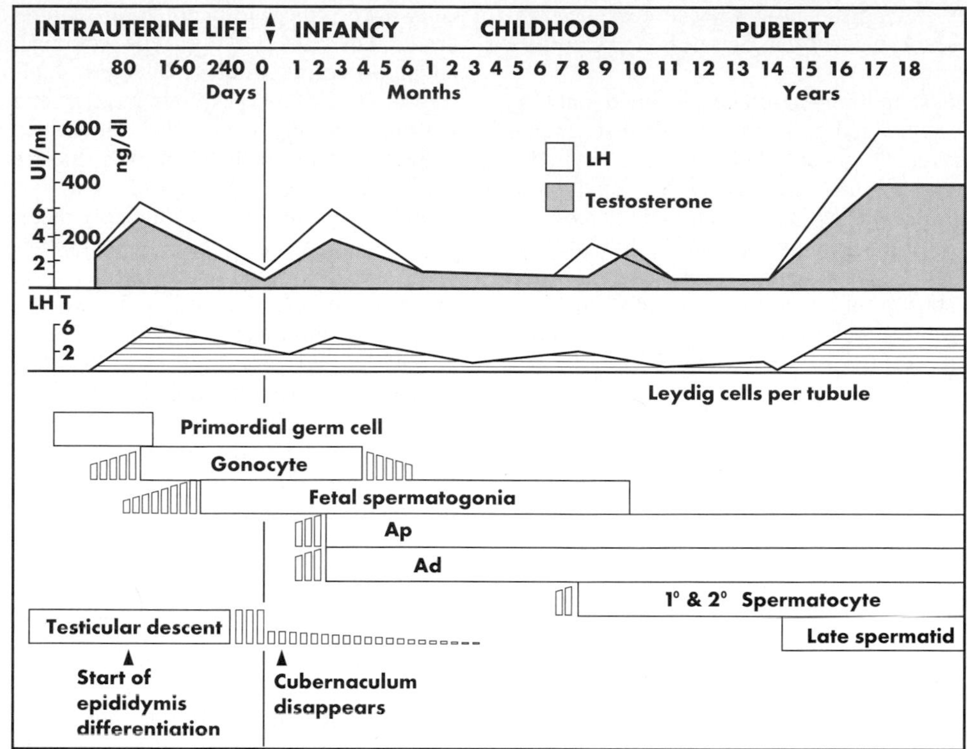

Fig. 67-1 Testicular development in relationship to luteotropic hormone and testosterone secretion in early life. (From Hadziselimovic F: Cryptorchidism. In Gillenwater JY et al, editor: *Adult and pediatric urology*, ed 2, St. Louis, 1991, Mosby.)

ferences must be taken into account when evaluating prepubertal testicular biopsy specimens and when attempting to distinguish changes related to cryptorchidism from those that are expected in a given age group.[6]

Normal anatomy. Normal adult testes weigh approximately 20 g and measure 4.5 × 3 × 2.5 cm. The right testis is usually larger than the left, except in *situs inversus,* a condition in which the left testis is larger. Asians have significantly smaller testes than whites and blacks do. The size of the testis may be measured clinically and constitutes part of the typical workup for infertility.

The testes are enveloped by the *tunica albuginea,* which is composed of fibrous tissues and covered externally with a layer of mesothelium. An identical epithelial layer lines the opposing surface of the tunica vaginalis, which is an extension of the mesothelium forming a sac that encloses the testis. The connective tissue of the tunica albuginea extends into the testis at the hilus. This area, also known as the "mediastinum of the testis," is the site where blood vessels, nerves, and lymphatics enter and also the site where the testis connects to the epididymis. The connective tissue extending from the hilus toward the periphery subdivides the testis into some 250 lobules, each of which contains convolutions of seminiferous tubules, a corresponding vascular supply, and supporting loose connective tissue rich in Leydig cells.

The convoluted *seminiferous tubules* connect to the rete testis at the hilus by means of a straight part *(pars recta). Rete testis* come together in the efferent ductules of the head of epididymis, where they form a single major epididymal duct. The *epididymal duct* is convoluted and forms a 2- to 3-cm-long paratesticular body that can be divided into three segments: the head, the body, and the tail. The tail of the epididymis, which is typically located caudaly to the head and the body, extends upward into the vas deferens. The *vas deferens* is a fibromuscular tube that connects the epididymis with the ejaculatory duct. It lies in the *spermatic cord* surrounded by the spermatic artery, the pampiniform venous plexus, and the efferent testicular lymphatics. The spermatic cord is partially encased on the outside by the cremaster muscle.

Histology. *The seminiferous tubules* are the most prominent component of the testis. Each tubule measures approximately 200 μm in its transverse diameter and is enclosed by a basement membrane. The epithelium is multilayered and consists of spermatogenic and Sertoli cells. In spermatogenesis, *spermatogonia* mature into *spermatozoa* by going through several stages typical of meiosis (Fig. 67-2), each of which can be identified morphologically.[6] *Sertoli cells* can be recognized by their elongated nuclei, which are arranged perpendicular to the basement membrane of the seminiferous tubules, and by their prominent nucleoli. In the normal adult testis the ratio of Sertoli cells to germ cells is 1:11.[7] Approximately 60% to 70% of tubules contain spermatozoa in their lumen.

The *basement membranes* of all tubules are composed of collagen type IV, laminin, and proteoglycans. Although there is some difference in the composition of the basement membrane lining the convoluted portion and pars recta of the seminiferous tubules,[8] ultrastructurally all testicular basement membranes have the same typical features as those in other anatomic sites. External to the basement membrane is a layer of smooth muscle cells, which in turn is surrounded by an amorphous extracellular matrix as well as by scattered connective tissue cells and Leydig cells. Leydig cells can be recognized by their round nuclei, and well-developed eosinophilic cytoplasm. Their cytoplasm may be vacuolated as a result of a high lipid content or may appear brown because of the presence of lipofuscin. The typical *Reinke crystals* are seen in a minority of Leydig cells.

Pars recta of the seminiferous tubules is lined only by Sertoli cells. *Rete testis* is lined by cuboidal cells that are flattened initially but ultimately become taller and even cylindrical as they reach the epididymis. The ducts of the epididymis are lined by pseudostratified cylindrical epithelium covered on the apical side with long microvilli that can be seen by light microscopy. The *vas deferens* is lined by cuboidal epithelium. Its wall consists of smooth muscle cells.

Electron microscopy. Electron microscopy is of limited diagnostic value in the study of testicular cells. Only Leydig cells have typical ultrastructural features. Like other steroid-producing cells, Leydig cells contain an abundant smooth endoplasmic reticulum and large mitochondria with vesicular cristae. The Reinke crystals have a characteristic appearance but are relatively scarce. The ultrastructural features of germ cells and Sertoli cells are less distinctive and of limited diagnostic significance. Sertoli cells may contain typical Charcot-Böttcher crystals, but unfortunately these are uncommon.

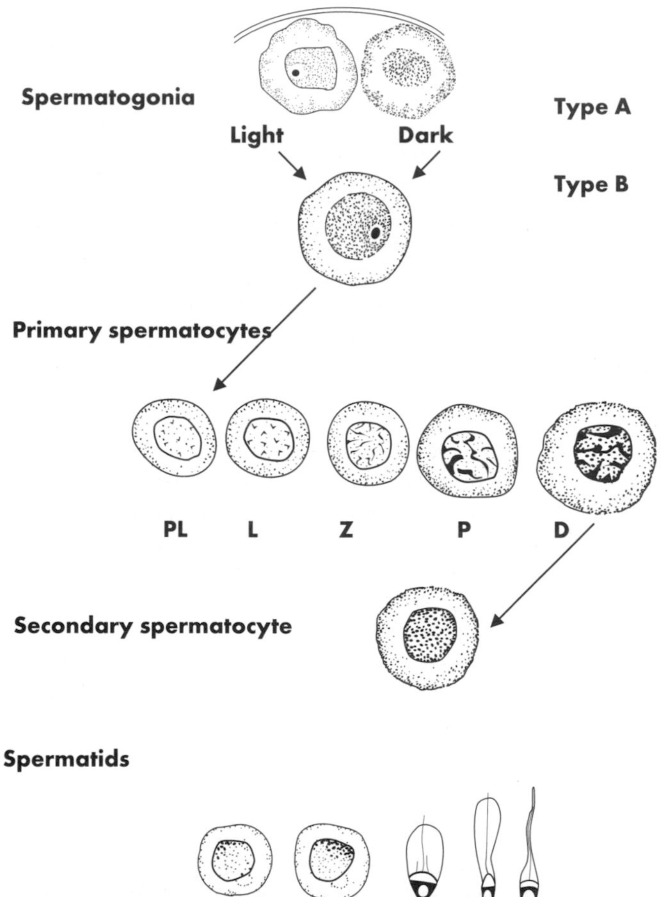

Fig. 67-2 Spermatogenesis. Stem cell spermatogonia of a light and a dark type lie against the basement membrane. The large cell have round nuclei with finely dispersed chromatin surrounded by clear cytoplasm. The activated spermatogonia show chromatin condensation. Primary spermatocytes pass sequentially through preleptotene *(PL)*, leptotene *(L)*, zygotene *(Z)*, pachytene *(P)*, and diplotene *(D)* stages to reach the stage of secondary spermatocytes. Secondary spermatocytes are the end-product of first meiotic division and are recognized by their round nuclei filled uniformly with granular chromatin. These cells are relatively sparse because their life span is only 8 hours, after which they enter into their second meiotic division. Second meiotic division produces round spermatids. These cells have round nuclei that condense and become darker and smaller. Finally the round spermatids transform into elongated spermatids, which lose cytoplasm, acquire a tail, and become spermatozoa. (Modified from Trainer TD: *Am J Surg Pathol* 11:797, 1987)

Physiology. The seminiferous epithelium of the testis differentiates into spermatozoa under the influence of the hormones of the hypothalamic-pituitary-testicular axis. These are commonly abbreviated to "sperm." Sperm production begins at puberty and persists in most healthy men until the end of their life. The sperm matures in the epididymis and is mixed with seminal fluids produced by the epididymis, seminal vesicles, and the prostate. Under normal conditions 1 ml of ejaculated semen contains an average of 60 million spermatozoa. If the ejaculate contains less than 20 million sperm per milliliter, this is called *oligospermia.*

The Leydig cells of the testes are the major source of androgens such as testosterone. The secretion of androgens is regulated by pituitary luteotropic hormone (LH). The pituitary also secretes the follicle-stimulating hormone (FSH), which stimulates the Sertoli cells. It has been estimated that the Sertoli cells secrete some one hundred distinct polypeptides important for spermatogenesis. The secretion of FSH and LH is regulated by the hypothalamic gonadotropin-releasing hormone (GnrH). Inhibin produced by Sertoli cells and testosterone have a negative-feedback effect on the pituitary-inhibiting secretion of GnrH, FSH, and LH.

Testicular biopsy

Pathologists usually receive two types of testicular samples: orchiectomy specimens and biopsy specimens. Orchiectomy is typically performed for the removal tumors or because of chronic inflammation resistant to medical treatment. Castration is commonly performed in patients with prostate carcinoma to reduce the level of testosterone in the body. Biopsies of the testes are mostly performed during the workup to determine the cause of infertility[9,10] (Table 67-1). Fine-needle aspiration biopsy, advocated as a substitute for surgical biopsy,[11] is rarely performed in the United States.

Optimal results are obtained by nontraumatic incisional surgical biopsy. The specimen, measuring 2 to 3 mm and removed without compression or squeezing with a forceps,

Table 67-1 Indications for testicular biopsy*

Absolute
Azoospermia
Oligozoospermia
Teratozoospermia
Atypical cells in ejaculate
Relative
Varicocele
Cryptorchidism
Chronic infection

*Elevation of follicle-stimulating hormone level to three times more than normal is considered sufficient evidence of primary hypogonadism to obviate the need for biopsy.

should be immersed immediately in a fixative that contains caustic salts (for examples mercury chloride) or picric acid, such as Stieve's fixative or Bouin's solution. A cytologic touch preparation air dried, fixed in alcohol, and stained routinely can be prepared at the same time. Formalin is not recommended for testicular biopsies because it produces undue artifacts and does not preserve adequately the architecture of seminiferous tubules. Tissue submitted for electron microscopy study is fixed in 1% glutaraldehyde.

The pathologist evaluating the testicular biopsy specimens should follow the recommendations I have outlined at length before.[12] It is important to assess the overall morphology of the testicular tissue. Spermatogenesis is best evaluated using either the criteria of Johnsen[13] or other less popular methods compared in my review.[12]

The mean Johnsen score for normal testes is 9.39 ± 0.24 on a scale of from 0 to 10. The Johnsen score for biopsy specimens from patients with oligozoospermia is 5.3 ± 2.1; that for pituitary hypogonadism is 3.95 ± 1.4 and that for Klinefelter's syndrome is 1.3 ± 0.3 (Fig. 67-3). This approach is time-consuming and may not always be warranted. Experienced pathologists may thus rely on subjective assessment and describe the abnormalities rather than quantitate them. Silber and Rodriguez-Rigau[14] have noted that one can adequately assess spermatogenesis by counting the round spermatids. These cells are located toward the center of tubules and are easily recognized because of their small, round, dark nuclei, which have this appearance even in suboptimally formalin fixed specimens. Normal testes contain at least 20 round spermatids per tubule, and a reduced number of these cells is indicative of oligospermia. A reduction in the sperm count correlates with a reduction in the number of round spermatids per tubule.

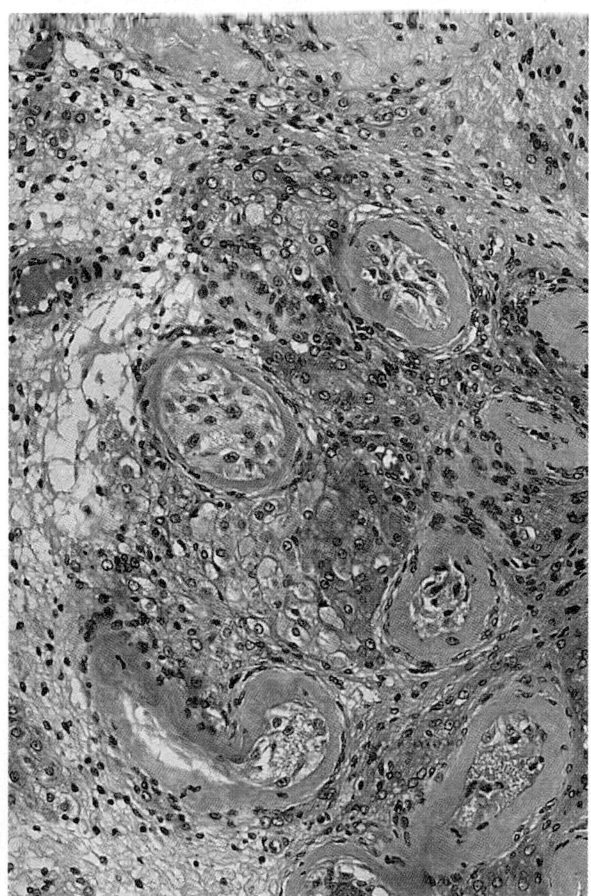

Fig. 67-3 Klinefelter's syndrome. There is marked tubular atrophy. (Courtesy Drs. N. Skakkebaek and A. Giwercman, Copenhagen, Denmark.)

Developmental anomalies

The abnormal development of the testis may result in:

1. Abnormal positioning of the testis—cryptorchidism, testicular ectopia, or dystopia
2. Numerical aberrations—anorchism, monorchism, polyorchidism
3. Structural malformations of testes or epididymis
4. Gonadal dysgenesis, which is almost always associated with sex chromosome abnormalities or intersexualism

Except for cryptorchidism, which is diagnosed in 1% to 2% of all male infants, all other developmental abnormalities are rare.

Cryptorchidism

The term *cryptorchidism,* derived from the Greek words *cryptos,* for "hidden," and *orchis,* for "testis," is generally used as a synonym for undescended testes. In true cryptorchidism, which requires surgical correction, the testes may be located in the abdominal cavity or in the inguinal canal, that is, along the normal pathway of testicular descent; or the testes may be located in ectopic sites, such as the femoral canal or suprapubic subcutaneous tissue. Undescended testes should be distinguished from retractile testes, which represent a physiologic variant found in 10% of newborn boys and 20% to 30% of those born prematurely.[3,4] These retractile testes are withdrawn into the open inguinal canal by a cremasteric reflex but can be repositioned in the scrotum. The closure of the inguinal canal that typically takes place during the first 3 months of life limits testicular mobility, and retraction cannot be induced thereafter. So that cryptorchidism is not misdiagnosed as retractile testes, most authorities delay the final diagnosis of cryptorchidism until the patient reaches 1 year of age. Surveys of populations have shown that the incidence of cryptorchidism diagnosed in 1-year-old boys ranges from 1% to 2%.[5] A slight increase in incidence has been reported recently in England and Wales.[4,15]

The etiology and pathogenesis of cryptorchidism are still matters of controversy. Although it has been generally accepted that cryptorchidism reflects disturbances in testicular descent during intrauterine life,[16] the reasons for the abnormal descent are not known. According to one view the testes themselves are abnormal and this prevents them from reaching their normal scrotal location. Others maintain that mechanical and endocrine factors impede the descent of the testis, thus hindering normal development of the testes.

Many disturbances of gonadal development are associated with cryptorchidism.[17] Cryptorchidism often occurs in association with developmental anomalies of the urogenital tract.[17] However, most children who have cryptorchidism have no other anomalies. An increased incidence of cryptorchidism has been noted in association with exposure to diethylstilbestrol in utero,[18] but it is doubtful whether endogenous hyperestrinism in the mother or the fetus could have a similar adverse effect.

The main issues surrounding the pathogenetic controversy that have been debated since John Hunter described cryptorchidism in 1786 apparently remain unresolved.

Cryptorchidism is most often unilateral, but it may be bilateral in a small number of patients.[19] Such testes are most often located high in the scrotum or retained in the connective tissue between the inguinal canal and scrotal inlet. In approximately 20% of patients the testis is in the inguinal canal and in 10% it is intraabdominal.[20] Dystopic testes, which may be found in a variety of other sites, are rare.

Undescended testes are usually smaller than normal testes, and they remain smaller even after orchiopexy. Abdominal testes are smaller than inguinal intracanalicular testes. The size of high scrotal testes is altered the least.[21] The histologic features vary depending on the age of the patient, the location of the testis, and the treatment that has been carried out. According to Nistal et al,[22] the histologic changes are minimal in 26% of the patients. Marked germinal hypoplasia is found in 24%, diffuse tubular hypoplasia in 33%, and severe atrophy in 17%. Approximately 25% of contralateral descended testes show changes that are similar to those in the undescended testis. Cryptorchidism is often associated with epididymal abnormalities.[23]

Undescended testes, including those that have been surgically repositioned in the scrotum, contain fewer spermatogenic cells[24] (Fig. 67-4). Blumer and Hedinger[25] could find no germ cells in 52% of surgically removed undescended testes and in 46% of those they examined after orchiopexy. In adults, approximately 2% to 3% of undescended testes contain carcinoma in situ (CIS),[24] which predictably gives rise to invasive germ cell tumors. Orchiopexy does not decrease the risk of cancer.

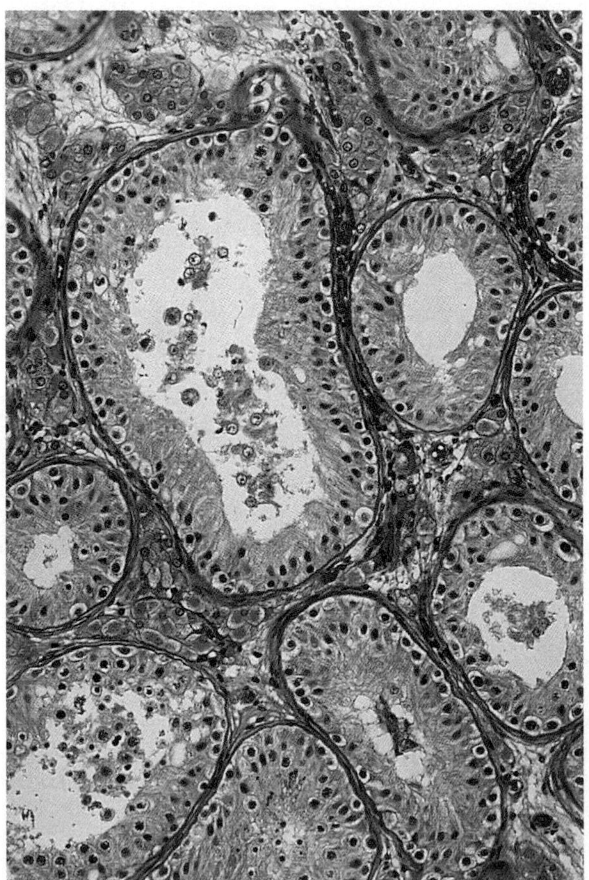

Fig. 67-4 Undescended testis. There is hypospermatogenesis.

Numerical aberrations

Normal males have two testicles. Bilateral absence of the testicles is called *anorchism. Monorchism* denotes a condition in which one testicle is missing. *Polyorchidism* is characterized by supernumerary testicles. Anorchism occurs in 1 in 20,000 males, monorchism in 1 in 5000.[26] Polyorchidism is rare; there are less than 60 cases on record. These rare conditions may cause infertility and are often associated with other urogenital anomalies, summarized in a recent monograph.[12]

Structural abnormalities

Abnormal development of the seminiferous epithelium results in azoospermia. In its most severe form the seminiferous tubules are lined by Sertoli cells and lack spermatogonia or their derivatives. This *germ cell aplasia,* also known as *Sertoli only syndrome* or *del Castillo's syndrome,* is found in approximately 10% to 20% of biopsy specimens obtained from infertile men. The defect is irreversible and cannot be treated.

Structural abnormalities of the epididymis may also cause infertility, especially if bilateral. Scorer and Farrington[20] classified these abnormalities into several groups, the most important of which are *aplasia, obstruction,* or *interruption* of the epididymis. These may be associated with cystic changes or ectopia of the epididymal tissue and if bilateral may result in obstructive azoospermia. The vas deferens may also be obliterated or interrupted. Congenital bilateral absence of the vas deferens occurs in association with renal malformations and is a constant feature of Potter's syndrome (bilateral renal agenesis). A genetic absence of the epididymis has been documented recently in patients with cystic fibrosis.[27] One-sided agenesis of the vas deferens is in 80% of cases associated with ipsilateral renal agenesis.[28]

Minor structural abnormalities of the epididymis present as embryonic rests and cysts,[12] some of which are considered normal anatomic variants. These are classified as *appendix testes,* which are derived from the proximal part of the müllerian duct; *appendix epididymis,* representing the remnant of the wolffian duct; and *aberrant ducts of Haller,* derived from the incompletely involuted mesonephric ducts. These appendages normally produce no symptoms but may undergo cystic dilatation or torsion. Cysts may also form in the testis and on the tunica albuginea.[29]

Choristomas of the testis and the epididymis include adrenal rests and splenic tissue fused with the gonad.[12] *Adrenal rests* (Fig. 67-5) are typical of the adrenogenital syndrome, in which they may assume tumorlike proportions.[30] An otherwise normal spermatic cord may contain ectopic Leydig cells, which may form microscopic nests but not grossly visible nodules.

Gonadal dysgenesis

Dysgenetic gonadal development is almost invariably associated with numerical or structural abnormalities of the Y chromosome.[31] The phenotype of affected patients varies,[12] and the gonadal pathologic characteristics are also quite variable.[32] A whole spectrum of changes can be found. The seminiferous tubules are usually atrophic and incompletely formed. Some

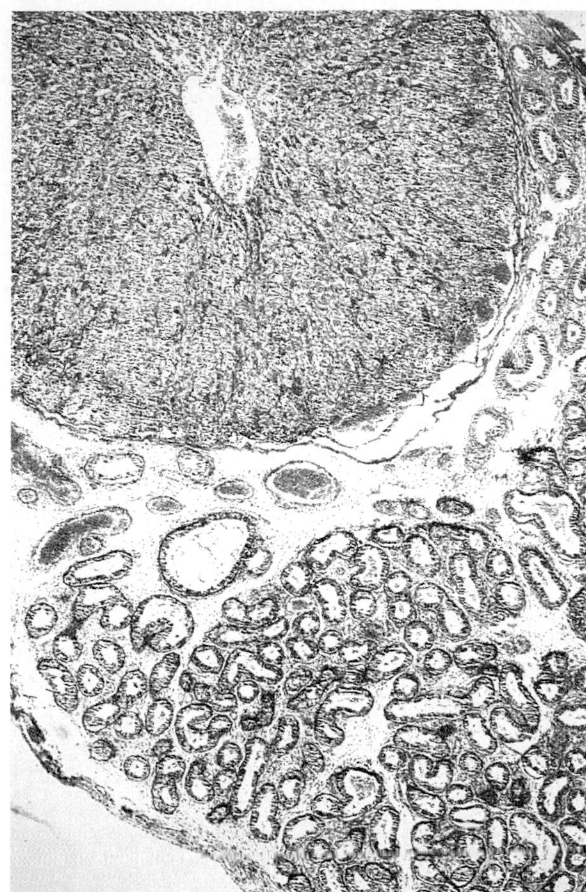

Fig. 67-5 Adrenal rest choristoma in the testis.

Table 67-2 Causes of epididymoorchitis

Bacteria
Sexually transmitted
Neisseria gonorrhoeae
Treponema pallidum
Uropathogens
Escherichia coli
Mixed flora
Mycobacteria
Mycobacterium tuberculosis
M. leprae
Rare blood-borne pathogens
Haemophilus influenzae
Salmonella sp.
Brucella sp.
Fungi
Histoplasma capsulatum
Blastomyces dermatitidis
Coccidioides immitis
Parasites
Wuchereria bancrofti
Schistosoma haematobium
Echinococcus granulosus
Viruses
Mumps virus
Adenovirus
Coxsackie virus B
Cytomegalovirus
Idiopathic or immune
Sarcoidosis
Malakoplakia
(Granulomatous orchitis)

gonads contain ovarian tissue, and these are classified as *ovotestes*.[33] Gonadoblastomas are found in some dysgenetic gonads.[32]

Gonadal dysgenesis occassionally does not occur in relation to chromosomal abnormalities. A unique developmental anomaly of the seminiferous tubules resembling annulate tubules of the ovary has been observed recently in the setting of the Peutz-Jeghers syndrome.[34]

Inflammation

Owing to the anatomic proximity of the testis and epididymis, *orchitis,* the inflammation of the testis, and *epididymitis* rarely occur in isolation but usually arise as inseparable components of a single inflammatory process—*epididymoorchitis*.[35] These infections are classified on the basis of various criteria, as follows:

1. Duration: acute or chronic
2. *Etiology:* bacterial, viral, fungal, protozoal, or parasitic
3. *Route of infection:* ascending (canalicular), hematogenous, lymphatic, or transcutaneous
4. *Morphology:* suppurative, interstitial, granulomatous, or fibrosing

Etiology and pathogenesis. The causes of epididymoorchitis are reviewed in greater detail in my monograph[12] and are listed in Table 67-2. This table also contains several histologically distinct forms of orchitis, such as malakoplakia, granulomatous orchitis, and sarcoidosis, the etiology and pathogenesis of which remain unknown. The immunologically mediated form of orchitis,[36] anticipated in human subjects on the basis of the autoimmune orchitis that can be easily induced in experimental animals, remains poorly defined and has not been definitively accepted as a distinct entity.[37]

The causes of epididymoorchitis have changed over the years but generally result from the transmission of various pathogens in populations at risk.[38] The etiology of infections also depends on the age, social habits, sexual orientation, and general health of each person.

Most *bacterial infections* are transmitted sexually and are therefore rare in children but prevalent in promiscuous adults. Recurrent urinary tract infections are the usual cause of epididymoorchitis in the elderly with hyperplasia of the prostate. *Neisseria gonorrhoeae* and *Chlamydia* and *Mycoplasma* organisms predominate as the cause in men under 35 and the coliform bacteria in those over 60 years of age. Untreated gonococcal infection is the major cause of male infertility in Africa.[12] In *Treponema pallidum* infection, which was common in the preantibiotic era, usually chronic interstitial lymphocytic orchitis or typical gummas are the presenting findings. *Mycobacterium tuberculosis* infections that typically cause caseating granulomas in the epididymis are also less common today. Granulomatous orchitis caused by *Mycobacterium leprae* infection is typical of the lepromatous leprosy

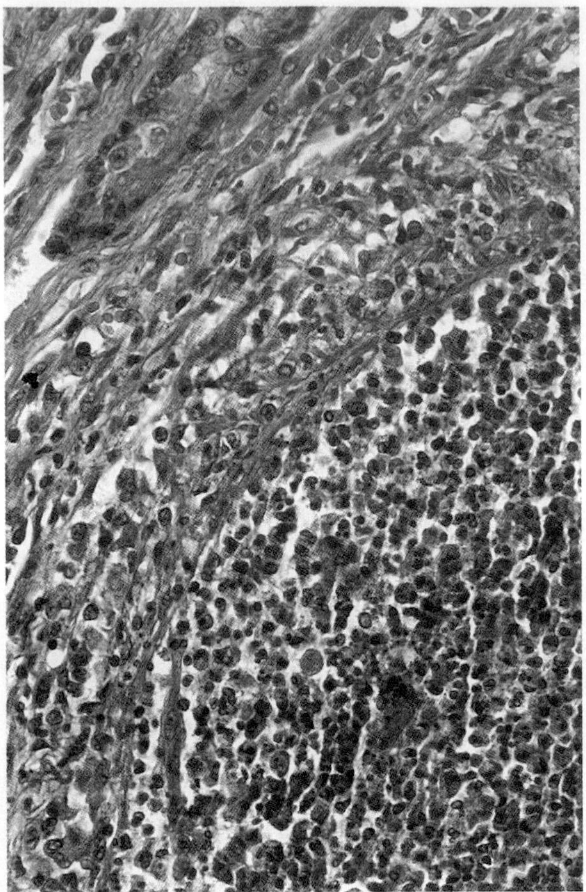

Fig. 67-6 Suppurative epididymitis.

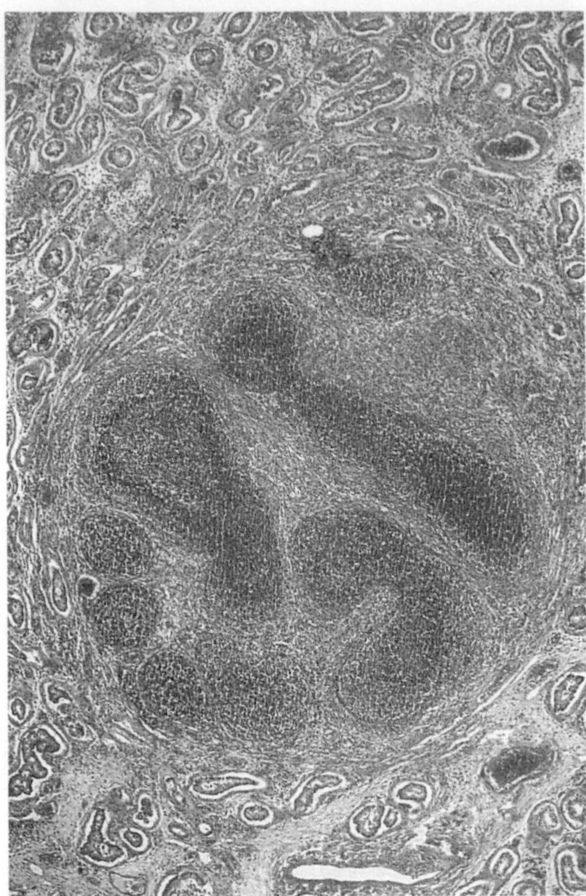

Fig. 67-7 Abscess of the testis.

that occurs in the populations of Africa and Asia, which is, however, rare in the United States. Lepra bacilli apparently proliferate best at lower temperatures, and thus the testis represents a favorite site of infection.[39]

Viral infections reach the scrotum by the hematogenous route. Accordingly most orchitides are noted during a bout of systemic viremia, and although sometimes suspected clinically, the infection of the testis is rarely documented morphologically. The best-known viral infection affecting the testes and epididymis is mumps,[40] but other viruses such as the Epstein-Barr virus, echovirus, and cytomegalovirus (CMV) have also been shown to produce similar changes.

Fungal epididymoorchitis is rare outside the tropics. The only exception is histoplasmosis, which may produce intrascrotal granulomas during systemic dissemination. Fungemia caused by other opportunistic pathogens that occur in men with the acquired immunodeficiency syndrome (AIDS) or in men in a medically induced immunosuppressed state may result in the development of testicular or epididymal lesions, but these are rarely of clinical significance. *Parasitic* infections are exceptionally rare outside the tropics.

Acute ascending bacterial infections typically cause a suppurative inflammation that spreads to the epididymis from the seminal ducts. Spreading infection may result in the formation of abscesses. The infection is often accompanied by the transudation of fluid into the peritesticular space *(hydrocele),* which may become infected and purulent. If this is left untreated, the entire scrotum may become filled with pus. In chronic stages of the infection the pus is replaced by granulation tissue and fibrosis, which obliterates all normal structures of the scrotum.

Pathology. The presenting features of epididymoorchitis may take several forms. The morphology of lesions may provide some clues to their causes, but the final diagnosis usually requires bacteriologic confirmation. This may be impossible in men with chronic lesions, many of which are bacteriologically sterile.

Suppurative inflammation is typically caused by an ascending bacterial infection. In this condition, bacteria and pus fill the duct of the epididymis and spread into the testis and the scrotal tissues (Fig. 67-6). Abscesses may then form, which may replace parts of the testis (Fig. 67-7). If the inflammation extends into the peritesticular space, collections of pus will form between the layers of the tunica vaginalis. Ultimately the entire scrotum could become filled with pus.

Abscesses may persist for some time. Healing results in extensive fibrosis, which obliterates all the intrascrotal structures and destroys the testis. If the condition is bilateral, this obviously leads to infertility. However, even lesser infections may cause obstructive infertility by destroying parts of the excretory duct system or by causing fibrotic obliteration as a result of the scarring that occurs during healing.

An *interstitial inflammation* typical of viral infection is most prominent in the testis (Fig. 67-8), but it often extends into the rete testis and epididymis. Focal interstitial orchitis is found quite often in testicles removed at autopsy or in those removed from prostate cancer patients, but the cause of this

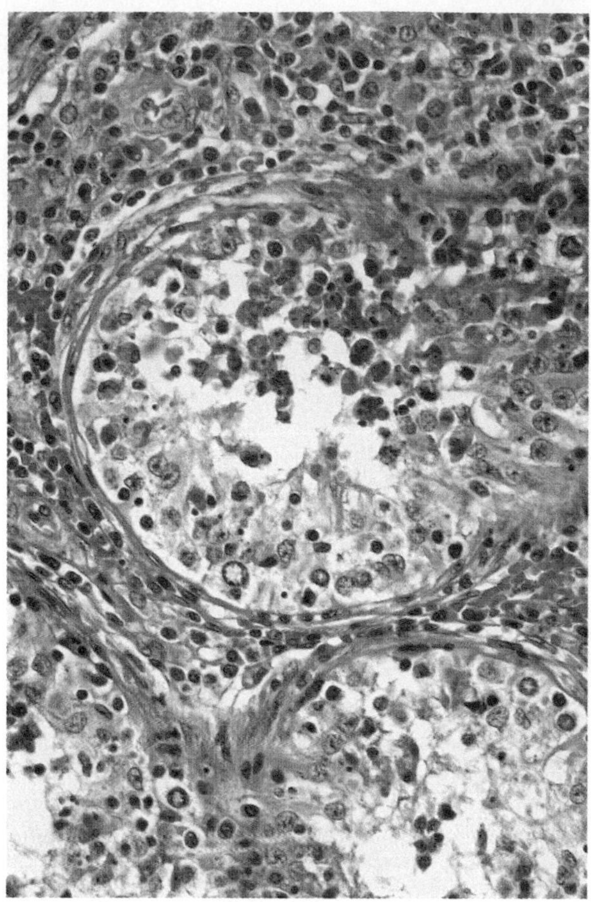

Fig. 67-8 Interstitial orchitis caused by mumps.

inflammation is usually not known. Severe interstitial orchitis is associated with atrophy of the germinal epithelium and if bilateral may result in infertility.

Granulomatous inflammation. Granulomas of the testis may be caused by bacteria or fungi.[35] Noninfectious granulomas are morphologic evidence of the existence of a cell-mediated immunity to foreign or endogenous antigens. Caseating granulomas typical of *M. tuberculosis* infection and fungal infection like *histoplasmosis* usually contain pathogens demonstrable with special stains. The granulomas of leprosy also contain acid-fast bacilli but are usually less discrete and show less necrosis. The gummas of syphilis that show a central necrotic area surrounded by epithelioid cells, lymphocytes, and scattered plasma cells are usually devoid of stainable spirochetes. In sarcoidosis, "naked" epithelioid granulomas with no necrosis are the presenting finding.

Malakoplakia, also known as *granulomatous orchitis,* is a morphologically distinct form of chronic infection.[41] In this disease the seminiferous tubules are infiltrated with numerous histiocytes, lymphocytes, and plasma cells (Fig. 67-9). The histiocytes have a prominent eosinophilic cytoplasm filled with residues of phagocytosed bacteria and concentrically calcified inclusions called *Michaelis-Gutmann bodies.* Testicular lesions have the same features as malakoplakia in the more common sites, such as the urinary bladder.

Chronic fibrosing epididymoorchitis is the end stage of acute and protracted infections.[35] As in any other end-stage organ lesions, the histopathologic characteristics provide few clues to the etiology or pathogenesis of the disease that has caused it. Occasional residues, such as the ova of parasites or persistent eosinophilic leukocytes, may provide some clues, but rarely if ever definitive evidence indicating the identity of the preexisting disease.

Testicular changes in AIDS. Infection with the human immunodeficiency virus causes profound testicular changes, even though it is not known whether the virus has a predilection

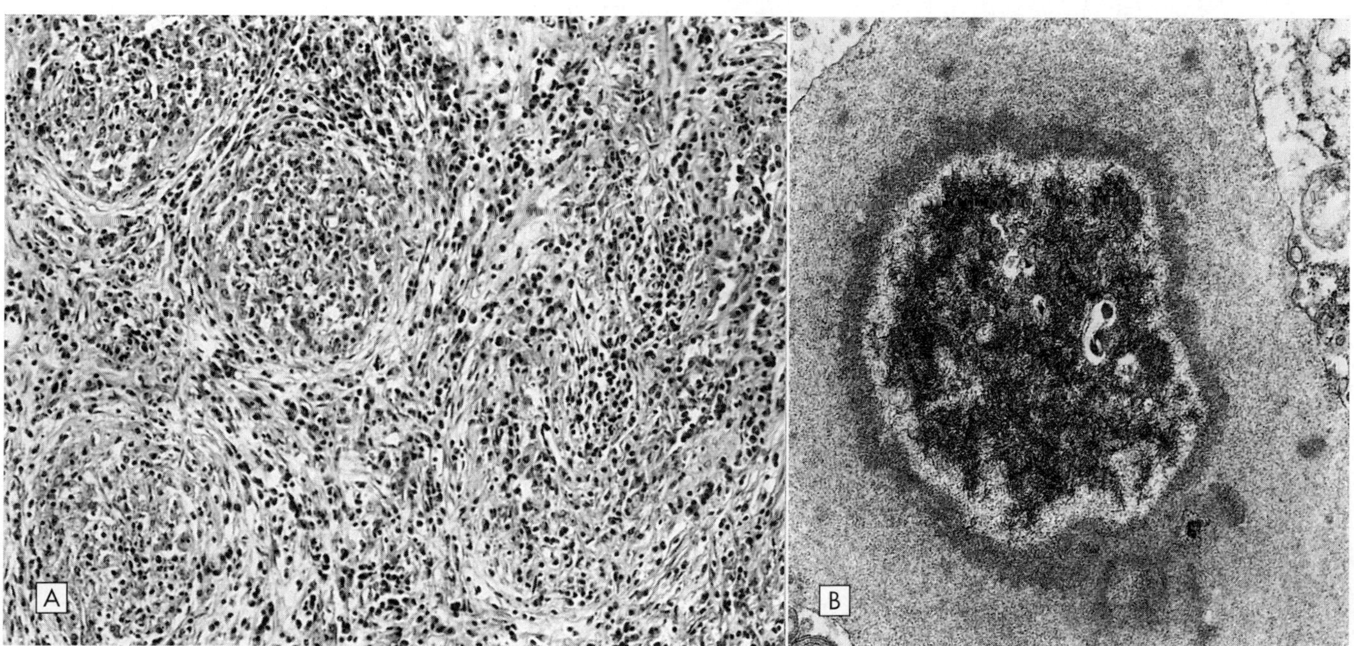

Fig. 67-9 Malakoplakia. **A,** By light microscopy the tubules and the interstitium have been obliterated by mononuclear cells. **B,** Electron micrograph of a typical Michaelis-Gutmann body.

for growing in intact testicular cells.[42,43] The testes may show atrophy of the germinal epithelium, tubular hyalinization, interstitial fibrosis, a reduced number of Leydig cells, and focal infiltrates of lymphocytes (Fig. 67-10). The testes may be colonized by the opportunistic pathogens prevalent in AIDS, such as *Mycobacterium avium–intracellulare, M. tuberculosis,* CMV, *Toxoplasma gondii,* and various fungi. Kaposi sarcoma may involve the testis, but it is more common on the scrotum.

Vascular disturbances

The testes have a complex blood supply.[12] The most important aspects of this circulation are as follows: *First,* the spermatic artery and the venous pampiniform plexus are situated near the spermatic cord, which makes it possible for the venous plexus to serve as a countercurrent cooling mechanism for the arterial blood. This ensures the maintenance of a low scrotal temperature, which is 2° to 3° C below the temperature of the rest of the body. On the other hand, stagnant venous blood may cause the intrascrotal temperature to increase and contribute to the development of infertility. *Second,* the right spermatic vein enters directly into the vena cava, whereas the left vein is confluent with the left renal vein. Accordingly the higher back pressure in the left vein, transmitted to the pampiniform plexus, accounts for the more common occurrence of varicocele on the left side. *Third,* the spermatic cord contains not only the blood vessels but also the vas deferens and the connective tissue that serves as a suspensory medium for the testis. The rotation of the testis may twist the spermatic cord, and this torsion may interrupt the blood flow to and from the testis, leading to infarction or hemorrhage. Other causes of testicular hemorrhage and infarction are listed in Table 67-3.

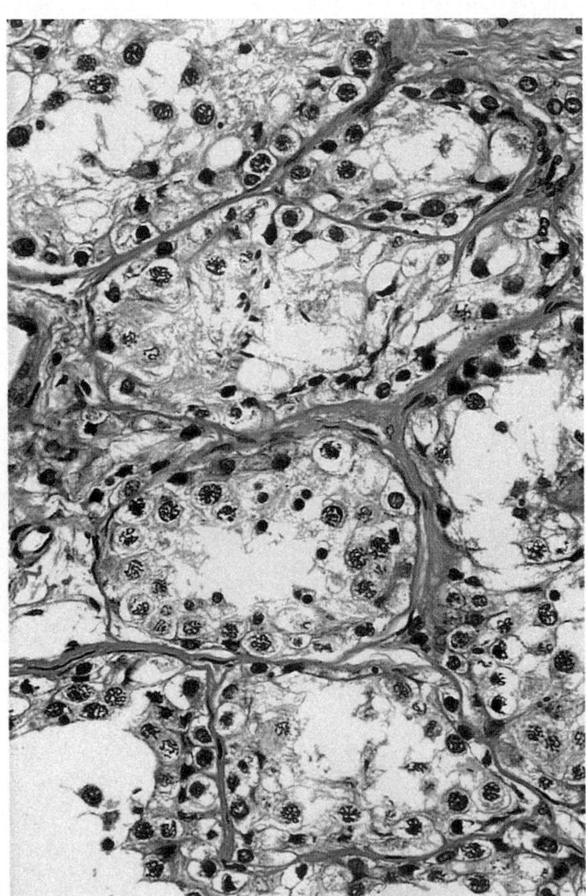

Fig. 67-10 Testis from the autopsy of a patient with AIDS shows cessation of spermatogenesis.

Torsion

Torsion of the testis around the spermatic cord can occur within the tunica vaginalis or external to it.[12] Intrascrotal torsions occur most often in the peripubertal period, less often in neonates, and only exceptionally in adults. The torsion is thought to be related to trauma, but there is often no history of any particular causative event. The torsion leads to the occlusion of blood vessels and infarction of the testis. Because the veins have thinner walls than the arteries and are therefore more easily compressed, venous congestion predominates initially, followed by an interruption of arterial blood flow. This typically results in a hemorrhagic infarction (Fig. 67-11), and unless the torsion is repaired surgically within 4 hours of occlusion, testicular function is permanently lost. Testes that have been ischemic for a short time can be salvaged by prompt surgical intervention.

Mikuz[44] has recommended grading the severity of histologic changes as follows:

1. Mild injury, typical of ischemia of less than 4 hours' duration. This is dominated by marked edema and some loss of seminiferous epithelium.
2. Interstitial hemorrhages and tubular necrosis, typically seen in testes 4 to 12 hours after the interruption of blood flow.
3. Hemorrhagic infarct, usually occurring in testes that have been ischemic for 12 hours or more.

The outcome of testicular torsion depends on the severity and duration of the ischemia. Irreversibly damaged testes are best resected.[45] If left in situ, the necrotic tissue may adversely affect spermatogenesis in the contralateral testis. Early resection of the damaged testis does not adversely influence fertility.

Table 67-3 Causes of testicular hemorrhage and infarction

Trauma
Torsion
Hematologic disorders
Coagulopathy
Polycythemia
Leukemia
Sickle cell anemia
Compression of blood vessels
Tumors
Hernia
Thromboembolism
Thrombosis of the vena cava, renal vein, or spermatic vein
Arterial emboli (for example, those resulting from endocarditis)
Vasculitis
Allergic vasculitis
Polyarteritis nodosa
Buerger's disease
Henoch-Schönlein purpura

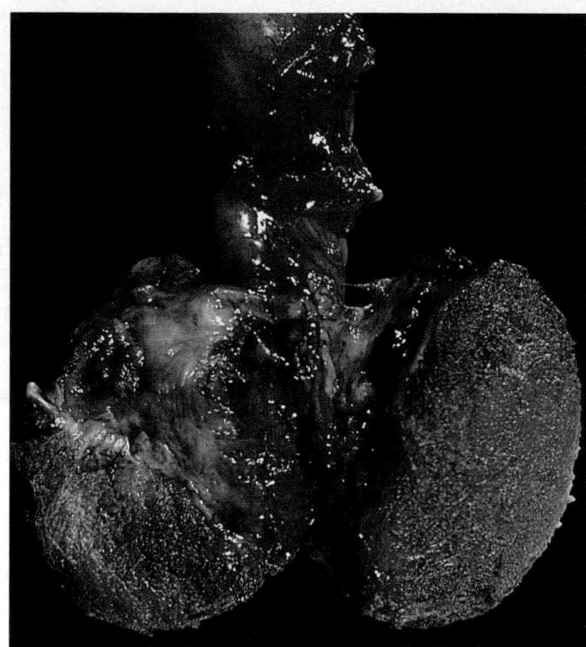

Fig. 67-11 Torsion of the testis. The testis appear dark red and partially necrotic owing to hemorrhagic infarction.

Varicocele

Varicocele is a dilatation of the testicular veins in the pampiniform plexus. It is most often located on the left side but is bilateral in about 10% to 15% of cases. A varicocele may be detected in as many as 25% of adults, but it appears to be more common in infertile men.[46] Overall it is considered to be the most common cause of infertility. Ligation of the varicocele may improve fertility in such cases.

The pathogenesis of varicocele remains poorly understood, but it appears to be related to an abnormal flow of venous blood from the scrotum. The confluence of the left spermatic vein and the renal vein may interfere with the drainage of venous blood on that side. The left vein is 10 cm longer than the right vein, which explains in part the increased back pressure on the left side. Compression of the left spermatic vein between the superior mesenteric artery and the aorta may be another contributing factor. The absence of valves in the internal spermatic veins facilitates the back flow of blood. A varicocele adversely affects spermatogenesis and is often associated with oligospermia and infertility. Relative intrascrotal hyperthermia, the reflux of renal and adrenal venous blood into the testis, altered testicular metabolism, hypoxia, and mechanical compression of scrotal structures by the dilated veins have all been proposed as causes of varicocele.[12]

Pathology. Dilated veins can be seen on the lateral side of the scrotum and are often palpable. Since the clinically assessed extent of the varicosities correlates well with the degree of hypospermatogenesis,[12] there is usually no need for testicular biopsy. The tissue containing the varicose veins is rarely submitted for histologic examination.

The testicular histologic changes vary from one patient to another and are nonspecific. In most cases there is some focal tubular atrophy, peritubular sclerosis, and fibrosis. Decreased spermatogenesis with maturation arrest and degeneration of the adluminal Sertoli cells may also be seen. The likelihood of the infertility being reversed depends on the extent of the testicular changes. Testicular biopsy is rarely done because fertility can be predicted on the basis of the spermiogram findings, the serum FSH level, and the testicular volume.[12]

Vasculitis

Testicular lesions are found at autopsy, in approximately 70% of patients with polyarteritis nodosa, but the disease is only exceptionally limited to the testis.[47] Henoch-Schönlein purpura, systemic lupus erythematosus, Wegener's granulomatosis, Buerger's disease, and hypersensitivity vasculitis[48] have also been found to affect the testis.

Amyloidosis

In systemic amyloidosis the testicular arteries and arterioles contain amyloid. This has few consequences and is rarely recognized clinically. In addition to deposits of amyloid in blood vessels, tubular basement membranes may be involved as well.[49]

Iatrogenic lesions

Radiation therapy and chemotherapy

Radiation therapy and cytoxic drugs used in the treatment of cancer often adversely affect the seminiferous epithelium of the testis. The final outcome depends on the age of the patient, the duration of therapy, and the treatment used.[50] Radiation-induced necrosis of the germinal epithelium results in its rapid depletion. The spermatogenic arrest persists for a variable time and may be irreversible depending on the dose of radiation administered.[12] Radiation does not significantly affect the Leydig cells.

Cytotoxic drugs may also deplete the germinal epithelium. The multidrug therapy used for Hodgkin's disease, combining nitrogen mustard, vincristine, procarbazine, and prednisone, usually results in the irreversible depletion of germ cells. Triple therapy with bleomycin, *cis*-platinum, and vinblastine sulfate, the most popular treatment for testicular cancer, causes temporary infertility, but 75% of patients regain fertility within 18 months of diagnosis.[51]

The fertility of men who were treated for childhood cancer can be predicted by the serum FSH level and testicular size.[52] These measurements correlate with the degree of drug-induced injury, and thus obviate the need for testicular biopsy.

Vasectomy

By extrapolating the data of the World Health Organization collected through 1987, it is possible to estimate that more than 50 million men will have undergone voluntary vasectomy so far. Surgical ligation of the vas deferens is still one of the most efficient, least expensive forms of contraception. It is reversible in a large number of men, it produces almost no side effects, and it is associated with only minor local complications.[12] These occur in approximately 3% of vasectomized men and include minor lesions resulting from technical problems arising during surgery, delayed healing, and late sequelae of vas transection. The most frequent complication resulting from technical surgical problems is bleeding at the site of incision or transection of the vas. Inadequate healing has been reported in 0.5% of patients. Complications include adhesions between the vas deferens and the skin, fistula formation, or the development of abscesses as a result of intraoperative infection. Recanalization may occur if the resected segment is too short.

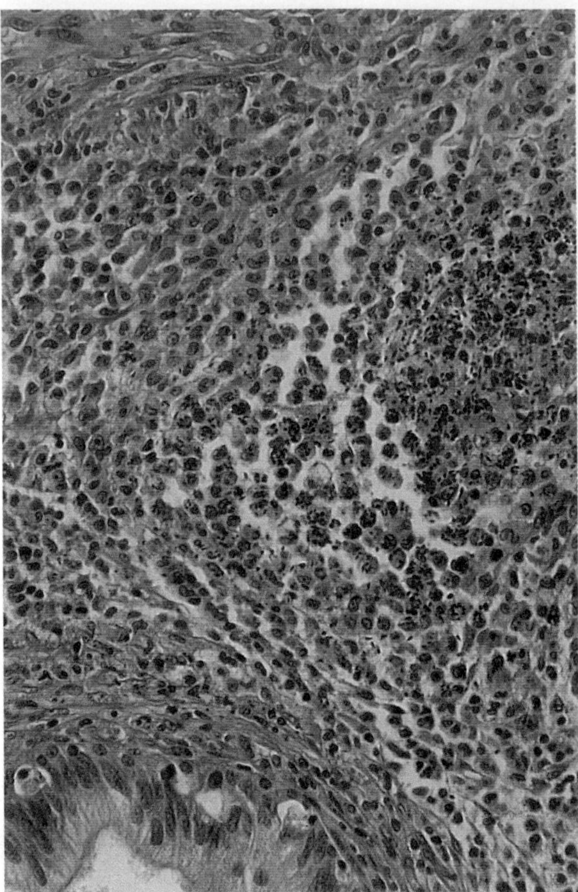

Fig. 67-12 Sperm granuloma.

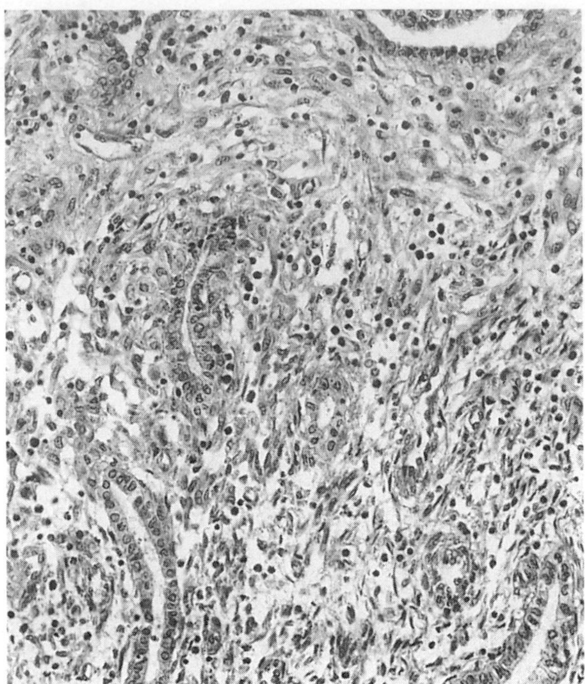

Fig. 67-13 Vasitis nodosa.

Sperm granulomas represent a reaction to sperm extravasated from the caudal part of the transected vas deferens. The lesions are typically nodular and measure 2 to 20 mm in diameter. Histologically the lesion is composed of macrophages, lymphocytes, and remnants of spermatozoa in the muscular wall of the epididymis (Fig. 67-12). Sperm granulomas are four times more common after surgical ligation than after fulguration of the opposing ends of the transected vas deferens. A foreign body granuloma that forms in reaction to the suture material also probably contributes to the development of sperm granulomas.[53] However, sperm granulomas may occur even without vasectomy and are probably caused by some other form of obstruction, such as postinflammatory stenosis or obliteration of the vas deferens.

Vasitis nodosa is a sign of epithelial regeneration and occurs in two thirds of all vasectomized men. The proliferating cells form anastomosing, epithelium-lined spaces often containing sperm (Fig. 67-13). These ductules may extend through the entire thickness of the vas deferens and into the surrounding connective tissue and nerves.[54] Vasitis nodosa may occur even in men who have not had a vasectomy. In such cases it is probably a complication of epididymitis or is a congenital structural defect resulting in diverticulosis of the epididymal duct.

Testicular changes in infertility

The causes of infertility are classified as pretesticular, testicular and posttesticular[55-57] (Table 67-4). Pretesticular causes include various disturbances of the hypothalamic-pituitary–gonadal and adrenal hormonal axis. These diseases are usually considered under the heading of hypogonadotropic hypogonadism. Testicular causes include idiopathic conditions affecting spermatogenesis and secondary testicular injury caused by inflammation, cryptorchidism, radiation therapy, drugs, or varicocele. Posttesticular causes include various disorders that obstruct the outflow of sperm.

Table 67-4 Causes of male infertility

Pretesticular causes
Disorders of the hypothalamus or pituitary
Endocrine diseases (thyroid or adrenal disorders or diabetes)
Metabolic disorders (renal or liver diseases)
Chronic infection
Drugs
Testicular causes
Idiopathic hypospermatogenesis or aspermatogenesis
Developmental and genetic disorders
Circulatory—varicocele or torsion
Inflammatory lesions—infectious or immune
Iatrogenic—chemical, radiation, or surgical
Environmental
Genital, posttesticular causes
Congenital anomalies of excretory ducts and accessory glands
Inflammatory lesions of the excretory ducts and accessory glands
Iatrogenic or posttraumatic lesions of the excretory ducts, accessory glands, or ejaculatory nerve plexus

Hypogonadotropic hypogonadism

Congenital or acquired lesions of the hypothalamus and pituitary affect the development and function of testes.[12] Such hypogonadotropic hypogonadism may be caused by tumors (for example, craniopharyngioma or pituitary adenoma), inflammation (for example, pituitary apoplexy), or genetic and developmental syndromes (for example, the Prader-Willi syndrome or Kallmann's syndrome). Various drugs, trauma, or irradiation of the hypothalamus may have the same consequences. All these conditions are characterized by low levels of serum gonadotropins. The testes are small and never attain the normal adult size. The seminiferous tubules are small and lined with immature Sertoli cells that have round nuclei and inconspicuous nucleoli (Fig. 67-14). The germ cells are sparse, and there is no evidence of spermatogenesis. Treatment with GnrH given in a pulsatile manner may initiate and maintain spermatogenesis and cure infertility.[58]

Testicular causes of infertility

Testicular causes of infertility are classified as either primary or secondary. Primary conditions are idiopathic, that is, the causes for the interruption of spermatogenesis are not evident. In secondary conditions, spermatogenesis is interrupted or perturbed by some identifiable external cause, such as inflammation, irradiation, or drugs. In either case the spermiogram shows either no living sperms (*azoospermia*) or fewer than 20 million sperm per milliliter (*oligospermia*) and such a patient is infertile or subfertile.

On the basis of testicular morphology, primary disturbances of spermatogenesis can be subdivided into three groups: germ cell aplasia, maturation arrest of spermatogenesis, and hypospermatogenesis.

Germ cell aplasia, or Sertoli only syndrome, is the most severe of these disturbances and is invariably accompanied by azoospermia. This finding is noted in 10% to 20% of all testicular biopsy specimens obtained from infertile men.[55-57] In this condition the seminiferous tubules are smaller than normal and are lined by a single layer of Sertoli cells (Fig. 67-15). The oval nuclei of the Sertoli cells are typically located in the midportion of their cytoplasm, with their longitudinal diameter perpendicular to the basement membrane of the tubule. The tubular basement membranes are typically thin, and there is no evidence of spermatogenesis. If the tubules with complete germ cell aplasia are admixed with tubules that show spermatogenesis, this finding is classifed as mixed germ cell aplasia with focal spermatogenesis.[56]

Maturation arrest of spermatogenesis is characterized by incomplete spermatogenesis. The maturation arrest can be at any stage of spermatogenesis but most often occurs at the level of the primary spermatocytes. The tubules in this setting usually show identical morphologic changes, in that all appear arrested at the same stage of spermatogenesis (Fig. 67-16). The term *incomplete maturation arrest* is used to refer to those cases in which the tubules show arrest at different stages of spermatogenesis. In such cases, some tubules show spermatogenic cells arrested at one stage (for example, spermatids) and adjacent tubules arrested at another stage (for example, primary spermatocytes).

Hypospermatogenesis is a quantitative reduction in the number of spermatozoa produced by spermatogenesis. It is associated with oligospermia in the range of from 2 to 20 million sperm per milliliter. Histologically the germinal epithelium may be hypoplastic and therefore thinner than normal. The lumens of the tubules appear dilated and conspicuously contain few mature spermatozoa (Fig. 67-17). In some cases the hypoplastic tubules are interspersed with normal seminiferous tubules. In some cases the spermatogenic cells occupy only a small portion of the entire circumference of the tubule, whereas other tubules contain only Sertoli cells. In some biopsy specimens normal tubules are interspersed with hypoplastic or immature tubules. Many genetic, toxic, infectious, and vascular disorders may produce the same morphologic changes (Table 67-5).

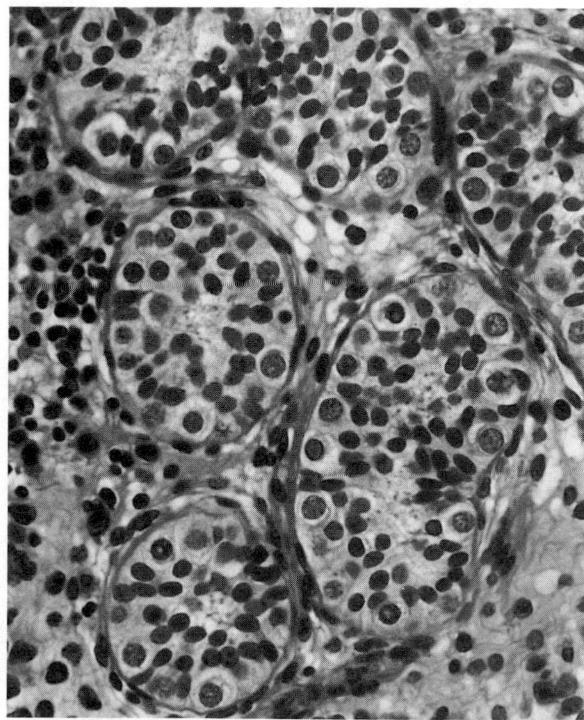

Fig. 67-14 Hypogonadotropic hypogonadism. The seminiferous tubules are immature and contain fetal Sertoli cells.

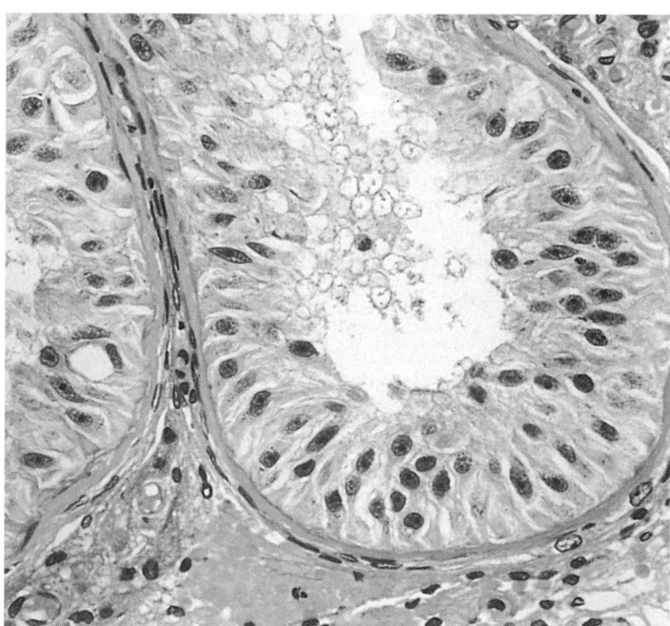

Fig. 67-15 Germ cell aplasia. The tubules contain only Sertoli cells. (Courtesy Drs. N. Skakkebaek and A. Giwercman, Copenhagen, Denmark.)

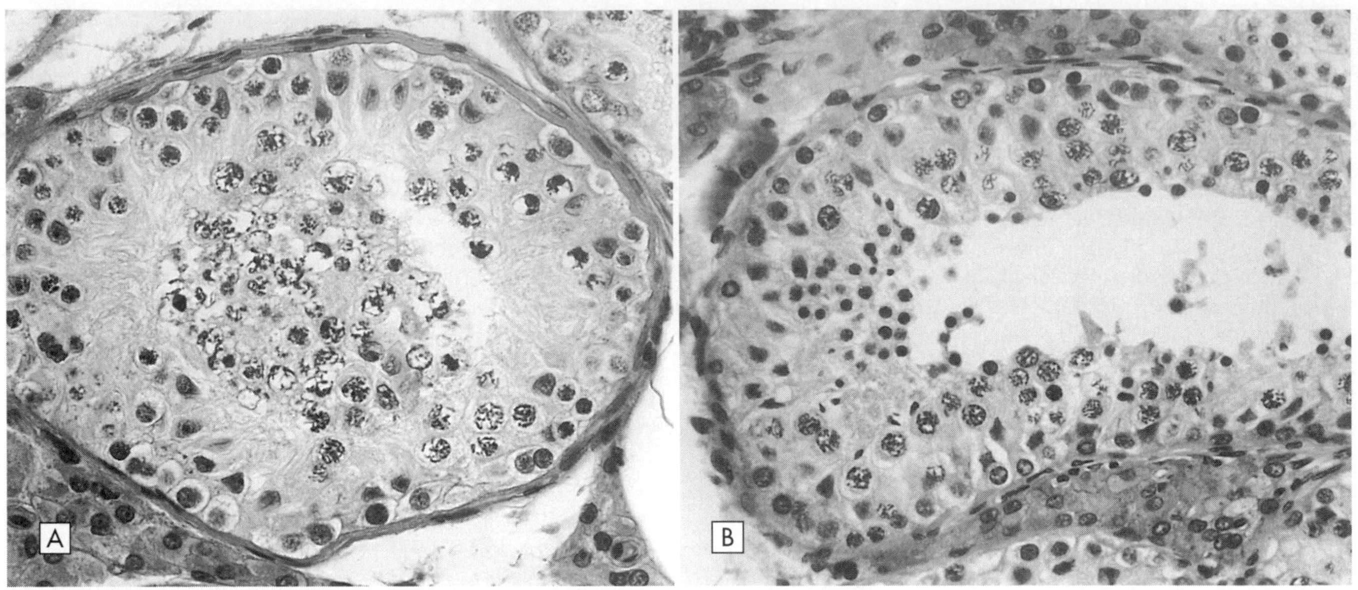

Fig. 67-16 Maturation arrest of spermatogenesis. **A,** Arrest at the stage of primary spermatocytes. **B,** Arrest at the stage of round spermatids. (Courtesy Drs. N. Skakkebaek and A. Giwercman, Copenhagen, Denmark.)

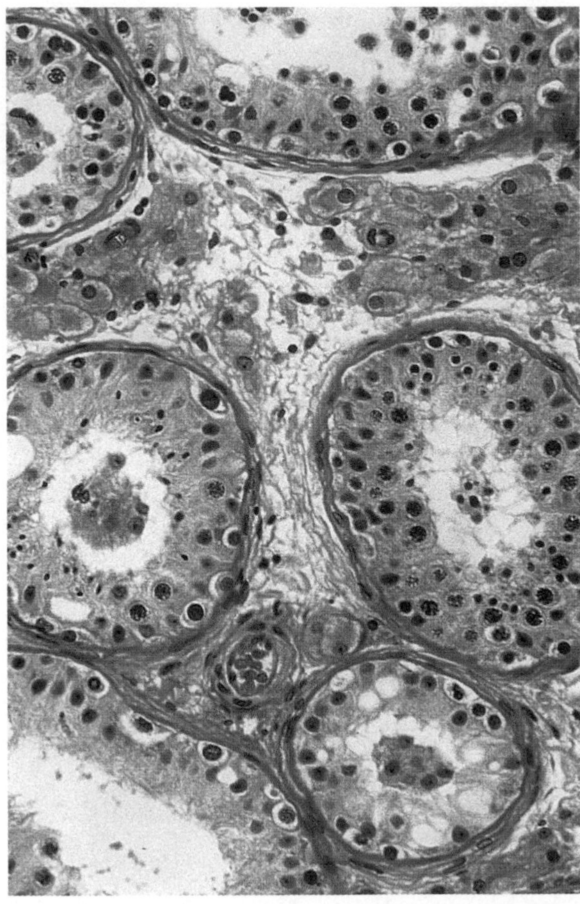

Fig. 67-17 Hypospermatogenesis.

Tubular hyalinization, also known as *tubular sclerosis* or *'end-stage' testis disease* is the end-product of many forms of tubular injury (Fig. 67-18). All disturbances of spermatogenesis may ultimately evolve into this end-stage disease. Hyalinization of the tubules is associated with a loss of germinal epithelium, obliteration of the lumens, and fibrosis of the interstitium. Foci of spermatogenesis may be seen in some of the preserved tubules, but even these tubules are probably obstructed by fibrous tissue and not connected to excretory ducts.

Table 67-5 Causes of hypospermatogenesis and aspermatogenesis

Idiopathic
Chromosomal anomalies
Sex chromosome defects (for example, Klinefelter's syndrome)
Down syndrome
Hormonal disturbances
Prolactinemia
Corticosteroid excess
Hypothyroidism
Hyperestrinism
Systemic diseases
Malnutrition
Metabolic diseases
Viral diseases
Iatrogenic
Chemotherapy
Radiation therapy

Posttesticular causes of infertility

Azoospermia or severe oligozoospermia in a patient whose testicular biopsy findings are normal is indicative of obstructive, posttesticular infertility.[12] The site of obstruction is best determined during surgical exploration or by a vasogram. According to Hendry et al,[59] who evaluated 370 patients with obstructive azoospermia, the obstruction is in the epididymis in approximately 50% of the cases (Fig. 67-19). In their

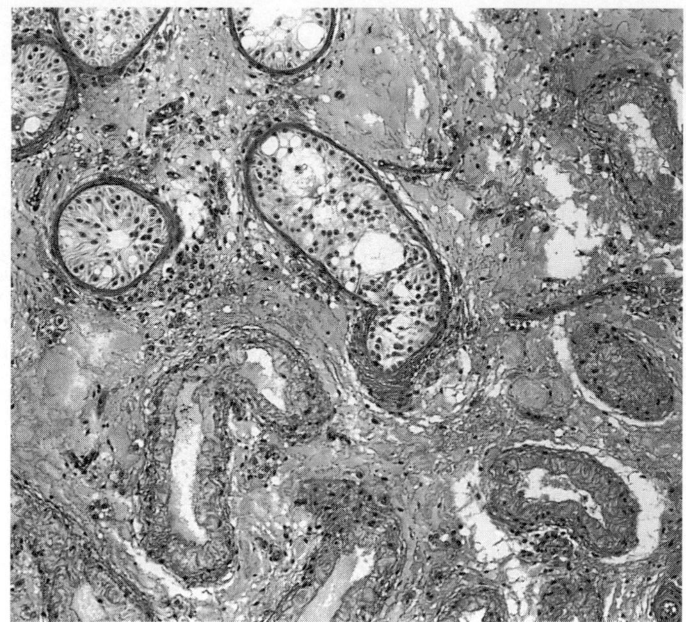

Fig. 67-18 Hyalinization of tubules in end-stage testis disease.

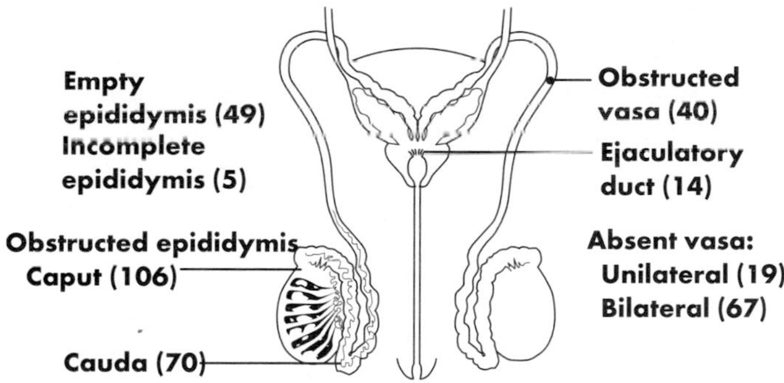

Fig. 67-19 Causes of obstructive azoospermia (From Hendry WF, Levison DA, Parkinson MC et al: *Ann R Coll Surg Engl* 72:396, 1990.)

remaining cases azoospermia resulted from absence of the vas deferens (23%), most of which were bilateral, or from obstruction of either the vas deferens (11%) or the ejaculatory duct (4%). Obstructions can be eliminated surgically in most cases using microsurgical techniques; and in those cases that are inoperable, the sperm can be aspirated from the epididymis for in vitro fertilization.

Neoplasms

More than 90% to 95% of all testicular tumors are of germ cell origin. Tumors originating from other components of the testis or epididymis and their tunics are considerably less common, and the various types of these tumors are listed in Table 67-6.

Germ cell tumors

Incidence. Overall, testicular cancer does not constitute more than 1% to 3% of all malignant tumors in men, but in men between 20 and 34 years of age, it accounts for almost 30% of all malignant tumors. New cases of testicular cancer are registered at the rate of 2 to 9 per 100,000 men in white populations and at a lower rate in men of other racial backgrounds.[60-62] The highest incidence recorded has been in the men of Denmark and neighboring Nordic countries. In Denmark the incidence has increased from 3.1 per 100,000 in 1945 to 8.9 in 1990.[61] The incidence of testicular cancer has been increasing in the men of other countries, including the United States. The incidence of testicular cancer is low among African Americans.[62]

Table 67-6 Classification of testicular and epididymal neoplasms

Germ cell tumors
Tumors of sex cord cells
Leydig cell tumors
Sertoli cell tumors
Mixed germ cell–sex cord cell tumors
Tumors of the rete testis
Tumors of the epididymal epithelium
Tumors of mesothelial origin
Tumors of nonspecific stromal cells
Tumors derived from epithelial rests and choristomas
Tumors of hematopoietic cells
Metastatic tumors

Etiology. The only known risk factors for testicular germ cell tumors are developmental disorders such as cryptorchidism, gonadal dysgenesis, and the androgen insensitivity syndrome. The risk of such cancer is 5 to 10 times higher in men with undescended testes than it is in the general male population.[63] Invasive cancer is preceded by CIS, also called "intratubular germ cell neoplasia," a premalignant lesion that predictably progresses to clinically apparent germ cell cancer. In Denmark the incidence of CIS in the population at large is 0.8%; it ranges from 2% to 3% in men with cryptorchidism, is 25% in men with the androgen insensitivity syndrome, and is close to 100% in those with gonadal dysgenesis.[63] Although such data do not provide clues to the etiology, all indications are that germ cell tumors result from developmental defects and can be traced to prenatal stages of gonadogenesis. The recently described finding of CIS in the gonad of an 18-week fetus lends additional support to this hypothesis.[64] However, neither cancer genes, nor a hereditary predisposition has been identified to explain these early neoplastic changes during gonadogenesis. Most testicular cancers are nonfamilial, and there is no evidence of the linkage of these tumors with any major gene.[65]

Pathogenesis. It sounds redundant to say that germ cell tumors originate from germ cells, but from a historical perspective it has not always been this obvious.[66] As shown in an exhaustive review published by Ewing in 1910,[67] many other cells have been considered the possible progenitors of the testicular tumors that today are called "germ cell tumors." It is also worth noting here that another concept, that of CIS of the testis, which was proposed by Niels Skakkebaek[68] and is today generally accepted, was initially received with incredulity and was not given credence for almost a decade.[69]

The pathogenesis of testicular germ cell tumors is still a controversial issue, and although there is general agreement that the tumors originate from germ cells, many issues remain unresolved.[66,70] CIS is found in the seminiferous tubules adjacent to most germ cell tumors in adults and is considered the preinvasive precursor to all these tumors. It is, however, not known how CIS becomes invasive, how long the preinvasive stage of tumorigenesis lasts, or at what stage of postnatal or possibly even prenatal life CIS becomes established. The cells giving rise to CIS have not been identified, but it has been proposed that CIS could evolve from either primordial germ cells, embryonic gonocytes, or adult spermatogonia. CIS is not found in the seminiferous tubules adjacent to yolk sac carcinomas of childhood, benign teratomas of children and adolescents, or spermatocytic seminomas, which indicates that these tumors may have a different pathogenesis than the seminomas and nonseminomatous germ cell tumors (NSGCT) of adult testes[71] (Fig. 67-20). Exceptions to this rule are occasionally reported,[72] indicating that even childhood germ cell tumors may follow the same developmental pathway as the tumors that affect adults.

It has been hypothesized that the germ cells in seminiferous tubules undergo an activation process similar to the parthenogenetic activation that affects oocytes in the ovary.[66] Activated cells that have not yet undergone malignant transformation could follow the normal embryonic pathway of development. A teratoma would form if these cells give rise to normal somatic tissues. A yolk sac tumor would develop if the descendants of the activated germ cells form only extraembryonic membranes of the yolk sac type. If these activated cells proliferate without further differentiation, a spermatocytic seminoma would form. If the "parthenogenetically activated" germ cells undergo malignant transformation as a result of a "second hit," CIS develops. It is not known how CIS becomes invasive, but one could postulate that a "third hit" occurs or that there is an epigenetic influence that causes noninvasive tumor cells to transform into invasive carcinoma cells.

CIS is found in the seminiferous tubules adjacent to almost all seminomas, embryonal carcinomas (EC), and other mixed germ cell tumors.[73] Although it is generally accepted that CIS is a direct precursor of seminoma, it has not been resolved whether CIS also gives rise to EC directly or whether a seminoma constitutes a prerequisite intermediate stage linking CIS and EC. The cells of CIS are tetraploid, whereas those of invasive germ cell tumors are hyperdiploid. Seminoma cells contain less chromosomes than the cells of CIS but more than the cells of EC, which led Oosterhuis et al[74] to propose a sequence of events in which CIS progresses to EC through an intermediate seminoma stage. The increasing malignancy that occurs in this sequence is apparently accompanied by a loss of chromosomes. However, in addition to this sequential evolution of EC, it also appears that CIS can give rise directly to EC and that seminoma as an intermediate step is not always required for all tumors to develop. In support of this view is the finding that CIS adjacent to a seminoma and CIS adjacent to other NSGCT appear to have different chromosomal markers and are distinct from each other, at least with regard to some tumors.[75] This indicates that some ECs could evolve directly from CIS without passing through the intermediate seminoma stage (Fig. 67-20).

EC cells, originally considered "more a concept than a cell type,"[76] are extremely important to our understanding of the cell biologic characteristics of germ cell tumors. The conceptual significance of these cells, which has been studied extensively in mice,[77,78] cannot be adequately addressed here. It is, however, important to realize the following:

1. EC cells correspond to developmentally pluripotent embryonic cells in the preimplantation stages of embryogenesis. This has been proved in the mouse and is most likely true for human tumors as well. Like embryonic cells, EC cells can differentiate into somatic and extraembryonic tissues. The somatic tissues correspond to derivatives of the classic embryologic germ layers—the ectoderm, endoderm, and mesoderm. The extraembryonic tissues correspond to the yolk sac and the chorionic epithelium of the placenta.

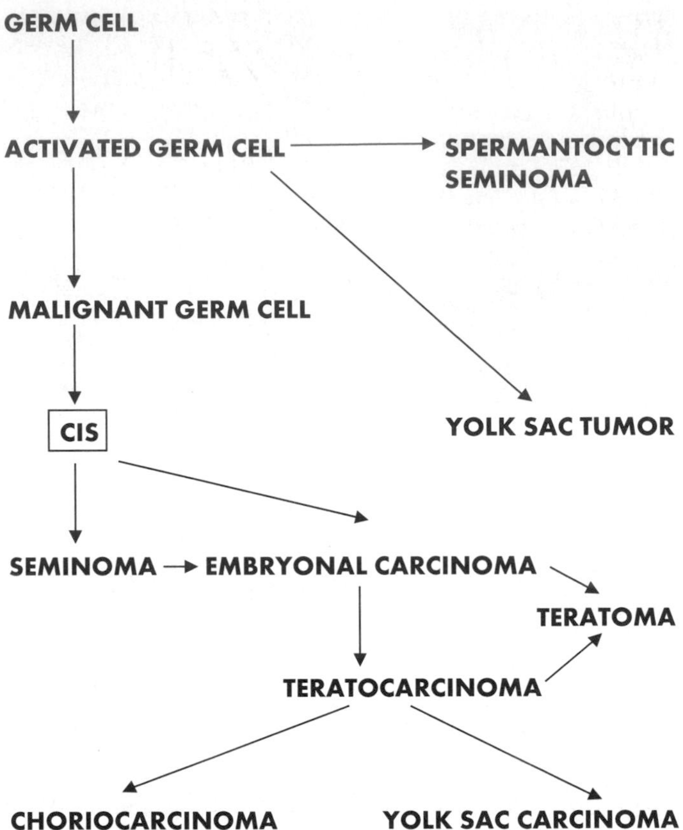

Fig. 67-20 Pathogenesis of germ cell tumors.

2. EC cells may occur in two forms: a developmentally pluripotent form and a developmentally nullipotent form. The developmentally pluripotent EC cells are the malignant stem cells of teratocarcinoma, which upon differentiation give rise to the terminally differentiated, nonproliferating "benign" tissues that forms the somatic parts of teratocarcinomas. Developmentally nullipotent EC cells form monomorphous tumors corresponding to pure EC. Because the EC cells represent the stem cells of both EC and teratocarcinoma, it is obvious that all tumors containing EC cells exhibit the same clinical features. These tumors show the same response to chemotherapy and the prognosis in affected patients is the same. In clinical practice it is thus customary to group all EC cell-containing tumors together as NSGCT and for therapeutic purposes to distinguish them from seminomas and other germ cell tumors, such as yolk sac tumor, teratoma, or spermatocytic seminoma (Table 67-7).

3. EC cells are embryonic cells that do not secrete specific products and morphologically do not express unique diagnostic features. However EC cells differentiate readily into alpha-fetoprotein (AFP)–producing yolk sac cells and human chorionic gonadotropin (hCG)–producing trophoblastic cells. These two tumor markers are thus present in the serum of 80% of patients with NSGCT.[79] The remaining 20% of NSGCT that

Table 67-7 Comparison of classifications of testicular germ cell tumors

Dixon and Moore,[76] 1953	British Testicular Tumor Panel (Pugh,[84] 1976)	Mostofi,[83] 1979
Seminoma	Seminoma	Seminoma
Group III	Teratoma	Teratoma, differentiated
Group IV: teratoma with carcinoma or sarcoma	Malignant teratoma, intermediate	Teratoma with malignant areas other than seminoma, embryonal carcinoma, or choriocarcinoma
Group IV: teratoma with embryonal carcinoma or choriocarcinoma	Malignant teratoma, intermediate	Embryonal carcinoma and teratoma (teratocarcinoma)
Group II: embryonal carcinoma	Malignant teratoma, undifferentiated	Embryonal carcinoma, adult type
Group V: choriocarcinoma	Malignant teratoma, trophoblastic	Choriocarcinoma, pure
Not listed	Yolk sac tumor	Infantile embryonal carcinoma
Not listed	Not listed	Polyembryoma

are AFP and hCG negative are composed of EC cells that have not differentiated into yolk sac and trophoblastic cells and are composed of nullipotent EC cells or EC and somatic tissues, such as epidermis or neural tissue which does not secrete AFP and hCG.

4. The nonproliferating derivatives of EC cells are in most cases differentiated terminally and therefore benign. This is best seen in metastatic foci of NSGCT treated with a combination of cytotoxic drugs. Chemotherapy destroys the malignant EC cells but does not affect their differentiated derivatives. The metastatic tumors remaining after chemotherapy are therefore composed predominantly of well differentiated "benign" tissues, such as bronchial epithelium, cartilage, bone, neural tissue, and squamous cysts.[80] However, some of these residual nodules may contain cytologically malignant tissues, and although these might not appear to proliferate, it is advisable to resect these tumors because of their potential maligant behavior.[81]

5. EC cells may give rise to malignant cells, which may proliferate on their own and form monomorphic tumors composed of a single cell type, such as a yolk sac carcinoma or choriocarcinoma.[82] Such secondary malignant tumors of extraembryonic type originating from EC cells are extremely rare in the adult testis. Secondary malignant tumors of the somatic cell type derived from EC cells, such as various sarcomas and carcinomas, are even more uncommon, although one might expect more of these tumors in patients treated with cytotoxic drugs.

Classification of germ cell tumors

Numerous schemes for classifying human germ cell tumors have been proposed on the basis of the tumors' presumed histogenesis or their predominant morphology.[83-86] The classification of Dixon and Moore[76] dominated for some time. The most widely used are the classifications proposed by Mostofi and accepted by the World Health Organization[83] and the British Testicular Tumor Panel.[84] These classifications are presented side by side in Table 67-7. Clinicians wary of the controversy among pathologists have adopted a more pragmatic approach and divide the germ cell tumors of adult testes (which account for 95% of all testicular tumors) into two groups: seminomas and nonseminomas (NSGCT).[87,88] Hence, the most important task for the pathologist is to distinguish seminoma from NSGCT. This is usually done by extensively sampling the tumor and by measuring the levels of the serologic markers AFP and hCG. AFP is not expressed in seminomas. Instead they contain hCG-positive trophoblastic cells, and an elevated concentration of hCG is measured in veins draining the tumor. However, the concentration of hCG in the systemic circulation is low, allowing one to distinguish seminomas from NSGCT.

Clinical evaluation of patients is essential for further staging of the tumors, which will determine the treatment and the prognosis.[89] Several staging systems are in use and are generally comparable. For prognostic purposes the tumors are divided into two groups: poor-risk and good-risk germ cell tumors.[90-92] In patients with good-risk tumors, complete remission can be achieved with current therapy, whereas the response of poor-risk tumors is less complete. An even better way of determining the prognosis can be done using a multivariate analysis of tumor parameters.[93] The most important factors are the size and number of lung metastatic lesions; whether there is a mediastinal mass, palpable abdominal mass ("bulky disease"), or visceral extrapulmonary metastatic lesions; the performance status of the patient; patient age; the serum hCG level; the serum AFP level; the serum lactic dehydrognase activity; the rate of marker decrease during chemotherapy; the growth rate of the tumor measured by the marker-production doubling time; whether prior treatment has been given and what it consisted of; and the time that has elapsed between diagnosis and the start of treatment.[89]

Carcinoma in situ. CIS, also known as *intratubular (testicular) neoplasia, intratubular germ cell neoplasia,* and *intratubular germ cell neoplasia, unclassified,* is the presumptive precursor of essentially all germ cell tumors of adult testes, except spermatocytic seminoma and benign teratoma. For the sake of simplicity I prefer the simpler term *CIS* as originally proposed Skakkebaek[68] and prefer to refrain from semantic discussions on the merits of other terms. Although the terms might not be important, the ominous ring of carcinoma, even if in situ, will more likely alert the clinician and the patients to the potential outcome of these lesions. Approximately 50% of the cases of CIS evolve into invasive carcinoma in 5 years, and there is no documented case of CIS that has regressed.[94] For practical purposes, CIS should be considered a premalignant lesion and treated by orchiectomy or irradiation.[94]

Incidence. The data collected in Denmark show that CIS occurs in 0.8% of all 20-year-old men, but its incidence decreases to less than 0.2% in men over 35 years of age.[94] Approximately 5% of men with germ cell tumors have CIS in the contralateral testis as well. In almost all cases CIS is found in the seminiferous tubules adjacent to invasive seminomas and NSGCT.[68]

Pathology. The testis affected by CIS shows no distinctive changes recognizable on gross examination. The neoplastic cells are usually diffusely distributed and may be found in many tubules, even in the rete testis. The distended tubules typically show thickening of the basement membrane and no spermatogenesis.

The diameter of the neoplastic cells is as much as twice that of normal spermatogonia. The cells are located along the basement membrane, displacing the Sertoli cells toward the lumen (Fig. 67-21). Neoplastic cells have a centrally located nucleus, which is irregularly shaped and hyperchromatic and contains a prominent nucleolus. The clear cytoplasm surrounding the nucleus is rich in glycogen and therefore appears clear in routine sections. Glycogen can be demonstrated by periodic acid–Schiff staining, but it may be washed out in routine sections. The neoplastic germ cells react immunohistochemically with antibodies to placental alkaline phosphatase (PLAP), which is similar to but nevertheless distinct from germ cell alkaline phosphatase,[95] from which it differs by only a few amino acids.

Several monoclonal antibodies have been found to react with CIS but are of limited diagnostic value because CIS expresses the same surface antigens as fetal gonocytes on one hand and as seminoma or EC cells on the other.[96] Ultrastructurally, CIS cells have also been found to be similar to fetal gonocytes and seminoma cells,[97] but in contrast to prespermatogenic intratubular cells, the adjacent CIS cells do not show intercellular bridges.

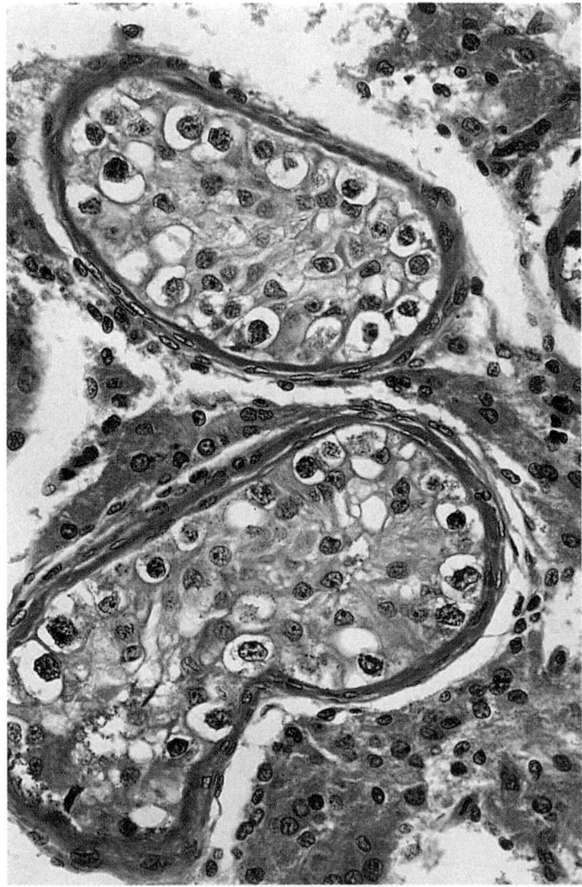

Fig. 67-21 Carcinoma in situ of the testis. The neoplastic cells are located along the basement membrane. They are large and have centrally located nuclei surrounded by clear cytoplasm.

Clinical features. CIS is a preinvasive form of testicular cancer and should be treated appropriately. Most cases are diagnosed in early adulthood, but there are reports of CIS occurring in children and even in fetal gonads.[69] Invasive neoplasia develops within 5 years in 50% of patients and after a longer period, even as much as 18 years, in the others.[94]

Seminoma. Seminoma is a malignant germ cell tumor composed of a monomorphous cell population. The term, coined in 1906 by the French pathologist Chevassu to indicate its derivation from the seminiferous epithelium, has been considered by some to be inaccurate, and alternative names such as "spermatocytoma," "germinoma," "gonocytoma," "spermatoblastoma," and "seminal carcinoma" have been proposed. None of these have been widely used, however. In current terminology *Dysgerminoma* is used to refer only to equivalent ovarian tumors.

Seminoma accounts for 35% to 45% of all testicular tumors. The tumor is most often diagnosed in men ranging in age from 30 to 50 years, and its incidence peaks at 40 years of age.[98] Seminomas do not occur before puberty and are rare in the elderly.

Pathology. On gross examination the involved testis appears enlarged and distorted, depending on the size of the tumor. The tumor is firm and usually lobulated. On cross sections it appears grayish white or yellow and homogeneous and has only minor areas of necrosis or discoloration, which are the result of focal necrosis or hemorrhage (Fig. 67-22). Owing to the expansile growth of seminoma the adjacent normal testicular tissue appears compressed and is usually sharply demarcated from the tumor. At the time of diagnosis the tumor is limited to the testis in more than 80% of cases. In 10% of

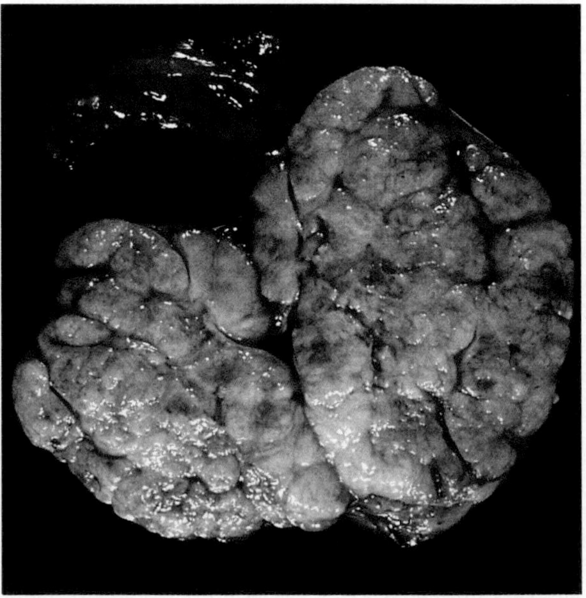

Fig. 67-22 Seminoma. On cross section the tumor appears yellowish and lobulated.

cases the tumor has invaded the epididymis or extended through the tunica albuginea.

Histologically a seminoma is composed of a uniform population of clear polyhedral large cells that measure 15 to 25 μm in diameter and are grouped into lobules surrounded by connective tissue septa (Fig. 67-23). The tumor cells have a glycogen-rich cytoplasm delimited sharply by a clearly visible plasma membrane. The centrally located nuclei are vesicular and contain finely dispersed chromatin and prominent nucleoli. The connective tissue septa are delicate but infiltrated with lymphocytes. Septa may also contain plasma cells and macrophages and even granulomas with giant cells. In most seminomas the cell populations are monotonous but some regional variation may be expected. Mitotic figures may also be more prominent in some parts of the tumor than in others.

Overall the nuclear pleomorphism and mitotic count noted for a seminoma have no prognostic value.[99] Designations such as "atypical," "undifferentiated," "anaplastic," or "high mitotic seminoma," which were previously in vogue, are therefore not justified. Approximately 20% of seminomas contain multinucleated syncytiotrophoblastic cells.[100] Because the spermatic vein effluent from seminomas usually contains elevated levels of hCG,[101] the syncytiotrophoblastic cells are probably more common than one would surmise from the routine pathology records. Such findings have no clinical significance, however. Giant cells should, however, not be confused with NSGCT elements.

Ultrastructurally seminoma cells resemble fetal gonocytes and CIS cells.[97] Immunohistochemically the tumor cell membrane reacts with antibodies to PLAP (Fig. 67-24) and the 200 kD glycoprotein known as TRA-1-60.[96] Most seminomas do not contain keratin tonofilaments and do not react with broad-spectrum antibodies to keratins, such as AE1/AE3. However, some cells express the low-molecular-weight keratin pair 8/18 and scattered cells may even express keratin 19 or other keratin polypeptides.[102] In paraffin sections the lack of reactivity to broad-spectrum antibodies to keratin and a positive reactivity to antibodies to PLAP identify a seminoma. These findings are useful for distinguishing seminomas from ECs, which are PLAP negative and keratin positive. Seminomas may contain hCG-positive cells reactive with antibody to keratin 7[103] but do not have AFP-positive cells.

In addition to the typical seminomas that account for more than 99% of all such tumors, there are occasional reports of unusual variants such as a cribriform sclerosing seminoma[104] and tubular seminoma.[105] These variants may contain few lymphocytes and could be confused with NSGCT. The most important issue, however, is to distinguish seminomas from other germ cell tumors, which may not always be simple.[106] Pure seminomas must be distinguished from the mixed germ cell tumors composed of seminoma and NSGCT elements. For practical reasons, such tumors, which account for approximately 15% of all testicular tumors, are treated clinically as NSGCT. An overabundance of lymphocytes may obscure a

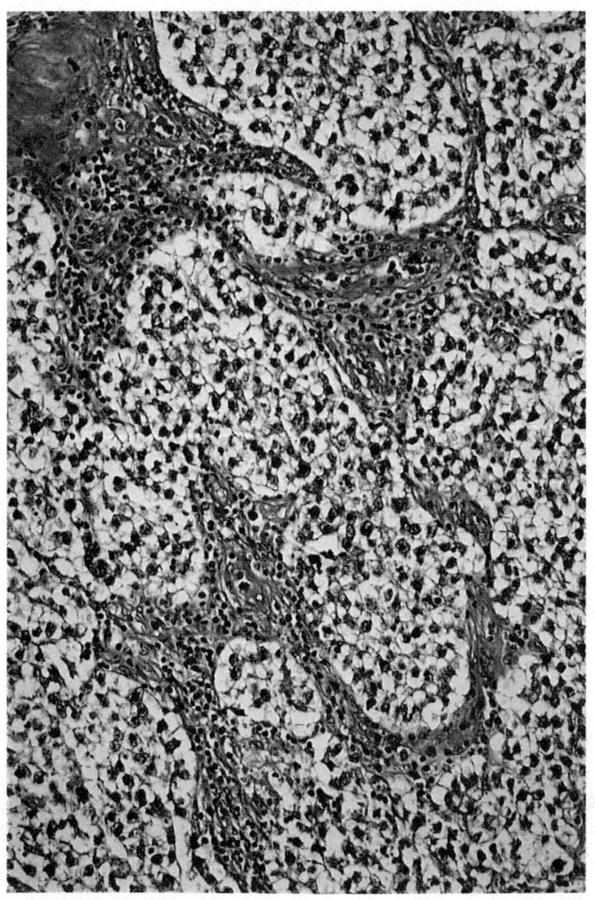

Fig. 67-23 Seminoma. Tumor cells are arranged into lobules surrounded by septa and infiltrated with lymphocytes.

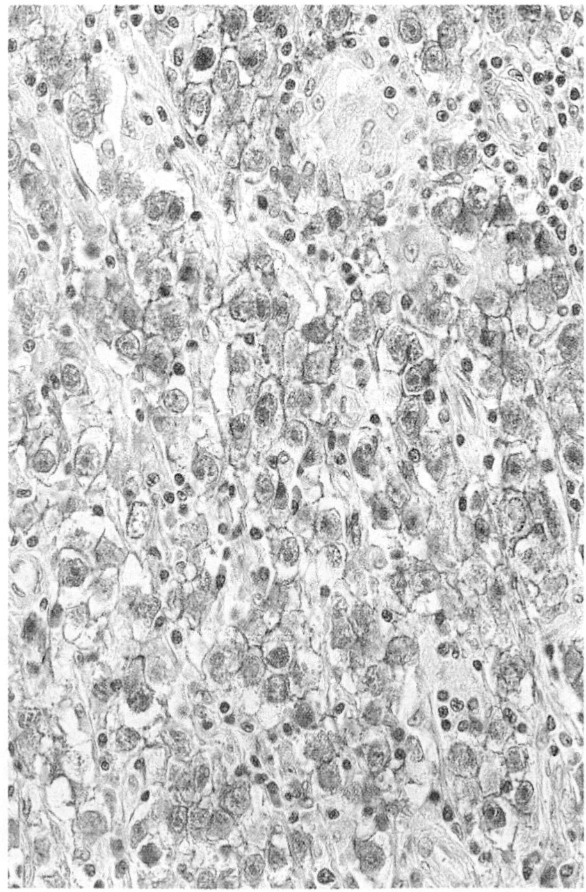

Fig. 67-24 Seminoma reactive with antibodies to placental alkaline phosphatase.

seminoma and lead to an erroneous diagnosis of lymphoma. It is worth remembering in this regard that lymphomas involve the testes more often in the elderly and very young than in middle aged men and they may be bilateral. Extensive granulomas may occasionally overshadow the tumor cells, and such seminomas could be mistaken for granulomatous orchitis.

Embryonal carcinoma. *Embryonal carcinoma* is the term theoretically reserved for NSGCT composed exclusively of EC cells. Clinically these tumors are negative for hCG and AFP. If one were to include in this category only tumors composed of developmentally nullipotent EC cells and exclude all tumors that show even some abortive differentiation, this subgroup would constitute only 2% to 10% of all testicular germ cell tumors. Mononuclear cytotrophoblastic cells and yolk sac carcinoma elements, which often develop from EC cells, are not routinely recognized in pathologic practice, and such "nonpure" tumors are therefore usually included in this group as well. Thus the incidence of ECs reported by different authors varies depending on the criteria used by the pathologist. For clinical purposes an EC is grouped with other NSGCT, and the discussion about whether the tumor is a "pure EC" or whether it shows occasional differentiation into yolk sac or cytotrophoblastic elements is of academic interest only.

Like patients with all other NSGCT, patients with ECs are younger by approximately 10 years than those with seminomas, the peak age at the time of diagnosis being 30 years.[98] In two thirds of the patients these are lymph node metastastic lesions at the time of diagnosis, even though the tumor is generally smaller than a seminoma (Fig. 67-25). The testicular mass is usually poorly demarcated from the remainder of the organ and may have satellite nodules. On cross sections the tumor varies from pale yellow to brown and contains prominent areas of hemorrhage and necrosis. Histologically the tumor is composed of malignant cells that have vesicular, irregularly shaped nuclei and a cytoplasm that has indistinct borders (Fig. 67-26). The nuclei typically show overcrowding and overlap one another. The chromatin is coarsely clumped along the nuclear membrane, and there is usually a prominent nucleolus. The cells are either arranged into sheets or form papillary and glandlike structures enclosed within a connective tissue stroma. There are numerous mitotic figures, many of which are abnormal. Secondary changes, such as solitary necrotic cells with clumped or karyorrhectic nuclei and smudged cells, also reflect the rapid growth of the tumor. Invasion into the surrounding testis and epididymis is common. The adjacent seminiferous tubules usually contain CIS and show decreased spermatogenesis.

Immunohistochemically, EC cells are keratin positive and AFP negative. Alkaline phosphatase has been demonstrated, at least focally, in almost all ECs.[107] However, because most permanent EC cell lines cultured in vitro do not express PLAP[108] but rather the other isoenzymes of alkaline phosphatase, it is not clear whether the commercial antibodies used in these pathologic studies recognize the unique PLAP gene product or cross-react with other alkaline phosphatases. Epithelial membrane antigen (EMA) is not expressed on typical EC cells.[107] Electron microscopy is of limited diagnostic value.[97]

Teratocarcinoma. Teratocarcinoma is a malignant tumor composed of undifferentiated stem cells and their more differentiated derivatives.[98] The stem cells of teratocarcinoma are equivalent to EC cells and by extrapolation to undifferentiated cells in the early embryo.[108] Developmentally they correspond to embryonic cells in the pregastrulation embryo before the separation of the embryonic from the extraembryonic lineages and before the formation of the germ layers. In accordance with this analogy it has been shown that the stem cells of tera-

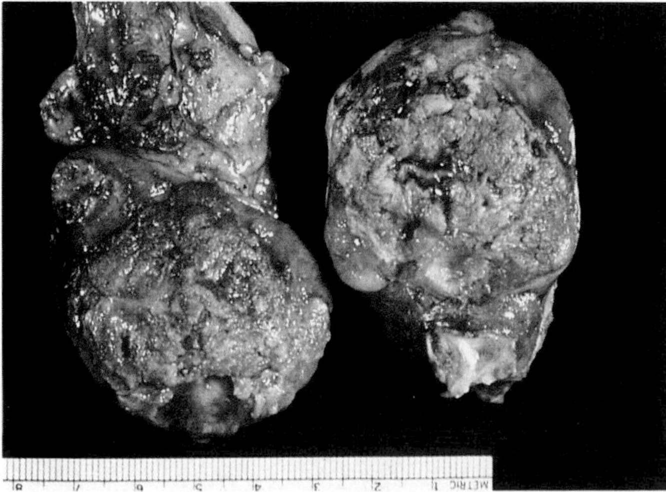

Fig. 67-25 Embryonal carcinoma. The tumor has a variegated appearance with focal areas of necrosis and hemorrhage.

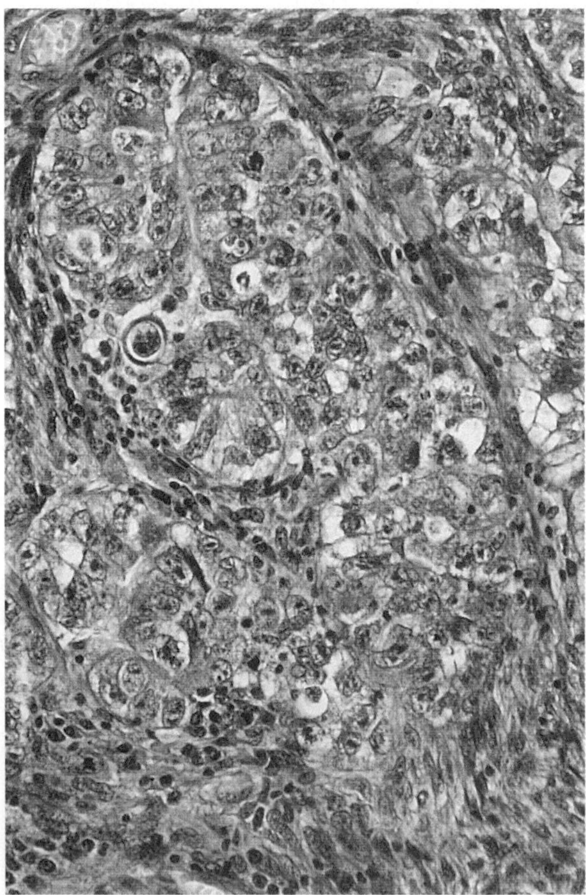

Fig. 67-26 Embryonal carcinoma. The crowding of nuclei and the indistinct cell borders are typical.

tocarcinoma may differentiate into embryonic tissue derived from all three germ layers on one hand and into extraembryonic cells on the other.[108] The stem cells of teratocarcinoma may also form embryoid bodies reminiscent of early human preimplantation stage embryos (Fig. 67-27).

Experimental studies have shown that human EC cell lines may differentiate into somatic tissues and under appropriate conditions lose their malignancy and cease proliferating.[109] After chemotherapy, teratocarcinoma stem cells can differentiate into nonproliferating somatic tissues, similar to the mature teratoma elements in primary tumors. In this respect, human teratocarcinoma cells resemble the better-studied mouse tumors of the same name.[78]

On gross examination, teratocarcinomas have a variegated appearance and may be solid or cystic (Fig. 67-28). Histologically the tumor invariably contains EC cells, which are the malignant tumor stem cells, and a variety of other tissues that histologically may appear immature or mature (Fig. 67-29). Choriocarcinomatous or yolk sac elements, or both, are found in the vast majority of tumors. Metastastic lesions are found in approximately two thirds of all patients. These lesions may contain not only EC cells but also other elements. Because the EC cells are more sensitive to chemotherapy, the metastatic lesions of treated patients may be composed of mature somatic tissues and devoid of EC cells.[80]

Choriocarcinoma. Choriocarcinoma is a malignant tumor composed of cytotrophoblastic and syncytiotrophoblastic cells. Pure choriocarcinomas in the testis are extremely rare. Most tumors diagnosed as choriocarcinoma are actually teratocarcinomas, the stem cell of which has given rise to malignant trophoblastic cells. In such tumors, malignant trophoblastic (choriocarcinoma) cells obliterate all other elements and even metastasize to distant sites. Careful examination of the primary tumor may reveal the presence of EC cells or other components of teratocarcinomas.

Choriocarcinomas are highly malignant. Distant metastatic lesions are present at the time of diagnosis even in patients with small primary tumors, which are typically hemorrhagic. Histologically the tumors are composed of mononuclear cytotrophoblastic and multinucleated syncytiotrophoblastic cells, surrounded by extravasated blood, fibrin clots, and necrotic tissues. In contrast to the terminally differentiated trophoblastic cells found in seminomas or teratocarcinomas and mixed germ cell tumors, choriocarcinoma cells are invasive, tend to destroy tissue, and penetrate into blood vessels. Syncy-

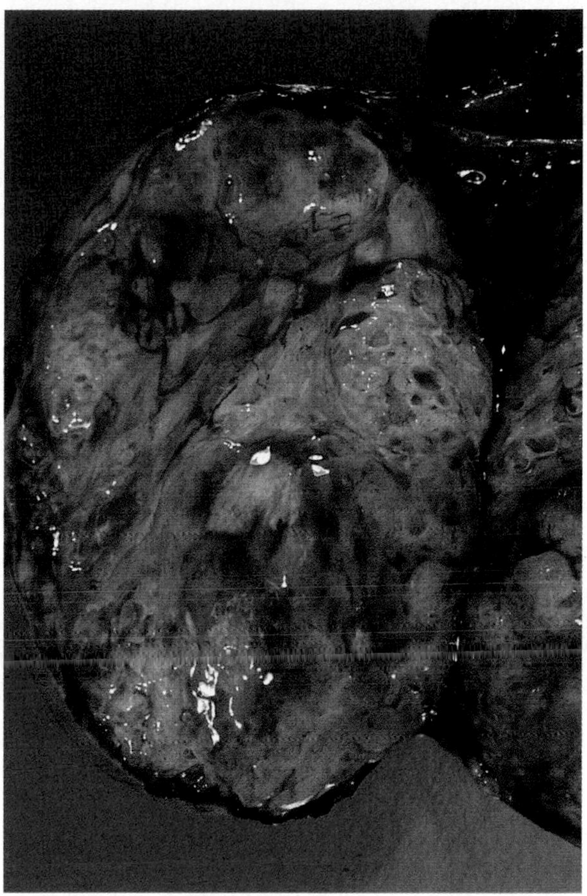

Fig. 67-28 Cross section of a teratocarcinoma showing solid and cystic components.

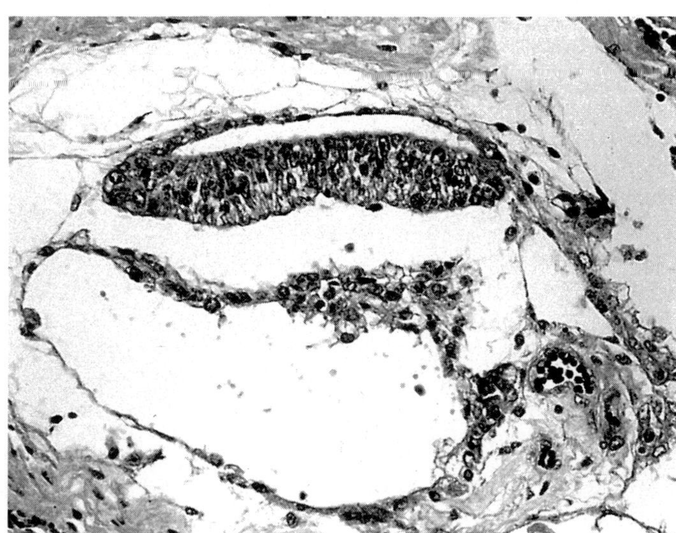

Fig. 67-27 Embryoid body in a teratocarcinoma.

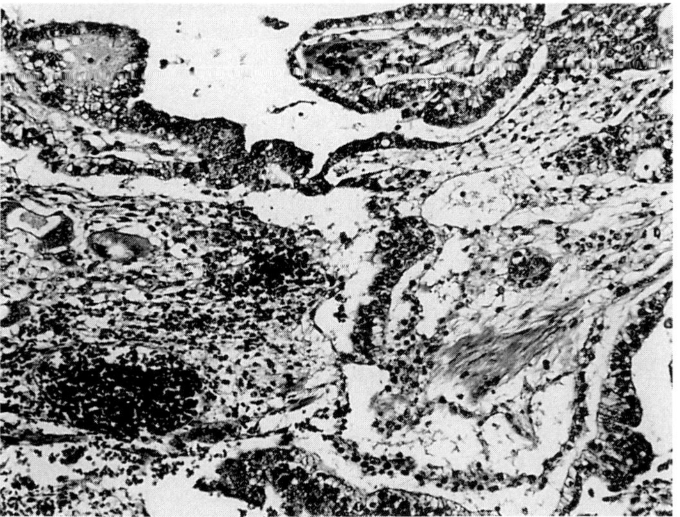

Fig. 67-29 Teratocarcinoma. The tumor consists of embryonal carcinoma cells and other elements.

tiotrophoblastic cells react with antibodies to hCG, whereas the cytotrophoblastic cells are unreactive. The serum contains high levels of hCG, but this usually produces no symptoms except occasionally those of hyperthyroidism.[110]

Teratoma. Teratomas are composed of well-differentiated benign tissues and occur in the testes in two biologically distinct forms. In adults, morphologically benign teratomas most likely represent the end-product of the differentiation of teratocarcinomas. Such tumors are devoid of malignant stem cells and carry an excellent prognosis, even though some tumors are associated with metastatic lesions.[111] One could assume that both the primary and the metastatic lesions have originated from EC cells that have undergone complete differentiation, both in the testis and at the metastatic site. The other form of teratomas that form in the testes occur in prepubertal boys; most of the tumors are benign, and affected children are under 4 years of age. Teratomas account for approximately 15% of all testicular tumors in that age group.[112] In both age groups, teratomas are multicystic tumors composed of various somatic tissues.

Yolk sac tumor. Yolk sac tumors, also known as an *endodermal sinus tumor* or Teilum's tumor, occur in the testes in two forms: as components of NSGCT and as tumors of childhood. The yolk sac components of adult NSGCT account for the AFP produced and secreted into the serum by these tumors but histologically are easily overlooked and apparently underdiagnosed.[113] Yolk sac tumors unassociated with other components of NSGCT are extremely rare in adults.

Yolk sac tumors of childhood account for only 2.5% of all testicular neoplasms but are the most common neoplasm of children under 4 years of age.[112] Histologically these tumors in children and adults may show the same variegated histologic appearance as yolk sac tumors of adult testes, ovaries, or extragonadal sites[114-116] (Fig. 67-30). The microcystic (reticular), solid, and macrocystic patterns predominate. Other patterns, termed "perivascular," "polyvesicular vitelline," or "endoderm sinus-like," as well as glandular, enteric, papillary, solid, myxomatous, sarcomatoid, hepatoid, and parietal yolk sac–like patterns, may also be found. The glomeruloid structures called "Schiller-Duval bodies," which are typical of the endodermal sinus pattern, and extracellular round hyaline bodies are often found, and their finding facilitates the diagnosis, but they are not present in all tumors. Immunohistochemical studies using antibodies to AFP may be useful in identifying tumors that do not have the typical histologic features.

Spermatocytic seminoma. Spermatocytic seminoma is a germ cell tumor of uncertain histogenesis. Despite its name, it is distinct from the classic seminomas and unrelated to other NSGCT. It occurs only in the testes and has no ovarian equivalent. It is rare, accounting for about 2% of all testicular neoplasms. It occurs in older men and is only exceptionally found in men under 30 years of age.[118] Unlike the classic seminomas, spermatocytic seminomas are never associated with other NSGCT. The adjacent seminiferous tubules do not contain CIS. Histochemically the tumor cells do not stain with antibodies to PLAP or keratin and do not contain either hCG-positive syncytiotrophoblastic cells or AFP-positive cells.[119] Spermatocytic seminoma is a benign lesion and metastasis occurs only exceptionally, unless the tumor contains a sarcomatoid component.[120]

Pathology. On gross examination, spermatocytic seminomas appear as multinodular intratesticular masses that may extend through the tunica albuginea and into the epididymis. The tumors are often large: the largest on record weighed 1500 g and measured 30 cm in its largest diameter.[121] On cross section the tumor is usually grayish white and has focal areas of necrosis and hemorrhage. The tissue may be cystic and often appears gelatinous.

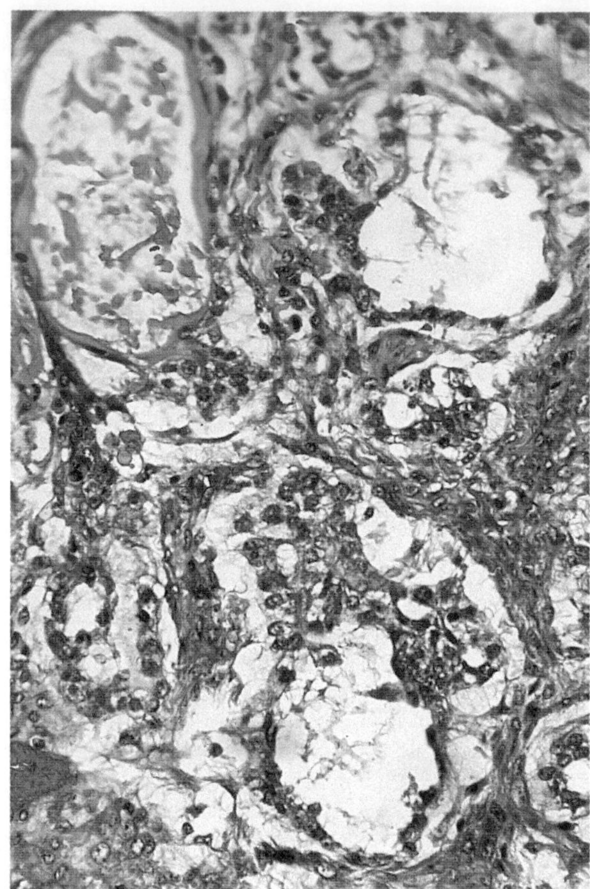

Fig. 67-30 Yolk sac carcinoma.

Histologically the tumors are composed of three cell types arranged into dense sheets. The medium-sized principal cells with round nuclei and scant cytoplasm predominate. Small cells that have round nuclei and resemble lymphocytes are scattered between these cells and are occasionally arranged into clusters. Giant cells, which may measure up to 100 μm in diameter, are the least common (Fig. 67-31). In the edematous tumors the cells may be grouped into larger nests or show a trabecular and glandlike arrangement. The tumor may extend into the tubules, but this intratubular growth should not be confused with CIS, which is never present. Spermatocytic seminomas never occur in combination with NSGCTs. However, a peculiar association with spindle cell sarcomatous tissue and rhabdomyosarcoma has been recognized recently.[120] These sarcomatous elements are prone to metastasize and may cause death.

Clinicopathologic correlations. The clinical significance of germ cell tumors is that most occur in the 20- to 50-year age group and thus affect men in the most productive years of their life. However, major advances in the chemotherapy for men with these previously often incurable tumors have been made, and a 5-year survival rate of close to 90% has been reached for most men with NSGCT of the testes.[87-93] Previously this could be achieved only for seminomas, which are radiosensitive.

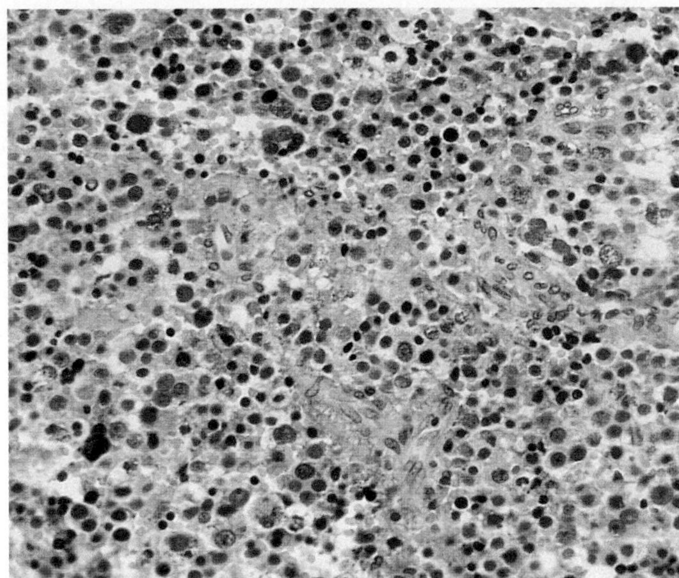

Fig. 67-31 Spermatocytic seminoma. There are three cell types: medium-sized prinicipal cells, small cells, and giant cells.

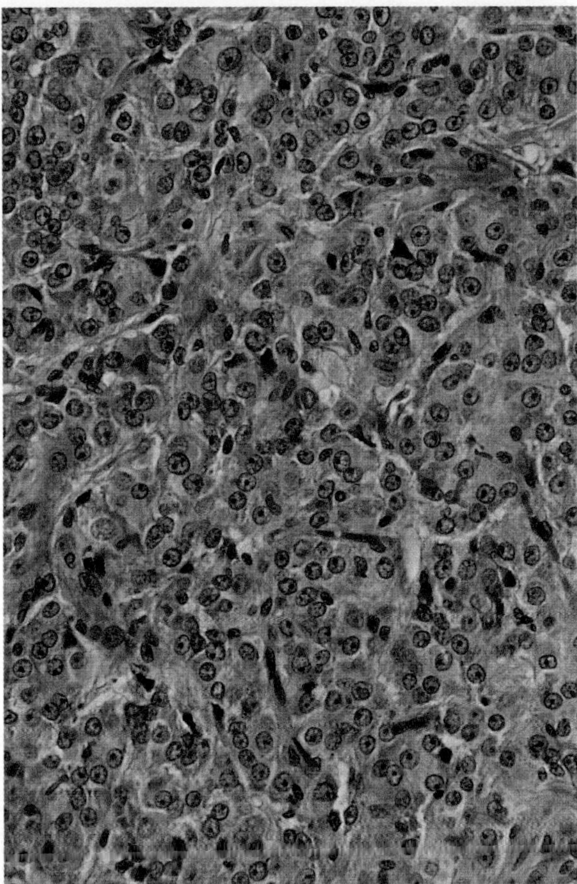

Fig. 67-32 Leydig cell tumor.

The prognosis depends on the stage of the tumor at the time of diagnosis and on other clinicopathologic variables used for multivariate analysis of the tumor response to therapy.[122] Histologic quantitation of the EC component has prognostic significance.[123] All malignant tumors of the testis metastasize through the same route, which typically involves the iliac, periaortic abdominal, and finally mediastinal lymph nodes. Surgical removal of the primary tumor is thus followed by a combination of chemotherapy and resection of metastases in all cases in which the tumor has spread beyond the testis.[124] Primary tumors limited to the testis are treated by surgical removal alone. The prognosis is excellent in infants and children under the age of 4 years who have germ cell tumors and undergo surgical resection, and they do not require chemotherapy.[112] The same is true for benign teratomas and spermatocytic seminomas, although there are occasional exceptions to this general rule.[120]

Sex cord stromal tumors

Tumors of specialized gonadal stroma include Leydig cell tumors, Sertoli cell tumors, and granulosa cell tumors. Leydig cell tumors account for 2% to 3% and, Sertoli cell tumors for 1% of all testicular neoplasms; granulosa cell tumors in the testis are extremely rare.

Leydig cell tumors. Leydig cell tumors are composed of cells that resemble Leydig cells and therefore may be hormonally active.[125] These tumors may occur at any age but most often in the 30- to 60-year age group. Approximately 20% of Leydig cell tumors occur in children. In prepubertal boys, Leydig cell tumors account for approximately 4% to 7% of all testicular tumors.[126]

The tumors vary in diameter from 0.5 to 10 cm and are usually well circumscribed, brownish yellow, firm, and sharply demarcated from the remainder of the testicular parenchyma. Extension into the rete testis or through the tunica albuginea occurs in about 15% of the cases, and metastatic lesions may be found in patients with malignant tumors.

Histologically, Leydig cell tumors are composed of well-differentiated polyhedral cells resembling normal Leydig cells (Fig. 67-32). These cells have round nuclei and well-developed eosinophilic granular cytoplasm. Fat vacuoles and lipofuscin granules are common. The typical Reinke crystal are sparse and found in only one third of tumors. The tumor cells are arranged into sheets or trabeculae, which are occasionally hypervascular, imparting an angiomatous appearance to the tumor. There are few mitotic figures, even in those tumors that have metastasized and are apparently malignant. Anaplastic cells with enlarged or multiple nuclei may be present. Most Leydig cell tumors are benign but 10% are malignant. The histologic criteria of malignancy are not reliable, and the finding of metastatic lesions is the only definitive proof that a tumor is malignant.[125]

Leydig cell tumors are usually hormonally active, and the nature of the symptoms depends on the predominant hormone synthesized in the tumor cells. Androgen-producing tumors in prepubertal boys may cause precocious puberty and macrogenitosomia, whereas the hormonal activity may be inconspicuous in adults. Estrogen-producing tumors in adults cause gynecomastia and other signs of feminization.

Sertoli cell tumors. Sertoli cell tumors are composed of cells resembling adult or fetal Sertoli cells. Tumors of this type are rare, accounting for 1% of testicular neoplasms. They occur in boys and men of all ages. Clinically they may be benign or malignant. Sertoli cell tumors assume several histologic patterns. Most often the cells line tubules (*"tubular adenoma* of Pick") or form cords (Fig. 67-33). The so-called

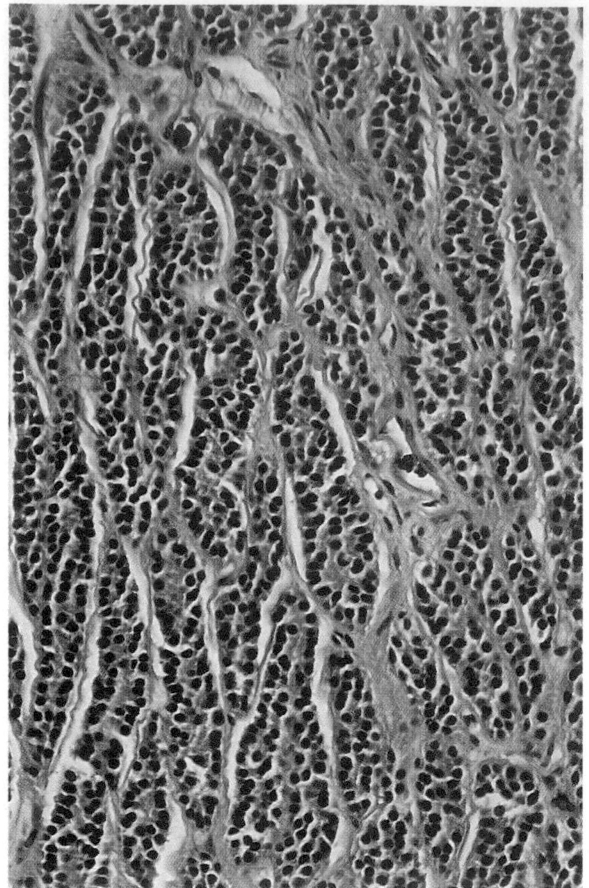

Fig. 67-33 Sertoli cell tumor.

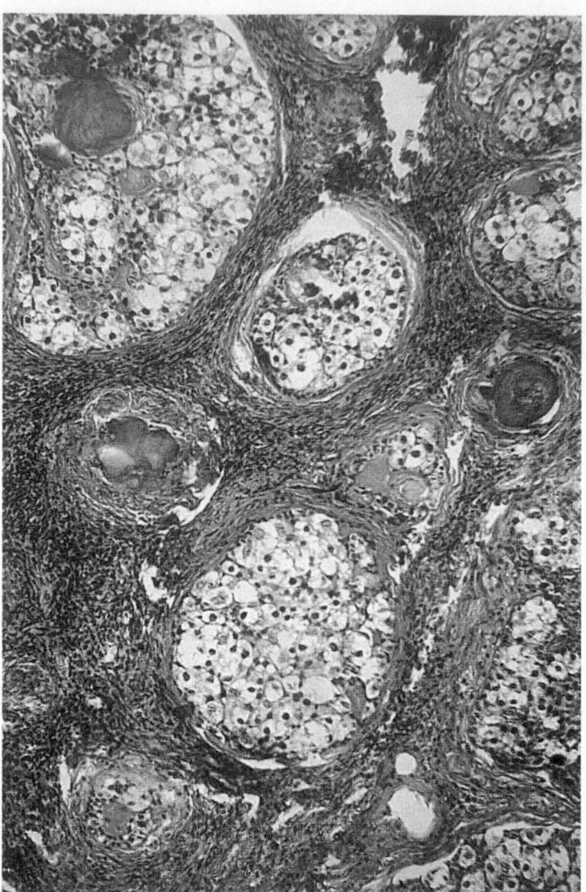

Fig. 67-34 Gonadoblastoma.

large-cell calcifying Sertoli cell tumors are composed of large polygonal cells enclosed by fibrous tissue with prominent foci of calcification.[127] *Sclerosing Sertoli cell tumors* are composed of cords and tubules of Sertoli cells embedded in a dense stroma.[128] Sertoli cell tumors resembling *ovarian sex cord tumors with annular tubules* are found in patients with the Peutz-Jeghers syndrome.[129] Approximately 10% of Sertoli cell tumors are malignant. Histologically such tumors are composed of pleomorphic and anaplastic cells and tend to invade locally and metastasize.[130]

Granulosa cell tumors. Granulosa cell tumors are rare and occur in the testis in two forms: adult and juvenile granulosa cell tumors.[131] Histologically these tumors resemble their more common ovarian counterparts. Juvenile granulosa cell tumors appear in the gonads of children who have sex cord abnormalities. These tumors are usually benign, but there are also several malignant ones on record.[133]

Mixed germ cell stromal tumors

Gonadoblastomas are tumors that arise in dysgenetic gonads and are composed of germ cells and sex cord cells arranged in an organoid pattern[134] (Fig. 67-34). Almost all persons harboring this lesion, which is considered a genetic malformation by some and a tumor by others, carry a Y chromosome. The stromal cells are considered to represent Sertoli and Leydig cells. Malignant tumors develop from gonadoblastomas with great regularity. Gonadoblastomas should therefore be treated as preinvasive lesions and removed as soon as diagnosed.

Mixed germ cell stromal tumors of adult testes are rare lesions that resemble the more common ovarian tumors that go by the same name.[136] These tumors are not associated with chromosomal abnormalities and are not malignant. Histologically three patterns can distinguished: trabecular, tubular, and solid.[137] In addition to germ cells these tumors contain stromal cells. The exact nature of these cells cannot be determined, although there is evidence that some are actually Sertoli cells.[136] All the tumors of this type described so far have been benign.

Tumors of nonspecific stroma

Benign and malignant mesenchymal tumors, composed of fats cells, capillaries, smooth muscle cells, or striated cells, may occur in the testis and epididymis[138-139] or in the spermatic cord.[138-140] These tumors correspond to similar lesions in other sites.

Rare lesions

The peritesticular tissue may contain cysts, hamartomas, and embryonic cysts that may be mistaken for true neoplasms.[141] *Cystic dysplasia of the rete testis,* a developmental anomaly encountered in children, may also present as an intrascrotal mass.[142] *Adenomatous hyperplasia of the rete testis,* presenting as tubulopapillary lesions of the testicular hilus, are found in adults.[143] These benign lesions must be distinguished from carcinoma of the rete testis.

Carcinoma of the rete testis is a rare testicular tumor that affects men more than 40 years old. There are about 50 cases of this rare lesion on record.[144] These malignant tumors also have papillary and tubular features, forming interconnecting, anastomosing channels within the normal rete testis (Fig. 67-35). Glomeruloid structures may also form im tumor cells, and calcifications are common. Nevertheless these tumors might be difficult to distinguish from metastatic adenocarcinomas.

Carcinoid tumors originating in the testis have been reported. These neoplasms have been considered possible derivatives of germ cell tumors because 15% are associated with teratomas. The exact origin of the others remains unknown.[145] *Primitive neurectodermal tumors*[146] and *melanotic neurectodermal tumor of infancy*[147] have been found in the scrotum. These tumors have the same features as equivalent tumors in other locations.

Metastatic neoplasms

Metastasis to the testis is not common. Most common secondary tumors of the testis are lymphomas and carcinomas of the urogenital tract, especially of the prostate and intestines, and melanoma.[98]

Tumors of the epididymis, tunica vaginalis, and spermatic cord

Tumors of the epididymis, tunica vaginalis, and spermatic cord may originate from epithelial and stromal components. They are rare, accounting for approximately 5% of all intrascrotal neoplasms.

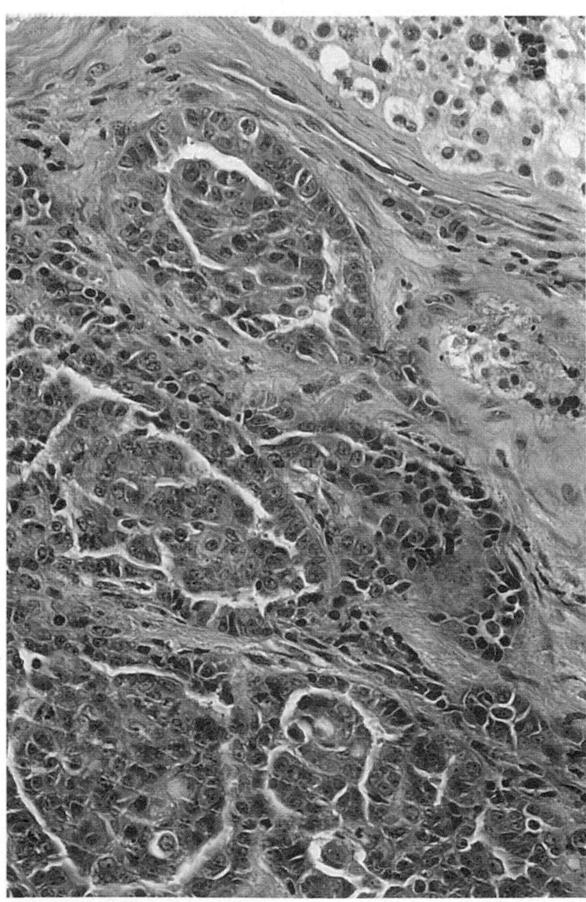

Fig. 67-35 Adenocarcinoma of the rete testis. (Courtesy Dr. L Nochomowitz, Washington, D.C.)

Mesothelial tumors

Adenomatoid tumor. Adenomatoid tumors are the most common paratesticular tumor, accounting for one third of all epididymal neoplasms. In 20% of the cases they are located within the testicular parenchyma.[148] The tumor is known under a variety of names, such as *mesothelioma, lymphangioma,* and *adenomyoma.* The ultrastructural and immunohistochemical data support the mesothelial derivation of these tumors. *Adenomatoid tumor,* a noncommittal term, is preferred to avoid the adverse connotation carried by "mesothelioma."

Most adenomatoid tumors are asymptomatic and discovered incidentally. Grossly they appear as small, firm, grayish white nodules that vary from a few millimeters to up to 6 cm in diameter. Histologically these tumors are composed of epithelial cells arranged into cords or strands or cells living glandlike or cystic spaces encased in an abundant connective tissue stroma (Fig. 67-36). The epithelial cells may be cuboidal, tall columnar, or flattened, and many are vacuolated. Several patterns, such as solid, tubular, canalicular, plexiform, and angiomatoid, have been recognized. Tumors displaying a mixed stromal-epithelial pattern, composed predominantly of fibroblasts, smooth muscle cells, and myofibroblasts, may be confused with primary connective tissue tumors. Lymphocytes and plasma cells are usually present in the stroma, but occasionally these cells may obscure the epithelial parts of the tumor and cause diagnostic problems. However, most adenomatoid tumors are easily diagnosed. Clinically they are benign.

Malignant mesothelioma of tunica vaginalis. Malignant mesothelioma of the tunica vaginalis is the malignant equivalent of benign adenomatoid tumors. These tumors originate from the mesothelial lining of the tunica vaginalis and are similar morphologically to the more common pleural and abdominal mesotheliomas,[148,149] although most tumors are unrelated to exposure to asbestos. Mesotheliomas of the tunica vaginalis are often papillary and may be indistinguishable from papillary cystadenomas of the epididymis.

Nodular and diffuse fibrous proliferation. The term "nodular and diffuse fibrous proliferation" (NDFP) was proposed[148] to include a variety of peculiar fibroblastic lesions

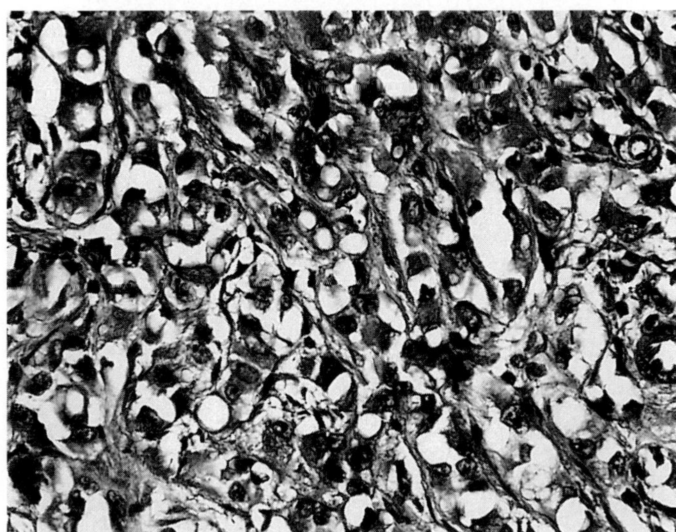

Fig. 67-36 Adenomatoid tumor. The widened spaces are lined by flattened tumor cells surrounded by connective tissue.

that arise as fibrous nodules of the testicular tunics and the surface of the testis and epididymis (Fig. 67-37). NDFPs is also known under a variety of other names, such as *nodular vaginalitis, pseudofibromatous periorchitis,* and *fibrous pseudotumors*. The nature of these lesions is not fully understood. In some cases there is a history of trauma, indicating that they might be reactive rather than neoplastic lesions. Histologically an NDFP is composed of fibroblasts, myofibroblasts, and various chronic inflammatory cells encased in a dense collagenous matrix. In contrast to fibrous mesotheliomas, with which they may be confused, an NDFP does not show any evidence of malignancy or epithelial differentiation.

Epithelial tumors of the epididymis. Tumors of the epididymal epithelium are rare. They may be benign or malignant. *Papillary cystadenoma* is a benign tumor composed of clear cells arranged into papillary folds and forming cavities that contain serous or mucinous fluid.[151] A high incidence of these tumors has been reported in men with the von Hippel–Lindau syndrome, in whom one third of the tumors seem to be bilateral. These tumors are benign but must be distinguished from well-differentiated adenocarcinomas or papillary mesotheliomas.

Müllerian-type tumors, which are classified as serous or mucinous adenocarcinomas, adenomas, or borderline tumors, have been identified in the epididymis.[150, 152] The diagnosis is usually made by excluding the possibility of metastasis from some other site and by recognizing the typical features, which are identical to those of the more common ovarian tumors of this type. Scrotal Brenner tumors have also been reported, some of which are even malignant.[153]

Spermatic cord neoplasms. Most of the tumors of the spermatic cord are of nonepithelial origin. Lipoma is the most common benign tumor, and rhabdomyosarcoma is the most common malignant tumor.[141] Malignant tumors predominate in children. Scrotal rhabdomyosarcomas of children are usually of the embryonal type. A good response to combined surgical and chemotherapeutic treatment[154] has been reported, with an 80% long-term survival.

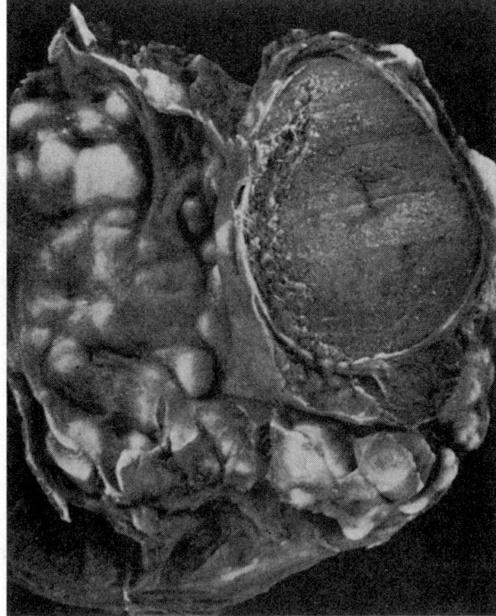

Fig. 67-37 Nodular and diffuse fibrous proliferation of tunica vaginalis. (Courtesy Dr. Robert S. Haukhol, Tampa, FL.)

PENIS AND SCROTUM

The penis is the main copulatory male organ, whereas the scrotum contains the testis and its appendages. The penis consists of the centrally located urethra surrounded by erectile tissue forming the corpora cavernosa. The proximal part of the urethra is lined by transitional epithelium and the terminal portion by squamous epithelium. The glans is covered with nonkeratinizing squamous epithelium, whereas the shaft of the penis and the scrotum are covered with keratinizing epithelium.

Developmental anomalies

Developmental anomalies of the penis and scrotum (Table 67-8) may occur in an isolated fashion or in association with other malformations of the urogenital tract and in the context of abnormal sexual differentiation. These variations from the norm may be severe, such as penile agenesis (*aphallia*), or mild, such as small penis (*micropenis*) and lateral and dorsal penile curvature.[12]

The most common penile anomaly is *phimosis*. In this congenital condition the prepuce has a narrow orifice and therefore it cannot be retracted over the glans. Obviously it is of no significance in countries where the circumcision rates are high. A retracted prepuce that cannot be rolled back over the glans is called "paraphimosis." Phimosis predisposes to the development of infections, and the infection may actually precipitate acute symptoms in patients with marginally patent prepuces. Paraphimosis may cause circulatory disturbances and necrosis of the penis.

Hypospadias refers to an opening of the external meatus of the urethra ventral to its normal position,[155] whereas *epispadias* refers to the opening on the dorsum of the penis. The incidence of hypospadias is 3% to 5% per 1000 male newborns, but epispadias are rare (1:100,000). The hypospadic urethral opening

Table 67-8 Anomalies of the penis and scrotum

Penis
Agenesis (aphallia)
Micropenis
Penile duplication (diphallia)
Penile torsion and curvatures
Phymosis
Penile Urethra
Hypospadias
Epispadias
Duplication
Urethral valves
Atresia and stenosis of the urethra
Scrotum
Scrotal hypoplasia
Scrotal ectopia
Bifid scrotum
Penoscrotal transposition

may be classified as anterior (65%), in the midshaft (15%), or posterior (20%). Affected children have problems with micturition and later on may have ejaculatory dysfunctions if the defect is not corrected surgically .

Scrotal anomalies typically result from the incomplete midline fusion of the fetal labioscrotal folds. They are common in various forms of intersexualism.

Mechanical trauma and hemodynamic disorders

Various mechanical traumatic lesions of the penis are known. Either direct force or a knife injury may result in avulsion of the penis and the entire scrotum and in complete or partial amputation of the penis. Laceration of the penis, rupture of the penis, and hemorrhagic suffusion are the consequences of blunt trauma.

Priapism, defined as consisting of persistent erection, penile congestion, and pain, may result from obstruction of the outflow of blood from the corpora cavernosa. The glans is usually spared. It is a complication of leukemia, hyperviscosity syndromes, and intravascular coagulation and may be associated with thrombosis of the penile veins. It is idiopathic in 40% of cases.

Inflammation

Inflammation of the penis usually involves the urethra or the mucosa of the glans *(balanoposthitis).* The infections can be transmitted sexually or acquired by other means, such as from dirty hands, orogenital contact, and dirty water and clothing. An excellent detailed discussion of various penile inflammatory lesions was recently published by Cubilla et al.[156]

Sexually transmitted diseases

Gonorrhea typically causes urethritis with a mucopurulent exudate. The primary lesion of *syphilis,* the *hard chancre,* is typically located on the glans penis. The presentomg finding is an ulcer that shows acute and chronic inflammation in its base. Plasma cell infiltrates are typically seen around the blood vessels. In *chancroid,* caused by *Haemophilus ducreyi,* ulcers on the glans, the penile shaft, or the prepuce are the presenting finding. The ulcer is necrotic and bleeds easily. Thus it is called "soft" in contradistinction to the "hard" ulcer of syphilis. Histologically the ulcer shows several layers: a surface layer of necrosis admixed with fibrin and polymorphonuclear leukocytes; an underlying zone of granulation tissue that also contains thrombosed vessels; and the layer of chronic inflammation consisting of dense infiltrates of lymphocytes and plasma cells.[157] In *Chlamydia trachomatis* infection, the presenting symptoms may be papules or shallow ulcers and an inguinal lymph node enlargement typical of lymphogranuloma venereum or more often a mild, nonspecific urethritis and balanitis.[158] *Herpesvirus* infection typically produces vesicles on the glans. *Human papillomavirus* (HPV) infection results in the formation of flat condylomas or condyloma acuminatum.

Noninfectious inflammatory lesions

Subcutaneous nodules on the shaft of the penis or scrotum are the presenting feature of *sclerosing lipogranuloma* (paraffinoma). It usually represents a reaction to paraffin, presumably injected for cosmetic reasons. Histologically the tissue shows fibrosis and contains numerous vacuoles from within which lipid has been removed during processing of the tissue (Fig. 67-38).

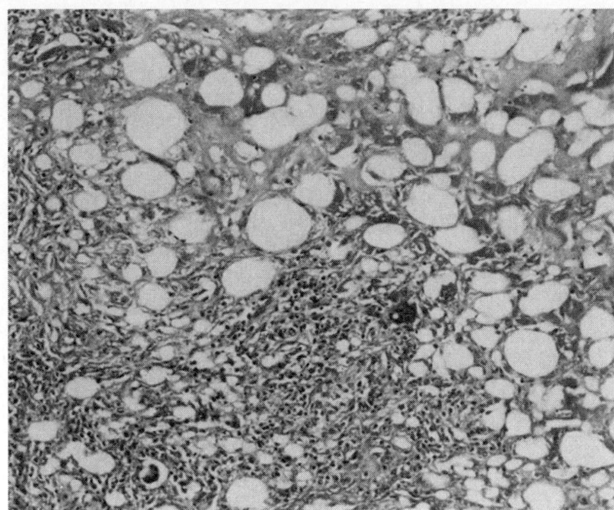

Fig. 67-38 Paraffinoma of testis.

Plastic induration of the penis (Peyronie's disease) is a form of fibromatosis of unknown origin. The lesion involves Buck's fascia of the penile shaft, thus causing deformities and pain during erection. Histologically the penile lesions resemble those of other forms of fibromatosis, such as palmar fibromatosis (Dupuytren's contracture), with which it may be associated. In addition to proliferating fibroblasts and a dense collagenous stroma, there may be calcification[159] and even extraosseous bone formation (Fig 67-39).

Balanitis xerotica obliterans is characterized by atrophy of the epidermis of the glans and prepuce and a bandlike lymphocytic infiltrate in the underlying connective tissue. It corresponds to vulvar lichen sclerosus.

Neoplasms

Penile neoplasms may originate from the mucosa of the glans and prepuce, the skin of the shaft, the penile urethra, and less often the mesenchymal components of the shaft.[160-165]

Benign lesions

Condyloma acuminatum is a HPV-induced papilloma that is most often located on the glans and foreskin. There may be either solitary or multiple lesions. It varies from 1 to 10 mm in diameter and typically appears as either a shiny, flesh-colored papule or a wartlike excrescence. Small, flat lesions may be imperceptible on physical examination. Histologically there is papillomatosis, hyperkeratosis, and parakeratosis. The surface keratinocytes typically show vacuolization of their cytoplasm. HPV can be demonstrated in these lesions either by immunohistochemical methods or by in situ hybridization.[162] Serologic types 6 and 11 of HPV predominate. Condylomas tend to recur after removal but do not evolve into cancer.

Bowenoid papulosis is a disease of young men, with multiple flat lesions the presenting features. The flat or slightly raised lesions on the glans measure a few millimeters in diameter and are pink to red-brown. Histologically there is acanthosis, hyperkeratosis, focal hypergranulosis, and vacuolization of superficial keratinocytes. The upper layers of the epithelium show orderly maturation, the scattered hyperchromatic, dysplastic, and irregularly shaped cells notwithstanding. These

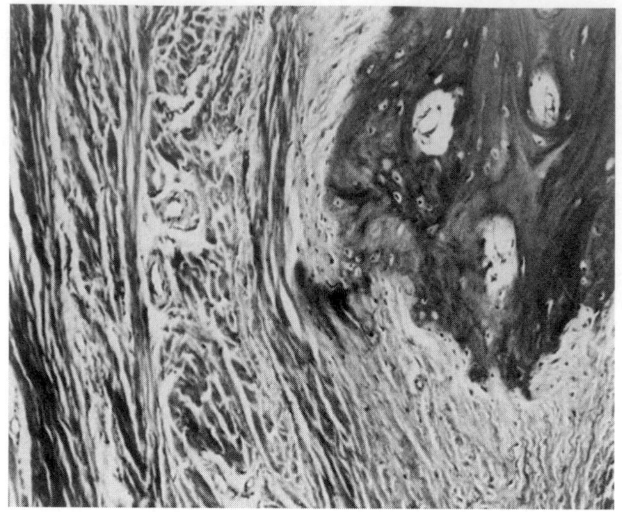

Fig. 67-39 Peyronie's disease with ectopic ossification.

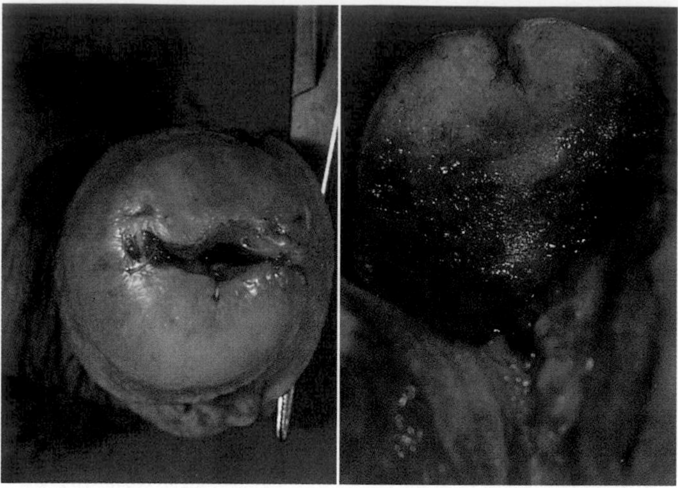

Fig. 67-40 Carcinoma of penis. The tumor is invasive, as seen on the cross-section of the glans.

atypical keratinocytes are, however, not seen throughout the entire thickness of the epithelium, which distinguishes this lesion from CIS.

HPV, which causes the lesions, can be detected by immunohistochemical and in situ hybridization. In addition to the low-risk serologic types 6, 11, 31, and 33 of HPV, bowenoid papulosis is usually associated with the high-risk types 16 and 18. Nevertheless, most lesions disappear spontaneously and are probably not direct precursors of cancer.[156]

Premalignant lesions

Erythroplasia of Queyrat is a pink, flat lesion of the glans that histologically represents CIS. The epidermis in patients with the disorder is thickened and shows hyperkeratosis, parakeratosis, and papillomatosis. The elongated rete ridges contain infiltrates of chronic inflammatory cells. Atypical and dysplastic cells are seen in all layers of the epithelium, but the tumor does not invade through the basement membrane.

Bowen's disease is also a CIS that presents as a plaquelike lesion but instead on the glans it is located on the skin of the shaft of the penis. Histologically it resembles CIS of the skin in other sites.

Carcinoma of the penis

Carcinoma of the penis accounts for 2% to 5% of all urogenital cancers and for less than 1% of all malignant tumors of males.[156] It is thus relatively rare in the United States and Western Europe, but it is among the most common malignant tumors in other parts of the world. In some countries of South America it constitutes 10% to 12% of the malignant tumors in males.[156, 160]

Etiology and pathogenesis. The search for the causes of penile cancer has revealed a beneficial effect of circumcision and a possible link with HPV. Carcinoma of the penis rarely occurs in circumcised men and is much more common in those who have not been circumcised. It is believed that the absent prepuce plays a protective role. It is not known how the prepuce promotes neoplasia, but it could be that the smegma that accumulates under the prepuce is transformed by coincidental infections into a potentially carcinogenic substance. HPV serologic types 16 and 18 have been found in at least two thirds of the cases of penile cancer.[163] Because HPV can be detected in the penile tissue of the partners of women with HPV-induced cervical lesions, it is possible that the cancerogenic virus is being transmitted as a venereal disease.[156]

Pathology. Almost all penile carcinomas are squamous cell carcinomas. Several subtypes have been recognized, such as superficial spreading, nodular, ulcerative, verrucous, and multicentric.[156,160] Most carcinomas are solitary, and there is vertical growth invasion in 80% of cases at the time of diagnosis (Fig. 67-40). Verrucous carcinoma, known as *Buschke-Löwenstein tumor* and *multifocal carcinoma,* is rare.[161]

Histologically the tumors vary with regard to the degree of differentiation. Well-differentiated keratinizing tumors predominate.[164] Histologic grading of the tumors may be important for determining the prognosis.[164] Despite their enormous size, verrucous carcinomas are only locally invasive. These tumors do not metastasize and the prognosis in affected patients is excellent.[161]

Prognosis. The progrosis in men with pentile carcinomas depends primarily on the extent of tumor spread and the clinical stage.[165] Carcinoma of the penis affects adult men, and its incidence increases with age. Approximately 50% of patients have inguinal lymph node metastatic lesions at the time of diagnosis. Surgical therapy combined with irradiation and chemotherapy is effective in eradicating tumors that show no clinical evidence of metastasis to lymph nodes, although some 20% of these patients will actually be found to have histologic evidence of tumor in the lymph nodes. Once the tumor has spread to the lymph nodes, complete cure can rarely be achieved. Nevertheless, multimodal therapy is associated with a 5-year posttreatment survival in approximately 55% of patients.[166]

Other malignant tumors

All other malignant tumors of the penis except squamous cell carcinoma are rare. There are, however, sporadic reports of melanomas, basal cell carcinomas, and Kaposi's sarcoma. Metastasis to the penis is uncommon.[167]

Neoplasms of the scrotum

In 1775 Sir Percival Pott described scrotal cancer in chimney sweeps and for the first time documented that human cancer could be caused by adverse environmental influences. Because of adequate prophylaxis, scrotal cancer is no longer a bane of chimney sweeps as in those days and is actually quite rare in the general population. Essentially all cases of cancer of the scrotum are squamous cell carcinomas. Other tumors are even less common. Six melanomas in this site have been reported so far.[168]

REFERENCES

Testis and epididymis

Normal anatomy and physiology

1. Jegou B: The Sertoli-germ cell communication network in mammals, *Int Rev Cytol* 147:1, 1993.
2. Pelliniemi LJ, Frojdman K, Paranki J: Cell biology of testicular development. In de Kretser D, editor: *Molecular biology of the male reproductive system,* New York, 1993, Academic Press.
3. Hadziselimovic F: *Cryptorchidism: management and implications,* Berlin, 1983, Springer Verlag.
4. John Radcliffe Hospital Cryptorchidism Study Group (JRHCSG): Boys with late descending testes: the source of patients with retractile testes undergoing orchidopexy, *Br Med J* 293:189, 1986.
5. Hadziselimovic F: Cryptorchidism. In Gillenwater JY et al, editors: *Adult and pediatric urology,* 2nd ed, St Louis, 1991, Mosby–Year Book.
6. Trainer TD: Histology of the normal testis, *Am J Surg Pathol* 11:797, 1987.
7. Johnson L: Spermatogenesis and aging in the human, *J Androl* 7:331, 1986.
8. Leu F-J, Engvall E, Damjanov I: Heterogeneity of basement membranes of the human genito-urinary tract revealed by sequential immunofluorescence staining with monoclonal antibodies to laminin, *J Histochem Cytochem* 34:483, 1986.
9. Pesce CM: Testicular biopsy in the evaluation of male fertility, *Semin Diagn Pathol* 4:264, 1987.
10. Magid MS, Cash KL, Goldstein M: The testicular biopsy in the evaluation of infertility, *Semin Urol* 8:51, 1990.
11. Papic Z, Katona G, Skrabalo Z: The cytologic identification and quantification of testicular cell subtypes: reproducibility and relation to histologic findings in the diagnosis of male infertility, *Acta Cytol* 32:697, 1988.
12. Damjanov I: *Pathology of infertility,* St. Louis, 1993, Mosby.
13. Johnsen SG: Testicular biopsy score count—method for registration of spermatogenesis in human testes: normal values and results in 335 hypogonadal males, *Hormones* 1:2, 1970.
14. Silber SJ, Rodriguez-Rigau LJ: Quantitative analysis of testicular biopsy: determination of partial obstruction and production of sperm count after surgery for obstruction, *Fertil Steril* 36:480, 1981.

Developmental anomalies

15. Chilvers C, Pike MC, Forman D et al: Apparent doubling of frequency of undescended testes in England and Wales in 1962-81, *Lancet* 2:330, 1984.
16. Hutson JM, Donahoe PK: The hormonal control of testicular descent. *Endocr Rev* 7:270, 1986.
17. Fram RJ, Garnick MB, Retik A: The spectrum of genitourinary abnormalities in patients with cryptorchidism, with emphasis on testicular carcinomas, *Cancer* 50:2243, 1982.
18. Gill WB, Schumacher GFB, Bibbo M et al: Association of diethylstilbestrol exposure in utero with cryptorchidism, testicular hypoplasia and semen abnormalities, *J Urol* 122:36, 1979.
19. Davies TW, Williams DRR, Whitaker RH: Risk factors for undescended testis, *Int J Epidemiol* 15:197, 1986.
20. Scorer CG, Farrington GH: *Congenital deformities of the testis and epididymis,* New York, 1971, Appleton-Century-Crofts.
21. Puri P, Sparnon A: Relationship of primary site of testis to final testicular size in cryptorchid patients, *Br J Urol* 66:208, 1990.
22. Nistal M, Paniagua R, Diez-Pardo JA: Histologic classification of undescended testes, *Hum Pathol* 11:666, 1980.
23. Koff WJ, Scaletscky R: Malformation of the epididymis in undescended testis, *J Urol* 143:340, 1990.
24. Giwercman A, Bruun E, Frimodt-Moller C et al: Prevalence of carcinoma *in situ* and other histopathological abnormalities in testes of males with history of cryptorchidism, *J Urol* 142:998. 1989.
25. Blumer CF, Hedinger CE: Vorkommen von Keimzellen in adulten kryptorchen Hoden, *Pathologe* 10:3, 1989.
26. Kogan SJ, Gill B, Bennett B: Human monorchidism: a clinico-pathological study of unilateral absent testes in 65 boys, *J Urol* 135:758, 1986.
27. Anguiano A, Oates RD, Amos JA et al: Congenital bilateral absence of the vas deferens: a primary genital form of cystic fibrosis, *JAMA* 267: 1794, 1992.
28. Donahue RE, Fauver HE: Unilateral absence of the vas deferens: a useful clinical sign. *JAMA* 261:1180, 1989.
29. Nistal M, Iniguez, Paniagua R: Cysts of the testicular parenchyma and tunica albuginea. *Arch Pathol Lab Med* 113:902, 1989.
30. Rutgers JL, Young RH, Scully RE: The testicular "tumor" of the adrenogenital syndrome: a report of six cases and review of the literature on testicular masses in patients with adrenocortical disorders. *Am J Surg Pathol* 12:503, 1988.
31. Wallace TM, Levine HS: Mixed gonadal dysgenesis: a review of 15 patients reporting single cases of malignant intratubular germ cell neoplasia of the testis, endometrial adenocarcinoma, and a complex vascular anomaly, *Arch Pathol Lab Med* 114:679, 1990.
32. Scully RE: Gonadal pathology of genetically determined diseases. In Kraus FT, Damjanov I, Kaufman N, editors: *Pathology of reproductive failure,* Baltimore, 1991, Williams & Wilkins.
33. Berkowitz GD, Fechner PY, Zacur HW et al: Clinical and pathologic spectrum of 46, XY gonadal dysgenesis: its relevance to the understanding of sex differentiation, *Medicine* 70:375, 1991.
34. Coen P, Kulin H, Bazlantine T et al: An aromatase-producing sex-cord tumor resulting in prepubertal gynecomastia, *N Engl J Med* 310:317, 1991.

Inflammation

35. Mikuz G, Damjanov I: Inflammation of the testis, epididymis, peritesticular membranes and scrotum, *Pathol Annu* 17:101, 1982.
36. Salomon F, Saremeslani P, Jakob M et al: Immune complex orchitis in infertile men: immunoelectron microscopy of abnormal basement membrane structures, *Lab Invest* 47:4555, 1982.
37. Tung SK, Lu CY: Immunologic basis of reproductive failure. In Kraus FT, Damjanov I, Kaufman N, editors: *Pathology of reproductive failure,* Baltimore, 1991, Williams & Wilkins.
38. Malekos ME, Asbach HW: Epididymitis: aspects concerning etiology and treatment, *J Urol* 138:83, 1987.
39. Aktar M, Ashraf M, Mackey DM: Lepromatous leprosy presenting as orchitis, *Am J Clin Pathol* 73:712, 1980.
40. Gall AE: The histopathology of mumps orchitis, *Am J Pathol* 23:637, 1947.
41. Damjanov I, Katz SM: Malakoplakia, *Pathol Annu* 16:103, 1981.
42. DaSilva M, Shevchuk MM, Cronin WJ et al: Detection of HIV related protein in testes and prostate of patients with AIDS, *Am J Clin Pathol* 93:196, 1990.
43. dePaepe ME, Waxman M: Testicular atrophy in AIDS: a study of 57 autopsy cases, *Hum Pathol* 20:210, 1989.

Vascular disturbances

44. Mikuz G: Testicular torsion: simple grading for histological evaluation of tissue damage, *Appl Pathol* 3:134, 1985.
45. Nistal M, Paniagua R: Primary testicular lesions in the twisted testis, *Fertil Steril* 57:381, 1992.
46. Pryor JL, Howards SS: Varicocele, *Urol Clin North Am* 14:499, 1987.
47. Shurbaji MS, Epstein JI: Testicular vasculitis: implications for systemic disease, *Hum Pathol* 19:186, 1988.
48. Baer HM, Gerber WL, Kendall AR et al: Segmental infarct of the testis due to hypersensitivity angiitis, *J Urol* 142:125, 1989.
49. Nistal M, Santamaria L, Codesl J et al: Secondary amyloidosis of the testis: an electron microscopic and histochemical study, *Appl Pathol* 7:2, 1989.

Iatrogenic lesions

50. Averette HE, Boike GM, Jarrell MA: Effects of cancer chemotherapy on gonadal function and reproductive capacity, *CA Cancer J Clin* 40:199, 1990.

51. Lange PH, Narayan P, Vogelzang NJ et al: Return of fertility after treatment for noseminomatous testicular cancer: changing concepts, *J Urol* 29:1131, 1982.
52. Siimes MA, Rautonen J: Small testicles with impaired production of sperm in adult male survivors of childhood malignancies, *Cancer* 65:1303, 1990.
53. Taxy JB, Marshall FF, Ehrlichman RJ: Vasectomy: subclinical pathologic changes, *Am J Surg Pathol* 5:767, 1981.
54. Zimmerman KG, Johnson PC, Paplanus SH: Nerve invasion by benign proliferating ductules in vasitis nodosa, *Cancer* 51:2066, 1983.

Infertility

55. Wong TW, Strauss FH II, Jones TM et al: Pathological aspects of infertile testes, *Urol Clin North Am* 5:503, 1978.
56. Levin HS: Testicular biopsy in the study of male infertility: its current usefulness, histologic techniques, and prospects for the future, *Hum Pathol* 10:569, 1979.
57. Wheeler JE: Histology of the fertile and infertile testis. In Kraus FT, Damjanov I, Kaufman N, editors: *Pathobiology of reproductive failure,* Baltimore, 1991, Williams & Wilkins.
58. Conn PM, Crowley WF Jr: Gonadotropin-releasing hormone and its analogues, *N Engl J Med* 24:324, 1991.
59. Hendry WF, Levison DA, Parkinson MC et al: Testicular obstruction: clinicopathologic studies, *Ann R Coll Surg Engl* 72:396, 1990.

Neoplasms of testis

60. Swerdlow AJ: The epidemiology of testicular cancer, *Eur Urol* 23(suppl): 35, 1993.
61. Moller H: Clues to the aetiology of testicular germ cell tumors from descriptive epidemiology, *Eur Urol* 23:8, 1993.
62. Van den Eden SK, Weiss NS: Is testicular cancer incidence in blacks increasing? *Am J Public Health* 79:1553, 1989.
63. Giwercman A, von der Maase H, Skakkebaek NE: Epidemiological and clinical aspects of carcinoma *in situ* of the testis, *Eur Urol* 23:104, 1993.

GERM CELL TUMORS

64. Jacobsen GK, Hendricksen OB, von der Maase H: Carcinoma in situ of testicular tissue adjacent to malignant germ cell tumors, *Cancer,* 47:2660, 1981.
65. Forman D, Oliver RTD, Brett AR et al: Familial testicular cancer: a report of the UK family register, estimation of risk and an HLA class I sib-pair analysis, *Br J Cancer* 65: 225, 1992.
66. Damjanov I: Pathobiology of human germ cell tumors, *Recent Results Cancer Res* 123:1, 1991.
67. Ewing J: Teratoma testis and its derivatives, *Surg Gynecol Obstet* 12:230, 1911.
68. Skakkebaek NE: Possible carcinoma-in-situ of the testis, *Lancet* 2:516, 1972.
69. Jacobsen GK, Henriques UV: A fetal testis with intratubular germ cell neoplasia (ITGCN), *Mod Pathol* 5:547, 1993.
70. Damjanov I: Pathogenesis of testicular germ cell tumors, *Eur Urol* 23:2, 1993.
71. Skakkebaek NE, Berthelsen JG, Giwercman A et al: Carcinoma-in-situ of the testis: possible origin from gonocytes and precursor of all types of germ cell tumours except spermatocytoma, *Int J Androl* 10:19, 1987.
72. Stamp IM, Barlebo H, Rix M et al: Intratubular germ cell neoplasia in an infantile testis with an immature teratoma, *Histopathology* 22:69, 1993.
73. Jacobson GK, Hendrickson OB, von der Maase H: Carcinoma in situ of testicular tissue adjacent to malignant germ cell tumors, *Cancer* 47:2660, 1981.
74. Oosterhuis JW, Castedo SMMM, deJong B et al: Ploidy of primary tumors of germ cell tumors of testis, *Lab Invest* 60:14, 1989.
75. Gillis AJM, Looijenga LHJ, de Jong B et al: Clonality of combined testicular germ cell tumors of adults, *Lab Invest* 71:874, 1994.
76. Dixon FJ Jr, Moore RA: Testicular tumors: a clinicopathologic study, *Cancer* 6:427, 1953.
77. Solter D, Damjanov I: Teratocarcinoma and the expression of oncodevelopmental genes, *Methods Cancer Res* 18:277, 1979.
78. Martin GR: Teratocarcinomas and mammalian embryogenesis, *Science* 209:768, 1980.
79. Mostofi FK, Sesterhenn IA, Davis CJ Jr: Immunopathology of germ cell tumors of the testis, *Semin Diagn Pathol* 4:320, 1987.
80. Moran CA, Travis WD, Carter D et al: Metastatic mature teratoma in lung following testicular embryonal carcinoma and teratocarcinoma, *Arch Pathol Lab Med* 117:641, 1993.
81. Ulbright TM, Loehrer PJ, Roth LM et al: The development of non-germ cell malignancies within germ cell tumors: a clinicopathologic study of 11 cases, *Cancer* 54:1816, 1984.
82. Damjanov I: Teratocarcinoma stem cells, *Cancer Surv* 9:303, 1990.
83. Mostofi FK: Comparison of various clinical and pathological classifications of tumors of testis, *Semin Oncol* 6:26, 1979.
84. Pugh RCB, editor: *Pathology of the testis,* Blackwell Scientific Oxford, 1976.
85. Srigley JR, Toth P, Edwards V: Diagnostic electron microscopy of male genital tract tumors, *Clin Lab Med* 7:91, 1987.
86. Grigor KM: A new classification of germ cell tumours of the testis, *Eur Urol* 23:93, 1993.
87. Einhorn LH: Testicular cancer: a new and improved model, *J Clin Oncol* 8:1777, 1990.
88. Murphy BR, Breeden ES, Donohue JP et al: Surgical salvage of chemorefractory germ cell tumors, *J Clin Oncol* 11:324, 1993.
89. Droz J-P, Kramar A, Rey A: Prognostic factors in metastatic disease, *Semin Oncol* 19:181, 1992.
90. Motzer RJ, Bajorin DF, Bosl GJ: "Poor risk" germ cell tumors: current progress and future directions, *Semin Oncol* 19:206, 1992.
91. Garrow GC, Johnson DH: Treatment of "good risk" metastatic testicular cancer, *Semin Oncol* 19:159, 1992.
92. Bosl GJ: Prognostic factors for metastatic testicular germ cell tumors: the Memorial Sloan-Kettering cancer model, *Eur Urol* 23:182, 1993.
93. Kramer A, Droz JP, Rey A et al: Prognostic factors in non-seminomatous germ cell tumours of the testis, *Eur Urol* 23:188, 1993.
94. Giwercman A, von der Maase H, Skakkebaek NE: Epidemiological and clinical aspects of carcinoma in situ of the testis, *Eur Urol* 23:104, 1993.
95. Hoffman MC, Millan JL: Developmental expression of alkaline phosphatase genes: reexpression in germ cell tumours and in vitro immortalized germ cells, *Eur Urol* 23:38, 1993.
96. Jorgensen N, Giwercman A, Muller J et al: Immunohistochemical markers of carcinoma in situ of the testis also expressed in normal infantile germ cells, *Histopathology* 22:373, 1993.
97. Gondos B: Ultrastructure of developing and malignant germ cells, *Eur Urol* 23:68, 1993.
98. Damjanov I: Tumors of the testis and epididymis. In Murphy WM, editor: *Urological pathology,* Philadelphia, 1989, Saunders.
99. von Hochstetter AR: Mitotic count in seminomas: an unreliable criterion for distinguishing between classical and anaplastic types, *Virchows Arch [A]* 390:63, 1981.
100. Mostofi FK, Sesterhenn I, Davis CJ Jr: Developments in histopathology of testicular germ cell tumors, *Semin Urol* 6:171, 1988
101. Memperow E, Hartmann M: Spermatic cord beta human chorionic gonadotropin levels in seminoma and their clinical implications, *J Urol* 147:1041, 1992.
102. Fogel M, Lifschitz-Mercer B, Moll R et al: Heterogeneity of intermediate filament expression in human testicular seminomas, *Differentiation* 45:242, 1990.
103. Damjanov I, Osborn M, Miettinen M: Keratin 7 is a marker for a subset of trophoblastic cells in human germ cell tumors, *Arch Pathol Lab Med* 114:81, 1990.
104. Damjanov I, Niejadlik DC, Rabuffto JF et al: Cribriform and sclerosing seminoma devoid of lymphoid infiltrates, *Arch Pathol Lab Med* 104:527, 1980.
105. Young RH, Finlayson N, Scully RE: Tubular seminoma: report of a case, *Arch Pathol Lab Med* 113:414, 1989.
106. Damjanov I, Horvat B, Gibas Z: Retinoic acid–induced differentiation of the developmentally pluripotent human germ cell tumor–derived cell line, NCCIT, *Lab Invest* 68:220, 1993.

107. Niehans GA, Manivel JC, Copland GT et al: Immunohistochemistry of germ cell and trophoblastic neoplasms, *Cancer* 62:1113, 1988.
108. Andrews PW: Human teratocarcinomas, *Biochim Biophys Acta* 948:17, 1988.
109. Trojanowski JQ, Mantione JR, Lee JH et al: Neurons derived from a human teratocarcinoma cell line establish molecular and structural polarity following transplantation into rodent brain, *Exp Neurol* 122:283, 1993.
110. Giralts S, Dexeus F, Amato R et al: Hyperthyroidism in men with germ cell tumors and high level of beta-human chorionic gonadotropin, *Cancer* 69:1286, 1992.
111. Cameron-Strange A, Horner J: Differentiated teratoma of testis metastasizing as differentiated teratoma in adult, *Urology* 33:481, 1983.
112. Kaplan GW, Cromie WC, Kelalis PP et al: Prepubertal yolk sac testicular tumors—report of the testicular tumor registry, *J Urol* 140:1109, 1988.
113. Sesterhenn IA, Weiss RB, Mostofi FK et al: Prognosis and other clinical correlates of carcinoma: a report from the Testicular Cancer Intergroup Study, *J Clin Oncol* 10:69, 1992.
114. Ulbright TM, Roth LM, Brodhecker CA: Yolk sac differentiation in germ cell tumors: a morphological study of 50 cases with emphasis on hepatic, enteric and parietal yolk sac features, *Am J Surg Pathol* 10:151 1986.
115. Jacobsen GK: Histogenetic considerations concerning germ cell tumours: morphological and immunohistochemical comparative investigation of the human embryo and testicular germ cell tumors, *Virchows Arch [A]* 408:509, 1986.
116. Talerman A: Germ cell tumors. In Talerman A, Roth LM, editors: *Pathology of the testis and its adnexa,* New York, 1986, Churchill-Livingstone.
117. Talerman A: Spermatocytic seminoma: clinicopathologic study of 22 cases, *Cancer* 45:2169, 1980.
118. Burke, AP, Mostofi FK: Spermatocytic seminoma: a clinicopathologic study of 79 cases, *J Urol Pathol* 1:21, 1993.
119. Cummings OW, Ulbright TM, Eble JN et al: Spermatocytic seminoma: an immunohistochemical study, *Hum Pathol* 25:54, 1994.
120. True LD, Otis CN, Delpado W et al: Spermatocytic seminoma of testis with sarcomatous transformation: a report of five cases, *Am J Surg Pathol* 12:75, 1988.
121. Thackray AC, Crane WAJ: Seminoma. In Pugh RCB, editor: *Pathology of the testis,* Oxford, 1976, Blackwell.
122. Stoter G, Sleijfer DT, Kaye SB et al: Prognostic factors in metastatic nonseminomatous germ cell tumours: an interim analysis of EORTC GU-group experience, *Eur Urol* 23:202, 1993.
123. Moul JW, McCarthy WF, Fernandez EB et al: Percentage of embryonal carcinomas and of vascular invasion predicts pathological stage in clinical stage I nonseminomatous testicular cancer, *Cancer Res* 54:362, 1994.
124. Bajorin DF, Herr H, Motzer RY et al: Current perspectives on the role of adjunctive surgery in combined modality treatment for patients with germ cell tumors, *Semin Oncol* 19:1148, 1992.

SEX CORD TUMORS

125. Kim I, Young RH, Scully RE: Leydig cell tumors of the testis: a clinicopathological study of 40 cases and review of the literature, *Am J Surg Pathol* 9:177, 1985.
126. Kaplan GW, Cromi WJ, Kelalis PP et al: Gonadal stromal tumors: a report of the Prepubertal Testicular Tumor Registry, *J Urol* 136:300, 1986.
127. Proppe KH, Scully RE: Large cell calcifying Sertoli cell tumor of the testis, *Am J Clin Pathol* 74:607, 1980.
128. Zukerberg LR, Young RH, Scully RE: Sclerosing Sertoli cell tumor of the testis: a report of 10 cases, *Am J Surg Pathol* 15:829, 1991.
129. Wilson DM, Pitts WC, Hintz RL et al: Testicular tumors with Peutz-Jeghers syndrome, *Cancer* 57:2238, 1986.
130. Nielsen K, Jacobsen GK: Malignant Sertoli cell tumour of the testis: an immunohistochemical study and a review of the literature, *APMIS* 96:755, 1988.
131. Nistal M, Lazaro R, Garcia J et al: Testicular granulosa cell tumor of the adult type, *Arch Pathol Lab Med* 116:284, 1992.
132. Jimenez-Quintero LP, Ro JY, Zavala-Popma et al: Granulosa cell tumors of the adult testis: a clinicopathologic study of seven cases and a review of the literature, *Hum Pathol* 24:1120, 1993.
133. Matoska J, Ondrus D, Talerman A: Malignant granulosa cell tumor of the testis associated with gynecomastia and long survival, *Cancer* 69:1769, 1992.
134. Scully RE: Gonadoblastoma: a review of 74 cases, *Cancer* 25:1340, 1970.
135. Rutgers JL: Advances in pathology of intersex syndromes, *Hum Pathol* 22:884, 1991.

OTHER TUMORS OF TESTIS AND EPIDIDYMIS

136. Matoska J, Talerman A: Mixed germ cell-sex cord stroma tumor of the testis: a report with ultrastructural findings, *Cancer* 64:2146, 1989.
137. Talerman A: Pathology of gonadal neoplasms composed of germ cells and sex cord stroma derivatives, *Pathol Res Pract* 180:24, 1980.
138. Yachia D, Auslaender L: Primary leiomyosarcoma of the testis, *J Urol* 141:955, 1989.
139. Zuckerber LR, Young RH: Primary testicular sarcoma: a report of two cases, Hum Pathol 21:932, 1990.
140. Fözesi L, Rixen H, Kirschner-Hermanns R: Cytologic findings in a metastasizing primary testicular chondrosarcoma, *Am J Surg Pathol* 17:738, 1993.
141. Srigley JR, Hartwick RWY: Tumors and cysts of the paratesticular region, *Pathol Annu* 25: 51, 1990.
142. Glantz L, Hansen K, Caldamone A et al: Cystic dysplasia of the testis, Hum Pathol 24:1142, 1993.
143. Hartwick RW, Ro JY, Srigley JR et al: Adenomatous hyperplasia of the rete testis: a clinicopathologic study of nine cases, *Am J Surg Pathol* 15:350, 1991.
144. Drozco RE, Murphy WM: Carcinoma of the rete testis: case report and review of the literature, *J Urol* 150:974, 1993.
145. Zavala-Pompa A, Ro JY, El-Naggar A et al: Primary carcinoid tumor of the testis: immunohistochemical, ultrastructural, and DNA flow cytometric study of three cases with review of the literature, *Cancer* 72:1726, 1993.
146. Nistal M, Paniagua R: Primary neuroectodermal tumor of the testis, *Histopathology* 9:1351, 1985.
147. Ricketts RR, Majmudar B: Epididymal melanotic neuroectodermal tumor of infancy, *Hum Pathol* 16:416, 1985.
148. Walker AN, Mills SE: Surgical pathology of the tunica vaginalis testis and embryologically related mesothelium, *Pathol Annu* 25:125, 1988.
149. Grove A, Jensen ML, Donna A: Mesothelioma of the tunica vaginalis and hernial sac, *Virchow Arch [A]* 415:283, 1989.
150. DeNictolis M, Tommasoni S, Fabris G et al: Intratesticular serous cystadenoma of borderline malignancy: a pathological, histochemical and DNA study of a case with long-term follow-up, *Virchows Arch [A]* 423:221, 1993.
151. Wernert N, Goebbels R, Prediger L: Papillary cystadenoma of the epididymis, *Pathol Res Pract* 181:260, 1986.
152. Young RH, Scully RE: Testicular and paratesticular tumors and tumor-like lesions of ovarian common epithelial and mullerian types, *Am J Clin Pathol* 86:146, 1986.
153. Cacamo D, Solcia M, Truchet C: Malignant Brenner tumor of the testis and epididymis, *Arch Pathol Lab Med* 115:524, 1991.
154. LaQuaglia MP, Ghavimi F, Heller G et al: Mortality in pediatric paratesticular rhabdomyosarcoma: a multivariate analysis, *J Urol* 142:473, 1989.

Penis and scrotum

155. Welch KJ: Hypospadias. In Benson CD et al, editors: *Pediatric surgery,* Chicago, 1962, Year Book.
156. Cubilla AL, Barreto JE, Ayala G: The penis. In Sternberg SS, editor: *Diagnostic surgical pathology,* ed 2, New York, 1994, Raven Press.
157. Sheldon WH, Heyman A: Studies on chancroid: observations of the histology with an evaluation of biopsy as a diagnostic procedure, *Am J Pathol* 22:415, 1946.
158. Shafer M-A, Schacter J, Moncada J et al: Evaluation of urine-based screening strategies to detect *Chlamydia trachomatis* among sexually active asymptomatic males, *JAMA* 270:2065, 1993.
159. Gelbrand MK: Dystrophic penile calcification in Peyronie's disease, *J Urol* 139:738, 1988.

160. Cubilla AL, Bareto J, Cabalero C et al: Pathologic features of epidermoid carcinoma of the penis: a prospective study of 66 cases, *Am J Surg Pathol* 17:753, 1993.
161. Masih AS, Stoler MH, Farrow GM et al: Penile verrucous carcinoma: a clinicopathologic, human papilloma—virus typing and flow cytometric analysis, *Mod Pathol* 5:48, 1992.
162. Nuovo GJ, Hochman HA, Ellizri YD et al: Detection of human papillomavirus DNA in penile lesions histologically negative for HPV, *Am J Surg Pathol* 14:829, 1990.
163. Varma VA, Sanchez-Lanier M, Under EP et al: Association of human papillomavirus with penile cancer: a study using polymerase chain reaction and in situ hybridization, *Hum Pathol* 22:908, 1991.
164. Maiche AG, Pyrhonen S, Karkinen M: Histological grading of squamous cell carcinoma of the penis: a new scoring system, *Br J Urol* 67:522, 1990.
165. Maiche AG, Pyrhonen S: Clinical staging of cancer of the penis: by size? By location? Or by depth infiltration? *Eur J Urol* 18:16, 1990.
166. Fair WR, Perez CA, Anderson T: Cancer of the urethra and penis. In De Vita VT Jr, Hellman S, Rosenberg SA, editors: *Cancer: princicples and practice of oncology,* ed 3, Philadelphia, 1989, JB Lippincott.
167. Bosch PC, Forbes KA, Kollin J et al: Secondary carcinoma of the penis, *J Urol* 132:990, 1984.
168. Konstadoulakis MM, Ricaniadis N, Karakousis CP: Malignant melanoma of the scrotum: report of 2 cases, *J Urol* 151:161, 1994.

B. PROSTATE AND SEMINAL VESICLES

David G. Bostwick
Mahul B. Amin

PROSTATE

Normal prostate

Embryology

The prostate arises during the third month of gestation as epithelial buds within the urogenital sinus. The stroma plays an inductive role in this process, converting testosterone to the required hormone dihydrotestosterone.[1]

Zonal anatomy

The urethra serves as a reference landmark for the study of prostatic anatomy.[2] There is a single 35-degree bend in the center of the prostatic urethra, creating proximal and distal segments of equal length. The verumontanum bulges from the posterior wall at the urethral bend and tapers distally to form the crista urethralis. Most prostatic ducts and the ejaculatory ducts empty into the urethra in this part of the distal prostatic urethra, whereas the small periurethral glands have ducts throughout the length of the urethra. Just proximal to the verumontanum is a müllerian remnant, the utricle, a small 0.5-cm-long, epithelium-lined cul-de-sac. The urethra and large periurethral prostatic ducts are lined by a distinctive urothelium surmounted by a single layer of luminal secretory cells. A circumferential sleeve of muscle surrounds the entire urethra, including a proximal preprostatic sphincter of smooth muscle which prevents retrograde ejaculation, and a distal sphincter of striated and smooth muscle at the apex, which is important in the control of micturition.

The prostate is composed of three distinct zones: the peripheral zone, central zone, and transition zone (Fig. 67-41). The *peripheral zone* constitutes approximately 70% of the prostate and is the most common site of prostatic intraepithelial neoplasia and carcinoma. Peripheral zone glands tend to be simple, small, and rounded and are set in a loose stroma of smooth muscle and collagen. Left and right "lobes" are usually palpated during digital rectal examination of the prostate. This finding is produced by an indentation in the midline (the median furrow) which divides the peripheral zone into left and right halves. The *central zone* makes up approximately 25% of the prostate, forming a cone-shaped area that includes the entire base of the prostate and encompasses the ejaculatory ducts. Central zone glands tend to be large and complex, with intraluminal ridges, papillary infoldings, and occasional epithelial arches and cribriform glands mimicking prostatic intraepithelial neoplasia. The ratio of epithelium to stroma is higher in the central zone than in other parts of the prostate, and the stroma is composed of compact, interlacing smooth muscle bundles. The *transition zone* is the smallest aspect of the normal prostate, approximately 5%, but can enlarge together with the anterior fibromuscular stroma to become massive as a result of benign prostatic hyperplasia. In this condition it can dwarf the remainder of the prostate. Transition zone glands tend to be simple, small, and rounded and are set in a compact stroma that forms a distinctive boundary with the loose stroma of the peripheral zone. The central and peripheral zones are often referred to together as the outer prostate or "nontransition zone," whereas the transition zone and anterior fibromuscular stroma are often referred to together as the inner prostate.

The *capsule* of the prostate consists of an inner layer of smooth muscle and an outer covering of collagen, with marked variability in the relative amounts of each in different areas. At the apex the glandular elements become sparse and the capsule becomes ill-defined, composed of a mixture of fibrous connective tissue, smooth muscle, and striated muscle. As a result, the prostatic capsule cannot be regarded as a well-defined anatomic structure showing constant features.[3]

Abbreviations

AAH	Atypical adenomatous hyperplasia
BCG	Bacille Calmette-Guérin
BPH	Benign prostatic hyperplasia
EGF	Epidermal growth factor
PAP	Prostatic acid phosphatase
PIN	Prostatic intraepithelial neoplasia
PSA	Prostate-specific antigen
TGF	Transforming growth factor
TURP	Transurethral resection of the prostate

The nerve supply of the prostate is furnished by paired neurovascular bundles that run along the posterolateral edge of the prostate from the apex to the base. When these structures are spared during radical prostatectomy, sexual potency may be preserved.[4] Autonomic ganglia are clustered near these neurovascular bundles, and small nerve trunks originating at this site arborize over the surface of the prostate, penetrating through the capsule and branching to form an extensive network of nerve "twigs" within the prostate, which are often in intimate contact with the walls of ducts and acini. Caution is warranted when interpretating perineural space invasion as an absolute criterion for the diagnosis of cancer, because this can be seen, albeit rarely, in benign glands.

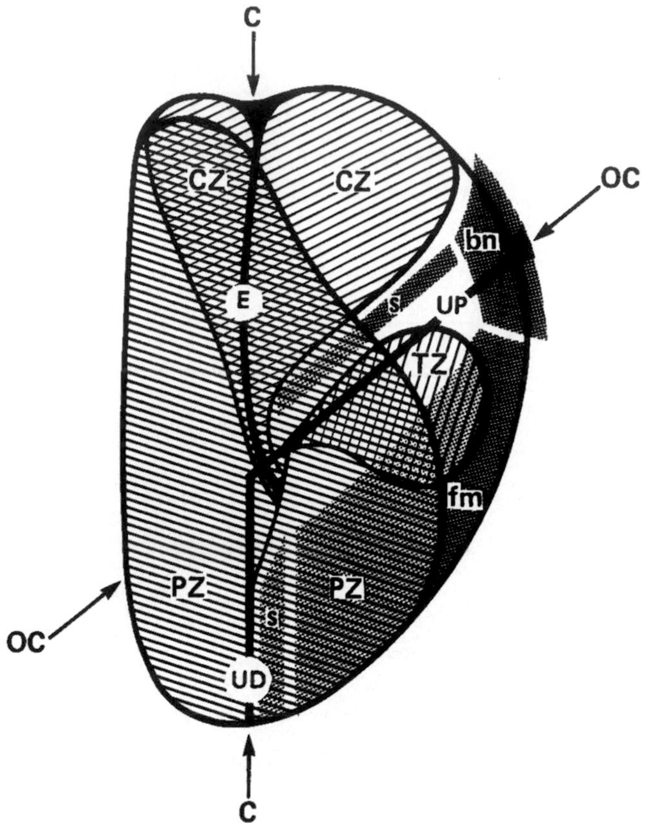

Fig. 67-41 Zonal anatomy of the prostate: the peripheral zone (*PZ*), central zone, (*CZ*),and transition zone (*TZ*). (From McNeal JE, Bostwick DG: Anatomy of the prostate: implications for disease. In Bostwick DG, editor: *Pathology of the prostate,* New York, 1990, Churchill Livingstone.)

The blood supply of the prostate is furnished by one of the branches of the internal iliac artery. Veins drain directly into the prostatic plexus, and an extensive arborizing network is present in the capsule. The venous drainage eventually empties into the internal iliac vein. Lymphatics from the prostate drain mainly into the internal iliac lymph nodes, with lesser drainage into the external iliac and sacral lymph nodes.

Cowper's glands are small, paired bulbomembranous urethral glands that may be mistaken for prostatic carcinoma in biopsy specimes. These glands are composed of lobules of closely packed, uniform acini lined by cytologically bland cells with abundant apical mucinous cytoplasm. Their nuclei are inconspicuous. Carcinoma of Cowper's glands is very rare and is characterized by frank anaplasia of the tumor cells.

Histology

The epithelium of the glandular prostate is composed of three principal cell types (Fig. 67-42). The **secretory luminal cells** are cuboidal to columnar and have pale to clear cytoplasm. Despite having the lowest proliferative activity, these terminally differentiated cells produce prostate-specific antigen (PSA), prostatic acid phosphatase (PAP), and scant amounts of mucin. The **basal cells** of the prostate form a flattened, attenuated layer of inconspicuous, horizontally disposed elongated cells at the periphery of the glands that surmount the basement membrane. These cells possess the highest proliferative activity of the prostatic epithelium, albeit low, and are thought to act as stem cells that repopulate the secretory cell layer. Basal cells are selectively labeled with antibodies to high-molecular-weight keratins such as clone 34-β-E12, a property that is exploited immunohistochemically distinguishing benign glan-

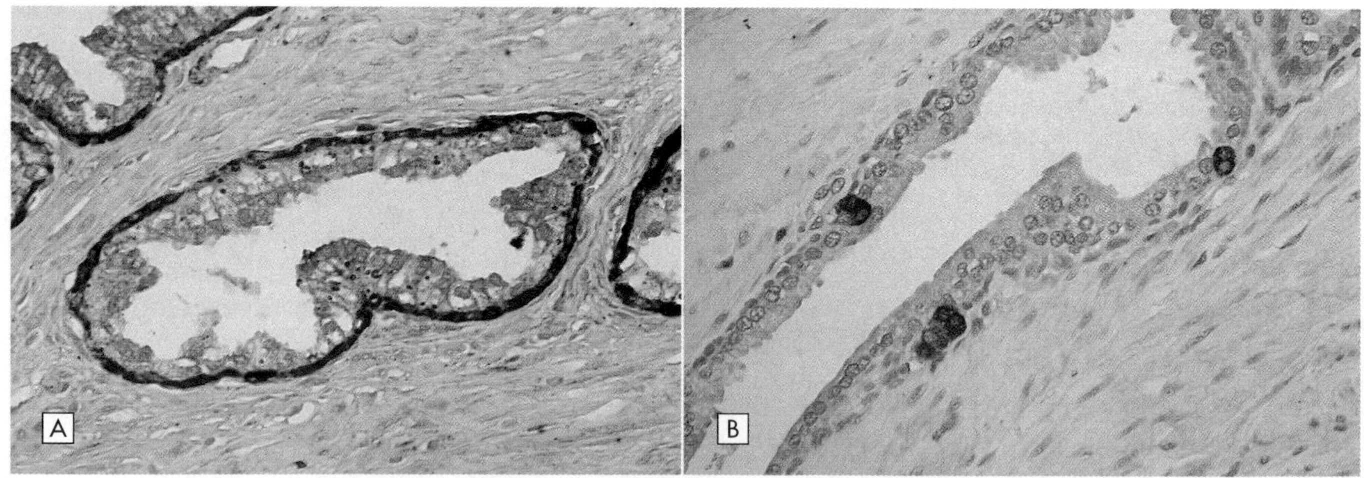

Fig. 67-42 Normal epithelial cells of the prostate. **A,** The basal cell layer shows cytoplasmic immunoreactivity for high-molecular-weight keratin, as shown by the dark reaction product (immunoperoxidase stain using monoclonal antibody 34-βE12). **B,** Neuroendocrine cells of the prostate are infrequent and may only be visible with immunoperoxidase stains (immunoperoxidase stain for chromogranin).

dular processes such as atrophy, which retains a basal cell layer, from adenocarcinoma, which lacks a basal cell layer. Basal cells contain little or no PSA, PAP, or mucin. The **neuroendocrine cells** are the least common cell type of the prostatic epithelium and are usually not identified in routine hematoxylin-eosin–stained sections, except for rare cells with large eosinophilic granules (formerly referred to as the "Paneth cell–like change"[5]). Although their function is unknown, neuroendocrine cells probably play an endocrine-paracrine regulatory role in growth and development, similar to the role of neuroendocrine cells in other organs, and contain multiple neuropeptides that can modulate cell growth and proliferation.[6-9] Androgen deprivation therapy does not appear to influence the number or distribution of neuroendocrine cells in the normal or neoplastic prostate.[6] Neuroendocrine cells coexpress PSA[6] and androgen receptors,[10] indicating a possible common cell of origin for both epithelial and neuroendocrine cells in the prostate. The preferential localization of neuroendocrine cells near the verumontanum is analogous to the cell clustering that occurs at branch points in the benign pulmonary bronchial tree, indicating they play a possible role in luminal constriction and dilatation.[8] Serotonin and chromogranin are the best immunohistochemical markers of neuroendocrine cells in formalin-fixed sections of the prostate.[8,9]

Melanin-like (Fontana-Masson–positive) and lipofuscin–like (Ziehl-Neelsen–positive, S-100 protein–negative) **pigment** is frequently found in scattered foci in the normal and hyperplastic prostate. It is a granular, golden yellow pigment within the epithelium or stroma, and the amount is rarely as great as that seen in the ejaculatory ducts or seminal vesicles.[11] This pigment probably represents a "wear-and-tear" or "old age" pigment resulting from endogenous cellular by-products of the prostate epithelium. It is present in all zones of the prostate, random in its distribution, and variable in amount.

Examination of specimens

Needle core biopsy

The introduction of the automated spring-loaded, 18-gauge core biopsy gun in the past decade began a new era in the sampling of the prostate for histologic diagnosis. The narrow 18-gauge needle offers numerous advantages over the traditional wider 14-gauge needle. The rate of postbiopsy infection declined to 0.81% from an earlier rate of from 7% to 39%, and there was a decrease in the incidence of significant hemorrhage with urinary clot retention of from 3.2% to less than 1%.[12] The false-negative rate declined to 11% from a previous rate of from 11% to 25%, and there was an increase in the quality of the tissue sample obtained, with little or no compression artifact at the lateral edges of the specimens. In addition, the 18-gauge needle allows systematic sextant biopsies of the prostate to be performed with minimal patient discomfort.[13-15] The main disadvantage of the 18-gauge needle is that it acquires less than half the amount of tissue per needle core of the traditional 14-gauge needle.

When the findings from needle core biopsy specimens are compared with those from matched prostatectomy specimens, it has been found that the tumor grade is underestimated in 33% to 45% of the cases and overestimated in 4% to 32%.[12,16,17] Grading errors are greatest when small amounts of tumor are obtained and when the tumors are low grade. These grading errors are probably the result of a sampling error, tumor heterogeneity, and undergrading of the needle biopsy finding. There is no correlation between biopsy grading error and clinical staging error.[12,18] In one study the accuracy of the findings yielded by biopsy was highest for the Gleason primary pattern, but a secondary pattern appeared to be sufficiently accurate in predicting the prostatectomy specimen grade to provide useful predictive information, particularly when combined with the primary pattern to create the Gleason score; we recommend use of the Gleason score in the evaluation of all needle biopsy specimens,[12] even when small, similar to the original recommendations of Gleason[19] (Fig. 67-43).

Fine-needle aspiration

Fine-needle aspiration (FNA) remains popular for cytologic examination of the prostate in parts of Europe, but interest in this method in the United States has waned in recent years because of the ease of acquisition and interpretation possible with the 18-gauge needle core biopsy. The sensitivity of both techniques in the diagnosis of prostate cancer is similar, and both are limited by small sample size; they are best considered as complementary techniques.[20,21] Complications of FNA occur in less than 2% of cases and are similar to those encountered in men who undergo needle core biopsy. They include epididymitis, transient hematuria, hemospermia, fever, and sepsis.

FNA yields clusters and small sheets of epithelial cells without stroma.[20] This enrichment of the epithelium allows the evaluation of single-cell morphology and the relationship between cells. In benign and hyperplastic prostatic epithelium there are orderly sheets of cells with distinct margins, creating a honeycomb-like pattern. Benign nuclei are uniform and contain finely granular chromatin and indistinct nucleoli; basal cells are often present at the edge. Prostatic carcinoma is distinguished from benign epithelium by the findings of increased cellularity, loss of cell adhesion, variation in nuclear size and shape, and nucleolar enlargement.

Transurethral resection

The regions of the prostate sampled by transurethral resection (TURP) and needle biopsy tend to differ.[22] TURP specimens consist of tissue from the transition zone, urethra, periurethral area, bladder neck, and anterior fibromuscular stroma. Studies of radical prostatectomies performed after TURP revealed that the resection tissue does not usually include tissue from the central or peripheral zones and not all of the transition zone is removed. Most needle biopsy specimens consist only of tissue from the peripheral zone, seldom including the central or transition zone.

Well-differentiated cancer found incidentally in TURP chips usually represents cancer that has arisen in the transition zone.[23] These tumors are frequently small and may be completely resected by TURP. Poorly differentiated cancer in TURP chips usually represents part of a larger tumor that has invaded the transition zone after arising in the peripheral zone.

The optimal number of chips from a TURP specimen to submit for histologic evaluation remains controversial, with some experts advocating complete submission, even of large specimens that would require many cassettes.[24-27] The Cancer Committee of the College of American Pathologists recommends a minimum of six cassettes prepared for the first 30 g of tissue and one cassette for every 10 g thereafter.[28] At a World Health Organization consensus conference it was recommended that at least 10 g of tissue be embedded and an additional cassette prepared for every 5 g thereafter; in addi-

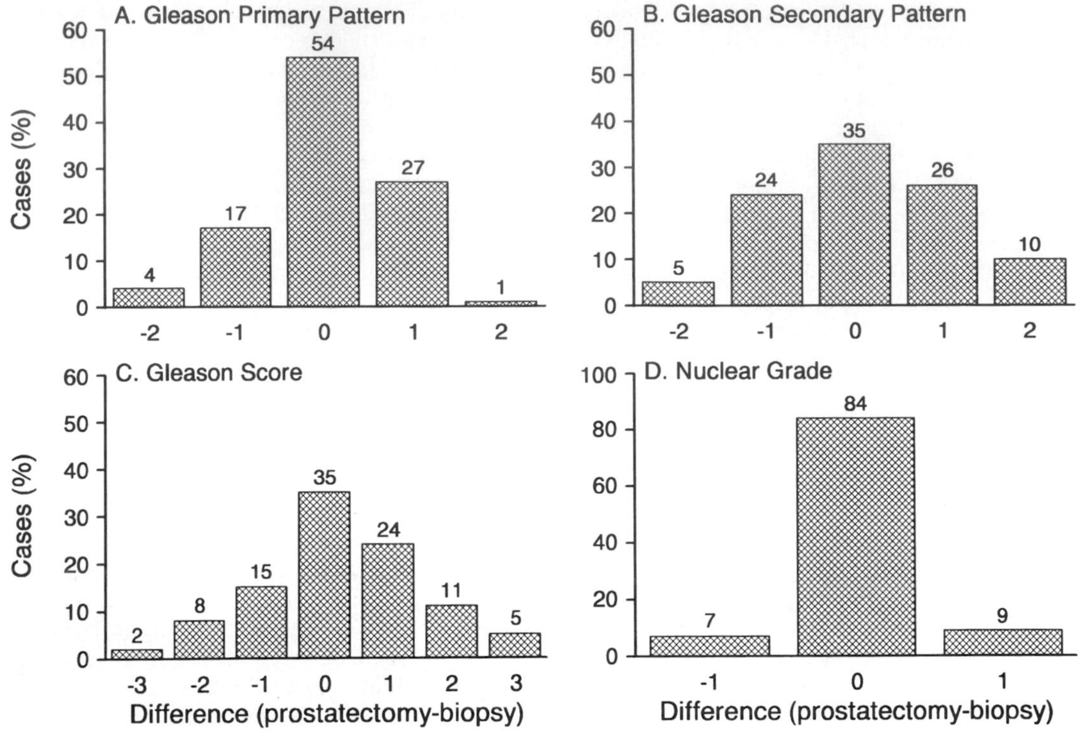

Fig. 67-43 Distribution of grading differences between prostatectomy and needle biopsy specimens. (From Bostwick DG: *Am J Surg Pathol* 18:796-803, 1994.)

tion, all tissue from patients 60 years of age or younger should be embedded.[29]

Simple prostatectomy and adenectomy

In patients with massive benign prostatic hyperplasia, open surgical excision (transvesical) may be preferred to TURP. The specimen then usually consists exclusively of transition zone tissue and periurethral tissue with grossly visible nodules.

Radical prostatectomy

There are two surgical approaches to radical prostatectomy. The first, retropubic prostatectomy, is the most popular method in the United States; it allows regional lymphadenectomy with frozen section evaluation to be performed before removal of the prostate. Many urologists do not proceed with prostatectomy if there are lymph node metastatic tumors. The second surgical approach, perineal prostatectomy, does not usually allow lymph node removal during the same operation because of the anatomic approach employed.

The completeness of pathologic sectioning performed at prostatectomy can affect the determination of pathologic stage of a tumor.[30,31] In one study the results of limited sectioning (sections of palpable tumor and two random sections of apex and base) were compared with the results of complete sectioning (whole-organ, step-sectioning procedure) and a significant increase in positive surgical margins (12% versus 59%, respectively) and pathologic stage was found in association with the complete approach.[32] In addition, the presence and extent of extraprostatic extension in clinical stage T2 (B) cancer (and hence clinical staging error) is related to the number of prostate slices submitted for examination.[33] The Cancer Committee of the College of American Pathologists has recently published guidelines for the examination of specimens removed from patients with prostate cancer, including TURP and radical prostatectomies.[28]

Complete and careful submission of tissue for histologic evaluation allows the following to be accomplished: (1) unequivocal determination of the orientation of the specimen and tumor (for example, left, right; transition zone, peripheral zone; anterior, mid, posterior; apex, base); (2) thorough evaluation of the extent and location of positive surgical margins; (3) thorough assessment and quantitation of the extent and location of capsular perforation and seminal vesicle invasion; (4) the provision of quality control data for the surgeon, particularly with regard to the status of the surgical margins in patients who have undergone nerve-sparing prostatectomy; (5) postoperative measurement of tumor volume for correlation with the findings from imaging studies, and the like; (6) complete evaluation of tumor for grading (for examples the percentage of poorly differentiated cancer); (7) fulfillment of all the recommendations made by the Cancer Committee of the College of American Pathologists[28]; and (8) comparison of results with the published results of prostatectomy studies. The Mayo Clinic protocol for handling prostatectomies and a sample case are presented in the box on p. 2203.[30]

Prostatic inflammation

Patchy acute and chronic inflammation is present in the prostates of most adult men and is considered a normal finding.[34] When the inflammation is severe and extensive or clinically apparent, the term *prostatitis* is warranted. There is a wide spectrum of prostatitides.[35]

Patients with **acute bacterial prostatitis** initially suffer the sudden onset of fever, chills, irritative voiding symptoms, and

Mayo clinic protocol for radical prostatectomy

Protocol for whole-mount sectioning

1. Weigh intact specimen.
2. Measure prostate and separately measure seminal vesicles.
3. Ink the right side in black and the left side in any other color.
4. Place specimen intact into neutral buffered formalin for overnight fixation (if fresh or frozen tissue is desired for molecular genetics, proceed to step 6 immediately; note location of tissue saved for such studies to allow correlation with light microscopy findings in adjacent sections).
5. Handle pelvic lymph nodes as frozen sections.
6. Cut off 4-mm-thick slice of *apex* and orient in quadrants as shown (urethra is central) with inked side facing up:

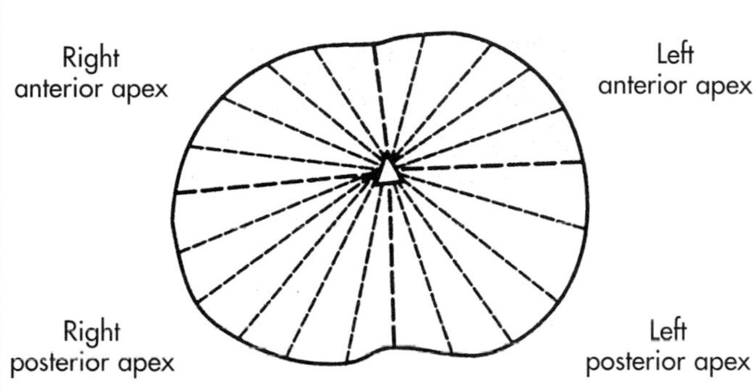

• Submit entire apex after cutting it *perpendicular* to the surgical margin (similar to cervical conization); submit for frozen section analysis *only* if requested by the urologist.

• If distal urethra forms a sleeve (easily distinguished from apex), then submit the margin for frozen section analysis.

7. Repeat step 6 for bladder base, noting the following differences:
   a. The specimen is frequently small, so bisection rather than quadrantectomy with submission of 2 cassettes is usually sufficient (left and right base).
   b. The slice should be perpendicular to the long axis of the urethra at that site; because of the 35-degree bend at the verumontanum, the urethral angle at the base is different from the apex.
8. Section the prostate from apex to base every 3 to 5 mm at right angles to the apical prostatic urethra; then section the seminal vesicles parallel to the junction with the prostate.

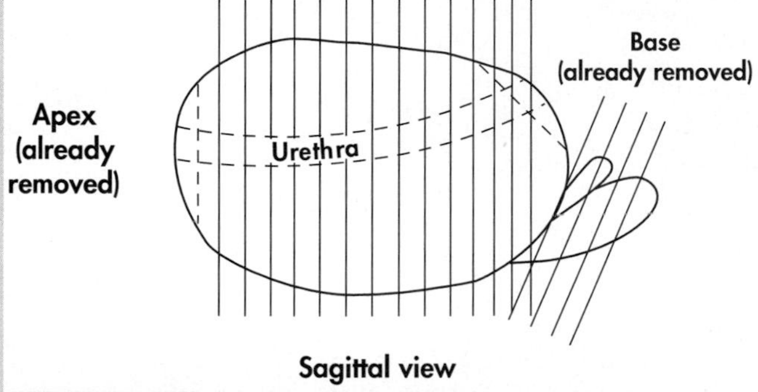

9. Orient sections with apical side facing up.
10. Place sections in large cassettes with apical faces up and fill out routine cassette section sheet with sections submitted in order from apex to base. (The histotechnologists are instructed to embed the sections with the apical face down, thereby resulting in sections of the apical face desired—ensures precise orientation.)
11. Submit to histology laboratory no later than 10 A.M. the morning after surgery.

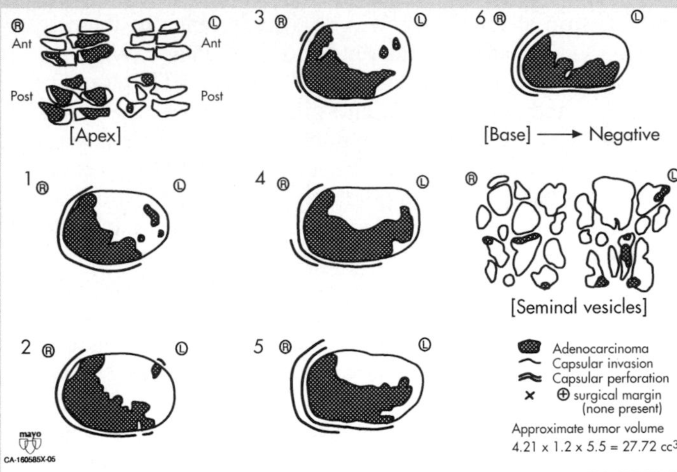

Fig. 67-44 Sample map of prostate cancer.

Report of findings

Tissue description

Prostate (5.5 × 3.8 × 3.5 cm) and seminal vesicles (4 × 3.2 × 1 cm) are submitted and weigh 40 and 15 g respectively. Tumor is identified grossly as involving both sides of the prostate extensively, chiefly on the right. Pelvic lymphadenectomy tissue (right, 5.5 × 3 × 1 cm and 3 × 1 × 1 cm; left 4.5 × 2 × 1 cm and 3 × 0.5 × 0.5 cm) submitted separately.

Diagnosis

Radical retropubic prostatoseminovesiculectomy—Mayo grade 3 (of 4) adenocarcinoma (Gleason grade, 4 + 5 = 9).
Size: About 27.72 cc.
Location: Bilateral peripheral zone and transition zone.
Resection margins: Negative.
Perineural invasion: Extensive.
Involvement of capsule: Bilateral invasion and extensive multifocal right-sided perforation.
Premalignant change: Patchy high-grade prostatic intraepithelial neoplasia.
Pelvic lymph nodes: Metastases to 2 of 9 right and 1 of 6 left pelvic lymph nodes.
Apex: Involvement of the right anterior and posterior and left posterior quadrants without extension to the margin.
Bladder base: Negative.
Gleason grade 4 pattern: 80%.
Gleason grade 5 pattern: 10%.
Vascular/lymphatic invasion: Extensive.
Clear cell change: 20%.
Other: Nodular hyperplasia. Focal papillary growth in the peripheral zone cancer.
DNA content (flow cytometry): Tetraploid (block C8: 60% cancer).
TNM (1992 revision) stage (pathologic): T3cN2Mx. ("M" is best determined by review of clinical chart.)

From Bostwick DG, Myers RP, Oesterling JE: *Semin Surg Oncol* 10:60, 1994.

pain in the lower back, rectum, and perineum. The prostate is swollen, firm, tender, and warm. Microscopically there are sheets of neutrophils surrounding prostatic glands, often with marked tissue destruction and cellular debris. The stroma is edematous and hemorrhagic, and microabscesses may be present. Diagnosis is based on the findings yielded by the culture of urine and expressed prostatic secretions, and biopsy is contraindicated because of the potential for sepsis. Most cases of acute prostatitis are caused by bacteria responsible for other urinary tract infections, including *Escherichia coli* (80% of infections); other *Enterobacteriaceae*, such as *Pseudomonas, Serratia, and Klebsiella* (10% to 15%); and enterococci (5% to 10%). Although prostatitis due to *Neisseria gonorrhoeae* was common in the preantibiotic era, it is rare today. Most patients with acute prostatitis respond to antibiotics. The formation of an abscess is a rare complication, usually occurring in immunocompromised patients such as those with the acquired immune deficiency syndrome.

Chronic bacterial prostatitis is a common cause of relapsing urinary tract infection and is usually caused by *E. coli*. Clinical diagnosis is difficult, often requiring the acquisition of multiple urine cultures obtained after prostatic massage. Treatment is also vexing because of the inability of most intravenous antibiotics to enter the prostate and prostatic fluids when the prostate is overrun with a chronic inflammatory infiltrate. In addition, prostatic calculi may contain bacteria embedded in the mineral matrix and this serves as a nidus of recurring infection. The secretory products of the inflamed prostate are alkaline, with decreased levels of zinc, citric acid, spermine, cholesterol, antibacterial factors, and certain enzymes.

Chronic abacterial prostatitis is more common than bacterial prostatitis and rarely follows infection elsewhere in the urinary tract. Patients often complain of painful ejaculation. Cultures of urine and expressed prostatic secretions yield negative findings. The etiologic agent is unknown, but *Chlamydia, Ureaplasma,* and *Trichomonas* infection have all been proposed. This form of prostatitis has a prolonged, indolent course characterized by relapses and remissions. There appears to be no relationship between chronic prostatitis and the pathogenesis of benign prostatic hyperplasia.[36]

Granulomatous prostatitis is a group of morphologically distinct chronic prostatitides, the pathogenesis of which cannot always be determined. Possible causes include infections, tissue disruption after biopsy, and others listed in Table 67-9.[35,37,38] Most of patients have a history of urinary tract infection. The prostate is often hard, fixed, and nodular, and cancer is usually suspected clinically. Urinalysis often shows pyuria and hematuria. Granulomatous prostatitis is probably caused by the blockage of prostatic ducts and the stasis of secretions, regardless of its etiology. The epithelium is destroyed, and cellular debris, bacterial toxins, and prostatic secretions such as corpora amylacea, sperm, and semen escape into the stroma, eliciting an intense localized inflammatory response. Tissue eosinophilia may be prominent in prostates infected with parasites, systemic allergic or autoimmune disease, iatrogenic post-TURP prostatitis, or nonspecific granulomatous prostatitis.

Idiopathic (nonspecific) granulomatous prostatitis ("of unknown cause") makes up the majority of cases. The granulomas are usually noncaseating and associated with parenchymal loss and marked fibrosis. Induration may persist for years even though there are no specific clinical symptoms. **Xanthoma** is a rare form of idiopathic granulomatous prostatitis and is characterized by a localized collection of cholesterol-laden histiocytes; it may also be seen in patients with hyperlipidemia[39] (Fig. 67-45). Xanthoma occurs in older men and is usually an incidental finding in patients undergoing TURP or needle biopsy, although it can appear as a palpable nodule. In rare cases there may be areas of typical granulomatous prostatitis and it is appropriate to identify such cases as **xanthogranulomatous prostatitis.** Distinction from clear cell carcinoma ("hypernephroid" pattern) may be difficult, and immunohistochemical stains for PSA and PAP often assist with this diagnostic concern.[40]

Infectious granulomatous prostatitis caused by bacteria, fungi, parasites, and viruses is uncommon (Table 67-9). *Mycobacterium tuberculosis* infection of the prostate only occurs after pulmonary infection or miliary dissemination. Small 1 to 2-mm caseating granulomas coalesce within the prostatic parenchyma, forming yellow nodules and streaks. Caseation and cavitation can be extensive. Brucellosis can mimic tuberculosis both clinically and pathologically. Mycotic infections of the prostate are rare and invariably follow fungemia. Most of the deep mycoses induce necrotizing and nonnecrotizing granulomas and fibrosis, but *Candida albicans* is usually associated with acute inflammation. Granulomas caused by *Schistosoma haematobium* are frequently found in the prostate as well as in the bladder and seminal vesicles in endemic areas such as Egypt. The organisms lodge in vesicular and pelvic venous plexuses as the final habitat. The adult female schistosome migrates into the submucosa of the urinary bladder and prostatic stroma where she lays eggs that induce granuloma formation and fibrosis. Rare cases of herpes zoster infection occurring in association with granulomatous prostatitis have been reported, usually in association with a sacral eruption.

Malakoplakia, a granulomatous disease associated with the defective intracellular lysosomal digestion of bacteria, occasionally occurs in the prostate.[34] In this condition the prostate is diffusely hard, a finding suggestive of prostatic carcinoma. *E. coli* is commonly isolated from urine cultures.

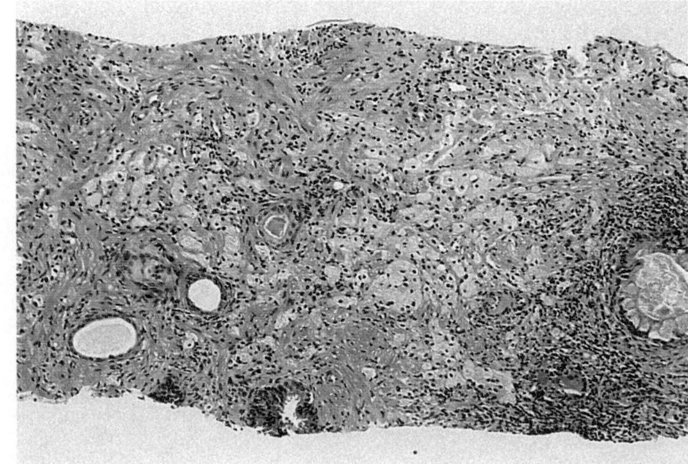

Fig. 67-45 Prostatic xanthoma showing a cohesive cluster of histiocytes with clear cytoplasm mimicking the clear cell pattern of adenocarcinoma.

Table 67-9 Classification of granulomatous prostatitis

Idiopathic ("nonspecific")
Typical idiopathic granulomatous prostatitis
Xanthoma and xanthogranulomatous prostatitis
Infectious
Bacterial
Tuberculosis
Brucellosis
Syphilis
Fungal
Coccidioidomycosis
Cryptococcosis
Blastomycosis
Histoplasmosis
Paracoccidioidomycosis
Parasitic
Schistosomiasis
Echinococcosis
Enterobiasis
Viral
Herpesvirus infection
Malakoplakia
Iatrogenic
Postsurgical
After radiation therapy
BCG associated
Systemic Diseases
Sarcoidosis
Rheumatoid arthritis
Wegener's granulomatosis
Polyarteritis nodosa
Churg-Strauss syndrome

(Modified from Lopez-Plaza I, Bostwick DG: Prostatitis. In Bostwick DG, editor: *Pathology of the prostate,* New York, 1990, Churchill Livingstone. *BCG,* Bacille Calmette-Guérin.)

Microscopically the prostate is effaced by sheets of macrophages admixed with lymphocytes and plasma cells. Intracellular and extracellular Michaelis-Gutmann bodies are identified, appearing as sharply demarcated, spherical structures with concentric "owl's eyes" measuring 5 to 10 μm in diameter.

Iatrogenic granulomatous prostatitis can be caused by surgery, radiation therapy, and bacille Calmette-Guérin (BCG) therapy for bladder cancer. **Postsurgical granulomatous prostatitis** can be identified up to 5 years after TURP and is caused by cauterization and surgical disruption of tissues[41,42] (Fig. 67-46). The granulomas are characteristically circumscribed and rimmed by palisading histiocytes with central fibrinoid necrosis. Multinucleated giant cells are frequently present. The striking histologic resemblance of postsurgical granulomatous prostatitis to rheumatoid nodules indicates the possible existence of a hypersensitivity reaction or a cell-mediated immune response. Tissue eosinophilia is present in many cases. No treatment is necessary for postsurgical prostatitis. **Postirradiation granulomatous prostatitis** is a rare complication of radiation therapy. **BCG-induced granulomatous prostatitis** occurs in virtually all patients treated with intravesicular BCG immunotherapy for superficial transitional cell carcinoma of the bladder.[43] The granulomas are characteristically discrete and often contain numerous acid-fast bacilli. No therapy is required.

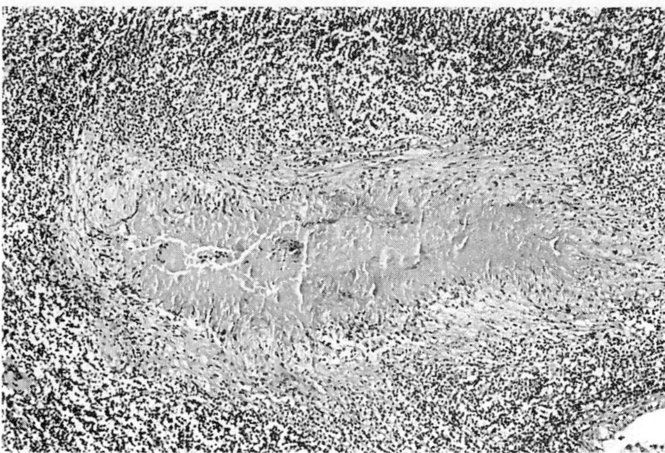

Fig. 67-46 Postsurgical granulomatous prostatitis showing fibrinoid necrosis and multinucleated giant cells.

Allergic ("eosinophilic") granulomatous prostatitis is a component of the Churg-Strauss syndrome. It should be diagnosed only in a patient with a history of asthma or allergy who has peripheral eosinophilia and systemic lesions. Histologically it exhibits granulomatous prostatitis, infiltrates of eosinophils, fibrinoid necrosis, and vasculitis.[35,37,38] Allergic granulomatous prostatitis is treated with steroids.

Other rare forms of granulomatous prostatitis include sarcoidosis, rheumatoid nodules, Wegener's granulomatosis, polyarteritis nodosa, and silicone-induced prostatitis.

Benign prostatic hyperplasia

Enlargement of the prostate, or benign prostatic hyperplasia (BPH), involves the overgrowth of the epithelium and fibromuscular tissue of the transition zone and periurethral area. Symptoms are caused by interference with muscular sphincteric function and by obstruction of urine flow through the prostatic urethra. These symptoms include urgency, difficulty in starting urination, diminished stream size and force, increased frequency, a sensation of incomplete bladder emptying, and nocturia.

Epidemiology

BPH is extremely common, accounting for approximately 400,000 partial prostatectomies annually, the most common form of surgery in American men.[44] There is a rapid increase in the prevalence of BPH beginning in the fourth decade of life and culminating in a nearly 100% prevalence in the ninth decade. The age-specific prevalence is remarkably similar in populations throughout the world.

Advanced age and an intact androgen supply are the only undisputed risk factors for BPH.[45,46] BPH does not occur in men castrated before puberty. Castration may relieve symptomatic BPH in older men. The risk of BPH is lower in patients with androgen resistance or deficiencies, including those with 5-α-reductase deficiency or hypopituitarism before 40 years of age. Antiandrogens, gonadotropin-releasing hormone agonists, and 5-α-reductase inhibitors also reduce the symptoms of BPH, underscoring the importance of androgens in the pathogenesis of hyperplasia.

The search for other risk factors of BPH has been unsuccessful. Most epidemiologic studies of environmental and lifestyle risk factors have yielded equivocal results, including studies of medical history, sexual history, smoking, alcohol use, socioeconomic status, and occupational exposure.

Pathogenesis

The development of BPH includes three pathologic changes: nodule formation, diffuse enlargement of the transition zone and periurethral tissue, and enlargement of nodules. In men under 70 years of age, diffuse enlargement predominates. This is attributed by McNeal[47] to a reawakening of the embryonic processes in stromal cells that allows them to act as an inductive force for reactivating adjacent epithelium-lined glands and causing them to proliferate. In men over 70 years of age, the prostatic enlargement characteristic of BPH is dominated by epithelial proliferation and the expansile growth of existing nodules, probably as the result of androgenic and other hormonal stimulation. The development of symptomatic BPH depends on the proportion of epithelium to stroma.[48]

The primary hormonal mediator of BPH is probably dihydrotestosterone. This androgen is the major intracellular metabolite of testosterone after its conversion by 5-α-reductase. Testosterone and dihydrotestosterone bind to nuclear androgen receptors in stromal and epithelial cells in the prostate, although dihydrotestosterone has a fivefold higher affinity. The nuclear androgen receptor content of BPH is greater than that of normal prostatic tissue. There may also be a synergistic stimulation of the growth of BPH produced by dihydrotestosterone and estrogens such as estradiol. It is likely that other biochemical growth factors are involved in the development of BPH.

Pathology

Grossly, BPH is characterized by variably sized nodules which are soft or firm, rubbery, and yellow-gray and bulge from the cut surface upon transection (Fig. 67-47). If there is prominent epithelial hyperplasia in addition to stromal hyperplasia, the abundant luminal spaces create soft and grossly spongy nodules from which oozes a pale white, watery fluid. If the BPH is predominantly fibromuscular, there may be diffuse enlargement or numerous trabeculations without a prominent nodularity. Degenerative changes include calcification and infarction. BPH usually involves the transition zone, but occasionally nodules arise from the periurethral tissue at the bladder neck.

Microscopically, BPH is typically nodular and is composed of varying proportions of epithelium and stroma (fibrous connective tissue and smooth muscle) (Fig. 67-48). The most common nodules are adenomyofibromatous nodules, which contain all elements.

Vascular insufficiency probably accounts for the **infarction** of BPH nodules, seen in up to 20% of resected cases. The center of the nodule undergoes hemorrhagic necrosis, often accompanied by reactive changes in the residual epithelium at the periphery, including **squamous metaplasia and transitional cell metaplasia.** These forms of metaplasia involve replacement of the normal glandular epithelium and may also be seen after estrogen therapy, androgen deprivation therapy, radiation therapy, trauma, and prostatitis.

Association of BPH and prostate cancer

There are many similarities between BPH and cancer.[45] Both display a parallel increase in prevalence with increasing patient age according to the results of autopsy studies, although cancer lags by 15 to 20 years. Both require androgens for growth and development to occur, and both may respond to androgen deprivation treatment. Most cancers arise in prostates together with BPH, and cancer is found incidentally in a significant number (10%) of TURP specimens. BPH may be related to prostate cancer arising in the transition zone, perhaps in association with certain forms of hyperplasia, but BPH is not a premalignant lesion or a precursor of carcinoma.

Variants of hyperplasia and associated benign lesions

Atrophy is a common microscopic finding and is characterized by small distorted glands with a flattened epithelium, hyperchromatic nuclei, and stromal fibrosis (Fig. 67-49, *A*). It is usually

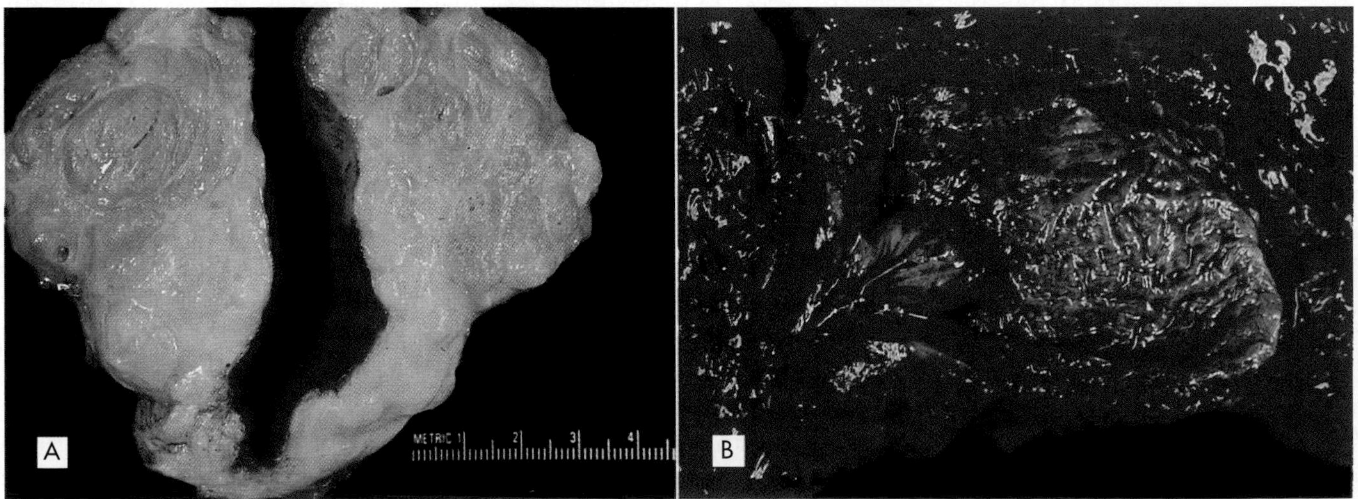

Fig. 67-47 Gross appearance of benign prostatic hyperplasia (BPH). **A,** Typical enlargement of the transition zone resulting from bulging nodules of varying size. **B,** BPH involving the prostatic glands at the bladder neck may cause polypoid protrusion into the bladder, with the mass acting as a ball valve causing severe urinary obstructive symptoms.

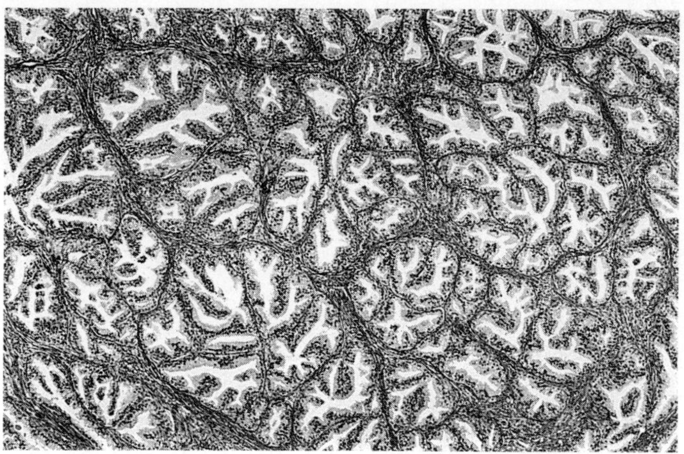

Fig. 67-48 Microscopic appearance of benign prostatic hyperplasia (BPH). Mixed epithelial-stromal nodules are typical of clinically apparent BPH.

idiopathic, and its prevalence increases with advancing age. In **postatrophic hyperplasia** there are benign proliferating luminal cells with small amounts of clear cytoplasm in an atrophic background. The cells often show mild cytologic atypia, and luminal mucin may be identified. Both of these lesions tend to show lobular organization at low-power magnification.

Basal cell hyperplasia is characterized by basal cell proliferation, in which layers composed of two or more cells are formed at the periphery of prostatic glands and acini[49,50] (Fig. 67-49, *B*). This proliferation sometimes appears as small, round, solid aggregates surrounded by a few concentric layers of compressed stroma. Frequently the site of proliferation is more than two cells thick and protrudes into the gland lumen, retaining the overlying secretory luminal epithelium. The hyperplastic basal cells are usually larger than the normal elongated or spindled basal cells, and often there is also nuclear enlargement. **Atypical basal cell hyperplasia** is basal cell hyperplasia in which the nucleoli are prominent.[50,51] **Basal cell adenoma** consists of a large, round, circumscribed nodule or nodules that contain uniformly spaced aggregates of hyperplastic basal cells varying from small solid nests to cystically dilated glands.[50] Stromal connective tissue often traverses the adenomatous nodule, creating incomplete lobulation in some cases. **Adenoid basal cell tumor,** also called **adenoid cystic–like tumor**, consists of basaloid cell nests of varying size that infiltrate the stroma. In contrast to basal cell adenoma, this lesion is not circumscribed.[49,50,52] The cell nests are frequently large and round to angular. Peripheral basaloid cells have elongated nuclei and often show palisading. Cell crowding is prominent. The luminal spaces surrounded by such cells vary in size. In rare cases there is perineural invasion and extension into the periprostatic soft tissues, but there are no metastatic lesions.

Cribriform hyperplasia, including **clear cell cribriform hyperplasia,** consists of a nodule composed of glands arranged in a distinctive cribriform pattern. The cells from such glands usually have pale to clear cytoplasm and small uniform nuclei with inconspicuous nucleoli[53,54] (Fig. 67-49, *C*).

Atypical adenomatous hyperplasia (adenosis) is a localized and circumscribed proliferation of small glands within the prostate that may be mistaken for carcinoma (see later discussion).

Sclerosing adenosis differs from atypical adenomatous hyperplasia in that it shows striking myoepithelial metaplasia of the basal cell compartment as well as an exuberant stroma composed of fibroblasts and loose ground substance[55-58]. The basal cells in this condition show positivity for S-100 protein and muscle-specific actin and are seen to have thin filament collections and dense bodies on electron microscopy. This phenotype is unusual in the prostate because normal prostatic basal cells do not demonstrate myoepithelial differentiation[59]; consequently, most authors believe that sclerosing adenosis is a form of metaplasia.

Stromal hyperplasia with atypia is characterized by stromal nodules that occur in the setting of BPH but show increased cellularity and nuclear atypia.[60,61] (Fig. 67-49, *D*). These may appear as solid stromal nodules (often referred to as **atypical leiomyoma**) or with atypical cells interspersed with benign glands. The stromal nuclei are large, hyperchromatic, and rarely multinucleated or vacuolated and contain inconspicuous nucleoli. There are no mitotic figures and no necrosis. Stromal hyperplasia with atypia has no malignant potential, and the atypical cells are considered degenerative.

Phyllodes tumor is a rare neoplasm of adults. It is a fibroadenoma that shows increased cellularity and cytologic atypia, reminiscent of phyllodes tumor of the breast[62-64] (Fig. 67-49, *E*). The glandular epithelium is distorted and lines slit-like spaces surrounded by a variably cellular proliferative stroma composed of fibroblasts and smooth muscle cells. Benign and malignant phyllodes tumors are distinguished on the basis of a number of factors, including the ratio of stroma to epithelium, the degree of stromal cellularity, mitotic activity, and cytologic atypia.[64-67]

Prostate cancer

Prostate cancer is the most common form of cancer among men in the United States and is second only to lung cancer as a cause of cancer-related death. In 1995 an estimated 40,4000 men will have died of prostate cancer and 244,000 new cases will have been diagnosed.[68] Although most prostate cancers are relatively slow growing and remain clinically unrecognized, their course is often unpredictable in terms of its speed of progression, perhaps because of the considerable heterogeneity of the histologic grade and a multitude of other factors that influence tumor growth. Despite an autopsy prevalence of up to 80% in men by the age of 80 years, the clinical incidence is much lower, indicating that most men die *with* prostate cancer rather than *of* prostate cancer. Little is known about the causes of prostate cancer despite its high incidence and prevalence.

Epidemiology

The incidence of prostate cancer has risen dramatically in the past decade, probably owing to early detection programs, reduced mortality resulting from other causes, and increased longevity, all of which allow prostate cancer to become clinically apparent in elderly men. The probability of clinically apparent prostate cancer increased from 6.1% in 1985 to 8.7% in 1986 for white American men, and the lifetime risk of a man dying of prostate cancer is 2.6% for white and 4.3% for black Americans.[69-71]

Prostate cancer is rare before 40 years of age, but the incidence rises quickly thereafter. Autopsy studies of thoroughly evaluated prostates from men without clinical evidence of cancer have shown an extraordinarily high level of latent cancer,

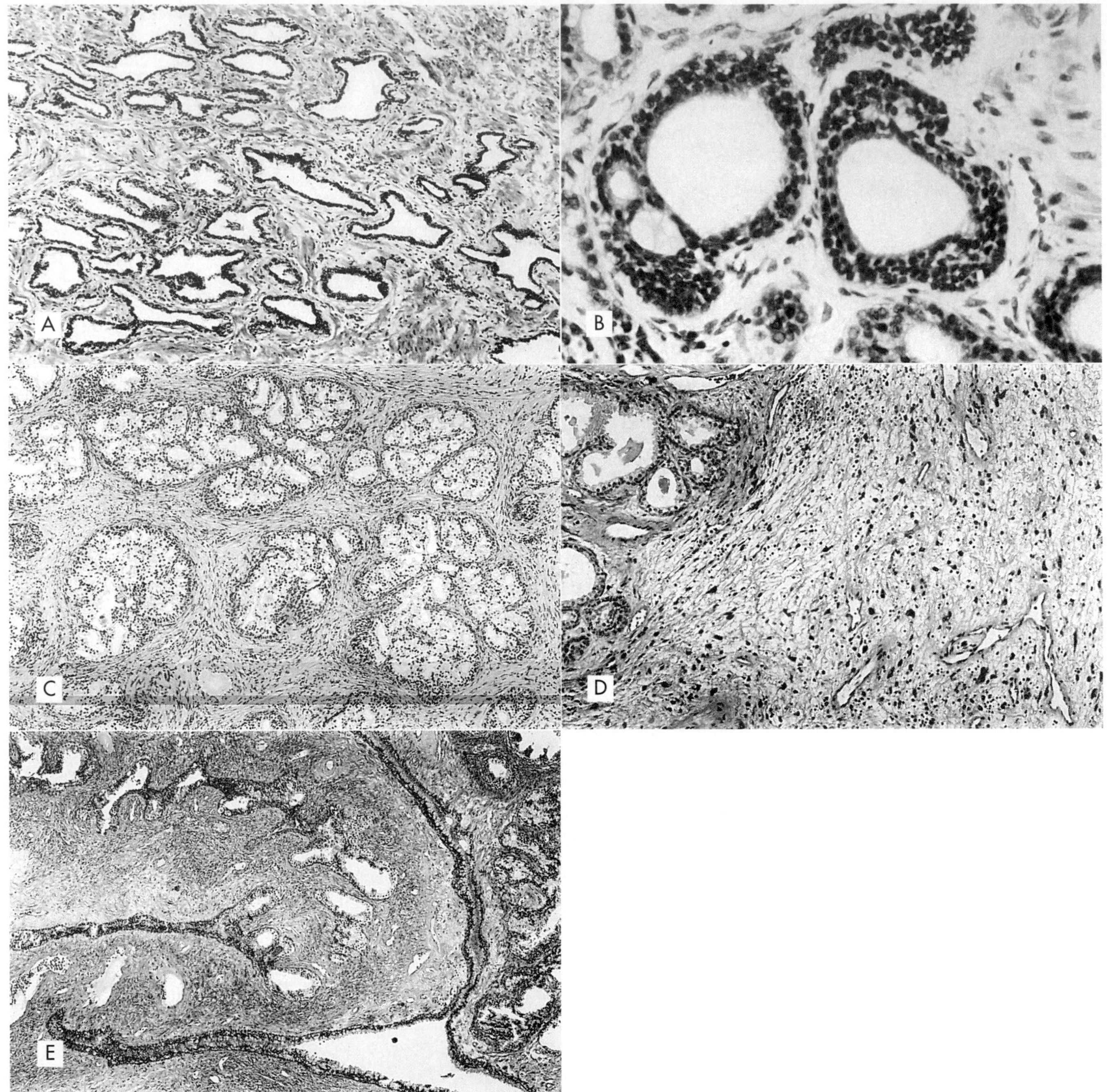

Fig. 67-49 Variants of benign prostatic hyperplasia and associated benign lesions. **A,** Atrophy. **B,** Basal cell hyperplasia. **C,** Clear cell cribriform hyperplasia. **D,** Stromal hyperplasia with atypia. **E,** Phyllodes tumor.

increasing from about 10% at 50 years of age to 80% by 80 years of age.[45] The incidence of prostate cancer is much higher in blacks (100 per 100,000) than in whites (70.1 per 100,000), and black men in the United States have the highest mortality from prostate cancer worldwide.[69,72-74] The incidence is low in American Indians, Hispanics, and Asians. Interestingly, the prevalence of latent cancer in different geographic groups is similar despite a wide variation in the clinical incidence.[45,72]

Pathogenesis

Hormones are essential for the development of prostate cancer. The normal epithelium and stroma require stimulation by testosterone and its metabolite dihydrotestosterone for growth and development to occur, and these androgens are also essential for tumor cell maintenance and growth.

There are no proven risk factors for the development of prostate cancer, but many factors have been proposed (Table 67-10). A familial predisposition with an early onset of prostate cancer probably accounts for about 9% of cases, with increasing risk as the number of affected relatives increases.[75-79] A man's risk is twofold higher if a first-degree relative such as a father or brother has prostate cancer, and the risk is fivefold to elevenfold higher if two or three first-degree relatives have cancer. Heredity appears to be one of

Table 67-10 Proposed risk factors for prostate cancer

Prostatic intraepithelial neoplasia
Family history
Diet
Fat
Cadmium
Zinc
Obesity
Alcohol
Hormones
Smoking
Sexual activity
Early sexual activity
Multiple sexual partners
Occupational exposure
Agricultural fertilizers and pesticides
Cadmium
Rubber
Zinc
Ionizing radiation
Venereal diseases
Herpesvirus type 2
Cytomegalovirus
Vasectomy
Benign prostatic hyperplasia

the most consistent and strongest risk factors for the development of prostate cancer.

According to cross-cultural comparisons, dietary fat may also cause prostate cancer, perhaps resulting in part from the influence of diet on the production of sex hormones, but the relationship is complex and ill-defined.[80] Obesity and alcohol abuse may also be risk factors. The data linking smoking, sexual activity, and occupational exposure with prostate cancer are inconclusive. The findings from early studies that implicated venereal diseases such as gonorrhea as a cause have been refuted. Viral diseases such as herpesvirus type 2 and cytomegalovirus have been implicated, but the data are not conclusive.

Vasectomy has been proposed as a risk factor for prostate cancer, but reports to date have been affected by patient selection bias.[81,82] BPH is frequently seen in association with prostate cancer, and there are numerous compelling similarities, including an increasing incidence and prevalence with age, a concordant natural history, and hormonal requirements for growth and development to take place, but no causal relationship has been established.[45]

Patients with prostatic intraepithelial neoplasia are at increased risk for prostate cancer, and many are found to have cancer on repeat biopsy; it is uncertain whether this represents an etiologic link or association.

Proposed premalignant lesions

Two histopathologic lesions in the prostate have been proposed as being premalignant: prostatic intraepithelial neoplasia, characterized by severe cytologic changes within preexisting ducts and acini, and atypical adenomatous hyperplasia, characterized by architectural changes with the proliferation of small glands but without significant cytologic atypia.

Prostatic intraepithelial neoplasia (PIN) represents the putative precancerous end of the morphologic continuum of cellular proliferations that occur within prostatic ducts, ductules, and acini.[83-86] The term *PIN* was proposed in 1987[84] and endorsed by consensus at a 1989 international conference[87] to replace other synonymous terms used in the literature, including "intraductal dysplasia,"[83] "large acinar atypical hyperplasia,"[85] "atypical primary hyperplasia," "hyperplasia with malignant change," "marked atypia," and "duct-acinar dysplasia." This consensus group also agreed that PIN be divided into two grades (low grade and high grade) to replace the previous three grade system: PIN 1 is considered low grade, and PIN 2 and 3 are considered high grade. At a subsequent consensus conference held by the American Cancer Society, PIN was declared the most likely precursor of prostate cancer.[88]

The continuum that culminates in high-grade PIN and early invasive cancer is characterized by basal cell layer disruption, progressive loss of the markers of secretory differentiation, increasing nuclear and nucleolar abnormalities, increasing proliferative potential, and increasing variation in DNA content (aneuploidy). Results of clinical studies indicate that PIN possibly predates carcinoma by 10 years or more, with low-grade PIN first emerging in men in the third decade of life.[85,86] PIN is often found in the vicinity of carcinoma; its identification in biopsy specimens of the prostate warrants a further search for concurrent invasive carcinoma.

In low-grade PIN (formerly known as PIN 1), the cells within ducts and acini are heaped up, crowded, and irregularly spaced and there is considerable variation in nuclear size (anisonucleosis) (Table 67-11). Elongated hyperchromatic nuclei and small nucleoli are also observed, but these are not usually prominent features. A combination of both cytologic and architectural characteristics must be identified for PIN to be diagnosed, and lesions displaying some but not all of these characteristics are considered atypical but not dysplastic. High-grade PIN (formerly considered PIN 2 and 3) exhibits features similar to those of low-grade PIN, although cell crowding and stratification are usually more pronounced and there is less variability in nuclear size because most of the nuclei are enlarged; the presence of prominent nucleoli, often multiple, is of greatest diagnostic value (Fig. 67-50).

High-grade PIN displays four architectural patterns: tufting, micropapillary, cribriform, and flat[89] (Fig. 67-51). The patterns often merge, although fields with only a single pattern may be present. Familiarity with these patterns aids in the recognition of PIN and averts potential diagnostic pitfalls.

PIN spreads through prostatic ducts in three different ways, similar to the manner of spread of prostatic carcinoma. In the first pattern, neoplastic cells replace the normal luminal secretory epithelium but the basal cell layer and basement membrane are preserved. Foci of high-grade PIN are usually indistinguishable from ductal spread of carcinoma on routine light microscopy studies. In the second pattern, there is direct invasion through the ductal or acinar wall and disruption of the basal cell layer and the basement membrane. In the third pattern, neoplastic cells invade between the basal cell layer and columnar secretory cell layer ("pagetoid spread"), but this is a very uncommon finding.

The peripheral zone of the prostate, the area in which most prostatic carcinomas occur (70%), is also the most common location for PIN. Cancer and PIN are frequently multifocal in the peripheral zone, indicating the existence of a "field" effect similar to the multifocality of papillary urothelial carcinoma and carcinoma in situ of the bladder. About 20% to 25% of the cases of prostate cancer occur in the transition zone and peri-

Table 67-11 Prostatic intraepithelial neoplasia (PIN): diagnostic criteria

	Low-grade PIN (formerly PIN 1)	High-grade PIN (formerly PIN 2 and 3)
Architecture	Epithelial cell crowding and stratification, with irregular spacing	Similar to low-grade PIN; more crowding and stratification; 4 patterns: tufting, micropapillary, cribriform, and flat
Cytology		
Nuclei	Enlarged, with considerable size variation	Enlarged; some size and shape variation
Chromatin	Normal	Increased density and clumping
Nucleoli	Rarely prominent	Occasionally to frequently large and prominent, similar to invasive carcinoma; sometimes multiple
Basal cell layer	Intact	May show some disruption
Basement membrane	Intact	Intact

(Modified from Bostwick DG, Brawer MK: *Cancer* 59:788, 1987.)

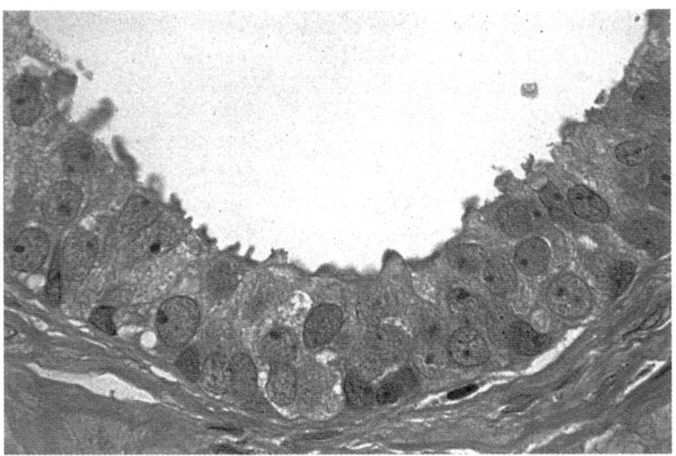

Fig. 67-50 High-grade prostatic intraepithelial neoplasia, flat pattern, in a needle biopsy specimen.

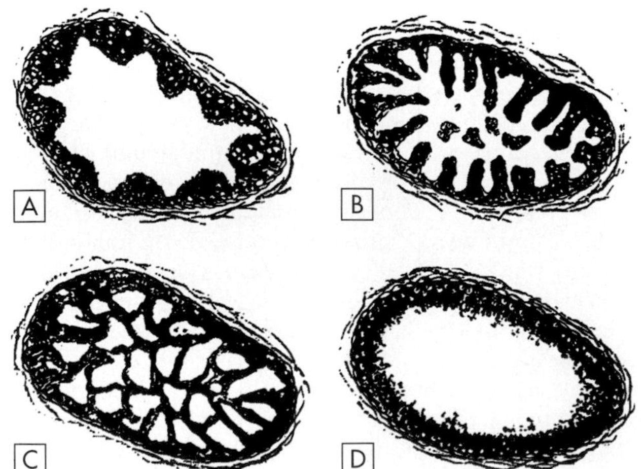

Fig. 67-51 The architectural patterns assumed by high-grade prostatic intraepithelial neoplasia. **A,** Tufting pattern. **B,** Micropapillary pattern. **C,** Cribriform pattern. **D,** Flat pattern. (From Bostwick DG, AminTB, Dundore P et al: *Hum Pathol* 24:298, 1993.)

urethral area, the anatomic areas where nodular hyperplasia occurs; these areas harbor faci of PIN in only 8% of cases.[90] By contrast, atypical adenomatous hyperplasia is found in up to 24% of transition zone specimens.

Increasing grades of PIN are associated with progressive disruption of the basal cell layer.[84] Antibodies directed against high-molecular-weight keratins (for example, clone 34-β-E12) have been employed immunohistochemically to selectively label the prostatic basal cell layer.[91] Tumor cells consistently fail to react with this antibody, whereas normal prostatic epithelium is consistently labeled, with a continuous intact circumferential basal cell layer observed in most instances. Disruption of the basal cell layer is present in 56% of the cases of high-grade PIN, more commonly in glands adjacent to sites of invasive carcinoma than in distant glands. The extent of disruption also increases with increasing grades of PIN, with loss of more than one-third of the basal cell layer in 52% of the foci of high-grade PIN. Early invasive carcinoma occurs at sites of glandular outpouching and basal cell disruption.[84] A model of prostatic carcinogenesis has been proposed based on the morphologic continuum of PIN and the multistep theory of transformation[84] (Fig. 67-52).

The frequency of PIN in cancerous prostates is significantly greater than its frequency in noncancerous prostates.[90,92-94] PIN was found in 82% of the step-sectioned cancerous prostates but in only 43% of the noncancerous prostates from patients of similar age. PIN is more extensive in lower-stage tumors, presumably because of the overgrowth or obliteration of PIN by larger high-stage tumors. The severity of PIN in cancerous prostates was significantly worse than its severity in noncancerous prostates.

In a study of 429 step-sectioned whole prostates, Kovi et al[85] found that the prevalence of PIN in cancerous prostates increased with age, predating the onset of carcinoma by more than 5 years. Sakr et al[86] studied young men and found PIN in 9% and 22% of men in their twenties and thirties respectively; most foci of PIN in young men were low grade, but the frequency of high-grade PIN increased with advancing age. The prevalence of PIN was similar in blacks and whites. Lee et al[95] studied 256 specimens of hypoechoic lesions of the prostate obtained by ultrasound-guided biopsy, and identified 103 cases of cancer and 27 cases of PIN; the mean age of those with PIN (65 years) was significantly lower than the age of the men with cancer (70 years).

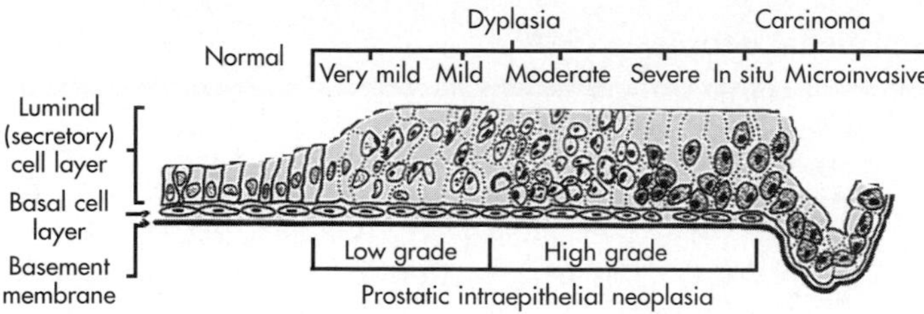

Fig. 67-52 Morphologic continuum from normal prostatic epithelium through increasing grades of prostatic intraepithelial neoplasia (PIN) to early invasive carcinoma, according to the disease continuum concept. Low-grade PIN (formerly grade 1) corresponds to very mild to mild dysplasia. High-grade PIN (formerly grades 2 and 3) corresponds to moderate to severe dysplasia and carcinoma in situ. The precursor state ends when malignant cells invade the stroma; this invasion occurs where the basal cell layer is disrupted. Notice that the dysplastic changes occur in the superficial (luminal) secretory cell layer, perhaps in response to luminal carcinogens. Disruption of the basal cell layer accompanies the appearance of the architectural and cytologic features of high-grade PIN and appears to be a necessary prerequisite for stromal invasion. (From Bostwick DG, Brawer MK: *Cancer* 59: 788, 1987.)

There is a progressive loss of the markers of secretory differentiation with increasing grades of PIN, indicating progressive impairment of cell differentiation and regulatory control with advancing stages of prostatic genesis.[96-100] With rare exceptions the expression of a wide variety of secretory proteins, cytoskeletal proteins, and glycoproteins in PIN differs from the histochemical makeup of normal epithelium but is similar to that of invasive prostatic carcinoma. Nagle et al[100] suggested that changes in the type of cytoskeletal proteins in PIN may affect the transport of cell products, accounting for the differences in the distribution of secretory proteins. McNeal et al[96] found that a reduction in the expression of cytoplasmic differentiation markers during the preinvasive phase may be followed by abrupt reexpression at the site of microinvasion. Other studies have shown an increased expression of type IV collagenase in the settings of both PIN and cancer.[101]

Virtually all measures of nuclear abnormality done by computer-based image analysis reveal a similarity of PIN to cancer, in contrast with the characteristics of normal and hyperplastic epithelium.[102-104] These changes include the nuclear area, the DNA content, the chromatin content and distribution, and the nuclear perimeter, diameter, and roundness. In addition, most measures of nucleolar abnormality show the similarity of PIN to cancer, in contrast with the nucleolar characteristics of normal epithelium.[104-108] These cumulative data indicate that the continuum from PIN to cancer is characterized by progressive nuclear and nucleolar changes.

These morphologic changes are accompanied by progressive changes in DNA ploidy.[104,109-111] Montironi et al[104] suggested that two successive phases occur: the first occurs in hyperplastic epithelium and low-grade PIN, and is characterized by DNA duplication without nuclear division, resulting in euploidy (diploidy or tetraploidy); the second phase occurs only in high-grade PIN and cancer and results in the emergence of aneuploid elements (triploidy, hyperdiploidy, hypotetraploidy, and aneuploidy). Similar results have been reported by other investigators.[109-111]

Biopsy remains the definitive method for detecting PIN and early invasive cancer, but noninvasive methods are being evaluated. Transrectal ultrasound (TRUS) imaging has shown PIN to be hypoechoic and thus indistinguishable from carcinoma.[112] TRUS-directed biopsy allows localization of the needle and tissue being sampled. In a case-control study conducted by Davidson et al,[113] of 100 patients with PIN identified on the basis of prostate biopsy findings, 33 (33%) had carcinoma identified in subsequent specimens; these results were confirmed in other studies[114-116] (Table 67-12). If all procedures fail to identify coexistent carcinoma, close surveillance and follow-up appear to be indicated. Follow-up examination at 6-month intervals for 2 years is suggested; thereafter follow-up examinations should be scheduled at 12-month intervals for life.[117] Most authors agree that the identification of premalignant lesions in the prostate should not influence or dictate the therapeutic decisions. PIN also offers promise as an intermediate end-point in studies of the chemoprevention of prostatic carcinoma.[117]

Atypical adenomatous hyperplasia (AAH) is a localized proliferation of small glands within the prostate that may be mistaken for carcinoma[118-124] (Fig. 67-53). The lesions form a morphologic continuum ranging from proliferations with minimal architectural and cytologic atypia (AAH) to those with a high degree of atypia easily mistaken for well-differentiated adenocarcinoma. An international consensus group has recommended use of the term "AAH" rather than "adenosis" to refer to these lesions to create a standard for comparison among different institutions, which would allow study of the prognostic significance of this finding.

AAH varies in incidence from 24% in an autopsy series consisting of 20- to 40-year-old men[123] to 23% in men with cancer who underwent radical prostatectomy.[124] It occurs throughout the prostate but is usually found near the apex and in the transition zone and periurethral area.[121-123] AAH is distinguished from well-differentiated carcinoma by its inconspicuous nucleoli, infrequent crystalloids, lack of basophilic mucin, and a fragmented basal cell layer, as seen with antibodies to high-molecular-weight keratins (Table 67-13). Despite the utility of these features, the absolute distinction between AAH and carcinoma is still problematic in some cases, and those cases may be best classified as atypical small

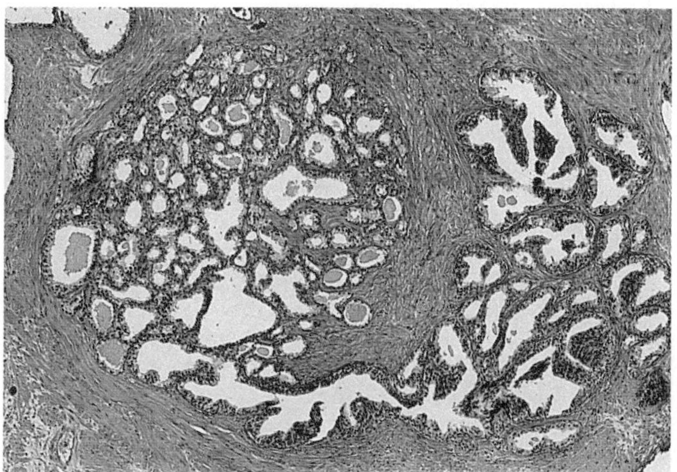

Fig. 67-53 Atypical adenomatous hyperplasia.

Table 67-12 Clinical follow-up results of prostatic intraepithelial neoplasia (PIN)

Author	Number of cases	Numbers (%) with cancer on follow-up study	Follow-up*
Brawer et al[114]	21	12 (57%)†	Immediate rebiopsy
Weinstein et al[115]	19‡	10 (53%)	Immediate rebiopsy
Davidson et al[113]	100	33 (33%)	Up to 4 years
Markham[116]	32	13 (41%)	Up to 1.5 years

*Follow-up indicates length of time from diagnosis of PIN to repeat biopsy.
†Includes cases with low-grade and high-grade PIN; other studies only included high-grade PIN.
‡Of 33 cases presented, first biopsy findings showed 19 had PIN without cancer.

glandular proliferation of uncertain significance (see later discussion).

Nucleoli are found in virtually all cells but are not usually considered "prominent" or enlarged in the prostatic epithelium and at the site of AAH until their diameter measures greater than 1.0 to 1.5 μm in routine formalin-fixed sections.[121] The prognostic significance and diagnostic utility of nucleolar area and size in the evaluation of prostatic carcinoma have been demonstrated by various methods, including scanning electron microscopy and computerized image analysis.[104,124-129] Nucleoli in AAH are intermediate in size between the size of the nucleoli in nodular hyperplasia and that of the nucleoli in well-differentiated adenocarcinoma and that only in cancerous tissue were there two or more nucleoli in an individual cell. The authors of other reports found that nucleolar prominence was the finding that distinguished AAH from carcinoma.[118,125,126]

Immunohistochemical techniques are also valuable in the diagnosis of AAH. The basal cell layer is characteristically discontinuous and fragmented in AAH, whereas in carcinoma there is an absent basal cell layer, and this diagnostic feature can be demonstrated immunohistochemically in routine formalin-fixed sections with antibodies against high-molecular-weight keratins (34-βE12).[91,118,127-131] Other phenotypic markers such as acidic mucin may also be of value in distinguishing AAH from carcinoma, but the finding of acidic mucin is not specific for malignancy.[130,132-134]

The greatest difficulty in distinguishing AAH from carcinoma is with lesions containing nucleoli intermediate in size between the nucleoli typical of benign tissue and malignant tissue. To accommodate this borderline group, the authors of a recent report recommended separating small glandular proliferations into AAH (probably benign) and atypical small glandular proliferation of uncertain significance (possibly benign, but having some features of carcinoma).[118] In view of the uncertainty about the nature of this lesion, some pathologists may prefer a noncommittal term such as *atypical small acinar proliferation, not further classified*.

Differential diagnosis. Histologic mimics of AAH include simple lobular atrophy, postatrophic hyperplasia, sclerosing atrophy, basal cell hyperplasia, atypical basal cell hyperplasia, and metaplastic changes associated with irradiation, infarction, and prostatitis (Table 67-14). Many of these mimics can display architectural and cytologic atypia, including nucleolomegaly; thus, caution is warranted in the interpretation of scant specimens, cauterized or distorted specimens, and specimens submitted with an incomplete patient history. AAH may be uncommonly associated with sclerosis, but further study is needed to determine the relationship of this lesion to sclerosing adenosis.

Is AAH a precursor of adenocarcinoma? It has been proposed that it is a premalignant lesion because of the following findings: an increased incidence in association with carcinoma (15% in 100 noncancerous prostates at autopsy and 31% in 100 cancerous prostates at autopsy)[119,121,123,135]; its topographic relationship with small acinar carcinoma[121]; an age peak incidence that precedes that of carcinoma[121]; an increasing silver-reactive nucleolar organizer region count[136,137]; increased nuclear area and diameter[138]; and a proliferative cell index that is similar to that of small acinar carcinoma and significantly greater than that of normal and hyperplastic prostatic epithelium. However, some authors claim that the link between cancer and AAH is an epiphenomenon and that the data are insufficient for it to be concluded that AAH is a premalignant lesion.[122] It has also been suggested that AAH may be related to the subset of cancers that arise in the transition zone in association with benign prostatic hyperplasia.[45] Although the biologic significance of AAH is uncertain, its light microscopic appearance and immunophenotype allow it to be distinguished from carcinoma.

When AAH is encountered in prostatic specimens, all tissue should be embedded and made available for examination; serial sections of suspicious foci may be useful. Unfortunately, needle biopsy specimens frequently fail to show the suspicious focus at deeper levels, confounding the diagnostic dilemma. The identification of AAH should not influence or dictate therapeutic decisions.

Clinical features

Prostate cancer exhibits no specific presenting symptoms and is usually clinically silent, although it may cause urinary obstructive symptoms mimicking BPH. As a consequence, cancer is often initially manifested in metastatic sites such as cervical lymph nodes and bone. The diagnosis may be made in the following clinical instances: (1) routine surveillance for prostate cancer in men over 40 years of age—digital rectal examination shows a nodular or diffusely enlarged prostate; the serum PSA level is greater than 4 g/ml; and TRUS findings and biopsy specimens are positive for malignancy (lesion-directed, random, or systematic sextant needle biopsy specimens); (2) incidental carcinoma in transurethral resectates (stage A or T1a carcinoma); (3) adenocarcinoma of unknown primary; and (4) carcinoma of the prostate presenting as a rectal mass—prostate cancer rarely produces an eccentric or circumferential rectal and perirectal mass, with or without mucosal involvement of the rectum.

Table 67-13 Diagnostic criteria for atypical adenomatous hyperplasia and comparison with low-grade adenocarcinoma

Feature	Atypical adenomatous hyperplasia	Carcinoma (Gleason grades 1 and 2)
Architectural and associated features		
Low power	Circumscribed or limited infiltration	Circumscribed or limited infilitration
Lesion size	Variable	Variable
Gland size	Variable	Less variable
Gland shape	Variable	Less variable
Crystalloids	Infrequent (16%)	Frequent (75%)
Corpora amylacea	Frequent (32%)	Infrequent (13%)
Basophilic mucin	Infrequent	Frequent
Nuclear features		
Nuclear size variation	Less variable	Variable
Chromatin	Uniform/granular	Uniform or variable
Parachromatin clearing	Infrequent	Frequent
Nucleoli	Inconspicuous	Prominent
Nucleoli (largest)	2.5 μm (rare)	3.0 μm
Nucleoli (mean)	<1.0 μm	1.8 μm
Nucleoli >1 μm	18%	77%
Basal cell layer		
Hematoxylin-eosin staining	Inconspicuous	Absent
Antikeratin staining (high molecular weight)	Fragmented	Virtually absent

From Bostwick DG, Srigley J, Grignon D, et al: *Hum Pathol* 24:819, 1993.

Table 67-14 Differential diagnosis of small glandular proliferations in the prostate

- Atypical adenomatous hyperplasia
- Typical and atypical basal cell hyperplasia
- Adenoid basal cell tumor
- Sclerosing adenosis
- Nephrogenic metaplasia
- Atrophy
  - Simple lobular atrophy
  - Cystic atrophy
  - Sclerotic atrophy
  - Postatrophic hyperplasia
- Seminal vesicles
- Paraganglionic tissue
- Cowper's glands
- Florid hyperplasia of mesonephric remnants
- Xanthoma

Pathology

Gross identification of prostate cancer may be difficult or impossible, and definitive diagnosis requires microscopic examination. In TURP specimens, unless it is extensive, cancer is rarely identified grossly because of the confounding macroscopic features of BPH. In prostatectomy specimens, cancer tends to be multifocal, with a predilection for the peripheral zone.[23] Grossly apparent tumor foci are at least 5 mm in their greatest dimension and appear yellow-white with a stony-hard consistency resulting from the stromal desmoplasia (Fig. 67-54). Some tumors appear as yellow granular masses, which contrast sharply with the normal spongy prostatic parenchyma. These could resemble lesions caused by tuberculosis, granulomatous prostatitis, and florid acute and chronic prostatitis.

Microscopically, prostatic adenocarcinoma in most cases consists of a proliferation of small glands exhibiting a myriad of patterns. Evaluation of these glandular proliferations can be a major challenge, particularly when the specimen or suspicious focus is small. Diagnosis relies on the combination of architectural and cytologic findings exhibited and may be aided by ancillary studies such as immunohistochemical analyses. The **architectural features** can be assessed at low- to medium-power magnification and include irregular glandular contours, which deviate from the smoothly sculpted, rounded contours of normal prostatic glands. The arrangement of the glands is useful for diagnosis: malignant glands often exhibit an irregular, haphazard arrangement, sometimes with splitting or distortion of muscle fibers in the stroma. A variation in gland size can also be of value, particularly when there are small, irregular, abortive glands with primitive lumens, usually at the periphery. Comparison with the adjacent uninvolved prostatic glands is always of value.

The histologic pattern of prostate cancer correlates strongly with the biologic behavior of malignancy, a finding exploited by more than thirty grading systems proposed during this century. All systems successfully identify well-differentiated cancer, which progresses slowly, and poorly differentiated cancer, which progresses rapidly; however, they are less successful in subclassifying the great majority of moderately differentiated cancers, which have an intermediate clinical and biologic potential.[139] The Gleason grading system, based on the Veterans Administration Cooperative Urological Research Group study of more than 4000 patients between 1960 and 1975, is the de facto grading standard in the United States and other parts of the world[140,141] (Table 67-15; Fig. 67-55); the only other system in widespread use internationally is the Mostofi[142] (World Health Organization) system. Both systems are clinically useful, correlating the various grades with patterns of tumor progression, including tumor volume; the pres-

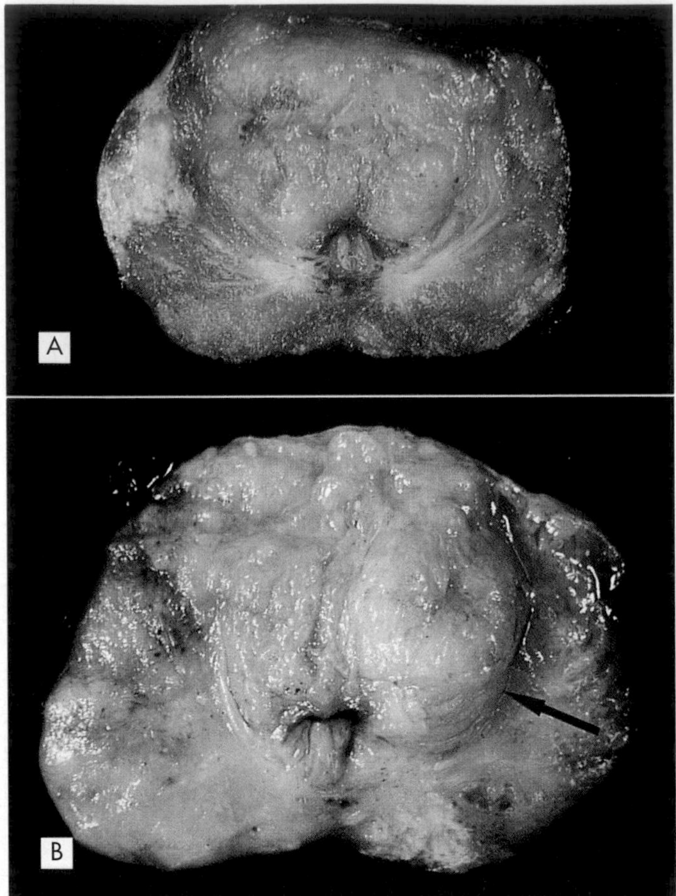

Fig. 67-54 Gross appearance of prostatic adenocarcinoma. **A,** The main tumor is present in the lateral peripheral zone as a firm, circumscribed, yellow-white mass, but multiple microscopic foci were present bilaterally in the periphery. Compare with **B,** showing transition zone cancer characterized by a bulging asymmetrical mass, which is present in association with benign prostatic hypertrophy (*arrow*).

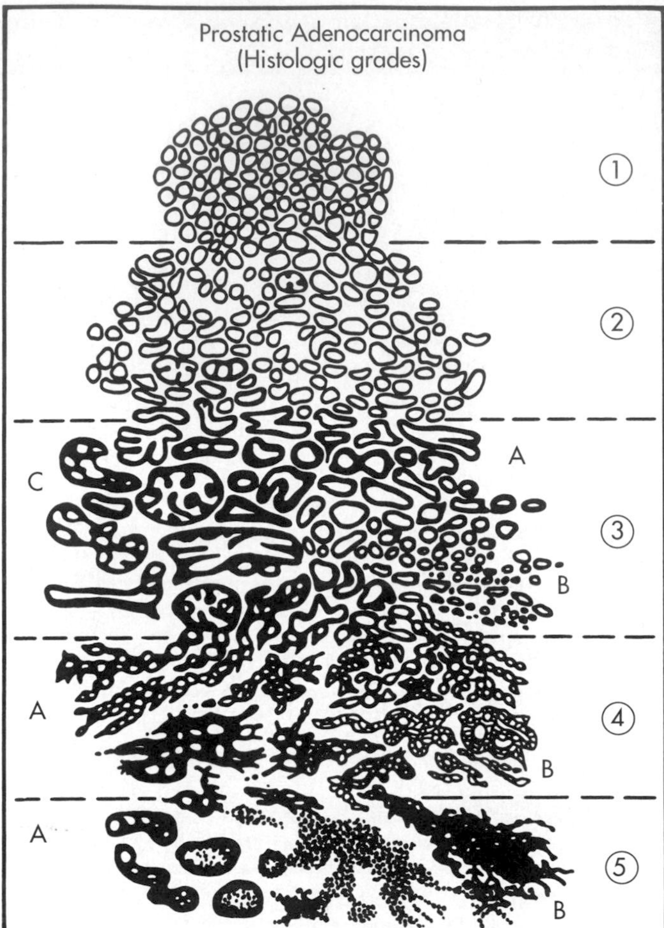

Fig. 67-55 Gleason grading system of prostatic adenocarcinoma.

ence of pelvic lymph node metastatic lesions; the serum concentration of PSA; and the likelihood of tumor recurrence after surgical and radiation therapy. The Gleason system is easier to use according to some advocates because only low or intermediate magnification needs to be employed.

The Gleason grading system is based on the degree of glandular differentiation, accommodating tumor heterogeneity by assigning a primary pattern for the dominant grade and a secondary pattern for the nondominant grade; the histologic score is derived by adding these two patterns. The success of the Gleason system is the result of four factors: (1) histologic patterns are identified by their degree of glandular differentiation without reliance on morphogenetic or histogenetic models (Fig. 67-56); (2) a simplified and standardized drawing was created by Gleason (see Fig. 67-55); (3) the Veterans Administration Cooperative Urologic Research Group study provided invaluable prospective information that allowed the objective development of this self-defining grading system; and (4) unlike any other tumor grading system in the body, the Gleason system provided for tumor heterogeneity by identifying primary and secondary patterns.

Cytologic features of cancer such as nuclear and nucleolar enlargement are also important for the diagnosis of malignancy. Enlargement should be seen in most of the suspicious cells. It is important to remember that every cell has a nucleolus, so one searches for "prominent" nucleoli, which are at least 1.25 to 1.50 μm in diameter or larger.[118] The identification of more than one nucleolus is virtually diagnostic proof of malignancy according to Helpap[126]; the nucleoli of cancer cells are frequently also eccentrically located in the nucleus, although this is a difficult feature to evaluate objectively.

The status of the **basal cell layer** is also critical in the diagnosis of adenocarcinoma.[91] Compressed stromal fibroblasts can mimic basal cells but are usually only seen focally at the periphery of the glands; an intact basal cell layer is present at the periphery of benign glands, whereas carcinoma entirely lacks a basal cell layer. Sometimes small foci of adenocarcinoma cluster around larger glands, which have an intact basal cell layer, thus compounding the difficulty. In problematic cases, it may be useful to employ monoclonal antibodies directed against high-molecular-weight keratin (for example 34-β-E12) to evaluate the basal cell layer.

Other ancillary histologic features may aid in the diagnosis of adenocarcinoma (Fig. 67-57). **Perineural invasion** is common in cancer and represents strong presumptive evidence of malignancy but is not pathognomonic because it has been noted rarely in benign glands.[143-145] However, circumferential

Table 67-15 Gleason grading system for prostatic adenocarcinoma: histologic patterns

Pattern	Peripheral borders	Stromal invasion	Appearance of glands	Size of glands	Architecture of glands	Cytoplasm
1	Circumscribed, pushing, expansile	Minimal	Simple, round, monotonously replicated	Medium, regular	Closely packed, rounded masses	Similar to benign epithelium
2	Less circumscribed; early infiltration	Mild, with definite separation of glands by stroma	Simple, round, some variability in shape	Medium, less regular	Loosely packed, rounded masses	Similar to benign epithelium
3A	Infiltration	Marked	Angular, with variation in shape	Medium to large	Variably packed, irregular masses	More basophilic than patterns 1 and 2
3B	Infiltration	Marked	Angular, with variation in shape	Small	Variably packed, irregular masses	More basophilic than patterns 1 and 2
3C	Smooth, rounded	Marked	Papillary and cribriform	Irregular	Round to elongated masses	More basophilic than patterns 1 and 2
4A	Ragged infiltration	Marked	Microacinar, papillary, and cribriform	Irregular	Fused, with chains and cords	Dark
4B	Ragged infiltration	Marked	Microacinar, papillary, and cribriform	Irregular	Fused, with chains and cords	Clear ("hypernephroid")
5A	Smooth, rounded	Marked	Comedocarcinoma	Irregular	Round to elongated masses	Variable
5B	Ragged infiltration	Marked	Difficulty to identify gland lumens	Fused sheets and masses		Variable

impingement or intraneural invasion are only seen in the setting of malignancy. Perineural invasion often indicates tumor spread along planes of least resistance that accompany intraprostatic nerves but does not represent lymphatic invasion. **Acidic sulfated and nonsulfated mucin** is seen in many cases of adenocarcinoma, appearing as wispy, faintly basophilic luminal material on hematoxylin- eosin–stained sections. This mucin stains with alcian blue and is best demonstrated at pH 2.5, whereas the normal prostatic epithelium contains periodic acid–Schiff–reactive, neutral mucin. The finding of acidic mucin is not specific for carcinoma, having been identified in the settings of PIN, AAH, sclerosing adenosis, and rarely BPH.[99,133,134] **Crystalloids** are needlelike, brightly eosinophilic, and sharp-edged structures that are often present in the lumens of well-differentiated and moderately differentiated carcinoma.[146,147] Ultrastructurally they are composed of electron-dense material that lacks the periodicity of crystals; thus the term *crystalloids* rather than *crystals* is appropriate in reference to these structures. X-ray microanalysis has demonstrated uniformly high sulfur peaks with small sodium peaks.[147] Their pathogenesis is uncertain, but it is probably the result of abnormal protein and mineral handling by malignant glands. Crystalloids are not a finding specific to carcinoma, having been found in the settings of PIN, AAH, BPH, and normal prostatic epithelium. **Collagenous micronodules** are an incidental finding in mucin-producing prostatic adenocarcinoma and consist of microscopic nodular masses of paucicellular, eosinophilic, fibrillar stroma that impinge on gland lumens; they probably result from the extravasation of acidic mucin into the stroma.[148,149] Despite being present in less than 13% of the cases of cancer, collagenous micronodules are found exclusively in association with cancer and are not present in benign epithelium, BPH, or PIN. **Microvascular invasion** is a strong indicator of malignancy, and its presence has been directly correlated with histologic grade, although it is sometimes difficult to distinguish from fixation-associated retraction artifact of glands.[150-151] The finding of **tumor within adipose tissue** is indicative of extraprostatic extension (capsular perforation), although this is a rare finding in biopsy specimens.

It is important to note **inflammation** when evaluating small glandular proliferations, particularly when the architectural features are equivocal and one is relying on the cytologic findings of nucleomegaly and nucleolomegaly to make the diagnosis of carcinoma. Reactive atypia within glands may result from inflammation, irradiation, infarcts, and other insults to the prostate. In addition, granulomatous prostatitis is a vexing problem and caution is warranted in the interpretation of biopsy specimens in which it is found.

Variants of prostatic carcinoma

Many interesting and unusual morphologic variants of prostatic carcinoma have been identified, accounting for less than 10% of cases[49,50,52,152-164] (Fig. 67-58). It is important to recognize and accurately diagnose special variants and to understand the criteria that distinguish these from benign mimics. Unusual tumors arising in the prostate raise questions concerning tumor origin, particularily whether the tumor represents a

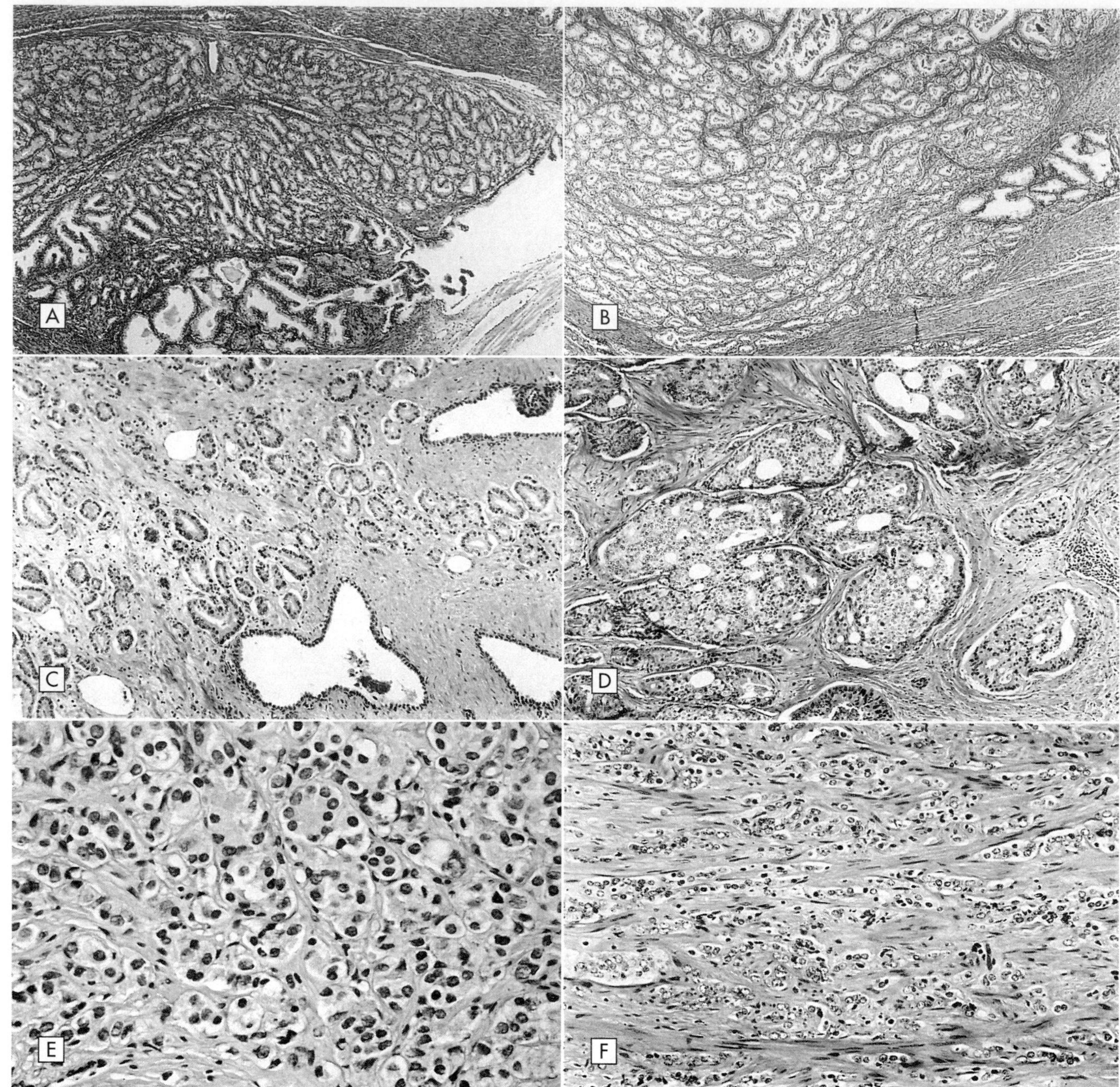

Fig. 67-56 Prostatic adenocarcinoma. **A,** Gleason pattern 1. **B,** Gleason pattern 2. **C,** Gleason pattern 3, small-gland subtype. **D,** Gleason pattern 3, cribriform subtype. **E,** Gleason pattern 4, with fused glands. **F,** Gleason pattern 5, with little or no glandular differentiation.

metastatic lesion from another site. The clinical behavior of morphologic variants may also differ from that of usual prostatic adenocarcinoma, carrying either a better or worse prognosis, but data on this are limited. The clinical and pathologic features are summarized in Table 67-16; these tumors are usually associated with typical acinar adenocarcinoma, rarely occurring in a pure form.

Diagnostic and prognostic markers

PSA is the most important, accurate, and clinically useful biochemical marker in the prostate because it is, for all practical purposes, produced by and specific to prostatic tissue. This 34 kD serine protease is manufactured by the epithelial cells and secreted into the prostatic ductal system, where it catalyzes the liquefaction of the seminal coagulum after ejaculation. Serum concentration is normally less than approximately 4.0 ng/ml but vary according to patient age[165] (Table 67-17); any process that disrupts the normal architecture of the prostate allows PSA to diffuse into the stroma, where it gains access to the blood through the microvasculature. Elevated serum PSA concentration is seen in the setting of prostatitis and BPH and transiently after biopsy, but the most clinically important ele-

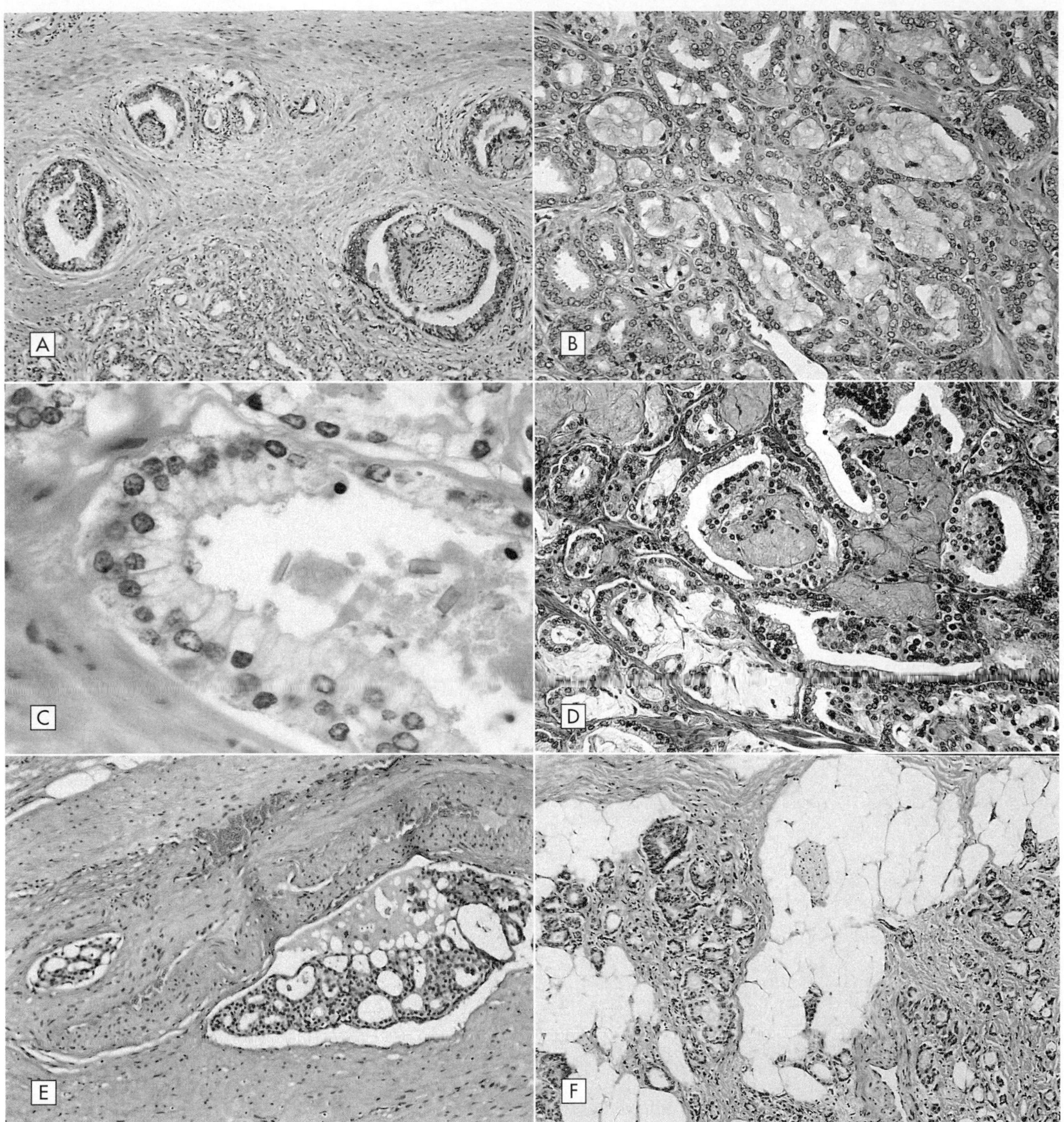

Fig. 67-57 Associated features in adenocarcinoma. **A,** Perineural invasion. **B,** Acidic mucin within lumens. **C,** Luminal crystalloids. **D,** Collagenous micronodules. **E,** Microvascular invasion. **F,** Extraprostatic extension into adipose tissue.

vation is seen in men with prostatic adenocarcinoma. Although cancer produces less PSA *per cell* than benign epithelium does, the greater number and density of malignant cells and the associated stromal disruption account for the elevated serum PSA concentration.[166] The clinical utility of PSA as a biochemical marker has been reviewed recently.[167,168] For greater accuracy PSA can be correlated with other parameters and expressed as PSA density (PSA level adjusted for prostatic volume), PSA velocity (rate of change in PSA concentration over time), and the PSA cancer density (PSA concentration adjusted for the prostatic and cancer volumes).[166-168]

The major form of measurable PSA in the serum is a complex between the PSA molecule and alpha-1-antichymotrypsin; there is a higher proportion of complexed PSA in the serum of patients with cancer than in other patients, and this serum fractionation may be diagnostically useful.[169] New microassays for serum PSA allow detectability to levels as low as 0.1 ng/ml.[170]

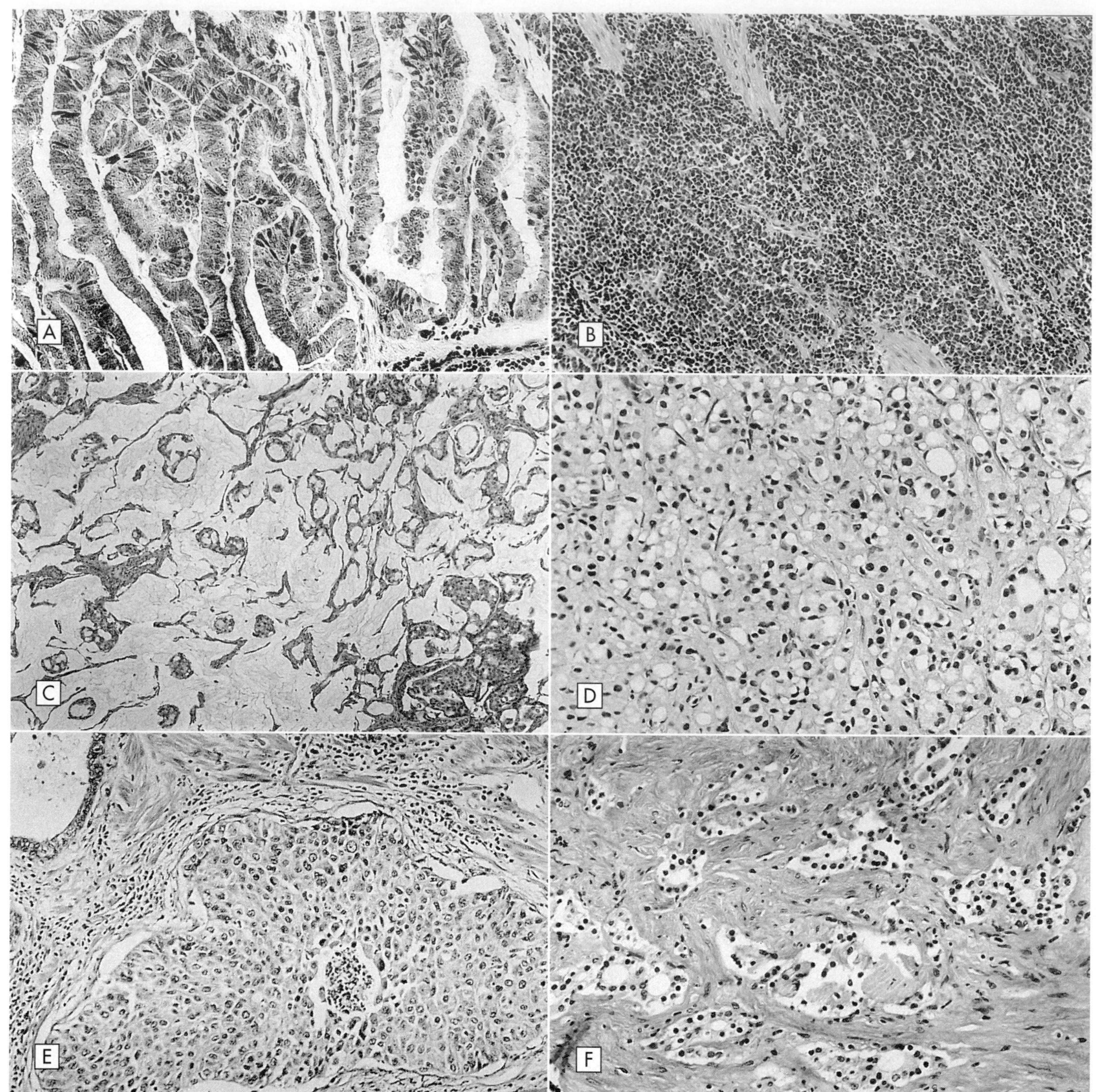

Fig. 67-58 Variants of prostatic carcinoma. **A,** Ductal (endometrioid) carcinoma. **B,** Small-cell carcinoma. **C,** Mucinous (colloid) adenocarcinoma. **D,** Signet-ring cell carcinoma. **E,** Urothelial carcinoma of the prostate. **F,** Adenocarcinoma after androgen deprivation therapy.

The degree of the immunohistochemical expression of PSA is diagnostically helpful for the pathologist in distinguishing high-grade prostate cancer from urothelial carcinoma, colonic carcinoma, granulomatous prostatitis, lymphoma, and other histologic mimics. It also allows identification of the site of tumor origin of metastatic adenocarcinoma (Fig. 67-59). PSA expression is generally greater in low-grade tumors than in high-grade tumors, but there is significant heterogeneity from cell to cell. A small number (1.6%) of poorly differentiated cancers express neither PSA nor PAP.[171,172]

PAP was at one time found to be useful for identifying the presence and extent of prostate cancer before PSA came into widespread use as a biochemical marker but has fallen into disfavor in recent years because of the inherent problems in the accuracy of its measurement, including the need for special handling because of enzyme instability, diurnal fluctuation, variation induced by prostatic digital examination and biopsy, and cross-reactivity with nonprostatic serum acid phosphatases produced by liver, bone, kidney, and blood cells. At present, the serum PAP activity has little or no clinical util-

Table 67-16 Variants of prostate adenocarcinoma

Ductal (endometrioid) adenocarcinoma
Histologic features: Florid papillary, cribriform, or solid epithelial proliferation in large periurethral prostatic ducts.
Clinical features: Often presents at an advanced stage without elevation of serum PSA level.

Small-cell, undifferentiated carcinoma (high-grade neuroendocrine carcinoma)
Histologic features: Identical to counterpart in lung and other sites.
Clinical features: Very poor prognosis, with mean survival less than 2 years; may be associated with paraneoplastic syndromes such as Cushing's syndrome, inappropriate antidiuretic hormone secretion, and others.

Mucinous (colloid) carcinoma
Histologic features: At least 25% of tumor is composed of extracellular mucin, some with extraglandular mucin and mucin lakes. Rare variant includes colonic-type carcinoma of the prostate, but this pattern is usually a result of contiguous spread from rectal cancer.
Clinical features: Similar or slightly worse than those of conventional adenocarcinoma.

Signet-ring cell carcinoma
Histologic features: Typical signet-ring cell features, with tumor cells showing PAP and PSA immunoreactivity; mucin may or may not be present; usually mixed with typical acinar adenocarcinoma.
Clinical features: Very rare in pure form; very poor prognosis.

Squamous cell carcinoma of the prostate
Histologic features: Most commonly seen as mixed adenosquamous carcinoma but may be pure squamous cell carcinoma with typical malignant features.
Clinical features: Mixed adenosquamous and pure squamous cell carcinoma pattern may appear after radiation or hormonal therapy for typical acinar adenocarcinoma. Pure squamous cell carcinoma is rare and carries a very poor prognosis; it is refractory to androgen deprivation therapy.

Sarcomatoid carcinoma of the prostate
Histologic features: Spindle cell carcinoma, usually with typical acinar carcinoma; immunohistochemical results may be positive for PSA, PAP, keratin proteins, and other epithelial markers; main differential diagnosis is carcinosarcoma, and some authors do not make this distinction.
Clinical features: Poor prognosis; death in less than 48 months

Carcinosarcoma
Histologic features: Adenocarcinoma with sarcomatous elements (for example, cartilage, bone, and smooth muscle).
Clinical features: Poor prognosis; apparently the same as sarcomatoid carcinoma.

Transitional cell carcinoma of the prostate
Histologic features: May be primary in the prostate or prostatic urethra but is usually secondary to bladder involvement. Tumor may be in situ or invasive within the prostate; look for pagetoid spread, which rarely can extend along the ejaculatory ducts through the prostate to the seminal vesicles.
Clinical features: Unfavorable prognosis; important to distinguish from adenocarcinoma because tumor is refractory to androgen deprivation therapy.

Adenoid basal cell tumor (adenoid cystic carcinoma or basal cell carcinoma)
Histologic features: Nests of basaloid round to oval cells, often with a cribriform pattern; look for luminal mucin and eosinophilic basement membrane-like material.
Clinical features: Very rare, with no definite metastatic tumors or deaths.

Lymphoepithelioma–like carcinoma
Histologic features: Islands of closely packed glands set in a dense lymphocytic stroma.
Clinical features: Only one reported case; unknown prognostic significance.

Adenocarcinoma after androgen deprivation therapy
Histologic features: Shrunken, closely packed glands with optically clear cytoplasm and inconspicuous nucleoli.
Clinical features: Unknown; no long-term follow-up studies of this histologic pattern.

PAP, Prostatic acid phosphatase; *PSA,* prostate-specific antigen.

ity, but this marker is valuable for immunohistochemical staining when used in combination with stains for PSA.[173]

Androgen receptors are present within both androgen-responsive and androgen-unresponsive cells in prostate cancer specimens. These receptors are widely distributed in the basal cell layer of the normal prostate and in BPH[174] and can be identified in localized and metastatic prostatic carcinoma.[175] The percentage of cancer cells with androgen receptors cannot be used to predict the time to progression after androgen deprivation therapy,[176] but greater heterogeneity in the androgen receptor immunoreactivity was seen in malignant tissue from patients who responded poorly to therapy.[175]

Neuroendocrine cells may be present in large numbers in cancer. The claim that this indicates a poor prognosis, perhaps as a result of insensitivity to hormonal growth regulation,[177] has been refuted.[6,178,179] The progressive loss of markers of neuroendocrine differentiation with increasing grades of PIN and cancer indicates that cell differentiation and regulatory control are progressively impaired with advancing stages of prostatic carcinogenesis.[8,9,180] Early studies indicated that neuroendocrine differentiation was present in only a minority of cases of adenocarcinoma, but recent studies have identified at least focal staining in most if not all cases, with variable findings resulting from the use of different fixatives, a variable

Table 67-17 Age-adjusted reference ranges for prostate-specific antigen

Age (yr)	PSA range (ng/ml)*	Age (yr)	PSA range (ng/ml)*
40	2.0	60	3.8
41	2.1	61	4.0
42	2.2	62	4.1
43	2.3	63	4.2
44	2.3	64	4.4
45	2.4	65	4.5
46	2.5	66	4.6
47	2.6	67	4.7
48	2.6	68	4.9
49	2.7	69	5.1
50	2.8	70	3.3
51	2.9	71	3.4
52	3.0	72	3.6
53	3.1	73	3.8
54	3.2	74	6.0
55	3.3	75	6.2
56	3.4	76	6.4
57	3.5	77	6.6
58	3.6	78	6.8
59	3.7	79	7.0

From Oesterling JE, Jacobsen SJ, Chute CG et al: *JAMA* 270:860, 1993.
*From 0.0 to the specified value.
PSA, Prostate-specific antigen.

number of sections stained, and a smaller number of antibodies employed.[8,9] Aprikian et al[6] found neuroendocrine cells in 77% of the specimens of untreated prostate cancers, 60% of the cases of hormone-refractory cancers, and 52% of the metastatic lesions, with a small number of dispersed positive cells in each of these cases. Berner et al[179] found no difference in neuron-specific enolase expression in pre-treatment and posttreatment specimens from 47 patients with hormone-resistant prostate cancer.[179] "Paneth cell–like metaplasia," present in 10% of the cases of prostatic adenocarcinoma, represents neuroendocrine differentiation, and the recommended term for this finding is "neuroendocrine cells with large eosinophilic granules."[5] Neuroendocrine differentiation is downregulated in prostatic carcinogenesis, with intermediate levels of expression in PIN compared with the level of expression in normal cells and carcinoma.[180] Further studies are needed to evaluate the function and prognostic utility of neuroendocrine cells in the evaluation of the normal and neoplastic prostate.

Peptide growth factors appear to control the development of normal and neoplastic prostatic epithelium by acting as paracrine mediators of epithelial–stromal interaction and growth.[181-184] The epidermal growth factor (EGF) family of peptides includes EGF, transforming growth factor–alpha (TGF-α) and other factors that act through the same transmembrane glycoprotein receptor and tyrosine kinase. Prostate cancer cells synthesize TGF-α, and this stimulates epithelial and fibroblastic proliferation. The transforming growth factor–beta (TGF-β) family of peptides, including TGF-β_1 and TGF-β_2, appear to be regulators of cell differentiation and proliferation.[182,185-187] Expression of the TGF-beta receptor appears to be under negative androgenic regulation, indicating that TGF-β may play a role in cell death after androgen deprivation. The TGF-β–binding protein is produced in benign and

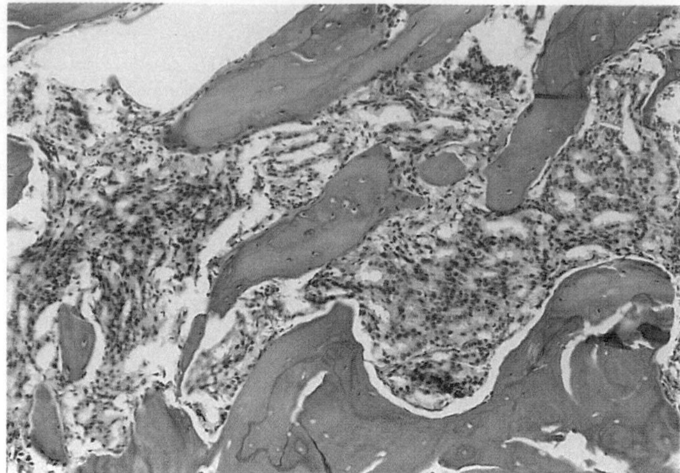

Fig. 67-59 Metastatic adenocarcinoma to the thoracic spine.

hyperplastic tissue but not in malignant tissue.[187] The growth factors operating in the context of prostate cancer have recently been reviewed.[181]

There are numerous other investigational tumor markers that may find use in the evaluation of prostate cancer.[188,189] **Prostate-associated glycoprotein complex,** a sialic acid–based group of glycoproteins identified by the monoclonal antibody TURP-27, appears to be a differentiation antigen, expressed in only 10% of normal prostatic epithelial cells but in up to 100% of BPH and malignant cells, including metastastic cancer. **Prostate mucin antigen,** a high-molecular-weight, non–sialic acid glycoprotein identified by the monoclonal antibody PD41, is expressed only in PIN and prostate cancer cells but not in benign or hyperplastic epithelial cells; maximal expression is seen in poorly differentiated cancer tissue and metastatic lesions. The antigen recognized by the monoclonal antibody **7E11-C5** is a mixture of unique glycoproteins expressed on normal and neoplastic prostatic tissues, with the greatest intensity seen in malignant and metastatic tumors. This antigen is not affected by androgen deprivation therapy; clinical trials are currently under way to evaluate the utility of this marker for the purposes of radioimmunodetection and radioimmunotherapy of prostate cancer.

Molecular biology of prostate cancer

DNA content analysis of prostate cancer by flow cytometry and static-image analysis may provide independent prognostic information that supplements that furnished by histopathologic examination. Patients with diploid tumors have a more favorable outcome than those with aneuploid tumors; for example, among patients with lymph node metastatic tumors treated with radical prostatectomy and androgen deprivation therapy, those with diploid tumors may survive 20 years or more, whereas those with aneuploid tumors die within 5 years[190] (Fig. 67-60). However, the ploidy pattern of prostate cancer is often heterogeneous, creating potential problems with sampling errors. At an international DNA Cytometry Consensus Conference, the literature was reviewed and participants concluded that the clinical significance and biologic basis of DNA ploidy need further investigation.[191]

Allelic loss is a common finding in prostatic adenocarcinoma, present in more than 50% of cases on chromosomes 8p,

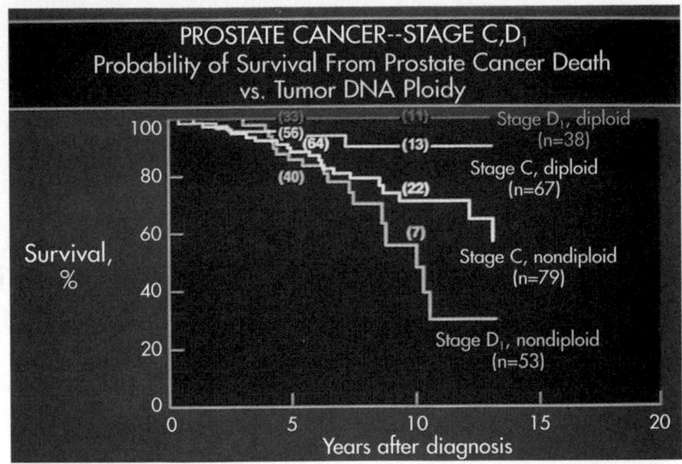

Fig. 67-60 Cause-specific survival related to tumor stage and DNA ploidy of patients with clinical stages C and D1 prostatic adenocarcinoma after radical prostatectomy. Numbers in parentheses denote number of patients at risk. (From Nativ O, Winkler HZM, Raz Y et al: *Mayo Clin Proc* 64:911, 1989.

10q, and 16q.[192-195] One or more tumor suppressor genes appear to be present on chromosome 8p, which may be involved in carcinogenesis.[193,194] Allelic loss appears to be more common in high-grade tumors.[193] Fluorescent in situ hybridization studies using centromere-specific probes for chromosomes 7, 8, 11, and 12 have shown that gains of chromosomes 7 and 8 are consistent numerical alterations and may be markers of tumor aggressiveness, and hence predictors of the prognosis.[196]

The tumor suppressor gene *p53,* located on chromosome 17p, is inactivated in as many as 25% of the cases of advanced prostate cancer, but this is rare in early cancers, indicating that it may play a role in the late progression stage.[197-199] Another tumor suppressor gene **DCC** shows allelic deletion and loss of expression in 45% of cases, indicating that it is a frequent feature of prostate cancer.[200] Loss of expression of the **retinoblastoma gene** on chromosome 13q is seen in a minority of patients with prostate cancer, usually in advanced stages.[201] Activated oncogenes such as *ras* appear to be infrequent in early prostate cancers.[202] Overexpression of **c-*erbB*-2** (HER-2/*neu*), present in normal basal cells and in the setting of PIN and many cancers, was found to be an independent predictor of poor prognosis in some studies but not in others.[203]

Clinical and pathologic staging

The staging of prostate cancer involves determination of the anatomic extent and burden of tumor based on the best available data. Two major systems are currently used: the modified American system and the TNM system (primary tumor, T; regional lymph node, N; and metastases, M)[204,205] (Table 67-18). These two systems are similar, although the TNM system contains a greater number of subdivisions for most stages. The TNM classification, revised in 1992, is considered the international standard for prostate cancer staging. Both systems stratify patients according to the method of tumor detection, separating nonpalpable "incidental" prostate cancer detected during TURP from clinically benign prostatic hyperplasia and palpable cancer detected by digital rectal examination. This reliance on the palpability of the tumor is unique among the organ staging systems and is hampered by the low sensitivity, low specificity, and low positive predictive value of digital rectal examination.[206] These staging systems also recognize nonpalpable tumors detected by an elevated serum PSA concentration or abnormal TRUS image.[207] Current staging is limited by a considerable level of clinical understaging (as much as 59%) and overstaging (as much as 5%), as shown by comparison with the results from the pathologic examination of resected specimens.[205]

Imaging studies that could assess tumor volume and extent would be invaluable for clinical staging, but the current utility of such methods is limited; for example, the accuracy of TRUS in correctly identifying extraprostatic extension is 63%,[208] that of body coil magnetic resonance imaging (MRI) is 71%,[208] and that of endorectal and surface coil MRI is 83%.[209]

Stage T1 (A) carcinoma, defined as incidentally detected and clinically inapparent tumor, is inadequately staged by TURP alone. Only 28% of T1 (A) carcinomas are detected by this technique, and 60% of patients with T1a (A1) cancers will be found to have residual tumor on repeat TURP, with upstaging of tumor in at least 26%. In 92%, residual cancer, as determined by examination of radical prostatectomy specimens, is at the apex or at the periphery of the gland, regions inaccessible to the TURP procedure.[210,211] The subdivision into T1a and T1b seems justified because the progression rates differ substantially (8% and 63%, respectively).[29]

Thorough examination of radical prostatectomy specimens is critical, allowing the pathologic stage as well as the Gleason score, tumor volume, and surgical margin status to be accurately determined.[212-217] The pathologic stage is assessed by determining whether there has been capsular perforation, seminal vesicle invasion, and lymph node metastasis. Seminal vesicle involvement by prostate cancer correlates with Gleason score, tumor volume, and capsular perforation and is predictive of a poor prognosis. Pelvic lymph node involvement by carcinoma is also an adverse prognostic sign.

The usual sites of metastasis of prostatic adenocarcinoma are the pelvic lymph nodes, bone (chiefly osteoblastic metastases), and the lungs[218] (Fig. 67-61). However, many unusual sites of metastasis have been described, including the kidneys, breast, brain, and other sites. Comparison of the metastatic pattern seen for men in Japan and America has revealed no important differences.[219,220] De La Monte[219] found no significant difference in the number of metastatic sites between patients who received estrogen therapy and those who did not, although patients who received estrogens had more frequent metastatic tumors to the central nervous system. Cluster analysis of the metastatic tumors revealed a subset of predominantly black men who suffer distant metastasis without much local spread of the tumor.

Treatment

The treatment of prostate cancer remains controversial, consisting of one or more of four major options: radical prostatectomy, radiation therapy, androgen deprivation therapy, and active surveillance (watchful waiting); there is currently no role for conventional chemotherapy. The choice of treatment is based on the patient's age, health, and life expectancy; the clinical stage of the cancer; the serum PSA concentration; and the tumor grade. The clinical management of prostate cancer is addressed in a recent review.[221]

Table 67-18 Comparison of staging systems for prostate cancer

Type	American system	TNM†
Nonpalpable cancer		
≤5% of TURP tissue*	A1	T1a
>5% of TURP tissue*	A2	T1b
Cancer detected by biopsy (for example, elevated PSA level)	B0	T1c
Palpable or visible cancer clinically confined within the capsule		
≤Half of one lobe	B1	T2a
>Half of one lobe, but not both lobes	B1	T2b
Both lobes	B2	T2c
Cancer with local extracapsular extension		
Unilateral	C1	T3a
Bilateral	C1	T3b
Seminal vesicle invasion	C2	T3c
Invasion of bladder neck, rectum, or external sphincter	C2	T4a
Invasion of levator muscle or pelvic wall	C2	T4b
Metastatic cancer		
Single regional lymph node, ≤2 cm in greatest dimension	D1	N1‡
Single regional lymph node, 2-5 cm, or multiple regional lymph nodes, ≤5 cm	D1	N2
Single regional lymph node, >5 cm	D1	N3
Distant metastasis	D2	M1
Nonregional lymph node(s)	D2	M1a
Bone(s)	D2	M1b
Other sites	D2	M1c

PSA, Prostate-specific antigen; *TURP,* transurethral prostatectomy.
*Different definitions exist for substaging A1 and A2 cancers.
†N_0 or N_x M_0 for T1-T4.
‡*Nx,* Regional lymph nodes are not assessable; M_x, distant metastatis is not assessable.

It is difficult to compare precisely the efficacy of different treatments and the outcomes in victims of prostate cancer because of the significant clinical staging error, the paucity of rigorous prospective and randomized clinical trials, and the lengthy follow-up period needed to obtain results of treatment for a relatively slow growing tumor such as prostate cancer. The 10-year cancer-specific survival rate for all stages of cancer is about 51%, with an estimated "cure" rate of 32%[74] (Table 67-19). Men with clinically localized cancer can expect the most favorable outcome. The risk of long-term progression of untreated stage T1a (A1) cancer varies from 8% to 37%, with the risk of progression increasing with additional years of follow-up; the survival rate at 10 years is 95%, similar to the age-specific survival rate, prompting the suggestion that treatment for cancer at this stage may be unnecessary. Patients with larger organ-confined cancers (T1b and T2) and those with local extraprostatic extension (T3 and T4) show progressively lower survival and "cure" rates, but the worst outcomes are observed in patients with cancer that has metastasized to regional lymph nodes (T1-4N+M0) (40% survival at 10 years) and distant organs (M+) (10% survival at 10 years). There are insufficient data available for stage T1c (B0) cancer, to allow determination of outcome because it has only recently been described.[207]

Other tumors and miscellaneous lesions

Benign soft-tissue tumors and tumorlike lesions

Several benign stromal tumors and tumorlike proliferations arise in the prostate. Although most benign stromal tumors are variants of BPH, there are two recently described lesions with overlapping histologic features that mimic sarcoma: **postoperative spindle cell nodules** and **inflammatory pseudotumor.**[222,223] Postoperative spindle cell nodules represent a reactive process occurring in the genitourinary tract after instrumentation. The nodules are usually small, measuring from 5 mm to 4 cm in diameter, and rarely produce symptoms. Histologically, postoperative spindle cell nodules resemble nodular fasciitis, characterized by a poorly circumscribed proliferation of spindle cells interspersed with abundant small blood vessels and chronic inflammation. Mitotic figures range in number from 1 to 15 per ten high-power fields, but atypical forms are not identified. These tumors are benign and do not recur. **Inflammatory pseudotumor** (pseudosarcomatous fibromyxoid tumor or atypical fibromyxoid tumor) was first found in the urinary bladder, and about 35 cases in the male genitourinary system have been reported.[223] Although histologically similar to postoperative spindle cell nodules, inflammatory pseudotumor arises spontaneously, unrelated to previous instrumentation. This spindle cell proliferation is variably cellular, usually with a prominent myxoid stroma, and has infiltrative borders (Fig. 67-62). Mitotic figures are present, and bizarre straplike and tadpole-shaped cells may be seen. Immunohistochemical and ultrastructural studies show the cells to have features of fibroblasts and myofibroblasts. Inflammatory pseudotumor rarely recurs, and surgical excision appears adequate; metastasis has not been reported. Clinical recurrence of a tumor originally classified as inflammatory pseudotumor strongly indicates the possibility of a underdiagnosis of sarcoma.

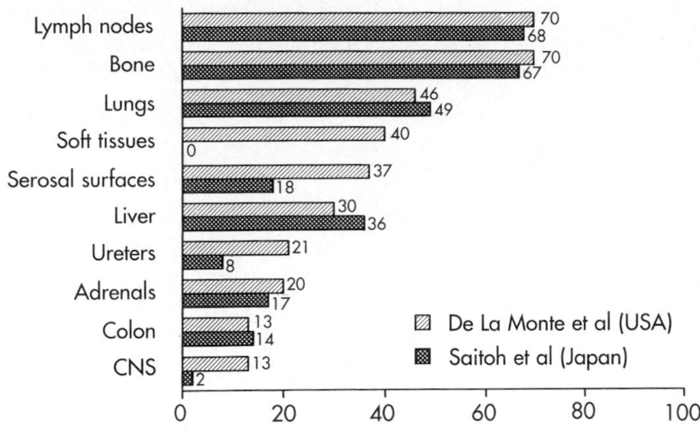

Fig. 67-61 Ten most common sites of metastasis of prostatic adenocarcinoma. (From Bostwick DG, Eble JN: *J Urol Pathol* 1:193, 1993.)

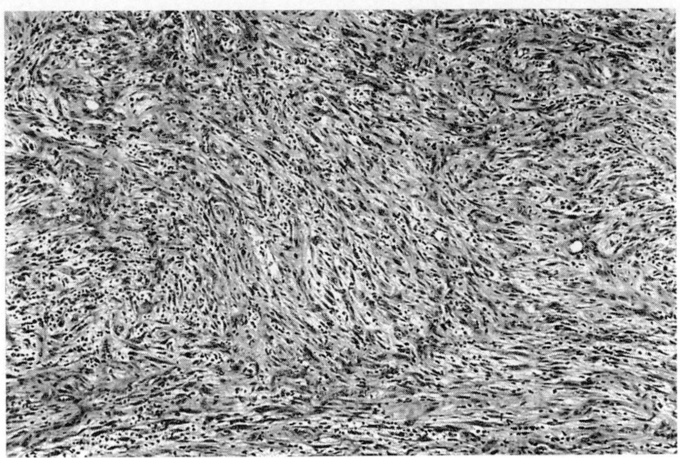

Fig. 67-62 Inflammatory pseudotumor of the prostate.

Table 67-19 Prostate cancer: diagnosis, risk of death, and cure rate by clinical stage

Percentage of patients	Stage	Prognosis	10-year cancer-specific survival rate (%)	Estimated cure rate (%)
10	T 1a (A1)	Treatment "unnecessary"	95	85
30	T 1b-T2 (A2-B2)	Often curable	80	65
10	T 3-4 (C1-2)	Occasionally curable	60	25
20	N+ (D1)	Rarely curable	40	<5
50	M+ (D2)	Incurable	10	<1
100	All stages		51	32
	excluding T1a (stage A1)		45	25

From Scardino PT, et al: 1992.

Melanotic lesions

Melanin in the prostatic stroma, known as **prostatic melanosis,** is rare and should be distinguished from **blue nevus,** an equally rare lesion resembling its cutaneous counterpart. The latter is characterized by an accumulation of dense brown melanin within fusiform dendritic bipolar cells.[224,225] **Malignant melanoma** may become clinically apparent in the prostate gland but is invariably a metastatic lesion or results from contiguous spread from neighboring viscera.

Sarcomas

Sarcomas of the prostate are rare and account for less than 0.1% of the primary prostatic neoplasms. One third of the cases occur in children under 10 years of age, and most of these are rhabdomyosarcomas. Leiomyosarcoma is the most common sarcoma in adults and accounts for 26% of all prostate sarcomas. Other rare sarcomas found in the prostate include malignant phyllodes tumors, fibrosarcoma, osteosarcoma, malignant fibrous histiocytoma, angiosarcoma, chondrosarcoma, neurofibrosarcoma, and undifferentiated sarcoma. Sarcomatoid carcinoma, carcinosarcoma, and metaplastic carcinoma, although not truly mesenchymal, must be included in the differential diagnosis of pleomorphic spindle cell neoplasms showing necrosis and significant mitotic activity. The recognition of the transition of carcinoma to sarcomatous differentiation and the findings yielded by immunostaining with cytokeratin, PSA, and PAP may be helpful.

The incidence of **rhabdomyosarcoma** of the prostate peaks between birth and 6 years of age, although rare cases in men over 50 years of age have been reported.[226] Combination chemotherapy together with surgery and radiotherapy has led to an improvement in patient outcome in the past two decades, with the median survival time increasing from 4 months to 3 years. The survival rate is better for children than for older patients.

Leiomyosarcoma of the prostate presents as a large, bulky mass that replaces most of the prostate and periprostatic tissues (Fig. 67-63). The mean patient age is 59 years, with a range of 40 to 71 years.[227] The histologic findings are typical of those of leiomyosarcoma at other sites; although the criteria for distinguishing between leiomyoma and low-grade leiomyosarcoma in the prostate have not been precisely defined, they are probably similar to those for leiomyosarcoma in other organs, including the degree of cellularity and cytologic anaplasia, the mitotic activity, the presence or absence of necrosis and vascular invasion, and size. Local recurrence and distant metastasis are frequent in patients with these tumors, and the prognosis for survival is poor.

Lymphoma and leukemia

Malignant lymphoma and **leukemia** are rare, involving the prostate gland either primarily or as secondary site of involve-

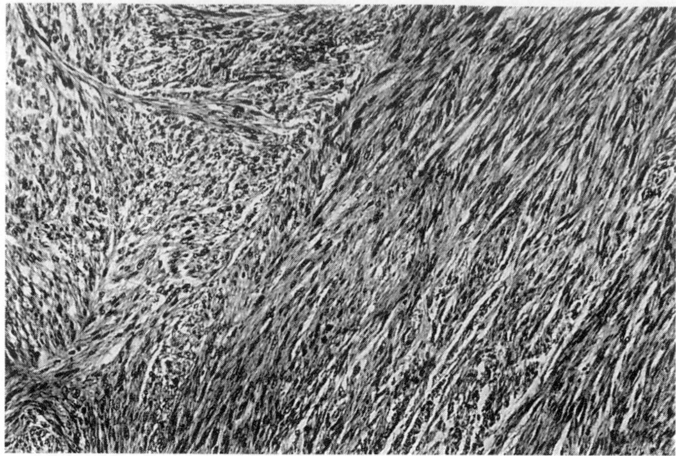

Fig. 67-63 High-grade leiomyosarcoma of the prostate.

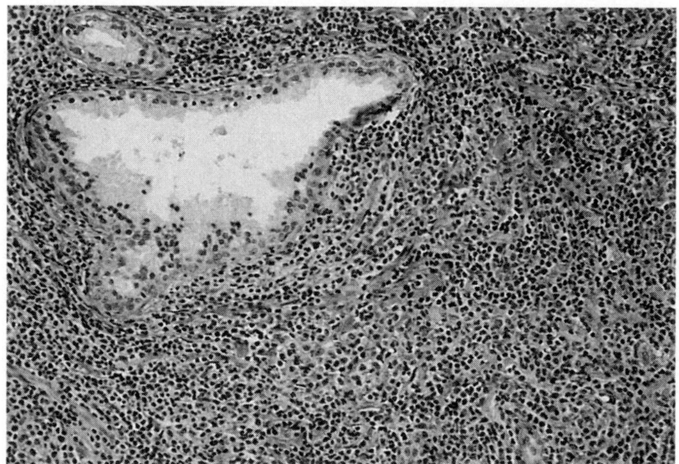

Fig. 67-64 Chronic lymphocytic leukemia involving the prostate.

ment of systemic or disseminated lymphoma or leukemia.[228,229] Criteria for primary lymphoma of the prostate include: (1) symptoms attributable to prostatic enlargement; (2) lymphoma chiefly involving the prostate with or without involvement of adjacent tissues; and (3) lack of liver, spleen, lymph node and peripheral blood involvement within 1 month of diagnosis.[228] Patients are usually older men (mean age, 61 years), and urinary obstructive symptoms are the presenting features. These include urgency, frequency, acute urinary retention, urinary tract infections, or hematuria, or a combination of these symptoms. Grossly the prostate gland is diffusely enlarged, nontender, and firm or rubbery on palpation. Microscopically the infiltrate may be diffuse or patchy within the stroma with distinctive preservation of the prostatic glands; by contrast, granulomatous prostatitis causes glandular destruction. The most frequent lymphomas are diffuse non-Hodgkin's lymphoma of small cleaved-cell, large-cell, and mixed-cell types. **Chronic lymphocytic leukemia** is the most common leukemic process involving the prostate, with more than a hundred cases reported (Fig. 67-64). The prognosis for patients with lymphoma and leukemia involving the prostate is usually poor regardless of their age, the stage of the tumor, the histologic classification, the type of involvement (primary or secondary), and the type of therapy employed. More than 60% of the patients die of the disease, although survival of up to 10 years is possible with combination chemotherapy.

SEMINAL VESICLES

Normal seminal vesicles

The seminal vesicles arise as outpouchings of the lower mesonephric ducts during the thirteenth week of development. They are bounded by the prostate distally, the base of the bladder anteriorly, and Denonvilliers' fascia and the rectum posteriorly. Their anatomic distribution in this region is variable, and they are occasionally found within the capsule of the prostate gland. The seminal vesicles may be palpable on digital rectal examination and when intimately associated with the prostate may be mistaken for prostatic nodularity or induration. As much as 20% of the prostate biopsy specimens obtained for the evaluation of nodularity contain fragments of seminal vesicle epithelium, a potential source of diagnostic confusion. In adults the seminal vesicles are approximately 6 cm long and 2 cm wide, although there is wide variation in size and shape.

The **mucosa** displays complex papillary folds and irregular convoluted lumens, and the lining consists of a nonciliated, pseudostratified tall columnar cell epithelium (Fig. 67-65). The cells are predominantly secretory and contain microvesicular lipid droplets and characteristic lipofuscin pigment granules. The pigment is golden brown and refractile, increasing in amount with age. Like the prostatic epithelial cells, these cells express androgen receptors. Secretory products include glycoproteins, fructose, prostaglandins, and ascorbic acid. As much as 85% of the seminal fluid (normally 2 to 5 ml) originates in the seminal vesicles. The **muscular wall** consists of a thick circumferential coat of smooth muscle and is thought to serve a contractile function. The **ducts** of the seminal vesicles merge with the vas deferens on each side to form the ejaculatory ducts, and they enter the central zone of the prostate and converge before terminating at the verumontanum and the prostatic urethra.

Age-associated changes

There is progressive flattening of the epithelial lining cells of the seminal vesicules with advancing age. Tall columnar cells account for most of the mucosa in young men but constitute only 50% in men in the fifth decade of life and 2% in men in the eighth decade, replaced over time by flattened cuboidal cells. With advancing patient age, the stroma of the seminal vesicles becomes hyalinized and fibrotic. Pronounced **cytologic atypia** accompanies the flattening of the epithelium, with the emergence of "monstrous" cells in up to 75% of the specimens from older men[230] (Fig. 67-66). These nuclear abnormalities are probably the result of degenerative changes or hormonal influences and are not observed in men under the age of 20 years. When encountered in needle biopsy specimens, such "pseudomalignant" cytologic atypia may lead to a mistaken diagnosis of prostatic carcinoma. Difficulty may also be encountered in the cytologic evaluation of prostatic fluids because these cells are frequently shed intact into the vesicular lumens, although the distinctive lipochrome pigment they contain is helpful in identifying them. Aneuploidy is found in 6.7% of seminal vesicles.[231] Consequently,

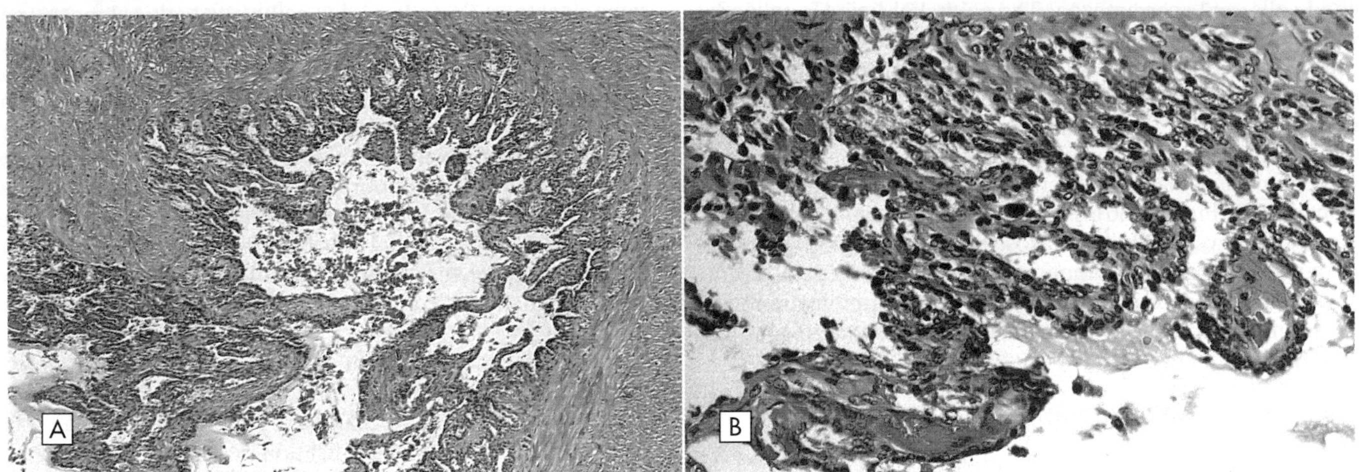

Fig. 67-65 Normal seminal vesicle epithelium. **A,** Low-power view. **B,** High-power view showing distinctive lipofuscin pigment and atypical cells.

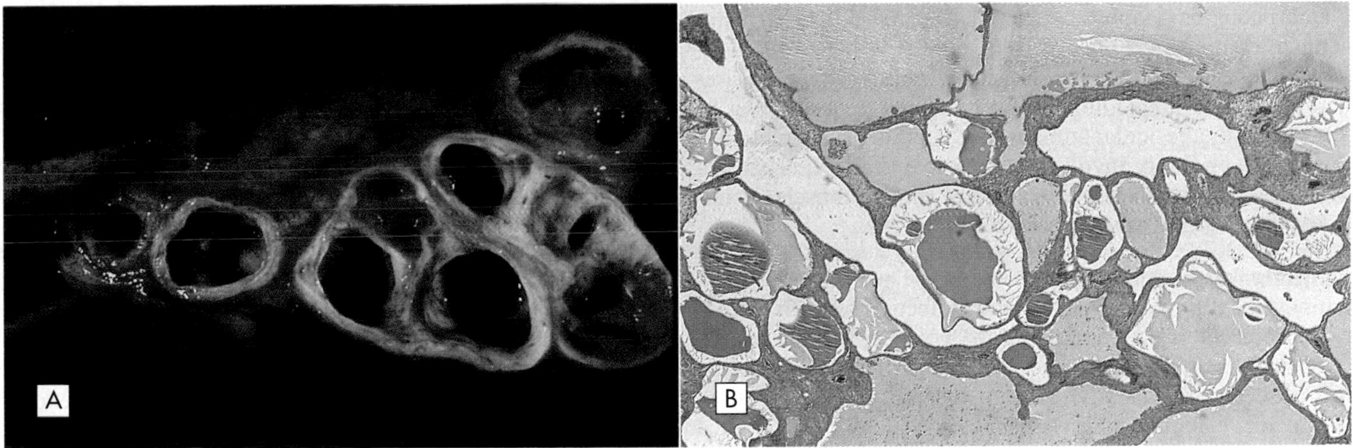

Fig. 67-66 Cystadenoma of the seminal vesicles. **A,** Gross appearance. **B,** Microscopic findings.

care must be taken to prevent the contamination of prostatic cancer specimens by seminal vesicular tissue obtained for DNA analysis.

Within the interstitium of the muscular wall of the seminal vesicles, small 15- to 20-μm eosinophilic **stromal hyaline bodies** can be observed. These round to oval structures probably represent hyaline degeneration of smooth muscle fibers, and special stains indicate smooth muscle derivation; transitional forms can be seen arising from smooth muscle cells.

Seminal vesicular cells are found as contaminants of female cervical smears in 10% of specimens with spermatozoa and may cause diagnostic confusion.[232]

Congenital and acquired malformations, including cysts

Malformations of the seminal vesicles are frequently observed in association with the abnormal development of other mesonephric derivatives, although isolated **hypoplasia, agenesis, duplication, stricture, and cyst formation** are observed. **Unilateral absence** may be associated with ipsilateral renal agenesis and infertility.[233] **Bilateral dilatation** or **absence** of the seminal vesicles is sometimes observed in patients with cystic fibrosis, reportedly resulting from failure of development. Maldevelopment of the ureteric bud results in **ureteral ectopy,** with the ureters terminating in the seminal vesicles, prostatic urethra, vas deferens, epididymis, or ejaculatory ducts.

Seminal vesicle cysts are rare and may be congenital or acquired. Symptoms are vague and include perineal pain during ejaculation or defecation, dysuria, urinary retention, and recurrent epididymitis. **Congenital cysts** are commonly seen in association with ipsilateral renal agenesis and ureteral ectopia or agenesis.[233,234] The ureteric bud is closely associated with the mesonephric duct during embryogenesis, accounting for the development of such paired anomalies. Patients with congenital cysts range in age from 18 to 41 years at the time of diagnosis, the period of maximal sexual and reproductive activity. The cysts are usually unilateral and unilocular and located lateral to the midline. Enlargement results from insufficient drainage with the accumulation of seminal fluid. **Acquired cysts** are usually associated with inflammation and obstruction of the ejaculatory ducts and seminal vesicles. These fluctuant cysts may be palpable on digital rectal examination and contain red blood cells, white

39. Sebo TJ, Bostwick DG, Farrow GM et al: Prostatic xanthoma: a mimic of prostatic adenocarcinoma, *Hum Pathol* 25:386, 1994.
40. Presti B, Weidner N: Granulomatous prostatitis and poorly differentiated adenocarcinoma: their distinction with the use of immunohistochemical methods, *Am J Clin Pathol* 95:330. 1991.
41. Mies C, Balogh K, Stadecker M. Palisading prostate granulomas following surgery, *Am J Surg Pathol* 8:217, 1984.
42. Koplovic J, Rivkind A, Sherman Y: Granulomatous prostatitis with vasculitis: a sequel of transurethral prostatic resection, *Arch Pathol Lab Med* 108:732, 1984.
43. Oates RD, Stilmant MM, Fredlund MC et al: Granulomatous prostatitis following bacillus Calmette-Guérin immunotherapy of bladder cancer, *J Urol* 140:751, 1988.

Benign prostatic hyperplasia

44. *National hospital discharge data tapes*. Hyattsville, Md, 1987, National Center for Health Statistics.
45. Bostwick DG, Cooner WH, Denis L et al: The association of benign prostatic hyperplasia and cancer of the prostate, *Cancer* 70:291, 1992.
46. Guess HA: Benign prostatic hyperplasia: antecedents and natural history, *Epidemiol Rev* 14:131, 1992.
47. McNeal JE: The pathobiology of nodular hyperplasia. In Bostwick DG, editor: *Pathology of the prostate*, New York, 1990, Churchill Livingstone.
48. Shapiro E, Becich MJ, Hartanto V et al: The relative proportion of stromal and epithelial hyperplasia is related to the development of symptomatic benign prostatic hyperplasia, *J Urol* 147:1293, 1992.
49. Grignon DJ, Ro JY, Ordonez NG et al: Basal cell hyperplasia, adenoid basal cell tumor, and adenoid cystic carcinoma of the prostate gland: an immunohistochemical study, *Human Pathol* 19:1425, 1988.
50. Devaraj LT, Bostwick DG: Atypical basal cell hyperplasia of the prostate: immunophenotypic profile and proposed classification of basal cell proliferations, *Am J Surg Pathol* 17:645, 1993.
51. Epstein JI, Armas OA: Atypical basal cell hyperplasia of the prostate, *Am J Surg Pathol* 16:1205, 1992.
52. Young RH, Frierson HF Jr, Mills SE et al: Adenoid cystic-like tumor of the prostate gland: a report of two cases and review of the literature on "adenoid cystic carcinoma" of the prostate, *Am J Clin Pathol* 89:49, 1988.
53. Ayala AG, Srigley JR, Ro JY et al: Clear cell cribriform hyperplasia of prostate, *Am J Surg Pathol* 10:665, 1986.
54. Frauenhoffer E, Ro JY, El-Naggar AK et al: Clear cell cribriform hyperplasia of the prostate: immunohistochemical and flow cytometric study, *Am J Clin Pathol* 95:446, 1991.
55. Young RH, Clement PB: Sclerosing adenosis of the prostate, *Arch Pathol Lab Med* 11:363, 1987.
56. Jones EC, Clement PB, Young RH: Sclerosing adenosis of the prostate gland: a clinicopathologic and immunohistochemical study of 11 cases, *Am J Surg Pathol* 15:1171, 1991.
57. Collina G, Botticelli AR, Martinelli AM et al: Sclerosing adenosis of the prostate: report of three cases with electronmicroscopy and immunohistochemical study, *Histopathol* 20:505, 1992.
58. Grignon DJ, Ro JY, Srigley JR et al: Sclerosing adenosis of the prostate gland: a lesion showing myoepithelial differentiation, *Am J Surg Pathol* 16:383, 1992.
59. Srigley JR, Dardick I, Hartwick RWJ et al: Basal epithelial cells of human prostate gland are not myoepithelial cells: a comparative immunohistochemical and ultrastructral study with human salivary gland, *Am J Surg Pathol* 136:957, 1990.
60. Leong SS, Vogt PF, Yu GM: Atypical stroma with muscle hyperplasia of prostate, *Urology* 31:163, 1988.
61. Eble JN, Tejada E: Prostatic stromal hyperplasia with bizarre nuclei, *Arch Pathol Lab Med* 115:87, 1991.
62. Reese JH, Lombard CM, Krone K et al: Phyllodes type of atypical hyperplasia: a report of 3 new cases, *J Urol* 138:623, 1987.
63. Ito H, Ito M, Mitsuhata N et al: Phyllodes tumor of the prostate: a case report, *Jpn J Clin Oncol* 19:299, 1989.
64. Bostwick DG, Halling AC, Jones EC et al: Prostatic phyllodes tumors: report of 7 cases with follow-up, (submitted).
65. Manivel C, Shenoy BV, Wick MR et al: Cystosarcoma phyllodes of the prostate, *Arch Pathol Lab Med* 110:534, 1986.
66. Lopez-Beltran A, Gaeta JF, Huben R, Croghan GA: Malignant phyllodes tumor of the prostate, *Urology* 35:164, 1990.
67. Young JF, Jensen PE, Wiley CA: Malignant phyllodes tumor of the prostate: a case report with immunohistochemical and ultrastructural studies, *Arch Pathol Lab Med* 116:296, 1992.

Prostate cancer

68. Wingo PA, Tong T, Bolden S: Cancer statistics, 1995, *CA Cancer J Clin* 45:8, 1995.

EPIDEMIOLOGY

69. Seidman H, Mushinski MH, Gelb SK, Silverberg E: Probabilities of eventually developing or dying of cancer—United States, 1985, *CA Cancer J Clin* 35:36, 1985.
70. Miller BA, Ries LAG, Hankey BF et al: *Cancer statistics review: 1973-1989*, Bethesda, Md, 1992, National Cancer Institute, NIH publication 92-2789.
71. Silverberg E: Statistical and epidemiologic data on urologic cancer, *Cancer* 60:692, 1987.
72. Morra MN, Das S: Prostate cancer: epidemiology and etiology. In Das S, Crawford ED, editors: *Cancer of the prostate*, New York, 1993, Marcel Dekker.
73. Nomura AMY, Kolonel LN: Prostate cancer: a current perspective, *Am J Epidemiol* 13:200, 1991.
74. Scardino PT: Early detection of prostate cancer, *Urol Clin North Am* 16:635, 1989.

PATHOGENESIS

75. Carter BS, Bova GS, Beaty TH et al: Hereditary prostate cancer: epidemiologic and clinical features, *J Urol* 150:797, 1993.
76. Cannon L, Bishop D, Skolnick M et al: Genetic epidemiology of prostate cancer in the Utah Mormon genealogy, *Cancer Surv* 1:47, 1982.
77. Steinberg G, Carter B, Beaty T et al: Family history and the risk of prostate cancer, *Prostate* 17:337, 1990.
78. Keetch D, Catalona W: Familial aspects of prostate cancer: a case-control review, *J Urol* 145:250A, 1991.
79. Spitz M, Currier R, Fueger J et al: Familial patterns of prostate cancer: a case-control analysis, *J Urol* 146:1305, 1991.
80. Pienta KJ, Esper PS: Is dietary fat a risk factor for prostate cancer? *J Natl Cancer Inst* 85:1538, 1993.
81. Giovannucci E, Ascherio A, Rimm E et al: A prospective cohort study of vasectomy and prostate cancer in U.S. men, *JAMA* 269:873, 1993.
82. Giovannucci E, Tosteson TD, Speizer FE et al: A retrospective cohort study of vasectomy and prostate cancer in U.S. men, *JAMA* 269:878, 1993.

PROPOSED PREMALIGNANT LESIONS

83. McNeal JE, Bostwick DG: Intraductal dysplasia: a premalignant lesion of the prostate, *Hum Pathol* 17:64, 1986.
84. Bostwick DG, Brawer MK: Prostatic intra-epithelial neoplasia and early invasion in prostate cancer, *Cancer* 59:788, 1987.
85. Kovi J, Mostofi FK, Heshmat MY et al: Large acinar atypical hyperplasia and carcinoma of the prostate, *Cancer* 61:555, 1988.
86. Sakr WA, Haas GP, Cassin BJ et al: The frequency of carcinoma and intraepithelial neoplasia of the prostate in young male patients, *J Urol* 150:379, 1993.
87. Drago JR, Mostofi FK, Lee F: Introductory remarks and workshop summary, *Urology* 34(suppl):2, 1989.
88. Graham SD Jr, Bostwick DG, Hoisaeter A et al: Report of the Committee on Staging and Pathology, *Cancer* 70(suppl):359, 1992.
89. Bostwick DG, Amin MB, Dundore P et al: Architectural patterns of high grade prostatic intraepithelial neoplasia, *Hum Pathol* 24:298, 1993.
90. Qian J, Wollan P, Bostwick DG: The extent and multicentricity of high grade prostatic intraepithelial neoplasia in clinically localized prostatic adenocarcinoma, *Hum Pathol* (in press).
91. Brawer MK, Peehl DM, Stamey TA et al: Keratin immunoreactivity in benign and neoplastic human prostate, *Cancer Res* 45:3665, 1985.
92. Troncosco P, Babaian RJ, Ro JY et al: Prostatic intraepithelial neoplasia and invasive prostatic adenocarcinoma in cystoprostatectomy specimens, *Urology* 24(suppl):52, 1989.
93. De La Torre, Haggman M, Brandstedt S et al: Prostatic intraepithelial neoplasia and invasive carcinoma in total prostatectomy specimens: distribution, volume and DNA ploidy, *Br J Urol* 72:207, 1993.

94. Quinn BD, Cho KR, Epstein JI: Relationship of severe dysplasia to stage B adenocarcinoma of the prostate, *Cancer* 65:2328, 1990.
95. Lee F, Torp-Pedersen ST, Carroll JT et al: Use of transrectal ultrasound and prostate-specific antigen in diagnosis of prostatic intraepithelial neoplasia, *Urology* 24(suppl):4, 1989.
96. McNeal JE, Alroy J, Leav I et al: Immunohistochemical evidence for impaired cell differentiation in the premalignant phase of prostate carcinogenesis, *Am J Clin Pathol* 90:23, 1988.
97. McNeal JE, Leav I, Alroy J et al: Differential lectin staining of central and peripheral zones of the prostate and alterations in dysplasia, *Am J Clin Pathol* 89:41, 1988.
98. Perlman EJ, Epstein JI: Blood group antigen expression in dysplasia and adenocarcinoma of the prostate. *Am J Surg Pathol* 14:810, 1990.
99. Humphrey PA: Mucin in severe dysplasia in the prostate, *Surg Pathol* 4:137, 1991.
100. Nagle RB, Brawer MK, Kittelson J et al: Phenotypic relationship of prostatic intraepithelial neoplasia to invasive prostatic carcinoma, *Am J Pathol* 138:119, 1991.
101. Stearns ME, Wang M: Type IV collagenase (M 72,000) expression in human prostate: benign and malignant tissue, *Cancer Res* 53:878, 1993.
102. Montironi R, Braccischi A, Matera G et al: Quantitation of prostatic intra-epithelial neoplasia: analysis of the nuclear size, number and location, *Pathol Res Pract* 187:307, 1991.
103. Petein M, Michel P, Van Velthoven R et al: Morphonuclear relationship between prostatic intraepithelial neoplasia and cancer as assessed by digital cell image analysis, *Am J Clin Pathol* 96:628, 1991.
104. Montironi R, Scarpelli M, Sisti S et al: Quantitative analysis of prostatic intraepithelial neoplasia on tissue sections, *Anal Quant Cytol Histol* 12:366, 1990.
105. Helpap B: Observations on the number, size and location of nucleoli in hyperplastic and neoplastic prostatic disease, *Histopathology* 13:203, 1988.
106. Min KW, Jin J-K, Blank J et al: AgNOR in the human prostatic gland, *Am J Clin Pathol* 95:508, 1990.
107. Layfield LJ, Goldstein NS: Morphometric analysis of borderline atypia in prostatic aspiration biopsy specimen, *Anal Quant Cytol Histol* 13:288, 1991.
108. Deschenes J, Weidner N: Nucleolar organizer regions (NOR) in hyperplastic and neoplastic prostate disease, *Am J Surg Pathol* 14:1148, 1990.
109. Amin MB, Schultz DS, Zarbo RJ et al: Computerized static DNA ploidy analysis of prostatic intraepithelial neoplasia, *Arch Pathol Lab Med* 117:794, 1993.
110. Weinberg DS, Weidner N: Concordance of DNA content between prostatic intraepithelial neoplasia and concomitant carcinoma: evidence that prostatic intraepithelial neoplasia is a precursor of invasive prostatic carcinoma, *Arch Pathol Lab Med* 117:1132, 1993.
111. Crissman JD, Sakr WA, Hussein ME et al: DNA quantitation of intraepithelial neoplasia and invasive carcinoma of the prostate, *Prostate* 22:155, 1993.
112. Shinohara K, Scardino PT, Carter SSC et al: Pathologic basis of the sonographic appearance of the normal and malignant prostate, *Urol Clin N Am* 16:675, 1989.
113. Davidson D, Bostwick DG, Qian J et al: Prostatic intraepithelial neoplasia is a risk factor for adenocarcinoma in needle biopsies: predictive accuracy, *J Urol* (in press).
114. Brawer MK, Bigler SA, Sohlberg OE et al: Significance of prostatic intraepithelial neoplasia on prostate needle biopsy, *Urology* 38:103, 1991.
115. Weinstein MH, Epstein JI: Significance of high grade prostatic intraepithelial neoplasia on needle biopsy, *Hum Pathol* 24:624, 1993.
116. Markham CW: Prostatic intraepithelial neoplasia: detection and correlation with invasive cancer in fine-needle biopsy, Urology 24(suppl):57, 1989.
117. Bostwick DG: High grade prostatic intraepithelial neoplasia: the most likely precursor to prostate cancer, *Cancer* 75:1823, 1995.
118. Bostwick DG, Srigley J, Grignon D et al: Atypical adenomatous hyperplasia of the prostate: morphologic criteria for its distinction from well-differentiated carcinoma, *Hum Pathol* 24:819, 1993.
119. Brawn PN: Adenosis of the prostate: a dysplastic lesion that can be confused with prostate adenocarcinoma, *Cancer* 49:826, 1982.
120. Gleason DF: Atypical hyperplasia, benign hyperplasia, and well-differentiated adenocarcinoma of the prostate, *Am J Surg Pathol* 9:53, 1985.
121. Kovi J: Microscopic differential diagnosis of small acinar adenocarcinoma of prostate, *Pathol Ann* 20:157, 1985.
122. Bostwick DG, Algaba F, Amin MB et al: Consensus statement on terminology: recommendation to use atypical adenomatous hyperplasia in place of adenosis of the prostate, *Hum Pathol* 25:840, 1994.
123. Brawn PN, Speights VO, Contin JU et al: Atypical hyperplasia in prostates of 20 to 40 year old men, *J Clin Pathol* 42:383, 1989.
124. Bostwick DG, Qian J: Atypical adenomatous hyperplasia of the prostate: relationship with carcinoma in 217 whole mount radical prostatectomies, *Am J Surg Pathol* 19:506, 1995.
125. Kelemen PR, Buschmann RJ, Weisz-Carrington P: Nucleolar prominence as a diagnostic variable in prostatic carcinoma, *Cancer* 65:1017, 1990.
126. Helpap B: Observations on the number, size, and localization of nucleoli in hyperplastic and neoplastic prostatic disease, *Histopathology* 13:203, 1988.
127. O'Malley FP, Grignon DJ, Shum DT: Usefulness of immunoperoxidase staining with high-molecular-weight cytokeratin in the differential diagnosis of small-acinar lesions of the prostate gland, *Virchows Arch[A]* 417:191, 1990.
128. Hedrick L, Epstein JI: Use of keratin 903 as an adjunct in the diagnosis of prostate carcinoma, *Am J Surg Pathol* 13:389, 1989.
129. Sakamoto N, Tsuneyoshi M, Enjoji M: Sclerosing adenosis of the prostate: histopathologic and immunohistochemical analysis, *Am J Surg Pathol* 15:660, 1991.
130. Jones EC, Clement PB, Young RH: Sclerosing adenosis of the prostate gland: a clinicopathologic and immunohistochemical study of 11 cases, *Am J Surg Pathol* 15:1171, 1991.
131. Amin MB, Schultz DS, Zarbo RJ: Analysis of cribriform morphology in prostate neoplasia using antibody to high molecular weight cytokeratins, *Mod Pathol* 5:50A, 1992.
132. Ro JY, Grignon DJ, Troncoso P et al: Mucin in prostatic adenocarcinoma, *Semin Diagn Pathol* 5:273, 1988.
133. Epstein JI, Fynheer J: Acidic mucin in the prostate: can it differentiate adenosis from adenocarcinoma? *Hum Pathol* 23:1321, 1992.
134. Goldstein NS, Qian J, Bostwick DG: Acid mucin in atypical adenomatous hyperplasia, (in press).
135. Tsukakitamoto T, Kumamoto Y, Masumori N et al: Studies on incidental carcinoma of the prostate, *Nippon Hinyokika Gakkai Zasshi* 81:1343, 1990.
136. Deschenes JH, Weidner N: Nucleolar organizer regions (NOR) in hyperplastic and neoplastic prostate disease, *Am J Surg Pathol* 14: 1148, 1990.
137. Ghazizadeh M, Sasaki Y, Oguro T et al: Silver staining of nucleolar organizer regions in prostatic lesions, *Histopathology* 19:369, 1991.
138. Aragona F, Franco V, Rodolico V et al: Interactive computerized morphometric analysis of the differential diagnosis between dysplasia and well differentiated adenocarcinoma of the prostate, *Urol Res* 17:35, 1989.

CLINICAL FEATURES

139. Murphy GP, Whitmore WF: A report of the workshop on the current status of the histologic grading of prostate cancer, *Cancer* 44:1490, 1979.
140. Gleason DF: Classification of prostatic carcinomas, *Cancer Chemother Rep* 50:125, 1966.
141. Gleason DF: Histologic grading of prostatic carcinoma. In Bostwick DG, editor: *Pathology of the prostate,* New York, 1990, Churchill-Livingstone.
142. Mostofi FK: Grading of prostatic carcinoma, *Cancer Chemother Rep,* 59 (part I):111, 1975.
143. Bastacky SI, Walsh PC, Epstein JI: Relationship between perineural tumor invasion on needle biopsy and radical prostatectomy capsular penetration in clinical stage B adenocarcinoma of the prostate, *Am J Surg Pathol* 17:336, 1993.
144. Hasson MO, Maksem J: The prostatic perineural space and its relation to tumor spread: an ultrastructural study; *Am J Surg Pathol* 4:143, 1980.

145. McIntire TL, Franzina DA: The presence of benign prostate glands in perineural spaces, *J Urol* 135:507, 1986.
146. Holmes EJ: Crystalloids of prostatic carcinoma: relationship to Bence-Jones crystals, *Cancer* 29:2073, 1977.
147. Del Rosario AD, Bui HX, Abdulla M et al: Sulfur-rich prostatic intraluminal crystalloids: a surgical, pathologic and electron probe x-ray microanalytic study, *Hum Pathol* 24:1159, 1993.
148. McNeal JE, Alroy J, Villers A et al: Mucinous differentiation in prostatic adenocarcinoma, *Hum Pathol* 22:979, 1991.
149. Bostwick DG, Adlakha H: Collagenous micronodules in prostate cancer: a specific but infrequent diagnostic finding, *Arch Pathol Lab Med* 119:444, 1995.
150. Bahnson RR, Dresner SM, Gooding W et al: Incidence and prognostic significance of lymphatic and vascular invasion in radical prostatectomy specimens, *Prostate* 15:149, 1989.
151. Napalkov P, Watts L, Gansler T et al: Microvascular invasion of the seminal vesicles in adenocarcinoma of the prostate: prognostic value, (in press).

VARIANTS

152. Amin MB, Ro JY, Ayala AG: The clinical relevance of histologic variants of prostate cancer, *Cancer Bull* 45:403, 1993.
153. Dhom G: Unusual prostatic carcinomas, *Pathol Res Pract* 186:28, 1990.
154. Ro JY, Grignon DJ, Ayala AG et al: Mucinous adenocarcinoma of the prostate: histochemical and immunohistochemical studies, *Hum Pathol* 21:593, 1990.
155. Alline KM, Cohen MB: Signet-ring cell carcinoma of the prostate, *Arch Pathol Lab Med* 116:99, 1992.
156. Moyana TN: Adenosquamous carcinoma of the prostate, *Am J Surg Pathol* 11:402, 1987.
157. Sarma DP, Weilbaecher TG, Moon TD: Squamous cell carcinoma of prostate, *Urology* 37:260, 1991.
158. Wernert N, Goebbels R, Bonkhoff H et al: Squamous cell carcinoma of the prostate, *Histopathology* 17:339, 1990.
159. Shannon RL, Ro JY, Grignon DJ et al: Sarcomatoid carcinoma of the prostate: a clinicopathologic study of 12 cases, *Cancer* 69:2676, 1992.
160. Lauwers GY, Shevchuk M, Armenakas N et al: Carcinosarcoma of the prostate, *Am J Surg Pathol* 17: 342, 1993.
161. Wick MR, Young RH, Malvesta R et al: Prostatic carcinosarcomas: clinical, histologic, and immunohistochemical data on two cases, with a review of the literature, *Am J Clin Pathol* 92:131, 1989.
162. Wood DP Jr, Montie JE, Pontes JE et al: Transitional cell carcinoma of the prostate in cystoprostatectomy specimens removed for bladder cancer, *J Urol* 141:346, 1989.
163. Wishnow KI, Ro JY: Importance of early treatment of transitional cell carcinoma of prostatic ducts, *Urology* 32:11, 1988.
164. Mahadevia PS, Koss LG, Tar IJ: Prostatic involvement in bladder cancer: prostate mapping in 20 cystoprostatectomy specimens, *Cancer* 58:2095, 1986.

DIAGNOSTIC AND PROGNOSTIC MARKERS

165. Oesterling JE, Jacobsen SJ, Chute CG et al: Serum prostate-specific antigen in a community-based population of healthy men: establishment of age-specific reference ranges, *JAMA* 270: 860, 1993.
166. Blackwell KL, Bostwick DG, Myers RP et al: Combining prostate specific antigen with cancer and gland volume to more reliably predict pathologic stage: the influence of PSA-cancer density, *J Urol* 151: 1565, 1994.
167. Ruckle HC, Klee GG, Oesterling JE: Prostate-specific antigen: critical issues for the practicing physician, *Mayo Clin Proc* 69:59, 1994.
168. Ruckle HC, Klee GG, Oesterling JE: Prostate-specific antigen: concepts for staging prostate cancer and monitoring response to therapy, *Mayo Clin Proc* 69:69, 1994.
169. Lilja H: Significance of different molecular forms of serum PSA: the free, noncomplexed form of PSA versus that complexed to alpha-1-antichymotrypsin, *Urol Clin North Am* 20: 681, 1993.
170. Vessella RL, Lange PH: Issues in the assessment of PSA immunoassays, *Urol Clin North Am* 20:607, 1993.
171. Ellis DW, Leffers S, Davies JS et al: Multiple immunoperoxidase markers in benign hyperplasia and adenocarcinoma of the prostate, *Am J Clin Pathol* 81:279, 1984.
172. Svanholm H: Evaluation of commercial immunoperoxidase kits for prostate specific antigen and prostatic specific acid phosphatase, *Acta Pathol Microbiol Immunol Scand [A]* 94:7, 1986.
173. Lowe FC, Trauzzi SJ: Prostatic acid phosphatase in 1993: its limited clinical utility, *Urol Clin North Am* 20: 589, 1993.
174. Bonkhoff H, Remberger K: Widespread distribution of nuclear androgen receptors in the basal cell layer of the normal and hyperplastic human prostate, *Virchows Arch* [A] 422:35, 1993.
175. Sadi MV, Barrack ER: Image analysis of androgen receptor immunostaining in metastatic prostate cancer, *Cancer* 71:2574, 1993.
176. Sadi MV, Walsh PC, Barrack ER: Immunohistochemical study of androgen receptors in metastatic prostate cancer: comparison of receptor content and response to hormonal therapy, *Cancer* 67:3057, 1991.
177. Cohen RJ, Glezerson G, Haffejee Z et al: Prostatic carcinoma: histological and immunohistological factors affecting prognosis, *Br J Urol* 66:405, 1990.
178. Wright C, Grignon D, Shum D et al: Neuroendocrine differentiation in prostatic adenocarcinoma is not an independent prognostic indicator, *Mod Pathol* 5:60A, 1992.
179. Berner A, Nesland JM, Waehre H et al: Hormone resistant prostatic adenocarcinoma: an evaluation of prognostic factors in pre- and post-treatment specimens, *Br J Cancer* 68: 380, 1993.
180. Bostwick DG, Dousa M, Wollan P et al: Neuroendocrine differentiation in prostatic intraepithelial neoplasia and adenocarcinoma, *Am J Surg Pathol* 18:1240, 1994.
181. Steiner MS: Role of peptide growth factors in the prostate: a review, *Urology* 42:99, 1993.
182. Myers RB, Kudlow JE, Grizzle WE: Expression of transforming growth factor-alpha, epidermal growth factor and the epidermal growth factor receptor in adenocarcinoma of the prostate and benign prostatic hyperplasia, *Mod Pathol* 6: 733, 1993.
183. Harper ME, Goddard L, Glynne-Jones E et al: An immunocytochemical analysis of TGF-alpha expression in benign and malignant prostatic tumors, *Prostate* 23:9, 1993.
184. Maygarden SJ, Strom S, Ware JL: Localization of epidermal growth factor receptor by immunohistochemical methods in human prostatic carcinoma, prostatic intraepithelial neoplasia, and benign hyperplasia, *Arch Pathol Lab Med* 116: 269, 1992.
185. Kyprianou N, Isaacs JT: Identification of a cellular receptor for transforming growth factor-beta in rat ventral prostate and its negative regulation by androgens, *Endocrinology* 27: 2124, 1988.
186. Thompson TC, Truong LD, Timme TL et al: Transforming growth factor beta-1 as a biomarker for prostate cancer, *J Cell Biochem* (suppl 16H):54, 1992.
187. Eklov S, Funa K, Nordgren H et al: Lack of the latent transforming growth factor beta binding protein in malignant, but not benign prostatic tissue, *Cancer Res* 53: 3193, 1993.
188. Schellhammer PF, Wright GL Jr: Biomolecular and clinical characteristics of PSA and other candidate tumor markers, *Urol Clin North Am* 20: 597, 1993.
189. Bostwick DG, Choi CC: Prognostic factors in early prostate cancer, *Urol Annu* 6: 63, 1992.

MOLECULAR BIOLOGY

190. Zincke H, Bergstrahl EJ, Larson-Keller JJ et al: Stage D1 prostate cancer treated by radical prostatectomy and adjuvant hormonal treatment: evidence for favorable survival in patients with DNA diploid tumors, *Cancer* 70(suppl 1):311, 1992.
191. Shankey TV, Kallioniemi O-P, Koslowski JM et al: Consensus review of the clinical utility of DNA content cytometry in prostate cancer, *Cytometry* 14: 497, 1993.
192. Sandberg AA: Chromosomal abnormalities and related events in prostate cancer, *Hum Pathol* 23: 368, 1992.
193. MacGrogan D, Levy A, Bostwick D et al: Loss of chromosome 8p loci in prostate cancer: mapping by quantitative allelic balance, *Genes Chromosom Cancer* 10: 151, 1994.
194. Bova GS, Carter BS, Bussemakers MJG et al: Homozygous deletion and frequent allelic loss of chromosome 8p22 loci in human prostate cancer, *Cancer Res* 53: 3869, 1993.

195. Bergerheim USR, Kunimi K, Collins VP et al: Deletion mapping of chromosomes 8, 10, and 16 in human prostatic carcinoma, *Genes Chromosom Cancer* 3: 215, 1991.
196. Takahashi S, Qian J, Brown JA et al: Potential markers of prostate cancer aggressiveness detected by fluorescence in situ hybridization in needle biopsies, *Cancer Res* 54: 3574, 1994.
197. Bookstein R, MacGrogan D, Hilsenbeck SG et al: p53 is mutated in a subset of advanced-stage prostate cancers, *Cancer Res* 53: 3369, 1993.
198. Effert PJ, McCoy RH, Walther PJ et al: p53 gene alterations in human prostate carcinoma. *J Urol,* 150:257, 1993.
199. Van Veldhuizen PJ, Sadasivan R, Garcia F et al: Mutant p53 expression in prostate carcinoma, *Prostate* 22:23, 1993.
200. Gao X, Honn KV, Grignon D et al: Frequent loss of expression and loss of heterozygosity of the putative tumor suppressor gene DCC in prostatic carcinomas, *Cancer Res* 53: 2723, 1993.
201. Bookstein R, Rio P, Madreperla S et al: Promoter deletion and loss of retinoblastoma gene expression in human prostate carcinoma, *Proc Natl Acad Sci USA* 87:7762, 1990.
202. Moul JW, Friedrichs PA, Lance RS et al: Infrequent RAS oncogene mutations in human prostate cancer, *Prostate* 20:327, 1992.
203. Bostwick DG. c-erbB-2 oncogene expression in prostatic intraepithelial neoplasia: mounting evidence for a precursor role, *J Natl Cancer Inst* 86:1108, 1994.

CLINICAL AND PATHOLOGIC STAGING

204. Shröder FH, Hermanek P, Denis L et al: The TNM classification of prostate carcinoma, *Prostate* 4(suppl):129, 1992.
205. Bostwick DG, Myers RP, Oesterling JE: The staging of prostate cancer, *Semin Surg Oncol* 10:60, 1994.
206. Friedman GD, Hiatt RA, Quesenberry CP et al: Case-control study of screening for prostate cancer by digital rectal examinations, *Lancet* 337:1526, 1991.
207. Oesterling JE, Suman VJ, Zincke H et al: PSA-detected (clinical stage T1c or B0) prostate cancer, *Urol Clin North Am* 20:687, 1993.
208. Rifkin MD, Zerhouni EA, Garsonis CA et al: Comparison of magnetic resonance imaging and ultrasonography in staging early prostate cancer: results of a multi-institutional cooperative trial, *N Engl J Med* 323:621, 1990.
209. Ramchandani P, Schnall MD: Magnetic resonance imaging of the prostate, *Semin Roentgenol* 28:74, 1993.
210. Greene DR, Egawa S, Neerhut G et al: The distribution of residual cancer in radical prostatectomy specimens in stage A prostate cancer, *J Urol* 145:324. 1991.
211. Epstein JI, Oesterling JE Walsh PC: The volume and anatomical location of residual tumor in radical prostatectomy specimens removed for stage A1 prostate cancer, *J Urol* 139:975, 1988.
212. Stamey TA, Villers AA, McNeal JE et al: Positive surgical margins at radical prostatectomy: importance of the apical dissection, *J Urol* 143:1166, 1990.
213. Ohori M, Scardino P, Lapin S et al: The mechanisms and prognostic significance of seminal vesicle involvement by prostate cancer, *Am J Surg Pathol* 17:1252, 1993.
214. Paulson DF, Stone AR, Walther PJ et al: Radical prostatectomy: anatomical predictors of success or failure, *J Urol* 136:1041, 1986.
215. Hering F, Rist M, Roth J et al: Does microinvasion of the capsule and/or micrometastases in regional lymph nodes influence disease-free survival after radical prostatectomy? *Br J Urol* 66:177, 1990.
216. Brawn P, Kuhl D, Johnson C III et al: Stage D1 prostate carcinoma: the histologic appearance of nodal metastases and its relationship to survival, *Cancer* 65:538, 1990.
217. McNeal JE: Cancer volume and site of origin of adenocarcinoma in the prostate: relationship to local and distant spread, *Hum Pathol* 66:177, 1992.
218. Bostwick DG, Eble JN: Prostatic adenocarcinoma metastatic to inguinal hernia sac, *J Urol Pathol* 1:193, 1993.
219. De La Monte SM, Moore GW, Hutchins GM: Metastatic behavior of prostate cancer: cluster analysis of pattern with respect to estrogen treatment, *Cancer* 58: 985, 1986.
220. Saitoh H, Hida M, Shimbo T et al: Metastatic patterns of prostatic cancer: correlation between sites and number of organs involved, *Cancer* 54:3078, 1984.

TREATMENT AND OUTCOME

221. See WA, Williams RD: Management of prostate cancer: stage by stage. In Das S, Crawford ED, editors: *Cancer of the prostate,* New York, 1993, Marcel Dekker.

Soft-tissue tumors and miscellaneous lesions

222. Proppe KH, Scully RE, Rosai J: Postoperative spindle cell nodules of genitourinary tract resembling sarcomas: a report of eight cases, *Am J Surg Pathol* 8:101, 1984.
223. Ro JY, El-Naggar AK, Amin MB et al: Pseudosarcomatous fibromyxoid tumor of the urinary bladder and prostate: immunohistochemical, ultrastructural, and DNA flow cytometric analyses of nine cases, *Hum Pathol* 24:1203. 1993.
224. Ro JY, Grignon DJ, Ayala AG et al: Blue nevus and melanosis of the prostate: electronmicroscopic and immunohistochemical studies, *Am J Clin Pathol* 90:530. 1988.
225. Martinez CJ, Garcia GR, Castaneda CA: Blue nevus of the prostate: report of two new cases with immunohistochemical and electron microscopic studies, *Eur Urol* 24:339, 1992.
226. Ghavimi F, Herr H, Jereb B et al: Treatment of genitourinary rhabdomyosarcoma in children, *J Urol* 132:313, 1984.
227. Witherow R, Molland E, Oliver T et al: Leiomyosarcoma of prostate and superficial soft tissue, *Urology* 15:513, 1980.

LYMPHOMA AND LEUKEMIA

228. Bostwick DG, Mann RB: Malignant lymphomas involving the prostate: a study of 13 cases, *Cancer* 56:2932, 1985.
229. Amin MB, Osborne B, Discigel G et al: Malignant lymphoma involving the prostate: report of 52 cases, *Mod Pathol* 6:54A, 1993.

Seminal vesicles

230. Kuo T, Gomez LG: Monstrous epithelial cells in human epididymis and seminal vesicles, *Am J Surg Pathol* 5:483. 1981.
231. Arber DA, Speights VO: Aneuploidy in benign seminal vesicular epithelium: an example of the paradox of ploidy studies, *Mod Pathol* 4:687, 1991.
232. Meisels A, Ayotte D: Cells from the seminal vesicles: contaminants of the V-C-E smear, *Acta Cytol.* 20:211, 1976.
233. Rappe BJM, Meuleman EJH, Debruyne FMJ: Seminal vesicle cyst with ipsilateral renal agenesis, *Urol Int* 50:54, 1993.
234. Ornstein MH, Kershaw DR: Cysts of the seminal vesicle are mullerian in origin, *J Royal Soc Med* 78:1050, 1985.
235. Genovois PA, Van Sinoy ML, Sintzoff SA et al: Cysts of the prostate and seminal vesicles: MR findings in 11 cases, *AJR* 155:1021, 1990.
236. Shabsigh R, Lerner S, Fischman IJ: The role of transrectal ultrasonography in the diagnosis and management of prostatic and seminal vesicle cysts, *J Urol.* 141:12061, 1989.
237. Mazzucchelli L, Studer UE, Zimmermann A: Cystadenoma of the seminal vesicle: case report and literature review, *J Urol* 147:1621. 1992.
238. Bahn DK, Brown RKJ, Shei KY et al: Sonographic findings of leiomyoma of seminal vesicle, *J Clin Ultrasound* 18:517, 1990.
239. Ramchandani P, Schnall MD, LiVolsi VA et al: Senile amyloidosis of the seminal vesicles mimicking metastatic spread of prostatic carcinoma on MR images, *AJR* 161: 99, 1993.
240. Khan SM, Birch PJ, Bass PS et al: Localized amyloidosis of the lower genitourinary tract: a clinicopathological and immunohistochemical study of nine cases, *Histopathology* 21:143. 1992.
241. Seidman JD, Shmookler BM, Connolly B et al: Localized amyloidosis of seminal vesicles: report of three cases in surgically obtained material, *Mod Pathol* 2:671, 1989.
242. Pitkanen P, Westermark P, Cornwell GG III et al: Amyloid of the seminal vesicles: a distinctive and common localized form of senile amyloidosis, *Am J Pathol* 110:64, 1983.
243. Chandra I, Doringer E, Sarica K et al: Bilateral seminal vesicle abscesses, *Eur Urol* 20:164. 1991.
244. Maglione M, Nardi A, Cranz C et al: Acute vesiculitis and its prostatic complications caused by *E. coli* in the rat, *Urol Res* 14:265. 1986.
245. Tanaka T, Takeuchi T, Oguchi K et al: Primary adenocarcinoma of the seminal vesicle, *Hum Pathol* 18:200, 1987.

246. Benson RC Jr, Clark WR, Farrow GM: Carcinoma of the seminal vesicle, *J Urol* 132:483. 1984.
247. Ro JY, Ayala AG, El-Naggar A et al: Seminal vesicle involvement by in situ and invasive transitional cell carcinoma of the bladder, *Am J Surg Pathol* 11:951, 1987.
248. Schned AR, Ledbetter JS, Selikowitz SM: Primary leiomyosarcoma of the seminal vesicle, *Cancer* 57:2202, 1986.
249. Chiou R-K, Limas C, Lange PH: Hemangiosarcoma of the seminal vesicle: case report and literature review, *J Urol* 134:371. 1985.
250. Fain JS, Cosnow I, King BF et al: Cystosarcoma phyllodes of the seminal vesicles, *Cancer* 71:2055, 1993.
251. Laurila P, Leivo I, Makisalo H et al: Mullerian adenosarcomalike tumor of the seminal vesicle: a case report with immunohistochemical and ultrastructural observations, *Arch Pathol Lab Med* 116:1072, 1992.

68 Female Reproductive System

Jaime Prat

NORMAL FEMALE GENITAL TRACT

Knowledge of the embryology of the female genital tract is helpful in understanding various malformations as well as the histogenesis of many tumors and their classification. A brief summary is supplied as a basis for such an understanding; for more detailed descriptions see standard texts.[1]

Gonadal differentiation. In humans, the karyotype XY genetically determines the male sex, whereas XX determines the female sex. Regardless of the number of X chromosomes, the presence of a single Y determines the male sex. The gene that regulates testicular development is called *SRY (sex-determining region Y)* gene, located in the region 1A1 at the distal end of the short arm of the Y chromosome.[2,3] Without *SRY* gene expression, the gonads differentiate as ovaries and the embryo develops as a female. The timely expression of the *SRY* gene is crucial to the development of male sex.[4]

Genital ridges and ducts. Except for the germ cells, which are of endodermal origin, the internal genitalia arise from the mesoderm (celomic epithelium and underlying mesenchyme) of the posterior body wall. Bilateral urogenital ridges are formed parallel to the body axis. In a 6 mm embryo (about 5 weeks of gestation) each of these has become divided longitudinally into a lateral wolffian (mesonephric) ridge and a medial genital ridge.

By the end of the sixth week the primitive gonad is represented by proliferating surface epithelial cells and an inner blastema of loose mesenchymal cells. A lateral groove forms in the surface epithelium of each urogenital ridge, rolls inward, and closes to form the müllerian (paramesonephric) duct on each side. Although lateral to the cranial aspect of the wolffian ducts, the müllerian ducts cross over caudally to lie medial to them as they enter the pelvis. The cranial ends remain open and eventually become the fimbriated open ends of the uterine tubes. The caudal ends adjoin the posterior wall of the urogenital sinus immediately between the two orifices of the wolffian ducts. The meeting point, transiently marked by a swelling named "Müller's tubercle," defines the site of the future vaginal orifice, the hymenal membrane. At this point begins the proliferation of the vaginal plate, a column of squamous epithelial cells that subsequently line the vagina.[5] By about the eighth week of embryonic life, the distal ends of the müllerian ducts fuse to become the uterus, cervix, and upper vagina. The myometrium and endometrial stroma differentiate from the surrounding mesenchyma (Fig. 68-1).

In a 60 mm (11 weeks) embryo the ovary is suspended by its mesovarium from the ventral surface of the mesonephros, which is still prominent. The mesonephric ducts are functional at this time and pass into the urogenital sinus through the lateral walls of the developing myometrium.

Ovary. Each ovarian blastema is covered by a surface layer of celomic epithelium, closely related but not identical to the cells that form the müllerian ducts. Perhaps because of this close relationship in early development, the adenocarcinomas that arise from ovarian surface epithelium closely resemble typical adenocarcinomas of the tube, endometrium, cervix, and vagina. As a result of this similarity, it has become customary to regard the common ovarian epithelial tumors as müllerian, even though the ovary does not actually form from the müllerian duct. Pelvic mesothelium and the underlying mesenchyme also maintain the capacity to generate, rarely, primary epithelial and stromal neoplasms identical to those of the uterus, tubes, and ovaries.[6]

The primordial germ cells originate in the yolk sac endoderm near the hindgut and about 3 weeks after fertilization migrate through the primitive hindgut mesentery and finally settle in the blastemas of the primitive ovaries.[7] The segregation of an occasional straggler along the way may explain some retroperitoneal germ cell tumors and the development of heterotopic ovarian tissue along the trail of this migration. This migration is completed by the tenth week. The germ cells begin to proliferate by mitosis on arrival, notably after the eighth week; by the twelfth week some begin the first meiotic division. At birth, germ cell mitosis has ceased, and most ova, at this time called "oogonia," are in the dictyotene stage of meiosis. The adjacent stromal cells differentiate into a single layer of flattened granulosa cells, forming a primary follicle. The granulosa cells proliferate; a cavity, the antrum, appears, forming a graafian follicle; follicles may be numerous, and some are large at birth. The ovaries descend into the pelvis attached to connective tissue strands, the gubernacula, which will become the medial ovarian ligaments and the round ligaments, extending from the uterine horns to the labia majora.

Müllerian ducts. The separate proximal portions of the müllerian ducts develop into the uterine (fallopian) tubes. The fused middle and distal portions complete their merger by the twelfth week, forming the uterus and upper part of the vagina respectively. The myometrium differentiates from the surrounding mesenchyme, enveloping the adjacent segments of the regressing mesonephric ducts.

Between the eighth and eleventh weeks the primitive vagina is a solid cord of epithelial cells ending distally in the urogenital sinus at Müller's tubercle. Evaginations of the urogenital sinus on either side of Müller's tubercle enlarge, fuse, and merge to form the hymen and distal vaginal wall. The lining of the vagina is formed by proliferation of epithelial cells from the dorsum of the urogenital sinus, extending cephalad toward the cervix, which is a crucial period for female infants exposed in utero to the drug diethylstilbestrol and its derivatives.

Vulva. The primitive hindgut, urinary ducts, and genital ducts empty into a common chamber, the cloaca. By the sixth week the urorectal septum has formed as a transverse ridge separating the urogenital sinus and rectum. Müller's tubercle moves progressively caudad. The urinary bladder forms from the allantois, so that the müllerian and urinary orifices empty as separate orifices into the shallow remains of the urogenital sinus, now the vestibule of the vulva.

The development of the vulva begins at a sexually indeterminate stage. At about 36 days (9 mm) the external structures are represented by a genital tubercle (a conic anterior midline protuberance) and the labioscrotal swellings (two broad lateral elevations located just caudad to the genital tubercle on either side of the cloacal groove) (Fig. 68-2). The cloacal groove at first is closed by the cloacal membrane. After the urorectal septum grows down to meet it, the cloacal membrane becomes divided into an anterior urogenital groove, closed by the urogenital membrane, and a posterior anal membrane. The urogenital membrane disintegrates at about 42 days; a glans become evident on the genital tubercle in the 46-day-old (19 mm) embryo. The urogenital groove extends anteriorly on the caudal aspect of the phallus thus formed. A sexual distinction is made evident by the urethral groove, which extends onto the phallus from the urogenital groove; the urethral groove extends distally onto the glans in the male but not in the female. This distinction is probably not a reliable indicator of sex until after the eleventh week (50 mm). The urethral folds lateral to the urethral groove fuse to form the male penile urethra; they persist as separate structures, the labia minora, in the female. The labioscrotal swellings enlarge to form the labia majora; they fuse posteriorly at the posterior commissure at about 50 mm. In the 4-month-old (100 mm) embryo the prepuce forms around the glans of the clitoris.

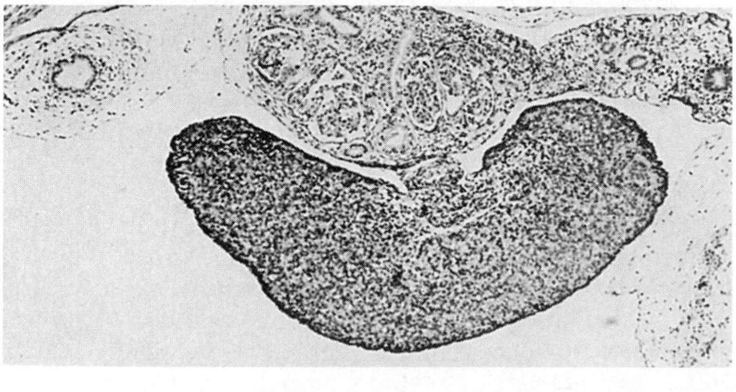

Fig. 68-1 Transverse section of ovary and adjacent mesonephros. Mesonephric glomeruli persist at this 60 mm stage. (From Kraus FT: *Gynecologic pathology*, St. Louis, 1967, Mosby.)

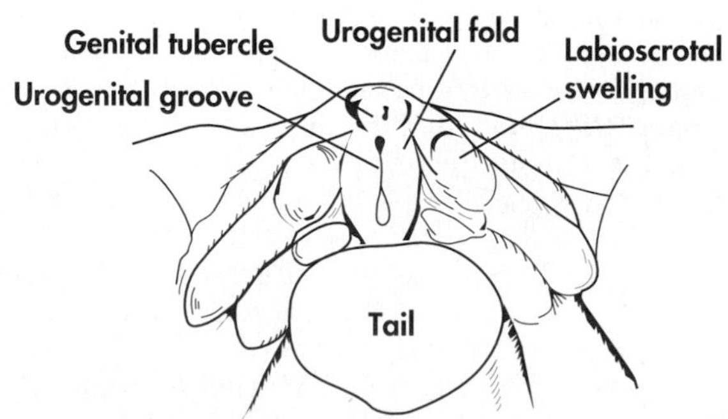

Fig. 68-2 External genitalia at about 7 weeks are sexually indeterminate. (Modified from Arey, LB: *Developmental anatomy*, ed 6, Philadelphia, 1954, Saunders.)

The most significant events in the embryologic development of the female genital tract are summarized in Table 68-1. This timetable of development is useful in relating malformations to possible teratogenic events such as maternal infection with a virus or exposure to a teratogenic drug.

Sexual differentiation: male and female. Female genital developmental anomalies often involve some degree of substitution of male-directed organogenesis. Therefore genital development in the male is basic to any understanding of the anatomy and physiology of intersex states in children or adults reared as females. In the absence of a Y chromosome the embryo develops (at least transiently) ovaries, müllerian ducts and their derivatives, vagina, vulva, and a basically female phenotype. Full expression of all female secondary sexual characteristics and development of a functional ovary require a second X chromosome.

The gonadal blastemas begin similarly in both sexes and at first are morphologically indistinguishable from one another. The definitive ovary and testis have been identified in 23 mm embryos at 42 days of age.[10] In the female the müllerian ducts and vulva develop appropriately, even when the ovaries are absent. In males, however, the persistence and development of the wolffian (mesonephric) ductal system, together with regression of the müllerian ducts and the structures that form from them, are dependent on two factors; a local-acting müllerian inhibiting substance (MIS) and circulating testosterone, both produced by the testis.[11,12]

Testosterone induces the formation of epididymis, vas deferens, and seminal vesicle from the mesonephric duct. Leydig cells appear in the testis around days 54 to 64 and immediately begin to produce testosterone. Dihydrotestosterone, produced from testosterone by the action of 5-alpha-reductase within the cells of the perineal tissues, stimulates fusion of labioscrotal folds, closure of the median raphe, and growth of the glans and shaft of the penis, enclosed penile urethra, and scrotum. External genital development is complete by the eighteenth to twentieth week. Male structures fail to develop when the somatic cells of a fetus are unresponsive to testosterone, which occurs in androgen-insensitivity (resistance) syndromes.

Because MIS acts locally, it must be produced in adequate amounts by both testes to prevent completely the development of both tubes, uterus, and upper portion of the vagina. Therefore an individual with a testis on one side and a streak (no gonad), an ovary, or ovotestis on the other usually will have a uterus and upper vagina and possibly a tube on the side opposite the testis.

Table 68-1 Correlation of age, size, and sequence of development of female urogenital organs

Age (approximately*)	Crown-rump length (mm)	Developmental levels in female urogenital tract
23-25 days	2.5	Limb buds appear
25 days		Pronephros formed; pronephric ducts grow caudad as blind tubes; cloaca and cloacal membrane present; embryo has 14 somites
25-28 days	5	Closure of neural tube
32 days		Pronephros degenerated; mesonephric tubules forming; pronephric (now mesonephric) ducts reach cloaca; metanephric bud forms at distal end of mesonephric duct
30-35 days	8	Retinal pigment appears
35 days		Genital ridge bulges; ureteric and renal pelvic primordia formed
35-36 days	13	Finger plate appears
40 days		Urorectal septum begins to subdivide cloaca; genital tubercle and labioscrotal swelling evident; müllerian duct begins to form
37-45 days	22	Elbow appears
40-46 days		Knee appears
7 weeks		Urogenital membrane dissolves; cloaca separated into urogenital sinus and rectum; glans of phallus is evident
8 weeks	30	Testis and ovary become recognizable as such; müllerian ducts approach urogenital sinus and begin to fuse (distal portion) to become uterovaginal primordium
10 weeks	46	Mesonephric ducts atrophy; glands of urogenital sinus (vulvourethral and vestibular glands) appear.
12 weeks	56	Uterine horns absorbed; muscular walls appear in uterus, vagina, and fallopian tubes; distinction of sex from external genitalia becomes possible
16 weeks	112	Uterus and vagina become distinctive structures
5 months	150	Primary ovarian follicles are found; vagina develops lumen; urogenital sinus becomes shallow vestibule
7 months	230	Uterine glands appear

*There is no accurate way of determining embryonic age from the length; the figures given represent a composite or average and are based on the stages described in several standard texts.[8-10]

In the strongly estrogenic maternal environment, genital development is female but independent of the presence of a fetal ovary. Therefore at birth a fetus with no gonadal tissue on either side (bilateral streaks or bilateral agenesis) will have a uterus, vagina, tubes, and the female appearance of external genitalia. Individuals with abnormal (dysgenetic) testes, which may not produce either MIS or testosterone in adequate amounts, will have some degree of müllerian tract development and either female external genitalia or incompletely formed male external genitalia. A single testis might be expected to inhibit müllerian development on the same side but not to inhibit that on the opposite side or the entire uterus; however, it could generate enough dihydrotestosterone to masculinize the external genitalia.

ABNORMAL SEXUAL DEVELOPMENT

Because of the importance of sex in social development, intersexual disorders have a devastating effect. Recent advances in chromosome analysis and molecular biology have permitted early detection and prompt therapy of the intersexual patient. In this chapter, intersexual conditions are conveniently divided into two broad groups: (1) those associated with an abnormal sex chromosome constitution and (2) those structural and localized developmental abnormalities, associated with normal sex chromosomes, in which one of the processes of the growth, fusion, canalization, or separation of developing tubular structures is incomplete. A detailed classification of abnormal sexual development that correlates the gonadal and genital anatomy with the chromosomal findings and specific genetic or metabolic defects has been developed.[13,14]

Intersexual states and cytogenetic abnormalities

Because normal sexual development is determined first of all by the presence in the zygote of a normal set of sex chromosomes, the initial factor in many sexual disorders is the contribution of abnormal or deficient genetic material by one of the gametes. Alternatively, during the first division of the zygote some genetic material may be lost or unevenly distributed in the daughter cells (nondisjunction), resulting in a mixture (mosaic) of two or more types of cells as the organism develops further. Although the loss, severe alteration, or duplication of an autosome is usually lethal, most sex chromosomal abnormalities exert their most notable effects in the form of altered genital structure and function.

A bewildering array of intersex states has been described, together with associated cytogenetic analyses and deranged endocrine physiologic processes. This discussion is limited to a brief description of the usual findings in some of the more common syndromes, which are summarized in Table 68-2. This table is a generalization. Certain commonly used terms require definitions, as follows:

hermaphrodite—an inexact term indicating that an individual has some kind of mixture of both male and female gonads, external genitalia, and sexual characteristics. A true hermaphrodite has both ovarian and testicular tissue, either or both of which may be functional.

pseudohermaphrodite—an inexact, confusing, and often unnecessary general term for an individual with gonads and genotype of one sex and external genitalia more consistent with the opposite sex. A male pseudohermaphrodite has testes but otherwise appears to be female (typically represented by the androgen-insensitivity syndrome) (Fig. 68-3). A female pseudohermaphrodite has ovaries, but the external genitalia are masculinized (typically represented by congenital adrenal hyperplasia). It is nearly always possible, desirable, and sufficient to name the specific condition or syndrome.

genotype—an expression of the genetic characteristics of an individual cell as determined by analysis of the number and morphologic characteristics of the chromosomes examined at metaphase; for example, 46, XX indicates that the individual has 44, normal autosomes and two normal X chromosomes, the genotype of a normal female; 46, XY is the normal male genotype; and 45, XO indicates 44 autosomes, one X, and deletion of the second sex chromosome, as seen in Turner's syndrome.

phenotype—the external habitus and general appearance of the individual. In intersex states, it refers more specifically to the appearance of the external genitalia (male or female). In the postpubertal individual it generally also includes secondary sexual characteristics such as hair distribution, wide or narrow hips, laryngeal enlargement.

dysgenetic gonad—an ovary or testis that has been abnormal from the beginning, usually as the result of the absence or other abnormality of a sex chromosome complement of the cells. The streak gonad (as in Turner's syndrome) can be regarded as a dysgenetic ovary. Neoplasms, especially gonadoblastoma, are likely to occur in dysgenetic gonads.[14-16]

gonadal dysgenesis—the gonads are streaks composed of fibrous ovarian stroma with no follicles and no ova. The phenotype is female, and fallopian tubes, uterus, and vagina are present. Patients with associated short stature, webbing of the neck, widely spaced nipples, and, less frequently, coarctation of the aorta and red-green color blindness are said to have Turner's syndrome. Those with the gonadal lesion only are classified as having pure gonadal dysgenesis. In Turner's syndrome, the cytogenetic lesion is usually (57%) absence of the second sex chromosome, critical for normal ovarian development and reproductive function, in at least some of the cells. Typically the karyotype is 45, XO, but mosaic forms are frequent. The remaining 43% have other abnormalities. The absence of the second X chromosome leads to an accelerated loss of oocytes.

Hilar cells, mesonephric duct remnants, and a fibrous stroma reminiscent of ovarian stroma usually are identifiable (Fig. 68-4). The presence of a few ova indicates that the patient may be a mosaic. Pure gonadal dysgenesis is most often associated with either a 46, XY or a 46, XX karyotype. Cordlike structures similar to an immature testis support the existence of at least a few Y chromosomes. When a chromosome Y is present, gonadoblastoma and other germ cell tumors may develop.[14]

mixed gonadal dysgenesis—second most common cause of sexual ambiguity. One gonad is a fibrous streak, as in Turner's syndrome, and the other is a testis (Fig. 68-5), usually an immature or rudimentary testis, but occasionally the dysgenetic gonad opposite the streak is replaced by a tumor (frequently a gonadoblastoma and other germ cell tumors).[14,17,18] The internal genitalia include a uterus, upper portion of a vagina, and, despite the influence of the testis, usually two fallopian tubes. The phenotype varies considerably, from normal male to normal female, with variable degrees of ambiguity in many instances; there is usually asymmetry of the labioscrotal swelling (Fig. 68-6), and a few have the appearance of those with Turner's syndrome. The chromosomal lesion varies but commonly includes mosaicism with both 45, XO and 46, XY stem lines. Approximately two thirds of the patients are reared as females.[14,17]

Table 68-2 Intersex syndromes affecting females, apparent females, or female genitalia

Syndrome	Gonads	Karyotype (genotype)	Inheritance	Internal genitalia	External genitalia	Habitus (phenotype)	Comment
Pure gonadal dysgenesis with abnormal karyotype	Bilateral streaks	XX/XO; XO/XY	No	Vagina uterus, and tubes		Female	
Pure gonadal dysgenesis with normal karyotype	Streaks	XX	Autosomal recessive	Female	Female	Female	Some with nerve deafness
Pure gonadal dysgenesis with male karyotype (Swyer syndrome)	Bilateral streaks	XY	X-linked recessive or autosomal dominant	Vagina, uterus, and tubes	Female	Female	Gonadal neoplasms; virilization
Turner's syndrome	Bilateral streaks	XO, mosaics	No	Vagina, uterus, and tubes	Female	Female	Multiple malformations
Gonadal agenesis	Absent	XY	Uncertain	Rudimentary tubal structures; no uterus or vagina	Ambiguous or female	Female	Minor malformations in some cases
Mixed gonadal dysgenesis	Streak and dysgenetic testis	XO/XY	No	May be uterus and tubes	Variable male-female	Female	Gonadal neoplasms; virilization at puberty
True hermaphrodite	Ovary and testis Ovotestis Ovotestis with ovary or testis	Majority XX Some XY Many mosaics	No	Usually vagina, uterus, and tubes	Ambiguous variable	Variable male-female	
Female pseudohermaphrodite (chiefly adrenogenital syndrome)	Ovaries	XX	Autosomal recessive	Vagina, uterus, and tubes	Ambiguous	Female	Some infants virilized by iatrogenic androgens
47, XXX syndromes	Ovaries	XXX, XXXX, and a variety of mosaics	No	Uterus, vagina, and tubes	Female	Female	Some have been mentally retarded
Male XX	Testes	XX	No	Male	Male		Similar to Klinefelter's syndrome (see Chapter 67)
Male pseudohermaphrodite with normal male karyotype							
1. Defect in testosterone synthesis	Testes	XY	Autosomal recessive	Male—may be rudimentary	Variable	Variable	
2. Defect in testosterone synthesis	Testes	XY	Autosomal recessive	Male	Ambiguous	Female	Virilization at puberty
3. Müllerian inhibitory substance (MIS) failure	Testes	XY	?	Female—no male structures	Male	Male	
Testicular feminization syndrome	Testes	XY	?	Male	Female	Female	

Courtesy Dr. Robert H. Shikes, Denver.

gonadal agenesis—gonads and internal genitalia are completely absent. Phenotype is female; genotype is XY. This is an extremely rare condition, the absence of müllerian duct derivatives is unexplained.

True hermaphroditism

Recognizable ovarian and testicular tissues are both present, together in the same gonad (an *ovotestis*), on opposite sides, or in combinations such as an ovotestis on one side with an ovary or a testis on the other. There is nearly always a uterus. The side with a testis has a vas deferens; the side with an ovary has a tube. A wide variety of internal genitalia combinations occurs, and the phenotypes and external genitalia are also extremely variable. Most patients have a 46, XX karyotype (60%), but 46, XY and a variety of mosaics have been reported. Some testes (but no ovotestes) have produced sper-

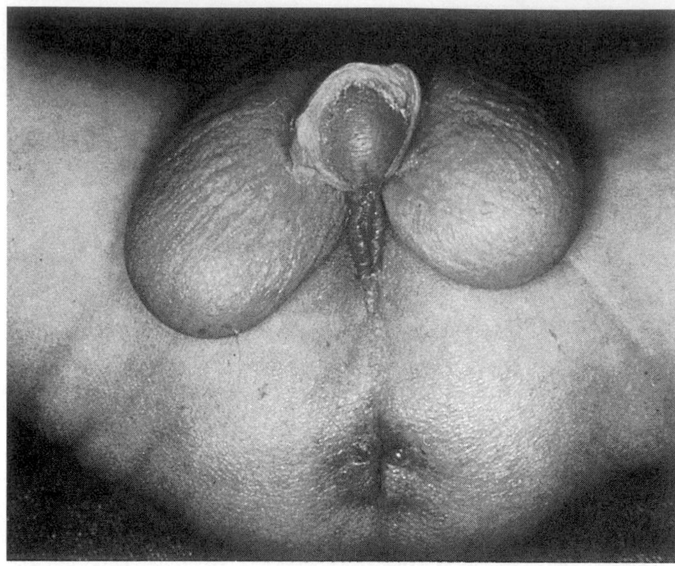

Fig. 68-3 External genitalia of a 46, XY male pseudohermaphrodite.

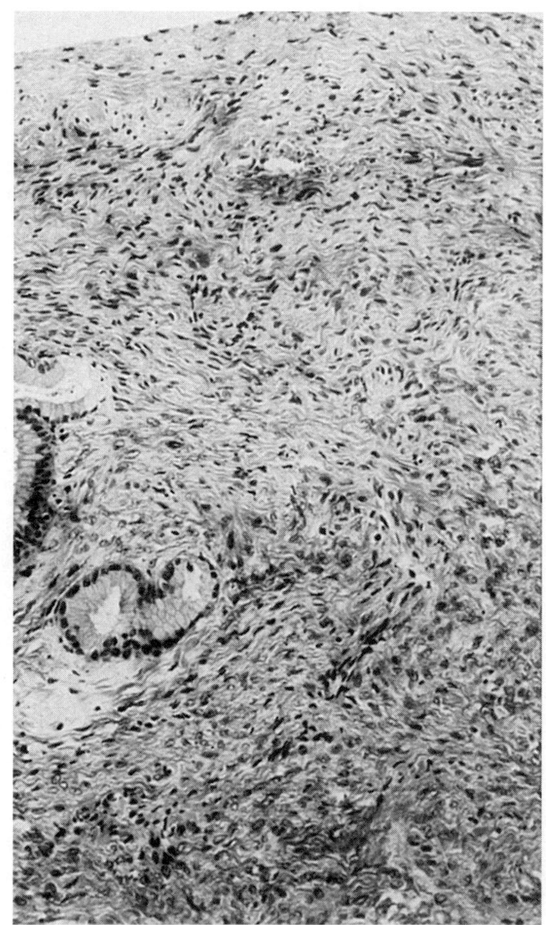

Fig. 68-4 Streak gonad in Turner's syndrome. Tiny müllerian cysts (lower left) and hilar Leydig cells are occasionally evident, but germ cells and follicles are absent after birth.

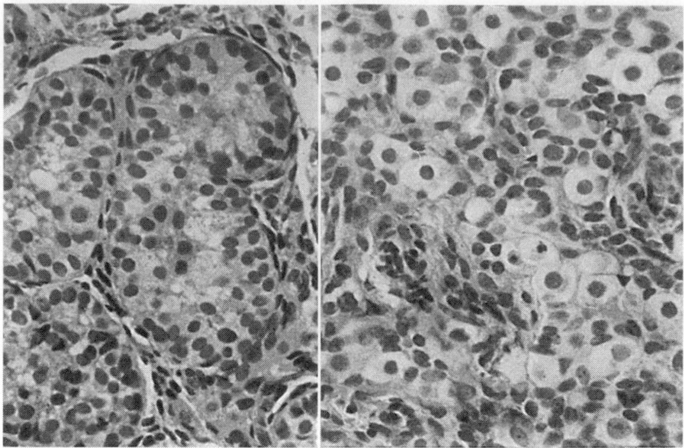

Fig. 68-5 Mixed gonadal dysgenesis. Testicular tissue *(left)* and streak gonad *(right)*.

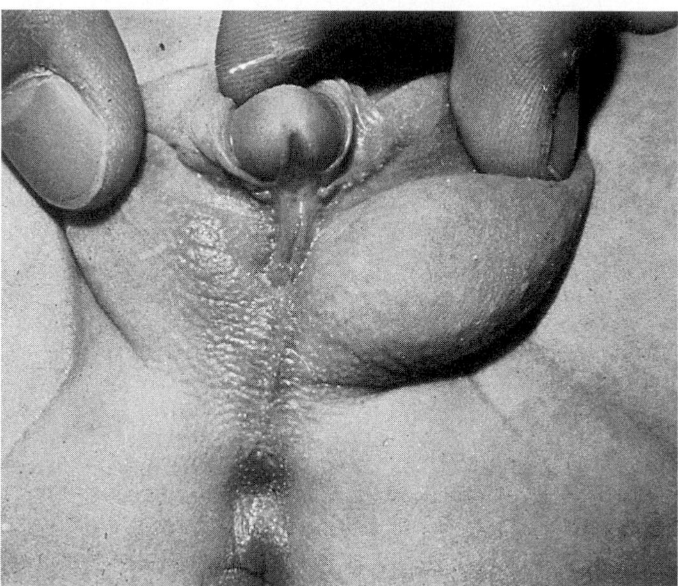

Fig. 68-6 External genitalia in mixed gonadal dysgenesis. The left testis has descended into the scrotum; the right streak was in the abdomen.

matozoa; there have been rare pregnancies.[19] Gonadal tumors, usually germinomas, occur in less than 3% of the patients.[20,21]

Androgen-insensitivity syndromes (testicular feminization) and other forms of male pseudohermaphroditism

End-organ abnormalities result in varying degrees of deficiency of masculinization. Androgen-insensitivity syndromes are the most common cause of male pseudohermaphroditism; there are three groups, all with XY genotypes and testes.[14,18,22,23] In the first group, (familial incomplete male pseudohermaphroditism, type 2) absence of the intracellular enzyme 5-alpha-reductase blocks formation of dihydrotestosterone, on which development of external genitalia depends: the external genitalia appear to be female. At puberty testicular androgens induce masculine habitus and phallus enlargement. The second category, *testicular feminization,* is a generalized insensitivity to all androgens (Figs. 68-7 and 68-8); not only are the external genitalia female, but also at puberty the breasts enlarge and a typical general female body habitus with normal female self-image develops. The vagina is short and ends blindly. The third, somewhat variable group may be lumped together as Reifenstein's syndrome (familial incomplete male pseudohermaphroditism, type 1). The predominant phenotype is male, and external genitalia appear male but with defects, notably hypospadias. Gynecomastia occurs at puberty. The testes are small and immature, spermatogenesis is defective, and infertility is the rule.

Hamartomas develop in 63% of the cases of androgen insensitivity syndrome, and Sertoli cell adenomas in 23%. Malignant tumors occur in about 9% of these patients.[23] Rare instances of deficient testosterone synthesis result in incomplete development of wolffian duct derivatives and female or ambiguous external genitalia. Finally, ineffective MIS secretion results in a phenotypic male with testes (often cryptorchid), male internal and external genitalia, and uterus (Fig. 68-9) and fallopian tubes.

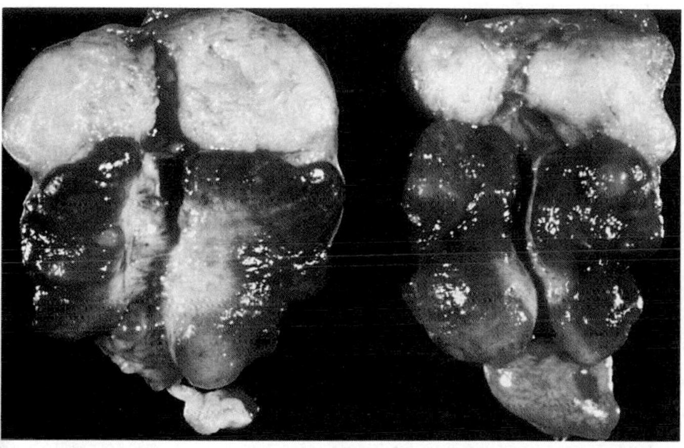

Fig. 68-7 Testes in the complete form of androgen insensitivity (testicular feminization) syndrome. The bisected nodules at the upper poles are muscle bodies; the testes appear dark and contain discrete harmartomas.

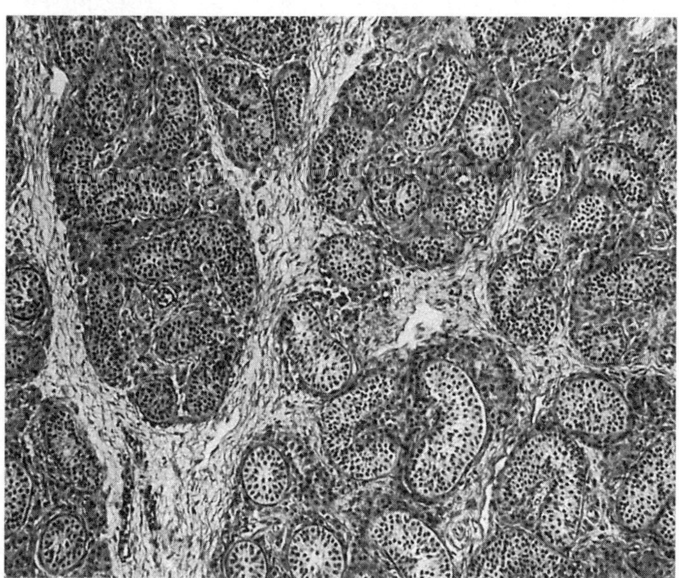

Fig. 68-8 Androgen insensitivity (testicular feminization) syndrome. The testis shows immature solid tubules filled with Sertoli cells and stroma resembling ovarian stroma.

Congenital adrenal hyperplasia and other hormonally induced causes of female pseudohermaphroditism

Congenital adrenal hyperplasia is fundamentally an adrenal abnormality in which defective hydrocortisone synthesis leads to androgen excess. The gonads are normal ovaries; the uterus and tubes are likewise normal. The morphologic genital defect involves the external genitalia only and is the result of excessive androgen production by hyperplastic adrenal glands. This is the most common cause of ambiguous genitalia; it is also the most effectively treatable so that fertility and all other aspects of a normal sex role can usually be achieved. Because of the hydrocortisone deficiency, it is also likely to be fatal if unrecognized and is therefore the most important abnormality of sexual development to recognize at birth.

Rarely a similar masculinization of the external genitalia has been caused by the androgenic effect of progestogens administered to pregnant women in the hope of preventing abortion.

Other chromosomal syndromes

Other cytogenetic abnormalities affecting the sex chromosomes are less likely to be seen as malformations of female genitalia. The female with one or more extra X chromosomes (such as 47, XXX) is phenotypically normal; some have mental retardation. Klinefelter's syndrome (usually 47, XXY) involves a malformation of the male genitalia.

Localized malformations

Ovary. An ovary may be absent. The tube and uterine horn on the same side usually are also absent, and, of great clinical

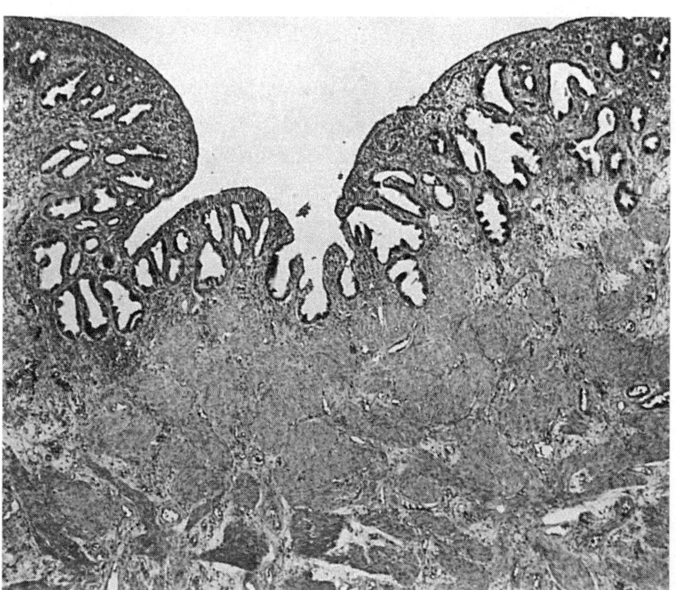

Fig. 68-9 Persistent müllerian duct syndrome (hernia uteri inguinalis) secondary to deficiency of müllerian inhibiting substance (MIS). Endomyometrium present in a hernia sac of a phenotypic male.

significance, the kidney and ureter on the affected side may be absent as well. Supernumerary ovaries and accessory ovarian tissue are most commonly found adjacent to a normally situated ovary. In rare instances ovarian tissue has been identified in the retroperitoneum, posterior bladder wall, and omentum and sigmoid mesentery.[24] Occasionally a cystic teratoma has arisen at such a site.

Fallopian tube. Duplication and atresia of the fallopian tubes occur rarely. Small patches of mucinous and endometrial epithelium may occur, especially when there is inflammation or endometriosis, and so it may not be clear whether this change in the tubal lining is congenital or acquired by metaplasia. Unilateral absence of a tube is uncommon and is associated with ureteral and renal abnormalities, including absence of ipsilateral kidney and ureter.

Uterus, vagina, and vulva. The most common anomaly of the uterus, vagina, and vulva is the result of failure of fusion of some or all of the lower müllerian ducts. All gradations may occur, from complete separation causing the development of two complete genital tracts, to minimum failure with an incomplete sagittal septum at the uterine fundus. In the presence of a complete double vagina, a double cervix and uterus are usual, but duplication of a distal structure such as the cervix does not invariably indicate that the uterine corpus is duplicated. Pregnancy may occur in either side or both.

Anomalies involving failure of fusion or establishment of patency in the lower müllerian system are often associated with urinary tract anomalies, including unilateral renal agenesis and misplaced ureters that discharge into the bladder at an abnormal site such as the uterus or vagina.

Transverse septa and atresias in the vagina probably result from the failure to canalize the distal end of the müllerian duct. Retention of fluid (hydrocolpos or hematocolpos) is usually caused by a transverse septum situated proximally to a patent hymen.

Nearly all patients with congenital absence of the vagina have no uterus; however, when the vagina is apparently absent and accumulated menstrual blood forms a bulging cystic mass, the obstruction is almost always below the cervical level.

An extreme degree of hypoplasia of the cervix—or apparent absence or atresia of the cervix—occasionally also causes a cystic accumulation of menstrual blood in the normally formed uterine corpus; successful term pregnancy is possible after surgical reconstruction.[25]

Associated with internal duplications, there may be even more rarely a duplication of the external genitalia, including both labia, the clitoris, and the urethra.[26] Congenital fistulas between the anus or rectum and vestibule have been described.[27]

VULVA

Anatomy and physiology

The vulva is an anatomic site of transition from the skin to the vaginal squamous mucosa. It is composed of the labia majora, labia minora, mons veneris, clitoris, vestibule, hymen, Bartholin's glands, and minor vestibular glands. The entire vulva is covered by keratinized squamous epithelium, which meets medially with the nonkeratinized glycogenated vaginal mucosa and anteriorly with the transitional epithelium of the urethral meatus. The mons veneris and labia majora have the gross and microscopic characteristics of skin with hair follicles, sebaceous glands, and sweat glands, including apocrine sweat glands. The inner surfaces of the labia majora, labia minora, and vestibule have sebaceous glands but no hair and are covered by a less keratinized epithelium. They are not really mucous membranes histologically. The vulva is profusely permeated by lymphatics that cross the midline extensively so that a lesion on one side is very likely to affect the lymph nodes on the opposite side. Lymph from the labia flows to the superficial inguinal nodes; lymph from the vestibule and clitoris may flow directly through the lymphatics of the urethra and anterior bladder plexus into the pelvic or deep femoral nodes. The vulvar epithelium that extends between the hymen and the edges of the labia minora is of endodermal origin, whereas the remaining outer portion of the vulva derives from the ectoderm, just like the skin.

To establish the correct histologic diagnosis of vulvar diseases, the pathologist must be familiar with diseases of both skin and mucous membranes, since the diseases of the vulva are essentially identical to those of the extravulvar skin and mucous membranes.

Infectious diseases

The vulva represents the portal of entry and the lesional site of most venereal infections. Many inflammatory lesions of the vulva are ulcerated and painful or pruritic. The infectious lesions of the vulva prevalent in North America and Europe include condylomata acuminata, herpes genitalis, syphilis, and molluscum contagiosum.[28] Two granulomatous diseases occurring preferably in tropical areas deserve a brief mention: granuloma inguinale, caused by *Calymmatobacterium granulomatis,* a gram-negative enterobacterium that appears as intracellular Donovan bodies; the lesions assume gigantic size and can be mistaken for carcinoma.[29-31] Lymphogranuloma venereum, caused by *Chlamydia* organisms, spreads through lymphatics and produces painful lymphadenopathy and fibrosis.[32,33] The specific pathologic features of venereal diseases and other infectious disease of the vulva are described in the chapters devoted to bacterial diseases (Chapter 33), viral diseases (Chapter 36), and fungal diseases (Chapter 37). Crohn's disease of the intestinal tract (Chapters 54 and 56) may produce destructive vulvar granulomas and abscesses.[34] Amebiasis may simulate carcinoma grossly and microscopically.[35]

Herpes genitalis

Herpetic vulvitis is caused by a distinctly specific strain of virus (herpesvirus, type 2) that is indigenous to the genital tract.[36] It is characterized by multiple painful vesicles that ulcerate, and heal in about 2 weeks (Fig. 68-10). Herpesvirus has been implicated by epidemiologic data as having some oncogenic potential, however its role has been overshadowed by that of human papillomavirus (HPV).[37] Active vulvar herpes infections are especially threatening during pregnancy because transmission to the newborn at parturition is usually fatal.[38]

Squamous cells with viral inclusions are round and exhibit the typical nuclear molding when multinucleated. They are easily identifiable at the margins of vulvar vesicles or ulcers (Tzank prep) and in vaginocervical smears.

Molluscum contagiosum

Molluscum contagiosum is a moderately contagious venereal disease caused by a large DNA-pox virus. The lesions are

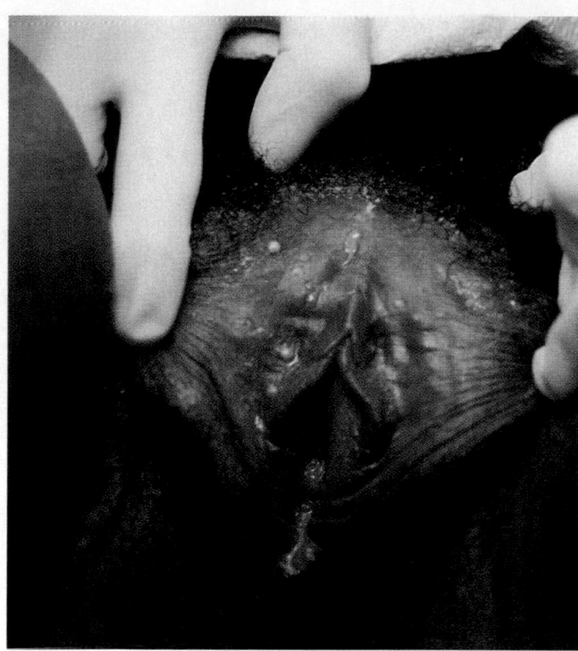

Fig. 68-10 Herpesvirus infection of vulva. The mucosa shows numerous vesicles. (Courtesy Dr. Cynthia Caputo, Philadelphia.)

small papulonodules with central umbilication. The characteristic bodies begin two or three cells above the basal cell layer as pink inclusions that become basophilic in upper layers of the epidermis. Eosinophilic inclusions are Feulgen negative, and the basophilicones are Feulgen positive.[39]

Bartholin's gland cyst and abscess

Bartholin's glands may be infected by any bacterial agent; the ducts may become dilated behind an obstruction, and so an abscess, which may be acutely swollen and painful, is produced. A less severe chronic bacterial infection may evolve more slowly into a fluid-filled cyst. The most common cause of Bartholin's gland abscesses and cysts is gonorrhea, but other pathogenic bacteria can cause the same reactions. The mass must be distinguished from a neoplasm, and therefore a biopsy at the time of drainage is desirable, especially in the absence of any prior symptoms of acute inflammation.

Nonneoplastic epithelial disorders

The vulvar epithelium is subject to a group of chronic conditions of unknown origin, chiefly affecting older women. The skin appears white, mottled red and white, or, less commonly, red. There are variable degrees of atrophy of the subcutaneous tissue, and so at an advanced stage the labia become obliterated and the introitus becomes stenotic. Pruritus is common and may be severe and unremitting. The perineum and perianal skin may also be affected. The word *dystrophy*, which means 'defective nutrition,' was proposed to simplify the designation of these intractable vulvar lesions.[40,41]

For many years, vulvar dystrophies were subclassified into two groups, those with or without atypia. Recently, this classification has been considered totally inadequate. The main reason is that a variety of inflammatory dermatoses of no or unknown malignant potential were classified together with the premalignant lesions of the vulvar epithelium. Specific dermatoses such as psoriasis and lichen planus affect the vulva, usually as a part of a more generalized process on other cutaneous surfaces, but occasionally are confined to the vulva.

Similarly, the term *leukoplakia* which means 'white plaque,' often is used by clinicians to describe the patchy areas of whitened skin or mucous membranes. As the result of extremely varied usage in the past, both terms (dystrophy and leukoplakia) have no specific pathologic diagnostic meaning at this time. Their use by a pathologist now is undesirable. The microscopic evaluation of the clinically abnormal area is crucial because a variety of vulvar lesions of different biologic significance and premalignant potential may appear either white or red, hypertrophic or atrophic.

In 1986, the International Society for the Study of Vulvar Diseases (ISSVD) in collaboration with the International Society of Gynecological Pathologists (ISGYP) proposed a new nomenclature that allowed a distinct separation of the premalignant and nonneoplastic epithelial lesions of the vulva.[42] The use of the term *dystrophy* was discontinued, and the nonneoplastic epithelial disorders of the vulvar skin and mucosa were subdivided into lichen sclerosus (lichen sclerosus et atrophicus), squamous cell hyperplasia (formerly hyperplastic dystrophy), and other dermatoses (such as lichen planus, psoriasis, seborrheic dermatitis, allergic contact dermatitis, and candidiasis). All these nonneoplastic lesions can present as leukoplakic vulvitis.

Lichen sclerosus (lichen sclerosus et atrophicus)

Lichen sclerosus is a nonneoplastic lesion of vulvar epithelium. It is not confined to the vulva and may affect both sexes at any age. However, the majority of patients are postmenopausal women whose lesion and symptoms are either confined to the vulva or associated with circumanal and perineal involvement.

The lesions appear first as small coalescent macules. There is progressive shrinkage of the vulvar connective tissues, and so the skin becomes smooth, shiny, and thin. Eventually, stenosis of the introitus develops. The microscopic appearance is characteristic, but it can vary considerably related to age of the lesion and treatment. In cross section, the epidermis of an advanced lesion is a thin atrophic band without rete ridges. The surface layer is hyperkeratotic. The most distinctive feature is the amorphous homogeneous degenerative change in the dermal collagen, usually in a wide band beneath the epidermis (Fig. 68-11). Elastic fibers are absent; the collagen that remains may stain densely or faintly and is relatively acellular, except for scattered lymphocytes. A band of lymphocytes with a few plasma cells lies beneath, in the middle of the dermis.

Ultrastructurally, elastic fibers become clumped, amorphous, and reduced in number.[43] Collagen metabolism has been found to be abnormally active. An excessive elastase activity and collagenase inhibitor may explain the altered elastic tissue components.[44,45] Premature maturation of all cells above the basal layer has been reported based on their high concentration of involucrin.[46] The cell cycle protein Ki-67 is present in basal and parabasal cells, and the uptake of tritiated thymidine is greater than normal, despite the lack of mitoses.[47,48] Many patients respond to topical testosterone applications. Recent studies have reported good results with topical, high-potency corticosteroids.[49]

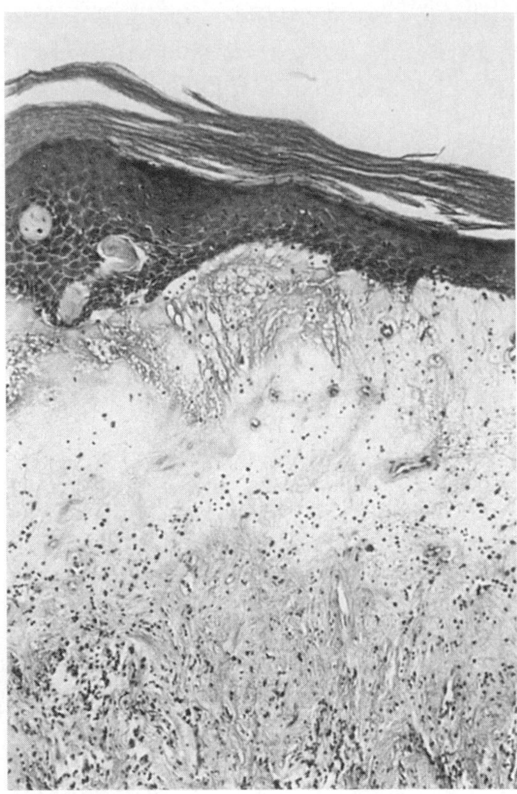

Fig. 68-11 Lichen sclerosus. Epidermis is thin and atrophic; underlying dermal collagen is hyalinized and edematous. Beneath this area is moderate chronic inflammation. There is surface hyperkeratosis.

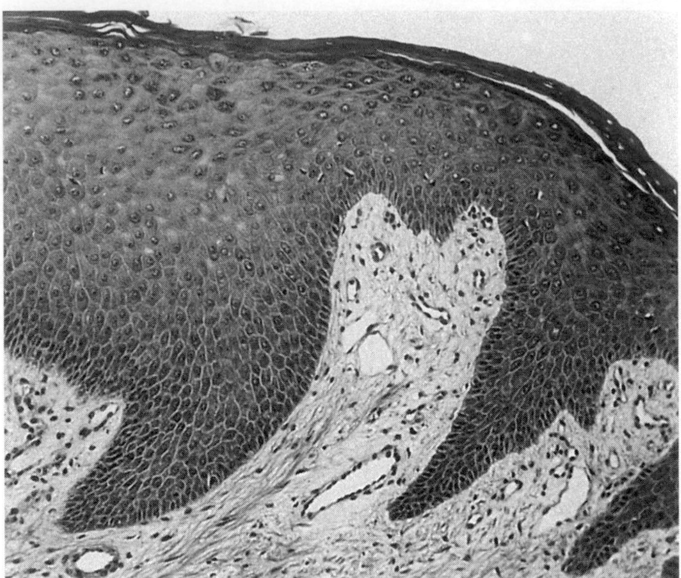

Fig. 68-12 Squamous hyperplasia (hyperkeratosis). Notice keratin layer at surface. Cytologic features are benign.

Squamous hyperplasia (lichen simplex chronicus)

The term *squamous hyperplasia* is used descriptively for a variety of nonneoplastic proliferative lesions of the vulva. Some of these lesions represent a response to hormonal influences, whereas others are induced by exposure to exogenous irritants.

Microscopically there is a thick layer of surface keratin, hyperplastic but cytologically benign squamous epithelium, and a mixture of chronic inflammatory cells distributed through the underlying dermis (Fig. 68-12). Scratching adds trauma and chronic inflammation and thereby probably reinforces pruritus. The microscopic pattern is often indistinguishable from the condition known to dermatologists as "lichen simplex chronicus" at other cutaneous locations.

Symptomatic relief has resulted from use of topical creams containing hydrocortisone or other corticoid hormone preparations. Lesions that include cells with atypical cytologic abnormalities are classified as vulvar intraepithelial neoplasia, as discussed later in this chapter.

Vulvar dermatoses

Vulvar dermatoses include, among others, lichen planus; psoriasis; contact, seborrheic and atopic dermatitis; fixed drug eruption; Fox-Fordyce disease; bullous diseases; and pigment disorders. The clinicopathologic features of these lesions are discussed in Chapter 71. Vulvar vestibulitis deserves special mention. It is a disorder of unknown cause associated with inflammation of the vulvar vestibule, tenderness to pressure, and dyspareunia. An infectious cause has been excluded. Microscopically there is mild to moderate superficial chronic inflammation, predominantly lymphocytic, but plasma cells are usually present. Minor vestibular glands appear surrounded by the inflammatory process. Topical therapy with testosterone obtains some relief. Management is long term and supportive.[50,51]

Clinicopathologic correlation. Lichen sclerosus and squamous hyperplasia may occur together and in the vicinity of precancerous lesions and carcinomas. Multiple biopsies are necessary for evaluation of an extensive lesion, especially if its appearance varies from place to place.

The frequency of subsequent malignant change has been much debated. In a series of 350 women whose original lesion was lichen sclerosus, subsequent malignant change has been uncommon; only 3.5% of these patients developed squamous cell carcinomas (SCC).[52] When lichen sclerosus is associated with SCC, squamous hyperplasia is usually found adjacent to the carcinoma.[53] Aneuploidy by flow cytometry has been reported in 4 of 17 cases of lichen sclerosus.[54]

Benign tumors and tumorlike conditions

Cysts and ectopic tumors

Bartholin cyst and abscess has been discussed. *Keratinous* cysts, usually located on the labia majora, are superficial and range in size from 2 to 5 mm. Some of them may be secondary to occlusion of sebaceous glands that subsequently undergo squamous metaplasia. *Mucous cysts* are encountered in the vestibule and are lined by mucus-secreting cuboidal to columnar epithelium. In contrast to the results from mesonephric cysts, Alcian blue and mucicarmine stains of mucous cysts show positive results. These cysts probably result from occlusion of minor vestibular glands and are believed to derive from urogenital sinus endoderm.[55] *Ciliated cysts,* lined by columnar epithelium resembling müllerian (tubal-endometrial) epithelium have been reported in the vulvar vestibule. They are believed to be acquired, since the müllerian ducts do not contribute to the formation of the vulvar vestibule. In contrast to endometriotic cysts no endometrial stroma or hemosiderin-laden macrophages are found. *Mesonephros-like cysts,* lined by cuboidal, nonciliated, mucin-negative epithelium, can be found on the lateral aspects of the vulva and vagina.[56] *Mesothelial cysts* of the canal of Nuck occur in the upper aspect of the labia majora and are believed to originate from peritoneal inclusions at the insertion of the round ligament into the labia majora. They are analogous to the hydrocele of the spermatic cord.[57] Ectopic breast tissue may develop within the labia majora, can be focal or bilateral and extensive, and has been observed to lactate during puerperium.[58] Fibrocystic disease, fibroadenomas, lactating adenomas, intraductal papillomas, and adenocarcinomas have been described.[59-61] Ectopic salivary gland tissue has also been described in the vulva.[62]

Hidradenoma papilliferum

Papillary hidradenoma is a small neoplasm that forms a nodule less than 2 cm in size in the subcutaneous tissue of the vulva. The papillary fronds are covered by epithelial and myoepithelial cells, supported by a delicate fibrovascular stalk, an arrangement that resembles intraductal papilloma of the breast (Fig. 68-13). Occasional large and pale cells with apocrine features are seen. Papillary hidradenoma is believed to derive from sweat glands. Most tumors are located in the labia, but some of the reported cases occurred in the circumanal region.[63]

Condyloma acuminatum (genital warts)

Condyloma acuminatum is a sexually transmitted benign papillary neoplasm composed of squamous epithelium that occurs chiefly as multiple soft warty masses. They may be large or small and may involve the anus, perineum, vaginal wall, and cervix, as well as the vulva (Fig. 68-14). Small lesions are best appreciated after application of 3% to 5% acetic acid for 3 to 5 minutes and colposcopic examination. Condylomas are commonly associated with sexual activity with multiple partners, immunosuppression, pregnancy, and diabetes mellitus.[64,65] Approximately 30% to 50% of women with vulvar condyloma acuminatum have associated cervical HPV infection.[66] Virologic studies have confirmed a high rate of transmission between sexual partners even in the absence of clinically obvious condylomas. Furthermore, it appears that juvenile laryngeal papillomatosis is often transmitted to infants from maternal condylomas, presumably at parturition.[67] In the United States the incidence of patients seeking treatment rose by over 400% between 1966 and 1981; two thirds of the patients were between 15 and 29 years of age.

The squamous epithelium that covers the papillary fronds is histologically benign and is supported by a uniformly distributed fibrovascular stroma that ramifies into all the papillary projections. Many epithelial cells have typical perinuclear cytoplasmic halos ("koilocytosis") and raisin-like pyknotic nuclei. Scattered cells may have enlarged, darkly stained nuclei related to polyploidy and arrested mitoses.

HPV infections of the vulva usually follow a long course and are influenced by immunologic factors. Regression after pregnancy has been observed. Progression of condyloma acuminatum to vulvar intraepithelial neoplasia and squamous cell carcinoma has also been documented.[68]

The etiologic agent is a papovavirus closely related to the virus of the ordinary cutaneous wart. Most lesions respond to podophyllin, cautery, excision, or freezing. Over 60 strains of HPV have been identified, and the numbers continue to increase. Types 6 and 11 have been recovered from most condylomas.[69-71] In contrast, similar-appearing lesions with dysplastic nuclear changes and many carcinomas (in situ and invasive) are associated with distinctly different strains of the virus (types 16, 18, and 31).[69] Latent virus may be present in normal-appearing skin adjacent to a condyloma, which may account for the high frequency of local recurrence after treatment. Lesions are often multicentric, and the same patient may be infected by more than one viral subtype. Variations in histologic pattern, size, and location indicate that host response can vary and that the appearance of a lesion may represent focal breakdown of host resistance within a larger field of latent HPV infection. Electron microscopic studies have demonstrated the presence of the intranuclear viral particles in condylomas.[72,73] HPV is also identifiable in tissue sections by immunohistochemical methods and by in situ hybridization (Fig. 68-15).

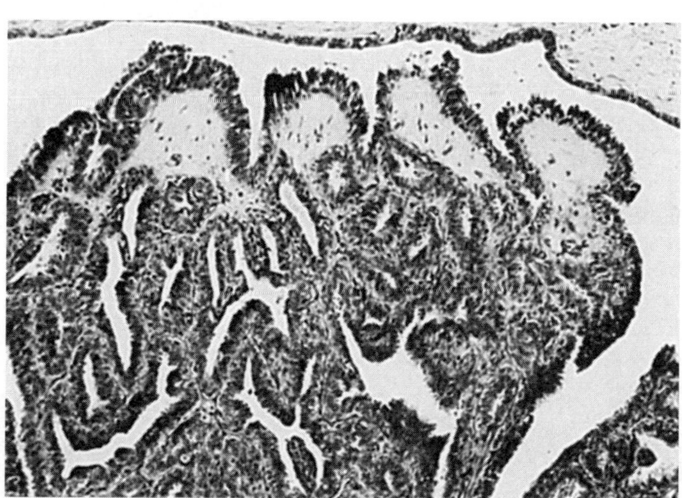

Fig. 68-13 Hidradenoma papilliferum. All the papillary processes have a delicate fibrovascular support, and there is a double layer of epithelial cells covering each of the papillary processes.

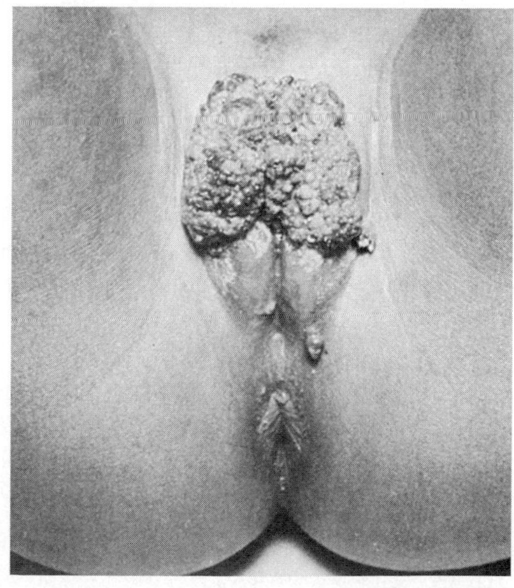

Fig. 68-14 Condyloma acuminatum. Exuberant keratotic papillary processes may cover and obliterate large areas of vulva.

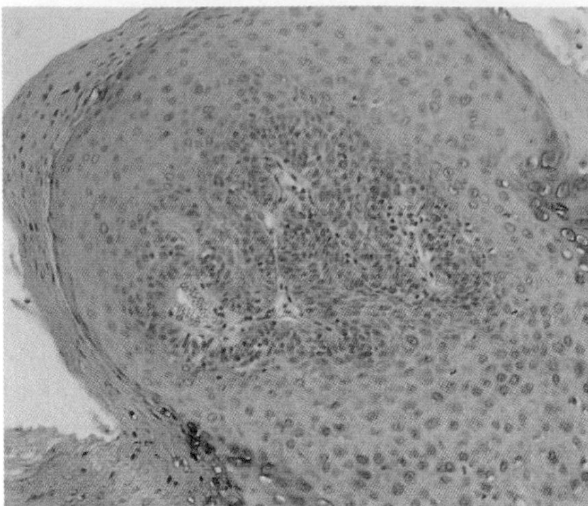

Fig. 68-15 Condyloma acuminatum. Human papilloma virus 6/11 demonstrated in infected cells. In situ hybridization. Virus is localized in the brown-colored nuclei.

Granular cell tumor

Although it is more commonly found in other sites such as the tongue, breast, and respiratory tract, granular cell tumor occasionally produces a poorly circumscribed indurated gray or yellow solid mass in the subcutaneous tissue of the vulva. The tumor cells are large, with abundant pink granular cytoplasm and benign, uniform, round nuclei.

The ultrastructural features are like those occurring in Schwann cells during wallerian degeneration. Secondary lysosomes and large granular structures, called "angulate bodies," appear packed with fibrillar material. Immunohistochemical reactions indicate the presence of S-100 protein and myelin basic protein.[74] Infiltration at the margins and in nearby nerves should not be taken as evidence of malignant behavior but may explain an occasional recurrence. In approximately 50% of these tumors, the overlying squamous epithelium shows pseudoepitheliomatous hyperplasia, which can closely mimic an invasive SCC. Pronounced squamous cell atypia is usually absent in pseudocarcinomatous hyperplasia.[75] The malignant counterpart of granular cell tumor exists but is rare.[76,77]

Fibroepithelial polyps

Cutaneous polyps are invested externally by an orderly epidermis that covers a loose fibrous connective tissue stroma with a variable component of adipose tissue and vessels. Ultrastructurally the stromal cells resemble fibroblasts and myofibroblasts. Their common association with pregnancy may represent a local exuberant response to some stimulating factor.[78]

Rarely a vulvar stromal polyp may include scattered large multinucleated giant cells of the type encountered more commonly in vaginal polyps that simulate sarcoma botryoides. Immunohistochemical studies indicate that the giant cells may derive from fibroblasts and histiocytes.[79]

Aggressive angiomyxoma

Locally, aggressive angiomyxoma may develop in the vulva as a mass within the labia. It occurs in adult women usually under 40 years of age and frequently involves contiguous sites including the vagina and pelvis; it may even reach the retroperitoneum. Grossly, aggressive angiomyxoma presents as a large soft myxoid and apparently well-circumscribed mass

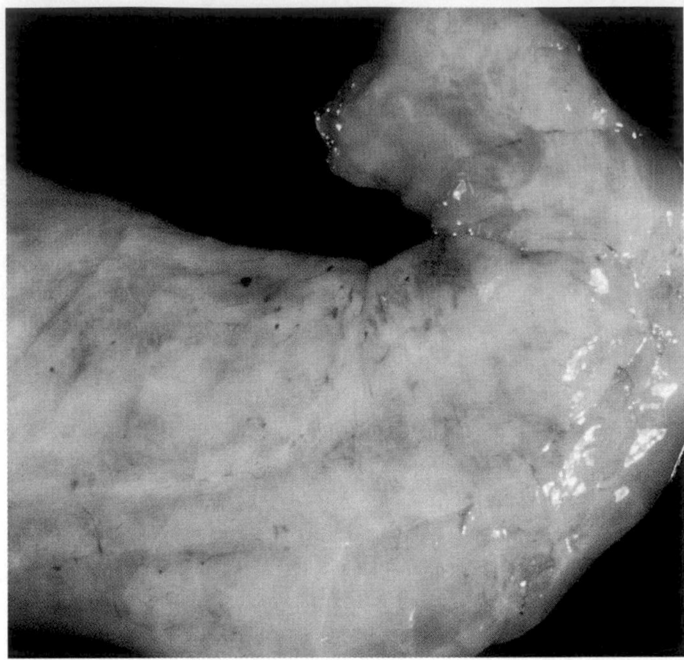

Fig. 68-16 Aggressive angiomyxoma. Large soft myxoid and well-circumscribed mass.

(Fig. 68-16). The microscopic pattern is distinctive and is characterized by hypocellular myxoid tissue with numerous muscular medium-sized vessels (Fig. 68-17). The tumor cells are spindle cell fibroblasts and myofibroblasts that lack significant nuclear atypia and mitotic activity. The cells are immunoreactive to muscle actin but do not show S-100 protein. Ultrastructurally they resemble fibroblasts or myofibroblasts. Differential diagnosis should be established with the myxoid variant of malignant fibrous histiocytoma, which exhibits a storiform pattern and higher degree of nuclear atypia. Although its behavior is benign, aggressive angiomyxoma infiltrates local tissue and local recurrences are common. Metastasis has not been reported. Wide local excision is the treatment of choice.[80,81]

Miscellaneous benign neoplasms

Miscellaneous benign neoplasms include fibromas, benign fibrous histiocytomas, nodular fasciitis, lipomas, hemangiomas, neurofibromas, schwannomas, leiomyomas, rhabdomyomas, ganglioneuromas, and lymphangiomas. Infiltrating margins and numerous mitoses are the most reliable indicators of aggressive behavior of smooth muscle tumors.[82] Cases of pleomorphic adenoma and various types of sweat gland adenomas have been described in the vulva. Cutaneous lesions such as pyogenic granuloma, seborrheic keratosis, nevi of various types, and single squamous papillomas have no distinctive features when encountered in the vulva and are discussed in Chapter 71.

Endometriosis occurs in the vulva usually as the result of implantation of endometrial tissue in minor operative wounds, notably episiotomy scars.

Premalignant lesions of the vulvar epithelium

The precancerous lesions of the squamous epithelium of the vulva are morphologically similar to those of the cervix and vagina, consistent with the observation that all these organs

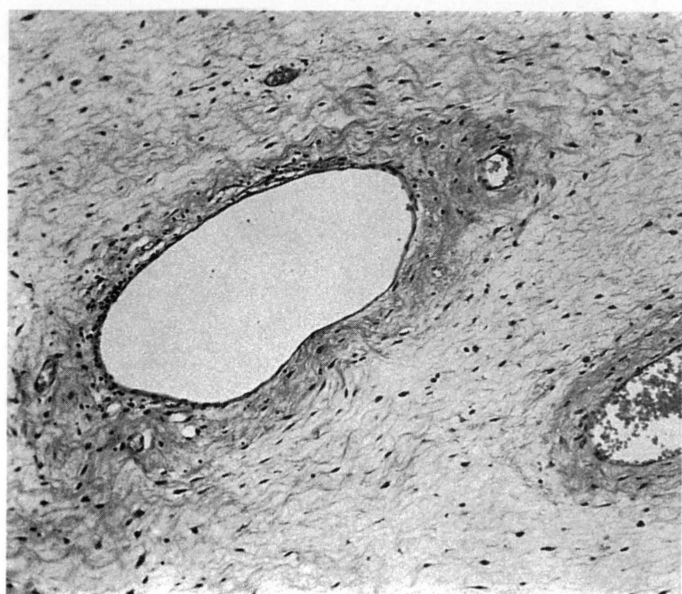

Fig. 68-17 Aggressive angiomyxoma is characterized microscopically by hypocellular myxoid tissue with numerous medium-sized blood vessels.

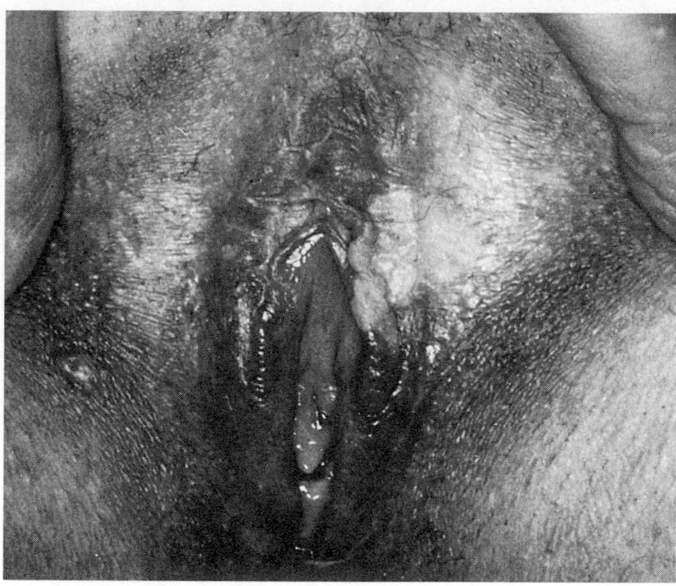

Fig. 68-18 Vulvar intraepithelial neoplasia (VIN). The lesion is white and well circumscribed. It involves the left labium minus.

are susceptible to infection by certain viruses that are known to play a role in carcinogenesis, mainly HPV. The simultaneous or consecutive development of precancerous or cancerous lesions in two or more sites (cervix, vagina, vulva, and circumanal skin) in the same patient is quite common. This field change in the epithelium of the lower female genital tract is of practical importance because it implies that once a precancerous or cancerous lesion has occurred in any of these sites the other sites are at increased risk and the patient requires close follow-up study. There are, however, striking differences histologically and biologically between the precancerous lesions of these organs. For example, lesions of the cervix usually begin in the transformation zone and have a strong tendency to invade. In contrast, those of the vulva arise from native squamous epithelium, exhibit much greater cellular maturation, may remain stable for many years, and may even regress.[41]

In the vulva, the term *carcinoma in situ* has been used in different ways by different investigators. For many years, four varieties were distinguished: Bowen's disease, erythroplasia of Queyrat, squamous cell carcinoma in situ, and extramammary Paget's disease.[83] As with the corresponding cervical lesions, premalignant vulvar lesions exhibiting lesser degrees of nuclear atypicality than carcinoma in situ were referred to with subjective and nonspecific terms such as *atypia* and *dysplasia*. They were also graded as mild, moderate, and severe based on the number of layers of atypical keratinocytes present in the epidermis.

Vulvar intraepithelial neoplasia

All the aforementioned terms (carcinoma in situ, atypia, and dysplasia) have recently fallen into disuse. All premalignant lesions of the squamous epithelium of the vulva are now grouped together under the single heading of *vulvar intraepithelial neoplasia (VIN)*,[42] accepted by both the ISSVD and the ISGYP, as well as by the World Health Organization (WHO). Vulvar intraepithelial neoplasia can be defined as an abnormal growth of vulvar epithelium exhibiting lack of cellular maturation and crowding of cells within the epithelium.[42] Nuclear hyperchromatism, variable nuclear pleomorphism, and abnormal mitoses are usually present. Both Paget's disease and melanoma in situ fall within the VIN category. Three histologic grades of VIN are recognized: VIN I, which corresponds to mild atypia; VIN II, which is equivalent to moderate atypia; and VIN III, which includes both severe atypia and carcinoma in situ.[42]

The acceptance of the VIN terminology was mainly attributable to the knowledge that in many cases the cells in the mild or moderate atypias are nondiploid and that there is no clear correlation between the ploidy value and the degree of maturation in the abnormal epithelium.[84] Almost all carcinomas in situ of the vulva are also nondiploid[84,85] and, apparently, nondiploid atypias and carcinoma in situ are simply different steps of progression of a single biologic entity.

Most studies of the clinical and biologic behavior of VIN have been concerned exclusively with VIN III, the biologic nature of which has been elucidated only recently.[86] It is now universally recognized that the incidence of VIN III is increasing, particularly in women younger than 35 years of age.[86-88] Although most patients complain of pruritus, approximately 40% are asymptomatic, and the VIN III is detected incidentally in patients being treated for condyloma or cervical intraepithelial neoplasia (CIN).[86] Clinically, the lesions are macular-papular, white, and multifocal in approximately 70% of the cases[86] (Fig. 68-18). The most common locations are the labia minora and the perineal region.[86] The vagina may be involved by local extension in about 10% of the cases.[89] About 15% to 30% of the patients have a history of condyloma acuminatum, which in 12% of the cases contain HPV 16, the HPV subtype most commonly associated with VIN and invasive carcinoma.[90] HPV 16 has been detected by Southern transfer hybridization in 81% of the HPV-related VIN cases.[90] HPV types 18 and 31 are less commonly identified.[90]

The diagnosis of VIN can be established only by biopsy, and the multifocal nature of the lesions requires that multiple biopsies be performed. Microscopically the keratinocytes show evidence of abnormal maturation with a high nuclear-to-cytoplasmic ratio, increased mitotic activity, and hyperchromatism. The cells may appear pyknotic and individually keratinized, or there may be formation of intraepithelial pearls within the thickened rete ridges. Multinucleation and atypical mitoses are common. When these changes are limited to the lower third of the epithelium, the lesion is diagnosed as VIN I. VIN II is reported when the changes involve over one third, but not greater than two thirds, of the epithelial thickness. If the cytologic abnormalities involve more than two thirds of the full thickness of the epithelium (excluding the keratin layer), the lesion is designated VIN III. VIN III is subclassified into three types: warty (condylomatous), basaloid (usual type), and differentiated (simplex type). Warty VIN is characterized by considerable proliferation, hyperkeratosis, and parakeratosis. The thickened epithelium has a warty or condylomatous appearance (Fig. 68-19). Although abnormal, the cells show evidence of maturation. Hyperchromatic shrunken nuclei surrounded by clear cytoplasms are typical. Basaloid VIN shows lesser degrees of hyperkeratosis and is almost entirely composed of immature parabasal cells. The picture resembles that of CIN III. Finally, there are rare differentiated cases with little evidence of surface epithelial atypia, the principal abnormality being in the base of the rete ridges where keratin pearls may be found.[89]

Involvement of the skin appendages by VIN occurs in more than 55% of the cases and should not be confused with early invasion. The risk of VIN evolving into an invasive carcinoma is not accurately known but is probably very low. Invasion is more common in elderly women and in those who are immunosuppressed.[86-88,91,92]

The AE1 keratin immunostaining may serve to differentiate hyperplastic lesions from early VIN. Whereas the hyperplastic epithelium shows a suprabasal and uniform stain, the dysplastic cells of VIN I-II lesions are negative, and only the most superficial and mature cell layers are stained. In contrast to VIN I and II, VIN III and invasive SCC exhibit an intense but patchy positive stain (Fig. 68-20). Thus, in vulvar epithelium, transition from VIN I-II to VIN III-SCC is associated with striking changes in keratins recognized by AE1.[41,93]

Frequently, transitional areas from typical condyloma acuminatum to VIN III are identified.[89] Such findings should not be surprising, since it is recognized that the majority of VIN lesions are associated with HPV. In these cases viral capsid antigen can be demonstrated within the condylomas by immunoperoxidase techniques in about 50% of the cases.[94] On the other hand, less than 10% of the cases of VIN III are immunoreactive.[94] Topical podophyllin results in mitotic arrest, and abnormal mitoses may be seen. In contrast to VIN there is nuclear disruption and cellular swelling, but the nuclei remain relatively uniform.

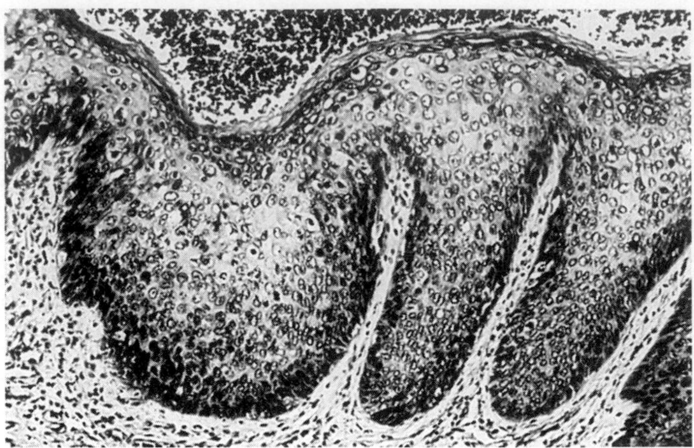

Fig. 68-19 VIN-III, warty type. Many scattered atypical cells through all layers of the epidermis and little evidence of maturation. Notice the koilocytotic atypia.

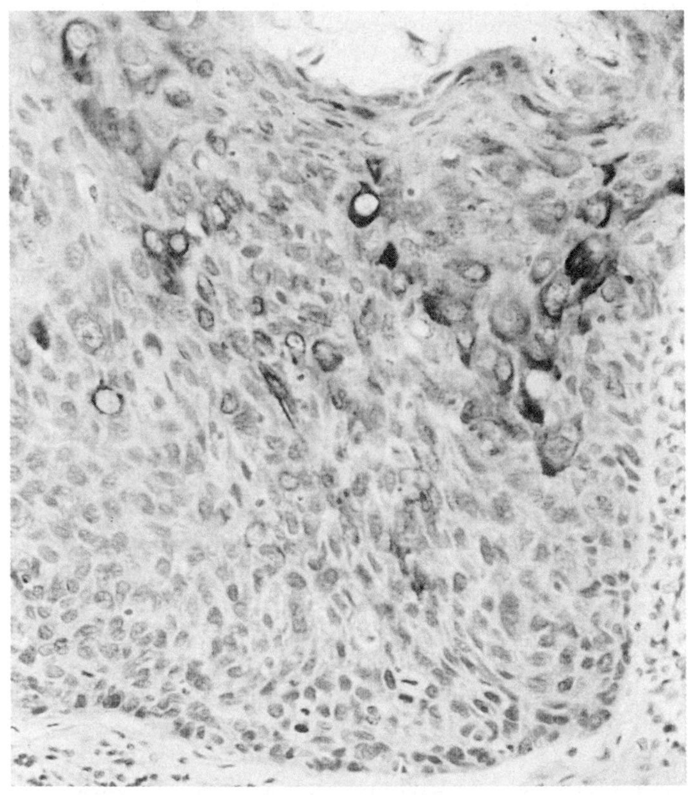

Fig. 68-20 VIN-III, warty type. Patchy reactivity with anti-keratin monoclonal antibody AE1 (Immunohistochemistry).

Bowenoid papulosis

The term *bowenoid papulosis* has been applied to a vulvar lesion characterized by an architectural pattern of condyloma acuminatum and cytologic features of VIN III.[95] These lesions usually present as pigmented papules in young females, often during pregnancy. In several cases, the papules spontaneously regressed, whereas lesions with identical microscopic features but with different gross appearances did not.[89] Some investigators[96] have suggested that bowenoid papulosis could be distinguished from VIN by the lack of pilosebaceous involvement and nuclear uniformity observed in the majority (94%) of cases of the former lesion. However, this distinction was not always obvious in approximately 20% of the cases within the study group.

Virtually every criterion suggested as helpful for the differential diagnosis between bowenoid papulosis and VIN is debatable. Spontaneous regression has been documented in a variety of VIN lesions, even in a case known to be aneuploid.[86] Regression has been recognized as an immunologic phenomenon mediated by T-lymphocytes.[97] In contrast, cases accepted as examples of bowenoid papulosis have been observed to progress both to VIN and to invasive carcinoma.[69,98] Furthermore, recent studies have identified HPV (including HPV 16) with approximately equal frequency in both lesions.[90,99] Skin appendage involvement by VIN is similar to endocervical gland involvement by CIN, and it lacks prognostic significance. VIN lesions exhibiting nuclear uniformity have often been demonstrated to be aneuploid or to show at least low aneuploidy.[84]

According to the ISGYP Committee on Nomenclature of Vulvar Diseases the term *bowenoid papulosis* should not be used as a histopathologic diagnosis. When the characteristic clinical features are present, the following statement could be made in the pathology report: "The pathologic findings are consistent with the clinical diagnosis of bowenoid papulosis."

Extramammary Paget's disease

Vulvar Paget's disease is an intraepidermal neoplasm with features of adenocarcinoma. Treatment and prognosis depend on the presence or absence of associated invasive carcinoma. Grossly, it is characterized by red eczematoid lesions with irregular discrete borders and white keratotic areas. The lesions usually begin in the labia majora, eventually involving labia minora, perineum, the pubic area, thighs, or sacral region.

The epidermis is infiltrated by large pale and vacuolated adenocarcinoma cells, scattered between compressed but normal appearing squamous epithelial cells (Fig. 68-21). The epithelium of hair follicles and apocrine sweat glands is characteristically involved. This is almost always associated with overlying epidermal involvement. Many of the Paget cells contain stainable epithelial mucin and occasionally gland spaces are formed within cells groups. Various types of cytologic differentiation, resembling eccrine, apocrine, and squamous cells, have been described in ultrastructural studies. Immunohistochemical stains consistently identify low-molecular-weight keratin, epithelial membrane antigen (EMA), casein, B72.3, carcinoembryonic antigen (CEA), and fibrocystic disease fluid protein (GCDFP-15).[100,101] The latter appears to be a reliable marker for apocrine epithelium.[102] Immunoreactivity for S-100 and melanoma antigen (HMB-45) is not found. These reactions help to distinguish Paget's disease from VIN and malignant melanoma. Most probably, Paget cells differentiate in situ from multipotential epidermal precursors.[103]

If there is no invasion, the prognosis is good. Treatment of choice varies from wide local excision to simple vulvectomy depending on the extension of the lesions. Margins are difficult to see, and local recurrence is therefore common.

Approximately one patient in three has an underlying infiltrating adenocarcinoma, usually poorly differentiated; foci of squamous differentiation are commonly present. In the presence of invasion, metastases are likely, and the prognosis is very poor.[104]

Malignant tumors

The most common malignant tumor of the vulva is SCC (at least 96%). Malignant melanoma accounts for another 2%, and the rest are rare adenocarcinomas, soft-tissue sarcomas, and occasional basal cell carcinomas. Vulvar carcinomas constitute less than 1% of all cancers and 3.5% to 8% of genital tract cancers in women.

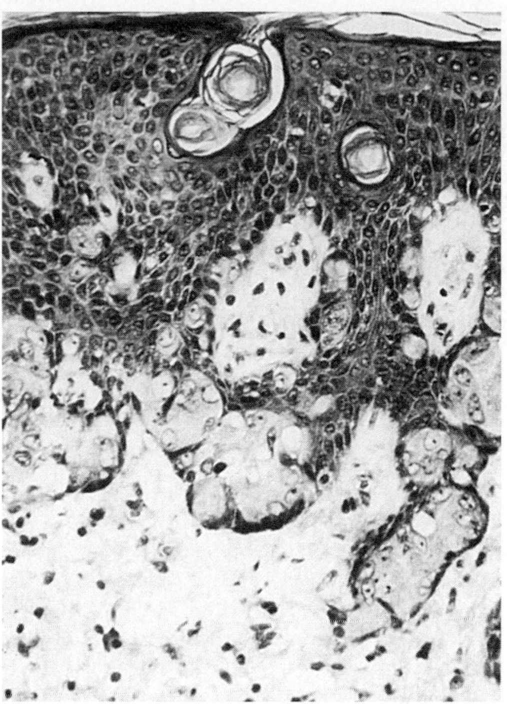

Fig. 68-21 Vulvar Paget's disease. Neoplastic cells infiltrate epidermis individually and in small clumps. Squamous cells of epidermis itself are histologically benign and compressed by tumor. There is no infiltration of underlying dermis.

Superficially invasive squamous cell carcinoma

In the cervix, the term *microinvasive carcinoma* is used to designate a subset of superficially invasive cancers in which the risk of metastasis to regional lymph nodes is negligible. Attempts to similarly define an early form of invasive carcinoma of the vulva have not met with success.

First, it was proposed that vulvar carcinomas less than 2 cm in size and 5 mm in depth were not associated with metastases to the inguinal nodes or recurrence and should be classified as microinvasive carcinomas.[105] Soon, it became increasingly clear that approximately 15% of patients with tumor invasion to a depth of 5 mm or less have inguinal node metastases at the time of vulvectomy.[106-110] Other investigators limited the depth of invasion to 3 mm, but such lesions were found to be associated with inguinal lymph node metastasis in 12% of the cases.[107-109] It has now become apparent that only those tumors that invade to a depth of 1 mm or less (Fig. 68-22) are unassociated, for practical purposes, with any risk of lymph node involvement.[109-113] There are some differences of opinion about where the superficial point of measurement should be made to determine the depth of invasion. According to Wilkinson and colleagues,[109] measurement from the epithelial stromal junction of the adjacent, most superficial dermal papilla has the advantage that an adjacent dermal papilla can be found in all sites in the vulva, and measurement will not be influenced by hyperkeratosis, tumor surface ulceration, or adjacent epithelial neoplasia or hyperplasia.

In 1984, the ISSVD accepted the concept of superficially invasive SCC of the vulva (stage IA), defined as a single lesion measuring 2 cm or less in diameter and with a depth of invasion of 1 mm or less. In patients with stage IA tumors, recommended therapy is wide local excision of the lesion,

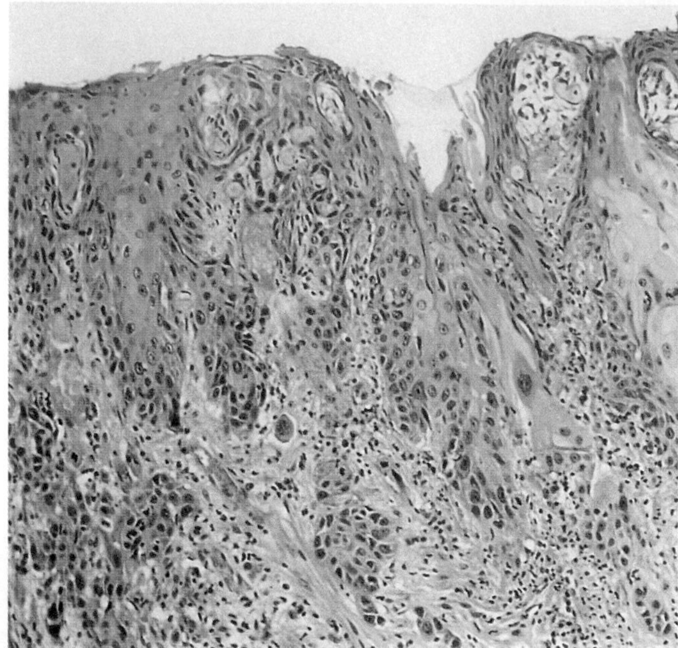

Fig. 68-22 Superficially invasive squamous cell carcinoma. The stroma is invaded by numerous tongues of well-differentiated tumor cells and shows inflammatory changes.

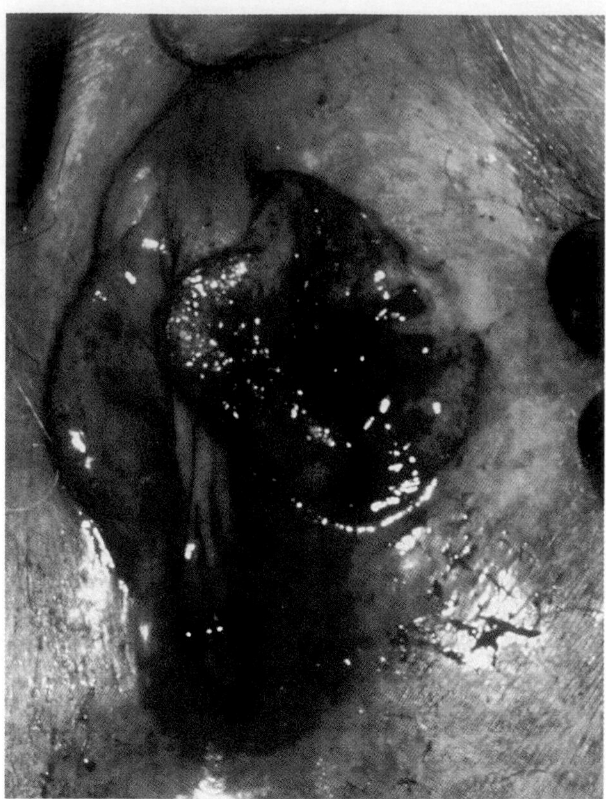

Fig. 68-23 Squamous cell carcinoma of the vulva. Tumor appears as an ulcerated and hemorrhagic mass. The labia are edematous.

without vulvectomy. Modified radical hemivulvectomy with ipsilateral superficial inguinal lymphadenectomy has been recently proposed by the Gynecologic Oncology Group (GOG) as an alternative treatment to traditional radical operation for vulvar carcinomas invading from 1.1 to 5 mm in depth (stage I).[114] The ISGYP committee did not endorse the use of the term "microinvasion," but recommended that the depth of invasion (in millimeters) and the thickness of the tumor (in millimeters) be reported.

Invasive squamous cell carcinoma

Invasive SCC is chiefly a disease of older women (mean age, 77 years) (Fig. 68-23). Approximately 65% of these tumors are well-differentiated SCC that rarely contain HPV.[115,116] The patients often have associated nonneoplastic epithelial lesions, particularly lichen sclerosus or squamous hyperplasia.[115,117,118] In tropical areas, association with chronic granulomatous disease is common. Other risk factors include cigarette smoking, immunosuppression, and diabetes mellitus.[119-121]

A smaller group of vulvar carcinomas (approximately 35%) occurs in younger women (mean age, 55 years) who frequently have associated VIN and even CIN. HPV 16 is detected in approximately 75% of these tumors. These patients are usually heavy cigarette smokers, and their tumors are predominantly of the warty or basaloid types. Squamous hyperplasia of the adjacent epithelium is present in only 17% of these cases.[115,116]

The usual location of vulvar SCC is the labia majora, especially the inner aspect; most tumors begin on the anterior two thirds of the vulva.

Well-differentiated SCC keratinize and have well-circumscribed margins. Lesions with this pattern are more likely to remain localized and have a better prognosis. Poorly differentiated carcinomas have a more diffusely infiltrating pattern, invade nerve sheaths and lymphatics, grow in narrow strands, and have a more aggressive natural history.

Microscopically, warty carcinoma is reminiscent of verrucous carcinoma; it shows multiple papillary projections with keratinized epithelial surfaces and fibrovascular cores. Koilocytotic atypia, dyskeratotic cells, and keratin pearls are frequent. The tumor has a favorable clinical course. However, lymph node metastases can occur. The prognosis appears intermediate between verrucous carcinoma and SCC.[115,116]

Basaloid carcinomas are frequently associated with adjacent VIN (usually of the basaloid type), as well as with SCC of the cervix and vagina.[115,116] Microscopically, these tumors show minimal, if any, squamous maturation. The histologic picture is reminiscent of carcinoma in situ of the cervix.

Some investigators have suggested the implication of HPV in the pathogenesis of warty and basaloid carcinomas.[115,116] It has been demonstrated that cells infected with HPV produce a viral protein (E6) that binds to and causes rapid degradation of the tumor-suppressor protein p53.[122,123] On the other hand, well-differentiated SCC, which are usually HPV-negative tumors, have been recently found to have point mutations of p53.[124]

The presence of inguinal lymph node metastasis in patients with vulvar carcinoma is the crucial prognostic factor. Patients with such metastases have a survival rate of 25% to 52% at 3 to 5 years postoperatively compared with a survival of 76% to

98% at 3 to 5 years in patients without lymph node involvement.[28,125-131] The International Federation of Gynecologists and Obstetricians (FIGO) staging of vulvar carcinoma classifies those carcinomas of the vulva that are 2 cm or less in diameter with clinically negative lymph nodes as stage I.[132] Approximately 50% of the women with vulvar carcinomas are clinically stage I[108] and yet 9% of them have metastatic tumor in the inguinal lymph nodes.[133] It is important to emphasize that a physical examination is an unreliable indicator of metastatic spread; even an experienced examiner is likely to miss metastases or overdiagnose their presence in about 40% of patients.[134]

The risk of lymph node metastasis is influenced by the location of the tumor. Tumors that involve the clitoris or perineal body have a higher risk of nodal metastasis as compared to those occurring in the labia and are more likely to spread to deeper (pelvic, iliac) lymph nodes.[133,135] A large collaborative study by the GOG found that the most significant predictive indicators of node metastases were tumor thickness, palpable nodes, lymphatic space invasion, midline location, and poorly differentiated histologic pattern. Predictive value in an individual case is enhanced when one considers all the above factors together.[133]

Lymph node metastases commonly appear in the opposite side of the vulva, and so bilateral inguinal lymph node dissections are necessary.

Verrucous carcinoma

Verrucous carcinoma is an extremely well-differentiated SCC that seems to push and compress the underlying tissue without any apparent infiltration (Fig. 68-24). Local recurrences are frequent, but metastases to regional lymph nodes do not occur. Aggressive behavior occurs only when the tumor has undergone anaplastic change, frequently after radiation therapy.[136] The vulva is the most common site of genital verrucous carcinoma, but it also occurs in the vagina and cervix.[137]

Although their histologic and cytologic patterns appear similar, it is possible to distinguish verrucous carcinoma from condyloma acuminatum by the larger size and uneven distribution of the fibrovascular stromal support in the former. The term *giant condyloma of Buschke-Löwenstein* is now considered to be a synonym for verrucous carcinoma.

The AE1 keratin–staining pattern of verrucous carcinoma appears uniform and homogeneous everywhere, in contrast to that of SCC, which exhibits a disorganized and patchy staining pattern.[138]

Adenocarcinoma and Bartholin's gland carcinoma

Adenocarcinomas of the vulva are uncommon; they may arise in Bartholin's gland or the minor vestibular glands. The initial appearance is a subcutaneous lump. The microscopic pattern may be that of an adenoid cystic carcinoma, papillary adenocarcinoma, mucoepidermoid carcinoma, or mucinous adenocarcinoma. About one third of Bartholin's gland carcinomas are SCC.

The principles of treatment are the same as those for other vulvar carcinomas. Many patients are premenopausal, and about half of the reported tumors have been originally underestimated as Bartholin's gland cysts.[139] Prognosis is poor because of the rich lymphatic supply to the region, the occult site of involvement, and the delay in diagnosis. The 5-year survival is approximately 33%.[139] Adenoid cystic carcinomas characteristically do not metastasize to lymph nodes but invade widely along nerve sheaths; hematogenous spread occurs late.[140]

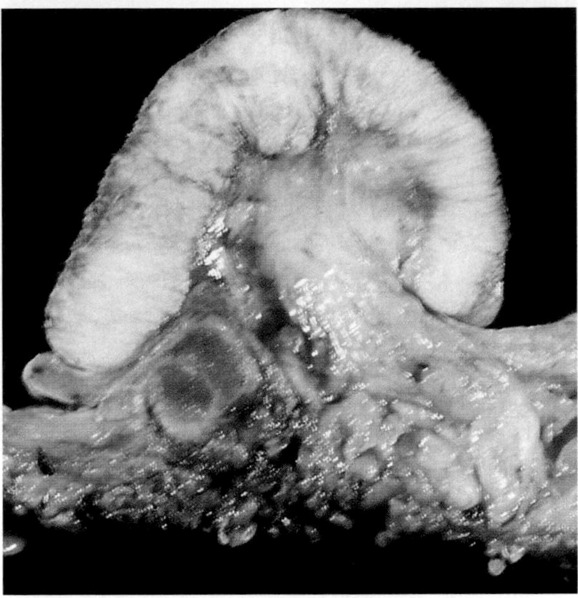

Fig. 68-24 Verrucous carcinoma of vulva in sagittal section. Large, papillary exophytic growth.

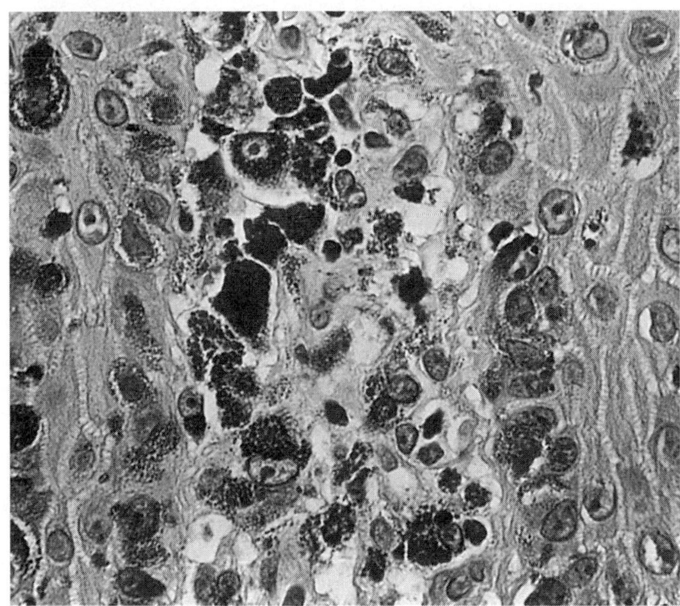

Fig. 68-25 Malignant melanoma of the acral lentiginous type. The epidermis appears infiltrated by pigmented dendritic cells.

Malignant melanoma

Melanomas account for less than 5% of all vulvar malignancies and occur predominantly in the sixth and seventh decades of life. Most tumors are located anteriorly near the midline.

Those arising from the vulvar mucosa are usually of the acral lentiginous type (63%), with junctional clusters of spindle cells[141] (Fig. 68-25), whereas melanomas of the vulvar skin have the pagetoid intracutaneous pattern of superficial spreading melanomas. Depth of invasion is the single most important indicator of prognosis.[142,143] Patients with lesion depths of 1.49 mm or smaller usually have no nodal metastases and may be treated with wide local excision; in contrast, patients with thicker tumors have a high frequency of local recurrence and poor survival and should be treated by radical vulvectomy and bilateral inguinofemoral lymphadenectomy.[143,144]

Metastatic carcinoma

Metastatic carcinoma accounts for approximately 8% of vulvar tumors.[145] The most common primary tumors are from cervix (46%) and endometrium (28%). Metastatic cancers from the colon, breast, and ovary are also found in the vulva and should not be mistaken for primary vulvar cancer. There is usually extensive vascular involvement in deep tissues.[146]

Rare malignant neoplasms

Malignant fibrous histiocytoma, leiomyosarcoma, rhabdomyosarcoma, and malignant lymphoma may occur in the soft tissues of the vulva.[28,147] Malignant rhabdoid tumor, an aggressive neoplasm with aberrant differentiation, has been confused with epithelioid sarcoma.[148] Basal cell carcinomas of the vulvar skin resemble those occurring in more common cutaneous locations.[149] Four yolk sac carcinomas of the vulva have been described.[150]

VAGINA

Anatomy and physiology

The vagina is a collapsed cylinder situated between the vestibule externally and the cervix internally. It has an inner lining of nonkeratinized squamous epithelium surrounded by a layer of connective tissue stroma, all supported by a double layer of smooth muscle. There are no glands, but small glandular remnants of the mesonephric ducts occasionally persist and may form cysts.

The histologic and cytologic features of the squamous epithelium are affected by hormonal stimuli. During the reproductive years estrogens increase the thickness of the epithelium and the amount of cytoplasmic glycogen. The epithelium is thin in childhood and atrophic after menopause, when estrogen stimulation is minimal.

Cytologic patterns, as seen in the vaginal smear, vary with age and undergo cyclic changes with the menstrual cycle. During the first 14 days of the menstrual cycle, a period of estrogen predominance, the exfoliated cells, called "superficial cells," are large and flattened and have pyknotic nuclei. After ovulation, under the superimposed influence of progesterone, the nuclei are larger and vesicular, and the cell margins are folded; these are called "intermediate cells" (Fig. 68-26). The amount of cytoplasmic glycogen is greatly increased, and cytoplasmic margins are dense and accentuated in pregnancy. In childhood, after menopause, and after childbirth the mucosa is atrophic and the predominant exfoliated cells are small, round or oval, parabasal cells that have little glycogen. Small amounts of estrogen administered at these times induce maturation to the estrogenic pattern of superficial cell predominance.

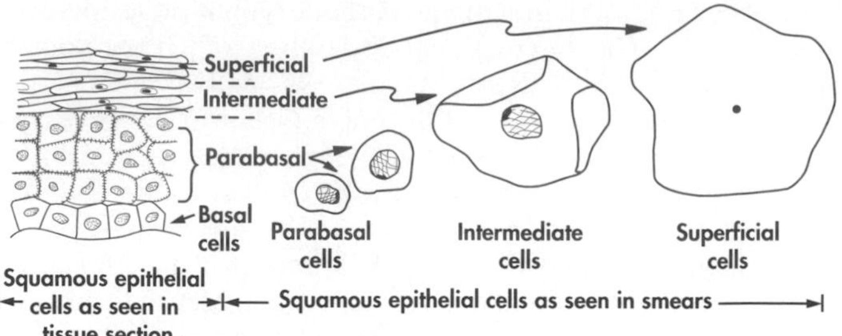

Fig. 68-26 Diagram of relationship between squamous mucosa of vagina and exocervix and parabasal, intermediate, and superficial cells exfoliated and seen in smears. Superficial cells predominate in estrogenic smears of first 2 weeks of menstrual cycle, and intermediate cells predominate in second 2 weeks after ovulation under influence of progesterone. (Modified from Frost JK: *Concepts basic to general cytopathology*, Baltimore, 1972, Johns Hopkins University Press).

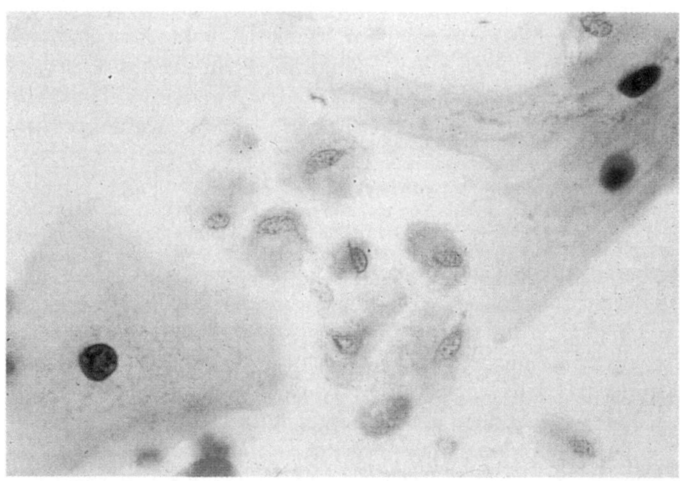

Fig. 68-27 *Trichomonas vaginalis* in cervicovaginal smear. (Courtesy Dr. Karen van Hoeven, Philadelphia.)

Knowledge of the normal cytologic variations is important in the identification of neoplastic cells and other pathologic states.

Cytopathology (infectious diseases)

Bacterial vaginosis, a condition affecting 5% to 10% of women, is caused by *Gardnerella vaginalis,* probably in association with other vaginal bacteria. It is associated with malodorous leukorrhea.

The most common causes of symptomatic vaginitis are a fungus, *Candida albicans,* and a protozoon, *Trichomonas vaginalis*. Hyphae of *Candida* species and are easily identified in smears (Fig. 68-27). In *Trichomonas* infections the vagina has a red punctate appearance with abundant frothy discharge. Candidiasis is associated in typical cases with white patches of mycelia attached to an inflamed mucosa and is more common in pregnant and diabetic women.[151] The vulva and cervix are usually involved simultaneously. In patients with intrauterine devices, infections by *Actinomyces israelii* may occur. In such cases, the vaginal discharge is foul-smelling and contains sul-

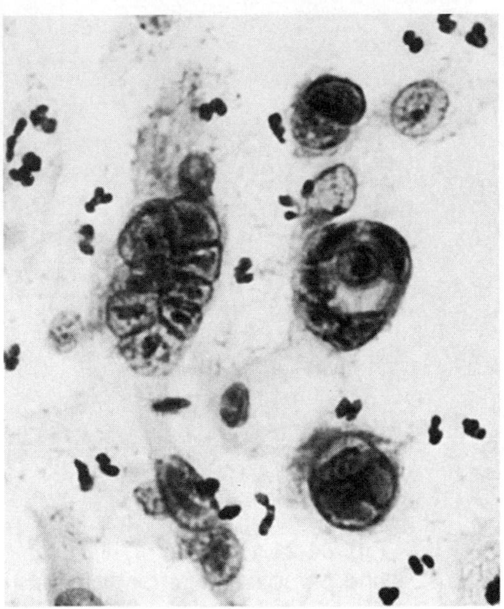

Fig. 68-28 Vaginal smears showing epithelial cells containing typical inclusions of herpesvirus. Notice clustering of nuclei.

fur granules. Actinomycosis has been implicated in upper genital tract infections.

The least common, but much more serious, are the shallow ulcers that result from the use of vaginal tampons when they occur in association with a specific form of staphylococcal infection. Absorption of enterotoxin F and exotoxin C produced by *Staphylococcus aureus* of phage group 1 results in the toxic shock syndrome, characterized by fever, erythematous rash, and shock, with a mortality of nearly 6%.[152]

The most important viral pathogen identifiable by vaginal cytologic examination is herpesvirus. The infected epithelial cells form a multinucleated syncytium (Fig. 68-28).

Cysts and fistulas

A variety of cysts may be found in the vagina, including epidermal inclusion cysts, cysts of müllerian type (cystic adenosis), and cysts of mesonephric (Gärtner's duct) origin, which are typically located in the anterolateral or lateral vaginal wall and are lined by low cuboidal epithelium. Rarer cysts of the vagina include those of Bartholin's duct or endometriotic origin.[153,154]

Mucinous cysts, considered to be of urogenital sinus origin, seem to be more commonly situated near the vestibule.[55,155] Endometriosis of the vagina forms multiple blue mucosal cysts, which may rupture and bleed during menses. The usual cause is implantation of endometrium in an incision, especially an episiotomy.

Vesicovaginal and ureterovaginal fistulas may occur as complication of hysterectomy resulting from ischemic necrosis secondary to interruption of the vascular supply.[156]

Benign tumors

Fibroepithelial polyp (stromal polyp)

The lesion fibroepithelial polyp, or stromal polyp, may be asymptomatic or associated with postcoital bleeding and occurs at an older age than sarcoma botryoides. Approximately 40% of the patients are pregnant or are receiving hormones.[154] Vaginal polyps are usually 4 cm or less in greatest dimension. Microscopic examination shows intact squamous epithelium overlying an edematous myxoid stroma. Occasionally, vaginal polyps contain atypical stromal cells, which may cause misdiagnosis of these polyps as sarcoma botryoides.[157-160] The absence of a cambium layer is a important point of distinction, but it should be remembered that a cambium layer may be present only focally in sarcoma botryoides. The bizarre cells in the stroma of vaginal polyps resemble activated fibroblasts and have sharply tapered cytoplasmic processes (Fig. 68-29). The cytoplasm may be granular and slightly eosinophilic, but cross striations and longitudinal fibrils are absent. Ultrastructural and immunohistochemical studies have shown evidence of fibroblastic or smooth muscle differentiation and localization of desmin but not smooth muscle actin.[78,161] Although mitoses, even abnormal forms, may be present in these polyps they are usually sparse.[160] Polyps of this type also occur rarely in the cervix.[162]

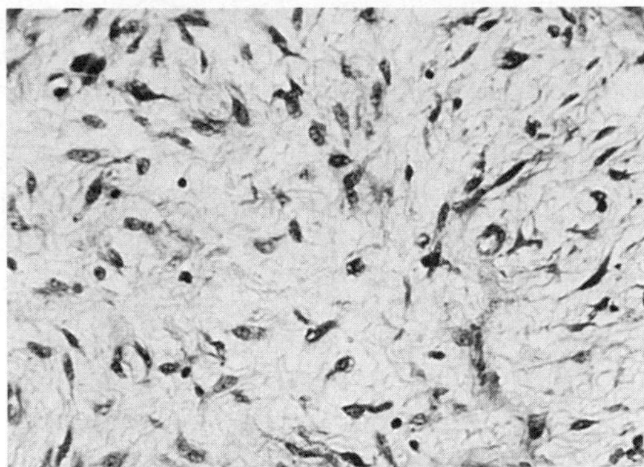

Fig. 68-29 Stromal polyp of vagina has loose myxoid appearance. Cells are spindle shaped or stellate and may be multinucleated.

Müllerian papilloma

The lesion müllerian papilloma, which may also arise in the cervix, typically occurs in young girls and is characterized by numerous branching papillae with central fibrovascular cores lined by epithelial cells with the occasional formation of gland lumens. Although at one time considered of mesonephric origin, a müllerian origin is now favored for these benign tumors.[163]

Leiomyoma

The most common benign mesenchymal tumor of the vagina is the leiomyoma. Such tumors are similar in appearance to leiomyomas found elsewhere. As with uterine smooth muscle tumors, a mitotic rate of over 5 per 10 high-power fields (HPF) is the single best criterion for distinguishing benign from malignant tumors. The presence of an infiltrative margin and cellular atypia are also of significance.[164] Only five of a series of 60 smooth muscle tumors of the vagina recurred and only one metastasized.

Mixed tumor

Mixed tumor, a benign tumor of the vagina, is rare but may be confused with a sarcoma.[165,166] The median age of the patients is 31 years; most of the tumors have been encountered on routine pelvic examination. They are typically located in or just above the hymenal ring and are usually small, from 1 to 5 cm in diameter, circumscribed, nonencapsulated, soft, submucosal nodules. The majority are unattached to the overlying vaginal mucosa and are separated from it by a band of unremarkable submucosa. Microscopically these tumors are clearly cellular and composed of bland stromal cells admixed with epithelial elements (Fig. 68-30). The stromal cells, most of which are spindle shaped, are small and arranged in a whorled pattern or as intersecting fascicles. The epithelial component consists of islands of squamous and well-differentiated glandular epithelium. The proximity of these tumors to the hymen is suggestive of a derivation from urogenital remnants. Both light and electron microscopic studies indicate that the tumor cells may arise from a single multipotential cell. A recent study has shown evidence of epithelial differentiation in both the epithelial and spindle cells.[167] This lesion has been associated with a benign course in all but one patient who developed a local vaginal recurrence 8 years after its original removal.[168] Local excision is the recommended therapy.

Postoperative spindle cell nodules and other iatrogenic lesions

Postoperative spindle cell nodules mimic sarcoma and occur after trauma or surgical procedures, often in episiotomy sites. Grossly, the lesions are polypoid. Microscopically they are composed of randomly arranged spindle cells separated by edematous or vascularized stroma. Mitotic figures are often present, but abnormal forms and pronounced cellular pleomorphism are not usually identified.[154]

Occasionally after a hysterectomy the tubal fimbria may herniate into the vaginal apex, simulating a neoplasm.[169]

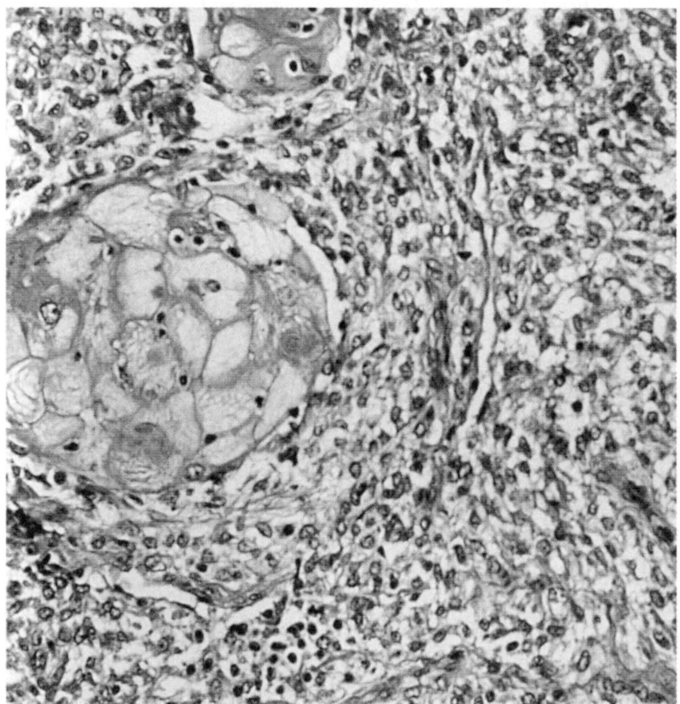

Fig. 68-30 Benign mixed tumor of the vagina. A nest of well-differentiated squamous cells is present within a cellular stroma without significant atypia.

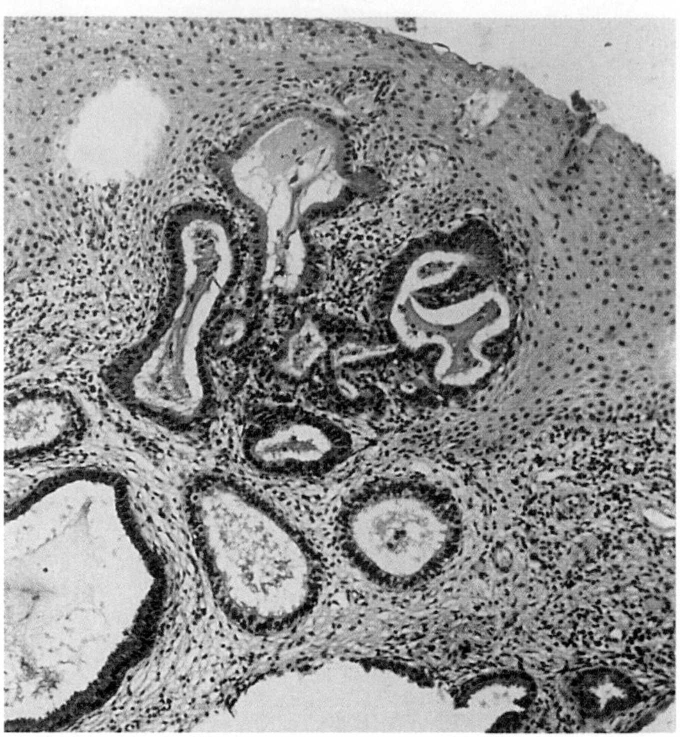

Fig. 68-31 Vaginal adenosis. The mucosa of the exocervix and adjacent vagina contains mucinous glands in place of normal squamous epithelium. (PAS.)

Granulation tissue, which may contain rapidly proliferating blood vessel sprouts, can produce sizable lumps at the vaginal apex after surgery.

Intrauterine diethylstilbestrol exposure: adenosis and clear cell adenocarcinoma

The term *adenosis* refers to the presence of histologically benign epithelium of endocervical or tuboendometrial types in the vaginal mucosa that is normally covered by stratified squamous epithelium. The lesion may be focal or virtually replace the entire vaginal lining epithelium.

Vaginal adenosis has a reddened, velvety appearance, in contrast to the more opaque pale pink of the normal squamous mucosa. Focal lesions require a colposcope for identification; larger patches are visible in ordinary physical examination.

The epithelium of adenosis is composed of a single layer of mucinous columnar epithelial cells (Fig. 68-31). Occasional patches of epithelium are composed of ciliated columnar cells without mucin vacuoles, resembling tubal mucosa.[170] Some degree of squamous metaplasia is often present, beginning as a proliferation of reserve cells beneath the gland cell layer, as in the cervix; a complete conversion to a squamous epithelial lining eventually occurs in most cases.

Adenosis in adolescent girls received considerable notoriety after the demonstration of a causal relationship with intrauterine exposure to diethylstilbestrol (DES) ingested by the mother. It has been shown that the crucial period of exposure is before the eighteenth week of gestation. After this time formation of the vagina is completed, and susceptibility to the effects of DES is apparently lost. DES-induced adenosis may also occur in the mucosa of the portio vaginalis. About one third of the patients have an anomalous ridge, or "hood," of muscular connective tissue surrounding the cervix. This and other upper genital tract changes have adverse effects on pregnancy.[171,172] Many of the structural anomalies occurring in humans exposed to DES have been reproduced in animal models[173] and provided insights into the normal embryology of the vagina.

The incidence of adenosis in DES-exposed infants is probably very high if minute areas are searched for carefully with a colposcope. A much more significant but fortunately less common association is clear cell adenocarcinoma of the vagina and cervix.[174,175] Both the epithelium of adenosis and clear cell adenocarcinomas are of müllerian duct origin.

Over 580 cases of clear cell adenocarcinoma of the vagina or cervix in young girls and women had been accessioned by the beginning of 1992 by the Registry for Research on Hormonal Transplacental Carcinogenesis.[176] Approximately 60% of the patients have had documented exposure in utero to DES; another 12% were exposed to an unknown medication, usually for a high-risk pregnancy.

The median age at the time of diagnosis is 19 years. Although a rare patient has been as young as 7 years of age, only after 14 years of age does the age-incidence curve rise sharply. It plateaus between 17 and 21 years and then declines rapidly. Clear cell adenocarcinoma develops in about 0.014% to 0.14% of exposed girls and women up to 24 years of age. The greatest number of DES-exposed patients with these tumors were born in the period of 1951 through 1953, the years when the drug was prescribed most frequently for pregnancy support.[176]

The tumor may involve any portion of the vagina or cervix. Approximately 60% of lesions have been confined to the vagina (Fig. 68-32). The remainder have been limited to the cervix or involved both the cervix and vagina.[175] Most vaginal tumors arise on the anterior wall, usually in the upper third, corresponding to the most frequent site of adenosis. Small tumors are usually asymptomatic and have been detected only as more young women have sought examination because of their known exposure to DES. Most cancers are superficial and invade only a few millimeters into the vaginal or cervical wall.[175]

By light and electron microscopy, the DES-associated clear cell adenocarcinoma is identical to those of the ovary and endometrium.[175] Several histologic subtypes may be found. In the most characteristic form the tumor consists of glycogen-rich clear cells arranged into solid sheets. The second and the most frequent form is tubulocystic, characterized by tubules lined by hobnail cells or by flat cells (Fig. 68-33). Flat tumor cells often appear innocuous. When only this type of epithelium is present in a small biopsy, it may be difficult to differentiate the tumor from adenosis. Less common patterns include the papillary and the one resembling endometrial carcinoma. Mitoses usually are rare. In any of these patterns, the gland lumen may contain mucin; the cytoplasm, however, is mucin free. By electron microscopy, the neoplastic cells contain glycogen and show prominent microvilli.[177]

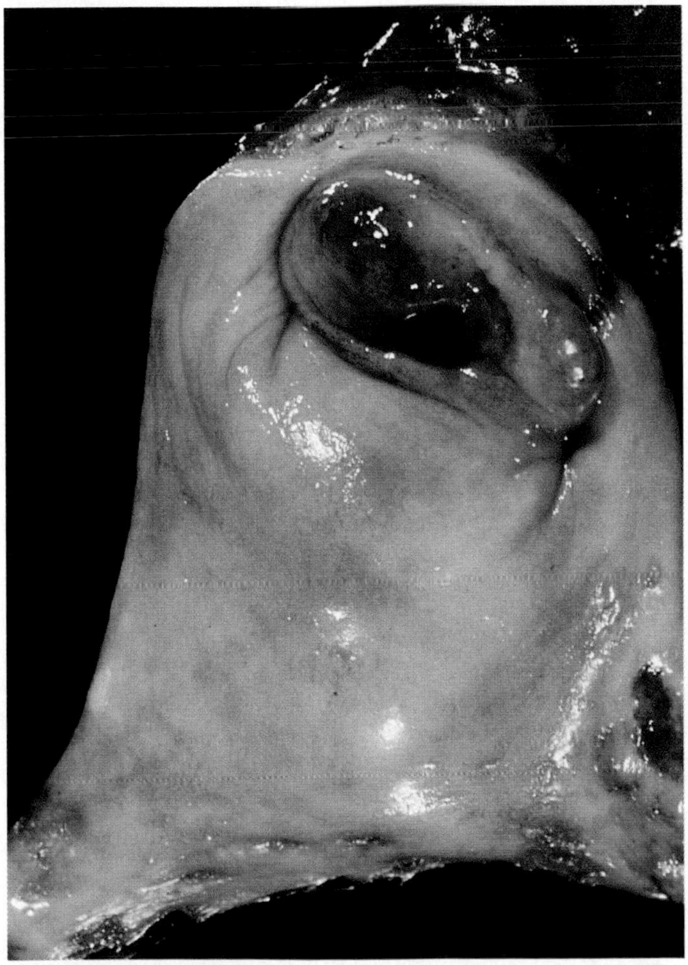

Fig. 68-32 Clear cell adenocarcinoma of vagina subsequent to in utero exposure to diethylstilbestrol. Carcinoma appears as an ulcerated nodule (*lower right*). The cervix (*upper center*) shows an abnormal configuration.

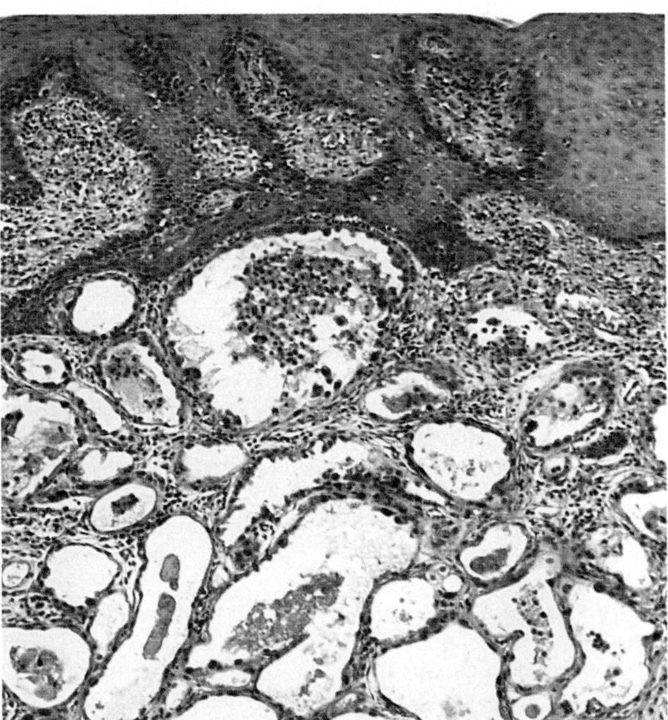

Fig. 68-33 Clear cell adenocarcinoma arising in vaginal adenosis from a young woman exposed in utero to diethylstilbestrol. Tubulocystic pattern.

Atypical adenosis, characterized by glands with cellular stratification and nuclear pleomorphism, has been identified near the periphery of most clear cell carcinomas after extensive pathologic sampling. The common finding of the tuboendometrial type of cells and the rarity of the mucinous cells adjacent to the tumors indicate that the clear cell adenocarcinoma may arise from the tuboendometrial cells.[178,179]

Differential diagnosis should be established with microglandular hyperplasia, a benign condition usually associated with the use of oral contraceptives or pregnancy. Some cases of microglandular hyperplasia arising in foci of vaginal adenosis have been described. Most of the patients had histories of exposure prenatally to DES.[180] Microscopic examination demonstrates many small, closely packed glands devoid of intervening stroma. A clue to the diagnosis is the presence of clefts lined by mucinous epithelium that traverse the metaplastic squamous epithelium.

Although usually seen in the endometrium, the *Arias-Stella reaction* has been observed in the endocervix and occasionally in vaginal adenosis of the tuboendometrial type. Characteristically, hypersecretory glands are lined by cells with considerably enlarged nuclei resembling hobnail cells. However, the hobnail-like nuclei in the Arias-Stella reaction commonly lack mitotic activity and appear to be degenerative.

The clear cell adenocarcinoma spreads locally and also metastasizes via lymphatics and blood vessels. Approximately one sixth of tumors confined clinically to the vagina or cervix (stage I) are discovered on exploration to have metastasized to the pelvic lymph nodes. The frequency of nodal involvement reaches approximately 50% when stage II tumors are considered.[181] Clear cell carcinoma extends outside the abdominal cavity more frequently than SCC of the vagina or cervix does. Thirty-six percent of the initial recurrences of clear cell carcinomas are in the lung or a supraclavicular lymph node, in contrast to less than 10% for SCC.[181]

The 5-year actuarial survival rates for patients with clear cell adenocarcinoma is high. It is about 93% at 5 years and 87% at 10 years when the tumor is in stage I.[176] Recurrences develop most often within 3 years after primary therapy; however, they may occur as late as 19 years after treatment.[181,182] After treatment of the recurrence, approximately one fifth of the patients survive 3 additional years or more.[181]

Other malignant tumors

Most cancers encountered in the vaginal wall are metastatic. According to the definition adopted by FIGO, a tumor that extends to the cervical os is classified as a cancer of the cervix, and a tumor that extends to the vulva is a vulvar carcinoma. The remaining true primary vaginal carcinomas represent slightly less than 1% of female genital cancers. Over 95% of vaginal cancers are SCC; of these, 10% have not invaded the vaginal wall. The remaining 5% are adenocarcinomas, malignant melanomas, and sarcomas.

Squamous cell dysplasia/carcinoma in situ (vaginal intraepithelial neoplasia, VAIN)

Dysplasia or SCC in situ occur less frequently in the vagina than in the cervix or vulva.[183-185] The mean age range of the patients is 50 to 55 years, and most lesions are detected on Pap smears. Many patients have a history of or coexisting preinvasive or invasive cervical carcinoma. The majority of the lesions involve the upper third of the vagina, and many are multifocal. The frequency of recurrent disease is influenced strongly by involvement of the margins in the initial surgical specimen. On microscopic examination VAIN is essentially similar to CIN, and similar criteria can be used to grade these lesions. As with CIN there may be concomitant koilocytosis making pathologic interpretation more difficult. One should diagnose koilocytosis of the vagina only when unequivocal HPV changes (perinuclear haloes and obvious nuclear atypia) are present, since 63% of unequivocal koilocytotic lesions contain HPV DNA, whereas only 14% of histologically equivocal vaginal lesions contain HPV DNA.[186,187] A recent study[188] has demonstrated that 9% of VAIN will progress to invasive carcinoma, 13% of lesions will persist and 78% will regress if treated only by biopsy.

Invasive squamous cell carcinoma

Invasive SCC of the vagina accounts for less than 2% of all gynecologic malignancies,[189-193] usually occurs between 45 and 70 years of age and is commonest in the upper third of the vagina, posteriorly. Extension from a cervical carcinoma should always be excluded clinically. In about one fourth of the cases there is a history of prior cervical carcinoma. The morphology of these tumors is similar to SCC occurring elsewhere in the female genital tract; verrucous carcinomas and carcinomas with a sarcoma-like stroma may be encountered;[194] rare carcinomas may evolve from a preexistent condyloma.[195] The DNA content and proliferative index of these tumors do not have prognostic importance.[196] HPV type 16 has been demonstrated in 20% to 60% of these tumors.

Adenocarcinoma

Adenocarcinomas of the vagina are about one fifth as common as SCC. They are of endometrioid or mucinous type and may have a prominent papillary component. Clear cell carcinoma associated with DES exposure in utero has already been discussed. It should be remembered that clear cell carcinoma unassociated with DES exposure also occasionally occurs in the vagina[197] and may be associated with endometriosis. When examining an adenocarcinoma of the vagina, one should always bear in mind the possibility of a metastasis from another site.[198,199] Tumors of true mesonephric origin have been reported in the vagina on rare occasions.[200] Adenocarcinoma in situ of the vagina has been rarely reported.[201,202]

Embryonal rhabdomyosarcoma (sarcoma botryoides)

Sarcoma botryoides (embryonal rhabdomyosarcoma) is the commonest malignant vaginal tumor of children. This tumor almost always occurs under 5 years of age, and the average age at diagnosis is about 3 years.[203] A polypoid grapelike appearance is characteristic (Fig. 68-34). On microscopic examination squamous epithelium overlies a prominently edematous myxoid tissue with focally hypercellular areas composed of malignant spindle cells. Beneath the epithelium is the so-called cambium layer composed of closely packed small round to spindle-shaped cells with hyperchromatic nuclei and scant cytoplasm. The immaturity of these cells and the occasional identification of cross striations should be suggestive of the diagnosis of rhabdomyosarcoma (Fig. 68-35). Cross striations, however, are not required to make the diagnosis. Invasion of the overlying epithelium by tumor cells may be helpful. Mitoses are usually numerous. This tumor has occasionally been treated successfully only by surgery, but radiation therapy and chemotherapy are also employed currently.

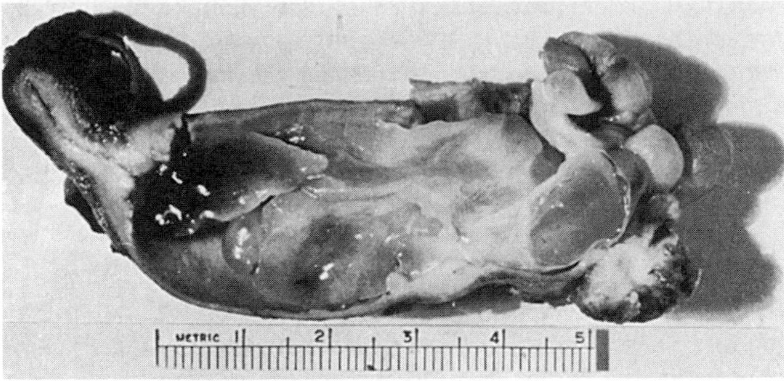

Fig. 68-34 Embryonal rhabdomyosarcoma of vagina (sarcoma botryoides) in sagittal section. Tumor arose in and filled vagina of 16-month-old infant and invaded adjacent pelvic tissues including base of urinary bladder. (Courtesy Dr. Sidney Farber, Boston.)

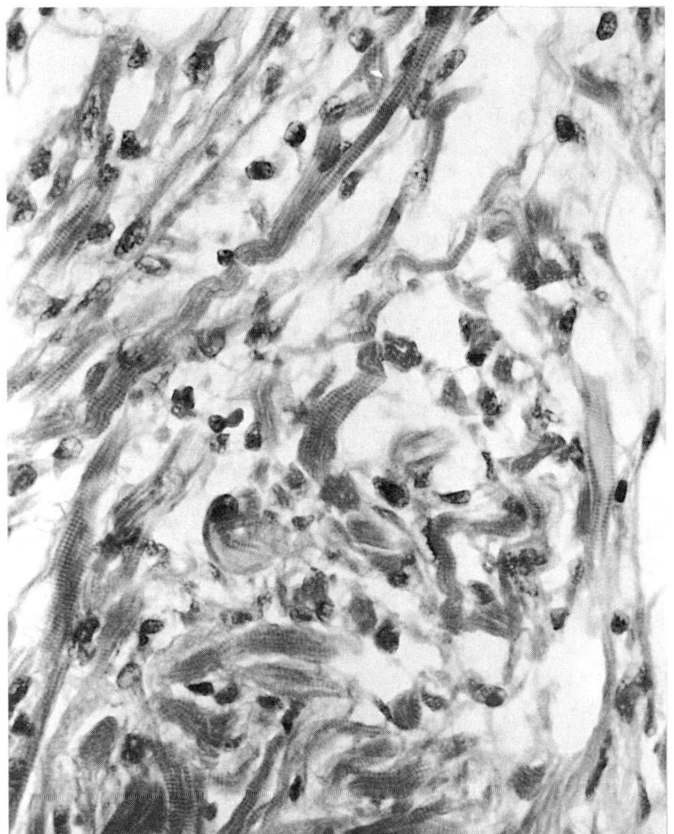

Fig. 68-35 Embryonal rhabdomyosarcoma. Typical strap cells with obvious cross-striations.

Sarcoma botryoides also occurs in the cervix.[203,204] The cervical tumors occur in an older age group than their vaginal counterparts do and more commonly contain cartilaginous foci. In some cases the tumor has been successfully treated by conservative surgery with preservation of fertility. It has a better prognosis than sarcoma botryoides of the vagina.

Yolk sac tumor (endodermal sinus tumor)

A yolk sac tumor is by far the most common primary germ cell tumor of the vagina and accounts for most extraovarian yolk sac tumors in the female genital tract; approximately 56

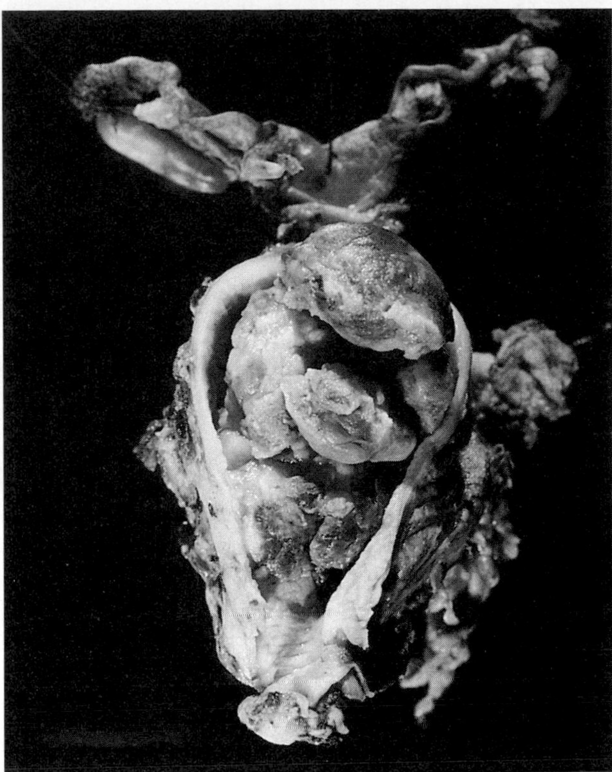

Fig. 68-36 Yolk sac tumor of vagina of 11-month-old infant.

vaginal yolk sac tumors have been reported in detail.[205,206] These tumors may be sessile or polypoid (Fig. 68-36) and, in the latter cases, are occasionally considered grossly to be examples of sarcoma botryoides. They appear similar microscopically to the yolk sac tumors of other sites and like them may be misdiagnosed as clear cell carcinomas. The age of the patient is of help because the yolk sac tumors have always arisen in children 3 years old or younger.

The prognosis and therapy of the yolk sac carcinomas of the vagina and other sites have changed greatly in recent years because of the introduction of effective chemotherapeutic agents.[205] Conservative surgical management of this tumor is now recommended in an effort to conserve fertility.[206]

Other neoplasms

Rare instances of leiomyosarcoma[164] and malignant melanoma[207] have been reported. The pathologic features do not differ significantly from those of similar tumors in more common locations.

CERVIX

Anatomy and physiology

The cervix is located in the distal part of the uterus and shows a cylindric shape. The portion that projects into the vagina is termed the "portio vaginalis," or "exocervix." It is surrounded by a reflection of the vaginal wall referred to as the "fornix" and is centered by the external os, which is circular in the nulligravida and shows a slitlike shape in multiparous women. The cervical canal or endocervix is an elliptical cavity that contains longitudinal mucosal ridges and multiple oblique folds arranged in a treelike pattern. The endocervix communicates with the endometrial cavity at an ill-defined internal os.

The *exocervix* is covered by nonkeratinizing stratified squamous epithelium, the proliferation and maturation of which is stimulated by estrogens and inhibited by progesterone. It is divided into three zones: (1) the *basal layer,* composed of one or two rows of basal cells; (2) the *midzone,* or *stratum spinosum,* which contains several layers of parabasal and intermediate cells; and (3) the *superficial zone,* composed of large eosinophilic superficial cells with small pyknotic nuclei. The *endocervix* is lined by a single layer of mucin-producing columnar epithelium. The endocervical mucosa contains a complex system of deep cleftlike infoldings of the surface epithelium into the underlying stroma. The border between the squamous and the columnar epithelia of the cervix is the *squamocolumnar junction.* The location of the squamocolumnar junction varies according to the hormonal status of the woman. In the fetus, the columnar epithelium extends onto the exocervix, whereas in postmenopausal women the junction is usually located above the external os. The cervical mucosa bounded by the original and the new squamocolumnar junction is termed the *transformation zone (T-zone).* In most women during the reproductive period, the columnar epithelium extends to the exocervix as a red velvety tissue, showing an eroded appearance. This condition is termed *erosion, ectopia,* or more properly *ectropion,* or *eversion.*

Nonneoplastic conditions

Squamous metaplasia

Squamous metaplasia is the phenomenon by which the columnar epithelium is replaced by stratified squamous epithelium. It usually represents a physiologic response to local factors such as pH and hormones.[208] Changes in the pH of the vagina, which lead to inactivation of the buffering effect of the mucin that protects the columnar epithelium, seem to play a significant role in such process. Squamous metaplasia begin by the proliferation of reserve cells, primitive bipotential cells located between the endocervical cells and the basement membrane. Subsequently the epithelium appears replaced by immature cells larger than reserve cells. This immature squamous metaplastic epithelium is characterized by lack of surface maturation and cytoplasmic glycogen (Fig. 68-37). Finally, the cells differentiate into basal, parabasal, intermediate, and even superficial cells with an appearance indistinguishable from the native squamous epithelium. Nabothian cysts are formed when the lumens of the preexisting endocervical clefts become obliterated by the metaplastic squamous epithelium.

Microglandular hyperplasia

Microglandular hyperplasia, very characteristic pattern of gland cell hyperplasia, occurs in young women taking oral contraceptives.[209,210] The larger lesions are polypoid. They show a mixure of small endocervical cells, reserve cells, and foci of squamous metaplasia, all creating an intricate but recognizable pattern that simulates carcinoma (Fig. 68-38). Similar changes occur in pregnancy. Less commonly, gland cells with large, dark, but cytologically benign polyploid nuclei may be found. This change is analogous to the secretory gestational hyperplasia described in the endometrium by Arias-Stella.[211] There is no evidence that birth control pills have any direct carcinogenic effect on the cervix.[212] Atypical variants of microglandular hyperplasia have been recently described.[213] Other nonneoplastic glandular lesions of the endocervix may occasionally be confused with malignancy. These include tunnel clusters, deep nabothian cysts, diffuse laminar endocervical hyperplasia, and various types of metaplasia.[214]

The cells of the subepithelial stroma are often multinucleated and occasionally have a prominent appearance, which should not be mistaken for a neoplasm.[215] Similar cells may be found in polyps and occasionally contain inclusions like those of infantile digital fibroma.[216] The function of these cells is unknown.

Vestigial and heterotopic structures

Remnants of the mesonephric ducts commonly persist in the lateral walls of the cervix and can be numerous. They are distinguished from well-differentiated adenocarcinoma by the absence of cytoplasmic mucin and their benign cytologic appearance. Occasionally, the remnants may become cystic.[217]

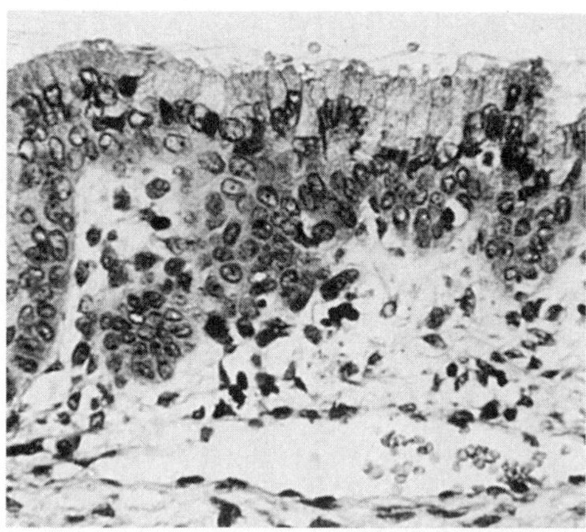

Fig. 68-37 Squamous metaplasia of cervix begins by proliferation of reserve cells beneath columnar epithelium. This new layer thickens, increases its glycogen content, and will become a squamous mucosa when surface gland cells ultimately are sloughed away.

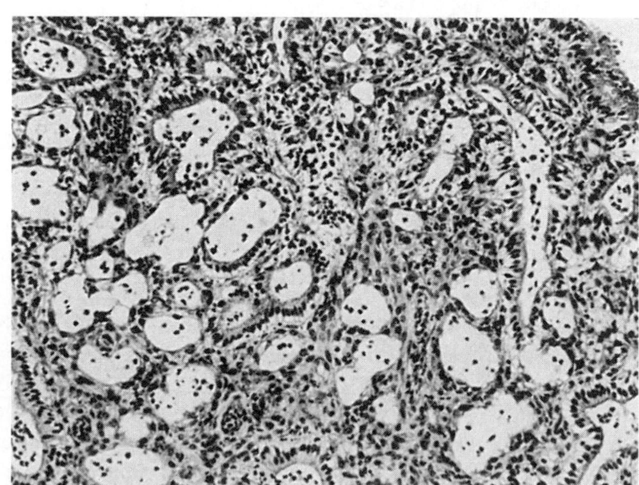

Fig. 68-38 Microglandular hyperplasia of cervix has complex architecture: small glandular spaces are surrounded by immature reserve cells and squamous epithelial cells, intermixed with inflammatory cells.

Less frequently, mesonephric remnants show a range of hyperplastic changes that have been classified as lobular, diffuse, and ductal types of mesonephric hyperplasia.[218] Carcinomas and carcinosarcomas arising from preexisting mesonephric remnants have been described.[218,219]

Heterotopic hyaline cartilage has been encountered in the cervix.[220] Benign endocervical polyps containing well-differentiated skeletal muscle, similar to that found in vaginal rhabdomyomas,[221] also occur. In most instances it is possible to show that apparent heterotopic tissues are the result of implantation of aborted fetal tissues.[222,223] Endometriosis of the cervix may appear as one or more blue hemorrhagic nodules or blisters on the portio vaginalis.

The startling occurrence of sebaceous glands, hair, and sweat glands[224] is harder to explain in this tissue of mesodermal derivation. Lesions with a similar appearance, called "Fordyce's spots," occurred simultaneously in the mouth of the patient.[225]

Infectious diseases

Acute cervicitis may be associated with an acute gonococcal infection or puerperal sepsis. Caustic substances used as abortifacients, such as potassium permanganate, produce extensive ulceration and hemorrhage. Occasionally, a biopsy of a primary chancre will be performed to exclude carcinoma. Acute cervicitis occurs also with herpes simplex infection; the characteristic multinucleated cells and intranuclear viral inclusions can be demonstrated. Ulcerated lesions may resemble cancer on visual inspection.[226,227] The relationship between HPV infections and cervical cancer is discussed below.

Cervical infection caused by *Chlamydia trachomatis* has been identified with increasing frequency as cultural techniques become more widely available. Although not all infected women are symptomatic, approximately 45% have extensive inflammation in the T-zone, as seen with the colposcope, and severe histologic changes, including intraepithelial microabscesses, epithelial necrosis, and ulceration.[228] The presence of chlamydial organisms in infected cells can be demonstrated by immunohistochemical techniques, with endocervical cells being most commonly affected.[229] Some patients also have had cervical dysplasia.

"Chronic cervicitis" is so common in sexually active women that the term is essentially useless as an informative pathologic diagnosis. Characteristically the everted endocervical mucosa may have a slightly papillary appearance, and the stroma is infiltrated by lymphocytes and plasma cells. The epithelium is intact, and usually some degree of squamous metaplasia is in progress, at least focally.

Rare infectious diseases

Amebiasis may cause painful ulcerative lesions in the cervix and vagina.[230] Schistosomiasis is common in some areas of Africa;[231] the finding of calcified ova in the cervical stroma is characteristic. The tiny vessels in which they are lodged may be difficult to identify in most histologic preparations.

Polyps and papillomas

Endocervical polyps represent the growth of redundant folds of endocervical mucosa, including both stroma and epithelium. There is often squamous metaplasia of the epithelium, especially at the tip. Much of the substance of the polyp may be the result of cystic dilatation of endocervical glands. Stromal polyps of the cervix resemble those in the vagina.

Condyloma acuminatum may occur as a typical papilloma in the cervix, but flattened lesions with cytologic features of condyloma are more common and have been recognized with increasing frequency.[232] The cytologic hallmark in cervical scrapings or histologic sections is koilocytic atypia: nuclei are enlarged, appear wrinkled, stain densely but evenly, and are surrounded by a clear halo.[233] Viral particles appear in affected cells when studied by electron microscopic, immunohistochemical, and in situ hybridization techniques.[234]

The application of recombinant DNA techniques to genital neoplasms has resulted in the identification of more than 20 subtypes of HPV,[37] many of which are associated with distinctive lesions. The usual condyloma acuminatum frequently contains type 6 or 11, whereas most carcinomas are associated with types 16, 18, or 31.[235] Virus subtypes can be identified by hybridization with labeled DNA probes. Southern blot hybridization applied to tissue homogenates is more sensitive, whereas the technique applied to microscopic sections or smears (in situ hybridization) is less sensitive but has the advantage of localizing viral DNA within the cells.[236] Polymerase chain reaction (PCR) is a useful tool for HPV detection in those lesions containing small numbers of viral DNA copies.[237]

Benign neoplasms

Leiomyomas of the cervix resemble those in the myometrium, described later. They may cause cervical stenosis with secondary pyometra or hematometra. Adenomyomas are polypoid smooth muscle tumors containing an admixture of endocervical or endometrial glands, characteristically occur in the lower uterine segment, and can exhibit architectural and cytologic atypicality.[238]

Rarely a papilloma, said to be of mesonephric duct origin, has been described in children.[239] The stroma is inconspicuous, and the epithelial component is flat cuboidal and cytologically benign. It is now considered a lesion of müllerian origin. Hemangiomas include the cervix in their ubiquitous distribution; the cervix itself is very vascular, and many reported "hemangiomas" are nothing more than a conspicuous demonstration of local vascularity.

Squamous intraepithelial lesions

In some women the replacement of the glandular epithelium by squamous metaplasia in the T-zone does not proceed in an orderly manner to form mature stratified squamous epithelium. Instead, the proliferating epithelium contains many cells that resemble carcinoma cells. The abnormal cells are confined to the epithelium and do not invade the stroma. The term *carcinoma in situ* was applied to those lesions in which, throughout their whole thickness, no differentiation took place. All other disturbances of differentiation (less severe than carcinoma in situ) were defined as *dysplasia* and graded as slight, moderate, and severe.[240] The classification of noninvasive lesions into dysplasia and carcinoma in situ was based exclusively on arbitrary morphologic differences, which were often subtle. Subsequently, several studies suggested that the cellular changes of dysplasia and carcinoma in situ were similar, and the intraepithelial lesions were regarded as a single disease process termed *cervical intraepithelial neoplasia* (CIN).[241] It was similarly graded from I to III (Figs. 68-39 to 68-41).

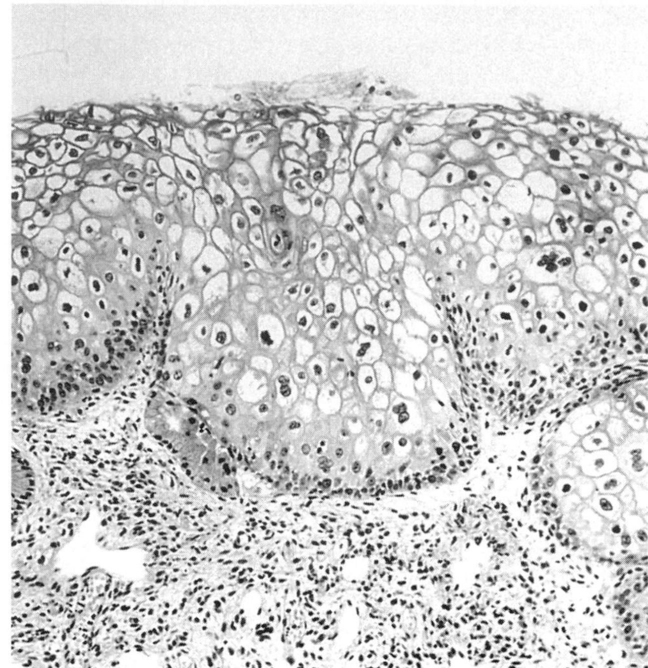

Fig. 68-39 Low-grade squamous intraepithelial lesion (cervical intraepithelial neoplasia I), or LSIL (CIN I), of cervix. This lesion, also known as "flat condyloma," is characterized by koilocytotic atypia and is usually related to HPV 6/11 infection.

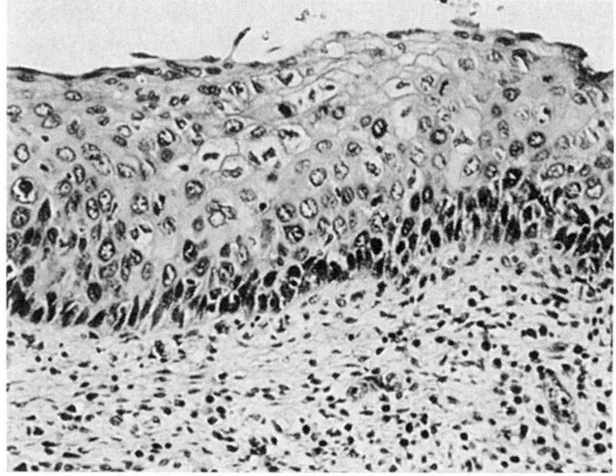

Fig. 68-40 High-grade SIL, or HSIL (CIN II) of cervix. Abnormal squamous epithelial cells appear atypical, but they vary considerably in size and shape and have a relative abundance of cytoplasm. Maturation is evident at surface.

According to this scheme, CIN I was the equivalent of slight dysplasia, and CIN III included severe dysplasia and carcinoma in situ.[241] CIN III was considered to be a precursor lesion with high risk of progression to invasive carcinoma; it usually predates invasive carcinoma by about 10 years. CIN may occur within endocervical glands; this may represent a separate focus of involvement but is not evidence of invasion. The estimated prevalence of CIN III in the United States is 1.8 out of 1000 Pap smears.[242]

Over the past 15 years, epidemiologic investigations, as well as the application of recombinant DNA analysis for the study of cervical cancer and its precursor lesions, have

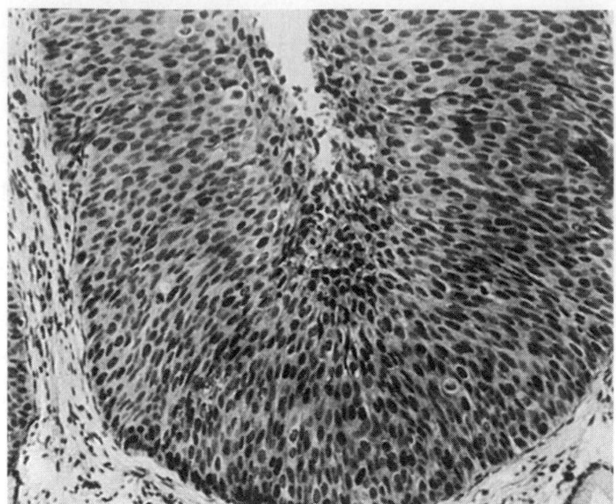

Fig. 68-41 HSIL (CIN III) of cervix. Abnormal cells have uniform size and shape and relatively scant cytoplasm. There is no evidence of maturation.

revealed that specific types of HPV that infect the anogenital tract play a crucial role in the carcinogenesis.[243]

Recently, the National Cancer Institute has proposed a new diagnostic terminology for cervicovaginal cytopathology reports.[244] According to this system (called the Bethesda System), the three-grade CIN scheme should be reduced to two grades of squamous intraepithelial lesion (SIL). The lesions formerly designated as CIN I, mild koilocytotic dysplasia, and simply koilocytosis would be classified under the term *low-grade squamous intraepithelial lesion* (LSIL) (Fig. 68-39), whereas those lesions previously called CIN II and CIN III would be encompassed under the designation *high-grade squamous intraepithelial lesion* (HSIL) (Figs. 68-40 and 68-41). The main reason for the proposal of this new terminology is the apparent differential distribution of HPVs. Whereas HPV 6 and 11 account for 70% to 90% of the HPVs associated with flat and exophytic condylomas, HPV 16 is found in nearly half of CIN III and invasive carcinomas.[235] Furthermore, many lower-grade lesions have been characterized as diploid or polyploid in DNA content and frequently regress.[245] In contrast, higher-grade lesions are mostly aneuploid and more likely progress.[246] It is now accepted that CIN do not represent a single disease process but rather two separate biologic entities; that is, a productive viral infection (LSIL) and a true neoplastic intraepithelial lesion (HSIL).

Several investigators have recommended the adoption of the Bethesda System; however, there is no general agreement about the real value of this new classification. Most of the criticism has been centered on the potential overtreatment of CIN II.[247,248]

Pathogenesis

Epidemiologic analyses of large populations of women with carcinoma of the cervix have identified several potential risk factors, which include early sexual activity, especially with multiple partners, cigarette smoking, oral contraceptive use, interval since the last Pap smear, a history of abnormal Pap smear, immunosuppression, and infection with herpes simplex virus type 2 (HSV-2) or HPV types 16 and 18.[249-255] An interesting study of the potential role of the male as a carrier found that the subsequent wives of men whose first spouse had cervical carcinoma are themselves at greater risk of developing cervical carcinoma.[256] This finding supports the concept that a transmissible agent is responsible, in part, for the pathogenesis of cervical cancer.

More recently, a dominant role has been ascribed to HPV, implicating a specific set of HPV types (most commonly 16, 18, 31, 33, and 35) as opposed to the types usually found in condylomas (types 6 and 11).[37,235] Viral localization studies consistently identify HPV in many but not all cervical dysplasias and squamous carcinomas[234-237] (Fig. 68-42). The consistent finding of specific strains of virus in cancers (as opposed to condylomas) strengthens the concept of a central role for HPV. On the other hand, the subject cannot be regarded as settled because some patients and even individual lesions are colonized by multiple types of virus. Virus can be recovered from morphologically normal squamous epithelium, and all patients with viral lesions do not develop carcinoma. It would appear that HPV may be an important initiator and that other factors such as herpesvirus, age, oncogenes, and toxic exposure (smoking) may serve as promoters or cocarcinogens.

In the cervical epithelium, the HPV life cycle is linked to squamous cell differentiation (Fig. 68-43). Once infection occurs, the virus may enter a dormant phase without further replication (latent infection) or undergo intranuclear replication with synthesis of viral particles, though remaining extrachromosomal (episomal state). Under certain circumstances, the viral genome may become incorporated into the cellular genome. This integration results in failure of transcription of the late genes, and viral particles are not produced. On the other hand, this integration disrupts the viral genome and produces uncontrolled transcription of E6-E7 genes leading to cell immortalization.[257]

Normal human cervical keratinocytes can be "immortalized" (that is, continue to grow and divide in tissue cultures for many generations beyond the usual survival time of normal

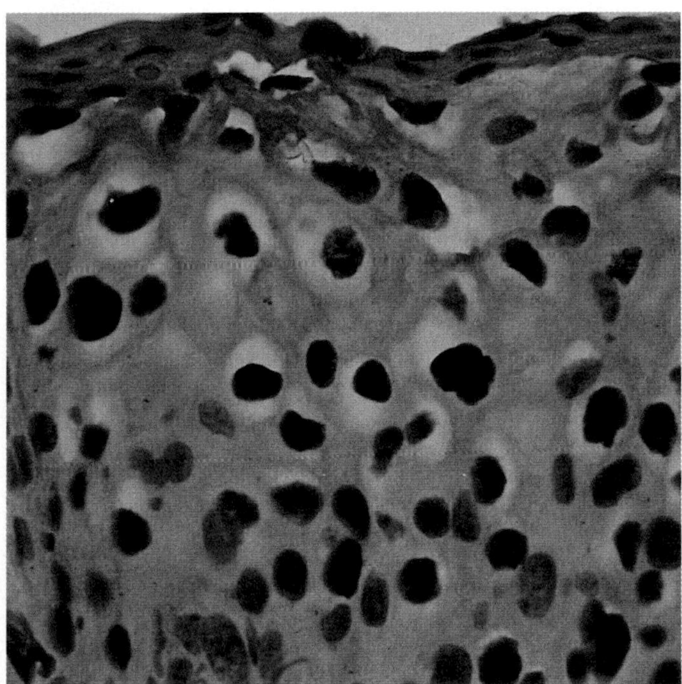

Fig. 68-42 HSIL of cervix. Human papillomavirus 31/33/51 demonstrated in keratinocytes. (In situ hybridization).

cells in vitro) by insertion of HPV 16 and 18 DNA. These cells are not tumorigenic when injected into nude mice; it appears therefore that HPV 16 and 18 may not be carcinogenic without some assistance.[258] Other studies have indicated some potential cofactors. One study used a cell line already immortalized by transfection with HSV-2; further transfection with HPV 16 and 18 produced cell lines that were fully tumorigenic in nude mice. This result indicates a possible initiator role for HSV-2 and a promotor role for HPV 16 and 18. Of great interest is the fact that persistence of the integrated viral sequences in tumor cell DNA does not appear necessary once oncogenic transformation is complete.[259] Furthermore, the HPV E6 and E7 genes, which seem to be the active viral component in carcinogenesis, can cooperate with the *ras* oncogene to transform primary rat cells.[260] Another interesting observation is that the E7 protein can complex and thereby probably inactivate the protein encoded by the retinoblastoma (Rb) gene in vitro.[261] The Rb gene and the protein encoded by it appear to be "tumor-suppressor" factors that are absent in some cancer cells.

Similarly, the HPV 16 and 18 E6 proteins bind to p53 tumor-suppressor phosphoprotein, whereas the E6 proteins from HPV types 6 and 11 fail to bind to p53 to a detectable extent.[122,123] Recently, it has been demonstrated that the transcriptional transactivation function of p53 can be inhibited by the HPV 16 E6 protein.[262] It has been suggested that p53 plays and important role in cervical tumorigenesis either by inactivation through interaction with HPV E6 protein or by mutation. In fact, p53 point mutations have been demonstrated in human cervical cancers, and there is an inverse correlation with HPV infections; HPV-unrelated carcinomas showing the highest incidence of p53 mutations.

Some interesting diagnostic applications arise from recombinant-DNA techniques. The HPV DNA can be demonstrated directly by use of PCR, capable of remarkable sensitivity, detecting less than one virus genome per cell. Target DNA sequences are selectively amplified by repeated cycles of denaturation, annealing with oligomer primers complementary to flanking regions of target DNA sequence, and primer extension with DNA polymerases. Final reaction products are detected by dot blot or Southern blot analyses using a ^{32}P-labeled probe. The potential of these techniques for detecting cells that have escaped intracellular control mechanisms shows promise in helping to distinguish dysplasias that can or will progress to cancers from those that cannot, thus allowing identification of the patients at greatest risk.

Colposcopy. The use of the colposcope has remarkably improved the accuracy of physical diagnosis of lesions of the cervix.[223] Based chiefly on differences in vascular pattern, distinctions can be made between squamous metaplasia, SIL (CIN), and early invasive carcinoma (Figs. 68-44 and 68-45). Used with cytologic studies, biopsy, and conization, the colposcope has significantly improved the accuracy of diagnosis and the effectiveness of local treatment.[263]

Clinical significance of SIL (CIN). Opinions about the significance of SIL vary widely. Accepted forms of treatment include local excision (conization) designed to excise most of the transformation zone, some form of cautery (laser, freezing, loop electrosurgical excision), and hysterectomy. The results are remarkably similar.

LSIL (CIN I), left undisturbed, may progress to HSIL (CIN II and III).[264] If there is no intervention of any sort, the

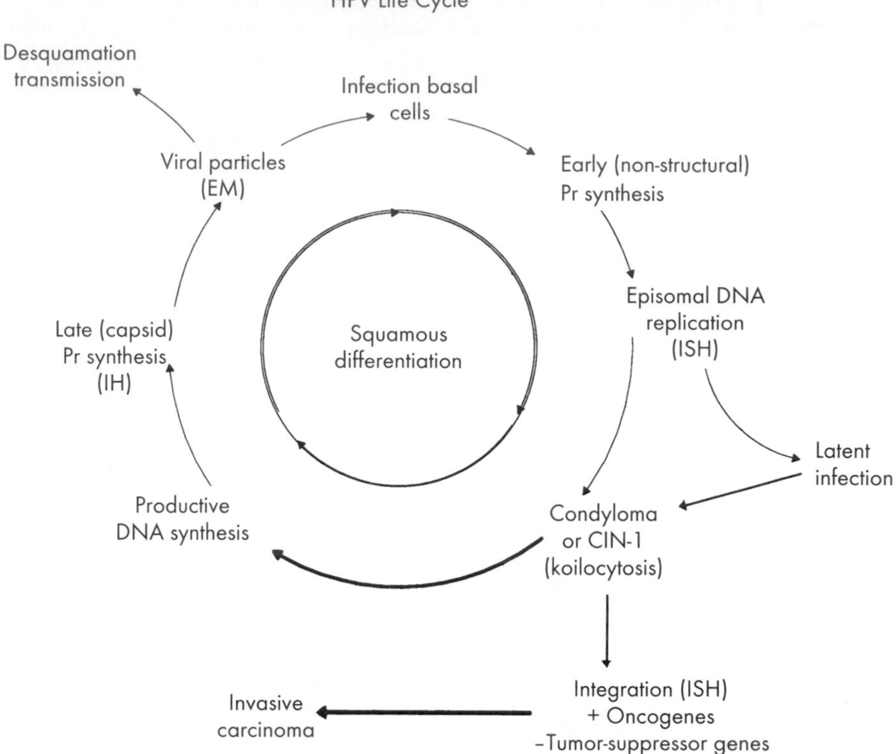

Fig. 68-43 Life cycle of human papillomavirus. (Modified from Ambros RA, Kurman RJ: *Semin Diagn Pathol* 7:158, 1990.) *EM*, Electron microscopy; *IH*, immunohistochemistry; *ISH*, in situ hybridization; *Pr*, protein.

observed conversion of SIL to invasive carcinoma is nearly constant: 21% in 5 years, 28% in 10 years, 33% in 15 years, and 38% in 20 years.[265,266] However, local treatment in the form of conization or cautery effectively interrupts the process in a high percentage of patients.[263,267-269] Residual CIN III (HSIL) has been identified in as much as one third of hysterectomy specimens obtained after cervical conization.[268] Those patients who require more extensive treatment can be identified by colposcopy and cytologic studies if one assumes that meticulous follow-up examinations will be carried out.[269] Ignoring cytologic evidence of carcinoma carries an unacceptably high risk of invasive carcinoma and death.[265] In a carefully conducted long-term study of 1121 women with CIN III (HSIL), subsequent invasive carcinoma was found in 2.1% of those treated by hysterectomy and in 0.9% of those treated only by conization.[270]

The screening of large populations of women has identified hundreds of cases with CIN III (HSIL), as well as early invasive carcinomas. Treatment of the lesion at this stage has considerably reduced the number of patients with advanced cervical cancer, for which treatment is much less effective, and has improved survival. The desirability of annual mass screening has been debated.[271] Success has been notable only in programs that include groups at greatest risk.[272,273] Persistence of the cervical lesion as shown by cytologic or colposcopic abnormalities is very significant regardless of the treatment selected. In a group of 949 women followed closely for 5 to 28 years, 86% had consistently normal cytologic features and among these 12 (1.5%) ultimately developed invasive carcinoma. By comparison, of the 131 who continued to have abnormal cytologic characteristics, 29 (22%) developed invasive carcinoma; the carcinomas occurred with approximately the same frequency whether the patients were initially treated by conization or by hysterectomy.[274]

Recently a prospective study has shown that 28% of women with normal cervical smears but with HPV DNA detected in cervical swabs developed CIN II/III (HSIL) within 2 years without ever manifesting CIN I (LSIL).[275] These findings suggest that high-grade lesions may develop de novo, rather than evolving from low-grade lesions.

There is also a definite but apparently small group of invasive cervical carcinomas that originate from the basal layer of histologically normal squamous epithelium. There may be no detectable surface abnormality at any point in the cervix, until (presumably) the lesion ulcerates, sloughing the surface and exposing the cancer beneath.[276] Approximately 10% of cervical carcinomas may arise in this manner.[277]

Adenocarcinoma in situ

Adenocarcinoma in situ is a rare lesion characterized by replacement of the gland cells of endocervical mucosa and its crypts by cytologically malignant gland cells. The columnar pattern is usually retained, but the basal polarity of the nuclei is lost, the cytoplasmic mucin is replaced by amphophilic cytoplasm, and the nuclei have malignant cytologic features. If involved, gland-space outlines resemble those lined by normal epithelium in the same cervix, and if only part of the gland-space lining is affected, it is reasonable to conclude that stroma invasion has not occurred. Associated SCC in situ is often present. In nearly every case the lesion is discovered when malignant gland cells are found in the cervical cytologic smear.[278]

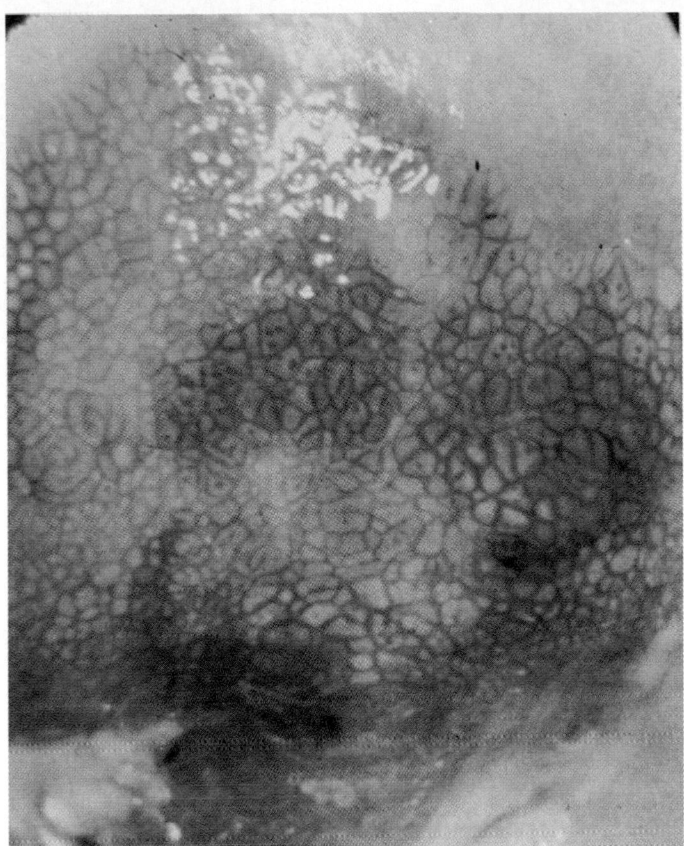

Fig. 68-44 Colposcopic photograph of HSIL of cervix. This mosiac pattern and accentuated punctate vessels emphasized against a background of opaque whitened epithelium are characteristic.

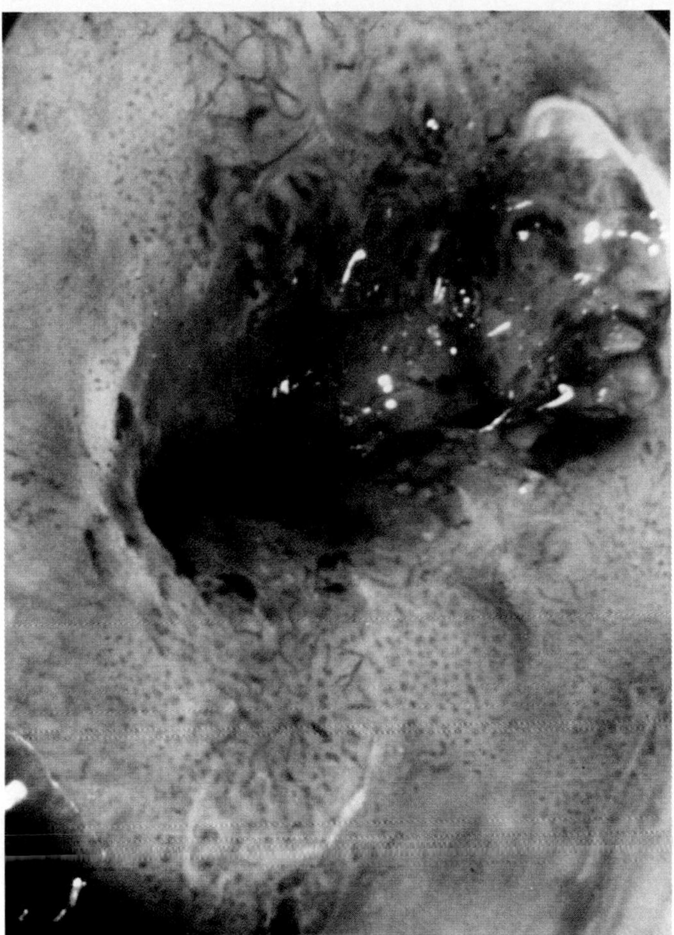

Fig. 68-45 Invasive carcinoma of cervix. Irregular tortuous blood vessels across the surface of the lesion are features of an invasive tumor.

Adenocarcinoma in situ is most likely a precursor to invasive adenocarcinoma because it has been invariably found with very small (microinvasive) adenocarcinomas.[279,280] Adenocarcinoma in situ is also located higher in the endocervix; a residual lesion remains in the resected uterus after conization in 66% of cases, which implies that conization for this lesions is probably an inadequate treatment. Recently, several investigators have reported the presence of high-risk HPV types (16 and 18) in cases of adenocarcinoma in situ of the uterine cervix, an indication that HPV infection may also be an important factor in cervical glandular carcinogenesis.[281]

Microinvasive carcinoma

Microinvasive carcinoma is a small cancer that has invaded the cervical stroma to a limited extent. The earliest invasive changes have the appearance of tiny irregular sprouts of neoplastic epithelial cells projecting into the cervical stroma, usually beneath an area of carcinoma in situ. The cells at the interface between infiltrating epithelium and stroma appear more differentiated, have abundant cytoplasm, and are often degenerated. The adjacent stroma is infiltrated by lymphocytes and plasma cells. No regional lymph node metastases or deaths from such lesions have been reliably documented.

The last classification system for microinvasive carcinomas of the cervix reported by FIGO[282] considers stage IA1 those tumors with stromal invasion to a depth of 1 mm from the point of origin; tumors with invasive component 5 mm or less in depth and 7 mm or less in horizontal spread are designated as stage IA2.* The risk of lymph node metastasis and recurrence for patients with stage IA1 is minimal. However, although patients with tumors classified as FIGO stage IA also have a very low incidence of nodal metastasis, the risk is greater in those with invasion between 3, 1, and 5 mm.[283] The Society of Gynecologic Oncologists (SGO) defines microinvasion as invasion of the stroma from the point of origin to a depth of less than 3 mm; lesions with vascular-lymphatic invasion are excluded from this category.

Involvement of the cone margin by invasive carcinoma or even by high-grade SIL precludes a diagnosis of microinvasive carcinoma, because deeper invasion may exist higher in the endocervix.

Invasive carcinoma of cervix

In contrast to the remarkable increase in the numbers of women treated for CIN, it was estimated that the number of patients with invasive cervical carcinoma had decreased to

*At the FIGO Congress, which was in September 1994, microinvasive cervical carcinomas invading less than 3 mm in depth with less than a 7 mm horizontal spread were reclassified as stage IA1. Tumors with depth of invasion from 3 to 5 mm were redesignated stage IA2.

12,900 in 1988 from 19,000 in 1975 and 20,000 in 1970.[284] After several decades as the most common gynecologic cancer, cervical carcinoma is now encountered less often than endometrial carcinoma, which has increased to first place in many institutions in the United States.

Gross appearance. Cervical carcinomas large enough to be visible and palpable have one of three growth patterns, sometimes in combination. The *ulcerating* type has an infiltrative pattern of growth and eventually becomes necrotic in the center and sloughs, leaving a cavity surrounded by invasive cancer. The *exophytic* type is often papillary and may form a bulky mass of considerable size while still confined to the superficial portions of the cervix. The *nodular* type originates typically in the endocervix, forming multiple firm masses that expand the cervix and isthmus. The mass may be large, and when it is distributed circumferentially, it has been called the *barrel-shaped cervix.* The gross relationships are important clinically because they affect the placement of radioactive sources used in treatment.

Clinical stages. The extent of involvement of the cervix and pelvic tissues is determined by physical examinations. The clinical staging of the extent of disease must be determined before treatment is begun. It is in part the basis of selection of the best treatment for the patient and forms the standard for comparing the results of treatment of large groups of patients.

Definitions of the different clinical stages in carcinoma of the cervix uteri, as established by the Cancer Committee of FIGO,[285] are given in Table 68-3.

Table 68-3 Clinical staging of carcinoma of the cervix

Stage 0	Preinvasive carcinoma (intraepithelial carcinoma, carcinoma in situ).
Stage I	Carcinoma strictly confined to the cervix (extension to the corpus should be disregarded)
IA	Preclinical carcinomas of the cervix, i.e., diagnosed only by microscopy, but showing:
IA1*	Minimal microscopically evident stromal invasion
IA2*	Lesions detected microscopically that can be measured. The upper limits of the measurement should not show a depth of invasion of more than 5 mm taken from the base of the epithelium, either surface or glandular, from which it originates; and a second dimension, the horizontal spread, must not exceed 7 mm. Larger lesions should be staged as Ib.
IB	Lesions of greater dimensions than stage Ia2, whether seen clinically or not. Preformed space involvement should not alter the staging but should be recorded specifically to determine whether it should affect treatment decisions in the future.
Stage II	Invasive carcinoma that extends beyond the cervix but has not reached either lateral pelvic wall; involvement of the vagina is limited to the upper two thirds
Stage III	Invasive carcinoma that extends to either lateral pelvic wall or the lower third of the vagina, or both
Stage IV	Invasive carcinoma that involves urinary bladder or rectum or extends beyond the true pelvis

*At the FIGO congress (September 1994), microinvasive cervical carcinomas invading less than 3 mm in depth with less than a 7 mm horizontal spread were reclassified as stage IA1. Tumors with depth of invasion from 3 to 5 mm were redesignated stage IA2.

Microscopic appearance. The majority of invasive cervical carcinomas, about 80%, are SCC; adenocarcinomas constitute about 10%, and the remainder is a variety of unusual adenocarcinomas or mixtures.[285,286]

Squamous cell carcinoma. The moderately differentiated, nonkeratinizing, large cell SCC (Fig. 68-46) is the most common histologic subtype (70%) and in some series, at least, has the best prognosis. Well-differentiated keratinizing SCC occurs less frequently (25%); small cell undifferentiated carcinoma is uncommon (about 5%) and has a distinctly poor prognosis.[285,286]

Adenocarcinoma. Although they are much less common than SCC, the proportion of cervical carcinomas arising from endocervical type cells doubled in the decade from 1960 to 1970.[281,287] The patterns vary from a well-differentiated mucinous adenocarcinoma (Fig. 68-47), sometimes papillary, to a clear cell pattern containing glycogen but no mucin. Many resemble endometrial adenocarcinoma. A mixed adenosquamous carcinoma apparently arises from subcolumnar reserve cells capable of both squamous and gland cell differentiation.

Spread of carcinoma of cervix. It is important to recognize simultaneous involvement of the cervix and endometrium because this distribution affects principles of treatment; the prognosis is not so good as that for carcinoma limited to the cervix. Hysterectomy with radiotherapy improves the results, probably because the more extensive distribution of some lesions interferes with the spatial arrangement of intrauterine radiation sources.

Carcinoma of the cervix spreads by direct extension into contiguous tissues, through lymphatics to regional lymph nodes, and less often by blood vessel invasion to embolize throughout the body. Because of their close anatomic relationship to the cervix, the ureters may be obstructed; secondary hydronephrosis, pyelonephritis, and renal failure remain the most common causes of death.[288] Distant metastases to lungs and liver are found in about 25% of fatal cases at autopsy. In patients dying of cancer of the cervix, central pelvic recurrences are more common after radiotherapy.[288] Less than 2% of patients with stage I or IIa carcinoma of the cervix treated by megavoltage radiotherapy with adequate dosage and distribution of the radiation will have a central pelvic recurrence.[289]

Local recurrence occurs in 5% of patients with stage IIb disease, 7.5% with stage IIa, 17% with stage IIIa, and 17% with stage IIIb. Over half the distant metastases become evident within the first year after treatment, and 95% appear by the end of the fifth year after treatment. Because most of the patients without evidence of cancer 5 years after treatment die of unrelated causes, this follow-up period is customarily used in evaluating the effectiveness of therapy.

Rare tumors

Verrucous carcinoma, an extremely well-differentiated form of SCC, resembles and behaves like the same lesion in the vulva. Clear cell adenocarcinomas identical to those in the vagina also occur occasionally in the cervix after intrauterine expo-

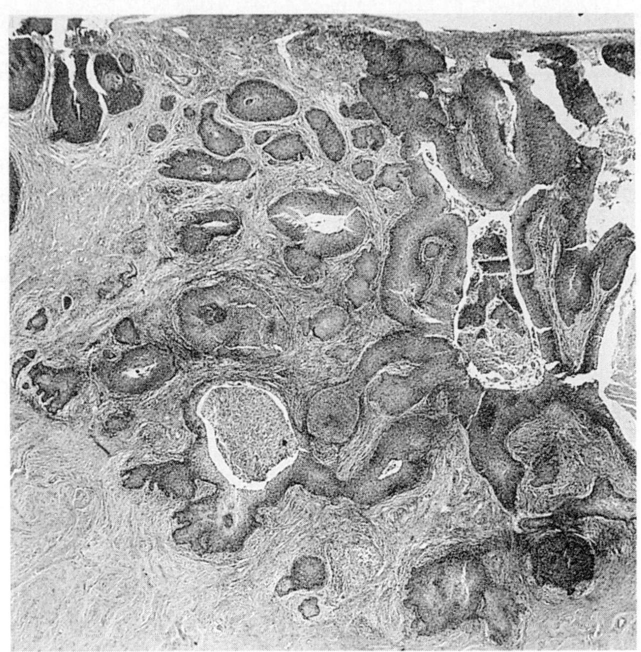

Fig. 68-46 Squamous cell carcinoma of cervix. This well-differentiated, nonkeratinizing tumor is the most common histologic type.

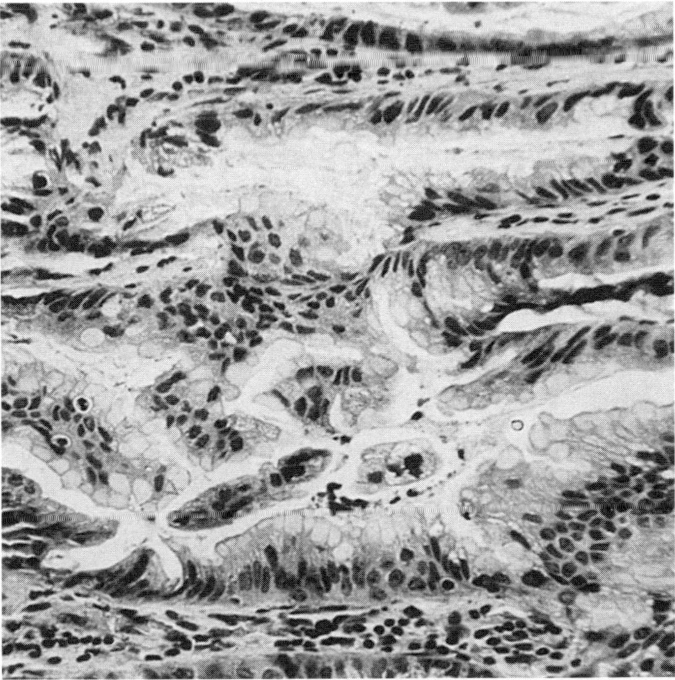

Fig. 68-47 Well-differentiated adenocarcinoma of cervix. Epithelial cells form bridges without stromal support.

sure to DES. Rarely a cervical adenocarcinoma may have a histologic pattern similar to that of adenoid cystic carcinoma, which is highly specific and more common in the salivary glands. This lesion in the cervix is highly aggressive, occurs in older women, and nearly always is associated with a more conventional SCC or adenosquamous carcinoma pattern.[290] As seen in the cervix, adenoid cystic carcinoma is clearly different from the similar tumor of the salivary gland; it should be distinguished also from adenoid basal cell carcinoma, which has a much better prognosis.[291]

An extremely well-differentiated mucinous adenocarcinoma (so-called adenoma malignum) may be difficult to recognize because the epithelial pattern closely resembles that of benign endocervical epithelium, even in metastases. With adequate treatment the prognosis is probably the same as that of any adenocarcinoma at the same stage.[292] These tumors have distinctive histologic features and produce cytoplasmic carcinoembryonic antigen, which may be diagnostically helpful.[293]

Recently a new variant of cervical adenocarcinoma has been described: the villoglandular papillary adenocarcinoma, characterized by exophytic growth pattern, elongated fibrovascular papillae, and well differentiated slightly atypical cells. It has been suggested that this particular type of tumor is associated with a good prognosis[294,295]

Malignant mixed müllerian tumors, carcinosarcomas, and leiomyosarcomas of the cervix resemble those occurring in the endometrium and share the same unfavorable prognosis.[296] Carcinoid tumors occur in the cervix as distinctly aggressive neoplasms. Like other tumors of the diffuse endocrine system, they contain argyrophil and neurosecretory granules.[297] The less-differentiated cases resemble oat cell carcinoma in the lung; one cervical carcinoma of this type produced ACTH, causing Cushing's syndrome.[298] Melanin is rarely evident in basal cells of the cervix. Blue nevi and primary malignant melanomas are rare.[299] Botryoid sarcoma in the cervix resembles the vaginal lesion described above but tends to occur at a somewhat older age and may have a better prognosis, especially with chemotherapy.[300] Some patients having polypoid tumors have been cured by "polypectomy" or cervical conization.[204]

Metastatic adenocarcinoma in the cervix is not common, but one should not mistake it for a primary lesion, thereby exposing the patient to a lengthy, painful, and expensive treatment that would be inappropriate. A cervical metastasis is usually the harbinger of rapid dissemination and death. The most common primary sites have been the ovary, colon, and breast.[301]

ENDOMETRIUM

The function of the normal endometrium is to produce a satisfactory substrate in which a healthy blastocyst may implant and flourish. Many of the pathologic changes that occur in the endometrium reflect its responsiveness to either hormonal stimulation or the lack of it.

The uterine lining can be divided into two regions: the mucosa of the lower uterine segment (itshmus) and the mucosa of the corpus proper. The isthmic mucosa is thinner than the fundal mucosa and often lags behind the rest of the endometrium in its development. The corpus mucosa is also divided into two layers: The lowermost basalis and the overlying functionalis. The weekly proliferative basalis shows dense spindled stroma in the vicinity of the myometrium. It plays an essential role as the "reserve cell layer" of the endometrium and is responsible for regeneration after menstruation. The functionalis exhibits the morphologic changes characteristic of the normal endometrium.[302] Both the proliferative and secretory types of epithelial cells stain for cytokeratin (AE1-3 and

CAM 5.2) and vimentin. Stromal cells react with vimentin and smooth muscle–related antigens.[303]

The sampling techniques available include the *endometrial curettage* and the *endometrial biopsy.* The former (cervical dilatation and endometrial curettage: D&C) alludes to the removal of almost the entire uterine mucosa by scraping with a curette, whereas the latter involves removal of a more limited sample of tissue. If an endometrial carcinoma is suspected clinically, a thorough curetting of the endocervical canal should be performed before cervical dilatation and endometrial curettage. Although the sample obtained by endometrial biopsy is smaller, the accuracy of diagnosis almost equals that of the D&C. The principal limitation of the endometrial biopsy lies in its potential to missing focal lesions; therefore, when carcinoma is suspected clinically, a complete D&C must be done.[302]

Endometrial cycle

In women of reproductive age, the endometrium undergoes a series of physiologic events and morphologic changes that occur regularly, approximately every month. The changes include proliferation, secretion, menstruation, and regeneration of the uterine mucosa. Under the influence of the pituitary follicle-stimulating hormone (FSH) and luteinizing hormone (LH), an ovarian follicle develops, an oocyte is expulsed, and the follicle is transformed into a corpus luteum. Estradiol (E_2) production by the enlarging ovarian follicle progressively rises during the first 2 weeks of the usual 28-day menstrual cycle. It reaches a peak just before ovulation and then falls and again begins to rise to a plateau at the end of the third week; these E_2 levels, however, are lower than those of the preovulatory period and, lastly, fall 3 to 4 days before the onset of menstruation. Ovulation is mediated by the *LH surge,* a synchronous burst of LH and FSH secretion that occurs on the fourteenth day of the cycle. Progesterone (P), produced by the corpus luteum, rises throughout the last half of the menstrual cycle to fall to basal levels just before the onset of menstrual bleeding.

The corpus luteum secretes both E_2 and large quantities of P characteristic of the ovarian luteal phase and corresponding to the endometrial secretory phase. Steroid hormone effect on endometrial epithelial, stromal, and endothelial cells is mediated by estrogen receptors (E_2R) and progesterone receptors (PR) concentrated in the nuclei of endometrial cells.[304] The mitogenic action of E_2 is indirectly determined (paracrine control) by a polypeptide growth factor, epidermal growth factor (EGF).[305] Regulation of EGF receptor content is achieved by ovarian E_2 and P secretion (autocrine control). The mechanisms of steroid hormone–receptor effect on target cells include the following steps: (1) circulating and unbound steroid hormone molecules are incorporated into the cell through the cytoplasmic membrane, probably by cytoplasmic receptors; (2) the steroid hormone molecules enter the nucleus, which contains about 90% to 95% of the cellular receptors; (3) the intranuclear hormone molecules induce conversion of the inactive 4S form of receptor to the active 5S form of receptor; (4) the 5S receptor binds to acceptor genes in the nucleus and stimulates RNA polymerase and messager RNA transcription; and (5) the manufactured mRNA is transported to the cytoplasm, where it is translated into proteins as well as new receptors. Therefore, sex hormones activate intranuclear receptors that subsequently initiate a series of events that alter target cells.[306] E_2 stimulates the development of organ-elles in endometrial cells. These structures provide a protein matrix, energy, and synthesis of enzymes such as lactate dehydrogenase, hexokinase, pyruvate kinase, and glucose-6-phosphatase.[306]

The typical 28-day endometrial cycle can be divided into menstrual, proliferative, and secretory phases with a distinctive ovarian secretory profile and characteristic endometrial morphologic features. The first day of menstrual bleeding is designated day 1 of the cycle. The menstrual phase lasts an average of 4 days, during which a variable amount of tissue is sloughed. Ovulation occurs typically on day 14. The relatively constant part of the cycle is the luteal phase (approximately 14 days long), whereas the follicular phase can vary considerably in length from one individual to another and from one cycle to another in the same individual. Furthermore, there is sufficient variation in the morphologic changes that occur during the secretory phase to make possible its division into 14 recognizable patterns. Morphologic changes are not obvious during the proliferative phase, therefore proliferative endometrium phases are classified only as early, mid-, or late proliferative.[307]

During the early proliferative phase (days 5 to 7), rising estrogen levels result in synchronous proliferation of glands, stroma, and vessels. The endometrial glands are sparse, straight, and narrow and are lined by columnar epithelium with few mitoses and little pseudostratification. The stroma is dense. From days 8 to 10 (midproliferative phase) the rate of growth of vessels and glands surpasses that of the stroma, and as a result glands and vessels become coiled (Fig. 68-48, *A*). The glandular epithelium shows increasing pseudostratification and numerous mitoses. The stroma is then loosened by edema. The stromal cells are of the "naked nuclei" type and exhibit narrow rim of cytoplasm and thin cytoplasmic projections. The spiraling of glands and vessels is intensified on days 11 to 14 and the stroma again becomes denser. There is an interval period of approximately 48 hours between ovulation and the appearance of glycogen vacuoles in gland-lining cells indicative of postovulation day 16 (Fig. 68-48, *B*). Mitoses are still abundant and the stroma is dense. Over the next 2 or 3 days the vacuoles change from a subnuclear to a supranuclear location and by day 19 most of the secretion has been discharged into the gland lumen. By this time mitoses have disappeared. Ultrastructurally, ovulation is associated with the appearance of a unique and specific nucleolar channel system formed by infolding of the nuclear membrane into the nucleolar substance.[308] Giant mitochondria, with increased numbers of tubular cristae develop in response to the increased demand for energy from glycogen metabolism.[309] Immunohistochemically, staining for B72.3 and the very late antigen-1 can be demonstrated.[306]

From days 19 to 23 there is increased distention and serration of glands and the epithelial cells become flatter with blurred epithelial borders. By days 20 to 21 the stroma is loosened by edema and the stromal cells have the appearance of "naked nuclei" (Fig. 68-48, *C*). These changes are mediated by prostaglandin F_2(PGF_2) and PGE_2, which increase vascular permeability.[310,311] The peak of glandular secretion corresponds to day 21, when implantation of the blastocyst occurs if fertilization takes place. The stromal edema that reaches its maximum around day 22 abates on days 23 to 25 when progressive predecidual change is seen in the stratum compactum (Fig. 68-48, *D*). Perivascular decidual cuffs develop and mitoses reappear in the stroma. This stromal predecidualization occurs almost simultaneously to stromal infiltration by granulocytes; these hematolymphoid cells represent either a subpopulation of T-lymphocytes or macrophages[312-316] and are a source of relaxin, an autocrine-paracrine hormone involved in collagenolysis.[306] By this time the glands typically have the serrated appearance sometime referred to as "secretory exhaustion." As the late secretory effect progresses, pyknotic epithelial nuclei appear and the stroma shows increasing leukocytic infiltration. Endometrial desquamation (day 28 to day 2) is the result of a complex series of vascular and hemodynamic changes. The endometrial spiral arteries respond to varying hormone levels by intermittent contraction resulting in ischemic necrosis of the stratum functionale and its subsequent sloughing. The fall of E_2 and P by day 25 allows the release of lysosomal enzymes, which destroy endometrial and endothelial cells. These changes are probably mediated by prostaglandin and thromboxane. Plasmin, present in the menstrual fluid, prevents clotting of menstrual blood.

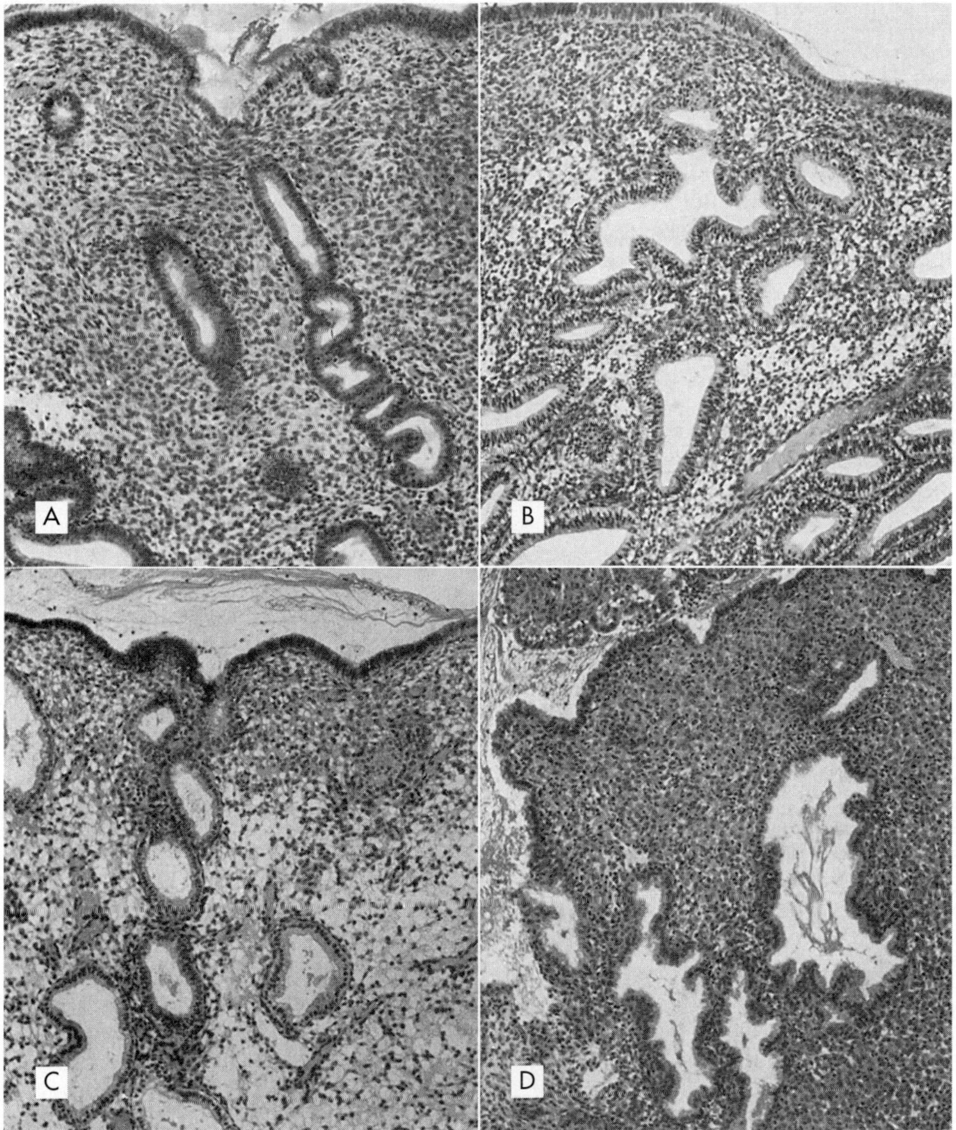

Fig. 68-48 **A**, Late proliferative endometrium at or about time of ovulation. Tortouous, pseudostratified glands with many mitoses are characteristic. Stroma, without predecidual reaction, may have variable degree of edema. **B**, Sixteen-day secretory endometrium. This early postovulatory endometrium is characterized by tortuous growing glands with irregular vacuolization caused by accumulation of glycogen in cytoplasm beneath nuclei. **C**, Twenty-two day secretory endometrium. Significant features of this stage are massive stromal edema, tortuousity of glands nearing secretory exhaustion, thin-walled blood vessels, and absence of predecidual cells. This coincides with peak of corpus luteum activity during which time the ovum is in process of implanting. **D**, Premenstrual endometrium. This phase is characterized by nearly complete predecidual transformation of stroma, secretory exhaustion of glands (which have serrated pattern), and inspissation of secretion. There is also leukocytic infiltration—both polymorphonuclear and monocytic. (From Noyes, RW, Hertig, AT, Rock, J: *Fertil Steril* 1:3, 1950.)

From days 3 and 4 regeneration takes place; the endometrium appears limited to the stratum basale and exhibits reepithelialization by extension of the residual glandular epithelium over the denuded surface. Endometrial stromal cells, which are similar to myofibroblasts, participate in wound healing. The basal layer and the thin overlying layer of loose connective tissue appear covered by flat to cuboid epithelium. Isolated mitoses are seen.

If pregnancy occurs, glandular secretion surges again and stromal edema persists. The developing decidua is gradually converted to a mature decidua after 14 days of conception. The transformation is completed by the end of the first month of gestation. Decidual cells stain with vimentin and desmin but not with cytokeratins or epithelial membrane antigen.[306] The infiltration of the decidua and the underlying myometrium by trophoblasts has been designated the placental site reaction.

Pregnancy is sometimes associated with the distinctive glandular change emphasized by Arias-Stella.[211] Most commonly this change is encountered in the endometrial glands but occasionally may be present in foci of endometriosis or adenomyosis, in endocervical glands, in fallopian tube epithelium, or in the glands within polyps.[302,317] The Arias-Stella phenomenon usually involves a focus of closely packed glands. The glandular epithelial cells exhibit pronounced nuclear pleomorphism and hyperchromatism. The nuclei typically have a smudged appearance. The cytoplasm is vacuolated and clear or may be densely eosinophilic. Mitotic figures are rarely present. The uninvolved endometrium usually exhibits typical gestational changes, that is striking decidualization. The *Arias-Stella reaction* is a glandular cell hypertrophy resulting from hyperstimulation induced by high levels of chorionic gonadotropin (hCG), estrogen, and progesterone.[317] It can be seen in normal intrauterine pregnancy, extrauterine pregnancy, gestational trophoblastic disease, and persistent corpus luteum.[317,318] It may also be produced by the administration of ovulation-inducing drugs or progestational agents and because of the pronounced nuclear atypia and the closely packed glands, the phenomenon can be confused with adenocarcinoma, particularly clear cell carcinoma. However, the phenomenon occurs in a secretory setting, glandular mitotic figures are not prominent, and typically there is nuclear polyploidy.[319] On the other hand, clear cell carcinoma develops almost exclusively in postmenopausal women, and usually contains near diploid or aneuploid nuclear DNA.[306]

Effects of hormones

Estrogens, progestins, or both are administered most frequently to alleviate the symptoms of estrogen deficiency (especially after menopause) and to control conception. The morphologic changes that result in the endometrium vary with the dosage and the sequence with which different combined preparations are used.

Estrogens. Estrogens stimulate the endometrium and are responsible for the characteristic changes of the proliferative phase. The E_2 produced by the ovarian follicle and synthetic estrogens have similar effects. In pathologic states, duration of exposure is more important than dose. High doses of estrogen in animal experiments actually cause endometrial atrophy. Unopposed estrogen stimulation as a result of anovulatory cycles characteristically occurs at menarche and at menopause or in patients with polycystic ovarian disease (Stein-Leventhal syndrome). In such cases proliferative activity continues, producing a typical histologic pattern with extensive fragmentation of proliferative endometrial glands and condensed stroma *(glandular-stromal breakdown)* (Fig. 68-49). The spiral arterioles do not develop adequately, the thin-walled ectatic venules undergo thrombosis, and there is random stromal necrosis with irregular shedding. The bleeding pattern therefore is variable. After months or years of unopposed estrogen stimulation different types of metaplasias, hyperplasia, and carcinoma can be produced.

Progestins. Progesterone or artificial progestins cause estrogen-primed endometrial glands to differentiate into a secretory pattern, and further growth is inhibited. This effect is produced if the endometrium has become hyperplastic, even in the case of complex atypical hyperplasia. The secretory changes induced are followed by regression, gland cell atrophy, and decidua-like transformation of the stroma.

Estrogens and progestins. If dosages and sequences are regulated carefully, it is possible to reproduce physiologic

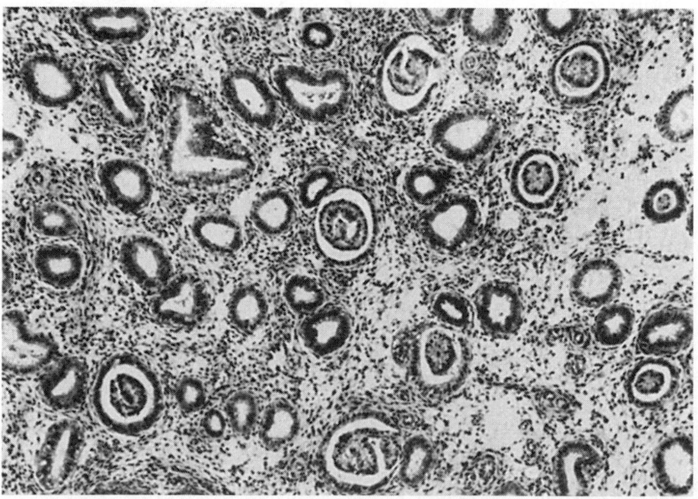

Fig. 68-49 Anovulatory endometrium. Irregular gland outlines are frequently found after anovulatory cycles, especially at time of menopause. The intraluminal protrusions of epithelium are belived to be an artifact caused by dilation and curettage procedure.

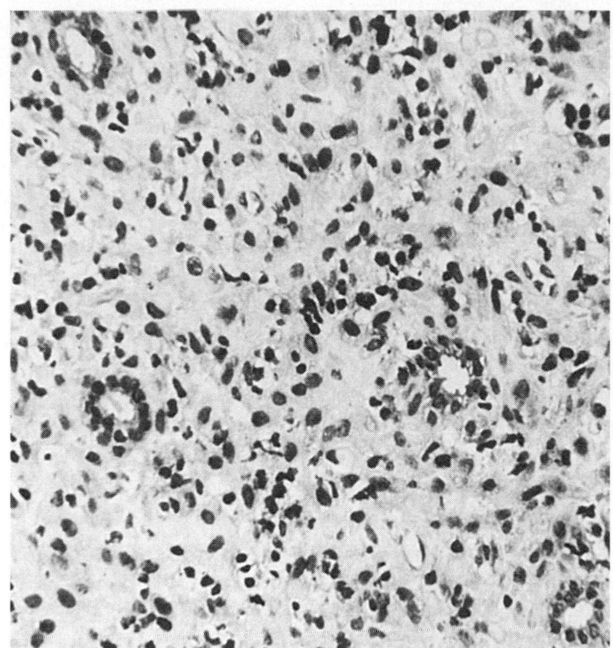

Fig. 68-50 Secretory atrophic pattern after long-term exposure to combination type of contraceptive hormonal preparation. Stromal cells are large and decidua-like; glands are small and atrophic with faint traces of secretion.

cycles with a normal endometrial morphology. Therefore, estrogen-progestin combination regimens are applied in the treatment of dysfunctional bleeding, endometriosis, menopausal symptoms, infertility, and some intersex states.

Unquestionably the most common application of hormonal therapy in gynecology is in conception control. The progestational agent in the combination pill prevents ovulation by inhibiting LH secretion through a negative-feedback effect on the hypothalamus.[320] In the endometrium, progestin-estrogen agents produce secretion at an early point in the cycle, arresting the proliferative stimulus of estrogen at an incompletely developed state. Continuation of the same stimulus leads to further gland atrophy, with a relatively pronounced deciduation-like stroma reaction at the end of the cycle. Estrogen-progestin sequential regimens operate in a different manner. The estrogen stimulus is carried past the time of ovulation and implantation so that secretion is delayed until about day 25 and does not exceed the early secretory pattern of endometrium of day 18. Predecidual stroma changes do not appear.

After several months of cyclic therapy with combination agents the endometrial glands become small and appear lined by low columnar cells with traces of cytoplasmic secretion (Fig. 68-50). Stromal cells are plump, with abundant cytoplasm. Vessels are small.

The atrophy is less pronounced after long-term exposure to sequential agents. Perhaps because of the proliferative effect of estrogen, hyperplasia and even carcinoma have developed in occasional patients at a relatively young age after long-term exposure to sequential agents,[321] which are no longer used or produced for this reason.

Tamoxifen. Tamoxifen is an estrogen receptor agonist paradoxically acting as antiestrogen in patients with breast cancer. This differential effect is probably secondary to a tissue-specific response to tamoxifen.[322] An increased risk of endometrial carcinoma has been reported.[323,324]

Danazol. Danazol acts on the endometrium as a weak progestin. It is used in the treatment of endometriosis.[325]

Clomiphene citrate. The nonsteroidal synthetic estrogen clomiphene citrate inhibits estrogen receptor replacement in the hypothalamus. Decreased endogenous estrogen levels cause secretion of gonadotropin-releasing hormone and subsequent pituitary secretion of FSH and LH. In secretory endometrium, a decreased gland-to-stroma ratio[326] and a discrepancy in the maturation of glands and stroma[327] have been described after administration of clomiphene citrate.

Dysfunctional uterine bleeding

Uterine bleeding that occurs at irregular intervals in excessive or scant amounts, especially when prolonged, is said to be dysfunctional when there is no easily assignable cause such as polyps, hyperplasia, neoplasm, trauma, blood dyscrasia, pregnancy, or hormone administration.

Anovulatory cycles are the most common cause of dysfunctional uterine bleeding in women of reproductive age. Less frequently, bleeding results from abnormal progesterone stimulation of the endometrium; either because of its insufficient secretion by the corpus luteum (inadequate luteal phase) or because of the failure of the corpus luteum to involute at the appropriate time (irregular shedding).

Inadequate luteal phase, also referred to as *luteal phase defect,* occurs (perhaps in 3% of infertile women) when the corpus luteum either fails to develop adequately or regresses prematurely.[328,329]

In a large proportion of women the basic disorder may be pituitary overproduction of prolactin, which in excess suppresses progesterone production. Rarely the endometrium lacks progesterone receptors.[330] The diagnosis is customarily based on an endometrial biopsy specimen, which shows a lag in development of more than 2 days from the expected day of the cycle. The syndrome is ill defined, appears to have many causes, and responds variably to progesterone replacement.

Irregular shedding is characterized by the presence of a mixed proliferative and secretory patterns. In curettings obtained 5 days after the onset of bleeding, early proliferative glands appear admixed with irregular star-shaped secretory glands. Menstrual bleeding is prolonged and heavy.

The most common cause of postmenopausal bleeding is *atrophy* of the endometrium. The glands are lined by flattened epithelium without mitotic activity and usually undergo pronounced cystic dilatation.

Some women with *unexplained menorrhagia* have regular ovulatory cycles. Bleeding seems to be secondary to focal hemostatic factors.[331] Abnormal platelet aggregation caused by a shift in prostaglandin synthesis has been suggested as the most likely mechanism.[332]

Infections

Chronic endometritis

Chronic endometritis is diagnosed in 3% to 10% of patients undergoing an endometrial biopsy for irregular vaginal bleeding.[333] It represents an intermediate stage of pelvic inflammatory disease from cervicitis to salpingitis.[334] Most endometritis result from ascending infection through the cervix after abortion, parturition, and instrumentation. Association with salpingitis and intrauterine devices (IUD) has been described in 25% and 14% of the cases respectively.[335] Most patients have menstrual disturbances, and about half may have pelvic pain or tenderness.

The finding of an infiltrate of plasma cells in the endometrial stroma is the pathologic basis for the diagnosis of chronic endometritis. However, plasma cells may be scant and difficult to distinguish from endometrial stromal granulocytes. The typical spindle-cell change of the stroma and the difficulty to decide whether the glands are proliferative or secretory, may be of help for establishing the diagnosis.

The microorganisms most commonly implicated are *Chlamydia trachomatis* and *Neisseria gonorrhoeae*.[336] *Mycoplasma* and *Listeria* organisms are relevant causes of endometrial infection in patients with infertility of repeated abortion.

The finding of hyalinized thick-walled stromal vessels and stellate glands with moderate secretory changes is sufficiently characteristic to identify a recent abortion as the most likely cause, even in the absence of villi.

Tuberculous endometritis is rare in the United States in comparison with other countries. Granulomas are usually small, sparse, and without caseation (Fig. 68-51). A reactive and atypical proliferation of the endometrial glands may simulate carcinoma. Patients are usually sterile; tubal infections typically occur first. Histologic diagnosis may be difficult, since the granulomas take up 2 weeks to develop, and the endometrium is shed every 4 weeks.[337]

Viral endometritis are produced by HSV and cytomegalovirus (CMV). In HSV infections the epithelial cells contain round pink inclusions surrounded by a halo. There is necrosis, acute inflammation, and multinucleated giant cells.[338] CMV endometritis occurs predominantly in immunocompromised women[339] but also during pregnancy, where it has been considered a cause of spontaneous abortion.[340] The inflammatory infiltrate is composed of plasma cells and lymphocytes. The characteristic inclusions are large, round, and basophilic. They are found within the nucleus and cytoplasm of the epithelial cells.

Infection with *Actinomyces israelii* gram-positive bacteria with fungal features, is associated with IUD use. The characteristic sulfur granules, formed by masses of hyphae surrounded by radiating filaments, can be found in Pap smears.[341] Tuboovarian abscess is a rare complication.[342]

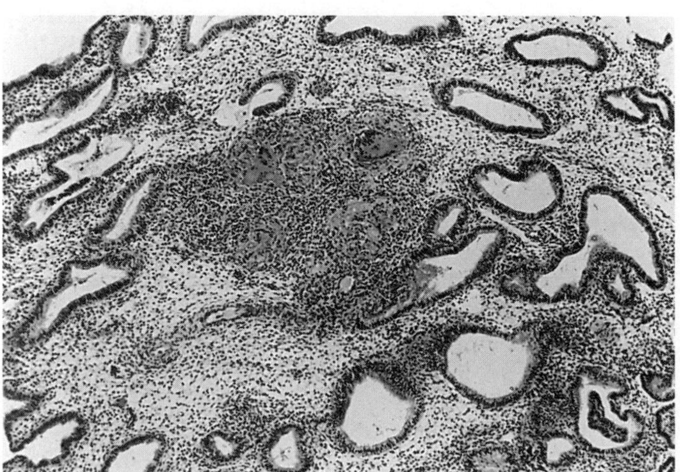

Fig. 68-51 Tuberculous endometritis. The granulomas contain several giant multinucleated cells.

Acute endometritis

The most significant form of acute endometritis is postpartum bacterial sepsis originating in the endometrium. The pathologic lesion is an acute suppurative infection with progressive infiltration of the endometrium, myometrium, and parametrium by polymorphonuclear leukocytes. The portal of entry is the vagina. The classic agents are *Streptococcus* and *Staphylococcus,* but anaerobic bacteria, notably *Bacteroides* species, have been implicated. Histologic diagnosis is based on finding extensive acute inflammation in nonbleeding endometrium.[343]

Benign polypoid lesions

Endometrial polyps are composed of a mixture of endometrial glands and stroma forming a circumscribed mass that protrudes into the endometrial cavity. They are usually solitary, but about 25% are multiple. The prevalence of polyps in the general population is approximately 25%. The histologic pattern usually resembles that of so-called cystic hyperplasia. There may be variable degrees of stromal fibrosis, traces of smooth muscle are commonly present, and stromal vessels are thick-walled and disproportionately large. When smooth muscle is abundant, the lesion is classified as a pedunculated adenomyoma.

Squamous metaplasia in an *atypical polypoid adenomyoma* (APA) produces a complex pattern that is easily confused with cancer.[238] APA occurs in the reproductive period and typically involves the lower uterine segment. The focal nature of this lesion and the presence of smooth muscle around glands distinguish APA from complex atypical hyperplasia. Invasive adenocarcinoma is associated with a desmoplastic or fibrous stroma. Despite its atypical histologic features, APA follows a benign course, and curettage may be curative. A case of endometrial adenocarcinoma in association with an APA has been reported.[344]

Endometrial polyps may be a source of abnormal uterine bleeding. An isolated carcinoma arising in an endometrial polyp is rare; patients who have focal carcinoma in polyps usually also have a carcinoma elsewhere in the endometrium.

Metaplasia

The replacement of typical endometrial epithelium by another type not found normally in the endometrium may occur in association with several benign lesions, such as endometritis and polyps, and in hyperplasia and carcinoma.[345] Endometrial metaplasia, often related to unopposed estrogen stimulation, may be focal or diffuse. Although pure metaplasia is a benign change without prognostic significance, its occurrence in association with hyperplasia may be the source of confusion with carcinoma.[346] On the other hand, metaplasia is often encountered in cancerous endometria, and its recognition should not be interpreted as evidence that the underlying endometrial changes are necessarily benign. In these cases, it is the nature of the associated process—polyp, hyperplasia, or carcinoma—that determines the diagnosis.[345]

One of the most characteristic forms of endometrial metaplasia is *squamous metaplasia* or *acanthosis.* It usually appears as "morules" of immature but cytologically bland squamous cells (Fig. 68-52), which may show focal keratinization and may undergo central necrosis. There is a tendency for it to be more common in the more atypical endometrial proliferations and is found in approximately 25% of atypical hyperplasias. The metaplastic change may be extensive and confluent and may lead to an erroneous diagnosis of adenoacanthoma when adequate attention is not paid to the cytologic features of the underlying glandular epithelium.[346-349]

The most common form of metaplasia is *ciliated (tubal) metaplasia*. Ciliated cells are occasionally observed in normal proliferative and postmenopausal endometria or in polyps. They may, however, constitute the predominant or sole cell type, particularly in cases of hyperplasia.[346] The absence of atypical nuclear features separates ciliated metaplasia from rare examples of ciliated cells and ciliated adenocarcinomas.[350]

In *mucinous metaplasia*, the endometrial surface or glands are lined by columnar mucinous epithelium resembling that of the endocervix. In contrast to secretory endometrium, the cell cytoplasms stain with PAS-diastase and mucicarmine but do not contain glycogen.[351] Rare cases may be associated with mucinous tumors of the ovary. In *eosinophilic metaplasia*, inactive or hyperplastic glands are lined by nonciliated cells with abundant eosinophilic cytoplasm. The uniformity of the round central nuclei and absence of mitotic figures distinguish eosinophilic metaplasia from atypical hyperplasia or adenocarcinomas.[346] *Papillary syncytial metaplasia* typically occurs on the surface of the endometrium and within the mouths of the endometrial glands of a regenerative epithelium that may have a papillary architecture. It is seen most often in the postmenstrual phase of the cycle and during regeneration after bleeding from a proliferative or a hyperplastic endometrium. The superficial location and the benign appearance of the nuclei distinguish this type of metaplasia from papillary carcinoma.[352]

Hobnail cell or *clear cell metaplasia* may be seen as isolated phenomena with no apparent cause, after hormonal medication or, most commonly, in patients with an intrauterine or ectopic pregnancy. Hobnail cell hyperplasia related to pregnancy is generally referred to as the *Arias-Stella* phenomenon.

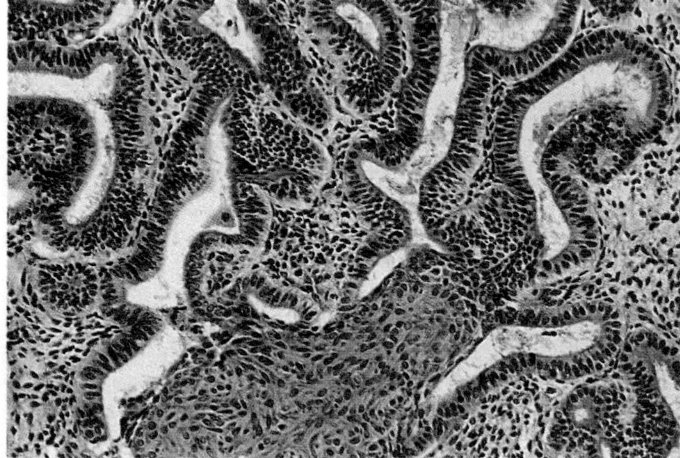

Fig. 68-52 Complex hyperplasia with squamous metaplasia. A morule lacking cytologic atypia is present.

More exotic tissues such as cartilage, bone, and glial tissue probably also arise as metaplastic foci sometimes, but implanted aborted fetal tissue may be the most common cause.

Mixtures of different types of metaplasias are common. Metaplasia occurs often in postmenopausal women who receive exogenous estrogens and in young women with persistent anovulation. The frequent association of endometrial metaplasia with hyperplasia is probably attributable to the fact that both are often associated with hyperestrogenism. The importance of recognizing endometrial metaplasia lies in not confusing this benign lesion with carcinoma.

Hyperplasia

Endometrial hyperplasias form a morphologic continuum of abnormal epithelial and stromal proliferation ranging from focal glandular crowding or simple hyperplasia to well-differentiated adenocarcinoma. It encompasses a variety of patterns, some of which are characterized by varying degrees of cellular atypia. For many years, pathologists have been concerned about the malignant potential of the various types of endometrial hyperplasia. Much of the confusion in the literature has resulted from different uses of the terms "adenomatous hyperplasia," "atypical hyperplasia," and "carcinoma in situ" to describe lesions in the borderline area. Also, there has been an absence of follow-up data. Recently, ultrastructural and DNA studies have indicated that cytologic atypia represents a more serious change than structural abnormalities from the viewpoint of risk of developing carcinoma.[353-355]

In 1977, it was first recommended to evaluate the architectural and cytologic abnormalities separately, to learn more about their own malignant potential. The following working classification was proposed: cystic hyperplasia, architectural atypia (mild to severe), and cytologic atypia (mild to severe).[353]

Cystic hyperplasia is characterized by large dilated glands with rounded profiles lined by nonproliferating or minimally proliferating epithelium, separated by an abundant and cellular stroma. The increased amounts of stroma account for the cystic dilatation of the glands. There is also dilatation and thrombosis of sinusoids and focal necrosis (Fig. 68-53).

The *complex forms of hyperplasia* exhibit a more distinctly proliferative pattern; the gland outlines are irregular because of outpouchings and papillary infoldings of the epithelium. In those cases with predominantly architectural abnormalities (formerly "adenomatous hyperplasia"), the glands are lined by columnar epithelial cells with large nuclei often exhibiting stratification, but nuclear polarity is generally maintained (Fig. 68-54). The stroma is dense, cellular, and compact. There are numerous mitoses in both glands and stroma. In higher grades of hyperplasia (formerly "atypical hyperplasia") striking architectural abnormalities are commonly associated with varying degrees of cellular atypia and the cytologic features—large cells and large irregular nuclei and nucleoli—are more like those of adenocarcinoma (Fig. 68-55). The cells that line the glands lose their polarity, and the cytoplasm often appears densely eosinophilic.

The new classification formulated by the WHO committee on endometrial tumors[356] breaks down endometrial hyperplasia into four subtypes: *simple hyperplasia without atypia* (SH), *simple hyperplasia with atypia* (SAH), *complex hyperplasia without atypia* (CH), and *complex hyperplasia with atypia*

(CAH). The term *atypia* refers to cellular atypia, and the term *complexity* refers to severe architectural abnormality close to that seen in cases of well-differentiated adenocarcinoma.[354] *Simple* includes cystic hyperplasia and mild and moderate degrees of architectural abnormality. SH is not significantly precancerous. Similarly, CH is also not demonstrably precancerous. There is not enough follow-up information about SAH to indicate that it is precancerous; this lesion, therefore, deserves further investigation. Finally, when CAH is diagnosed in a biopsy specimen, a well-differentiated adenocarcinoma is discovered in the hysterectomy specimen in 15% to 20% of the cases, or the lesion will eventually be followed by carcinoma in approximately 30% of the patients.[357,358]

It is unquestionable that estrogen administration produces endometrial hyperplasia. Prolonged periods of anovulation with steady and unopposed estrogen secretion have a similar effect, even in young women.[359,360] CAH apparently responds completely to the differentiating effect of progestins. Those lesions that do not respond to treatment (progestins, discontinued estrogen therapy, and D & C) are most likely to occur in women with polycystic ovarian disease, pronounced obesity, or both.[354] In obese women without polycystic ovarian disease, hyperplasia results from peripheral conversion of androstenedione to estrone in adipose tissue. The carcinomas that develop in this clinical setting are usually well differentiated, confined to the uterus, and associated with hyperplasia; they have an excellent prognosis.[358]

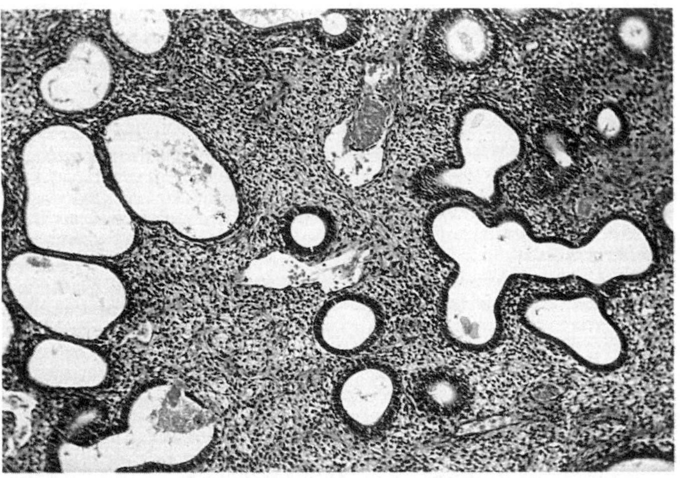

Fig. 68-53 Simple (cystic) hyperplasia. Endometrial glands are dilated and cystic. Stroma between the glands is abundant. Thrombosis of vessels is present.

Atypical hyperplasia versus well-differentiated adenocarcinoma

In curettage specimens, well-differentiated adenocarcinoma is often difficult to distinguish from CAH because the histologic criteria for both lesions are highly subjective. Recently, criteria for making this differential diagnosis have been proposed by two groups of investigators.[358,361] These criteria were validated by the findings in hysterectomy specimens, including the presence or absence of myometrial invasion, after a diagnosis of either CAH or well-differentiated adenocarcinoma had been made on biopsy specimens. The first group[361] underlined various architectural and cytologic abnormalities, some of which may be absent in individual cases, leaving the final decision to the overall evaluation of the lesion. Both, pronounced architectural atypia and at least moderate cytologic abnormality were required for the diagnosis of adenocarcinoma.[361]

In contrast, the second group of investigators proposed strict criteria emphasizing architecture, qualitative stromal changes, and quantitative features.[358] They used as their primary criterion for adenocarcinoma the presence or absence of stromal invasion, which is defined arbitrarily by the presence of at least one of the following features: (1) desmoplastic stromal response in the vicinity of infiltrating glands, (2) confluent or cribriform glandular pattern, (3) extensive papillary pattern, and (4) replacement of stroma by squamous epithelium.[358] To qualify as invasion, the last three changes are required to

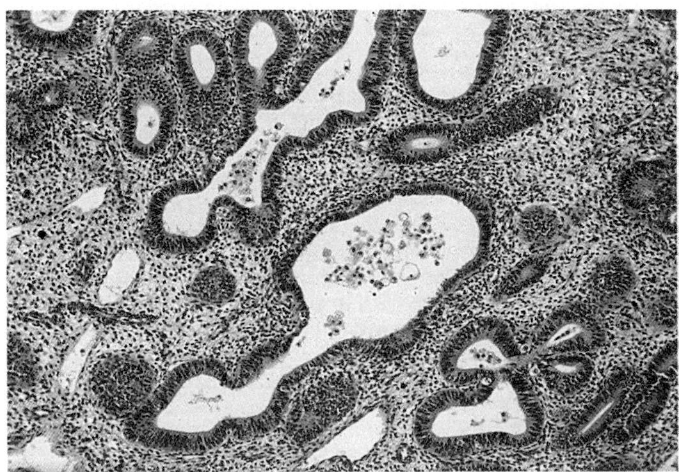

Fig. 68-54 Complex hyperplasia (adenomatous hyperplasia). The glands are fairly widely separated by stroma but exhibit architectural complexity. Cytologic atypia is absent.

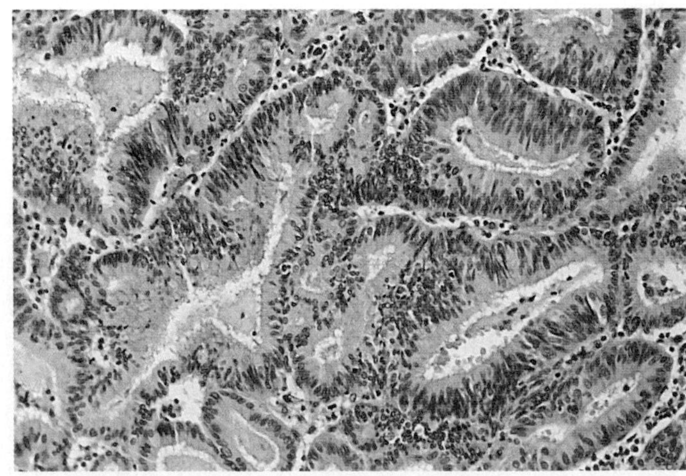

Fig. 68-55 Complex atypical hyperplasia. Closely packed glands show a lack of polarity with stratification and nuclear atypia. Changes are close to those of well-differentiated adenocarcinoma.

occupy at least half (2.1 mm) of a low-power microscopic field 4.2 mm in diameter. Using these criteria, when stromal invasion was absent in the endometrial curettings (and a diagnosis of CAH had been made), invasive adenocarcinoma was present in the hysterectomy specimen in 17% of the cases. The carcinomas in these cases were well differentiated and confined to the endometrium or were only superficially invasive.[358] In contrast, when stromal invasion was present in the curettings, residual carcinoma was identified in the uterus in 50% of the cases and, of these, one third were moderately or poorly differentiated, and one quarter deeply invaded the myometrium.[358]

Although the criteria proposed in the first study[361] are imprecise and somewhat subjective, those of the second[358] are too strict. This should not be surprising, since the differential diagnosis of CAH and well-differentiated adenocarcinoma is difficult and sometimes impossible. These lesions represent a morphologic continuum, and their separation depends on subjective weighing of various inexact criteria.[345] Usually, when a truly desmoplastic stroma is present, the diagnosis of carcinoma is already quite obvious for other reasons. On the other hand, biopsy sampling of the endometrial cavity is most frequently incomplete and, therefore, quantitative criteria are not justified.

In practice, the differential diagnosis of CAH and well-differentiated adenocarcinoma of the endometrium is usually not of great clinical importance. In the young patient who wishes to maintain her fertility, conservative therapy has been successful in the treatment of both lesions. When a borderline lesion occurs in a menopausal or postmenopausal woman who is not a poor surgical risk, the usual therapy is hysterectomy.

Malignant neoplasms

Adenocarcinoma

Endometrial carcinoma occurs primarily in menopausal and postmenopausal women. As previously discussed, unopposed estrogen effect leads to endometrial hyperplasia and in some cases to adenocarcinoma. Other important predisposing factors include obesity, infertility, late menopause, diabetes, and hypertension. In industrialized countries, endometrial carcinoma has become increasingly common and has finally surpassed the incidence of cervical carcinoma.[362,363] The incidence rate increased in the 1970s when unopposed estrogen replacement therapy was used and decreased in the 1980s after the addition of progestins.[364,365] In the United States, about 1 women in 100 will develop the disease. Despite its high frequency, endometrial cancer usually presents clinically as abnormal vaginal bleeding, which permits early detection and cure.

Continuous estrogen stimulation of the endometrium may produce a CAH difficult to distinguish from a well-differentiated carcinoma. Such a lesion can be associated with exogenous estrogens and endogenous estrogens from ovarian neoplasms, particularly granulosa and theca cell tumors. Lesions of this type have a favorable prognosis and may regress when the stimulus is removed.

Tamoxifen, a nonsteroidal hormone with antiestrogenic effect in the reproductive age, has a weak estrogenic effect in postmenopausal women. Recently, over 80 cases of endometrial adenocarcinoma in women with breast cancer who have been treated with tamoxifen have been described.[324]

From a pathogenetic viewpoint, two different forms of endometrial carcinoma with distinct clinicopathologic features have been identified: A low-grade ("endometrioid") carcinoma, which is estrogen-related, is usually associated with endometrial hyperplasia, and occurs in younger, perimenopausal women, and a second, more aggressive type (serous, adenosquamous, and clear cell carcinomas), unrelated to estrogen stimulation that occurs in older women.[366]

Gross features. Endometrial adenocarcinoma forms large irregular masses of friable, granular, gray-tan tissue that protrude into the endometrial cavity (Fig. 68-56). Myometrial invasion is identified in cut sections by the presence of softer bulging masses of granular tissue that replaces the smooth muscle.[367-369] Extension to the cervix is common.

Microscopic features. The new classification of endometrial carcinomas proposed by the WHO[356] is based primarily on the cell type of the tumor (Table 68-4), reflecting that tumor cell type, as well as histologic grade, and the degree of myometrial invasion has an important effect on biologic behavior.

Endometrioid carcinoma. Over 80% of endometrial adenocarcinomas are composed of tubular glands lined by stratified non–mucin containing epithelium.[370-372] In the rare cases in which basal vacuolization or supranuclear vacuolization are present, a diagnosis of secretory endometrioid adenocarcinoma is appropriate. Separation of adenoacanthomas and adenosquamous carcinomas has been based on whether the squamous component of the tumor is cytologically benign (Fig. 68-57) or cytologically malignant and invasive of the stroma, independently of the glandular component.[373-375] Recently the WHO committee has concluded that such a distinction was not reproducible because of the frequency of tumors in an intermediate category. The term "adenocarcinoma with squamous differentiation," modified by the grade of the tumor, has been recommended. A granulomatous response may be encountered in the pelvic peritoneum, secondary to keratin exfoliation in cases of adenocarcinomas with squamous differentiation. These granulomas have no prognostic significance.[376] High-grade endometrioid carcinomas may contain a trophoblastic component and are associated with the production of hCG.

Mucinous adenocarcinoma. Mucinous adenocarcinoma is characterized by the presence of a significant amount of

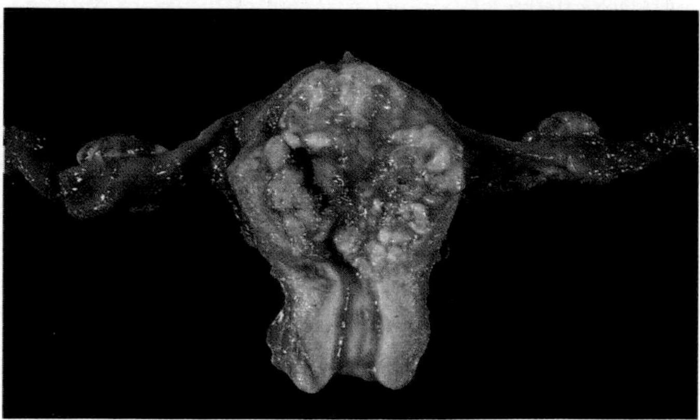

Fig. 68-56 Adenocarcinoma of endometrium. Tumor fills the endometrial cavity. Obvious myometrial invasion is seen.

Table 68-4 Classification of endometrial carcinoma*

Endometrioid
Typical
Variants
With squamous differentiation
Secretory carcinoma
Ciliated carcinoma
Serous papillary adenocarcinoma
Clear cell adenocarcinoma
Mucinous adenocarcinoma
Squamous cell carcinoma
Mixed carcinoma†
Undifferentiated carcinoma

*Modified from the World Health Organization and International Society of Gynecological Pathologists classifications of endometrial carcinoma.[356]
†A carcinoma containing more than 10% of a second cell type.

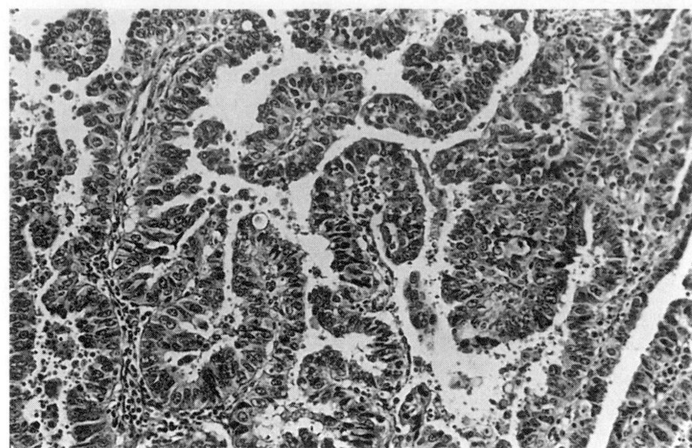

Fig. 68-58 Serous papillary adenocarcinoma of endometrium. Thick papillae are lined by stratified anaplastic cells.

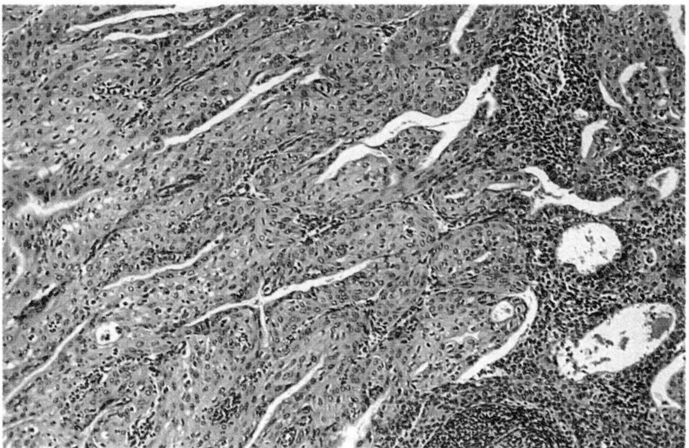

Fig. 68-57 Adenocarcinoma of endometrium with squamous differentiation (adenoacanthoma). The squamous component appears benign.

intracellular mucin in a significant number of the tumor cells.[377] Admixture of a few mucinous cells to an otherwise typical endometrioid adenocarcinoma does not warrant a diagnosis of mucinous adenocarcinoma. Mucinous adenocarcinoma of the endometrium may be difficult to distinguish from mucinous adenocarcinoma of the endocervix in a curettage specimen. In the endometrial tumor there is usually an admixture with endometrioid neoplastic glands, whereas in the endocervical tumor there is often a dense fibrous stroma. In some cases, however, the differential diagnosis may be impossible.

Serous papillary adenocarcinoma. Serous papillary adenocarcinoma is characterized by microscopic features similar to those of serous carcinoma of the ovary, that is, a fine and irregular papillary pattern with cellular budding, pronounced nuclear pleomorphism, slitlike and irregular glandular spaces, and occasionally psammoma bodies[378] (Fig. 68-58). The papillary pattern of the serous carcinoma is to be distinguished from the typical villoglandular papillary pattern that is sometimes found in endometrioid carcinomas. The differential diagnosis is important because the serous carcinoma of the endometrium is associated with a poor prognosis related to the frequency of deep myometrial invasion and peritoneal dissemination, whereas the villoglandular endometrioid carcinoma is associated with a good prognosis, similar to that of the nonpapillary endometrioid adenocarcinoma. The finding of c-*myc* amplification, immunoreactivity for p53 (Fig. 68-59) and c-*erb* B-2 and aneuploidy in this type of endometrial cancer is consistent with its aggressive behavior.[379,380]

Clear cell carcinoma. Clear cell carcinoma of the endometrium again is identical histologically to the clear cell carcinoma of the ovary.[381,382] Ultrastructural studies indicate a müllerian histogenesis.[383] It may be characterized by clear cells filled with glycogen, hobnail cells protruding into glandular lumens, or both. It may be highly papillary. This tumor, like the serous carcinoma, tends to occur in older women and to be associated with a poor prognosis.

There are occasional reports of endometrial squamous cell carcinoma.[384] Small-cell carcinomas of the endometrium are aggressive tumors with a propensity for systemic spread and a poor prognosis.[385]

Prognostic factors. Prognosis in endometrial carcinoma is related to tumor stage, tumor grade, and histologic type. The new FIGO staging system (Table 68-5) requires assessment of the pelvic and para-aortic lymph nodes, adnexae and peritoneal fluid cytologic findings.[386]

Pathologic analysis includes evaluation of the histologic grade, depth of myometrial invasion, and determination of endocervical involvement.[387] Nearly 90% of women with endometrial cancer limited to the endometrium survive 5 years. As invasion extends to the inner half of the myometrium, survival falls to 70%, and with cancer spread outside the uterus, survival is less than 15%. Endometrial carcinomas that involve the cervix are more likely to metastasize to pelvic lymph nodes, with a similar distribution to that of cervical carcinoma.[387]

Histologic grading is based on both the proportion of solid areas and the degree of nuclear atypia.[386] In grade 1 carcinoma, 5% or less of the tumor is composed of solid nonsquamous tissue, whereas this type of tissue composes 6% to 50% in grade 2 carcinomas and over 50% in grade 3 carcinomas. Nuclear atypia exceeding that expected for grade 1 or grade 2 carcinoma raises the grade by one. Adenocarcinomas with

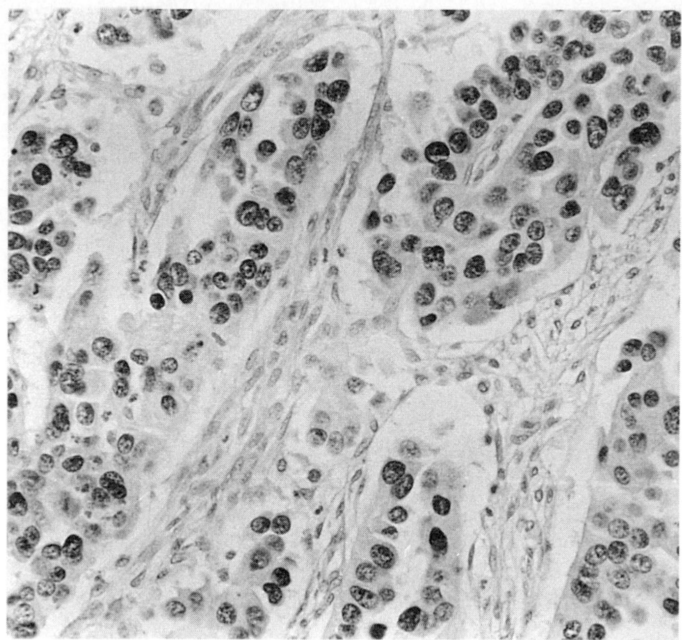

Fig. 68-59 Serous papillary adenocarcinoma of endometrium. Diffuse nuclear staining for p53-associated protein. (Immunohistochemistry.)

Table 68-5 FIGO staging of endometrial adenocarcinoma (1988)

Stage I	Carcinoma is confined to the corpus uteri itself
Stage Ia	Tumor limited to the endometrium
Stage Ib	Invasion to < ½ of the myometrium
Stage Ic	Invasion to > ½ of the myometrium
Stage II	Carcinoma has involved the corpus and the cervix
Stage IIa	Endocervical glandular involvement only
Stage IIb	Cervical stromal invasion
Stage III	Carcinoma has extended outside the uterus but not outside the true pelvis
Stage IIIa	Tumor invades serosa and/or adnexae and/or positive peritoneal cytology
Stage IIIb	Vaginal metastases
Stage IIIc	Metastases to pelvis and/or para-aortic lymph nodes
Stage IV	Carcinoma has extended outside the true pelvis or has obviously involved the mucosa of the bladder or the rectum
Stage IVa	Tumor invasion of bladder and/or bowel mucosa
Stage IVb	Distant metastases including intra-abdominal and/or inguinal lymph nodes

squamous differentiation are graded according to the nuclear grade of the glandular component. Serous, clear cell, and pure squamous carcinomas are graded only by nuclear features.

Vascular invasion is an important predictor of recurrence, particularly in stage I endometrioid carcinoma.[388] Progesterone receptor status is a more important risk factor than estrogen receptor status.[389,390] Approximately half of the tumors that recur are aneuploid,[391] but S-phase fraction is a stronger prognostic indicator.[392] K-*ras* abnormalities may be involved in the hyperplasia-to-carcinoma sequence in human endometrium.[393,394] In contrast, inactivation of p53 occurs as a later event in endometrial carcinogenesis.[380,395,396] Overexpression of c-*erb*-B-2 has been found in 15% of endometrial carcinomas.[397]

The conventional treatment for endometrial carcinomas is hysterectomy and bilateral salpingo-oophorectomy. Postoperative chemotherapy or radiotherapy are used in patients with unfavorable prognostic factors.

Endometrial stromal tumors

Endometrial stromal tumors include benign nodules, low-grade sarcomas and high-grade sarcomas.[398] Benign endometrial stromal nodules form single, well-circumscribed masses that can often be distinguished grossly from leiomyomas by their yellow color and softer consistency. Most are in the myometrium, but some protrude into the endometrial cavity (Fig. 68-60). The histologic appearance closely resembles that of normal endometrial stroma, with numerous evenly distributed small vessels.[399] Stromal lesions of similar origin that have a distinct trabecular architecture have also been called "plexiform tumorlets." The endometrial stroma can form a variety of glandlike structures, some of which mimic ovarian sex cord–stromal tumors. The epithelial elements appear benign; they may occur in stromal nodules as well as low-grade and high-grade stromal sarcomas, including those with prominent intravascular components. When these sex cord–like elements predominate, the designation "uterine tumor resembling ovarian sex cord tumor" has been used.[400] Most of these tumors have a benign clinical course.

Low-grade endometrial stromal sarcomas occur as grossly circumscribed nodules with or without extensive intravascular extensions ("endolymphatic stromal myosis"). The most characteristic feature is the presence of numerous wormlike masses of stromal tissue that extrude from vascular channels when the uterine wall is cut. The microscopic pattern resembles a stromal nodule, but the margins may infiltrate adjacent myometrium (Fig. 68-61), and mitotic figures are common and may be numerous. The tumor cells, however, closely resemble the stromal cells of the proliferative endometrium and are separated by a network of small blood vessels.[398,401,402] (Fig. 68-62).

The clinical course is usually benign, but incompletely resected lesions may recur slowly in the pelvis, and in an occasional patient pulmonary metastases develop. Some metastatic lesions have regressed after progestin therapy.[403-405] Similar stromal lesions may arise in the pelvic retroperitoneum.[406]

High-grade endometrial stromal sarcoma is a malignant tumor that characteristically forms one or more polypoid endometrial masses. Margins are indistinct as the result of diffuse infiltration of the myometrium by poorly differentiated small cells that bear little resemblance to endometrial stromal cells.[401,403] The characteristic vascular pattern of the low-grade tumors is usually absent. Mitoses are numerous; usually more than 10 mitotic figures (MF) per 10 HPF. The histologic appearance of the tumor is a more reliable index of behavior than the mitotic rate is.[402]

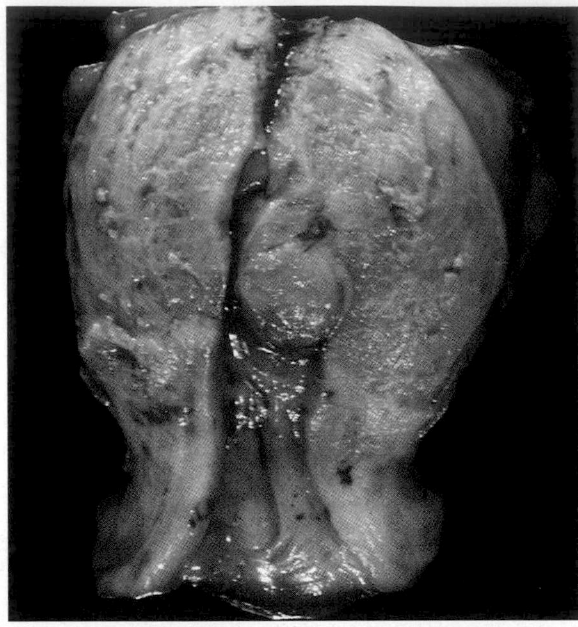

Fig. 68-60 Endometrial stromal nodule. Cross section of a well-circumscribed nodule protruding into the endometrial cavity. The tumor was limited to the endometrium. (From Lloreta J, Prat J: *Int J Pathol* 11:293, 1992.)

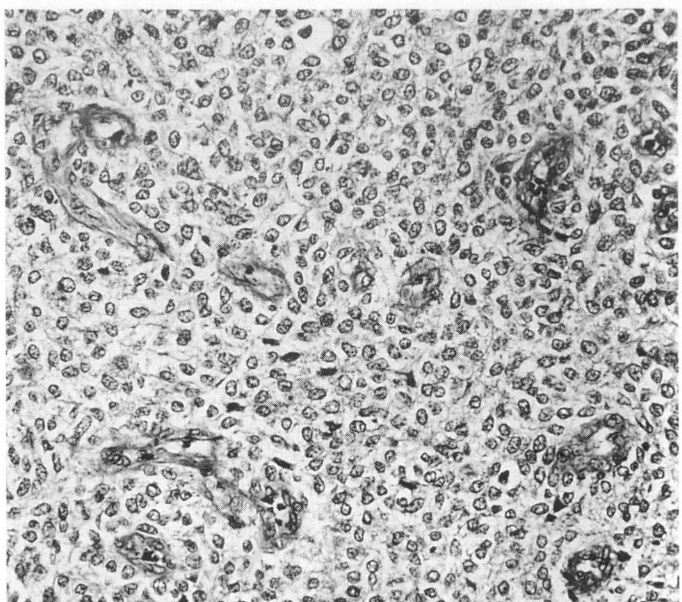

Fig. 68-62 Low-grade endometrial stromal sarcoma. Tumor cells resemble endometrial cells of proliferative endometrium and are separated by a network of small blood vessels.

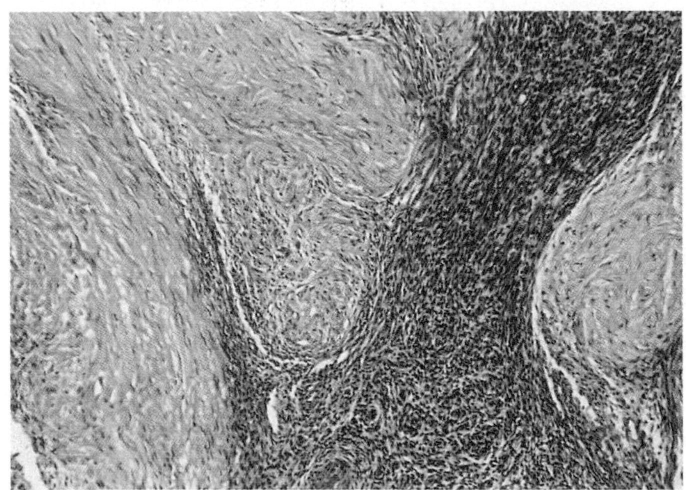

Fig. 68-61 Low-grade endometrial stromal sarcoma. Myometrium appears infiltrated by irregularly contoured aggregates of tumor cells resembling endometrial stromal cells.

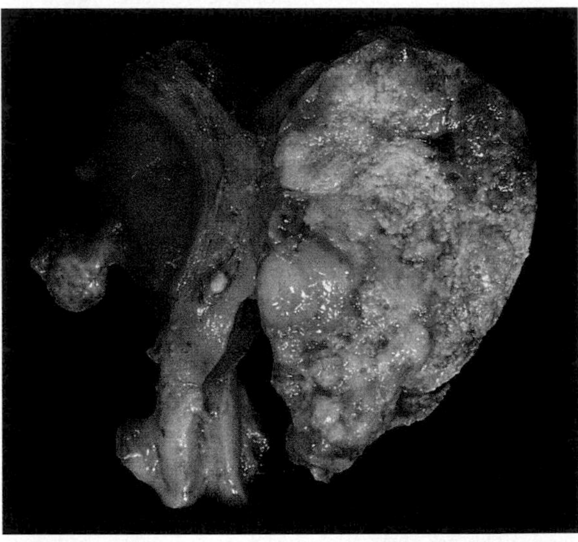

Fig. 68-63 Malignant mixed müllerian tumor. Large polypoid tumor with obvious malignant gross features.

Mixed müllerian tumors (lesions with mixed epithelial and stromal elements)

An uncommon and highly malignant group of endometrial cancers is composed of a mixture of carcinoma and sarcoma. The patients are usually elderly and postmenopausal. A large proportion of them have received prior radiotherapy.[407,408]

Abnormal bleeding is the most common symptom; the tumor may appear as a large polyp protruding through the cervical canal (Fig. 68-63). The carcinoma component includes the full range of histologic variants of endometrial adenocarcinoma. Poorly differentiated (often papillary serous) endometrial adenocarcinoma is usually predominant (Fig. 68-64). If the stromal component is an undifferentiated sarcoma, the tumor is said to be homologous mixed müllerian tumor or carcinosarcoma. Heterologous mixed müllerian tumors are those that also contain chondrosarcoma, osteosarcoma, or rhabdomyosarcoma.

Because of the simultaneous expression of epithelial and mesenchymal markers in both tumor tissue components, it has been suggested that these tumors may represent metaplastic carcinomas.[409,410]

The prognosis is extremely poor. Metastases occur early. The few survivors have had small lesions confined to the uterus, but even with such limited involvement the tumor

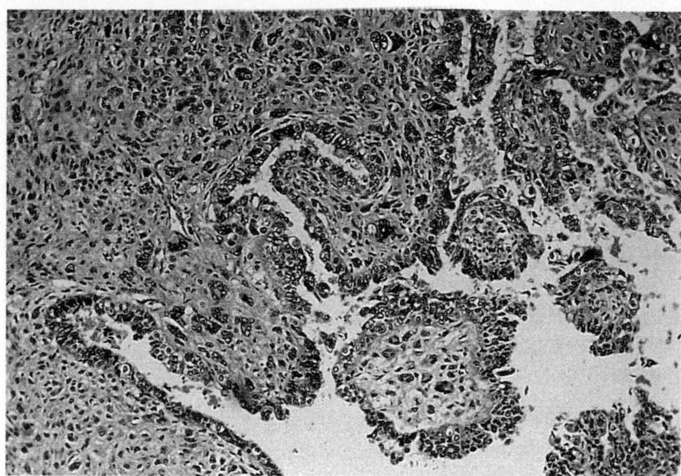

Fig. 68-64 Malignant mixed müllerian tumor. The carcinomatous component is of the papillary serous type.

often may disseminate widely, rapidly, and fatally.[411] The presence or absence of heterologous elements has not affected the prognosis significantly in most series. Radiotherapy may control localized lesions.[412]

An uncommon variant with a benign epithelial component mixed with a sarcomatous stroma has been called "müllerian adenosarcoma."[413] Mitoses among the stromal cells usually exceed 4 per 10 HPF; the most aggressive lesions are those that invade the uterine wall.

Adenofibroma, the rare benign extreme in the continuum of mixed müllerian tumor of the uterus, is distinguished by its circumscribed growth and fewer than 4 MF per 10 HPF among the stromal cells. Its histologic appearance resembles that of the more common ovarian adenofibroma.[414,415] Other rare lesions with mixed components, including carcinofibroma and adenomyoma also occur.[408]

Metastatic carcinoma

Metastatic carcinoma from distant sites is rare in the endometrium. The most common origin noted is breast cancer usually identified at autopsy.[416] Gastrointestinal cancer has also been reported and may be identified in endometrial curettage. The simultaneous finding of carcinoma in the endometrium together with cancer of the ovary may occasionally represent a metastasis, but in most instances it probably has a multifocal origin. Although conventional pathologic features are crucial to establish the differential diagnosis, DNA flow cytometry may also be of some value.[417]

Primary malignant lymphomas originating in the cervix and corpus have a relatively good prognosis when confined to the uterus.[418] Follicular lymphomas were more often localized and had the best prognosis.[419]

THE MYOMETRIUM

The myometrium provides a tough envelope for the developing fetus and propels it into independent life at parturition. The bulk of the myometrium is composed of smooth muscle cells. There are also extracellular components such as collagen and elastin.

Adenomyosis

Adenomyosis is characterized by an abnormal distribution of nests of histologically benign endometrial tissue within the myometrium. It may be focal or diffuse. The involved portions of myometrium are hypertrophied.

The uterus is enlarged and globular, often with lateral humps at the horns. The cut surface of areas of adenomyosis bulges and has ill-defined margins and a coarse trabecular appearance. The scattered foci of endometrial tissue appear depressed, soft, and occasionally hemorrhagic.

The islands of ectopic endometrium appear normal on histologic examination, except that an orientation of the glands is lacking. Both glands and stroma are present. Recent hemorrhage and hemosiderin in macrophages, indicating past hemorrhage, are usually found only in occasional areas. Both glands and stroma may respond to hormonal stimulation but not in all cases or in all parts of the same lesion.

The minimum criteria for diagnosis are vague. Most texts refer to the depth of more than 1 low-power microscopic field as the borderline beyond which endometrium qualifies for the diagnosis of adenomyosis. The presence of associated muscle hypertrophy is characteristic. The common extensions of endometrium that retain continuity with the surface but reach a depth of 1 to 2 mm are probably not significant.

The symptoms ascribed to adenomyosis are pain, especially with menstrual periods, cramps, and abnormally prolonged and profuse menstrual bleeding.[420]

The pathogenesis is unexplained. Adenomyosis is not seen in children and is much less common in young women, a finding indicating that it is unlikely to be a congenital malformation. The most popular concept is that the endometrium extends into the myometrium; a metaplasia of the myometrium is equally tenable. Estrogen simulation may be an important etiologic factor. Adenomyosis is not usually associated with endometriosis, even when the endometriosis is extensive. It does seem to occur more frequently in women with endometrial hyperplasia or endometrial carcinoma.[421] In such cases the foci of adenomyosis may occasionally also appear hyperplastic or neoplastic, in step with the endometrial lesion.

Smooth muscle tumors

Leiomyoma

The most common lesion of the myometrium is a benign neoplasm composed of smooth muscle with a variable fibrous tissue component. Leiomyomas are well circumscribed, rounded, firm or hard, rubbery masses of gray-white tissue with a characteristic whorled appearance on a cut surface. They are often multiple and vary considerably in size (Fig. 68-65). Most occur during the years of active reproductive life; growth may be stimulated by pregnancy or hormonal therapy. Their size decreases when the patient is treated with a gonadotropin-releasing hormone (GnRH) agonist.[422] Chromosomal aberrations may play a role in their pathogenesis.[423]

Symptoms vary with location. *Subserosal* leiomyomas may impinge on the bladder or the sacral plexus, for example, causing urinary frequency or pain. *Submucous* leiomyomas that protrude into the endometrial cavity cause abnormal bleeding. Rarely very large leiomyomas have been associated with polycythemia.[424,425] Leiomyomas undergoing infarction or hemorrhage may be painful.

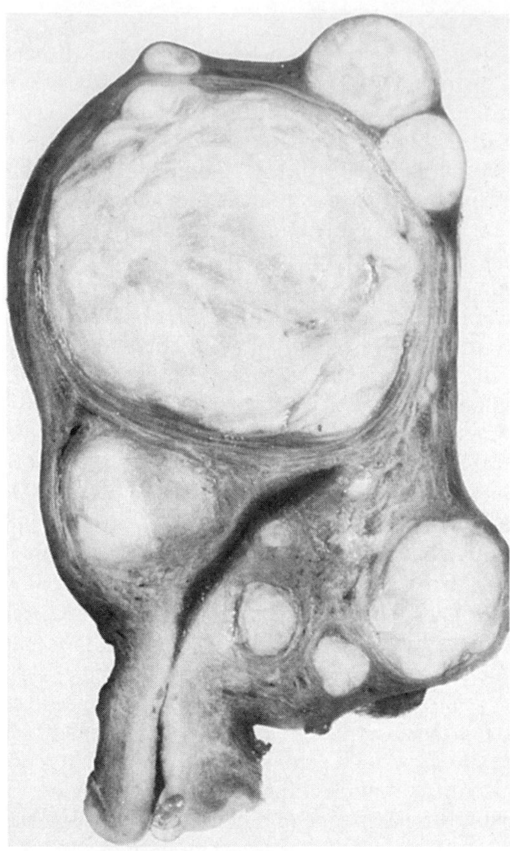

Fig. 68-65 Multiple leiomyomas in sagittal section. Typical, well-circumscribed, solid, light gray nodules distort uterus.

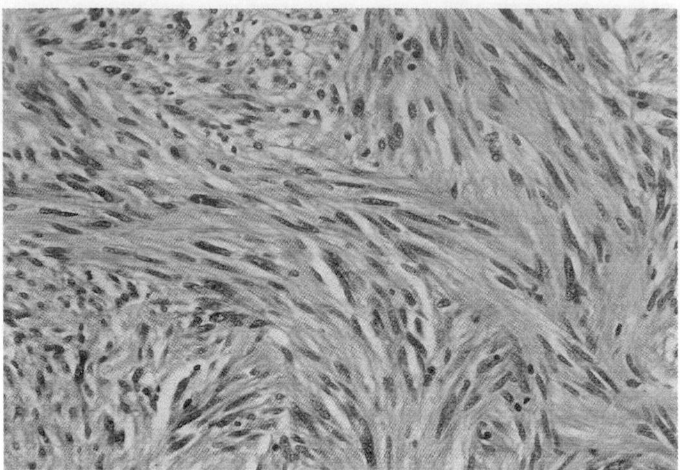

Fig. 68-66 Leiomyoma. Elongated cells in a typical interlacing pattern.

The histologic pattern is familiar, with streaming masses of smooth muscle separated by strands or masses of collagen (Fig. 68-66). Some remarkable variations occur, with pronounced edema or massive calcification or hyalinization. Leiomyomas that have a sizable adipose tissue component have been called *lipoleiomyomas*.

Cellular leiomyomas are unusually cellular but otherwise typical. They may resemble endometrial stromal nodules, but the presence of fusiform nuclei, a fascicular growth pattern, and the lack of extensive vascular network indicate the correct diagnosis.[403]

Bizarre (*symplastic*) *leiomyomas* have a frightening microscopic appearance because of the many large giant cells with very large, cytologically malignant-looking nuclei, which may be multiple. These lesions, which occur at premenopausal age, lack the mitoses that characterize leiomyosarcoma and have proved to be benign.[403,426,427] Occasional association with exogenous progestins occurs.[403,428]

Epithelioid leiomyomas (leiomyoblastomas) are rare uterine counterparts of a similar tumor found in the stomach,[429] characterized histologically by abundant clear cytoplasm. Nearly all are benign; the few aggressive lesions contained more numerous mitoses.[430]

Unusual smooth muscle neoplasms related to leiomyomas

Rarely smooth muscle tumors may behave in an aggressive manner that belies their benign microscopic appearance.[403]

Peritoneal leiomyomatosis. Peritoneal leiomyomatosis refers to the extensive proliferation of histologically benign nodules of smooth muscle about the peritoneal surfaces but limited to the peritoneal cavity. There seems to be a close relationship to pregnancy; it is probable that the origin is metaplastic rather than metastatic from the uterus.[431,432] Regression occurs in most cases after the stimulatory hormonal factors have been withdrawn.[403]

Metastasizing leiomyoma. Rarely a histologically benign leiomyoma may seem to be the source of lymph nodal or pulmonary metastases.[433-435] Mitoses are not seen. In some cases progression seems related to hormonal factors, including pregnancy.[436] Intravenous extensions of the uterine tumor are absent. Estrogen receptors have been identified in an aggressive metastasizing leiomyoma; regression occurred after termination of pregnancy.[437] Other smooth muscle lesions (pulmonary lymphangiomyomatosis) have appeared to respond to endocrine manipulation.[438] It has been thought that most or all "multiple pulmonary fibroleiomyomas" are actually metastatic uterine smooth muscle tumors, despite admixed (entrapped) glandular components.[434]

Intravenous leiomyomatosis. Intravenous leiomyomatosis is a benign smooth muscle neoplasm characterized by the presence of grossly visible intravenous proliferations that produces histologically benign smooth muscle into pelvic veins. Mitoses are absent. The prognosis is good even if all the intravenous extensions cannot be resected.[439-441] The changes are dramatic when extensive; less obvious cases are probably often overlooked.

Recently, it has been shown that otherwise typical or cellular leiomyomas with up to 15 MF per 10HPF have a benign course (even when treated by myomectomy), provided that they are benign by other clinical and pathologic criteria. Such tumors are typically small (<10 cm) and have a grossly benign appearance. The terms *mitotically active leiomyoma* (MAL)[442-444] or *leiomyoma with increased mitotic figures*[403] have been suggested for such tumors. In contrast to leiomyosarcomas, MALs almost invariably occur in women of reproductive age, are associated with the secretory phase of the menstrual cycle, pregnancy, or the use of exogenous progestins. These observations indicate that the mitotic activity in at least some MALs may be attributable to an exogenous or endogenous progestational effect.[443-446]

Leiomyosarcoma

Leiomyosarcoma accounts for one third of uterine sarcomas. It has been estimated that 1 of every 800 smooth muscle tumors of the uterus is a leiomyosarcoma.[447] Although an origin from a leiomyoma is possible and associated leiomyomas are present in a minority of cases, it is unusual to be able to prove such an occurrence.[403,448,449] The mean age of patients at the time of diagnosis in most series is over 50, with a range of 40 to 80 years. The clinical presentation is nonspecific. The main symptoms are uterine enlargement and abnormal uterine bleeding; only occasionally does tissue obtained by curettage establish a preoperative diagnosis.

Most leiomyosarcomas are intramural, solitary, large and soft masses; the yellow or tan color, lack of a trabeculated pattern, at least in some areas, and poorly circumscribed margins may indicate the diagnosis on gross inspection (Fig. 68-67).

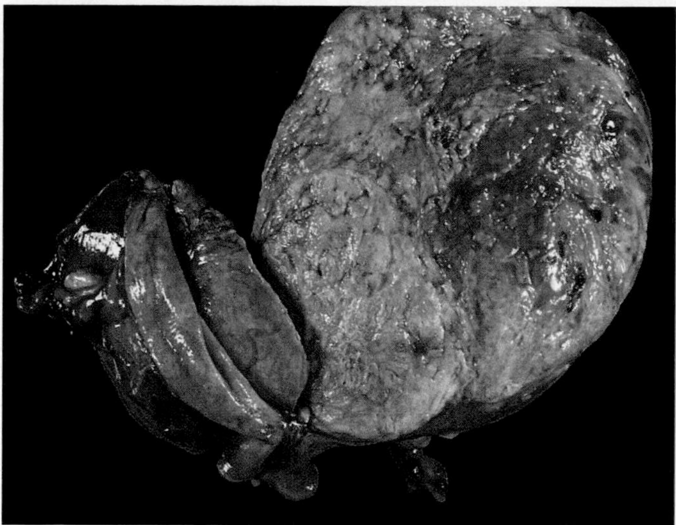

Fig. 68-67 Leiomyosarcoma of uterus. Intramural, solitary mass with foci of necrosis.

Microscopically, it is characterized by fascicles of spindle-shaped smooth muscle cells with ample eosinophilic cytoplasm containing identifiable myofibrils. The grouping of hypercellularity, remarkable degrees of nuclear atypia, and high mitotic rates establishes the diagnosis (Fig. 68-68). Nuclei are usually large and hyperchromatic with irregularly clumped chromatin.

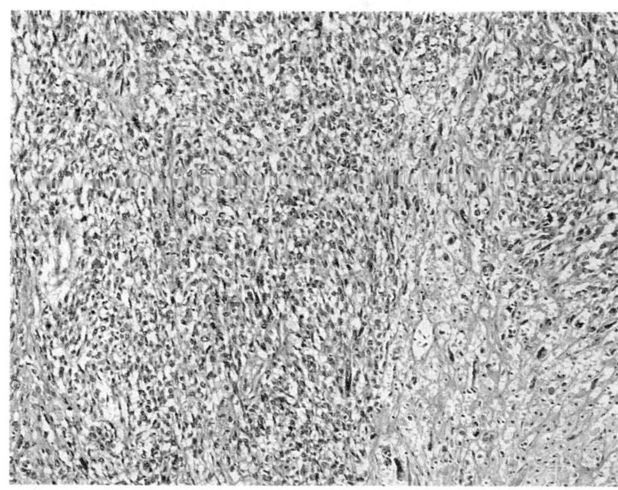

Fig. 68-68 Leiomyosarcoma. Hypercellularity, nuclear pleomorphism, and coagulative tumor necrosis are striking. Mitotic figures were numerous.

Traditionally the most significant indicator of malignant behavior has been mitotic index.[418] Over 75% of leiomyosarcomas contain atypical nuclei and have 10 or more MF per 10 HPF. The minimal pathologic criteria that justify a diagnosis of leiomyosarcoma are more problematic. The combining results of 8 series from the literature revealed that lesions containing 5 or more MF per 10 HPF and cytologic atypia should be designated as "leiomyosarcomas."[426] Hypercellular smooth muscle tumors with no cytologic atypia but more than 5 MF per 10 HPF are designated as "mitotically active leiomyomas."[426]

One or more supportive clinical or pathologic features are also commonly present, including perimenopausal or postmenopausal age, extrauterine extension of tumor, a diameter over 10 cm, an infiltrating border, coagulative tumor necrosis (Fig. 68-68), and atypical mitotic figures.[403,426,427,442] Vascular invasion is identified in 10% to 20% of leiomyosarcomas. A recent study has indicated that the presence of coagulative necrosis in a moderately atypical tumor justifies the diagnosis of leiomyosarcoma regardless of the mitotic count.[450]

Extension beyond the uterus is associated with a fatal prognosis. Chemotherapy with doxorubicin (Adriamycin) has seemed to produce a transient antitumor effect in a few patients.[451] Most leiomyosarcomas are aneuploid.[452,453]

Other neoplasms

Lipomas, composed entirely of adipose tissue, are rare and probably result from metaplasia in smooth muscle or stromal cells. *Adenomatoid tumor* is an uncommon benign nodular mass that resembles a leiomyoma grossly but microscopically has a microcystic honeycomb appearance caused by numerous small spaces lined by vacuolated cells.[403,454,455] Similar lesions occur in the fallopian tube.[456] Ultrastructural and histochemical studies support a mesothelial origin.[457]

Rarely primitive neuroectodermal tumors develop in the uterus.[458,459]

FALLOPIAN TUBES

Anatomy and physiology

The paired fallopian tubes are divided into specific regions with different functions. The interstitial portion is a narrow channel through the cornual wall of the uterine fundus. The isthmic portion, about 2 to 3 cm long, is immediately distal to the tubouterine junction and probably functions as a sphincter. The ampullary portion, about 5 to 8 cm long, has a much wider lumen and a extensive mucosa with complex folds, or plicae. The infundibulum is the trumpetlike distal portion that terminates in the tubal fimbriae; it also has the capacity to act as a sphincter.

The tubal mucosa is composed of three types of cells. The ciliated cells have an obvious function in transport through the tube. The secretory cells are columnar and become actively secreting during the secretory half of the menstrual cycle. Also present are narrow, dark intercalated or inactive cells. The outer serosal covering is a mesothelial structure.

The fallopian tubes are complex structures that represent more than conduits from ovary to endometrial cavity. The fimbriae are actively approximated to the ovary at ovulation. Coordination of muscular activity, epithelial proliferation, ciliary activity, and mucosal secretion is under endocrine control and varies with the phases of the menstrual cycle. Spermatozoa are conveyed to the ampullary portion of the tube, where fertilization takes place.

Infectious diseases

Acute salpingitis and pelvic inflammatory disease

Acute salpingitis originates chiefly as a complication of venereally transmitted infection of the lower genital tract. Puerperal or postabortal salpingitis occurs especially after intrauterine instrumentation. Intra-abdominal infections such as appendicitis with peritonitis may secondarily affect the tube. Hematogenous spread is important in the pathogenesis of tuberculosis of the tube and some cases of pneumococcal salpingitis occurring in children.

The most common infectious organism is *Chlamydia trachomatis*,[460] followed closely by the still very significant *Neisseria gonorrhoeae*. The frequency with which salpingitis and pelvic inflammatory disease occur after exposure is probably 50%.[461] Subsequently, with the formation of more extensive pelvic tubo-ovarian abscess, numerous other organisms, notably anaerobes, have been cultured, usually species of *Bacteroides, Clostridium, Mycoplasma hominis* and *Ureaplasma urealyticum*.[462] IUDs may increase the risk of salpingitis and more extended pelvic infection after lower genital tract infections.[462-465]

The fallopian tubes are nearly always affected bilaterally. The fimbriated ends are sealed by organizing inflammatory exudate, and the lumens are dilated, especially the ampullary portion, producing a retort-shaped deformation (Fig. 68-69). The serosa is red and covered with purulent exudate, which extends to the ovaries and pelvic wall. Loculated pockets of pus may accumulate, producing a tubo-ovarian abscess, with the tube, uterus, broad ligament, and ovary forming parts of the surrounding abscess wall.

Microscopically the lumen of the tube is filled with polymorphonuclear leukocytes, which also extensively infiltrate the tubal mucosa and wall. The mucosal epithelium may be focally ulcerated but generally remains intact.

Complication of acute salpingitis include peritonitis, disseminated systemic infections, usually gonococcal, and rarely death when there is a rupture of an adnexal abscess.[462]

Chronic salpingitis

After approximately 10 days, plasma cells, macrophages, and lymphocytes begin to dominate the inflammatory exudate. Fibrosis becomes progressively more apparent as the exudate organizes. The tubal plicae form adhesions in many areas, sometimes producing a complicated multiglandular structure. As the inflammatory process finally resolves, this arrangement persists and has been termed *follicular salpingitis*.

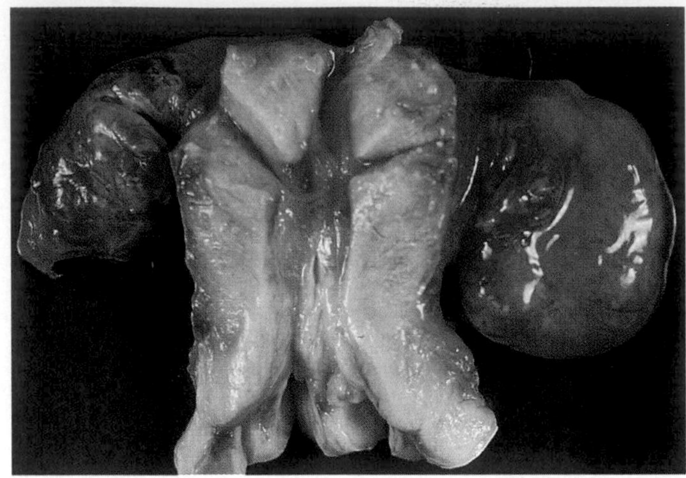

Fig. 68-69 Chronic salpingitis. Bilateral, retort-shaped, swollen, sealed tubes and adhesions of ovaries are typical of salpingitis.

The causative organisms, often anaerobes, may be difficult to culture, but they are and can be identified and treated effectively. Anaerobes are especially likely to be present in the most serous and life-threatening pelvic infections.

Granulomatous salpingitis is most commonly caused by *Mycobacterium tuberculosis*. The tube is dilated, with a thickened wall. The exudate within the lumen usually appears purulent rather than caseous. Typical caseating granulomas are identified in microscopic section, however. The glandlike pattern produced by the combination of adhesions of plicae and epithelial hyperplasia may be remarkably proliferative and has been mistaken for adenocarcinoma. Tubal tuberculosis was invariably present when any part of the female genital tract is affected; two thirds of the women are between 25 and 35 years of age, and the most common initial complaint is infertility (94%). The diagnosis of tubal tuberculosis is based on the demonstration of acid-fast bacilli in the tissues or by positive cultures or guinea pig inoculation.[337]

Foreign-body granulomas in the tube may occur after instillation of oily contrast media used in hysterosalpingography, and talc granulomas have occurred after laparotomy. Rare instances of sarcoidosis, actinomycosis, and schistosomiasis have been reported.

It has been proposed that pseudoxanthomatous salpingiosis is related to ovarian endometriosis and develops after an episode of acute salpingitis during which actively bleeding ovarian endometriosis leaks blood into the lumen of the fallopian tube. Lipofuscin-laden macrophages are located in lamina propria.[466]

Endometriosis

Ectopic growth of endometrial glands and stroma can occur in all parts of the tube. Serosal implants appear as small red or red-brown patches or nodules with hemorrhage and fibrous adhesions. They are usually part of more generalized pelvic endometriosis. The anatomic distribution of the disease is consistent with retrograde menstruation; lesions are more common in the pelvis, and one or both tubes present implants in approximately 6% of cases and adhesions in about 25%.[467] Involvement of the muscular wall stimulates muscle proliferation, and a nodular enlargement results. The tubal mucosa is affected in 10% of the cases. Endometriosis is associated with infertility, pelvic pain, or dysmenorrhea.[468]

In pregnancy, focal decidual reaction may involve the serosa or mucosal stroma, especially in the plicae of the ampullary portion of the tube. The cells closely resemble endometrial decidual cells; they must not be confused with granulomas or metastatic carcinoma.

Salpingitis isthmica nodosa

The characteristically bilateral nodular enlargements of salpingitis isthmica nodosa are located in the tubal isthmus and may be multiple. They vary from a few millimeters to a few centimeters in diameter, are firm, and appear gray, yellow, or brown on the cut surface.

Microscopically the nodules are composed of channels or spaces, lined by benign tubal epithelium separated by bundles of smooth muscle, which forms the major component of the mass. Inflammatory changes are inconspicuous or absent. The glandular channels communicate with the tubal lumen and therefore can be demonstrated by hysterosalpingography.[469] The lesions apparently are acquired, but the pathogenesis is unknown. Most patients are sterile.

Ectopic pregnancy

Implantation of a fertilized ovum may occur in the tube, especially when tubal structure or function has been altered or impaired by inflammation. Chronic salpingitis, follicular salpingitis, and salpingitis isthmica nodosa appear to be the major factors associated with recurrent tubal gestation.[470] The muscular wall is weakened by trophoblastic infiltration and attenuated because the lumen is distended by hemorrhage (Fig. 68-70). Vascular invasion by trophoblast is invariably present.

The diagnosis is not always easy because only a minority of the patients report the typical clinical picture or amenorrhea, pain, and vaginal bleeding, but today early diagnosis can be achieved after a combination of clinical and laboratory tests.[471] Salpingectomy is done to control the massive hemorrhage that often results from rupture of the tube. Repeat tubal pregnancy occurs in about 10% of patients.

Attempts to enhance future fertility by excision of the ectopic gestation by means of a linear salpingostomy may be successful,[471] but the procedure carries a high rate of repeated ectopic pregnancy. This risk is worth consideration when future pregnancy is desired because the expectation of an intrauterine pregnancy is about 50%. Occasionally the residual trophoblast may persist, requiring reoperation.[472]

Sequelae of tubal sterilization

Immediate clinical complications are well documented.[473-475] Pregnancy occurs on the average of 0.37 per 100 women-years in the first poststerilization year and 0.10 per 100 women-years subsequently;[476] the relative frequency of tubal pregnancies is significantly higher than expected.[477] Regardless of the procedure of sterilization, the blind proximal stump shows luminal dilatation, flattening of the fronds, intraluminal polyps, and a higher mitotic rate. Other common changes are epithelial inclusions and mucosal endometriosis related to menstrual reflux.[462]

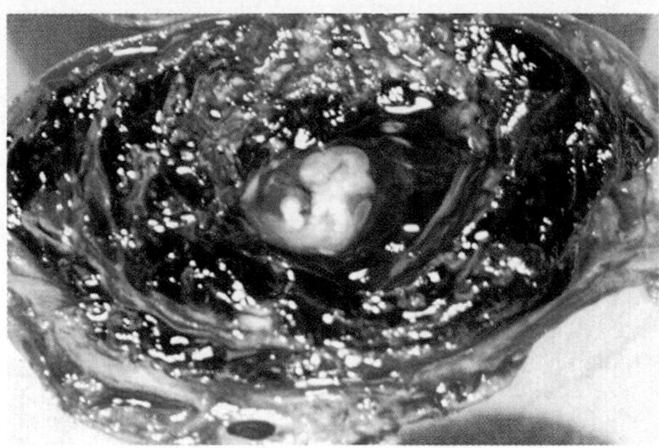

Fig. 68-70 Tubal ectopic pregnancy. Placental villi have infiltrated muscular wall, forming a hemorrhagic mass.

Benign tumors and cysts

Hydatids of Morgagni are unilocular, thin-walled cysts that hang from the tubal fimbriae. The epithelium is like that of the tube and undergoes cyclic changes in step with tubal epithelium; these are true tubal cysts.[478]

Mesonephric (paratubal or parovarian) *cysts* are also unilocular thin-walled cysts filled with clear straw colored fluid. The epithelium of these cysts resembles that of the mesonephric duct remnants of the mesovarium and does not undergo cyclic changes as tubal epithelium does.[478]

Adenomatoid tumors of the tube are histologically identical to those in the uterine wall. In the tube they form a well-circumscribed nonencapsulated small nodular mass that compresses the tubal lumen to one side. It is important to recognize the pseudoglandular pattern to avoid a mistaken diagnosis of adenocarcinoma.[456]

Papillomas of fallopian tube are rare.[479] Occasionally, papillary proliferation composed of large polygonal cells with vesicular nuclei and abundant acidophilic cytoplasm have been reported under the name of "metaplastic papillary tumor."[480] The clinical course is benign, and the pathogenesis is uncertain but is believed to be the consequence of a reactive change found in postpartum women at the time of tubal ligation. Leiomyomas of the tube are surprisingly rare in view of their common occurrence in the adjacent uterus and the smooth muscle origin of both organs. Of the 60 or 80 cases reported, a few have been remarkably large.[481]

Rarely, *teratomas* have originated from within the tube.[482] Most are intraluminal and cystic and resemble ovarian cystic teratomas (dermoid cysts). A few have been solid. Rare cases of malignant teratoma have been recorded.[483] The histogenesis of these lesions is much debated.

Malignant tumors

Adenocarcinoma

Tubal adenocarcinoma, the least common of female genital tract carcinomas, is also one of the most aggressive. It usually arises in old women with a wide range of age and a mean of 52.7 years.[484] The main symptoms are pain and vaginal discharge, which are more characteristic of tubal inflammation. Both tubes are affected in 20% of the cases.

Because of the nonspecific symptoms, the diagnosis is rarely made before laparotomy. The affected tube resembles a distorted sausage and tends to feel firm instead of fluctuant (Fig. 68-71). The appearance of the tumor in the opened tube is usually papillary but may be soft or solid. Simultaneous involvement of tube and ovary may occur, in which case the lesion is considered by convention to be of ovarian origin.

The histologic appearance closely resembles that of papillary serous adenocarcinoma of the ovary (Fig. 68-72). Better-differentiated lesions may contain psammoma bodies. Invasion of the tubal wall is common. Other tumors have endometrioid differentiation, and some of them may resemble neoplasms of probable wolffian origin.[485]

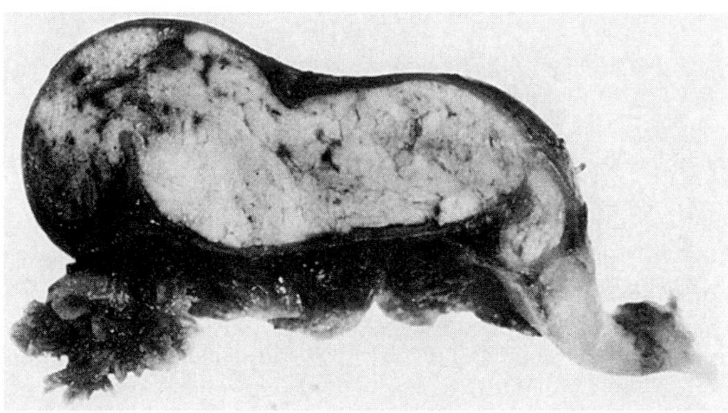

Fig. 68-71 Adenocarcinoma of fallopian tube, distending tubal lumen with soft gray tissue.

The prognosis is poor; only 33% of the patients survive 5 years after the diagnosis is established.[486] The few survivors usually have well-differentiated lesions confined to the tubal mucosa, situated within a sealed tube.[487]

Malignant mixed müllerian tumor of the tube is extremely rare. It has no gross distinguishing features. The histologic appearances and clinical correlations are similar to those described for carcinosarcoma and malignant mixed müllerian tumors of the endometrium. The prognosis is very poor.[488,489]

Metastatic tumors involving the tube are more common than primary carcinomas. The most frequent primary sites are the ovary and endometrium; breast and gastric adenocarcinoma are also encountered. The conspicuous lymphatic involvement and lack of neoplastic change in the tubal epithelium easily distinguish metastatic from primary carcinomas.

OVARY

The main function of the ovary is to produce eggs to implant after fertilization in the endometrium, the preparation of which is coordinated afresh each time by the ovarian hormones.

Anatomy and physiology

The ovaries are paired pelvic organs that lie on either side of the uterus close to the lateral pelvic wall, behind the broad ligament, and anterior to the rectum. The mesovarium joins the ovary to the posterior aspect of the broad ligament; the ovarian ligament to the ipsilateral uterine cornu, and the suspensory ligament to the lateral pelvic wall.[490] Adult ovaries are ovoid, measure approximately 3 to 5 cm in greatest dimension, and weigh 5 to 8 g. However, size and weight vary considerably depending on age and content in follicular derivates.[490] The

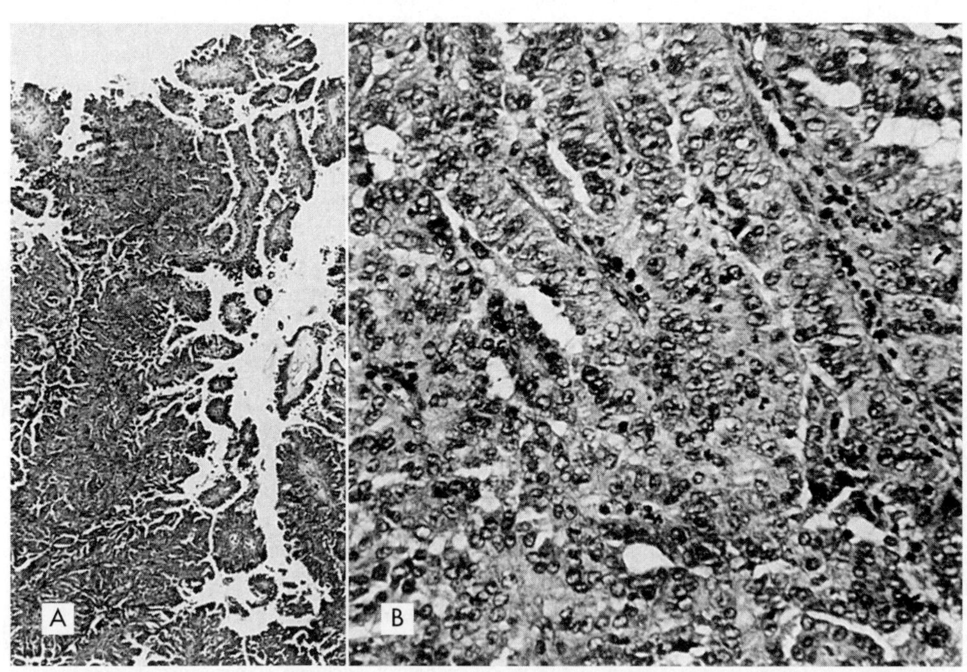

Fig. 68-72 Adenocarcinoma of fallopian tube. **A,** Typical papillary pattern. **B,** Higher magnification showing poorly differentiated adenocarcinoma. (From Kraus FT: *Gynecologic pathology*, St. Louis, 1967, Mosby.)

blood vessels and lymphatics enter and leave through the lateral suspensory ligaments and thence through long channels to terminate at the level of the kidneys. The major lymphatic drainage of the ovary is therefore cephalad toward the para-aortic nodes.

Cells of the ovary

Germ cells. At birth the germ cells are represented by oocytes, in a resting stage of the first meiotic division, a process that will not be completed until ovulation occurs and fertilization is in process.[491] Germ cells have the potential for reproducing tissues of all germ layers and are considered to be the cell of origin of teratomas. They do not themselves produce ovarian hormones but organize the cells that do; adjacent ovarian stromal cells are induced to specialize and form the granulosa and theca cells that produce estrogens and progestagens.

Granulosa cells. In the primary follicle of an infant the granulosa cells lie in a single layer around the oocyte. Under the influence of FSH they proliferate, forming a fluid that contains the precursor of the zona pellucida, a dense capsule that surrounds the maturing oocyte. Cytoplasmic projections of granulosa cells extend through the zona pellucida and abut on the oocyte cell membrane. As the graafian follicle enlarges, a fluid-filled space, the antrum, forms. The oocyte, surrounded by a hillock of granulosa cells, lies eccentrically near the wall of the follicle (Fig. 68-73). Small round masses of dense pink material surrounded by a rosette of granulosa cells are usually evident in sections; these *Call-Exner bodies* are a specific product of granulosa cells, normal and neoplastic. The granulosa layer is avascular until ovulation. Granulosa cells can synthesize estrogen (estrone) and various intermediates, including dehydroepiandrosterone.[492] At the time of ovulation they enlarge and form the corpus luteum, described subsequently.

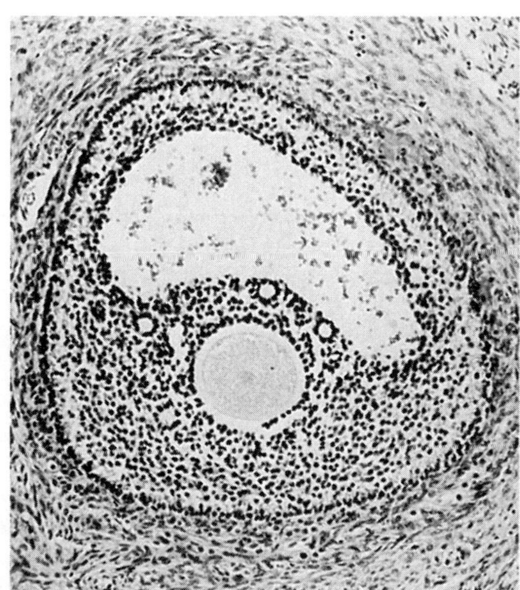

Fig. 68-73 Ovarian follicle. Large ovum is surrounded by mass of granulosa cells in which four Call-Exner bodies can be seen. Concentrically arranged plump spindle cells surrounding the follicle margin compose theca externa.

Theca cells. As the maturing graafian follicle enlarges, the immediately surrounding stromal cells also enlarge and become rounded and plump. This change in an ovarian stromal cell is called *luteinization.* The luteinized theca layer becomes noticeably more vascular than the adjacent stroma. Follicle-associated theca cells thus activated produce estrogen (both estrone and estradiol) and are considered to be the primary source of estrogen in the preovulatory stage of the menstrual cycle.

Corpus luteum. In response to the midcycle peak of pituitary LH (and with local help from prostaglandins),[493] the graafian follicle ruptures, expels the oocyte, and rapidly becomes a corpus luteum. The granulosa layer becomes vascularized, and the granulosa cells enlarge; they are then said to be luteinized. This transformation probably results from LH stimulation alone.[494] High content of LH receptors has been identified within the granulosa-lutein cells.[495] FSH receptors have also been identified in the early corpus luteum. Electron micrographs show abundant cytoplasmic agranular reticulum and mitochondria with tubular cristae typical of steroid hormone–producing cells.[496] The corpus luteum is the principal source of progesterone (which stimulates the secretory endometrium) but also synthesizes estrone and E_2, as well as androgens, mostly androstenedione.[497]

After ovulation, LH, FSH, and E_2 levels fall, but the LH concentration is sufficient to maintain the corpus luteum, producing a midluteal peak in P and E_2 concentrations. If fertilization does not occur, the increased levels of P and E_2 through negative feedback result in a fall of LH and FSH to basal levels, a reduction in LH and FSH receptors within the corpus luteum, and a sharp decline in P and E_2 synthesis after day 22 of the cycle.[495,498-500] These changes are reflected by the regression of the corpus luteum and the onset of menses.

After fertilization, placental hCG stimulates P production by the granulosa-lutein cells. Progesterone concentration within the corpus luteum increases sixfold, while the E_2 level drops to 10% of that within the preovulatory follicle.[501,502] Although reduced amounts remain, P production by the corpus luteum of pregnancy begins to decline by the end of the second month of gestation as its production is largely assumed by the placenta. There is a rapid decline in function during the puerperium, reflecting falling hCG levels during this period.[490] Relaxin, a polypeptide hormone, is also produced during gestation and the puerperium by the corpus luteum, probably under the control of hCG.[503,504]

Nonspecific ovarian stroma. The unspecialized ovarian stroma is a deceptively innocent-appearing mass of spindle-shaped cells. They produce collagen and also are capable of responding to gonadotropic stimuli to become luteinized producers of steroid hormones. They are considered to be the cells of origin from which hyperplastic lesions and stromal tumors (such as granulosa-theca cell and Sertoli-Leydig cell) arise. The ovarian stroma also contains smooth muscle fibers, which respond to prostaglandins, cholinergic agents, and oxytocin.

Surface mesothelium. The ovary is invested with a mesothelial covering, like other organs of the abdominal cavity. It is the mesothelium of the urogenital ridge from which the müllerian ducts arise; the surface covering of the ovary seems to share or retain some specialized potential for differentiation with the related müllerian cells that form the lining of tube, endometrium, cervix, and upper part of the vagina. This relationship seems to be the basis for the close similarity between the epithelial cell types found in hyperplastic, metaplastic, and neoplastic growths that occur in or on the ovary.

Focal decidual reaction is regularly present on the surface of the ovaries in pregnancy and may be extensive on peritoneal surfaces generally. Rarely a similar change is seen in postmenopausal women.

Hilum cells (hilar Leydig cells). Clusters of large cells with abundant pink cytoplasm are commonly associated with nonmyelinated nerve fibers in the hilum of the ovary at the insertion of the mesovarium. Hilum cells regularly contain crystalloids of Reinke, a feature shared with testicular Leydig (interstitial) cells but not with luteinized stromal cells in the ovary. The physiologic significance of hilum cells in the ovary has not been demonstrated; they are increased in the newborn in association with pregnancy complications such as toxemia, diabetes, and multiple pregnancy, perhaps as a response to increased amounts of placental chorionic gonadotropin.[505]

Vestigial structures. Traces of the mesonephros persist as isolated small ducts in the mesovarium; a more plexiform glandular structure, the rete ovarii, is situated at the margin of the ovarian-hilar junction. It is homologous with the rete testis. Tiny nodules of heterotopic adrenocortical tissue occur in the ovarian suspensory ligament, broad ligament, and mesovarium.

Ovarian senescence and disorders of ovarian failure

The ovary at birth contains about a half million oocytes. Between 300 and 400 oocytes may mature as potential gametes. Some of the rest form small follicles, which undergo atresia, but the majority lyse and disappear.

As the age of menopause approaches, the number of oocytes diminishes and the number of anovulatory cycles increases.

The postmenopausal ovary is composed chiefly of stroma, which remains biochemically active and may be slightly or moderately hyperplastic. It produces chiefly the androgenic steroids dehydroepiandrosterone, androstenedione, and testosterone; it does not aromatize androgens to estrogen.

Premature ovarian failure results from a variety of disorders that cause secondary amenorrhea and infertility before 35 years of age. If one excludes gonadal lesions associated with chromosomal abnormalities and surgical, radiation-induced, or drug-induced ablation of the ovaries, at least three disorders are associated with premature ovarian failure: premature follicle depletion (true premature menopause); resistant ovary; and autoimmune oophoritis. In true premature menopause the ovaries are small, lack primordial or developing follicles, and resemble postmenopausal ovaries.

The resistant ovary syndrome is found in approximately 20% of patients with premature ovarian failure and is characterized by primary or secondary amenorrhea, high gonadotropin levels, and resistance to both endogenous and exogenous gonadotropins, even when administered in massive doses.[506-509] The pathogenesis of the disorder is unknown, but a deficiency of FSH and LH receptors in the follicles, the presence of antibodies to these receptors, and a postreceptor defect have all been implicated.

The ovaries typically have a normal prepubertal or adult appearance. Microscopically there is an appropriate number of normal-appearing primordial follicles but a complete, or nearly complete, absence of developing follicles beyond the antral stage. Stromal luteinization and hilum cell hyperplasia may result from a high level of LH and be associated with virilization. In autoimmune oophoritis, the ovarian failure is often accompanied by one or more of the following disorders, most of which are believed to be on an autoimmune basis: Addison's disease, idiopathic hypoparathyroidism, Hashimoto's disease, hypothyroidism, hyperthyroidism, myasthenia gravis, juvenile-onset diabetes mellitus, juvenile rheumatoid arthritis, sicca syndrome, pernicious anemia, autoimmune hemolytic anemia, idiopathic thrombocytopenia purpura, and mucocutaneous candidiasis.[510-512] On gross examination, the ovaries are usually of normal size. On histologic examination, inflammatory cells infiltrate the theca cell layer (Fig. 68-74).

Nonneoplastic lesions

Epithelial inclusion cysts

Surface epithelial inclusion cysts arise from cortical invaginations of surface epithelium that have lost their connection with the surface perhaps as the result of contraction after ovulation. They are most numerous in postmenopausal women and may measure up to 1 cm in diameter, but most are incidental, microscopic findings, scattered singly or in clusters throughout the superficial cortex. They are typically lined by a single layer of columnar epithelium, which may be ciliated; psammoma bodies may be present. Less commonly their lining is a single layer of endometrioid or endocervical type of epithelium.[513] Occasionally in adults and typically in fetal and premenarchal ovaries, the cysts have a flat, cuboidal, or columnar lining. The occasional finding of dysplastic epithelium lining the cysts supports the hypothesis that surface epithelial carcinomas may arise from them.[514]

Solitary cysts of follicular origin

Solitary follicle cysts are particularly common after the menarche and in the perimenopausal period.[515-517] *Corpus luteum cysts* occur during the reproductive age. *Follicle cysts* may be incidental findings or manifestations related to increased estrogen production such as isosexual precocity,[518] menstrual disturbances[519] or endometrial hyperplasia.[516] An uncommon presen-

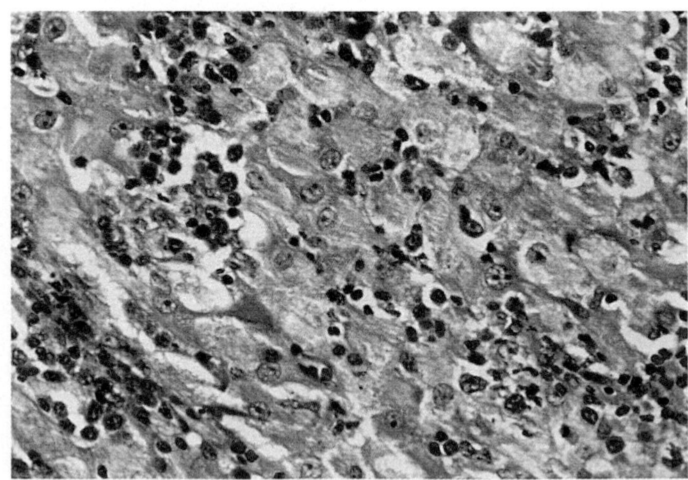

Fig. 68-74 Autoimmune oophoritis. Ovarian follicle is infiltrated by lymphocytes and plasma cells.

tation of both types of cyst is rupture with hemoperitoneum. A corpus luteum cyst arising in residual ovarian tissue is the most frequent finding in the ovarian remnant syndrome.

Most follicle cysts result from gonadotropin stimulation. Isosexual pseudoprecocity caused by autonomous follicle cysts may regress spontaneously and may also be reversed by removal of the cyst.[520] Autonomous cysts may be single or multiple and in the McCune-Albright syndrome[521] may be accompanied by corpora lutea and a potential for pregnancy.

A rare type of solitary follicle cyst, the *large solitary luteinized follicle cyst of pregnancy and the puerperium,* is presumably related to hCG stimulation.[522] The patients present with a palpable adnexal mass or with a unilateral ovarian cyst discovered at cesarean section. None had clinical evidence of an endocrine disturbance.[522]

Follicle cysts and corpus luteum cysts are unilocular, smooth surfaced, and thin walled and rarely exceed 8 cm in diameter. The wall of corpus luteum cyst is usually yellow and convoluted. The large luteinized cyst of pregnancy, however, has a median diameter of 25 cm. On microscopic examination, follicle cysts are lined by an inner layer of granulosa cells and an outer layer of theca internal cells. Distinction between the two layers can be facilitated by a reticulin stain that reveals a dense network in the theca cell layer but sparse or absent reticulum in the granulosa cell layer.

The large solitary luteinized cyst of pregnancy appears lined by large luteinized cells that typically exhibit pronounced nuclear pleomorphism and hyperchromatism. The corpus luteum cyst of pregnancy contains hyaline bodies and foci of calcification.

Polycystic ovarian disease, stromal hyperplasia, and stromal hyperthecosis

Physiopathologic studies have shown that polycystic ovarian disease, stromal hyperplasia, and stromal hyperthecosis, which may be associated with evidence of androgen excess, estrogenic manifestations, or both, are part of a continuum and that clear-cut distinctions cannot always be made among them.

Polycystic ovarian disease (PCOD) occurs in approximately 3.5% to 7% of the female population.[523] The pathogenetic and endocrinologic features of the disease are complex.[524,525] Theoretically, increased secretion of LH stimulates the theca lutein cells of the follicles, resulting in excessive production of androgens (androstenedione), which is subsequently converted to estrone. It is believed that the ovarian and hormonal changes are secondary to asynchronous release of LH by the pituitary caused by hypothalamic dysfunction.

The patients typically present in their third decade with a history of oligomenorrhea (rarely primary amenorrhea), infertility, and hirsutism; frank virilization is rare. The ovaries may be palpably enlarged. The endometrium may be hypoactive and proliferative, or may contain a well-differentiated adenocarcinoma.[526,527] Typically, the ovaries have a white surface, with cysts less than 1 cm in diameter visible just below the surface Fig. (68-75). The central portion of the ovary is composed of stroma without corpora lutea or corpora albicantia.[528]

Microscopically the ovarian cortex resembles a fibrous capsule. The cystic follicles have an inner lining of nonluteinized granulosa cells and a prominent outer layer of luteinized theca interna cells (follicular hyperthecosis).[523,529] Primordial follicles are normal in number and appearance.[529] Although corpora lutea are typically absent, they have been described in up

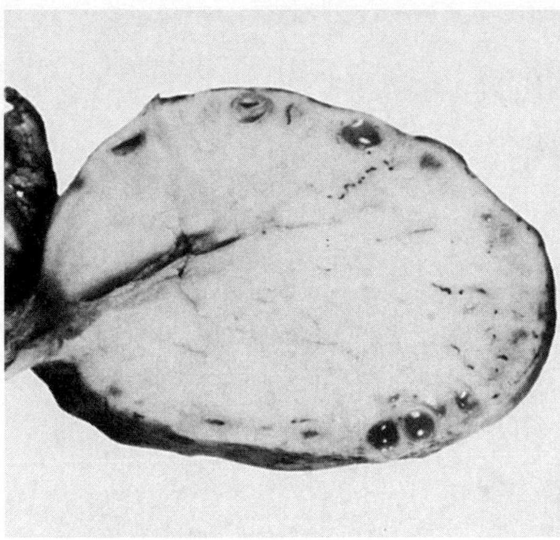

Fig. 68-75 Enlarged ovary from young woman with polycystic ovary (Stein-Leventhal) syndrome. Notice abundant central stroma and peripheral subcapsular follicles.

to 30% of otherwise typical cases of PCOD.[528,529] The deeper cortical and medullary stroma is often hyperplastic and may exhibit hyperthecosis.

PCOD is currently managed medically by regulation of the menstrual cycle or induction of ovulation.

The amount of ovarian stroma varies and may be abundant at the menopause and thereafter. Stromal hyperthecosis refers to the presence within the ovarian stroma, almost always a hyperplastic stroma, of luteinized stromal cells. *Stromal hyperplasia* is most common in patients in the sixth and seventh decades.[530] It may be associated with androgen hypersecretion as well as obesity, hypertension, and disorders of glucose metabolism.[530] An association with endometrial adenocarcinoma has been described.[531] Androgen production by nonluteinized ovarian stromal cells is consistent with their content of oxidative enzymes, the so-called enzymatically active stromal cells.[532]

Stromal hyperthecosis usually occurs in patients in the sixth to ninth decades.[530] Younger patients may present with noticeable virilization, obesity, hypertension, and decreased glucose tolerance.[533] Stromal hyperthecosis (or occasionally, PCOD) typically accompanies the *HAIR-AN syndrome,* which encompasses hyperandrogenism (HA), insulin resistance (IR), and acanthosis nigricans (AN).[534] As in cases of PCOD, estrogenic manifestations such as endometrial hyperplasia or carcinoma may be present.[533,535] The disorder may be familial.[536]

Both stromal hyperplasia and hyperthecosis produce bilateral ovarian enlargement, with each gonad measuring up to 8 cm in diameter, and thus may simulate an ovarian tumor. The cut surface is homogeneous, firm, and white to yellow.[537]

On microscopic examination, both the cortical and the medullary stroma may be hyperplastic. In hyperthecosis, luteinized stromal cells appear singly, in small clusters, or in nodules (Fig. 68-76).

Massive edema and fibromatosis

Massive enlargement of one or both ovaries secondary to an accumulation of edema fluid within the ovarian stroma is referred to as "massive ovarian edema;[538] approximately 50 cases of this disorder have been reported.[539] A lesion desig-

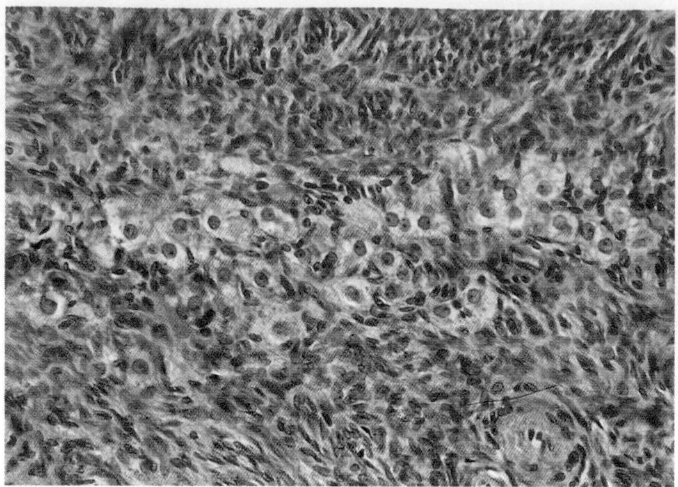

Fig. 68-76 Stromal hyperthecosis of ovary. Nests of luteinized stromal cells.

nated *ovarian fibromatosis* has clinical and pathologic features that overlap with those of massive edema, indicating a probable relationship between the two entities.[539] The patients have ranged in age from 6 to 33 years, with an average of 21 years. Three fourths of them have presented with abdominal or pelvic pain, menstrual irregularities, evidence of androgen excess, or both. Pelvic examination typically reveals a palpable adnexal mass. At operation the ovarian enlargement (5 to 35 cm) is unilateral in about 90% of the cases. Partial or complete torsion of the involved ovary has been present in at least half the cases. The involved ovary has a shiny, white, smooth surface and a tan, homogeneous cut surface exuding watery fluid. The presence of cystic follicles and corpora lutea within the edematous tissue is strongly suggestive of the diagnosis of massive edema. The striking microscopic finding is diffuse stromal edema that spares the fibrotic cortex. In approximately 40% of cases, luteinized stromal cells are present. Associated findings include vascular and lymphatic dilatation.

Ovarian fibromatosis is also usually unilateral, and in 15% of the cases the involved ovaries have undergone torsion.[539]

The ovaries, 6 to 12 cm in diameter, exhibit firm, white, and solid surfaces. Microscopic examination reveals bundles of spindle cells producing variable amounts of collagen, with a focal storiform pattern and bands of dense collagen.[539] The process typically surrounds normal follicular structures. Foci of stromal edema are present in approximately half the cases.

Endometriosis

Ectopic endometrium in the ovary is troublesome because it forms fibrous adhesions and hemorrhagic cysts, which are painful and a cause of infertility. Accumulated hemorrhage results from stromal breakdown at the time of menstrual bleeding. Cysts may become large and typically are filled with semisolid, dark brown, altered blood. Endometrial tissue usually can be found somewhere in the fibrous wall, but a search may be necessary. Smaller foci of hemorrhage organize and contract, leaving a characteristic puckered scar tinged yellow-brown with hemosiderin (Fig. 68-77). The pathogenesis has been debated. Implants from a reflux of menstrual blood have been shown to occur. Serosal metaplasia is another possibility and almost certainly has been the cause in some cases.

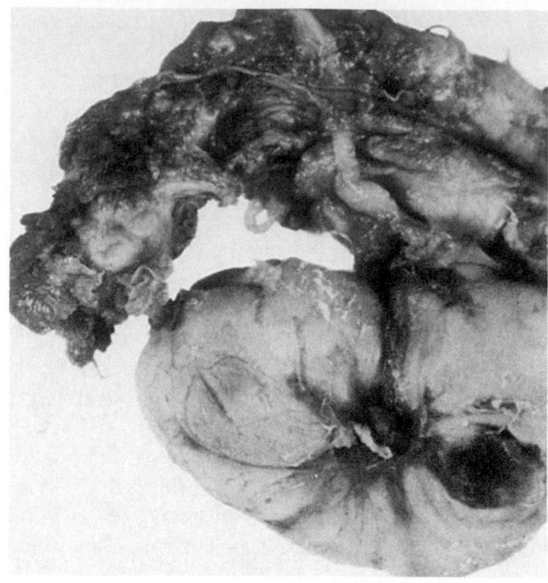

Fig. 68-77 Ovarian endometriosis forming characteristic puckered hemorrhagic scar and extensive tubal adhesions.

Pregnancy-related lesions

Pregnancy luteoma

The pregnancy luteoma is likely related to hCG stimulation. Most patients have been in their third or fourth decades, black, and multiparous. The lesion is usually discovered incidentally during cesarean section or postpartum tubal ligation. In approximately 25% of the cases there is hirsutism or virilization; two thirds of female infants born to virilized mothers are also virilized.[540] Regression of the enlarged ovaries usually begins within days after delivery, and they become normal in size within several weeks.

The lesions range from small nodules to masses up to 20 cm in diameter, with soft, brown cut surfaces. They may be bilateral or multiple.

The cells resemble luteinized granulosa cells, mitotic figures range up to 7 per 10 HPF, and occasional atypical forms may be seen[541] (Fig. 68-78, *A*). Ultrastructural examination has shown the characteristic features of steroid-producing cells.[542] Postpartum examination of the lesions reveals lipid accumulation in the cells, round cell infiltration, and fibrosis[543] (Fig. 68-78, *B*). This lesion should be distinguished from metastatic carcinoma, especially a Krukenberg tumor.

Hyperreactio luteinalis. Hyperreactio luteinalis is characterized by multiple bilateral luteinized follicle cysts and is most commonly associated with disorders of pregnancy in which there are high levels of circulating hCG, such as hydatidiform moles, choriocarcinoma, fetal hydrops, and multiple gestations,[544-546] but has also been reported during otherwise uncomplicated pregnancies.[545] Hyperreactio luteinalis typically regresses in the postpartum period but may persist for up to 6 months. An iatrogenic form of hyperreactio luteinalis, the *ovarian hyperstimulation syndrome,* develops in women undergoing ovulation induction, typically with FSH followed by hCG, or less often with Clomid alone.[547,548] Patients with this disorder may also have ascites and occasionally hydrothorax of acute onset (acute Meigs' syndrome).

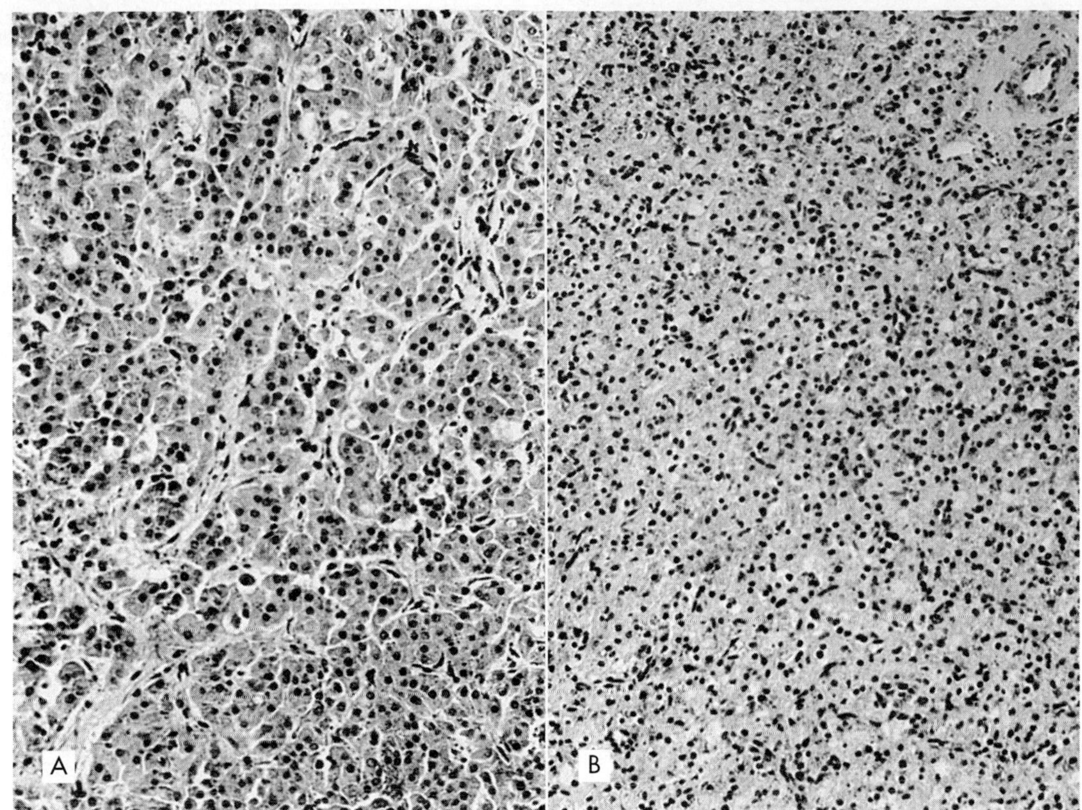

Fig. 68-78 **A,** Pregnancy luteoma composed of large luteinized stroma cells occurred as multiple red-brown nodules, identified at cesarean section. Female infant was temporarily masculinized. **B,** Section from ill-defined yellow area in opposite ovary 2 months later. (Courtesy Drs. LR Malmak and George V. Miller).

Hilum cell hyperplasia

Hilum cell hyperplasia may be seen during pregnancy as a result of hCG administration and in postmenopausal women in whom the process is presumably related to elevated pituitary gonadotropins.[530] Androgenic and estrogenic manifestations have been reported.[549] Multiple, yellow, hilar nodules, usually less than 2 mm in diameter may be seen.[541]

Decidual reaction

An ovarian decidual reaction is usually a response of the stromal cells to high circulating or local levels of estrogen and progesterone.[530] The process is seen most commonly during pregnancy, occurring as early as the ninth week of gestation, and is present in almost all ovaries at term.[550,551] Less often it is associated with trophoblastic disease or occurs in patients treated with progestins. Most frequently, the decidual foci are incidental findings on microscopic examination. Florid examples can simulate metastatic carcinoma, particularly if the decidual cells show focal cytologic atypia.

Ovarian changes secondary to cytotoxic drugs and radiation

Cytotoxic drugs may be associated with a variety of histologic changes in the ovary. These include a reduction or depletion of follicles, impaired follicular maturation, and focal or diffuse cortical fibrosis.[552] In occasional cases, the ovarian failure may be reversible after the cessation of the therapy.

The ovary is among the most radiosensitive of organs, and ovarian failure occurs in the majority of patients who receive pelvic irradiation.[552] Relatively low doses of irradiation (500 to 600 roentgens) to the ovaries are associated with complete or nearly complete disappearance of primordial and developing follicles, fibrosis of the ovarian stroma, and vascular sclerosis in over 90% of patients. The ovarian stroma appears to be more radioresistant than the follicles and may continue to secrete androgens after irradiation.

Neoplasms

Ovarian cancer is the fifth most common malignant tumor among women in the United States, with an annual incidence of 22,000 new cases.[553] It affects predominantly postmenopausal women and is responsible for about 13,300 deaths per year. This high mortality is attributed to the lack of symptoms in most patients with early stages of disease. In approximately 70% of the patients the tumor has spread outside of the pelvis at the time of presentation. Extensive surgery is often insufficient to eliminate the intraabdominal tumor, and response to chemotherapy is only partial in many of these patients.[554]

Etiology and pathogenesis. The malignant transformation of the ovarian surface epithelium has been explained by the incessant ovulation theory, according to which ovulation disrupts the surface epithelium and is followed by reparative proliferation. The newly formed epithelial cells are capable of proliferating in response to additional trauma caused by subsequent ovulations. Continuous reparation may trigger mutations and activation of oncogens or elimination of tumor-suppressor genes.[555]

The epidemiologic data supporting this theory include the increased risk (1.5 to 3.2) associated with nulliparity, the decreased risk in women using oral contraceptives (0.4 to 0.7), and the increased incidence of ovarian cancer in patients who have received drugs that induce ovulation but have not become pregnant.[556]

Most ovarian carcinomas apparently arise from epithelial inclusion cysts that result from downgrowth of the surface epithelium after repair. It has also been postulated that elevated gonadotropin levels may contribute to malignant transformation. Oral contraceptives cause a reduction in pituitary gonadotropins.[557]

The principal risk factor, however, is a family history of ovarian cancer, particularly when two or more first-degree relatives have been affected.[558] Three hereditary familial ovarian cancer syndromes have been described: the ovary-specific syndrome, the breast-ovary syndrome, and the Lynch II syndrome, in which cancer may develop in the ovary, endometrium, and colon (in the absence of polyposis coli). Familial ovarian cancer accounts for 5% to 10% of the total. The gene responsible for the breast-ovary syndrome (BRCA 1) is located in the long arm of chromosome 17 at locus 17q12-q23.[559]

From a histogenetic viewpoint, ovarian cancer may develop de novo or may arise from preexisting benign epithelial tumors.[560] In favor of the latter hypothesis is (1) the higher average age of the patients with carcinomas (approximately 12 years) as compared with that of patients with benign epithelial tumors;[514] (2) the finding of a benign epithelial component in a high number of ovarian carcinomas, specially mucinous carcinomas, which often exhibit focal, abrupt transition from benign to malignant epithelium.[514]

The role of oncogens and tumor-suppressor genes in ovarian carcinogenesis is not well known.[561,562] Amplification or overexpression of c-*erb*-B-2 has been found in approximately 30% of ovarian cancers and correlate with low survival.[563,564] *ras* mutations are frequent in mucinous ovarian tumors.[565-567] About 50% to 80% of ovarian carcinomas show overexpression of the tumor-suppressor gene p53, which correlates with aneuploidy, high grade, advanced stage, and unfavorable prognosis.[568-570]

Determinations of the serum tumor marker CA-125 and pelvic ultrasonography are highly specific screening methods.

Classification

Because of their remarkable diversity, ovarian tumors may be bewildering. Natural history and response to treatment vary considerably from one tumor group to another. The best therapeutic approach including chemotherapy and radiotherapy may be highly specific for a single type of neoplasm; accordingly, accurate histologic diagnosis is often a critical factor in achieving an optimum treatment response.

The histogenetic classification in Table 68-6 is a simplified version of the one proposed by the ISGYP in 1993 and subsequently accepted by the WHO.[356]

The relative frequency with which different types of ovarian neoplasms occur is summarized in Table 68-7. The proportions indicated are approximate and represent a synthesis of numerous reports.

Table 68-6 WHO classification of ovarian tumors

1. **Surface epithelial-stromal tumors**
   - Serous tumors
     - Benign (cystadenoma)
     - Of borderline malignancy
     - Malignant (serous cystadenocarcinoma)
   - Mucinous tumors, endocervical-type and intestinal-type
     - Benign
     - Of borderline malignancy
     - Malignant
   - Endometrioid tumors
     - Benign
     - Of borderline malignancy
     - Malignant
     - Epithelial-stromal
       - Adenosarcoma
       - Mesodermal (müllerian) mixed tumor
   - Clear cell tumors
     - Benign
     - Of borderline malignancy
     - Malignant
   - Transitional cell tumors
     - Brenner tumor
     - Brenner tumor of borderline malignancy
     - Malignant Brenner tumor
     - Transitional cell carcinoma (non-Brenner-type)
   - Undifferentiated carcinoma
2. **Sex cord–stromal tumors**
   - Granulosa-stromal cell tumors
     - Granulosa cell tumors
     - Tumors of the thecoma-fibroma group
   - Sertoli-stromal cell tumors (androblastomas)
   - Sex-cord tumor with annular tubules
   - Gynandroblastoma
   - Steroid (lipid) cell tumors
3. **Germ cell tumors**
   - Dysgerminoma
   - Yolk sac tumor (endodermal sinus tumor)
   - Teratoma
     - Immature
     - Mature (adult)
     - Solid
     - Cystic (dermoid cyst)
   - Monodermal (e.g., struma ovarii, carcinoid)
   - Mixed germ cell tumors
4. **Gonadoblastoma**
5. **Tumors not specific to ovary**
6. **Unclassified**
7. **Metastatic tumors**

Certain clinical or gross features may provide important diagnostic clues. One of the most important clinical features is the age of the patient. For example, within the surface epithelial category, borderline tumors are seen often in women in their thirties and less frequently in younger women, whereas invasive tumors in this category are rare in women under 40 years of age. On the other hand, germ cell tumors are almost never found in women over 50 years of age.

The stage and laterality of ovarian tumors also indicate their nature. For example, tumors in the sex cord–stromal category are almost always confined to a single ovary. On the other hand, approximately 65% of the metastatic tumors are bilateral.

Table 68-7 General classification of primary ovarian neoplasms

Cell of origin (representative tumor types)	Relative proportion, all ovarian neoplasms (%)*	Relative proportion, malignant neoplasms only (%)
Surface epithelium (serous, mucinous, endometrioid, clear cell, etc.)	65	94
Germ cells (dysgerminoma, cystic teratoma, etc.)	20	1
Stromal cells (sex cords) (granulosa-theca cells, Sertoli-Leydig cells, steroid cells, fibroma, etc.)	12	2
Tumors in dysgenetic gonads (gonadoblastoma)	1	—
Unclassified (chiefly undifferentiated carcinoma)	2	3

*The relative proportion of figures noted here represents an approximation.

Surface epithelial-stromal tumors (common epithelial tumors)

Surface epithelial tumors form the most common group of ovarian neoplasms and include the majority (90%) of ovarian carcinomas (Table 68-7). They originate from the celomic mesothelium that covers the ovary, which, after neoplastic transformation, seems to retain the capacity to recapitulate the epithelial components of the müllerian ducts. For example, the epithelium of serous tumors resembles that lining the tube, whereas the cells that line mucinous cystadenomas resemble those of the endocervical mucosa. These tumors usually have a prominent cystic component with single or multiple loculations, a variable amount of fibrous stroma, and an epithelial lining that often is thrown into papillary tufts.

On the basis of histologic features and clinical behavior, these tumors are divided into benign, borderline (low malignant potential, LMP), and malignant categories. Benign cystic tumors are lined by a single layer of well-oriented columnar epithelial cells; papillary projections, if present, are supported by fibrovascular stromal stalks and covered by the same type of epithelium (Fig. 68-79). Obviously malignant tumors have an anaplastic epithelial component that invades the underlying stroma in addition to forming the epithelial lining. The epithelial cells are usually several layers thick and have anaplastic nuclei, with a loss of polarity. The prognosis is poor; about 15% of patients survive 5 years.

Tumors in the borderline (LMP) category are characterized by epithelial proliferation greater than that seen in benign tumors of the same cell type but an absence of "destructive" invasion of the stroma.[571-578] Despite their lack of an invasive potential within the ovary, these tumors can implant on peritoneal surfaces, and the implants often invade the underlying tissue; rarely, these tumors spread through the lymphatics and, exceptionally, through blood vessels. The diagnosis, however, is based on pathologic examination of the primary ovarian tumor itself without knowledge of whether spread beyond the ovary has taken place.

Although the behavior of borderline tumors is unpredictable in individual cases, as a group they have a much better prognosis than their malignant counterparts. Approximately 70% are stage I, with spread within the pelvis (stage II) or upper abdomen (stage III) being present in the remainder. One third of the tumors are bilateral.

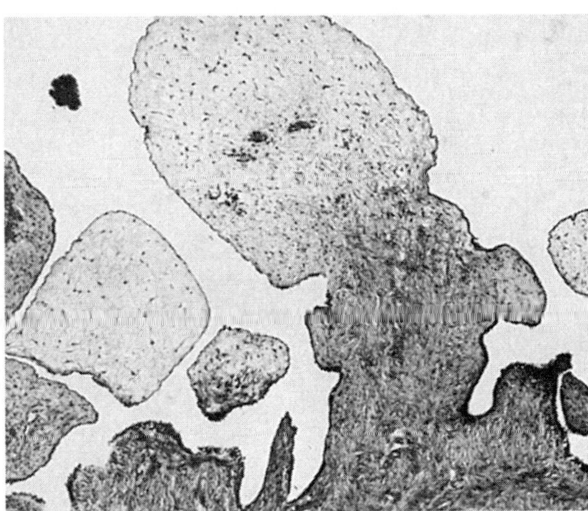

Fig. 68-79 Benign papillary serous tumor, with abundant fibrous stroma covered by single layer of stromal flattened epithelial cells.

The 5-year survival for borderline and malignant tumors confined to the ovary is 100% and 70%, whereas the 5-year survival for the same tumors involving the peritoneum is approximately 90% and 25%, respectively. Recurrences of borderline tumors typically appear after several years, if at all; the minority of tumors that have a malignant course tend to progress slowly.

Borderline tumors are best treated by removal of the uterus and adnexa as well as by use of indicated biopsies for complete staging. However, in young women with stage I tumors, unilateral adnexectomy may be acceptable. The risk that another tumor will develop in a normal-appearing ovary in these circumstances is about 15% in a 5- to 7-year period.[579] Furthermore, the tumors that do recur consistently maintain their borderline clinical and pathologic characteristics, including an excellent prognosis.

Various tumor-associated antigens may circulate in the blood of women with borderline and malignant tumors of common epithelial type. CA-125 antigen is most commonly associated with serous and endometrioid tumors; mucinous tumors often produce CEA, as colon cancers do. Monitoring the appropriate antigen titers is very useful in identification of occult metastases,[580] monitoring of therapeutic response,[581] and detection of asymptomatic recurrence at an early stage.

Serous tumors. Benign serous cysts and cystadenomas may form single or multiple loculations, lined by low columnar epithelium, which is sometimes ciliated and resembles tubal epithelium (Fig. 68-79). The cyst fluid is watery or viscous and contains a variety of mucins; however, the epithelial cells that secrete the fluid do not have the characteristic vacuolated appearance of mucinous epithelium. Papillary processes are common and may be complex. The epithelial component of serous tumors, unlike other neoplasms of surface epithelium, may appear on the external surfaces. It is common to find tiny round laminated calcific concretions called *psammoma bodies* in the stroma of the papillary processes. Papillary and cystic tumors with a prominent or abundant fibrous stromal component are designated "papillary adenofibromas and cystadenofibromas." Borderline serous tumors are often multilocular and have a more complex papillary pattern (Fig. 68-80); fine papillae, closely packed, may resemble solid epithelial proliferation. Variable degrees of cell stratification, nuclear atypia, and mitotic activity are present (Fig. 68-81).

Otherwise typical serous borderline tumors may contain foci of *microinvasion*.[582,583] Such tumors have a prognosis similar to that of serous borderline tumors without this feature, and conservation of the contralateral ovary and uterus may be acceptable.

Serous borderline tumors are associated in from about 30% of the cases with *peritoneal implants*, which may vary greatly in their histologic appearance.[577,584] It should be remembered that in these cases the designation of the tumor depends on the appearance of the primary neoplasm. The peritoneal implants have been classified into noninvasive and invasive categories, with the former being further subdivided into epithelial and desmoplastic subtypes.[585] In the epithelial subtype of noninvasive implant, papillary proliferations of atypical serous cells are present on the surface of the peritoneum (Fig. 68-82). In contrast, the desmoplastic subtype of noninvasive implant, is characterized by a predominant stromal reaction to the tumor,

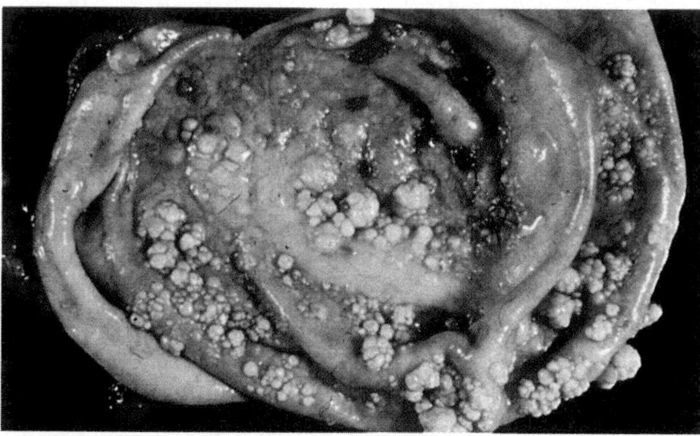

Fig. 68-80 Borderline serous tumor of ovary. The inside of the cyst is studded with papillary epithelial masses.

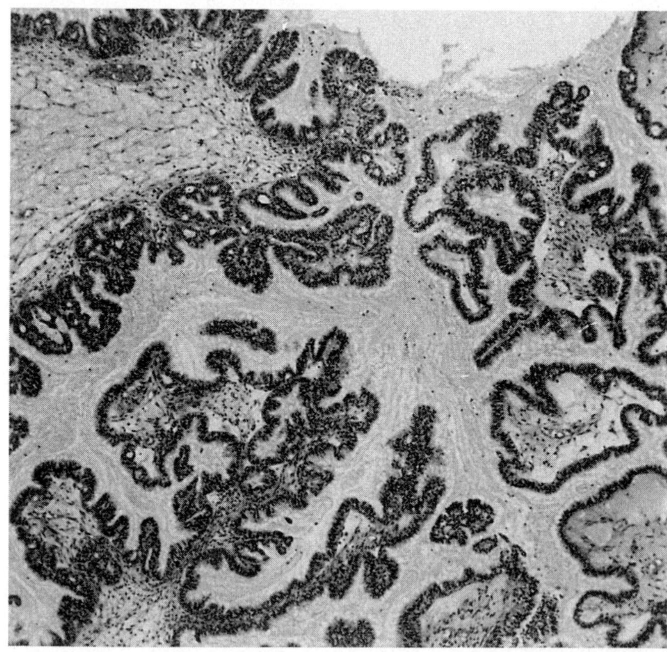

Fig. 68-81 Serous borderline tumor of ovary. Prominent papillary epithelial proliferation without destructive stromal invasion. (From de Nictolis M et al: *Cancer* 70:152, 1992.)

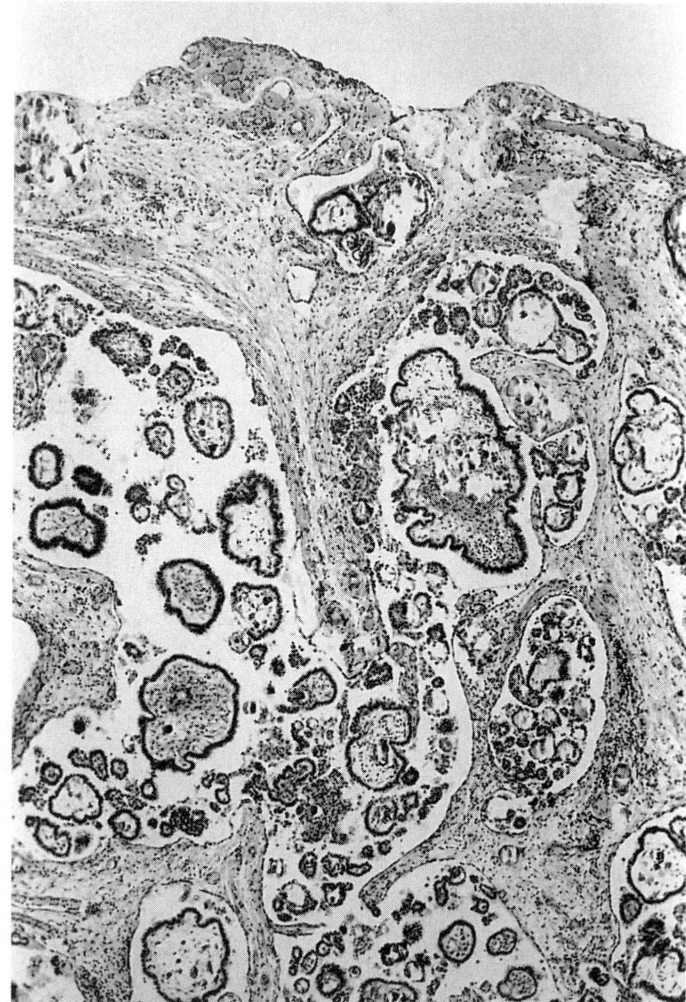

Fig. 68-82 Omental implant of serous borderline tumor of noninvasive epithelial type. Papillae fill submesothelial invaginations. (From de Nictolis M et al: *Cancer* 70:152, 1992.)

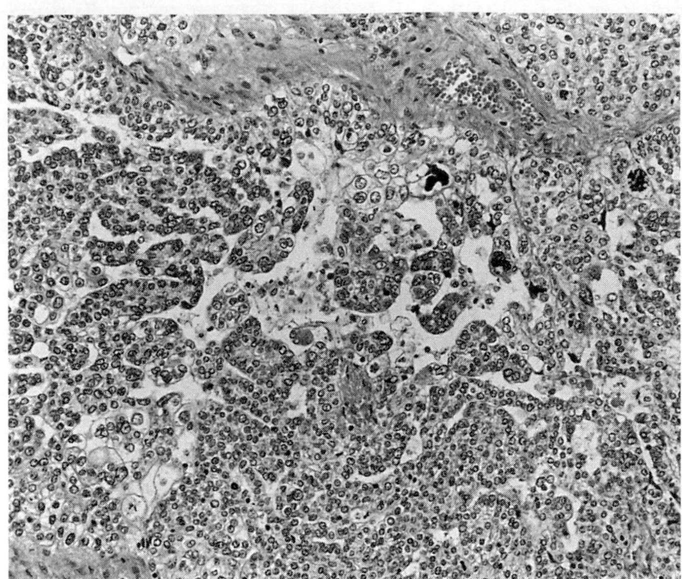

Fig. 68-83 Serous carcinoma of ovary showing typical papillary architecture with scattered large anaplastic cells.

which is layered upon serosal surfaces. Invasive implants are characterized by an irregular infiltration of a normal tissue, such as the omentum. They resemble histologically a serous adenocarcinoma (Fig. 68-83); pronounced cytologic atypia may be present. Three recent studies have shown that the presence of invasion in implants is strongly related to progression of the disease.[577,584,585] Aneuploidy of the invasive implants seems to have an unfavorable prognostic significance.[577]

Tumors with a morphology identical to that of serous borderline tumors may arise as *primary neoplasm of the peritoneum* with no, or only minimal, involvement of the ovarian surfaces.[586] A tumor that shares many features with the serous borderline tumor is the rare *serous psammocarcinoma*.[587] This diagnosis is made when the following microscopic features are present: (1) destructive invasion of ovarian stroma or vascular space invasion, or deep invasion of intraperitoneal viscera; (2) no more than moderate nuclear atypia; (3) no significant solid epithelial proliferation; (4) at least 75% of the papillae or nests are associated with or completely replaced by psammoma bodies. The clinical behavior of these tumors more closely resembled that of a borderline serous tumor than that of a serous carcinoma.

Mucinous tumors. Mucinous tumors are typically large unilocular or multilocular cystic masses. The epithelium that lines the cysts is composed of tall columnar cells with basal nuclei and prominent mucin vacuoles; it may resemble endocervical mucosa *(endocervical type)*. Most frequently, the epithelium appears like intestinal epithelium, including goblet cells, argentaffin cells argyrophil cells and even Paneth's cells *(intestinal type)*. Mucinous intestinal tumor may occasionally produce enough gastrin to cause the Zollinger-Ellison syndrome.[588-590] Since about 5% of mucinous tumors are associated with cystic teratomas, it has been suggested that some, at least, originate from germ cells; an intestinal metaplasia of these exotic cell types seems more likely.[591] A larger number, however, may have endometrioid or serous elements, the presence of which supports their classification with surface epithelial tumors.

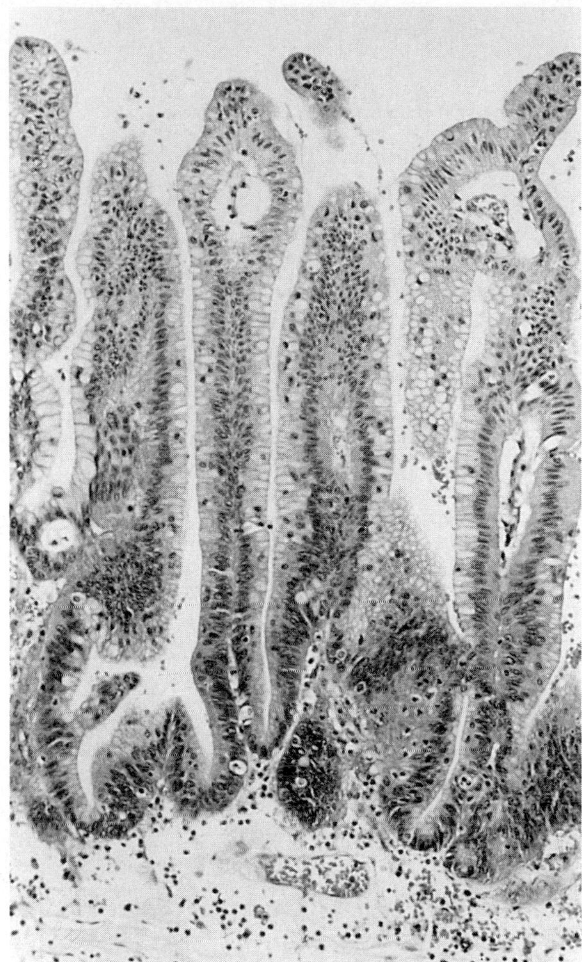

Fig. 68-84 Intestinal mucinous borderline tumor with slender papillae and short glands. It resembles intestinal mucosa. (From de Nictolis M et al: *Int J Gynecol Pathol* 13:10, 1994.)

Mucinous borderline tumors are almost as common as serous borderline tumors and account for 40% to 50% of all mucinous malignant tumors[592] and for 71% of those that are in stage I.[571] Approximately 85% of the cases are of the intestinal type.[593]

It is often difficult to decide whether a mucinous tumor is a borderline or a low-grade carcinoma. The main reason for this is the difficulty of determining stromal invasion in many cases of carcinoma, since the stroma, instead of being desmoplastic, may resemble ovarian stroma and is often luteinized. The criteria for the diagnosis of carcinoma include height of four or more epithelial cells,[593] fingerlike projections of solid cellular masses without connective tissue supports (Fig. 68-84) or cribriform pattern[571] (Fig. 68-85). Other investigators rely mostly on the nuclear features of the tumor cells.[592] Recently, separation of intestinal mucinous borderline tumors from well-differentiated carcinomas has been achieved by quantitative nuclear morphologic analysis.[594]

Extraovarian spread of the intestinal-mucinous borderline tumors typically appears as mucinous ascites ("pseudomyxoma peritonei"). Patients with an ovarian borderline mucinous tumor and pseudomyxoma peritonei often prove to have a similar tumor of the appendix.[595] The synchronous presentation, the histologic similarity, the frequency of bilaterality of the

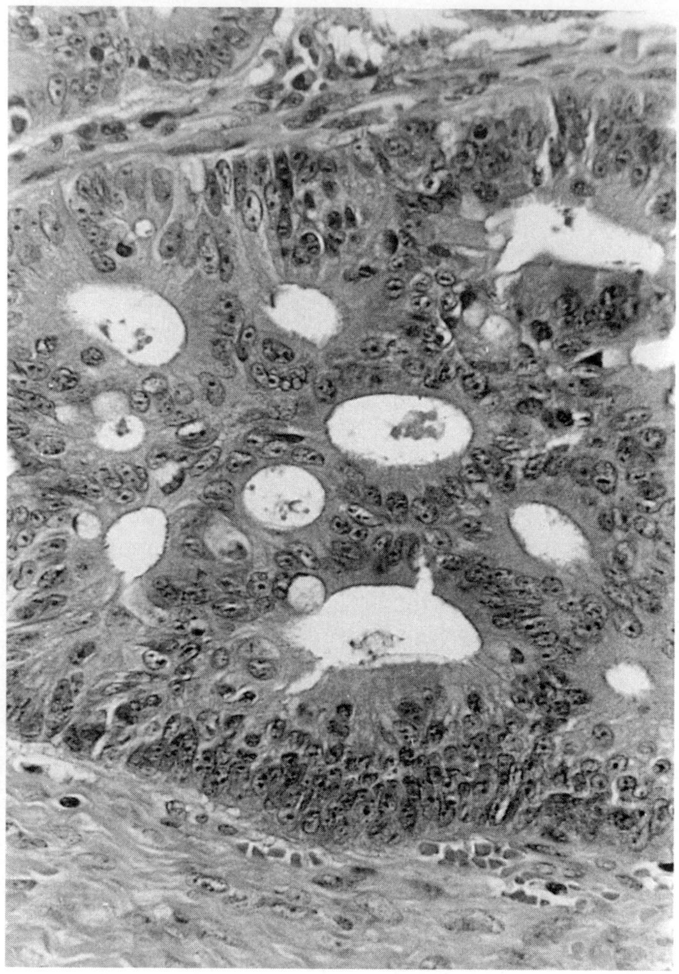

Fig. 68-85 Well-differentiated intestinal mucinous carcinoma without obvious invasion but exhibiting cribriform pattern.

ovarian tumors, and the predominance of right-sided ovarian involvement, point toward the probable metastatic nature of the ovarian tumors in such cases.[595]

Borderline mucinous tumors of endocervical type have a distinctly better prognosis than the more common mucinous tumors of intestinal type, even in the presence of extraovarian spread.[596] They are frequently associated with endometriosis.[596]

Mucinous cystic tumors, benign, borderline or carcinomas, may contain one or more solid mural nodules composed occasionally of anaplastic carcinomas,[597] rarely of sarcoma,[598] and more often of a sarcoma-like proliferation that has been associated with an uneventful follow-up study in all cases.[599-601]

Endometrioid tumors. Endometrioid carcinomas are so named because the histologic pattern closely resembles that of uterine endometrial adenocarcinomas. The distinction is most easily made in well-differentiated carcinomas. Less-differentiated lesions may have a typical endometrioid appearance only in focal areas or foci of squamous metaplasia as the only clues to their identity. They probably constitute between 15% and 20% of ovarian cancers. The benign counterpart is probably represented by cystic endometriosis of the ovary. Criteria for the diagnosis of a borderline endometrioid tumor are controversial,[602-604] though such lesions are rare.

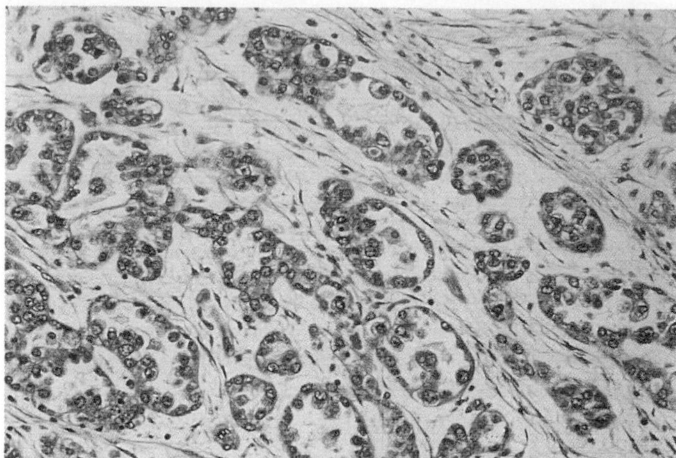

Fig. 68-86 Clear cell adenocarcinoma. Tubulocystic pattern is identical to that found in clear cell carcinomas of vagina, cervix, and endometrium.

Endometrioid carcinomas are often partly cystic with prominent solid areas; the cyst fluid is brown or bloody. Association with endometriosis is demonstrable in about one third of the cases, but its presence is not required for the diagnosis. Endometriosis is even more frequently encountered together with clear cell tumors. Unusual histologic appearances of endometrioid carcinomas that may cause confusion with sex cord–stromal tumors have been described.[605,606] Distinguishing endometrioid carcinoma from an occasional metastatic adenocarcinoma from the large intestine may be difficult.[607]

The prognosis for well-differentiated carcinomas is good; about 60% of patients survive for 5 years, compared to 23% survival for poorly differentiated carcinomas.

In about one third of the patients there is a coexistent adenocarcinoma of the endometrium. It is generally accepted that both lesions are separate primary cancers because the survival rate in the presence of endometrial involvement is not appreciably lower.[608] Furthermore, both the absence of extragenital tumor and the presence of endometrial hyperplasia favor a multifocal process. In contrast, simultaneous uterine and ovarian involvement by common epithelial carcinomas of other types such as papillary serous or clear cell carcinomas is usually associated with a poor prognosis.[608] In some cases, DNA flow cytometry may help distinguishing metastatic from synchronous tumors.[417]

Other endometrioid neoplasms such as stromal sarcoma,[609,610] malignant mixed müllerian tumor,[611] and adenosarcoma[612] have been reported rarely as primary tumors of the ovary. The histologic features and prognosis do not differ significantly from those of similar lesions occurring in the endometrium.

Clear cell tumors. The gross appearance of clear cell tumors is often a combination of solid and cystic components much like that of endometrioid carcinoma. The cyst is usually unilocular, the fluid is commonly brown, and the solid areas form nodular masses that protrude into the lumen.

Microscopically these tumors are characterized by masses of large epithelial cells with abundant clear cytoplasm, supported by delicate hyalinized stroma. The cytoplasm contains abundant glycogen. The most common pattern, however, is that of small tubules and cysts lined by a single layer of large hobnail cells (Fig. 68-86); the cell nuclei are bulbous and protrude into the lumens of the tubules. Hyaline bodies are present in 25% of the cases.[613] The cytologic features, absence of lymphocytes, and lower or negative serum values of alpha-fetoprotein (AFP) help to distinguish clear cell carcinoma from dysgerminoma and yolk sac tumor.

Less than 10% of clear cell tumors are bilateral. Benign and borderline clear cell tumors occur rarely, mainly as adenofibromas. Association with endometriosis is six times as great as with ovarian carcinoma in general.[614] Clear cell carcinomas of the ovary and identical neoplasms of the endometrium, cervix, and vagina are closely related to tumors of müllerian origin, particularly endometrioid tumors.[615] Endometrioid and clear cell components may occur together in ovarian and endometrial carcinomas, and clear cell tumors have been shown to arise in patients with endometriosis.[615] Survival rates are in an intermediate range; 37% of the patients survive 5 years.

Transitional cell tumors. The recently recognized transitional cell carcinomas of the ovary can be divided into two groups: those that arose from a preexisting Brenner tumor and those that are surface epithelial origin.[616-618]

Brenner tumors account for 2% to 3% of all ovarian tumors,[619-621] and less than 2% of them are borderline (proliferative) or malignant.[621-625] Benign Brenner tumors are typically small and mostly solid; 10% to 25% appear as small, firm nodules in the wall of a mucinous cystadenoma. Borderline tumors are predominantly cystic with papillomatous masses protruding into the locules.

Microscopically the benign tumor is composed of round nests of epithelial cells lying within an abundant fibrous stroma (Fig. 68-87). The nests may be solid or have a central lumen that contains dense eosinophilic material or mucin. The tumor cells are polygonal and have clear cytoplasm and grooved nuclei. The cells lining the lumens often contain mucin. The stromal component may be focally hyalinized, and calcification is common.

The epithelial component of the borderline tumors resembles a grade I papillary carcinoma of the urinary bladder. No invasion of the stroma is observed, and a benign component is also found in most cases. In malignant Brenner tumors, the epithelial component has, at least in part, the typical features of higher grade transitional cell carcinoma or squamous cell carcinoma.

Transitional cell carcinoma of the ovary is rare;[616,618] it apparently responds much better to chemotherapy than most other surface epithelial carcinomas at all stages. A common problem is the distinction of these tumors from poorly differentiated carcinomas, which typically exhibit central necrosis.

Mixed forms. Surface epithelial tumors often include a combination of the foregoing types. Unless two or more components are prominent, the tumor is classified after the predominant cell type.

Undifferentiated carcinoma. About 3% to 6% of ovarian carcinomas are undifferentiated. Clinically they resemble serous carcinoma, and about 50% are bilateral. Most are stage III tumors at presentation.[626] Many are composed of small cells of nearly uniform size. Mitoses are numerous; nuclei are pleomorphic. Occasionally, undifferentiated carcinomas resemble superficially granulosa cell tumors. Because of the considerable differences in prognosis, an accurate histologic diagnosis is important.[614]

A distinctive type of undifferentiated carcinoma that is associated with hypercalcemia in approximately two thirds of the cases occurs predominantly in young women (average 22 years). It has been designated *small cell carcinoma.*[627,628] The histogenesis of this aggressive tumor remains unknown.[628,630] Hypercalcemia has been attributed to tumor production of parathyroid hormone–related substance.[631] All tumors have been diploid.

Extragenital tumors with müllerian histologic features. Neoplasms resembling any of the foregoing tumor types may develop in the peritoneal and retroperitoneal tissues of the female pelvis without involvement of the uterus, tubes, or ovaries. This versatile tissue has been referred to as the "secondary müllerian system."[632]

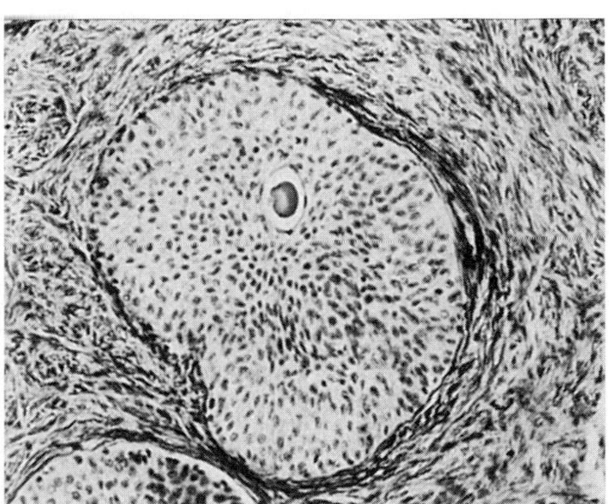

Fig. 68-87 Brenner tumor. Typical sharply circumscribed nest of uniform cytologically benign cells surrounded by dense fibrous stroma. (AFIP 305334-1-4-2.)

Sex cord-stromal tumors

The sex cord–stromal tumors arise from ovarian stromal cells specialized in steroid hormone production; they account for most functioning tumors with endocrine manifestations.[633] The designation of sex cord–stromal tumors is favored because the assumption that the embryonic sex cords and their derivatives are mesenchymal (stromal) derivatives (rather than celomic epithelium) remains unproved.

Granulosa cell tumors. Granulosa cell tumors are mostly estrogenic (75%), but rare cases, usually large cystic tumors, are associated with androgenic manifestations.[634,635] The tumors are cystic and solid and characteristically contain blood clots.

Granulosa cells have uniform, oval, rounded, or angulated pale nuclei, with a cleft in the nuclear membrane. Mitotic activity is not conspicuous. The cells are haphazardly distributed in masses with little intervening stroma. Characteristic rosette-like structures, or Call-Exner bodies, are almost always present (Fig. 68-88); they are rounded masses of eosinophilic material surrounded by a circular row of typical granulosa cells and resemble the normal graafian follicle. The nuclei tend to lie adjacent to the inner rim of the space.

A variety of microscopic patterns occur; microfollicular and macrofollicular tumors resemble clusters of small or large graafian follicles. The descriptive terms *trabecular*, *insular*, and *gyriform*, are often applied without significant clinical correlations. The diffuse, or "sarcomatoid," variety, char-

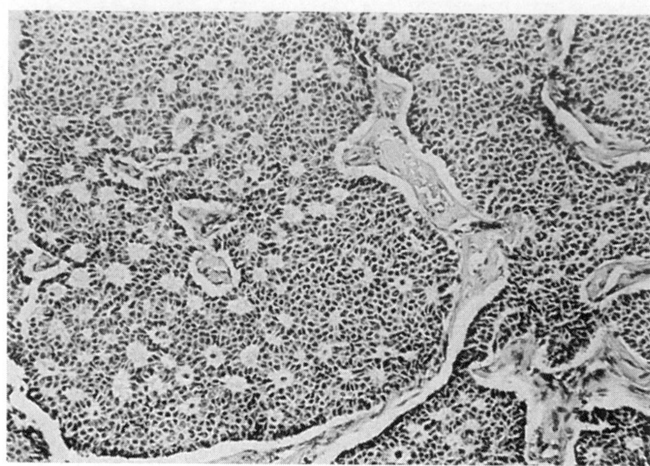

Fig. 68-88 Granulosa cell tumor. Many rounded spaces (Call-Exner bodies) containing amorphous eosinophilic material are scattered among uniform small cells with compressed-appearing nuclei. Strands of hyalinized stroma are a characteristic feature.

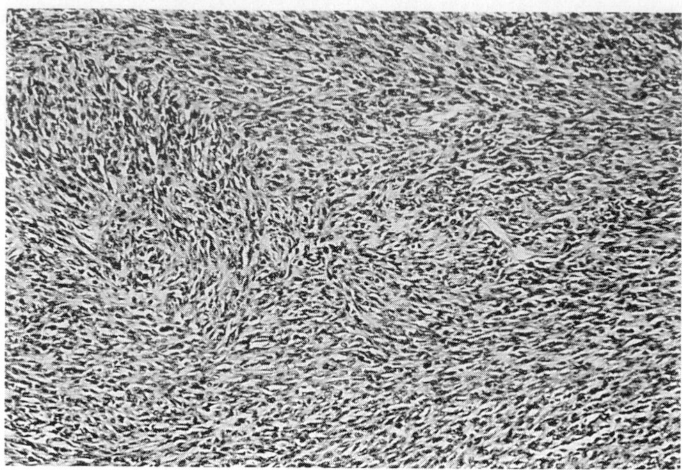

Fig. 68-90 Cellular fibroma of ovary. Mitotic index of less than 3 MF per 10 HPF, lack of nuclear atypia, and absence of adhesions help to separate this lesion from fibrosarcoma.

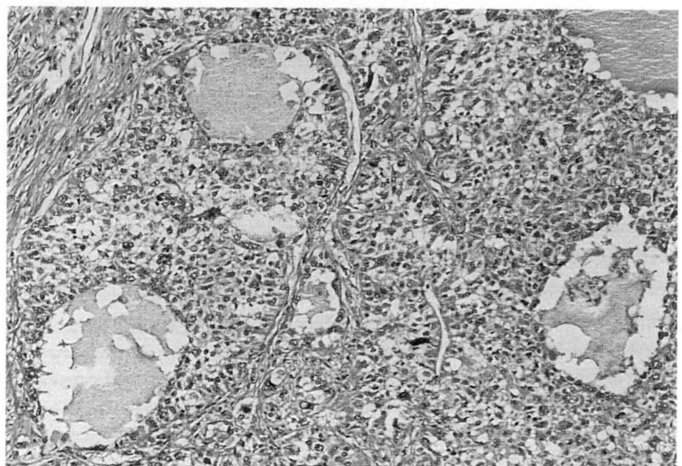

Fig. 68-89 Juvenile granulosa cell tumor of ovary. Rudimentary follicles and cytologic atypia. Both granulosa cell and theca cell components appear luteinized.

acterized by somewhat spindle-shaped cells, may have a more aggressive behavior.

The juvenile type, chiefly prepubertal, has distinctive microscopic features such as rudimentary follicles, rarely grooved hyperchromatic nuclei, and striking luteinization of both granulosa and thecal components.[636-638]

The most consistent indicator of aggressive behavior has been the presence of metastases or invasion of structures outside the ovary at the time of diagnosis. Also unfavorable but less significant factors are large tumor size, increasing age, poorly differentiated tumors with a high mitotic rate, and tumor rupture[636,639-641] (Fig. 68-89).

Juvenile granulosa cell tumors may produce precocious sexual development in prepuberal girls. In adult women, however, the most common symptom is uterine bleeding as a result of endometrial hyperplasia. Well-differentiated endometrial adenocarcinoma occurs in 10% to 25% of the cases in postmenopausal women. These adenocarcinomas usually have a remarkably good prognosis, possibly because most of them are highly estrogen dependent and therefore fail to progress when the source of estrogen is withdrawn.

Less than 5% of granulosa cell tumors are bilateral. Over 90% of the patients survived for 10 years, and some had residual tumor. Recurrences continue to appear as late as 30 years postoperatively. It is reasonable to conserve the opposite ovary and uterus of a young woman with a small tumor confined to one ovary.

Fibroma. Fibrous tumors of the ovary without clinical or morphologic evidence of endocrine activity are relatively common and account for 6% of all ovarian tumors. Densely collagenized fibrous tissue forms a monotonous histologic pattern occasionally broken by areas of calcification.[642] In rare cases, large fibromas may be associated with benign ascites and pleural effusion, which disappear when the tumor is resected (Meigs' syndrome).[643] Cellular fibromas with only slight mitotic activity (3 or less MFs per 10 HPF) and mild to moderate nuclear atypia are almost always benign unless they are adherent or ruptured[644] (Fig. 68-90). Fibrosarcomas typically exhibit higher mitotic rate and pronounced nuclear pleomorphism; they are extremely rare.[644]

Thecomas. Thecomas are less common than granulosa cell tumors. They are frequently associated with estrogenic manifestations and are bilateral in only 3% of the cases.[645-647] About 80% of the patients are postmenopausal (mean age, 59 years). Grossly, thecomas are typically solid yellow masses of about 7 cm in diameter. Microscopical examination reveals large rounded cells with abundant vacuolated cytoplasm containing lipid. The nuclei are round without significant atypia. Hyaline plaques are frequent, and there is often a fibrous component separating the nests of theca cells; focal calcification may be observed.[648] Severe atypia, high mitotic activity, and malignant behavior are extremely rare.

Luteinized thecoma has the appearance of a fibroma or typical thecoma with foci of lutein cells.[649] They typically occur in young women and, although estrogenic in about half the cases, are occasionally associated with androgenic manifestations.[650] The *sclerosing stromal tumor* is a distinctive tumor that occurs at a younger average age than the typical thecoma or fibroma; over 80% of the patients are less than 30 years old (average age, 27 years).[651,652] Low-power microscopic examination typically shows ill-defined cellular pseudolobules separated by stroma. It can be mistaken with a Krukenberg tumor because of the presence of vacuolated lutein cells.

Sertoli-Leydig cell tumors (Sertoli-stromal cell tumors). The rare Sertoli-Leydig cell tumors occur in all age groups, but they peak during reproductive years (average age, 25 years). They are bilateral in only 3% of the cases. Although Sertoli-Leydig cell tumors often produce androgens and masculinize the patient, many are nonfunctioning, and some even have estrogenic effects.[653] Testosterone and a variety of androgenic precursors may be secreted in variable proportions. Their histologic appearance resembles that of the developing testis.

Five histologic categories are distinguished: (1) well-differentiated tumors that form tubular structures composed of Sertoli cells, separated by a fibrous stroma, and intermixed with nests of large round Leydig cells; (2) tumors of intermediate differentiation in which large eosinophilic Leydig cells are separated by a spindly stroma; abortive tubule formation resembles early sex cords of the embryonic testis (Fig. 68-91); (3) sarcomatoid variant, composed of spindle cells with vague trabecular arrangement. Leydig cells may or may not be present; (4) Sertoli-Leydig cell tumors with heterologous elements such as neoplastic mucinous glands, cartilage, and skeletal muscle.[654,655] Heterologous elements are found in 25% of these tumors; (5) retiform Sertoli-Leydig cell tumor mimics histologically the rete of the ovary or testis.[656]

About half the well-differentiated tumors, three fourths of intermediate tumors, and all sarcomatoid tumors are androgenic. Pure Sertoli cell tumors occur in younger women and children; most cause hyperestrinism, including isosexual precocious puberty in children, but few have caused virilization.[657]

Almost all Sertoli-Leydig cell tumors are benign The rare malignant cases were all poorly differentiated or had mesenchymal heterologous elements.[655] Intra-abdominal spread but no distant metastases were recorded in such cases.

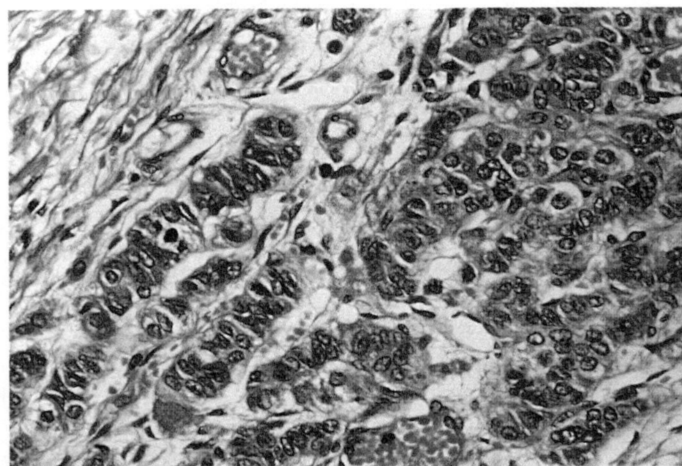

Fig. 68-91 Moderately differentiated intermediate type of Sertoli-Leydig cell tumor. Large, dense, eosinophilic Leydig cells are intermixed with cordlike strands of smaller Sertoli cells in a loose, sparsely cellular stroma.

Sex cord tumor with annular tubules (SCTAT). A sex cord tumor with annular tubules has distinctive morphologic features that are intermediate between a granulosa cell tumor and a Sertoli cell tumor. One third of the cases are associated with the Peutz-Jeghers syndrome.[658] Most cases have a favorable clinical course.

Gynandroblastoma. Rarely, a sex cord–stromal tumor may include both granulosa-theca cell and Sertoli-Leydig cell patterns.[659] Most have been benign. Those with hormonal function have produced androgens.

Steroid (lipid) cell tumors. Steroid cell tumors are a distinctive group of neoplasms that occur in the form of soft yellow or yellow-brown nodules. These tumors are divided into stromal luteomas,[660] (hilum) cell tumors,[661] and steroid cell tumors not otherwise specified (NOS).[662] The tumor cells are large, rounded, or polyhedral cells resembling lutein cells, Leydig cells, and adrenocortical cells. Although most of them contain abundant intracellular fat, some do not. Ultrastructure is consistent with ovarian stromal origin; cytoplasmic organelles resemble those of steroid-secreting cells.[663] Stromal luteomas are located within the ovarian stroma, lack crystalloids of Reinke, and are rarely androgenic.[660] In contrast, (hilum) cell tumors are often androgenic and typically contain crystalloids of Reinke. Both tumors occur in postmenopausal women and are benign. Steroid cell tumors NOS occur in patients younger than those having the other two forms and may be malignant (25% to 40%). When functioning, these tumors are typically androgenic.[662] Malignant behavior is indicated by the presence of 2 MF per HPF, necrosis, large size, and nuclear atypia.[662] A few have caused Cushing's syndrome.

Germ cell tumors

Germ cell tumors are composed of cells derived from oocytes.[664] Although germ cell tumors of the ovary are morphologically similar to testicular germ cell tumors, they may not necessarily have an identical histogenesis.[665] Some tumors may arise from preexisting somatic neoplasms of the female genital tract.[666-668] Recent evidence has indicated that even germinomas are not necessarily end-stage tumors, as previously believed, but composed of cells capable of differentiation.[669,670]

Morphologic overlapping between early developmental forms of germ cell tumors, such as embryonal carcinoma, dysgerminoma, and yolk sac tumor, supports the view that these tumors constitute a closely related group of neoplasms capable of extraembryonal or intraembryonal differentiations.[671,672] These new concepts have been represented in a tridimensional tetrahedron model of interrelationships between the different components.[673]

Dysgerminoma. Dysgerminoma, the most common malignant germ cell tumor of the ovary,[659] is morphologically identical to testicular seminoma. Grossly, these neoplasms are large, solid, encapsulated masses of soft, gray-white tissue (Fig. 68-92). They are composed of large rounded or polygonal cells resembling primordial germ cells.[674] The tumor cells are distributed in large masses separated by delicate fibrous trabeculas. The fibrous stroma is almost always infiltrated by lymphocytes and may contain sarcoid granulomas (Fig. 68-93). The presence of calcification is suggestive of an underlying gonadoblastoma. About 80% are stage I, and 10% are grossly bilateral. The opposite ovary may contain microscopic foci of dysgerminoma even when it appears grossly normal (10%); if

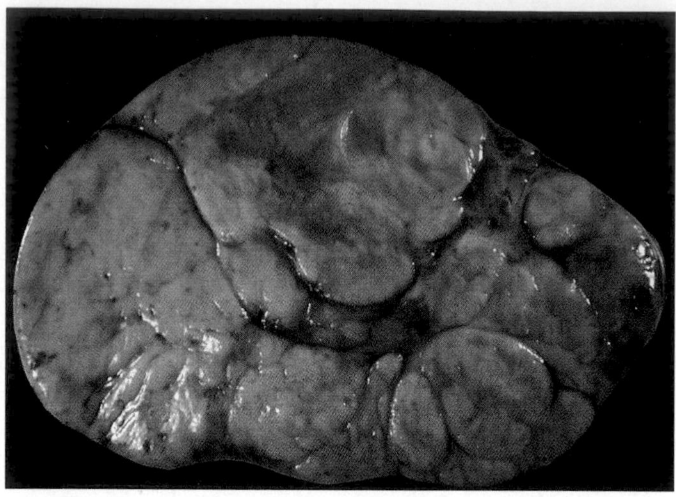

Fig. 68-92 Dysgerminoma. Large, solid, lobulated tumor from a 6-year-old girl.

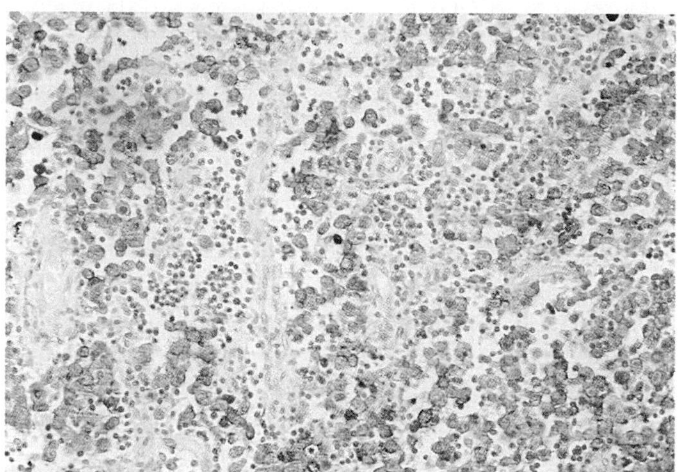

Fig. 68-93 Dysgerminoma. Masses of large uniform germ cells are separated by fibrous trabeculas that are infiltrated by lymphocytes. Positive stain for placental alkaline phosphatase. (Immunohistochemistry.)

it is to be preserved, biopsy with frozen-section examination is desirable.[675-677]

Dysgerminoma is an extremely radiosensitive tumor, but, currently, cisplatin-based chemotherapy has become the treatment of choice. The tumor is curable even in the presence of metastases. The 5-year survival rate is between 70% and 90%. For pure stage I dysgerminoma, the 5-year survival rate approaches 95% for patients treated with unilateral salpingo-oophorectomy. The occasional dysgerminoma that contains syncytiotrophoblastic giant cells (about 3%) does not behave more aggressively than the ordinary dysgerminoma.[678] These tumors may produce hCG, which can serve as a tumor marker.

Yolk sac tumor (YST). In the age group under 20 years, YST are almost as common as dysgerminoma. They consistently produce alpha-fetoprotein, which can be demonstrated in tissue sections by immunohistochemical techniques and in the patient's serum. This substance, which is normally produced in the yolk sac of the developing embryo, may serve as a tumor marker in evaluating the course of the patient after treatment.[679]

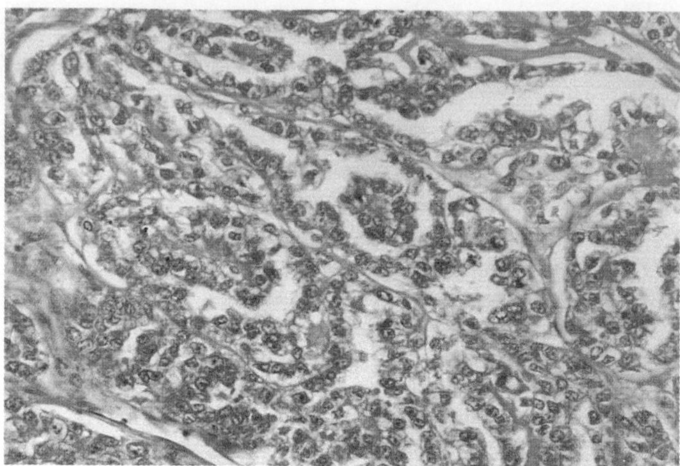

Fig. 68-94 Yolk sac tumor. There is a tangle of papillary processes with central blood vessel, usually covered by a single layer of anaplastic epithelial cells; stroma is inconspicuous.

The gross appearance may be similar to that of dysgerminoma except for the more extensive yellow and red areas of hemorrhage and necrosis and the common presence of cysts. The typical microscopic features are highly variable and include several distinct patterns, such as reticular, microcystic, tubular, and so forth. Glomeruloid Schiller-Duval bodies are typical (Fig. 68-94). Another distinctive feature is the presence of PAS-positive, diastase-resistant hyaline globules partly composed of AFP and alpha-1-antitrypsin. Some tumors contain multiple gland spaces with hourglass constrictions resembling yolk sac vesicles, a pattern designated as *polyvesicular vitelline tumor.*[680] Hepatic and enteric (glandular differentiation) may predominate in rare tumors.[681-684]

Before the use of combination chemotherapy, the prognosis of YST was very poor; remissions have occurred in some patients treated postoperatively with multiple chemotherapeutic agents. For patients with stage I tumors, survival rates have approached 80%.

Embryonal carcinoma. Embryonal carcinoma is an uncommon ovarian germ cell tumor that has been confused with YST, which it resembles.[685] From a histogenetic viewpoint, embryonal carcinoma has been considered a pluripotent stem cell tumor capable of differentiating along different pathways.[686] The patients are young, present with an abdominal mass, and consistently have a positive pregnancy test as a result of hCG production by the tumor.[685] Premenarchal girls undergo precocious puberty. Histologically, it resembles testicular embryonal carcinoma: large primitive anaplastic cells form solid masses interspersed with glandlike cleft and scattered giant cells. Multinucleated giant cells of syncytiotrophoblastic type immunoreactive for hCG are common. Similarly, mononuclear embryonal cells stain for alpha-fetoprotein. Both substances can be used as tumor markers.[687] Although these tumors are highly malignant, chemotherapy has resulted in some long-term survivors. Most tumors are unilateral, and salpingo-oophorectomy is the recommended surgical procedure.

Polyembryoma. Some germ cell tumors contain large numbers of embryoid bodies, closely resembling early embryos, typically distributed in a primitive mesenchymal stroma.[688,689]

Choriocarcinoma. Nongestational primary choriocarcinoma of the ovary is rare and malignant. The histologic picture and clinical correlations are similar to those of gestational choriocarcinoma, except that the remarkable response to chemotherapy usually does not occur. Choriocarcinomatous differentiation, usually interpreted as "retrograde differentiation," has been reported in ovarian carcinomas.[668]

Teratomas. Teratomas are composed of recognizable tissues of ectodermal, mesodermal, and endodermal origin, in any combination. They are common and usually benign and inert but rarely produce remarkably bizarre and varied syndromes, reflecting the diverse potentials of the germ cells.

Benign cystic teratoma (dermoid cyst). Cystic teratomas are composed of a great variety of mature somatic tissues. Most cysts are unilocular, and the tissue that forms the lining is usually skin. The desquamated keratin and secretions, notably from sebaceous glands, accumulate with masses of hair to fill the lumen of the cyst (Fig. 68-95). This mixture is liquid at body temperature but solidifies when chilled. Other common components are salivary gland; bronchus; fat; smooth muscle; cartilage; bone; neural tissue, including ganglia, glia, and choroid plexus; retina; pancreas; thyroid; and teeth. Characteristically, a protuberance from the inner surface is the locus of growth of most of the hair and teeth. Uncommon tissues are skeletal and cardiac muscle, kidney, and liver.

Bilaterality occurs in 8% to 15% of cases. Cystic teratomas constitute 20% of all ovarian tumors in adults and 50% of all ovarian tumors in children. Most patients are between 20 and 40 years, but the tumors occur at all ages.

The pathogenesis of teratomas has always excited speculation because of their exotic composition. Cytogenetic analysis using chromosome-banding techniques has indicated that ovarian teratomas are parthenogenetic tumors that must originate from a single germ cell after its first miotic division.[690]

The most serious complication of a mature cyst teratoma is malignant change. Almost any component may become malignant, but squamous cell carcinoma accounts for 90% of the cases.[691] Sweat gland carcinoma, thyroid carcinoma, malignant melanoma, and various sarcomas, including osteosarcoma, occur rarely.

Solid teratomas (teratomas with abundant solid tissue and relatively small cysts) are nearly all malignant (as discussed subsequently), but a few benign solid teratomas have been reported.[692]

Immature teratoma (malignant teratoma). Malignant teratoma, the third most common ovarian germ cell tumor, usually presents in young adults and children (median age 18 years) as a unilateral solid mass with a heterogeneous appearance on cut surface. Grossly evident dermoid cysts are present in 25% of the cases.[693] The histologic appearance is also extremely variable; the immature tissue is predominantly neuroectodermal tissue in the form of rosettes and tubules and cellular foci of glia with numerous mitoses (Fig. 68-96). Islands of immature cartilage, bone, and glandular structures are distributed through a poorly differentiated stroma. Bilateral involvement in patients with stage I malignant teratoma is extremely rare, but a dermoid cyst is present in the contralateral ovary in 10% of the cases.[693]

The relative amount of primitive neuroepithelial tissue is an important factor in grading and determining the prognosis.

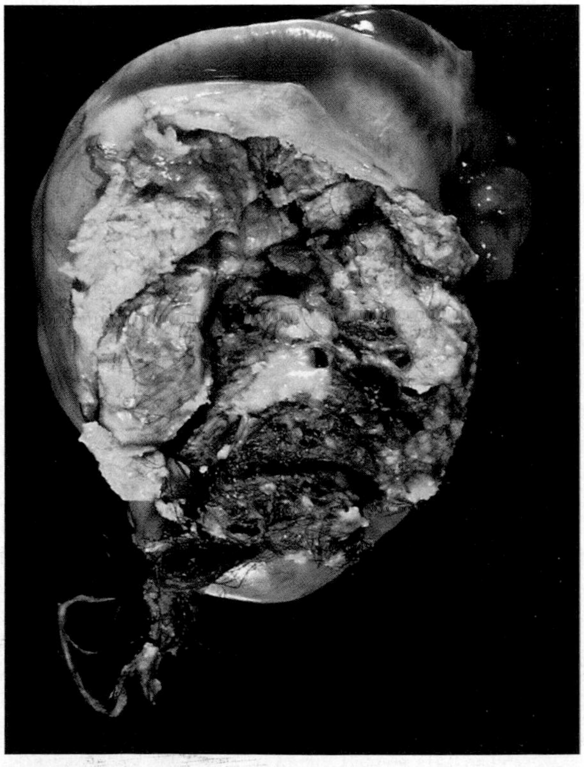

Fig. 68-95 Benign cystic teratoma (dermoid cyst). The cavity is filled with sebaceous material and hair.

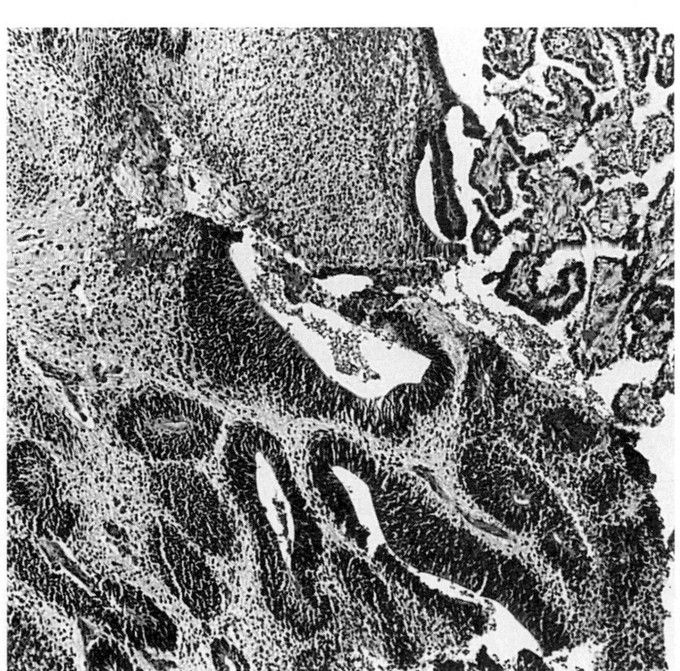

Fig. 68-96 Immature teratoma. Immature neuroectodermal tissue. There are several neuroepithelial rosettes in the vicinity of choroid plexus.

"Grade 1" has been applied to tumors with rare foci of immature neural tissue occupying less than 1 low power field (LPF) per slide, "grade 2" to tumors with moderate quantities of immature neural tissue filling more than one but 3 or fewer LPF per slide, and "grade 3" to tumors with large amounts of immature neural tissue occupying 4 or more LPF per slide. Patients with relatively mature (grade 1) malignant teratomas have a good prognosis, whereas for those with immature teratomas (grade 3) the prognosis is poor.[694-698] AFP, once believed to be an exclusive marker for YST, is also secreted by the immature endodermal tissues in immature teratomas.

About one third of immature teratomas are found in stage II or III at the time of laparotomy and are usually associated with peritoneal implants. The neural component, even in the implants, may mature, leaving well-differentiated glial vestiges on the peritoneal surfaces. Mature glial implants are innocuous and not an indication for radical treatment.[694] Therefore the grading of metastases, once they have occurred, is also prognostically important.[695] In contrast to the dismal results obtained by surgery or radiation in the past, combination chemotherapy has produced remarkable effect resulting in over 70% survival.[698] Chemotherapy induces maturation of the implants.

Specialized teratomas. Rare teratomas composed exclusively of thyroid tissue are usually benign but may function and even cause thyrotoxicosis. Carcinoid tumors with the insular pattern typical of midgut derivatives[699,700] and trabecular carcinoids of the foregut and hindgut type also occur as primary ovarian tumors.[701,702] The latter type may be mixed with thyroid tissue *(strumal carcinoid).*[703,704] Both are nearly always unilateral and benign; insular carcinoids, especially if large, may cause the carcinoid syndrome. On the other hand, intestinal carcinoids metastatic to the ovary are usually bilateral and have a poor prognosis. It is especially important to distinguish them from granulosa cell tumors and Sertoli-Leydig cell tumors, as well as from primary ovarian carcinoids.[705] Several primitive neuroectodermal tumors, similar to neoplasms of the central nervous system (medulloepithelioma, neuroblastoma, ependymoblastoma and medulloblastoma) have been described in the ovary. Prognosis is poor.[706,707]

Mixed forms. Germ cell tumors occur in various combinations. Malignant mixed germ cell tumors (stage I) have a poor prognosis if more than one third of the tumor consists of endodermal sinus tumor, choriocarcinoma, or grade 3 teratoma. Tumors that contain less than one third of these components or contain combinations of dysgerminoma, embryonal carcinoma, or grade 1 or 2 teratoma have a good prognosis. Patients with tumors less than 10 cm in diameter are more likely to survive regardless of tumor composition.[708]

Gonadoblastoma

Gonadoblastoma is a rare tumor that may arise in a dysgenetic gonad. The patients are usually phenotypic females, but nearly all are genotypic males (that is, have a Y chromosome). The tumor contains both immature germ cells and sex cord–stromal cells, which resemble granulosa or Sertoli cells, arranged in small islands and intermixed with rounded pink hyaline bodies (Fig. 68-97). Leydig cells or lutein cells are distributed through the intervening stroma in about two thirds of the cases and are responsible for the endocrine manifestations. Small calcifications may be extensive and may be detected by x-rays. Most gonadoblastomas are benign, but dysgerminomas and other malignant germ cell tumors develop occasionally from them.[15]

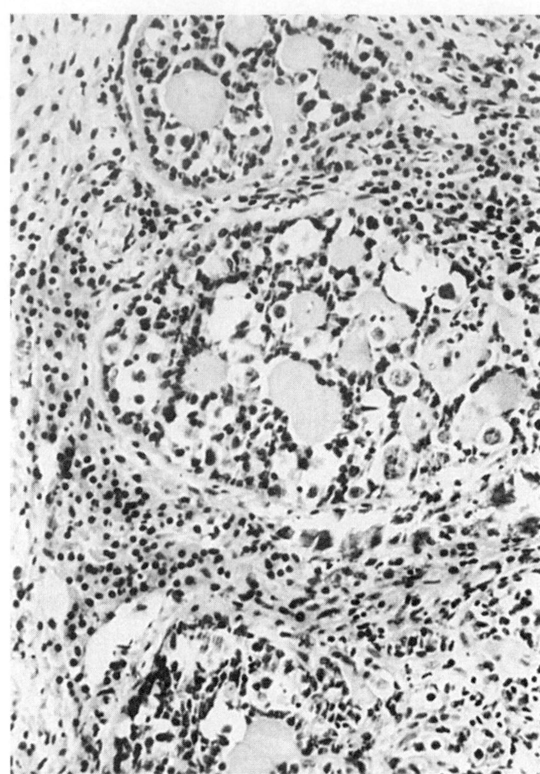

Fig. 68-97 Gonadoblastoma. Large germ cells and hyaline globules are intermixed with smaller granulosa cells, forming islands or nests. Clumps of Leydig cells are scattered through intervening stroma (Courtesy Dr. Jerry Teter, Warsaw, Poland. From Scully RE: Androgenic lesion of the ovary. In Grady HG, Smith DE, editors: *The ovary*, Baltimore, 1963, Williams & Wilkins.)

Metastatic tumors

Metastases to the ovary are common. Approximately 10% of all malignant tumors involving the ovary are actually metastatic, but their nature is frequently unsuspected by gynecologists and even by pathologists, particularly when the tumors are cystic.[709-711] Metastases often mimic primary ovarian tumors and may even be the first manifestation of disease. In most cases, the primary site is the breast, colon, or stomach, but the original tumor may be small and difficult to detect, even when the ovarian metastases are large.

The routes of spread vary, but lymphatic and hematogenous dissemination to the ovaries is the most common mechanism.[709-711] Direct extension is also frequent, particularly for tumors arising from adjacent organs such as the uterus, fallopian tube, and sigmoid colon. Transtubal spread of uterine cancers may also occur. Tumors from abdominal organs, such as the appendix, may also reach the ovary by the transcelomic route. Embolic spread results in the development of multiple intraovarian tumor nodules, and, in these cases, vascular invasion is frequently found microscopically in the ovarian hilum.[709-711]

The most helpful gross and microscopic clues in the diagnosis of metastatic tumors to the ovary are bilaterality, the finding of small (often microscopic) and superficial tumor nodules, extensive extraovarian dissemination, unusual patterns of spread, infrequent histologic features, vascular invasion, and prominent desmoplastic reaction.[709-711]

Colonic adenocarcinomas probably account for most metastatic tumors to the ovary that are microscopically confused with endometrioid carcinoma.[710,711] Frequently, the ovarian and primary tumors are discovered synchronously or the intestinal tumors have been resected months or years previously without the pathologist's knowledge.[711] Occasionally, the colonic primary tumor is discovered several months after resection of the ovarian tumor. About 75% of them arise in the rectum or sigmoid colon.[710, 711] Features favoring a metastasis are large cysts filled with necrotic material, abundant eosinophilic debris ("dirty necrosis"), focal segmental necrosis of the glands, occasional presence of goblet cells, and absence of müllerian features (squamous differentiation, or association with endometriosis).[710,711] Strong immunoreactivity for CEA favors colonic origin.

The ovarian stroma may be stimulated to secrete estrogenic, androgenic, or progestogenic hormones in the presence of metastatic carcinoma, particularly those from the gastrointestinal tract. In these ovarian tumors with functioning stroma, hCG or hCG-like substances produced by the neoplastic cells may be responsible.[712,713]The *Krukenberg tumor* is almost invariably secondary from a primary gastric or, less frequently, intestinal adenocarcinoma. Grossly, the tumors are bilateral in about 60% of the cases, and typically large, solid, and multinodular. The basis for the selective enhancement of growth is unknown. Most patients are premenopausal, about a decade younger than those with primary ovarian adenocarcinoma; the phenomenon may be hormone dependent. The term *Krukenberg tumor* is usually reserved for this typical clinicopathologic presentation when the tumor cells have large eccentric mucin vacuoles (signet-ring cells) and the primary site is the stomach (Fig. 68-98). Stromal proliferation may resemble a fibromatous tumor (fibroma, thecoma, or sclerosing stromal tumor).[711] A misdiagnosis of Krukenberg tumor can be made in rare cases of primary mucinous carcinoid tumor of the ovary. Chromogranin, synaptophysin, and Grimelius stains may be of help. The tubular variant, commonly associated with stromal luteinization, can be confused with sex cord–stromal tumors, particularly with Sertoli-Leydig cell tumors (Fig. 68-99). PAS-diastase and mucicarmine stains are of great value.[714] Metastatic tumors from the pancreas, biliary tract[715] and appendix[595] simulate primary ovarian mucinous tumors.

Breast carcinoma is the most common metastatic tumor to the ovaries but only occasionally presents itself as a primary ovarian tumor.[709,711] It may exhibit an endometrioid appearance, an insular pattern simulating a carcinoid tumor, or even a diffuse pattern mimicking granulocytic sarcoma or lymphoma. Positive immunostaining for EMA, S-100 and E_2R protein and negativity for CA 12.5 and CA 19.9 can be useful.

Metastatic renal cell carcinomas and melanomas may be interpreted as clear cell carcinomas and granulosa cell or lipid cell tumors.[711,716]

Lymphomas and *leukemias* frequently involve the ovaries late in the course of the disease (25%) but rarely present initially as ovarian tumors (0.2%).[717-721] The tumor cells are often distributed in single-file rows, producing a histologic picture reminiscent of metastatic lobular carcinoma of the breast. Large cell lymphomas may simulate several primary tumors, such as dysgerminoma. The appearance of the cell nuclei is very important. Immunohistochemical analysis for lymphoid markers and placental alkaline phosphatase are helpful. In some cases, carcinoid tumors, granulosa cell tumors or small cell carcinoma can resemble lymphomas.

The ovaries, like the facial bones and orbital tissue, are common sites of involvement in Burkitt's lymphoma, including the American variety.[719] In rare cases, myelogenous leukemia appears initially as an ovarian tumor (so-called granulocytic sarcoma).[719] Only a few tumors contain sufficient myeloperoxidase to have a green color on gross inspection (chloroma). Chloroacetate esterase, muramidase and Factor VIII immunostains are helpful.[719]

Pathologic factors affecting prognosis

The foregoing discussion has emphasized that each different type of ovarian neoplasm is in fact a separate disease. There are, however, some general characteristics that also affect the outcome of treatment.

Established prognostic factors include FIGO stage (Table 68-8), histologic type, and tumor grade, and clinical-surgical parameters include residual disease after debulking surgery,

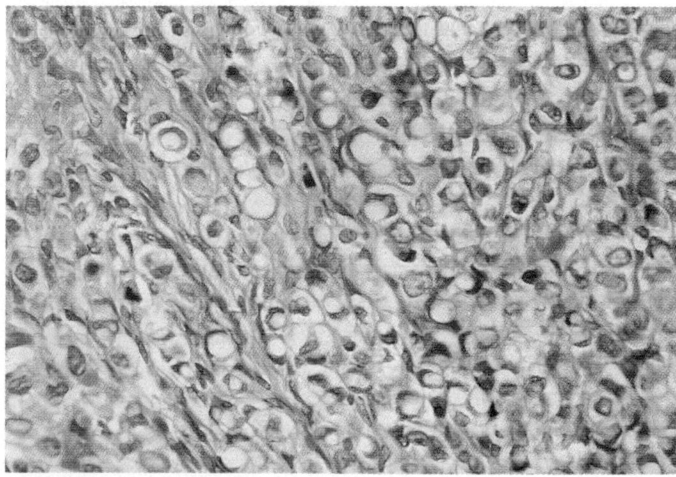

Fig. 68-98 Krukenberg tumor. The ovary is infiltrated with signet-ring cells. (Courtesy Dr. Peter A. McCue, Philadelphia.)

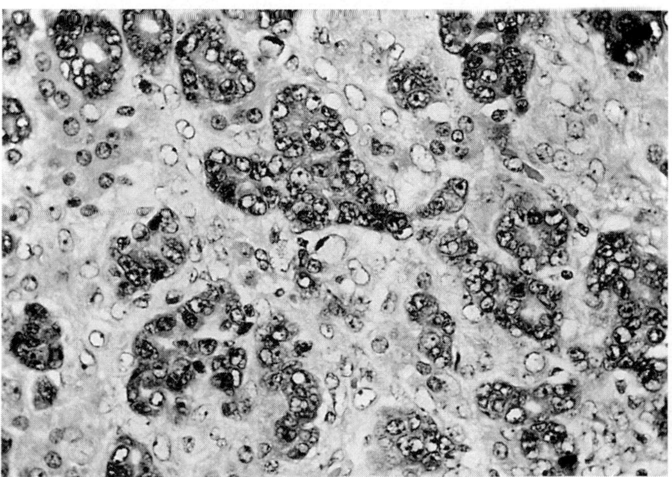

Fig. 68-99 Tubular Krukenberg tumor. Ovarian tumor with functioning stroma simulating Sertoli-Leydig cell tumors.

Table 68-8 FIGO staging of ovarian cancer

Stage I: Growth limited to the ovaries.
- **Stage Ia:** Growth limited to one ovary; no ascites. No tumor on the external surface; capsule intact.
- **Stage Ib:** Growth limited to both ovaries; no ascites. No tumor on the external surface; capsules intact.
- **Stage Ic:** Tumor either stage Ia or stage Ib but with tumor on the surface of one or both ovaries; or with capsule ruptured; or with ascites present containing malignant cells; or with positive peritoneal washings.

Stage II: Growth involving one or both ovaries with pelvic extension.
- **Stage IIa:** Extension and/or metastases to the uterus and/or tubes.
- **Stage IIb:** Extension to other pelvic tissues.
- **Stage IIc:** Tumor either stage IIa or IIb but with tumor on the surface of one or both ovaries; or with capsule or capsules ruptured; or with ascites present containing malignant cells; or with positive peritoneal washings.

Stage III: Tumor involving one or both ovaries, with peritoneal implants outside the pelvis and/or positive retroperitoneal or inguinal nodes. Superficial liver metastasis qualifies as stage III.
- **Stage IIIa:** Tumor grossly limited to true pelvis, with negative nodes but with histologically confirmed microscopic seeding of abdominal peritoneal surfaces.
- **Stage IIIb:** Tumor of one or both ovaries with histologically confirmed implants of abdominal peritoneal surfaces, none exceeding 2 cm in diameter. Nodes are negative.
- **Stage IIIc:** Abdominal implants greater than 2 cm in diameter and/or positive retroperitoneal or inguinal nodes.

Stage IV: Growth involving one or both ovaries with distant metastases. If pleural effusion is present, there must be positive cytologic findings to allot a case to stage IV. The presence of parenchymal liver metastases equals stage IV.

Special category

Unexplored cases that are believed to be ovarian carcinoma. Stage is based on findings at clinical examination and surgical exploration. The final histology after surgery is to be considered in the staging, as well as cytology as far as effusions are concerned.

Ascites is peritoneal effusion that, in the opinion of the surgeon, is pathologic and/or clearly exceeds normal amounts.

the presence or absence of ascites, performance status, and age.[722-724] Of these, FIGO stage is the most important independent prognostic factor. Five-year survival for stage I tumors (limited to the ovary) is 60% to 80%; 45% to 60% for stage II (spread to the pelvis); 15% for stage III (intra-abdominal or lymph node metastases); and less than 10% for stage IV disease (distant or parenchymal liver metastases). Survival rates vary somewhat among the histologic types of epithelial-stromal tumors; for example, serous cystadenocarcinomas have a lower survival rate than endometrioid cystadenocarcinomas. This difference is most likely dependent on grade, because most endometrioid cystadenocarcinomas are well or moderately differentiated, whereas serous tumors are more often poorly differentiated. Tumor grade is related to survival rates, though this is not an independent prognosticator when controlled for stage. Because these pathologic and clinical parameters present an incomplete profile of the behavior of ovarian carcinomas, the search for prognostic factors continues.

Ploidy is an independent prognostic factor, with a decreased rate and length of survival in aneuploid ovarian carcinomas.[725] Ploidy is also related to stage, because 60% to 80% of stage III and stage IV tumors are aneuploid, compared to 45% to 60% of stage I and stage II tumors. Analyses of cells in the S-phase fraction and other proliferation markers generally parallel those for ploidy; an S-phase fraction above 10% is a marker of aggressivesness.[726]

OC-125 is a monoclonal antibody that recognizes a glycoprotein, CA-125, present on more than 80% of nonmucinous ovarian tumors.[727] Serum OC-125 is elevated above 35 U/ml in more than 80% of ovarian carcinoma patients and is most often elevated in higher-stage disease. CA125 can be measured in the peritoneal fluid as well.[728] Newer markers, such as the soluble tumor necrosis factor receptor, which are elevated in peritoneal fluid in up to 84% of ovarian cancer patients, seem to be even better for monitoring these patients.[728]

Studies of oncogenes and antioncogenes in ovarian carcinoma have begun to outline their role in carcinogenesis and have identified several genes that are of prognostic significance, though this work is still considered investigational.[729]

ACKNOWLEDGMENTS

The author acknowledges the generosity of Doctor Frederick T. Kraus, Professor of Pathology, Washington University, St. Louis, Missouri, and skillful writer of the previous editions of this chapter for graciously providing all his material.

REFERENCES

Normal female genital tract and abnormal sexual development

1. Sadler TW: *Langman's medical embryology,* ed 5, Baltimore, 1985, Williams & Wilkins.
2. Harley VR, Jackson DI, Hextall PJ et al: DNA binding activity of recombinant SRY from normal males and XY females, *Science* 255:453, 1992.
3. Sinclair AH, Berta P, Palmer MS et al: A gene for the human sex determining region encodes a protein with homology to a conserved DNA binding motif, *Nature* 346:240, 1990.
4. McLaren A: Development of the mammalian gonad: the fate of the supporting cell lineage, *Bioessays* 13:151, 1991.
5. Forsberg JG: Origin of vaginal epithelium, *Obstet Gynecol* 25:687, 1965.
6. Ulbright TM, Kraus FT: Endometrial stromal tumors of the extra-uterine tissue, *Am J Clin Pathol* 76:371, 1981.
7. Pinkerton JH, McKay DG, Adams EC, Hertig AT: Development of the human ovary: a study using histochemical techniques, *Obstet Gynecol* 18:152, 1961.
8. Hamilton WJ, Boyd JD, Mossman HW: *Human embryology,* ed 4, Baltimore, 1972. Williams & Wilkins.
9. Kalousek DK, Poland BJ: Embryonic and fetal pathology of abortion. Chapter 2 in Perrin VDK, editor: *Pathology of the placenta,* New York, 1984, Churchill Livingstone.
10. Van Wagenen G, Simpson ME: *Embryology of the ovary and testis: Homo sapiens and Macaca mulatta,* New Haven, Conn, 1965, Yale University Press.
11. Donahoe PK: Müllerian inhibiting substance in reproduction and cancer, *Mol Reprod Dev* 32:168, 1992.
12. Kuroda T, Lee MM, Ragin RC et al: Müllerian inhibiting substance production and cleavage is modulated by gonadotropins and steroids, *Endocrinology* 129:2985, 1991.
13. Robboy SJ, Bernhardt PF, Parmley T: Embryology of the female genital tract and disorders of abnormal sexual development In Kurman RJ, editor: *Blaustein's pathology of the female genital tract,* New York, 1994, Springer-Verlag.
14. Scully RE: Gonadal pathology of genetically determined diseases In Kraus FT, Damjanov I, editors *The pathology of reproductive failure,* Inter-

national Academy of Pathology, Monogr no 33 Baltimore, 1991, Williams & Wilkins.

15. Scully RE: Gonadoblastoma: a review of 74 cases, *Cancer* 25:1340, 1970.
16. Page DC: Hypothesis: a Y-chromosomal gene causes gonadoblastoma in dysgenetic gonads, *Development* 101(suppl):151, 1987.
17. Robboy SJ, Miller T, Donahoe PK et al: Dysgenesis of testicular and streak gonads in the syndrome of mixed gonadal dysgenesis: perspective derived from a clinicopathologic analysis of twenty-one cases, *Hum Pathol* 13:700, 1982.
18. Rutgers JL: Advances in the pathology of intersex conditions, *Hum Pathol* 22:884, 1991.
19. Tegenkamp TR, Brazzell JW, Tegenkamp I, Labidi F: Pregnancy without benefit of surgery in a bisexually active true hermaphrodite, *Am J Obstet Gynecol* 135:427, 1979.
20. Talerman A, Verp MS, Senekjian E et al: True hermaphrodite with bilateral ovotestes, bilateral gonadoblastomas and dysgerminomas, 46 XX/46 XY karyotype, and a successful pregnancy *Cancer* 66:2668, 1990.
21. Van Niekerk WA: True hermaphroditism: an analytic review with a report of three cases, *Am J Obstet Gynecol* 126:890, 1976.
22. Griffin JE: The syndromes of androgen resistance, *N Engl J Med* 302:198, 1980.
23. Rutgers JL, Scully RE: The androgen insensitivity syndrome (testicular feminization): a clinicopathologic study of 43 cases, *Int J Gynecol Pathol* 10:126, 1991.
24. Prinz JL, Choate JW, Townes, PL, Harper RC: The embryology of supernumerary ovaries, *Obstet Gynecol* 41:246, 1973.
25. Farber M, Marchant DJ: Congenital absence of the uterine cervix, *Am J Obstet Gynecol* 121:414, 1975.
26. Fanning J: Double vulva: a case report, *J Reprod Med* 32:297, 1987.
27. Stephens FD: The female anus, perineum, and vestibule: embryogenesis and deformities, *Aust NZ J Obstet Gynaecol* 8:55, 1968.

Vulva

28. Wilkinson EJ: Diseases of the vulva. In Kurman RJ, editor: *Blaustein's pathology of the female genital tract.* ed 4 New York, 1994, Springer-Verlag.
29. Dodson RF, Fritz GS, Hubler WR et al: Donovanosis: a morphologic study, *J Invest Dermatol* 62:611, 1974.
30. Rosen T, Tschen JA, Ramsdell W et al: Granuloma inguinale, *J Am Acad Dermatol* 11:433, 1984.
31. Sehgal VN, Shyamprasad AL, Beohar PC: The histopathological diagnosis of donovanosis *Br J Vener Dis* 60:45, 1984.
32. Douglas CP: Lymphogranuloma venereum and granuloma inguinale of the vulva, *J Obstet Gynecol Br Common* 69:871, 1962.
33. Morse SA: *Atlas of sexually transmitted diseases.* Philadelphia, 1990, Lippincott.
34. Devroede G, Schlaeder G, Sánchez G, Haddad H: Crohn's disease of the vulva, *Am J Clin Pathol* 63:348, 1975.
35. Majmudar B, Chaikeu ML, Lee KU: Amebiasis of clitoris mimicking carcinoma, *JAMA* 236.1145, 1976.
36. Kaufman RH, Dreesman GR, Burek J et al: Herpes-induced antigens in squamous cell carcinoma in situ of the vulva, *N Engl J Med* 305:483, 1981.
37. zur Hausen H: Papillomaviruses in human cancer, *Cancer* 59:1692, 1987.
38. Amstey MS, Monif GR, Nahmias AJ, Josey WE: Cesarean section and genital herpes infection, *Obstet Gynecol* 53:641, 1979.
39. Reed RJ, Parkinson RP: The histogenesis of molluscum contagiosum, *Am J Surg Pathol* 1:161, 1977.
40. Jeffcoate TNA, Woodcock AS: Premalignant conditions of the vulva with particular reference to chronic epithelial dystrophies, *Br Med J* 2:127, 1961.
41. Prat J: Pathology of vulvar intraepithelial lesions and early invasive carcinoma, *Hum Pathol* 22:877, 1991.
42. Wilkinson EJ, Kneale B, Lynch PJ: Report of the ISSVD Terminology Committee, *J Reprod Med* 31:973, 1986.
43. Kint A, Geerts ML: Lichen sclerosus et atrophicus: an electron microscopic study, *J Cutan Pathol* 2:30, 1975.
44. Mann PR, Cowan MA: Ultrastructural changes in four cases of lichen sclerosus et atrophicus, *Br J Dermatol* 89:223, 1973.
45. Godeau C, Frances C, Hornebeck D et al: Isolation and partial characterization of an elastase-type protease in human vulva fibroblasts: its possible involvement in vulvar elastic tissue destruction of patient with lichen sclerosus et atrophicus, *J Invest Dermatol* 78:270, 1982.
46. de Oliveira M, Saleiro V: Involucrin expression in vulvar lesions, *J Reprod Med* 31:828, 1986.
47. Hendricks JB, Wilkinson EJ et al: Ki-67 expression in lichen sclerosus of the vulva. 1994. (Unpublished.)
48. Kaufman RH, Friedrich EG Jr, Gardner HL: *Benign diseases of the vulva and vagina.* St. Louis, 1990, Mosby. 1990.
49. Dalziel KL, Mallard R, Wojnarowska F: The treatment of vulvar lichen sclerosus with very potent topical steroid (clobetasol propionate 0.05%) cream, *Br J Dermatol* 124:461, 1991.
50. Friedrich EG Jr: Vulvar vestibulitis syndrome, *J Reprod Med* 32:110, 1987.
51. McKay M, Frankman O, Horowitz B et al: Vulvar vestibulitis and vestibular papillomatosis. Report of the ISSVD Committee on vulvodynia, *J Reprod Med* 36:413, 1991.
52. Ridley CM: *The vulva,* Philadelphia, 1975, Saunders.
53. Rodke G, Friedrich EG Jr, Wilkinson EJ: Malignant potential of mixed vulvar dystrophy (lichen sclerosis associated with squamous cell hyperplasia), *J Reprod Med* 33:545, 1988.
54. Newton JA, Camplejohn RS, McGibbon DH: A flow cytometric study of the significance of DNA aneuploidy in cutaneous lesions, *Br J Dermatol* 117:169, 1987.
55. Robboy SJ, Ross JS, Prat J et al: Urogenital sinus origin of mucinous and ciliated cysts of the vulva, *Obstet Gynecol* 51:347, 1978.
56. Junard TA, Thomas SM: Cysts of the vulva and vagina: a comparative study, *Int J Gynecol Obstet* 19:239, 1981.
57. Kucera PR, Glazer J: Hydrocele of the canal of Nuck: a report of four cases, *J Reprod Med* 30:439, 1985.
58. García JJ, Verkauf BS, Hochberg CJ, Ingram JM: Aberrant breast tissue of the vulva: a case report and review of the literature, *Obstet Gynecol* 52:225, 1978.
59. Floushee JH, Pruitt AB Jr: Vulvar fibroadenoma from aberrant breast tissue: report of 2 cases, *Obstet Gynecol* 29:819, 1967.
60. O'Hara MF, Page DL: Adenoma of the breast and ectopic breast under lactational influences, *Hum Pathol* 16:707, 1985.
61. Rickert RR: Intraductal papilloma arising in supernumerary vulvar breast tissue, *Obstet Gynecol* 55:84, 1980.
62. Marwah S, Bergman ML: Ectopic salivary gland in the vulva (choristoma): report of a case and review of the literature, *Obstet Gynecol* 56:398, 1980.
63. Basta A, Madej JG Jr: Hydradenoma of the vulva: incidence and clinical observations, *Eur J Gynecol Oncol* 11:185, 1990.
64. Lowell DM, LiVolsi VA, Ludwig ME: Genital condyloma virus infection following pelvic radiation therapy: report of seven cases, *Int J Gynecol Pathol* 2:294, 1983.
65. von Krogh G: Warts: immunologic factors of prognostic significance, *Int J Dermatol* 18:195, 1979.
66. Walker PG, Colley NV, Grubb C et al: Abnormalities of the uterine cervix in women with vulvar warts: a preliminary communication, *Br J Vener Dis* 59:120, 1983.
67. Majmudar B, Hallden C: Juvenile laryngeal papillomatosis and maternal condyloma, *Lab Invest* 52:40A, 1985.
68. Kovi J, Tillman RL, Lee SM: Malignant transformation of condyloma acuminatum: a light microscopic and ultrastructural study, *Am J Clin Pathol* 61:702, 1974.
69. Bergeron C, Nayhashfar A, Canaan C et al: Human papillomavirus type 16 in intraepithelial neoplasia (Bowenoid papulosis) and coexistent invasive carcinoma of the vulva, *Int J Gynecol Pathol* 6:1, 1987.
70. Gissmann L, deVillers EM, zur Hausen H: Analysis of human warts (condylomata acuminata) and other genital tumors for human papilloma virus type 6 DNA, *Int J Cancer* 29:143, 1982.
71. Gissmann L, Wolnik L, Ikenberg H et al: Human *Papillomavirus* types 6 and 11 DNA sequences in genital and laryngeal papillomas and in some cervical cancers, *Proc Natl Acad Sci* 80:560, 1983.
72. Oriel JD, Almeida JD: Demonstration of virus particles in human genital warts, *Br J Vener Dis* 46:37, 1970.
73. Oriel JD: Natural history of genital warts, *Br J Vener Dis* 47:1, 1971.
74. Nadji M, Ganjei P, Penneys NS, Morales AR: Immunohistochemistry of vulvar neoplasms: a brief review, *Int J Gynecol Pathol* 3:41, 1984.

75. Wolber RA, Talerman A, Wilkinson EJ, Clement PB: Vulvar granular cell tumors with pseudocarcinomatous hyperplasia: a comparative analysis with well-differentiated squamous carcinoma, *Int J Gynecol Pathol* 10:59, 1991.
76. Majmudar B, Castellano PZ, Wilson RW, Siegel RJ: Granular cell tumors of the vulva, *J Reprod Med* 35:1008, 1990.
77. Robertson AJ, McIntosh W, Lamont P, Guthrie W: Malignant granular cell tumor (myoblastoma) of the vulva: report of a case and review of the literature, *Histopathology* 5:69, 1981.
78. Mucitelli DR, Charles EZ, Kraus FT: Vulvovaginal polyps: histologic appearance, ultrastructure, immunocytochemical characteristics and clinicopathologic correlations, *Int J Gynecol Pathol* 9:20, 1990.
79. Östör AG, Fortune D, Riley CB: Fibroepithelial polyps with atypical stromal cells (pseudosarcoma botryoides) of vulva and vagina: a report of 13 cases, *Int J Gynecol Pathol* 7:351, 1988.
80. Steeper T, Rosai J: Aggressive angiomyxoma of the female pelvis and perineum: report of nine cases, *Am J Surg Pathol* 7:463, 1983.
81. Bëgin LR, Clement PB, Kirk ME et al: Aggressive angiomyxoma of pelvic soft parts: a clinicopathologic study of nine cases, *Hum Pathol* 16:621, 1985.
82. Tavassoli FA, Norris HJ: Smooth muscle tumors of the vulva, *Obstet Gynecol* 53:213, 1979.
83. Kaufman RH, Gardner HL: Intra-epithelial carcinoma of the vulva, *Clin Obstet Gynecol* 8:1035, 1965.
84. Fu YS, Reagan JW, Townsend DE et al: Nuclear DNA study of vulvar intraepithelial and invasive squamous neoplasms, *Obstet Gynecol* 57:643, 1981.
85. Wilkinson EJ, Fiedrich EG Jr, Fu YS: Multicentric nature of vulvar carcinoma in situ, *Obstet Gynecol* 58:69, 1981.
86. Friedrich EG Jr, Wilkinson EJ, Fu YS: Carcinoma in situ of the vulva: a continuing challenge, *Am J Obstet Gynecol* 136:830, 1980.
87. Crum CP, Liskow A, Petras P et al: Vulvar intraepithelial neoplasia (severe atypia and carcinoma in situ), *Cancer* 54:1429, 1984.
88. Powell LC, Dinh TV, Rajaraman S et al: Carcinoma in situ of the vulva: a clinicopathologic study of 50 cases, *J Reprod Med* 31:808, 1986.
89. Wilkinson EJ: Vulvar intraepithelial neoplasia and squamous cell carcinoma with emphasis on new nomenclature. In Damjanov I, Cohen A, Mills SE, et al, editors: *Progress in reproductive and urinary tract pathology,* vol 2. Philadelphia, 1990, Field & Wood.
90. Buscema J, Naghashfar Z, Sawada E et al: The predominance of human papillomavirus type 16 in vulvar neoplasia, *Obstet Gynecol* 71:601, 1988.
91. Buscema J, Woodruff JD, Parmley TH et al: Carcinoma in situ of the vulva, *Obstet Gynecol* 55:225, 1980.
92. Jones I, Buntine D: Progression of vulvar carcinoma in situ, *Aust NZ J Obstet Gynaecol* 18:274, 1978.
93. Esquius J, Brisigotti M, Matías-Guiu X, Prat J: Keratin expression in normal vulva, non-neoplastic epithelial disorders, vulvar intraepithelial neoplasia, and invasive squamous cell carcinoma, *Int J Gynecol Pathol* 10:341, 1991.
94. Crum CP, Braun LA, Shah KV et al: Vulvar intraepithelial neoplasia: correlation of nuclear DNA content and the presence of a human papilloma virus (HPV) structural antigen, *Cancer* 49:468, 1982.
95. Wade TR, Kopf AW, Ackerman AB: Bowenoid papulosis of the genitalia, *Arch Dermatol* 115:306, 1979.
96. Ulbright TM, Stehman FB, Roth LM et al: Bowenoid dysplasia of the vulva, *Cancer* 50:2910, 1982.
97. Aiba S, Rokugo M, Tagami H: Immunohistologic analysis of the phenomenon of spontaneous regression of numerous flat warts, *Cancer* 58:1246, 1986.
98. De Villez RL, Stevens CS: Bowenoid papules of the genitalia: a case progressing to Bowen's disease, *J Am Acad Dermatol* 3:149, 1980.
99. Twiggs L, Okagaki T, Clark B et al: A clinical, histopathologic, and molecular biologic investigation of vulvar intraepithelial neoplasia, *Int J Gynecol Pathol* 7:48, 1988.
100. Michael H, Roth LM: Congenital and acquired cysts, benign and malignant skin adnexal tumors, and Paget's disease of the vulva. In Wilkinson EJ, editor: *Contemporary issues in surgical pathology: pathology of the vulva and vagina,* New York, 1987, Churchill Livingstone.
101. Olson DJ, Fujimura M, Swanson P, Okagaki T: Immunohistochemical features of Paget's disease of the vulva with and without adenocarcinoma, *Int J Gynecol Pathol* 10:285, 1991.
102. Mazoujian G, Pinkus GS, Haagensen DE Jr: Extramammary Paget's disease: evidence for apocrine origin, *Am J Surg Pathol* 8:43, 1984.
103. Roth LM, Lee SC, Ehrlich CE: Paget's disease of the vulva: a histogenetic study of five cases including ultrastructural observations and review of the literature, *Am J Surg Pathol* 1:193, 1977.
104. Hart WR, Millman JB: Progression of intraepithelial Paget's disease of the vulva to invasive carcinoma, *Cancer* 40:2333, 1977.
105. Wharton JT, Gallager S, Rutledge FN: Microinvasive carcinoma of the vulva, *Am J Obstet Gynecol* 118:159, 1974.
106. Barnes AE, Crissman JD, Schellhas HF et al: Microinvasive carcinoma of the vulva: a clinicopathologic evaluation, *Obstet Gynecol* 56:234, 1980.
107. Wilkinson EJ: Superficial invasive carcinoma of the vulva, *Clin Obstet Gynecol* 28:188, 1985.
108. Wilkinson EJ: Superficially invasive carcinoma of the vulva. In Wilkinson EJ, editor: *Contemporary issues in surgical pathology: pathology of the vulva and vagina.* New York, 1987, Churchill Livingstone.
109. Wilkinson EJ, Rico MJ, Pierson KK: Microinvasive carcinoma of the vulva, *Int J Gynecol Pathol* 11:29, 1982.
110. Sedlis A, Homesley H, Bundy BN et al: Positive groin lymph node in superficial squamous cell vulvar cancer, *Am J Obstet Gynecol* 156:1159, 1987.
111. Kneale BL: Microinvasive cancer of the vulva: report of the International Society for the Study of Vulvar Disease Task Force, *J Reprod Med* 29:454, 1983.
112. Dvoretsky PM, Bonfiglio T, Helmkamp F et al: The pathology of superficially invasive, thin vulvar squamous cell carcinoma, *Int J Gynecol Pathol* 3:331, 1984.
113. Hoffman JS, Kumar NB, Morley GW: Microinvasive squamous cell carcinoma of the vulva: search for a definition, *Obstet Gynecol* 61:615, 1983.
114. Stehman FB, Bundy BN, Dvoretsky PM, Creasman WT: Early stage I carcinoma of the vulva treated with ipsilateral superficial inguinal lymphadenectomy and modified radical hemivulvectomy: a prospective study of the Gynecologic Oncology Group, *Obstet Gynecol* 79:490, 1992.
115. Kurman RJ, Toki T, Schiffman MH: Basaloid and warty carcinomas of the vulva: Distinctive types of squamous cell carcinoma frequently associated with HPV, *Am J Surg Pathol* 17:133, 1993.
116. Toki T, Kurman RJ, Park JS et al: Probable nonpapillomavirus etiology of squamous cell carcinoma of the vulva in older women: a clinicopathologic study using in situ hybridization and polymerase chain reaction, *Int J Gynecol Pathol* 10:107, 1991.
117. Crum CP: Carcinoma of the vulva: epidemiology and pathogenesis, *Obstet Gynecol* 79:448, 1992.
118. Hart WR, Norris HJ, Helwig EB: Relation of lichen sclerosus et atrophicus of the vulva to development of carcinoma, *Obstet Gynecol* 45:369, 1975.
119. Mabuchi K, Bross DS, Kessler II: Epidemiology of cancer of the vulva: a case control study, *Cancer* 55:1843, 1985.
120. Caterson RJ, Furber J, Murray J, et al: Carcinoma of the vulva in two young renal allograft recipients, *Transplant Proc* 16:559, 1984.
121. Newcomb PA, Weiss NS, Daling JR: Incidence of vulvar carcinoma in relation to menstrual, reproductive and medical factors, *J Natl Cancer Inst* 73:391, 1981.
122. Scheffner M, Werness BA, Huibregtse JM et al: The E6 oncoprotein encoded by human papillomavirus types 16 and 18 promotes the degradation of p53, *Cell* 63:1129, 1990.
123. Werness BA, Levine AJ, Howley PM: Association of human papillomavirus type 16 and 18 E6 proteins with p53, *Science* 248:76, 1990.
124. Lee YY, Wilczynski SP, Chumakov A et al: Carcinoma of the vulva: HPV and p53 mutations, *Oncogene* 9:1655, 1994.
125. Donaldson ES, Powell DE, Hanson MB, van Nagell JR: Prognostic parameters in invasive vulvar cancer, *Gynecol Oncol* 11:184, 1981.
126. Curry SL, Wharton JT, Rutledge F: Positive lymph nodes in vulvar squamous carcinoma, *Gynecol Oncol* 9:63, 1980.
127. Morley GW: Cancer of the vulva: a review, *Cancer* 48:597, 1981.

128. Jafari K, Castnick EN: Microinvasive squamous cell carcinoma of the vulva, *Gynecol Oncol* 4:158, 1976.
129. Iversen T, Abeler V, Aalders J: Individualized treatment of stage I carcinoma of the vulva, *Obstet Gynecol* 57:85, 1981.
130. Iversen T, Aalders JG, Christensen A, Kalstad P: Squamous cell carcinoma of the vulva: a review of 424 patients, 1956-1974, *Gynecol Oncol* 9:271, 1980.
131. Hacker NF, Berek JS, Lagasse LD et al: Individualization of treatment for stage I squamous cell vulvar carcinoma, *Obstet Gynecol* 63:155, 1984.
132. FIGO news: annual report on the results of treatment in gynecological cancer, *Int J Gynecol Obstet* 28:189, 1989.
133. Sedlis A, Homesley H, Bundy BN et al. Positive groin lymph nodes in superficial squamous cell vulvar cancer (a Gynecologic Oncology Group study), *Am J Obstet Gynecol* 156:1159, 1987.
134. Way S, Benedet JL: Involvement of inguinal lymph nodes in carcinoma of the vulva: a comparison of clinical assessment with histological examination, *Gynecol Oncol* 1:119, 1973.
135. Sedlis A, Homesley H, Marshall R, Bundy BN: Evaluating risk factors for vulvar cancer, *Contemp Obstet Gynecol* 67:74, 1988.
136. Kraus FT, Pérez-Mesa C: Verrucous carcinoma: a clinical and pathologic study of 105 cases involving oral cavity, larynx, and genitalia, *Cancer* 19:26, 1966.
137. Isaacs JH: Verrucous carcinoma of the female genital tract, *Gynecol Oncol* 4:259, 1976.
138. Brisigotti M, Moreno A, Murcia C et al: Verrucous carcinoma of the vulva: a clinicopathologic and immunohistochemical study of five cases, *Int J Gynecol Pathol* 8:1, 1989.
139. Leuchter RS, Hacker NF, Voet RL et al: Primary carcinoma of the Bartholin gland: a report of 14 cases and review of the literature, *Obstet Gynecol* 60:361, 1982.
140. Wheelock JB, Goplerud DR, Dunn LJ, Oates JF: Primary carcinoma of the Bartholin gland: a report of ten cases, *Obstet Gynecol* 63:820, 1984.
141. Benda JA, Platz CE, Anderson B: Malignant melanoma of the vulva: a clinical-pathologic review of 16 cases, *Int J Gynecol Pathol* 5:202, 1986.
142. Chung AF, Woodruff JM, Lewis JL Jr: Malignant melanoma of the vulva: a report of 44 cases, *Obstet Gynecol* 45:638, 1975.
143. Podratz KC, Gaffey TA, Symmonds RE et al: Melanoma of the vulva: an update, *Gynecol Oncol* 16:153, 1983.
144. Johnson TL, Kumar NB, White CD, Morley GW: Prognostic features of vulvar melanoma: a clinicopathologic analysis, *Int J Gynecol Pathol* 5:110, 1986.
145. Mazur MT, Hsueh S, Gersell DJ: Metastases to the female genital tract: analysis of 325 cases, *Cancer* 53:1978, 1984.
146. Cohen R, Margolius KA, Guidoszi F: Non gynaecological metastases to the vulva and vagina, *S Afr Med J* 6:159, 1988.
147. Di Saia PJ, Rutledge R, Smith JP: Sarcoma of the vulva: report of 12 patients, *Obstet Gynecol* 38:180, 1971.
148. Perrone T, Swanson PE, Twiggs L et al: Malignant rhabdoid tumor of the vulva: is distinction from epithelioid sarcoma possible? A pathologic and immunohistochemical study, *Am J Surg Pathol* 13:848, 1989.
149. Cruz-Jiménez PR, Abell MR: Cutaneous basal cell carcinoma of the vulva, *Cancer* 36:1860, 1975.
150. Dudley AG, Young RH, Lawrence WD, Scully RE: Endodermal sinus tumor of the vulva in an infant, *Obstet Gynecol* 61:76s, 1983.

Vagina

151. Gardner HL, Kaufman RH: *Benign diseases of the vulva and vagina*. St. Louis, 1969, Mosby.
152. Wagner JP: Toxic shock syndrome: a review, *Am J Obstet Gynecol* 146:93, 1983.
153. Pradham S, Tobon H: Vaginal cysts: a clinicopathological study of 41 cases, *Int J Gynecol Pathol* 5:35, 1986.
154. Robboy SJ, Welch WR. Selected topics in the pathology of the vagina, *Hum Pathol* 22:868, 1991.
155. Friedrich EG, Wilkinson EJ: Mucous cysts of the vulvar vestibule, *Obstet Gynecol* 42:407, 1973.
156. Mascasaet MA, Lu T, Nelson JH: Ureterovaginal fistula as a complication of radical pelvic surgery, *Am J Obstet Gynecol* 124:757, 1976.
157. Norris HJ, Taylor HB: Polyps of the vagina: a benign lesion resembling sarcoma botryoides, *Cancer* 19:227, 1966.
158. Chirayil SJ, Tobon H: Polyps of the vagina: a clinicopathological study of 18 cases, *Cancer* 47:2904, 1981.
159. Miettinen M, Wahlström T, Vesterinen E, Saksela E: Vaginal polyps with pseudosarcomatous features: a clinicopathologic study of seven cases, *Cancer* 51:1148, 1983.
160. Mitchell M, Talerman A, Sholl J et al: Pseudosarcoma botryoides in pregnancy: report of case with ultrastructural observations, *Obstet Gynecol* 70:522, 1987.
161. Hartmann CA, Sperling M, Stein H: So-called fibroepithelial polyps of the vagina exhibiting an unusual but uniform antigen profile characterized by expression of desmin and steroid hormone receptors but no muscle-specific actin or macrophage markers, *Am J Clin Pathol* 93:604, 1990.
162. Elliott GB, Elliott JDA: Superficial stromal reactions of lower genital tract, *Arch Pathol* 95:100, 1973.
163. Ulbright TM, Alexander RW, Kraus FT: Intramural papilloma of the vagina, *Cancer* 48:2260, 1981.
164. Tavassoli FA, Norris HJ: Smooth muscle tumors of the vagina, *Obstet Gynecol* 53:689, 1979.
165. Sirota RL, Dickersin GR, Scully RE: Mixed tumor of the vagina. A clinicopathological analysis of eight cases, *Am J Surg Pathol* 5:413, 1981.
166. Chen KTK: Benign mixed tumor of the vagina, *Obstet Gynecol* 57:89s, 1981.
167. Branton PA, Tavassoli FA: Spindled cell epithelioma, the so-called mixed tumor of the vagina: a clinicopathologic, immunohistochemical, and ultrastructural analysis of 28 cases, *Am J Surg Pathol* 17:509, 1993.
168. Wright RG, Buntine DW, Forber KL: Recurrent benign mixed tumor of the vagina, *Gynecol Oncol* 40:84, 1991.
169. Silverberg SG, Frable WJ: Prolapse of fallopian tube into vaginal vault after hysterectomy, *Arch Pathol* 97:100, 1974.
170. Scully RE, Robboy SJ, Herbst AL: Vaginal and cervical abnormalities, including clear cell adenocarcinoma, related to prenatal exposure to diethylstilbestrol, *Am Clin Lab Sci* 4:222, 1974.
171. Kaufman RH, Adam E, Binder GL, Gerthoffer E: Upper genital tract changes and pregnancy outcome in offspring exposed in utero to diethylstilbestrol, *Am J Obstet Gynecol* 137:299, 1980.
172. Robboy SJ, Kaufman RH, Prat J et al: Pathologic findings in young women enrolled in national cooperative diethylstilbestrol adenosis (DESAD) project, *Obstet Gynecol* 53:309, 1979.
173. Taguchi O, Cunha GR, Robboy SJ: Experimental study of the effect of diethylstilbestrol (DES) on the development of the human female reproductive tract, *Biol Res Pregnancy Perinatol* 4:56, 1983.
174. Herbst AL, Green TH Jr, Ulfelder H: Primary carcinoma of the vagina: an analysis of 68 cases, *Am J Obstet Gynecol* 106:210, 1970.
175. Herbst AL, Robboy SJ, Scully RE, Poskanzer DC: Clear cell adenocarcinoma of the vagina and cervix in girls: analysis of 170 registry cases, *Am J Obstet Gynecol* 119:713, 1974.
176. Herbst AL: Vaginal clear cell cancer: incidence, survival and screening. In *Long-term effects of exposure to diethylstilbestrol (DES),* NIH Workshop, April 22-24, 1992, Falls Church, Va., p119.
177. Dickersin GR, Welch WR, Erlandson R, Robboy SJ: Ultrastructure of 16 cases of clear cell adenocarcinoma of the vagina and cervix in DES-exposed young women, *Cancer* 45:1615, 1980.
178. Robboy SJ, Welch WR, Young RH et al: Topographic relation of adenosis, clear cell adenocarcinoma and other related lesions of the vagina and cervix in DES-exposed progeny, *Obstet Gynecol* 60:546, 1982.
179. Robboy SJ, Young RH, Welch WR et al: Atypical (dysplastic) adenosis: forerunner and transitional state to clear cell adenocarcinoma in young women exposed in utero to diethylstilbestrol, *Cancer* 54:869, 1984.
180. Robboy SJ, Welch WR: Microglandular hyperplasia in vaginal adenosis associated with oral contraceptives and prenatal diethylstilbestrol (DES) exposure, *Obstet Gynecol* 49:430, 1977.
181. Zaino RJ, Robboy SJ, Bentley R, Kurman RJ: Diseases of the vagina. In Kurman RJ, editor: *Blaustein's pathology of the female genital tract,* ed 4, New York, 1994, Springer-Verlag.

182. Burks RT, Schwarz AM, Wheeler JE, Antonioli D: Late recurrence of clear cell adenocarcinoma of the cervix: case report, *Obstet Gynecol* 76:525, 1990.
183. Benedet JL, Sanders BH: Carcinoma in situ of the vagina, *Am J Obstet Gynecol* 148:695, 1984.
184. Audet-Lapointe P, Body G, Vauclair R et al: Vaginal intraepithelial neoplasia, *Gynecol Oncol* 36:232, 1990.
185. Lenehan PM, Meffe F, Lickrish GM: Vaginal intraepithelial neoplasia: biologic aspects and management, *Obstet Gynecol* 68:333, 1986.
186. Nuovo GJ: Correlation of histology with human papillomavirus DNA detection in the female genital tract, *Gynecol Oncol* 31:176, 1988.
187. Nuovo GJ, Blanco JS, Silverstein SJ, Crum CP: Histologic correlates papillomavirus infection in the vagina, *Obstet Gynecol* 72:770, 1988.
188. Aho M, Vesterinen E, Meyer B et al: Natural history of vaginal intraepithelial neoplasia, *Cancer* 68:195, 1991.
189. Marcus RB, Million RR, Daly JW: Carcinoma of the vagina, *Cancer* 42:2507, 1978.
190. Houghton CRS, Iverson T: Squamous cell carcinoma of the vagina: a clinical study of the location of the tumor, *Gynecol Oncol* 13:365, 1982.
191. Rasmussen J, Diernaes E: Neoplasia in the vagina following hysterectomy for dysplasia or carcinoma in situ of the uterine cervix, *Acta Obstet Gynecol Scand* 62:437, 1983.
192. Peters WA, Kumar NB, Morley GW: Microinvasive carcinoma of the vagina: a distinct clinical entity? *Am J Obstet Gynecol* 153:505, 1985.
193. Gallup DG, Talledo E, Shah KJ, Hayes C: Invasive squamous cell carcinoma of the vagina: a 14-year study, *Obstet Gynecol* 69:782, 1987.
194. Steeper TA, Piscioli F, Rosai J: Squamous cell carcinoma with sarcoma-like stroma of the female genital tract: clinico-pathologic study of four cases, *Cancer* 52:890, 1983.
195. Beck I, Clayton JK: Vaginal carcinoma arising in vaginal condylomata: case report, *Br J Obstet Gynaecol* 91:503, 1984.
196. Punnonen R, Kallioniemi OP, Mattila J et al: Primary invasive and in situ vaginal carcinoma: flow cytometric analysis of DNA aneuploidy and cell proliferation from archival paraffin-embedded tissue, *Eur Obstet Gynecol Reprod Biol* 32:247, 1989.
197. Novak E, Woodruff JD, Novak ER: Probable mesonephric origin of certain female genital tumors, *Am J Obstet Gynecol* 68:1222, 1954.
198. Way S: Vaginal metastases of carcinoma of the body of the uterus, *J Obstet Gynaecol Brit Emp* 58:558, 1951.
199. Wright VC: Vaginal metastases of hypernephroma: case report and summary of world literature, *Can Med Assoc J* 100:816, 1969.
200. Shevchuk MM, Fenoglio CM, Lattes R et al: Malignant mixed tumor of the vagina probably arising in mesonephric rests, *Cancer* 42:214, 1978.
201. Clement PB, Benedet JL: Adenocarcinoma in situ of the vagina: a case report, *Cancer* 43:2479, 1979.
202. Cullimore JE, Luesley DM, Rollason TP et al: A case of glandular intraepithelial neoplasia involving the cervix and vagina, *Gynecol Oncol* 34:249, 1989.
203. Copeland LJ, Gershenson DM, Saul PB et al: Sarcoma botryoides of the female genital tract, *Obstet Gynecol* 66:262, 1985.
204. Daya D, Scully RE: Sarcoma botryoides of the cervix in young women: a clinicopathological study of 13 cases, *Gynecol Oncol* 29:290, 1988.
205. Young RH, Scully RE: Endodermal sinus tumor of the vagina: a report of nine cases and review of the literature, *Gynecol Oncol* 18:380, 1984.
206. Copeland LJ, Sneige N, Ordóñez NG et al: Endodermal sinus tumor of the vagina and cervix, *Cancer* 55:2558, 1985.
207. Berman MC, Tobon H, Surti U: Primary malignant melanoma of the vagina, *Am J Obstet Gynecol* 139:963, 1981.

Cervix

208. Graham CE: Uterine cervical epithelium of fetal and immature females in relation to estrogenic stimulation, *Am J Obstet Gynecol* 97:1033, 1967.
209. Taylor HB, Irey NS, Norris HJ: Atypical endocervical hyperplasia in women taking oral contraceptives, *JAMA* 202:637, 1967.
210. Kyriakos M, Kempson RL, Konikov NF: A clinical and pathologic study of endocervical lesions associated with oral contraceptives, *Cancer* 22:99, 1968.
211. Arias-Stella J: Atypical endometrial changes produced by chorionic tissue, *Hum Pathol* 3:450, 1972.
212. Worth AJ, Boyes DA: A case control study of the possible effects of birth control pills on pre-clinical carcinoma of the cervix, *J Obstet Gynaecol Br Commonw* 79:673, 1972.
213. Young RH, Scully RE: Atypical forms of microglandular hyperplasia of the cervix simulating carcinoma: a report of 5 cases and review of the literature, *Am J Surg Pathol* 13:50, 1989.
214. Young RH, Clement PB: Pseudoneoplastic glandular lesions of the uterine cervix, *Semin Diagn Pathol* 8:234, 1991.
215. Clement PB: Multinucleated stromal giant cells of the uterine cervix, *Arch Pathol Lab Med* 109:200, 1985.
216. Cachaza JA, Caballero JL, Fernández JA, Salido E: Endocervical polyp with pseudosarcomatous pattern and cytoplasmic inclusions: an electron microscopic study, *Am J Clin Pathol* 85:633, 1986.
217. Sherrick JC, Vega JG: Congenital intramural cysts of uterus, *Obstet Gynecol* 19:486, 1962.
218. Ferry JA, Scully RE: Mesonephric remnants, hyperplasia, and neoplasia in the uterine cervix, *Am J Surg Pathol* 14:1100, 1990.
219. Clement PB, Young RH, Scully RE: Mesonephric carcinomas and carcinosarcomas of the uterine cervix. (In preparation.)
220. Roth E, Taylor HB: Heterotopic cartilage in the uterus, *Obstet Gynecol* 27:838, 1966.
221. Ceremsak RJ: Benign rhabdomyoma of the vagina, *Am J Clin Pathol* 52:604, 1969.
222. Ayers LR, Drosman S, Saltzstein SL: Iatrogenic paracervical implantation of fetal tissue during therapeutic abortion: a case report, *Obstet Gynecol* 37:755, 1971.
223. Coppleson M, Pixley E, Reid B: *Colposcopy: a scientific and practical approach to the cervix in health and disease,* Springfield, Ill., 1971, Charles C Thomas, Publisher.
224. Willis RA: *The borderland of embryology and pathology.* ed 2, Washington, D.C., 1962, Butterworth.
225. Watson AA, Cochran AJ: Sebaceous glands of the cervix uteri and buccal mucosa, *J Pathol Bacteriol* 98:87, 1969.
226. Kaufman RH, Gardner HL, Rawls WE et al: Clinical features of herpes genitalis, *Cancer Res* 33:1446, 1973.
227. Naib ZM, Nahmias AJ, Josey WE, Zaki SA: Relation of cytohistopathology of genital herpesvirus infection to cervical anaplasia, *Cancer Res* 33:1452, 1973.
228. Paavonen J, Meyer B, Vesterinen E, Saksela E: Colposcopic and histological findings in cervical chlamydial infection, *Lancet* 2:320, 1980.
229. Crum CP, Mitao M, Winkler B et al: Localizing chlamydial infection in cervical biopsies with the immunoperoxidase technique, *Int J Gynecol Pathol* 3:191, 1984.
230. Cohen C: Three cases of amoebiasis of the cervix uteri, *J Obstet Gynaecol Br Commonw* 80:476, 1973.
231. Berry A: A cytopathological and histopathological study of bilharziasis of the female genital tract, *J Pathol Bacteriol* 91:325, 1966.
232. Reid R, Laverty CR, Coppleson M et al: Noncondylomatous cervical wart virus infection, *Obstet Gynecol* 55:476, 1980.
233. Meisels A, Fortin R, Roy M: Condylomatous lesions of the cervix. II. Cytologic, colposcopic, and histopathologic study, *Acta Cytol* 21:379, 1977.
234. Gupta J, Gendelman HE, Naghashfar Z et al: Specific identification of human papillomavirus type in cervical smears and paraffin sections by in situ hybridization with radioactive probes, *Int J Gynecol Pathol* 4:211, 1985.
235. Crum CP, Mitao M, Levine RU, Silverstein S: Cervical papillomaviruses segregate within morphologically distinct precancerous lesions, *J Virol* 54:675, 1985.
236. Crum CP, Nagi N, Levine RU, Silverstein S: In situ hybridization analysis of HPV 16 DNA sequences in early cervical neoplasia, *Am J Pathol* 123:174, 1986.
237. Margall N, Matías-Guiu X, Chillón M et al: Detection of human papillomavirus 16 and 18 DNA in epithelial lesions of the lower genital tract by *in situ* hybridization and polymerase chain reaction. Cervical scrapes are not substitutes for biopsies, *J Clin Microbiol* 31:924, 1993.
238. Mazur MT: Atypical polypoid adenomyomas of the endometrium, *Am J Surg Pathol* 5:473, 1981.

239. Janovski NA, Kasdon EJ: Benign mesonephric papillary and polypoid tumors of the cervix in childhood, *J Pediatr* 63:211, 1963.
240. Bettinger HF, Reagan JW: Proceedings of the International Committee on Histologic Terminology for lesions of the Uterine Cervix. In Wied GL, editor: *Proceedings of the First International Congress of Exfoliative Cytology,* Philadelphia, 1962, Lippincott.
241. Richart RM: Cervical intraepithelial neoplasia: a review, *Pathol Annu* 8:301, 1973.
242. Sadeghi SB, Sadeghi A, Robboy SJ: Prevalence of dysplasia and cancer of the cervix in a nation wide, planned parenthood population, *Cancer* 61:2359, 1988.
243. zur Hausen H: Human papillomaviruses and their possible role in squamous cell carcinomas, *Curr Top Microbiol Immunol* 78:1, 1977.
244. National Cancer Institute Workshop Report. The 1988 Bethesda system for reporting cervical/vaginal cytologic diagnoses, *JAMA* 262:931, 1989.
245. Fu YS, Braun L, Shah KV et al: Histologic, nuclear DNA and human papillomavirus study of cervical condylomas, *Cancer* 52:1705, 1989.
246. Fu YS, Huang I, Beaudenon S et al: Correlative study of human papillomavirus DNA, histopathology and morphology in cervical condyloma and intraepithelial neoplasia, *Int J Gynecol Pathol* 7:297, 1988.
247. Richart RM: A modified terminology for cervical intraepithelial neoplasia, *Obstet Gynecol* 75:131, 1990.
248. Herbst AL: The Bethesda system for cervical/vaginal cytologic diagnoses: a note of caution, *Obstet Gynecol* 76:449 1990.
249. Brinton LA: Epidemiology of cervical cancer—an overview. In Muñoz N, Bosch FX, Shah K, Meheus A, (editors), *The epidemiology of cervical cancer and human papillomavirus,* Lyon, 1992, IARC Scientific Publication.
250. Gram IT, Austin H, Stalsberg H: Cigarette smoking and the incidence of cervical intraepithelial neoplasia, grade III, and cancer of the cervix, *Am J Epidemiol* 135:341, 1992.
251. Gram IT, Macaluso M, Stalsberg H: Oral contraceptive use and the incidence of cervical intraepithelial neoplasia, *Am J Obstet Gynecol* 167:40, 1992.
252. Hildesheim A, Mann V, Brinton LA et al: Herpes simplex virus type 2: a possible interaction with human papillomavirus types 16/18 in the development of invasive cervical cancer, *Int J Cancer* 49:335, 1991.
253. Jones CJ, Brinton LA, Hamman RF et al: Risk factors for in situ cervical cancer: results from a case-control study. *Cancer Res* 50:3657, 1990.
254. La Vecchia C, Franceschi S, DeCarli A et al: Sexual factors, venereal diseases, and the risk of intraepithelial and invasive cervical neoplasia, *Cancer* 58:935, 1986.
255. zur Hausen H: Human papillomaviruses in the pathogenesis of anogenital cancer, *Virology* 184:9, 1991.
256. Kessler II: Etiologic concepts of cervical carcinogenesis, *Gynecol Oncol* 12 (suppl):7, 1981.
257. Ambros RA, Kurman RJ: Current concepts in the relationship of human papilloma virus infection to the pathogenesis and classification of precancerous lesions of the uterine cervix, *Semin Diagn Pathol* 7:158, 1990.
258. Woodworth CD, Bowden PE, Doniger J et al: Characterization of normal human exocervical epithelial cells immortalized in vitro by papillomavirus types 16 and 18 DNA, *Cancer Res* 48:4620, 1988.
259. Iwasaka T, Yokoyama M, Hayashi Y, Sugimori H: Combined herpes simplex virus type 2 and human papillomavirus type 16 or 18 deoxyribonucleic acid leads to oncogenic transformation, *Am J Obstet Gynecol* 150:1251, 1988.
260. Banks L, Crawford L: Analysis of human *Papillomavirus* type 16 polypeptides in transformed primary cells, *Virology* 165:326, 1988.
261. Dyson N, Howley PM, Munger K, Harlow E: The human papillomavirus 16 E7 oncoprotein is able to bind to the retinoblastoma gene product, *Science* 243:934, 1989.
262. Mietz JA, Unger T, Huibregtse JM, Howley PM: The transcriptional transactivation function of wild-type-p53 is inhibited by SV40 large T-antigen and by HPV-16 E6 oncoprotein, *EMBO J* 11:5013, 1992.
263. Chanen W, Hollyock VE: Colposcopy and the conservative management of cervical dysplasia and carcinoma in situ, *Obstet Gynecol* 43:527, 1974.
264. Richart RM, Barron BA: A follow-up study of patients with cervical dysplasia, *Am J Obstet Gynecol* 105:386, 1969.
265. Kinlen LJ, Spriggs AL: Women with positive cervical smears but without surgical intervention, *Lancet* 2:463, 1978.
266. Sorensen HM, Petersen O, Nielson J et al: The spontaneous course of premalignant lesions on the vaginal portion of the uterus, *Acta Obstet Gynecol Scand* 43(suppl 7):103, 1964.
267. Green GH, Donovan JW: Natural history of carcinoma in situ of the cervix, *J Obstet Gynaecol Br Commonw* 77:1, 1970.
268. Selim MA, So-Bosita J, Neuman MR: Carcinoma in situ of cervix uteri, *Surg Gynecol Obstet* 139:697, 1974.
269. Knapp RC, Feldman GB: The problem of optimal management of cervical carcinoma in situ, *Clin Obstet Gynecol* 13:889, 1970.
270. Kolstad P, Kelm V: Long term follow up of 1121 cases of carcinoma in situ, *Obstet Gynecol* 48:125, 1976.
271. Love RR, Camilli AE: The value of screening, *Cancer* 48:489, 1981.
272. Boyes DA, Worth AJ, Fidler HK: The results of treatment of 4389 cases of pre-clinical cervical squamous carcinoma, *J Obstet Gynaecol Br Commonw* 77:769, 1970.
273. Christopherson WM, Scott MA: Trends in mortality from uterine cancer in relation to mass screening, *Acta Cytol* 21:5, 1977.
274. McIndoe WA, McLean MR, Jones RW, Mullins PR: The invasive potential of carcinoma in situ of the cervix, *Obstet Gynecol* 64:451, 1984.
275. Koutsky LA, Holmes KK, Critchlow CW et al: A cohort study of the risk of cervical intraepithelial neoplasia grade 2 or 3 in relation to papillomavirus infection, *N Engl J Med* 327:1272, 1992.
276. Nangle R, Berger M, Levin M: Variations in the morphogenesis of squamous carcinoma of the cervix, *Cancer* 16:1151, 1963.
277. Abell MR: Invasive carcinomas of the cervix. In Norris HJ, Hertig AT, Abell MR, editors: *The uterus,* Baltimore, 1973, Williams & Wilkins.
278. Qizilbasch AH: In situ and microinvasive adenocarcinoma of the uterine cervix: a clinical, cytologic, and histologic study of 14 cases, *Am J Clin Pathol* 64:155, 1975.
279. Christopherson WM, Nealon N, Gray LA Sr: Noninvasive precursor lesions of adenocarcinoma and mixed adenosquamous carcinoma of the cervix uteri, *Cancer* 44:975, 1979.
280. Jaworski RC: Endocervical glandular dysplasia, adenocarcinoma in situ, and early invasive (microinvasive) adenocarcinoma of the uterine cervix. In Clement PB, Young RH, guest editors: Pathology of the uterine cervix, *Semin Diagn Pathol* 7:190, 1990.
281. Alejo M, Macedo I, Matías-Guiu X, Prat J: Adenocarcinoma in situ of the uterine cervix: clinicopathological study of 9 cases with detection of human papilloma virus DNA by in situ hybridization and the polymerase chain reaction, *Int J Gynecol Pathol* 12:219, 1993.
282. Burghardt E, Girardi F, Lahouser M et al: Microinvasive carcinoma of the uterine cervix (International Federation of Gynecology and Obstetrics stage IA), *Cancer* 67:1037, 1991.
283. Kolstad P, Abeler V, Iverson T et al: Microinvasive carcinoma of the cervix: definition and treatment problems, *Clin Oncol* 1:335, 1982.
284. Silverberg E, Lubera JA: *Cancer statistics,* CA, 38:5, 1988.
285. Benda JA: Pathology of cervical carcinoma and its prognostic implications, *Semin Oncol* 21:3, 1994.
286. Ng ABP, Atkin NB: Histological cell type and DNA value in the prognosis of squamous cell cancer of the uterine cervix, *Br J Cancer* 28:322, 1973.
287. Abell MR, Gosling JRG: Gland cell carcinoma (adenocarcinoma) of the uterine cervix, *Am J Obstet Gynecol* 83:729, 1962.
288. Badib AO, Kurohara SS, Webster JH, Pickren JW: Metastasis to organs in carcinoma of the uterine cervix, *Cancer* 21:434, 1968.
289. Paunier JO, Delclos L, Fletcher GH: Causes, time of death, and sites of failure in squamous cell carcinoma of the uterine cervix on intact uterus, *Radiology* 88:555, 1967.
290. Miles PA, Norris HJ: Adenoid cystic carcinoma of the cervix: an analysis of 12 cases, *Obstet Gynecol* 38:103, 1971.
291. Ferry JA, Scully RE: "Adenoid cystic" carcinoma and adenoid basal carcinoma of the uterine cervix, *Am J Surg Pathol* 12:134, 1988.
292. Silverberg SG, Hurt GW: Minimal deviation adenocarcinoma ("adenoma malignum") of the cervix: a reappraisal, *Am J Obstet Gyneol* 121:971, 1975.
293. Michael H, Grawe L, Kraus FT: Minimal deviation endocervical adenocarcinoma: clinical and histologic features, immunohistological staining for

carcinoembryonic antigen, and differentiation from confusing benign lesions, *Int J Gynecol Pathol* 3:261, 1984.
294. Young RH, Scully RE: Villoglandular papillary adenocarcinoma of the uterine cervix, *Cancer* 63:1773, 1989.
295. Jones MW, Silverberg SG, Kurman RJ: Well differentiated villoglandular adenocarcinoma of the uterine cervix: a clinicopathological study of 24 cases, *Int J Gynecol Pathol* 12:1, 1993.
296. Abell MR, Ramírez JA: Sarcomas and carcinosarcomas of the uterine cervix, *Cancer* 31:1176, 1973.
297. Albores-Saavedra J, Larrazo O, Poucell S, Martínez HAR: Carcinoid of the uterine cervix, *Cancer* 38:2328, 1976.
298. Jones HW III, Plymate S, Gluck FB et al: Small cell non-keratinizing carcinoma of the cervix associated with ACTH productions, *Cancer* 38:1629, 1976.
299. Hall DJ, Schneider V, Gopelrud DR: Primary malignant melanoma of the uterine cervix, *Obstet Gynecol* 56:525, 1980.
300. Brand E, Berek JS, Nieberg RK, Hacker NF: Rhabdomyosarcoma of the cervix: sarcoma botryoides, *Cancer* 60:1552, 1987.
301. LeMoine NR, Hall PA: Epithelial tumors metastatic to the cervix, *Cancer* 57:2002, 1986.

Endometrium

302. Hendrickson MR, Kempson RL: Uterus and fallopian tubes. In Sternberg SS, editor: *Histology for pathologists,* New York, 1992, Raven Press.
303. Dabbs DJ, Geisinger KR, Norris HT: Intermediate filaments in endometrial and endocervical carcinomas: the diagnostic utility of vimentin patterns, *Am J Surg Pathol* 10:568, 1986.
304. Katzenellenbogen BS: Dynamics of steroid hormone receptor action, *Annu Rev Physiol* 42:17, 1980.
305. Taketani Y, Masahiko M: Evidence for direct regulation of epidermal growth factor receptors by steroid hormones in human endometrial cells, *Hum Reprod* 6:1365, 1991.
306. Ferenczy A: Anatomy and histology of the uterine corpus. In Kurman RJ, editor: *Blaustein's pathology of the female genital tract,* ed 4, New York, 1994, Springer-Verlag.
307. Noyes RW: Normal phases of the endometrium. In Norris HJ, Hertig AT, Abell MR, editors: *The uterus,* Baltimore, 1973, Williams & Wilkins.
308. More IAR, Armstrong EM, McSeveney D, Chatfield WR: The morphogenesis and fate of the nucleolar channel system in the human endometrial glandular cells, *J Ultrastruct Res* 47:74, 1974.
309. Wilkinson N, Buckley CH, Chawner L, Fox H: Nucleolar organiser regions in normal, hyperplastic and neoplastic endometrium, *Int J Gynecol Pathol* 9:55, 1990.
310. Ferenczy A: Regeneration of the human endometrium. In Fenoglio CM, Wolff M, editors: *Progress in surgical pathology,* vol 1, New York, 1980, Masson Publishing.
311. Smith SK, Abel MH, Baird DT: Effect of 17 β-estradiol and progesterone on the levels of prostaglandin $F_{2\alpha}$ and E_2 in human endometrium, *Prostaglandins* 27:591, 1984.
312. Bulmer JN, Sunderland CA: Bone-marrow origin of endometrial granulocytes in the early human placental bed, *J Reprod Immunol* 5:383, 1983.
313. Press MF, King WJ: Distribution of peroxidase and granulocytes in the human uterus, *Lab Invest* 54:188, 1986.
314. Marshall RJ, Jones DB: An immunohistochemical study of lymphoid tissue in human endometrium, *Int J Gynecol Pathol* 7:225, 1988.
315. Kamat BR, Isaacson PG: The immunocytochemical distribution of leukocytic subpopulations in human endometrium, *Am J Pathol* 127:66, 1987.
316. Bulmer JN, Lunny DP, Hagin SV: Immunohistochemical characterization of stromal leucocytes in nonpregnant human endometrium, *Am J Reprod Immunol Microbiol* 17:83, 1988.
317. Silverberg SG, Arias-Stella J: Phenomenon in spontaneous and therapeutic abortion, *Am J Obstet Gynecol* 112:777, 1972.
318. Kjer JJ, Eldon K: The diagnostic value of the Arias-Stella phenomenon, *Zentralbl Gynäkol* 104:753, 1982.
319. Wagner D, Richart RM: Polyploidy in the human endometrium with the Arias-Stella reaction, *Arch Pathol* 85:475, 1968.
320. Speroff L, Glass RH, Kase NG: *Clinical gynecological endocrinology and infertility,* ed 4, Baltimore, 1989, Williams & Wilkins.
321. Silverberg SG, Makowski EL: Endometrial carcinoma in young women taking oral contraceptive agents, *Obstet Gynecol* 46:503, 1975.
322. Gottardis MM, Robinson SP, Satyaswaroop PG, Jordan VC: Contrasting actions of tamoxifen on endometrial and breast tumor growth in the athymic mouse, *Cancer Res* 48:812, 1988.
323. Fornander T, Rutqvist LE, Cedermark B et al: Adjuvant tamoxifen in early breast cancer: occurrence of new primary cancers, *Lancet* 1:117, 1989.
324. Seoud MA-F, Johns J, Weed JC Jr: Gynecologic tumors in tamoxifen-treated women with breast cancer, *Obstet Gynecol* 82:165, 1993.
325. Speroff L, Glass RH, Kase NG: *Clinical gynecological endocrinology and infertility,* ed 3, Baltimore, 1983, Williams & Wilkins.
326. Benda JA: Clomiphene's effect on endometrium in infertility, *Int J Gynecol Pathol* 11:273, 1992.
327. Deligdisch L: Effects of hormone therapy on the endometrium, *Mod Pathol* 6:94, 1993.
328. Jones GS: The luteal phase defect, *Fertil Steril* 27:351, 1976.
329. Andrews WC: Luteal phase defects, *Fertil Steril* 32:501, 1979.
330. Laatikainen T, Anderson B, Kärkkäinen J et al: Progestin receptor levels in endometria with delayed or incomplete secretory changes, *Obstet Gynecol* 62:592, 1983.
331. Hourihan HM, Sheppard BL, Bonnar J: The morphologic characteristics of menstrual hemostasis in patients with unexplained menorrhagia, *Int J Gynecol Pathol* 8:221, 1989.
332. Adelanto JM, Rees MRP, Lopez Bernal A, Turnbull AC: Increased uterine prostaglandin E receptors in menorrhagic women, *Br J Obstet Gynaecol* 99:162, 1988.
333. Greenwood SM, Moran JJ: Chronic endometritis: morphologic and clinical observations, *Obstet Gynecol* 58:176, 1981.
334. Paavonen J, Aine R, Teisala K et al: Comparison of endometrial biopsy and peritoneal fluid cytologic testing with laparoscopy in the diagnosis of acute pelvic inflammatory disease, *Am J Obstet Gynecol* 151:645, 1985.
335. Cadena D, Cavanzo FJ, Leone GL, Taylor HB: Chronic endometritis: a comparative clinicopathologic study, *Obstet Gynecol* 41:733, 1973.
336. Kiviat NB, Eschenbach DA, Paavonen JA et al: Endometrial histopathology in patients with culture-proved upper genital tract infection and laparoscopically diagnosed acute salpingitis, *Am J Surg Pathol* 14:167, 1990.
337. Nogales-Ortiz F, Tarancón I, Nogales FF Jr: The pathology of female genital tuberculosis: A 31-year study of 1436 cases, *Obstet Gynecol* 53:422, 1979.
338. Duncan DA, Varner RE, Mazur MT: Uterine herpes virus infection with multifocal necrotizing endometritis, *Hum Pathol* 20:1021, 1989.
339. Sayage L, Gunby R, Gonwa T, et al: Cytomegalovirus endometritis after liver transplantation, *Transplantation* 49:815, 1990.
340. Ledger WJ: *Infection in the female,* Philadelphia, 1977, Lea & Febiger.
341. Bhagavan BS, Gupta PK: Genital actinomycosis and intrauterine contraceptive devices, *Hum Pathol* 9:567, 1978.
342. Niebyl JR, Parmley TH, Spence MR, Woodruff JD: Unilateral ovarian abscess associated with the intrauterine device, *Obstet Gynecol* 52:165, 1978.
343. Poropatich C, Rojas M, Silverberg SG: Polymorphonuclear leukocytes in the endometrium during the normal menstrual cycle, *Int J Gynecol Pathol* 6:230, 1987.
344. Staros EB, Shilkitus WF: Atypical polypoid adenomyoma with carcinoma transformation: a case report, *Surg Pathol* 4:157, 1991.
345. Scully RE: Atypical hyperplasia and carcinoma of the endometrium. *Pathology: postgraduate course in gynecologic and obstetric pathology with clinical correlation,* syllabus, Boston, 1992, Harvard Medical School.
346. Hendrickson MR, Kempson RL: Endometrial epithelial metaplasias—proliferations frequently misdiagnosed as adenocarcinoma: report of 89 cases and proposed classification, *Am J Surg Pathol* 4:525, 1980.
347. Crum CP, Richart RM, Fenoglio CM: Adenoacanthosis of the endometrium: a clinicopathologic study in premenopausal women, *Am J Surg Pathol* 5:15, 1981.
348. Blaustein A: Morular metaplasia misdiagnosed as adenoacanthoma in young women with polycystic ovarian disease, *Am J Surg Pathol* 6:223, 1982.
349. Lauchlan S: Metaplasias and neoplasias of Müllerian epithelium, *Histopathology* 8:543, 1984.

350. Hendrickson M, Kempson R: Ciliated carcinoma: a variant of endometrial adenocarcinoma: a report of 10 cases, *Int J Gynecol Pathol* 2:1, 1983.
351. Demopoulos R, Greco M: Mucinous metaplasia of the endometrium: ultrastructural and histochemical characteristics, *Int J Gynecol Pathol* 1:383, 1983.
352. Zaman S, Mazur M: Endometrial papillary syncytial change: A nonspecific alteration associated with active breakdown, *Am J Clin Pathol* 99:741, 1993.
353. Welch WR, Scully RE: Precancerous lesions of the endometrium, *Hum Pathol* 8:503, 1977.
354. Kurman RJ, Kaminski PF, Norris HJ: The behavior of endometrial hyperplasia: a long term study of "untreated" hyperplasia in 170 patients, *Cancer* 56:403, 1985.
355. Ferenczy A, Gelfand M: The biologic significance of cytologic atypia in progestogen-treated endometrial hyperplasia, *Am J Obstet Gynecol* 160:126, 1989.
356. Scully RE, Poulson H, Sobin L: Histological typing of the female genital tract tumors, Berlin, 1994, Springer-Verlag.
357. Tavassoli F, Kraus FT: Endometrial lesions in uteri resected for atypical endometrial hyperplasia, *Am J Clin Pathol* 70:770, 1978.
358. Kurman RJ, Norris HJ: Evaluation of criteria for distinguishing atypical endometrial hyperplasia from well differentiated carcinoma, *Cancer* 49:2547, 1982.
359. Chamlian DL, Taylor HB: Endometrial hyperplasia in young women, *Obstet Gynecol* 36:659, 1970.
360. Vellios F: Endometrial hyperplasias, precursors of endometrial carcinoma, *Pathol Annu* 7:201, 1972.
361. Hendrickson MR, Ross J, Kempson RL: Toward the development of morphologic criteria for well-differentiated adenocarcinoma of the endometrium, *Am J Surg Pathol* 7:819, 1983.
362. American Cancer Society: Cancer statistics, *CA* 41:1, 1991.
363. Parazzini F, La Vecchia C, Bocciolone L, Franceschi S: The epidemiology of endometrial cancer, *Gynecol Oncol* 41:1, 1991.
364. Gusberg SB: Editorial: The rise and fall of endometrial cancer, *Gynecol Oncol* 35:124, 1989.
365. Walker AM, Jick H: Declining rates of endometrial cancer, *Obstet Gynecol* 56:733, 1980.
366. Bokhman JV: Two pathogenetic types of endometrial carcinoma, *Gynecol Oncol* 15:10,1983.
367. Doering DL, Barnhill DR, Weiser EB et al: Intraoperative evaluation of depth of myometrial invasion in Stage I endometrial adenocarcinoma, *Obstet Gynecol* 74:930, 1989.
368. Fanning J, Tsukada Y, Piver MS: Intraoperative frozen section diagnosis of depth of myometrial invasion in endometrial adenocarcinoma, *Gynecol Oncol* 37:47, 1990.
369. Goff BA, Rice LW: Assessment of depth of myometrial invasion in endometrial adenocarcinoma, *Gynecol Oncol* 38:46, 1990.
370. Connelly PJ, Alberhasky RC, Christopherson WM: Carcinoma of the endometrium. III. Analysis of 865 cases of adenocarcinoma and adenoacanthoma, *Obstet Gynecol* 59:569, 1982.
371. Eifel P, Ross J, Hendrickson M et al: Adenocarcinoma of the endometrium: analysis of 262 cases with disease limited to the uterine corpus: treatment comparisons, *Cancer* 52:1026, 1983.
372. Hendrickson M, Ross J, Eifel PJ et al: Adenocarcinoma of the endometrium: analysis of 256 cases with carcinoma limited to the uterine corpus: pathology review and analysis of prognostic variables, *Gynecol Oncol* 13:373, 1982.
373. Abeler VM, Kjørstad KE: Endometrial adenocarcinoma with squamous cell differentiation, *Cancer* 69:488, 1992.
374. Alberhasky RC, Connelly PJ, Christopherson WM: Carcinoma of the endometrium. IV. Mixed adenosquamous carcinoma: a clinical-pathological study of 68 cases with long-term follow-up, *Am J Clin Pathol* 77:655, 1982.
375. Ng ABP, Reagan JW, Storaasli JP, Wentz MB: Mixed adenosquamous carcinoma of the endometrium, *Am J Clin Pathol* 59:765, 1973.
376. Kim K-R, Scully RE: Peritoneal keratin granulomas with carcinomas of endometrium and ovary and atypical polypoid adenomyoma of endometrium, *Am J Surg Pathol* 14:925, 1990.
377. Ross JC, Eifel PJ, Cox RS et al: Primary mucinous adenocarcinoma of the endometrium: a clinicopathologic and histochemical study, *Am J Surg Pathol* 7:715, 1983.
378. Hendrickson MR, Ross J, Eifel P et al: Uterine papillary serous carcinoma: a highly malignant form of endometrial adenocarcinoma, *Am J Surg Pathol* 6:93, 1982.
379. Sasano H, Comerford J, Wilkinson DS et al: Serous papillary adenocarcinoma of the endometrium: analysis of proto-oncogene amplification, flow cytometry, estrogen and progesterone receptors, and immunohistochemistry, *Cancer* 65:1545, 1990.
380. Prat J, Oliva E, Lerma E et al: Uterine papillary serous adenocarcinoma: a 10-case study of p53 and c-*erb*B-2 expression and DNA content, *Cancer* 74:1778, 1994.
381. Christopherson WM, Alberhasky RC, Connelly PJ: Carcinoma of the endometrium. I. A clinicopathological study of clear cell carcinoma and secretory carcinoma, *Cancer* 49:1511, 1982.
382. Kurman RJ, Scully RE: Clear cell carcinoma of the endometrium: an analysis of 21 cases, *Cancer* 37:872, 1976.
383. Silverberg SG, DiGeorgi LS: Clear cell carcinoma of the endometrium, *Cancer* 31:1127, 1973.
384. Bibro MC, Kapp DS, LiVolsi VA, Schwartz PE: Case report: squamous carcinoma of the endometrium with ultrastructural observations and review of the literature, *Gynecol Oncol* 10:217, 1980.
385. Huntsman DG, Clement PB, Gilks CB, Scully RE: Small-cell carcinoma of the endometrium: a clinicopathological study of sixteen cases, *Am J Surg Pathol* 18:364, 1994.
386. Creasman WT: Announcement, FIGO stages: 1988 revisions, *Gynecol Oncol* 35:125, 1989.
387. Morrow CP, Bundy BN, Kurman RJ et al: Relationship between surgical-pathological risk factors and outcome in clinical stage I and II carcinoma of the endometrium: a Gynecologic Oncology Group study, *Gynecol Oncol* 40:55, 1991
388. Ambros RA, Kurman RJ: Combined assessment of vascular and myometrial invasion as a model to predict prognosis in Stage I endometrioid adenocarcinoma of the uterine corpus, *Cancer* 69:1424, 1992.
389. Creasman WT, Soper JT, McCarty KS Jr et al: Influence of cytoplasmic steroid receptor content on prognosis of early stage endometrial carcinoma, *Am J Obstet Gynecol* 151:922, 1985.
390. Palmer DC, Muir IM, Alexander AI et al: The prognostic importance of steroid receptors in endometrial carcinoma, *Obstet Gynecol* 72:388, 1988.
391. Van Dam PA, Watson JV, Lowe DG, Shepherd JH: Flow cytometric DNA analysis in gynecological oncology, *Int J Gynecol Cancer* 2:57, 1992.
392. Stendahl U, Strang P, Wagenius G et al: Prognostic significance of proliferation in endometrial adenocarcinomas: a multivariate analysis of clinical and flow cytometric variables, *Int J Gynecol Pathol* 10:271, 1991.
393. Enomoto T, Inoue M, Perantoni AO et al: K-*ras* activation in neoplasms of the human female reproductive tract, *Cancer Res* 50:6139, 1990.
394. Enomoto T, Fujita M, Inoue M et al: Alterations of the p53 tumor suppressor gene and its association with activation of the c-K-*ras*-2 protooncogene in premalignant and malignant lesions of the human uterine endometrium, *Cancer Res* 51:5308, 1991.
395. Bur ME, Perlman C, Edelmann L et al: p53 expression in neoplasms of the uterine corpus, *Am J Clin Pathol* 98:81, 1992.
396. Kohler MF, Berchuck A, Davidoff AM et al: Overexpression and mutation of p53 in endometrial carcinoma, *Cancer Res* 52:1622, 1992.
397. Berchuck A, Rodrigues G, Kinney RB et al: Overexpression of HER-2/*neu* in endometrial cancer is associated with advanced stage disease, *Am J Obstet Gynecol* 164:15, 1991.
398. Norris HJ, Taylor HB: Mesenchymal tumors of the uterus. I. A clinical and pathological study of 53 endometrial stromal tumors, *Cancer* 19:755, 1966.
399. Lloreta J, Prat J: Endometrial stromal nodule with smooth and skeletal muscle components simulating stromal sarcoma, *Int J Gynecol Pathol* 11:293, 1992.
400. Clement PB, Scully RE: Uterine tumors resembling ovarian sex-cord tumors: a clinicopathologic analysis of fourteen cases, *Am J Clin Pathol* 66:512, 1976.

401. Evans HL: Endometrial stromal sarcoma and poorly differentiated endometrial sarcoma, *Cancer* 50:2170, 1982.
402. Chang KL, Crabtree GS, Lim-Tan SK et al: Primary uterine endometrial stromal neoplasms: a clinicopathologic study of 117 cases, *Am J Surg Pathol* 14:415, 1990.
403. Kempson RL, Hendrickson MR: Pure mesenchymal neoplasms of the uterine corpus: selected problems, *Semin Diagn Pathol* 5:172, 1988.
404. Thatcher SS, Woodruff JD: Uterine stromatosis: a report of 33 cases, *Obstet Gynecol* 59:428, 1982.
405. Katz K, Merino MJ, Sakamoto H, Schwartz PE: Endometrial stromal sarcoma: a clinicopathologic study of 11 cases with determination of estrogen and progestin receptor levels in three tumors, *Gynecol Oncol* 26:87, 1987.
406. Ulbright TM, Kraus FT: Endometrial stromal tumors of extra-uterine tissue, *Am J Clin Pathol* 76:371, 1981.
407. Norris HJ, Roth E, Taylor HB: Mesenchymal tumors of the uterus. II. A clinical and pathological study of 31 mixed mesodermal tumors, *Obstet Gynecol* 28:57, 1966.
408. Clement PB, Scully RE: Uterine tumors with mixed epithelial and mesenchymal elements, *Semin Diagn Pathol* 5:199, 1988.
409. Bitterman P, Chun B, Kurman RJ: The significance of epithelial differentiation in mixed mesodermal tumors of the uterus: a clinicopathologic and immunohistochemical study, *Am J Surg Pathol* 14:317, 1990.
410. Silverberg SG, Major FJ, Blessing JA et al: Carcinosarcoma (malignant mixed mesodermal tumor) of the uterus: a gynecologic oncology group pathologic study of 203 cases, *Int J Gynecol Pathol* 9:1, 1990.
411. Barwick KW, LiVolsi VS: Malignant mixed müllerian tumors of the uterus: a clinicopathologic assessment of 34 cases, *Am J Surg Pathol* 3:125, 1979.
412. Perez CA, Askin F, Baglan RJ et al: Effects of radiation on mixed müllerian tumors of the uterus, *Cancer* 43:1274, 1979.
413. Clement PB, Scully RE: Mullerian adenosarcomas of the uterus: a clinicopathologic analysis of 100 cases with a review of the literature, *Hum Pathol* 21:363, 1990.
414. Zaloudek CJ, Norris HJ: Adenofibroma and adenosarcoma of the uterus: a clinicopathologic study of 35 cases, *Cancer* 48:354, 1981.
415. Clement PB, Scully RE: Mullerian adenofibroma of the uterus with invasion of myometrium and pelvic veins, *Int J Gynecol Pathol* 9:363, 1990.
416. Klaer W, Holm-Jensen S: Metastases to the uterus, *Acta Pathol Microbiol Scand* 80:835, 1972.
417. Prat J, Matías-Guiu X, Barreto J: Simultaneous carcinoma involving the endometrium and the ovary: a clinicopathological, immunohistochemical and DNA flow cytometric study of 18 cases, *Cancer* 68:2455, 1991.
418. Chorlton I, Karnei RF Jr, King FM, Norris HJ: Primary malignant reticuloendothelial disease involving the vagina, cervix, and corpus uteri, *Obstet Gynecol* 44:735, 1974.
419. Harris NL, Scully RE: Malignant lymphoma and granulocytic sarcoma of the uterus and vagina: a clinicopathologic analysis of 27 cases, *Cancer* 53:2530, 1984.
420. Emge LA: The elusive adenomyosis of the uterus: its historical past and its present state of recognition, *Am J Obstet Gynecol* 83:1541, 1962.
421. Marcus CC: Relationship of adenomyosis uteri to endometrial hyperplasia and endometrial carcinoma, *Am J Obstet Gynecol* 82:408, 1961.
422. Adamson GD: Treatment of uterine fibroids: current findings with gonadotropin releasing hormone agonist, *Am J Obstet Gynecol* 166:746, 1992.
423. Fletcher JA: Chromosome aberrations in uterine smooth muscle tumors: potential diagnostic relevance and cytogenetic instability, *Cancer Res* 50:4092, 1990.
424. Paranjothy D, Vaish SK: Polycythemia associated with leiomyoma of the uterus, *J Obstet Gynaecol Br Commonw* 74:603, 1967.
425. Rothman D, Rennard M: Myoma erythrocytosis syndrome: report of a case, *Obstet Gynecol* 21:102, 1963.
426. Zaloudek CJ, Norris HJ: Mesenchymal tumors of the uterus. In Fenoglio CM, Wolff M, editors: *Progress in surgical pathology,* vol 3, New York, 1981, Masson Publishing.
427. Evans HL, Chawla SP, Simpson C, Finn KP: Smooth muscle tumors of the uterus other than ordinary leiomyoma: a study of 46 cases, with emphasis on diagnostic criteria and prognostic factors, *Cancer* 62:2239, 1988.
428. Fechner RE: Atypical leiomyomas and synthetic progestin therapy, *Am J Clin Pathol* 49:697, 1968.
429. Stout AP: Bizarre smooth muscle tumors of the stomach, *Cancer* 15:400, 1962.
430. Kurman RJ, Norris HJ: Mesenchymal tumors of the uterus. VI. Epithelioid smooth muscle tumors including leiomyoblastoma and clear-cell leiomyoma: a clinical and pathological analysis of 26 cases, *Cancer* 37:1853, 1976.
431. Parmley TH, Woodruff JD, Winn K et al: Histogenesis of leiomyomatosis peritonealis disseminata (disseminated fibrosing deciduosis), *Obstet Gynecol* 46:511, 1975.
432. Tavassoli FA, Norris HJ: Peritoneal leiomyomatosis (leiomyomatosis peritonealis disseminata): a clinicopathologic study of 20 cases with ultrastructural observations, *Int J Gynecol Pathol* 1:59, 1982.
433. Tench WD, Dail D, Gmelich JT, Matani N: Benign metastasizing leiomyomas: a review of 21 cases (Abstract), *Lab Invest* 38:37, 1978.
434. Wolff M, Silva F, Kaye G: Pulmonary metastases (with admixed epithelial elements) from smooth muscle neoplasms, *Am J Surg Pathol* 3:325, 1979.
435. Rigaud C, Bogomoletz W: Leiomyomatosis in pelvic lymph node, *Arch Pathol Lab Med* 107:153, 1983.
436. Boyce CR, Buddhdev HN: Pregnancy complicated by metastasizing leiomyoma of the uterus, *Obstet Gynecol* 42:252, 1973.
437. Cramer SF, Meyer JS, Kraner JF et al: Metastasizing leiomyoma of the uterus: S-phase, fraction, estrogen receptor, and ultrastructure, *Cancer* 45:932, 1980.
438. Banner AS, Carrington CB, Emory WB et al: Efficacy of oophorectomy in lymphangiomyomatosis and benign metastasizing leiomyoma, *N Engl J Med* 305:204, 1981.
439. Norris HJ, Parmley T: Mesenchymal tumors of the uterus. V. Intravenous leiomyomatosis: a report of 14 cases, *Cancer* 36:2164, 1975.
440. Clement PB: Intravenous leiomyomatosis, *Pathol Annu* 23:153, 1988.
441. Clement PB, Young RH, Scully RE: Intravenous leiomyomatosis of the uterus: a clinicopathologic analysis of 16 cases with unusual histologic features, *Am J Surg Pathol* 12:932, 1988.
442. Perrone T, Dehner LP: Prognostically favorable "mitotically active" smooth-muscle tumors of the uterus: a clinicopathologic study of 10 cases, *Am J Surg Pathol* 12:1, 1988.
443. O'Connor DM, Norris HJ: Mitotically active leiomyomas of the uterus, *Hum Pathol* 21:223, 1990.
444. Prayson RA, Hart WR: Mitotically active leiomyomas of the uterus, *Am J Clin Pathol* 97:14, 1992.
445. Tiltman AJ: The effect of progestins on the mitotic activity of uterine fibromyomas, *Int J Gynecol Pathol* 4:89, 1985.
446. Kawaguchi K, Fujii S, Konishi I et al: Mitotic activity in uterine leiomyomas during the menstrual cycle, *Am J Obstet Gynecol* 160:637, 1989.
447. Leibsohn S, d'Ablaing G, Mischell DR Jr, Schlaerth JB: Leiomyosarcoma in a series of hysterectomies performed for presumed uterine leiomyomas, *Am J Obstet Gynecol* 162:968, 1990.
448. Taylor HB, Norris HJ: Mesenchymal tumors of the uterus. IV. Diagnosis and prognosis of leiomyosarcomas, *Arch Pathol* 82:40, 1966.
449. Christopherson WM, Williamson EO, Gray LA: Leiomyosarcoma of the uterus, *Cancer* 29:1512, 1972.
450. Bell SW, Kempson RL, Hendrickson MR: Problematic uterine smooth muscle neoplasms: a clinicopathologic study of 213 cases, *Am J Surg Pathol* 18:535, 1994.
451. Barlow JJ, Piver MS, Chuang JT et al: Adriamycin and bleomycin, alone and in combination, in gynecologic cancers, *Cancer* 32:735, 1973.
452. Malmström H, Schmidt H, Persson PG et al: Flow cytometric analysis of uterine sarcoma: ploidy and S-phase rate as prognostic indicators, *Gynecol Oncol* 44:172, 1992.
453. Peters WA III, Howard DR, Andersen WA, Figge DC: Deoxyribonucleic acid analysis by flow cytometry of uterine leiomyosarcomas and smooth muscle tumors of uncertain malignant potential, *Am J Obstet Gynecol* 166:1646, 1992.
454. Christensen C: Adenomatoid tumors of the uterus, *Eur J Gynecol Oncol* 11:85, 1190.
455. Quigley JC, Hart WR: Adenomatoid tumors of the uterus, *Am J Clin Pathol* 76:627, 1981.

456. Youngs LA, Taylor HB: Adenomatoid tumors of the uterus and fallopian tube, *Am J Clin Pathol* 48:537, 1967.
457. Suzuki T, Yoshida Y, Kaku T et al: Adenomatoid tumor of the uterus: ultrastructural, histochemical, and immunohistochemical analysis, *Arch Pathol Lab Med* 109:1049, 1985.
458. Daya D, Lukka H, Clement PB: Primitive neuroectodermal tumors of the uterus: a report of four cases, *Hum Pathol* 23:1120, 1992.
459. Hendrickson MR, Scheithauer BW: Primitive neuroectodermal tumor of the endometrium: report of two cases, one with electron microscopic observations, *Int J Gynecol Pathol* 5:249, 1986.

Fallopian tube

460. Washington AE, Johnson RE, Sanders LL Jr: *Chlamydia trachomatis* infections in the United States. What are they costing us? *JAMA* 257:2070, 1987.
461. Platt R, Rice PA, McCormack WM: Risk of acquiring gonorrhea and prevalence of abnormal adnexal findings among women recently exposed to gonorrhea, *JAMA* 250:3205, 1983.
462. Honoré LH: Pathology of the fallopian tube. In Fox H, editor: *Haines and Taylor's obstetrical and gynaecological pathology,* Churchill Edinburgh, 1987, Livingstone.
463. Friberg J, Confino E, Suarez M, Gleicher N: *Chlamydia trachomatis* attached to spermatozoa recovered from the peritoneal cavity of patients with salpingitis, *J Reprod Med* 32:120, 1987.
464. Keith LG, Berger GS, Edelman DA et al: On the causation of pelvic inflammatory disease, *Am J Obstet Gynecol* 149:215, 1984.
465. Pungetti D, Lenzi M, Muzzi Rossi P et al: *Chlamydia trachomatis,* pelvic inflammatory diseases and sterility, *Minerva Ginecol* 45:95, 1993.
466. Seidman JD, Oberer S, Bitterman P, Aisner SC: Pathogenesis of pseudoxanthomatous salpingiosis, *Mod Pathol* 6:53, 1993.
467. Jenkins S, Olive DL, Haney AF: Endometriosis: pathogenic implications of the anatomic distribution, *Obstet Gynecol* 67:335, 1986.
468. Olive DL, Schwartz LB: Endometriosis, *N Engl J Med* 328:1759, 1993.
469. Thomas ML, Rose DH: Salpingitis isthmica nodosa demonstrated by hysterosalpingography, *Acta Radiol* 14:295, 1973.
470. Stock RJ: Histopathology of fallopian tubes with recurrent tubal pregnancy, *Obstet Gynecol* 75:9, 1990.
471. Carson SA, Buster JE: Ectopic pregnancy, *N Engl J Med* 329:1174, 1993.
472. Rivlin ME, Meeks FR, Cowan BD, Bates GW: Persistent trophoblastic tissue following salpingostomy for unruptured ectopic pregnancy, *Fertil Steril* 43:323, 1985.
473. Frenkel Y, Oelsner G, Ben-Baruch G, Menczer J: Major surgical complications of laparoscopy, *Eur J Obstet Gynecol Reprod Biol* 12:107, 1981.
474. DeStefano F, Peterson HB, Layde PM, Rubin GL: Risk of ectopic pregnancy following tubal sterilization, *Obstet Gynecol* 60:326, 1982.
475. Peterson HB, DeStefano F, Greenspan JR, Ory JW: Mortality risk associated with tubal sterilization in United States hospitals, *Am J Obstet Gynecol* 143:125, 1982.
476. Vessey M, Huggins G, Lawless M et al: Tubal sterilization: findings in a large prospective study, *Br J Obstet Gynaecol* 90:203, 1983.
477. Wolf GC, Thompson NJ: Female sterilization and subsequent ectopic pregnancy, *Obstet Gynecol* 55:17, 1980.
478. Ferenczy A, Richart RM: *Female reproductive system: dynamics of scan and transmission electron microscopy,* New York, 1974, Wiley & Sons.
479. Kanbour AI, Burges F, Salazar H: Intramural adenofibroma of the fallopian tube: light and electron microscopy, *Cancer* 31:1433, 1973.
480. Keeny GL, Thrasher TV: Metaplastic papillary tumor of the fallopian tube: a case report with ultrastructure, *Int J Gynecol Pathol* 7:86, 1988.
481. Woodruff JD, Pauerstein CJ: *The fallopian tube,* Baltimore, 1969, Williams & Wilkins.
482. Mazzarella P, Okagaki T, Richart RM: Teratoma of the uterine tube: a case report and review of the literature, *Obstet Gynecol* 39:381, 1972.
483. Sweet RI, Selinger HE, McKay DG: Malignant teratoma of the uterine tube, *Obstet Gynecol* 45:553, 1975.
484. Yoonessi M: Carcinoma of the fallopian tube, *Obstet Gynecol Surv* 34:257, 1979.
485. Daya D, Young RH, Scully RE: Endometrioid carcinoma of the fallopian tube resembling an adnexal tumor of probable Wolffian origin: a report of six cases, *Int J Gynecol Pathol* 11:122, 1992.
486. Eddy GLL, Copeland LJ, Gershenson DM et al: Fallopian tube carcinoma, *Obstet Gynecol* 64:546, 1984.
487. Rosen A, Klein M, Lahousen M et al: Primary carcinoma of the fallopian tube—a retrospective analysis of 115 patients, *Br J Cancer* 68:605, 1993.
488. Weber AM, Hewett WF, Gajewski WH, Curry SL: Malignant mixed müllerian tumors of the fallopian tube, *Gynecol Oncol* 50:239, 1993.
489. Carlson JA, Ackerman BL, Wheeler JE: Malignant mixed müllerian tumor of the fallopian tube, *Cancer* 71:187, 1993.

Ovary

490. Clement PB: Ovary. In Sternberg SS, editor: *Histology for pathologists,* New York, 1992, Raven Press.
491. Baca M, Zamboni L: The fine structure of the human follicular oocyte, *J Ultrastruct Res* 19:354, 1967.
492. Ryan KJ, Petro Z, Kaiser J: Steroid formation by isolated and recombined ovarian granulosa and thecal cells, *J Clin Endocrinol* 28:355, 1968.
493. Behrman HR, Caldwell BV: Role of prostaglandins in reproduction. In Greep RO, editor: *Reproductive physiology: M.T.P. International Review of Science,* vol 8, Baltimore, 1974, University Park Press.
494. Keyes PL: Luteinizing hormone: action of the Graafian follicle in vitro, *Science* 164:846, 1969.
495. Shima K, Kitayama S, Nakano R: Gonadotropin binding sites in human ovarian follicles and corpora lutea during the menstrual cycle, *Obstet Gynecol* 69:800, 1987.
496. Adms EC, Hertig AT: Studies on the human corpus luteum. II. Observation on the ultrastructure of luteal cells during pregnancy, *J Cell Biol* 41:716, 1969.
497. LeMarie WJ, Conly PW, Moffett A et al: Function of the human corpus luteum during the puerperium: its maintenance by exogenous human chorionic gonadotropin, *Am J Obstet Gynecol* 110:612, 1971.
498. Erickson GF: Normal ovarian function, *Clin Obstet Gynecol* 21:31, 1978.
499. Centola GM: Structural changes: follicular development and hormonal requirements. In Serra GB, editor, *The ovary,* New York, 1983, Raven Press.
500. Rao CV: Receptors for gonadotropins in human ovaries. In *Recent advances in fertility research. Part A: Developments in reproductive endocrinology,* New York, 1982, Alan R Liss, p 123.
501. McNatty KP: Follicular determinants of corpus luteum function in the human ovary. In Channing CP, Marsh JM, Sadler WA, editors: *Ovarian follicular and corpus luteum function: advances in experimental medicine and biology,* vol 112, New York, 1978, Plenum Press.
502. McNatty KP: Cyclic changes in antral fluid hormone concentrations in humans, *Clin Endocrinol Metab* 7:577, 1978.
503. Weiss G, O'Byren EM, Steinetz BG: Relaxin: a product of the human corpus luteum of pregnancy, *Science* 194:948, 1976.
504. Schmidt CL, Black VH, Sarosi P, Weiss G: Progesterone and relaxin secretion in relation to the ultrastructure of human luteal cells in culture: effects of human chorionic gonadotropin, *Am J Obstet Gynecol* 155:1209, 1986.
505. Zondek LH, Zondek T: Leydig cells of the foetus and newborn in various complications of pregnancy, *Acta Obstet Gynaecol Scand* 46:392, 1967.
506. Koninckx PR, Brosens IA: The "gonadotropin-resistant ovary" syndrome as a cause of secondary amenorrhea and infertility, *Fertil Steril* 28:926, 1977.
507. Gloor E, Juillard E, Curchod A et al: Ovarian hypoplasia with follicular calcifications, *Am J Clin Pathol* 78:857, 1982.
508. Talbert LM, Raj MHG, Hammond MG et al: Endocrine and immunologic studies in a patient with resistant ovary syndrome, *Fertil Steril* 42:741, 1984.
509. Massachusetts General Hospital Case Records: Case 46-1986: Resistant-ovary syndrome, with hyalinization of preantral follicles, *N Engl J Med* 315:1336, 1986.
510. Biscotti CV, Hart WR, Lucas JG: Cystic ovarian enlargement resulting from autoimmune oophoritis, *Obstet Gynecol* 74:492, 1989.
511. Bannatyne P, Russell P, Shearman RP: Autoimmune oophoritis: a clinicopathologic assessment of 12 cases, *Int J Gynecol Pathol* 9:191, 1990.
512. Lonsdale RN, Roberts PF, Trowell JE: Autoimmune oophoritis associated with polycystic ovaries, *Histopathology* 19:77, 1991.

513. Mulligan RM: A survey of epithelial inclusions in the ovarian cortex of 470 patients, *J Surg Oncol* 8:61, 1976.
514. Scully RE: Ovary. In Henson DE, Albores-Saavedra J, editors: *The pathology of incipient neoplasia,* Philadelphia, 1986, Saunders.
515. Landrum B, Ogburn PL Jr, Feinberg S et al: Intrauterine aspiration of a large fetal ovarian cyst, *Obstet Gynecol* 68:11S, 1986.
516. Stevens ML, Plotka ED: Functional lutein cyst in a postmenopausal woman, *Obstet Gynecol* 50:27S, 1977.
517. Strickler RC, Kelly RW, Askin FB: Postmenopausal ovarian follicle cyst: an unusual case of estrogen excess, *Int J Gynecol Pathol* 3:318, 1984.
518. Kosloske AM, Goldthorn JF, Kaufman E et al: Treatment of precocious pseudopuberty associated with follicular cysts of the ovary, *Am J Dis Child* 138:147, 1984.
519. Piver MS, Williams LJ, Marcuse PM: Influence of luteal cysts on menstrual function, *Obstet Gynecol* 35:740, 1970.
520. Monteleone JA, Monteleone PL, Danis RK: Pseudoprecocious puberty associated with isolated follicle cyst of the ovary, *J Pediatr Surg* 8:949, 1973.
521. Danon M, Robboy SJ, Kim S et al: Cushing syndrome, sexual precocity and polyostotic fibrous dysplasia (Albright's syndrome) in infancy, *J Pediatr* 87:917, 1975.
522. Clement PB, Scully RE: Large solitary luteinized follicle cyst of pregnancy and puerperium, *Am J Surg Pathol* 4:431, 1980.
523. Futterweit W: *Polycystic ovarian disease,* New York, 1985, Springer-Verlag.
524. Biggs JSG: Polycystic ovarian disease—current concepts, *Aust NZ J Obstet Gynaecol* 21:26, 1981.
525. Yen SSC: The polycystic ovary syndrome, *Clin Endocrinol* 12:177, 1980.
526. Gallup DG, Stock RJ: Adenocarcinoma of the endometrium in women 40 years of age or younger, *Obstet Gynecol* 64:417, 1984.
527. Ramzy I, Nisker JA: Histologic study of ovaries from young women with endometrial adenocarcinoma, *Am J Clin Pathol* 71:253, 1979.
528. Green JA, Goldzieher JW: The polycystic ovary. IV. Light and electron microscope studies, *Am J Obstet Gynecol* 91:173, 1965.
529. Hughesdon PE: Morphology and morphogenesis of the Stein-Leventhal ovary and of so-called "hyperthecosis," *Obstet Gynecol Surv* 37:59, 1982.
530. Boss, JH, Scully RE, Wegner KH et al: Structural variations in the adult ovary—clinical significance, *Obstet Gynecol* 25:747, 1965.
531. Snowden JA, Harkin PJR, Thornton JG, Wells M: Morphometric assessment of ovarian stromal proliferation—a clinicopathological study, *Histopathology* 14:369, 1989.
532. Scully RE, Cohen RB: Oxidative-enzyme activity in normal and pathologic human ovaries, *Obstet Gynecol* 24:667, 1964.
533. Madeido G, Tieu TM, Aiman J: Atypical ovarian hyperthecosis in a virilized postmenopausal woman, *Am J Clin Pathol* 83:101, 1985.
534. Barbieri RL, Ryan KJ: Hyperandrogenism, insulin resistance, and acanthosis nigricans syndrome: a common endocrinopathy with distinct pathophysiologic features, *Am J Obstet Gynecol* 147:90, 1983.
535. Stearns HC, Sneeden VD, Fearl JD: A clinical and pathologic review of ovarian stromal hyperplasia and its possible relationship to common diseases of the female reproductive system, *Am J Obstet Gynecol* 119:375, 1974.
536. Judd HL, Scully RE, Herbst AL et al: Familial hyperthecosis: comparison of endocrinologic and histologic findings with polycystic ovarian disease, *Am J Obstet Gynecol* 117:976, 1973.
537. Nagamani M, Lingold JC, Gomez JR et al: Clinical and hormonal studies in hyperthecosis of the ovaries, *Fertil Steril* 36:326, 1981.
538. Kalstone CE, Jaffe RB, Abell MR: Massive edema of the ovary simulating fibroma, *Obstet Gynecol* 34:564, 1969.
539. Young RH, Scully RE: Fibromatosis and massive edema of the ovary, possibly related entities: a report of 14 cases of fibromatosis and 11 cases of massive edema, *Int J Gynecol Pathol* 3:153, 1984.
540. Hensleigh PA, Woodruff JD: Differential maternal-fetal reponse to androgenizing luteoma or hyperreactio luteinalis, *Obstet Gynecol Surv* 33:262, 1978.
541. Norris HJ, Taylor HB: Nodular theca-lutein hyperplasia of pregnancy (so-called "pregnancy luteoma"): a clinical and pathologic study of 15 cases, *Am J Clin Pathol* 47:557, 1967.
542. García-Buñuel R, Brandes D: Luteoma of pregnancy: ultrastructural features, *Hum Pathol* 7:205, 1976.
543. Malinak LR, Miller GV: Bilateral multicentric ovarian luteomas of pregnancy associated with masculinization of a female infant, *Am J Obstet Gynecol* 91:251, 1965.
544. Girouard DP, Barclay DL, Collins CG: Hyperreactio luteinalis: review of the literature and report of 2 cases, *Obstet Gynecol* 23:513, 1964.
545. Barad DH, Gimovsky ML, Petrie RH et al: Diagnosis and management of bilateral theca lutein cysts in a normal term pregnancy, *Diagn Gynecol Obstet* 3:27, 1981.
546. Wajda KJ, Lucas JG, Marsh WL: Hyperreactio luteinalis: benign disorder masquerading as an ovarian neoplasm, *Arch Pathol Lab Med* 113:921, 1989.
547. Haning RV Jr, Strawn EY, Nolten WE: Pathophysiology of the ovarian hyperstimulation syndrome, *Obstet Gynecol* 66:220, 1985.
548. Golan A, Ron-el R, Herman A et al: Ovarian hyperstimulation syndrome: an update review, *Obstet Gynecol Surv* 44:430, 1989.
549. Meldrum DR, Frumar AM, Shamonki IM et al: Ovarian and adrenal steroidogenesis in a virilized patient with gonadotropin-resistant ovaries and hilus cell hyperplasia, *Obstet Gynecol* 56:216, 1980.
550. Bersch W, Alexy E, Heuser HP et al: Ectopic decidua formation in the ovary (so-called deciduoma), *Virchows Arch [A] (Pathol Anat)* 360:173, 1973.
551. Herr JC, Heidger PM Jr, Scott JR et al: Decidual cells in the human ovary at term. I. Incidence, gross anatomy and ultrastructural features of merocrine secretion, *Am J Anat* 152:7, 1978.
552. Clement PB: Nonneoplastic lesions of the ovary. In Kurman RJ, editor: *Blaustein's pathology of the female genital tract,* ed 4, New York, 1994, Springer-Verlag.
553. Boring CC, Squires TS, Tong T: Cancer statistics, *CA Cancer J Clin* 43:7, 1993.
554. Cannistra SA: Cancer of the ovary, *N Engl J Med* 329:1550, 1993.
555. Hamilton TC: Ovarian cancer. Part I: Biology, *Curr Probl Cancer* 16:3, 1992.
556. Whittemore AS, Harris R, Ithyre J: Collaborative ovarian cancer group: characteristics relating to ovarian cancer risk: collaborative analysis on 12-case control studies. II. Invasive epithelial ovarian cancers in white women, *Am J Epidemiol* 136:1184, 1992.
557. Negri E, Franceschi S, Tzonou A: Pooled analysis of 3 European case-control studies. I. Reproductive factors and risk of epithelial ovarian cancer, *Int J Cancer* 49:50, 1991.
558. Lynch HT, Lynch JF: Hereditary ovarian carcinoma, *Hematol Oncol Clin North Am* 6:783, 1992.
559. Narod SA, Feunteun J, Lynch HT et al: Familial breast-ovarian cancer locus at chromosome 17q12-q23, *Lancet* 338:82, 1991.
560. Bell DA, Scully RE: Early de novo ovarian carcinoma: a study of 14 cases, *Cancer* 73:1859, 1994.
561. Berchuck A, Kohler MF, Bast RC Jr: Oncogenes in ovarian cancer, *Hematol Oncol Clin North Am* 6:813, 1992.
562. Sasano H, Garrett CT: Oncogenes in gynecological tumors, In *Curr Top Pathol* 85:357, 1992.
563. Berchuck A, Kamel A, Whitaker R et al: Overexpression of HER-2/*neu* is associated with poor survival in advanced epithelial ovarian cancer, *Cancer Res* 50:4087, 1990.
564. Slamon DJ, Godolphin W, Jones LA: Studies of the Her-2/*neu* protooncogene in human breast and ovarian cancer, *Science* 244:707, 1989.
565. Enomoto T, Weghorst CM, Inoue M et al: K-*ras* activation occurs frequently in mucinous adenocarcinomas and rarely in other common epithelial tumors of the human ovary, *Am J Pathol* 139:777, 1991.
566. Ichikawa Y, Nishida M, Suzuki H et al: Mutation of K-*ras* protooncogene is associated with histological subtypes in human mucinous ovarian tumors, *Cancer Res* 54:33, 1994.
567. Prat J, Cuatrecasas M, Matías-Guiu X et al: K-*ras* mutations in ovarian mucinous tumors, *Mod Pathol* 7:94A, 1994 (Abstr).
568. Marks JR, Davidoff AM, Kerns BJ et al: Overexpression and mutation of p53 in epithelial ovarian cancer, *Cancer Res* 51:2979, 1991.
569. Kohler MF, Kernes B-J M, Humphrey PA et al: Mutation and overexpression of p53 in early-stage ovarian cancer, *Obstet Gynecol* 81:643, 1993.
570. Frank TS, Bartos RE, Haefner HK et al: Loss of heterozygosity and overexpression of the p53 gene in ovarian carcinoma, *Mod Pathol* 7:3, 1994.

571. Hart WR: Ovarian epithelial tumors of borderline malignancy (carcinomas of low malignant potential), *Hum Pathol* 8:541, 1977.
572. Russell P: The pathological assessment of ovarian neoplasms. II: The proliferating "epithelial" tumours, *Pathology* 11:251, 1979.
573. Barnhill D, Heller P, Brzozowski P et al: Epithelial ovarian carcinoma of low malignant potential, *Obstet Gynaecol* 65:53, 1985.
574. Tasker M, Langley FA: The outlook for women with borderline epithelial tumours of the ovary, *Br J Obstet Gynaecol* 92:969, 1985.
575. Bostwick DG, Tazelaar HD, Ballon SC et al: Ovarian epithelial tumors of borderline malignancy: a clinical and pathologic study of 109 cases, *Cancer* 58:2052, 1986.
576. Padberg B-C, Arps H, Franke U et al: DNA cytophotometry and prognosis in ovarian tumors of borderline malignancy: a clinicomorphologic study of 80 cases, *Cancer* 69:2510, 1992.
577. De Nictolis M, Montironi R, Tommasoni S et al: Serous borderline tumors of the ovary: a clinicopathologic, immunohistochemical and quantitative study of 44 cases, *Cancer* 70:152, 1992.
578. Julian GC, Woodruff JD: The biological behavoir of low-grade papillary serous carcinoma of the ovary, *Obstet Gynecol* 40:860, 1972.
579. Tazelaar HD, Bostwick DG, Ballon SC et al: Conservative treatment of borderline ovarian tumors, *Obstet Gynecol* 66:417, 1985.
580. Finkler NJ, Kopnick SJ, Griffiths CT, Knapp RG: Elevated CA-125 serum levels in epithelial ovarian cancer metastatic to retroperitoneal lymph nodes, *Gynecol Oncol* 29:356, 1988.
581. Lavin PT, Knapp RC, Malkasian C et al: CA-125 for the monitoring of ovarian carcinoma during primary therapy, *Obstet Gynecol* 69:223, 1987.
582. Tavassoli FA: Serous tumor of low malignant potential with early stromal invasion (serous LMP with microinvasion), *Mod Pathol* 1:407, 1988.
583. Bell DA, Scully RE: Ovarian serous borderline tumors with stromal microinvasion: a reported of 21 cases, *Hum Pathol* 21:397, 1990.
584. McCaughey WTE, Kirk ME, Lester W, Dardick I: Peritoneal epithelial lesions associated with proliferative serous tumors of ovary, *Histopathology* 8:195, 1984.
585. Bell DA, Weinstock MA, Scully RE: Peritoneal implants of serous borderline tumors: histologic features and prognosis, *Cancer* 62:2212, 1988.
586. Bell DA, Scully RE: Serous borderline tumors of the peritoneum, *Am J Surg Pathol* 14:230, 1990.
587. Gilks CB, Bell DA, Scully RE: Serous psammocarcinoma of the ovary and peritoneum, *Int J Gynecol Pathol* 9:110, 1990.
588. Bollen ECM, Lamers CBHW, Jansen JMBJ et al: Zollinger-Ellison syndrome due to a gastrin-producing ovarian cystadenocarcinoma, *Br J Surg* 68:776, 1981.
589. Matson PN, Mackem SM, Norton JA et al: Ovarian carcinoma as a cause of Zollinger-Ellison syndrome: natural history secretory products, and response to provocative test, *Gastroenterology* 97:468, 1989.
590. Primrose JN, Maloney M, Wells M et al: Gastrin-producing ovarian mucinous cystadenomas: a cause of the Zollinger-Ellison syndrome, *Surgery* 104:830, 1988.
591. Fenoglio CM, Ferenczy A, Richart RM: Mucinous tumors of the ovary: ultrastructural studies of mucinous cystadenomas with histogenetic considerations, *Cancer* 36:1709, 1975.
592. Bell DA, Rutgers JL, Scully RE: Ovarian epithelial tumors of borderline malignancy. In Damjanov I, Cohen AH, Mills SE, Young RH, editors: *Progress in reproductive and urinary tract pathology,* vol 1, Philadelphia, 1989, Field & Wood.
593. Hart WR, Norris HJ: Borderline and malignant mucinous tumors of the ovary: histologic criteria and clinical behavior, *Cancer* 31:1031, 1973.
594. De Nictolis M, Montironi R, Tommasoni S et al: Benign, borderline and well-differentiated malignant intestinal mucinous tumors of the ovary: a clinicopathologic, histochemical, immunohistochemical and nuclear quantitative study of 57 cases, *Int J Gynecol Pathol* 13:10, 1994.
595. Young RH, Gilks CB, Scully RE: Mucinous tumors of the appendix associated with mucinous tumors of the ovary and pseudomyxoma peritonei: a clinicopathological analysis of 22 cases supporting an origin in the appendix, *Am J Surg Pathol* 15:415, 1991.
596. Rutgers JL, Scully RE: Ovarian müllerian mucinous papillary cystadenomas of borderline malignancy: a clinicopathologic analysis of 30 cases, *Cancer* 61:340, 1988.
597. Prat J, Young RH, Scully RE: Ovarian mucinous tumors with foci of anaplastic carcinoma, *Cancer* 50:300, 1982.
598. Prat J, Scully RE: Sarcomas in ovarian mucinous tumors: a report of two cases, *Cancer* 44:1327, 1979.
599. Prat J, Scully RE: Ovarian mucinous tumors with sarcoma-like mural nodules: a report of seven cases, *Cancer* 44:1332, 1979.
600. Matías-Guiu X, Aranda I, Prat J: Immunohistochemical study of sarcoma-like mural nodules in a mucinous cystadenocarcinoma of the ovary, *Virchows Arch [A]* 419:89, 1991.
601. Baergen RN, Rutgers JL: Mural nodules in common epithelial tumors of the ovary, *Int J Gynecol Pathol* 13:62, 1994.
602. Roth LM, Czernobilsky B, Langley FA: Ovarian endometrioid adenofibromatous and cystadenofibromatous tumors: benign, proliferating, and malignant, *Cancer* 48:1838, 1981.
603. Bell DA, Scully RE: Atypical and borderline endometrioid adenofibromas of the ovary, *Am J Surg Pathol* 9:205, 1985.
604. Snyder RR, Norris HJ, Tavassoli F: Endometrioid proliferative and low malignant potential tumors of the ovary: a clinicopathologic study of 46 cases, *Am J Surg Pathol* 12:661, 1988.
605. Young RH, Prat J, Scully RE: Ovarian endometrioid carcinomas resembling sex cord–stromal tumors: a clinicopathologic analysis of 13 cases, *Am J Surg Pathol* 6:513, 1982.
606. Roth LM, Liban E, Czernobilsky B: Ovarian endometrioid tumors mimicking Sertoli and Sertoli-Leydig cell tumors: sertoliform variant of endometrioid carcinoma, *Cancer* 50:1322, 1982.
607. Lash RH, Hart WR: Intestinal adenocarcinoma metastatic to the ovaries: a clinicopathological evaluation of 22 cases, *Am J Surg Pathol* 11:114, 1987.
608. Eifel P, Hendrickson M, Ross J et al: Simultaneous presentation of carcinoma involving the ovary and the uterine corpus, *Cancer* 50:163, 1982.
609. Young RH, Prat J, Scully RE: Endometrioid stromal sarcomas of the ovary: a clinico-pathologic analysis of 23 cases, *Cancer* 53:1143, 1984.
610. Chang KL, Crabtree GS, Lim-Tan SK: Primary extrauterine endometrial stromal neoplasms: a clinicopathologic study of 20 cases and a review of the literature, *Int J Gynecol Pathol* 12:282, 1993.
611. Terada KY, Johnson TL, Hopkins M, Roberts JA: Clinicopathologic features of ovarian mixed mesodermal tumors and carcinosarcomas, *Gynecol Oncol* 32:228, 1989.
612. Clement PB, Scully RE: Extrauterine mesodermal (müllerian) adenosarcoma, *Am J Clin Pathol* 69:276, 1978.
613. Klemi PJ, Meurmann L, Gronroos M et al: Clear cell (mesonephroid) tumor of the ovary with characteristics resembling endodermal sinus tumor, *Int J Gynecol Pathol* 1:95, 1982.
614. Scully RE: Recent progress in ovarian cancer, *Hum Pathol* 1:73, 1970.
615. Scully RE, Barlow JF: "Mesonephroma" of ovary: the tumor of müllerian nature related to the endometrioid carcinoma, *Cancer* 20:1405, 1967.
616. Austin RM, Norris HJ: Malignant Brenner tumor and transitional cell carcinoma of the ovary: a comparison, *Int J Gynecol Pathol* 6:29, 1987.
617. Robey SS, Silva EG, Gershenson DM et al: Transitional cell carcinoma in high-grade high-stage ovarian carcinoma, *Cancer* 63:839, 1989.
618. Silva EG, Robey-Cafferty SS, Smith TL et al: Ovarian carcinomas with transitional cell carcinoma pattern, *Am J Clin Pathol* 93:457, 1990.
619. Silverberg SG: Brenner tumor of the ovary: a clinicopathologic study of 60 tumors in 54 women, *Cancer* 28:588, 1971.
620. Fox H, Agrawal K, Langley FA: The Brenner tumour of the ovary: a clinicopathological study of 54 cases, *J Obstet Gynecol Br Commonw* 79:661, 1972.
621. Trebeck CE, Friedlander ML, Rusell P et al: Brenner tumors of the ovary: a study of the histology, immunohistochemistry and cellular DNA content in benign, borderline and malignant ovarian tumors, *Pathology* 19:241, 1987.
622. Hallgrímson J, Scully RE: Borderline and malignant Brenner tumours of the ovary: a report of 15 cases, *Acta Pathol Microbiol Scand [A]* 233:56, 1972.
623. Miles PA, Norris HJ: Proliferative and malignant Brenner tumors of the ovary, *Cancer* 30:174, 1972.
624. Roth LM, Dallenbach-Hellweg G, Czernobilsky B: Ovarian Brenner tumors. I. Metaplastic, proliferating, and of low malignant potential, *Cancer* 56:582, 1985.
625. Roth LM, Czernobilsky B: Ovarian Brenner tumors. II. Malignant, *Cancer* 56:592, 1985.

626. Silva EG, Tornos C, Bailey MA, Morris M: Undifferentiated carcinoma of the ovary, *Arch Pathol Lab Med* 115:377, 1991.
627. Dickersin GR, Kline IW, Scully RE: Small cell carcinoma of the ovary with hypercalcemia: a report of eleven cases, *Cancer* 49:188, 1982.
628. Young RH, Oliva E, Scully RE: Small cell carcinoma of the ovary, hypercalcemic type: a clinicopathological analysis of 150 cases, *Am J Surg Pathol* 18:1102, 1994.
629. Aguirre GR, Thor AD, Scully RE: Ovarian small cell carcinoma: histogenetic considerations based on immunohistochemical and other findings, *Am J Clin Pathol* 92:140, 1989.
630. McMahon JT, Hart WR: Ultrastructural analysis of small cell carcinomas of the ovary, *Am J Clin Pathol* 90:523, 1988.
631. Matías-Guiu X, Prat J, Young RH et al: Human parathyroid hormone–related protein (PTHrp) in ovarian small cell carcinomas: an immunohistochemical study, *Cancer* 73:1878, 1994.
632. Lauchlan SC: The secondary müllerian system, *Obstet Gynecol Surv* 27:133, 1972.
633. Young RH, Scully RE: Ovarian sex cord–stromal tumors: recent advances and current status, *Clin Obstet Gynaecol* 11:93, 1984.
634. Norris HJ, Taylor HB: Virilization associated with cystic granulosa cell tumors, *Obstet Gynecol* 34:629, 1969.
635. Nakashima N, Young RH, Scully RE: Androgenic granulosa cell tumors of the ovary: a clinicopathologic analysis of 17 cases and review of the literature, *Arch Pathol Lab Med* 108:786, 1984.
636. Young RH, Dickersin GR, Scully RE: Juvenile granulosa cell tumor of the ovary: a clinicopathologic analysis of 125 cases, *Am J Surg Pathol* 8:575, 1984.
637. Lack EE, Pérez-Atayde AR, Murty ASK et al: Granulosa theca cell tumors in premenarchal girls: a clinical and pathologic study of ten cases, *Cancer* 48:1846, 1981.
638. Zaloudek C, Norris HJ: Granulosa tumors of the ovary in children: a clinical and pathologic study of 32 cases, *Am J Surg Pathol* 6:503, 1981.
639. Stenwig JT, Hazekamp JT, Beecham JB: Granulosa cell tumors of the ovary: a clinicopathological study of 118 cases with long term follow-up, *Gynecol Oncol* 7:136, 1979.
640. Fox H, Agrawal K, Langley FA: A clinicopathologic study of 92 cases of granulosa cell tumor of the ovary with special reference to the factors influencing prognosis, *Cancer* 35:231, 1975.
641. Björkholm E, Silfverswärd C: Prognostic factors in granulosa-cell tumors, *Gynecol Oncol* 11:261, 1981.
642. Dockerty MB, Masson JC: Ovarian fibromas: a clinical and pathologic study of two hundred and eighty-three cases, *Am J Obstet Gynecol* 47:741, 1944.
643. Meigs JV: Fibroma of the ovary with ascites and hydrothorax—Meigs' syndrome, *Am J Obstet Gynecol* 67:962, 1954.
644. Prat J, Scully RE: Cellular fibromas and fibrosarcomas of the ovary: a comparative clinicopathological analysis of 17 cases, *Cancer* 47:2663-2670, 1981.
645. Banner EA, Dockerty MB: Theca cell tumors of the ovary: a clinical and pathologic study of twenty-three cases (including thirteen new cases) with a review, *Surg Gynecol Obstet* 81:234, 1945.
646. Sternberg WH, Gaskill CJ: Theca-cell tumors: with a report of twelve new cases and observations on the possible etiologic role of ovarian stromal hyperplasia, *Am J Obstet Gynecol* 59:575, 1950.
647. Björkholm E, Silfverswärd C: Theca-cell tumors: clinical features and prognosis, *Acta Radiol Oncol Radiat Phys Biol* 19:241, 1980.
648. Young BH, Clement PB, Scully RE: Calcified thecomas in young women: a report of four cases, *Int Gynecol Pathol* 7:343, 1988.
649. Roth LM, Sternberg WH: Partly luteinized theca cell tumor of the ovary, *Cancer* 51:1697, 1983.
650. Zhang J, Young RH, Arseneau J, Scully RE: Ovarian stromal tumors containing lutein or Leydig cells (luteinized thecomas and stromal Leydig cell tumors): a clinicopathological analysis of fifty cases, *Int J Gynecol Pathol* 1:270, 1982.
651. Chalvardjian A, Scully RE: Sclerosing stromal tumors of the ovary, *Cancer* 31:664, 1973.
652. Gee DC, Rusell P: Sclerosing stromal tumours of the ovary, *Histopathology* 3:367, 1979.
653. Young RH, Scully RE: Ovarian Sertoli-Leydig cell tumors: a clinicopathological analysis of 207 cases, *Am J Surg Pathol* 9:543, 1985.
654. Young RH, Prat J, Scully RE: Ovarian Sertoli-Leydig cell tumors with heterologous elements: (1) mucinous and carcinoid components: a clinicopathologic analysis of thirty-six cases, *Cancer* 50:2448, 1982.
655. Prat J, Young RH, Scully RE: Ovarian Sertoli-Leydig cell tumors with heterologous elements: (2) with cartilaginous and skeletal muscle components: a clinico-pathologic analysis of twelve cases, *Cancer* 50:2465, 1982.
656. Young RH, Scully RE: Ovarian Sertoli-Leydig cell tumors with a retiform pattern: a problem in histopathologic diagnosis: a report of 25 cases, *Am J Surg Pathol* 77:755, 1983.
657. Young RH, Scully RE: Ovarian Sertoli cell tumors: a report of ten cases, *Int J Gynecol Pathol* 2:349, 1984.
658. Young RH, Welch WR, Dickersin GR, Scully RE: Ovarian sex cord tumor with annular tubules: review of 74 cases including 27 with Peutz-Jeghers syndrome and 4 with adenoma malignum of the cervix, *Cancer* 50:1384, 1982.
659. Scully RE: Tumors of the ovary and maldeveloped gonads. In *Atlas of tumor pathology,* series 2, fasc 16, Washington, D.C., 1979, Armed Forces Institute of Pathology.
660. Hayes MC, Scully RE: Stromal luteoma of the ovary: a clinico-pathological analysis of 25 cases, *Int J Gynecol Pathol* 6:313, 1987.
661. Paraskevas M, Scully RE: Hilus cell tumor of the ovary: a clinicopathological analysis of 12 Reinke crystal–positive and nine crystal-negative cases, *Int J Gynecol Pathol* 8:299, 1989.
662. Hayes MC, Scully RE: Ovarian steroid cell tumor (not otherwise specified): a clinicopathological analysis of 63 cases, *Am J Surg Pathol* 11:835, 1987.
663. Kempson RL: Ultrastructure of ovarian stromal cell tumors: Sertoli-Leydig cell tumor and lipid cell tumor, *Arch Pathol* 86:492, 1968.
664. Pierce GB: Teratocarcinoma: a model for developmental concept of cancer, *Curr Top Dev Biol* 2:223, 1967.
665. Damjanov I: Pathobiology of human germ cell neoplasia, *Recent Results Cancer Res* 123:1, 1991.
666. Rutgers JL, Young RH, Scully RE: Ovarian yolk sac tumor arising from endometrioid carcinoma, *Hum Pathol* 18:1296, 1987.
667. Mazur MT, Talbot WH Jr, Talerman A: Endodermal sinus tumor and mucinous cystadenofibroma of the ovary: occurrence in an 82 year old woman, *Cancer* 62:2011, 1988.
668. Oliva E, Andrada E, Pezzica E, Prat J: Ovarian carcinomas with choriocarcinomatous differentiation, *Cancer* 72:2441, 1993.
669. Oosterhuis JW, Castedo SMMJ, de Jong B et al: Ploidy of primary germ cell tumors of the testis; pathogenetic and clinical relevance, *Lab Invest* 60:14, 1989.
670. Damjanov I: Is seminoma a relative or a precursor of embryonal carcinoma? *Lab Invest* 60:1, 1989.
671. Walt H, Arrenbrecht S, DeLozier-Blanchet CD et al: A human testicular germ cell tumor with borderline histology between seminoma and embryonal carcinoma secreted beta-human chorionic gonadotropin and alpha-fetoprotein only as a xenograft, *Cancer* 58:139, 1986.
672. Pera MF, Cooper S, Bennett W, Crawford-Bryce K: Human embryonal carcinoma and yolk sac carcinoma in vitro: cell lineage relationships and possible paracrine regulatory interactions, *Recent Results Cancer Res* 123:51, 1991.
673. Srigley JR, Mackay B, Toth P, Ayala A: The ultrastructure and histogenesis of male germ cell neoplasia with emphasis on seminoma with early carcinomatous features, *Ultrastruct Pathol* 12:67, 1988.
674. Gondos B: Comparative studies of normal and neoplastic ovarian germ cells 2. Ultrastructure and pathogenesis of dysgerminoma, *Int J Gynecol Pathol* 6:124, 1987.
675. De Palo G, Lattuada A, Kenda R et al: Germ cell tumors of the ovary: the experience of the national cancer institute of Milan. I. Dysgerminoma, *Int J Radiat Oncol Biol Phys* 13:853, 1987.
676. Thomas GM, Dembo AJ, Hacker NF et al: Current therapy for dysgerminoma of the ovary, *Obstet Gynecol* 70:268, 1987.
677. Björkholm E, Lundell M, Gyftodimos A, Silfverswärd C: Dysgerminoma: the Radiumhemmet series 1927-1984, *Cancer* 65:38, 1990.

678. Zaloudek CJ, Tavassoli FA, Norris HJ: Dysgerminoma with syncytiotrophoblastic giant cells: a histologically and clinically distinctive subtype of dysgerminoma, *Am J Surg Pathol* 5:361, 1981.
679. Kurman RJ, Norris HJ: Endodermal sinus tumor of the ovary: a clinical and pathologic analysis of 71 cases, *Cancer* 38:2404, 1976.
680. Nogales FF Jr, Matilla A, Nogales-Ortiz F et al: Yolk sac tumors with pure and mixed polyvesicular vitelline patterns, *Hum Pathol* 9:553, 1978.
681. Prat J, Bhan AK, Dickersin GR et al: Hepatoid yolk sac tumor of the ovary (endodermal sinus tumor with hepatoid differentiation): a light microscopical, ultrastructural and immunohistochemical study of seven cases, *Cancer* 50:2355, 1982.
682. Ulbright TM, Roth LM, Brodhecker CA: Yolk sac differentiation in germ cell tumors: a morphologic study of 50 cases with emphasis on hepatic, enteric, and parietal yolk sac features, *Am J Surg Pathol* 10:151, 1986.
683. Clement PB, Young RH, Scully RE: Endometrioid-like variant of ovarian yolk sac tumor: a clinicopathological analysis of eight cases, *Am J Surg Pathol* 11:767, 1987.
684. Nakashima N, Fukatsu T, Nagasaki T et al: The frequency and histology of hepatic tissue in germ cell tumors, *Am J Surg Pathol* 11:682, 1987.
685. Kurman RJ, Norris HJ: Embryonal carcinoma of the ovary: a clinicopathologic entity distinct from endodermal sinus tumor resembling embryonal carcinoma of the adult testis, *Cancer* 38:2420, 1976.
686. Pierce GB, Dixon FJ: Testicular teratomas. I. The demonstration of teratogenesis by metamorphosis of multipotential cells, *Cancer* 12:573, 1958.
687. Nakakuma K, Tashiro S, Uemura K et al: Alpha-fetoprotein and human chorionic gonadotropin in embryonal carcinoma of the ovary: an 8-year survival case, *Cancer* 52:1470, 1983.
688. Prat J, Matías-Guiu X, Scully RE: Hepatic yolk sac differentiation in an ovarian polyembryoma, *Surg Pathol* 2:147, 1989.
689. Takeda A, Ishizuka T, Goto T et al: Polyembryoma of ovary producing alpha-fetoprotein and HCG: immunoperoxidase and electron microscopic study, *Cancer* 14:1878, 1982.
690. Lindner D, McCaw BK, Hecht F: Parthenogenic origin of benign ovarian teratomas, *N Engl J Med* 292:63, 1975.
691. Pantoja E, Noy MA, Axtmayer RW et al: I. Ovarian dermoids and their complications: comprehensive historical review, *Obstet Gynecol Surv* 30:1, 1975.
692. Thurlbeck WM, Scully RE: Solid teratoma of the ovary: a clinicopathological analysis of 9 cases, *Cancer* 13:804, 1960.
693. Yanai-Inbar I, Scully RE: Relations of ovarian dermoid cysts and immature teratomas: an analysis of 350 cases of immature teratoma and 10 cases of dermoid cyst with microscopic foci of immature tissue, *Int J Gynecol Pathol* 6:203, 1987.
694. Robboy SJ, Scully RE: Ovarian teratoma with glial implants on the peritoneum, *Hum Pathol* 1:643, 1970.
695. Kurman RJ, Norris HJ: Malignant germ cell tumors of the ovary, *Hum Pathol* 8:551, 1977.
696. Norris HJ, Zirkin HJ, Benson WL: Immature (malignant) teratoma of the ovary: a clinical and pathologic study of 58 cases, *Cancer* 37:2359, 1976.
697. Nogales FF Jr, Favara BE, Major FJ et al: Immature teratoma of the ovary with a neural component ("solid" teratoma): a clinicopathologic study of 20 cases, *Hum Pathol* 7:625, 1976.
698. Gershenson DM, Del Junco G, Silva EG et al: Immature teratoma of the ovary, *Obstet Gynecol* 68:624, 1986.
699. Robboy SJ, Norris HJ, Scully RE: Insular carcinoid primary in the ovary: a clinicopathologic analysis of 48 cases, *Cancer* 36:404, 1975.
700. Talerman A: Carcinoid tumors of the ovary, *J Cancer Res Clin Oncol* 107:125, 1984.
701. Robboy SJ, Scully RE, Norris HJ: Primary trabecular carcinoid of the ovary, *Obstet Gynecol* 49:202, 1977.
702. Talerman A, Okagaki T: Ultrastructural features of primary trabecular carcinoid tumor of the ovary, *Int J Gynecol Pathol* 4:153, 1985.
703. Robboy SJ, Scully RE: Strumal carcinoid of the ovary: an analysis of 50 cases of a distinctive tumor composed of thyroid tissue and carcinoid, *Cancer* 46:2019, 1980.
704. Snyder RR, Tavassoli FA: Ovarian strumal carcinoid: immunohistochemical, ultrastructural, and clinicopathologic observations, *Int J Gynecol Pathol* 5:187, 1986.
705. Robboy SJ, Scully RE, Norris HJ: Carcinoid metastatic to the ovary: a clinicopathologic analysis of 35 cases, *Cancer* 33:798, 1974.
706. Aguirre P, Scully RE: Malignant neuroectodermal tumor of the ovary, a distinctive form of monodermal teratoma: report of five cases, *Am J Surg Pathol* 6:283, 1982.
707. Kleinman GM, Young RH, Scully RE: Primary ovarian neuroectodermal tumors: a report of 25 cases, *Am J Surg Pathol* 17:764, 1993.
708. Kurman RJ, Norris HJ: Malignant mixed germ cell tumor of the ovary: a clinical and pathologic analysis of 30 cases, *Obstet Gynecol* 48:579, 1976.
709. Ulbright TM, Roth LM, Stehman FB: Secondary ovarian neoplasia: a clinicopathologic study of 35 cases, *Cancer* 53:1164, 1984.
710. Lash RH, Hart WR: Intestinal adenocarcinomas metastatic to the ovaries: a clinicopathologic evaluation of 22 cases, *Am J Surg Pathol* 11:114, 1987.
711. Young RH, Scully RE: Metastatic tumors of the ovary. In Kurman RJ, editor: *Blaustein's pathology of the female genital tract,* ed 4, New York, 1994, Springer-Verlag.
712. Young RH, Scully RE: Sex cord–stromal, steroid cell and other ovarian tumors with endocrine, paraendocrine and paraneoplastic manifestation. In Kurman RJ, editor: *Blaustein's pathology of the female genital tract,* ed 4, New York, 1994, Springer-Verlag.
713. Matías-Guiu X, Prat J: Ovarian tumors with functioning stroma: an immunohistochemical study of 100 cases with human chorionic gonadotropin monoclonal and polyclonal antibodies, *Cancer* 65:2001, 1990.
714. Bullon A, Arseneau J, Prat J et al: Tubular Krukenberg tumor: a problem in histopathologic diagnosis, *Am J Surg Pathol* 5:225, 1981.
715. Young RH, Hart WR: Metastases from carcinoma of the pancreas simulating primary mucinous tumors of the ovary: a report of seven cases, *Am J Surg Pathol* 13:748, 1989.
716. Young RH, Scully RE: Malignant melanoma metastatic to the ovary: a clinicopathologic analysis of 20 cases, *Am J Surg Pathol* 15:849, 1991.
717. Chorlton I, Norris HJ, King FM: Malignant reticuloendothelial disease involving the ovary as a primary manifestation: a series of 19 lymphomas and 1 granulocytic sarcoma, *Cancer* 34:397, 1974.
718. Osborne BM, Robboy SJ: Lymphomas or leukemia presenting as ovarian tumors: an analysis of 42 cases, *Cancer* 52:1933, 1983.
719. Ferry JA, Young RH: Malignant lymphoma, pseudolymphoma, and hematopoietic disorders of the female genital tract, *Pathol Annu* 26(Pt 1):227, 1991.
720. Monterosso V, Jaffe ES, Merino MJ, Medeiros LJ: Malignant lymphomas involving the ovaries: a clinicopathologic analysis of 39 cases, *Am J Surg Pathol* 17:154, 1993.
721. Fox H, Langley FA, Govan ADT et al: Malignant lymphoma presenting as an ovarian tumour: a clinicopathologic analysis of 34 cases, *Br J Obstet Gynaecol* 95:386, 1988.
722. de Souza PL, Friedlander ML: Prognostic factors in ovarian cancer, *Hematol Oncol Clin North Am* 6:761, 1992.
723. Saksela E: Prognostic markers in epithelial ovarian cancer, *Int J Gynecol Pathol* 12:156, 1994.
724. Hendrickson MR, Longacre TA, Kempson RL: Clinicopathology of malignant surface epithelial neoplasms of the ovary. In Hendrickson MR, editor: *Pathology: state of the art reviews,* vol 1, no. 2, Philadelphia 1993, Hanley & Belfus.
725. Iversen O-E: Prognostic value of the flow cytometric DNA index in human ovarian carcinoma, *Cancer* 61:971, 1988.
726. Henriksen R, Strang P, Bäckström T et al: Ki-67 immunostaining and DNA flow cytometry as prognostic factors in epithelial ovarian cancers, *Anticancer Res* 14:603, 1994.
727. Jacobs I, Bast RC: The CA 125 tumour–associated antigen: a review of the literature, *Hum Reprod* 4:1, 1989.
728. Onsrud M, Shabana A, Austgulen R et al: Comparison between soluble tumor necrosis factor receptors and CA125 in peritoneal fluids as a marker for epithelial ovarian cancer, *Gynecol Oncol* 57:183, 1995.
729. Ozols RF: Research directions in epithelial ovarian cancer, *Gynecol Oncol* 55:S168, 1994.

69 Placenta

Carolyn M. Salafia
Edwina J. Popek

NORMAL PLACENTA

The placenta's basic function is to provide fetal nutrients and remove fetal wastes. Battaglia and Meschia describe the factors determining placental function: "maternal and fetal blood flows, the pattern of placental perfusion, the surface, thickness and physicochemical properties of the placental membrane, the metabolic activity of the placenta, the various mechanisms of transfer which are available (e.g., diffusion, carrier mediated transfer, active transfer), and regional differences in placental histology and function."[1]

To establish an intrauterine pregnancy, trophoblast must anchor to and invade decidualized endometrium[2] (Fig. 69-1), and the uterine vasculature must change to allow progressive increases in blood flow.[3] Endovascular trophoblast invades the fibromuscular decidual spiral vessels in 2 waves.[4-6] The first is completed by the end of the first trimester, and the second by the early second trimester when extravillous trophoblast penetrates to the superficial one third of the myometrium.[4-7] Converted decidual vessels, no longer responsive to vasomotor stimuli (Fig. 69-2),[8] empty into the intervillous space. Before uterine vascular conversion, endometrial flow is a low capacitance-high resistance system. After conversion, the intervillous space is a high capacitance-low resistance circuit. Decreased trophoblastic invasion results in reduced decidual vascular conversion.[4,7,9] Thus the placental margins are less well perfused, less functional zones that contribute little to fetal nutrition. Routine sampling of placental margins is not useful.

Three types of trophoblast are defined by their anatomic location: (1) villous trophoblast, which lines the intervillous blood space with cytotrophoblast "stem cells" producing mature syncytiotrophoblast, (2) anchoring (mononuclear) trophoblast, and (3) invasive interstitial and endovascular trophoblast. Interstitial trophoblast cells fuse after decidual vascular conversion is complete, becoming multinucleate "placental bed giant cells."[9]

Villous morphology reflects placental growth and functional maturation (Figs. 69-3 and 69-4). By the fifth or sixth week of gestation, nucleated erythrocytes from the yolk sac fill the fetoplacental circulation (Fig. 69-3, *A*). Villous macro-

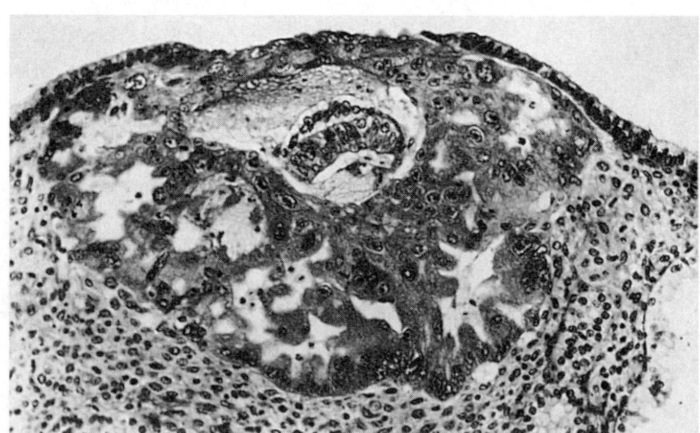

Fig. 69-1 Blastocyst of approximately 9 days, implantation onto the endometrium with early differentiation of the cytotrophoblast and syncytiotrophoblast. The villi do not yet have a mesenchymal core. No maternal blood supply is developed at this time. The endometrium covers the blastocyst at this stage.

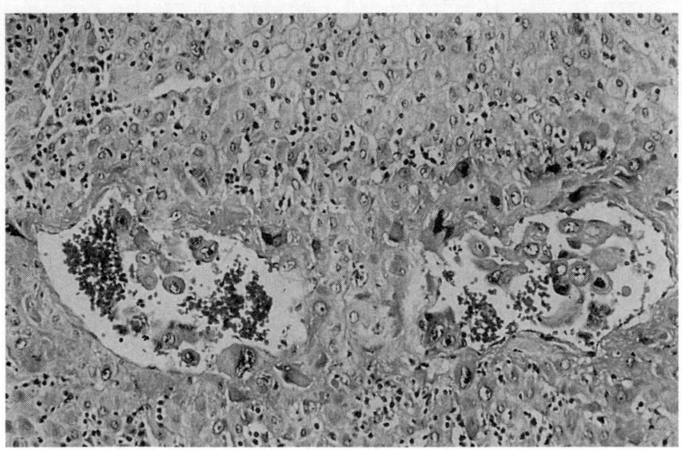

Fig. 69-2 The spiral artery of the endometrium shows invasion and destruction of the muscular wall by intermediate trophoblasts. There are trophoblast microthrombi in the vessel lumen. A usual component of maternal lymphocytes are seen scattered in the decidua.

phages (Hofbauer cells) are numerous throughout gestation (40% of stromal cells),[10] although at term they may be less conspicuous, with a spindled appearance. Villi arborize by mesenchymal invasion of syncytial sprouts (Fig. 69-3, *B*)[11] Sprouts can be deported into the maternal circulation, where they may influence maternal tolerance of the conceptus. Villi originally develop over the entire sphere of the conceptus, but they atrophy over the extraplacental membranes by the end of the first trimester. Remnants of ghost villi can be seen on the free membranes *(chorion laeve)* even at term (Fig. 69-4, *E, F*). The chorion frondosum then becomes the placental disk.

Early villous vessels are located deep in the villous stroma, with mean distance from intervillous space to villous vessel of 24 to 27 μm[12] (Fig. 69-3, *A, B*). The early conceptus is relatively oxygen poor.[1] Placental growth slows by the end of the second trimester.[13] Fetal growth continues disproportionate to the mass of the nurturing placenta because of increased placental diffusion efficiency. Progressive reduction in trophoblast thickness, villous size, and distance between the intervillous space and the fetoplacental capillary are the recognizable features responsible for greater placental efficiency (Fig. 69-3, *C*). The placental vasculature increases in complex-

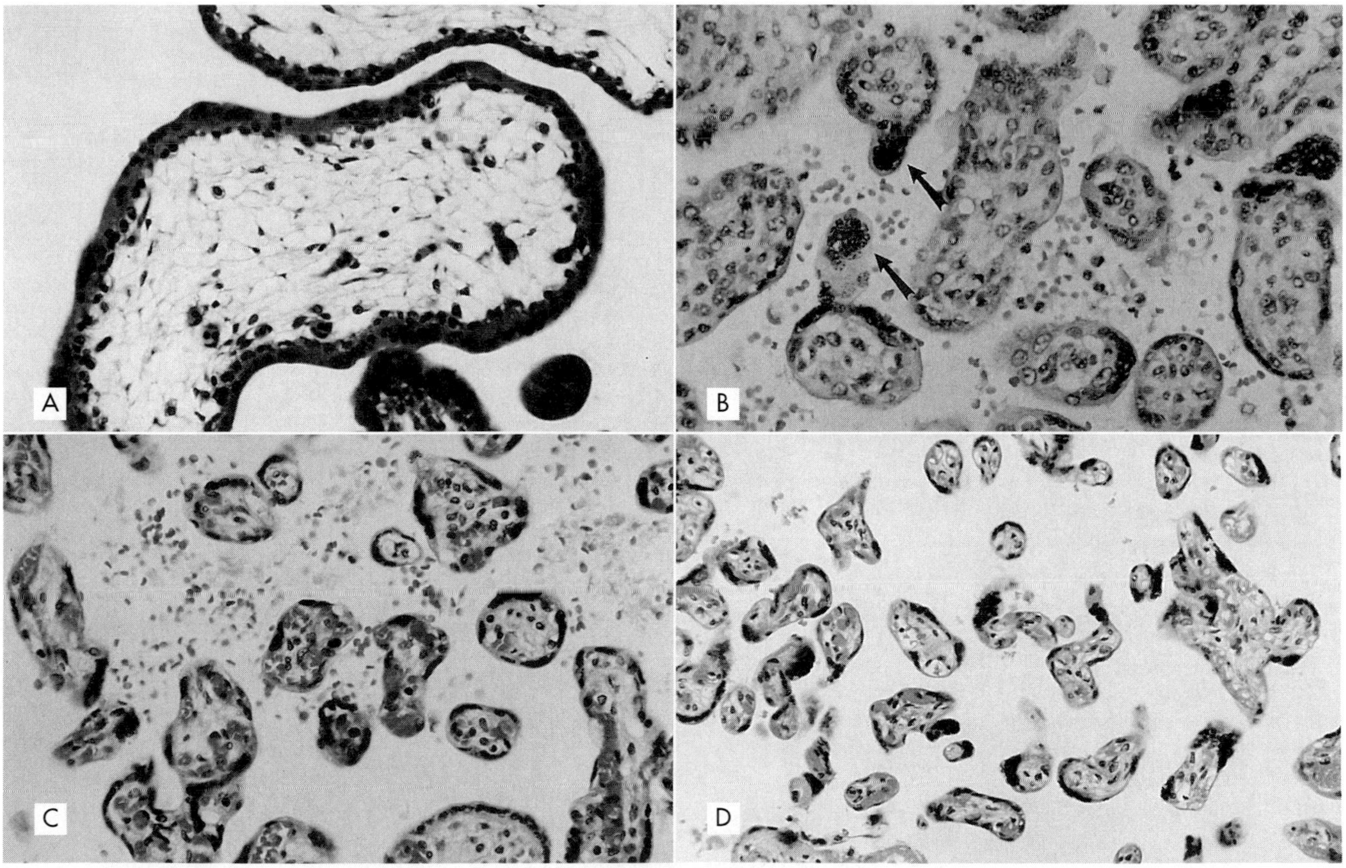

Fig. 69-3 **A,** First trimester villi measure 170 μm in diameter and are covered by two cell layers, an outer syncytiotrophoblast and an inner cytotrophoblast layer. **B,** Second trimester villi are smaller, 70 μm in diameter, and the cytotrophoblasts are less conspicuous. Outgrowths of syncytial nuclei, sprouts *(arrows),* form into the intervillous space and develop into new villi or break loose into the maternal intervillous space and may be carried to the lung. **C,** Third trimester villi are 40 μm in diameter and have few visible cytotrophoblasts. Vasculosyncytial membranes form by clumping of the nuclei, which results in nucleus-free cytoplasm of the syncytiotrophoblast, which nearly fuses with the capillary basement membrane, **D,** Postterm villi are smaller and may have stromal fibrosis and exaggerated syncytial knots.

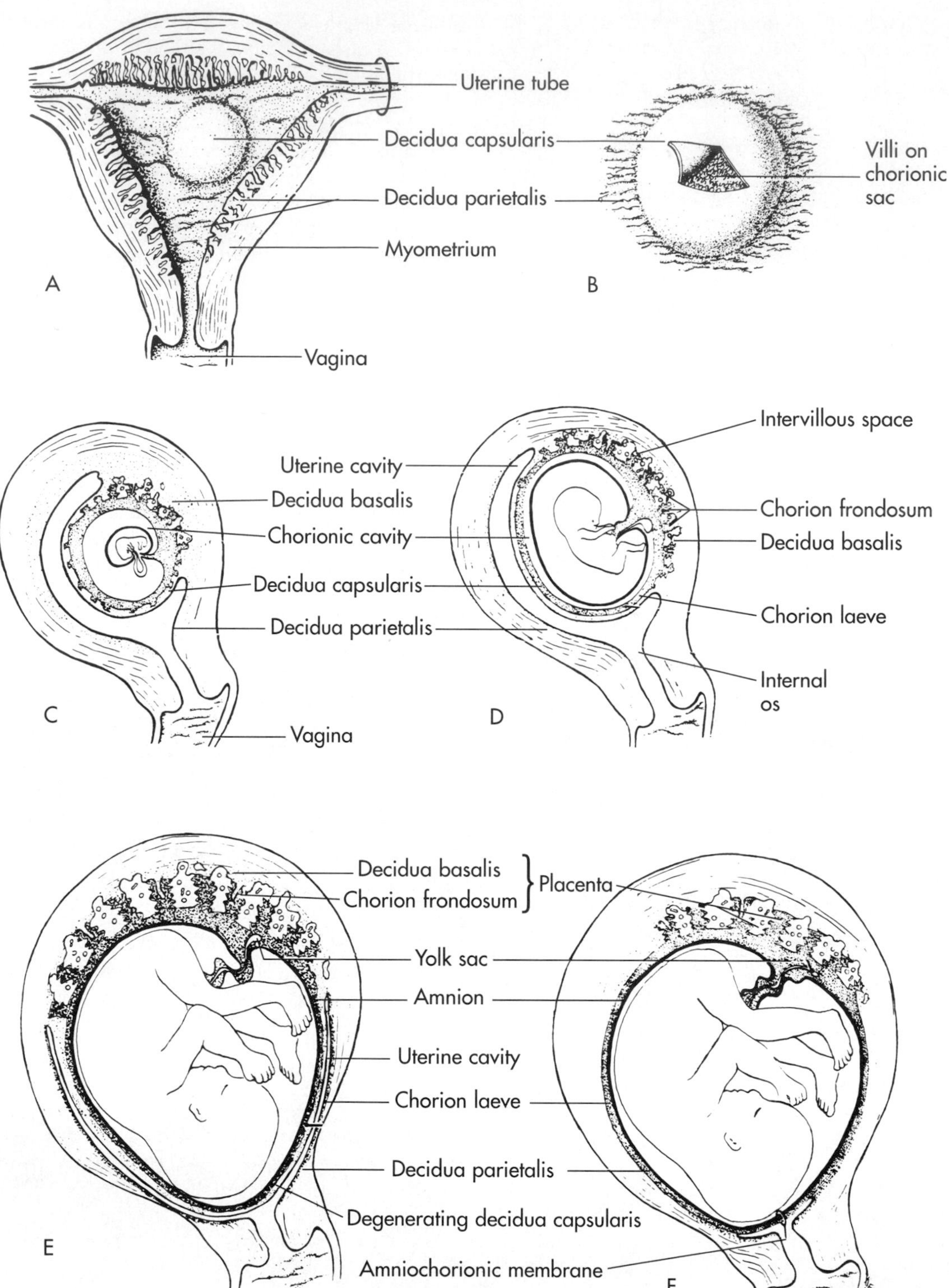

Fig. 69-4 **A, B,** Drawing of a frontal section of the uterus showing the elevation of the decidua capsularis caused by the expanding chorionic sac of a 4-week embryo. **C–F,** Drawings of sagittal sections of the gravid uterus from the fifth to twenty-second weeks, showing the changing relationship of the fetal membranes to the decidua. In **F,** the amnion and chorion are closely approximated but never quite fuse with each other and the decidua parietalis, thereby obliterating the uterine cavity. Note in **D** to **F** that the chorionic villi thrive only where the chorion is associated with the decidua basalis; here they form the chorion frondosum, and the chorion laeve will show persistence of ghostlike atrophic villi seen even at term on the free membranes. (Modified from Moore KL, Persaud TVN: *The developing human, clinically oriented embryology,* ed 5, Philadelphia, 1993, Saunders.)

ity (more capillary outlines per villus) until about week 36 of gestation.[14,15] The mature villous functional unit is a barrel, with the staves formed by the large fetal stem vessels, and the villous tree arborizing toward the center. The "youngest," or most recently formed, villi are in the center.[16] Sections through these areas of the villous tissue allow some assessment of the growth capacity of the placenta. The postmaturity syndrome is thought to be caused by progressive insufficiency of the aging placenta[17] (Fig. 69-3, *D*) but some placental growth continues until late in gestation.[18] If a placenta at greater than week 42 of gestation shows healthy terminal villi and active villous sprouting, a cause for fetal/neonatal compromise other than placental insufficiency should be sought.

In vasculosyncytial membranes, which develop late in gestation, villous capillaries abut the trophoblast basement membrane. Syncytiotrophoblast nuclei cluster at the margins of the mature vasculosyncytial membrane (Fig 69-3, *C*). The membrane itself measures only 0.5 to 1.0 μm in thickness; the capillary basal lamina and trophoblastic basal lamina may focally fuse.[13] A mature placenta forming vasculosyncytial membranes may be similar to the lung, maturation of which involves progressive approximation of alveolar air spaces and capillary networks. The maternal cardiac blood flow to the term placenta is 500 ml per minute.

Placental examination

All placentas should be considered potentially infectious and should be handled accordingly. Gross examination can be performed when the specimen is received fresh, or it may be performed 1 to 2 days after immersion of the placenta in formalin. We prefer gross examination of fresh placentas with tissue samples fixed in formalin overnight before trimming. Placentas from stillborn fetuses should not be fixed in formalin because placental fibroblasts may be needed for cytogenetic or other metabolic analyses. Microbial cultures should be performed in the labor and delivery suite, and not in the pathology laboratory hours after birth.

Placentas must be weighed and measured. Different approaches to placental weighing (removing cord, removing extraplacental membranes, or draining maternal intervillous blood) may be taken, but one method must be used consistently and documented in the pathology report. The fetoplacental weight ratio increases throughout gestation, and abnormally high or low ratios are likely indicators of fetoplacental pathology (Table 69-1).

An approach to tissue sampling of the placenta is presented in Fig. 69-5. The placental parenchyma is grossly examined by slicing perpendicular to the maternal surface and chorionic plate at approximately 1 cm intervals, leaving the chorionic plate intact. Each surface of each slice is examined for obvious lesions (e.g., infarct or intervillous thrombi) or subtle lesions, such as increased villous granularity (e.g., villous swelling or chronic villitis). Villous tissue should be uniform in color; dark and pale areas may mark microscopic pathology. Examination of decidual vasculature is important and often overlooked in placental evaluation. Especially in the fixed placenta, decidual spiral vessels can be seen as small irregularities or an S shape on the maternal surface. Several thin slices of the basal plate may be placed in one cassette and generally yield at least one decidual vessel for examination. A minimum of two samples of villous parenchyma from grossly normal villi, plus sections from any lesions, will permit identification of most lesions.

Table 69-1 Expected fetal-to-placental weight ratios

Weeks of gestation	Placental weight (g)	Fetal weight (g)	F:P
8	6	1.1	0.18
10	14	5	0.36
12	26	17	0.65
14	42	30	0.71
16	65	60	0.92
18	90	130	1.44
20	115	250	2.17
22	150	400	2.67
24	185	560	3.03
26	210	750	3.57
28	250	1000	4.00
30	285	1260	4.42
32	315	1550	4.92
34	355	1900	5.35
36	390	2300	5.90
38	425	2750	6.47
40	470	3400	7.23

From Molteni RA: *Semin Perinatol* 8:94, 1984; and Benirschke K, Kaufman P, editors: *Pathology of the human placenta,* New York, 1990, Springer-Verlag. *F:P,* Fetal-placental weight ratio.

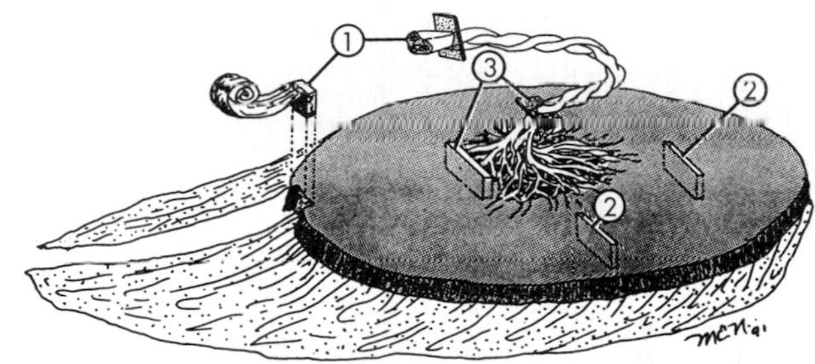

Fig. 69-5 Recommended minimum sections include a membrane roll, which included the zone of rupture and a marginal portion of the placental disk for orientation. There are two sections of umbilical cord, one from the fetal end and the other from the placental end, 2 to 3 cm from the insertion. It has been shown that the majority of placental abnormalities can be detected in four sections of placental tissue, and these should include midzonal full thickness sections and a central section. Both the fetal and maternal surfaces should be submitted, which may necessitate dividing the tissue into two blocks. Additional sections should be submitted from grossly abnormal areas and additional sections in cases of specific disorders should be considered (i.e., thin sections from the maternal surface to evaluate maternal decidual arteries in cases of PIH). (Computer-generated diagram by Martin E. Nau.)

Suggested criteria for selection of placentas for pathologic examination are presented in Table 69-2.

PLACENTAL EXAMINATION IN MATERNAL DISEASE

There is no "one-to-one" relationship between placental lesions and specific maternal conditions or fetal outcomes. Almost no placental lesions are pathognomonic for a maternal condition or fetal outcome. Almost no maternal and fetal/neonatal conditions have a single placental histology. The

Table 69-2 Which placentas should be examined by a pathologist?

	Recommended	Optional (depending on clinical conditions)
Fetus/newborn/maternal considerations		
Intrauterine fetal demise (IUFD)	*	
Intrapartum or neonatal death	*	
Preterm delivery (<34 completed weeks)	*	
Delivery between 35 and 37 weeks		*
Postterm delivery (≥42 weeks)		*
Intrauterine growth retardation (IUGR)	*	
Large for gestational age fetus/newborn		*
Discordant growth in length versus weight	*	
Major congenital anomalies	*	
Hydrops fetalis or severe fetal anemia HCT <35	*	
Admission to the neonatal intensive care unit	*	
Depressed fetus (5-minute Apgar <7, pH <7, mechanical ventilation greater than 10 minutes)	*	
Neonatal neurologic problems/seizures	*	
Suspected fetal or maternal infection (intrapartum or recent fever)	*	
History of primary or untreated syphilis	*	
Multiple gestations	*	
Oligohydramnios (unexplained)	*	
Polyhydramnios		*
Vaginal bleeding late in pregnancy (unexplained)	*	
Maternal systemic disease with clinical concern for mother or baby	*	
Maternal illicit drug use	*	
History of previous poor pregnancy outcome		*
Placental considerations		
Abnormally small or large placentas	*	
Visible or palpable abnormalities infarcts, abruption, tumors, surface vessel thromboses, abnormal shape with velamentous vessels or associated hemorrhage	*	
Heavy meconium staining with thick meconium	*	
Amnion nodosum	*	
Umbilical cord abnormalities thrombosis, torsions, true knots, SUA, absent Wharton's jelly	*	
Abnormally short (<32 cm) or long (>100 cm) cord at term	*	
Placenta previa		*

Guidelines based on recommendations made by the College of American Pathologists Committee on Practice Guidelines, Placental Pathology Task Force.

"end-stage" histologic features seen in the placenta nevertheless provide clues about pathogenesis that may direct further clinical and laboratory testing. A brief guide to the interpretation of placental lesions and their correlations with clinical conditions is given in Table 69-3. Pregnancy induces widespread systemic maternal changes, including a physiologic anemia caused by 50% increase in plasma volume disproportionate to increase in erythrocyte number, increased cardiac output and glomerular filtration, and the endocrine changes of pregnancy. These adaptive and reactive changes in the maternal organism are physiological responses, and their goal is the optimal support of the developing conceptus. Common maternal diseases that may be associated with placental lesions are listed in Table 69-4.[19-48]

Hypertensive diseases

Generally placentas in uncomplicated chronic hypertension are well grown and without significant lesions, and their fetuses are healthy.[49] Poor pregnancy outcome in chronic hypertension is due to the greater risk of superimposed preeclampsia. No specific vascular pathology distinguishes pure chronic hypertension from preeclampsia, chronic hypertension with superimposed preeclampsia, or hypertension associated with maternal diabetes mellitus.

Preeclampsia, prematurity, and idiopathic intrauterine growth retardation (IUGR) each often show abnormal, incomplete, or failed uterine vascular adaptation.[50,51] In vessels with absent, incomplete, or failed adaptation, there is variable persistence of vascular muscle and elastic lamina. This leads to increased uterine vascular resistance, decreased capacitance, and decreased total blood flow to the placenta. These lesions are classically described in placental bed (myometrial) biopsy specimens[52] but are seen in endometrial decidual vessels delivered with the placenta.[53] Doppler and isotope studies in the human suggest uteroplacental flow is decreased to 50% to 70% of normal, which may explain the often associated fetal IUGR.[54,55] Other common decidual lesions are thrombosis, fibrinoid necrosis of the vessel wall with mural foamy cells ("atherosis"), and chronic vasculitis. Decidual lesions carry increased risk of "decidual vascular accidents" such as placental infarcts or abruption[56] (Fig. 69-6, *A, B, C*). When a decidual vessel is occluded, intervillous flow ceases, the intervillous space collapses, and villi become compressed and undergo ischemic necrosis. In abruption, the placenta is forcibly sepa-

Table 69-3 Gross and microscopic placental lesions and their obstetric associations

Tissue	Aspects of gross and microscopic diagnosis	Clinical correlation	Events associated with placental lesions
Extraplacental membranes	Blood attached to decidual surface	Suspicion of abruption	Preeclampsia and medical conditions associated with vascular pathology, cocaine use, after elevated midtrimester maternal serum AFP testing
	Opacity	Ascending intraamniotic infection	Prematurity, preterm labor, preterm membrane rupture, decreased biophysical profile score, increased cord systolic/diastolic pressure, abnormal fetal heart rate
	Color	Green membranes indicate meconium staining, yellow staining amniotic hyperbilirubinemia and possible intraamniotic bleed	Green: stress significance mainly in preterm; often "normal" in normal term infants. In preterms, bacterial pigments may tint membranes green or yellow Yellow: intrauterine hemolysis, including Rh isoimmunization, congenital viral infection. Red-brown: abruption, vasa previa or chorionic trauma, prolonged retention in utero after fetal demise
Site of rupture	1. At placental margin	1. Placental edge may have been in cervical area, or low lying	1. Placenta previa, vasa previa, low-lying implantation
	2. >10 cm from margin	2. Implantation site was likely fundal	2. Normal
Membrane insertion	1. Marginal	1. Normal	
	2. Circummarginate	2. Probable normal variant	
	3. Circumvallate	3. Placental margin is undermined, and chorionic plate is smaller than placental disk. Chorionic plate is delimited by band of necrotic decidua and fold of membranes	3. Chronic oligohydramnios, amnion rupture, maternal smoking, and other conditions of uterine vascular insufficiency
	4. Membranacea	4. Failure of bald chorion to regress with no chorion free of vascularized villi	4. Antepartum or postpartum hemorrhage, IUGR prematurity
Umbilical cord length	1. Long (>100 cm)	1. ? Increased fetal movement	1. Greater risk of cord accident including multiple nuchal cords, cord prolapse or funic presentation
	2. Normal (54–61 cm)	2. Normal	2. Normal
	3. Short (<32 cm)	3. Decreased fetal movement	3. Chronic intrauterine constriction, amnion band syndrome, body stalk anomalies, extensive neonatal blood sampling with removal of cord segments for venipuncture, failure to include complete cord with pathology specimen
Cord thickness/ edema	1. Increased: >2 cm thick at term; >1.5 cm <32 weeks	1. Focal: umbilical angioma or other focal intrafunicular lesion. Diffuse: fetal volume expansion, change in cord permeability	1. Focal: intrafunicular lesion may reduce venous return. Diffuse: acute intraamniotic infection, hydrops fetalis, maternal diabetes, recipient of twin transfusion syndrome
	2. Decreased: <1 cm at term, <0.8 cm <32 weeks	2. Fetal volume depletion	2. IUGR, preeclampsia
	3. Decreased, focal	3. ?Torsion, stricture, compression	3. ? IUFD
Cord vessels	1. Three-vessel cord	1. Normal	1. Normal
	2. Two-vessel cord (single umbilical artery)	2. Atresia of second artery vs. agenesis	2. Fetal anomalies and ?abnormal fetoplacental hemodynamics. Often an isolated abnormality in an IUGR infant; higher incidence of twins
	3. More than three vessels	3. Cord varicosities, persistent vitelline vessels allantoic duct, umbilical angiomas, conjoined twins	3. Mass lesions causing increased intrafunicular pressure would lead to decreased blood flow
Umbilical cord insertion on chorionic plate	1. Central/eccentric	1. Normal/normal variant	
	2. Marginal	2. ?Greater ease of cord compression because unstable location at junction of extraplacental and plate chorion.	2. ?IUGR, fetal heart rate abnormalities, fetal demise

(continued)

Table 69-3 Gross and microscopic placental lesions and their obstetric associations—cont'd

Tissue	Aspects of gross and microscopic diagnosis	Clinical correlation	Events associated with placental lesions
	3. Velamentous	3. Velamentous vessels susceptible to mechanical compression (fluctuating fetoplacental perfusion), laceration (vasa previa)	3. Intrauterine crowding (multiple gestation or uterine septi) or stillbirth (in vasa previa)
Cord knots	1. Loose, without deformation of Wharton's jelly	1. No functional significance	
	2. Tight, with deformation of Wharton's jelly	2. Placental side of cord edematous—?increased venous resistance Fetal side of cord hemorrhagic —increased arterial resistance and intrafunicular hemorrhage	2. Pulled tight because of underlying abnormality of fetoplacental hemodynamics and exacerbated underlying pathology; postmortem event after drop in cord turgor
Maternal surface	1. Complete		
	2. Incomplete	2. Retained villous placenta	2. Risk for postpartum hemorrhage or endometritis. ? abruption or other traumatic placental detachment
Retroplacental hemorrhage	1. None/nonadherent	1. Normal/artifact of specimen handling	
	2. Adherent/organized	2. Decidual vascular accident/ abruption	2. Preeclampsia, cocaine use, IUGR, stillbirth, or induced delivery for termination of pregnancy
Amnion epithelium	1. Flat/low cuboidal	1. Normal preterm	
	2. Tall columnar, apical blebbing	2. Normal term, or preterm with chronic pathology	2. Preterm IUGR, preeclampsia, or chronic oligohydramnios
	3. Absent	3. Necrotic epithelium	3. PROM or oligohydramnios
	4. Amnion nodosum	4. Amorphous debris embedded in amnion, reephithelialized (easily scraped off)	4. Prolonged, severe oligohydramnios
	5. Hyperplastic	5. Pseudostratified	5. Meconium staining
	6. Squamous metaplasia	6. Metaplasia	6. Normal—seen most commonly on cord and near insertion, does not scrape off ("sign of maturity")
Meconium staining	1. Amnion only	1. Relatively light volume and short exposure	Significance ?at term, due to maturation of fetal bowel. In preterms, suggests fetal stress
	2. Chorionic staining	2. Larger volume or longer exposure	Rule out infection or hemosiderin
	3. Cord staining	3. Prolonged exposure	
Acute ascending infection	1. Maternal response	1. Histology depends on duration of infection, severity, and host response to organism	Bacterial invasion of amniotic fluid space and intrauterine tissues is associated with preterm labor, PROM, fetal/neonatal/maternal infectious sequelae, decreases in measures of fetal well-being, increased systolic/diastolic ratio in cord, ? alteration of fetoplacental hemodynamics, or bacterial toxin-induced fetal damage
	(a) Choriodecidua and amnion	(a) Free chorion and amnion are avascular; all PMNs are maternally derived. If inflammation is based in decidua, PMNs remain in decidua ("necrotizing inflammation"). If inflammation is based in amniotic fluid, PMNs "marginate"	
	(b) Chorionic plate	(b) PMN's marginate within subchorionic fibrin and ultimately penetrate up to full thickness of chorion connective tissue	
	2. Fetal response (a) Umbilical vessels (b) Chorionic vessels	2. Histology depends on duration of infection, severity, and maturity of fetal immune system's capacity for response to organism (gestational age); it is more indicative of	

(continued)

Table 69-3 Gross and microscopic placental lesions and their obstetric associations—cont'd

Tissue	Aspects of gross and microscopic diagnosis	Clinical correlation	Events associated with placental lesions
		(a) positive intraamniotic bacterial culture[150] and (b) PMN margination to surface of umbilical cord. Eosinophilic and immature myeloid forms marginate more commonly preterm (rarely at term), reflecting myeloid reserve depletion or immature/aberrant response to organism	
Syncytiotrophoblast basophilia	Trophoblast nuclei are intensely basophilic with no nuclear detail	Nonspecific response to changes in maternal or fetal perfusion	Stillbirth, vicinity of infarcts and other circulatory lesions, avascular villi (intraplacental vaso-occlusion)
Reduced mean villous diameters	Throughout gestation terminal villous diameters decrease. Excessively small villi for gestational age at delivery, often with numerous vasculo-syncytial membranes (if vascularized) or fibrosis/hypovascularity	? Precocious placental maturation due to intrauterine stress, failure of normal placental growth, or destruction of normally forming villous structures (e.g., fibrosis/hypovascularity)	Chronic uterine vascular insufficiency states (see Decidual vascular pathology)
Infarct	1. Location	1.	1.
	(a) Marginal	(a) A lesion based on the maternal surface located within outer 10% of placental surface	(a) Present in 10% of normal term deliveries, significance increased in preterm birth
	(b) Central/eccentric	(b) A maternal surface-based lesion within inner 90% of the placental surface	(b) Decidual vascular pathology, uterine vascular insufficiency
	2. Size/number	2.	2.
		(a) < 1 cm^3	(a) One 1-cm^3 lesion is present in 10% of normals at term, increased significance in preterms and for either larger or multiple lesions
		(b) > 1 cm^3	(b) Decidual vascular pathology, uterine vascular insufficiency, preeclampsia, IUGR
	3. Color	3.	3.
		(a) Red to maroon granular	(a) Early, occurring probably <2–3 days prior
		(b) Pale pink	(b) Subacute, occurring probably 3–5 days prior
		(c) White to tan	(c) Old, occurring probably at least 1 week prior
Intervillous thrombi	Location	(a) A parabasal lesion located within outer 10% of placental surface	(a) Present in 10% of normal term deliveries, significance increased in preterm birth
		(b) A parabasal lesion within inner 90% of placental surface	(b) Decidual vascular pathology, uterine vascular insufficiency
		(c) Nonparabasal or centric	(c) ?Locus of fetal maternal transfusion, increased incidence in immune and nonimmune hydrops fetalis
	Size		
	(a) <1 cm^3	(a) Normal at term, increased significance in preterms	(a) One 1-cm^3 lesion is present in 10% of normal at term, increased significance in preterms
	(b) >1 cm^3	(b) Decidual vascular pathology, uterine vascular insufficiency	(b) Decidual vascular pathology, uterine vascular insufficiency, preeclampsia, IUGR
	Color	(a) Red to maroon, early laminations	(a) Early, occurring probably <2–3 days prior
		(b) Pale pink	(b) Subacute, occurring probably 3–5 days prior
		(c) White to tan, well-established laminations	(c) Old, occurring probably at least 1 week prior

(continued)

Table 69-3 Gross and microscopic placental lesions and their obstetric associations—cont'd

Tissue	Aspects of gross and microscopic diagnosis	Clinical correlation	Events associated with placental lesions
Chorangioma			
1. Number	(a) Solitary or multiple	Associated with fetal angiomas in skin, brain, liver, or other viscera	Intrauterine demise, with or without fetal hydrops. Solitary or several small lesions may present clinically as fetal tachycardia, or fetal distress. Neonatal thrombocytopenia, especially in infarcted chorangiomas, due to thrombosis and platelet consumption within tumor. Associated with elevated maternal serum AFP; may be detected on ultrasound
2. Color	(a) Red/maroon (b) Pink (c) Tan/myxoid	Color indicates lesion vascularity or lesion infarct Infarcted lesion may calcify	
Maternal floor infarction	Extent of parenchymal involvement	Uniform tan-white lesion based on maternal surface, often thickest in central placenta with marginal sparing, often grossly evident normal and patent decidual vessels, may resemble exaggerated Nitabuch's fibrin	Recurrent poor pregnancy outcome, fetal demise An immunologic etiology has been suggested
Perivillous fibrin deposition	Location and extent 1. Focal	1. Isolated focus or small foci in 5% to 10% of normal term placentas	1. May represent focal basalis defects (such as S/P cesarean section or implantation over locus of fallopian tube attachment into uterus
	2. Diffuse/ Multifocal	2. Abnormal trophoblast damage with secondary coagulation, or primary uteroplacental coagulopathy	2. Associated with idiopathic recurrent spontaneous abortion, may be seen in certain patients with clinical or subclinical autoimmunity including antiphospholipid antibody syndrome
"X-cells"	1. Focal 2. Diffuse	Proliferation of cytotrophoblastic cells believed to reflect trophoblast ischemia; intermediate cytotrophoblast contribute to placental septal cysts	1. Small foci in many normal term placentas 2. Often associated with perivillous coagulation
Subchorionic fibrinoid	Decreased or increased	Uncommon in preterm, but becomes more prominent towards term—probably a response to "injury" of subchorionic space	Amount is a relative reflection of fetal movement. decreased amounts at term are abnormal
Subchorionic hematoma	Breus' mole > 1 cm thick	Will laminate over time	Often IUFD; lesion can be seen on ultrasound
Placental intravascular thrombi and related lesions	1. Mural thrombi in chorionic or large fetal stem vessels	1. Mural desposition of fibrin with endothelial loss, often in inflamed vessels (acute ascending or chronic villitis)	1. Acute ascending infection, placental sepsis, chronic villitis, ? cocaine related, related to abnormal placental perfusion
	2. "Hemorrhagic endovasculitis/ endovasculosis"	2. May affect any level of placental circulation. In larger vessels, it is a vaso-occlusive process with endothelial damage, fibroblast proliferation, scalloping of vessel outline, and red cell fragmentation and extravasation into vessel wall and villous stroma. At capillary level, only erythrocyte fragmentation and endothelial disruption are present	2. Initially reported as a cause of stillbirth, in some cases reflects vascular degeneration related to prolonged retention in utero after fetal death; seen nearby infarct, chorangioma, and other lesions of abnormal placental perfusion. Associated with abnormal fetal heart rate, fetal distress
	3. Avascular terminal villi "fetal infarct"	3. Avascular villi with densely basophilic trophoblast, stromal fibrosis and mineralization	3. May reflect "burnout" areas of old placental vaso-occlusion. Tiny foci in 15% of normal term deliveries, increased in twin-transfusion, intrauterine shock, "fetal infarct"

(continued)

Table 69-3 Gross and microscopic placental lesions and their obstetric associations—cont'd

Tissue	Aspects of gross and microscopic diagnosis	Clinical correlation	Events associated with placental lesions
Villous stromal hemorrhage	1. Focal vs. diffuse 2. "Age"	1. Terminal villous capillary rupture with stromal bleeding. 2. Hemosiderin deposition occurs in 24–48 hours after bleed	1. Abruption, induced delivery, severe villous edema 2. May permit distinction between antepartum and intrapartum events
Chronic villitis	1. Anchoring villi only 2. Terminal (nutrient) villi 3. Intervillous chronic inflammation	1. A chronic inflammatory infiltrate within villi or the intervillous space; immunohistochemically, macrophages and T-cells with rare B-cells. Occasionally villous Langhans'-type cells and plasma cells are present.	1-3. Etiology classically is congenital infection by TORCH entities; recently suggested to reflect a maternal immune rejection of the placentation process or the conceptus proper. Intervillous cells are presumed to be of maternal origin. Intravillous cells may be of mixed (fetal and maternal) origin
Decidual vascular pathology	1. Incomplete or absent physiologic conversion	1. Persistence of prepregnancy spiral vascular media/ intima, failure of replacement of media/intima with normal eosinophilic material and embedded trophoblasts seen in decidua basalis and parietalis	1. Classic lesion of preeclampsia, in which context abnormal trophoblast invasion and conversion of spiral vessels was first described. Either the first (weeks 6-7 to 16) or second (week 18 to approximately 22) wave of trophoblast migration may be abnormal. In tertiary care centers, most common in preterm preeclampsia. In low-risk context, associated with IUGR, stillbirth, preterm labor, nonhypertensive abruption
	2. Decidual vasculitis	2. Intramural lymphocytic infiltrates; must be carefully distinguished from normal perivascular cuffing	2. Frequently seen in patients with subclinical or clinical autoimmunity. May be seen in <5% of uncomplicated term births
	3. Decidual thrombi	3. Mural and/or occlusive thrombi of decidual vessels	3. Multifocal and extensive thrombi are considered reflective of antiphospholipid antibody syndrome, but may accompany other subclinical autoimmune serologies or be present in serologically negative women. Small mural thrombi (<10% stenosis) are common at term
	4. Fibrinoid necrosis/atherosis	4. Replacement of vessel wall with fibrinoid necrosis with embedded foamy macrophages (atherosis). May occur in parietal vessels. Is believed to occur only in vessels lacking physiologic conversion	4. The only decidual vascular lesion that may be characteristic of preeclampsia, this is still not specific for preeclampsia and indicates abnormal vascular conversion with vessel wall damage associated with immunoglobulin and complement deposition. Seen in preeclampsia, unexplained stillbirth, idiopathic IUGR, and occasionally in non-preeclamptic conditions of prematurity
	5. Decidual plasma cells	While normal decidua contains lymphocytes, plasma cells are not normal. Tend to aggregate adjacent to anchoring villi or to converted decidual vessels	Antibody-forming cells in the intrauterine compartment is seen in severe Rh isoimmunization, occasionally with documented congenital viral infections, and most commonly in women with clinical or subclinical pregnancy compromise
	6. Acute vasculitis	PMN infiltrate in decidual vessel wall, often with necrotizing deciduitis	Seen in severe acute ascending infection, and with abruption
Fibrinoid necrosis	May be difficult to distinguish from perivillous fibrin; acellular masses of dense eosinophilic material form a lump on the trophoblast basement membrane, covered at least partly by trophoblast; fibrinoid replaces the villous stroma	Fox described "fibrinoid" to contain immunoglobulins	Up to 3% villous involvement is likely part of normal placental "wear and tear," increased in uteroplacental insufficiency, acute ascending infection (?direct endotoxin effect on trophoblast

AFP, Alpha-fetoprotein; *IUFD*, intrauterine fetal demise; *IUGR*, intrauterine growth retardation; *PMN*, polymorphonuclear leukocytes; *PROM*, premature rupture of membranes.

Table 69-4 Common maternal conditions associated with placental lesions

Maternal conditions	Maternal/fetal neonatal conditions	Placental lesions
Cervical carcinoma[19]	? Higher incidence of invasion, 1st trimester conization, 15% to 33% spontaneous loss (0.6% incidence of loss after colposcopic biopsy). Vaginal delivery does not spread disease	None reported
Metastic malignancies[20,21]	Generally reflect extent of maternal disease; maternal-fetal metastases are rare but reported	Intervillous metastases reported in melanoma (melanin-postive), breast carcinoma and oat cell carcinoma
Postchemotherapy[22]	No increase in spontaneous loss or anomalies in pregnancies after completion of chemotherapy or during treatment	None reported
Leiomyoma[23]	Abnormal implantation (low-lying or previa), accreta, or fenestrated placenta, abruption	Occasionally mild uterine vascular insufficiency (due to poor pericervical perfusion), incomplete placenta with myofibers within the delivered basal plate, abnormal shape, extra lobes, abnormally thin
Abdominal trauma[24,26]	Fetal demise in 20%, related to severity of maternal injury, maternal hypoperfusion and fetal hypoxemia, abruption (in 6% to 66% of major abdominal trauma), premature birth, preterm labor or membrane rupture, and fetal fractures	Increased trophoblast basophilia due to maternal hypoperfusion, typical changes in abruption, often small abruption-like lesions are seen in preterm labor/birth after trauma
Thyroid disease[27]	Hypothyroidism: infertility, and increased spontaneous loss, congenital anomalies, stillbirth if untreated Hypothyroidism: IUGR, fetal tachycardia, hyperkinesis and neonatal thyrotoxicosis	None reported
Skin disease[28]	Dermatopathic melanosis	Melanin deposted in Hofbauer cells, areas of calcification
Asthma[29]	Increased risk of prematurity, perinatal death; transplacental theophylline may cause fetal tachycardia; epinephrine decreases uteroplacental flow and is linked to congenital anomalies	None reported
Hemoglobinopathy (especially sickle cell disease)[30,31]	Reports of IUGR and spontaneous abortions with sickle trait but more common in disease	Any HbS will lead to intervillous sickling; homozygous HbS or HbS paired with another abnormal Hb, acceleration of villous maturity, infarcts, abruptions and villous edema
Maternal anemia High-altitude effects[32]	Folic acid deficiency may lead to abruption, rarely associated with "nonimmume" hydrops fetalis	Placentomegaly, increased syncytial knotting
Maternal diabetes mellitus	Increased incidence of preeclampsia, late fetal death, congenital anomalies, fetal macrosomia, neonatal hypoglycemia, fetal asphyxia, fetal trauma and dystocia/abnormal labor due to large fetus	Placentomegaly, increased intervillous space, increased villous tissue Placentomegaly, immature villi with diffuse edema, numerous tortuous vessels, uterine vascular insufficiency when diabetic vasculopathy is present
Inflammatory bowel disease[33]	No change in disease course	None reported
Maternal obesity[34]	Excessive fetal growth, increased risk of diabetes mellitus, preeclampsia, and medical complications such as wound dehiscence, thrombophlebitis, dystocia, dysfunctional labor, fetal trauma, twins	Placentomegaly, abnormal (delayed) villous maturation
Renal disease/transplantation[33]	Infertility, preeclampsia, infection	May be normal, may have vasculopathy, probably related to cause of renal failure

(continued)

Table 69-4 Common maternal conditions associated with placental lesions—cont'd

Maternal conditions	Maternal/fetal neonatal conditions	Placental lesions
Liver disease[35-38]	May occur due to pregnancy (HELLP syndrome); acute fatty liver occurs in third trimester, mild prodrome, jaundice, hepatic encephalopathy, and high maternal and fetal mortality	None reported, although in HELLP syndrome, liver dysfunction may accompany histology otherwise consistent with preeclampsia
Maternal heart disease	Reduced uteroplacental blood flow, with ?IUGR	Villous hypoperfusion changes, fibrosis, intervillous thombosis, and reduced villous surface exchange area
Alcohol abuse[39,40]	IUGR, mental retardation, dysmorphisms, short umbilical cord	Reported lesions include acute ascending infection, meconium staining, but may be related to socioeconomics of ethanol abuse
Cocaine[41,42]	Abruptio placentae, IUGR, neonatal hypertension, learning disability	Lesions may reflect effects of severe maternal vasoconstriction (retroplacental hematoma meconium), but no lesions may be seen
Maternal hyper-coagulability[43]	Systemic arterial or venous thrombi, pregnancy wastage	Decidual thrombi, placental infarction, ?chronic villitis
Maternal connective tissue disorders[44]	SLE associated with fetal cardiac arrhythmia due to conduction system damage; scleroderma associated with abortion, stillbirth, prematurity	Often chronic villitis, and changes consistent with preeclampsia. In scleroderma, there are reports of "maternal floor infarct"
Maternal heart disease	Reduced uteroplacental blood flow, with ?IUGR	Villous hypoperfusion changes, fibrosis, intervillous thombosis, and reduced villous surface exchange areas
Tobacco abuse[45,46]	Increased spontaneous abortions, low birth weight, single umbilical artery; passive smoking may have similar effects	Reduced placental weight, fibrosis/hypovascularity and/or hypervascularity (? dose effect) decidual necrosis, small infarcts degeneration of endothelium with thrombosis of umbilical vessels
Idiopathic thrombocytopenic purpura (ITP)[47]	Rarely bleeding under 50,000/μl rare intraventricular hemorrhage thrombocytopenia in 50% of neonates	Intervillous thrombi, infarcts, and decidual vascular lesions may be present
Thrombotic thrombocytopenic purpura (TTP)[48]	High mortality rate for both fetus and mother	Hyaline thrombi in maternal decidual vessels resembling atheroma

IUGR, Intrauterine growth retardation; *SLE*, systemic lupus erythematosus.

rated from the uterine wall by retroplacental hemorrhage from abnormal decidual vessels.[57] Separation from the uterine lining precludes effective blood flow to the involved placental area, acutely reducing fetoplacental oxygen availability.[57] Placental compression by a retroplacental hematoma increases fetal blood volume and may be associated with the visceral and germinal matrix hemorrhages commonly seen in abruption.[57] Basal intervillous thrombi are primarily maternal blood;[58] these lesions may be mild forms of abruption-type pathology. Scarred, shrunken, fibrotic, and hypovascular villi, with reduced number or caliber of placental capillaries (Fig. 69-7, *A*), result from destruction of growing villous capillaries by abnormal uteroplacental flow.[59] Villous capillary damage may lead to fetomaternal hemorrhage, which is more frequent in hypertensive pregnancies in the second trimester.[60] Since 500 ml/min of maternal blood is directed to the placenta, a reduced villous capillary bed may increase fetal cardiac work. An indirect reflection of placental resistance is the umbilical systolic/diastolic (S/D) ratio. The S/D ratio approaches infinity and end-diastolic flow in the umbilical artery may be negative when the placental capillary bed is reduced.[61] If fetoplacental volume is decreased, reduced fetal glomerular filtration rate may cause oligohydramnios and may be associated with fetal distress.[62]

Maternal and fetal effects of preeclampsia may not be evident until many weeks after uterine vascular conversion is complete (22 to 24 weeks). The chronic subclinical effects of

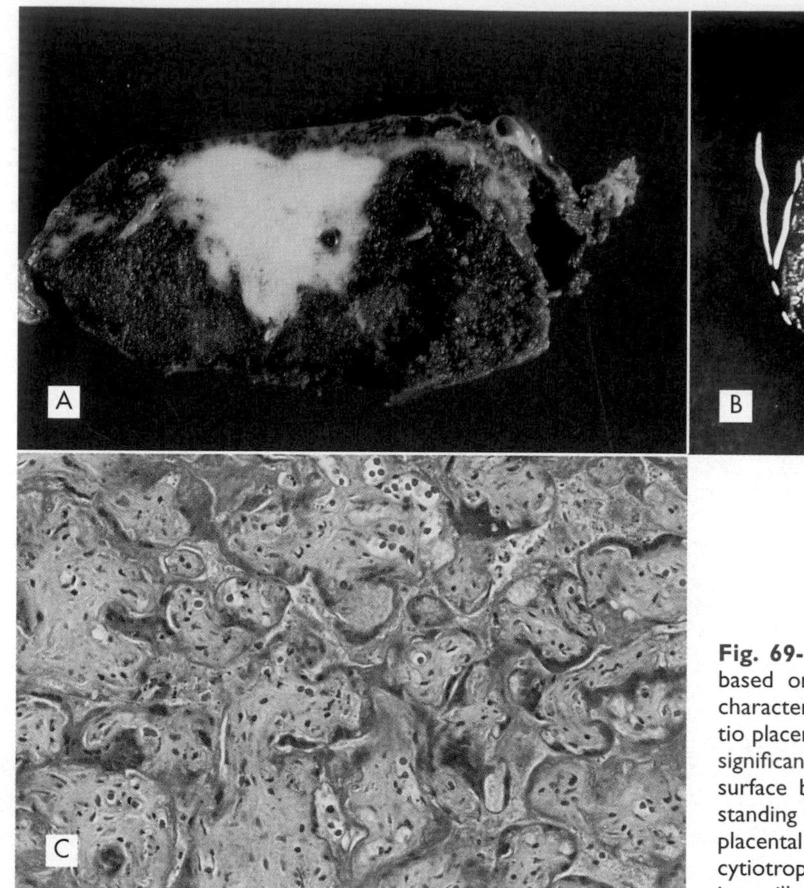

Fig. 69-6 **A,** Wedge-shaped infarct of several days duration based on the white coloration. **B,** Retroplacental hematoma characteristic of one third of cases clinically suspected of abruptio placentae. The central location seen in this case is much more significant than a marginal location. Indentation of the placental surface by the well-formed hematoma is consistent with long standing and is usually associated with infarction of the overlying placental villi. **C,** Infarct shows ghost-like villi with smudged syncytiotrophoblasts and cellular debris in the collapsed maternal intervillous space.

decidual vasculopathy on the fetus and placenta may be extensive (Table 69-5).

Hypercoagulable states

Maternal hypercoagulable states may damage maternal vasculature, and they carry increased risk of pregnancy failure.[63-67] The characteristic pathology of pregnancy loss in these conditions, decidual thrombosis and placental infarction,[68] is not pathognomonic. Hypercoagulability may accompany maternal autoimmune diseases (e.g., systemic lupus erythematosus) or may occur in clinically healthy patients. Serologic definition of these states is controversial[69,70] but includes detection of the "lupus anticoagulant" and anticardiolipin and antiphospholipid antibodies. Many mechanisms have been proposed to explain their thrombogenic properties, but antiphospholipid antibodies may be mere epiphenomena of other primary disorders.[71] The uterine vasculature is particularly susceptible to thrombosis; its endothelium is normally eroded, and its basement membranes and decidual stromal collagen are normally exposed to circulating maternal platelets, for up to 24 weeks. Fetal death associated with antiphospholipid antibodies and the typical decidual thromboses and placental infarctions occur in the second trimester.[68,72] Deficiencies in protein C, S[13,73] and antithrombin III may cause hypercoagulability during pregnancy, fetal wastage, and similar placental findings.

Smoking and cocaine use

These common maternal habits can affect placental growth and development and are associated with greater likelihood of poor pregnancy outcome. Maternal smoking increases circulating nicotine levels, causing uterine vasoconstriction and reduced uteroplacental flow for minutes after a cigarette has been smoked.[74] Structural changes in the placenta have been described.[75,76] Maternal smoking increases the concentrations of thiocyanate, carboxyhemoglobin, and carcinogens.[77,78] Smoking may reduce fetal prostacyclin production[79] and acutely cause fetal tachycardia.[80]

Cocaine is an even more powerful vasoconstrictor. There is a reported increase of abruptions, a "decidual vascular accident," in mothers using cocaine.[81] Placental transfer of cocaine also may directly affect fetoplacental hemodynamics.[82] Indirect effects of cocaine on the conceptus may include maternal ischemia and reperfusion producing oxygen free radicals. Oxygen free radicals may be potent inducers of fetal damage.[83]

Diabetes mellitus

Abnormal placental vascular development is commonly related to maternal diseases, including diabetes mellitus. In maternal diabetes mellitus, abnormal growth factor expression and effect may be associated with overgrowth of the placental vessels (Fig. 69-7, *B*), as well as a wide range of direct fetal effects, including macrosomia, polycythemia, and late fetal death.[84] Vascular proliferation may be seen in other conditions, including IUGR[85] and twin gestations, in which case two fetuses are competing for a single volume of uterine blood flow. In maternal diabetes mellitus, fetal IUGR, and multiple gestation, capillary proliferation may be an endothelial response to decreased oxygen availability.[85] Capillary proliferation may increase placental microvascular resistance, the dif-

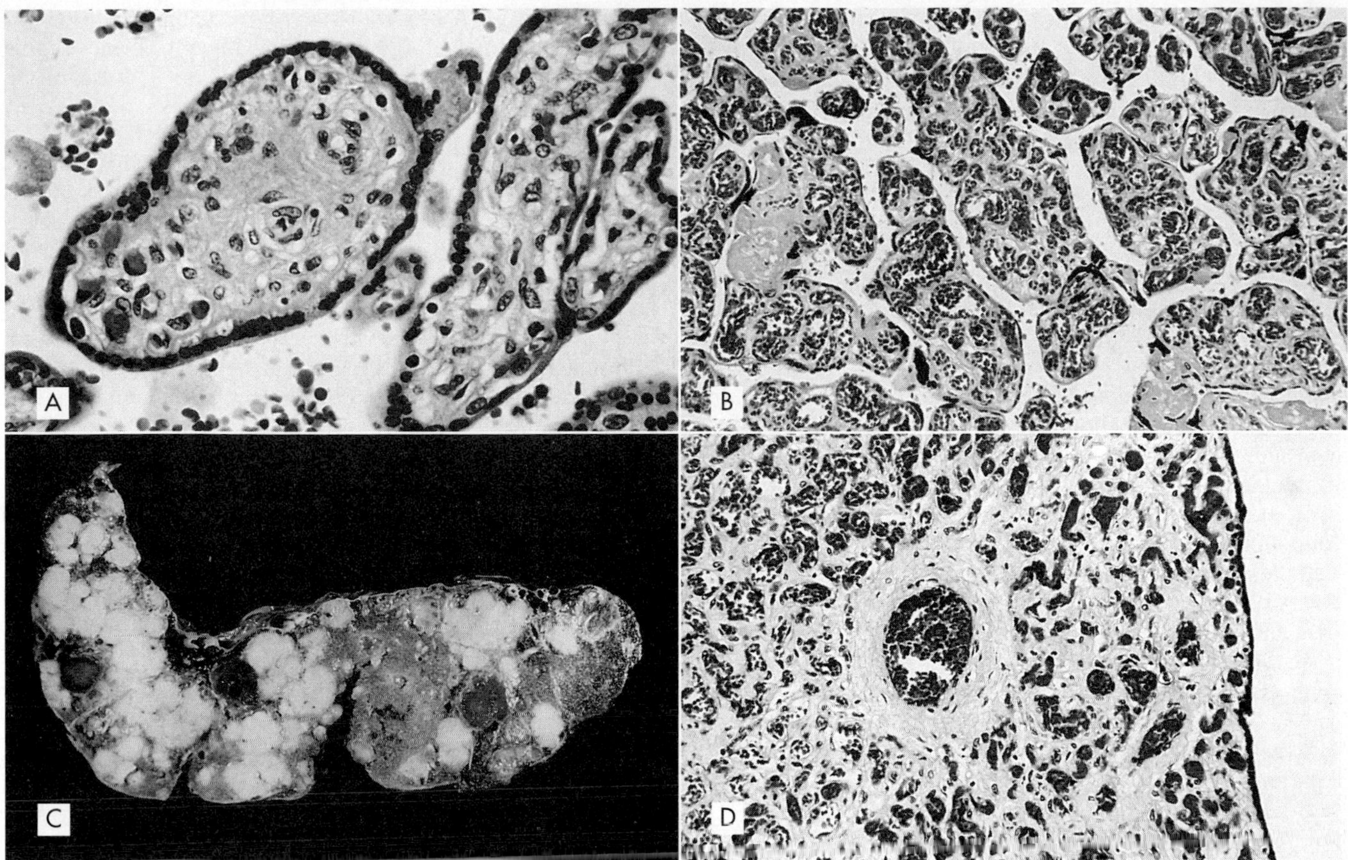

Fig. 69-7 **A,** Hypovascular villi are characterized by smaller than expected or more centrally placed vessels rather than a reduction in number. **B,** Chorangiosis is defined as villi with greater than 10 vessels, in 10 villi, in 10 fields at 10× power. At term the normal villus has 2 to 6 vessels. **C,** Chorangioma is a true benign tumor of the placenta. More often occurring singly, multiple chorangiomas may be associated with placentomegaly. (Courtesy Bahig M. Shehata, M.D., and The Toledo Hospital, Toledo, Ohio.) **D,** Chorangiomas are hemangiomas that are usually covered by trophoblasts and may be loosely associated with the placenta and therefore amenable to infarction.

Table 69-5 Effects of decidual vascular pathologic conditions on placenta and fetus

Placental effects	Fetal effects
Intervillous thrombosis Villous infarcts Decreased capillary number Reduced capillary diameter Hypertrophy of vascular smooth muscle Increased trophoblast knots Increased perivillous fibrin Increased fibrinoid necrosis "X-cell" proliferation	Few direct effects; indirect effects are related to extent of placental damage and reduced placental function. Indirect effects include impaired fetal metabolism and fetal growth, fetal hypoxia, abnormal placental and umbilical hemodynamics
Intraplacental coagulation	
Hemorrhagic endovasculitis	Placentofetal embolic damage
Placental intravascular thrombi	Rare fetomaternal bleeding, fetal anemia, hydrops
Capillary destruction and villous stromal hemorrhage	
Abruption	IUFD, due to acute asphyxia Visceral and germinal matrix hemorrhages Necrotizing enterocolitis

IUFD, Intrauterine fetal demise.

fusion distance for nutrients to cross the placental membrane, fetoplacental intravascular volume, and fetal cardiac work. Umbilical S/D ratios generally remain within normal limits (CS, unpublished observations). Chorangioma (Fig. 69-7, *C, D*), a focal placental vascular tumor or malformation, occurs singly or multifocally and may function as an arteriovenous malformation or vascular shunt. This lesion may present with stillbirth, hydrops fetalis caused by congestive heart failure, or unexplained fetal tachycardia.

ABNORMAL PLACENTAL IMPLANTATION

Placenta previa, implantation of the placenta partially or completely over the cervical os, is the most common cause of antepartum hemorrhage. Other causes are shown in Table 69-6. Predisposing factors for abnormal site of implantation include maternal age, parity, anatomic uterine abnormality (leiomyoma, septate uterus), and previous uterine surgery (curettage, cesarean section, or myomectomy).[86] The delivered placenta previa may show basal decidual hemosiderin or focal villous atrophy in the area of previa.

Placenta accreta is a generic term for an abnormally deep trophoblast invasion into the uterine wall. This results in difficult placental delivery. Either retention of placental fragments or uterine damage by areas of accreta may cause postpartum hemorrhage. *Placenta increta* extends into the myometrium, and *placenta percreta* completely through the wall, even into the bladder. The lower uterine segment, endocervix, and fallopian tube do not transform into decidua. By definition, implantation in these sites results in placenta accreta. Placenta accreta and placenta previa frequently occur together. Most cases are clinically diagnosed. Diagnosis of placenta accreta may be difficult from gross placental examination alone. Most indicative of placenta accreta is focal absence of cotyledons, but absent cotyledons, especially at the placental margins, may be overlooked. The true depth of placental implantation is determined only when the rare hysterectomy is performed following peripartum hemorrhage. Histologically there is absent decidua and the villi are implanted on or into the myometrium or tubal muscle (Fig. 69-8). The amount of Nitabuch's fibrinoid is usually decreased. There may be absent placental septae.

Circumvallate membrane insertion may result from abnormally deep implantation in the normal location (the uterus). In some cases, circumvallate membrane insertion is believed to reflect a healed injury to the amnion and chorion. It is associated with maternal bleeding, preterm delivery, and, possibly, IUGR and must be distinguished from circummarginate membrane insertion, which is not associated with any abnormal fetal outcome.

Table 69-6 Abnormal placental implantation resulting in maternal hemorrhage

Placental findings	Incidence	Significance
Placenta accreta (increta, percreta) absent decidua	0.4%	AP and PP hemorrhage Uterine rupture Maternal and fetal mortality
Placenta previa	5% to 28% 0.3% to 3%	Early pregnancy, common Term delivery, less common May be partial or complete AP hemorrhage Maternal and fetal mortality
Low-lying placenta	?	Placenta accreta PP hemorrhage
Abruptio placentae	0.17% to 3.75%	Fetal mortality (30% to 65%) AP bleeding Tonic uterine contractions 33% are associated with a retroplacental hematoma Placental infarct
Circumvallate placenta	1% to 5%	AP bleeding Premature delivery Associated with abruptio placenta

AP, Ante partum; *PP,* post partum.

PLACENTAL EXAMINATION IN FETAL DISEASE

Multiple gestation

Multiple gestations carry higher risk to both maternal and fetal well-being. Maternal risks are most often the result of increased pregnancy hormone levels (e.g., gestational diabetes mellitus), expanded blood volume (anemia), uterine overdistention (e.g., preterm labor and postpartum hemorrhage), and increased placental mass (some cases of preeclampsia).[88-93] Despite advances in neonatal care, perinatal mortality in twins is 14%. The risk varies with type of placentation. Although only 1% of twin placentas are monochorionic monoamniotic, they account for 54% of the deaths.

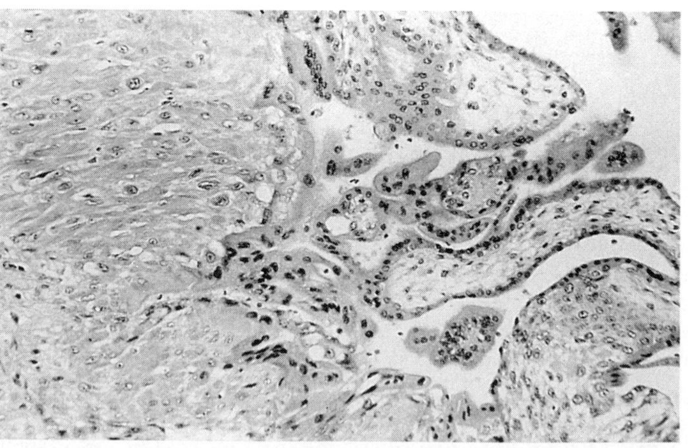

Fig. 69-8 Placenta accreta showing absent decidualized endometrium with implantation of the villi directly onto the myometrium with deficiency of Nitabuch's fibrinoid.

Monochorionic diamniotic placentation accounts for 30% of twins and 27% of total mortality. Therefore monochorionic placentation accounts for 31% of twins but 71% of twin mortalities.[88,92]

Twinning is the most common naturally occurring type of multiple gestation. The incidence of monozygotic twinning (identical or monovular twins) is stable worldwide (3 to 5/1000 births). The etiology is unknown but may be a teratogenic event. There is a 1% recurrence risk. Dizygotic twinning (fraternal or binovular twins) in the United States occurs in approximately 8/1000 births, but this incidence varies with populations. When twinning is familial, it is dizygotic, due to an inherited propensity to multiple ovulations. Twinning is more frequent with advanced maternal age and increased parity.[87] Rarely, dizygotic twins may be conceived at nearly the same time (*superfecundation*) or be conceived at different times (*superfetation*), and possibly by different fathers. Twenty percent of dichorionic twins are monozygous. Zygosity can be determined in 55% to 60% of twins by a combination of placental examination and knowledge of the sex of the babies.[94] All monochorionic twins are monozygous, and all opposite-sexed twins are dizygotic. Slightly more than half of dichorionic placentas are associated with like-sex babies; of these, additional testing will reveal one third to be monozygous.[94] Whether dichorionic placentas are separate or fused is not predictive of zygosity because this is determined by proximity of implantation of the two blastocysts. Placentation with monozygous twins is determined by the time of zygote or blastocyst division. In earlier division, the placentas are more separate. Late division (occurring after postovulation day 13) results in conjoined twins.[93]

The pathologist should examine the chorion to determine number, locate vascular anastomoses, and identify other abnormalities. It is useful to have the obstetrician label which umbilical cord was associated with twin A (born first) and which with twin B (born second). Twin A is usually nearest the birth canal and more susceptible to ascending (transcervical) infection. Twin B is more likely to be growth retarded, have congenital malformations, or suffer from perinatal asphyxia than twin A. This accounts for the convention that twin B has a worse perinatal outcome. In the long term, twin B does not fare worse than twin A if all other circumstances are taken into consideration (e.g., IUGR, single umbilical artery, and congenital malformations).[88] If the placenta is received in pathology without labeled cords, the pathologist should identify the different cords, placental regions, and membranes as twin 1 and twin 2.

Monochorionic twins share a single placental disk. However, the placental zones surrounding each umbilical cord should be treated separately and sections submitted for each. Separate or partly fused placentas are examined identically to singleton placentas. For a single placental disk, a membrane roll from the dividing membrane or its junction on the placental surface (the "T-zone") is the single most important section. Gross examination of the dividing membrane usually reveals the number of amnions and chorions. Membranes in different types of placentation are shown in Fig. 69-9. The vascular bed associated with an individual umbilical cord (vascular equator) may not be the same as the division of the placental disk made by the dividing membrane. Discordant placental sizes may not be the sole determinant of discordant twin growth. The normal weight of the singleton placenta for a given gestational age has been established, but similar standards have not been published for twin placentas. In dichorionic diamniotic separate placentas, the weight is not double that expected for a singleton at the same gestational age. From personal experience, monochorionic placentas are usually 1½ times heavier than expected for a singleton placenta. Cord length is shorter in twins, due in part to confined space in the uterus.[95]

Superficial *vascular anastomoses* are seen in most monochorionic placentas and are easy to identify by injecting air or milk into the vessels. The vessels involved can be distinguished by their orientation on the chorionic plate. Arteries always cross over veins, and in each placental area there should be a paired artery and vein. Deep anastomoses, the so-called third circulation, most commonly involve an outflow artery-to-vein anastomosis balanced by a vein-to-artery inflow anastomosis. When unbalanced, the outflow vessel may be large, calcified, and not paired with a vessel returning to the same cord. Careful dissection may reveal the cotyledon, which is supplied by one twin and drained by the other twin.

More accurate identification of these anastomoses requires cumbersome injection studies. For such studies, the placenta must be submitted intact, unfixed, and at room temperature. The blood clots must be flushed from the circulation. The chorionic vessels may then be injected with a water-soluble dye, milk, or radiopaque fluid[96] (Fig. 69-9, *B*). This technique is generally used only for research purposes and only exceptionally in routine pathology practice. The common indications for extensive evaluation of the placental circulation are death of one or both twins, discordance of intrauterine growth or fetal well-being, and fetal anomalies.

Fetal death is a common complication of multiple gestation. Cord accidents, including cord entanglement, complicate 50% of fetal demise in single sac twins. Prolapse of the umbilical cord of twin B during delivery of twin A[97] is more common in monoamniotic placentas, but may occur in any type of placentation as the dividing membrane ruptures. During the first trimester, as many as 21% of twins may be lost.[97] In early fetal losses, there may be no evidence of the fetus at the time of delivery (the "vanishing twin").[97] Fetal loss in the second or third trimester occurs in 0.5% to 6.8%.[98] A fetus papyraceous forms following fetal death after 13 weeks of gestation (Fig. 69-10). Radiologic confirmation of suspected fetus papyraceous will show skeletal remains. Death of one twin may be followed by death of the co-twin because they may share a "hostile environment," or premature delivery of the living twin. Although maternal coagulopathy may occur with a retained dead fetus, it is rare if only one of the pair dies. Focal embolic or thrombotic damage of brain, skin, kidneys, and intestine of the living co-twin may occur. This may be related to passage of thromboplastins derived from dead tissue into the circulation of the surviving twin through placental vascular anastomoses. Alternatively, after the demise of the co-twin, the circulation of the dead twin loses vasomotor tone. The drop in blood pressure across anastomoses may cause hypovolemic/hypotensive ischemia and damage to the surviving twin.[99-101] When one of a twin pair dies, the placenta of the dead twin is initially normal but will eventually atrophy from hypoperfusion unless the living co-twin continues to perfuse its capillary bed through anastomoses.[102]

Prematurity, acute chorioamnionitis, premature rupture of membranes, and IUGR of one or both twins are all more com-

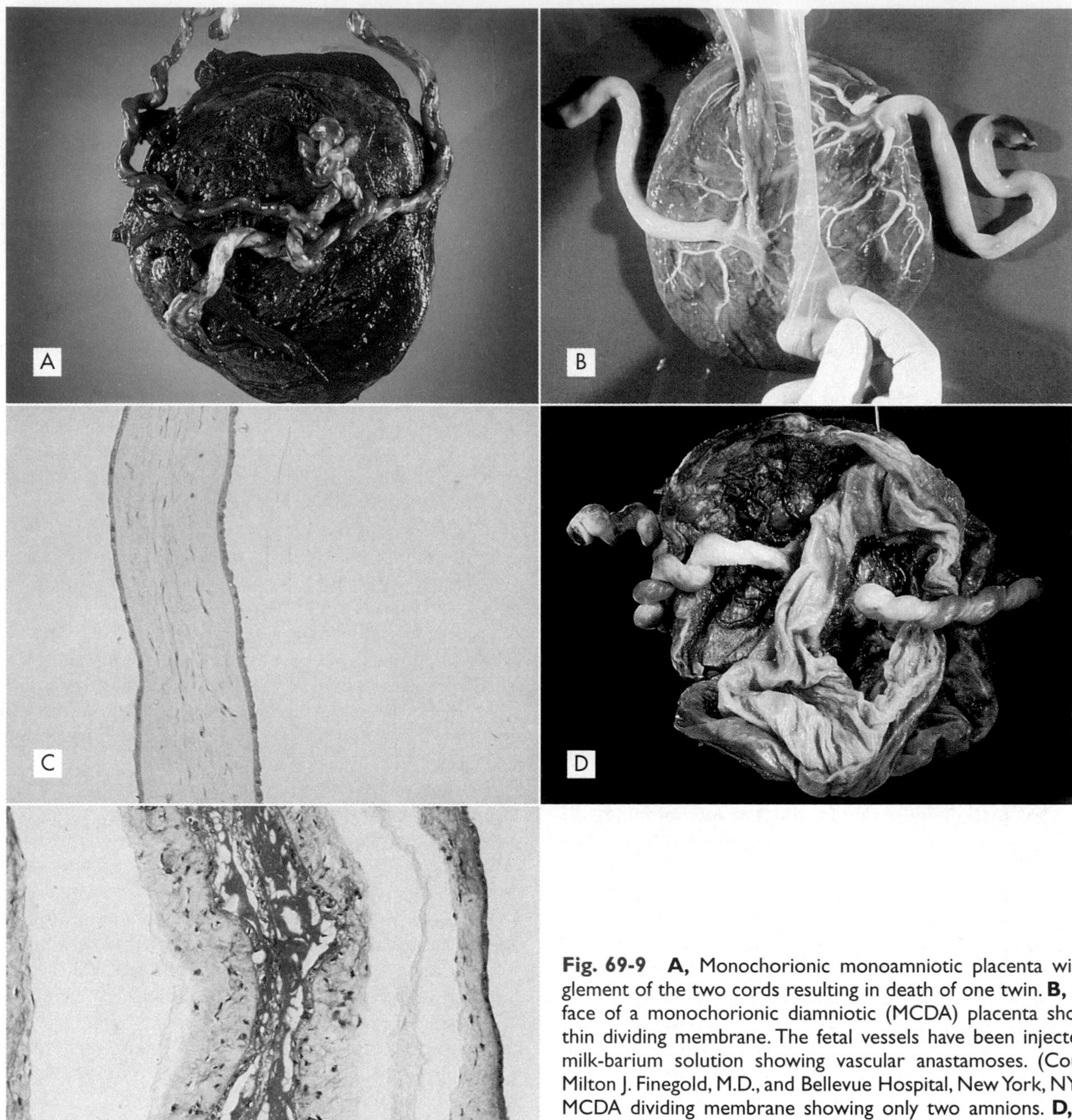

Fig. 69-9 **A,** Monochorionic monoamniotic placenta with entanglement of the two cords resulting in death of one twin. **B,** Fetal surface of a monochorionic diamniotic (MCDA) placenta showing the thin dividing membrane. The fetal vessels have been injected with a milk-barium solution showing vascular anastamoses. (Courtesy of Milton J. Finegold, M.D., and Bellevue Hospital, New York, NY.) **C,** The MCDA dividing membrane showing only two amnions. **D,** Dichorionic diamniotic (DCDA) placenta showing the very thick dividing membrane. **E,** The dividing membrane showing two amnions separated by cellular chorion, which gives the membranes their thick gross appearance and which also contains a few ghostlike villi.

mon in multifetal gestations and carry risk for immediate and long-term morbidity and mortality. At the beginning of twin gestation, the weight and size of both fetuses are equal and appropriate for gestational age. Twins follow the growth curves of singletons until the third trimester, when their rate of growth slows. This may be due to uterine crowding, decreased placental reserve, or abnormal blood flow to one twin.[103] The IUGR is usually asymmetric, with "head sparing." *Discordant growth* of monozygous twins may be due to unequal division of cytoplasmic mass during the equal division of the genetic material or the twin transfusion syndrome (discussed in subsequent paragraphs). Discordant growth is seen almost as commonly in dizygous twins. Chronic villitis, intraplacental thrombi, fibrosis, villous hypovascularity, villous infarcts, and maternal decidual vasculopathy are seen more commonly in the smaller dichorionic twin.[104] IUGR and fetal compromise are more common with velamentous cord insertion. Congenital malformations occur in approximately 10% of monochorionic twins.[105,106] Single umbilical artery (SUA) is seen in 2.5% to 4% of twins as compared with approximately 1% in singletons. SUA is seen in 20% of acardiac twins.[107] Abnormal cord insertions are seen in 16% of all twins, compared with 1% in singletons. Marginal insertion is seen in 14% of monochorionic and 4% of dichorionic placentas. Velamentous

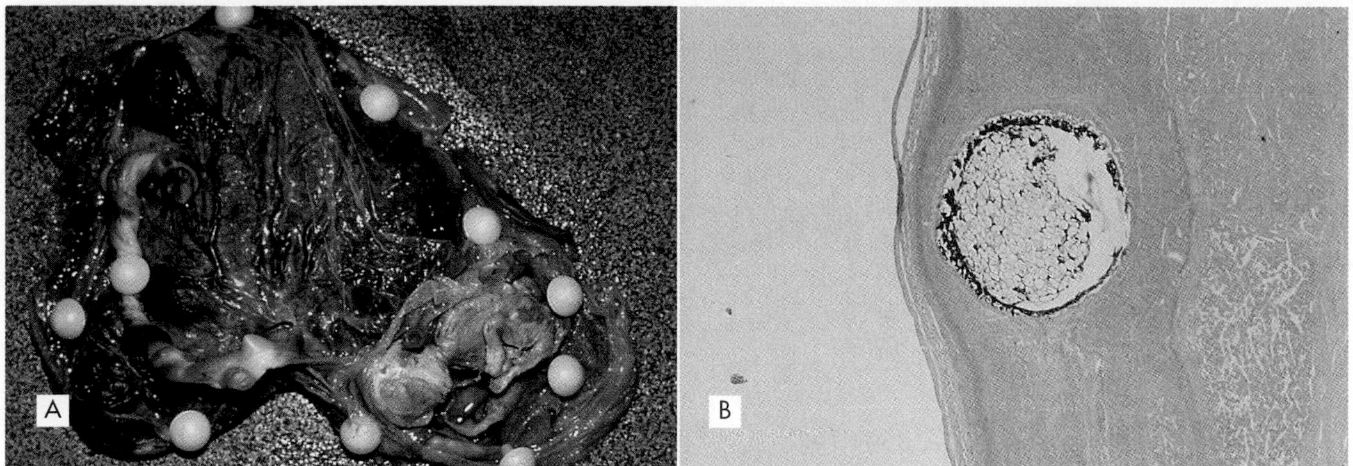

Fig. 69-10 **A,** Fetus papyraceous showing a small fetus in separate amniotic sac at the margin of an otherwise normal placenta **B,** A plaquelike lesion was noted on the placental surface of this singleton placenta, which on sectioning, demonstrated fetal tissues, bone, and remnants of intestines, consistent with the "vanishing twin."

insertion is seen in 9% of monochorionic and 5% of dichorionic placentas.[107] There is a higher incidence of loss of chromosomal material and midline defects, including neural tube defects, facial clefts, tracheoesophageal fistulas, and sirenomelia.[106]

Although nearly all monochorionic placentas have vascular anastomoses, *twin transfusion syndrome (TTS)* occurs in from 7.5% to 30%.[88,92] Chronic TTS occurs most often in monochorionic diamniotic placentas, infrequently in monochorionic monoamniotic placentas (possibly caused by nearly complete sharing of the placental substance), and rarely in dichorionic diamniotic fused placentas.[108] TTS is the result of chronic unidirectional vascular "steal," from the artery of one twin (donor) through the "third circulation" to the vein of the other twin (recipient). When one twin's cord is inserted velamentously, the fetal vessels are adjacent to the rigid myometrium and are not on the chorionic plate, and thus are more subject to compression. This twin is more likely to become the donor.[109] The donor is growth retarded and anemic, with delayed organ maturation and oligohydramnios.[110,111] The recipient becomes plethoric and is overgrown.[110] Polyhydramnios and congestive heart failure (caused by volume overload) and polycythemia may occur.[110] Although the criteria for clinical diagnosis of TTS remain controversial, TTS should be considered when monochorionic twins have >20% discordance in their weights and >5 g/dl difference in hemoglobin levels.[112] However, discordance of weight and hematocrit of equal or greater severity can occur in cases without TTS.[112] The placenta reflects the fetal abnormalities (Fig. 69-11, *A, B*).[113]

Acute TTS may occur at the time of fetal demise, during delivery, or rarely, in conjunction with chronic TTS.[114] Placentas examined after selective feticide in cases of severe TTS show sclerosis of the chorionic circulation of the terminated twin.[115] Laser ablation of anastomotic vessels results in yellow-tan nodules, which are either confined to the chorionic surface or may extend the full thickness of the placenta. Injection studies show no or very small residual anastomotic channels.[115,116]

Acardia is a rare malformation restricted to monozygotic twins of either monoamniotic or diamniotic placentation. Its occurrence is estimated at 1/35,000 births.[93,117] Acardia is caused by reversal of blood flow, most commonly through superficial vascular anastomoses. The acardiac twin loses direct vascular connection with the placental villi and receives its entire blood supply from the pump twin. Close proximity of the two umbilical cords on a common chorion and discordant development between the twins must be present for reversal of arterial blood flow to occur. Deoxygenated, low-pressure blood from the pump twin, which would normally return to the placenta, instead flows directly to the acardiac twin, causing a wide array of structural abnormalities. Chromosomal abnormalities have been reported in more than 50% of the acardiac twins studied.[117,118] Mortality of the pump twin is 50% to 75%, usually the result of heart failure, and of course 100% of acardiac fetuses die.[119] The acardiac twin may be amorphous, and a diagnosis of placental teratoma may be considered. The absence of umbilical cord or axial skeleton is consistent with a teratoma (Fig. 69-12).[120]

Conjoined twins are a rare malformation of monochorionic monoamniotic twinning occurring in 1/50,000 to 100,000 live births. Conjoined twins presumably result from late division of the blastocyst.[121] They may have umbilical cords that are branched or fused, often with an abnormal number of vessels.

Higher-order multiple births (triplets, quadruplets, etc.) are more frequent in recent years, due to delayed childbearing, use of fertility drugs, and in vitro fertilization techniques. Naturally occurring higher-order multiple births are infrequent (triplets 1/10,000 births, quadruplets 1/100,000 births).[122] Higher-order multiple births may be a combination of monozygous and dizygous siblings. The placenta is evaluated as described previously, with particular attention paid to the number of chorions and amnions. Monochorionic placentation means monozygosity of those offspring, independent of other placental features.

Early fetal loss

Approximately 50% of spontaneous abortions are caused by fetal karyotypic abnormalities. Discordance of genetic composition of the trophoblast and the conceptus and placental postmitotic errors may lead to confined placental mosaicism, and

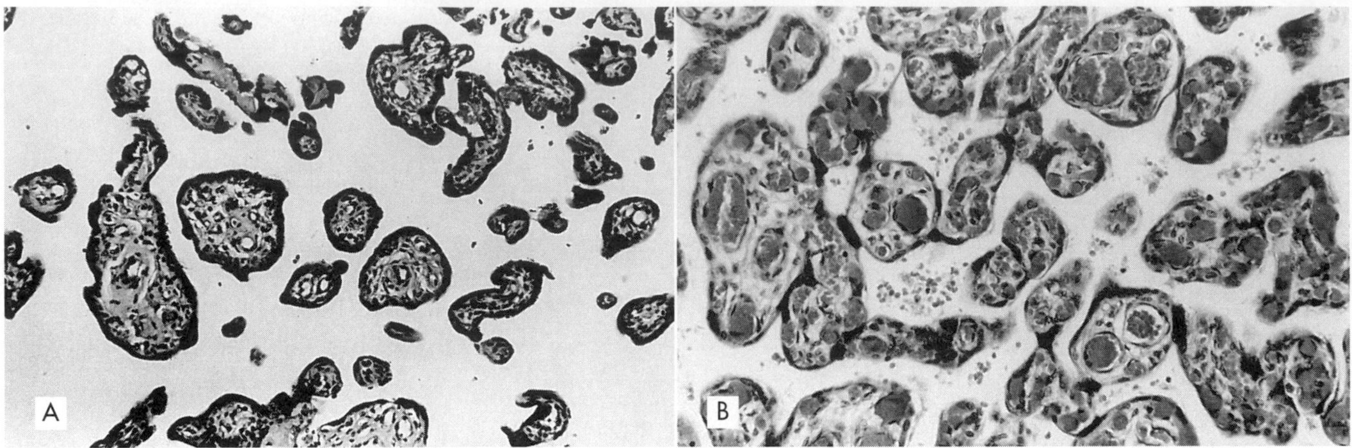

Fig. 69-11 The placenta in twin transfusion syndrome shows placental differences consistent with the changes seen in the fetuses. **A,** the donor villi are more immature than expected for gestation. The villous vessels are empty or contain nucleated red blood cells. Perivillous/intervillous fibrinoid may be increased; only a small portion is seen here. **B,** The recipient villi are more mature, usually appropriate for gestation, with a few syncytial knots and dilated and congested vessels.

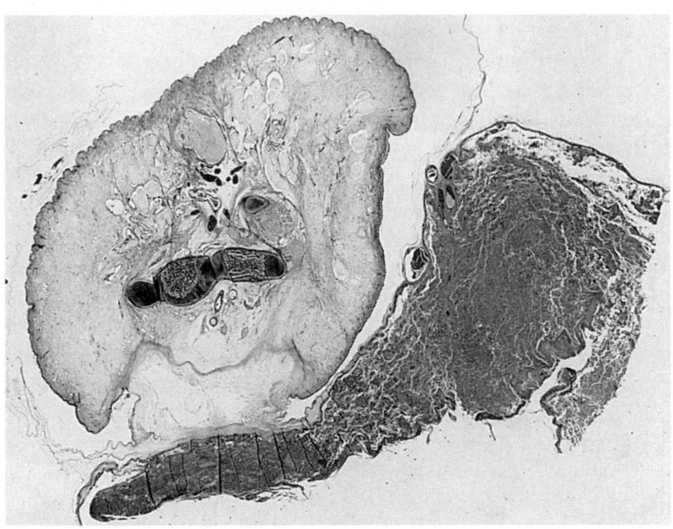

Fig. 69-12 A nodule noted at the periphery of the placental disk is probably a placental teratoma rather than an acardiac because of the absent umbilical cord and lack of a well-developed axial skeleton.

discordance between fetal and placental karyotype on chorionic villous sampling.[123] If examination of the chromosomes of spontaneously aborted fetuses shows an abnormal fetal karyotype, the risk of subsequent pregnancy loss is less than if the karyotype were normal. If the karyotype is normal, additional studies might be indicated, especially if there were prior pregnancy losses or "habitual abortion." In women receiving therapy for recurrent spontaneous abortions, fetal karyotype is helpful in deciding if treatment has failed or if that particular pregnancy would have been lost despite treatment. Pathologic examination of products of conception (POC) should include but not be limited to tissue documentation of the *fact* of pregnancy, since examination of POC can contribute data relevant to patient counseling and future therapy.[124-126]

The pathologic examination of POC is performed to determine the cause of pregnancy failure and retrospectively to evaluate placental and decidual integrity and fetal viability. In genetically normal conceptuses, the tissues often reveal an embryo viable for most of the gestation. Abortion can be related to abnormalities of the placenta, decidua, or both. In genetically abnormal conceptions, the embryo/fetus may be abnormal or have failed to form at all, and placental and decidual lesions are caused by embryo/fetal demise.

Fetal viability may be estimated by the type of erythroid elements in the placental circulation. Nucleated erythrocytes are produced in the yolk sac and circulate in the early weeks of pregnancy. With hepatic hematopoiesis (week 7 to 9), anucleate erythrocytes begin to circulate. The proportion of nucleated erythrocytes is closely correlated with crown-rump length (Table 69-7).[127] A greater proportion of nucleated erythrocytes than expected for fetal age indicates an abnormal hematopoietic stress. This occurs in a variety of conditions, including chromosomal aberrations (in particular, triploidy and trisomies), hydrops fetalis, antiphospholipid antibody production, and massive placental infarction, and in recurrent midtrimester losses with dense chronic intervillous inflammation.

In a study of spontaneous loss,[124] we grouped karyotype as euploid and aneuploid and evaluated the histologic features presented in Table 69-8. Decreasing maternal age and increasing gestational age at loss, villous circulation indicative of fetal life to 10+ weeks, decidual vasculitis, chronic intervillositis, and villous infarcts were significantly associated ($p < 0.01$) with euploid and viable conceptions. Because almost all spontaneous abortions are retained in utero for some time following fetal demise and preceeding onset of clinical symptoms, there is a great deal of "baseline pathology" in all tissues of failed pregnancies regardless of etiology. Preliminary data indicate that multiple spontaneous abortions from the same mother will have similar histology and are likely to demonstrate a viable embryo/fetus.

Examination of POC passed spontaneously or removed by curettage must also determine the fact of an intrauterine gestation, confirming that any maternal symptoms are not due to a potentially life-threatening extrauterine gestation. Intrauterine gestation is diagnosed by presence of chorionic villi or decidual trophoblasts on hematoxylin and eosin stain or immuno-

Table 69-7 Correlation of crown-rump length (CRL) and calculated gestational age (EGA) with estimated percentage of nucleated red blood cells (NRBC)

CRL (mm)	EGA (days)	Estimated % NRBC
10	48	97
15	53	75
20	59	58
25	63	42
30	69	28
35	71	18
40	76	10
45	78	4
50	81	1

From Salafia CM, Weigl CA, Foye JG: *Pediatr Pathol* 8:495, 1988.

histochemistry using antibodies to human placental lactogen or cytokeratin.[128,129] The amount of tissue obtained at uterine evacuation increases with gestational age. Discordance between tissue volume and estimated gestational age of a pregnancy may suggest incomplete uterine evacuation. The completeness of evacuation, however, is not a pathologic diagnosis.

Late fetal loss

Genest and others[130-132] have described placental features associated with different times of in utero retention after demise (Table 69-9). In summary, after cessation of the fetal heart, the villous circulation collapses, becoming obliterated. The degeneration of the villous circulation after fetal death is characterized by intraplacental coagulation and endothelial disruption (Fig. 69-13). The circulatory lesions, therefore, are not specific to stillbirth because they may be caused by any process that damages fetoplacental endothelium, including cocaine-induced vasospasm, viral infection, fluctuating perfusion (hypoperfusion/reperfusion), and cessation of perfusion (stillbirth). However, the lesions are generally more diffuse and extensive in stillbirth than in, for example, preeclampsia

Table 69-8 Villous (*n*-221) and decidual (*n*-175) features of nonrecurrent spontaneous losses with normal and abnormal chromosome number

		Normal chromosome number	Abnormal chromosome number
Villous circulation	Absent circulation	43 (46%)	77 (59%)
	Moderate/severe degeneration	24 (26%)	38 (29%)
	Mild degeneration	14 (16%)	15 (11%)
	Intact circulation	9 (10%)	1 (0.07%)
Percentage of nucleated erythrocytes*	**100% (7 weeks)**	**48 (53%)**	**105 (80%)**
	>50% (7-9 weeks)	**7 (8%)**	**8 (6%)**
	5-50% (9-11 weeks)	**5 (5%)**	**9 (7%)**
	<5% (>11 weeks)	**30 (33%)**	**9 (7%)**
Hydropic changes	Not present	41 (46%)	42 (32%)
	Mild/moderate	31 (35%)	56 (43%)
	Severe	18 (20%)	33 (24%)
Perivillous fibrin deposition	Mild	33 (37%)	50 (39%)
	Moderate	50 (55%)	72 (55%)
	Severe	7 (8%)	9 (7%)
Villous infarct	**Not present**	**76 (84%)**	**125 (95%)**
	Present	**14 (16%)**	**6 (6%)**
Chronic intervillositis	**Not present**	**77 (86%)**	**122 (93%)**
	Present	**13 (14%)**	**9 (7%)**
Decidual vascular adaptation	Only normal vessels	36 (48%)	56 (56%)
	Any abnormal	31 (18%)	33 (18%)
Decidual thrombosis	Not present	47 (63%)	72 (72%)
	Present	28 (37%)	28 (28%)
Decidual vasculitis	**Not present**	**43 (57%)**	**68 (68%)**
	Present	**32 (43%)**	**32 (32%)**
Excessive decidual necrosis	Not present	42 (56%)	58 (58%)
	Present	33 (44%)	42 (42%)
	Not present	72 (96%)	96 (96%)
	Present	3 (4%)	4 (4%)
	Not present	43 (57%)	56 (56%)
	Present	52 (43%)	44 (44%)

From Salafia CM, Maier D, Vogel C et al: *Obstet Gynecol* 82:295, 1993.
*Bolded features show significant differences ($p < 0.05$) between pregnancy losses with normal and abnormal chromosome numbers.

Table 69-9 Histologic features as individual markers of time of fetal death

Histologic feature	Time of fetal death (before birth)	Sensitivity	Specificity	Positive predictive value
Good predictors				
Intravascular karyorrhexis	≥6 hr	0.935	1.000	1.000
Stem vessel luminal abnormalities				
Multifocal	≥48 hr	0.944	1.000	1.000
Extensive	≥14 days	0.777	0.976	0.875
Extensive villous fibrosis	≥14 days	1.000	0.928	0.750
Poor predictors				
Stromal "dusty" calcification	≥24 hr	0.478	0.969	0.916
Wharton jelly necrosis	≥48 hr	0.733	0.843	0.688
Trophoblast basement membrane calcification/thickening	≥48 hr	0.333	0.928	0.667
Cord vascular necrosis	≥7 days	0.600	1.000	1.000

From Genest D et al: *Obstet Gynecol* 80:585, 1992.

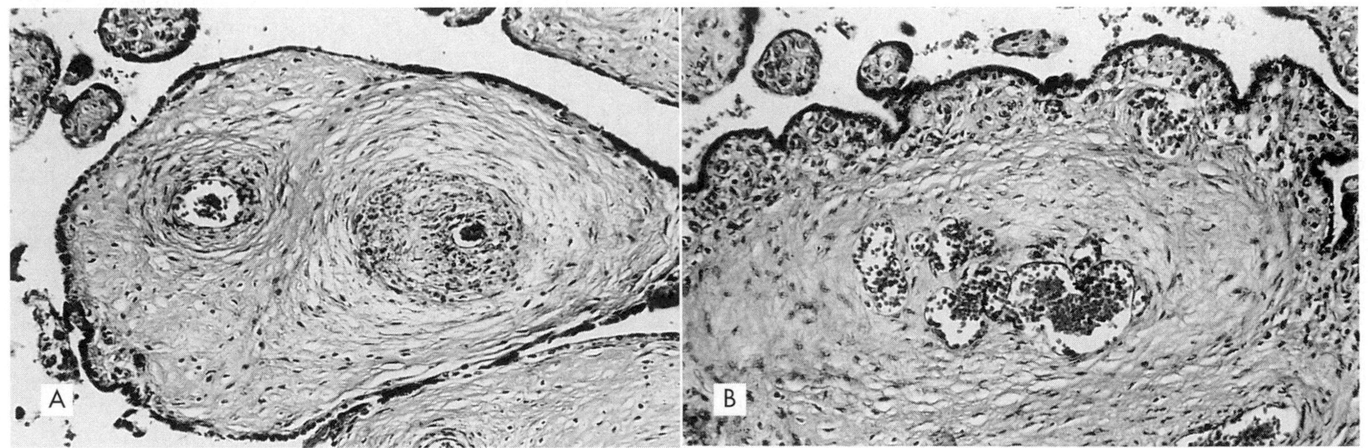

Fig. 69-13 A, The fetal vascular changes referred to as hemorrhagic endovasculosis form a continuum beginning with endothelial vacuolation, muscular proliferation, vessel obliteration, and extravasation of red blood cells. **B,** The vessels may appear to be recanulized.

or IUGR. Villous vaso-occlusion with fetal red cell fragmentation and intravillous bleeding was first described in placentas from stillborn fetuses and was termed "hemorrhagic endovasculitis."[133] This lesion is not a true vasculitis; in stillborn fetuses it may be a postmortem event rather than a cause of death and may occur in in vitro organ cultures[134] or in retained secundines. It is associated with circulatory instability[135] and may be found adjacent to foci of chronic villitis, at the periphery of infarcts and intervillous thrombi, and in infarcted chorangiomas. Chorionic and fetal stem vessel thrombi and avascular terminal villi are related lesions. Intraplacental vaso-occlusion may accompany antiphospholipid antibody-related pregnancy compromise (CS, unpublished observations) or intraamniotic infection by endotoxin-producing organisms.[136] Placental venous thrombi may lead to fetal thromboemboli and cerebral damage. After the fetus dies, the villous stroma also becomes denser and more fibrotic, villous diameter is reduced, and trophoblast basophilia increases.

It is useful for the pathologist to know the clinically estimated time of fetal demise and to have relevant data from postmortem fetal examination.[137,138] Clinically, causes of "late fetal demise" differ with gestational age at demise. In the second trimester, fetal death in utero may be reflect fetal aneuploidy (e.g., Turner's syndrome), "incompetent cervix," or acute intraamniotic infection. Although fetal demise may be caused by intraamniotic infection, fetal sepsis is uncommon in this country, at least in the community hospital. In the last trimester, uteroplacental insufficiency, cord accidents, and diffuse chronic villitis/congenital viral infection are most common. Fetal chromosomal abnormalities are uncommon causes of late fetal death. Abnormal uterine vascular adaptation chronically restricts fetal nutrients before fetal decompensation and death; many such fetuses are IUGR or have a low weight-to-length ratio ("ponderal index"), indicating abnormal weight gain before death. Chronic villitis may suggest congenital viral infection[139-141] or maternal immune-related pathology.[142-144]

Placental lesions reflective of antemortem fetoplacental disease can point to a cause of death in many cases, but some lesions in placentas of dead fetuses are caused by fetal death. As with "hemorrhagic endovasculitis," the dividing line between antemortem lesions and postmortem changes is not always clear. Often the difference among the placentas of a dead fetus, a damaged newborn, and a healthy newborn is the extent of the histologic lesion.

Elective termination of pregnancy

Elective termination of pregnancy causes detachment of the placenta from the uterine lining before any natural messages have signaled that it is time for labor and parturition to begin. Uterotonins employed to induce pregnancy expulsion are extremely effective in initiating uterine contractions, but the contractions of an immature myometrium may be poorly coordinated or extremely intense. Prostaglandin-induced abortion in particular is almost universally associated with abruption and villous stromal hemorrhage. Intervillous coagulation and subchorionic congestion are common.

Low-birth-weight infants

Low birth weight (LBW) is a leading cause of perinatal morbidity and mortality. LBW is also associated with increased mortality in the early postnatal period and during infancy. LBW is due either to premature delivery or to IUGR. LBW is defined as birth weight less than 2500 g and very low birth weight (VLBW) as birth weight less than 1500 g.

Major clinical factors resulting in premature delivery include (1) placenta previa, (2) premature rupture of membranes (before the onset of labor), (3) preterm labor (preterm regular uterine contractions with cervical effacement and dilation with intact membranes at the onset of labor), (4) preeclampsia (hypertension defined as blood pressure of at least 140/90 or increases of 30 mm Hg systolic or 15 mm Hg diastolic, with proteinuria, edema or laboratory abnormalities sufficient to warrant preterm delivery), and (5) nonhypertensive abruption (antepartum vaginal bleeding judged clinically to be sufficient to cause preterm delivery).

Any placenta delivered spontaneously or iatrogenically before term is not a normal placenta. In a study of 249 infants with birth weight <1500 g,[150] more placental and decidual lesions were seen in preterm cases than at term (Table 69-10). No lesion is specific for a particular clinical setting. Acute inflammation was more frequent in premature labor or premature membrane rupture than in preeclampsia. Defective placentation (generally characteristic of preeclampsia) and lesions of chronic placental inflammation are seen in 49% of placentas of infants born at <1500 g to nonhypertensive mothers and may be linked to IUGR.[145]

In nonhypertensive LBW pregnancies, a low placental weight and chronic villitis are related to impaired fetal growth. In preeclamptic LBW cases, the cumulative burden of all decidual vascular lesions and not the presence of any individual lesion type is significantly related to reduced birth weight. IUGR is more common in preterm infants than infants born at term,[146] and the growth failure may begin at any gestational age.[147] It may predict distress during a normal labor and delivery.[148] Long-term effects may include suboptimal neurodevelopmental outcome.[149]

The factors that preclude a genetically intact fetus from reaching full growth potential are not always obvious. Those that can be recognized by examining the placenta include (1) congenital viral infection, classically of TORCH origin and manifested by chronic villitis; (2) reduced nutrient provision, classically seen in preeclampsia and related to decidual vascular pathology; and (3) confined placental mosaicism, in which a chromosomally abnormal placenta with impaired growth and function may compromise fetal growth. This latter may be an extremely subtle finding. The most common placental changes identified in growth-retarded infants born prematurely and born at term are listed in Table 69-11.

Maternal serum alpha-fetoprotein (MSAFP) elevations associated with structurally normal fetuses carry increased risk of IUGR, as well as abruption, preeclampsia, and fetal death. Many common placental lesions have been associated with elevated MSAFP levels. The lesions are not specific for elevated MSAFP levels, and it is not clear how many cases of unexplained elevated MSAFP levels can be attributed to placental lesions (Table 69-12).

Trisomy 18, trisomy 13, and trisomy 21 (in order of decreasing severity of effect) each are related to LBW, and most autosomal aneuploidies or heteroploidies are associated with LBW infants. The growth failure tends to symmetrically involve both the fetus and placenta. A single umbilical artery is frequent in trisomy 18. Trisomic placentas may have irregularly shaped villi and atypical stromal migrating trophoblasts (Fig. 69-14).[150] There is a reduction of small muscular arteries in the stem villi and reduced small muscular artery/villous ratio, but absolute villous count is normal.[151] The villi are immature, with histology lagging about 4 weeks. No specific gross features have been described in monosomy X, wherein villi show lack of structural uniformity; they tend to be small, with increased intervillous space, and are either acellular and fibrotic or irregularly hypercellular. The villous trophoblastic layer is hypoplastic without syncytial budding. The gross and microscopic features of the triploid partial mole are discussed later in this chapter. Triploid conceptions,

Table 69-10 Incidences of specific placental lesions according to clinical complications leading to preterm birth and the term population for comparison

	PROM (n = 116)	PTL (n = 55)	PIH (n = 54)	ABR (n = 241)	TERM (n = 214)
Acute inflammation, maternal	89 (77%)	38 (69%)	2 (4%)	11 (46%)	47 (21%)
Acute inflammation, fetal	65 (56%)	23 (42%)	1 (2%)	4 (17%)	22 (10%)
Abnormal conversion of spiral arteries	35 (30%)	15 (27%)	21 (39%)	4 (17%)	33 (15%)
Decidual vasculitis	5 (4%)	7 (13%)	6 (11%)	3 (13%)	11 (6%)
Fibrinoid necrosis	2 (2%)	1 (2%)	12 (23%)	1 (4%)	1 (0.5%)
Abruption	25 (22%)	17 (31%)	12 (23%)	15 (63%)	25 (12%)
Chronic inflammation	2 (2%)	4 (7%)	4 (8%)	2 (8%)	51 (23%)

PROM, Premature rupture of membranes; *PTL*, preterm labor; *PIH*, pregnancy-induced hypertension; *ABR*, abruption.
From Salafia CM, Ernst L, Pezzullo JP et al: *Am J Perinatol* 10:135, 1993.

Table 69-11 Distribution of lesions among intrauterine growth retardation (IUGR) infants

Placental vascular thrombosis	Chronic villitis	Hemorrhagic endovasculitis	Placental infarction	Total number
−	−	−	−	57
−	−	−	+	17
−	−	+	−	5
−	+	−	−	20
+	−	−	−	4
+	−	−	+	3
+	−	+	−	1
+	+	−	−	2
−	−	+	+	3
−	+	+	−	7
−	+	−	+	5
−	+	+	+	2
+	−	+	+	0
+	+	+	−	1
+	+	−	+	1
+	+	+	+	0

From Salafia CM et al: *Am J Perinatol* 9:181, 1992.

Table 69-12 Placental causes of elevated maternal serum alpha-fetoprotein

Intervillous hematoma/thrombi
Subchorionic hemorrhage
Chorangioma
Increased perivillous fibrinoid
Presence of sonolucent spaces in placenta
Chronic villitis
Infarcts
Abruption
Amnion rupture sequence
Cord hemangioma/hematoma
Hydropic placenta (hydrops fetalis) cord edema
Vanishing twin/fetus papyraceus
Placenta accreta

especially those with a diploid maternal genome (digyny), may be nonmolar. In these cases there is usually scant tissue (less than expected for dates). Microscopic features may be relatively normal, without trophoblastic proliferation. Occasional enlarged villi may vaguely resemble partial mole. Tetraploidy may rarely have acute intervillous hematomas and infarcts.[140] Tetraploid villi are large, round, and without trophoblastic proliferation.

Hydrops fetalis

Hydrops fetalis of any cause is almost always reflected by placental hydrops,[152-155] and placental abnormalities (e.g., chorangioma or vascular obstruction) may be primarily responsible for fetoplacental hydrops. Placental findings in hydrops fetalis are summarized in Table 69-13. Microscopically, there may be increased mitoses in cytotrophoblasts, thickened trophoblastic basement membranes, increased fibrinoid necrosis of villi and syncytial knotting, and swelling of endothelial cells. Excess nucleated erythrocytes may be seen in either immune and nonimmune hydrops fetalis (Fig. 69-15). There is often hemosiderin pigment in membranes, trophoblasts, Hofbauer cells, endothelium, villous stroma, and on basement membrane. Increased amounts of both intravillous and extravillous calcification are seen with cardiac failure, intrauterine fetal demise, or when there is less demand for calcium because of fetal disease, such as osteogenesis imperfecta.

Oligohydramnios

Decreased amniotic fluid production (e.g., decreased urine output in renal agenesis or lower urinary tract obstructions) or chronic amniotic fluid leak will result in *amnion nodosum*. Amnion nodosum develops most often after vernix has accumulated (by 32 weeks). Small, finely granular or greasy plaques are seen on the fetal surface, and much less often on free/reflected membranes or umbilical cord (Fig. 69-16). These nodules are easily scraped off the placental surface. Mechanical trauma to the amnion from decreased amniotic volume may cause amnion degeneration, which may be the only feature of early lesions. Amnion

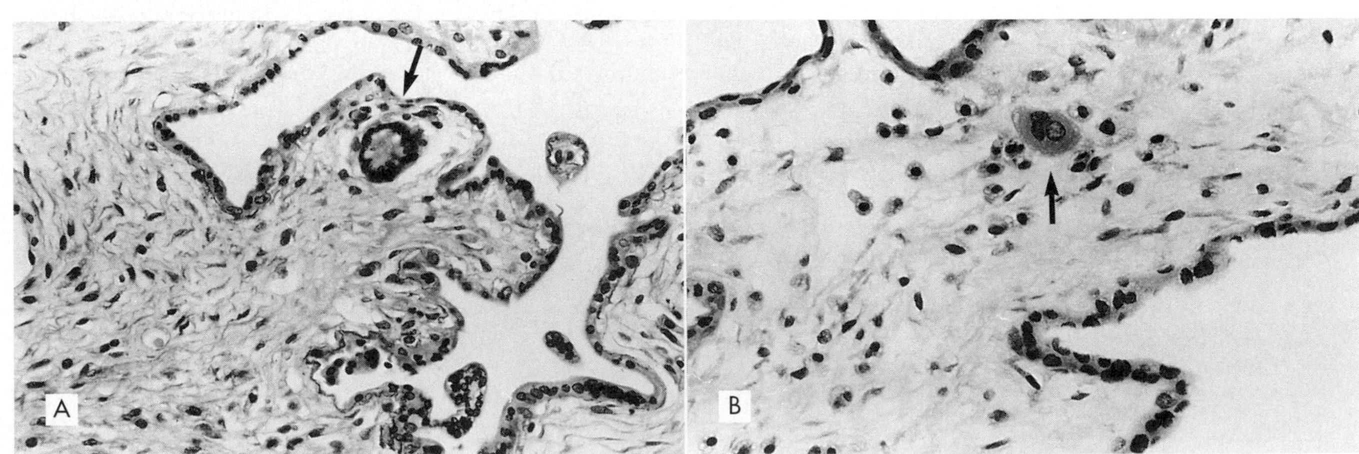

Fig. 69-14 **A,** Placenta from trisomy 13 showing a dimorphic two-villus population, mild villus scalloping, and trophoblastic inclusion similar to those seen in partial hydatidiform moles. **B,** Atypical migrating villous trophoblasts, which stain as intermediate trophoblasts, are commonly seen in trisomies and more commonly in molar gestations (*arrow*).

Table 69-13 Placental findings in hydrops fetalis

Increased placental weight (>50% expected for gestation)
Fetal to placental ratio 4:1
Bulky, maybe pale, easily fragmented
Short cord (fetal immobility)
Umbilical vein dilated
Increased Hofbauer cells
Intervillous fibrin and thrombi
Increased calcification (in usual locations)
Increased erythroblasts, even in cases not associated with anemia
Storage product in syncytiotrophoblasts or Hofbauer cells (rare)
Chorangioma
Polyhydramnios/oligohydramnios
Preterm labor

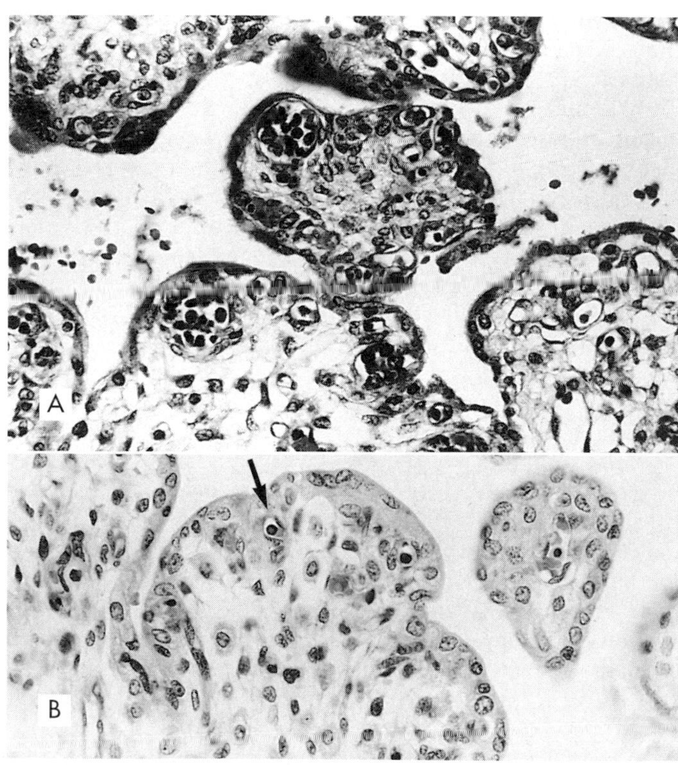

Fig. 69-15 **A,** The classic placental change seen in erythroblastosis fetalis caused by alloimmunization by anti-D; massive erythroblastosis. **B,** Other causes of hydrops also may have erythroblastosis, as in this case of parvovirus infection showing villous edema and a viral inclusion in the nucleus of a nucleated red blood cell *(arrow)*.

nodosum should be distinguished from squamous metaplasia, a normal feature of mature placentas that occurs near the umbilical cord insertion and is not easily removed (Fig. 69-16, *C*).

Other fetal anomalies

Gastroschisis, a fetal abdominal wall defect of vascular origin, is associated with fine, uniform, extensive vacuolation of the

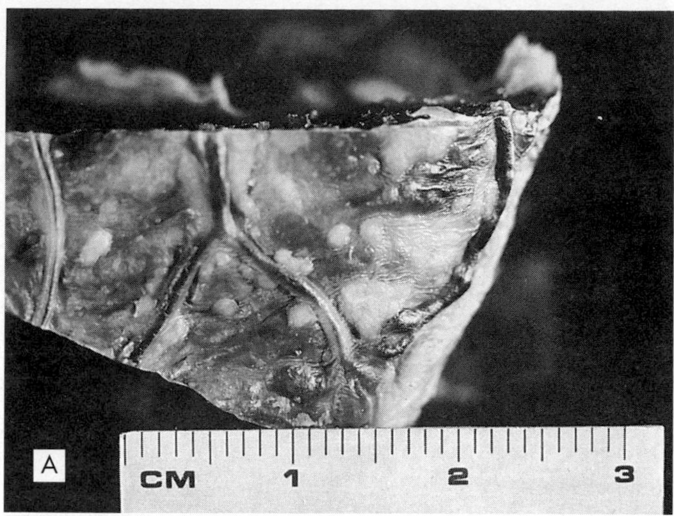

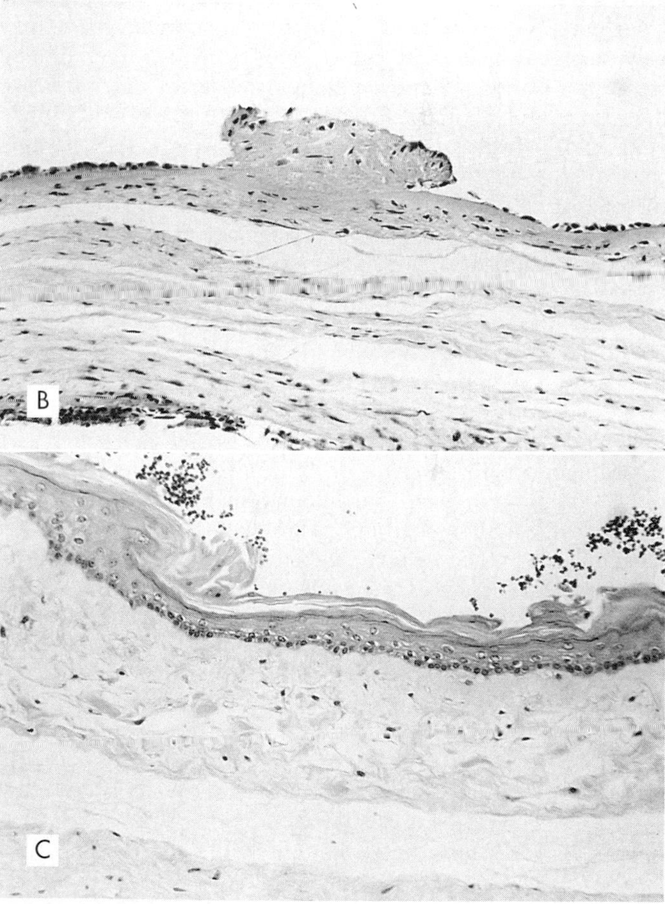

Fig. 69-16 **A,** Amnion nodosum characteristically forms dull plaques on the surface of the placenta. **B,** Microscopically amnion nodosum is cellular debris, degenerating cellular walls, hair, and squamous cells without reactive amnion. There may rarely be reepithelization by amnion over the top of a nodule of amnion nodosum. **C,** Squamous metaplasia also forms dull plaques on the surface of the placenta, usually near the cord insertion, but it is distinguished microscopically as normal cuboidal amnion replaced by metaplastic squamous cells, often with granular layer and keratinization.

amnion.[156] Lipid accumulates by unknown mechanisms in the amniotic epithelium, causing a vacuolated appearance. However, amniotic vacuoles can be seen in the absence of abdominal wall defects.

Genetic defects in the synthesis of collagen types I, III and V, the major types in fetal membranes, could be expected to cause increased fragility of placental membranes.[157] However, no specific gross or microscopic features have been described in placentas of fetuses with these collagen defects. Ehlers-Danlos syndrome has been associated with premature rupture of membranes and amniotic bands.[158] Osteogenesis imperfecta has been linked with amniotic bands and premature rupture of membranes, but this relationship may be fortuitous.

Tumors metastatic to placenta

Neuroblastoma is the most frequent tumor involving the placenta. Eight percent of neuroblastomas are congenital. Not all are stage IV or IV-S and potentially metastatic to the placenta. Congenital neuroblastoma in monozygous twin pairs may have poorer prognosis.[159] Tumor cells are usually seen in fetal stem arteries and villous capillaries and rarely extend out of the fetal vessels to invade villous stroma (Fig. 69-17)[160] When congenital neuroblastoma occurs in twins, particular attention should be paid to anastomotic circulations, through which metastases could be passed from twin to twin. Distribution of neuronspecific enolase, synaptophysin, and chromogranin may be focal or diffuse.

In cases of congenital giant nevi, nevus cells in the stroma of stem villi may represent aberrant migration because the nevus cells do not show cytologic atypia.[161] Fetal melanoma has rarely been reported to metastasize to the placenta. Either of these lesions may have small, grossly pigmented lesions in the villous parenchyma.[162]

Malignant cells in cases of congenital fetal leukemia are most commonly found in fetoplacental vessels but may infiltrate the villous stroma. The diagnosis of congenital leukemia is made when leukemic cells infiltrate nonhematopoietic tissues. These cells must be distinguished from neonatal leukemoid reaction. Most congenital leukemia is acute nonlymphoblastic.[163] There is a high association of trisomy 21 with both transient leukemoid reaction and true leukemia.

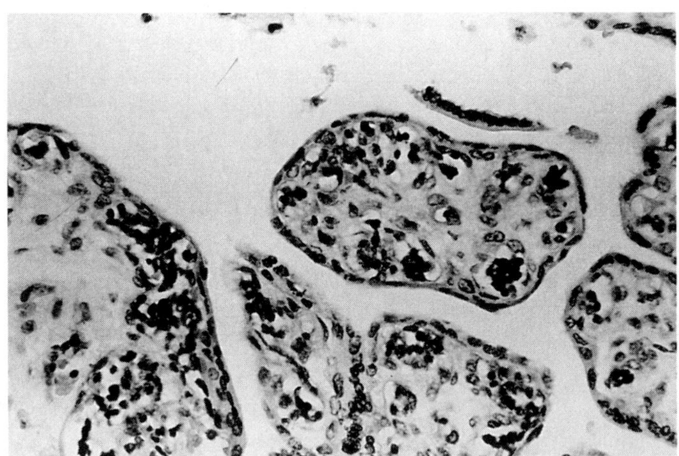

Fig. 69-17 Congenital neuroblastoma metastatic to the placenta. Neuroblastoma cells are seen in the fetal capillaries and must be differentiated from other nucleated cells such as nucleated red blood cells or other immature hematopoietic cells.

The early amnion rupture sequence

The early amnion rupture sequence (TEARS) occurs in its severe form in 1/25,000 and in its mild form in 1/10,000 live births. TEARS is much more frequent in previable fetuses (estimated incidence as high as 1/53)[164,165] and is underdiagnosed in small or fragmented specimens. The sequence begins with amnion rupture. The detaching amnion draws fibrous strands from the chorionic extraembyronic mesoderm, which entangle body parts or umbilical cord[166] or are swallowed or aspirated. The stripped chorion is more water permeable, leading to oligohydramnios and fetal compression. Immature fetal skin (devoid of surface keratin layers) may adhere to the denuded and sticky chorion, tethering and tearing the body.[167] Such secondary defects include neural tube defects, craniofacial clefts, primary body wall defects, caudal regression, and limb reduction defects (Fig 69-18, *A*).[168] Effects of amnion rupture vary depending on the time in gestation of rupture. Early rupture (<45 days) carries high risk of cerebral and limb abnormalities.[164] Later rupture is usually associated with limb abnormalities and a lower incidence of central nervous system abnormalities.[164] Limb anomalies tend to be irregular, asymmetric, and "vertical," with proximal structures relatively normal. Constricting bands without amputation may be seen. Pathologic findings may overlap with those of the abdominal wall/absent umbilical cord syndrome. The TEARS placenta lacks amnion and shows prominent bands (Fig. 69-18, *B, C*). Any residual amnion is usually attached to the insertion of the cord. Strands should be mostly acellular, without an amnionic epithelium.

Amnion rupture is generally of obscure etiology, but it may be related to connective tissue disorders (Ehlers Danlos IV or osteogenesis imperfecta) or blunt abdominal trauma,[169-171] or may follow amniocentesis. It rarely recurs. Environmental factors may be responsible for reports of clustering. TEARS is more frequent in twins, with SUA, and with short cords. Recently, similar fetal morphology has been seen with normal amnions, prompting another theory of maldevelopment related to a defect in the genes responsible for embryonal organization.[172]

Storage disorders

Accumulation of metabolites in fetal and placental tissues may cause hydrops fetalis. In these large pale, bulky placentas, abnormal materials may be seen in distended syncytiotrophoblastic, intermediate trophoblastic, Hofbauer, or endothelial cells or in fetal leukocytes in placental capillaries.[173-175] The amount of stored material may be greater in the placenta than in the fetus, primarily because abnormal storage occurs mainly in functional (differentiated) cells and, to a lesser extent, in germinative, immature, or reserve cells. Placental lesions in different storage disorders are virtually indistinguishable, and the specific metabolic defect cannot be identified without genetic enzyme analysis. The most common placental changes in various storage diseases are listed in Table 69-14. Many of these substances are water soluble (glycogen or gangliosides) or soluble in xylene

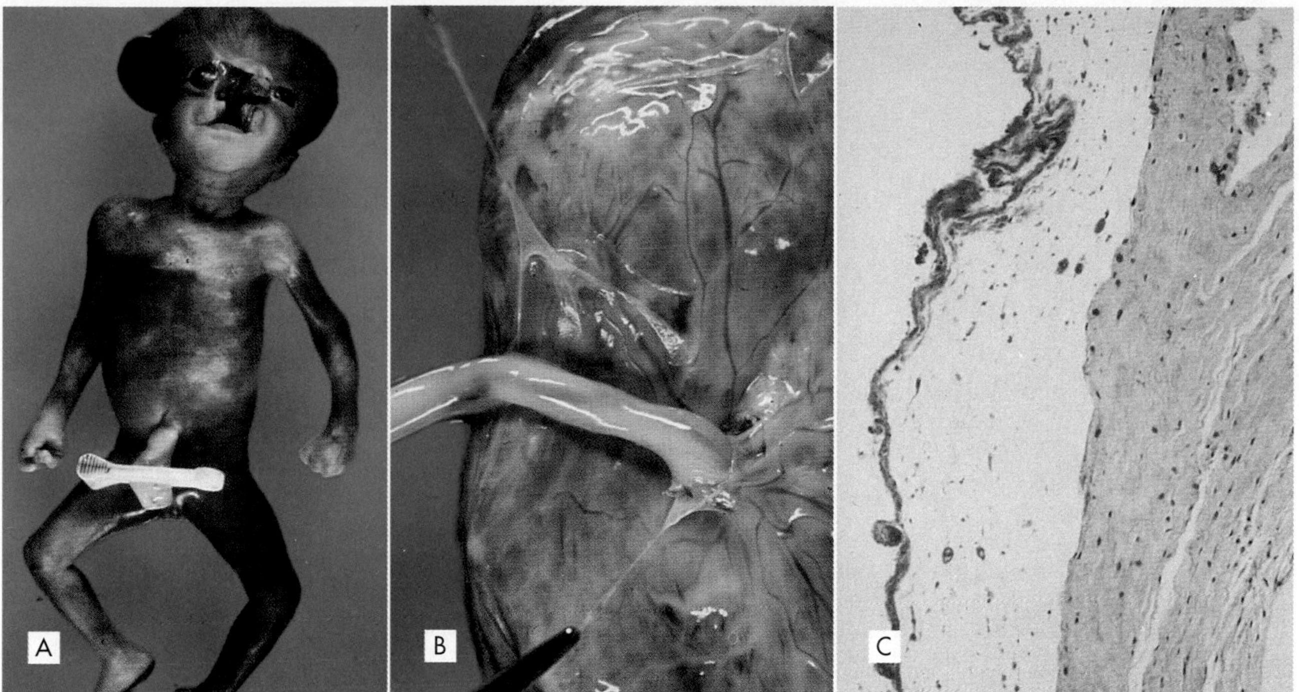

Fig. 69-18 **A,** The early amnion rupture sequence (TEARS) results in a wide variety of severe fetal malformations usually affecting the head, face, and extremities, as seen here. **B,** The gross placenta shows a dull denuded chorionic surface with thin bands of tissue protuding from the surface. (**A** and **B,** courtesy Sherrie A. Caldwell, M.D., The Children's Hospital, Denver, Colo.) **C,** Microscopically the amnion is absent and the chorion is thickened and cellular.

(lipids), leaving only empty vacuoles on routine fixed tissues.

Fetal distress

No consensus exists regarding the highly controversial diagnosis of fetal distress. The relationship of meconium passage to "fetal distress" is also disputed. Fetal distress may be defined differently by the same obstetrician under different circumstances, and it is imperative to understand what the clinician means in any particular case. Events that can mean "fetal distress" include (1) "meconium," from simple meconium passage immediately before birth or during the act of delivery to meconium staining of amniotic fluid during labor, at spontaneous membrane rupture, or on amniocentesis; (2) abnormal antepartum testing, including reduced biophysical profile score[176] and fetal heart rate abnormalities (e.g., severe variable decelerations, late decelerations, extended bradycardia, reduced beat-to-beat variability, and sustained tachycardia);[177] and (3) fetal acidosis on scalp blood sample.

The significance of meconium passage is different at different gestational ages. The fetal gut matures progressively, moving meconium ever closer to the terminal colon. Meconium passage at term, therefore, may reflect a trivial and unsustained stressful event without fetal or neonatal repercussions. In the term infant, meconium passage in the absence of the stress during labor or before membrane rupture (e.g., at diagnostic amniocentesis) may be more significant. On the other hand, passage of meconium in a preterm fetus may imply a significant, possibly protracted stress sufficient to move meconium over a greater colonic distance. Midtrimester passage of meconium may be associated with acute ascending infection, causing a fetal gastroenteritis and diarrhea. Acute meconium soilage, occurring immediately preceding or during delivery, can be easily washed off the surface of the amnion. Meconium that sits on the amnion surface will begin to cause amnion damage. The initial change is individual cell necrosis, followed by amnion hyperplasia, pseudostratification, and vacuolation (Fig. 69-19, *A*). Meconium is phagocytosed by macrophages (Fig. 69-19, *B*) in the membranes and eventually cleared from the amnion fluid. What time is required to clear meconium from the amniotic fluid and whether meconium is ever cleared from cells of the extraplacental membranes are unknown.

A commonly performed antepartum test is a biophysical profile, a "fetal Apgar score" in which fetal tone, breathing movements, activity, heart rate, amniotic fluid volume, and placental ultrasonographic features are assessed. A biophysical profile score of <7 or a drop in biophysical profile score from a previous study imply diminished fetal well-being, and may be an early marker of nascent intraamniotic infection.[176] Fetal heart rate patterns that may (in some cases) raise concerns of fetal jeopardy include (1) severe variable decelerations, believed to reflect cord compression, during which times umbilical circulation may be impaired; (2) late decelerations that occur after the end of a labor contraction, considered to indicate "placental insufficiency;" (3) extended bradycardia; and (4) sustained tachycardia, either from intraamniotic infection or as a cardiac response to stress or fetal anemia.[177] It is worth recalling that all prenatal health care measures including routine antepartum fetal heart monitoring performed regularly for the last decade have not reduced the incidence of cerebral palsy or mental retardation when appropriately adjusted for

Table 69-14 Placental lesions in metabolic disorders

Metabolic disorders	Syncytiotrophoblast	Cytotrophoblast	Invasive trophoblast	Hofbauer cells	Endothelium	Stroma	Amnion
G_{M1}-gangliosidosis	+	–	+	+		–	–
G_{M2} (Tay-Sachs, type 1)	+	+*	+*			+*	
G_{M2} (Sandhoff, type 2)	+*				+*	+*	
Mucopolysaccharidosis I		+*			+*	+*	
MPS III	+*			+			
MPS IV	–	–	–	+	–	–	
MPS VII	–			+			
Sialidosis	+*	–	+	+	+	+	+
Mucolipidosis II (I-cell)	+	–	+	+	–	–	
Mucolipidosis IV	–		+				
Salla's disease	+	–	–	+	–	–	–
Gaucher's disease							
Wolman's disease	–			–			
Pompe's disease (GSD II)	+/–*	+*	–	*	+/–*	+/–*	
Ceroid lipofuscinosis	*			*			
Zellweger syndrome				*			*
Niemann-Pick disease	+	–	+	+	?	+*	+

+ or – Changes on light microscopy, *changes on EM only, ? variable reports of fetal leukocytes in capillaries, blank = not reported.

gestational age of observed populations.[178] Fetal heart rate patterns cannot predict future neurologic integrity. In our experience, more "ominous" heart rate patterns generally occur in a fetus with a chronically damaged placenta (e.g., chronic villitis or defective placentation). Fetal acidosis can be diagnosed as a fetal scalp blood pH of <7.20. Only when acidosis is extreme (pH < 6.99) can any significant association of low pH and poor long-term neurological outcome be seen. Even at this extreme, only 40% of such infants demonstrate long-term damage. Fetal acidosis may indicate some abnormality in placental gas exchange, maternal blood flow, placental perfusion or fetoplacental metabolism, but it is not diagnostic of a damaged child.[179]

Neuromuscular disorders

The most common neuromuscular disorder, cerebral palsy, is a chronic nonprogressive disorder of movements or posture that appears early in childhood. Cerebral palsy is often accompanied by spasticity or paralysis and can be further classified as quadriplegic or nonquadriplegic.

Many maternal and fetal circumstances and placental lesions are recognized as antecedents in cases of cerebral palsy. However, most often the cause remains obscure. Some cases are seen in patients with congenital malformations or syndromes. In cases of cerebral palsy related to genetic, chromosomal, and teratogenic factors, there is often mental retardation as well. Complications of prematurity and postnatal cerebral infections account for another 10%. However, only one third of infants with cerebral palsy have a history of low birth weight,[180] and most infants with postnatal cerebral infections do not develop cerebral palsy. Maternal cocaine use during pregnancy is, with increasing frequency, recognized as an antecedent event in cerebral palsy. Birth asphyxia has been associated with 6% to 20% of neurologic complications with cerebral palsy.[180] Such claims are often incompletely documented. The isolated finding of meconium in the amniotic fluid has not been a reliable

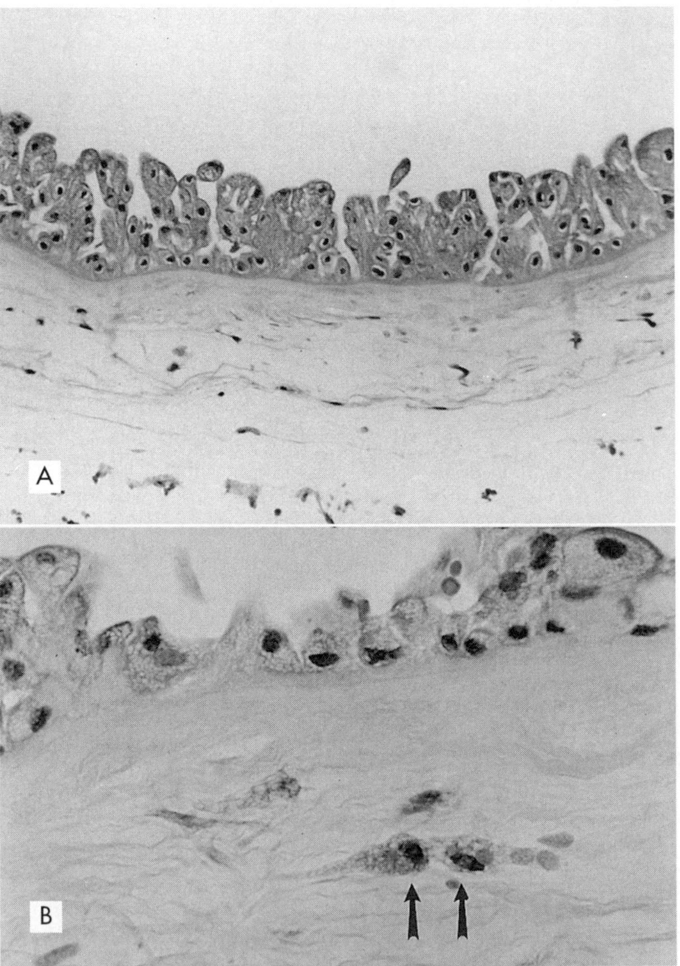

Fig. 69-19 **A,** Early meconium changes usually show hyperplasia with pseudostratification of the amnion. **B,** The smooth, golden-brown meconium is phagocytized by macrophages *(arrow)* in the membranes and is eventually cleared from the amniotic fluid. The time necessary for these changes to occur is still speculative.

marker for asphyxia or distress. The overwhelming majority of infants born with meconium in amniotic fluid are normal. Although putative "explanations" for fetal and neonatal compromise may be offered by clinical or placental review, the lack of sensitivity and specificity of both clinical and placental findings betrays incomplete understanding of critical pathophysiology in many cases of fetal damage. The usual history of a child with cerebral palsy is noncontributory, and it has been stated that at least half, if not more, of all brain-damaged infants and children have no scientifically or clinically based explanations for their problems.[180] Examination of placentas may increase our understanding of the causes of nongenetic, nonsyndromal cerebral palsy and mental retardation. However, studies have been inconclusive. Placental features associated with neuromuscular disorders are listed in Table 69-15.[181]

Umbilical cord disorder

Umbilical cord disorder is an important consideration in cases of fetal distress because compromise of these vessels clearly affects fetal well-being. Thrombosis, knots, hematomas, body wraps, torsion, or strictures may occur and infrequently cause fetal distress or demise.[182-186]

The normal umbilical cord epithelium is continuous with amniotic epithelium. It is tightly adherent to the underlying mucoid and compressible Wharton's jelly. The cord has no vasa vasorum, lymphatics, or nerves. Abundant mast cells in Wharton's jelly may protect against umbilical thrombosis. Meconium staining and cord trauma (e.g., cordocentesis) may be accompanied by pigment-laden cells in Wharton's jelly. These may be histiocytes or stromal cells capable of assuming macrophagic activities. The umbilical vein has a well-developed internal elastic lamina, whereas the arteries have elastic tissue only in the media. The vascular muscle is a decussating helix of smooth muscle fibers. The umbilical arteries anastomose within the first 2 or 3 cm of cord proximal to the chorionic plate, which may facilitate uniform placental perfusion.

Table 69-15 Placental findings in neuromuscular disorders*

Placental findings	Proposed etiology/mechanism
Short umbilical cord	Decreased fetal movement
Decreased subchorionic fibrinoid	Decreased fetal movement
Meconium	Asphyxia
Umbilical cord compression	Asphyxia
Thrombosis of umbilical cord vessels	Decreased placental fetal blood flow
Fetal stem vessel abnormalities	Decreased placental fetal blood flow
Uneven villous maturity	Decreased uteroplacental blood flow
Villous edema, diffuse/severe	Acidosis
Retroplacental hematoma (abruptio)	Decidual vasculopathy

Data from Mann LI: *Am J Obstet Gynecol* 155:6, 1986; and Naeye RL: *Disorders of the placenta, fetus and neonate: diagnosis and clinical significance,* St Louis, 1992, Mosby.
*Quadriplegic cerebral palsy.

Absence of one artery may be due to failure of formation or regression with a residual calcified remnant.[187,188] Recently it has been proposed that meconium may cause umbilical vasospasm and degeneration of the smooth muscle of the vessel walls and may be causally related to cerebral damage.[189,190] Embryonic remnants occur most commonly near the fetal end of the cord and are of little clinical significance.[191] Umbilical cord length is in part a reflection of fetal growth and in utero fetal activity[192] (Fig. 69-20). Umbilical cord pathology and some guides to clinical correlation are presented in Table 69-16.

Intrauterine infections

Acute ascending infection

Intrauterine infection may follow ascending, hematogenous, transabdominal, or transfallopian pathways. Most commonly, infectious agents ascend from the perineum, vagina, and cervix. The causative organisms may be of low virulence, part of normal flora, or obvious pathogens (e.g., *Escherichia coli*). The infectious agent crosses intact or ruptured membranes into the amniotic fluid. The maternal immune response to bacteria or their toxins in the amniotic fluid results first in neutrophil margination in the subchorionic space, and then neutrophilic migration across the chorion and amnion into the amniotic fluid (so-called amniotrophic movement, Fig. 69-21 *A*). Amniotic fluid neutrophils may be aspirated or swallowed by the fetus. Mild chorioamnionitis may be missed on gross inspection of the membranes, but in severe infection membranes are opacified, discolored, and, depending on the organisms, foul smelling. Microscopic examination should include samples from the zone of rupture of the membranes, the first area affected when infection ascends (Fig. 69-21, *B*).

Premature rupture of membranes for greater than 18 hours may lead to chorioamnionitis, but membranes most often rupture because they are already infected. Acute intraamniotic infection may "cause" as many as 50% of premature deliveries, and only 8% to 25% of mothers are symptomatic.[193,194] Intraamniotic bacteria may cause congenital pneumonia, gastroenteritis, otitis media, and meningitis. Few infants are septic at the time of delivery.[194] Decreased fetal well-being (as assessed by biophysical profile score), abnormal fetal heart rate, and, possibly, increased umbilical systolic/diastolic ratio

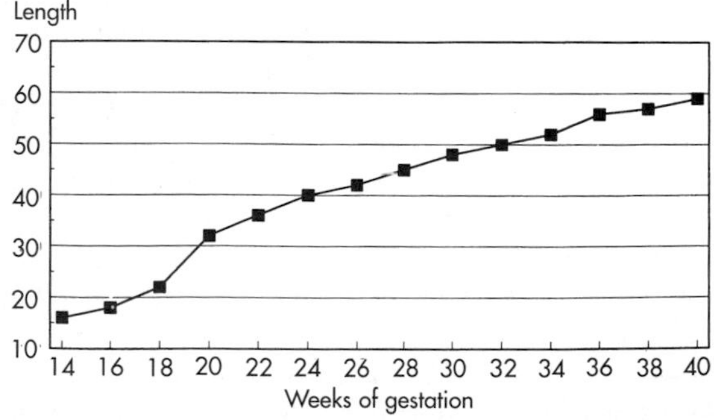

Fig. 69-20 Expected umbilical cord length. The umbilical cord length is a reflection of fetal growth and movement. At term the cord is normally 60 cm long; less than 32 cm is considered short, greater than 100 cm, long. (Modified from Benirschke D, Kaufmann P: *Pathology of the human placenta,* New York, 1990, Springer-Verlag.)

Table 69-16 Umbilical cord abnormalities

Abnormality	Incidence	Significance
SUA	1% 2.5% stillborn	20% congenital malformations, IUGR, small placenta, twins, trisomy 18, maternal diabetes
Supernumerary vessels	Rare	Section taken within 3 cm of placental insertion, conjoined twins, vessel remnants
Short cords	?	<32 cm, decreased fetal movement and neurodevelopmental abn, musculoskeletal abn, difficult delivery, congenital malformations, twins, breech presentation
Long cords	?	>100 cm, increased fetal movement, thrombosis, entanglements, torsions
Edema	2.7%	Hydrops fetalis, preeclampsia, acute chorioamnionitis
Thin cord	0.2%	IUGR, fetal malformations, increased prolapse and compression
Omphalomesenteric duct	1.5%	Near surface of cord, muscle in wall, intestinal-type mucosa, rarely ulceration of gastric mucosa, ? association with Meckel's diverticulum or intestinal atresia
Allantoic duct	15%	Located between the arteries, connective tissue wall, transitional-type epithelium, ? patent urachus or cyst
Vitelline vessels	7%	Usually central, usually capillary-like, rarely with muscular wall, origin of hematoma or hemangioma
Teratoma	Rare	Benign
Hematoma	2%	Rupture of umbilical vein, iatrogenic most common, short cords
True knots	0.5% to 1%	Rarely tighten during labor, rare cause of in utero hypoxia
False knots	Frequent	Vascular redundancies, varicosities, rare thrombosis
Thrombosis	0.7%	Associated with perinatal death, more common in vein, reported to be more significant in arteries, congenital hypercoagulable states, acute chorioamnionitis, funisitis, vigorous fetal motor activity, commonly associated with true knot
Strictures	?	Focal deficiency of WJ, rarely due to "amniotic bands"
Torsion	?	Exaggerated spiraling, increased fetal movement; most occur after fetal demise
Decreased spiraling	?	SUA, decreased fetal movement
Cord rupture	2% to 4%	Short cord, velamentous or marginal insertion
Marginal insertion	5% to 7%	Compression of vessels, thrombosis, rupture, twins
Velamentous insertion	0.3% to 2%	Compression of vessels, thrombosis, avulsion of cord, rupture of vasa previa, twins, diabetes, congenital malformation
Cord prolapse	2% to 4%	Long cords, multiple gestations
Funisitis	?	Fetal reaction to infection or cord compression, margination, angiitis, funisitis (polys in WJ), rare before 26 WGA candidiasis, plaques on surface
Necrotizing funisitis	Rare	Syphilis, herpes, toxoplasmosis often associated with villitis and chorioamnionitis
Calcification	Rare	Necrotic inflammatory debris, muscle fibers, etiology known
Muscle degeneration	Rare (live births) Common	<1% of meconium-stained placentas After fetal demise, autolysis begins at fetal end of cord

See also Table 69-3.
ABN, Abnormalities; *SUA*, single umbilical artery; *IUGR*, intrauterine growth retardation; *WGA*, weeks of gestation; *WJ*, Wharton's jelly; *abn*, abnormalities.

are associated with subclinical acute ascending infections.[195-197]

The histologic pattern of acute inflammation in amnion, umbilical cord, chorionic plate, and chorion decidua is strongly associated with ascending bacterial infection, does not occur secondary to intrauterine fetal demise, and is not caused by meconium staining. Inflammation in the subchorionic fibrin (margination of maternal cells) is the earliest sign of infection; however, it is not often associated with a positive amniotic fluid culture.[198] Variables affecting extent of histologic inflammation include the intraamniotic bacterial load, bacterial virulence, maternal immune competence, antibiotic therapy, and duration of exposure to the infectious agents. Therefore, timing of onset of infection cannot be determined from histologic examination of tissue alone. Acute inflammation is more common and more severe in more premature placentas.

Organisms may not be recovered by routine culture methods. The addition of cultures for anaerobic bacteria, *Mycolasma*, and *Ureaplasma* will recover organisms in over 75% of cases; many are mixed infections. *Fusobacterium* spp. are anaerobic filamentous bacteria that cause necrosis of the amnion and is often associated with preterm delivery.[199] (Fig. 69-21, *C*). *Group B Streptococcus* may result in "clouds" of bacteria without an appropriate maternal inflammatory response, especially in chronic carrier states.[200,201] (Fig. 69-21, *D*) Patterns of placental inflammation for various organisms are listed in Table 69-17.

As the fetus responds to intraamniotic infection, marginating fetal leukocytes are seen in umbilical cord and chorionic vessels (Fig. 69-22, *A*). Initially inflammation begins at the placental end of the cord, almost always begining in the vein with later arterial involvement. Umbilical vasculitis is a more specific histologic predictor of a positive amniotic fluid culture.[198] Inflammation is not seen in the intraabdominal umbilical vein or ductus venosus. Umbilical cord inflammation may be described, in order of increasing severity, as margination, angitis, and funisitis once the inflammation has extended to Wharton's jelly. Pathologic diagnoses should describe the fetal infiltrate in terms of location, intensity, and cell types. Because

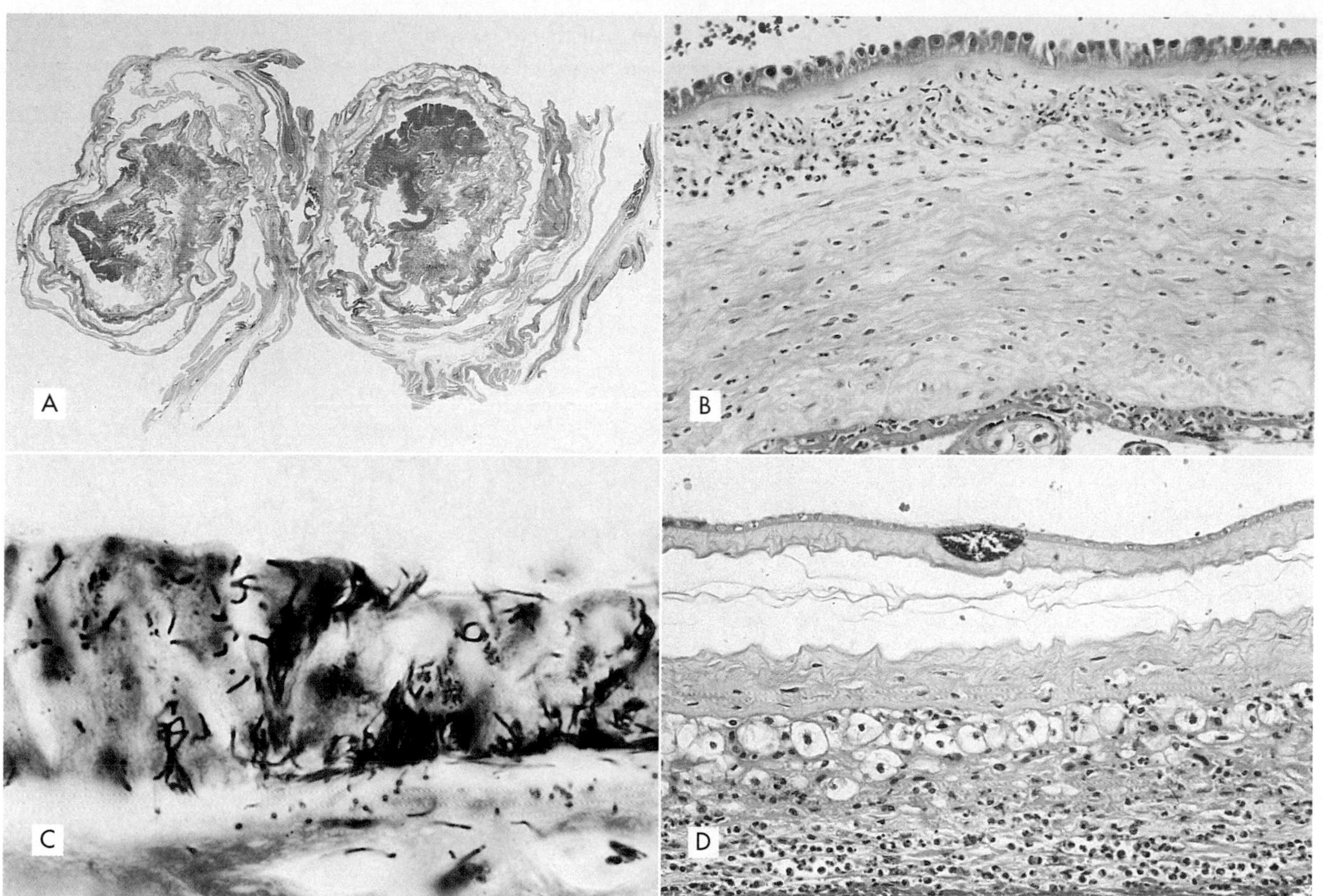

Fig. 69-21 **A,** Acute chorioamnionitis showing significantly more inflammation at the center of the membrane roll nearest the cervical os. **B,** Polymorphonuclear leukocytes of maternal origin extending from the maternal intervillous space at the subchorionic space into the chorion. **C,** Fusobacterium, a common cause of preterm labor, is seen "standing on end" in the amnion. (Warthin-Starry stain.) **D,** "Bacterial cloud" consistent with group B Streptococcus is seen without much inflammation, a feature suggestive of inadequate maternal response.

the fetal white cell pool is relatively small, in severe infections there may be many immature neutrophils and numerous eosinophils. Sclerosing (necrotizing) funisitis is caused by long-standing intraamniotic infection in which the fetal inflammatory cells have lysed and become calcified (Fig. 69-22, *B-D*). Funisitis is uncommon before 24 weeks because of the relative immunoincompetence of the fetus.[202] For this reason, the intensity of fetal inflammation relative to maternal inflammation at any gestational age varies and may be abnormal when mother is immunoincompetent (e.g., maternal HIV infection).

Villous edema is commonly seen with acute ascending infections. Villous edema is generally more severe in placentas delivered earlier in gestation, and it has been suggested to be associated with increased perinatal morbidity.[203] Edema is a nonspecific response to any change in trophoblast permeability/integrity, intravascular pressure, and capillary integrity (Fig. 69-23). Both perivillous fibrin deposition and villous fibrinoid necrosis (Fig. 69-24, *A, B*) are lesions that develop external to at least the trophoblast basement membrane[16] and are more common in acute ascending infection. Fibrinoid necrosis of individual villi occurs in 3% of villi in normal term placentas.[16]

Hematogenous infection

Hematogenous infections are most often associated with either acute or chronic villitis. Acute villitis and decidual and villous microabscesses are caused by maternal bacterial sepsis (Fig. 69-25, *A*). Viral infections are more often associated with chronic villitis or with chronic chorioamnionitis,[204] although chronic chorioamnionitis may be caused by a previously treated ascending acute chorioamnionitis or a chronic bacterial infection (e.g., syphilis). In chronic villitis, the inflammatory cell type may help determine the etiologic agent. Plasma cells in decidua and villi can be associated with cytomegalovirus,[205] herpes, and syphilis (Fig. 69-25, *B*). Cytomegalovirus, and syphilis also damage villous endothelium, and affected villi may have variable amounts of hemosiderin. Granulomatous villitis may be due to various viruses, mycobacteria, fungus, or parasitic agents (Fig. 69-25, *C*). Chronic umbilical vasculitis may also be caused by viral and chronic bacterial infections.[206,207]

Both chronic villitis and chronic chorioamnionitis may be of undetermined or obscure etiology; such lesions have been termed "villitis of undetermined etiology" or "VUE."[208] In some cases, it can be argued that infectious agents have left no clinical or histologic "footprints." However, chronic villi-

Table 69-17 Organisms implicated in in utero infections and the placental features, if known

Organism	Membranitis	Villitis	Funisitis	Deciduitis	Miscellaneous
Bacteria					
Gram-positive cocci					
Streptococcus group A,B,D,	A	A	A	A	Bacterial "clouds"
Staphylococcus (coagulase +/–)	A	A	A	A	
Gram-positive rods					
Listeria monocytogenes	A	A (abscess)		A	
Corynebacterium (diptheroids)	A		A		
Gram-negative cocci					
Neisseria gonorrhoeae	A	A (rare)	A		
Gram-negative rods					
Haemophilus influenzae	A				
Pseudomonas aeruginosa	A				
Enterobacteriaceae *(E. coli,*	A	A (abscess)	A		
Klebsiella)	A				
Gardnerella vaginalis					
Campylobacter sp.		A, C, Nec			
Anaerobic bacteria					
Fusobacterium nucleatum	A				Necrosis of amnion
Bacteroides					
Peptococcus/Peptostreptococcus					
Clostridium	A				
Miscellanous bacteria					
Mycobacterium tuberculosis		C			
Treponema pallidum	C	C	C, Nec	PC	
Mycoplasma hominis	A				
Ureaplasma urealyticum	A				
Chlamydia trachomatis	A				
Virus					
DNA					
Herpes simplex 1 and 2	A, C	C, subacute	C	LP	Inc
Cytomegalovirus		A, C, PC		PC	Hemosiderin, Inc
Adenovirus					
Varicella-zoster (chickenpox)		C, Nec, LP, G			
Variola (smallpox)	C	C, G			
Vaccinia (roseola)		G			
Epstein-Barr virus		LP		N	
Parvovirus B-19					Inc in RBC
Human papilloma virus (HPV)					
Hepatitis B					Bilirubin in HB
RNA					
Enterovirus		A			
Coxsackievirus		A, Nec			Vasculitis
Echovirus		Nec		A	Vasculitis
Polio					
Rubella		A, C			Inclusions
Measles		C, giant cells			
Mumps		C, G, Nec			
Influenza				C	Vasculitis
Retrovirus					
Human immunodeficiency virus	A	C			
Protozoa					
Toxoplasma *gondii*	C	C, G	C		Oraganisms in HB
Malaria					Organisms in IVS RBC
Trypanosoma (Chagas' disease)		C, G			Organisms in HB
Fungus					
Candida albicans		A	A (rare)	A, abscess	
Coccidioides immitis		C			

A, Acute; *C,* chronic; *G,* granulomatous; *HB,* Hofbauer cells; *Inc,* inclusions; *IVS,* intervillous space; *LP,* lymphocytic; *Nec,* necrotizing; *PC,* plasmacytic.

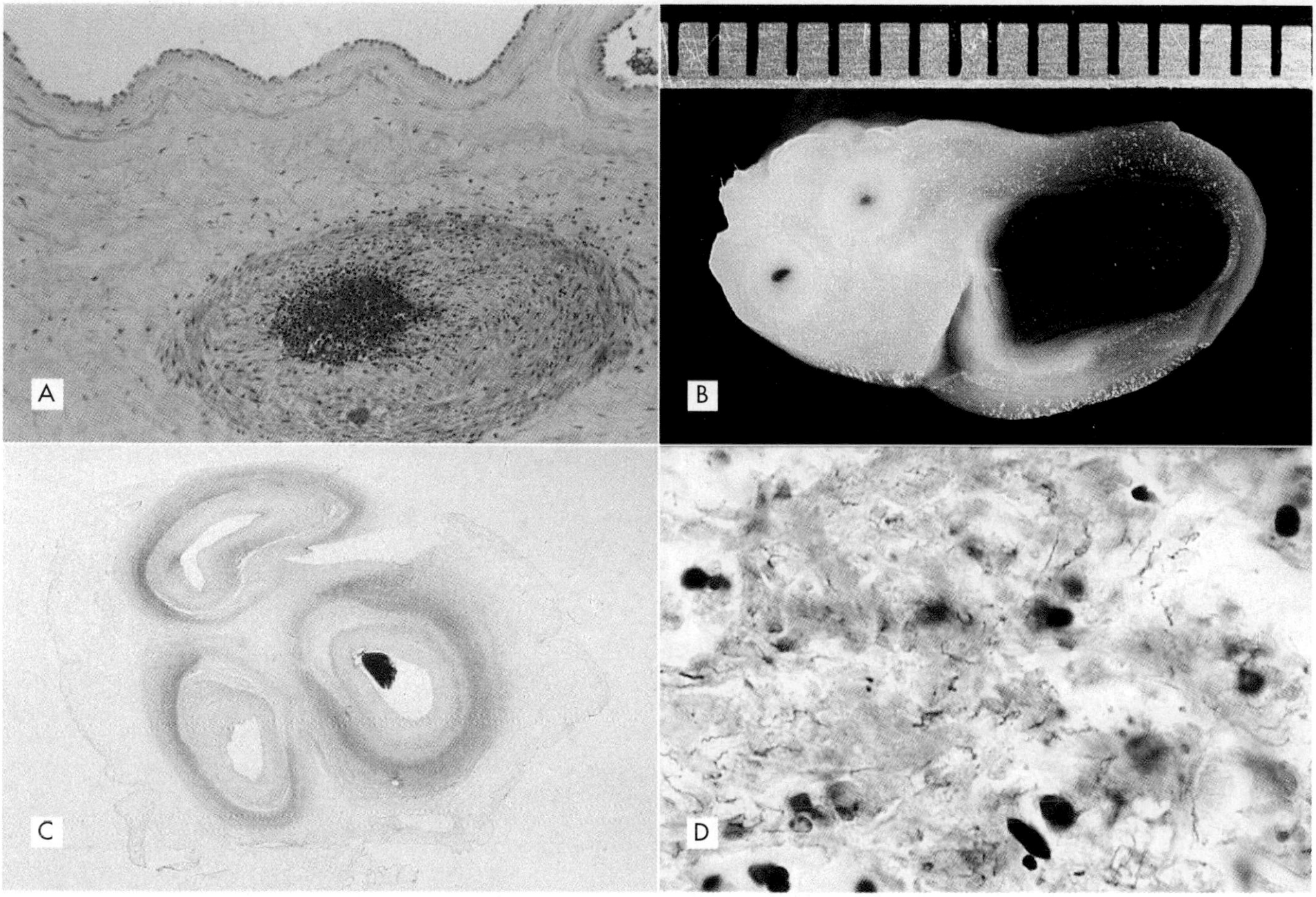

Fig. 69-22 **A,** Fetal reaction to infection may be seen in the large chorionic vessels. There is no maternal response in this case of fetal sepsis after therapeutic cordocentesis. **B,** More commonly the umbilical cord is involved, beginning as margination, progressing to angiitis and then funisitis with inflammation extending into Wharton's jelly, here showing a dense white accumulation around the umbilical vessels. **C,** The microscopic pattern of amniotrophic inflammation, here showing necrosis; thus the distinctive name necrotizing or sclerosing funisitis. **D,** The etiology in some, but not all, cases of necrotizing funisitis is syphilis; the spirochetes are seen here. (Warthin-Starry stain.)

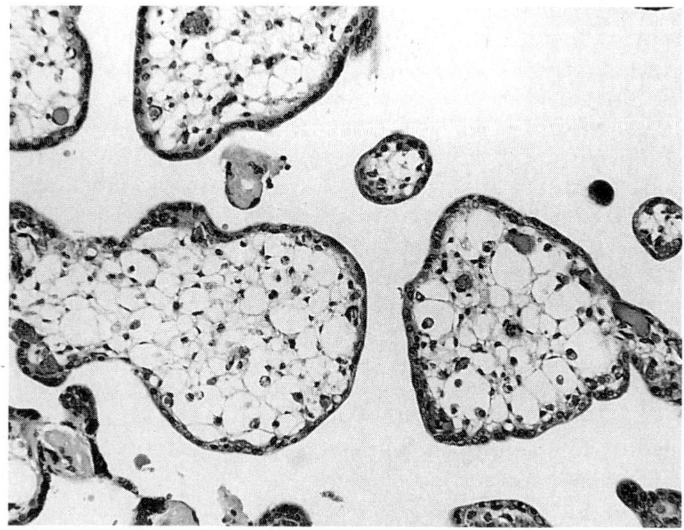

Fig. 69-23 Villous edema may be focal or diffuse. Accumulation of intervillous fluid results in "holes" in the villus stroma, resulting in a prominence of Hofbauer cells.

tis without positive viral cultures must be considered as of undetermined etiology (Fig. 69-25, *D*) and may raise a question of maternal immunologic disorders.[209,210] Chronic villitis is seen in cases of recurrent pregnancy failure.[209] The implications of chronic villitis for future pregnancies depends on intercurrent maternal disease and past pregnancy outcome. Grading of chronic villitis considers the relative volume and the spatial extent of villous involvement. "Grade 1" is a solitary focus of chronic villitis in any one of four slides of villi. "Grade 2" describes two foci of chronic villitis on one slide. "Grade 3" describes multiple foci on at least two different slides. Higher grades (up to six) are assigned subjectively based on estimated percent of inflamed villi. Chronic villitis will be seen in approximately 15% of normal term placentas. Over 90% will be Grade 1 or Grade 2. In uncomplicated term deliveries, more severe grades of chronic villitis are rare.

A few decidual lymphocytes are normally present. Dense chronic decidual inflammation may accompany decidual vascular lesions. Plasma cells are not normally in the decidua and are seen in congenital infections, such as cytomegalovirus,

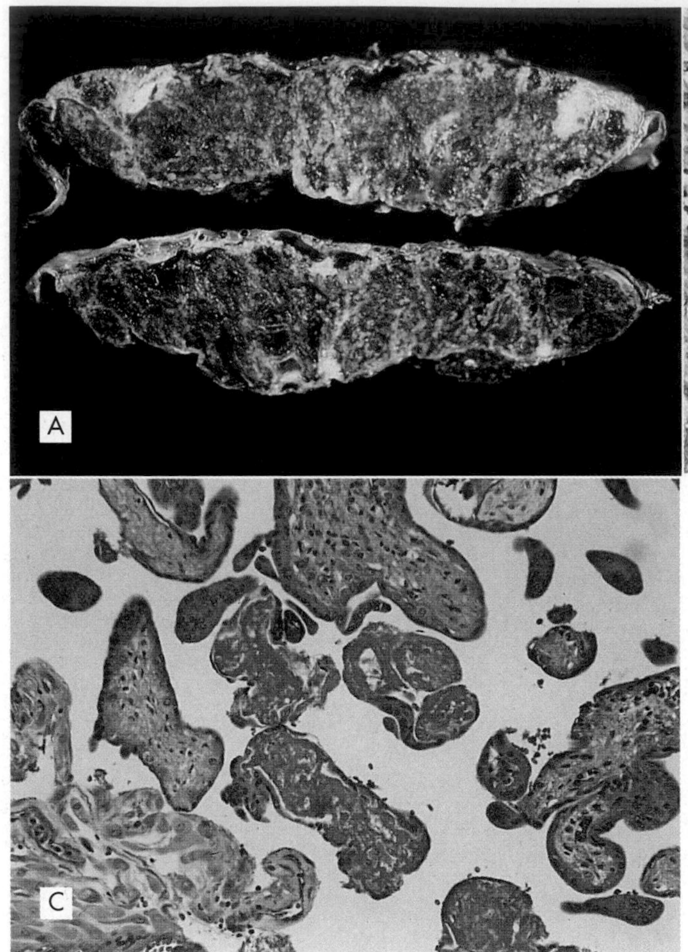

Fig. 69-24 **A,** Perivillous fibrinoid results in firm consistency of the placental substance and a glassy gross appearance. (Courtesy Craig Zupan, M.D., Loma Linda University Medical Center, Loma Linda, Calif.) **B,** Acellular eosinophilic material surrounds the villi. In contrast to an infarct, the syncytiotrophoblasts have disappeared, leaving proliferating cytotrophoblasts and fetal vessels, features of ischemia. **C,** Fibrinoid necrosis of individual villi, seen in 3% of villi at term, is the result of acellular eosinophilic material being deposited underneath the trophoblasts and eventually occupying the entire villus.

herpes, and syphilis, and with maternal immunologic disorders. Chronic lymphohistiocytic inflammation of the intervillous space is termed "chronic intervillositis"[210] (Fig. 69-26) and is often associated with trophoblastic necrosis. Chronic intervillositis has been seen in cases of maternal malaria.[211] In this country, it is more often seen in cases of maternal immunological diseases and may represent a maternal response to placental alloantigens or to autoantigens common to mother and placenta.[210] It is almost always seen with chronic villitis but may be an isolated finding in preterm placentas. Acute intervillositis is seen with maternal sepsis or severe intraamniotic infection.

GESTATIONAL TROPHOBLASTIC DISEASE

(GTD) has been recently defined by the World Health Organization-International Society of Gynecologic Pathologists and comprises several different entities: complete hydatidiform mole, partial hydatidiform mole, invasive mole, placental site trophoblastic tumor, choriocarcinoma, and other miscellaneous trophoblastic lesions.[212]

Hydatidiform mole

This nonspecific term *hydatidiform mole* (HM) includes two entities: complete HM and partial HM, typical features of which are listed in Table 69-18.[212-216] The diagnosis of HM is used only if a distinction between complete and partial HM cannot be made by gross, histologic, and karyotypic data. Most HM are characterized by elevations of serum B-human chorionic gonodotrophin (BhCG) levels. HM occurs in the United States in 1/2000 deliveries. Worldwide, the incidence varies from 1/200 (Mexico) to 1/4369 (Paraguay) and is more common in women of Asian descent.[13] Partial HM is underdiagnosed and is probably more common than complete HM. A differential diagnosis includes hydropic abortus in chromosomally normal or abnormal conceptuses. Risk for choriocarcinoma or recurrence of HM in a subsequent pregnancy differs among types of GTD. Adequate sectioning, a minimum of 5 to 10 blocks of placental tissue and anything suspicious of membranes or fetal tissues is recommended.[217-219] Suction curettage and formalin fixation collapses hydropic villi. A brief submergence in water will rehydrate them and clarify morphology.

Complete hydatidiform mole (CHM) develops when an empty ovum is fertilized by two sperm (heterozygotic, dispermic diandrogenetic fertilization) or by one diploid sperm (homozygotic, monospermic, diandrogenetic fertilization).[220] CHM is classically described as a mass of grapelike vesicles (Fig 69-27, *A*). Histologically, enlarged villi show central edema and circumferential proliferation of syncytiotrophoblasts and intermediate and cytotrophoblasts (Fig

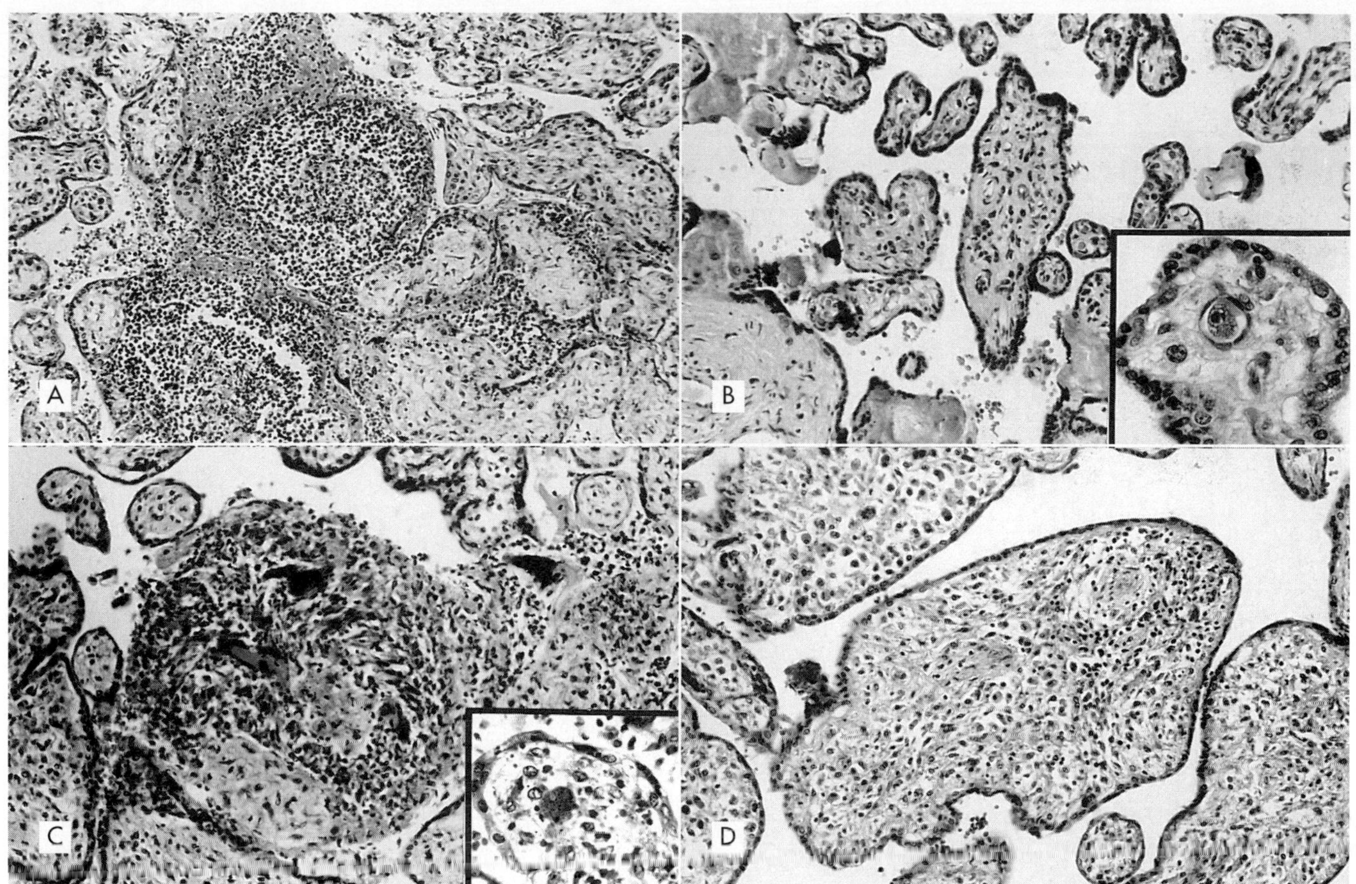

Fig. 69-25 Villitis presents in several forms. **A,** Acute vasculitis, usually caused by maternal bacteremia, in this case *Listeria.* **B,** Chronic lymphoplasmacytic villitis, characteristic of cytomegalovirus, with hemosiderin in villi and (inset) showing cytomegalovirus inclusions in a cell within a villus vessel. **C,** Granulomatous villitis with palisading histiocytes surrounding a central zone of necrosis, which in this case is due to *Toxoplasma gondii.* Inset shows the characteristic cyst. **D,** Chronic lymphohistiocytic villitis, characteristic of the villitis, of undetermined etiology (VUE).

69-27, *B*). Nuclear atypia may be considerable but is without prognostic significance.[221] A fetus is generally absent unless there is a concurrent nonmolar twin pregnancy. Residual blood vessels empty of erythrocytes are common in villi before 10 weeks of gestation. Risk of persistent disease or transformation into choriocarcinoma is 10% to 20% and 2% to 8%, respectively. There may be increased risk of choriocarcinoma in the 6% to 9% of CHM that result from dispermic fertilization.[219,222-224]

Partial hydatidiform mole (PHM), incorrectly referred to as a "transitional mole," is the result of fertilization of a normal ovum by either two sperm (dispermic, diandrogenetic fertilization) or one diploid sperm (diandrogenetic fertilization).[214] A diploid ovum may be fertilized by a normal haploid sperm (dygynic fertilization), resulting in a triploid abortus without partial molar features.[225] The tissue may be more abundant than expected for gestational age and usually includes membranes, rarely an umbilical cord or fetus. Only some villi are enlarged (Fig. 69-28, *A*) resulting in a dual villous population. Histologically, the large villi are distinct from those of CHM (Fig. 69-28, *B*). In PHM, the trophoblastic proliferation is not circumferential but patchy, and confined to syncytiotrophoblast only. In CHM, the trophoblast proliferation is generally circumferential and involves all types of trophoblast. Because molar gestations are now diagnosed earlier on ultrasound and curetted, these features may be less well evolved and the distinction among complete and partial moles and even hydropic abortus may be more difficult. The final diagnosis may depend on special studies, including flow cytometry and immunohistochemistry.

Choriocarcinoma is a rare complication of PHM. The several case reports[226-228] often fail to completely describe the preceding molar lesion.

Invasive hydatidiform mole occurs frequently in CHM and rarely in PHM. "Invasive" implies that molar villi and trophoblasts have extended more deeply and widely than the normal uterine implantation.[229] (Fig. 69-29). Invasive HM is more common in patients over age 40. Invasive HM forms an irregular hemorrhagic mass that raggedly penetrates the myometrium; extrauterine sites have also been identified. The villi are usually smaller than those in the intracavitary HM and are overshadowed by a variable proliferation of syncytiotrophoblasts and cytotrophoblasts. There is no higher risk for choriocarcinoma when HM is invasive.[230,231] The differential diagnosis includes choriocarcinoma and placenta accreta.

Table 69-18 Gestational trophoblastic disease: clinical, gross, microscopic, and flow cytometric features

Features	CHM	PHM	HA	PSTT	Choriocarcinoma
Clinical					
Maternal age	<20, >40	27	n/r	28	n/r
Weeks gestation	12	15	11	Postpartum	Postpartum
Clinical diagnosis	Mole	Missed AB, 10% mole	SAB	Incomplete AB, Dysfunctional bleeding	Bleeding
Hyperemesis	50%	Rare	No	No	n/r
Theca-lutein cysts	20% to 50%	Rare	No	No	Rare
Preeclampsia	25%	Rare	No	No	No
Ultrasound	"Snowstorm"	Rare cysts	Rare cysts	Submucosal mass	mass
βhCG (mIU/ml)	160,000	27,000-80,000	19,000	<1,000	>150,000
Gross					
Villi	Yes	Yes	Yes	No	No
Gross vesicles	All	Focal	Rare	n/a	n/a
Vesicle size	5-20 mm	3-6 mm	3 mm	n/a	n/a
Fetus	No	Yes	Yes	No	No
Amount of tissue	200 g	150 g	50 g	Scant	Abundant
Membranes	No	Yes	Yes	No	No
Microscopic					
Villus size	Uniform	Dual population	Uniform	None	None
shape	Round	Scalloped	round		
Cisterns	Many	Few	Rare		
Stroma	Necrobiosis	No necrobiosis Trophoblastic Inclusions	Necrobiosis		
Vessels	Rare	Yes	Yes	None	None
NRBC	No	Yes (>50%)	Yes	n/a	n/a
Trophoblast					
Proliferation	Mod-marked	Min-mod	Atrophic/polar	Marked	Marked
Trophoblast type	ST,CT,IT	ST	ST,IT	IT, rare ST	ST, CT, rare IT
Location	Circumferential	Focal	Polar	Diffuse	Bilaminar
Necrosis	Yes	Yes	No	Rare	Yes
Lacy vacuolation	Yes	Yes	No	No	Yes
Karyotype					
	96% 46,XX 4% 46,XY	58% to 70% 69,XXY 27% to 40% 69,XXX 2% to 4% 69,XYY	20% abnormal	n/r	46,XY, plus Miscellaneous abnormalities
Flow cytometry					
	60% to 80% diploid 2% to 43% tetraploid 10% aneuploid Rare triploid	80% to 100% triploid 0% to 20% diploid 10% aneuploid 2% tetraploid 2% haploid	80% to 85% diploid 6% to 10% triploid 4% aneuploid 4% tetraploid	Diploid, triploid Tetraploid	Diploid
Risk for malignancy					
Recurrence	1%	Possible	Unknown	Unknown	n/a
Persistent disease	10% to 20%	4% to 13%	Unknown	Yes	n/a
Choriocarcinoma	2% to 8%	Case reports	1/160,000	20%	n/a

From Popek EJ: ASCP check sample AP 94-7(AP-241), "Partial hydatidiform mole," American Society of Clinical Pathologists, 1994. *AB*, Abortion; *CHM*, complete hydatidiform mole; *CT*, cytotrophoblast; *HA*, hydropic abortus; *IT*, intermediate trophoblast; *n/a*, not applicable; *n/r*, none reported; *NRBC*, nucleated red blood cells; *PHM*, partial hydatidiform mole; *PSTT*, placental site trophoblastic tumor; *SAB*, spontaneous abortion; *ST*, syncytiotrophoblast.

Hydropic abortus must be included in the differential diagnosis of molar gestation. The classic features are amphophilia of the villous stroma and atrophy of the trophoblasts. Trophoblastic proliferation, if present at all, is polar, representing a normally implanting villus (Fig. 69-30).

Immunohistochemistry may be useful in differentiating various forms of molar gestations. Placental markers such as hCG, placental alkaline phosphatase, and human placental lactogen have shown variability of syncytiotrophoblast staining in normal gestation compared with all molar pregnancies,[232,233] as summarized in Table 69-19. Cytotrophoblasts stain with proliferative cell nuclear antigen.[239]

Flow cytometry is useful in confirming a diagnosis of PHM by determining DNA ploidy. Although either fresh or forma-

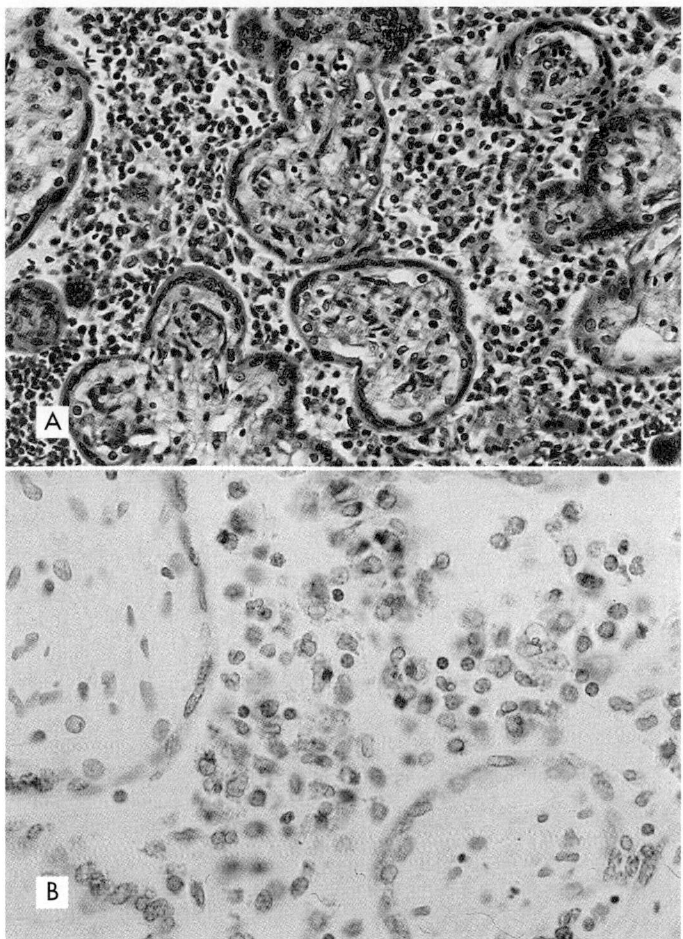

Fig. 69-26 **A,** Massive intervillositis evidenced by the presence of maternal macrophages. The etiology may by infectious (seen in malaria and toxoplasmosis), or an abnormal maternal response to autoantibodies or alloantibodies probably manifested on the trophoblast. **B,** The maternal cells stain positively with antibodies to KP-1, a monocyte/macrophage marker.

lin-fixed paraffin-embedded tissue may be used,[219,235-237] fixed tissue allows selective analysis of villi. The technique is fast, easy, reproducible, and measures many cells. The technique and interpretation of flow cytometry histograms has been reviewed elsewhere.[237-240] Aneuploid cells must compose 6% to 10% of the total cells to be seen as a separate peak.[237] The limit of sensitivity variation is 2 or 3 chromosomes.[138] Trisomies, monosomy, or translocations are not detected with the current methodology. Flow can also be used to determine an S-phase fraction, giving a rough estimate of the number of proliferating cells, which may or may not have value in predicting which cases will go on to persistent disease.[219]

Placental site trophoblastic tumor

Formerly called trophoblastic pseudotumor, this is not a molar pregnancy but a persistent proliferation of intermediate trophoblasts in the placental implantation site[241,242] (Fig. 69-31). Decidual vascular invasion occurs normally. "Excessive" invasion is a highly subjective assessment. The lesion follows a normal pregnancy or miscarriage in 95% of cases and molar gestation in 5%;[212] 10% to 23% have malignant behavior.[243-245] One third of patients have a positive pregnancy test.[243,246] The presenting symptoms are summarized in Table 69-18. The differential diagnosis includes the "exaggerated implantation site" and the placental nodule (Fig. 69-32). The histologic feature most suggestive of malignant behavior is 5 or more mitoses per 10 high-power fields; necrosis and clear, sparsely granular cytoplasm has also been described.[212,215] The malignant lesion is less responsive to chemotherapy than other GTD and is usually treated with hysterectomy.[243,244] Hematogenous metastases may develop in lung, brain, liver, lower genital tract, and abdomen. Few tumors have been studied by flow cytometry; most have been diploid.[247]

Choriocarcinoma

Choriocarcinoma is preceded by CHM in 50%, miscarriage in 25%, normal pregnancy in 24%, an ectopic pregnancy

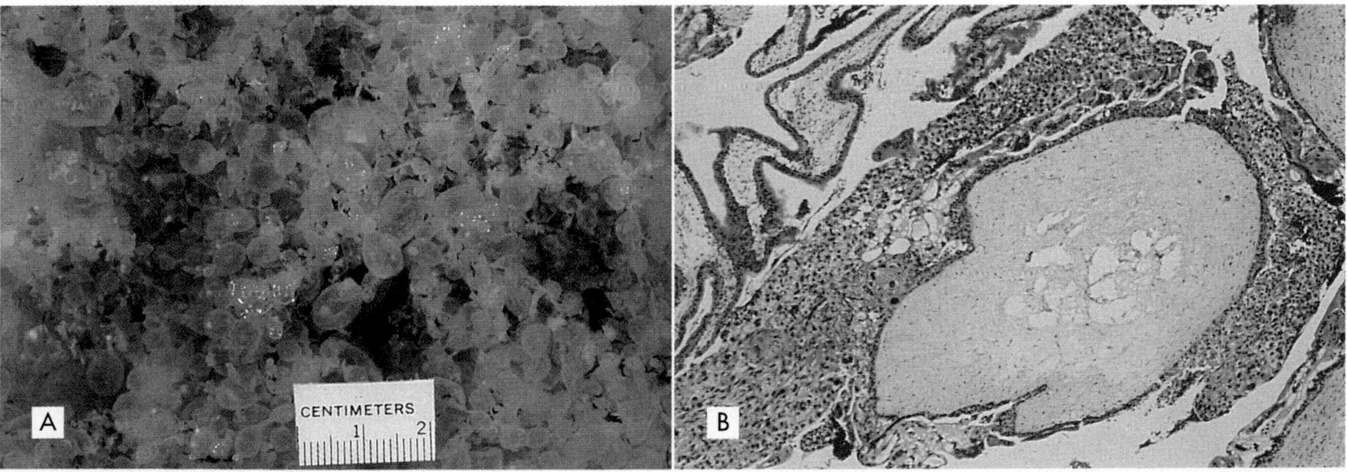

Fig. 69-27 **A,** Complete hydatidiform mole (CHM) immersed in water to redistend the vesicles. Nearly all villi are enlarged and are connected to one another by thin nonedematous cordlike structures. **B,** Greatly enlarged villus with incompletely formed central cistern. Circumferential proliferation of syncytiotrophoblasts, cytotrophoblasts, and intermediate trophoblasts, some showing eosinophilic necrosis and vacuolation.

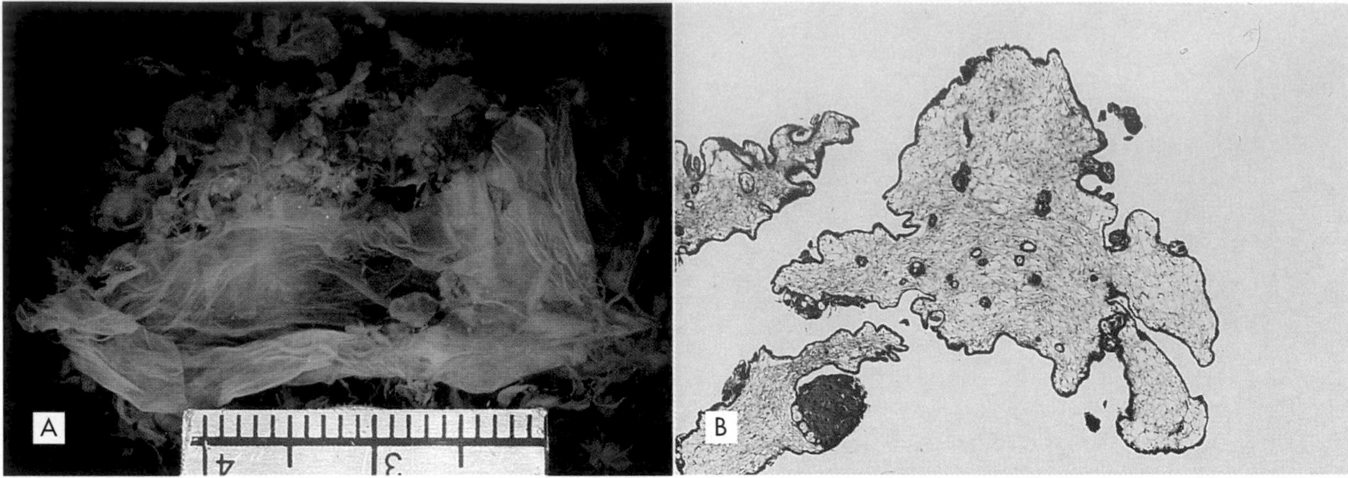

Fig. 69-28 Partial hydatidiform mole (PHM) immersed in water and showing only focal hydropic change. Less than 20% of villi affected. Fetal membranes are seen at the bottom. **B,** Enlarged villus with pronounced scalloping resulting in pseudoinclusions, islands of trophoblasts in the villus stroma. "Knuckles" of proliferating syncytiotrophoblasts have undergone eosinophilic necrosis.

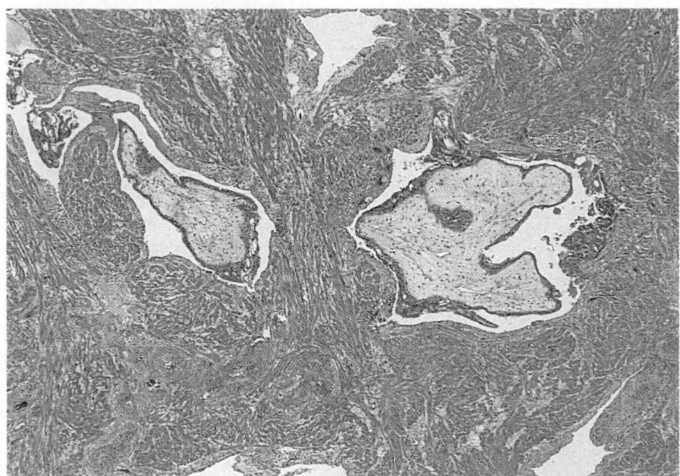

Fig. 69-29 Invasive CHM showing enlarged villi with trophoblastic proliferation deeply invasive into the myometrium.

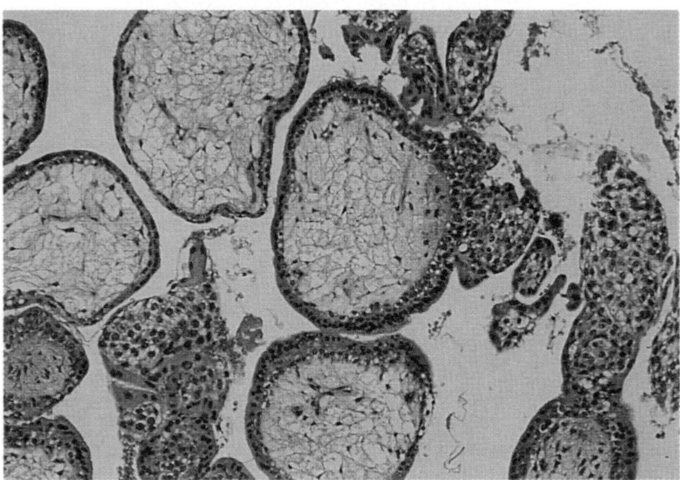

Fig. 69-30 Hydropic abortus (HA) with enlarged edematous villi with amphophilic stroma, few residual blood vessels, and polar trophoblastic proliferation of anchoring villi.

in 1.5% of cases, and only exceptionally by PHM.[248] Cytogenetically the vast majority are 46,XY, often with additional chromosomal numerical or structural abnormalities.

Grossly the tumor is hemorrhagic and friable. Classically devoid of villi, a rare case of choriocarcinoma in situ has been reported in a normal placenta.[249] Choriocarcinoma is a bilaminar tumor with a central core of cytotrophoblasts surrounded by a covering of syncytiotrophoblasts with a few intermediate trophoblasts (Fig. 69-33). The tumor widely invades maternal vessels, with extensive hemorrhage and necrosis. Degree of cytologic atypia has not proven to be of prognostic significance, but associated with worse outcome are maternal age, location, and extent of metastases.[248,250,251]

LEGAL ASPECTS OF PLACENTAL EXAMINATION

Legal defense of alleged malpractice in unfavorable pregnancy outcome has increasingly relied on evidence of subclinical intrauterine pathology revealed by careful placental study.[84,252-260] Physicians' malpractice liability insurance companies have been heavy promoters of placental examination. The information gleaned from placental examination has also proved useful to plaintiffs' attorneys. The delivered placenta can be dissected and examined more extensively than a living neonate. Placental lesions can be looked at as a record of some aspects of intrauterine life. Not all pathologic abnormalities seen in the placenta carry risk of adverse outcome, but the information gained through good gross and microscopic examination may be invaluable contributions to understanding causes of adverse maternal, fetal, or neonatal outcomes. Conversely, severe and chronic fetal damage may occur in the absence of placental lesions (e.g., fetal alcohol syndrome). Even when placental lesions are identified, it may not always be possible to determine the nature of possible cause-and-effect relationships between placental lesions and maternal, fetal, or neonatal outcome. Not every pathologist who examines placentas is or should be considered an expert, but an adequate gross examination and submission of standard sections will allow involved parties to seek a consultation.

Table 69-19 Immunohistochemistry (IHC) of normal and molar syncytiotrophoblasts

Diagnosis	IHC	6-10 WG	11-15 WG	16-24 WG
Normal	hCG	+++	+	+
	PlAP	–	+/++	+++
	hPL	++	+++	++++
HA	hCG	++++	++	++
	PlAP	+	–	–
	hPL	++/+++	+++/++++	+++
CHM	hCG	++++	++++	++++
	PlAP	–/+	–/+	+
	hPL	++	++/+++	++/+++
PHM	hCG	+++/++++	++	+
	PlAP	++	+/++	++++
	hPL	++++	+++/++++	++++

hCG, Human chorionic gonadotrophin; *PIAP,* placental alkaline phosphatase; *hPL,* human placental lactogen; *WG,* weeks of gestation; % of cells staining: no staining, –; 1% to 25%, +; 25% to 50%, ++; 50% to 75%, +++; 75% to 100%, +++.

Data from Popek EJ: ASCP check sample AP 94-7 (AP-241), "Partial hydatidiform mole," American Society of Clinical Pathologists, 1994.

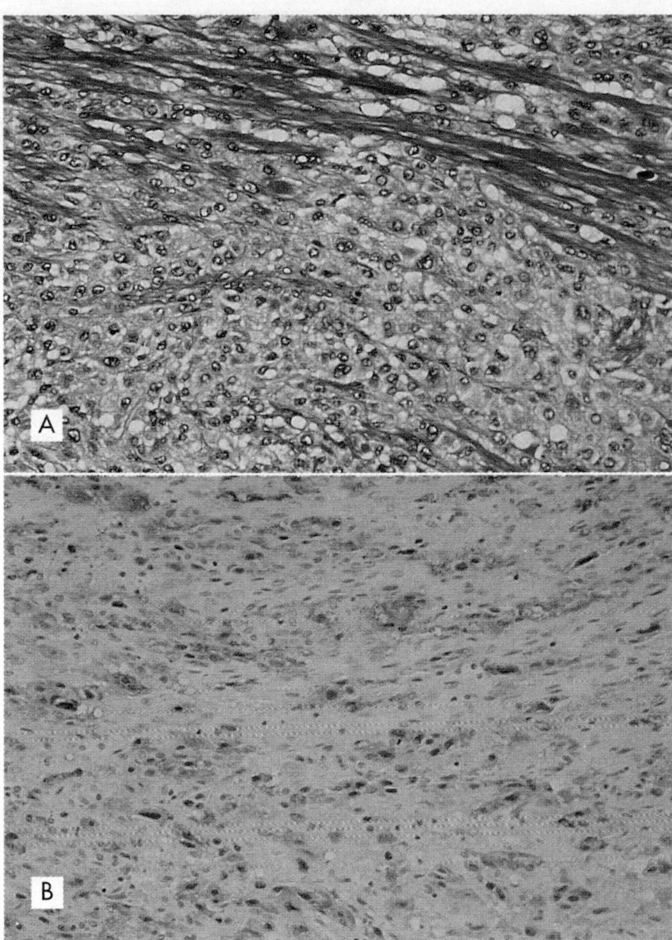

Fig. 69-31 Placental site trophoblastic tumor (PSTT). **A,** Sheets of uniform, polygonal intermediate trophoblasts with only a rare multinucleated cell seen invading between myometrial fibers. **B,** The cells show variable staining with immunohistochemistry for human placental lactogen.

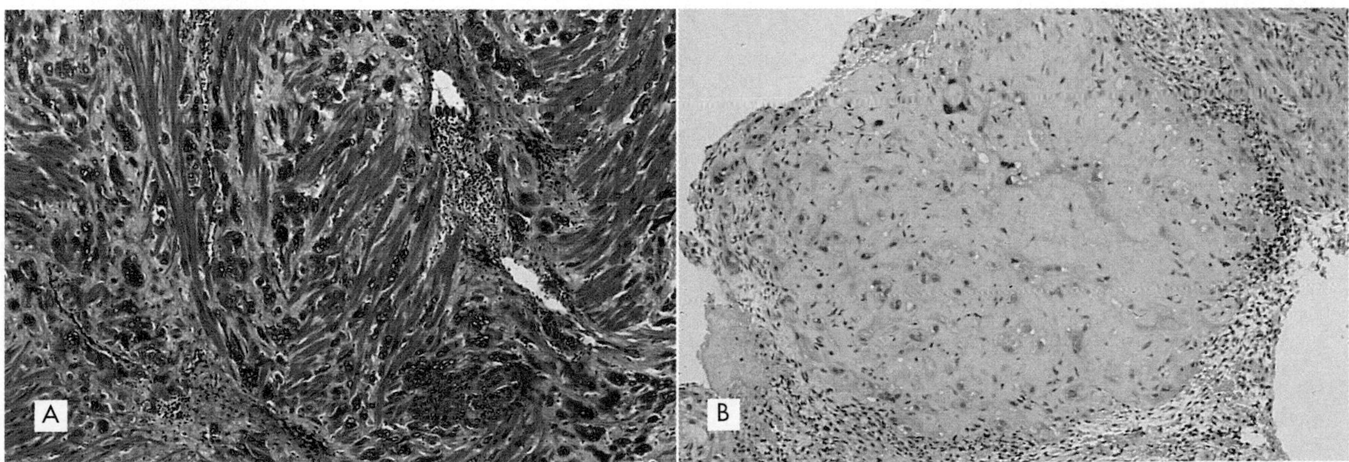

Fig. 69-32 Lesions easily confused with PSTT. **A,** Exaggerated implantation site with numerous mononuclear cells within the maternal myometrium. Normal invasion of the uterus by trophoblasts is extensive in early pregnancy and may be underappreciated. **B,** Placental nodule is residua from a previous pregnancy; well circumscribed, it has a central acellular or sclerotic region surrounded by a few viable intermediate trophoblasts. The last documented pregnancy in this case was several years before this curettage.

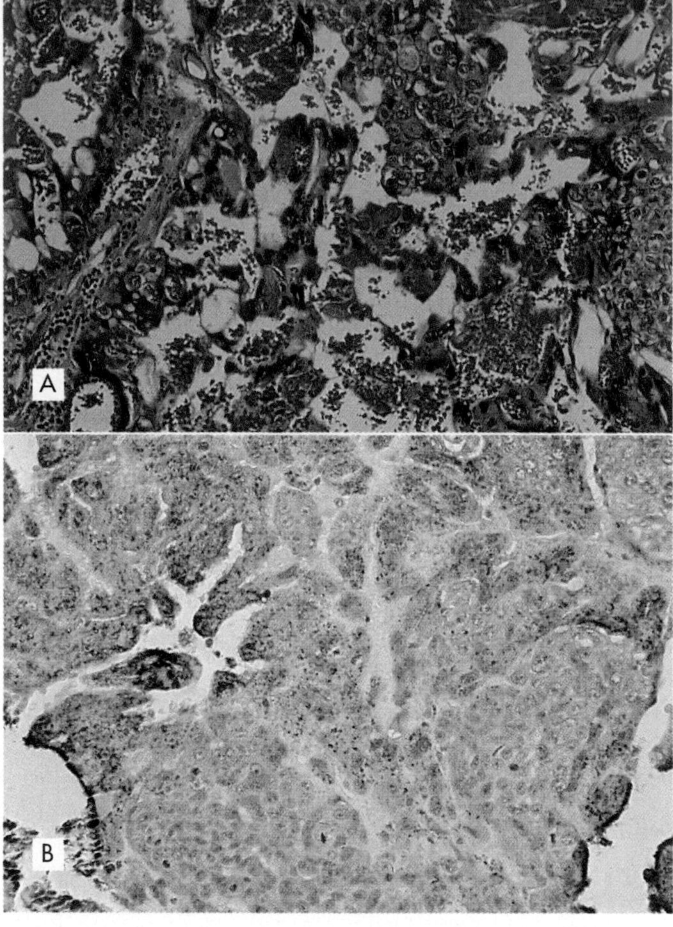

Fig. 69-33 **A,** Choriocarcinoma, hemorrhage, and focal necrosis. The bilaminar appearance of positive-staining syncytiotrophoblasts covering unstained cytotrophoblasts is better demonstrated on **B.** Stained with immunohistochemistry for human chorionic gonadotrophin (hCG).

REFERENCES

Normal placental anatomy and physiology

1. Battaglia FC, Meschia G, editors: *An Introduction to fetal physiology,* London,1986, Academic Press.
2. Feinberg RF, Kliman HJ, Lockwood CJ: Is oncofetal fibronectin a trophoblast glue for human implantation? *Am J Pathol* 138:537, 1991.
3. Enders AC: Trophoblast differentiation during the transition from trophoblastic plate to lacunar stage of implanation in the rhesus monkey and human, *Am J Anat* 186:85, 1989.
4. Pijnenborg R, Dixon G, Robertson WB et al: Trophoblastic invasion of human decidua from 8 to 18 weeks of pregnancy, *Placenta* 1:3, 1980.
5. Pijnenborg R, Robertson WB, Brosens I et al: Review article: trophoblast invasion and the establishment of haemochorial placentation in man and laboratory animals, *Placenta* 2:71, 1981.
6. Brosens I, Robertson WB, Dixon HG: The physiological response to the vessels of the placental bed to normal pregnancy, *J Pathol Bacteriol* 93:570, 1967.
7. Robertson WB, Brosens I, Dixon G: The Robertson-Brosens-Dixon hypothesis: evidence for the role of haemochorial placentation in pregnancy success, *Br J Obstet Gynaecol* 98;1195, 1991.
8. DeWolf F, DeWolf-Peters C, Brosens I et al: The human placental bed: electron microscopic study of trophoblastic invasion of spiral arteries, *Am J Obstet Gynecol* 137:58, 1980.
9. Pijnenborg R, Bland JM, Robertson WB et al: The pattern of interstitial trophoblastic invasion of the myometrium in early human pregnancy, *Placenta* 2:303, 1981.
10. Goldstein J, Braverman M, Salafia C et al: The phenotype of human placental macrophages and its variation with gestational age, *Am J Pathol* 133:648, 1988.
11. Cantle SJ, Kaufmann P, Luckhardt M et al: Interpretation of syncytial sprouts and bridges in the human placenta, *Placenta* 8:221, 1987.
12. Benirschke K, Kaufmann P, *Pathology of the human placenta,* ed 3, New York, 1995, Springer-Verlag.
13. Molteni RA: Placental growth and fetal/placental weight (F/P) ratios throughout gestation–their relationship to patterns of fetal growth, *Semin Perinatol* 8: 94, 1984.
14. Teasdale F, Jean-Jacques G: Morphometric evaluation of the microvillous surface enlargement factor in the human placenta from mid-gestation to term, *Placenta* 6:375, 1985.
15. Teasdale F: Gestational changes in the functional structure of the human placenta in relation to fetal growth: a morphometric study, *Am J Obstet Gynecol* 137:560, 1980.
16. Fox H, editor: *Pathology of the placenta,* London, 1978, Saunders.
17. Vorherr H: Placental insufficiency and postmaturity, *Eur J Obstet Gynecol Reprod Biol* 5:109, 1975.
18. Sands J, Dobbing J: Continuing growth and development of the third-trimester human placenta, *Placenta* 6:13, 1985.

Placental examination in maternal disease

19. Hacker NF, Berek JS, Lagasse LD et al: Carcinoma of the cervix associated with pregnancy, *Obstet Gynecol* 59:735, 1982.
20. Delerive C, Locquet F, Mallart A et al: Placental metastasis from maternal bronchial oat cell carcinoma, *Arch Pathol Lab Med* 113:556, 1989.
21. Anderson JF, Kent S, Machin GA: Maternal malignant melanoma with placental metastasis: a case report with literature review, *Pediatr Pathol* 9:35, 1989.
22. Zuazu J, Julia A, Sierra J et al: Pregnancy outcome in hematologic malignancies, *Cancer* 67:703, 1991.
23. Rice JP, Kay HH, Mahony BS: The clinical significance of uterine leiomyomas in pregnancy, *Am J Obstet Gynecol* 160:1212, 1989.
24. Rosenfeld JA: Abdominal trauma in pregnancy: when is fetal monitoring necessary? *Postgrad Med* 88:89, 1990.
25. Newberger EH, Barkan SE, Lieberman ES et al: Abuse of pregnant women and adverse birth outcome, current knowledge and implications for practice, *JAMA* 267:2370, 1992.
26. Scorpio RJ, Esposito TJ, Smith LG et al: Blunt trauma during pregnancy: factors affecting fetal outcome, *J Trauma* 32:213, 1992.
27. Reid RL, Thomas R: Thyroid disease and pregnancy: effects on the mother, fetus and newborn, *Fam Pract Recertif* 10:45,1988.
28. Ishizaki Y, Belter LF: Melanin deposition in the placenta as a result of skin lesions (dermatopathic melanosis of placenta), *Am J Obstet Gynecol* 79:1074, 1960.
29. Hernandez E, Angell CS, Johnson JW: Asthma in pregnancy: current concepts, *Obstet Gynecol* 55:739, 1980.
30. Koshy M, Burd L, Wallace D et al: Prophylactic red-cell transfusions in pregnant patients with sickle cell disease: a randomized cooperative study, *N Engl J Med* 319:1447, 1988.
31. Blattner P, Dar H, Nitowsky HM: Pregnancy outcome in women with sickle cell trait, *JAMA* 238:1392, 1977.
32. Jackson MR, Mayhew TM, Haas JD: The volumetric composition of human term placentae: altitudinal, ethnic and sex differences in Bolivia, *J Anat* 152:173, 1987.
33. Baldwin VJ: Morphologic pathology of fetomaternal interaction, *Contr Gynecol Obstet* 9:1, 1982.
34. Kliegman R, Gross T: Perinatal problems of the obese mother and her infant, *Obstet Gynecol* 66:299, 1985.

35. Rolfes DB, Ishak KG: Liver disease in pregnancy, *Histopathology* 19:555, 1986.
36. Kaplan MM: Acute fatty liver of pregnancy, *N Engl J Med* 313:367, 1985.
37. Fisk NM, Storey ENG: Fetal outcome in obstetric cholestasis, *Br J Obstet Gynaecol* 95:1137, 1988.
38. Costoya AL, Leontic EA, Rosenberg HG et al: Morphologic study of placental terminal villi in intrahepatic cholestasis of pregnancy: histochemistry, light and electron microscopy, *Placenta* 1:361, 1980.
39. Baldwin VJ, MacLeod PM, Benirschke K: Placental findings in alcohol abuse in pregnancy, *Birth Defects* 18:89, 1982.
40. Kaminski M, Rumeau-Rouquette C, Schwartz D: Effects of alcohol on the fetus, *N Engl J Med,* 298:55, 1978.
41. Chasnoff IJ, Burns WJ, Schnoll SH, Burns KA: Cocaine use in pregnancy, *N Engl J Med,* 313:666, 1985.
42. Page DV, Brady K, Ward S: The placental pathology of substance abuse, *Mod Pathol* 2:69A, 1989.
43. Vogel JJ, DeMoerloose PA, Bounameaux H: Protein C deficiency and pregnancy: a case report, *Obstet Gynecol* 73:455, 1989.
44. Abramowsky CR, Vegas ME, Swinehart G, Gyves M: Decidual vasculopathy of the placenta in lupus erythematosus, *N Engl J Med* 303:668, 1980.
45. Teasdale F, Chislaine JJ: Morphological changes in the placentas of smoking mothers: a histomorphometric study, *Biol Neonate* 55:251, 1989.
46. Rubin DH, Krasilikoff PA, Leventhal JM et al: Effects of passive smoking on birth-weight, *Lancet* 2:415, 1986.
47. Kaibara M, Kobayashi T, Matsumoto S: Idiopathic thrombocythemia and pregnancy: report of a case, *Obstet Gynecol* 65:18S, 1985.
48. Mercer B, Drouin J, Jolly E, D'Anjou G: Primary thrombocythemia in pregnancy: a report of two cases, *Am J Obstet Gynecol* 159:127, 1988.

Hypertensive diseases

49. Mabie WC, Pernoll ML, Biswas MK: Chronic hypertension in pregnancy, *Obstet Gynecol* 67:197, 1986.
50. DeWolf F, Brosens I, Renaer M: Fetal growth retardation and the maternal arterial supply of the human placenta in the absence of sustained hypertension, *Br J Obstet Gynaecol* 87:678, 1980.
51. Robertson WB, Brosens I, Dixon HG: The pathological response of the vessels of the placental bed to hypertensive pregnancy, *J Pathol Bacteriol* 93:581, 1967.
52. Robertson WB, Khong TY, Brosens CB et al: The placental bed biopsy: review from three European centers, *Am J Obstet Gynecol* 155:401, 1986.
53. Khong TY, Chambers HM: Alternative method of sampling placentas for the assessment of uteroplacental vasculature, *J Clin Pathol* 45:925, 1992.
54. Trudinger BJ, Giles WB, Cook CM: Uteroplacental blood flow velocity-time waveforms in normal and complicated pregnancy, *Br J Obstet Gynaecol* 92:39, 1985.
55. Lunell NO, Lewander R, Mamoun I et al: Uteroplacental blood flow in pregnancy induced hypertension, *Scand J Clin Lab Invest suppl* 169:28, 1984.
56. Brosens I, Renaer M: On the pathogenesis of placental infarcts in preeclampsia, *J Obstet Gynaecol Br Commonw* 79:794, 1972.
57. Singer DB, MacPherson T: Fetal death and the macerated stillborn fetus. In Wigglesworth J, Singer DB, editors: *Textbook of fetal and perinatal pathology,* Cambridge, Mass, 1991, Blackwell Scientific.
58. Batcup G, Tovey LAD, Longster G: Fetomaternal blood group incompatibility studies in placental intervillous thrombosis, *Placenta* 4:449, 1983.
59. Giles W, Trudinger B, Cook C, et al: Placental microvascular changes in twin pregnancies with abnormal umbilical artery waveforms, *Obstet Gynecol* 81:556, 1993.
60. Los FJ, DeWolf BT, Huisjes HJ: Raised maternal serum-alpha fetoprotein levels and spontaneous fetomaternal transfusion, *Lancet* 2:1210, 1979.
61. Giles WB, Trudinger BJ, Baird PJ: Fetal umbilical artery flow velocity waveforms and placental resistance: pathological correlation, *Br J Obstet Gynaecol* 92:31, 1985.
62. Groome LJ, Owen J, Neely CL et al: Oligohydramnios: antepartum fetal urine production and intrapartum fetal distress, *Am J Obstet Gynecol* 165:1077, 1991.

Hypercoagulable states

63. Gleicher N, Fribert J: IgM gammopathy and the lupus anticoagulant syndrome in habitual aborters, *JAMA* 253:3278, 1985.
64. Carreras LO, Vermylen J, Spitz B et al: "Lupus" anticoagulant and inhibition of prostacyclin formation in patients with repeated abortion, intrauterine growth retardation and intrauterine death, *Br J Obstet Gynaecol* 88:890, 1981.
65. Petri M, Golbus M, Anderson R et al: Antinuclear antibody, lupus anticoagulant, and anticardiolipin antibody in women with idiopathic habitual abortion, *Arthritis Rheum* 30:601, 1987.
66. Branch DW, Scott JR, Kochenour KK, Hershgold E: Obstetric complications associated with the lupus anticoagulant, *N Engl J Med* 313:1322, 1985.
67. Triplett A, Harris EN: Antiphospholipid antibodies and reproduction, *Am J Reprod Immunol* 21:123, 1989.
68. DeWolf F, Carreras LO, Moerman P et al: Decidual vasculopathy and extensive placental infarction in a patient with repeated thromboembolic accidents, recurrent fetal, and a lupus anticoagulant, *Am J Obstet Gynecol* 142:829, 1982.
69. Feinstein DI: Lupus anticoagulant, thrombosis, and fetal loss, *N Eng J Med* 21:1348, 1985.
70. Cowchock S, Smith JB, Gocial B: Antibodies to phospholipids and nuclear antigens in patients with repeated abortions, *Am J Obstet Gynecol* 155:1002, 1986.
71. Triplett DA: Pathogenic mechanisms of action: effects on the coagulation system, Fifth International Symposium on Antiphospholipid Antibodies, San Antonio, Texas, 1992.
72. Out H, Kooijman CD, Bruinse HW, Derksen R: Histopathological findings in placentae from patients with intrauterine fetal death and antiphospholipid antibodies, *Eur J Obstet Gynecol Reprod Biol* 41:179, 1991.
73. Griffun JH: Clinical studies of protein C, *Semin Thromb Hemost* 10:162, 1984.

Smoking and cocaine use

74. Andersen KV, Hermann N: Placenta flow reduction in pregnant smokers, *Acta Obstet Gynecol Scand* 63:707, 1984.
75. Van Der Velde WJ, Peereboom-Stegeman JC et al: Basal lamina thickening in the placentae of smoking mothers, *Placenta* 6:329, 1985.
76. Jauniaux E, Burton GJ: The effect of smoking in pregnancy on early placental morphology, *Obstet Gynecol* 79:645, 1992.
77. Saloojee Y, Vesey CJ, Cole PV, Russell M: Carboxyhaemoglobin and plasma thiocyanate: complementary indicators of smoking behaviour? *Thorax* 37:521, 1982.
78. Rush D, Kristal A, Blanc W et al: The effects of maternal cigarette smoking on placental morphology, histomorphometry and biochemistry, *Am J Perinatol* 3:263, 1986.
79. Busacca M, Balconi G, Pietra A et al: Maternal smoking and prostacyclin production by cultured endothelial cells from umbilical arteries, *Am J Obstet Gynecol* 148:1127, 1984.
80. Sorensen KE, Borlum KG: Acute effects of maternal smoking on human fetal heart function, *Acta Obstet Gynecol Scand* 66:217, 1987.
81. Dombrowski MP, Sokol RJ: Cocaine and abruption, *Contemp Obstet Gynecol* 35:13, 1990.
82. Woods JR, Plessinger MA: Maternal, placental, and fetal pathophysiology of cocaine exposure during pregnancy, *Clin Obstet Gynecol* 36:267, 1993.
83. Zimmerman EF, Potturi RB, Resnick E, Fisher JE: Role of oxygen free radicals in cocaine-induced vascular disruption in mice, *Teratology* 49:192, 1994.

Diabetes mellitus

84. Salafia CM: Fetal and placental pathology in diabetic patients. in Reece EA, Coustan DR, editors: *Diabetes mellitus in pregnancy: principles and practice,* New York, 1988, Churchill Livingstone.
85. Altshuler G: Some placental considerations related to neurodevelopmental and other disorders, *J Child Neurol* 8:78, 1993.

Abnormal placental implantation

86. Mashiah N, Levit A, Sherer DM et al: Two rare complications of simultaneously occurring placenta previa and placenta percreta, *Acta Obstet Gynecol Scand* 67:655, 1988.

Placental examination in fetal disease

Multiple gestations

87. Wenstrom KD, Gall SA: Incidence, morbidity and mortality, and diagnosis of twin gestations, *Clin Perinatol* 15:1, 1988.
88. Bronsteen R, Goyert G, Bottoms S: Classification of twins and neonatal morbidity, *Obstet Gynecol* 74:98, 1989.
89. Johnson SF, Driscoll SG: Twin placentation and its complications, *Semin Perinatol* 10:9, 1986.
90. McCulloch K: Neonatal problems in twins, *Clin Perinatol* 15:141, 1988.
91. Newton ER: Antepartum care in multiple gestations, *Semin Perinatol* 10:19, 1986.
92. Kleinman JC, Fowler MG, Kessel SS: Comparison of infant mortality among twins and singletons: United States 1960 and 1983, *Am J Epidemiol* 133:133, 1991.
93. Benirschke K, Kim CK: Multiple pregnancy (first of two parts), *N Engl J Med* 188:1276, 1973.
94. Baldwin VJ: Pathology of multiple gestation. In Wigglesworth J, Singer DB, editors: *Textbook of fetal and perinatal pathology,* Cambridge, Mass, 1991, Blackwell Scientific.
95. Soernes T, Bakke T: The length of the human umbilical cord in twin pregnancies, *Am J Obstet Gynecol* 157:1229, 1987.
96. Robertson EG, Neer KJ: Placental injection studies in twin gestation, *Am J Obstet Gynecol* 147:170, 1983.
97. Landy HJ, Weiner S, Corson SL et al: The "vanishing twin": ultrasonographic assessment of fetal disappearance in the first trimester, *Am J Obstet Gynecol* 147:170, 1983.
98. Dudley DKL, D'Alton ME: Single fetal death in twin gestation, *Semin Perinatol* 10:65, 1986.
99. Cherouny PH, Hoskins IA, Johnson TRB et al: Multiple pregnancy with late death of one fetus, *Obstet Gynecol* 74:318, 1989.
100. Patten RM, Mack LA, Nyberg DA et al: Twin embolization syndrome: prenatal sonographic detection and significance, *Radiology* 173:685, 1989.
101. Benirschke K: Intrauterine death of a twin: mechanisms, implications for surviving twin, and placental pathology, *Semin Diagn Pathol* 10:222, 1993.
102. Enbom JA: Twin pregnancy with intrauterine death of one twin, *Am J Obstet Gynecol* 131:267, 1978.
103. Naeye RL, Benirschke K, Hagstrom JWC et al: Intrauterine growth in twins as estimated from liveborn birth weight data, *Pediatrics* 37:409, 1966.
104. Eberle AM, Levesque D, Vintzileos AM et al: Placental pathology in discordant twins, *Am J Obstet Gynecol* 169:931, 1993.
105. Benirschke K, Kim CK: Multiple pregnancy (second of two parts), *N Engl J Med* 188:1329, 1979.
106. Little J, Bryan E: Congenital anomalies in twins, *Semin Perinatol* 10:50, 1986.
107. Heifetz SA: The placenta. In Stocker JT, Dehner LP, editors, *Pediatric pathology,* Philadelphia, 1992, Lippincott.
108. Lage JM, Vanmarter LJ, Mikhail E: Vascular anastomoses in fused, dichorionic twin placentas resulting in twin transfusion syndrome, *Placenta* 10:55, 1989.
109. Fries MH, Goldstein RB, Kilpatrick SJ et al: The role of velamentous cord insertion in the etiology of twin-twin transfusion syndrome, *Obstet Gynecol* 81:569, 1993.
110. Blickstein I: The twin-twin transfusion syndrome, *Obstet Gynecol* 76:714, 1990.
111. Genest DR, Lage JM: Absence of normal-appearing proximal tubules in the fetal and neonatal kidney: prevalence and significance, *Hum Pathol* 22:147, 1991.
112. Danskin WH, Neilson JP: Twin-to-twin transfusion syndrome: what are appropriate diagnostic criteria? *Am J Obstet Gynecol* 161:365, 1989.
113. Sala MA, Matheus M: Placental characteristics in twin transfusion syndrome, *Arch Gynecol Obstet* 246:51, 1989.
114. Bendon RH, Siddiqi T: Clinical pathology conference: acute twin-to-twin in utero transfusion, *Pediatr Pathol* 9:591, 1991.
115. Baldwin VJ, Wittmann BK: Pathology of intragestational intervention in twin-to-twin transfusion syndrome, *Pediatr Pathol* 10:79, 1990.
116. DeLia JE, Cruckshank DP, Kete WR: Fetoscopic neodynium: YAG laser occlusion of placental vessels in severe twin-twin transfusion syndrome, *Obstet Gynecol* 75:1047, 1990.
117. Van Allen MI, Smith DW, Shepard TH: Twin reversed arterial perfusion (TRAP) sequence: a study of 14 twin pregnancies with acardius, *Semin Perinatol* 7:285, 1983.
118. Wolf HK, MacDonald J, Bradford WB et al: Acardius anceps with evidence of intrauterine vascular occlusion: report of a case and discussion of the pathogenesis, *Pediatr Pathol* 11:143, 1991.
119. Moore TR, Sale SA, Benirschke K: Perinatal analysis of forty-nine pregnancies complicated by acardiac twinning, *Am J Obstet Gynecol* 163:907, 1990.
120. Stephens TD, Spall R, Urfer AG et al: Fetus amorphus or placental teratoma, *Teratology* 40:1, 1989.
121. The International Clearinghouse for Birth Defects Monitoring Systems: Conjoined twins—an epidemiological study based on 312 cases, *Acta Genet Med Gemellot (Roma)* 40:235, 1991.
122. Kiely JL, Kleinman JC, Kiely M: Triplets and higher-order multiple births, time, trends, and infant mortality, *Am J Dis Child* 146:862, 1992.
123. Kalousek DK: The role of confined chromosomal mosaicism in placental function and human development, *Growth Gen Horm* 4:1, 1988.

Early fetal loss

124. Salafia CM, Maier D, Vogel C et al: Placental and decidual histology in spontaneous abortions: detailed description and correlations with chromosome number, *Obstet Gynecol* 82:295, 1993.
125. Jauniaux E, Hustin J: Histological exam of the first trimester spontaneous abortions: the impact of materno-embryo interface features, *Histopathology* 21:409, 1992.
126. Khong TY, Liddell HS, Robertson WB: Defective haemochorial placentation as a cause of miscarriage: a preliminary study, *Br J Obstet Gynaecol* 94:649, 1987.
127. Salafia CM, Weigl CA, Foye GJ: Correlation of placental erythrocyte morphology and gestational age, *Pediatr Pathol* 8:495, 1988.
128. Daya D, Sabel T: The use of cytokeratin as a sensitive and reliable marker for trophoblastic tissue, *Am J Clin Pathol* 95:137, 1991.
129. Kaspar HG, To T, Dinh TV: Clinical use of immunoperoxidase markers in excluding ectopic gestation, *Obstet Gynecol* 78:433, 1991.

Late fetal loss

130. Genest DR: Estimating the time of death in stillborn fetuses. II. Histologic evaluation of the placenta, a study of 71 stillborns, *Obstet Gynecol* 80:585, 1992.
131. Fox H: Morphological changes in the human placenta following fetal death, *J Obstet Gynaecol Br Commonw* 75:839, 1968.
132. Ornoy A, Crone K, Altshuler G: Pathological features of the placenta in fetal death, *Arch Pathol Lab Med* 100:367, 1976.
133. Sander CH, Stevens NG: Placental hemorrhagic endovasculitis: risk factors and impact on pregnancy outcome, *Int J Obstet Gynecol* 22:393, 1984.
134. Silver M, Yeger H, Lines L: Hemorrhagic endovasculitis-like lesion induced in placental organ culture, *Hum Pathol* 19:251, 1988.
135. Shen-Schwarz S, MacPherson TA, Mueller-Heubach E: The clinical significance of hemorrhagic endovasculitis of the placenta, *Am J Obstet Gynecol* 159:48, 1988.
136. Bakker WW, Timmerman W, Poelstra K, Schuiling GA: Endotoxin induced intraplacental thrombotic tendency and decreased vascular ADPase in the pregnant rat, *Placenta* 13:281, 1992.
137. Genest DR, Singer DB: Estimating the time of death in stillborn fetuses: III. External fetal examination; a study of 86 stillborns, *Obstet Gynecol* 80:593, 1992.
138. Genest DR, Williams MA, Greene MF: Estimating the time of death in stillborn fetuses: I. Histologic evaluation of fetal organs; an autopsy study of 150 stillborns, *Obstet Gynecol* 80:575, 1992.
139. Garcia AGP, Marques RLS, Lobato YY et al: Placental pathology in congenital rubella, *Placenta* 6:281, 1985.
140. Perrin EVDK, editor: *Pathology of the placenta,* New York, 1984, Churchill Livingstone.
141. Labarrere C, Althabe O, Caletti E, Muscolo D: Deficiency of blocking factors in intrauterine growth retardation and its relationship with chronic villitis, *Am J Reprod Immunol Microbiol* 10:14, 1986.
142. Labarrere C, Althabe O: Chronic villitis of unknown aetiology and intrauterine growth retarded infants of normal and low ponderal index, *Placenta* 6:369, 1985.

143. Labarrere C: Allogeneic recognition and rejection reactions in the placenta, *Am J Reprod Immunol* 21:94, 1989.
144. Gersell DJ: Chronic villitis, chronic chorioamnionitis and maternal floor infarction, *Semin Diagn Pathol* 10:251, 1993.

Low birth weight infants

145. Salafia CM, Ernst L, Pezzullo JP et al: The very low birth weight infant: maternal complications leading to preterm birth, placental lesions, and intrauterine growth, *Am J Perinatol* 10:135, 1993.
146. Yogman MW, Kraemer HC, Kindlon D et al: Identification of intrauterine growth retardation among low birth weight preterm infants, *J Pediatr* 115:799, 1989.
147. Villar J, Belizan JM: The timing factor in the pathophysiology of the intrauterine growth retardation syndrome, *Obstet Gynecol Surv* 37:499, 1982.
148. Starfield B, Shapiro S, McCormick M, Bross D: Mortality and morbidity in infants with intrauterine growth retardation, *J Pediatr* 101:978, 1982.
149. Villar J, Smeriglio V, Martorell R et al: Heterogeneous growth and mental development of intrauterine growth-retarded infants during the first 3 years of life, *Pediatrics* 74:783, 1984.
150. Honore LH, Dill FJ, Poland BJ: Placental morphology in spontaneous human abortuses with normal and abnormal karyotypes, *Teratology* 14:151, 1976.
151. Rochelson B, Kaplan C, Guzman E et al: A quantitative analysis of placental vasculature in the third trimester fetus with autosomal trisomy, *Obstet Gynecol* 75:59, 1990.

Hydrops fetalis

152. Machin GA: Hydrops revisited: literature review of 1414 cases published in the 1980's, *Am J Med Genet* 34:366, 1989.
153. Nakamura Y, Komatus Y, Yano H et al: Nonimmune hydrops fetalis: a clinicopathological study of 50 autopsy cases, *Pediatr Pathol* 7:19, 1987.
154. Nicolaides KH: Studies on fetal physiology and pathophysiology in rhesus disease, *Semin Perinatol* 13:328, 1989.
155. Harman CR: Fetal monitoring in the alloimmunized pregnancy, *Clin Perinatol* 16:691, 1989.

Other fetal anomalies

156. Grafe MR, Benirschke K: Ultrastructural study of the amniotic epithelium in a case of gastroschisis, *Pediatr Pathol* 10:95, 1990.
157. Young ID, Lundenbaum RHJ, Thompson EM, Pembrey ME. Amniotic bands in connective tissue disorders, *Arch Dis Child* 60:1061, 1985.
158. Barabas AP: Ehlers-Danlos syndrome associated with prematurity and premature rupture of foetal membranes, *Br Med J* 2:682, 1966.

Tumors metastatic to placenta

159. Mancini AF, Rosito P, Faldella G et al: Neuroblastoma in a pair of identical twins, *Med Pediatr Oncol* 10:45, 1982.
160. Perkins DG, Koop CM, Haust MD: Placental infiltration in congenital neuroblastoma: a case study with ultrastructure, *Histopathology* 4:383, 1980.
161. Sotelo-Avila C, Graham M, Hanby DE, Rudolph AJ: Nevus cell aggregated in the placenta, *Am J Clin Pathol* 89:395, 1988.
162. Schneiderman H, Wu AYY, Campbell WA et al: Congenital melanoma with multiple prenatal metastases, *Cancer* 60:1371, 1987.
163. Las Heras J, Leal G, Haust MD: Congenital leukemia with placental involvement, *Cancer* 58:2278, 1986.

The early amnion rupture sequence

164. Higginbottom MC, Jones KL, Hall BD, Smith DW: The amniotic band disruption complex: timing of amniotic rupture and variable spectra of consequent defects, *J Pediatr* 95:544, 1979.
165. Kalousek D: Amniotic band syndrome in previable fetuses, *Pediatr Pathol* 7:488, 1987.
166. Heifetz SA: Strangulation of the umbilical cord by amniotic bands: report of 6 cases and literature review, *Pediatr Pathol* 2:285, 1984.
167. Miller ME, Graham JM, Higginbottom MC, Smith DW: Compression defects from early amnion rupture: evidence for mechanical teratogenesis, *J Pediatr* 98:292, 1981.
168. Seeds JW, Cafelo RC, Herbert WP: Amniotic band syndrome, *Am J Obstet Gynecol* 144:243, 1982.
169. Irving WL, Doublestein GL: Congenital amniotic band syndrome: report of a familial recurrence, *J Am Osteopathic Assoc* 88:891, 1988.
170. Moessinger AC, Bland WA, Byrne J et al: Amniotic band syndrome associated with amniocentesis, *Am J Obstet Gynecol* 141:589, 1981.
171. Lockwood C, Ghidini A, Romero R, Hobbins JC: Amniotic band syndrome: reevaluation of its pathogenesis, *Am J Obstet Gynecol* 160:1030, 1989.
172. Bamforth JS: Amniotic band sequence: Streeter's hypothesis reexamined, *Am J Med Genet* 44:280, 1992.

Storage disorders

173. Dimmick JE, Applegarth DA: Inborn metabolic diseases of the perinatal infant. In Wigglesworth J, Singer DB, editors: *Textbook of fetal and perinatal pathology,* Cambridge, Mass, 1991, Blackwell Scientific.
174. Jones CJP, Mehroo L, Chawner LE, Jauniaux E: Ultrastructure of the human placenta in metabolic storage disease, *Placenta* 11:395-411.
175. Roberts DJ, Ampola MG, Lage JM: Diagnosis of unsuspected fetal metabolic storage disease by routine placental examination, *Pediatr Pathol* 11:647, 1991.

Fetal distress

176. Vintzileos AM, Campbell WA, Ingardia CJ, Nochimson NJ: The fetal biophysical profile and its predictive value, *Obstet Gynecol* 62:271, 1983.
177. Freeman RK, Garite TJ, Nageotte MP: In Brown CL, editor: *Fetal heart rate monitoring,* ed 2, Baltimore, 1991, Williams & Wilkins.
178. Nelson KB, Ellenberg JH: The asymptomatic newborn and risk of cerebral palsy, *Am J Dis Child* 141:1333, 1987.
179. Low JA, Galbraith RS, Muir D et al: Intrapartum fetal asphyxia: a preliminary report in regard to long-term morbidity, *Am J Obstet Gynecol* 130:525, 1978.

Neuromuscular disorders

180. Mann LI: Pregnancy events and brain damage, *Am J Obstet Gynecol* 155:6, 1986.
181. Naeye RL: *Disorders of the placenta, fetus and neonate: diagnosis and clinical significance,* St Louis, 1992, Mosby.
182. McLennan H, Price E, Urbanska M et al: Umbilical cord knots and encirclements, *Aust N Z J Obstet Gynaecol* 28:116, 1988.
183. Glanfield PA, Watson R: Intrauterine fetal death due to umbilical cord torsion, *Arch Pathol Lab Med* 110:357, 1986.
184. Kiley KC, Perkins CS, Penney LL: Umbilical cord stricture associated with intrauterine fetal demise: a report of two cases, *J Reprod Med* 31:154, 1986.
185. Heifetz SA: Thrombosis of the umbilical cord: analysis of 52 cases and literature review, *Pediatr Pathol* 8:37, 1988.
186. Hankins GDV, Snyder RR, Hauth JC et al: Nuchal cords and neonatal outcomes, *Obstet Gynecol* 70:687, 1987.
187. Heifetz SA: Single umbilical artery: a statistical analysis of 237 autopsy cases and review of the literature, *Perspect Pediatr Pathol* 8:345, 1984.
188. Byrne J, Blanc WA: Malformations and chromosome anomalies in spontaneously aborted fetuses with single umbilical artery, *Am J Obstet Gynecol* 151:340, 1985.
189. Altshuler G, Hyde S: Meconium-induced vasocontraction: a potential cause of cerebral and other fetal hypoperfusion and of poor pregnancy outcome, *J Child Neurol* 4:137, 1989.
190. Altshuler G, Arizawa M, Molnar-Nadasdy G: Meconium induced umbilical vascular necrosis and ulceration: a potential link between the placenta and poor pregnancy outcome, *Obstet Gynecol* 79:760, 1992.
191. Jauniaux E, DeMunter C, Vanesse M et al: Embryonic remnants of the umbilcal cord: morphologic and clinical aspects, *Hum Pathol* 20:458, 1989.
192. Naeye RL: Umbilical cord length: clinical significance, *J Pediatr* 107:278, 1985.

Intrauterine infections

ACUTE ASCENDING INFECTION

193. Romero R, Sirtori M, Oyarzun E et al: Infection and labor v. prevalance, microbiology and clinical significance of intraamniotic infection in women with preterm labor and intact membranes, *Am J Obstet Gynecol* 16:817, 1989.
194. Guzick DS, Winn K: The association of chorioamnionitis with preterm delivery, *Obstet Gynecol* 65:11, 1985.

195. Salafia CM, Mangam HE, Weigl CA et al: Abnormal fetal heart rate patterns and placental inflammation, *Am J Obstet Gynecol* 160:140, 1989.
196. Fleming AD, Salafia CM, Vintzileos AM et al: The relationships amongst umbilical arterial velocimetry, fetal biophysical profile and placental inflammation in preterm premature rupture of the membranes, *Am J Obstet Gynecol* 164:38, 1991.
197. Salafia CM, Silberman L: Placental pathology and abnormal fetal heart rate patterns in gestational diabetes, *Pediatr Pathol* 9:513, 1989.
198. Romero R, Baumann P, Gomez R et al: The relationship between spontaneous rupture of membranes, labor, and microbial invasion of the amniotic cavity and amniotic fluid concentrations of prostaglandins and thromboxane B_2 in term pregnancy, Am J Obstet Gynecol 168:1654, 1993.
199. Altshuler G: Fusobacteria, an important cause of chorioamnionitis, *Arch Pathol Lab Med* 109:739, 1985.
200. Novak RW, Platt MS: Significance of placental findings in early onset group B streptococcal neonatal sepsis, *Clin Pediatr* 24:256, 1985.
201. Ariel I, Singer DB: Streptococcus viridans infections in mid-gestation, *Pediatr Pathol* 11:75, 1991.
202. Burgio GR, Ugazio AG, editors: *Immunology of the neonate,* Heidelberg, 1987, Springer-Verlag.
203. Naeye RL, Maisels J, Lorenz RP et al: The clinical significance of placental villous edema, *Pediatrics* 71:588, 1983.

HEMATOGENOUS INFECTION

204. Kaplan C: The placenta and viral infections, *Semin Diagn Pathol* 10:222, 1993.
205. Garcia AGP, Fonseca EF, Marques RLdeS, Lobato YY: Placental morphology in cytomegalovirus infection, *Placenta* 10:1, 1989.
206. Fojaco RM, Hensley GT, Moskowitz L: Congenital syphilis and necrotizing funisitis, *JAMA* 261:1788, 1989.
207. Qureshi F, Jacques SM, Reyes MP: Placental histopathology in syphilis, *Hum Pathol* 24:779, 1993.
208. Russell P: Inflammatory lesions of the human placenta. III. The histopathology of villitis of unknown aetiology, *Placenta* 1:227, 1980
209. Redline RW, Abramowsky CR: Clinical and pathologic aspects of recurrent placental villitis, *Hum Pathol* 16:727, 1985.
210. Labarrere C, Mullen E: Fibrinoid and trophoblastic necrosis with massive chronic intervillositis: an extreme variant of villitis of unknown etiology, *Am J Reprod Immunol Microbiol* 15:85, 1987.
211. Bulmer JN, Rasheed RN, Francis N et al: Placental malaria. I. Pathological classification, *Histopathology* 22:211, 1993.

Gestational trophoblastic disease

212. Kurman RJ: The morphology, biology and pathology of intermediate trophoblast: a look back to the present, *Hum Pathol* 22:847, 1991.
213. Vassilakos P, Kajii T: Hydatidiform mole: two entities, *Lancet* 1:259, 1976.
214. Vassilakos P, Riotton G, Kajii T: Hydatidiform mole: two entities, a morphologic and cytogenetic study with some clinical considerations, *Am J Obstet Gynecol* 127:167, 1977.
215. Szulman AE, Surti U: The syndromes of hydatidiform mole. I. cytogenetic and morphologic correlation, *Am J Obstet Gynecol* 131:655, 1987.
216. Szulman AE, Surti U: The syndromes of hydatidiform mole. II. morphologic evolution of the complete and partial mole, *Am J Obstet Gynecol* 132:20, 1978.
217. Lage JM: Diagnostic dilemmas in gynecologic and obstetric pathology, *Semin Diagn Pathol* 7:146, 1990.
218. Szulman AE: Trophoblastic disease: clinical pathology of hydatidiform moles, *Obstet Gynecol Clin North Am* 15:443, 1988.
219. Conran RM, Hitchcock CL, Popek EJ et al: Diagnostic considerations in molar gestations, *Hum Pathol* 24:41, 1993.
220. Kajii T, Ohama K: Androgenetic origin of hydatidiform mole, *Nature* 268:633, 1977.
221. Genest DR, Oaborde O, Berkowitz RS et al: A clinicopathologic study of 153 cases of complete hydatidiform mole (1980–1990): histologic grade lacks prognostic significance, *Obstet Gynecol* 78:402, 1991.
222. Surti V: Genetic concepts and techniques. In Sulzman AE, Buchsbaum HJ, editors: *Gestational trophoblastic disease,* New York, 1987, Springer Verlag.
223. Lawler SD, Fisher RA, Dent J: A prospective genetic study of complete and partial hydatidiform moles, *Am J Obstet Gynecol* 164:1270, 1991.
224. Wake N, Jujino T, Hoshi S et al: The propensity to malignancy of dispermic heterozygous moles, *Placenta* 8:319, 1987.
225. Szulman AE, Philippe E, Boue JG, Boue A: Human triploidy: association with partial hydatidiform moles and nonmolar conceptuses, *Hum Pathol* 12:1016, 1981.
226. Gardner HAR, Lage JM: Choriocarcinoma following a partial hydatidiform mole: a case report, *Hum Pathol* 23:468, 1992.
227. Heifetz SA, Czaja J: In situ choriocarcinoma arising in partial hydatidiform mole: implications for the risk of persistent trophoblastic disease, *Pediatr Pathol* 12:601, 1992.
228. Bagshawe KD, Lawler SD, Paradinas FJ et al: Gestational trophoblastic tumors following initial diagnosis of partial hydatidiform mole, *Lancet* 335:1074, 1990.
229. Garger LW, Redline RW, Mostoufi-Zadeh M, Driscoll SG: Invasive partial mole, *Am J Clin Pathol* 85:722, 1986.
230. Kanazawa K, Suzuki T, Sasgawa M et al: Clinical problem of invasive hydatidiform moles in patients aged 40 or more, *Gynecol Oncol* 28:330, 1987.
231. Takeuchi S: Nature of invasive mole and its rational treatment, *Semin Oncol* 16:410, 1989.
232. Sabet LM, Daya D, Stead R et al: Significance and value of immunohistochemical localization of pregnancy specific proteins in feto-maternal tissue throughout pregnancy, *Mod Pathol* 2:227, 1989.
233. Brescia RJ, Kurman RJ, Main CS et al: Immunocytochemical localization of chorionic gonadotropin, placental lactogen, and placental alkaline phosphatase in the diagnosis of complete and partial hydatidiform moles, *Int J Gynecol Pathol* 6:213, 1987.
234. Wolf HK, Michalopoulos GK: Proliferating cell nuclear antigen in human placenta and trophoblastic disease, *Pediar Pathol* 12:147, 1992.
235. Lage JM, Mark SD, Roberts DJ et al: A flow cytometric study of 137 fresh hydropic placentas: correlation between types of hydatidiform moles and nuclear DNA ploidy, *Obstet Gynecol* 79:403, 1992.
236. Lage JM, Popek EJ: The role of DNA flow cytometry in evaluation of partial and complete hydatidiform moles and hydropic abortions, *Semin Diagn Pathol* 10:267, 1993.
237. Hitchcock CL, Conran RM, Griffin JL: Hydatidiform moles and use of flow cytometry in their diagnosis. In: Rosenberg HS, Bernstein J, editors: *Perspectives in pediatric pathology: pediatric molecular pathology,* Basel, Switzerland, 1991, Karger.
238. Koss LG, Czerniak B, Herz F et al: Flow cytometric measurements of DNA and other cell components in human tumors: a critical apprasial, *Hum Pathol* 20:528, 1989.
239. Barclay IDR, Debbagh L, Babiak J, Poppema F: DNA analysis (ploidy) of molar pregnancies with image analysis on paraffin tissue sections, *Am J Clin Pathol* 100:451, 1993.
240. Wersto RP, Liblit RL, Koss LG: Flow cytometric DNA analysis of human solid tumors: a review of the interpretation of DNA histograms, *Hum Pathol* 22:1085, 1991.
241. Duncan DA, Manzur MT: Trophoblastic tumors: ultrastructural comparison of choriocarcinoma and placental site trophoblastic tumor, *Hum Pathol* 20:370, 1989.
242. Fukunaga M, Ushigome S: Malignant trophoblastic tumors: immunohistochemical and flow cytometric comparison of choriocarcinoma and placental site trophoblastic tumors, *Hum Pathol* 24:1098, 1993.
243. Lathrop JC, Lauchlan S, Nayak R, Ambler M: Clinical characteristics of placental site trophoblastic tumor (PSTT), *Gynecol Oncol* 31:32, 1988.
244. Eckstein RP, Russell P, Friedlander ML et al: Metastasizing placental site trophoblastic tumor: a case study, *Hum Pathol* 16:632, 1985.
245. Gloor E, Dialdas J, Hurlimann J et al: Placental site trophoblastic tumor (trophoblastic pseudotumor) of the uterus with metastases and fatal outcome, clinical and autopsy observations of a case, *Am J Surg Pathol* 7:483, 1983.
246. Finkler NJ: Placental site trophoblastic tumor: diagnosis, clinical behavior and treatment, *J Reprod Med* 36:27, 1991.
247. Kotylo PK, Michael H, Davis TE et al: Flow cytometric DNA analysis of placental site trophoblastic tumor, *Int J Gynecol Pathol* 11:245, 1992.

248. Nishikawa Y, Kaseki S, Tomoda Y et al: Histopathologic classification of uterine choriocarcinoma, *Cancer* 55:1044, 1985.
249. Brewer JI, Mazur MT: Gestational choriocarcinoma, its origin in the placenta during seemingly normal pregnancy, *Am J Surg Pathol* 5:267, 1981.
250. Lewis JL: Diagnosis and management of gestational trophoblastic disease, *Cancer* 71:1639, 1993.
251. Smith DB, O'Reilly SM, Newlands ES: Current approaches to diagnosis and treatment of gestational trophoblastic disease, *Curr Opin Obstet Gynecol* 5:84, 1993.

Legal aspects of placental examination

252. Salafia CM, Vintzileos AM: Why all placentas should be examined by a pathologist in 1990, *Am J Obstet Gynecol* 163:282, 1990.
253. Altshuler G: A conceptual approach to placental pathology and pregnancy outcome, *Semin Diagn Pathol* 10:204, 1993.
254. Craighead JE: The pathologist as an expert witness, *Arch Pathol Lab Med* 116:488, 1992.
255. Towbin A: Obstetric malpractice litigation: the pathologist's view, *Am J Obstet Gynecol* 155:927, 1986.
256. Tsuda R, Kimura H: Prognostic value of the placenta in medico-legal practice, *Forensic Sci Int* 40:79, 1989.
257. Benirschke K: The placenta in the litigation process, *Am J Obstet Gynecol* 162:1445, 1990.
258. Cordry RD: Placental evidence in malpractice litigation, *Arch Pathol Lab Med* 115:682, 1991.
259. MacPherson T: Fact and fancy; what can we really tell from the placenta? *Arch Pathol Lab Med* 115:672, 1991.
260. Schindler NR: Importance of the placenta and cord in the defense of neurologically impaired infant claims, *Arch Pathol Lab Med* 114:685, 1991.

70 Breast

Francis E. Sharkey
D. Craig Allred
Philip T. Valente

INTRODUCTION

Carcinoma of the breast is the most common malignancy in adult women, and attention to it often overshadows that given other breast lesions. However, noncancerous conditions of the breasts are far more common than cancer; for example, 10% to 15% of women experience discomfort in their breasts at the time of menstruation; also, there are many benign lesions of the breast that would be of concern to patient and clinician alike even if the incidence of mammary carcinoma were zero. It is essential, therefore, not to downplay these other conditions in the face of the overwhelming attention paid to breast cancer in both the science laboratory and the popular media.

The frequency with which various lesions are encountered can be stated only in general terms, because it depends greatly upon clinical presentation (Table 70-1). Palpable masses that are biopsied are over twice as likely to be malignant as those discovered by mammography, though mammography itself greatly increases the frequency with which malignant lesions are found in a noninvasive state.[1] In the physician's office, cysts make up approximately one third of palpable masses,[2] but surgical biopsy of these lesions is progressively being replaced by fine-needle aspiration biopsy.[3] The prevalence of lesions also varies among age groups and among different ethnic populations.[4,5]

In addition to this clinical variability, mammary anatomy and pathomorphology also vary considerably among women, among different areas of the same breast, and even within the same lesion. It is therefore important for the reader to realize that the descriptions and frequencies that follow represent the most common, the most prominent, or the most typical and that variants are common and frequently coexist. It also justifies the generous sampling of breast lesions that is traditionally practiced in the surgical pathology laboratory.

Table 70-1 Relative incidence of breast lesions in different clinical populations

Diagnosis	Surgically biopsied[1] Palpable	Surgically biopsied[1] Nonpalpable*	Fine-needle aspiration[2]
Benign	71%	88%	90%
Cyst	n/a	n/a	29%
Malignant	29%	12%	10%
Noninvasive	1%	5%	n/a
Invasive	28%	7%	n/a

*Discovered by mammogram only.
n/a, Not applicable.

GROWTH, DEVELOPMENT, AND NORMAL ANATOMY

The breast forms as a conical projection between the subcutaneous tissue of the chest and the greater pectoral muscle. The upper outer quadrant contains 40% to 50% of the mammary tissue, with variable lateral extension as far as the axilla in some women; the remainder is approximately equally divided among the other three quadrants. Lymphatic drainage of breast tissue lateral to the nipple is toward the axilla, but the medial breast drains into the internal mammary chain.[6]

The mammary tissue is divided into 15 to 25 ill-defined lobes, each approximately pyramidal in shape and having its apex at the areola.[6] The glandular tissue of each lobe terminates in a single collecting duct that forms a subareolar dilatation (known as the lactiferous sinus) before emerging at the nipple (Fig. 70-1). Within the mammary tissue the ducts ramify as straight, symmetrically dividing tubular structures. Along the lengths of these ducts arise lobular units consisting of a central terminal duct and outer alveolar ducts (ductules), all embedded in a loose connective tissue stroma. The lumens of both the ducts and the lobular units are lined by a continuous single layer of cuboidal to low columnar epithelium surrounded by a basket-weave array of myoepithelial cell processes.[6] Scattered neuroendocrine cells are also present.[7] Immunohistochemistry identifies estrogen receptors in a small minority of epithelial cells, but not in stromal cells.[8] Except for the breasts of oral contraceptive users, it is unclear whether true acini are present in the nonlactating adult breast.[6] However, since even ductal epithelium may undergo lactational change, this may be a moot point.[9]

In utero, the milk line appears bilaterally at the fifth week of gestation, and differentiates into individual globular structures at about 7 to 8 weeks.[10] Epithelial buds can be seen at 10 to 12 weeks of gestation, and ducts grow progressively during the second and third trimesters. At birth, simple ducts, branched ducts, and a few lobular units may be seen, but there is considerable individual variation in their relative proportions.[9] Many newborns display mammary secretion that appears to arise from a generalized response of the mammary ductal epithelium to maternal hormones; this response regresses during the first months postpartum.[9]

There is no discernible difference between the breast tissue of males and females from the time of conception up to puberty.[9,10] At puberty, however, females display lengthening and further branching of ducts, development of lobules, and proliferation of accompanying fibrous stroma and fat.[10,11] Breast development reaches a maximum by about 20 years of age and displays considerable individual variation at both the gross and microscopic levels[12] (Fig. 70-1). After the third decade, epithelial proliferative activity decreases but the overall proportion of epithelium increases progressively until menopause (Fig. 70-2). During and after the menopause, there is progressive epithelial atrophy, increased density of collagen, and a proportionate increase in fat.[13]

Adult breast tissue displays a distinctive response to the hormonal milieu of the menstrual cycle (Fig. 70-3), though there is considerable variability both among women and even within the same breast.[14,15] In the late post-ovulatory phase of the cycle and in women taking oral contraceptives, proliferation of ductal and lobular lining cells occurs and is at its highest.[15-17] Themyoepithelial cells do not proliferate.[18] The postovulatory lobule also displays vacuolization of myoepithelial cells, lymphocytosis, and edema of the intralobular stroma (Fig. 70-4) that accounts for much of the increase in breast size during this time.[19] With the onset of menstruation, there is apoptosis and sloughing of duct epithelium, involution of the stroma, and reduction in breast volume. Estrogen receptor levels also vary, being highest during days 5 to 8 of the the menstrual cycle.[20] Secretory immunoglobulin can be detected at any stage, particularly in women taking oral contraceptives.[17]

Pregnancy is accompanied by extensive proliferation of the epithelium (Fig. 70-5, *A*), primarily by growth and division of terminal ducts during the first half of pregnancy, followed by additional ductal growth and the formation of secretory acini during the second half.[10] During lactation, there is little mor-

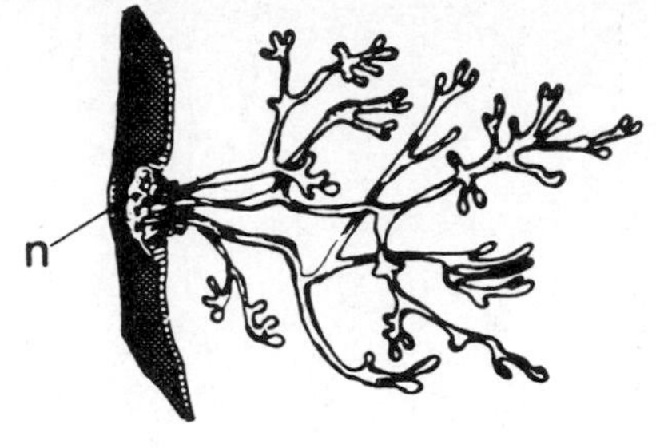

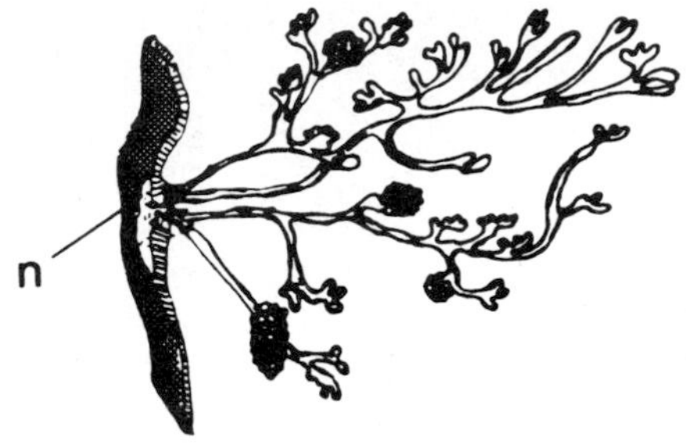

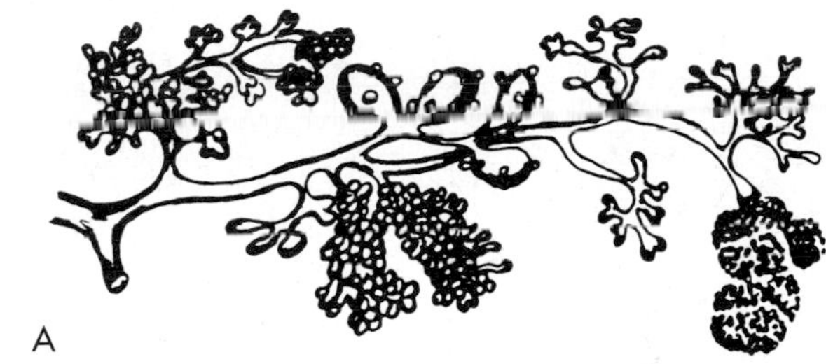

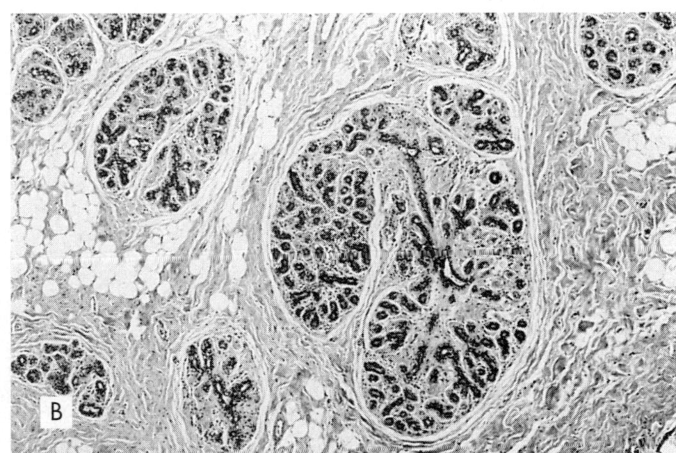

Fig. 70-1 **A,** Development of mammary ducts and lobules (n, nipple). *Upper,* Birth; *middle,* early adolescence; *lower,* adult. **B,** Adult breast illustrating typical variability in size and development of lobules. (**A** from Russo J, Russo IH: Development of the human mammary gland. In Neville MC, Daniel CW, editors: *The mammary gland: development, regulation, and function,* New York and London, 1987, Plenum Press.)

phologic change, though the secretory activity is extensive and striking. Weaning brings on progressive involution, primarily because of cellular autolysis and collapse of acinar structures, with a relative increase in perilobular connective tissue and fat.[6,10] Although acini regress completely, the parous breast retains more glandular tissue after weaning than if pregnancy had not occurred.[10] Localized secretory changes in breast epithelium occasionally accompany normal menstrual cycling, a fact that must be considered in the evaluation of breast biopsy tissue so that these epithelial changes are not misinterpreted as hyperplasia.

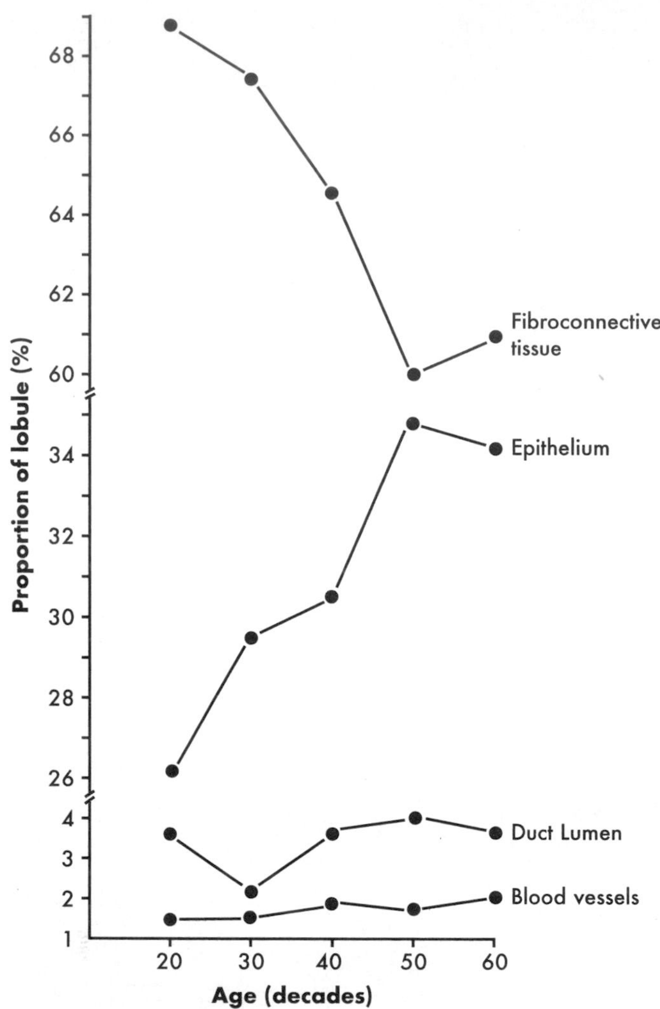

Fig. 70-2 Relative proportions of lobular tissues during a woman's lifespan. (From Hutson SW, Cowen PN, Bird CC: *J Clin Pathol* 38:281, 1985.)

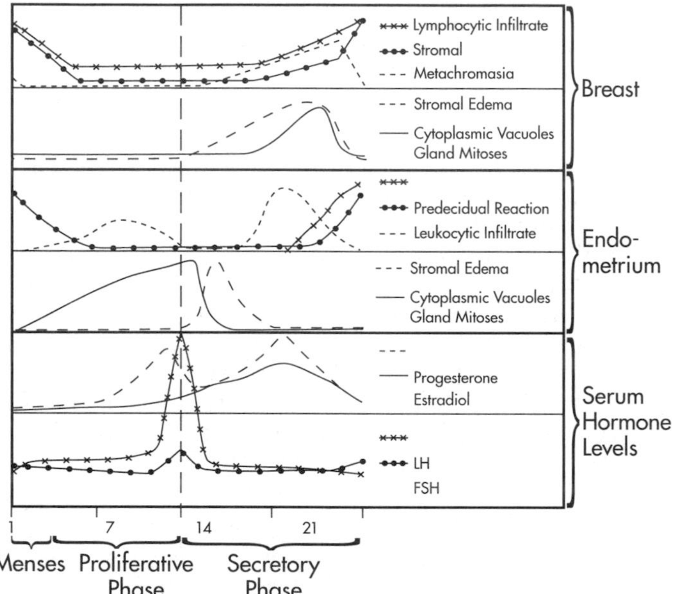

Fig. 70-3 Comparative response of breast and endometrium to serum hormone levels. (From Longacre TA, Bartow SA: *Am J Surg Pathol* 10:382, 1986.)

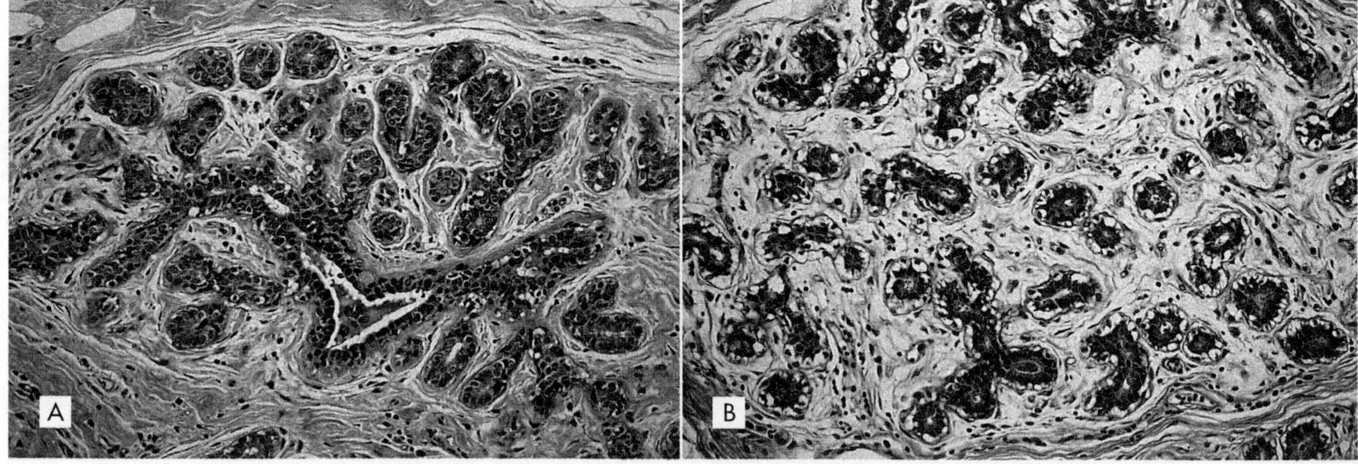

Fig. 70-4 **A,** Lobule during follicular phase of menstrual cycle. **B,** Lobule during luteal phase of menstrual cycle illustrating myoepithelial prominence, lymphocytosis, and stromal edema.

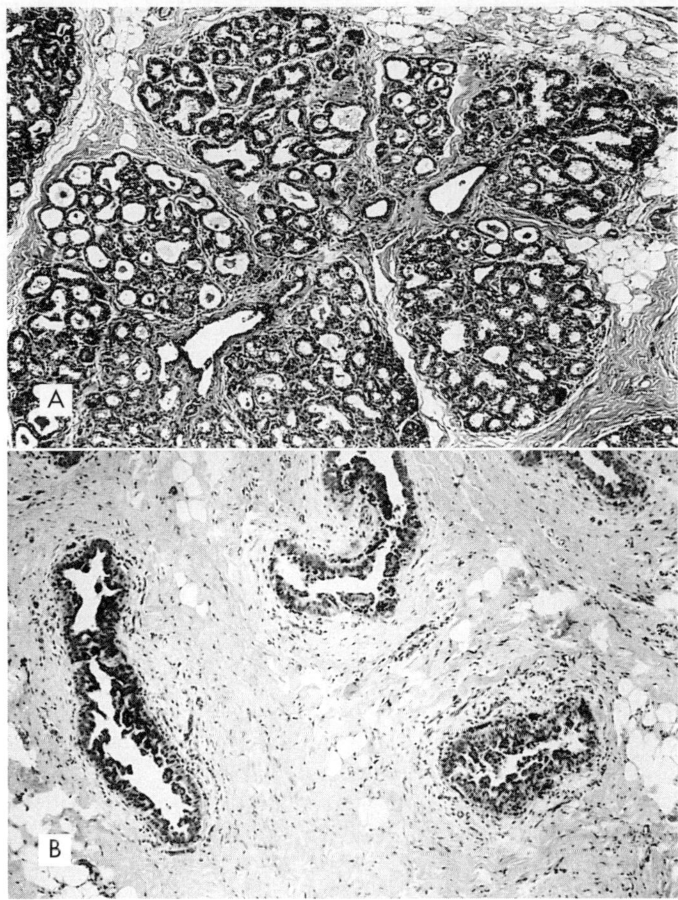

Fig. 70-5 **A,** Lactational changes with expansion of lobules by development of acini; the latter contain secretions. **B,** Gynecomastia with periductal edema, intraductal epithelial proliferation, and absence of lobules.

HYPERTROPHIES AND HYPERPLASIAS

Gynecomastia

Gynecomastia refers to expansion of the subareolar breast bud in men and peaks at three distinct stages: birth, puberty, and older adulthood.[21] In many cases, the cause appears to be a change in the ratio of estrogens to androgens. Both male and female infants normally display mild expansion of breast tissue at birth that is caused by maternal estrogens that cross the placenta; as a result a form of colostrum may also be produced.[9] During early puberty, the normal estrogen levels in males rise more rapidly than do androgen levels, which typically peak later in puberty; in some men, gynecomastia results. In adults, the condition is commonly idiopathic; other causes are therapeutic drugs, hypogonadism, cirrhosis, malnutrition and endocrinologically active neoplasms.[21]

The proliferation involves both the ductal epithelium and the surrounding stroma (Fig. 70-5, *B*). The ducts divide and increase in length, but the formation of lobular units is very rare.[22] The surrounding fibrous stroma is edematous and concentrically arranged around the ducts; this accounts for most of the increase in volume of the involved breast tissue. The ducts often display papillary intraluminal hyperplasia of the lining epithelium, a feature that may occasionally be confused with intraductal carcinoma.

Juvenile hypertrophy

Juvenile hypertrophy is a rare, bilateral, massive symmetrical enlargement of the breasts that develops shortly after menarche in most cases. Growth of the breasts can be extremely rapid, particularly during the first 3 to 6 months, and can result in postural abnormalities and in severe venous engorgement and necrosis in dependent portions of the breasts. Sex hormone levels and other aspects of sexual development appear to be normal in these patients, and the abnormality appears to be a hyperresponsiveness of the breast tissue.[23] The condition may recur after surgical reduction.

The process is actually a hyperplasia, though it is called "juvenile hypertrophy." The histologic appearance is strikingly similar to that of gynecomastia because it involves the proliferation of the ducts and the surrounding connective tissue; lobular units are infrequently observed.[24] The connective tissue is particularly abundant. The ducts are often dilated and display papillary hyperplasia of the lining epithelium into the lumen. The histologic appearance is similar to that of juvenile fibroadenoma discussed later in this chapter, which in some instances has been erroneously reported as juvenile hypertrophy. Although fibroadenomas in this age group may be massive, they are usually unilateral and the affected breast is asymmetrical.[23]

NONNEOPLASTIC LESIONS

Inflammations

Inflammatory lesions of the breast are common and of diverse origins. Although these lesions are considered to be of clinical significance mainly because of the potential for confusing them with cancer, some, such as an inadequately treated abscess, can result in significant morbidity and even disfigurement.

Acute mastitis

Acute infections of the breast are separable into those that occur during the puerperium and those that are unrelated to pregnancy and lactation.[25,26] Puerperal abscesses are in the minority, typically occur 2 to 3 weeks after birth, and are associated with lactation. They are mainly caused by staphylococci, and respond promptly to antibiotic therapy; breast feeding need not be interrupted. If the infection is unresponsive to treatment, or if it is not treated early enough, an abscess may result; this may require surgical drainage. The gross and microscopic features of mastitis are those of an abscess in fatty tissue: there is an abundance of free lipid and foamy macrophages together with a mixed inflammatory cell infiltrate.

Nonpuerperal breast infections that occur at the periphery of the breast are similar to those of the puerperium, but those occurring in the subareolar region are quite different. In addition to staphylococci, anaerobes are commonly recovered, and polymicrobial infections are not uncommon. Despite treatment with antibiotics or surgical drainage, these infections often recur, and excision of the subareolar ducts may be necessary. Preexisting duct ectasia (see next section) is believed to be the underlying cause of many infections.[25,27]

Mammary duct ectasia and periductal mastitis

Ectasia of subareolar ducts is a common incidental finding in the breast.[4] Clinically apparent lesions occur most commonly in the subareolar ducts, and patients present with nipple discharge or a subareolar mass. Periductal mastitis, a chronic inflammatory and fibrosing condition of the periductal tissues, is also often present. The cause of duct ectasia is in dispute, some believing that there is spontaneous blockage of the ducts, which leads to leakage of inspissated duct contents and inflammation, whereas others believe that inflammation is the primary process.[28] Bacteriologic examination of the duct contents has revealed pathogenic organisms, supporting the notion that the lesion may be etiologically related to nonpuerperal subareolar abscess.[27]

The involved ducts are filled with grumous material and display attenuation of the epithelium rather than hyperplasia. There may be calcifications and extravasation of the duct contents. The surrounding connective tissue displays chronic inflammation and fibrosis, and nipple inversion may result. Foamy macrophages may be present both within the duct and in the surrounding tissue; with fine-needle aspiration biopsy specimens the presence of these may lead to confusion of this condition with fat necrosis. A subareolar location, however, favors the diagnosis of duct ectasia.

Fat necrosis

Clinical confusion of fat necrosis with invasive mammary carcinoma has been recognized for many years.[29] Although it forms a hard mass, fat necrosis is painless, with perhaps a history of rapid growth. Some cases may also display skin or nipple retraction. A history of trauma to the breast is usually present.[30]

The gross appearance mimics the hard, stellate appearance of invasive carcinoma, but typically there is chalky streaking and often a central translucent region of necrotic fat. The microscopic appearance is quite variable, and depends on the size of the lesion and the time elapsed since the originating trauma. Initially, there is infarctlike necrosis of fat, with an acute inflammatory cell reaction, release of free lipid, and a foreign-body giant cell reaction. With time, the acute inflammatory cells are replaced by mononuclear inflammatory cells including foamy macrophages, and eventually there is fibrosis and focal calcification. The surrounding ducts may display reactive epithelial hyperplasia that should not be mistaken for atypical ductal hyperplasia or intraductal carcinoma. Similar findings may be seen in breasts that have undergone a biopsy. Fat necrosis is a self-limited lesion and will heal with scarring. Successful diagnosis using fine-needle aspiration has replaced open biopsy in many patients.[3]

Other forms of mastitis

Several other uncommon chronic, inflammatory lesions affect the breast. Sarcoidosis and granulomatous inflammation, caused by organisms such as mycobacteria, fungi, and actinomycetes, are usually seen only as a manifestation of systemic disease.[31] There is idiopathic form of granulomatous mastitis that is typically discovered when a biopsy is performed for suspected carcinoma. These patients respond to treatment with steroids.[32] Rare cases of fibrosis related to diabetes mellitus[33] and suspected autoimmunity[34] have also been described.

Lesions related to mammary prostheses

Breast implants made of silicone provoke a foreign-body reaction in surrounding tissues; this results in the formation of a fibrous capsule that is so dense that the prosthesis may become contracted and misshapen. Examination of the fibrous capsule reveals the presence of silicone that has leaked from the prosthesis.[35] Although in a small proportion of prostheses the envelope ruptures, a more significant problem is the slow bleeding of microdroplets of the gel filling through an intact envelope.[36] The histologic appearance is one of dense fibrosis, with varying concentrations of fibroblasts, mononuclear inflammatory cells, and scattered foreign-body giant cells. The silicone gel may also migrate to axillary lymph nodes.[37]

It is controversial whether patients with silicone prostheses are more likely to develop connective tissue diseases, particularly scleroderma, but evidence is currently against this hypothesis.[38] The evaluation of these kinds of complications has been hindered by the large number of manufacturers, the variety of designs, and the lack of a central registry for reporting and collating data. Patients are not at increased risk for developing mammary carcinoma, but cancer may be detected incidentally in residual breast tissue in patients treated by subcutaneous mastectomy and silicone prosthesis reconstruction.

Fibrocystic change

Fibrocystic change is a complex of lesions that includes fibrosis, epithelial proliferation, and cyst formation.[39] The relative proportions of these lesions vary both among the women affected and among different areas of the same breast. By menopause, most women have some of these changes,[4,5] which are therefore considered by some physicians to be normal, or minor variations of these changes.[40,41] Nevertheless, approximately 10% of women experience pain or other discomfort, and fibrocystic change may also be clinically confused with cancer. As a result, 10% to 15% of women undergo breast biopsy by 50 years of age,[42] though the use of open biopsy appears to be decreasing in institutions where other diagnostic techniques, such as mammography and fine-needle aspiration biopsy, are well developed.[3]

The epidemiology of fibrocystic change is similar to that of breast cancer though not all studies are in agreement. A significant methodologic weakness has been the tendency to consider all benign breast lesions as a single entity, rather than analyzing them separately.[43] The presence of epithelial hyperplasia is the most important risk factor for subsequent malignancy. Fibrocystic changes increase progressively in women through the childbearing years, reach a peak during the perimenopausal period, and regress after menopause.[4,5,42,43] The relative incidence of these changes differs among population groups,[5] being lower in oriental populations, though recent studies show that the frequency of benign proliferative breast lesions is increasing in Japan, particularly among young women.[44]

Risk factors include early menarche, nulliparity or low parity, and late age at birth of first child. In some studies, these same risk factors also apply to the development of benign breast tumors.[42,45] Oral contraceptives earned a reputation for having a protective effect on the development of fibrocystic changes, but more recent studies suggest that the current formulations, with relatively low progestogen concentration, have no effect.[46] Neither oral contraceptives nor unopposed estrogen results in an increased incidence of atypia in breast biopsy specimens.[47,48] Attempts to relate the incidence of fibrocystic changes to concentrations of endogenous estrogens in serum or breast fluid have yielded conflicting results.[49] The consumption of caffeine and other methylxanthines, however, does seem to increase the risk of benign breast disease to some extent.[50]

Although the various components of fibrocystic change are usually found together, it has become increasingly clear that this is a heterogeneous group of lesions that should be diagnosed separately.[41,51] The extent and type of epithelial proliferation found in these biopsy specimens is a major predictor for the subsequent development of mammary carcinoma, whereas the other components are of little significance in that regard.[52,53] In addition, epidemiologic similarities to breast cancer apply most consistently to the subset of patients with significant epithelial atypia.[45] In the discussion that follows, therefore, the fibrocystic complex will be separated into its three major components: cystic disease, fibrosis, and epithelial proliferative disease.

Cystic disease

Cysts are the most common feature of the fibrocystic complex to become clinically apparent.[31] They are also the most easily treated, because simple aspiration of fluid suffices in most cases.[54] Cystic change can be induced in experimental animals by manipulation of estrogens and progestogens. It is assumed, therefore, that human breast cysts are the result of ovarian dysfunction, but the exact mechanism has not been clarified.[55] A variety of bioactive substances are secreted into cyst fluid, including polypeptide hormones and both the male and the female sex steroid hormones. Some investigators have attempted to relate these to the development of both proliferative changes and mammary cancer.[56] By themselves, cysts have little or no premalignant significance.[52,53]

Cysts develop most commonly in terminal ducts and lobules,[57] and should be differentiated from ectasia of subareolar ducts. The largest cysts are associated with atrophy of the remaining lobular elements, whereas small cysts typically develop as multiple dilatations within the same lobule. Solitary cysts are usually lined by simple cuboidal epithelium, whereas multiple cysts are more likely to be lined by the apocrine type of epithelium (apocrine metaplasia). The latter may display considerable nuclear atypia, but this does not appear to convey any premalignant significance.

Fibrosis

In adult women, mammary fibrous tissue increases progressively up until menopause and regresses thereafter. The fibrosis that occurs in association with cysts and epithelial proliferative lesions, therefore, is probably a normal process. Fibrous nodules, however, occur in a younger age group than the other fibrocystic lesions, and are the sole abnormality in approximately 5% of benign breast biopsy specimens.[58]

Epithelial proliferative disease

Included in this category are such morphologically diverse lesions as sclerosing adenosis, radial scar, and the lobular and ductal hyperplasias. Among the various lesions of the fibrocystic complex, it is these that have the greatest epidemiologic similarity to breast carcinoma and place a woman most at risk for the development of carcinoma.

Sclerosing adenosis displays enlargement of one or more lobular units because of a great increase in the number of alveolar ducts, along with an increase in the density of intralobular fibrous tissue. Although most are grossly inapparent, some may appear as stellate lesions measuring up to 1.0 cm in diameter. Occasionally, a mass is produced by aggregation of adjacent lobules or less commonly by massive enlargement of a single lobule. Microscopically the alveolar ducts are elongated and are organized into concentrically swirling groups, sometimes with a dilated central terminal duct (Fig. 70-6, *A*). The normal double cell layer is preserved, but the lumen is attenuated and may contain microcalcifications. In some examples, the lumen is dilated (Fig. 70-6, *B*); this has been called "blunt duct adenosis" [59] or "microglandular adenosis."[60] Perineural invasion has been reported.[61] The low-power architecture of the lesion is so characteristic that, in excisional biopsies, the experienced pathologist will rarely confuse it with well-differentiated carcinoma. The differential diagnosis, however, can be a problem in core-needle biopsies and with frozen sections.

Ductal hyperplasia occurs predominantly in terminal ducts and lobular units[57] and is characterized by increased numbers of cells within the lumen of the structures involved. It involves most or all of each affected lobule and associated ducts, though the degree of proliferation within each lobule varies. Ductal hyperplasia includes a continuum of changes ranging from a trivial increase in cellularity to features resembling in situ ductal carcinoma; in the latter case, a diagnosis of *atypical* ductal hyperplasia is made.[60]

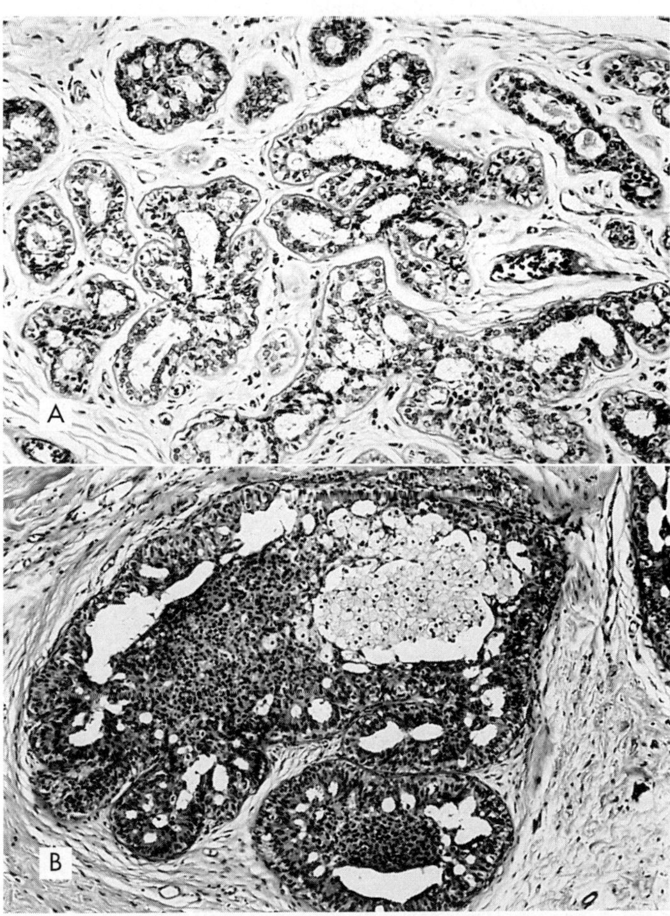

Fig. 70-6 A, Mild duct hyperplasia involving an entire lobule. **B,** Florid duct hyperplasia involving adjacent ducts.

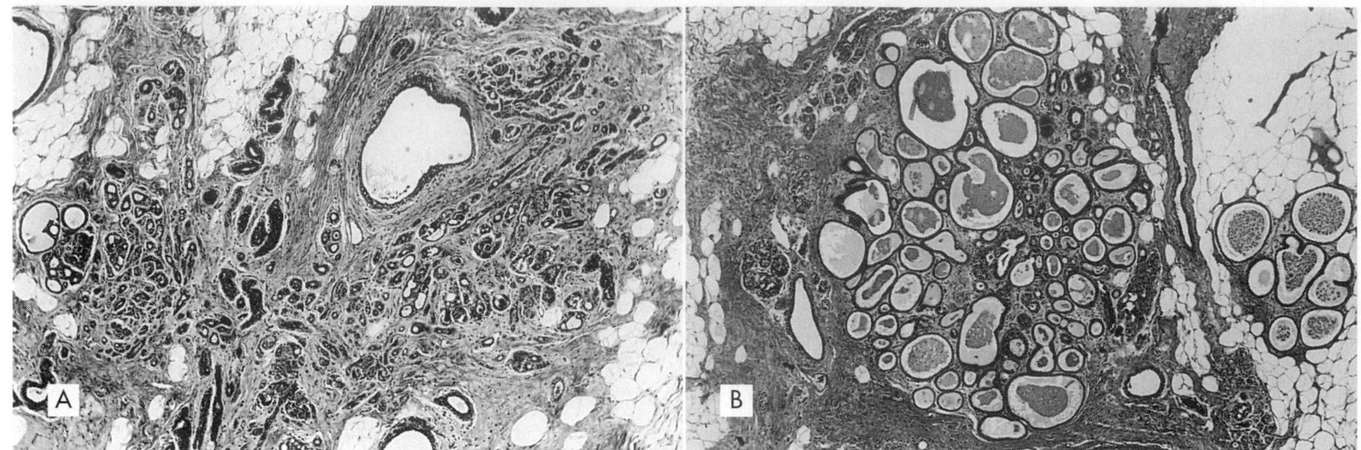

Fig. 70-7 **A,** Sclerosing adenosis involving two adjacent lobules. **B,** Blunt duct adenosis with dilatation of all lobular elements.

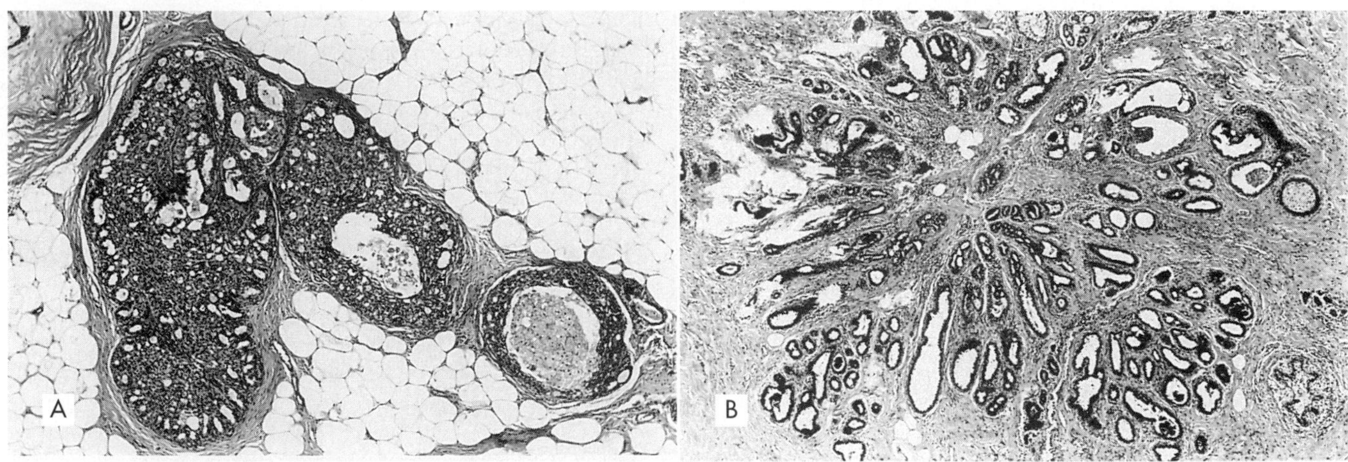

Fig. 70-8 **A,** Florid duct hyperplasia with massive expansion of ducts by proliferated epithelium. **B,** Radial scar with centripetal proliferation of ductlike structures and central fibrosis.

Mild hyperplasia exists when there are one or two extra, but often incomplete, layers of epithelial cells, with little or no dilatation of the lumen. Moderate and florid hyperplasia describe increasing degrees of epithelial proliferation, with progressive expansion and filling of the structures affected (Figs. 70-7 and 70-8, *A*). Attempts have been made to define the boundaries between these varying degrees of hyperplasia more precisely,[51] but studies of interobserver reproducibility show only moderate agreement, even among experienced pathologists.[62] With problem cases, reference to a well-illustrated textbook is common practice.[60]

Radial scar has been recognized under a variety of names, such as "radial sclerosing lesion" and "sclerosing papillary proliferation."[63] It consists of an irregular radial proliferation of duct-like mammary epithelial structures, with dense central fibrosis (Fig. 70-8, *B*). The lesions typically range in size from 0.2 to 1.5 cm in diameter and may be multiple. The appearance in mammograms and also the gross and microscopic appearance can cause it to be confused with infiltrating ductal carcinoma. The epithelial features consist predominantly of ductal hyperplasia, but any type of mammary epithelial proliferation may be present, including sclerosing adenosis, apocrine change, and lobular hyperplasia. The epithelial proliferation is often quite florid, but atypical hyperplasia is uncommon. The central fibrosis is quite dense, with prominent elastic fibers. The epithelial structures, particularly toward the center, may be small and teardrop shaped, resembling tubular carcinoma, but the presence of the usual types of ductal hyperplasia and the absence of in situ ductal carcinoma provide reassurance that the lesion is benign. Also, myoepithelial cells are present in radial scar, but not in tubular carcinoma. The premalignant significance is related to the degree of atypia of any epithelial hyperplasia, which should be quantified and included in the surgical pathology report.

Lobular hyperplasia refers to proliferation of small, uniform cells in the lumen of lobular units. Usually all structures within each lobular unit are uniformly affected, and the process may also extend up into ducts in a histologically characteristic manner. When the degree of proliferation and dilatation approaches that of lobular carcinoma in situ, a diagnosis of *atypical* lobular hyperplasia is made. Some authors do not recognize mild degrees of lobular hyperplasia but instead use the diagnosis of atypical lobular hyperplasia to cover all but the most minimal degrees of proliferation.[60]

Although both lobular hyperplasia and ductal hyperplasia affect the lobular unit predominantly,[57] lobular hyperplasia differs histologically in several ways: The cells are more uniform; the proliferating cells are present between the basement membrane and the cells that normally line the lumen both within the lobular unit and most distinctively within ducts; the residual lumen, if any, is lined by the original cuboidal epithelium rather than by the proliferating cells; and there is only mild to moderate dilatation of the structures affected. Because of these differences, the cell of origin was once believed to be the myoepithelial cell, but a variety of studies, including electron microscopy and immunohistochemistry, have been unable to confirm this hypothesis.

NEOPLASTIC LESIONS

Stromal neoplasms

The connective tissue of the breast can give rise to the full range of benign and malignant stromal neoplasms, but they are uncommon. An interesting and unanswered question regarding these lesions is their origin. Breast tissue contains both hormonally responsive and unresponsive connective tissue, the intralobular and the extralobular connective tissue respectively. Some neoplasms, particularly the fibroepithelial growths, display a propensity for development or increased growth during puberty and pregnancy. However, in general, despite the occasional case report to the contrary, they are unresponsive to hormonal treatment, and their overall response to the hormonal milieu is inconsistent.

Benign stromal neoplasms

The most frequently encountered benign stromal neoplasms are lipoma and hemangioma, though many other types have also been reported. Mammography has significantly increased the number of lesions detected because some lesions, such as hemangiomas, may not produce a palpable mass.[64]

The frequency of lipoma is hard to determine, because well-delineated nodules of adipose tissue are found quite commonly in the breast. If the diagnosis of lipoma requires that encapsulation, gross distinction from surrounding adipose tissue, and hypervascularity be present, then lipoma would be a rare condition. The occasional case of "lipoadenoma" probably represents lobular breast tissue that is enclosed within a well-demarcated mass of adipose tissue.

Hemangiomas are most frequently encountered as incidental lesions and are important because they need to be differentiated from low-grade angiosarcomas. They most commonly occur in the perilobular tissues and are almost always smaller than 2 cm in diameter.[65] Some display atypical features, such as prominence or budding of the endothelial lining cells, but the absence of necrosis and destructive invasion should point to a benign diagnosis.[64]

Granular cell tumor is even more uncommon but is significant for its ability to mimic both the gross and histologic appearance of mammary carcinoma.[66] These tumors often display stellate extensions into the surrounding breast tissue, and they may be hard and gritty on the cut surface. Microscopically, the tumors resemble granular cell tumors in other sites, but may present a diagnostic problem in a frozen section.

Malignant stromal neoplasms

Although constituting less than 1% of breast malignancies, the full histologic continuum of sarcomas occurs in the breast. Angiosarcoma is the most common, with the remainder being made up mainly of fibrous neoplasms. Because these tumors appear to be derived from the extralobular connective tissue and are usually not responsive to hormonal therapy, it is recommended that the term *stromal sarcoma* be discarded and that the nomenclature for these neoplasms be the same as that for extramammary soft tissue neoplasms.[67]

Mammary angiosarcomas develop primarily in women of childbearing age and may even be diagnosed during pregnancy.[68] They have only rarely been reported in men. Experience with mammary angiosarcoma indicates that these can be histologically separated into low-grade and high-grade varieties, though even the former may metastasize in a minority of patients.[68] Peripheral regions of a high-grade tumor may display a low-grade histologic features, and so it is important that a diagnostic biopsy sample be taken from deep within the tumor. Surgery is used as primary therapy. The efficacy of adjuvant chemotherapy is uncertain, though it is likely to be tried for high-grade tumors because of their poor prognosis (approximately 15% 5-year survival). A few survivors may develop other forms of mammary cancer, but there are too few cases to estimate whether the risk for such tumors is increased. Primary mammary angiosarcoma should not be confused with postmastectomy angiosarcoma (Stewart-Treves syndrome). The latter develops in the arm or axilla of patients with chronic lymphedema and often occurs 10 to 20 years after the original axillary lymph node dissection.[68a]

Fibrous neoplasms range morphologically from fibromatosis to fibrosarcoma and malignant fibrous histiocytoma. These tumors are grossly and histologically identical to their counterparts in other tissues, and display the same tendency for recurrence and metastasis.[69,70] Fibromatosis may be mistaken for mammary carcinoma in patients with skin or nipple retraction. Fibrosarcoma and malignant fibrous histiocytoma have been separated into low-grade and high-grade varieties on the basis of mitotic activity and nuclear atypia.[70] With this system, only high-grade lesions tended to metastasize, though recurrence occurred in over half of the cases with low-grade tumor. Immunohistochemical markers may help distinguish these lesions from pseudosarcomatous variants of mammary carcinoma. As with fibrous neoplasms in other locations in the body, surgery is the primary treatment.

Complex stromal-epithelial neoplasms

Fibroadenoma

Fibroadenoma is the most common breast mass encountered in young women, constituting the majority of lesions found at biopsy in women up to 25 years of age.[71] The incidence decreases thereafter, but it still accounts for 25% of lesions biopsied during the fourth decade. Fibroadenomas occur more frequently and are more likely to be multiple in blacks and during pregnancy. The etiology is not well understood, but the association with endocrine surges during adolescence and pregnancy cannot be ignored and has led some authors to consider fibroadenomas to be localized hyperplasias rather than neoplasms. Regressive changes are common after 30 years of age, and in post menopausal women they may be found incidentally as hyalinized nodules with atrophic epithelium.[72] The risk factors for development of fibroadenoma have some similarity to those of mammary carcinoma.[42,45] However, there is only a small increase in risk for patients with fibroadenoma to develop carcinoma.[73]

Fibroadenomas are sharply circumscribed, rubbery masses that are grossly distinct from the surrounding tissues (Fig. 70-9, *A*). The size range is enormous, with individual lesions ranging from less than 1 mm to tens of centimeters in diameter. The latter are referred to as "giant fibroadenoma," but they are clinically and pathologically similar to their smaller cousins. The cut surface is lobulated with slitlike spaces and ranges from rubbery to hard on palpation. Microscopically, there is a balanced proliferation of ducts and stroma. The proportion of these two elements is substantially similar throughout even the largest regions, but varies greatly from patient to patient. Myxoid stroma predominates in younger patients (Fig. 70-10, *A*), but fibrous stroma is more common in older patients. In some lesions, the stroma is somewhat more cellular near the ducts, and mitoses are also more common at the stroma-epithelium interface, suggestive of an epithelial-stromal interaction.[74]

The epithelial-stromal growth displays two distinct patterns (intracanalicular and pericanalicular) but both usually occur in the same lesion. The ductal epithelium is typically double layered but may be either greatly attenuated by the surrounding stroma or may display papillary intraductal hyperplasia. The latter condition has been designated "juvenile fibroadenoma" by some authors,[75] but this designation is best reserved for the lesion that develops in adolescents (see next section).

Fibroadenomas appear to arise from lobules,[57] and lobular structures may be identified within even the largest examples of this lesion. The epithelium may undergo changes similar to those in lobules elsewhere in the breast, including sclerosing adenosis, apocrine metaplasia, and lactational changes, but this typically involves only isolated foci. Atypical ductal and lobular hyperplasia may occur; although these changes may be quite florid, their occurrence is so uncommon that the premalignant significance is uncertain.[75]

Even more uncommon is the development of carcinoma within a fibroadenoma. Most of these contain in situ carcinoma only, mostly of the lobular type.[76,77] Multifocal involvement of breast tissue outside the fibroadenoma occurs in at least 20% of cases, but the risk of developing invasive mammary carcinoma later has not been shown to be greatly elevated. Secondary involvement of a preexisting fibroadenoma by invasive carcinoma from the surrounding breast may also occur.

Juvenile fibroadenoma

Juvenile fibroadenoma is an uncommon variant of fibroadenoma that occurs as a large, rapidly growing mass in adolescent females. Its gross appearance differs from the usual fibroadenoma in that the cut surface is yellow-tan and homogeneous, rather than lobulated (Fig. 70-9, *B*). Microscopically the stroma is more cellular and displays more mitoses. There is a greater tendency toward papillary intraductal hyperplasia, and lobules are typically present.[78,79] Some authors regard these lesions as histologically indistinguishable from juvenile hypertrophy.[60] Juvenile fibroadenomas typically are solitary and unilateral and do not recur after excision. However, in a minority of patients multiple or bilateral lesions occur, and

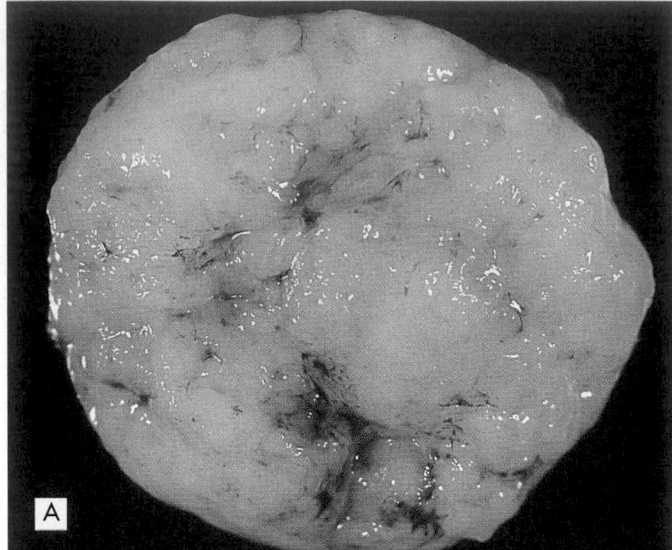

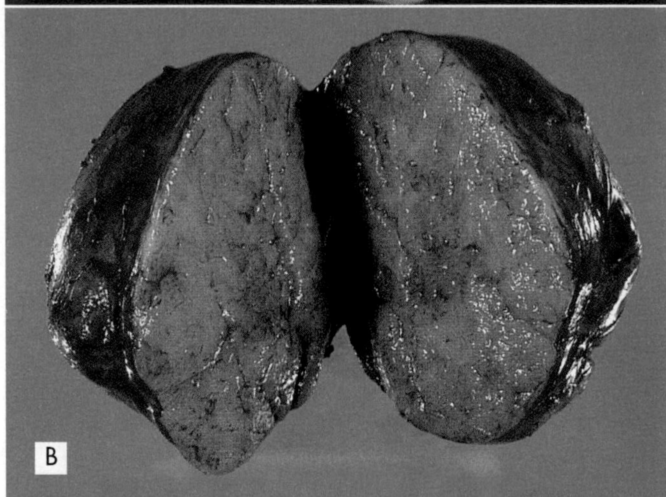

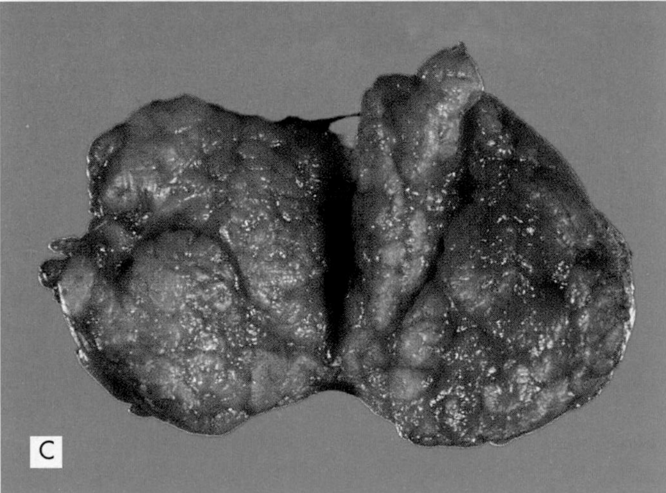

Fig. 70-9 **A,** Myxoid type of fibroadenoma showing pale, lobulated, translucent tissue. **B,** Juvenile fibroadenoma showing well-circumscribed mass of tan, fleshy, lobulated tissue. **C,** Lactation adenoma showing poorly circumsribed margins and lobulated, fleshy tissue.

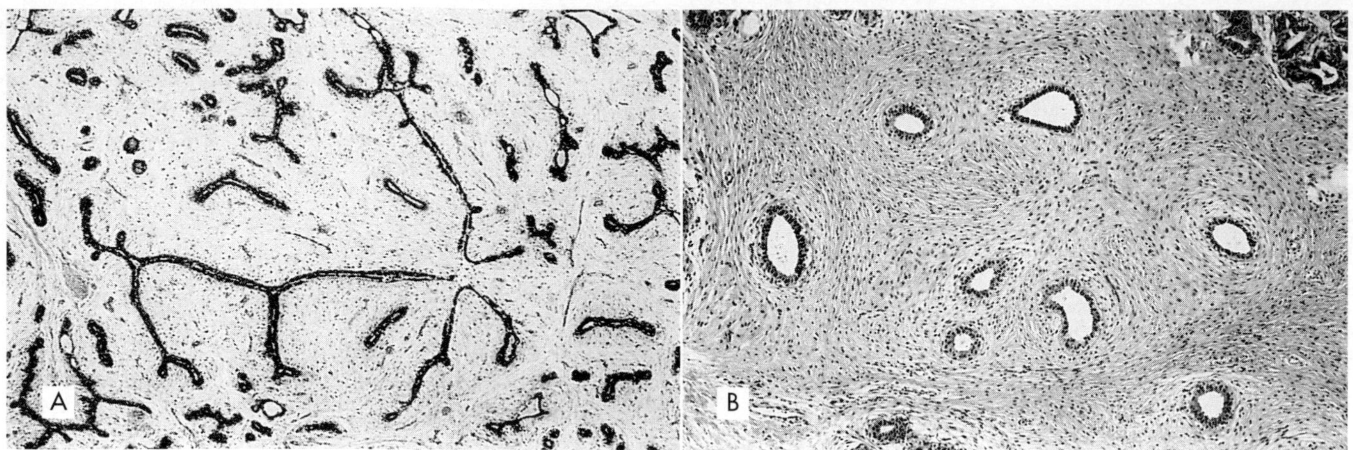

Fig. 70-10 **A,** Intracanalicular type of fibroadenoma with myxoid stroma. **B,** Pericanalicular type of fibroadenoma showing circumductal proliferation of stroma.

development of new lesions after initial excision is more likely under those circumstances.[78]

Phyllodes tumor

Phyllodes tumor, like the fibroadenoma, is a combined proliferation of ductal epithelium and stroma, but the resemblance ends there because the phyllodes tumor may display behavior that ranges from the locally aggressive to the frankly malignant. The peak incidence is in the fifth decade, with a population range extending from adolescents to the very elderly. Malignancy is more common in older patients but is exceedingly rare in adolescents. Men are affected in less than 1% of cases.

At presentation, phyllodes tumors are on the average larger than fibroadenomas and commonly have a history of rapid growth. The excised specimen is firm and rubbery and may separate into leaflike structures (Greek: *phyllon* 'leaf'; *eidos* 'form'[80]). The cut surface of low-grade tumors is quite variegated, in contrast to the more homogeneous appearance of fibroadenomas (Fig. 70-11). The epithelial element of the phyllodes tumor resembles that of the fibroadenoma, and may infrequently display atypical hyperplasia or in situ carcinoma.[81] On the other hand, the stroma is considerably more cellular and resembles that of fibrous tumors ranging from nodular fasciitis through extra-abdominal desmoid tumor to fibrosarcoma (Fig. 70-12). In malignant cases, the stroma tends to overwhelm the epithelium, and in some cases there may be a gradient of transformation from a lower to a higher grade. Other stromal elements, such as fat or cartilage, may occasionally coexist.

Predicting the behavior of a phyllodes tumor is a major challenge for the pathologist, and many studies on this topic have been published.[82] Although malignant tumors tend to be larger and more infiltrative, the prognosis is most consistently related to the histologic characteristics of the stromal element—cellularity, nuclear atypia, mitotic activity, necrosis, and the presence of focal histologic transformation—and is similar to that of the fibrous neoplasm that the stroma most resembles. In some studies, the presence of stromal overgrowth, the presence of other malignant histologic phenotypes, or the presence of both features has been the most specific indicator of a poor outcome.[83] Quantitation of DNA and measurement of the S-phase fraction of cells has yielded inconsistent prognostic results.[81] With adequate sampling and reliance upon the parameters outlined above, most tumors can be separated into the benign and malignant categories, with approximately 15% remaining borderline. Because of this prognostic range, the pathologist should not simply diagnose "phyllodes tumor," but should also append the appropriate qualifier—benign, borderline, or malignant.

Treatment has a significant influence on prognosis, since even "benign" tumors must be excised with a surrounding rim of normal tissue for prevention of recurrence. In the case of very large tumors or of frank histologic malignancy, mastectomy may be the only practical treatment. The occasional enlargement of axillary lymph nodes is usually a reactive change as a result of tumor necrosis or other complicating factors, and lymph node metastases are rare.[82] Metastasis is almost exclusively by the blood-borne route and includes only the stromal component.

Since these tumors may be clinically mistaken for a fibroadenoma, the initial excision is often inadequate. In addition, many published studies of this tumor originate from referral centers, with both primary and referred cases being grouped together. It is therefore difficult to determine the true frequency of malignancy, or even of recurrence after an initial adequate excision. Nevertheless, it appears that only about 20% of cases are histologically malignant, and less than half of these ever metastasize.[81] Use of the older term *cystosarcoma phyllodes* should therefore be discouraged because it is confusing and may mislead the unwary clinician.

Hamartoma

Hamartoma is a discrete mass lesion that occurs in middle-aged women. Clinically, a fibroadenoma is usually expected. The gross appearance may resemble that of a fibroadenoma or of a sharply demarcated region of fibrocystic change, depending on the amount of epithelium and the cellularity of the intervening stroma. Although usually less than 5 cm in diameter, hemartomas up to 17 cm in diameter and weighing 1400 g have been reported.[84,85]

This lesion is uncommon, but its exact definition varies among studies, with corresponding variation in its frequency.

In general, however, the lesion should include lobular breast tissue with or without fibrocystic changes, along with varying amounts of adipose tissue; smooth muscle and cartilage are less frequent. Some authors also include lesions in which the lobular tissue assumes the appearance of a fibroadenoma, as long as one or more of the other elements (usually adipose tissue) is present. The term *hamartoma* may not be fully appropriate because many examples do not display abnormal growth,[85] but the name has persisted.

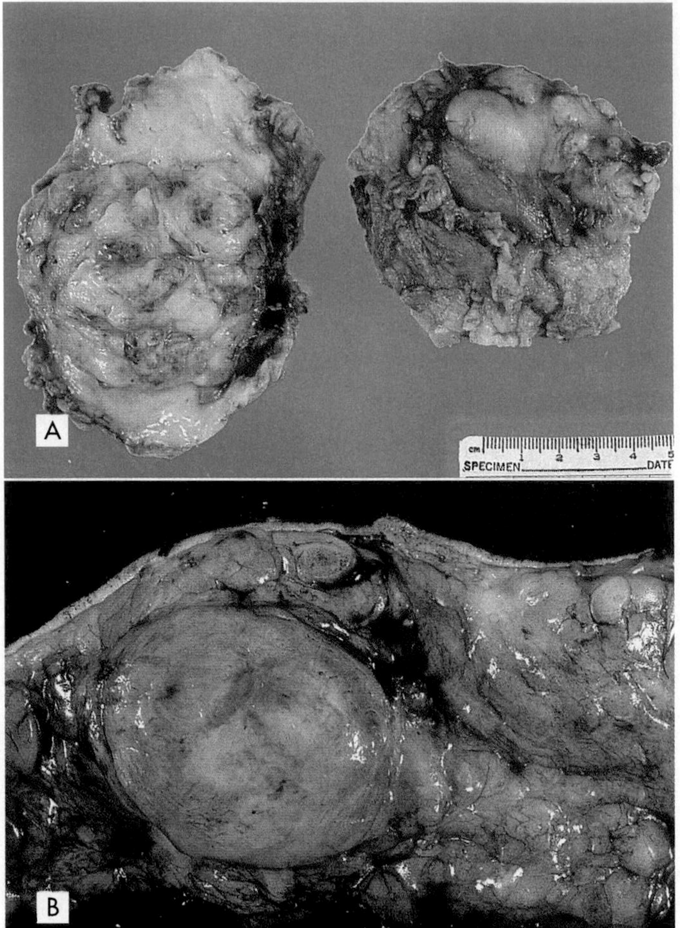

Fig. 70-11 **A,** Low-grade phyllodes tumor showing variegated red-tan and white cut surface and lack of encapsulation. **B,** High-grade phyllodes tumor showing homogenous fleshy mass.

Benign epithelial neoplasms

Adenoma

Considering the relative frequency of fibroadenoma and mammary carcinoma, it is surprising that adenomas of the breast are so infrequent. Most are classified as either tubular or lactating adenomas (Fig. 70-9, *C*), and the latter may simply be tubular adenomas that develop lactational changes during pregnancy or breast-feeding.[86,87] Patients are almost exclusively in their childbearing years, but there does not appear to be any relationship to oral contraceptive use.[86] Both types of adenoma produce distinct masses within the breast, though the lactating adenoma tends to be less well circumscribed, and both types are composed of closely packed terminal ducts with little surrounding stroma. Myoepithelial cells are present external to the ductal lining epithelium.

The tubular and lactating adenomas should be differentiated from the so-called nipple adenoma in which there is a mixed ductal and stromal cell proliferation that produces a mass immediately beneath the nipple.[88] The frequent presence of erosion of the surface epithelium leads to clinical confusion with mammary Paget's disease. Microscopically there is prominent ductal and intraductal proliferation, along with a densely fibrous stroma. This proliferation may be complex and papillary, but the presence of two cell types—epithelial and myoepithelial—confirms the benign nature of the process. Also, single cells infiltrating the surface epithelium, the so-called pagetoid extension, does not occur.

Adenomyoepithelioma

Adenomyoepithelioma is a recently described form of adenoma in which the myoepithelial component is unusually prominent.[89] Earlier studies tended to classify this lesion with tumors that mimicked salivary or skin appendage neoplasms. The lesion may display considerable associated fibroplasia, making it less well circumscribed than the tubular adenoma, and it appears in the age group most commonly affected by

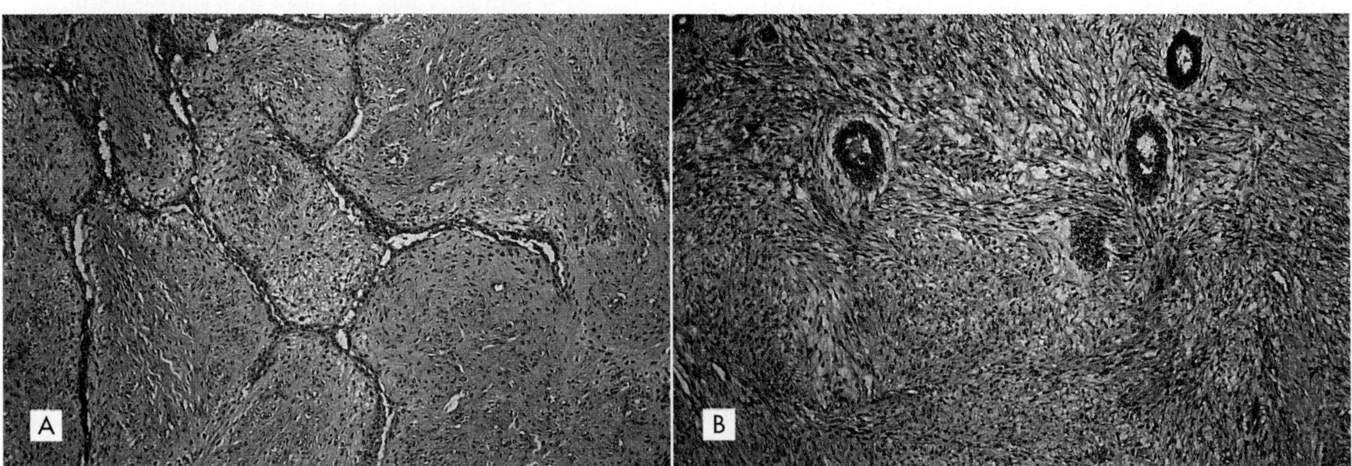

Fig. 70-12 **A,** Low-grade phyllodes tumor showing low-grade stromal hypercullularity. **B,** High-grade phyllodes tumor with strongly atypical stromal elements.

carcinoma. Such characteristics may lead to clinical confusion with cancer. The lesion may recur if incompletely excised.

Papilloma

Papilloma is a benign, largely intraductal lesion that reaches clinical attention primarily because of nipple discharge, though a minority also produce a palpable mass. Patients affected are in the same age range as those that develop fibrocystic changes, and some papillomas display histologic features similar to those of epithelial proliferative disease. Most papillomas develop in the large collecting ducts, though 20% to 25% occur more peripherally and appear to be multiple.

The gross appearance varies considerably. Most lesions range from 0.5 to 2 cm in diameter and occupy a single dilated duct. However, accompanying fibroplasia is common, both around and within the lesion, and this may obscure the gross papillary appearance. Multiple papillomas display considerable surrounding sclerosis and may be mistaken for comedocarcinoma. Microscopically the hallmark of the papilloma is the presence of papillary intraductal proliferation of epithelial fronds *that contain fibrovascular cores* (Fig. 70-13, *A*). A diagnosis of papilloma should not be made in the absence of the latter feature. These lesions also display a propensity for degeneration and necrosis, which accounts for the nipple discharge and may also account for the frequent occurrence of dense, hyalinized scarring around the lesion. Epithelial elements trapped in this scar may be mistaken for invasive carcinoma but the absence of associated intraductal carcinoma is a clue to the benign nature of the lesion. Papillomas that appear to involve multiple ducts have been shown by three-dimensional reconstruction to be part of the same duct complex (Fig. 70-13, *B*), though domains of normal ductal epithelium may intervene.[90]

Papilloma must be differentiated from papillary carcinoma, an indolent malignancy of older women that is also largely intraductal but displays definitive features of malignancy, including a cribriform pattern, nuclear anaplasia, and intraductal papillary proliferation *without* fibrovascular stalks.[91,92] A difficult diagnostic problem arises when on rare occasions features of both papilloma and papillary carcinoma are present in the same lesion.

Papillomas as a group confer a slightly elevated risk for the subsequent development of mammary carcinoma. Some authors have found that this risk is largely confined to patients with multiple papillomas.[31,91,93] However, it has also been pointed out that multiple lesions are more commonly associated with atypical patterns of epithelial proliferative disease, and the of risk should therefore be predicated on the degree of atypia.[60]

CARCINOMA OF THE BREAST

Epidemiology

Carcinoma of the breast is overwhelmingly a disease of females (female to male ratio of approximately 200 to 1). It is particularly common in women from more affluent countries, including those in North America, Western Europe, and Scandinavia.[94] However, there are notable exceptions, such as Japan, where the incidence is only 20% of that in the United States. This indicates that there are important genetic, cultural, and environmental factors involved in the development of this disease.[94,95]

The figures for incidence and mortality of breast cancer in the United States are staggering. For 1993, 183,000 new cases and 46,000 deaths are anticipated, making it the most common (35% of all cases) and the second most lethal (18% mortality) female cancer.[96,97] The incidence of breast cancer changes significantly with age (Fig. 70-14). In the United States it is very rare in women less than 25 years of age, rare in women less than 50 years of age, and common in women over 60 years of age, a finding emphasizing a prominent increase after menopause.[98,99] The current overall risk of developing breast cancer during an 80-year life-span is about 10%.[99]

Although the age-standardized incidence of breast cancer in the United States has nearly doubled during the past four decades, the mortality has remained remarkably stable[94,98] (Fig. 70-15). The reasons for this disparity are not entirely known but certainly include more accurate record keeping, earlier detection, and advances in treatment. Major improvements in each of these areas have been widely used clinically for the past decade, yet the incidence relative to mortality con-

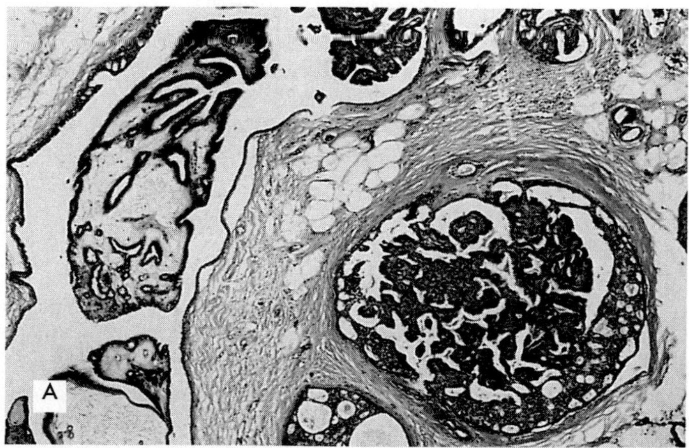

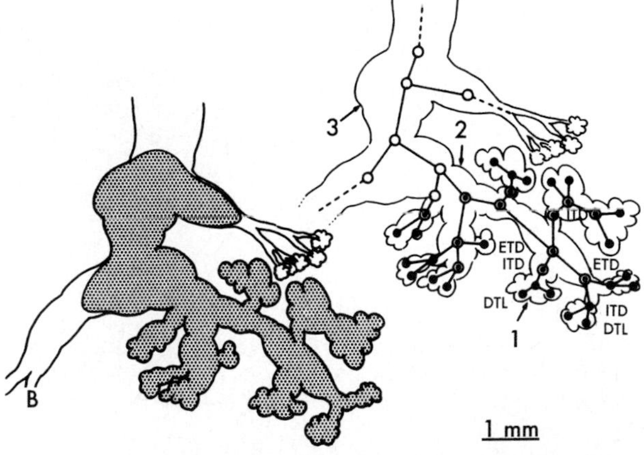

Fig. 70-13 **A,** Papilloma showing involvement of multiple adjacent ducts. **B,** three-dimensional reconstruction showing that an apparently multifocal papilloma, as seen in two-dimensional histologic sections, may actually be a single lesion. (**B** from Ohuchi N, Abe Rikiya, Takahashi T, and Tezuka F: *Breast Cancer Res Treat* 4:117, 1984.)

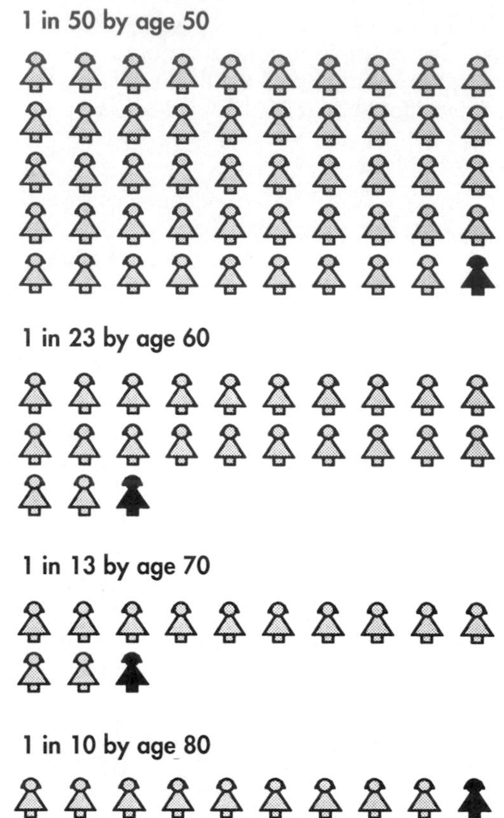

Fig. 70-14 Age-related incidence of breast cancer.

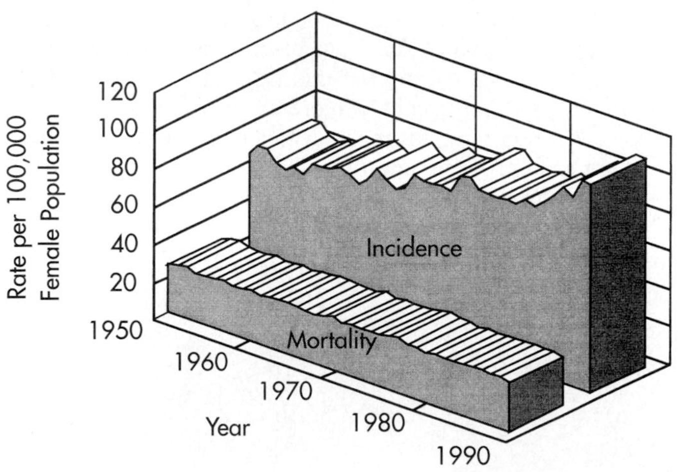

Fig. 70-15 Increased incidence of breast cancer but stable mortality over the past 40 years.

tinues to rise, indicating that there is an ongoing absolute increase in the incidence of breast cancer attributable largely to unknown factors.[94]

Etiology and risk factors

Genetic alterations leading to the initiation, transformation, and progression of normal cells to malignant neoplastic cells are the ultimate causes of all cancers. These genetic alterations, most of which are still unknown, may be inherited or acquired. Epidemiologic observations, such as the increasing rate of disease occurrence seen in populations migrating from regions of low incidence to those of high incidence, indicate that a significant proportion of breast cancer may be related to cultural and environmental factors. The identification of these risk factors is important because they provide insight into the causes of breast cancer and opportunities to reduce its incidence.

Table 70-2 Risk factors for developing breast cancer

Factor	Relative risk*
Family history[94,100]	
Mother affected before 60 years of age	2.0
Two first-degree relatives affected	4.0-6.0
Excess estrogen exposure	
Early menarche[101]	
(before 14 years of age)	1.3
Late childbearing[102]	
(nulliparous or after 30 years of age)	1.9
Late menopause[103]	
(after 55 years of age)	1.5
Postmenopausal estrogen therapy[104]	1.4
Oral contraceptive use[105]	1.5
Radiation exposure	
Atomic bomb[106]	3.0
Repeated fluoroscopy[107]	1.5-2.0
Benign breast disease[53,108,109]	
Hyperplasia	1.5-2.0
Atypical hyperplasia	4.0-5.0
Obesity[110]	1.2
Alcohol abuse[111]	1.4-2.0

*Relative risk is the incidence of breast cancer in persons with the factor, divided by the incidence in otherwise similar persons without the factor.

Factors known to be associated with a significantly elevated risk are listed in Table 70-2.[53,94,100-111] Family history and previous atypical hyperplasia are among the strongest risk factors. Women whose mothers had breast cancer before 60 years of age have twice the risk (relative risk of 2.0) of developing the disease as women whose mothers do not have breast cancer. The relative risk increases to 4.0 to 6.0 if two first-degree relatives (such as a mother and a sister) have breast cancer. Women with previous atypical hyperplasia also have relative risks in the range of 4.0 to 5.0, and the risk doubles if they also have a strong family history of that condition. Several weaker risk factors appear to be directly related to total lifetime estrogen exposure (such as early menarche and late menopause). Unfortunately, even women without identifiable risk factors still have an appreciable lifetime risk of developing breast cancer (approximately 6% by age 80).[100]

Atypical hyperplasia

This section is a detailed discussion of atypical hyperplastic lesions because they are such strong risk factors for the development of breast cancer, because they may represent precursor lesions for breast cancer, and because accurate diagnosis is a major challenge to pathologists. Two categories of hyperplasia are recognized: atypical ductal hyperplasia and atypical lobular hyperplasia.

Atypical ductal hyperplasia (ADH) accounts for less than 3% of all breast lesions found at biopsy. This is probably an underestimate of its incidence because it lacks distinctive features that would bring it to medical attention. It is most common in postmenopausal women. Several studies have shown that women with diagnosed ADH have a relative risk of 4.0 to 5.0 for the subsequent development of invasive carcinoma.[53,108,109]

A common criticism is that the reproducibility of diagnosing ADH is low, and this has been attributed to a lack of consensus regarding its histologic criteria.[112] Recent studies have taken an empirical approach to defining ADH that is based on evaluating the association between "worrisome" proliferative lesions (irrespective of traditional concepts of dysplasia) and the clinical outcome.[52,53,108] Reproducible diagnostic criteria have been defined,[113] and these have been used repeatedly to validate ADH as a strong risk factor for breast cancer.[53,108,109]

There is a controversy regarding whether ADH is merely a risk factor, or also a precursor lesion for breast cancer. Some authors have suggested that ADH is a small noninvasive carcinoma, basing their speculation on the close histologic resemblance between them. However, noninvasive carcinoma has a twofold to threefold stronger association than ADH does with the subsequent development of invasive carcinoma, and this risk is ipsilateral for noninvasive carcinoma,[114,115] but bilateral for ADH.[108,109] Noninvasive carcinoma is also often seen in continuity with concurrent invasive disease, whereas ADH is not. These data and observations indicate that noninvasive carcinoma may be both a risk factor and a nonobligatory precursor for invasive carcinoma, though ADH may only be a marker of increased risk.[116] However, this issue is far from settled, and is likely to remain so until more is known about the biology of breast cancer evolution.

ADH is usually an incidental finding associated with other benign breast disease. Microscopically, it is represented by an intraductal epithelial proliferation showing either the growth pattern or the cytologic features characteristic of noninvasive carcinoma but neither in fully developed form. The growth patterns mimicked by ADH are those of noncomedo ductal carcinoma in situ and include the cribriform, micropapillary, solid, or mixed subtypes. Regularity of pattern, regardless of the specific cellular arrangement, is an important theme of ADH. The cytologic features mimicked by ADH are also those of noncomedo ductal carcinoma in situ and include relatively small, round cells with distinct borders, moderate-to-scant amounts of cytoplasm, uniform round-to oval nuclei with delicate, occasionally hyperchromatic chromatin, small nucleoli, and rare mitotic figures

One can imagine that the various permutations of growth patterns and cytologic features diagnostic of ADH are quite large. Representative examples of ADH are shown in Fig. 70-16 to illustrate the perplexing similarities as well as the variability of these lesions. Fig. 70-16, *A* demonstrates a uniform growth pattern and cytologic features approaching cribriform

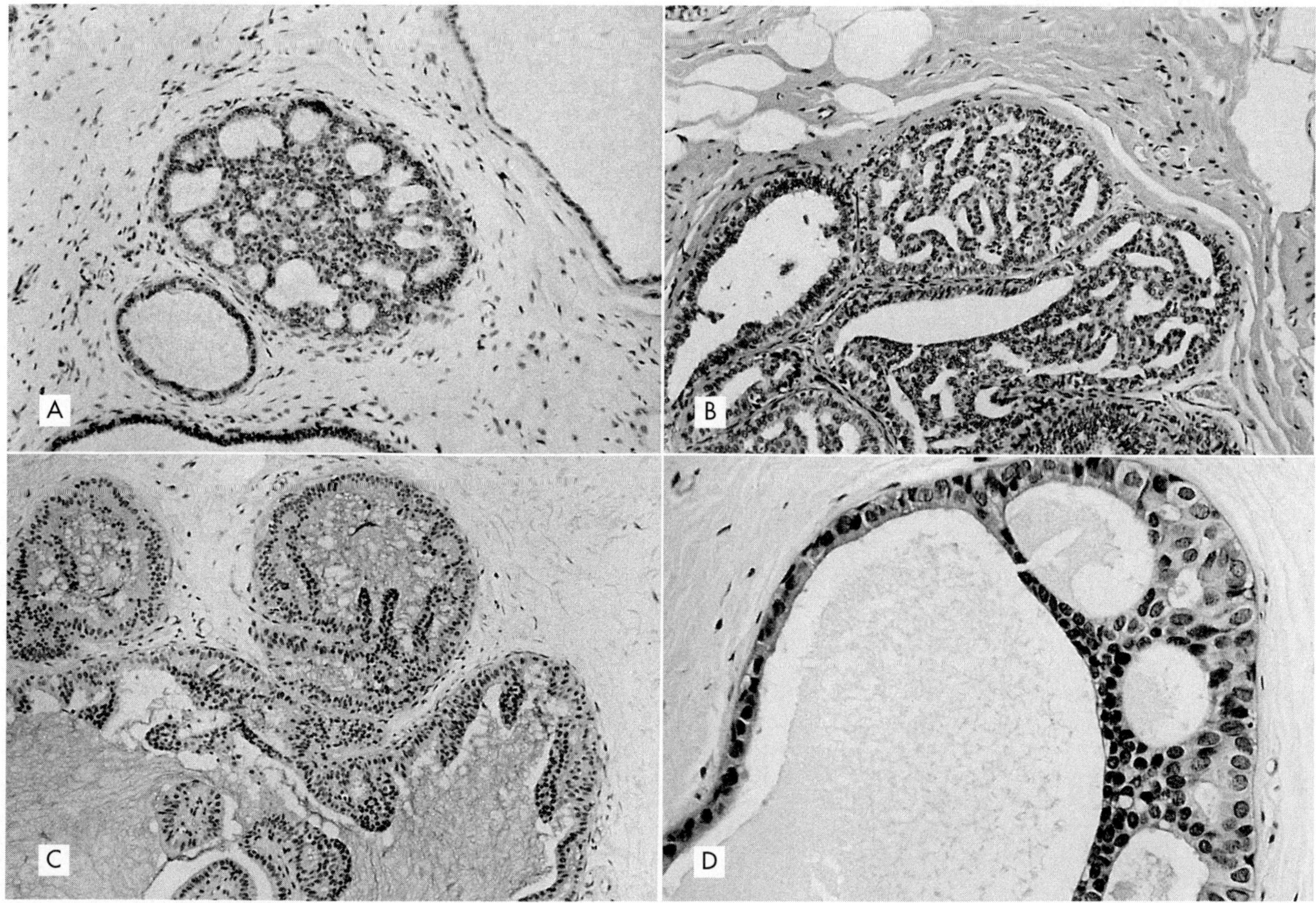

Fig. 70-16 Examples of ADH showing **A,** cribriform; **B,** fenestrated; **C,** micropapillary; and **D,** partial cribriform growth patterns.

ductal carcinoma in-situ. Fig. 70-16, *B*, shows an example of ADH composed of monotonous cells in an evenly distributed fenestrated pattern. Other frequent features include micropapillary proliferation of uniform-looking cells with trabecular bridging and partial involvement of ducts by cribriform proliferation of monotonous cells as shown in Fig. 70-16, *C* and *D*, respectively.

Currently there is no consensus regarding the treatment of ADH and most patients are only counseled and followed closely. Prophylactic mastectomies may be considered in women with ADH and a strong family history of breast cancer where the relative risk of developing invasive carcinoma is very high (more than tenfold).

Atypical lobular hyperplasia (ALH) accounts for less than 1% of all breast lesions biopsied and is more common in premenopausal women. Studies have shown that women diagnosed with ALH have a relative risk of 4.0 to 5.0 for the subsequent development of invasive breast cancer and that the risk is bilateral.[117,118] It is rarely associated with invasive carcinoma, and when invasive lesions develop in women with previous ALH, they are more often ductal than lobular. For these reasons, ALH is generally considered to be a marker of increased cancer risk rather than a precursor of invasive disease.

ALH has no distinguishing clinical or mammographic features and is usually an incidental finding associated with other benign disease. The microscopic features of ALH are distinctive. They show an intralobular epithelial proliferation distending a portion of the acini of a lobular unit (Fig. 70-17). The cells are uniform, small, and round-to-polygonal in shape, contain moderate-to-scant amounts of cytoplasm, have round regular nuclei with delicate chromatin and small nucleoli, and show rare mitoses. ALH is frequently multicentric.

The clinical and histologic features of ALH are qualitatively the same as those of lobular carcinoma in situ, and they have collectively been referred to as "lobular neoplasia" based on the belief by some authors that they represent the same lesion at different stages of progression.[117,118] At present the treatment for ALH is similar to that described for ADH.

Classification of breast carcinoma

The classification of breast carcinoma is continually evolving. Useful systems stratify breast cancer into categories based on distinct histologic, biologic, and clinically important features. Table 70-3 shows a classification distilled from several large studies.[62,119-122]

Noninvasive carcinoma

Noninvasive carcinoma of the breast accounts for about 10% of all breast cancer, though the incidence may vary from one clinical setting to another. The two major categories currently recognized are referred to as "ductal carcinoma in situ" (DCIS) and "lobular carcinoma in situ" (LCIS). Although both are believed to arise from transformed cells located in terminal ducts,[94,119] they are lesions with important histologic, biologic, and clinical distinctions. DCIS is further subdivided into comedo, cribriform, micropapillary, solid, and papillary subtypes. Recent studies have shown that, relative to the other subtypes of DCIS, comedo DCIS is associated with many aggressive biologic and clinical features. These observations have motivated a further simplification of nomenclature recognizing only comedo and noncomedo subtypes.

Comedo ductal carcinoma in situ accounts for 3% to 5% of all breast carcinomas and 35% to 50% of solitary noninvasive carcinomas.[119,123-126] The natural history of DCIS is poorly understood because until recently it was treated by total mastectomy resulting in 98% to 100% long-term survival.[94] Some insights into the biologic features of these lesions have been provided by studies showing that DCIS is present concurrently in 48% of breasts contralateral to breasts containing invasive carcinoma,[127] and that up to 10% of breasts contralateral to one with an invasive carcinoma eventually develop invasive carcinoma,[128] indicating that a significant proportion of DCIS have the ability to progress to invasive disease. Similar conclusions come from retrospective studies showing a high incidence (at least 30%) and relative risk (about tenfold) of developing invasive breast carcinoma in the same breast as previously excised DCIS.[114,115,129] Recent studies of comedo DCIS treated by lumpectomy report local recurrence rates of 7% to 20% with half the recurrences being invasive.[123,125,127,128,130] This clinical aggressiveness is consistent with the aggressive biologic features associated with comedo DCIS, including absence of hormone receptors,[131] a high proliferation rate,[132] and an aneuploid DNA content.[133]

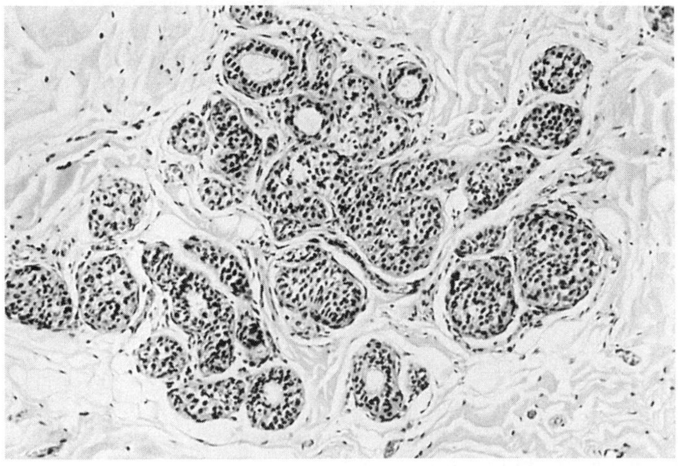

Fig. 70-17 Atypical lobular hyperplasia showing low-grade uniform cells distending a portion of the acini of a lobular unit.

Table 70-3 Major histologic types of breast carcinoma and their relative incidences for all stages combined[119-122]

Subtype	Incidence (%)
Noninvasive carcinoma	10
Ductal	8
Noncomedo	5
Comedo	3
Lobular	2
Invasive carcinoma	90
Ductal—not otherwise specified	60
Special types—classical and variants	30
Lobular	15
Medullary	7
Tubular	5
Mucinous	3
Unusual/rare types	<1

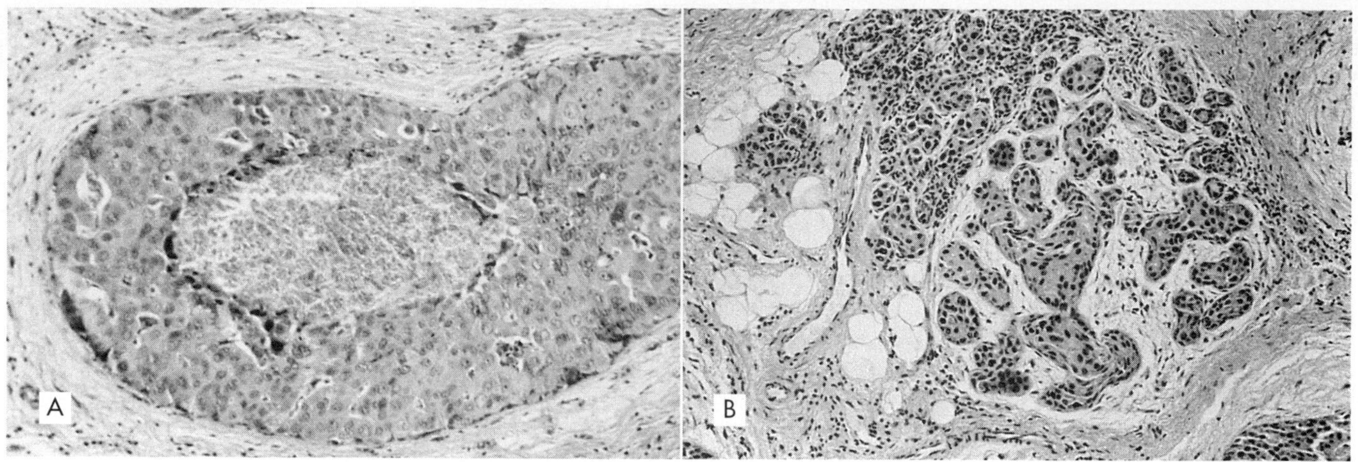

Fig. 70-18 Examples of comedo ductal carcinoma in situ showing **A,** distended ducts with central necrosis and **B,** "cancerization" of lobular acini.

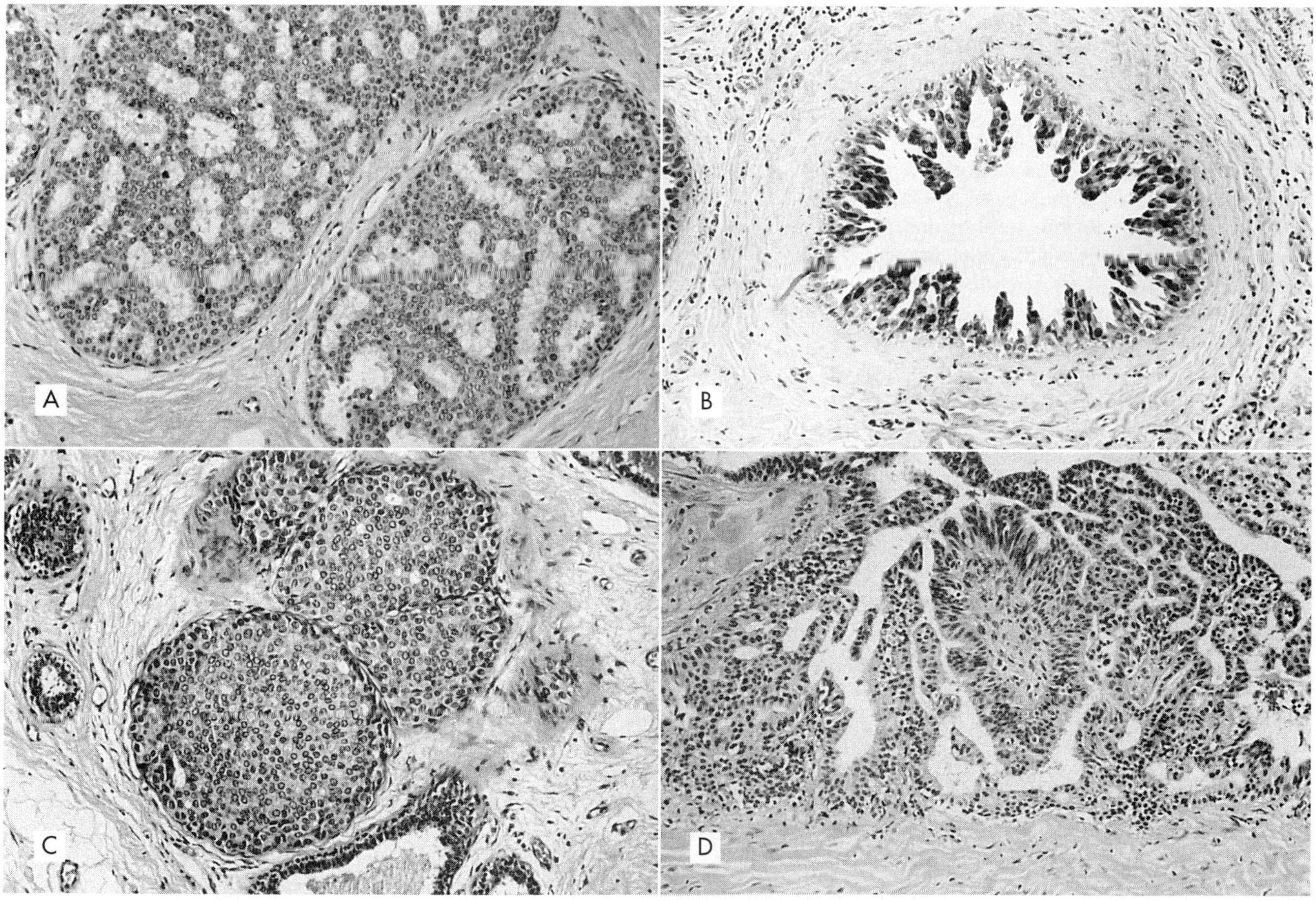

Fig. 70-19 Noncomedo ductal carcinoma in situ showing **A,** cribriform; **B,** micropapillary; **C,** solid; and **D,** papillary growth patterns.

The majority of comedo DCIS present as palpable masses averaging 2 to 3 cm in diameter, though lesions larger than 5 cm are common. On gross examination they are relatively well circumscribed and characteristically exude cheesy, "comedo-like," necrotic debris from distended ducts.

Microscopically comedo DCIS is characterized by noninvasive tumor cells distending the ducts to as much as 10 times their normal diameter (Fig. 70-18, *A*); and retrograde extension into lobules ("cancerization") is common (Fig. 70-18, *B*). Although occasional ducts may demonstrate a solid growth pattern, most show prominent central necrosis, with viable cells being present only at the periphery in solid or perforated arrangements. Cytologic and nuclear features are generally those of a high-grade tumor. They include large, irregularly shaped cells with abundant cytoplasm. Nuclei are large, pleomorphic, contain dark condensed chromatin, prominent nucleoli, and numerous mitotic figures that are often atypical.

The major problem in differential diagnosis involves distinguishing cancerization of lobules from microinvasive carcinoma. This problem can be minimized by adoption of the conservative strategy of requiring the invasive cells to extend beyond the specialized intralobular connective tissue.

Noncomedo ductal carcinoma in situ accounts for 5% to 8% of all breast carcinomas and 50% to 70% of solitary noninvasive carcinomas.[123,124,126,134] It is considered to be a less aggressive lesion than comedo DCIS, with lower short-term recurrence rates (less than 5%) after local excision[125] and strong associations with favorable biologic features such as presence of hormone receptors,[131] low proliferation rates,[132] and diploid DNA content.[133] However, the unequivocal malignant potential of noncomedo DCIS is underscored in retrospective studies showing long-term local recurrence rates of up to 30% after incomplete surgical excision, together with invasiveness in half of the recurrences.[114,115,126]

The majority of noncomedo DCIS are nonpalpable and are initially called to attention by small microcalcifications seen on mammograms.[134] A minority are found incidentally in breasts on which biopsies are done for other reasons.

There are several subtypes of noncomedo DCIS, each having distinctive microscopic features. They are often found together in the same lesion, though one pattern usually predominates. The cribriform subtype is composed of cells forming evenly spaced, uniform, roundish microacini in moderately distended ducts (Figure 70-19, *A*). Extension of tumor into the lobules is rare. Central necrosis of cells within ducts may be present and is occasionally prominent. Cytologic and nuclear features are generally of low grade. They include uniform, small, round cells with distinct surface membranes and scant-to-moderate amounts of cytoplasm. Nuclei are typically small to intermediate in size and round to oval in shape and contain relatively homogeneous chromatin and small nucleoli. Mitotic figures are rare. Micropapillary noncomedo DCIS is characterized by small papillary projections of cells without fibrovascular cores (Fig. 70-19, *B*). The micropapillae are similar in length and smooth in outline and have slightly bulbous tips. Cytologic features are the same as these described for the cribriform subtype. Solid noncomedo DCIS is characterized by uniform cells with the same cytologic features but which distend ducts as a solid proliferation without forming discernible acini or micropapillae (Fig. 70-19, *C*).

Noninvasive papillary carcinoma is rarer than the other forms of noncomedo DCIS. It usually presents as a 1 to 3 cm palpable mass with an "intracystic" appearance.[135] Microscopically it is composed of elongated branching papillae with fibrovascular cores lined by columnar cells showing variable degrees of atypia (Fig. 70-19, *D*). Papillae may fuse, forming solid or cribriform cellular arrangements. Other patterns of noncomedo DCIS (such as the cribriform subtype) are commonly found adjacent to the intracystic papillary mass and may be of help in distinguishing papillary carcinoma from intraductal papilloma.

Lobular carcinoma in situ accounts for 1% to 3% of all breast carcinomas and 10% to 30% of solitary noninvasive carcinomas. It is a nonpalpable microscopic lesion nearly always encountered as an incidental finding in the breasts of premenopausal women.[117] The risk of developing invasive carcinoma in a breast with previously excised LCIS increases about 1% per year, a rate that translates to a greater than tenfold relative risk and a 20% absolute risk after 20 years.[117,118,136] This risk is bilateral, and most invasive cancers that develop are ductal rather than lobular, an indication that LCIS may be a marker for the development of invasive breast cancer rather than a precursor.

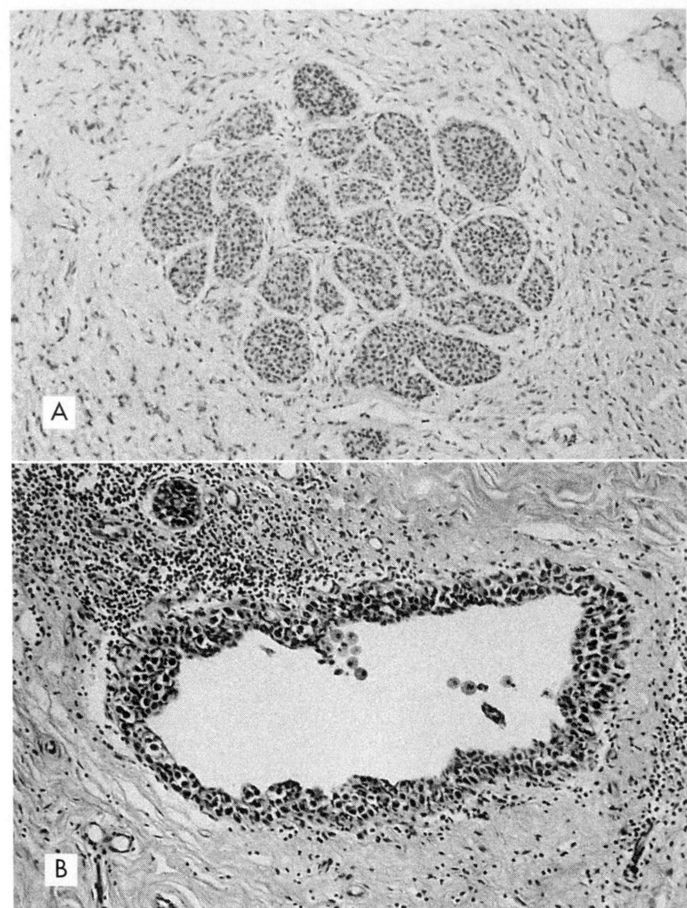

Fig. 70-20 Lobular carcinoma in situ (LCIS). **A,** LCIS showing uniform cells distending all acini of a lobular unit. **B,** LCIS extending into proximal ducts in a pagetoid fashion.

Microscopically LCIS is usually multicentric and characterized by lobular units in which all acini are filled and distended by loosely cohesive cells with generally low-grade cytologic and nuclear feature (Fig. 70-20, *A*). The cells are small, round, or polygonal and have distinct cell membranes and moderate amounts of relatively clear cytoplasm. They may have prominent cytoplasmic vacuoles imparting a signet-ring appearance. Nuclei are typically round or oval and contain homogeneous dark chromatin and small or inconspicuous nucleoli. Mitotic figures are rare. LCIS has a tendency to spread beneath the epithelium of proximal large ducts in a pagetoid fashion (Fig. 70-20, *B*).

Invasive carcinoma

Invasive carcinomas account for about 90% of all breast cancers. Modern taxonomy attempts to subdivide them into categories with distinct morphologic, biologic, and clinical charac-

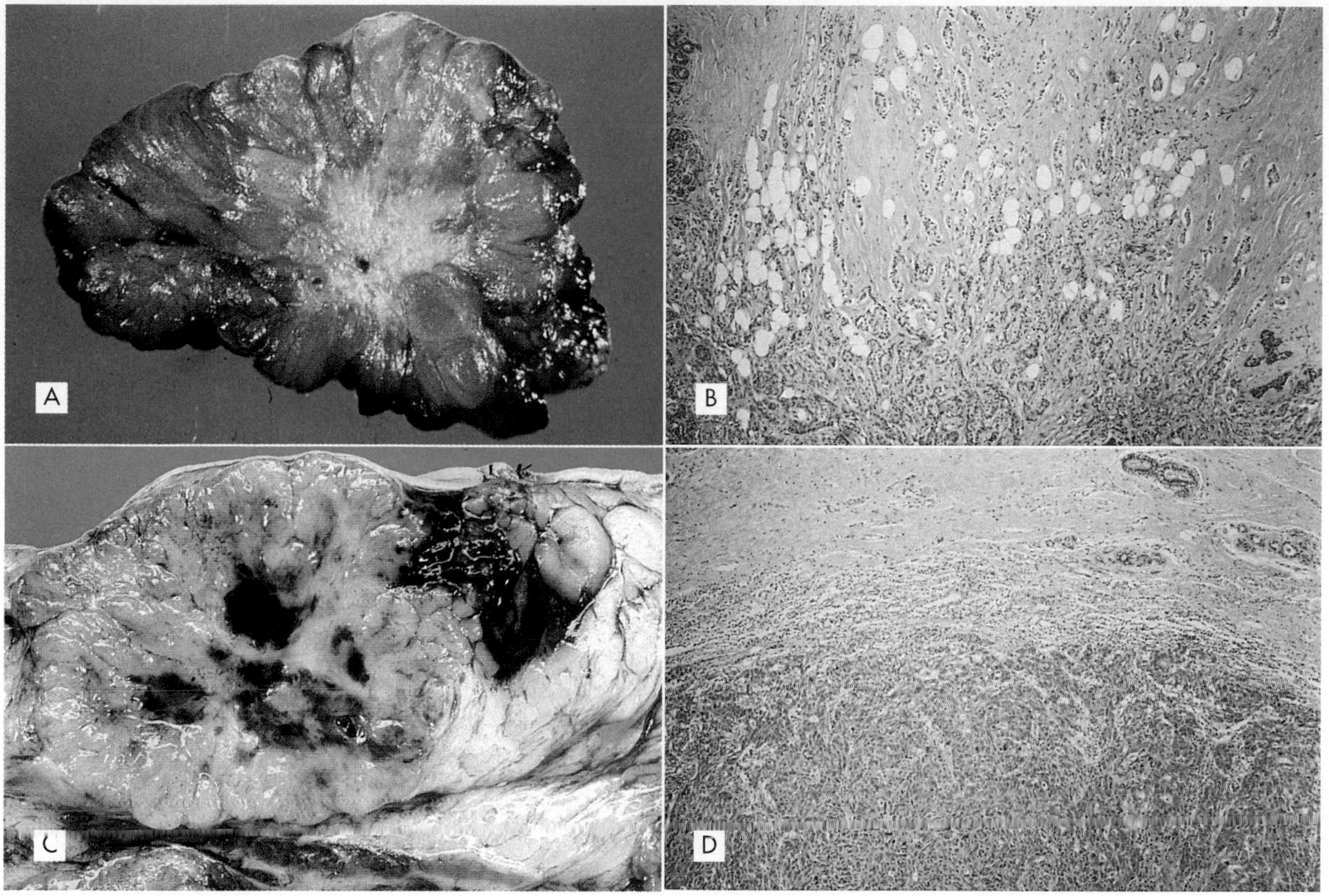

Fig. 70-21 Infiltrating ductal carcinoma (IDC-NOS) **A,** Macroscopically stellate reflecting an infiltrative growth front microscopically, **B. C,** Macroscopically circumscribed IDC-NOS, reflecting a blunt pushing growth front microscopically, **D.** Combined patterns are encountered frequently.

teristics. In practice this has been difficult because these characteristics are quite heterogeneous in the majority of invasive carcinomas. The system of nomenclature adopted in this chapter (see Table 70-3) is a compromise derived from several studies.[120-122]

Infiltrating ductal carcinoma not otherwise specified (IDC-NOS) is a heterogeneous group of lesions characterized by a relative absence of the histologic features that define the special types of invasive carcinoma and, in this sense, is the result of a diagnosis by exclusion. It accounts for about 60% of all breast carcinomas and 70% of invasive carcinomas, though its relative incidence varies with clinical stage. It is biologically and clinically more aggressive than the special types of invasive carcinoma. The median 5-year survival for patients with IDC-NOS for all stages combined is only about 60%, compared to 80% to 95% for the special types.[120,122,137] IDC-NOS usually presents as a hard, palpable mass averaging 2 to 3 cm in greatest dimension. Typical mammograms show an irregular density with internal microcalcifications, features that are nearly always interpreted as either consistent with or highly suspicious of cancer.

Macroscopically IDC-NOS is usually whitish gray and firm to palpation and has a gritty texture. Shapes vary from those with an irregular stellate outline (Fig. 70-21, *A*), reflecting an infiltrative growth front microscopically (Fig. 70-21, *B*), to those with a lobulated or circumscribed contour (Fig. 70-21, *C*), reflecting a blunt pushing growth front microscopically (Fig. 70-21, *D*).

IDC-NOS has no typical features microscopically. Some lesions may be solid and highly cellular (Fig. 70-22, *A*), whereas others may be solid but paucicellular and accompanied by a prominent desmoplastic stroma (Fig. 70-22, *B*). Acinus or tubule formation may dominate (Fig. 70-22, *C*) or be combined with solid tumor (Fig. 70-22, *D*). Combinations of growth patterns are the rule, though one pattern usually predominates.

The cytologic and nuclear features of IDC-NOS are also heterogeneous. Cells may be small, intermediate, or large; they may be round, pleomorphic, or intermediate in shape. The amount of cytoplasm is highly variable. Nuclear features (including size, shape, chromatin, and nucleoli) may show mild, moderate, or severe atypia (Fig. 70-23). The number of mitotic figures is highly variable, and their conformation may be normal or atypical.

Over the years several histological grading systems have been developed that represent an attempt to order the enormous histologic variability of infiltrating ductal carcinomas into a few manageable categories with some meaningful relationship to clinical outcome.[138] One of the most useful methods is the Elston modification[139] of the much earlier Bloom-Richardson grading system.[140] As shown in Table 70-4,

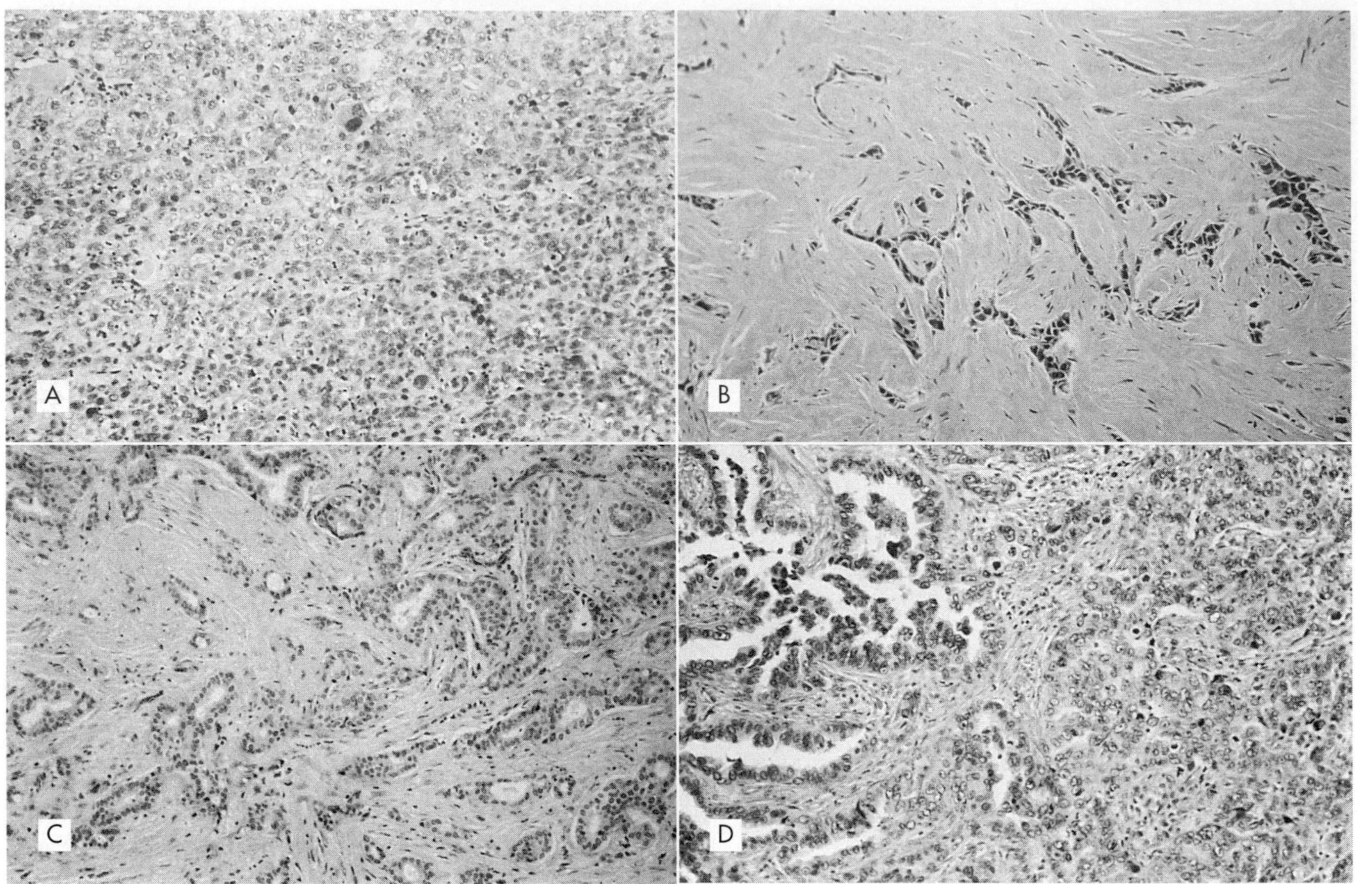

Fig. 70-22 Infiltrating ductal carcinoma (IDC-NOS). Highly variable growth patterns of IDC-NOS are shown. **A,** Common patterns are solid and highly cellular; **B,** solid, desmoplastic, and paucicellular; **C,** entirely acinar; or **D,** acinar and solid.

numerical scores are assigned to each of three major histologic features: the percentage of tubule formation, the degree of nuclear pleomorphism, and the number of mitoses per 10 high-power fields, based on a thorough microscopic evaluation of the entire lesion. The scores for each feature are then added to determine the histologic grade, which is directly related to differentiation. Using this grading system in a prospective study involving more than 1800 patients with invasive breast cancer, median 10-year survivals of 90%, 60%, and 40% were associated with grade I, grade II, and grade III lesions, respectively.[139] Although these data were not corrected for stage, the differences in survival were highly significant and emphasize the usefulness of grading breast cancer. An important challenge for pathology is to devise an optimum and universally acceptable grading system.

The major problem in the differential diagnosis of IDC-NOS involves distinguishing it from special types of invasive carcinoma. Thus, familiarity with the histologic features of the latter neoplasm is a prerequisite. In general, if less than 75% of a lesion shows the features of a special subtype, it should be diagnosed as IDC-NOS because its prognosis is likely to be worse than that for the special type. Classical lobular carcinoma rarely presents a problem, though its variants may be confused with IDC-NOS.

Infiltrating lobular carcinoma (ILC), including both the classical and the variant subtypes, accounts for about 15% of all invasive breast cancer.[120,122,141] Classical ILC is the most common (75% of cases),[141] and studies of this subtype have reported 7- to 10-year survivals of 80% to 90% for all stages.[120,141,142] Despite these favorable statistics, there is an appreciable risk of late systemic relapse, even after 10 years of disease-free survival. The prognosis of ILC variants is similar to that of IDC-NOS,[137] but their recognition remains important because all subtypes of ILC are associated with significant rates of concurrent (10% to 15%) or subsequent (20% to 35%) contralateral invasive breast cancer.[143-145]

Patients with ILC may present with a palpable mass or a diffuse lesion that is not detectable by palpation or mammography. Macroscopically some lesions are discrete, firm, and stellate, whereas others appear as an ill-defined thickening identifiable as cancer only under the microscope.

Microscopically, classical ILC is characterized by uniform, small, round, poorly cohesive cells with low-grade nuclear features growing in short, straight, single-file arrangements ("Indian file") (Fig. 70-24, *A*) or swirling around vessels, ducts, and lobules ("targetoid" pattern). Signet-ring cells may be common. LCIS is present in 80% to 90% of classical ILC.[146]

Variants of ILC include solid, alveolar, mixed, and pleomorphic subtypes. The cytologic features of the solid, alveolar, and mixed variants are the same as in classical ILC, and they are distinguished by their growth patterns. The solid variant grows in sheetlike cellular arrangements (Fig. 70-24, *B*). The

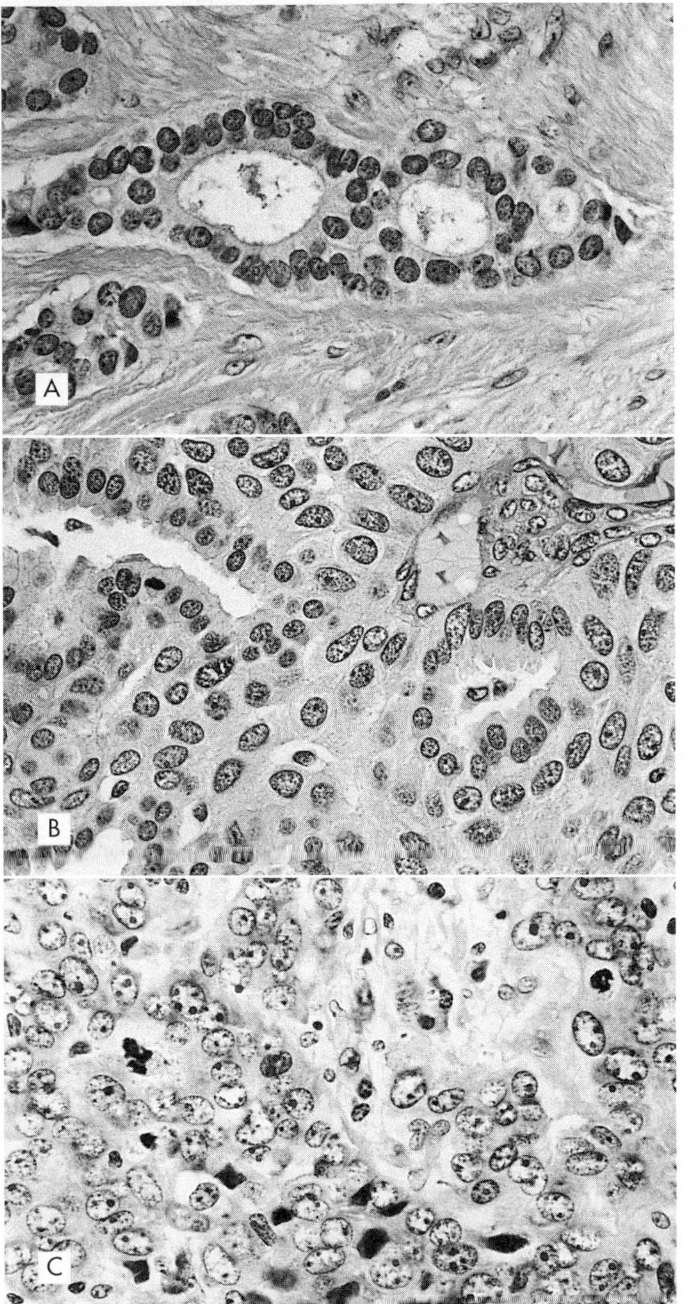

Fig. 70-23 Degrees of atypia of nuclear features of breast carcinoma cells. **A,** mild atypia. **B,** moderate atypia. **C,** severe atypia. The degree of nuclear atypia or pleomorphism is evaluated in the histologic grading of breast carcinoma.

Table 70-4 Histologic grading of breast carcinoma[139]

Feature		Feature score
Percent tubule formation*		
>75		1
10-75		2
<10		3
Nuclear pleomorphism*†		
Mild (small and uniform)		1
Intermediate		2
Severe (pronounced variation)		3
Mitotic counts per 10 high-power fields (HPFs)*		
≤9 mitoses/10 HPFs		1
10-19 mitoses/10 HPFs		2
≥20 mitoses/10 HPFs		3
Total score	**Grade**	
3-5	I (well differentiated)	
6-7	II (moderately differentiated)	
8-9	III (poorly differentiated)	

*The percentage of tubule formation is based on assessment of the entire tumor. However, nuclear pleomorphism is assessed in the worst area, and mitotic counts at the leading edge of tumor growth.

†Mild, intermediate, and severe nuclear pleomorphism are illustrated in Fig. 70-23.

alveolar variant is characterized by small, crowded, solid nests of cells (Fig. 70-24, *C*). The mixed variant shows combinations of classical, solid, and alveolar patterns. Pleomorphic ILC has a diffuse growth pattern and is distinguished by its high-grade nuclear atypia (Fig. 70-24, *D*). LCIS is present in less than 50% of ILC variants.[146]

The diagnosis of classical ILC is usually straightforward, though an occasional lesion may be missed if it is very small or contains lymphocytes in Indian-file arrangements. Microscopic deposits of metastatic ILC in axillary lymph nodes are notoriously difficult to recognize because of their resemblance to lymphocytes and sinus histiocytes. The solid variant of ILC may be confused with lymphoma and requires special stains (such as immunohistochemical stains) to resolve. All variants may be misdiagnosed as IDC-NOS or as "combined ductal-lobular carcinomas," which is potentially a serious problem if screening for contralateral disease is neglected.

Medullary carcinoma accounts for about 7% of all breast cancer.[120,121] This includes both the typical and the variant subtypes, which are about equally frequent.[147] Typical medullary carcinoma has a better prognosis than IDC-NOS with reports of 10-year survival of 80% to 90%.[147-150] The prognosis of the variant subtype, also referred to as atypical medullary carcinoma,[150] is controversial, with reports of only slightly higher[141,149] or equivalent[147,150] survival relative to IDC-NOS.

Medullary carcinoma usually presents as a palpable, mobile, circumscribed mass ranging from 2 to 3 cm in greatest dimension, though lesions larger than 5 cm may be encountered. Gross pathologic features reflect the clinical presentation. Lesions are well circumscribed, lobulated, tan-white, relatively soft, and homogeneous in consistency (resembling the tumor shown in Fig. 70-21, *C*).

The microscopic features of typical medullary carcinoma include a blunt or pushing leading edge, solid-syncytial groups of cells with high-grade nuclei, scanty loose stroma, and a prominent interstitial lymphocytic infiltrate (Fig. 70-25). These features must be well developed and compose more than 90% of the lesion. Bizarre tumor giant cells and foci of squamous metaplasia are occasionally encountered. There may be a minor in situ component that is usually solid or of the comedo type. Medullary carcinoma variant has these same features, but constituting only 75% to 90% of the lesion. Lesions with similar features in less than 75% of the tumor should be diagnosed as IDC-NOS, because they will generally have the poorer prognosis associated with this type.

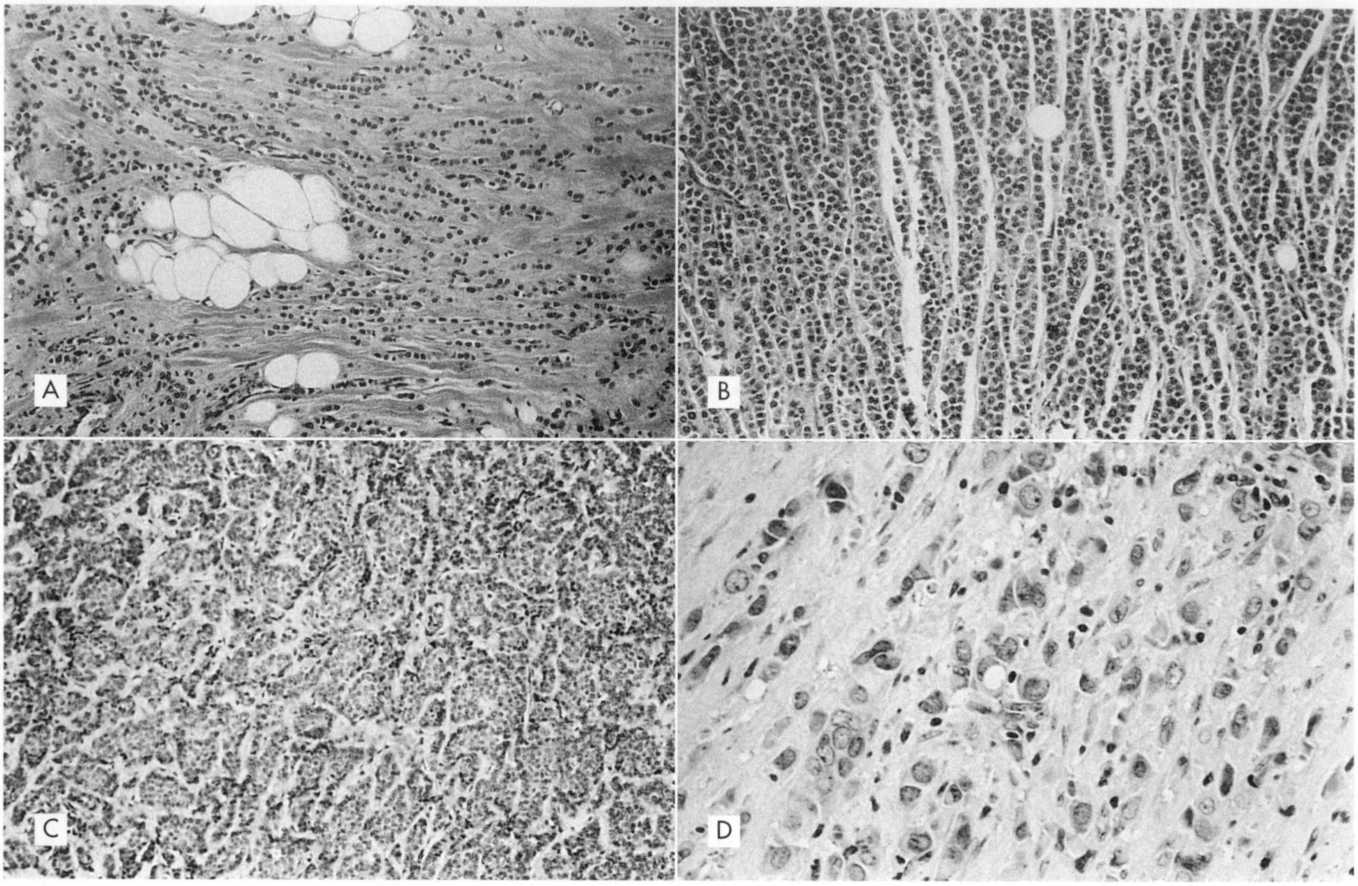

Fig. 70-24 Subtypes of infiltrating lobular carcinoma. **A,** Classical. **B,** Solid. **C,** Alveolar. **D,** Pleomorphic.

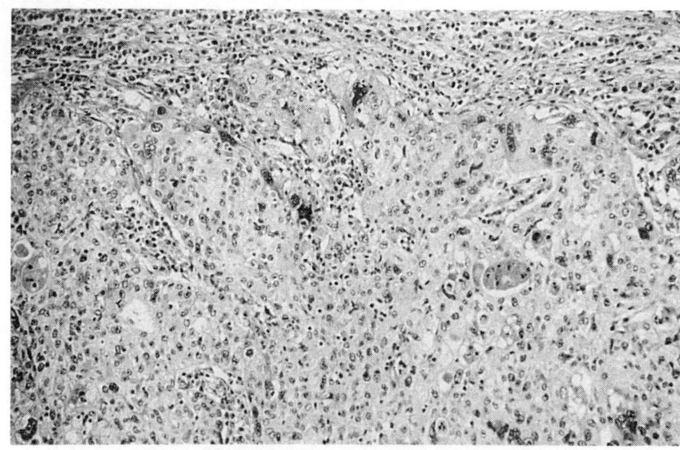

Fig. 70-25 Medullary carcinoma showing atypical cells with a solid-syncitial growth pattern, delicate stroma, prominent lymphocytic infiltrate, and circumscribed leading edge.

Tubular carcinoma, including typical and variant subtypes, accounts for about 5% of all breast cancers, though the incidence varies with the clinical setting and is higher among lesions detected by mammography.[151] The typical subtype has the best prognosis of all the special types of invasive breast carcinoma with reports of 5-year survival of 95% to 100%.[152,153] Five-year survivals of 90% have been reported for the variant pattern.[153] Concurrent or subsequent contralateral invasive breast cancer may be present in up to 20% of patients with tubular carcinoma.[154,155]

Tubular carcinoma may present as a hard palpable mass, but average diameter is approximately 1 cm,[152] and the majority of tumors are detected by mammography. They typically have a firm, white, stellate appearance on gross examination. Microscopically they are composed of small glands or tubules with round, oval, or angular ("teardrop") shapes (Fig. 70-26, *A*). The glands are uniformly distributed in a centrally dense fibrous stroma with prominent elastosis. The stroma is less dense near the periphery where isolated glands may invade adjacent adipose tissue. A single layer of cuboidal or columnar cells with low-grade cytologic and nuclear features line the malignant glands. Cribriform or micropapillary DCIS may be present in up to 65% of tubular carcinomas.[152]

Tubular carcinoma may be confused with focal sclerosing adenosis and radial scar. Sclerosing adenosis is distinguished by its lobular distribution, circumscribed border, absence of elastosis, absence of DCIS, and flattened tubules lined by both a myoepithelial and an epithelial layer. Radial scar can be differentiated by its lobulated smooth border, absence of DCIS, patent glands with myoepithelial and epithelial layers, and absence of glandular infiltration beyond the central scar into adjacent fat.

Invasive cribriform carcinoma is a recently described histologic entity that is biologically similar to tubular carcinoma.[156] Its appearance is that of infiltrating islands of low-grade cells perforated by small acini in a cribriform

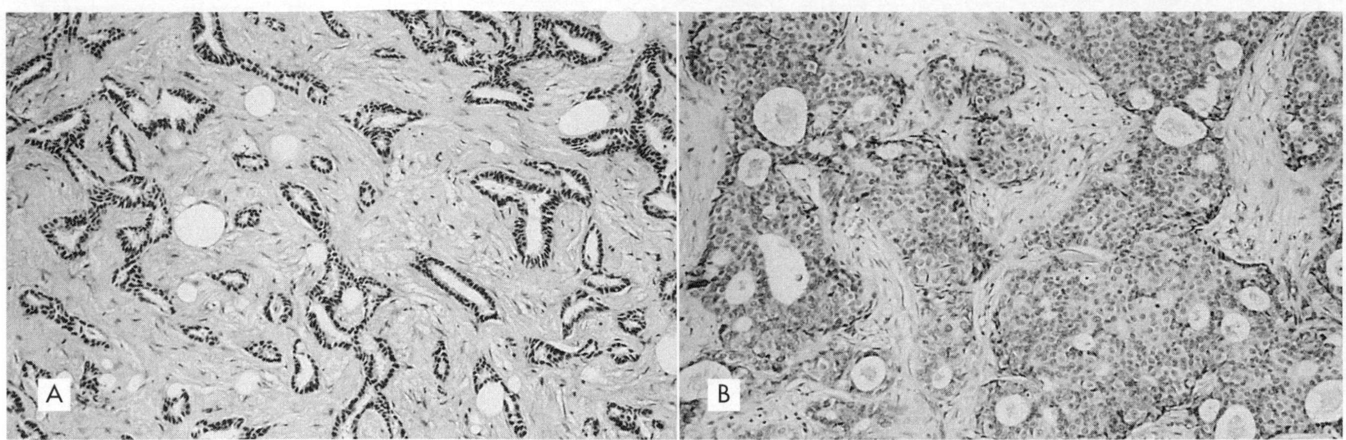

Fig. 70-26 **A,** Tubular carcinoma showing characteristic small angular glands that are evenly distributed in a dense fibrous stroma. **B,** Cribriform carcinoma displaying features similar to those in **A.**

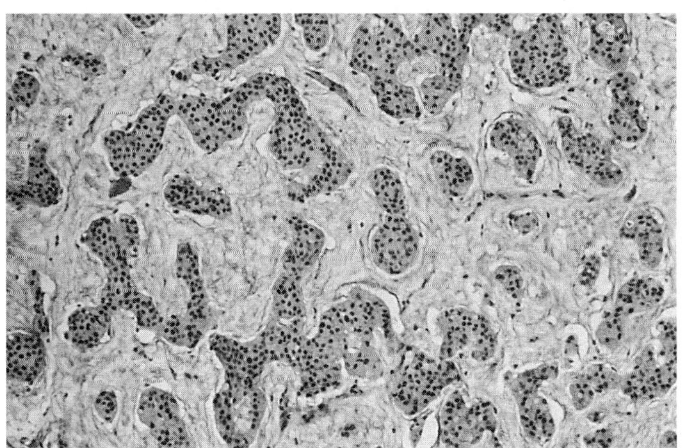

Fig. 70-27 Mucinous carcinoma showing characteristic clusters of well-differentiated cells suspended in a pool of interstitial mucinous material.

arrangement (Fig. 70-26, *B*). This pattern may appear in pure form, or more commonly, be combined with the features of tubular carcinoma.

Mucinous carcinoma, also known as colloid carcinoma, has typical and variant subtypes collectively accounting for only 2% to 3% of all breast carcinomas.[121,122] The variant is three times more common than the typical subtype[141] and both are more common in older women.[157] Typical mucinous carcinoma has a very good prognosis, with survival in the range of 85% to 90% at 10 years, compared with only 70% to 80% for the variant subtype.[158,159] Recurrences after mastectomy are relatively rare, and 50% of these occur after 10 years of disease-free survival.[160]

Mucinous carcinomas present as soft palpable masses with vague, nonspecific, findings on mammograms. Gross pathologic features include an average diameter of 2 to 3 cm, a circumscribed shape, glistening tan color, and soft gelatinous texture (resembling the tumor shown in Fig. 70-21, *C*). Microscopically they are composed of small islands of malignant cells suspended in a contiguous pool of extracellular mucinous material[121] (Fig. 70-27). The tumor border is blunt rather than infiltrative. An in situ component is rare. Cell groups may be solid or perforated by acinar spaces. Cytological and nuclear features are of a low-grade to intermediate-grade tumor. For a lesion to be diagnosed as typical mucinous carcinoma, these combined features should constitute more than 90% of the tumor. In the variant subtype they account for only 75% to 90% of the lesion. If less than 75% of the tumor contains these features it should be categorized as IDC-NOS.

Although rare mucocele-like tumors of the breast can be mistaken for mucinous carcinoma,[161] they are nearly always less than 5 mm in diameter and composed of a mucin pool with rare cells located at the outer edge rather than suspended internally. They are probably reactive and result from obstruction in a proximal duct.

Unusual presentations of breast carcinoma

Two unusual presentations of otherwise common breast cancer are Paget's disease of the nipple[162] and inflammatory carcinoma.[163] Paget's disease is a clinical and pathologic diagnosis characterized by an eczematous lesion of the nipple caused by intraepidermal spread of malignant cells from an underlying comedo DCIS or high-grade invasive ductal carcinoma (Fig. 70-28, *A*). Inflammatory carcinoma is a clinical diagnosis referring to red, warm, edematous skin overlying an invasive breast carcinoma. Usually there is invasion of dermal blood vessels and embolization of dermal lymphatics (Fig. 70-28, *B*). This clinical sign indicates a poor prognosis.

Rare types of breast carcinoma

Several exceptionally rare types of invasive carcinomas collectively account for less than 1% of all breast cancer. Metaplastic carcinomas are in this group and include squamous cell carcinoma[164] and pseudosarcomatous carcinomas.[165,166] Because focal squamous metaplasia is frequent in the common types of breast carcinoma, lesions diagnosed as squamous carcinoma must show unequivocal squamous differentiation throughout. Pseudosarcomatous lesions must be composed of at least 20% metaplastic elements, which most commonly are fibrous, chondroid, or osseous. They have a very poor prognosis.

Also included among the rare malignant epithelial lesions are signet-ring cell carcinoma,[167] invasive papillary carcinoma,[168] carcinoid tumor,[169] salivary gland like carcinomas,[170]

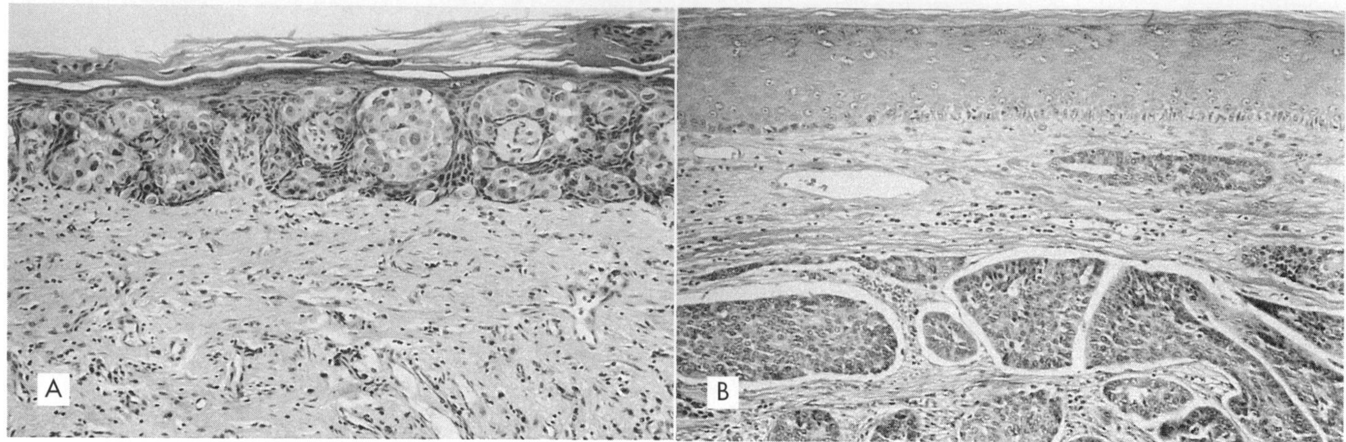

Fig. 70-28 **A,** Paget's disease of the nipple with characteristic intraepidermal spread of underlying carcinoma. **B,** Inflammatory carcinoma. Breast carcinoma cells have formed emboli in dermal lymphatics.

secretory carcinoma,[171] and clear cell carcinoma.[172] Signet-ring cell carcinoma must contain more than 20% signet-ring cells to qualify for this diagnosis; it has a diffuse ILC-like growth pattern, and has a very poor prognosis. Invasive papillary carcinoma is circumscribed and composed of papillae with true fibrovascular cores lined by cells with intermediate-grade to high-grade atypia. They usually have a favorable outcome. Lesions with light microscopic, ultrastructural, and biochemical features of carcinoid tumors occur in the breast, but it is controversial whether they represent true neuroendocrine neoplasms. Malignant salivary gland like tumors include mucoepidermoid and adenocystic carcinomas, with the latter being most common.

Metastasis of breast carcinoma

Approximately 30% of breast cancer patients have metastatic implants in regional axillary lymph nodes when they are first diagnosed, and another 10% have distant metastatic disease. The clinical assessment of lymph node status is extremely inaccurate and error rates of up to 30% have been reported in studies comparing clinical to histopathologic evaluation.[173] There may also be a significant error in the routine histopathologic evaluation of nodes for metastatic disease, since studies have shown that more extensive serial sectioning or immunostaining with antibodies to epithelial components detect micrometastases in up to 10% of patients originally diagnosed as having negative nodes.[174,175] Large studies have shown a 10% reduction in 5-year survival associated with such occult micrometastastic tumor.[174]

Distant metastatic disease is the first sign in about 50% of women with previously excised breast cancer who relapse.[176] Nearly all patients dying of breast cancer have widely disseminated metastatic disease, with lung, liver, and bone being the favored sites.[177] The treatment of metastatic disease based on clinical evaluation alone can be a problem because of the high error rate for clinical evaluation alone in detecting metastatic disease when compared with autopsy results in the same patients.[177]

Cancer metastatic to the breast

Nearly every type of cancer has metastasized to the breast at one time or another, though collectively it is quite rare. When it occurs, it is usually late in the clinical course of widely disseminated disease.[178] Non-Hodgkin's lymphomas, myeloid leukemias, and systemic myeloma are among the most frequent tumors that metastasize to the breast,[178,179] and each may be problematic in differentiating from ILC. Lymphomas may also be primary in the breast but are exceedingly rare (less than 0.1% of all breast cancer).[180] Lung carcinomas and malignant melanoma are the most common solid cancers that metastasize to the breast.[178,179]

Prognosis

There are well-documented historical studies describing the untreated natural history of breast cancer. For example, Bloom and colleagues[181] collected survival data for 250 women with breast cancer followed up at London Middlesex Hospital from 1804 to 1933. Over 80% presented with a breast mass as their initial symptom. The median survival of these women was only 2.7 years and less than 1% were alive 15 years later, an indication that nearly all women with invasive breast cancer will eventually die if not treated.

The duration of survival with breast cancer is closely associated with the extent of disease at diagnosis, and several "staging" systems have been developed to express this extent. The most widely used is the TNM clinical-pathologic staging system as endorsed by the International Union Against Cancer and the American Joint Committee on Cancer.[182] As discussed in Chapter 3, the TNM is a code where the *T* value designates the increasing size or local extension of the primary tumor, the *N* value conveys the extent of metastatic disease in regional lymph nodes, and the *M* value indicates the presence or absence of distant metastases. TNM combinations with a similar prognosis are grouped into one of four stages (I to IV), with the higher numbers reflecting increasingly widespread disease and reduced survival probabilities. Table 70-5 presents data for the United States and compares 5-year survival in the 1940s and in the 1980s for breast cancer patients stratified by tumor stage.[97] Both time periods show the expected strong indirect association between stage and outcome. The comparison also shows that survival for only local stage disease has improved during this 40-year interval.

The TNM staging parameters are currently the most powerful prognostic factors allowing prediction of survival in breast

Table 70-5 Survival of patients with breast carcinoma stratified by stage[97]

Stage		5-Year survival (%) 1940s	1983-1987
Localized	(stage I-II)	78	93
Regional	(stage III)	71	71
Advanced	(stage IV)	18	18

cancer patients.[183] Of all the factors, the presence of distant metastases, which occur in about 10% of women presenting with breast cancer, has the strongest association with reduced survival. Nodal status is the second most powerful factor, and, in the absence of distant metastases, survival is poorer in the 20% to 30% of women presenting with positive axillary nodes than in the 60% to 70% with negative nodes.[183] In the absence of distant or nodal metastases, tumor size is the factor most strongly associated with clinical outcome.[138,183]

During the past 30 years, basic research on the development and progression of breast cancer has identified many biologic factors that influence or are associated with prognosis. These factors arise from the abnormal expression or suppression of genes regulating the ability of tumor cells to differentiate, proliferate, invade, and metastasize.

For example, more than 20 years ago it was learned that normal breast epithelium contains receptors for estrogen and progesterone and that the interaction between these receptors and hormones stimulated cells to differentiate and proliferate.[184] Sixty percent to 70% of breast carcinomas also express estrogen receptors (ER) or progesterone receptors (PgR), and these manifestations of differentiation are associated with modestly prolonged survival.[138,184] Paradoxically, ER-positive or PgR-positive tumors may also be stimulated to proliferate by interacting with circulating endogenous hormones. There have been developed drugs that interfere with hormone binding in ER-positive or PgR-positive tumors and thereby inhibit tumor cell proliferation, prolong patient survival, and even reduce the size of existing tumors.[184]

The histologic grading of ductal carcinomas and the recognition of special cancer types are other expressions of differentiation with strong associations to clinical outcome.[122,139,183] pS2 is a recently discovered estrogen-induced protein which, in preliminary studies, is associated with prolonged disease-free survival and response to antiestrogen drug therapy.[185]

Several different measures can be used to assess the proliferation of breast cancer cells. Some values, such as the mitotic index (determined by light microscopy) and the percentage of S-phase cells (determined by DNA flow cytometry) represent the overall proliferation rate. High values detected by either method are associated with a relatively poor prognosis.[138,173,186,187] Recently discoved proliferation-associated molecules, such as Ki-67, have been measured in cells by immunohistochemistry and have been shown to be associated with reduced survival when expressed in a high percentage of cells.[188] Overexpression of the epidermal growth factor receptor, a proto-oncogene product, has, in preliminary studies, also been associated with poor outcome.[189] HER-2/*neu,* also known as c-*erb*B-2, is another proto-oncogene product and probable growth factor receptor associated with reduced survival when amplified and overexpressed in breast cancer.[190,191] Another example is p53, a tumor-suppressor gene normally involved in suppression of the cell cycle. Recent studies have shown that p53 is mutated and over-expressed in about 50% of breast cancers and that these genetic alterations are strongly associated with an increased tumor proliferation rate and poor clinical outcome.[192]

Invasion-related factors with demonstrated or potential prognostic significance include several enzymes that, when expressed by tumor cells or by the adjacent stroma, may promote local invasion or distant metastasis leading to reduced survival. These include such recently identified factors as laminin receptor,[193] cathepsin D,[194] stromolysin 3,[195] and urokinase-plasminogen activator.[196]

Metastasis-related factors overlap to a degree with invasion-related factors because the ability to invade is necessary for metastasis. For example, recent studies have shown an association with cathepsin D expression and a higher probability of metastasis in breast cancer.[197] High vascular density within a primary tumor has also been associated with a stronger likelihood of nodal metastases and a poor prognosis.[198] In preliminary studies, mutations of the recently discovered *nm*23 gene are associated with breast cancer metastasis, a finding indicating that it may function normally as a metastasis-suppressor gene.[199]

The role of pathologists is central to breast cancer prognostication. Their most important responsibilities are to provide accurate diagnosis and pathologic staging. The need for accurate reporting of the size of the tumor, the histologic type, and the nuclear grade cannot be overemphasized. Immunohistochemical analysis is being increasingly employed by pathologists to measure unreported prognostic factors, including ER, PgR, pS2, Ki-67, HER-2/*neu,* and p53 (Fig. 70-29). Although these tests will undoubtedly play an important role in the future, they have yet to be technically and clinically validated before they become part of routine practice.[200,201]

Treatment of breast carcinoma

If treatment is loosely defined as any attempt to improve the survival of breast cancer patients, all efforts by patients and health care professions that involve the detection, diagnosis, and eradication of breast cancer qualify as treatment.

Screening. The detection of a breast mass by comprehensive physical examination or by mammography are the screening methods that bring most breast cancers to medical attention. The strategy behind any screening is to decrease mortality through the early detection of small cancers before they have metastasized and while they are still amenable to cure by surgical excision.

Since the 1960s, there have been significant improvements in the guidelines for breast physical examination (for both health care professionals and patients). This cost-effective screening method has undoubtedly contributed to the increased detection of small breast cancers. Since the 1970s, mammography has become routinely available, and technical advances have improved its sensitivity to the point where nonpalpable lesions smaller than 1.0 cm are easily detected (Fig. 70-30). The overall increased incidence of breast cancer since 1980 has been dominated by small Tis and T1 stage lesions, a finding attributed largely to mammography.[202] Results from prospective clinical trials indicate that mammography may reduce absolute breast cancer mortality by as much as 25%, a major therapeutic achievement by any standard.[94,202,203]

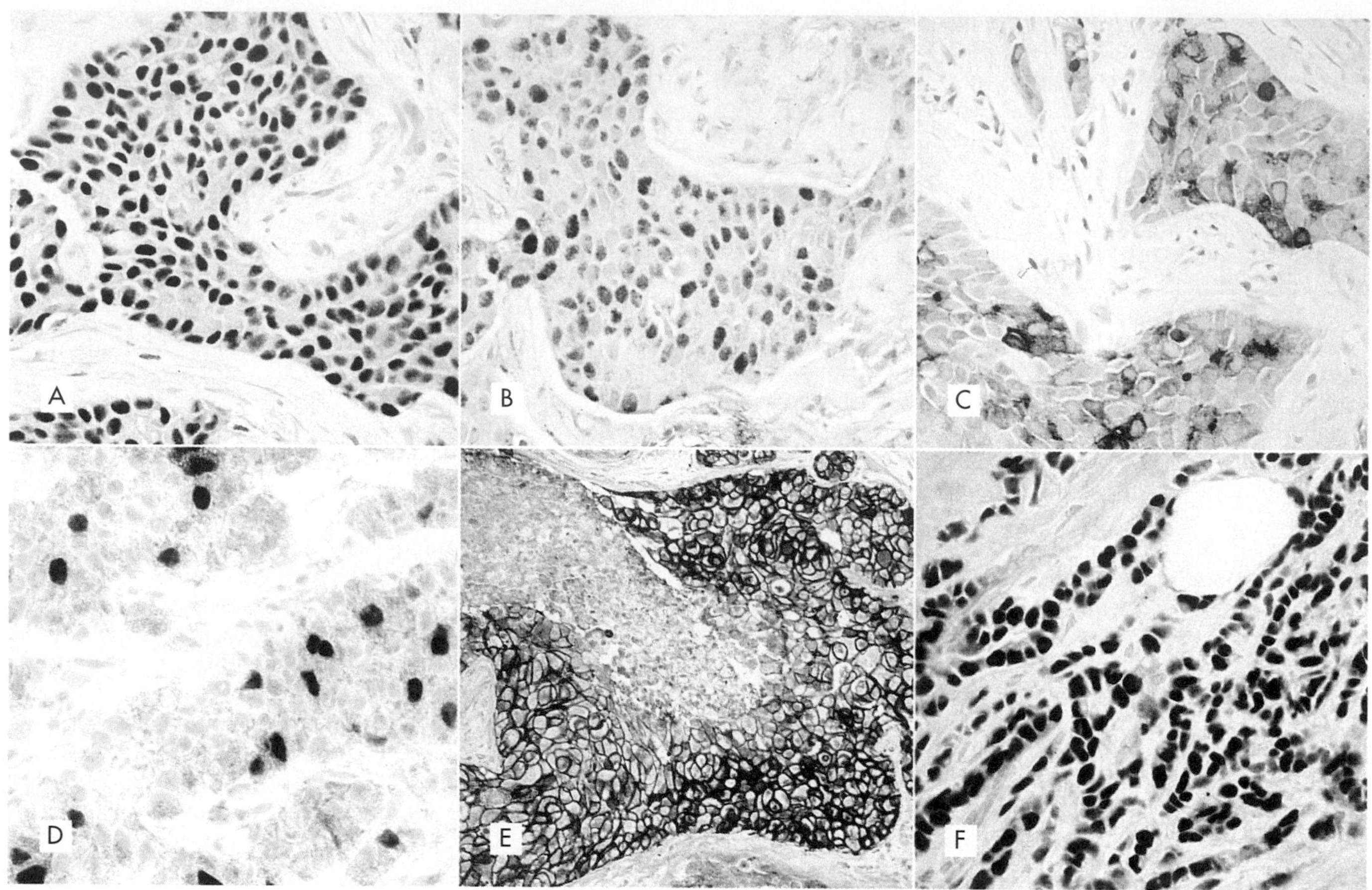

Fig. 70-29 Immunohistochemistry of breast cancer. **A,** estrogen receptors; **B,** progesterone receptors; **C,** estrogen-induced protein pS2; **D,** proliferation-associated marker Ki-67; **E,** HER-2/*neu* oncoprotein; and **F,** p53 tumor-suppressor gene product.

Diagnosis. Pathologists evaluating breast cancer are responsible for providing an accurate diagnosis, staging the tumor, and performing or facilitating special studies for prognostic factors. A comprehensive diagnostic evaluation and report should provide information on specimen size, tumor size, macroscopic appearance, histologic type, histologic grade, extent of in situ disease, lymphatic or vascular invasion, and status of surgical margins.[204] If axillary nodes have been excised, the proportion containing metastatic disease must also be reported based on meticulous sampling and examination.

Today, lumpectomies are encountered as often as mastectomies. If a breast biopsy is done for mammography-detected calcifications or for a small (less than 1 cm) mass, frozen-sections should be avoided. Presurgical and postsurgical mammograms should be compared for assessment of the adequacy of excision in the frozen-section room, and the entire specimen should be submitted for preparation of permanent sections and microscopic examination. For lesions 1 cm or larger, frozen sections are appropriate, and adequate tissue should be processed for routine histologic examination and then distributed (usually in the fresh-frozen state) to laboratories performing flow cytometry and assays for hormone receptors and other prognostic factors. Pathologists must remember that they are guardians of specimens owned by patients and must be open to distributing tissue if it is the patients' desire and in their best interest.

Surgical and medical treatment. Breast cancer treatment is based primarily on clinicopathologic staging. Only a general outline of current surgical and medical management is provided, and we refer you to recent reviews for comprehensive discussion of these controversial and rapidly evolving issues.[205]

Currently there is no consensus regarding the treatment of stage 0 breast cancer. Options include lumpectomy with local irradiation or simple mastectomy, except for very large comedo DCIS in which lower axillary nodes may also be excised. Stage I disease is usually treated by either modified radical mastectomy or by lumpectomy with axillary dissection together with local breast irradiation. These strategies are considered to be equally effective, and adjuvant medical therapy is not usually employed. The surgical management of most stage II to stage III breast cancer also involves either modified radical mastectomy or lumpectomy with local irradiation and axillary dissection, but adjuvant medical therapy is nearly always employed. In premenopausal or postmenopausal ER- and PgR-negative women this usually involves cytotoxic chemotherapy using combinations of several drugs (the most common are cyclophosphamide, methotrexate, 5-fluorouracil, and doxorubicin). Antihormonal drugs (such as tamoxifen) are used in ER-positive or PgR-positive postmenopausal women. Preoperative or neoadjuvant chemotherapy may be given to a few patients with very large or locally extensive lesions to reduce the tumor size before surgery. Stage IV breast cancer is usually treated med-

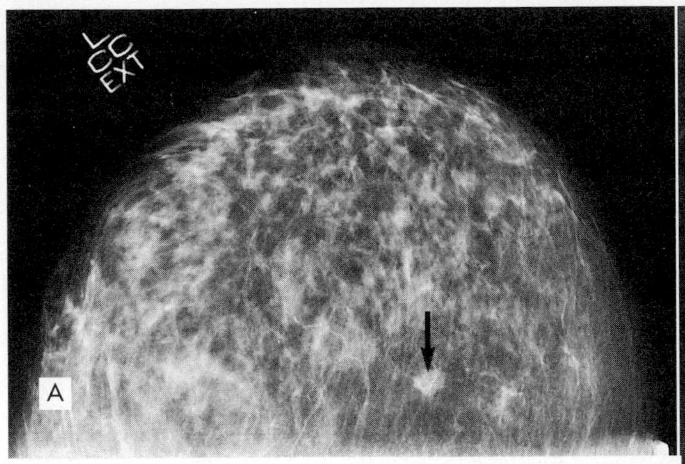

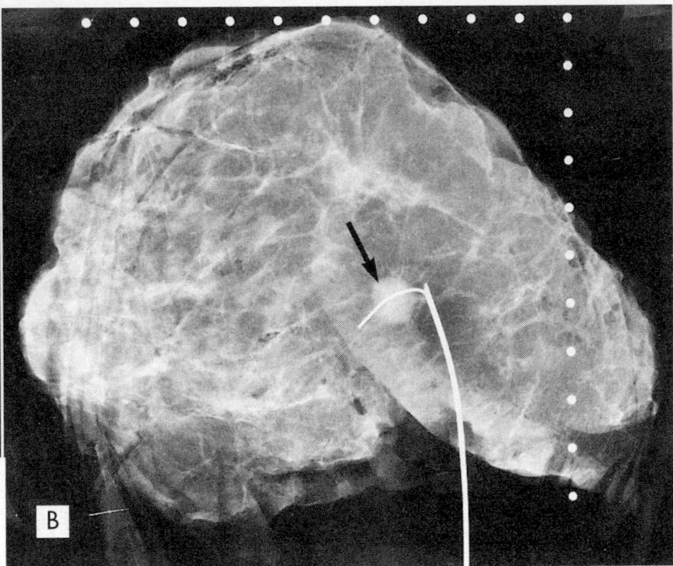

Fig. 70-30 Infiltrating ductal carcinoma (nonpalpable, 0.8 cm) treated by a needle-directed excision. **A,** Presurgical mammogram. **B,** Postsurgical mammogram.

ically. Surgery is not an option except in situations where a large tumor is excised for cosmetic or hygienic reasons.

FINE-NEEDLE ASPIRATION OF THE BREAST

Cytologic examination was first widely applied to the breast in the evaluation of exfoliated cells in nipple discharges.[206] Although a wide variety of physiologic and endocrinologic disturbances lead to a discharge from the nipple, it is occasionally caused by neoplasms such as intraductal papillomas or carcinomas. The diagnostic yield of cells is quite low, however. One large study showed only 4% of bloody discharges to contain cytologically malignant cells whereas less than 1% of serous, watery, or milky discharges revealed malignant cells.[207]

In contrast, the application of fine-needle aspiration (FNA) in the evaluation of breast lesions has had a major influence on patient management.[208] FNA offers a safe and rapid diagnostic approach, which may be employed as an office procedure without anesthesia. Prompt diagnosis relieves patient anxiety and allows time to plan definitive treatment. FNA may also be used to document recurrent or metastatic tumor or to acquire a sample for steroid receptor analysis or DNA ploidy studies.[209,210]

Procedure

Palpable lesions are readily accessible to aspiration with a 22- to 25-gauge needle attached to a disposable syringe. Some smears should be alcohol fixed and stained by the Papanicolaou method and others should be air-dried and stained with a rapid modified Wright's stain (DiffQuik). DiffQuik-stained smears allow for an immediate assessment of the procedure so that additional aspirations can be performed if necessary. Complications are minimal. Occasional hematomas may occur but are rare in the absence of a bleeding disorder. Seeding of the needle tract has never been demonstrated in FNA of the breast[211] and therapeutic measures subsequent to a diagnosis of malignancy, that is, surgery or radiation, further minimize this consideration. Pneumothorax may occur rarely, and deep-seated lesions should therefore be aspirated by a lateral approach.[212]

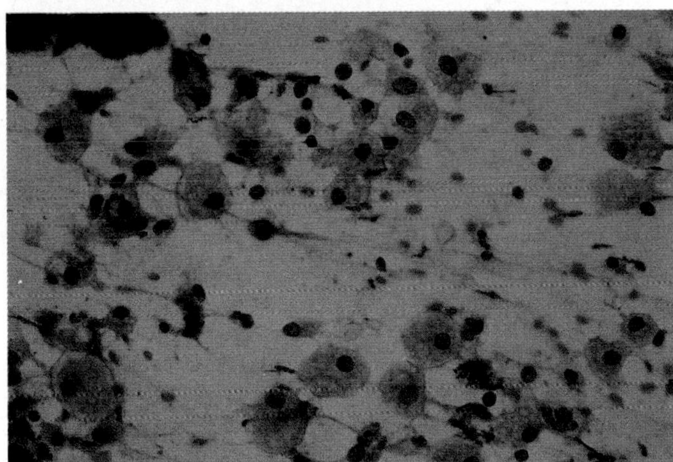

Fig. 70-31 Cystic changes with numerous foam cells. (Papanicolaou)

Major diagnostic categories

An in-depth treatment of diagnostic criteria in FNA cytology of the breast is beyond the scope of this chapter, and we refer you to other comprehensive discussions of the subject.[211,213,214]

Cysts are common and often disappear after aspiration. The cyst fluid usually contains numerous foam cells, such as those seen in nipple secretions (Figure 70-31). Pale yellow or light green fluids tend to be benign, whereas blood-tinged or turbid fluids may reflect a serious lesion and should always be submitted for cytologic examination.[215] In addition, any residual mass after cyst aspiration must itself be aspirated or removed by surgical biopsy.

Fibrocystic changes are frequently characterized by foam cells and by flat sheets of large polygonal cells with abundant granular cytoplasm, uniform round nuclei, and prominent nucleoli (Fig. 70-32). The latter cells are diagnostic of apocrine metaplasia, a common feature of fibrocystic change. Cohesive clusters of ductal epithelial cells are often present, reflecting epithelial hyperplasia. Naked bipolar nuclei are

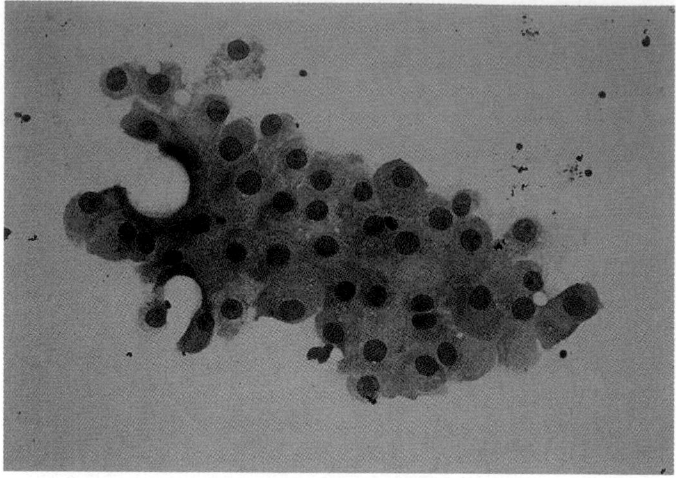

Fig. 70-32 Apocrine metaplasia with flat sheets of uniform cells with abundant granular cytoplasm. (DiffQuik)

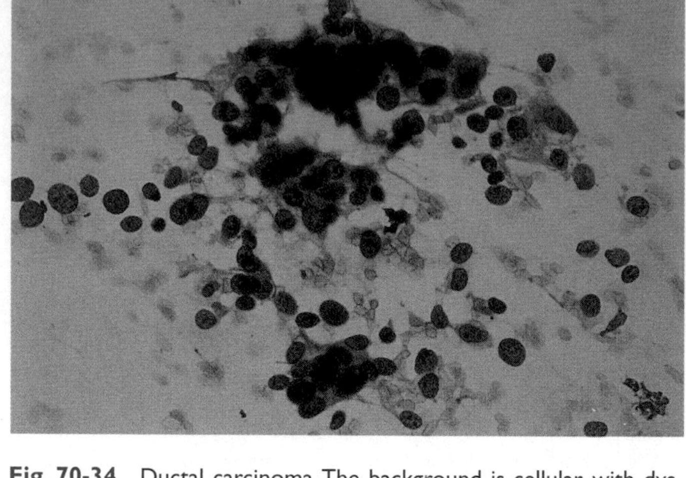

Fig. 70-34 Ductal carcinoma. The background is cellular, with dyshesive clusters of neoplastic cells. (Papanicolaou).

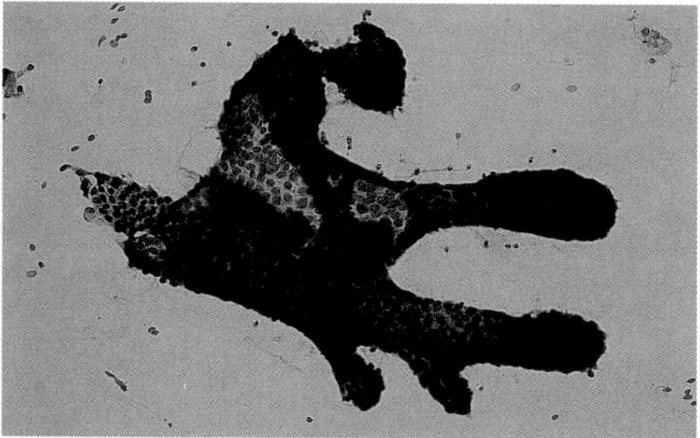

Fig. 70-33 Fibroadenoma displaying branching "antler"-like arrangements of epithelial cells. (Papanicolaou)

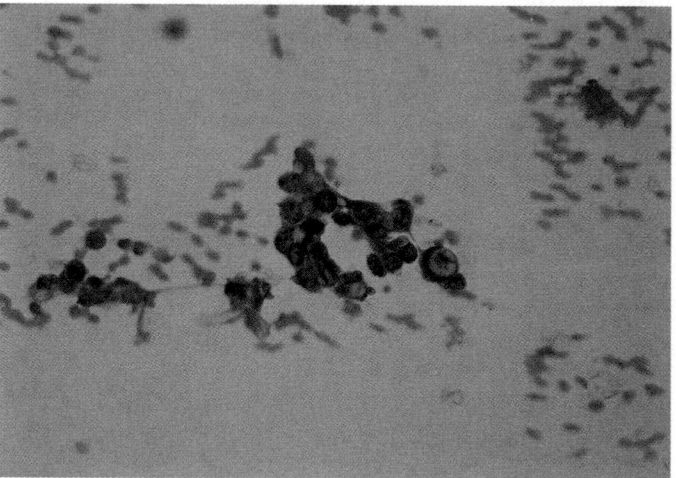

Fig. 70-35 Infiltrating lobular carcinoma. FNA specimens are often hypocellular. Some cells may have mucin vacuoles. (Papanicolaou)

prominent, both in fibrocystic change and in fibroadenoma, and are generally absent from aspirates containing malignant cells. These cells are believed to be derived from myoepithelial cells, but some have suggested a stromal origin.[216] The proliferative component of fibrocystic change, ranging from benign to atypical epithelial hyperplasia, may be recognized in FNA specimens,[217] and in some cases it may be possible to distinguish between atypical ductal hyperplasia and ductal carcinoma in situ.[218] However, any lesion with atypical cytologic features requires histopathologic examination.

Fibroadenoma aspirates are moderately cellular and are characterized by epithelial aggregates with branching, rounded fingerlike projections that have been described as resembling antlers (Fig. 70-33). Naked bipolar nuclei similar to those seen in fibrocystic change are usually numerous. Epithelial nuclei are usually uniform, but nucleoli may be prominent. Stromal fragments are present in about 40% of aspirates.[219] Increased stromal cellularity and atypia may indicate a phyllodes tumor.[220] Variant patterns may be encountered, including hypercellular specimens with epithelial atypia and dyshesion. These may mimic carcinoma.[221]

Carcinoma. Aspirates from infiltrating ductal carcinomas are hypercellular and composed of pleomorphic cells in loosely cohesive overlapping clusters (Fig. 70-34). Many single malignant cells are present, but naked bipolar nuclei are generally absent. A granular or bloody background, sometimes referred to as "tumor diathesis," may be seen. In well-differentiated tumors, nuclei may be more uniform, but malignant features are nevertheless present. Nuclear grading, similar to that for surgical biopsies, may be applied to FNA material.[210] It should be noted, however, that FNA cannot reliably distinguish between invasive ductal and intraductal carcinoma.[222] This point is especially relevant for aspirates of small, mammographically detected lesions, which are more likely to have an entirely intraductal component than larger palpable lesions.

Infiltrating lobular carcinoma poses a particularly difficult challenge.[214] Because of prominent associated desmoplasia, aspirates are often hypocellular, resulting in a false-negative diagnosis in as many as 37% of cases.[2] When tumor cells are present, they are often bland and single or in small clusters and rows. Small mucin vacuoles, when present, are diagnostically relevant (Fig. 70-35).

Other subtypes, such as medullary carcinoma and mucinous carcinoma, have characteristic features on FNA, but papillary and tubular carcinomas are more difficult to subclassify. The five-needle aspiration cytologic testing of a wide variety of less common breast tumors, such as metaplastic carcinoma, primary sarcomas, and adenoid cystic carcinoma, has also been described.[223-225] The aspirated lesion may be a tumor metastatic to the breast, and it is important to recognize such unusual aspirate patterns so that unnecessary therapy for primary breast carcinoma is avoided.[226]

Male breast lesions may also be examined by FNA. Aspirates of gynecomastia contain cohesive clusters of epithelial cells, which may show distinct nucleoli and some crowding.[227] Breast carcinomas in men have cytologic features similar to those in women.

Several clinical and pathologic settings present pitfalls for the cytologic diagnosis of breast lesions. In women of reproductive age, the hypercellularity, nuclear enlargement, and dyshesion associated with lactational changes mimic malignancy. Abundant vacuolated cytoplasm and knowledge of the clinical history will help to avoid a false-positive diagnosis of a malignancy.[228] Occasionally, hypercellularity, epithelial atypia, and cellular dispersion occur in fibroadenomas or phyllodes tumors and are falsely suggestive of carcinoma.[221,229] Clusters of small cells from intraductal papilloma or epithelial hyperplasia associated with fat necrosis can also mimic malignancy.[230] On the other hand, ductal carcinomas rarely produce a fibroadenoma-like pattern.[231]

Accuracy and pitfalls

Despite the many diagnostic challenges in breast cytology, FNA biopsy of this organ is a highly accurate diagnostic procedure. Although false-negative results have ranged from 1% to 31%, a recent interinstitutional survey found an average rate of false-negative findings of 7.8%.[232] In experienced hands, a 10% rate of false-negative results should not be exceeded. A negative FNA result should always be cautiously interpreted and viewed in its clinical context because it may simply represent sampling error. This is particularly important for stereotactically guided FNA applied to mammographically detected lesions.[233] In general, any clinically suspicious lesion must be examined through biopsy. Aspirates of infiltrating lobular carcinomas, as noted earlier, are especially likely to have false-negative results. The rates for false-positive diagnoses have ranged from 0% to 4%, with the great majority of aspirates having been falsely labeled "suspicious." False-positive diagnoses are of course unacceptable because they could lead to unnecessary mastectomy. In many settings, confirmation with frozen sections may be required until the cytopathologist acquires the level of expertise necessary for making a defin-itive diagnosis of primary carcinoma. Many cytopathologists, however, have achieved a high level of diagnostic accuracy, and FNA biopsy of the breast will continue to progress as an important procedure.

REFERENCES

Introduction

1. Symonds DA, Copeland BE, Drane A et al: Pathologic correlation in mammographically directed breast biopsies, *Arch Pathol Lab Med* 116:28, 1992.
2. Kline TS, Joshi LP, Neal HS: Fine-needle aspiration of the breast: diagnoses and pitfalls: a review of 3545 cases, *Cancer* 44:1458, 1979.
3. Linell F, Ostberg G, Rank F: Changes in diagnostic pattern in breast pathology, *Lancet* 335:1402, 1990.
4. Frantz VK, Pickren JW, Melcher GW, Auchincloss H Jr: Incidence of chronic cystic disease in so-called "normal breasts": a study based on 225 postmortem examinations, *Cancer* 4:762, 1951.
5. Bartow SA, Pathak DR, Black WC et al: Prevalence of benign, atypical and malignant breast lesions in populations at different risk for breast cancer: a forensic autopsy study, *Cancer* 60:2751, 1987.

Growth, development and normal anatomy

6. Fawcett DW: Mammary gland. In Bloom & Fawcett: *A textbook of histology*, Philadelphia, 1976, Saunders.
7. Bussolati G, Gugliotta P, Sapino A et al: Chromogranin-reactive endocrine cells in argyrophilic carcinomas ("carcinoids") and normal tissue of the breast, *Am J Pathol* 120:186, 1985.
8. Petersen OW, Hoyer, van Deurs B: Frequency and distribution of estrogen receptor-positive cells in normal, nonlactating human breast tissue, *Cancer Res* 47:5748, 1987.
9. Anbazhagan R, Bartek J, Monaghan P, Gusterson BA: Growth and development of the human infant breast, *Am J Anat* 192:407, 1991.
10. Russo J, Russo IH: Development of the human mammary gland. In Neville MC, Daniel CW, editors: *The mammary gland: development, regulation, and function*, New York and London, 1987, Plenum Press.
11. Monaghan P, Perusinghe NP, Cowen P, Gusterson BA: Peripubertal human breast development, *Anat Rec* 226:501, 1990.
12. Rudland PS: Histochemical organization and cellular composition of ductal buds in developing human breast: evidence of cytochemical intermediates between epithelial and myoepithelial cells, *J Histochem Cytochem* 39:1471, 1991.
13. Hutson SW, Cowen PN, Bird CC: Morphometric studies of age related changes in normal human breast and their significance for evolution of mammary cancer, *J Clin Pathol* 38:281, 1985.
14. Vogel PM, Georgiade NG, Fetter BF et al: The correlation of histologic changes in the human breast with the menstrual cycle, *Am J Pathol* 104:23, 1981.
15. Longacre TA, Bartow SA: A correlative morphologic study of human breast and endometrium in the menstrual cycle, *Am J Surg Pathol* 10:382, 1986.
16. Anderson TJ, Ferguson DJP, Raab GM: Cell turnover in the "resting" human breast: influence of parity, contraceptive pill, age and laterality, *Br J Cancer* 46:376, 1982.
17. Going JJ, Anderson TJ, Battersby S, Macintyre CCA: Proliferative and secretory activity in human breast during natural and artificial menstrual cycles, *Am J Pathol* 130:193, 1988.
18. Joshi K, Smith JA, Perusinghe N, Monoghan P: Cell proliferation in the human mammary epithelium: differential contributions by epithelial and myoepithelial cells, *Am J Pathol* 124:199, 1986.
19. Fowler PA, Casey CE, Cameron GG et al: Cyclic changes in composition and volume of the breast during the menstrual cycle, measured by magnetic resonance imaging, *Br J Obstet Gynaecol* 97:595, 1990.
20. Silva JS, Georgiade GS, Dilley WG et al: Menstrual cycle-dependent variations of breast cyst fluid proteins and sex steroid receptors in the normal human breast, *Cancer* 51:1297, 1983.

Hypertrophies and hyperplasias

21. Braunstein GD: Gynecomastia, *N Engl J Med* 328:490, 1993.
22. Bannayan GA, Hajdu SI: Gynecomastia: clinicopathologic study of 351 cases, *Am J Clin Pathol* 57:431, 1972.
23. Kupfer D, Dignman D, Broadbent R: Juvenile breast hypertrophy: report of a familial pattern and review of the literature, *Plast Reconstr Surg* 90:303, 1992.
24. Oberman HA: Breast lesions in the adolescent female, *Pathol Annu* 14(pt 1):175, 1979.

Nonneoplastic lesions

Inflammatory lesions

25. Scholefield JH, Duncan JL, Rogers K: Review of a hospital experience of breast abscesses, *Br J Surg* 74:469, 1987.
26. Rogers K: Breast abscesses and problems with lactation. In Smallwood JA, Taylor I, editors: *Benign breast disease*, Baltimore, 1990, Urban & Schwarzenberg.
27. Bundred NJ, Dixon JMJ, Lumsden AB et al: Are the lesions of duct ectasia sterile? *Br J Surg* 72:844, 1985.

28. Smith BL: Duct ectasia, periductal mastitis, and breast infections. In Harris JR, Hellman S, Henderson IC, Kinne DW, editors: *Breast diseases*, Philadelphia, 1991, Lippincott.
29. Lee BJ, Adair F: Traumatic fat necrosis of the female breast and its differentiation from carcinoma, *Ann Surg* 72:188, 1920.
30. Adair F, Munzer J: Fat necrosis of the female breast, *Am J Surg* 74:117, 1947.
31. Haagensen CD: *Diseases of the breast*, ed 3, Philadelphia, 1986, Saunders.
32. Jørgensen MB, Nielsen DM: Diagnosis and treatment of granulomatous mastitis, *Am J Med* 93:97, 1992.
33. Tomaszewski JE, Brooks JSJ, Hicks D, LiVolsi VA: Diabetic mastopathy: a distinctive clinicopathologic entity, *Hum Pathol* 23:780, 1992.
34. Schwartz IS, Strauchen JA: Lymphocytic mastopathy: an autoimmune disease of the breast? *Am J Clin Pathol* 93:725, 1990.
35. Thomsen JL, Christensen L, Nielsen M et al: Histologic changes and silicone concentrations in human breast tissue surrounding silicone breast prostheses, *Plast Reconstr Surg* 85:38, 1990.
36. Barker DE, Retsky MI, Schultz S: "Bleeding" of silicone from bag-gel breast implants and its clinical relation to fibrous capsule reaction, *Plast Reconstr Surg* 61:836, 1978.
37. Hausner RJ, Schoen FJ, Mendez-Fernandez MA et al: Migration of silicone gel to axillary lymph nodes after prosthetic mammoplasty, *Arch Pathol Lab Med* 105:371, 1981.
38. Independent Advisory Committee on Silicone-Gel-Filled Implants: Summary of the report on silicone-gel–filled breast implants, *Can Med Assoc J* 147:1141, 1992.

Fibrocystic change

39. Foote FW, Stewart FW: Comparative studies of cancerous versus noncancerous breasts, *Ann Surg* 121:6, 1945.
40. Love SM, Gelman RS, Silen W: Fibrocystic "disease" of the breast: a nondisease? *N Engl J Med* 307:1010, 1982.
41. Hutter RVP: Goodbye to "fibrocystic disease," *N Engl J Med* 312:179, 1985.
42. Cole P, Elwood JM, Kaplan SD: Incidence rates and risk factors of benign breast neoplasms, *Am J Epidemiol* 108:112, 1978.
43. Ernster VL: The epidemiology of benign breast disease, *Epidemiol Rev* 3:184, 1981.
44. Schnitt SJ, Jimi A, Kojiro M: The increasing prevalence of benign proliferative breast lesions in Japanese women, *Cancer* 71:2528, 1993.
45. Parazzini F, La Vecchia C, Franceschi S et al: Risk factors for pathologically confirmed benign breast disease, *Am J Epidemiol* 120:115, 1984.
46. McGonigle KF, Huggins GR: Oral contraceptives and breast disease, *Fertil Steril* 56:799, 1991.
47. Berkowitz GS, Kelsey JL, LiVolsi VA et al: Exogenous hormone use and fibrocystic breast disease by histopathologic component, *Int J Cancer* 34:443, 1984.
48. LiVolsi VA, Stadel BV, Kelsey JL et al: Fibrocystic breast disease in oral-contraceptive users: a histopathological evaluation of epithelial atypia, *N Engl J Med* 299:381, 1978.
49. Ernster VL, Wrensch MR, Petrakis NL et al: Benign and malignant breast disease: initial study results of serum and breast fluid analyses of endogenous estrogens, *J Natl Cancer Inst* 79:949, 1987.
50. Vecchia CL, Franceschi S, Parazzini F et al: Benign breast disease and consumption of beverages containing methylxanthines, *J Natl Cancer* Inst 74:995, 1985.
51. Hutter RVP, Albores-Saavedra J, Anderson E et al: Is 'fibrocystic disease' of the breast precancerous? *Arch Pathol Lab Med* 110:171, 1986.
52. Page DL, Vander Zwaag R, Rogers LW et al: Relation between component parts of fibrocystic disease complex and breast cancer, *J Natl Cancer Inst* 61:1055, 1978.
53. Dupont WD, Parl FF, Hartmann WH et al: Breast cancer risk associated with proliferative breast disease and atypical hyperplasia, *Cancer* 71:1258, 1993.
54. Sterns EE: The natural history of macroscopic cysts in the breast, *Surg Gynecol Obstet* 174:36, 1992.
55. Bässler R: The morphology of hormone induced structural changes in the female breast, *Curr Top Pathol* 53:1, 1970.
56. Greenblatt RB, Mahesh VB, Sullivan D: Gross cystic disease of the breast, *Maturitas* 9:171, 1987.
57. Wellings SR, Jensen HM, Marcum RG: An atlas of subgross pathology of the human breast with special reference to possible precancerous lesions, *J Natl Cancer Inst* 55:231, 1975.
58. Rivera-Pomar JM, Vilanova JR, Burgos-Bretones JJ, Arocena G: Focal fibrous disease of breast: A common entity in young women, *Virchows Arch [A] Pathol Anat Histol* 386:59, 1980.
59. Azzopardi JG: Problems in breast pathology. In Bennington JL, consulting editor: *Major problems in pathology*, Philadelphia, 1987, Saunders.
60. Page DL, Anderson TJ: *Diagnostic histopathology of the breast*, New York, 1987, Churchill Livingstone.
61. Taylor HB, Norris HJ: Epithelial invasion of nerves in benign diseases of the breast, *Cancer* 20:2245, 1967.
62. Schnitt SJ, Connolly JL, Tavassoli FA et al: Interobserver reproducibility in the diagnosis of ductal proliferative breast lesions using standardized criteria, *Am J Surg Pathol* 16:1133, 1992.
63. Anderson JA, Carter D, Linell F: A symposium of sclerosing duct lesions of the breast, *Pathol Annu* 21(pt 2):145, 1986.

Neoplastic lesions

Stromal neoplasms

64. Hoda SA, Cranor ML, Rosen PP: Hemangiomas of the breast with atypical histologic features: further analysis of histological subtypes confirming their benign character, *Am J Surg Pathol* 16:553, 1992.
65. Jozefczyk MA, Rosen PP: Vascular tumors of the breast, *Am J Surg Pathol* 9:491, 1985.
66. DeMay RM, Kay S: Granular cell tumor of the breast, *Pathol Annu* 19(pt 2):121, 1984.
67. Callery CD, Rosen PP, Kinne DW: Sarcoma of the breast: a study of 32 patients with reappraisal of classification and therapy, *Ann Surg* 201:527, 1985.
68. Rosen PP, Kimmel M, Ernsberger D: Mammary angiosarcoma: the prognostic significance of tumor differentiation, *Cancer* 62:2145, 1988.
68a. Stewart FW, Treves N: Lymphangiosarcoma in post-mastectomy lymphoedema: a report of six cases in elephantiasis chirurgica, *Cancer* 1:64, 1948.
69. Wargotz ES, Norris HJ, Austin RM et al: Fibromatosis of the breast: a clinical and pathological study of 28 cases, *Am J Surg Pathol* 11:38, 1987.
70. Jones MW, Norris HJ, Wargotz ES, Weiss SW: Fibrosarcoma-malignant fibrous histiocytoma of the breast: a clinicopathological study of 32 cases, *Am J Surg Pathol* 16:667, 1992.

Complex stromal-epithelial neoplasms

71. Ferguson CM, Powell RW: Breast masses in young women, *Arch Surg* 124:1338, 1989.
72. Kern WH, Clark RW: Retrogression of fibroadenomas of the breast, *Am J Surg* 126:59, 1973.
73. Carter CL, Corle DK, Micozzi MS et al: A prospective study of the development of breast cancer in 16,692 women with benign breast disease, *Am J Epidemiol* 128:467, 1988.
74. Sawhney N, Garrahan N, Douglas-Jones AG, Williams ED: Epithelial-stromal interactions in tumors: a morphologic study of fibroepithelial tumors of the breast, *Cancer* 70:2115, 1992.
75. Mies C, Rosen PP: Juvenile fibroadenoma with atypical epithelial hyperplasia, *Am J Surg Pathol* 11:184, 1987.
76. Fondo EY, Rosen PP, Fracchia AA, Urban JA: The problem of carcinoma developing in a fibroadenoma: recent experience at Memorial Hospital, *Cancer* 43:563, 1979.
77. Diaz NM, Palmer JO, McDivitt RW: Carcinoma arising within fibroadenomas of the breast: a clinicopathologic study of 105 patients, *Am J Clin Pathol* 95:614, 1991.
78. Pike AM, Oberman HA: Juvenile (cellular) adenofibromas, *Am J Surg Pathol* 9:730, 1985.
79. Ashikari R, Farrow JH, O'Hara J: Fibroadenomas in the breast of juveniles, *Surg Gynecol Obstet* 132:259, 1971.
80. *Dorland's illustrated medical dictionary*, ed 28, Philadelphia, 1994, Saunders.
81. Grimes MM: Cystosarcoma phyllodes of the breast: histologic features, flow cytometric analysis, and clinical correlations, *Mod Pathol* 5:232, 1992.

82. Keelan PA, Myers JL, Wold LE et al: Phyllodes tumor: clinicopathologic review of 60 patients and flow cytometric analysis in 30 patients, *Hum Pathol* 23:1048, 1992.
83. Hawkins RE, Schofield JB, Fisher C et al: The clinical and histologic criteria that predict metastases from cystosarcoma phyllodes, *Cancer* 69:141, 1992.
84. Jones MW, Norris HJ, Wargotz ES: Hamartomas of the breast, *Surg Gynecol Obstet* 173:54, 1991.
85. Linell F, Östberg G, Söderström J et al: Breast hamartomas: an important entity in mammary pathology, *Virchows Arch [A] (Pathol Anat Histol)* 383:253, 1979.

Benign epithelial neoplasms

86. Hertel BF, Zaloudek C, Kempson RL: Breast adenomas, *Cancer* 37:2891, 1976.
87. O'Hara MF, Page DL: Adenomas of the breast and ectopic breast under lactational influences, *Hum Pathol* 16:707, 1985.
88. Diaz NM, Palmer JO, Wick MR: Erosive adenomatosis of the nipple: histology, immunohistology, and differential diagnosis, *Mod Pathol* 5:179, 1992.
89. Rosen PP: Adenomyoepithelioma of the breast, *Hum Pathol* 18:1232, 1987.
90. Ohuchi N, Abe Rikiya, Takahashi T, Tezuka F: Origin and extension of intraductal papillomas of the breast: a three-dimensional reconstruction study, *Breast Cancer Res Treat* 4:117, 1984.
91. Murad TM, Contesso G, Mouriesse H: Papillary tumors of large lactiferous ducts, *Cancer* 48:122, 1981.
92. Kraus FT, Neubecker RD: The differential diagnosis of papillary tumors of the breast, *Cancer* 15:444, 1962.
93. Carter D: Intraductal papillary tumors of the breast: a study of 78 cases, *Cancer* 39:1689, 1977.

Carcinoma of the breast

Epidemiology

94. Harris JR, Lippman ME, Veronesi U, Willett W: Breast Cancer, *N Engl J Med* 327:319,390,473, 1992.
95. Armstrong B, Doll R: Environmental factors and cancer incidence and mortality in different countries with special reference to dietary practices, *Int J Cancer* 15:617, 1975
96. Boring CC, Squires TS, Tong T: Cancer statistics: 1993, CA *Cancer J Clin* 43:7, 1993.
97. *Cancer facts and figures—1993*, Atlanta, 1993, American Cancer Society.
98. Holford TR, Roush GC, McKay LA: Trends in female breast cancer in Connecticut and the United States, *J Clin Epidemiol* 44:29, 1991.
99. Miller BA, Feuer EJ, Hankey BF: Recent incidence trends for breast cancer in women and the relevance of early detection: an update, *CA Cancer J Clin* 43:27, 1993.

Etiology and risk factors

100. Gail MH, Brinton LA, Byar DP et al: Projecting individualized probabilities of developing breast cancer for white females who are being examined annually, *J Natl Cancer Inst* 81:1879, 1989.
101. Kampert JB, Whittemore AS, Paffenbarger RS Jr: Combined effect of childbearing, menstrual events, and body size on age-specific breast cancer risk, *Am J Epidemiol* 128:962, 1988.
102. White E: Projected changes in breast cancer incidence due to the trend toward delayed childbearing, *Am J Public Health* 77:495, 1987.
103. Trichopoulos D, MacMahon B, Cole P: Menopause and breast cancer risk, *J Natl Cancer Inst* 48:605, 1972.
104. Colditz GA, Stampfer MJ, Willett WC et al: Prospective study of estrogen replacement therapy and risk of breast cancer in postmenopausal women, *JAMA* 264:2648, 1990.
105. Romieu I, Willett WC, Colditz GA et al: Prospective study of oral contraceptive use and risk of breast cancer in women, *J Natl Cancer Inst* 81:1313, 1989.
106. McGregor DH, Land CE, Choi K et al: Breast cancer incidence among atomic bomb survivors, Hiroshima and Nagasaki, 1950-1969, *J Natl Cancer Inst* 59:799, 1977.
107. Boice JD Jr, Monson RR: Breast cancer in women after repeated fluoroscopic examination of the chest, *J Natl Cancer Inst* 59:823, 1977.
108. Dupont WD, Page DL: Risk factors for breast cancer in women with proliferative breast disease, *N Engl J Med* 312:146, 1985.
109. London SJ, Connolly JL, Schnitt SJ, Colditz GA: A prospective study of benign breast disease and the risk of breast cancer, *JAMA* 267:941, 1992.
110. Tretli S: Height and weight in relation to breast cancer morbidity and mortality: a prospective study of 570,000 women in Norway, *Int J Cancer* 44:23, 1989.
111. Longnecker MP, Berlin JA, Orza MJ, Chalmers TC: A meta-analysis of alcohol consumption in relation to risk of breast cancer, *JAMA* 260:652, 1988.
112. Rosai J: Borderline epithelial lesions of the breast, *Am J Surg Pathol* 15:209, 1991.
113. Schnitt SJ, Connolly JL, Tavassoli FA et al: Interobserver reproducibility in the diagnosis of ductal proliferative breast lesions using standardized criteria, *Am J Surg Pathol* 16:1133, 1992.
114. Rosen PP, Braun DW, Kinne DE: The clinical significance of pre-invasive breast carcinoma, *Cancer* 46:919, 1980.
115. Page DL, Dupont WD, Rogers LW, Landenberger M: Intraductal carcinoma of the breast: follow-up after biopsy only, *Cancer* 49:751, 1982.
116. Connolly JL, Schnitt SJ: Benign breast disease: resolved and unresolved issues, *Cancer* 71:1187, 1993.
117. Haagensen CD, Lane N, Lattes R, Bodian C: Lobular neoplasia (so-called lobular carcinoma in situ) of the breast, *Cancer* 42:737, 1978.
118. Page DL, Kidd TE Jr, Dupont WD et al: Lobular neoplasia of the breast: higher risk for subsequent invasive cancer predicted by more extensive disease, *Hum Pathol* 22:1232, 1991.

Noninvasive breast carcinoma

119. Page DL, Anderson TJ, Lowell WR: Carcinoma in situ (CIS). In Page DL, Anderson TJ, editors: *Diagnostic histopathology of the breast,* Edinburgh, 1987, Churchill Livingstone.
120. Simpson JF, Page DL: Prognostic value of histopathology of the breast, *Semin Oncol* 19:254, 1992.
121. Page DL, Anderson TJ, Sakamoto G: Infiltrating carcinoma: major histological types. In Page DL, Anderson TJ, editors: *Diagnostic histopathology of the breast,* Edinburgh, 1987, Churchill Livingstone.
122. Page DL: Prognosis and breast cancer: recognition of lethal and favorable prognostic types, *Am J Surg Pathol* 15:334, 1991.
123. Lagios MD, Margolin FR, Westdahl PR, Rose MR: Mammographically detected duct carcinoma in situ: frequency of local recurrence following tylectomy and prognostic effect of nuclear grade on local recurrence, *Cancer* 63:618, 1989.
124. Patchefsky AS, Schwartz GF, Finkelstein SD et al: Heterogeneity of intraductal carcinoma of the breast, *Cancer* 63:731, 1989.
125. Silverstein MJ, Cohlan BF, Gierson ED et al: Duct carcinoma in situ: 227 cases without microinvasion, *Eur J Cancer* 28:630, 1992.
126. Bellamy COC, McDonald C, Salter DM et al: Noninvasive ductal carcinoma of the breast: the relevance of histologic categorization, *Hum Pathol* 24:16, 1993.
127. Alpers CE, Wellings SR: The prevalence of carcinoma in situ in normal and cancer-associated breasts, *Hum Pathol* 16:796, 1985.
128. Robbins GF, Berg JW: Bilateral primary breast cancers: a prospective clinicopathological study, *Cancer* 17:1501, 1964.
129. Page DL, Anderson TJ, Rogers LW: Epithelia hyperplasia. In Page DL, Anderson TJ, editors: *Diagnostic histopathology of the breast,* Edinburgh, 1987, Churchill Livingstone.
130. Solin LJ, Recht A, Fourquet A et al: Ten-year results of breast-conserving surgery and definitive irradiation for intraductal carcinoma (ductal carcinoma in situ) of the breast, *Cancer* 68:2337, 1991.
131. Poller DN, Snead DRJ, Roberts EC et al: Oestrogen receptor expression in ductal carcinoma in situ of the breast: relationship to flow cytometric analysis of DNA and expression of the c-erbB-2 oncoprotein, *Br J Cancer* 68:156, 1993.
132. Meyer JS: Cell kinetics of histologic variants of in situ breast carcinoma, *Breast Cancer Res Treat* 7:171, 1986.
133. Aasmundstad TA, Haugen OA: DNA ploidy in intraductal breast carcinomas, *Eur J Cancer* 26:956, 1990.
134. Schwartz GF, Finkel GC, Garcia JC, Patchefsky AS: Subclinical ductal carcinoma in situ of the breast, *Cancer* 70:2468, 1992.

135. Carter D, Orr SL, Merino MJ: Intracystic papillary carcinoma of the breast after mastectomy, radiotherapy or excisional biopsy alone, *Cancer* 52:14, 1983.
136. Rosen PP, Kosloff C, Lieberman PH et al: Lobular carcinoma in situ of the breast: detailed analysis of 99 patients with average follow-up of 24 years, *Am J Surg Pathol* 2:225, 1978.

Invasive breast carcinoma

137. Dixon JM, Page DL, Anderson TJ et al: Long-term survivors after breast cancer, *Br J Surg* 72:445, 1985.
138. McGuire WL, Tandon AK, Allred DC et al: How to use prognostic factors in axillary node-negative breast cancer patients, *J Natl Cancer Inst* 82:1006, 1990.
139. Elston CW, Ellis IO: Pathological prognostic factors in breast cancer. I. The value of histological grade in breast cancer: experience from a large study with long-term follow-up, *Histopathology* 19:403, 1991.
140. Bloom HJG, Richardson WW: Histological grading and prognosis in breast cancer, *Br J Cancer* 11:359, 1957.
141. Anderson TJ, Lamb J, Donnan P et al: Comparative pathology of breast cancer in a randomized trial of screening, *Br J Cancer* 64:108, 1991.
142. Poen JC, Tran L, Juillard G et al: Conservation therapy for invasive lobular carcinoma of the breast, *Cancer* 69:2789, 1992.
143. Dixon JM, Anderson TJ, Page DL et al: Infiltrating lobular carcinoma of the breast: an evaluation of the incidence and consequence of bilateral disease, *Br J Surg* 70:513, 1983.
144. Wheeler JE, Enterline HT: Lobular carcinoma of the breast in situ and infiltrating, *Pathol Annu* 11(pt 2):161, 1976.
145. Neuman W: Lobular carcinoma of the female breast, *Ann Surg* 164:305, 1966.
146. Dixon JM, Anderson TJ, Page DL et al: Infiltrating lobular carcinoma of the breast, *Histopathology* 6:149, 1982.
147. Rapin V, Contesso G, Mouriesse H et al: Medullary breast carcinoma: a reevaluation of 95 cases of breast cancer with inflammatory stroma, *Cancer* 61:2503, 1988.
148. Wargotz ES, Silverberg SG: Medullary carcinoma of the breast: a clinicopathologic study with appraisal of current diagnostic criteria, *Hum Pathol* 19:1340, 1988.
149. Ridolfi RL, Rosen PP, Port A et al: Medullary carcinoma of the breast: a clinicopathologic study with 10 year follow-up, *Cancer* 40:1365, 1977.
150. Fisher ER, Kenny JP, Sass R et al: Medullary cancer of the breast revisited, *Breast Cancer Res Treat* 16:215, 1990.
151. Patchefsky AS, Shaber GS, Schwartz GF et al: The pathology of breast cancer detected by mass population screening, *Cancer* 40:1659, 1977.
152. McDivitt RW, Boyce W, Gersell D: Tubular carcinoma of the breast: clinical and pathological observations concerning 135 cases, *Am J Surg Pathol* 6:401, 1982.
153. Deos PH, Norris HJ: Well-differentiated (tubular) carcinoma of the breast. A clinicopathologic study of 145 pure and mixed cases, *Am J Clin Pathol* 78:1, 1982.
154. Cooper HS, Patchefsky AS, Krall RA: Tubular carcinoma of the breast, *Cancer* 42:2334, 1978.
155. Taylor HB, Norris HJ: Well-differentiated carcinoma of the breast, *Cancer* 25:687, 1970.
156. Venable JG, Schwartz AM, Silverberg SG: Infiltrating cribriform carcinoma of the breast: a distinctive clinicopathologic entity, *Hum Pathol* 21:333, 1990.
157. Rosen PP, Lesser ML, Kinne DW: Breast carcinoma at the extremes of age: a comparison of patients younger than 35 years and older than 75 years, *J Surg Oncol* 28:90, 1985.
158. Norris HJ, Taylor HB: Prognosis of mucinous (gelatinous) carcinoma of the breast, *Cancer* 18:879, 1965.
159. Silverberg SG, Kay S, Chitale AR, Levitt SH: Colloid carcinoma of the breast, *Am J Clin Pathol* 55:355, 1971.
160. Clayton F: Pure mucinous carcinomas of breast: morphologic features and prognostic correlates, *Hum Pathol* 17:34, 1986.
161. Rosen PP: Mucocele-like tumours of the breast, *Am J Surg Pathol* 10:464, 1986.
162. Ashikari R, Park K, Huvos AG, Urban JA: Paget's disease of the breast, *Cancer* 26:680, 1970.
163. Jaiyesimi IA, Buzdar AU, Hortobagyi G: Inflammatory breast cancer: a review, *J Clin Oncol* 10:1014, 1992.
164. Wargotz ES, HJ Norris: Metaplastic carcinomas of the breast. IV. Squamous cell carcinoma of ductal origin, *Cancer* 65:272, 1990.
165. Wargotz ES, Deos PH, Norris HJ: Metaplastic carcinomas of the breast. II. Spindle cell carcinoma, *Hum Pathol* 20:732, 1989.
166. Wargotz ES, Norris HJ: Metaplastic carcinomas of the breast. III. Carcinosarcoma, *Cancer* 64:1490, 1989.
167. Merino MJ, LiVolsi VA: Signet ring carcinoma of the female breast: a clinicopathologic analysis of 24 cases, *Cancer* 48:1830, 1981.
168. Fisher ER, Palekar AS, Redmond C et al: Pathologic findings from the national surgical adjuvant breast project (protocol no. 4). VI. Invasive papillary cancer, *Am J Clin Pathol* 73:313, 1980.
169. Bussolati G, Papotti M, Sapino A et al: Endocrine markers in argyrophilic carcinomas of the breast, *Am J Surg Pathol* 11:248, 1987.
170. Peters GN, Wolff M: Adenoid cystic carcinoma of the breast: report of 11 new cases, review of the literature and discussion of biological behavior, *Cancer* 52:680, 1982.
171. McDivitt RW, Stewart FW: Breast carcinoma in children, *JAMA* 195:388, 1966.
172. Hull MT, Priest JB, Broadie TA et al: Glycogen-rich clear cell carcinoma of the breast: a light and electron microscopic study, *Cancer* 48:2003, 1981.
173. Fisher ER: The impact of pathology on the biologic, diagnostic, prognostic and therapeutic considerations in breast cancer, *Surg Clin North Am* 64:1073, 1984.
174. International (Ludwig) Breast Cancer Study Group: Prognostic importance of occult axillary lymph node micrometastases from breast cancers, *Lancet* 335:1565, 1990.
175. Raymond WA, Leon ASY: Immunoperoxidase staining in the detection of lymph node-metastases in stage I breast cancer, *Pathology* 21:11, 1989.
176. Lee YTM: Patterns of metastasis and natural courses of breast carcinoma, *Cancer Metastasis Rev* 4:153, 1985.
177. Hagemeister FB, Buzdar AU, Luna MA, Blumenschein GR: Causes of death in breast cancer: a clinicopatholigic study, *Cancer* 46:162, 1980.
178. Nielsen M, Andersen JA, Henriksen FW et al: Metastases to the breast from extramammary carcinomas, *Acta Pathol Microbiol Scand (A)* 89:251, 1981.
179. McCrea ES, Johnston C, Haney PJ: Metastases to the breast, *Am J Roentgenol* 141:685, 1983.
180. Mambo NC, Burke JS, Butler JJ: Primary malignant lymphomas of the breast, *Cancer* 39:2033, 1977.

Prognosis

181. Bloom HJG, Richardson WW, Harries EJ: Natural history of untreated breast cancer (1805-1933): comparison of untreated and treated cases according to histological grade of malignancy, *Br Med J* 2:213, 1962.
182. Spiessl B, Beahrs OH, Hermanek P et al, editors: *TNM atlas: illustrated guide to the TNM/pTNM-classification of malignant tumours,* ed 3, New York, 1989, Springer-Verlag.
183. Fisher ER: Prognostic and therapeutic significance of pathological features of breast cancer, *NCI Monogr* 11:29, 1986.
184. Osborne CK: Receptors. In Harris JR, Hellman S, Henderson IC, Kinne DW, editors: *Breast diseases,* Philadelphia, 1991, Lippincott.
185. Foekens JA, Rio M-C, Seguin P et al: Prediction of relapse and survival in breast cancer patients by pS2 protein status, *Cancer Res* 50:3832, 1990.
186. Simpson JF, Dutt PL, Page DL: Expression of mitoses per thousand cells and cell density in breast in breast carcinoma: a proposal, *Hum Pathol* 23:608, 1992
187. Clark GM, Dressler LG, Owens MA et al: Prediction of relapse or survival in patients with node-negative breast cancer by DNA flow cytometry, *N Engl J Med* 320:627, 1989.
188. Veronese SM, Gambacorta M, Gottardi O et al: Proliferation index as a prognostic marker in breast cancer, *Cancer* 71:3926, 1993.
189. Sainsbury JRC, Farndon JR, Needham GK et al: Epidermal-growth-factor receptor status as predictor of early recurrence of and death from breast cancer, *Lancet* 1:1398, 1987.

190. Tandon AK, Clark GM, Chamness GC et al: HER-2/*neu* oncogene protein and prognosis in breast cancer, *J Clin Oncol* 7:1120, 1989.
191. Allred DC, Clark GC, Tandon AK et al: HER-2/*neu* in node-negative breast cancer: prognostic significance of overexpression influenced by the presence of in situ carcinoma, *J Clin Oncol* 10:599, 1992.
192. Allred DC, Clark GC, Elledge R et al: Association of p53 protein expression with tumor cell proliferation rate and clinical outcome in node-negative breast cancer, *J Natl Cancer Inst* 85:200, 1993.
193. Martignone S, Menard S, Bufalino R et al: Prognostic significance of the 67-kilodalton laminin receptor expression in human breast carcinomas, *J Natl Cancer Inst* 85:398, 1993.
194. Thorpe SM, Rochefort H, Garcia M et al: Association between high concentrations of Mr 52,000 cathepsin D and poor prognosis in primary human breast cancer, *Cancer Res* 49:6008, 1989.
195. Basset P, Bellocq JP, Wolf C et al: A novel metalloproteinase gene specifically expressed in stromal cells of breast carcinomas, *Nature* 348:699, 1990.
196. Foekens JA, Schmitt M, van Putten WLJ et al: Prognostic value of urokinase-type plasminogen activator in 671 primary breast cancer patients, *Cancer Res* 52:6101, 1992.
197. Spyratos F, Maudelonede T, Brouillet JP et al: Cathepsin D: an independent prognostic factor for metastasis of breast cancer, *Lancet* 2:1115, 1989.
198. Weidner N, Semple JP, Welch WR, Folkman J: Tumor angiogenesis and metastasis-correlation in invasive breast carcinoma, *N Engl J Med* 324:1, 1991.
199. Bevilacqua G, Sobel ME, Liotta LA, Steeg PS: Association of low nm23 RNA levels in human primary infiltrating ductal breast carcinomas with lymph node involvement and other histopathological indicators of high metastatic potential, *Cancer Res* 49:5185, 1989.
200. McGuire WL: Breast cancer prognostic factors: evaluation guide-lines, *J Natl Cancer Inst* 83:54, 1991.
201. Allred DC: Should immunohistochemical examination replace biochemical hormone receptor assays in breast cancer? *Am J Clin Pathol* 99:1, 1993.
202. Miller AB: Early detection of breast cancer. In Harris JR, Hellman S, Henderson IC, Kinne DW, editors: *Breast diseases*, ed 2, Philadelphia, 1991, Lippincott.
203. Rutqvist LE, Miller AB, Andersson I et al: Reduced breast cancer mortality with mammography screening: an assessment of currently available data, *Int J Cancer* 5(suppl):76, 1990.
204. Schnitt SJ, Connolly JL: Processing and evaluation of breast excision specimens: a clinically oriented approach, *Am J Clin Pathol* 98:125, 1992.
205. Fisher B, Osborne CK, Margolese R, Bloomer W: Neoplasms of the breast. In Holland JF, Frei E, Bast RC et al, editors: *Cancer medicine*, Philadelphia, 1993, Lea & Febiger.

Fine-needle aspiration of the breast

206. Koss LG: *Diagnostic cytology and its histopathologic bases*, ed 4, Philadelphia, 1992, Lippincott.
207. Ciatto S, Bravotti P, Caraggi P: Significance of nipple discharge clinical patterns in the selection of cases for cytologic examination, *Acta Cytol* 30.17, 1986.
208. Silverman JF, Lannin DR, O'Brien K, Norris HT: The triage role of fine needle aspiration biopsy of palpable masses: diagnostic accuracy and cost-effectiveness, *Acta Cytol* 31:731, 1987.
209. Masood S: Fluorescent cytochemical detection of estrogen and progesterone receptors in breast fine-needle aspirates, *Am J Clin Pathol* 95:35, 1991.
210. Davey DD, Banks ER, Jennings D, Powell DE: Comparison of nuclear grade and DNA cytometry in breast carcinoma aspirates to histologic grade in excised cancers, *Am J Clin Pathol* 99:708, 1993.
211. Orell SR, Sterrett GF, Walters MN-I et al: *Manual and atlas of fine needle aspiration cytology*, ed 2, New York, 1992, Churchill Livingstone.
212. Catania S, Boccato P, Bono A et al.: Pneumothorax: a rare complication of fine needle aspiration of the breast, *Acta Cytol* 32:140, 1989.
213. Koss LG, Woyke S, Olszewski W: *Aspiration biopsy: cytologic interpretation and histologic bases*, New York, 1992, Igaku-Shoin.
214. Silverman JF: Breast. In Bibbo M, editor: *Comprehensive cytopathology*, Philadelphia, 1992, Saunders.
215. Ciatto S, Cariaggi P, Bulgaresi P: The value of routine cytologic examination of breast cyst fluids, *Acta Cytol* 31:301, 1987.
216. Tsuchiya SI, Maruyama Y, Koike Y et al: Cytologic characteristics and origin of naked nuclei in breast aspirate smears, *Acta Cytol* 31:285, 1987.
217. Marshall CJ, Schumann GB, Ward JH et al: Cytologic identification of clinically occult proliferative breast disease in women with a family history of breast cancer, *Am J Clin Pathol* 95:157, 1991.
218. Abendroth CS, Wang HH, Ducatman BS: Comparative features of carcinoma in situ and atypical ductal hyperplasia of the breast on fine-needle aspiration biopsy specimens, *Am J Clin Pathol* 96:654, 1991.
219. Dejmek A, Lindholm K: Frequency of cytologic features in fine needle aspirates from histologically and cytologically diagnosed fibroadenomas, *Acta Cytol* 35:695, 1991.
220. Dusenbery D, Frable WJ: Fine needle aspiration cytology of phyllodes tumor: potential diagnostic pitfalls, *Acta Cytol* 36:215, 1992.
221. Benoit JL, Kara R, McGregor SE, Duggan MA: Fibroadenoma of the breast: diagnostic pitfalls of fine needle aspiration, *Diagn Cytopathol* 8:643, 1992.
222. Wang HH, Ducatman BS, Eick D: Comparative features of ductal carcinoma in situ and infiltrating ductal carcinoma of the breast on fine-needle aspiration biopsy, *Am J Clin Pathol* 92:736, 1989.
223. Pettinato G, Manivel JC, Petrella G et al: Primary osteogenic sarcoma and osteogenic metaplastic carcinoma of the breast: immunocytochemical identification in fine needle aspirates, *Acta Cytol* 33:620, 1989.
224. Gorczyca W, Olszewski W, Tuziak T et al: Fine needle aspiration cytology of rare malignant tumors of the breast, *Acta Cytol* 36:918, 1992.
225. Galed-Placed I, García-Ureta E: Fine-needle aspiration biopsy diagnosis of adenoid cystic carcinoma of the breast: a case report, *Acta Cytol* 36:364, 1992.
226. Silverman JF, Feldman PS, Covell JL, Frable WJ: Fine-needle aspiration cytology of neoplasms metastatic to the breast, *Acta Cytol* 31:291, 1987.
227. Bhagat P, Kline TS: The male breast and malignant neoplasms: diagnosis by aspiration biopsy cytology, *Cancer* 65:2338, 1990.
228. Novotny DB, Maygarden SJ, Shermer RW, Frable WJ: Fine-needle aspiration of benign and malignant breast masses associated with pregnancy, *Acta Cytol* 35:676, 1991.
229. Maygarden SJ, McCall JB, Frable WJ: Fine-needle aspiration of breast lesions in women aged 30 and under, *Acta Cytol* 35:687, 1991.
230. Kline TS: Masquerades of malignancy: a review of 4241 aspirates from the breast, *Acta Cytol* 25:263, 1981.
231. Rogers LA, Lee KR: Breast carcinoma simulating fibroadenoma or fibrocystic change by fine-needle aspiration. a study of 16 cases, *Am J Clin Pathol* 98:155, 1992.
232. Zarbo RJ, Howanitz PJ, Bachner P: Interinstitutional comparison of performance in breast fine-needle aspiration cytology: a Q-probe quality indicator study, *Arch Pathol Lab Med* 115:743, 1991.
233. Bibbo M, Scheiber M, Cajulis R et al: Stereotaxic fine-needle aspiration cytology of clinically occult malignant and premalignant breast lesions, *Acta Cytol* 32:193, 1988.

Part Eight

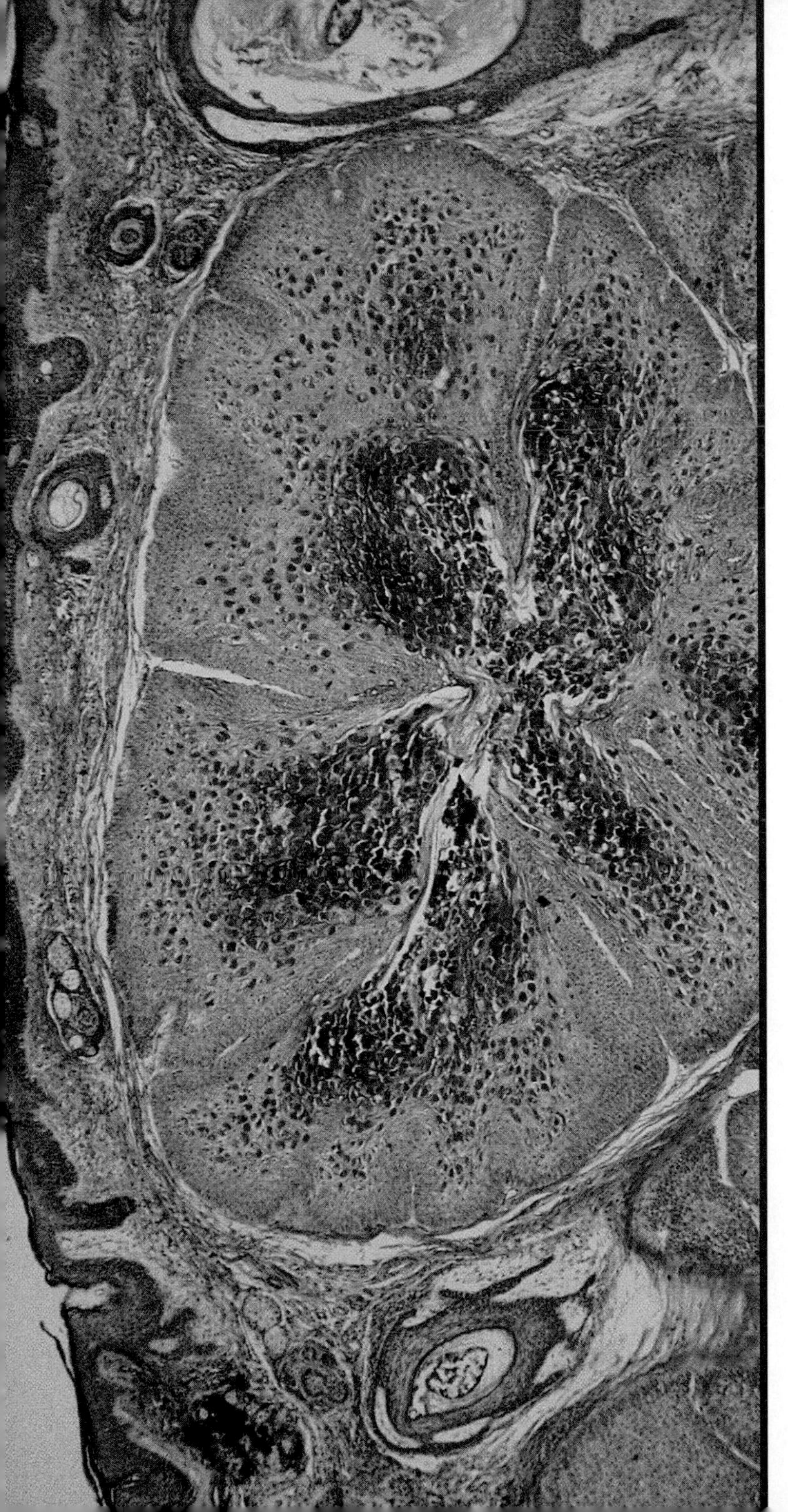

DISEASES OF THE SKIN AND CONNECTIVE TISSUES

71 Skin

Neil Scott McNutt
Bruce R. Smoller
Félix Contreras

INTRODUCTION AND NORMAL SKIN

A schema of the anatomy of normal skin is presented in Fig. 71-1. A detailed discussion of the normal histology is available in several excellent specialty texts that deal with this subject.[1,2] The skin is a laminated or layered structure, with each layer having its distinctive structures, functions, and diseases. A systematic approach to the diagnosis of the skin biopsy must include an evaluation of the skin in all of its layers. This chapter is divided so that one can concentrate on those diseases that affect the particular skin layers of interest, such as those layers that appear abnormal in a particular microscopic slide. Cross-referencing is needed for the diseases that affect more than one layer of the skin during the progression of the disease. For convenience adnexal tumors are presented in the section on tumors affecting both the epidermis and dermis.

Brief glossary of dermatopathology terms

Related terms and contrasting terms are identified by the number at the end of the definition.

1. **acantholysis** Detachment of keratinocytes from each other because of loss of intercellular contacts, usually with rounding of the cell profile in sections. (9, 42)
2. **acanthosis** Increase in thickness of spinous layer; may be described as papillomatous, psoriasiform, etc. (31, 37)
3. **adventitial dermis** The connective tissue composed of fine collagen fibers and delicate blood and lymphatic vessels that surround the epidermal appendages. It is continuous with the papillary dermis. (30, 40)
4. **apoptosis** Individual cell death; in skin, it often leads to formation of residual bodies which contain many condensed keratin filaments. (8, 12)
5. **ballooning degeneration** Intracellular edema and cellular swelling, often secondary to viral injury or nutritional deficiency. (42, 44)
6. **Birbeck granule** A distinctive vesicle within the cytoplasm of intraepidermal Langerhans' cells. The vesicle is partially flattened, and in the flattened zone, by electron microscopy, there is a proteinaceous material that forms a central layer with a 10 nm periodicity. The vesicles are often associated with the Golgi apparatus but also can be found in continuity with the plasma membrane and may contain the CD1a antigen.
7. **bulla** (pl. **bullae**) A circumscribed, fluid-filled, elevated lesion, greater than 5 mm in diameter. (38, 45, 46)
8. **Civatte body** A dead keratinocyte usually in the basal layer or in the papillary dermis. It consists of anuclear cytoplasm rich in keratin with fragments of other organelles. (4, 12)
9. **corps ronds** Rounded acantholytic cells with a perinuclear ring of keratin filaments. (1)
10. **crust** Serum, blood, or pus on the skin surface. (18, 33, 41)
11. **Darier-Pautrier microabscess** Collections of five or more atypical lymphocytes in the epidermis in well-demarcated cavities usually with little spongiosis or necrosis of the epidermis. These are proliferation centers for the atypical lymphocytes, which usually contain Langerhans' cells also. They can be found in

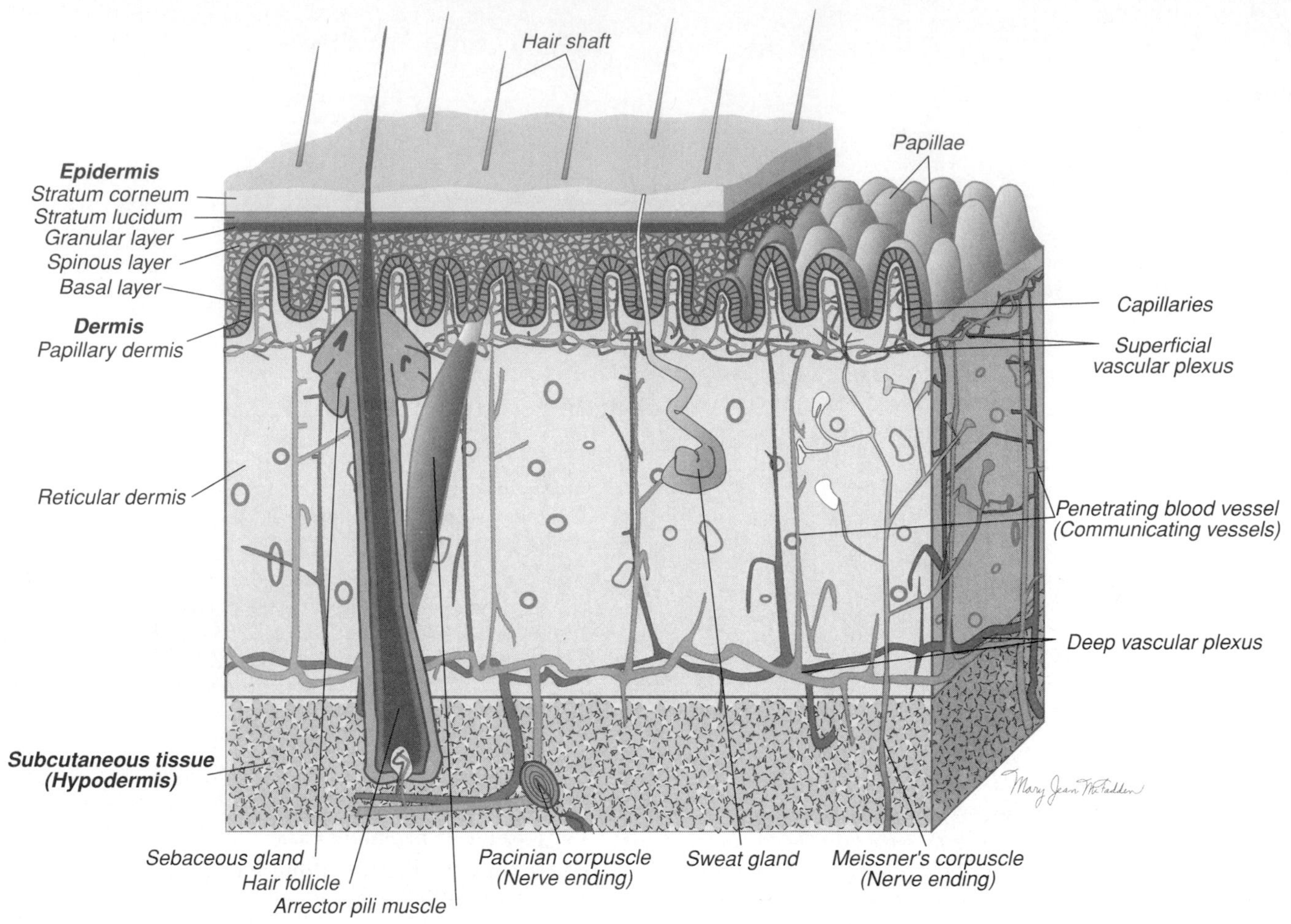

Fig. 71-1 Drawing of normal skin.

mycosis fungoides, lymphomatoid papulosis, and chronic actinic dermatitis. (39)

12. **dyskeratosis** Cell death associated with premature keratinization below the level of the stratum granulosum. (4, 8)
13. **erosion** A moist, circumscribed, usually depressed lesion that results from loss of all or a portion of the viable epidermis; may heal without scarring. (14, 43)
14. **excoriation** A traumatic erosion or ulcer that often is linear, such as a deep scratch. (13, 43)
15. **exocytosis** Emigration of inflammatory or neoplastic cells into the epidermis.
16. **grains** Enlarged ovoid parakeratotic cells. (33)
17. **herpetiform** Clusters of vesicles resembling those of herpes simplex or zoster infection. (47)
18. **hypergranulosis** Increase in thickness of the granular layer. (2)
19. **hyperkeratosis** Thickening of stratum corneum whether attributable to normal or abnormal keratinocytes. (28, 33)
20. **Koebner phenomenon** The tendency for lesions to form at sites of trauma.
21. **lentigo** A pigmented lesion that histologically has elongated rete ridges that are hyperpigmented and has a slightly increased number of melanocytes distributed individually along the dermoepidermal junction. The adjective **lentiginous** has been used to describe these findings.
22. **lichenification** Plaque with accentuated skin markings, usually secondary to chronic rubbing.
23. **Lupus band test** Deposition of immunoglobulin in a granular form along the dermoepidermal junction. This is seen by direct immunofluorescence in lesional skin of patients with lupus erythematosus and also in nonlesional skin of some patients with the systemic form of lupus erythematosus.
24. **macule** A circumscribed, flat lesion differing in color from the surrounding skin; may be of any size. (27, 32, 34, 35)
25. **melanophage** Macrophage that has ingested melanin pigment lost from the melanocytes or keratinocytes. (36)
26. **Merkel cell** Neuroendocrine cells of the epidermis and possibly of the sweat glands; they have contact with very fine nerve endings.
27. **nodule** A palpable, solid, round, or ellipsoidal lesion, usually more than 1 cm in diameter. (24, 32, 34, 35)

28. **orthokeratosis** Process of normal keratinization that leads to the production of anucleate squames in the stratum corneum. (19, 33)
29. **panniculitis** Inflammation of the adipose tissue and supporting connective tissues of the subcutis.
30. **papillary dermis** The upper portion of the dermis that consists of the dermal papillae and the underlying dermis down to and including the superficial vascular plexus at the upper border of the reticular dermis. (3, 40)
31. **papillomatosis** Formation of projections from the surface of the skin that are composed of keratinocytes and usually also of elongated dermal papillae; typical example is a wart. (2)
32. **papule** A small, solid, elevated lesion, less than 1 cm in diameter, usually superficial and mostly projecting from the surface. (24, 27, 34, 35)
33. **parakeratosis** Process of keratinization in which the superficial keratinocytes retain their nuclei; abnormal in skin, normal in mucous membranes. (19, 28)
34. **patch** A large, flat macule, more than 1 cm, usually with a fine scale. (24, 27, 32, 35)
35. **plaque** A mesa-like elevation that occupies a relatively large surface area (more than 1 cm), or a large area of induration or even atrophy of the skin. (24, 27, 32, 34)
36. **poikiloderma** Usually a plaque (less often a macule) that has the combination of atrophy, telangiectasia, and pigmentary alteration (hyperpigmentation or hypopigmentation, or both). There is also a fine scale.
37. **psoriasiform epidermal hyperplasia** Increase in keratinocytes with elongation of rete ridges and elongation of dermal papillae; a typical example is psoriasis. (2)
38. **pustule** A circumscribed, vesicular, or bullous lesion containing many neutrophils and occasionally eosinophils. (7, 45)
39. **rete ridges** The portion of the epidermis projecting toward the dermis. These form an interlocking zone of attachment between the epidermis and dermal papillae and are composed of basal and spinous layer keratinocytes. (2)
40. **reticular dermis** The portion of the dermis that extends from the superficial vascular plexus down to the subcutis. It contains larger collagen bundles than the papillary dermis. (3, 30)
41. **scale** Dry, horny, platelike excrescence, usually composed of stratum corneum keratinocytes, which may be parakeratotic. (10, 18, 33)
42. **spongiosis** Widening of the intercellular spaces between keratinocytes because of edema fluid, with retention of desmosomal contacts except in vesicles and bullae.
43. **ulcer** A loss of epidermis and at least superficial dermis. It usually heals with scarring. (13, 14)
44. **vacuolar change (vacuolization)** The formation of fluid-filled vacuoles within cells or in the basement membrane zone. (5, 42)
45. **vesicle** A circumscribed lesion, 5 mm in diameter or less, that is elevated and contains fluid. (7, 38, 46)
46. **wheal** A rounded or flat-topped elevated lesion that is characteristically evanescent, disappearing within hours; also called an urticarial lesion. (7, 27, 32, 38, 45)
47. **zosteriform** Clusters of lesions within a dermatome. (17)

DISEASES MAINLY INVOLVING THE EPIDERMIS

Genodermatoses and developmental disorders

Epidermolysis bullosa, epidermal type

Epidermolysis bullosa (EB) is a complex group of genetic disorders that is characterized by increased mechanical fragility of the skin, usually presenting at birth.[3,4] The exact anatomic and biochemical causes are different in the different forms of the disease (Table 71-1). EB, epidermal type, includes three entities that affect primarily the epidermis; they are inherited as autosomal dominant traits. EB, simplex type, has a generalized distribution. The Weber-Cockayne variant is limited to the hands and feet. The Dowling-Meara variant is generalized, can be severe, may be lethal early in life, and can be detected by fetal skin biopsy in the twentieth week of pregnancy. The patients all present with blisters since birth and developing after slight mechanical trauma.

PATHOLOGY. The skin biopsy shows total or partial separation of the epidermis from the dermis in a vesicle or bulla. There is disruption of the subnuclear cytoplasm in the basal keratinocytes. An anuclear portion of the cytoplasm remains attached to the basement membrane. Acantholysis is absent.

Table 71-1 Types of epidermolysis bullosa (EB)

Type	Level of splitting
Epidermal	
EB simplex	Generalized; through base of basal keratinocytes
Weber-Cockayne	Hands and feet; through basal cells
Dowling Meara	Generalized; as above; clumped tonofilaments
Junctional	
Junctional EB (lethalis)	Generalized; lamina lucida split
Dermal	
Recessive dystrophic EB	Generalized; subbasal lamina split; loss of type VII collagen fibrils, or "anchoring fibrils"
Dominant dystrophic EB	Generalized or localized; subbasal lamina split; decreased numbers of type VII collagen fibrils
Acquired EB	Generalized; IgG antibody against type VII collagen, with loss of anchoring fibrils
Bart's syndrome	Congenital; localized; epidermal, junctional and dermal types have been described

There is usually very little if any inflammation and generally scarring is absent. In EB, simplex type, electron microscopy (EM) shows a lack of basal tonofilament bundles, whereas in the Dowling-Meara variant, the tonofilaments are coarsely clumped in the cytoplasm. These changes may be related to abnormality in the production of keratins 5 and 14 in the basal cells in the epidermal forms of EB.

The differential diagnosis includes a common friction blister, but this has a split just below the stratum granulosum, whereas epidermal types of EB split through the basal keratinocytes. Of course, severe friction can produce an erosion or an ulcer.

Epidermolysis bullosa, junctional and dermal types

In junctional EB blisters are formed because of defects in the attachment of cells to the basement membrane, whereas in dermal EB the blisters result from abnormalities in the structure of the basement membrane itself (see Table 71-1). In general, junctional EB (and EB simplex) do not produce scarring ("nondystrophic"), whereas dermal EB does scar ("dystrophic").

PATHOLOGY. In routine histologic preparations, junctional and dermal forms of EB often cannot be distinguished, and special techniques may be necessary to classify the forms of EB. By EM, junctional EB has a split in the lamina lucida portion of the basement membrane, and immunofluorescence studies reveal that the proteins laminin and type IV collagen are in the floor of the blister. Junctional EB has a reduction in formation of hemidesmosomes, but the bullous pemphigoid antigen, which is associated with hemidesmosomes, is in the roof of the blister. Laminin and type IV collagen are in the floor of the blister. In contrast, the dermal forms of EB have the split below the lamina lucida on EM and are associated with an absence or severe depletion of anchoring fibrils. By immunofluorescence microscopy, dermal EB has laminin, type IV collagen, and the bullous pemphigoid antigen in the roof of the blister. In acquired EB, the split is below the lamina densa, and most of the patients have deposition of IgG in a linear pattern along the dermoepidermal junction. Acquired EB has laminin in the roof of the blisters, whereas the disease bullous pemphigoid has laminin in the floor of the blisters.

Patients with acquired EB have antibodies to type VII collagen, which is a component of the anchoring fibrils. Some patients with a form of lupus erythematosus called "subacute bullous lupus erythematosus" also have autoantibodies to type VII collagen.

Darier's disease

Darier's disease (also known as "Darier-White disease," or "keratosis follicularis") is a rare disease of keratinization that is transmitted as an autosomal dominant trait with variable penetrance.[5] It is symmetrical on the scalp, neck, and upper chest in a distribution resembling seborrheic dermatitis but can be widespread and can involve the nails and the mucous membranes, such as the hard palate. The basic lesion is a 1 to 3 mm papule that has a dirty gray-tan, keratotic surface (Fig. 71-2). These papules become confluent, thereby forming plaques. Secondary infection is common. The differential diagnosis includes a form of epidermal nevus with the histology of Darier's disease and transient acantholytic dermatosis "Grover's disease."

PATHOLOGY. Histologically, the basic lesion consists of a broad zone of hyperkeratosis with parakeratosis, suprabasal acantholysis, and rounded cells *(corps ronds)* (Fig. 71-3). The parakeratotic cells, called "grains," often have an ovoid, slightly flattened appearance. In well-developed lesions, the basal layer forms projections, or "villi," in the acantholytic cleft. The dermal inflammatory infiltrate contains lymphocytes and macrophages. Eosinophils are more common in transient acantholytic dermatosis than in true Darier's disease. A well-developed solitary lesion with this histologic characterization is called **warty dyskeratoma.**

Hailey-Hailey disease (familial benign pemphigus)

Hailey-Hailey disease presents with small vesicles on an erythematous base and is transmitted as an autosomal dominant trait.[6] The vesicles become confluent, producing irregular plaques (Fig. 71-4) that frequently involve the axillae, neck, and intertriginous zones, that is, areas predisposed to friction and excessive moisture. Superficial bacterial infections also trigger or exacerbate lesions, which become crusted and fissured.

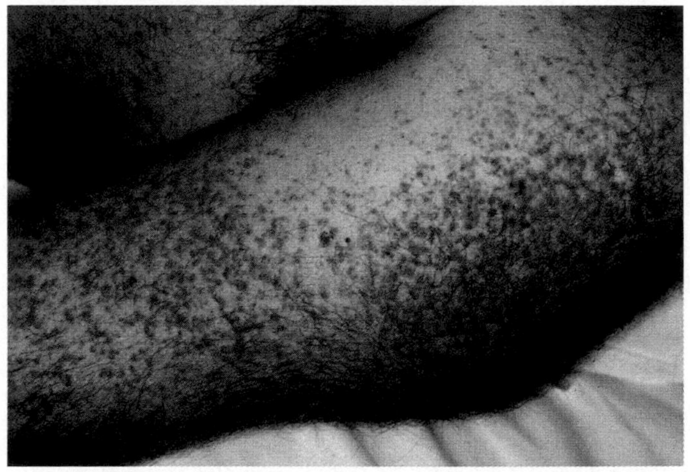

Fig. 71-2 Darier's disease. There are brown scaly papules that aggregate into groups on the lateral surface of the shoulder.

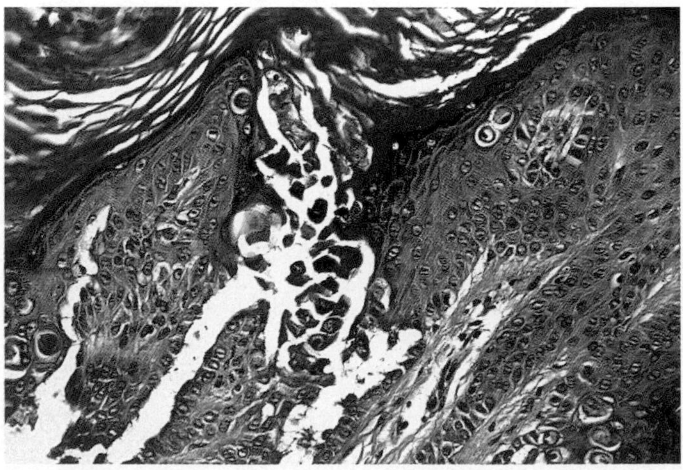

Fig. 71-3 Darier's disease. Microscopically there is acantholysis, with the formation of rounded cells (*"corps ronds"*) and oval, individually keratinized cells ("grains").

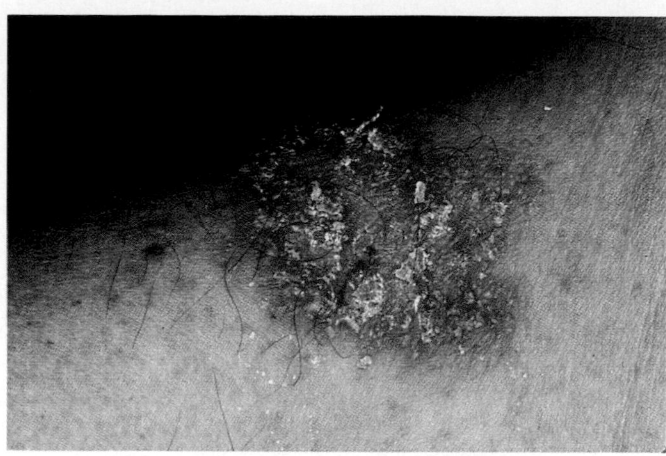

Fig. 71-4 Hailey-Hailey disease. The papules and vesicles have fused to form a fissured plaque with a scaly surface.

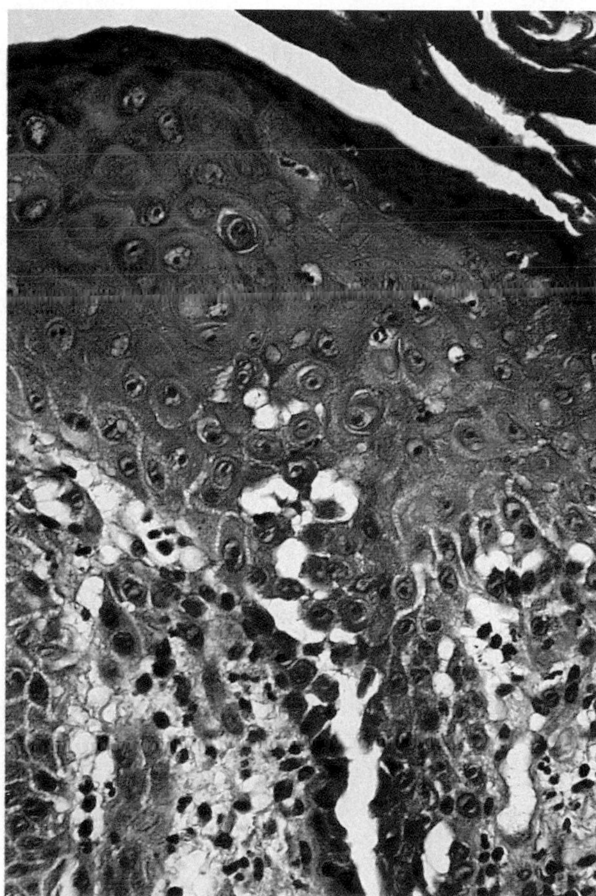

Fig. 71-5 Hailey-Hailey disease. Notice the partial acantholysis separating the cells in the suprabasal region.

PATHOLOGY. The lesions have pronounced partial acantholysis in the lower stratum spinosum (Fig. 71-5). A suprabasal cleft is formed with groups of cells and a few individual cells floating in the cavity. Dermal inflammation is minimal.

Small pruritic lesions with these histologic features also occur in transient acantholytic dermatosis, that is, Grover's disease. Immunofluorescence is negative. The epidermis in the roof of the Hailey-Hailey blister has much more partial acantholysis than the blister roof in pemphigus vulgaris.

Ichthyosis

The ichthyoses are a complex group of disorders of keratinization that form a scale on the skin surface (Table 71-2).[7] The diseases usually are hereditary, but there is an acquired form. The name "ichthyosis" is derived from the appearance of the scales that have a polygonal appearance and resemble fish scales. *Ichthyosis vulgaris* (Fig. 71-6) is a rather common disease that is transmitted as an autosomal dominant trait. It is not present at birth but develops within the first few years of life. It is symmetrical and involves the extensor surfaces of the limbs and also the trunk, often with follicular hyperkeratosis. *Acquired ichthyosis* closely resembles ichthyosis vulgaris but develops in adult life in patients with lymphomas, carcinomas, sarcoidosis, acquired immunodeficiency syndrome (AIDS), or after ingestion of cholesterol-lowering drugs. *Pityriasis rotunda* is a rare form of acquired ichthyosis that is named for its large round lesions. *X-linked recessive ichthyosis* occurs in male children, often is present at birth, and spares the palms and soles. *Lamellar ichthyosis* has recessive transmission, with thick scale. Often the children are born enclosed within a parchment-like keratinous membrane, the "collodion membrane."

Two types of ichthyosis are classically associated with severe erythema of the skin. The first is *nonbullous congenital ichthyosiform erythroderma,* which produces a fine branny scale. The second is *bullous congenital ichthyosiform erythroderma* (epidermolytic hyperkeratosis) that produces a thick, dirty scale and forms large flaccid bullae, often with secondary infection. A limited form of this disease also occurs as a type of epidermal nevus, called ichthyosis hystrix.

PATHOLOGY. All forms of ichthyosis have hyperkeratosis. In ichthyosis vulgaris and acquired ichthyosis, the granular layer is diminished or absent and the residual keratohyalin granules are very small. There is compact orthokeratosis within the plates of the scale. In contrast, both X-linked ichthyosis and lamellar ichthyosis retain their granular layer and have an orthokeratotic compact scale. Nonbullous congenital ichthyosiform erythroderma has a thinner scale, which can be parakeratotic. The dermis contains dilated vessels and a slight increase in lymphocytes. Bullous congenital ichthyosiform erythroderma ("epidermolytic hyperkeratosis") has hyperkeratosis that is dense, orthokeratotic, and somewhat coarse and slightly granular in appearance and keratinocytes with coarse large polygonal keratohyalin granules and with vacuolated cytoplasm. The vacuolization begins above the basal layer and is most pronounced in the granular layer. There is vasodilatation and a sparse lymphocytic infiltrate in the papillary dermis.

The hyperkeratosis may be a consequence of the retention of scale without increased proliferation, as in ichthyosis vulgaris, or augmented epidermal proliferation, as in congenital bullous ichthyosiform erythroderma. By EM, X-linked recessive ichthyosis cells lack membrane-coating granules, or Odland bodies. This is associated with a generalized lack of steroid sulfatase, not only in the epidermis, but also in other cells as well.

Epidermal nevi, warts, and a small solitary lesion named *epidermolytic acanthoma* can have epidermolytic hyperkeratosis, which can also be an incidental subclinical finding in very small regions, possibly because of localized defects in the for-

Table 71-2 Types of ichthyosis

Type	Inheritance	Distribution	Histology
Ichthyosis vulgaris	Autosomal dominant	Flexures spared	Decreased or absent granular layer
Acquired ichthyosis	None	Flexures spared	Decreased or absent granular layer
X-linked ichthyosis	X-linked recessive	Flexures involved	Normal granular layer
Lamellar ichthyosis	Autosomal recessive	Flexures involved	Thick scale, thickened granular layer
Nonbullous congenital ichthyosiform erythroderma	Autosomal recessive	Flexures involved	Fine scale; variable granular layer occasionally parakeratosis
Bullous congenital ichthyosiform erythroderma	Autosomal dominant	Flexures involved	Thick coarse scale; vacuolated granular and spinous layer
Ichthyosis hystrix	Unknown	Localized	As bullous CIE above

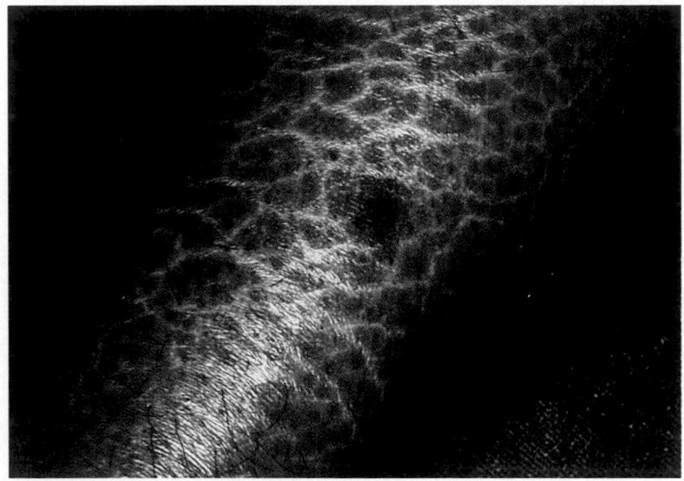

Fig. 71-6 Ichthyosis vulgaris. The dark polygonal scales that tend to be on extensor surfaces are characteristic.

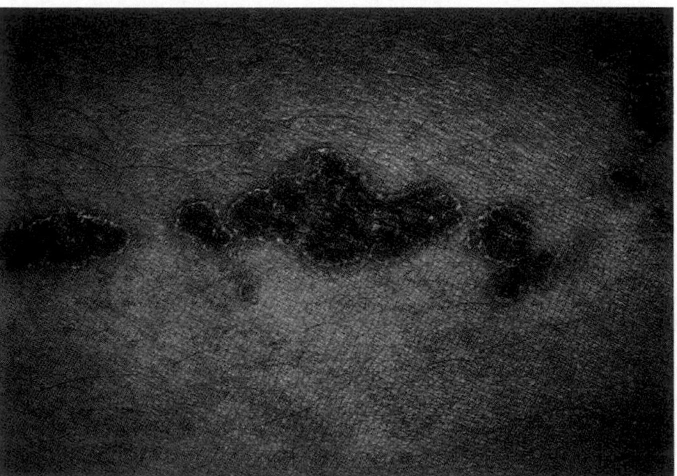

Fig. 71-7 Porokeratosis. Notice the hyperpigmented lesions with a pearly discrete scaly rim around them.

mation of keratins 1 or 10.[8,9] The ichthyotic character of the lesions is not explained solely by the keratin abnormality but seems to involve the lipid permeability barrier as well.[10]

Porokeratosis

There are several clinical forms of porokeratosis, all of which begin as a small papule with a surface scale and then enlarge to form a sharply demarcated ring of hyperkeratosis often with an atrophic center (Fig. 71-7). Men are affected more than women. Autosomal dominant transmission has been suggested for the variant known as "porokeratosis of Mibelli."

PATHOLOGY. The stratum corneum has a discrete column of hyperkeratosis that is parakeratotic, which has been given the name "cornoid lamella" (Fig. 71-8) and which forms the edge of the ring of hyperkeratosis seen clinically. There is a lymphocytic infiltrate underlying the epidermis at the cornoid lamella.

The term *porokeratosis* originally implied an association with the sweat pore, but the disease can affect all the epidermis as the ring migrates centrifugally. Squamous cell carcinomas arise in some lesions of porokeratosis, especially in porokeratosis of Mibelli. Cytogenetic studies have detected abnormal ploidy in some lesions of porokeratosis.[11]

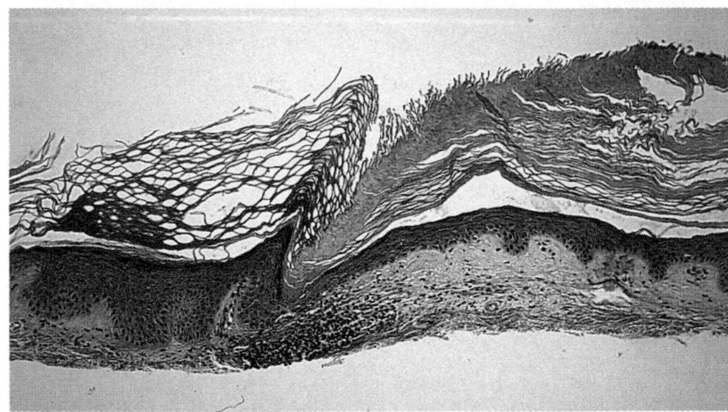

Fig. 71-8 Porokeratosis. The cornoid lamella is a column of parakeratosis overlying slightly vacuolated keratinocytes that have migrated slowly centrifugally, here from the right toward the left.

Xeroderma pigmentosum

The term *xeroderma pigmentosum* (XP) includes several diseases all of which are characterized by defective repair of ultraviolet (UV) radiation–induced DNA damage.[12] The main type of XP lacks an endonuclease enzyme needed to excise the pyrimidine dimers formed by UV irradiation. Other more rare forms of the disease attributable to deficiencies in other steps of DNA repair have been described. At an early age, the affected children develop many lentigines, solar keratoses, squamous and basal cell carcinomas, and malignant melanomas on their sun-exposed skin. Such lesions develop after minimal sun exposure and are associated with very little solar elastosis. Deep dermal tumors and soft-tissue tumors are also slightly increased in incidence.

The UV damage affects many genes and chromosomes. One is the N-*ras* oncogene, in which the codon 61 has been shown to be sensitive to ultraviolet radiation. Cells transfected with such a mutant form of N-*ras* are capable of producing malignant tumors.[13] Also UV radiation has been shown to induce mutations in the p53 tumor suppressor gene that are detectable in squamous cell carcinomas.[14]

Inflammatory, metabolic, and traumatic disorders

Acropustulosis of infancy

Acropustulosis of infancy, also known as "infantile acropustulosis," begins shortly after birth and produces superficial pustules, 1 to 5 mm in diameter, on the distal extremities.[15,16] The pustules are sterile and pruritic and often resolve spontaneously by 3 years of age.

PATHOLOGY. A biopsy specimen shows a subcorneal pustule filled with neutrophils. The dermis has a sparse superficial perivascular lymphocytic infiltrate with a few neutrophils also. In the differential diagnosis, one must consider various infections, particularly scabies, dermatophytosis, candidiasis, or impetigo, as well as pustular psoriasis affecting palms and soles, subcorneal pustular dermatosis, and transient neonatal pustular melanosis.

Subcorneal pustular dermatosis

The rare disease subcorneal pustular dermatosis (also known as "Sneddon-Wilkinson disease") produces superficial, subcorneal pustules. Often it affects middle-aged women.[17] Lesions appear on the trunk and proximal extremities, usually as papules with central pustules that coalesce and form irregular serpiginous and circinate lesions with central clearing.

PATHOLOGY. A biopsy specimen shows a pustule filled with neutrophils just below the stratum corneum, often with very little spongiosis in the adjacent epidermis. A parakeratotic scale is formed containing neutrophils. There is only slight acanthosis accompanied by a minimal superficial perivascular lymphoid infiltrate in the dermis. Special stains for fungi and bacteria are negative.

This disease may be a form of psoriasis, since it is histologically so similar to acute pustular psoriasis. Differences from psoriasis include distribution of lesions, lack of Koebner's phenomenon, and the fact that some patients have an IgA monoclonal gammopathy or an IgA-producing myeloma.

Pemphigus

The term *pemphigus* encompasses several diseases characterized by formation of intraepidermal blisters caused by the binding of an antibody to surface epitopes of the keratinocytes (Table 71-3).[18] The keratinocytes detach from each other and form rounded acantholytic cells. The most common form, *pemphigus vulgaris,* produces clear flaccid blisters that rupture and leave reddened eroded skin (Fig. 71-9). Approximately half of the cases start with lesions in the mouth. There is an association with HLA-A13, with HLA-DR4, and with other autoimmune diseases such as lupus erythematosus or myasthenia gravis. The patients are at risk of dying from secondary infection and sepsis. *Pemphigus vegetans* has a similar immunopathogenesis, but the lesions have a thickened verrucous or hyperkeratotic appearance.

Pemphigus foliaceus has flaccid blisters also, but the oral cavity is spared. The blisters and erosions of the epidermis are more superficial and more easily broken and are less debilitating that those of pemphigus vulgaris. The autoantibody binds to an antigen that occurs in the upper part of the epidermis. *Pemphigus erythematosus* is a variant of pemphigus foliaceus.

Paraneoplastic pemphigus (Fig. 71-9) clinically resembles pemphigus vulgaris or erythema multiforme but occurs in association often with lymphomas such as non-Hodgkin's lymphoma, chronic lymphocytic leukemia, and Castleman's

Table 71-3 Acantholytic disorders

Disease	Level of cleft	Antibody	Comment
For primary acantholysis			
Pemphigus vulgaris	Just suprabasal	IgG	Most common
Pemphigus vegetans	Just suprabasal	IgG	Epidermal hyperplasia
Pemphigus foliaceus	Near granular layer	IgG	Uncommon
Pemphigus erythematosus	Near granular layer	IgG	May have systemic lupus erythematosus
Folgo selvagem	Near granular layer	IgG	Brazilian jungle
Paraneoplastic pemphigus	Just suprabasal	IgG	Necrotic keratinocytes
Darier's disease	Just suprabasal	None	Dyskeratosis
Grover's disease	Just suprabasal	None	Variable dyskeratosis
For secondary acantholysis			
Impetigo	Above granular layer	None	Minimal acantholysis
Subcorneal pustular dermatosis	Above granular layer	None	Minimal acantholysis
Staphylococcal scalded-skin syndrome	Just below granular layer	None	Staphylococcal exotoxin
Herpetic vesicles	Irregular	None	Multinucleation
For solitary lesions			
Warty dyskeratoma	Just suprabasal	None	Like Darier's disease
Acantholytic acanthoma	Just suprabasal	None	Like Grover's disease
Actinic keratosis	Suprabasal	None	Cytologic atypia and parakeratosis
Squamous cell carcinoma	Suprabasal	None	Cytologic atypia

skin. The clinical lesions have a greasy, fine branlike scale (furfuraceous scale) and occur mainly on the trunk, neck, and face.

Tinea nigra is an infection of the upper epidermis by *Cladosporium* organisms. This infection principally occurs in the tropics, commonly after a superficial abrasion. The fungus contains a brown pigment and produces generally round, brown or black, sharply marginated lesions with slight scaling or erythema. Clinically the lesion may be mistaken for a junctional nevus.

PATHOLOGY. The fungal growth in the stratum corneum varies in its effect on the thickness of the epidermis or on the amount of inflammation in the dermis. The mixture of yeasts and hyphal forms, 1 to 3 μm in diameter, in tinea versicolor produces a distinctive appearance (Fig. 71-15). The fungi of tinea nigra have hyphae with a slightly larger diameter, and contain brown pigment. Periodic acid–Schiff (PAS) stains are recommended to help identify fungi, especially if they are not obvious.

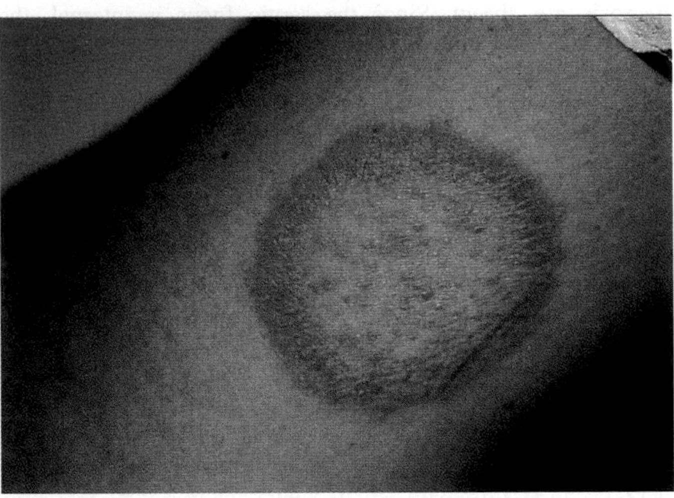

Fig. 71-14 Tinea infection. A common appearance is an annular, scaly erythema, or "ringworm," but there are many varied types of lesions.

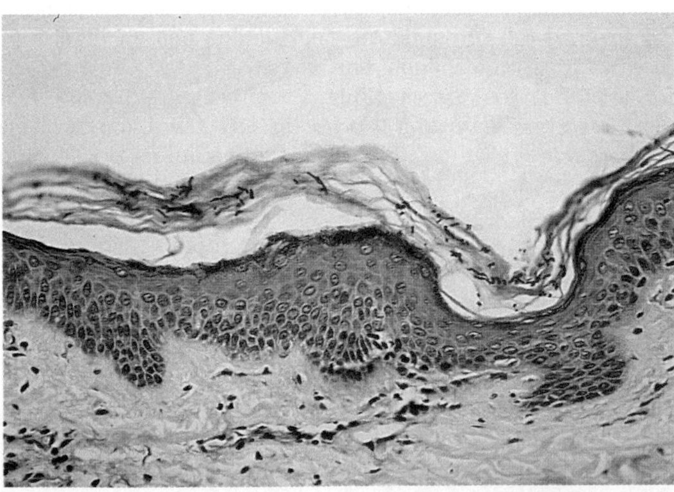

Fig. 71-15 Tinea versicolor. The dermatophyte infection of the stratum corneum produces both branching hyphae and spores, usually with little inflammation.

Papillomavirus infections

Certain types of human papillomavirus (HPV) infections are very common, occur at any age, and can begin very early in life.[1,30] Currently, more than 55 types of HPV have been identified, based on molecular genetic analysis. The members of the HPV family share at least 50% nucleotide homology (Table 71-4).

The clinical lesions vary from the very protuberant lesions such as the common wart, *verruca vulgaris,* to very flat lesions that seem to affect only the epidermis, such as the flat versions of genital warts, *condyloma acuminatum* and *bowenoid papulosis.* Other very flat lesions are *verruca plana* (Fig. 71-16) and *epidermodysplasia verruciformis,* which are often very widespread. Verruca plana are associated mainly with HPV 3. HPV 5 is believed to have the potential for malignant transformation in epidermodysplasia verruciformis. See a later section for a discussion of large lesions involving both epidermis and dermis and the chapter on penis and vulvar pathology for a discussion of bowenoid papulosis and its association with HPV 16 or 18[31-33] and condylomata acuminata, which are associated with HPV types 6 and 11.

PATHOLOGY. The epidermis of all HPV-induced lesions is acanthotic. In the flat lesions there is very little participation of the dermis. The epidermis in verruca plana shows prominent vacuolization of the cytoplasm of the cells of the stratum granulosum and upper stratum spinosum (Fig. 71-17). Kerato-

Table 71-4 Human papillomavirus (HPV) lesions

Lesion	Major HPV types
Verruca plantaris	1
Verruca vulgaris	2, 4
Verruca plana	3, 10, 27-29
Butcher's warts	7
Epidermodysplasia verruciformis	5, 8, 9, 10, others
Condyloma acuminatum	6, 11
Bowenoid papulosis	16, 18, 31, 33-35, others

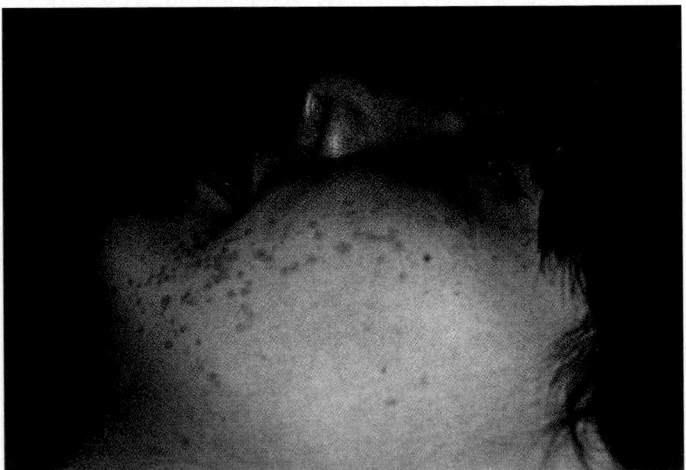

Fig. 71-16 Verruca plana. This viral infection can produce numerous slightly hyperpigmented lesions that are only minimally elevated. The face is a common site.

hyalin granules are enlarged and round. Similar lesions on the skin of the genitalia are early condylomata acuminata, if they have at least a slightly papillomatous shape and vacuolization of keratinocytes in the upper stratum spinosum. In the granular layer, nuclei are swollen and contain viral particles.

Neoplasms of the epidermis

Keratinocytic lesions

Seborrheic keratosis. Seborrheic keratosis, a very common benign lesion, also known as "verruca seborrheica," occurs in elderly persons of either sex.[34,35] The lesions are sharply demarcated, flat to raised papules or plaques, often with a flesh-colored (Fig. 71-18) or slightly yellow or hyperpigmented appearance (Fig. 71-19). Generally they are small and are totally exophytic lesions a few millimeters in diameter but can achieve a large size. Often there is very little inflammation, but they may itch and can become traumatized through scratching. There is a type that develops prominent lymphocytic infiltration, and it is discussed with benign lichenoid keratosis in the section on tumors affecting both epidermis and dermis. The lesions are common on the trunk and proximal extremities but can occur anywhere, except on the palms, soles, or oral mucosa. This indicates a probable relationship to hair follicles.

PATHOLOGY. The lesions consist of acanthotic epidermis usually without cytologic atypia of the keratinocytes (Fig. 71-20). Even in early lesions, the papillary dermis immediately beneath the lesion is sclerotic. The earliest lesions of seborrheic keratosis show elongation and interconnection of rete ridges. The basal keratinocytes are slightly to heavily pigmented. When these are the only findings, the diagnosis often is "reticulated seborrheic keratosis." As the lesions thicken, they develop papillomatosis or greater degrees of acanthosis. The papillomatous lesions are sometimes called "stucco keratoses" and may lack the horn pseudocysts of the acanthotic type. These pseudocysts contain orthokeratin and are formed by the fusion of globules of orthokeratin within the thickened

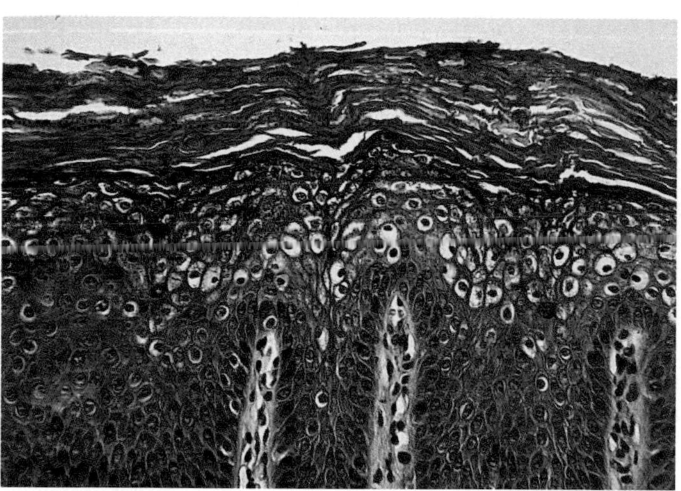

Fig. 71-17 Verruca plana. Characteristically, vacuolization is prominent in the keratinocytes of the upper spinous layer and granular layer. Keratohyalin granules are coarse.

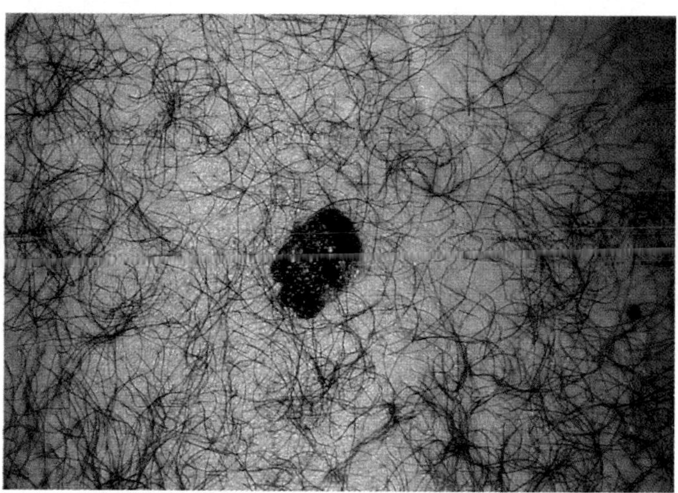

Fig. 71-19 Seborrheic keratosis. Hyperpigmented variants with an irregular outline and irregular pigment distribution can resemble melanocytic nevi or melanomas.

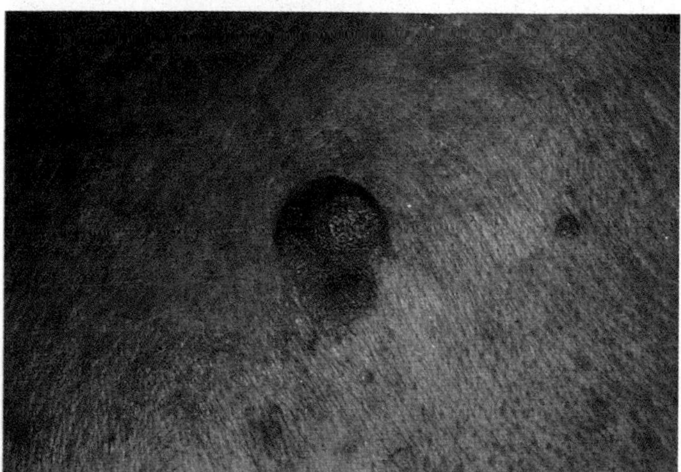

Fig. 71-18 Seborrheic keratosis. Usually this is an exophytic lesion that has a slightly yellow color and a rugose surface.

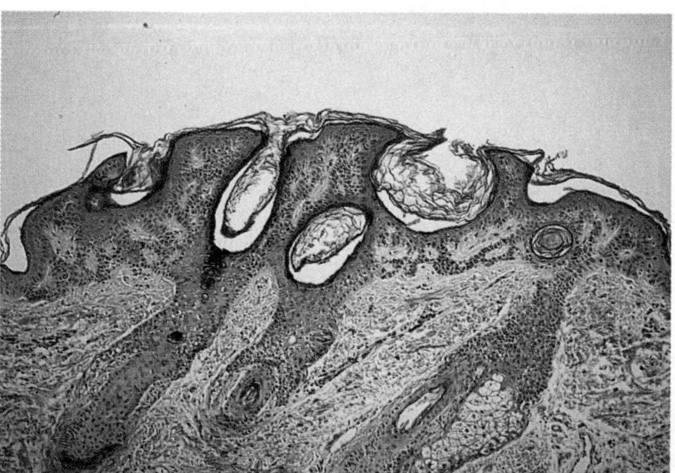

Fig. 71-20 Seborrheic keratosis. The epidermis is acanthotic with interconnected rete ridges, and the dermal papillae are fibrotic. Small intraepidermal collections of keratin are "horn pseudocysts."

epidermis. They are pseudocysts because the fused keratin masses often form a channel to the surface of the lesion. Seborrheic keratoses can become infected by fungi or bacteria in the pseudocysts and develop considerable inflammation. Another histologic pattern in early seborrheic keratoses is sometimes called "clonal seborrheic keratosis" because of focal groups of keratinocytes in the epidermis that maintain evidence of polarity (Fig. 71-21). These foci develop in irritated seborrheic keratoses or as a primary phenomenon, but there is no definite evidence that they represent true clones of keratinocytes. When the groups of keratinocytes lack polarity and are atypical cytologically, the lesion is classified as intraepidermal squamous cell carcinoma in situ. A variant of pigmented seborrheic keratosis is called a *melanoacanthoma* because it has prominent dendritic melanocytes containing abundant pigment with poor pigment transfer to the adjacent keratinocytes. It occurs in older patients, whites more than blacks, with a slow onset and no spontaneous resolution.

The differential diagnosis includes warts. Most seborrheic keratoses are histologically distinct from warts and HPV has not been demonstrated in them. However, they may become infected by wart virus, as demonstrated in histologically typical seborrheic keratoses in the groin that contain HPV from nearby condyloma acuminatum. In a very young person, under 20 years of age, an epidermal nevus is in the differential diagnosis.

A controversial observation is that patients with internal malignancies can develop many inflamed seborrheic keratoses acutely over the upper trunk and sometimes in peculiar whorled patterns. This has been called the "sign of Leser and Trélat" and may be associated with a variety of carcinomas of the stomach, lung, and colon, as well as lymphomas.[36,37]

Pale cell acanthoma of Degos. The uncommon, benign, well-circumscribed tumor pale cell acanthoma of Degos (also known as "clear cell acanthoma") tends to occur on the lower extremities as a solitary tumor in middle-aged or elderly individuals. There may be multiple tumors. A surface scale and erythema often are present with punctate bleeding points in the surface of the lesion.

PATHOLOGY. The lesion has a very sharply demarcated zone of acanthosis, with many of the keratinocytes having a pale to clear cytoplasm, that is strongly PAS-positive and sensitive to diastase digestion. The epidermis above the dermal papillae (suprapapillary plate) is considerably thinned. There is a parakeratotic scale containing neutrophils. The blood vessels in the dermal papillae are prominent and thin walled. The keratinocytes lack nuclear atypism.

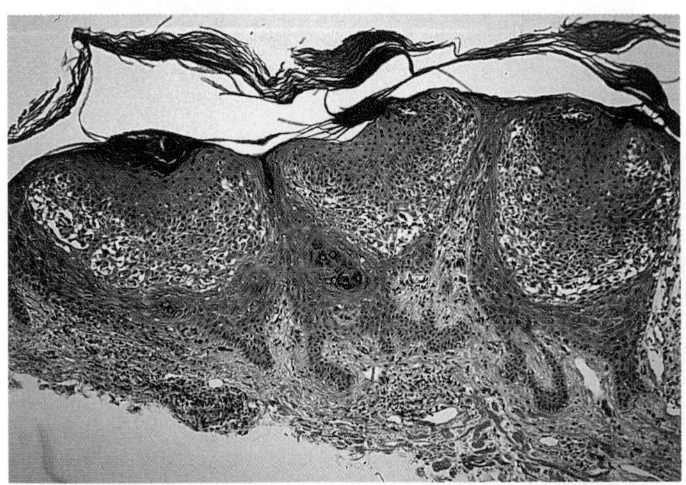

Fig. 71-21 Seborrheic keratosis. Intraepidermal nests of keratinocytes form in response to irritation. They maintain a polarity within the nests and lack cytologic atypia.

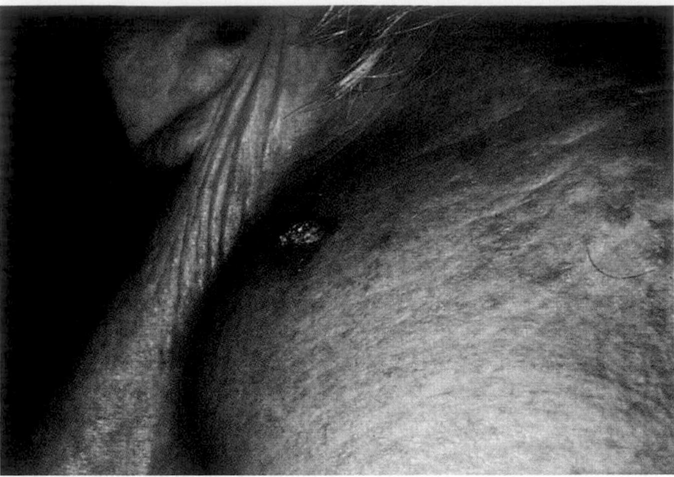

Fig. 71-22 Actinic keratosis. The lesions often are discrete erythematous papules that have a yellow hyperkeratotic surface.

This lesion resembles psoriasis in many features, except that it is distinguishable because of the pale to clear cytoplasm of cells in the lesion that is sharply demarcated from the adjacent epidermis. Psoriasis has cells with more basophilic cytoplasm. The basic defect seems to be the lack of a phosphorylase that is needed in the degradation of glycogen.[1]

Warty dyskeratoma. Warty dyskeratoma is a solitary, keratotic, slightly verrucous papule, usually on the head and neck, and less often elsewhere.[1,38]

PATHOLOGY. The lesion shows suprabasal acantholysis, villous basal protrusions, corps ronds, and grains. The lesion may be relatively flat or may project downward into the dermis slightly. There is often sparse dermal lymphocytic inflammatory infiltrate.

Small lesions are indistinguishable from Grover's disease, and large lesions resemble Darier's disease. Small papules with similar changes are found as an incidental finding in large excision specimens of clinically normal skin. The diagnosis of warty dyskeratoma should be reserved for solitary nonpruritic lesions several millimeters in diameter.

Actinic keratosis. Actinic keratosis, also known as "senile keratosis" and "solar keratosis," is one of the most common neoplasms of whites, generally presenting as a scaly, erythematous patch (Fig. 71-22) on a sun-exposed part of the body.[36,38] The lesions can be hyperpigmented and can become extensive and confluent (Fig. 71-23). They are directly related to the total cumulative dose of UV radiation, particularly UVB (280 to 320 nm wavelength). Other forms of ionizing radiation can produce similar keratoses. In contrast, patients exposed to excessive levels of inorganic arsenic compounds develop similar keratoses, but they also occur on skin not exposed to the sun and even on palms and soles. Actinic keratoses are part of a progressive sequence that can lead to carcinoma in situ.[1]

PATHOLOGY. The lesions begin as enlarged basal keratinocytes with nuclear enlargement and hyperchromatism in an irregular pattern along the dermoepidermal junction (Fig. 71-24). Subsequently acanthosis develops as well as the spread of obviously atypical cells to upper layers of the epidermis. In contrast, some lesions remain atrophic. Often there is parakeratosis and hyperkeratosis, except for orthokeratosis over the appendages. In advanced lesions, the epidermis becomes more completely replaced by atypical cells. If the atypical cells permeate the full thickness of the epidermis and particularly if the lesion is large and obliterates the orifices of the hair follicles and sweat ducts, the diagnosis of squamous cell carcinoma in situ is warranted. The dermis usually has abundant solar elastosis; if this is lacking, the possibility of an arsenical keratosis should be considered.

Actinic keratosis may have acantholysis in the suprabasal region (Fig. 71-24), mimicking primary acantholytic disorders (Table 71-3), which, however, lack cytologic atypism of the basal cells and the overlying parakeratotic scale. *Pigmented actinic keratosis* has hyperpigmentation because of increased melanin in the basal keratinocytes with very little increase in the size or number of the melanocytes among the atypical keratinocytes. *Lichenoid actinic keratoses* have a dense inflammatory infiltrate of lymphocytes and plasma cells in the dermis, which makes them lesions in which both the epidermis and dermis are involved. *Hyperplastic actinic keratosis* is a term used to designate lesions with features intermediate between ordinary thin actinic keratoses and squamous cell carcinoma in situ. *Large cell acanthoma* usually is a variant of an actinic keratosis that lacks a surface parakeratotic scale and has nuclei of the basal keratinocytes that are enlarged to twice to three times normal size.[38]

Actinic keratosis is squamous cell neoplasia in situ. Invasion deep down into follicles or full-thickness atypism of epidermis over a broad area with obliteration of follicle demarcation are expressions of advanced stages of tumor progression, that is, squamous cell carcinoma in situ. Lesions on the progression between early actinic keratosis and squamous cell carcinoma in situ also have been divided into three categories based on the amount of cytologic atypism and the degree of replacement of the epidermis. Early lesions with a relatively low degree of cytologic atypism restricted to the basal region are called *squamous intraepidermal neoplasia* (SIN), grade 1, or SIN-I (Fig. 71-25).[39,40] Lesions in which the atypical cells replace much of the lower half of the epidermis are SIN-II (Fig. 71-26). Lesions with full-thickness atypia and appendages that extend down are "bowenoid actinic keratoses," that is, squamous cell carcinoma in situ or SIN-III (Fig. 71-27). Paradoxically, SIN-III lesions may remain in an in situ phase longer than some SIN-I and SIN-II lesions, and invasion into the dermis by squamous cell carcinoma can arise from lesions with less than full-thickness atypism of keratinocytes.

Mutations in the p53 gene, a tumor-suppressor gene, occur in response to UV radiation and may be involved in some aspect of the production of squamous cell carcinomas in sun-damaged skin.[14] Overexpression of p53 has been found in some actinic keratoses as well, and this may reflect a mutation occurring during the early stages of the development of actinic keratoses and squamous cell carcinomas.[41]

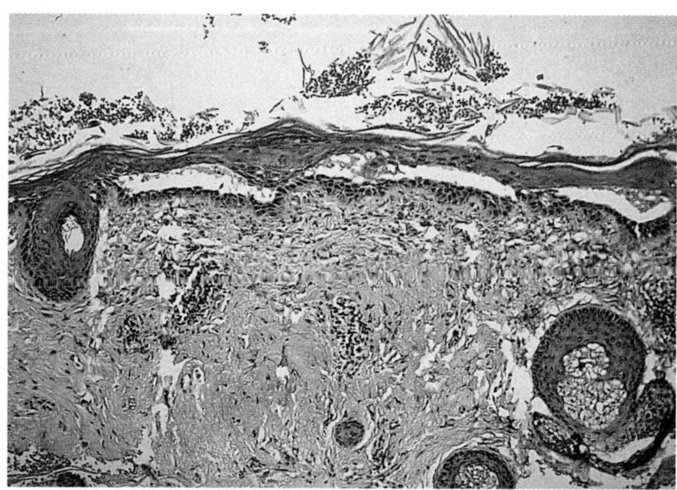

Fig. 71-24 Actinic keratosis. This lesion has a layer of atypical keratinocytes replacing most of the normal basal layer. A decrease of adhesive junctions between cells leads to increased mechanical fragility and acantholytic clefts.

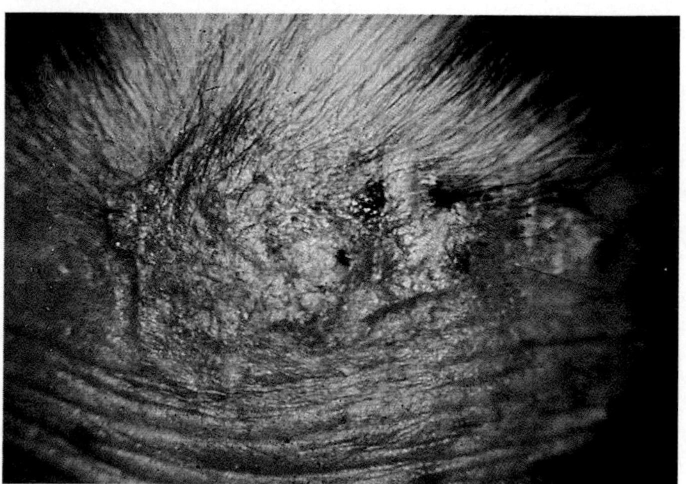

Fig. 71-23 Actinic keratosis. Actinic damage is diffuse and actinic keratoses can be confluent. Mechanical fragility of the epithelium causes an increased tendency to ulcerate and bleed.

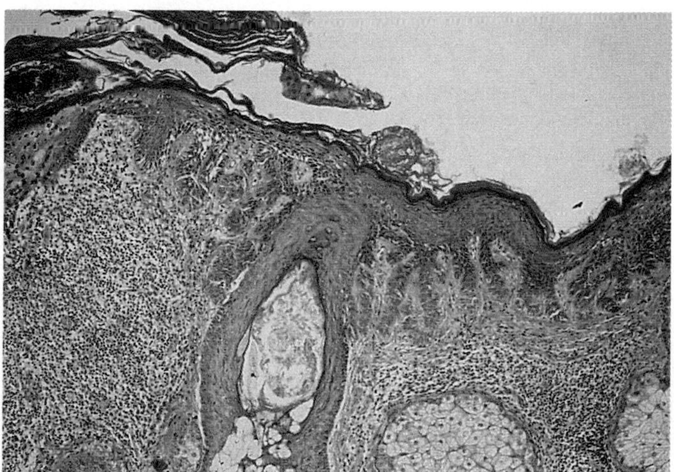

Fig. 71-25 Actinic keratosis (SIN-I). The basal layer has been increased by protrusions of atypical cells into the papillary dermis.

Squamous cell carcinoma in situ Squamous cell carcinoma in situ occurs not only in sun-damaged skin, but also on sun-protected regions. It has been given special names when it appears on various body sites, for example, "erythroplasia of Queyrat," when it appears on the penis, and "Bowen's disease," when the lesions are mainly erythematous plaques on sun-protected skin (Fig. 71-28).[38] In all these lesions the skin has a surface scale that is slight or may be thick. Radiation, chemical exposure, certain papillomaviruses (HPV 5, 16, and 18), and nonhealing ulcers, have all been suggested causes of squamous cell carcinoma. At times the lesions can have a very verrucous appearance, particularly in the oral cavity, near the anus and genitalia, and on the soles of the feet. This form has been called "verrucous carcinoma," with special names given for lesions in the oral cavity (oral florid papillomatosis), in the genital region *(giant condyloma of Buschke and Loewenstein),* and on the soles *(carcinoma cuniculatum).* Immunosuppression leads to rapid progression from in situ to invasive lesions. The invasive lesions are discussed later in the section on tumors affecting both the epidermis and dermis.

PATHOLOGY. The histologic hallmark of this disorder is severe cytologic atypism of the keratinocytes through the full thickness of the epidermis, with obliteration and sometimes invasion of the epidermal appendages. However, large lesions with only basal cytologic atypia in the epidermis should be considered squamous cell carcinomas in situ (Fig. 71-29) if there is obliteration of or invasion down the appendages. Just as in actinic keratoses, these lesions correspond to SIN-I. SIN-II lesions have more extensive cytologic atypia, often with large cells migrating upward in the epidermis (Fig. 71-30). SIN-III corresponds to full-thickness severe atypia in the epidermis (Fig. 71-31). In contrast, verrucous carcinoma often has very little if any nuclear atypism but is considerably thickened, with a papillomatous surface, and has broad bulbous protrusions into the dermis. Some areas may manifest more severe cytologic atypia, particularly if they are in a lesion that is invasive. There usually is a lymphocytic inflammatory infiltrate in the dermis. Lesions may be hyperpigmented because of increased melanin in basal keratinocytes.

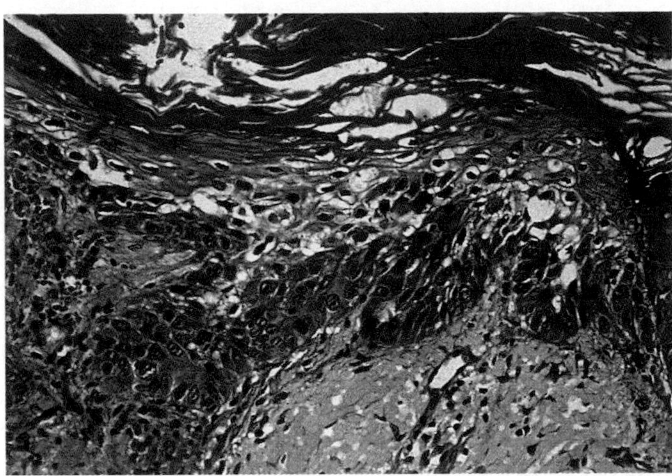

Fig. 71-26 Actinic keratosis (SIN-II). The lower half of the epidermis has been extensively replaced by atypical keratinocytes.

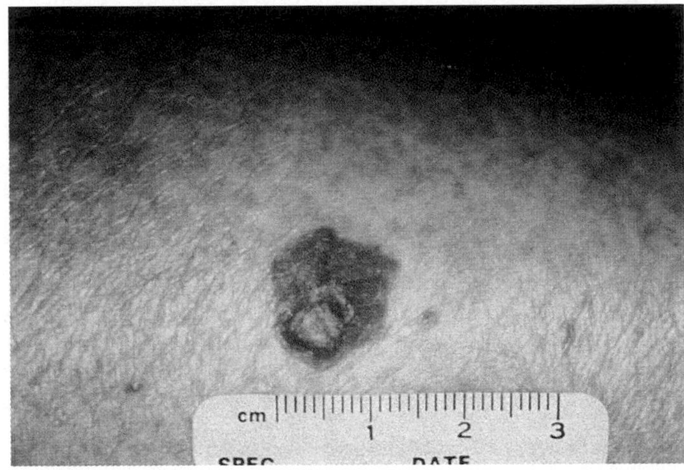

Fig. 71-28 Bowen's disease. This irregular, scaly, well-demarcated, erythematous patch on sun-protected skin is squamous cell carcinoma in situ.

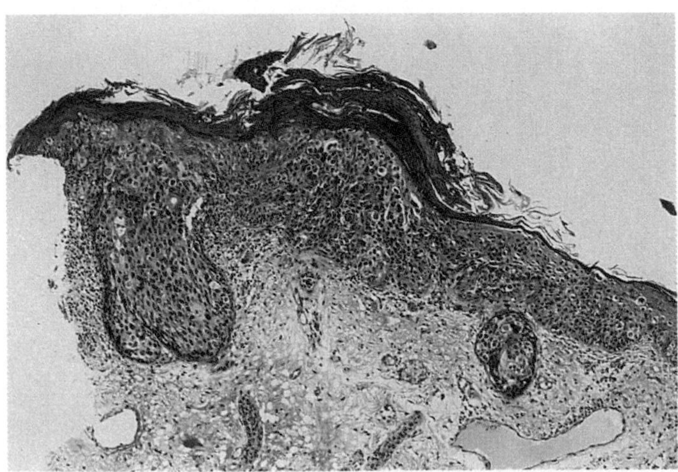

Fig. 71-27 Actinic keratosis (SIN-III). This lesion is equivalent to carcinoma in situ. The epidermis has atypical keratinocytes throughout its thickness, and there is extension down the appendages.

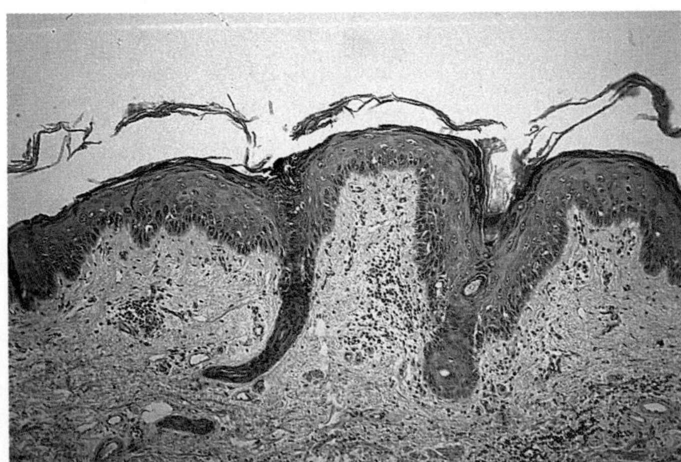

Fig. 71-29 Bowen's disease (SIN-I). The presence of cytologic atypism of keratinocytes may be only in the basal region of the epidermis in some lesions, which are recognizable as Bowen's disease because of their large size.

Small biopsy specimens are very difficult to classify, particularly in the case of verrucous carcinoma versus verruca vulgaris. By immunoperoxidase techniques, the production of virus protein in the nucleus of the keratinocytes is much more typical of wart than it is of verrucous carcinoma. EM fails to detect virus particles in the nuclei of verrucous carcinoma but demonstrates the intranuclear virus particles in warts, particularly if the cytoplasm is somewhat vacuolated, corresponding to *koilocytosis*. EM of Bowen's disease shows a partial to complete obliteration of the normal basement membrane structures, with cytoplasmic protrusions, called "pseudopodia," extending into the basement membrane zone. In contrast, the basement membrane zone of verrucous carcinoma usually is indistinguishable from normal epidermis, except in invasive regions. Amplification of the viral DNA by the polymerase chain reaction followed by DNA hybridization methods provides the most sensitive approach for detection of the papillomaviruses.

Paget's disease. The term *Paget's disease* includes mammary and extramammary Paget's disease. Clinically the disease presents as an erythematous, eroded plaque on the breast or other skin site[42] (Fig. 71-32). The lesions of the breast very frequently involve the nipple. Other sites are areas with apocrine sweat glands, such as the axilla, periumbilical region, scrotum or vulva, and perianal region. The skin can resemble that seen in spongiotic dermatitis ("eczema"), but the sharp demarcation and centrifugal enlargement of the lesion are important clues to Paget's disease.

PATHOLOGY. In the epidermis, there is an infiltrate of atypical cells, often dispersed individually (Fig. 71-33), and occasionally forming glandular structures in the epidermis. The atypical cells are large, with prominent nuclear hyperchromasia and pleomorphism, as well as abundant, usually clear, cytoplasm. The Paget's cells tend to crush down the normal basal keratinocytes against the basement membrane but also can replace them. Melanin pigment occasionally is transferred to the cytoplasm of Paget's cells. Special stains can reveal PAS-positive, diastase-resistant components of the cytoplasm. Alcian blue (at pH 2.5) or colloidal iron will stain strongly the mucins containing sialic acid in the cytoplasm. Aldehyde-

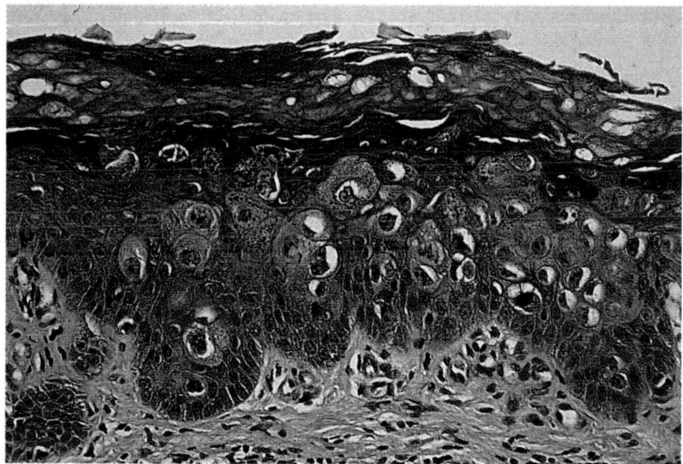

Fig. 71-30 Bowen's disease (SIN-II). Migration of large atypical cells individually in the epidermis is present here. They may also replace the lower epidermal keratinocytes in SIN-II.

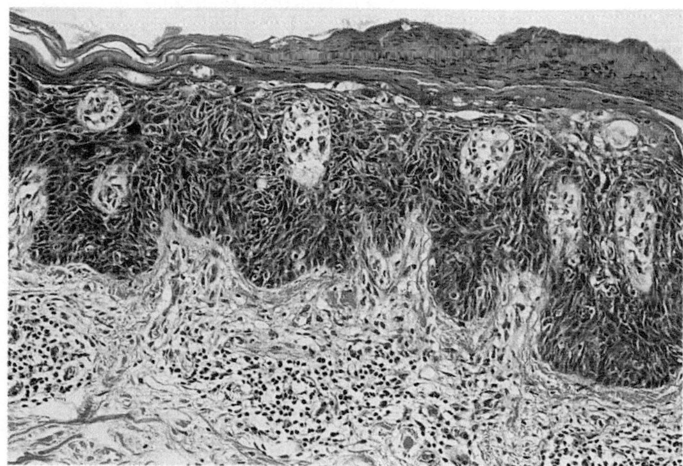

Fig. 71-31 Bowen's disease (SIN-III). This group has readily recognizable cytologic atypia throughout the full thickness of the epidermis and is clearly squamous cell carcinoma in situ.

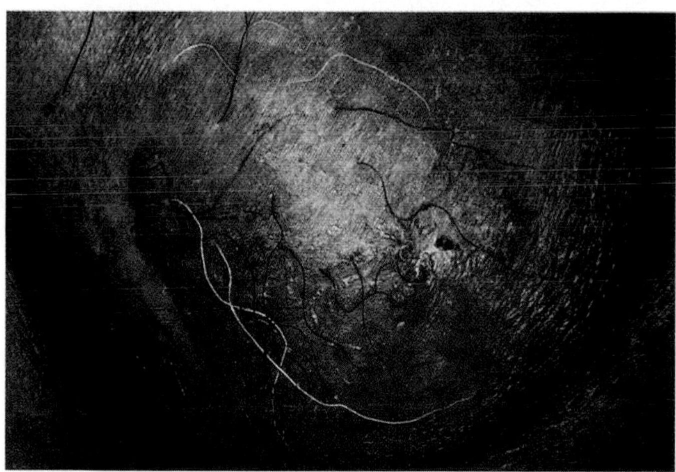

Fig. 71-32 Paget's disease. Extramammary Paget's disease, here of the scrotum, is a well-demarcated, erythematous region, which may or may not be scaly.

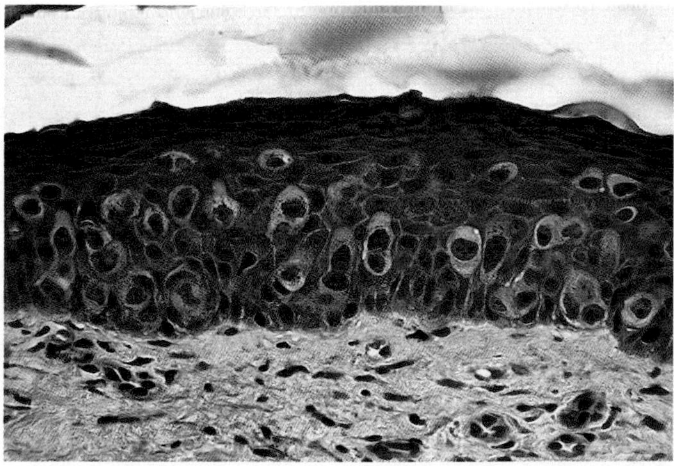

Fig. 71-33 Paget's disease. The migration of large, pale atypical cells in the epidermis usually spares the basal layer.

fuchsin with PAS stains intracytoplasmic mucin a purplish color.

Carcinoembryonic antigen (CEA) can be demonstrated by immunohistochemistry in the cytoplasm of Paget's cells[43] (Fig. 71-34) and is useful for differentiating them from malignant melanoma. CEA positivity is a feature of the eccrine or apocrine duct and secretory glandular epithelium, as well as breast carcinoma cells and adenocarcinomas in general. The presence of melanin pigment does not distinguish melanoma from Paget's disease, since melanin can be transferred from normal melanocytes to Paget's cells. Intraepidermal malignant melanomas stain for S-100 protein and vimentin and usually for HMB-45 antigen, which are not features of Paget's cells. An underlying ductal carcinoma of the breast is almost always found in Paget's disease of the nipple, and adenocarcinoma of the rectum can be the cause of perianal Paget's disease. In the purely skin lesions, the Paget's cells can arise from an underlying sweat gland carcinoma or from aberrant differentiation of the keratinocytes in surface epidermis. Other tumors that can produce an intraepidermal pattern of migration mimicking Paget's disease are eccrine porocarcinoma and sebaceous carcinoma, particularly on the eyelid.

Melanocytic lesions

Freckle. Freckles, or ephelids, are small discrete, nearly round macules that are less than 5 mm in diameter and have a uniform brown color.[44] They appear in areas exposed to UV radiation. The tendency to form freckles is transmitted as an autosomal dominant trait.

PATHOLOGY. The freckle is characterized by an increased amount of melanin in the basal keratinocytes. Melanocytes are not increased in number. The dendrites of the melanocytes may be prominent.

A freckle fades with sun protection but a lentigo does not. "Freckling" has been described in several diseases, but these do not have true freckles and actually have lentigines. Axillary "freckling" is a marker for neurofibromatosis. "Freckling" of the oral mucosa and facial skin can be a marker of Peutz-Jeghers syndrome. Many "freckles" in children can also be found in XP.

Café-au-lait spot. In contrast to a freckle, a café-au-lait spot is larger and more irregular in outline, but the color is uniform, light tan.[44] The size can be as much as 20 cm in diameter. A few small café-au-lait macules, less than 3, can be found in 10% of the normal population. They are found in almost 100% of patients with neurofibromatosis. The presence of 5 or more café-au-lait macules that are more than 5 mm in diameter in a child under the 5 years of age is indicative of neurofibromatosis until proved otherwise. Café-au-lait macules also occur in Albright's syndrome (polyostotic fibrous dysplasia, endocrine dysfunction, and melanotic macules).

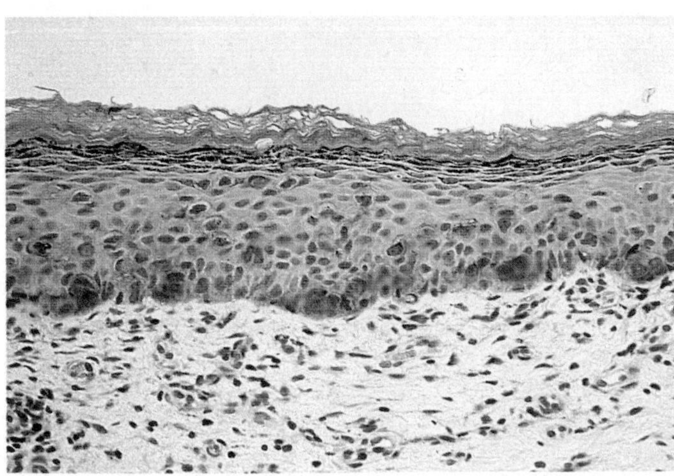

Fig. 71-34 Paget's disease. Staining for carcinoembryonic antigen is positive on the malignant cells of Paget's disease and negative on cells of Bowen's disease.

PATHOLOGY. A café-au-lait macule has hyperpigmentation of basal keratinocytes with very little increase in the number of melanocytes in the basal epidermis. The melanocytes often contain macromelanosomes, which can be seen in the light microscope as round pigment globules, 0.5 to 2 μm in diameter. Macromelanosomes may be seen, however, in lentiginous nevi and nevi with architectural disorder and thus are not diagnostic of café-au-lait macules.

Melanotic macule, reactive type. Simple hyperpigmentation of basal keratinocytes may occur in response to epidermal injury. This is common after UV exposure as well as in response to trauma or to hormones, as in melasma or Addison's disease. Oral mucosa may also respond to trauma with hyperpigmentation, which has been named *mucosal melanotic macule, reactive type*.[45] This can present as a relatively large area of dark brown hyperpigmentation of the oral mucosa that has to be distinguished from malignant melanoma. The onset is acute, a history of prior trauma is common, and the lesions tend to spontaneously resolve by 6 months. The lesions are more frequent in black than in white patients.

PATHOLOGY. There is an upward migration of heavily pigmented, dendritic melanocytes in the mucosal epithelium, without cytologic atypia. It is important to note that the basal layer of the epithelium lacks any evidence of melanocytic proliferation.[45]

Lentigo and lentiginous melanocytic lesions. Lentigo is a discrete, round to oval, hyperpigmented lesion (Fig. 71-35) characterized by elongation of rete ridges and increased melanin pigment in the basal keratinocytes (Fig. 71-36). Clinically, lentigines have been divided on the basis of associated findings such as evidence of sun damage *(solar lentigo)*, or the unilateral occurrence of the pigmentation in association with hypertrichosis often on the shoulder of young men *(Becker's nevus)*, or with polyps of the gastrointestinal tract *(Peutz-Jeghers syndrome)*.[36,44] Without these associations, a similar small lesion of hyperpigmentation is called *simple lentigo*, or *lentigo simplex*. Sometimes the name "lentigo" is used as the adjective "lentiginous" to refer to a proliferation of individual melanocytic cells along the dermoepidermal junction associated with elongation of rete ridges. Clinically a lentigo simplex often is a macular, uniformly tan to dark brown, sharply demarcated lesion, approximately 3 to 5 mm in diameter. Lentigo simplex may be present at birth or may be acquired. In large numbers they are associated with several syndromes; for example, perioral lentigines are associated with intestinal polyps in Peutz-Jeghers syndrome. In the LEOPARD syndrome, the acronym stands for the first letters of each of the following: *l*entigines, *e*lectrocardiographic abnormalities, *o*cular disorders including hypertelorism, *p*ulmonary stenosis, *a*bnormalities in genitalia, *r*etardation of growth, *d*eafness caused by an inner-ear defect. Solar lentigines are often slightly larger lesions, which may be up to 1 cm in diameter, and are slightly irregular in outline but are a uniform light tan or brown color.

PATHOLOGY. The lesions consist of a combination of both keratinocyte and melanocyte growth to produce acanthosis and elongation of rete ridges as well as varying degrees of enlargement and increase in number of melanocytes (Fig. 71-36). In Becker's nevus, a complex hamartoma of the epidermis and dermis, the epidermal histologic characteristics are similar to those of a lentigo simplex, in which the melanocytes are small and are not increased much in number.[44] Unique aspects of Becker's nevus are enlarged hair follicles and smooth muscle hamartomas in the dermis. In ordinary forms of lentigo simplex, the melanocytes often are minimally enlarged and not particularly increased in number, though there is variation in opinion on this description.[36,44,46] In contrast, in solar lentigo ("senile lentigo"), the melanocytes are slightly increased in size and in number. An important characteristic of solar lentigo is that the rete ridges are elongated, indicating a preservation of the epidermal-melanin unit. Upward migration of individual melanocytes in the epidermis is absent. When lentigines are induced by psoralen and ultraviolet radiation (PUVA) therapy, the melanocyte enlargement may be striking and the borders of the lesion are irregular.[47] For lesions in which individually dispersed melanocytes have increased greatly in number on the elongated rete ridges, the term *simple lentigo* may be used,[44] but the term *nevoid lentigo* seems preferable. When the melanocytes have formed rounded nests of nevus cells on the elongated rete ridges, the preferable term is "lentiginous junctional melanocytic nevus."[36] In some enlarged nevi with irregular pigmentation (Fig. 71-37), the rete ridges are elongated and distorted and the papillary dermis is fibrotic; thus the lentiginous junctional nevus has architectural disorder (Figs. 71-38 to 71-40). These lesions can be graded based on the amount of cytologic atypism of melanocytes.[48,49] One may use adjectives or roman numerals[39] to express these grades of atypia in nested populations of melanocytes in the basal portion of the epidermis. "Mild," or minimal, atypism corresponds to an irregular architecture with melanocytes that have condensed nuclei without prominent nucleoli (melanocytic intraepidermal neoplasia, or MIN-I) (Fig. 71-38); "moderate" atypism has enlarged

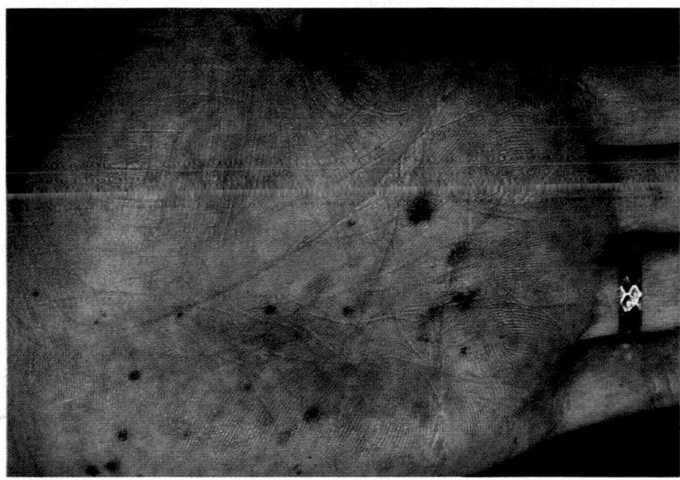

Fig. 71-35 Lentigo. This patient has multiple small round pigmented lentigos on the palm, an unusual site.

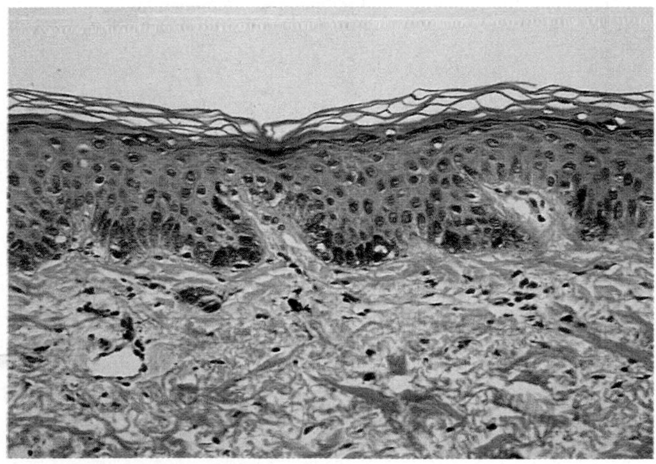

Fig. 71-36 Lentigo. There is slight thickening of rete ridges, increased prominence of a few melanocytes, and hyperpigmentation of basal keratinocytes at the bases of rete ridges.

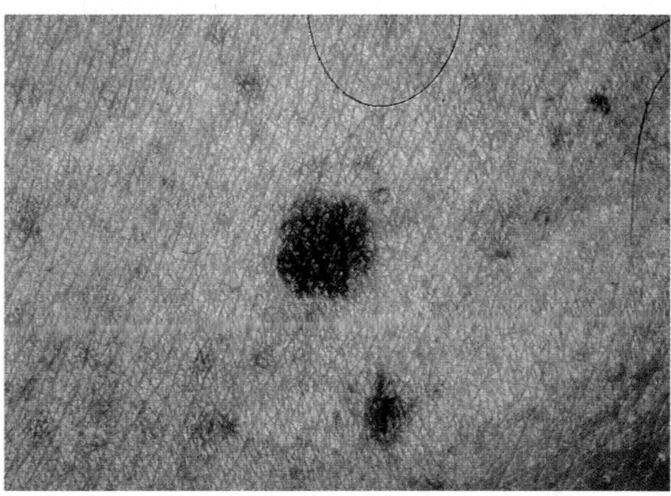

Fig. 71-37 Junctional nevus with architectural disorder, formerly dysplastic nevus." This lesion is larger than 6 mm in diameter and has irregular pigmentation as well as inflammatory erythema around the periphery.

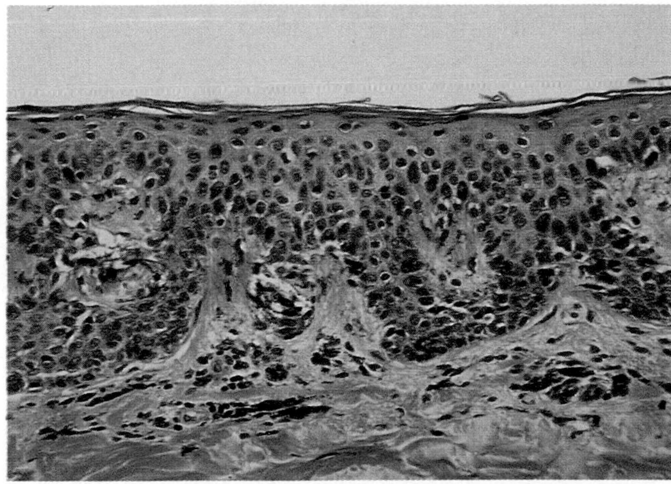

Fig. 71-38 Lentiginous junctional nevus with minimal architectural disorder and cytologic atypism (MIN-I). Nests of nevus cells are present as well as individual melanocytes on slightly distorted rete ridges. The papillary dermis is fibrotic. The nevus cell nuclei are small, and nucleoli are not visible.

polygonal, hyperchromatic nuclei, often with visible nucleoli (MIN-II) (Fig. 71-39); "severe" atypism is characterized by enlarged nuclei with vesicular chromatin and prominent nucleoli (MIN-III) (Fig. 71-40). MIN-III is not always separable from malignant melanoma in situ.[48] These nested melanocytic lesions with nuclear atypism formerly were called "dysplastic junctional melanocytic nevi," but the current suggested name is "junctional melanocytic nevus with architectural disorder and atypism of melanocytes"[50] (Table 71-5).

Lentiginous lesions may be static or unchanging over time, or they may progress from simple lentigines to various lentiginous nevi. Consequently the definitions represent fixed points on a dynamic range of changes, and various authors have divided this range somewhat differently. However, all these lesions have the participation of the epidermal keratinocytes that form the elongated rete ridges. In contrast, malignant melanoma in situ often has lost this pattern of keratinocyte proliferation, and the atypical melanocytes migrate upward in

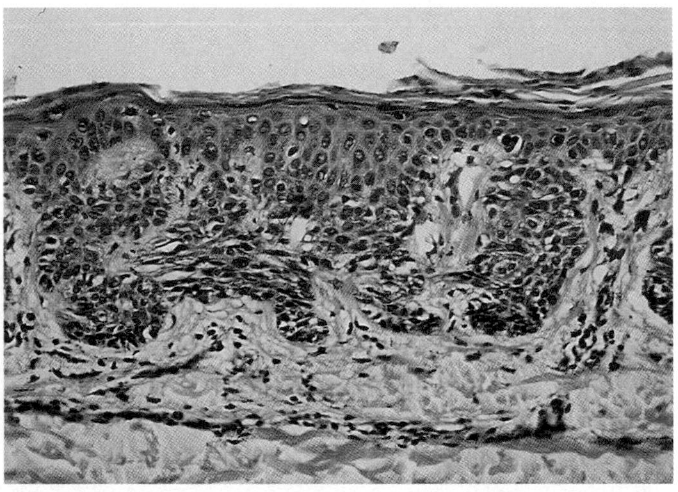

Fig. 71-39 Lentiginous junctional nevus with moderate architectural disorder and cytologic atypism (MIN-II). The nests of nevus cells distort the rete ridges more than those in Fig. 71-38. The nuclei are larger, and a few cells have visible nucleoli.

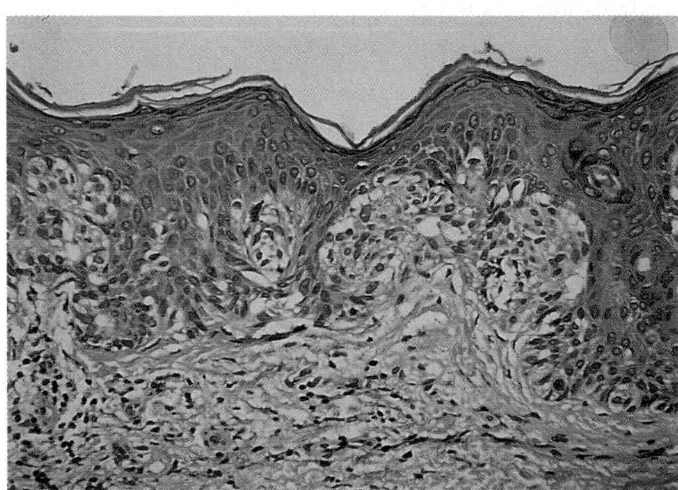

Fig. 71-40 Junctional melanocytic nevus with severe architectural disorder and cytologic atypism (MIN-III). The nests of nevus cells are almost confluent on the distorted rete ridges. The nuclei are enlarged and nucleoli are prominent. Intraepidermal upward migration of individual atypical melanocytes is absent.

Table 71-5 Comparison of melanocytic lesions*

	Nevi		Melanoma		
Histologic feature	**Compound**	**Disordered**	**Spitz**	**In situ**	**Invasive**
Acanthosis	+	+	++	+/–	+/–
Elongated rete ridges	+	++	++	+/–	+/–
Distorted rete ridges	+/–	+++	+/–	+/–	+/–
Pagetoid migration	+/–†	+/–	+	++	++
Lesion symmetry‡	++	+	+++	+/–	+/–
Sharp circumscription	++	+	+	+/–	+/–
Uniform nests	+	–	+	–	–
Vertical nests	+/–	+/–	++	+/–	+/–
Cytologic atypia	+/–	+	+	++	+++
Mitoses in epidermis	+	+	+	++	++
Mitoses at dermal base	–	–	+/–	–§	++
Cells smaller at base	++	++	+	–	–
Nuclear atypia at base	–	+/–	+/–	–§	++
Junctional beyond dermal	+/–	++	+/–	–§	++
Dermal fibrosis	+	++	+	+‖	++
Lamellar fibroplasia	–	++	–	+/–¶	+/–¶

*, Meaning of scale: – = absent; +/– = rare or uncommon; + = common; ++ = present in almost all lesions; +++ = very striking feature in almost all lesions.
†, At birth, occasionally in acral nevi in young patients, and in some recurrent junctional components of nevi after surgery or trauma.
‡, Nodular melanomas, small melanomas, and metastatic melanomas may have symmetry.
§, Melanoma in situ does not have a dermal component.
‖, Regression of the dermal portion of a lesion can lead to fibrosis.
¶, Lamellar fibroplasia at the tips of rete ridges can be a residual component in melanomas that arise in disordered nevi.

an epidermis that is nearly normal in thickness or is atrophic. Despite controversy over the criteria for the definition of "dysplastic nevus," indeed there is a familial syndrome in which the patients have irregular nevi and a high risk for the development of melanoma. This syndrome has been called the "familial atypical multiple mole and melanoma (FAMMM) syndrome" or the "dysplastic nevus syndrome."

Malignant melanoma in situ. It is of the utmost importance to recognize this lesion.[44,50,51] Clinically, melanomas in situ are often irregular macules with poor circumscription and blurred margins (Fig. 71-41). Usually there are irregularities in color also, with a light tan interspersed with dark brown and black. Gray color may be present in areas of lesion regression. Erythema indicates inflammation that is frequent in the dermis adjacent to these lesions. Some lesions do not have any melanin coloration visible grossly and are purely erythematous macules. Others have a slight scale, making differentiation from an inflamed actinic keratosis impossible without microscopic examination. Also the pigmentation may be uniformly dark and difficult to differentiate from that of a nevus. Although "malignant melanoma in situ" is the preferred term for many of the lesions, other names historically have been applied to these lesions, for example, malignant melanoma in situ on sun-damaged atrophic skin of the face was called "Hutchinson's melanotic freckle," or "lentigo maligna" (Fig. 71-42).[36] When the same lesion occurred on acral sites, it was called "acral lentiginous malignant melanoma in situ." There has been disagreement concerning the use of these terms, and in some opinions the simple designation "malignant melanoma in situ" is preferable. Lesions that have black or red thickened areas are suspicious for having developed invasion. The invasive forms of these lesions are discussed in the section on tumors affecting both the epidermis and dermis.

PATHOLOGY. The degree of cytologic atypia of melanocytes and their scatter in the epidermis are both greater in malignant melanoma in situ than in lentigines and lentiginous nevi.[44] Melanomas often show upward migration of atypical melanocytes beyond the basal layer and over the suprapapillary plates as well as on the rete ridges (Fig. 71-43). This migration ("pagetoid upward migration") can continue even to the stratum granulosum and stratum corneum, where the melanocytes appear as rounded balls of pigment in the surface keratin without connection to the surrounding keratinocytes. However, not all melanomas in situ have prominent upward migration, especially the lentigo maligna type (Fig. 71-44). Another exception is that some benign lesions show upward migration of melanocytes, as in compound nevi shortly after birth, in junctional Spitz's nevi, and in regenerating junctional components of nevi over a scar. Usually melanoma cells are enlarged and have cytologic atypia, such as irregular chromatin patterns and prominent nucleoli. The cytoplasm may be prominent and often contains irregular small and large granules of pigment.

In occasional lesions, the melanoma cells are small and show very little individual cell migration upward in the epidermis. Such melanoma cells have hyperchromatic, condensed, irregularly shaped nuclei without prominent nucleoli. These

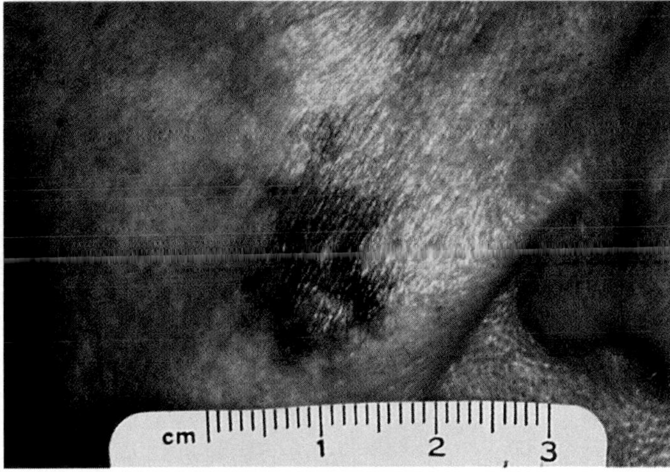

Fig. 71-42 Malignant melanoma in situ. This irregularly shaped and pigmented lesion is on the sun-damaged skin of the cheek in an elderly person. It is the "lentigo maligna" type of melanoma in situ. Notice the presence of pseudopod-like extensions of the lesion into the adjacent epidermis.

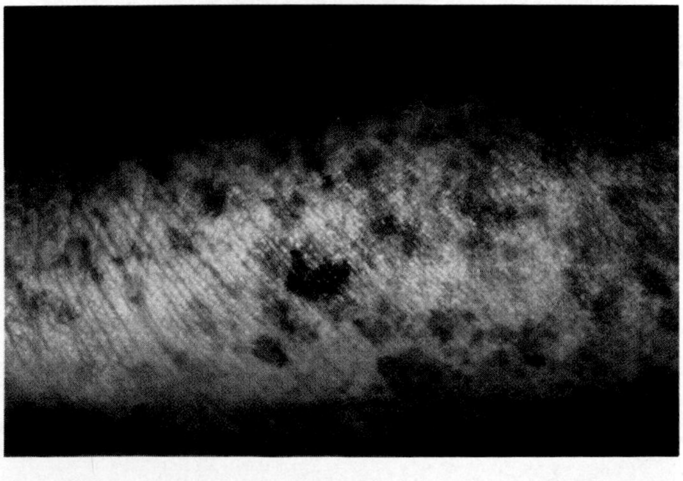

Fig. 71-41 Malignant melanoma in situ. The black irregular lesion on the forearm was a malignant melanoma in situ histologically. It is arising on skin with numerous tan-brown macules that are solar lentigines.

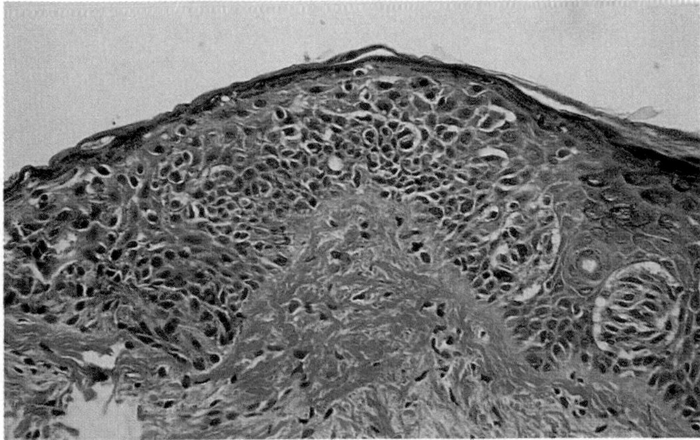

Fig. 71-43 Malignant melanoma in situ. There is a diffuse proliferation of atypical melanocytes, singly and in irregular nests, with extensive intraepidermal upward migration.

features may be hard to distinguish from a traumatized or a desiccated nevus. These melanomas that mimic nevi have been called "minimal deviation melanoma," or "nevoid melanoma."[36,52]

Malignant melanoma in situ typically evokes very little keratinocyte reaction. Thus proliferation of melanocytes in an atrophic epidermis is very suspect of being a melanoma in situ, particularly if that is in sun-damaged skin, without the scar of a previous biopsy site. A recurrent junctional component of a nevus after partial biopsy can have extensive proliferation of individual melanocytes in the epidermis that is very difficult to distinguish from melanoma in situ. A review of any previous biopsy slide is very helpful. If there is any suggestion of a lesion either being or containing an area of malignant melanoma in situ, a conservative reexcision of the lesion can be recommended so that one can be sure that all the atypical melanocytes are removed.

Immunohistochemistry may be needed in problematic cases to determine whether the malignant cells are melanocytes or pigmented keratinocytes.[53-56] S-100 protein and HMB-45 antigen (found in premelanosomes) (Fig. 71-45) are good markers of melanocytes and are useful in distinguishing melanoma from Bowen's disease or Paget's disease. Melanocytes also contain vimentin in contrast to keratinocytes and Paget's disease cells that express cytokeratins. In Paget's disease, the tumor cells express low molecular weight keratins, such as keratins 8 and 18, more than in Bowen's disease.

Junctional melanocytic nevus and Spitz's nevus, junctional type. In contrast to lentiginous nevi, ordinary junctional melanocytic nevi are common in children and young adults but are quite rare after 50 years of age, and they become increasingly rare with greater age.[44] Clinically these lesions are frequently of recent onset. They present as macules that may enlarge up to 6 mm in diameter, are well circumscribed, and have a relatively uniform tan to dark brown pigmentation. Some lesions have very little pigment and appear red, because of slight vasodilatation and inflammation associated with the lesion. Also melanosomes may contain abundant pheomelanin, which has a red color. Junctional nevi on the palms and soles often have a slightly irregular outline (Fig. 71-46) and can be difficult to distinguish from early malignant melanoma in situ. Junctional nevi tend to progress with time to compound nevi by migration of cells into the dermis. Compound nevi and intradermal nevi are discussed later.

PATHOLOGY. Junctional nevi have in common a proliferation of rounded melanocytic cells in circumscribed aggregates at the dermoepidermal junction (Fig. 71-47). These cells are called nevus cells, or "nevomelanocytes," since they differ from normal melanocytes by their lack of dendrites and their tendency to aggregation. The junctional nevus characteristically has sharply defined lateral edges. Upward migration of individual melanocytes is minimal to absent but can be prominent in newborn children in the first few months of life. The cells are uniform round to oval cells, with delicate chromatin patterns and often nucleoli of moderate and similar sizes. The cytoplasm is more abundant than in normal melanocytes and contains fine pigment granules. Junctional nevi on the palms and soles of children can show prominent upward migration of individual cells and be very difficult to distinguish from early malignant melanoma in situ on histologic grounds alone.

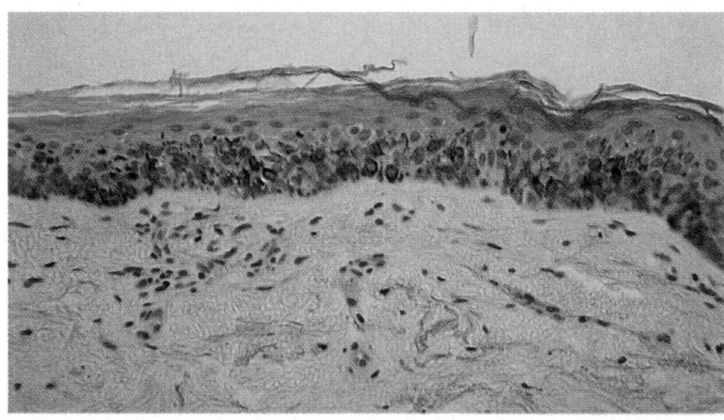

Fig. 71-45 Malignant melanoma in situ. Staining with HMB-45 can reveal the extensive proliferation of melanocytes (labeled by the brown reaction product) within the epidermis; keratinocytes and lymphoid cells do not stain.

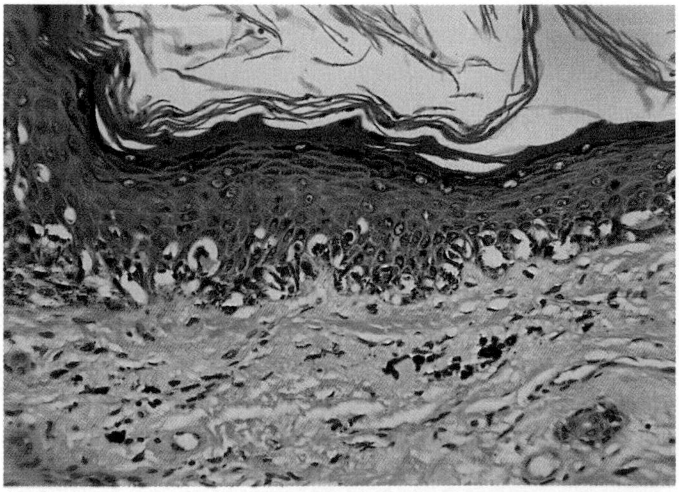

Fig. 71-44 Malignant melanoma in situ, lentigo maligna type. The epidermis is atrophic, and rete ridges are effaced. There is a proliferation of atypical melanocytes individually along the dermoepidermal junction. Melanophages are in the dermis.

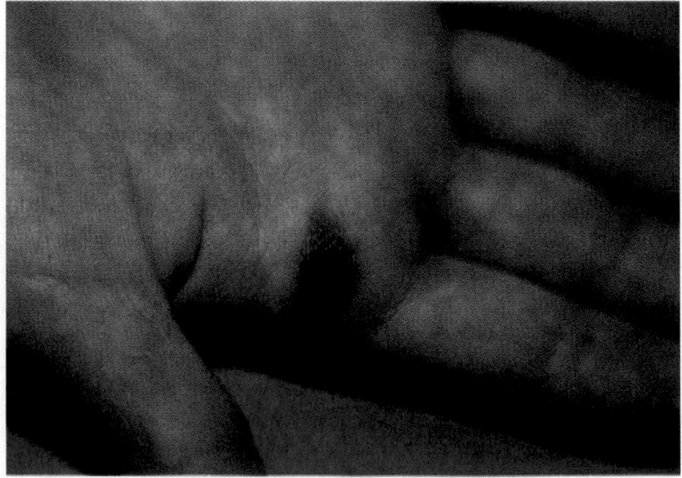

Fig. 71-46 Acral junctional nevus. This lesion in a child is congenital. It has an irregular outline with speckled pigmentation near its edge.

The junctional Spitz's nevus differs from the above description in that the nevus cells form large nests that contain a mixture of spindle and epithelioid cells (Fig. 71-48).[44] Although nuclear atypia may be striking focally, usually the nuclei are simply more enlarged than those in ordinary junctional nevus cells and have more prominent nucleoli. However, the chromatin patterns remain delicate, and the thickness of nuclear envelopes is uniform. Furthermore, epidermal hyperplasia often is present in Spitz's nevi. The junctional nests may be demarcated by small clefts between the nevus cell nests and the adjacent epidermis because of shrinkage during processing. In junctional Spitz's nevi, upward migration of individual cells can be a striking finding, particularly in the center of the lesion. Whole nests of nevus cells also may be eliminated into the stratum corneum. The distinction from malignant melanoma in situ is based on the sharp circumscription, small size, and symmetry of the junctional type of Spitz's nevus.

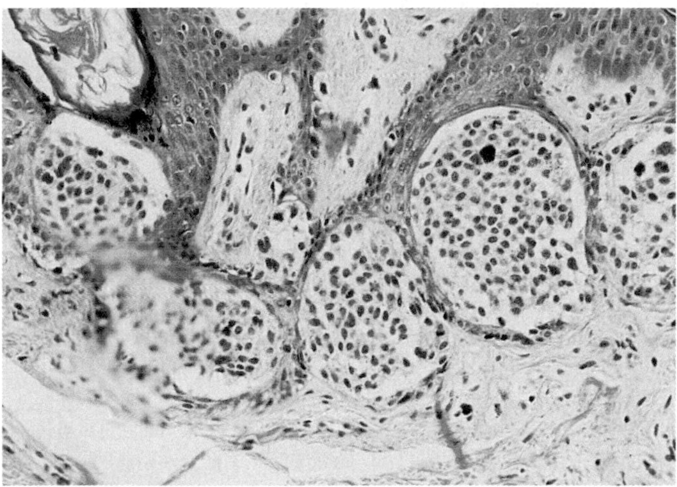

Fig. 71-47 Junctional nevus. The melanocytic cells are in discrete rounded nests near the base of the epidermis and have very little cytologic atypism.

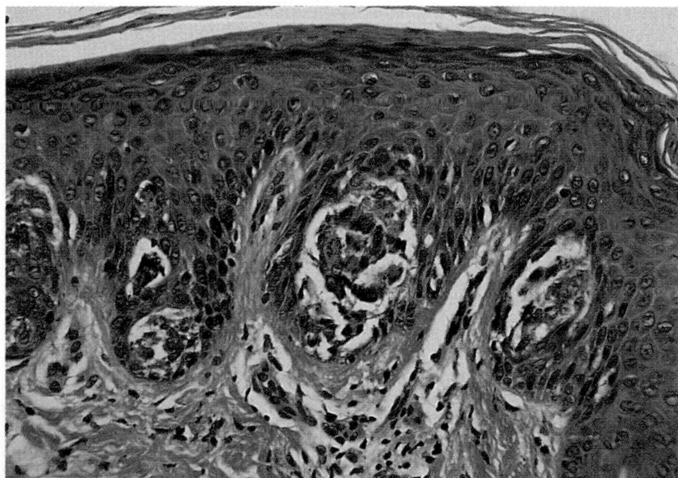

Fig. 71-48 Junctional Spitz's nevus. The nevus cells are large with abundant eosinophilic cytoplasm with variable degrees of pigmentation. Nests of nevus cells are sharply delimited, and the lesion is symmetrical and well circumscribed.

Malignant melanoma is very rare in children under 10 years of age. In contrast, Spitz's nevi are most common in children but may continue to be formed into the fourth decade of life, and so age alone does not distinguish these lesions from melanoma. Malignant melanoma on volar skin is extremely rare in children but begins to appear during middle age and is most frequent in elderly patients.

Lymphoid lesions

Epidermotropic T-cell lymphoma. Early cutaneous T-cell lymphoma (CTCL) often has its initial manifestation as lymphocytic infiltration in the epidermis ("epidermotropism") without much infiltration into the dermis.[57,58] This disease is also known under the historic (but etymologically incorrect) term "mycosis fungoides" (MF). The initial flat macules evolve over a period of years into slightly elevated patches, more elevated plaques, and finally nodular tumors. Clinically the lesions present as poorly circumscribed, irregular macules and patches of erythema, occasionally with a fine surface scale. There may be hypopigmentation (Fig. 71-49), but symmetry and complete depigmentation are not found. Favored sites are sun-protected areas of the body, such as the buttocks and upper thighs and lower abdomen. The patches may start small, only several centimeters in diameter, and can slowly enlarge to 10 or 20 cm in diameter. Central clearing because of regression can occur, giving the lesions irregular arcuate and ring shapes. Pruritus is common and may be severe. Tumors arise within these relatively flat lesions or at distant sites; the thick lesions with prominent dermal infiltration are discussed in a subsequent section. Most of the other neoplastic lymphocytic infiltrates involve the dermis and are also discussed in later sections.

PATHOLOGY. The initial lesions contain hyperchromatic, slightly enlarged lymphocytes scattered through the lower portion of the epidermis (Fig. 71-50). In approximately 50% of patients, the lymphocytes aggregate to form *Darier-Pautrier microabscesses,*[59-61] which are spherical aggregates of atypical lymphocytes in the epidermis, with five to eight nuclei per plane of section. These microabscesses may be purely basal in

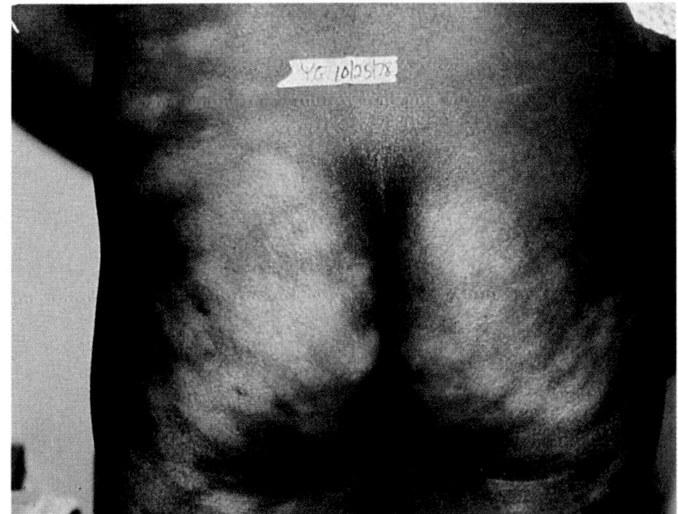

Fig. 71-49 Mycosis fungoides. This patient had very early lesions that produced partial irregular depigmentation of the epidermis. The tendency to involve the buttocks area is common.

location but often migrate upward in the epidermis. The lymphocytes have irregular nuclei with deep irregular convolutions of the nuclear envelope, which may require examination of skin or blood under oil immersion or in the electron microscope (Fig. 71-51). Small nucleoli often are visible. Usually there is very little spongiosis. Slight spongiosis can be found in some patients, particularly in lesions that have been scratched. Parakeratotic scales are common. Melanocytes appear partially disrupted by the lymphoid infiltrate particularly in hypopigmented lesions. Langerhans' cells are increased in number in early lesions and have been suggested to act as foci for aggregation of the lymphocytes in the Darier-Pautrier microabscesses. Mitoses occur in the lymphocytes in the epidermis.

Immunohistochemistry has shown that the neoplastic intraepidermal lymphocytes are T-cells.[62] They express CD4 and HLA-DR but frequently lack certain pan T-cell antigens, such as Leu-8 antigen and CD7.[63,64] CD2, CD3, and CD5 may also show partial loss. The cells are negative for S-100 protein, which distinguishes them from melanocytes and Langerhans' cells in the epidermis. Reactive $CD8^+$ cells and B-lymphocytes may be present also, particularly in cases with spongiosis.

Woringer-Kolopp disease. Woringer-Kolopp disease, also known as "pagetoid reticulosis," is an unusual form of CTCL, which is distinct from mycosis fungoides only in that the patients have a single lesion.[1] The lesion is an erythematous, scaly macule ("patch") or thin plaque that may be eroded. Patients tend to have the lesions on acral sites. Some patients have been cured by local excision or radiation.

PATHOLOGY. The histologic characteristics of this lesion are distinctive because of the extreme epidermotropism of the T-lymphocytes, usually with a diffuse pattern of infiltration in the epidermis. The cells often are large and pale staining, with large nuclei and nucleoli. Nuclear membrane convolutions may be prominent. These cells are rather large T-lymphocytes that are $CD4^+$ or $CD8^+$, and some are $Ki\text{-}1^+$ ($CD30^+$).[65]

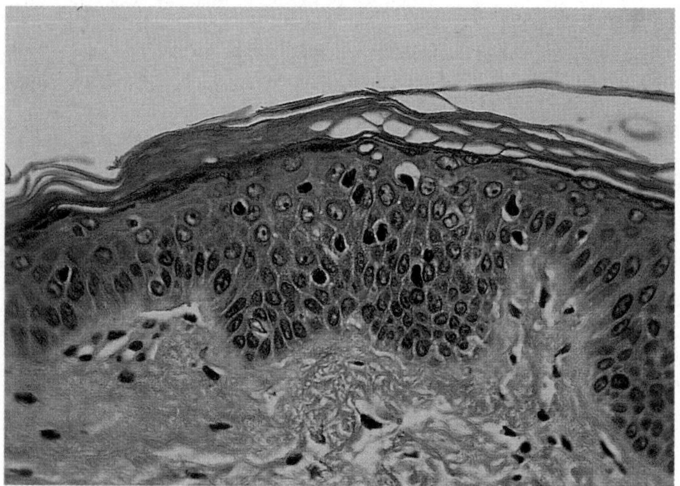

Fig. 71-50 Mycosis fungoides. Very early lesions have small numbers of atypical lymphocytes, often with epidermotropism.

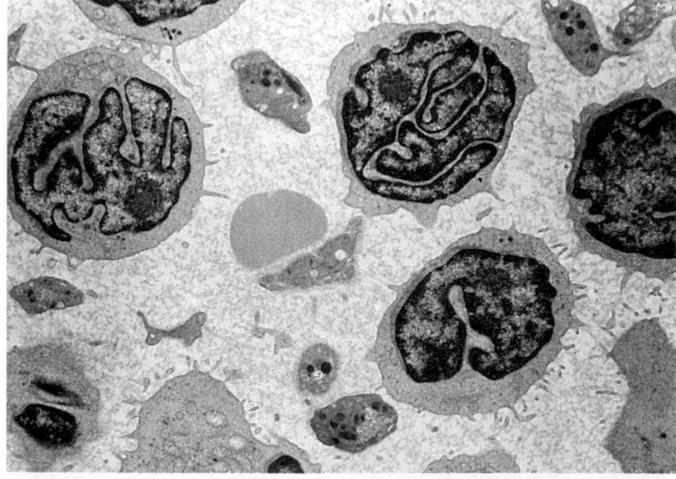

Fig. 71-51 Mycosis fungoides in a leukemic form (Sézary's syndrome). Electron micrograph of T-lymphocytes shows deep irregular indentations of the nuclear envelope with prominent nucleoli. The lymphocytes may be small or may be enlarged.

DISEASES INVOLVING BOTH EPIDERMIS AND DERMIS

Genodermatoses

Incontinentia pigmenti

Incontinentia pigmenti is a rare X-linked dominant disease that occurs almost exclusively in female children, since it is usually lethal in males.[66] The disease has three phases and has its onset near the time of birth. The first stage can begin in utero or even occur entirely in utero. The child has unusual streaks of erythema that contain linear or grouped clear vesicles on the trunk or extremities (Fig. 71-52). The second stage has papules that are warty in appearance and are also in linear or grouped arrays, the location of which may be different from that of the vesicles. The third stage is characterized by hyperpigmented streaks, which result from the regression of the inflammatory and verrucous lesions. The child usually evolves through these stages over several years. Approximately half the children have other congenital malformations, of teeth, eyes, or central nervous system.

PATHOLOGY. The various stages of the disease are distinctive histologically. The early inflammatory phase has spon-

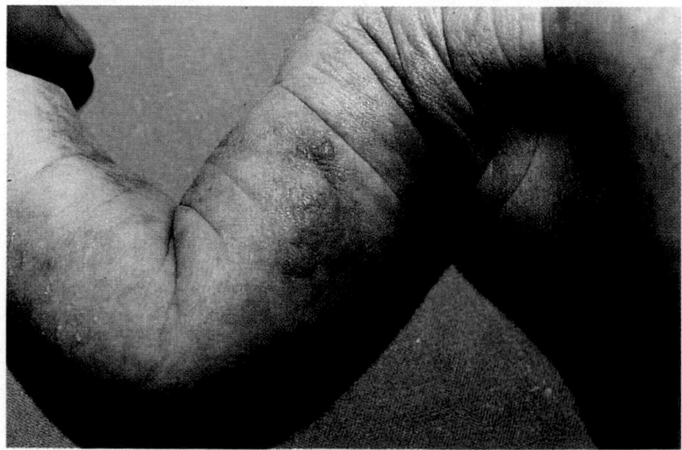

Fig. 71-52 Incontinentia pigmenti. This child has irregular patches of erythema with vesicles on the arm. The patches are often in a linear arrangement.

giosis and a superficial perivascular dermal infiltrate of lymphocytes and eosinophils (Fig. 71-53). The eosinophils are abundant in the epidermis in the spongiotic zones, which can form small vesicles. In the midphase, or "warty" phase, the lesions have hyperkeratosis, acanthosis, and many individual necrotic keratinocytes in the epidermis. The dermis has a superficial perivascular lymphocytic infiltrate with few eosinophils. The final phase of hyperpigmentation is attributable to melanin in macrophages in the papillary dermis, which could be the remainder after resolution either of the inflammatory lesions or the keratinocyte necrosis in the warty lesions.

This disease is in the differential diagnosis of spongiotic dermatitis in newborns. Another disease in newborns that is associated with eosinophils in the epidermis is erythema toxicum neonatorum, which involves the follicles, whereas incontinentia pigmenti has no such predilection. A type of verrucous epidermal nevus can have the histologic features of the warty lesions, can occur in males, and needs to be distinguished from true incontinentia pigmenti.

Inflammatory, metabolic, and traumatic disorders

Vesicular and bullous disorders

Intraepidermal spongiotic vesicles and bullae. Under the heading "intraepidermal spongiotic vesicles and bullae" we have included diseases that clinically can present with large plaques or even small papules. There is usually a surface keratotic scale. The amount of spongiosis is variable, but lesions with vesicles grossly have a weeping of fluid that was called "eczema," a clinical term that should be avoided, since it includes many types of spongiotic dermatitides such as contact dermatitis, atopic dermatitis, and seborrheic dermatitis, in the work of some authors both in the United States and in Europe. The following diseases and reactions have this histologic appearance, which is discussed below for the group as a whole.

Contact dermatitis can be on the basis of direct irritation ("irritant contact dermatitis") or from an allergic reaction ("allergic contact dermatitis").[67] Clinically, it may be difficult to distinguish these two forms from each other. Tense spongiotic vesicles tend to be somewhat more frequent in the allergic form. Both have erythema and can have weeping of fluid from the skin surface (Fig. 71-54). Chronic contact dermatitis leads to thickening of the skin, erythema, and surface scaling. In the chronic form, the amount of fluid lost through the epidermis may be minimal. Contact dermatitis often can be recognized clinically by the distribution of lesions to particular anatomic sites and the unusual linearity of lesions, such as that attributable to brushing against a plant such as poison ivy or poison oak. However, the persistence of antigens in the environment and unusual routes of exposure, such as airborne antigens, can produce confusion clinically with numerous other inflammatory disorders.

Atopic dermatitis is a complex disorder in which young children are the most frequently affected.[68] There is skin inflammation and evidence of altered immunity, particularly hyperreactivity to certain antigens, such as foods, house dust, pollens, and animal hairs. The children often have elevated IgE levels in the blood during exacerbations of the disease and a decreased number of CD8-positive lymphocytes in the peripheral circulation in severely affected children. Atopic dermatitis resolves spontaneously in many patients during the first 5 years of life, but in a few it persists throughout life. An early manifestation in children is pruritus that can lead to rubbing and scratching of the face (Fig. 71-55) and secondary impetiginization of lesions. Later in life, as in adolescence, many of the patients experience pruritus in antecubital fossae (Fig. 71-56), and the chronic rubbing leads to secondary lesions having thickened skin with accentuated skin markings

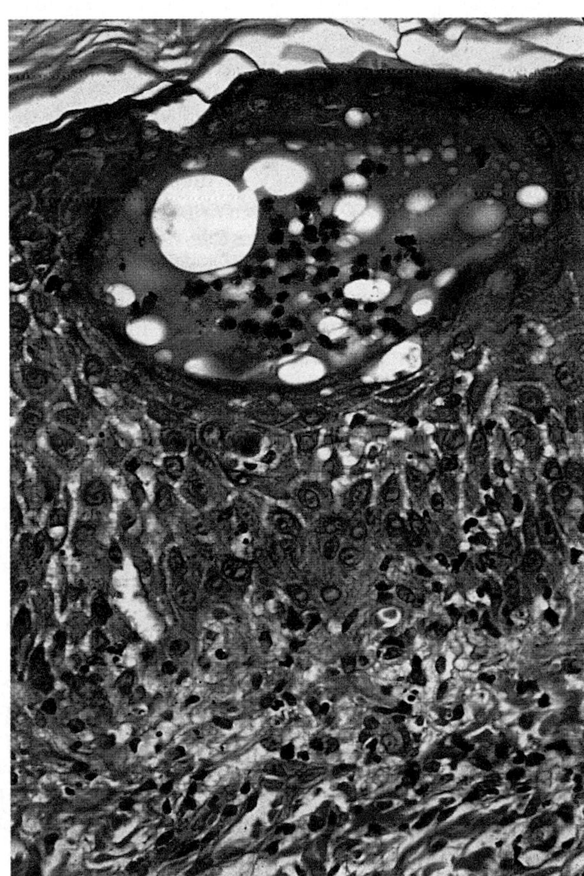

Fig. 71-53 Incontinentia pigmenti. Spongiotic microvesicles are in the epidermis with many eosinophils.

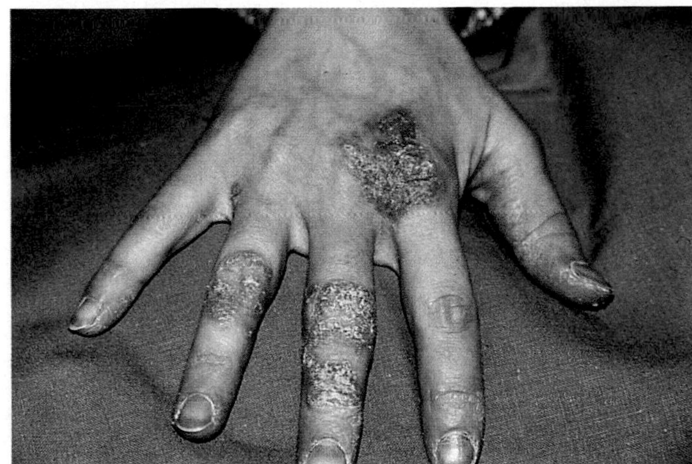

Fig. 71-54 Contact dermatitis. An allergen has led to vesicles and scaling at the sites of contact with the hand.

skin, the dermoepidermal junction lacks immunoglobulin deposits, which is a feature that can help distinguish this disease from SLE.

Graft-versus-host disease. Graft-versus-host disease (GVHD) is an inflammatory syndrome that affects multiple organs and develops in immunodeficient patients who are injected with normal immunocompetent lymphocytes, as during bone marrow transplantation.[125-127] Reactions to differences in minor histocompatibility antigens are likely causes.[128] The gastrointestinal tract, liver, and skin are primary targets of attack by these grafted lymphoid cells. The earliest and most minimal skin lesions present as macular erythema or erythematous papules with some scale. Follicle-based reactions are also frequent in the early stages.[129] Later lesions may resemble those of lupus erythematosus or systemic scleroderma.[130] Lichenoid papules can resemble lichen planus. In very severe reactions, epidermal necrosis and sloughing is prominent.

PATHOLOGY. The histopathologic manifestations of GVHD are diverse. The early lesions have few lymphoid cells at the dermoepidermal junction associated with a few necrotic keratinocytes (Fig. 71-88). The close attachment and even stretching of the lymphocytes over the surface of the target cell is indicative of the phenomenon called "satellitosis," suggestive of direct lymphocyte-mediated cytotoxicity. The keratinocytes at the bases of rete ridges seem to be preferential early targets. Lichenoid lesions contain more infiltrate and show epidermal hyperplasia. The late scarred lesions often have sclerosis throughout the dermis with very few lymphoid cells. They are indistinguishable from late lesions of systemic scleroderma. The finding of necrotic keratinocytes in the hair follicles and sweat glands helps distinguish acute GVHD from erythema multiforme.

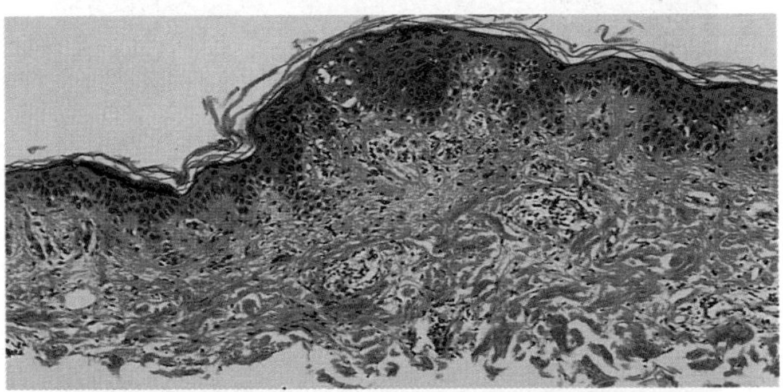

Fig. 71-87 Dermatomyositis. This acute lesion shows slight lymphocytic infiltration into the epidermis with focal necrosis of keratinocytes. A superficial perivascular lymphocytic infiltrate is present in an edematous dermis.

Other papulonodular and plaque lesions.

Lichen simplex chronicus. This disorder, which historically was called "neurodermatitis," presents as thickening of the epidermis and papillary dermis at the site of chronic irritation and rubbing.[36] The lesions are raised plaques (Fig. 71-89) with hyperkeratosis, accentuation of the skin markings ("lichenification"), and hyperpigmentation. Some lesions consist of coalescent small whitish papules (called "lichenoid frictional dermatitis"). When the patient picks instead of rubs one spot consistently, the skin develops a more hyperkeratotic, nodular lesion, called "prurigo nodularis," or "picker's nodule." The diagnosis of prurigo nodularis or lichen simplex chronicus should always elicit a search for an underlying cause of pruritus. A verruca vulgaris, actinic keratosis, or even mild spongiotic dermatitis can provide a focus for rubbing. Systemic causes of pruritus include renal failure, hepatic disease, and lymphomas. Patients with atopy have a tendency to develop these lesions (Fig. 71-56).

PATHOLOGY. The skin lesions show a thickened and compact stratum corneum with a mixture of orthokeratosis and parakeratosis and with hypergranulosis (Fig. 71-58). A stratum lucidum can be present. Both lichen simplex chronicus and prurigo nodularis have irregular acanthosis and fibrosis of the papillary dermis. Fibrin and extravasated erythrocytes are present at the tips of dermal papillae, which are characteristic findings attributable to trauma. The dermis has a superficial perivascular lymphocytic infiltrate.

Reactive perforating collagenosis. Reactive perforating collagenosis is a rare disease that is characterized by a focal transepidermal elimination of dermal collagen. Clinically the

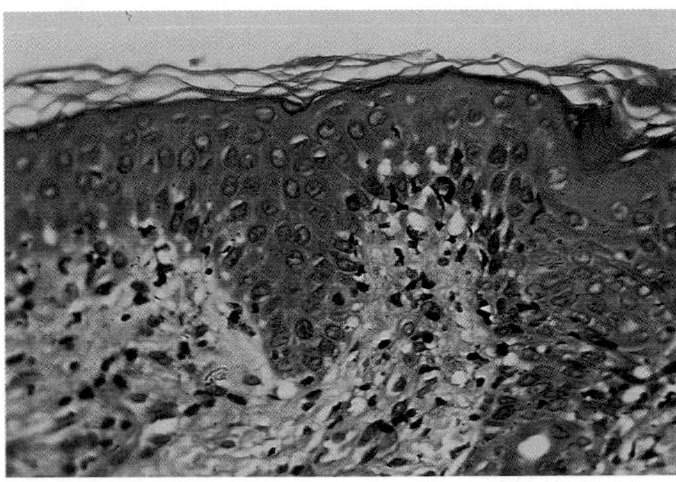

Fig. 71-88 Acute graft-versus-host disease. Lymphocytes infiltrate into the epidermis and are stretched over the surface of keratinocytes that are undergoing necrosis.

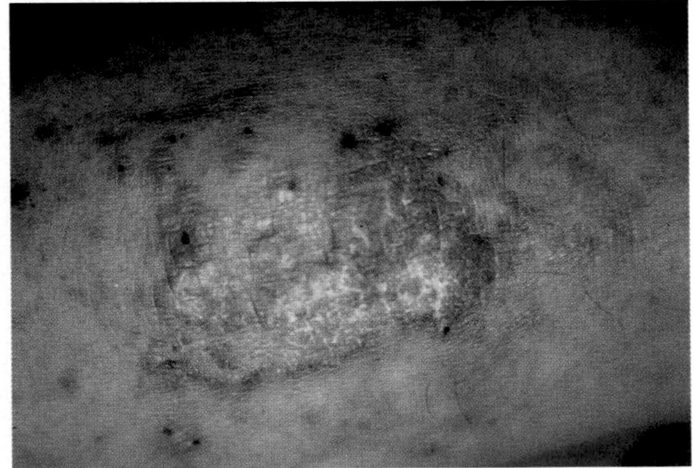

Fig. 71-89 Lichen simplex chronicus. A raised plaque of thickened skin has a keratotic scaly surface, accentuated skin lines, and irregular hyperpigmentation.

unit lesion is an umbilicated papules in the center of which is a small tuft of dermal collagen protruding through the epidermis.[131,132] In the genetically determined form of the disease (autosomal recessive), the lesions appear after minor trauma during childhood. An acquired form can affect adults with an underlying chronic renal disease and has been named perforating disorder of renal disease. Similar lesions can appear in diabetic patients. On a microscopic slide, the differential diagnosis includes prurigo nodularis, which can have focal protrusion of microscopic amounts of collagen through the epidermis into the overlying crust during wound healing. The formation of the small papules in linear arrays at the sites of minor trauma is a key observation. It is peculiar that the patients heal surgical wounds normally.

PATHOLOGY. The lesions typically have a deposition of fibrin in the papillary dermis, as one would expect after minor trauma. In early lesions, there may be a lymphocytic and macrophage response at the site. Eventually the epidermis becomes hyperplastic, and collagen fibers can be seen penetrating through the epidermis. By EM, the collagen fibrils have a normal banding pattern.

Elastosis perforans serpiginosa. Elastosis perforans serpiginosa is a rare dermatosis in which the epidermis has elastin perforating through it.[131-133] The clinical appearance is that of grouped papules sometimes in an annular or circinate pattern. The disease may appear without other associations or can be seen in patients with Down syndrome, Ehlers-Danlos syndrome, pseudoxanthoma elasticum, or Marfan's syndrome, or in those given penicillamine.

PATHOLOGY. There is hyperkeratosis and irregular acanthosis of the epidermis around an irregularly shaped channel containing refractile elastic fibers. Elastic tissue stains are positive on the elastin in the crust and also frequently reveal a concentration of elastic fibers near the epidermal basement membrane in a manner not seen in perforating folliculitis or reactive perforating collagenosis. The perforating channel may be distorted and irregular in shape, and so serial sections are needed to trace its path through the epidermis.

Chondrodermatitis nodularis helicis. The common disorder chondrodermatitis nodularis helicis is characterized by the development of a painful nodule on the helix or antihelix of the ear at the site of chronic trauma, particularly pressure (Fig. 71-90).[134] There is a central ulcer surrounded by a hyperkeratotic surface.

PATHOLOGY. The skin is focally ulcerated (Fig. 71-91) and there is deposition of fibrin at the dermoepidermal junction adjacent to the ulcer. In the ulcer bed, granulation tissue, and fibrosis are prominent. A deep biopsy specimen shows that the ear cartilage (elastic cartilage) has undergone degeneration and has an eosinophilic matrix. Transepidermal elimination of the fibrin and degenerated cartilage can be found. This lesion should be distinguished from an actinic keratosis or a squamous carcinoma in situ.

Pruritic urticarial papules and plaques of pregnancy. The uncommon disorder pruritic urticarial papules and plaques of pregnancy (PUPPP) presents in the third trimester of pregnancy with intense pruritus and erythematous papules and plaques involving the abdomen and proximal extremities.[135,136] The lesions often are in the lines of striae distensae, a finding that helps to rule out an adverse reaction to a medication.

PATHOLOGY. The epidermis is slightly acanthotic, and there is a thin parakeratotic scale. Mild spongiosis is common. The dermis has a superficial to a superficial and deep perivascular lymphocytic infiltrate with a scattered population of eosinophils. Papillary dermal edema is present but there is no separation of the epidermis from the dermoepidermal junction. The histologic picture is only diagnostic when both the epidermal and dermal changes are present. Immunofluorescence may be definitive in separation of this disease from pemphigoid gestationis, since there is no deposition of immune complexes in

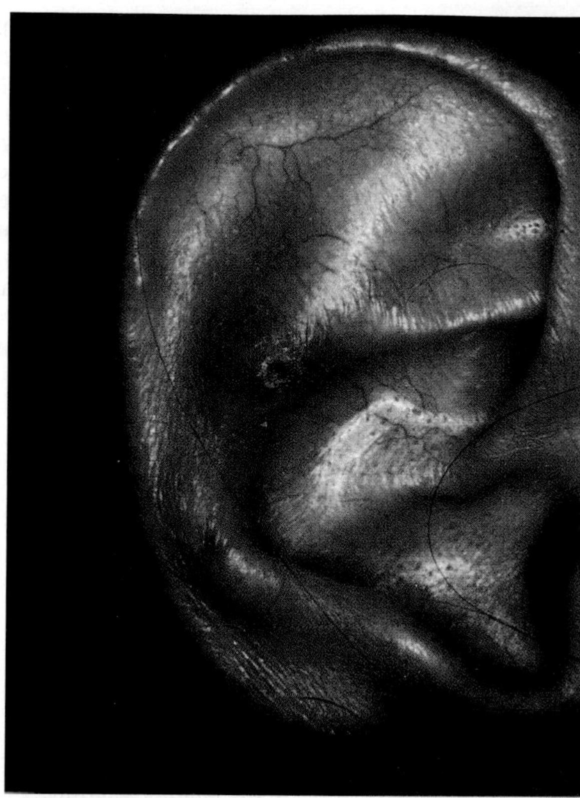

Fig. 71-90 Chondrodermatitis nodularis helicis. At the site of chronic trauma, a painful scaly nodule develops with eventual ulceration.

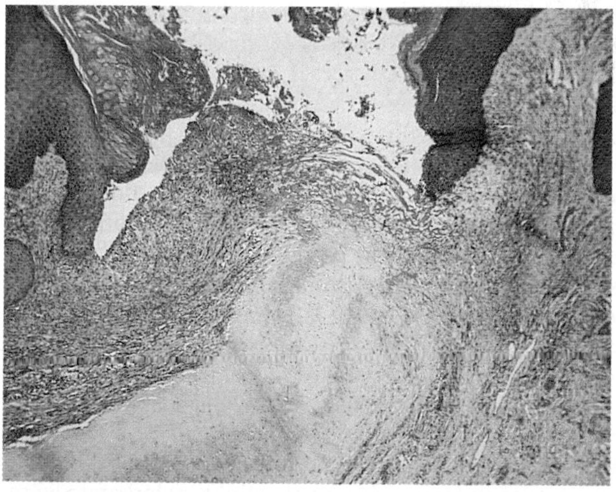

Fig. 71-91 Chondrodermatitis nodularis helicis. At the site of chronic ulceration, extrusion of fibrin and degenerated cartilage occur.

tion of the stratum corneum with the stratum granulosum.[159] At the leading edge of the burrow, the fertilized females feed and deposit eggs and feces. The lesions tend to be on moist skin surfaces, such as interdigital web spaces, breast, umbilicus, and penis, but can involve even the thick stratum corneum of the palms and soles. As immunity develops, the ensuing hypersensitivity reaction causes extreme pruritus and erythema. Secondary effects of scratching are frequent. The site of the burrow can be recognized as a short linear vesicular lesion with a black dot at the leading edge. After death of the scabies mite because of treatment, a deep dermal nodule may persist as a result of a hypersensitivity reaction without intact mites being present, is called the "persistent scabies nodule," and can mimic a lymphoma or pseudolymphoma.

PATHOLOGY. Burrows are found in the stratum corneum, and near the leading edge, they may contain fertilized eggs with refractile cuticles, feces, or parts of mites. There is usually a striking dermal response, because of a perivascular lymphocytic infiltrate that is distributed in both the superficial and deep dermis. Eosinophils are abundant and often are in the interstitium of the reticular dermis. Plasma cells also may be present. Endothelial cells are swollen.

In patients with normal immune status, the number of mites is low, and so a careful search for mites may be necessary in step sections of the tissue block. Other *arthropod bites and stings* tend to have a similar histologic pattern, often with spongiosis near the center of the lesion and occasionally with focal slight hemorrhages where the bite was located. The follicle mite, *Demodex folliculorum,* has the same length as the scabies mite (approximately 0.3 mm) but is much more slender. *Demodex folliculorum* has been implicated in rosacea, but it is not clear whether this widespread mite is pathogenic in this disease.

Neoplasms

Keratinocytic lesions

Invasive squamous cell carcinoma. Clinically, invasive squamous cell carcinoma frequently presents as a nodular lesion on sun-damaged skin that is prone to bleeding and ulceration (Fig. 71-104).[169] Both the invasive and the in situ forms can have abundant hyperkeratosis, occasionally so thick as to produce a *cutaneous horn* ("cornu cutaneum"). More than 90% of cutaneous squamous cell carcinomas are related to solar damage. These lesions often have a relatively good prognosis that is not very different from that of basal cell carcinoma, except that there is a slightly greater risk of metastases from squamous cell carcinoma. However, squamous cell carcinomas that arise in scars, in chronic radiodermatitis, and in the margins of long-standing ulcers ("Marjolin's ulcer") have a much higher tendency for metastasis and more frequently are poorly differentiated tumors histologically. Metastasis tends to be by lymphatic channels. HPV-16 and HPV-18 have been associated with certain squamous cell carcinomas of the skin as well as the genital tract. Mutations in the p53 gene play a role in the development of squamous cell carcinomas on sun-damaged skin.[14,170,171]

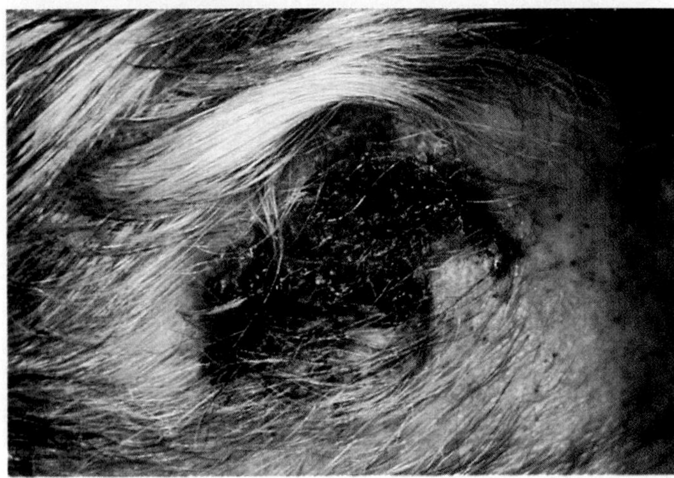

Fig. 71-104 Squamous cell carcinoma. This irregular raised plaque on the forehead has a hyperkeratotic and hemorrhagic crust.

PATHOLOGY. Invasive squamous cell carcinomas infiltrate the dermis usually as nests of neoplastic keratinocytes (Fig. 71-105) with prominent nuclear atypia, enlarged nucleoli, and moderately abundant eosinophilic cytoplasm. Intercellular "bridges" often can be found. Occasionally, the cells are small and produce small amounts of keratin (Fig. 71-106) or even assume a spindle-cell shape with increased collagenous stroma. These spindle-cell and desmoplastic squamous cell carcinomas can be difficult to recognize without additional studies. Immunohistochemically the malignant cells contain both low and high molecular weight keratins. Spindle cell forms of squamous cell carcinoma often contain vimentin as well.

Primary skin tumors need to be distinguished from metastatic squamous cell carcinomas. Primary tumors usually are con-

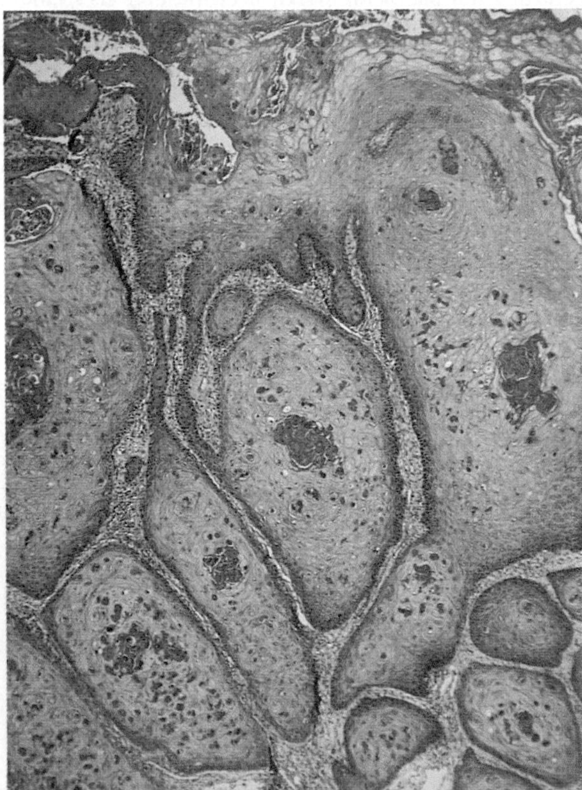

Fig. 71-105 Invasive, well-differentiated squamous cell carcinoma. The invasive tumor nests contain enlarged cells with abundant eosinophilic cytoplasm. Necrosis of cells and individual cell keratinization are prominent in this example. Cytologic atypism of nuclei can be minimal.

nected to the overlying epidermis; however, metastatic squamous cell carcinomas can reestablish contact with the overlying epidermis but usually lack an extensive intraepidermal component.

Keratoacanthoma. Keratoacanthoma is a solitary, round, symmetrical nodular lesion with a central keratotic plug (Fig. 71-107) that usually occurs on sun-damaged skin of elderly patients. It characteristically grows rapidly, and the typical nodule develops in a few weeks to months. However, the appearance does not exclude a squamous cell carcinoma, since a few lesions with these clinical features have metastasized, particularly in immunosuppressed patients.[172] Keratoacanthomas undergo three phases of growth: first, rapid growth as a sharply-circumscribed, round, erythematous, hard nodule; secondly, slower growth with formation of a prominent central keratin plug; and third, involution. A depressed region that has lost its central keratin can persist for several years. The lesions can be multiple. They usually involve hair-bearing skin and do not penetrate deeply, such as not to the fascia. Occasionally, keratoacanthomas have been described on the vermilion border of the lip and in the nail beds.

PATHOLOGY. An elliptical excision specimen is important for proper evaluation. Keratoacanthomas at low magnification have symmetry histologically just as they have symmetry grossly (Fig. 71-108). The lesion is sharply circumscribed and does *not* extend in the adjacent epidermis as carcinoma in situ. The surface is hyperkeratotic, with a mixture of orthokeratosis and parakeratosis, often with orthokeratosis predominating. In the regions of orthokeratosis, hypergranulosis is present, and the keratohyalin granules are often coarse and round, similar to those found in verruca vulgaris. In the dermis, the lesion has a nearly spherical shape that rarely penetrates around nerves and into blood vessels. The keratinocytes in the lesion are large and pale staining and remain closely adherent to each other (Fig. 71-109); primary acantholysis is not a feature of keratoacanthoma but is found in squamous cell carcinoma. Intraepidermal neutrophilic abscesses frequently are present.

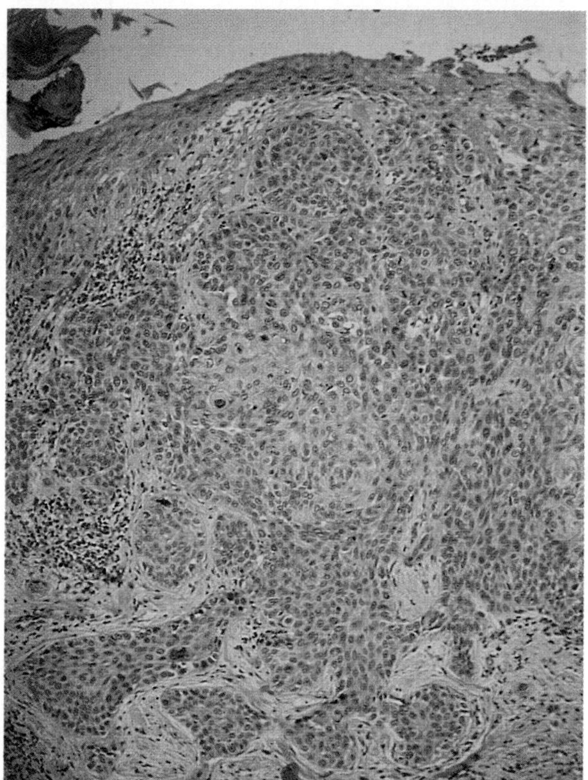

Fig. 71-106 Invasive, poorly differentiated squamous cell carcinoma. The keratinocytes in the invasive nests are small, with a high ratio of nucleus to cytoplasmic size. Lack of definite peripheral palisading, cleft formation, and distinctive mucinous stroma are differences from basal cell carcinoma.

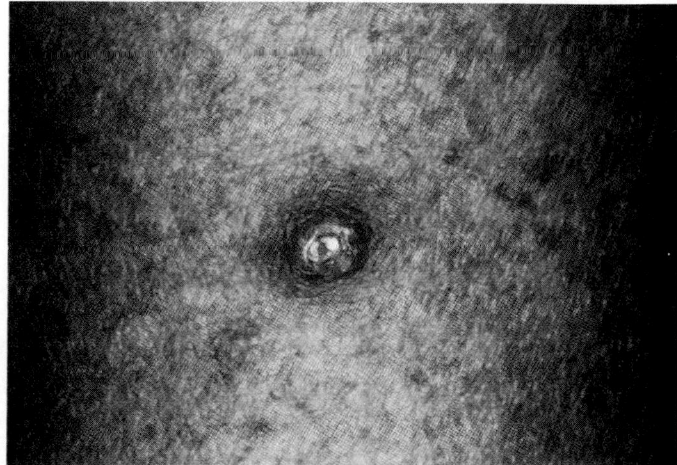

Fig. 71-107 Keratoacanthoma. This tumor is round and symmetrical in appearance and, in well-developed examples, has a visible central keratin plug.

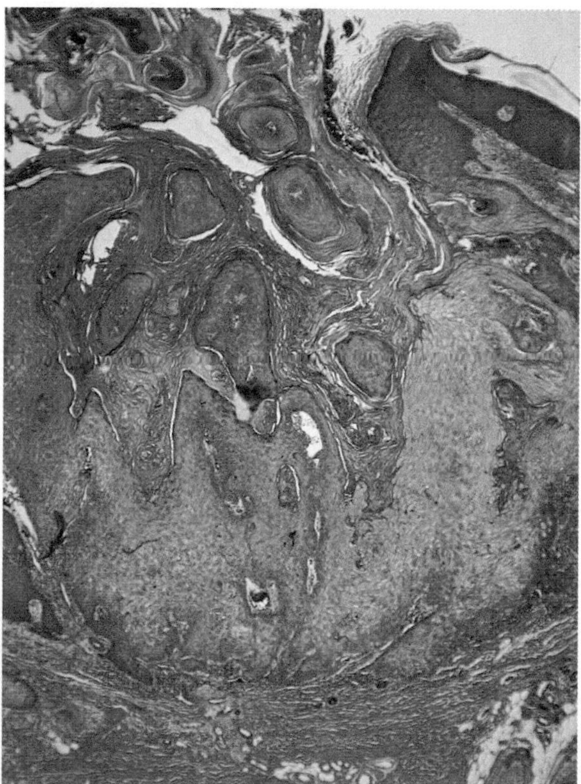

Fig. 71-108 Keratoacanthoma. At low magnification, there are often papillomatous projections into the central keratin plug. Histologically, symmetry is maintained.

There is debate as to whether these lesions represent a distinct entity or are just squamous carcinomas with a propensity to spontaneous regression. In our view, these lesions are a distinctive clinicopathologic entity that can be recognized when all the characteristics are present; however, those "keratoacanthomas" with atypical features, such as asymmetry, deep penetration, primary acantholysis, or perineural or vascular invasion, are better considered to be well-differentiated squamous cell carcinomas.

Basal cell carcinoma. Basal cell carcinoma is the most common malignant tumor of whites, and in most cases it occurs in the elderly and is directly related to excessive exposure to ultraviolet radiation in sunlight. However, basal cell carcinomas may appear at a young age in patients with a genetic predisposition and in the so-called basal cell nevus syndrome, and it may occur in adults in sites not commonly exposed to sunlight. Clinically, there are three types of tumors: (1) *Nodular basal cell carcinoma* is an opalescent, or "pearly," firm nodule often with adjacent telangiectatic blood vessels (Fig. 71-110). (2) *Superficial basal cell carcinoma* is a scaly, erythematous, flat lesion with a distinct sometimes "pearly" border (Fig. 71-111). (3) *Morpheic basal cell carcinoma* is a flat, sometimes depressed, white plaque with adjacent erythema (Fig. 71-112); this appearance is similar to lesions of morphea. Each of these types of tumors usually enlarges very slowly but can grow quickly and ulcerate and bleed. Inexorable local extension is common, but metastasis is extremely rare. Pigmented basal cell carcinomas have very abundant melanin and can be mistaken for malignant melanomas. Cystic basal cell carcinomas are nodular basal cell carcinomas with a bluish appearance clinically. Basal cell carcinomas are less likely than squamous cell carcinomas to have abundant keratin or cutaneous horns on the surface of the tumor.

A unique and complex dependency exists between the tumor and its stroma. Epithelial islands of basal cell carcinoma transplanted without their stroma into the reticular dermis resulted in no growth, whereas if stroma was included, the nests grew. Collagenase produces microscopic clefts between

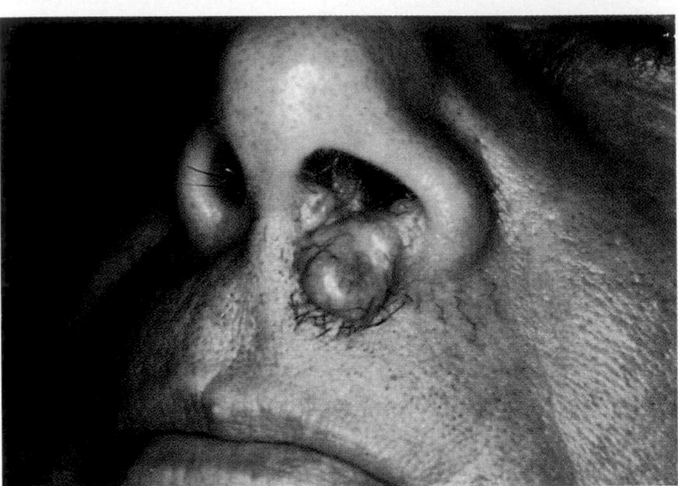

Fig. 71-110 Basal cell carcinoma, nodular type. At the nasal orifice is a nodular opalescent tumor with prominent telangiectatic blood vessels.

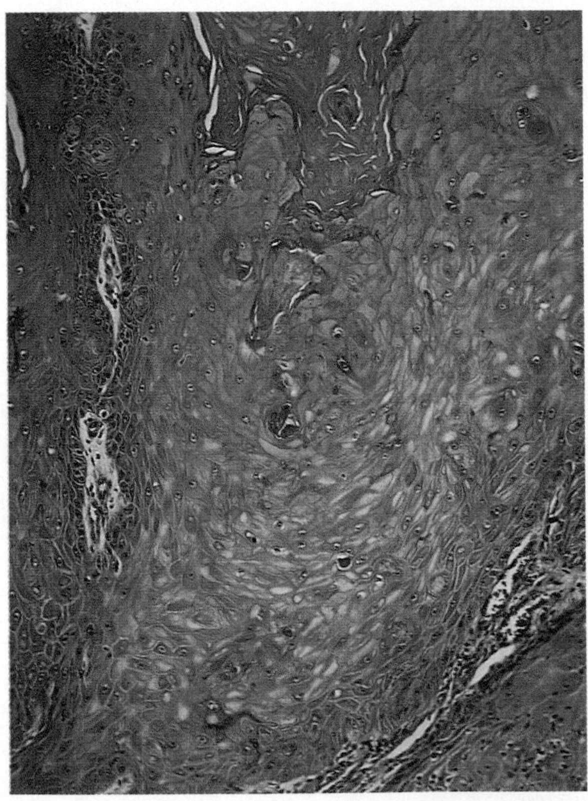

Fig. 71-109 Keratoacanthoma. Coherent masses of large pale-staining keratinocytes without noticeable cytologic atypism are the most common features. There is no primary acantholysis.

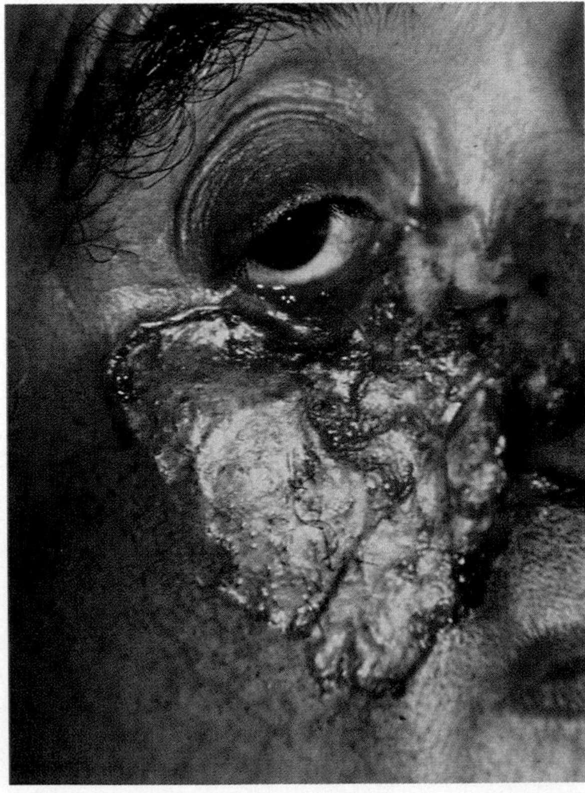

Fig. 71-111 Basal cell carcinoma, superficial type. This extensive tumor has a threadlike, "pearly," raised border, with adjacent telangiectasia.

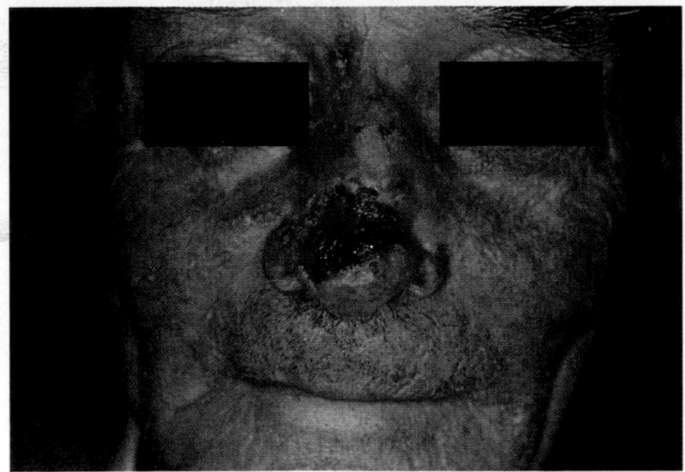

Fig. 71-112 Basal cell carcinoma, morpheic type. This tumor has a flattened appearance with a mottled erythema and whitish appearance. It has extensively infiltrated this patient's nose, cheeks, and periorbital skin.

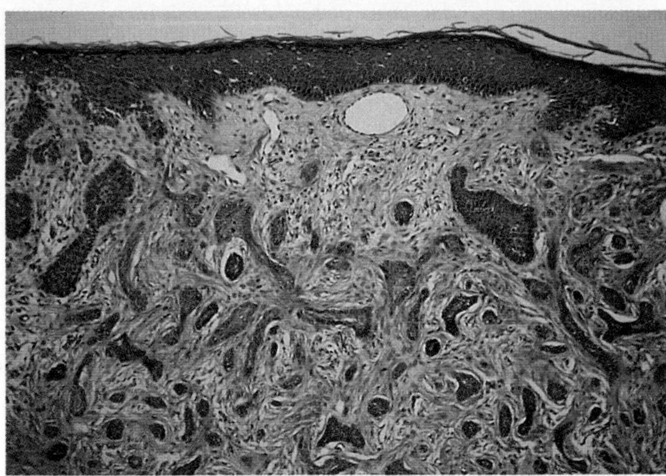

Fig. 71-113 Basal cell carcinoma, morpheic type. Basaloid cells infiltrate as thin ribbons of cells in an abundant, distinctive, cellular, and mucinous stroma. Regions of contact with the overlying epidermis are present.

epithelium and stroma in the tumor and on a larger scale could account for the erosive properties of the tumor.[173,174] The underlying genetic causes of basal cell carcinoma are unknown, but increased production of p53 protein has been demonstrated in some basal cell carcinomas and may be related to mutations produced by ultraviolet radiation.[41,175-177] A fourfold increase in the *bcl*-2 protein has been reported also and could increase the number of proliferating cells by inhibition of apoptosis. E-cadherin expression is reduced focally in basal cell carcinomas and could contribute to the cell surface abnormalities associated with invasion by infiltration.[178]

PATHOLOGY. Basal cell carcinomas can present in several histologic forms, and such a variety reflects the fact that basal keratinocytes are the precursors of all epidermal and adnexal structures in the developing skin. Superficial basal cell carcinoma has nests of basal keratinocytes that project downward to involve the papillary dermis while maintaining close contact with the surface epidermis. Nodular and morpheic basal cell carcinomas invade both the papillary and reticular dermis and also have areas of contact with the overlying epidermis or the follicular epithelium (Fig. 71-113).

Basal cell carcinomas often have at least four of the following six features (Fig. 71-114): (1) Basaloid cells, which resemble those of the basal row of keratinocytes in the epidermis, except for slight nuclear enlargement and more hyperchromatism; (2) peripheral palisading, which is an expression of residual polarity of the basal cells; (3) Mitotic figures; (4) individual necrotic keratinocytes, which by apoptosis balance the increased mitoses in this tumor that grows slowly; (5) an unusual cellular stroma composed of spindle cells in a mucinous matrix with fine collagen fibrils and many mast cells; (6) cleft formation that separates the nests of basal cell carcinoma from their stroma, attributable to collagenase activity, mucin deposition, and a reduction in the number of hemidesmosomes.[179] However, morpheic basal cell carcinomas often lack peripheral palisading and show very little cleft formation. In some tumors, the stroma focally is filled with dense collagen or amyloid. In areas of ulceration or trauma, frequently there are microscopic foci of keratinization.

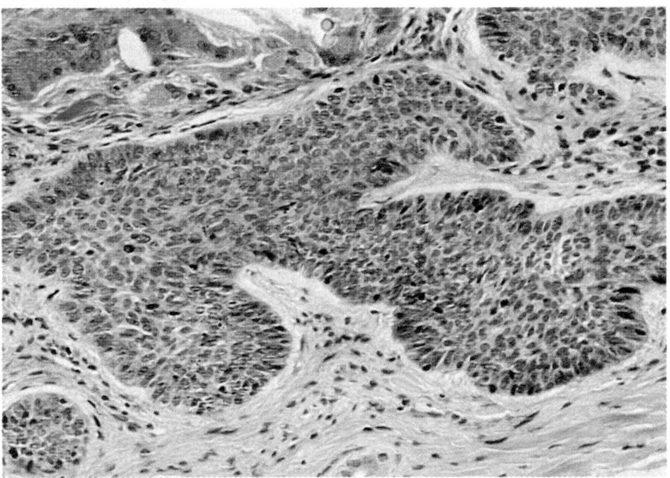

Fig. 71-114 Basal cell carcinoma, nodular type. Nests of basaloid cells show peripheral palisading, clefts at the interface between tumor epithelium and stroma, prominent mitoses, and individual necrotic cells.

Keratinization can proceed to complete keratin production in the "keratotic basal cell carcinoma," and at times they can resemble squamous cell carcinomas. When areas become indistinguishable from squamous cell carcinoma, the terms *basosquamous carcinoma* or *metatypical basal cell carcinoma* have been used for such tumors.[180] Also there can be focal areas of sebaceous differentiation or even formation of tubules resembling sweat ducts. Pigmentation is attributable to the proliferation of dendritic, heavily pigmented melanocytes along with the keratinocytes and the transfer of pigment to those keratinocytes, most often in superficial basal cell carcinoma. Basal cell carcinoma-like changes may occur over dermatofibromas.[181]

The presence of three or more of the following histologic features has been associated with a greatly increased tendency for the tumor to recur after surgical resection, in addition to demonstrated positive resection margins: an infiltrative, morpheic, or superficial growth pattern; "spiky" shape of cell groups; infiltrating advancing edge; poorly formed peripheral palisades; and high degree of nuclear pleomorphism.[182]

Actinic keratoses, hyperplastic and lichenoid types. Most actinic keratoses are flat and seem limited to the epidermis. Certain types of actinic keratoses have more dermal reaction. In hyperplastic actinic keratoses the lesions are thick and indurated. Lichenoid actinic keratosis has such a dense lymphoid inflammatory response that the lesion gives the clinical impression of invasion into the dermis.

PATHOLOGY. Hyperplastic actinic keratosis shows acanthosis and extension of atypical keratinocytes into the hair follicles and sweat ducts, usually only the same distance as the elongated acanthotic rete ridges. Inflamed or lichenoid actinic keratosis has a dense lymphocytic infiltrate in the dermis just beneath the lesion. Often the lymphocytes invade the epidermis and produce necrosis of basal keratinocytes, which results in colloid bodies among the lymphoid cells. Plasma cells may be abundant, particularly in lesions on the face, in periorificial regions, and in lesions that have invasive squamous carcinomas in other planes of section.

This lesion often is in the histologic differential diagnosis of lichen planus on sun-damaged skin. They differ in that the lichen planus-like actinic keratosis has more parakeratosis and more cytologic atypism of the keratinocytes than lichen planus itself.[183,184]

Melanocytic lesions

Compound melanocytic nevus. Compound melanocytic nevi are formed by the proliferation of nevus cells in the epidermis followed by the extension of these cells, with certain cytologic modifications, into the dermis.[46,185] Most compound nevi are acquired after birth, and only 1% of all whites are born with a congenital compound melanocytic nevus. Grossly, the compound nevus is slightly raised above the skin surface and has palpable thickening of the skin. In addition, congenital nevi often have slight thickening and darkening of any hairs that emerge from the nevus. Most acquired compound nevi remain less than 6 mm in diameter, have a smooth outline, and are round-to-oval, symmetrical lesions, with rather uniform brown pigmentation (Fig. 71-115). In contrast congenital nevi can achieve a very large size, covering whole segments of the body in the so-called giant congenital nevi that are over 20 cm in diameter. Intermediate-sized congenital nevi are ones that are from 1.5 to 20 cm in diameter. Small congenital nevi are less than 1.5 cm in diameter. Congenital compound melanocytic nevi often have slightly irregular outlines with peripheral speckling of the pigmentation (Fig. 71-116).

The risk of melanoma is greatest in the giant nevi, much less in the intermediate congenital nevi, and indeterminate in the small nevi. Paradoxically, because there are so many small congenital nevi, it is more common for melanomas to arise in association with small congenital nevi. However, the overall risk of melanoma in any given small nevus is very low.

PATHOLOGY. Compound melanocytic nevi have sharply circumscribed lateral borders (Table 71-5). In the epidermis, there is a proliferation of melanocytes (or "nevomelanocytes") in nests at the dermoepidermal junction (Fig. 71-117), but some compound nevi may have an increased number of individual melanocytes along the dermoepidermal junction on elongated rete ridges. These epidermal changes have already been discussed as "lentiginous nevi" because of the similarity to solar lentigo. After the first few months of life, upward migration of nevus cells is rare but may be present in a small focus near the center of a lesion, or at sites of trauma or regeneration. The edges of a nevus in adults (other than recurrent nevus after incomplete excision) do not have upward migration of melanocytes in the epidermis, and such a feature is far more typical of a malignant melanoma. Nests of nevus cells can be quite large, occasionally spanning the entire thickness of the stratum spinosum in young children. The nests are well circumscribed, and the nevus cells are cohesive within the nests.

When the nests of nevus cells enter the papillary dermis, often there is not much change in the cytologic features when compared with those in the overlying epidermis. However, as the nevus cells migrate farther down in the dermis, they become smaller both in the amount of cytoplasm and in the size of the nucleus. The size of the nests of nevus cells is also reduced, and the cells tend to disperse in a fine collagenous matrix. Particularly in congenital nevi, progressive descent in

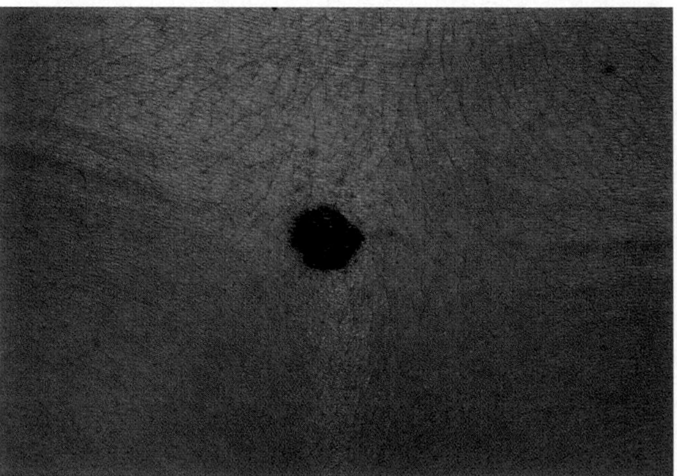

Fig. 71-115 Acquired compound melanocytic nevus. This is a small, elevated, sharply circumscribed lesion, with a smooth outline and variable degrees of pigmentation but usually uniformly colored.

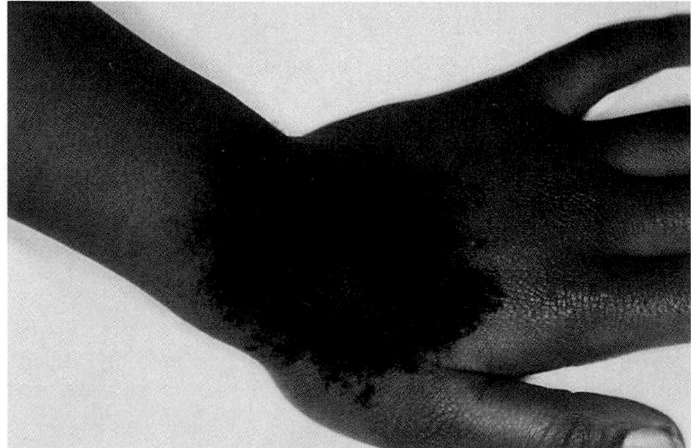

Fig. 71-116 Congenital compound melanocytic nevus. This is an intermediate-sized lesion that shows peripheral speckling of pigmentation.

the dermis converts the nevus nests into arrays of spindle-shaped thin nevus cells dispersed individually in the collagenous stroma of the nevus. These cytologic changes have been described as a conversion of the "type A," or epithelioid, nevus cells into "type B" nevus cells, which are nearly the size of lymphocytes, and finally into "type C" nevus cells, which have a spindle shape and resemble cells in a neurofibroma. Type C nevus cells show schwannian differentiation and can form structures resembling Meissner's corpuscles in the lower portion of nevi. In congenital and some acquired compound nevi,[186] the nevus cell nests penetrate down eccrine ducts or the infundibulum or hair follicles for a short distance, but deep penetration of benign nevus cells in these structures is found only in congenital nevi. In large congenital nevi, nevus cells often penetrate into the lower third of the reticular dermis, into the arrector pili muscles, and lie within the basement membrane of sebaceous glands and hair follicles. They also aggregate in the wall of small lymphatics and in nerves. As these cells migrate farther from the stratified squamous epithelium, they become smaller, lose prominence of nucleoli, and sharply decrease mitosis. The nuclei usually have smooth outlines, but intranuclear pseudoinclusions are common in some nevi and represent occasional deep indentations of the nuclear envelope that contain portions of the Golgi zone and other cytoplasmic organelles.

In the papillary dermis, mitoses are quite rare in compound nevi; in the portions of the lesions in the reticular dermis, mitoses are so rare that they cannot be found in most instances. Proteins associated with cell proliferation, such as Ki-67 and cyclin, have been studied in compound nevi, and sharp declines in the amounts of these proteins occur with progressive descent of nevus cells in the dermis. However, cyclin is overexpressed in the dermal portion of some nevi even without mitoses.

In compound nevi with architectural disorder and cytologic atypism of melanocytes (so-called compound dysplastic nevi), there is extension of the junctional component for many rete ridges beyond the region of the dermal component (Fig. 71-118).[187,188] The epidermal changes have been discussed previously (Figs. 71-38 to 71-40). The dermal changes also include fibrosis of the dermis at the tips of rete ridges to produce collagen fibers and cells parallel to the epidermal surface *(lamellar fibroplasia)* (Fig. 71-119). Also dense eosinophilic collagen accumulates around the elongated rete ridges (so-called concentric eosinophilic fibrosis).

Spitz's nevus is another variant of a compound nevus.[189,190] (Table 71-5). It has all the features of the compound nevus but in addition is composed of large cells, with large nuclei, often having delicate chromatin and thin nuclear envelopes and a single large round nucleolus (Figs. 71-120 and 71-121). There usually is a mixture of spindle and epithelioid melanocytes. Mitoses can be common in the upper part but not in the lower part of the lesion. When the nevus is heavily pigmented and restricted to the epidermis and papillary dermis, the name "pigmented spindle cell nevus of Reed" is sometimes applied

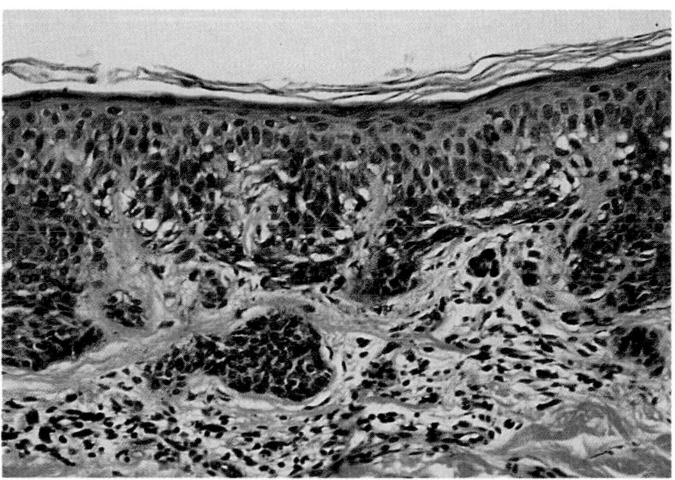

Fig. 71-118 Compound melanocytic nevus with architectural disorder. Frequently the epidermal component extends many rete ridges beyond the dermal component, with irregular nests of nevus cells and distortion of the rete ridges.

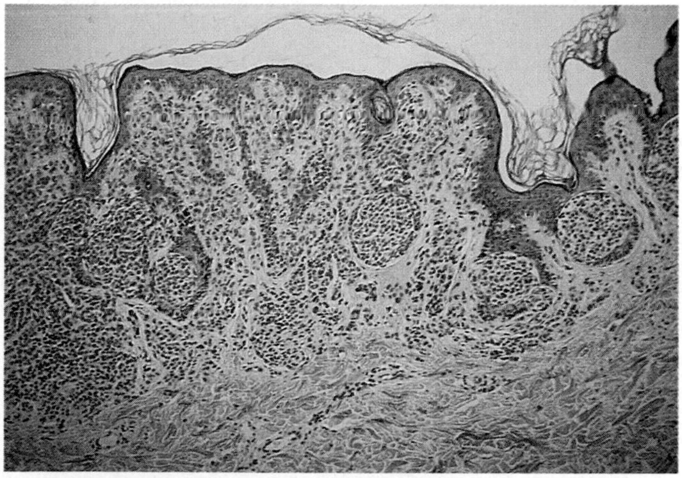

Fig. 71-117 Compound melanocytic nevus. As nests of melanocytic nevus cells descend into the dermis, each nest is surrounded by a fibrillar basement membrane. The cells become dispersed in this fibrous matrix with deeper descent into the dermis, usually with a decrease in cell and nuclear size also.

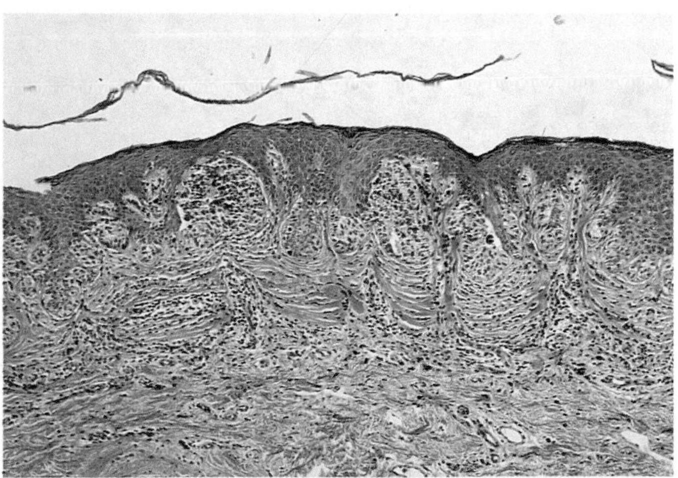

Fig. 71-119 Junctional portion of a compound melanocytic nevus with architectural disorder. A prominent dermal change is "lamellar fibroplasia," which is the deposition of collagen fibers and reactive cells parallel to the epidermal surface and at the bases of rete ridges.

to this variant of a Spitz nevus.[191] Spitz's nevi, as all growing nevi, are usually in children and young adults. The pigmented spindle cell nevus is usually on the thighs of women. Spitz's nevi and their variants sometimes are difficult to distinguish from invasive malignant melanoma.[190]

Another variant of compound nevus is the *balloon cell nevus*. More than 50% of cells in this nevus have very enlarged and vacuolated cytoplasm. This ballooning is attributable to swollen and incompletely melanized melanosomes. When a compound nevus induces an intense lichenoid lymphocytic infiltrate, the dermal portion of the nevus may be partially vacuolated or destroyed, and the destruction of adjacent melanocytes in the epidermis produces clinical depigmentation around the nevus, which has been called the "halo nevus."

Invasive malignant melanoma. Melanoma is a malignant neoplasm of melanocytes. The clinical appearances of invasive malignant melanomas can be quite diverse and can vary in their degree of pigmentation from very hyperpigmented (black) to amelanotic (white to red). Often great variation in the degree of pigmentation is visible within a lesion even when it is small. This variation reflects the disorderly growth that is so characteristic of melanoma. Melanomas in the epidermis do not have very regular or smooth borders and often extend in an asymmetric fashion. Melanomas also may arise within a preexisting nevus as a focal change that does not alter the outlines of the lesion.[192] The prognosis of the patient is determined by the characteristics of the dermal growth phase, or "vertical growth phase."

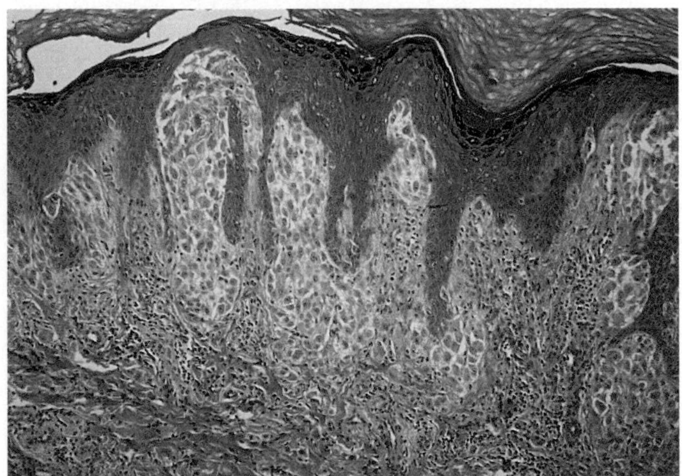

Fig. 71-120 Compound Spitz's nevus. Epidermal hyperplasia is associated with a proliferation of large epithelioid and spindle-shaped melanocytic nevus cells in nests at the dermoepidermal junction. Smaller groups of cells have descended into the dermis.

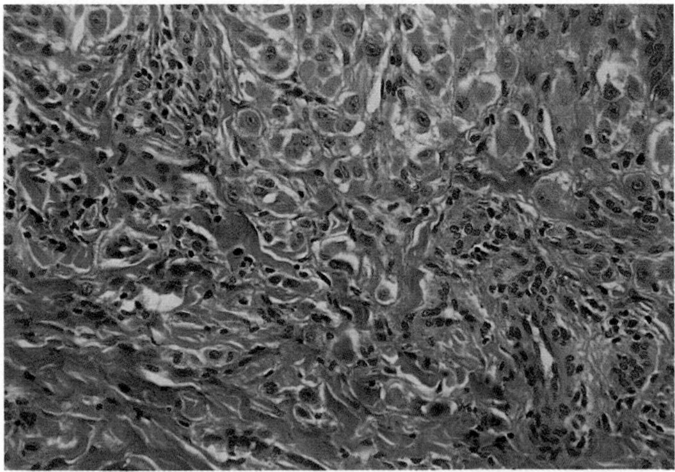

Fig. 71-121 Compound Spitz's nevus. At the base of the lesion, the cells decrease in size, become dispersed between the collagen bundles, and cease mitotic proliferation.

Malignant melanomas occur in all age groups, including newborn children, but they increase in frequency with advancing age of the individual.[193] Among all cancers, the incidence of melanoma is one of the most rapidly increasing in whites, and may reach a lifetime risk of 1 out of every 70 persons by the year 2000. Certain patterns of clinical presentation have been defined.[46] One of them *lentigo maligna melanoma* (LMM), occurs most often on the face of elderly persons with very sun-damaged skin, in approximately 15% of melanoma cases (Fig. 71-122). It characteristically has a long in situ, intraepidermal growth phase, which was discussed previously as "lentigo maligna." When it eventually invades into the dermis, the invasive form is called "lentigo maligna melanoma," and in the dermis it often forms a spindle cell nodule (Fig. 71-123). The most frequent clinical pattern (in approximately 60% of cases) is *superficial spreading malignant melanoma* (SMM), which is an irregular maculopapular lesion with varied pigmentation (Fig. 71-124) and tends to grow rapidly and extensively within the epidermis but also to enter the dermis relatively early in its course. They are most frequent on the

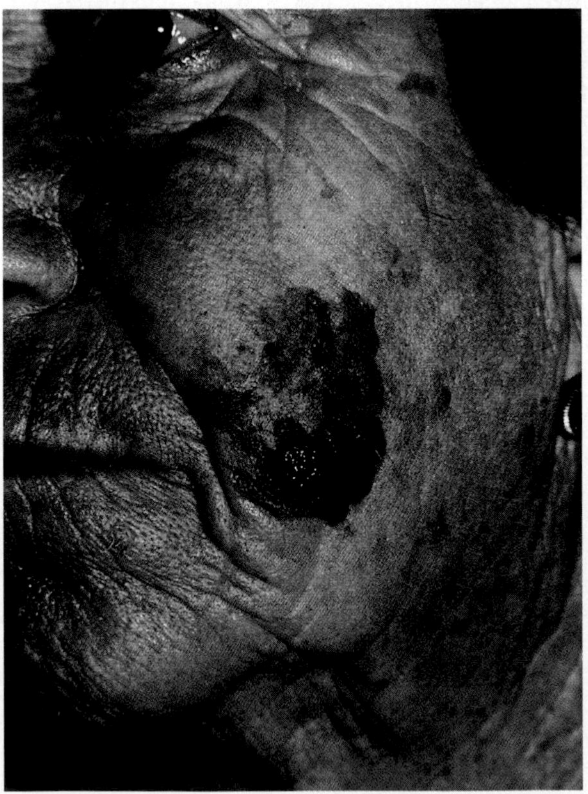

Fig. 71-122 Lentigo maligna melanoma. This form of lentiginous melanoma has invaded into the dermis, which grossly is correlated with increased nodularity in the lesion or with ulceration.

trunk, particularly the midback of both men and women, on the proximal extremities, and on the posterior calf region of women. The relation to sunlight exposure is dependent on intermittent intense sun exposure, particularly in childhood, and the tumor often arises on skin that does not appear very sun damaged in the adult. Another clinical pattern (in approximately 15% of cases) is *nodular melanoma* (NM), a well-circumscribed nodule (Fig. 71-125) that arises quickly and enters an intradermal growth phase very early with only a very limited spreading phase in the epidermis. A fourth clinical pattern accounting for approximately 5% of cases is called *acral lentiginous melanoma,* which has its origin on the distal area of the extremities (Fig. 71-126). These four types of presentations of melanomas have their histologic correlates also.

PATHOLOGY. Histologic sections of invasive malignant melanoma usually contain an intraepidermal component of atypical melanocytes in the overlying epidermis[50,194,195] (Fig. 71-127). In nodular melanomas this is quite focal, but it is extensive in LMM and in SSM. In LMM the atypical cells tend to remain closely associated with the dermoepidermal junction, but in comparison to lentigo maligna, there is more upward migration in the epidermis in invasive lesions. The cells can be large or small in size, often have dendritic cytoplasmic extensions, and proliferate both as individual cells and in nests at the dermoepidermal junction. In SSM the melanoma cells have prominent upward migration in the epidermis and the cells have moderately abundant cytoplasm with irregular fine pigment granules, and have nuclei with open chromatin and one or more prominent irregular nucleoli. However, the cell size is variable from small epithelioid to large epithelioid to balloon cell types. The cytoplasm often is rounded, and dendrites are not prominent. Pigmentation may be very dense to absent. Likewise in NM, the cells may have the same range of cytologic features just described for LMM and SSM. One distinctive type of melanoma, named "desmo-

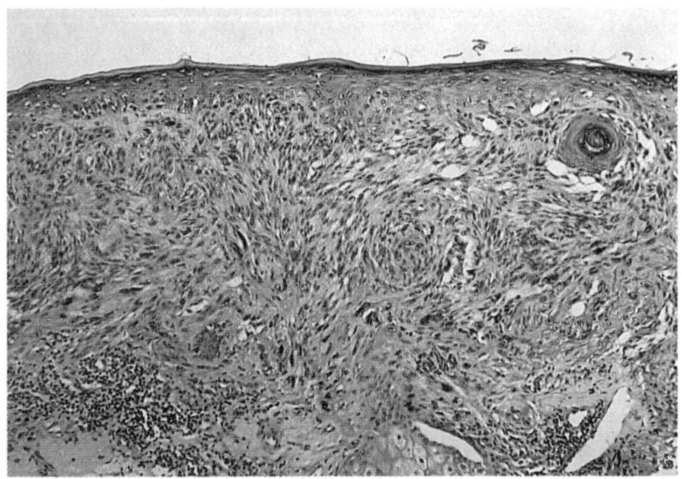

Fig. 71-123 Lentigo maligna melanoma. The invasive nodules that form are frequently composed of spindle-shaped atypical melanocytes. The degree of pigmentation varies.

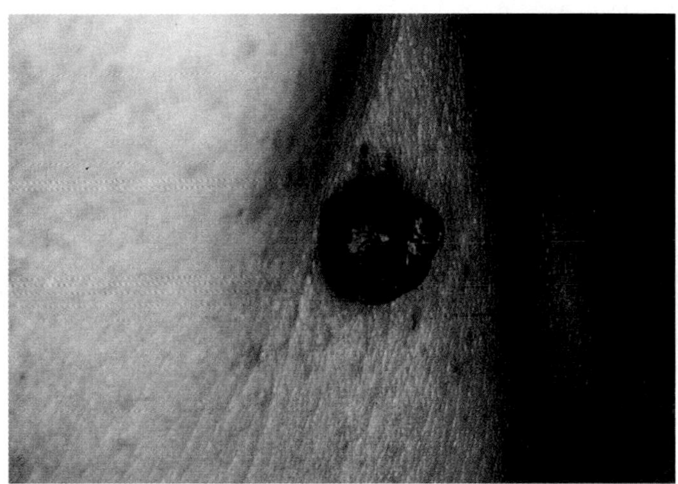

Fig. 71-125 Nodular melanoma. This tumor is a well-circumscribed nodule that is mainly intradermal and has very little tendency to spread into the adjacent epidermis. Polypoid masses are typical examples.

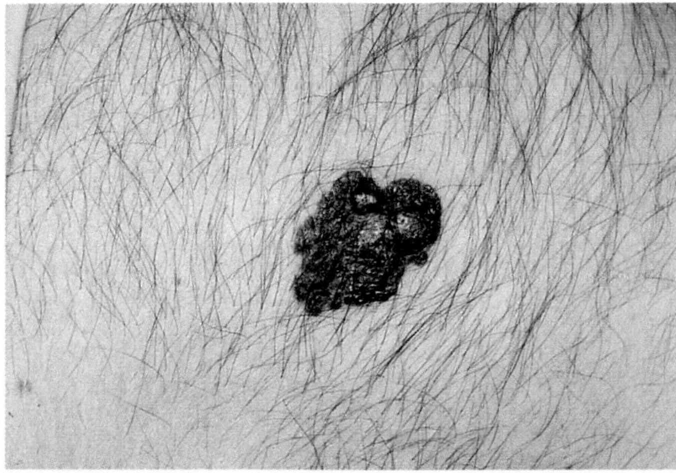

Fig. 71-124 Superficial spreading malignant melanoma, invasive. Grossly, there is evidence of multinodularity in the lesion with some areas of atrophy or regression as indicated by a pale gray scaly portion of the lesion.

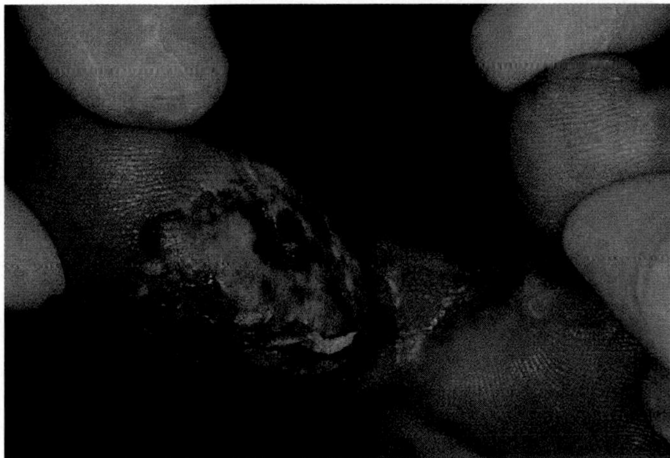

Fig. 71-126 Acral lentiginous melanoma. This type is closely related to superficial spreading melanoma in that it has a prolonged intraepidermal growth phase. It arises in relatively sun-protected sites and may be pigmented or amelanotic.

plastic melanoma,"[196-198] usually has a minimal lentiginous proliferation of atypical melanocytes in the epidermis and an extensive proliferation of spindle-shaped, amelanotic cells in a fibrous and myxoid stroma (Fig. 71-128). It can be extremely difficult to recognize and to distinguish from a scar. When desmoplastic melanoma forms structures that resemble nerves or invades down nerves in the dermis, the term "neurotropic melanoma" is applied.[199] Acral lentiginous melanoma has the growth pattern of a lentigo maligna melanoma or a superficial spreading melanoma but characteristically has an abundance of highly dendritic and often small melanoma cells (Fig. 71-129).

In contrast to nevus cells, melanoma cells usually do not become smaller with progressive invasion into the dermis. Actually the deep portion of the dermal component often contains the largest and most atypical cells. Mitoses are present in both the upper and lower portions of the lesions. Atypical mitoses such as tripolar mitoses occur and are extremely rare in any other melanocytic lesion. A lymphocytic inflammatory infiltrate with variable numbers of plasma cells is common. Macrophages can be very abundant; they ingest melanin pigment from the melanoma cells, making it difficult at times to distinguish between a melanoma cell and a pigmented macrophage, or "melanophage." In general, the melanoma cells form aggregates with mitoses, and the melanophages are rounded cells with very little tendency to form aggregates in the stroma. Melanophages can have prominent nucleoli, but mitoses are not found in macrophages containing pigment. Groups of melanoma cells often infiltrate into lymphatics or blood vessels in the dermis.

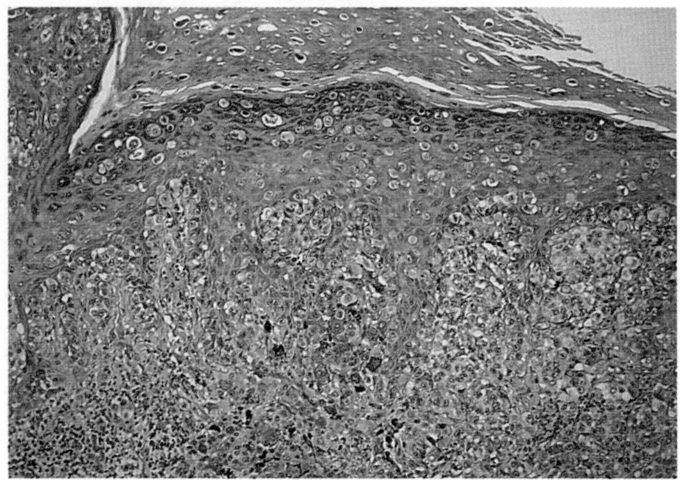

Fig. 71-127 Superficial spreading malignant melanoma, invasive. Often the epidermis has atypical melanocytes scattered upward into the granular layer or stratum corneum as well as infiltrating into the dermis.

The prognosis of these invasive lesions is related mainly to the depth of penetration of the tumor in the dermis[46] (Table 71-6). The most unambiguous method for assessing this depth has been to measure the thickness of the tumor with an ocular micrometer from the top of the granular layer to the base of the lesion at its deepest point, which is called the "Breslow thickness."[200] It is related not only to the anatomic depth of penetration into the dermis, but also to tumor volume. A system of estimating the anatomic level of penetration is called "Clark's level." Clark's level I corresponds to a lesion that is purely intraepidermal. Clark's level II describes a melanoma that extends into the papillary dermis. At Clark's level III, a melanoma fills and expands the papillary dermis without invading below the level of the superficial vascular plexus that defines the border between the papillary and reticular dermis. Clark's level IV corresponds to a melanoma that extends into the reticular dermis (at least five collagen bundles below the superficial vascular plexus). At Clark's level V, melanomas extend into the subcutaneous fat. Clark's levels have a general relationship to Breslow thickness. Clark's level II lesions are generally less than 0.75 to 0.86 mm in thickness and have a relatively good prognosis. Clark's level III lesions may be quite thick, and level IV lesions can be either very thick or thin. Level V lesions are thick, often more than 2 mm. Level IV and V lesions have a bad prognosis, which correlates best with the measured thickness. When lesions of LMM, SSM, and NM are matched for thickness and anatomic site, the prognoses are similar. Other important prognostic factors include mitotic rate per

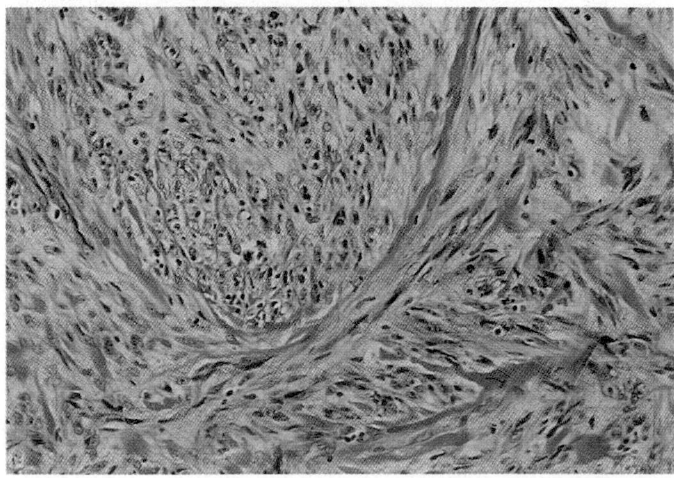

Fig. 71-128 Desmoplastic melanoma. There is a proliferation of spindle cells with nuclear atypism and usually without pigment production but with prominent fine collagen deposition.

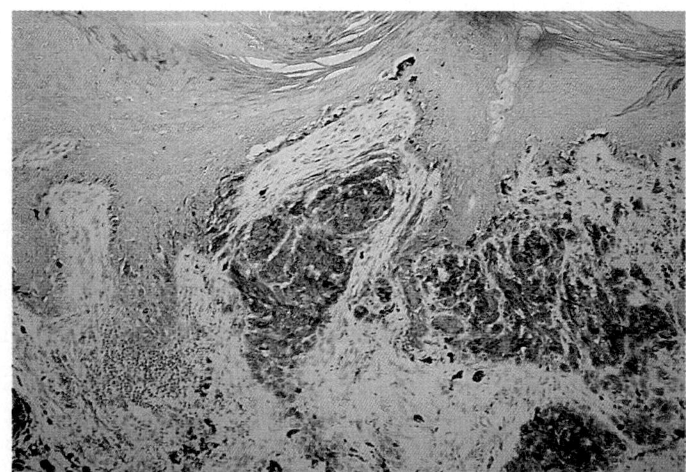

Fig. 71-129 Acral lentiginous melanoma, invasive. This preparation has been stained with HMB45 to show the dendritic melanocytes in the epidermis as well as the nodule of tumor cells in the dermis. Lymphocytic infiltration is present.

square millimeter, ulceration, and microsatellites, which actually are intracutaneous metastases.[50,201] It is important to excise completely any malignant melanoma, since the effective treatment is complete, early surgical removal of the primary lesion. Reexcisions are recommended to be sure that the primary tumor and any possible microsatellites are removed.[50]

The unusual variants of melanoma may not have the same prognosis by these measurements as the more frequent melanoma types, since these rare tumors have not been collected into sufficiently large series of cases. Desmoplastic melanomas often are deep, but survivals seem to be longer than for other NM at the same depth. When desmoplastic melanomas form metastases, they usually are not desmoplastic and are high-grade malignancies. Likewise, in the primary lesions, minimal deviation melanoma 202 and "nevoid melanoma" [203] are composed of small cells that do not have much cytologic atypism and architecturally mimic compound nevi. However, the prognosis seems to be similar to other NM, despite the minimal anaplasia.[52,203] Metastases from these lesions also can be high-grade anaplastic tumors.

Malignant melanomas arise within very large, or "giant," congenital nevi; however, estimates of risk are difficult to determine but may be as high as 10%. Histologic evidence of dysplasia has been found in up to 50% of giant congenital nevi.[204]

Table 71-6 Evaluation of histologic levels and depth of invasion in invasive malignant melanomas

Clark's levels of invasion

Level I: Tumor cells are confined to the epidermis or its extensions as appendages. The tumor has not penetrated through the basement membrane to grow in the dermis.

Level II: Tumor cells extend singly or in nests into the papillary dermis, or into the adventitial dermis around appendages. When the nests are larger in the dermis than in the epidermis or have mitoses in them, the dermal growth phase can be recognized.

Level III: Groups of tumor cells fill and expand the papillary dermis. The tumor does not extend below the superficial vascular plexus.

Level IV: Tumor cells penetrate into the reticular dermis at least five collagen bundles below the superficial vascular plexus.

Level V: Tumor cells are present in the subcutaneous fat, as a continuous process of extension rather than as a detached metastasis.

Breslow's thickness

With an ocular micrometer, the depth of invasion is measured in millimeters from the top of the granular layer to the deepest melanoma cell. If ulcerated, the base of the ulcer excluding crust is the top.

0.0 to 0.75 mm: Low-risk lesions; most of these are also Clark's level II.

0.75 to 1.50 mm: Intermediate-risk; most lesions are Clark's level II or III, though some tumors may be early level IV.

1.50 mm or more: High-risk lesions; most are Clark's level IV or V lesions.

Other important factors for assessing prognosis include mitotic rate, width of ulceration, regression, and presence of microsatellites.

Modified from Elder DE, Murphy GF: *Melanocytic tumors of the skin. Atlas of tumor pathology,* series 3, fasc 2, Washington, DC, 1991, Armed Forces Institute of Pathology.

Lymphoid lesions, including cutaneous T-cell lymphomas

Mycosis fungoides is the most common form of cutaneous T-cell lymphoma (CTCL).[57,62,205] Its incidence in the general population is similar to that of Hodgkin's disease, making it one of the most frequent types of lymphoma overall. The patients are usually elderly males, more than females, often with lesions that begin in the region of the lower trunk, buttocks, and upper thighs. The initial intraepidermal stages have been presented. As the lymphocytes infiltrate the dermis as well as the epidermis, the irregular, erythematous, well-demarcated macules become more elevated and indurated plaques (Fig. 71-130). Also they can involute partially to produce irregular serpiginous regions of erythema and scaling, interspersed with varied hyperpigmentation and hypopigmentation, with atrophy of the epidermis; this grouping of features has been called "poikiloderma." Plaques can become tumors, by convention more than 5 mm in thickness, but tumors can arise directly from previously uninvolved skin. The tumors have a deep erythema, almost purple in color, and ulceration is common (Fig. 71-131).

Sézary's syndrome is a variant of CTCL.[206] The symptoms and signs include generalized erythroderma, pruritus, hyperkeratosis of the palms and soles, edema of the lower extremities, lymphadenopathy, hepatosplenomegaly, and circulating blood lymphocytes with nuclei that are enlarged, hyperchromatic, and hyperconvoluted. Patients with Sézary's syndrome occasionally have antecedent lesions of mycosis fungoides. Lymphomatous infiltration of the skin can be secondary to a T-cell lymphoma arising in lymph nodes or other internal sites; the patients with such a "peripheral T-cell lymphoma" have a worse prognosis than those with classical mycosis fungoides.

Infection by human T-cell lymphotrophic virus type 1 (HTLV-I) can produce lesions resembling the tumor stage of mycosis fungoides or the erythroderma of Sézary's syndrome.[207,208] HTLV-I–associated CTCL characteristically is resistant to therapy and often has a rapidly lethal course.

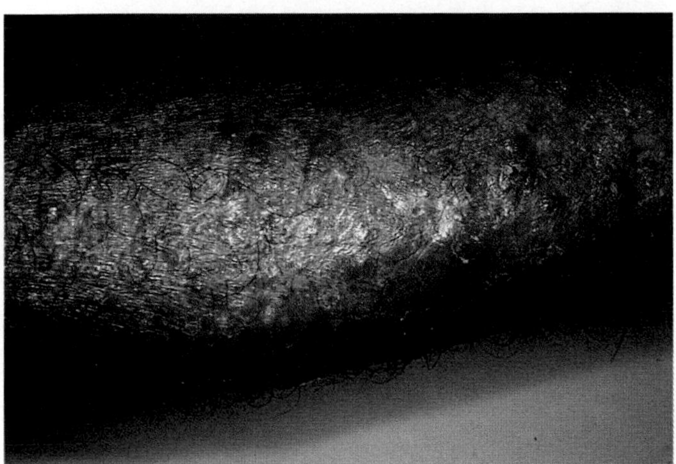

Fig. 71-130 Mycosis fungoides, plaque lesion. Both the epidermis and the dermis are infiltrated by atypical lymphocytes in this irregular, indurated region of the forearm. Follicular mucinosis also is present, with white material at several follicular orifices.

Hypercalcemia and osteolytic bone lesions are present in half of the patients. The cause of mycosis fungoides is unknown. However, the similarity between patients with CTCL caused by HTLV-I and some patients with mycosis fungoides or Sézary's syndrome has led to a search for viruses that may cause this disease. Hall and colleagues have described several patients with a defective form of HTLV-I that have had clinical diagnoses of mycosis fungoides.[209] Molecular probes have shown that mycosis fungoides is a proliferation of T-cells with a clonal rearrangement of the beta chain of the T-cell antigen receptor.[210-212] Probes have also been developed by which an individual patient's T-cell lymphoma can be identified both prospectively and retrospectively in tissues.[213] Immunophenotypic studies are less specific but have shown that T-cell lymphomas can be suspected by abnormalities in the pattern of T-cell differentiation antigens in approximately 48% of patients with mycosis fungoides.[214-216]

PATHOLOGY. Cutaneous lymphomas often are composed of cytologically atypical lymphoid cells infiltrating the epidermis and dermis (Fig. 71-132).[58] In the early macular stages, there is an infiltrate of atypical lymphoid cells in the epidermis, with a few cells present in the dermis around the blood vessels of the superficial vascular plexus. However, as mycosis fungoides progresses, there is a shift toward more proliferation in the dermis. A mixture of reactive T- and B-lymphocytes can accompany the lymphoma cells. Thick indurated lesions have lymphoma cells in the dermis or subcutis that often replace or obliterate the dermal structures. Often the lymphocytes have enlarged hyperchromatic nuclei with deep irregular indentations in the nuclear envelope[217-219] (Fig. 71-133). In the late tumor stage lesions, nuclei frequently are greatly enlarged and lack most of the nuclear indentations or "convolutions."

Precursor lesions for mycosis fungoides include *large plaque parapsoriasis,* which has atrophic plaques in a distribution similar to mycosis fungoides, but it lacks atypical lymphocytes by routine histology and lacks prominent epidermotropism or Darier-Pautrier microabscesses.[57,214] At least 10% of patients with large plaque parapsoriasis go on to develop obvious lymphoma.[96] Other patients present with papular lesions that have a transient course of several weeks but histologically contain large atypical lymphocytes that are CD30 positive.[220-222] This disease, called *lymphomatoid papulosis,* progresses to obvious lymphoma in approximately 10% of cases. Kadin and colleagues have reported that this progression is associated with a loss of the receptors for transforming growth factor-beta on the surfaces of the lymphocytes.[223,224] *Lymphomatoid granulomatosis* has occasionally been considered a precursor of CTCL but is rather a subtle form of *angiocentric T-cell* (or B-cell) *lymphoma* that begins as a lymphocytic vasculitis with variable degrees of atypia of the lymphocytes (Fig. 71-134).[225,226] It progresses to vascular and tissue destruction because of infiltration of blood vessel walls by atypical lymphocytes with thrombosis and infarction of the abnormal and normal tissue that these vessels supply. Lymphomatoid granulomatosis affects the lung and skin of the extremities often.[227] In contrast, a similar disease called *lethal midline granuloma* affects the sinuses and skin of the central face.[225]

The differential diagnosis includes infiltrates of Langerhans' cells, which exhibit epidermotropism and produce papules, nodules or plaques. These disorders, now termed

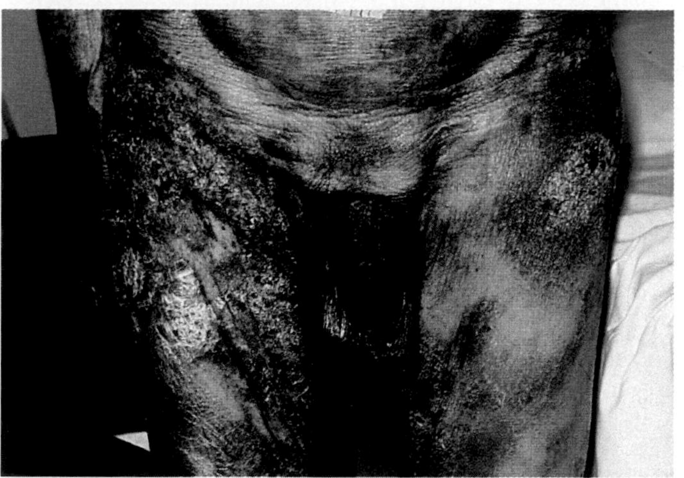

Fig. 71-131 Mycosis fungoides, tumor stage. Progressive thickening of the plaques leads to tumors, frequently with ulceration. Hyperpigmentation, crusting, and a deep violaceous erythema are striking findings.

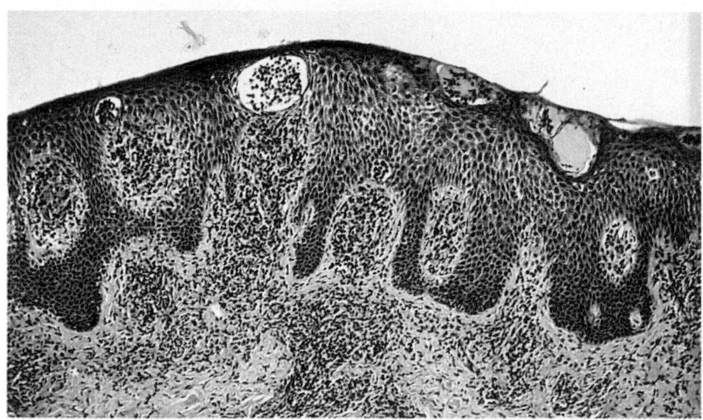

Fig. 71-132 Mycosis fungoides, plaque lesion. In addition to the well-demarcated Darier-Pautrier microabscesses in the epidermis, there is significant infiltration of atypical lymphocytes into the dermis around the blood vessels and in the interstitium.

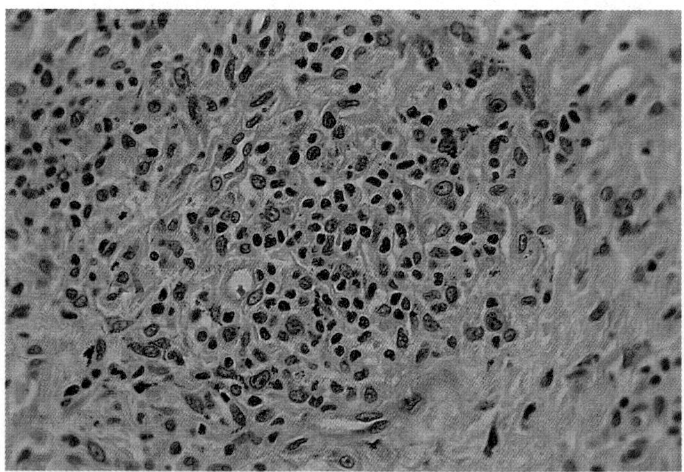

Fig. 71-133 Mycosis fungoides, plaque lesion. At higher magnification, the mixture of lymphoid cells in the dermis contains atypical lymphocytes with deep irregular indentations of their nuclei.

"Langerhans' cell histiocytosis,"[228] are discussed later with the diseases involving mainly the dermis. These cells are S-100$^+$ and CD1a$^+$ and contain Birbeck granules visible by EM.[229,230]

Hair follicle tumors

Clinically these lesions present as nodules in the deep dermis (Fig. 71-135) without surface epidermal change, except for the occasional presence of a central comedone in a dilated follicular orifice in the center of the lesion. They are often soft, nontender, and flesh colored, but if they are traumatized, the keratinous contents that are released into the dermis induce inflammation.

PATHOLOGY. These disorders can be divided into true cysts and more solid neoplasms.[38] Most cysts of the skin are derived from the hair follicle. The wall of the cyst often has differentiation toward some part of the normal epithelium of the hair follicle.[36,231-233] One type has been named "infundibular cyst" when it mimics the differentiation of the infundibular portion of the hair follicle, by having a granular layer and loosely packed keratin contents. Another common cyst, often of the scalp, is the *isthmus cyst* (also called "pilar cyst," or "trichilemmal cyst"), which mimics the differentiation of the isthmus portion of the hair follicle, particularly in the catagen phase of the normal hair cycle (Fig. 71-136). These cysts show abrupt keratinization without the formation of a granular layer and form very dense keratin in the lumen of the cyst. *Steatocystoma multiplex* is a genetic disorder with autosomal dominant inheritance in which affected members have many cysts of the hair follicle that mimic the sebaceous duct and have sebaceous epithelium in the wall of the cyst, very oily contents, and have a surface refractive cuticle similar to that of the normal sebaceous duct. Other types of cysts include eruptive vellus hair cyst, milia, dilated pore of Winer, true dermoid cyst, and true epidermal inclusion cyst that forms after surface epidermis has been displaced into the dermis by trauma. The more solid tumors of the hair follicle are quite varied. The most common of the solid tumors is the *trichoepithelioma* [1,38] (Fig. 71-137) which can mimic most of

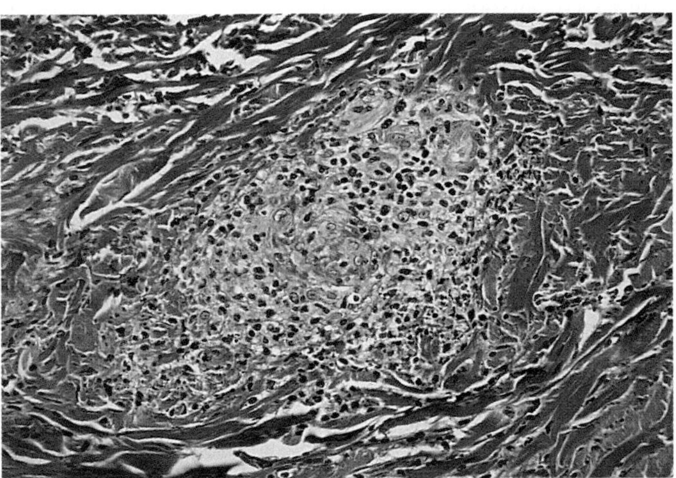

Fig. 71-134 Angiocentric T-cell lymphoma. The atypical lymphocytes have infiltrated the small blood vessels and led to necrosis and thrombosis in this form of lymphocytic vasculitis.

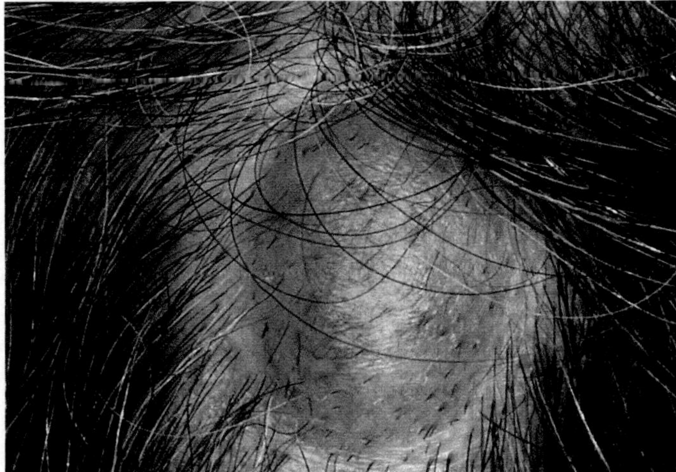

Fig. 71-135 Isthmus-catagen cyst. This cyst is common on the scalp and is usually deep seated in the dermis or subcutis. Rupture can lead to severe local inflammation.

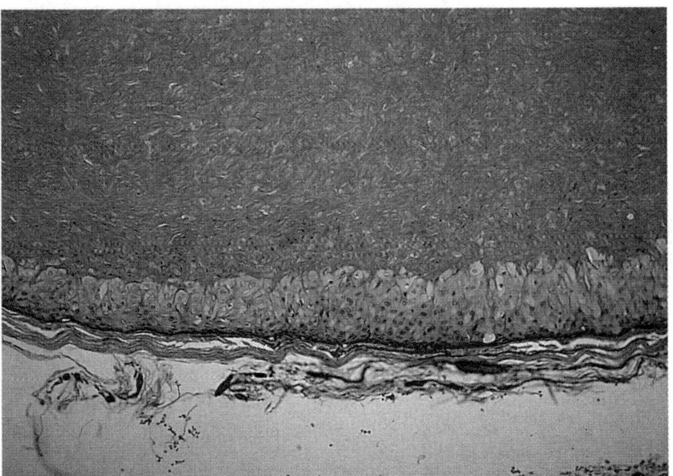

Fig. 71-136 Isthmus-catagen cyst. The cyst wall is stratified squamous epithelium with abrupt keratinization without a granular layer and very dense keratin in the center of the cyst. This appearance is similar to that in the isthmus portion of the hair follicle during catagen.

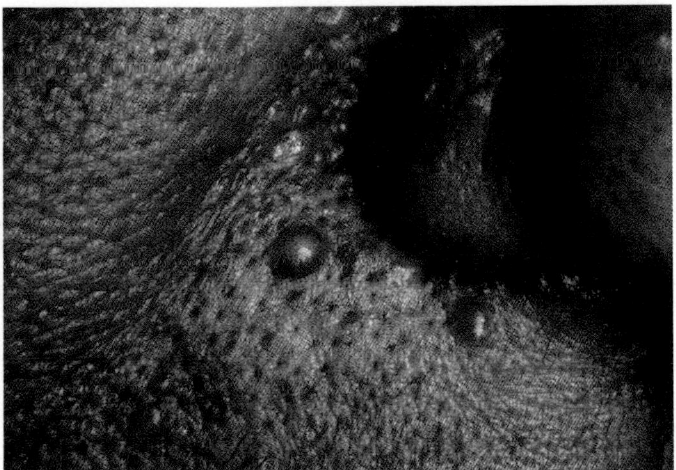

Fig. 71-137 Trichoepithelioma. These tumors often are multiple small papular lesions that are flesh colored. The central face is a common site.

the regions of the hair follicle but does not produce terminal or vellus hairs from the lesion. Trichoepitheliomas vary in the degree of differentiation but usually contain both keratotic areas as well as basaloid regions (Fig. 71-138). They are very slow growing tumors with very low mitotic rates and do not have the erosive character of basal cell carcinoma. They lack the collagenolytic clefts between epithelium and stroma. Basaloid cells and fibroblastic cells form "papillary mesenchymal bodies" that resemble the epithelial and mesenchymal arrangement of the anagen hair bulb (Fig. 71-139). In contrast, a *trichilemmoma* has many cells with clear cytoplasm that resemble the glycogen-rich outer root sheath of the hair follicle and have peripheral palisading, as well as basement-membrane thickening reminiscent of the thickened basement membrane of the catagen follicle. These tumors may have coarse keratohyalin at the surface, and some dermatopathologists have considered them to be warts affecting vellus hair follicles. Trichilemmomas may be important to identify, since, when multiple, they can be a marker for Cowden's syndrome, which among other cutaneous and visceral abnormalities has an increased incidence of breast and thyroid cancers. Three other tumors also form a range of disease: *proliferating tricholemmal cyst, pilar tumor of the scalp,* and *trichilemmal carcinoma*. The proliferating cyst has thickening of the wall of an isthmus-catagen cyst with retention of the polarity of the epithelium in relation to the stroma. The pilar tumor of the scalp is an infiltrative lesion that lacks sharp circumscription and has lost the polarity of the epithelium, which keratinizes both toward residual lumens as well as toward the stroma. Both of these lesions lack the cytologic atypia of true trichilemmal carcinoma. Mitoses may be present in all three of the lesions. At times, the differentiation between pilar tumor and trichilemmal carcinoma may be impossible on histologic grounds alone.

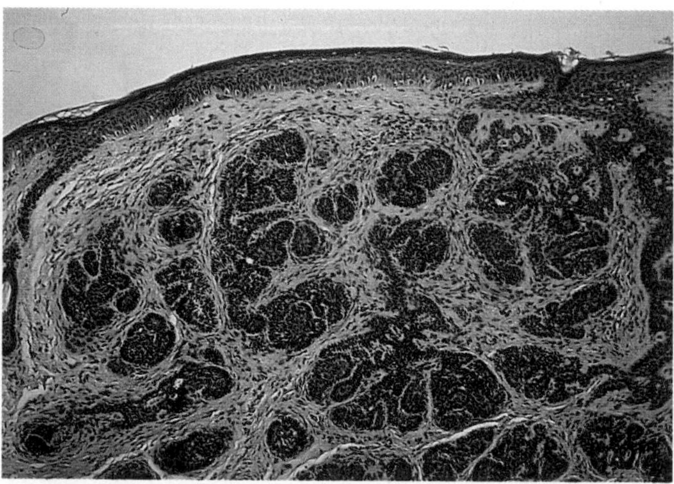

Fig. 71-138 Trichoepithelioma. Groups of basaloid cells are present in a cellular stroma, but they differ from basal cell carcinoma in the lack of clefts, a low mitotic rate, and absence of confluent areas of necrosis.

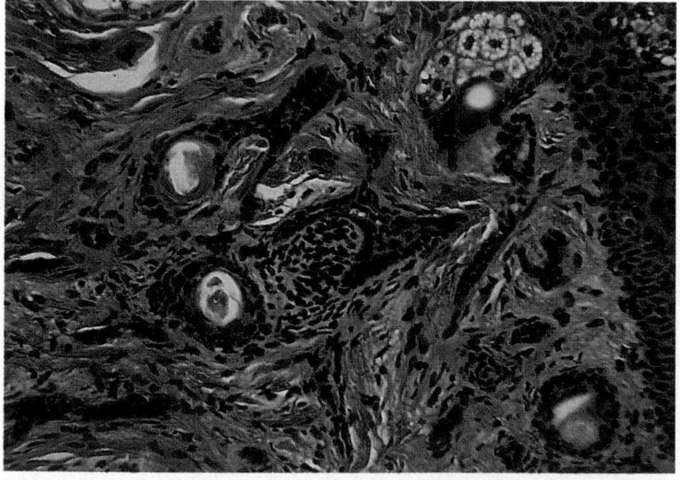

Fig. 71-139 Desmoplastic trichoepithelioma. The stroma can be quite sclerotic, and the tumor epithelium can be compressed into thin strands. Aggregations of stromal cells in relation to indentations in the epithelium are distinctive "papillary-mesenchymal bodies" and help to differentiate this tumor from morpheic basal cell carcinoma.

Sebaceous tumors

Clinically, only two of sebaceous tumors have a distinctive presentation in the patient, and all the others are simply firm intradermal to subcutaneous nodules.[1,38] One distinctive lesion, *sebaceous hyperplasia*, is most common on the face and has a widely dilated orifice of a sebaceous follicle around which there is a symmetrical, ringlike elevation that is soft and yellow. There may be adjacent telangiectatic blood vessels reminiscent of those associated with basal cell carcinoma. At the opposite end of the disease manifestation is sebaceous carcinoma, which presents as a dermal nodule. Particularly in the eyelid, it often spreads in the epidermis overlying the nodule to produce a red scaly lesion resembling squamous cell carcinoma in situ.

PATHOLOGY. These tumors have been divided on the basis of whether they maintain the overall architecture of the lobules of sebaceous glands, the degree of admixture of the basaloid and lipidized sebaceous cells within the lobules, and the degree of cytologic atypism. *Sebaceous hyperplasia* has well-formed, enlarged sebaceous lobules that are high in the papillary dermis instead of in their normal middermal location. The germinative layer is around only the periphery of the lobules and is no more than one to two cells layers in thickness. Cytologic atypism is absent. *Sebaceous adenoma* has a mixture of mature sebaceous cells and basaloid germinative cells in the lobules, and so the ratio of basaloid to lipidized cells may approach up to 50% of the cells in the lobules. Some lobules have the basaloid cells only near the basement membrane region, whereas others have them admixed throughout the lobule. In contrast, *sebaceous epithelioma* is synonymous with basal cell carcinoma with sebaceous differentiation. In sebaceous epithelioma, more than 50% of the cells are basaloid germinative cells and at least some of the lobules show features of basal cell carcinoma with peripheral palisading, mitoses, necrosis, and stromal changes adjacent to the lobules. *Sebaceoma* is similar but lacks peripheral palisading and abundant mitoses.[36] These features are different from those of sebaceous carcinoma, which has more cytologically atypical sebaceous cells often with eosinophilic cytoplasm and striking nuclear atypism.

Sebaceous carcinoma is a poorly circumscribed lesion that infiltrates the dermis and occasionally the epidermis as well in a pattern that resembles Paget's disease or squamous cell carcinoma in situ. Cytoplasmic lipid vacuoles that indent the nuclear outline may be an important clue to sebaceous differentiation. Sebaceous carcinomas can vary in their degree of differentiation, with some areas mimicking sebaceous adenomas, sebaceous epitheliomas, or sebaceomas but differing from them in greater cytologic atypism and an infiltrative pattern of growth (Fig. 71-140). Complete excision of sebaceous adenomas and carcinomas is recommended to judge the degree of infiltration of the skin and the range of histologic appearances within the tumor. In patients over 50 years of age, a sebaceous neoplasm, other than sebaceous hyperplasia, can be associated with internal malignancy (Muir-Torre syndrome).

A congenital hamartomatous malformation of the skin, usually of the scalp, has been called *nevus sebaceus of Jadassohn.* The malformation lacks hair follicles and sebaceous glands often insert directly into the epidermis. At puberty the sebaceous glands enlarge. The hamartoma involves both epidermal and adnexal structures of the skin. The epidermis often has a verrucous hyperplasia that can resemble a wart. Apocrine glands are common. After puberty, nevus sebaceus gives rise to a number of tumors including basal cell carcinomas (in approximately 10%), syringocystadenoma papilliferum (in approximately 10%), as well as a variety of apocrine and eccrine tumors.

Apocrine tumors

Clinically the presentation of these tumors is that of a dermal to subcutaneous nodule.[1,38] Some of the lesions have a bluish color, and the benign ones are freely mobile. They may be solitary or multiple. *Syringocystadenoma papilliferum* occurs as an isolated tumor or in association with a nevus sebaceus of Jadassohn; it is often on the scalp or face and has crusted papillomatous surface (Fig. 71-141).

PATHOLOGY. Histologically, apocrine differentiation often is evident in a columnar to cuboidal lining cell that has prominent apical cytoplasm that tends to be quite eosinophilic. In some instances this apical cytoplasm protrudes prominently into the lumen to give the impression of so-called "decapitation secretion." This differentiation can be present in simple cysts called "apocrine hidrocystomas," or in complex cysts called "apocrine cystadenomas," which can be tubular or papillary. One of the papillary forms, that is, *hidradenoma papilliferum*, occurs on the vulva, or perineal or circumanal regions. *Syringocystadenoma papilliferum* is another papillary tumor that has papillae projecting into a deep cystic cavity or onto the skin surface and has many plasma cells in the stroma (Fig. 71-142). *Cylindroma* is a tumor that is often considered to be of apocrine differentiation, though this is disputed. Nests of basaloid cells are surrounded by a thick basement membrane of type IV collagen. Some of the nests have small tubular lumens with PAS-positive, diastase-resistant material in the lumen. There are two cell types—the smaller cells are often near the periphery of the lobules, and the larger cells are near the lumen. There is a high nuclear to cytoplasmic ratio, and mitoses are not common. Malignancy is extremely rare. *Apocrine carcinoma* does occur and is usually a tubular adenocarcinoma with atypical glandular lining cells that lack a surrounding layer of myoepithelial cells and that have abundant eosinophilic cytoplasm.

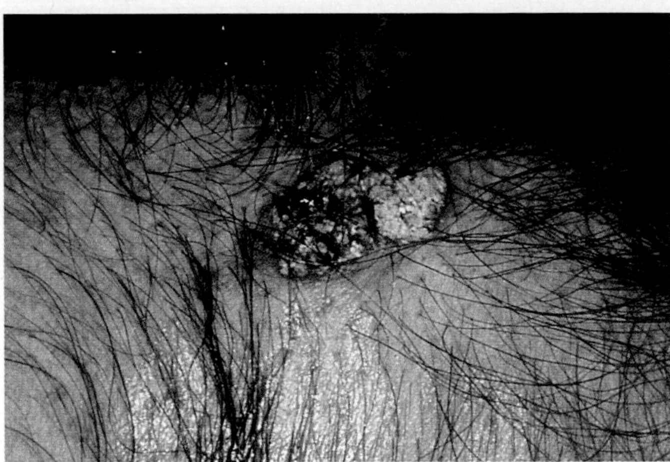

Fig. 71-141 Syringocystadenoma papilliferum. This solitary crusted tumor on the scalp has papillomatous projections on the surface. Production of a thin fluid is common.

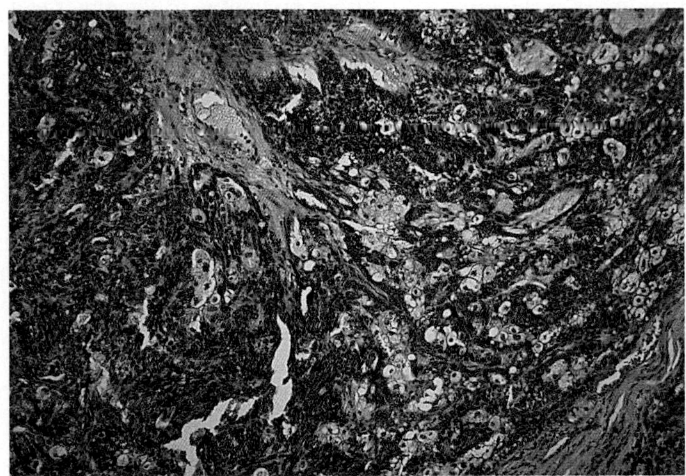

Fig. 71-140 Sebaceous carcinoma. This region of a well-differentiated sebaceous carcinoma has features similar to those of sebaceous adenoma except for greater atypism of the basaloid cells and a high mitotic rate. This tumor also diffusely infiltrated the dermis and subcutis.

Eccrine tumors

Almost all these tumors present as dermal or subcutaneous nodules.[1,38,234] Although they can occur anywhere, some have common locations; for example, syringoma often occurs on the face around the eye. Eccrine poroma is usually on the lower legs below the knee. Sclerosing sweat duct carcinoma ("microcystic adnexal carcinoma") is usually in the skin of the central face.

PATHOLOGY. These tumors are quite varied in morphologic patterns and in their location in the skin. *Eccrine poroma* is a benign tumor of keratinocytes which mimic the uppermost portion of the eccrine duct as it penetrates through the epidermis, that is, the acrosyringium. The keratinocytes have small nuclei, moderate amounts of eosinophilic cytoplasm, and a rather uniform cell size. Central cysts or cavities contain fluid. The cell surfaces lining the cysts have a PAS-positive, diastase-resistant, glycoprotein coat that is positive also for carcinoembryonic antigen. The tumor may be purely intraepidermal and form nests of cells in the epidermis *(hidroacanthoma simplex)*, or

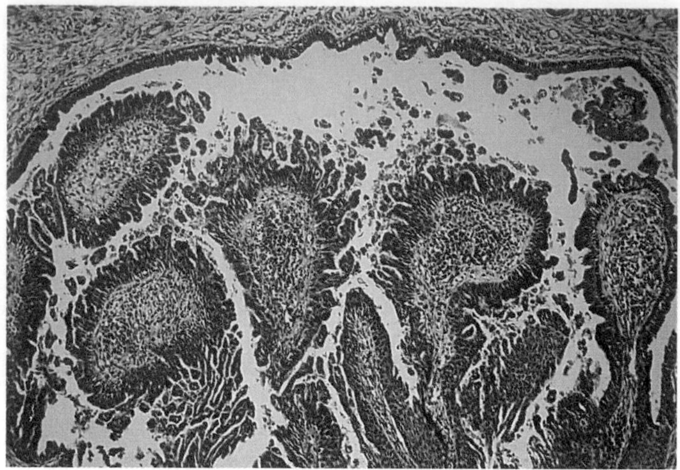

Fig. 71-142 Syringocystadenoma papilliferum. Deep within the dermis is a epithelium-lined cyst with papillomatous processes and many plasma cells in the stroma.

may infiltrate into the dermis while maintaining continuity with the epidermis. *Eccrine porocarcinoma* has greater cytologic atypism, may infiltrate the epidermis diffusely like Paget's disease, and often infiltrates into the dermis.

A related but deeper benign tumor is *eccrine acrospiroma* (synonyms are "nodular hidradenoma," "clear cell hidradenoma," "epidermoid hidradenoma," and "solid-cystic hidradenoma"). It is composed of keratinocytes that mimic the fetal acrosyringium in the formation of tubular lumens by the fusion of small cytoplasmic vacuoles. In the dermis, characteristically this tumor forms nodular masses of keratinocytes with relatively uniform nuclei and moderate amounts of eosinophilic cytoplasm. The nodules have glandular lumens containing PAS-positive, diastase-resistant material. The keratinocytes can vary from those with prominent eosinophilic cytoplasm, to ones with glycogen-rich clear cytoplasm, and to spindle-shaped cells. Carcinoembryonic antigen is usually positive in the lumens and on the surfaces of some of the cells. Malignant eccrine acrospiroma (nodular hidradenocarcinoma) has prominent mitoses, necrosis in tumor nodules, and a multinodular pattern of growth in the dermis. Cytologic atypism can be subtle.

Syringoma is a benign tumor formed by keratinocytes that produce small glands in the dermis, often associated with prominent sclerosis or fibrosis of the dermis. The glands have small lumens and cords of cells that have the appearance of "tadpole-shaped tails." Nuclear atypism is minimal, and the glands formed have at least a bilayered epithelium. Malignant syringoma, or so-called *sclerosing sweat duct carcinoma* or *microcystic adnexal carcinoma,* is a tubular adenocarcinoma often with solid cords or glands with an irregular and possibly single layer of lining cells. Infiltration can be deep and perineural, and cytologic atypism can be minimal.

Chondroid syringoma (mixed tumor of the skin) is similar to the mixed tumor or pleomorphic adenoma of the salivary glands. There is an admixture of tubular glandular components with stromal components including small nests of epithelial cells and cartilaginous stroma. These are malignant versions of this tumor that have increased nuclear atypism, mitoses, and necrosis in the tumor lobules.

Eccrine epithelioma is a basal cell carcinoma with areas of eccrine differentiation. These tumors have a greater propensity for metastasis than ordinary basal cell carcinomas. Eccrine differentiation is evident in the formation of tubules lined by atypical epithelium but with classical basal cell carcinoma elsewhere.

Eccrine spiradenoma is a tumor of small basaloid cells deep in the dermis usually without any connection to the epidermis. The cells form small nodules without prominent eosinophilic basement membranes around them, which helps to differentiate them from cylindroma. Otherwise the cells tend to resemble the small cell components of the cylindromas, with some larger cells and small lumens in most tumors. A few patients with both multiple cylindromas and eccrine spiradenomas have been described. Adenocarcinomas very rarely arise in association with eccrine spiradenoma and are aggressive, atypical tubular adenocarcinomas that are not subtle mimics of eccrine spiradenoma.

Adenoid cystic carcinomas and primary mucinous carcinomas of the sweat glands occur and resemble those of the salivary gland. The distinction between metastatic adenocarcinoma and primary sweat gland carcinoma can be very difficult.

It is important to recognize sweat gland carcinomas, since they may metastasize widely. Other sweat gland tumors include acrosyringeal nevus and syringofibroadenoma (Mascaro tumor).

DISEASES INVOLVING MAINLY THE DERMIS

The dermal group of disorders has its major manifestations in the dermis, with only minor changes in the epidermis. Slight degrees of acanthosis can be a reaction to dermal inflammation or can be attributable to scratching or other trauma to the lesion.

Genodermatoses and developmental abnormalities

Many genetic disorders alter the arrangement or proportions of the connective tissues of the dermis. Those that present as tumors are included in the sections on tumors of the major cell type. Textbooks of dermatology and dermatopathology need to be consulted on many of these disorders, since we consider here only four.

Elastic tissue abnormalities

Cutis laxa. The patients often present with sagging skin that hangs in folds, usually on the trunk. Internal organs can be affected also, producing hernias, diverticuli, and emphysema. It is an autosomal dominant trait but can be acquired.

PATHOLOGY. Routine histologic sections show no obvious abnormality. Elastic tissue stains reveal fragmentation and loss of elastic fibers.

Slack skin can occur as an aging phenomenon, particularly as a result of actinic damage to elastic tissue. Acquired elastolysis can present a similar picture also.

Pseudoxanthoma elasticum. Pseudoxanthoma elasticum is a rare but devastating disease in which the patients develop white to yellow soft plaques of loose, wrinkled skin, on the sides of the neck and in the axillae and groin. Retinal hemorrhages occur as a result of ruptures of Bruch's membrane, an elastic lamina between the retina and choroid layers. Atherosclerosis is accelerated as a result of the degenerative changes in the elastic laminas of arteries, leading to angina pectoris, myocardial infarction, and intermittent claudication. Transmission usually is autosomal recessive, but autosomal dominant disease has been reported. Also there are patients with only partial expression of the disease.

The cause of this disease is not known but seems related to defective formation of elastin or the protein fibrillin, a component of microfibrils that surround the elastin core.[235] The elastic fibers are both structurally and biochemically abnormal. Treatment should minimize the calcification of the elastic fibers and reduce the risk of atherosclerotic vascular occlusions.

PATHOLOGY. The sections of involved skin reveal fragmentation and irregular clumping of elastic fibers in the reticular dermis. Tangled masses of small, calcified elastic fibers are found. The calcium phosphate deposits can be demonstrated with the von Kossa silver stain. Similar changes occur in the elastic fibers of blood vessel walls. The calcification precedes the fragmentation and distortion of the elastic fibers. In routine sections, the hematoxylin stains the altered elastic fibers a gray-blue color.

Collagen abnormalities

Connective tissue nevus. A connective tissue nevus is a hamartoma of the dermal fibrous tissue that often is present near the time of birth but can be noticed later in life. It usually is an asymptomatic firm nodule in the dermis. Often the lesion is small, only a few millimeters in diameter, but lesions can be up to many centimeters, and they may be multiple. Solitary lesions often do not imply an inherited syndrome. Multiple lesions occur in the familial cutaneous collagenoma syndrome that has been associated with an idiopathic progressive cardiomyopathy. A large plaque lesion on the lower back occurs in patients with tuberous sclerosis and is called a "shagreen patch." Lesions with increased large elastic fibers also are found in the Buschke-Ollendorf syndrome, which is associated with osteopoikilosis.

PATHOLOGY. The connective tissue nevus consists of enlarged collagen bundles that produce thickening of the dermis. The arrangement of the collagen can seem normal or can be abnormal, with many parallel collagen bundles in the deep dermis. Elastic tissue often is decreased but can be normal. It is increased in Buschke-Ollendorf lesions. A congenital form of connective tissue nevus with many perivascular adipose tissue cells occurs in a zosteriform distribution in the nevus lipomatosis of Hoffman and Zurhelle. A similar histologic appearance is found in an acquired polypoid lesion called "fibroma molle," which is better named a "dermatolipoma."

Mastocytosis

Mastocytosis is a group of disorders characterized by an excessive accumulation of mast cells, particularly in the skin but also in internal organs. *Urticaria pigmentosa*, the cutaneous form of mastocytosis, is usually a disease of children. The skin lesions are hyperpigmented, reddish-brown papules and macules usually on the trunk or proximal extremities. Stroking of the lesions causes a surrounding flare of erythema (Darier's sign), and bullae may form. The mast cell accumulations often produce multiple papules, or rarely plaques and nodules, or they can form a solitary nodule ("mastocytoma"). The lesions regress by puberty in most patients. In adults the lesions usually are flat hyperpigmented macules with associated telangietasia ("telangiectasia macularis eruptiva perstans," TMEP), which is a form with less tendency to spontaneous regression than the childhood forms.

PATHOLOGY. Mast cells form perivascular collections of cells that have round to ovoid shapes, central nuclei, and grayish, slightly granular cytoplasm in standard sections. The cytoplasmic granules are metachromatic with Giemsa or toluidine blue stains, and are positive on periodic acid–Schiff and naphthol AS-D chloracetate esterase (Leder) stains. The TMEP form can be very subtle, with only a slight increase in size and number of spindle-shaped mast cells around telangiectatic blood vessels and hair follicles and in the interstitium of the dermis. Systemic mast cell disease is almost always present if the patient has a diffuse erythroderma as a result of mast cell infiltration. In such cases, the bone marrow often has fusiform collections of mast cells adjacent to bony trabeculae, and such collections are associated with bone resorption.

Inflammatory, metabolic, and traumatic disorders

Perivascular infiltrates

Urticaria. Urticaria is a dermal vascular reaction that characteristically is transient and produces smooth-surfaced, edematous, erythematous macules to plaques that are pruritic. The edema and vascular congestion in an individual lesion slowly resolve after several hours and rarely persist more than 12 to 24 hours. When there is massive or deep edema of the subcutis also, the term *angioedema* is used. Urticaria is divided into acute and chronic forms. The causes are diverse and are physical agents, exogenous urticariogenic chemicals, and immune reactions, including complement-mediated and complement-independent forms and both IgE-dependent and IgE-independent forms. Frequent causes of immunologically mediated urticaria are inhalants, ingestants, injected material, infections, contactants, and medications. The cause in most chronic cases remains unknown, since "chronic idiopathic urticaria" is the diagnosis of 80% to 90% of patients with urticaria lasting more than 6 weeks.[236]

PATHOLOGY. Acute urticaria, such as physical urticaria from mechanical or thermal stimuli, shows varying degrees of perivascular edema in the papillary and reticular dermis. There is widening of the perivascular spaces and the distances between collagen bundles and cells in the area, with partial mast cell degranulation and without much inflammatory infiltration. The more complex forms of urticaria, secondary to complement activation or immune mechanisms, produce mast cell degranulation that can be partial or complete in Giemsa stains. Infiltration by eosinophils and neutrophils can be prominent. Chronic idiopathic urticaria often has more perivascular infiltration of lymphocytes and eosinophils as well as a few neutrophils, along with perivascular and papillary dermal edema.

Immunofluorescent staining in acute urticaria shows fibrin (or fibrinogen leakage) around blood vessels in the affected area, without deposition of immunoglobulins or complement. Chronic urticaria often has deposition of small amounts of complement in the blood vessel walls and perivascular fibrin.

Urticarial vasculitis. Patients with transient lesions that resemble urticaria but have persistance of individual lesions for slightly more than 24 hours can have urticarial vasculitis.[237,238] When initially introduced, this term included disorders with severe necrotizing vasculitis with either neutrophilic or lymphocytic infiltrates. Gradually the name has become applied to milder forms of vasculitis, with prolonged but transient lesions, without the clinical appearance of a hemorrhagic and necrotizing leukocytoclastic vasculitis.[239]

PATHOLOGY. Biopsy specimens of urticarial vasculitis contain a minimal neutrophilic infiltrate in the walls of venules usually near the superficial vascular plexus. Small amounts of fibrin are present in the vessel walls, and the neutrophils undergo karyorrhexis to form nuclear fragments ("nuclear dust"). Hemorrhage is minimal. Endothelial cells are swollen but are not necrotic. Consequently, urticarial vasculitis corresponds to a mild form of leukocytoclastic vasculitis. The mildest forms of this reaction have very little karyorrhexis and have been called "neutrophilic urticaria," which seems to correspond to the histologic characteristics of the so-called toxic erythema seen, for example, in juvenile rheumatoid arthritis, and other collagen-vascular diseases. The histologic pattern of neutrophilic urticaria has been reproduced by injections of the patient's own serum into the skin, an indication of a possible role for blood coagulation factors and nonimmune complement activation. Immunofluorescence studies of urticarial vasculitis generally show fibrin and small amounts of granular complement and IgM or IgG in the walls of affected vessels.

Leukocytoclastic vasculitis. Leukocytoclastic vasculitis is a hypersensitivity, type III, immune-mediated vasculitis that occurs in serum sickness, essential mixed cryoglobulinemia, reactions to medications, lupus erythematosus, and other diseases with circulating immune complexes. Erythema elevatum diutinum and granuloma faciale are peculiar localized, chronic forms of leukocytoclastic vasculitis.[240] Septicemia can produce a "septic vasculitis" that is a necrotizing, neutrophilic vasculitis with thrombi in the lumen of the vessels. IgA-mediated leukocytoclastic vasculitis is the basis of Schönlein-Henoch purpura. The lesions of leukocytoclastic vasculitis present as papules to nodules with hemorrhage or deep persistent erythema[241] (Fig. 71-143). Necrosis of the epidermis and ulceration can occur. The lesions are most common on the dependent portions of the body, such as the lower legs of ambulatory patients. This type of vasculitis is most commonly attributable to circulating immune complexes that elicit a type III immune reaction initially in the walls of postcapillary venules. Severe reactions can affect a greater variety of types of vessels. Hypocomplementemia can occur.

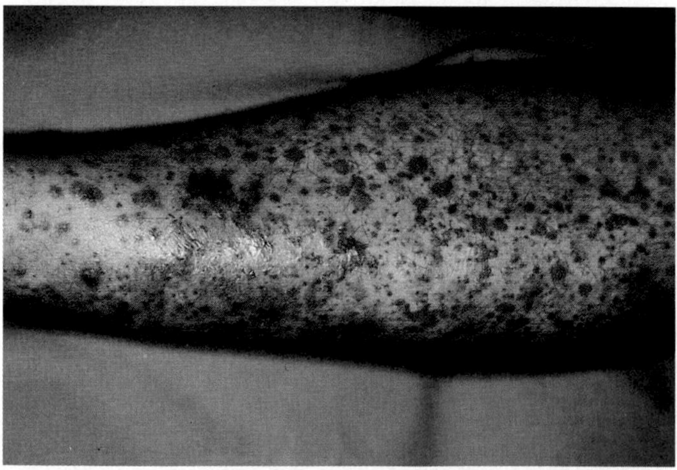

Fig. 71-143 Leukocytoclastic vasculitis. Focal regions of superficial venulitis produce small punctate hemorrhages that can become confluent and necrotic.

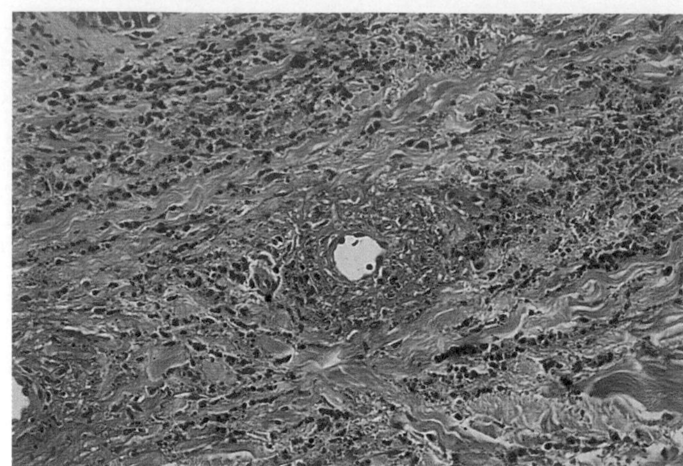

Fig. 71-144 Leukocytoclastic vasculitis. Thin-walled postcapillary venules often are surrounded by fibrin-containing neutrophils and fragments of neutrophil nuclei. Hemorrhage is common but is variable in extent.

PATHOLOGY. Histologic features that define this entity are neutrophils and their nuclear fragments in association with blood vessel walls that contain fibrin and have endothelial swelling or necrosis, and have extravasation of erythrocytes (Fig. 71-144). In histologic sections, the necrosis of the vessels often obliterates their architecture. When this process affects thick-walled blood vessels, particularly arteries, the disease is named *polyarteritis nodosa*, which can exist in a skin-limited phase for months to years or can be a systemic disease with skin involvement.[242] Immunofluorescence studies reveal deposition of immune complexes in the blood vessel walls in biopsy specimens taken during the first few days of the lesion. The pattern most frequently encountered is deposition of fibrin and complement along with IgM, IgG, or IgA, in descending order. When there are many thrombi in the small vessels, a search for organisms can reveal infection in cases of septic vasculitis (Fig. 71-145).

Delayed-hypersensitivity reaction. Patients with a type IV, or delayed hypersensitivity reaction, present with irregular erythematous plaques in a distribution similar to urticaria (Fig. 71-146) but with persistance of individual lesions for more than 24 to 48 hours and more palpable induration. Causes include a variety of circulating antigens, including medications, foodstuffs, chemicals, and infectious agents. The lesions are multiple, with a propensity to involve the trunk and proximal extremities, but some patients have relatively few lesions, and the face and other acral sites can also be involved. In the past it has been typical to classify this disorder as the dermal type of erythema multiforme;[1] however, the lack of epidermal necrosis separates the dermal type IV hypersensitivity reaction from erythema multiforme. Lesions having an annular shape with central pallor can occur in urticaria, in dermal hypersensitivity reactions, and in erythema multiforme, and in the latter condition they can go on to form a subepidermal blister with necrosis of the epidermis. Other names for the dermal hypersensitivity reaction are "urticarial allergic eruption"[243] and "urticarial or morbilliform drug eruptions."[244]

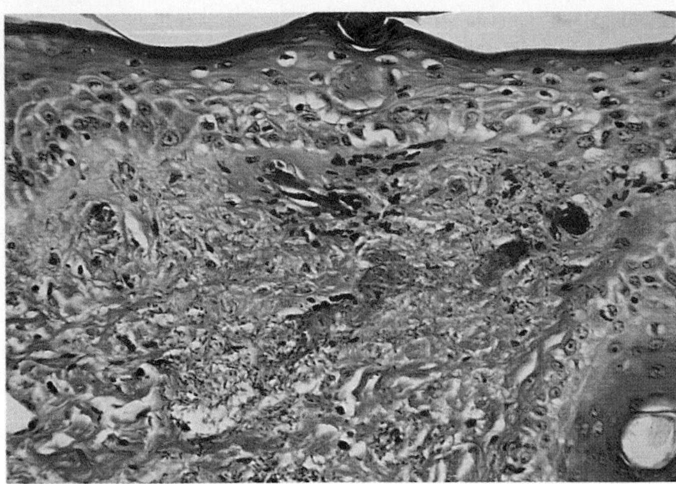

Fig. 71-145 Septic vasculitis. The focal hemorrhages with necrosis and many thrombi in the vessel lumens is due to *Candida albicans sepsis.*

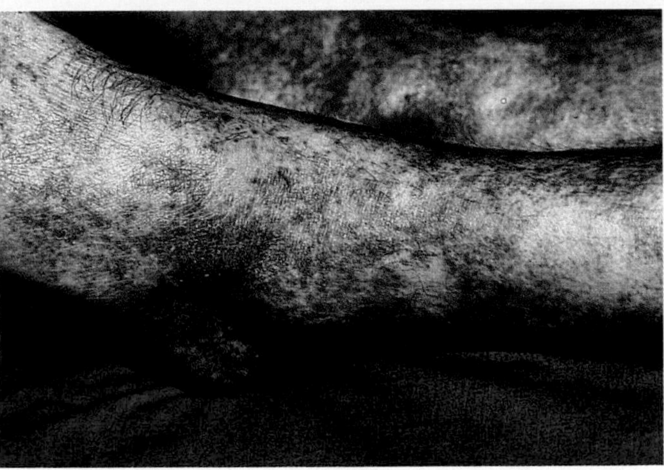

Fig. 71-147 Pigmented purpura, Schamberg' disease type. There are hemorrhagic papules bilaterally on the lower extremities with extensive brown hemosiderin pigmentation in the surrounding skin. This must be differentiated from stasis dermatitis.

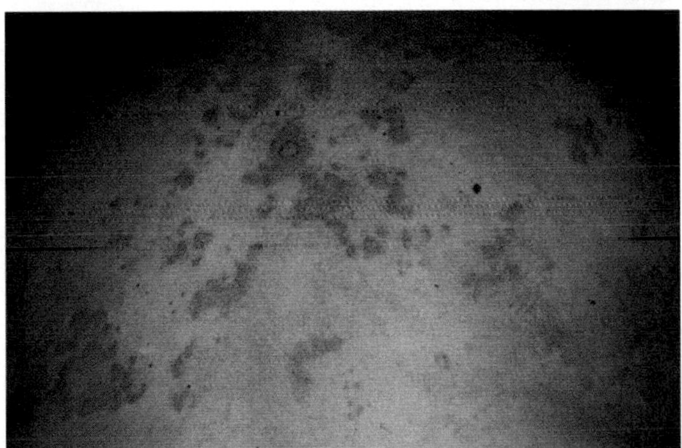

Fig. 71-146 Delayed hypersensitivity reaction. Irregular regions of erythema and edema are present, but they lack the focal hemorrhages of leukocytoclastic vasculitis (compare that in Fig. 71-143).

PATHOLOGY. The lesion is characterized by an infiltrate of lymphocytes, eosinophils, and occasional neutrophils around vessels to produce the patterns either of superficial or superficial and deep perivascular inflammation. Endothelial cells often are swollen. However, vascular wall necrosis and necrosis of keratinocytes are not found. Slight extravasation of erythrocytes is present in some patients, particularly in biopsy specimens from lower extremity lesions. Plasma cells can be present but are in small numbers.

Immunofluorescence findings include deposits of fibrin or fibrinogen around the blood vessels. There are no immunoglobulin deposits, and only trace amounts of granular complement are occasionally found in walls of small dermal vessels. In patients with slight spongiosis of the epidermis, trace amounts of granular complement can be found at the dermoepidermal junction without immunoglobulin.

Lymphocytic vasculitis. Clinically, acute lymphocytic vasculitis resembles leukocytoclastic vasculitis, with some exceptions. The lesions can be slower in their development with more epidermal reaction. Several diseases with lymphocytic vasculitis have been considered previously, such as pityriasis lichenoides (Fig. 71-77), acute graft-versus-host disease, secondary syphilis, lymphomatoid papulosis, lymphomatoid granulomatosis, and midline facial granuloma, as well as angiocentric and angiodestructive T-cell lymphoma (Fig. 71-134). In addition, Rocky Mountain spotted fever (tick borne) and rickettsialpox (rodent mite borne) are two diseases in which an angiodestructive lymphocytic infiltrate is present in reaction to infection of endothelial cells by *Rickettsia rickettsii* or *Rickettsia akari,* respectively. Another form of lymphocytic vasculitis is produced by exposure of skin to damp cold conditions so that erythematous nodules are produced in *pernio* (chilblains), which usually affects the hands and feet.

PATHOLOGY. The lesions are characterized by lymphoid infiltrates in the blood vessel walls associated with vascular necrosis and thrombosis.[241] Extravasation of erythrocytes is common. Macrophages also are involved in the destructive process. In pernio, there is a superficial and deep perivascular infiltrate with many lymphocytes in blood vessel walls. Blisters and necrotic ulcers develop because of vascular occlusion.

Several diseases need to be discussed here, since they are *not* examples of lymphocytic vasculitis but are commonly mistaken for it clinically or histologically. *Pigmented purpuric eruptions* are hemorrhagic diseases (Fig. 71-147) of unknown cause that often do not have any epidermal manifestations and seem restricted to the dermis. The blood vessels of the superficial vascular plexus are not necrotic and have only slight endothelial swelling, but extravasation of erythrocytes is prominent in the areas of lymphocytic infiltration (Fig. 71-148). Hemosiderin in present in lesions more than 48 hours old. There is no evidence of a disorder of blood coagulation. Various clinical forms include *Schamberg's disease* (usually bilaterally on the lower extremities) (Fig. 71-147), the *Gougerot-Blum* form (also affects the upper trunk and has more lichenoid lymphocytic infiltrate near the epidermis), and *lichen aureus* (a few large lesions usually on the lower extremities). Some patients were reported previously to have a lymphocytic vasculitis as the basis for "urticarial vasculitis," but

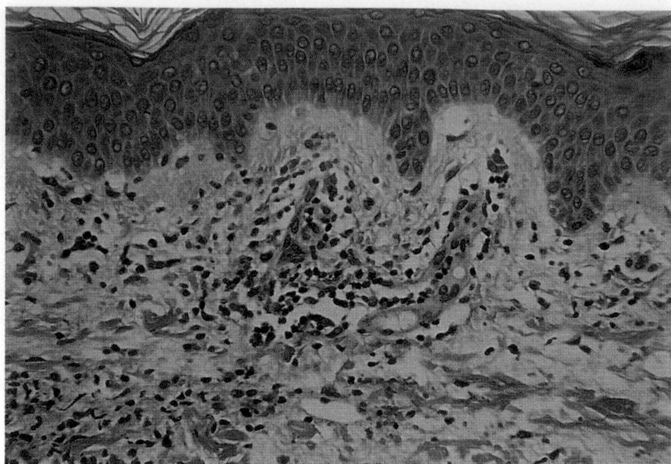

Fig. 71-148 Pigmented purpura, Schamberg's disease type. Extravasated erythrocytes and lymphocytes are around the superficial dermal vessels, but there is no vascular necrosis.

this interpretation is diminishing with better definitions separating ordinary, nonnecrotizing, type IV dermal hypersensitivity reactions from true necrotizing lymphocytic vasculitis. Livedoid vasculitis also has been reported to be a lymphocytic vasculitis but is better regarded as an obliterative vasculitis.[241] Leukocytoclastic vasculitis begins as a neutrophilic vasculitis, and as the lesions begin to resolve, they have more infiltration by lymphocytes and macrophages, and so late lesions can resemble a lymphocytic vasculitis. Residual neutrophil fragments in the cytoplasm of macrophages is a clue to the prior neutrophilic vasculitis, rather than a primary lymphocytic vasculitis.[241]

Obliterative vasculitis. In obliterative vasculitis, the vascular occlusive component of the lesion is much more prominent histologically than the inflammatory component.[241] Vascular occlusion can be attributable to fibrin, cholesterol emboli, red blood cells, cryoglobulins, or fibrous tissue. Patients with disorders in this group have a variety of clinical presentations depending on the underlying causes of the vascular obliterative reaction.

PATHOLOGY. The lesions are characterized by occlusion of the lumen of blood vessels often with a relatively sparse inflammatory infiltrate of lymphocytes and occasional neutrophils. Fibrin is the occlusive agent in the vascular lumen after thromboembolism or thrombotic thrombocytopenic purpura. Fibrin accumulation restricts the diameter of the lumen and thickens the wall of the vessels in *livedoid vasculitis*, which usually is secondary to hypercoagulability and vascular stasis. The lower extremities are the main sites of involvement. *Cholesterol emboli* are most common in the lower extremities secondary to atheromatous disease of the abdominal aorta and particularly after vascular surgery. Cholesterol emboli can also be in other locations.[245] The characteristic histologic feature is occlusion and distortion of the vascular lumen by needle-like clefts that remain after the cholesterol has been extracted by the routine processing. *Sickle-cell anemia* can occlude small blood vessels with sickled red blood cells and produce cutaneous infarction. Patients with myelomas that produce large amounts of cryoglobulins can have these proteins form occlusive precipitates in peripheral blood vessels. Fibrous tissue occlusion of the lumen of vessels results from organization of thrombi or can occur as a primary phenomenon in *Degos's disease* (malignant atrophic papulosis), a disease of unknown but possibly infectious cause.

Granulomatous infiltrates

Granulomatous vasculitis. Granulomatous vasculitis can have vascular as well as extravascular granulomas.[241] Clinical forms of granulomatous vasculitis include Wegener's granulomatosis, allergic granulomatosis (Churg-Strauss syndrome), lymphomatoid granulomatosis, secondary syphilis, temporal arteritis, and Takayasu's arteritis (giant cell arteritis). Rarely patients with acute sarcoidosis can have involvement of blood vessel walls with sarcoidal granulomas, along with uveoparotid fever and erythema nodosum. Necrobiosis lipoidica rarely can have a granulomatous vasculitis. Another disease that has granulomatous involvement of the small vessels of the skin is cheilitis granulomatosa (Melkersson-Rosenthal syndrome). The correct diagnosis depends on clinicopathologic correlation.

PATHOLOGY. Typical lesions consist of well-formed aggregates of macrophages that form granulomas in the walls of the vessels and the perivascular connective tissue. Eosinophils are abundant in allergic granulomatosis. Plasma cells are found in granulomatous secondary syphilis. Multinucleated giant cells with partially lysed elastic fibers are in temporal and Takayasu's arteritis. The lesions must be separated from angiocentric T-cell or B-cell lymphomas, which are distinguished by the presence of many atypical lymphocytes.

Sarcoidosis. Sarcoidosis is a multisystem granulomatous disease of unknown cause that involves the skin in 25% of cases. Cutaneous sarcoidosis presents with lesions commonly on the face, near the nose and eyes (Fig. 71-149), and on the trunk. The lesions have a variety of clinical appearances, including lichenoid papules, plaques, deep nodules, annular lesions with central atrophy, and infiltration of old scars. Approximately 20% of patients with systemic sarcoidosis develop erythema nodosum as a nonspecific manifestation of acute sarcoidosis but one that usually indicates a relatively good prognosis. Patients with an insidious onset of sarcoidosis, without erythema nodosum, have a worse prognosis.

PATHOLOGY. Sarcoidosis in the skin usually resembles that seen in lymph nodes and shows noncaseating granulomas that tend to remain discrete (Fig. 71-150). Distinctive features in the skin are the tendency to involve the papillary as well as the reticular dermis and subcutis. Granulomas in the papillary dermis abut on the overlying epidermis and often lead to hypopigmentation at that site probably by destruction of melanocytes. Although sarcoidosis generally has relatively few lymphocytes associated with the deep granulomas, those lesions near the body orifices can have a pronounced lymphocytic infiltrate often with plasma cells as well. For the final diagnosis, one should exclude mycobacterial, fungal, and bacterial infections. The tissue should be examined under polarized light to detect foreign material. In selected cases, tissue may have to be analyzed chemically for beryllium or zirconium, which also can produce granulomas.

Granuloma annulare. Granuloma annulare refers to an annular arrangement of papules in the dermis (Fig. 71-151) that on biopsy have granulomatous features in that there is an aggregation of macrophages. The cause is unknown. Patients often have lesions on the hands and feet, and over joints, but

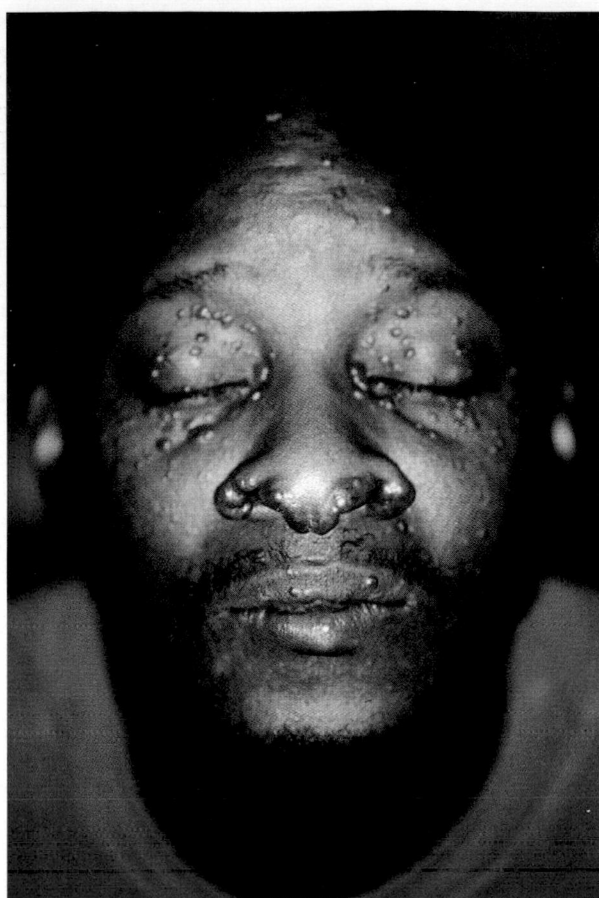

Fig. 71-149 Sarcoidosis. Destructive papules and nodules are present around the nose, mouth, and eyes.

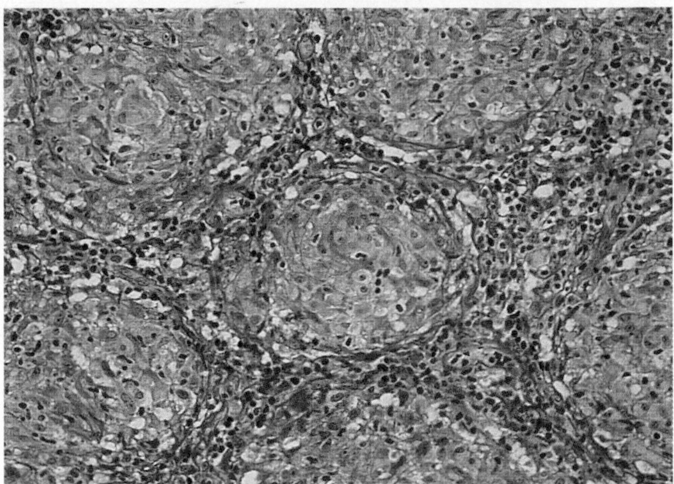

Fig. 71-150 Sarcoidosis. Discrete granulomas formed by enlarged macrophages ("epithelioid cells") without necrosis and with variable numbers of lymphocytes.

they can be generalized. Trauma, sun exposure, and diabetes have been suggested to predispose to granuloma annulare. The disease usually persists for 1 to 2 years, and lesions often regress after biopsy or freezing of lesions.

PATHOLOGY. Granuloma annulare is characterized by a focal dermal infiltrate of macrophages in between and around collagen bundles (Fig. 71-152). The centers of lesions contain abundant "dermal mucin" (hyaluronic acid). Smaller amounts of fibrin are present in the centers of lesions also and coat the surface of collagen bundles. The dermal involvement is characteristically focal and usually superficial. Both nonpalisaded and palisaded granulomas occur, the latter resembling a rheumatoid nodule when in the deep dermis and subcutis. These pseudorheumatoid nodules contain abundant hyaluronic acid, which is useful in their recognition as granuloma annulare. Resolution of granuloma annulare generally does not leave residual depressed scars. Multinucleated giant cells are few, and intimal proliferation in blood vessels is not part of this disease.

Necrobiosis lipoidica. The disease necrobiosis lipoidica diabeticorum (NLD) is known as such because of its association with diabetes mellitus in at least half of the cases and up to two thirds if blood chemical evidence of prediabetes is included.[246,247] Either the remaining patients may develop diabetes later, or they may have a lesion that histologically mimics NLD, such as Miescher's granulomatosis disciformis,

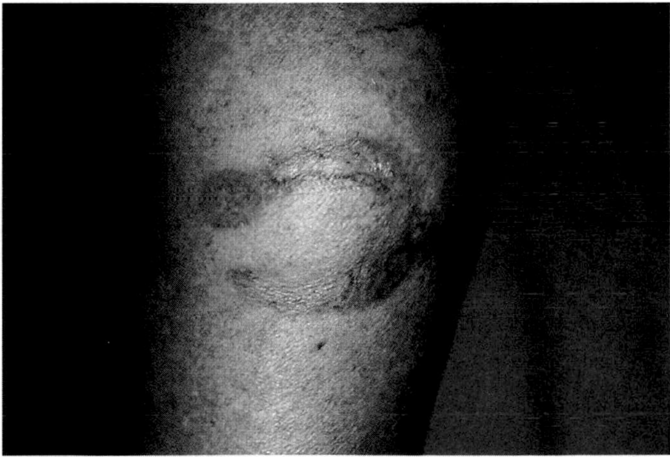

Fig. 71-151 Granuloma annulare. Dermal papules may form annular configurations or be isolated papules or plaques. The extremities are favored sites.

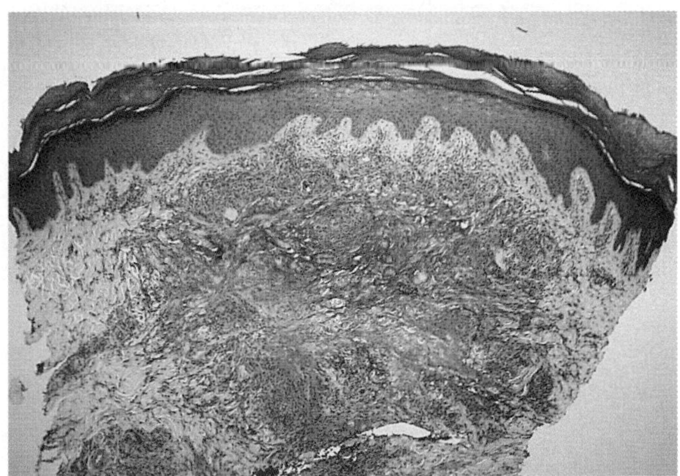

Fig. 71-152 Granuloma annulare. Focal areas of dermal mucin and fibrin deposition are surrounded by macrophages between collagen bundles.

which occurs on the lower extremities or elsewhere, including on the face. The lesions are infiltrated plaques which are irregular in outline and are sharply demarcated (Fig. 71-153). The earliest changes are those of erythema, and later the centers of the lesions develop atrophy with telangiectasia, a yellow-brown color, and induration. The lesions have a predilection to occur on the shins but also elsewhere especially calves, distal upper extremity, face, and scalp.

PATHOLOGY. The lesions show two types of histologic appearances. The *necrobiotic type* has extensive and rather diffuse necrosis of the superficial and deep dermis (Fig. 71-154). Blood vessels often have thickened sclerotic walls (Fig. 71-155), which are not found in granuloma annulare. Diabetic vasculopathy and the necrobiosis lipoidica itself seem responsible. Scattered macrophages, multinucleated giant cells, and plasma cells lie between sclerotic collagen bundles (Fig. 71-156). Lipid deposits such as cholesterol crystals and foamy macrophages are abundant if the biopsy is from the center of a well-developed lesion. The *granulomatous type* has more well-demarcated granulomas and giant cells along with sclerosis but not extensive necrosis. This second form resembles sarcoidosis and Miescher's granulomatosis disciformis.

Biopsy specimens from the centers of well-developed lesions on the lower extremities are not recommended, since the wounds heal very slowly. The differential diagnosis includes Miescher's granulomatosis disciformis, annular elastolytic granuloma, sarcoidosis, necrobiotic xanthogranuloma with paraproteinemia, and mycobacterial infection.

Xanthomas. *Xanthoma* is a term applied to nodules composed of macrophages containing abundant lipid. Xanthomas occur in various metabolic disorders and can also be neoplasms. Hyperlipoproteinemias often are associated with certain of these xanthomatous infiltrates. Hypertriglyceridemia is associated with eruptive xanthomas, which are soft yellow papules that occur at sites of pressure, such as the buttocks and posterior area of the thighs. Increased low density lipoproteins (LDL, beta-lipoproteins) are associated with tuberous xanthomas, which present clinically as nodules or plaques on the buttocks, knees, elbows, and fingers and also with tendon xanthomas. Dystrophic xanthomatosis occurs in the skin after

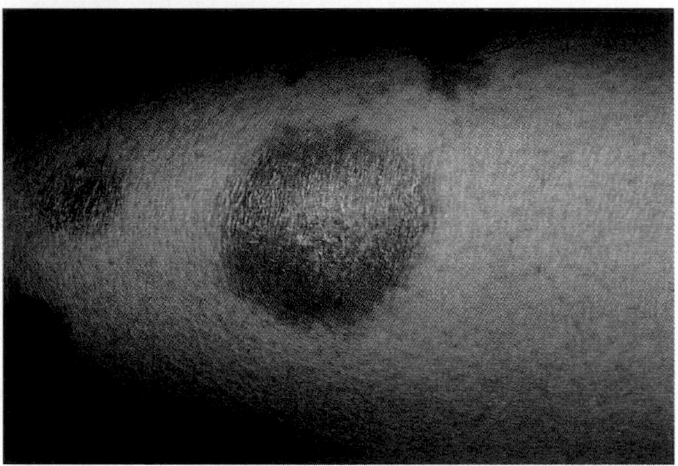

Fig. 71-153 Necrobiosis lipoidica. Irregular erythematous plaques are often on the shins.

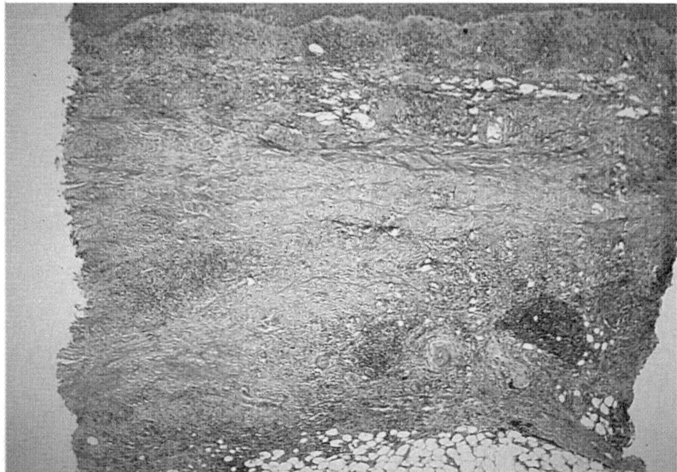

Fig. 71-154 Necrobiosis lipoidica. Broad zones of dermal fibrosis are present with surrounding infiltration by macrophages and multinucleated giant cells.

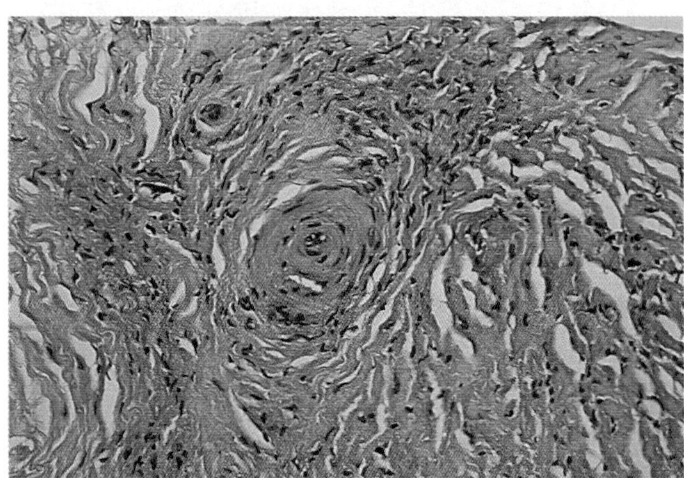

Fig. 71-155 Necrobiosis lipoidica. Sclerosis of small blood vessels is common and helps distinguish this disease from granuloma annulare.

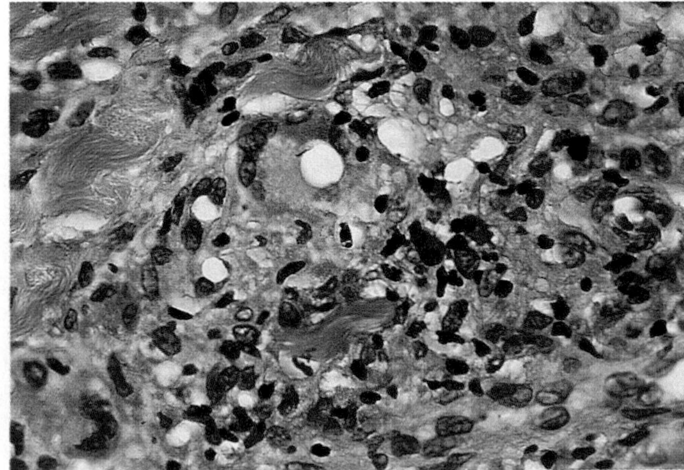

Fig. 71-156 Necrobiosis lipoidica. Lipid deposition with multinucleated giant cells and plasma cells are common.

severe inflammation, blistering diseases, mycosis fungoides, or burns and is associated either with hyperlipidemia or normal blood lipid levels. Xanthelasma are yellowish papules to plaques on the eyelids that are associated with hypertriglyceridemia or hypercholesterolemia in approximately 50% of patients. It is important to distinguish these diseases from necrobiotic xanthogranuloma, which is associated with an IgG monoclonal paraprotein and occasionally with myeloma. This disease often has periorbital plaques, which can undergo ulceration and can perforate the sclera. Lesions may also occur elsewhere, as on the trunk. There are numerous rare lipid disorders that are associated with xanthomatous infiltrates, such as Tangier's disease, Farber's disease, Niemann-Pick disease, and Gaucher's disease.

PATHOLOGY. The biopsy specimens show an accumulation of macrophages with many small fat droplets filling the cytoplasm. In *xanthelasma,* the lesions lack any fibrosis and have very little admixture of inflammatory cells. The cell accumulations are both perivascular and interstitial in the reticular dermis. Multinucleated giant cells are rare. In contrast, in *eruptive xanthomas,* the lesions have fatty macrophages with a mixture of lymphocytes and occasionally neutrophils as well, usually in a perivascular location. *Tuberous xanthomas* have more massive nodular accumulations of fatty macrophages, with fibrosis and breakdown of the cells to leave cholesterol deposits with needle-like clefts in the fibrous tissue. *Necrobiotic xanthogranuloma* differs in having extensive vertically oriented zones of hyaline necrosis of the fat, with the massive accumulations of xanthoma cells. Multinucleated giant cells with peripheral lipidization (Touton giant cells) are abundant.

Various accumulations

A variety of metabolic diseases or disturbances can result in accumulations of material abnormally in the dermis. The patients present clinically with thickening and induration of the skin.

PATHOLOGY. Examples include *solar elastosis*, which is secondary to excessive sunlight or radiation exposure that results in the excess deposition of degenerated and fragmented elastic material in the papillary and upper reticular dermis.

Amyloidosis can present as hemorrhagic papules in the skin as a result of increased vascular fragility caused by perivascular amyloid deposits in patients with systemic amyloidosis. Localized, skin-limited amyloidosis can show amyloid accumulations in the papillary dermis that arise from excessive keratinocyte necrosis and conversion of keratin proteins to amyloid. This type of amyloidosis occurs after excessive heat or rubbing of the skin in susceptible patients.

Calcification in the skin can be associated with the vascular walls, particularly when it is a result of hypercalcemia (metastatic calcification), but it can also be diffuse in the dermis. Calcification diffusely in the dermis or in scars can also be secondary to trauma in the presence of normal calcium levels (dystrophic calcification). The calcification can progress to ossification.

Mucin deposition in the dermis is attributable to excessive accumulation of hyaluronic acid between collagen bundles. This mucin can be very focal and an incidental degenerative finding or else reflect an underlying systemic disorder. Pretibial mucinosis is associated with hyperthyroidism. Diffuse mucinosis is found in myxedema. Both of these have very little inflammation. More inflammation is associated with the mucinosis in lupus erythematosus. In papular mucinosis (lichen myxedematosus, or scleromyxedema), there is increased mucin and an increase in fibroblastic spindle cells in the mucinous papules. The latter patients have an eruption of many small papules that often are located on the upper back, face, and arms and are associated with a polyclonal IgG paraprotein. In scleredema, there is increased dermal mucin with thickening of the amount of dermal collagen as well but very little increase in fibroblastic cells or inflammatory infiltration. Scleredema may follow an upper respiratory tract infection or may be part of the skin changes of diabetes mellitus. Myxoid degeneration of tumors such as neurofibromas is in the differential diagnosis of solitary myxoid lesions.

Fibrotic disorders

Scleroderma and *morphea* are diseases of unknown cause that present with deep induration of the skin and varied degrees of hyperpigmentation, hypopigmentation, or erythema of the skin surface. When the disease forms a localized plaque with a rim of deep erythema (violaceous ring), the disease has been called "morphea" (Fig. 71-157). In patients with systemic sclerosis there can be localized lesions of morphea, disseminated lesions of morphea, or distinctive diffuse sclerosis of the skin, often affecting the acral parts of the body (Fig. 71-158), including the nose and circumoral region of the face to produce tight, nonsmiling facies with an atrophic, beaked nose. Certain patients present with disease that resembles scleroderma or morphea in some respects but have distinctive clinical or pathologic aspects. For example, *atrophoderma of Pasini and Pierini* has circumscribed areas of atrophy with loss of dermal collagen and later can develop typical lesions of morphea. *Eosinophilic fasciitis* (Schulman's syndrome) is a symmetrical acral sclerosis which often appears after strenuous exercise or is related to ingestion of impure preparations of L-tryptophan. The panniculus and fascia are involved as well as the dermis. There is often a peripheral blood eosinophilia. Eosinophilic fasciitis responds to steroid treatment more than ordinary scleroderma.

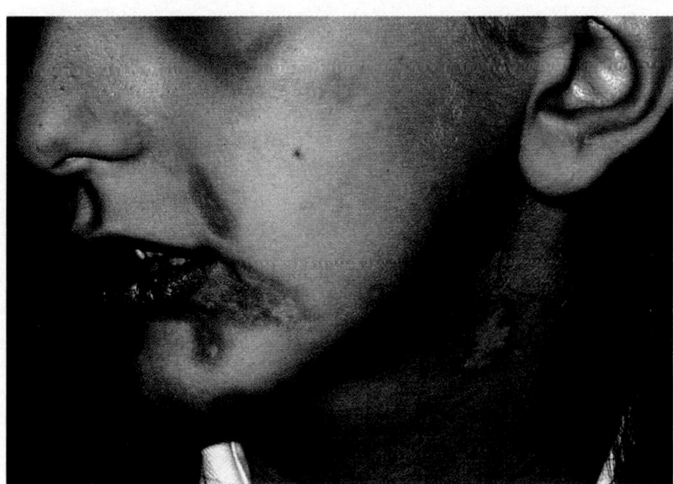

Fig. 71-157 Morphea. Sclerotic plaques with violaceous borders are characteristic lesions, here affecting the lower lip, cheek, and neck.

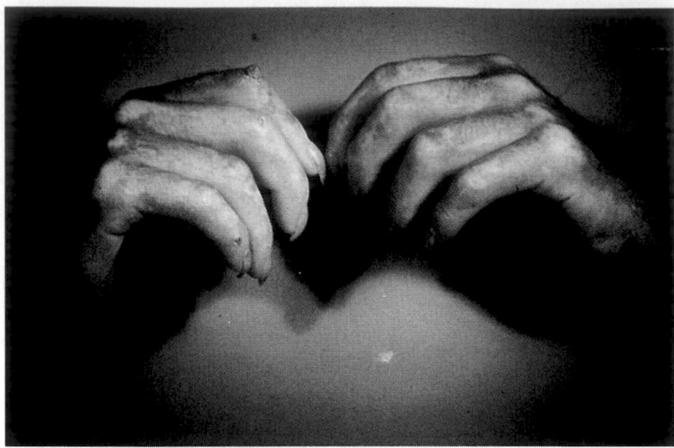

Fig. 71-158 Scleroderma, acral sclerosis. The hands have become immobilized by sclerosis. The excrescences are perforations because of calcifications.

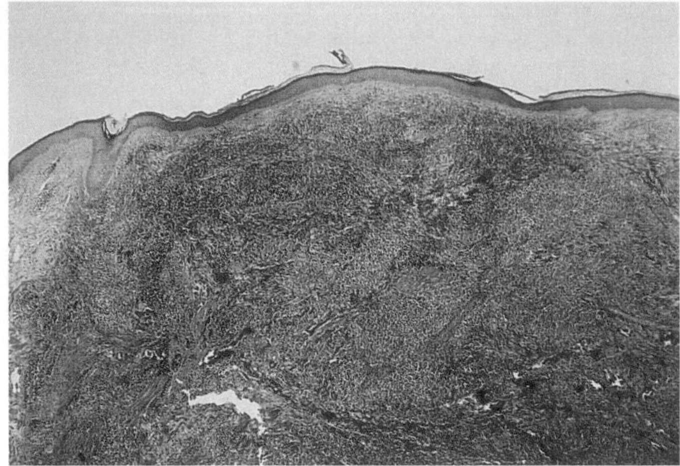

Fig. 71-160 Lymphocytoma cutis. A diffuse nodular infiltrate of lymphocytes is the most common histologic pattern.

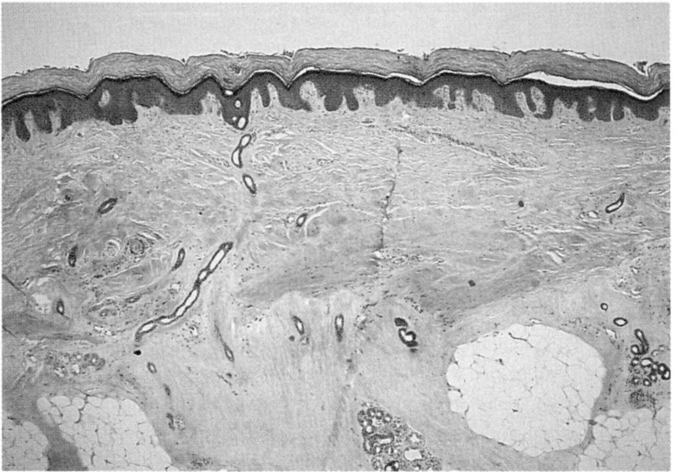

Fig. 71-159 Scleroderma. Thickened collagen bundles in a relatively acellular deep dermis are distinctive.

PATHOLOGY. The lesions show an evolution from inflammatory to densely sclerotic lesions, with the most characteristic lesions being those that have almost acellular, avascular, hyalinized, sclerotic collagenous connective tissue (Fig. 71-159). The deep dermis is affected preferentially. Late lesions often have very little lymphocytic infiltration. In contrast, the earlier inflammatory stages of morphea or scleroderma have a superficial and deep perivascular lymphocytic infiltrate with very few if any eosinophils. Plasma cells often are in the deep portions of the lesions and can be found in the lymphocytic infiltrate at the junction of the deep reticular dermis and subcutis. Eosinophilic fasciitis has mucin deposition in the dermis, with or without eosinophils in the dermal infiltrate. In each of these disorders, lymphocytes infiltrate between dermal collagen bundles that focally are thickened and fused because of the filling of the interspaces between the bundles with small collagen fibers. The vascularity is decreased. Atrophoderma of Pasini and Pierini appears very similar to early inflammatory lesions of morphea, but the degree of sclerosis is slight. The lymphocytic infiltrates consist mostly of helper T-lymphocytes,[248] but in contrast to CTCL, the lymphocytes in these sclerotic disorders do not show cytologic atypia.

Lymphoid infiltrates

Lymphocytoma cutis. Lymphocytoma cutis, also known as "pseudolymphoma," or "lymphadenosis benigna cutis," is a benign nodular lesion formed by a dense accumulation of lymphocytes. The patients present with a dermal to subcutaneous nodule having a smooth epidermal surface, without ulceration. The lesions are firm and indurated but are well-circumscribed and movable lesions. They are erythematous to violaceous in color and are usually tender, solitary, and on the trunk, proximal extremities, and head and neck. Itching is variable. Although the lesions commonly are considered to be benign neoplasms, in some of these patients there is evidence of response to antibiotic therapy and of *Borrelia* organisms in the lesions.

PATHOLOGY. The most common histologic patterns are a superficial and deep perivascular lymphocytic infiltrate and a nodular diffuse infiltrate (Fig. 71-160). Both of these patterns can occur after arthropod bites, depending on the intensity of the immune reaction and on the exact level of sectioning with regard to the center of the lesion. The perivascular pattern is in the milder reactions and is at the periphery of the nodular pattern. The infiltrate usually is a mixed one, with lymphocytes, macrophages, and a variable number of eosinophils and plasma cells but occasionally is almost monomorphous (Fig. 71-161). Often, some of the lymphocytes are enlarged and resemble germinal center or follicular center cells. Well-demarcated follicular centers are formed in the nodular regions of the infiltrate. The perivascular infiltrates can have loose clusters of follicular center cells along the adventitial dermis of the blood vessels, which require special immunostains to visualize. At times, the follicular center pattern is irregular, and the infiltrate is rather purely lymphocytic. Such lesions are suspicious for lymphoma of the follicular type even when the cytologic features of the lymphocytes are not atypical. Special techniques are needed to rule out lymphoma.

On immunostaining, the main cells in the germinal centers are B-cells and the surrounding cells are T-cells. The T-cell infiltrate can predominate, and indeed in lymphocytic infiltra-

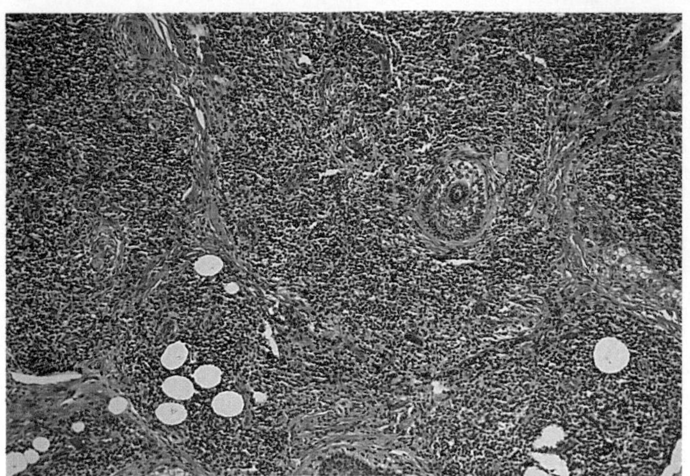

Fig. 71-161 Lymphocytoma cutis. Cytologic atypism of lymphocytes is rare. The infiltrate can be relatively monomorphous with few eosinophils or plasma cells.

tion of Jessner the perivascular infiltrate is entirely composed of T-cells. In our view, lymphocytic infiltration of Jessner is a diagnosis of exclusion and should not contain abundant eosinophils or immune deposits. Mucin can be present in the dermis in the areas of Jessner's infiltration. When the lesion contains many eosinophils, Jessner's infiltration is only a localized or an "erythema perstans" type of dermal hypersensitivity reaction, type IV. When immune deposits are present at the dermoepidermal junction, these patients usually have lupus erythematosus and not lymphocytic infiltration of Jessner.

The pattern of T-cell zones surrounding B-cell zones is similar to that found in the normal lymph node as well as in some follicular lymphomas. Cutaneous B-cell lymphomas are usually monoclonal with regard to kappa and lambda light chains but can coexpress certain B-cell and T-cell antigens, such as those reactive with the monoclonal antibodies L26 (CD20) and Leu-22 (CD43), for example. T-cell lymphomas often have an abnormal phenotype because of deletions of certain pan–T-cell antigens. The lesions of lymphocytoma cutis do not have such abnormalities initially, but a few cases have been found to undergo a slow progressive evolution to a primary cutaneous lymphoma.[249] Consequently, follow-up study with sequential biopsy specimens of persistent lesions is very important. Recently, the *bcl*-2 gene has been shown to suppress apoptosis and to be activated in the follicular centers of some B-cell lymphomas but not in benign lymphocytoma cutis.

Alopecia areata. Alopecia areata is an immunologically mediated disease characterized by circumscribed regions of acute hair loss without surface scale or erythema. Hair loss in a few areas of the crown has a better prognosis than hair loss in the ophiasis pattern, that is, around the lower edge of the scalp. Related conditions are alopecia totalis that involves the whole scalp and alopecia universalis in which there is hair loss over the entire body surface. Occasionally the patients have dysesthesia in an area of incipient hair loss, and a biopsy specimen in that location will show the most characteristic changes. The hair follicles are not destroyed initially but go into a long telogen phase and on occasion are stimulated to grow again. The greater the degree of initial hair loss, the less likely is regrowth. The cause is unknown, but alopecia areata has been reported to be associated with Hashimoto's thyroiditis, vitiligo, pernicious anemia with autoimmune gastritis, and Addison's disease.

PATHOLOGY. The skin contains lymphocytic infiltrates mainly in the deep dermis and concentrated around the follicular sheath at the base of the hair apparatus. Eosinophils and plasma cells are absent. The blood vessels in the deep dermis near the hair follicles have a perivascular lymphocytic infiltrate also. The lymphocytes penetrate into the follicular epithelium of the hair bulbs, but necrosis of the keratinocytes is very limited. Instead, the follicles are triggered to go into a phase of regression resembling catagen but with less glassy membrane, more irregularity in the outline of the follicle epithelium, and individual apoptotic cells above the hair bulb. The lymphocytes are a mixture of CD4-positive helper T-cell and CD8-positive suppressor T-cells. Routine immunofluorescence studies do not show a deposition of immunoglobulins.

Light eruptions. The term *light eruption* refers to a group of inflammatory reactions of the skin to light that cause disease because an erythematous response is triggered by an antigen that is produced in the skin even when it is exposed to low doses of light, usually UVB, but also UVA, and rarely even visible light. Consequently, in areas of sun exposure, the patients develop irregular erythematous macules, papules, and plaques. Blisters can form. Initially the lesions appear only in sun-exposed areas, and the wavelengths of UVB that trigger the lesions are in a narrow range. With progression of persistent light reaction, the wavelengths broaden to include UVA and can even extend into the visible range. *Polymorphous light reaction* is considered to be a type IV delayed hypersensitivity reaction to an unknown component of skin that is modified or produced by the skin in the presence of light. In patients, who are considered "persistent light reactors," this disease can become debilitating with a burning sensation on exposure, thickening and fissuring of the exposed skin, and therapeutic unresposiveness unless the eliciting wavelengths are blocked. In some persistent light reactors there is an exogenous or endogenous chemical to which the skin is exposed that, even in minute quantities, can trigger an allergic reaction on exposure to light. Examples of substances that are photosensitizing compounds include medications (thiazides, chlorpromazine, tetracyclines) and porphyrins, furocoumarins (psoralens), and chromates.

PATHOLOGY. The skin biopsy specimen has varying degrees of change depending on the course and the nature and number of previous reactions. In the most acute form, *solar urticaria*, there is an intense urticarial reaction of the skin within the first 10 to 15 minutes of sun exposure with diminution of the reaction in 1 to 2 hours. There is only perivascular edema with a very sparse cellular infiltrate within this time course.

The subacute form, *polymorphous light reaction,* has lesions that develop within hours to days after exposure to light. There is a superficial and deep perivascular lymphocytic infiltrate in well-developed lesions and a superficial infiltrate in the earliest ones. The papillary dermis and perivascular spaces have edema, endothelial swelling, and occasionally extravasation of erythrocytes. Necrosis of keratinocytes is not prominent. A few eosinophils may be present, particularly in a photoallergic reaction to a medication.

With repeated episodes of polymorphous light reaction, the papillary dermis becomes thickened and fibrotic; rubbing of the lesions by the patient may accentuate these changes as well as acanthosis. In such lesions, there is a minimal superficial perivascular lymphocytic infiltrate during the times between acute reactions. A papulovesicular form of polymorphous light eruption has spongiosis in the epidermis and is peculiar in its predilection to involve the upper extremities and to spare the face.

The most severe, chronic form, *actinic reticuloid,* has significant thickening and fissuring of the skin. There is a dense lymphocytic infiltrate in the papillary and upper reticular dermis, with epidermal hyperplasia and fibrosis of the papillary dermis. The lymphocytes infiltrate into the epidermis and in some patients form a few small collections of cells in the base of the epidermis that resemble small Pautrier microabscesses. Cytologically atypical lymphocytes with hyperconvoluted nuclei can also be present but usually are few in number.

Immunologic characterization of the lymphocytes has been performed in the lesions of patients with "chronic actinic dermatitis," a category that represents a combination of patients with persistent light reactions attributable to photocontact allergy, repeated polymorphous light reactions, and actinic reticuloid. The lymphocytes are mainly CD8-positive cytotoxic suppressor T-cells. In severely affected patients, the CD4-to-CD8 ratio in the peripheral blood can be decreased and can resemble the values obtained with AIDS.[250] Patients with AIDS have been described with actinic reticuloid.[251] Blood smears also may contain atypical cells.[108,252] These lesions must be differentiated from the lesions of lupus erythematosus, which also can present with profound photosensitivity of the skin, and a superficial and deep perivascular lymphocytic infiltrate. The lesions of lupus have immune complexes at the dermoepidermal junction and have more epidermal atrophy and necrosis of keratinocytes than the lesions of polymorphous light eruption. Mucin is also more abundant in the dermis in lupus. Other lesions in the differential diagnosis include Jessner's lymphocytic infiltrate of the skin and cutaneous T-cell lymphoma of the CD8-positive type.

Infectious diseases

Many of the infectious diseases that affect mainly the dermis resemble those that occur in other organs as well and are described in other parts of this textbook. We emphasize here some of those with very distinctive skin manifestations.

Borrelia *infection*

Lyme disease is a tick-borne zoonosis caused by *Borrelia burgdorferi*. In 90% of the humans that become infected, a characteristic skin lesion develops at the site of the tick bite and consists of erythema with slight elevation and induration. The lesions initially are uniform in color but develop central clearing as they enlarge. The ringlike lesion can enlarge to 52 cm in diameter.[253] It may last from 3 days to 1½ years and is named *erythema chronicum migrans*. In Europe, *Borrelia* spirochetes are responsible also for *acrodermatitis chronica atrophicans,* an erythematous lesion that persists for many months and causes severe dermal atrophy. Especially in Europe, *Borrelia*-like organisms have also been implicated in other skin diseases, such as localized morphea, lichen sclerosus et atrophicus, and lymphocytoma cutis.

PATHOLOGY. The lesions of erythema chronicum migrans have a superficial and deep perivascular lymphocytic infiltrate. Plasma cells are found in 50% of biopsy specimens of the erythematous ring. Endothelial cells are swollen. Eosinophils are not prominent. Secondary lesions of erythema migrans can have spongiosis in the epidermis also. Lesions of acrodermatitis chronica atrophicans have a thin and flattened epidermis overlying severe thinning of the dermis because of loss of collagen and elastin as well as dermal appendages.

There is less thickening of individual collagen bundles in erythema chronicum migrans than in morphea and there is not the edematous collagen in the papillary dermis that is so characteristic of lichen sclerosus et atrophicus. In sections, the *Borrelia* spirochete itself has a more variable size and shape than the more familiar *Treponema pallidum spirochete*.[115] In tissue sections, the size of the organism is approximately 0.2 to 0.3 μm in width and 10 to 35 μm in length.[253]

Mycobacterial infection

Mycobacterial infections produce two types of skin lesions, that is, granulomas caused by direct infection of the skin and granulomatous lesions named *tuberculids,* which are delayed hypersensitivity (type IV) reactions to mycobacterial antigens. *Mycobacterium tuberculosis* is the most common pathogen. Primary inoculation into the skin occurs when skin with a broken permeability barrier comes into contact with blood or secretions containing viable mycobacteria. The skin also can be infected directly by extension of tuberculous abscesses from the lungs or bones into the subcutaneous tissues and dermis as well as by spread through the blood circulation, which produces miliary tuberculosis. In skin, there several distinctive tuberculids, such as *erythema induratum, papulonecrotic tuberculid, lupus miliaris disseminata faciei,* and *lichen scrofulosorum*.[254-256] Erythema induratum is discussed in the section on diseases of the subcutis.

PATHOLOGY. Tuberculosis of the skin forms noncaseating or caseating granulomas depending on the immune status of the host. The cellular composition of the granulomas in the skin resembles that in other organs. Papulonecrotic tuberculid is a form of necrotizing lymphocytic vasculitis that produces regions of epidermal and dermal necrosis without well-formed granulomas. In contrast, lupus miliaris disseminata faciei has necrotizing granulomas with caseous necrosis. Lichen scrofulosorum is distinctive in the perifollicular location of the granulomas without caseation. Intact bacilli are not identified by routine histologic methods in the tuberculids.

Mycobacterium avium–intercellulare infections of the skin can cause the same types of tuberculid reactions that are seen with *M. tuberculosis*. Among the other nontuberculous mycobacteria, direct skin infection by *Mycobacterium marinum* is frequent and produces granulomatous nodules at sites of trauma in fish tanks and other aquatic situations. In immunodeficient patients, the skin inoculation site often has numerous neutrophils, few granulomas, and numerous acid-fast organisms. *Mycobacterium haemophilum* produces similar lesions.

Rochalimaea henselae *infection*

The cutaneous manifestations of infection by the primitive archibacterium *Rochalimaea henselae* are distinctive and usually are in immunosuppressed patients. The organism is closely related genetically to *Rochalimaea quintana*, the rickettsial organism of trench fever,[257] but produces vascular lesions very similar to those produced by *Bartonella bacilliformis*, the organisms of verruga peruana in Carrion's disease.[258] Grossly the lesions in the skin resemble pyogenic granulomas or even lesions of Kaposi's sarcoma.

PATHOLOGY. The lesions appear as vascular nodules composed of capillaries surrounded by a stroma containing granular purple material and many neutrophils. The granular deposits are aggregates of bacilli that are positive on Warthin-Starry silver stains[259] and bind antibodies to *Rochalimaea henselae*.[260] Because of the proliferations of endothelial cells and pericytes in well-formed vessels, the lesions resemble pyogenic granulomas rather than to Kaposi's sarcoma.

Protozoal infections

Two most important protozoal infections of the skin are cutaneous *leishmaniasis* and *Chagas disease*.[261,262] Direct inoculation and subsequent growth of organisms in the skin occur in both of these diseases. Travel to endemic areas brings the human host into contact with *Phlebotomus* sand flies carrying *Leishmania* organisms or with triatomid (reduviid) bugs that are infected with *Trypanosoma cruzi,* the organism of Chagas disease. Cutaneous leishmaniasis usually is a self-limited disease without notable internal organ involvement, except in the case of *Leishmania mexicana* infection, which can be both mucocutaneous and visceral in its manifestations.

PATHOLOGY. Both organisms grow inside macrophages as 2 to 4 μm, round, amastigote forms that have a stainable nucleus and a kinetoplast that distinguishes them from *Histoplasma capsulatum.* Although both organisms infect macrophages, *T. cruzi* also infects smooth muscle of blood vessels and arrector pili muscles, whereas *Leishmania* organisms show no tendency to infect these cells.[263] In the primary infections, early lesions are composed of lymphocytes with only a few macrophages containing few parasites,[264] but later lesions are more granulomatous and have many parasites. In patients with chronic systemic forms of these diseases, who become immunosuppressed, dermal lesions of dense lymphocytic infiltrates or granulomas appear with varying but small numbers of organisms, in both leishmaniasis and in Chagas disease.[263]

Neoplasms

Keratinocytic tumors

Keratinocytic tumors that mainly involve the dermis include metastatic or recurrent squamous or basal cell carcinomas and a variety of adnexal tumors that were discussed previously. A frequent problem is the decision as to whether a particular dermal tumor is a metastasis from an unknown visceral primary. Both metastatic squamous carcinomas and adenocarcinomas can form attachments to the overlying epidermis, but this is not very common because metastatic nodules usually lie deep in the dermis. They infiltrate the dermis; small cell and signet-ring variants can mimic dermatofibromas, granuloma annulare, or other histiocytic infiltrates. A sclerotic PAS-positive stroma often accompanies primary sweat gland carcinomas but not metastatic adenocarcinomas. Regardless, a careful examination for a visceral primary tumor and review of any previous histologic material are warranted.

Melanocytic lesions

Intradermal nevus of small epithelioid cells. The most common type of purely dermal melanocytic lesion is the small acquired intradermal nevus (Unna's nevus), composed of small epithelioid cells. Congenital intradermal nevi can be small to very large in size; these latter ones are called "giant congenital" or "bathing trunk nevi." Most acquired lesions are less than 6 mm in diameter and are symmetrical in distribution of pigment. In contrast, congenital intradermal nevi often have enlarged hairs within them and irregular outlines with speckled pigmentation, most evident at the periphery.

PATHOLOGY. Intradermal nevi of the common type have a progressive maturation of the cells with descent in the dermis, away from the local influence of the epidermis or appendages. This maturation is manifest in a decrease in size of nevus cell nuclei and nucleoli. Mitoses are very rare and are not present in the deep dermal part of these nevi. There is a progressive dispersion of the cells in the dermal collagen as they enter into the reticular dermis, with a loss of melanin pigmentation and loss of binding with the antibody HMB-45.

Blue nevus. Pigmented spindle cells form blue nevi and cellular blue nevi. Clinically common blue nevi (Fig. 71-162) are small and symmetrical in appearance on the skin surface and have a dark blue-black color because the melanin pigment is deep in the dermis and reflects most efficiently those wavelengths of light near the blue end of the spectrum.

PATHOLOGY. The most common form of blue nevus has dendritic and spindle cells that contain a large amount of rather coarsely distributed melanin pigment. The nuclei are ovoid and usually have only a small nucleolus. Mitoses are very rare. The lesions are strongly HMB-45 positive.[265,266] Melanophages often are present.

Cellular blue nevus. Cellular blue nevi are rare and occur on the lower back or buttocks, the dorsal surfaces of the hands and feet, scalp, and occasionally in other areas as well (Fig. 71-163). They can be large, greater than 1 to 1.5 cm in diameter.

PATHOLOGY. Cellular blue nevi have a compact population of cells (Fig. 71-164) that contain spindle-shaped or dendritic cells with very abundant melanin pigment in their cytoplasm admixed with groups of ovoid cells that have less pigmentation and with melanophages (Fig. 71-165). The nevus cells form fascicles that extend deep in the dermis and often produce bulbous protrusions into the subcutis. The ovoid pale cells often are in the centers of the deep aggregates with the pigmented dendritic cells at the periphery. Necrosis, ulcera-

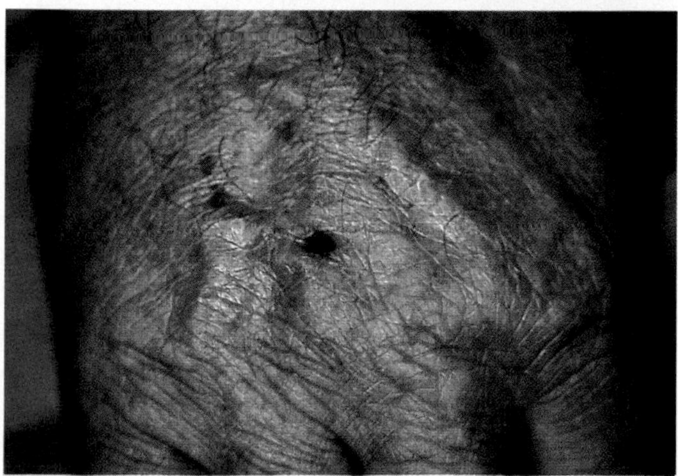

Fig. 71-162 Blue nevus, common type. The nevus is a dark blue-black color and is small and symmetrical.

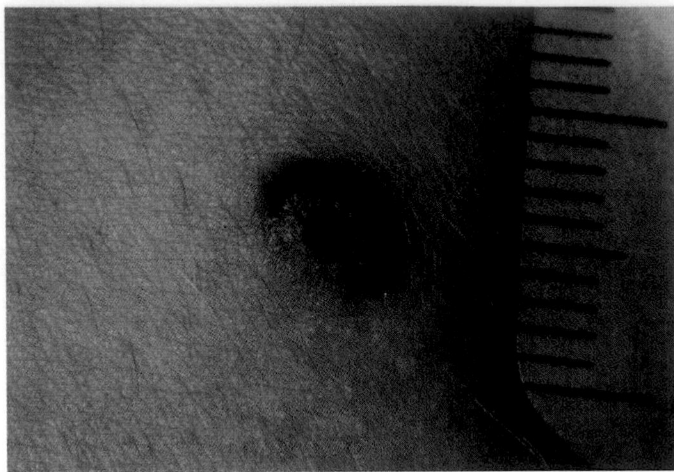

Fig. 71-163 Cellular blue nevus. This nevus is larger than a common blue nevus but is relatively symmetrical and well circumscribed laterally. It is a dark blue-brown to black lesion that is difficult to distinguish from nodular melanoma.

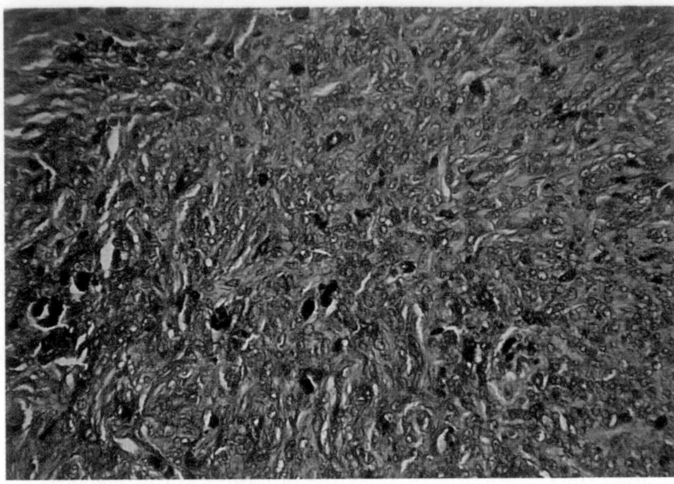

Fig. 71-165 Cellular blue nevus. A mixture of slender dendritic pigmented cells, ovoid cells, and melanophages compose this lesion. The less pigmented cells may be segregated into the center of the lesion, and mitoses often can be found.

Fig. 71-164 Cellular blue nevus. The dermis is densely packed with cells containing variable amounts of brown melanin pigment.

tion, cytologic atypia, and atypical mitoses are indications of malignant degeneration of cellular blue nevi.[267] Ordinary mitoses can be present in the lower part of benign lesions. Cellular blue nevi rarely have spread to local lymph nodes as small deposits of cells in the capsular region. The nevus cells bind the antibody HMB-45.[54,266]

Dermal Spitz's nevus. Spitz's nevi also present as purely intradermal nodules that clinically resemble dermatofibromas in being round, well circumscribed, firm, and symmetrical, usually less than 1 cm in diameter. In their purely intradermal form, Spitz's nevi presumably have undergone a maturation from the intraepidermal and compound types to leave a residual population of dermal nevus cells.

PATHOLOGY. The lesions of the dermal type of Spitz's nevus may have a few nests in the upper portion of the lesions and cells are dispersed between collagen bundles in the lower part. The cytology of the nevus cells resembles that in the compound Spitz's nevus. Mitoses are very rare.

Malignant melanoma. Malignant melanomas can present as purely intradermal nodules or as predominantly intradermal nodules with a small and rather inconspicuous intraepidermal component.[193,203,268] There may be evidence of regression of a previous epidermal component. Clinically these melanomas often grow rapidly but maintain a symmetrical nodular appearance, have variable degrees of pigmentation, and can ulcerate.[269]

PATHOLOGY. Nodular melanomas without an epidermal component usually show highly atypical melanocytic cells that form closely packed groups of anaplastic cells or confluent sheets of atypical cells in the dermis. Mitoses can be found both in the upper and lower portions of the tumor. Nodular melanoma that is purely dermal is difficult to distinguish from metastatic melanoma.

Rarely dermal nodular melanomas are composed of spindle-shaped cells with very little pigment and a stroma filled with mucinous matrix or with collagen. One example is *desmoplastic melanoma*, which clinically and histologically can mimic hypertrophic scars[196,198] (Fig. 71-128). Perineural invasion is frequent and such tumors are sometimes classified as *neurotropic melanomas*.[199]

Malignant blue nevus is a rare nodular melanoma that reaches a bulky size and tends to ulcerate. Microscopically, the lesions have pronounced anaplasia and often necrosis as well. The tumor cells often are elongated, are heavily pigmented, and aggregate into groups sometimes mimicking a cellular blue nevus. Atypical mitoses provide an important clue to malignant blue nevus.[270]

In contrast, there are purely dermal forms of malignant melanoma that are very subtle lesions in which the cytologic transformation of the melanocytes is rather incomplete. These tumors have been named "minimal deviation melanomas," or "nevoid melanomas." Minimal deviation melanoma was proposed as a category of melanomas that have relatively little cytologic atypia but have the architectural features of melanomas.[52,202] Nevoid melanomas are included in this category by some authors but differ in that they have the architectural features of common nevi and little cytologic atypism but some subtle cytologic characteristics of melanoma.[203] It has not been possible to establish definitively whether minimal deviation melanomas have any different prognosis compared to standard melanomas with severe cytologic atypism. However, the largest study of nevoid melanomas up to now has indicated that they are just as malignant as ordinary nodular melanomas of similar thickness.[203] Nevoid melanomas mimic congenital intradermal or compound nevi and even papillomatous intradermal nevi (Fig. 71-166). They are recognized by their confluent nests or sheetlike patterns of growth in the dermis (Figs. 71-167 and 71-168), failure of maturation in the dermis, enlarged nucleoli and mitoses, and failure to lose HMB-45 antigen at the base of the lesion.[54,271] These are uncommon lesions.

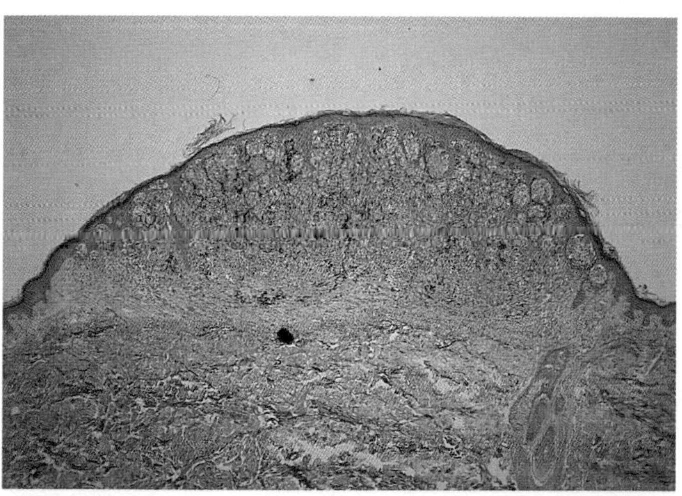

Fig. 71-166 Nevoid melanoma. This lesion is a type of nodular melanoma that is well circumscribed and at low magnification mimics the architecture of a nevus.

Lymphoid lesions

There are many types of lymphoid lesions that involve the dermis with only minimal extension into the epidermis. Although B-cell infiltrates are the majority of these tumors, there are T-cell lesions as well. The clinical appearance is generally a nodule or plaque with induration and a dark red to violaceous color (Fig. 71-169). The overlying epidermis is stretched and occasionally becomes ulcerated in malignant lesions.

PATHOLOGY. The benign lymphoid infiltrates in the dermis have been discussed previously under the category of *lymphocytoma cutis* in the case of B-cell infiltrates and *Jessner's lymphocytic infiltration* when composed of T-cells.[57,109,272,273] In routine sections, the cytologic features of malignant lymphoid infiltrates range from very little atypism to anaplastic tumors. *Granulomatous slack skin* has a neoplastic T-cell infiltrate also with large multinucleated giant cells and pronounced elastolysis in the dermis.[274,275] Although the T-cells do not appear very atypical cytologically, the lesions are clonal and are associated with progression to T-cell lymphoma or Hodgkin's disease. In nonepidermotropic T-cell infiltrates, the cytologic features of the tumors are the clue to their malignant phenotype. Many T-cell lymphomas based in peripheral lymph nodes can secondarily affect the skin to produce either diffuse dermal infiltrates or perivascular ones and even angiodestructive infiltrates. In the case of *pleomorphic T-cell lymphoma* (Fig. 71-170), the large lymphoid cells show the presence of the CD30 activation antigen.[221,276] *Angioimmunoblastic lymphadenopathy* affecting the skin presents clinically as a maculopapular eruption that histologically has deep perivascular infiltrates of atypical lymphocytes mixed with small lymphocytes without destruction of the vessels. Usually there is coexistant lymphadenopathy.[277] *Angiocentric T-cell lymphoma* has a similar pattern but with vascular necrosis and thrombosis leading to ischemic necrosis of both lymphoma cells and adjacent normal tissues.[225] *B-cell lymphomas* of the skin have the

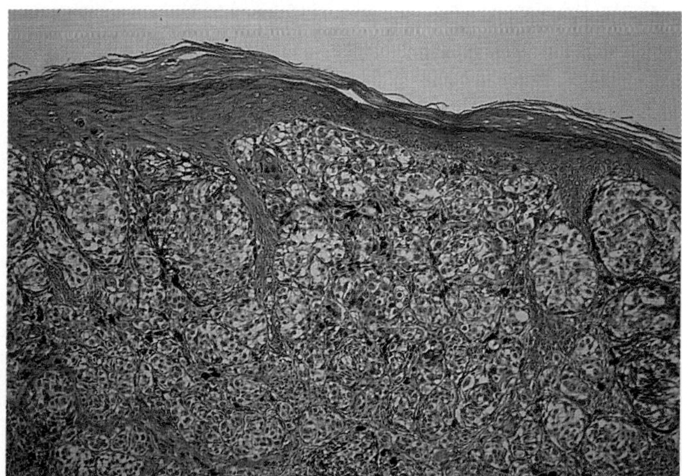

Fig. 71-167 Nevoid melanoma. The nests of melanoma cells are large and closely packed. There is no pagetoid upward migration of individual melanoma cells.

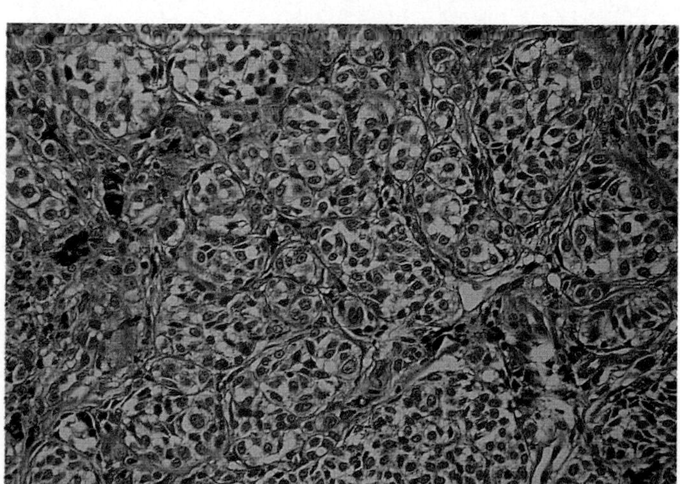

Fig. 71-168 Nevoid melanoma. Even at the base of the lesion there is no maturation of the cells toward smaller cell types. Nucleoli are prominent. Mitoses are few but can be found.

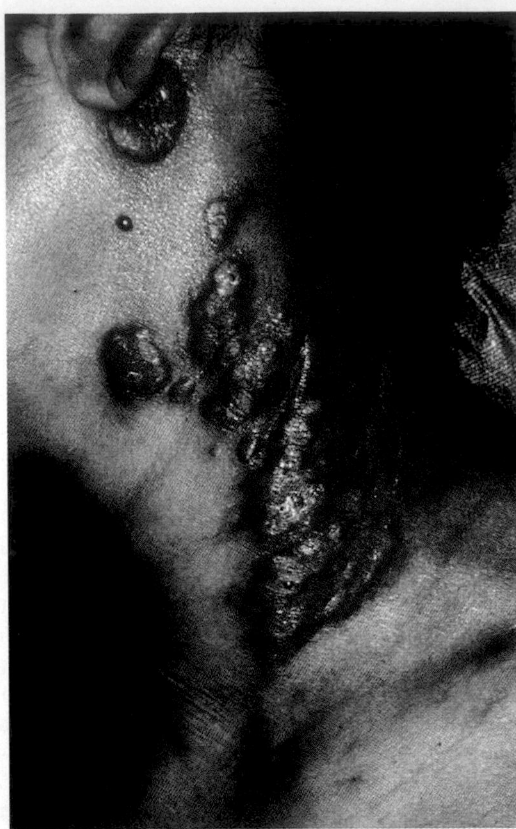

Fig. 71-169 Pleomorphic T-cell lymphoma. This appearance of a dermal erythematous plaque to tumor without epidermal scaling or ulceration can be produced either by B-cell or T-cell lymphomas.

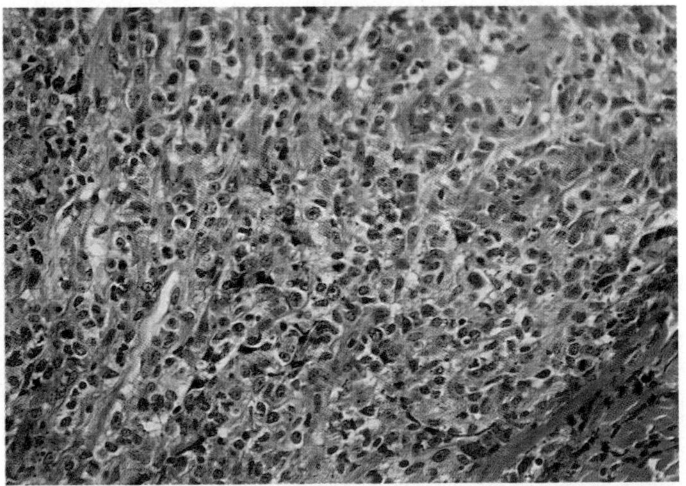

Fig. 71-170 Pleomorphic T-cell lymphoma. This is a large cell lymphoma that cannot be distinguished from a B-cell lymphoma except by special methods. The large cells with prominent nucleoli and abundant eosinophilic cytoplasm are often CD30 positive.

same variations in their appearance as those found in the lymph nodes.[57,278] The classification of the tumors into follicular versus diffuse is best performed on the lymph nodes, since follicular lymphomas in the nodes can have diffuse infiltrates in the skin. However, a well-formed follicular or germinal center pattern in the skin can be classified as a follicular lymphoma, which constitute the majority of cutaneous B-cell lymphomas[278-280] (Fig. 71-171). The presence of sheets of atypical large lymphoid cells is diagnostic of lymphoma (Fig. 71-172). When less atypia is present, the feature that best separates B-cell lymphoma from lymphocytoma cutis is clonality on B-cell gene rearrangements for kappa or lambda light chains. In general, clonality roughly correlates histologically with a monomorphous population of lymphocytes having poorly formed germinal centers in a predominantly deep distribution in the skin ("bottom heavy"). Both pleomorphic T-cell and B-cell lymphomas tend to spare the epidermis and a thin zone of papillary dermis ("grenz zone"). *Leukemic infiltration* of the skin is generally diffuse rather than perivascular and often involves the subcutis as well as the dermis.[281,282] The cells in the skin are very similar to those in bone marrow and other organs. Monocytic leukemia in the skin has to be distinguished from T-cell lymphoma, since both have the CD4 antigen.

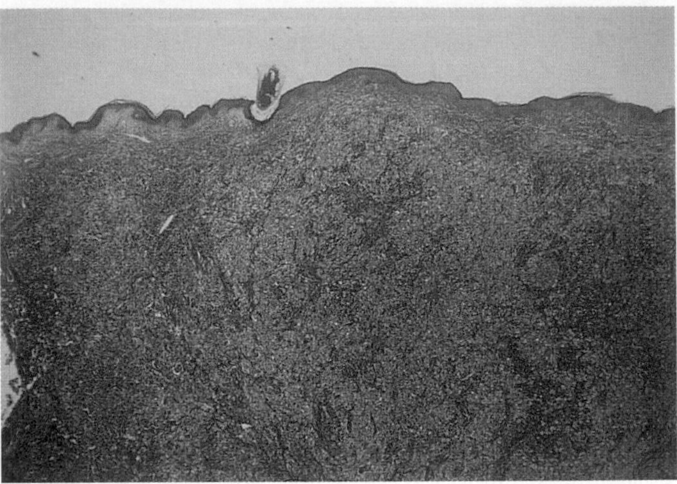

Fig. 71-171 B-cell lymphoma. Notice that the infiltrate spares the epidermis and a thin zone of papillary dermis. Germinal center patterning is present.

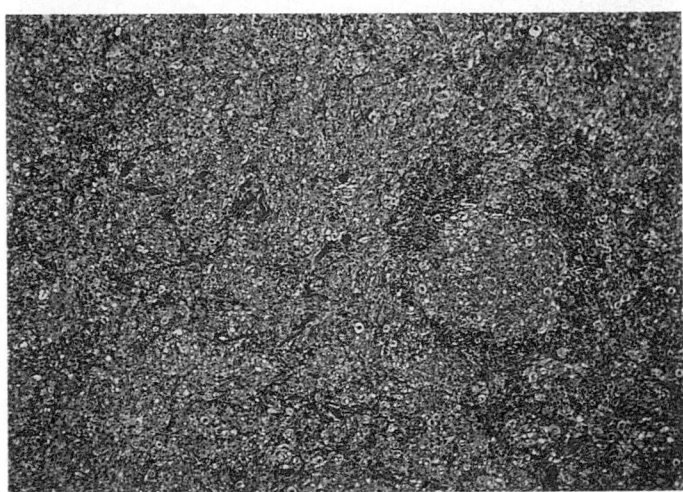

Fig. 71-172 B-cell lymphoma. Sheets of atypical large lymphoma cells are present with similar cells in the pseudogerminal centers.

Histiocytic lesions

Dermal *histiocytic infiltrates* are divided into those composed of Langerhans' cells and their relatives and those formed by non-Langerhans' cells. Clinically, they are often not distinguishable from each other and resemble the lymphoid infiltrations described above except for a more orange to yellow color, when the lesions contain abundant lipid, and a more brown color, when the lesions have epidermal hyperplasia and hyperpigmentation overlying them. In newborn children, Langerhans' cell infiltrations may mimic seborrheic dermatitis but have a hemorrhagic character (Fig. 71-173).

PATHOLOGY. Langerhans' cells and their variants are recognized as cells with eccentric nuclei often with a central depression or groove and eosinophilic cytoplasm (Fig. 71-174). With immunohistochemical methods these cells show the presence of S-100 protein (Fig. 71-175), CD1a, and HLA-DR, as well as binding of peanut agglutinin.[229,283] EM shows Birbeck's granules in the cytoplasm of mature Langerhans' cells. A subgroup of macrophages, so-called indeterminate cells, have S-100 protein but lack Birbeck's granules and form infiltrates in the skin.[284] When these S-100-positive macrophages also phagocytize lymphocytes and neutrophils and have a plasma cell infiltrate without many eosinophils, the diagnosis is *Rosai-Dorfman disease,* also known as "sinus histiocytosis with massive lymphadenopathy."[285-287] When these cells have all the markers of Langerhans' cells without hemophagocytosis or plasma cell infiltration, the diagnosis of *Langerhans' cell histiocytosis* is used.[288] The disorders of Langerhans' cells are clonal proliferations, probably neoplastic,[289] and constitute a range of clinical aggressiveness from the occasionally lethal Letterer-Siwe disease, usually of infants, to the Hand-Schüller-Christian disease of adolescents, and the eosinophilic granulomas of adults. Letterer-Siwe disease in the skin is a hemorrhagic maculopapular rash in a seborrheic distribution, thus mimicking some aspects of seborrheic dermatitis in infants. The prognosis of the patient depends on how many organs are involved and the severity of the internal organ involvement. A related disease of Langerhans' cells is present at birth, is generally limited to the skin, and often regresses spontaneously, and so has been named "congenital self-healing histiocytosis" (Hashimoto-Pritzker disease).[230]

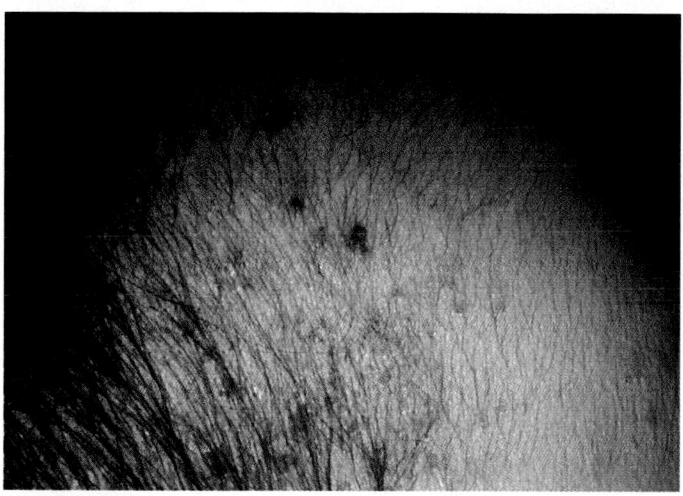

Fig. 71-173 Langerhans' cell histiocytosis (Letterer-Siwe type). This child has scaly slightly hemorrhagic papules mimicking seborrheic dermatitis.

Juvenile xanthogranuloma. Juvenile xanthogranuloma (JXG) is a distinctive nodular infiltrate composed of non-Langerhans' cell histiocytes that have no S-100 protein but have markers of lysosomes, macrophages, and monocytes.[290] This entity presents as single or multiple nodules, usually in children, from birth to early teens.[288] Also it does occur in adults. The nodules are usually up to 1 cm in diameter and are protuberant because of their rather superficial location in the skin (Fig. 71-176). Their color varies from erythematous to yellow-orange, depending on the amount of lipid deposition, which increases with the age of the lesion. They often regress spontaneously. Internal involvement can occur, including in the eye, where it is very important to distinguish JXG from a malignant tumor. Deep forms have been reported, and there are forms with very little lipid deposition. Uncommon associations are with neurofibromatosis and with juvenile myeloid leukemia. Serum lipid abnormalities have not been reported.

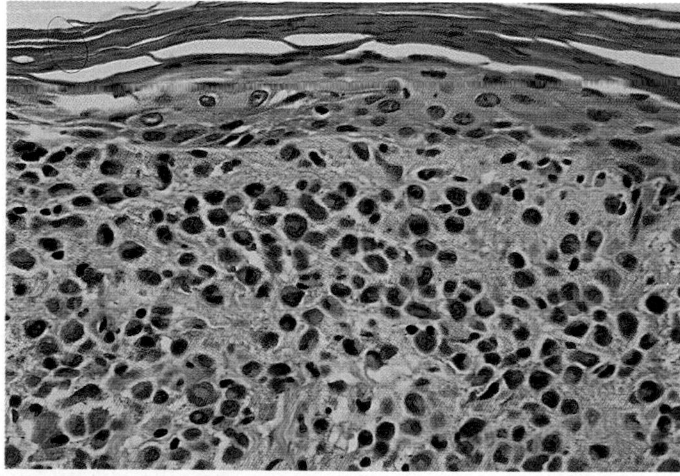

Fig. 71-174 Langerhans' cell histiocytosis. The infiltrating cells in the dermis often extend into the epidermis as well and consist of cells with eccentric nuclei, a central nuclear indentation, and eosinophilic cytoplasm.

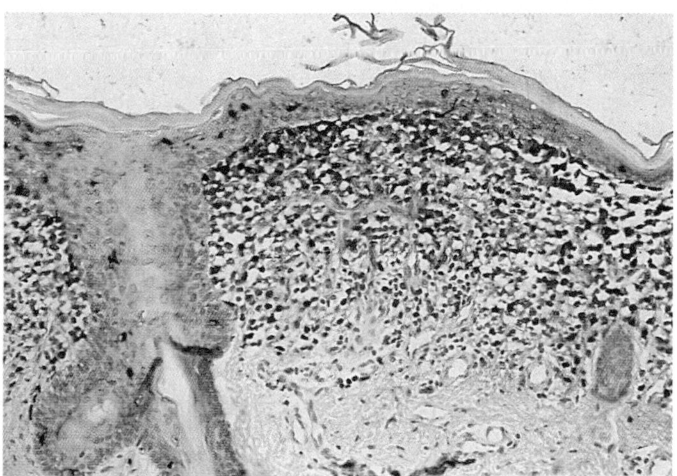

Fig. 71-175 Langerhans' cell histiocytosis. Immunohistochemical staining for S-100 protein is strongly positive on the infiltrating Langerhans' cells.

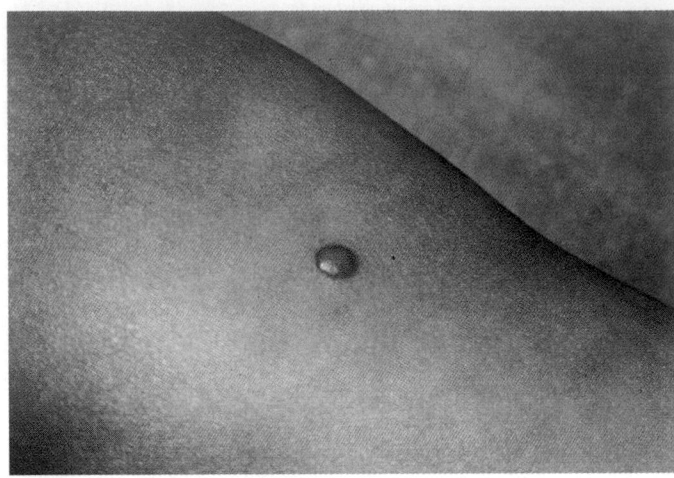

Fig. 71-176 Juvenile xanthogranuloma. The typical lesion is a protuberant slightly orange-colored papule or nodule.

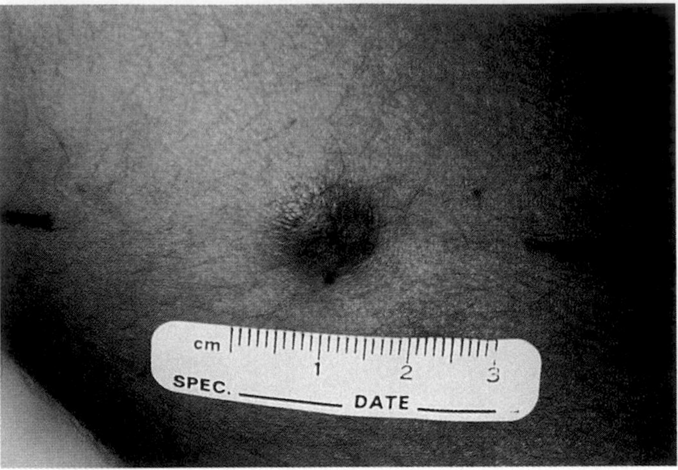

Fig. 71-178 Dermatofibroma. The usual clinical presentation is a firm symmetrical nodule in the dermis with overlying hyperpigmentation.

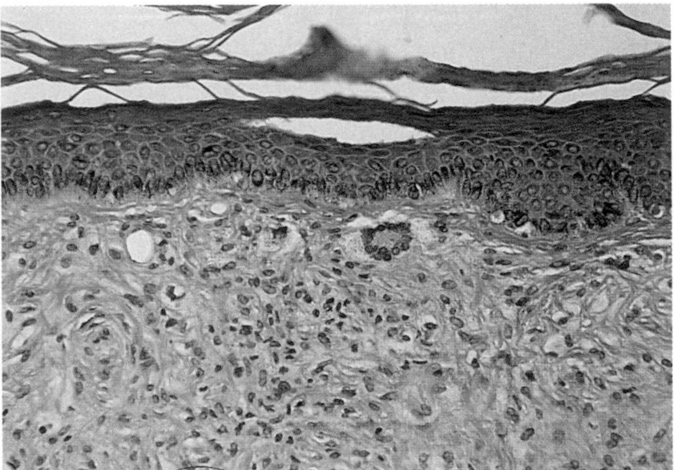

Fig. 71-177 Juvenile xanthogranuloma. This well-developed lesion has many lipidized mononuclear cells as well as multinucleated "Touton" giant cells.

PATHOLOGY. JXG presents somewhat different appearances depending on whether the lesion is studied at its earliest developing stages or in the mature lesions. The early lesions consist of numerous macrophages (histiocytes) that form a dense infiltrate in the interstitial spaces of the dermis, with extension into the subcutis in some cases. At low magnification, the lesion usually has a symmetrical appearance and does not infiltrate into the epidermis. In very early lesions, lipid-laden or foam cells are uncommon and multinucleated cells are rare. As the lesions mature, the amount of lipid increases in the mononuclear cells as well as in the peripheral cytoplasm of the multinucleated giant cells (Fig. 71-177). These lipidized giant cells (Touton giant cells) have a central zone of the cytoplasm containing the Golgi apparatus and other organelles, an intermediate zone containing the multiple nuclei, and a peripheral zone with many lipid droplets. Although they are seen frequently in JXG, they are not pathognomonic, since they also occur in necrobiotic xanthogranuloma with paraproteinemia, Langerhans' cell granulomatosis of the Hand-Schüller-Christian type, occasional benign fibrous histiocytomas, xanthoma disseminatum, and rarely tuberous and tendinous xanthomas. Benign cephalic histiocytosis may belong in the range of early lesions of JXG.[291]

Special studies of JXG have shown that dendritic S-100–positive cells can infiltrate near the edge of the lesions, but most of the cells are of macrophage lineage and are not S-100 positive.[290] The macrophages show the presence of lysozyme and alpha-1-antichymotrypsin. Only scattered dendritic cells are positive for the blood coagulation factor XIIIa.

Fibrous tumors

Dermatofibroma. Dermatofibroma is a benign tumor that presents as a round, firm nodule that has overlying hyperpigmentation (Fig. 71-178). The lesion is very sharply circumscribed, though it is not encapsulated. They occur mostly in young to middle-aged adults and have a propensity to form on the anterior thighs of women.

PATHOLOGY. Dermatofibroma often is a superficial tumor just below the epidermis but can be a deep tumor that involves the deep dermis and subcutis. In the superficial form, epidermal hyperplasia and hyperpigmentation are common (Fig. 71-179), but the deep lesions often lack these epidermal findings. Both superficial and deep forms have a central focus of fibrosis in the dermis, often with thickened, eosinophilic collagen bundles at the periphery of the lesion. Other components are blood vessels, spindle-shaped fibroblastic cells, and macrophages containing variable degrees of melanin pigment, lipid, or hemosiderin. Mitoses may be abundant but are not atypical.

Some pathologists consider dermatofibroma to be a reactive fibrous proliferation secondary to trauma or wound healing but with a distinctive evolution and histologic pattern. Some of them evolve through a lymphocytic and histiocytic stage and then partially regress to a fibrous with few histiocytes. However, some lesions progressively but slowly enlarge, contain an admixture of histiocytic and fibroblastic cells, and are best classified as true tumors of fibrohistiocytes.

Dermatofibrosarcoma protuberans. Dermatofibrosarcoma protuberans (DFSP) is a low-grade malignant tumor of the dermis. It begins as a small, symmetrical tumor but usually is

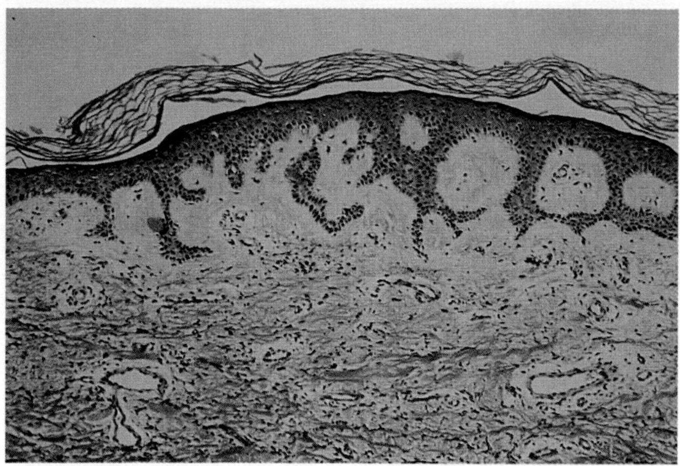

Fig. 71-179 Dermatofibroma. The epidermis is acanthotic in an irregular pattern, and the central area of fibrosis is in the reticular dermis. Dendritic cells are present between thickened collagen bundles.

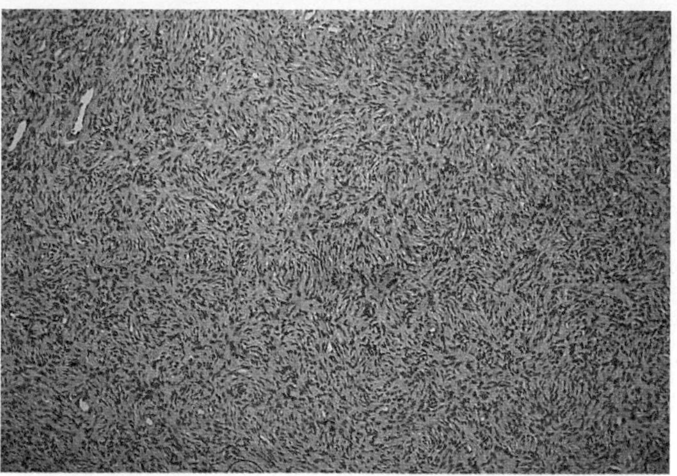

Fig. 71-180 Dermatofibrosarcoma protuberans. There is a uniform population of thin spindle cells in a delicate myxoid fibrous stroma. Whirling arrays of cells form "storiform arrays."

detected when it has reached a size greater than 1 cm in diameter. It is a tumor with a flat macular component and a focal nodular component. Ulceration of the nodules leads to superficial infection. The lesion has a slow growth pattern and occurs mostly on the trunk and proximal extremities of young to middle-aged adults. DFSP has a high rate of local recurrence because of incomplete surgical excision initially. These tumors must be excised with margins that extend beyond any regions in which there is consideration of tumor versus scar. They tend to recur locally before they metastasize to the lungs and regional lymph nodes.

PATHOLOGY. DFSP differs from dermatofibroma in that very rarely are epidermal hyperplasia and hyperpigmentation present, unless the lesion has been rubbed or traumatized. The tumor itself is formed by delicate elongated spindle cells in a fine fibrous stroma composed of small collagen fibers in a myxoid matrix (Fig. 71-180). Polarizable collagen is rare. In the flat macular region, the tumor cells spread through the dermis with thinning of the dermis. In nodular regions, the tumor cells form poorly circumscribed nodules in the dermis, which infiltrate diffusely into the fat in the subcutis. Usually mitoses are uncommon and cellular pleomorphism is not striking. Both dermatofibroma and DFSP can have spindle cells in whirling arrays, or "storiform arrays" (Fig. 71-180). DFSP is composed of a single cell type, whereas dermatofibroma contains spindle-shaped fibroblastic cells admixed with macrophages. When broad fascicles of spindle cells develop, the DFSP is said to have undergone fibrosarcomatous transformation.[292,293]

Immunoperoxidase staining has revealed important differences between dermatofibroma and DFSP. Dermatofibromas contain a prominent admixture of cells of macrophage lineage that stain for CD68. Also many of the tumor cells contain factor XIIIa and are negative for CD34. In contrast, DFSP does not show factor XIIIa and but shows CD34 (Fig. 71-181).

Other dermal fibrous lesions include the innocuous acrochordon (skin tag, soft fibroma, fibroepithelial polyp), scars, hypertrophic scars, keloids, fibrous papules (with and without associated tuberous sclerosis), atypical fibroxanthoma, epithelioid sarcoma, and various mucinous accumulations.

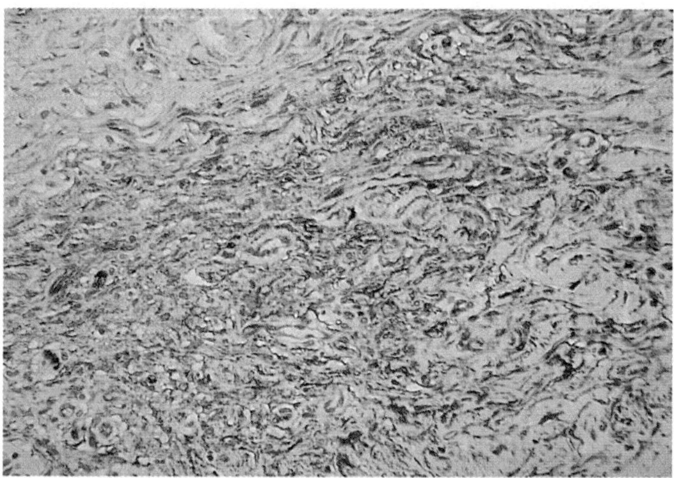

Fig. 71-181 Dermatofibrosarcoma protuberans. Immunostaining shows that the cells and their fine processes stain for CD34.

Vascular tumors

Many of the vascular tumors of the skin are the same entities that occur in the deep soft tissues and are presented in other chapters. Several distinctive benign skin lesions occur and need to be distinguished from malignant vascular tumors, which may appear primarily in the skin.

Pyogenic granuloma. The so-called pyogenic granuloma, which is better considered a form of *lobular capillary hemangioma,*[294,295] is a common, usually solitary nodule, up to 1 cm in diameter, composed of highly vascular tissue that bleeds easily on slight trauma (Fig. 71-182). It forms rapidly and often is ulcerated in the early stages of its development. If incompletely excised, it can recur rapidly and can have satellite nodules as well. It is most common on body surfaces exposed to trauma, such as the hands and feet, but also occurs on the gingiva, particularly of pregnant women.

PATHOLOGY. The lesion is a protuberant nodule of ulcerated granulation tissue, with a lobular pattern to the proliferating vessels (Fig. 71-183). The lobules are irregularly formed but have large vessels near the center and small vessels, some-

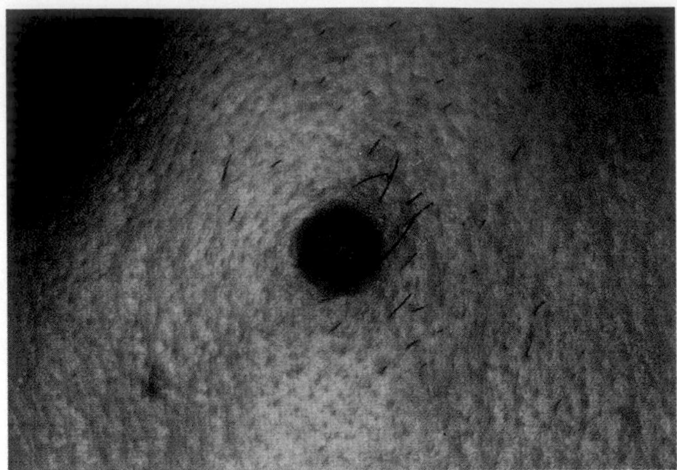

Fig. 71-182 Pyogenic granuloma. This lesion is a well-circumscribed, red nodule that bleeds easily on trauma and often has a collarette of epidermis.

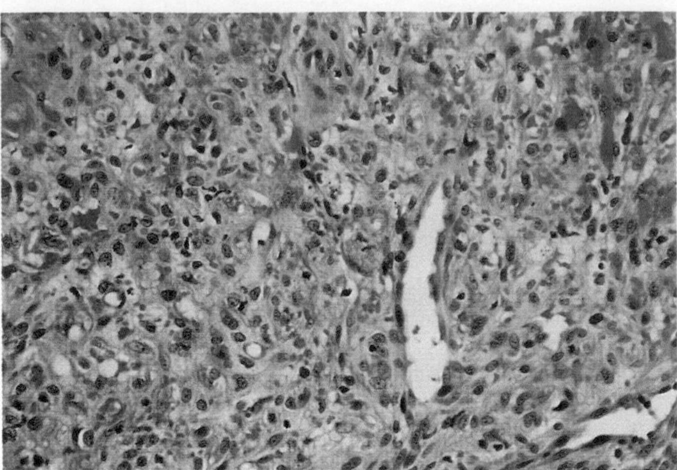

Fig. 71-184 Pyogenic granuloma. At higher magnification the thin-walled vessels and the capillaries have delicate walls, and extravasated erythrocytes are common. The interstitium is edematous.

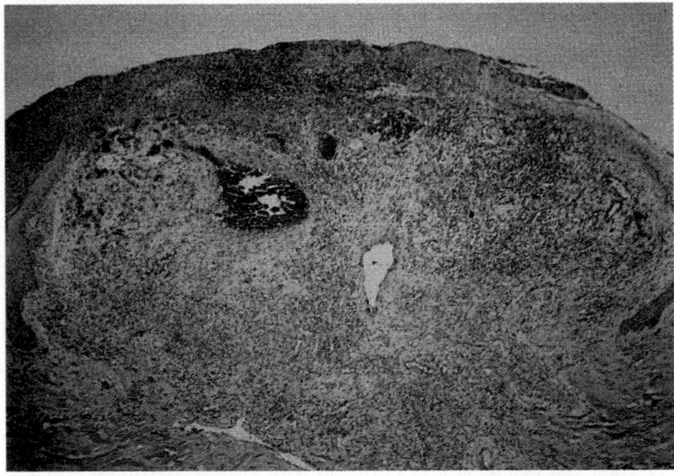

Fig. 71-183 Pyogenic granuloma. At low magnification the epidermal surface is ulcerated, and the underlying granulation tissue has prominent dilated thin-walled vessels as well as adjacent capillaries with small lumens.

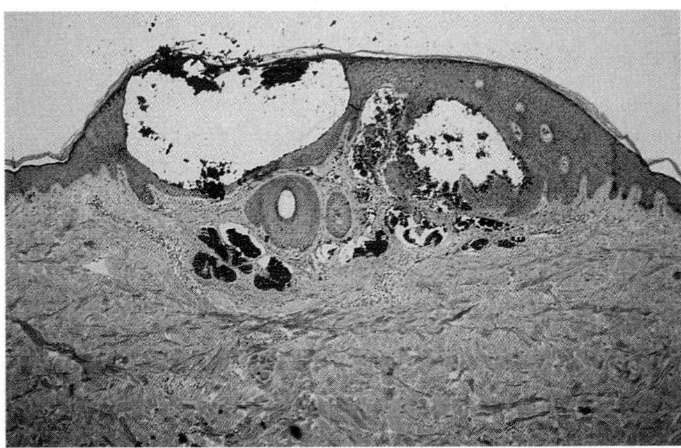

Fig. 71-185 Angiokeratoma. Dilated thin-walled blood vessels are closely associated with epidermal hyperplasia. Thrombosis and transepidermal elimination of blood is common.

times with inapparent lumens, near the periphery (Fig. 71-184). These lobules are separated by thin fibrous septa. Near the surface, the stroma between the vessels is edematous and neutrophils form a crust on the surface.

In the differential diagnosis are lesions of *bacillary angiomatosis,* which resemble pyogenic granulomas, but in the stroma, there is gray-purple granular material that consists of aggregates of *Rochalimaea henselae*. Similar cutaneous lesions of trench fever contain *Rochalimaea quintana*;[296] and similar skin lesions of Oroya fever, or Carrion's disease, or bartonellosis have been called "verruga peruana" and contain *Bartonella bacilliformis*. The ulcerated surface of ordinary pyogenic granulomas often contain staphylococci or streptococci. One hypothesis has been that these organisms cause an overgrowth of granulation tissue because of a retardation of reepithelialization of a wound. Circulating angiogenic factors can also play a role, particularly in pregnancy.

Angiokeratoma. Angiokeratoma is a vascular lesion of the papillary dermis that characteristically is closely associated with epidermal hyperplasia (Fig. 71-185). In patients with Fabry's disease, it is related to the deposition of a sphingolipid in the endothelial cells and presents as many small, 1 to 2 mm in diameter, keratotic superficial angiomas in a widespread distribution (*angiokeratoma corporis diffusum*). Solitary and localized forms of angiokeratoma also occur, without any relationship to Fabry's disease.

PATHOLOGY. The epidermis is hyperplastic in a region containing widely dilated, thin-walled blood vessels in the papillary dermis (Fig. 71-185). Occasionally the vascular abnormalities also involve the reticular dermis.[297] Thrombosis and transepidermal elimination of hemorrhagic material are common.

Other benign vascular lesions. *Angiomyxomas* of the skin present as 1 or 2 cm in diameter nodules with myxoid stroma, prominent vascular proliferation, and occasionally with epidermal strands or cysts.[298] In some patients, they are part of Carney's syndrome, which includes atrial myxomas, lentigines, blue nevi, and endocrine abnormalities.

Epithelioid hemangiomas (synonym: angiolymphoid hyperplasia with eosinophilia) resemble some aspects of Kimura's disease, except epithelioid hemangiomas are superficial lesions, lack associated peripheral eosinophilia, and have more prominent enlargement of the endothelial cells in thick-walled blood vessels.[299]

In some instances, the organization of a thrombus within a hemangioma or in an extravascular hematoma develops a papillary pattern (*intravascular papillary endothelial hyperplasia of Masson*) that needs to be distinguished from angiosarcoma.[300,301] This is usually possible in those lesions confined to a thrombus in a well-demarcated blood vessel.

Other benign vascular lesions of the skin include capillary and cavernous hemangiomas and a variety of mixed hemangiomas that have been subdivided into acquired tufted angioma,[302] targetoid hemosiderotic hemangioma,[303] and microvenular hemangioma.[304]

Kaposi's sarcoma. Kaposi's sarcoma is a low-grade, multifocal malignant vascular tumor that often begins in the skin but can involve many internal organs. The cause is unknown. It is increased in incidence in elderly men of Mediterranean origin, renal transplant patients on immunosuppressive therapy, and homosexual males with AIDS.[305] The patients present with purplish macules on the skin, often bilaterally on the feet in the classic form, or "old-age" form, of Kaposi's sarcoma. In patients with HIV-1 infection and CD4 counts below 200 cells/mm^3 of peripheral blood, lesions often are in a more generalized distribution, including the oral cavity. The macules initially resemble bruises but become elevated and are soft on palpation. Large tumors can form and ulcerate (Fig. 71-186). Systemic involvement is common but seems to be the result of multicentric formation of tumor rather than metastasis.[306]

PATHOLOGY. The early lesions of Kaposi's sarcoma consist of irregular dilatation of vessels in the reticular dermis in areas around the penetrating blood vessels or the adnexal structures.[307] These vessels have very thin walls that in areas consist only of endothelium with discontinuous linings, thereby resembling lymphatic spaces; however, they are filled with blood[138,308-310] (Fig. 71-187). Well-developed lesions have proliferations of spindle cells adjacent to these irregular vessels, with entrapment and phagocytosis of erythrocytes (Fig. 71-188). Hemosiderin is notable particularly in lesions on the dependent parts of the body. Nuclear atypism is minimal. Mitoses are present. Rapidly growing lesions also contain apoptotic endothelial cells.[138]

In tumoral lesions of Kaposi's sarcoma, the spindle cells predominate. Many special studies have been devoted to the origin of the spindle cell population, but there continues to be disagreement about this subject. In contrast, there is general agreement that the cells lining the vessels are endothelial cells. In studies utilizing sensitive methods, the spindle cells have been found to contain factor VIII–related antigen and CD34 antigen, which are both markers for endothelial cells.[311,312] Recently, a role for factor XIIIa-positive dendritic cells has been postulated in the development of early lesions.[313-315] There is controversy also over whether Kaposi's sarcoma is a true malignancy or a multifocal overgrowth of diploid endothelial cells.

The differential diagnosis in the early stages of the disease include the usual form of *angiosarcoma*, which occurs most frequently in the skin of the head and neck area of elderly

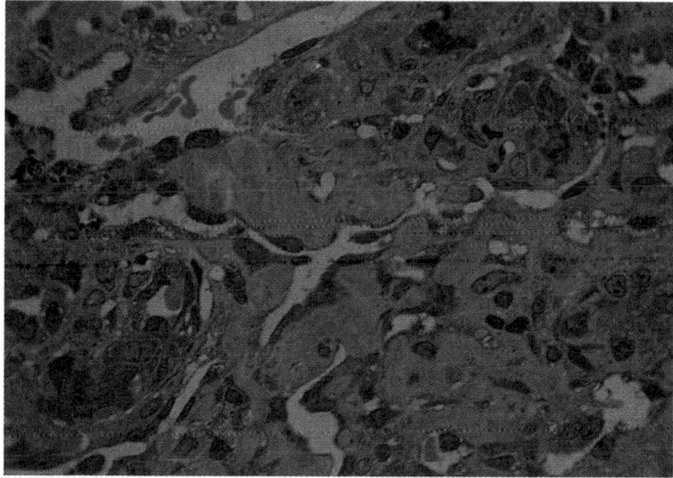

Fig. 71-187 Kaposi's sarcoma. 1 μm thick plastic section of an early lesion shows the permeation of the dermal collagen by thin-walled irregular blood vessels lined by endothelium without many pericytes.

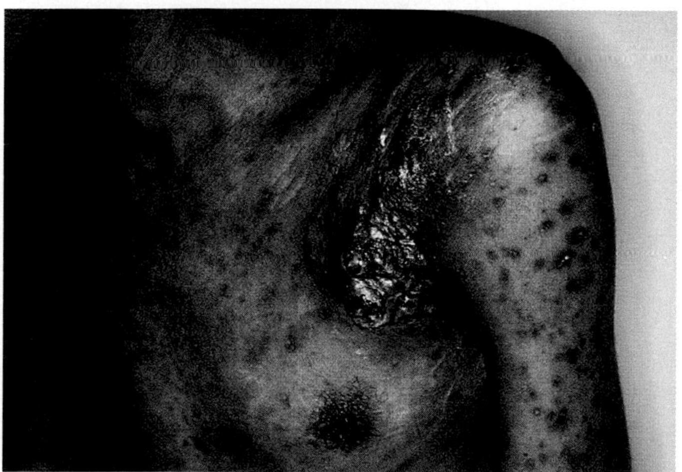

Fig. 71-186 Kaposi's sarcoma. Purplish nodules have formed and are ulcerated. Numerous other small ovoid macular lesions resemble small bruises but are also Kaposi's sarcoma in this AIDS patient.

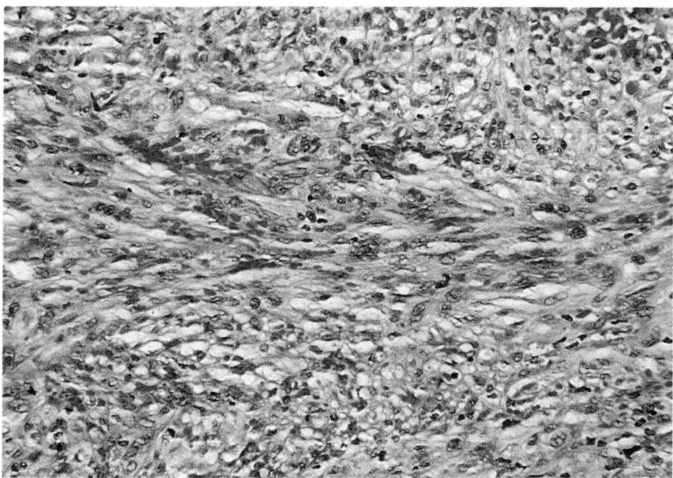

Fig. 71-188 Kaposi's sarcoma. A lesion with many spindle cells shows entrapment of erythrocytes in slitlike spaces between the cells.

individuals and in lymphedematous extremities after mastectomy or lymph node dissections.[316] These forms are presented in Chapter 73, as are glomus tumors.

Tumors of muscle and fat

Tumors composed of smooth muscle cells and fat cells are not rare in the skin. Although the general aspects are discussed in Chapter 73, several aspects are peculiar to the skin.

Leiomyoma. Leiomyoma is a benign tumor of smooth muscle. Clinically, leiomyomas present as papules to nodules in the dermis and may be tender and painful. They generally are small, may be multiple, and show no tendency to ulcerate or grow rapidly.

PATHOLOGY. Leiomyomas of the skin can be divided into those that arise from arrector pili muscles and those that arise from vascular structures, such as the walls of veins. The pilar leiomyomas are poorly circumscribed in the dermis and are composed of fascicles of spindle-shaped smooth muscle cells with moderately abundant eosinophilic cytoplasm. Epithelioid and clear cell variants are very rare. Pilar leiomyomas generally lack cytologic atypism and mitoses. If the tumor has prominent nuclear atypism, a very careful search at multiple levels of sectioning is needed to rule out a *leiomyosarcoma.* Only 2 mitoses per 10 high-power fields is one suggested threshold for the diagnosis of cutaneous leiomyosarcoma. Another feature of malignancy is infiltration into the fat. This must be distinguished from the fascicles of myofibroblasts, which resemble smooth muscle, which occur at the junction of the dermis and subcutis in the disease *infantile myofibromatosis.*[317] A similar lesion is *dermatomyofibroma*, which occurs as a solitary plaque lesion in young individuals and often near the axilla of women.[318] The differential diagnosis also can include smooth muscle *hamartoma* such as that found in association with hyperpigmentation of the epidermis and enlargement of hairs in *Becker's nevus*, which usually occurs on the upper trunk in males. Smooth muscle hamartomas can also occur as a congenital abnormality in the lumbosacral area, without hyperpigmentation.

Lipoma. Lipoma is a benign tumor of adipose tissue cells that contain either unilocular or multilocular fat droplets in the cytoplasm. A lesion unique to the skin is the *dermatolipoma*, in which there is a infiltration of fat cells in the dermis, usually around blood vessels but occasionally diffusely in the reticular dermis. Dermatolipoma may present in newborns as a localized plaque of thickened skin as a hamartoma known as *nevus lipomatosus of Hoffman and Zurhelle*. It may also be an acquired lesion, usually on the lower trunk and thigh region, of middle-aged adults. The lesions are often protuberant fleshy polyps that are relatively asymptomatic unless traumatized. The acquired form of dermatolipoma is quite common and has been given various names including "fibroma molle," "soft fibroma," and "nevus lipomatosus." The occurrence of these lesions is not necessarily correlated with obesity.

PATHOLOGY. In dermatolipoma, unilocular adipose tissue cells extend along perivascular connective tissue sheaths to involve the dermis up to the level of the superficial vascular plexus. Infiltration between collagen bundles also can be prominent in well-developed lesions. Cytologic atypism and mitoses are not seen. Macrophage infiltration and myxoid degenerative change can occur in lesions subjected to chronic trauma. Fatty infiltration can also occur in melanocytic nevi.

Neural tumors

A few aspects of peripheral nerve tumors deserve mention here because of distinctive features in the skin. However, most of the lesions described in Chapter 73 as peripheral nerve sheath tumors also occur in the skin.

Palisaded encapsulated neuroma. Palisaded encapsulated neuroma (PEN) is a distinctive cutaneous nodular lesion often in the region of the central face.[319] The lesions are benign and are not associated with neurofibromatosis. Although they may be related to trauma, they differ from the classical traumatic neuroma.

PATHOLOGY. The lesion is composed of fascicles of spindle cells that are schwannian in derivation and are accompanied by numerous axons, at least focally (Fig. 71-189). It is this profusion of axons that distinguishes PEN from neurofibromas and schwannomas. Also the spindle cells usually do not form as good palisaded arrangements (Fig. 71-190), or Verocay bodies, as those seen in the schwannoma. PEN are circumscribed but are not truly encapsulated. They may extend in a dumbbell fashion into the deep dermis or subcutis. PEN show the presence of S-100 protein and neurofilament proteins in the axons.

Neurothekeoma. Neurothekeoma is a rare tumor, but when it occurs, the skin is a common site.[320-322] Synonyms for it

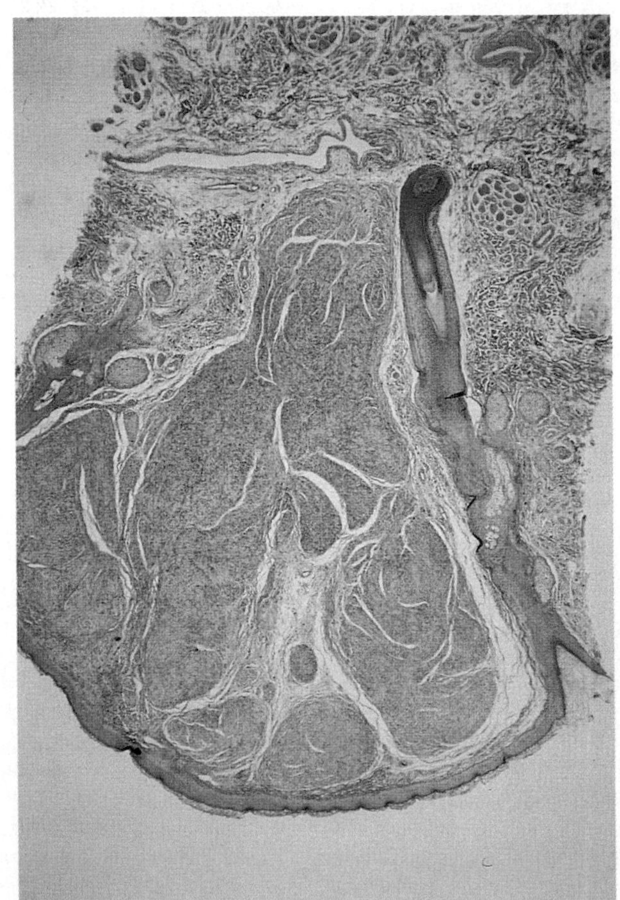

Fig. 71-189 Palisaded encapsulated neuroma. This generally superficial tumor forms a circumscribed nodule formed by groups of fascicles of spindle cells.

include "nerve sheath myxoma," "lobular neuromyxoma," and "pacinian neurofibroma." The lesion is solitary and has a predilection to occur on the extremities or face of young adults, often females. There is no definite association with neurofibromatosis, though the lesion can be confused with myxoid neurofibromas.

PATHOLOGY. Many neurothekeomas contain well-circumscribed and even encapsulated fascicles of stellate and spindle cells in a myxoid stroma. The upper portion of the lesion can have little encapsulation. The tumor extends down existing nerves at the periphery of the lesion. Nuclear pleomorphism can be present, but mitoses are rare. The degree of cellularity can vary from sparse to dense. The myxoid types of neurothekeoma contain detectable S-100 protein on routine immunoperoxidase stains, whereas the most cellular variants are negative. This has led to controversy about the true nature of "cellular neurothekeoma," but the S-100 negativity is useful diagnostically in differentiating it from malignant melanoma. Neurothekeoma is an important benign tumor to recognize, since nuclear atypism can be prominent and can lead to a mistake in diagnosis of malignancy.

Neuroendocrine carcinoma of the skin. Neuroendocrine carcinoma of the skin, also known as Merkel cell carcinoma, is a malignant tumor of uncertain origin.[323-326] Various hypotheses include origin from the dark cells of the sweat glands or from the Merkel cells in the epidermis. They present clinically as deep nodular tumors, often with rapid growth, in late middle-aged or elderly patients, on sun-exposed skin. The head and neck and extremities are common sites, but they can occur in other locations, such as the buttock. This is a highly malignant tumor with a high rate of recurrence and metastasis.[327]

PATHOLOGY. Merkel cell tumor often is deep in the dermis and is composed of rather uniform cells with a very high nucleus to cytoplasm ratio (Fig. 71-191). The nuclei have a distinctive dispersed chromatin with small nucleoli. Mitoses usually are numerous. The cells aggregate into trabeculae or cords of cells indicative of their epithelial origin.

The differential diagnosis of Merkel cell tumors includes Burkitt's lymphoma and metastatic oat cell carcinoma of the lung. A distinction from lymphoma can be made by immunoperoxidase findings of positivity of Merkel cell carcinoma cells for paranuclear dotlike whorls of low molecular weight cytokeratin (Fig. 71-192) and also the frequent presence of neuron-specific enolase. Although metastatic oat cell carcinoma often has a diffuse cytokeratin staining, the primary lesions in the lung can also have a dotlike staining.

Other malignant tumors of peripheral nerve origin occur in the skin and include *malignant peripheral nerve sheath tumor,* which encompasses both neurofibrosarcoma and malignant schwannoma. Also both benign and malignant types of *granular cell tumors* of schwannian origin occur in the skin.

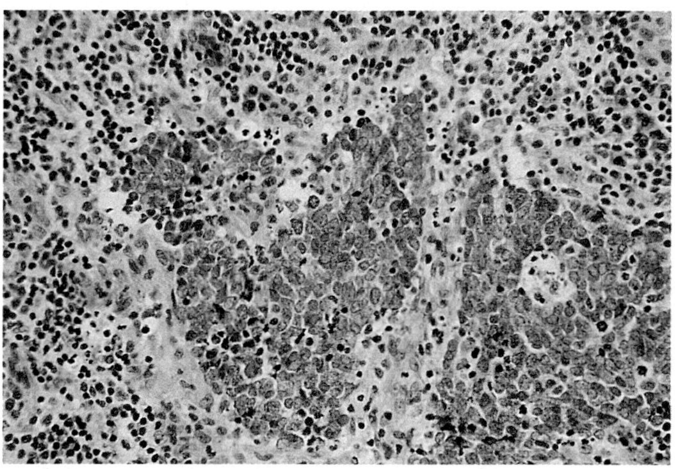

Fig. 71-191 Merkel cell carcinoma. These small cells have round nuclei with dispersed chromatin and many small nucleoli. The mitotic rate is high.

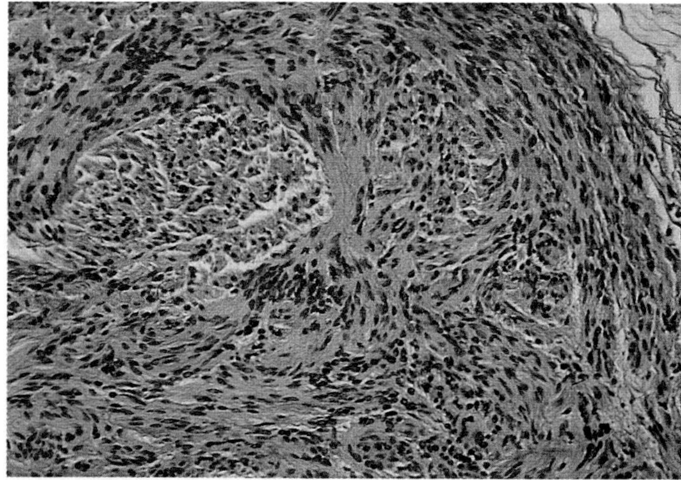

Fig. 71-190 Palisaded encapsulated neuroma. The spindle cells have a delicate wavy stroma and form nuclear palisades mimicking those in schwannoma. Special stains reveal many axons.

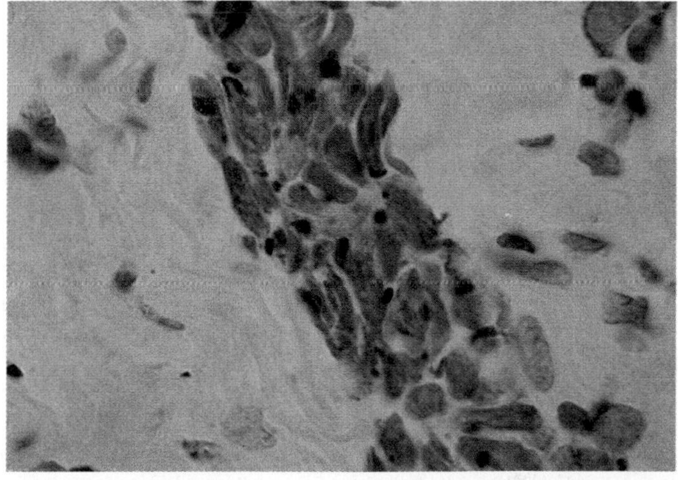

Fig. 71-192 Merkel cell carcinoma. Typical dotlike staining with antibodies to cytokeratin. These dots correspond to cytoplasmic aggregates of cytokeratin filaments.

DISEASES INVOLVING MAINLY THE SUBCUTIS AND FASCIA

The classification of diseases of this region follows the anatomic distribution of its component parts. The subcutis is divided into fat lobules that are separated by fibrous septa. The largest blood vessels and nerves run in the septa. Certain diseases are distinctive to the subcutaneous fat and clinically do not involve the fat elsewhere in the body.[328] These are emphasized here.

Inflammatory and traumatic disorders

Erythema nodosum

Erythema nodosum is an inflammatory lesion of the subcutis that has widening of the septa and inflammation generally centered at the junction of the septa and the fat lobules. Clinically the disease most typically presents as erythematous painful nodules on the anterior shins (Fig. 71-193) but may spread to involve other areas of the legs, the hands, and even the face. When the nodules are over a joint, an inflammatory arthritis can be mimicked. Many of the patients have fever and a mild leukocytosis. The causes of erythema nodosum are many, but leading causes are streptococcal infection and sarcoidosis, and many other infectious diseases and drugs can cause erythema nodosum. These causes have in common the ability to elicit a type IV delayed hypersensitivity reaction, which may be the basis for the lesions, though circulating immune complexes have been found in some patients.[329,330] Delayed hypersensitivity skin tests with antigens can cause a flare of erythema nodosum. The lesions of erythema nodosum resolve clinically without scarring in 4 to 8 weeks. There are patients with recurrent crops of lesions and with persistent lesions that represent special subgroups.[331]

PATHOLOGY. The initial lesions have edema of the septa, with only a few lymphocytes, neutrophils, and eosinophils in the septa.[332] Focal small hemorrhages occur commonly in the septa and give the lesions a bruise-like appearance. Later in the evolution of the lesions, more lymphocytes and macrophages infiltrate the septa, which become widened and have increased collagen deposition (Fig. 71-194). Small granulomas often can be found in the septa. The inflammatory infiltrate concentrates near the borders between the fat lobule and the septa and extends into the lobule from this region. Necrosis of the fat is very rare. Necrotizing vasculitis is very rare also but does occur, sometimes in association with recurrent episodes of erythema nodosum related to medications.

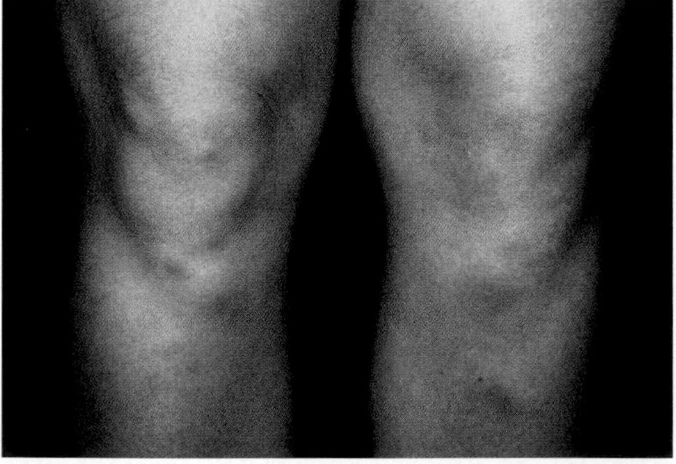

Fig. 71-193 Erythema nodosum. The shins are a favored site for the formation of these erythematous deep subcutaneous nodules. They may also be in other acral sites.

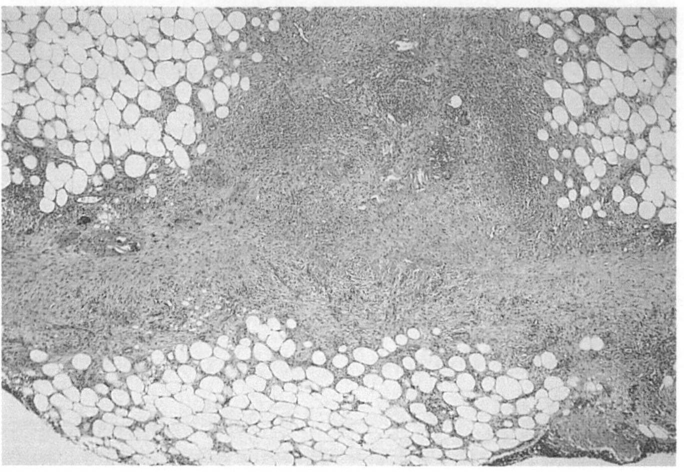

Fig. 71-194 Erythema nodosum. In the subcutis, the septa are widened and become fibrotic with a lymphocytic inflammatory infiltrate at the edges of the septa. Multinucleated giant cells and eosinophils are common in fully developed lesions.

The pathogenesis of erythema nodosum has not been elucidated fully. The localization may be at sites of sluggish blood flow and trauma, which result in the release and trapping of antigens or immune complexes of a particular size in the adipose tissue and septa. This in turn could trigger a type III or a type IV delayed hypersensitivity response. Chronic or persistent lesions or those in unusual locations are suspect for mycobacterial infection, which may need cultures to identify small numbers of organisms.[333]

Erythema induratum

Erythema induratum is one of the classic "tuberculids,"[36] that is, hypersensitivity reactions that occur in patients with mycobacterial infection, in which intact organisms have not been identified by special stains or by cultures. The patients present with firm, erythematous nodules that are painful and occur most frequently on the lower legs (Fig. 71-195), with a predilection for the posterior calf region. The lesions often ulcerate and resolve with scarring. They respond to treatment with antituberculous therapy. *Nodular vasculitis* is a similar lesion in terms of its localization, but it is not related to tuberculosis. Nodular vasculitis is subcutaneous *polyarteritis nodosa,* which can be caused by many possible antigen sources including streptococcal infection, medications, and hepatitis B antigens. Cutaneous polyarteritis nodosa in some patients is limited to the skin for a prolonged time, but some patients have evidence of systemic polyarteritis also.[241,242]

PATHOLOGY. Both erythema induratum and nodular vasculitis have a necrotizing vasculitis that affects arteries and veins in the fat lobules (Fig. 71-196). In our experience, there is more extensive caseous necrosis of the fat and more granuloma formation in erythema induratum than in nodular vasculitis.

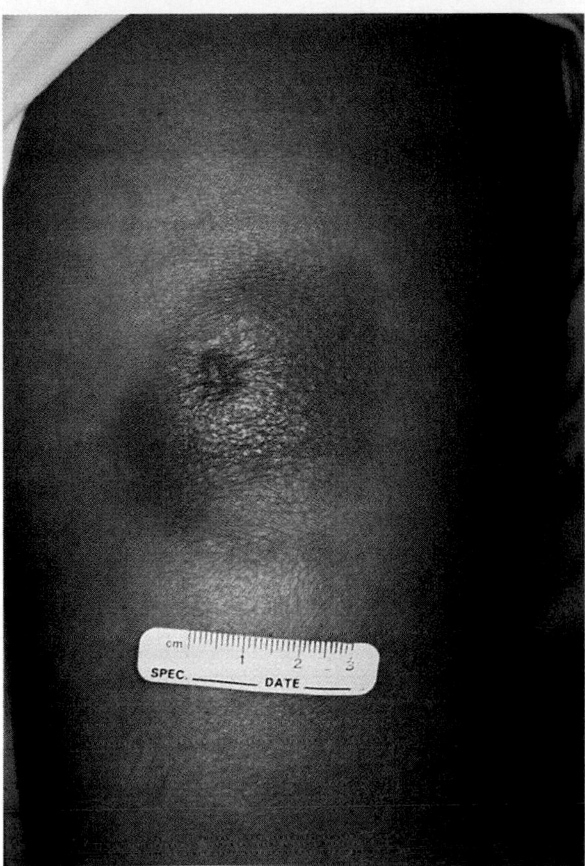

Fig. 71-195 Erythema induratum. Deep erythematous nodules are formed on the legs with less predilection for the shins than erythema nodosum. The underlying vasculitis leads to more necrosis and ulceration and leaves depressed scars.

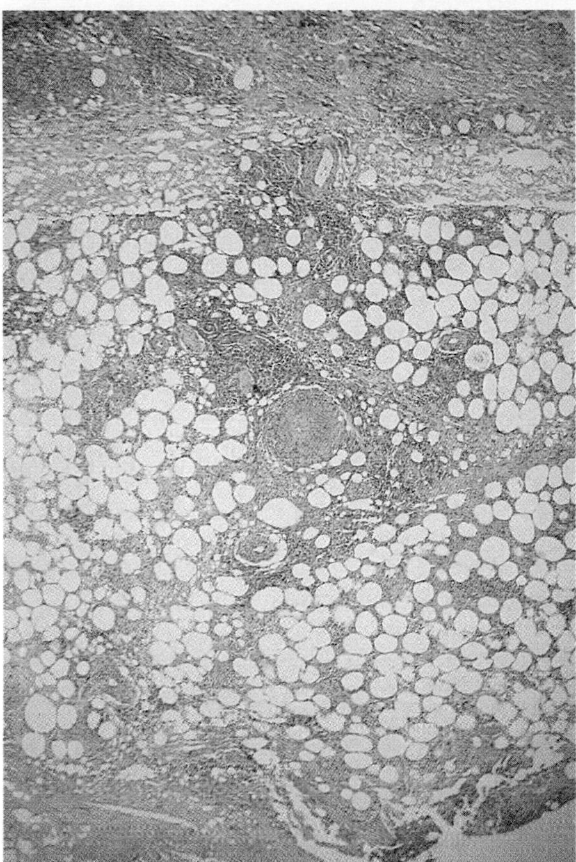

Fig. 71-196 Nodular vasculitis. The inflammation is centered around medium-sized arteries in the fat lobules. Lymphocytic infiltrates predominate in the fat. In subcutaneous polyarteritis nodosa, neutrophils infiltrate in segments of the walls of the arteries.

Histiocytic cytophagic panniculitis

Histiocytic cytophagic panniculitis is a rare form of panniculitis that can be fatal and usually affects middle-aged patients and approximately twice as many females as males. The patients have nodules and plaques in the subcutaneous fat, which tend to ulcerate. They have fever, hepatosplenomegaly, lymphadenopathy, anemia, thrombocytopenia, and elevation of products of degradation of fibrin in the blood. The disease results in death in approximately 70% of patients, usually from massive gastrointestinal hemorrhage and liver failure.[334-336] The cause is unknown.

PATHOLOGY. The subcutaneous lesions contain an inflammatory infiltrate that involves both the septa and the lobules of adipocytes. The infiltrate consists of small lymphocytes, macrophages, and often hemorrhage and necrosis, which obscures the distinctive changes. The characteristic finding is the presence of many macrophages that are enlarged and contain fragments of phagocytized lymphocytes, erythrocytes, neutrophils, and other inflammatory cells.

The differential diagnosis includes sinus histiocytosis with massive lymphadenopathy (*Rosai-Dorfman disease*),[337] which may involve the subcutaneous tissues in approximately 8% of patients.[338] It also has distinctive large phagocytic histiocytes containing lymphocytes and plasma cells. In contrast, the macrophages of Rosai-Dorfman disease contain S-100 protein, whereas the macrophages of histiocytic cytophagic anniculitis do not show S-100 protein. The histiocytes of both of these diseases lack cytologic atypia that is present in malignant histiocytosis. The relationship to terminal *hemophagocytic syndromes* associated with subcutaneous T-cell lymphomas[339] and infections[340] is controversial,[341,342] but these postinfectious syndromes usually do not have panniculitis.

Panniculitis secondary to systemic connective tissue disease

Lupus erythematosus. *Lupus erythematosus* can involve the panniculus without inflammation in the overlying dermis.[343] These patients present with deep, indurated, painful nodules that have slight overlying erythema and tend to resolve with depressed scars.

PATHOLOGY. There is a lymphocytic infiltrate in the lobules of the subcutis and often in the septa as well, with frequent formation of germinal centers. Plasma cells are also observed. The fat undergoes necrosis and has a eosinophilic amorphous ("hyalin") material between the necrotic cells. The overlying skin has deposition of immunoglobulins at the dermoepidermal junction in approximately 50% of cases.

Rheumatoid nodule. Rheumatoid arthritis patients develop *rheumatoid nodules* in the subcutis at pressure points, such as the elbows, hands, and feet. They are movable, deep nodules up to several centimeters in diameter.

PATHOLOGY. The subcutis contains a zone of extensive necrosis filled with fibrin and cellular debris and surrounded by numerous macrophages that usually form a palisade around the regions of necrosis. Mucin accumulation is not evident in routine sections, and instead the necrosis has a deep red color on eosin staining. In some patients, the lesions may extend into the dermis and can ulcerate. This lesion has to be differentiated from "pseudorheumatoid nodule," that is, *granuloma annulare*. Nonpalisaded forms of rheumatoid nodule also occur and can mimic a neutrophilic dermatosis.[344]

Scleroderma and morphea. Scleroderma and morphea can start in the septa of the subcutis, with induration and immobility of the skin.

PATHOLOGY. The lesions show homogeneous, thickened collagen bundles in widened septa in the subcutis. In most cases, the disease also involves the deep reticular dermis in a similar fashion. Fibrin and mucin deposition are generally inapparent in routine sections. The differential diagnosis includes *eosinophilic fasciitis* (Shulman's syndrome).[345-348]

Other causes of panniculitis

Pancreatic enzyme–induced fat necrosis is caused by circulating lipases released from an inflamed pancreas. The fat necrosis can occur in many locations including the subcutis. The fat cells undergo necrosis and lysis of their nuclei and cytoplasm. The lipases convert the triglycerides into fatty acids and glycerol. The fatty acids bind calcium and also stain with hematoxylin to produce a bluish color to the necrotic adipose tissue. A neutrophilic inflammatory infiltrate is an early response.

Traumatic or factitial panniculitis has rupture of the fat cells with release of the fat into the extracellular spaces and connective tissue, where a macrophage reaction is elicited. Lipases are not sufficiently involved to convert the triglycerides into the bluish deposits seen in the pancreatic enzyme-induced panniculitis. Clues to the diagnosis of factitial panniculitis are in the presence of coagulative necrosis of the overlying epidermis, thrombosis of blood vessels, and the deposition of polarizable foreign material at injection sites.

In newborns, two types of distinctive lobular panniculitis can occur. One is catastrophic and is named "sclerema neonatorum." In this disease, the infant often is born prematurely, and the crystallization temperature of the fat is near to room temperature. The fat hardens quickly, with rupture of the fat cells. The children usually die rather quickly in a few days, and so secondary changes of inflammation are rather sparse. Histologic sections show fat cells with many radiating arrays of crystals within them. The other form is minor and is named subcutaneous fat necrosis of the newborn. This is related to birth trauma, and nodules of fat necrosis appear within a few days of birth. On histologic examination, there is a mixed inflammatory infiltrate in the lobules, containing macrophages and lymphocytes with rare neutrophils. A few fat cells also contain radiating arrays of crystals, indicating that some of the fat contains saturated fatty acids with crystallization temperatures near room temperature.

Neoplasms

The neoplastic diseases of the subcutaneous fat are generally the same as those that affect fatty tissues throughout the body and are described in Chapter 73. Several distinctively cutaneous lesions do occur and are described briefly here.

Subcutaneous T-cell lymphoma

Subcutaneous T-cell lymphoma is an unusual form of T-cell lymphoma that causes deep nodules in the subcutis without particular involvement of the overlying dermis.[339,349,350] These nodules are movable, painless tumors that may spontaneously regress and reappear over a course of many years before showing systemic involvement.

PATHOLOGY. The lesions have a dense lymphoid infiltrate in the lobules and in the septa of the panniculus, without the hyalinized necrosis of lupus erythematosus. The identification of this "panniculitis" as a lymphoma is based on cytologic atypism of the lymphocyte nuclei and on gene rearrangement studies that have shown clonal rearrangements of the T-cell receptor beta-chain gene. If a hemophagocytic syndrome occurs, these lesions resemble histiocytic cytophagic panniculitis except for the greater atypism of the lymphocyte nuclei in subcutaneous T-cell lymphoma.

Leukemic panniculitis

"Leukemic panniculitis" refers to extensive infiltration of the panniculus by leukemic cells, either of myeloid or lymphoid origin.[281] The patients present with induration and erythema of the skin.

PATHOLOGY. The lesions show a diffuse infiltration throughout the adipose tissue lobules by leukemic cells. There is very little if any necrosis of the fat lobules, which distinguishes these infiltrations from a true panniculitis. Most of these leukemias differ from hypersensitivity reactions to medications by their cellular atypia and by the leukemic infiltrate being very diffuse, whereas the hypersensitivity reactions are concentrated around the blood vessels.[282]

ACKNOWLEDGMENTS

We thank Dr. Eduardo Fonseca-Capdevila, Servicio de Dermatología, Hospital "La Paz," Madrid for his generous contributions of clincial photographs for our chapter. We also thank Dr. Herschel S. Zackheim, University of California, San Francisco, for clinical photographs of patients with mycosis fungoides.

REFERENCES

General

1. Lever WF, Schaumburg-Lever G: *Histopathology of the skin,* ed 7, Philadelphia, 1990, Lippincott.
2. Farmer ER, Hood AF: *Pathology of the skin,* Norwalk, Conn., 1990, Appleton & Lange.

Diseases mainly involving the epidermis

Genodermatoses and developmental disorders

3. Pearson RW: Clinicopathologic types of epidermolysis bullosa and their nondermatologic complications, *Arch Dermatol* 124:718, 1988.
4. Lin AN, Carter DM: *Epidermolysis bullosa: basic and clinical aspects,* New York, 1992, Springer-Verlag.
5. Rand R, Baden HP: Commentary: Darier-White disease, Arch Dermatol 119:81, 1983.
6. Steffen CG: Familial benign chronic pemphigus, *Am J Dermatopathol* 9:58, 1987.
7. Williams ML: The ichthyoses—pathogenesis and prenatal diagnosis: a review of recent advances, *Pediatr Dermatol* 1:1, 1983.
8. Ishida-Yamamoto A, McGrath JA, Judge MR et al: Selective involvement of keratins K1 and K10 in the cytoskeletal abnormality of epidermolytic

hyperkeratosis (bullous ichthyosiform erythroderma), J Invest Dermatol 99:19, 1992.
9. Fuchs E: Genetic skin disorders of keratin, *J Invest Dermatol* 99:671, 1992.
10. Williams ML, Elias PM: From basket weave to barrier: unifying concepts for the pathogenesis of disorders of cornification, *Arch Dermatol* 129:626, 1993.
11. Otsuka F, Shima A, Ishibashi Y: Porokeratosis as a premalignant condition of the skin: cytologic demonstration of abnormal DNA ploidy in cells of the epidermis, *Cancer* 63:891, 1989.
12. Kraemer KH, Lee MM, Scotto J: Xeroderma pigmentosum: cutaneous, ocular and neurologic abnormalities in 830 published cases, *Arch Dermatol* 123:241, 1987.
13. Bos JL: *ras* oncogenes in human cancer: a review, *Cancer Res* 49:4682, 1989.
14. Brash DE, Rudolph JA, Simon JA et al: A role for sunlight in skin cancer: UV-induced p53 mutations in squamous cell carcinoma, *Proc Natl Acad Sci USA* 88:10124, 1991.

Inflammatory, metabolic, and traumatic disorders

15. Kahn G, Rywlin AM: Acropustulosis of infancy, *Arch Dermatol* 115:831, 1979.
16. Jarratt M, Ramsdell W: Infantile acropustulosis, *Arch Dermatol* 115:834, 1979.
17. Sneddon IB, Wilkinson DS: Subcorneal pustular dermatosis, *Br J Dermatol* 100:61, 1979.
18. Dugan EM, Anhalt GJ, Diaz LA: Pemphigus. In Jordon RE, editor: *Immunologic diseases of the skin,* East Norwalk, Conn., 1991, Appleton & Lange.
19. Jensen PJ, Baird J, Morioka S et al: Epidermal plasminogen activator is abnormal in cutaneous lesions, *J Invest Dermatol* 90:777, 1988.
20. Hu C-H, Michel B, Farber EM: Transient acantholytic dermatosis (Grover's disease): a skin disorder related to heat and sweating, *Arch Dermatol* 121:1439, 1985.
21. Brownstein MH: Acantholytic acanthoma, *J Am Acad Dermatol* 19:783, 1988.
22. Brown J, Winkelmann RK: Acanthosis nigricans: a study of 90 cases, *Medicine* 47:33, 1968.
23. Rendon MI, Cruz PD Jr, Sontheimer RD, Bergstresser PR: Acanthosis nigricans: A cutaneous marker of tissue resistance to insulin, *J Am Acad Dermatol* 21:461, 1989.
24. Hamilton D, Tavafoghi V, Shafer JC, Hambrick GW Jr: Confluent and reticulated papillomatosis of Gougerot and Carteaud. Its relation to other papillomatoses, *J Am Acad Dermatol* 2:401, 1980.
25. Nordlund JJ: Vitiligo. In Thiers BH, Dobson RL, editors: *Pathogenesis of skin disease,* New York, 1986, Churchill Livingstone.

Infectious diseases

26. Barton LL, Freidman AD: Impetigo: a reassessment of etiology and therapy, *Pediatr Dermatol* 4:185, 1987.
27. Elias PM, Fritsch P, Epstein EH Jr: Staphylococcal scalded skin syndrome: clinical features, pathogenesis, and recent microbiological and biochemical developments, *Arch Dermatol* 113:207, 1977.
28. Lyell A: The staphylococcal scalded skin syndrome in historical perspective: emergence of dermopathic strains of *Staphylococcus aureus* and discovery of the epidermolytic toxin, *J Am Acad Dermatol* 9:285, 1983.
29. Kwon-Chung KJ, Bennett JE: *Medical mycology,* Philadelphia, 1992, Lea and Febiger.
30. Lutzner MA: The human papillomaviruses, *Arch Dermatol* 119:631, 1983.
31. Wade TR, Kopf AW, Ackerman AB: Bowenoid papulosis of the genitalia, *Arch Dermatol* 115:306, 1979.
32. Patterson JW, Kao GF, Graham JH, Helwig EB: Bowenoid papulosis: a clinicopathologic study with ultrastructural observations, *Cancer* 57:823, 1986.
33. Gross G, Hagedorn M, Ikenberg H et al: Bowenoid papulosis: presence of human papillomavirus (HPV) structural antigens and of HPV 16–related DNA sequences, *Arch Dermatol* 121:858, 1985.

Neoplasms of the epidermis

34. Braun-Falco O: Zur Histogenese der Verruca seborrhoica. I. Mitteilung: Einleitung, histologische, und histochemische Befunde, *Arch Klin Exp Dermatol* 216:615, 1963.
35. Braun-Falco O, Kint A, Vogell W: Zur Histogenese der Verruca seborrhoica. II. Mitteilung: elektronenmikroskopische Befunde, *Arch Klin Exp Dermatol* 217:627, 1963.
36. Weedon D: Systemic pathology, In *The skin,* vol 9, New York, 1992, Churchill Livingstone.
37. Rampen FHJ, Schwengle LEM: The sign of Leser-Trélat: does it exist, *J Am Acad Dermatol* 21:50, 1989.
38. Murphy GF, Elder DE: *Atlas of tumor pathology: non-melanocytic tumors of the skin,* Washington, DC, 1991, Armed Forces Institute of Pathology.
39. Crum CP: Vulvar intraepithelial neoplasia: the concept and its application, *Hum Pathol* 13:187, 1982.
40. Voet RL: Classification of vulvar dystrophies and premalignant squamous lesions, *J Cutan Pathol* 21:86, 1994.
41. Shea CR, McNutt NS, Volkenandt M et al: Overexpression of p53 protein in basal cell carcinomas of human skin, *Am J Pathol* 141:25, 1992.
42. Jones RE, Austin C, Ackerman AB: Extramammary Paget's disease: a critical reexamination, *Am J Dermatopathol* 1:101, 1979.
43. Guarner J, Cohen C, DeRose PB: Histogenesis of extramammary and mammary Paget cells: an immunohistochemical study, *Am J Dermatopathol* 11:313, 1989.
44. Maize JC, Ackerman AB: *Pigmented lesions of the skin: clinicopathologic correlations,* Philadelphia, 1987, Lea & Febiger.
45. Horlick HP, Walther RR, Zegarelli DJ et al: Mucosal melanotic macule, reactive type: a simulation of melanoma, *J Am Acad Dermatol* 19:786, 1988.
46. Elder DE, Murphy GF: *Melanocytic tumors of the skin. Atlas of tumor pathology,* series 3, fasc 2, Washington, DC, 1991, Armed Forces Institute of Pathology.
47. Rhodes AR, Harrist TJ, Momtaz-T K: The PUVA-induced pigmented macule: a lentiginous proliferation of large, sometimes cytologically atypical, melanocytes, *J Am Acad Dermatol* 9:47, 1983.
48. Tong AKF, Murphy GF, Mihm MC Jr: Dysplastic nevus: a formal histogenetic precursor of malignant melanoma. In Mihm MC Jr, Murphy GF, Kaufman N, editors: *Pathobiology and recognition of malignant melanoma,* Baltimore, 1988, Williams & Wilkins.
49. Mihm MC Jr, Googe PB: *Problematic pigmented lesions: a case method approach,* Philadelphia, 1990, Lea & Febiger.
50. NIH Consensus Development Panel on Early Melanoma: NIH Consensus Conference: Diagnosis and treatment of early melanoma, *JAMA* 268:1314, 1992.
51. Koh HK: Cutaneous melanoma, *N Engl J Med* 325:171, 1991.
52. Phillips ME, Margolis RJ, Merot Y et al: The spectrum of minimal deviation melanoma: a clinicopathologic study of 21 cases, *Hum Pathol* 17:796, 1986.
53. Wick MR, Swanson PE, Rocamora A: Recognition of malignant melanoma by monoclonal antibody HMB-45: an immunohistochemical study of 200 paraffin-embedded cutaneous tumors, *J Cutan Pathol* 154:201, 1988.
54. McNutt NS, Urmacher C, Hoss DM, Lugo JR: La utilidad del anticuerpo monoclonal HMB-45 en el diagnóstico de las lesiones melanocíticas, *Patología* 24:93, 1991.
55. Skelton HG III, Smith KJ, Barrett TL et al: HMB-45 staining in benign and malignant melanocytic lesions: a reflection of cellular activation, *Am J Dermatopathol* 13:543, 1991.
56. Smoller BR: Immunohistochemistry in the diagnosis of malignant melanoma, *Clin Dermatol* 9:235, 1991.
57. Burg G, Braun-Falco O: *Cutaneous lymphomas, pseudolymphomas, and related disorders,* Berlin, 1983, Springer-Verlag.
58. Sánchez JL, Ackerman AB: The patch stage of mycosis fungoides: criteria for histologic diagnosis, *Am J Dermatopathol* 1:5, 1979.
59. Darier J, Sabouraud R, Gougerot R et al: *Nouvelle Pratique dermatologique,* Paris, 1936, Masson et cie, pg. #1/286.
60. Degos R: *Dermatologie,* Paris, 1953, Flammarion Medecine-Sciences, p 906a.
61. Besnier E, Brocq L, Jacquet L: *La pratique dermatologique,* Paris, 1902, Masson et cie, p #3/547.
62. Edelson RL: Cutaneous T-cell lymphoma: mycosis fungoides, Sézary syndrome and other variants, *J Am Acad Dermatol* 2:89, 1980.

63. Wood GS, Weiss LM, Warnke RA, Sklar J: The immunopathology of cutaneous lymphomas: immunophenotypic and immunogenotypic characteristics, *Semin Dermatol* 5:334, 1986.
64. Wood GS, Hong SR, Sasaki DT et al: Leu-8/CD7 antigen expression by CD3 + T-cells: comparative analysis of skin and blood in mycosis fungoides/Sézary syndrome relative to normal blood values, *J Am Acad Dermatol* 22:602, 1990.
65. Smoller BR, Stewart M, Warnke R: A case of Woringer-Kolopp disease with Ki-1 (CD30)$^+$ cytotoxic/suppressor cells, *Arch Dermatol* 128:526, 1992.

Diseases involving both the epidermis and dermis

Genodermatoses

66. Roberts WM, Jenkins JJ, Moorhead ELII, Douglass EC: Incontinentia pigmenti, a chromosomal instability syndrome, is associated with childhood malignancy, *Cancer* 62:2370, 1988.

Inflammatory, metabolic, and traumatic disorders

67. Baer RL: The mechanisms of allergic contact sensitivity. In Fisher AA, editor: *Contact dermatitis*, ed. 3, Philadelphia, 1986, Lea & Febiger.
68. Hanafin JM: Atopic dermatitis, *J Am Acad Dermatol* 6:1, 1982.
69. Arnold HA Jr, Odom RB, James WD: *Andrew's diseases of the skin: clinical dermatology*, ed 8, Philadelphia, 1990, Saunders.
70. Gollhausen R, Ring J: Allergy to coined money: nickel contact dermatitis in cashiers, *J Am Acad Dermatol* 25:365, 1991.
71. Sirot G: Nummular eczema, *Semin Dermatol* 2:68, 1983.
72. Kligman AM, Leyden JJ: Seborrheic dermatitis, *Semin Dermatol* 2:57, 1983.
73. Gammon WR: Bullous pemphigoid. In Jordon RE, editor: *Immunologic diseases of the skin*, Norwalk, Conn., 1991, Appleton & Lange.
74. Gammon WR, Kowalewski C, Chorzelski TP et al: Direct immunofluorescence studies of sodium choride–separated skin in the differential diagnosis of bullous pemphigoid and epidermolysis bullosa acquisita, *J Am Acad Dermatol* 22:664, 1990.
75. Fine J-D: Cicatricial and localized pemphigoid. In Jordon RE, editor: *Immunologic diseases of the skin*, Norwalk, Conn., 1991, Appleton & Lange.
76. Shornick JK: Herpes gestationis, *J Am Acad Dermatol* 17:539, 1987.
77. Zone JJ: Dermatitis herpetiformis. In Jordon RE, editor: *Immunologic diseases of the skin*, Norwalk, Conn., 1991, Appleton & Lange.
78. Karpati S, Meurer M, Stolz W et al: Dermatitis herpetiformis bodies: ultrastructural study on the skin of patients using direct preembedding immunogold labeling, *Arch Dermatol* 126:1469, 1990.
79. Baden LA, Apovian C, Imber MJ, Dover JS: Vancomycin-induced linear IgA bullous dermatosis, *Arch Dermatol* 124:1186, 1988.
80. Ackerman AB, Penneys NS, Clark WH Jr: Erythema multiforme exudativum: distinctive pathological process, *Br J Dermatol* 84:554, 1971.
81. Patterson JW, Parsons JM, Blaylock WK et al: Eosinophils in skin lesions of erythema multiforme, *Arch Dermatol* 113:36, 1989.
82. Tonnesen MG, Harrist TJ, Wintroub BU, Mihm MC Jr et al: Erythema multiforme: microvascular damage and infiltration of lymphocytes and basophils, *J Invest Dermatol* 80:282, 1983.
83. Avakian R, Flowers FP, Araujo OE, Ramos-Caro FA: Toxic epidermal necrolysis: a review, *J Am Acad Dermatol* 25:69, 1991.
84. Bastuji-Garin S, Rzany B, Stern RS et al: Clinical classification of cases of toxic epidermal necrolysis, Stevens-Johnson syndrome, and erythema multiforme, *Arch Dermatol*129:92, 1993.
85. Van Voorhees A, Stenn KS: Histological phases of Bactrim-induced fixed drug eruption: the report of one case, *Am J Dermatopathol* 9:528, 1987.
86. Smoller BR, Luster AD, Krane JF et al: Fixed drug eruptions: evidence for a gamma-interferon mediated process, *J Cutan Pathol* 18:13, 1991.
87. Shiohara T, Nickoloff BJ, Sagawa Y et al: Fixed drug eruption: expression of epidermal keratinocyte intercellular adhesion molecule-1 (ICAM-1), *Arch Dermatol* 125:1371, 1989.
88. Braun-Falco O, Plewig G, Wolff HH, Winkelmann RK: *Dermatology*, Berlin, 1991, Springer-Verlag.
89. Soeprono FF, Schinella RA, Cockerell CJ, Comite SL: Seborrheic-like dermatitis of acquired immunodeficiency syndrome: a clinicopathologic study, *J Am Acad Dermatol* 14:242, 1986.
90. McNutt NS, Urmacher C: Las erupciones papuloescamosas del síndrome de inmunodeficiencia adquirida (SIDA), *Patología* 23:3, 1990.
91. Smoller BR, McNutt NS, Gray MH et al: Detection of interferon-gamma–induced protein 10 in psoriasiform dermatitis of acquired immunodeficiency syndrome, *Arch Dermatol* 126:1457, 1990.
92. Gottlieb AB: Immunologic mechanisms in psoriasis, *J Am Acad Dermatol* 18:1376, 1988.
93. Gottlieb AB, Kreuger JG: HLA region genes and immune activation in the pathogenesis of psoriasis, *Arch Dermatol* 126:1083, 1990.
94. Gibson LE, Perry HO: Papulosquamous eruptions and exfoliative dermatitis. In Moschella SL, Hurley HJ, editors: *Dermatology*, ed 3, Philadelphia, 1992, Saunders.
95. Griffiths WAD: Pityriasis rubra pilaris, *Clin Exp Dermatol* 5:105, 1980.
96. Samman PD: The natural history of parapsoriasis en plaques (chronic superficial dermatitis) and prereticulotic poikiloderma, *Br J Dermatol* 87:405, 1972.
97. King-Ismael D, Ackerman AB: Guttate parapsoriasis/digitate dermatosis (small plaque parapsoriasis) is mycosis fungoides, *Am J Dermatopathol* 14:518, 1992.
98. Bennaman O, Sánchez JL: Comparative clinicopathological study on pityriasis lichenoides chronica and small plaque parapsoriasis, *Am J Dermatopathol* 10:189, 1988.
99. Longley J, Demar L, Feinstein RP et al: Clinical and histologic features of pityriasis lichenoides et varioliformis acuta in children, *Arch Dermatol* 123:1335, 1987.
100. Ashworth J, Paterson WD, MacKie RM: Lymphomatoid papulosis/pityriasis lichenoides in two children, *Pediatr Dermatol* 4:238, 1987.
101. Muhlbauer JE, Bhan AK, Harrist TJ et al: Immunopathology of pityriasis lichenoides acuta, *J Am Acad Dermatol* 10:783, 1984.
102. Benmaman O, Sánchez JL: Comparative clinicopathological study on pityriasis lichenoides chronica and small plaque parapsoriasis, *Am J Dermatopathol* 10:189, 1988.
103. Danbolt N: Acrodermatitis enteropathica, *Br J Dermatol* 100:37, 1979.
104. Niemi KM, Anttila PH, Kanerva L, Johannson E: Histopathological study of transient acrodermatitis enteropathica due to decreased zinc in breast milk, *J Cutan Pathol* 16:382, 1989.
105. Kheir SM, Omura EF, Grizzle WE et al: Histologic variation in the skin lesions of the glucagonoma syndrome, *Am J Surg Pathol* 10:445, 1986.
106. Feingold KR, Elias PM: Endocrine-skin interactions. cutaneous manifestations of pituitary disease, thyroid disease, calcium disorders, and diabetes, *J Am Acad Dermatol* 17:921, 1987.
107. Ive FA, Magnus IA, Warin RP, Wilson Jones E: "Actinic reticuloid": a chronic dermatosis associated with severe photosensitivity and histological resemblance to lymphoma, *Br J Dermatol* 81:469, 1969.
108. Norris PG, Morris J, Smith NP et al: Chronic actinic dermatitis: an immunohistologic and photobiologic study, *J Am Acad Dermatol* 21:966, 1989.
109. Kerl H, Smolle J: Pseudolymphomas of the skin. In Friedman RJ, Rigel DS, Kopf AW, et al, editors: *Cancer of the skin*, Philadelphia, 1991, Saunders.
110. Thomsen K: The development of Hodgkin's disease in a patient with actinic reticuloid, *Clin Exp Dermatol* 21:109, 1977.
111. Boyd AS, Neldner KH: Lichen planus, *J Am Acad Dermatol* 25:593, 1991.
112. Patterson JW: The spectrum of lichenoid dermatitis, *J Cutan Pathol* 18:67, 1991.
113. Ridley CM: Lichen sclerosis et atrophicus, *Semin Dermatol* 8:54, 1989.
114. Patterson JAK, Ackerman AB: Lichen sclerosis et atrophicus is not related to morphea, *Am J Dermatopathol* 6:323, 1984.
115. Aberer E, Stanek G: Histological evidence for spirochetal origin of morphea and lichen sclerosis et atrophicans, *Am J Dermatopathol* 9:374, 1987.
116. García-Bravo B, Sánchez-Pedreño P, Rodríguez-Pichardo A, Camacho F: Lichen sclerosis et atrophicus: a study of 76 cases and their relation to diabetes, *J Am Acad Dermatol* 19:482, 1988.
117. Sontheimer RD, Euwer RL, Geppert TD, Cohen SB: Connective tissue diseases. In Moschella SL, Hurley HJ, editors. *Dermatology*, ed 3, Philadelphia, 1992, Saunders.
118. Provost TT, Talal N, Harley JB et al: The relationship between Anti-Ro (SS-A) antibody-positive Sjögren's syndrome and Anti-Ro (SS-A) antibody-positive lupus erythematosus, *Arch Dermatol* 124:63, 1988.
119. Jerdan JS, Hood AF, Moore GW, Callen JP: Histopathologic comparison of the subsets of lupus erythematosus, *Arch Dermatol* 126:52, 1990.

120. Harrist TJ, Mihm MC Jr: The specificity and clinical usefulness of the lupus band test, *Arthritis Rheum* 23:479, 1980.

121. Gilliam JN, Prystowsky SD: Mixed connective tissue disease syndrome, *Arch Dermatol* 113:583, 1977.

122. Bentley-Phillips CB, Geake TMS: Mixed connective tissue disease characterized by speckled epidermal nuclear IgG deposition in normal skin, *Br J Dermatol* 102:529, 1980.

123. Dalakas MC: Polymyositis, dermatomyositis, and inclusion body myositis, *N Engl J Med* 325:1487, 1991.

124. Callen JP, Hyla JF, Bole GG Jr, Kay DR: The relationship of dermatomyositis and polymyositis to internal malignancy, *Arch Dermatol* 116:295, 1980.

125. Hood AF, Soter NA, Rappeport J, Gigli I: Graft-versus-host reaction: cutaneous manifestations following bone marrow transplantation, *Arch Dermatol* 113:1087, 1977.

126. Mauduit G, Claudy A: Cutaneous expression of graft-vs-host disease in man, *Semin Dermatol* 7:149, 1988.

127. Hymes SR, Hood AF, Farmer ER: Graft-versus-host disease. In Jordon RE, editor: *Immunologic diseases of the skin,* Norwalk, Conn., 1991, Appleton & Lange.

128. Guillen FJ, Ferrara J, Hancock WW et al: Acute cutaneous graft-versus-host disease to minor histocompatibility antigens in a murine model: evidence that large granular lymphocytes are effector cells in the immune response, *Lab Invest* 137:1874, 1986.

129. Friedman KJ, LeBoit PE, Farmer ER: Acute follicular graft-vs-host reaction: a distinct clinicopathologic presentation, *Arch Dermatol* 124:688, 1988.

130. Spielvogel RL, Goltz RW, Kersey JH: Scleroderma-like changes in chronic graft vs host disease, *Arch Dermatol* 113:1424, 1977.

131. Patterson JW: The perforating disorders, *J Am Acad Dermatol* 10:561, 1984.

132. Patterson JW: Progress in the perforating dermatoses, *Arch Dermatol* 125:1121, 1989.

133. Mehregan AH: Elastosis perforans serpiginosa: a review of the literature and report of 11 cases, *Arch Dermatol* 97:381, 1968.

134. Santa Cruz DJ: Chondrodermatitis nodularis helicis: a transepidermal perforating disorder, *J Cutan Pathol* 7:70, 1980.

135. Yancey KB, Hall RP, Lawley TJ: Pruritic urticarial papules and plaques of pregnancy: clinical experience with twenty-five patients, *J Am Acad Dermatol* 10:473, 1984.

136. Black MM: Prurigo of pregnancy, papular dermatitis of pregnancy, and pruritic folliculitis of pregnancy, *Semin Dermatol* 8:23, 1989.

137. Earhart RN, Aeling JA, Nuss DD, Mellette JR: Pseudo-Kaposi's sarcoma, *Arch Dermatol* 110:907, 1974.

138. McNutt NS, Fletcher V, Conant MA: Early lesions of Kaposi's sarcoma in homosexual men: an ultrastructural comparison with other vascular proliferations in skin, *Am J Pathol* 111:62, 1983.

139. Shalita AR, Leyden JE Jr, Pochi PE, Strauss JS: Acne vulgaris, *J Am Acad Dermatol* 16:410, 1987.

140. Norris JFB, Cunliffe WJ: A histological and immunocytochemical study of early acne lesions, *Br J Dermatol* 118:651, 1988.

141. Helm KF, Menz J, Gibson LE, Dicken CH: A clinical and histopathologic study of granulomatous rosacea, *J Am Acad Dermatol* 25:1038, 1991.

142. Nunzi E, Rebora A, Hamerlinck F, Cormane RH: Immunopathological studies on rosacea, *Br J Dermatol* 103:543, 1980.

143. Manna V, Marks R, Holt P: Involvement of immune mechanisms in the pathogenesis of rosacea, *Br J Dermatol* 107:203, 1982.

144. Ofuji S, Atsuhiko O, Horio T et al: Eosinophilic pustular folliculitis, *Acta Dermatol Venereol (Stockh)* 50:195, 1970.

145. Ofuji S: Eosinophilic pustular folliculitis, *Dermatologica* 174:53, 1987.

146. Buchness MR, Lim HW, Hatcher VA et al: Eosinophilic pustular folliculitis in the acquired immunodeficiency syndrome: treatment with ultraviolet B phototherapy, *N Engl J Med* 318:1183, 1988.

147. Rosenthal D, LeBoit PE, Klumpp L, Berger TG: HIV-associated eosinophilic folliculitis: a unique dermatosis associated with advanced HIV infection, *Arch Dermatol* 127:206, 1990.

148. Nickoloff BJ, Wood C: Benign idiopathic versus mycosis-fungoides–associated follicular mucinosis, *Pediatr Dermatol* 2:201, 1985.

149. Gibson LE, Muller SA, Leiferman KM, Peters MS: Follicular mucinosis: clinical and histopathological study, *J Am Acad Dermatol* 20:441, 1989.

150. Sentis HJ, Willemze R, Scheffer E: Alopecia mucinosa progressing into mycosis fungoides: a long term follow-up study of two patients, *Am J Dermatopathol* 10:478, 1988.

Infectious diseases

151. Tunnessen WW Jr: Practical aspects of bacterial skin infections in children, *Pediatr Dermatol* 2:255, 1985.

152. Greene SL, Su WPD, Muller SA: Ecthyma gangrenosum: report of clinical, histopathologic, and bacteriologic aspects of eight cases, *J Am Acad Dermatol* 11:781, 1984.

153. Fleming MG, Milburn PB, Prose NS: *Pseudomonas* septicemia with nodules and bullae, *Pediatr Dermatol* 4:18, 1987.

154. Shatin H, Canizares O, Ladany E: Reiter's syndrome and keratosis blennorrhagica, *Arch Dermatol* 81:551, 1960.

155. Keat A: Reiter's syndrome and reactive arthritis in perspective, *N Engl J Med* 309:1606, 1983.

156. Duvic M, Johnson TM, Rapini RP, Freese T et al: Acquired immunodeficiency syndrome–associated psoriasis and Reiter's syndrome, *Arch Dermatol* 123:1622, 1987.

157. Reveille JD, Conant MA, Duvic M: Human immunodeficiency virus–associated psoriasis, psoriatic arthritis, and Reiter's syndrome: a disease continuum, *Arthritis Rheum* 33:1574, 1990.

158. Roberts DT, Tuyp E: Onychomycosis, *Semin Dermatol* 4:222, 1985.

159. Moschella SL, Hurley HJ: *Dermatology,* ed 2, Philadelphia, 1985, Saunders.

160. Piot P, Plummer FA, Mhalu FS et al: AIDS: an international perspective, *Science* 239:573, 1988.

161. Kaplan MH, Sadick NS, McNutt NS et al: Dermatologic findings and manifestations of acquired immunodeficiency syndrome (AIDS), *J Am Acad Dermatol* 16:485, 1987.

162. Sadick NS, McNutt NS: Cutaneous hypersensitivity reactions in patients with AIDS, *Int J Dermatol* 32:621, 1993.

163. Kaplan MH, Sadick NS, McNutt NS et al: Acquired ichthyosis in concomitant HIV-1 and HTLV-II infection: a new association with intravenous drug abuse, *J Am Acad Dermatol* 29:701, 1993.

164. Cooper DA, Gold J, MacLean P et al: Acute AIDS retrovirus infection: definition of a clinical illness associated with seroconversion, *Lancet* 1:537, 1985.

165. Tschachler E, Groh V, Popovic P et al: Epidermal Langerhans cells: a target for HTLV-III/LAV infection, *J Invest Dermatol* 88:233, 1987.

166. Cameron PU, Freudenthal PS, Barker JM et al: Dendritic cells exposed to human immunodeficiency virus type-1 transmit a vigorous cytopathic infection to CD4[+] T-cells, *Science* 257:383, 1992.

167. Spiegel H, Herbst H, Niedobitek G et al: Follicular dendritic cells are a major reservoir for human immunodeficiency virus type 1 in lymphoid tissues facilitating infection of CD4[+] T-helper cells, *Am J Pathol* 140:15, 1992.

168. Pantaleo G, Graziosi C, Fauci AS: The immunopathogenesis of human immunodeficiency virus infection, *N Engl J Med* 328:327, 1993.

Neoplasms

169. Kwa RE, Campana K, Moy RL: Biology of cutaneous squamous cell carcinoma, *J Am Acad Dermatol* 26:1, 1992.

170. Campbell C, Quinn AG, Ro Y-S et al: p53 mutations are common and early events that precede tumor invasion in squamous cell neoplasia of the skin, *J Invest Dermatol* 100:746, 1993.

171. Nagano T, Ueda M, Ichihashi M: Expression of p53 protein is an early event in ultraviolet light-induced cutaneous squamous cell carcinogenesis, *Arch Dermatol* 129:1157, 1993.

172. Hodak E, Jones RE, Ackerman AB: Solitary keratoacanthoma is a squamous cell carcinoma: three examples with metastases, *Am J Dermatopathol* 15:332, 1993.

173. Tsuboi R, Yamaguchi T, Kurita Y et al: Comparison of proteinase activities in squamous cell carcinoma, basal cell epithelioma, and seborrheic keratosis, *J Invest Dermatol* 90:869, 1988.

174. McArdle JP, Roff BT, Müller HK: Characterization of retraction spaces in basal cell carcinoma using an antibody to type IV collagen, *Histopathology* 8:447, 1984.

72 Soft-Tissue Tumors

Markku Miettinen
Sharon W. Weiss

INTRODUCTION

Soft tissue is defined as the nonskeletal connective tissues of the body, excluding supporting tissues of the internal organs, glia, and hematopoietic tissues. Soft-tissue tumors are generally classified according to their resemblance to the presumptive normal mesenchymal cell counterparts (Table 72-1). They arise nearly everywhere in the body, the most important locations being the extremities, trunk, and abdominal cavity. Soft-tissue tumors originating in internal organs are discussed in the appropriate respective chapters.

It is presumed that sarcomas arise from uncommitted mesenchymal cells that have the potential to differentiate along a given cell line. In some instances the tumors recapitulate the development of normal differentiated mesenchymal cell types. For example, leiomyosarcomas arising in the smooth muscles of internal organs apparently arise from the same precursor cells as the smooth muscle cells. In other instances the sarcoma assumes a phenotype unrelated to the cells found in the local tissues. For example, rhabdomyosarcoma of the urinary bladder does not have a local normal-cell counterpart.

Most sarcomas arise deep in soft tissue and grow in an expansile fashion, flattening normal tissue around them creating a so-called pseudocapsule. In actuality the pseudocapsule is often penetrated by tumor cells that extend well beyond the visible tumor mass. Such multiple satellite tumor cells are the source of local recurrences when tumors are simply shelled out or enucleated during surgical removal. Sarcomas spread by way of hematogenous rather than lymphatic routes, and the most common site of metastatic lesions is the lungs, with the liver and bones the next most common sites.

Incidence. Benign soft-tissue tumors such as lipomas, hemangiomas, and dermatofibromas (benign fibrous histiocytomas) are among the most common neoplasms in human beings. Their incidence is difficult to determine because these lesions do not necessarily come to medical attention. In the hospital-based population they outnumber malignant tumors by 100 to 1.

Soft-tissue sarcomas are rare. The American Cancer Society estimated that about 6000 new cases of cancer of connective tissue would be diagnosed in 1992; of these, 3300 (55%) would be fatal.[1] If sarcomas of internal organs are added to these numbers, soft-tissue sarcomas would then constitute approximately 1% of all malignant tumors. In comparison, 181,000 cases of breast carcinomas and 120,000 cases of lung cancer were projected for 1992. The recent increase in the incidence of soft-tissue sarcomas in the western world appears to be explained by the increase incidence of acquired immune deficiency syndrome (AIDS)–associated Kaposi's sarcoma.[2]

Soft-tissue sarcomas occur in subjects of all ages, but the overall incidence rises with advancing age. Congenital sarcomas are rare. However, certain types of sarcomas (rhabdomyosarcoma and small round cell sarcoma) are seen predominantly in children and adolescents. Others are most prevalent in young adults (synovial sarcoma and clear cell sarcoma), and malignant fibrous histiocytoma, the most common type of sarcoma, is usually seen in older persons. A slight male predominance (55%-60%) has been observed in many population-based series of patients with sarcoma.

Table 72-1 The World Health Organization classification of soft tissue tumors*

Fibrous tissue tumors
Benign
Fibroma
Keloid
Nodular fasciitis
Proliferative fasciitis
Proliferative myositis
Elastofibroma
Fibrous hamartoma of infancy
Myofibromatosis, solitary and multicentric
Fibromatosis colli
Calcifying aponeurotic fibroma
Hyalin fibromatosis
Fibromatosis
Superficial fibromatosis
  Palmar and plantar fibromatosis
  Infantile digital fibromatosis (digital fibroma)
Deep fibromatosis
  Abdominal fibromatosis (desmoid tumor)
  Extraabdominal fibromatosis (desmoid tumor)
  Intraabdominal and mesenteric fibromatosis
  Infantile fibromatosis
Malignant
Fibrosarcoma
  Adult fibrosarcoma
  Congenital or infantile fibrosarcoma
Fibrohistiocytic tumors
Benign
Fibrous histiocytoma
  Cutaneous histiocytoma (dermatofibroma)
  Deep histiocytoma
Juvenile xanthogranuloma
Reticulohistiocytoma
Xanthoma
Intermediate
Atypical fibroxanthoma
Dermatofibrosarcoma protuberans
Pigmented dermatofibrosarcoma protuberans (Bednar tumor)
Giant cell fibroblastoma
Plexiform fibrohistiocytic tumor
Angiomatoid fibrous histiocytoma
Malignant
Malignant fibrous
  Storiform-pleomorphic type
  Myxoid type
  Giant cell type
  Xanthomatous (inflammatory) type
Lipomatous tumors
Benign
Lipoma
Lipoblastoma (fetal lipoma)
Lipomatosis
Angiolipoma
Spindle cell lipoma/pleomorphic lipoma
Angiomyolipoma
Myelolipoma
Hibernoma
Atypical lipoma
Malignant
Well-differentiated liposarcoma
  Lipoma-like type
  Sclerosing type
  Inflammatory type
Myxoid liposarcoma
Round cell liposarcoma (poorly differentiated myxoid liposarcoma)
Pleomorphic liposarcoma
Dedifferentiated liposarcoma
Smooth muscle tumors
Benign
Leiomyoma
Angiomyoma
Epithelioid leiomyoma
Leiomyomatosis peritonealis disseminata
Malignant
Leiomyosarcoma
Epithelioid leiomyosarcoma
Skeletal muscle tumors
Benign
Rhabdomyoma
  Adult
  Genital
  Fetal
Malignant
Rhabdomyosarcoma
  Embryonal rhabdomyosarcoma
  Botryoid rhabdomyosarcoma
  Spindle cell rhabdomyosarcoma
  Alveolar rhabdomyosarcoma
  Pleomorphic rhabdomyosarcoma
  Rhabdomyosarcoma with ganglionic differentiation (ectomesenchymoma)
Endothelial tumors of blood and lymph vessels
Benign
Papillary endothelial hyperplasia
Hemangioma
  Capillary hemangioma
  Cavernous hemangioma
  Venous hemangioma
  Epithelioid hemangioma (angiolymphoid hyperplasia, histiocytoid hemangioma)
  Pyogenic granuloma (granulation tissue–type hemangioma)
  Acquired tufted hemangioma (angioblastoma)

(continued)

Etiology. Little is known about specific causes of soft-tissue sarcomas, although numerous physical and chemical factors have been implicated. Etiologic factors or clinical associations of pathogenetic significance are known for only a small percentage of the cases of soft-tissue sarcomas.

Ionizing radiation is probably the most important known external etiologic factor linked to the development of soft-tissue (and bone) sarcomas. In approximately 1%-3% of patients undergoing radiation therapy, a sarcoma will develop 5 to 15 years later. Histologically these tumors are of diverse types; the most common types are malignant fibrous histiocytoma, fibrosarcoma, and extraskeletal osteosarcoma.[3,4] Occasional angiosarcomas, chondrosarcomas, and peripheral nerve sheath sarcomas have been reported. The use of Thorothrast, an x-ray contrast medium containing radioactive thorium oxide, has been followed by the development of hepatic angiosarcoma in many patients; other forms of liver cancer have also been found in these patients. Although Thorotrast is

Table 72-1 The World Health Organization classification of soft tissue tumors*—cont'd

Lymphangioma	Malignant granular cell tumor
Lymphangiomyoma, lymphangiomyomatosis	Clear cell sarcoma (malignant melanoma of soft parts)
Angiomatosis, lymphangiomatosis	Malignant melanotic schwannoma
Intermediate: hemangioendothelioma	Neuroblastoma
Spindle cell hemangioendothelioma	Ganglioneuroblastoma
Endovascular papillary angioendothelioma (Dabska tumor)	Neuroepithelioma (peripheral neuroectodermal tumor, peripheral neuroblastoma)
Epithelioid hemangioendothelioma	**Paraganglionic tumors**
Malignant	Benign paraganglioma
Angiosarcoma (including lymphangiosarcoma)	Malignant paraganglioma
Kaposi's sarcoma	**Cartilage and bone tumors**
Perivascular tumors	***Benign***
Benign	Panniculitis ossificans
Benign hemangiopericytoma	Myositis ossificans
Glomus tumor	Fibrodysplasia (myositis) ossificans progressiva
Malignant	Extraskeletal chondroma
Malignant hemangiopericytoma	Extraskeletal osteochondroma
Malignant glomus tumor	Extraskeletal osteoma
Synovial tumors	***Malignant***
Benign	Extraskeletal chondrosarcoma
Tenosynovial giant cell tumor	Well-differentiated chondrosarcoma
Localized	Myxoid chondrosarcoma
Diffuse (extra-articular pigmented villonodular synovitis)	Mesenchymal chondrosarcoma
Malignant	Dedifferentiated chondrosarcoma
Malignant tenosynovial giant cell tumor	Extraskeletal osteosarcoma
Neural tumors	**Pluripotential mesenchymal tumors**
Benign	Benign mesenchymoma
Traumatic neuroma	Malignant mesenchymoma
Morton's neuroma	**Miscellaneous tumors**
Neuromuscular hamartoma	***Benign***
Nerve sheath ganglion	Congenital granular cell tumor
Schwannoma (neurilemoma)	Tumoral calcinosis
Plexiform schwannoma	Myxoma
Cellular schwannoma	Cutaneous myxoma
Degenerated (ancient) schwannoma	Intramuscular myxoma
Neurofibroma	Angiomyxoma
Diffuse neurofibroma	Amyloid tumor
Plexiform neurofibroma	Parachordoma
Pacinian neurofibroma	Ossifying fibromyxoid tumor
Epithelioid neurofibroma	Juvenile angiofibroma
Granular cell tumor	Inflammatory myofibroblastic tumor (inflammatory fibrosarcoma)
Melanocytic schwannoma	***Malignant***
Neurothekeoma (nerve sheath myxoma)	Alveolar soft-part sarcoma
Ectopic meningioma	Epithelioid sarcoma
Ectopic ependymoma	Extraskeletal Ewing's sarcoma
Ganglioneuroma	"Synovial" sarcoma, biophasic, and monophasic fibrous type
Pigmented neuroectodermal tumor of infancy (retinal anlage tumor, melanotic progonoma)	Malignant (extrarenal) rhabdoid tumor
Malignant	Desmoplastic small round cell tumor of children and young adults
Malignant peripheral nerve sheath tumor (MPNST) (malignant schwannoma, neurofibrosarcoma)	
MPNST with rhabdomyosarcoma (malignant Triton tumor)	
MPNST with glandular differentiation	
Epithelioid MPNST	

Mesothelial tumors are excluded from this table.

no longer used, late side effects are still occasionally encountered.[5,6]

Numerous *chemicals* have been either suspected on epidermiologic grounds or proved to be linked to the development of sarcomas. Chlorophenoxyacetic acid herbicides, including 2,4-D and 2,4,5-T, and dioxins present as their contaminants, have been suggested to have a role in the development of sarcoma on the basis of epidemiologic evidence. However, results from studies of larger cohorts of patients such as American soldiers exposed to dioxin-contaminated phenoxyherbicides (Agent Orange in Vietnam) have not confirmed such a risk.[7,8] Vinyl chloride, used in rubber manufacturing, has been linked to the development of angiosarcoma of the liver.[6]

Animal tumor models have shed some light on the nature of chemical carcinogenesis, but the extrapolation of experimental data to the setting of human cancer should be done with caution. Known carcinogens, such as polycyclic hydrocarbons and hydroxyquinolines may cause sarcomas in laboratory rodents. Ethylnitrosourea has been used to produce experimental tumors in both the central and peripheral nervous system.[9]

Trauma has been anecdotally implicated in the pathogenesis of sarcomas, but in most of these cases the trauma may have only called attention to a preexisting tumor. Rarely, severe blunt or sharp trauma has been followed by the local development of a sarcoma with a delay between the time of the injury and development of the tumor in keeping with a possible etiologic relationship. Sarcomas have been noted to develop in chronic tropical ulcers[10] and occasionally at sites of implanted foreign bodies such as shrapnel and bullets.[11]

Viral carcinogenesis has not been documented in human cases of sarcoma. Although the viral origin of chicken fibrosarcoma was demonstrated by Rous in the early 1900s, no viruses have been isolated so far from human sarcomas. However, very recently herpesvirus-like sequences have been demonstrated in AIDS-associated Kaposi's sarcoma, but the etiologic role of the virus remains to be proved.[12]

Chronic lymphedema, either congenital or acquired, may precede the local development of angiosarcoma. Most commonly this occurs after mastectomy for breast carcinoma (Stewart-Treves syndrome). It has been suggested that diseases or conditions causing lymphedema with poor flow in lymphatics leads to impaired circulation of lymphocytes and faulty local immunosurveillance, permitting the proliferation of the malignant cells. Alternatively, the retention of carcinogens in the obstructed lymphatics has been implicated.[13]

A *hereditary predisposition* to the development of soft-tissue sarcomas may be more common than previously thought, as revealed by recent genetic research. Neurofibromatosis type 1 (von Recklinghausen's disease) is a relatively common hereditary condition inherited in an autosomal dominant fashion. The gene for neurofibromatosis type 1, shown to be a tumor suppressor gene, has been localized to chromosome 17. This disease is associated with the development of multiple neurofibromas, and nerve sheath sarcomas may develop in 1% to 5% of affected patients.[14] In a familial cancer syndrome (Li-Fraumeni syndrome), there is a high incidence of various carcinomas and other malignant tumors in the relatives of children with soft-tissue sarcoma, usually rhabdomyosarcoma. Germline deletion of the tumor suppressor gene p53 has been identified in patients with this syndrome.[15] Certain benign tumors are associated with hereditary conditions, such as hemihypertrophy (lipomas) and Gardner's syndrome (mesenteric desmoid tumors plus gastrointestinal tract adenomatosis).

Acquired genetic alterations are evidently the root cause of most cases of malignant transformation. These changes are gradually being discovered as the specific gene lesions responsible for the chromosomal changes are being identified. A common theme for many sarcomas such as alveolar rhabdomyosarcoma and Ewing's sarcoma is the formation of a fusion gene and a pathologic fusion transcript as a result of the chromosomal translocation. Many of the genes involved are transcriptional regulators.[16]

Specimen handling and reporting

Open biopsy usually precedes the radical surgical removal of soft-tissue sarcomas. Needle biopsy and fine-needle aspiration biopsy yield limited material, which may be satisfactory for the evaluation of recurrent or metastatic lesions, but this usually does not permit a comprehensive evaluation of an unknown process. Intraoperative frozen sections are used most successfully to evaluate the adequacy of biopsy material and excision margins but are used less frequently as a guide to the immediate definitive treatment of a previously undiagnosed tumor.

In all instances, the need for special diagnostic techniques should be anticipated upon arrival of the specimen. Aliquots of tissue snap-frozen or fixed in glutaraldehyde ensure the availability of optimal material for immunohistochemical studies or electron microscopy (EM), respectively. Snap-frozen (or fresh) tissue is also the optimal preparation for DNA flow cytometry, and fresh tissue placed in cell culture media is the optimal preparation for cytogenetic analysis.

The exterior surface of the resection specimen should be marked with ink to facilitate evaluation of the surgical margins when pertinent. Gross examination should include measurement of the tumor and determination of its location and growth pattern in relation to normal tissue components (bones, major nerves, and vessels, when applicable). The tumor should be sliced systematically, and the presence of grossly different components and necrosis should be noted and these included in the histologic samples. Ideally one block per each centimeter of the tumor diameter should be examined. This routine should be followed at least for those tumors for which the differential diagnosis includes benign and malignant tumor.

Ancillary diagnostic procedures

Although many tumors can be diagnosed on the basis of the findings yielded by hematoxylin-eosin staining, special studies are often necessary for the accurate diagnosis of soft-tissue tumors. The most useful auxiliary techniques are immunohistochemical studies, cytogenetic analysis, staining with selected histochemical stains, and EM.

Histochemical stains. The relative importance of many histochemical stains has decreased since more specific methods, such as immunohistochemical techniques, have become available. Periodic acid–Schiff (PAS) staining with and without diastase digestion can determine whether and how much glycogen is present, which varies in different sarcomas. Ewing's sarcoma, rhabdomyosarcoma, leiomyosarcoma, and cartilage tumors are rich in glycogen, but fibroblastic, fibrohistiocytic, and neural tumors typically do not contain it. The reticulin fibers assume a characteristic pattern, as demonstrated by various silver impregnation methods in some types of tumors such as hemangiopericytoma. Masson-Fontana staining for melanin may help in the identification of metastatic melanoma and clear cell sarcoma, although immunohistochemical tests are now more specific and sensitive. Argyrophilic stains such as Grimelius' stain can be used to demonstrate neuroendocrine granules in neural and neuroendocrine tumors. Differences between fibrous and muscular tissue can be highlighted with trichrome stains such as van Gieson's and Masson's trichrome stains.

Electron microscopy. EM is most useful in the identification and differential diagnosis of particular types of neoplasms, such as small round cell tumors, muscle cell tumors (rhabdomyosarcoma and leiomyosarcoma), and Schwann cell tumors[17,18] (Table 72-2). In addition to purely diagnostic applications, EM provides information about the nature of many tumors. Structures of diagnostic significance include neuroen-

Table 72-2 The most important ultrastructural features of soft-tissue tumors

Fibrohistiocytic tumors
Features of other specific cell types excluded
Fibroblasts and myofibroblasts in variable numbers, some cells with multiple lysosomes
Histiocytes (representing reactive components)
Liposarcoma
Cytoplasmic lipid droplets, variably developed basement membranes, fibroblast-like general features
Endothelial neoplasms
Weibel-Palade bodies (progressive loss in poorly differentiated tumors), pinocytic vesicles, abundant intermediate filaments, vasoformation
Leiomyosarcoma
Actin filaments with dense bodies, variably developed basement membranes, pinocytic vesicles, intermediate filaments, glycogen
Rhabdomyosarcoma
Combination of thin and thick filaments, variably developed sarcomeres, glycogen, basement membranes
Schwannoma
Cell processes with prominent, often reduplicated basement membranes, fibroblast-like cytoplasmic features
Clear cell sarcoma
Melanosomes (often), basement membranes possible
Chondrosarcoma
Scalloped margins of cells, prominent rough endoplasmic reticulum, cytoplasmic glycogen
Synovial sarcoma
Biphasic: glands surrounded by basement membranes and lumens lined by microvilli
Monophasic: frequent cell junctions, primitive glandular formations
Epithelioid sarcoma
Abundant intermediate filaments, keratin-like bundles of filaments, complex cellular outlines

docrine granules, basement membrane material, pinocytic vesicles, actin filaments, Z-bands, accumulations of glycogen, melanosomes, Weibel-Palade bodies, and specific crystals. Unfortunately, only limited numbers of cellular and extracellular components are specific to the cell type and may be lost in less-differentiated tumors. In addition, sampling of diagnostic components is of critical importance but may be difficult in a practical sense. Although the reliable identification of melanosomes and Weibel-Palade bodies requires that material be optimally fixed, cytoplasmic filaments such as those in rhabdomyosarcoma are resistant to damage caused by tissue processing and can be identified in specimens reprocessed from paraffin-embedded tissue.

Immunohistochemical tests. Antigens that are more or less specific for epithelial, endothelial, muscle, and neural cells are among the most useful markers in the evaluation of soft-tissue tumors.[19] The most important antigens and their distribution in soft-tissue sarcomas are summarized in Table 72-3. The application of panels of antibodies that address the different diagnostic possibilities is highly recommended. The specificity and sensitivity of each marker should be acknowledged. For example, although keratins are markers for epithelial differentiation and are consistently seen in synovial sarcoma and epithelioid sarcoma, they may be present in other sarcomas as well. Many antigens, formerly endorsed as histiocytic markers, such as alpha$_1$-antitrypsin and alpha$_1$-antichymotrypsin, are widespread, limiting their value in the identification of histiocytic tumors. Specific applications of immunohistochemical tests are cited in the discussion of different tumors.

DNA flow cytometry. The assessment of DNA-ploidy and S-phase volume (synthesis phase during which chromosome replication occurs) has been shown to provide prognostically useful information for some types of soft-tissue sarcoma. For example, aneuploidy has been proved to be a negative prognostic indicator in cases of synovial sarcoma and in cases of certain high-grade sarcoma. Well-differentiated tumor types, which show only chromosomal translocations and not numerical alterations of chromosomes, are uniformly diploid, and flow cytometry is thus less useful in evaluating them. DNA flow cytometry cannot differentiate between benign and malignant tumors.

Cytogenetics. The development of accurate chromosomal identification and short-term cell culture techniques has enabled the collection of voluminous cytogenetic data on soft-tissue tumors during the past 10 years.[20,21] Successful use of these techniques requires the availability of viable tumor tissue for cell culture and the subsequent evaluation of chromosomal preparations of mitotic cells. Typical clonal (nonrandom) chromosomal translocations have been found in many soft-tissue tumors, and some of these are constant enough to be considered diagnostic of certain tumor entities, for example, the translocation t(12;16) in myxoid liposarcoma (Table 72-4). Cytogenetic data are not only helpful in the diagnosis of certain tumor types but also contribute to a better understanding of the neoplastic process as the specific gene alterations responsible for the cytogenetic changes are identified. Many sarcomas, such as malignant fibrous histiocytoma and leiomyosarcoma, show complex cytogenetic changes; in such situations it has not yet been possible to pinpoint any pathogenetically important or primary genetic changes. Numerical changes in the chromosomal pattern and a few other changes in tumors can be detected in tissue sections or cell smears of tumors by fluorescent in situ hybridization using specific gene probes.

Molecular genetics. In some cases the specific genetic changes can be analyzed using DNA or RNA isolated from the tumor tissue. Many translocations in sarcomas lead to the formation of a fusion transcript by two intact genes and also lead to the expression of a pathologic fusion protein. Many such fusion transcripts, such as the *EWS-FLI1* from the t(11;22) translocation in Ewing's sarcoma and the *PAX3-FKHR* from the t(2;13) translocation in alveolar rhabdomyosarcoma, can be used as diagnostic markers and identified by the reverse transcriptase polymerase chain reaction, starting with RNA extracted from the tumor tissue[16,22].

Grading and staging of sarcomas

The histologic grade should be provided as a part of each sarcoma diagnosis, because this is used to guide decisions concerning adjuvant therapy. Several histologic grading schemes for sarcomas have been proposed, but none is uniformly accepted.[23-29] They employ various combinations of criteria, such as the degree of cellularity, the mitotic index, the presence or absence of necrosis, and the level of cellular atypia, as judged by light microscopy. However, in most grading

Table 72-3 The most important immunohistochemical markers in soft-tissue tumors and their patterns of reactivity

Vimentin
Intermediate-filament protein of mesenchymal cells in general
Nearly ubiquitous in soft-tissue tumors
Suggested as a marker for evaluation of the preservation of immunoreactivity
Desmin
Intermediate-filament protein of the muscle cell type
Most smooth muscle cells and striated muscle cells positive, some myofibroblasts, some cells in fibromatosis
Almost all leiomyosarcomas and rhabdomyosarcomas positive, also heterologous striated muscle in multidirectional tumors (Triton tumors)
Desmoplastic small round cell tumor
Actins
A family of ubiquitous microfilament proteins. Different subsets have cell type–selective distribution
Alpha-actins specific for smooth muscle
Sarcomeric actin in striated muscle and rhabdomyosarcomas
Muscle actin antibodies react with alpha- and gamma-actins (HHF-35)
Smooth and striated muscle, leiomyosarcomas and rhabdomyosarcomas
Myofibroblasts and their tumors also positive
Glial fibrillary acidic protein
Intermediate-filament protein of glial cells, present in some benign schwannomas
Keratins (cytokeratins)
A group of intermediate-filament proteins typically present in epithelial cells but now also known to be present in some mesenchymal cells, including transformed fibroblasts and smooth muscle cells (keratins 8, 18, and 19)
Synovial sarcoma (mainly epithelium-like cells), epithelioid sarcoma, chordoma, rhabdoid tumor regularly positive
Leiomyosarcomas variably positive
Many tumors such as malignant peripheral nerve sheath sarcoma and epithelioid angiosarcoma and some malignant fibrous histiocytomas may contain positive cells
Epithelial membrane antigen
Relatively widespread in different epithelia, perineurial cells, and perineurial cell tumors
Synovial sarcoma, epithelioid sarcoma positive, sporadic reactivity in leiomyosarcoma, myxoid chondrosarcoma
S-100 protein
Schwann cells, melanocytes
Infiltrating Langerhans' cells (small numbers present in most tumors)
Schwannoma, neurofibroma (focal), granular cell tumor
Malignant peripheral nerve sheath sarcoma (variably positive)
Clear cell sarcoma, malignant melanoma
Liposarcoma (variable, present in differentiated cells and lipoblasts)
Cartilaginous components of soft-tissue tumors, chordoma
Melanoma-specific antigen (HMB-45 antibody)
Neoplastic and proliferative melanocytes
Clear cell sarcoma malignant melanoma
Smooth muscle component of angiomyolipoma and lymphangiomyoma
von Willebrand factor (factor VIII–related antigen)
Endothelial cells
Well-differentiated endothelial cell tumors
Some angiosarcomas
CD31 (platelet endothelium cell adhesion molecule)
Endothelial cells, hemangiomas, angiosarcoma, Kaposi's sarcoma
CD34 (myeloid progenitor cell antigen)
Endothelial cells, some fibroblasts
Angiosarcoma, Kaposi's sarcoma, epithelioid sarcoma, dermatofibrosarcoma protuberans, solitary fibrous tumor, gastrointestinal tract stromal tumors, some leiomyosarcomas
CD68 (KP1 and PG-M1 antibodies)
Histiocytes, myeloid cells
Some malignant fibrous histiocytomas, some melanomas
Granular cell tumor, pheochromocytoma
Angiomatoid fibrous histiocytoma
CD99 (HBA71 antibody, p30/32 antigen)
Cortical thymocytes (T-cells), Langerhans islet cells
Ewing's sarcoma, lymphoblastic lymphoma
Neuron-specific enolase
Neural cells, neuroblastic and paraganglionic tumors, some (smooth) muscle cells and their tumors
Clear cell sarcoma, malignant melanoma

Table 72-4 Typical chromosome translocations in soft-tissue sarcomas and the resulting corresponding gene fusions

Tumor type	Translocation	Resulting gene fusion	Reference
Extraskeletal Ewing's sarcoma	t(11;22)(q24;q12)	*EWS-FLI1**	16, 22, 398, 406
	t(21;22)(q22;q12)	*EWS-ERG**	16
Desmoplastic small round cell tumor	t(11;22)(p13;q12)	*EWS-WT1**	16, 415
Alveolar rhabdomyosarcoma	t(2;13)(q35;q14)	*PAX3-FKHR**	16, 22
	t(1;13)(p36;q14)	*PAX7-FKHR**	16, 22
Myxoid liposarcoma	t(12;16)(q13;p11)	*CHOP-TLS*	165
Synovial sarcoma	t(X;18)(p11,2;q11.2)	*SYT-SSX*	435
Clear cell sarcoma	t(12;22)(q13;q12.2-12.3)	None known	367a
Extraskeletal myxoid chondrosarcoma	t(9;22)(q22;q12)	None known	391

*Reverse transcription polymerase chain reaction test available for diagnosis of the translocation. Note that Ewing's sarcoma and alveolar rhabdomyosarcoma have two alternative translocations.

schemes the histologic type by itself grades the tumor, obviating the need for further analysis of the histologic features. For example, pure myxoid liposarcoma is uniformly a low-grade tumor, whereas alveolar rhabdomyosarcoma and Ewing's sarcoma are high-grade tumors. A full spectrum of grades can be observed for fibrosarcoma, leiomyosarcoma, and peripheral nerve sheath sarcoma.

Clinical staging consists of the clinical evaluation of the extent of tumor spread as well as radiologic assessment using computed tomography and magnetic resonance imaging. The essential features include tumor size, the pattern of local spread, and the presence of local or distant metastastic tumors. Whether the tumor is confined to a soft-tissue compartment defined by fascial planes (compartmental or extracompartmental) is also important to the planning of the surgical strategy. In some staging schemes, a high histologic grade connotes a higher-stage tumor.

FIBROBLASTIC LESIONS

Benign fibroblastic tumors and tumorlike lesions

Fibroblastic tumors encompass a variety lesions ranging from purely reactive conditions secondary to injury to fibrosarcomas having the ability to both recur and metastasize. Fibromatoses fall midway in the spectrum and have the ability to recur locally but do not metastasize.

Fibroma is the designation for lesions composed of relatively mature fibroblasts that occur in several clinical settings. A *nuchal fibroma* is a collagen-rich benign fibroblastic lesion that arises in the subcutis of the posterior aspect of the neck. *Fibroma of the tendon sheath* is a nodular, sometimes polypoid tumorlike proliferation within the tendon sheath. The lesion occurs in the hands and feet of adults, and although entirely benign, it may recur locally.[30-32] Histologically it consists of nodules of scattered to moderately dense uniform fibroblasts embedded in a dense collagen matrix. Slitlike vascular spaces are typical and may divide the lesion into lobules. EM shows a mixture of fibroblasts and myofibroblasts, as is seen in many other fibroblastic lesions. Because transitional forms between this tumor and giant cell tumor of the tendon sheath and nodular fasciitis occur, fibroma of the tendon sheath has been proposed in some cases to represent a late stage of nodular fasciitis or giant cell tumor of the tendon sheath.[30]

Solitary/localized fibrous tumor (fibroma) of the pleura may develop in soft tissues other than those on serous surfaces, especially in the mediastinum and the head and neck area. This tumor is usually benign and is discussed in detail among the tumors of the pleura.

A *keloid* is an exaggerated scar that forms at sites of minor trauma, chronic inflammation, surgical scars or burn injuries.[33] The single most common site is the earlobe and develops after ear piercing. Keloids have a greater tendency to develop in blacks. Keloids vary in size from a small nodule to a lesion up to several centimeters in diameter. This nonneoplastic lesion consists of sparse fibroblasts and thick bundles of glassy, eosinophilic collagen fibers in a slightly myxoid stroma.

Nodular fasciitis is the designation for a tumorlike reactive spindle cell proliferation that can be confused with a sarcoma.[34-38] It is more common in young adults but also occurs in older adults. Typically it first appears as a small (1-3 cm in diameter), rapidly enlarging, mildly painful subcutaneous nodule in the upper extremity, especially the forearm. Although most lesions are superficial, they may extend to the fascia or present as an intramuscular mass that may be confused with a soft-tissue sarcoma.

Histologically, nodular fasciitis is composed of enlarged spindled to rounded cells in a richly vascular myxoid background containing extravasated erythrocytes, variable lymphocytic infiltration, and newly formed collagen fibers (Fig. 72-1, *A*). The cells resemble tissue culture fibroblasts in that they have enlarged but regular nuclei with prominent nucleoli. Multinucleated giant cells may occur. Mitotic figures may be numerous, but atypical forms are seldom present. The histologic appearance changes as the lesion ages. A lesion of short duration is likely to show a more cellular appearance with brisk mitotic activity, whereas older lesions are less cellular, hyalinized, and cystic. EM reveals myofibroblastic features in a large proportion of tumor cells.[39] Immunohistochemically the cells are positive for muscle-specific types of actin, which is consistent with their myofibroblastic nature.[40]

Variants of nodular fasciitis have been described that differ principally in their manner of presentation. These include *cranial fasciitis,* which involves the scalp of infants and may cause erosion of the underlying skull bone.[41] *Parosteal fasciitis* occurs adjacent to bones,[42] and *intravascular fasciitis* develops within the lumen of veins,[43] usually in the head and neck

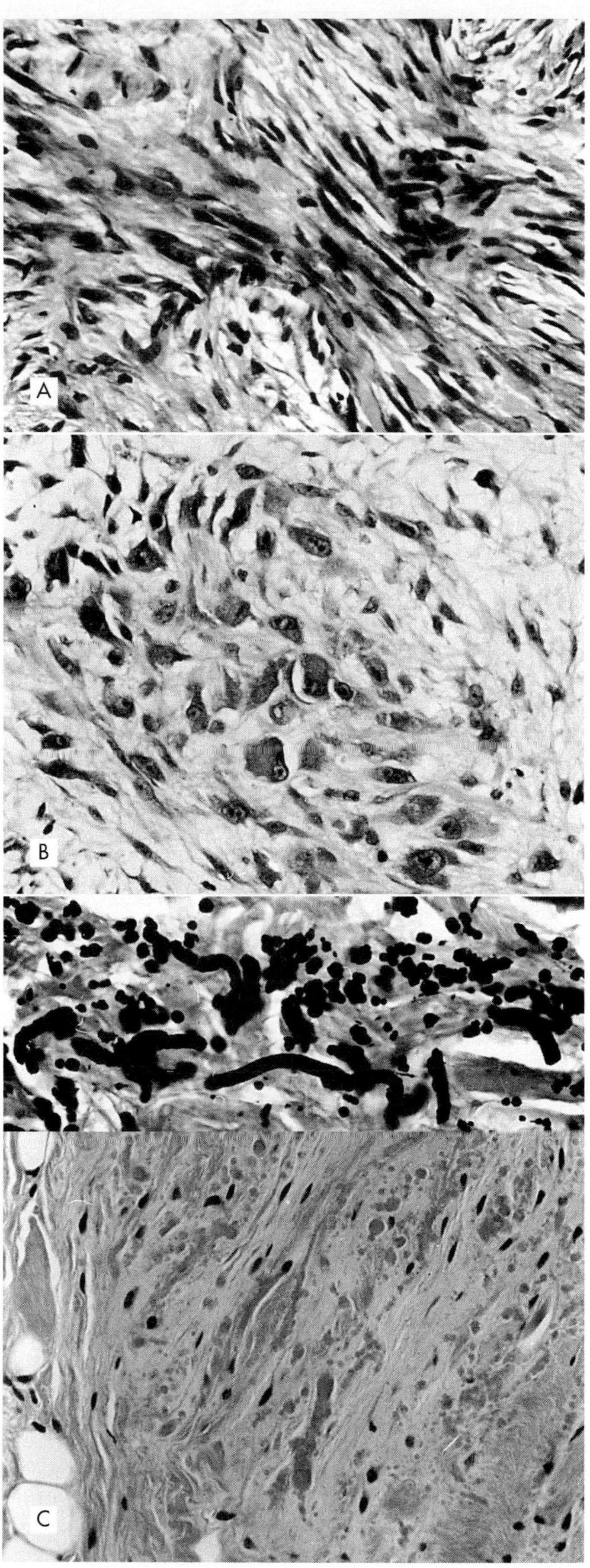

area. It should be noted that *eosinophilic fasciitis* is not a variant of nodular fasciitis but a peculiar inflammatory lesion characterized by infiltrates of eosinophilic granulocytes in fascia. It is associated with scleroderma.[44,45]

Proliferative fasciitis and proliferative myositis are reactive fibrous lesions that have similar histologic features.[46-48] The former arises at the fascial level, the latter within the muscles, typically in middle-aged persons. These lesions resemble nodular fasciitis in their proliferative spindle cell component and myxoid background but also contain ganglion cell–like cells with large nuclei and prominent nucleoli (Fig. 72-1, *B*). These cells appear to be modified fibroblasts containing ultrastructurally prominent rough endoplasmic reticulum.[49]

Retroperitoneal fibrosis is a midline sclerosing process that binds the retroperitoneal structures and may cause ureteral obstruction.[50] Historically methysergide use was linked to the development of retroperitoneal fibrosis in some cases. In patients with aortic aneurysms, retroperitoneal fibrosis has been thought to develop as an autoallergic reaction to atheromatous material. Histologically the lesion contains variably cellular, densely collagenous fibrous tissue mixed with an inflammatory infiltrate rich in plasma cells and lymphocytes. Mediastinal fibrosis (sclerosing mediastinitis) and Riedel's fibrosing thyroiditis are believed to be closely related lesions.

Elastofibroma is a nonneoplastic, probably degenerative condition that typically and almost exclusively occurs on the thoracic wall at the lower end of the scapula.[51-53] The lesion is seen in adults, mostly elderly women. Manual labor that involves repetitive movement of the scapula has been proposed as the cause. An autopsy study revealed that similar lesions of microscopic size exist in up to 15% of the population.[54] Elastofibroma forms an ill-defined tumorlike mass, which histologically consists of scattered fibroblasts, collagen fibers, fat cells, and large amounts of coarse, serrated elastic fibers of variable sizes that can be highlighted with elastin stains (Fig. 72-1, *C*).

Fibrous hamartoma of infancy usually occurs in the axillary soft tissue or in the proximal parts of the extremities during the first year of life, more commonly in boys.[55] The lesion is poorly circumscribed and usually measures 3 to 5 cm in diameter. Histologically it consists of collections of cellular fibrous tissue traversing fibroadipose tissue and of nodules of immature-appearing fibroblasts in a myxoid stroma (Fig. 72-2, *A*). There is no mitotic activity, and the lesion is completely benign, although it may occasionally recur.

Myofibroma presents as small (1-2 cm in diameter) solitary or multiple (myofibromatosis), dermal, subcutaneous, or sometimes deep intramuscular nodules, usually in small children; rarely similar lesions have been noted in adults.[56] An autosomal dominant mode of inheritance has been suggested on the basis of its familial occurrence in some cases.[57] The condition is almost always benign and self-limited, but generalized forms with internal organ involvement occur rarely. In such cases the tumor may compromise pulmonary function and be lethal; such variants have been previously classified as "generalized fibrosarcoma." Histologically the lesions consist

Fig. 72-1 **A,** Nodular fasciitis showing cellular spindle cell proliferation with myxoid stroma. **B,** Proliferative fasciitis showing ganglion cell–like cells in a fibromyxoid stroma. **C,** Elastofibroma composed of coarse, fragmented elastic fibers in fibrofatty tissue. Detail shows elastic fibers outlined with elastica–van Gieson stain.

of a peripheral zone of spindle cells resembling smooth muscle cells and arranged in nodules. These zones blend with a central zone composed of fibroblast-like cells sometimes showing a hemangiopericytoma-like pattern. Immunohistochemical evidence (desmin positivity) has been interpreted as a sign of its smooth muscle cell differentiation.[58]

Calcifying aponeurotic fibroma (Keasbey's tumor) is a rare tumor that is usually located in the palms and fingers and typically occurs in children and young adults.[59,60] Its locally aggressive behavior can be accounted for by its infiltration into the subcutis and muscle. It does not metastasize, however. The tumor usually measures less than 3 cm in diameter and grossly is ill-defined. Microscopically it shows focal calcifications or cartilage-like areas surrounded by rounded cells that are sometimes arranged in a cordlike fashion (Fig. 72-2, *B*). A fibromatosis-like spindle cell component may also be present.[60]

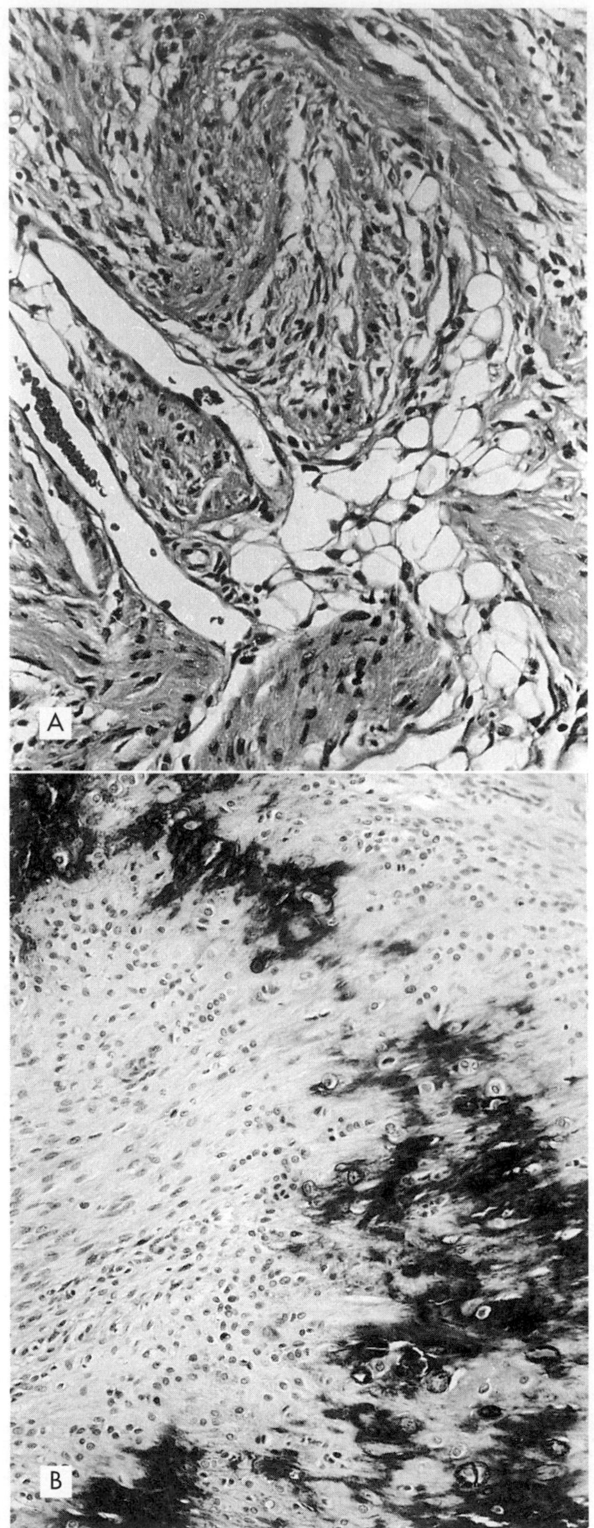

Fig. 72-2 **A,** Fibrous hamartoma of infancy showing cellular fibrous proliferation with streaks of fat cells and less-differentiated mesenchymal cells. **B,** Calcifying aponeurotic fibroma shows calcified foci surrounded by round and spindle cells in a fibrous background. The lesion bears slight resemblance to cartilage.

Fibromatoses

Fibromatosis is the term given to a group of differentiated fibroblastic lesions with locally infiltrative features.[61] Fibromatoses in adults are divided into two groups: a deep (desmoid tumor) and a superficial (palmar and plantar) form that vary in their clinical presentation and biologic behavior.

Desmoid (aggressive or musculoaponeurotic fibromatosis), previously commonly classified as low-grade fibrosarcoma, has three distinct clinicopathologic variants that are distinguished on the basis of their location.[62-66] Approximately half of the cases are abdominal desmoids and typically occur in young women in the rectus abdominis muscles. Extraabdominal desmoids occur in both women and men, most commonly between 30 and 40 years of age. The most common locations include the shoulder girdles, chest wall, and thigh. Some mesenteric desmoids occur in patients with Gardner's syndrome (autosomal dominant inheritance) together with colonic adenomatosis, epidermal inclusion cysts, and osteomas of the skull. Although there may be multiple recurrences over the years, metastasis does not occur.

Fibromatosis typically arise within muscles. On sectioning they are firm gray-white masses with a rubbery consistency and a trabeculated surface. The periphery may have an infiltrating or sharply demarcated appearance. Histologically all fibromatosis appear identical and are composed of long, sweeping fascicles of differentiated fibroblastic cells with ill-defined cytoplasmic borders, delicately staining nucleoli, and only rare mitoses (Fig 72-3, *A*). Broad bands of collagen, similar to those seen in keloids, may be present. Slightly dilated blood vessels with a variably prominent endothelium and muscular walls are typical. The lesion is often surrounded by compressed atrophic muscle fibers which may also be invaded by proliferating fibroblasts. The microscopic tumor infiltration beyond the margins explains the common recurrence of locally excised desmoids.

EM studies of fibromatosis show a mixture of fibroblasts with a prominent dilated rough endoplasmic reticulum and myofibroblasts that have both a prominent dilated rough endoplasmic reticulum and bundles of actin filaments with focal densities, the latter feature also seen in smooth muscle cells. Immunohistochemically, desmoids show varying numbers of muscle actin–positive and desmin-positive myofibroblastic cells but are generally negative for S-100 protein, which distinguishes a fibromatosis from a schwannoma, a common differential diagnosis for extraabdominal desmoids. Cytogenetic abnormalities seen in desmoid tumors include telomeric associations and loss of the Y-chromosome.[67,68]

Infantile (desmoid-type) fibromatosis is usually encountered in small children and occurs in the head and neck region. Histologically it consists of round fibroblast-like cells that appear less mature than the cells in desmoids and that form less collagen, although some lesions may appear indistinguishable from the desmoids that occur in adults. The lesion may be locally infiltrative and often recurs after primary excision.

Palmar fibromatosis (Dupuytren's contracture) is a fibrous proliferation that may lead to contracture of the fingers. The lesion consists of multiple subcutaneous indurations in the palmar aspect of the hand that typically occur in elderly men. Palmar fibromatosis has an unexplained association with diabetes, epilepsy, alcohol use, and human immune deficiency virus (HIV) infection. Local recurrence after surgical excision is relatively common.[69-72] Histologically, several stages reflecting the maturation of the lesion can be recognized. In the early cellular stages large numbers of plump myofibroblasts are seen. In the later stages an amorphous fibrosis with inconspicuous fibroblasts predominates.

Plantar fibromatosis usually occurs in patients younger than those with palmar fibromatosis and is histologically and clinically similar to its palmar counterpart. It may occur locally after excision.

Infantile digital fibromatosis is a rare, peculiar fibrous lesion; it is a subcutaneous nodule of up to 3 cm in diameter that mainly is found in the fingers and toes of infants.[73-74,74a] This lesion is benign but often recurs locally. Histologically it consists of intersecting fascicles of plump polygonal fibroblasts and myofibroblasts in a collagenous stroma. A characteristic of this condition is the presence of small globular eosinophilic cytoplasmic inclusions, which are fuchsinophilic on trichrome staining. By EM these inclusions are seen to consist of whorls of microfilaments, most likely representing actin.

Fibrosarcoma

Fibrosarcoma is a rare type of soft-tissue sarcoma composed of malignant fibroblast-like spindle cells. It accounts for less than 10% of all sarcomas.[75,76] Many tumors classified as fibrosarcoma in the past actually represent various forms of fibromatosis and malignant fibrous histiocytoma, or even reactive lesions such as nodular fasciitis. It is diagnosed after other spindle cell sarcomas, such as monophasic synovial sarcoma, malignant schwannoma, and the spindle cell type of rhabdomyosarcoma, have been excluded by immunohistochemical findings and the results of other ancillary techniques. Numerous fibrosarcomas arise after radiation therapy, most commonly for malignant lymphoma or breast carcinoma. These sarcomas typically appear 5 to 15 years after irradiation. Postirradiation fibrosarcomas are usually of high-grade malignancy and the prognosis in such patients is poor. The overall 5-year survival for patients with fibrosarcoma is 40% to 50%, but it is better in patients with lower-grade tumors.[76]

By definition fibrosarcomas are composed of relatively uniform spindle-shaped cells resembling fibroblasts that are arranged in long fascicles, often in a chevron or herringbone pattern (Fig. 72-3, *B*). The distinction between fibrosarcoma and malignant fibrous histiocytoma is arbitrary in some instances. By convention, tumors showing less pleomorphism

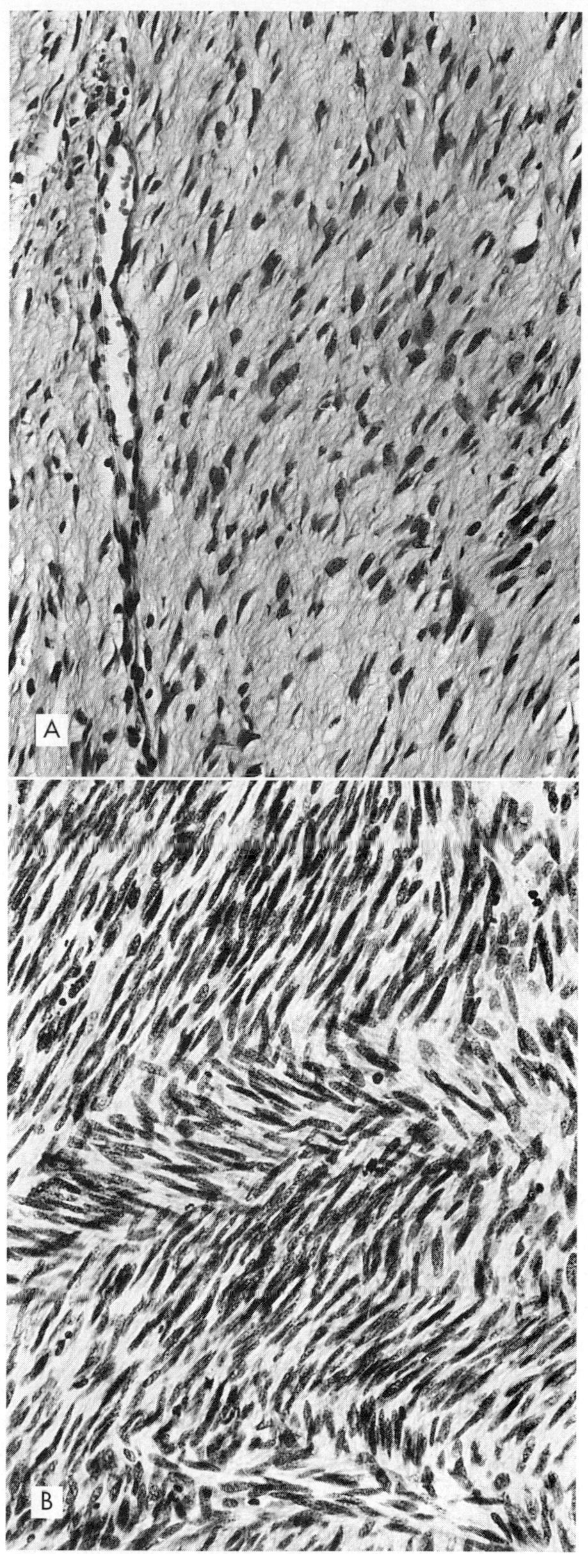

Fig. 72-3 **A,** Desmoid tumor showing moderately cellular mature fibrous tissue with prominent blood vessels. **B,** Fibrosarcoma composed of a highly cellular spindle cell proliferation. Notice the perivascular grouping of the tumor cells that gives the lesion a herringbone pattern.

are classified as fibrosarcoma and those showing more pleomorphism, as malignant fibrous histiocytoma. Grading is based on the mitotic activity and the cellularity; thus they range from low-grade tumors resembling benign fibromatosis to high-grade spindle cell sarcomas. Low-grade fibrosarcomas with myxoid stroma have been termed *low-grade fibromyxoid sarcoma.*[77] There are no immunohistochemical markers specific for fibroblastic differentiation and fibrosarcoma. EM typically shows both fibroblasts and myofibroblasts, similar to those seen in fibromatosis.

Infantile fibrosarcoma is a spindle cell sarcoma that affects small children.[78,79] Approximately half of these tumors are congenital, and the other half appear mostly during the first year of life. These tumors range from being low-grade malignant lesions resembling fibromatosis to being highly cellular and high-grade malignant tumors with abundant mitoses. However, clinically all cases of infantile fibrosarcoma appear to have a relatively favorable course, despite their sometimes ominous histologic appearance. These tumors often recur locally after an unsatisfactory excision but metastasis is exceptionally rare. Trisomies of chromosomes 11, 20, and others have been found consistently in tumor cells of infantile fibrosarcoma.[80,81]

Inflammatory fibrosarcoma (inflammatory myofibroblastic tumor) occurs predominantly in children, most commonly in the mesentery and retroperitoneum.[82] This tumor recurs commonly but usually does not metastasize; therefore some authors prefer to call it "inflammatory myofibroblastic tumor." Histologically this tumor consists of fascicles and clusters of plump fibroblasts and myofibroblasts intermingled with lymphocytes and plasma cells.

FIBROHISTIOCYTIC TUMORS

The concept of fibrohistiocytic tumors was introduced in the early 1960s to refer to lesions that were believed to be derived from histiocytes that under certain circumstances could acquire fibroblast-like features and produce collagen (facultative fibroblasts). Results of recent immunophenotypic studies have not confirmed the assumption that fibrohistiocytic tumors are derived from histiomonocytic cells (macrophages) but rather point to their fibroblastic nature. The historic term *fibrohistiocytic* persists for the sake of convenience and to facilitate clinicopathologic communication. It includes both benign and malignant fibrous histiocytoma as well as intermediate (borderline) tumors such as dermatofibrosarcoma protuberans and angiomatoid fibrous histiocytoma (formerly known as "angiomatoid malignant fibrous histiocytoma").

Benign fibrohistiocytic tumors

Benign fibrous histiocytoma (dermatofibroma, sclerosing hemangioma) most commonly occurs as an elevated red-brown tumor of the skin of extremities in young to middle-aged persons.[83-86] Most commonly it consists of a more or less circumscribed proliferation of plump spindle cells arranged in a crisscross pattern that is usually confined to the dermis, with occasional involvement of the subcutis. Although these tumors can be highly cellular and show mitotic activity, the cells are uniform and soft-tissue infiltration is limited. Some benign fibrous histiocytomas contain a mixture of spindle cells, siderophages, xanthoma cells, and Touton giant cells. Interstitial and perivascular fibrosis may be striking in some cases.

Juvenile xanthogranuloma (see Chapter 71) is a superficial histiocytic tumor composed of multinucleated giant cells of the Touton type, often with a prominent eosinophilic infiltrate. Usually this condition occurs in the skin of children but is occasionally seen in deep soft tissue.[87,88]

Reticulohistiocytoma is a rare, benign cutaneous histiocytic proliferation. Histologically the lesions show a mixture of histiocyte-like cells (multinucleated giant cells with an eosinophilic cytoplasm), neutrophils, and lymphocytes. The histiocytic component may show moderate pleomorphism, but mitotic activity is absent. There is no association with lipid disorders.[89,90] Multicentric reticulohistiocytosis occurs in association with multifocal superficial soft tissue tumors and destructive arthritis, and is probably unrelated to solitary forms of reticulohistiocytosis.

A *xanthoma* is an accumulation of lipid-laden histiocytes that occurs in skin and soft tissues in association with different types of hyperlipidemias. Xanthomas arise commonly in the skin and tendons of the hands and feet and are characterized by sheets of foamy histiocytes admixed with occasional giant cells and lymphocytes.[91] "Cholesterol clefts," elongated spaces previously occupied by cholesterol crystals, are a characteristic feature of this condition.

Fibrohistiocytic tumors of intermediate malignancy

Dermatofibrosarcoma protuberans (DFSP) is a superficial tumor of intermediate (low-grade) malignancy. This tumor occurs primarily in young adults and develops as a cutaneous mass, most commonly on the chest wall or trunk. Initially developing as a plaque or small nodule, it may grow to a large size, ulcerate, and give rise to satellite nodules.[92-95]

Histologically it is composed of slender fibroblastic cells often arranged in a repetitive storiform pattern. Although most lesions are quite cellular, hyalinization or a myxoid change of the stroma may supervene to obscure the typical appearance (Fig. 72-4, *A*). The cells seldom display significant mitotic activity. The tumors show an infiltrative pattern of growth into subcutaneous fat, a feature accounting for the high frequency of recurrences after conservative local excision. It has been estimated that up to 50% of these tumors recur, but metastasis, mainly to the lymph nodes and lungs, occurs in only 5% of cases. The cell lineage of DFSP has not been conclusively proved, although results of older studies have indicated a possible fibrohistiocytic differentiation.[96] Areas resembling fibrosarcoma or malignant fibrous histiocytoma, with increased cellularity, pleomorphism, and mitotic activity, may occur in DFSP. Such a change appears to confer an increased risk of distant metastasis.[92] Immunohistochemically, DFSP is positive for vimentin and often for CD34 antigen but is negative for muscle cell markers and S-100 protein. Some EM studies have indicated a possible peripheral nerve sheath cell differentiation. Cytogenetic studies have shown ring chromosomes, trisomy of chromosome 8, and additional copies of other chromosomes.[97,97a]

There are two rare variants of DFSP: *pigmented DFSP* (Bednar tumor)[98,99] and *giant cell fibroblastoma.*[100-102] The former is identical in all respects to DFSP, except that it includes scattered melanin-bearing spindle cells containing melanosomes. The latter is an unusual tumor of childhood characterized by spindle-shaped and giant cells lining sinusoidal pseudovascular spaces. Giant cell fibroblastoma is believed to be a juvenile variant of DFSP because it exhibits overlapping histologic features.

The differential diagnosis of DFSP includes diffuse neurofibroma, a tumor that can infiltrate subcutaneous fat in a fashion similar to that of DFSP, but does not show the cartwheel-like pattern typical of DFSP. Polypoid benign fibrous histiocytomas (dermatofibromas) that are cytologically uniform and microscopically only slightly infiltrative should be distinguished from DFSP.

Angiomatoid fibrous histiocytoma (formerly known as "angiomatoid malignant fibrous histiocytoma") is a rare distinctive tumor occurring predominantly in children and young adults.[103,104] It presents as a relatively small, often subcutaneous nodule (up to 5 cm in diameter) and is usually found in the extremities. Systemic symptoms, including fever, anemia, and weight loss, may be encountered. They occur locally in 20% of the cases, but metastasis occurs only exceptionally (less than 1% of the cases).

Histologically the tumor is composed of round to spindle-shaped, medium-sized, uniform cells separated by cystic "angiomatoid" blood-filled spaces, which, however, are not lined by endothelial cells. A cufflike peripheral lymphocytic infiltrate with germinal centers is often seen within the fibrous pseudocapsule and may give the lesion a lymph node metastasis-like appearance (Fig. 72-4, *B*). Findings from some studies have indicated that angiomatoid fibrous histiocytoma may show a myofibroblastic differentiation,[105] whereas those from other studies have indicated the tumor cells resemble primitive mesenchymal cells.[106]

Plexiform fibrohistiocytic tumor occurs in the superficial soft tissues of the extremities of children and young adults, most commonly in the shoulder and upper extremities.[107] Histologically the tumor consists of multiple nodules that infiltrate into subcutaneous fat and are composed of rounded histiocytic and multinucleated osteclast-like cells circumscribed by fibromatosis-like spindle cell areas. The tumor recurs commonly, but metastasis is exceptional and such lesions have been found only in regional lymph nodes.

Malignant fibrous histiocytoma

Malignant fibrous histiocytoma (MFH; also called "fibroxanthosarcoma" and "malignant fibroxanthoma") is composed of fibroblast and histiocyte-like cells typically showing significant pleomorphism, although several morphologic variants occur. MFH was described in the 1960s as a new tumor entity encompassing tumors that had previously been classified as pleomorphic fibrosarcoma or rhabdomyosarcoma.[108] Currently it is one of the most common types of soft-tissue sarcoma.[109-112] MFH was originally believed to be a histiocytic tumor, the cells of which could acquire features of fibroblasts.[113] However, immunohistochemical observations have not confirmed its histiocytic nature but have rather led to the conclusion that MFH cells show a fibroblastic or primitive mesenchymal cell differentiation.[114-118] MFH cells do not contain leukocyte common antigen (CD45) and are negative for most histiocytic markers such as CD14. However, some authors have reported that MFH cells are variably positive for CD68, an antigen present in histiomonocytic cells.[119] The significance of this observation in relation to the possible histiocytic differentiation of MFH remains to be determined. Other histiocytic markers, α-1-antitrypsin and α-1-antichymotrypsin, seem to be even less specific, and therefore posi-

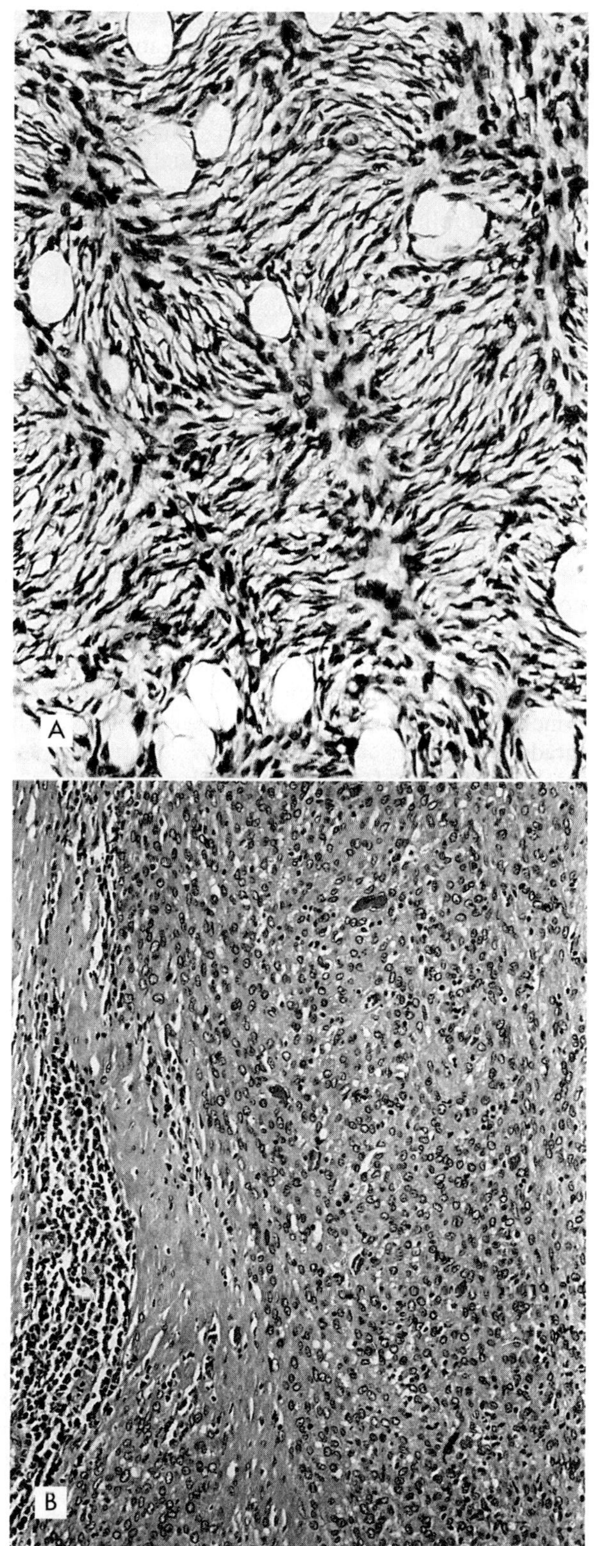

Fig. 72-4 A, Dermatofibrosarcoma protuberans composed of uniform spindle cells in a repetitive cartwheel pattern. Notice the diffuse infiltration in the subcutaneous fat. **B,** Angiomatoid fibrous histiocytoma composed of uniform round cells. Notice the lymphocytic infiltration in the area surrounding the tumor *(lower left corner).*

Grossly and microscopically, lipomas resemble normal subcutaneous fat. They are irregularly lobulated by delicate fibrous septa containing small capillaries. Those lipomas with prominent fibrous septa can be designated *fibrolipomas*. Several variants of benign lipoma are known, and many of these have distinctive clinicopathologic features. Benign lipomas commonly show reactive changes that may create a superficial resemblance to liposarcomas. These include fat necrosis, atrophy, and myxoid changes.

Intramuscular lipoma (intermuscular lipoma, infiltrating lipoma) occurs in adults as a deeply located tumor in the large muscles of the proximal extremities, usually in the thigh or shoulder region.[140-142] These tumors can become very large and measure up to 20 cm in diameter. Histologically the muscle is replaced by mature adipose tissue, creating an alternating checkerboard pattern of fat and striated muscle cells. The tumors recur in approximately 15% of cases, and this result from the diffuse nature of the lesion, which makes complete surgical excision difficult.

Perineural fibrolipoma (fibrolipomatous hamartoma of nerves) is a probable hamartoma that causes disfiguring enlargement of the fingers and the flexor side of hands in young people.[143] The lesion is characterized by an excess of mature adipose tissue surrounding the digital nerves, which often display concentric perineural fibrosis.

Angiolipoma arises as a small subcutaneous, occasionally painful nodule usually measuring 1 to 3 cm in diameter. Most patients are young adults, and the tumors are sometimes multiple.[144] The forearm is the most common site. This tumor consists of mature fat tissue containing an admixture of dilated capillaries, some of which contain fibrin thrombi (Fig. 72-6, *A*). Hypercellular variants of angiolipoma in which the vascular component obliterates the adipose tissue may resemble sarcoma. However, these tumors are invariably small and encapsulated, consisting of blood cells.

Spindle cell lipoma usually occurs in the subcutaneous tissue of the posterior aspect of the neck or shoulder of middle-aged men.[145] It is a circumscribed tumor composed of mature adipose tissue interspersed with short fascicles of bland spindle cells in a matrix containing bands of collagen and occasional mast cells (Fig. 72-6, *B*). Mitotic activity is absent. The tumor is readily cured by local excision.

Pleomorphic lipoma, having identical clinical features to spindle cell lipoma, is considered a closely-related lesion.[146,147] The tumor typically contains spindled, rounded, and multinucleated floret-like giant cells, so named because their multiple radially arranged nuclei resemble the petals of flowers. Its superficial location and sharp circumscription distinguish it from liposarcoma. Transitional forms between spindle cell and pleomorphic are occasionally seen.

Angiomyolipoma is a benign and probably hamartomatous lesion usually occurring within or in close association with the kidney in the perirenal soft tissue. Rare tumors have been encountered in the liver or lung. The lesion may occur in the setting of tuberous sclerosis, sometimes as a bilateral kidney mass. Most angiomyolipomas are asymptomatic and discovered incidentally, typically in adults, but some cause intraabdominal hemorrhage after the rupture of tumoral vessels. Grossly, angiomyolipoma appears as a lipomatous tumor, often bulging outward from the kidney surface, Histologically it consists of a mixture of mature adipose tissue and dilated

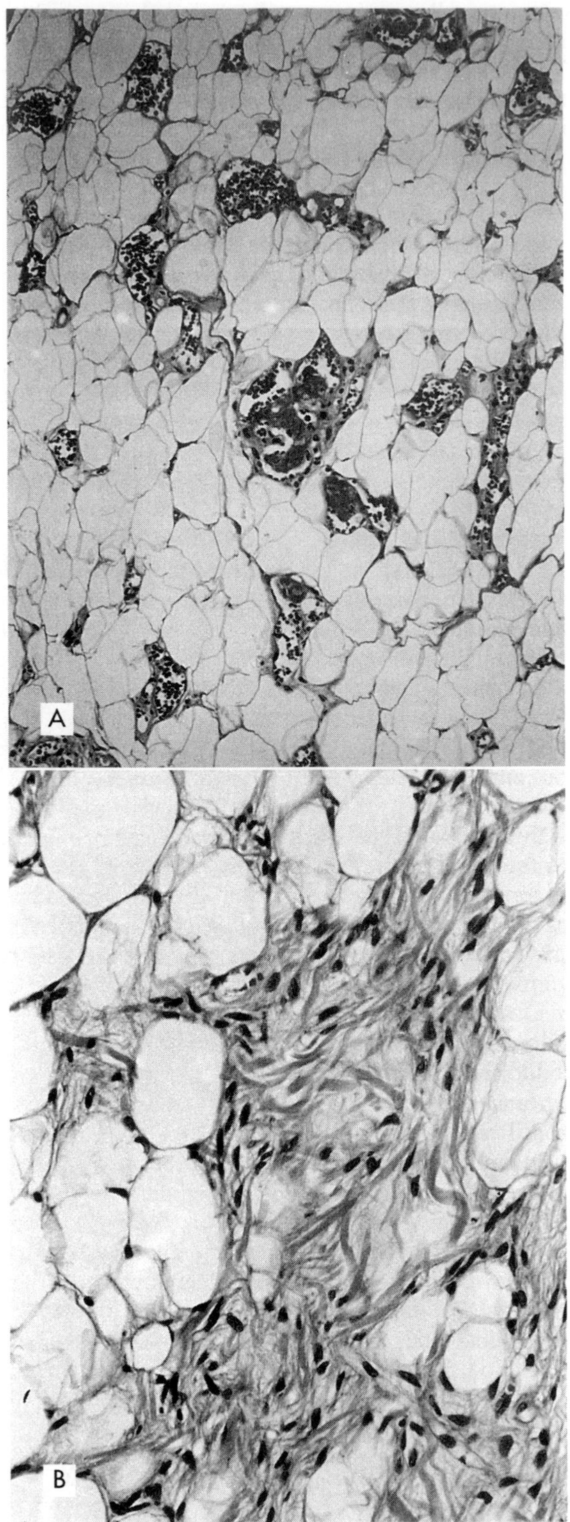

Fig. 72-6 A, Angiolipoma showing fatty tissue with numerous blood vessels, some of which contain microthtrombi. **B,** Spindle cell lipoma showing fatty tissue with an intervening uniform spindle cell proliferation.

blood vessels that are surrounded by sheets of well-differentiated smooth muscle cells.

Myelolipoma is a tumor of the adrenal, which rarely may present extraadrenally in the retroperitoneum. It is composed of normal bone marrow–like fatty and hematopoietic elements and is discussed with the tumors of adrenal.

Hibernoma is a rare tumor composed of brown fat cells (cells that produce body heat in hibernating animals through the uncoupling of mitochondrial oxidative phosphorylation).[148] Brown fat is present mainly in the posterior neck and retroperitoneum and is sometimes seen in axillary dissections. Hibernomas occur most commonly in the shoulder and back but sometimes also develop in the thigh. Affected patients are younger than those with lipomas. The tumor, which is circumscribed and usually measures 5 to 10 cm in diameter, is cured by local excision. Histologically, hibernomas are lobulated and contain multivacuolated brown fat–like cells with a granular, variably eosinophilic cytoplasm and small nuclei (Fig. 72-7, *A*). There are also often areas of white fat.

Lipoblastoma is a benign tumor composed of immature fetal fat. It occurs chiefly on the trunk of infants and is composed of lobules of immature fat. Because of their arborizing vascular pattern, myxoid stroma, and the presence of lipoblasts, these tumors resemble myxoid liposarcoma (Fig. 72-7, *B*). However, liposarcomas rarely if ever occur in infants and lack the lobular organization seen in lipoblastoma.[149] Cytogenetic studies of patients with lipoblastoma have consistently shown a trisomy of chromosome 8.[149a]

Lipoblastomatosis is the term used to refer to diffuse lipoblastoma, which may recur locally.[150,151]

Liposarcoma

Liposarcomas are malignant tumors made up of cells resembling to a variable degree adipose tissue cells. Liposarcomas are among the most common types of soft-tissue sarcomas and occur almost exclusively in adults, although rare cases have been documented in children.[152] There are several clinicopathologically distinct types of liposarcoma: well differentiated (lipoma-like and sclerosing), myxoid, round cell, pleomorphic, and dedifferentiated.[153,154] The first two are low-grade sarcomas, whereas the last three are high-grade sarcomas with a significant potential for metastasizing. Approximately one half of the tumors are located in the lower extremity, and 20% develop in an intraabdominal location. Typically liposarcomas are located in deep soft tissues, in contrast to the subcutaneous location of most benign lipomas (Fig. 72-8, *A*).

Well-differentiated liposarcoma occurs principally in late adult life and is both grossly and microscopically reminiscent of normal adipose tissue or benign lipoma. The designation "atypical lipoma" has been used as a synonym for well-differentiated liposarcoma when it occurs in the subcutaneous fat, to indicate its limited morbidity.[155,156] The most common locations are the deep soft tissues of the extremities and the retroperitoneum.[154,155,157,158]

The biologic behavior of the well-differentiated liposarcomas depends on their location. Although these lesions are nonmetastasizing, approximately 50% of tumors in the extremities recur locally. However, patients rarely die of their tumor. On the other hand, intraabdominal tumors recur in about 90% of patients and at least one third die of the local effects of the tumor. Approximately 10% of well-differentiated liposarcomas of the deep soft

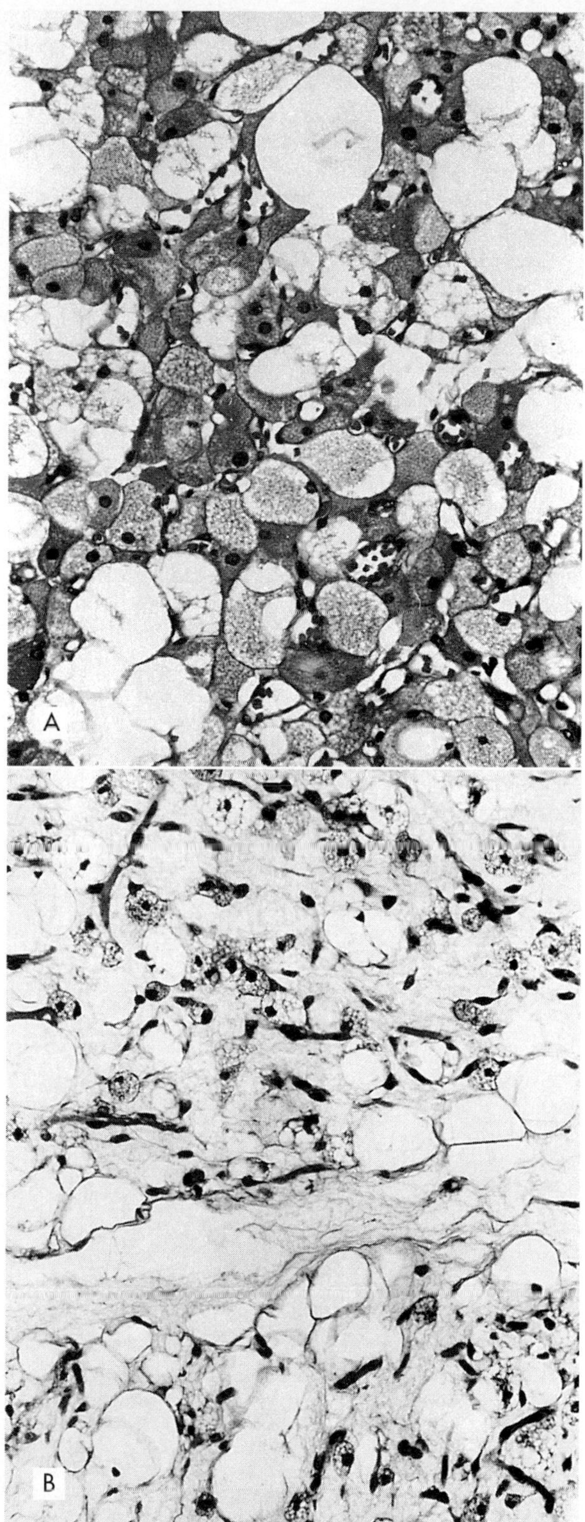

Fig. 72-7 A, Hibernoma consisting of multivacuolated cells that resemble brown fat. **B,** Lipoblastoma. Immature, richly vascular fat tissue with a lobular arrangement can be seen.

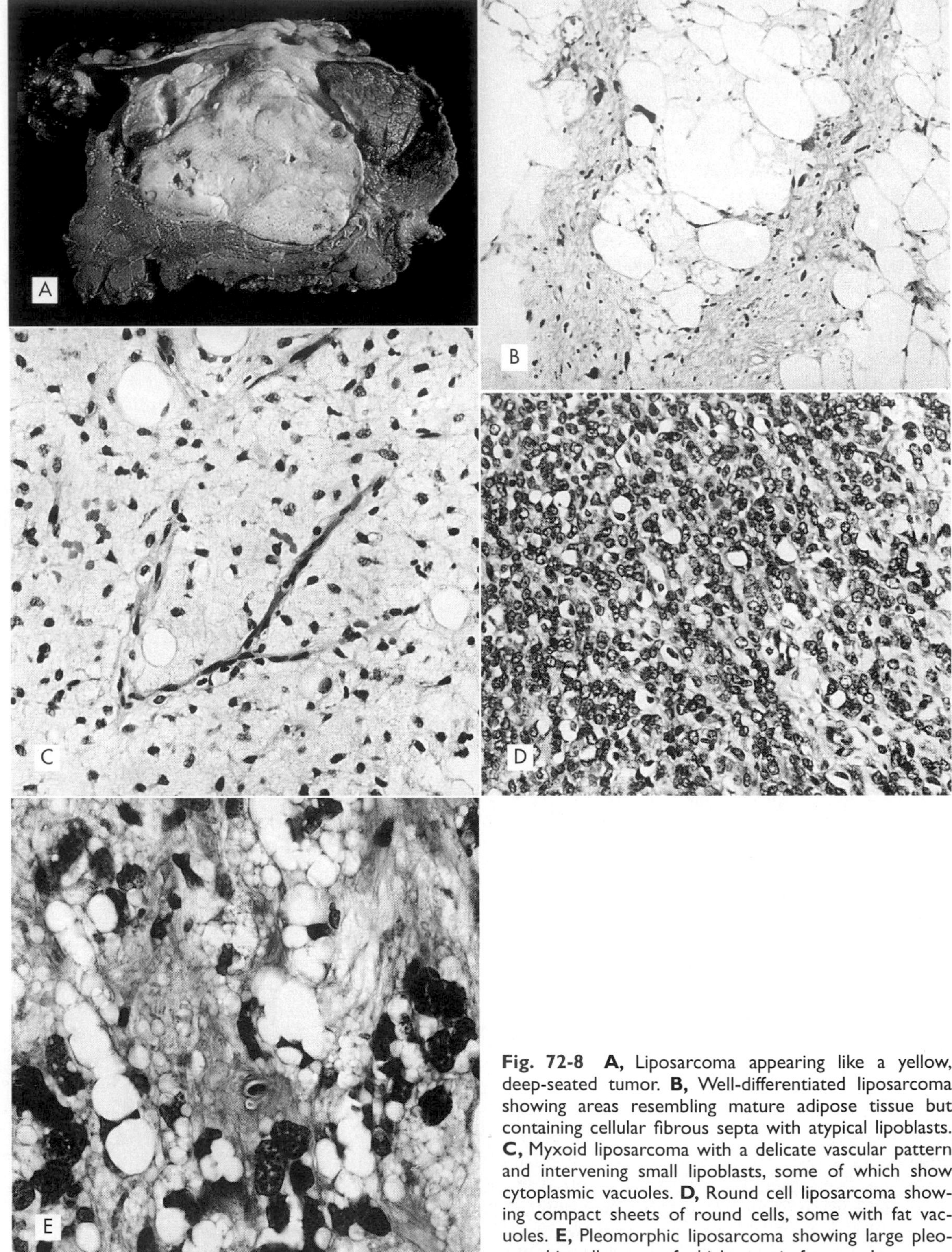

Fig. 72-8 **A,** Liposarcoma appearing like a yellow, deep-seated tumor. **B,** Well-differentiated liposarcoma showing areas resembling mature adipose tissue but containing cellular fibrous septa with atypical lipoblasts. **C,** Myxoid liposarcoma with a delicate vascular pattern and intervening small lipoblasts, some of which show cytoplasmic vacuoles. **D,** Round cell liposarcoma showing compact sheets of round cells, some with fat vacuoles. **E,** Pleomorphic liposarcoma showing large pleomorphic cells, many of which contain fat vacuoles.

tissues or body cavities with time become a higher-grade lesion, designated a "dedifferentiated liposarcoma" and resembling MFH.[159,160] This progression signifies the existence of a more aggressive tumor with metastatic potential.

Microscopically, well-differentiated liposarcomas differ minimally from mature adipose tissue but are identified as liposarcomas by virtue of their atypical hyperchromatic septal cells and lipoblasts. The latter are immature fat cells that typically contain one or more fat vacuoles which indent or scallop the nucleus (Fig. 72-8, *B*). A subtype known as "well-differentiated sclerosing liposarcoma" shows near-normal to normal adipose tissue with hypercellular fibrous septa containing mildly atypical fibroblast-like tumor cells. Lymphocytic infiltration is common, especially in abdominal liposarcomas.

Lipoma-like and sclerosing appearances are commonly seen within the same tumor. Well-differentiated liposarcomas show chromosomal changes, including telomeric associations, ring chromosomes, and large marker chromosomes.

Myxoid liposarcoma is the most common histologic variant of liposarcoma. It usually occurs in middle-aged persons and develops in deep soft tissues of the extremities, less often in the retroperitoneum. Typically, myxoid liposarcoma recurs locally; infrequently there is distant metastasis.[156,158,161,162]

Grossly, myxoid liposarcoma is a soft, mucoid, gray-white to yellow lesion with small cysts. Microscopically this tumor shows a typical architectural pattern with abundant branching fine capillaries and uniform small tumor cells suspended in a hyaluronic acid–rich matrix and traversed by a delicate arborizing capillary vasculature. (Fig. 72-8, *C*). Pools of mucoid material surrounded by tumor cells are commonly seen. Varying numbers of lipoblasts are present, and these range in appearance from multivacuolated cells to cells with a single large vacuole, an appearance imitating that of mature fat cells. Cytoplasmic lipid vacuoles and complete basement membranes are typical EM findings.[163]

Myxoid liposarcoma is characterized by a consistent nonrandom chromosomal translocation t(12,16)(q13;p11).[164] The translocation causes the fusion of genes *CHOP* and *TLS* and leads to the formation of the corresponding fusion transcript, potentially diagnosable by the reverse transcriptase polymerase chain reaction.[165] Interestingly, the *CHOP* gene codes for a transcription factor involved in adipocyte differentiation.[166] The trisomy of chromosome 8 found in many cases has been suggested to represent a secondary change.[167]

Round cell liposarcoma represents the cellular or poorly differentiated variant of myxoid liposarcoma and occurs in a similar age group and location as myxoid liposarcoma. It may coexist as a minor component in an otherwise typical myxoid liposarcoma; in such cases the tumor is associated with increased aggressiveness.[161] The presence of areas of lipoblastic differentiation is a diagnostic finding. Histologically, round cell liposarcomas contain uniform primitive round cells with a high nuclear-to-cytoplasmic ratio (Fig. 72-8, *D*). There is commonly a hemangiopericytoma-like pattern. The differential diagnosis of this form of liposarcoma includes other round cell sarcomas and lymphoma, and in problem cases immunohistochemical tests can aid in establishing the diagnosis.

Pleomorphic liposarcoma is actually a relatively rare tumor when strict diagnostic criteria are applied. These tumors develop in the extremities and retroperitoneum of elderly patients. This tumor shows an aggressive growth pattern, and it has a considerable metastatic potential. Histologically it is composed of pleomorphic tumor cells, including highly atypical multinucleated giant cells, many of which show multiple lipid vacuoles. In many respects the lesion resembles an MFH, except for the presence of lipoblastic differentiation which can also be documented by EM (Fig. 72-8, *E*). There may be few lipoblasts, and finding them may require extensive sampling. The histochemical evaluation of fat is of limited value because of the common existence of fat vacuoles in other types of sarcomas, including MFH. Cytogenetically, pleomorphic liposarcomas are heterogeneous and show variable complex chromosomal changes.[168]

Dedifferentiated liposarcoma contains areas of well-differentiated liposarcoma and high-grade MFH-like spindle cells or pleomorphic sarcoma. It is believed that the anaplastic cells develop from the well-differentiated component as a manifestation of tumor progression. These tumors occur at sites typical of other liposarcomas and are aggressive clinically. The "dedifferentiated" component has a tendency to metastasize to the lungs.

VASCULAR TUMORS

Vascular tumors are among the most common soft-tissue tumors, and the overwhelming majority of them are benign. Benign vascular tumors occur primarily in superficial soft tissue and most develop during childhood.[169] Sarcomas of endothelial lineage are rare and, in contrast to benign lesions, almost exclusively arise in adults.

Hemangiomas and related tumors

Hemangiomas are benign soft-tissue tumors that usually occur in skin and subcutaneous tissue. Depending on their size, location, and histologic appearance, they may exhibit a variety of clinical patterns, such as port-wine nevus, cherry nevus, or flame nevus. Some of these conditions occur in young patients, and some may regress during childhood; others may persist during adult life. Many hemangiomas are actually hamartomas and not neoplasms, and some may even be reactive lesions.

Capillary hemangiomas consist of narrow capillary-like vascular slits lined by regular or hyperplastic endothelial cells. Typically, larger capillary hemangiomas are made up of capillary vessels forming sharply demarcated lobules separated by connective tissue septa. Capillary hemangiomas may be very cellular and show significant mitotic activity, especially those found in small children.

Cavernous hemangiomas are composed of dilated vessels filled with blood. This condition may occur in skin and superficial soft tissue, but it is also common in the liver and in deep soft tissue sites. The cavernous vessels are lined by flat to mildly hyperplastic endothelia and correspond to dilated capillaries or venules. Some blood spaces may show signs of extramedullary hematopoiesis with the formation of erythrocyte precursors and megakaryocytes.

Intramuscular hemangioma appears as a locally infiltrative deep soft tissue tumor which can recur locally if incompletely excised. Histologically the tumor can resemble cavernous or capillary hemangioma, and have the features of a vascular malformation showing dilated vein–like vascular lumens.[170,171]

Epithelioid hemangioma (angiolymphoid hyperplasia with eosinophilia) is a benign tumor that forms in the skin and less commonly in the subcutaneous tissue and shows well-formed vascular lumens lined by plump epithelioid-appearing endothelial cells with abundant eosinophilic cytoplasm. This lesion is typically infiltrated by eosinophils and aggregates of lymphocytes.[172,173]

Angiomatosis is basically a hemangioma growing in a diffuse fashion such that it involves a large segment of the body or multiple tissue planes within the same general area of the body. *Lymphangiomatosis* is a similar process involving the lymphatics.

Bacillary angiomatosis is the designation for a reactive tumorlike, florid capillary proliferation that occurs in the skin and soft tissues of AIDS patients and is probably triggered by an opportunistic bacterial infection with *Rochalimaea henselae*.[175,176]

Pyogenic granuloma is the clinical designation for a benign, probably reactive capillary proliferation that resembles granulation tissue in appearance.[177,178] It may be associated with trauma or may occur on the gums during pregnancy (granuloma gravidarum). Grossly the lesions are mostly small cherry red, exophytic nodules that bulge into the skin or mucosal surfaces in the head and neck area. Secondary ulceration is common. An intravascular location has been reported.[178a] Microscopically, pyogenic granulomas resemble capillary hemangiomas in that they show sprouting capillaries grouped around a parent vessel. Such a highly organized lobular architecture and the lack of atypia distinguish pyogenic granuloma from angiosarcoma (Fig. 72-9, *A*). The capillary endothelial cells may have large nuclei, and mitotic activity is common. Necrosis is limited to ulcerated mucosal surfaces. The lesions are often infiltrated by inflammatory cells, including granulocytes, plasma cells, and lymphocytes, but the extent of the infiltration varies from case to case.

Intravascular papillary endothelial cell hyperplasia (Masson's hemangioma) is an exuberant intravascular, reactive endothelial cell proliferation that occurs as a response to organizing thrombi. Histologically, papillary tufts of reactive endothelium are intimately associated with thrombus material. The purely intravascular location, the absence of significant soft-tissue invasion, and the absence of solid areas, atypia, and significant necrosis distinguish this lesion from angiosarcoma[179-181] (Fig. 72-9, *B*).

Lymphangioma usually occurs in children and young adults; many lesions appear in newborns, indicating they may represent hamartomas or malformations.[182] The lesions may occur in both superficial and deep soft tissues, including the abdominal cavity. Histologically, lymphangioma usually consists of clusters of cystically dilated lymphatics lined by an attenuated endothelium and often containing lymph and lymphocytes. Lymphoid aggregates are often seen between the vessels (Fig. 72-10, *A*). Many lymphangiomas are locally infiltrative, which makes their complete excision difficult and results in a moderate frequency of recurrence after their surgical removal.

Cystic lymphangioma (cystic hygroma) is usually discovered as a neck mass in infants and small children. It has also been found in spontaneously aborted fetuses, many of which have shown a 45,XO karyotype typical of Turner's syndrome.[183] Cystic lymphangiomas that are located intraabdominally have to be distinguished from so-called multicystic peritoneal mesothelioma, which has keratin-positive mesothelial cells lining the cystic spaces.

Lymphangiomyoma (previously also called "lymphangiopericytoma") is a rare hamartomatous lesion that involves the proliferation of smooth muscle cells in the walls of lympatics and within the major lymphatic ducts and lymph nodes of the retroperitoneum and thoracic cavity; it is usually associated with a chylous pleural effusion or ascites.[184-188] This condition occurs exclusively in women of reproductive age. Some patients respond to hormone therapy; both progesterone and antiestrogenic treatment have been used with some success to induce tumor regression. The presence of multiple minute pulmonary nodules of lymphangiomyoma is referred to as *lymphangiomyomatosis*. This systemic form can result in death

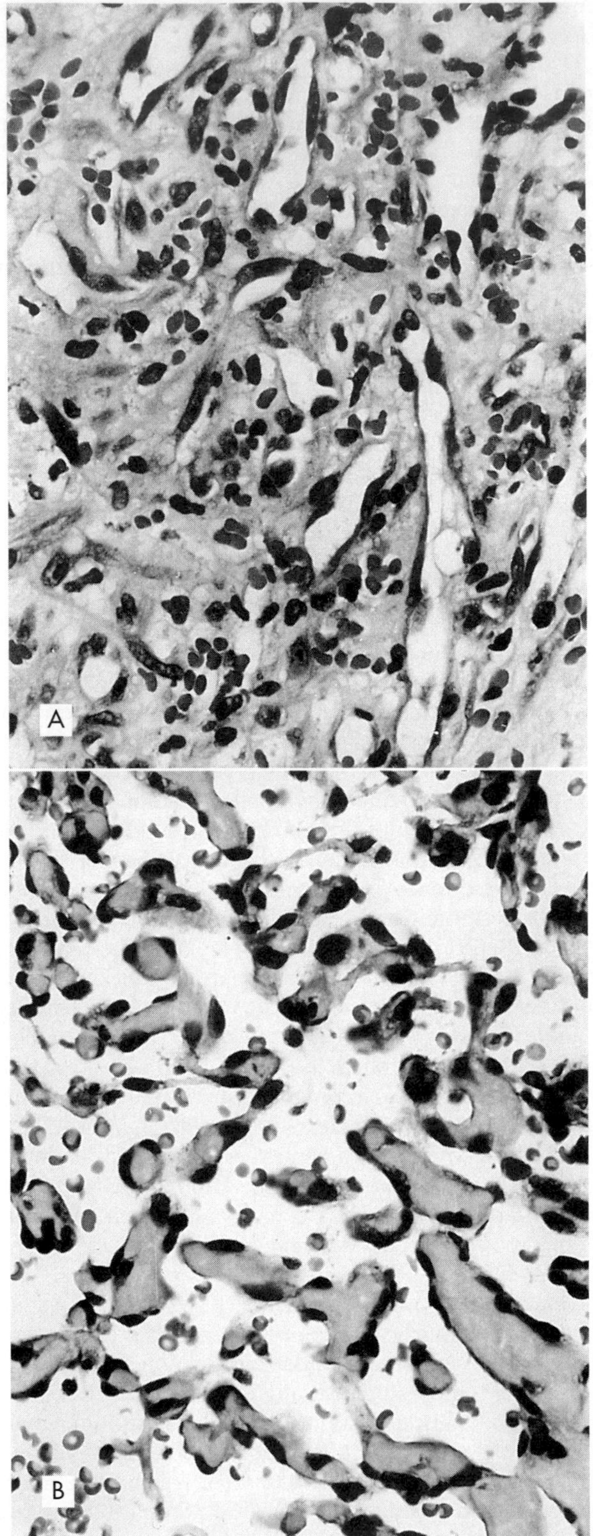

Fig. 72-9 **A,** Pyogenic granuloma. A vascular proliferation consisting of a meshwork of delicate capillaries can be seen. **B,** Masson's hemangioma, which is composed of a papillary endothelial cell proliferation.

because of the progressive pulmonary insufficiency it causes and may be associated with the tuberous sclerosis syndrome.

Hemangioendothelioma

Hemangioendotheliomas are endothelial cell neoplasms of intermediate (borderline) malignancy; three variants are discussed here.[189-200a]

Epithelioid hemangioendothelioma includes lesions previously called "histiocytoid hemangiomas" and typically is composed of endothelial cells with an ample eosinophilic cytoplasm that resemble histiocytes.[189,193,197] These tumors may arise in superficial or deep soft tissue and mainly affect adults. Similar tumors are seen in the lungs, liver, and bone. More than one half of epithelioid hemangioendotheliomas of soft tissue arise from the walls of vessels, and they produce the symptoms of vascular thrombosis. Although most lesions behave in a benign fashion, as many as a third eventually metastasize to the lungs, liver, or regional lymph nodes.[198]

Histologically the typical lesion contains cords and clusters of plump epithelioid endothelial cells in a fibromyxoid stroma. Intracellular vacuoles representing miniature vascular lumens and often containing erythrocytes are a characteristic feature (Fig. 72-10, *B*). Mitoses and necrosis are uncommon. The endothelial cell differentiation of these tumors can be confirmed both by EM (with the finding of Weibel-Palade bodies, basement membranes, and pinocytic vesicles) and by immunohistochemical tests (with the finding of von Willebrand factor, CD34, and vimentin positivity, and usually keratins negativity).[200] Metastatic carcinoma and melanoma should be considered in the differential diagnosis.

Spindle cell hemangioendothelioma is a rare vascular tumor occurring mainly in young adults.[194,195,199] The tumor is typically located in the subcutis of distal parts of the extremities, the hands being the most common location. Recurrence or multifocal disease develops in approximately a third of the cases, but distant metastasis does not occur. Histologically this tumor is characterized by cavernous blood spaces juxtaposed with bland spindle cells, an appearance somewhat reminiscent of that of Kaposi's sarcoma; a reactive origin to the lesion has been suggested.[191]

Kaposiform hemangioendothelioma is a rare childhood tumor that may develop in either superficial or deep soft tissue.[196,200a] It is composed of nodules of capillary-sized vessels, some of which show spindling of the cells that focally resemble the features of Kaposi's sarcoma. This tumor may be associated with lymphangiomatosis and the *Kasabach-Merritt* syndrome. The latter is the designation for the condition when vascular tumors trap circulating platelets and cause thrombocytopenia and hemorrhagic diathesis. This syndrome mainly afflicts children.

Angiosarcoma

Angiosarcoma is a clinically heterogeneous group of soft-tissue sarcomas that exhibit endothelial cell differentiation. Angiosarcomas can be divided into four clinically distinct groups according to the site where they arise and their manner of presentation: (1) cutaneous tumors occurring without preexisting lymphedema, (2) cutaneous tumors arising in lymphadematous extremities, (3) angiosarcomas of the breast, and (3) angiosarcomas of deep soft tissue. When strictly defined, angiosarcomas are very rare compared with their benign vas-

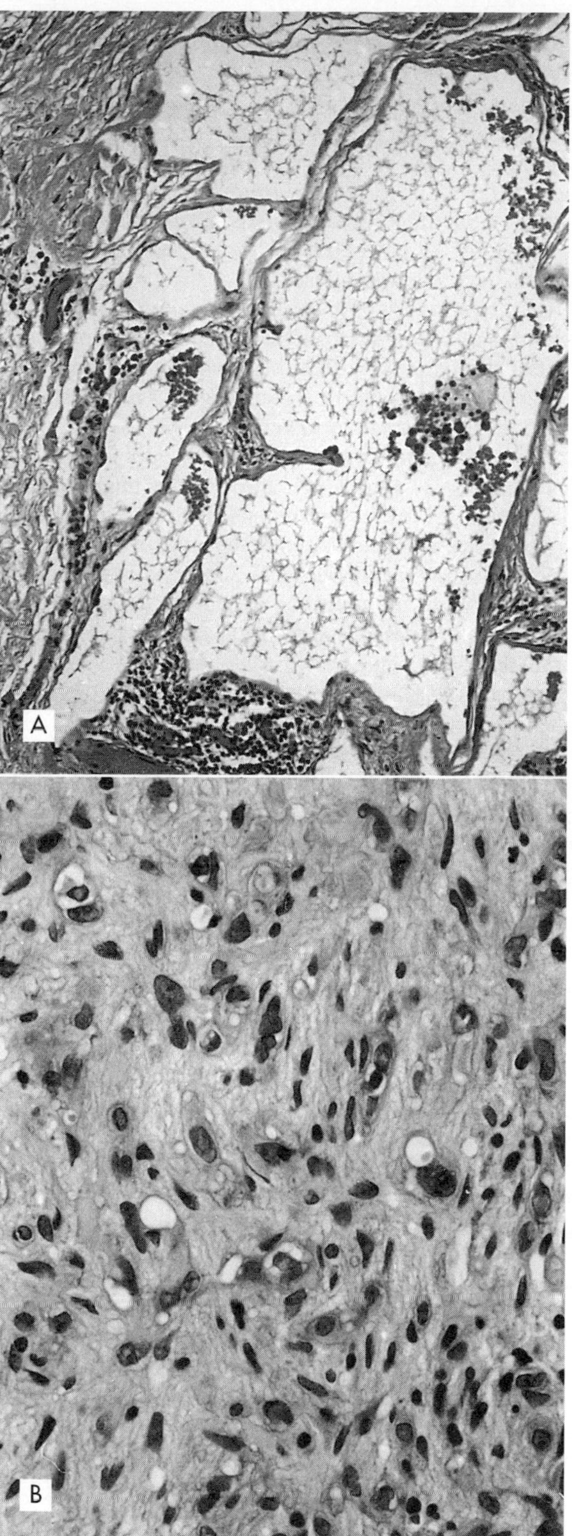

Fig. 72-10 **A,** Lymphangioma in which there are multiple dilated vascular channels that contain lymph and lymphocytes. **B,** Epithelioid hemangioendothelioma. Cords and clusters of epithelioid tumor cells in a fibromyxoid stroma can be seen. Notice the vacuoles that represent microlumens. The entire lesion is located inside a small vein.

cular counterparts, and they appear to be easily overdiagnosed, at the expense of both other malignant tumors and benign vascular tumors.

Cutaneous angiosarcomas are usually found in the head and neck area of elderly patients, particularly in the scalp and on the face.[201-203] The tumors have the appearance of ill-defined plaques or diffusely infiltrative nodules that often extend to subcutaneous tissue. The growth of cutaneous angiosarcomas cannot be easily controlled locally, and lethal metastasis occurs in most cases.

Angiosarcomas arising in lymphedematous extremities are morphologically similar to other cutaneous angiosarcomas.[204] They occur in patients with either congenital or acquired lymphedema, most commonly after mastectomy that included lymph node dissection followed by radiation therapy (postmastectemy angiosarcoma, Stewart-Treves syndrome). Their clinical behavior is aggressive, and death as the result of widespread metastasis to internal organs is the rule. Angiosarcoma in the presence of lymphedema typically grows as multiple cutaneous and subcutaneous coalescent plaques and nodules. Their grade of differentiation varies from areas that simulate benign hemangioma to solid sheets of undifferentiated cells that may resemble metastatic carcinoma.

Lymphangiosarcoma does not appear in the current classification of soft-tissue tumors; sarcomas arising in connection with lymphedema are simply classified as angiosarcomas because thay do not differ from other cutaneous angiosarcomas and there is no proof of their lymphatic vascular origin.

Angiosarcomas of the breast are ill-defined hemorrhagic nodules and masses.[205-207] They occur only in women and mostly in those who are premenopausal (30 to 50 years of age). These tumors may be extremely well differentiated and at times simulate the appearance of benign vascular tumors.

Angiosarcomas of deep soft tissues are rare.[207a] They present as combined hemorrhagic and necrotic masses and are mostly found deep in the extremities or in the retroperitoneum. Angiosarcomas also occur in internal organ sites, including the liver, heart, lungs, and gastrointestinal tract and may arise intraluminally in the major vessels.

Histologically all angiosarcomas show a wide spectrum of differentiation. The well-differentiated tumors show irregular anastomosing, blood-filled vascular channels lined by variably atypical endothelial cells which often show papillary, intraluminal tufting. In the skin the vascular channels typically dissect the collagen fibers and often extend to the subcutaneous fat. The less-differentiated tumors may show solid sheets of undifferentiated-appearing cells that may resemble a carcinoma or a lymphoma, and the diagnosis of angiosarcoma has to be made on the basis of the presence of differentiated vasoformative components or on the basis of immunohistochemical findings (Fig. 72-11).

The diagnosis of angiosarcomas often requires immunohistochemical or EM confirmation. The ultrastructural hallmark of endothelial cell differentiation is the finding of Weibel-Palade bodies, which, however, are found only in the better-differentiated tumors. A focal basement membrane, abundant pinocytic vesicles, and prominent cytoplasmic intermediate filaments are common but less specific features. Many immunohistochemical markers for endothelial cells and their tumors can be applied to formaldehyde-fixed and paraffin-embedded material. Von Willebrand factor (factor VIII–related antigen) is specific for endothelial cells. This antigen, however, is present only in the more-differentiated angiosarcomas. CD31 and CD34 antigens are sensitive markers, but the latter is not specific and is also present in a subset of perivascular mesenchymal cells, many epithelioid sarcomas, and subsets of leiomyosarcomas and dermatofibrosarcomas[208,209] (Fig. 72-11, *B*). *Ulex europaeus* lectin and antibodies such as BNH9, which recognize similar carbohydrate structures (H antigen), are sensitive but relatively nonspecific endothelial cell markers that react with a variety of carcinomas.[208,210,211]

Malignant angioendotheliomatosis is a historical term for a condition originally believed to represent a disseminated endothelial cell neoplasm. It has been shown conclusively that this lesion constitutes a peculiar intravascular manifestation of lymphoma.[212]

Kaposi's sarcoma is a morphologically characteristic spindle cell, vascular proliferation that occurs primarily in the skin but may also occur in deeper sites and in parenchymal organs. It arises in several different clinical settings.[213,214]

Sporadic Kaposi's sarcoma was originally described as a cutaneous tumor that developed in the distal extremities of elderly patients. This form is clinically indolent, although it may be multifocal, locally invasive, and sometimes recurrent.

Endemic Kaposi's sarcoma, which affects the population of equatorial Africa, has long been known in this part of the world as a skin tumor that involves lymph node and internal organ dissemination. It affects persons of all ages and is not necessarily associated with HIV infection.

Kaposi's sarcoma in transplant recipients is associated with an immunosuppressed state and has been observed during the past 30 years.

In the *Kaposi's sarcoma associated with AIDS,* it is not known how the HIV infection is associated with the development of the tumors and why the tumors occur mainly in homosexually transmitted cases as opposed to cases transmitted by intravenous drug use. Interestingly, NIH-T3 fibroblasts formed a Kaposi's sarcoma-like tumor in nude mouse inoculations after treatment with HIV-infected lymphocytes.[215] This finding may indicate the role of a transmissible viral factor not necessarily related to HIV. In AIDS patients the Kaposi's sarcoma may appear as multiple plaques and tumors in the skin and gastrointestinal tract and may also disseminate in the lungs and other parenchymal organs.[215a]

Histologically different stages are recognized in the development of the lesions of Kaposi's sarcoma. In the early stage a plaque consisting of telangiectatic vessels and chronic inflammation forms and may be histologically difficult to diagnose. It is followed by the progressive formation of vascular slits surrounded by mitotically active spindle cells with extravasated erythrocytes. In the late stages there may be a nearly pure spindle cell sarcomatous proliferation resembling fibrosarcoma. The spindle cells often show PAS-positive hyaline globules. Although the histogenesis of Kaposi's sarcoma has not been fully defined, current evidence points to the significant participation of endothelial cells in the development of the lesion. The spindle cells express two antigens, CD31 and CD34, which are also expressed by normal endothelia and a variety of endothelial cell tumors.[208] Other endothelial cell markers have been variably reported. Some authors have suggested that Kaposi's sarcoma represents a neoplastic proliferation of lymphatic capillaries.[216,217]

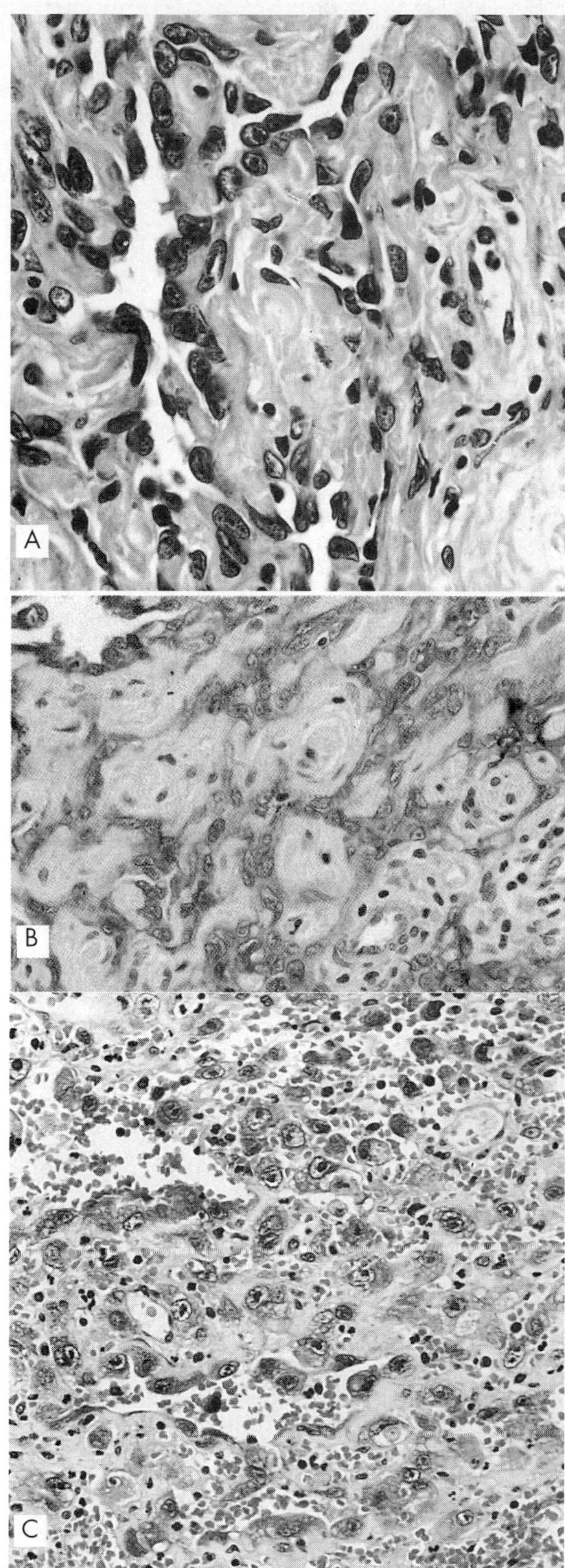

Fig. 72-11 **A,** Cutaneous angiosarcoma showing anastomosing vascular channels lined by atypical endothelial cells. **B,** Immunohistochemically the angiosarcoma cells are positive for CD31 (PECAM-1). **C,** Angiosarcoma of deep soft tissue consisting of vascular spaces lined by highly atypical neoplastic cells.

PERIVASCULAR TUMORS

The new World Health Organization classification assigns glomus tumors and hemangiopericytomas to the new group of perivascular tumors.

The development of a *glomus tumor* recapitulates the appearance of the cells of the normal glomus bodies that represent specialized arteriovenous anastomoses regulating the blood flow in the distal body parts. Glomus tumors usually present as a small painful superficial soft tissue nodule in adults but can occasionally reach several centimeters in diameter.[218] Among the most common locations where they arise are the nailbeds of the fingers and the palms, feet, legs, and forearms. In some cases there are multiple tumors.[219] Glomus tumors identical to their peripheral soft-tissue counterparts have been found in internal organs, such as the lungs and stomach, which are not known to contain glomus structures.[220] Simple local excision is the treatment of choice. The peripheral tumors recur locally in 10% of the cases.

Histologically, glomus tumors are composed of uniform, round to polygonal cells arranged in sheets and cords. The nuclei are round and regular, and the cell borders are sharp because basement membranes encircle the cells; these can be highlighted with PAS and reticulin stains or with immunostains for basement membrane components (Fig. 72-12 *A*). A myxoid stromal change is common, and the tumors typically contain numerous mast cells. Histologic variants include *glomangioma,* in which the tumor cells are distributed as thin collars around dilated vessels; this variant is associated with multiple tumors showing a familial predisposition.[10] In another variant, *glomangiomyoma,* there are round glomus tumor cells together with vascular smooth muscle cells and features of both glomus tumors and angiomyomas.

Glomus tumor cells are vascular smooth muscle cells and show ultrastructural features typical of smooth muscle cells, with bundles of actin filaments, cytoplasmic dense bodies, well-developed basement membranes, and pinocytic vesicles at the membranes.[221,222] Immunohistochemically, glomus tumor cells are positive for vimentin and actins, specifically alpha-actins, and are negative for keratins and desmin.[223-225]

Malignant variants of glomus tumor have been described recently. These rare tumors are hypercellular and may show a focal spindle cell pattern. They show mitotic activity and local invasion, but metastasis has not been reported.[226]

Special studies may be necessary to distinguish glomus tumors from solid variants of hidradenomas; the latter are epithelial neoplasms that have keratins as a constituent. A glomus tumor has to be distinguished conceptually from head and neck paragangliomas, sometimes referred to as "glomus tympanicum tumors," "glomus jugulare tumors," and "glomus caroticum tumors." All of these have a neuroendocrine phenotype, in contrast to the vascular smooth muscle features of the glomus tumor of soft tissues.

Hemangiopericytoma is a rare soft-tissue tumor characterized by spindle-shaped, uniform tumor cells grouped around dilated vascular channels and slits, appearing as if the cells were originating from the vessel walls. The relationship of hemangiopericytoma to normal pericytes, however, has not been established. In fact, the actin subset pattern of pericytes differs from that of hemangiopericytoma, indicating a possible nonpericytic origin for hemangiopericytomas.[224,225]

Hemangiopericytoma develop in deep soft tissues, especially those of the extremities or retroperitoneum, and affect middle-aged patients.[227-231] Results of recent studies have indicated that "angioblastic meningioma" and hemangiopericytoma may be closely related, if not identical.[232-235] Most hemangiopericytomas are borderline or low-grade malignant tumors that show some likelihood of local recurrence, but the incidence of metastasis is low and such lesions may appear in the lungs or skeleton. It is difficult to histologically predict the course of these tumors in individual patients.

Histologically, hemangiopericytoma consists of uniform spindled or rounded cells embedded in a moderately collagenous stroma and arranged around dilated vascular lumens. A reticulin stain shows abundant fibers surrounding each tumor cell and arranged radially perpendicular to the vessels (Fig. 72-12, *B*). The mitotic activity is usually low, but malignant variants with brisk mitotic activity do occur. The latter should be distinguished from other soft-tissue sarcomas that may have a hemangiopericytoma-like architectural pattern. These especially include synovial sarcoma and mesenchymal chondrosarcoma, which can be differentiated from hemangiopericytoma by their epithelial or cortiloginous elements respectively.[236]

There are no immunohistochemical markers typical of hemangiopericytoma. The tumor cells are positive for vimentin and negative for muscle actins, desmin, and endothelial cell markers, although tumor cells may be CD34 positive.[223,224] Ultrastructurally the tumor cells do not show specific features, but complex interdigitating basement membranes are typical.[237] Multiple complex abnormalities seem to be the most common clonal chromosomal abnormalities in hemangiopericytoma, although a simple translocation t(12;19) has also been reported.[238]

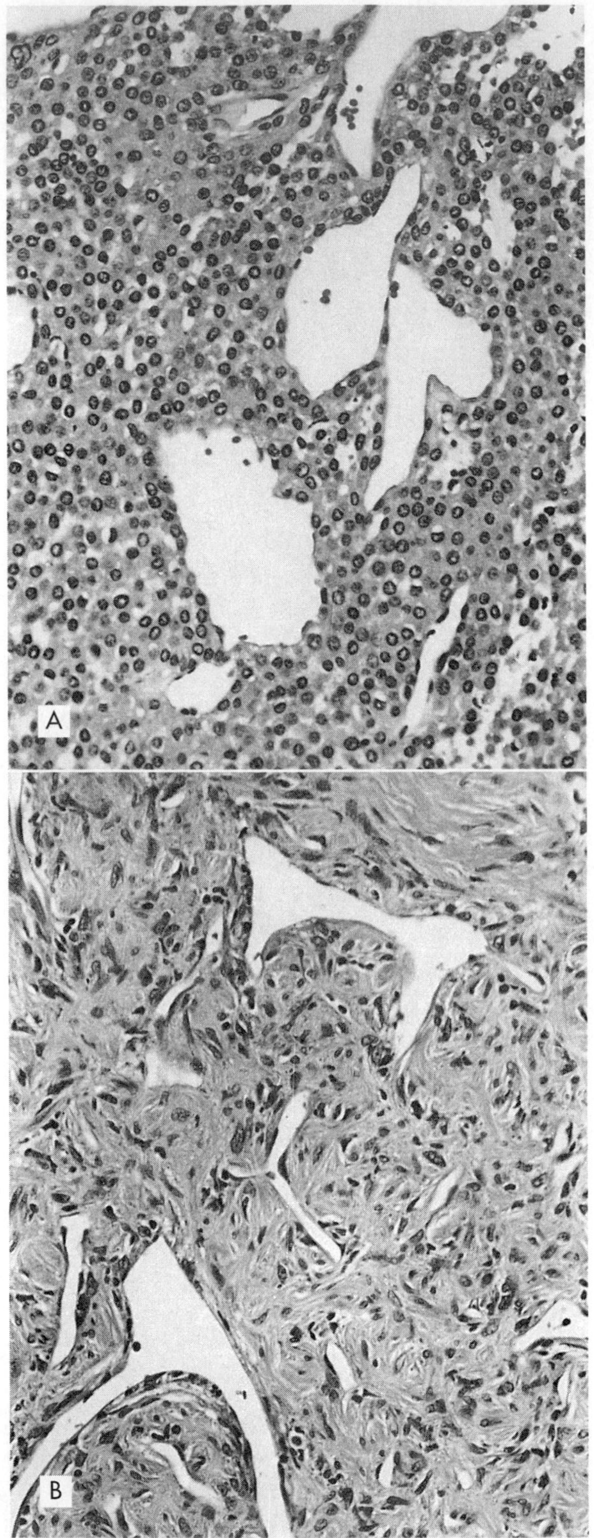

Fig. 72-12 **A** Glomus tumor showing small round or polygonal cells surrounding blood vessels in a collarlike pattern. **B** Hemangiopericytoma consisting of uniform spindle cells and prominent dilated vascular spaces in between.

TUMORS OF SMOOTH MUSCLE

Leiomyoma

Benign tumors of smooth muscle cells can be grouped into four clinicopathologic categories.

Piloleiomyomas are cutaneous tumors that arise from arrector pili muscles and present as small (up to 1 cm to 2 cm in diameter) often multiple chronically painful skin nodules. Piloleiomyomas are most common in the extremities and typically occurs in young or middle-aged persons. They are composed of radially arranged bundles of mature smooth muscle fibers, and the lesions often have irregular margins.

Genital leiomyomas are rare, solitary, usually small (1 cm to 2 cm) spherical smooth muscle nodules that most commonly arise in the vulva or scrotum (tunica dartos) in adults. Similar tumors may arise from the smooth muscle of the nipple. These leiomyomas are not painful.

Angiomyoma (angioleiomyoma, vascular leiomyoma) is a benign, relatively common subcutaneous tumor that has a predilection for the lower extremities, especially the legs and ankles.[239] These tumors occur in middle-aged and elderly patients, more commonly in women, and are typically painful. Most tumors are small (up to 1 cm to 2 cm in diameter), sharply demarcated spherical nodules and consist of mature smooth muscle cells arising from the walls of multiple adjoining vessels, which are variably occluded as the result of the proliferation of vascular smooth muscle cells. The vessels of angiomyomas with their thick, muscular walls resemble arteries, but elastic laminae are absent. These lesions may undergo hyalinization and calcification.

Leiomyomas of the deep soft tissues are rare. They arise in the extremities and retroperitoneum and often show considerable regressive changes, including calcification and hyalinization.

Histologically all leiomyomas show a spindle cell pattern with blunt-ended, cigar-shaped, usually uniform nuclei and scant or absent mitotic activity (Fig. 72-13, *A*). Although routine stainings are usually sufficient for diagnosis, smooth muscle differentiation can be documented by trichrome staining, EM, and immunohistochemical tests using markers such as (smooth) muscle actins and desmin, which usually, although not always show positivity). The most important differential diagnoses are benign and malignant fibrous histiocytoma, desmoid, neurofibroma, and schwannoma. These tumors are distinguished from leiomyosarcomas on the basis of the

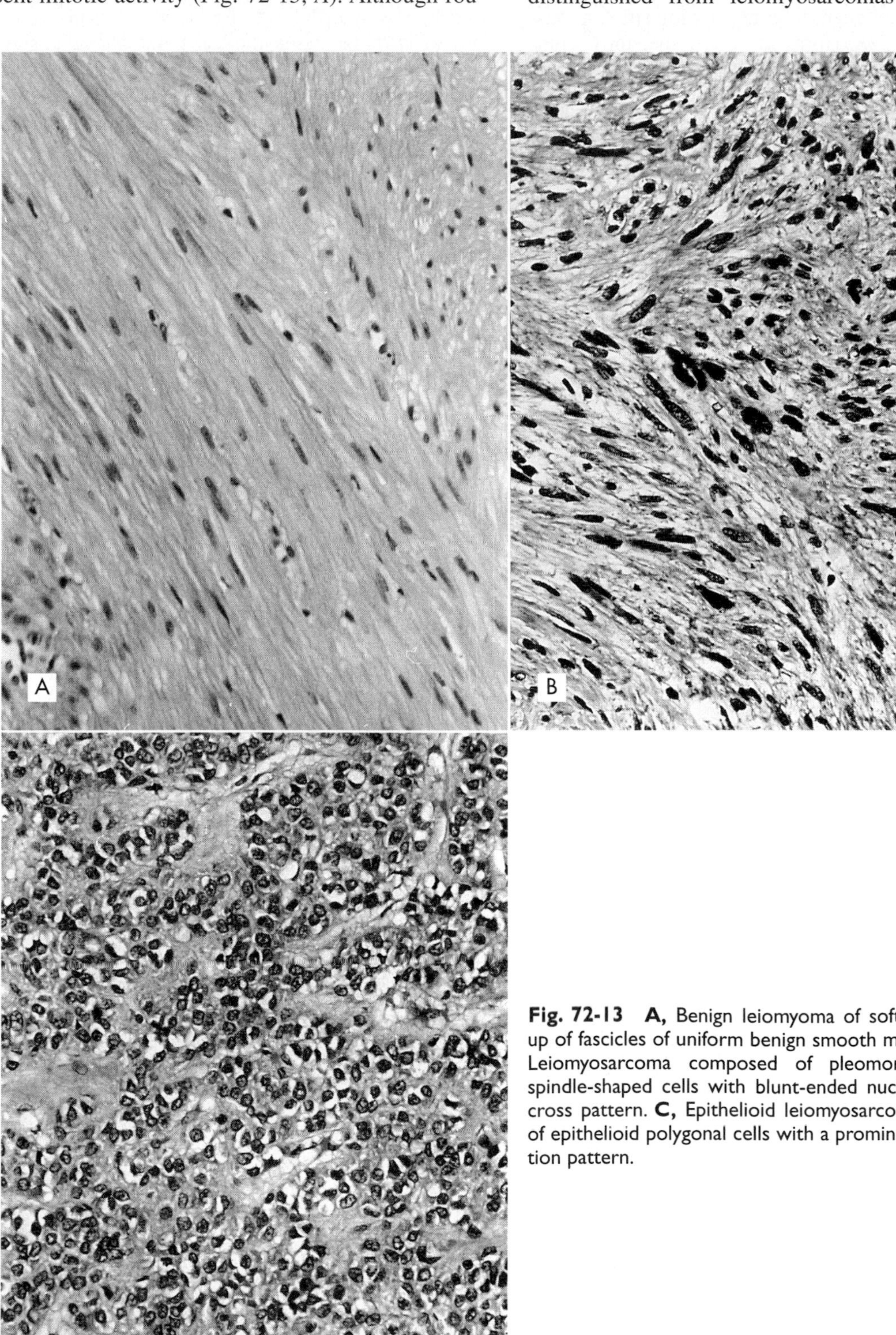

Fig. 72-13 **A,** Benign leiomyoma of soft tissue made up of fascicles of uniform benign smooth muscle cells. **B,** Leiomyosarcoma composed of pleomorphic, mostly spindle-shaped cells with blunt-ended nuclei in a crisscross pattern. **C,** Epithelioid leiomyosarcoma consisting of epithelioid polygonal cells with a prominent vacuolization pattern.

mitotic count and atypia. Generous sampling is necessary in order not to miss the mitotically active sarcomatous areas. Sarcomas are more common in retroperitoneal locations than benign leiomyomas are, except for the pelvic area, where intraligamentary and parauterine benign leiomyomas, comparable to their uterine counterparts, are relatively common.

Leiomyosarcoma

Leiomyosarcomas are malignant tumors showing smooth muscle cell differentiation. They form in soft tissue, most commonly in the skin, deep soft tissues of the extremities, and the retroperitoneum. The possibility of metastasis from a primary tumor in a deep internal organ has to be considered when there are multiple superficial leiomyosarcomas.

Cutaneous leiomyosarcomas usually occur in late adult life.[240-243] These tumors are usually small, and patients have a good prognosis because these tumors are generally diagnosed at an early stage when they are superficial and local. They may arise from vascular walls or arrector pili muscles. In contrast, deep soft tissue and retroperitoneal leiomyosarcomas follow a far more aggressive course.[244-246] Leiomyosarcomas in the deep soft tissues of extremities often arise in the walls of veins, and a multinodular intravascular growth may be seen at gross examination.[242,247,248] Numerous cases of leiomyosarcomas have been described as arising in the inferior vena cava, mostly in women. There are scattered reports of leiomyosarcomas involving the great vessels of the thorax.[249]

Histologically all leiomyosarcomas show essentially similar features, regardless of their location. They are composed of spindle cells arranged in fascicles that intersect obliquely or perpendicular to one another. The cells have blunt-ended, cigar-shaped nuclei that vary in the degree of pleomorphism (Fig. 72-13, *B*). The cytoplasm is variably eosinophilic and may contain clumped eosinophilic material representing the dense bundles of cytoplasmic filaments. In some cases the cytoplasm is clear or vacuolated. Necrosis is usually prominent in large tumors, but the mitotic activity varies and is an important feature when assessing the malignancy of the lesion. Nonetheless, the site of the lesion is also an important factor determining the biologic behavior. For example, retroperitoneal leiomyosarcomas may have as few as one mitosis per 50 high-power fields and still behave in a malignant fashion.[245]

Immunohistochemically, leiomyosarcomas are typically positive for muscle-specific actins (including alpha-actin) and desmin.[250,251] However, well-documented cases of desmin negativity do occur, paralleling the desmin negativity of subpopulations of smooth muscle cells.[250] Keratins and epithelial membrane antigen are found in a significant number of cases, the former paralleling the observation that keratins also occur in some normal smooth muscle cells, such as those in the myometrium.[252-254]

Ultrastructurally, shows leiomyosarcomas contain cytoplasmic bundles of actin filaments with dense bodies; the latter at the cell membrane are referred to as "attachment plaques." The tumor cells are variably surrounded by basement membranes and show pinocytic vesicles. Cytogenetic studies of leiomyosarcomas have not established any typical pattern but have shown complex morphologic and numerical chromosomal changes.[254a]

Epithelioid leiomyosarcoma (leiomyoblastoma, bizarre leiomyoblastoma) occurs more commonly in the gastrointestinal tract and uterus but may also arise intraabdominally without any connection to parenchymal organs.[255] The usual sites in such cases are the omentum, mesentery, and pelvic cavity. The tumor size is an important determinant of malignancy: tumors more than 6 cm in diameter and those with mitotic counts greater than per/10 high-power fields are usually malignant.

Histologically the tumors are composed of sheets of polygonal cells containing a cytoplasm that varies from being clear to deeply eosinophilic. Cytoplasmic vacuolization is common, and in extreme cases the cells may have a signet-ring cell appearance (Fig. 72-13, *C*). Because the cytologic features are not typical of smooth muscle cells, the diagnosis may be difficult. In addition, immunohistochemical evaluation and EM reveal features of smooth muscle cells in only a small percentage of tumor cells.

TUMORS OF STRIATED MUSCLE

Rhabdomyoma

Rhabdomyomas are benign tumors showing a striated muscle differentiation. These tumors can be divided into four clinicopathologic groups.

Adult rhabdomyoma is a very rare, slowly growing tumor occurring primarily in the oral cavity and pharynx in men over 40 years of age.[256-257a] The tumor may recur in the span of more than 30 years. Grossly the tumor is a brown, often multilobular mass usually measuring 1 to 5 cm in diameter. Histologically the tumor cells are large and polygonal and resemble normal skeletal muscle cells in cross section (Fig. 72-14). Compared with hyperplastic muscle, rhabdomyoma cells are

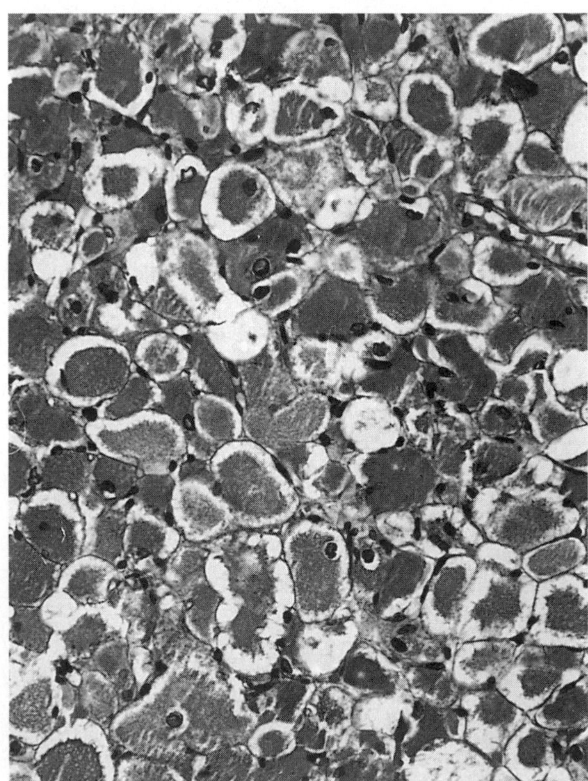

Fig. 72-14 Adult rhabdomyoma, which is composed of large polygonal, mature rhabdomyoblasts with small nuclei.

larger and often show cytoplasmic vacuolization. The nuclei are small and mitoses are not seen. In keeping with the low growth potential of these tumors, cell-labeling studies show that cellular replication is extremely slow, indicating that it may take 10 years for the tumor to reach 1 cm in diameter.

Adult rhabdomyoma can hardly be confused with any other tumor. Immunohistochemically the cells are positive for myoglobin, desmin, and muscle actins, confirming its striated muscle nature. EM shows the presence of Z-bands typical of striated muscle tissue. Some tumors show crystallike material similar to that seen in a muscle disease known as "nemaline myopathy." The neoplastic nature of rhabdomyoma has been debated, but recent findings of cytogenetic abnormalities in cases of rhabdomyoma occurring in adults favor a neoplastic as opposed to a hyperplastic process.

Rhabdomyoma of the female genitals usually arises as a small vaginal or vulvar polyp in adults.[260] Histologically it is composed of fibroblast-like cells admixed with clusters of elongated spindle-shaped cells showing the ultrastructural and immunohistochemical features of well-differentiated striated muscle cells. This tumor is entirely benign. The smallness of the lesions, their limited cellularity, and the fact that the tumor affects adults set it apart from botryoid rhabdomyosarcoma.

Fetal rhabdomyoma is a very rare tumor that affects small children and is composed of well-differentiated elongated rhabdomyoblasts.[258] The absence of mitotic activity and sharp circumscription distinguish it from embryonal rhabdomyosarcoma, but a recent study showing progression of recurrent fetal rhabdomyoma to embryonal rhabdomyosarcoma indicates that these entities may overlap.

Cardiac rhabdomyoma is a distinctive, probably hamartomatous proliferation that arises in the heart muscle of infants and small children.[259] It is associated with the tuberous sclerosis syndrome and is discussed further in Chapter 44.

Rhabdomyosarcoma

Rhabdomyosarcomas are malignant tumors showing a striated muscle–like differentiation. Previously believed to be among the most common soft-tissue sarcomas in subjects of all ages, rhabdomyosarcoma is now recognized as a tumor affecting mainly children and adolescents.[260] However, rhabdomyosarcoma-like heterologous components are commonly seen in the malignant mixed müllerian tumors of the female genitals that occur during adult life and occasionally in germ cell tumors. Five clinicopathologically distinct types are recognized: embryonal, botryoid, spindle cell, alveolar, and pleomorphic, although some overlap may exist among them. The overall survival rate in patients with the different types of rhabdomyosarcomas has improved significantly during the past 5 years because of the effectiveness of multimodality chemotherapy and now ranges from 80% to 90% in patients with the histologically favorable types.[261]

The cells that make up *embryonal rhabdomyosarcoma,* the most common type of rhabdomyosarcoma (75% of all cases), bear an either greater or lesser resemblance to early fetal striated muscle cells.[262-264] The incidence peaks in the first years of life, and the urogenital organs (paratesticular and scrotal as well as the bladder) and the head and neck area (orbit, sinonasal region, and middle ear) are the most common sites. Some tumors occur in the soft tissues of the trunk, whereas only a few arise in the extremities. Occasional well-documented cases of embryonal rhabdomyosarcoma in older patients and even in elderly ones are reported.[265] All embryonal rhabdomyosarcomas are regarded as high-grade malignant tumors, but the prognosis is favorable because of the effectiveness of the currently available chemotherapy.[261,263,264,266,267]

Grossly, embryonal rhabdomyosarcoma typically appears as a myxoid, gray-white mass (Fig. 72-15, *A*). Histologically it consists of a mixture of undifferentiated round cells and immature striated muscle-like cells with abundant eosinophilic cytoplasm (rhabdomyoblasts) (Fig. 72-15, *B*). The proportion of rhabdomyoblasts varies from case to case; the tumor composition ranges from one in which primitive-appearing round cells dominate to one in which there is extensive rhabdomyoblastic differentiation. (Fig 72-15, *C*) The degree of rhabdomyoblastic differentiation appears to be positively correlated with the prognosis. In some cases loose myxoid areas alternate with the cellular areas in a trabecular pattern.

Immunohistochemical evaluation of muscle-specific proteins is of prime importance in the identification and documentation of rhabdomyosarcoma.[268,273] Of these, desmin and muscle actins are consistently present in many of the tumor cells, including undifferentiated-appearing cells. Keratins have also been found in some cases. Myoglobin is restricted to more-differentiated rhabdomyoblasts and is generally absent in primitive round cells. Chemotherapy has been reported to cause an increase in the number of differentiated rhabdomyoblasts in some cases, probably through selection of the nonproliferating component.[274] MyoD1, a nuclear antigen typical of cells of striated muscle lineage, has been suggested as a new marker for rhabdomyosarcoma.[275] EM shows alternating thin and thick filaments that may form sarcomeric units; the presence of the former constitutes the minimum ultrastructural criteria for rhabdomyosarcoma[276] (Fig. 72-15, *D*).

Ectomesenchymoma is a term used to refer to an embryonal rhabdomyosarcoma that contains mature ganglion cells. This extremely rare tumor has been encountered in children.[277]

Botryoid rhabdomyosarcoma, previously considered a type of embryonal rhabdomyosarcoma, has clinicopathologic features distinctive enough to warrant its classification as a separate entity. It mainly affects infants, but occasional cases in adults have been reported. This tumor usually presents in the urogenital tract, including the vagina, uterine cervix, and urinary bladder, as a polypoid, myxoid, exophytic mass resembling a bunch of grapes. Bile ducts and the upper respiratory tract are rare additional locations.[278, 279] With the treatments currently available, prognosis is excellent.

Microscopically, botryoid rhabdomyosarcoma consists of undifferentiated rounded and spindled cells admixed with more differentiated elongated rhabdomyoblasts which often show distinctive cross striations. The cells are typically embedded in a highly myxoid stroma that is condensed beneath the subepithelial, densely cellular zone called the "cambium layer."

Spindle cell rhabdomyosarcoma is a rare well-differentiated variant of childhood rhabdomyosarcoma is composed of uniform spindle cells which correspond to the myotube stage of fetal striated muscle cells.[280,281] This type, previously classified as an embryonal rhabdomyosarcoma and also called "leiomyosarcomatous rhabdomyosarcoma," occurs in the urogenital organs in the paratesticular, prostatic, and parauterine regions. Patients with this variant have an excellent prognosis, with a 5-year survival rate of more than 90%. Spindle cell rhabdomyosarcoma can be distinguished

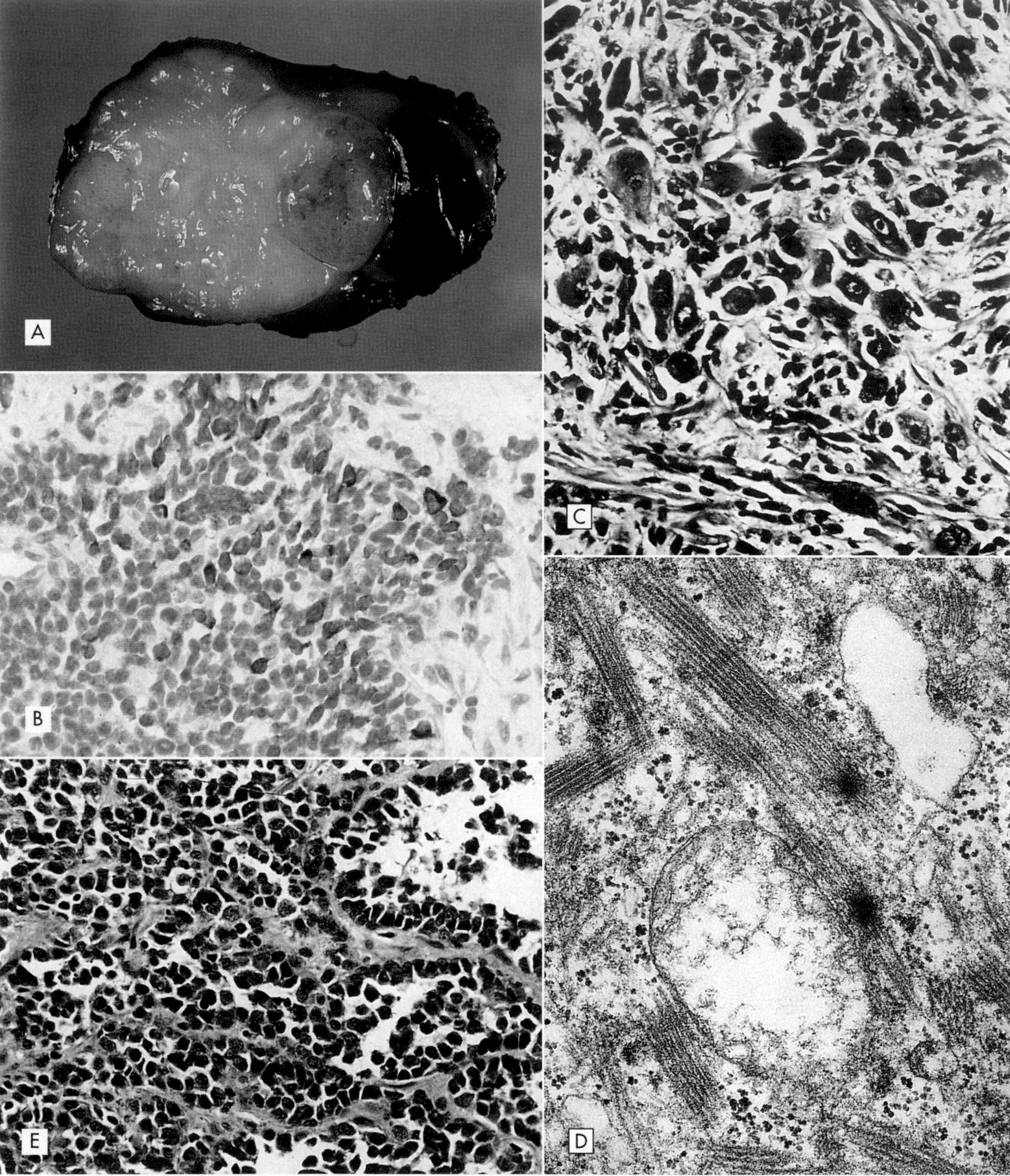

Fig. 72-15 **A,** Rhabdomyosarcoma appearing as a myxoid mass. **B,** Embryonal rhabdomyosarcoma consisting of primitive round cells and foci of large rhabdomyoblasts. **C,** Embryonal rhabdomyosarcomas composed of larger rhabdomyoblastic cells are desmin positive. **D,** Electron micrograph showing a rhabdomyosarcoma in which thin and thick filaments are coaligned with Z-band–like densities *(lower center)*. **E,** Alveolar rhabdomyosarcoma consisting of undifferentiated round cells with the formation of aveolar spaces between fibrous septa.

from other spindle cell sarcomas by the presence of striated muscle differentiation, as verified by immunohistochemical and EM findings.

Alveolar rhabdomyosarcoma is a clinically and histologically distinct variant of rhabdomyosarcoma that accounts for 10% to 20% of all cases. It occurs mainly in adolescents; it is rare in small children and exceptional in old persons.[282,283] The preferential locations are the distal parts of the extremities and head and neck. Rarely it occurs in the female genitals.[284] This tumor is a high-grade malignant lesion that was usually uniformly lethal before the advent of the current methods of chemotherapy. It is still, however, considered a prognostically unfavorable type of rhabdomyosarcoma. The primary tumor may be small and remain undetected even though the tumor has metastasized widely. Unlike many other sarcomas, alveolar rhabdomyosarcoma has a tendency to spread to regional lymph nodes. Superficial soft tissues, including the breasts of women, are also common metastatic sites.

Histologically, alveolar rhabdomyosarcoma shows nests of neoplastic cells separated by fibrovascular septa. These are lined by undifferentiated round cells and small numbers of multinucleated giant cells with an eosinophilic cytoplasm (Fig. 72-15, *E*). Poor cellular cohesion and degeneration of the tumor cells create the "alveolar" spaces. Variants with no alveolar spaces are named "solid variant of alveolar rhabdomyosarcoma"; these may resemble other small round cell tumors.[285] Desmin and muscle actins can be readily demonstrated by immunohistochemical tests, but myoglobin is present only in differentiated rhabdomyoblasts.[271,272] Because of the minimal cell differentiation, the striated muscle nature of the tumor cells cannot be easily demonstrated by EM.[286]

A balanced chromosomal translocation t(2;13)(q35;q14) is a typical cytogenetic finding and can be considered diagnostic of alveolar RMS. Variant translocations t(1;13) and t(8;13) have been noted in some cases. Numerical chromosomal alterations often accompany the typical translocation, and tetraploidy is common.[287-289] The typical, t(2;13), or less common, t(1;13), chromosomal translocations involve *PAX3* and *FKHR* or *PAX7* and *FKHR* genes and create a fusion gene that leads to the formation of a chimeric transcript and fusion protein; the presence of these translocations can be diagnosed by the reverse transcriptase polymerase chain reaction. Interestingly, a mutation of the *PAX3* gene has been found in an unrelated disorder, Waardenburg's syndrome,which is associated with a hereditary sensorineural hearing loss.

Pleomorphic rhabdomyosarcoma, once believed to be a common sarcoma occurring in the extremities of adults, is now believed to be very rare.[290-292] Well-documented and immunohistochemically or ultrastructurally defined cases occur in the extremities of adults, and generally the prognosis is poor. Histologically, pleomorphic rhabdomyosarcoma bears some resemblance to MFH of the storiform-pleomorphic type but shows definite rhabdomyoblastic differentiation. The diagnosis usually has to be based on the ultrastructural and immunohistochemical findings.

NEURAL TUMORS

Benign neural and nerve sheath tumors

Nerve sheath tumors include those lesions that show nerve sheath cell differentiation (neurofibroma, schwannoma) as well as those that display neuronal features (ganglioneuroma). Tumors in the former group may contain Schwann cells, perineurial cells, and perineurial fibroblasts. Most of these tumors are benign, and many of them are common.

Traumatic neuroma is the designation for the hyperplastic disordered regeneration of a peripheral nerve.[293] Clinically it presents as a small painful nodule at the site of previous trauma or surgery, such as an amputation stump, hence its alternative term *amputation neuroma.* The lesion is continuous with the proximal end of the lacerated or transected nerve. Histologically a traumatic neuroma consists of interwoven small-nerve fascicles surrounded by myelin sheaths. Each of the substructures resembles normal nerve at the level of cellular organization. In contrast, neurofibromas show a disorderly proliferation of subsets of nerve sheath cells.

Morton's neuroma is a clinically distinct condition causing paroxysmal pain in the foot.[294] The lesion is usually located between the roots of the third and fourth toes and clinically appears as a mild tumorlike swelling. External compression and repeated minor trauma resulting from unsuitable footwear are believed to be the causes. Histologically the plantar digital nerve is marked by circumferential perineural fibrosis and degenerative changes in the soft tissue.

Neurofibroma (solitary neurofibroma) is a common benign tumor of the peripheral nerves composed of haphazardly arranged fibroblasts, perineurial cells, and Schwann cells.[293,295] It presents most commonly as either a small dermal nodule or a broad-based polypoid skin lesion, but it may occur in deeper sites such as the subcutis, mediastinum, and retroperitoneum. It may occur sporadically or in the setting of neurofibromatosis type 1. Histologically, neurofibromas are unencapsulated lesions consisting of slender spindle cells intermingled with wavy collagen bundles. The stroma may vary from myxoid to collagenous (Fig. 72-16, *A*). Cutaneous neurofibromas apparently arise in small-nerve endings, and their connection with normal nerves cannot be demonstrated histologically. Some subcutaneous neurofibromas may contain tactile bodies (Wagner-Meissner corpuscles)[296] (Fig. 72-16, *B*).

Diffuse neurofibroma occurs predominantly in children and young adults. It forms diffuse neurofibromatous growths in superficial soft tissues chiefly in the head and neck area. Some cases are associated with neurofibromatosis type I (see later discussion). The subcutaneous infiltration of diffuse neurofibroma should not be confused with DFSP, which usually exhibits a more distinct storiform pattern.

Plexiform neurofibroma is composed of one or more adjoining nerves that have been transformed into neurofibromas, sometimes becoming large tortuous masses. Small nerves with multiple plexiform neurofibromas alternating with normal stretches of the nerve may clinically resemble a chain of lymph nodes or beads in a string. Except for its distincive gross appearance, it is microscopically identical to ordinary neurofibroma and is considered virtually diagnostic of neurofibromatosis type 1.

Neurofibromatosis includes two different hereditary diseases involving nerves. In neurofibromatosis type 1 (von Recklinghausen's disease), varying numbers of cutaneous and plexiform neurofibromas develop that may form mutilating tumors and involve both superficial and deep soft tissues. Lightly pigmented (café au lait) spots on the skin and Lisch nodules of the iris are additional diagnostic features. Neurofibromatosis type 1 is one of the most common genetic diseases. It is inherited in an autosomal dominant fashion, and it occurs in 1 in 4000 births in the population of the United States. The genetic lesion has been localized to chromosome 17, and it is believed to cause impairment of the production or function of a growth regulatory protein, neurofibromin.[297] This condition carries a 1% to 5% risk of progressing to malignant peripheral nerve sheath tumors.[298,299]

Neurofibromatosis Type 2 is manifested as bilateral acoustic nerve schwannomas and is not associated with subsequent malignancy. The genetic lesion has been localized to chromosome 22.[300]

Nerve sheath myxoma (neurothekeoma) is a benign tumor usually occurring as a small cutaneous or subcutaneous nodule in children and young adults. Histologically it is composed of multiple round or oval lobules of spindle cells in a myxoid stroma separated by fibrous septa (Fig. 72-16, *C*). Cellular, less myxoid variants have also been described. The tumor shows variable S-100 protein positivity, and EM has shown the presence of basement membranes, indicating possible Schwann cell differentiation.[301-303]

Perineurioma is a rare benign soft-tissue tumor in which slender spindle cells are arranged in a fascicular or storiform pattern. These lesions have been principally identified by immunohistochemical tests as epithelial membrane antigen–positive and S-100 antigen–protein–negative spindle cell proliferations recapitulating the immunophenotype of normal perineurial cells.[304-309]

Schwannoma (neurilemoma, neurinoma) is a benign tumor composed of well-differentiated Schwann cells.[293,310] It is among the most common benign, deeply located soft-tissue tumors and typically occurs in young and middle-aged adults. Schwannoma arises eccentrically from a nerve, displacing it to one side. Common locations include the head, neck, mediastinum, and retroperitoneum. It also arises intracranially, most commonly from the acoustic (eighth) and trigeminal (fifth) cranial nerves and has been found in the gastronintestinal tract.[311] There is a weak association of schwannoma with neurofibromatosis type 1 (generalized); bilateral acoustic schwannomas are pathognomonic of neurofibromatosis type 2.

Schwannomas are typically circumscribed, if not encapsulated, tumors that vary in size from a few millimeters to 15 cm in diameter. The largest tumors occur in body cavities, where they grow unnoticed and therefore become large. On cross section schwannomas are grossly yellow-white. The large tumors often show central cystic degeneration.

Histologically they are characterized by cellular Antoni A areas alternating with myxoid, loose degenerative Antoni B areas. The cellular areas consist of sheets of spindle cells with palisaded nuclei that may form columns around amorphous matrix (Verocay bodies) (Fig. 72-16, *D*). The myxoid, loose degenerative areas show haphazardly arranged Schwann cells admixed with sheets of foamy macrophages (xanthoma cells) and lymphocytes. Hyalinization and regressive changes, including vascular thrombosis, are common. Nuclear atypia and monster giant cells may be present. Tumors with such degenerative atypia have been called *ancient schwannoma*.[312] Some benign schwannomas consist predominantly or exclusively of Antoni A areas without Verocay bodies and occasionally with considerable mitotic activity. Such tumors may be mistaken for fibrosarcoma or leiomyosarcoma and have been named *cellular schwannomas*. They are more often seen in the mediastinum and retroperitoneum. Although a cellular schwannoma is benign, occasional recurrences have been reported.[313-315]

Immunohistochemical evaluation is useful in the differential diagnosis of schwannoma and other spindle cell tumors. Schwannomas typically show diffuse and rather intense S-100 protein positivity in the cellular areas. They also stain strongly for basement membrane components such as laminin and collagen type IV. Glial fibrillary acidic protein is present in some benign schwannomas.[316-318]

EM shows the presence of typical Schwann cell features, which include cells with interdigitating cytoplasmic processes surrounded by complete basement membranes[295](Fig. 72-16, *E*). Deposits of extracellular, long-spacing collagen (Luse bodies) are typical but not specific to schwannomas.

Cytogenetic features of schwannomas include common monosomy of chromosome 22. This change occurs both in sporadic cases and in those associated with neurofibromatosis type 2.[300,319]

A plexiform schwannoma is a schwannoma that has a multinodular growth pattern, either grossly or microscopically. Most cases have been found in superficial soft tissues. Unlike plexiform neurofibroma, this tumor is not associated with neurofibromatosis.[320,321]

Melanotic schwannoma is a rare variant of schwannoma; containing melanin pigment and often psammoma bodies.[322] This tumor occurs in the midline, most commonly in the chest wall and paraspinal region, but also occasionally in the gastrointestinal tract. More than half of the cases, are linked with a hereditary condition associated with spotty pigmentation, endocrine hyperactivity, and cardiac myxoma (Carney's complex). Most of these tumors are benign, but the ones that show marked mitotic activity may be malignant and metastasize. Histologically, melanotic schwannoma consists of highly cellular, sometimes mildly pleomorphic spindle cells arranged in a fascicular pattern. Melanin is usually abundant, and psammoma bodies are common. Ultrastructurally the cells resemble Schwann cells, but they also contain melanosomes.

Ganglioneuroma is a mature tumor of the autonomic nervous system that occurs predominantly in young adults but may be encountered in patients of all ages. These tumors usually arise in the posterior mediastinum, retroperitoneum, or the adrenals and may be large encapsulated masses that grossly appear myxoid. Histologically, ganglioneuroma is composed of bundles of Schwann cells and nerves with an appearance reminiscent of that of a neurofibroma. Mature and immature ganglion cells are scattered throughout (Fig. 72-16, *F*). Adequate sampling should be done so that the presence of immature neuroblastic component can be excluded.

Paraganglioma and pheochromocytoma are paraganglionic tumors of the autonomic nervous system that show true neural differentiation. The former is usually found in the head and neck and the latter in the adrenals or retroperitoneum.

Neuroblastoma and ganglioneuroblastoma are immature tumors of the sympathetic nervous system typically found in the adrenals or mediastinum of infants and small children. They are discussed among neoplasms of the adrenals (Chapter 63).

Granular cell tumor was originally described as a "granular cell myoblastoma." EM and immunohistochemical findings have convincingly established its relationship to other peripheral nerve sheath tumors. Granular cell tumor occurs as a small, superficial dermal or subcutaneous nodule (1 cm to 3

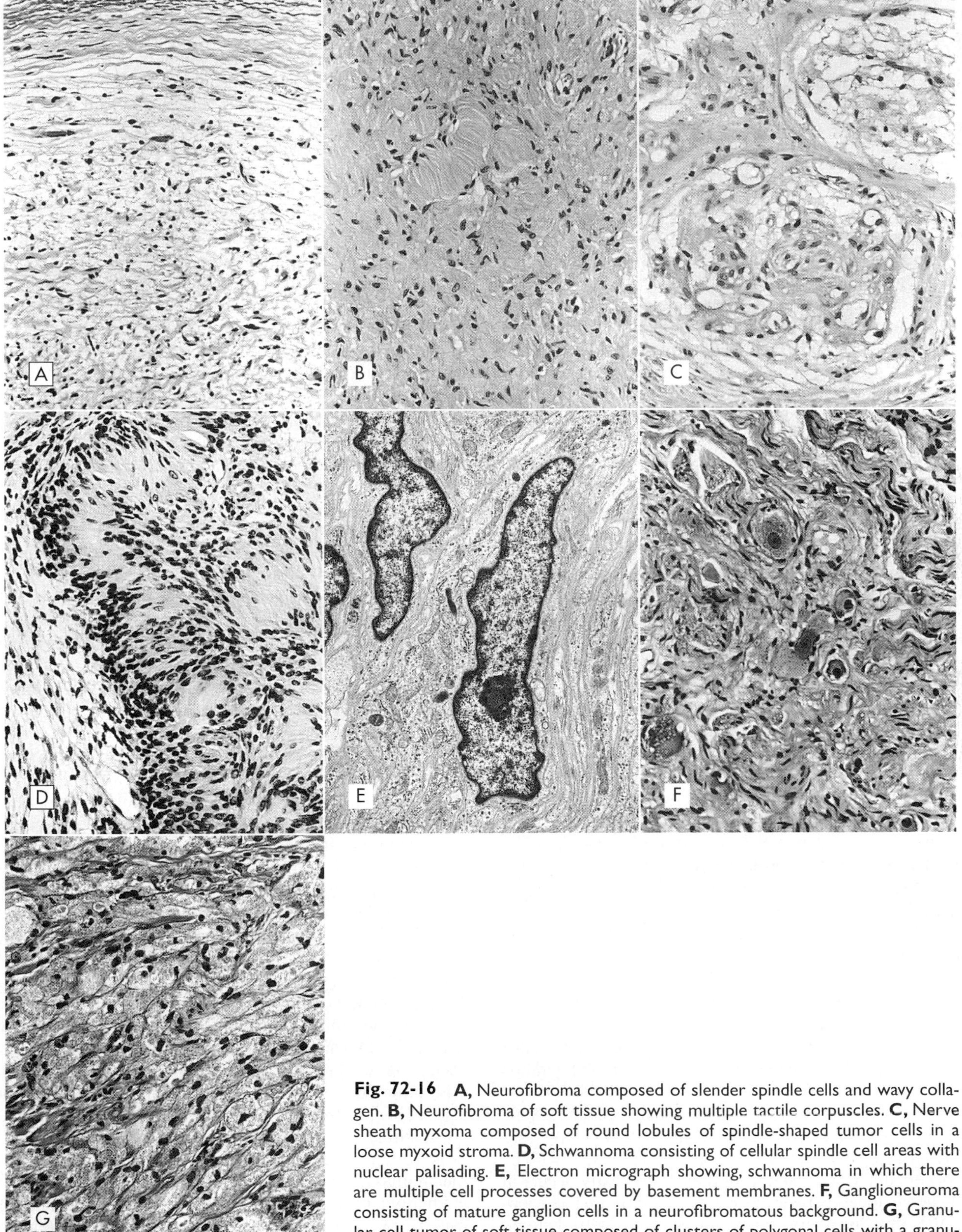

Fig. 72-16 **A,** Neurofibroma composed of slender spindle cells and wavy collagen. **B,** Neurofibroma of soft tissue showing multiple tactile corpuscles. **C,** Nerve sheath myxoma composed of round lobules of spindle-shaped tumor cells in a loose myxoid stroma. **D,** Schwannoma consisting of cellular spindle cell areas with nuclear palisading. **E,** Electron micrograph showing, schwannoma in which there are multiple cell processes covered by basement membranes. **F,** Ganglioneuroma consisting of mature ganglion cells in a neurofibromatous background. **G,** Granular cell tumor of soft tissue composed of clusters of polygonal cells with a granular appearance.

cm in diameter) on the extremities or trunk or in the tongue, and occasionally in the respiratory tract and esophagus. In the female breast it may present as an induration that clinically and grossly may look like carcinoma.[323,337] Occasionally granular cell tumors are multiple. Most patients are middle-aged, and it tends to occur in women. Most granular cell tumors are benign, and local recurrences are rare. Well-documented malignant variants are found in 1% to 2% of the cases.[325,326] These can be distinguished from their benign counterparts by the presence of mitoses, atypia, and a destructive growth pattern.

Granular cell tumors appear grossly as yellowish poorly circumscribed nodules. Histologically they show ragged margins that infiltrate muscle or connective tissue. The large polygonal tumor cells have small, dark nuclei and are arranged in irregular nests and clusters surrounded by collagenous septa (Fig. 72-16, *G*). The tumor cells contain abundant, finely granular, PAS-positive cytoplasm. Superficial tumors often show pseudoepitheliomatous hyperplasia of the overlying epithelium that should not be mistaken for squamous cell carcinoma.

Immunohistochemically granular cell tumors are positive for S-100 protein, vimentin, and myelin basic protein.[327-329] These findings, together with the fact that some granular cell tumors are closely associated with small nerves, support their relationship to Schwann cell neoplasms.[330] Ultrastructurally the cytoplasmic granules correspond to clusters of secondary lysosomes showing autophagic vacuoles. The presence of so-called angulate bodies, which are polygonal structures filled with microtubules, is typical. Basement membranes around the cells are less prominent than they are in schwannomas.[330]

Granular cell tumor of the gingiva of the newborn seems to constitute an entity distinct from other granular cell tumors.[331] These tumors are typically found in the anterior alveolar ridge in female newborns, more commonly in the upper jaw. Histologically they are made up of ballooned cells with rounded contours and a granular cytoplasm interspersed with a prominent capillary pattern. Lack of S-100 protein combined with ultrastructural data indicate that this tumor is unrelated to granular cell tumor of the peripheral soft tissues and is probably of fibroblastic derivation. These lesions may be nonneoplastic and spontaneously involute.

Granular cell histiocytic reactions at sites of previous trauma or surgery[332] and histiocytic pseudotumors caused by *Mycobacterium avium-intracellulare* infection in AIDS patients have to be distinguished from granular cell tumors. In addition, smooth muscle cells of the gastrointestinal tract and urinary bladder can acquire a focal granular cell appearance under certain conditions; such lesions do not represent genuine granular cell tumors.[333]

Meningioma and *ependymoma* occasionally occur as soft-tissue tumors outside the central nervous system, supposedly arising from ectopic tissue or developmental rests.[334,335] The former occurs in the scalp and face; the latter usually occurs in a subcutaneous location over the sacrococcygeal area and represents the myxopapillary type. Although usually benign, some soft-tissue ependymomas (as much as 20%) eventually metastasize to the lungs during the protracted course of the disease.

Pigmented neuroectodermal tumor of infancy (retinal anlage tumor, melanotic progonoma) is a rare tumor that usually occurs in the jaws of small children, but similar tumors have been seen in the epididymis. Although most of these tumors are benign, occasional ones have behaved aggressively. Histologically the tumor is composed of clusters of melanin-pigmented and nonpigmented epithelioid cells that may line alveolar-like spaces set amidst a fibrous background. Immunohistochemically the epithelioid cells are positive for melanoma-associated antigen (HMB-45) and vimentin and focally for keratins but are negative for S-100 protein.[335a]

Malignant nerve sheath tumors

Malignant peripheral nerve sheath tumor [MPNST] malignant schwannoma, neurofibrosarcoma) accounts for less than 10% of all sarcomas. Approximately 50% arise in patients with neurofibromatosis type 1 through the malignant transformation of nerve trunk neurofibromas; the remainder occur sporadically.[336-340] However, this tumor almost never arises from a benign schwannoma. A few cases have been described as postirradiation sarcomas.[341] Tumors not arising in nerve trunks may be deemed MPNST on the basis of Schwann cell features, as revealed by EM and immunohistochemical tests. Most patients are middle-aged, but the tumor may also develop in young persons and occasionally in children, especially in the setting of neurofibromatosis. Multiple simultaneous or synchronous tumors at different sites occur in some patients. The prognosis is relatively poor, with the 5-year survival rate of approximately 40%. Although the prognosis in patients with tumors arising in neurofibromatosis has usually been considered more unfavorable then those occurring sporadically, recent evidence suggests that this may not be true.[342]

Those tumors arising from major nerve trunks expand the nerve in a fusiform fashion, and remnants of plexiform neurofibroma can often be found (Fig. 72-17, *A*). Histologically, MPNST usually resembles fibrosarcoma, except that the spindle cells tend to have an irregular, buckled shape reminiscent of the shape of normal Schwann cell and are arranged in fascicles that alternate in cellularity (Fig. 72-17, *B*). Some tumors may be highly pleomorphic and have MFH-like features. Heterologous components such as cartilage and bone may be present. Immunohistochemically, vimentin and S-100 protein are variably present. Ultrastructural evidence of Schwann cell differentiation may be minimal or absent altogether[343-347] (Fig. 72-17, *C*). Thus the findings from special studies indicate that most of these tumors may be poorly differentiated sarcomas which have arisen within the confines of a nerve sheath or a benign nerve sheath tumor may have features of Schwann cells, perineural cells, or fibroblasts.

Malignant epithelioid schwannoma is a peculiar variant of nerve sheath sarcoma that usually arises within the nerve trunks of middle-aged patients. A minority of patients with this tumor have also had neurofibromatosis. The tumor consists of sheets or cords of large polygonal cells with a deeply eosinophilic cytoplasm. These cells are positive for S-100 protein and vimentin but are negative for keratins and melanoma-associated antigen (HMB-45).[348,349] Malignant epithelioid (and other types of malignant) schwannoma can usually be differentiated from metastatic melanoma on the basis of the clinical context and the immunohistochemical profile.

Malignant Triton tumor is the designation for peripheral nerve sheath sarcomas that contain rhabdomyoblasts, and their existence illustrates the capacity of multipotential differentiation.[350-352] As with other malignant schwannomas, Triton

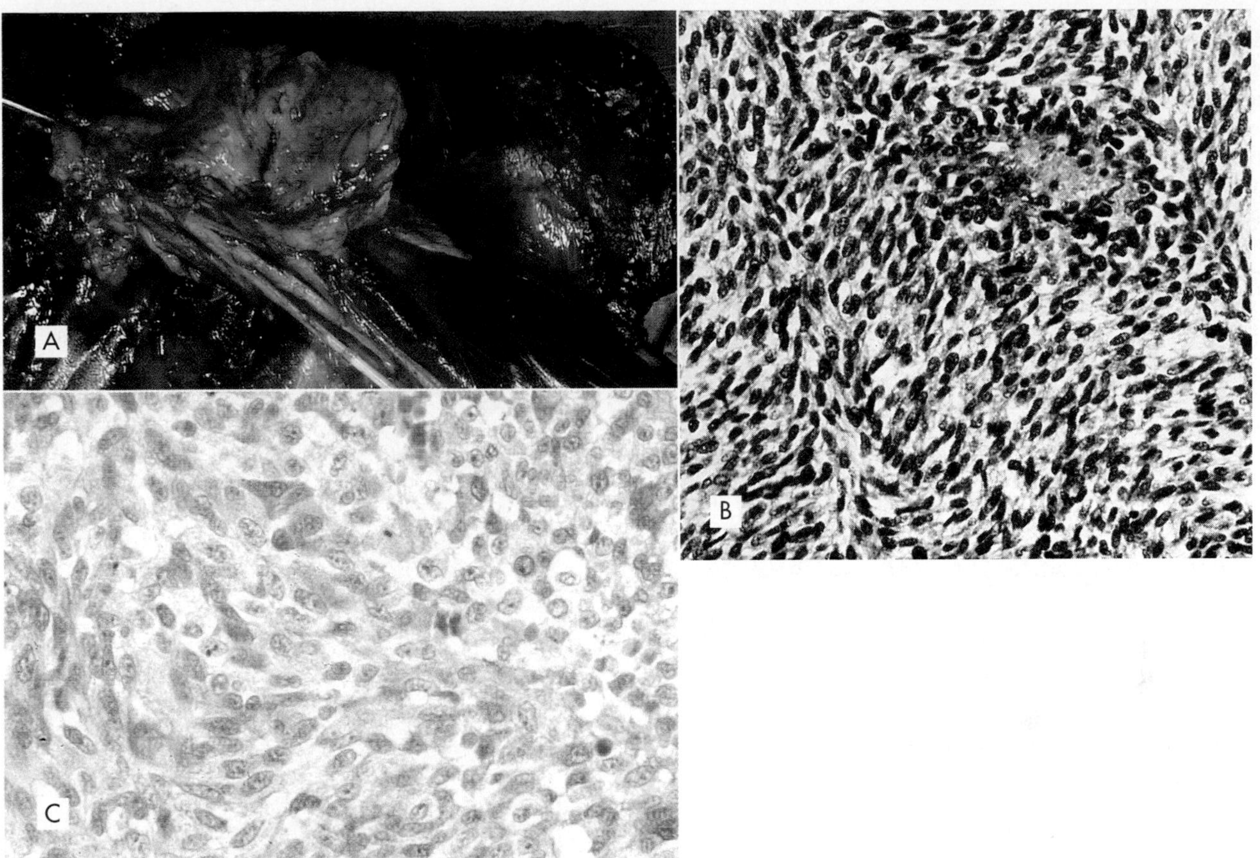

Fig. 72-17 **A,** Peripheral nerve sheath sarcoma arising from the ulnar nerve. **B,** Histologic appearance of peripheral nerve sheath sarcoma showing a spindle cell pattern. **C,** S-100 protein immunoreactivity in scattered spindle cells of a malignant schwannoma.

tumors are associated with neurofibromatosis type 1. Rare benign variants with a similar constellation of well-differentiated components have been reported; they are called as *neuromuscular hamartoma* or "benign Triton tumor."[353]

Glandular malignant schwannoma is the designation for a very rare peripheral nerve sheath sarcoma containing glands lined by cuboidal or occasionally by goblet cell–containing epithelium. Most of these tumors are high-grade malignant lesions and occur in young adults in the context of neurofibromatosis type 1.[354]

Clear cell sarcoma is a rare melanocytic soft-tissue tumor originally described by Enzinger in 1965. Although the term "melanoma of soft parts" has been proposed as an alternative term, significant differences between this tumor and conventional cutaneous melanoma exist, such that this lesion should be considered a distinct entity.[355, 356] Clear cell sarcoma of the tendons and aponeuroses is unrelated to clear cell sarcoma of the kidney, a childhood tumor.

Clear cell sarcoma occurs predominantly in young adults.[355-361] A slight preponderance of cases in female patients has been reported in many series. The tumor occurs predominantly in the distal extremities, most commonly in the feet and ankles. Less common sites are the hand, wrist, knee area, and shoulder. Typically the tumor involves tendon sheaths and arises as a slowly enlarging, painless mass, often of long duration (up to several years in 20% of cases). Metastasis to the lungs, bones, and lymph nodes occurs in nearly half of the cases, and the 5-year survival rate is approximately 50% to 60%. Large tumor size and the presence of necrosis have been identified as adverse prognostic factors.[358,361]

Grossly the tumor is a circumscribed, lobular, or multinodular mass that is usually less than 5 cm in diameter and displays a gray-white homogeneous surface on sectioning. Some cases show gross pigmentation. Microscopically, clear cell sarcoma consists of large, irregularly shaped packets and fascicles of tumor cells separated by variably sized fibrous septa, which often cross at sharp angles (Fig. 72-18). Further compartmental organization can be demonstrated with reticulin stain, which shows the existence of fibers surrounding clusters of tumor cells. Most tumor cells are uniformly polygonal or fusiform, but multinucleated cells resembling Touton giant cells may be seen. The nuclei are vesicular and contain a single prominent basophilic nucleolus. Mitotic activity is typically scant. The cytoplasm varies from being mildly eosinophilic to clear and contains glycogen. More than half of the tumors contain melanin.

Immunohistochemically, clear cell sarcoma is positive for vimentin, S-100 protein, melanoma-associated antigen (HMB-45), and neuron-specific enolase, characteristics similar to those of cutaneous melanoma.[362,363] The cell surface characteristics also resemble those of melanoma.[364] The absence of keratins helps to distinguish this tumor from metastatic clear cell carcinoma.[365] Typical ultrastructural features include the presence of (pre)melanosomes in most of cases. Basement

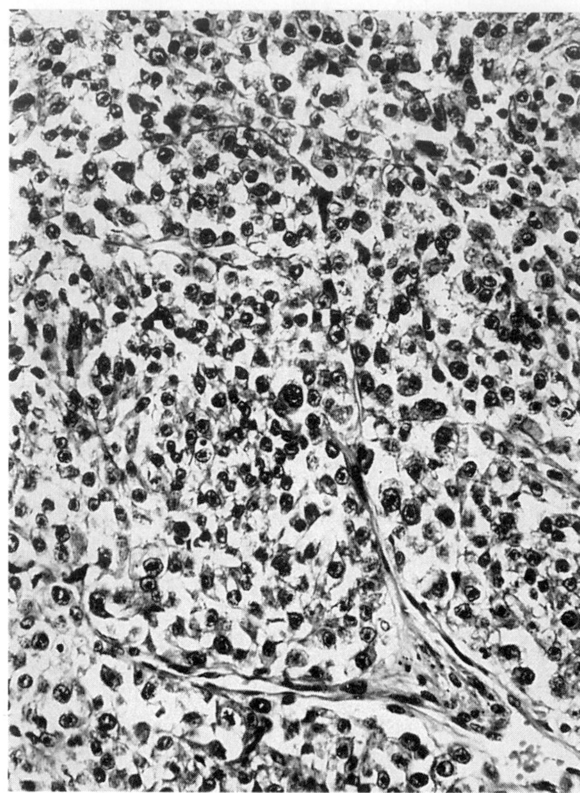

Fig. 72-18 Clear cell sarcoma composed of sheets of polygonal and spindle-shaped cells with large nucleoli.

membranes usually surround the clusters of tumor cells but sometimes also the individual tumor cells, in which case the tumor then resembles a melanotic schwannoma.[362,366,367]

Clear cell sarcoma has a specific cytogenetic abnormality, translocation t(12;22)(q13;q12), which is not seen in melanoma.[367a] The genes involved in this translocation are not yet known. However, some of the numerical chromosomal changes noted for clear cell sarcoma resemble those seen in melanoma.[368-371]

CARTILAGE AND BONE-FORMING SOFT-TISSUE TUMORS

Myositis ossificans is a pseudoneoplastic condition marked by the formation of reactive bone.[372-374] This tumorlike condition is a painful soft-tissue swelling that typically occurs in young adults, especially in athletically active men. Local trauma often precedes this lesion, but such a history is not elicited in all cases. The lesion is usually located in the extremities, most commonly in the anterior muscles of the thigh or in the buttock.

Grossly a mature lesion is typically sharply demarcated and shows a peripheral shell of variably calcified bone with trabeculas radiating inward. The center of the lesion may consist of trabecular immature bone, osteoclast-like giant cells, and fascicles of proliferative fibroblasts (Fig. 72-19). Such a zonal pattern is typical of this condition. Somewhat similar lesions without typical zonation and located in the distal parts of the extremities have been termed *fibroosseous pseudotumor of the digits*[375] and *florid reactive periostitis*.[376] The early lesion con-

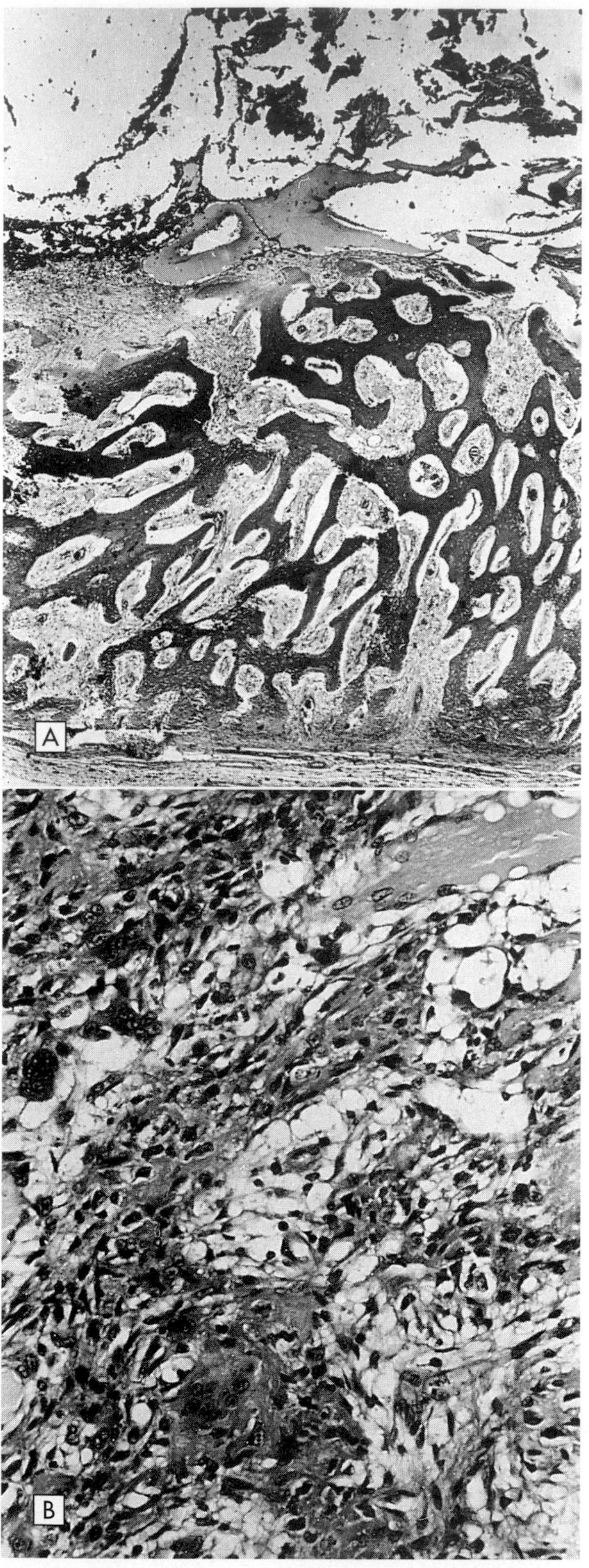

Fig. 72-19 **A,** The periphery of myositis ossificans showing trabeculae tuberculae of newly formed bone, resembling a callus. **B,** The central portion of myositis ossificans in which there are immature osteoid and osteoclast-like giant cells.

sists of sheets of fibroblasts and giant cells with scattered, disorganized bony trabeculae tuberculae. Malignant transformation of myositis ossificans has been reported anecdotally, but these cases more likely represent extraskeletal osteosarcomas with well-differentiated areas that may simulate the appearance of myositis ossificans. Metaplastic bone may also form in a variety of soft-tissue tumors, such as malignant fibrous histiocytoma, synovial sarcoma, and malignant schwannoma.

Fibrodysplasia (myositis) ossificans progressiva is a rare hereditary condition inherited in an autosomal dominant fashion.[377,378,378a] The nature of the genetic defect is unknown, but involvement of the genes that code for bone morphogenetic proteins has been suggested. This crippling condition is usually diagnosed in children before they are 10 years of age. Multifocal and slowly progressive, tumor-forming, calcifying soft-tissue ossifications develop first in the upper part of the body and later extend caudally, ultimately mechanically restricting movement and respiratory function. Congenital anomalies, including absence of the great toes, are typical clinically. The patients have a shortened life span, mainly resulting from the respiratory complications. Histologically, the lesions show metaplastic bone formation, but in contrast to myositis ossificans, the bone occurs in the center of the lesion; aspects of the early lesions may resemble the histologic appearance of fibromatosis or nodular fasciitis. Surgical trauma may promote metaplastic bone formation and should be avoided. No therapy has proved effective.

Osteosarcoma can present as a primary soft-tissue tumor (extraskeletal osteosarcoma). In contrast to its skeletal counterpart, extraskeletal osteosarcoma occurs mostly in adults over 40 years of age.[379-382] Deep muscle compartments of the extremities and retroperitoneum are the most common sites. Most extraskeletal osteosarcomas are high-grade sarcomas, and metastasis to the lungs is the rule. Histologic evidence of osteoid formation by the tumor cells with or without the presence of malignant cartilage is required to establish the diagnosis. The common appearance of extraskeletal osteosarcoma is that of a pleomorphic sarcoma resembling a malignant fibrous histiocytoma in which areas of tumor show the definite production of lacy or trabecular osteoid. Some tumors may be extensively ossified and calcified. The histologic variants of skeletal osteosarcoma are infrequently seen in extraskeletal osteosarcomas. These include small cell, telangiectatic, and low-grade parosteal osteosarcoma-like variants.[383]

Ossifying fibromyxoid tumor is the designation for a peculiar rare generally benign, superficial soft tissue tumor of adults. Typically it consists of nodules of S-100 protein– and vimentin-positive bland round cells in a variably myxoid stroma, usually together with peripheral spicules of metaplastic bone. Schwann cell as well as chondroid differentiation has been suggested but not proved.[384]

Chondromas of soft tissues are benign pure cartilaginous tumors, which are typically well circumscribed and located in the subcutaneous tissues at various sites.[385,386] Chondromas are composed of multiple nodules of mature hyaline cartilage containing cells situated in lacuna-like spaces (Fig. 72-20, *A*). Some tumors can be quite cellular. Synovial chondromatosis may cause a sizable soft-tissue mass to form around joints; this condition is discussed in Chapter 75.

Extraskeletal myxoid chondrosarcoma (ESMC) is a rare histologically distinctive tumor referred to by some as "chor-

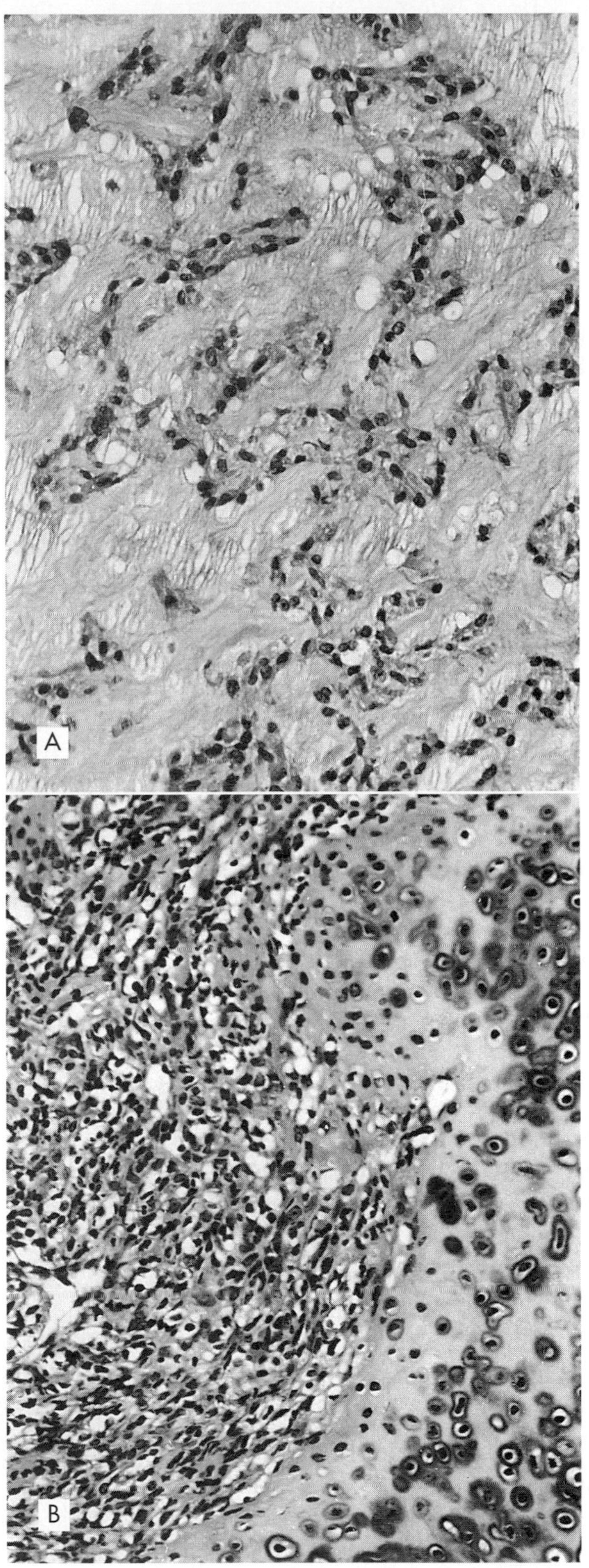

Fig. 72-20 **A,** Extraskeletal myxoid chondrosarcoma consisting of trabeculas of spindle cells in a myxoid stroma. **B,** Mesenchymal chondrosarcoma of soft tissue consisting of primitive-appearing round cells in fibrous stroma showing abrupt transition to differentiated cartilage.

doid sarcoma."[387,388] ESMC presents as a deeply located soft-tissue tumor in the extremities or retroperitoneum and typically affects middle-aged patients. Grossly the tumor is gray and gelatinous. Histologically it consists of oval or spindle-shaped, mitotically inactive cells arranged in anastomosing cords in a myxoid matrix of chondroitin sulfate. The cords and clusters of polygonal cells in this tumor may resemble chordoma (Fig. 72-20, *A*). Hyaline cartilage, a typical finding in skeletal chondrosarcoma, is only rarely seen as occasional foci. Although the clinical course in most patients with these tumors is slow, lung metastasis eventually occurs in as much as 30% of the cases.

These tumors have to be distinguished from myxoid liposarcoma, which has a different architectural pattern consisting of randomly scattered cells in a highly vascular myxoid background. In contrast to chordoma or mixed tumor of the skin, ESMC does not show epithelial differentiation and does not react with antibodies to keratins or with epithelial membrane antigen.[389] Ultrastructurally the polygonal tumor cells have scalloped outer margins like the margins of normal chondroblasts. Clusters of microtubules inside the rough endoplasmic reticulum have been repeatedly observed, although this is not a specific finding.[390] The chromosomal translocation t(9;22)(q22;q12) seems to be a typical cytogenetic finding.[391,392]

Mesenchymal chondrosarcoma occurs very rarely in soft tissues and is histologically similar to its osseous counterpart.[388,393] Many patients are relatively young. The most common sites are the thigh and meninges, and imaging studies typically show the existence of a calcified mass. The clinical course is that of a highly malignant tumor, and lung metastasis regularly occurs. The tumor consists of primitive round cells in a collagenous stroma arranged in a hemangiopericytoma-like pattern and punctuated by demarcated islands of differentiated cartilage (Fig. 72-20, *B*). The latter but not the former component is S-100 protein positive, similar to the immunohistochemical reactivity of normal cartilage.

SMALL ROUND CELL TUMORS

Small round cell tumors are a group of sarcomas that usually occur in children and consist of small, round "blue" cells. They include rhabdomyosarcoma, Ewing's sarcoma, neuroblastoma, and other primitive neuroepithelial tumors, as well as desmoplastic small round cell tumor. In addition, certain lymphomas (lymphoblastic lymphoma) and carcinomas (small cell carcinoma) also enter this differential diagnosis depending on the age of the patient. Immunohistochemical studies, EM, and more recently cytogenetic studies are important in the differential diagnosis.

Ewing's sarcoma, occurring in an extraosseous location without bone involvement, is termed *extraskeletal Ewing's sarcoma.*[394-396] Skeletal Ewing's sarcoma is much more common, and it may appear clinically as a large soft-tissue mass associated with a small primary focus in the adjacent bone. Extraskeletal Ewing's sarcoma presents as a deep soft tissue mass, it primarily affects adolescents and young adults and is rarely encountered in subjects after 40 years of age. The most common locations are the paravertebral area and the extremities. With advanced chemotherapy a moderate cure rate has been achieved in patients with this disease. A 40% 5-year survival rate has been reported by the Mayo Clinic, and the Intergroup Rhabdomyosarcoma Study has documented a 75% 3-year survival rate. Wide surgical resection and adjuvant radiotherapy improve the chances of survival in affected patients, but a pelvic location is an unfavorable prognostic factor.[397]

Grossly these tumors are multinodular gray masses usually measuring 5 to 10 cm. Histologically, extraskeletal Ewing's sarcoma is similar to its skeletal counterpart and is composed of sheets of uniform small round cells with centrally placed nuclei and scant, faintly staining cytoplasm. The nuclei have a fine chromatin pattern with inconspicuous nucleoli. The tumor has a rich vascular pattern, and in some cases the septa contain thick-walled vessels. The mitotic rate is variable, and necrosis is striking. The cytoplasmic glycogen can be demonstrated with PAS staining, with and without diastase. Because of its solubility, glycogen can be better demonstrated in alcohol-fixed or briefly formalin fixed tissue.

Immunohistochemically, Ewing's sarcoma cells are positive for vimentin and show reactivity for CD99 (antibody HBA71 recognizing a 30/32 kD T-cell and neuroendocrine antigen, a product of the *MIC2* gene).[398,399] Keratins 8 and 18 are often present in scattered tumor cells, which are uniformly negative for desmin, endothelial markers, and leukocyte antigens.[400,401] Neuron-specific enolase immunoreactivity is variable, neurofilament proteins are occasionally present, and results of cell culture studies have indicated the possibility of neural differentiation.[402] On EM studies the tumor is identical to Ewing's sarcoma of bone, showing cytoplasmic aggregates of glycogen particles and zonula adherens–type cell junctions.[403]

Cytogenetically, Ewing's sarcoma is characterized by a chromosomal translocation t(11,22)(q24;q12). This finding is consistent enough for it to be used as a diagnostic test, although related translocations may occur in other tumors such as desmoplastic small round cell tumor.[398,404,405] The typical translocation in Ewing's sarcoma leads to the formation of an *EWS-FLI1* fusion gene and fusion transcript; the latter can be detected by the reverse transcriptase polymerase chain reaction. Another translocation t(21;22) leads to fusion of the *EWS* and *ERG* genes and can also be diagnosed by the reverse transcriptase polymerase chain reaction.[406]

Peripheral neuroepithelioma is a tumor that has features of both Ewing's sarcoma and neuroblastoma.[398,407,408] It occurs chiefly in children and young adults at varying peripheral soft tissue sites, usually in association with the nerve trunks, and is a high-grade malignant lesion. Histologically it is composed of sheets, cords, and nests of small round cells, but usually the tumors show more nuclear variability than Ewing's sarcoma and often show distinct neural rosettes. However, in contrast to neuroblastoma, these tumors almost invariably do not display neurofibrillary material or ganglion cells. Immunohistochemically these tumors are positive for neuron-specific enolase and ultrastructurally contain dense-core (neuroendocrine) granules, although catecholamine production is rarely measurable. Cytoplasmic glycogen is a common but not consistent finding. The fact that it shows a chromosomal translocation, t(11;22)(q24;q12), identical to that found in Ewing's sarcoma indicates a possible close relationship of the two tumors.[409]

Askin's tumor (small cell tumor of the thoracopulmonary region) is a another high-grade, small round cell malignant lesion occurring in the chest wall of children and young adults.

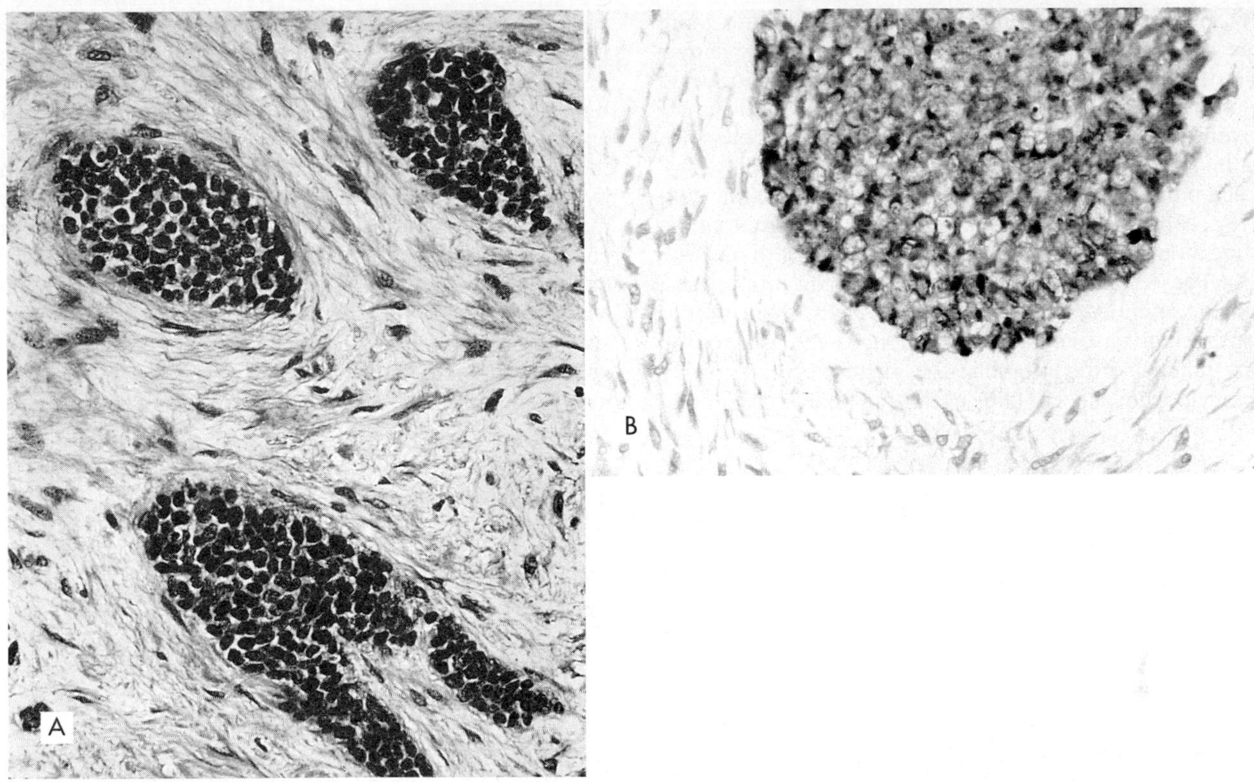

Fig. 72-21 **A,** Intraabdominal desmoplastic small round cell tumor showing clusters of round cells in a cellular desmoplastic stroma. **B,** The tumor cells of intraabdominal desmoplastic small round cell tumors are positive for keratin.

Most likely it represents a variant of peripheral neuroepithelioma.[410-412]

Intraabdominal desmoplastic small round cell tumor (DSRCT) is a distinctive high-grade malignant tumor that usually affects boys under 15 years of age (less than 20% of patients are female).[413] The tumor usually arises in the abdominal cavity, where it may form single or multiple peritoneal, omental, or retroperitoneal nodules. It has also been found in the pleural cavity.[414] Most patients have died within 1 to 5 years of diagnosis despite systemic chemotherapy using soft-tissue sarcoma or neuroblastoma protocols.

Histologically, DSRCT shows clusters and sheets of small round to epithelioid-appearing, diffusely hyperchromatic cells embedded in a desmoplastic and in places a richly vascular stroma (Fig. 72-21, *A*). Cellular pleomorphism is occasionally present. A typical and nearly unique feature of this tumor is its dual expression of desmin and cytokeratins (Fig. 72-21, *B*). The tumor cells are also positive for epithelial membrane antigen, variably positive for neuron-specific enclase, but typically negative for S-100 protein. They are negative for CD99.[413] Ultrastructurally the tumor cells have epithelial features with well-developed cell junctions and occasional neuroendocrine dense-core granules.

The precise cell lineage of DSRCT is unknown. Interestingly, fetal mesothelial cells express desmin and keratins, indicating the possibility that DSRCT is a primitive mesothelial neoplasm, a "mesothelioblastoma." Cytogenetic studies have revealed chromosomal translocation t(11;22)(p13;q12). Molecular genetic analysis has shown associated rearrangement of the *EWS* (Ewing's sarcoma) and *WT1* (Wilms' tumor) genes.[415]

TUMORS OF UNKNOWN HISTOGENESIS

Synovial sarcoma is a distinctive soft-tissue sarcoma showing a dual epithelial and spindle cell mesenchymal differentiation, previously believed to reflect a synovial tissue differentiation. Because of its perceived similarity to developing synovium, this tumor was so named, but over the years it has become clear that it bears little or no relationship to synovium, either histologically or histogenetically.[416] Yet the name of this tumor has been retained for historical reasons. No benign counterpart is known.

Synovial sarcoma occurs mainly in young adults (25-35 years), more commonly in men, and accounts for about 10% of all soft-tissue sarcomas.[417-420] Occasional cases in children and elderly patients are on record. The most common sites are the deep soft tissues of the popliteal area, knee, thigh, feet, hands, and forearm. Rare cases in the head, neck, upper aerodigestive tract, abdominal wall, and mediastinum have been described. Clinically the tumors are often painful and radiographically often show spotty calcifications. Small tumors in peripheral parts of extremities may clinically simulate ganglion cysts or other benign lesions. Some tumors are grossly cystic, but this is not believed to indicate its origin from bursae or other synovial structures.

The 5-year survival rate in patients with synovial sarcoma is approximately 50%, but further tumor-related deaths occur during extended follow-up. The tumor metastasizes most commonly to the lungs and pleural cavity. Smaller tumors (less than 5 cm in diameter), those in peripheral locations, and those with low mitotic activity seem to be associated with a more favorable prognosis.[420-422] DNA flow cytometry has shown most synovial sarcomas to be diploid; aneuploidy appears to be an unfavorable sign associated with increased tumor aggressiveness.[423] The data on the prognostic significance of different histologic variants are contradictory.

Histologically the typical biphasic synovial sarcoma consists of two components: epithelial glandular structures and an intervening uniform, highly cellular spindle cell stroma (Fig. 72-22, *A*). These components are seen in varying proportions. Although the spindle cell component is usually more prominent, and in many cases extensive sampling is required to find areas of epithelial differentiation. The glandular lumens may be well developed and contain a PAS-positive secretion. In well-differentiated cases, the glands are surrounded by basement membranes. In other cases the epithelium-like cells form less apparent slitlike structures or clusters and strands of lighter-staining cells lacking distinctive glandular lumens. The epithelial cells range from high columnar to cuboidal. Squamous cell differentiation may occur.[424,425] Calcification and hyalinization are commonly seen in the spindle cell compartments. Occasionally, synovial sarcoma shows massive stromal calcification; such tumors seem to be more common in the extremities and may be associated with a better prognosis.[426] Metaplastic bone may also form. Tumors that show only a spindle cell component are called "monophasic (fibrous type) synovial sarcoma" (Fig. 72-22, *B*). They are at least as common as the biphasic forms. Tumors with only epithelial cells,

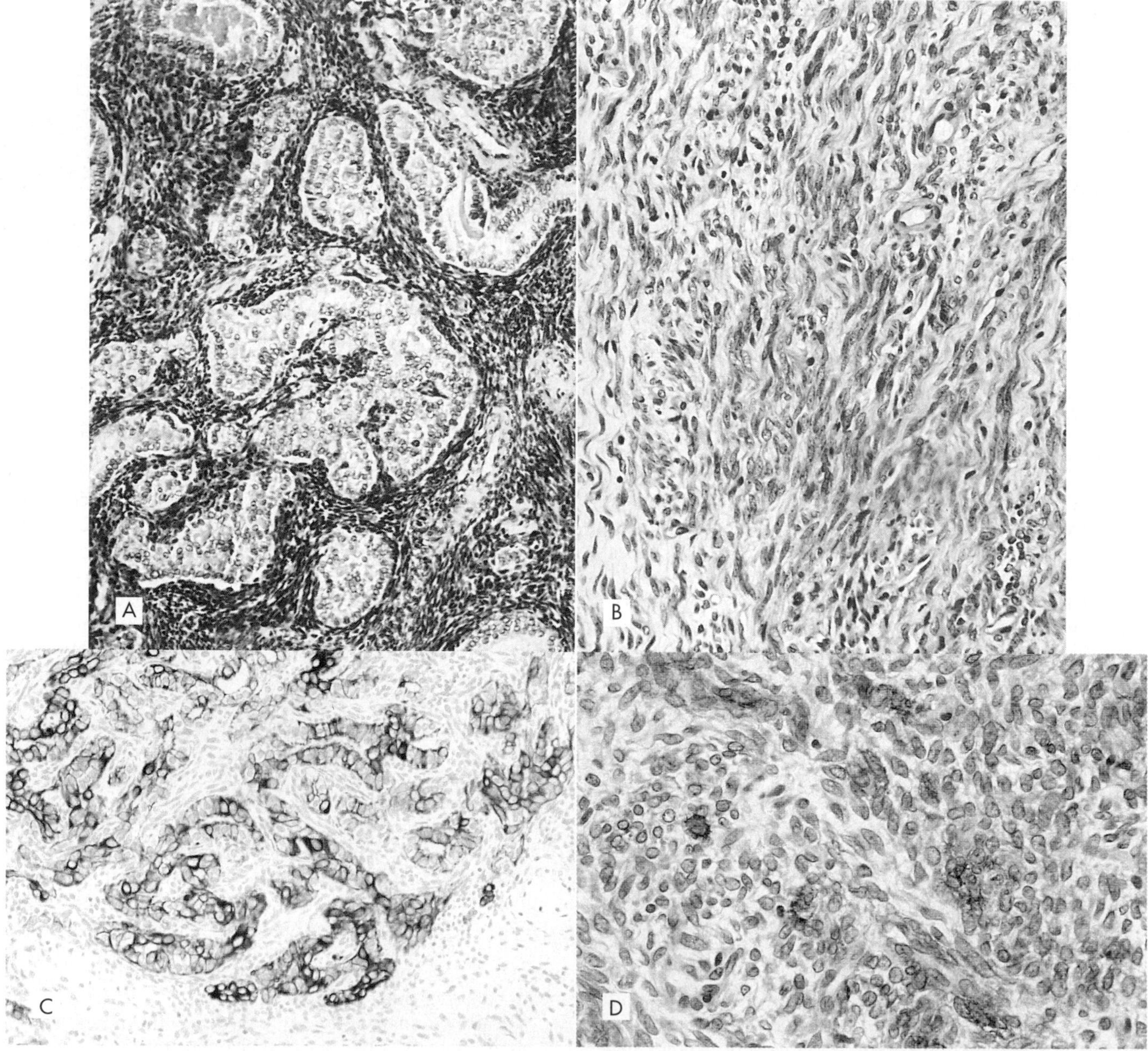

Fig 72-22 **A,** Biphasic synovial sarcoma with glandlike spaces and intervening uniform spindle cells. **B,** Monophasic synovial sarcoma of spindle cell type is composed of nearly uniform spindle cells with focal whorl formations. **C,** Biphasic synovial sarcoma in which keratin-positive epithelial slits can be seen. **D,** Monophasic synovial sarcoma with epithelial membrane antigen immunoreactivity in scattered spindle cells.

without spindle cells (monophasic epithelial type), are very unusual and are difficult to distinguish from carcinomas.

Immunohistochemically the dondulor structures as well as some spindle cells are positive for epithelial markers, including keratins 8, 18, and 19, and others and epithelial membrane antigen.[427,448] The demonstration of epithelial markers is diagnostically helpful in identifying monophasic synovial sarcomas of the fibrous type and those with a subtle epithelial component (Fig. 72-22, *C* and *D*). However, it should be noted that keratins (mostly numbers 8 and 18) may be present in other types of sarcomas. The monophasic tumors generally also show foci positive for keratins, epithelial membrane antigen, or both. Ultrastructurally the epithelial component is surrounded by a basement membrane, similar to the ultrastructure of true epithelium. The spindle cells in monophasic synovial sarcoma appear to be closely related to the epithelial cells of the biphasic tumors, and these tumors represent poorly differentiated biphasic tumors.[429-431]

The typical diagnostically significant cytogenetic finding in synovial sarcoma is a balanced translocation t(18;X)(p11,2;q11,2). Additional more complex and numerical chromosomal changes have been seen in anaplastic variants.[432-434] Similar translocations occur in both biphasic and monophasic variants, supporting their close relationship. Recently genes named *SYT* and *SSX* were identified in a synovial sarcoma translocation that apparently lead to the formation of a pathologic fusion transcript, like many other translocations in soft-tissue sarcomas.[435]

Epithelioid sarcoma is a rare soft-tissue sarcoma having characteristic clinicopathologic features.[436,437] This tumor typically occurs in young adults (median age, 30-35 years) and occasionally in children and arises in the distal parts of the extemities, such as the fingers, hands, and ankles. Male patients outnumber female patients in most series.[438-440] This tumor presents as a superficial nodule or sometimes as a nonhealing ulcer. The neoplastic nature of the lesion may elude the clinician and the pathologist alike. Epithelioid sarcoma may histologically simulate necrotizing granuloma or carcinoma, as pointed out by Enzinger[437] in his original description. Metastasis to the lymph nodes, lungs, and skin (the scalp in particular) occurs in about half of the patients. The 5-year survival rate is 70%, but the rate falls to 50% at 10 years.[9,5,18]

Epithelioid sarcomas typically grow along the tendon sheaths and fascial planes and microscopically are often found to be more extensive than anticipated clinically. Therefore exact measurement of the tumor size may be impossible. The dominant tumor mass usually measures up to 3 to 6 cm in diameter, but some epithelioid sarcomas appear as small dermal nodules, clinically simulating benign skin tumors. Histologically, epithelioid sarcoma consists of sheets and clusters of large polygonal cells with an eosinophilic cytoplasm that may assume a spindled shape and merge with the collagenous stroma (Fig. 72-23, *A*). The nuclei of the tumor cells have complex outlines and the cytoplasm is deeply eosinophilic. Central necrosis is common in larger clusters of tumor cells. Mitoses are present but are usually not numerous. Tumor size of more than 3 cm in diameter, deep location, and the presence of necrosis, vascular invasion, and lymph node metastastastic lesions have been identified as adverse prognostic signs.[439,441]

Immunohistochemically, epithelioid sarcoma is typically positive for vimentin, keratins, and epithelial membrane antigen, and occasionally also for carcinoembryonic antigen.[442-445] Most epithelioid sarcomas are positive for CD34, a myeloid progenitor cell antigen also present in endothelial cells, but other endothelial cell markers are not present (Fig. 72-23, *B* and *C*).[438] Desmin and neurofilaments have been found in some cases indicating the possibility of multidirectional differentiation.[446] Immunohistochemical analysis helps

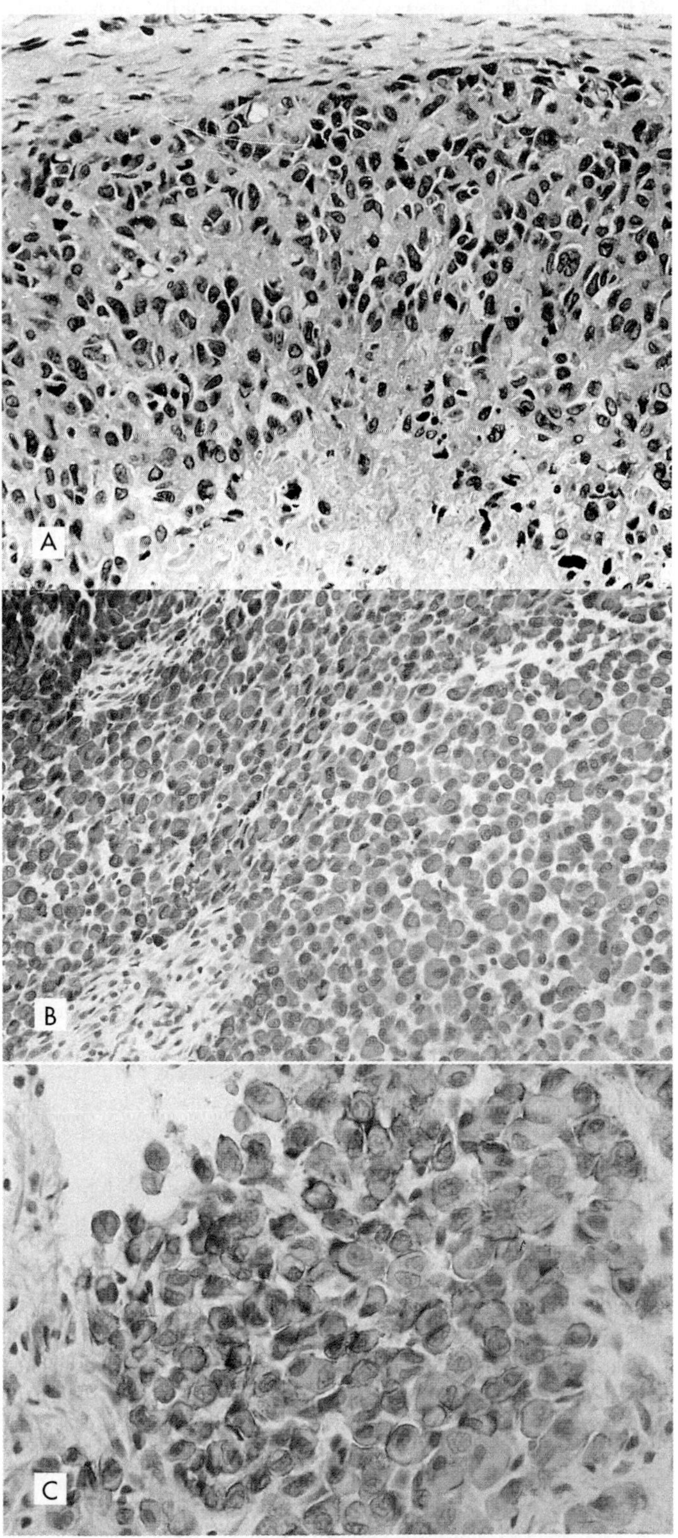

Fig. 72-23 **A,** Epithelioid sarcoma showing sheets of epithelioid tumor cells with a necrotic zone. **B,** The epithelioid sarcoma cells are uniformly positive for cytokeratin. **C,** The cells show membrane staining for CD34.

differentiate epithelioid sarcoma from melanoma and necrobiotic collagen granuloma resembling rheumatoid nodules; the latter lacking epithelial markers.[447] Epithelioid sarcoma must also be distinguished from metastatic and primary skin adnexal carcinoma.[448] EM reveals prominent cytoplasmic filaments, which may resemble bundles of keratin tonofilaments or form whorls corresponding to eosinophilic cytoplasmic inclusions similar to those present in so-called rhabdoid tumors. The cellular outlines are complex and may show filopodial protrusions into intercellular lumens.[445,449] Deletion of the short arm of chromosome 1 has been reported as a cytogenetic characteristic of epithelioid sarcoma, but the chromosomal data are scant.[450]

Epithelioid sarcoma may overlap with extrarenal rhabdoid tumors,[451] and the question has been raised whether some vulvar epithelioid sarcomas are better classified as rhabdoid tumors than as epithelioid sarcomas, which in this location are known to be clinically more aggressive.[452]

Malignant rhabdoid tumor of soft tissue (extrarenal rhabdoid tumor) is the designation for a soft-tissue sarcoma with histologic features identical to those of the corresponding kidney tumor, originally regarded as a variant of the Wilms' tumor complex.[453-458] This tumor is highly malignant and usually seen in children or young adults. The tumor cells are large and polygonal with vesicular nuclei and prominent nucleoli. Because of their deeply eosinophilic cytoplasm, the tumor cells may resemble rhabdomyoblasts. However, the cytoplasm does not contain myofilaments but instead contains inclusions of intermediate filaments, which immunohistochemically contain both keratins and vimentin. Desmin has been found in occasional cases, indicating a possible complex differentiation pattern. Other sarcomas (epithelioid sarcoma, synovial sarcoma) that show focal rhabdoid features should not be classified as rhabdoid tumors.

Malignant mesenchymoma is the designation introduced by Stout to refer to soft-tissue sarcomas that contain two differentiated sarcoma types together with a nonspecific fibrosarcoma-like component. Today this designation is rarely used, and other sarcomas with such multiple components are more common, including Triton tumor and malignant mixed müllerian tumor (see Chapter 68). The most common combination seen in malignant mesenchymomas is osteosarcoma/chondrosarcoma and rhabdomyosarcoma, but numerous different combinations are possible. Malignant mesenchymoma reflects the divergent differentiation potential of primitive mesenchymal cells. The demographic features of this tumor parallel those of MFH. Most tumors occur in middle-aged or elderly patients. The least-differentiated or highest-grade component usually determines the outcome.

Alveolar soft-part sarcoma (ASPS) is an architecturally distinct, rare soft-tissue sarcoma occurring mainly in children and adolescents. ASPS was described as a new entity by Christopherson et al[459] in 1952, who considered it a malignant organoid granular cell tumor or paraganglioma.

ASPS is most commonly located in the deep soft tissues of the thigh but has been found in a wide variety of locations in the extremities, trunk, neck, and head, in the orbit in particular.[460-463] Single cases in internal organs such as the stomach and in the genitals, including the uterine cervix and vagina, have been reported.[464,465] Most of the patients are young and there is a preponderance of cases in female patients. Although the clinical course of ASPS is slow, there

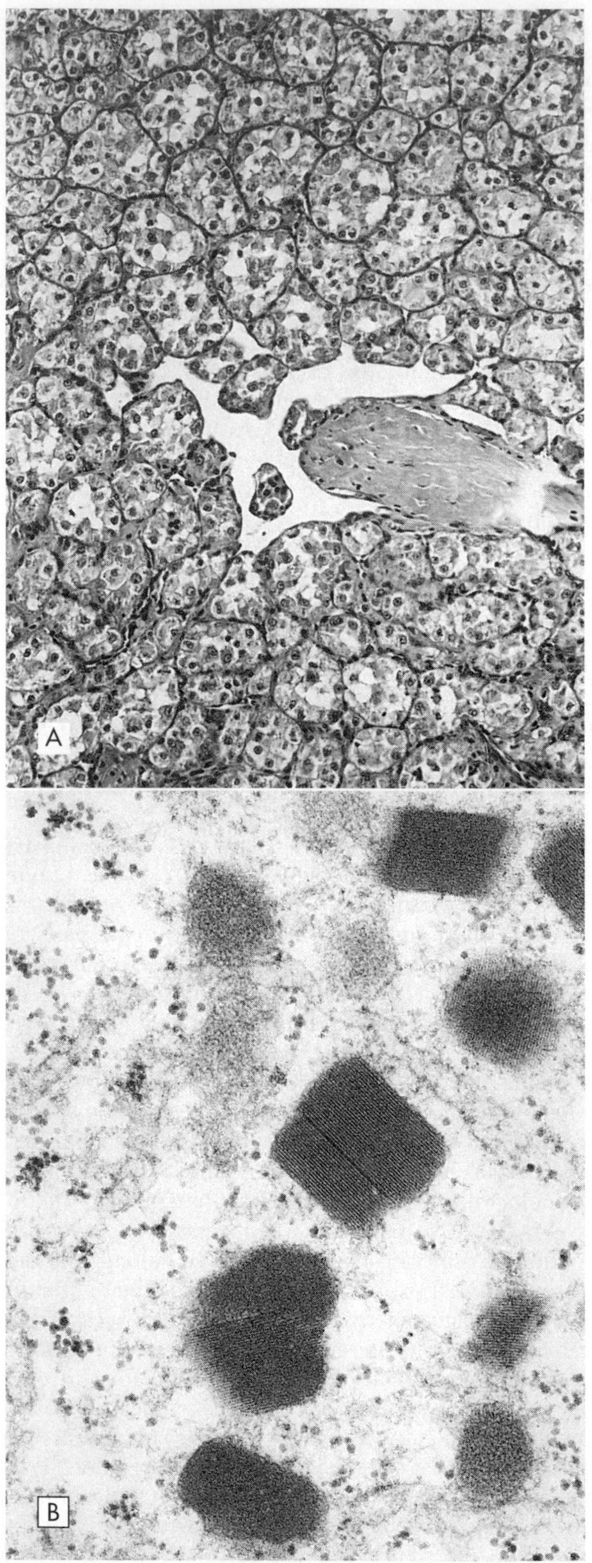

Fig. 72-24 **A,** Alveolar soft-part sarcoma. Round organoid clusters of uniform polygonal tumor cells can be seen. **B,** Electron micrograph showing alveolar soft-part sarcoma. Rhomboid crystals with a latticelike pattern with a regular periodicity can be seen.

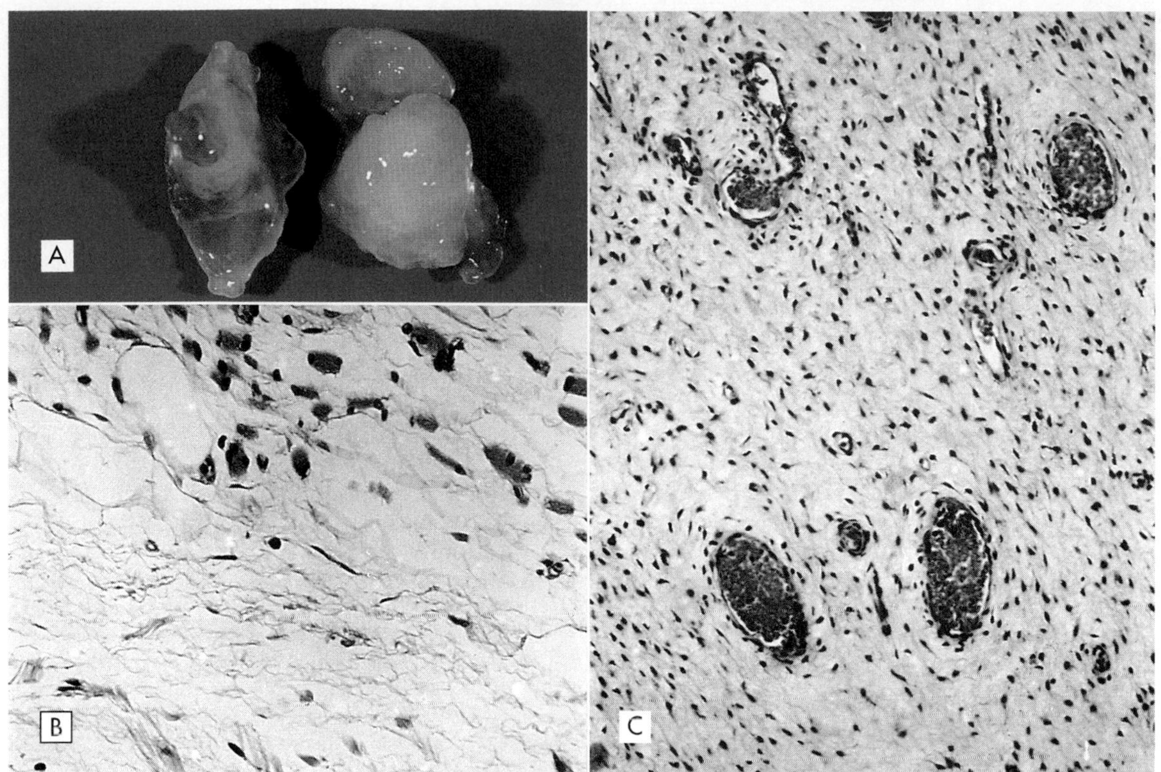

Fig. 72-25 **A,** Intramuscular myxoma. **B,** The tumor shows a loose myxoid texture and infiltrates into the muscle in the periphery of the tumor. **C,** Angiomyxoma of the pelvis showing scattered small polygonal cells in a myxoid stroma rich in dilated small vessels.

is relentless disease progression, with late recurrences and metastases during a disease course of 10 to 20 years. Numerous patients have metastatic lesions at the time presentation.[462]

Histologically, ASPS has a distinctive organoid structure consisting of nests of tumor cells surrounded by delicate or coarse collagenous fibrovascular septa. The cellular areas usually, but not invariably, have a central open "alveolar" space created by the degeneration of tumor cells. The cells are uniform and polygonal with small nuclei and abundant, variably eosinophilic cytoplasm. The cytoplasm may contain PAS-positive crystals that ultrastructurally have a typical latticelike periodicity (Fig. 72-24). Mitoses are rare. Variants with a less developed compartmental structure have been described and may be more aggressive.[466] Necrosis occurs in larger tumors, and vascular invasion is common.

The nature of ASPS remains a mystery, but recent immunohistochemical observations have suggested a possible striated muscle differentiation. The immunoreactivity of ASPS for sarcomeric muscle actins, desmin, and Myo-D protein, a gene product of striated muscle cells, suggests that the cells that make up ASPS are related to striated muscle cells.[467-475] However, both the clinical and ultrastructural features are different from those of rhabdomyosarcoma. The markers for neural differentiation (as would be seen in paraganglioma) are absent, and histochemical features, including the lack of formaldehyde-induced fluorescence, differ from those of paraganglioma.[476] A cytogenetic study in one case has shown multiple complex chromosomal abnormalities.[477]

The differential diagnosis of ASPS especially includes (metastatic) renal carcinoma, melanoma, and paraganglioma, all of which may show an alveolar pattern resembling that of ASPS. The demonstration of epithelial markers in renal carcinoma and of S-100 protein and melanoma-associated antigen (HMB-45) in melanoma is helpful. Alveolar rhabdomyosarcoma, a high-grade round cell tumor, is not likely to be confused histologically with ASPS.

Miscellaneous benign soft-tissue tumors

Intramuscular myxoma is a rare benign tumor of deep soft tissues that occurs in middle-aged or old patients, more commonly in women. The most common locations are the large muscles of the thigh, leg, and shoulder.[478-481] This tumor is benign and does not recur after simple local excision. Multiple intramuscular myxomas are present in some patients, and there is a rare association with fibrous dysplasia of adjacent bone. An increased frequency of minor bone abnormalities has also been reported.

Grossly the tumor is myxoid and appears a gelatinous gray-white on sectioning; it measures from 2 to 3 cm to as much as 10 cm in diameter (Fig. 72-25, *A*).

Histologically, intramuscular myxoma consists of scattered elongated or stellate-shaped cells embedded in a loose myxoid matrix with scattered collagen fibers (Fig. 72-25, *B*). The nuclei are uniformly small and oval, and there is practically no mitotic activity. The tumor cells may show cytoplasmic vacuoles. The vasculature is poorly developed, and there is no cellular density around the vessels. The lesions typically blend with adjacent atrophic muscle fibers at the periphery. The myxoma cells show the ultrastructural features of fibroblasts and myofibroblasts. Cytoplasmic vacuoles corresponding to hugely dilated sacs of rough endoplasmic reticulum and are apparently filled with the mucinous material, which histochemically are shown to contain hyaluronic acid.

Intramuscular myxoma must be differentiated from low-grade sarcomas with myxoid stroma. Myxoid MFH and liposarcoma, are more cellular and show a prominent vascular pattern. In imaging studies intramuscular myxoma is found to be hypovascular, in contrast to the richly vascular myxoid liposarcoma and myxoid MFH.[480]

Aggressive angiomyxoma is a benign but potentially recurring myxoid soft-tissue tumor that typically occurs in the vulvar and lower pelvic area of young women but has also been observed in men in the lower pelvic and perineoscrotal area.[482,483] Grossly the tumor has a rubbery, gelatinous consistency and is multinodular and unencapsulated. Histologically it consists of uniform round or stellate-shaped fibroblasts embedded in a loose myxoid matrix containing abundant dilated blood vessels. Mitotic activity is absent or scant (Fig. 72-25, *C*).

Tumoral calcinosis is a rare disorder in which there are focal and multifocal periarticular soft-tissue calcifications. Small nodules consisting of amorphous calcifications with a histiocytic giant cell reaction surrounding them occur in superficial soft tissues, most commonly in the hands, feet, and elbow area. This condition is a benign hereditary disorder and occurs mostly in young adults, with cases sometimes showing a familial clustering. Histologically similar lesions occur in patients with chronic renal disease and secondary hyperparathyroidism.

Amyloid tumor is a localized nodular mass formed of amyloid with a surrounding foreign body, giant cell reaction. Most commonly it is associated with generalized amyloidosis in patients with plasma cell neoplasia or chronic disease but has been rarely been encountered as a primary soft-tissue lesion in the absence of systemic disease.

REFERENCES

Introduction, epidemiology, and etiology

1. *Cancer facts and figures 1992,* Atlanta, 1992, American Cancer Society.
2. Ross JA, Severson RK, Davis S, Brooks JJ: Trends in the incidence of soft tissue sarcomas in the United States from 1973 through 1987, *Cancer* 72:486, 1993.
3. Laskin WB, Silverman TA, Enzinger FM: Postirradiation soft tissue sarcomas: an analysis of 53 cases, *Cancer* 68:524, 1991.
4. Wiklund TA, Blomqvist CP, Räty J et al: Postirradiation sarcoma: analysis of a nationwide cancer registry material, *Cancer* 68:524, 1991.
5. Ito Y, Kojiro M, Nakashima T, Mori T: Pathomorphologic characteristics of 102 cases of Thorotrast related hepatocellular carcinoma, cholangiocarcinoma, and hepatic angiosarcoma, *Cancer* 62:1153, 1988.
6. Popper H, Thomas LB, Telles NC et al: Development of hepatic angiosarcoma in man induced by vinyl chloride, Throrotrast, and arsenic: comparison with cases of unknown etiology, *Am J Pathol* 92:349, 1978.
7. Kelly SJ, Guidotti TL: Phenoxyacetic herbicides and chlorophenols and the etiology of lymphoma and soft tissue neoplasms, *Publ Health Rev* 17:1, 1989-1990.
8. McClay EF: Epidemiology of bone and soft tissue sarcomas, Semin Oncol 16:264, 1989.
9. Cardesa A, Ribalta T, von Schilling B et al: Experimental model of tumors associated with neurofibromatosis, *Cancer* 63:1737, 1989.
10. Fletcher CD: Soft tissue sarcomas apparently arising in chronic tropical ulcers, *Histopathology* 11:501, 1987.
11. Jennings TA, Peterson L, Axiotis CA et al: Angiosarcoma associated with foreign body material: a report of three cases, *Cancer* 62:2436, 1988.
12. Chang Y, Cesarman E, Pessin M et al: Identification of herpesvirus-like DNA-sequences in AIDS-associated Kaposi's sarcoma, *Science* 266:1865, 1994.
13. Schreiber H, Barry FM, Russell WC et al: Stewart-Treves syndrome: a lethal complication of postmastectomy lympedema and regional immune deficiency, *Arch Surg* 114:82, 1979.
14. O'Connell P, Cawthon R, Xy GH et al: The neurofibromatosis type I (NF1) gene: identification and partial characterization of a putative tumor suppressor gene, *J Dermatol* 19:881, 1992.
15. Strong LC, Williams WR, Tainsky MA: The Li-Fraumeni syndrome: from clinical epidemiology to molecular genetics, *Am J Epidermal* 135:190, 1992.
16. Barr FG, Chatten J, D'Cruz CM et al: Molecular assays for chromosomal translocations in the diagnosis of pediatric soft tissue sarcomas, *JAMA* 273:553, 1995.

Ancillary diagnostic procedures

17. Erlandson RA: Diagnostic transmission electron microscopy of human tumors, New York, 1981, Masson.
18. Mackay B: Electron microscopy of soft tissue tumours. In Fletcher CDM, McKee PH, editors: *Pathobiology of soft tissue tumours,* London, 1990, Churchill Livingstone.
19. Miettinen M: Immunohistochemistry of soft tissue tumors: possibilities and limitations in surgical pathology, *Pathol Annu* 23 (part 1):1, 1990.
20. Fletcher JA, Kozakewich HP, Hoffer FA et al: Diagnostic relevance of clonal cytogenetic aberrations in malignant soft tissue tumors, *N Engl J Med* 324:436, 1991.
21. Sandberg AA, Bridge J: *Cytogenetics of soft tissue and bone tumors,* Boca Raton, Fla, 1994, CRC Press.
22. Downing JR, Khandekar A, Shurtleff SA et al: Multiplex RT-PCR assay for the differential diagnosis of alveolar rhabdomyosarcoma and Ewing's sarcoma, *Am J Pathol* 146:626, 1995.

Grading and staging

23. Angervall L, Kindblom LG, Rydholm A, Stener B: The diagnosis and prognosis of soft tissue tumors, *Semin Diagn Pathol* 3:240, 1986.
24. Coindre JM, Trojani M, Contesso G et al: Reproducibility of histological grading system for adult soft tissue sarcoma, *Cancer* 58:306, 1986.
25. Coindre JM, Nguyen BB, Bonichon F et al: Histologic grading in spindle cell soft tissue sarcomas, *Cancer* 61:2305, 1988.
26. Costa J, Wesley RA, Glatstein E et al: The grading of soft tissue sarcomas: results of a clinicohistopathologic correlation in a series of 163 cases, *Cancer* 53:530, 1984.
27. Costa J: The grading and staging of soft tissue sarcomas. In Fletcher CDM, McKee PH, editors: *Pathobiology of soft tissue tumours,* London, 1990, Churchill Livingstone.
28. Markhede G, Angervall L, Stener B: A multivariate analysis of the prognosis after surgical treatment of malignant soft tissue tumors, *Cancer* 49:1721, 1982.
29. Russel WO, Cohen J, Enzinger FM et al: A clinical and pathological staging system for soft tissue sarcomas, *Cancer* 40:1562, 1977.

Benign fibroblastic tumors and tumorlike lesions

30. Chung EM, Enzinger FM: Fibroma of tendon sheath, *Cancer* 41:1945, 1979.
31. Pulitzer DR, Martin PC, Reed RJ: Fibroma of tendon sheath: a clinicopathologic study of 32 cases, *Am J Surg Pathol* 13:472, 1989.
32. Satti MB: Tendon sheath tumours: a pathological study of the relationship between giant cell tumour and fibroma of tendon sheath, *Histopathology* 20:213, 1992.
33. Datubo-Brown DD: Keloids: a review of the literature, *Br J Plast Surg* 43:70, 1990.
34. Allen PW: Nodular fasciitis, *Pathology* 4:9, 1972.
35. Bernstein KE, Lattes R: Nodular (pseudosarcomatous) fasciitis, a nonrecurrent lesion: clinicopathologic study of 134 cases, *Cancer* 49:1668, 1982.

36. Hutter RV, Stewart FW, Foote FW: Fasciitis: a report of 70 cases with follow-up proving the benignity of the lesion, *Cancer* 15:992, 1962.
37. Iwasaki H, Enjoji M: Nodular fasciitis: a clinicopathologic study of 84 cases, *Jpn Cancer Clin* 18:793, 1972.
38. Shimizu S, Hashimoto H, Enjoji M: Nodular fasciitis: an analysis of 250 patients, *Pathology* 16:161, 1984.
39. Wirman JA: Nodular fasciitis, a lesion of myofibroblasts: an ultrastructural study, *Cancer* 38:2378, 1976.
40. Montgomery EA, Meis JM: Nodular fasciitis: its morphological spectrum and immunohistochemical profile, *Am J Surg Pathol* 15:942, 1991.
41. Lauer DH, Enzinger FM: Cranial fasciitis in childhood, *Cancer* 45:401, 1980.
42. Hutter RV, Foote FW, Francis KC, Higinbotham N: Parosteal fasciitis: a self-limited benign process that simulates malignant neoplasm, *Am J Surg* 104:800, 1962.
43. Patchefsky AS, Enzinger FM: Intravascular fasciitis: a report of 17 cases, *Am J Surg Pathol* 5:29, 1981.
44. Cramer SF, Kent L, Abramowsky C, Moskowitz RW: Eosinophilic fasciitis: immunopathology, ultrastructure, literature review, and consideration of its pathogenesis and relation to scleroderma, *Arch Pathol Lab Med* 106:85, 1982.
45. Michet C, Doyle J, Ginsburg W: Eosinophilic fasciitis: report of 15 cases, *Mayo Clinic Proc* 56 :271, 1988.
46. Chung EM, Enzinger FM: Proliferative fasciitis, *Cancer* 36:1450, 1975.
47. Enzinger FM, Dulcey F: Proliferative myositis: report of 33 cases, *Cancer* 20:2213, 1967.
48. Kern WH: Proliferative myositis: a pseudosarcomatous reaction to injury, *Arch Pathol* 69:209, 1960.
49. Rose AG: An electron microscopic study of the giant cells in proliferative myositis, *Cancer* 33:1543, 1974.
50. Mitchinson MJ: Retroperitoneal fibrosis revisited, *Arch Pathol Lab Med* 110:784, 1986.
51. Järvi OH, Saxén E, Hopsu-Havu V et al: Elastofibroma—a degenerative pseudotumor, *Cancer* 23:42, 1969.
52. Kindblom LG, Spicer SS: Elastofibroma: a correlated light and electron microscopic study, *Virchows Arch [A]* 396:127, 1982.
53. Nagamine N, Nohara Y, Ito E: Elastofibroma in Okinawa: a clinicopathologic study of 170 cases, *Cancer* 50:1794, 1982.
54. Järvi OH, Länsimies PH: Subclinical elastofibromas in the scapular region in an autopsy series, *Acta Pathol Microbiol Scand* 83:87, 1975.
55. Enzinger FM: Fibrous hamartoma of the infancy, *Cancer* 18:241, 1965.
56. Chung EM, Enzinger FM: Infantile myofibromatosis, *Cancer* 48:1807, 1981.
57. Jennings TA, Duray PH, Collins FS et al: Infantile myofibromatosis: evidence for an autosomal dominant disorder, *Am J Surg Pathol* 8:529, 1984.
58. Fletcher CD, Achu P, van Noorden S, McKee PH: Infantile myofibromatosis: a light microscopic, histochemical and immunohistochemical study suggesting true smooth muscle differentiation, *Histopathology* 11:245, 1987.
59. Allen PW, Enzinger FM: Juvenile aponeurotic fibroma, *Cancer* 26:857, 1970.
60. Goldman RL: The cartilage analogue of fibromatosis (aponeurotic fibroma): further observations based on 7 new cases, *Cancer* 26:1325, 1970.

Fibromatoses

61. Allen P: The fibromatoses: a clinicopathologic classification based on 140 cases, *Am J Surg Pathol* 1:255, 1977.
62. Enzinger FM, Shiraki M: Musculoaponeurotic fibromatosis of the shoulder girdle, *Cancer* 20:1131, 1967.
63. Häyry P, Reitamo J, Totterman S et al: The desmoid tumor. II. Analysis of factors possibly contributing to the etiology and growth behavior, *Am J Clin Pathol* 77:665, 1982.
64. Posner MC, Shiu MH, Newsome JL et al: The desmoid tumor: not a benign disease, *Arch Surg* 124:191, 1989.
65. Reitamo JJ, Häyry P, Nykyri E, Saxen E: The desmoid tumor. I. Incidence, sex-, age- and anatomocal distribution in the Finnish population, *Am J Clin Pathol* 77:665, 1982.
66. Taylor LJ: Musculoaponeurotic fibromatosis: a report of 28 cases and review of the literature, *Clin Orthoped* 224:294, 1987.
67. Bridge JA, Sreekantaiah C, Mouron B et al: Clonal chromosomal abnormalities in desmoid tumors: implications for histopathogenesis, *Cancer* 69:430, 1992.
68. Karlsson I, Mandahl N, Heim S: Complex chromosome rearrangements in an extraabdominal desmoid tumor, *Cancer Genet Cytogenet* 34:241, 1988.
69. Iwasaki H, Muller H, Stutte HJ, Brennscheidt U: Palmar fibromatosis (Dupuytren's contracture: ultrastructural and enzyme histochemical studies of 43 cases, *Virchows Arch [A]* 405:41, 1989.
70. Murrell GA: An insight into Dupuytren's contracture, *Ann R Coll Surg Engl* 74:156, 1992.
71. Paletta FX: Dupuytren's contracture, *Am Fam Phys* 23:85, 1981.
72. Ushijima M, Tsuneyoshi M, Enjoji M: Dupuytren type fibromatosis: a clinicopathological study of 62 cases, *Acta Pathol Jpn* 34:991, 1984.
73. Iwasaki H, Kikuchi M, Mori R et al: Infantile digital fibromatosis: ultrastructural, histochemical, and tissue culture observations, *Cancer* 46:2238, 1980.
74. Iwasaki H, Kikuchi M, Ohtsuki I et al: Infantile digital fibromatosis: identification of actin filaments in cytoplasmic inclusions by heavy meromyosin binding, *Cancer* 52:1653, 1983.

74a. Mukai M, Torikata C, Iri H et al: Immunohistochemical identification of aggregated actin filaments in formalin-fixed, paraffin-embedded sections: a study of infantile digital fibromatosis by a new pretreatment, *Am J Surg Pathol* 16:110, 1992.

Fibrosarcoma

75. Iwasaki H, Enjoji M: Infantile and adult fibrosarcomas of the soft tissues, *Acta Pathol Jpn* 29:377, 1979.
76. Scott SM, Reiman HM, Pritchard DJ, Ilstrup DM: Soft tissue fibrosarcoma: a clinicopathologic study of 132 cases, *Cancer* 64:925, 1989.
77. Evans HL: Low grade fibromyxoid sarcoma: a report of 12 cases, *Am J Surg Pathol* 17:595, 1993.
78. Balsaver AM, Butler JJ, Martin RG: Congenital fibrosarcoma, *Cancer* 20:1607, 1967.
79. Chung EB, Enzinger FM: Infantile fibrosarcoma, *Cancer* 38:729, 1976.
80. Adam LR, Davison EV, Malcolm AJ et al: Cytogenetic analysis of a congenital fibrosarcoma, *Cancer Genet Cytogenet* 52:37, 1991.
81. Dal Cin P, Brock P, Casteels-van Daele M et al: Cytogenetic characterization of congenital or infantile fibrosarcoma, *Eur J Pediatr* 150:579, 1991.
82. Meis JM, Enzinger FM: Inflammatory fibrosarcoma of the mesentery and retroperitoneum: a tumor closely simulating infllammatory pseudotumor, *Am J Surg Pathol* 15:1146, 1991.

Benign fibrohistiocytic tumors

83. Gonzalez S, Duarte I: Benign fibrous histiocytoma of the skin: a morphologic study of 290 cases, *Pathol Res Pract* 174:379, 1982.
84. Katenkamp D, Stiller D: Cellular composition of the so-called dermatofibroma (histiocytoma cutis), *Virchows Arch [A]* 367:325, 1975.
85. Meister P, Konrad E, Krauss F: Fibrous histiocytoma: a histological and statistical analysis of 155 cases, *Pathol Res Pract* 162:361, 1978.
86. Niemi KM: The benign fibrohistiocytic tumours of the skin, *Acta Dermatovenerol* 50 (suppl 63):1, 1970.
87. Helwig EB, Hackney VC: Juvenile xanthogranuloma (nevoxanthoendothelioma), *Am J Pathol* 30:625, 1954.
88. Sonoda T, Hashimoto H, Enjoji M: Juvenile xanthogranuloma: clinicopathologic analysis and immunohistochemical study of 57 patients, *Cancer* 56:2280, 1985.
89. Ehrlich GE, Young I, Nosheny SZ, Katz WA: Multicentric reticulohistiocytosis (lipoid dermatoarthritis: a multisystem disorder), *Am J Med* 52:830, 1972.
90. Taylor DR: Multicentric reticulohistiocytosis, *Arch Dermatol* 113:330, 1977.
91. Wilkes LL: Tendon xanthoma in type IV hyperlipoproteinemia, *South Med J* 70:254, 1977.
92. Connelly JH, Evans HL: Dermatofibrosarcoma protuberans: clinicopathologic review with emphasis on fibrosarcomatous areas, *Am J Surg Pathol* 16:921, 1992.

93. Fletcher CDM, Evans BJ, Macartney JC et al: Dermatofibrosarcoma protuberans: a clinicopathological and immunohistochemical study, and review of the literature, *Histopathology* 9:921, 1985.
94. McPeak CJ, Cruz T, Nicastri AD: Dermatofibrosarcoma protuberans: an analysis of 86 cases—five with metastasis, *Ann Surg* 166:803, 1967.
95. Taylor HB, Helwig EB: Dermatofibrosarcoma protuberans: a study of 115 cases, *Cancer* 1962;15:717.
96. Ozzello L, Hamels J: The histiocytic nature of dermatofibrosarcoma protuberans: tissue culture and electron microscopic study, *Am J Clin Pathol* 65:136, 1976.
97. Bridge JA, Neff JR, Sandberg AA: Cytogenetic analysis of dermatofibrosarcoma protuberans, *Cancer Genet Cytogenet* 49:199, 1990.
97a. Stephenson CF, Berger CS, Leong SP et al: Ring chromosome in dermatofibrosarcoma protuberans, *Cancer Genet Gytogenet* 58:52, 1992.

Fibrohistiocytic tumors of intermediate malignancy

98. Bednar B: Storiform neurofibromas of the skin, pigmented and non-pigmented, *Cancer* 10:368, 1957.
99. Dupree WB, Langloss JM, Weiss SW: Pigmented dermatofibrosarcoma protuberans (Bednár tumor): a pathologic, ultrastructural, and immunohistochemical study, *Am J Surg Pathol* 9:630, 1985.
100. Beham A, Fletcher CD: Dermatofibrosarcoma protuberans with areas resembling giant cell fibroblastoma: report of two cases, *Histopathology* 17:165, 1990.
101. Dymock RB, Allen PW, Stirling JW et al: Giant cell fibroblastoma: a distinctive, recurrent tumor of childhood, *Am J Surg Pathol* 11:263, 1987.
102. Shmookler BM, Enzinger FM, Weiss SW: Giant cell fibroblastoma: a juvenile form of dermatofibrosarcoma protuberans, *Cancer* 64:2154, 1989.
103. Costa MJ, Weiss SW: Angiomatoid malignant fibrous histiocytoma: a follow-up study of 108 cases with evaluation of possible histologic predictors of outcome, *Am J Surg Pathol* 14:1126, 1990.
104. Enzinger FM: Angiomatoid malignant fibrous histiocytoma: a distinctive fibrohistiocytic tumor of children and young adults simulating a vascular neoplasm, *Cancer* 44:2147, 1979.
105. Fletcher CD: Angiomatoid "malignant fibrous histiocytoma": an immunohistochemical study indicative of myoid differentiation, *Hum Pathol* 22:563, 1991.
106. Smith ME, Costa MJ, Weiss SW: Evaluation of CD68 and other histiocytic antigens in angiomatioid malignant fibrous histiocytoma, *Am J Surg Pathol* 15:757, 1991.
107. Enzinger FM, Zhang R: Plexiform fibrohistiocytic tumor presenting in children and young adults: an analysis of 65 cases, *Am J Surg Pathol* 12:818, 1988.

Malignant fibrous histiocytoma

108. O'Brien JE, Stout AP: Malignant fibrous xanthomas, *Cancer* 17:1445, 1964.
109. Enzinger FM: Malignant fibrous histiocytoma 20 years after Stout, *Am J Surg Pathol* 10(suppl 1):43, 1986.
110. Kearney MM, Soule EH, Ivins JC: Malignant fibrous histiocytoma: a retrospective study of 167 cases, *Cancer* 45:167, 1980.
111. Meister P: Malignant fibrous histiocytoma: history, histology, histogenesis. *Pathol Res Pract* 183:1, 1988.
112. Weiss SW: Malignant fibrous histiocytoma: a reaffirmation, *Am J Surg Pathol* 6:773, 1982.
113. Fu YS, Gabbiani G, Kaye GI, Lattes R: Malignant soft tissue tumors of probable fibrohistiocytic origin (malignant fibrous histiocytomas): general considerations and electron microscopic and tissue culture studies, *Cancer* 35:176, 1975.
114. Iwasaki H, Isayama T, Johzaki H, Kikuchi M: Malignant fibrous histiocytoma: evidence of perivascular mesenchymal cell origin: immunocytochemical studies with monoclonal anti-MFH antibodies, *Am J Pathol* 128:528, 1987.
115. Iwasaki H, Yoshitake K, Ohjimi Y et al: Malignant fibrous histiocytoma: proliferative compartment and heterogeneity of "histiocytic" cells, *Am J Surg Pathol* 16:735, 1992.
116. Roholl PJM, Kleyne J, Elbers J, van Unnik JA: Characterization of tumour cells in malignant fibrous histiocytomas and other soft tissue tumors, in comparison with malignant histiocytes. II. Immunoperoxidase study on cryostat sections, *Am J Pathol* 121:269, 1985.
117. Roholl PJM, Kleyne J, van Basten CDH et al: A study to analyze the tumor cells in malignant fibrous histiocytomas: a multiparametric characterization, *Cancer* 56:2809, 1985.
118. Wood GS, Beckstead JH, Turner RR et al: Malignant fibrous histiocytoma tumor cells resemble fibroblasts, *Am J Surg Pathol* 10:323, 1986.
119. Soini Y, Miettinen M: Immunohistochemical markers of histiomonocytic cells in malignant fibrous histiocytoma: a monoclonal antibody study, *Pathol Res Pract* 186:759, 1990.
120. Lawson CW, Fisher C, Gatter KC: An immunohistochemical study of differentiation in malignant fibrous histiocytoma, *Histopathology* 11:375, 1987.
120a. Fletcher CD: Pleomorphic malignant fibrous histiocytoma—fact or fiction? A critical reappraisal based on 159 tumors diagnosed as pleomorphic sarcoma, *Am J Surg Pathol* 16:213, 1992.
121. Lagacé R: The ultrastructural spectrum of malignant fibrous histiocytoma, *Ultrastruct Pathol* 11:153, 1987.
122. Tsuneyoshi M, Enjoji M, Shinohara N: Malignant fibrous histiocytoma: an electron microscopic study of 17 cases, *Virchows Arch [A]* 392:135, 1981.
123. Becker RL, Venzon D, Lack EE et al: Cytometry and morphometry of malignant fibrous histiocytoma of the extremities: prediction of metastasis and mortality, *Am J Surg Pathol* 15:87, 1991.
124. Bertoni F, Capanna R, Biagini R et al: Malignant fibrous histiocytoma of soft tissue: an analysis of 78 cases located and deeply seated in the extremities, *Cancer* 56:356, 1985.
125. Enjoji M, Hashimoto H, Tsuneyoshi M, Iwasaki H: Malignant fibrous histiocytoma: a clinicopathologic study of 130 cases, *Acta Pathol Jpn* 30:727, 1980.
126. Rydholm A, Syk I: Malignant fibrous histiocytoma of soft tissue: correlation between clinical variables and histologic malignancy grade, *Cancer* 57:2323, 1986.
127. Weiss SW, Enzinger FM: Malignant fibrous histiocytoma: an analysis of 200 cases, *Cancer* 41:2250, 1978.
128. Fretzin DF, Helwig EB: Atypical fibroxanthoma of the skin: a clinicopathologic study of 140 cases, *Cancer* 31:1541, 1973.
129. Hudson AW, Winkelmann RK: Atypical fibroxanthoma of the skin: a reappraisal of 19 cases in which the original diagnosis was spindle-cell squamous carcinoma, *Cancer* 29:413, 1972.
130. Weiss SW, Enzinger FM: Myxoid variant of malignant fibrous histiocytoma, *Cancer* 39:1672, 1977.
131. Merck C, Angervall L, Kindblom LG, Oden A: Myxofibrosarcoma: a malignant soft tissue tumor of fibroblastic-histiocytic origin. A clinicopathologic and prognostic study of 110 cases using multivariate analysis, *Acta Pathol Microbiol Immunol Scand* 282(suppl):1, 1983.
132. Guccion JG, Enzinger FM: Malignant giant cell tumor of soft parts: an anaylsis of 32 cases, *Cancer* 29:1518, 1972.
133. Kyriakos M, Kempson RL: Inflammatory fibrous histiocytoma: an aggressive and lethal lesion, *Cancer* 37:1584, 1976.
134. Isoda M, Yasumoto S: Eosinophil chemotactic factor derived from a malignant fibrous histiocytoma, *Clin Exp Dermatol* 11:253, 1986.

Synovial tumors

135. Rao AS, Vigorita VK: Pigmented villonodular synovitis (giant cell tumor of the tendon sheath and synovial membrane): a review of eighty-one cases, *J Bone Joint Surg [Am]* 66a:76, 1984.
136. Ushijima M, Hashimoto M, Tsuneyoshi M, Enjoji M: Giant cell tumor of tendon sheath (nodular tenosynovitis): a study of 207 cases to compare the large joint group with the common digit group, *Cancer* 57:875, 1986.

Lipoma and related benign tumors

137. Rydholm A, Berg NO: Size, site, and clinical incidence of lipoma: factors in the differential diagnosis of lipoma and sarcoma, *Acta Orthop Scand* 54:929, 1983.
138. Sreekantaiah C, Leong SP, Chu D, Sandberg AA: Translocation (X;12)(q27;q14) in a lipoma, *Cancer Genet Cytogenet* 49:235, 1990.

139. Sreekantaiah C, Leong SP, Sandberg AA: Complex cytogenetic changes in benign neoplasms: report of six lipomas. *Cancer Genet Cytogenet* 47:113, 1990.
140. Bjerregaard P, Hagen K, Daugaard S, Kofoed H: Intramuscular lipoma of the lower limb: long term follow-up after local resection, *J Bone Joint Surg [Br]* 71:812, 1989.
141. Fletcher CD, Martin-Bates E: Intramuscular and intermuscular lipoma: neglected diagnoses, *Histopathology* 12:275, 1988.
142. Kindblom LG, Angervall L, Stener B, Wickbom I: Intermuscular and intramuscular lipomas and hibernomas: clinical, roentgenologic, histologic, and prognostic study of 46 cases, *Cancer* 33:754, 1974.
143. Silverman TA, Enzinger FM: Fibrolipomatous hamartoma of nerve: a clinicopathologic analysis of 26 cases, *Am J Surg Pathol* 9:7, 1985.
144. Dionne GP, Seemayer TA: Infiltrating lipomas and angiolipomas revisited, *Cancer* 33:732, 1974.
145. Enzinger FM, Harvey DA: Spindle cell lipoma, *Cancer* 36:1852, 1975.
146. Azzopardi JG, Iocco J, Salm R: Pleomorphic lipoma—a tumor simulating liposarcoma, *Histopathology* 7:511, 1983.
147. Shmookler BM, Enzinger FM: Pleomorphic lipoma: A benign tumor simulating liposarcoma. A clinicopathologic analysis of 48 cases, *Cancer* 47:126, 1981.
148. Gaffney EF, Hargreaves HK, Semple E, Vellios F: Hibernoma: distinctive light and electron microscopic features and relationship to brown adipose tissue, *Hum Pathol* 14:677, 1983.
149. Bolen JW, Thorning D: Benign lipoblastoma and myxoid liposarcoma: a comparative light and electron microscopic study, *Am J Surg Pathol* 4:163, 1980.
149a. Fletcher JA, Kozakewich HP, Schoenberg ML, Morton CC: Cytogenetic findings in pediatric adipose tumors: consistent rearrangement of chromosome 8 in lipoblastoma, *Genes Chromosom Cancer* 6:24, 1993.
150. Chung EB, Enzinger FM: Benign lipoblastomatosis: an analysis of 35 cases, *Cancer* 32:482, 1973.
151. Vellios F, Baez JM, Shumacker HB: Lipoblastomatosis: a tumor of fetal fat different from hibernoma. Report of a case, with observations on the embryogenesis of human adipose tissue, *Am J Pathol* 34:1149, 1958.

Liposarcoma

152. Shmookler BM, Enzinger FM: Liposarcoma occurring in children: an analysis of 17 cases and review of the literature, *Cancer* 52:567, 1983.
153. Bolen JW, Thorning D: Liposarcomas: a histogenetic approach to the classification of adipose tissue neoplasms, *Am J Surg Pathol* 8:3, 1984.
154. Enzinger FM, Winslow DJ: Liposarcoma: a study of 103 cases, *Virchows Arch [A]* 335:367, 1962.
155. Evans HL: Liposarcomas and atypical lipomatous tumors: a study of 66 cases followed for a minimum of 10 years, *Surg Pathol* 3:169, 1990.
156. Hashimoto H, Enjoji M: Liposarcoma: a clinicopathologic subtyping of 52 cases, *Acta Pathol Jpn* 32:933, 1982.
157. Azumi N, Curtis J, Kempson RL, Hendrickson MR: Atypical and malignant neoplasms showing lipomatous differentiation: a study of 111 cases, *Am J Surg Pathol* 11:161, 1987.
158. Evans HL: Liposarcoma: a study of 55 cases with a reassessment of its classification, *Am J Surg Pathol* 3:507, 1979.
159. Snover DC, Sumner HW, Dehner LP: Variability of histologic pattern in recurrent soft tissue sarcomas originally diagnosed as liposarcoma, *Cancer* 49:1005, 1982.
160. Weiss SW, Rao VK: Well-differentiated liposarcoma (atypical lipoma) of deep soft tissue of the extremities, retroperitoneum, and miscellaneous sites: a follow-up study of 92 cases with analysis of the incidence of "dedifferentiation," *Am J Surg Pathol* 16:1051, 1992.
161. Kindblom LG, Angervall L, Svendsen P: Liposarcoma: a clinicopathologic, radiographic, and prognostic study, *Acta Pathol Microbiol Scand* 253:(suppl) 1, 1975.
162. Reszel PA, Soule EH, Coventry MB: Liposarcoma of the extremities and limb girdles: a study of 222 cases, *J Bone Joint Surg [Am]* 48:229, 1966.
163. Battifora H, Nunez-Alonso C: Myxoid liposarcoma: study of 10 cases, *Ultrastruct Pathol* 1:157, 1980.
164. Turc-Carel C, Limon J, Dal Cin PD et al: Cytogenetic studies on adipose tissue tumors. II. Recurrent reciprocal translocation t(12;16)(q13;p11) in myxoid liposarcomas, *Cancer Genet Cytogenet* 23:291, 1986.
165. Crozat A, Aman P, Mandahl N, Ron D: Fusion of CHOP to a novel RNA-binding protein in human myxoid liposarcoma, *Nature* 363:640, 1993.
166. Aman P, Ron D, Mandahl N et al: Rearrangement of the transcription factor gene CHOP in myxoid liposarcomas with t(12;16)(q13;p11), *Genes Chromosom Cancer* 5:278, 1992.
167. Sreekantaiah C, Karakousis CP, Leong SP, Sandberg AA: Trisomy 8 as a non-random secondary change in myxoid liposarcoma, *Cancer Genet Cytogenet* 51:195, 1991.
168. Sreekantaiah C, Karakousis CP, Leong SP, Sandberg AA: Cytogenetic findings in liposarcoma correlate with histopathologic subtypes. *Cancer* 69:2484, 1992.

Hemangioma, lymphangioma and related benign tumors

169. Coffin CM, Dehner LP: Vascular tumors in children and adolescents: a clinicopathologic study of 228 tumors in 222 patients, *Pathol Annu* 281, (part 1):97, 1993.
170. Allen PW, Enzinger FM: Hemangioma of skeletal muscle: an analysis of 89 cases, *Cancer* 29:8, 1972.
171. Angervall L, Nielsen JM, Stener B, Svendsen P: Concomitant AV-malformation in skeletal muscle: a clinical, angiographic and histological study, *Cancer* 44:232, 1979.
172. Castro C, Winkelmann RK: Angiolymphoid hyperplasia with eosinophilia in the skin, *Cancer* 34:1696, 1974.
173. Mehregan AH, Shapiro L: Angiolymphoid hyperplasia with eosinophilia, *Arch Dermatol* 103:50, 1971.
174. Rao VK, Weiss SW: Angiomatosis of soft tissue: an analysis of the histologic features and clinical outcome in 51 cases, *Am J Surg Pathol* 16:764, 1992.
175. Cotell SL, Noskin GA: Bacillary angiomatosis: clinical and histologic features, diagnosis, and treatment. *Arch Intern Med* 154:524, 1994.
176. Le Boit PE: Bacillary angiomatosis: a systemic opportunistic infection with prominent cutaneous manifestations, *Semin Dermatol* 10:194, 1991.
177. Bhaskar SN, Jacoway JR: Pyogenic granuloma—clinical features, incidence, histology, and results of treatment: report of 242 cases, *J Oral Surg* 24:391, 1966.
178. Patrice SJ, Wiss K, Mulliken JB: Pyogenic granuloma (lobular capillary hemangioma): a clinicopathologic study of 178 cases, *Pediatr Dermatol* 8:267, 1991.
178a. Cooper PH, McAllister HA, Helwig EB: Intravenous pyogenic granuloma: a study of 18 cases, *Am J Surg Pathol* 3:221, 1979.
179. Clearkin KP, Enzinger FM: Intravascular papillary endothelial hyperplasia, *Arch Pathol Lab Med* 100:441, 1976.
180. Hashimoto H, Daimaru Y, Enjoji M: Intravascular papillary endothelial hyperplasia: a clinicopathologic study of 91cases, *Am J Dermatopathol* 5:539, 1983.
181. Kuo TT, Sayers CP, Rosai J: Masson's "vegetant intravascular hemangioendothelioma": a lesion often mistaken for angiosarcoma. Study of seventeen cases located in the skin and soft tissues, *Cancer* 38:1227, 1976.
182. Flanagan BP, Helwig EB: Cutaneous lymphangioma, *Arch Dermatol* 113:24, 1977.
183. Byrne J, Blanc WA, Warburton D, Wigger J: The significance of cystic hygroma in fetuses, *Hum Pathol* 15:61, 1984.
184. Carey WD: Pulmonary lymphangiomyomatosis, *Chest* 85:796, 1984.
185. Urban T, Kuttenn F, Gompel A et al: Pulmonary lymphangiomyomatosis: follow-up and long-term outcome with antiestrogen therapy: a report of eight cases, *Chest* 102:472, 1992.
186. Vazquez JJ, Fernandez-Cuervo L, Fidalgo B: Lymphangiomyomatosis: morphogenetic study and ultrastructural confirmation of the histogenesis of the lung lesion, *Cancer* 37:2321, 1976.
187. Wolff M: Lymphangiomyoma: Clinicopathological and ultrastructural confirmation of its histogenesis, *Cancer* 31:988, 1973.

188. Cornog JL, Enterline HT: Lymphangiomyoma: a benign lesion of chyliferous lymphatics synonymous with lymphangiopericytoma, *Cancer* 19:1909, 1966.

Hemangioendothelioma

189. Allen PW, Ramakrishna B, MacCormak LB: The histiocytoid hemangiomas and other controversies, *Pathol Annu* 27(part 2):51, 1992.
190. Ellis GL, Kratochvil FJ: Epithelioid hemangioendothelioma of the head and neck: A clinicopathologic report of twelve cases, *Oral Surg Oral Med Oral Pathol* 61:61, 1986.
191. Imayama S, Murakamai Y, Hashimoto H, Hori Y: Spindle cell hemangioendothelioma exhibits the ultrastructural features of reactive vascular proliferation rather than of angiosarcoma, *Am J Clin Pathol* 97:279, 1992.
192. Niedt GW, Greco MA, Wieczorek R et al: Hemangioma with Kaposi's sarcoma–like features: report of two cases, *Pediatr Pathol* 9:567, 1989.
193. Rosai J, Gold J, Landy R: The histiocytoid hemangiomas: a unifying concept embracing several previously described entities of skin, soft tissue, large vessels, bone and heart, *Hum Pathol* 10:707, 1979.
194. Scott GA, Rosai J: Spindle cell hemangioendothelioma: report of seven additional cases of a recently described vascular neoplasm, *Am J Dermatopathol* 10:281, 1988.
195. Terashi H, Itami S, Kurata S et al: Spindle cell hemangioendothelioma: report of three cases, *J Dermatol* 18:104, 1991.
196. Tsang WY, Chan JK: Kaposi-like infantile hemangioendothelioma: a distinctive vascular neoplasm of the retroperitoneum, *Am J Surg Pathol* 15:982, 1991.
197. Weiss SW, Enzinger FM: Epithelioid hemangioendothelioma: a vascular tumor often mistaken for a carcinoma, *Cancer* 50:970, 1982.
198. Weiss SW, Ishak KG, Dail DH et al: Epithelioid hemangioendothelioma and related lesions, *Semin Diagn Pathol* 3:259, 1986.
199. Weiss SW, Enzinger FM: Spindle cell hemangioendothelioma: a low grade angiosarcoma resembling a cavernous hemangioma and Kaposi's sarcoma, *Am J Surg Pathol* 10:521, 1986.
200. Wick MR, Manivel JC: Epithelioid sarcoma and epithelioid hemangioendothelioma: an immunocytochemical and lectin histochemical comparison, *Virchows Arch [A]* 410:309, 1987.
200a. Zukerberg LR, Nickoloff BJ, Weiss SW: Kaposiform hemangioendothelioma of infancy and childhood: an aggressive neoplasm associated with Kasabach-Merritt syndrome and lymphangiomatosis, *Am J Surg Pathol* 17:321, 1993.

Angiosarcoma

201. Holden CA, Spittle MF, Jones EW: Angiosarcoma of the face and scalp: prognosis and treatment, *Cancer* 59:1046, 1987.
202. Maddox JC, Evans HL: Angiosarcoma of skin and soft tissue: a study of 44 cases, *Cancer* 48:1907, 1981.
203. Rosai J, Sumner HW, Kostianovsky M, Perez-Mesa C: Angiosarcoma of the skin: a clinicopathologic and fine structural study, *Hum Pathol* 7:83, 1976.
204. Kindblom LG, Stenman G, Angervall L: Morphological and cytogenetic studies of angiosarcoma in Stewart-Treves syndrome, *Virchows Arch [A]* 419:439, 1991.
205. Merino MJ, Carter D, Berman M: Angiosarcoma of the breast, *Am J Surg Pathol* 7:53, 1983.
206. Rosen PP, Kimmel M, Ernsberger D: Mammary angiosarcoma: the prognostic significance of tumor differentiation, *Cancer* 62:2145, 1988.
207. Donnell RM, Rosen PP, Lieberman PH et al: Angiosarcoma and other vascular tumors of the breast: pathologic analysis as a guide to prognosis, *Am J Surg Pathol* 5:629, 1981.
207a. Fletcher CD, Beham A, Bekir S et al: Epithelioid angiosarcoma of deep soft tissue: a distinctive tumor readily mistaken for an epithelial neoplasm, *Am J Surg Pathol* 15:915, 1991.
208. Miettinen M, Lindenmayer AE, Chaubal A: Immunohistochemical diagnosis of endothelial cell tumors: comparison of CD31, CD34, and BNH9 antibody to H-antigen with von Willebrand's factor, *Mod Pathol* 8:31, 1994.
209. Traweek ST, Kandalaft PL, Mehta P, Battifora H: The human hematopoietic progenitor cell antigen (CD34) in vascular neoplasia, *Am J Clin Pathol* 96:25, 1991.
210. Berry CL, Amerigo J: Blood group antigens in vascular tumors, *Virchows Arch [A]* 388:167, 1980.
211. Ordóñez NG, Batsakis JG: Comparison of *Ulex europaeus* lectin and factor VIII–related antigen in vascular lesions, *Arch Pathol Lab Med* 108:129, 1984.
212. Carroll TJ, Schelper RL, Goeken JA, Kemp JD: Neoplastic angioendiotheliomatosis: immunopathologic and morphologic evidence for intravascular malignant lymphomatosis, *Am J Clin Pathol* 85:169, 1986.
213. Friedman-Kien AE, Saltzman BR: Clinical manifestations of classical, endemic African, and epidemic AIDS-associated Kaposi's sarcoma, *J Am Acad Dermatol* 22:1237, 1990.
214. Wahman A, Melnick SL, Rhame FC, Potter JD: The epidemiology of classic, African, and immunosuppressed Kaposi's sarcoma, *Epidemiol Rev* 13:178, 1991.
215. Lo S-C, Liotta LA: Vascular tumors produced by NIH/3T3 cells transfected with human AIDS Kaposi's sarcoma DNA, *Am J Pathol* 118:7, 1985.
215a. Ensoli B, Barillari G, Gallo RC: Cytokines and growth factors in the pathogenesis of AIDS-associated Kaposi's sarcoma, *Immunol Rev* 127:147, 1992.
216. Beckstead JH, Wood GS, Fletcher V: Evidence for the origin of Kaposi's sarcoma from lymphatic endothelium, *Am J Pathol* 119:294, 1985.
217. Dorfman RF: Kaposi's sarcoma: evidence supporting its origin from the lymphatic system, *Lymphology* 21:45, 1988.
218. Tsuneyoshi M, Enjoji M: Glomus tumor: a clinicopathologic and electron microscopic study, *Cancer* 50:1601, 1982.
219. Conant MA, Wiesenfield SL: Multiple glomus tumors of the skin, *Arch Dermatol* 103:481, 1971.
220. Appelman HD, Helwig EB: Glomus tumors of the stomach, *Cancer* 23:1969, 1969
221. Toker C: Glomangioma: an ultrastructural study, *Cancer* 23:48, 1969.
222. Venkatachalam MA, Greally JG: Fine structure of glomus tumor: similarity of glomus cells to smooth muscle cells, *Cancer* 23:1176, 1969.
223. Miettinen M, Lehto V-P, Virtanen I: Glomus tumor cells—evaluation of smooth muscle cell and endothelial cell properties, *Virchows Arch [B]* 43:139, 1983.
224. Porter PL, Bigler SA, McNutt M, Gown AM: The immunophenotype of hemangiopericytomas and glomus tumors, with special reference to muscle protein expression: an immunohistochemical study and review of the literature, *Mod Pathol* 4:46, 1990.
225. Schürch W, Skalli O, Lagace R et al: Intermediate filament proteins and actin isoforms as markers for soft tissue tumor differentiation and origin. III. Hemangiopericytomas and glomus tumors, *Am J Pathol* 136:771, 1990.
226. Gould EW, Manivel JC, Albores-Saavedra J, Monforte H: Locally infiltrative glomus tumors and glomangiosarcomas: a clinical, ultrastructural, and immunohistochemical study, *Cancer* 65:310, 1990.
227. Croxatto JO, Font RL: Hemangiopericytoma of the orbit: a clinicopathologic study of 30 cases, *Hum Pathol* 13:199, 1972.
228. Enzinger FM, Smith BH: Hemangiopericytoma: an analysis of 106 cases, *Hum Pathol* 7:61, 1976.
229. Goldman SM, Davidson AJ, Neal J: Retroperitoneal and pelvic hemangiopericytomas: clinical, radiologic, and pathologic correlation, *Radiology* 168:13, 1988.
230. McMaster M, Soule E, Ivins J: Hemangiopericytoma—clinicopathologic study and long term follow-up of 60 patients, *Cancer* 36:2232, 1975.

Perivascular tumors

231. Angervall L, Kindblom LG, Nielsen JM et al: Hemangiopericytoma: a clinicopathologic, angiographic and microangiographic study, *Cancer* 42:2412, 1978.
232. Gurthrie BL, Ebersold MJ, Scheithauer BW, Shaw EG: Meningeal hemangiopericytoma: histopathologic features, treatment, and long-term follow-up of 44 cases, *Neurosurgery* 25:514, 1989.
233. Iwaki T, Fukui M, Takeshita I et al: Hemangiopericytoma of the meninges: a clinicopathologic and immunohistochemical study, *Clin Neuropathol* 7:93, 1988.
234. Jääskeläinen J, Servo A, Haltia M et al: Meningeal hemangiopericytoma. In Schimidek HH, editor: Meningiomas and their surgical management. Philadelphia, 1992, Saunders.

235. Mena H, Ribas JL, Pezeshkpour GH et al: Hemangiopericytoma of the central nervous system: a review of 94 cases, *Hum Pathol* 22:84, 1991.
236. Tsuneyoshi M, Daimaru Y, Enjoji M: Malignant hemangiopericytoma and other sarcomas with hemangiopericytoma-like pattern, *Pathol Res Pract* 178:446, 1984.
237. Dardick I, Hammar SP, Scheithauer BW: Ultrastructural spectrum of hemangiopericytoma: a comparative study of fetal, adult, and neoplastic pericytes, *Ultrastruct Pathol* 13:111, 1989.
238. Sreekantaiah C, Bridge JA, Rao UN et al: Clonal chromosomal abnormalities in hemangiopericytoma, *Cancer Genet Cytogenet* 54:173, 1991.

Leiomyoma and leiomyosarcoma

239. Hachisuga T, Hashimoto H, Enjoji M: Angioleiomyoma: a clinicopathologic reappraisal of 562 cases, *Cancer* 54:126, 1984.
240. Dahl I, Angervall L: Cutaneous and subcutaneous leiomyosarcoma—a clinicopathologic study of 47 patients, *Pathologia Eur* 9:307, 1974.
241. Fields JP, Helwig EB: Leiomyosarcoma of the skin and subcutaneous tissue, *Cancer* 47:156, 1981.
242. Hashimoto H, Daimaru Y, Tsuneyoshi M, Enjoji M: Leiomyosarcoma of the external soft tissues: a clinicopathologic, immunohistochemical and electron microscopic study, *Cancer* 57:2077, 1986.
243. Stout AP, Hill WT: Leiomyosarcoma of the superficial soft tissue, *Cancer* 11:844, 1958.
244. Kay S, McNeill DD: Leiomyosarcoma of retroperitoneum, *Surg Gynecol Obstet* 129:285, 1969.
245. Shmookler BM, Lauer DH: Retroperitoneal leiomyosarcoma: a clinicopathologic analysis of 36 cases, *Am J Surg Pathol* 7:269, 1983.
246. Wile AG, Evans HL, Romsdahl MM: Leiomyosarcoma of soft tissue: a clinicopathologic study, *Cancer* 48:1022, 1981.
247. Berlin O, Stener B, Kindblom LG, Angervall L: Leiomyosarcoma of venous origin in the extremities: a correlated clinical, roentgenologic, and morphologic study with diagnostic and surgical implications, *Cancer* 54:2147, 1984.
248. Leu HJ, Makek M: Intramural venous leiomyosarcomas, *Cancer* 57:1395, 1986.
249. Baker PB, Goodwin RA: Pulmonary artery sarcomas: a review and report of a case, *Arch Pathol Lab Med* 109:35, 1985.
250. Schürch W, Skalli O, Seemayer TA, Gabbiani G: Intermediate filament proteins and actin isoforms as markers for soft tissue tumor differentiation and origin. I. Smooth muscle tumors, *Am J Pathol* 128:91, 1987.
251. Tsukada T, McNutt MA, Ross R, Gown AM: HHF35, a muscle actin–specific monoclonal antibody. II. Reactivity in normal, reactive, and neoplastic tissues, *Am J Pathol* 127:389, 1987.
252. Brown DC, Theaker JM, Banks PM et al: Cytokeratin expression in smooth muscle and smooth muscle cell tumors, *Histopathology* 11:477, 1987.
253. Miettinen M: Immunoreactivity for cytokeratin and epithelial membrane antigen in leiomyosarcoma, *Arch Pathol Lab Med* 112:637, 1988.
254. Norton AJ, Thomas JA, Isaacson PG: Cytokeratin specific monoclonal antibodies are reactive with tumors of smooth muscle derivation: an immunocytochemical and biochemical study using antibodies to intermediate filament cytoskeletal proteins, *Histopathology* 11:487, 1987.
254a. Sreekantaiah C, Davis JR, Sandberg AA: Chromosomal abnormalities in leiomyosarcoma, *Am J Pathol* 142:293, 1993.
255. Lavin P, Hajdu SI, Foote FW: Gastric and extragastric leiomyoblastoma, *Cancer* 29:305, 1972.

Rhabdomyoma and rhabdomyosarcoma

256. DiSant'Agnese PA, Knowles DM: Extracardiac rhabdomyoma: a clinicopathologic study and review of the literature, *Cancer* 46:780, 1980.
257. Fu YS, Perzin KH: Non-epithelial tumors of the nasal cavity, paranasal sinuses, and nasopharynx: a clinicopathological study. V. Skeletal muscle tumors (rhabdomyoma and rhabdomyosarcoma), *Cancer* 37:364, 1976.
257a. Gibas Z, Miettinen M: Recurrent parapharyngeal rhabdomyoma: evidence of neoplastic nature of the tumor from cytogenetic study, *Am J Surg Pathol* 16:721, 1992.
258. Dehner LP, Enzinger FM, Font RL: Fetal rhabdomyoma: an analysis of nine cases, *Cancer* 30:160, 1972.
259. Burke AP, Virmani R: Cardiac rhabdomyoma: a clinicopathologic study, *Mod Pathol* 4:70, 1991.
260. Gaiger AM, Soule EH, Hewton WA et al: Pathology of rhabdomyosarcoma: experience of the Intergroup Rhabdomyosarcoma Study, 1972-1978, *Natl Cancer Inst Monogr* 56:19, 1981.
261. Rodary C, Gehan EA, Flamant F et al: Prognostic factors in 951 nonmetastatic rhabdomyosarcomas in children: a report from the International Rhabdomyosarcoma Workshop, *Med Pediatr Oncol* 19:89, 1991.
262. Bale PM, Parsons RE, Stevens MM: Diagnosis and behavior of juvenile rhabdomyosarcoma, *Hum Pathol* 14:596, 1983.
263. Raney RB, Tefft M, Lawrence W et al: Paratesticular sarcoma in childhood and adolescence: a report from the Intergroup Rhabdomyosarcoma Studies I and II, 1973-1983, *Cancer* 60:2337, 1987.
264. Schmidt D, Reimann O, Treuner J, Harms D: Cellular differentiation and prognosis in embryonal rhabdomyosarcoma: a report from the cooperative Soft Tissue Sarcoma Study 1981 (CWS 81), *Virchows Arch [A]* 409:183, 1986.
265. LLoyd RV, Hajdu SI, Knapper WH: Embryonal rhabdomyosarcoma in adults, *Cancer* 51:557, 1983.
266. Flamant F, Hill C: The improvement in survival associated with combined chemotherapy in childhood rhabdomyosarcoma, *Cancer* 53:2417, 1984.
267. Maurer HM, Beltangady M, Genhan EA et al: The Intergroup Rhabdomyosarcoma Study. I. A final report, *Cancer* 61:209.1988.
268. Altmannsberger M, Weber K, Droste R, Osborn M: Desmin a specific marker for rhabdomyosarcomas of human and rat origin, *Am J Pathol* 118:85, 1985.
269. DeJong AS, van Kessel-van Vark M, Albus-Lutter CE et al: Skeletal muscle actin as tumor marker in the diagnosis of rhabdomyosarcoma in childhood, *Am J Surg Pathol* 9:467, 1985.
270. Eusebi V, Ceccarelli C, Gorza L: Immunocytochemistry of rhabdomyosarcoma: the use of four different markers, *Am J Surg Pathol* 10:293, 1986.
271. Miettinen M, Rapola J: Immunohistochemical spectrum of rhabdomyosarcoma and rhabdomyosarcoma-like tumors: the common presence of keratins and the 68kD neurofilament, *Am J Surg Pathol* 13:120, 1989.
272. Parham DM, Webber B, Holt H et al: Immunohistochemical study of childhood rhabdomyosarcomas and related neoplasms: results of an Intergroup Rhabdomyosarcoma Study project, *Cancer* 67:3072, 1991.
273. Skalli O, Gabbiani G, Babai F et al: Intermediate filament proteins and actin isoforms as markers for soft tissue tumor differentiation and origin. II. Rhabdomyosarcomas, *Am J Pathol* 130:515, 1988.
274. Molenaar WM, Oosterhuis AM, Kamps WA: Cytological "differentiation" in childhood rhabdomyosarcoma following polychemotherapy, *Hum Pathol* 15:973, 1984.
275. Dias P, Parham DM, Shapiro DN et al: Myogenic regulatory protein (MyoD1) expression in childhood solid tumors: diagnostic utility in rhabdomyosarcoma, *Am J Pathol* 137:1283, 1990.
276. Erlandson RA: The ultrastructural distinction between rhabdomyosarcoma and other undifferentiated "sarcomas", *Ultrastruct Pathol* 11:83, 1988.
277. Kawamoto EH, Weidner N, Agostini RM, Jaffe R: Malignant ectomesenchymoma of soft tissues: report of two cases and review of the literature, *Cancer* 59:1791, 1987.
278. Davis GL, Kissane JM, Ishak KG: Embryonal rhabdomyosarcoma (sarcoma botryoides) of the biliary tree: report of five cases and review of literature, *Cancer* 24:333, 1969.
279. Lack EE, Perez-Atayde AR, Schuster SR: Botryoid rhabdomyosarcoma of the biliary tree, *Am J Surg Pathol* 5:143, 1981.
280. Cavazzana AO, Schmidt D, Ninfo V et al: Spindle cell rhabdomyosarcoma: a prognostically favorable variant of rhabdomyosarcoma, *Am J Surg Pathol* 16:229, 1992.
281. Leuschner I, Newton WA, Schmidt D et al: Spindle cell variants of embryonal rhabdomyosarcoma in the paratesticular region: a report of the Intergroup Rhabdomyosarcoma Study, *Am J Surg Pathol* 17:221, 1993.
282. Enterline HT, Horn RC: Alveolar rhabdomyosarcoma: a distinctive tumor type, *Cancer* 9:356, 1958.

283. Enzinger FM, Shiraki M: Alveolar rhabdomyosarcoma: an analysis of 110 cases, *Cancer* 24:18, 1969.
284. Copeland LJ, Sneige N, Stringer CA et al: Alveolar rhabdomyosarcoma of the female genitalia, *Cancer* 56:849, 1985.
285. Tsokos M ,Webber BL, Parham DM et al: Rhabdomyosarcoma: new classification scheme related to prognosis, *Arch Pathol Lab Med* 116,847, 1992.
286. Churg A, Ringus J: Ultrastructural observations on the histogenesis of alveolar rhabdomyosarcoma, *Cancer* 41:1355, 1978.
287. Biegel JA, Meek RJ, Parmiter AH et al: Chromosomal translocation t(1;13)(p36;q14) in a case of rhabdomyosarcoma. *Genes Chromosom Cancer* 3:483,1991.
288. Douglass EC, Valentine M, Etcubanas E et al: A specific chromosomal abnormality in rhabdomyosarcoma, *Cytogenet Cell Genet* 45:148, 1987.
289. Douglass EC, Rowe ST, Valentine M et al: Variant translocations of chromosome 13 in alveolar rhabdomyosarcoma, *Genes Chromosom Cancer* 3:480, 1991.
290. DeJong AS, van Kessel-van Vark M, Albus-Lutter CE: Pleomorphic rhabdomyosarcoma in adults: immunohistochemistry as a tool for its diagnosis, *Hum Pathol* 18:298, 1987.
291. Gaffney EF, Dervan PA, Fletcher CDM: Pleomorphic rhabdomyosarcoma in adulthood: analysis of 11 cases with definition of diagnostic criteria, *Am J Surg Pathol* 17:601, 1993.
292. Molenaar WM, Oosterhuis AM, Ramaekers FC: The rarity of rhabdomyosarcoma in the adult: a morphologic and immunohistochemical study, *Pathol Res Pract* 180:400, 1985.
293. Harkin JC, Reed RJ: Tumors of the peripheral nervous system. In *Atlas of tumor pathology,* Washington, DC, 1969, Armed Forces Institute of Pathology, second series, fascicle 3.
294. Reed RJ, Bliss BO: Morton neuroma: regressive and productive intermetatarsal elastofibrositis, *Arch Pathol* 95:123, 1973.
295. Erlandson RA, Woodruff JM: Peripheral nerve sheath tumors: an electron microscopic study of 43 cases, *Cancer* 49:273, 1982.
296. Kaiserling E, Geerts ML: Tumour of Wagner-Meissner touch corpuscles: Wagner-Meissner neurilemmoma, *Virchows Arch [A]* 409:241, 1986.
297. Barker D, Wright E, Nguyen K et al: Gene for von Recklinghausen neurofibromatosis is in the pericentromeric region of chromosome 17, *Science* 236:1100, 1987.
298. Brasfield RD, das Gupta TK: von Recklinghausen's disease: a clinicopathological study, *Ann Surg* 175:86, 1972.
299. Sorensen SA, Mulvihill JJ, Nielsen A: Long-term follow-up of von Recklinghausen neurofibromatosis: survival and malignant neoplasms, *N Engl J Med* 290:626, 1986.
300. Bijlsma EK, Brouwer-Mladin R, Bosch DA et al: Molecular characterization of chromosome 22 deletions in schwannomas, *Genes Chromosom Cancer* 5:201, 1992.

Benign neural tumors

301. Angervall L, Kindblom LG, Haglid K: Dermal nerve sheath myxoma: a light and electron microscopic, histochemical, and immunohistochemical study, *Cancer* 53:1752, 1984.
302. Fletcher CDM, Chan JK, McKee PH: Dermal nerve sheath myxoma: a study of three cases, *Histopathology* 10:135, 1986.
303. Gallager RL, Helwig EB: Neurothekeoma: a benign cutaneous tumor of nerve sheath origin, *Am J Clin Pathol* 74:759, 1980.
304. Ariza A, Bilbao JM, Rosai J: Immunohistochemical detection of epithelial membrane antigen in normal perineurial cells and perineurioma, *Am J Surg Pathol* 12:678, 1988.
305. Erlandson RA: The enigmatic perineurial cell and its participation in tumors and in tumorlike entities, *Ultrastruct Pathol* 15:335, 1991.
306. Lazarus SS, Trombetta LD: Ultrastructural identification of a benign perineurial cell tumor, *Cancer* 41:1823, 1978.
307. Perentes E, Nakagawa Y, Ross GW et al: Expression of epithelial membrane antigen in perineurial cells and their derivatives: an immunohistochemical study with multiple markers, *Acta Neuropathol* 75:160, 1987.
308. Tsang YW, Chan JKC, Chow LTC et al: Perineurioma: an uncommon soft tissue neoplasm distinct from localized hypertrophic neuropathy and neurofibroma, *Am J Surg Pathol* 16:756, 1992.
309. McDonald DM, Wilson-Jones E: Pacinian neurofibroma, *Histopathology* 1:247, 1977.
310. Das Gupta TK, Brasfield RD, Strong EW et al: Benign solitary schwannomas (neurilemomas), *Cancer* 24:355, 1979.
311. Daimaru Y, Kido H, Hashimoto H, Enjoji M: Benign schwannoma of the gastrointestinal tract: a clinicopathologic and immunohistochemical study, *Hum Pathol* 19:257, 1988.
312. Dahl I: Ancient neurilemmoma (schwannoma), *Acta Pathol Microbiol Scand* 85:812, 1977.
313. Lodding P, Kindblom LG, Angervall L, Stenman G: Cellular schwannoma: a clinicopathologic study of 29 cases, *Virchows Arch [A]* 416,237, 1990.
314. White W, Shiu MH, Rosenblum MK et al: Cellular schwannoma: a clinicopathologic study of 57 patients and 58 tumors, *Cancer* 66:1266, 1990.
315. Woodruff JM, Godwin TA, Erlandson RA et al: Cellular schwannoma: a variety of schwannoma sometimes mistaken for a malignant tumor, *Am J Surg Pathol* 5:733, 1981.
316. Gould VE, Moll R, Moll I et al: The intermediate filament complement of the spectrum of nerve sheath neoplasms, *Lab Invest* 55:463, 1986.
317. Kawahara E, Oda Y, Ooi A: Expression of glial fibrillary acidic protein (GFAP) in peripheral nerve sheath tumors: a comparative study of immunoreactivity of GFAP, vimentin, S-100 protein and neurofilament in 38 schwannomas and 18 neurofibromas, *Am J Surg Pathol* 12:115, 1988.
318. Nakajima T, Watanabe S, Soto Y et al: An immunoperoxidase study of S-100 protein distribution in normal and neoplastic tissues, *Am J Surg Pathol* 6:715, 1982.
319. Stenman G, Kindblom LG, Johansson M, Angervall L: Clonal chromosomal abnormalities and in vitro growth characteristics of classical and cellular schwannomas, *Cancer Genet Cytogenet* 57:121, 1991.
320. Fletcher CDM, Davies SE: Benign plexiform (multinodular) schwannoma: a rare tumor unassociated with neurofibromatosis, *Histopathology* 19:971, 1986.
321. Woodruff JM, Marshall ML, Godwin TA et al: Plexiform (multinodular) schwannoma: a tumor simulating the plexiform neurofibroma, *Am J Surg Pathol* 7:691, 1983.
322. Carney JA: Psammomatous melanotic schwannoma: a distinctive, heritable tumor with special associations, including cardiac myxoma and the Cushing syndrome, *Am J Surg Pathol* 14:206, 1990.
323. Lack EE, Worsham GF, Callihan MD et al: Granular cell tumor: a clinicopathologic study of 110 patients, *J Surg Oncol* 13:301, 1980.
324. Paskin DL, Hull JD: Granular cell myoblastoma: a comprehensive review of 15 years' experience, *Ann Surg* 175:501, 1972.
325. Kindblom LG, Olsson K-M: Malignant granular cell tumor: a clinicopathologic and ultrastructural study of a case, *Pathol Res Pract* 172:384, 1981.
326. Robertson AJ, McIntosh W, Lamont P, Guthrie W: Malignant granular cell tumour (myoblastoma) of the vulva: report of a case and review of the literature, *Histopathology* 5:69, 1981.
327. Miettinen M, Lehtonen E, Lehtola H et al: Histogenesis of granular cell tumour–an immunohistochemical and ultrastructural study, *J Pathol* 142:221, 1984
328. Mukai M: Immunohistochemical localization of S-100 protein and peripheral nerve myelin proteins (P2 protein and PO protein) in granular cell tumors, *Am J Pathol* 112:139, 1983.
329. Nakazato Y, Ishizeki J, Takahashi K et al: Immunohistochemical localization of S-100 protein in granular cell myoblastoma, *Cancer* 49:1624, 1982.
330. Sobel H, Marquet E: Granular cells and granular cell lesions, *Pathol Annu* 9:43, 1974.
331. Lack EE, Worsham GF, Callihan MD et al: Gingival granular cell tumor of the newborn (congenital "epulis"): a clinical and pathologic study of 21 patients, *Am J Surg Pathol* 5:37, 1981.
332. Sobel H, Arvin E, Marquet E et al: Reactive granular cells in sites of trauma, *Am J Clin Pathol* 61:223, 1974.
333. Christ ML, Ozzello L: Myogenous origin of a granular cell tumor of the urinary bladder, *Am J Clin Pathol* 56:736, 1971.
334. Bain GO, Shnitka TK: Cutaneous meningioma (psammoma), *Arch Dermatol* 74:590, 1956.

335. Helwig EB, Stern JB: Subcutaneous sacrococcygeal myxopapillary ependymoma: a clinicopathologic study of 32 cases, *Am J Clin Pathol* 89:156, 1984.

335a. Raju U, Zarbo RJ, Regezi JA et al: Melanotic neuroectodermal tumors of infancy: intermediate filament-, neuroendocrine-, and melanoma-associated antigen profiles, *Appl Immunohistochem* 1:69, 1993.

Malignant neural tumors

336. D'Agostino AN, Soule EH, Miller RH: Primary malignant neoplasms of nerves (malignant neurilemomas) in 2 patients without manifestations of multiple neurofibromatosis (von Recklinghausen's disease), *Cancer* 16:1003, 1963.

337. D'Agostino AN, Soule EH, Miller RH: Sarcomas of the peripheral nerves and somatic soft tissues associated with multiple neurofibromatosis (von Recklinghausen's disease), *Cancer* 16:1015, 1963.

338. Ducatman BS, Scheithauer BW, Piepgras DG et al: Malignant peripheral nerve sheath tumors: a clinicopathologic study of 120 cases, *Cancer* 57:2006, 1986.

339. Guccion JG, Enzinger FM: Malignant schwannoma associated with von Recklinghausen's neurofibromatosis, *Virchows Arch [A]* 383:43, 1979.

340. Trojanowski JQ, Kleinman GM, Proppe KH: Malignant tumors of nerve sheath origin, *Cancer* 46:1202, 1980.

341. Ducatman BS, Scheithauer BW: Postirradiation neurofibrosarcoma, *Cancer* 51:1028, 1983.

342. Hruban RH, Shiu MH, Senie RT, Woodruff JM: Malignant peripheral nerve sheath tumors in the buttock and lower extremity: a study of 43 cases, *Cancer* 66:1253, 1990.

343. Daimaru Y, Hashimoto H, Enjoji M: Malignant peripheral nerve sheath tumors (malignant schwannomas): an immunohistochemical study of 29 cases, *Am J Surg Pathol* 9,434, 1985.

344. Herrera GA, deMoraes HP: Neurogenic sarcomas in patients with neurofibromatosis (von Recklinghausen's disease): light, electron microscopy and immunohistochemistry study, *Virchows Arch [A]*, 403:361, 1984.

345. Matsunou H, Shimoda T, Kakimoto S et al: Histopathologic and immunohistochemical study of malignant tumors of peripheral nerve sheaths (malignant schwannoma), *Cancer* 56:2269, 1985.

346. Tsuneyoshi M, Enjoji M: Primary malignant peripheral nerve sheath tumors (malignant schwannomas): a clinicopathologic and electron microscopic study, *Acta Pathol Jpn* 29:363, 1979.

347. Wick MR, Swanson PE, Scheithauer BW, Manivel JC: Malignant peripheral nerve sheath tumor: an immunohistochemical study of 62 cases, *Am J Clin Pathol* 87:425, 1987.

348. Laskin WB, Weiss SW, Bratthauer GL: Epithelioid variant of malignant peripheral nerve sheath tumor (malignant epithelioid schwannoma), *Am J Surg Pathol* 15:1136, 1991.

349. Lodding P, Kindblom LG, Angervall L: Epithelioid malignant schwannoma: a study of 14 cases, *Virchows Arch [A]* 409:433, 1986.

350. Brooks JS, Freeman M, Enterline HT: Malignant "triton" tumors: natural history and immunohistochemistry of nine new cases with literature review, *Cancer* 55:2543, 1985.

351. Daimaru Y, Hashimoto H, Enjoji M: Malignant "triton" tumors: a clinicopathologic and immunohistochemical study of nine cases, *Hum Pathol* 15:768, 1984.

352. Woodruff JM, Chernik NL, Smith MC et al: Peripheral nerve sheath tumors with rhabdomyosarcomatous differentiation (malignant "triton" tumors), *Cancer* 32:426, 1973.

353. Markel SF, Enzinger FM: Neuromuscular hamartoma—a benign "triton tumor" composed of mature neural and striated muscle elements, *Cancer* 49:140, 1982.

354. Ducatman BS, Scheithauer BW: Malignant peripheral nerve sheath tumor with divergent differentiation, *Cancer* 54:1049, 1984.

Clear cell sarcoma

355. Chung EB, Enzinger FM: Malignant melanoma of soft parts: a reassessment of clear cell sarcoma, *Am J Surg Pathol* 7:405, 1983.

356. Enzinger FM: Clear-cell sarcoma of tendons and aponeuroses: an analysis of 21 cases, *Cancer* 18:1163, 1965.

357. Eckardt JJ, Pritchard DJ, Soule EH: Clear cell sarcoma: a clinicopathologic study of 27 cases, *Cancer* 52:1482, 1983.

358. Lucas DR, Nascimento AG, Sim FH: Clear cell sarcoma of soft tissues: Mayo Clinic experience with 35 cases. *Am J Surg Pathol* 16:1197, 1992.

359. Montgomery EA, Meis JM, Ramos AG et al: Clear cell sarcoma of tendons and aponeuroses: a clinicopathologic study of 58 cases with analysis of prognostic factors, *Int J Surg Pathol* 1:89, 1993.

360. Pavlidis NA, Fisher C, Wiltshaw E: Clear-cell sarcoma of tendons and aponeuroses: a clinicopathologic study. Presentation of six additional cases with review of the literature, *Cancer* 54:1412, 1984.

361. Sara AS, Evans HL, Benjamin RS: Malignant melanoma of soft parts (clear cell sarcoma): a study of 17 cases, with emphasis on prognostic factors, *Cancer* 65:367, 1990.

362. Hasegawa T, Hirose T, Kudo E, Hizawa K: Clear cell sarcoma: an immunohistochemical and ultrastructural study, *Acta Pathol Jpn* 39:321, 1989.

363. Swanson PE, Wick MR: Clear cell sarcoma: an immunohistochemical analysis of six cases and comparison with other epithelioid neoplasms of soft tissue, *Arch Pathol Lab Med* 113:55, 1989.

364. Epstein AI, Martin AO, Kempson R: Use of a newly established human cell line (SU-CCS-1) to demonstrate the relationship of clear cell sarcoma to malignant melanoma, *Cancer Res* 44:1265, 1984.

365. Benson JD, Kraemer BB, Mackay B: Malignant melanoma of soft parts: an ultrastructural study of four cases, *Ultrastruct Pathol* 8:57, 1985.

366. Mukai M, Torikata C, Iri H, et al: Histogenesis of clear cell sarcoma of tendons and aponeuroses: an electron microscopic, biochemical, enzyme histochemical, and immunohistochemical study, *Am J Pathol* 114:264, 1984.

367. Kindblom LG, Lodding P, Angervall L: Clear cell sarcoma of tendons and aponeuroses: an immunohistochemical and electron microscopic analysis indicating neural crest origin, *Virchows Arch [A]* 401:109, 1983.

367a. Mrozek K, Karakousis CP, Perez-Mesa C, Bloomfield CD: Translocation t(12;22)(q13;q12.2-12.3) in clear cell sarcoma of tendons and aponeuroses, Genes Chromosom Cancer 6:249, 1993.

368. Bridge JA, Sreekantaiah C, Neff JR, Sandberg AA: Cytogenetic findings in clear cell sarcoma of tendons and aponeuroses: malignant melanoma of soft parts, *Cancer Genet Cytogenet* 52:101, 1991.

369. Rodriguez E, Sreekantaiah C, Reuter VE et al: t(12;22)(q13;q13) and trisomy 8 are nonrandom aberrations in clear cell sarcoma, *Cancer Genet Cytogenet* 64:107, 1992.

370. Stenman G, Kindblom LG, Angervall L: Reciprocal translocation t(12;22)(q13,q13) in clear cell sarcoma of tendons and aponeuroses, *Genes Chromosom Cancer* 4:122, 1992.

371. Travis JA, Bridge JA: Significance of both numerical and structural chromosomal abnormalities in clear cell sarcoma, *Cancer Genet Cytogenet* 64:104, 1992.

Bone- and cartilage-forming soft-tissue tumors

372. Ackerman LV: Extra-osseous localized non-neoplastic bone and cartilage formation (so-called myositis ossificans): clinical and pathological confusion with malignant neoplasms, *J Bone Joint Surg [Am]* 40a:279, 1958.

373. Campanacci M, Gardini GF, Giunti A, Donati U. Pseudo-tumoral ossification of the muscles and/or periosteum: a study of 57 cases, *Italian J Orthop Traumatol* 6:385, 1980.

374. Sumiyoshi K, Tsuneyoshi M, Enjoji M: Myositis ossificans: a clinicopathologic study of 21 cases, *Acta Pathol Jpn* 35:1109, 1985.

375. Dupree WB, Enzinger FM: Fibro-osseous pseudotumor of the digits, *Cancer* 58:2103, 1986.

376. Spjut HJ, Dorfman HD: Florid reactive periostitis of the tubular bones of the hands and feet: a benign lesion which may simulate osteosarcoma, *Am J Surg Pathol* 5:423, 1981.

377. Connor JM, Evans PA Fibrodysplasia ossificans progressiva: the clinical features and natural history of 34 patients, *J Bone Joint Surg [Br]* 64:76, 1982.

378. Kaplan FS, Tabas JA, Zasloff MA: Fibrodysplasia ossificans progressiva: a clue from the fly? *Calcif Tissue Int* 47:117, 1990.

378a. Kaplan FS, Tabas JA, Gannon FH et al: The histopathology of fibrodysplasia ossificans progressiva: an enchondral process, *J Bone Joint Surg [Am]* 75:220, 1993.

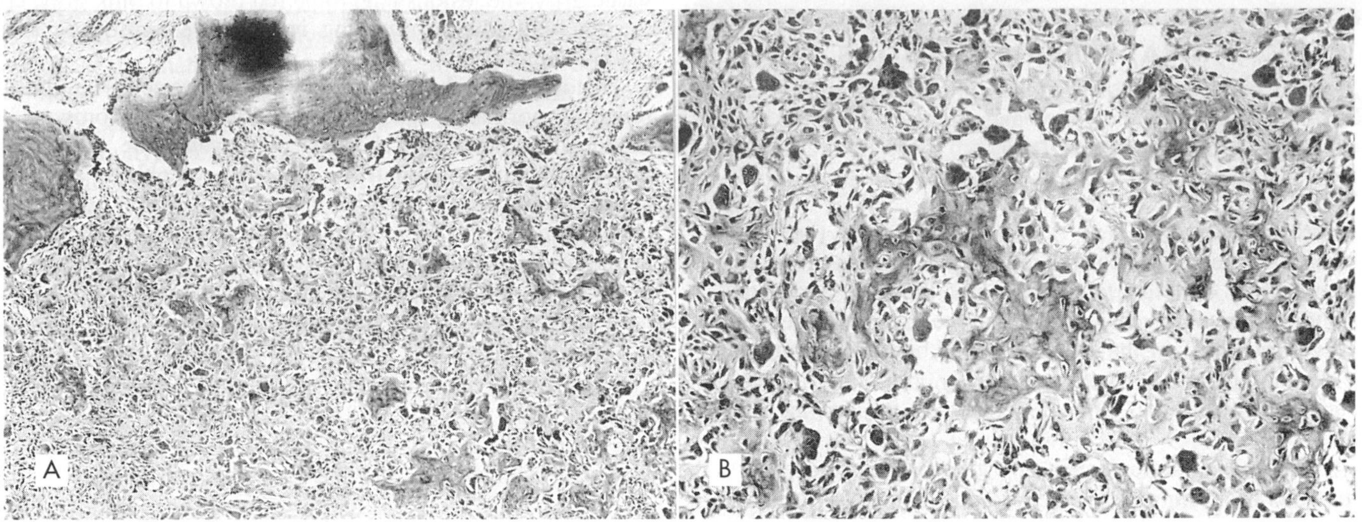

Fig. 73-4 Histology of osteoid osteoma. **A,** Low-power view of nidus. **B,** On higher magnification fibro-osseous proliferation with bone spicules lined by large osteoblasts is present.

TREATMENT AND PROGNOSIS. Treatment is surgical and directed to complete extirpation of the lesion. Failure to remove the lesion completely results in recurrence of symptoms.[7]

Even in the best of hands, the nidus can be missed in some cases, necessitating reoperation. Several techniques have been employed successfully to detect the nidus during surgery. One technique incorporates the use of a radionuclide that localizes in areas of high bone turnover. A Geiger counter is brought into the operating room, and the lesion is curetted until there is no evidence of radioactivity left in the surgical bed.[8,9] We have adopted an alternative that takes advantage of two properties of tetracycline: its localization in areas of new bone formation and its fluorescence in ultraviolet radiation.[10] The patient is given tetracycline 1 or 2 days preoperatively. The lesion is curetted and the resulting specimen examined in a dark room under an ultraviolet radiation lamp. The nidus shows a finely granular yellow-green fluorescence, whereas the surrounding tissue is manifested by a dull yellow-white appearance. Both the Geiger counter and ultraviolet-radiation techniques have been reported to be highly successful in identifying the nidus at the time of surgery and allowing judgments regarding the necessity of additional surgery.

Osteoblastoma

Osteoblastoma, another benign bone-producing neoplasm, accounts for approximately 1% of all primary bone tumors.[1-4] It occurs most often in the second and third decades of life, and males are affected approximately thrice as often as females are.[1-4]

Pain is generally the presenting symptom and is usually described as "deep," "aching," or "boring," in contrast with the severe pain of osteoid osteoma. Symptoms may also be attributable to mass effects that result in compression of vital structures. Osteoblastoma is not a disease of limited growth potential. By definition, an osteoblastoma is larger than 2 cm; it may attain an enormous size.

Although osteoblastoma may arise in any bone, it occurs most often in the spine, particularly the posterior elements (transverse and spinous processes).[11] The distribution of osteoblastoma in the spine has been described to be about equal for the different anatomic locations,[1-4] but large series have revealed some variation. In the study of Nemoto and colleagues[12] of 75 cases of osteoblastoma of the spine, 29 occurred in the cervical spine, 16 in the thoracic spine, 17 in the lumbar spine, and 13 in the sacral spine (Fig. 73-5), whereas in Boriani amd colleagues's series of 30 cases, 16 (53%) occurred in the lumbar spine.[13]

Radiographically, osteoblastoma presents as a mixed lytic/blastic lesion. With time and increased lesional size,

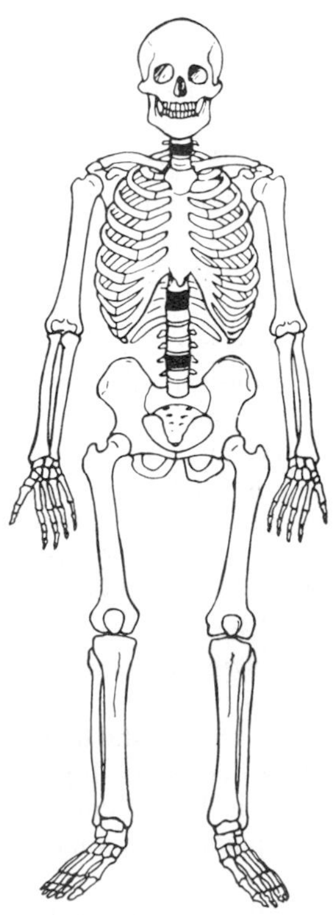

Fig. 73-5 Osteoblastoma. Anatomic distribution in the spine.

osteoblastoma may result in cortical thinning and eventual cortical expansion. Extension through cortex into the soft tissues is an extremely rare event. On CT scan examination the extent of the tumor and delineation of the margin, sometimes depicted as a thin bony shell, is often better ascertained than with plain radiographs.[14] MRI offers findings similar to those of CT scan and may help to differentiate tumor tissue from edema.[14]

PATHOLOGY. Grossly, osteoblastoma consists of finely granular and hemorrhagic bone. There may be extensive intralesional hemorrhage and large cavernous hemorrhagic cystic areas characteristic of secondary aneurysmal bone cyst change.[1-4]

Histologically, osteoblastoma is composed of randomly anastomosing trabeculas of osteoid and woven bone that are lined by a nearly continuous population of osteoblasts and occasional osteoclasts and are set in a capillary-rich stroma (Fig. 73-6). The osteoblasts are uniform; they have been likened to soldiers in a row or crows on a fence. No other histologic elements are present; the presence of heterogeneous elements should alert the observer to the possibility that the lesion is something other than osteoblastoma (in particular, osteosarcoma). However, Bertoni and colleagues[15] recently described a series of 18 osteoblastomas containing cartilage. The finding of cartilage was rare, however; these 18 cases were found during review of 325 cases of osteoblastomas treated or seen in consultation by the authors.

Histologically, osteoblastoma is indistinguishable from osteoid osteoma. Although histologically similar entities, the two types of lesions are distinguished by clinicopathologic criteria: symptoms, skeletal location, radiographic appearance, and most important size.

TREATMENT AND PROGNOSIS. The treatment of choice for osteoblastoma is curettage and packing with autologous bone chips. The local relapse rate is about 15%,[1-4,14] even with incomplete curettage; second curettage is almost always curative. Malignant transformation is rare but has been well described.

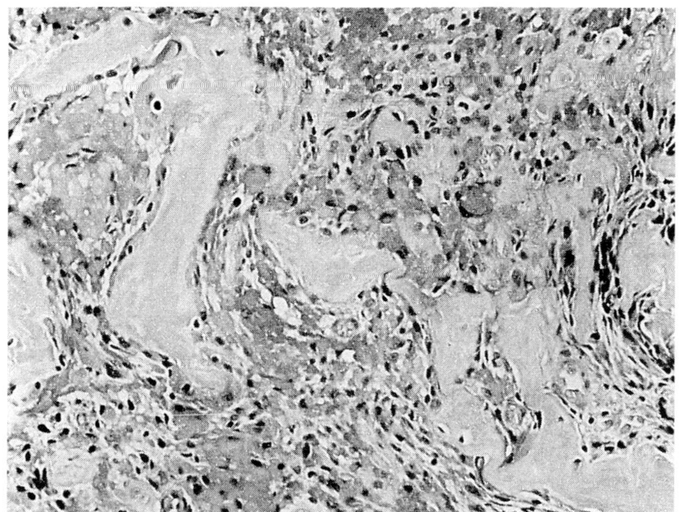

Fig. 73-6 Histologically, osteoblastoma shows proliferation of bone with mature bone spicules and fibrovascular stroma.

Aggressive osteoblastoma

Aggressive osteoblastoma has been referred to by a variety of terms: aggressive osteoblastoma,[16] malignant osteoblastoma,[17] and osteosarcoma resembling osteoblastoma.[18]

Aggressive (epithelioid) osteoblastoma is a rare osseous producing lesion similar to osteoblastoma except that the aggressive form typically contains large plump osteoblasts that often have a large nucleolus and some degree of mitotic activity; large collections of "epithelioid" osteoblasts are commonly seen. Clinically this lesion has a tendency for local growth and local recurrence. We have seen one example of this lesion in which there developed pulmonary metastases that resulted in the patient's death. In our opinion, these lesions are best viewed as a form of low-grade osteosarcoma. At M.D. Anderson Cancer Center patients with aggressive osteoblastoma are treated with an osteosarcoma protocol.

Malignant

Osteosarcoma

With the accrual of large numbers of cases, it has become apparent that osteosarcoma (OS) is a complex family of biologically diverse pathologic entities that share a single histologic finding: the production of bone or osteoid (a form of collagen that constitutes unmineralized bone) by malignant cells.[1-4] Histologic features alone might allow identification of an almost limitless number of patterns in OS. However, there appear to be a relatively limited number of subtypes that define biologically unique entities.

Although the finer points of such classification may better fall within the domain of the ultraspecialist, a few things are of importance. It should be recognized that there is a classification system and that it does have biologic significance. This system divides OS into its "conventional" ("classical," "textbook") forms and "variants." Conventional OS constitutes most of the OSs (65% to 75%).[1-4] The remaining 25% to 35% of OSs are made up of variants that are defined by clinical setting and by morphologic and histologic parameters. The variants frequently have prognoses that are significantly different from conventional OS. The most important contribution of such classification systems is to emphasize the predictably intrinsic biologic diversity within OS. The use of such systems allows intelligent comparison of data derived from various treatment strategies. Because of the significant differences in prognosis most studies compare results of treatment of conventional OS and leave the variants to independent reporting.

Conventional osteosarcoma. The most common and possibly the most important of the OSs is conventional, or medullary, OS.[1-4] Before the 1970s conventional OS was a devastating disease with limited treatment options and had a nearly uniformly fatal prognosis; 80% to 90% of patients with conventional OS who underwent an immediate ablative procedure developed systemic metastases within 9 to 18 months, and of these, all died within 18 to 36 months.[19-21] If 80% to 90% of patients were dying of systemic disease despite early radical surgery, they must have had systemic metastases at the time of presentation, merely at a level undetectable by conventional staging methods. Recognition of the subclinical micrometastases was the point that allowed multidisciplinary therapy into the treatment of conventional OS about 1975.[22,23] Thereafter the survival of this disease began to change dramatically.[24-28] Patients still die of this disease, but early diagnosis and management with chemotherapy and surgery have afforded a chance for life and for limb preservation.[29-32]

Although conventional OS may occur at any age, it is most frequently seen in the second and third decades of life[1-4]; its occurrence in any patient over the age of 40 years of age should at least alert the observer to possible underlying predisposing factors[1-4] (such as radiation exposure,[33] Paget's disease of bone,[34,35] bone infarct[36,37]). Males are affected approximately twice as often as females. Although any part of any bone may be affected, conventional OS most frequently arises in the distal area of the femur and the proximal areas of the tibia, humerus, and femur (Fig. 73-7). It almost exclusively arises within the metadiaphysis: about 91% arise in the metaphysis and 9% in the diaphysis. Epiphyseal involvement is virtually always either secondary to direct extension from a metaphyseal primary or a metastasis; primary epiphyseal involvement is extraordinarily rare (<0.1%).[38] Although it is the most common primary bone malignancy, exclusive of myeloma, there are fewer than 1000 new cases per year within the United States.

The clinical hallmark of conventional OS is severe, unrelenting pain. Pain may be accompanied by other findings such as tenderness, localized warmth, interference with normal function, and symptoms referable to mass effect. A history of trauma is frequently associated with symptomatic onset in conventional OS. However, there is no causal relationship between trauma and conventional OS; the pain merely brings attention to a preexistent lesion.[1-4]

Radiographically, conventional OS presents as a highly aggressive and destructive lesion with a diverse range of roentgenographic findings. Conventional OS may be purely radiopaque, extending into soft tissue and having an overall "sunburst" appearance, or it may be purely radiolucent. However, most cases are a mixture of radiopacity and radiolucency with cortical destruction and extension into soft tissue. There may be periosteal reactive bone formation and periosteal elevation (Codman's triangle). There are no specific radiographic features that are themselves prognostically significant.[39]

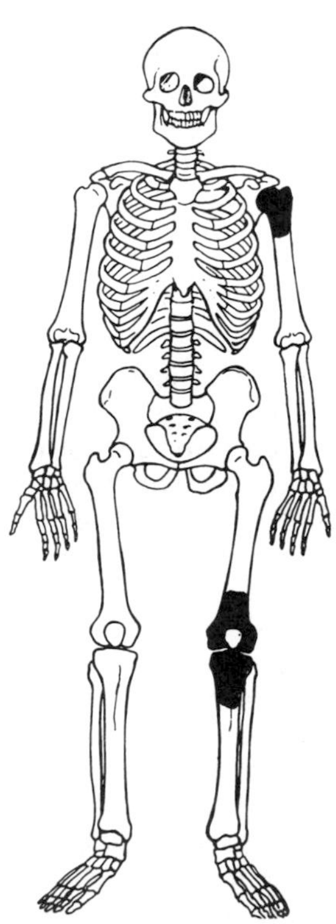

Fig. 73-7 Conventional osteosarcoma. Skeletal distribution of most common locations of this tumor.

CT[40,41] and MRI[42,43] provide two complementary ways of analyzing this type of sarcoma. CT provides detailed information regarding the interaction between mineralized structures, tumor, normal cortex, cancellous bone, and reactive bone. In contrast, MRI provides detailed information regarding interaction between interface or nonmineralized structures and thereby allows precise and quantitative estimation of extent of disease. T_1-weighted images, in which the tumor has a dark signal compared with normal fatty marrow, provide detailed information regarding the extent of medullary cavity involvement by the tumor. T_2-weighted images, in which the tumor has a bright signal and the interface between tumor and normal structures has a dark signal, provide detailed information regarding extension of the tumor outside the confines of the bone and its precise relationship with overlying soft-tissue structures.

Additional tests provide additional information. Radionuclide scintigraphy ("bone scan") utilizes an isotope that has an affinity for areas of bone metabolism.[44] It can identify the primary tumor, areas of tumor within the involved bone that are discontinuous with the primary tumor ("skip metastases"), and metastases. Skeletal survey is used to examine all bones within the body for the presence of disease and establish a base line for the future. A CT of the chest provides information regarding the status of the lungs.

Arteriographically, conventional OS is a hypervascular lesion. Response to preoperative chemotherapy corresponds to an involution of such neovascularity.[45]

Although radiographic examination is almost diagnostic in most cases, a biopsy is mandatory. It is recommended that the surgeon involved in the procedure be part of the management team. An inappropriately placed incision may determine radical surgical management for an otherwise salvageable extremity. At The University of Texas M.D. Anderson Cancer Center, needle biopsies are the diagnostic procedure of choice for any bone tumors.[46,47] These are done by an interventional radiologist under fluoroscopic guidance. A cytopathologist and a cytotechnician are always available to make smears and make sure the specimen is adequate. If the biopsy and smears are not adequate or if there is any question in regard to the diagnosis, an open biopsy is done.[46-48]

PATHOLOGY. The gross appearance of conventional OS is highly variable and dependent on the relative contribution of various tissue constituents. When osteoid and bone are the predominant finding, the lesions tend to be dense, granular, and sclerotic and may vary from yellow-brown to ivory-white (Fig. 73-8). If there is a significant amount of cartilage, the tumor may have an overall gray-blue, lobulated chondroid appearance. If little matrix is present, the tumors tend to be gray-tan; hemorrhage may occur and impart additional features.[1-4]

Microscopically, the production of osteoid or bone by malignant cells, even if only in small amounts, constitutes the single diagnostic criterion of conventional OS (Fig. 73-9). Osseous matrix may be the dominant histologic finding, or it may be present in only small amounts. In addition, other matrix forms may also be present, such as cartilage or fibrous tissue. Although unequivocal separation from nonosseous col-

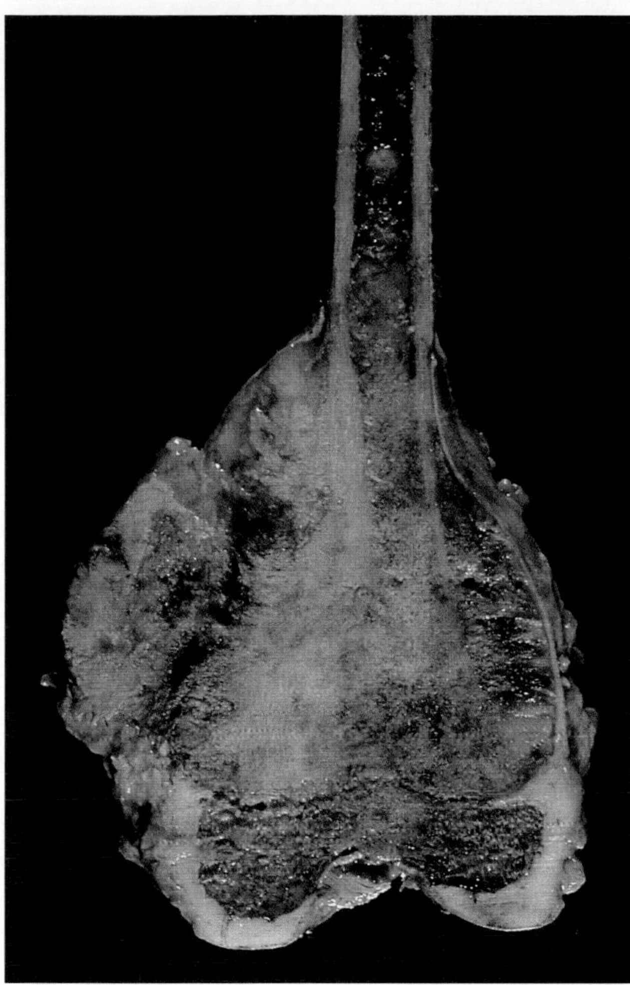

Fig. 73-8 Osteosarcoma. Distal femur shows a large mass involving the metaphysis of the bone; the tumor has destroyed the cortex, forming a large, soft-tissue component. Whitish areas represent sclerotic component of tumor. Notice a "skip" metastasis in the medullary cavity manifested as a small white nodule present in the shaft right above the tumor.

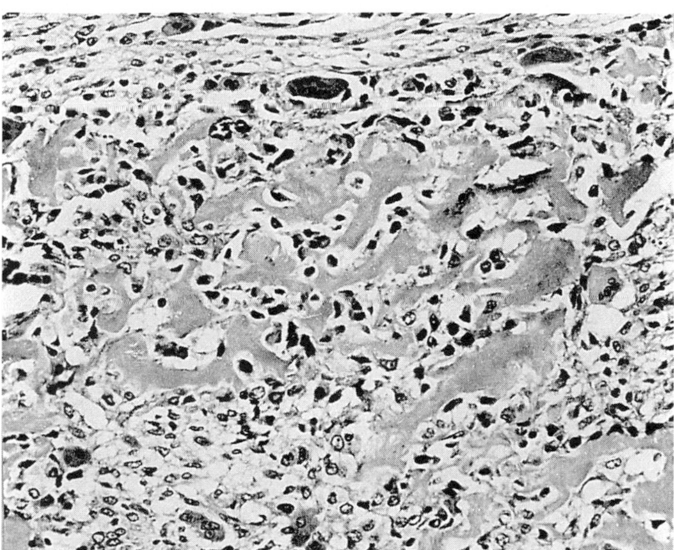

Fig. 73-9 Osteosarcoma. Notice typical lace-like osteoid formation surrounded by anaplastic cells at center. A few osteoclastic giant cells are also present.

lagen may be difficult at times, there are many features that are helpful. Osteoid is a dense, uniform, eosinophilic intercellular material. It tends to lack the delicate internal longitudinal lamellations of nonosseous collagen. Whereas nonosseous collagen tends to compress parallel to the axis of highly cellular tumors, osteoid tends to remain curvilinear as if it retains some primitive potential for lacunar formation.[1-4] Conventional OS has been traditionally divided into three cell types: osteoblastic, chondroblastic, and fibroblastic. Most tumors are a mixture of cells, but the predominance of one component would put the tumor in one of the above categories.

Since the evaluation of the specimen will reflect the results of the chemotherapy, the specimen, whether an en bloc resection or an amputation, should be handled with a uniform method of processing. The examination of the specimen should begin with the review of the last x-ray study, especially the angiogram, which will provide information as to the site in the tumor of hypervascularity; if any, the transection of the bone should be in the plane that will maximally demonstrate the suspected areas of malignancy. A slab section is then obtained and entirely cut into small sections suitable for histologic processing with each being properly labeled. These sections will provide histologic information of the tumor in a single plane. In addition, multiple random sections are also submitted from the remaining hemispheres of bone.[49]

TREATMENT AND PROGNOSIS. Regimens that employ a multidisciplinary team approach incorporating chemotherapy and surgery have become the standard treatment of conventional OS.[27-29] It must be emphasized that excellent chemotherapy must be complemented by excellent surgery. Complete surgical extirpation of the entire area involved by tumor remains the treatment of choice for control of the primary tumor.

Chemotherapy is given in both the preoperative and postoperative settings. No single chemotherapeutic agent has been found universally effective in the treatment of conventional OS; currently, the most effective agents are adriamycin, cisplatin, ifosfamide, and methotrexate.[21-29] Several parameters have been found to be of prognostic significance, including patient age, sex, site of tumor, size of tumor, duration of symptoms, and tumor classification. However, histologic evidence of response to preoperative chemotherapy is the most powerful prognostic indicator. In effect, preoperative chemotherapy provides an in vivo test of a specific agent, or combination of agents, against a specific tumor within the idiosyncratic, physiologic milieu of a specific patient. Most studies indicate that tumor necrosis ≥90% induced by preoperative chemotherapy is associated with a long-term survival of 80% to 90%, but tumor necrosis <90% is generally associated with a poorer prognosis (10% to 40%).[27,28,49,50] On an individual patient basis, response to preoperative chemotherapy is used to "tailor" postoperative chemotherapy. That is, if a good response is achieved by preoperative chemotherapy, it is assumed that the tumor is sensitive to the preoperative chemotherapy agents and they should be continued in the postoperative setting. However, if response to preoperative therapy is poor, the chemotherapy regimen must be changed in the postoperative setting.

The use of such multidisciplinary protocols has resulted in some benefits to the patient with conventional OS. Long-term, overall disease-free survival has increased from 10% to 20% to 65% to 80%.[21-29] Ablative surgery is no longer necessary in the most cases. As a result of the local effects of tumor shrinkage and consolidation, ≥90% of patients with conventional OS involving the extremities are able to undergo limb-salvage procedures without risk of decreased survival; if pulmonary metastases occur, these are frequently resected.

Surface osteosarcoma

Parosteal osteosarcoma. Parosteal OS is a form of low-grade OS arising on the surface of the bone. It occurs most frequently in young and middle-aged adults (third to fifth decades), and women are affected twice as often as men. It is almost exclusively a disease of the long bones of the appendicular skeleton, with the posterior aspect of the distal femur being by far the most frequent primary site (Fig. 73-10). The patients typically present with a long history of a slowly growing, painless mass. Radiographically, the tumor appears as a radiopaque, lobulated mass seemingly applied to the surface of the involved bone. Tumor generally grows along the surface of the bone, both linearly and longitudinally, without involvement of the medullary cavity.

PATHOLOGY. The tumor arises from the surface and generally tends to be large. Occasionally the tumor encircles the major vessels (Fig. 73-11).

Histologically, it is composed of relatively innocuous spindle-fibroblastic cells that produce well-formed lamellar bone (Fig. 73-12). A cartilaginous cap may be present.

Open or needle biopsies are discouraged because the findings may be confusing. Since management depends on the clinical presentation, it is preferable to do an en bloc excision when feasible. An amputation is reserved for large tumors that involve nerves or large vessels.

When the initial diagnosis and treatment are appropriate, long-term survival in excess of 90% can be expected. Intralesional subtotal resection is absolutely contraindicated, as it is associated with a 100% local relapse rate that may be accompanied by a change in histologic features and a considerable worsening of prognosis.

A variant of parosteal OS is dedifferentiated parosteal OS.[51] It is a tumor that shows the typical clinical and radiologic features of parosteal OS, including the innocuous histologic morphology, but contains a high-grade sarcoma (osteosarcoma, malignant fibrous histiocytoma, or an unclassified high-grade sarcoma). It is more commonly seen in young and middle-aged adults between the third and fifth decades of life, and women are affected more frequently than men. Like parosteal OS, it affects commonly the posterior distal femur and radiologically shows a large blastic lesion seated on the surface of the bone. In addition there are large areas of lucency that on arteriograms

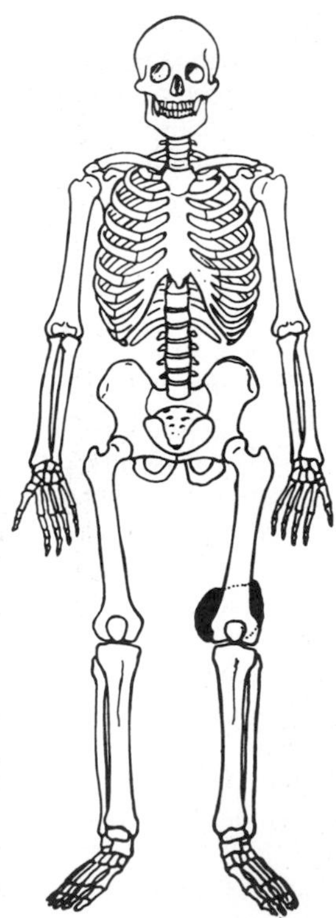

Fig. 73-10 Parosteal osteosarcoma. The surface of the posterior aspect of the femur is by far the most common location of this tumor.

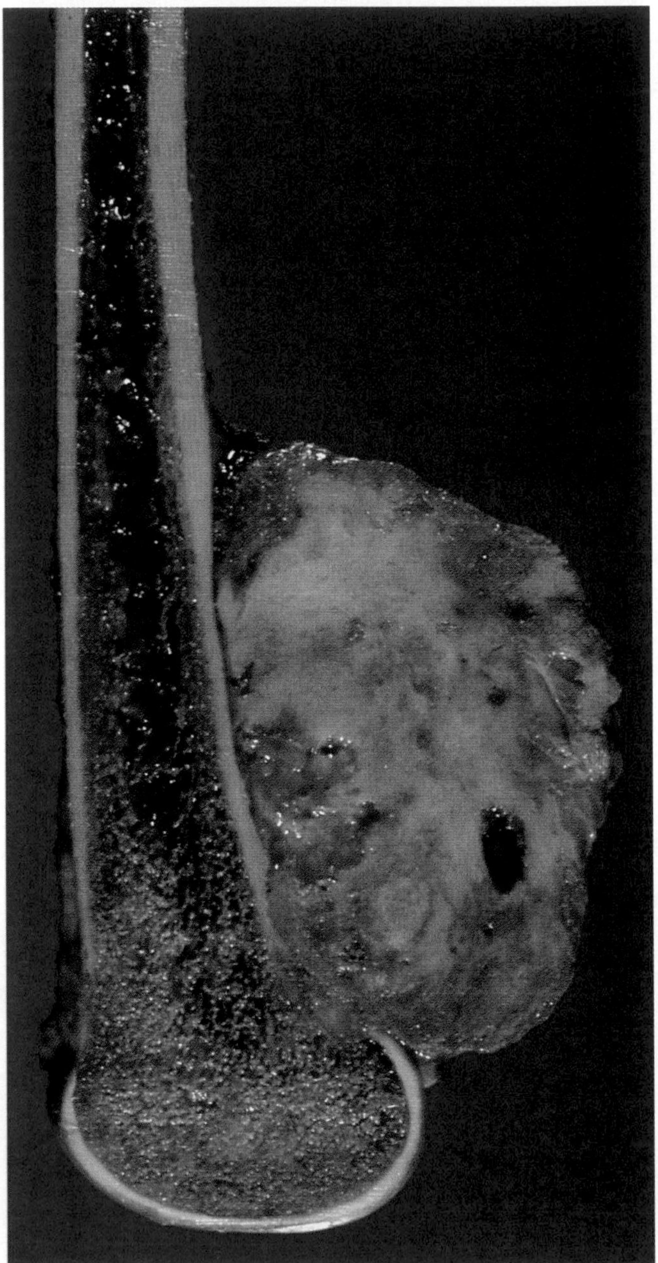

Fig. 73-11 Longitudinal section of femur showing a surface tumor in posterior distal end of femur typical of parosteal osteosarcoma.

are hypervascular.[52,53] It is important to recognize this type of OS because it requires aggressive therapy.

Periosteal osteosarcoma. Periosteal OS is characterized by the presence of cartilage as the predominant histologic component.[54,55] Because of this predominance, this type of surface OS was initially referred to as a "juxtacortical chondrosarcoma."[56] This lesion occurs in the second and third decades of life, and men are affected more frequently than women. Unlike parosteal OS, periosteal OS affects the diaphysis or metadiaphysis of the long bones, especially the femur and the tibia[1-4,54,55] (Fig. 73-13). Radiologically, it may involve part of the surface or, like parosteal OS, the entire circumference of the tubular bone. A spiculated-sunburst appearance is commonly found.[57]

PATHOLOGY. Grossly this lesion arises from the diaphysis or metadiaphysis of the long bone; it has a broad base with fusiform elevation of the periosteum. (Fig. 73-14). Microscopically, it shows a high grade chondroblastic osteosarcoma.

PROGNOSIS. The survival for this sarcoma treated surgically is approximately 50% at 5 years.

High-grade osteosarcoma on the surface. High-grade OS is the least common of the surface OSs.[58] It occurs most frequently in the second and third decades of life, and men are more frequently affected than women.[1-4] The femur is the most commonly affected bone. Histologically it contains a high-grade OS, usually an osteoblastic OS. Aggressive chemotherapy is required because it has the same biologic behavior as conventional OS.

Special types of osteosarcoma

Intracortical osteosarcoma. Rarely an OS may arise in the cortex of bone. The histologic features are similar to those of a conventional OS.[1-4,59-61]

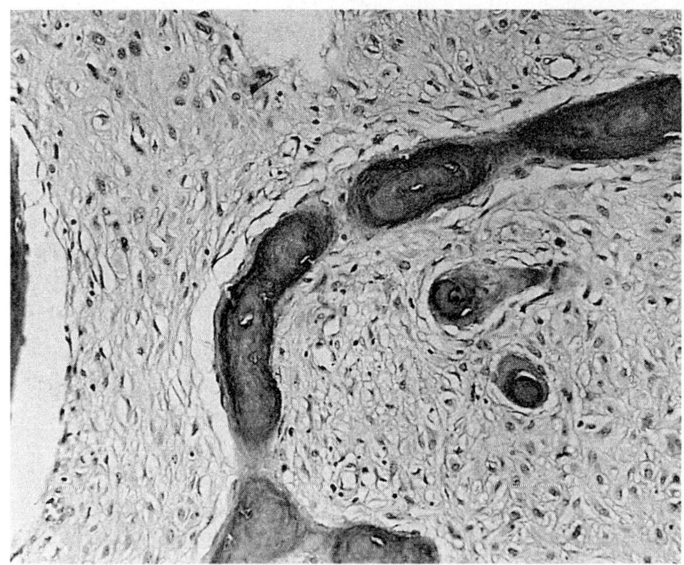

Fig. 73-12 Microscopically, parosteal osteosarcoma shows mature bony spicules and a bland fibroblastic stroma.

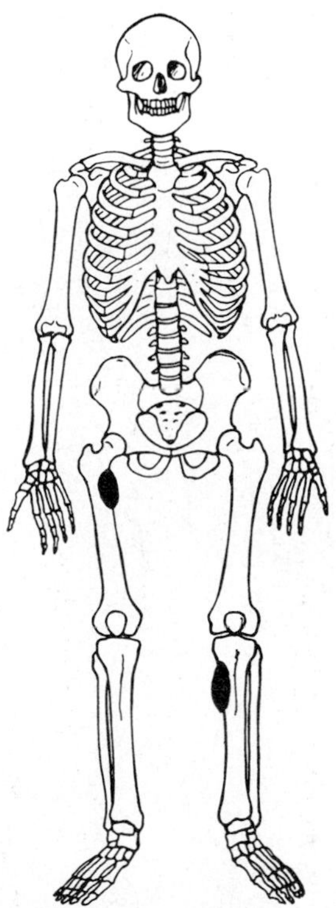

Fig 73-13 Periosteal osteosarcoma. The surface of the diaphysis of the femur and the proximal metaphysis of the tibia are the most common locations of this tumor.

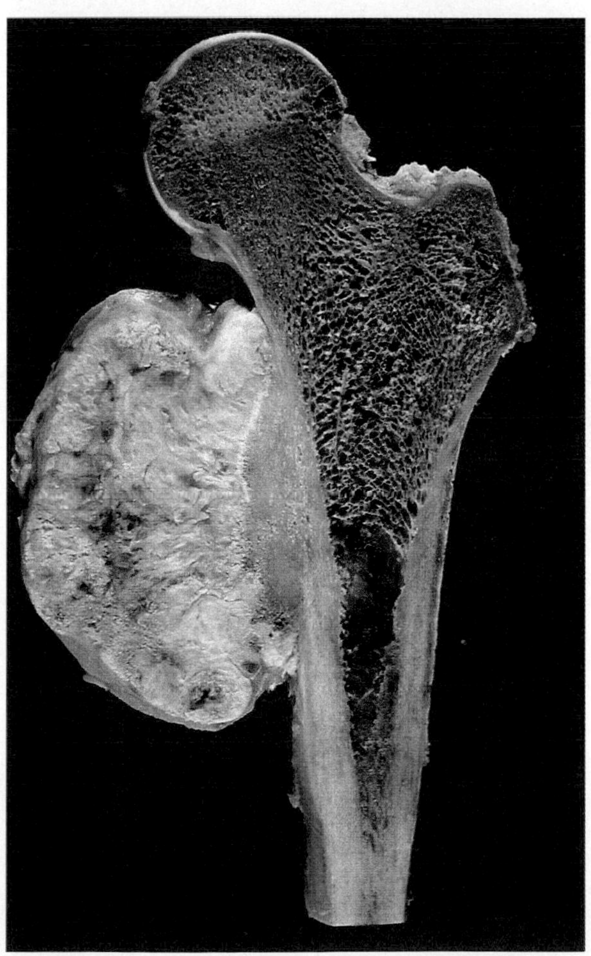

Fig. 73-14 Periosteal osteosarcoma. A surface lesion arises from the shaft of the femur. Medullary cavity is intact.

Intraosseous well-differentiated osteosarcoma. Intraosseous well-differentiated OS (IOWDOS) is extremely rare. It affects women more commonly than men, and the mean age is in the third decade. The tumor has a strong predilection for the long bones of the extremities, especially the metaphysis, but may occur in the diaphysis. Radiologically the lesion shows nondistinctive features often simulating fibrous dysplasia or desmoplastic fibroma.

PATHOLOGY. Grossly the lesion shows a mixed blastic and lytic pattern and is often confined within the medullary cavity in the bone. However, the older lesion frequently extends beyond the cortex (Fig. 73-15). Histologically, IOWDOS shares the innocuous histologic features and the low-grade behavior of its surface counterpart, the parosteal osteosarcoma (Fig. 73-16). En bloc resection is the therapy of choice.[1-4,62,63] This type may also undergo dedifferentiation.

Telangiectatic osteosarcoma. Telangiectatic OS has the same clinical features as conventional OS but differs from conventional OS in three ways: (1) it is cystic and thus radiologically appears as a purely lytic lesion (Fig. 73-17), (2) grossly the lesion simulates an aneurysmal bone cyst (Fig. 73-18), and (3) histologically it has a complex vascular pattern with a high-grade morphology and little uncalcified or focally calcified osteoid (Fig. 73-19). Recognition of this variant is important because if treated with surgery alone, most patients

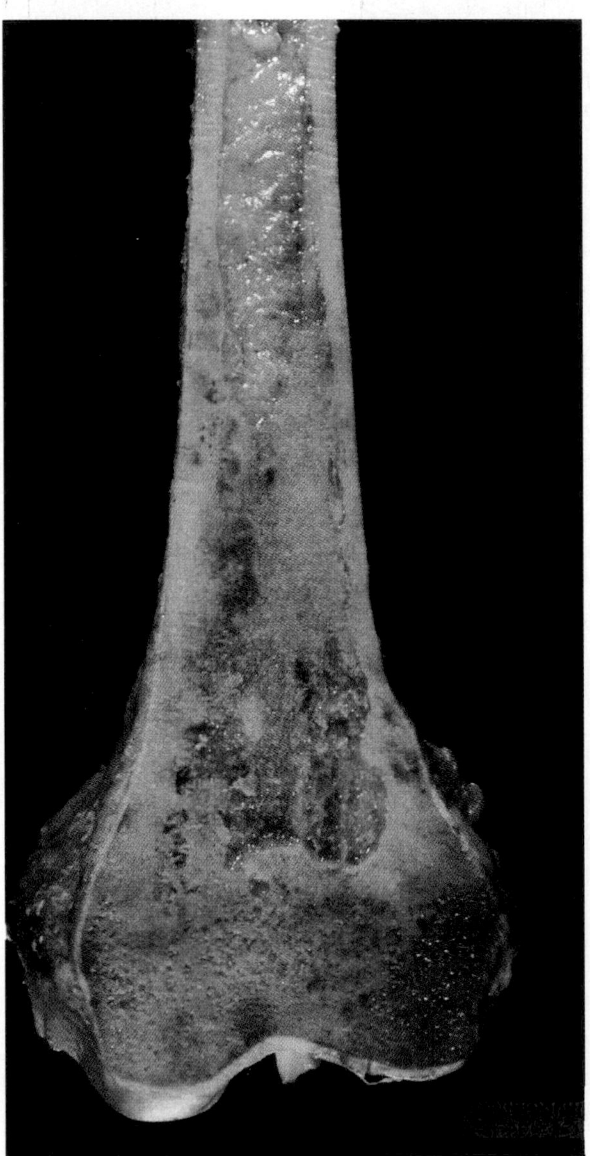

Fig. 73-15 Gross specimen of intraosseous well-differentiated osteosarcoma (IOWDOS) of distal femur..

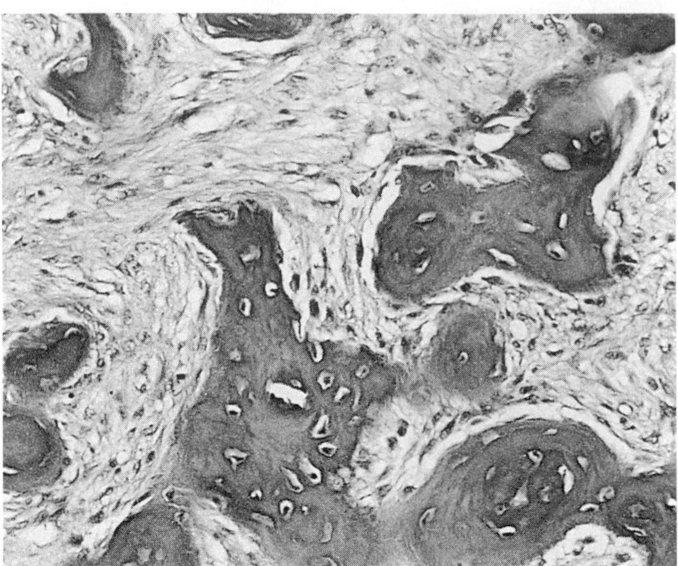

Fig. 73-16 Microscopically, intraosseous well-differentiated osteosarcoma shows numerous mature bone spicules associated with an innocuous fibrous proliferation that contains rare mitoses.

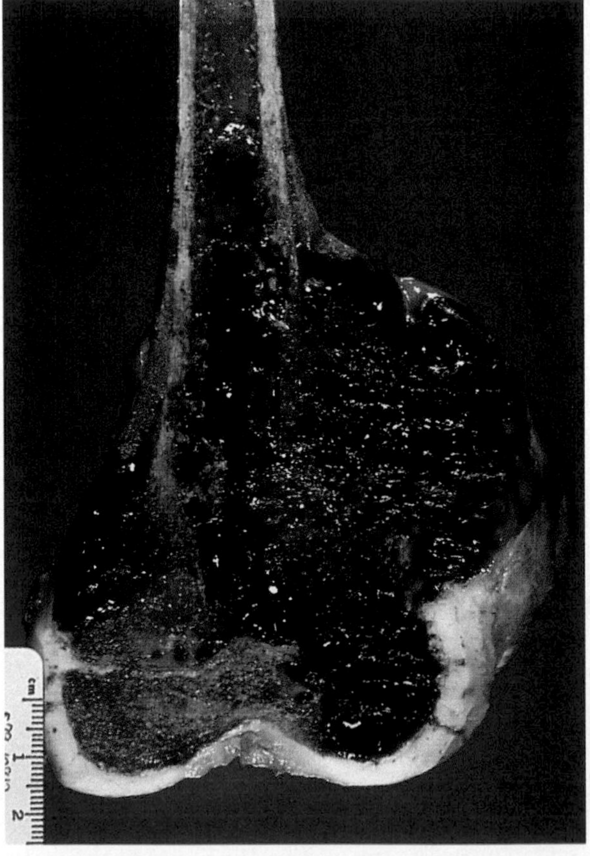

Fig. 73-17 Telangiectatic osteosarcoma. Grossly a large hemorrhagic mass occupies the distal epimetaphysis of the femur extending beyond the cortex of the bone.

die, but if treated with combined surgery and chemotherapy, the survival may be excellent.[1-4,64]

Small cell osteosarcoma. The incidence of small cell osteosarcoma (SCO) varies from 1.1% to 4.0%[65-67] and affects predominantly people in the second decade of life. As in conventional OS, the metaphyses of the long bones are affected. Histologically the tumor is made up of small cells that generally resemble those of Ewing's sarcoma, but the tumor cells may be spindle shaped or may simulate the cells of large cell lymphoma. The majority of the cases show clear-cut osteoid production, which is the sine qua non finding for the diagnosis. There are no specific cell markers for SCO. The value of immunohistochemistry resides in the utilization of leukocyte-common antigen, S-100 protein, and HBA-71 (Ewing's sarcoma marker), which do not occur in this tumor, but if they do occur, they help to identify other small cell tumors of bone such as lymphoma, mesenchymal chondrosarcoma, and Ewing's sarcoma.[68] The prognosis of this type of OS seems to be the same as or slightly worse than that of conventional OS.[67]

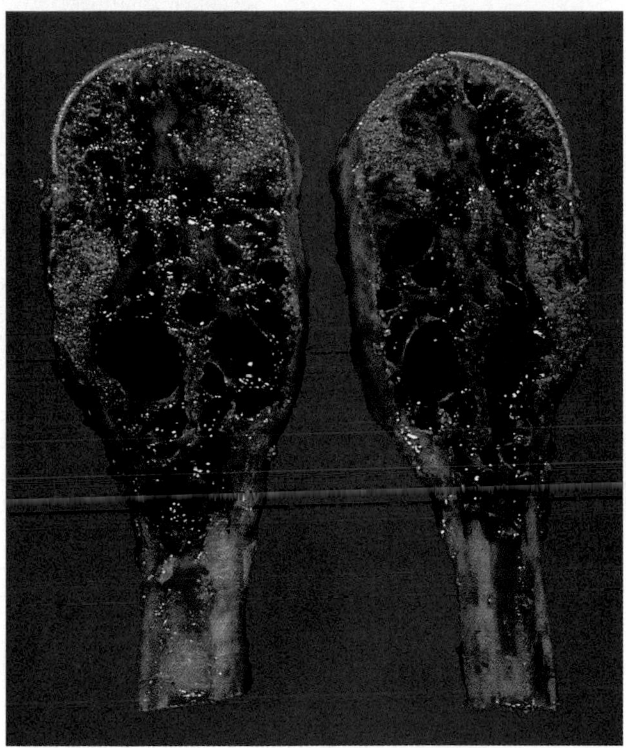

Fig. 73-18 En bloc resection shows multiple cystic areas involving the proximal metaphysis of the bone. This is a postchemotherapy specimen.

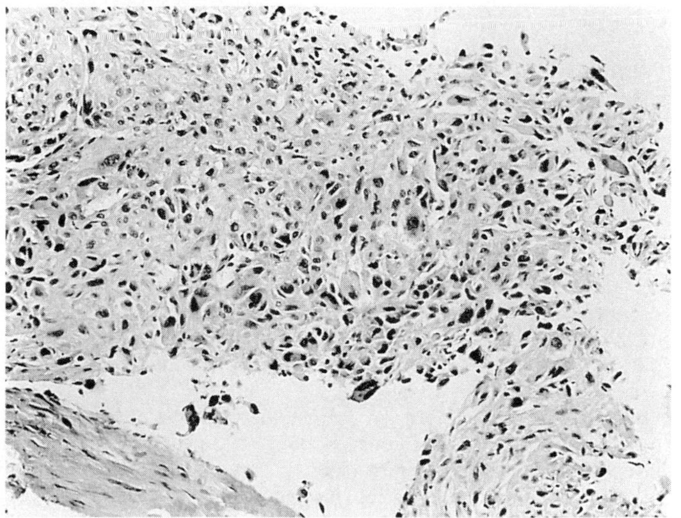

Fig. 73-19 Anaplastic features of telangiectatic osteosarcoma.

Other variants of osteosarcoma. Multicentric OS is a rare presentation. Generally, several bones are involved but without evidence of disease in the lung.[1-4,69]

Other cell types of OS have been mentioned in the literature, including the malignant fibrous histiocytoma type,[70] and the epithelioid types of OSs.[71,72]

OS of the jaw bones occurs most commonly in the third and fourth decade of life and shows a slight predilection for males.[1-4,73] The most common site of involvement is the body of the mandible and the infrastructure of the maxilla.[73] The chondroblastic histologic type is the most commonly seen.[73] The treatment of choice for mandibular OS is radical surgery.[73] Unfortunately, postoperative adjuvant chemotherapy has not shown a significant influence on the survival of these patients.[73] The prognosis for mandibular OS has been reported to be better than that for OS of the maxilla, but in the series of Goepfert and colleagues, the survival rate was similar.[73] Systemic metastases occur in about 35% of cases.[73]

Secondary osteosarcoma. OS may develop on benign neoplastic and nonneoplastic lesions of bone. The most common of these lesions include Paget's disease, fibrous dysplasia, bone infarction, and chronic osteomyelitis. Postradiation OS has also been reported.

OS arising in Paget's disease is a well-recognized entity. Late in the course of Paget's disease of bone a sarcomatous transformation may occur. The patients are usually in the seventh decade of life, and any bone affected with Paget's disease may be the seat of the malignant transformation: the most commonly affected bones are the femur, humerus, and pelvis. OS is the most common neoplasm developing in Paget's disease, but a spindle cell sarcoma or rarely a chondrosarcoma may also occur. When the radiologic features of Paget's disease change by becoming more exuberant, a sarcomatous transformation should be suspected. The survival is worse than the historic survival of patients with conventional OS.[1-4,34,35]

The incidence of sarcomatous transformation in fibrous dysplasia is about 1%. The sarcoma is either an osteosarcoma or a fibrosarcoma. Since bone infarcts are rare, only a relatively few cases of sarcomatous transformation have been reported; although osteosarcoma occurs, malignant fibrous histiocytoma is the more likely tumor to develop on a bone infarction.

Chronic osteomyelitis may also transform into a malignancy. Squamous carcinoma is the usual type of malignancy, but osteosarcoma may also develop.

The incidence of postradiation sarcomas varies from 3.6% to 5.5%.[1-4] To be considered as a postradiation sarcoma the tumor should develop within the irradiated field and an interval of at least 3.5 years should have occurred between the time of irradiation and the development of the sarcoma. The amount of irradiation is usually in the neighborhood of 5000 rad though some cases have been reported to occur with less radiation. The prognosis for these patients is extremely poor, with a 5-year survival rate of approximately 20%.

CARTILAGE-FORMING TUMORS

The most troublesome lesions to interpret are the tumors of cartilaginous origin. Some are strictly benign (such as osteochondroma, enchondroma, periosteal chondroma, chondroblastoma), some are locally aggressive (such as chondromyxoid fibroma of bone), and some are highly malignant (such as high-grade chondrosarcoma, dedifferentiated chondrosarcoma). But the borderline cartilaginous lesions (those with low-grade malignant potential) are the ones that cause diagnostic and therapeutic difficulties for the interpreting pathologist and the clinician.

Benign

Osteochondroma

Osteochondroma is the most common benign cartilaginous tumor of the bone.[1,74] It arises from the cortex of the bone, and it owes its name to growing out by enchondral proliferation. In the Mayo Clinic's experience, it constitutes 35.8% of all benign bone tumors.[1]

Most of these lesions develop in children and adolescents, and their tumors grow in similar fashion as the growth plates do, including ceasing growth when the epiphyses close.[1,74] There is a slight male predominance of osteochondroma patients, about 1.5 males per 1 female. These lesions are usually asymptomatic, but symptoms can occur as a result of fractures or complications of tumor growth, such as impingement of nerves and vessels.

The most frequent site of occurrence is the metaphysis of the long bones, and these lesions typically tend to grow away from the nearest joint (Fig. 73-20).

The theory to explain the pathogenesis of osteochondroma goes as far back as 1891, when Virchow postulated that osteochondroma arises from a displaced epiphyseal plate.[75] D'ambrosia and Ferguson have produced experimental osteochondromas in rabbits by placing fragments of epiphyseal plate cartilage in the cortex of the metaphysis, supporting Virchow's theory.[76]

Radiographically osteochondromas arise from the metaphysis of the long bone and grow toward the opposite direction of the nearest joint. The lesions project from the cortical surface and have a small to broad stalk. The cortex and medullary cavity of the long bone are continuous with the body of the osteochondroma, a feature that is diagnostic of this process.

PATHOLOGY. Grossly these lesions arise from the cortex of the bone and may be sessile or pedunculated. A cartilaginous cap is present and may be up to 3 cm in thickness (Fig. 73-21). Histologically the cartilaginous cap is cellular in young patients but becomes attenuated and may disappear in older patients. The cap is similar in morphology to the epiphyseal growth plate, exhibiting actively growing chondrocytes arranged in parallel columns. As the cartilaginous cap grows, the cortex of the bone is pulled carrying the cancellous bone with its medullary contents, a feature that can be seen in radiographic examination.

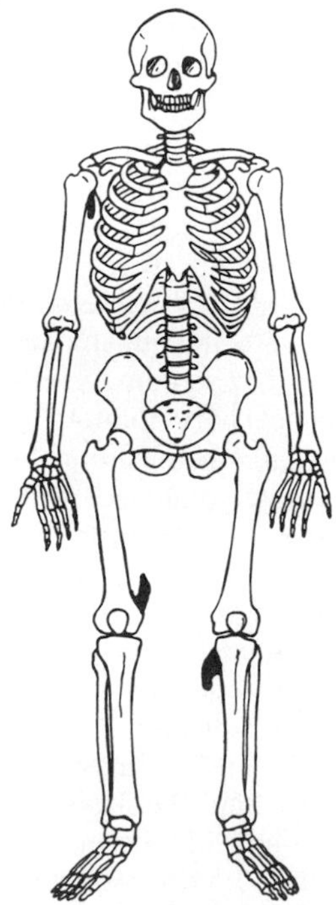

Fig. 73-20 Osteochondroma. Most common anatomic locations for this tumor.

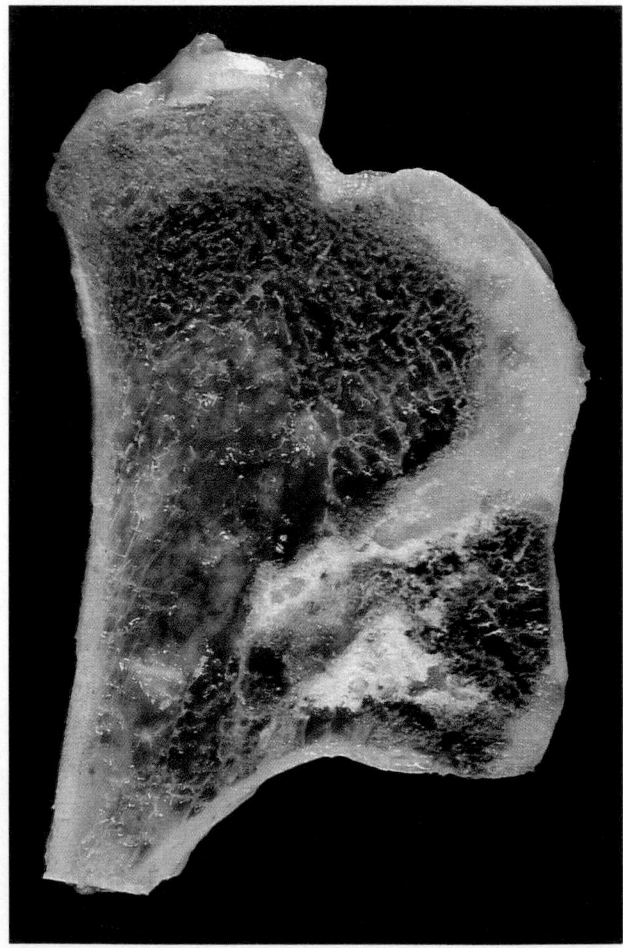

Fig. 73-21 Gross specimen of an osteochondroma. Proximal fibula shows a broad-based osteochondroma. Cancellous bone forms the body of the lesion. Whitish band of tissue covering the body of the mass is the cartilaginous cap. Notice that the cortex is continuous with the lesion.

An osteochondroma is not resected unless there is a fracture or the lesion compresses adjacent organs or continues to grow after puberty. Sarcomatous transformation in osteochondroma has been reported[77] but is extremely rare when one considers the common occurrence of osteochondroma. However, sarcomatous transformation does occur in patients bearing multiple osteochondromatosis.

In addition to the typical osteochondroma, there are a few other benign cartilaginous lesions that merit mention. Subungual exostoses[78,79] typically arise in the distal parts of the phalanges and are usually associated with trauma, and so they are often referred to as "traumatic osteochondromas." Unlike the typical osteochondroma, these lesions are histologically more proliferative; the advancing edge is generally a proliferating osteocartilaginous element, sometimes with a fibrous complex that often shows mitoses and high cellularity, raising the question of malignancy.

A rare lesion is the "bizarre parosteal osteochondromatous proliferation of the hands and feet."[80,81] This lesion arises in the proximal aspect of the phalanges, and the cartilaginous component may be very cellular, simulating a chondrosarcoma. The clues for diagnosis of these lesions are the characteristic location and the radiographic appearance.

Enchondroma

Although the term *enchondroma* has been applied to lesions occurring in both the large long bones and small bones, it is preferred to categorize these lesions separately based on the locations, since they are biologically different; the former are discussed in the section on chondrosarcoma.

Enchondromas of the small bones of the hand and foot are rare benign lesions that frequently occur in adults. They may be solitary or multiple. When multiple and unilateral, they are referred to as *Ollier's disease*. If multiple and associated with angiomas of the soft tissues, they are termed *Maffucci's syndrome*.

Solitary enchondroma is the most common of all tumors occurring in the short tubular bones of the hands. In order of frequency, the most common sites are the phalanges of the fingers, metacarpal bones, phalanges of the toe, and metatarsal bones.[82]

These tumors arise from the medullary cavity, usually the metaphyseal region of the bone, and often extend the length of the bone, expanding it and inducing cortical thinning. Although most enchondromas are initially asymptomatic, pain or swelling develops eventually.

Radiographically a well-demonstrated, usually expansile radiolucent medullary cavity lesion with stippled calcifications is seen; the endosteum may be scalloped, and if the lesion is left untreated, it may break through the cortex.

PATHOLOGY. Histologically, these lesions consist of hyaline cartilage. Innocuous lesions show poorly cellular areas with chondrocytes containing small, dark nuclei. Often the lesions are cellular, exhibiting numerous binucleated chondrocytes with nuclei that are larger than a mature lymphocyte; the nuclei show a fine chromatin pattern and small nucleoli may be seen. Despite this appearance, the lesions do not metastasize.

TREATMENT AND PROGNOSIS. The treatment of choice for enchondromas is curettage and bone packing. Although the incidence of recurrence is high, conservative management is preferred even after the lesion recurs.

Periosteal chondroma

Periosteal chondroma is a benign, slow-growing, cartilaginous lesion that arises from the surface of a bone under the periosteum.[3] Like the enchondromas of the hands and feet, its histologic features can be alarming, yet its behavior is benign. There have been 165 cases reported in the literature[83] and according to Mirra and colleagues,[3] periosteal chondroma accounts for 0.5% of the biopsy specimens analyzed for primary bone tumors.

Of 165 cases reported, 94 patients were male and 57 were female; in the remainder, no sex was indicated.[83] The peak incidence is in the second and third decades of life, but this lesion has been reported in the seventh and eighth decades of life.[83,84]

The most common location of periosteal chondroma is the metaphyseal region of a long tubular bone. The upper end of the humerus, phalanges of the hand, distal femur, proximal tibia, and proximal femur, in descending order, are the most common sites of occurrence for this lesion.[2,3]

Radiologically, most of the lesions appear small (1 to 3 cm). Typically, a lesion is seen on the surface of a bone, inducing a saucer-shaped appearance with a dense rim of reactive bone tissue. The lesion usually protrudes into the soft tissue, but it is well delimited by the periosteum, which may form a thin eggshell ossification around it. In addition, most tumors contain matrix calcification shaped in the form of ringlets or popcorn.[83-85] On x-rays films this appearance is diagnostic of a periosteal chondroma.

PATHOLOGY. Grossly, these lesions show typical lobulated cartilage, which on the cortical surface is surrounded by a rim of bone. The periphery is usually covered by periosteum, which may be calcified. Histologically, the lesions may appear as innocuous proliferations of hyaline cartilage containing relatively few cells with small, dark pyknotic nuclei, but the lesions are also commonly cellular with binucleated cells and nuclei with a fine chromatin pattern. This histologic pattern is similar to that of a low-grade chondrosarcoma (Fig. 73-22), but periosteal chondroma is not a malignant tumor. Therefore, radiologic correlation is of utmost importance in the histologic interpretation of this lesion.

The differential diagnosis includes periosteal (juxtacortical) chondrosarcoma and periosteal osteosarcoma. The latter is easy to rule out, since it shows histologically a high-grade chondroblastic osteosarcoma. Periosteal chondrosarcoma is much more difficult to rule out, but large-size, infiltrative borders and high nuclear grade should be helpful in making a correct diagnosis.[86]

TREATMENT AND PROGNOSIS. Curettage or en bloc resection (marginal or intralesional excision) is the therapy of choice for periosteal chondroma.[83,84] A 3.5% recurrence rate has been reported for this lesion.[83]

Chondromyxoid fibroma of bone

Chondromyxoid fibroma (CMF) of bone is a peculiar, rare, locally aggressive but benign tumor of bone. It accounts for less than 0.5% of benign bone tumors.[1]

CMF of bone occurs in a wide range of ages, from 4 to 70 years,[87] but it is more commonly seen in the second and third decades of life; Gherlinzoni and colleagues[88] noted a second peak of incidence in the seventh decade of life, and Zillmer and Dorfman[87] noted a second peak in the sixth decade. The male-to-female ratio of incidence was reported in one series as 1:1[87] and in another as almost 2:1.[1]

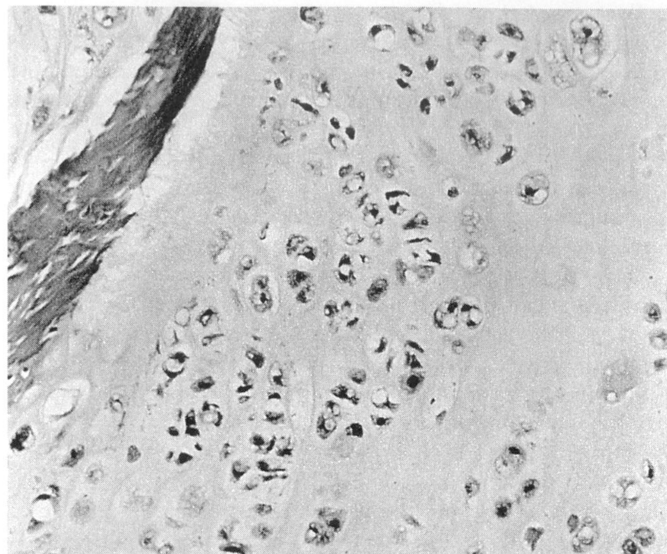

Fig. 73-22 Microscopically, periosteal chondroma consists of a cellular hyaline cartilage proliferation with large atypical nuclei.

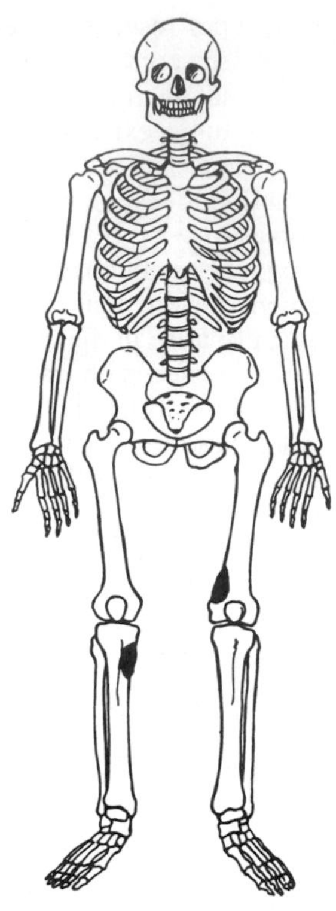

Fig. 73-23 Chondromyxoid fibroma of bone. Most common anatomic locations of this lesion.

In the series of Zillmer and Dorfman,[87] 42% of CMF cases were found in the long bones, 25% in the flat bones, 20% in the small tubular bones, 8% in the vertebrae, and 5% in the ribs.

The most common site of involvement for this tumor is the metaphyseal region of a long tubular bone, with the proximal tibia and the distal end of the femur being the most commonly affected bones[87,89] (Fig. 73-23). In a review of the literature by Wilson and colleagues,[89] of 356 cases reported, 126 were located in the tibia, 50 in the femur, 28 in the fibula, 26 in the ilium, 61 in the foot (26 in the metatarsal bone, 21 in the tarsal, and 14 in the phalanges), and 65 in other sites.

Localized pain with or without tenderness is the usual presenting symptom in the majority of patients (86% in one series[87]), but swelling may be seen in cases in which the bone lesion is in contact with the skin. The duration of symptoms varies from a few days to 20 years.[87]

Radiographically the lesion is an eccentric radiolucent area surrounded by a sclerotic rim of dense bone, imparting a geographic appearance.[89-92] A CMF is commonly localized in the metaphysis and often has cortical expansion; the cortex is often destroyed. However, the lesion is generally well delimited by the periosteum. In the small tubular bones a CMF is usually round, less lobulated, and more centrally located, often filling the entire medullary canal.[89] Unlike other cartilaginous tumors, matrix calcifications are rarely seen; in one series[91] 13% of CMFs showed calcification, whereas in another series calcification was found in only one of 38 cases.[89]

PATHOLOGY. Grossly this tumor has a glistening myxoid, lobulated, cartilaginoid appearance; in resected specimens, a thick sclerotic rim of dense bone is often seen (Fig. 73-24). Microscopically the tumor contains lobules of myxoid tissue surrounded by condensation of cells at the periphery of the lobulations (Fig. 73-25). The myxoid areas are poorly cellular, containing stellate, triangular-shaped, or sometimes spindle or round cells. Hyaline cartilage differentiation is not seen. In recurrent lesions the cells may develop a globoid appearance. At the periphery of the lobules there is a condensation of medium-sized cells; many of them resemble chondroblasts. Some of the cells are osteoclast-like giant cells, and others are spindle cells. Mitoses are rare. The least common component is fibrous tissue, which can be found in the periphery of the lobules. Aneurysmal bone cyst formation may be present occasionally, and microcalcifications have been reported to occur in 14%[93] and 27%[94] of cases.

Ultrastructurally, CMF contains cells with irregular cell processes, indented nuclei, and thick nuclear lamina.[93] Abundant fibrils have also been described.[94]

Determination of the cartilaginous origin is based on the histologic characteristics, including the presence of mixed chondroblastoma and CMF components, similarity of histochemical reactions to those of normal cartilage, and a positive reaction for S-100 protein, a marker that stains cartilage.[92-98]

TREATMENT AND PROGNOSIS. En bloc resection of the lesion is the management strategy of choice, but if it is not feasible, a curettage should be attempted. In the series of Gherlinzoni and associates,[88] local recurrence was seen in 27% of the cases treated by curettage; with curettage alone there was an 80% recurrence rate but when curettage was combined with corticocancellous bone grafting, the recurrence rate decreased to 7%. In Zillmer and Dorfman's series[87] the recurrence rate was 22%.

Although malignancy has been cited in the literature, most authors believe it has not been convincingly documented. Implantation in the soft tissue, though rare, has occurred.[99]

Chondroblastoma

Chondroblastoma is a well-known, albeit relatively rare, benign cartilaginous tumor that has typical clinicopathologic features. It accounts for approximately 1% of the benign tumors of bone.[1,74]

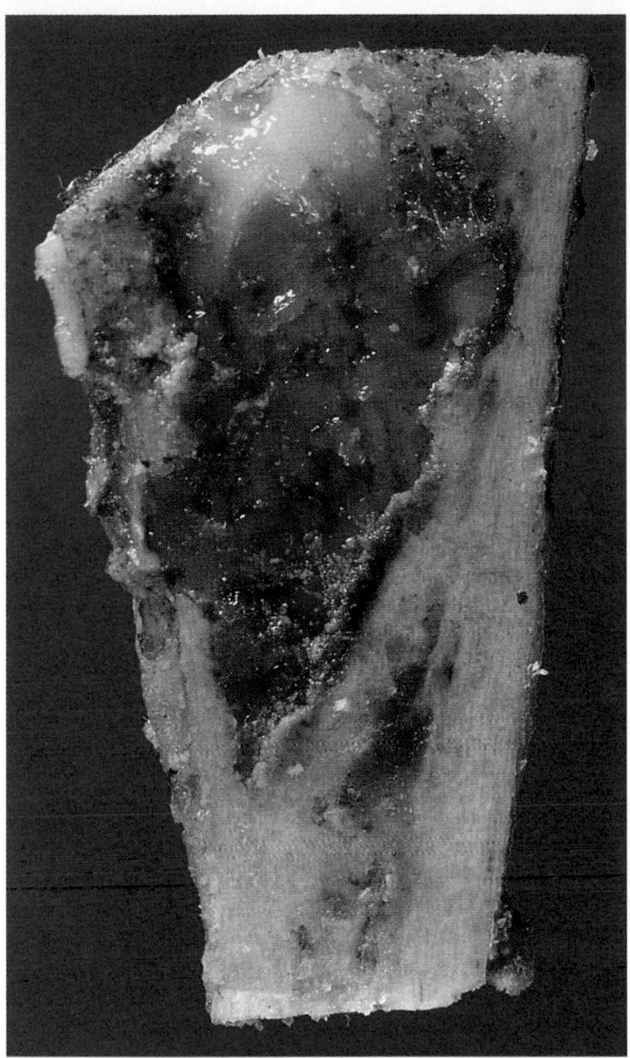

Fig. 73-24 Chondromyxoid fibroma specimen shows a thick sclerotic rim of bone and a central lobulated cartilaginous lesion.

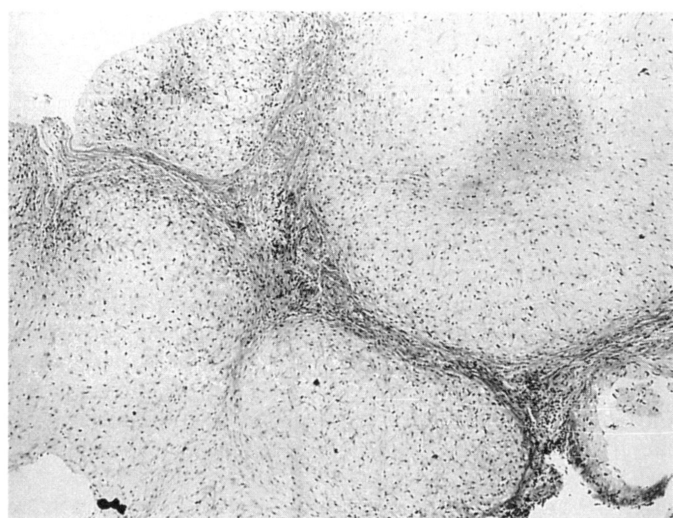

Fig. 73-25 Myxoid cartilaginous tumor consists of lobules separated by fibrous septa.

Although chondroblastoma can occur in most decades of life, it is most common in the second decade.[1,3,74] It is slightly more common in males than in females,[1] and pain is a constant symptom of this lesion. In the series of the Rizzoli Orthopedic Institute,[100] and from the Netherlands[101] 83% and 95%, respectively, of the patients complained of pain. The pain is attributable to irritation of the synovial membrane and may appear before classic radiologic features are established. Effusion of a joint may also be present.

Chondroblastoma affects the epiphyses of the long bones, and as it grows, it extends into the metaphysis. Any apophysis may also be a site of origin, and the greater trochanter is not an uncommon site. Metaphyseal origin is distinctly rare but has been reported.[102]

The most common sites for the occurrence of this tumor are the distal end of the femur, the proximal end of the humerus, the tibia, and other areas of the femur[1-4,100,101,103] (Fig. 73-26). Other not uncommon locations include the innominate bone and the talus.

Radiographically, the lesion is eccentric in 75% of cases[101] and may be located in the epiphysis only or may have traversed the growth plate (50% of cases).[100] Chondroblastoma has a geographic pattern of bone destruction with a sclerotic rim of dense bone tissue at the periphery of the lesion, a sign that indicates chronicity or a long history in any benign bone lesion. The central aspect of the lesion may be lytic or may contain calcified matrix, which appears as ringlets or "popcorn" formations typical of any cartilage lesion. Cortical changes present in most cases manifest as endosteal erosion, local destruction of the cortex, or formation of new cortex by the periosteum.[101] Minor pathologic fractures may occur.

PATHOLOGY. Grossly these lesions consist of reddish brown hemorrhagic tissue, possibly with small calcifications that impart a gritty consistency. Histologically there are several characteristic components of this lesion: (1) chondroblasts, (2) islands of cartilage, (3) giant cells, and (4) calcifications (Fig. 73-27). The chondroblasts are polygonal or round cells containing an indented or grooved nucleus without a nucleolus and abundant light tan-pink cytoplasm. These cells stain with the S-100 protein.[104-106] Mitotic figures are seen in 77% of the chondroblastomas, ranging from 1 to 3 per 10 high-power fields.[107] Nuclear atypia and focal necrosis may be found, but these changes alone do not imply malignancy.[107]

The cartilage is usually found as small islands of tissue haphazardly arranged within the chondroblasts and is present in 95% of the tumors.[107] It is not typical hyaline cartilage but appears as ill-defined amorphous pink tissues that often resemble osteoid formation. Mirra and associates[3] have referred to it as "chondroid" because of its appearance, richness in collagen, and depletion of proteoglycans. Giant cells are of the osteoclastic type, and their number varies from case to case; some tumors have a few giant cells, and others have many. Historically, Codman described chondroblastoma as an epiphyseal chondromatous giant cell tumor of the proximal humerus.[108] Calcifications are of two types: small, irregular, ill-defined calcifications and those of the "chicken-wire" type. The latter are lacelike calcifications that are deposited at the periphery of the chondroblasts and impart a honeycomb appearance. Ossification is present in 5% of the chondroblastomas and rarely is so extensive that the tumor simulates an osteoblastoma.[107]

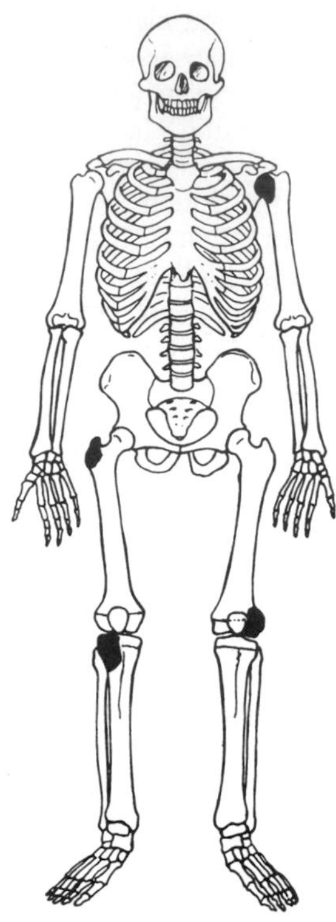

Fig. 73-26 Chondroblastoma. Skeletal distribution of the most common locations of this tumor. The epiphysis of distal end of femur, proximal end of tibia, and proximal end of humerus are the most common locations for this tumor. Chondroblastoma may also arise in an apophysis, such as the greater trochanter.

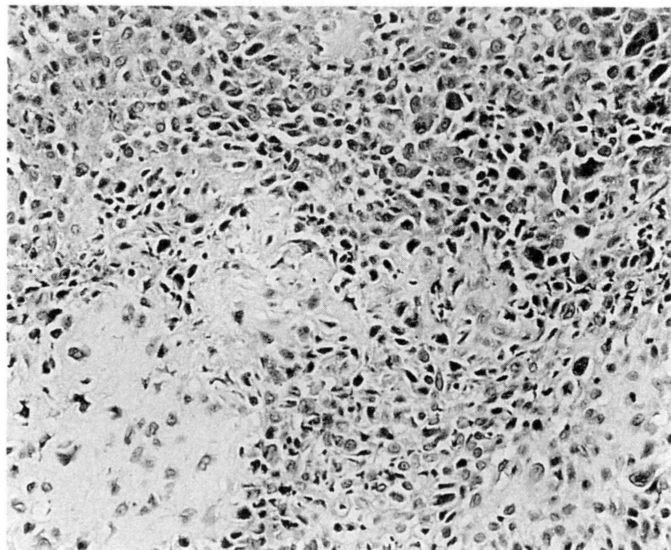

Fig. 73-27 Chondroblastoma consists of cartilage in the right and left lower corners, scattered giant cells, and numerous chondroblasts in the center.

A secondary phenomenon is the presence of an aneurysmal bone cyst component; it can be microscopic or can be grossly visible. Although in one study the presence of aneurysmal bone cysts was associated with a higher number of recurrences,[107] other studies have not confirmed this implication.[100,101]

Chondroblastoma can be easily diagnosed on fine-needle aspiration (FNA). Fanning and colleagues[109] reported 12 patients so diagnosed. On FNA there are three major components: mononuclear cells (chondroblasts), multinucleated osteoclast-like giant cells, and chondroid matrix components. The chondroblasts are scattered individually, creating a pebbled appearance, have round to oval nuclei with an evenly distributed fine nuclear chromatin, and show longitudinal nuclear grooves.[109]

Chondroblastomas may occur in the cranial bones, of which the temporal bone is the most common site, followed by the mandible.[110] Significant clinical differences have been reported for lesions in the cranial bones. The patients are older, generally over 30 years of age. Chondroid differentiation, although present, is not always clearly seen, and approximately half of these patients develop a recurrence after curettage.[110]

TREATMENT AND PROGNOSIS. Conservative management including a thorough curettage, and bone packing of the lesion is the therapy of choice. Recurrences may be expected in up to 16% of cases.[3]

Malignant chondroblastoma,[111,112] reported as metastasizing chondroblastomas with benign- or malignant-looking histology, has been reported, but such cases are extremely rare. Another rarity is the occurrence of chondroblastoma in the soft tissue.[113]

Malignant

Chondrosarcomas of the bone represent a range of malignant tumors of cartilage that includes the classic or conventional chondrosarcoma, dedifferentiated chondrosarcoma, clear cell chondrosarcoma, mesenchymal chondrosarcoma, and malignant chondroblastoma.

Classic chondrosarcoma (central and peripheral chondrosarcoma)

With myeloma excluded, classic chondrosarcoma, or simply chondrosarcoma, is the second most common malignant neoplasm of bone after osteosarcoma.[1]

Chondrosarcoma is subclassified as central (medullary) if it is located within the medullary cavity or peripheral (juxtacortical) if its origin is on the surface of the bone.[1,2] Chondrosarcomas may arise de novo or secondarily from preexisting benign cartilage lesions such as the osteochondromas in multiple osteochondromatosis or the enchondromas of Ollier's disease[1,2] (Fig. 73-28).

High-grade chondrosarcomas are not difficult to diagnose. However, low-grade tumors may present significant problems to the interpreting pathologist, largely because the most innocuous histologic pattern is the common denominator for lesions that have clinicoradiologic signs of benignity (so-called enchondromas), for lesions that show aggressive features (such as expansion of the bone, scalloping of the endosteum, thinning of the cortex), and for lesions that break through the cortex and are generally interpreted as chondrosarcomas. Furthermore, the presence of pain in an otherwise histologically and radiologically benign cartilage lesion has been interpreted clinically as a sign of malignancy.

Because of these problems, in this section, we discuss lesions that may be interpreted as enchondromas, together with true malignant tumors of hyaline cartilage.

The following discussion is largely based on M.D. Anderson Cancer Center experience with 171 cases of chondrosar-

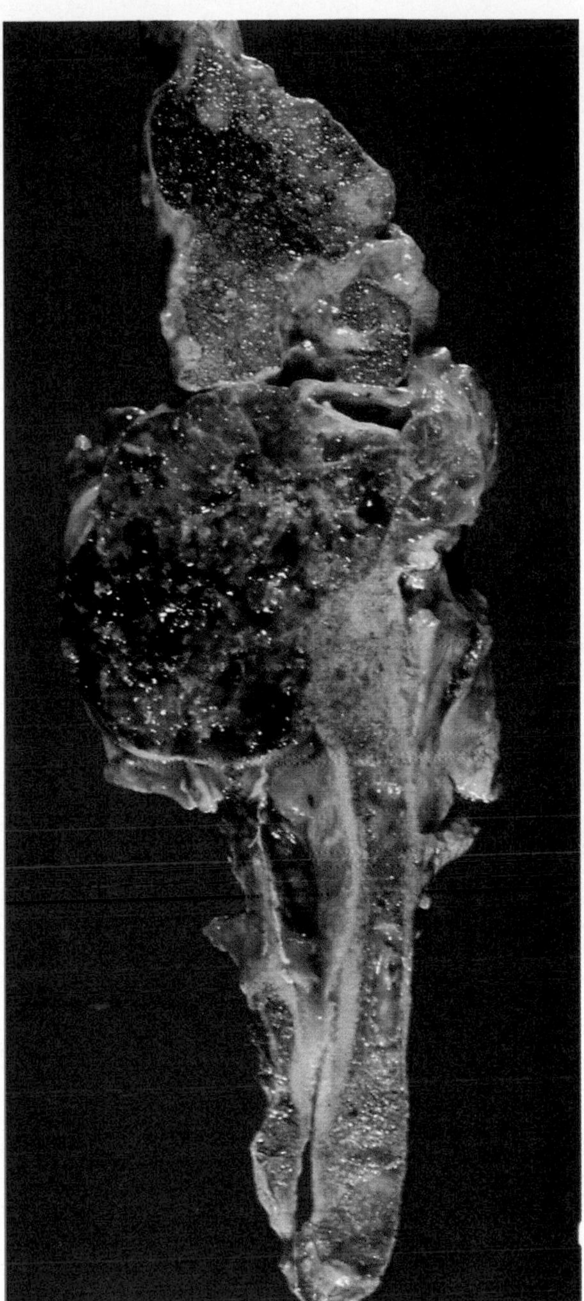

Fig. 73-28 Ollier's disease. A lower extremity showing a chondrosarcoma of the proximal end of tibia. Notice several enchondromas in the distal end of the femur.

coma.[114] This study included lesions that ranged from clinicoradiographically benign lesions (enchondroma and large osteochondromatous lesions) to aggressive lesions (intramedullary lesions showing scalloping of endosteum or expansion, and large osteochondromatous lesions with a thick cartilaginous cap) to lesions that break through the cortex and have definitive clinicopathologic evidence of malignancy.

Chondrosarcoma is a malignant tumor of hyaline cartilage that arises in the medullary cavity or on the surface of a bone.[1-4] It is a tumor of adults generally between 20 and 70 years of age, perhaps more common in the fourth to the sixth decades of life.[1-4,114,115] In children or adolescents the tumor is distinctly rare.[116,117] Males are affected more often than

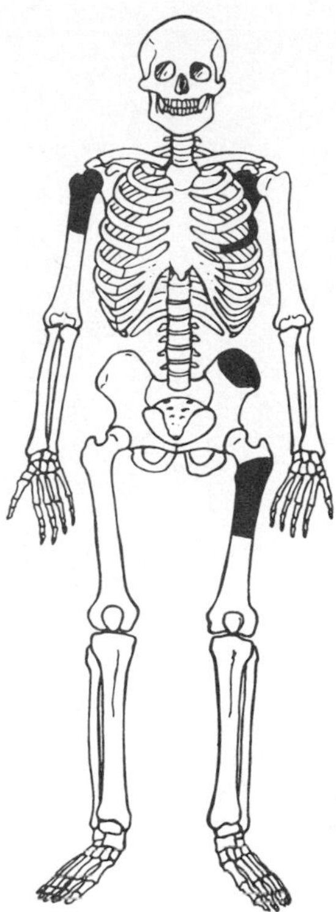

Fig. 73-29 Skeletal distribution of conventional chondrosarcoma. Common locations of this lesion.

females.[1-4,114,115] The most common sites of involvement are the pelvis, femur, scapula, humerus, and ribs (Fig. 73-29). Pain is the most common complaint of patients, but a painless mass (as in the scapula) is not an uncommon presentation.[1-4,114,115] Some lesions attain large sizes before they become symptomatic, however.

Radiographic findings indicate the cartilaginous nature of a tumor when typical calcifications are present. Matrix calcifications have been variously described as annular, punctate, popcorn-like, ringlet-like, stippled, or small ill-defined radiodense formations. These features identify a tumor as having a cartilaginous nature but do not discriminate benign from malignant tumors.

PATHOLOGY. Grossly the tumors show the typical glistening lobulated appearance of cartilage whether they are within the medullary cavity or on the surface of a bone[1] (Figs 73-30). Within the medullary cavity, the tumors may sit in the cancellous bone, may enlarge the cavity, or may induce scalloping of the endosteum and finally break through the cortex. On the surface, they are often sessile but may be pedunculated; as they grow, they tend to push tissues, and large lesions can trap adjacent tissue.

One of the most important parameters is the histologic evaluation and grading of a cartilaginous lesion.[114,115] Chondrosarcomas span from histologic benignity to histologic malignancy. Borderline or low-grade lesions are made up of hyaline cartilage with sparse cellularity and rare binucleated cells in the lacunae. As the grade increases, the tumor becomes more cellular and the nucleus enlarges and develops a fine nuclear chromatin pattern with occasional nucleoli. The number of binucleated cells increases. High-grade tumors show nuclear atypia, pleomorphism, and mitotic activity.

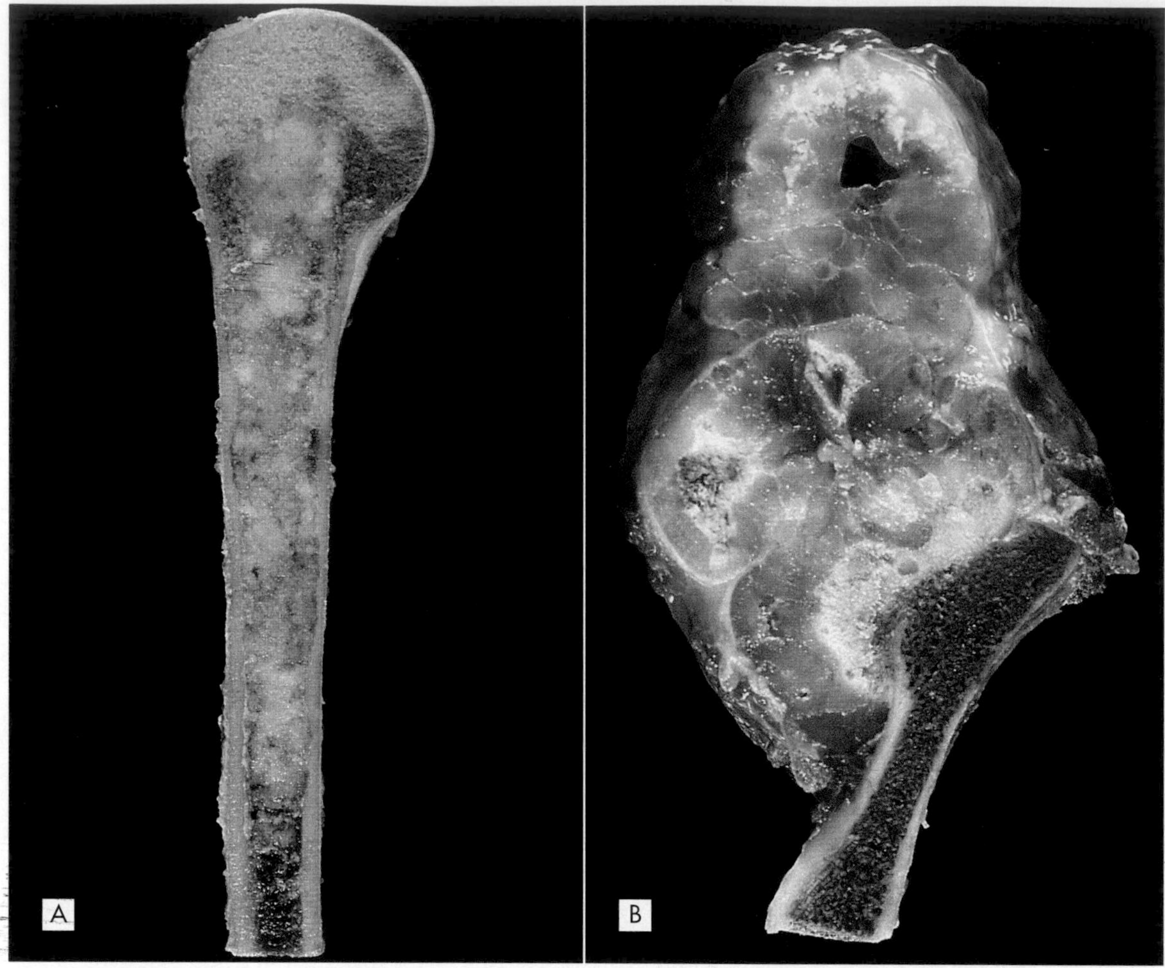

Fig. 73-30 **A,** Gross picture of chondrosarcoma of humerus. There is extensive diaphyseal and metaphyseal involvement with scalloping of endosteum. **B,** Surface chondrosarcoma of ilium. Notice the typical lobulations of cartilaginous neoplasm.

There are several different systems to grade cartilaginous tumors. The M.D. Anderson Cancer Center uses a modification of the grading system[114] proposed by Evans and colleagues[115] in 1976. Grade 1 lesions are those that contain innocuous hyaline cartilage manifested by sparse cellularity. The cells typically contain dark, pyknotic nuclei no larger than the nucleus of a mature lymphocyte; a small percentage of cells (no more than 20%) may contain larger nuclei with a fine nuclear chromatin pattern. Mitoses are not seen in this grade (Fig. 73-31, *A*).

Grade 2 lesions are divided into two subtypes, A and B, according to cellularity and nuclear atypia. Grade 2A lesions are slightly more cellular than grade 1 lesions are, and more than 20% of their nuclei are larger than the nucleus of a mature lymphocyte. The nuclei of these cells show a fine nuclear chromatin pattern and may contain nucleoli; binucleated cells are easily found, but mitoses are not seen in this grade (Fig. 73-31, *B*). Grade 2B lesions are cellular lesions with numerous binucleated cells per lacuna and nuclear atypia manifested by large nuclei, occasionally bizarre nuclear shapes, nuclear spindling, and, in general, variation in nuclear size. The cellular areas tend to concentrate at the periphery of the lobules. Mitoses may be found, but these should not be more than 1 per 10 high-power fields.

Grade 3 lesions differ from grade 2B lesions in that they contain at least two or more mitoses per 10 high-power fields counted in the most cellular areas (Fig. 73-31, *C*).

CLINICAL SIGNIFICANCE OF GRADING. Grade 1 lesions are often found in the so-called enchondromas, aggressive intramedullary lesions of the long bones and in some cases where the tumor breaks through the cortex. These lesions do not metastasize but may recur if they are incompletely excised. The possibility of dedifferentiation exists in this grade if the lesion is left untreated.

Grade 2A lesions parallel the behavior of grade 1 lesions in that they recur if they are incompletely resected but do not metastasize.

Grade 2B lesions recur and have the capacity for distant metastasis.

Grade 3 lesions have the highest potential for distant metastasis, and patient survival is approximately 55% at 10 years.

Grading is the most important parameter of diagnosis because it helps to prognosticate the outcome of the lesion. For grading to be prognostically significant it has to be done after the tumor has been completely removed and the pathologist has the opportunity to take many samples of the lesion to be studied histologically. In general, one section per centime-

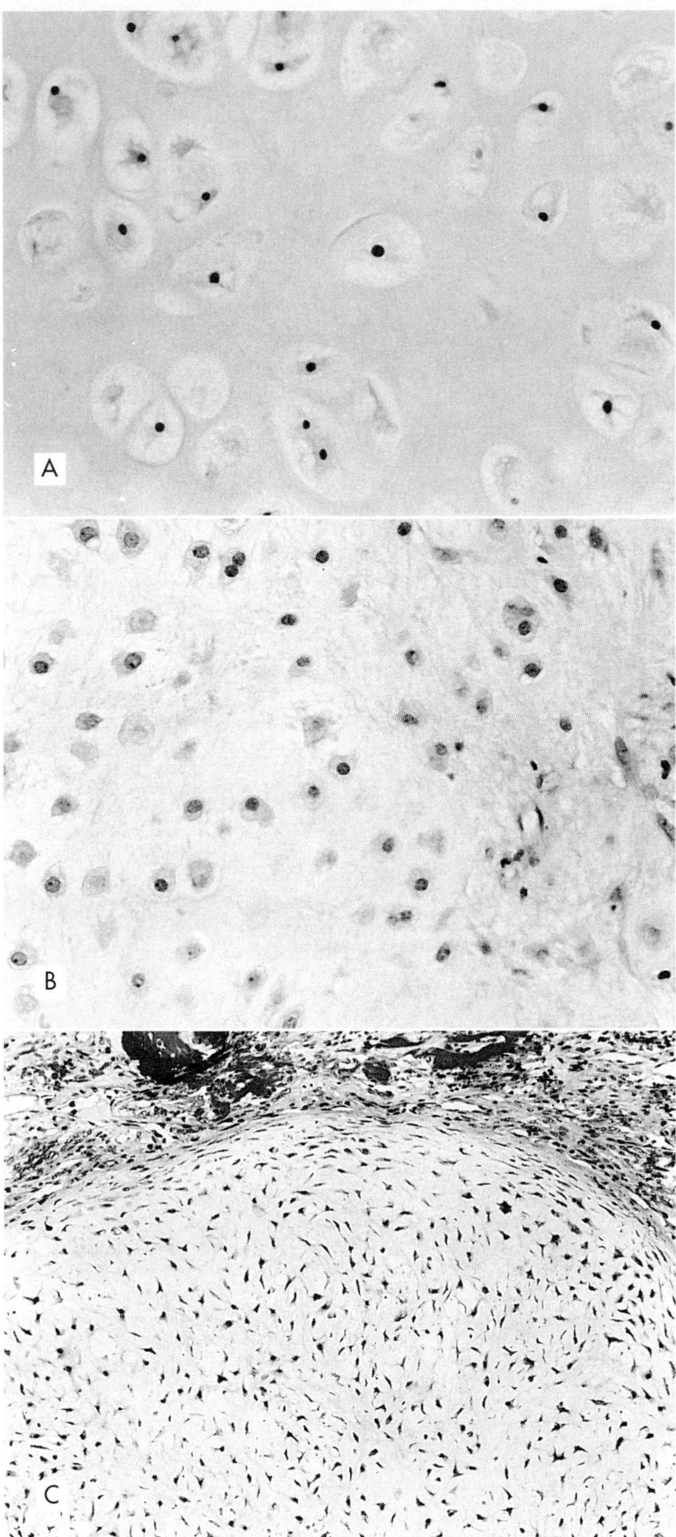

Fig. 73-31 Chondrosarcoma. **A,** Grade 1, showing hyaline tumor containing cells with small and dark nuclei. Tumors of this type do not metastasize. **B,** Grade 2A, consisting of cartilaginous cells showing enlargement of nuclei that exhibit a fine nuclear chromatin pattern and occasional small nucleoli. **C,** Grade 3, consisting of increased cellularity and obvious nuclear anaplasia. The difference between grade 2B and grade 3 is the presence of at least 2 mitoses per 10 high-power fields in grade 3 tumors.

ter of the diameter of the lesion should be sufficient; however, should there be any questionable areas, especially myxoid areas, they should also be included in the sampling.

Should there be a biopsy? If the tumor can be identified on radiologic examination as a cartilaginous tumor, a biopsy should not be done. However, if the lesion is identifiable as cartilaginous in nature but presents alarming radiologic features, such as a lytic component, the biopsy should be done and should be directed to the lytic areas of the tumor, presumably the area containing a high-grade malignancy.

Medullary cavity lesions are commonly found in the proximal humerus and in the area of the greater trochanter and shaft of the femur. When intramedullary, the lesions may cause no change to the bone, may cause expansion of the bone or may induce scalloping of the endosteum. Scalloping of the endosteum is manifested by the presence of small scooped-out areas of the inner aspect of the cortex that do not break through the cortex. A medullary cavity lesion can also break through the cortex and extend into the soft tissues.

Surface tumors usually contain typical chondroid calcifications and appear as sessile or pedunculated polypoid tumors. Much has been written on the thickness of the cartilaginous cap of the surface lesions; some authors claim that a thickness of more than 1 cm is diagnostic of malignancy.

The acetabular region of the pelvis is also a common site for the development of chondrosarcoma; in this location the initial presentation may be a totally lytic tumor.

TREATMENT AND PROGNOSIS. The management of chondrosarcoma is surgical; the amount of surgery depends on the clinical presentation. Painless lesions that cause no scalloping or remodeling of the bone can be carefully watched with frequent follow-up examinations; however, if the patient may not come back for follow-up examinations (because of unreliability or living too far away to travel), the lesion should be removed by curettage and the area filled with cement. If the lesion is not removed, the patient should be informed that there is a remote chance of developing dedifferentiated chondrosarcoma. Aggressive intramedullary tumors can be either curettaged and packed with cement or removed by an en bloc resection. Lesions that break through the cortex can be excised locally with bone reconstruction. The histologic grade of the tumor should not be a factor in deciding the management strategy, but the most important factor should be the location and extent of the lesion. A major amputation should be the last resort when conservative therapy cannot be used.

Chemotherapy has no effect in chondrosarcoma, but radiotherapy may be used as a palliative procedure.

Chondrosarcoma variants

Dedifferentiated chondrosarcoma. A dedifferentiated chondrosarcoma has the worst prognosis of all the chondrosarcomas; practically all patients reported in most series with this disease died of it.[1-4] The concept of dedifferentiation was introduced in 1971 by Dahlin and Beabout[118] who postulated that low-grade cartilaginous lesions may transform (dedifferentiate) into a high-grade sarcoma. Their concept has been accepted by most investigators, though other authors believe that these tumors are formed by the synchronous differentiation of two separate clones of cells.[119,120]

Very few cases of dedifferentiated chondrosarcoma are seen in early adulthood; most occur in the sixth decade of life.[1-4,119,121,122] The patient distribution by sex is about equal. The site of tumor is most often the bones of the pelvis, followed by the femur;[1-4,119,121,122] the tumor can occur in other locations but does so with less frequency. Pain is the common initial symptom, but some cases have the history of a long-standing indolent cartilage tumor (enchondroma).[119,121,122]

Radiologically these tumors may show foci of typical cartilaginous calcifications, denoting the low-grade component, and a large lytic component, which usually has a significant soft-tissue mass component. However, a good number of tumors do not present the calcifications of the low-grade component, but only the large noncalcified mass. In the follow-up study of seemingly benign low-grade cartilage tumors, the finding of a lytic component should raise the suspicion of a dedifferentiated component; a biopsy of the questionable area is mandatory in these cases.

PATHOLOGY. Grossly these tumors are large infiltrative lesions that not only involve the bone but also extend into the adjacent soft tissues. Foci of cartilage may be seen on gross inspection.

Histologically the diagnosis is made when one finds areas of hyaline cartilage tumor and high-grade sarcoma[118,119] (Fig. 73-32).

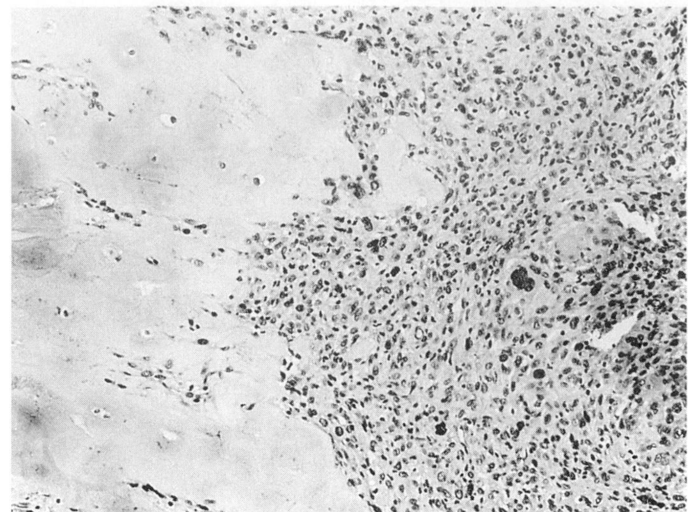

Fig. 73-32 The combination of a low-grade chondrosarcoma and a high-grade sarcoma as depicted here is diagnostic of dedifferentiated chondrosarcoma.

The hyaline cartilage component is a low-grade tumor (grade 1 or grade 2A); if the cartilage is high grade, the tumor should not be considered in the dedifferentiated category.

The high-grade sarcoma usually takes the shape of pleomorphic malignant fibrous histiocytoma or of an unclassified spindle cell sarcoma; osteosarcoma and rhabdomyosarcoma have also been reported to be sarcomatous components of dedifferentiated chondrosarcoma.[119]

Zalupski and associates[123] have reported rearrangement and translocation at the same band on chromosome 1 in two cases of dedifferentiated chondrosarcoma.

Dedifferentiation of a surface cartilage lesion may also occur.[124] Bertoni and associates found five previously reported cases and reported seven of their own.[124] The survival rate of these patients was as poor as that of patients with medullary dedifferentiated chondrosarcomas.

TREATMENT AND PROGNOSIS. The management strategy of this lesion is surgical ablation and intensive chemotherapy.[119] However, despite radical management, the survival rate is dismal.

Mesenchymal chondrosarcoma. Mesenchymal chondrosarcoma is another variant of chondrosarcoma that has been described both in the bones and in the soft tissue.[1-4,125-128] This tumor is rare, accounting for 0.33% to 0.5% of all primary malignant neoplasms of bone.[1,3] It is rare in children under 10 years of age, but 80% of cases are diagnosed before 40 years of age. The peak incidence is in the second decade of life.

The initial symptom is usually pain that has been present for a short time or for several years. Swelling or a mass may also be seen.

Radiologically there is nothing characteristic for this tumor. On the other hand, if calcified cartilage matrix is present, the tumor may look like a conventional chondrosarcoma.

Any bone may be involved. Huvos[2] reported 31% of mesenchymal chondrosarcoma in the lower extremity, 17% in the pelvic girdle, and 14% in the cranial bones.

PATHOLOGY. Grossly this tumor may show nodules of cartilage admixed with a meaty red-brown hemorrhagic tumor.

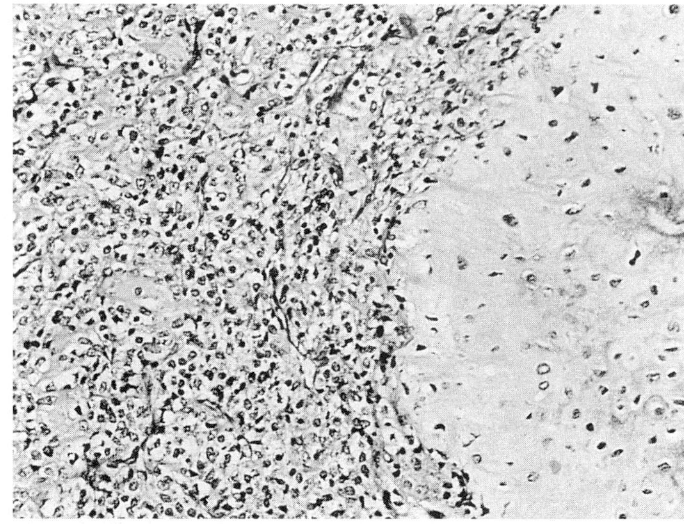

Fig. 73-33 Mesenchymal chondrosarcoma. There is a nodule of hyaline cartilage of low-grade malignancy associated with a small cell sarcoma.

Histologically, there are two basic components: a primitive small cell neoplasm and areas of hyaline cartilage of benign status or low-grade malignancy. The small cell component shows round to oval or spindle cells, with little cytoplasm, growing in a rich vascular capillary bed. The pattern may simulate that of Ewing's sarcoma or of hemangiopericytoma (Fig. 73-33). Mitosis may be seen. The nodules of hyaline cartilage have innocuous histologic features ranging from benign pattern (low cellularity and small pyknotic nuclei) to low-grade malignancy (cellular lesions with large nuclei exhibiting a fine chromatin pattern and numerous double nuclei per lacuna). The cartilage eventually ossifies to form mature bone spicules.

TREATMENT. The management for this type of lesion is surgical. Some cases have also benefited from chemotherapy.

Clear cell chondrosarcoma. The clear cell variant of chondrosarcoma, unlike dedifferentiated chondrosarcoma, has a

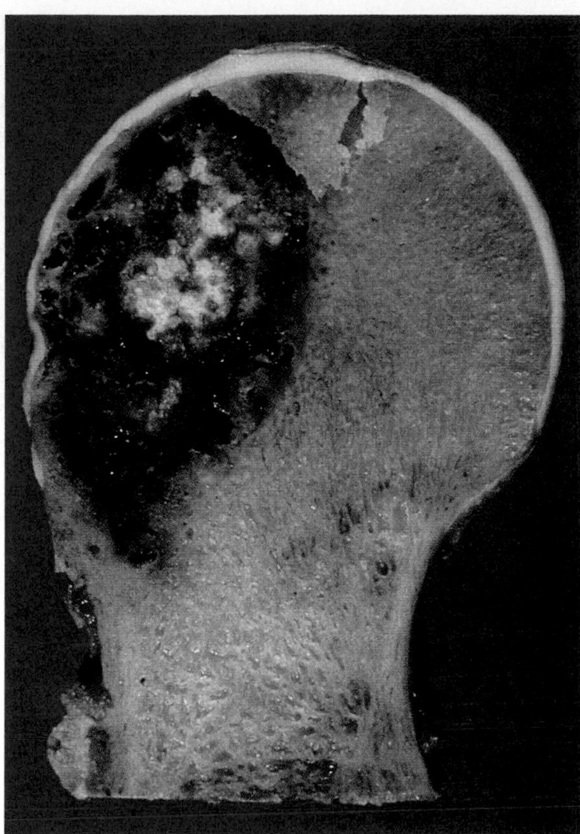

Fig. 73-34 Clear cell chondrosarcoma. Head of femur shows central whitish calcified areas surrounded by darker tissue. The lesion reaches but does not penetrate the articular surface.

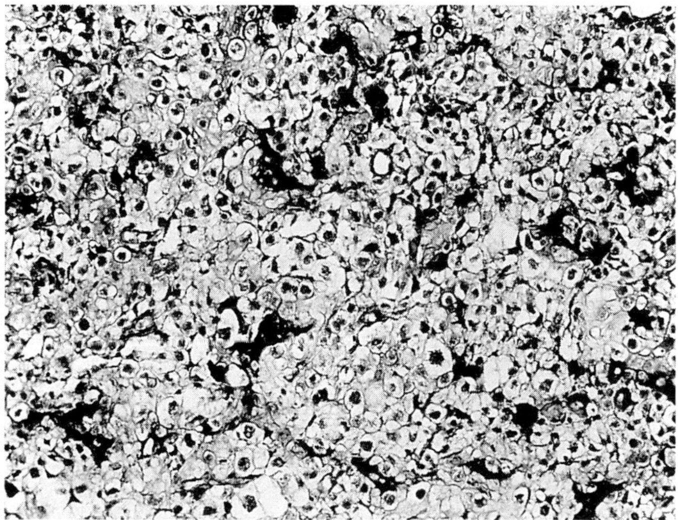

Fig. 73-35 Clear cell chondrosarcoma. Microscopically this lesion exhibits large clear cells associated with mature bone formation.

relatively good prognosis. Clear cell chondrosarcoma is extremely rare; in the Mayo Clinic's experience, there were only 12 cases of a total of 545 primary chondrosarcomas.[1]

In the Mayo Clinic experience, patients ages ranged from 14 to 84 years, with a slight peak in the third and fourth decades of life.[1] There was a male predominance; the male-to-female ratio was 2.5 to 1.[1,129]

Radiologically this lesion is seen in the epiphysis of the long bones, especially the head of the femur which is the most common location;[129] most of these tumors contain typical cartilaginous calcifications. Some clear cell chondrosarcomas, especially small tumors, may be difficult if not impossible to differentiate from chondroblastoma.[1,129,130]

PATHOLOGY. Grossly, clear cell chondrosarcomas show multiple calcifications and focal ossified areas alternating with glistening myxoid cartilaginoid tissue (Fig. 73-34). In general, most lesions are confined within the bone, but some may be large, not only expanding the bone, but also breaching its confines and reaching the soft tissues.

Histologically, components of this type of lesion are (1) clear cells, (2) areas of ossification and calcification, (3) osteoclastic giant cells, and (4) not uncommonly, aneurysmal bone cysts. The clear cells are large cytoplasmic cells with round to oval nuclei that may contain a nucleolus. The cytoplasmic borders are usually seen, and the overall growth imparts a lobulated characteristic (Fig. 73-35). Fine capillaries traverse these cells. Osteoclastic giant cells are not numerous but may be seen in clusters of a few cells or scattered individually throughout the tumor. There is definite osteoid and mature bone production, which may cause a small microscopic change or formation of large bone spicules. Focal calcification may be seen around some of the cells as is seen in chondroblastomas, but this feature is not prominent. Some cases also show foci of hyaline cartilage.

TREATMENT AND PROGNOSIS. The management strategy for clear cell chondrosarcoma is en bloc resection with a margin of normal bone and soft tissue.[129] The 5-year survival is 85%.[129]

FIBROUS LESIONS OF BONE

Fibrous neoplasms of bone include those that are typically benign, such as fibrous cortical defect/nonossifying fibroma of bone, fibrous histiocytoma, xanthoma, osteofibrous dysplasia/fibrous dysplasia, aggressive lesions such as desmoplastic fibroma (desmoid tumor of bone), and malignant fibrous histiocytoma.

Benign

Fibrous cortical defect and nonossifying fibroma

The two benign fibrous lesions of bone, fibrous cortical defect and nonossifying fibroma, are closely related if not the same entity: they share a fibrous histologic nature and the self-healing that eventually occurs, but the sizes of the lesions differ.[1-4]

Fibrous cortical defect is an asymptomatic lesion that occurs in young children. The lesion is usually recognized radiologically and appears as a small radiolucent change in the cortical aspect of the metaphysis of a long bone.[1-4]

Grossly and microscopically this lesion is fibrous in morphology, consisting of fibroblasts with collagen fibers and rare vessels.

Since fibrous cortical defect involutes, with the area becoming sclerotic, no therapy is needed.

Nonossifying fibroma (NOF) is a lesion of children, and over 80% of cases are discovered before 20 years of age; although NOF may persist beyond the second decade of life, it usually undergoes involutional changes. The lesion is asymptomatic; consequently it is usually discovered incidentally during x-ray examinations done for other reasons. Pathologic fracture is not an uncommon presentation, especially in large lesions. The lesion is more commonly seen in males than in females, with a ratio of 1.6:1,[3] and the most commonly affected bones are the femur, the tibia, and the fibula in descending order of frequency.

Radiologically NOF is an eccentric, metaphyseal, radiolucent lesion that shows loculi; its periphery is rimmed by a zone of sclerosis. Large lesions may induce a bulge in the bone or expansion of the medullary cavity. As the lesion involutes, increasing areas of ossification develop, and the area shrinks and may eventually disappear.[1-4]

PATHOLOGY. On gross examination this lesion has a yellowish to rusty brown appearance, depending on the amount of lipid and hemosiderin. A sclerotic peripheral rim of reactive bone may be appreciated. Histologic examination reveals fibroblasts and histiocytic cells. The fibroblastic component shows bland nuclear features and no mitotic activity or rare mitoses; a storiform arrangement of the cells is the rule (Fig. 73-36). The histiocytic cells usually contain lipid that imparts a foamy vacuolated appearance to the cytoplasm. Hemosiderin is usually present between the fibroblastic cells.[1-4]

TREATMENT AND PROGNOSIS. Treatment of NOF is not required because the lesion self-heals. However, painful lesions, large lesions that are not 100% radiologically typical, and lesions that continue to grow after puberty should be removed. The management strategy is usually curettage with bone packing.[3]

Fibrous histiocytoma of bone

There are cases in which a tumor shows the same morphology as NOF does but is located in a different site from the usual site of NOF.[131] Lesions of this type do not regress with time but may behave in an aggressive manner. The term *atypical fibrous histiocytoma* has been applied to some of these lesions when they exhibit cytologic atypia and an increased number of mitotic figures.[2-3]

At the Mayo Clinic, Wold[132] described 38 cases of benign and atypical fibrous histiocytoma of bone. The age distribution for the group spanned from the first decade to the eighth decade with a slight peak in the fourth decade of life. The pelvis and the femur were the most commonly involved bones.

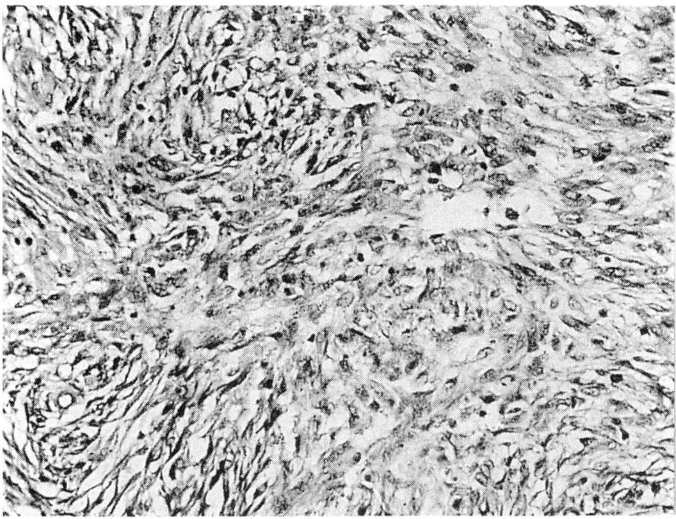

Fig. 73-36 Nonossifying fibroma. There is a fibrous neoplasm with a storiform pattern.

Radiologically, these lesions produce a radiolucent change and may have a peripheral sclerotic rim of dense bone tissue. In other cases, they are purely lytic; for example, in the epiphysis and metaphysis of a long bone, the radiologic appearance may be similar to that of a giant cell tumor of bone.

From the gross and histologic points of view, the lesions do not differ from NOF.

Management should be conservative involving curettage and bone packing and possibly cement packing, depending on the clinical aggressiveness of the lesion.

Xanthoma (fibroxanthoma)

Another fibrous histiocytic lesion is one that is extremely rare, xanthoma or fibroxanthoma of bone. In this lesion the foamy histiocytes predominate. Some authors deny its existence, speculating that it is a degenerative process replacing a benign bone lesion.[1-4] There is no question that xanthomatous changes occur in many benign lesions, including fibrous dysplasia, giant cell tumor of bone, and nonossifying fibroma of bone, but purely fibroxanthomatous lesions also occur.[133]

Osteofibrous dysplasia (cortical fibrous dysplasia, ossifying fibroma)

Osteofibrous dysplasia is an interesting lesion of the tibia and fibula of children that, unlike fibrous dysplasia, arises in the cortex of the bone.[1-4,134,135] It is also called "cortical fibrous dysplasia" and "ossifying fibroma of bone."[134,136] It is extremely rare, accounting for about 0.2% of primary bone tumor biopsy specimens.[3]

Osteofibrous dysplasia is a disease of children; over 50% of cases are diagnosed at or under 5 years of age and almost all under 10 years of age. Pain and swelling of the tibia are the most common presentation. The tibia is the most frequently involved bone (78%).[3] Both the tibia and the fibula may be simultaneously involved (12%), and the fibula alone is less common (7%). Bilateral involvement of the tibias may also be seen.[3]

Radiologically this lesion is an eccentric cortical and diaphyseal lesion. It begins in the cortex, spreading in the long axis. It can be purely lytic or may have a ground-glass appearance, and there is usually a sclerotic reaction around the lesion. In some advanced lesions the tibia may show an anterior bowing. Pathologic fracture may also occur.

PATHOLOGY. Grossly the lesion is fibrous and has a gritty consistency. Histologically, it is a fibro-osseous proliferation showing immature woven bone as in fibrous dysplasia and bone spicules arising directly from osteoblastic activity. The fibrous component may have a faint storiform arrangement; although focally cellular, it does not show cellular atypia.

According to Campanacci and Laus,[135] if the lesion is left untreated, it becomes quiescent and stops growing after puberty. Therefore they recommend that these lesions be left alone, especially in children under 5 years of age. Pathologic fractures should be treated with a cast; if bowing is present, it can be treated at any age by osteotomy.

The finding of keratin-positive cells in the spindle stroma of cases of osteofibrous dysplasia has led some investigators to postulate that osteofibrous dysplasia is intimately related to adamantinoma.[137] Czerniak and colleagues[137] proposed that osteofibrous dysplasia is a differentiated (regressing) adamantinoma. A study by Sweet and colleagues[138] of osteofibrous dysplasia demonstrated the presence of keratin in the spindle cells of 28 of 30 osteofibrous dysplasia cases; none of the cases progressed to adamantinoma.

Czerniak and colleagues'[137] concept is of academic interest in regard to the histogenesis of both adamantinoma and osteofibrous dysplasia. The finding of keratin positive cells in a case of osteofibrous dysplasia has, so far, no clinical significance, since no case has shown progression to full-blown adamantinoma.[138]

Desmoplastic fibroma

Desmoplastic fibroma of bone is a locally aggressive, benign, rare entity characterized by proliferating fibrous tissue similar to desmoid fibromatosis of the soft tissues.[139] Approximately 150 cases have been reported.[140] Although the lesion has been reported in the metaphysis of the long bones, it is more commonly seen in the maxilla and mandible of children and adolescents.[140,141]

About 74% of cases occur before 30 years of age, and there is a male predominance of approximately 2.4 per 1 female.[140] Pain and swelling are the most common presenting symptoms. In the maxilla and mandible, desmoplastic fibroma usually presents as a painless mass that grows slowly, invading the masseter and pterygoid muscles and leading to the appearance of trismus. The mass may become large.

Radiologically the metaphysis of a long bone involved by this tumor shows a lytic lesion that has a trabeculated bubbly appearance. There is usually expansion of the bone, and large lesions may permeate through the cortex. A soft-tissue component is the rule in lesions of the mandible.

After surgery alone, recurrences are common; about 42% of patients treated with curettage alone have recurrent disease. Chemotherapy with doxorubicin HCl (Adriamycin) and DTIC for the head and neck lesions has shown to reduce the size of the lesion and make it amenable to more conservative surgery.[141]

The term *periosteal desmoid* has been utilized to denote (1) a desmoplastic fibroma (desmoid tumor) arising in the cortex or periosteum of a bone and (2) a benign fibrous cortical defect. Although it is extensively used in radiologic language, we discourage its use in pathology, preferring the terms *desmoid fibromatosis* for the aggressive bone surface lesion and *fibrous cortical defect* for the benign lesion of the cortex.

Fibrous dysplasia

Fibrous dysplasia (FD) is a relatively common benign disorder affecting children and young adults. Considered a developmental anomaly rather than a neoplasm, FD consists of a fibro-osseous proliferation replacing the normal marrow spaces. It may affect a single bone (monostotic FD) or multiple bones (polyostotic FD).[1-4] The monostotic form is more common than the polyostotic type.

About two thirds of FD cases are diagnosed before 30 years of age. The sex distribution is about equal,[1-4] though in the Armed Forces Institute of Pathology series there was a 2:1 male predominance for the monostotic variant and a 1.3:1 male predominance for the polyostotic form.[142] Usually, monostotic FD is asymptomatic and diagnosed when incidental radiographs are made. Pain, swelling, and stress or pathologic fracture may occur.[1-4,142] Skin discoloration in the trunk may coexist (café-au-lait spots). Multiple endocrine abnormalities have also been described in patients with FD. The triad of polyostotic FD (typically unilateral), café-au-lait spots, and endocrine dysfunction (precocious puberty in females) constitute Albright's syndrome. Other endocrine disorders such as Cushing's syndrome, hyperparathyroidism, hyperthyroidism, acromegaly, and diabetes mellitus have also been reported to occur with FD.[1-4,142] Intramuscular myxomas may also coexist with FD. Cherubism, an autosomal dominant disorder, is a special form of FD. Patients with cherubism present with symmetrical involvement of the mandible and maxilla.

Radiologically, FD shows the typical "ground-glass" pattern that denotes the fibro-osseous content of the lesion. The epicenter of the lesion is in the medullary cavity and may be eccentric, but these lesions do not form in cortical locations.[142] Older lesions may undergo expansion and thinning of the cortex. The shepherd's crook deformity, a strong curvature of the proximal femur, can appear in long-standing cases of FD.

Although FD may involve any bone, the ribs, femur, and cranial bones are the areas most frequently affected.[142]

PATHOLOGY. Histologically, FD consists of a fibro-osseous proliferation. The bone varies in makeup from small, thin trabeculas without osteoblastic rimming to large, thick bone spicules, the latter especially in older lesions (Fig. 73-37). Under polarizing-lens examination, the bone trabeculas of FD show an irregularly woven pattern that is different from the lamellar bone pattern present in normal bone. Because of the complicated irregular outlines, forming short, curved, serpiginous, curlicue shapes, the bone fragments of FD have been likened to Chinese letters or an alphabetic soup. A hyaline cartilage component has also been described in FD.[143] Secondary aneurysmal bone cyst formation may also occur.[144]

FD tends to stop growing at puberty; therefore, therapy should be conservative.

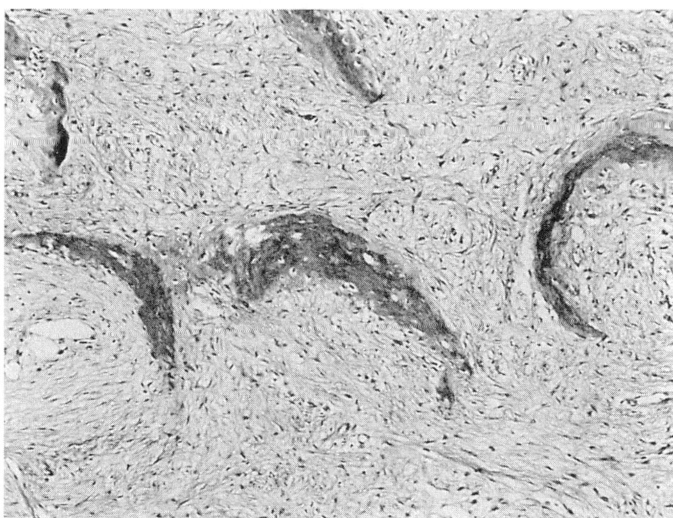

Fig. 73-37 Microscopically, fibrous dysplasia shows bone produced directly from fibrous tissue and, consequently, no osteoblastic activity. The bony spicules of fibrous dysplasia resembles Chinese characters.

Malignant transformation of FD occurs rarely, in less than 0.5% of patients.[1-4,142,145] Osteosarcoma, chondrosarcoma, or malignant fibrous histiocytoma may develop.

Malignant

Malignant fibrous histiocytoma

Malignant fibrous histiocytoma (MFH) is a rare malignant tumor of bone that has histologic features similar to those of its soft-tissue counterpart.[1-4] Before 1970 most non–matrix producing sarcomas of bone were classified under the term *fibrosarcoma*, but the description of MFH in the soft tissues and bones has largely replaced the term *fibrosarcoma*. The rarity of this tumor is attested by the finding of only 52 cases of MFH among 6514 primary malignant tumors of bone in the Mayo Clinic experience, though in the New South Wales Bone Tumor Registry the incidence was higher: 38 cases of 506 malignant bone tumors.[146]

The age of presentation ranges from the first to the eighth decades of life without any significant peaks among the decades. It more often affects males than females, at about a ratio of 1.5:1.[147,148] The metaphysis of the long bones is the preferred site for this tumor, with the femur, proximal tibia, and pelvis being the most commonly affected bones[1-4,146-149] (Fig. 73-38).

There are no characteristic features on radiographic examination, except for radiologic signs of malignancy; these include large lytic areas without matrix production, ill-defined borders, and extension of the tumor through the cortex, often with a large soft-tissue mass component.

PATHOLOGY. Grossly, these tumors have the meaty appearance of a soft-tissue sarcoma with focal areas of hemorrhage and necrosis. Histologically, MFH is composed of spindle fibroblastic cells with variable nuclear pleomorphism and numerous mitoses, many of which are abnormal. Matrix is not seen, but reactive osteoid formation may be present. Huvos and colleagues[148] subclassified MFH of bone into fibrous (62%), histiocytic or xanthomatous (30%), and malignant giant cell (8%) types.

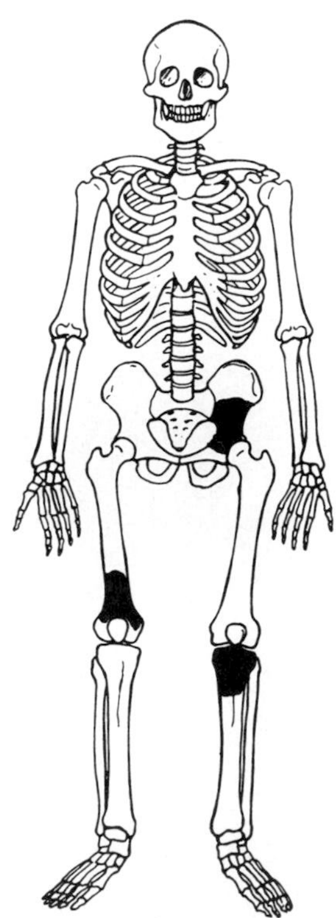

Fig. 73-38 Malignant fibrous histiocytoma. Skeletal localization of common sites of involvement.

About 28% of MFHs arise secondarily to bone infarction or Paget's disease of bone or as a result of irradiation.[148,149]

The differential diagnosis on radiologic and microscopic examinations includes osteosarcoma in children or in young adults and metastatic disease in adults. For children a diagnosis of spindle cell sarcoma is sufficient in a difficult case, since MFH and osteosarcoma are so far treated with the same approach. In adults the finding of a pleomorphic spindle cell sarcoma in the bone always raises the need for differential between sarcoma and metastatic sarcomatoid carcinoma, especially from primaries in the kidney or the lung. The use of keratin immunostaining may help to characterize the tumor, but unfortunately MFH may also coexpress keratin immunoreactivity. A chest x-ray films and a CT scan of the kidney become necessary.

TREATMENT AND PROGRESS. Metastasis to the lung is the usual pathway of spread for MFH. The overall survival at 5 years has been reported to be 34%[147] to 53%.[146,148,150] The management requires a combination of surgery, radiotherapy, and chemotherapy.[147]

Leiomyosarcoma

Leiomyosarcoma of bone is an extremely rare form of bone sarcoma[3] with approximately 50 cases reported.[151] It occurs primarily in adults and is slightly more common in men than in women. The most common location is the distal femur, followed by the proximal tibia and proximal humerus.

The radiographic findings are nonspecific. A lytic lesion without matrix formation involving the medullary cavity with extension into the soft tissue is the usual finding. The lesion may involve the diaphysis or the metaphyseal area of a long bone.[3]

PATHOLOGY. Histologically leiomyosarcoma shows the interlacing bundles typical of a smooth muscle neoplasm. The cells are immunoreactive to smooth muscle actin and rarely to desmin, though these muscle markers are not specific because they can be expressed in malignant fibrous histiocytomas.[152]

The most important differential diagnosis is a metastatic leiomyosarcoma, especially from the uterus. Therefore a detailed clinical history is very important when one is evaluating a smooth muscle neoplasm involving a bone.

TREATMENT AND PROGNOSIS. The mortality is approximately 48% and the average survival from the time of diagnosis is 3.4 years.[151] Management is surgical excision of the lesion.

GIANT CELL TUMOR OF BONE

Benign

Giant cell tumor (GCT) of bone is a benign lesion that affects the epiphysis and metaphysis of the long bones. It is a relatively common neoplasm, accounting for 21% of the benign tumors of bone.[1] Because of its high incidence of recurrence, at least 50% after curettage,[153] GCT was considered by many authorities a low-grade malignant tumor.

Newer techniques of treatment, however, have reduced the recurrence rate.

With a few exceptions GCTs occur after completion of maturation of the skeleton, especially in the third, fourth, and late half of the second decades of life; 80% of the GCT patients are between 20 and 40 years of age.[2,3,153] The disease is more common in women than in men, with a ratio of 3:2.[1-4,153] Although it has been reported in children,[154] the tumor is essentially a lesion of postpubertal patients;[2,3] when confronted with a possible GCT in a child, the pathologist and or clinician must prove that it is indeed a GCT of the bone and not another type of giant cell–rich tumor.

The lesions usually attain a large size before they become symptomatic; pain, swelling, or a pathologic fracture are generally the presenting symptoms. A mass may be seen, and large lesions may present a bruit at auscultation because of the vast vascularity of this tumor.

The most common site of involvement is the distal end of the femur; second most common is the proximal end of the tibia.[1-4,153] About 50.5% of GCT cases occur in these areas.[153] Other common sites include the distal end of the radius, proximal humerus, proximal femur, and sacrum[1-4,153-157] (Fig. 73-39). An extremely rare site is the skull.[158]

Radiologically GCT involves the epiphysis of the long bones and extends into the metaphysis of the bones.[155,156] Since the lesions grow quickly and there is no growth plate barrier, at initial presentation most have already involved both the epiphyseal and metaphyseal areas of the bone.

On plain films GCT presents as a radiolucent lesion involving the end of the bone, reaching its articular cartilage.[2-4,155,156] This important characteristic is present in nearly all GCTs of the bone. The periphery of the lesion seldom shows a sclerotic reaction though focal sclerosis (less than 5%) is occasionally present.[2] On the cortical side, the tumor destroys the cortex and grows out; the periosteum stretches out, serving as a temporary barrier, but finally it is breached in large, neglected lesions. Although the radiologic features are not pathognomonic, when they are present in a skeletally mature patient, especially in a woman between 20 and 35 years of age, they are almost diagnostic.

In the vertebral column GCT usually involves the body of the vertebra. A giant-cell lesion in the posterior elements of the vertebrae is more likely to be an aneurysmal bone cyst than a GCT.[2]

Nonepiphyseal origin of GCT is rarely seen. In the series of Fain and colleagues[159] 14 of 1682 cases of GCT of bone presented with nonepiphyseal origins; 10 were metaphyseal, 2 were metadiaphyseal, and 2 were diaphyseal. The tibia (6 of 14 cases) and the radius (3 of 14 cases) were the most commonly involved bones.

Angiographic studies of GCTs demonstrate extensive vascularity and the presence of numerous arteriovenous fistulas.[160] No correlation has been found between angiographic findings and histologic aggressiveness of the tumor.[161]

Multicentricity of GCT rarely occurs.[162,163] Dahlin[163] reported its occurrence in 3 of 407 patients with GCT.

PATHOLOGY. On gross examination, GCT of bone has a red-brown appearance, which reflects its noticeable vascularity;[1-4] focal areas of yellowish discoloration are usually present, reflecting either focal necrosis or lipid accumulation in the histiocytes (Fig. 73-40). A common component is an aneurysmal bone cyst, which is manifested by small or large cavernous spaces containing blood. Some GCTs of the bone may be almost totally replaced by the aneurysmal bone cyst component.

On histologic examination, a GCT has two components: giant cells and stroma (Fig.73-41). The giant cells are of the osteoclastic type, containing from a few nuclei to about 300 nuclei. The quantity of giant cells varies in relation to the stroma; most GCTs of the bone have an overabundance of giant cells. Mitotic figures are not seen in the giant cells.

The stroma, on the other hand, consists of round to spindle-shaped cells that contain a moderate degree of cytoplasm. The nuclei are generally round or elongated and occasionally

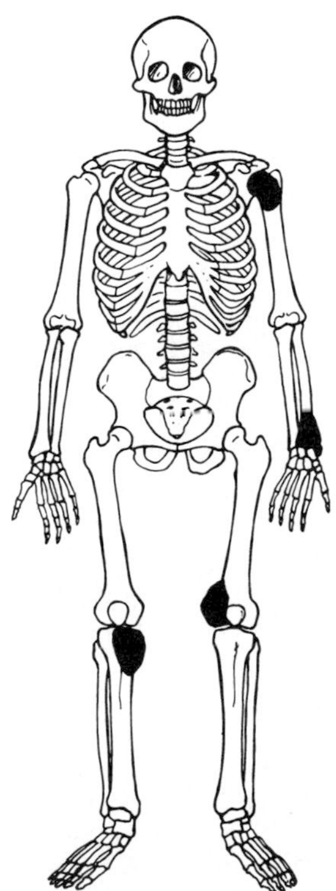

Fig. 73-39 Giant cell tumor of bone. The most common skeletal localizations of this tumor are the distal end of the femur, proximal end of the tibia, proximal end of the humerus and distal radius.

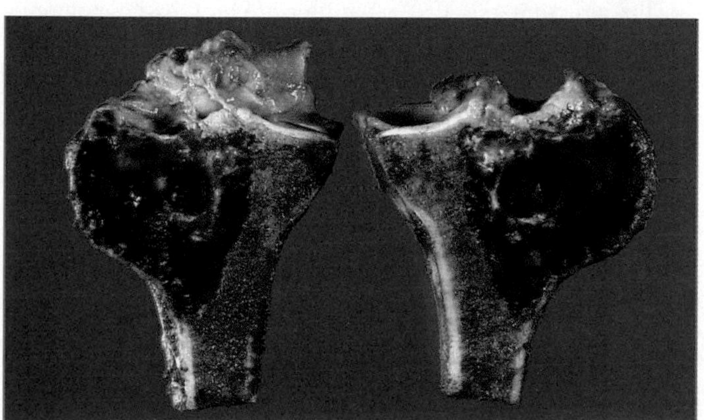

Fig. 73-40 Gross picture of giant cell tumor of bone. The epimetaphysis shows a meaty tumor that destroys the cortex and expands the periosteum. Notice tumor at articular cartilage.

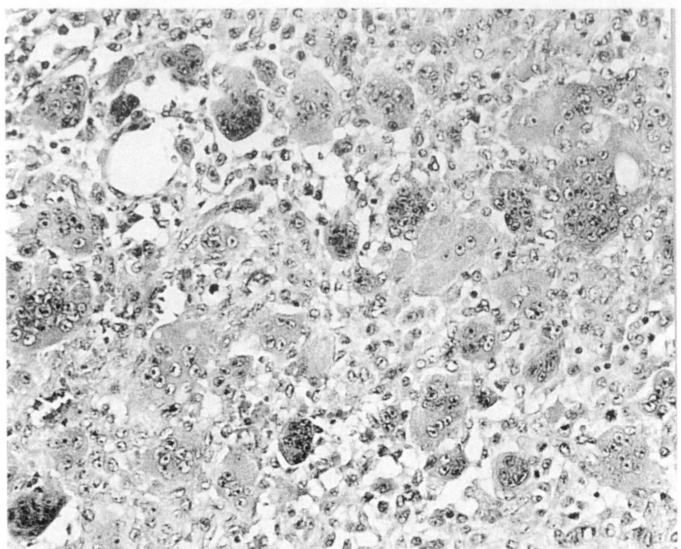

Fig. 73-41 Low-power view of giant cell tumor of bone. Many multinucleated giant cells characterize this lesion.

indented. Mitotic activity is variable; some tumors may have a significant amount of mitosis. The mitotic activity, however, is always of the normal type; if abnormal mitoses are present, the lesion is most likely not a GCT. There may be areas containing stromal spindle cells without giant cells; these areas should not be interpreted as a sign of malignant transformation of this tumor. Hemosiderin deposition is usually present in GCTs because of the significant vascularity of the tumor and its inherent focal hemorrhages. Some of the stromal cells are histiocytes and may contain significant amounts of lipid. Collections of these xanthomatous cells give the yellowish appearance of this tumor. Sometimes the quantity of xanthomatous cells is significant, occupying a great portion of the tumor; however, the xanthomatous component has no clinical significance. For tumors showing a predominant spindle cell component along with histiocytic cells and only a focal classic GCT component, Mirra and associates have proposed the term *fibrous histiocytoma–like variant of GCT*.[3]

Cytologic diagnosis of GCT can be also made with FNA.[164] Sheets of osteoclastic giant cells and stromal cells are seen in GCTs; although the FNA findings are not pathognomonic, when put in context with the clinicoradiologic findings they are extremely helpful.

GCTs of the bone tend to keep growing if left alone. They can penetrate through the cortex and invade the adjacent soft tissues, sometimes freezing a joint. Fortunately, most tumors are resected before they reach this state.

Immunohistochemically, GCTs react with histiocytic markers. Ling and associates[165] found a positive reaction for alpha-1-antitrypsin in both the giant cells and the mononuclear stromal cells. Regezi and associates[166] also observed positive reactions for alpha-1-antitrypsin and for alpha-1-antichymotrypsin in both giant and mononuclear cells. S-100 protein stained the mononuclear cells of two of six cases but did not stain the giant cells.[166]

DNA analysis has demonstrated aneuploidy in some GCTs.[167-169] In a study by Sara and colleagues,[168] 16 of 60 cases (27%) of GCT of the bone demonstrated an aneuploid pattern. Relapse was more common in aneuploid tumors than in diploid lesions, but the relapse was related to the treatment modality employed rather than the ploidy status. Fukunaga and associates[169] also concluded that DNA analysis has a limited utility in predicting the biologic behavior of GCT of bone.

TREATMENT AND PROGNOSIS. Current management of GCT includes a thorough curettage followed by cementation with methyl methacrylate of the cavity.[170] Lesions located in "expendable" bones (such as the fibula) are resected. Freezing of the GCT bed with liquid nitrogen has also been utilized to destroy any tumor left after curettage.[171]

GCT of the sacrum is generally difficult to treat because it is nearly impossible to eradicate all of the tumor in that area. Some institutions have utilized a radical management strategy that includes arterial occlusion.[172] Infarcted lesions tend to consolidate in the periphery and to become stable.[172]

Malignant

A primary (de novo) malignant GCT[173] (also called dedifferentiated GCT[174]) of bone is the combination of an untreated, radiologically typical, histologically benign GCT with a synchronous sarcomatous component. Nascimiento and colleagues[173] described eight such cases; the age range was 17 to 76 years, with four patients being 50 years or older. The bones of the knee were most commonly affected.

Malignancy in a GCT may also result from irradiation of a benign GCT.[175] Since most of the reported cases of postradiation sarcomas occurring in GCT are from the older literature, it is believed that sarcomatous transformation was probably caused by utilization of old-fashioned equipment. Sarcomatous transformation of a GCT has also been reported after a long period of latency or after repeated recurrences.[175]

Other malignant GCTs of the bone includes the benign metastasizing GCT. Rock and associates[176] found eight patients with metastasizing GCT in a series of over 400 cases of GCT; four of these tumors originated from the radius. Murray and colleagues[157] found that one of 16 cases of radial GCT metastasized to the lung.

MARROW TUMORS ("ROUND CELL TUMORS")

Ewing's sarcoma

Ewing's sarcoma is a primitive malignant small cell tumor of bone and soft tissue that has a very poor prognosis.[1-4] It encompasses a range of tumors that include the classic Ewing's sarcoma, atypical Ewing's sarcoma, and peripheral neuroectodermal (neuroepithelioma) tumor (PNET), which are linked by a constant chromosomal translocation, t(11;22)(q24;q12).[177-180] Since the clinicoradiologic aspects of these tumors are the same, they are considered together under the general term of *Ewing's sarcoma*.

Ewing's sarcoma accounts for 6% to 14.2% of the primary malignant tumors of bone,[1,181] making it the third most common malignant tumor of bone, exceeded only by osteosarcoma and chondrosarcoma.[1]

Ewing's sarcoma occurs in males twice as often as in females, and it is a disease of children and young adults, with a peak incidence in the second decade of life.[1-4] Ewing's sarcoma may be seen in children under 3 years of age[182,183] or in adults about 40 years of age or older; in these situations, other diseases have to be considered in the differential diagnosis, including neuroblastoma, leukemia/lymphoma in the young children, and metastatic small cell carcinoma in adults. Ewing's sarcoma is essentially a disease of white persons; the incidence in blacks has been reported to be less than 2% of all Ewing's sarcomas.

Most Ewing's sarcomas affect the bones of the lower extremities, with the femur, pelvis, and tibia being the most common sites[1-4] (Fig. 73-42). Any other bones, however, may be affected by this disease.

The initial presentation of this disease may be pain, swelling, or a combination of both; pain is the presenting symptom in over 95% of cases.[1-4] Fever, which has been attributed to tumor necrosis, is not an uncommon accompanying symptom,[184] but some patients with rather large tumors may be asymptomatic. By the time Ewing's sarcoma is detected, it has usually formed a large mass, attesting to its rapid growth.

From the radiologic point of view, Ewing's sarcoma presents as an intramedullary and extramedullary mass that shows a permeative, mottled, or "moth-eaten" radiologic pattern.[1-4] In a long bone the tumor may produce a diffuse fusiform swelling extensively involving the medullary cavity and not uncommonly the entire length of the bone. Generally, there is a large soft-tissue component with an ill-defined margin; the periosteum may give an onionskin appearance, which is not a pathognomonic radiologic sign, since it can also be seen in reactive processes such as osteomyelitis. Another important feature of Ewing's sarcoma is the presence of reactive bone within the medullary cavity. Such change must not be confused with osteosarcoma; the lack of matrix formation in the extraosseous component of the tumor should be a clue that one is dealing with a small cell tumor rather than an osteosarcoma. A periosteal origin has also been described[185] as well as origin in the soft tissues.[186,187] The so-called Askin tumor, representing small cell tumors involving the chest wall, is also within the range of Ewing's sarcoma–peripheral neuroectodermal tumor.[188,189]

CT scan and MRI techniques are of great value in the evaluation of the extent of the lesion, with MRI being the most sensitive.

PATHOLOGY. On gross examination, Ewing's sarcomas have a whitish, glistening, homogeneous appearance that permeates between bony spicules, breaks through the cortex, distends the periosteum and may infiltrate into the adjacent soft tissues (Fig. 73-43). Reactive osteosclerosis may be present within the medullary cavity. Outside the medullary cavity, there may be a spiculated, sunburst response of the periosteum as it is lifted from the bone.

Histologically, Ewing's sarcoma is a primitive round cell tumor with histologic changes ranging from the typical Ewing's sarcoma pattern to the atypical (large cell) Ewing's sarcoma to the peripheral neuroectodermal tumor. The growth pattern in the typical Ewing's sarcoma manifests as a monotonous proliferation of small cells that have round to oval nuclei and scanty cytoplasm. The nuclei show a finely dispersed chromatin pattern and may contain a small nucleolus. The cytoplasm is moderate in amount, but distinct cytoplasmic borders are generally not seen, since the cells overlap one another (Fig. 73-44). Cytoplasm is clear because of its high content of glycogen.[1-4] Atypical (large cell) Ewing's sarcoma[190,191] consists of a round cell proliferation that resembles

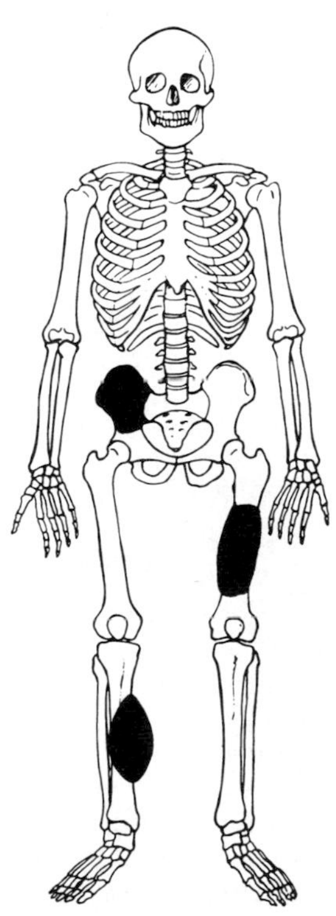

Fig. 73-42 Ewing's sarcoma. Most common anatomic sites of involvement by this tumor.

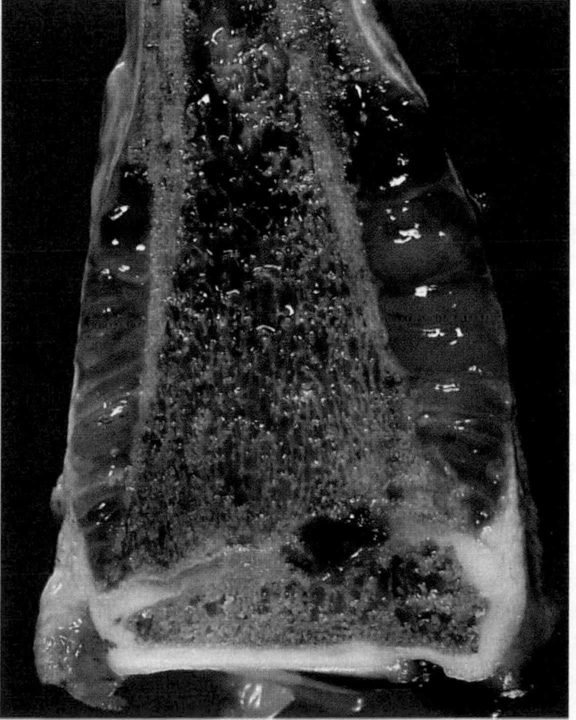

Fig. 73-43 Close-up view of Ewing's sarcoma. The distal end of the tibia shows a permeative glistening tumor in the medullary cavity that extends into the soft tissue but it is still covered by the periosteum.

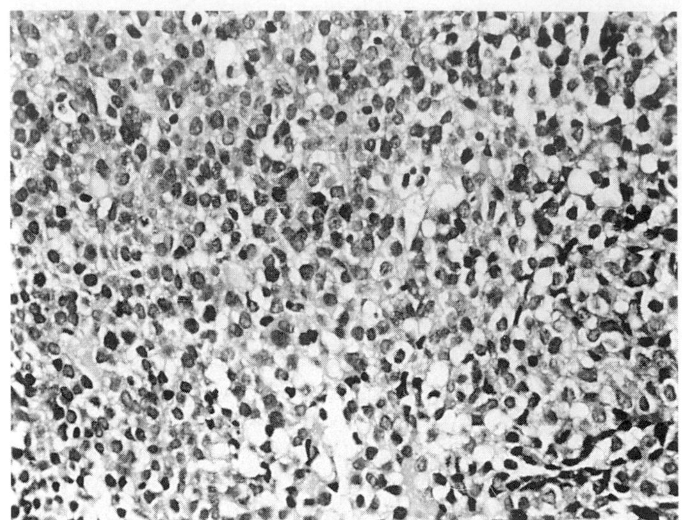

Fig. 73-44 Microscopically, Ewing's sarcoma is characterized by a monotonous proliferation of undifferentiated small cells.

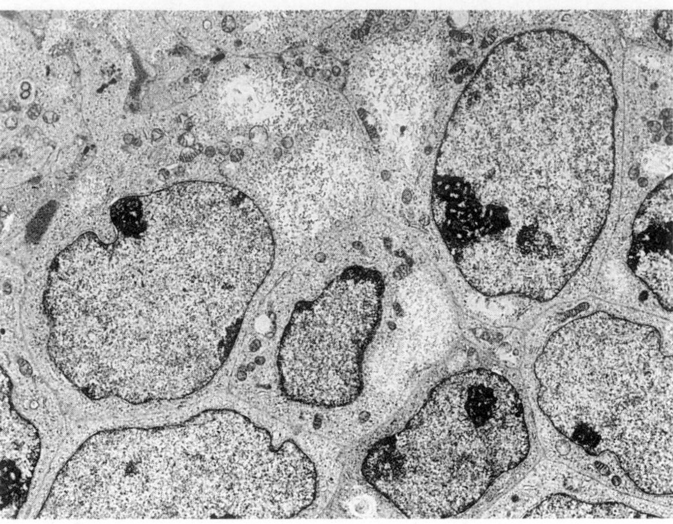

Fig. 73-45 Ultrastructurally the cells of Ewing's sarcoma show round-to-oval nuclei with a fine nuclear chromatin pattern and one or two small nucleoli. The cytoplasm shows very few organelles and some lakes of glycogen.

classic Ewing's sarcoma but shows nuclear pleomorphism, lacks glycogen (glycogen may be seen in electron micrographs), has an increased number of mitoses (more than 2 per high-power field), and has evidence of neoplastic vascular formation.[191]

At the other end of the scale is the PNET that on special procedures (immunohistochemistry and EM) shows neural differentiation but is histologically similar to classic Ewing's sarcoma.

Immunohistochemical profiles in PNET demonstrate immunoreactivity for neuron-specific enolase, neuroblastoma cell surface antigen, neuron cell surface antigen, neurofilament, HNK-1, and HBA71.[192,193] S-100 protein has also been found in PNET, but it is not constant.[180] These markers, however, stain both classic Ewing's sarcoma and PNET.[192,193] At present there are no markers specific for PNET, and its diagnosis has to be based on ultrastructure.

The HBA71 antigen, a cell surface glycoprotein, is expressed in Ewing's sarcoma but apparently not in other small cell neoplasms; it can be detected by use of the monoclonal antibody HBA71 or p30/32^{MIC2} through an immunohistochemical reaction.[194-197]

Fluorescence in situ hybridization, a technique used for gene mapping and ordering probes on interphase and metaphase preparations, has been utilized to diagnose Ewing's sarcoma and PNET.[198] In the future this application may prove to be a simple diagnostic test.

Under the electron microscope, the cells of classic Ewing's sarcoma reflect its histologic pattern. The monotonous nuclei are round to oval and contain a fine chromatin pattern with some small nucleoli. The cytoplasm contains very few organelles and abundant glycogen (Fig. 73-45). Between the cells there are small attachments, but true desmosomes are not seen. Atypical Ewing's sarcoma shows similar changes except for pleomorphic nuclear profiles.[3,4,199]

PNET differs from Ewing's sarcoma in that it contains neurosecretory granules and neural processes. The neurosecretory granules are dense core granules with 120 to 150 nm in diameter.

The diagnosis of Ewing's sarcoma can be made by FNA, a core needle biopsy, or an open biopsy. At the M.D. Anderson Cancer Center, interventional radiologists do core or FNA biopsies. The initial step is to aspirate the tumor and submit it to the cytopathologist for evaluation. If it is a small cell tumor, the radiologist is immediately notified so that additional aspirations can be made for (1) diagnosis, (2) EM, and (3) cytogenetic analysis.

TREATMENT AND PROGNOSIS. The management strategy for Ewing's sarcoma is primary chemotherapy. Chemotherapy can destroy most of the tumor, and once the tumor is clinically deleted, the area of the origin in the bone should be resected surgically. Radiotherapy is also utilized in combination with chemotherapy, though many oncologists would rather utilize radiation for consolidation of the chemotherapy. In the first intergroup Ewing's sarcoma study of patients with disease localized to the bone (1973-1978), the treatment regimen was a combination of cyclophosphamide, vincristine, dactinomycin, Adriamycin (doxorubicin), and radiation therapy to the tumor. At 5 years the disease-free survival was 60% and the survival rate was 65%. However, the survival for patients with metastatic disease was very poor.[200]

Lymphoreticular neoplasms

Non-Hodgkin's lymphoma

Lymphoma of bone was described over 50 years ago, but much of the knowledge of lymphoma of the lymphatic system and of bone has been acquired within the last decade. Primary non-Hodgkin's lymphoma of bone may be defined as an extranodal lymphoma histologically similar to its nodal counterpart, affecting bone that may or may not subsequently develop systemic or multicentric disease. For the tumor to be categorized as primary bone lymphoma, there must be an interval of 4 to 6 months between the onset of the osseous manifestation and the development of systemic disease.

The age of patients with malignant lymphoma of bone ranges from 1 to 91 years, but well over half of patients are over 40 years of age.[1-4] A slight predominance of males has been reported (a male-to-female ratio of 1.6:1).[2,201-203] Lymphoma may develop in almost any bone of the body, but particular sites are commonly affected: the femur (21.9%) and sacrum and pelvis (19.4%).[2,201-203] The long bones of the extremities are more commonly involved than the bones of the axial skeleton are. Lymphomas of bone may be multifocal; the incidence of multifocality varies from 11% to 38%.[2,201-203]

Pain is the most common initial manifestation of disease, but tenderness or swelling may also be presenting signs. Fever is uncommon, in contrast with Ewing's sarcoma, in which fever is common.[1-4,201-203]

The radiologic features of malignant lymphoma are similar to those of Ewing's sarcoma or any other small cell lesion.[204,205] There is a permeative pattern of infiltration, and there may be a soft-tissue component; when this occurs, the soft-tissue component does not present any matrix formation. A not-uncommon feature is the presence of dense sclerotic bone reaction within the medullary cavity, which may simulate an osteosarcoma. The so-called ivory vertebra often harbors malignant lymphoma. The intraosseous advancing tumor edge of lymphoma is usually ill defined. CT scans and MRI are invaluable in establishing the degree of soft-tissue involvement. MRI also helps to evaluate the degree of bone marrow involvement.[1-4,201-203]

PATHOLOGY. Grossly, malignant lymphoma is similar to Ewing's sarcoma in its color and infiltrative pattern. The cut surface shows a grayish white tumor with a fish-flesh appearance permeating the cancellous bone or producing a "moth-eaten" pattern of destruction. The medullary cavity may show bone sclerosis. Permeation of the cortex with spread outside the bone is common, though malignant lymphoma may remain confined to the bone.

Histologically, malignant lymphoma of bone may be represented by any of the special cell types. However, large or mixed large and small cell types are by far the most common types seen in bones.[2,201-203] Most are the diffuse B-cell type of lymphomas,[206-208] and tumors composed of large cleaved cells appear to have a better prognosis than those of large noncleaved cells or of the immunoblastic type.[202,203]

Immunohistochemistry is very valuable in the differential diagnosis of lymphoma from other small cell tumors. Immunohistochemical profiles are used to confirm a diagnosis of lymphoma and to characterize the cell lineage. Leukocytic common antigen (LCA) is an overall marker for lymphoid lesions, and a positive reaction in the tumor cells is indicative of a lymphoma. A commonly utilized pan–B-cell marker L26 (CD20) is also extremely helpful. These markers have the advantage of being effective in paraffin-embedded tissues. In addition to the above markers, a pan–T-cell marker often utilized is the UCHL1 (CD45). T-cell lymphoma and anaplastic Ki-1 lymphomas rarely occur within the bone. The role of gene rearrangement studies has not been established so far in the study of bone lymphoma.

TREATMENT. Management has been irradiation to the bone involved, but approximately 50% of the cases relapse. Consequently current management includes both radiotherapy and chemotherapy.[209]

Hodgkin's lymphoma

Although Hodgkin's disease has been reported to occur as a primary bone lesion,[201] it is extremely rare. However, secondary bone involvement is known to occur in patients who have histories of the nodular sclerosing type of Hodgkin's disease.

Solitary plasmacytoma

Multiple myeloma is not discussed in this chapter, since it is not a true primary bone tumor. However, solitary plasmacytoma of bone often presents its initial course as a primary lesion of bone.

Solitary plasmacytoma of bone is a localized plasma cell tumor unaccompanied by evidence of systemic disease. It is rare, occurring in 5% of patients with plasma cell myeloma.[210] Men are affected in about 70% of cases, and the median ages of incidence reported range from 50 to 58 years.[211] Any bone may be affected, but one third of cases occur in the spine.[211] Pain is the most common presenting symptom.[212]

Required diagnostic criteria include (1) solitary bone lesion, (2) a negative skeletal survey, (3) the absence of plasma cell infiltrate in random bone marrow samples, (4) a lack of anemia, hypercalcemia, or renal involvement, and (5) presence in a biopsy specimen of a monoclonal plasma cell proliferation.[211] Meis and colleagues reported that nuclear immaturity and the presence of nucleoli appear to be the best indicators to predict the development of multiple myeloma.[213]

The management strategy for solitary plasmacytoma is radiotherapy. Adjuvant therapy has been utilized, but no convincing benefit has been shown to result.[211] Although long-term control can be achieved with radiotherapy, in most patients (85%) the disease eventually progresses to multiple myeloma.[211]

VASCULAR TUMORS

Benign

Hemangioma

Hemangioma is a benign lesion composed of vessels, which may be capillaries or large cavernous venous vessels, or a combination of both.[1-4] Histologically they are similar to soft-tissue hemangiomas.[1-4]

Hemangiomas are rare and occur at any age but are commonly seen after middle age. Women are affected more commonly than are men.

Most hemangiomas are asymptomatic unless they compromise adjacent organs. If symptoms develop, they are usually insidious.

The spine is the most common location, followed by the skull, though a hemangioma may occur at any site. Lymphangiomas may also occur in bones, but they are rarer than hemangiomas.

Skeletal angiomatosis and lymphangiomatosis

Skeletal angiomatosis and lymphangiomatosis is a rare disorder; less than 100 cases have been reported. It may be solitary or multicentric. A bone may be involved without soft-tissue compromise, but some cases may have extensive soft-tissue involvement, and some patients may even have visceral involvement.[1-4]

Disappearing bone disease (Gorham's disease)

Gorham's disease is another benign vascular lesion of the bone characterized clinically by the virtual disappearance of the bone affected by a hemangiomatous proliferation.[1-4,214,215]

Glomus tumor (glomangioma)

Glomus tumor, or glomangioma, is a benign lesion of bone that occurs most commonly in the medullary cavity of a distal phalanx. Histologically, it consists of uniform cells with round nuclei that are associated with vascular structures, sometimes around small vessels and occasionally arising from or infiltrating the wall of thicker vessels.[1-4]

Malignant

There has been a significant amount of confusion in regard to the terminology for malignant tumors of vessel origin. However, even in early articles on malignant tumors, it was recognized that there were two types of malignant vascular tumors: some with a low-grade behavior and some with a high-grade behavior.[216-219] The work of Rosai and collaborators[220] in regard to vascular lesions of soft tissue and bone has shed significant light on these tumors. These investigators postulated that vascular tumors containing large, plump histiocytoid cells have a good prognosis and collectively named such tumors "histiocytoid hemangiomas." Tsuneyoshi and colleagues,[221] based on an article on soft-tissue lesions,[222] introduced the term *epithelioid hemangioendothelioma* for bone lesions. In this chapter we discuss three types of vascular lesions: hemangioendothelioma, which represents a range of benign/low-grade vascular tumors characterized by histiocytoid/epithelioid cells; the high-grade vascular tumor referred to as "angiosarcoma"; and hemangiopericytoma.

Hemangioendothelioma

Hemangioendothelioma of bone encompasses vascular lesions that have as a common denominator the presence of large histiocytoid and epithelioid cells; the size of these lesions range from small lesions, termed "epithelioid hemangiomas,"[223] that are similar to angiolymphoid hyperplasia of the skin[224,225] to lesions, called "epithelioid hemangioendotheliomas," that are cellular and may be confused with other neoplasms.[221,222] These lesions may be solitary or multicentric.[221,225,226]

Hemangioendothelioma of bone has been described in the second, third, fourth, fifth, and sixth decades with about equal frequency, but it is extremely rare under 10 years of age.[219,221,225,226] It is slightly more common in males than in females and can occur in almost any bone. When it is multicentric, it tends to affect one extremity, and the lesions seldom skip beyond the extremity; when the tumor is solitary, it tends to involve the epiphysis and metaphysis of the long bones but has also been seen in the diaphysis of the bones.

From the radiologic point of view, these lesions manifest themselves as osteolytic lesions that generally show areas of peripheral sclerosis, attesting to their slow growth. Angiography shows that they are vascular tumors.

PATHOLOGY. On gross examination, the tumors are red-brown and hemorrhagic, reflecting the vascularity present throughout the tumor. At times the surgeon finds a large-caliber feeding vessel.

Histologically, this tumor consists of a proliferation of small vessels lined by characteristic large, plump histiocytoid and epithelioid cells that have round to oval nuclei, often containing nucleoli, and abundant cytoplasm[220] (Fig. 73-46). In some areas the endothelial cells are so prominent that they occlude the lumen of the vessels. The morphology is best appreciated at the periphery of the tumor, where single capillaries containing plump endothelial cells are easily seen. Although most of the benign and low-grade lesions do not show mitotic activity, 2 to 10 mitotic figures per 10 high-power fields may be seen. Another cell that often appears in this tumor is the eosinophil. This inflammatory cell is often seen scattered or in clumps within a hemangioendothelioma. The histologic features of multicentric tumors are identical to those of unicentric tumors.

For tumors in which the vascular proliferation becomes solid, no longer forming vascular spaces but instead forming anastomosing cords or nests or fascicles of large vacuolated cells, usually over a myxoid background, the term *epithelioid hemangioendothelioma* has been used.[221] This growth pattern may be mistaken for metastatic carcinoma, chordoma, chondrosarcoma, chondromyxoid fibroma, or other neoplasms.[221,222] Despite this alarming histologic pattern, only one of 14 patients developed metastasis (in the abdomen from a vertebra primary) in the series of Tsuneyoshi and colleagues.[221]

TREATMENT AND PROGNOSIS. Unicentric tumors can be controlled with curettage and bone packing or cement packing. However, in a relatively low percentage of patients, the tumor may recur in the same site; management for the recurrent lesions should also be conservative. Since multicentric lesions are difficult to control, a major amputation may be needed.

High-grade angiosarcoma

The high-grade angiosarcomas in bone do not differ in histology from the high-grade angiosarcomas seen in soft tissues. Histologically, they show typical anastomosing vascular channels and high-grade pleomorphism of the individual cells. These tumors often have solid areas with no vascular differentiation. These tumors are rare and have been described in many bones; there does not seem to be a particularly preferred site. Management strategies for these lesions include surgery, chemotherapy, and radiotherapy.

Hemangiopericytoma

Hemangiopericytoma of the bone is an extremely rare vascular tumor that accounts for 0.08% of all primary bone tumors and 0.1% of all primary malignant bone tumors.[1,2,227]

The age of presentation ranges from the second to the ninth decade of life; and there is a peak incidence in the fourth and

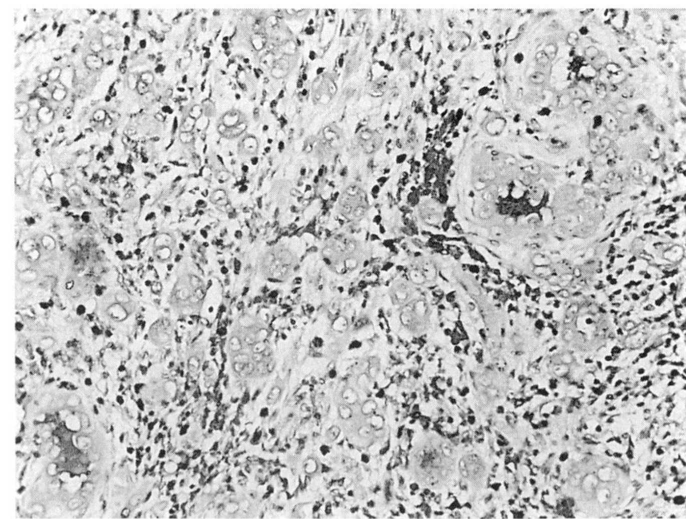

Fig. 73-46 Hemangioendothelioma of bone. The tumor consists of numerous vessels lined by large, plump, endothelial cells.

fifth decades.[1,2,227,228] The male-to-female ratio is about 1.8:1.[229] Pain is the most common presenting complaint, though some cases may manifest a mass that persists from weeks to years. The most common location of this tumor is within the bones of the pelvis and lower extremities.[2,229] The lesions usually affect the medullary cavity, though rarely they may arise in a periosteal location.[229]

Radiographically, hemangiopericytomas show a lytic type of bone destruction that is nonspecific. CT scans and MRI may be valuable in demonstrating the extent of the tumor but are not diagnostic.[229]

Histologically, hemangiopericytoma is similar to its soft-tissue counterpart. There are sheets of closely packed spindle cells surrounding capillaries. Typical staghorn-like vascular spaces are a prominent finding.

This lesion is treated surgically by en bloc excision with clean margins or by an amputation. The reported survivals in this group of patients at 5 and 10 years are 75% and 44% respectively.[229] Metastasis occurs most often in the lung.

MISCELLANEOUS TUMORS

Adamantinoma of the long bones

Adamantinoma of the long bones is a rare low-grade malignant lesion that shows both epithelial and mesenchymal differentiation. The name refers to the strong resemblance of the histologic pattern of this tumor to adamantinoma arising in the jaws, but there is nothing in common between these two types of tumors.[1-4]

This lesion is extremely rare, accounting for less than 1% of all primary malignant tumors of bone. The incidence of this lesion is equally distributed among males and females or slightly higher in males, and the tumor is most commonly seen in the second, third, and fourth decades of life. Nearly all adamantinomas (90%) involve the shaft of the tibia, but the lesion has also been described in other bones.[230-232] Pain is the most common initial complaint and is of long duration (many months or even years) in some patients, attesting to the chronicity of the tumor.[1]

From the radiologic point of view, adamantinoma has a typical appearance, which has been described as a soap-bubble pattern; this pattern consists of multiple sharply circumscribed, radiolucent areas of different sizes that contain a rim of sclerotic bone. These radiolucent areas are usually eccentrically located in the shaft of the tibia; early lesions may be localized, but long-standing lesions may show a diffuse involvement of the bone. The lesion also induces remodeling of the bone, manifested by dilatation of the medullary cavity. Scalloping and breakthrough of the cortex may be also present.[1,3]

PATHOLOGY. On gross examination, adamantinoma of bone appears lobulated. The cut surface of the tumor is whitish and glistening, denoting the high content of fibrous connective tissue. Multiple cystlike spaces are present and surrounded by thick sclerotic bone. At the cortex there may be scooped-out endosteal areas, or the cortex may be totally destroyed (Fig. 73-47).

On histologic examination, adamantinoma contains epithelial and stromal elements.[233] The epithelial component may show different patterns; one of these, resembling a basal cell carcinoma of the skin, consists of nests of darkly staining cells that have a peripheral palisading of these cells (Fig. 73-48). Another pattern simulates a vascular tumor; cords of cells focally containing a lumenlike formation may form an anastomosing pattern simulating the appearance of an angiosarcoma. In addition, adamantinomas may show squamoid or glandular change. Expression of keratin is found in the epithelial cells of adamantinoma.[234] The stroma is generally fibroblastic, and its fibrous tissue varies from loose to very cellular.

A fibrous dysplasia–like component is also a well-known component of adamantinoma.[1-4,233] Occasionally it may be the predominant component of an adamantinoma. Some tibial lesions do not show an epithelial component but only a fibro-osseous proliferation otherwise typical of osteofibrous dysplasia; these lesions may exhibit keratin expression in the spindle cells. The term *differentiated (regressing) or juvenile adamantinoma* has been applied to such lesions.[3,137] Whether these

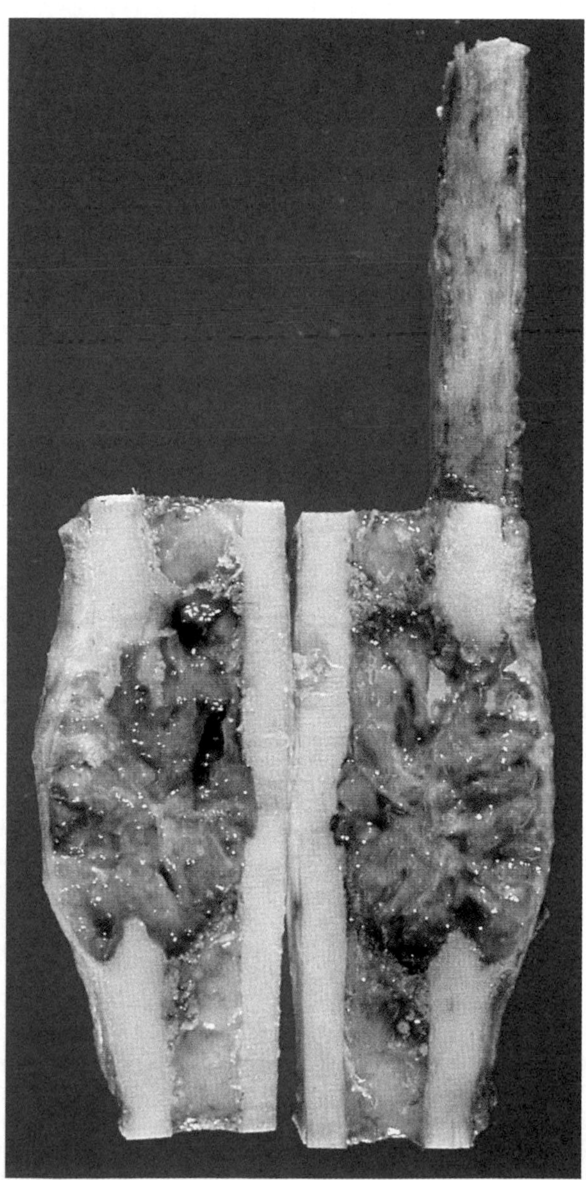

Fig. 73-47 A bivalved segment of the tibia showing a medullary tumor that is destroying the cortex and is elevating the periosteum. The thin segment of cortical bone was resected because small lytic areas of tumor growth were present.

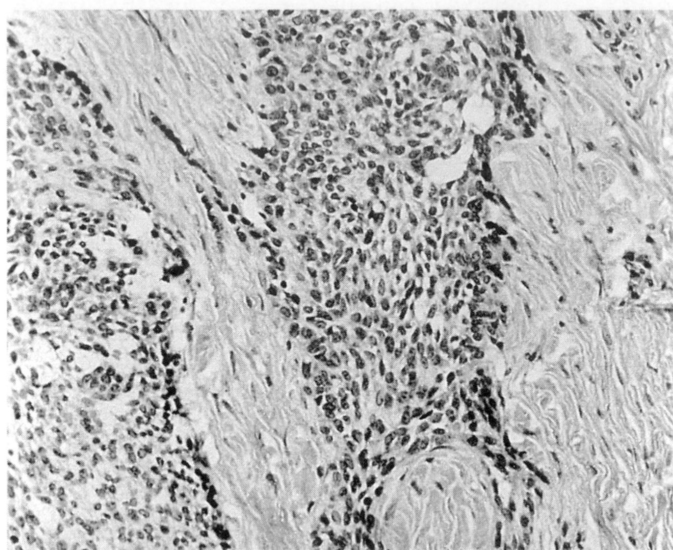

Fig. 73-48 Adamantinoma. Notice the dark basaloid cells separated by a dense fibrous stroma.

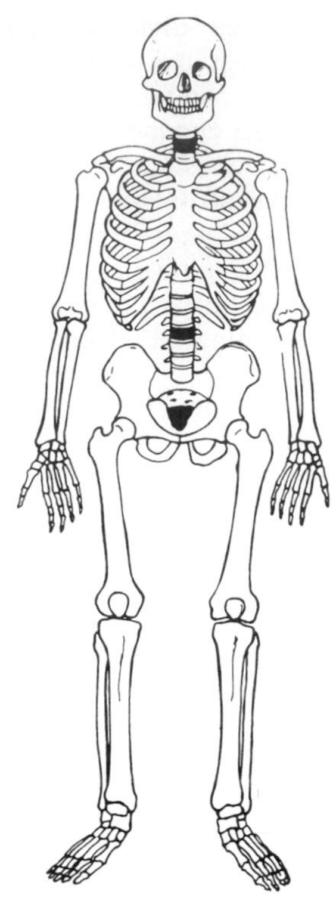

Fig. 73-49 Chordoma. Spinal axis distribution of this tumor.

lesions are true adamantinomas or variants of osteofibrous dysplasia or a link between the two remains to be proved, but so far no case of this lesion has shown malignant progression to adamantinoma (see also the discussion of osteofibrous dysplasia).

TREATMENT AND PROGNOSIS. The management of adamantinoma is surgical. Resection with clear margins is the therapy of choice, and whether an en bloc resection or an amputation is necessary will depend on the extent of the lesion.

The incidences of recurrence and lung metastasis are about 30% and 15% respectively, and regional lymph node metastasis may also occur.[232] Metastatic disease may occur many years after the initial surgery; in the series reported by Keeney and associates,[232] 13 of 85 patients developed lung metastasis, and 6 of 85 patients developed lymph node metastasis, an average of 8.2 and 5.8 years respectively after the initial diagnosis. Therefore a long-term follow-up study should be planned for patients with this disease.

Chordoma

Chordoma is not an uncommon tumor; it accounts for about 4% of the primary malignant bone tumors seen at the Mayo Clinic.[1] It is a lesion of the midline of the spinal column that originates from primitive notochord.[1-4]

The peak incidence for this lesion is in the sixth decade of life.[1-4] The lesion is distinctly uncommon in children and affects more males than females (1.8:1).[1-4] About half of the tumors occur in the sacrococcygeal region and 37% at the base of the skull in the spheno-occipital region. The cervical, lumbar, and thoracic regions are involved in descending order of frequency (Fig. 73-49).

The symptoms are related to the destruction and compromise of the regions affected by the tumor. Pain is a common initial symptom in sacrococcygeal tumors, and as the tumor grows, invading nerve roots and compressing the rectum, additional discomfort and constipation may occur.[1-4] Spheno-occipital lesions cause nerve-related symptoms and, if they grow inside the cranial cavity, may cause increased intracerebral pressure.

Radiologically a sacrococcygeal chordoma exhibits a mass that destroys the sacrum and may protrude into the pelvic cavity; although lytic, it may contain amorphous residual osseous tissue or dystrophic calcifications. Plain films may not demonstrate the lesion, but CT and MRI provide invaluable information, especially the extension and relation of the lesion to the pelvic anatomic structures. In the skull there are invariably lytic changes in the region of the clivus. Vertebral lesions tend to show asymmetric destruction of the bone with an adjacent soft-tissue mass.[235]

PATHOLOGY. On gross examination chordoma is a gray-white tumor with myxoid areas, focal necrosis, and focal hemorrhage. The tumor is lobulated and usually well delimited, but the advancing margin is ill defined, especially the bone margin. The lesions affecting the clivus are similar. Because of the myxoid matrix of chordomas, lesions may grossly resemble a mucus-producing adenocarcinoma or a myxoid chondrosarcoma.[1-4]

Histologically the tumor appears lobulated; the lobules vary in size and shape and are separated by bands of connective tissue. Within the nodules there is a myxoid background, over which there is a cellular network arranged in strands of cells interconnecting with each other. The cells of chordoma are round, sometimes spindle shaped, and not uncommonly gigantic. Most cells show numerous vacuoles, but the characteristic chordoma cell is a large multivacuolated cell that resembles a jellyfish, the physaliferous cell (Fig. 73-50). The nuclei are generally round, but the cytoplasm may be elongated, angu-

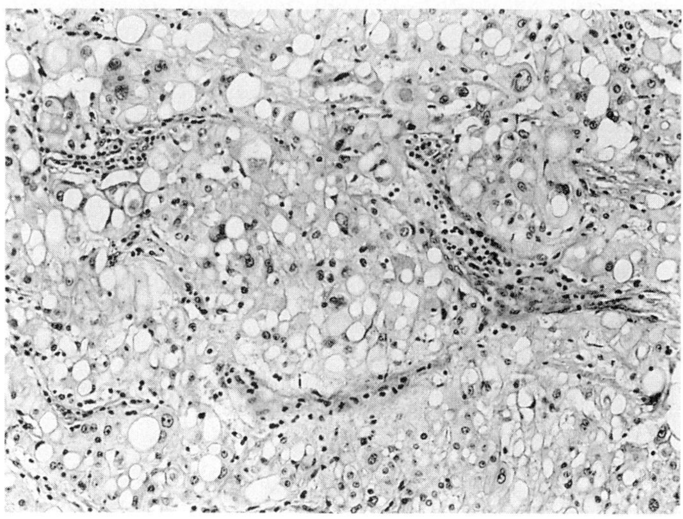

Fig. 73-50 Chordoma. Over a myxoid background there are cords of large cells with vacuolated cytoplasm.

lated, or rounded. The elongated cells join each other by tails of their cytoplasm; cellular areas, however, show indistinct cell borders. Mitotic activity is meager, but some tumors may be mitotically active.[1-4]

Chordomas contain cytoplasmic glycogen and mucopolysaccharides.[236] On immunohistochemistry study, chordomas coexpress cytokeratin, epithelial membrane antigen, vimentin, and the S-100 protein.[237,238] These features provide invaluable information for the differential diagnosis.

Chordomas arising in the base of the skull may contain a low-grade hyaline cartilage; these are designated chondroid chordomas. In the Mayo Clinic series, about one third of these tumors are partially or almost completely made up of chondroid tissue.[1,239]

TREATMENT AND PROGNOSIS. The management of chordoma is surgical. Sacral lesions are resected and then treated with radiotherapy to the bed, especially if it was difficult to obtain clean margins. In the base of the skull, resection of all the tumor should be attempted.[1-4]

Although surgery cures some patients, especially patients with small resectable lesions, most chordomas recur; the sacral lesions progress to form large pelvic masses that eventually spread to the peritoneum. Distant metastasis may develop late in the course of the disease.[1-4]

In the spheno-occipital region the chondroid chordomas have a slow-growing relatively long indolent behavior.[239-241]

Chordomas may transform to high-grade sarcomas usually with the pattern of malignant fibrous histiocytoma or that of a high-grade unclassified spindle cell sarcoma.[242-244] The term *dedifferentiated chordoma* has been applied to this variant.[244] When this transformation occurs, the behavior of this tumor worsens, and metastatic disease is likely to develop shortly in the course of the disease requiring aggressive chemotherapy.[2,245,246]

Parachordoma (chordoma periphericum)

In 1977 Dabska[247] described a rare tumor that resembled chordoma histologically; unlike chordoma, however, it arose outside the spinal column, where there is no notochord. This lesion, called "parachordoma," is identical or nearly identical in morphology to chordoma and shares the same immunohistochemical reactions. In the soft tissues it arises deep within tendons or aponeuroses, usually in contact with the periosteum. It may also arise from bone, and when it does, it involves the cortical surface. Management of this lesion is surgical. Parachordoma has a much better prognosis than chordoma does. Incompletely excised tumors may recur, but the recurrence is late (within a few years). So far no case has shown distant metastasis, though the number of cases has been too small to enable a definitive statement.

NONNEOPLASTIC TUMOROUS CONDITIONS

There are several lesions that show radiologic features simulating neoplastic lesions of bone. In general the histopathologic features of these lesions are those of reactive bone changes, but such changes may be misinterpreted for a bone tumor.

The most common pseudoneoplastic lesions occurring in normal bones include unicameral bone cyst, aneurysmal bone cyst, eosinophilic granuloma, exuberant fracture callus, stress fracture, Charcot's disease of the joints, hemophiliac pseudotumor, osteomyelitis, brown tumor of hyperparathyroidism, osteitis condensans of the clavicle, mastocytosis, and others. Some of these lesions are discussed in detail, whereas others are only briefly mentioned.

Simple bone cyst (unicameral bone cyst)

Although simple cysts of bone were known before the turn of the century,[248] Jaffe and Lichtenstein in 1942 elegantly described the epidemiology, radiologic features, and pathology of these lesions.[249] The cause of simple cysts is still unknown.[1-4,248,249]

Simple cysts are common in children and adolescents[2,3] and usually begin to form at about 4 years of age. A simple bone cyst is asymptomatic and generally is diagnosed as a result of a pathologic fracture or of an incidental trauma to the area.[2,3]

Early lesions develop at or beneath the epiphyseal plate, and as the bone grows in length, the cyst tends to migrate to the diaphysis; hence older lesions are large and occupy a significant portion of the bone.[2,3,249]

Radiologically a unicameral bone cyst presents as a radiolucent change with expansion of the bone beginning at the epiphyseal line and extending into the diaphysis; healed or fresh fractures may be present.[2,3]

PATHOLOGY. Grossly, the wall of a simple cyst consists of a thin fragment of connective tissue. The cavity has a clear pink fluid that contains elevated levels of prostaglandin[250] and extracellular lysosomal enzymes.[251] Both of these substances have been implicated in the pathogenesis of this lesion. Histologically the cyst wall consists of a thin layer of fibrous connective tissue with few or no osteoclastic giant cells.[2,3] Reparative new bone formation secondary to the fracture may also be seen.

TREATMENT AND PROGNOSIS. The current management technique is instillation of methylprednisolone acetate into the cavity.[252] Under this treatment reparative connective tissue fills the cavity and is later replaced by bone. A 70% healing rate occurs with this treatment.[253] In contrast, with curettage and bone packing, the healing rate is 53%.[253]

Aneurysmal bone cyst

There are two types of aneurysmal bone cyst (ABC), those that arise de novo (primary ABC), and those that arise on a preexisting bone lesion (secondary ABC).

Primary ABC

Primary ABC is a relatively uncommon bone lesion, accounting for 1% to 6% of all bone lesions.[1-4] It was recognized over 50 years ago,[254,255] and there are numerous publications on the subject. Its importance derives from the fact that it is a lesion in children and young adults and affects the metaphysis of the long bones, characteristics that are shared with conventional osteosarcoma.[1-4]

The peak age of incidence of this lesion is the second decade of life.[256,257] ABC may be seen in adults, but children less than 15 years old are most commonly affected; a study at the M.D. Anderson Cancer Center found an average age of 16.6 years in 22 males and 26 females with ABC.[256] A slightly higher incidence in females is also reflected in the literature.[255-258] Almost any bone may be affected, but the extremities, particularly the femur and proximal tibia are by far the most common sites[1-3,256,257] (Fig. 73-51). As with conventional osteosarcoma, the metaphysis is the location affected by this lesion, a fact that should be kept in mind when one is evaluating a bone lesion.

Radiologically, the lesion involves the metaphysis of long and short tubular bones,[256,257] especially the metadiaphyseal area, in most cases. A large, blown-out eccentric lytic lesion producing an aneurysm-like change is typically found. The inner aspect of an ABC may show a sclerotic rim of bone tissue, but the peripheral advancing edge usually destroys the cortex, producing a large bulging effect. The periosteum, however, contains this lesion. If the periosteum is calcified, an eggshell-like appearance may be seen; if not, the advancing edge may look infiltrative. CT scan becomes very valuable, since it can clearly demonstrate the sharp periosteal margin. The main differential diagnosis on x-ray films is from telangiectatic osteosarcoma.[257]

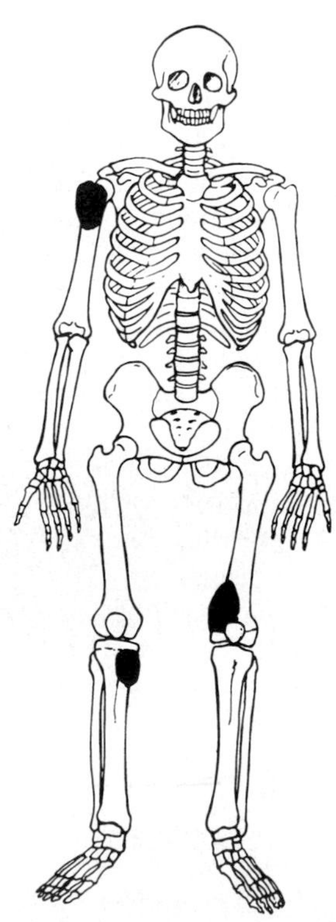

Fig. 73-51 Primary aneurysmal bone cyst (ABC). ABC affects the metaphysis of the long bones, with the proximal end of the humerus, distal end of the femur, and proximal end of the tibia being the most common locations.

PATHOLOGY. Grossly, ABC consists of multiple hemorrhagic cysts and a solid component. Microscopically the cysts are lined by connective tissue that contains stroma and few giant cells (Fig. 73-52); not uncommonly, the cyst walls contain a few slender spicules of reactive bone. Mitotic figures may be seen, but none of them are atypical.[256,257] In the usual situation, the solid component is not prominent. When present, it is usually located in the advancing edges of the lesion. It consists of a reactive fibro-osseous proliferation with active osteoblastic proliferation and osteoid formation. One should be aware of this change to avoid mistaking ABC for osteosarcoma. Reactive fibroblastic proliferation may also be seen. These reactive changes are similar to those seen in myositis ossificans or in nodular fasciitis.

Some ABCs may be almost totally composed of a solid component, an observation that has given origin to the term "solid ABC."[259] In general most solid ABCs do have a minimal typical cystic component.

The cause of ABC is uncertain. One of the most widely held views is that a local vascular disturbance attributable to either trauma or a preexisting lesion results in an arteriovenous shunt.[2] Dahlin and McLeod[260] have proposed that ABC is a purely reparative proliferation similar to other reparative lesions such as myositis ossificans and reparative granuloma. Other theories involve a developmental error or an aberrant overgrowth of pluripotential cells.[261,262] Dodd and associates[256] recently found two near-diploid aneuploid lesions of 27 examples of ABC. This finding, along with the recent description of chromosomal abnormalities in ABC,[263,264] is sugges-

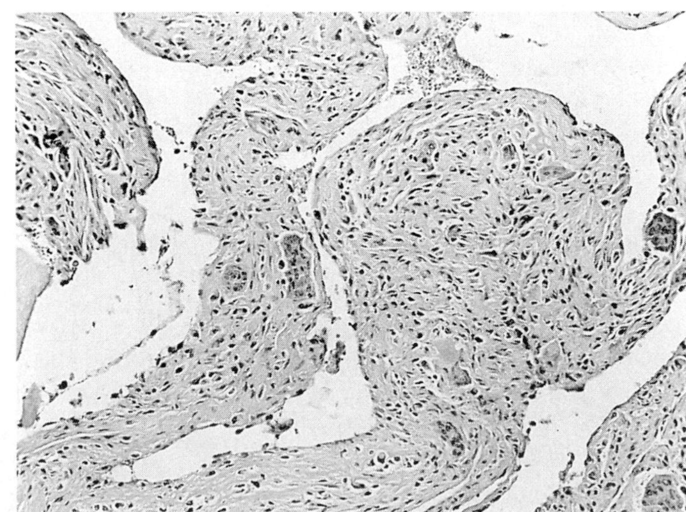

Fig. 73-52 Thin membranous walls of the multiple cystic areas of an ABC.

tive of a neoplastic origin for ABC. Because of the limited material, a conclusive statement cannot be made.

TREATMENT AND PROGNOSIS. The management strategy for primary ABC is curettage with bone packing. With this treatment, recurrence rates have been reported to be as high as 40%.[256] Recurrence of ABC in the majority of cases appears within 2 years of the initial treatment. Recurrences are treated identically, with curettage and bone packing.[256,257] Malignant transformation of ABC has also been reported.[265]

Secondary ABC

Most benign lesions of bone may have a secondary ABC; giant cell tumor and chondroblastoma are the tumors most commonly affected by a secondary ABC. The solid pattern of GCT of bone may be almost totally replaced by the typical multicystic hemorrhagic change of ABC. In a curettage it may be impossible to distinguish between primary ABC and secondary ABC. The location in the bone (metaphysis for primary ABC and epiphysis for GCT of bone with secondary ABC), usually gives the clue to the diagnosis. Chondroblastoma may have a significant amount of ABC component, and the differential diagnosis may be difficult from a biopsy specimen. However, on curetted specimens the differential diagnosis is not difficult; the cell composition (in particular the grooved nuclei of the chondroblasts) allows one to give the diagnosis. There is no clinical significance of an ABC component in GCT of bone. However, some investigators believe that an ABC component in chondroblastoma imparts a higher tendency for recurrence than chondroblastoma without an ABC component.[2]

Other lesions associated with secondary ABC include fibrous dysplasia, osteofibrous dysplasia of Campanacci, nonossifying fibroma, and fibrous histiocytoma.[1-4]

Eosinophilic granuloma

Eosinophilic granuloma of bone is a benign, solitary, or multiple tumorlike disorder of children or young adults.[1-4] It is part of the range of Langerhans histiocytosis that also includes the fatal Letterer-Siwe disease of children and the chronic form of Hand-Schüller-Christian disease seen in adults. This triad of diseases was also known by the collective name of "histiocytosis X." Lichtenstein and Jaffe coined the name of "eosinophilic granuloma."[266]

Solitary eosinophilic granuloma occurs in children and young adults; about half of the cases occur in the first decade of life. Rare cases may be encountered in patients over 30 years of age. There is a slight predominance in females both in the solitary and in the multifocal disease.

Pain is the usual initial manifestation of the disease, though some patients may present with limping if the lesion is located in the lower extremities. The polyostotic form of the disease may be associated with exophthalmos or diabetes insipidus. Almost any bone may be involved.

Radiologically the solitary lesion presents an alarming lytic aspect that may be confused with Ewing's sarcoma. The lytic region usually occurs in the medulla of a bone but may start in the cortex. MRI findings are nonspecific and may also simulate malignancy.[267]

PATHOLOGY. Histologically the basic proliferation is of Langerhans' histiocytes, which are accompanied by a variable number of eosinophils; chronic inflammatory cells may be focally present (Fig. 73-53). The histiocytes are positive for S-100 protein and for peanut agglutinin, which are the most commonly used markers for this disease. Ultrastructurally, the Langerhans' histiocyte shows Birbeck granules; these are rod-shaped structures, some of which exhibit a tennis-racket shape. The rods contain a central striated lamella, creating an overall picture resembling a zipper (Fig. 73-54).

Cytologic diagnosis is easily made.[268,269] Smears show histiocytes with grooved or infolded nuclei and numerous eosinophils. Other cells such as multinucleated giant cells, foamy histiocytes, lymphocytes, and plasma cells may also be seen.[269]

TREATMENT AND PROGNOSIS. The current management technique for eosinophilic granuloma is the intralesional injection of steroids.[270] Curettage or radiotherapy also gives good results.

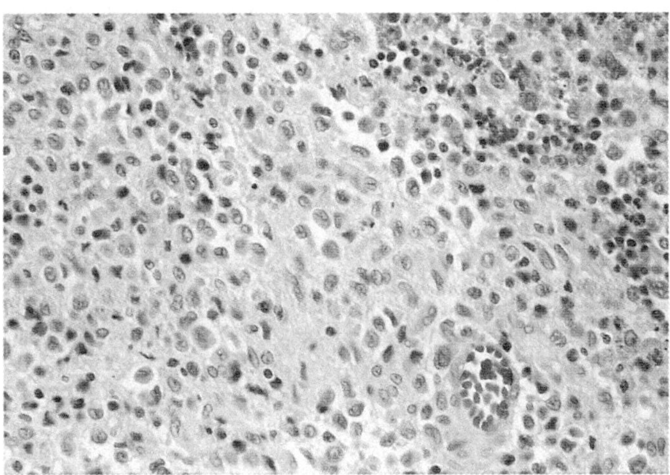

Fig. 73-53 Histologically, eosinophilic granuloma consists of a proliferation of histiocytes (Langerhans' cells) depicted here as the large collection of cells with abundant cytoplasm and a variable number of inflammatory cells including eosinophils.

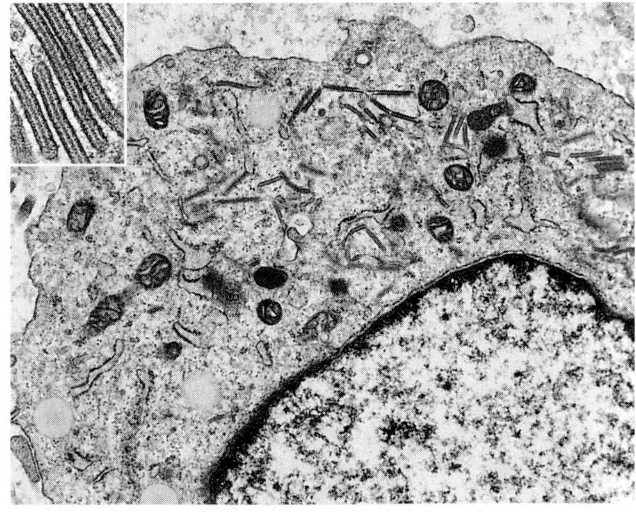

Fig. 73-54 Ultrastructurally the Langerhans' cells contain Birbeck granules, which are seen in the cytoplasm of the cell and in the inset.

Fracture callus

An exuberant callus developing in a fractured bone may pose a significant diagnostic problem. When a fracture develops, several sequential steps occur in the process of healing. Initially there is hemorrhage, edema, necrosis, and fibrin exudation followed by granulation tissue with an intense mesenchymal proliferation of primitive spindle cells that will differentiate into osteoblasts and chondroblasts. Osteoid, produced by the osteoblasts, begins to develop around the seventh day after the fracture. When osteoid is formed, it appears as irregular single or interlacing cords of a pink amorphous material initially without cells but becoming cellular as time passes; the cells are large osteoblasts containing rounded or ovoid nuclei often with a prominent nucleolus. As the tissue matures, the osteoblasts rim the osteoid, which eventually undergoes calcification. The cartilaginous proliferation is cellular and as a general rule the amount of cartilage increases with the instability of the fracture. If a biopsy is taken during repair of a fracture, the histopathologic changes may be suggestive of an osteosarcoma or a chondrosarcoma. A zonation effect does occur: the periphery matures earlier than the central portion of the fracture. Thus maturing bone is present at the periphery, whereas the center shows immature cellular proliferation. The history and good radiologic findings are essential for a correct diagnosis.

Stress fracture

A stress fracture may occur in healthy or diseased bones. It is usually secondary to minor but repeated trauma such as that which occurs in jogging, long-distance walking or marching, or competitive sports. Pain is the usual complaint with a stress fracture and appears from 1 to 3 weeks after the occurrence of the fracture.

Any bone may be affected; the tibia and fibula are affected in joggers, jumpers, and long-distance walkers, whereas the second and third metatarsal bones are commonly affected in walkers or marchers. Stress fractures are also seen in debilitated bones. Osteoporosis/osteomalacia, osteopetrosis, and Paget's disease of bone are not uncommonly the sites of stress fractures.

Radiologically there is a periosteal reaction that varies in its size according to the evolution of the lesion. An undisplaced hairline fracture may be seen, but often a CT study may be necessary to demonstrate the fracture.

PATHOLOGY. Histologically the tissue shows reactive new bone formation with numerous capillaries. Reactive cartilage may be present. Management should be conservative.

Charcot's joints

The impairment of proprioceptive and pain sensations is the basic cause of Charcot's joints, which represent complications of syringomyelia, paraplegia, quadriplegia, diabetes mellitus, and tabes dorsalis. The latter two processes are the most common causes of Charcot's joint.

Radiologic features reflect severe degrees of destruction and disorganization of the joints involved. Often a joint shows massive destruction of the articular surface and adjacent bone with associated edematous and inflammatory changes.

PATHOLOGY. Histologically there is abundant granulation tissue with edematous changes and the presence of cellular debris not uncommonly represented by spicules of dead bone.

TREATMENT. There is no effective management for this condition other than symptomatic treatment of the joint involved and treatment of the basic disease.

Hemophiliac pseudotumor

Hemorrhage in hemophiliac patients often occurs in the joints and in bone and, when severe, may produce a pseudotumor. In these cases a joint or a bone is the seat of a severe effusion, hemosiderotic synovitis, and degenerative arthritis. Hemorrhages occurring within the bone may produce large lytic changes within the medullary cavity of a bone or large tumorous elevation of the periosteum. The femur, tibia, iliac wing, and calcaneus are the most commonly affected bones.

Histologically there is evidence of recent and old hemorrhage with secondary bone changes such as reactive bone formation and fibrosis.

Brown tumor of hyperparathyroidism

A complication of hyperparathyroidism is the development of bone lesions known as "osteitis fibrosa cystica" and "brown tumor" when a mass develops.[1-4]

Radiologically a brown tumor may affect any part of the bone that usually shows a lytic aspect. Older lesions remodel the bone expanding the medullary cavity, which often displays a bubbly appearance. A brown tumor may be solitary or multicentric, though the latter occurrence is more common. In addition, other associated radiologic signs of hyperparathyroidism are usually present, including subperiosteal resorption and generalized osteopenia.

PATHOLOGY. Histologically a brown tumor consists of a giant cell proliferation of osteoclastic type over a hemosiderin-rich background. This background imparts the brownish discoloration characteristic of these lesions.

Giant cell tumor of bone is the main differential diagnosis for lesions situated in the epiphysis of a long bone. Although a brown tumor may be confused with a giant cell tumor of bone, there are differences between the two that help to separate them. The clinical manifestations of chronic hyperparathyroidism such as asthenia, muscular hypotonia, mental changes including psychosis, renal lithiasis, renal insufficiency, bone pain, and fractures are generally present; rarely osteitis fibrosa cystica may simulate metastatic disease.[271] Most important of all is the presence of hypercalcemia; therefore, determination of serum calcium should be done.

Giant cell reparative granuloma

Giant cell reparative granuloma (GCRG) is a proliferation of giant cells over a reactive fibrovascular stroma.

This lesion was initially described in the jaws and later in the small bones of the hand and feet. The solid phase of aneurysmal bone cyst has also been likened to GCRG.

In the hand and foot the lesion may affect patients from the first to the seventh decade of life, but it is more common in the second decade of life.[4] It has an equal sex distribution, and pain and swelling are common complaints.

Radiographically the lesion involves the shaft or metaphysis of the phalanges and metacarpal or metatarsal bones. A radiolucent fusiform expansion of the bone without peripheral sclerosis and well-demarcated ends are usually seen.

PATHOLOGY. Since most cases are the product of a curettage, gross lesions are not readily obvious. Microscopically the lesion shows a prominent fibrovascular proliferation with associated hemorrhage and a variable number of giant cells. The latter usually contain less nuclei than those of giant cell tumor of bone. A reactive fibro-osseous proliferation is also present in the majority of these lesions.

The differential diagnosis includes brown tumor of hyperparathyroidism and giant cell tumor of bone. Since it is histologically indistinguishable from brown tumor, a parathyroid serum profile should be done. GCT of bone always involves an epiphysis reaching the articular joint surface and is usually more destructive than a GCRG. Histologically the features overlap, but GCT of bone has more giant cells and the giant cells are larger than those of a GCRG.[4]

TREATMENT AND PROGNOSIS. Curettage with or without bone packing is the treatment of choice. The lesions are self-limited.

Osteomyelitis

Osteomyelitis either acute or chronic may simulate a bone neoplasm. Acute osteomyelitis is usually attributable to the common bacterial organisms such as *Staphylococcus, streptococcus, Escherichia coli, Aerobacter,* and *Haemophilus, etc.* Clinically bone pain and fever are common complaints.

In the acute phase, the bone lesions may simulate a malignant round cell tumor on radiologic examination. The reaction of the periosteum in layers (onionskin) may be associated with a lytic lesion of the bone. As the lesion progresses from acute to chronic, fragments of dead bone are left behind (sequestrum). Chronic lesions involve large parts of the bone often forming fistulous tracts that open into the skin or adjacent organs.

A characteristic subacute or chronic presentation of osteomyelitis is the localized form of the disease known as "Brodie's abscess." This is usually a small circumscribed lesion containing reactive osteosclerotic margins. It is nearly always caused by *Staphylococcus* organisms.

Brodie's abscess occurs predominantly in the long bones with the tibia and the femur being the most commonly involved bones. The metaphysis is the preferred site, but it may occur in the epiphysis or in the metadiaphyseal area of the bone.

Radiologically this lesion appears as a lytic area surrounded by a sclerotic margin. When the lesion is small, the radiologic appearance is similar to that of an osteoid osteoma. When the lesion is large, it may be confused with chondromyxoid fibroma of bone, chondroblastoma, fibrous dysplasia, nonossifying fibroma, simple bone cyst, and others.[272]

PATHOLOGY. Histologically the lesion is an abscess with severe acute and chronic inflammatory changes present.

TREATMENT. Management of this lesion is its removal and coverage with appropriate antibiotics.

Another form of chronic osteomyelitis is the sclerosing osteomyelitis of Garré, which is characterized by the formation of dense sclerosis. It is rare and likely to occur in the bones of the jaws.

Osteomyelitis is the great imitator of benign and malignant bone tumors. Therefore, when dealing with any bone lesion, no matter what the clinicoradiologic diagnosis is, the orthopedic surgeon should always take cultures.

Specific osteomyelitis

Tuberculous and fungal osteomyelitis do occur but are extremely rare. The histologic findings in the bone are similar to those seen in other locations.

METASTATIC BONE TUMORS

Metastatic tumors to the skeleton are more common than primary bone lesions especially in adults and elderly patients. Carcinomas are the most common type[3,4,273] (80%).

From the radiologic point of view metastatic disease may appear as a lytic or as a blastic process. Purely lytic lesions occur frequently, but not infrequently a metastatic tumor may express a combination of a lytic and a blastic process together or in different bones; breast and lung adenocarcinomas are good examples of this occurrence and less commonly lesions originating in the gastrointestinal tract (gastric, colon, and gallbladder). Purely lytic lesions are usually produced by renal and thyroid carcinomas; melanoma and gastrointestinal carcinomas may also produce lytic metastases. Purely blastic lesions are generally produced by metastatic prostate carcinoma, carcinoid tumor, and medulloblastoma. Mucinous tumors not infrequently develop calcifications that may simulate a cartilaginous malignancy.

"Ivory vertebrae" as a name refers to the finding of a densely blastic radiologic change on vertebrae. Prostate, breast, and pancreas tumors and lymphoma are common tumors that induce this type of change. Benign processes, however, may also induce ivory vertebrae; these include Paget's disease of bone, osteomyelitis, a healing fracture, and renal osteodystrophy. Rarely, multiple ivory vertebrae may be found in some patients because of carcinomatosis, lymphoma, and Paget's disease, amongst other causes.

A metastasis from a sarcomatoid renal or lung carcinoma may simulate a primary bone sarcoma, both histologically and radiographically; histologically the sarcomatoid change may have a malignant fibrous histiocytoma or an angiosarcoma pattern. Therefore, when confronted with an adult patient who presents a lesion that looks like a malignant fibrous histiocytoma of bone, clinical efforts should be made to rule out a kidney or a lung primary by means of chest x-ray films and a CT scan of the kidneys. Melanoma may also show a sarcomatoid change. Therefore the history is very important for the final diagnosis.

Immunohistochemistry is of value in the evaluation of metastatic disease, but in the case of a tumor with differential diagnosis between metastatic sarcomatoid carcinoma (lung or renal) and malignant fibrous histiocytoma, it may not help, since the latter may express keratin immunoreactivity. EM may also be of help.

REFERENCES

General aspects

1. Dahlin DC, Unni KK: *Bone tumors: general aspects and data on 8,542 cases*, ed 4, Springfield, Ill., 1986, Charles C Thomas Publisher.
2. Huvos AG: *Bone tumors: diagnosis, treatment, and prognosis*, ed 2, Philadelphia, 1991, Saunders.
3. Mirra J, Picci P, Gold RH: *Bone tumors: clinical, radiologic, and pathologic correlations*, Philadelphia, 1989, Lea & Febiger.
4. Fechner RE, Mills SE: *Tumors of the bones and joints. Atlas of tumor pathology*, ser 3, fasc 8, Washington, DC, 1993, Armed Forces Institute of Pathology.

Primary bone tumors

Osteoma

5. Järvinen HJ, Peltokallio P, Landtman M et al: Gardner's stigmas in patients with familial adenomatosis coli, *Br J Surg* 69:718, 1982.

6. Chang CH, Piatt ED, Thomas KE et al: Bone abnormalities in Gardner's syndrome, *Am J Roentgenol Radium Ther Nucl Med* 103:645, 1968.

Osteoid osteoma

7. Sim FH, Dahlin DC, Beabout JW: Osteoid-osteoma: diagnostic problems, *J Bone Joint Surg* 57A:154, 1975.
8. Gelman B, Thompson FM, Arnold WD: Intraoperative radioactive localization of an osteoid osteoma: case report, *J Bone Joint Surg* 63A:826, 1981.
9. Gelman B, Vigorita VJ: Post-operative radionuclide evaluation of osteoid osteomas, *Radiology* 144:509, 1983.
10. Ayala AG, Murray JA, Erling MA, Raymond AK: Osteoid-osteoma: intraoperative tetracycline-fluorescence demonstration of the nidus, *J Bone Joint Surg* 68A:747, 1986.

Osteoblastoma

11. Lucas DR, Unni KK, McLeod RA et al: Osteoblastoma: clinicopathologic study of 306 cases, *Hum Pathol* 25:117, 1994.
12. Nemoto O, Moser RP, Van Dam BE et al: Osteoblastoma of the spine: a review of 75 cases, *Spine* 15:1273, 1990.
13. Boriani S, Capanna R, Donati D et al: Osteoblastoma of the spine, *Clin Orthop* 278:37, 1992.
14. Kroon HM, Schurmans J: Osteoblastoma: clinical and radiologic findings in 98 new cases, *Radiology* 175:783, 1990.
15. Bertoni F, Unni KK, Lucas DR et al: Osteoblastoma with cartilaginous matrix: an unusual morphologic presentation in 18 cases, *Am J Surg Pathol* 17:69, 1993.

Aggressive osteoblastoma

16. Dorfman HD, Weiss SW: Borderline osteoblastic tumors: problems in the differential diagnosis of aggressive osteoblastoma and low-grade osteosarcoma, *Semin Diagn Pathol* 1:215, 1984.
17. Schajowicz F, Lemos C: Malignant osteoblastoma, *J Bone Joint Surg* 56B:202, 1976.
18. Bertoni F, Unni KK, McLeod RA et al: Osteosarcoma resembling osteoblastoma, *Cancer* 55:416, 1985.

Osteosarcoma

19. Friedman MA, Carter SK: The therapy of osteogenic sarcoma: current status and thoughts for the future, *J Surg Oncol* 4:482, 1972.
20. Uribe-Botero, G, Russell WO, Sutow WW, Martin RG: Primary osteosarcoma of bone: a clinicopathologic investigation of 243 cases, with necropsy studies in 54, *Am J Clin Pathol* 67:427, 1977.
21. Rosen G, Tan C, Sanmaneechai A et al: The rationale for the multiple drug chemotherapy in the treatment of osteogenic sarcoma, *Cancer* 35:936, 1975
22. Sutow WW, Sullivan MP, Fernbach DJ et al: Adjuvant chemotherapy in primary treatment of osteogenic sarcoma: a South West Oncology Group study, *Cancer* 36:1598, 1975.
23. Jaffe N, Frei E III, Traggis D, Watts H: Weekly high-dose methotrexate-citrovorum factor in osteogenic sarcoma: pre-surgical treatment of primary tumor and of overt metastases, *Cancer* 39:45, 1977.
24. Link MP, Goorin AM, Miser AW et al: The effect of adjuvant chemotherapy on relapse-free survival in patients with osteosarcoma of the extremity, *N Engl J Med* 314:1600, 1986.
25. Link MP, Goorin AM, Horowitz M et al: Adjuvant chemotherapy of high-grade osteosarcoma of the extremity: updated results of the multi-institutional osteosarcoma study, *Clin Orthop* 270:8, 1991.
26. Rosen G, Marcove RC, Huvos AG et al: Primary osteogenic sarcoma: eight year experience with adjuvant chemotherapy, *J Cancer Res Clin Oncol* 106(suppl):55, 1983.
27. Benjamin RS, Chawla SP, Carrasco CH et al: Preoperative chemotherapy for osteosarcoma with intravenous adriamycin and intra-arterial *cis*-platinum, *Ann Oncol* 3(suppl):3, 1992.
28. Hudson M, Jaffe MR, Jaffe N et al: Pediatric osteosarcoma: therapeutic strategies, results, and prognostic factors derived from a 10-year experience, *J Clin Oncol* 8:1988, 1990.
29. Bacci G, Picci P, Ruggieri MD et al: Primary chemotherapy and delayed surgery (neoadjuvant chemotherapy) for osteosarcoma of the extremities. The Istituto Rizzoli experience in 127 patients treated preoperatively with intravenous methotrexate (high versus moderate doses) and intraarterial cisplatin, *Cancer* 65:2539, 1990.
30. Bacci G, Picci P, Ferrari S et al: Primary chemotherapy and delayed surgery for nonmetastatic osteosarcoma of the extremeties: results in 164 patients preoperatively treated with high dose methotrexate followed by cisplatin and doxorubicin, *Cancer* 72:3227, 1993.
31. Murray JA, Jessup K, Romsdahl M et al: Limb savage-surgery in osteosarcoma: early experience at M.D. Anderson Hospital and Tumor Institute, *Cancer Treat Symp* 3:131, 1985.
32. Marcove RC, Rosen G: En bloc resections for osteogenic sarcoma, *Cancer* 45:3040, 1980.
33. Huvos AG, Woodard HQ, Cahan WG et al: Postradiation osteogenic sarcoma of bone and soft tissues: a clinicopathologic study of 66 patients, *Cancer* 55:1244, 1985.
34. Hadjipavlou A, Lander P, Srolovitz H, Enker IP: Malignant transformation in Paget's disease of bone, *Cancer* 70:2802, 1992.
35. Haibach H, Farrell C, Dittrich FG: Neoplasms arising in Paget's disease of bone: a study of 82 cases, *Am J Clin Pathol* 83:594, 1985.
36. Torres FX, Kyriakos M: Bone infarct–associated osteosarcoma, *Cancer* 70:2418, 1992.
37. Resnick CS, Aisner SC, Young JWR, Levine A: Case Report 767: osteosarcoma arising in bone infarct, *Skeletal Radiol* 22:58, 1993.
38. Raymond Ak, Murphy GF, Rosenthal DI: Case report 425: (epiphyseal osteosarcoma, *Skeletal Radiol* 16:336, 1987.
39. Edeiken J, Dalinka M, Karasick D: Osteosarcoma. In *Edeiken's Roentgen diagnosis of diseases of bone*, vol. 1, ed 4, Baltimore, 1990, Williams & Wilkins.
40. Heller M, Jend HH, Bucheler E et al: The role of CT in diagnosis and follow-up of osteosarcoma, *J Cancer Res Clin Oncol* 106(suppl):43, 1983.
41. Shirhoda A, Jaffe N, Wallace S et al: Computed tomography of osteosarcoma after intraarterial chemotherapy, *Am J Radiol* 144:95, 1985.
42. O'Flanagan SJ, Stack JP, McGee HMJ, Dervan P: Imaging of intramedullary tumor spread in osteosarcoma: a comparison of techniques, *J Bone Joint Surg* 73B:998, 1991.
43. Boyko OB, Cory DA, Cohen MD et al: MR imaging of osteogenic and Ewing's sarcoma, *Am J Radiol* 148:317, 1987.
44. Knop J, Montz R: Bone scintigraphy in patients with osteogenic sarcoma: study group COSS 80, *J Cancer Res Clin Oncol* 106(suppl):49, 1983.
45. Carrasco CH, Charnsangavej C, Raymond AK et al: Osteosarcoma: angiographic assessment of response to preoperative chemotherapy, *Radiology* 170:839, 1989.
46. Ayala AG, Zornoza J: Primary bone tumors: percutaneous needle biopsy: radiologic-pathologic study of 222 biopsies, *Radiology* 149:675, 1983.
47. Ayala AG, Raymond AK, Ro JY et al: Needle biopsy of primary bone lesions, *Pathol Annu*, 24(pt 1):219, 1989.
48. White VA, Fanning CV, Ayala AG et al: Osteosarcoma and the role of fine needle aspiration: a study of 51 cases, *Cancer* 62:1238, 1988.
49. Raymond AK, Chawla SP, Carrasco CH et al: Osteosarcoma chemotherapy effect: a prognostic factor, *Semin Diagn Pathol* 4:212, 1987.
50. Picci P, Bacci G, Campanacci M et al: Histologic evaluation of necrosis in osteosarcoma induced by chemotherapy: regional mapping of viable and nonviable tumor, *Cancer* 56:1515, 1985.
51. Wold LE, Unni KK, Beabout JW et al: "Dedifferentiated" parosteal osteosarcoma, *J Bone Joint Surg* 66A:53, 1984.
52. Raymond AK, Ayala A, Carrasco H et al: Parosteal osteosarcoma vs. dedifferentiated: preoperative identification, *Lab Invest* 54:53A, 1986.
53. Raymond AK: Surface osteosarcoma, *Clin Orthop* 270:140, 1991.
54. Unni KK, Dahlin DC, Beabout JW: Periosteal osteogenic sarcoma, *Cancer* 37:2476, 1976.
55. Spjut HJ, Ayala AG, de Santos LA, Murray JA: Periosteal osteosarcoma. In *Management of primary bone and soft tissue tumors*, St. Louis 1977, Mosby.
56. Schajowicz F: Juxtacortical chondrosarcoma, *J Bone Joint Surg* 59B:473, 1978.
57. de Santos LA, Murray JA, Finkelstein JB, Ayala AG: The radiographic spectrum of periosteal osteosarcoma, *Radiology* 127:123, 1978.
58. Wold LE, Unni KK, Beabout JW, Pritchard DJ: High-grade surface osteosarcoma, *Am J Surg Pathol* 8:181, 1984.

59. Kyriakos M: Intracortical osteosarcoma, *Cancer* 46:2525, 1980.
60. Vigorita VJ, Jones JK, Ghelman B, Marcove RC: Intracortical osteosarcoma, *Am J Surg Pathol* 8:65, 1984.
61. Kyriakos M, Gilula LA, Becich MJ, Schoenecker PL: Intracortical osteosarcoma, *Clin Orthop* 279:269, 1992.
62. Kurt AM, Unni KK, McLeod DJ: Low-grade intraosseous osteosarcoma, *Cancer* 65:1418, 1990.
63. Bertoni F, Bacchini P, Babbri N et al: Osteosarcoma: low-grade intraosseous-type osteosarcoma, histologically resembling parosteal osteosarcoma, fibrous dysplasia, and desmoplastic fibroma, *Cancer* 71:338, 1993.
64. Rosen G, Huvos AG, Marcove R, Niremberg A: Telangiectatic osteogenic sarcoma: improved survival with combination chemotherapy, *Clin Orthop* 207:164, 1986.
65. Sim FH, Unni KK, Beabout JW, Dahlin DC: Osteosarcoma with small cells simulating Ewing's tumor, *J Bone Joint Surg* 61A:207, 1979.
66. Ayala AG, Ro JY, Raymond AK et al: Small cell osteosarcoma: clinicopathologic study of 27 cases, *Cancer* 64:2162, 1989.
67. Ayala AG, Ro JY, Papadopoulos NK et al: Small cell osteosarcoma. In Humphrey G.B, editor: *Osteosarcoma in adolescents and young adults,* Boston, 1993, Kluwer Academic Publishers.
68. Davaney R, Vinh TN, Sweet D: Small cell osteosarcoma of bone: an immunohistochemical study with differential diagnostic considerations, *Hum Pathol* 24:1211, 1993.
69. Parham DM, Pratt CB, Parvey LS et al: Childhood multifocal osteosarcoma: clinicopathologic and radiologic correlates, *Cancer* 55:2653, 1985.
70. Ballance WA, Mendelsohn G, Carter JR et al: Osteogenic sarcoma: malignant fibrous histiocytoma type, *Cancer* 62:763, 1988.
71. Hasegawa T, Shibata T, Hirose T et al: Osteosarcoma with epithelioid features: an immunohistochemical study, *Arch Pathol Lab Med* 117:295, 1993.
72. Kramer K, Hicks DG, Palis J et al: Epithelioid osteosarcoma of bone: immunohistochemical evidence suggesting divergent epithelial and mesenchymal differentiation in a primary osseous neoplasm, *Cancer* 71:2977, 1993.
73. Goepfert H, Raymond AK, Spires JR et al: Osteosarcoma of the head and neck, *Cancer Bull* 42:347, 1990.

Osteochondroma

74. Spjut HJ, Dorfman HD, Fechner RE et al: *Tumors of bone and cartilage.* In *Atlas of tumor pathology,* series 2 Washington, DC, 1970, Armed Forces Institute of Pathology.
75. Virchow R: Ueber multiple Exostosen mit Vorlegung von Präparaten, *Klin Wochenschr* 28:1082, 1891.
76. D'ambrosia R, Ferguson AB: The formation of osteochondromas by epiphyseal cartilage transplantation, *Clin Orthop* 61:103, 1968.
77. Garrison RC, Unni KK, McLeod RA et al: Chondrosarcoma arising in osteochondroma, *Cancer* 49:1890, 1982.
78. Evison G, Price CHG: Subungual exostosis, *Br J Radiol* 39:451, 1966.
79. Miller-Breslow A, Dorfman HD: Dupuytren's (subungual) exostosis, *Am J Surg Pathol* 12:368, 1988.
80. Nora F, Dahlin DC, Beabout JW: Bizarre parosteal osteochondromatous proliferations of the hands and feet, *Am J Surg Pathol* 7:245, 1983.
81. Meneses MF, Unni KK, Swee RG: Bizarre parosteal osteochondromatous proliferation of bone (Nora's lesion), *Am J Surg Pathol* 17:691, 1993.

Enchondroma

82. Perlman MD, Gild ML, Schor AD: Enchondroma: a case report and literature review, *J Foot Surg* 27:556, 1988.

Periosteal chondroma

83. Lewis MM, Kenan S, Yabut SM et al: Periosteal chondroma: a report of ten cases and review of the literature, *Clin Orthop* 256:185, 1990.
84. Boriani S, Bachinni P, Bertoni F, Campanacci M: Periosteal chondroma: a review of twenty cases, *J Bone Joint Surg* 65A:205, 1983.
85. de Santos L, Spjut HJ: Periosteal chondroma: a radiologic spectrum, *Skeletal Radiol* 6:15, 1981.
86. Nojima T, Unni KK, McLeod R, Pritchard D: Periosteal chondroma and periosteal chondrosarcoma, *Am J Surg Pathol* 9:666, 1985.

Chondromyxoid fibroma

87. Zillmer DA, Dorfman HD: Chondromyxoid fibroma of bone: Thirty-six cases of clinico-pathologic correlation, *Hum Pathol* 20:952, 1989.
88. Gherlinzoni F, Rock M, Picci P: Chondromyxoid fibroma: the experience at the Istituto Ortopedico Rizzoli, *J Bone Joint Surg* 65A:198, 1983.
89. Wilson AJ, Kyriakos M, Ackerman LV: Chondromyxoid fibroma: radiographic appearance in 38 cases and in a review of the literature, *Radiology* 179:513, 1991.
90. Lodwick GS: *The bones and joints: An atlas of tumor radiology: radiologic concepts,* vol 1, Chicago, 1971, Mosby.
91. Beggs IG, Stoker DJ: Chondromyxoid fibroma of bone, *Clin Radiol* 33:671, 1982.
92. Rahimi A, Beabout JW, Ivins JC, Dahlin DC: Chondromyxoid fibroma: a clinico-pathologic study of 76 cases, *Cancer* 30:726, 1972.
93. Steiner GC: Ultrastructure of benign cartilaginous tumors of intraosseous origin, *Hum Pathol* 10:71, 1979.
94. Ushigome S, Takakuwa T, Shinagawa T et al: Chondromyxoid fibroma of bone: an electron microscopic observation, *Acta Pathol Jpn* 32:113, 1984.
95. Schajowicks F, Gallardo H: Chondromyxoid fibroma (fibromyxoid chondroma) of bone, *J Bone Joint Surg* 53B:198, 1971.
96. Weiss APC, Dorfman HD: S-100 protein in human cartilage lesions, *J Bone Joint Surg* 68A:521, 1986.
97. Bleiweiss IJ, Klein MJ: Chondromyxoid fibroma: report of six cases with immunohistochemical studies, *Mod Pathol* 3:664, 1990.
98. Ushigome S, Takakuwa T, Shinigawa T et al: Ultrastructure of cartilaginous tumors and S-100 protein in the tumors with reference to the histogenesis of chondroblastoma, chondromyxoid fibroma and mesenchymal chondrosarcoma, *Acta Pathol Jpn* 34:1285, 1984.
99. Troncoso A, Ro JY, Edeiken J et al: Case report 798: Recurrent chondromyxoid fibroma in connective tissue, *Skeletal Radiol* 22:445, 1993.

Chondroblastoma

100. Springfield DS, Capanna R, Gherlinzoni F et al: Chondroblastoma. A review of 70 cases, *J Bone Joint Surg* 67A:748, 1985.
101. Bloem JL, Mulder JD: Chondroblastoma: a clinical and radiological study of 104 cases, *Skeletal Radiol* 14:1, 1985.
102. Sotelo-Avila C, Sundaram M, Kyriakos M et al: Case report 373: diametaphysical chondroblastoma of the upper portion of the left femur, *Skeletal Radiol* 15:387, 1986.
103. Kurt AM, Unni KK, Sim FH, McLeod RA: Chondroblastoma of bone, *Hum Pathol* 20:965, 1989.
104. Weiss APC, Dorfman HD: S-100 protein in human cartilage lesions, *J Bone Joint Surg* 68A:521, 1986.
105. Breches ME, Simon MA: Chondroblastoma: an immunohistochemical study, *Hum Pathol* 19:1043, 1988.
106. Ushigome S, Takakuwa T, Shinigawa T et al: Ultrastructure of cartilaginous tumors and S-100 protein in the tumors with reference to the histogenesis of chondroblastoma, chondromyxoid fibroma and mesenchymal chondrosarcoma, *Acta Pathol Jpn* 34:1285, 1984.
107. Huvos AG, Marcove RC: Chondroblastoma of bone: a critical review, *Clin Orthop* 95:300, 1973.
108. Codman EA: Epiphyseal chondromatous giant cell tumors of the upper end of the humerus, *Surg Gynecol Obstet* 52:543, 1931.
109. Fanning CV, Sneige NS, Carrasco CH et al: Fine needle aspiration cytology of chondroblastoma of bone, *Cancer* 65:1847, 1990.
110. Bertoni F, Unni KK, Beabout JW et al: Chondroblastoma of the skull and facial bones, *Am J Clin Pathol* 88:1, 1987.
111. Kyriakos M, Land VJ, Penning L, Parker SG: Metastatic chondroblastoma, *Cancer* 55:1770, 1985.
112. Knuze E, Graewe TH, Peitsch E: Histology and biology of metastatic chondroblastoma: report of a case and review of the literature, *Pathol Res Pract* 182:113, 1987.
113. Abdul-Karim F, Ayala AG, Spjut HJ: Case report 321: extraosseous chondroblastoma in the subcutaneous tissues of the right shoulder, *Skeletal Radiol* 14:73, 1985.

Classic chondrosarcoma

114. Ayala AG, Ro JY, Han W et al: Chondrosarcoma: a clinicopathologic study of 173 cases with a minimal 5 years follow-up, *Lab Invest* 64:2A, 1991 (Abst 3).
115. Evans HL, Ayala AG, Rombsdahl MM: Prognostic factors in chondrosarcoma of bone: a clinicopathologic analysis with emphasis on histologic grading, *Cancer* 40:818, 1977.
116. Huvos AG, Marcove RC: Chondrosarcoma in the young: a clinicopathologic analysis of 79 patients younger than 21 years of age, *Am J Surg Pathol* 11:930, 1987.
117. Young CL, Sim FH, Unni KK, McLeod RA: Chondrosarcoma of bone in children, *Cancer* 66:1641, 1990.

Chondrosarcoma variants

118. Dahlin DC, Beabout JW: Dedifferentiation of low-grade chondrosarcomas, *Cancer* 28:461, 1971.
119. Johnson S, Tetu B, Ayala AG, Chawla SP: Chondrosarcoma with additional mesenchymal component (dedifferentiated chondrosarcoma). I. A clinicopathologic study of 26 cases, *Cancer* 58:278, 1986.
120. Tetu B, Ordóñez NG, Ayala AG, Mackay B: Chondrosarcoma with additional mesenchymal component (dedifferentiated chondrosarcoma). II. An immunohistochemical and electron microscopic study, *Cancer* 58:287, 1986.
121. Frassica FI, Unni KK, Beabout JW, Sim FH: Dedifferentiated chondrosarcoma: a report of the clinicopathologic features and treatment of seventy-eight cases, *J Bone Joint Surg* 68A:1197, 1986.
122. Campanacci M, Bertoni F, Capanna R: Dedifferentiated chondrosarcomas, *Ital J Orthop Traumatol* 3:331, 1979.
123. Zalupski MM, Ensley JF, Ryan J et al: A common cytogenetic abnormality and DNA content alterations in dedifferentiated chondrosarcoma, *Cancer* 66:1176, 1990.
124. Bertoni F, Present D, Bachinni P et al: Dedifferentiated peripheral chondrosarcomas: a report of seven cases, *Cancer* 63:2054, 1989.
125. Shapeero LG, Vanel D, Couanet D et al: Extraskeletal mesenchymal chondrosarcoma, *Radiology* 186: 819, 1993.
126. Swanson PE, Lillemoe TJ, Manivel JC, Wick MR: Mesenchymal chondrosarcoma: an immunohistochemical study, *Arch Pathol Lab Med* 114:943, 1990.
127. Bertoni F, Bacchini P, Picci P, Gherlinzoni F: Case report 517: mesenchymal chondrosarcoma of the femur, *Skeletal Radiol* 18:221, 1989.
128. Jacobs JL, Merriam JC, Chadburn et al: Mesenchymal chondrosarcoma of the orbit: report of three new cases and review of the literature, *Cancer* 73:339, 1994.
129. Bjornsson J, Beabout JW, Unni KK et al: Clear cell chondrosarcoma of bone: observations in 47 cases, *Am J Surg Pathol* 8:223, 1984.
130. Wang LT, Liu TC: Clear cell chondrosarcoma of bone: a report of three cases with immunohistochemical and affinity histochemical observations, *Pathol Res Pract* 189:411, 1993.

Benign fibrous lesions

131. Bertoni F, Calderoni P, Bacchini P et al: Benign fibrous histiocytoma of bone, *J Bone Joint Surg* 68A:1225, 1986.
132. Wold LE: Fibrous histiocytic tumors of bone, Unni KK, editor: *Bone tumors,* New York, 1988, Churchill Livingstone.
133. Bertoni F, Unni KK, McLeod RA et al: Xanthoma of bone, *Am J Clin Pathol* 90:377, 1988.
134. Johnson LC: Congenital pseudoarthrosis, adamantinoma of long bone, and intracortical fibrous dysplasia of the tibia, *J Bone Joint Surg* 54A:1355, 1972.
135. Campanacci M, Laus M: Osteofibrous dysplasia of the tibia and fibula, *J Bone Joint Surg* 63A:367, 1981.
136. Kempson R: Ossifying fibroma of the long bones: a light and electron microscopic study, *Arch Pathol* 82:218, 1966.
137. Czerniak B, Rojas-Corona RR, Dorfman HD: Morphologic diversity of long bone adamantinomas: the concept of differentiated (regressing) adamantinoma and its relationship to osteofibrous dysplasia, *Cancer* 64:2319, 1989.
138. Sweet DE, Tuyethoa NV, Devaney K: Cortical osteofibrous dysplasia of long bone and its relationship to adamantinoma: a clinicopathologic study of 30 cases, *Am J Surg Pathol* 16:282, 1992.
139. Jaffe HL: Desmoplastic fibroma and fibrosarcoma. In Jaffe HL, editor: *Tumors and tumorous conditions of bones and joints,* Philadelphia, 1958, Lea & Febiger.
140. Inwards CY, Unni KK, Beabout JW, Sim FH: Desmoplastic fibroma of bone, *Cancer* 68:1978, 1991.
141. Ayala AG, Ro JY, Goepfert H et al: Desmoid fibromatosis: a clinicopathologic study of 25 children, *Semin Diagn Pathol* 3:138, 1986.
142. Kransdorf MJ, Moser RP, Gilkey FW: Fibrous dysplasia, *Radiographics* 10:519, 1990.
143. Ishida T, Dorfman HD: Massive chondroid differentiation in fibrous dysplasia of bone (fibrocartilaginous dysplasia), *Am J Surg Pathol* 17:924, 1993.
144. Wojno KJ, McCarty EF: Fibro-osseous lesions of the face and skull with aneurysmal bone cyst formation, *Skeletal Radiol* 23:15, 1994.
145. Ruggieri P, Sim FH, Bond JR, Unni KK: Malignancies in fibrous dysplasia, *Cancer* 73:1411, 1994.

Malignant fibrous tumors

146. Little DC, McCarthy SW: Malignant fibrous histiocytoma of bone: the experience of the New South Wales Bone Tumour Registry, *Aust NZ J Surg* 63:346, 1993.
147. Capanna R, Bertoni F, Bacchini P et al: Malignant fibrous histiocytoma of bone: the experience at the Rizzoli Institute: report of 90 cases, *Cancer* 54:177, 1984.
148. Huvos AG, Heilweil M, Bretski SS: The pathology of malignant fibrous histiocytoma: a study of 130 patients, *Am J Surg Pathol* l9:853, 1985.
149. Cossetto D, Nade S, Blackwell J: Malignant fibrous histiocytoma of bone: a report of seven cases, *Aust NZ J Surg* 62:52, 1992.
150. Yokoyama R, Tsuneyoshi N, Enjoji M et al: Prognostic factors of malignant fibrous histiocytoma of bone: a clinical and histopathologic analysis of 34 cases, *Cancer* 72:1902, 1993.
151. Myers JL, Arocho J, Bernreuter W et al: Leiomyosarcoma of bone: a clinicopathologic, immunohistochemical, and ultrastructural study of five cases, *Cancer* 67:1051, 1991.
152. Hirose T, Kudo E, Hasegawa T et al: Expression of intermediate filaments in malignant fibrous histiocytomas, *Hum Pathol* 20:871, 1989.

Giant cell tumor of bone

153. Goldenberg RR, Campbell CJ, Bonfiglio M: Giant-cell tumor of bone: an analysis of two hundred and eighteen cases, *J Bone Joint Surg* 52A:619, 1970.
154. Schütte HE, Taconis WK: Giant cell tumor in children and adolescents, *Skeletal Radiol* 22:173, 1993.
155. Jacobs P: The diagnosis of osteoclastoma (giant cell tumour): a radiological and pathological correlation, *Br J Radiol* 45:121, 1972.
156. MacIntyre RS, Latourette HB, Hodges FG: Radiologic aspects of giant cell-tumor of bone, *Clin Orthop* 7:82, 1956.
157. Murray JA, Schlafly B: Giant-cell tumors in the distal end of the radius, *J Bone Joint Surg* 68A:687, 1986.
158. Bertoni F. Unni KK, Beabout JW, Ebersold MJ: Giant cell tumor of the skull, *Cancer* 70:1124, 1992.
159. Fain JS, Unni KK, Beabout JW, Rock MG: Nonepiphyseal giant cell tumor of the long bones: clinical, radiologic, and pathologic study, *Cancer* 71:3514, 1993.
160. Lundström B, Lorentzon R, Larsson SE et al: Angiography in giant-cell tumors of bone, *Acta Radiol (Diagn)* 18:541, 1977.
161. Prando A, de Santos LA, Wallace S et al: Angiography in giant-cell bone tumors, *Radiology* 130:323, 1979.
162. Peimer CA, Schiller AL, Mankin HJ, Smith RJ: Multicentric giant-cell tumor of bone, *J Bone Joint Surg* 62A:652, 1980.
163. Dahlin DC. Giant cell tumor of bone: highlights of 407 cases, *Am J Radiol* 144:955, 1985.
164. Sneige N, Ayala AG, Carrasco CH et al: Giant cell tumor of bone: a cytologic study of 24 cases, *Diagn Cytopathol* 1:111, 1985.
165. Ling L, Klein MJ, Sissons HA, Steiner GC: Lysozyme and alpha-1-antitrypsin in giant-cell tumor of bone and in other lesions that contain giant cells, *Arch Pathol Lab Med* 110:713, 1986.
166. Regezi JA, Zarbo RJ, Lloyd RV: Muramidase, alpha-1-antitrypsin, alpha-1-antichymotrypsin, and S-100 protein immunoreactivity in giant cell lesions, *Cancer* 59:64, 1987.

167. Mankin H, Matsuno T, Gebhardt M et al: Flow cytometry in the management of bone tumors. In Unni KK, editor: *Bone tumors,* New York, 1988, Churchill Livingstone.
168. Sara AS, Ayala AG, El-Naggar A et al: Giant cell tumor of bone: a clinicopathologic and DNA flow cytometric analysis, *Cancer* 66:2186, 1990.
169. Fukunaga M, Nikaido T, Shimoda T et al: A flow cytometric DNA analysis of giant cell tumor of bone including two cases with malignant transformation, *Cancer* 70:1886, 1992.
170. Pearson BM, Ekelund L, Lovdahl R, Gunterberg B: Favourable results of acrylic cementation for giant cell tumors, *Acta Orthop Scand* 55:209, 1984.
171. Marcove RR, Weis LD, Vaghaiwalla MR, Pearson R: Cryosurgery in the treatment of giant cell tumors of bone: a report of 52 consecutive cases, *Clin Orthop* 134:275, 1978.
172. Chuang VP, Soo CH, Wallace S, Benjamin RS: Arterial occlusion: management of giant cell tumor and aneurysmal bone cyst, *Am J Radiol* 136:1127, 1981.
173. Nascimiento AG, Huvos AG, Marcove RC: Primary malignant giant cell tumor of bone: a study of eight cases and review of the literature, *Cancer* 44:1393, 1979.
174. Meis JM, Dorfman HD, Nathanson D et al: Primary malignant giant cell tumor of bone: "dedifferentiated" giant cell tumor, *Mod Pathol* 2:541, 1988.
175. Rock, MG, Sim FH, Unni KK et al: Secondary malignant giant-cell tumor of bone: clinicopathologic assessment of nineteen patients, *J Bone Joint Surg* 68A:1073, 1986.
176. Rock MG, Pritchard DJ, Unni KK: Metastases from histologically benign giant-cell tumor of bone, *J Bone Joint Surg* 66A:269, 1984.

Ewing's sarcoma

177. Turc-Carel C, Philip T, Berger MP et al: Chromosome study of Ewing's sarcoma (ES) lines: consistency of a reciprocal translocation t(11:22)(q24:q12), *Cancer Genet Cytogenet* 12:1,1984.
178. Turc-Carel C, Aurias A, Mugneret F et al: 1. An evaluation of 85 cases and remarkable consistency of a reciprocal translocation of t(11:22)(q24;q12), *Cancer Genet Cytogenet* 32:229, 1988.
179. Whang-Peng J, Triche TJ, Knutsen T et al: Chromosome translocation in peripheral neuroepithelioma, *N Engl J Med* 30:584, 1989.
180. Dehner LP: Primitive neuroectodermal tumor and Ewing's sarcoma, *Am J Surg Pathol* 17:1, 1993.
181. Larsson SE, Boquist L, Bergdahl L: Ewing's sarcoma: a consecutive series of 64 cases diagnosed in Sweden, 1958-1967, *Clin Orthop* 95:263, 1973.
182. Maygarden SJ, Askin FB, Siegal SP et al: Ewing's sarcoma of bone in infants and toddlers, *Cancer* 71:2109, 1993.
183. Glass AG, Fraumeni JF Jr: Epidemiology of bone cancer in children, *J Natl Cancer Inst* 44:187, 1970.
184. Wilkins RM, Pritchard DJ, Burgeret EO Jr, Unni KK: Ewing's sarcoma of bone: experience with 140 patients, *Cancer* 58:2551, 1986.
185. Bator SM, Bauer TW, Marks KE, Norris DG: Periosteal Ewing's sarcoma, *Cancer* 58:1781, 1986.
186. Rud MP, Reiman HM, Pritchard DJ et al: Extraosseous Ewing's sarcoma: a study of 42 cases, *Cancer* 64:1548, 1989.
187. Llombart-Bosch A, Carda C, Peydro-Olaya A et al: Soft tissue Ewing's sarcoma, *Cancer* 66:2589, 1990.
188. Askin FB, Rosai J, Sibley RK et al: Malignant small cell tumor of the thoracopulmonary region in childhood: a distinctive clinicopathologic entity of uncertain histogenesis, *Cancer* 43:2438, 1979.
189. Contesso G, Llombart-Bosch A, Terrier P et al: Does malignant small cell tumor of the thoracopulmonary region (Askin tumor) constitute a clinicopathologic entity? An analysis of 30 cases with immunohistochemical and electron-microscopic support treated at the Institute Gustave Roussy, *Cancer* 69:1012, 1992.
190. Nascimiento AG, Unni KK, Pritchard DJ et al: A clinicopathologic study of 20 cases of large cell (atypical) Ewing's sarcoma of bone, *Am J Surg Pathol* 4:29, 1980.
191. Hartman KR, Triche TJ, Kinsella TJ, Miser JS: Prognostic value of histopathology in Ewing's sarcoma, *Cancer* 67:163, 1991.
192. Ushigome S, Shimoda T, Takaki K et al: Immunocytochemical and ultrastructural studies of the histogenesis of Ewing's sarcoma and putatively related tumors, *Cancer* 64:52, 1989.
193. Moll R, Lee I, Gould VE et al: Immunocytochemical analysis of Ewing's tumors, pattern of expression of intermediate filaments and desmosomal proteins indicate cell type heterogeneity and pluripotential differentiation, *Am J Pathol* 127:288, 1987.
194. Fellinger EJ, Garin-Chesa P, Glaser DB et al: Comparison of cell surface antigen HBA71 (p30/32^{MIC}), neuron-specific enolase, and vimentin in the immunohistochemical analysis of Ewing's sarcoma of bone, *Am J Surg Pathol* 16:746, 1992.
195. Fellinger EJ, Garin-Chesa P, Su SL et al: Biochemical and genetic characterization of HBA71 Ewing's sarcoma cell surface antigen, *Cancer Res* 51:336, 1991.
196. Fellinger EJ, Garin-Chesa P, Triche TJ et al: Immunohistochemical analysis of Ewing's sarcoma cell surface antigen p30/32^{MIC32}, *Am J Pathol* 139:275, 1991.
197. Perlman EJ, Dickman PS, Askin FB et al: Ewing's sarcoma-routine diagnostic utilization of MIC2 analysis: a Pediatric Oncology Group/Children's Cancer Group Intergroup Study, *Hum Pathol* 25:304,1994.
198. Taylor C, Patel K, Jones T et al: Diagnosis of Ewing's sarcoma and peripheral neuroectodermal tumour based on detection of t(11;22) using fluorescence in situ hybridisation, *Br J Cancer* 67:128, 1993.
199. Mawad JK, Mackay B, Raymond AK, Ayala AG: Electron microscopy in the diagnosis of small round cell tumors, *Ultrastruct Pathol* 18:263, 1994.
200. Nesbitt ME, Gehan EA, Burgert EO et al: Multimodal therapy for the management of primary, non-metastatic Ewing's sarcoma of bone: a long term follow-up of the first intergroup study (IESS-I), *J Clin Oncol* 8:1664, 1990.

Lymphoma

201. Ostrowski ML, Unni KK, Banks PM et al: Malignant lymphoma of bone, *Cancer* 58:2646, 1986.
202. Dosoretz DE, Raymond AK, Murphy GF et al: Primary lymphoma of bone: the relationship of morphologic diversity to clinical behavior, *Cancer* 50:1009, 1982.
203. Clayton F, Butler JJ, Ayala AG et al: Non-Hodgkin's lymphoma in bone: pathologic and radiographic features with clinical correlates, *Cancer* 60:2494, 1987.
204. Braunstein EM, White SJ: Non-Hodgkin's lymphoma of bone, *Radiology* 135:59, 1980.
205. Phillips WC, Kattapuram SV, Dosoretz DE et al: Primary lymphoma of bone: relationship of radiographic appearance and prognosis, *Radiology* 144:285, 1982.
206. Pettit CK, Zukerberg LR, Gray MH et al: Primary lymphoma of bone: a B-cell neoplasm with a high frequency of multilobated cells, *Am J Surg Pathol* 14:329, 1990.
207. Radaszkiewicz T, Hansmann ML: Primary high-grade malignant lymphomas of bone, *Virchows Arch [A]* 413:269, 1988.
208. Falini B, Binazzi R, Pileri S et al: Large cell lymphoma of bone: a report of three cases of B-cell origin, *Histopathology* 12:177, 1988.
209. Baar J, Burkes RL, Bell R et al: Primary non-Hodkgin's lymphoma of bone: a clinicopathologic study, *Cancer* 73:1194, 1994.

Plasmacytoma

210. Knowling MA, Harwood AR, Bersagel DE: Comparison of extramedullary plasmacytomas with solitary and multiple plasma cell tumors of bone, *J Clin Oncol* 1:255, 1983.
211. Dimopoulos MA, Moulopoulos A, Delasalle K, Alexanian R: Solitary plasmacytoma of bone and asymptomatic multiple myeloma, *Hematol Oncol Clin North Am* 6:359, 1992.
212. Kayrouz T, Jose B, Chu AN, Scott RM: Solitary plasmacytoma, *J Surg Oncol* 24:46, 1983.
213. Meis JM, Butler JJ, Osborne BM, Ordóñez NG: Solitary plasmacytomas of bone and extramedullary plasmacytomas: a clinicopathologic and immunohistochemical study, *Cancer* 59:1475, 1987.

Vascular tumors

214. Gorham LW, Stout AP: Massive osteolysis (acute spontaneous absorption of bone, phantom bone, disappearing bone): its relation to hemangiomatosis, *J Bone Joint Surg* 37A:985, 1955.

215. Gorham LW, Wright AW, Schultz HH et al: Disappearing bones: a rare form of massive osteolysis: report of two cases, one with autopsy findings, *Am J Med* 17:674, 1954.
216. Stout AP: Hemangioendothelioma: a tumor of blood vessels featuring vascular endothelial cells, *Ann Surg* 118:445, 1943.
217. Hartman WH, Stewart FW: Hemangioendothelioma of bone: unusual tumor characterized by indolent course, *Cancer* 15:846, 1962.
218. Otis J, Hutter RVP, Foot FW et al: Hemangioendothelioma of bone, *Surg Gynecol Obstet* 127:295, 1968.
219. Dorfman HD, Steiner GC, Jaffe HL: Vascular tumors of bone, *Hum Pathol* 2:253, 1971.
220. Rosai J, Gold J, Landy R: The histiocytoid hemangiomas: a unifying concept embracing several previously described entities of skin, soft tissue, large vessels, bone and heart, *Hum Pathol* 10:707, 1979.
221. Tsuneyoshi M, Dorfman HD, Bauer TW: Epithelioid hemangioma of bone: a clinicopathologic, ultrastructural, and immunohistochemical study, *Am J Surg Pathol* 10:754, 1986.
222. Weiss SW, Enzinger FW: Epithelioid hemangioendothelioma: a vascular tumor often mistaken for a carcinoma, *Cancer* 50:970, 1982.
223. O'Connell JX, Kattapuram SV, Mankin HJ et al: Epithelioid hemangioma of bone: a tumor often mistaken for low-grade angiosarcoma or malignant hemangioendothelioma, *Am J Surg Pathol* 17:610, 1993.
224. Castro C, Winkelmann RK: Angiolymphoid hyperplasia with eosinophilia in the skin, *Cancer* 34:1696, 1974.
225. Srigley JR, Ayala AG, Ordóñez NG, van Nostrand AWP: Epithelioid hemangioma of the penis, *Arch Pathol Lab Med* 109:51, 1985.
226. Campanacci M, Boriani S, Giunti A: Hemangioendothelioma of bone: a study of 29 cases, *Cancer* 46:804, 1980.
227. Vang PS, Falk E: Hemangiopericytoma of bone, *Acta Orthop Scand* 51:903, 1980.
228. Bollinger BK, Laskm WB, Knight CB: Epithelioid hemangioendothelioma with multiple site involvement, *Cancer* 73:610, 1994.
229. Tang JSH, Gold RH, Mirra JM, Eckardt J: Hemangiopericytoma of bone, *Cancer* 62:848, 1988.

Adamantinoma

230. Moon NF: Adamantinoma of the appendicular skeleton: a statistical review of reported cases and inclusion of 10 new cases, *Clin Orthop* 43:189, 1965.
231. Moon NF, Mori H: Adamantinoma of the appendicular skeleton-updated, *Clin Orthop* 204:215, 1986.
232. Keeney GL, Unni KK, Beabout JW, Pritchard DJ: Adamantinoma of long bones: a clinicopathologic study of 85 cases, *Cancer* 64:730, 1989.
233. Weiss SW, Dorfman HD: Adamantinoma of long bone: an analysis of nine new cases with emphasis on metastasizing lesions and fibrous dysplasia–like changes, *Hum Pathol* 8:141, 1977.
234. Hazelbag HM, Fleuren GC, Broeck LJCM et al: Adamantinoma of the long bones: keratin subclass immunoreactivity pattern with reference to histogenesis, *Am J Surg Pathol* 17:1225, 1993.

Chordoma and parachordoma

235. Pinto RS, Lin JP, Firooznia H et al: The osseous and angiographic manifestations of vertebral chordoma, *Neuroradiology* 9:231, 1975.
236. Uhrenholt L, Stimpel H: Histochemistry of sacrococcygeal chordoma, *Acta Pathol Microbiol Scand* 93:203, 1985.
237. Meis JM, Giraldo AA: Chordoma: an immunohistochemical study of 20 cases, *Arch Pathol Lab Med* 112:553, 1988.
238. Abenoza P, Sibley RK: Chordoma: an immunohistochemical study, *Hum Pathol* 17:744, 1986.
239. Heffelfinger MJ, Dahlin DC, MacCarty CS, Beabout JW: Chordomas and cartilaginous tumors at the base of the skull, *Cancer* 32:410, 1973.
240. Rosenberg AE, Brown GA, Bhan AK, Lee JM: Chondroid chordoma: a variant of chordoma: a morphologic and immunohistochemical study, *Am J Clin Pathol* 101:36, 1994.
241. Wojno KD, Aruban RH, Garin-Chesa P, Huvos AG: Chondroid chordomas and low grade chondrosarcomas of the craneospinal axis, *Am J Surg Pathol* 16:1144, 1992.
242. Miettinen M, Lehto VP, Virtanen I: Malignant fibrous histiocytoma within a recurrent chordoma, *Am J Clin Pathol* 82:738, 1984.
243. Belza MG, Urich H: Chordoma and malignant fibrous histiocytoma: evidence for transformation, *Cancer* 58:1082, 1986.
244. Meis JM, Raymond AK, Evans HL et al: "Dedifferentiated" chordoma: a clinicopathologic and immunohistochemical study of three cases, *Am J Surg Pathol* 11:516, 1987.
245. Hruban RH, Traganos F, Reuter VE, Huvos AG: Chordomas with malignant spindle cell components, *Am J Pathol* 137:435, 1990.
246. Fleming GF, Herman PS, Stephens JK et al: Dedifferentiated chordoma: response to aggressive chemotherapy in two cases, *Cancer* 72:714, 1993.
247. Dabska M: Parachordoma: a new clinicopathologic entity, *Cancer* 40:1586, 1977.

Nonneoplastic tumorous conditions

248. Virchow R: Ueber die Bildung von Knochenzysten: *Sitzungsb d Akad d Wissensch* (Berlin) 369, 1876.
249. Jaffe HL, Lichtenstein L: Solitary unicameral bone cyst with emphasis on the roentgen picture, pathological appearance, and pathogenesis, *Arch Surg* 44:1004, 1942.
250. Shindell R, Huurman WW, Lippiello L, Connolly JF: Prostaglandin levels in unicameral bone cysts treated by intralesional steroid injection, *J Pediatr Orthop* 9:516, 1989.
251. Gerasimov AM, Toporova SM, Furtseva LN et al: The role of lysosomes in the pathogenesis of unicameral bone cysts, *Clin Orthop* 256:53, 1991.
252. Scaglietti O, Marchetti PG, Bartolozzi P: Final results obtained in the treatment of bone cysts with methylprednisolone acetate (Depo-Medrol) and a discussion of results achieved in other bone lesions, *Clin Orthop* 165:33, 1982.
253. Farber JM, Stanton RP: Treatment options in unicameral bone cysts, *Orthopedics* 13:25, 1990.
254. Jaffe HL: Aneurysmal bone cyst, *Bull Hosp Jt Dis* 11:3, 1950.
255. Lichtenstein L: Aneurysmal bone cyst: observations in 50 cases, *J Bone Joint Surg* 39A:873, 1957.
256. Dodd LG, Ayala AG, Ro J et al: Aneurysmal bone cyst: a clinicopathologic and DNA flow cytometric study on 48 cases, *Lab Invest* 66:5A, 1992.
257. Vergel de Dios AM, Bond JR, Shives TC et al: Aneurysmal bone cyst: a clinicopathologic study of 238 cases, *Cancer* 69:2921, 1992.
258. Oda Y, Tsuneyoshi M, Shinohara N: "Solid" variant of aneurysmal bone cyst (extragnathic giant cell reparative granuloma) in the axial skeleton and long bones: a study of its morphologic spectrum and distinction from allied giant cell lesions, *Cancer* 70:2642, 1992.
259. Bertoni F, Bachinni P, Capanna R et al: Solid variant of aneurysmal bone cyst, *Cancer* 71:729, 1993.
260. Dahlin DC, McLeod RA: Aneurysmal bone cyst and other nonneoplastic conditions, *Skeletal Radiol* 8:243, 1982.
261. Edling NPG: Is the aneurysmal bone cyst a true pathological entity? *Cancer* 18:1127, 1965.
262. Clough JR, Price CHG: Aneurysmal bone cyst: pathogenesis and long term results of treatment, *Clin Orthop* 97:52, 1973.
263. Pfeifer FM, Bridge JA, Neff JR, Mouron BJ: Cytogenetic findings in aneurysmal bone cysts, *Genes Chromosom Cancer* 3:416, 1991.
264. Mouron BJ, Bridge JA, Pfeifer FM, Neff JR: Chromosomal "normality" in aneurysmal bone cyst. *The Fourth International Workshop On Chromosomes in Solid Tumors,* Tucson, Ariz, Feb 24-26, 1991.
265. Kyriakos M, Hardy D: Malignant transformation of aneurysmal bone cyst, with an analysis of the literature, *Cancer* 68:1770, 1991.
266. Lichtenstein L, Jaffe HL: Eosinophilic granuloma of bone with report of case, *Am J Pathol* 16:595, 1940.
267. Beltran J, Aparisi F, Bonmati LM et al: Eosinophilic granuloma: MRI manifestations, *Skeletal Radiol* 22:157, 1993
268. Katz RL, Silva EG, de Santos L, Lukeman JM: Diagnosis of eosinophilic granuloma of bone by cytology, histology, and electron microscopy of transcutaneous bone-aspiration biopsy, *J Bone Joint Surg* 62A:1284, 1980.
269. Shabb N, Fanning CV, Carrasco CH et al: Diagnosis of eosinophilic granuloma of bone by fine-needle aspiration with concurrent institution

therapy: a cytologic, histologic, clinical, and radiologic study of 27 cases, *Diagn Cytopathol* 9:1, 1993.

270. Nauert C, Zornoza J, Ayala AG, Harle TS: Eosinophilic granuloma of bone: diagnosis and management, *Skeletal Radiol* 10:227, 1983.
271. Bassler T, Wong ET, Brymes RK: Osteitis fibrosa cystica simulating metastatic tumor: an almost forgotten relationship, *Am J Clin Pathol* 100:697, 1993.
272. Azouz EM, Greenspan A, Marton D: C.T. evaluation of primary epiphyseal bone abscesses, *Skeletal Radiol* 22:17, 1993.

Metastatic bone tumors

273. Rougraft BT, Kneisl JS, Simon MA: Skeletal metastasis of unknown origin: a prospective study of a diagnostic strategy, *J Bone Joint Surg* 75A:1276, 1993.

74 Metabolic and Nontumorous Bone Disorders

Lorraine A. Fitzpatrick

MACROARCHITECTURE AND MICROARCHITECTURE OF NORMAL BONE

Structure and composition

The skeleton is a specialized structure composed of multiple tissues, including bone, cartilage, fat, connective tissue, hematopoietic bone marrow, nerves, and vessels. These tissues serve three major functions: to provide mechanical support, to protect vital organs, and to serve as a metabolic reserve of calcium and phosphate.

Bone is classified as either *cortical,* which predominates in the appendicular skeleton, or as *cancellous* (or trabecular), which predominates in the axial skeleton (pelvis and vertebrae). Although cortical and cancellous bone consist of the same cellular elements and matrix proteins, there are distinct structural and functional differences between the two. Cortical bone is dense and compact and makes up 60% of the skeleton. Structural stability is provided by cortical bone, which is largely present in the shafts of long bones. Cancellous bone constitutes 20% of the skeleton. However, because cancellous bone is more metabolically active and contains a higher surface area, the respective metabolic contributions of cortical and cancellous bone to the maintenance of calcium homeostasis are approximately equal.[1]

Anatomically there are two types of bone, and these derive from two distinct types of histogenesis: *flat bones* (the skull, scapula, mandible, and ilium), which are formed by intramembranous calcification, and *long bones* (the tibia, femur, and humerus), which are formed by endochondral ossification. Intramembranous formation occurs de novo from undifferentiated connective tissue (Fig. 74-1). The formation of endochondral bones is preceded by the formation of cartilage (Fig. 74-2).

Bone consists of specialized cells and an extracellular matrix. The fibrous matrix of bone is predominantly composed of type I collagen, which provides the structural framework for calcification.[2] Breakdown products of type I collagen include pyridinoline and deoxypyridinoline. These urinary metabolites are currently the primary biochemical markers used in the assessment of bone resorption.[3]

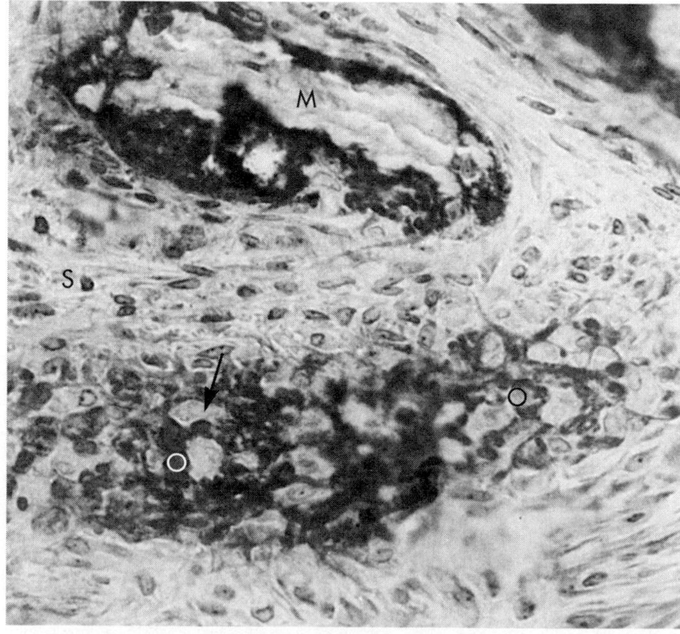

Fig. 74-1 Membranous ossification. Stromal mesenchymal cells *(S)* give rise to osteoblasts *(arrow),* which begin to secrete osteoid matrix, O. *M,* Mineralized bone spicule.

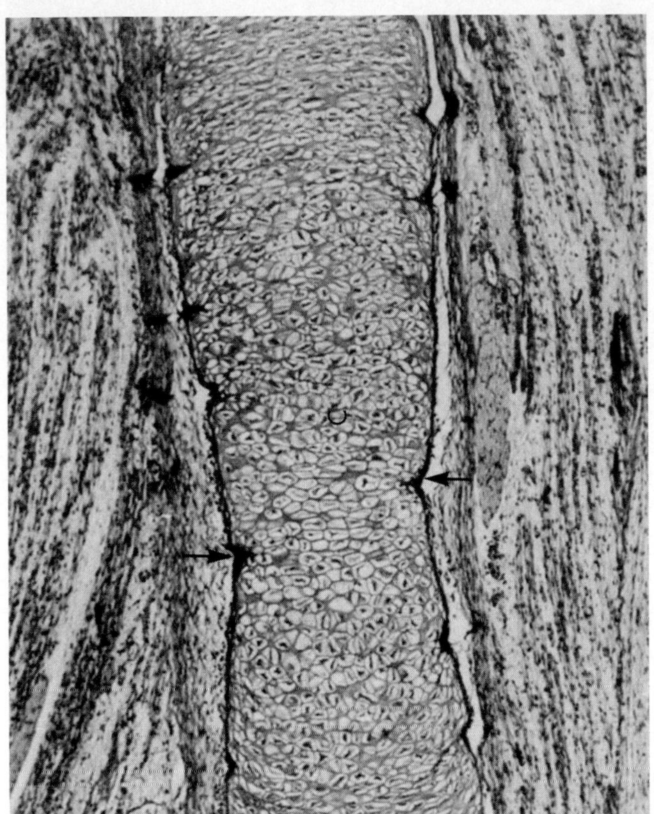

Fig. 74-2 Endochondral ossification. The primary ossification center is initiated by the formation of a periosteal collar of bone *(arrows)*.

The ground substance of bone consists of proteoglycans and glycoproteins that have a high ion-binding capacity and are important to calcification. Additional noncollagenous matrix proteins (10% to 15% of the matrix) such as osteopontin, bone sialoprotein, osteocalcin, osteonectin, biglycan, and decorin have been isolated. These proteins serve important functions in bone modeling and remodeling. A fourth of these noncollagenous proteins is derived from the serum and becomes bound to the hydroxyapatite component of bone. Although these proteins have been isolated and characterized biochemically, little is known about their physiologic roles in bone remodeling. *Bone sialoprotein,* a phosphorylated glycoprotein, constitutes 15% of noncollagenous bone matrix proteins. It is important in cell attachment, avidly binds calcium, and is found in normal mineralized tissue. *Osteopontin* is a phosphorylated glycoprotein that, like bone sialoprotein, contains the integrin-binding tripeptide sequence Arg-Gly-Asp (RGD) common to proteins of the cell attachment type. Both bone sialoprotein and osteopontin have a high affinity for mineral. *Osteonectin* is a phosphorylated glycoprotein that is synthesized and secreted by osteoblasts. It is responsible for the deposition of mineral into the matrix and for regulation of the crystal growth rate. *Osteocalcin* is a 6 kD glutamic acid–containing protein that inhibits mineralization and promotes bone resorption. It is chemotactic for certain types of cell, especially osteoclasts. It has been proposed that this protein plays an important role in the regulation of the remodeling sequence that occurs with aging.[4,5]

Proteoglycans are macromolecules that contain acidic polysaccharide charges (glycosaminoglycans) attached to a central protein core.[6] Two types are found in bone: chondroitin sulfate and heparin sulfate. Chondroitin sulfate is composed of three separate core proteins, each with a separate gene product. PG-1, or biglycan, is more abundant in fetal bone than in adult bone. PG-2, or decorin, binds to collagen and regulates collagen fibrillogenesis. The activation of PG-1 may indicate that osteoblast growth is taking place and may be of significance in understanding the nature of the cellular changes in growth and differentiation that occur during calcification. Heparin sulfate is important in facilitating the interaction between osteoblasts and heparin-binding growth factors[7] (Table 74-1).

The preferential organization of collagen fibrils alternates in adult bone, resulting in bone having a lamellar appearance when examined under polarized light (Fig. 74-3). This organization confers the highest density of collagen per unit volume of tissue. Lamellae deposited in a concentric fashion in cortical bone forms the haversian system, which is composed of cervical lamellar bone centered on a blood vessel. Osteocytes are dispersed in a regular fashion with their long axes parallel to the collagen lamellae. Long processes within microscopic lacunae connect adjacent osteocytes but do not cross adjacent osteons (Fig. 74-4). Tight junctions are an additional mechanism of cellular communication and may regulate the transfer of calcium from bone to the extracellular fluid.[8]

Woven bone is a fine sponge of cancellous bone that is not formally organized. Under polarized light, woven bone has the appearance of mesh (Fig. 74-5). Woven bone composes the immature bone found in the embryo, growing prepubertal bone, and bone that forms at sites of repair and in areas of malformation associated with metabolic bone disease. Noncollagenous proteins constitute a greater proportion of the matrix in woven bone than that in mature bone. Osteocytes are distributed randomly.

Bones can mineralize in one of two ways. In the cartilage of growing bones and woven bone (such as fracture callus), lipid-rich matrix vesicles derived from osteoblasts or chondroblasts serve as a nidus for the deposition of mineral. In lamellar bone, mineralization is initiated in association with the formation of collagen fiber–noncollagenous protein complexes. The mechanism that governs calcification and the role of various initiators and inhibitors are both poorly understood. Mineralization is slower in lamellar bone than in woven bone. Because the mineral and the collagen fibers in lamellar bone are closely situated, this type of bone is less elastic and its tensile strength and rigidity are greater than those of woven bone.

Cellular and matrix components

Osteoblasts are responsible for the production of collagenous and noncollagenous proteins that form unmineralized bone (osteoid). Like other osteoprogenitor cells, osteoblasts derive from primitive mesenchymal cells. "Active" osteoblasts cover the bone surface and appear as columnar cells containing amphophilic to basophilic cytoplasm and eccentrically located nuclei (Fig. 74-6). Ultrastructurally the cytoplasm of osteoblasts contains a well-developed Golgi apparatus and an extensive network of rough endoplasmic reticulum, which is predominantly under the plasma membrane. The existence of rough endoplasmic reticulum indicates the presence of ribosomes associated with messenger RNA and also reflects the active secretory state of the cell. Mature, functioning

Table 74-1 Noncollagenous proteins of bone matrix

Protein	Gene location	Potential function
Osteopontin	Chromosome 4	Osteoclast attachment via $\alpha V\beta 3$, osteogenesis, bone remodeling
Osteocalcin	Chromosome 1	Avidly binds Ca^{2+}, remodeling signal, 3γ-carboxyglutamic acid residues, vitamin K–dependent protein
Osteonectin	Chromosome 5	Avidly binds Ca^{2+}, tissue remodeling
Matrix Gla protein	Chromosome 12 (short arm)	Vitamin K–dependent protein
Bone sialoprotein	Chromosome 4	Cell attachment, binds integrin $\alpha_V\beta_3$, binds hydroxyapatite, RGD site
Biglycan (proteoglycan I)	Chromosome Xq27-qter	—
Decorin (proteoglycan II)	Chromosome 12q21-q22	Collagen fibrogenesis, binds transforming growth factor-beta
Thrombospondin	Thrombospondin I on chromosome 15q15; II on 6q27; III on 1q21-24	Cell attachment, migration, proliferation
Fibronectin	Chromosome 2	Cell attachment and migration, regulation of cell growth and differentiation

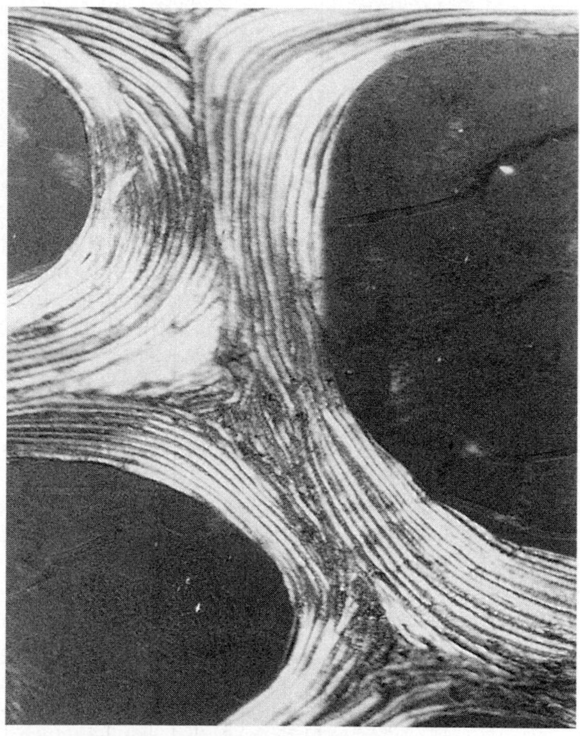

Fig. 74-3 Example of normal lamellar cancellous bone as viewed with polarized light microscopy.

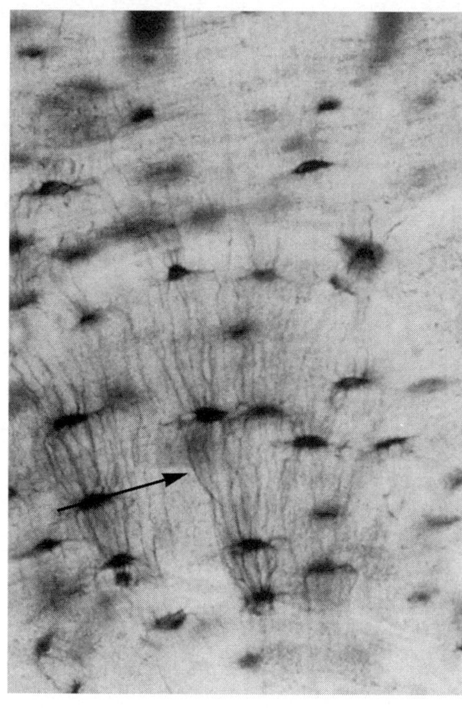

Fig. 74-4 Canaliculi *(arrow)* extending from osteocytic lacuna to osteocytic lacuna in a fresh, unembedded ground section.

osteoblasts are unable to divide, and if mitotic forms are noted, then by convention that cell represents an osteoblast precursor.

Osteoblasts contain a specific isoform of alkaline phosphatase that can be localized to the plasma membrane of the osteoblast. This ectoenzyme is utilized as a histologic marker, and its function is debated. Hypotheses regarding its role in mineralization have been suggested, and a clear association between enzymatic activity and bone formation has been noted. Measurement of the serum level of the isoenzyme of alkaline phosphatase specific to bone can aid in the diagnosis of various metabolic bone diseases, and elevated enzyme activity is considered a marker of bone formation. Increased enzyme activity is associated with the growth and repair of bone and is physiologic during the rapid period of skeletal growth that takes place during puberty. A series of sequential steps is associated with bone formation.[9] The osteoblast regulates these processes, which include the synthesis and internal processing of type I collagen; the secretion and extracellular processing of the collagen; the formation of microfibrils, fibrils, and fibers from the collagen; matrix maturation; and the nucleation of hydroxyapatite crystals. Regulation of the bone-forming activity of osteoblasts is an intense area of investigation, and numerous local factors have been isolated

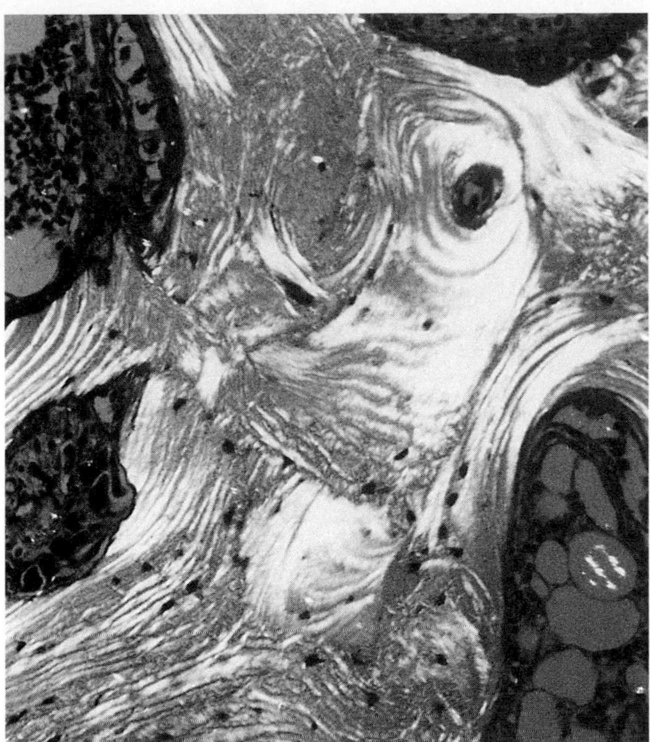

Fig. 74-5 Example of woven bone frequently seen in the high-turnover state. In this specimen, the final diagnosis of hyperparathyroidism is consistent with the high-turnover state noted on histomorphometric analysis.

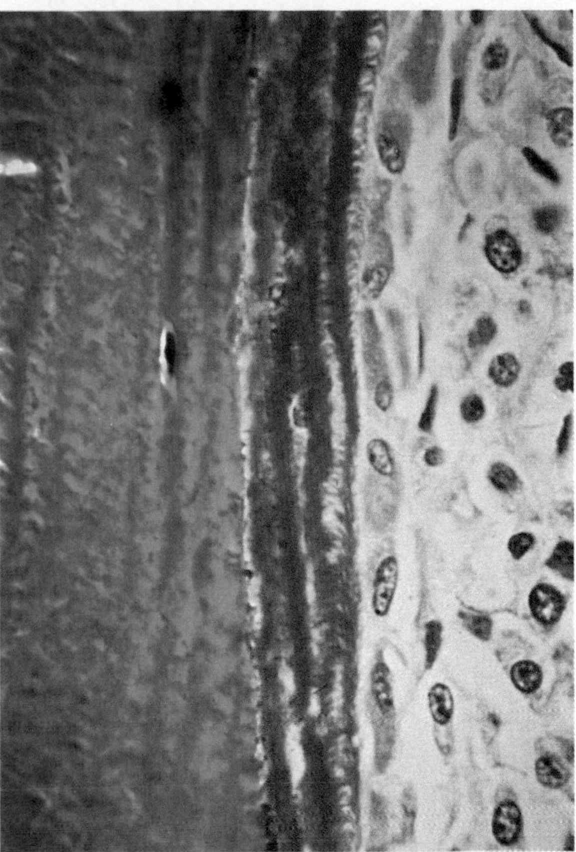

Fig. 74-6 Osteoblasts are responsible for the production of collagenous and noncollagenous proteins that compose osteoid. Active osteoblasts are lined up on the osteoid. Notice the eccentrically located nuclei.

that participate in the control of bone formation. Recently it has become evident that the matrix has an important role in the regulation of bone formation at both the cellular and molecular levels.

As the rate of bone formation decreases, osteoblasts become flattened and fusiform, reflecting their decreased secretory activity. These inactive cells line bone surfaces and play an important role in the regulation of calcium flux across the bone surface in response to hormonal stimuli.[10]

Osteocytes are inactive osteoblasts incorporated into the matrix. Contact between them is maintained by cellular processes that traverse mineralized tissue through the canalicular space. The long axis of the osteocyte is aligned in parallel with collagen fibers, and the spatial distribution of the osteocytes is a reliable criterion for distinguishing woven from lamellar bone. Osteocytes are probably responsible for the exchange of ions that takes place within the calcified bone matrix.

Osteoclasts are multinucleated cells that are largely responsible for bone resorption. It is generally accepted that osteoclast progenitor cells belong to the monocyte-macrophage lineage, though the possible existence of a separate stem cell committed to osteoclast formation is disputed. It is generally accepted that osteoclasts form by the fusion of progenitor cells.[11] Osteoclasts are 40 to 100 μm in diameter and contain an average of 10 to 15 nuclei. The cell is highly polarized, with the nuclei congregating away from the bone surface. Cytoplasm is amphophilic on light microscopy studies, and abundant Golgi complexes are found scattered among the nuclei. The ruffled border is a specialized area of membrane that is rich in actin and is composed of numerous fingerlike projections that are juxtaposed to the bone surface. The complexity and extent of the ruffled border increase during bone resorption.

Normally osteoclasts are directly apposed to the bone surface (Fig. 74-7). Actual osteoclast attachment to the bone surface is essential for resorption to occur. This attachment is mediated, at least in part, by cell surface proteins called "integrins" that interact with the RGD sequence (Arg-Gly-Asp) on several noncollagenous bone matrix proteins. After a period of active resorption, the osteoclasts are found in pits called "Howship's lacunae."[12,13]

Embryology

The neuroderm in the embryo is made up of connective tissue (mesenchyme) and gives rise to the skeleton. Mesenchyme can differentiate into fibroblasts, osteoblasts, chondroblasts, and other connective tissue precursors. The first bone in the embryo derives from one of two precursor tissues, mesenchyme or cartilage.

The skeleton develops by means of either intramembranous or endochondral ossification. Endochondral ossification uses a collagen template that originates from undifferentiated mesenchymal cells. In contrast, intramembranous ossification, or "membranous bone," arises directly in the mesenchyme. In the embryo cells are organized into vascularized connective tissue aggregates. Mesenchymal cells give rise to osteoblasts, which lay down a mat of interlacing fibers composed of collagen called "osteoid." This woven bone becomes mineralized and

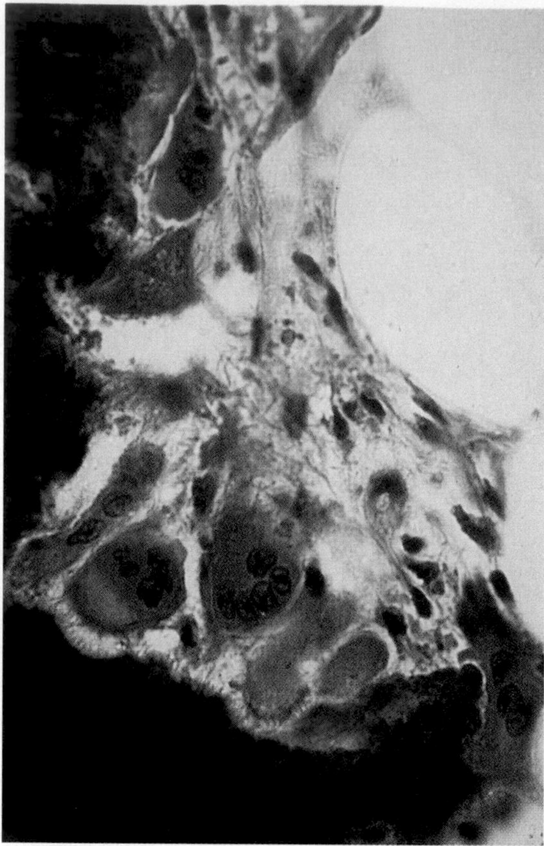

Fig. 74-7 Osteoclasts actively resorbing mineralized tissue. The scalloped surface in which the multinucleated osteoclasts rest is termed "Howship's lacunae."

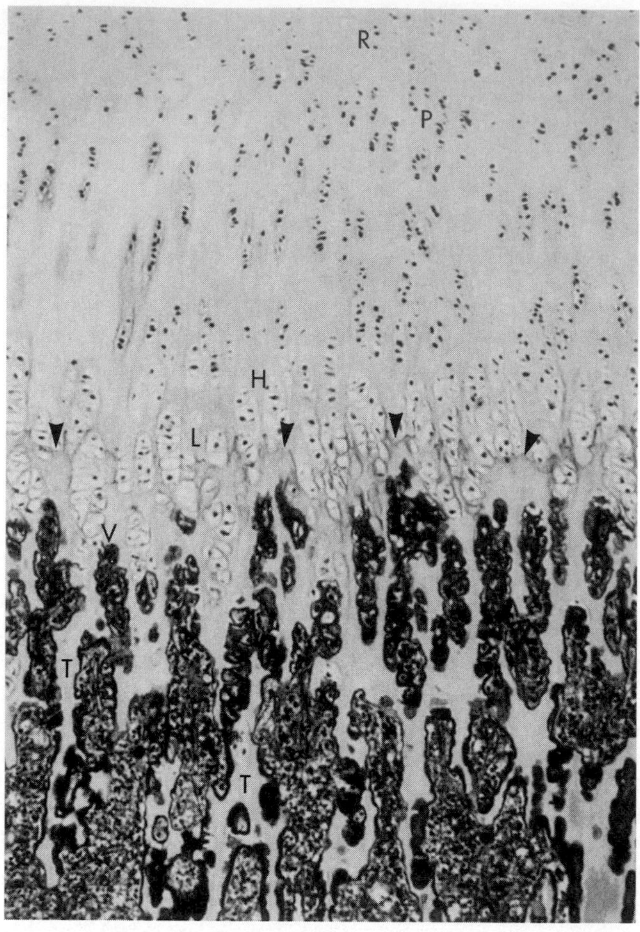

Fig. 74-8 Zones of epiphyseal growth plate. The resting cartilage *(R)* gives rise to the proliferating zone of chondrocytes *(P)*, recognized by the vertical orientation of the cartilage cells. Expanding cells force the cartilage matrix into longitudinal columns *(L)*. This cartilage matrix calcifies in the zone of provisional calcification *(arrowheads)* and is soon invaded by blood vessels, *V. T,* Primary trabeculae, consisting of cartilage bars, are surrounded by bone matrix. *H,* Hypertrophic chondrocyte zone.

eventually organizes into broad, flat plates of compact bone that enclose an inner space composed of marrow and trabecular bone. Further growth occurs radially by means of the periosteal apposition of new bone and concomitant endosteal resorption along the medullary cavity. The endosteal formation associated with periosteal resorption allows the inner table to grow, and with maturation the bone becomes lamellar.

Endochondral ossification begins in cartilage formed from mesenchymal cells that differentiate into chondroblasts. The ability of cartilage to grow throughout and the apposition of perichondral cells such that they form chondrocytes enable it to serve as a scaffold for bone growth. The skeleton of the 8-week-old embryo is composed of a template of cartilage that has the crude configuration of the adult skeleton. The initial formation of bone begins as a shaft surrounded by undifferentiated mesenchyme that eventually develops into a periosteum. Growth occurs through the production and accumulation of extracellular matrix: type II collagen is predominant, with types IX, X, XI, and XIII collagens and proteoglycans making up the remainder. Distinct zones form as the cartilaginous skeleton enlarges. The chondrocytes in the primary center of ossification become increasingly hypertrophied and deposit type X collagen, and mineralization begins. The cartilage in the central portion degenerates and is invaded by vascular endothelial cells. The calcified debris is removed by osteoclasts, leaving behind a cavity filled with loose connective, adipose, and hematopoietic tissue. By birth most long bones have ossified throughout the major portion of their length.

After the cartilage in the central region has been supplanted by spicules of bone, the endochondral replacement of cartilage is predominantly limited to the diaphyseal-epiphyseal junction, where it forms the *epiphyseal growth plate,* or physis (Fig. 74-8). This structure consists of several zones characterized by a regular pattern of progressive cartilage maturation and its replacement by bone. The first zone consists of a resting zone of chondrocytes that merges into a proliferative zone of cells. Additional matrix is synthesized in the next region, the area of chondrocyte hypertrophy. The third zone is characterized by calcification and the formation of primary trabeculae. The calcified cartilage is invaded by vessels growing into the diaphysis. In diseases in which mineralization is impaired or in areas where matrix formation is limited, the organization of these primary trabeculae is chaotic.

In long bones the secondary center of ossification arises in the epiphysis. The maturation and replacement of the cartilage anlage are identical to those taking place in the diaphysis, except that they proceed rapidly from the center to the periphery.[14]

The final shape of the bone is determined by external mechanical factors and Wolff's law.[15,16] Mechanical forces exerted by attached muscles alter the rate and final shape of bone. Modeling is defined as the shaping of growing bone to conform to its genetically determined shape. As the diaphysis elongates, a new cylinder of bone develops at the adjacent growth plate. This area of "sleeve-bone" extension, called the "ring of Ranvier," determines the directional growth of bone.

Endochondral growth is mediated by several peptide and steroid hormones until puberty. Low doses of androgens and estrogens secreted during puberty increase cell proliferation and the rate of cartilage maturation, the result of which is the so-called growth spurt. Toward the end of puberty the growth plates close, and thereafter additional growth is only appositional.

Most of the bone mass in adults is produced through the lateral growth of bone from the shaft in the periosteal region of the diaphysis. Concentric lamellae of bone around the haversian canal create the primary osteon. The osteon is the basic structural and metabolic unit of mature cortical bone. New osteons (secondary osteons) are created to accommodate changes in stress and strain. The existing bone is removed by the osteoclasts that resorb the bone along the course of the blood vessel, enlarging the vascular channel into a cutting cone. The cavity of the cutting cone is filled in by osteoblasts that secrete matrix in parallel successive layers. These cutting cones may extend across osteons, and after several cycles of remodeling, interstitial fragments become more numerous. The age of the skeleton can be estimated from the number of interstitial osteonal fragments and the number of rings, or lamellae, within the completed osteons.

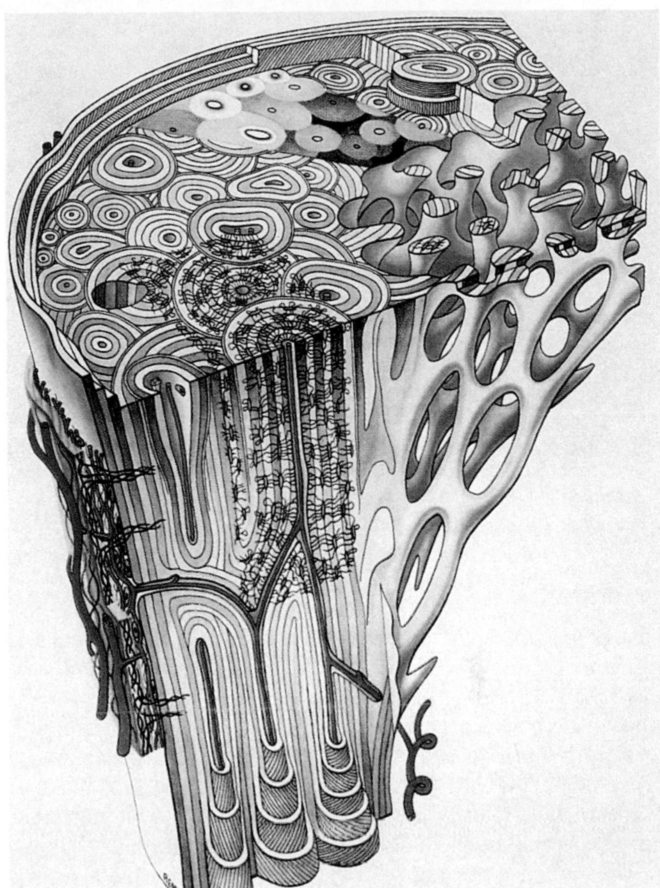

Fig. 74-9 Appearance of bone in transverse and longitudinal sections. This model depicts the general construction of osteons, osteocyte lacunae, haversian canals, and areas of resorption. (From Warwick, Williams, editors: *Grays anatomy*, Philadelphia, 1975, WB Saunders.)

Bone envelopes

A bone envelope is a broad surface area of the skeleton that contains similar cells that perform coordinated functions. The metabolic activities that occur within an envelope are different, and therefore envelopes are distinct functionally.

The *periosteal envelope* encases the entire skeleton on its outer margin. It is covered by a layer of undifferentiated cells, which is further covered by a sheath of fibrous connective tissue. The layers are not present in areas where tendons and ligaments attach. The periosteal envelope enlarges throughout life in human beings and plays an important role in fracture healing and in the response of bone to mechanical usage.

The *haversian envelope* encompasses compact or cortical bone (Fig. 74-9). The center of each haversian system contains vessels and a nerve, which lie within a fibroblast network surrounded by a membrane opposed to the bone surface. The walls of Volkmann's canals are also part of this envelope. Primary osteons are the first haversian systems that form. Secondary osteons form later and leave parts of primary osteons between them. Neither spaces nor voids develop in the haversian envelopes of subjects with metabolic bone disease, but the haversian envelope does shrink with age.

The *cortical-endosteal envelope* limits the outermost boundary of the medullary canal. It is interrupted by trabeculas that connect with the cortex.

The *trabecular or endosteal envelope* is the interface between the marrow and the trabecular bone. The ratio of the endosteal surface to the trabecular volume is greater than the surface-to-volume ratio of other envelopes. The greater the volume of bone, the greater is the metabolic activity; thus, because this is a predominantly bone-losing envelope, the metabolic activity in it is relatively high. The *transitional envelope* is an ill-defined area adjacent to the cortical-endosteal envelope and occupies a third of the medullary cavity between the cortical-endosteal surfaces. It is often included within the endosteal envelope, but because it is an area where trabecular bone remodeling is highest, it is considered by some to be functionally distinct.[14]

Regulation of bone formation and resorption

Bone is a dynamic tissue that undergoes constant remodeling. Remodeling is important to the renewal of the skeleton and also to the regulation of calcium homeostasis. *Bone remodeling units* (BRUs) are groups of cells that occur at discrete locations and at different phases of bone growth. The changes in bone matrix and mineral content that take place during normal development and aging are functions of BRUs. In some disease states abnormalities in the BRUs cause an imbalance between bone formation and resorption.[17-19]

In the classic view of remodeling, the remodeling cycle consists of three phases: activation, resorption, and formation

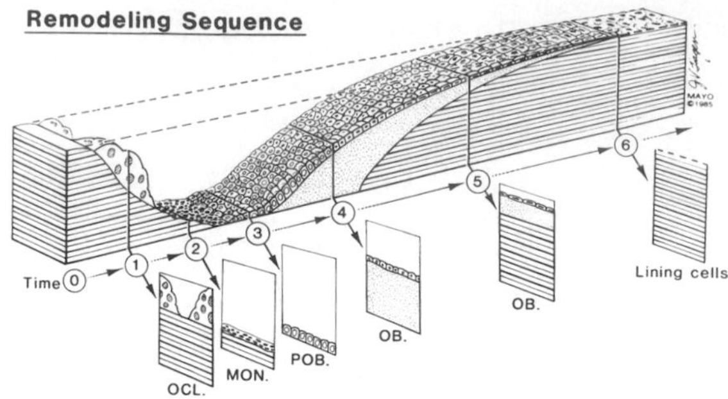

Fig. 74-10 Longitudinal and cross-sectional representation of the bone remodeling unit in cancellous bone. Five phases are distinguishable: *1*, osteoclast-mediated bone resorption; *2*, resorption by mononuclear cells; *3*, migration of preosteoblasts and differentiation into osteoblasts; *4*, osteoid deposition; and *5*, mineralization. *MON.*, mononuclear cells; *OB.*, osteoblasts; *OCL.*, osteoclasts; *POB.*, preosteoblasts. (Courtesy Mayo Foundation, 1985.)

(Fig. 74-10). The cycle is initiated by the activation of osteoclast precursors, which become osteoclasts and begin resorbing bone. During a reversal phase a densely staining metachromatic band termed a "reversal" or "cement line," forms at the limits of the resorption focus. The area is subsequently invaded by preosteoblasts that differentiate into osteoblasts. These cells form a new matrix that becomes mineralized. In the normal skeleton, the complete remodeling cycle takes 100 days in cortical bone and 200 days in trabecular bone.[20,21]

The linked activation of osteoclast-mediated bone resorption and bone formation by osteoblasts is termed "coupling." In the quantum theory of Frost, it is hypothesized that changes in bone mass result from an imbalance between the amount of bone resorbed and the amount of bone formed. Normally, coupling ensures that the amount of bone removed is deposited again during the formation phase. The amount of bone remodeled per unit of time depends on the cellular activity at each BRU and on the number of active remodeling sites per unit of bone volume. The rate at which BRUs are formed is called the *"activation frequency."*[22]

Bone remodeling is regulated systemically by polypeptide, steroid, and thyroid hormones and by numerous locally produced cytokines and growth factors. Growth factors are also present in the circulation and like hormones act as systemic regulators. These hormones, growth factors, and cytokines[23,24] are listed in Table 74-2.

Table 74-2 Growth factors, cytokines, and hormones that regulate bone formation and resorption

Peptide hormones
Parathyroid hormone
Parathyroid hormone–related peptide
Calcitonin
Insulin
Growth hormone
Steroid hormones
Estrogens
Androgens
1,25-Dihydroxyvitamin D
Glucocorticoid hormones
Thyroid hormones
Growth factors
Insulin-like growth factors I and II
Insulin-like growth factor–binding proteins
Acidic and basic fibroblast growth factors
Platelet-derived growth factor
Transforming growth factors
Cytokines and other factors
Interleukins
Tumor necrosis factor
Colony-stimulating factors
Lymphotoxin
Prostaglandins

Polypeptide and steroid hormones

Parathyroid hormone (PTH) is a polypeptide that is secreted in response to low concentrations of ionized calcium in the serum. PTH stimulates osteoclasts to resorb bone, acting primarily on osteoblasts. The way in which signals are transmitted from osteoblasts to osteoclasts is not fully understood. Various growth factors, hormones, and bone matrix proteins have been implicated. Osteoclasts do not contain receptors for PTH, and thus it is believed that PTH acts directly on the osteoblast, perhaps causing a local factor to be produced that enhances osteoclast-mediated bone resorption. PTH also augments the renal tubular resorption of calcium and enhances the excretion of phosphate. PTH stimulates the production of 1,25-dihydroxyvitamin D—1,25$(OH)_2D_3$—by the kidney, which in turn stimulates intestinal calcium absorption. Osteoclast-mediated bone resorption is stimulated at supraphysiologic doses of 1,25$(OH)_2D_3$. These processes act in concert to raise the serum concentrations of ionized calcium, which in turn inhibits the release of PTH.

The effect of PTH on the osteoblast varies with the dose and timing of administration. Continuous stimulation of bone by PTH directly inhibits the formation of collagen at the transcriptional level. Intermittent treatment with PTH, however, stimulates the formation of collagen and bone. The anabolic effect of PTH is mediated, at least in part, by insulin-like growth factor-I (IGF-I).[25]

Calcitonin inhibits bone formation through its effects on the osteoclasts. Most of calcitonin's actions have been observed at pharmacologic doses, and its role as a physiologic regulator of bone remodeling is poorly understood.

Insulin greatly stimulates the formation of the bone matrix, and normal mineralization cannot occur without it. This is the reason skeletal mineralization and growth are impaired in persons with untreated diabetes mellitus. The role of insulin differs from that of insulin-like growth factors (IGFs), in that IGFs stimulate cell proliferation.[24]

Growth hormone (GH) from the pituitary has no effect on bone resorption, and its role in the formation of bone is debated. In vivo GH is necessary for maintaining normal bone mass, but its actual role in the local production of IGFs is unknown, making it difficult to differentiate between the direct and indirect effects of GH.[26,27]

Thyroid hormones are necessary for normal growth and development and mostly influence cartilage formation. They do not alter bone cell replication or matrix formation but can stimulate bone resorption. Excessive amounts of endogenous or exogenous thyroid hormone can cause osteopenia, but the clinical significance of this bone loss remains controversial.[28-30]

Estrogens and androgens play a critical role in the maturation of the skeleton and in the prevention of bone loss. In vivo estrogens cause a decrease in bone resorption and perhaps a decrease in the synthesis of cytokines such as interleukin-6 that are present in the bone microenvironment. Results of other studies indicate that estrogen may stimulate the production of a variety of growth factors, including transforming growth factor-beta (TGFβ), IGF-I, and IGF-II. Estrogens may decrease the sensitivity of the skeleton to PTH. Additional mechanisms that control the interaction between estrogen deficiency and bone loss have been proposed; thus there may be several mechanisms responsible for the changes in bone remodeling that occur in postmenopausal women. Androgens can inhibit PTH-stimulated cyclic adenosine monophosphate production in bone cells, and osteopenia is a common clinical sequela of hypogonadism in men.[31]

Glucocorticoids directly inhibit bone resorption, both in vivo and in vitro. They transiently augment the formation or function of osteoclasts, but with time, bone resorption is reduced because fewer precursor cells are recruited. The increased bone resorption caused by the impaired calcium absorption brought about by glucocorticoids results in secondary hyperparathyroidism. The effects of glucocorticoid on bone formation are complex and may stem from its short-term versus long-term effects and its concentration. Its long-term effects on collagen synthesis are inhibitory and may result from a decrease in the recruitment of preosteoblastic cells. Glucocorticoids inhibit the synthesis of IGF-I by bone cells, which may indirectly inhibit bone formation.[32,33]

$1,25(OH)_2D_3$ stimulates bone resorption. It is necessary for normal bone growth and mineralization but does not directly stimulate bone formation. Its complex effects on bone formation may be related to a variety of actions, including the direct inhibition of collagen synthesis. An increased binding of IGF-I to its receptor in osteoblast-like cells and the synthesis of selected IGF-binding proteins by glucocorticoids may modify the actions of IGF.[34]

Growth factors and cytokines

Under some conditions, *IGF-I* itself may act as a systemic agent, but the local (that is, produced) IGFs probably have a more important regulatory role. For example, IGF-I directly modulates the differentiation of osteoblasts and augments matrix production. There are at least six IGF-binding proteins in bone cells, and these proteins are important because they neutralize or enhance the biologic activities of the IGFs.[34] The TGFβs are abundant in bone tissue. Several subtypes have been isolated, but as a group they stimulate the replication of osteoblast-like cells and matrix formation.[35] These effects on the proliferation and differentiation of osteoblast-like cells may in turn stimulate bone formation. TGFβ also inhibits bone resorption. Other acidic polypeptides, which are similar to TGFβ in terms of their amino acid sequence and effects on bone cells and matrix, include osteoinductive factors such as osteogenin and other bone morphogenic proteins, several of which have been isolated and characterized.

Acidic and basic fibroblast growth factors stimulate osteoblast replication, thus increasing the number of cells that can produce bone matrix. These factors are manufactured locally in the bone and are believed to play a critical role in healing and bone repair. *Platelet-derived growth factor* is secreted by normal bone cells in the form of the platelet-derived growth factor AA dimer and stimulates bone cell replication and resorption. Like the fibroblast growth factors, this polypeptide may be important in the repair process.[24]

Recent research has been focused on the role of various cytokines synthesized by bone cells and present in the bone microenvironment and on their activity. The interleukins, macrophage- and granulocyte-macrophage colony–stimulating factors, and tumor necrosis factor influence bone remodeling and stimulate bone resorption.

In summary, bone remodeling is a dynamic and complex process that is regulated by numerous systemic hormones and local factors. The direct action of these agents on cellular proliferation and differentiation profoundly affects the remodeling cycle and can alter the activation frequency. Other factors promote bone repair or have a specific role in the pathogenesis of metabolic bone disease. Bone remodeling is essential for removing aged, microdamaged bone and for rearranging bone architecture to meet the varying demands for the mechanical support required of the skeleton.[36]

Bone biopsy and bone histomorphometry

Histologic sections can be prepared either from decalcified bone or from intact bone embedded in plastic without having been decalcified. The latter approach is especially suitable when investigating the nature of metabolic bone diseases because the processing does not alter the basic structure of bone. Several important technical advances have facilitated the examination of bone and hence the diagnosis of metabolic bone disease. Previously it was necessary to decalcify bone specimens in preparation for paraffin embedding and sectioning. With the development of reproducible, reliable methods of plastic embedding, ultrathin sections of undecalcified tissue, which thus preserved the basic structure of bone, could be prepared.

Another important advance was the discovery that orally administered tetracycline antibiotics are permanently incorporated into sites of bone formation (Fig. 74-11). With this it became possible to histologically quantitate bone formation, allowing dynamic indices of bone formation to be assessed. In addition, a safe and relatively noninvasive method of obtaining bone specimens from the anterior iliac crest with the patient under local anesthesia, performed as an outpatient procedure, permitted widespread performance of bone biopsy as part of the diagnosis of disease and assessment of therapy.[19,37,38]

There are limitations to the clinical utility of bone biopsy specimens. Only samples of a single skeletal site are obtained, but there is regional variation in some disorders. Frequently this variation stems from the severity of the disorder, such that a diagnosis cannot always be rendered on the basis of the findings yielded by the small specimen of bone obtained. An additional limitation is that the current rate of bone remodeling may be normal, and the cause of bone loss may thus not be apparent on the biopsy specimen. Histomorphometry does not consistently adequately estimate the rate of bone resorption, and this is an additional limitation. It is assumed that bone formation and resorption are closely coupled, and the rate of bone formation is therefore utilized as an index of skeletal turnover.

Tetracycline binds in an irreversible manner to hydroxyapatite at the mineralization front. To "label" bone, one administers tetracycline for 3 days; this is followed by 12 to 14 drug-free days, after which the drug is administered for an

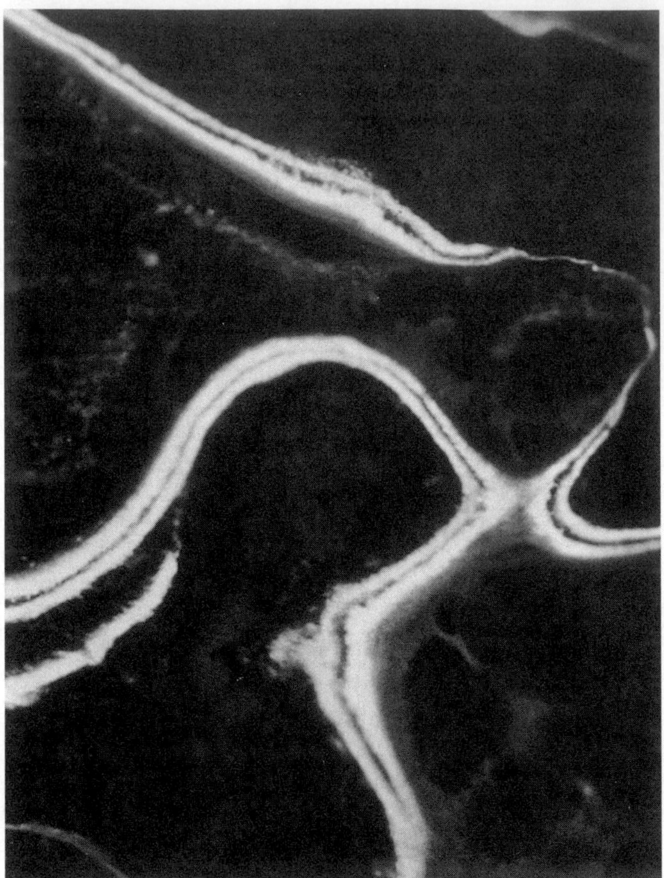

Fig. 74-11 Tetracycline label as viewed by fluorescent microscopy. Tetracycline was administered before bone biopsy. A double label is present; by measuring the distance between the two labels, the rate of bone formation can be calculated.

additional 3 days (3:12:3 sequence). The biopsy is performed on the fourth or fifth day after the last dose of tetracycline has been administered.[39] When the biopsy section is viewed under blue or violet light, a thin fluorescent line is seen at the mineralization front. The use of two different tetracyclines (demeclocycline, tetracycline hydrochloride, or oxytetracycline), though not necessary, may aid in identifying the label because of the two different colors of fluorescence that are yielded. Tetracycline should not be given to children or pregnant women because it is incorporated into growing teeth and can cause discoloration. The tetracycline should be taken on an empty stomach because dairy products and other foods or medications that contain calcium, aluminum, or magnesium will bind the medication. Patients taking the medication should avoid direct exposure to sunlight or ultraviolet rays to prevent the phototoxicity associated with the antibiotics.

The iliac crest is the preferred site for biopsy because of its accessibility, the inclusion of both cortical and trabecular bone in the sample, and the large amount of histomorphometric data that has been yielded by specimens from this site.[40] The usual biopsy site is 2 cm posterior to the anterior superior iliac spine, immediately inferior to the crest. A standard trephine with an internal diameter of at least 7.5 mm is recommended to ensure that an adequate sample is obtained. With mild sedation and careful local anesthesia, patient tolerance is excellent and discomfort minimal. Complications are rare, and in an international multicenter study of 9131 transiliac crest biopsies, only 0.7% of the patients experienced complications. These complications included pain at the biopsy site that persisted for more than 7 days, which is usually treatable with nonnarcotic analgesics. Rarely, hematoma, wound infections, osteomyelitis, or fracture through the iliac crest has been reported.[41]

The specimens are fixed in 70% ethanol to preserve the tetracycline label and then embedded in methyl methacrylate. Plastic-embedded tissue is cut with a tungsten-carbide–edged knife. The methyl methacrylate is flexible but adequately supports the undecalcified section. The 5 to 10 μm thick sections can be stained with a variety of dyes to distinguish bone marrow and mineralized and unmineralized matrix. Unstained sections are used to assess the extent of the tetracycline label under ultraviolet radiation. Specimens are examined under polarized light to determine whether the bone is woven or lamellar.

Quantitative bone histomorphometry is the only method that can distinguish alterations in cell activity from changes in cell number.[42] It is performed using standard stereologic techniques such as point counting or computerized planimetry. There are two types of histomorphometric indices: static ones that are measured directly and dynamic ones. Static indices provide information on the amount of bone and the proportion of the bone surface involved in a particular phase of remodeling. Dynamic indices provide information on the cell-mediated aspect of bone remodeling (Table 74-3). Tetracycline labeling is necessary when one is assessing the dynamic indices. Assessment of the dynamic indices may be very important in a particular patient because an increase in the resorption surface area (a static index) may not accurately reflect an increase in the resorption rate (a dynamic index). The standard nomenclature for the static and dynamic indices of bone and their abbreviations are summarized in Table 74-3.

The indications for bone biopsy may vary, and these are expected to change as new treatments for metabolic bone diseases come available. Some of the current indications for transiliac bone biopsies are listed in Table 74-4.

SKELETAL DEVELOPMENTAL AND GENETIC DISORDERS

Chondrodysplasias

Chondrodysplasias are a heterogeneous group of disorders associated with abnormalities in the size and shape of bones and are manifested by a disproportionate shortness in stature. They are typically named after the part of the bone that is affected, such as epiphyseal, metaphyseal, or diaphyseal dysplasia. If the spine is involved, the prefix "spondylo-" is added, and if the skull is affected, the prefix "cranio-" is used. Other names refer to the appearance of the bone itself, such as "diastrophic" ('twisted'), "thanatophoric" ('death-bearing'), and "metatropic" ('changing'). Although these represent a heterogeneous group of disorders that have been segregated on the basis of clinical characteristics, a family history of the disease is obligatory. The evolving nomenclature and the distinction in the pathogenesis have been the topics of several recent reviews.[43,44]

Table 74-3 Terminology of bone histomorphometry

Proposed term	Abbreviation	Units
Bone volume	BV/TV	%
Osteoid volume	OV/BV	%
Osteoid volume	OV/TV	%
Osteoid surface	OS/BS	%
Osteoblast surface	Ob.S/BS	%
Osteoid thickness	O.Th	μm
Eroded surface	ES.BS	%
Osteoclast surface	Oc.S/BS	%
Osteoclast number	N.Oc/T.A	$/mm^2$
Bone surface	BS/TV	mm^2/mm^3
Mineralizing surface	MS/BS	%
Mineralizing surface	MS/OS	%
Mineral opposition rate	MAR	μm/d
Trabecular thickness	Tb.Th	μm
Trabecular number	Tb.N	/mm
Trabecular separation	Tb.Sp	μm
Adjusted apposition rate	Aj.AR	μm/d
Bone formation rate	BFR/BS	$\mu m^3/\mu m^2/d$
Bone formation rate	BFR/BV	%/y

Table 74-4 Clinical indications for bone biopsy and histomorphometry

Renal osteodystrophy
Osteomalacia
Undiagnosed bone disease
Bone disease refractory to standard treatment
Ruling out secondary causes of osteoporosis

In patients with chondrodysplasias that involve primarily metaphyseal defects, the radiologic appearance of the growth plates may be confused with the appearance exhibited by metabolic bone diseases. However, serum levels of biochemical markers are normal, the skeleton is well mineralized, and the radiographic appearance of the metaphyseal defects can be correctly identified by an experienced radiologist.

Achondroplasia

Achondroplasia is the most common cause of a disproportionately short stature. It occurs in 1 of 40,000 live births and is inherited in an autosomal dominant manner. The homozygous form of the disease is uniformly fatal, either at birth or within the first few months of life. Usually the head is large, the frontal region is protuberant, and the nasal bridge is depressed. Lordosis and dorsal lumbar kyphosis are present, and there is an anteroposterior flattening of the pelvic inlet, leading to reproductive problems in the female offspring. Eighty percent of the cases are sporadic.

The histologic appearances are variable, but overall it is generally agreed that the physical appearance reflects the failure of normal endochondral ossification at the level of the proliferating and maturing cartilage (Figs. 74-12 and 74-13). Bones that calcify through endochondral ossification are the only bones affected. Therefore the base of the skull is hypoplastic, the calvarium is normal in size, and there is a characteristic facial appearance. Minor abnormalities have been noted in some areas of the growth plate, consisting of clumps of proliferating chondrocytes separated by fibrosepta. Other investigators have noted that the hypertrophic zone is attenuated and the number of chondrocytes is diminished. This has led to confusion about the actual histologic appearance because originally well-organized growth plates with normal columns of chondrocytes were described. The differentiation from thanatophoric dysplasia and other dysplasias is usually made on clinical radiologic and histologic grounds. Periosteal overgrowth results in the cupping of the epiphyseal region in both the heterozygous and homozygous forms of achondroplasia.

Achondrogenesis

Two syndromes that involve severe failure of growth are classified as achondrogenesis. Affected infants are either stillborn or do not survive the immediate neonatal period. The two syndromes are known as achondrogenesis I (Parenti-Fraccaro) and achondrogenesis II (Langer-Saldino). Achondrogenesis I may be associated with congenital heart defects. There is absolutely no ossification in the skull and vertebral bodies. Histopathologic studies have shown that endochondral ossi-

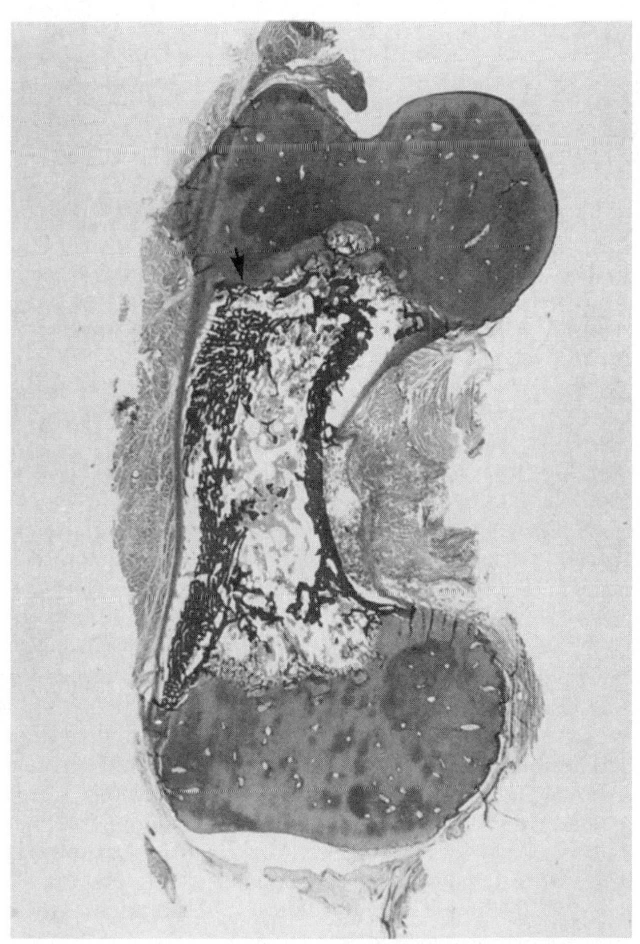

Fig. 74-12 Macrosection of achondroplastic bone. Lack of cartilage maturation results in greatly shortened long bones. Normal periosteal bone growth with narrowed growth plate is seen, and there is infolding and apposition of the periosteum and perichondrium at the level of the perichondrial rim *(arrow)*.

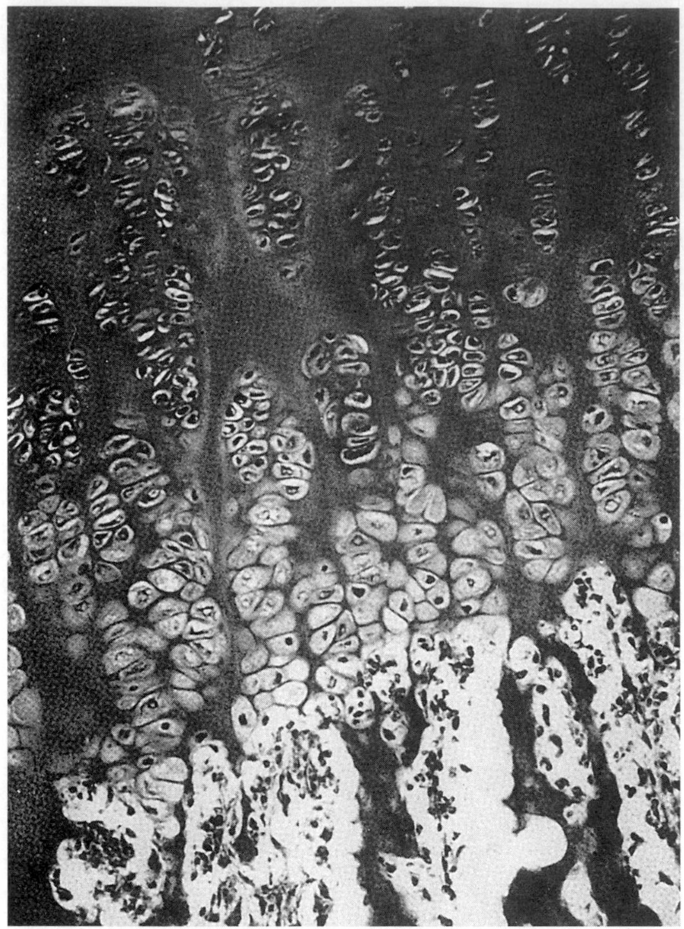

Fig. 74-13 Hematoxylin and eosin–stained section from a patient with achondroplasia of costochondral junction growth plate showing relatively normal endochondral ossification with cartilage column formation. (From Revell PA, editor: *Pathology of bone,* Berlin, 1986, Springer-Verlag.)

fication is very abnormal, manifesting as hypercellularity throughout the growth plate.

Achondrogenesis II is clinically different, and those with the disorder have shortened limbs and a disproportionally large head. Radiographically, underdeveloped ossification centers are found in the vertebral bodies and pelvis. Ossification in the cranial belt, however, is well developed. Histopathologically, achondrogenesis II is very different from other chondroplasias. The epiphyseal cartilage is lobulated and shows increased vascularity. The reserve cartilage is hypercellular, and hypertrophic chondrocytes are separated by small amounts of matrix. Endochondral ossification at the growth plate is completely disorganized, and there is no column formation. Primary trabeculae are sometimes arranged horizontally, and they are irregular and decreased in number.

Thanatophoric dysplasia

Infants with thanatophoric dysplasia are either stillborn or die of respiratory distress during the neonatal period. The pattern of inheritance is unknown, and most cases are sporadic. The length of the trunk is normal, but the head is large and there is cranial-facial disproportion. Anomalies in both the cardiovascular and central nervous systems are not unusual, and the diagnostic radiologic features are pronounced platyspondyly of the lumbar vertebrae with an inverted U appearance, curvature of the femurs with medial and lateral spikes at their low ends, and short, flared ribs. Histologically the resting cartilage is fairly normal and is made up of round or spindle-shaped cells contained in a homogeneous matrix. Endochondral ossification is disrupted at the growth plate, and there is no regular column formation.

Other chondrodysplasias

Several other chondrodysplasias fall into the category of lethal neonatal skeletal dysplasia. One such syndrome is the *short rib–polydactyly syndrome.* This autosomal recessive disorder is difficult to differentiate from a fixating thoracic dysplasia. Histologically, abnormal chondro-osseous development has been reported, consisting of reduced numbers of chondrocytes with disorganized column formation.

Chondroectodermal dysplasia (Ellis-van Creveld syndrome) is characterized by short-limb dwarfism. Consanguinity is an important factor in the acquisition of this dysplasia, which includes narrowing of the rib cage, congenital heart disease, and ectodermal abnormalities affecting the hair, teeth, and nails. It is inherited in an autosomal recessive manner, and its radiographic appearance resembles that of asphyxiating thoracic dysplasia. In the Ellis-van Creveld syndrome, there is acromelic micromelia (shortening of the distal segment of the limb). The histologic appearances are inconsistent, and some have described nuclear abnormalities of the chondrocytes in islands of bone in the metaphyseal cartilage.

In *asphyxiating thoracic dysplasia* (Jeune's syndrome), there is a severe narrowing of the chest and immobility. Early death caused by respiratory distress and infection is the usual outcome, but milder forms are compatible to life. In later childhood the shape of the thorax reverts toward normal, and there are case reports of adult patients. The femoral heads in affected neonates often show growth of the epiphyses. The sternum may be incompletely ossified, and varied histologic abnormalities have been described. They include a reduction in the number of proliferating chondrocytes, irregular vascularization during periods of endochondral ossification, and the presence of islands of cartilage in the metaphyses.

Stippled epiphyses and chondrodysplasia punctata are striking features seen on radiographic studies. These are features of a number of different disorders, including multiple epiphyseal dysplasia, the mucolipidoses, the mucopolysaccharidoses, trisomy 18, trisomy 21, anencephaly, cretinism, and peripheral resistance to thyroxine. Three types of congenital dysplasia that involve stippling of the epiphyses and manifest as chondrodysplasia punctata of the autosomal dominant and autosomal recessive types and the sex-linked variant. No histopathologic studies have been performed in patients with the sex-linked form of chondrodysplasia punctata.

Sclerosing bone dysplasias

In addition to dietary, metabolic, endocrine, and hematologic disorders, many dysplastic conditions assume the form of a focal or generalized osteosclerosis. These uncommon conditions are primarily hereditary.

Osteopetrosis

Osteopetrosis, also called "marble bone disease," was first described in 1904 by Albers-Schönberg.[45] The autosomal dominant form of the syndrome is considered benign, in that there are few or no symptoms; the autosomal recessive form is considered malignant because it is typically fatal during infancy or early childhood.[46,47] An intermediate autosomal recessive form has been described, but it has not been well characterized. The fourth clinical type, an autosomal recessive syndrome of osteopetrosis, renal tubular acidosis (RTA), and cerebral calcification, results from carbonic anhydrase-II deficiency. Although the clinical types appear diverse, the pathogenesis of all forms involves defective osteoclast function that impairs skeletal resorption. As a result, the primary spongiosa persists during adult life and characteristic histologic changes take place.

In victims of the malignant form of osteopetrosis, which is inherited as an autosomal recessive trait, there is an increased incidence of parental consanguinity. Malformation of the mastoid and paranasal sinuses may be an early symptom. Cranial foramina do not widen fully, and there may be palsies of the optic, ocular motor, and facial nerves. Eruption of dentition is delayed. Although bones appear dense on radiographs, they are actually fragile and may fracture. Retinal degeneration with blindness, recurrent infection together with spontaneous bruising and bleeding resulting from the myelophthisis occurring in dense bone, hypersplenism, and hemolysis are other presenting features. The autosomal dominant form of osteopetrosis is considered benign because it is a developmental condition and most affected subjects are asymptomatic. The long bones are brittle, and associated clinical problems such as compromised vision or hearing, carpal tunnel syndrome, and osteoarthritis have been described. Adult patients may be asymptomatic, but pathologic fractures can occur because the dense bone and calcified cartilage are so brittle.

The defective osteoclastic bone resorption results in a pronounced increase in calcified skeletal tissue, which radiographically appears dense. At the growth plate the primary spongiosa is not converted to more mature trabecular bone and the central calcified bars of cartilage are surrounded by woven bone. The medullary space may be filled by calcified skeletal tissue to the exclusion of normal bone marrow elements (Fig. 74-14).

The radiologic features of osteopetrosis are diagnostic in most cases.[48] The failure of osteoclasts to resorb skeletal tissue constitutes a pathognomonic histologic finding.[49] The number of osteoclasts may be increased, normal, or decreased. In the malignant autosomal recessive form these multinucleated cells are usually abundant, their nuclei are especially numerous, and the characteristic ruffled border of clear zones is absent.[50] There may be increased amounts of osteoid in the benign form of the disease. The osteoclasts can be few and lack ruffled borders, or they can be numerous and enlarged.[51,52]

One of the molecular defects identified in patients with this disorder is carbonic anhydrase-II deficiency (Table 74-5). Abnormalities in the microenvironment or in the osteoclast stem cell itself, in the mature osteoclast, or in the bone matrix are other potential defects. A primary lysosomal defect may be present in a few patients with the osteopetrosis associated with neuronal storage disease (characterized by an accumulation of ceroid lipofuscin). In other patients, viruslike inclusions have been found in the osteoclasts, but the significance of these findings is uncertain.[53] The factors responsible ultimately impair bone resorption, and skeletal fragility and the defective remodeling of woven bone to compact bone are the consequences. In an osteopetrotic (op/op) mouse model, the lack of macrophage colony–stimulating factor (M-CSF or CSF-I) produces a syndrome similar to that seen in humans.[54] Treatment of rats with one of these osteopetrotic mutations using CSF-I was found to alleviate the skeletal problems, but the metaphyseal sclerosis

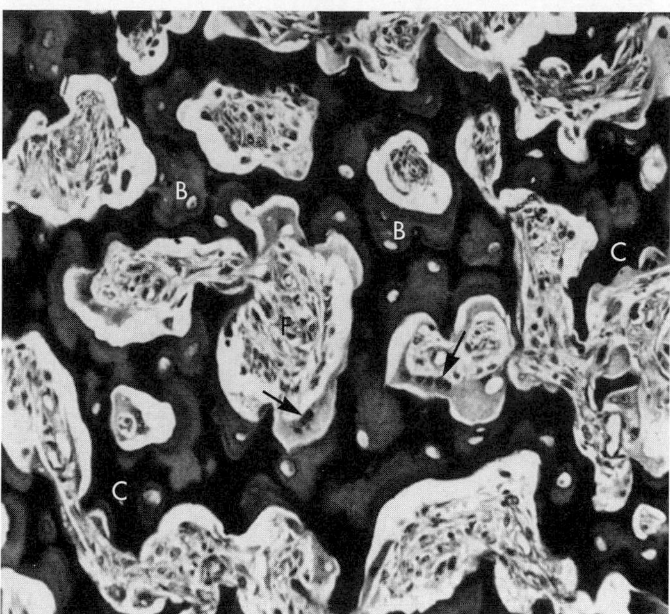

Fig. 74-14 Histologic appearance of infantile malignant osteopetrosis. The bone is sclerotic because of the preservation of the primary spongiosa, which consists of calcified cartilage bars *(C)* surrounded by bone *(B)*. The marrow is fibrotic *(F)*. The osteoclast morphologic appearance is abnormal *(arrows)*.

Table 74-5 Molecular defects in developmental skeletal disorders

Clinical syndrome	Molecular defect
Chondrodystrophies	Genetic linkage of insulin-like growth factor-I gene at chromosome 12q23*
Osteogenesis imperfecta	Collagen gene defects† (see Table 74-6)
Osteopetrosis	*His* to *Tyr* missense mutation or an intron 5 splice acceptor mutation of the carbonic anhydrase-II gene‡
Sclerosing bone disorders	Animal model: transgenic overexpression of *fos*§

*From Mullis PE, Patel MS, Brickell PM et al: *Clin Endocrinol* 34:265, 1991.
†From Lee B, D'Alessio M, Ramírez F: *Crit Rev Eukaryotic Gene Expression* 1:173, 1991.
‡From Roth DE, Venta PJ, Tashian RE, Sly WS: *Proc Natl Acad Sci USA* 89:1804, 1992.
§From Ruther U, Garber C, Komitowski D et al: *Nature* 325:412, 1987.

persisted.[55] Knockout experiments of the *Src* proto-oncogene in mice was observed to cause osteopetrosis, with failure of the *Src* mutant osteoclast to form ruffled borders.[56]

Intermediate osteopetrosis is relatively benign, and spontaneous gradual resolution of the osteosclerosis may occur in infants or young children with carbonic anhydrase-II deficiency. Bone marrow transplantation has brought about considerable improvement in a few patients with malignant osteopetrosis,[57] but not all patients may benefit from it because there is a variety of defects, not all of which are intrinsic to the osteoclast. Therapy by means of large doses of calcitriol and limited calcium intake has been shown to prevent hypercalciuria; occasionally hypercalcemia abates in patients with malignant osteopetrosis. Calcitriol may stimulate dormant osteoclast activity, and the long-term infusion of PTH was helpful in one infant.[58] High-dose glucocorticoid therapy stabilizes the condition of patients with pancytopenia and hepatomegaly resulting from malignant osteopetrosis.

In 1983 the autosomal recessive syndrome of osteopetrosis, RTA, and cerebral calcification was discovered to be caused by a deficiency in the carbonic anhydrase-II isoenzyme.[59] Although there is considerable clinical variability in the syndrome among affected families, the subjects may suffer fractures or show failure to thrive, developmental delay, or short stature. Compression of the optic nerves and dental malocclusion are additional complications. Although fracture is unusual, recurrent breaks in long bones may result in considerable morbidity.

The osteopetrosis stemming from carbonic anhydrase-II deficiency resembles other forms, except that cerebral calcification develops during childhood. The defects in skeletal modeling and the osteosclerosis may diminish spontaneously over the course of years.[60] The cerebral calcification is developmental, appears between 2 and 5 years of age, increases during childhood, and is similar if not identical to that which arises in the settings of idiopathic hypoparathyroidism and pseudohypoparathyroidism. Bone marrow biopsy findings are unremarkable. Metabolic acidosis occurs in the neonatal period, and both proximal and distal forms of RTA have been described. There is no aminoaciduria or glycosuria.

The carbonic anhydrase-II isoenzyme accelerates the first step in the conversion of carbon dioxide and water to bicarbonate. Accordingly these isoenzymes are important in acid-base regulation and carbonic anhydrase-II is widely distributed in a diversity of tissues. Defects in the carbonic anhydrase-II gene, which has been localized to the short arm of chromosome 8 in human beings, have been identified in several patients.[61,62] RTA and the underlying carbonic anhydrase-II deficiency have been treated with bicarbonate supplementation, but the long-term effects of this therapy are unknown.

Progressive diaphyseal dysplasia (Camurati-Engelmann disease)

Progressive diaphyseal dysplasia is a rare autosomal dominant disorder characterized by the formation of new bone at both the periosteal and endosteal surfaces of the long bones. Descriptions of more than 100 cases show that the clinical penetrance is variable and that some carriers have no radiologically detected abnormalities. Some cases have been described as autosomal recessive ("Ribbing's disease").

The disorder usually is manifested in childhood, and because of the antalgic gait, leg pain, and fat and muscle wasting, it may be mistaken for a form of muscular dystrophy. The clinical course, including the age of onset and progression, is variable. The head may be enlarged and show proptosis and a prominent forehead; the bony defects are associated with cranial nerve palsies. Biochemical markers of bone turnover are usually normal in quantity. In some patients the serum alkaline phosphatase activity, urinary hydroxyproline levels, and erythrocyte sedimentation rate are elevated. Modest hypocalcemia and hypocalciuria have been described and attributed to the positive calcium balance.

The most commonly involved bones are the tibias and femurs. A bone scan reveals focally increased uptake, but findings may appear discordant because of the presence of notable but quiescent disease on radiographs. The principal radiographic feature of progressive diaphyseal dysplasia is cortical hyperostosis as a result of new bone proliferation on the endosteal and periosteal surfaces of long bones. The epiphyses are spared, and sclerosis is relatively symmetrical.

Histologically, new bone formation is often disorganized, in that woven bone undergoes centripetal maturation and is incorporated into the cortex. Recently, defects in the differentiation of the monocyte-macrophage line have been suggested as the pathogenetic basis for the disease. Glucocorticoid therapy has successfully ameliorated the pain associated with this disorder, and surgical removal of the local affected area through a "cortical window" has been effective.[63]

Endosteal hyperostosis

Hyperostosis corticalis generalisata was described by van Buchem and colleagues in 1955. This set of disorders has been broadened to include both a clinically severe autosomal recessive type and a benign autosomal dominant form (Worth type). Recent evidence indicates that van Buchem disease and sclerostenosis may reflect similar genetic defects. Van Buchem disease begins with the progressive enlargement of the mandible during puberty. The jaw angles are widened, resulting in prognathism or dental malocclusion. Recurrent facial nerve palsy, deafness, or optic nerve compression may occur. Endosteal thickening produces a dense and homogeneous diaphyseal cortex together with narrowing of the medullary canal, and this is the major radiographic feature. The hyperostosis is selectively endosteal, and generalized osteosclerosis may include the base of the skull, facial bones, vertebrae, pelvis, and ribs. The serum level of alkaline phosphatase of bone origin may be elevated, but the levels of other biochemical markers of bone remodeling are unremarkable. Surgical decompression of the narrowed foramina or surgical reconstruction of the mandible may be palliative.[63]

Sclerostenosis, a variant of van Buchem disease, is defined as cortical hyperostosis with syndactyly. This disorder involves the same gene defect as van Buchem disease and is distinguished by the presence of syndactyly, noted as early as at birth. This autosomal recessive form occurs in the Afrikaners of South Africa as well as other persons of Dutch ancestry. Physical features similar to those described for van Buchem disease are noted, and raised intracranial pressure may be the sequela of a small cranial cavity. Intelligence is normal, fractures are rare, and the life expectancy may be shortened. The principal radiographic feature is the progressive bony thickening with widening of the skull and prognathism. Syndactyly most commonly involves the index and long fingers. The vertebral pedicles, pelvis, and ribs may become dense. Histomorphometric findings indicate dense, thickened trabeculas and osteoidosis with increased rates of bone formation. The indices of bone resorption indicate quiescence. Treatment is by surgical repair of the bony defect.[63]

Osteopoikilosis

Osteopoikilosis is a benign disorder characterized by the presence of numerous foci of sclerosis in cancellous bone ("spotted bones"). It is inherited as an autosomal dominant trait and exhibits high penetrance. The bone changes are asymptomatic and are found incidentally on radiographs (Fig. 74-15). The foci remain unchanged for decades and show no increased uptake of radionucleotides. The foci consist of thickened sclerotic lamellar bone that is merging imperceptibly with the trabeculas of surrounding normal bone. Mature lesions appear to remodel. No treatment is required.[63]

Osteopathia striata

Osteopathia striata is characterized by linear striations at the ends of long bones and in the ilium. In its isolated form, which is a radiographic curiosity, it is transmitted as an autosomal dominant trait. However, the disorder may be associated with other syndromes, such as cranial sclerosis, that lead to cranial nerve palsies or focal dermal hypoplasia, a serious X-linked recessive disorder.

Radiographic features include gracile linear striations in the cancellous regions of the skeleton, particularly in the epiphyseometaphyseal portions of long bones and the periphery of iliac bones. Scintigraphy shows no excessive radionucleotide accumulation. The histopathologic features have not been well defined as yet. No treatment is required.[63]

Melorheostosis

The sporadic disorder melorheostosis is characterized by hyperostosis of the limb bones. Radiographically it has been likened to the appearance of melted wax that has dripped down the side of a candle, hence its Greek name *melos* meaning 'limb' and *rhoē* meaning 'flowing' (Fig. 74-16). It is rarely bilaterally symmetrical, and cutaneous changes can occur at sites over the affected skeletal regions. The condition may be associated with fibromas, fibrolipomas, capillary hemangiomas, lymphangiectasis, and arterial aneurysms. The distribution and associated soft tissue lesions in sclerotomes, myotomes, and dermatomes implies the existence of a segmentary embryogenetic defect. The major symptoms are pain and stiffness; contractures in the affected joint can occur. Skeletal changes progress most rapidly during childhood, and the disease process appears to slow or halt during adulthood.

Eccentric, dense hyperostosis occurs and affects the cortices and adjacent medullary canal of a single bone. The lower extremities are more commonly involved than the upper extremities. The increased blood flow that is associated with the "dripping candle wax" appearance avidly accumulates radionucleolide during imaging. The levels of the biochemical markers of bone resorption are normal.

The typical histologic finding in affected children is endosteal thickening; new periosteal bone forms during adult-

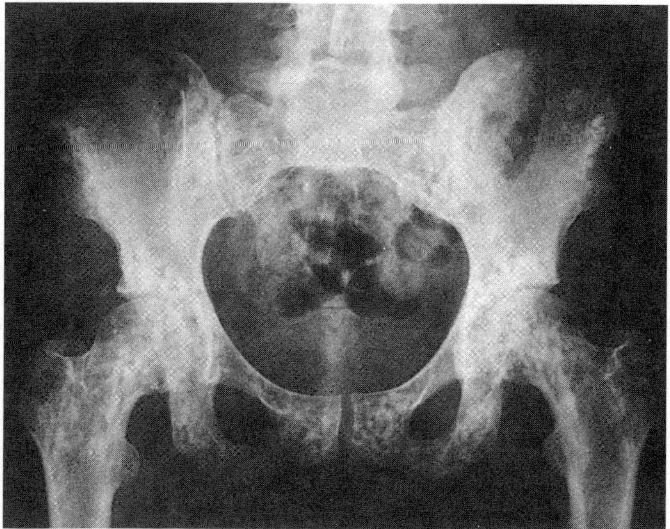

Fig. 74-15 Osteopoikilosis. Notice the typical "spotted bones" appearance of this benign disorder. (From Favus MJ, editor: *Primer on the metabolic bone diseases and disorders of mineral metabolism,* ed 2, New York, 1993, Raven Press.)

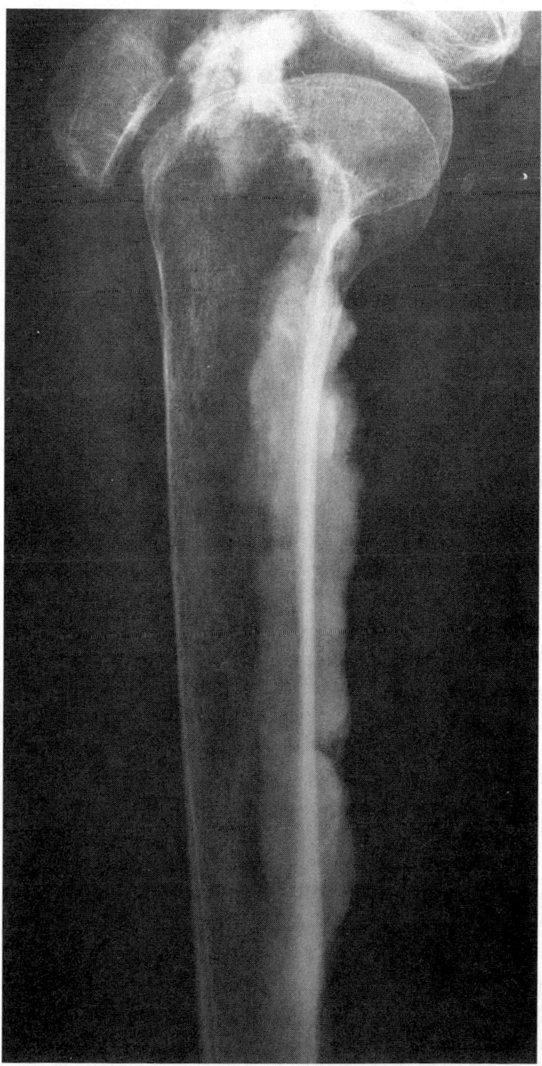

Fig. 74-16 Melorheostosis. The appearance has been likened to that of wax melted down the side of a candle. (Courtesy Dr. Alan Hoffman, Mayo Clinic and Mayo Foundation, Rochester, Minn.)

hood, and pain may be the presenting symptom of this process. The thickened irregular lamellae may occlude haversian systems and produce marrow fibrosis. The collagen of the sclerodermatous skin lesions is normal in appearance. Surgical repair of the contractions has often led to recurrent deformity, and so far no treatment has proved completely satisfactory.[63]

Mixed sclerosing bone dystrophy

Mixed sclerosing bone dystrophy is a rare skeletal dysplasia that exhibits the combined radiographic features of osteopoikilosis, osteopathia striata, melorheostosis, and cranial sclerosis, as well as additional defects. Symptoms may be related to any one of the disorders. The cause remains uncertain, especially in view of the fact that some disorders (osteopoikilosis) are heritable and others (melorheostosis) are sporadic.

Axial osteomalacia

Fewer than 20 cases of axial osteomalacia have been reported. Typically there is coarsening of the trabecular pattern of the axial but not the appendicular skeleton. The symptoms are nonspecific and usually manifest as dull, vague, and chronic pain involving the axial skeleton. The cervical spine and ribs are the most severely affected. Looser's transformation zones, a radiographic hallmark of osteomalacia, have not been reported. Serum biochemical findings are nonspecific and variable; low serum phosphate levels have been noted in a few patients, and the activity of the bone isoenzymes of serum alkaline phosphatase may be increased.

On histologic examination of iliac crest specimens, distinct corticomedullary junctions and wide and porous cortices are found. Under polarized light microscopy, collagen has a lamellar appearance. Osteoid seams are widened on trabecular surfaces, and results of tetracycline-labeling studies confirm that skeletal mineralization is defective. The osteoblasts appear flat and inactive and have reduced Golgi complexes and rough endoplasmic reticulum; staining for alkaline phosphatase is not intense. Although an effective medical treatment has not been reported, the natural history of the disorder indicates that it is relatively benign.[64]

Fibrogenesis imperfecta ossium

Fibrogenesis imperfecta ossium is a rare sporadic disease of unknown cause that afflicts middle-aged persons who typically complain of gradually increasing, intractable pain. Bony tenderness is considerable, and patients become bedridden. The clinical course is debilitating and leads to progressive immobility. Fibrogenesis imperfecta ossium may be an acquired disorder of collagen synthesis affecting lamellar bone. Radiographic abnormalities are found throughout the skeleton except in the skull.

Initially the radiographic appearance is similar to that of osteopenia, but as the disorder progresses, the coarse and dense appearance of trabecular bone is consistent with that of osteomalacia. The corticomedullary junctions become indistinct as cortices are replaced by trabecular bone that exhibits an abnormal pattern. Mixed lytic and sclerotic lesions may appear. As the cortices thin, the remaining trabeculas become coarse and dense and have a "fishnet"-like appearance. Pseudofractures may develop, and some patients have a "rugger jersey" spine that may be confused with similar findings encountered in patients with osteopetrosis or renal osteodystrophy. Periosteal reactions may occur on the shafts of long bones. Serum alkaline phosphatase activity may be increased, and acute agranulocytosis and macroglobulinemia have been reported. Serum calcium and phosphate levels are normal.

Histopathologically the bone biopsy specimen has features of osteomalacia, though the amount of affected bone is variable. Aberrant collagen deposits are found in the regions where the mineralization patterns are abnormal. Osteoid seams are thick, and no birefringence is noted in the abnormal collagen when the bone specimen is viewed under polarized light microscopy. Electron microscopy studies have revealed the presence of thin collagen fibrils that are randomly organized. Collagen synthesis in nonosseous tissues appears normal. The distinction between osteoporosis or osteomalacia and fibrogenesis imperfecta ossium can be made only when one views the specimen under polarized light or by electron microscopy. There is no specific medical therapy. Ectopic calcification occurred in one patient treated with high-dose vitamin D_2 therapy; synthetic salmon calcitonin, sodium fluoride, and $24,25(OH)_2D$ have shown no apparent benefit.[65]

Pachydermoperiostosis

Hypertrophic osteoarthropathy, or pachydermoperiostosis, is characterized by clubbing of the digits, hyperhydrosis, thickening of the skin especially around the face and forehead, and periosteal new bone formation, predominantly in the distal limbs. The disease is inherited as an autosomal dominant trait that exhibits variable penetrance or as an autosomal recessive trait. Men are more severely affected than women; blacks, more commonly than whites. No gene defects have been identified yet. The clinical expression occurs slowly over the course of a decade, and then the disease may become quiescent. Progressive enlargement of the hands and feet have led to an agromegaloid appearance in affected patients. Pseudogout can occur, and chondrocalcinosis was encountered in one patient. There can be stiffness and limited mobility of both the appendicular and axial skeleton.

Radiographically, severe periostosis results in thickening and sclerosis of the distal portions of the tubular bones (tibia, fibula, radius, and ulna). Acro-osteolysis can occur. The differential diagnosis includes secondary hypertrophic osteoarthropathy, but the periosteal reaction in this disorder typically assumes a smooth, undulating appearance. The periosteal proliferation in pachydermoperiostosis is irregular and often involves the epiphysis. Bone scintigraphy reveals regular uptake of radionucleotide along the cortical margins of bones, resulting in a "double stripe" sign.

Subsequently the newly formed osseous tissue undergoes cancellous compaction and can be difficult to distinguish from the original cortex. Mild cellular hyperplasia near the synovial membranes and thickening of the synovial membranes are noted.[66]

Osteogenesis imperfecta

The so-called brittle bone disease comprises a group of hereditary disorders involving defects in the synthesis or structure of collagen type I (see Table 74-5). The severity of the clinical expression varies; the cardinal features include osteopenia associated with recurrent fracture and skeletal deformity (Fig. 74-17). Patients also have dental defects manifesting as dentinogenesis imperfecta and defective dentine formation as well as abnormalities of other tissues containing type I collagen (ligaments, skin, and sclerae). Recent molecular findings have provided new insight into the mode of inheritance, and the heterogeneous clinical manifestations and prognoses in patients with the disease are beginning to be understood.[67,68]

The severity of osteogenesis imperfecta can vary from stillbirth to a lifelong absence of symptoms, and this diversity may be present within a given kindred. The recurrent fractures that bring infants and children to medical attention may result from congenital indifference to pain or from child abuse. Patients with osteogenesis imperfecta can usually be distinguished from those patients with these other disorders by the fact that they suffer ligamentous laxity with joint hypermobility, excessive diaphoresis, easy bruisability, dentinogenesis imperfecta, and hearing loss. The deafness may stem from either conductive or sensorineural hearing loss. The sclerae of these patients may have a blue or gray tint. Other features of osteogenesis imperfecta include a high-pitched voice, short stature, scoliosis, hernias, and a head that is disproportionately large for the body size.

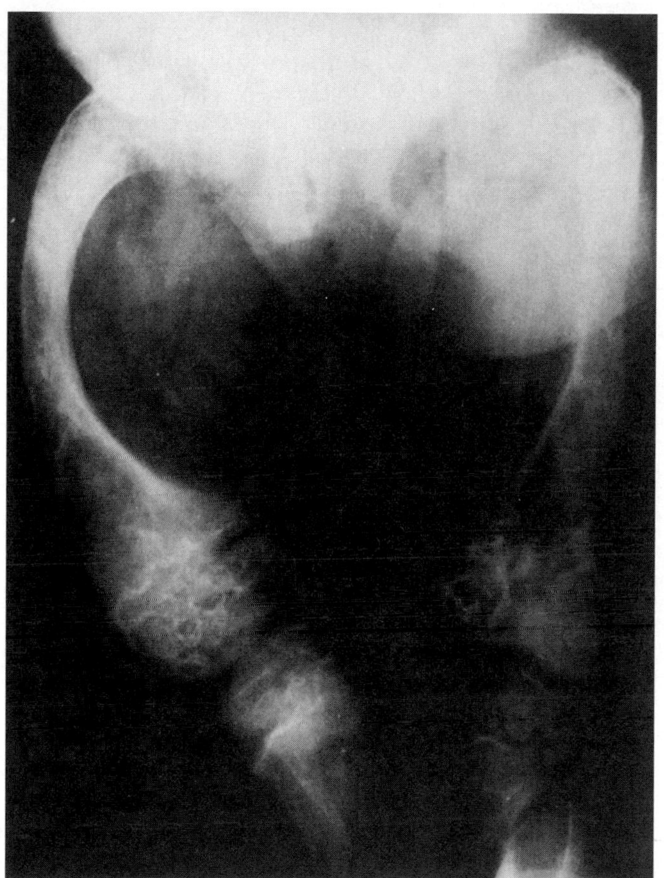

Fig. 74-17 Osteogenesis imperfecta congenita. Radiographic changes showing the typical bowing deformities and severe osteopenia of the bones.

A classification system based on the clinical phenotype was devised by Sillence.[69] Now that the modes of transmission have been clarified and the molecular defects and associated heterogeneity defined, this system has proved limited.[67,68,70] However, it is still useful because it organizes the types according to the clinical features (Table 74-6).

Patients with type I disease experience mild osteopenia with recurrent fracture, and their sclerae are blue. Deafness is common (30% incidence) and adult height is normal. In the older female patient this form may be confused with postmenopausal osteoporosis. Bone histomorphometry may reveal that there are more cortical osteocytes than are typically found in patients with postmenopausal osteoporosis. Type IA and type IB osteoporosis imperfecta are distinguished on the basis of the absence or presence, respectively, of dentinogenesis imperfecta. Approximately a third of all new cases are new mutations resulting in a decreased production of type I collagen, and these are transmitted in an autosomal dominant manner.

Type II osteogenesis imperfecta is often fatal within the first few days or weeks of life. Infants are often premature, have short bowed limbs and a small thoracic cavity that compromises respiratory function, and suffer numerous fractures.

Type III disease is characterized by skeletal deformity resulting from recurrent fractures. Other manifestations include dental abnormalities and short stature. A frameshift mutation prevents the incorporation of pro-alpha-2(I) into a collagen helix. Point mutations in the alpha-1 or alpha-2 chain have also been described.

Osteogenesis imperfecta type IV is transmitted as an autosomal dominant trait and is considered rare. It has recently been suggested that it may account for multigenerational dis-

Table 74-6 Osteogenesis imperfecta: biochemical, genetic, and clinical features

Type	Inheritance	Biochemical/genetic defect	Clinical features
I	Autosomal dominant	Decreased production of type I procollagen; substitution of amino acid residue in triple helix of α1(I)	Normal stature; blue sclerae; hearing loss (50%); dentinogenesis imperfecta (rare)
II	Autosomal dominant (new mutation)	Rearrangements in COL1A1 and COL1A2 genes; substitutions for glycyl residues in triple helix of α1(I)α2(I) chain	Lethal in perinatal period; minimal calvarial mineralization, compressed femurs, platyspondylisis, beaded ribs
	Autosomal recessive (rare)	Deletion in α2(I)	—
III	Autosomal recessive	Frameshift mutation prevents incorporation of pro α2(I) into molecules dentinogenesis imperfecta and hearing loss common	Short stature; progressive deformity, sclerae variable in color;
	Autosomal dominant	Point mutations in α1(I) or α2(I) chain	
IV	Autosomal dominant	Point mutations in α2(I) chain. Point mutations in α1(I) chain; deletions in α2(I) chain.	Mild to moderate bone deformity and variable short stature; dentinoimperfecta common; hearing loss occurs occasionally

ease.[67] Patients can suffer dental disease, hearing loss, and skeletal deformity, but their sclerae are usually a normal color.

The cardinal features of osteogenesis imperfecta are modeling defects of the long bones and deformity resulting from fractures stemming from the generalized osteopenia. Defective periosteal bone formation that retards the circumferential growth of bone, resulting in characteristically thin cortices, and recurrent fractures in deformed vertebrae and long bones are other abnormalities. Numerous large wormian bones are frequently seen in the skull but are not pathognomonic of the disease. Platybasia and excessive pneumatization of the frontal and mastoid sinuses are found in severely affected persons. "Popcorn calcifications" are unusual developmental defects in the epiphyses and metaphyses of the major long bones of patients with type III disease. These may result from traumatic fragmentation and disordered maturation of growth plate cartilage. They resolve after puberty as the growth plates fuse with the mineralized aspect of cartilage.

Biochemical findings are typically unremarkable. In some patients the serum alkaline phosphatase activity is elevated and the urinary levels of hydroxyproline are increased. Recently, hypercalciuria has been found in severely affected children with osteogenesis imperfecta.

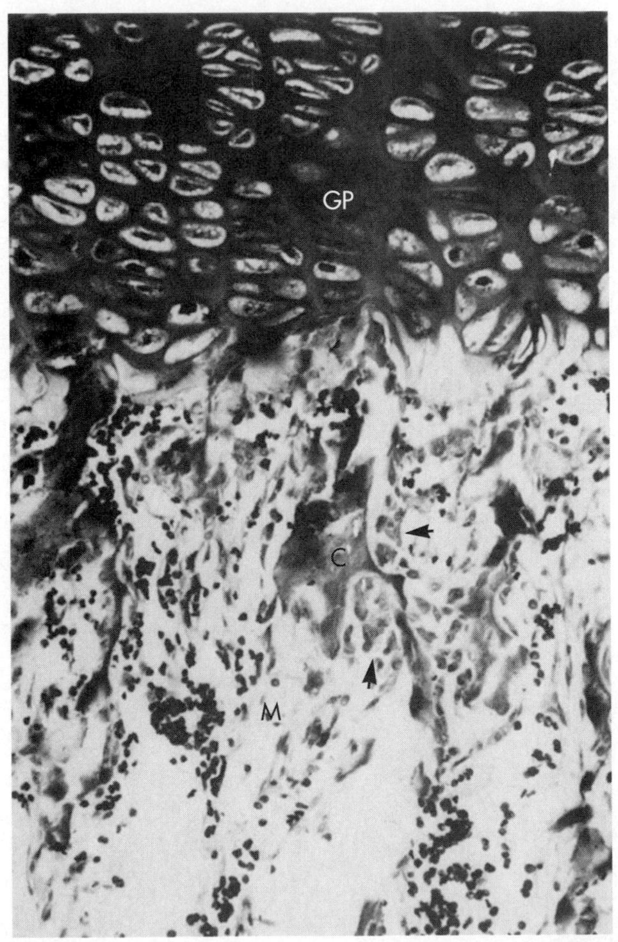

Fig. 74-18 Histologic appearance of a fatal case of osteogenesis imperfecta congenita. The growth plate *(GP)* is normal, and there is normal cartilage development. The calcified cartilage bars *(C)*, however, do not become enveloped by bone. In the metaphysis *(M)* osteoblasts *(arrows)* are present, but bone collagen deposition is absent.

The histologic appearance of bone reflects the abnormal skeletal matrix. The most pronounced changes are seen in the bones of infants who die at birth. The growth plate cartilage is normal in these infants, but the cartilaginous bars formed by vascular invasion of the metaphyses do not become enveloped by bone (Fig. 74-18). Cortical bone is almost nonexistent (Fig. 74-19). Osteoblasts are present, but matrix production is drastically reduced. The changes are less pronounced in the less severe form of the disease. The number of osteocytes may be increased per unit volume of bone, and the remodeling of growing bones may be abnormal. The bones appear less mature because the transformation of cancellous bone into cortical bone has been retarded. The bone trabeculas remain irregularly shaped, the cortex remains porous, and the osteon formation is defective (Fig. 74-20). Polarized light microscopy may reveal an abundance of disorganized woven bone and abnormally thin collagen bundles in lamellar bone. The overall rate of skeletal turnover can be rapid, as indicated by in vivo tetracycline labeling studies.

Considerable progress has been made in identifying the biochemical and molecular defects associated with osteogenesis imperfecta, but up to now there is no established medical therapy.[71] Supportive treatment requires orthopedic, rehabilitative, and dental intervention to manage the various manifestations of the disorder. Genetic counseling should be available, especially in view of the rapid progress that has been made in identifying the genetic defects responsible for the disorder. Prenatal diagnosis has been successful.[72] Support groups are an important source of information and comfort for patients and their families.[67]

METABOLIC BONE DISEASES

In adult humans, metabolic bone disease is a disorder of the bone remodeling system. One can directly examine these systems by histomorphometrically analyzing microscopic sections of trabecular bone obtained by transiliac bone biopsy. In some instances a genetic defect has been linked to the bone disease (Table 74-7).

Osteoporosis

Osteoporosis is defined as the loss of normally mineralized bone and has been diagnosed more commonly clinically with the advent of noninvasive radiographic techniques that measure bone density. Overall the bones are structurally weak, and this is associated with the loss of trabecular bone, enlargement of the medullary space, cortical porosity, and a reduction in cortical thickness. The reduction in bone mass and the changes in bone architecture are associated with an increased risk of fracture and result in pain and deformity. The generalized osteoporoses represent a heterogeneous group of conditions that encompass many pathogenetic mechanisms associated with low, normal, or increased bone remodeling rates. Osteopenia is the fundamental disease in primary osteoporosis. An underlying clinical disease, medical condition, or medication is associated with the development of osteopenia in secondary osteoporosis.

Low bone mass and nontraumatic or atraumatic fractures are features of osteoporosis. The excessive bone loss that characterizes the pathogenesis of osteoporosis results from abnormalities in the bone-remodeling cycle. Osteopenia is the fundamental problem in primary osteoporosis, and the devel-

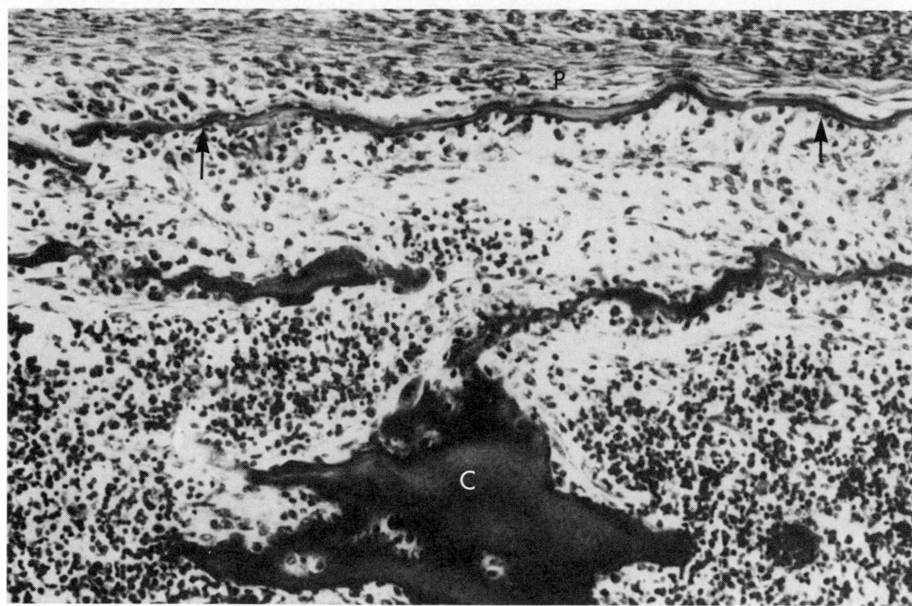

Fig. 74-19 Fatal case of osteogenesis imperfecta congenita. Cortical bone is virtually absent. The periosteum *(P)* contains only a thin ribbon of poorly formed bone *(arrows)*. *C,* Calcified cartilage.

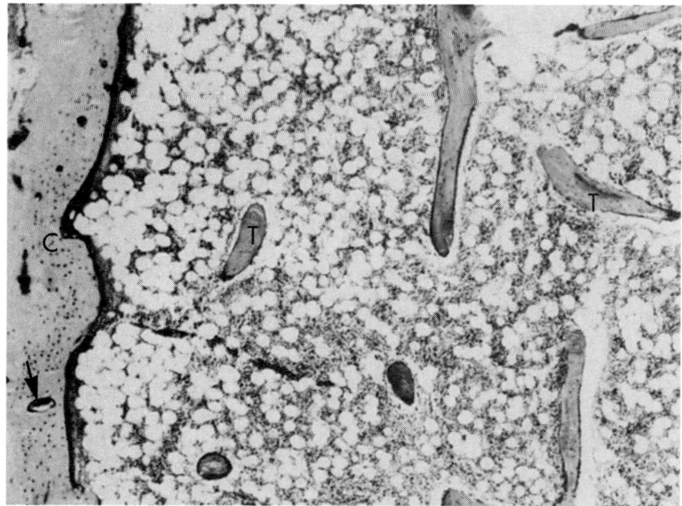

Fig. 74-20 Osteogenesis imperfecta tarda. The histologic organization of the bone is immature, as revealed by the poorly formed cortical bone *(C)* with minimal incorporation of the trabecular bone *(T)* into the cortex. Cortical bone osteons *(arrow)* are also rudimentary.

opment of primary osteoporosis is associated with the specific risk factors listed in Table 74-8. Secondary osteoporosis results from a clearly identifiable etiologic mechanism (Table 74-9).

Primary osteoporosis

Postmenopausal osteoporosis Once the peak adult bone mass has been attained in the third or possibly fourth decade of life, age-related bone loss occurs, and this is a universal phenomenon. With each bone remodeling cycle, there is an imperceptible deficit in bone formation. With the increased rate of the activation phase of bone remodeling, the proportion of skeleton undergoing remodeling at any one time, and hence the rate of bone loss, increases. With normal aging the progressive impair-

Table 74-7 Molecular defects in metabolic bone diseases

Clinical syndrome	Defect
Hypophosphatasia	Multiple missense mutations of the alkaline phosphatase gene
Marfan's syndrome	*Cys* to *ser* missense mutation of the fibrillin gene
McCune-Albright syndrome	Activating mutations of the alpha subunit of stimulatory guanine nucleotide regulatory protein
Osteomalacias	
Hypophosphatemic vitamin D–resistant rickets	Genetic linkage to Xp22.1-22.2
Vitamin D renal hydroxylase deficiency	Genetic linkage to 12q14
Vitamin D receptor disorders	Mutations of the vitamin D receptor
Osteoporosis	Association with allelic differences in 3′untranslated end of vitamin D receptor in select populations

Table 74-8 Risk factors for primary osteoporosis

Genetic factors
Sex
Race
Body weight
Low calcium intake
Sedentary life-style
Smoking
Excessive alcohol consumption
Sex steroid deficiency

Table 74-9 Secondary causes of osteoporosis

Endocrine disorders
Diabetes mellitus
Hyperparathyroidism
Hyperthyroidism
Cushing's syndrome
Acromegaly
Drugs
Anticonvulsant medication
Glucocorticoids
Immobilization
Hepatic disease
Mastocytosis
Gastrointestinal diseases
Malignant tumors
Starvation hemochromatosis

ment of coupling between bone resorption and formation becomes progressively impaired, such that the deficit between resorption and formation becomes exaggerated.[73-75]

Bone loss is an asymptomatic process, and the key to the prevention of osteoporosis is early identification of those patients at greatest risk. In addition, the microarchitecture within cancellous bone is disrupted. Several findings support the concept that the initial bone mass may be an important factor in determining the susceptibility to osteoporosis. The peak bone mass is primarily under genetic control and variance in bone mass does not change with age. This may explain why fracture prevalence and incidence are greatest in those with a low bone mass at any age[76] (Fig. 74-21).

As already mentioned, the bone loss that occurs in patients with osteoporosis results from an increase in the rate of the activation phase of the bone-remodeling cycle. This is termed "high-turnover osteoporosis," and the deficit per BRU is apparently constant. Secondary causes of osteoporosis are also frequently associated with an increased in the rate of the activation phase of the remodeling cycle.

Osteoporosis in the absence of fractures is otherwise asymptomatic. Osteoporosis per se does not result in delayed fracture union, and if nonunion or delayed union occurs, conditions other than osteoporosis should be considered. Osteoporotic vertebral fractures may occur in the absence of acute symptoms. If acute symptoms do occur, as manifested by intense pain and limitation of motion, immobilization and appropriate analgesia are the mainstays of treatment. Vertebral fractures are associated with a loss of stature and progressive kyphosis. Anatomic changes become more pronounced as more vertebral bodies fracture. The abdomen and in severe cases the lower hips protrude, and this reflects the changes in the pelvic rim. This distorted body image may result in an altered self-image and vague gastrointestinal problems.

The biochemical profile in the setting of osteoporosis is unremarkable but it is important to determine it to rule out secondary causes of the osteoporosis. Measuring the biochemical markers of bone formation and resorption may be useful in predicting future rates of bone loss and in monitoring a patient's response to therapy.

The histologic characteristics of osteoporosis are consistent with the loss of bone mineral density that takes place (Fig. 74-22). The mineralization of bone is normal, as shown by the pattern of tetracycline deposition. If defective mineralization

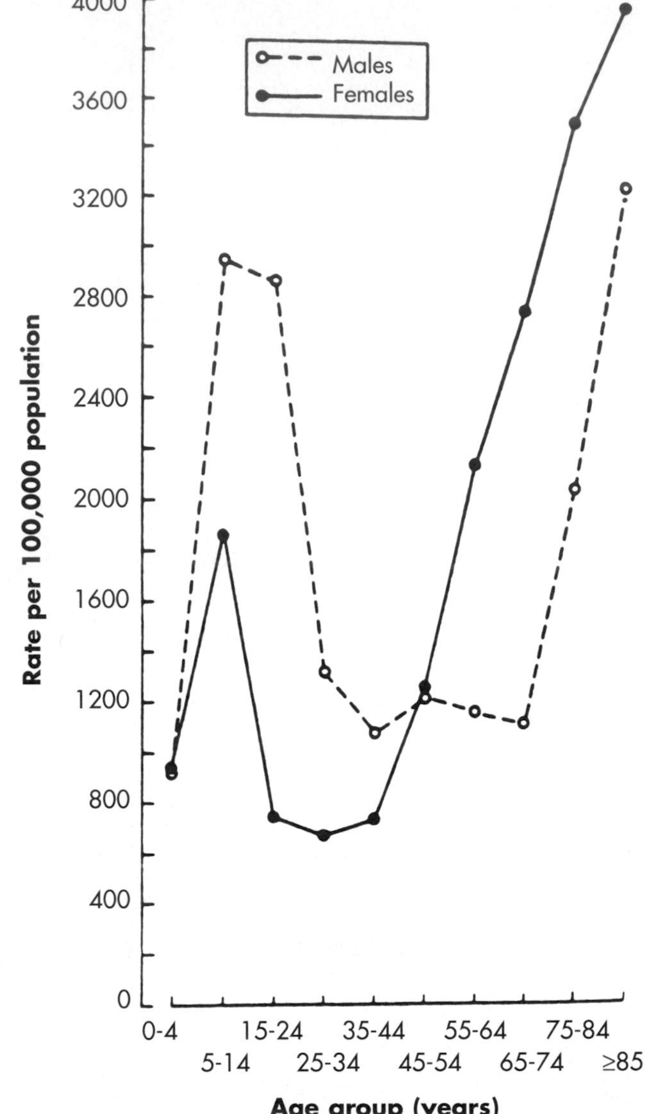

Fig. 74-21 Rates of limb fracture among male and female patients as a function of age in Rochester, Minnesota. (From Garroweg JC et al: *Mayo Clinic Proc* 54:701, 1979.)

is detected, by definition this is a diagnostic feature of osteomalacia. Histologic evidence of increased bone resorption and formation (accelerated turnover) in conjunction with suppressed bone cell activity is also a diagnostic feature of osteoporosis.

In states of low bone turnover, the rate of bone formation is normal to reduced, and small amounts of osteoid are present. Osteoid surface areas are decreased, and osteoid width may also be normal or decreased (Fig. 74-23). The fraction of tetracycline-labeled trabecular bone is decreased, with a predominance of single labels (Fig. 74-24). Mineralization rates are reduced. Bone resorption indices indicate a decrease in resorption surface areas and in the numbers of osteoclasts.

In high-turnover osteoporosis, the osteoid surface areas may be increased (Fig. 74-25), and the osteoid width is usually normal. The fraction of the tetracycline-labeled surface is increased, and the mineralization rate is normal or increased (Fig. 74-26). The bone resorption indices also show increases.

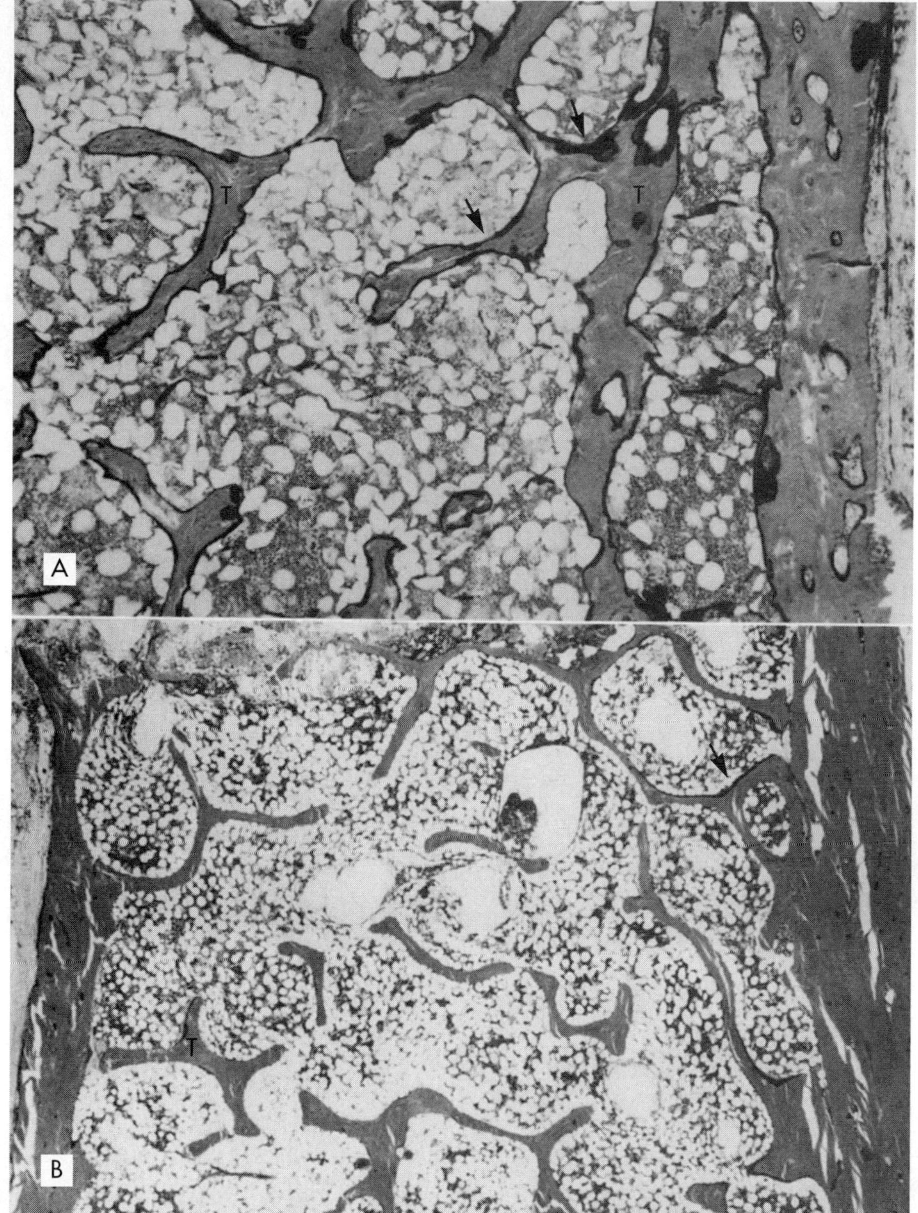

Fig. 74-22 **A,** Histologic appearance of active osteoporosis compared with, **B,** a normal bone specimen. *T,* Trabecular bone; *arrows,* osteoid.

The resorptive surface area and the number of osteoclasts may be normal or slightly elevated.

The genetic component of postmenopausal osteoporosis and its relationship to the peak bone mass have recently been described. In a recent study, the common allelic variance in the gene encoding the vitamin D receptor was used to predict differences in bone density and was found to account for as much as 75% of the total genetic effect on bone density in healthy persons.[77] The genotype associated with a lower bone density was overrepresented in postmenopausal women with bone densities more than 2 standard deviations below the values in normal young women. Allelic differences in the 3′ untranslated end of the vitamin D–receptor gene may alter messenger RNA levels and may be responsible for governing the molecular mechanisms that regulate bone density. Although these findings await further confirmation in other populations, they could be used to develop and target prophylactic interventions.

Juvenile osteoporosis Idiopathic juvenile osteoporosis is a rare disorder of unknown cause. Patients come to medical attention before puberty and show a progressive form of osteoporosis that later becomes stable. Bone formation is believed to proceed normally, and osteoclastic activity is increased. The osteoporosis becomes most evident in the thoracic and lumbar spine, and manifests as anterior wedging and concave deformities of the vertebral bodies. The condition should be distinguished from the juvenile apophysitis that occurs in Scheuermann's disease. Slipped-capital femoral epiphyses may be present. The disorder is usually self-limited, laboratory values are typically normal, and the diagnosis is made by exclusion.

Symptoms in a child with idiopathic juvenile osteoporosis begin with the insidious onset of pain in the lower back, hips,

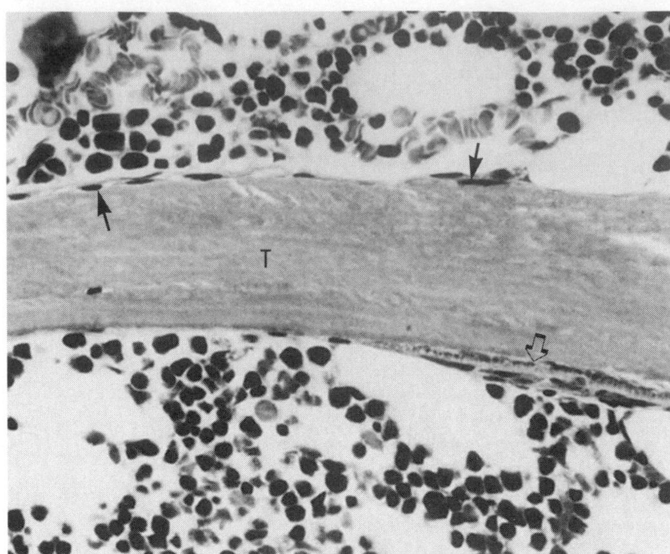

Fig. 74-23 Inactive osteoporosis. Histologic appearance of an inactive, smooth trabecular bone surface *(T)* with a minimal osteoid lining *(open arrow)* and covered only by flattened lining cells *(solid arrows).*

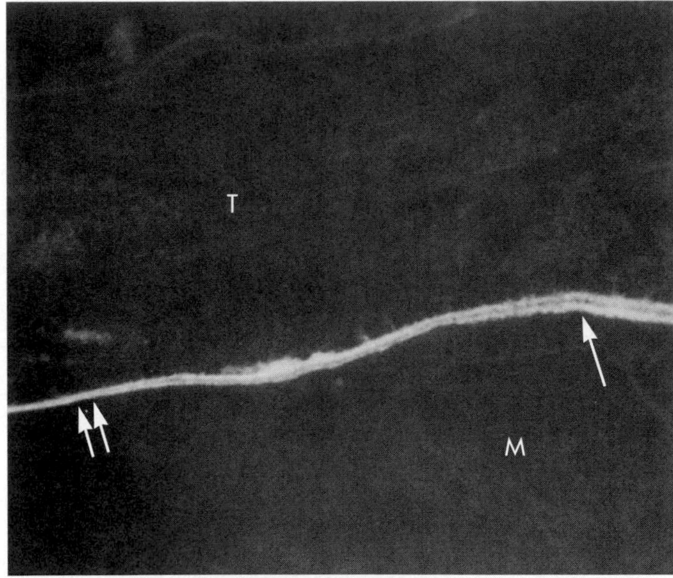

Fig. 74-24 Inactive osteoporosis. Histologic expression of reduced bone synthesis as shown by tetracycline label and viewed by fluorescent microscopy. Notice that, when present, the double labels are narrowly placed *(single arrow)* and are often fused, resulting in the formation of a single thin label *(double arrows). M,* Marrow; *T,* trabecular bone.

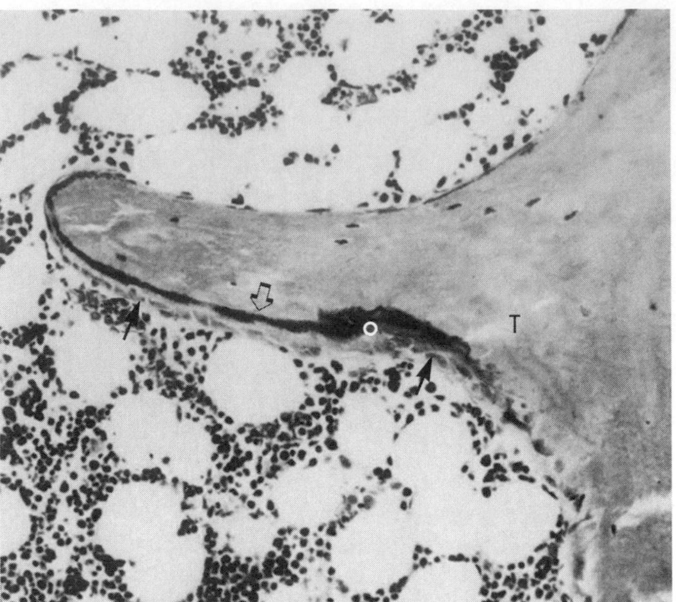

Fig. 74-25 Active osteoporosis. Histologic appearance of bone-forming surfaces with a trabecular bone spicule *(T)* lined by osteoblasts *(solid arrows)* and secreting osteoid matrix *(open arrow* and *O).*

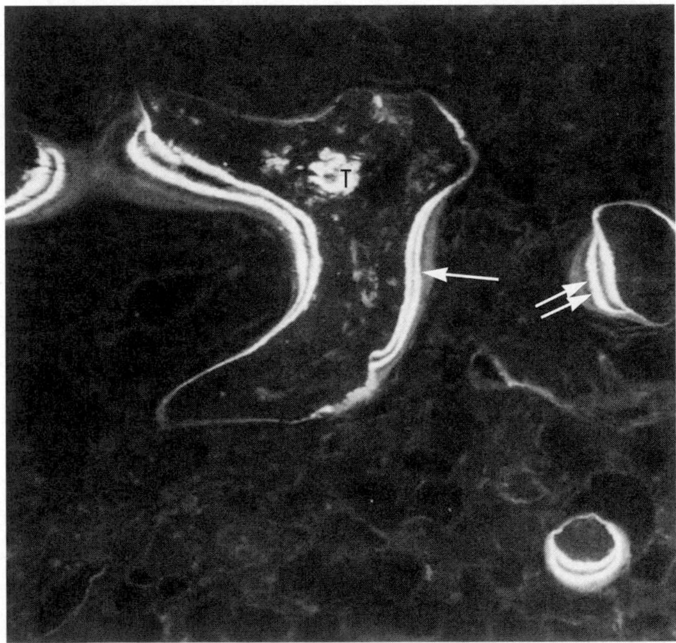

Fig. 74-26 Active osteoporosis. Histologic appearance of active bone-forming surfaces as shown by tetracycline label and viewed by fluorescent microscopy. Notice the increase in the surface area of trabecular bone *(T)* lined by double labels *(arrow)* and those surfaces exhibiting an increased distance between the labels *(double arrows),* indicating an increase in the bone appositional rate.

and feet and of difficulty in walking. There may also be knee and ankle pain and fractures of the lower extremities. Both sexes are affected equally; family and dietary histories yield no relevant findings. Few qualitative or quantitative studies of bone tissue have been performed in the setting of childhood osteoporosis. Increased bone resorption has been reported.[78,79] Smith[80] found indirect evidence of decreased bone formation. Diagnosis early in the disease is important, though there are no specific medical or surgical therapies. Supportive care is instituted promptly in anticipation of spontaneous recovery with the onset of puberty. Except for a few patients who suffer progressive deformities of the lower extremities, spine, and chest wall and are confined to wheelchairs or bed, the prognosis is generally excellent.

Osteoporosis in men The causes of age-related bone loss in women have been extensively investigated, but the pathogenesis of age-related bone loss in men has received less attention.[81,82] A fourth to a third of all hip fractures and a seventh of all vertebral compression fractures occur in men, resulting in significant morbidity, mortality, and cost to society. In men trabecular bone loss at the hip is greater than that in the spine;[82] thus men suffer more hip than vertebral fractures. Unlike women, men lose less bone in the spine with aging because of the compensatory subperiosteal cortical bone formation and less endocortical bone resorption that take place.[83] Although many men with osteoporosis have at least one identifiable secondary cause, many do not. The age-related bone loss that occurs in men is multifactorial, and overall the lower incidence of osteoporosis in men stems from the fact that their peak bone mass is higher, their life expectancy is shorter, and they have no distinct menopause equivalent that accelerates bone loss. Studies of bone mass and density in aging men have shown a gradual decline in bone mineral content that is similar to but slower than that in women. Most studies of bone mass show that the bone mineral content at cortical sites is lost at a rate of 3% to 4% per decade after 40 years of age; the loss at cancellous sites occurs at a rate of 7% to 12% after 30 to 35 years of age. Cancellous bone with its greater surface area and metabolic activity therefore appears to be lost at a greater rate. Recently examination of the three-dimensional trabecular microstructure has shown that loss of this component of bone may greatly alter bone strength.[84] Reduction in osteoblast function with aging, resulting from decreased osteoblast longevity or impaired regulation of activity, may have synergistic effects on the skeleton. Decreased mechanical loading, exercise, and muscle mass in the elderly may also cause remodeling to be impaired.

Long-standing testosterone deficiency is predicted to be present in approximately 30% of the men with spinal osteoporosis.[85] Testosterone deficiency may be a significant risk factor for hip fracture in elderly men and contributes to the bone loss associated with secondary factors. The detection of hypogonadism may be a challenging search because testosterone-deficient men may be capable of adequate sexual functions and secondary sex characteristics usually do not regress once they are established after puberty. Histomorphometrically, bone turnover is increased, and the effects are reversible with testosterone replacement therapy. Significant increases in cortical bone density have been demonstrated in hypoprolactinemic hypogonadal men who have undergone such therapy.[86] Recent evidence indicates that adrenal androgens may also play a role in the bone loss that takes place in the normal aging process in men.[87]

Regional osteoporosis Local osteoporosis has been noted as an incidental finding on radiographs. This may be found in patients with the reflex sympathetic dystrophy syndrome or in patients with limbs that have been immobilized for more than 4 weeks. Pain and swelling of the affected limb occur in patients with the reflex sympathetic dystrophy syndrome. The pathogenesis of the osteoporosis is unclear, but injured axons show an increased sensitivity to norepinephrine and other substances, and this may offer a clue to the underlying process. Biochemical markers are normal, except for a sedimentation rate that may be elevated. A technetium 99m bone scan can demonstrate affected areas.[87]

Secondary osteoporosis

Secondary osteoporosis is a bone loss resulting from specific well-defined clinical disorders. These disorders are diverse, ranging from disorders related to the close apposition of cancellous and endocortical surfaces to the bone marrow, to systemic disorders such as Cushing's disease in which a glucocorticoid excess results in osteoporosis.[88]

Secondary osteoporosis associated with drug therapy

Glucocorticoids. Skeletal decalcification was recognized as a clinical feature of Cushing's disease as early as 1932. The bone loss stemming from the glucocorticoid excess is diffuse and affects both the cortical and axial skeleton. Glucocorticoids affect trabecular bone more than they do cortical bone, perhaps because of the greater surface area of trabecular bone. The osteopenia is brought about by several mechanisms: the suppression of osteoblast function; the inhibition of intestinal calcium absorption, leading to secondary hyperparathyroidism; and the increased osteoclast-mediated bone resorption. Bone loss is also promoted by the direct stimulation of renal excretion of calcium by glucocorticoids and the hypogonadism associated with the suppressive effects of glucocorticoids on the hypothalamic-pituitary axis.

Glucocorticoids directly affect osteoblasts by inhibiting the differentiation of preosteoblasts. Glucocorticoid receptors have been demonstrated on bone cells, and the direct effects of glucocorticoids have been analyzed in cell culture systems. These studies have shown that glucocorticoids inhibit the growth of osteoblast-like cells, citrate decarboxylation, alkaline phosphatase activity, and the synthesis of collagen and noncollagenous proteins.

Glucocorticoids cause a decrease in the net intestinal calcium absorption, but the mechanism responsible for this is unknown. Only active intestinal absorption is inhibited; the passive diffusion of calcium is not altered. Up to now the mechanism by which glucocorticoids interfere with intestinal calcium absorption is not agreed upon, but the net effect of reduced calcium absorption is the development of secondary hyperparathyroidism.

Glucocorticoids alter the levels of gonadal hormones in both men and women. Glucocorticoid therapy also reduces the level of sex hormone–binding globulin, and there is a concurrent reduction in the total testosterone level, resulting in reduced bioactive free testosterone levels in male patients.

Bone density is reduced in 40% to 60% of the patients with an endogenous glucocorticoid excess, and pathologic fractures have been observed in 16% to 67% of them. Short-term studies have shown that glucocorticoid-induced bone loss appears to be greater in the first 6 to 12 months of therapy. The minimum dose of glucocorticoids associated with rapid bone loss is not established. Some studies indicate that as little as 7.5 mg of prednisone per day produces considerable bone loss. The traditional risk factors associated with osteoporosis are believed to operate in the context of glucocorticoid-induced osteoporosis. In addition, osteoporosis is more severe in patients younger than 15 years and those older than 50 years as well as in postmenopausal women.

Histomorphometrically, dynamic indices of bone formation show a profound reduction, indicating that remodeling has been uncoupled. The number of osteoid seams is reduced and the mineral oppositional rate is low, as shown by tetracycline-labeling studies. The mean wall thickness of trabecular osteons is decreased in steroid-treated patients, and this has been hypothesized to reflect the decreased longevity of active osteoblasts within each BRU. Overall, there is a reduction in the volume of cancellous bone.

Results of calcium kinetic studies and histomorphometric analysis support the hypothesis that glucocorticoids promote bone resorption. An increased number of resorption lacunae in osteoclasts is frequently observed, and, overall, bone turnover is increased. Divergent results have been noted, and this may stem from the possibility that glucocorticoids have a biphasic dose effect on the differentiation of the function of osteoclasts.

Serum and urine biochemical indices in patients with glucocorticoid-induced osteopenia are generally normal. Serum immunoreactive PTH levels may be normal or mildly elevated. Serum alkaline phosphatase (bone fraction) activity and osteocalcin levels decline steadily after the initiation of glucocorticoid therapy. Urinary calcium excretion may be increased during the first several months to years of steroid therapy, and this results from the direct calciuric effect of glucocorticoids on the kidney. After several years of glucocorticoid therapy, urinary calcium excretion is usually within the normal range.[33]

Anticonvulsant medications. The bone disease associated with anticonvulsant therapy has been considered a form of osteomalacia. However, it has recently become clear that a high-turnover osteoporosis is also present. In its most florid form, there are bone changes such as osteopenia and fractures that are associated with hypocalcemia, hypophosphatemia, and muscle weakness. Rickets has been observed in children taking anticonvulsant medication. Commonly, however, only minimal biochemical abnormalities have been demonstrated, including increased circulating levels of PTH and skeletal changes such as deficits in the cortical bone mass.[88]

A recent study of 20 epileptic adults treated with anticonvulsant agents for at least 10 years disclosed substantial reductions in the serum and urinary calcium levels and elevated serum alkaline phosphatase activities.[89] The trabecular bone volume noted on bone biopsy specimens was similar to control values, but the relative osteoid volume, the prevalence of bone-forming surfaces, and the degree of tetracycline labeling were significantly increased. Resorptive surface areas were also increased. In a second study of 120 epileptic patients who had been taking anticonvulsant medication for an average of 18 years, the trabecular bone volume was normal and the osteoid volume and surface area were significantly increased. The osteoid seam width was normal, and the mineralization rates were consistently increased.[90] The results of both of these studies indicate that anticonvulsant-induced bone disease may reflect a rapid remodeling state. Alterations in the hepatic metabolism of vitamin D, such that inactive polar metabolites are produced, have been demonstrated in epileptic subjects. A decrease in the available stores of 25-hydroxyvitamin D, leading to decreased intestinal calcium absorption, could explain a compensatory secondary hyperparathyroidism that occurs. Despite this attractive explanation, however, recent studies have shown that 25-hydroxyvitamin D levels in patients taking anticonvulsant medication may not differ from control values. Multiple confounding variables, including the geographic location of the patients and the amount of ultraviolet-radiation exposure, make interpretation of these results difficult.

Heparin. Heparin enhances PTH-dependent bone resorption. Recently it has been suggested that heparin stimulates osteoblast collagenase activity. Although the possible links between collagenase production and bone resorption are disputed, it is acknowledged that osteoblast synthesis and the secretion of collagenase, prostaglandins, and other agents that contribute directly to resorption or assist in the recruitment of osteoclasts may be affected by heparin administration. In animal studies, heparin has been found to decrease the conversion of tritiated proline to hydroxyproline, indicating that bone formation may be inhibited. The extraskeletal actions of heparin may be involved in the osteoporosis induced by this medication. Anecdotal accounts of alterations in the vitamin D axis have been reported.[88]

Miscellaneous medications associated with osteoporosis. Other medications have also been associated with the development of osteoporosis. Methotrexate has been implicated as a cause of bone loss, but most studies of its effects are confounded by the fact that other drugs have been administered or the gonadal status of the subjects has been altered. Prolonged administration of methotrexate in an animal model has been observed to result in the suppression of osteoblast activity and stimulation of bone resorption. The zealous administration of exogenous thyroid hormone has also been associated with osteopenia. The clinical relevance of the osteoporosis has recently been examined in terms of the development of fractures, but the data remain controversial.[91]

Endocrine disorders associated with secondary osteoporosis

Hyperthyroidism. Thyroid insufficiency and excess lead to alterations in bone mass. The primary effect of thyroid hormone is to increase the creation of new BRUs, accompanied by an overall increase in the remodeling activity taking place in an enlarged remodeling space. Thyrotoxicosis is associated with increased bone resorption. Trabecular bone volume may be low but is often normal in bone biopsy material. Resorption indices show increases, and the osteoid surfaces are also increased. However, the increased mineral apposition rate and the increase in the fraction of tetracycline-labeled surfaces excludes osteomalacia. In a detailed analysis of resorption versus formation in the setting of hyperthyroidism, Erickson and coworkers[26] found that bone resorption was much faster than normal (3.8 versus a normal value of 1.1 mm/day). The total formation period was significantly shortened, but directly obtained measurements of the mean wall thickness were normal. Whether the bone mass deficit is reversible remains uncertain. There has been some indication that the bone mineral content returns to normal after treatment, particularly in younger patients.[28] Even mildly excessive doses of thyroid hormone may prevent bone loss, and this has recently raised the clinical specter of iatrogenic hyperthyroidism. The published evidence overall indicates that minimally excessive long-term thyroid hormone replacement can bring about a decrease in the cortical bone mass.[92]

Primary hyperparathyroidism. PTH is responsible for stimulating calcium homeostasis in mammals through its action on the target cells in the bone and kidney. The maintenance of calcium homeostasis and the response to PTH involve the transport of calcium to the extracellular environment by osteocytes or lining cells on bone surfaces, or by both types of cells. PTH also causes a release of calcium from bone by stimulating osteoclast-mediated resorption. PTH mobilizes calcium as early as 3 hours after its administration, and in a second phase, which occurs 24 hours later, both the number and metabolic activity of osteoclasts are increased.[25]

Primary hyperparathyroidism is a common disorder and is usually asymptomatic; it is usually detected by routine screening by use of a multichannel chemistry panel. PTH itself has devastating effects on the skeleton, though severe bone involvement is now uncommon. The findings yielded by bone histomorphometry in the setting of primary hyperparathyroidism have been extensively studied in order to gain an understanding of the microarchitecture of bone.

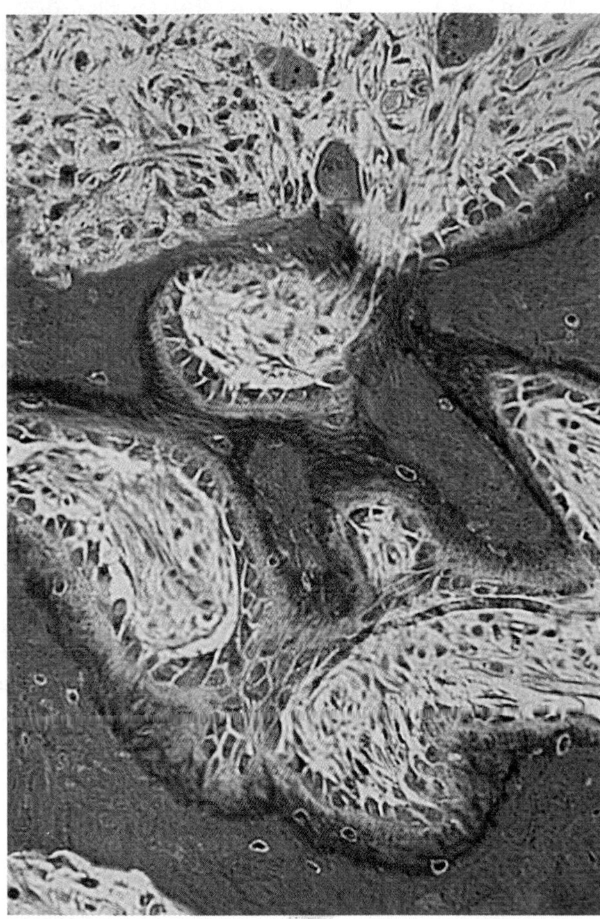

Fig. 74-27 Active bone remodeling seen in the settings of primary or secondary hyperparathyroidism. Notice the active osteoblasts surmounted on red-stained osteoid. Marrow fibrosis is present.

The hallmark of the skeletal involvement in primary hyperparathyroidism is an increase in the bone turnover rate (Fig. 74-27). The osteoid surface area, osteoid volume, mineralizing surface area, and tissue-based bone formation rates correlate well with the levels of PTH, as determined by midmolecule radioimmunoassay.[91] The eroded and mineralizing surface areas correlate with the serum calcium and urinary adenosine monophosphate levels respectively. These correlates reflect the response of the skeleton to PTH, and abnormal values are detectable even when the clinical manifestations are minimal. The physiologic action of PTH has a preference for cortical bone (Fig. 74-28). Cortices are thin or excessively porous and the cancellous bone volume is relatively well maintained in primary hyperparathyroidism. This increase in cancellous bone volume is reflected in a greater compressive strength, and this indicates that in mild primary hyperparathyroidism cancellous bone may be preserved and cortical bone may be preferentially lost. Trabecular plates are somewhat thinner than those in normal subjects, and trabecular separation increases as a function of age in normal subjects but not in patients with primary hyperparathyroidism.[93]

A technique of two-dimensional trabecular strut analysis permits the number of connecting points or nodes between trabecular segments to be quantitated. The free ends of unconnected trabeculae are terminuses, and the relative lengths of trabecular struts show various degrees of connectivity and the total length of all trabecular struts. Using this method, the indices of connectivity have been found to be greater in patients with primary hyperparathyroidism than in normal subjects. These findings are consistent with the higher cancellous bone volume and the greater degree of trabecular connectivity noted in patients with hyperparathyroidism as compared with normal subjects. Several hypotheses have been advanced in attempt to define the mechanism responsible for the maintenance of bone volume and structure in the cancellous compartment. Erickson[94] has suggested that bone remodeling is

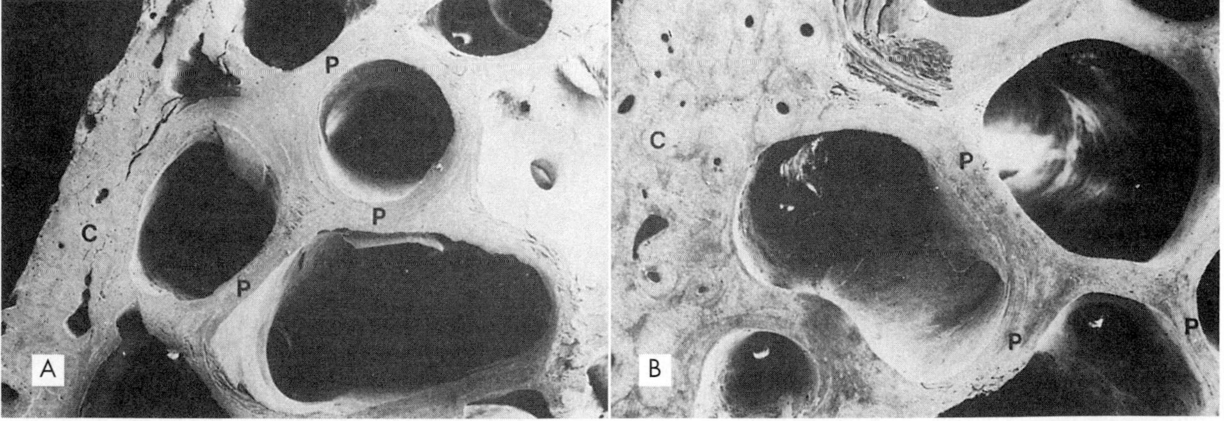

Fig. 74-28 Scanning electron micrographs of bone obtained from a patient with primary hyperparathyroidism **(A)** and from an age and sex matched normal subject **(B).** Notice the loss of cortical bone *(C)* in primary hyperparathyroidism compared with the appearance of normal bone. This is in sharp contrast to the abnormalities that occur in other disease states such as osteoporosis or Paget's disease. Notice the preservation of the trabecular plates *(P)*. (From Becker KL, editor: *Principles and practice of endocrinology and metabolism,* Philadelphia, 1990, Lippincott.)

increased in patients with primary hyperparathyroidism with a resultant decrease in the final erosion depth and thickness of the rows of completed structural units. Overall, there is an increased bone balance. In this model, a smaller amount of bone is exchanged during the remodeling sequence and this loss is compensated for by an increased bone turnover at the tissue level. This contrasts with the events that occur in hyperthyroidism, in which a normal erosion depth and a decrease in the estimated complete wall thickness result in a net negative balance between erosion and formation at the conclusion of each remodeling cycle.[95]

Christiansen and colleagues[96] suggest that at the cellular level there is a twofold increase in the activation frequency with a substantial enlargement of the remodeling space. The change in osteoclast behavior results in a tangential pattern of "sleeping" erosion as opposed to the more traditional tunneling erosion that takes place. The effects of PTH on osteoclast recruitment or activity, or both, differ between the cortical and cancellous envelopes.

Hypoparathyroidism. There are multiple causes of hypoparathyroidism, though the most common is surgical removal of the glands. Damage to the parathyroid glands is brought about by the diminished vascular supply of the glands and may result in the decreased release of PTH. Acquired hypoparathyroidism can be induced by various drugs, sepsis, irradiation, or infiltrative diseases of the parathyroids. In addition, there are rare sporadic and familial developmental disorders that also cause hypoparathyroidism. Finally, hypoparathyroidism is part of an autoimmune polyglandular failure syndrome.[97]

Baseline levels of $1,25(OH)_2D_3$ are reduced in patients with hypoparathyroidism. However, findings from many studies indicate that the lack of PTH in patients with hypoparathyroidism is responsible for preserving the overall bone density, though it is difficult to assess whether the increased bone mineral density stems from the lack of PTH itself or from the treatment for the condition. The total body calcium content, as determined by neutron-activation analysis together with measurement of the vertebral mineral content or by dual-photon absorptiometry, is greater than that in age-matched controls. These findings may reflect the decreased bone turnover that occurs in patients with hypoparathyroidism. The trabecular bone mineral content, as determined by quantitative computerized tomography, is not increased, and such a lack of change indicates that the cortical bone may be preferentially preserved in these patients. Biochemical markers of bone turnover have been measured in patients with hypoparathyroidism. The serum alkaline phosphatase activity and osteocalcin concentration (both indices of bone formation) and the urinary ratio of hydroxyproline to creatinine (a measure of bone resorption) are decreased in patients with hypoparathyroidism.

Extensive ligamentous and tendinous ossifications and soft-tissue calcification have been noted in patients with idiopathic hyperparathyroidism. These skeletal changes are indistinguishable from those exhibited by patients with diffuse idiopathic skeletal hyperostosis.[97]

Acromegaly. Elevated concentrations of GH cause bone turnover to be accelerated. In patients with acromegaly, the frequency of osteoporosis or fractures does not appear to be increased. In some studies bone mass has been proved to be increased, and this has included a thickened cortical bone and augmented trabecular bone volume. Elevations in the $1,25(OH)_2D_3$ level have been noted in patients, and the augmentation in intestinal calcium absorption associated with this may also contribute to the features of active remodeling noted on bone biopsy specimens. These observations have provided the impetus for the establishment of clinical trials investigating the use of GH in the treatment of primary osteoporosis.

Recent findings have indicated that osteoporosis can occur in acromegaly, and the bone in this setting shows an unusual architecture and composition. In this study, histomorphometry revealed a very low trabecular bone volume, and the mean trabecular plate thickness was strikingly increased.[98]

Cushing's syndrome. Hypercortisolism is a well-recognized risk factor for the development of osteoporosis. As also occurs in exogenous or iatrogenic hypercortisolism, more trabecular bone than cortical bone tends to be lost. If Cushing's syndrome is cured surgically, some of the bone loss can be reversed.[33]

Insulin-dependent diabetes mellitus. Recent studies have indicated that low bone mineral density is associated with insulin-dependent diabetes mellitus. No increase in the incidence of fracture versus the incidence in the nondiabetic population has been noted, but the incidence of stress fractures in the foot bones is higher in diabetic patients than that in nondiabetic subjects. Bone histomorphometric analyses of cortical and cancellous bone obtained from the iliac crest have confirmed that bone formation rates are low in patients with diabetes mellitus. Such low rates are associated with low levels of osteocalcin. This reduction in the bone turnover rate could cause bone to be more fragile and explain the ensuing risk of fracture seen in a subset of such patients.[99]

Miscellaneous causes of secondary osteoporosis

Immobilization. Immobilization causes a rapid and diffuse bone loss. The nature and the mechanics of normal bone stress have been intensely studied. When healthy adults are placed on a regimen of bed rest, hypercalciuria develops and persists for months. The calcium loss approximates a −200 mg per day, with a whole body mineral loss of about 0.5% per month. Remineralization begins once ambulation is resumed. The critical importance of gravitational stress is shown by the data generated during space flights. Despite frequent strenuous exercise, astronauts in a weightless orbit suffer an impressive hypercalciuria and a negative calcium balance. A few weeks of simple "therapeutic" bed rest is sufficient to foster significant loss of the axillary bone mineral. The lumbar spine mineral content decreases by 0.9% per week in bed-ridden patients; this is equivalent to a 45% loss per year. Once the subjects started walking again, the axillary mineral content is restored within 4 months. The hormonal and metabolic consequences of immobilization have been partially characterized. Fasting and 24-hour urinary calcium excretions are grossly elevated, and the serum inorganic phosphate levels are elevated. Both immunoreactive PTH and $1,25(OH)_2D_3$ excretions are suppressed. This reduction indicates that the primary loss of mineral from bone stems from a suppressed parathyroid–vitamin D access. Most of the patients remained normocalcemic, but hypercalcemia may develop in children and young adults.

Histomorphometric data from immobilized patients are derived primarily from studies of patients who have suffered spinal cord trauma. Trabecular bone loss is very rapid in these patients, and resorption activity appears to be increased in the first few months. Resorption activity normalizes later, but the static and dynamic indices of bone-forming activity show profound reductions.[100]

Vitamin A and vitamin E. Hypervitaminosis A results in weakness, emotional lability, musculoskeletal pain, headache, pseudotumor cerebri, and osteopenia. The periosteal new bone formation in close apposition to the cortex assumes the appearance of hyperostosis. This is most commonly observed in the ulnar, metacarpal, and metatarsal bones and in the skull. Biochemically, the serum alkaline phosphatase activity is elevated because a combination of both hepatic and bone enzymes is present. Hypercalcemia may be seen in children. In rib biopsy specimens obtained from a patient before and after the ingestion of massive doses of vitamin A, a severalfold increase in the resorption area was noted on the initial biopsy specimen, and this was found to be resolved on the second specimen. Bone formation rates were normal initially but showed a sevenfold increase in the second specimen. The cellular basis for the effects of vitamin E on the skeleton is unclear. Both retinol and calcitriol stimulate bone resorption and inhibit bone collagen synthesis. Both agents increase the production of interleukin-1 (IL-1), a potent bone resorber, by macrophages and monocytes.[88]

Marrow-related disorders. Cancellous and endocortical bone surfaces are in close opposition to bone marrow, and for this reason disorders of bone marrow can produce profound changes in bone. Plasma cell dyscrasias, such as multiple myeloma and macroglobulinemia, are associated with several bone disorders. Osteolytic lesions are associated with multiple myeloma, and a number of bone resorbing cytokines (IL-1, tumor necrosis factor, and lymphotoxin) have been implicated as agents that promote bone destruction. PTH-related peptide may also enhance resorption. Systemic mastocytosis, an abnormal proliferation of mast cells, results in mixed sclerotic-porotic lesions. Histomorphometric analysis of bone in patients with systemic mastocytosis reveals a high-turnover state. Other disorders, such as leukemia and lymphomas, can also result in osteoporosis. The generalized osteoporosis with hypercalcemia associated with lymphoma has been proposed to result from the production of $1{,}25(OH)_2D_3$. Chronic anemias, such as sickle cell disease and beta-thalassemia, are associated with bone loss, and bone disease is a common feature of Gaucher's disease and Niemann-Pick disease. In these later instances, remodeling fails and generalized osteoporosis results from the operation of an unknown mechanism.[101]

Metabolic bone disease associated with disorders of the gastrointestinal and biliary tracts. Impaired absorption or catabolism, or both, of vitamin D and its metabolites and malabsorption of calcium can occur in subjects with gastrointestinal tract disorders. Secondary hyperparathyroidism occurs and is characterized by an increased surface area and volume of osteoid, but its thickness is normal. Osteomalacia is defined by an osteoid thickness of more than 15μm and a mineralization lag time of more than 100 days. Both the surface volume and thickness of osteoid are increased in this setting. The most common finding in patients with gastrointestinal tract disorders and bone disease is low-turnover osteoporosis. Protein and other micronutrient deficiencies may contribute to this, and biochemical abnormalities are infrequent. In this subset of patients, the osteoid thickness is normal or reduced and bone formation rates are reduced.

Secondary hyperparathyroidism is a consistent feature in these vitamin D–deficient patients with an accelerated loss of cortical bone. The postmenopausal osteoporosis that may accompany vitamin D–related bone disease does not respond to therapy with vitamin D or its metabolites. In this instance examination of a transiliac bone biopsy specimen obtained after tetracycline labeling is a definitive way to determine the nature of the underlying bone disease.[102,103]

Renal osteodystrophy

In patients suffering from advanced renal failure, osteodystrophy is a major cause of morbidity and bone pain is the most common clinical manifestation of this. Other problems in such patients include spontaneous fractures, aseptic necrosis of the hip, and myopathy. These abnormalities are termed collectively "renal osteodystrophy." Several histologic subclasses of renal osteodystrophy exist and are distinguished by their respective rate of bone turnover. These include high-turnover osteodystrophy *(osteitis fibrosa),* low-turnover osteodystrophy *(osteomalacia),* and *mixed or mild uremic bone disease,* which has the features of both high-turnover and low-turnover osteodystrophy.

PTH and $1{,}25(OH)_2D_3$ are two of the most important hormonal regulators of bone metabolism. In high-turnover disease, the serum levels of PTH are persistently high. Low-turnover disease may stem from an excess bone aluminum deposition, and the serum PTH levels are normal or reduced. A patient may have more than one type of metabolic bone disease, and the histopathologic manifestations represent the effects of a combination of both the high-turnover and low-turnover states.

High-turnover osteodystrophy is the most prevalent disorder in patients with renal osteodystrophy, and it is often the result of secondary hyperparathyroidism. Phosphorus retention and hyperphosphatemia have been recognized for many years as important factors in the pathogenesis of secondary hyperparathyroidism. In addition, a decrease in the number of vitamin D receptors on the parathyroid cell may contribute to the alterations in calcium-regulated PTH secretion that occur in the context of chronic renal failure. A combination of low levels of $1{,}25(OH)_2D_3$, hyperphosphatemia, hypocalcemia, and alterations in the secretion or activity of PTH is the hallmark of the disorder.

High-turnover bone disease. Osteitis fibrosa is a common manifestation of the high-turnover lesions of renal osteodystrophy (Fig. 74-29). There is histologic evidence of active resorption, as shown by increases in the number and size of osteoclasts and the percentage of the surface eroded. Fibrous tissue may be found immediately adjacent to the bony trabeculas and accumulates throughout the marrow space. In advanced cases the bone marrow is partially or completely replaced by fibrous tissue. Osteoblast activity is increased, and the rate of bone formation is above the upper limits of normal. The number of osteoblasts is substantially increased, and a greater proportion of cancellous bone is covered with newly formed osteoid. Osteoid seams may appear woven and may reflect changes in the arrangement of collagen fibrils. Both the biochemical and roentgenographic manifestations of secondary hyperparathyroidism are present.

Subperiosteal erosions are one of the most consistent radiographic findings in patients with secondary hyperparathyroidism. Patchy osteosclerosis is also common and accounts for the classic "rugger jersey" appearance of the spine on lateral views of thoracic vertebrae and for the

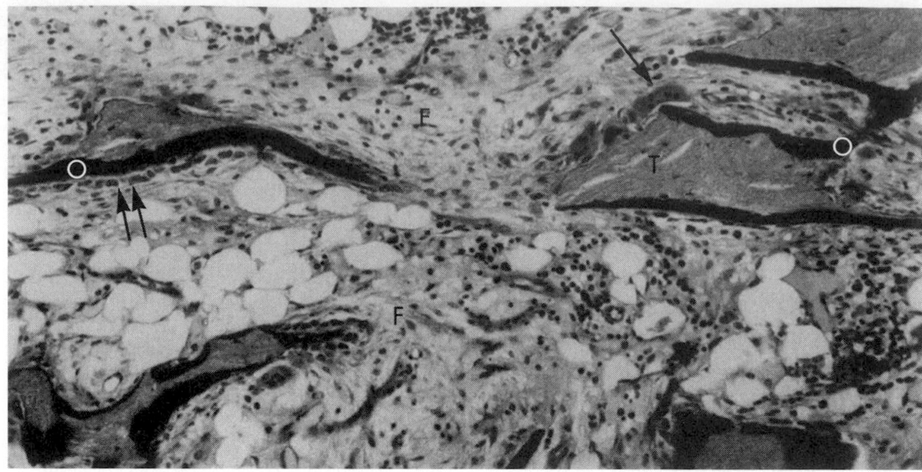

Fig. 74-29 Histologic appearance of the osteitis fibrosa that occurs in secondary hyperparathyroidism. Notice the deposition of fibrous tissue *(F)* the increased osteoclastic activity *(arrow)*, and the increased osteoblastic activity *(double arrows)*. Osteoid *(O)* is therefore increased along the trabecular bone surface *(T)*.

"salt-and-pepper" appearance of the skull. Slipped epiphyses are the most striking clinical and radiographic manifestations of renal osteodystrophy in children, but the site affected depends on the age of the child. The epiphyseal slippage that occurs in preschool children can lead to gross deformities of the skeleton together with ulnar deviation of the hands and gait abnormalities.

Low-turnover bone disease. Low-turnover osteodystrophy can be subdivided on the basis of the osteoid volume into osteomalacia and aplastic bone disease. The histologic features of osteomalacia secondary to renal disease are the same as those characteristics of other forms of osteomalacia.

Aluminum toxicity is the most common cause of osteomalacia in the setting of the aplastic bone disease that afflicts patients undergoing long-term dialysis. Recently the number of patients with adynamic bone lesions who have no evidence of bone aluminum deposition has increased substantially and has been attributed to the increased use of vitamin D steroids and calcium, both of which suppress parathyroid cell function.

There are two possible sources of the aluminum overload in patients with renal failure. The use of aluminum-contaminated dialysate can cause severe bone disease and dialysis-related encephalopathy, but the therapeutic ingestion of aluminum-containing phosphate-binding agents has been implicated as the primary source of the aluminum overload. Clinical manifestations include bone pain, fractures, and a proximal myopathy.

Depositions of aluminum are found within the mineralization front of bone in patients with aluminum-related renal osteomalacia or adynamic bone disease. This site arises coincidentally with the site where newly formed bone collagen is calcified. Aluminum impedes mineralization directly by slowing the formation of hydroxyapatite crystals. Aluminum can also directly affect the osteoblasts, and this accounts for the increase in osteoclast numbers noted in this disorder. Mineralization lags behind collagen synthesis, leading to osteoid accumulation and thickened osteoid seams. Osteoid seams often have a multilamellar appearance. The histologic severity of osteomalacia generally corresponds to the amount of surface-stainable aluminum in bone (Fig. 74-30).

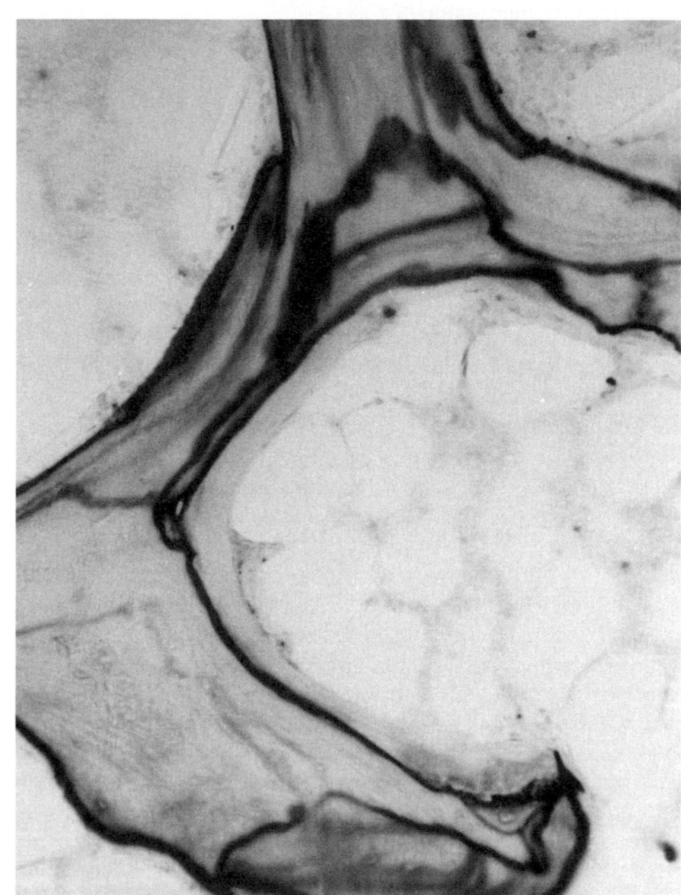

Fig. 74-30 Osteomalacia. Aluminum was stained with acid solochrome. Notice the intense staining of the mineralization front and cement lines.

In another group of patients with symptomatic bone disease, a normal or reduced amount of osteoid, the absence of tissue fibrosis, and diminished numbers of osteoblasts and osteoclasts are noted. This histologic appearance has been termed the "adynamic" or "aplastic lesion of renal osteodystrophy," and aluminum deposition along the bone surfaces is a common finding.

The pattern of bone deformity varies with the age of onset of renal failure. In children, the rapid rates of bone growth and skeletal remodeling result in deformities in either the axial or appendicular skeleton. Children with chronic renal failure invariably exhibit growth retardation. Only the axial skeleton is deformed in adults with aluminum-related bone disease. Lumbar scoliosis, kyphosis, and distortion of the thoracic cage may occur.

Soft-tissue calcification in patients with renal failure can be detected by radiographic examination. Tumoral or periarticular calcifications are seen most frequently and are common when the serum phosphorus concentrations exceed 8 to 9 mg/dl or when the calcium-phosphorus ion product exceeds 75. The soft-tissue calcifications regress with sustained reductions in the serum phosphorus concentrations. Vascular calcification occurs and is localized to the medial layer of small and medium-sized arteries (Mönckeberg's sclerosis). Rarely, ischemic necrosis of the skin, muscle, or subcutaneous tissue occurs, and this is termed "calciphylaxis." Visceral calcifications are infrequent.

Pseudofractures are the most pathognomonic radiographic finding in patients with osteomalacia. These straight, wide radiolucent bands in the cortex are perpendicular to the longitudinal axis of bone. Ricketslike lesions have been noted in children with aluminum-related bone disease in the setting of osteomalacia, and these may result from deferoxamine treatment. The rachitic lesions in children are not pathognomonic for any particular histologic lesions, and bone biopsy specimens are often needed to distinguish between high- and low-turnover bone disease.

Currently renal osteodystrophy is treated in several ways.[104] Normal serum calcium and phosphorus levels must be maintained to prevent hyperplasia of parathyroid glands; exposure to toxic agents such as aluminum is avoided; extraskeletal calcifications are prevented; and vitamin D steroids are used judiciously. Chelating agents such as deferoxamine are also administered as appropriate to treat aluminum intoxication.

Osteomalacia and rickets

Osteomalacia represents a group of metabolic bone diseases resulting from defective mineralization of the trabecular and cortical bone matrix.[105] Rickets stems from defective mineralization of the epiphyseal growth plate cartilage. Skeletal disease in children is therefore a combination of rickets and osteomalacia, provided the growth plates remain open. In contrast, adults may manifest osteoid (bone) changes only after the epiphyses close. The resulting bone mass may be decreased, normal, or increased (that is, osteosclerosis). The most common forms of osteomalacia and rickets are associated with a decreased serum calcium-phosphate product (Ca × P), such that mineralization is not supported. Consequently, defective mineralization of the skeletal matrices may result directly from disorders that influence calcium homeostasis or phosphate metabolism. Indirectly, calcium and phosphate deficiency may be mediated by secondary mechanisms such as deficiencies in vitamin D or in other agents that regulate mineral metabolism.

The osteomalacia that occurs in adults is a common complication of chronic renal failure, as already described. The most common form of osteomalacia in adults is that arising from secondary vitamin D deficiency, that is, vitamin D–deficiency states secondary to an abnormality in vitamin D metabolism despite adequate vitamin D intake. Thus osteomalacia may be further subclassified on the basis of the abnormality in vitamin absorption or bioactivation. Of the postmenopausal women with osteopenia as a presenting symptom, as many as 20% have osteomalacia, not osteoporosis. In this group, chronic gastrointestinal malabsorption is the clinical condition most often associated with the development of vitamin D–deficiency osteomalacia. Other causes of osteomalacia are listed in Table 74-10.

Rickets. Growth is impaired in children with mineralization disorders, and height is consequently below the third percentile. The head is abnormal because the skull is soft and may deform (craniotabes). The frontal bones are prominent, resulting in frontal bossing. Flaring and deformity of the ribs, with nodular swelling of the costochondral junctions resulting in the rachitic rosary appearance, are noted during the chest examination. In addition to pectus excavatum, the thorax may be indented where the diaphragm inserts into the lower ribs, a finding referred to as "Harrison's groove." Because of the structural compromise of the thorax, frequent respiratory infections and a chronic cough are likely. Along with the chest abnormality, the spine is deformed, resulting in thoracic kyphosis; this in turn produces a protuberant abdomen (rachitic potbelly). The rapidly growing regions of the extremities also manifest the changes produced by defective mineralization, with symmetric enlargement or swelling of the elbows, wrists, and knees. The legs may be bowed (genu varum) or less frequently knock kneed (genu valgum).

The histologic appearance of the growth plate cartilage is characteristic. The rachitic growth plate is wide and irregular, and the architecture is abnormal. The columnar arrangement of the hypertrophic chondrocytes is lost, and the zone of provisional calcification disappears. Cartilage extends deep into the metaphysis, where it becomes surrounded by osteoid, which fails to mineralize (Fig. 74-31). In affected children, cup-shaped growth plate indentations and bowed legs develop

Table 74-10 Clinical classification of osteomalacia

Vitamin D deficiency
Primary
Secondary
Vitamin D dependency types I and II
Hypophosphatemic states
X-linked hypophosphatemia (vitamin D–resistant rickets)
Sporadic hypophosphatemia
Antacid-induced hypophosphatemia
Oncogenic osteomalacia
Drugs
Aluminum deposition
Sodium fluoride toxicity
Diphosphonate toxicity
Chronic renal failure and renal osteodystrophy
Hypophosphatasia
Hepatobiliary disease
Small bowel disease
Pancreatic insufficiency

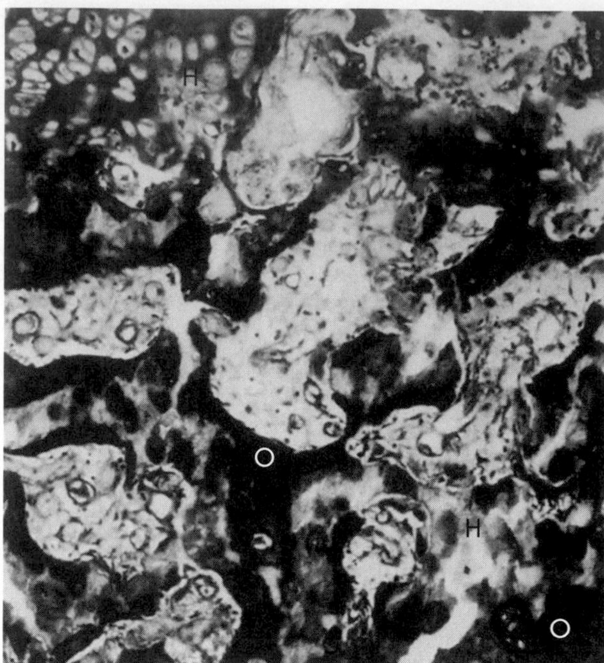

Fig. 74-31 Detailed histologic appearance of bone in rickets. Disorganization of the lower zones of the growth plate is apparent, and there are irregular columns of hypertrophic chondrocytes *(H)* and cartilage that has failed to mineralize. The bone that is deposited on this cartilage is also unmineralized and therefore appears as an increased quantity of osteoid *(O)*.

because of the structural weakness of the widened epiphyses and the osteomalacic bone.

Osteomalacia. Adults with osteomalacia complain of generalized weakness, diffuse bone pain, easy fatigability, and malaise. The physical findings may be minimal, in contrast to the findings noted in rickets; they manifest as bony tenderness and a waddling gait attributable to a proximal muscle myopathy. The gait produced is an abductor-lurch one, the so-called Trendelenburg gait. Curvature of the long bones and spine may occur, resulting in bowing with coxa vara and kyphosis.

Histologically, osteomalacia is usually characterized by excessive quantities of osteoid because of the failed matrix calcification despite continued matrix synthesis by the osteoblasts (Fig. 74-32). Pronounced increases in the thickness of the osteoid seams is characteristic, such that the seams are often more than 24 μm in width, or as a rough guide, the seams are thicker than the collagen lamellae. In addition, the total quantity of osteoid may be increased because of an increase in the osteoid surface area, that is, the fraction of trabecular bone surfaces lined by osteoid. In severe cases of osteomalacia, the osteoid surface area may exceed 60% and may even reach 100%, with the total trabecular surface enveloped by abnormally thick osteoid seams.

Although osteomalacia is usually characterized by osteoid excess, it may also be associated with normal or even reduced quantities of osteoid. Because active osteoporosis is associated with increased quantities of osteoid, it may be indistinguishable from milder cases of osteomalacia. In contrast to the static indices of bone formation (that is, the osteoid surface area, osteoid seam width, and osteoblastic surface area), in vivo tetracycline-labeling studies permit evaluation of the kinetic indices of formation (that is, the fraction of the double tetracycline–labeled trabecular bone surface, the fraction of osteoid-labeled surfaces, and the rate of bone matrix mineralization). As the mineralization defect increases, the percentage of the osteoid seams that bear normal tetracycline labels decreases (often below 20% to 40%). This is seen on fluorescent microscopy studies either as osteoid surfaces that fail to assimilate tetracycline or as seams that are diffusely fluorescent. Usually normal double tetracycline labels are absent, such that the fraction of double tetracycline-labeled trabecular bone surfaces is zero. In any areas showing double labels the distance between the labels is reduced, and such a reduction indicates that the mineralization rate is reduced. The differences between osteomalacia and osteoporosis in terms of the bone formation indices are listed in Table 74-11.

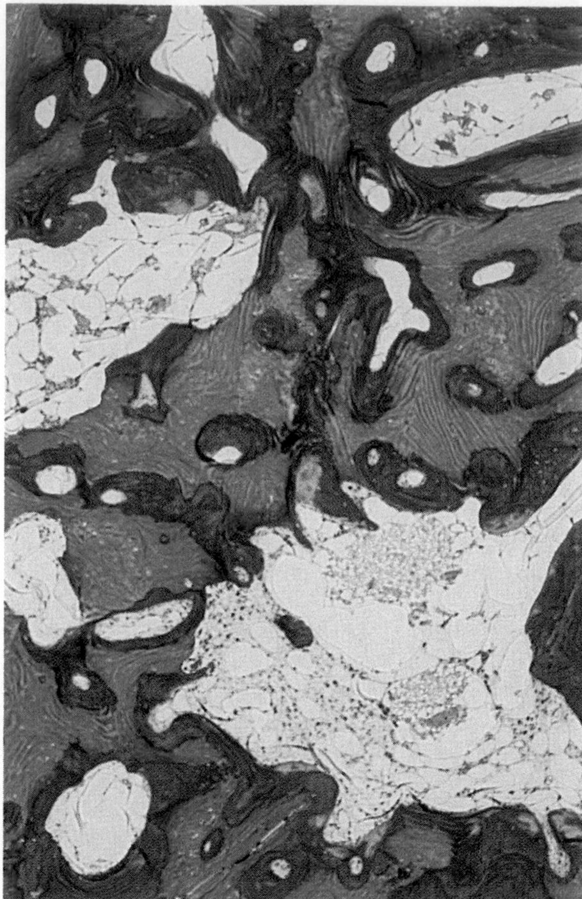

Fig. 74-32 Osteomalacia. Thick seams of osteoid cover the bone trabeculas.

Table 74-11 Histologic differential diagnosis: osteoporosis versus osteomalacia

Index	Osteoporosis	Osteomalacia
Osteoid volume	<4%	Often >20%
Osteoid seam width	<24 μm; <3 lamellae wide	Often >24 μm; >4 lamellae wide
Tetracycline labeling	Single and double labels	Unlabeled or diffusely labeled seams

TRAUMA

Fracture repair

When trauma occurs, the skeleton attempts to restore functional and anatomic integrity. The general principles of the repair process are not unique to bone. As with any injured tissue, adult bone tissue must revert to the basic undifferentiated mesenchymal tissue, the blastema, which is followed by wound closure and scar formation. What is unusual, however, is that the scar tissue of bone is bone, and thus repair of any skeletal tissue is essentially a recapitulation of the many steps that make up normal bone development and growth. Fracture repair can be thought of as a microcosm of endochondral and membranous bone formation occurring within the stabilizing skeletal wound tissue; the initial repair tissue formed is called *callus,* which is ultimately modeled into normal bone. Like growing bone, the callus is dynamic and undergoes rapid structural changes. Callus is composed of fibrous tissue, woven bone, and cartilage (Fig. 74-33). All these components are derived from a common endosteal or periosteal progenitor cell. Mechanical stress and oxygen tension are important in determining whether these cells differentiate into osteoblasts or chondroblasts. For example, intermittent stress favors cartilage formation. Predominantly membranous bone forms, in suitably immobilized fractures, whereas endochondral bone forms in free fractures.

Fracture healing can be divided into three general phases: inflammatory, reparative, and modeling. The *inflammatory phase* begins after the moment of trauma, and as in other inflammatory processes occurring elsewhere in the body, cellular and vascular events take place. Trauma sufficient to fracture a bone also damages the overlying muscle, tendon, periosteum, associated blood vessels, and marrow, resulting in hematoma formation. During the first 5 days after injury, the necrotic and damaged tissue generates an inflammatory cellular response. Surviving cells and new mesenchymal cells brought in by the ingrowth of granulation tissue create the blastema. The granulation tissue invades and eventually replaces ("organizes") the hematoma. A rich vascular network develops around the fracture zone. Peripherally, reactive hyperemia occurs as blood flow around the fracture increases. Centrally in the region of injury, dilated capillary spaces become engorged with blood; with stasis, passive congestion develops. In the congested central region, osteoid secretion is stimulated by osteoblasts arising from the blastema. Immature woven bone is deposited, and the first signs of mineralization are visible radiographically after 14 days. The development of this primitive tissue from the blastema represents the primary callus.

The *reparative phase* of fracture healing is characterized by the more orderly secretion of callus, the removal and replacement of the immature woven bone through the process of cartilage differentiation, and endochondral ossification. Several types of callus have been identified and have been named primarily on the basis of their location in the healing bone; they should not be considered as separate entities with distinct functions. A buttressing callus is adjacent to the outer cortical surface and is formed by the periosteum and skeletal muscle. A sealing callus fills the medullary cavity, and the cellular elements arise from the marrow to seal the fracture site. A bridging callus unites the gap between the two buttressed ends. The uniting callus joins the cortical portions of the fractured bone. Clinical union is achieved when the callus is sufficiently developed to allow weight-bearing or similar stress, usually at around 4 weeks after injury. The fracture continues to strengthen during the modeling phase.

The *modeling phase* involves the realignment and mechanical shaping of the bone and callus along lines of stress. It

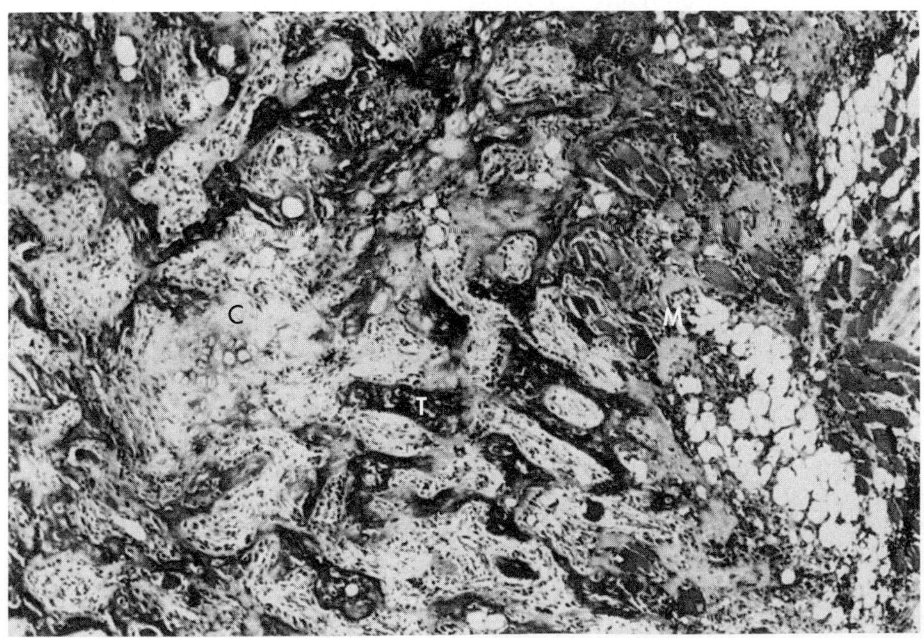

Fig. 74-33 Early fracture repair with immature callus formation. A rich mesenchymal proliferation with trilineage differentiation is seen, which includes cartilage *(C)*, mineralized trabecular bone *(T)*, and fibrous tissue. *M*, Trapped skeletal muscle.

involves the deposition of extra bone in stress lines and removal of bone in areas where stress is not applied, in accordance with the postulates of Wolff's law. This final stage of fracture healing results in restoration of the medullary cavity and bone marrow. Clinical healing precedes anatomic reconstitution. Extensive modeling will continue for years, and anatomic reconstitution usually occurs as a consequence of extensive osteoclastic resorption and osteoblast formation of bone according to the mechanical demands of that bone. Thus exact replacement of the fractured bone fragments is not required for complete healing.

The sequence of events that take place in the healing of a fracture are of practical consequence in the subsequent management of patients with fractures. Although the hematoma is not essential for fracture healing, it plays a metabolic role in inducing the formation of granulation tissue. The greater the hematoma formation, the more cellular and robust is the callus that is formed. Therefore the hematoma should not be disturbed. Large necrotic bone fragments must be removed by osteoclastic activity and may impede callus formation. Large sequestered bone fragments may have to be removed surgically. The injury itself induces a vascular response, which results in an increased vascularity in the damaged area, and, as a result of the subsequent metabolic changes that occur, promotes callus formation. Skeletal muscle is richly vascular and contributes extensively to the development of the callus. Therefore injured soft tissue should not be disturbed. In fact, poor fracture healing typically occurs in those superficial bones that have little or no adjacent musculature, such as the tibia.

Complications of fracture healing

Nonunions. The time it takes for most fractures to heal is surprisingly uniform. When fractures take longer than usual to heal but show signs of progressive healing, this is considered a *delayed union.* A *nonunion* is present when the fracture remains unhealed and shows no signs of further healing. Numerous factors may contribute to delayed union or nonunion; these include the location of the fracture, soft-tissue damage, tissue interposition, bone loss, and wound contamination or infection. The incidence of delayed union is unknown, but nonunion is estimated to occur in 5% of all long bone fractures. Nonunion rarely occurs in bones of the axial skeleton, the skull, ribs, vertebrae, scapulas, and pelvis.

Fibrous union. Bones with a relatively poor blood supply and little associated subcutaneous tissue and muscle, such as the distal pretibia and carpal navicular bone, have difficulty establishing the normal vascular network at the fracture zone. Poor blood supply to a fracture site promotes primitive scar tissue rather than callus formation. The bridge between the two fractured bone fragments is consequently filled in with an avascular fibrous connective tissue rather than the usual bone and cartilage elements of a callus. Electrical stimulation to the fracture site has dramatically improved the response of these fibrous nonunions to treatment.

INFLAMMATORY BONE DISORDERS

Osteomyelitis

Osteomyelitis (infection of bone) may be classified according to several factors, including (1) its duration—acute, subacute, or chronic; (2) the nature of the exudate—hemorrhagic, purulent, or nonsuppurative; (3) its location—bone, periosteum, or epiphysis; and (4) the etiologic agent—*Staphylococcus aureus, Mycobacterium tuberculosis,* and so on.[106,107]

Invasion of tissue by bacteria is followed by vascular and cellular responses. This process is modified by the rigid wall of the bony cortex and by the baffle system created by the trabeculas of the cancellous bone, in that increased tissue pressure cannot be dissipated into the soft tissue and consequently the traditional swelling, or "tumor," component of the inflammatory triad is absent. The capillaries and sinusoids of the marrow are compressed as a result of the increased intramedullary pressure, producing infarction of the marrow fat, hematopoietic elements, and bone. There is active hyperemia at the edge of the infarction zone. This increased blood flow is associated with increased osteoclastic activity, resulting in the removal of bone and localized osteoporosis (Fig. 74-34). An inflammatory exudate gathers at the margin of the infarct zone. The inflammatory process penetrates through the cortex into the subperiosteal area through Volkmann's canals. In infants and older children the periosteum has very few anchoring fibers (Sharpey's fibers), and consequently the periosteum is readily stripped from the bone surface by the increased periosteal pressure. This causes the periosteal component of the blood supply to the cortex to be disrupted, producing cortical bone infarction. The cortical bone infarction results in the formation of the classic sequestrum. The isolated or sequestered bone wall retains its original radiographic density until revascularization takes place, and osteoclastic activity may then ensue. A rim of reactive new bone, or involucrum, is formed by the periosteum around the dead (sequestered) fragment.

Histologically, acute osteomyelitis exhibits the features typically associated with acute inflammation (Fig. 74-34). The most sensitive indicator of skeletal disease is the loss of the normal marrow architecture. Normal hematopoietic elements and fat are replaced by the leukocytic infiltrate. The nature of the leukocytic infiltrate may vary with the type of infection, but generally polymorphonuclear leukocytes are found. A fibrous wall is created to sequester the infarcted areas, and a chronic inflammatory cell infiltrate ultimately predominates. Small collections of polymorphonuclear leukocytes, however, persist as microabscesses, and the designation of acute versus chronic osteomyelitis is not meaningful on a histologic basis.

The goals of therapy are to reduce the intraosseous pressure and prevent infarction. In principle, this is accomplished by drainage and specific therapy directed against the particular etiologic agent. Antibiotics, however, are limited in their ability to combat organisms harbored within either abscess cavities or infarcted tissue. Despite rigorous antibiotic therapy, recurrent infections are the rule, particularly in patients with *S. aureus* infections. Ultimately the osteomyelitis resolves, and because the scar tissue of bone is bone, fibrous tissue is replaced by dense bone. The disease may be chronic from the outset and manifest as a sharply localized reaction to the inflammatory stimulus but without the usual abscess formation. In these rare instances the only findings are dense, scarred bone and few clinical symptoms. This silent condition in which there is radiographic evidence of new bone formation is termed "chronic sclerosing osteomyelitis of Garré." Osteomyelitis may also be sharply limited to one site, with the formation of an abscess cavity surrounded by a rim of sclerotic bone, a condition known as "Brodie's abscess."

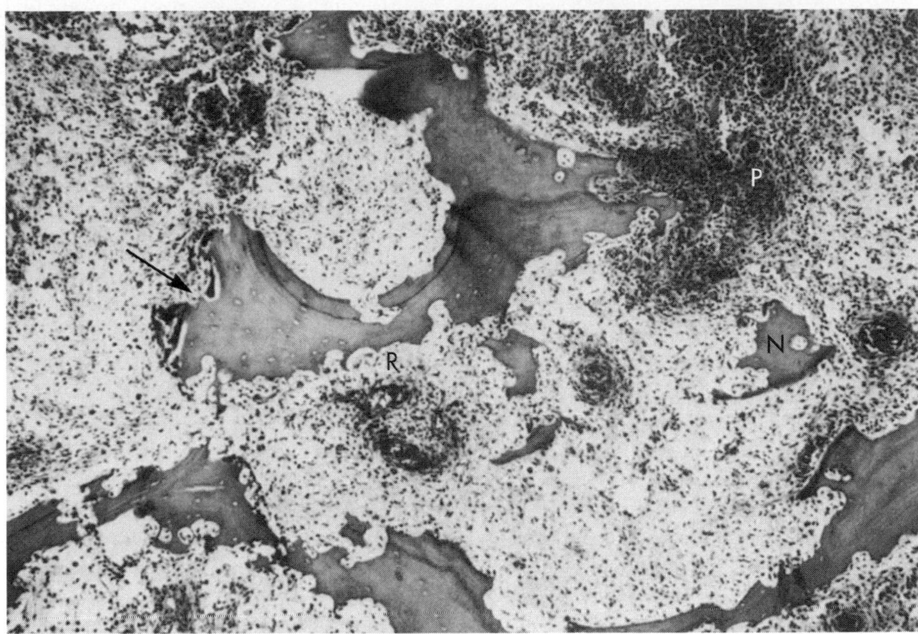

Fig. 74-34 Histologic appearance of osteomyelitis. Necrotic bone *(N)* and bone undergoing extensive resorption *(R)* by osteoclasts *(arrow)* are adjacent to the purulent *(P)* inflammatory infiltrate of the infectious process.

The most common cause of osteomyelitis is coagulase-positive *Staphylococcus* organisms (60% to 90%). The second most common organism, particularly in infants, is *Streptococcus. Pneumococcus, Escherichia coli, Klebsiella, Salmonella,* and *Bacteroides* organisms are also occasionally isolated in patients with hematogenous osteomyelitis. In postoperative osteomyelitis and osteomyelitis contracted by contiguous spread, *Staphylococcus, Streptococcus, Pseudomonas, Proteus,* and *E. coli* organisms are often encountered.

Salmonella osteomyelitis may follow typhoid fever in about 1% of patients with typhoid fever. The most important association, however, is that of *Salmonella* osteomyelitis with hemoglobinopathies. In sickle cell anemia, focal necrosis and bone infarction are common after a sickle cell crisis. The exact mechanism of and reason for the *Salmonella* bacteremia, however, remain unclear. For some reason, *Salmonella* organisms have an unusual predilection for the bone marrow in these patients. The hand-and-foot syndrome manifests as infarction of the small bones of the hands and feet, followed by *Salmonella* osteomyelitis. In some instances *Salmonella* organisms appear to inhibit the systemic granulocyte response, producing leukopenia. Within bone the lack of polymorphonuclear leukocytes combined with a pronounced lymphocytic-plasmacytic response, the inflammatory response, may be mistaken for multiple myeloma.

In contrast to bacterial osteomyelitis, fungal osteomyelitis is rare. However, when systemic dissemination of a fungal infection occurs, seeding may take place in the skeleton. The portal of entry is usually the respiratory tract, and organisms reach the bone through the circulation. Although any bone can be involved, the small bones of the hands and feet are favored sites. The tissue response is a chronic suppurative inflammation with granuloma formation. Because the granulomatous reaction is nonspecific, the organism must be identified for the diagnosis to be confirmed. Organisms that have been associated with fungal osteomyelitis produce the following pathoses: coccidioidomycosis, blastomycosis, paracoccidioidomycosis, cryptococcosis, histoplasmosis, sporotrichosis, mucormycosis, actinomycosis, and nocardiosis.

Tuberculosis

The tubercle bacillus, *Mycobacterium tuberculosis,* is a nonmotile organism that prefers areas of high oxygen pressure. The hematogenously spread organisms therefore commonly lodge in the synovium, producing an erosive, deforming arthritis, and they involve the associated epiphyseal and metaphyseal portions of the bones on either side of the joint by means of the common blood supply. The granulomatous inflammatory reaction to the organisms with the associated caseating necrosis often involves the subchondral portion of a joint, replacing the trabecular bone support such that the contiguous articular surface is destroyed. With continued inflammatory destruction, sequestrum forms in the subchondral bone and articular cartilage; this may occur on both sides of the involved joint, resulting in the formation of a "kissing" sequestrum. The increased vascularity associated with the inflammatory process results in the development of localized osteoporosis, a bone loss that is often out of proportion to the degree of associated infection.

A very common site of skeletal tuberculosis is the spine *(Pott's disease).* The infection is not contained to one vertebral body but rather spreads to adjacent disks and the spinal canal, ultimately resulting in soft-tissue extension and fistula formation.

Sarcoidosis

Sarcoidosis is a noncaseating granulomatous process that may manifest in the skeleton as small lytic and sclerotic foci in the bones of the hand. Large areas of destruction such as those seen in tuberculosis are not typically found. Sarcoidosis is considered in the differential diagnosis of all granulomatous inflammatory reactions.

PAGET'S DISEASE OF BONE (OSTEITIS DEFORMANS)

Paget's disease of bone (osteitis deformans)[108-109] is a common chronic osteolytic and osteosclerotic disease of uncertain cause that may involve one or more bones and results in pain, skeletal deformities, and occasionally sarcomatous transformation. Approximately 120 years ago Sir James Paget[110] described the 20-year clinical course and autopsy findings in a man who suffered from an apparently rare, progressively deforming bone disease.

The increasingly routine performance of serum chemical assays (alkaline phosphatase activity) and the widespread availability and use of diagnostic radiologic methods have resulted in the frequent detection of patients with limited skeletal involvement and asymptomatic Paget's disease of bone. It became apparent that Paget's disease is in fact not rare and afflicts approximately 3% of the white population over 40 years of age. The incidence increases with age, with men more frequently affected than women. Most patients (80% to 90%) are asymptomatic. Unfortunately, it is not possible to predict which patients will experience progression of disease. Symptoms include deformity, fracture, deafness, and arthritis. Although many bones may be affected (a *polyostotic* manifestation), involvement is typically either asymmetric or limited to one bone *(monostotic)*. The hematopoietically active flat bones and acral areas of the long bones (sacrum, spine, pelvis, skull, femurs, clavicles, tibias, ribs, and humeruses) are common skeletal sites of involvement.

There are many reports of the familial clustering of Paget's disease, whereby several siblings of one family or various members of several generations of a given family may be affected.

Histopathology. Paget's disease can be divided into three phases: an active resorptive phase, an active formation phase, and a quiescent, inactive phase. Paget's disease is initiated when normal marrow is replaced by a richly vascular, loose fibrous connective tissue. Isolated clusters of chronic inflammatory cells may be seen. Osteoclasts congregate on the existing bone trabeculas and within the cortex, resulting in the formation of large resorbing fronts. The osteoclasts are morphologically abnormal, with many attaining enormous proportions, and each may contain an excessive number of nuclei, as many as 100 per cell (Fig. 74-35).

After the wave of osteoclastic activity, osteoblastic activity is triggered (Fig. 74-36). The newly formed bone is woven. Repeated episodes of removal and formation result in the appearance of innumerable small, irregularly shaped bone fragments that appear to be joined in a chaotic jigsaw or mosaic pattern, the histologic hallmark of Paget's disease (Fig. 74-37). The osteoblastic phase dominates as the disease progresses. As excessive formation occurs, bone becomes more compact and dense, but structurally and morphologically this

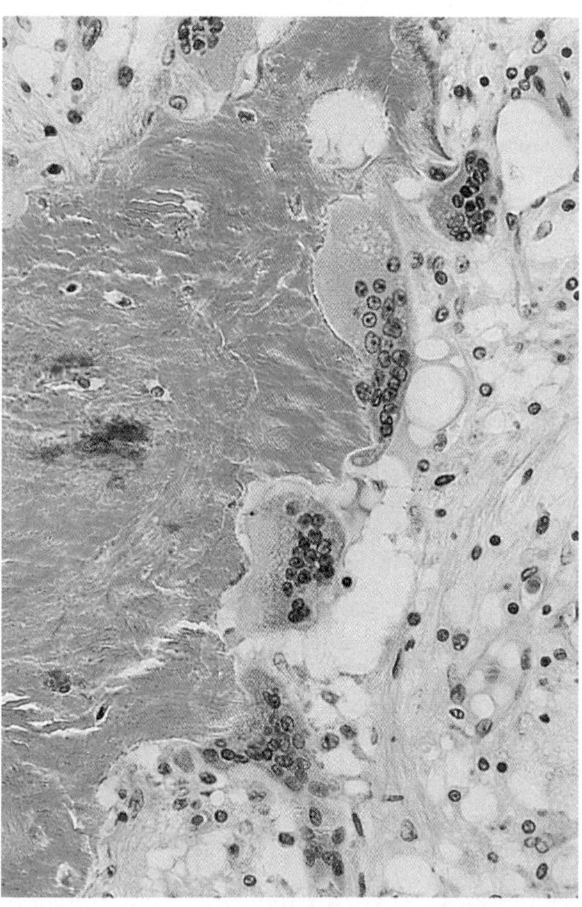

Fig. 74-35 Paget's disease. Abnormal multinucleated osteoclasts are seen apposed to the bone. The marrow is fibrotic.

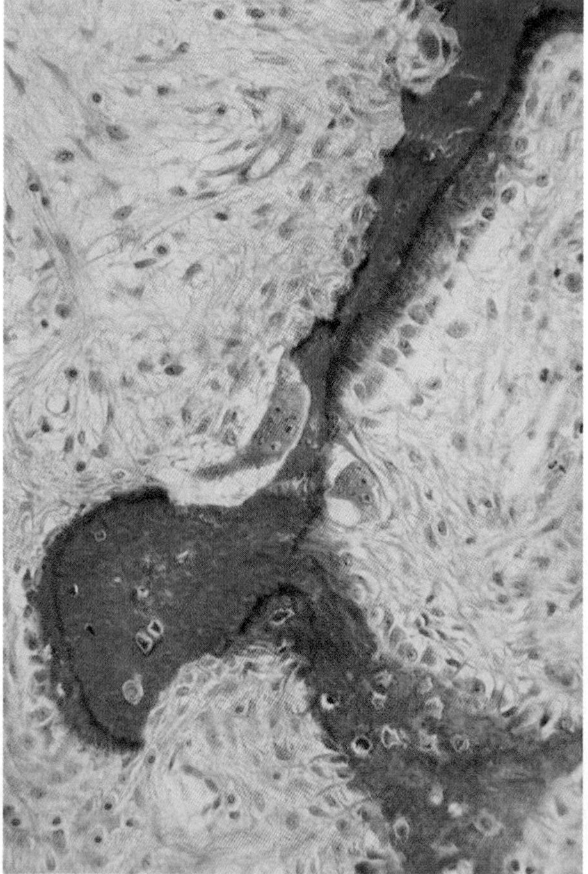

Fig. 74-36 Paget's disease. Bone resorption is accompanied by bone formation. The marrow is fibrotic.

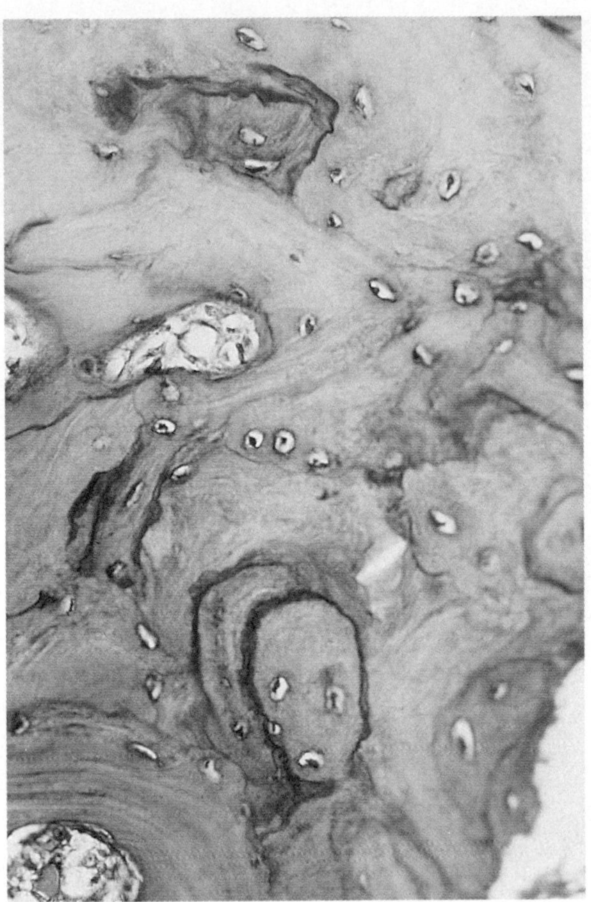

Fig. 74-37 Mosaic pattern of cement lines characteristic of the sclerotic phase of Paget's disease.

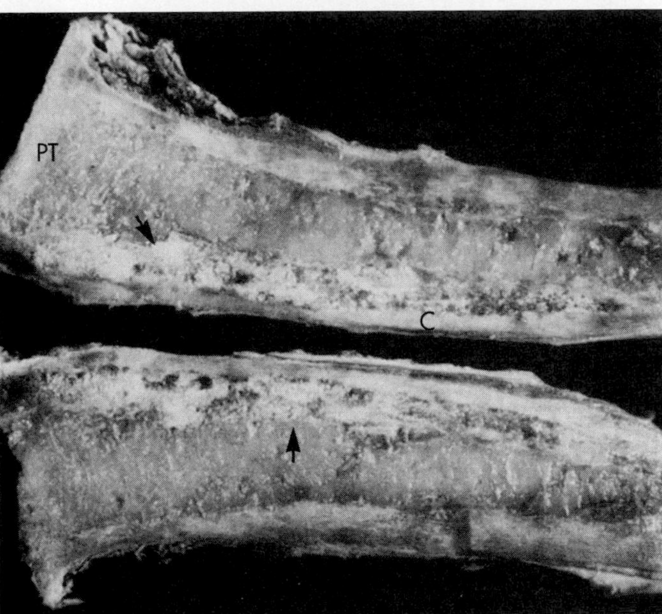

Fig. 74-38 Gross appearance of bone in Paget's disease. The sagittal section of this proximal tibial bone *(PT)* shows dense deposits of new bone with the consistency of lava rock, hence the term "pumice bone" *(arrows)*. In addition, as is characteristic, the entire bone shaft is enlarged, the cortex is thickened *(C)* and there is anterior bowing.

tissue is abnormal. Grossly it resembles the gritty but brittle texture of pumice or lava rock (Fig. 74-38). Radiologically this formation results in a flocculant, radiopaque deposit that has been likened to cotton wool. The remaining trabeculas become thicker or more dense as the trabecular spicules oriented along lines of stress is wider. The cortical bone becomes irregularly thickened as the bone enlarges. The cortical trabecular bone junction at the endosteum becomes indistinct. The clinical and radiographic features are easily detected, given this underlying pathologic process. Besides pain, a common complication of Paget's disease is deformity, manifested as either bowing of a weight-bearing long bone or enlargement of the skull. Hypervascularity with gross dilatation of the superficial vessels in bone was originally described by Paget, and increased blood flow to an affected extremity with resultant warmth and erythema may be seen.

The disease in long bones is usually initially characterized by the lytic "blade-of-grass" lesion. A wave of osteoclastic activity produces an advancing edge of lysis, which begins at the epiphyseometaphyseal ends of the bone and extends toward the diaphysis. The advancing wedge causes the diameter of the long bone to increase because of the subsequent periosteal reinforcement of the cortex. Deformities of the long bones are confined to the bones in the lower extremity. The bowing deformity of the femur and tibia may be severe. Nevertheless, the involved bone may be weak and prone to pathologic fracture.

The pelvis is a common site of involvement. The osteolytic phase of the disorder is not usually appreciated, perhaps because of its asymptomatic nature. The osteoblastic phase may on occasion be confused with metastatic osteosclerotic (blastic) carcinomas.

Reflecting the elevated level of bone turnover, the serum alkaline phosphatase activity and osteocalcin level are both elevated, representing osteoblastic activity. As a measurement of bone resorption, the urinary excretion of hydroxyproline, pyridinoline and deoxypyridinoline is also elevated.

Paget observed malignant transformation in five of his 23 patients. Because the disease involves the osteoblastic, osteoclastic, and fibroblastic cell lines, tumors that arise in this setting not surprisingly are osteosarcomas, fibrosarcomas, and giant cell malignant fibrous histiocytomas.

DEGENERATIVE DISEASES OF BONE (OSTEONECROSES)

Osteonecrosis is a family of disorders characterized by infarction of bone, typically involving the femoral head. Although all forms of this disorder are characterized by necrotic bone, the natural history and pathologic expression of the various entities may vary.[11]

Although there are many classification schemes, there are three generic categories of osteonecrosis: postfracture, idiopathic, and renal transplant associated. Most commonly the infarction occurs after a fracture of the femoral neck, with interruption of the retinacular blood supply. In this setting osteonecrosis may also be called *avascular necrosis of bone*. Osteonecrosis may also occur in persons who do not have vascular insufficiency. Although there may be an associated systemic illness in some of these patients, such as alcoholism, hyperlipidemia, or hyperuricemia, the cause of the infarction remains unknown, and this form of the disorder may best be referred to as "idiopathic osteonecrosis." In a third broad category are patients who are receiving immunosuppressive agents, particularly corticosteroids. Renal transplant recipients who require therapy involving the use of multiple immunosuppressive agents are particularly at risk.

Although the pathogenesis of the infarction is unknown in the latter two clinical groups, all the various osteonecroses may be related by their associated lipid abnormalities. Enlargement of the individual adipocytes within the marrow may increase the intramedullary pressure and occlude sinusoids and blood vessels. Increasing intraosseous pressure is also believed to play a role in the development of osteonecrosis in the miscellaneous marrow-packing disorders, such as Gaucher's disease. In these disorders marrow infiltration by foamy histiocytes may produce an intramedullary pressure that exceeds the vascular perfusion pressure.

The earliest histologic change occurring in any of the forms of osteonecrosis is death of the bone and the surrounding hematopoietic and fatty marrow. After a fracture, all the remaining pathologic changes seen in infarction reflect the repair process, and it is by the exuberance of these events that the various clinical forms of osteonecrosis differ. For example, idiopathic osteonecrosis, particularly that associated with corticosteroid therapy, undergoes a less pronounced repair process; woven bone does not form about the dead trabeculas, and so the degree of bone sclerosis may not be very great. Otherwise, the infarcted tissue incites the same inflammatory response as that seen with any other infarct at any other site in the body. The infarcted tissue is sharply demarcated from the viable tissue, which has maintained a blood supply (Fig. 74-39). In the immediate vicinity of the infarcted zone, a band of variable width containing ischemic but not infarcted tissue is seen. This ischemic zone is composed of dense fibrous tissue. Outside this zone is a hyperemic reactive zone from which granulation tissue enters the edges of the infarcted regions. Fibroblastic proliferation, accompanied by the formation of new blood vessels and osteoclasts, removes dead bone. Osteoblasts then differentiate from this connective tissue, and new bone is deposited on top of some of the preexisting necrotic trabeculas. This removal of old bone and deposition of additional bone on a scaffolding of dead bone is termed "creeping substitution." It is the ability of the granulation tissue to form new bone on the scaffolding of the preexisting bone that is the basis for the success of bone grafts used in orthopedic surgery in general and in the core decompression with grafting therapy of avascular necrosis, in particular.

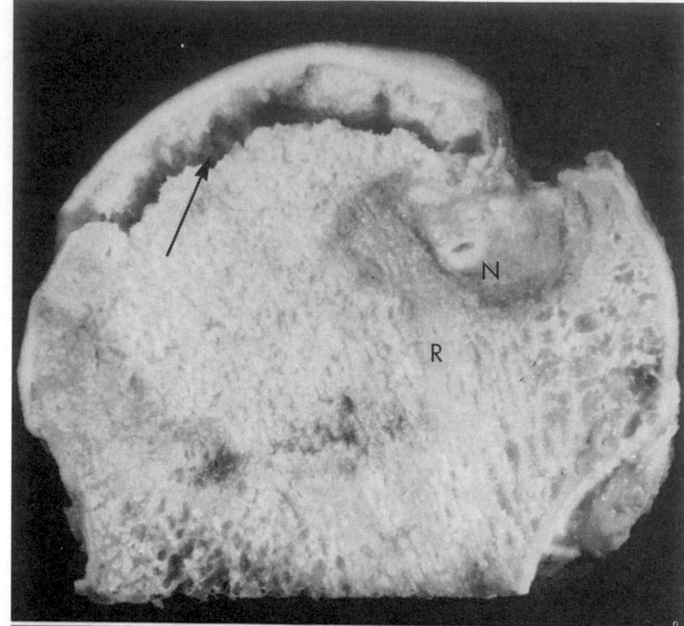

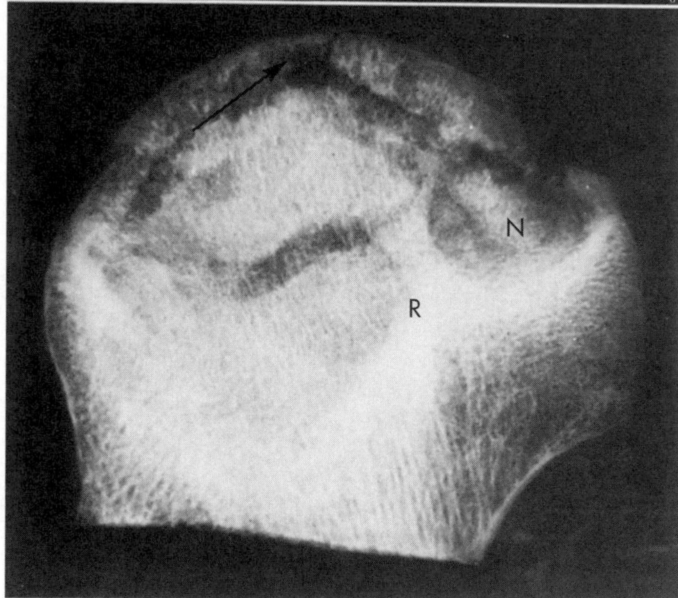

Fig. 74-39 **A,** Sagittal section and, **B,** radiograph of femoral head excised for the treatment of advanced avascular necrosis. Notice the subchondral lucent zone *(arrow),* the destruction and collapse of the articular cartilage, and the sclerotic zone of repair *(R)* surrounding the necrotic focus *(N).*

The consequences of infarction may vary from none to severe secondary degenerative joint disease. If the infarct is of limited size and the blood supply can be reestablished, recovery will occur without any persistent damage to the structural integrity of the bone. The dead bone cannot resist or transmit stress. Continued use of the affected limb will result in multiple small fractures of the infarcted trabeculas. These small fractures are of particular importance to the subcondral plate of a major weight-bearing bone such as the femoral head. With continued use there is impaction of the dead bone, which compresses the trabeculas into a smaller volume, resulting in a relative increase in radiodensity. A separation, or fracture cleft, ultimately forms between the impacted fragments and the overlying subchondral plate, which can be recognized radiographically in the femoral head as the crescent sign (Fig. 74-40). This radiolucent subchondral fracture is often the first diagnostic feature to be recognized on plain film radiographs. At the moment of infarction, however, dead bone does not exhibit any radiographic change. Radiographs will reveal only areas that have undergone secondary structural changes, long after the infarction has occurred.

In addition to the crescent sign, the radiographic diagnosis of osteonecrosis is based on subsequent changes in bone density. In general the density of bone may be increased, decreased, or unchanged. Increased and decreased density are relative concepts, depending on what happens to the adjacent viable bone.

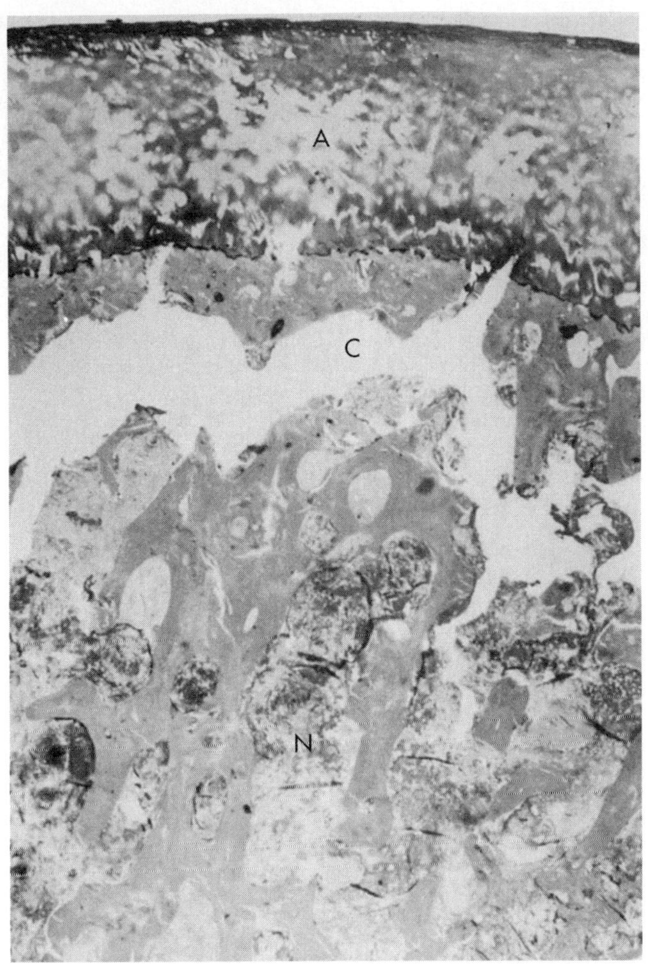

Fig. 74-40 Histologic appearance of avascular necrosis of the femoral head. The articular cartilage *(A)* is separated from the underlying necrotic bone *(N)* resulting in a fracture line or the so-called crescent sign *(C)*.

The diagnosis of bone infarct is classically made on the basis of the appearance of increased density within the necrotic region. In reality the infarcted bone itself is unchanged. Without a blood supply there can be no cellular activity and thus no change—increase or decrease—in bone substance.

Once the subchondral bone is resorbed or the necrotic tissue becomes impacted or crushed, the overlying joint surface becomes unstable. This instability leads to femoral head collapse and considerable distortion of the articular cartilage surface, eventuating in degenerative joint disease. The pathologic and corresponding radiographic changes seen in avascular necrosis are depicted in Fig. 74-40.

ACKNOWLEDGMENTS

The authors wish to acknowledge that some of the illustrative material used in this chapter was derived from the teaching collections of our former affiliations: The Health Science Center, Winnipeg, Canada; The Medical University of South Carolina; Columbia University College of Physicians and Surgeons; and especially Albert Einstein College of Medicine. We also thank Linda Crandall and Barbara Rockafellow for their secretarial expertise and Phil Verzola for photographic assistance.

REFERENCES

Normal bone

1. Parfitt AM: The physiologic and clinical significance of bone histomorphometric data. In Recker R, editor: *Bone histomorphometry: techniques and interpretation,* Boca Raton, Fla., 1983, CRC Press.
2. Burgeson RE, Nimni ME: Collagen types: molecular structure and tissue distribution, *Clin Orthop* 282:250, 1992.
3. Delmas PD: Biochemical markers of bone turnover [Review]. *J Bone Miner Res* 8:S549, 1993.
4. Robey PG, Fedarko NS, Hefferan TE et al: Structure and molecular regulation of bone matrix proteins, *J Bone Miner Res* 8:S483, 1993.
5. Anderson HC: Recent advances in methods for inducing bone formation, *Curr Opin Ther Patients* 4:17, 1994.
6. Ruoslahti E: Structure and biology of proteoglycans, *Annu Rev Cell Biol* 4:229, 1988.
7. Termine JD: Bone matrix proteins and the mineralization process. In Favus MJ, editor: *Primer on the metabolic bone diseases and disorders of mineral metabolism,* New York, 1993, Raven Press.
8. Talmage RV, Grubb SA: A laboratory model demonstrating osteocyte-osteoblast control of plasma calcium concentration, *Clin Orthop* 122:299, 1977.
9. Gehron Robey P, Bianco P, Termine JD: The cellular biology and molecular biochemistry of bone formation. In Coe FL, Favus MJ, editors: *Disorders of bone and mineral metabolism,* New York, 1992, Raven Press.
10. Raisz LG: Bone cell biology: new approaches and unanswered questions, *J Bone Miner Res* 8:S457, 1993.
11. Teitelbaum SL: Bone remodeling and the osteoclast, *J Bone Miner Res* 8:S523, 1993.
12. Zaidi M, Pazianas M, Shankar VS et al: Osteoclast function and its control, *Exp Physiol* 78:721, 1993.
13. Suda T, Takahashi N, Martin TJ: Modulation of osteoclast differentiation, *Endocr Rev* 13:66, 1992.
14. Recker RR: Embryology, anatomy and microstructure of bone. In Coe FL, Favus MJ, editors: *Disorders of bone and mineral metabolism,* New York, 1992, Raven Press.
15. Wolff J: Das Gesetz der Transformation der Knochen, Berlin, 1892, A Hirschwald (English translation: Berlin, 1986, Springer-Verlag).
16. Carter DR: Mechanical loading history and skeletal biology, *J Biomech* 20:1095, 1987.
17. Frost HM: *Bone modeling and skeletal modeling errors,* Springfield, Ill, 1973, Charles C Thomas.
18. Väänänen HK: Mechanism of bone turnover, *Ann Med* 25:353, 1993.
19. Ericksen EF, Axelrod DW, Melsen F: *Bone histomorphometry,* New York, 1994, Raven Press.
20. Canalis E: Regulation of bone remodeling. In Favus MJ, editor: *Primer on the metabolic bone diseases and disorders of mineral metabolism,* New York, 1993, Raven Press.
21. Dempster DW: Bone remodeling. In Coe FL, Favus MJ, editors: *Disorders of bone and mineral metabolism,* New York, 1992, Raven Press.
22. Parfitt AM: The physiologic and pathogenetic significance of bone histomorphometry. In Coe FL, Favus MJ, editors: *Disorders of bone and mineral metabolism,* New York, 1992, Raven Press.
23. MacDonald BR, Gowen M: The cell biology of bone, *Baillieres Clin Rheumatol* 7:421, 1993.
24. Canalis E: Systemic and local factors and the maintenance of bone quality, *Calcif Tissue Int* 53:S90, 1993.
25. Fitzpatrick LA, Coleman DT, Bilezikian JP: The target tissue actions of parathyroid hormone. In FL Coe Favus MJ, editors: *Disorders of bone and mineral metabolism,* New York, 1992, Raven Press.
26. Eriksen EF, Kassem M, Brixen K: Growth hormone and insulin-like growth factors as anabolic therapies for osteoporosis, *Horm Res* 40:95, 1993.
27. Slootweg MC: Growth hormone and bone, *Horm Metab Res* 25:335, 1993.
28. Allain TJ, McGregor AM: Thyroid hormones and bone, *J Endocrinol* 139:9, 1993.
29. Raisz LG: Local and systemic factors in the pathogenesis of osteoporosis, *World Rev Nutr Diet* 72:92, 1993.

30. Mosekilde L, Eriksen EF, Charles P: Effects of thyroid hormones on bone and mineral metabolism, *Endocrinol Metab Clin North Am* 19:35, 1990.
31. Oursler MJ, Landers JP, Riggs BL, Spelsberg TC: Oestrogen effects on osteoblasts and osteoclasts [review], *Ann Med* 25:361, 1993.
32. Lukert BP, Raisz LG: Glucocorticoid-induced osteoporosis: pathogenesis and management, *Ann Intern Med* 112:352, 1990.
33. Fitzpatrick LA: Glucocorticoid-induced osteoporosis. In Marcus R, editor: *Osteoporosis,* Boston, 1994, Blackwell Scientific Publications.
34. Canalis E, Centrella M, McCarthy TL: The role of insulin-like growth factors in bone remodeling and bone metabolism: basic and clinical aspects. In *Excerpta medica,* vol 11, Amsterdam, 1992, Elsevier.
35. Ingram RT, Park YK, Clarke BL, Fitzpatrick LA: Age and gender-related changes in the distribution of osteocalcin in the extracellular matrix of normal male and female bone: possible involvement of osteocalcin in bone remodeling, *J Clin Invest* 93:989, 1994.
36. Price JS, Oyajobi BO, Russell RG: The cell biology of bone growth, *Eur J Clin Nutr* 48:S131, 1994.
37. Weinstein RS: Clinical use of bone biopsy. In Coe FL, Favus MJ, editors: *Disorders of bone and mineral metabolism,* New York, 1992, Raven Press.
38. Dempster DW, Shane E: Bone quantification and dynamics of turnover. In Becker KL, editor: *Principles and practice of endocrinology and metabolism,* Philadelphia, 1990, Lippincott.
39. Recker RR: Bone biopsy and histomorphometry in clinical practice. In Favus MJ, editor: *Primer on the metabolic bone diseases and disorders of mineral metabolism,* New York, 1993, Raven Press.
40. Rao SR: Practical approach to bone biopsy. In Recker R, editor: *Bone histomorphometry: techniques and interpretation,* Boca Raton, Fla., 1983, CRC Press.
41. Rao DS, Matkovic V, Duncan H: Transiliac bone biopsy: complications and diagnostic value, *Henry Ford Hosp Med J* 28:112, 1980.

Skeletal developmental and genetic disorders

42. Parfitt AM, Drezner MK, Glorieux FH et al: Bone histomorphometry: standardization of nomenclature, symbols, and units, *J Bone Miner Res* 2:595, 1987.
43. Rimoin DL, Lachman RS: The chondrodysplasias. In Emery AEH, Rimoin DL, Sofaer JA, editor: *Principles and practice of medical genetics,* London, 1983, Churchill Livingstone.
44. Wynne-Davies R, Hall CM, Apleg AG: *Atlas of skeletal dyscrasias,* Edinburgh, 1985, Churchill Livingstone.
45. Albers-Schönberg H: Röntgenbilder einer seltenen Knochenerkrankung, *Münch Med Wochenschr* 51:365, 1904.
46. Johnson CC Jr, Lavy N, Lord T et al: Osteopetrosis: a clinical, genetic metabolic and morphologic study of the dominantly inherited, benign form, *Medicine* 47:149, 1968.
47. Loria-Cortes R, Quesada-Calvo E, Cordero-Chaverri E: Osteopetrosis in children: a report of 26 cases, *J Pediatr* 91:43, 1977.
48. Resnick D, Niwagama G: *Diagnosis of bone and joint disorders,* ed 2, Philadelphia, 1988, Saunders.
49. Revell PA: *Pathology of bone,* Berlin, 1986, Springer-Verlag.
50. Helfrich MH, Aronson DC, Everts V et al: Morphologic features of bone in human osteopetrosis, *Bone* 12:411, 1991.
51. Bollersleu J, Steiniche T, Melsen F, Mosekilde L: Structural and histomorphometric studies of iliac crest trabecular and cortical bone in autosomal dominant osteopetrosis: a study of two radiological tests, *Bone* 10:19, 1989.
52. Bollerslev J, Mosekilde L: Autosomal dominant osteopetrosis, *Clin Orthop* 294:45, 1993.
53. Mills BG, Yabe H, Singer FR: Osteoclasts in human osteopetrosis contain renal nucleocapsid-like nuclear inclusions, *J Bone Miner Res* 3:101, 1988.
54. Lee TH, Fevold KL, Muguruma Y et al: Relative roles of osteoclast colony-stimulating factor and macrophage colony-stimulating factor in the course of osteoclast development, *Exp Hematol* 22:66, 1994.
55. Marks SC, Mackay CA, Jackson ME et al: The skeletal effects of colony-stimulating factor-1 in toothless (osteopetrotic) rats: persistent metaphyseal sclerosis and the failure to restore subepiphyseal osteoclasts, *Bone* 14:675, 1993.
56. Boyce BF, Chen H, Soriano P, Mundy GR: Histomorphometric and immunocytochemical studies of *src*-related osteopetrosis, *Bone* 14:335, 1993.
57. Kaplan FS, August CS, Fallon MD et al: Successful treatment of infantile malignant osteopetrosis by bone-marrow transplantation: a case report, *J Bone Joint Surg [Am]* 70:617, 1988.
58. Glorieux FH, Pettifor JM, Mane PJ et al: Induction of bone resorption by parathyroid hormone in congenital malignant osteoporosis, *Metab Bone Dis Rel Res* 3:143, 1981.
59. Sly WS, Hewett-Emmett D, Whyte MP et al: Carbonic anhydrase II deficiency identified as the primary defect in the autosomal recessive syndrome of osteopetrosis with renal tubular acidosis and cerebral calcification, *Proc Natl Acad Sci USA* 80:2752, 1983.
60. Whyte MP, Murphy WA, Fallon MD et al: Osteopetrosis, renal tubular acidosis, and basal ganglia calcification in three sisters, *Am J Med* 69:64, 1980.
61. Roth DE, Venta PJ, Tashian RE, Sly WS: Molecular bases of human carbonic anhydrase II deficiency, *Proc Natl Acad Sci USA* 89:1804, 1992.
62. Whyte MP: Carbonic anhydrase II deficiency, *Clin Orthop* 294:52, 1993.
63. Whyte MP: Sclerosing bone dysplasias. In Favus MJ, editor: *Primer on the metabolic bone diseases and disorders of mineral metabolism,* ed 2, New York, 1993, Raven Press.
64. Whyte MP, Fallon MD, Murphy WA et al: Axial osteomalacia: clinical, laboratory and genetic investigation of an affected mother and son, *Am J Med* 71:1041, 1981.
65. Swan CHJ, Shah K, Brewer DB et al: Fibrogenesis imperfecta ossium, *Q J Med* 45:233, 1976.
66. Matucci-Cerinic M, Lott T, Jajic I et al: The clinical spectrum of pachydermoperiostosis (primary hypertrophic osteoarthropathy), *Medicine* 70:208, 1991.
67. Byers PH, Steiner RD: Osteogenesis imperfecta, *Annu Rev Med* 43:269, 1992.
68. Hollister DW: Molecular bases of osteogenesis imperfecta, *Curr Probl Dermatol* 17:76, 1987.
69. Sillence D: Osteogenesis imperfecta: an expanding panorama of variants, *Clin Orthop* 159:11, 1981.
70. Prockop DJ, Colige A, Helminen H et al: Mutations in type I procollagen that cause osteogenesis imperfecta: effects of the mutations on the assembly of collagen into fibrils, the basis of phenotypic variations, and potential antisense therapies, *J Bone Miner Res* 8:S489, 1993.
71. Marini JC: Osteogenesis imperfecta: comprehensive management, *Adv Pediatr* 35:391, 1988.
72. Thompson EM: Non-invasive prenatal diagnosis of osteogenesis imperfecta, *Am J Med Genet* 45:201, 1993.

Metabolic bone diseases

73. Cooper C, Aihie A: Osteoporosis: recent advances in pathogenesis and treatment, *Q J Med* 87:203, 1994.
74. Belchetz PE: Hormonal treatment of postmenopausal women [review], *N Engl J Med* 330:1062, 1994.
75. Sowers MR, Galuska DA: Epidemiology of bone mass in premenopausal women [review], *Epidemiol Rev* 15:374, 1993.
76. Consensus Development Conference: Prophylaxis and treatment of osteoporosis, *Osteoporosis Int* 1:114, 1991.
77. Morrison NA, Qi JC, Tokita A et al: Prediction of bone density from vitamin D receptor alleles, *Nature* 367:284, 1994.
78. Cloutier MD, Hayles AB, Riggs BL et al: Juvenile osteoporosis: report of a case including a disruption of some metabolic and microradiographic studies, *Pediatrics* 40:649, 1967.
79. Jowsey J, Johnson KA: Juvenile osteoporosis: bone findings in seven patients, *J Pediatr* 81:511, 1972.
80. Smith R: Idiopathic osteoporosis in the young, *J Bone Joint Surg [Br]* 62:417, 1980.
81. Clarke BL, Ebeling PR, Jones JD et al: Increased bone turnover with aging in men is not due to testosterone deficiency, Las Vegas, Nev., 1993, Proceedings of the annual meeting of the Endocrine Society.
82. Meier DE, Orwoll ES, Jones JM: Marked disparity between trabecular and cortical bone loss with age in healthy men: measurement by vertebral computed tomography and radial photon absorptiometry, *Ann Intern Med* 101:605, 1984.

83. Seeman E: Osteoporosis in men: epidemiology, pathophysiology and treatment possibilities, *Am J Med* 95:22S, 1993.
84. Parfitt AM: Age-related structural changes in trabecular and cortical bone: cellular mechanisms and biochemical consequences, *Calcif Tissue Int* 36:S123, 1984.
85. Jackson JA, Kleerekoper M, Parfitt M et al: Bone histomorphometry in hypogonadal and eugonadal men with spinal osteoporosis, *J Clin Endocrinol Metab* 65:53, 1987.
86. Greenspan SL, Oppenheim DS, Klibanshi A: Importance of gonadal steroids to bone mass in men with hyperprolactinemic hypogonadism, *Ann Intern Med* 110:526, 1989.
87. Duncan H: Regional osteoporosis. In Favus MJ, editor: *Primer on the metabolic bone diseases and disorders of mineral metabolism,* New York, 1993, Raven Press.
88. Marcus R: Secondary osteoporosis. In Coe FL, Favus MJ, editors: *Disorders of bone and mineral metabolism,* New York, 1992, Raven Press.
89. Mosekilde L, Melsen F: Dynamic differences in trabecular bone remodeling between patients after jejuno-ileal bypass for obesity and epileptic patients receiving anticonvulsant therapy, *Metab Bone Dis Rel Res* 2:77, 1980.
90. Weinstein RS, Bryce GF, Sappington LJ et al: Decreased serum ionized calcium and normal vitamin D metabolite levels with anticonvulsant drug treatment, *J Clin Endocrinol Metab* 58:1003, 1984.
91. Parisien M, Silverberg SJ, Shane E et al: Bone disease in primary hyperparathyroidism, *Endocrinol Metab Clin North Am* 19:19, 1990.
92. Wartofsky L: Use of sensitive TSH assay to determine optimal thyroid hormone therapy and avoid osteoporosis, *Annu Rev Med* 42:341, 1991.
93. Parisien M, Silverberg SJ, Shane E et al: The histomorphometry of bone in primary hyperparathyroidism: preservation of cancellous bone structure, *J Clin Endocrinol Metab* 70:930, 1990.
94. Erickson EF: Normal and pathological remodeling of human trabecular bone: three dimensional reconstruction of the remodeling sequence in normals and in metabolic bone disease, *Endocrine Rev* 7:379, 1986.
95. Parisien M, Dempster DW, Shane E, Bilezikian JP: Histomorphometric analysis of bone in primary hyperparathyroidism. In Bilezikian JP, Marcus J, Levine M, editors: *The parathyroids, basic and clinical concepts,* New York, 1994, Raven Press.
96. Christiansen P, Steiniche T, Vesterby A et al: Primary hyperparathyroidism: iliac crest trabecular bone volume, structure, remodeling and balance evaluated by histomorphometric methods, *Bone* 13:41, 1992.
97. Fitzpatrick LA, Arnold A: Hypoparathyroidism. In DeGroot LJ, editor: *Endocrinology,* ed 3, Philadelphia, 1995, Saunders.
98. Diebold J, Batge B, Stein H et al: Osteoporosis in longstanding acromegaly: characteristic changes of vertebral trabecular architecture and bone matrix composition, *Virchows Archiv [A] (Pathol Anat)* 419:209, 1991.
99. Krakauer J, McKenna MJ, Rao DS et al: Low bone turnover in diabetes mellitus accounts for preservation of bone mineral density, *Diabetologia* 35:A192, 1992.
100. Elias AN, Gwinup G: Immobilization osteoporosis in paraplegia, *J Am Paraplegia Soc* 15:163, 1992.
101. McKenna MJ: Miscellaneous causes of osteoporosis. In Favus MJ, editor: *Primer on the metabolic bone diseases and disorders of mineral metabolism,* New York, 1993, Raven Press.
102. Parfitt AM, Miller MJ, Frame B et al: Metabolic bone disease after intestinal bypass for treatment of obesity, *Ann Intern Med* 88:193, 1978.
103. Morgan DB, Hunt G, Paterson CR: The osteomalacia syndrome after stomach operations, *Q J Med* 39:395, 1970.
104. Goodman WG, Coburn JW, Ramírez JA et al: Renal osteodystrophy in adults and children. In Favus MJ, editor: *Primer on the metabolic bone diseases and disorders of mineral metabolism,* New York, 1993, Raven Press.
105. Teitelbaum SL: Pathological manifestations of osteomalacia and rickets, *Clin Endocrinol Metab* 9:43, 1980.

Osteomyelitis

106. Kelly PJ: Osteomyelitis in the adult, *Orthop Clin North Am* 6:983, 1975.
107. Morrey BF, Peterson HA: Hematogenous pyogenic osteomyelitis in children, *Orthop Clin North Am* 6:935, 1975.

Paget's disease

108. Gallacher SJ: Paget's disease of bone, *Curr Opin Rheumatol* 5:351, 1993.
109. Kanis JA: Treatment of Paget's disease—an overview, *Semin Arthritis Rheum* 23:254, 1993.
110. Paget J: On a form of chronic inflammation of bones (osteitis deformans), *Trans Med Chir Soc Lond* 60:37, 1877.

Osteonecroses

111. Jacobs B: Epidemiology of traumatic and nontraumatic osteonecrosis, *Clin Orthop* 130:51, 1978.

75 Joints

Aubrey J. Hough Jr.

BASIC CONCEPTS

The 206 bones of the human skeleton articulate by means of several hundred joints of varying structure and function. Several classification systems for joints have been advanced,[1] but the one that is most widely employed is based on the type of movement at the joint. Immovable joints firmly joined by fibrous or cartilaginous elements are called *synarthroses*. Slightly movable joints, or *amphiarthroses*, are characterized by flattened disks of fibrocartilage connecting the articular surfaces without a true joint cavity. This pattern is seen in the intervertebral disks between the vertebral bodies. Freely movable joints, or *diarthroses*, are characterized by two opposed hyaline cartilage surfaces separated by a cavity lined by synovium and supported by ligaments. This last type of joint constitutes the majority of those present in the extremities. Considerable variety exists among the subtypes of diarthrodial joints depending on the motion required.[2] Some joints, where both hinge and rotary types of motion are experienced, also contain stabilizing fibrocartilaginous disks. Examples of these include the knee, sternoclavicular, and temporomandibular joints.

Diarthrodial joints

Development

The development of the joint tissues begins early in embryonic life, shortly after the emergence of the primitive limb buds (days 26 to 28 of gestation).[2] Cartilage is the principal skeletal tissue during embryonic and fetal life and can be identified in the limb buds by the seventh week after conception (fifth postovulatory week).[3] Whereas embryonic bones develop as linear condensations from the primordial blastema, joints develop as cartilaginous expansions at the sites of future articulations, usually at the ends of bones, where they are continuous with the adjacent cartilaginous growth centers.[4] The primordial joint structures of the hip are clearly discernible at the 17 mm stage of development. All joints begin as solid condensations of cartilaginous material. Those destined to differentiate into the true synovial or diarthrodial joints typically demonstrate a trilayered structure composed of two chondrogenic zones and a central layer of mesenchymal material. The central layer undergoes cavitation during the early fetal stages of development,[4,5] with concomitant differentiation of synovial, ligamentous, and tendinous structures (Fig. 75-1). Denervation by either mechanical or chemical means abolishes joint cavitation in

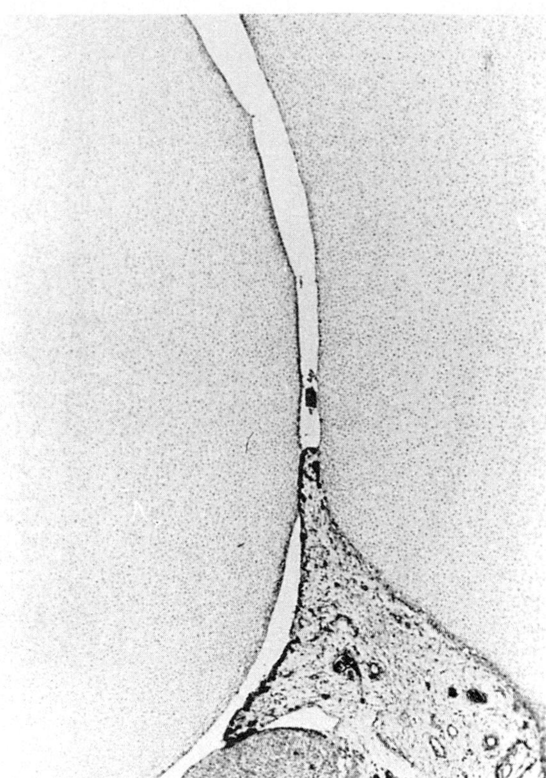

Fig. 75-1 Fetal knee joint after formation of joint cavity. Synovial primordium is at lower right.

experimental models,[5] and such cavitation indicates that fetal movement plays a role in the process.

Function

The normal diarthrodial joint is a complex structure composed of two opposed articular surfaces lined by hyaline cartilage. Underlying the hyaline cartilage is a transitional zone of calcified cartilage and a subchondral bony plate. The joint cavity and any internally disposed ligaments, fibrocartilaginous disks, or connecting bursae are also lined by synovium. The bones are maintained in approximation primarily by a fibrous joint capsule and extra-articular ligaments. These structures complement one another to allow movement while permitting absorption of forces. The synovium provides lubrication, nutrients, and cytokines to maintain the cartilage.[2]

Hyaline articular cartilage is sparsely cellular, but those cells that are present are organized into distinct zones (Fig. 75-2) with biomechanical implications.[2] A superficial zone of elongated chondrocytes with their long axes arranged tangentially to the articular surface is adjacent to a transitional or intermediate zone where the chondrocytes are oriented more randomly in small groups. Most of the cartilage consists of a deep radial zone where chondrocytes are oriented perpendicularly to the surface. A thin zone of calcified cartilage lies between the deep zone and the subchondral bone. This calcified cartilage zone contains a sinuous hematoxyphilic line, called the "tidemark" (Fig. 75-2) that may act to limit the extension of calcification into the deep zone.[6-8]

Articular chondrocytes are metabolically active and capable of cell division under pathologic stimuli.[9] These metabolic activities are essential to maintain the biomechanical properties of the cartilage.[2] Electron microscopy (Fig. 75-3) demonstrates the presence of organelles typical of cells engaged in protein synthesis and secretion, including rough endoplasmic reticulum, Golgi apparatus, aggregated free ribosomes, and cell membrane vesicles.[10] Because articular cartilage is avascular, the chondrocytes receive sustenance by absorption of nutrients from the synovial fluid, which is a dialysate of plasma.[2] The chondrocytes of the basal calcified zone may derive some nutrition from the vasculature at the bone cartilage junction.[8]

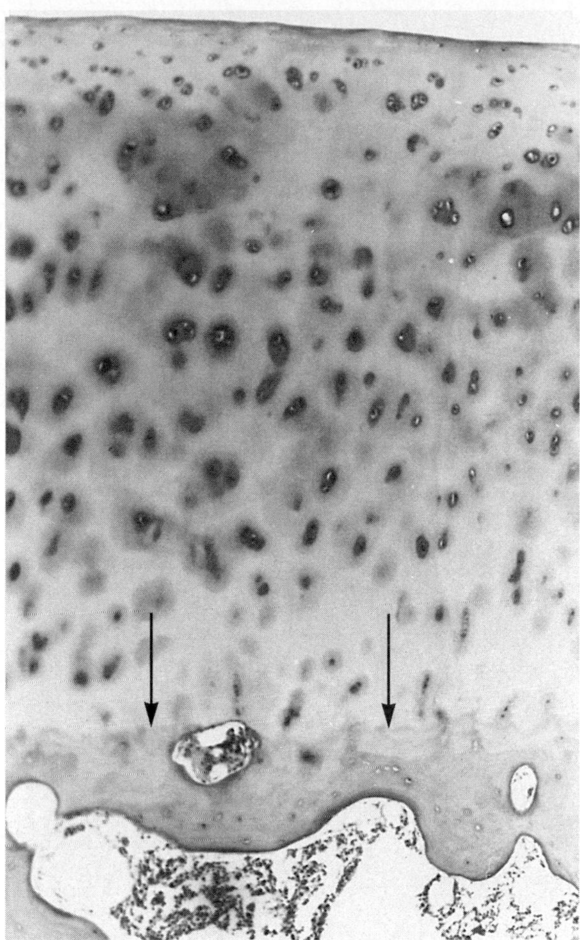

Fig. 75-2 Normal adult articular cartilage demonstrates three clearly defined zones; tidemark (*arrows*) marks extent of calcification.

The collagenous matrix accounts for approximately 55% of the dry weight of articular cartilage.[11] Like the chondrocytes the superficial collagen fibers are oriented tangentially to the surface. The fibers of the transitional or intermediate zone appear to be randomly oriented, whereas those of the deep and calcified zones are approximately perpendicular to the joint surface.[2] Although many molecular species of collagen are found in articular cartilage, 80% to 90% of the total is type II collagen, a monomeric fibrillar collagen found only in cartilage, nucleus pulposus, and the ocular vitreous material.[12] Three other collagens are found only in cartilage (types IX, X, and XI). Type X collagen is associated with enchondral ossification and thus persists in the basal calcified zone near the

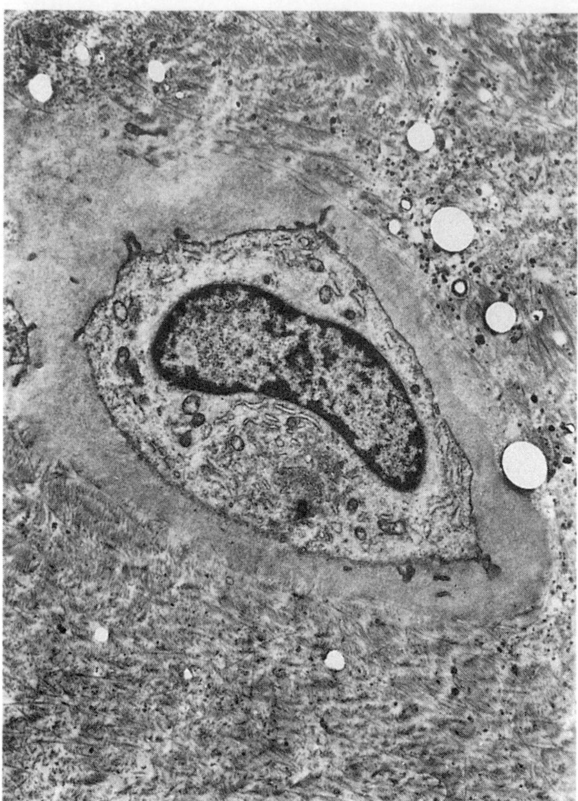

Fig. 75-3 Electron micrograph of articular chondrocyte from deep zone demonstrates prominent Golgi apparatus and fine perilacunar collagenous matrix.

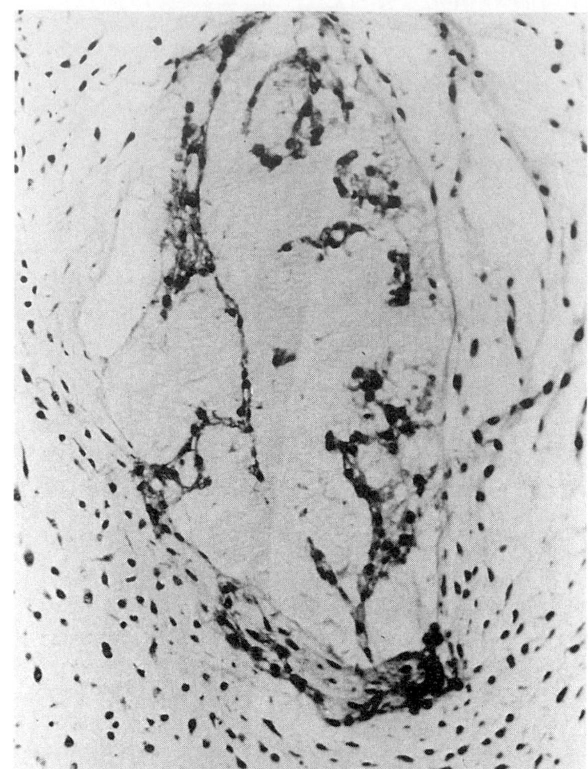

Fig. 75-4 Fetal intervertebral disk at 16 weeks gestation. Notochordal remnant is clearly visible in nucleus pulposus.

osteochondral junction.[13] Collagen types IX and XI are associated with type II fibers and are not localized to any one zone.[12] There is accumulating evidence that changes in the distribution and content of these minor collagens may be involved in subsequent breakdown of the type II collagenous matrix.[13]

The remainder of the articular cartilage matrix is composed of a protein polysaccharide gel, accounting for approximately 29% of the dry weight of the cartilage.[11] The composition of this gel is complex, with core proteins, chondroitin sulfates A and C, and keratan sulfate bound to high molecular weight hyaluronic acid molecules.[13,14] Approximately 70% of the weight of fresh articular cartilage is water that is trapped in the highly charged protein polysaccharide gel and held by the collagenous framework.[15] This structure is therefore responsible for the viscoelastic behavior of articular cartilage under repetitive compressive loading,[16] where the cartilage can be reversibly compressed to as little as 20% of its original height by the expelling of water.[2] The proteoglycans of articular cartilage are continuously being renewed by the metabolic activities of the chondrocytes.[13] Both qualitative and quantitative changes in the proteoglycans occur with aging,[17] but the role such changes play in contributing to disease is controversial.

The synovial membrane is composed of an inner secretory zone lined by a discontinuous layer of specialized cells with both secretory and phagocytic functions. Under certain circumstances, synovial cells perform antigen-processing functions similar to those of macrophages. The outer layer is a loose connective tissue with considerable flexibility. The vasculature is located at the outer edge of the connective tissue layer at a considerable distance from the inner synovial layer.[2]

Vertebral joints

Development

The vertebral bodies develop from segmental embryonic somites arranged on each side of the notochord. Primordial vertebral bodies are visible by the fourth week of embryonic life.[3] Processes extend dorsally and laterally to begin formation of the neural arch and costal processes, and chondrification begins.[3] Ossification begins at 9 weeks with the formation of primitive costovertebral joints.[3] The notochord largely disappears during this process, but a portion remains in each intervertebral disk as the nucleus pulposus[2] (Fig. 75-4). The cartilaginous end plates remain after ossification to form a portion of each intervertebral disk bounded by the anulus fibrosus.

Function

The zygapophyseal, or facet, joints, costovertebral joints, and costotransverse joints are all true diarthroses of composition similar to that of the peripheral joints.[18] The uncinate, or Luschka, joints of the cervical spine are also true diarthrodial joints. The intervertebral disks are amphiarthroses, intermediate in both structure and capacity for movement between the diarthrodial joints and the synchondroses such as the sacroiliac joint.[1]

The intervertebral disks are composed of cartilaginous end plates of structure and composition similar to those of articular cartilage. Between the two disks lies a central zone of gelatinous cartilage known as the *nucleus pulposus*. This area is surrounded by a series of concentric fibrocartilaginous rings that insert into the margins of the cartilaginous end plates. Together the fibrocartilaginous rings constitute the *anulus fibrosus*.[2] Unlike the nucleus pulposus, the anulus fibrosus is heavily collagenized and contains considerable amounts of type I as well as type II collagen. The nucleus pulposus contains a higher ratio of proteoglycans to collagen than other cartilaginous tissues.[2] Because of the high proteoglycan content, the water content of the nucleus pulposus is greater than that of the anulus.[2] The resistance to axial loading of the spine is accomplished through compressibility of the nucleus pulposus, with consequent temporary loss of height and gain in the diameter of each disk.[19] In effect, the axial stress is transferred horizontally against the surrounding anulus fibrosus. Individually the intervertebral disks allow only slight movement, but the sum of the movements over the entire spine confers mobility while maintaining a strong resistance to displacement.[2] Nevertheless, the spine is the site of a wide range of pathologic conditions resulting from a broad range of causes.

Examination and sampling of joint tissues

Before the era of advanced surgical techniques, such as prosthetic and allograft joint replacement, pathologic material for study of joint disease was almost exclusively obtained from postmortem samples. Biopsy of adventitial, supporting, or underlying tissues of the joint is also a relatively recent innovation. Because many joint diseases necessarily evolve slowly over many years, understanding of initial changes characteristic of individual joint tissues was limited. In addition, histologic, electron microscopic, and immunocytologic studies of many joint tissues require decalcification of the tissues. Most commercial rapid decalcifying agents are highly extractive, and such extraction renders special techniques unreliable. Slower methods involving buffered solutions of formic acid or ethylenediaminetetraacetic acid (EDTA) preserve many antigens and even some enzymes for subsequent detection.[20] Specimens from whole-joint resections, as typified by the femoral head, are best studied by reproducible sawing of 1 cm slabs with use of a band saw, followed by radiography of the slabs with use of a commercial low-kilovoltage radiography cabinet. Whole-mount microscopic sections may then be compared with the corresponding slab section radiograph. Similar techniques are applicable to the study of spinal arthroses.[18,21] As with examination of bone diseases in general, joint pathology should be carefully correlated with findings on clinical examination, radiographs, and computerized tomography (CT) scans.[22,23] Magnetic resonance imaging can accurately depict intra-articular structures and has thus added a new dimension to radiologic-pathologic correlation, especially of the knee.[24]

Advanced immunocytochemical and molecular biologic techniques can be applied to the study of the supporting soft tissues of the joint. Where possible, contiguous synovial, capsular, ligamentous, and meniscal tissues should be studied histologically without decalcification. This requires excision from the hard tissues before processing. Specific techniques unique to the diagnosis of individual disease states are described with the respective conditions.

Common factors uniting joint diseases

The varied conditions that lay waste to the joints result from basic mechanisms of joint destruction. The conditions depicted

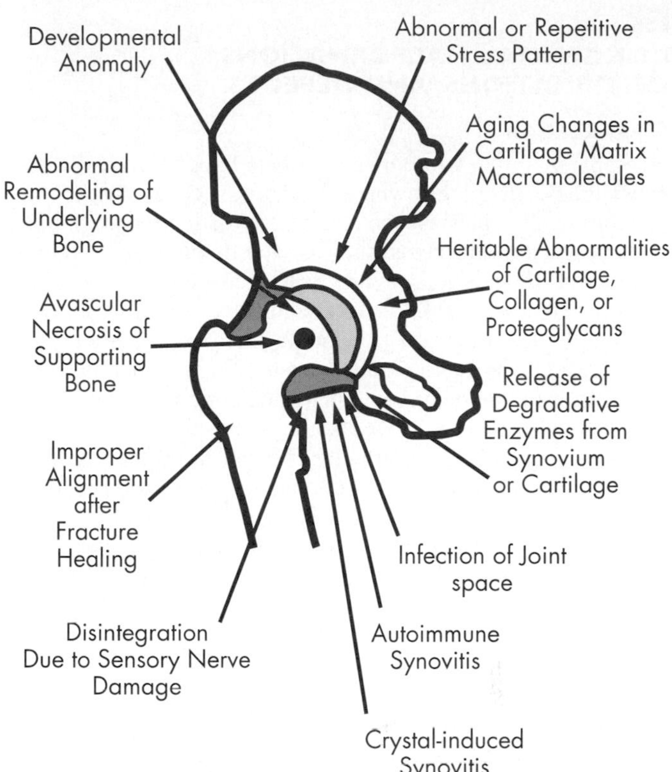

Fig. 75-5 Possible insults to joint structure and function are numerous and result in a high cumulative prevalence of joint disorders.

in Fig. 75-5 underlie the overwhelming number of diseases affecting the joints.

The molecular pathogenesis of many joint conditions has yet to be discovered, but a classification system developed from existing data would highlight the following variables. First, joint diseases[25] vary widely in prevalence from the ubiquitous (osteoarthritis), to the common (rheumatoid arthritis), to the rare (chondrodysplasias). Second, many joint conditions arise as primary diseases within the joints (osteoarthritis)[26,27] but others are clearly the manifestations of systemic disease states (rheumatoid arthritis),[28] with prominent extra-articular manifestations. Other joint diseases may fall into either category. Hence, calcium pyrophosphate deposition disease (chondrocalcinosis) may occur alone[29] but is also strongly associated with hemochromatosis[30] and primary hyperparathyroidism,[31] as well as with other systemic diseases.[32] The mechanisms by which systemic diseases affect the joints are highly variable. Examples include endocrine diseases such as acromegaly[33] and diabetes mellitus,[34] which alter cartilage metabolism or affect the surrounding connective and neural tissues. In autoimmune diseases, such as systemic lupus erythematosus and rheumatoid arthritis complement is fixed within the joint tissues, initiating an inflammatory response.[35] Third, many joint diseases pursue a "final common pathway" of progressive destructive changes leading to "burned-out" joints that may closely resemble primary degenerative joint disease. This is analogous to the "end-stage" kidney that may have resulted from numerous different mechanisms of immune, toxic, or metabolic injury. Thus, examining only late stages of joint disease can be misleading.

CONGENITAL MALFORMATIONS, DEFORMATIONS, AND DEFECTS

Classification

Heritable disorders of connective tissue have been reviewed in considerable detail elsewhere.[36] Many, such as the spondyloepiphyseal dysplasias, can result from distinctive point mutations in structural proteins, such as type II collagen.[37,38] Others result from defects in enzymes that exercise posttranslational control over the metabolism of connective tissues.[39,40] Other congenital disorders are true malformations, where primary structural defects have resulted from complex, but localized, disturbances in development during the period of fetal organogenesis that lasts up to 8 weeks after conception.[41] Many congenital defects, however, are classified as deformations. These structural abnormalities arise later in intrauterine life because of pathologic remodeling of previously normal organs.

The situation is actually somewhat more complex than these definitions would indicate. For example, renal malformations can and do cause joint deformations by a reduction in amniotic fluid volume. Thus either sporadic or heritable malformations can be associated clinically with deformations in a single syndrome.[41] An additional confounding factor is that mutations in structural proteins such as collagens or protein polysaccharides may not produce clinical joint disease until adult life, even though they are clearly heritable disorders.[38] In a broad sense, common disorders, such as rheumatoid arthritis[42] and generalized osteoarthritis[43] where definite genetic predispositions exist, could also be considered heritable.

Congenital disorders with known molecular pathogenesis

A full description of the congenital disorders producing arthropathy is beyond the scope of this work. At the level of clinical organ pathology congenital defects may be further classified as (1) bone related, (2) soft-tissue related, or (3) complex joint dysplasias involving both types of tissue. The most prominent diseases of the bone-related group are osteogenesis imperfecti (especially types I and III)[36] and achondroplasia.[36] Both are autosomal dominant disorders that produce joint degeneration secondary to deformity of underlying bone. In the former, soft-tissue laxity because of defects in type I collagen is an additional contributor to subsequent joint degeneration. In the latter, joint deformity and excessive weight borne on the small frame are likely to be contributing factors.[36] The specific molecular abnormality in achondroplasia is unknown.

Table 75-1 summarizes the principal congenital disorders producing joint disease in which a specific defect is known. Many are quite rare. An exception is the Stickler syndrome, an autosomal dominant disorder resulting in progressive degenerative arthropathy. This disorder occurs relatively frequently, affecting approximately 1 person per 10,000 in the population.[36] Of particular interest is thinking that some kindreds with the Stickler syndrome,[6] as well as others with spondyloepiphyseal dysplasia,[6,37,38] have various specific defects in the α 1(II) procollagen gene.

Other genetic diseases in soft tissues contribute to joint degeneration by inducing joint laxity with recurrent dislocations. In some diseases with joint laxity, specific defects of type I collagen in tendons and ligaments have been noted, as in osteogenesis imperfecti[44] and Ehlers-Danlos syndrome type VII.[45] In other congenital disorders the molecular basis of the syndrome is presently obscure. Table 75-2 lists miscellaneous congenital conditions with complex pathogenesis resulting in severe joint degeneration. Of particular interest is congenital hip dysplasia (dislocation). This common condition occurs at a frequency about 1.5 per 1000 live births,[46] occurring more frequently in females. The disorder is usually manifest at birth with bilateral poorly formed hip joints, usually with congenital dislocation.[47] Although much evidence indicates that deformation caused by fetal positioning may play a role,[48] equally strong evidence indicates a heritable,[47] generalized connective tissue defect.[49]

Table 75-1 Congenital disorders affecting the joints

Defect type	Syndrome	Clinical features	Inheritance
Structural protein disorders			
Type I collagen, defects of structure or production	Osteogenesis imperfecta types I and III	Brittle bones, recurrent fractures, recurrent joint dislocations	AD (Type I), AR and sporadic (Type III)
Type I collagen or procollagen peptidase defects	Ehlers-Danlos type VII	Multiple congenital dislocations leading to deformity	AR and AD forms
Type II collagen (some cases)	Stickler (progressive arthro-ophthalmopathy)	Retinal detachment, hearing loss, cleft palate, recurrent joint dislocation	AD
Type II collagen (some cases)	Spondyloepiphyseal dysplasia, congenital	Short stature, abnormal vertebrae, peripheral joint deformity,especially proximally	AD
Fibrillin (some cases)	Marfan	Tall stature, ectopia lentis, pronounced joint laxity	AD
Metabolic diseases			
Homogentisic acid oxidase deficiency	Ochronosis	Fragility of articular and intervertebral cartilage,profound degenerative disease	AR
L-Iduronidase deficiency	Hurler- Scheie (MPS I)	Stiff joints, spinal degeneration	AR
Iduronate-2-sulfatase deficiency	Hunter's (MPS II)	Stiff joints, spinal degeneration	X-R
N-Acetylgalactosamine-6-sulfatase deficiency	Morquio's (MPS IV)	Severe spinal degeneration	AR

AD, Autosomal dominant; *AR*, autosomal recessive, *MPS*, mucopolysaccharidosis, *X-R*, x-linked recessive.

Table 75-2 Multifactorial congenital disorders affecting the joints

Syndrome	Clinical description	Inheritance	Contributing factors
Arthrogryposis multiplex congenita	Rigid joints, fixed in fetal position	Some X-R, most sporadic	Deformation resulting from denervation
Familial articular hypermobility	Joint laxity without skin involvement	AD	None known, may include some cases of congenital hip dislocation
Osteochondrodysplasia with joint laxity (Larsen syndrome)	Multiple congenital dislocations	Both AD and AR forms	None known
Congenital hip dysplasia (dislocation)	Poorly formed femoral head and acetabulum	Complex, multifactorial inheritance possible	Deformation resulting from fetal positioning
Multiple epiphyseal dysplasia	Short stature, congenital, poorly formed epiphyses with stippled calcification	AD	Severe degenerative joint disease by early adult life
Arthropathies of cerebral palsy	Dislocated joints, especially hips, knees, ankles	Sporadic	Severe degenerative joint disease, especially hips
Achondroplasia	Short extremities, midfacial and skull abnormalities	AD	Excessive weight gain, premature degenerative joint disease

AD, Autosomal dominant; *X-R*, x-linked recessive; *AR*, autosomal recessive.

The influence of other environmental agents on the development of congenital hip dysplasia is illustrated by the increased prevalence of the disorder (along with other skeletal abnormalities) in offspring of diabetic mothers.[50,51] Even if corrected, degenerative disease of the hips frequently develops in early adult life. Some studies[52] have suggested that a forme fruste of this disorder contributes to hip osteoarthritis in the general population, but this is controversial.

Complex joint deformities and dislocations also occur in many cases of cerebral palsy. The prevalence of hip dislocation approaches 50% in neurologically immature, spastic quadriplegic children.[53] The subluxation and dislocation occur gradually in infancy, probably because of muscle imbalance.[53] Erosion of the cartilage may occur with replacement by fibrous tissue and periarticular bone. Neither eburnation nor subchondral bony cysts are ordinarily present. Thus the joint changes are distinct from those associated with secondary osteoarrthritis. Loss of muscular function that facilitates circulation of synovial fluid over the joint is one possible cause for the condition. Attributing the process entirely to neurologic dysfunction requires caution because both major[54] and minor[55] noncerebral malformations are increased in children with cerebral palsy. Dislocation and degeneration of other lower extremity joints and scoliosis are also common in cerebral palsy.

Multiple epiphyseal dysplasia is a disorder characterized by structurally abnormal epiphyses with punctate, stippled calcification noted on radiographs.[36] Diversity in inheritance pattern and clinical manifestations make the disorder heterogeneous. An autosomal dominant form is most common, with short stature, delayed ossification, and irregular shape in the appendicular growth centers. Premature bilateral degenerative arthritis, especially of the hips, is customary. The femoral hip demonstrates severe degenerative changes with considerable flattening and loss of cartilage (Fig. 75-6). The differential diagnosis includes bilateral congenital hip dislocation, Legg-Perthes disease (Fig. 75-7), and secondary osteoarrthritis associated with aseptic necrosis or osteomyelitis. Spondyloepiphyseal dysplasias can be excluded by absence of spinal involvement.[36]

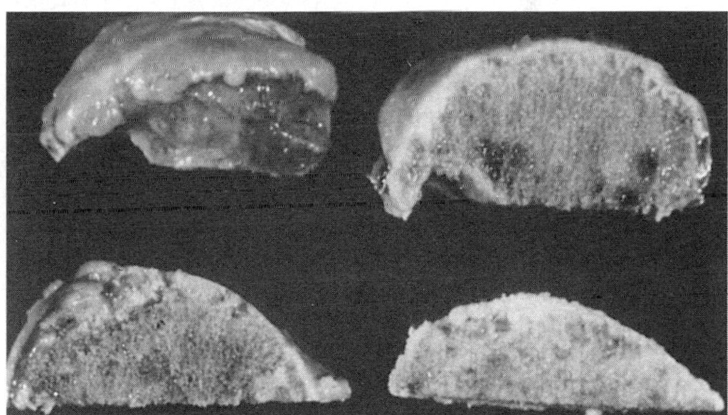

Fig. 75-6 Severe precocious secondary osteoarthritis of the hip in a young woman with multiple epiphyseal dysplasia. Femoral head is small and deformed without conspicuous osteophytes.

Arthrogryposis multiplex congenita is another disorder illustrating the complex interaction between heritable malformations and acquired deformations in the pathogenesis of a clinical syndrome. The condition presents in utero or at birth with multiple immovable joints fixed in a posture determined by fetal positioning.[36] In some cases fibrous tissue occupies the nonexistent joint spaces. Based on experimental models, denervation by mechanical, developmental, or pharmacologic means is postulated.[5] Other cases have shown X-linked inheritance.[56]

DEGENERATIVE AND TRAUMATIC JOINT DISEASES

The degenerative and traumatic joint diseases constitute a diverse collection of pathologic and clinical entities that develop at various times after either acute or repetitive trauma. Although many diseases can definitely be ascribed to a traumatic event, two cautionary comments are in order. The first is that many diseases were formerly erroneously ascribed to

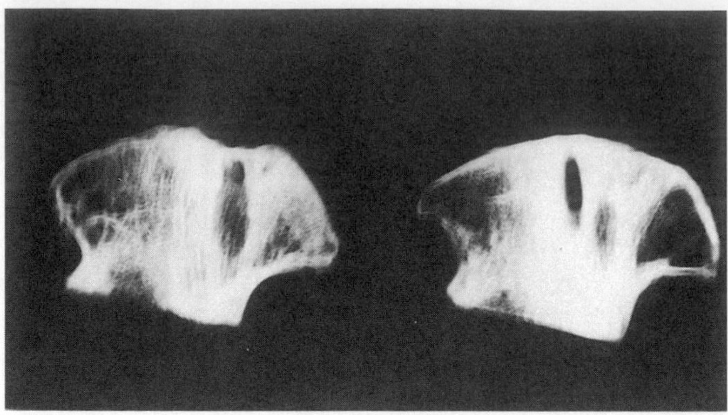

Fig. 75-7 Severe secondary osteoarthritis in early adult life as a result of Legg-Perthes disease of the femoral head. Reduction in height and bilateral beaklike osteophytes are characteristic.

trauma—including rheumatoid arthritis, gout, and ankylosing spondylitis.[57] The second is that minor trauma may actually induce joint disease in genetically susceptible individuals, as is the case with generalized osteoarrthritis.[43] Minor trauma may also exacerbate preexisting articular disease as in cases of acute gout occurring after joint trauma where uric acid deposits have ruptured into the joint space.

Although all components of the joint are capable of repairing injury, the capability of articular chondrocytes to repair defects is limited.[58] Superficial defects usually do not heal, whereas those reaching the subchondral bone are repaired by fibrous tissue components migrating from the bone marrow.[59] Thus the most optimistic outcome of a cartilaginous defect is replacement by fibrocartilage whose mechanical properties are not the same as those of native articular cartilage. This phenomenon is observed regularly in specimens obtained from joints that have undergone a previous arthroplasty.[60]

Injuries to the joints are of two types: acute injury produced by a single, relatively violent force and chronic injury occurring after minor but repetitive trauma. The former are easier to define pathogenetically.

Acute injuries

After acute force is exerted on a joint by means of rotational, longitudinal, or transverse application, swelling develops from acute traumatic synovitis. This results in joint effusion. The more rapid the swelling, the more likely that a hemarthrosis has developed.[57] In cases of acute joint injury with hemarthrosis, intra-articular fractures, ligamentous tears, and other major internal derangements are present in up to 75% of patients.[57] Any peripheral joint is a likely candidate for such acute injury, but the knee and ankle joints are particularly succeptable.

Severely injured joints may be permanently unstable, leading to aberrant motion, subluxation, or even recurrent dislocation, all leading to secondary degenerative disease. In fact, in the Pond-Nuki model of osteoarrthritis in dogs, osteoarrthritis occurs after sectioning of the anterior cruciate ligament.[61] In humans, injury to the menisci of the knee is common[62] and is associated with subsequent osteoarrthritis. Reflex sympathetic dystrophy or Sudeck's atrophy may occur after even minor acute joint trauma.[63] In this condition, pain, atrophy of soft tissues, and osteoporosis develop in the affected extremity. Hemorrhage into the joint usually resolves without organization into fibrous adhesions. Portions of bone or cartilage detached as a result of the trauma can result in continuing joint injury by both mechanical and inflammatory mechanisms, as malalignment of a joint can after fracture. In summary, a single acute joint injury does not ordinarily produce joint degeneration unless there is significant injury to the cartilage, underlying bone, or supporting ligaments.

Chronic trauma

Damage from repeated minor injuries, often so mild as to escape detection, has long been implicated in so-called wear-and-tear arthritis. Clear examples include elbow osteoarrthritis in foundry workers who use long tongs to lift crucibles and osteoarrthritis of the back in coal miners who must work in a stooped posture.[58] Other studies have shown no increase in osteoarrthritis of the knees in long-distance runners.[64,65] Studies in pneumatic hammer operators have shown both negative[66] and positive[67] correlation with osteoarrthritis of the upper extremities. Retired soccer players have a higher incidence of osteoarrthritis of the hips than age- and weight-matched controls do,[68] and osteoarrthritis of the knee is more common in individuals who perform heavy manual labor.[69]

The role of minor repetitive trauma in arthritis is obviously controversial. Some evidence favors damage to the underlying subchondral bone as the most important factor.[70] Perhaps more significant in the general population are the numerous examples of periarticular diseases, such as bursitis, tendinitis, and tenosynovitis that are associated with routine recreational and occupational use of joints. Tennis elbow (epicondylitis) and biceps tendinitis are two examples. Periarticular calcification resulting from these types of posttraumatic periarthritis is relatively common, and the crystals may induce further inflammation.[57]

Osteoarthritis

Definition. Osteoarthritis (OA) is a very common noninflammatory disorder of movable joints whose pathologic hallmarks are articular cartilage degeneration and new bone formation at the joint surfaces and margins. Despite the lack of evidence of an etiologic role for inflammation in most cases, the term *osteoarthritis* has not been supplanted by *osteoarthrosis* or the more general term *degenerative joint disease*.[58] Numerous other histopathologic events are seen in the disorder, some of which clearly are late reactive changes. However, the roles of other processes such as focal subchondral bone necrosis[71,72] and subchondral bone microfractures[70,73] in the disorder are controversial.[58] Epidemiologically, osteoarrthritis is associated with aging,[25,74] and the changes of the biochemical[13,17] and biomechanical properties of cartilage with age are well described,[2,75] but the relationship between the two is unclear. Many older individuals have no evidence of osteoarrthritis at necropsy.

Classification. Several distinct varieties of osteoarrthritis exist. Although differences in both the distribution and the character of pathologic lesions exist among the variants, the putative cause remains the strongest distinguishing factor in the current nosology. All subtypes, however, create in the affected joints, the cartilaginous and bony lesions that define OA. Osteoarthritis is customarily divided into primary and secondary types,[58,76] with numerous subtypes described under each. As noted in Table 75-3, primary OA can be further segregated into generalized and localized subtypes. Many specific conditions can be grouped under these headings. The

Table 75-3 Classification of primary osteoarthritis (OA)

Generalized types	Localized types
Generalized OA with Heberden's nodes	OA of hip (coxarthrosis)
Erosive OA	OA of knee (gonarthrosis)
Endemic OA	OA of spinal facet joints
OA with inborn type II procollagen defects	Chondromalacia patellae

Table 75-4 Classification of secondary osteoarthritis (OA)

GROUP I: Crystal deposition
Hyperparathyroidism
Hemochromatosis
Wilson's disease
Gout
Calcium pyrophosphate deposition disease
Basic calcium phosphate deposition disease
Oxalosis
GROUP II: Necrosis or abnormality in subchondral bone
Aseptic necrosis
Legg-Perthes disease
Slipped capital femoral epiphysis
Posttraumatic OA*
Paget's disease (osteitis deformans)
Steroid arthropathy
GROUP III: Abnormal joint laxity
Ehlers-Danlos syndrome (esp. Type VII)
Osteogenesis imperfecta (esp. Types I and III)
Marfan syndrome
GROUP IV: Abnormal cartilage growth or function
Acromegaly†
Achondroplasia
Spondyloepiphyseal dysplasias
Multiple epiphyseal dysplasias
Congenital hip dysplasia
Mucopolysaccharidoses
Ochronosis‡
Diabetes mellitus§
GROUP V: Synovial destruction of cartilage and bone
Postinflammatory OA
Postinfectious OA
Hemophilic arthropathy

* Group I and III also.
† Groups I, II, and III as well.
‡ Group I also.
§ Complex pathogenesis, including group II.

varieties of primary OA have in common the absence of an obvious external antecedent, whereas the varieties of secondary OA have a clear antecedent. From these observations, it has been inferred that primary OA results from intrinsic degenerative, regressive, or proliferative changes in the articular cartilage and subchondral bone.[27,58] Although localized severe primary OA of the hips and knees is a common clinical occurrence, there is evidence that many of these cases are localized exacerbations of generalized OA[77] rather than truly localized OA. Thus the subclassification of generalized OA is problematic, whereas that of the secondary variants is somewhat clearer.

Etiology and Pathogenesis. Any explanation for the cause of OA must reconcile conflicting biochemical[13,15,17] and biomechanical[27,78,79] evidence. Current evidence[27,76,79-82] suggests that several types of insults to cartilage or bone can result in a pathway of degradation of the articular cartilage-subchondral bone unit. Conceptually, primary OA results from a failure of biomaterials, either because of an intrinsically *abnormal* cartilage-subchondral bone unit that fails under normal loading or because of an intrinsically *normal* unit that fails under cumulative *abnormal* use.[27] Either the matrix or the cells may be the initial site of failure. Osteoarthritis with inborn type II collagen defects[37,38] is an example of the former, whereas rapidly progressive OA with subchondral osteocyte death illustrates the latter.[83] Most examples of secondary OA involve preexisting immune, metabolic, structural, or physiologic abnormalities of the involved joints (Table 75-4).

Traditional ideas that OA begins with fibrillation or denudation of the joint surface[58,82] do not explain the observation that age-related remodeling of the osteochondral junction may coexist with cartilage changes[27,79,81] and may precede subsequent generalized OA.[84] Perhaps it is best to consider the disease as the end product of an imbalance between osteocartilaginous damage and repair. Over the long periods of time required for the disease to evolve, minor discrepancies are translated into the conspicuous pathologic state seen in many specimens. The destructive and reparative processes are so interwoven that the actual precipitating event, if a single one exists, has not yet been established.[27,79] Nevertheless, the histopathologic and molecular events characterizing OA can be grouped into three phases: induction, progression, and augmentation. Such teleologic reasoning requires one to accept that certain mechanisms do, in fact, operate at more than one level in the sequence. These events are summarized in Fig. 75-8. In the early (*induction*) stages, matrix damage by either mechanical or biochemical means produces a cellular proliferative response. This response releases additional degradative enzymes.[85,86] As noted earlier, subchondral bone damage may precede the cartilaginous changes.[81,84] Likewise, microcrystal deposition in joint tissues may play a role as an initiating factor.[27,32,85] It has been established that in generalized OA there is an immunologic attack on cartilage.[86,87] During the *progression* phase, articular cartilage and bony changes coexist, as progressive loss of cartilage accelerates repair and remodeling attempts. There is proliferation of osteogenic tissue from the bone marrow at the site of the defects on the joint surface. During the *augmentation* phase, continued recruitment of synovial cytokines[79,88,89] and inflammatory mediators[79] may be of fundamental importance in producing the pronounced bone sclerosis and marginal bone overgrowth that are so characteristic of the disorder. There is undeniable evidence of focal subchondral bone necrosis with osteocytic death,[71,83,90,91] but most of the evidence indicates that this is a late secondary event in otherwise established OA. This process is distinct from the secondary OA that regularly follows geographic aseptic necrosis of the femoral head.

The various diseases culminating in secondary OA act through a few convergent mechanisms (Table 75-4). This allows categorization of the secondary OA along pathogenetic

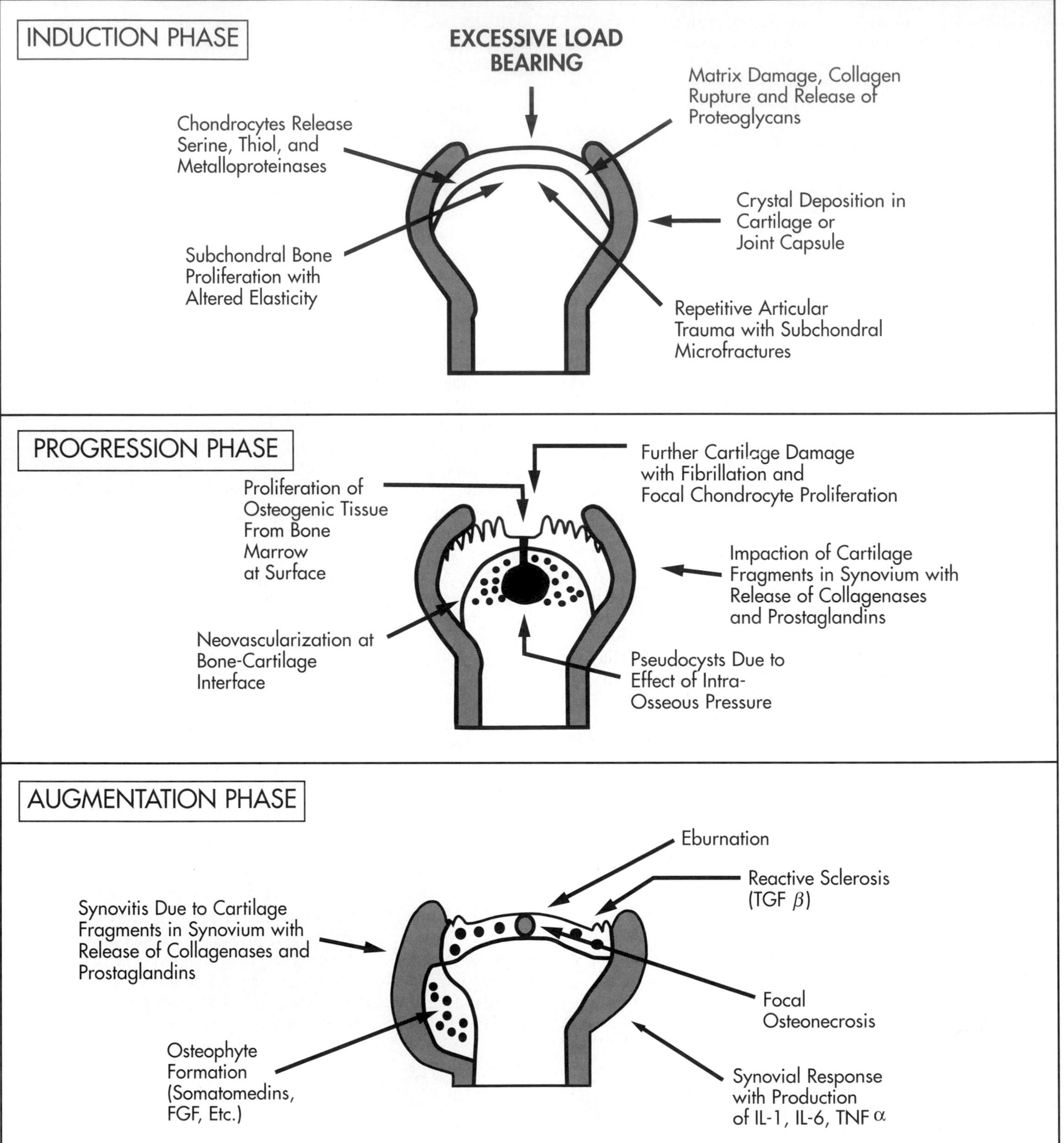

Fig. 75-8 Complex pathogenesis of OA reflects both biomechanical and biochemical injury to the joint.

lines. Many metabolic diseases (group I) produce direct or indirect cartilage damage by facilitating crystal deposition within joints, often inducing acute inflammatory attacks as well as chronic arthropathy. Others produce OA as a result of necrosis or abnormality of subchondral bone. A third group comprises diseases such as Ehlers-Danlos disease Type VII and Marfan syndrome that cause cartilage damage because of recurrent joint dislocations. A fourth group comprises diseases such as acromegaly and achondroplasia in which abnormal cartilage growth or function leads to premature joint degeneration. The fifth group comprises inflammatory conditions that induce chronic synovial pannus formation leading to cartilage destruction. Most antecedent conditions act by more than one mechanism. An example is acromegaly, classified in group IV but sharing mechanisms in common with the conditions in groups II and III as well. Ochronosis clearly causes direct cartilage damage by deposition of homogentisic acid polymers, but it also induces calcium pyrophosphate crystal deposition. In conditions such as diabetes mellitus, the evidence linking it to OA is largely by epidemiologic and clinical inference.[34] Available scientific evidence indicates that a variety of factors including nonenzymatic glycosylation of cartilage structural proteins, autoimmune disease, neuropathy, and growth hormone excess[89] may all contribute to OA in diabetics.

Primary Osteoarthritis

Pathology. Pathologic changes in OA provide a wide variety of destructive, reparative, and degenerative changes[58] (Table 75-5). Although some changes appear early in the process, it has not been possible to establish an unequivocal order of occurrence. Fibrillation of the joint surface, loss of metachromatic matrix material, and fragmentation of collagen fibrils occur early in OA (Fig. 75-9). Changes that are seen relatively late include pronounced subchondral bone sclerosis, eburnation of the joint surface, and secondary osteonecrosis. Many other changes are seen throughout the process. Included in this group are remodeling of the tidemark zone of calcified cartilage, formation of osteophytes, subchondral pseudocysts, and detritic synovitis from the shards of bone and cartilage embedded in the synovium (Fig. 75-10). The pathogenetic sequence is further complicated by the fact that the severity of change varies from one portion of the joint to another at any given time. Taken as a group, the pathologic findings in OA define an entity, even if they do not firmly establish the cause.

Clinical presentation. Primary OA is a disease occurring in the middle aged and older. Younger individuals who appear to have the disorder frequently have secondary OA resulting from one of the well-known antecedents (Table 75-4). A specialized form of generalized ostesarthritis (GOA) occurs almost exclusively in women who have prominent osteophytes of the distal interphalangeal joints (Heberden's nodes) (Fig. 75-11). These patients also develop widespread OA with osteophytes in the weight-bearing joints. An increased prevalence of HLA 1-B8 has been described in GOA patients.[25,43]

Another special variant of OA is erosive inflammatory OA.[43,76] This disorder, similar to GOA with Heberden's nodes, presents with hand involvement. In these cases, however, inflammatory changes, denudation of cartilage from the joint, and periarticular bone erosions may cause confusion with rheumatoid arthritis. Because of its overall frequency, rheumatoid arthritis is a relatively frequent diagnostic consideration in young adults with precocious or generalized OA. The absence of systemic or extra-articular manifestations, including rheumatoid factor, and the presence of distal interphalangeal involvement, serve to exclude rheumatord arthritis readily in most cases.[76]

Table 75-5 Pathology of primary osteoarthritis

Pathology of primary osteoarthritis
Fragmentation of cartilage collagen fibrils
Loss of metachromatic matrix material
Fibrillation of surface cartilage
Chondrocyte proliferation
Lacunar resorption by chondrocytes
Remodeling of tidemark
Subchondral pseudocysts
Detritic synovitis
Osteophytes
Eburnation
Subchondral bone sclerosis
Focal osteonecrosis in subchondral bone

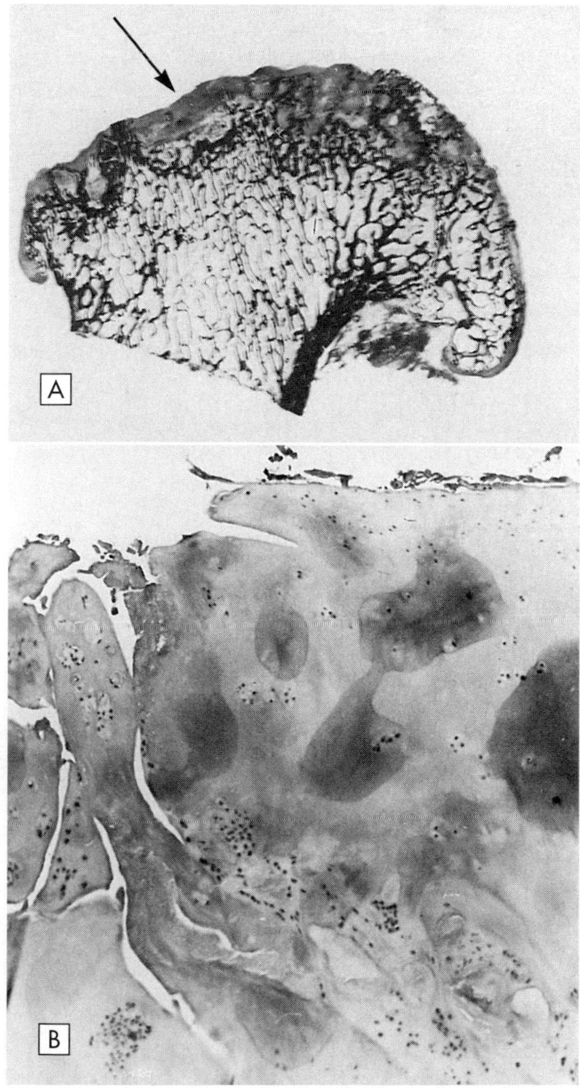

Fig. 75-9 Primary ostesarthritis of femoral head. **A,** Considerable loss of bone and cartilage. **B,** Fibrillation in remaining cartilage is accompanied by chondrocyte proliferation.

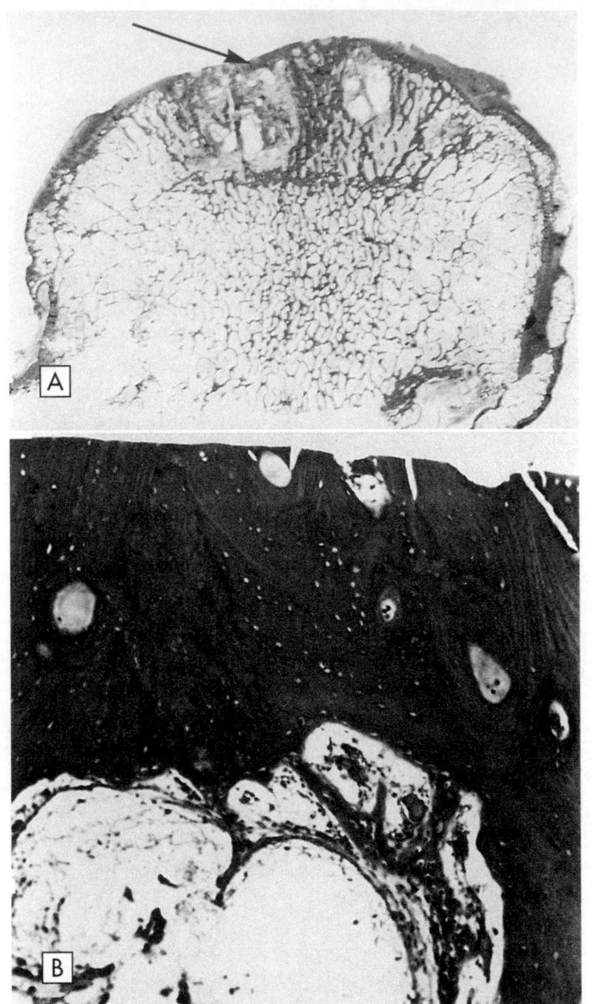

Fig. 75-10 Primary osteoarthritis of femoral head. **A**, Eburnation (*arrow*) is subchondral. **B**, Eburnated zone contains foci of dense cancellous bone.

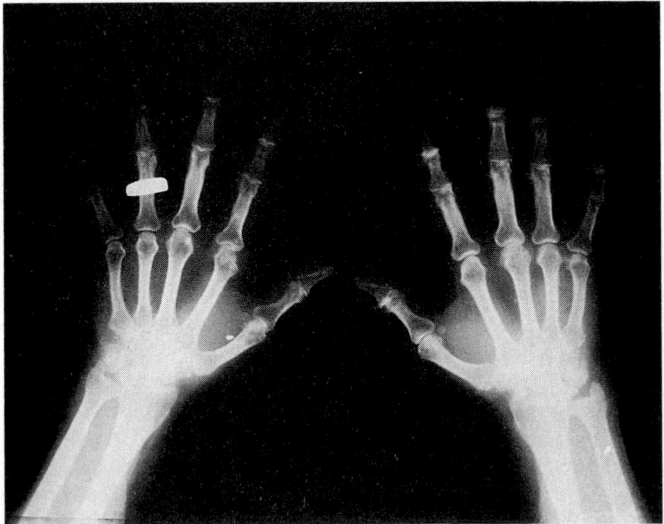

Fig. 75-11 Primary generalized osteoarthritis in a middle-aged woman. Osteophytes and bony sclerosis of both proximal and distal interphalangeal joints are present.

Another clinical presentation of OA is chondromalacia patellae.[76] This disorder is a precocious OA of the patellofemoral articular surface characterized by softening, fibrillation, and grossly apparent abrasion of the patellar articular cartilage.[58] Formerly considered a distinct clinicopathologic entity, it is now regarded as an early sign of OA of the knee.[76] An association with repetitive minor trauma has been described.[92]

Secondary osteoarthritis

Many chronic arthritic conditions (Table 75-4) progress in pathology to closely resemble primary OA. In some cases such as posttraumatic or acromegalic arthropathies, the changes leading to secondary OA are so similar that only historical information and knowledge of the overall pattern of multiple joint involvement allows distinction from primary OA. In many other types of secondary OA, additional pathologic findings beyond those encountered in primary OA allow specific diagnosis.[58]

Hemophilic arthropathy. This condition is a chronic destructive degenerative condition terminating in severe secondary OA.[93] It occurs in both hemophilia A (factor VIII deficiency) and hemophilia B (factor IX deficiency).[94] Although von Willebrand's disease (vascular hemophilia) is almost as common as Hemophilia A, hemarthroses and consequently chronic arthropathies are rarely encountered[93] in that disorder. Hemophilic hemarthroses follow trauma, which is often insignificant, and are especially common in individuals with levels of coagulant less than 3% of normal. Recurrent hemarthroses set in motion a self-sustaining synovitis leading to synovial hyperplasia, invasive pannus formation, and release of degradative enzymes.[95,96] Direct toxic effects of iron on chondrocytes may also be involved.[97] These processes destroy cartilage and produce severe deformity (Fig. 75-12). The synovium is hypertrophic and reddish brown grossly. As the disease progresses, the synovium becomes less hyperplastic and more fibrotic, with large amounts of iron present primarily in macrophages deep in the synovial layer. The original articular cartilage is destroyed early in the process and is replaced by a reparative fibrocartilage. Large subchondral cysts filled with hemosiderin-laden macrophages are also characteristic of the disorder. Unlike other variants of secondary OA, fibrous adhesions (ankylosis) between opposing joint surfaces are relatively common. The elbow, knee, and hip joints are most frequently affected.[93] The routine daily administration of factor VIII- and factor IX-containing blood products has greatly reduced the prevalence of severe hemophilic arthropathy in the United States in recent years.

Hemochromatosis. The autosomal recessive disorder hemochromatosis is characterized by excessive uptake of iron with deposition in multiple organs.[98] Up to 50% of the documented cases develop a degenerative arthropathy leading to secondary ostesarthritis.[40,99] Calcium pyrophosphate or basic calcium phosphate crystals have been identified in articular cartilage or synovium[100] in up to 60% of the cases. Inhibition of pyrophosphatase by ferric ions has been proposed as a mechanism for the calcium pyrophosphate deposition.[101] Involvement of the small joints of the hand is characteristic, but the knees, hips,[40] and spine may also be affected. The synovium is brownish red grossly because of deposition of iron in the form of hemosiderin. Microscopically the synovium shows mild degrees of hyperplasia with proliferation of fibroblasts. Iron is deposited within synovial cells, predominantly in perivascular locations.[102] Necrosis of chondrocytes and fibrillation of cartilage occur and are frequently associated with deposits of calcium pyrophosphate. This indicates that chondrocalcinosis may be involved in the degeneration of cartilage in this disorder.[100] Although iron is present in copious quantities in the synovium, deposition in the cartilage is confined to chondrocytes and to the tidemark of calcified cartilage. Deposition of iron in the tidemark is seen in other disorders of excessive iron deposition, such as hemophilia and thalassemia. As the arthropathy progresses, fibrillation of cartilage and prominent osteophytes, which are typical features of osteoarthritis, develop. Chondrocalcinosis may be detectable on routine radiographs.[40]

Wilson's disease (hepatolenticular degeneration. The rare autosomal recessive disorder Wilson's disease is characterized by copper deposition in multiple tissues, cirrhosis, degeneration in the basal ganglia, and renal tubular dysfunction.[40] Neurologic signs characteristically appear in childhood or adolescence, but joint symptoms are seen in approximately 50% of adults with the disorder.[40] Articular involvement is variable inseverity, with severe osteoarthritis at one end of the range.[103] Involvement of multiple sites including the hand, elbow, shoulder, hip, and knee joints is seen.[40] The early age of onset and prominent wrist involvement are suggestive of a pattern different from that of GOA.[76] As in patients with hemochromatosis, chondrocalcinosis has been described, as well as periarticular calcification.[40] Copper has been identified in articular cartilage by electron microscopy,[103] but the actual mechanism of cartilage injury is unclear. In one study the synovium showed only mild hyperplastic changes.[104] Osteochondritis dissecans has been noted in this arthropathy,[99] and it may be related to the chondrocalcinosis,[32] as it is relatively frequent in this disorder.[32,58]

Onchronotic arthropathy. Ochronotic arthropathy is the articular manifestation of alkaptonuria, an autosomal recessive disorder characterized by the absence of homogentisic acid oxidase.[40] As a consequence, polymers of homogentisic acid accumulate in connective tissues, particularly in cartilage, where they create a blue-black discoloration easily visible grossly[105,106] (Fig. 75-13). The homogentisic acid polymers interfere with the metabolism of cartilage, perhaps through inhibition of hydroxylysine formation.[107] The articular cartilage becomes brittle and is easily abraded from the joint surface. A generalized precocious arthropathy with some features of OA develops.[40,58] However, several important distinctions between primary OA and ochronotic arthropathy are present. In ochronotic arthropathy, involvement of the finger joints is not prominent, unlike OA. Also, a severe degenerative spondylosis with chondrocalcinosis in the intervertebral disks is frequent in ochronotic arthropathy[40,58] (Fig. 75-13). Large peripheral joints such as the knee, shoulder, and hip joints develop severe secondary osteoarthritic changes[40] as well. Inflammatory synovitis with shards of onchronotic cartilage embedded in the synovium is characteristic, as are loose bodies of pigmented cartilage.[40] In contrast to GOA, osteophyte formation is not characteristic of the disorder.[108] Because of the severity of the spondylosis, confusion with mucopolysaccharidoses, ankylosing spondylitis, and hyperostotic spondylosis is possible on clinical grounds.

Acromegalic arthropathy. Acromegalic arthropathy is a complex disorder resulting from a relative excess of growth hormone and consequently of somatomedin C (IGF-I) and

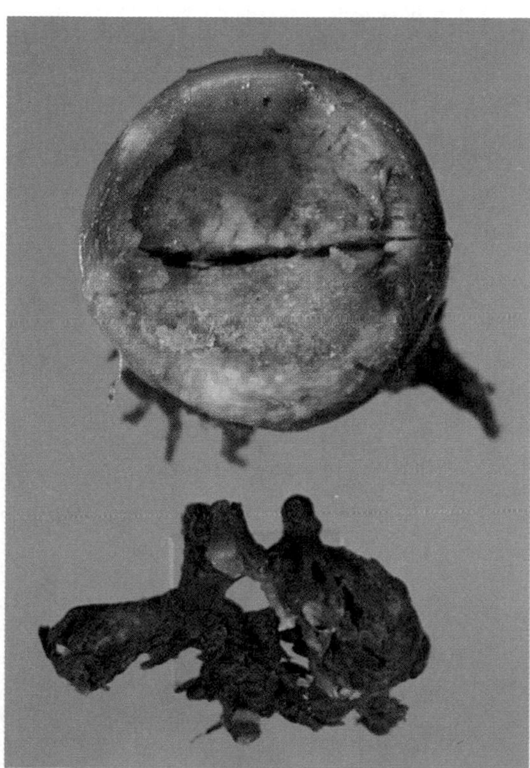

Fig. 75-12 Hemophilic arthropathy with destruction of joint surface. Discoloration of synovium results from iron deposits.

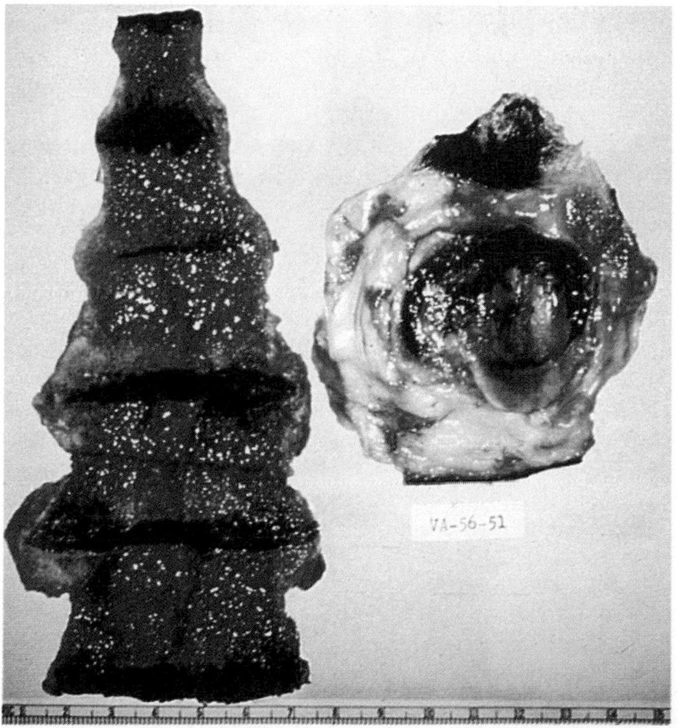

Fig. 75-13 Ochronotic arthropathy of patella and spine. Black discoloration of cartilage is characteristic (Courtesy Dr. W.A. Gardner, Mobile, Ala.)

somatomedin A (IGF-II).[109,110] It is probable that both biochemical and biomechanical factors are involved in the genesis of the arthropathy.[108] The overgrowth of the ends of the long bones in acromegaly results both from thickening of cartilage and from prominent osteophyte formation. The increased thickness of cartilage in the disorder results from a combination of cellular hyperplasia and increased matrix accumulation.[111] There is also extensive bone remodeling because of ingrowth of capillaries at the osteochondral junction leading to extensive osteophyte formation. The "arrowhead" configuration of the terminal phalanges resulting from bony outgrowth is characteristic of acromegalic arthropathy and serves to distinguish the disorder from GOA.[112] The knees, hips, and shoulders are characteristically involved as well.[110] The thickened cartilage is prone to fibrillation, with abrasion from the joint surface. Hypermobility of the joints also contributes to the pathogenesis of the arthropathy.[110] Relatively severe spinal osteophytosis develops, but unlike ankylosing hyperostosis, the spine is hypermobile, probably from the increased amounts of intervertebral disk tissue present.[109-111,113] Calcium pyrophosphate crystals have been described in joint tissues in acromegalic arthropathy and may contribute to episodes of acute synovitis seen in the disorder.[109]

Hyperparathyroid arthropathy. A grouping of rheumatic conditions accompanies hyperparathyroidism.[109,110] Multiple pathogenetic mechanisms involving calcium pyrophosphate deposition, hyperuricemia, subchondral bone erosions, and joint laxity contribute to the increased prevalence of OA-like changes in these patients.[109,110] Although degenerative disease can occur without chondrocalcinosis, more severe changes are associated with the presence of calcium pyrophosphate crystals.[110] The degenerative arthropathy is promoted by subchondral bone resorption, leading to cysts. This is usually most evident in the proximal humeral and hand joints.[109]

Secondary coxarthroses. Many local disturbances of growth and nutrition of the hip joints are associated with severe, progressive secondary OA. One such condition, congenital hip dysplasia (dislocation)[46-49] has been previously discussed. Several other distinct entities are relatively frequently encountered. Some investigation have maintained that up to 85% of localized OA of the hip is related to some type of preexisting disease,[52] but others have failed to substantiate this finding.[114,115]

Aseptic necrosis (avascular necrosis). The relatively common entity aseptic necrosis accompanies a wide variety of insults to the bone microcirculation.[116] Although numerous conditions, including hemoglobinopathies, corticosteroid administration, ethanolism, dysbarism, and trauma are associated with the disorder, all except for trauma, act by disruption of the microcirculation.[116] Evidence supports fat embolism as a precipitating event in microthrombosis in most of these disorders.[117] Although aseptic osteonecrosis may affect the subchondral bone of almost any joint, that in the femoral head[118] is most likely to result in secondary OA. Collapse of the underlying subchondral bone occurs in the later stages of the disease, creating a noncongruent articular surface (Fig. 75-14). Under these conditions, cartilage is rapidly abraded from the surface. Osteophytes form at joint margins, but eburnation usually does not occur. The process is distinct from secondary focal osteonecrosis that can develop in sclerotic bone in advanced OA[58,71,90,91] (Fig. 75-10).

Legg-Perthes disease. Legg-Perthes disease, a specialized form of osteonecrosis, occurs in the growth center of the femoral head of preadolescent children, predominantly in males.[119] Children characteristically present with a limp, with or without pain. The condition may be bilateral. The disease leads to severe disturbances of growth,[120] depending somewhat on the extent of necrosis of the epiphyseal plate area and results in a flattened femoral head with bilateral beaklike osteophytes (coxa plana) (Fig. 75-7). Severe OA frequently develops, especially if early treatment is not instituted. The pathogenesis is unclear, but minor trauma[57] and elevated intraarticular pressures caused by synovitis[121] have been suggested as the causes for obstruction of the microcirculation. Although a considerable body of literature on the pathology of the disorder exists,[122] early-stage specimens that might give more insight into the pathogenesis are rarely obtained.[123]

Slipped capital femoral epiphysis. Another childhood hip disorder with potentially devastating arthritogenic potential is slipped capital femoral epiphysis. Characteristically the presentation occurs at an age later than that of Legg-Perthes disease, with bilateral involvement in 5% to 25% of patients.[124] The disorder is a fracture through the growth plate that leads to variable degrees of inferior and posterior slippage of the femoral head,[125,126] hence the name "coxa vara" (Fig. 75-15). Complications ensue, including avascular necrosis, chondrolysis, and severe OA.[126] The extent of the sequelae relate to the degree of slippage. With incomplete slippage, the femoral head may be reattached relatively close to its original position. In more severe instances, the head may be positioned below the greater trochanter. In most cases, the condition is associated with trauma, but children are rarely seen in the acute stage of the disease.[124] Most pathologic material is therefore obtained from individuals with chronic degenerative arthritis occurring after a past acute episode.

Differential diagnosis. In the usual patient, OA presents characteristic clinical and radiographic signs localized to the joints. These are sufficient, when examined in context, to exclude rheumatoid arthritis. The major concern is the differentiation of primary from secondary OA.[22,25,58,74,76,80] In addition, many degenerative joint diseases other than OA must be excluded. Joints in primary OA usually demonstrate more extensive osteophyte formation than those with sec-

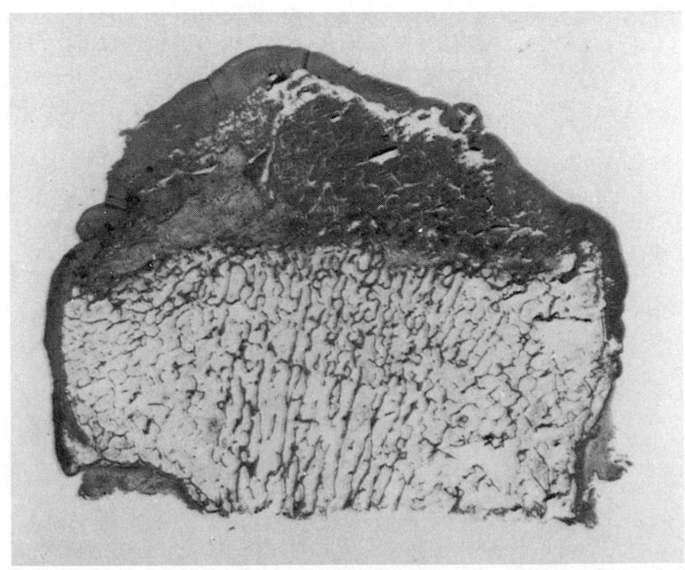

Fig. 75-14 Aseptic (avascular) necrosis of femoral head. Subchondral necrotic zone is sharply demarcated.

ondary OA do. This is especially true of ochronotic arthropathy[108] and postinflammatory OA, such as that occurring after rheumatoid arthritis[58] and infectious arthritis. Specialized variants of osteoarthritis, such as GOA with Heberden's nodes, must also be excluded.[76] Because chondrocalcinosis and OA present in the same age group, a distinction must frequently be made between the two conditions.[32,71] The situation is complicated by the observation that both calcium pyrophosphate and basic calcium phosphate deposition diseases can lead to secondary OA.

Endemic osteoarthritis. In certain parts of the world, distinctive, geographically localized forms of GOA are endemic.[127] One such clinical presentation is that of *Kashin-Beck disease*,[128] a severe GOA localized to parts of eastern Siberia and contiguous regions of China and North Korea. The disorder begins in childhood as a zonal necrosis of growth plate chondrocytes[127] leading to growth retardation and OA that become clinically manifest during adolescence.[129] An idea of the prevalence of this condition can be obtained from an estimate that 3 million persons are affected in China alone.[130] The cause has been ascribed variously to mycotoxins on grain,[129] dietary selenium deficiency,[131] and most recently to effects of fulvic acid in drinking water on procollagen II processing.[130] Chondrocyte growth in vitro has not been shown to be affected by the absence of selenium, providing no support for that hypothesis.[132]

A pathologically similar disorder called *Mseleni disease* occurs in portions of Zululand in southern Africa.[133] There, many young people are afflicted with a disabling OA. The disorder is polyarticular, but the hip is particularly susceptible.[134] Examination of surgical specimens has revealed joint surfaces covered by degenerative and regenerative cartilage without eburnation.[134] The disorder is associated with osteopenia and osteomalacia as well.[135] The cause is unknown, but some authors have suggested that the disorder is heterogeneous, with some cases being examples of spondyloepiphyseal dysplasia.[133] In this age of rapid intercontinental travel, knowledge of such diseases is of more than academic interest.

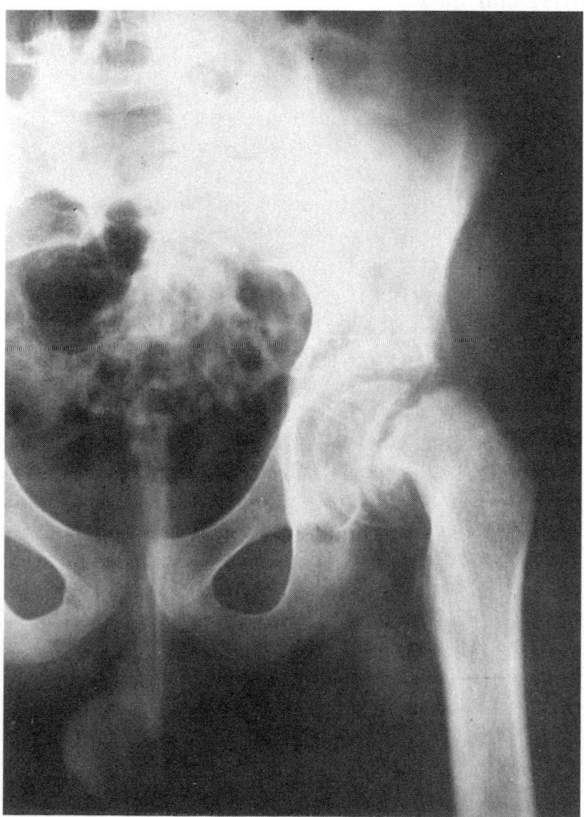

Fig. 75-15 Slipped capital femoral epiphysis. Separated portion of femoral head lies inferior and slightly posterior to the femoral neck.

Other degenerative joint diseases

Neuropathic arthropathy (Charcot's joint)

The destructive joint condition neuropathic arthropathy bears the name of the French neurologist, J.M. Charcot, who, in 1868, described the disease in patients with neurosyphilis. This extremely destructive joint disorder[136] develops in patients who have diseases that damage sensory innervation to the joint.[137] The prevalence of tertiary syphilis has declined with the widespread use of antibiotics, but other diseases have now become more frequent as antecedents of neuropathic arthropathy.[137] These include syringomyelia, amyloid and alcoholic neuropathies, and Hansen's disease (leprosy).

Diabetes mellitus is the most common predisposing condition in the United States.[138] The neuropathic arthropathy of diabetes occurs as a consequence of the neuropathy seen in most long-standing diabetics. The reason why only a small fraction of long-standing diabetics with neuropathy develop Charcot's joints is unclear, but those who do usually have clinical signs of neuropathy.[137] The neuropathic joints of diabetics are most commonly those of the feet, with obliteration of the outlines of the tarsal bones[138] and disintegration of the tarsometatarsal joints being a characteristic feature. Pathologic findings common to neuropathic arthropathy include fragmentation of the joint surface, with extensive detritic synovitis resulting from particles of bone and cartilage embedded in the synovium. Manifestations of inflamation, including pannus, are present. Osteochondromatosis of the synovium is not infrequent.[58] Eburnation and osteophytes are not seen. Calcium pyrophosphate deposition disease[32,139] may produce neuropathic arthropathy–like changes in the hips, knees, and shoulders. However, calcium pyrophosphate deposition has been described in neuropathic arthropathy and may contribute to the pathogenesis of the disorder.[137] Some studies have suggested that more subtle neuropathic changes accentuate established idiopathic OA.[140]

Amyloid arthropathy

Amyloid deposition occurs in numerous hereditary, neoplastic, hyperimmune, and degenerative states[141] (Chapter 20). A large number of different protein moieties may polymerize to form amyloid fibrils. Likewise, patterns of deposition, including those in the joint tissues, vary widely among the forms of systemic amyloidosis. Systemic amyloidosis of the amyloid A (AA) protein type occurs regularly in individuals with chronic inflammatory joint diseases, including rheumatoid arthritis, Still's disease, and the seronegative spondyloarthropathies.[141] However, amyloid deposition in the synovium and joint capsule does not occur in significant amounts, despite extensive involvement of the liver, spleen, and other viscera. On the other hand, in amyloidosis with amyloid light chain (AL) protein, associated with multiple myeloma, synovial amyloid deposition is frequent and may mimic rheumatoid arthritis,[142] with subcutaneous nodules and polyarticular involvement. In patients undergoing long-term hemodialysis, a destructive osteoarthropathy develops because of heavy deposition of amyloid in synovium, joint capsules, and subchondral bone marrow.[143,144] This type of amyloid is composed of polymerized β-2-microglobulin. The arthropathy is often quite severe and is frequently complicated by the osseous pathologic condition accompanying secondary hyperparathyroidism in these patients. Small amounts of amyloid have been found in the cartilage and synovium of patients with OA.[145] The significance of the finding is unclear because minute amounts of amyloid can be found in the joints of older individuals without joint disease.[146]

Hypertrophic osteoarthropathy

Hypertrophic osteoarthropathy, often called *pulmonary osteoarthropathy*, manifests as the clinical triad of (1) overgrowth of the ends of the digits (clubbing), (2) painful arthritis, and (3) periosteal new bone formation.[147] The overgrowth of the ends of the fingers and toes results from a combination of hyperemia, edema, fibroblastic proliferation, and periosteal new bone formation. The arthritis is usually symmetric and is characterized by sparse inflammatory cells in the synovium with a mucoid synovial fluid. Clubbing as an isolated finding occurs in association with cyanotic congenital heart disease, bacterial endocarditis, and chronic inflammatory bowel disease. The complete triad is usually seen in patients with chronic pulmonary disease, especially pulmonary neoplasia, including metastatic lesions to the lungs.[148] The cause of the disorder is presently obscure. A primary form of the disease, called *pachydermatoperiosteitis* has been described as an inherited autosomal dominant trait.[149] Unlike the frequent secondary variant, primary hypertrophic osteoarthropathy characteristically presents in childhood.

Osteochondrosis dissecans

Osteochondrosis dissecans is frequently called *osteochondritis dissecans*, a term that is inappropriate because no inflammation is involved. The lesions consist of variable numbers of loose bodies composed of bone and cartilage within the joint cavity (Fig. 75-16). These bodies, often called *joint mice* are ovoid, measuring up to 2 cm in diameter. Examination of the articular surfaces during surgical removal of the loose bodies often reveals grooves or discontinuities in the articular margin that presumably were sites of detachment of the loose bodies. The cartilage of the fragments may show oppositional growth, fibrillation, or calcification. The underlying bone is usually sclerotic. The condition is usually seen in the knees of young adults, more frequently in males,[57] but can be present in the hip, elbow, and shoulder joints as well.[150] Antecedent trauma is implicated in many cases,[57] but preexisting developmental or circulatory factors may also trigger the disorder.[57] Familial aggregation of cases has been noted.[151,152]

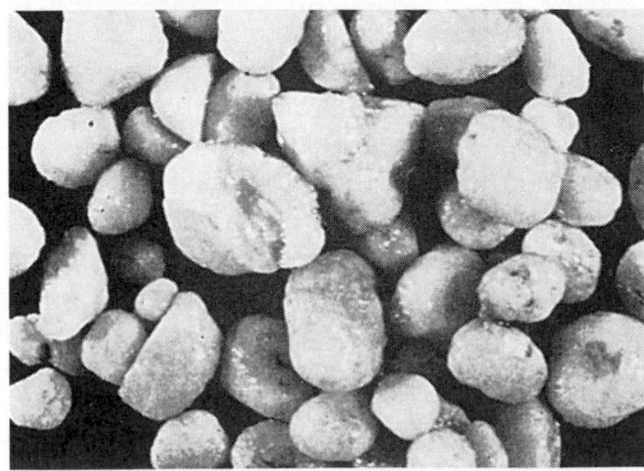

Fig. 75-16 "Joint mice" removed from shoulder joint.

Diabetic arthropathy

The increased prevalence of OA in diabetics has been noted on clinical and epidemiologic grounds.[34] Circulating levels of insulin are elevated in patients with OA as compared to controls.[89] The influence of neuropathic changes[137,138] on osteoarthritic disorders cannot be excluded. An additional complicating factor is the fibrositis syndrome associated with diabetes mellitus.[153] In diabetic fibrositis pronounced stiffness of the finger joints develops. Studies have shown a decreased mobility of major weight-bearing joints as well.[154] The syndrome may be related to chronic nonenzymatic glycosylation of collagen and other connective tissue proteins.[155-157] The arthropathies affecting diabetic patients are complex and involve multiple pathogenetic mechanisms.[156]

INFLAMMATORY JOINT DISEASE: INFECTIOUS ARTHRITIS

General concepts. Infectious arthritis is a potential complication of any infectious disease. In some circumstances the arthritis is a major clinical finding, an example being the chronic arthropathy of Lyme borreliosis.[158] At other times, an initial infection may predispose an individual to chronic arthritis by an immune mechanism as in Reiter's syndrome that occurs after chlamydial urethritis[159,160] or after a gram-negative enteric infection.[161,162] Even in the antibiotic era, infectious arthritis remains a serious problem because many joint infections arise in individuals with damaged joints or a deficient immune system.

Etiology and pathogenesis. Infection may reach the joint space by one of three principal mechanisms. The first and most common is by hematogenous or lymphatic spread to the synovial membrane.[163-165] Hematogenous spread is the mode for most forms of arthritis, especially the viral arthritides. The second mechanism is by direct entry into the joint space because of a penetrating injury. The third mechanism involves invasion of the joint space from a lesion in nearby bone or soft tissue. This is seen in mycobacterial and fungal infections involving joints. Bacterial and fungal arthritis are usually monarticular, whereas viral infections frequently involve multiple joints simultaneously.

Pathology. The synovial tissue reaction produced by infection depends on the pathogenicity of the organism involved. The inflammatory process within the joint is similar to that in other tissues, beginning with hyperemia of the synovium and continuing with infiltration with polymorphonuclear leukocytes, lymphocytes, and macrophages. The exudate that develops in the joint space may be serous, fibrinous, or purulent. More severe infections result in granulation tissue and adhesions between the normally movable components of the joint. In pyogenic bacterial infections, localized abscesses may be resistant to antibiotic therapy and may require surgical drainage.

Although most viral arthritides do not produce lasting damage, bacterial, mycobacterial, and fungal infections frequently result in permanent joint impairment by one of several mechanisms. These include the organization of adhesions into fibrous ankylosis of joint components, the destruction of stabilizing ligaments and intra-articular disks, and the formation of granulation tissue that erodes articular cartilage and subchondral bone, leading to secondary OA (group V, Table 75-4).

A characteristic feature of the inflammatory joint diseases is lysis of articular cartilage. This process is particularly prominent in bacterial, mycobacterial, and fungal arthritdes. Although granulation tissue, often called *pannus*, may contribute to chondrolysis, the process is actually mediated by substances that destroy the cartilage matrix directly or induce chondrocytes to release lytic enzymes.[166] Examples of cartilage-destroying agents include the granulocyte hydrolytic enzymes, and the lytic enzymes include the metalloproteinases such as collagenase and stromelysin.[166] The ongoing inflammatory reaction generates Interleukin-1-beta (IL-1 β) and tumor necroris factor-alpha (TNF-α), which act synergistically to induce the release of degradative enzymes from chondrocytes and inhibit the synthesis of matrix macromolecules. Other cytokines such as IL-6 and IL-8 are also involved in the process.[166] The result is visible lysis of cartilage. Severe inflamation can lead to rapid destruction of the articular surface, with severe secondary ostesarthritis in later years.

Viral arthritis

Many systemic viral diseases result in episodes of acute arthritis as a component of the clinical illness.[167] Because these diseases are ordinarily self-limited, descriptions of the joint tissue pathology are scarce.[150] Included in this group of diseases are rubella, mumps, infectious mononucleosis, variola, influenza, and pneumonia caused by parainfluenza virus and respiratory syncytial virus.[111,150,167] Among the most important clinically in this group is the arthritis that follows rubella in young women. Synovitis may persist for up to 28 days. The synovial joints of the knees, hands, and ankles are usually affected.[111] Chronic rubella arthritis has been reported,[150,168] as has joint involvement after rubella vaccination.[150] Arthralgia is an occasional component of the acute infectious mononucleosis syndrome occurring with Epstein-Barr virus (EBV) infection.[167] Molecular studies have implicated EBV as a possible promoting factor in rheumatoid arthritis in genetically susceptible individuals[169-171] because of induction of both B-lymphocyte proliferation and antibody production.[172] The arthralgic syndrome in infectious mononucleosis is, however, ordinarily self-limited and relatively brief.[167] Since many acute viral illnesses occur in children and adolescents, those that produce transient synovitis can be initially confused with Still's disease. This is especially true of infectious mononucleosis because of the presence of a rash and an enlarged spleen.[111] Pathologic findings in viral synovitis are nonspecific by routine histologic examination and manifest as edema, lymphocytic infiltration, and mild synovial hyperplasia.[111,150,167] Specialized immunocytochemical techniques can be used to identify specific viral proteins in synovium.[173]

It is well established that arthritis is a component of acute infection with hepatitis B virus,[174] and that viral antigens have been identified in synovial tissues in these cases of arthritis.[167] The arthritis is usually polyarticular and mild nonspecific synovitis is seen in biopsy specimens. More recently, a symmetric polyarthritis occurring after acute infection with parvovirus B19 has been described.[167] This organism is also the cause of erythema infectiosum that is seen in children and in which joint symptoms are rare.[167] Some adult patients develop chronic synovitis,[175] with persistence of parvoviral DNA in synovium.[176] The relationship of this chronic rheumatic disease to rheumatoid arthritis is currently a subject of considerable interest.[177]

Joint involvement may occur as a consequence of human immunodeficiency virus (HIV) infection, which is increasing in prevalence.[178] Although HIV has been inconsistently isolated from synovial cells of patients with HIV,[179] antibodies to retroviral antigens are implicated in the pathogenesis of several autoimmune disorders with arthritic components.[180] HIV infection may also be a potentiating factor in Reiter's syndrome.[181] In addition to these viral arthritides many arthropod-borne viruses of the alpha group cause acute arthritic manifestations, some severe, as a routine component of the respective illnesses.[167]

Bacterial arthritis

Arthritis caused by bacterial infection has remained an important clinical problem, despite the availability of antibiotics.[163] The clinical and pathologic characteristics vary widely with respect to host resistance, portal of entry, and type of organism involved. As with all bacterial infections age is an important factor in the pattern of infections observed in the joints.[182,183] Other factors include the presence of preexisting synovitis from rheumatoid arthritis,[184] crystal-deposition diseases,[185] or other destructive and inflammatory joint processes.[163] Individuals with either disease-induced or iatrogenic immunosuppression are also at increased risk for bacterial arthritis.[186] Some studies indicate that the elderly are also at increased risk.[163] A combination of crystal-induced and septic arthritis is not infrequent.[163] On the other hand, the young adult, sexually active population is particularly likely to acquire *Neisseria gonorrhea*–induced arthritis.[187] A wide range of organisms accompanies the septic arthritis seen in intravenous drug users. In this group of patients, involvement of the axial skeleton is more common than in the sporadic cases of septic arthritis.[163] The organisms normally present on the skin constitute the most frequent pathogens (staphylococci, streptococci, pseudomonads, and, less commonly, *Enterobacter* and *Serratia species*).[165] In children and the elderly, staphylococci remain the most common agents of bacterial arthritis.[188]

The extent of synovitis varies widely among pathogens. The synovial reaction is characterized by hyperemia, edema, surface deposits of fibrin, and infiltration by polymorphonuclear leukocytes (Fig. 75-17). In established bacterial arthritis, bacteria may usually be demonstrated in gram-stained smears of centrifuged synovial fluid sediment and in synovial biopsy specimens. Cultures are also usually positive. However, in presumed gonococcal arthritis, both direct staining and isolation techniques are frequently negative, and the extent of synovial inflammatory response is less than in other forms of bacterial arthritis.[187] The destruction of cartilage, bone, and supporting tissues resulting from nongonococcal arthritis can be very severe (Fig. 75-18) because of the release of enzymes and inflammatory mediators from the granulocytes that accumulate in the joint space. Staphylococcal arthritis constitutes a particularly destructive process, with long-term implications[189] for joint function.

Spirochetal arthritis

Musculoskeletal manifestations of various spirochetal diseases have become more apparent in recent years because of a vari-

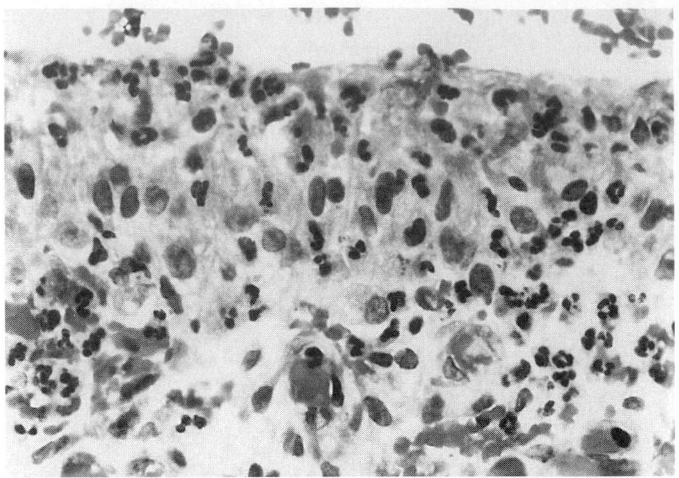

Fig. 75-17 Acute synovitis caused by staphylococcal arthritis after penetrating injury. Granulocytic infiltrate and congestion are present.

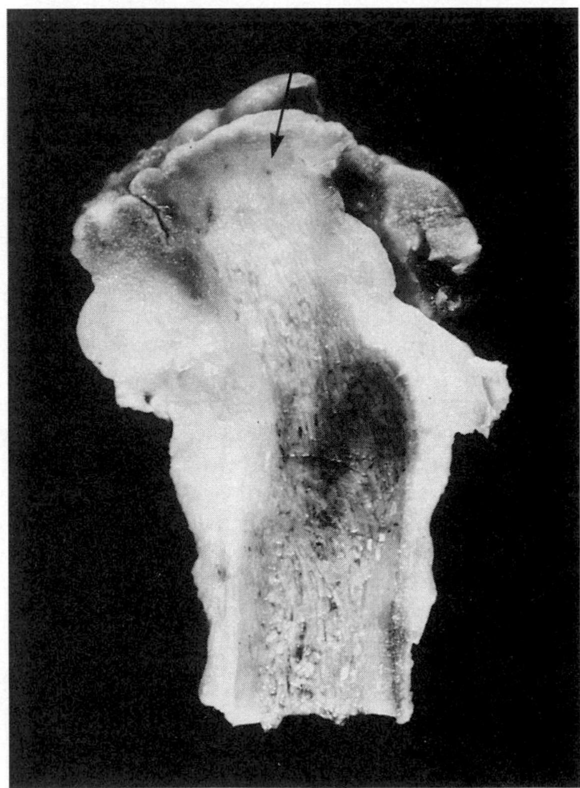

Fig. 75-18 Severe degenerative arthritis of the hip occurring after bacterial arthritis many years previously. Residual chronic hypertrophic synovitis lies adjacent to the deformed femoral head (*arrow*).

ety of circumstances. The prototype spirochetal disease is syphilis, whose great influence on Western civilization ranks with that of typhus, bubonic plague, smallpox, and tuberculosis. *Treponema pallidum,* the causative agent of syphilis, is responsible for several types of arthritis. Joint inflammation as a manifestation of primary or secondary syphilis is rare in immunocompetent hosts,[163] but syphilitic polyarthritis resembling that of systemic lupus erythematosus has been described in AIDS patients.[186,190] In tertiary syphilis, gummatous lesions of para-articular connective tissues may rupture into joint spaces. Such gummatous arthritis is characterized by a large quantity of painless effusion,[163] and must be distinguished from neuropathic arthropathy of tertiary neurosyphilis[137] where striking disintegration of the articular surface is the common finding. Histologic findings in the synovium are variable but include villous hypertrophy, perivascular lymphoid and plasma cell infiltrates, and endothelial proliferation. Actual gummas are quite rare.[191] Late changes include pannus formation and cartilaginous erosion similar to rheumatoid arthritis. In congenital syphilis, similar arthritic manifestations may occur.[191] Two other osteoarticular presentations are typical late manifestations of congenital syphilis. These are Parrot's pseudoparalysis, an osteochondritis of the epiphyseal and articular cartilages of the humerus and tibia, and Clutton's joints, a chronic hydrarthrosis of the knee joints.[163,191]

Nontreponemal spirochetal arthritis is typified by Lyme disease caused by *Borrelia burgdorferi.* Originally described in the northeastern United States, the disease has a wide distribution across North America, Europe, Asia, and Australia,[192] where ticks of the genus *Ixodes* serve as vectors. Although originally recognized as a cutaneous disease, joint symptoms occur in both the early and the late manifestations of the disease.[193] In many individuals with untreated Lyme disease, intermittent arthritis develops as late as 2 years after the onset of the acute illness.[192,193] In a few individuals, the arthritis becomes chronic and destructive, resembling rheumatoid arthritis clinically and histologically, with hypertrophic villous synovitis, pronounced lymphoid infiltration, and destructive pannus formation.[194] Some biopsy specimens have an obliterative endarteritis typical of a spirochetal illness.[158] Histologic identification of actual organisms has been rarely reported,[158] but cultural isolation from joint fluid of patients with chronic Lyme arthritis has been successful.[195] The arthritic symptoms may be overshadowed by chronic neurologic disease,[196] further illustrating the similarities to tertiary syphilis.

Mycobacterial arthritis

Evidence of osteoarticular tuberculosis can be seen in Egyptian mummies in the form of destructive spondylosis with paraspinal cold abscess formation.[197] Notwithstanding the recent increase in mycobacterial disease in HIV-positive individuals, mycobacterial arthritis remains an uncommon manifestation of tuberculosis.[198] However, failure to diagnose the tuberculous cause of a chronic inflammatory monoarthritis or oligoarthritis can be devastating,[199] because destruction of both articular and underlying bone by invasive pannus can occur. About half of all cases of tuberculous arthritis involve the spine,[199] and the large peripheral joints of the hip and knee are the next most commonly affected areas. There is no pathognomonic radiographic picture, but involvement of both joint space and underlying bone is usually present.[199] Although direct spread of mycobacteria to the synovium by either the hematogenous or the lymphogenous routes is possible, in most cases joint spread occurs from the underlying bone marrow, cartilage proving an ineffective barrier.[200] Because many patients with tuberculous arthritis do not have demonstrable pulmonary foci, dissemination to the bone marrow probably occurrs during the primary infection, perhaps many years earlier.[201] Definitive diagnosis is made by histologic examination (Fig. 75-19) and culture of a biopsy specimen from the affected joint , with either one or both tests being positive in 90% of the

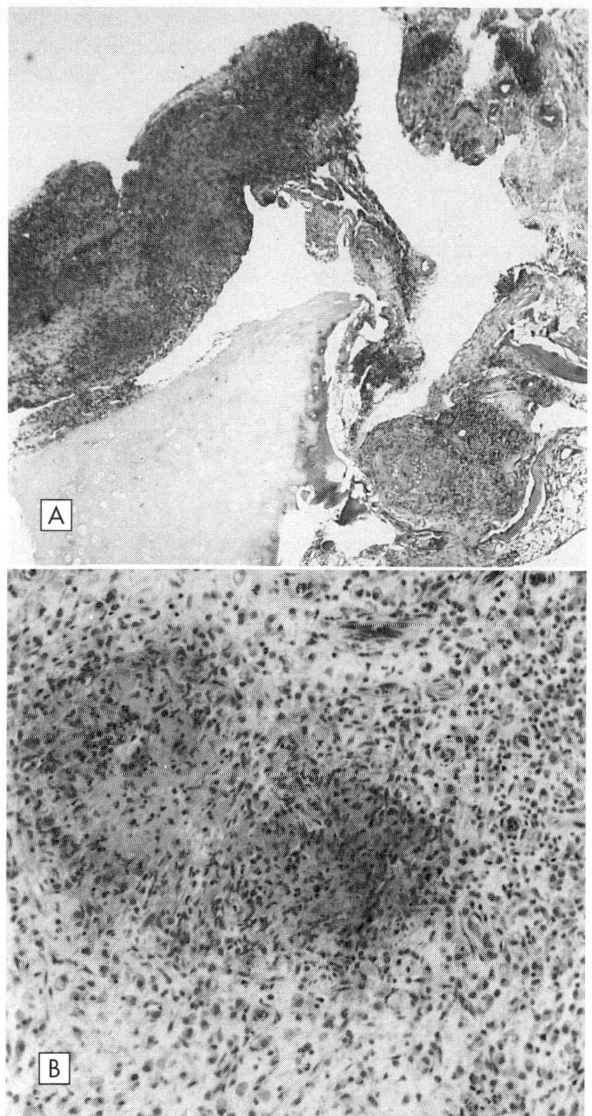

Fig. 75-19 Chronic arthritis of talocalcaneonavicular joint resulting from *Mycobacterium tuberculosis* infection. **A,**Destructive pannus, containing granulomas, undermines cartilage and destroys epithelioid bone. **B,** Resemblance to rheumatoid arthritis is obvious (see Fig. 75-23).

specimens.[202] The differential diagnosis includes atypical rheumatoid arthritis, crystal-induced arthropathy, and neuropathic arthropathy. Spinal involvement may lead to paraplegia because of vertebral collapse.

Even in the era of AIDS, most cases of articular mycobacterial infection are still caused by *Mycobaterium tuberculosis*, with *M. avium-intracellulare* causing predominantly diffuse bone marrow involvement,[203] rather than arthritis[204] in HIV-positive patients. Tenosynovitis can develop from both *M. avium–intracellulare* infection[205] and *M. tuberculosis* infection.[199] Other atypical mycobacteria can also cause arthritis in susceptible individuals.[199] The synovitis caused by *M. marinum* resembles that of rheumatoid arthritis histologically.[206] Before the widespread use of pasteurization, *M. bovis* was a common cause of gastrointestinal and spinal tuberculosus. Bacille Calmette-Guérin, a *M. bovis* strain used for immunization in many countries and for immunotherapy, may disseminate, causing arthritis.[207] *M. leprae,* the etiologic agent of Hansen's disease, historically known as leprosy, results in a variety of pathologic changes in the small joints of the hands and feet.[199] These include hypersensitivity reactions in periarticular tissues, as well as acute synovitis, possibly on an immune basis.[199] The bacilli can actually be found in subsynovial tissue in some cases of "swollen hands syndrome."[202] Disintegration of joints caused by neuropathic arthropathy is more common than actual inflammatory arthritis.[199,202]

Fungal arthritis

Fungal infection of joints is uncommon in the United States[199,202,208] because joint involvement is rare in the deep mycoses seen in the temperate zones. Infection may occur by any of the previously described mechanisms for gaining access to the joints. Most deep mycoses have one predominant mechanism of entry into the joints, but most, as in the case of *Blastomyces dermatitidis,* can cause arthritis by more than one means. In this case, either hematogenous dissemination or direct spread from involved bone[209] can be involved. Most individuals with fungal arthritis have predisposing factors, with immunosuppression being common. Fungal arthritis, in particular, is relatively rare in AIDS patients,[209] in comparison with the other infectious complications of the disease. When coccidioidomycosis, histoplasmosis, blastomycosis, or cryptococcosis develops in an HIV-positive patient, it is usually as a systemic process[199] with diffuse bone marrow involvement[203] rather than as a discrete focus of osteomyelitis or arthritis.

In coccidioidomycosis, two forms of arthropathy are seen. The first is an acute inflammatory polyarthritis associated with antigen-antibody reactions during the benign primary illness (so-called desert rheumatism). This resolves without deformity. The second is a chronic destructive monarthropathy resulting either from hematogenous dissemination or from direct spread from an osteomyelitic focus.[199,202] *Histoplasma capsulatum* causes a self-limited pulmonary disease that is endemic in the Ohio and lower Mississippi river basins.[199] Dissemination is rare, except in immunocompromised individuals who develop generalized bone-marrow involvement. However, *Histoplasma capsulatum* var. *duboisii,* the agent of African histoplasmosis, much more frequently causes discrete osteomyelitic lesions and secondary destructive arthritis.[210] Invasion of the joints by lymphatic spread from soft-tissue lesions has been described in sporotrichosis, but it is rarely seen and is difficult to diagnose on pathologic grounds.[199,202] Many different fungal organisms are implicated in the pathogenesis of mycetoma (Madura foot), a destructive soft-tissue process that eventually produces osteoarticular deformity as well.[199,210] This disorder is relatively common in certain tropical areas[199] but is rare in the temperate zones.

POSTINFECTIOUS ARTHRITIS

Many postinfectious arthritic conditions have been described. Basic mechanisms involve complement fixation in the synovium by antigen-antibody complexes, sometimes with microbial antigens that cross react with human ones. Delayed hypersensitivity has been implicated in some cases.[211] Both the severity and the pattern of arthritis varies among the clinical conditions. Most are self-limited and nondestructive. Examples include the arthritis accompanying acute hepatitis B infection, acute Lyme arthritis, Reiter's syndrome after chlamydial infection, reactive arthritis after *Yersinia enterocolitica* infection, and of course rheumatic fever.

Rheumatic fever arthritis

Rheumatic fever results from a complex of inflammatory and vasculitic lesions involving the heart, subcutaneous tissues, joints, skin, and brain.[212] The cardiac pathology, by far the most serious aspect of the disease, is considered in Chapter 45. Cases of acute rheumatic fever and hence the late sequelae have declined considerably[213] in the developed countries since the introduction of penicillin, though elimination of crowded living conditions may also be an important factor.[212] The disorder occurs within 2 to 3 weeks after a pharyngeal infection with one of certain selected strains of group A streptococci.[212,213] Most primary acute cases occur in children, but young adults can also develop initial attacks.[212] The arthritis is characteristically acute, polyarticular, migratory, and quite painful. Young adults generally have more severe articular manifestations. The joint disorder is an acute edematous synovitis with sterile effusions. Scattered mononuclear inflammatory cells are seen in the synovium but polymorphonuclear leukocytes predominate in the synovial fluid.[212] The exact pathogenesis is unclear, but increased levels of circulating immune complexes have been demonstrated.[212] Possibilities of genetic susceptibility related to either HLA-DR4[212] or to B-lymphocyte antigens[214] have been raised.

The arthritis is characteristically self-limited, disappearing within 1 month and leaving no permanent sequelae.[150] Subcutaneous nodules, characterized by palisading mononuclear cells surrounding eosinophilic zones of swollen, degenerated collagen, frequently occur in the vicinity of the joints.[111,150,212,213] These findings are seen more frequently in children and usually indicate that carditis is also present.[212] The rheumatic fever nodules superficially resemble early rheumatoid nodules but are less organized, more inflammatory, and less likely to contain areas of fibrinoid necrosis than rheumatoid nodules are.[215] The acellular center contains mucopolysaccharides and is surrounded by a margin of lymphocytes, monocytes, multinucleated giant cells, and occasionally eosinophils. Both the synovial and subcutaneous tissues may contain vasculitic lesions characterized by intimal proliferation and perivascular inflammation.[111,150] The nodules disappear within a few weeks, in contrast to those of rheumatoid arthritis, which may persist for months to years.

The differential diagnosis of acute rheumatic fever is most complicated in adolescents or young adults who do not manifest carditis. Thus adult rheumatoid arthritis, Still's disease (juvenile rheumatoid arthritis), gonococcal arthritis, viral arthritis, HIV-related arthropathy, and Reiter's syndrome are all possibilities to be excluded by appropriate clinical and laboratory examination. In adult patients with recurrent episodes of rheumatic fever, painless deformities of the hands have been rarely reported, presumably because of damage to the ligaments and tendons[216] with subluxation of the metacarpophalangeal joints.[215] Unlike rheumatoid arthritis, neither bony erosions nor systemic symptoms are seen.[213]

Rheumatoid arthritis

Definition. Rheumatoid arthritis (RA) is an idiopathic chronic inflammatory disorder with both systemic and articular manifestations. The arthritis is polyarticular, symmetric, and predisposed to involve the small joints of the hands and proximal fingers. The disorder affects an estimated 0.5% to 1.5% of the population of the United States.[172,217] The disorder increases in prevalence with increasing age, but the peak incidence falls between the fourth and the sixth decades of life.[218] Women are affected two to three times more frequently than are men. The prevalence is estimated to be 5% in women by 65 years of age.[218] RA is characterized by persistent inflammation in the synovium, bursae, tendon sheaths, and, in many patients, extra-articular tissues, including blood vessels, pericardium, pleura, lungs, and heart.

Classification. The diagnosis of RA, and the inference that a single disease state manifests in the wide variety of lesions encountered rest on histopathologic, radiologic, clinical, and laboratory findings.[172,219] Application of defined clinical criteria such as the American Rheumatism Association criteria,[25] the American College of Rheumatology criteria[25] and the New York[220] criteria is an attempt to standardize classification. Patients can be divided into two groups based on the presence or the absence of rheumatoid factors, which are antibodies (usually IgM) directed against epitopes on the Fc portion of IgG.[221] About 75% of RA patients have significant titers of rheumatoid factor when tested by conventional laboratory techniques.[221] More sensitive techniques increase this number to 85% or 95%.[150] Seropositive individuals are far more likely to develop severe erosive articular, extra-articular, and vasculitic disease.[219] Rheumatoid factors, however, can be detected in other types of autoimmune connective tissue disease,[221] in some infections, and in the asymptomatic elderly.

Etiology and pathogenesis. Rheumatoid arthritis has long been suspected to be the consequence of an ongoing infectious process.[176] Scientific, clinical, and epidemiologic evidence indicates that some type of acquired infectious agent precipitates RA in genetically susceptible individuals. Molecular studies have shown that individuals bearing the HLA-DR4 (HLA-DR1 in some populations)[172] haplotype with specific HLA-DQ and HLA-DP alleles[222,223] are more likely to develop severe RA. Individuals with RA also have decreased numbers of $CD4^+2H^+$ suppressor-inducer cells in the synovium[224] and thus may be unable to contain ongoing articular inflammation. The concordance of RA in identical twins, however, is only about 30%,[25] indicating that environmental factors are necessary to induce the disease.

Attempts to isolate bacteria from joints of RA patients have been unsuccessful,[172] and initial enthusiasm for mycoplasmas as etiologic agents, based on similarities between mycoplasma-induced disease in animals[225] to human RA, has also faded.[172] Speculation now centers on viruses as inducing agents. Rubella infection has long been suspected because of the ability of this virus to persist for long periods of time in joints[168] and to result in chronic polyarthritis,[226] even in children and adults with no previous history of rubella infection or immunization.[227]

More recently *Parvovirus* B-19 has been implicated in causing RA-like chronic disease,[174] and *Parvovirus* DNA has been detected with increased frequency in the synovium of RA patients.[175] Cytomegalovirus (CMV) has also been a candidate. Synovial cells in RA appear transformed and CMV DNA has been demonstrated in synovial fluid from RA patients.[228] CMV antigens have been isolated from antigen-antibody complexes in an RA patient.[172]

EBV is also postulated to play a role. Individuals with RA have increased numbers of $CD5^+$ B-cells.[229] This class of lymphocytes produces rheumatoid factor in vitro in response to EBV infection.[230,231] Furthermore, antibodies against an EBV-related antigen (RANA, or rheumatoid arthritis precipitin[232]) and to synthetic peptides from EBV nuclear antigen-1[233] occur with a higher frequency in RA patients. In addition, B-lymphocytes from RA patients develop lymphoblastoid colonies faster and produce more rheumatoid factor after in vitro EBV infection than B-lymphocytes of normal patients do.[172] However, attempts to recover intact EBV from synovium have not been successful.[172] Other observations have suggested that retroviruses[178,181] might be involved in the transformation[234] of synoviocytes observed in RA. Although several lines of investigation involving viral pathogenesis in RA appear promising, none has established a definite causal relationship. Likewise, studies of common antigenic structures among bacterial heat-shock proteins and human proteins are promising but have not established an etiologic relationship.[235] Thus, the cause of RA remains an enigma at present.

The joint destruction is promoted by degradative enzymes from polymorphonuclear leukocytic,[172] synovial cytokines,[236,237] and chondrocyte-derived degradative enzymes such as collagenase and stromelysin.[238] IL-6 released in response to IL-1 production has been shown to inhibit matrix synthesis by chondrocytes.[239] Bone destruction is also promoted by release of IL-1's and other cytokines such as TNF-α, TNF-β, and colony-stimulating factors.[240] The majority of the lymphocytes in the synovium in RA are activated T-cells, many of which have acquired reactivity against native chondrocyte membranes,[241] and so local cytotoxic effects are also possible. The pathogenesis of RA is depicted in schematic form in Fig. 75-20. The result is a persistent inflammatory response that produces the characteristic pathologic stigmas of RA.

Pathology. The pathologic lesions in RA vary in intensity and distribution among individual patients, but they are consistent regardless of the site from which the tissue is obtained. None of the histologic changes is individually pathognomonic, but taken as a whole, the changes are characteristic of the disease.[242] Rheumatoid lesions have in common lymphoid infiltration, as well as vasculitis with endothelial proliferation, fibrinoid necrosis of vessel walls, and perivascular mononuclear infiltrates.[243-245] In the synovium this process produces a hypertrophic villous synovitis (Fig. 75-21) with lymphoid aggregates.[111,246] Although rheumatoid synovium produces copious amounts of rheumatoid factor,[247] most of the lymphocytes are T-cells,[248] predominantly arranged deep to the synovial surface (Fig. 75-22). Several studies have shown an overall decrease in $CD8^+$ suppressor cells in the rheumatoid synovium.[249,250] The enormous increase in surface area produced by villous projections facilitates the exchange of inflammatory mediators across the synovium. Plasma cells may cluster near the synovial surface[242] in more chronic lesions. A vascularized pannus, complete with lymphocytes, monocytes, mast cells, plasma cells, and fibroblasts,[251-254] extends from the inflamed synovium onto the surface of the cartilage. Although the synovial fluid in RA usually contains large numbers of granulocytes, they are rare in rheumatoid synovium and pannus, except at the cartilage-pannus, junction.[255] The pannus erodes cartilage directly (Fig. 75-23) by several mechanisms. These include substances released by inflammatory cells of the pannus[172,255] and from transformed synoviocytes[256] into the synovial fluid. Near the pannus, the

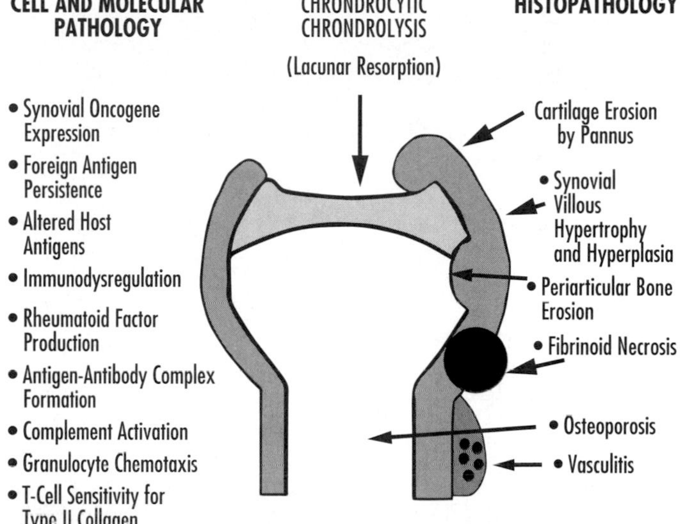

Fig. 75-20 Complex multifactorial pathogenesis of rheumatoid arthritis involves genetic susceptibility and environmental influences.

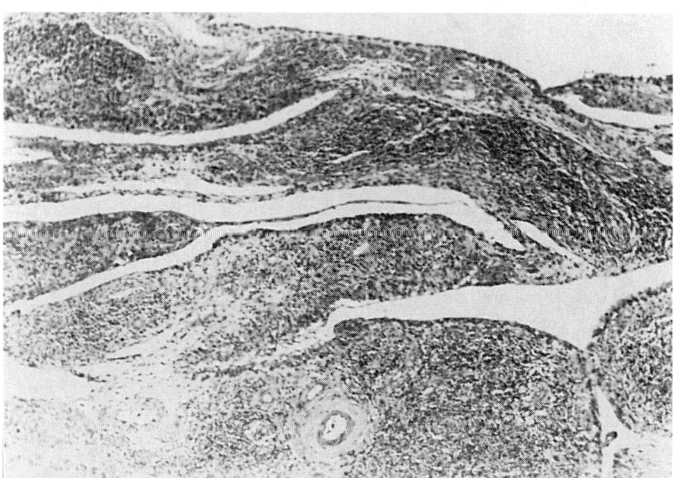

Fig. 75-21 Hypertrophic villous synovitis typical of rheumatoid arthritis. Dense lymphoid infiltrates are present in villi.

chondrocytes themselves resorb their matrix by releasing degradative enzymes.[172] Fibronectin is localized to the cartilage-pannus interface[257] and plays a role in attachment of the inflammatory cells within the pannus to the cartilage. As the pannus matures, it becomes more fibrotic, with formation of

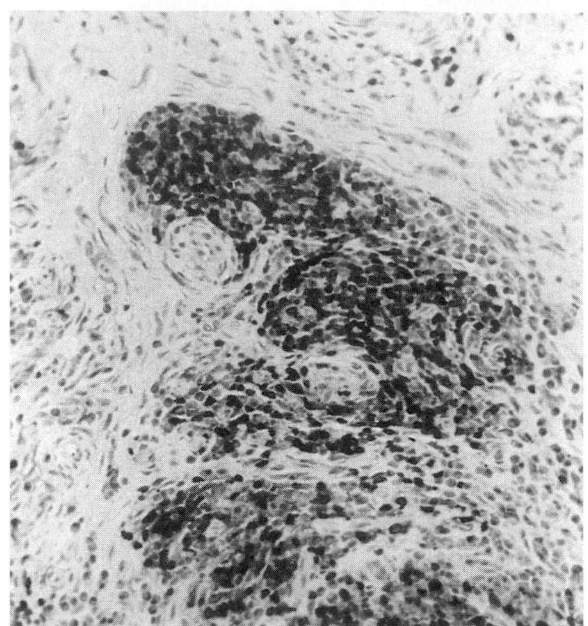

Fig. 75-22 Rheumatoid synovitis demonstrates large numbers of dark-staining T-lymphocytes targeted by UCHL-1 antibodies and visualized by a biotin-avidin technique.

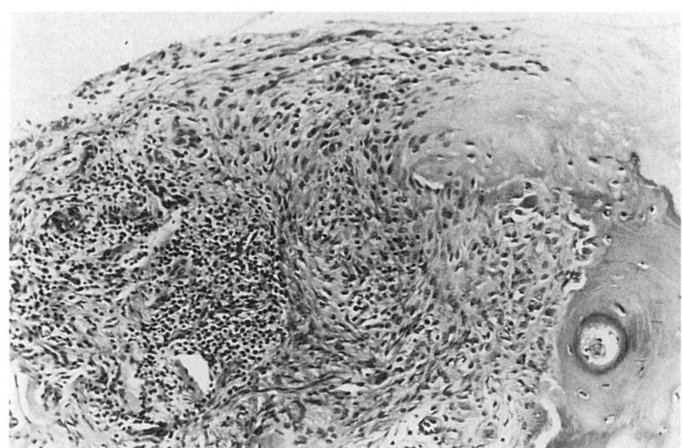

Fig. 75-23 Rheumatoid pannus. Granulation tissue replaces both articular cartilage and adjacent subchondral bone. Some preserved articular cartilage is seen at right.

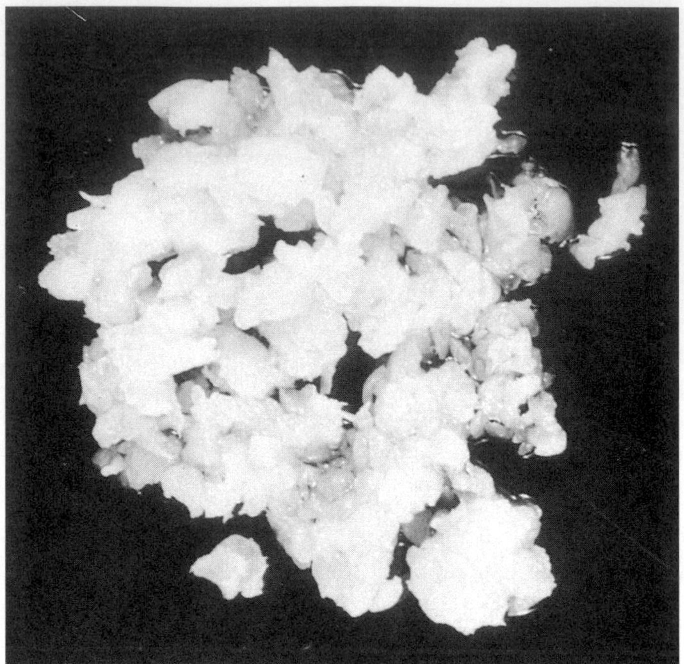

Fig. 75-24 Rice bodies removed from olecranon bursa of patient with rheumatoid arthritis. They are composed of necrotic tissue with admixtures of fibrin, immunoglobulin, fibronectin, and collagen.

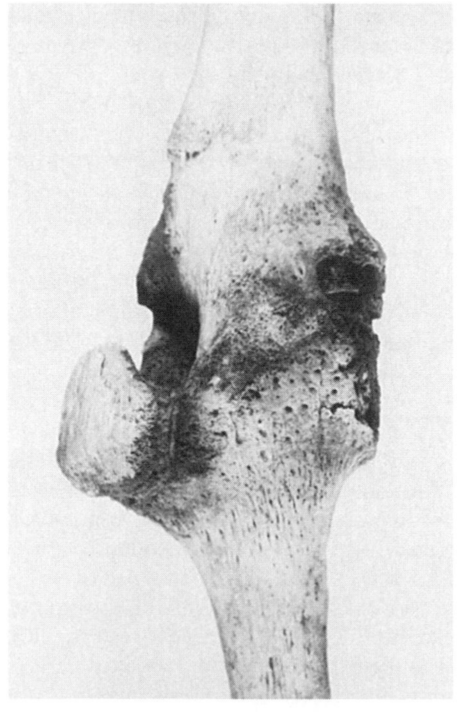

Fig. 75-25 Macerated specimen from knee joint. Advanced rheumatoid arthritis with bony fusion (ankylosis) of joint.

intra-articular and periarticular adhesions that produce dislocation and subluxation.[150]

The synovium frequently displays vasculitis with foci of fibrinoid necrosis. These necrotic zones are often extruded into the synovial cavity to form rice bodies[258,259] (Fig. 75-24). Similar inflammation and necrosis may involve the tendon sheaths in the hands and the feet because they are of synovial derivation, as the bursal lining cells are. The results of these processes are resorption of cartilage and periarticular bone, deformity with supervening secondary osteoarthritis, and, more rarely, fibrous or bony ankylosis (Fig. 75-25). The destruction of cartilage and the persistent inflammation produces profound deformity in the hands, characterized by fixed subluxation of the metacarpophalangeal and proximal interphalangeal joints with ulnar deviation (Fig. 75-26). Similar changes can occur in large peripheral joints. Osteoporosis develops locally near affected joints and may become generalized, especially in bedridden patients.

Several types of extra-articular lesions occur in RA (Fig. 75-27). The most common are the rheumatoid nodules of the

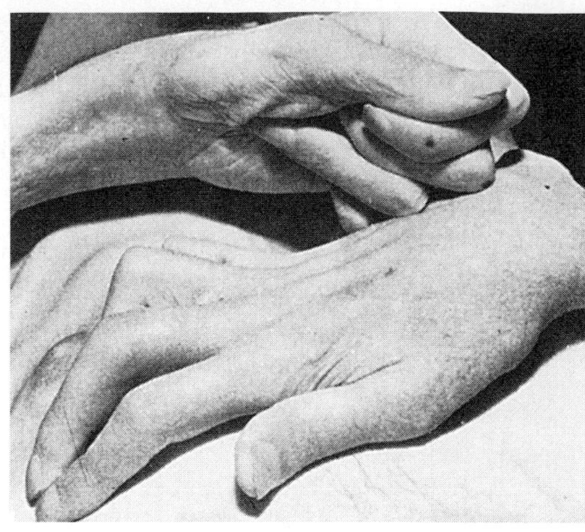

Fig. 75-26 Deformed hands in chronic rheumatoid arthritis. Fixed subluxation of metacarpophalangeal and proximal interphalangeal joints is accompanied by muscular atrophy.

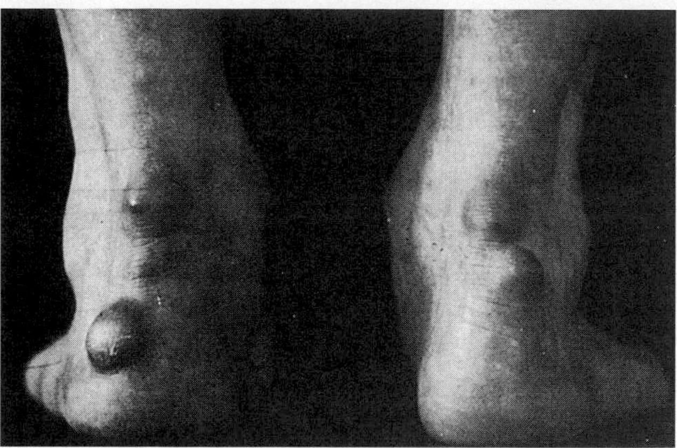

Fig. 75-28 Rheumatoid arthritis. Subcutaneous nodules over achilles tendon area are typical of RA (Courtesy Dr. F.A. Chandler, Atlanta, Ga.)

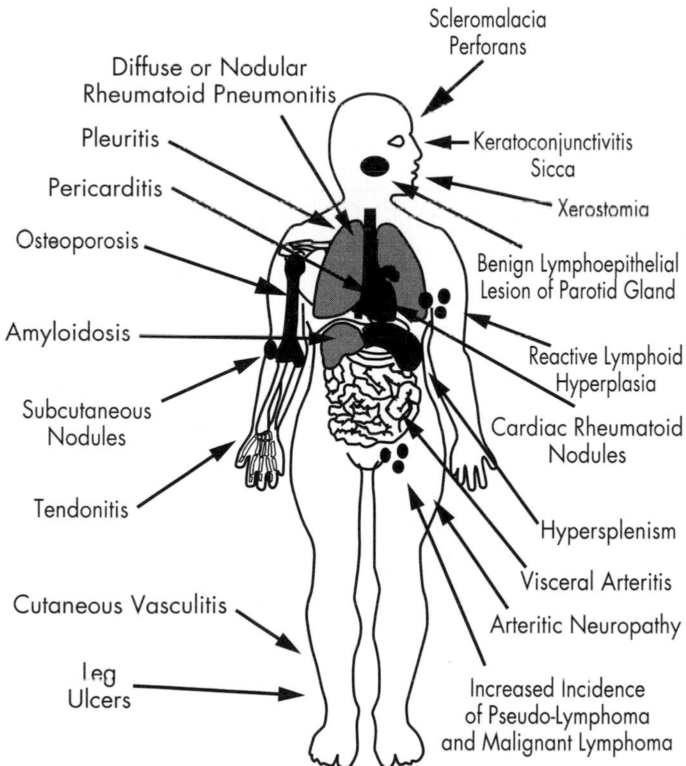

Fig. 75-27 A wide variety of extra-articular conditions is associated with rheumatoid arthritis. These contribute to the high mortality associated with RA.

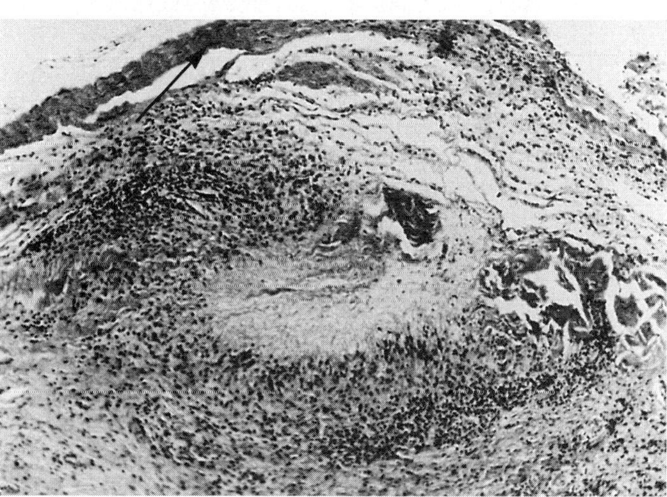

Fig. 75-29 Rheumatoid nodule of tendon sheath at wrist. Typical necrotic zone is surrounded by palisade of macrophages. Portion of tendon is seen (*arrow*).

subcutaneous tissue.[260,261] These usually occur at pressure points such as the olecranon, knee, or ankle areas (Fig. 75-28) and are firm, painless, and relatively slow to evolve. They are characterized in their early stages by an inflammatory vasculitis surrounded by a poorly organized inflammatory infiltrate. Later, the minute foci of necrosis and inflammation are transformed into stellate geographic zones of necrosis surrounded by palisading connective tissue cells that have been shown to be macrophages[262] (Fig. 75-29). Vasculitis is not apparent at this stage. Rheumatoid nodules may also occur on tendons and ligaments and in heart, skeletal muscle, lungs, lymph nodes, and spleen[242] (Fig. 75-30). Inflammation, apart from the rheumatoid nodules, is also seen in the tendon sheaths.

A frank vasculitis (Fig. 75-31) with deposition of immune complexes in the walls of small arterioles is occasionally seen, more often in patients with high titers of IgM rheumatoid factor.[263] Occlusion of vessels can result in ischemia and microinfarcts. Involvement of larger vessels can cause gangrene of the terminal phalanges. The long list of extra-articular lesions includes lymph node hyperplasia,[264,265] pulmonary lesions, including diffuse interstitial fibrosis,[266] parenchymal and pleural rheumatoid nodules,[267] silicofibrotic nodules (Caplan's syndrome),[268] and cardiac lesions. The latter include myocardial, pericardial, and valvular rheumatoid nodules,[269,270] as well as chronic pericarditis.[271] Scleritis that may lead to ocular perforation develops in about 1% of RA patients[272] and is associated with vasculitis. Immune complex deposits can also be demonstrated in the blood vessels of uninvolved skin in patients with seropositive RA.[273] Peripheral neuropathy result-

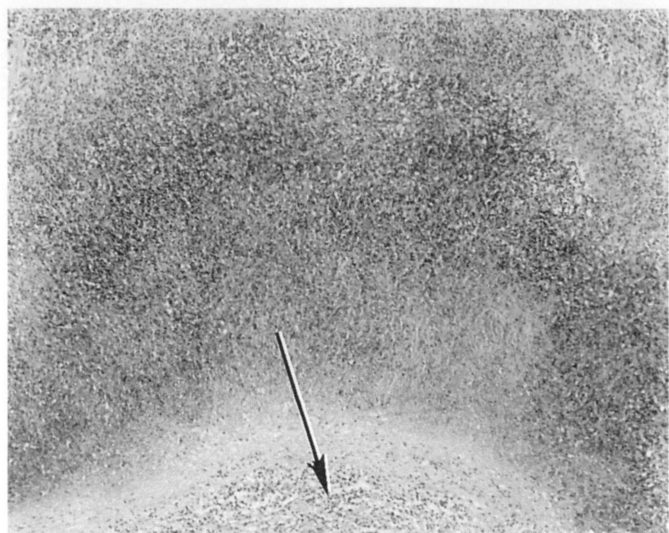

Fig. 75-30 Rheumatoid nodule in spleen closely resembles those seen in subcutaneous tissue with central zone of fibrinoid necrosis. Residual splenic parenchyma is adjacent (*arrow*).

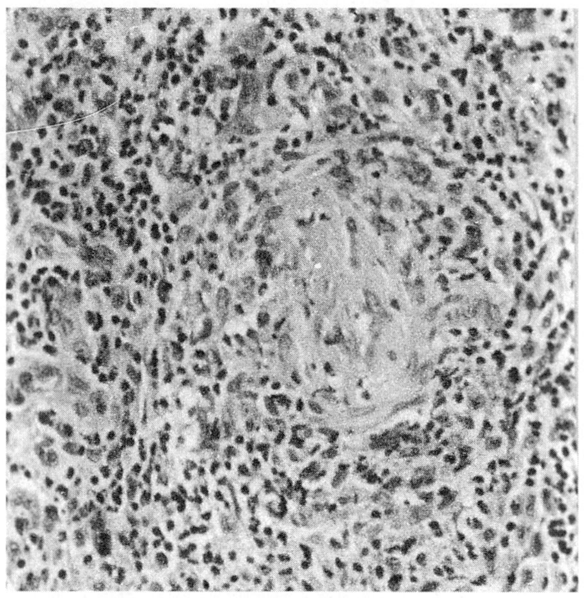

Fig. 75-31 Rheumatoid vasculitis in dermal arteriole. Fibrinoid necrosis with occlusion is accompanied by a dense inflammatory infiltrate.

ing from vasculitis (so-called mononeuritis multiplex) is an infrequent but serious problem.[274] Rarely, a necrotizing vasculitis with multiple small papules develops in the skin in a patient with RA (rheumatoid papulosis).[275] The lesions are histologically intermediate between the rheumatoid nodules and the rheumatoid vasculitis that is seen in deeper tissues.

RA may contribute to central as well as peripheral nervous system dysfunction. Rheumatoid granulomas not infrequently destabilize the ligaments of the upper cervical spine, resulting in acute and chronic myelopathy.[18,112] This is chiefly because of subluxation of the atlantoaxial articulation, though erosion in discovertebral joints and spinous processes[276,277] also occurs. The erosive nature of spinal disease is one of the important differences between RA and ankylosing spondylitis.

In addition to the articular and extra-articular pathologic lesions, several systemic conditions are associated with RA. Sjögren's syndrome (keratoconjunctivitis sicca) is a combination of seropositive but usually mild RA with inflammation of the lacrimal, salivary, and, less commonly, other exocrine glands. It develops in 10% to 15% of RA patients.[278] A primary form of Sjögren's syndrome associated with the HLA-B8 and HLA-DR3 haplotypes also exists.[279] Felty's syndrome is another RA-associated state involving splenomegaly, anemia, granulocytopenia, refractory leg ulcers, and severe rheumatoid arthritis.[280] Antinuclear antibodies are usually present, as are high titers of immune complexes. Large granular cell lymphocytosis and $CD3^+$ $CD8^+$ T-cell leukemia are seen with increased frequency in Felty's syndrome.[281] Systemic amyloidosis also regularly occurs in patients with long-standing RA. Past studies[150] cited cumulative frequencies in excess of 20%, but more recent studies[282] indicate that it is becoming less common. The amyloid is composed of AA protein, and cardiac, renal, hepatic, gastrointestinal, and splenic[141] involvement is the usual pattern. Deposition in the joints is not routinely seen with this type of amyloid.

Differential diagnosis. In its later stages RA presents a characteristic clinical picture. Numerous other conditions resemble RA in its early stages, and therefore careful attention to one of the sets of defined criteria for diagnosis is necessary.[25] The uncommon presentations of adult RA in childhood, Still's disease, ankylosing spondylitis, rheumatic fever, and Lyme disease are all diagnostic possibilities. In adolescents, systemic lupus erythematosus, Reiter's syndrome, gonorrheal arthritis, and HIV-associated arthritis also merit consideration. In young adults generalized osteoarthritis and psoriatic arthritis add to the customary listing of possibilities. In elderly adults, polymyalgia rheumatica should be considered. This disorder presents with generalized muscle and joint pain with mild synovitis but no joint destruction. Rheumatoid factor is usually not present, but the erythrocyte sedmentation rate is very high. An association with hypothyroidism has been described.[283] Some patients with polymyalgia rheumatica also have giant cell arteritis of the cerebral circulation (temporal arteritis).[284] Both of these conditions are not ordinarily associated with RA.[263]

Clinical presentation. Several types of presentation have been described.[219] A relatively sudden or acute onset is uncommon. An insidious onset with mild initial symptoms is more usual. Complaints of morning stiffness, possibly associated with fibrinous adhesions within joints and tendon sheaths and mild swelling, are common. The disease is characteristically symmetric and polyarticular, beginning in the hands and later proceeding to the large joints. The distal interphalangeal joints are spared. This is a point of distinction from both GOA and psoriatic arthritis. Rheumatoid subcutaneous nodules may be present, as well as splinter hemorrhages in the nail beds. Skin rashes, fever, and abnormalities of renal function are not seen, unlike lupus erythematosus. Later in the course of the disease, joint deformity, bone erosions, and generalized osteoporosis are usually present. Titers of rheumatoid factor may rise as the disease progresses or fall with aggressive therapy.[219] Rheumatoid arthritis is a serious disease with diminished life expectancy because of a variety of direct and indirect associations, including the increased likelihood of amyloidosis, diabetes mellitus, malignant lymphoma, and bacterial sepsis.[285]

Still's disease

General considerations. Still's disease is a complex of three distinct diseases classified by the type of initial presentation.[286] In the United States the term *juvenile rheumatoid arthritis* is used as a synonym for this condition, whereas in Europe *juvenile chronic arthritis* is preferred.[287,288]

Patients with more than five joints involved are considered to have the polyarticular variant, and a minority of these patients are rheumatoid factor positive at initial presentation. The prognosis for this group is mixed, with those who are seropositive being likely to develop severe joint erosions and rheumatoid nodules. The second subgroup consists of those patients with the pauciarticular variant, who present with fewer than four joints involved. These are usually weight-bearing joints in the lower extremities. This group contains some HLA-B27–positive patients, predominantly females, who are at risk for chronic iridocyclitis. Otherwise their prognosis is excellent. Others will develop rheumatoid factor and severe erosive polyarthritis in later life. The third variant manifests as a systemic presentation with fever, maculopapular skin rash, splenomegaly, and lymphadenopathy.[289] Patients with persistent systemic symptoms and elevated platelet counts are likely to develop chronic erosive disease.[290] One major difference between the American and European systems of classification is that obvious juvenile presentations of ankylosing spondylitis are excluded from the pauciarticular variant in the American system but expressly included in the European system.[287,288] Nevertheless, some patients with the American pauciarticular variant will develop ankylosing spondylitis at a later date.[291] Finally, patients with polyarticular disease who are seropositive are likely to be HLA-DR4 positive and thus represent true juvenile presentations of adult RA.[290]

Pathology. The pathologic findings are extremely variable, as would be expected. Mild, nonspecific synovitis is customary in the pauciarticular variant, but severe erosive pannus develops in the polyarticular variant. Severe joint deformity can occur by early adult life. Fibrous or bony ankylosis of hip and shoulder joints is more common than in classic adult RA. Involvement of the temporomandibular joint is particularly characteristic of the polyarticular variant. Not only is there erosive disease of the joint, but also involvement of the growth center can result in facial asymmetry.[289] Individuals who develop chronic polyarticular disease are also at increased risk for amyloidosis.

Seronegative spondyloarthropathies

Definition. The diseases in this group of chronic inflammatory joint disorders termed seronegative spondyloarthoropathies (SNSA) are considered together because of common clinical, pathologic, radiologic, and immunologic findings. They differ from RA in several important respects (Table 75-6). The main differences are the absence of rheumatoid factor and subcutaneous nodules and the prevalence of spinal ankylosis in SNSA. The percentage of SNSA patients positive for HLA-B27 varies from a low of 40% in psoriatic spondyloarthropathy to 90% in ankylosing spondylitis.[25] Reiter's syndrome and enteropathic spondyloarthritis demonstrate intermediate degrees of positivity for HLA-B27.

Etiology and pathogenesis. Numerous predisposing conditions, some with epidemiologic and immunologic evidence of a postinfectious cause, are associated with SNSA. In contrast to RA, where only a 5% concordance in dizygotic twins is noted,[25] the concordance for ankylosing spondylitis in first-degree relatives is approximately 20%.[292] Although SNSA, as a group, demonstrate strong hereditary tendencies, environmental influences are certain to play a major role in precipitating the arthropathy.[293] Recurrent bacterial infections are currently leading candidates as precipitating factors.[294–297] Although molecular mimicry of bacteria for human antigens has been suggested as a mechanism,[298] this hypothesis is by no means secure. Inflammation of the gastrointestinal or genitourinary tract appears to be a trigger mechanism for most SNSA. This includes gastrointestinal inflammation in ankylosing spondylitis,[299] enteropathic spondyloarthritis,[300] and reactive (post-*Yersinia*) spondyloarthritis.[301] Reiter's syndrome may be precipitated by either genitourinary chlamydial infection[159,297,302,303] or gram-negative bacterial dysenteric illnesses.[297] Increased fecal carriage of *Klebsiella spp.* is present in patients with ankylosing spondylitis.[298] IgA levels are elevated[304] as are IgA–alpha-1-antitrypsin immune complexes[305] in ankylosing spondylitis patients, providing additional evidence for mucosal abnormalities. In some way, the HLA-B-27–positive individual is prone to spondyloarthropathy after mucosal bacterial challenge. The pathogenesis of ankylosing spondylitis, the prototype SNSA, is depicted in Fig. 75-32.

Table 75-6 Comparison of rheumatoid arthritis (RA) and seronegative spondyloarthriopathies (SNSA)

Criterion	RA	SNSA
Spinal ankylosis	–	2–4+*
Iridocyclitis	–	2+
Sacroiliitis	–	4+
HLA–B27 prevalence	–	2–4+
GI, GU, or skin inflammation	–	3–4+
Peripheral joint destruction	3–4+	–
Rheumatoid factor	3–4+	–
HLA–DR4 prevalence	3+	–
Rheumatoid nodules	2+	–

*Prevalence: – = 0% = 1+ < 25% to 49%, 3+ – 50% to 75%, 4+ – >75%.
GI, Gastrointestinal; *GU*, genitourinary.

Classification. Many distinct seronegative spondyloarthropathies have been recognized. Most are classified according to the antecedent conditions that lead to subsequent arthritic manifestations, but broad overlap exists. Ankylosing spondylitis, formerly considered a "primary spondyloarthropathy," is now associated with inflammatory gut disease,[299,300] forming a link[292] with enteropathic spondyloarthritis, reactive or post-*Yersinia* spondyloarthritis, and gut-associated Reiter's syndrome. All spondyloarthritides have in common some degree of sacroiliitis.[306] Many patients subsequently develop variable degrees of bony ankylosis in the spine as well. Reiter's syndrome,[307] defined originally to include peripheral arthritis, conjunctivitis, and nongonococcal urethritis, also occurs after dysenteric illness caused by certain species of *Yersinia, Salmonella, Shigella,* or *Campylobacter*.[307,308] Thus it is really only a subtype of reactive postinfectious spondyloarthropathy. Furthermore, the skin rash that is common in Reiter's syndrome[307,309] is histologically indistinguishable from pustular[310] psoriasis. In psoriasis patients, two types of arthritis develop. In most, a

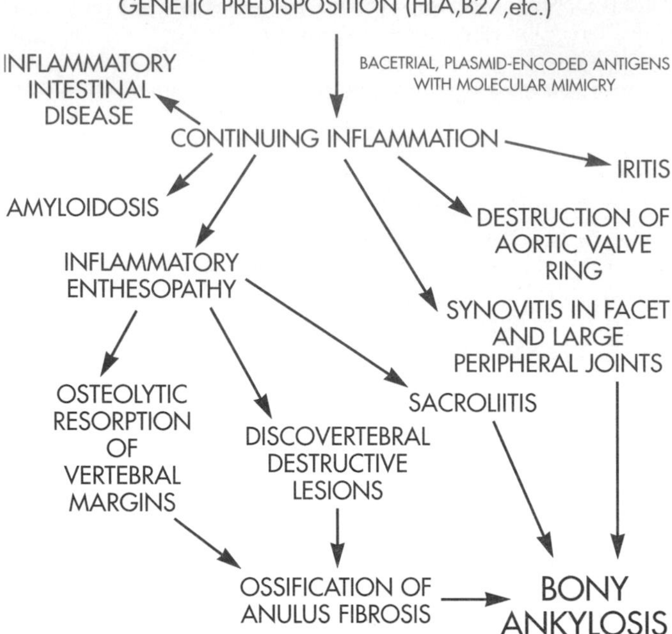

Fig. 75-32 Pathogenesis of ankylosing spondylitis, the prototype of the seronegative spondyloarthropathies.

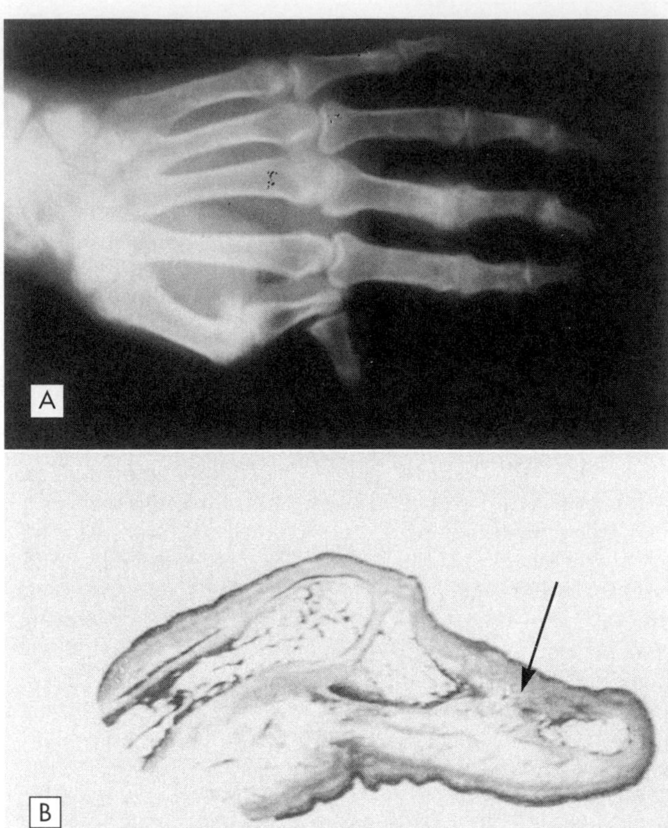

Fig. 75-33 Peripheral psoriatic arthropathy. **A,** Radiograph of hand shows distal interphalangeal involvement with sparing of metacarpophalangeal joints; notice dislocation in thumb. **B,** Resorption of bone in distal phalanx (*arrow*) is characteristic of peripheral psoriatic arthropathy.

destructive asymmetric peripheral arthritis[311] develops (Fig. 75-33), but in HLA-B27–positive psoriatics, a spondylitis with patchy, asymmetric ankylosis is common.[312] Enteropathic spondyloarthropathy, characterized by asymmetric spinal involvement, also predominantly occurs in HLA-B27–positive patients. It is also associated with cutaneous manifestations such as pyoderma gangrenosum and other dermatitides.[313] Clearly the syndromes merge with one another clinically and are best considered as a group[292] because of their common pathologic features.

Pathology. The osteoarticular pathologic state of the SNSA is characterized by synovitis in the peripheral joints, especially the large central joints of the lower extremities. Involvement of small joints can occur as well and is most characteristic of Reiter's syndrome, reactive spondyloarthritis, and psoriatic spondyloarthritis. Unlike RA, erosive pannus formation is rarely seen. Another characteristic feature is enthesopathy, or inflammation of ligaments and tendons at their insertion into bone, often followed by ossification. This feature may be the only obvious early manifestation of juvenile ankylosing spondylitis. Bony ankylosis of large peripheral joints such as the hip also occurs, most commonly in ankylosing spondylitis. The involvement of the vertebral column is described in the section dealing with that structure.

Differential diagnosis. The chief concern is separating the SNSA from RA and from postinfectious arthropathies such as hepatitis B–associated arthritis,[263] Lyme disease, and HIV-associated arthritis. Rheumatoid arthritis has a significantly different clinical presentation (Table 75-6). The history, immunologic features, and radiographic findings will usually distinguish the SNSA from the other arthropathies. Caution is required because HIV-positive patients with psoriasis develop more severe manifestations of their cutaneous and arthritic disease.[312] In juvenile spondyloarthropathies, some confusion with Still's disease is inevitable. The presence of radiographic sacroiliitis and enthesopathy in a HLA-B27–positive child is a strong indication that the arthritis will evolve into SNSA.[291,314]

Clinical presentation. As with many disease states, the manner of onset of the disease is a key factor in successful diagnosis.[315] The onset of ankylosing spondylitis is insidious. Therefore, patients are often undiagnosed until frank sacroiliitis or other spinal changes have become apparent on radiographs. On the other hand, reactive arthritis and Reiter's syndrome develop suddenly, with a history of recent antecedent illness. Rarely, psoriatic and enteropathic arthritis may precede the onset of clinical skin or bowel disease, but the progression to destructive peripheral or axial arthropathy is inconsistent and slow. Only a minority of individuals with reactive, Reiter's, psoriatic, or enteropathic arthritides develop spinal disease, and these individuals frequently have HLA-B27.[292,315] Finally the extra-articular disorder of most spondyloarthropathic conditions is, of itself, frequently diagnostic.

Other inflammatory arthritides

Behçet's syndrome

Behçet's syndrome is a multisystem inflammatory disorder presenting with circumscribed ulcers of the skin, iridocyclitis, and mucous membrane ulcerations. Mild asymmetric synovitis of the peripheral joints occurs in up to 90% of the patients.[316] Destructive pannus does not result, however. Synovial biopsy specimens have shown polymorphonuclear and lymphoid cellular infiltrates.[317] Vascular lesions, possibly resulting from immune complex–mediated injury, can develop.[318] The disorder does not result in sacroiliitis or spondylitis and is associated with HLA-B5 rather than with HLA-B27.[318] For these reasons it is not ordinarily grouped with the seronegative spondyloarthropathies.

Sarcoid arthropathy

Arthritis routinely accompanies acute sarcoidosis,[319] but is less common as a chronic disorder. The acute arthritic form demonstrates nonspecific mild synovitis in biopsy specimens, but the chronic variants may have noncaseating granulomas.[320] Arthritis is polyarticular but the ankles and knees are most commonly affected. Although focal cystic bone lesions may occur in chronic recurrent sarcoidosis, destructive arthritis is not often seen. The differential diagnosis includes rheumatic fever, Still's disease, Reiter's syndrome, reactive arthritis, and Lyme arthritis. RA does not characteristically present acutely, but some studies have indicated increased prevalence of rheumatoid factor in sarcoidosis patients.[319] Arthritis may also clinically precede the characteristic pulmonary lesions of sarcoidosy.[319]

Arthritis with primary immunodeficiency

Several types of congenital or acquired hypogammaglobulinemia are associated with symptoms resembling those of RA, including morning stiffness, joint effusions, and joint space narrowing.[321] Arthritis has been reported in up to 29% of patients with various types of immunoglobulin deficiency.[322] The pathologic findings are nonspecific and vary according to whether there is a total deficiency of all immunoglobulin classes or a selective deficiency.[263] In total deficiency, no plasma cells are present, but some have been identified in cases where an isolated immunoglobulin class is deficient.[323] Subcutaneous nodules have been described on several occasions, but they more closely resemble those found in Still's disease or rheumatic fever than those of rheumatoid arthritis.[263] The differential diagnosis includes not only rheumatoid disease, but the ever-present possibility of septic arthritis.

Relapsing polychondritis

Relapsing polychondritis[324] is remarkable for the suddenness with which structural abnormalities can appear in a wide variety of structures, the most serious being those in the tracheal and laryngeal cartilage and in the aortic valve ring.[325] Collapse of the nasal and aural cartilages is often the most prominent sign. Joint involvement is variable. Most published accounts[150] emphasize a RA-like appearance of the synovium with infiltration by lymphocytes and plasma cells and hyperplasia of synoviocytes. The cartilage matrix loses the normal basophilic staining pattern with hematoxylin and eosin, and staining for acid mucopolysaccharides by Alcian blue or toluidine blue is greatly reduced. Lymphocytic infiltration occurs in the extra-articular cartilages as well. Electron microscopy demonstrates degenerative changes in chondrocytes, with unusual bulbous bodies in cytoplasmic processes and large numbers of lysosomes and dense bodies.[150] The disease has a putative immune cause because of the presence of antibodies against native type II collagen in acute cases.[325]

Arthritis with generalized autoimmune diseases

Acute transitory arthritis is characteristic of several diseases of hyperimmunity, often known as *connective tissue diseases*.[111,150] These include systemic lupus erythematosus, erythema nodosum, progressive systemic sclerosis, and intergrade conditions such as the CREST syndrome. Several forms of vasculitis are also associated with arthritic manifestations.[326] A familial tendency for patients with systemic lupus erythematosus to develop *arthritis* has been noted.[327] Synovial histologic features in lupus synovitis show mild nonspecific changes with focal mononuclear infiltrates. There is no permanent articular damage from the synovitis, but aseptic necrosis is significantly increased in frequency in systemic lupus erythematosus,[328] possibly augmented by corticosteroid administration. Permanent articular disease does result from progressive systemic sclerosis (scleroderma). Resorption of the tufts of the terminal phalanges eventually results in joint disease. Occlusive disease of the small nutrient arteries produces avascular necrosis and progressive fibrosis of synovial and capsular structures.[329] The periarticular fibrosis must be distinguished from the fibrositis syndrome accompanying diabetes mellitus.

CRYSTAL-INDUCED ARTHRITIS

Crystal-induced arthritis as a group of diseases is characterized by crystal deposition in and around joints. Crystal-induced arthritis includes that resulting from deposition of monosodium urate,[330] calcium pyrophosphate,[32] basic calcium phosphate (hydroxyapatite),[331,332] and calcium oxalate. Although the epidemiologic pattern of each condition is varied, the articular pathophysiologic characteristics involves promotion of inflammation by both direct and indirect means. Mechanisms of inflammation include activation of complement, induction of the release of lysosomal emzymes and lipoxygenases from granulocytes, and inducing the release of IL-1, IL-6, IL-8, and TNF-α by macrophages and synovial lining cells.[333] Mast cells may also be involved. The result of recurrent bouts of inflammation can be severe secondary ostesarthritis. Because this group of diseases is strongly associated with metabolic dysfunction, they are often seen along with coexistent endocrine, toxic, and hereditofamilial biochemical diseases (see Table 75-4).

Gout (hyperuricemic arthropathy)

Definition. Gout is the articular manifestation of a systemic disorder caused by at least one of the following: (1) excessive purine synthesis, (2) excessive conversion of purines to uric acid, or (3) decreased renal clearance of urate. More often than not, one of these conditions is present in patients. The manifestations of gout[334-336] have long been the subject of inquiry and exegesis. Hippocrates, in keeping with his philosophy of holistic medicine, associated the disease with intemperance in food and drink. Claudius Galen and his legions of followers over the centuries ascribed gout to an imbalance in the body's humors.[150] Paracelsus (Theophrastus von Hohenheim) postulated that gout was casued by a substance called "tartar," which originated from food and combined with "synovia," an egg-white–like substance in joint fluid.[150] Sydenham, although a humoralist as were almost all physicians of his day, noted the connection between gout and urinary stones. The advances in chemistry in the late eighteenth and early nineteenth centuries saw the identification of uric acid in kidney stones from gout patients by Scheele in 1769 and of urates in tophi by Wollaston in 1797. Sir Alfred Baring Garrod, in a series of brilliant clinical investigations,[336] demonstrated in 1859 that patients with gout had hyperuricemia and that the joint fluid also contained urates. As so

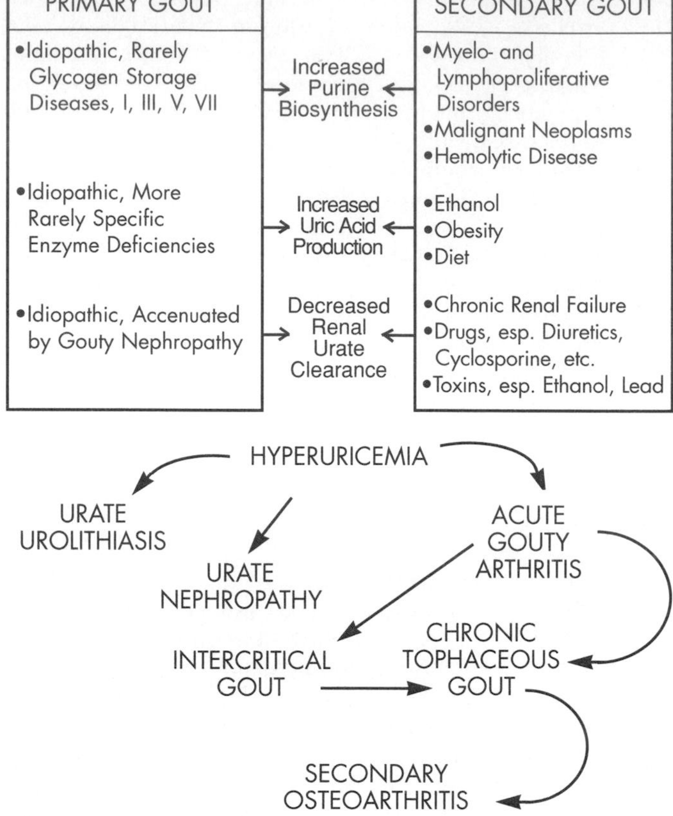

Fig. 75-34 Pathogenesis of gout, the prototype of crystal-induced arthropathy

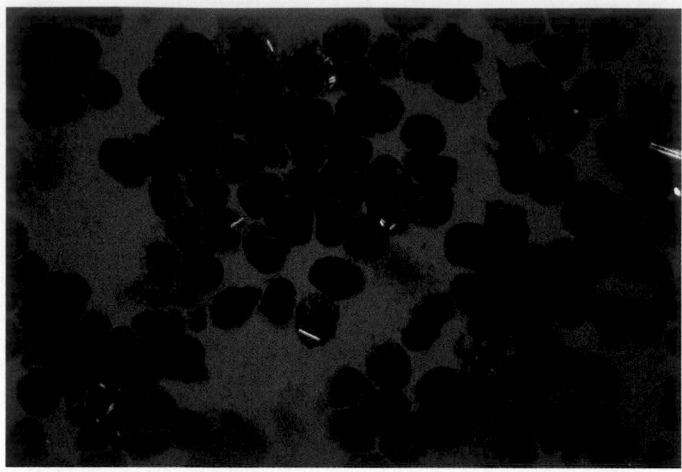

Fig. 75-35 Synovial fluid in acute gout. Polymorphonuclear leukocytes contain typical negatively birefringent needlelike crystals seen with plane-polarized light microscopy.

often happens, Garrod's work was largely ignored until McCarty and Hollander explained the pathogenesis of acute gout in 1961.[337]

Classification. In theoretical terms, gout can be separated into primary and secondary varieties. Patients have primary gout if they have acquired the disease as a consequence of one of several known metabolic defects or for idiopathic reasons. Idiopathic primary gout is by far the most common category. Secondary gout develops in individuals under a wide variety of circumstances (Fig. 75-34), such as use of diuretics, chemotherapy, intoxications, and immunosuppression with cyclosporin A.[330] Individuals with primary asymptomatic hyperuricemia (estimated at 5% to 8% of the adult male population in the United States[330] are at risk when challenged with one of the above conditions. Thus, in practical terms, the distinction between primary and secondary gout blurs in any given patient. Secondary gout of a serious nature is most frequently seen in elderly patients on thiazide diuretics and in children receiving chemotherapy for disseminated neoplastic disease.

Etiology and pathogenesis. There is a definite hereditary predisposition to primary idiopathic gout.[330] Individuals with clinical gout are more likely to have relatives with gout or asymptomatic hyperuricemia.[330] Young individuals who are identified with asymptomatic hyperuricemia appear particularly likely to have a family history of gout.[338] In population studies, gout is also strongly related to hyperuricemia, and has been shown to be about nine times as frequent in hyperuricemic as normouricemic men over a 14-year period of study.[339] However, the attack rate for gout in hyperuricemic males is as low as 2% to 3%.[150] There is also no evidence that asymptomatic hyperuricemia predisposes to renal disease, though the prevalence of cerebral thromboses, hypertension, and diabetes are all increased.[330] Asymptomatic hyperuricemia is predominantly a disease of adult males, as is idiopathic primary gout, 90% of which occurs in men. When primary gout occurs in women, it is almost always after the menopause.[330] However, secondary gout associated with thiazide-induced hyperuricemia is not uncommon in elderly women under treatment for hypertension or congestive heart failure.[340]

A complete deficiency of hypoxanthine-guanine phosphoribosyltransferase (HGPRT) results in the *Lesch-Nyhan syndrome,* characterized by severe hyperuricemia and hyperuricosuria, mental retardation, and self-mutilation.[330] Partial deficiencies of HGPRT result in hyperuricemia, gout, and uric acid urolithiases, presenting in adolescence or early adult life. Both of these rare disorders are X-linked, occurring only in males. Other enzyme abnormalities such as X-linked phosphoribosylpyrophosphate synthetase superactivity and autosomal recessive glucose-6-phosphatase deficiency[330] may lead to primary gout at an early age.

Pathology. Acute gout results from accumulation of urate crystals in the synovial fluid.[349] These crystals invoke an acute inflammatory response in the synovium. Polymorphonuclear leukocytes phagocytose the crystals, releasing lysosomal enzymes into the joint fluid (Fig. 75-35). Monosodium urate crystals also induce antibody formation.[341] Urate crystals are also found in synoviocytes,[150] where they induce release of other inflammatory mediators.[330] Free urate crystals can be found in the synovial fluid in most asymptomatic individuals who have previously had acute gout.[342] However, the presence of crystals within granulocytes is necessary to confirm an acute attack.[330] Chronic tophaceous gout is characterized by macroscopic deposits of urate crystals associated with a central core of proteinaceous material (Fig. 75-36). Foreign-body giant cells may also be seen. These nodules are found in the periarticular and subcutaneous tissues. They can be aspirated and visualized under plane-polarized light to confirm the cause of the nodule. However, only about 10% of patients with acute

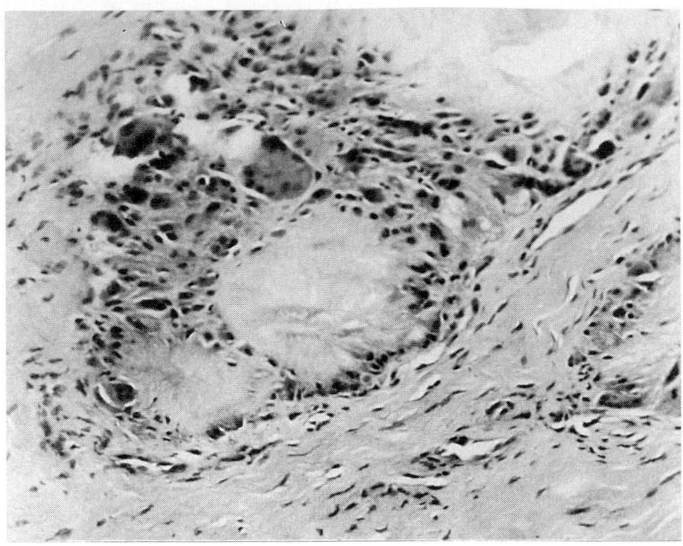

Fig. 75-36 Portion of a gouty tophus in periarticular tissue. Urate crystals originally present have been dissolved during tissue processing, leaving a proteinaceous matrix surrounded by granulation tissue and multinucleated giant cells.

gout will have tophi.[330] Urate crystals may be grossly apparent as chalklike deposits in the synovium, on the cartilage surface, or in the subchondral bone of individuals with chronic destructive gouty arthritis. The presence of urate crystals, either free or within granulocytes, does not exclude coexistent calcium pyrophosphate[32] or apatite[185] deposition diseases or septic arthritis.[330]

Differential diagnosis. Acute gout may be accompanied by mild fever suggesting an infectious process. In a typical case of acute monoarticular gout in a middle-aged male, septic arthritis, and calcium pyrophosphate or basic calcium phosphate arthropathy are to be excluded. The increasing prevalence of secondary gout in elderly women poses additional diagnostic considerations. Polyarticular presentations are more common in this group,[341] and gout can coexist with Heberden's nodes, which is suggestive of generalized or erosive OA. Alternatively, multiple tophi may simulate rheumatoid nodules in a patient with polyarticular gout. Secondary OA with eburnation and osteophytes may result from chronic gout.

Clinical presentation. Gout may be divided into three clinical presentations: (1) acute gouty arthropathy, (2) intercritical gout, and (3) chronic tophaceous gout. In untreated or inadequately treated patients, there is a definite tendency to progress from multiple acute episodes into chronic destructive disease.[330] For some unexplained reason, acute gout has a predilection for the proximal first metatarsal joint, but ankles, knees, wrists, and elbows are frequently involved.[330] Tophi are characteristically seen around the olecranon, knee, volar forearm, and the achilles tendon, but the helix of the ear is a classic location[330] as well.

Calcium pyrophosphate dehydrate (CPPD) deposition disease

Definition. The condition calcium pyrophosphate dehydrate deposition disease, commonly known as pseudogout, results from acute inflammation deposition of calcium prophosphate crystals in articular cartilage, synovium, ligaments, menisci, and intervertebral disks.[32] Unlike gout, the history of this relatively common condition is brief. Initially, chondrocalcinosis of cartilage was described radiologically.[31,343] Light microscopic, electronmicroscopic, and x-ray diffraction studies have established CPPD as the chemical species involved[330] in most cases.

Classification. A clear analogy to gout is present. Primary CPPD deposition disease occurs principally in the elderly,[344] where an association with osteoarthritis is often present.[27,58] Secondary CPPD disease is seen in association with hyperparathyroidism,[31] acromegaly,[108,109] hemochromatosis,[30,101] Wilson's disease,[104] ochronosis,[40] and neuropathic arthropathy.[137] CPPD crystals are frequently observed in osteoarthritic joints.[345] Whether this illustrates cause,[346] effect,[347] or no relationship[348] to osteoarthritis remains controversial.[58]

Etiology and pathogenesis. The CPPD crystals are present in articular cartilage, synovium, menisci, and ligaments of many asymptomatic elderly individuals (chondrocalcinosis). Under certain conditions, crystals accumulate in the synovial fluid, where an acute inflammatory reaction develops.[32] Granulocytes and macrophages phagocytose the crystals, releasing inflammatory mediators. Recurrent acute attacks can develop. This condition is known as pseudogout.

Pathology. In acute pseudogout the synovium first develops granulocytic, and then mononuclear infiltration. In some cases, polymorphonuclear leukocytes attach to the superficial cartilage near where degradation of matrix is occurring.[32] In chronic cases, chalklike deposits can be visible grossly, and microscopic deposits of typical biaxial crystals can be identified in synovium and other articular tissues (Fig. 75-37). The crystals show weak positive birefringence.

Differential diagnosis. CPPD crystal deposition disease must be distinguished from osteoarthritis, gout, RA, and neuropathic arthropathy. Septic arthritis is not excluded by the presence of CPPD crystals in synovial fluid. Gout coexists with pseudogout in about 5% of the cases.[32] The systemic metabolic diseases associated with CPPD crystal deposition must also be excluded.

Clinical presentation. CPPD crystal deposition disease may present as chronic osteoarthritis, as acute pseudogout, or as a variety of other arthritic conditions. The knee is by far the most commonly affected joint, but the wrist, hip, shoulder, and spinal joints can also be involved. The arthritis is usually symmetric when multiple joints are involved.[32]

Basic calcium phosphate crystal disease

These arthropathies also present with radiologic chondrocalcinosis.[332] They result from deposition of several chemical species of basic calcium phosphate (BCP), including hydroxyapatite, octacalcium phosphate, and tricalcium phosphate. Several clinical presentations, including calcific periarthritis and tendinitis, bursitis, erosive polyarticular disease, idiopathic destructive monarthritis (Milwaukee knee-shoulder syndrome), and Charcot-like articular degeneration, have all been described.[331,332] Accurate diagnosis is difficult because the individual crystals are too small to detect by conventional polarizing microscopy. Quantitative transmission electron microscopy, Fourier-transform infrared spectroscopy, or x-ray diffraction can be employed but are usually not practical. Alizarin red S staining of smears of centrifuged synovial fluid is often employed for screening, even though false-positive results are common.[332] Acute BCP destructive arthritis is characterized by granulocytic snyovial

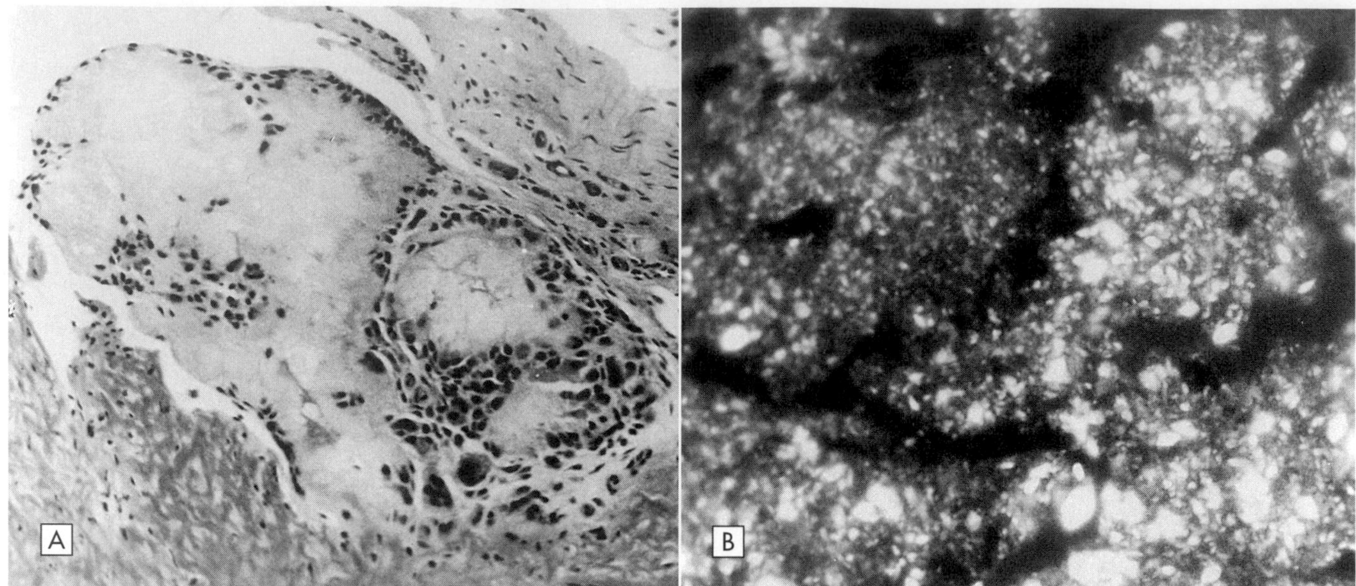

Fig. 75-37 Deposition of calcium pyrophosphate crystals in knee joint ligament (chondrocalcinosis). **A,** Routine light microscopic picture closely resembles a gouty tophus. **B,** Polarizing microscopy reveals positively birefringent biaxial crystals of calcium pyrophosphate dihydrate.

effusions and acute inflammation in the synovium. Confusion with OA is obvious because apatite crystals are commonly seen in joint tissues and synovial fluid in advanced OA.[332] Septic arthritis is an ever-present possibility in these patients.[185] The diagnosis should be suspected in patients with rapidly progressive destructive arthritis of the shoulder or knee joints, in association with extensive periarticular calcification.[332]

DISEASES OF BURSAE, TENDONS, AND FASCIAE

Bursitis

The bursae are lined by synovial cells. Their pathologic reaction to injury is therefore similar to that of the joint cavity synovial cells. Traumatic bursitis in the form of housemaid's knee is an inflammation of the prepatellar bursa caused by repeated minor trauma. More serious are the involvements of bursae by acute bacterial infections and by RA, the olecranon bursa being particularly susceptible to bacterial infection. Purulent bursitis is most commonly caused by staphylococci, which can reach the cavity by hematogeneous, lymphatic, or direct spread.

Tendinitis and tenovaginitis

Inflammation of tendons and tendon sheaths also frequently occurs after repetitive trauma, RA, and blood-borne infection. The tendon sheaths are of synovial derivation and demonstrate reactions resembling those of the true synovial lining cells. The pathologic state varies depending on the offending agent or disease process.[150] Acute inflammation occurs after bacterial infections with *Neisseria gonorrhoeae* and *Salmonella spp.* Granulomatous infection is seen with mycobacteria, including *M. tuberculosis, M. avium–intracellulare, M. leprae,* and *M. marinum,* the latter two reaching the tendon sheath by direct spread from contiguous soft tissues. Chronic stenosing tenosynovitis can result in greatly diminished mobility of tendons, especially at the wrist. This process occurs in RA and often contributes to loss of manual function.

Palmar aponeurotic fibromatosis

Palmar aponeurotic fibromatosis is also known as "Dupuytren's contracture," and a similar process can involve the plantar aponeuroses. The process can be divided into three phases: (1) proliferation of fibroblasts, (2) collagenization of the matrix, and (3) regression, with atrophy and greatly diminished cellularity.[150] The process is often nodular and may be confused with fibrosarcoma and nodular fasciitis during the cellular proliferation stage. The condition characteristically extends into the adjacent subcutaneous tissue and dermis, fixing the aponeuroses to the skin. The result is permanent flexion contracture of some combination of the fifth, fourth, and third digits. Men are affected more commonly than women, and bilaterality occurs in 50% of cases.[150] The proliferating cells are myofibroblasts[350] containing contractile proteins. This may be an explanation for the contractures that result from the process. Some cases appear to be hereditary.[150] An association with diabetes has been described,[351] but the syndrome of limited joint mobility in diabetes mellitus must first be differentiated.[153-157]

CYSTS OF JOINT TISSUES

Ganglion cysts

Ganglion cysts present as ovoid, movable subcutaneous nodules, most commonly on the volar surface of the wrist but also on the dorsal foot or about the knee. They are usually connected by an inconspicuous pedicle to a tendon sheath or subsynovial tissue. The pathologic state is characteristically bland (Fig. 75-38). The cysts are filled with clear mucoid material that contains delicate filaments and collagen fragments.[150] The lining of the cysts varies from a continuous layer of cells resembling synovium, to a partial lining or no lining at all. Some ganglia are not completely cystic, being composed partially of tissue resembling synovium. The histogenesis is obscure, with the dominant cause being ascribed to

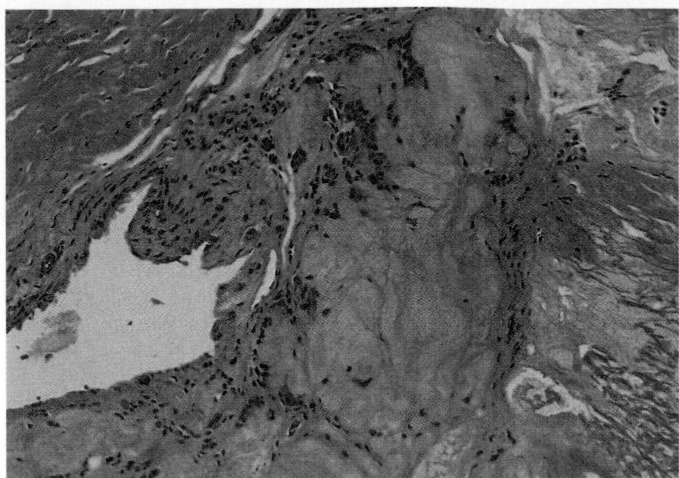

Fig. 75-38 Ganglion cyst of tendon sheath. Mucoid cyst has typical incomplete lining of flattened cells resembling synovium.

herniation or rupture of tendon sheath. They do not recur after complete excision.

Meniscal cysts

Cysts of the semilunar cartilages in the knee are relatively common.[62] They are usually located in the lateral meniscus near the anterior insertion into the synovium. Grossly they are composed of indistinct lobules filled with mucoid material. Microscopic sections resemble those of ganglion cysts, with an incomplete synovial lining and diffuse fraying of the fibrocartilage surrounding the lesion. Meniscal cysts are not seen in infants and young children, and it is therefore inferred that they are acquired, probably in a manner similar to ganglion cysts. They are not associated with either traumatic or degenerative tears of the menisci.[62]

Bursal cysts

Bursal cysts are true synovial cysts most commonly seen posterior to the knee joint. They are often associated with RA or other chronic inflammatory arthritides. In some cases the cysts communicate with the knee joint by a tortuous ductlike structure. At times a ball-valve type of mechanism can develop, allowing fluid to enter the cyst but not to return to the joint cavity. The term *Baker's cyst* is usually applied to these, though the original description by Baker in 1877 was of a variety of pathologic conditions.[352] As with any chronic inflammatory joint condition, bursal cysts may become superinfected with bacteria entering the synovium either hematogenously or directly from contiguous tissue.

TUMORS AND TUMORLIKE LESIONS OF THE JOINTS

Any component of the joint may theoretically give rise to a neoplasm. This includes the synovium, tendons, tendon sheaths, bursae, intra-articular disks, intra-articular ligaments, and even articular cartilage. In actual experience, neoplasms of the joint tissues are collectively quite rare. Some malignant neoplasms such as synovial and epithelioid sarcomas were formerly considered to arise from synovial rests. They occur within joints only on very rare occasions.[353] Evidence has accumulated that these are not of synovial derivation,[354] and they are therefore considered with the soft-tissue malignancies in Chapter 72. Likewise, the neoplasms arising in or on subchondral bone, such as osteochondroma, chondroblastoma, and giant cell tumor, are considered in Chaper 73. Narrowly defined in this manner, only a small number of primary neoplastic disorders of the joints remain (Table 75-7).

Table 75-7 Tumors of the joints

Benign
Pigmented villonodular synovitis (xanthofibroma)
Synovial chondromatosis
Synovial and tenosynovial hemangioma
Synovial lipoma (arborescens)
Tenosynovial fibroma
Malignant
Clear cell sarcoma of tendon sheath and aponeurosis
Synovial chondrosarcoma
Malignant tenosynovial giant cell tumor

Pigmented villonodular synovitis (xanthofibroma)

These tumorlike lesions exist in several forms, including the destructive synovial process known as diffuse pigmented villonodular synovitis, the localized nondestructive villonodular synovial variant, and nodular giant cell tumor of the tendon sheath. The diffuse variant occurs most commonly in young adults in whom the knee is the joint most frequently involved.[355] Occasionally other joints such as the hip, the ankle, or the shoulder may be the site. The involved joint is swollen and painful with limitation of movement. Radiographs frequently demonstrate thickening of the soft tissues without calcification, but erosion of cartilage and periarticular bone are not uncommon. Magnetic resonance imaging is particularly useful because the complex intra-articular relationships of the knee are well depicted. Grossly the lesions are villous, with brown discoloration. In the solid tissue deep to the villous surface, yellow and tan zones are frequent. These correspond to areas rich in lipid-containing macrophages and fibroblastic cells, respectively. The overall microscopic appearance[356] reveals sheets of small ovoid or spindle-shaped cells, multinucleated giant cells, macrophages, plasma cells, and a rich vascular plexus. Both the ratio between the cellular types and their distribution within the lesions is extremely variable (Fig. 75-39). Some lesions are highly cellular with demonstrable mitotic activity in the mononuclear cells. Others are sparsely cellular, being composed predominantly of fibrous tissue. The numbers of multinucleated giant cells and lipid-containing macrophages are also variable. Most lesions contain considerable numbers of pigment-laden cells staining positively with the Prussian blue reaction for ferric iron. Hemosiderin-like deposits can be found extracellularly as well.

Although the histologic appearance of the localized synovial villonodular synovitis is very similar to that of the diffuse variant, the natural history is quite different. In the localized variant, bone invasion does not occur, and recurrence after excision is uncommon, both behaviors being in contrast to the behavior of the diffuse variant.[356] Both diffuse and nodular

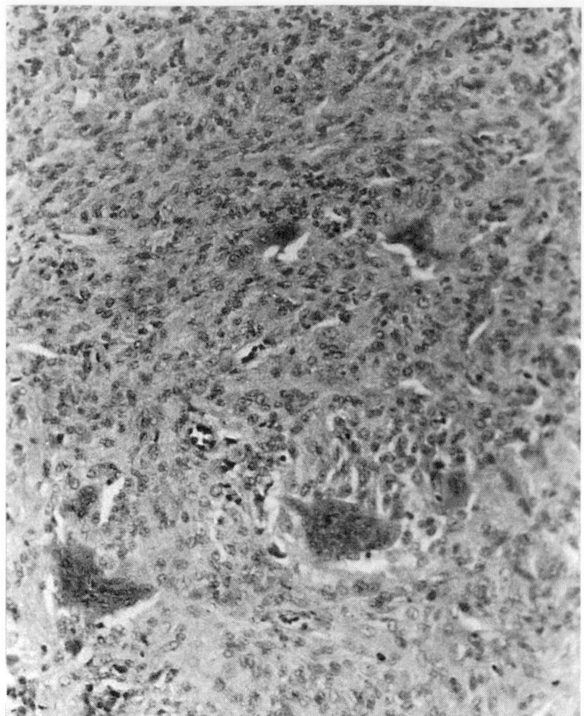

Fig. 75-39 Pigmented villonodular synovitis (xanthofibroma) of knee joint, diffuse articular type. Sheets of ovoid cells, inflammatory cells, and multinucleated giant cells are present.

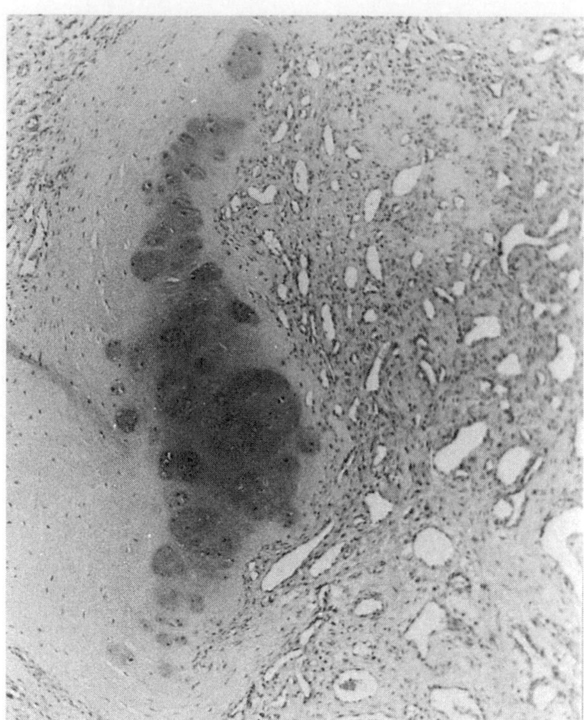

Fig. 75-40 Synovial chondromatosis. Cartilaginous nodule surrounded by zone of circumferential fibrous tissue lies in synovium. Multiple such nodules were present in the specimen.

variants frequently show areas of synovial differentiation characterized by irregular slitlike spaces lined by flattened or ovoid cells. Flow cytometric analyses of DNA content have shown that cells of the diffuse variant are frequently aneuploid, whereas those of the nodular counterpart are uniformly diploid.[357] This is in keeping with the concept that the aggressive diffuse variant is a true neoplasm.

The final and most frequent presentation of this lesion is as a "giant cell tumor" of the tendon sheath. These lesions closely resemble pigmented villonodular synovitis, with variable numbers of multinucleated giant cells, lipid-containing macrophages, and iron pigment-containing cells. These tumors present as discrete nodules, usually on the proximal digits. They occur in adults and are more common in women. Immunocytochemical studies[358] have shown both mononucleated and multinucleated cells in these lesions to have a macrophage differentiation pattern resembling that of osteoclasts. These giant cell tumors of the tendon sheath frequently contain hypocellular fibrous areas. Some authors have proposed that fibromas of the tendon sheath are actually giant cell tumors that have undergone regression.[359] Although these lesions are benign and self-limited, they may recur after inadequate excision[355] and may cause pressure erosion of adjacent bone.[360] Because of their clinical presentation, they may be confused with rheumatoid nodules, tendinous xanthomas, or infectious granulomas.[361]

Synovial chondromatosis

The unusual and rare condition synovial chondromatosis is characterized by multiple metaplastic nodules of cartilage that develop in the synovium. Some may show evidence of maturation into osseous tissue. In addition, others may detach to become loose bodies in the synovial cavity. The condition is usually seen as a monarticular disorder in young or middle-aged adults. The most common site is the knee joint,[362] but hip, elbow, and shoulder joint involvement also occurs. Unlike osteochondritis dissecans, the loose cartilaginous bodies are derived from the synovium, not from the articular surface. The pathogenesis has been examined by electron microscopy, which shows that perivascular cells accumulate at a basal lamina and subsequently display chondroid differentiation.[363] The definitive nodules are composed of mature cartilage surrounded by circumferential layers of fibrous tissue (Fig. 75-40). Severe cases may recur because of inadequate excision, and considerable disability may result. Malignant transformation to synovial chondrosarcoma has been reported[364] but is very rare.[361] Familial distribution in association with dwarfism has been described.[365] The differential diagnosis includes those conditions that cause loose bodies of the joint space and synovial nodularity, including neuropathic arthropathy, apatite arthropathy (Milwaukee shoulder-knee syndrome), CPPD disease, osteochondritis dissecans, and OA with detritic synovitis.[361]

Synovial hemangioma

The rare benign neoplasms called "synovial hemangioma" are composed of either diffuse or nodular overgrowths of blood vessels in the synovium. The knee joint is most commonly affected.[366] Because most patients are seen at adolescence, with a long history of symptoms, these tumors are believed to arise in childhood.[361] Recurrent hemarthrosis is the most common presentation. Some studies have advocated hemangiomas as a cause of some cases of pigmented villinodular synovitis.[367] At any rate, recurrent bleeding from intra-articular hemangiomas can cause degenerative joint disease resembling

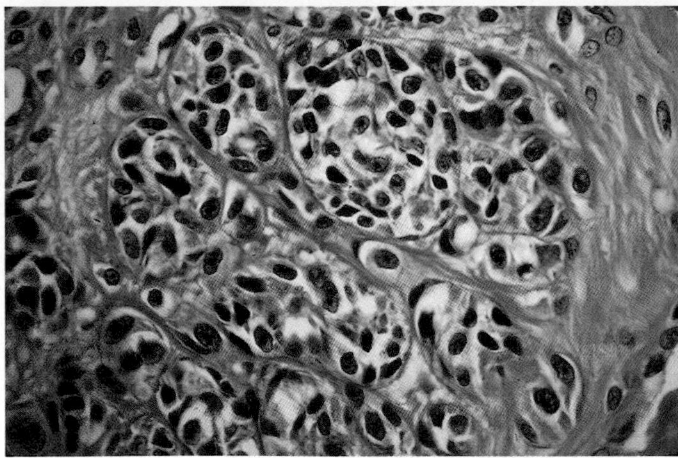

Fig. 75-41 Clear cell sarcoma of tendon sheath and aponeurosis presented as a mass on dorsum of foot. Epithelium-like ovoid cells with clear cytoplasm are characteristic.

hemophilic arthropathy.[368] The differential diagnosis includes pigmented villinodular synovitis, chronic infectious processes, and pauciarticular presentations of Still's disease. Histologically similar angiomas occur in tendon sheaths as well. Like the articular variants, they are frequently associated with cutaneous and soft-tissue hemangiomas.[361,366]

Synovial lipomas

True lipomas composed of localized nodules of mature adipose tissue are rare as an intra-articular phenomenon.[361] More common are lipomatous transformations of the synovium occurring in association with synovial hyperplasia. This condition is known as *lipoma arborescens* because of the villous appearance of the synovium. An association with osteoarthritis has been noted.[369]

Clear cell sarcoma of tendon sheaths and aponeuroses

These rare and histologically distinctive malignant neoplasms[370] are seen predominantly in young adults, and present as painless, slowly enlarging masses. The most common site is in the foot, often near the Achilles tendon or plantar aponeurosis, but the ankle, the knee, or the thigh can also harbor the neoplasm.[361] The microscopic appearance is that of nests of ovoid or fusiform, pale-staining cells with prominent nuclei (Fig. 75-41). The evidence for a neuroectodermal origin of these neoplasms is compelling. Even if melanin is not demonstrable by light microscopy, melanosomes[371,372] and S-100 protein[371-373] are present in almost all cases. Many authors regard these tumors as derived from deep melanocytic cells associated with the tendons and aponeuroses.[374] The tumor is discussed with other tumors of the joints because it is clearly associated with the tendons. The prognosis is relatively poor, with local recurrences being common and metastatic spread occurring in around 65% of patients in one recent report.[375] Unlike most other sarcomas, spread to regional lymph nodes is also frequent, occurring in about 30% of cases.[361]

Synovial chondrosarcoma

Despite the presence of articular cartilage in every joint, chondrosarcoma does not develop from this tissue. The rare articular chondrosarcomas that originate in the synovium[364] almost always do so in the setting of synovial chondromatosis[361] as previously described (Fig. 75-42).

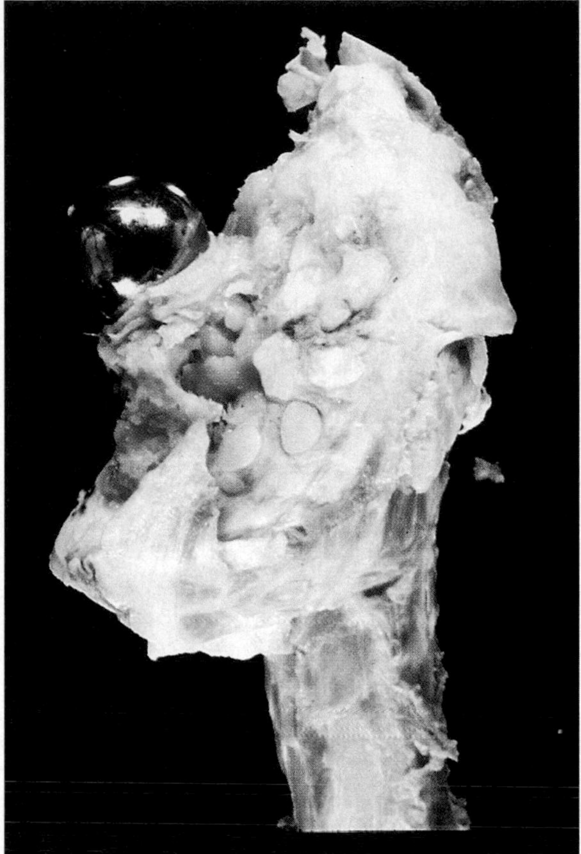

Fig. 75-42 Large chondrosarcoma arising within the hip joint cavity in a patient with long-standing, recurrent synovial chondromatosis.

Tenosynovial giant cell sarcoma

The rare neoplasm tenosynovial giant cell sarcoma[376,377] is the malignant counterpart of the much more common benign giant cell tumor of the tendon sheath. Because other neoplasms of soft tissues, such as clear cell sarcoma, fibrosarcoma, epithelioid sarcoma, and malignant fibrous histiocytoma, may resemble a malignant tenosynovial giant cell tumor, some authors reserve this diagnosis for a tumor that clearly originates as a benign giant cell tumor of the tendon sheath.[378] The histologic appearance is very similar to that of the benign counterpart, but giant cells are less numerous in malignant variants. Metastases to the lungs have been reported.[378] The relationship of abnormalities of chromosome 7, observed in some cases of nodular pigmented villinodular synovitis and tenosynovial giant cell tumor,[379] to subsequent aggressive behavior is unclear.

DISEASES OF THE VERTEBRAL COLUMN

Several types of disease may result in abnormal structure and function of the spine. Many of these conditions are primarily diseases of the bony vertebrae such as Paget's disease (osteitis deformans), osteoporosis, and osteitis fibrosa cystica (see

Table 75-8 Degenerative spondyloses

Heritable disorders
Mucopolysaccharidoses
Spondyloepiphyseal dysplasias
Osteogenesis imperfecta
Ochronotic spondylosis
Acquired disorders
Spinal osteophytosis
Hyperostotic spondylosis
Senile kyphoscoliosis
Intervertebral disk protrusion
Inflammatory spondyloses
Rheumatoid spondylitis
Ankylosing spondylitis (seronegative spondyloarthropathy, SNSA)
Infectious spondylitis

Chapter 74). Others involve heritable disorders of collagen or proteoglycan metabolism, as previously considered in this chapter. Other than chordoma (discussed in chapter 73), there are no neoplasms restricted to the vertebral column. A classification of the spinal diseases affecting the structure and function of the articulations of the spine is included in Table 75-8. Three types of gross deformity of the spine are relatively common: (1) kyphosis, or increased convexity in the anteroposterior direction; (2) lordosis, or increased concavity in the anteroposterior plane; and (3) scoliosis, or lateral deviation of the spine. Senile kyphoscoliosis is a complex disorder caused by a combination of uneven disk degeneration and frequent anterior collapse of vertebral bodies because of osteoporosis.

Disk disease

Deterioration of the intervertebral disks is very common, beginning in early adult life and progressing with age.[380] The pathologic changes are accompanied by loss of matrix metachromatic material,[58] water content,[381] and normal collagen fibrillar structure.[382] As a result, the normal mechanical properties of the disk are disturbed. There is decreased capacity of the anulus fibrosus to contain the nucleus pulposus under normal compressive loading.[2,19] Rupture of the disk material into the spinal canal, the spinal foramina, or the vertebral bodies is common, especially in the lower lumbar spine. Rupture into a vertebral body produces a bony reaction to the cartilage nodule, called a *Schmorl's node*.[383] Even without frank rupture, the reaction of the cartilaginous vertebral endplates to the process of degeneration produces a marginal osteophytosis that results in bony osteophytes projecting from the joint[382] (Fig. 75-43). This phenomenon can be seen over the length of the spine but is most likely to cause neurologic symptoms in the cervical spine.[18] There, posteriolateral osteophytes often compromise the dorsal spinal nerve roots, resulting in chronic pain (Fig. 75-44).

Hyperostotic spondylosis

The relatively frequently occurring condition hyperostotic spondylosis affects middle-aged to elderly males[58,76] and is more common in diabetics.[89] It is characterized by bony ankylosis along the anterior portions of the spine, accompanied by dense bony sclerosis of the contiguous portions of the vertebral bodies (Fig. 75-45). Unlike ordinary spinal osteophytosis, concomitant disk space degeneration is not present. A possible

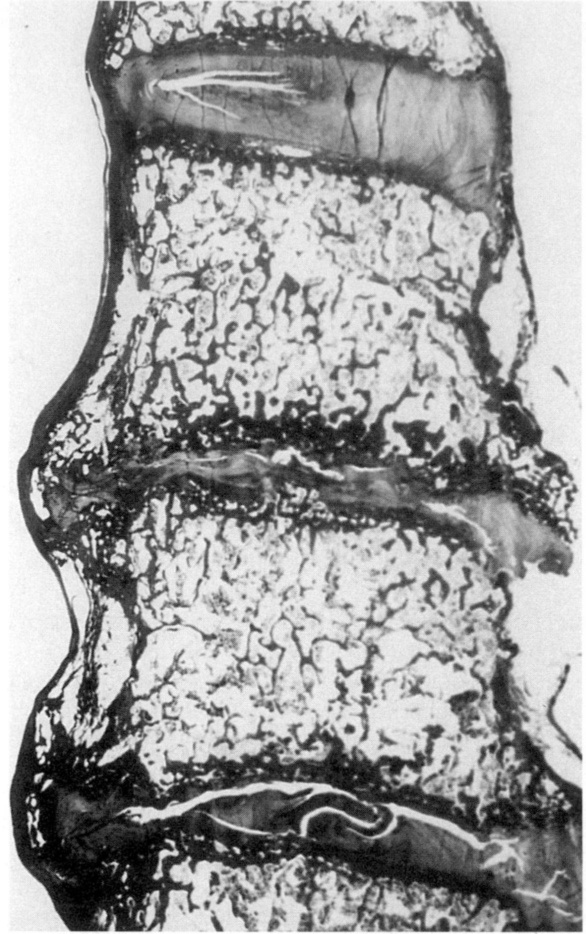

Fig. 75-43 Osteophytosis of lumbar spine. Degeneration of intervertebral disks is associated with both posterior and anterior osteophytes.

relationship to growth hormone excess has been advocated.[89] The condition is often associated with the syndrome of diffuse idiopathic skeletal hyperostosis (DISH) characterized by excessive osteophyte formation in peripheral joints.[384]

Inflammatory spinal disease

The principal diseases to be distinguished are rheumatoid spondylitis, ankylosing spondylitis (and other SNSA), and infectious spondylitis (especially that attributable to *M. tuberculosis*). The pathogenesis of these conditions has been discussed earlier in connection with disease of the peripheral joints. Rheumatoid arthritis causes distinctive discovertebral erosions,[276,277] especially in the upper cervical spine.[18] The diarthrodial joints contain destructive pannus as well[263,276] and ligament destruction predisposes to subluxation of the upper cervical vertebrae, often with devastating neurologic sequelae.[277] Ankylosis does not ordinarily develop.

On the other hand, ankylosing spondylitis begins with inflammation of the tendinous insertions (enthesopathy) at the junction with the vertebral end plates.[112] This causes initial osteolytic "squaring off" of the vertebra, followed by subsequent ossification across both the disk margin and the facet joints.[385] Thus, the two diseases are as distinct in their spinal manifestations as they are in the peripheral joints.

Tuberculous spondylitis is particularly likely to present with disease that is limited to one or two vertebrae, with

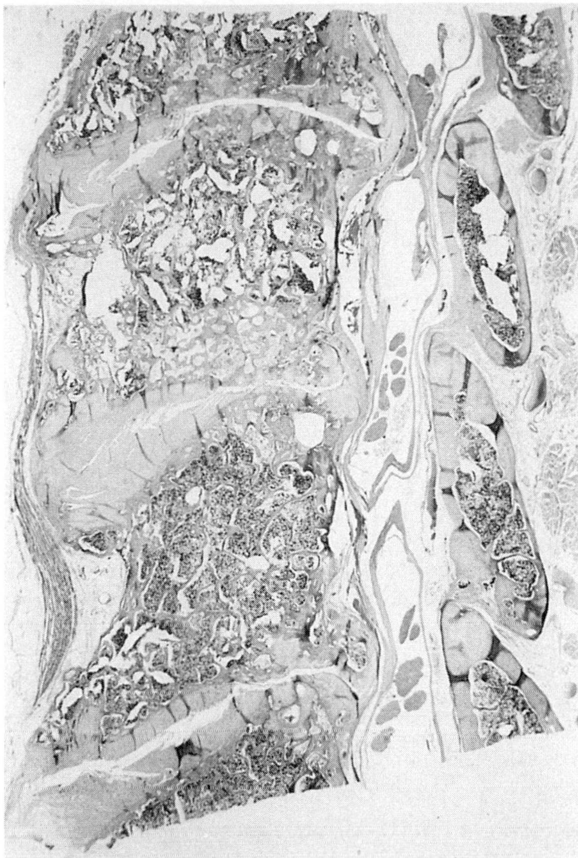

Fig. 75-44 Osteophytosis of cervical spine (cervical spondylosis). Posterior osteophytes compress the dorsal spinal nerves within the dural sheath.

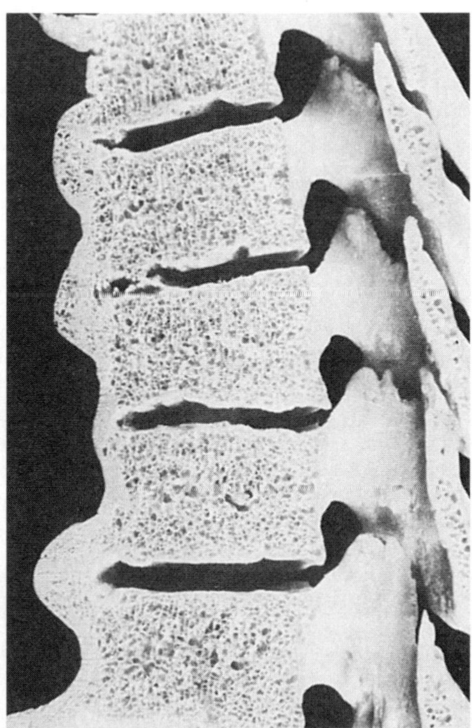

Fig. 75-45 Hyperostotic spondylosis, macerated specimen. Anterior fusion of vertebral bodies by osseous bridges. (Courtesy Dr. Max Aufdermaur, Lucerne, Switzerland).

destruction of both bone and disk tissues. Pathologic ossification and facet joint involvement are not characteristic, but gradual disappearance of the disk space is the rule.[112] Distinction of tuberculous from rheumatoid or ankylosing spondylitis is facilitated by the presence of prominent extraspinal manifestations in the latter two entities. Infection of the disk space by pyogenic bacteria is usually by hematogenous spread in immunosuppressed individuals. Unlike tuberculous spondylitis, contiguous osteomyelitis is usually not present, and the disk destruction is rapid.

REFERENCES

Development, structure, and function

1. Gray H: *Anatomy of the human body,* Clemente C, editor of edition 30, Philadelphia, 1985, Lea & Febiger.
2. Mankin HJ, Radin EL: Structure and function of joints. In McCarty DJ, Koopman WJ, editors: *Arthritis and allied conditions,* ed 12, Philadelphia, 1993, Lea & Febiger.
3. Urist M: The origin of cartilage: investigations in quest of chondrogenic DNA. In Hall BK, editor: *Cartilage,* vol 2, *Development, differentiation and growth,* New York, 1983, Academic Press.
4. O'Rahilly R, Gardner E: The embryology of movable joints. In Sokoloff L, editor: *The joints and synovial fluid,* vol 1, New York, 1978, Academic Press.
5. Thorogood P: Morphogenesis of cartilage. In Hall BK, editor: *Cartilage,* vol 2, *Development, differentiation and growth,* New York, 1983, Academic Press.
6. Redler I: The ultrastructure and biochemical significance of the tidemark of articular cartilage, *Clin Orthop* 112:357, 1975.
7. Revell PA, Pirie C, Amir G et al: Metabolic activity in the calcified zone of cartilage: observations on tetracycline labelled articular cartilage in human osteoarthritic hips, *Rheumatol Int* 10:143, 1990.
8. Oettmeier R, Abendroth K, Oettmeier S: Analyses of the tidemark on human femoral heads, *Acta Morphol Hung* 37:169, 1989.
9. Hirotani H, Ito T: Chondrocyte mitosis in the articular cartilage of femoral heads with various diseases, *Acta Orthop Scand* 46:979, 1975.
10. Ghadially FN: Fine structure of joints. In Sokoloff L, editor: *The joints and synovial fluid,* vol 1, New York 1978, Academic Press.
11. Prockop DJ, Williams CJ, Vandenberg P: Collagen in normal and diseased connective tissue. In McCarty DJ, Koopman WJ, editors: *Arthritis and allied conditions* ed 12, Philadelphia, 1993, Lea & Febiger.
12. Burgeson RE, Nimni ME: Collagen types: molecular structure and tissue distribution, *Clin Orthop* 282:250, 1992.
13. Kuettner KE: Biochemistry of articular cartilage in health and disease, *Clin Biochem,* 25:155, 1992.
14. Hardingham TE: Cartilage proteoglycans, *Ciba Found Symp* 124:30, 1986.
15. Grushko G, Schneiderman R, Maroudas A: Some biochemical and biophysical parameters for the study of the pathogenesis of osteoarthritis: a comparison between the processes of aging and degeneration in human hip cartilage, *Connect Tissue Res* 19:149, 1989.
16. Rosenberg L: Structure and function of cartilage proteoglycans. In McCarty DJ, Koopman WJ, editors: *Arthritis and allied conditions,* ed 12, Philadelphia, 1993, Lea & Febiger.
17. Hardingham TE, Bayliss M: Proteoglycans of articular cartilage: changes in aging and in joint disease, *Semin Arthritis Rheum* 205:12, 1990.
18. Bland JH: *Disorders of the cervical spine: diagnosis and medical management,* Philadelphia, 1987, Saunders.
19. Broberg KB: On the mechanical behavior of intervertebral discs, *Spine* 8:151, 1983.

Basic principles of methodology and diagnosis

20. Page KM, Stevens A, Lowe J et. al: Bone. In Bancroft JD, Stevens A, editors: *theory and practice of histological techniques,* ed 3, Edinburgh, 1990, Churchill Livingston.
21. Lestini WF, Wiesel SW: Pathogenesis of cervical spondylosis, *Clin Orthop* 239:69, 1989.

22. Milgram JW: Osteoarthritis (degenerative joint disease). In *Radiologic and histologic pathology of nontumorous diseases of bones and joints,* Northbrook, Ill., 1990, Northbrook Publishing.
23. Resnick D, Niwayama G: Degenerative joint diseases. In *Diagnosis of bone and joint disorders,* vol 2, Philadelphia, 1981, Saunders.
24. Monson NL, Haughton VM, Modl JM et al: Normal and degenerating articular cartilage: in vitro correlation of MR imaging and histologic findings, *J Magn Reson Imaging* 2:41, 1992.
25. Felson DT: Epidemiology of the rheumatic diseases. In McCarty DJ, Koopman WJ, editors: *Arthritis and allied conditions,* ed 12, Philadelphia, 1993, Lea & Febiger.
26. Hochberg MC, Lethbridge-Cejku M, Plato CC et al: Factors associated with osteoarthritis of the hand in males: data from the Baltimore longitudince study of aging, *Am J Epidemiol* 134:1121, 1991.
27. Howell DS, Pelletier J-P: Etiopathogenesis of osteoarthritis. In McCarty DJ, Koopman WJ, editors: *Arthritis and allied conditions,* ed 12, Philadelphia, 1993, Lea & Febiger.
28. Bernhard G: Extra-articular rheumatoid arthritis: clinical features and treatment overview. In Utsinger PD, Zvaifler NJ, Ehrlich GE, editors: *Rheumatoid arthritis,* Philadelphia, 1985, Lippincott.
29. McCarty DJ: The Heberden Oration 1982: Crystals, joints and consternation, *Ann Rheum Dis,* 42:243, 1983.
30. Adamson TC, Resnik CS, Guerra J et al: Hand and wrist arthropathies of hemochromatosis and calcium pyrophosphate deposition disease, *Radiology* 147:377, 1983.
31. Pritchard MH, Jessop JD: Chondrocalcinosis in primary hyperparathyroidism, *Ann Rheum Dis* 36:146, 1977.
32. Ryan LM, McCarty DJ: Calcium pyrophosphate crystal deposition disease, pseudogout, articular chondrocalcinosis. In McCarty DJ, Koopman WJ, editors: *Arthritis and allied conditions,* ed 12, Philadelphia, 1993, Lea & Febiger.
33. Layton, MW, Fudman EJ, Barker A et al: Acromegalic arthropathy: characteristics and response to therapy, *Arthritis Rheum* 31:1022, 1988.
34. Cimmino MA, Cutolo M: Plasma glucose concentration in symptomatic osteoarthritis: a clinical and epidemiological survey, *Clin Exp Rheumatol* 8:251, 1990.
35. Rothfield NF: Systemic lupus erythematosus: clinical aspects and treatment. In McCarty DJ, Koopman WJ, editors: *Arthritis and allied conditions,* ed 12, Philadelphia, 1993, Lea & Febiger.

Congenital malformations, deformations, and defects

36. Pyeritz RE: Heritable and developmental disorders of connective tissue and bone. In McCarty DJ, Koopman WJ, editors: *Arthritis and allied conditions,* ed 12, Philadelphia, 1993, Lea & Febiger.
37. Palotie A, Väisänen P, Ott J et al: Predisposition to familial osteoarthroses linked to type II collagen gene, *Lancet* 1:924, 1989.
38. Knowlton RG, Katzenstein PL, Moskowitz RW et al: Genetic linkage of a polymorphism in the type II procollagen gene (COL2A1) to primary osteoarthritis associated with mild chondrodysplasia, *N Engl J Med* 322:526, 1990.
39. Neufeld EF, Meunzer Z: The mucopolysaccharidoses. In Scriver CR, Beaudet AL, Sly WS, Valle D, editors: *The metabolic basis of inherited disease,* ed 6, New York, 1989, McGraw-Hill.
40. Schumacher HR: Ochronosis, hemochromatosis, and Wilson's disease. In McCarty DJ, Koopman WJ, editors: *Arthritis and allied conditions,* ed 12, Philadelphia, 1993, Lea & Febiger.
41. Wigglesworth JS: Principles of developmental pathology. In McGee JO, Isaacson PG, Wright NA, editors: *Oxford textbook of pathology,* vol 1, Oxford, 1992, Oxford University Press.
42. Weyand CM, Hicok KC, Conn DL et al: The influence of HLA-DRB1 genes on disease severity in rheumatoid arthritis, *Ann Intern Med* 117:801, 1992.
43. Pattrick M, Manhire A, Ward AM et al: HLA-A, B antigens and alpha$_1$-antitrypsin phenotypes in nodal generalized osteoarthritis and erosive osteoarthritis, *Ann Rheum Dis* 48:470, 1989.
44. Beighton PM, De Paepe A, Hall JG et al: Molecular nosology of the heritable disorders of connective tissue, *Am J Med Genet* 42:431, 1992.
45. Byers PH: Disorders of collagen biosynthesis and structure, In Scriver CR, Beaudet AL, Sly WS, Valle D, editors: *The metabolic basis of inherited disease,* ed 6, New York, 1989, McGraw-Hill.
46. Tredwell SJ: Neonatal screening for hip joint instability, *Clin Orthop* 281:63, 1992.
47. Wilkinson JA: Etiologic factors in congenital displacement of the hip and myelodysplasia, *Clin Orthop* 281:75, 1992.
48. Smith DW: Recognizable patterns of human deformation: identification and management of mechanical effects on morphogenesis, *Major Probl Clin Pediatr* 21:1, 1981.
49. Udén A, Lindhagen T et al: Inguinal hernia in patients with congenital hip dislocation, *Acta Orthop Scand* 59:667, 1988.
50. Silberberg R: The skeleton in diabetes mellitus: a review of the literature, *Diabetes Res* 3:329, 1986.
51. Hod M, Merlob P, Friedman S et al: Prevalence of congenital anomalies and neonatal complications in the offspring of diabetic mothers in Israel, *Isr J Med Sci* 27:498, 1991.
52. Stulberg SD: The etiology and natural course of osteoarthritis of the hip (coxarthrosis). In Moskowitz RW, Howell DS, Goldberg VM, Mankin HJ, editors: *Osteoarthritis: diagnosis and management,* Philadelphia, 1984, Saunders.
53. Gamble JG, Rinsky LA, Bleck EE: Established hip dislocations in cerebral palsy, *Clin Orthop* 253:90, 1990.
54. Nelson KB, Ellenberg JH: Antecedents of cerebral palsy: multivariate analysis of risk, *N Engl J Med,* 315:81, 1986.
55. Coorssen EA, Msall ME, Duffy LC: Multiple minor malformations as a marker for prenatal etiology of cerebral palsy, *Dev Med Child Neurol* 33:730, 1991.
56. Hall JG, Reed SD, Scott JG et al: Three distinct types of X-linked arthrogryposes seen in 6 families, *Clin Genet* 21:81, 1982.

Degenerative and traumatic joint diseases

Traumatic arthritis

57. Pinals RS: Traumatic arthritis and allied conditions. In McCarty DJ, Koopman WH, editors: *Arthritis and allied conditions,* ed 12, Philadelphia, 1993, Lea & Febiger.
58. Hough AJ: Pathology of osteoarthritis, In McCarty DJ, Koopman WJ, editors: *Arthritis and allied conditions,* ed 12, Philadelphia, 1993, Lea & Febiger.
59. Albright JA, Misra RP: Mechanisms of resorption and remodeling of cartilage. In Hall BK, editor: *Cartilage,* vol 3, *Biomedical aspects,* New York, 1983, Academic Press.
60. Milgram JW, Rana NA: The pathology of the failed cup arthroplasty, *Clin Orthop* 158:159, 1981.
61. Pond MJ, Nuki G: Experimentally-induced osteoarthritis in the dog, *Ann Rheum Dis* 32:387, 1973.
62. Hough AJ, Webber RJ: Pathology of the meniscus, *Clin Orthop* 252:3, 1990.
63. Silber TJ, Majd M: Reflex sympathetic dystrophy syndrome in children and adolescents: report of 18 cases and review of the literature, *Am J Dis Child* 142:1325, 1988.
64. Lane NE, Bloch DA, Hubert HB et al: Long-distance running, bone density, and osteoarthritis, *JAMA* 255:1147, 1986.
65. Konradsen L, Hansen E-MB, Sundergaard L: Long-distance running and osteoarthrosis, *Am J Sports Med* 18:379, 1990.
66. Burke MD, Fear EC, Wright V: Bone and joint changes in pneumatic drillers, *Ann Rheum Dis* 36:276, 1977.
67. Bovenzi M, Petronio L, DiMarino F: Epidemiological survey of shipyard workers exposed to hand-arm vibration, *Int Arch Occup Environ Health* 46:251, 1980.
68. Klunder KB, Rud B, Hansen J: Osteoarthritis of the hip and knee in retired football players, *Acta Orthop Scand* 51:925, 1980.
69. Lindberg H, Montgomery F: Heavy labor and the occurrence of gonarthrosis, *Clin Orthop* 214:235, 1987.
70. Koszyca B, Fazzalari NL, Vernon-Roberts N: Microfractures in coxarthrosis, *Acta Orthop Scand* 61:307, 1990.

Osteoarthritis

71. Ilardi CF, Sokoloff L: Secondary osteonecrosis in osteoarthritis of the femoral head: a pathological study, *Hum Pathol* 15:79, 1984.

72. Wong SYP, Evans RA, Needs C et al: The pathogenesis of osteoarthritis of the hip: evidence for primary osteocyte death, *Clin Orthop* 214:305, 1987.
73. Fazzalari NL, Vernon-Roberts B, Darracott J: Osteoarthritis of the hip: possible protective and causative roles of trabecular microfractures in the head of the femur, *Clin Orthop* 216:224, 1987.
74. Peyron JG: The epidemiology of osteoarthritis. In Moskowitz R, Howel DS, Goldberg V, Mankin H, editors: *Osteoarthritis: diagnosis and management,* Philadelphia, 1984, Saunders.
75. Kempson GE: Age-related changes in the tensile properties of human articular cartilage: a comparative study between the femoral head of the hip joint and the talus of the ankle joint, *Biochim Biophys* Acta 1075:223, 1991.
76. Moskowitz RW: Clinical and laboratory findings in osteoarthritis. In McCarty DJ, Koopman WJ, editors: *Arthritis and allied conditions,* ed 12, Philadelphia, 1993, Lea & Febiger.
77. Croft P, Cooper C, Wickham C, Coggon D: Is the hip involved in generalized osteoarthritis? *Br J Rheumatol* 31:325, 1992.
78. Radin EL, Rose RM: Role of subchondral bone in the initiation and progression of cartilage damage, *Clin Orthop* 213:34, 1986.
79. McDevitt CA, Miller RR: Biochemistry, cell biology, and immunology of osteoarthritis, *Curr Opin Rheumatol* 1:303, 1989.
80. Hamerman D: The biology of osteoarthritis, *N Engl J Med* 320:1322, 1989.
81. Sokoloff L: Osteoarthritis as a remodeling process, *J Rheumatol* 14 (suppl 14):7, 1987.
82. Soren A, Cooper NS, Waugh TR: The nature and designation of osteoarthritis determined by the histopathology, *Clin Exp Rheumatol* 6:41, 1988.
83. Mitrovic DR, Riera H: Synovial, articular cartilage and bone changes in rapidly destructive arthropathy (osteoarthritis) of the hip, *Rheumatol Int* 12:17, 1992.
84. Hutton CW, Higgs ER, Jackson PC et al: ^{99m}Tc-HMDP bone scanning in generalized nodal osteoarthritis: the four-hour bone scan image predicts radiographic change, *Ann Rheum Dis* 45:617, 1986.
85. Ali SY, Rees JA, Scotchford CA: Microcrystal deposition in cartilage and in osteoarthritis, *Bone Miner* 17:115, 1992.
86. Hopkinson ND, Powell RJ, Doherty M: Autoantibodies, immunoglobulins, and G_m allotypes in nodal generalized osteoarthritis, *Br J Rheumatol* 31:605, 1992.
87. Cooke TD: Which comes first: inflammation or osteoarthritis? Relationship of immune deposits in articular collagenous tissues to synovitis in osteoarthritis. In Cook TD, Dwosh I, Cossairt J, editors: Clinical Pathological Osteoarthritis Workshop, *J Rheumatol* 10(suppl 9):55, 1983.
88. Balblanc JC, Vignon E, Mathieu P et al: Cytokines, prostaglandin E_2, phospholipase A and metalloproteases in synovial fluid in osteoarthritis, *Rev Rhumatol Malad Osteo-Articulaires* 58:343, 1991.
89. Moskowitz RW, Boja B, Denko CW: The role of growth factors in degenerative joint disorders, *J Rheumatol* 27(suppl):147, 1991.
90. Streda A: Participation of osteonecrosis in the development of severe coxarthrosis, *Acta Univ Carol* [Med] (Praha) 46:103, 1971.
91. Ahuja SA, Bullough PG: Osteonecrosis of the knee: a clinicopathological study in twenty-eight patients, *J Bone Joint Surg* 60A:191, 1978.

Osteoarthritis with specific disease states

92. Dehaven KE, Dolan WA, Mayer PJ: Chondromalacia patellae in athletes, *Am J Sports Med* 7:1, 1979.
93. Weisman MH: Arthritis associated with hematologic disorders, storage diseases, disorders of lipid metabolism, and dysproteinemias. In McCarty DJ, Koopman WJ, editors: *Arthritis and allied conditions,* Philadelphia, 1993, Lea & Febiger.
94. Mosher DF: Disorders of blood coagulation. In Wyngaarden JB, Smith LH, Bennett JC, editors: *Cecil's textbook of medicine,* ed 19, Philadelphia, 1992, Saunders.
95. Mainardi CL, Levine PH, Werb Z, Harris ED: Proliferative synovitis in hemophilia: biochemical and morphological observations, *Arthritis Rheum,* 21:137, 1978.
96. McLarady-Smith PD, Ashton IK, Duthie RB: A tissue culture model of cartilage breakdown in haemophilic arthropathy, *Scand J Haematol* 40(suppl):215, 1984.
97. Hough AJ, Banfield WG, Sokoloff L: Cartilage in hemophilic arthropathy: ultrastructural and microanalytical studies, *Arch Pathol Lab Med* 100:91, 1976.
98. Cartwright GE, Edwards CQ, Kravitz K: Hereditary hemochromatosis: phenotypic expression of the disease, *N Engl J Med* 301:175, 1979.
99. Dymock IW, Hamilton EB, Laws JW et al: Arthropathy of hemochromatosis, *Ann Rheum Dis* 29:469, 1970.
100. Schumacher HR: Articular cartilage in the degenerative arthropathy of hemochromatosis, *Arthritis Rheum* 25:1460, 1982.
101. McCarty OJ, Pepe PF: Erythrocyte neutral inorganic pyrophosphatase in pseudogout, *J Lab Clin Med* 79:277, 1972.
102. Schumacher HR: Ultrastructural characteristics of the synovial membrane in idiopathic hemochromatosis, *Ann Rheum Dis* 31:465, 1972.
103 Menerey KA, Eider W, Brewer GJ et al: The arthropathy of Wilson's disease, *J Rheumatol,* 15:331, 1988.
104. Kaklamanis P, Spengos M: Osteoarticular change and synovial biopsy findings in Wilson's disease, *Ann Rheum Dis* 32:422, 1973.
105. Schumacher HR, Holdsworth DE: Ochronotic arthropathy I Clinicopathologic aspects, *Semin Arthritis Rheum* 6:207, 1977.
106. O'Brien WM, LaDu DN, Bunim JJ: Biochemistry, pathologic and clinical aspects of alkaptonuria, chronosis and ochronotic arthropathy, *Am J Med* 34:813, 1963.
107. Angeles AP, Badger R, Gruber H, Seegmiller JE: Chondrocyte growth inhibition induced by homogentisic acid and its partial prevention with ascorbic acid, *J Rheumatol,* 16:512, 1989.
108. Lagier R: The concept of osteoarthritic remodeling as illustrated by ochronotic arthropathy of the hip: an anatomicroradiological approach, *Virchows Arch [A]* 385:293, 1980.
109. Pritzker KPH: The articular-skeletal system: muscle, fat, and other connective tissues. In Kovacs K, Asa SL, editors: *Functional endocrine pathology,* vol 2, Boston, 1991, Blackwell Scientific.
110. Cronin ME: Rheumatic aspects of endocrinopathies. In McCarty DJ, Koopman WJ, editors: *Arthritis and allied conditions,* ed 12, Philadelphia, 1993, Lea & Febiger.
111. Bluestone R, Bywaters EGL, Hartog M et al: Acromegalic arthropathy, *Ann Rheum Dis* 30:243, 1971.
112. Gardner DL: General pathology of the peripheral joints. In Sokoloff L, editor: *The joints and synovial fluid,* vol 2, New York, 1980, Academic Press.
113. Bywaters EGL: The pathology of the spine. In Sokoloff L, editor: *The joints and synovial fluid,* vol 2, New York, 1980, Academic Press.
114. Solomon L: Patterns of osteoarthritis of the hip, *J Bone Joint Surg* 58B:176, 1976.
115. Meachim G, Whithouse GH, Pedley RD et al: An investigation of radiological, clinical, and pathological correlations in osteoarthrosis of the hip, *Clin Radiol* 31:565, 1980.
116. Jones JP Jr: Osteonecrosis. In McCarty DJ, Koopman WJ, editors: *Arthritis and allied conditions,* ed 12, Philadelphia, 1993, Lea & Febiger.
117. Jones JP Jr: Intravascular coagulation and osteonecrosis, *Clin Orthop* 277:41, 1992.
118. Ohzono K, Saito M, Takaoka K et al: Natural history of nontraumatic avascular necrosis of the femoral head, *J Bone Joint Surg* 73A:134, 1991.
119. Bowen JR, Foster BK, Hartzell CR: Legg-Calvé-Perthes disease, *Clin Orthop* 185:97, 1984.
120. Leitch JM, Patterson DC, Foster BK: Growth disturbance in Legg-Calvé-Perthes disease and the consequences of surgical treatment, *Clin Orthop* 262:178, 1991.
121. Soto-Hall R, Johnson LH, Johnson RA: Variations in the hip joint in injury and disease, *J Bone Joint Surg* 46A:509, 1964.
122. Caterall A, Pringle J, Byers PD et al: A review of the morphology of Perthes disease, *J Bone Joint Surg* 64B:269, 1982.
123. Milgram JW: Idiopathic osteonecorsis of the juvenile femoral head. In *Radiologic and histologic pathology of nontumorous diseases of bones and joints,* vol 2, Northbrook, Ill, 1990, Northbrook Publishing.
124. Aadalen RJ, Wiener DS, Hoyt W, Herndon CH: Acute slipped capital femoral epihysis, *J Bone Joint Surg* 56A:1473, 1974.
125. Milgram JW: Growth plate fractures. In *Radiologic and histologic pathology of nontumorous diseases of bones and joints,* vol 2, Northbrook, Ill, 1990, Northbrook Publishing.

126. Maussen JPG, Rozing PM, Obermann MD: Intertrochanteric osteotomy in slipped capital femoral epiphysis, *Clin Orthop* 259:100, 1990.
127. Sokoloff L: Endemic forms of osteoarthritis, *Clin Rheum Dis* 11:187, 1985.
128. Sokoloff L: The history of Kashin-Beck disease, *NY State J Med* 89:343, 1989.
129. Nesterov AI: The clinical course of Kashin-Beck disease, *Arthritis Rheum* 7:29, 1964.
130. Yang C, Bodo M, Holger N et al: Fulvic acid disturbs processing of procollagen II in articular cartilage of embryonic chicken and may also cause Kashin-Beck disease, *Eur J Biochem,* 202:1141, 1991.
131. Jiang YF, Xu GL: Selenium in biology and medicine. In Wendel A, editor: *Selenium in biology and medicine,* Berlin, 1989, Springer-Verlag.
132. Wei XQ, Wright GC, Sokoloff L: The effect of sodium selenite on chondrocytes in monolayer culture, *Arthritis Rheum* 29:660, 1986.
133. Solomon L: Distinct types of hip disorder in Mseleni joint disease, *S Afr Med J* 69:15, 1986.
134. Sokoloff L, Fincham JE, duToit GT: Pathological features of the femoral head in Mseleni disease, *Hum Pathol* 16:117, 1985.
135. Schnitzler CM, Pieczkowski WM, Fredlund V et al: Histomorphometric analysis of osteopenia associated with endemic osteoarthritis (Mseleni joint disease), *Bone* 9:21, 1988.

Other degenerative joint diseases

136. Brower AC, Allman RM: The neuropathic joint: a neurovascular bone disorder, *Radiol Clin North Am* 19:571, 1981.
137. Ellman MH: Neuropathic joint disease (Charcot joints). In McCarty DJ, Koopman WJ, editors: *Arthritis and allied conditions,* ed 12, Philadelphia, 1993, Lea & Febiger.
138. Raju UB, Fine G, Partemian JO: Diabetic neuroarthropathy (Charcot's joint), *Arch Pathol Lab Med* 106:349, 1982.
139. Menkes CJ, Simon F, Delrieu F et al: Destructive arthropathy in chondrocalcinosis articularis, *Arthritis Rheum,* 19 (suppl 3):329, 1976.
140. Connor BL, Palmoski MJ, Brandt KD: Neurogenic acceleration of degenerative joint lesions, *J Bone Joint Surg* 67A:562, 1985.
141. Cohen AS: Amyloidosis. In McCarty DJ, Koopman WJ, editors: *Arthritis and allied conditions,* ed 12, Philadelphia, 1993, Lea & Febiger.
142. Hickling P, Wilkens M, Newman GR: A study of arthropathy in multiple myeloma, Q J Med 200:417, 1981.
143. Sethi D, Naunton-Morgan TC, Brown EA et al: Dialysis arthropathy: a clinical, biochemical, radiological and histological study of 36 patients, *O J Med* 77:1061, 1990.
144. Bardin T, Kuntz D, Zingraff J et al: Synovial amyloidosis in patients undergoing long term hemodialysis, *Arthritis Rheum* 28:1052, 1985.
145. Egan MS, Goldenberg DL, Cohen AS, Segal D: The association of amyloid deposits and osteoarthritis, *Arthritis Rheum* 25:204, 1982.
146. Goffin YA, Thova Y, Potvliege PR: Micro-deposition of amyloid in the joints, *Ann Rheum Dis,* 40:27, 1981.
147. Altman RD: Hypertrophic osteoarthropathy. In McCarty DJ, Koopman WJ, editors: *Arthritis and allied conditions,* ed 12, Philadelphia, 1993, Lea & Febiger.
148. Schumacher HR: Articular manifestations of HPO in bronchogenic carcinoma: a clinical and pathologic study, *Arthritis Rheum* 19:629, 1976.
149. Martinez-Lavin M, Pineda C, Valdez T et al: Primary hypertrophic osteoarthropathy, *Semin Arthritis Rheum* 17:156, 1988.
150. Silberberg R: Diseases of joints. In Kissane JM, editor: *Anderson's pathology,* ed 9, St. Louis, 1990, Mosby.
151. Phillips HO, Grubb SA: Familial multiple osteochondritis dissecans, *J Bone Joint Surg* 67A:155, 1985.
152. Mubarak SJ, Carroll NC: Familial osteochondritis dissecans of the knee, *Clin Orthop* 140:131, 1979.
153. Pal B, Anderson J, Dick WC et al: Limitation of joint mobility and shoulder capsulitis in insulin- and non-insulin-dependent diabetes mellitus, *Br J Rheumatol* 25:147, 1986.
154. Sukenik S, Weitzman S, Buskila D et al: Limited joint mobility and other rheumatological manifestations in diabetic patients, *Diabetes Metab Rev* 13:187, 1987.
155. Monnier VM, Kohn RR, Cerami A: Accelerated age-related browning of human collagen in diabetes mellitus, *Proc Natl Acad Sci USA* 81:583, 1984.
156. Rosenbloom AL: Skeletal and joint manifestations of childhood diabetes, *Pediatr Clin North Am* 31:569, 1984.
157. Mitchell WS, Winocour PH, Gush RJ et al: Skin blood flow and limited joint mobility in insulin-dependent diabetes mellitus, *Br J Rheumatol* 28:195, 1989.

Infectious arthritis

158. Johnston YE, Duray PH, Steere AC et al: Lyme arthritis: spirochetes found in synovial microangiopathic lesions, *Am J Pathol* 118:26, 1985.
159. Keat AC, Thomas BJ, Hughes R, Taylor-Robinson D: *Chlamydia trachomatis* in reactive arthritis, *Rheumatol Int* 9:197, 1989.
160. Sieper J, Kingsley G, Palacios-Boix A et al: Synovial T-lymphocyte–specific immune response to *Chlamydia trachomatis* in Reiter's disease, *Arthritis Rheum* 34:588, 1991.
161. Merilahti-Palo R, Söderström K-O, Lahesmaa-Rantala R et al: Bacterial antigens in synovial biopsy specimens in yersinia triggered reactive arthritis, *Ann Rheum Dis* 50:87, 1991.
162. Keat A: Infections and the immunopathogenesis of seronegative spondyloarthropathies, *Curr Opin Rheumatol* 4:494, 1992.
163. Ho G Jr: Bacterial arthritis. In McCarty DJ, Koopman WJ, editors: *Arthritis and allied conditions,* ed 12, Philadelphia, 1993, Lea & Febiger.
164. Paterson MP, Hoffman EB, Roux P: Severe disseminated staphylococcal disease associated with osteitis and septic arthritis, *J Bone Joint Surg* 72B:94, 1990.
165. Brancos MA, Peris P, Miro JM et al: Septic arthritis in heroin addicts, *Semin Arthritis Rheum* 21:81, 1991.
166. Poole AR: Cartilage in health and disease. In McCarty DJ, Koopman WJ, editors: *Arthritis and allied conditions,* ed 12, Philadelphia, 1993, Lea & Febiger.
167. Ytterberg SR: Viral arthritis. In, McCarty DJ, Koopman WJ, editors: *Arthritis and allied conditions,* ed 12, Philadelphia, 1993, Lea & Febiger.
168. Ford OK, Reid GO, Tingle AJ et al: Sequential follow-up observations of a patient with rubella associated with persistent arthritis, *Ann Rheum Dis* 51:407, 1992.
169. Birkenfield P, Haratz N, Klein G et al: Cross-reactivity between EBNA-1 p107 peptide, collagen, and keratin: implications for the pathogenesis of rheumatoid arthritis, *Clin Immunol Immunopathol* 54:14, 1990.
170. Burastero SE, Cutolo M, Dessi V et al: Monoreactive and polyreactive rheumatoid factors produced by in vitro Epstein-Barr virus–transformed peripheral blood and synovial B-lymphocytes from rheumatoid arthritis patients, *Scand J Immunol* 32:347, 1990.
171. Peterson J, Rhodes G, Roudier J et al: Altered immune response to glycine-rich sequences of Epstein-Barr nuclear antigen-1 in patients with rheumatoid arthritis and systemic lupus erythematosus, *Arthritis Rheum* 33:993, 1990.
172. Zvaifler NJ: Etiology and pathogenesis of rheumatoid arthritis. In McCarty DJ, Koopman WJ, editors: *Arthritis and allied conditions,* ed 12, Philadelphia, 1993, Lea & Febiger.
173. McCormick JN, Wojtacha D, Edmond E: Detection of cytomegalovirus antigens in phagocytosed serum complexes from a patient with rheumatoid arthritis, vasculitis, peripheral neuropathy, cutaneous ulceration, and digital gangrene, *Ann Rheum Dis* 51:553, 1992.
174. Inman RD: Rheumatic manifestations of hepatitis B infection, *Semin Arthritis Rheum* 11:406, 1982.
175. Taylor HG, Borg AA, Dawes PT: Human parvovirus B19 and rheumatoid arthritis, *Clin Rheumatol,* 11:548, 1992.
176. Saal JG, Steidle M, Einsele H et al: Persistence of B19 parvovirus in synovial membranes of patients with rheumatoid arthritis, *Rheumatol Int* 12:147, 1992.
177. Inman RD: Infectious etiology of rheumatoid arthritis, *Rheum Dis Clin North Am* 17:859, 1991.
178. Weyand CM, Goronzy JJ: HIV infection and rheumatic diseases: autoimmune mechanisms in immunodeficient hosts, *Z Rheumatol* 51:55, 1992.
179. Hughes RA, Macatonia SE, Rowe JF et al: The detection of human immunodeficiency virus DNA in dendritic cells from the joints of patients with aseptic arthritis, *Br J Rheumatol* 29:166, 1990.
180. Ranki A, Kurki P, Riepponen S, Stephansson E: Antibodies to retroviral proteins in autoimmune connective tissue disease: relation to clinical manifestations and ribonucleoprotein autoantibodies, *Arthritis Rheum* 35:1483, 1992.

181. Espinoza LR, Aguilar JL, Berman A et al: Rheumatic manifestations associated with human immunodeficiency virus infection, *Arthritis Rheum* 32:1615, 1989.
182. Yagupsky P, Dagan R, Howard CW et al: High prevalence of *Kingella kingae* in joint fluid from children with septic arthritis revealed by the BACTEC blood culture system, *J Clin Microbiol* 30:1278, 1992.
183. Welkon CJ, Long SS, Fisher MC et al: Pyogenic arthritis in infants and children: a review of 95 cases, *Pediatr Infect Dis* 5:669, 1986.
184. Soria LM, Solé JM, Sacanell AR et al: Infectious arthritis in patients with rheumatoid arthritis, *Ann Rheum Dis* 51:402, 1992.
185. Jones A, Henderson MJ, Berman P, Doherty M: Septic arthritis complicating apatite associated destructive arthropathy, *Ann Rheum Dis* 49:1005, 1990.
186. Hughes RA, Rowe IF, Shanson D, Keat AC: Septic bone, joint and muscle lesions associated with human immunodeficiency virus infection, *Br J Rheumatol* 31:381, 1992.
187. Goldenberg DL: Gonococcal arthritis and other neisserial infections. In McCarty DJ, Koopman WJ, editors: *Arthritis and alied conditions*, ed 12, Philadelphia, 1993, Lea & Febiger.
188. Malawista SE: Infectious arthritis. In Wyngaarden JB, Smith LH Jr, Bennett JC, editors: *Cecil's textbook of medicine*, ed 19, Philadelphia, 1992, Saunders.
189. Bennett OM, Namnyak SS: Acute septic arthritis of the hip joint in infancy and childhood, *Clin Orthop* 281:123, 1992.
190. Burgoyne M, Agudelo C, Pisko E: Chronic syphilitic polyarthritis mimicking systemic lupus erythematosis/rheumatoid arthritis as the initial presentation of human immunodeficiency virus infection, *J Rheumatol* 19:31, 1992.
191. Jaffe HL: *Metabolic, degenerative, and inflammatory diseases of bones and joints*, Philadelphia, 1972, Lea & Febiger. pp 941-947.
192. Rahn DW, Malawista SE: Lyme disease. In McCarty DJ, Koopman WJ, editors: *Arthritis and allied conditions*, ed 12, Philadelphia, 1993, Lea & Febiger.
193. Szer IS, Taylor E, Steere AC: The long-term course of Lyme arthritis in children, *N Engl J Med* 325:159, 1991.
194. Steere AC, Dwyer E, Winchester R: Association of chronic Lyme arthritis with HLA-DR4 and HLA-DR2 alleles, *N Engl J Med* 323:219, 1990.
195. Snydman DR, Schenkein DP, Beradi VP et al: *Borrelia burgdorferi* in joint fluid in chronic Lyme arthritis, *Ann Intern Med* 104:798, 1986.
196. Pachner AR, Steere AC: The triad of neurologic manifestations of Lyme disease: meningitis, cranial neuritis, and radiculoneuritis, *Neurology* 35:47, 1985.
197. Lyons AS, Petrucelli RJ: *Medicine: an illustrated history*, New York, 1978, Abradale Press.
198. Alvarez S, McCabe WR: Extrapulmonary tuberculosis revisited: a review of experience at Boston City and other hospitals, *Medicine* 63:25, 1984.
199. Meissner RP: Arthritis due to mycobacteria, fungi, and parasites. In McCarty DJ, Koopman WJ, editors: *Arthritis and allied conditions*, ed 12, Philadelphia, 1993, Lea & Febiger.
200. Milgram JW: Tuberculosis of bones and joints. In *Radiologic and histologic pathology of nontumerous diseases of bones and joints*, Northbrook, Ill, 1990, Northbrook Publishing.
201. Wolinsky E: Tuberculosis. In Wyngaarden JB, Smith LH Jr, Bennett JC, editors: *Cecil's textbook of medicine*, ed 19, Philadelphia, 1992, Saunders.
202. Campion GV, Karakusis P, Schnitzer TJ: Tuberculous arthritis. In Schumacher HR, Klippel JH, Robinson DR: *Primer on the rheumatic diseases*, ed 9, Atlanta, 1988, Arthritis Foundation.
203. Nichols L, Florentine B, Lewis W et al: Bone marrow examination for the diagnosis of mycobacterial and fungal infections in the acquired immune deficiency syndrome, *Arch Pathol Lab Med* 115:1125, 1991.
204. Vinetz JM, Rickman LS: Chronic arthritis due to *Mycobacterium avium* complex infection in a patient with the acquired immunodeficiency syndrome [letter], *Arthritis Rheum* 34:1339, 1991.
205. Eggelmeijer F, Kroon FP, Zeeman RJ et al: Tenosynovitis due to *Mycobacterium avium–intracellulare:* case report and a review of the literature, *Clin Exp Rheumatol* 10:169, 1992.
206. Travis WD, Travis LB, Roberts GC et al: The histopathologic spectrum in *Mycobacterium marinum* infection, *Arch Pathol Lab Med* 109:1109, 1985.
207. Puett DW, Fuchs HA: Arthritis after bacillus Calmette-Guérin therapy [letter], *Ann Intern Med* 117:537, 1992.
208. Cuéllar ML, Silveira LH, Espinoza LR: Fungal arthritis, *Ann Rheum Dis* 51:690, 1992.
209. Rivera J, Monteagudo I, López-Longo J, Sánchez-Atrio A: Septic arthritis in patients with acquired immunodeficiency syndrome with human immunodeficiency virus infection, *J Rheumatol* 19:1960, 1992.
210. Binford CH, Dooley JR: Diseases caused by fungi and actinomycetes: deep mycoses. In Binford CH, Connor DH, editors: *Pathology of tropical and extraordinary diseases: an atlas*, vol 2, Washington, D.C., 1976, Armed Forces Institute of Pathology.

Postinfectious arthritis

211. Phillips PE, Inman RD: Infectious agents in chronic rheumatic disease. In, McCarty DJ, Koopman WJ, editors: *Arthritis and allied conditions*, ed 12, Philadelphia, 1993, Lea & Febiger.
212. Taranta A: Rheumatic fever. In McCarty DJ, Koopman WJ, editors: *Arthritis and allied conditions*, ed 12, Philadelphia, 1993, Lea & Febiger.
213. Pope RM: Acute rheumatic fever and Jaccoud's arthropathy. In Schumacher HR, Klippel JH, Robinson DR, editors: *Primer on the rheumatic diseases*, ed 9, Atlanta, 1988, Arthritis Foundation.
214. Froude J, Gibofsky A, Buskirk DR, et al: Cross-reactivity between streptococcus and human tissue: a model of molecular mimicry and autoimmunity, *Curr Top Microbiol Immunol* 145:5, 1989.
215. Fassbender HG: Rheumatic fever. In *Pathology of rheumatic diseases*, New York, 1975, Springer-Verlag.
216. Girigis FL, Popple W, Bruchner FE: Jaccoud's arthropathy: a case report and necropsy study, *Ann Rheum Dis* 37:561, 1978.

Rheumatoid arthritis

217. Smith CA, Arnett FC: Epidemiologic aspects of rheumatoid arthritis: current immunogenetic approach, *Clin Orthop* 265:23, 1991.
218. Praemer A, Furner S, Rice DP: *Musculoskeletal conditions in the United States*, Park Ridge, Ill., 1992, American Academy Orthopedic Surgeons.
219. McCarty DJ: Clinical picture of rheumatoid arthritis. In McCarty DJ, Koopman WJ, editors: *Arthritis and allied conditions*, ed 12, Philadelphia, 1993, Lea & Febiger.
220. Lawrence RC, Hochberg MC, Kelsy JL et al: Estimates of the prevalence of selected arthritic and musculoskeletal diseases in the United States, *J Rheumatol* 16:427, 1989.
221. Schrohenloher RE, Koopman WJ: Rheumatoid factor. In McCarty DJ, Koopman WJ, editors: *Arthritic and allied conditions*, ed 12, Philadelphia, 1993, Lea & Febiger.
222. Weyand CM, Hicok KC, Conn DL, Goronzy JJ: The influence of HLA-DRB1 genes on disease severity in rheumatoid arthritis, *Ann Intern Med* 117:801, 1992.
223. Ilonen J, Reijonen H, Arvilommi H et al: HLA-DR antigens and HLA-DQβ chain polymorphism in susceptibility to rheumatoid arthritis, *Ann Rheum Dis* 49:494, 1990.
224. Nakao H, Eguchi K, Kawakami A et al: Phenotypic characterization of lymphocytes infiltrating synovial tissue from patients with rheumatoid arthritis: analysis of lymphocytes isolated from minced synovial tissue by dual immunofluorescent staining, *J Rheumatol* 17:142, 1990.
225. Sokoloff L: Animal models of rheumatoid arthritis, *Int Rev Exp Pathol* 26:107, 1984.
226. Grahame R, Armstrong R, Simmons N et al: Chronic arthritis associated with the presence of intrasynovial rubella virus *Ann Rheum Dis* 42:2, 1983.
227. Chantler JK, Tingle AS, Petty R: Persistent rubella virus infection associated with chronic arthritis in children, *N Engl J Med* 313:1117, 1986.
228. Murayama T, Jisaki F, Ayata M et al: Cytomegalovirus genomes demonstrated by polymerase chain reaction in synovial fluid from rheumatoid arthritis patients, *Clin Exp Rheumatol* 10:161, 1992.
229. Einsele H, Steidle M, Müller CA et al: Demonstration of cytomegalovirus (CMV) DNA and anti-CMV response in the synovial membrane and serum of patients with rheumatoid arthritis, *J Rheumatol* 19:677, 1992.
230. Hardy RR, Hayakawa K, Shimizu B et al: Rheumatoid factor secretion from human Leu 1+ B-cells, Science 236:81, 1987.
231. Maini RN, Zyberk CP: The significance of $CD5^+$ B-cells in rheumatic diseases, *Scand J Rheum* 76 (suppl):237, 1988.
232. Catalano MA, Carson DA, Niederman JC et al: Antibody to the rheumatoid arthritis nuclear antigen: its relationship to in vitro Epstein-Barr virus infection, *J Clin Invest* 65:1238, 1980.
233. Kouri T, Petersen J, Rhodes G et al: Antibodies to synthetic peptides from Epstein-Barr nuclear antigen-1 in sera of patients with early

rheumatoid arthritis and in preillness sera, *J Rheumatol* 77:1442, 1992.

234. Trabandt A, Gay RE, Gay S: Oncogene activation in synovium, *Acta Pathol Microbiol Scand* 100:861, 1992.
235. Rook G, McCulloch J: HLA-DR4, mycobacteria, heat-shock proteins and rheumatoid arthritis, *Arthritis Rheum* 35:1409, 1992.
236. Kahle P, Saal JG, Schaudt K et al: Determination of cytokines in synovial fluids with diagnosis and histomorphological characteristics of synovial tissue, *Ann Rheum* Dis 51:73, 1992.
237. Westacott CI, Whicher JT, Barnes IC et al: Synovial fluid concentration of five different cytokines in rheumatic diseases, *Ann Rheum Dis* 49:676, 1990; comment: 50:405, 1991.
238. Gravallese EM, Darling JM, Ladd AL et al: In situ hybridization studies of stromelysin and collagenase messenger RNA expression in rheumatoid synovium, *Arthritis Rheum* 34:1076, 1991.
239. Nietfield JJ, Wilbrink B, Helle M et al: Interleukin-1-induced interleukin-6 is required for the inhibition of proteoglycan synthesis by interleukin–1 in human articular cartilage, *Arthritis Rheum* 33:1695, 1990.
240. Goldring MB and Goldring SR: Skeletal tissue response to cytokines, *Clin Orthop* 258:245, 1990.
241. Alsalameh S, Mollenhauer J, Hain N et al: Cellular immune response toward articular chondrocytes: T-cell reactivities against chondrocyte and fibroblast membranes in destructive joint diseases, *Arthritis Rheum* 33:1477, 1990.
242. Hough AJ, Sokoloff L: Pathology. In Utsinger PD, Zvaifler NJ, Ehrlich GE, editors: *Rheumatoid arthritis: etiology, diagnosis, management,* Philadelphia, 1984, Lippincott.
243. Rooney M, Whelan A, Feighery C, Bresnihan B: Changes in lymphocyte infiltration of the synovial membrane and the clinical course of rheumatoid arthritis, *Arthritis Rheum* 32:361, 1989.
244. Lindblad S: Recent progress in the study of synovitis by macroscopic and microscopic examination: a review, *Scand J Rheumatol* 76 (suppl):27, 1988.
245. Kennedy TD, Plater-Zyberk C, Partridge TA et al: Morphometric comparison of synovium from patients with osteoarthritis and rheumatoid arthritis, *J Clin Pathol* 41:847, 1988.
246. Gardner DL: The pathology of rheumatoid arthritis, Baltimore, 1972, Williams & Wilkins.
247. Wenick RM, Lipsky P, Marban-Acros E et al: IgG and IgM rheumatoid factor synthesis in rheumatoid synovial membrane cultures, *Arthritis Rheum* 28:742, 1985.
248. Nakao H, Eguchi K, Kawakami A et al: Phenotypic characterization of lymphocytes infiltrating synovial tissue from patients with rheumatoid arthritis: analysis of lymphocytes isolated from minced synovial tissue by dual immunofluorescent staining, *J Rheumatol* 17:142, 1990.
249. Padula SJ, Clark RB, Korn JH: Cell-mediated immunity in rheumatic disease, *Hum Pathol* 17:254, 1987.
250. Cush JJ, Lipsky PE: Phenotypic analysis of synovial tissue and peripheral blood lymphocytes isolated from patients with rheumatoid arthritis, *Arthritis Rheum* 31:1230, 1988.
251. Iguchi T, Kurosaka M, Ziff M: Electron study of HLA-DR and monocyte macrophage staining of cells in the rheumatoid synovial membrane, *Arthritis Rheum* 29:600, 1986.
252. Rooney M, Whelan A, Feighery C et al: The immunohistologic features of synovitis, disease activity and *in vitro* rheumatoid factor synthesis by blood mononuclear cells in rheumatoid arthritis, *J Rheumatol* 16:459, 1989.
253. Malone DG, Wilder RC, Saavedra-Delgado AM et al: Mast cell numbers in rheumatoid synovial tissues, *Arthritis Rheum* 30:130, 1987.
254. Ridley MG, Kingsley G, Pitzalis C et al: Monocyte activation in rheumatoid arthritis: evidence for *in situ* activation and differentiation in joints, *Br J Rheumatol* 29:84, 1990.
255. Menninger H, Putzier R, Mohr W: Granulocyte elastase at the site of cartilage erosion to rheumatoid synovial tissue, *J Rheumatol* 39:145, 1980.
256. Krane SM, Conca W, Stephenson ML et al: Mechanisms of matrix degradation in rheumatoid arthritis, *Ann NY Acad Sci* 580:340, 1990.
257. Shiozawa S, Yoshihara R, Kuroki Y et al: Pathogenic importance of fibronectin in the superficial region of articular cartilage as a local factor for the induction of pannus extension on rheumatoid articular cartilage, *Ann Rheum Dis* 51:869, 1992.
258. Gálvez J, Sola J, Guzman O et al: Microscopic rice bodies in rheumatoid synovial fluid sediments, *J Rheumatol* 19:1851, 1993.
259. Popert AJ, Scott DL, Wainwright AC et al: Frequency of occurrence, mode of development and significance of rice bodies in rheumatoid joints, *Ann Rheum Dis* 41:109, 1982.
260. Fukase M, Koizumi F, Wakaki K: Histopathologic analysis of sixteen subcutaneous nodules, *Acta Pathol Jpn* 30:87, 1980.
261. Athanasou NA, Quinn J, Woods CG et al: Immunohistology of rheumatoid nodules and rheumatoid synovium, *Ann Rheum Dis* 47:398, 1988.
262. Patterson JW: Rheumatoid nodule and subcutaneous granuloma annulare: a comparative histologic study, *Am J Dermatopathol* 10:1, 1988.
263. Hough AJ: Pathology of rheumatoid arthritis and allied disorders. In McCarty DJ, Koopman WJ, editors: *Arthritis and allied conditions,* ed 12, Philadelphia, 1993, Lea & Febiger.
264. Kondratowicz GM, Symmons DPM, Bacon PA et al: Rheumatoid lymphadenopathy: a morphological and immunohistochemical study, *J Clin Pathol* 43:106, 1990.
265. Wilkens FR, Roth GF, Husby G, Williams RC: Immunopathological studies in lymph nodes in rheumatoid arthritis and malignant lymphomas, *Ann Rheum Dis* 39:147, 1989.
266. Jurik AG, Davidsen D, Graudal H: Prevalence of pulmonary involvement in rheumatoid arthritis and its relationship to some characteristics of the patients: a radiological and clinical study, *Scand J Rheumatol* 11:217, 1982.
267. Walters MN, Ojeada VJ: Pleuropulmonary necrobiotic rheumatoid nodules, *Med J Aust* 144:648, 1986.
268. Klocklars M: Silica exposure and rheumatoid arthritis: a follow-up study of granite workers 1940-81, *Br Med J* 294:997, 1987.
269. Robinowitz M, Virmani R, McAllister HA: Rheumatoid heart disease: a clinical and morphologic analysis of 34 autopsy patients, *Lab Invest* 42:146, 1980.
270. Roberts WC, Kehoe JA, Carpenter OF, Golden A: Cardiac valvular lesions in rheumatoid arthritis, *Arch Intern Med* 122:141, 1968.
271. John JT, Hough AJ, Sergent JS: Pericardial disease in rheumatoid arthritis, *Am J Med* 66:385, 1979.
272. Foster CF, Forstot SL, Wilson LA: Mortality rate in rheumatoid arthritis patients developing necrotizing scleritis or peripheral ulcerative keratitis, *Ophthalmology* 91:1253, 1984.
273. Bernelot-Moens HJ, Ament HJW, Vroom TM, et al: Perivascular infiltration in normal skin of patients with rheumatoid arthritis: association with rheumatoid factors and HLA-DR antigens, *Ann Rheum Dis* 47:838, 1988.
274. Vollertsen RS, Conn DL: Vasculitis associated with rheumatoid arthritis, *Rheum Dis Clin North Am* 16:445, 1990.
275. Higaki Y, Yamashita H, Sato K et al: Rheumatoid papules: a report on four patients with histopathologic analysis, *J Am Acad Dermatol* 28:406, 1993.
276. Bywaters EGL: Rheumatoid and other disease of the cervical interspinous bursae, and changes in the spinous processes, *Ann Rheum Dis* 41:360, 1982.
277. Schils JP, Resnick D, Haghighi PN et al: Pathogenesis of discovertebral and manubriosternal joint abnormalities in rheumatoid arthritis: a cadaveric study, *J Rheumatol* 16:291, 1989.
278. Talal N: Sjögren's syndrome and connective tissue diseases associated with the immunologic disorders. In McCarty DJ, Koopman WH, editors: *Arthritis and allied conditions,* ed12, Philadelphia, 1993, Lea & Febiger.
279. Fox RI, Howell FV, Bone RC et al: Primary Sjögren syndrome: clinical and immunologic features, *Semin Arthritis Rheum* 14:77, 1984.
280. Rosenstein ED, Kramer N: Felty's and pseudo-Felty's syndromes, *Semin Arthritis Rheum* 21:129, 1991.
281. Loughran TP: Clonal diseases of large granular lymphocytes, *Blood* 82:1, 1993.
282. Husby G: Amyloidosis and rheumatoid arthritis, *Clin Exp Rheumatol* 3:173, 1985.
283. Bowness P, Shotliff K, Middlemiss A, Myles AB: Prevalence of hypothyroidism in patients with polymalagia rheumatica and giant cell arteritis, *Br J Rheumatol* 30:349, 1991.

284. Delecoeuillerie G, Joly P, Cohen de Lara A, Paolaggi JB: Polymyalgia rheumatica and temporal arteritis: a retrospective analysis of prognostic features and different corticosteroid regimes (11 year survey of 210 patients), *Ann Rheum Dis* 47:733, 1988.
285. Pincus T, Callahan LF: The "side effects" of rheumatoid arthritis: joint destruction, disability and early mortality, *Br J Rheumatol* 32(suppl 1):28, 1993.

Still's disease

286. Cassidy JT, Levinson JE, Bass JC et al: A study of classification criteria for a diagnosis of juvenile rheumatoid arthritis, *Arthritis Rheum* 29:274, 1986.
287. Anderson GB, Fasth A, Andersson J et al: Incidence and prevalence of juvenile chronic arthritis: a population survey, *Ann Rheum Dis* 46:277, 1987.
288. Ström H, Lindvall N, Hellström B, Rosenthal L: Clinical, HLA, and roentgenological follow-up study of patients with juvenile arthritis: comparison between the long term outcome of transient and persistent arthritis in children, *Ann Rheum Dis* 48:918, 1989.
289. Pachman LM, Poznanski AK: Juvenile rheumatoid arthritis. In McCarty DJ, Koopman WJ, editors: *Arthritis and allied conditions,* ed12, Philadelphia, 1993, Lea & Febiger.
290. Schneider R, Lang BA, Reilly BJ et al: Prognostic indicators of joint destruction in systemic-onset juvenile rheumatoid arthritis, *J Pediatr* 120:200, 1992.
291. Burgos-Vargas R, Petty RE: Juvenile ankylosing spondylitis, *Rheum Dis Clin North Am* 18:123, 1992.

Seronegative spondyloarthropathies

292. Kahn MA: An overview of clinical spectrum and heterogeneity of spondyloarthropathies, *Rheum Dis Clin North Am* 18:1, 1992.
293. Calin A, Elswood J: Relative role of genetic and environmental factors in disease expression: sib pair analysis in ankylosing spondylitis, *Arthritis Rheum* 32:77, 1989.
294. Leirisalo-Repo M: Inflammation in HLA-B27-associated diseases, *Scand J Rheumatol* 87(suppl):140, 1990.
295. Wagener D, Hammer M, Schedel I: Detection of endotoxin in synovial tissue of patients with inflammatory-rheumatic diseases, *Z Rheumatol* 48:200, 1989.
296. Mäki-Ikola D, Lehtinen K, Granfors K et al: Bacterial antibodies in ankylosing spondylitis, *Clin Exp Immunol* 84:472, 1992.
297. Keat A: Infections and the immunopathogenesis of seronegative spondyloarthropathies, *Curr Opin Rheumatol* 4:494, 1992.
298. Ball GV: Ankylosing spondylitis. In McCarty DJ, Koopman WJ, editors: *Arthritis and allied conditions,* ed 12, Philadelphia, 1993, Lea & Febiger.
299. Mielants H, Veys EM, Cuvelier C, De Vos M: Ileocolonoscopic findings in seronegative spondyloarthropathies, *Br J Rheumatol* 27(suppl 2):95, 1988.
300. Mielants H, Veys EM, Goemaere S et al: Gut inflammation in the spondyloarthropathies: clinical, radiologic, biologic, and genetic features in relation to type of histology: a prospective study, *J Rheumatol* 18:1542, 1991.
301. Nikkari S, Merilahti-Palo R, Saario R et al: *Yersinia*-triggered reactive arthritis: use of polymerase chain reaction and immunocytochemical staining in the detection of bacterial components from synovial specimens, *Arthritis Rheum* 35:682, 1992.
302. Taylor-Robinson D, Gilroy CB, Thomas BJ, Keat AC: Detection of *Chlamydia trachomatis* DNA in joints of reactive arthritis patients by polymerase chain reaction, *Lancet* 340:81, 1992.
303. Rahman MU, Cheema A, Schumacher HR, Hudson AP: Molecular evidence for the presence of chlamydia in the synovium of patients with Reiter's syndrome, *Arthritis Rheum* 35:521, 1992.
304. Peeters AJ, Daha MR, Smeets TJ, Breedvelt FC: Bone marrow IgA and IgA subclass syntheses in ankylosing spondylitis, *J Rheumatol* 19:751, 1992.
305. Struthers GR, Lewin IV, Stanworth DR: IgA-alpha-1 antitrypsin complexes in ankylosing spondylitis, *Ann Rheum Dis* 48:30, 1989.
306. Docherty P, Mitchell MJ, MacMillan L et al: Magnetic resonance imaging in the detection of sacro-iliitis, *J Rheumatol* 19:393, 1992.
307. Cush JJ, Lipsky PE: Reiter's syndrome and reactive arthritis. In McCarty DJ, Koopman WJ, editors: *Arthritis and allied conditions,* ed 12, Philadelphia, 1993, Lea & Febiger.
308. Stieglitz H, Fosmire S, Lipsky P: Identification of a 2-Md plasmid from *Shigella flexneri* associated with reactive arthritis, *Arthritis Rheum* 32:937, 1989.
309. Yu DTY, Hoffman RW: Reiter's syndrome. In Schumacher HR, Klippel JH, Robinson DR, editors: *Primer on the rheumatic diseases,* ed 9, Atlanta, 1988, Arthritis Foundation.
310. Gladman DD: Psoriatic arthritis: recent advances in pathogenesis and treatment, *Rheum Dis Clin* North Am 18:247, 1992.
311. Helliwell P, Marchesoni A, Peters M et al: A re-evaluation of the osteoarticular manifestations of psoriasis, *Br J Rheumatol* 30:339, 1991.
312. Bennett RM: Psoriatic arthritis. In McCarty DJ, Koopman WJ, editors: *Arthritis and allied conditions,* ed 12, Philadelphia, 1993, Lea & Febiger.
313. Mielants H, Veys EM: Enteropathic arthritis. In McCarty DJ, Koopman WJ, editors: *Arthritis and allied conditions,* ed 12, Philadelphia, 1993, Lea & Febiger.
314. Cabral DA, Oen KG, Petty RE: SEA syndrome revisited: a longterm followup of children with a syndrome of seronegative enthesopathy and arthropathy, *J Rheumatol* 19:1282, 1992.
315. Calin A: Ankylosing spondylitis and the spondyloarthropathies. In Schumacher HR, Klippel JH, Robinson DR, editors: *Primer on the rheumatic diseases,* ed 9, Atlanta, 1988, Arthritis Foundation.

Other inflammatory arthritides

316. Vernon-Roberts B, Barnes CG, Revell RA: Synovial pathology in Behçet's syndrome, *Ann Rheum Dis* 37:139, 1978.
317. Yurdakul S, Yazici H, Tüzün Y: The arthritis of Behcet's disease: a prospective study, *Ann Rheum Dis* 42:505, 1983.
318. Choi SJ: Behçet's syndrome. In Schumacher HR, Klippel JH, Robinson DR, editors: *Primer on the rheumatic diseases,* ed 9, Atlanta, 1988, Arthritis Foundation.
319. Schumacher HR: Sarcoidosis. In McCarty DJ, Koopman WJ, editors: *Arthritis and allied conditions,* ed 12, Philadelphia, 1993, Lea & Febiger.
320. Scott DGI, Porto LOR, Lovell CR, Thomas GD: Chronic sarcoid synovitis in the Caucasian: an arthroscopic and histological study, *Ann Rheum Dis* 40:121, 1981.
321. Barnett EV: Arthritis associated with immunodeficiency disease. In Schumacher HR, Klippel JH, Robinson DR, editors: *Primer on the rheumatic diseases,* ed 9, Atlanta, 1988, Arthritis Foundation.
322. Preston SJ, Buchanan WW: Rheumatic manifestations of immune deficiency, *Clin Exp Rheumatol* 7:547, 1989.
323. Grayzel AI, Marcus R, Stern R et al: Chronic polyarthritis associated with hypogammaglobulinemia: a study of two patients, *Arthritis Rheum* 20:887, 1977.
324. Michet CJ Jr, McKenna CH, Luthra HS, O'Fallon WM: Relapsing polychondritis: survival and predictive role of early disease manifestations, *Ann Intern Med* 104:74, 1986.
325. Trentham DE, Relapsing polychondritis. In McCarty DJ, Koopman WJ, editors: *Arthritis and allied conditions,* ed12, Philadelphia, 1993, Lea & Febiger.
326. Lie JT. Diagnostic histopathology of major systemic and pulmonary vasculitis syndromes, *Rheum Dis Clin North Am* 16:269, 1990.
327. Block SR, Winfield JB, Locskin MD et al: Studies of twins with systemic lupus erythematoses, *Am J Med* 59:533, 1975.
328. Klippel JH: Systemic lupus erythematosus: treatment-related complications superimposed on chronic disease, *JAMA* 263:1812, 1990.
329. Schumacher HR: Joint involvement in progressive systemic sclerosis (scleroderma), *Am J Clin Pathol* 60:593, 1973.

Crystal-induced arthritis

330. Levinson DJ, Becker MA: Clinical gout and the pathogenesis of hyperuricemia. In McCarty DJ, Koopman WJ, editors: *Arthritis and allied conditions,* ed 12, Philadelphia, 1993, Lea & Febiger.
331. Halverson PB, Garancis JC, McCarty DJ: Histopathologic and ultrastructural studies of Milwaukee shoulder syndrome: a basic calcium phosphate arthropathy, *Ann Rheum Dis* 43:734, 1984.
332. Halverson PB, McCarty DJ: Basic calcium phosphate (apatite, octacalcium phosphate, tricalcium phosphate) crystal deposition diseases. In McCarty DJ, Koopman WJ, editors: *Arthritis and allied conditions,* ed 12, Philadelphia, 1993, Lea & Febiger.

333. Terkeltaub RA: Pathogenesis and treatment of crystal-induced inflammation. In McCarty DJ, Koopman WJ, editors: *Arthritis and allied conditions,* ed 12, Philadelphia, 1993, Lea & Febiger.
334. Brick JE: Conquest of the gout, *WV Med J* 87:470, 1991.
335. Rodnan GP: Early theories concerning etiology and pathogenesis of gout, *Arthritis Rheum* 8:599, 1965.
336. Benedek TG: History of the rheumatic diseases. In Schumacher HR, Klippel JH, Robinson DR, editors: *Primer on the rheumatic diseases,* ed 9, Atlanta, 1988, Arthritis Foundation.
337. McCarty DJ, Hollander JL: Identification of urate crystals in gouty synovial fluid, *Ann Intern Med* 54:452, 1961.
338. Calabrese G, Simmonds HA, Cameron JS, Davies PH: Precocious familial gout with reduced fractional urate clearance and normal purine enzymes, *Q J Med* 78:441, 1990.
339. Hall AP, Barry PE, Dawber TR: Epidemiology of gout and hyperuricemia: a long-term population study, *Am J Med* 42:27, 1967.
340. Meyers OL, Monteagudo FSE: Gout in females an analysis of 92 patients, *Clin Exp Rheumatol* 3:105, 1985.
341. Kam M, Perl-Treues D, Caspi D, Addadi L: Antibodies against crystals, *FASEB J* 6:2608, 1992.
342. Pascual E: Persistence of monosodium urate crystals and low grade inflammation in the synovial fluid of patients with untreated gout, *Arthritis Rheum* 34:141, 1991.
343. Halvorsen PB, McCarty DJ: Patterns of radiographic abnormalities associated with basic calcium phosphate and calcium pyrophosphate dehydrate deposition in the knee, *Ann Rheum Dis* 45:603, 1986.
344. Felson DT, Anderson JJ, Naimark A et al: The prevalence of chondrocalcinosis in the elderly and its association with knee osteoarthritis: the Framingham Study, *J Rheumatol* 16:1241, 1989.
345. Sokoloff L, Varma AA: Chondrocalcinosis in surgically resected joints, *Arthritis Rheum* 31:750, 1988.
346. Menkes CJ, Decraemer W, Poste M, Forest M: Chondrocalcinosis and rapid destruction of the hip, *J Rheumatol* 12:130, 1985.
347. Dieppe PA, Watt I: Crystal deposition: opportunistic event? *Clin Rheum Dis* 11:367, 1985.
348. Pritzker KPH, Cheng PT, Renlund RC: Calcium pyrophosphate crystal deposition in hyaline cartilage: Untrastructural analysis and implications for pathogenesis, *J Rheumatol* 15:828, 1988.
349. Gordon C, Swan A, Dieppe P: Detection of crystals in synovial fluids by light microscopy: sensitivity and reliability, *Ann Rheum Dis* 48:737, 1989.

Cysts, tumors, and tumorlike lesions

350. Gabbiani G, Majno G: Dupuytren's contracture: fibroblast contraction? An untrastructural study, *Am J Pathol* 66:131, 1972.
351. Noble J, Heathcote JG, Cohen H: Diabetes mellitus in the aetiology of Dupuytren's disease, *J Bone Joint Surg* 66B:322, 1984.
352. Wigley RD: Popliteal cysts: variations on a theme by Baker, *Semin Arthritis Rheum* 12:1, 1982.
353. McKinney CD, Mills SE, Fechner RE: Intra-articular synovial sarcoma, *Am J Surg Pathol* 16:1017, 1992
354. Fisher C: Synovial sarcoma: ultrastructural and immunohistochemical features of epithelial differentiation in monophasic and biphasic tumors, *Hum Pathol* 17:996, 1986.
355. Myers BW, Masi AT, Feigenbaum SL: Pigmented villonodular synovitis and tenosynovitis: a clinical epidemiologic study of 166 cases and literature review, *Medicine* (Baltimore) 59:223, 1980.
356. Schumacher HR, Lothe P, Athreya B, Rothfuss S: Pigmented villonodular synovitis: light and electron microscopic studies. *Semin Arthritis Rheum* 12:32, 1982.
357. Abdul-Karim FW, El-Naggar AK, Joyce MJ et al: Diffuse and localized tenosynovial giant cell tumor and pigmented villonodular synovitis: a clinicopathologic and flow cytometric DNA analysis, *Hum Pathol* 23:729, 1992.
358. Wood GS, Beckstead JH, Medeiros LJ et al: The cells of giant cell tumor of tendon sheath resemble osteoclasts, *Am J Surg Pathol* 12:444, 1988.
359. Satti MB: Tendon sheath tumors: a pathological study of the relationship between giant cell tumor and fibroma of tendon sheath, *Histopathology* 20:213, 1992.
360. Sherry CS, Harms SE: MR evaluation of giant cell tumors of tendon sheath, *Magn Reson Imaging* 7:195, 1989.
361. Canoso JJ: Tumors of joints and related structures. In McCarty DJ, Koopman WJ, editors: *Arthritis and allied conditions,* ed 12, Philadelphia, 1993, Lea & Febiger.
362. Maurice H, Crone M, Watt I: Synovial chondromatoses, *J Bone Joint Surg* 70B:807, 1988.
363. Leu J-Z, Matsubara T, Hirohata K: Ultrastructural morphology of early cellular changes in the synovium of primary synovial chondromatosis, *Clin Orthop* 276:299, 1992.
364. Bertoni F, Unni KK, Beabout JW, Sim FH: Chondrosarcomas of the synovium, *Cancer* 67:155, 1991.
365. Felbel J, Gresser U, Lohmöller G, Zöllner N: Familial synovial chondromatosis combined with dwarfism, *Hum Genet* 88:351, 1992.
366. Enzinger FM, Weiss SW: Benign tumors and tumorlike lesions of blood vessels. In Enzinger FM, editor: *Soft tissue tumors,* ed 2, St. Louis, 1988, Mosby.
367. Juhl M, Krebs B: Arthroscopy and synovial hemangioma or giant cell tumor of the knee, *Arch Orthop Trauma Surg* 108:250, 1989.
368. Resnick D, Oliphant M: Hemophilia-like arthropathy of the knee associated with cutaneous and synovial hemangiomas, *Radiology* 114:323, 1975.
369. Hallel T, Lew S, Bansal M: Villous lipomatous proliferation of the synovial membrane (lipoma arborescens), *J Bone Joint Surg* 70A:264, 1988.
370. Enzinger FM: Clear-cell sarcoma of tendons and aponeuroses: an analysis of 21 cases, *Cancer* 18:1163, 1965.
371. Hasegawa T, Hirose T, Kudo E, Hizawa K: Clear cell sarcoma: an immunohistochemical and ultrastructural study, *Acta Pathol Jpn* 39:321, 1989.
372. Mii Y, Miyauchi Y, Hohnoki K et al: Neural crest origin of clear cell sarcoma of tendons and aponeuroses: ultrastructural and enzyme cytochemical study of human and nude mouse-transplanted tumours, *Virchows Arch [A]* 415:51, 1989.
373. Swanson PE, Wick MR: Clear cell sarcoma: an immunohistochemical analysis of six cases and comparison with other epithelioid neoplasms of soft tissue, *Arch Pathol Lab Med* 113:55, 1989.
374. Chung EB, Enzinger FM: Malignant melanoma of soft parts: a reassessment of clear cell sarcoma, *Am J Surg Pathol* 7:405, 1983.
375. Lucas DR, Nascimento AG, Sim FH: Clear cell sarcoma of soft tissues, *Am J Surg Pathol* 16:1197, 1992.
376. Kahn LB: Malignant giant cell tumor of tendon sheath, *Arch Pathol* 95:203, 1973.
377. Carstens HB, Howell RS: Malignant giant cell tumor of tendon sheath, *Virchows Arch [A]* 382:237, 1979.
378. Enzinger FM, Weiss SW: Benign tumors and tumorlike lesions of synovial tissue. In Enzinger FM, editor: *Soft tissue tumors,* ed 2, St. Louis, 1988, Mosby.
379. Ray RA, Morton CC, Lipinski KK et al: Cytogenetic evidence of clonality in a case of pigmented villonodular synovitis, *Cancer* 67:121, 1991.

Diseases of the vertebral column

380. Bishop PB, Pearce RH: The proteoglycans of the cartilaginous end-plate of the human intervertebral disc change after maturity, *J Orthop Res* 11:324, 1993.
381. Andersson GBJ: Measurements of loads of lumbar spine. In White AA, Gordon SL, editors: *American Academy of Orthopedic Surgeons symposium on low back pain,* St. Louis, 1982, Mosby.
382. Bullough PG, Boachie-Adjei O: *Atlas of spinal diseases,* Philadelphia, 1988, Lippincott.
383. Resnick D, Niwayama G: Intravertebral disk herniations: cartilaginous (Schmorl's) nodes, *Radiology* 126:57, 1978.
384. Resnick D, Shapiro RF, Wiesner KB et al: Diffuse idiopathic skeletal hyperostosis (DISH) (ankylosing hyperostosis of Forestier and Rotes-Querol), *Semin Arthritis Rheum* 7:153, 1978.
385. Ball J: Articular pathology of ankylosing spondylitis, *Clin Orthop* 143:30, 1979.

76 Skeletal Muscle

Reid R. Heffner, Jr.
Sydney S. Schochet, Jr.

NORMAL MUSCLE

Most striated muscles are partitioned into multiple fascicles, or bundles of fibers, each being surrounded by a connective tissue sheath, the perimysium, through which the intramuscular nerves and blood vessels are conveyed. Intramuscular nerve twigs are especially prominent in the muscle belly at the innervation zone. An individual twig consists of up to 10 myelinated nerve fibers inside a thin coat of perineurial fibrous connective tissue. Within the perimysium, muscle spindles also reside. These mechanoreceptors are present in all muscles, usually in the vicinity of the muscle belly, but are more prevalent in small muscles devoted to finely coordinated movements such as the interossei. The normal muscle spindle is composed of several intrafusal fibers that are enclosed by a lamellar fibrous capsule. The perimysial septa are projections from the epimysium, which in turn encircles groups of fascicles or the entire muscle. Thicker than the perimysial trabeculas and constructed of dense collagen, the epimysium is part of the mesenchymal scaffolding to which the fascia overlying the muscle and the tendons are connected. Each muscle fiber is invested with an endomysial envelope, normally an unobtrusive interconnecting meshwork of collagen, reticulin, and elastic fibers that support a rich capillary bed. The muscle fiber is a multinucleated, syncytium-like cell with a shape resembling that of a cylinder. Muscle fibers vary in length but typically extend for several centimeters, traversing the length of a fascicle without interruption or branching. In cross section, the normal adult myocyte is polygonal rather than rounded in configuration. The diameter of fibers measured in the transverse plane depends on several factors. Powerful, large, proximal muscles are composed of fibers with greater mean diameter (85 to 90 μm) than those of slender, distal, or ocular muscles (20 μm). In general, muscles designed for precisely coordinated activity like those of the eyes or digits have smaller fibers than muscles involved in less refined or postural movements like the glutei and quadriceps femoris. Fiber size in males exceeds that in females, presumably because of more strenuous physical demands and hormonal factors, though exercise induces fiber hypertrophy, regardless of sex. Muscle fibers in infants (mean diameter, 12 μm) and children are smaller than in healthy young adults. Some reduction in fiber size is also a legacy of advancing age.

In longitudinal sections, especially paraffin sections stained with phosphotungstic acid–hematoxylin or resin-embedded sections, striations within the sarcoplasm are visible, reflecting the arrangement of the contractile proteins that is seen better ultrastructurally. In hematoxylin and eosin–stained cross sections, the sarcoplasm has a somewhat homogeneous appearance without evidence of striations, unless the cut is tangential. The sarcolemmal nuclei are peripherally located and number four to six per fiber (Fig. 76-1). These nuclei are oriented parallel to the long axis of the fiber in longitudinal sections, and they are seen at intervals of 10 to 50 μm.

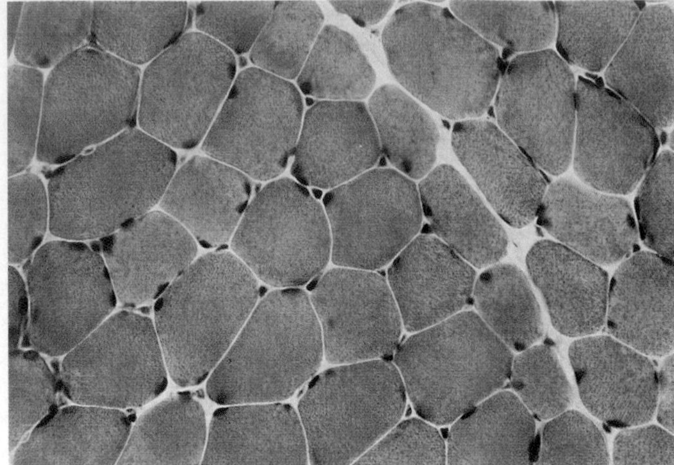

Fig. 76-1 Normal muscle. Fibers are polygonal in shape. The sarcolemmal nuclei are peripheral in location.

The ultrastructural examination of muscle is optimally conducted on longitudinal sections where any departure from normal striation is more easily appreciated than in transverse sections. The plasma membrane measures about 8 nm in width and may be difficult to visualize as a discrete entity. Externally and closely adherent to the plasmalemma is the broader, more conspicuous basement membrane, a moderately electron-dense, amorphous structure with a mean width of 20 to 30 nm. Satellite cells, with scant cytoplasm and devoid of cross striations, are deployed between the basement membrane and the plasmalemma of the muscle fiber. These cells cannot be distinguished from sarcolemmal nuclei in light microscopic sections. Their nuclei represent 5% to 10% of nuclei having a parasarcolemmal location. Satellite cells are considered to be quiescent stem cells with a penchant for responding to muscle fiber injury by participating in the enterprise of regeneration. Each muscle fiber is composed of a myriad of parallel subunits, the myofibrils, which are minute, virgate contractile elements with an average diameter of 1 μm. The myofibril is apportioned into an iterative series of identical segments known as "sarcomeres." The sarcomeres of each myofibril are of equal length and are aligned in register with those in neighboring myofibrils. The cross striations or periodicity of the muscle fiber is a function of the strict regimentation of the sarcomeres. The arrangement of the filaments within the sarcomere is responsible for the rectangular bands that are seen. The length of the sarcomeres, 2.5 to 3 μm, is the distance between consecutive Z bands, which constitute the lateral boundaries of the sarcomere (Fig. 76-2). The Z band (*Zwischenscheibe*), meaning 'intermediate disk,' is an extremely electron-dense linear disk perpendicular to the long axis of the myofibril. The Z band bisects the I (isotropic) bands of adjacent sarcomeres. Situated medial to the Z disks of a sarcomere, the I bands are more lightly stained and shorter in length than the central A (anisotropic) band. Inside the sarcomere are imbricating parallel filaments in the A and I band regions. The thick filaments, which are chiefly composed of myosin, measure 15 nm in diameter. The thin filaments, containing predominantly actin, have a diameter of 8 nm. The thick filaments, confined to the A band, dictate its length. The thin filaments extend from the Z band, to which they are attached, traverse the I band, where

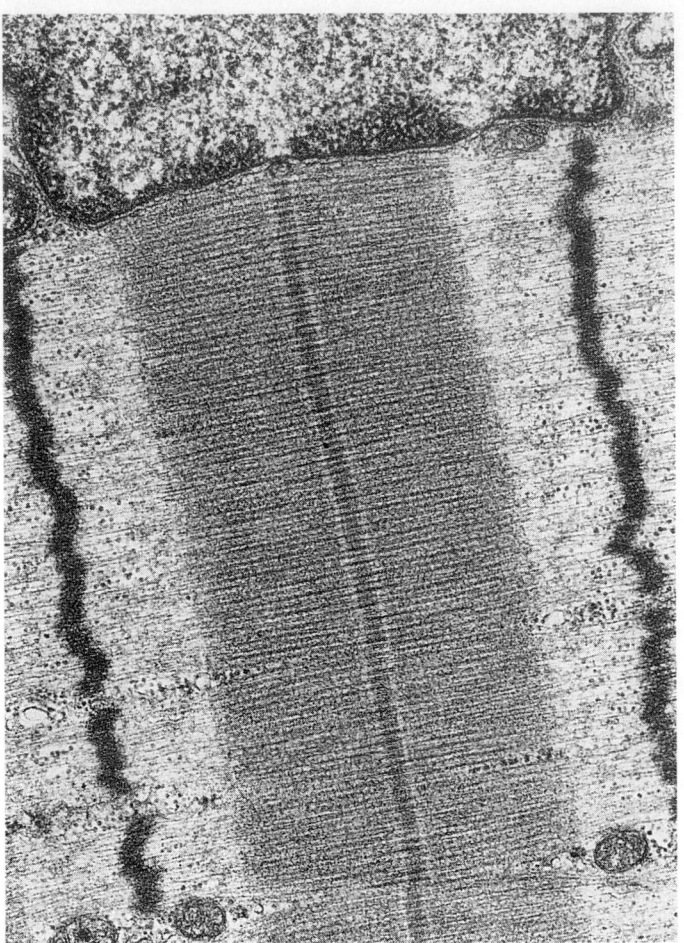

Fig. 76-2 Normal muscle. The sarcomere is composed of a central A band and lateral, more lightly stained I bands. The Z bands, which are the lateral boundaries of the sarcomere, bisect the I bands of adjacent sarcomeres and are very electron dense.

only thin filaments are present, and enter the A band to interdigitate with the thick filaments. The Z band, a major constituent of which is alpha-actinin, exhibits a gridlike or basketweave infrastructure. During muscular contraction, the Z bands are drawn toward the center of the sarcomere. The sarcomere length shortens as the thick and thin filaments slide past each other until the I bands are virtually obliterated. The organelles of the myofiber tend to congregate around the sarcolemmal nuclei and between the myofibrils. Glycogen granules, ranging from 15 to 30 nm in diameter, are found in greater concentration in type 2 fibers and are more prevalent in the I band regions. Lipid vacuoles and mitochondrial are more prominent in type 1 fibers. The majority of mitochondria are ovoid or elliptical with an average diameter of 1.0 μm. They are predictably situated adjacent to the Z bands with their long axes parallel to those of the myofibrils. The sarcotubular complex (SRT), a bipartite system composed of the sarcoplasmic reticulum (SR) and the transverse (T) tubules, is a distinctive ultrastructural component of striated muscle. The T tubules originate as invaginations from the plasmalemma and are distributed at regular intervals along the fiber at the junction of the A and I bands. Coursing in a generally transverse direction, they form a weblike network of tubules that is perforated by the longitudinally oriented myofibrils. Unlike the transverse

Table 76-1 Summary of fiber properties

	Type 1 fiber	Type 2 fiber
Physiology		
Function	Weight bearing	Sudden activity
Contraction	Sustained	Rapid
Electrical	Slow twitch	Fast twitch
Metabolism	Aerobic	Anaerobic
Histochemistry		
Oxidative enzymes	High	Low
Lipid	High	Low
Glycogen	Low	High
Phosphorylase	Low	High
ATPase (pH 9.4)	Low	High

tubular system, which communicates with the extracellular space, the sarcoplasmic reticulum is a closed, internalized array of vesicles that arborizes in all directions around the myofibrils. In routine electron microscopic sections, SR and T tubules appear as hollow, membrane-bound profiles. At the A-I band junctions, branches of the SRT come together into triads, composed of a pair of terminal cisternae of the SR between which is a centrally positioned tubule.

For a great many years it has been well known that there are physical and biochemical differences among skeletal muscles (Table 76-1). For example, in endothermic vertebrates, particularly some avian species, it is possible to distinguish between red (weight-bearing) and white (alar) muscles. The color of red muscles is bestowed upon them by their richer myoglobin content and increased capillary density. Red muscle, with its larger mitochondrial population and higher rate of blood flow, is more specialized for aerobic respiration and for postural or sustained activity. On the other hand, white muscle, endowed with fewer mitochondria, yet with abundant glycogen stores, is more suited to anaerobic respiration and is thus designed for sudden, intermittent activity. Although in lower vertebrates an entire muscle may be composed of either red or white fibers, human muscles are a mosaic of both fiber types, arranged in a pattern like that of a checkerboard. The proportion of type 1 and type 2 fibers depends on the function and anatomic location of the muscle, but the idealized muscle contains approximately 35% to 40% type 1 fibers and 60% to 65% type 2 fibers. Fiber typing, the demonstration of the histochemical properties of muscle fibers within a tissue sample, is determined through the use of enzyme histochemistry and is not evident in routine hematoxylin and eosin sections. Most laboratories utilize two complementary histochemical reactions carried out on fresh-frozen sections for this purpose. Oxidative enzyme reactions, such as NADH-TR or succinic dehydrogenase, display the density of mitochondria within the muscle fiber. With this method, darkly stained fibers are designated as type 1 (oxidative) and lighter fibers as type 2. Most oxidative enzyme reactions further segregate type 2 fibers into two subpopulations, with type 2B fibers being most lightly stained and type 2A fibers being intermediately stained. In the ATPase reaction, a range of staining intensities can be achieved by manipulation of the pH during the staining procedure. When the standard or alkaline ATPase reaction is conducted at a pH of 9.4, type 1 fibers appear light and type 2 fibers are dark (Fig. 76-3). Fibers with intermediate staining

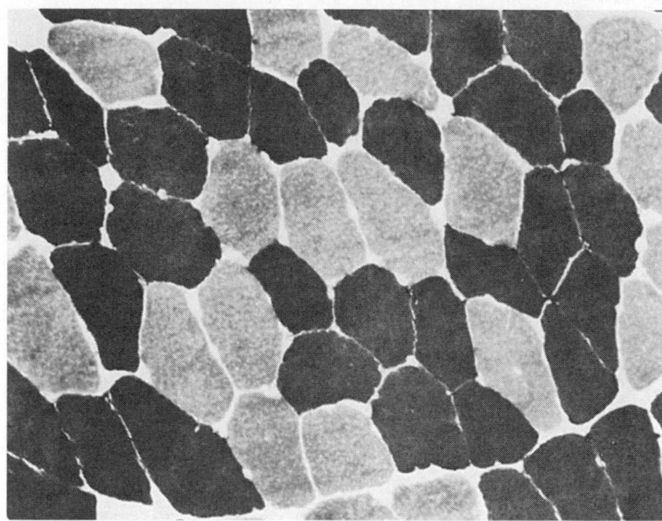

Fig. 76-3 Fiber typing using histochemistry. There are two fiber populations. The dark fibers are designated type 2. Light fibers are type 1. (ATPase, pH 9.4.)

properties are not apparent in the alkaline ATPase reaction. It is possible to reverse the staining reaction by altering the incubating solution to an acidic pH, usually about 4.6. In the reverse ATPase reaction, type 1 fibers are very darkly stained, type 2A fibers are very lightly stained, and type 2B fibers are intermediate in their staining attributes between the two. Some laboratories employ a histochemical reaction for phosphorylase, which is more abundant in type 2 (glycolytic) fibers, as a means of fiber typing. Although type 2 fibers should theoretically appear dark and type 1 fibers should appear light, in our experience this staining reaction is capricious and unreliable.

MUSCLE BIOPSY: PROCEDURES AND TECHNIQUES

Our knowledge of neuromuscular diseases has expanded in dramatic fashion during the past three decades. Much of this enlightenment has been a product of the application of modern pathologic technology to the study of muscle biopsy samples.

Unlike neoplasms of muscle, neuromuscular diseases are medical rather than surgical conditions, requiring that the pathologic examination of muscle tissue, which is only one piece of the total diagnostic effort in evaluating the patient, not be divorced from the patient's history, physical examination, and relevant laboratory tests. In the subsequent discussion of individual neuromuscular diseases, the role of clinical data will soon become obvious. For example, the temporal profile of disease is often informative, in that a rapid onset of symptoms is suggestive of an infectious or inflammatory myopathy, whereas insidious progression favors muscular dystrophy, metabolic myopathy, or a neurogenic process. The distribution of weakness is frequently an indication of whether the neuromuscular disorder is a primary myopathy, in which weakness tends to be proximal in location, or a denervating disease, in which weakness begins distally. Gross wasting of muscles is a sign of myotonic dystrophy or a denervating disorder. The medical record, specifically a familial history of muscle disease, may provide an important clue to the diagnosis of certain muscle diseases, such as the congenital myopathies, which are hereditary. The most revealing laboratory test is the serum level of a creatine kinase (CK), significant elevations of which are indicative of active muscle destruction and point toward a myopathic rather than an atrophic process. Electromyography (EMG) can be invaluable in demonstrating myotonia or myasthenia and in discriminating between myopathic and denervating disorders. Reports of EMG studies are helpful in putting the pathologic picture into the proper perspective in some cases.

In the collection of the biopsy specimen, specific aspects of the routine should be emphasized.[1, 2] A physician familiar with the patient is obligated to ensure that an appropriate muscle is sampled (Table 76-2). It is imperative that the biopsy sample be representative of the disease status. Accordingly, if symptoms are confined to the legs, biopsy findings of the upper extremity are not likely to reflect the disease process accurately. The biopsy sample should be obtained from a muscle in which the disease is active rather than from a severely affected muscle in which there is considerable weakness or atrophy, since the latter can be expected to reveal end-stage disease, which is difficult to interpret. Muscle subjected to previous trauma, such as needle EMG or intramuscular injections of therapeutic drugs, should not be subjected to biopsy. The residua of trauma—fiber necrosis, regeneration, inflammation, and endomysial fibrosis—mimic the stigmas of certain neuromuscular diseases and may confuse the pathologist. The biopsy specimen should be removed from the belly of the muscle at a distance from tendinous insertions where normal histologic features, specifically extreme variability in fiber diameters and numerous internal nuclei, simulate pathologically involved muscle.

In most laboratories two separate specimens, which are employed for different purposes, are routinely submitted. The first specimen is maintained in an isometric state by its insertion into a muscle clamp. Such a device prevents undesirable contraction artifact that results from excision of the specimen and immersion into fixative. Because of vigorous and unopposed contraction, the muscle fibers begin to pull themselves apart. This common artifact is more obvious in longitudinal sections in which dark perpendicular contraction bands and lucent tears occur within the sarcoplasm. In transverse sections, these tears look like irregular cracks within the fibers. Contraction artifact particularly jeopardizes tissue sent for electron microscopic study, since the normally striated architecture is destroyed by disruption and disorientation of the myofibrils.

The fixed specimen should measure a minimum of 1 cm in length and 0.5 cm in diameter. The fixed sample is dedicated to the preparation of routine paraffin, 1 to 2 μm resin-embedded, and ultrathin sections. A second specimen ideally measuring $1 \times 0.5 \times 0.5$ cm remains unfixed for the preparation of frozen sections. Different techniques have been advocated for tissue freezing. The most important consideration is extremely rapid freezing, usually obtained by immersion in liquid nitrogen. Serial frozen sections are generally subjected to a standard panel of stains including hematoxylin and eosin (H&E), rapid Gomori trichrome (RTC), and ATPase, and oxidative enzyme reactions such as NADH-TR or succinic dehydrogenase. As required, additional stains such as periodic acid–Schiff (PAS) for glycogen, oil red O or other suitable method for fat, phosphorylase, and additional histochemical reactions may be performed. Frozen tissue may also be utilized in selected cases for immunohistochemical or biochemical analysis.

Table 76-2 Clinical indications for muscle biopsy

General reasons
Weakness of uncertain cause
Generalized
Proximal
Floppy infant syndrome
Muscle pain, cramps, stiffness
Persistently elevated muscle enzymes (CK)
Specific reasons
Hereditary muscle disease in other family members
Carrier detection
Systemic connective tissue disease and vasculitis
Certain metabolic diseases such as storage disease
Suspicion of steroid myopathy in treated myositis
Exclude drug-induced myopathy
Suspected malignant hyperthermia (in vitro test only)
Conflicting clinical, EMG, or laboratory findings
Confirm/reinforce clinical diagnosis

GENERAL REACTIONS OF MUSCLE TO INJURY

Dysvoluminal changes. One of the fundamental manifestations of disease in skeletal muscle is a variation in fiber size, the basis of which may be atrophy or hypertrophy of fibers. Since the integrity of the muscle fiber is contingent upon neural and other homeostatic influences, any compromise of these trophic factors may underly fiber atrophy. Denervation is the most familiar example of atrophy in neuromuscular disease. Prolonged bed rest or orthopedic immobilization, which does not allow the muscle to engage in regular contraction, may engender disuse atrophy. A reduction in fiber size may represent a complication of malnutrition, aging[3] or ischemia.[4] Muscle hypertrophy, on the other hand, is principally attributable to increased muscular effort, either from exercise or as a compensatory adjustment of normal intact fibers to the process of atrophy among nearby counterparts. The technique of morphometric analysis may be especially useful when shifts in fiber diameters are minor and equivocal.[5] One can perform morphometry manually by taking measurements directly from a microscopic slide using an eyepiece micrometer or electronically using a computerized apparatus for image analysis. In order to garner statistically significant data, one should record measurements of the lesser diameter or circumference of each muscle fiber and the sample should consist of at least 200 fibers. In histochemical preparations, the atrophic or hypertrophic process may be selective, affecting mainly one fiber type, or nonselective, affecting all types.[6] Selective atrophy of type 1 fibers is seen in several of the congenital myopathies but is most commonly encountered in myotonic dystrophy. Type 2 fiber atrophy is most often a sequela of corticosteroid therapy (Fig. 76-4). It is also associated with myasthenia gravis, acute denervation, disuse, and malignancy as a paraneoplastic syndrome.[7]

Hypertrophy restricted to type 1 fibers occurs in normal athletes who participate in endurance training programs and in children with Werdnig-Hoffman disease. Type 2 fiber hypertrophy has been described in sprinters and, as a pathologic incident, in patients with congenital fiber type disproportion. Nonselective changes in fiber size are quite nonspecific. A large proportion of cases of nonselective atrophy are ascribable to denervation, though nonselective hypertrophy of fibers has also been reported in limb-girdle dystrophy, myotonia congenita, and acromegaly.

Reactions of the sarcolemmal nuclei. Quantitative studies have demonstrated that in cross sections of normal muscle the nuclei are peripheral or subsarcolemmal in 97% of fibers. Internalized nuclei are noted in many biopsy specimens from patients with neuromuscular disease (Fig. 76-5). Typically this change affects no more than 10% of fibers. However, scores of internal nuclei in the majority of fibers is highly suspicious for myotonic dystrophy. In contrast to nuclear internalization without compromise to the sarcoplasm, after sarcoplasmic damage the nuclei may no longer remain in a peripheral location. Sarcolemmal nuclei commonly migrate centripetally during the evolution of fiber necrosis and regeneration. Atrophic fibers may also harbor multiple, often pyknotic internal nuclei, which seem to escape significant harm, despite reduction in the sarcoplasmic volume.

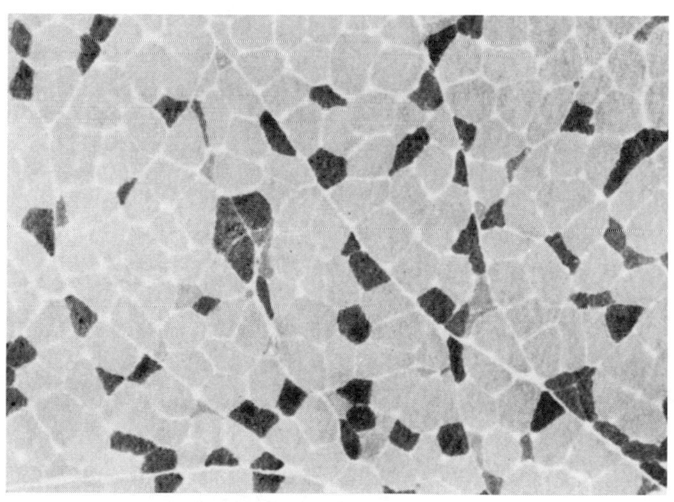

Fig. 76-4 Type 2 fiber atrophy in which small fibers are darkly stained. (ATPase, pH 9.4.)

Disfigurative changes. Abnormalities of the sarcoplasm, which are usually nonlethal, have been referred to as "disfigurative."[8] Such changes include hyaline, moth-eaten, ragged-red, ring, and target fibers as well as cores, rods, and vacuoles. These are discussed with the individual neuromuscular diseases where they take on the most importance. A common disfigurative alteration is vacuolization of muscle fibers. Vacuolar change after improper freezing or storage of the specimen is a vexing artifact. Vacuoles produced in this way may simulate bona fide pathologic change, as might be confronted in a vacuolar myopathy, or so distort pathologically affected fibers that accurate morphologic interpretation is impossible. Moreover, vacuoles may also represent abnormal accumulations of glycogen in the glycogenoses or lipid in the rather rare lipid storage diseases.

Fiber necrosis. Fiber necrosis, a minor part of the pathologic reaction in many muscle diseases, is widespread in the muscular dystrophies, particularly Duchenne muscular dystrophy, and in the inflammatory myopathies such as polymyositis (Fig. 76-6). In light microscopic sections stained with hematoxylin and eosin, the first warning of impending necrosis is a departure from the expected color of the sarcoplasm. The acutely necrotic fiber initially assumes a bright eosinophilic tone that is gradually converted to a pale shade of pink. During this interval, the sarcoplasm becomes coarsely granular, vacuolated, and finally fragmented. The sarcolemmal nuclei migrate internally and are pyknotic or karyorrhexic. As necrosis continues, phagocytosis of the dead cellular contents proceeds apace. The sarcoplasm is invaded by macrophages, but before the ingestion of all the necrotic debris, the process of restoration has ensued, and so myogenesis and phagocytosis may be observed in the same cell simultaneously.

Fiber regeneration. Fiber necrosis seems to serve as a stimulus for subsequent regeneration. Current evidence indicates that the regeneration of fibers may arise by two independent routes. If necrosis is segmental within the fiber, buds of myoplasm from the viable sarcomeres adjacent to the damaged segment are the mediators of the regenerative effort. A second source of regeneration is the satellite cell, which is probably a more important agent in regeneration than sarco-

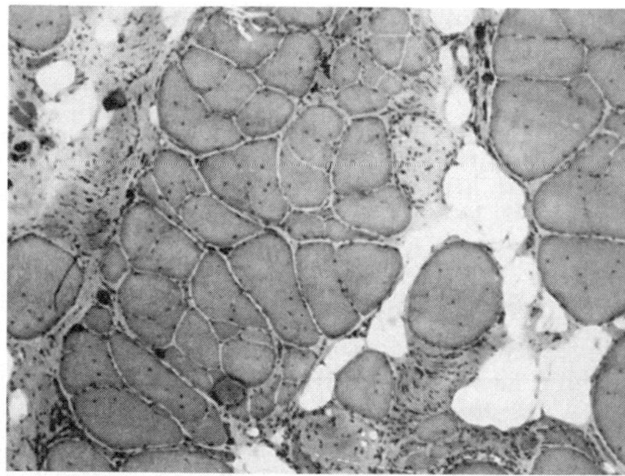

Fig. 76-5 Increased numbers of internal nuclei are seen within several fibers.

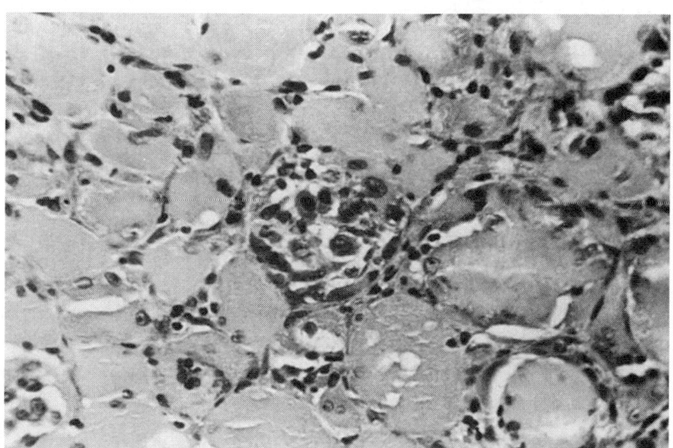

Fig. 76-6 Fiber necrosis in which the fiber at the center of the field is invaded by macrophages.

plasmic sprouting.[9] Satellite cells, prompted by cellular injury to transform into myoblasts, have the capacity to synthesize new muscle. Regenerating fibers are rapidly sighted in hematoxylin-and-eosin sections, wherein the basophilia of their sarcoplasm may be readily appreciated (Fig. 76-7). Ultrastructurally, the regenerating fiber is amply endued with ribosomes, a condition that accounts for its sarcoplasmic basophilia under the light microscope.[10] The nuclei of regenerating fibers are often internalized and numerically increased. They tend to be enlarged and to have dispersed chromatin with prominent nucleoli. The expression of neural cell adhesion molecule also appears to be a marker of fiber regeneration.[11]

Interstitial reactions. The interstitial compartment surrounding the muscle fibers may also sustain pathologic change. Interstitial inflammatory infiltrates are most often discernible in the immunologically mediated myopathies such as polymyositis and in the systemic connective tissue diseases, some of which are stigmatized by vasculitis. Particularly in the setting of chronic neuromuscular disease of either myopathic or neurogenic persuasion, fibrosis and fatty replacement of muscle tend to be prominent. At a point in the disease when they have attained significant proportions, the ardor of an active pathologic process has probably cooled and the likelihood of discovering specific pathologic changes is remote. The biopsy of an end-stage muscle that is not likely to provide relevant diagnostic information should be strongly discouraged.

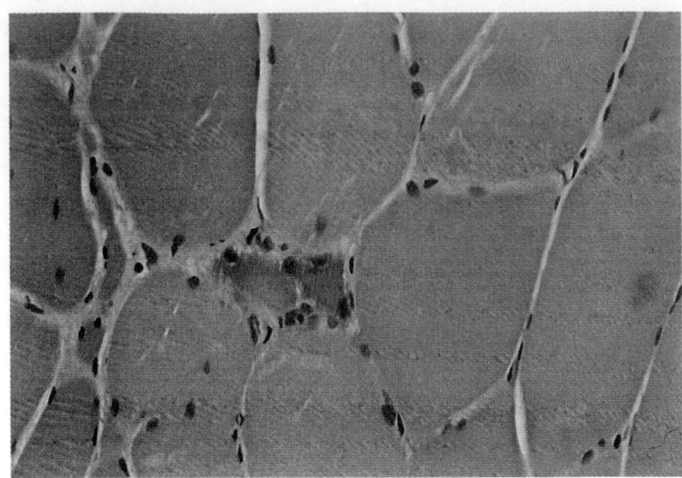

Fig. 76-7 Fiber regeneration is recognized by the presence of sarcoplasmic basophilia. Regenerating fibers may also have large vesicular nuclei with prominent nucleoli.

CONGENITAL MYOPATHIES

Congenital myopathies are most often manifest in childhood, though not all cases meet the definition of congenital, inasmuch as symptoms are not invariably apparent at birth (Table 76-3). Typically the patient has features of the floppy infant syndrome—a triad of adaxial weakness, hypotonia, and a poverty of spontaneous activity.[12] Being inherited diseases, the congenital myopathies usually display familial tendencies within a kinship. In contrast to the muscular dystrophies, the clinical course of congenital myopathies can be static, or progressive but at a largo tempo, or sometimes remitting. Conventionally, certain myopathies such as the lipid and glycogen storage diseases and the periodic paralyses, which are congenital disorders, are excluded from this disease category. Although the congenital myopathies are similar from a clinical standpoint, each is distinguished by morphologic features. As a result, the muscle biopsy is a valuable tool.

Table 76-3 Congenital myopathies

Central core disease
Multicore disease
Nemaline (rod) myopathy
Centronuclear (myotubular myopathy)
Congenital fiber type of disproportion
Fingerprint body myopathy
Cytoplasmic body myopathy
Zebra body myopathy
Spheroid body myopathy
Sarcotubular myopathy
Reducing body myopathy
Trilaminar fiber myopathy
Microfiber myopathy

Diseases in **bold type** are discussed in the text. Others below are less common and can be found in the sources listed in the Suggested Readings.

Central core disease

Central core disease was described in a seminal, now-famous publication as a benign, familial, congenital myopathy.[13] Central core disease is a myopathy of infants and children, causing a delay in the development of motor milestones.[14] Muscle involvement is mild, proximal, and nonprogressive. Within a carefully evaluated family, an autosomal dominant pattern of inheritance usually emerges. The gene locus in some cases appears to be on chromosome 19.[15] In sections of skeletal muscle, cores are visualized as regions of depleted or absent oxidative enzyme activity (Fig. 76-8).

Based on ultrastructural appearance, cores may be structured, in which the cross-banding pattern is maintained, or unstructured (Fig. 76-9), in which there is a myofibrillar disorganization resulting in an effacement of cross striations.[16] Structured and unstructured cores may coexist in the same specimen. Within the core there may be abnormalities of the organelles including the sarcotubular system.[17] In central core disease, cores are numerous and more prevalent in type 1 fibers. They are likely to be single and centrally positioned inside the fiber. Cores cannot be construed as a totally specific pathologic finding, in light of their occurrence in other diseases, most notably in chronic denervation. Cores, if they are a nonspecific reaction to injury, are confined to only a few fibers and tend to be large, eccentric, and at times multiple within the fiber.

Multicore myopathy

Multicore disease, also called "minicore disease,"[18] is a congenital, usually nonprogressive myopathy characterized by hypotonia, diffuse muscle weakness and delayed early motor milestones.[19] A family history is commonly present, and the disorder is more frequent in males. Nonobligate clinical features include kyphosis, scoliosis, and muscle contractures. The typical pathologic criteria are type 1 fiber predominance, disproportionately small type 1 fibers, and minute, corelike struc-

Classification of skeletal muscle diseases

Congenital myopathies
- Often, but not always congenital
- Onset usually in childhood, typically as floppy infant
- Hereditary diseases, often with a family history
- Weakness frequently generalized and mild
- Nonprogressive course
- Distinctive pathologic change (such as cores, rods)
- Most fibers are affected

Muscular dystrophies
- Usually not congenital
- Onset in childhood, young adults
- Hereditary diseases, often with a family history
- Weakness frequently severe, variable distribution
  - Proximal in Duchenne muscular dystrophy, Becker muscular dystrophy, limb-girdle dystrophy
  - Facial in fascioscapulohumeral dystrophy
  - Distal in distal myopathy and myotonic dystrophy
- Progressive course
- Fiber destruction pathologically
  - Damage is random, not all fibers are affected

Myotonic disorders
- Onset in childhood, young adults
- Hereditary disease in many cases
- Clinical picture variable
  - Distal weakness in myotonic dystrophy
  - Muscle hypertrophy in myotonia congenita
- Progressive course in many cases

Inflammatory myopathies
- Sporadic, nonhereditary diseases
- Age of onset variable, more often in adults
- Onset of weakness relatively sudden
  - Often generalized, associated with myalgia
- High elevations of serum creative kinase
- Inflammation and fiber necrosis seen pathologically

Glycogen storage disease
- Onset often in childhood
- Hereditary disorders
- Systemic involvement common
- Weakness often episodic
  - Exercise-induced with myalgia, cramps
- Ischemic exercise test positive
- Vacuolar myopathy with PAS-positive sarcoplasmic vacuoles

Lipid storage myopathies
- Onset often in children
- Hereditary diseases
- Systemic involvement in many cases
- Rhabdomyolysis, especially in carnitine palmityl transferase deficiency
- Symptoms may be worse during fasting
- Vacuolar myopathy
  - Vacuoles identified with fat stains
  - Mitochondria may be abnormal by electron microscopy

Mitochondrial myopathies
- Heterogeneous disease group
- Some are inherited
  - May have defect in mitochondrial genome
- Variable clinically
  - Ptosis is a common symptom
- Systemic involvement is common
  - CNS frequently affected
  - Ragged red fibers are present in rapid Gomori trichrome stains (frozen sections)
- Electron microscopy demonstrates abnormal mitochondria

Myasthenic disorders
- Congenital or immune-mediated
- Age of onset variable
- Ptosis, extraocular muscles affected in many cases
- Weakness fluctuates
- Slowly or nonprogressive course
- Electron mictroscopy demonstrates motor end-plate abnormalities

Denervating diseases
- Most common type of neuromuscular disease
- Weakness begins distally
- Muscle wasting and atrophy are common
- Muscle biopsy reveals grouped atrophy, type grouping, and targets

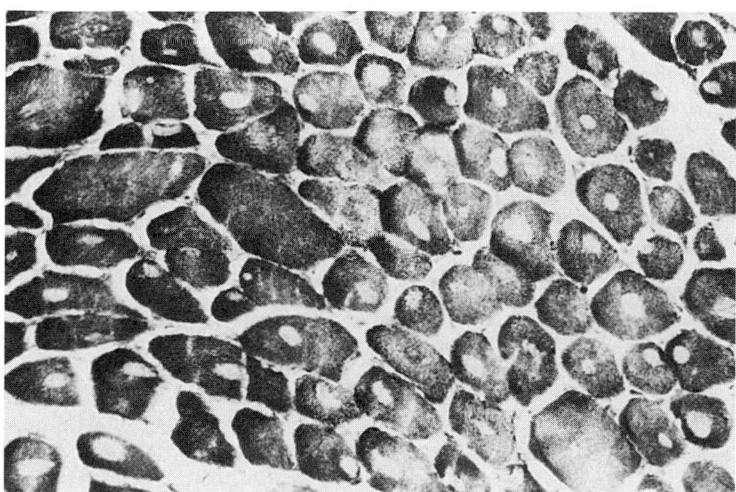

Fig. 76-8 Central core disease. Numerous areas of reduced enzyme activity (cores) are seen. (NADH-TR.)

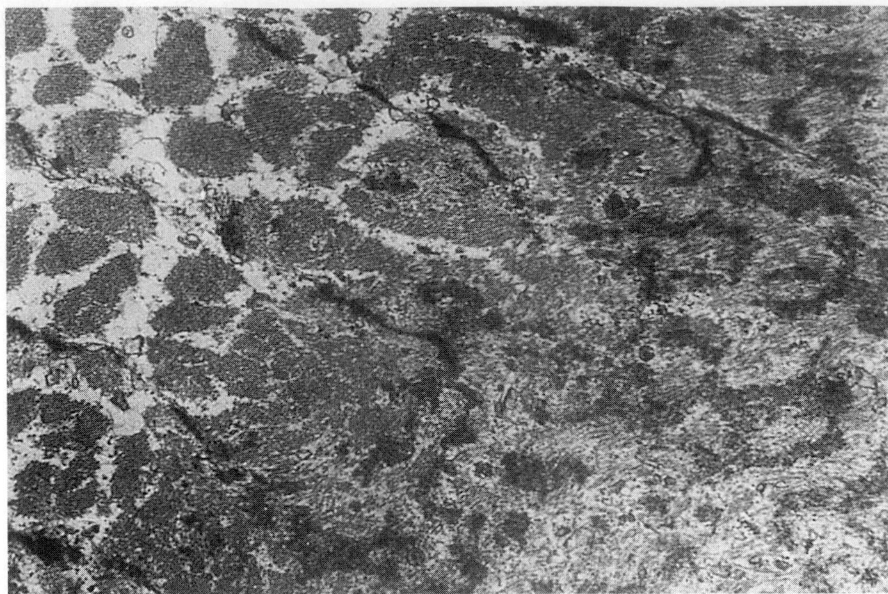

Fig. 76-9 Central core disease. Ultrastructurally, in the unstructured core, the orderly arrangement of the sarcomeres is lost because of disorganization of the myofilaments.

tures in the majority of muscle fibers. Multicores resemble central cores in that they are pale in most stains such as PAS, trichrome, and NADH-TR. They are numerous within each fiber and are oriented with their long axis perpendicular to the longitudinal dimension of the fiber so that they assume a disk shape in fibers that are sectioned lengthwise (Fig. 76-10). By electron microscopy, there is disorganization of the myofibrils within multicores, which also contain few organelles, particularly mitochondria and glycogen.

Nemaline (rod) myopathy

Nemaline myopathy may be passed on in accordance with mendelian dominant or recessive precepts and is inexplicably more common in girls. When seen by the pediatrician, the child will lament his or her inability to keep up with peers. During physical examination, a poor motor performance is more pronounced in the facial muscles and proximal muscles of the extremities. The diagnosis may be suspected in patients in whom facial dysmorphism is evident. This peculiar abnormality is a composite of facial elongation, prognathism of the mandible, and arching of the hard palate. The term *nemaline,* derived from the Greek word meaning 'threadlike,' was chosen to underscore the pathologic hallmark of this disease.[20] Rods are difficult to discern in hematoxylin-and-eosin sections and are ideally detected in rapid Gomori trichrome (RTC) stains on frozen sections and in resin sections (Fig. 76-11). Rods may be haphazardly distributed in the sarcoplasm but more commonly are found as focal subsarcolemmal collections. Ultrastructurally, rods are electron dense and rectangular or cylindrical in shape, having a maximum dimension of 6 to 7 μm (Fig. 76-12). They are in continuity with the Z bands and are believed by many authorities to arise as proliferations of Z-band material. Moreover, immunocytochemical studies have demonstrated that rods, like normal Z disks, are partly composed of alpha-actinin.[21] They have a lattice-like ultrastructure similar to that of the normal Z-band,[22] with an axial periodicity of 14 to 20 nm when viewed in the longitudinal plane.[23] After the original description of nemaline myopathy, it has become unavoidably clear that rods are not a unique pathologic attribute. Rods have been reported in many diverse conditions such as muscular dystrophy, polymyositis, peripheral neuropathy, and experimental tenotomy. However, in this context rods are sparse in number and located in only occasional fibers.

Centronuclear myopathy

In transverse microscopic sections, a central or paracentral nucleus is visible within almost every muscle fiber (Fig. 76-13). These abnormally situated nuclei are larger than normal and possess a vesicular chromatin pattern. The sarcoplasm in the immediate vicinity of the nucleus may be clearer, producing a rarefaction or halo that is poorly stained in paraffin sections. In some cases type 1 fiber hypotrophy has been reported.[24] This disease, described by Spiro and co-workers as "myotubular myopathy,"[25] has been considered by these authors and others to constitute an arrest of muscle maturation because of the resemblance of the muscle biopsy to the fetal myotube stage of muscle development. However, this embryologic explanation, though conceptually useful, has not been proved. Evincing genetic heterogeneity, centronuclear myopathy may be transmitted as a dominant, recessive, or X-linked abnormality.[26] The time of onset is difficult to date and may be delayed until middle age. There is a progression of weakness in some cases, but the extent of eventual disability is unpredictable. Extraocular and facial muscle palsies may accompany the loss of strength in the axial musculature.

Congenital fiber type disproportion

As defined by Brooke,[27] congenital fiber type disproportion has two essential pathologic features—type 1 fiber atrophy and enlargement of type 2 fibers. A predominance of type 1 fibers has been observed in some cases. The genetics in this condition are poorly understood, though congenital fiber type disproportion is presumably inherited in certain families. Both

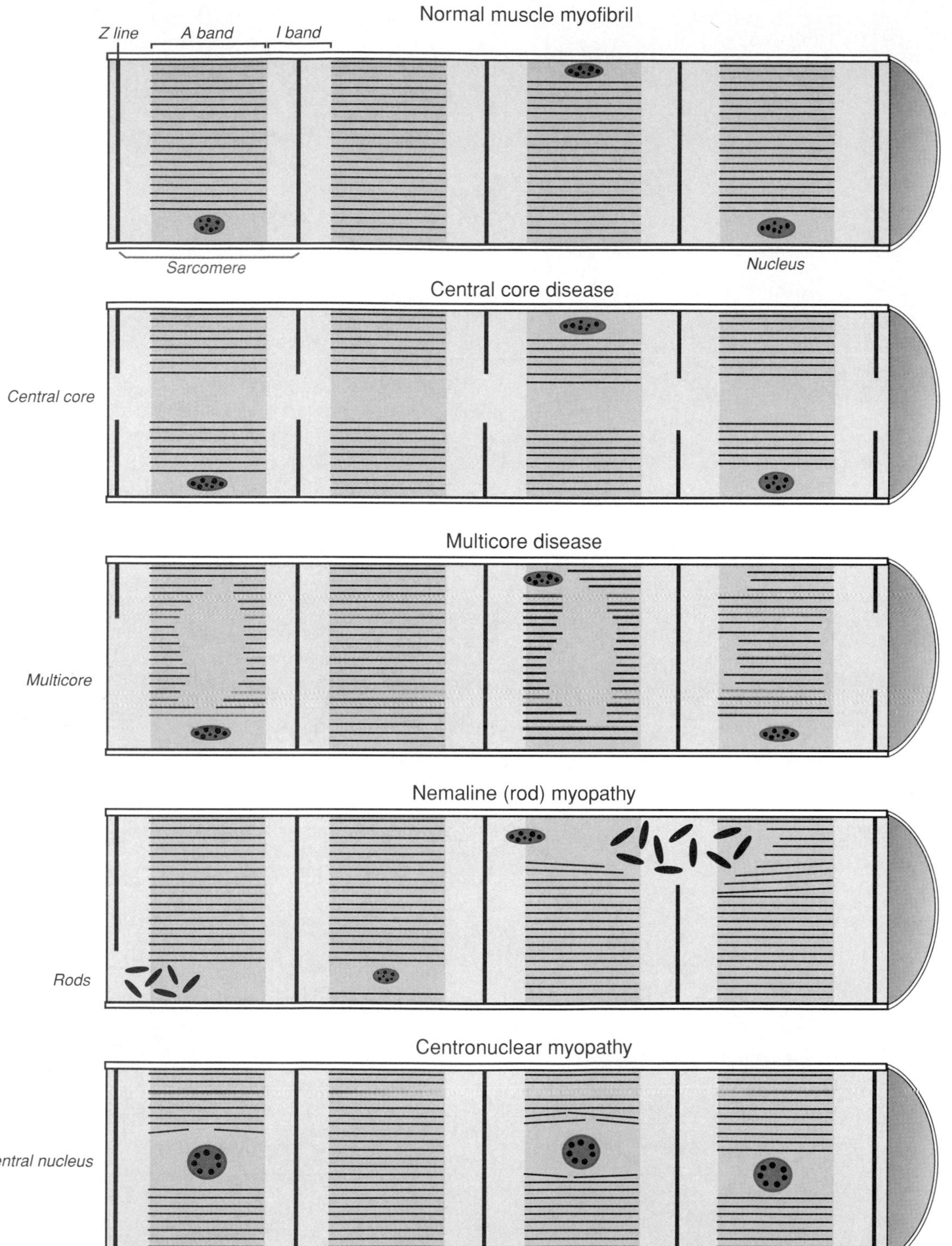

Fig. 76-10 Schema of four typical congenital myopathies. **A,** Central core disease. In this disorder, the core tends to be central and to run the length of the fiber. Cores have few organelles and often lack striations (unstructured). **B,** Multicore disease. Multicores are unstructured and devoid of organelles. They are somewhat disk shaped with their long axes perpendicular to the fiber length. **C,** Nemaline (rod) myopathy. Rods are often found in clusters beneath the sarcolemma. Many such clusters can be seen within the same fiber. **D,** Centronuclear myopathy. Very few if any subsarcolemmal nuclei are seen in this disorder. Multiple, somewhat enlarged, vesicular central nuclei are found within each fiber. Central nuclei are typically surrounded by a zone of sarcoplasm that is unstructured and lacks the normal architecture of the sarcomere. *N,* Normal nucleus; *S,* normal sarcomere.

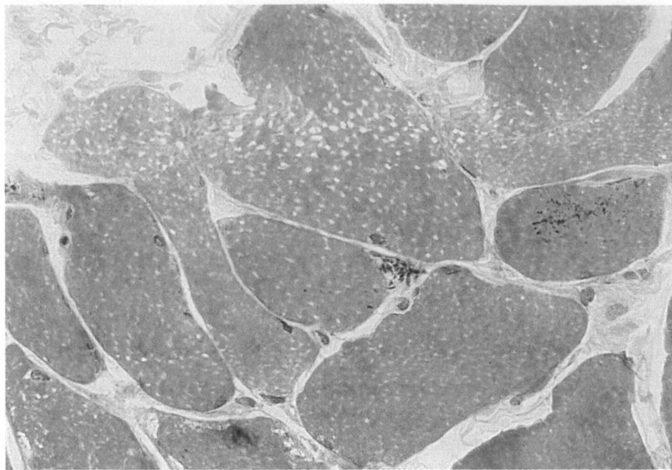

Fig. 76-11 Nemaline myopathy. Many darkly stained rods are seen. Rods may cluster in subsarcolemmal regions. (Rapid Gomori trichrome stain.)

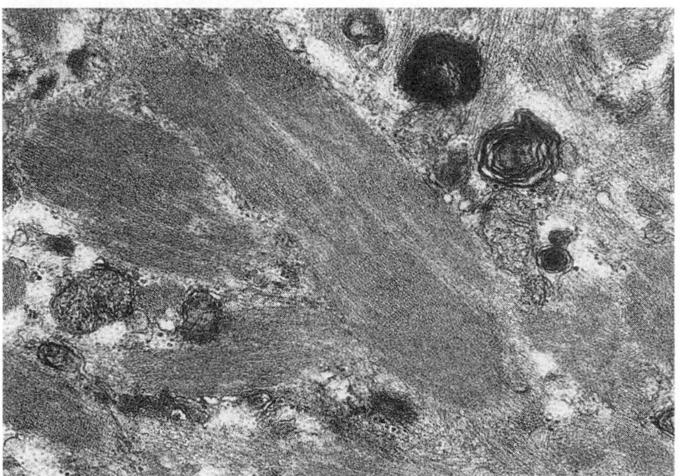

Fig. 76-12 Nemaline myopathy. At the electron microscopic level, rods are osmiophilic and resemble Z bands in staining characteristics and structure.

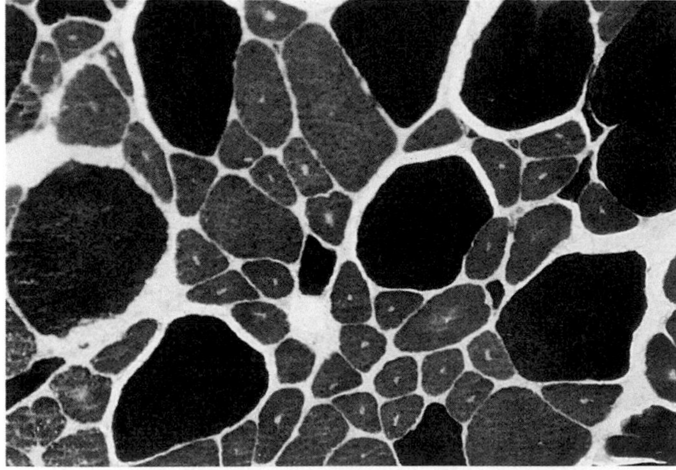

Fig. 76-13 Centronuclear myopathy. Type 1 fibers are abnormally small, and type 2 fibers are enlarged. Central nuclei are seen as unstained, clear regions within the fibers. (ATPase, pH 9.4.)

an autosomal recessive and an autosomal dominant mode of inheritance have been suggested. The clinical range is from a rapidly fatal disease of infants to an indolent myopathy of midlife adults.[28] Skeletal deformities such as kyphoscoliosis, hip dislocation, joint contractures, high-arched palate, and diminutive stature have been reported in over 50% of patients.[29]

THE MUSCULAR DYSTROPHIES

The rather unsophisticated term *dystrophy,* literally meaning 'poor nourishment,' was popularized at the close of the nineteenth century, perhaps in homage to the prevailing view of the pathogenesis of the muscular dystrophies. Although all the muscular dystrophies, which are collectively somewhat similar both clinically and pathologically, have traditionally been considered under a single rubric, this time-honored convention has foundered lately on such an erroneous oversimplification. In fact, each type of muscular dystrophy is a discrete entity. (Table 76-4). Nonetheless, in general, these diseases make their debut in childhood or early adulthood. The cardinal symptom is muscular weakness that worsens steadily and unremittingly. Most forms of dystrophy are genetically inherited, and so a family history of neuromuscular difficulties is likely to be elicited in many cases. The pathologic reactions unifying this group of myopathies—fiber necrosis, regenerative activity, and interstitial fibrosis—are more prominent in some types of dystrophy than in others.

Duchenne muscular dystrophy

With a prevalence rate of 1 per 3500 live male births, Duchenne muscular dystrophy (DMD) is the most common member of this disease category. It is inherited as an X-linked recessive disorder, in which genetic mapping studies have shown the DMD gene to be situated in band Xp21 on the short arm of the X chromosome.[30] Molecular studies have identified the gene as a 2500 kilo–base pair sequence containing over 70 exons, which appears to be the largest known human gene.[31] The high mutation rate in this type of dystrophy, accounting for about one third of new cases, is presumably related to the huge size of the DMD gene.[32] Investigations using cDNA probes indicate that 65% of patients with Duchenne dystrophy may have deletions in the DMD gene.[33] The remainder have

Table 76-4 Muscular dystrophies

Duchenne
Becker
Emery-Dreifuss
Facioscapulohumeral
Limb girdle
Distal
Myotonic*
Congenital
Ocular
Oculopharyngeal

Dystrophies in bold type are discussed in the text. Others may be found in the sources listed in the Suggested Readings.

*Myotonic dystrophy is also listed in many sources under the myotonic disorders (Table 76-5).

frameshift and point mutations. Moreover, identification of prenatal disease and of dystrophy carriers is now possible, based upon the detection of DMD gene deletions. Deletions are clustered at two areas of vulnerability in the proximal (30%) and distal (70%) regions of the gene. Proximal deletions are more likely to occur earlier in embryologic development with a greater chance of becoming an inherited mutation. Distal deletions occur later and are frequently manifest as a sporadic mutation.[34] Molecular research has demonstrated that patients with Duchenne dystrophy lack the DMD gene product dystrophin.[35] This 427 kD highly charged, rod-shaped, hinged protein molecule consists of 3685 amino acids. The protein is composed of four domains (Fig. 76-14) that are separated by proline-rich hinge regions that act as spacers and render the molecule more flexible.[36] The N-terminal domain is composed of 240 amino acids and has homology with the calcium binding region of α-actinin. The central domain is similar to spectrin and is constructed from 24 repeats, each consisting of 109 amino acids arranged in a triple helix. The third, cysteine-rich domain is composed of 280 amino acids. The C-terminal domain is composed of 420 amino acids. Dystrophin is a cytoskeletal, costameric protein that forms a lattice that encircles the muscle cell, attaching the sarcomeres at I bands and M lines to the sarcolemma. Dystrophin is not directly joined to the membrane but attaches by means of a dystrophin-glycoprotein complex composed of at least four subunits (Fig. 76-15). The oligomeric dystrophin complex is tightly bound to transmembrane glycoproteins 35 DAG (35 kD), 43 DAG (43 kD), and 50 DAG (50 kD) and an extracellular glycoprotein, 156 DAG (156 kD), as well as a cytoskeletal protein, 59 DAP (59 kD).[37] The extracellular 156 DAG is bound to the extracellular matrix protein, laminin. Within the muscle cell, the N-terminal of dystrophin is bound to F-actin, and the C-terminal is bound to 59 DAP. Of great interest is the fact that in DMD there is not only a loss of dystrophin, but also a dramatic reduction in the dystrophin-associated proteins including 43 DAG and 156 DAG. Dystrophin is most abundant in skeletal muscle, though the protein is not unique to myocytes. The 14 kb mRNA transcribed from the dystrophin gene can be alternatively spliced, and certain promoters operate with tissue specificity. Thus isoforms of dystrophin also exist in brain, smooth muscle, myocardium, and Schwann cells in lower concentrations. In skeletal muscle the association of dystrophin with the sarcolemmal membrane[38] is presumed to maintain sarcolemmal membrane stability, which may be most essential during muscular contraction.[39] It is postulated that the absence of dystrophin causes membrane destabilization, allowing an influx of calcium ions into the sarcoplasm.[40] The shift in calcium activates cellular proteases, which initiate cell necrosis.[41]

In normal muscle, monoclonal antibodies to the dystrophin molecule can demonstrate a positive reaction at the sarcolemmal membrane. The sarcolemma of almost all fibers of DMD patients

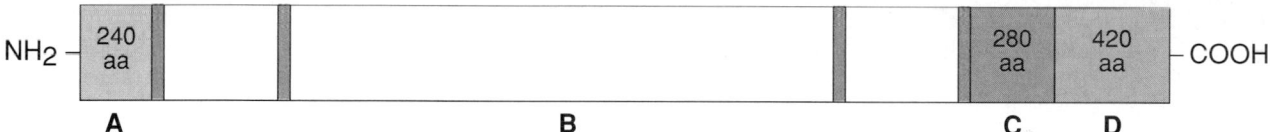

Fig. 76-14 *Dystrophin molecule.* Dystrophin is a rod-shaped molecule with four hinged regions *(H),* which give it increased flexibility. The N-terminal domain composed of 240 amino acids *(A)* is similar to the actin-binding region of alpha-actinin. The large central domain is similar to alpha-spectrin and consists of 24 triple helical repeats *(B).* All four hinges are associated with this domain, two being at either end of the helical structure. On the C-terminal side of the fourth hinge is a cysteine-rich domain containing 280 amino acids *(C)* with homology to the calcium-binding domain of alpha-actinin. The C-terminal domain is composed of 420 amino acids *(D)* and has an affinity for 59 DAP in the glycoprotein complex in the sarcolemma. (Modified from Rosenberg RN et al, editors: *The molecular and genetic basis of neurological disease,* Boston, 1993, Butterworth-Heinemann.)

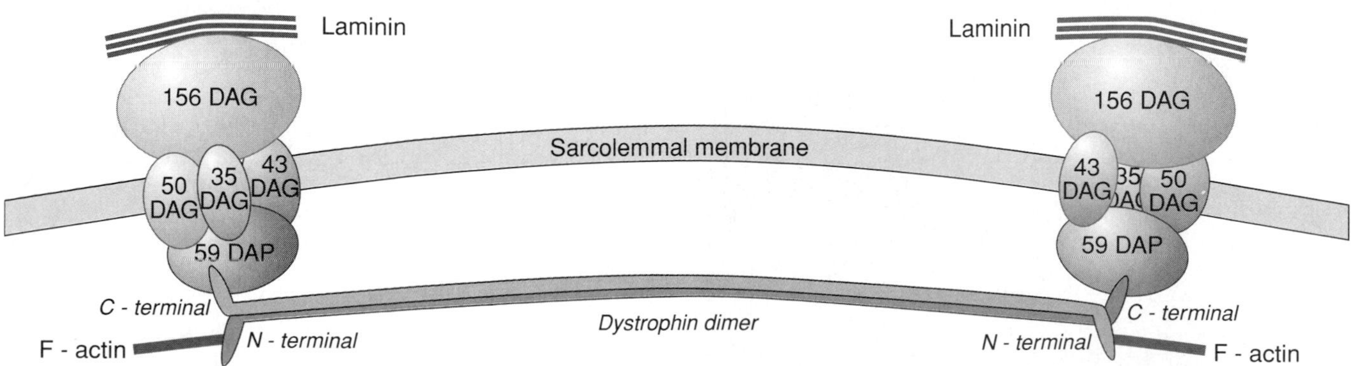

Fig. 76-15 The dystrophin-glycoprotein complex. The dystrophin molecule is considered to be a dimer that attaches the sarcomeres at actin-binding sites to the sarcolemmal membrane by joining to the transmembrane glycoprotein complex. This complex is composed of at least four subunits or dystrophin-associated glycoproteins with molecular weights of 35 kD (35 DAG), 43 kD (43 DAG), 50 kD (50 DAG), and 156 kD (156 DAG). The largest subunit, 156 DAG, is extracellular and bound to laminin. The glycoprotein complex is attached to a cytoskeletal dystrophin-associated protein with a molecular weight of 59 kD (59 DAP). The C-terminal of dystrophin is bound to 59 DAP.

are nonreactive for dystrophin. The occasional immunoreactive dystrophin-positive myocytes have recently been explained on the basis of second, or somatic, mutations.[42] There is now some hope that DMD may be treated in the future by gene therapy in which myoblast transfer would introduce dystrophin genes into dystrophic muscle.[43] With this technique, normal myoblasts are injected into dystrophin-deficient muscle where they are allowed to fuse with diseased myofibers. In the process, dystrophic cells acquire the nuclei of normal dystrophin-producing fibers and are no longer dystrophin deficient.

DMD occurs almost exclusively in young boys, the onset in most cases being before 5 years of age. The affected child shows no overt signs of diseases at birth, but by the time he begins to ambulate, clumsiness and frequent falling have already become a cause for concern. Weakness, initially in the shoulder, pelvic, and proximal appendicular muscles, is remorselessly progressive and eventually generalized, save for the extraocular, facial, and pharyngeal muscles. Pseudohypertrophy, particularly in muscles of the calves and buttocks, is highly suggestive of DMD. This adventitious enlargement of muscles, which are swollen by fat and fibrous tissue infiltration yet are weak and rubbery, is paradoxical. Cardiac-muscle along with striated-muscle impairment is not infrequent, giving rise to labile tachycardia and various cardiac arrhythmias. Diminished mental prowess (mean IQ 80) does not correlate with the measure of physical disability and is therefore considered to be an independent component of the disease. The most informative laboratory determination is the serum creatine kinase (CK), which soars to very high values early in this condition, preceding detectable pathologic changes in muscle in many cases. Pathologically, the most striking feature of DMD is necrosis and commensurate regeneration of muscle fibers, the intensity of which far surpasses that in other forms of muscular dystrophy. Hyaline or opaque fibers are also more conspicuous than in other dystrophies. These fibers are so named because they are dense and darkly stained in both paraffin and frozen sections (Fig. 76-16). Such fibers tend to be rounded and increased in diameter with smudged, homogeneous cytoplasm. The hyaline appearance has been shown to be secondary to hypercontraction in electron microscopic studies, perhaps incidental to excessive "irritability" of the fiber. The hyaline fiber is believed to represent a nascent phase of cell necrosis.[44] In serial sections of the same fiber, regions of necrosis and phagocytosis can be demonstrated adjacent to hyalinization. Patchy endomysial fibrosis, an expected nonspecific reaction to injury in chronic neuromuscular disease, develops almost from the outset and is disproportionately severe when compared with the destruction of muscle cells.

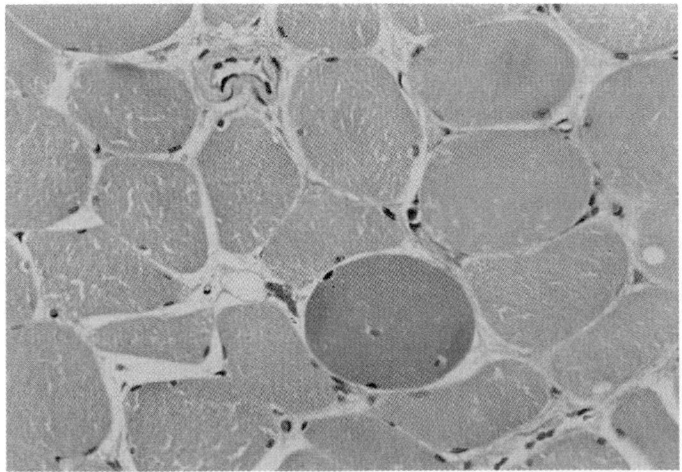

Fig. 76-16 Duchenne dystrophy. Hyaline fibers are rounded and deep red.

Becker muscular dystrophy

The incidence of the X-linked muscular dystrophy called "Becker muscular dystrophy" is approximately 10% of Duchenne muscular dystrophy. In contrast to DMD, Becker muscular dystrophy (BMD) is later in onset, less severe clinically, and slower in progression. Cardiac involvement is uncommon. As expected, the histologic findings resemble those in DMD but are mild. Hypercontracted hyaline fibers, necrotic myocytes, and regenerating fibers are present in fewer numbers. More advanced disease is characterized by numerous internal nuclei and split fibers. The gene for Becker dystrophy is also on the short arm of the X-chromsome and is allelic with the locus for Duchenne dystrophy. Approximately 60% of BMD patients have deletions of one or more exons in the dystrophin gene, but in most cases the deletions maintain the translational reading frame of mRNA, resulting in an abnormal, yet partially functional, dystrophin molecule and less severe clinical expression of the disease.[45] In Becker dystrophy, dystrophin is typically not greatly reduced in muscle, but its molecular weight is abnormal. Immunocytochemical techniques demonstrate that in comparison to DMD, where muscle fibers are unreactive with antibodies against dystrophin, in BMD some fibers exhibit patchy staining.

Emery-Dreifuss muscular dystrophy

The rare Emery-Dreifuss muscular dystrophy represents a third X-linked disorder and has been mapped to the Xq27-28 region. Onset is usually in adolescence with early involvement of the arms and shoulder girdle. The dystrophic process is slowly progressive, but cardiac disease may develop relatively early in the course and give rise to potentially fatal dysrhythmias.

Facioscapulohumeral dystrophy

Facioscapulohumeral (FSH) dystrophy with a prevalence of about 5 per 100,000 is a relatively mild disorder principally involving the muscles of the head and neck, shoulders, upper back, and arms. In most pedigrees this dystrophy follows an autosomal dominant mode of inheritance and is equally expressed in males and females. Genetic linkage analysis has established that the gene locus is in the 4q35 region.[46-48] FSH dystrophy starts to exact its toll in the second and third decades. Pseudohypertrophy, mental deficiency, and cardiac dysfunction are not part of the clinical picture. Pathologic review of muscle tissue reveals numerous atrophic and hypertrophic muscle fibers but little fiber necrosis or regeneration. A consistent observation in this disease is the moth-eaten or mottled fiber, which is most convincingly demonstrated in oxidative enzyme reactions (Fig. 76-17). The peculiar uneven staining reaction of fibers is produced by multiple, punctate zones of diminished enzyme activity that are randomly dispersed in the sarcoplasm. The fact that the ultrastructural integrity of the sarcoplasm between zones of mottling is maintained upholds the idea that the mottled fiber represents a form of reversible

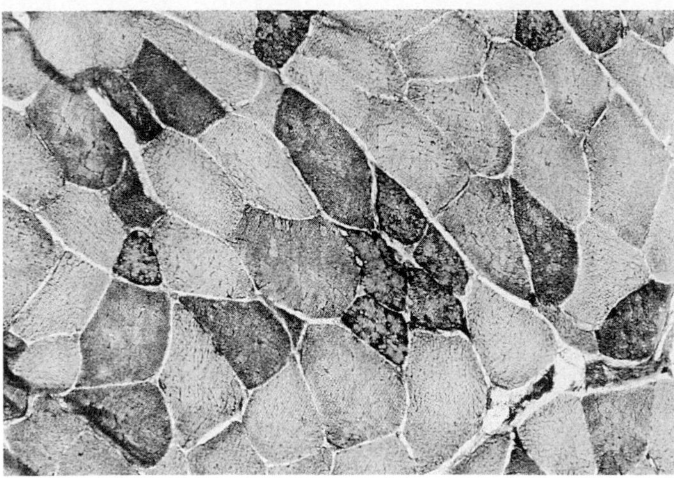

Fig. 76-17 Facioscapulohumeral dystrophy. Moth-eaten fibers are often darkly stained with multiple, small, poorly demarcated, unreactive sarcoplasmic areas. (NADH-TR.)

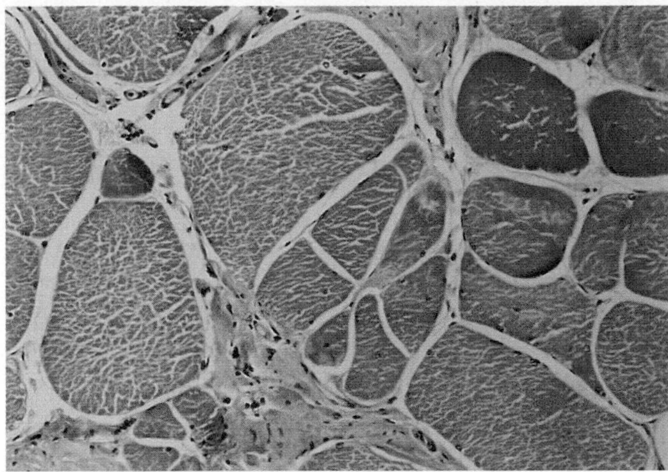

Fig. 76-18 Limb girdle dystrophy. Hypertrophic fiber at the center has split into six smaller segments.

cell injury. The identification of inflammatory cells, almost exclusively mature lymphocytes, serves to distinguish FSH dystrophy from other dystrophies where inflammation is absent. Inflammatory infiltrates within the endomysium and surrounding perimysial blood vessels are usually only noticeable during the ingravescent states of the illness.

Limb-girdle dystrophy

The hallmark of limb-girdle dystrophy is a decline in strength in the shoulder and pelvic girdles as well as in the proximal limbs.[49] The clinical course is one of steady deterioration, though the pace is slow, after the first manifestations of myopathy in late adolescence or young adulthood. Most cases are inherited through an autosomal recessive mechanism. Muscular pseudohypertrophy is a significant finding in approximately a third of patients. The pathologic theme of this disorder is epitomized by prominent internalization of sarcolemmal nuclei, fiber atrophy, and often florid fiber hypertrophy associated with widespread fiber splitting (Fig. 76-18). Fiber necrosis and regeneration tend to occur in chronic disease.

Distal myopathy

Distal myopathy is an unusual form of dystrophy because of its rather atypical clinical features. Muscle weakness and wasting affect primarily the acral muscles of the extremities, generally in males between 40 and 60 years of age. The largest cluster of cases has been reported in the Scandinavian countries where distal myopathy appears to be a dominantly transmitted infirmity. Pathologic examination of muscle shows excessive numbers of internal nuclei, selective atrophy of type 1 fibers, and minimal fiber necrosis and regeneration. In many cases so-called rimmed vacuoles, which ultrastructurally appear to be autophagic vacuoles, have been described.[50]

MYOTONIC DISORDERS

Myotonic muscular dystrophy

Myotonic muscular dystrophy (MyD) is a multisystem disorder that approaches DMD in incidence in certain geographic locations within the United States. The overall incidence in North America is approximately 1 per 8000 population.[51] MyD is therefore the most common dystrophy in adults and the most important of the myotonic disorders, which also include myotonia congenita, paramyotonia, chondrodystrophic myotonia (Schwartz-Jampel syndrome), and acquired myotonia, which may be drug-induced or associated with malignancy (Table 76-5). Linkage studies indicate that the MyD gene, a 200 kb interval, is located on the proximal long arm of chromosome 19 (19q13.2-13.3). Presymptomatic and prenatal diagnosis is possible using genetic markers CKMM and ApoC2, which are tightly linked to MyD.[52] More accurate diagnosis is now available with use of Southern blot analysis to detect the mutation.[53] The genetic basis for MyD involves a mutation causing the insertion of cytosine-thymidine-guanine (CTG) repeats. The number of repeats varies from 50 to several thousand trinucleotides compared with the normal gene having 5 to 40 repeats. Phenotypic expression is related to expansion of this region of the gene, much like triplet repeat expansions in X-linked spinal muscular atrophy and Huntington's disease.[54] Clinical symptoms often appear at a younger age and become increasingly severe in successive generations. This observation, known as "anticipation," tends to be accompanied by increasingly longer CTG repeat sequences. It has recently been discovered that the CTG repeats in the offspring of MyD patients may rarely normalize in length. In this

Table 76-5 Myotonic disorders

Myotonic dystrophy
Myotonia congenita
Paramyotonia
Chondrodystrophic myotonia
Periodic paralysis
Acquired myotonia
Drug-induced
Malignancy-associated

Diseases in **bold type** are discussed in the text. Others may be found in the Suggested Readings.

process of reverse mutation, offspring are healthy and unaffected by the disease.[55] This mutation interrupts the 3′untranslated region, which codes for an enzyme known as "myotonin protein kinase." It is not clear how reduced levels of this enzyme explain the clinical and pathologic findings in MyD, but protein kinases have a central role in the modulation of channel proteins, and their absence can lead to disruption of signal and amplification pathways.[56]

MyD is dominantly inherited with variable penetrance, making the age of onset and the clinical expression somewhat unpredictable. Congenital MyD is uncommon and is a severe disease with a significant mortality.[57] Symptoms become apparent in the average patient during the third or fourth decade. Muscular weakness and wasting are first confined to the face and distal portions of the extremities. Hence typical signs are ptosis, a vacant countenance, a slack transverse smile, and difficulty in swallowing. Myotonia is an early clue to the patient's condition and a prerequisite for the diagnosis of MyD. An inability of muscle to relax after contraction, myotonia is a consequence of muscle membrane instability and may be exacerbated during vigorous voluntary muscle contraction or at the bedside by percussion of the muscle with a reflex hammer. Electromyography may be necessary to document myotonia that is clinically silent. The classical systemic signs are embodied in ocular cataracts in 90% of patients, testicular atrophy, endocrine disturbances such as hyperinsulinism, cardiomyopathy, and dementia. There may be smooth muscle dysfunction in the esophagus, colon, urinary bladder, or uterus, which can be demonstrated with the assistance of appropriate physiologic and roentgenographic studies. In muscle biopsy specimens a multitude of internal nuclei and selective atrophy of type 1 fibers are found initially. Ring fibers, in which a group of peripherally located myofibrils are circumferentially oriented and encircle the normal internal portion of the fiber, are frequently identified without difficulty in MyD (Fig. 76-19). Ring fibers are considered to represent a bona fide pathologic disturbance in MyD, but they may reflect the phenomenon of hypercontractility, since they have been reported in muscle tissue specimens containing contraction artifact. In muscle samples from patients with long-standing disease, the features of dystrophic change—fiber necrosis, regeneration, and reactive fibrosis—are likely to supervene.

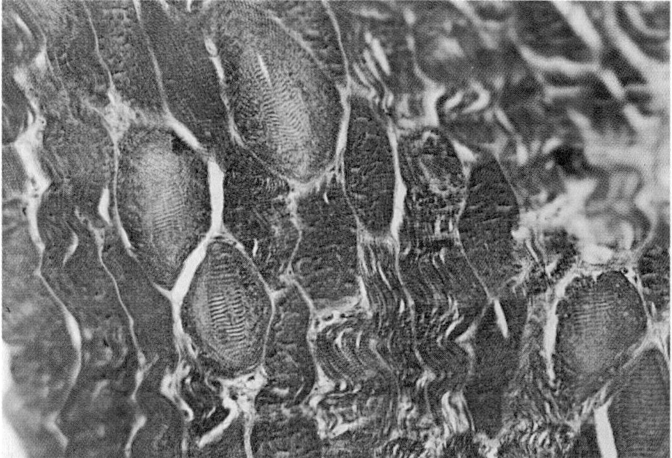

Fig. 76-19 Myotonic dystrophy. Illustrated are ring fibers in which the normal cross striations of the central portions of the fibers are enclosed by a ring of myofibrils that are not oriented longitudinally and lack striations. (Phosphotungstic acid–hematoxylin.)

Myotonia congenita

Myotonia congenita (Thomsen's disease) may be confused with myotonic dystrophy, despite the fact that this condition is neither a dystrophy, nor congenital in many cases. Onset ranges from the neonatal period to adolescence. Both autosomal dominant and recessive patterns of inheritance have been reported. Evidence suggests that the Thomsen's disease gene is linked to the T-cell receptor beta locus on chromosome 7q35.[58] Skeletal muscle is the only organ affected, and myotonia is the major symptom in many patients. Muscle weakness may develop later in the course of disease. In the muscle biopsy, a variation in fiber size is common and striking fiber hypertrophy may be seen. Abundant internal nuclei are found in the muscle fibers.

INFLAMMATORY MYOPATHIES

The inflammatory myopathies are a diverse group of diseases that are frequently infectious in origin or immune mediated[59] (Table 76-6). Typically the onset of symptoms is relatively sudden, weakness is associated with muscular pain, and serum CK is elevated.

Infectious myositis

Bacterial myositis

Bacterial infections of muscle are more prevalent in the tropics and subtropics than in the temperate global regions,[60] though they are becoming more common in patients with HIV infection worldwide. Bacterial myositis may be focal, typically an intramuscular abscess (pyomyositis), or the infection may be generalized with diffuse lesions. Generalized muscle infection arises by a hematogenous route rather than from a site of infection adjacent to the muscle, which is more likely to be the origin of a muscle abscess. Closed trauma to muscle precedes pyomyositis in some cases. Pyogenic organisms are often the

Table 76-6 Inflammatory myopathies

Inflammatory myopathies
Infectious
Bacterial
Fungal
Viral
Parasitic
Idiopathic
Polymyositis
Dermatomyositis
Inclusion body myositis
Collagen disease associated
Lupus erythematosus
Rheumatoid disease
Sjögren's syndrome
Polyarteritis
Drug-induced

Diseases in **bold type** are discussed in the text. Others may be found in the Suggested Readings.

pathogens in bacterial myositis, with *Staphylococcus aureus* being the agent that has attracted the most attention. Patients with generalized bacterial myositis are acutely ill with fever, bacteremia, and neutrophilic leukocytosis. Widespread necrosis is evident pathologically, involving not only muscle fibers but also the perimysium and blood vessels. The inflammatory infiltrate is pleomorphic, composed of both lymphocytes and neutrophils. Even with special stains, bacteria are elusive under the microscope.

Viral myositis

Innumerable viral syndromes are accompanied by myalgias and muscle weakness. Influenza and coxsackieviruses are well recognized causes of myositis in a systemic viral process. Viruses that are increasingly reported in the pathogenesis of myositis are parainfluenza, hepatitis B, and echoviruses. Viral myositis is characterized by severe muscle pain and swelling that tend to last 1 to 2 weeks and resolve spontaneously. Viral infection of muscle may result in rhabdomyolysis, notably in coxsackievirus, echovirus, and adenovirus infections. Patients with this potentially fatal complication are gravely ill, with nausea, vomiting, and profound muscular weakness. Myoglobinuria may lead to acute renal tubular necrosis and oliguric kidney failure.

Neuromuscular disease is common in the acquired immunodeficiency syndrome (AIDS) and is most often attributable to peripheral nerve disease. An immune-mediated inflammatory vasculopathy leading to red blood cell extravasation, erythrophagocytosis, and hemosiderin deposition in muscle has been reported in up to 50% of cases studied.[61] A few cases of myositis resulting from HIV infection have been reported.[62] Muscle involvement resembles polymyositis and is manifested by generalized muscular weakness, a rise in serum CK, and features of myositis on electromyography. Muscle fiber necrosis and lymphocytic, T-cell inflammation are visualized histologically. Multinucleated giant cells, similar to those described in the central nervous system of AIDS patients, have occasionally been reported in skeletal muscle. The present of nemaline rods in patients with HIV myopathy is of interest but of uncertain significance.[63] Epidemiologic studies of human T-cell leukemia virus type I (HTLV-1) indicate a probable association of this infection with polymyositis. In Jamaica, where the prevalence of HTLV-1 infection reaches 18%, a series of patients with polymyositis were found to be seropositive for HTLV-1.[64]

Chronic fatigue syndrome is of unknown cause, though it is postulated to be of viral origin. Epstein-Barr virus and coxsackievirus have been most frequently cited in the pathogenesis.[65] The syndrome affects young women who develop headache, sleep disturbances, pharyngitis, lymphadenopathy, fever, and lassitude. Patients typically report diffuse myalgias and muscular weakness, though muscle strength is not significantly impaired on physical examination.[66] The pathologic features of muscle disease in chronic fatigue syndrome are currently under investigation, but they may include inflammatory infiltrates.

Parasitic myopathies

The most important parasitic myopathies in North America are toxoplasmosis, trichinosis, and cysticercosis. Invasion of muscle by *Toxoplasma gondii* usually occurs in disseminated toxoplasmosis in patients who are immunocompromised.[67] Such individuals also exhibit signs of myocarditis, pneumonitis, and meningitis. Tissue samples of skeletal muscle may show inflammatory infiltrates composed of neutrophils, lymphocytes, plasmacytes, and histiocytes. The inflammatory cells surround necrotic muscle fibers or infiltrate the endomysial spaces. Organisms are often difficult to identify and may be located within cysts containing numerous bradyzoites. Toxoplasma may be best identified in Giemsa-stained sections or by use of anti-*Toxoplasma* antibodies that are appropriately labeled for visualization in tissue sections. There has been speculation that some cases of polymyositis may actually represent *Toxoplasma* infection. Elevated antibody titers to *Toxoplasma* organisms have been found in some patients with polymyositis.

The most common parasitic infestation of skeletal muscle is trichinosis, which is caused by the nematode *Trichinella spiralis*. Trichinosis is usually acquired after the ingestion of raw or inadequately cooked pork. Infection begins as larvae penetrate the mucosa of the small bowel, entering the bloodstream and disseminating systemically. With invasion of the musculature, there is intermittent myalgia and weakness that is variable in severity. Cutaneous involvement may manifest as a petechial or urticarial dermatitis. Trichinosis is suspected with the development of periorbital edema and subconjunctival hemorrhages. Cardiac and brain involvement may develop in severe disease. An eosinophilic leukocytosis is evident in the overwhelming majority of cases and may be the only manifestation in subclinical disease. Muscle fiber necrosis and inflammation are the result of larval invasion of skeletal muscle. In acute disease there is a brisk interstitial inflammatory reaction in which eosinophils may outnumber other inflammatory constituents including lymphocytes and plasma cells. Definitive diagnosis is based upon the demonstration of *Trichinella* organisms, which, in our experience, are infrequently identified in muscle biopsy specimens. Rather than coiled, encysted larvae, one is more likely to encounter the sequelae of parasitic invasion after organisms no longer remain viable. These include encapsulated cysts devoid of larvae, focal calcification, and granuloma formation.

Cysticercosis is most prevalent in eastern Europe, India, and Central America and Mexico. In the United States, infection is likely to be encountered only in recent immigrants. Like trichinosis, this disease is a consequence of eating uncooked or inadequately cooked pork which is contaminated with the encysted larvae of the cestode *Taenia solium*. Adult worms in the intestinal tract uncommonly cause clinical symptoms. The entrance of larvae into the blood of humans, who are the inadvertent intermediate host, is accompanied by fever, muscle pain, and peripheral eosinophilia. Any organ may be affected, but the most common sites are skeletal and cardiac muscle, brain, and the eyes. Skeletal muscle involvement may be associated with the appearance of palpable cysticerci in the subcutaneous tissues. A remarkable feature of this myopathy is muscular pseudohypertrophy, which may be seen in the tongue or the extremities, particularly the calf muscles.[68] Viable larvae generally cause little or no tissue reaction. However, death or rupture of a cysticercus produces an acute inflammatory response with an exudate composed of neutrophils and eosinophils. With the passage of time, cysts become encapsulated by fibrous tissue, which may eventually undergo calcification. Cystic structures are often surrounded by a chronic inflammatory reaction, which may be granulomatous.

Polymyositis

Polymyositis (PM) is the most important inflammatory myopathy of adults.[69] Based on epidemiologic information, polymyositis has a mean annual incidence of 5 to 10 cases per million population and is slightly more prevalent in black individuals. The average age of onset of symptoms is 35 to 40 years and the disease is more prevalent (2:1) in women. Muscular weakness often culminates abruptly over a period of several weeks. Proximal muscle groups are more severely involved, though weakness is generalized. In contrast to facial and extraocular muscles, which are seldom affected, distal muscles are clinically weak in many patients. Other symptoms that may be anticipated are fever, malaise, dysphagia from involvement of pharyngeal muscles, and myalgias. The clinical course, almost by definition, is characterized by remissions and exacerbations.

Laboratory data are useful and even essential for diagnosis. During the early or acute phase, there is an elevation of the erythrocyte sedimentation rate and a significant rise in plasma CK levels up to 50 times normal values. EMG recordings show small, brief, polyphasic motor units with increased insertional activity and spontaneous fibrillation potentials in over 90% of patients. A variety of antinuclear antibodies have been found in polymyositis. Antibodies reactive to PM-1, an extractable nuclear antigen, are present in more than 50% of patients with PM and in perhaps half that number in dermatomyositis. Antibodies against Jo-1 antigen, a subunit of histidine tRNA synthetase, are observed in patients with PM, particularly those with interstitial lung disease. Diffuse, chronic interstitial pulmonary disease develops in about 70% of patients with polymyositis in contrast to 30% of patients with dermatomyositis.

Polymyositis is an autoimmune disease in which the data support a cell-mediated mechanism of tissue damage. T-cells become sensitized to muscle cellular antigens, precipitating a cell-mediated attack on muscle fibers, resulting in cell necrosis. Although humoral mechanisms may also be involved in PM, their exact role in the pathogenesis of fiber destruction is unexplained. Although deposits of both immunoglobulins and complement as visualized by immunofluorescence microscopy have been reported in cases of polymyositis,[70] other studies indicate that such deposits are usually absent.[71] However, not only in PM, but also in other diseases with fiber necrosis like Duchenne dystrophy, the lytic C5b-9 complement components, or membrane attack complex (MAC), has been localized to necrotic fibers. Complement activation probably represents a nonspecific and poorly understood event during fiber necrosis in a variety of disease conditions.[72] The inflammatory cells in polymyositis infiltrate the interstitium, ultimately surrounding necrotic fibers and, to a lesser extent, the intramuscular blood vessels (Fig. 76-20). The inflammatory response consists primarily of mature lymphocytes and is virtually devoid of plasma cells, neutrophils, and eosinophils. Approximately 30% of the mononuclear cells encircling muscle fibers are macrophages, and the remainder are T-cells.[73] The majority of T-cells are $CD8^+$ cytotoxic/suppressor cells, many of which express Ia markers, indicating cellular activation. Major histocompatibility complex class I (MHC-I) expression is considered a requirement for antigen-specific T-cell–directed cytotoxicity. In immunocytochemical studies of PM, fibers under attack by $CD8^+$ cytotoxic lymphocytes express MHC-I antigen, which is not normally detectable in muscle cells. MHC-I

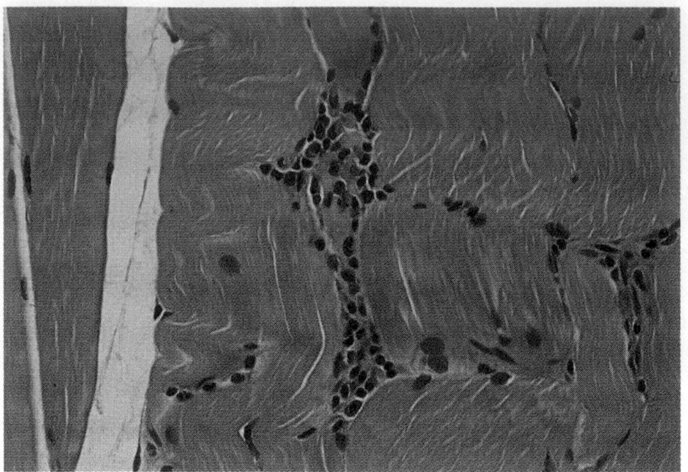

Fig. 76-20 Polymyositis. Necrotic fiber is surrounded and invaded by lymphocytes.

expression in muscle fibers is presumed to be modulated by interferons, which are released by inflammatory cells.[74] In the active phase of disease, many inflammatory cells and necrotic fibers are encountered. After a short time, the appearance of regenerating fibers is noted. Small, often angulated fibers become numerous with time and represent incomplete regeneration.[75] In chronic polymyositis, inflammatory infiltrates may be sparse or lacking, and fibrosis of the endomysium and perimysium are associated with widespread atrophy of fibers.

Dermatomyositis

Adult dermatomyositis (DM) is seen more often in women, though the female-to-male ratio (3:2) is below that in polymyositis (PM). The clinical manifestations of muscle involvement are very similar to those in polymyositis, such that some authorities consider both to be opposite ends of a range in a single disease process. In 90% to 95% of patients, a cutaneous rash is the first symptom. The dermatologic findings are variable, often starting as dusky erythematous lesions in a butterfly pattern on the face or as a purple rash on the eyelids with surrounding periorbital edema. A rash is also frequently present on the neck, shoulders, and extensor surfaces of the extremities and over the fingers and toes. Hyperemic, scaling lesions are seen on the knuckles in association with telangiectasia and periungual hyperemia. In many cases of childhood DM, the disease becomes a systemic vasculopathy involving, in addition to skin and muscle, the intestine, peripheral nerves, and subcutaneous tissues.[76] Calcifications develop in subcutaneous nodules, which ulcerate in vulnerable locations like knuckles, heels, and elbows. Angiitis of the alimentary tract produces mucosal ulcerations, at times with GI hemorrhage or perforation.

In contrast to polymyositis, the humoral rather than the cellular constituents of the immune system are more critical to the development of dermatomyositis. With direct immunofluorescence techniques, deposits of immunoglobulin (IgG, IgM) and complement, particularly C3, can be demonstrated in intramuscular vessels in most children and in many adults with DM and C5b-9 complement components, or membrane attack complexes, have been immunolocalized to blood vessels.[77] The granular appearance of the deposits by electron microscopy is also consistent with the presence of immune complexes. Nevertheless, the antigenic portion of the immune complexes has not been elucidated. Deposits are most often observed in perimysial venules and arterioles, which may become narrow and thickened but are generally free of acute inflammatory cells.

Lymphocytic inflammation tends to be most severe around blood vessels, as opposed to PM where infiltrates surround muscle fibers. Most of the lymphocytes are T-cells, but a larger proportion of $CD4^+$ and B-lymphocytes are present as compared with polymyositis. Ultrastructural studies reveal alterations in the intramuscular blood vessels that are not evident under the light microscope. The abnormalities are more concentrated in capillaries than in arterioles or venules. Swelling of endothelial cells with luminal narrowing is almost always present. Less predictably seen are endothelial cell necrosis and fibrin thrombi. Collections of viruslike undulating tubular profiles (Fig. 76-21) are identified in endothelial cells and pericytes.[78] Despite this observation, molecular studies have failed to establish that enteroviral or other viral nucleic acid sequences are detectable with any regularity in DM or PM.[77] As a result of vascular injury, a loss of capillaries is a consistent feature in the muscle of children with dermatomyositis.[80] The loss of capillaries is greater at the periphery of the fascicles. In adult dermatomyositis, the amount of vascular damage is more variable, and the depletion in intramuscular capillaries cannot be appreciated in some cases. Perifascicular atrophy is more extensive in advanced disease and occurs more frequently in pediatric cases (Fig. 76-22). The severity of fiber atrophy at the periphery of the fascicles is believed to be attributable to ischemia, which is secondary to vasculopathy. Ischemia is more intense in the distal vascular bed, which is presumed to be located at the fascicular margins.

Dermatomyositis and somewhat less frequently polymyositis are associated with malignant neoplasms. Based on statistical analysis of patients with inflammatory myopathies, the incidence of malignancy in patients with DM and PM is estimated to be 10% to 15%. In patients who are older than 55 years of age, the incidence of malignancy is higher, perhaps 25% to 30%. The most commonly associated malignancies are carcinomas arising in the lung, breast, and gastrointestinal tract. The malignancy may initially be occult and appear to be preceded by a myositis that is later discovered to be paraneoplastic. Moreover, a warning sign of recurrent tumor may be the development of dermatomyositis or polymyositis.

Inclusion body myositis

Since the first description of inclusion body myositis (IBM),[81] this disorder has emerged as an inflammatory myopathy distinct in many ways from polymyositis and dermatomyositis.[82] The typical patient is a male who is 50 to 70 years of age. The disease is generally indolent in its behavior but slowly progressive and resistant to steroid therapy. However, there is some evidence that IBM may be successfully treated with intravenous immunoglobulin.[83] Muscle involvement is painless and generalized, with weakness that is asymmetrical or greater distally. Dysphagia is said to be uncommon but is frequently overlooked.[84] Serum CK is normal or minimally elevated. Higher CK levels are reported in younger patients, especially women. Results of an electromyogram are usually interpreted as myopathic, but a neurogenic pattern may be observed. IBM may occasionally coexist with collagen vascular disease or malignancy.[85] Histologic examination of muscle tissue is suggestive of polymyositis in a minority of patients. Lymphocytic inflammation, fiber necrosis, and regeneration

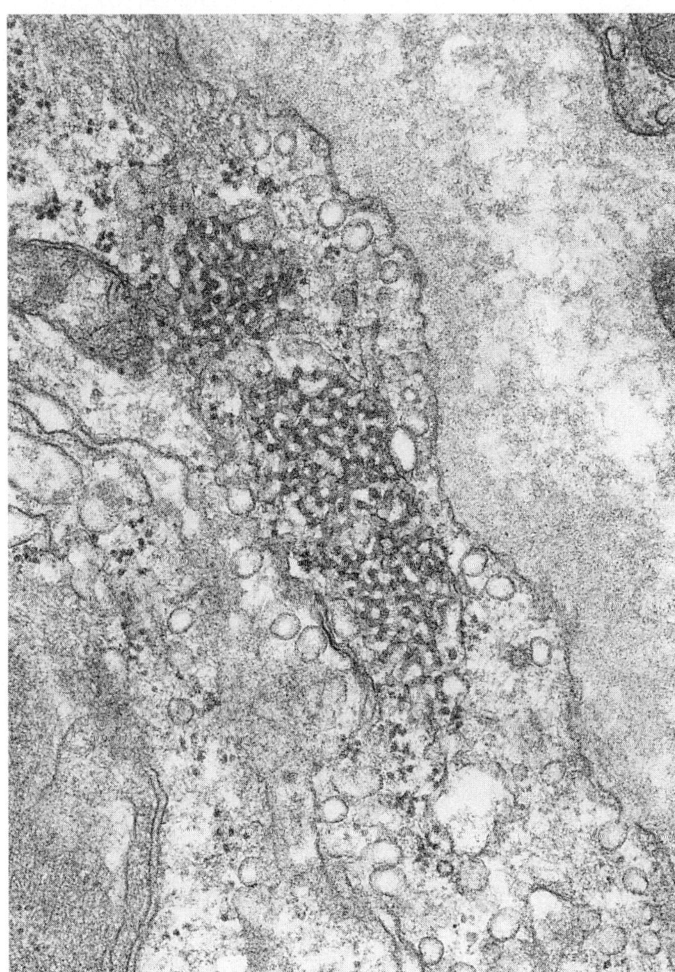

Fig. 76-21 Dermatomyositis. Undulating tubular profiles are seen in endothelial cells.

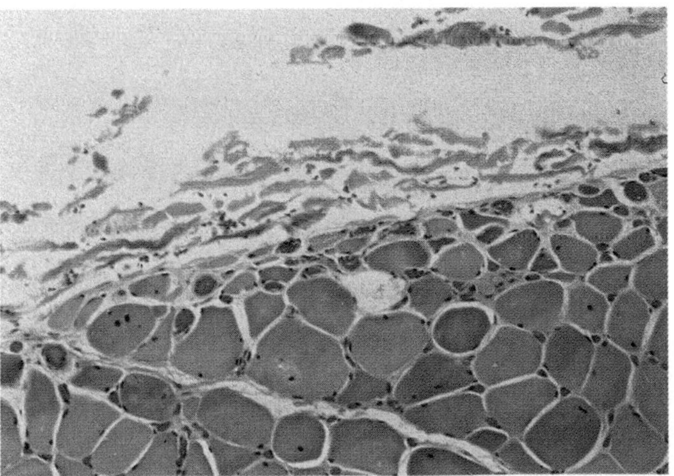

Fig. 76-22 Dermatomyositis. The edge of a fascicle at the top of the picture shows perifascicular atrophy.

are present in only 40% of cases. Enlarged fibers are more frequent than in PM or DM.[86] Cryostat sections are needed to identify the characteristic vacuoles containing small granules that are basophilic in H&E and red in RTC stains (Fig. 76-23). Classic rimmed vacuoles are lined by tiny granules at the margins of the vacuoles. Granules may not be marginated and may fill the vacuolar spaces. Ultrastructurally, the basophilic granules are composed of whorls of membranous profiles (Fig. 76-24). These profiles are usually located in aggregates beneath the sarcolemma, as well as with the vacuoles. By electron microscopy, masses of virus-like tubular filaments (inclusions) are detected within muscle fiber nuclei and in the sarcoplasm, often in association with rimmed vacuoles. The filaments are found in bundles and measure 15 to 18 nm in diameter. Often the filaments, which are present in only a few fibers, are difficult to locate. The nature of the filaments is controversial, but the possibility of a viral origin has been strongly considered. Immunohistochemical techniques have indicated that inclusion bodies contain mumps virus,[87] but in situ hybridization studies have not verified the presence of mumps virus nucleocapsid. Recent reports indicate that the filaments are made of beta-amyloid.[88,89] Ubiquitin has also been localized to vacuolated fibers, an indication of an intracellular degradation of abnormal tubular filaments.[90]

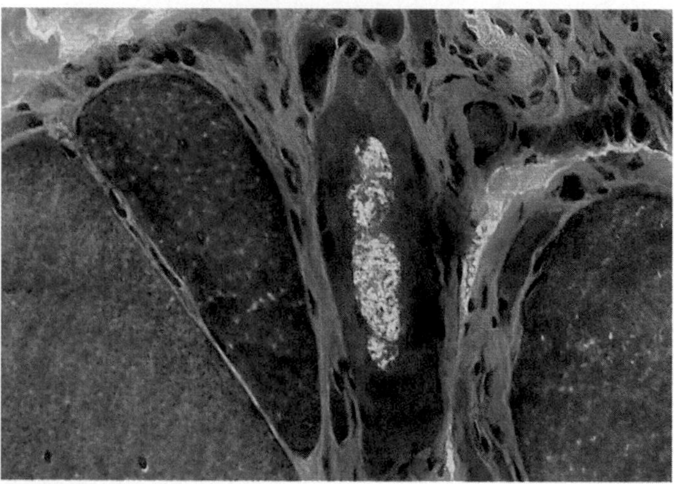

Fig. 76-23 Inclusion body myositis. Cryostat section showing characteristic vacuole containing numerous small red granules. (Rapid Gomori trichrome stain.)

Drug-induced inflammatory myopathy

The use of certain medications may be complicated by the onset of myositis. For many years D-penicillamine has been known to induce a polymyositis-like inflammatory myopathy. Other drugs that are potential causes of myositis include methyldopa, cimetidine, penicillin, certain diuretics, procainamide, and hydralazine. Drug-induced myositis is typically characterized by mild muscular weakness without myalgias. Serum CK is usually mildly elevated. In the muscle biopsy, necrosis of muscle fibers is minimal or absent. Inflammatory infiltrates are often perivascular and contain a disproportionate number of eosinophils[91] (Fig. 76-25). The presence of eosinophils should alert the pathologist to the possibility of drug-induced myositis or tryptophan myopathy. The latter disease has been reported in patients taking large amounts of the aminoacid L-tryptophan, which may be prescribed as a dietary supplement or as therapy for depression and insomnia. The high incidence of the eosinophilia myalgia syndrome (EMS) in individuals ingesting L-tryptophan led the Food and Drug Administration to ban tryptophan preparations from the market in 1989. It is now clear that the syndrome represents an allergic reaction to a contaminant in tryptophan preparations, an unusual dimeric form of the aminoacid. It has also been established that all cases of EMS were attributable to the ingestion of a product manufactured by one Japanese company. The hallmarks of EMS are diffuse muscle weakness, severe myalgias, fatigue, skin rash with edema and induration, and peripheral eosinophilia often in excess of 1000/mm^3.[92] Muscle biopsy reveals fascial and interstitial inflammation with infiltrates composed of a mixture of lymphocytes and some eosinophils.[93] EMS appears to be a T-cell–mediated disorder against fibroblasts and extracellular matrix components.[94]

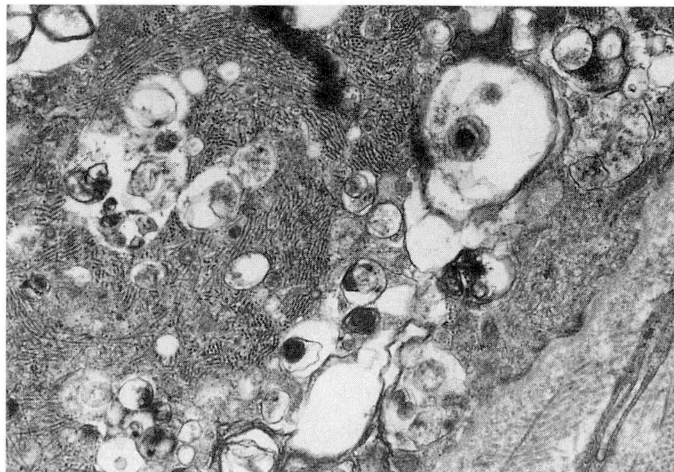

Fig. 76-24 Inclusion body myositis. Rimmed vacuole containing membranous profiles and bundles of viruslike tubulofilamentous structures.

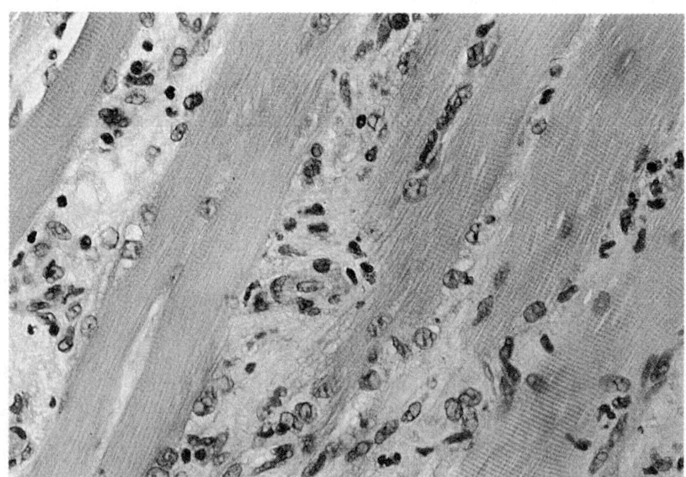

Fig. 76-25 Drug-induced myositis. Eosinophils are prominent in the inflammatory infiltrates.

STORAGE DISEASES

Carbohydrate storage diseases

Carbohydrate metabolism in muscle includes uptake of glucose, synthesis of glycogen, and degradation of glycogen. The muscle sarcolemma is not freely permeable to glucose and the rate of membrane transport limits the utilization of circulating glucose. Carbohydrate is stored in muscle in the form of glycogen and broken down to glucose when additional energy production is needed. The glycogen storage diseases include disorders of glycogen synthesis and degradation (Table 76-7). Traditionally, they have been designated by eponyms and numerals reflecting the order of their description. Classification according to their defective enzyme function is more precise. Several of the glycogenoses that affect muscle are manifested predominantly during periods of intense energy demand. Patients with some of the glycogenoses show impaired lactate production when subjected to an ischemic exercise test.

Acid maltase deficiencies (type II glycogenosis)

Acid maltase is a lysosomal enzyme that cleaves 1,4 and 1,6 alpha-glycosidic linkages. Since this hydrolytic enzyme is not in the main synthetic or degradative pathways for glycogen, some authors have suggested that this enzyme deficiency is an epiphenomenon rather than the basic metabolic defect. Acid maltase deficiency occurs in several forms. The varied expression in infants, children, and adults has been attributed to multiple genetic mutations and the level of residual enzyme activity.[95]

The infantile form, otherwise known as "Pompe's disease," is a systemic disease manifest by hypotonia, weak bulky muscles, macroglossia, cardiomegaly, and congestive heart failure. The disease is inexorably progressive and death occurs within 1 or 2 years. Abnormal storage of glycogen occurs in many organs including the central nervous system, heart, liver, and skeletal muscles. The intramuscular storage of glycogen is more severe in Pompe's disease than in the other glycogenoses.

Sections of skeletal muscle generally disclose severe vacuolation of the myofibers (Fig 76-26). The vacuolar contents are PAS positive and are extensively digested with diastase, reflecting the presence of glycogen. In addition, there are deposits of basophilic material that are PAS positive but resistant to diastase digestion. The latter material is believed to be a mucopolysaccharide. Stains for acid phosphatase activity are strongly positive in many of the vacuoles, reflecting the increased lysosomal activity secondary to the acid maltase deficiency.

Electron microscopy discloses massive accumulation of glycogen granules beneath the sarcolemma and between the myofibrils. Much of the glycogen is free in the sarcoplasm with only a portion confined within lysosomal membranes. The individual myofibrils often appear abnormally thin or atrophic. The myofiber damage has been attributed to leakage of acidic hydrolases from the abnormally distended lysosomes. Whether the free glycogen deposits result from rupture of distended lysosomes or other metabolic defects is uncertain.

The childhood and adult forms of acid maltase deficiency are manifested predominantly as myopathies. Patients with the childhood form have delayed development and weakness of the proximal limb and respiratory muscles. Some show calf hypertrophy and clinically resemble children with X-linked dystrophy. Most of these patients die by the end of the second decade of life from respiratory complications. Patients with the adult form typically present during the third or fourth decades. These patients have slowly progressive muscular weakness and clinically are often thought to have limb-girdle dystrophy or a chronic inflammatory myopathy. Some of the patients develop respiratory failure and die from the involvement of the intercostal muscles and diaphragm. The heart,

Table 76-7 Carbohydrate storage diseases

Carbohydrate storage diseases
Glycogen storage
Acid maltase deficiency (type II)
Debranching enzyme deficiency (type III)
Branching enzyme deficiency (type IV)
Myophosphorylase deficiency (type V)
Phosphofructokinase deficiency (type VII)
Disorders of glycolysis
Phosphoglycerate kinase deficiency
Phosphoglycerate mutase deficiency
Lactate dehydrogenase deficiency

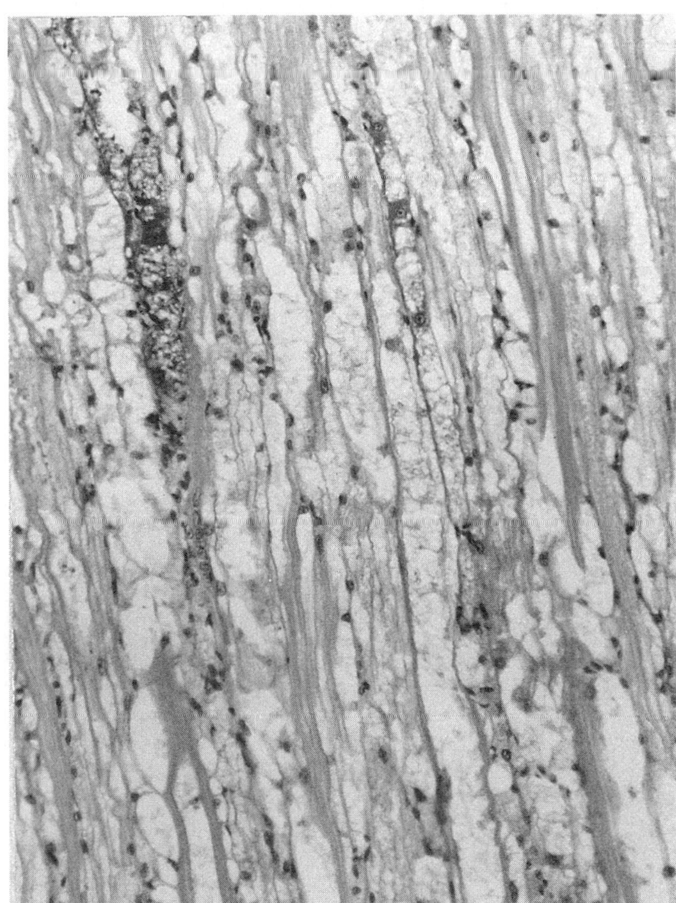

Fig. 76-26 Infantile acid maltase deficiency (Pompe's disease). Notice the severe vacuolation and dark deposits of basophilic mucopolysaccharide. (Paraffin-embedded section of Susa fixed tissue, H&E.)

liver, and central nervous system are generally uninvolved in the childhood and adult forms.

The vacuolation of muscle fibers is much less severe than in the infantile form of the disease (Fig. 76-27). The vacuolar contents are PAS positive and partially diastase digestible. The deposits of basophilic mucopolysaccharide that may be seen in the childhood cases are inconspicuous or absent in the adult cases. Increased acid phosphatase activity is demonstrable in the vacuoles and in scattered foci even within nonvacuolated myofibers. Electron microscopy discloses multiple, focal deposits of glycogen. The glycogen is both free in the sarcoplasm and membrane bounded where it is accompanied by granular osmiophilic and lamellar material.

Lysosomal glycogen storage disease with normal acid maltase activity

More recently, another form of glycogenosis with prominent autophagic vacuoles and normal acid maltase activity has been reported[96,97] These patients have proximal muscle weakness, hypertrophic cardiomyopathy, and mental retardation. Morphologic studies of skeletal muscle from these cases reveal a vacuolar myopathy. The vacuoles contain granular basophilic material that is at least partially PAS positive. Many of the vacuoles show increased acid phosphatase activity. By electron microscopy, free glycogen granules and fine fibrillar material are found in the subsarcolemmal and intermyofibrillar space. In addition, membrane-bound glycogen is contained in numerous small residual bodies along with osmiophilic lamellar and granular material. The biochemical basis for this disorder has not yet been elucidated.

Debranching enzyme deficiency (type III glycogenosis)

The debranching enzyme complex includes an oligotransferase that moves a three-carbon oligosaccharide and an alpha-1,6-glucosidase. Debranching enzyme deficiency, also known as "Forbes's disease," is most commonly manifest as a disorder of childhood dominated by hepatomegaly, delayed development, and only mild weakness. Because of their inability to catabolize glycogen properly, these children have mild fasting hypoglycemia, ketonuria, and hyperlipidemia. In most cases, there is considerable improvement or even total remission of symptoms during adolescence. Adults with debranching enzyme deficiency may be asymptomatic or have a late-onset myopathy with varying degrees of exercise intolerance, proximal muscular weakness, and distal muscular wasting.[98] These patients show no increase in serum glucose after administration of glucagon and little or no rise in serum lactate after ischemic exercise. Muscle specimens from adults with debranching enzyme deficiency show a vacuolar myopathy (Fig. 76-28). The vacuolation may affect the entire muscle fiber or may be predominantly subsarcolemmal in location. The vacuolar contents are PAS positive and at least partially digestible with diastase. Electron microscopy discloses numerous free glycogen granules beneath the sarcolemma and to a lesser extent within intermyofibrillar spaces. Some of the glycogen granules may be membrane bounded.

Branching enzyme deficiency (type IV glycogenosis)

The rare disorder branching enzyme deficiency, also known as "Andersen's disease," is the result of deficient activity of the branching enzyme, alpha-1,4-glucan:alpha-1,6-glycosyl transferase. Many tissues are affected and contain deposits of an abnormal carbohydrate that is biochemically similar to amylopectin. Some of the patients come to medical attention early in life with infantile hypotonia ("floppy infants"). This aspect of their illness is rapidly overshadowed by the development of

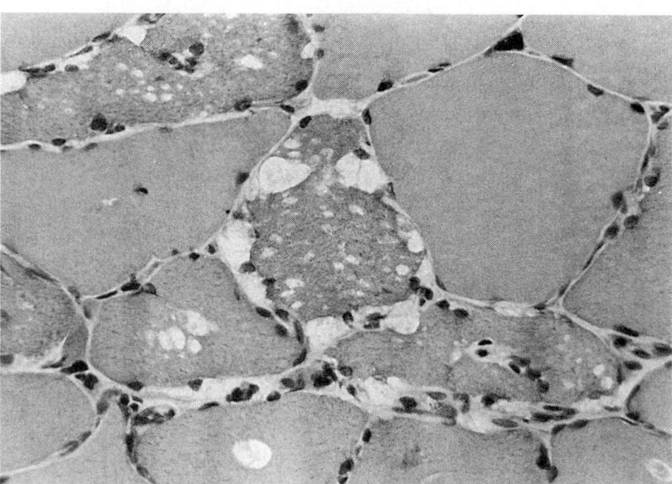

Fig. 76-27 Adult acid maltase deficiency. Notice the scattered vacuolated myofibers.

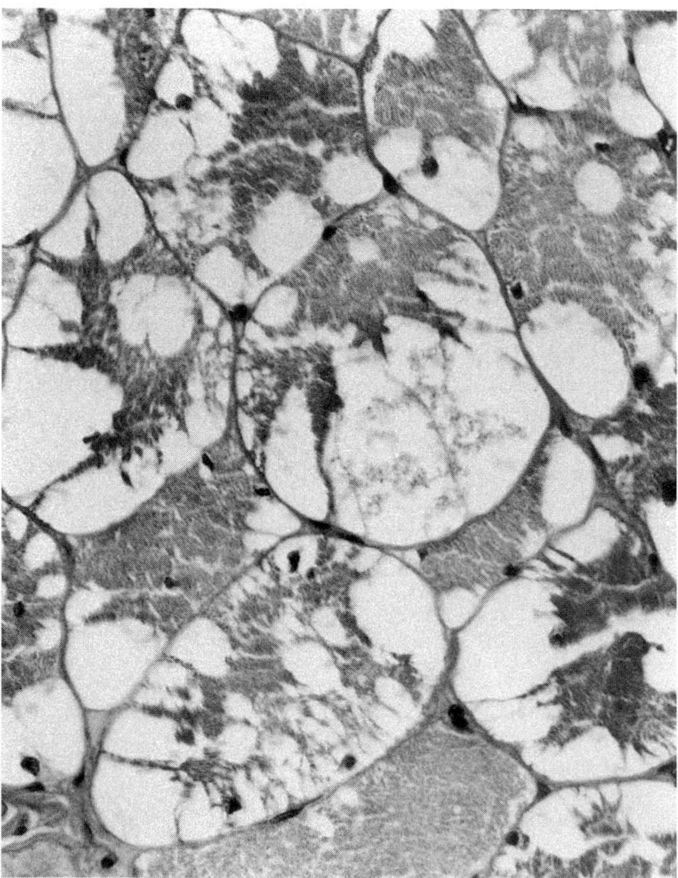

Fig. 76-28 Debranching enzyme deficiency (type III glycogenosis) in an adult. There are numerous large vacuoles. (Paraffin-embedded section of Susa fixed tissue, trichrome.)

hepatic dysfunction and cirrhosis. Death generally occurs within the first few years of life from hepatic failure or, occasionally, cardiac involvement.[99]

Abnormal deposits of polysaccharide have been described in the skeletal muscle in about half of the reported cases of branching enzyme deficiency.[100] The deposits consist of small collections of spheroidal or polyhedral granules that are often located at the periphery of the affected myofibers (Fig 76-29). The granules stain blue with H&E and are strongly PAS positive. By electron microscopy, the deposits appear as unbounded aggregates of osmiophilic branched fibrils and granular material. Ultrastructurally and to a lesser extent histochemically, these carbohydrate deposits are remarkably similar to Lafora bodies, polyglucosan bodies, corpora amylacea, and basophilic degeneration of the myocardium.

Adult polyglucosan body disease is a multisystem disorder with onset during the fifth or sixth decades. The clinical manifestations include upper and lower motor neuron involvement, sensory loss, neurogenic bladder, and in some cases dementia. Spheroidal or ellipsoidal polyglucosan bodies can be found in many tissues. The polyglucosan bodies are PAS positive and are partially or completely removed with alpha- and gamma-amylases. Ultrastructurally the inclusions consist of compact masses of filaments 6 to 8 nm in diameter. The diagnosis is often made by demonstration of the polyglucosan bodies in sural nerve biopsy specimens. At least some of these patients have branching enzyme deficiency.[101]

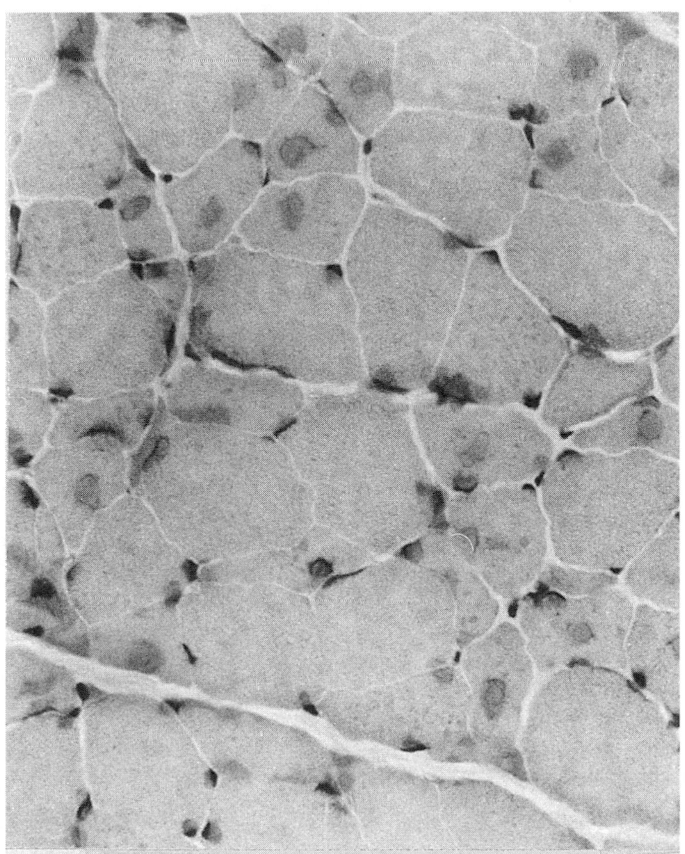

Fig. 76-29 Branching enzyme deficiency (type IV glycogenosis) in a young child. There are numerous polyglucosan bodies in muscle fibers.

Myophosphorylase deficiency (type V glycogenosis)

Myophosphorylase deficiency is commonly designated as "McArdle's disease." Myophosphorylase cleaves 1,4-alpha-glucosidic linkages, releasing glucose from glycogen chains. The deficient activity may result from absence of the enzyme or from the presence of a mutant form of the enzyme.[102] Since intramuscular glycogen cannot be utilized as a source of glucose for anaerobic glycolysis, the enzyme deficiency is manifested predominantly during brief periods of high energy demand. It also impedes less intense but sustained exercise. The deficient enzyme activity is reflected by a failure of venous lactate to increase during an ischemic exercise test. This laboratory finding is characteristic but not pathognomonic of myophosphorylase deficiency, since similar results can be seen with debranching enzyme deficiency and phosphofructokinase deficiency and the rare disorders of terminal glycolysis.

Most patients with myophosphorylase deficiency have a history of exercise intolerance dating back to childhood or adolescence. Initially, strenuous exercise produces muscle pain, stiffness, and fatigue that are relieved by periods of rest. Later in adulthood, overexertion may produce muscle cramps, episodes of myoglobinuria, and even renal failure. About one third of the patients eventually develop mild but persistent proximal muscle weakness. Rarely, adults with myophosphorylase deficiency present as a late-onset myopathy with progressive weakness but no cramps or myoglobinuria. There are also atypical cases that become manifest early in life. A rapidly progressive form leading to death from respiratory failure in infancy and an early childhood form with proximal muscle weakness resembling Duchenne muscular dystrophy have been reported.

Frozen sections and, less consistently, paraffin-embedded sections of skeletal muscle from adults with McArdle's disease usually disclose small subsarcolemmal vacuoles or blebs (Fig. 76-30). Smaller deposits in the form of minute vacuoles may be seen within the interior of the myofibers. The vacuolar contents are PAS positive and at least partially digestible with diastase.

Usually the diagnosis of McArdle's disease can be established by the histochemical evaluation of myophosphorylase

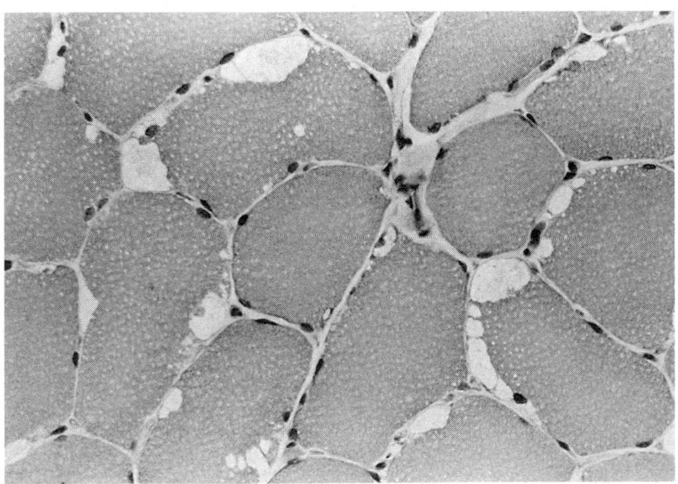

Fig. 76-30 McArdle's disease (type V glycogenosis). Notice the peripheral vacuoles.

activity in frozen sections. This procedure employs iodine to demonstrate the formation of glycogen chains by glucose-1-phosphate in the presence of myophosphorylase. The histochemical assay reaction is the reverse of the reaction normally catalyzed by myophosphorylase in vivo. In patients with myophosphorylase deficiency there is no staining of intact myofibers of either major type. Regenerating myofibers after rhabdomyolysis and smooth muscle fibers in vessel walls will be stained. The histochemical procedure can be monitored by having sections from a control and from the patient suspected of having McArdle's disease mounted on the same slide (Fig. 76-31). Rarely, patients with partial myophosphorylase deficiency may escape detection by this procedure, since as little as 10% of normal myophosphorylase activity will result in staining. The staining of regenerating myofibers has been attributed to the presence of the so-called fetal myophosphorylase isoenzyme. Electron microscopy reveals abnormal deposits of glycogen granules beneath the sarcolemma and to a lesser extent within the intermyofibrillar spaces.

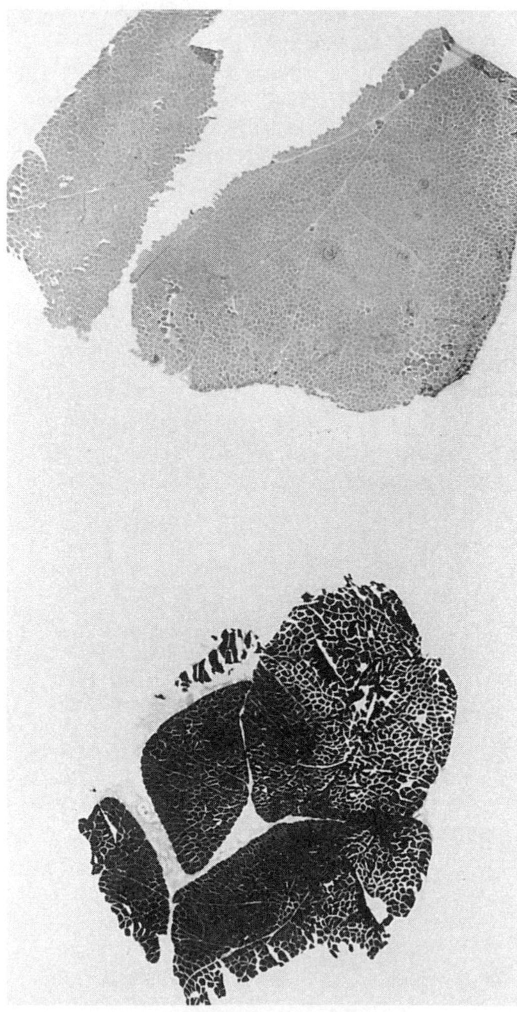

Fig. 76-31 Sections from a patient with McArdle's disease *(light)* and a control *(dark)*. (Myophosphorylase) (From Schochet SS Jr: *Diagnostic pathology of skeletal muscle and peripheral nerve,* Norwalk, Conn, 1986, Appleton-Century-Crofts.)

Phosphofructokinase deficiency (type VII glycogenosis)
Phosphofructokinase deficiency, a rare disorder of carbohydrate metabolism, also known as "Tarui's disease," is attributable to deficient phosphofructokinase activity. This enzyme catalyzes the conversation of fructose-6 phosphate to fructose-1,6-diphosphate and is one of the main rate-limiting steps of glycolysis. When the activity of this enzyme is deficient, neither glycogen nor glucose can be utilized as a source of energy. As in myophosphorylase deficiency, this is reflected by failure of ischemic exercise to elevate venous lactate.

Most patients with phosphofructokinase deficiency have clinical manifestations that are similar to McArdle's disease. Beginning in childhood, the patients have exercise intolerance, cramps, and occasionally myoglobinuria. Most patients also have a mild hemolytic anemia caused by an associated deficiency of erythrocyte phosphofructokinase activity. Occasional adults present as a late myopathy with progressive weakness but no cramps or episodes of myoglobinuria.[103] Rapidly progressive infantile cases also have been described.[104]

Frozen and paraffin-embedded sections of muscle from patients with phosphofructokinase deficiency usually contain scattered subsarcolemmal and intermyofibrillar vacuoles. The vacuolar contents are PAS positive and are at least partially digestible with diastase. Electron microscopy demonstrates morphologically normal glycogen particles. Scattered degenerating and regenerating myofibers will be present if the patient has had a recent episode of rhabdomyolysis and myoglobinuria. These morphologic features are virtually identical to those seen in cases of McArdle's disease. In some infantile cases, vacuoles and abnormal deposits of PAS-positive material are not evident in frozen sections but can be seen in epoxy-embedded sections. The diagnosis can be suggested by the histochemical demonstration of deficient phosphofructokinase activity and confirmed biochemically.

Polyglucosan bodies have been reported in muscle biopsy specimens from some patients with phosphofructokinase deficiency.[103,105] The inclusions are found individually and in groups in a small proportion of the myofibers. The polyglucosan bodies are PAS positive and stain brown with iodine. They are partially or completely removed with alpha-amylases and gamma-amylases. By electron microscopy, the inclusions are composed of compact masses of filaments 6 to 8 nm in diameter. These polyglucosan bodies have many morphologic, histochemical, and ultrastructural features in common with the polysaccharide deposits in branching enzyme deficiency. The polyglucosan bodies in phosphofructokinase deficiency may result from activation of glycogen synthetase by the elevated levels of glucose-6-phosphate.[105]

Disorders of glycolysis
Phosphoglycerate kinase deficiency, phosphoglycerate mutase deficiency, and lactate dehydrogenase deficiency are rare diseases affecting the glycolytic pathway. In all three of these diseases, ischemic exercise test results in mildly impaired production of venous lactate. Phosphoglycerate kinase deficiency is an X-linked recessive disorder that causes hemolytic anemia, mental retardation, and seizures in infants and young children. Rarely, this enzyme deficiency causes recurrent myoglobinuria in children and adults.[106] Biopsy specimens have shown structurally normal muscle with mildly increased lipid in type 1 myofibers but no vacuoles or focal accumulations of

PAS-positive material. Phosphoglycerate mutase deficiency is a very rare autosomal recessive disorder that may be responsible for recurrent myoglobinuria.[107] Muscle biopsy specimens have shown variation in myofiber size with occasional necrotic myofibers, tubular aggregates in type 2 myofibers, and a mild increase in PAS-positive material. Lactate dehydrogenase deficiency is another very rare autosomal recessive disorder that may cause myoglobinuria. During attacks, the serum creatine kinase is greatly elevated but the lactate dehydrogenase remains low.

Lipid storage myopathies

Skeletal muscle utilizes long-chain fatty acids as a major source of energy during fasting and during sustained exercise. The long-chain fatty acids must be combined with carnitine in order to pass through the mitochondrial membranes to the matrix compartment where they undergo beta-oxidation (Fig. 76-32). The carnitine used in this reaction is synthesized mainly in the liver and actively transported into the muscle against a concentration gradient. Free fatty acids, derived from circulating lipids and endogenous triglycerides, are first converted to acyl CoA compounds by the action of fatty acyl CoA synthetases. The long-chain acyl CoA compounds are then bound to carnitine by acylcarnitine transferases such as carnitine palmitoyltransferase (CPT I). This reaction occurs on the outer mitochondrial membrane. These acylcarnitine compounds are transferred across the inner membrane by the action of acylcarnitine translocase. Within the matrix compartment, other acylcarnitine transferases (CPT II) free the fatty acids from the carnitine. The long-chain fatty acids can then undergo beta-oxidation within the mitochondrial matrix compartment. Myopathies can result from lack of carnitine, from deficiency of the carnitine palmitoyl transferases, and defects in beta-oxidation of lipids (Table 76-8).

Carnitine deficiencies

Two more or less distinct disorders had been attributed to primary carnitine deficiency.[108] In so-called myopathic carnitine

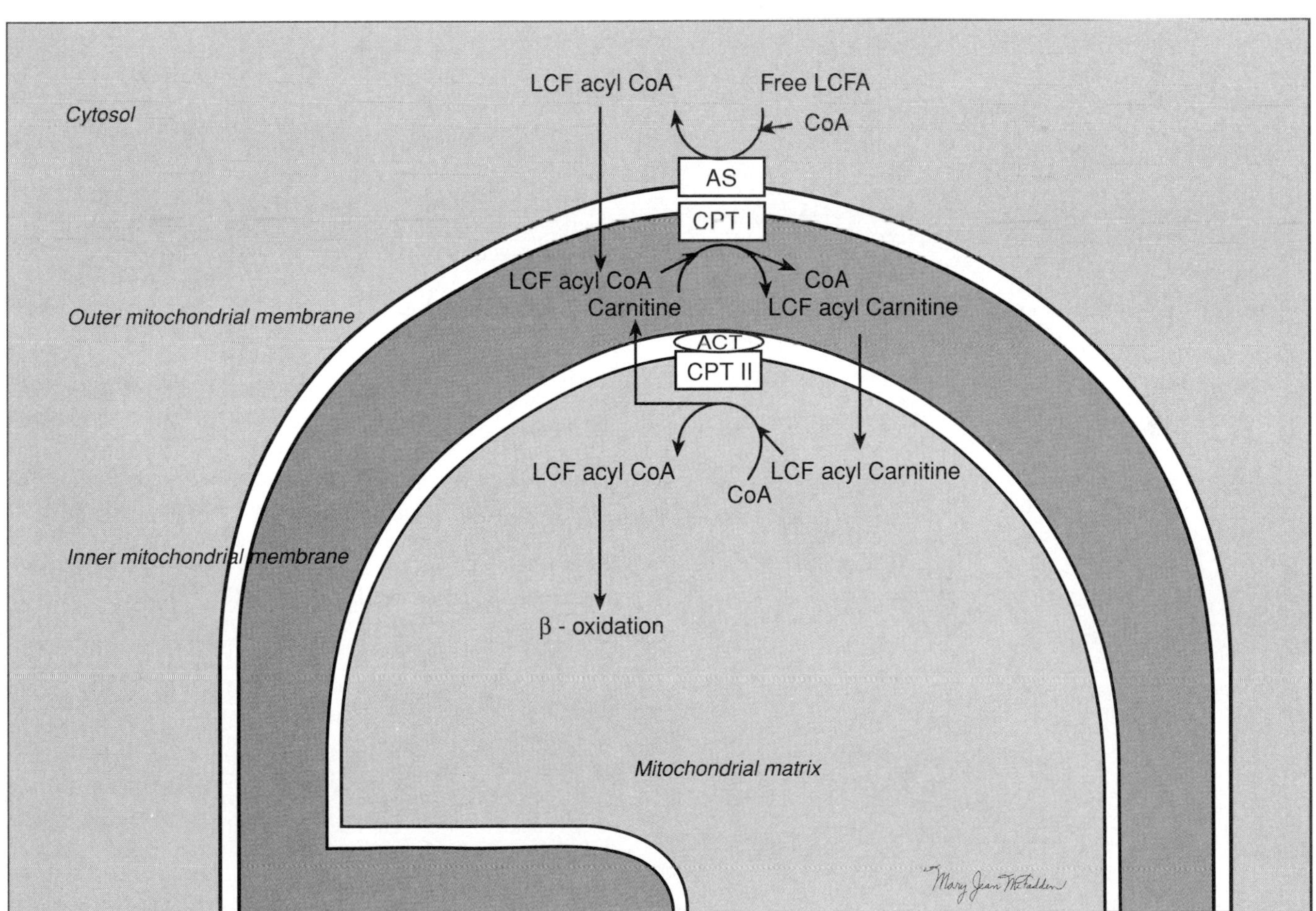

Fig. 76-32 Transport of long-chain fatty acids through the mitochondrial membrane. Free long-chain fatty acids (LCFA) are converted to acyl CoA compounds (LCFacylCoA) by acyl CoA synthetase (AS). LCFacylCoA can cross the outer mitochondrial membrane but are unable to penetrate the inner membrane. They must first be attached to their carrier, carnitine, by carnitine palmitoyltransferase I (CPT I) located on the inner face of the outer mitochondrial membrane. Acylcarnitines (LCFacylcarnitine) are transported across the inner membrane in exchange for carnitine by the catalyst carnitine-acylcarnitine translocase (ACT). Once inside the mitochondrial matrix, LCFacylcarnitine is combined with CoA and is restored to LCAacylCoA through the action of a second transferase (CPT II) located on the inner face of the mitochondrial inner membrane. These long-chain acyl CoA thioesters can then undergo beta-oxidation.

deficiency, muscle carnitine levels are greatly reduced while the liver and plasma carnitine levels are normal or only slightly decreased. The disease usually becomes manifest during childhood or early adult life and is characterized by progressive proximal muscle weakness, exertional myalgias, and rarely if ever myoglobinuria. Muscle biopsy specimens from these patients contain an increased number of lipid droplets especially in type 1 myofibers (Fig. 76-33). Electron microscopy shows the abnormal lipid accumulation accompanied by minimal or no increase in the number of mitochondria. The carnitine deficiency had been attributed to impaired active transport of this compound into the muscle.

Table 76-8 **Lipid storage myopathies**

Carnitine deficiency
Systemic
Myopathic
Carnitine palmitoyl transferase (CPT deficiency)
Defects of beta-oxidation
Acyl CoA dehydrogenase deficiency
Short chain
Medium chain
Long chain
Triglyceride storage disease

Diseases in **bold type** are discussed in the text. Others are found in selected references.[109,110]

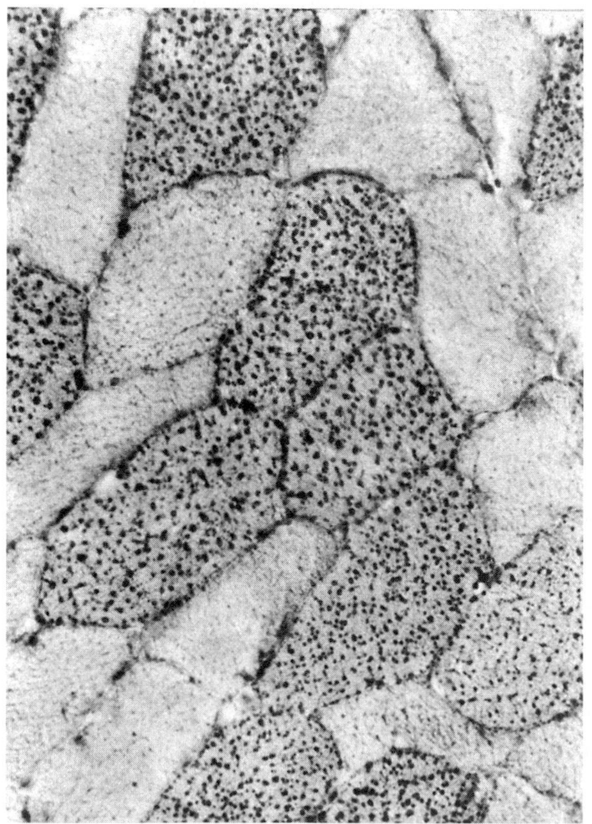

Fig. 76-33 Lipid storage myopathy in a patient with secondary carnitine deficiency. (Frozen section, osmium tetroxide–paraphenylene.)

In so-called systemic carnitine deficiency, the plasma, liver, and muscle carnitine levels are reduced. The disease becomes manifest in infancy or childhood and is characterized by progressive muscle weakness and episodes of hepatic and cerebral dysfunction that resemble Reye's syndrome. The encephalopathy may be precipitated by fasting. Death may result from an associated cardiomyopathy. Muscle biopsy specimens from these patients also show a prominent increase in the number of lipid droplets mainly within type 1 myofibers. The carnitine deficiency was variously attributed to deficient hepatic biosynthesis, impaired uptake by multiple organs, or excessive renal excretion. However, the distinction between "myopathic" and "systemic" carnitine deficiency has been challenged. Furthermore, many of the cases formerly considered to be primary systemic carnitine deficiency are now believed to be secondary to other metabolic diseases, especially medium-chain acyl CoA dehydrogenase deficiency.[95] Reduced levels of carnitine in serum or muscle or both have been encountered in association with many genetic and acquired diseases. The genetic causes include deficiency of one or more of the acyl CoA dehydrogenases involved in the metabolism of short-, medium-, and long-chain fatty acids.[109] Of these, medium-chain acyl CoA deficiency is the most common. These patients are generally children who have recurrent episodes of lethargy, vomiting, and hypoglycemia that are often precipitated by fasting. The clinical manifestations resemble Reye's syndrome. Other patients may have deficiency of multiple acyl CoA dehydrogenases.[110] Reduced carnitine levels are also found in patients with certain mitochondrial myopathies and advanced X-linked dystrophies. Among the acquired causes of secondary carnitine deficiency are hemodialysis for renal failure, total parenteral nutrition, and valproate therapy. Muscle biopsy specimens from patients with these various forms of secondary carnitine deficiency may show abnormal accumulation of lipid droplets predominantly in type I muscle fibers.

Carnitine palmitoyltransferase deficiency

Carnitine palmitoyltransferase deficiency is the most commonly identified metabolic cause of myoglobinuria in adults. Patients with carnitine palmitoyltransferase deficiency often have a history of recurrent episodes of rhabdomyolysis and myoglobinuria dating back to childhood.[111] Men are affected far more often than women. Most of the episodes of rhabdomyolysis are precipitated by prolonged exercise, especially when combined with exposure to cold or during fasting. Other cases are precipitated by concurrent infection. The patients have no premonitory cramps or contractures. Some have strikingly elevated plasma triglyceride levels and decreased ketone production during prolonged fasting. In addition to the usual adult disease, a lethal disorder in infants has been attributed to multiorgan deficiency of carnitine palmitoyltransferase II.[112]

Muscle biopsy specimens from adults with carnitine palmitoyltransferase deficiency may show no abnormalities. Scattered necrotic myofibers and an increased number of lipid droplets may be encountered if the biopsy specimen is obtained during or after an episode of rhabdomyolysis. Lipid storage, when present, is far less conspicuous than in the carnitine deficiency states. Increased numbers of lipid droplets have been observed in less than one third of the reported cases of carnitine palmitoyltransferase deficiency. The explanation for this striking contrast between these two categories of carnitine-related diseases is unknown.

Other lipid myopathies

There are other, less well-delineated lipid myopathies that are unrelated to abnormalities of carnitine metabolism. There is a multisystem triglyceride storage disease that is characterized by congenital ichthyosis, hepatosplenomegaly, vacuolated granulocytes, and myopathy.[113] Muscle biopsy specimens from these patients have shown increased numbers of lipid droplets in type 1 myofibers. Excess lipid is also present in numerous other tissues including liver, intestinal mucosa, fibroblasts, and leukocytes. A defect in triglyceride utilization has been suggested, but the metabolic basis for this entity has not been fully elucidated. Occasionally excess lipid storage may be encountered in muscle specimens from patients with various glycogenoses including Pompe's disease and in adult onset acid maltase deficiency.

MITOCHONDRIAL MYOPATHIES

Mitochondrial diseases are a heterogeneous group of disorders characterized by functionally abnormal mitochondria. The mitochondrial myopathies are a subset of these disorders.[114-117] Several categories of disease have been delineated under the heading of mitochondrial myopathies (Table 76-9). These include defects of substrate utilization, defects of oxidative phosphorylation, and respiratory chain defects. Unfortunately, morphologic features alone are not sufficient for the recognition and characterization of specific diseases. Some disorders with abnormal mitochondrial function show no corresponding structural abnormalities, and when present, the structural abnormalities do not uniquely characterize specific disorders. Furthermore, multiple defects may give rise to a single clinical entity.

In addition, occasional structurally aberrant mitochondria may be encountered in diseases that do not result primarily from mitochondrial dysfunction. When morphologically evident, mitochondrial abnormalities are generally manifest as abnormal accumulations of these organelles in subsarcolemmal and intermyofibrillar locations. The abnormal mitochondrial accumulations appear as granular deposits that stain blue with H&E and red with the modified trichrome stain (Fig. 76-34). The affected fibers are most often type 1 myofibers and are usually described as "ragged-red" fibers. The tentative identification of

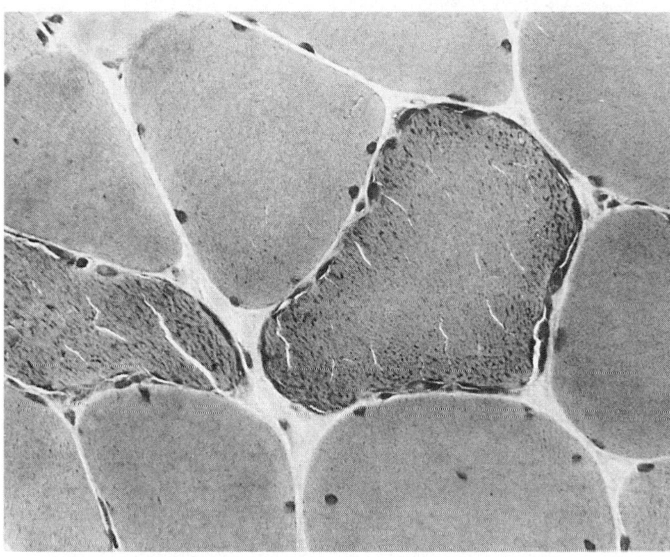

Fig. 76-34 Ragged-red fiber in a patient with a mitochondrial myopathy. (Rapid Gomori trichrome stain.)

Table 76-9 Mitochondrial myopathies

Defect in mitochondrial substrate transport
Carnitine deficiency
Carnitine palmitoyltransferase deficiency
Defect in mitochondrial substrate utilization
Fatty acid oxidation
Acyl CoA dehydrogenase deficiencies
Pyruvate oxidation
Pyruvate dehydrogenase deficiencies
Krebs cycle enzymes
Respiratory chain defects
Complex I
MELAS
Complex II
Complex III
Complex IV
MERRF
Kearns-Sayre
Leigh's disease
Defective energy conservation
Luft's disease

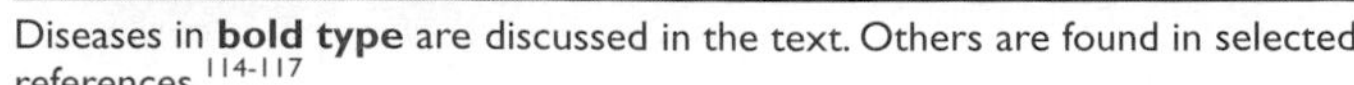

Diseases in **bold type** are discussed in the text. Others are found in selected references.[114-117]

MELAS, Mitochondrial myopathy, encephalopathy, lactic acidosis, and strokes; *MERRF*, myoclonus epilepsy with ragged red fibers.

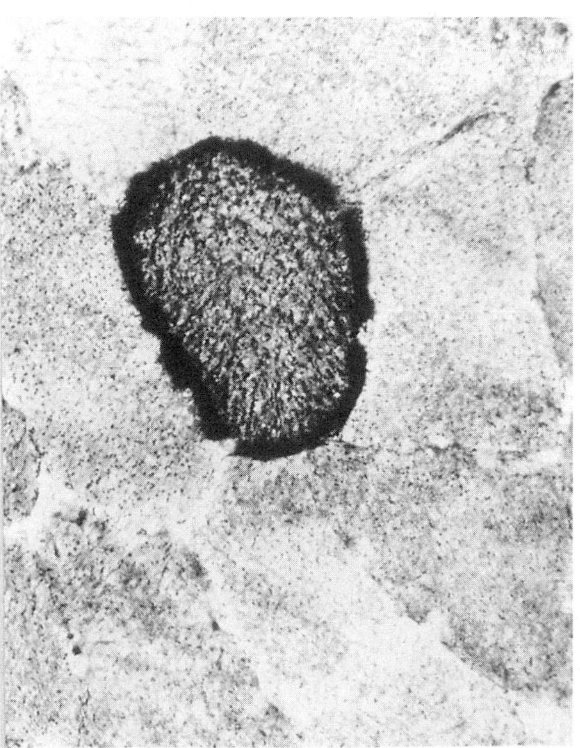

Fig. 76-35 Ragged-red fiber in a patient with a mitochondrial myopathy. (Frozen section, succinic dehydrogenase.)

mitochondrial deposits can be confirmed histochemically by the use of oxidative enzyme stains. The succinic dehydrogenase stain is especially suitable for this purpose. With this procedure, the abnormal mitochondrial deposits stain darkly (Fig. 76-35). The deposits of mitochondria also stain darkly with the NADH-TR reaction. However, this reaction is less specific, since normal and abnormal components of the sarcoplasmic reticulum also stain darkly with this technique. The cytochrome *c* oxidase stain is another histochemical technique that is useful in the evaluation of the mitochondrial myopathies. In some cases, the ragged-red fibers show deficient cytochrome *c* oxidase activity.

A wide variety of mitochondrial abnormalities may be seen by electron microscopy. In some cases, morphologically normal mitochondria may be present in excessive numbers. In other cases, the mitochondria may be abnormally large or may display aberrant orientation of their cristae (Fig. 76-36). The most distinctive structural abnormality is the presence of rectangular paracrystalline inclusions (Fig. 76-37). These are located within the intracristal spaces and between the inner and outer mitochondrial membranes. The paracrystalline masses are composed of parallel osmiophilic lines with periodic punctate densities. These inclusions are sometimes described as resembling a parking lot. Relatively little is known about the chemical composition and pathogenesis of these paracrystalline structures. It has been suggested that they may be biochemically inert.

Several relatively distinctive clinical syndromes are typically associated with abnormalities in mitochondrial DNA. The Kearns-Sayre syndrome is characterized by progressive external ophthalmoplegia, pigmentary degeneration of the retina, heart block, cerebellar ataxia, and increased cerebrospinal fluid protein. The disease has its onset in childhood or adolescence and is usually apparent before 20 years of age. Other clinical features that occasionally may be present include short stature, impaired hearing, vestibular dysfunction, intellectual impairment, and peripheral neuropathy. Death often results from the cardiac conduction defects. Mitochondrial DNA deletions have been demonstrated in the Kearns-Sayre syndrome and other cases of progressive external ophthalmoplegia that do not have all the features of the Kearns-Sayre syndrome.[118,119] Muscle specimens from patients with the Kearns-Sayre syndrome have shown few to many ragged-red myofibers. In addition, the ragged-red fibers in this disorder often show deficient cytochrome *c* oxidase activity. Diverse ultrastructural abnormalities, including numerous intracristal paracrystalline inclusions, are encountered among the mitochondria. Similar mitochondrial abnormalities have been demonstrated in other tissues including liver, skin, and brain.

The MELAS syndrome (mitochondrial myopathy, encephalopathy, lacticacidosis, and strokes) occurs predominantly in children. It is attributable to point mutations in mitochondrial DNA involving the $tRNA^{Leu\ (UUR)}$ gene, usually as an A to G mutation at base pair 3243, and is transmitted by maternal inheritance.[120] Children with this syndrome have stunted growth, seizures, intermittent vomiting, lacticacidosis, weakness, and recurrent strokes that can produce hemiparesis, aphasia, and cortical blindness. Diabetes mellitus and neurosensory hearing loss have also been reported.[121] Magnetic resonance imaging shows multiple areas of hyperintense signal that are predominantly cortical but do not conform precisely to perfusion beds. Muscle biopsy specimens usually contain ragged-red fibers and show increased succinic dehydrogenase activity in arterioles. Electron microscopy discloses abnormal numbers of mitochondria with proliferated cristae in the arteriolar smooth muscle. Brain specimens show status spongiosus (vacuolation) primarily in the cerebral white matter and mineralization of the basal ganglia.[122]

The MERRF syndrome (myoclonus epilepsy with ragged-red fibers) is attributable to a point mutation in mitochondrial DNA involving the $tRNA^{Lys}$ gene and is transmitted by maternal inheritance.[123,124] The disease is typically manifest in

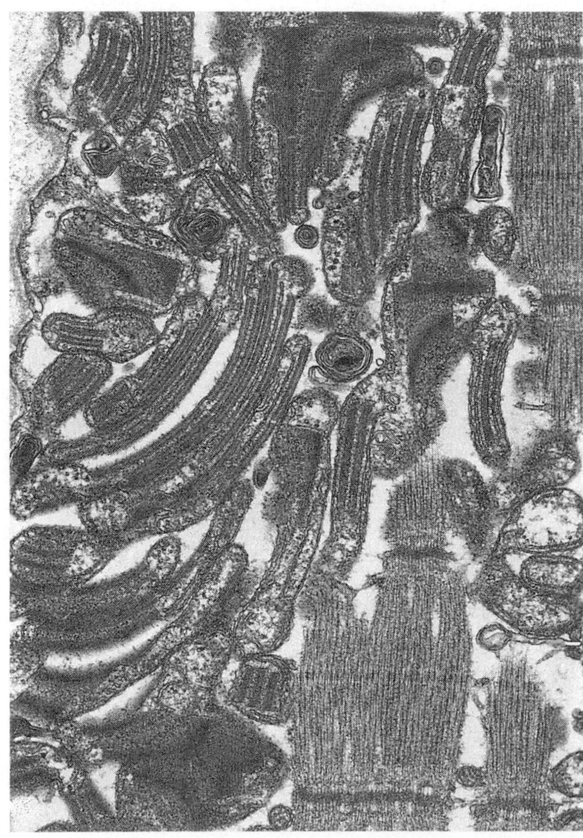

Fig. 76-36 Abnormal mitochondria in the periphery of a myofiber from a patient with Kearns-Sayre syndrome.

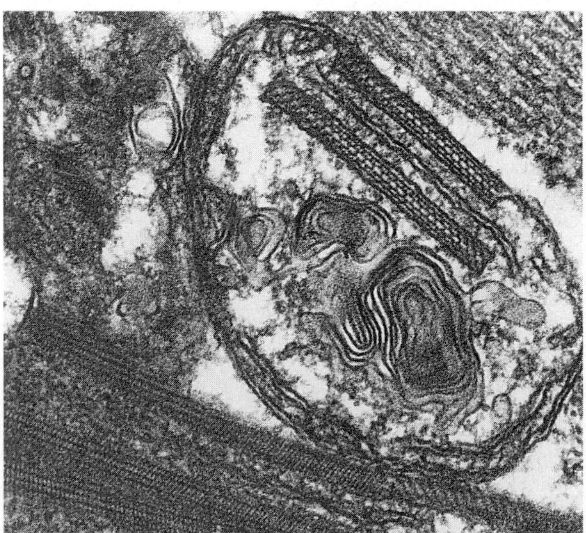

Fig. 76-37 Paracrystalline inclusion in a mitochondrion from a patient with Kearns-Sayre syndrome.

childhood but may vary in severity. Children with this syndrome usually present with myoclonus and ataxia and may have weakness, deafness, dementia, and seizures. Muscle biopsy specimens show numerous ragged-red myofibers. Some of the ragged-red fibers and occasionally non-ragged red fibers show deficient cytochrome *c* oxidase activity.

Cytochrome *c* oxidase deficiency results from nuclear and mitochondrial DNA abnormalities. The condition may be manifest as an infantile myopathy characterized by hypotonia, respiratory insufficiency, lacticacidosis, and variable degrees of renal and cardiac dysfunction.[117] Less often, the disease is manifest in adulthood. Muscle biopsy specimens show variable numbers of ragged red fibers, increased glycogen and lipid, and a paucity of staining for cytochrome *c* oxidase. A more benign form of cytochrome *c* oxidase deficiency has been determined to be the cause of so-called mitochondria-lipid-glycogen disease.[125]

MISCELLANEOUS METABOLIC MYOPATHIES

There are certain metabolic diseases in which morphologic abnormalities can be demonstrated in skeletal muscle specimens even though skeletal muscle is not the major target of the disease process. On the other hand, there are other conditions in which there are major functional abnormalities but only minimal morphologic manifestations.

Batten's disease (neuronal ceroid lipofuscinoses)

Batten's disease is a group of closely related neurodegenerative disorders that are characterized by the accumulation of autofluorescent lipopigments in various tissues. The major clinical manifestations include varying degrees of mental retardation, seizures, and visual impairment. The syndrome can be divided into four or more relatively distinct types based on the age at the onset and the rate of disease progression.[126] The infantile form is characterized by very early onset of blindness and rapid neurologic deterioration but relatively few seizures. The late-infantile form usually begins with seizures between 2 and 5 years of age. The disease progresses rapidly, with severe seizures and pronounced mental deterioration. Visual impairment is a relatively late manifestation. The juvenile type generally begins somewhat later and is dominated by visual impairment. The adult form progresses very slowly and is dominated by behavioral changes, dementia, movement disorders, and seizures. Vision is generally preserved.

Although the clinical manifestations of this group of diseases reflect predominantly the involvement of the central nervous system and eyes, muscle specimens may be used for morphologic diagnosis. Frozen sections stained by the routine histochemical procedures and paraffin-embedded sections usually show no evidence of abnormal lipopigment storage. Occasionally, examination with ultraviolet radiation will disclose abnormal deposits of autofluorescent material. The diagnosis is most readily demonstrated by electron microscopy. Muscle from patients with the infantile type of neuronal ceroid lipofuscinosis harbor deposits of finely granular osmiophilic material. In the late-infantile form, myofibers contain numerous membrane-bound deposits of curvilinear profiles beneath the sarcolemma (Fig. 76-38) and to a lesser extent between myofibrils. Similar deposits may be found in the endothelial cells of intramuscular capillaries. In the juvenile form, muscle fibers may contain deposits of identical curvilinear profiles or cytosomes with so-called rectilinear profiles. Curvilinear profiles have also been reported in muscle from patients with the adult form. Although electron microscopy of muscle biopsy specimens is an effective means of confirming a diagnosis of neuronal ceroid lipofuscinosis, it is less suitable for distinguishing among the various forms.

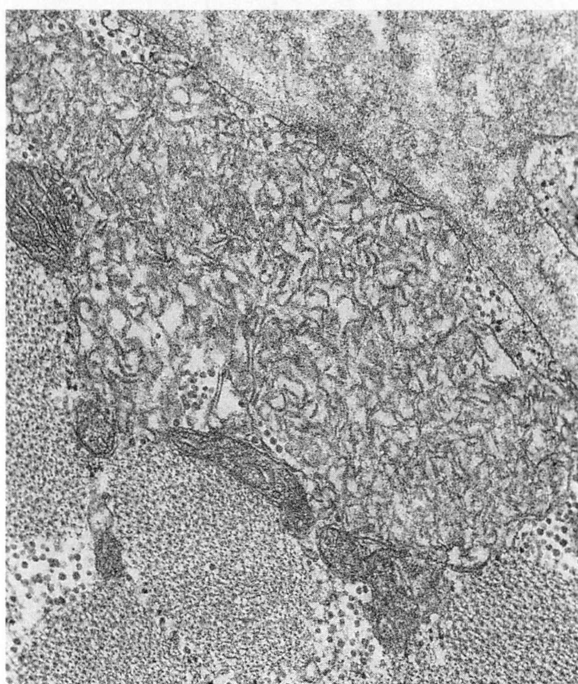

Fig. 76-38 Muscle biopsy from a child with Batten's disease.

The biochemical defect responsible for neuronal ceroid lipofuscinosis has not been fully elucidated. Some authors suggest that the pigments result from storage of dolichol compounds, whereas others emphasize the presence of subunit c of mitochondrial ATP synthetase.

Myoadenylate deaminase deficiency

Myoadenylate deaminase converts adenosine monophosphate to inosine monophosphate with the release of ammonia. This enzyme is abundant in skeletal muscle, where it is involved in replenishing ATP after exercise. Deficient activity of this enzyme was originally demonstrated in individuals with weakness, cramps, and exercise intolerance. The enzyme activity can be demonstrated biochemically and histochemically. Patients with myoadenylate deaminase deficiency show little or no staining of either major fiber type. Routine use of this technique has shown that the deficiency is common and encountered in as many as 2% of all muscle biopsy specimens. The demonstration of myoadenylate deaminase deficiency in diverse conditions such as motor neuron diseases, muscular dystrophies, inflammatory myopathies, and collagen vascular diseases has led to the proposal that there may be both primary and secondary forms of the deficiency state with only the primary form causing exercise-related symptoms.[127]

Amyloidosis

Amyloid is an abnormal, predominantly proteinaceous material that is derived from several different precursor proteins.

Various forms of amyloidosis are recognized as discussed in Chapter 20.

Rarely, amyloid deposition in skeletal muscles produces weakness and pseudohypertrophy.[128,129] Histopathologic studies on these patients have revealed deposits of amyloid within endomysial connective tissue as well as nerves and blood vessels. Although the deposits are outside of the sarcolemma, it has been suggested that the amyloid interferes with the propagation of action potentials along the surface of the muscle fibers.[81] Recently, several authors have reported amyloid fibrils, derived from beta-amyloid precursor protein, within the muscle fibers of patients with inclusion body myositis.[88,130]

Malignant hyperthermia

Malignant hyperthermia is a potentially lethal syndrome that is most frequently precipitated by the administration of halogenated anesthetics or succinylcholine.[131] The syndrome is inherited as an autosomal dominant trait and may be attributable to a mutation in the RYR1 gene, which codes for the calcium release channel of the sarcoplasmic reticulum. Susceptible individuals do not invariably develop malignant hyperthermia upon exposure to these agents, and many of those at risk have had previous anesthesia without overt disease. The clinical manifestations of the fully expressed syndrome include rapid rise in body temperature, tachycardia and cardiac arrhythmias, muscle rigidity, and rhabdomyolysis. Awareness of the syndrome and modern therapy has reduced the mortality to below 30%. The fundamental abnormality responsible for this condition has not been fully elucidated, though a major metabolic derangement appears to be an increase in intracytoplasmic calcium. This leads to abnormal contractions and loss of metabolic control in muscle. Because of the potential risk of anesthesia, much effort has been made to identify susceptible individuals. About two thirds of the patients at risk have increased serum creatine kinase (CK) levels. Routine histologic studies on muscle biopsy specimens from these individuals have shown only nonspecific alterations including increased numbers of internal nuclei, moth-eaten fibers, and occasional cores. In a few cases, malignant hyperthermia has been associated with central core disease. When present, the morphologic abnormalities seem to involve predominantly type 1 myofibers. However, it must be emphasized that susceptibility to malignant hyperthermia cannot be diagnosed histologically. In vitro studies of muscle contraction upon exposure to succinylcholine, caffeine, and halothane must be employed.

Type 2 myofiber atrophy and steroid myopathy

Type 2 myofiber atrophy is very commonly encountered in muscle biopsy specimens. It can been seen in frozen sections and in paraffin-embedded sections stained with a wide variety of techniques and appears as large numbers of small angular myofibers randomly dispersed among normal-sized myofibers. However, it can be diagnosed definitively only with fiber typing stains such as the ATPase reactions. Type 2 myofiber atrophy occurs in a wide variety of conditions including disuse, neurodegenerative diseases, myasthenia gravis, collagen vascular diseases, and Cushing's disease and after high-dose steroid therapy. In the last condition, it is often manifest by proximal muscular weakness and atrophy and is designated as "steroid myopathy." It is distinguished from neurogenic atrophy by the lack of involvement of type 1 myofibers.

Rhabdomyolysis and myoglobinuria

There are many circumstances in which skeletal muscle undergoes acute necrosis.[132-134] These can be broadly divided into exogenous and endogenous causes. Among the exogenous causes are mechanical trauma and muscle ischemia, fluid and electrolyte imbalances, hyperthermia or hypothermia, exposure to various myotoxic drugs and chemicals, infections, and inflammatory myopathies.[135] Included among the many endogenous causes are carnitine palmitoyltransferase deficiency, various disorders of carbohydrate metabolism, and malignant hyperthermia. Carnitine palmitoyltransferase deficiency is probably the most common cause of familial myoglobinuria.

The term *rhabdomyolysis* is often employed to indicate widespread necrosis of individual myofibers rather than whole muscles. When more than 200 g of muscle undergoes necrosis, myoglobin may appear in the urine. In some cases, the myoglobinuria may lead to renal failure.

Histologic examination generally shows multiple myofibers at a similar stage of injury, that is, undergoing necrosis, myophagocytosis, or regeneration. In some cases, there may be preferential involvement of one fiber type. Endomysial inflammation is often remarkably sparse. Additional pathologic changes may be present reflecting the specific cause of the rhabdomyolysis. However, at present, the cause of many cases remains undetermined.

TOXIC MYOPATHIES

There is a wide variety of chemical agents and drugs that directly or indirectly damage skeletal muscle. One of the more common is ethanol. Alcohol abuse can cause both acute and chronic myopathies.[136] They are probably the result of direct toxic effects of ethanol; however, the precise pathogenesis remains controversial. The manifestations vary from asymptomatic elevation of the creatine kinase to rhabdomyolysis with myoglobinuria. The acute myopathy is often the consequence of an alcoholic binge and is characterized by pain, tenderness, weakness, and muscle swelling. Histologic examinations disclose necrotic or regenerating myofibers depending on the time between intoxication and biopsy. Type 1 myofibers may be the more vulnerable. The chronic myopathy evolves over weeks to months and is characterized by weakness and atrophy especially of proximal muscles. Histologic studies show type 2 myofiber atrophy.

Chloroquine is a quinoline used as an antimalarial and in the treatment of certain collagen vascular diseases such as lupus erythematosus. The chronic administration of this drug produces slowly progressive weakness. Histologic studies have shown a vacuolar myopathy in which the vacuoles are partially filled with PAS-positive material. The vacuoles result from focal autophagic degeneration of the muscle fibers. Electron microscopy reveals myelin figures, lipofuscin granules, and curvilinear bodes similar to those in Batten's disease.[137]

Colchicine, used in the therapy of gout, can produce both neuropathy and myopathy.[138] Muscle biopsy specimens from patients who have taken this drug for a prolonged period of time show scattered vacuolated myofibers, targetoid fibers, and rare necrotic myofibers. Electron microscopy discloses myelin figures and autophagic vacuoles.

A myopathy occurring as a complication from the treatment of human immunodeficiency virus (HIV) infection with

Zidovudine (ZDV) has been reported with increasing frequency. Patients present with proximal weakness, myalgia, and elevated serum CK levels. A favorable clinical response often occurs after withdrawal of the drug.[139] ZDV myopathy is a mitochondrial myopathy characterized by the appearance of ragged-red fibers and greatly abnormal mitochondria ultrastructurally. Mitochondrial damage is the result of inhibition of muscle mitochondrial gamma-DNA polymerase by ZDV.[140] Mitochondrial dysfunction is associated with impaired cytochrome *c* oxidase activity.[141]

DISORDERS OF THE NEUROMUSCULAR JUNCTION

The neuromuscular junction consists of presynaptic (PRS) and postsynaptic (POS) regions separated by a narrow, intercellular space, the synaptic cleft (Fig. 76-39). At the PRS region, the myelinated motor nerve terminates as an unmyelinated axonal segment that contains numerous synaptic vesicles, 45 to 50 nm in diameter. The vesicles congregate around zones of increased electron density at the presynaptic membrane. Freeze-fracture electron microscopy has shown that at these electron-dense zones there are parallel pairs of double rows of intramembranous particles measuring 10 nm in diameter (Fig. 76-40). The particles are believed to represent voltage-sensitive calcium channels called "active zones." The POS region belonging to the muscle fiber is elevated above the cell surface as the so-called sole plate. Here the sarcoplasm is undulating, forming a series of postjunctional folds. The spaces or gutters between them are the secondary synaptic clefts. These clefts increase the area of the POS membrane, which is approximately 10 times greater than the PRS area.

The process of neuromuscular transmission occurs in 3 steps:

1. It is initiated by depolarization of the PRS axonal terminal of the motor nerve and an elevation of intracellular Ca^{2+}. Calcium enters the axon through calcium channels, which are the active zone particles in the PRS membrane.
2. The next event is the Ca^{2+} dependent fusion of acetylcholine (ACh)-containing PRS vesicles with the axolemma and subsequent release into the extracellular space.

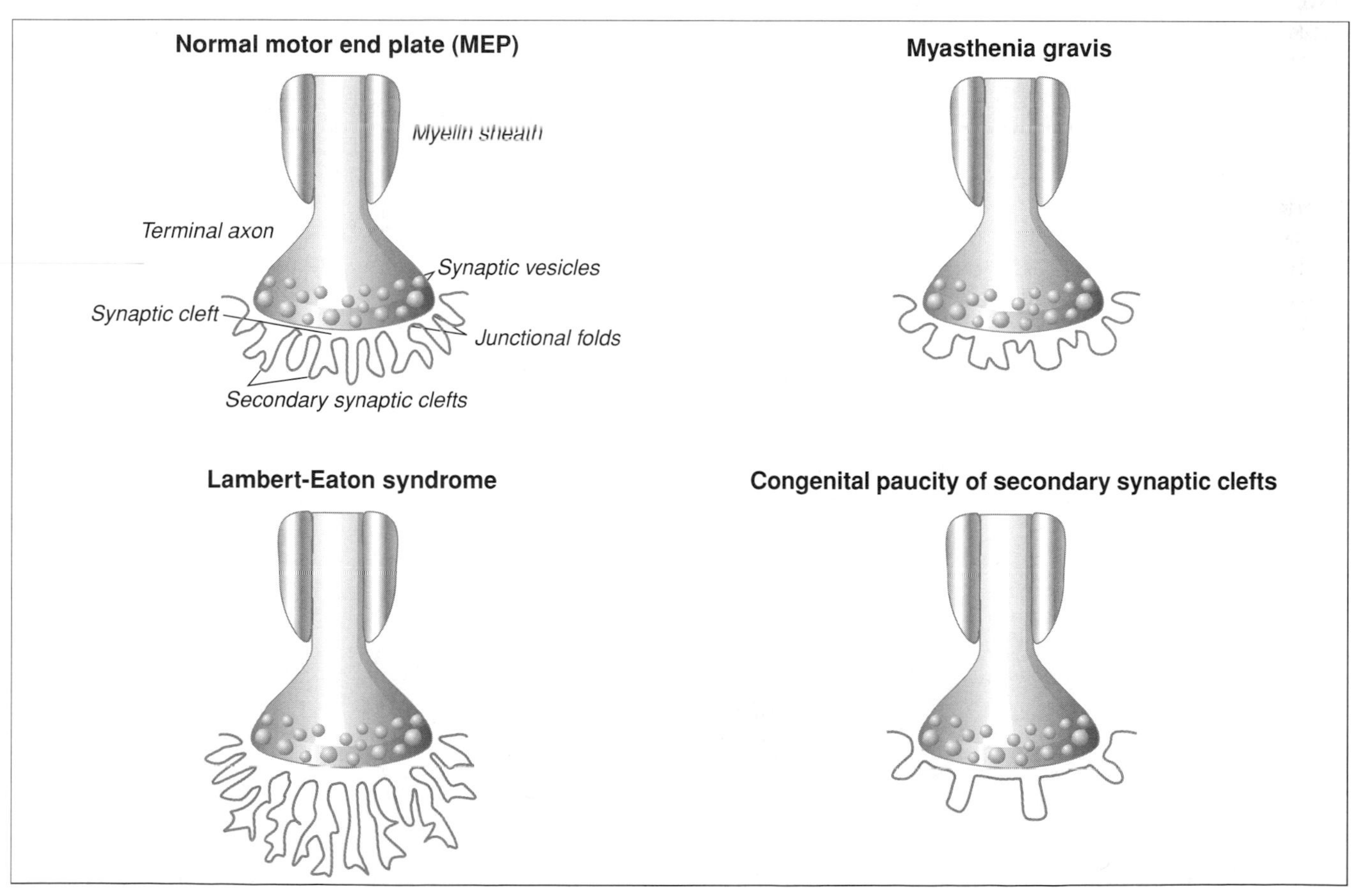

Fig. 76-39 Comparison of the normal motor end plate (MEP) with abnormal MEP in neuromuscular junction disease. **A,** Normal MEP. The terminal axon *(A)* with acetylcholine- containing synaptic vesicles *(SV)* forms the presynaptic portion of the neuromuscular junction. The synaptic cleft *(SC)* separates A from the postsynaptic portion where the junctional folds *(JF)*, between which are the secondary synaptic clefts *(SCC)*, are located. **B,** Myasthenia gravis. The postsynaptic region is simplified. The *SCC* are fewer in number, widened, and shallow. **C,** Lambert-Eaton syndrome. The postsynaptic region is abnormally complex. The JF and SCC are more convoluted and appear more numerous. **D,** Congenital paucity of secondary synaptic clefts. The SCC are rudimentary and reduced in number.

Normal motor end plate

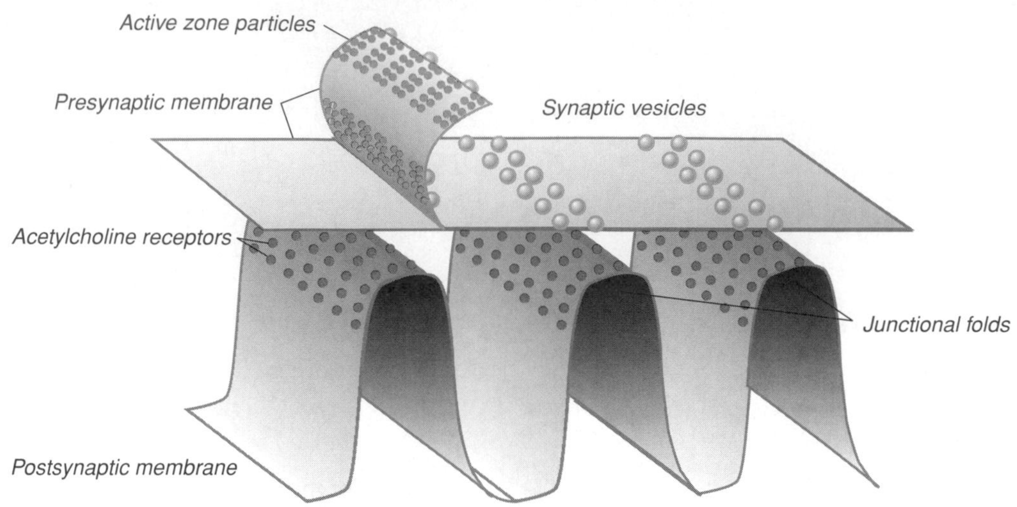

Lambert-Eaton syndrome

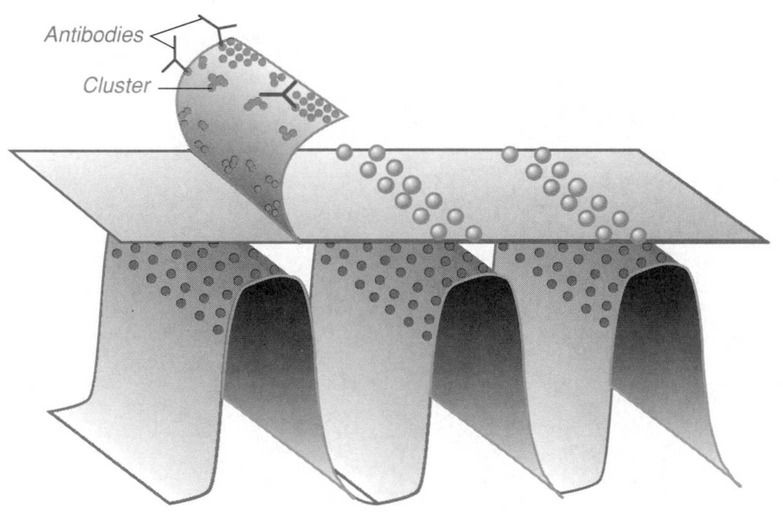

Myasthenia gravis

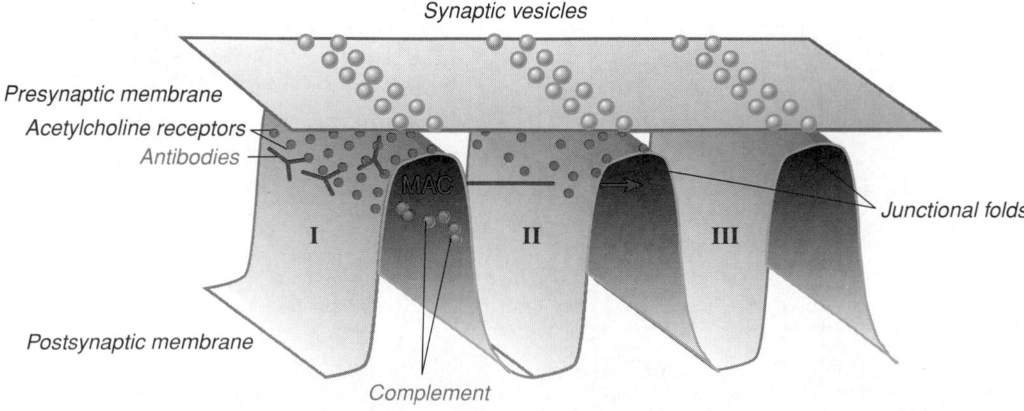

3. ACh molecules traverse the synaptic cleft and interact with cation channels of the acetylcholine receptors (AChR) on the POS membrane of the muscle fiber. AChR are known to be located primarily on the juxtaneural crests of the junctional folds. The AChR has a pentameric configuration, the subunits of which differ in embryonic and mature muscle. AChR in embryonic muscle is composed of α, β, γ, and δ subunits ($\alpha_2\beta\gamma\delta$). After innervation, the γ subunit is replaced by the Σ unit, so that the adult AChR is a $\alpha_2\beta\Sigma\delta$ oligomer.

4. As the cation channels open, membrane depolarization and activation of the T tubular system begin the process of muscle cell contraction.

5. ACh is quickly inactivated by acetylcholinesterase (AChE), which cleaves the neurotransmitter. In normal muscle, like AChR, AChE is localized to the postsynaptic region of the motor end plate.

Disorders of the neuromuscular junction include immune-mediated, congenital, and toxic conditions (Table 76-10). They are generally associated with defects in neuromuscular transmission.

Myasthenia gravis

Myasthenia gravis (MG) is a chronic, autoimmune disease that has received considerable attention throughout the past decade.[142,143] Recent research indicates that a humoral mechanism plays a pivotal role in the pathogenesis of myasthenia gravis, in that patients with this disease synthesize circulating antibodies against the postsynaptic acetylcholine receptor protein (AChR) at the motor end plate (MEP). These antibodies bind to the postsynaptic membrane of the MEP, blocking neuromuscular transmission and initiating the phenomenon of myasthenia. Furthermore, the binding of antibody at postsynaptic sites activates the complement cascade, and a complement-dependent destruction of the end-plate region ensues.[144] Patients with MG often have antibodies specific for the embryonic AchR that contains the γ subunit. There is now evidence that the γ subunit occurs in ocular but not in other skeletal muscle.[145] This finding explains the preferential involvement of extraocular muscles in MG. The ultrastructural evidence for this process is the eventual simplification of the junctional folds and a widening of the synaptic secondary clefts at the MEP.[146] In routine muscle biopsy specimens, examination of the MEP region by electron microscopy is generally impractical, since the end plates are primarily localized to the innervation zone of the muscle, which can be properly identified only by electrical stimulation while the biopsy is being performed. Experimentally the pathogenesis of human myasthenia gravis has been elucidated by injection of animals with purified acetylcholine receptor, resulting in the production of antibodies against the motor end plate and the development of autoimmune myasthenia gravis. MG can also be reproduced in animals by transfer experiments using serum from MG patients[147] or monoclonal anti-AChR antibodies.[148] More recently the immunopathologic characteristics of MG has been demonstrated in immune-deficient mice receiving peripheral blood lymphocytes from myasthenic patients.[149]

Myasthenia gravis with a prevalence rate of 3 per 100,000 is more common in young adult females with a peak age of onset before 40 years. Patients typically suffer from easy fatigability and muscular weakness that is worse at the end of the day. At first, symptoms predominate in the extraocular and facial muscles, prompting complaints of diplopia, dysphagia, and dysarthria. The clinical diagnosis depends heavily on a salutary response to anticholinesterase agents such as edrophonium and punctilious electromyographic examination during which a decrement in motor-action potentials evoked by repetitive stimulation is documented. The muscle biopsy sample is frequently unremarkable or characterized by a nonspecific atrophy. The well-known diagnostic parameter of moderate-to-severe type 2 fiber atrophy is present in only about 50% of cases. Its immune-oriented pathogenesis notwithstanding, myasthenia gravis is not a prototype of inflammatory myopathy. Small focal lymphocytic infiltrates are appreciated in muscle tissue, but they

Table 76-10 Neuromuscular junction disorders

Autoimmune
Myasthenia gravis
Lambert-Eaton syndrome
Congenital
Defect in acetylcholine synthesis
Acetylcholinesterase deficiency
Acetylcholine receptor deficiency
Congenital paucity of synaptic clefts
Abnormalities of ion channel closure
Slow channel syndrome
Toxic
Botulism
Drug-induced

Diseases in **bold type** are discussed in the text. Others may be found in Engel and Franzini-Armstrong and in Mastaglia and Walton (see Suggested Readings).

Fig. 76-40 Normal neuromuscular junction compared to junctional regions in myasthenia gravis and Lambert-Eaton syndrome. **A,** Normal motor end plate (MEP). The presynaptic membrane has been split to reveal the active zone particles *(AZP)* on the P face of the membrane. They are organized in pairs of double rows. Clusters of synaptic vesicles *(SV)* are seen adjacent to the presynaptic membrane. At the crests of the junctional folds *(JF)* the acetylcholine receptors *(AChR)* are seen. **B,** Myasthenia gravis. At the postsynaptic portion of the MEP, antibody *(Ab)* binds to the AChR *(I)*. The complement cascade is activated and the lytic membrane attack complex *(MAC)* produces focal destruction in the postsynaptic membrane *(II)*. There is a loss of AChR in the damaged membrane *(III)*. **C,** Lambert-Eaton syndrome. At the presynaptic portion of the MEP, antibody *(Ab)* binds to the AZP, presumably damaging these structures *(I)*. As a result, fewer AZP are found, and they appear to be reorganized. The AZP are less likely to occur in pairs of double rows, and the remaining AZP tend to occur in clusters. (Modified from Schmalbruch H: *Skeletal muscle,* Berlin, 1985, Springer-Verlag.)

are often not localized to end plates and are considered to be a nonspecific indicator of immune dysregulation.[150]

Lambert-Eaton syndrome

The Lambert-Eaton myasthenic syndrome (LEMS) is an autoimmune presynaptic disorder of neuromuscular transmission.[151] Myasthenic symptoms involve proximal limb muscles rather than ocular and bulbar muscles. Dry mouth, constipation, and impotence indicate coexisting autonomic nervous system disease in many patients. Neuromuscular transmission is defective at lower frequencies of electrical stimulation but paradoxically improves at high frequency. Dysfunctional neuromuscular transmission in LEMS is the result of a decrease in the amount of acetylcholine liberated from the motor nerve terminal, in that fewer synaptic vesicles are released with each action potential. Presynaptic quantities of acetylcholine are normal, as are postsynaptic responses to acetylcholine. Freeze-fracture electron microscopy discloses a diminution of the active zone particles, which represent the sites of calcium channels in the presynaptic membrane. The active zone particles that are seen on the P face of the membrane also appear to be reorganized. Fewer numbers of paired double rows are present, and the remaining particles are found in clusters, which are not evident in normal axon terminals. The reduction in quantal release of acetylcholine appears to be attributable to impaired calcium entry into the nerve terminal. Both nonneoplastic and paraneoplastic types of LEMS, 60% of which in the latter instance are discovered in patients with small cell lung carcinoma, are immune mediated. The essential features of the syndrome can be passively transferred to mice by intraperitoneal injections of IgG from patient's serum. In this model, freeze-fracture studies confirm changes in the active zones of the presynaptic membrane that are similar to those described in human Lambert-Eaton syndrome. The membrane alterations in LEMS are mediated by IgG, and the particles within the active zones are the targets of the autoimmune reaction.[152]

Congenital myasthenic syndromes

The heterogeneous category of genetic diseases called "congenital myasthenic syndromes" may be attributable to a defect in acetylcholine synthesis, a deficiency of acetylcholinesterase, an insufficiency of acetylcholine receptors, or to abnormally slow or rapid closure of ion channels.[153] The congenital paucity of secondary synaptic clefts (CPSC) syndrome and the slow-channel syndrome have received the most attention. CPSC syndrome is a familial disorder seen in children or young adults. It is nonprogressive and characterized by ptosis and extraocular muscular weakness. Acetylcholine receptors are reduced in number, leading to a diminution in the amplitude of miniature end-plate potentials (MEPPS), which are studied using in vitro microelectrode techniques.

Pathologically, the ratio of motor end-plates to muscle fibers is greater than normal, perhaps as a compensatory response.[154] The secondary synaptic clefts are undeveloped and resemble the clefts of fetal muscle.[155] They are reduced in number and shallow. Slow-channel syndrome is a familial disease, with onset in early adulthood. Weakness and fatigability are most severe in the neck, shoulders, and forearm.[156] Histochemical analysis of muscle reveals a predominance of type 1 fibers and fiber atrophy, involving type 1 and type 2 fibers. Electron microscopic studies show damage to the junctional folds, loss of acetylcholine receptor, and thickening of the motor end-plate basal lamina. Acetylcholinesterase is abundant in the neuromuscular junctions, and enzyme activity is unaffected. In the slow-channel syndrome, the acetylcholine-induced ion channels appear to remain open for an abnormally long period of time, and so there is increased influx of calcium into the neuromuscular junction. Newly formed motor end plates are characterized by the presence of slow channels. It is possible that the slow-channel syndrome is attributable to a defective gene that does not activate the synthesis of fast channels, which are normally found in innervated end plates.[157]

DENERVATING DISEASES

The welfare of the muscle fiber is intimately linked to the preservation of its nerve supply. Any disruption of these neural trophic influences will probably subject the myofiber to

Table 76-11 Denervating diseases

Denervating diseases
Central nervous system diseases
Amyotrophic lateral sclerosis
Infantile spinal muscular atrophies
ISMA I
ISMA II
ISMA III
Peripheral neuropathies
Hereditary
Metabolic
Diabetes mellitus
Chronic renal disease
Leukodystrophies
Refsum's disease
Amyloidosis
Toxic
Immune–mediated
Antimyelin antibodies
Vasculitis
Guillain-Barré syndrome

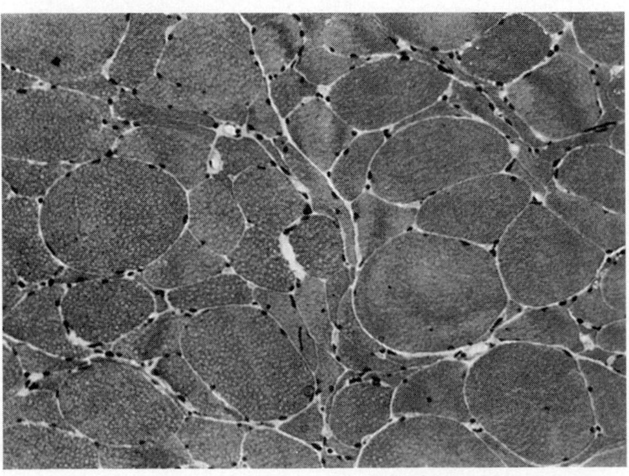

Fig. 76-41 Denervation atrophy. Atrophic fibers are angular in shape.

adverse dysvoluminal changes. Neurogenic atrophy may stem from disease of the anterior horn cell, exemplified by amyotrophic lateral sclerosis and Werdnig-Hoffmann disease, or from injury to its myelinated axon, most commonly against a clinical background of peripheral neuropathy. It should be pointed out that, statistically, the most important neuromuscular disorders are neurogenic in origin, more than 80% of which are attributable to some form of peripheral nerve disease. A detailed consideration of motor neuron diseases and peripheral neuropathies is a ambitious topic in itself, beyond the scope of the discussion here (Table 76-11).

Except for Werdnig-Hoffmann disease, the pathologic effects of denervation are essentially the same in all neurogenic atrophies.[158] During acute denervation, atrophic fibers are randomly scattered. Abnormally small fibers are angular or ensiform when cut transversely, with tapered or pointed, rather than gradually curving, edges (Fig. 76-41). Atrophic fibers appear flattened with the longer diameter even remaining that of a normal fiber while the shorter diameter is considerably reduced. At

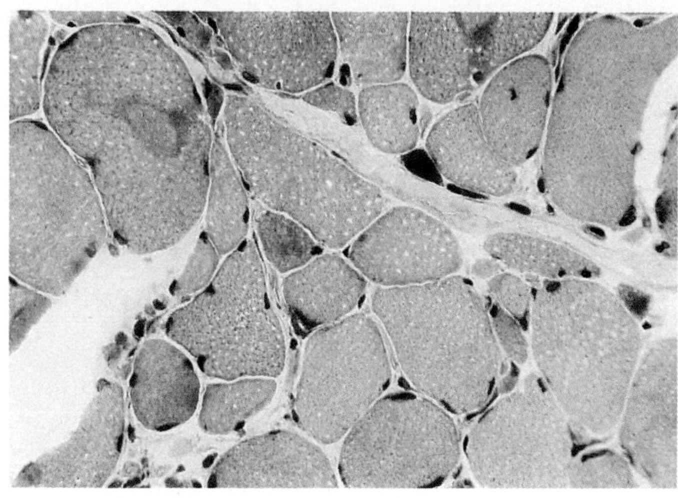

Fig. 76-42 Neurogenic atrophy. Atrophic denervated fibers stain dark brown, indicating increased esterase activity. (Esterase.)

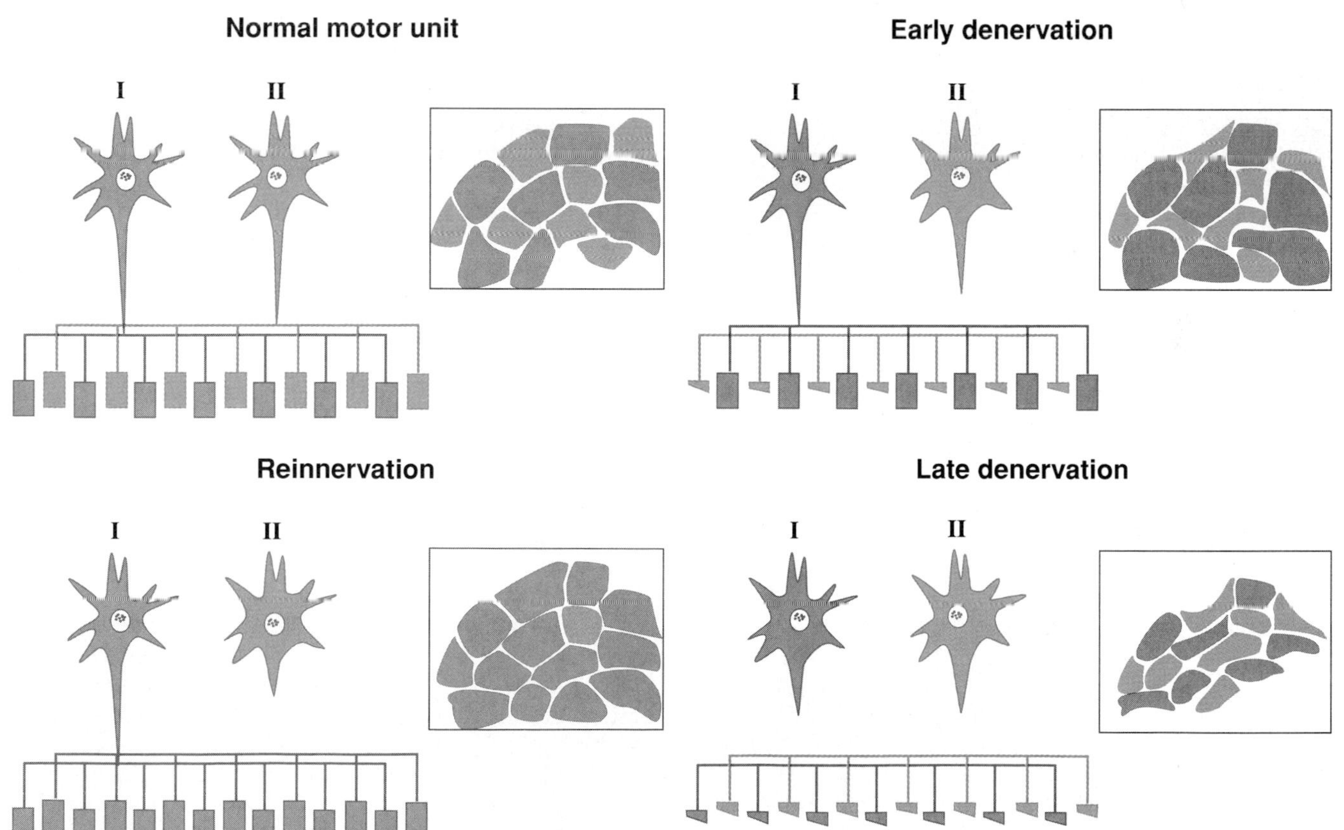

Fig. 76-43 Schema of the normal motor unit and three stages of denervation. **A,** Normal motor unit. Two oversimplified motor units are shown *(I* and *II)*. Each motor neuron *(MN)* innervates only muscle fibers of the same type. By neurotrophic influences, the motor neuron determines the fiber type within the motor unit. Notice that the fibers from each motor unit are geographically dispersed and are not grouped together. **B,** Early denervation. Atrophic fibers in the diseased motor unit II *(dark)* are angular and randomly distributed. **C,** Reinnervation. The remaining motor neuron I *(light)* has reinnervated the type 2, dark fibers by means of sprouting collateral axons. Notice that the previous type 2, dark fibers have been converted to type 1, light fibers, since the motor neuron governs the fiber type within the motor unit. This process of reinnervation leads to type grouping. **D,** Grouped atrophy. In chronic denervation, groups of atrophic fibers result from the process of denervation, reinnervation, and subsequent denervation of the reinnervated fibers.

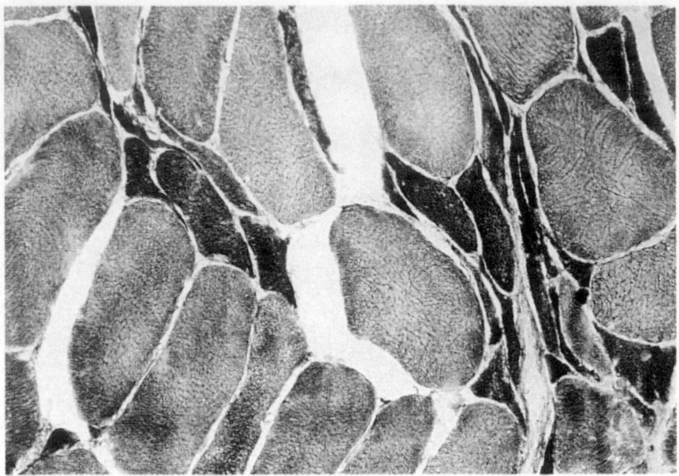

Fig. 76-44 Chronic neurogenic atrophy. Atrophic fibers are found in groups. Notice that they are also very darkly stained, a characteristic typical of denervated fibers. (NADH-TR.)

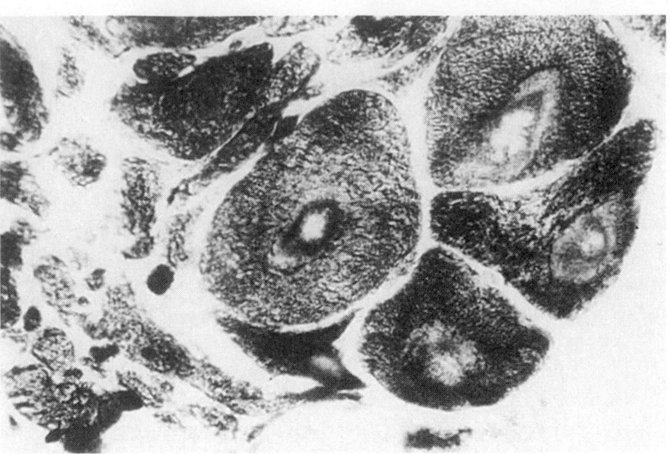

Fig. 76-46 Chronic denervation with target fibers. (NADH-TR.)

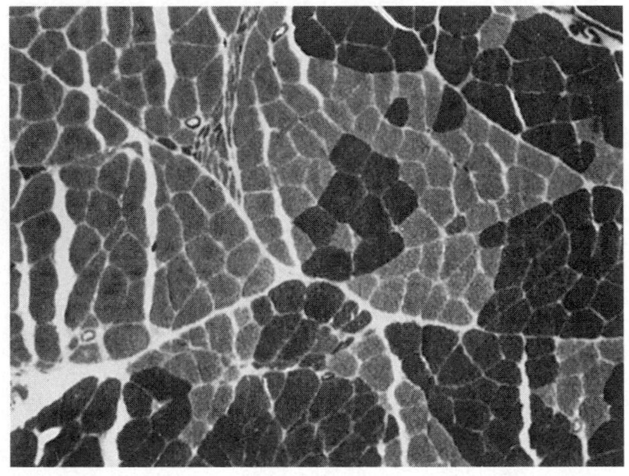

Fig. 76-45 Denervation with reinnervation. Type grouping replaces the normal checkerboard staining pattern. (ATPase, pH 9.4).

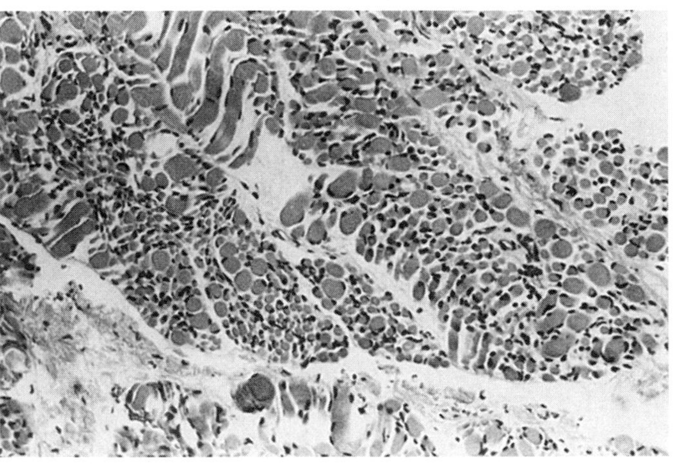

Fig. 76-47 Infantile spinal muscular atrophy. Many fibers in each fascicle are small and rounded in shape.

this stage, many or all of the atrophic fibers are glycolytic in type. Since these atrophic changes are not specific, staining frozen sections for esterase may be useful (Fig. 76-42). Denervated fibers are distinguished from atrophic fibers in most other disease conditions by positive esterase staining. If denervation continues unabated, the population of atrophic type 1 and type 2 fibers approaches parity. Advanced denervation is typified by a pattern of atrophy that progresses from one of random distribution to one in which there is grouping of affected fibers (Fig. 76-43). Grouped atrophy is usually recognized in the presence of multiple aggregations of five or more small, ensiform fibers in the tissue sample (Fig. 76-44). Fiber hypertrophy may occur in neurogenic diseases that are chronic and long standing. Hypertrophic fibers are believed to represent a compensatory reaction to the inefficiency of fibers that have undergone atrophy. The hypertrophic process is not type selective and involves both type 1 and type 2 fibers generally. At the same time, the normal checkerboard staining profile obtained in histoenzymatic reactions is distorted as a consequence of type grouping, denoted by unnaturally large congeries of muscle fibers having identical histochemical properties (Fig. 76-45). Type grouping occurs when residual, intact intramuscular nerve fibers send out collateral sprouts to reestablish innervation to denervated, atrophic fibers.[159] For practical purposes, target fibers are pathognomonic of chronic denervation,[160] though they are encountered in fewer than 25% of cases of neurogenic atrophy. Despite certain similarities, targets are not synonymous with cores. In contrast to the core, the target boasts a three-zone architecture (Fig. 76-46). The bull's-eye, or central zone, imitative of an unstructured core, is surrounded by an intermediate zone, a rim that is darkly stained in oxidative enzyme reactions. The intermediate zone, not part of a core lesion, is one of the pathologic transitions between the severely disrupted center zone and the third zone, which is the outer portion of the fiber composed of intact sarcoplasm.

In contrast to the atrophic pattern that characterizes adult denervation, neurogenic atrophy in infants has a different pathologic appearance, particularly in Werdnig-Hoffmann disease or type I infantile spinal muscular atrophy (ISMA I). Fiber atrophy in young infants tends to be severe and widespread. The numerous atrophic fibers within most fascicles, a finding known as "panfascicular atrophy," probably represents the infantile counterpart of grouped atrophy in older patients (Fig. 76-47). Instead of an angular shape, atrophic fibers are rounded, a paradoxical observation, since abnormally round fibers are otherwise typical of myopathies. Hypertrophic fibers are more consistently present in Werdnig-Hoffmann disease than in denervating diseases of adults. The hypertrophic process may be limited to type 1 fibers. Unlike adult denervation, for obscure reasons neurogenic disease in infants is not associated with type grouping or target fibers.

SUGGESTED READINGS

1. Bethlem J: *Myopathies*, ed 2, New York, 1980, Elsevier.
2. Carpenter S, Karpati G: *Pathology of skeletal muscle*, New York, 1984, Churchill-Livingstone.
3. Engel AG, Franzini-Armstrong C: *Myology*, New York, 1994, McGraw-Hill.
4. Heffner RR, editor: *Muscle pathology*, New York, 1984, Churchill-Livingstone.
5. Heffner RR: Muscle biopsy in neuromuscular disorders. In Sternberg SS, editor: *Diagnostic surgical pathology*, ed 2, New York, 1994, Raven Press.
6. Heffner RR: Diseases of skeletal muscle. In Nelson JS, Parisi JE, Schochet SS, editors: *Principles and practice of neuropathology*, St. Louis, 1993, Mosby.
7. Mastaglia FL, Walton JN: *Skeletal muscle pathology*, Edinburgh, 1992, Churchill-Livingstone.
8. Schochet SS: *Diagnostic pathology of skeletal muscle and nerve*, Norwalk, 1986, Appleton-Century-Crofts.
9. Walton JN, editor: *Disorders of voluntary muscle*, ed 2, Edinburgh, 1988, Churchill-Livingstone.

REFERENCES

Muscle biopsy

1. Bossen EH: Collection and preparation of the muscle biopsy. In Heffner RR, editor: *Muscle pathology*, New York, 1984, Churchill-Livingstone.
2. Pamphlett R: Muscle biopsy. In Mastaglia FL, Walton JN, editors: *Skeletal muscle pathology*, Edinburgh, 1992, Churchill-Livingstone.

General reactions of muscle to injury

3. Lacomis D, Chad DA, Smith TW: Myopathy in the elderly: evaluation of the histopathologic spectrum and the accuracy of clinical diagnosis, *Neurology* 43:825, 1993.
4. Regensteiner JG, Wolfel EE, Brass EP: Chronic changes in skeletal muscle histology and function in peripheral arterial disease, *Circulation* 87:413, 1993.
5. Bennington JL, Krupp M: Morphometric analysis of muscle. In Heffner RR, editor: *Muscle pathology*, New York, 1984, Churchill-Livingstone.
6. Engel WK: Selective and nonselective susceptibility of muscle fiber types: a new approach to human neuromuscular diseases, *Arch Neurol* 22:97, 1970.
7. Barron SA, Heffner RR: Weakness in malignancy: evidence for a remote effect of tumor on distal axons, *Ann Neurol* 4:268, 1978.
8. Kakulas BA, Adams RD: *Diseases of muscle*, Philadelphia, 1985, Harper & Row.
9. Chou SM, Nonaka I: Satellite cells and muscle regeneration in diseases human skeletal muscles, *J Neurol Sci* 34:131, 1977.
10. Mastaglia FL, Dawkins RL, Papadimitriou JM: Morphological changes in skeletal muscle after transplantation: a light and electron-microscopic study of the initial phase of degeneration and regeneration, *J Neurol Sci* 25:227, 1975.
11. Illa I, Leon-Monzon M, Dalakas MC: Regenerating and denervated human muscle fibers and satellite cells express neural cell adhesion molecule recognized by monoclonal antibodies to natural killer cells, *Ann Neurol* 31:46, 1992.

Congenital myopathies

12. Greenfield JG, Cornman T, Shy GM: The prognostic value of the muscle biopsy in the "floppy infant," *Brain* 81:461, 1958.
13. Shy GM, Magee KR: A new congenital non-progressive myopathy, *Brain* 79:610, 1957.
14. Shaib A, Paasuke RT, Brownell KW: Central core disease: clinical features in 13 patients, *Medicine* 66:389, 1987.
15. Haan EA, Freemantle CJ, McCure JA et al: Assignment of the gene for central core disease to chromosome 19, *Hum Genet* 86:187, 1990.
16. Neville HE, Brooke MH: Central core fibers structured and unstructured. In Kakulas BA, editor: *Proc of the Second International Congress on Muscle Diseases, Perth, Australia*, Amsterdam, 1973, Excerpta Medica.
17. Hayashi K, Miller RG, Brownell AK: Central core disease: ultrastructure of the sarcoplasmic reticulum and T-tubules, *Muscle Nerve* 12:95, 1989.
18. Paljärvi L, Kalimo H, Lang H et al: Minicore myopathy with dominant inheritance, *J Neurol Sci* 77:11, 1987.
19. Heffner RR, Cohen M, Duffner P et al: Multicore disease in twins, *J Neurol Neurosurg Psychiatry* 39:602, 1976.
20. Shy GM, Engel WK, Somers JE et al: Nemaline myopathy: a new congenital myopathy, *Brain* 86:793, 1963.
21. Hashimoto K, Shimizu T, Nonaka I et al: Immunochemical analysis of alpha-actinin of nemaline myopathy after two-dimensional electrophoresis, *J Neurol Sci* 93:199, 1989.
22. Heffner RR: Electron microscopy of disorders of skeletal muscle, *Ann Clin Lab Sci* 5:338, 1975.
23. Price HM, Gordon GB, Pearson CM et al: New evidence for excessive accumulation of Z-band material in nemaline myopathy, *Proc Natl Acad Sci USA* 54:1398, 1965.
24. Lo WD, Barohn RJ, Bobulski RJ et al: Centronuclear myopathy and type I hypotrophy without central nuclei, *Arch Neurol* 47:273, 1990.
25. Spiro AJ, Shy GM, Gonatas NK: Myotubular myopathy: persistence of fetal muscle in an adolescent boy, *Arch Neurol* 14:1, 1966.
26. Thomas NST, Sarfarazi M, Roberts K et al: x-linked myotubular myopathy, *Cytogenet Cell Genet* 46:704, 1987.
27. Dubowitz V, Brooke MH: *Muscle biopsy: a modern approach*, Philadelphia, 1974, Saunders.
28. Torres CF, Moxley RT: Early predictors of poor outcome in congenital fiber-type disproportion myopathy, *Arch Neurol* 49:855, 1992.
29. Clancy RR, Kelts KA, Oehlert JW: Clinical variability in congenital fiber type disproportion, *J Neurol Sci* 46:257, 1980.

Muscular dystrophies

30. Hejtnancik JF, Harris SG, Tsao CC et al: Carrier diagnosis of Duchenne muscular dystrophy using restriction fragment length polymorphisms, *Neurology* 36:1553, 1986.
31. Koenig M, Hoffman EP, Bertelson CJ et al: Complete cloning of the Duchenne muscular dystrophy (DMD) CDNA and preliminary genomic organization of the DMD gene in normal and affected individuals, *Cell* 50:509, 1987.
32. Prior TW: Genetic analysis of the Duchenne muscular dystrophy gene, *Arch Pathol Lab Med* 115:984, 1991.
33. Liechti-Gallati S, Koenig M, Kunkel LM et al: Molecular detection patterns in Duchenne and Becker type muscular dystrophy, *Hum Genet* 81:343, 1989.
34. Passos-Bueno MR, Bakker E, Kneppers ALJ et al: Different mosaicism frequencies for proximal and distal Duchenne muscular dystrophy (DMD) mutations indicate difference in etiology and recurrence risk, *Am J Hum Genet* 51:1150, 1992.
35. Hoffman EP, Fischbeck KH, Brown RH et al: Dystrophin characterization in muscle biopsies from Duchenne and Becker muscular dystrophy patients, *N Engl J Med* 318:1363, 1988.
36. Emery AEH: *Duchenne muscular dystrophy*, New York, 1993, Oxford University Press.
37. Ohlendieck K, Matsumura K, Ionasescu VV et al: Duchenne muscular dystrophy: Deficiency of dystrophin-associated proteins in the sarcolemma, *Neurology* 43:795, 1993.
38. Bonilla E, Samitt CE, Miranda AF et al: Duchenne muscular dystrophy: deficiency of dystrophin at the muscle cell surface, *Cell* 54:447, 1988.
39. Uchino M, Araki S, Miike T et al: Localization and characterization of dystrophin in muscle biopsy specimens from Duchenne muscular dys-

trophy and various neuromuscular disorders, *Muscle Nerve* 12:1009, 1989.

40. Cornelio F, Dones I: Muscle fiber degeneration and necrosis in muscular dystrophy and other muscle diseases: cytochemical and immunocytochemical data, *Ann Neurol* 16:694, 1984.
41. Fong P, Turner PR, Denetclaw WF et al: Increased activity of calcium leak channels in myotubes of Duchenne human and mdx mouse origin, *Science* 250:673, 1990.
42. Walgren-Pettersson C, Jasani B, Rosser LG et al: Immunohistochemical evidence for second or somatic mutations as the underlying cause of dystrophin expression by isolated fibres in Xp21 muscular dystrophy of Duchenne-type severity, *J Neurol Sci* 118:56, 1993.
43. Karpati G, Ajdukovic D, Arnold D et al: Myoblast transfer in Duchenne muscular dystrophy, *Ann Neurol* 34:8, 1993.
44. Cullen MJ, Fulthrope JJ: Stages in fiber breakdown in Duchenne muscular dystrophy, *J Neurol Sci* 24:179, 1975.
45. Gangopadhyay SB, Sherratt TG, Heckmatt JZ et al: Dystrophin in frameshift deletion patients with Becker muscular dystrophy, *Am J Hum Genet* 51:562, 1992.
46. Wijmenga C, Frants RR, Brouwer OF et al: Location of facioscapulohumeral muscular dystrophy gene on chromosome 4, *Lancet* 336:651, 1990.
47. Sarfarzi M, Wijmenga C, Upadhyaya M et al: Regional mapping of facioscapulohumeral muscular dystrophy gene on 4q35, *Am J Hum Genet* 51:396, 1992.
48. Upadhyaya M, Lunt P, Sarfarzi M et al: The mapping of chromosome 4q markers in relation to facioscapulohumeral muscular dystrophy (FSHD), *Am J Hum Genet* 51:404, 1992.
49. Chutkow JG, Heffner RR, Kramer AA et al: Adult-onset autosomal dominant limb-girdle muscular dystrophy, *Ann Neurol* 20:240, 1986.
50. Markesbery WR, Griggs RC, Herr B: Distal myopathy: electron microscopic and histochemical studies, *Neurology* 27:727-735, 1977.
51. Harper PS: *Myotonic dystrophy,* London, 1989, Saunders.
52. Pericak-Vance MA, Yamayoka LH, Assinder RIF et al: Tight linkage of apolipoprotein C2 to myotonic dystrophy on chromosome 19, *Neurology* 36:1418, 1986.
53. Shelbourne P, Davies J, Buxton et al: Direct diagnosis of myotonic dystrophy with a disease-specific DNA marker, *N Engl J Med* 328:471, 1993.
54. La Spada AR, Wilson EM, Lubahn DB et al: Androgen receptor gene mutations in X-linked spinal and bulbar muscular atrophy, *Nature* 352:77, 1991.
55. Brunner HG, Jansen G, Nillesen W et al: Reverse mutation in myotonic dystrophy, *N Engl J Med* 328:476, 1993.
56. Fu YH, Friedman DL, Richards S et al: Decreased expression of myotonin-protein kinase messenger RNA and protein in adult form of myotonic dystrophy, *Science* 260:235, 1993.
57. Hageman ATM, Gabreels FJM, Liem KD et al: Congenital myotonic dystrophy; a report on 13 cases and a review of the literature, *J Neurol Sci* 115:95, 1993.
58. Abdalla JA, Casley WL, Cousin HK et al: Linkage of Thomsen disease to the T-cell receptor beta (TCRB) locus on chromosome 7q35, *Am J Hum Genet* 51:579, 1992.

Inflammatory myopathies

59. Heffner RR: Inflammatory myopathies: a review, *J Neuropathol Exp Neurol* 52:339, 1993.
60. Kallen PS et al: Infectious myositis and related syndromes, *Semin Arthritis Rheum* 11(4):421, 1982.
61. Gherardi RK, Mhiri C, Baudrimont M et al: Iron pigment deposits, small vessel vasculitis, and erythrophagocytosis in the muscle of human immunodeficiency virus–infected patients, *Hum Pathol* 22:1187, 1991.
62. Simpson DM, Bender AN: HIV-associated myopathy: analysis of 11 patients, *Ann Neurol* 24:79, 1988.
63. Dwyer BA, Mayer RF, Lee SC: Progressive nemaline (rod) myopathy as a presentation of human immunodeficiency virus infection, *Arch Neurol* 49:440, 1992.
64. Morgan OS, Rogers-Johnson P, Mora C, Chat G: HTLV-I and polymyositis in Jamaica, *Lancet* 334:1184, 1989.
65. Gold D, Bowden R, Sixbey J et al: Chronic fatigue: a prospective clinical and virologic study, *JAMA* 264:48, 1990.
66. Warner C, Heffner RR, Cookfair D: Neuromuscular abnormalities in patients with chronic fatigue syndrome. In Hyde BM, editor: *Clinical and scientific basis of myalgic encephalomyelitis/CFS,* Ottawa, 1992, Nightingale.
67. Gherardi RK, Baudrimont M, Lionnet F et al: Skeletal muscle toxoplasmosis in patients with acquired immunodeficiency syndrome: a clinical and pathological study, *Ann Neurol* 32:535, 1992.
68. Jacob JC, Mathew NT: Pseudohypertrophic myopathy in cysticercosis, *Neurology* 18:767, 1968.
69. Dalakas MC: Polymyositis, dermatomyositis, and inclusion-body myositis, *N Engl J Med* 325:1487, 1991.
70. Oxenhandler R, Adelstein EH, Hart MN: Immunopathology of skeletal muscle: the value of direct immunofluorescence in the diagnosis of connective tissue disease, *Hum Pathol* 8:321, 1977.
71. Heffner RR, Barron SA, Jenis EH et al: Skeletal muscle in polymyositis: immunohistochemical study, *Arch Pathol Lab Med* 103:310, 1979.
72. Engel AG, Biesecker G: Complement activation in muscle fiber necrosis: demonstration of the membrane attack complex of complement in necrotic fibers, *Ann Neurol* 12:289, 1982.
73. Engel AG, Arahata K: Mononuclear cells in myopathies, *Hum Pathol* 17:704, 1986.
74. Emslie-Smith AM, Arahata K, Engel AG: Major histocompatibility complex class I antigen expression, immunolocalization of interferon subtypes, and T-cell–mediated cytotoxicity in myopathies, *Hum Pathol* 20:224-231, 1989.
75. Carpenter S, Karpati G: The pathological diagnosis of specific inflammatory myopathies, *Brain Pathol* 2:13, 1992.
76. Banker BQ, Victor M: Dermatomyositis (systemic angiopathy) of childhood, *Medicine* 45:261, 1966.
77. Kissel TJ, Mendell JR, Rammohan K et al: Microvascular deposition of complement membrane attack complex in dermatomyositis, *N Engl J Med* 314:329, 1986.
78. Banker BQ: Dermatomyositis of childhood: ultrastructural alterations of muscle and intramuscular blood vessels, *J Neuropathol Exp Neurol* 34:46, 1975.
79. Leon-Monzon M, Dalakas MC: Absence of persistent infection with enteroviruses in muscles of patients with inflammatory myopathies, *Ann Neurol* 32:219, 1992
80. Carpenter S, Karpati G, Rothman S et al: The childhood type of dermatomyositis, *Neurology* 26:952, 1976.
81. Chou SM: Myxovirus-like structures in a case of human chronic polymyositis, *Science* 158:1453, 1967.
82. Carpenter S, Karpati G, Heller I et al: Inclusion body myositis: a distinct variety of idiopathic inflammatory myopathy, *Neurology* 28:8, 1978.
83. Soueidan SA, Dalakas MC: Treatment of inclusion-body myositis with high-dose intravenous immunoglobulin, *Neurology* 43:876, 1993.
84. Riminton DS, Chambert ST, Parkin PJ et al: Inclusion body myositis presenting solely as dysphagia, *Neurology* 43:1241, 1993.
85. Ytterberg SR, Roelofs RI, Mahowald ML: Inclusion body myositis and renal cell carcinoma, *Arthritis Rheum* 36:416, 1993.
86. Verma A, Bradley WG, Soule NW et al: Quantitative morphometric study of muscle in inclusion body myositis, *J Neurol Sci* 112:192, 1992.
87. Chou SM: Inclusion body myositis: a chronic persistent mumps myositis? *Hum Pathol* 17:765, 1986.
88. Mendell JR, Sahenk Z, Gales T et al: Amyloid filaments in inclusion body myositis: novel findings provide insight into nature of filaments, *Arch Neurol* 48:1229, 1991.
89. Askanas V, Alvarez RB, Engel WK et al: β-Amyloid precursor epitopes in muscle fibers of inclusion body myositis, *Ann Neurol* 34:551, 1993.
90. Askanas, V, Serdaroglu P, Engel WK, Alvarez RB: Immunocytochemical localization of ubiquitin in inclusion body myositis allows its light-microscopic distinction from polymyositis, *Neurology* 42:460, 1992.
91. Heffner RR: Eosinophilic drug-induced myositis, *J Neuropathol Exp Neurol* 52:308, 1993.
92. Kamb ML, Murphy JJ, Jones JL et al: Eosinophilia-myalgia syndrome in L-tryptophan-exposed patients, *JAMA* 267:77, 1992.

93. Lin JD, Phelps RG, Gordon ML et al: Pathologic manifestations of the eosinophilia myalgia syndrome: analysis of 11 cases, *Hum Pathol* 23:429, 1992.
94. Illa I, Dinsmore S, Dalakas MC: Immune-mediated mechanisms and immune activation of fibroblasts in the pathogenesis of eosinophilia-myalgia syndrome induced by L-tryptophan, *Hum Pathol* 24:702, 1993.

Miscellaneous metabolic myopathies

95. DiMauro S, Bonilla E, Hays AP et al: Skeletal muscle storage diseases: myopathies resulting from errors in carbohydrate and fatty acid metabolism. In Mastaglia FL, Walton JN, editors: *Skeletal muscle pathology,* ed 2, Edinburgh, 1992, Churchill Livingstone.
96. Riggs JE, Schochet SS Jr, Gutmann L et al: Lysosomal glycogen storage disease without acid maltase deficiency, *Neurology* 33:873, 1983.
97. Hart ZH, Servidei S, Peterson PL et al: Cardiomyopathy, mental retardation, and autophagic vacuolar myopathy, *Neurology* 37:1065, 1987.
98. DiMauro S, Hartwig GB, Hays A et al: Debrancher deficiency: neuromuscular disorder in 5 adults, *Ann Neurol* 5:422, 1979.
99. Schochet SS Jr, McCormick WF, Zellweger H: Type IV glycogenosis (amylopectinosis): light and electron microscopic observations, *Arch Pathol* 90:354, 1970.
100. Servidei S, DiMauro S: Disorders of glycogen metabolism of muscle, *Neurol Clin* 7:159, 1989.
101. Bruno C, Servidei S, Shankse S et al: Glycogen branching enzyme deficiency in adult polyglucosan body disease, *Ann Neurol* 33:88, 1993.
102. Servidei, S, Shankse S, Zeviani M et al: McArdle's disease: biochemical and molecular genetic studies, *Ann Neurol* 24:774, 1988.
103. Danon MJ, Servidei S, DiMauro S et al: Late-onset muscle phosphofructokinase deficiency, *Neurology* 38:956, 1988.
104. Servidei S, Bonilla E, Diedrich RG et al: Fatal infantile form of muscle phosphofructokinase deficiency, *Neurology* 36:1465, 1986.
105. Hays AP, Hallett M, Delfs J et al: Muscle phosphofructokinase deficiency: abnormal polysaccharide in a case of late-onset myopathy, *Neurology* 31:1077, 1981.
106. Tonin P, Shanske S, Miranda AF et al: Phosphoglycerate kinase deficiency: biochemical and molecular genetic studies in a new myopathic variant (PGK Alberta), *Neurology* 43:387, 1993.
107. Kissel JT, Beam W, Bresolin N et al: Physiologic assessment of phosphoglycerate mutase deficiency: incremental exercise tests, *Neurology* 35:828, 1985.
108. Engel AG: Carnitine deficiency syndromes and lipid storage myopathies. In Engel AG, Banker BQ, editors: *Myology: basic and clinical,* vol 2, New York, 1986, McGraw-Hill.
109. Roe CR, Coates PM: Acyl-CoA dehydrogenase deficiencies. In Scriver CR, Beaudet AL, Sly WS et al, editors: *The metabolic basis of inherited disease,* vol 1, New York, 1989, McGraw-Hill.
110. Visser M, Schlote HR, Schutgens RBH et al: Riboflavin-responsive lipid storage myopathy and glutaric aciduria type II of early adult onset, *Neurology* 36:367, 1986.
111. DiMauro S, Papadimitriou A: Carnitine palmitoyltransferase deficiency. In Engel AG, Banker BQ, editors: *Myology: basic and clinical,* vol 2, New York, 1986, McGraw-Hill.
112. Hug G, Bove KE, Soukup S: Lethal neonatal multiorgan deficiency of carnitine palmitoyltransferase II, *N Engl J Med* 325:1862, 1991.
113. Angelini C, Philippart M, Borrone C et al: Multisystem triglyceride storage disorder with impaired long-chain fatty acid oxidation, *Ann Neurol* 7:5, 1980.
114. DiMauro S, Bonilla E, Zeviani M et al: Mitochondrial myopathies, *Ann Neurol* 17:521, 1985.
115. Morgan-Hughes JA: Mitochondrial diseases. In Mastaglia FL, Walton JN, editors: *Skeletal muscle pathology,* ed 2, Edinburgh, 1992, Churchill Livingstone.
116. Sparaco M, Bonilla E, DiMauro S, Powers JM: Neuropathology of mitochondrial encephalomyopathies due to mitochondrial DNA defects, *J Neuropathol Exp Neurol* 52:1, 1993.
117. Zeviani M, Nonaka I, Bonilla E et al: Fatal infantile mitochondrial myopathy and renal dysfunction caused by cytochrome *c* oxidase deficiency: immunological studies in a new patient, *Ann Neurol* 17:414, 1985.
118. Moraes CT, DiMauro S, Zeviani M et al: Mitochondrial DNA deletions in progressive external ophthalmoplegia and Kearns-Sayre syndrome, *N Engl J Med* 320:1293, 1989.
119. Yamamoto M, Clemens PR, Engel AG: Mitochondrial DNA deletions in mitochondrial cytopathies: observations in 19 patients, *Neurology* 41:1822, 1991.
120. Goto Y, Horai S, Matsuoka T: Mitochondrial myopathy, encephalopathy, lactic acidosis, and stroke-like episodes (MELAS): a correlative study of the clinical features and mitochondrial DNA mutation, *Neurology* 42:545, 1992.
121. Remes AM, Majamaa K, Herva R, Hassinen IE: Adult-onset diabetes mellitus and neurosensory hearing loss in maternal relatives of MELAS patients in a family with the $tRMA^{Leu(UUR)}$ mutation, *Neurology* 43:1015, 1993.
122. Sparaco M, Bonilla E, DiMauro S: Neuropathology of mitochondrial encephalomyopathies due to mitochondrial DNA defects, *J Neuropathol Exp Neurol* 52:1, 1993.
123. Rosing HS, Hopkins LC, Wallace DC et al: Maternally inherited mitochondrial myopathy and myoclonus epilepsy, *Ann Neurol* 17:228, 1985.
124. Graf WD, Sumi SM, Copass MK et al: Phenotypic heterogenity in families with the myoclonus epilepsy and ragged-red fiber disease point mutation in mitochondrial DNA, *Ann Neurol* 33:640, 1993.
125. DiMauro S, Nicholson JF, Hays AP et al: Benign infantile mitochondrial myopathy due to reversible cytochrome *c* oxidase deficiency, *Ann Neurol* 14:226, 1983.
126. Lake BD: Lysosomal and peroxisomal disorders. In Adams JH, Duchen LW, editors: *Greenfield's Neuropathology,* ed 5, New York, 1992, Oxford University Press.
127. Sabina RL, Swain JL, Holmes EW: Myoadenylate deaminase deficiency. In Scrivner CR, Beaudet AL, Sly WS et al, editors: *The metabolic basis of inherited disease,* ed 6, vol 1, New York, 1989, McGraw-Hill.
128. Whitaker JN, Hashimoto K, Quinones M: Skeletal muscle pseudohypertrophy in primary amyloidosis, *Neurology* 27:47, 1977.
129. Ringel SP, Claman HN: Amyloid-associated muscle pseudohypertrophy, *Arch Neurol* 39:413, 1982.
130. Askanas V, Engel WK, Alvarez RB: Light and electron microscopic localization of β-amyloid protein in muscle biopsies of patients with inclusion-body myositis, *Am J Pathol* 141:31, 1992.
131. Harriman DGF: The pathology of malignant hyperthermia. In Mastaglia FL, Walton JN, editors: *Skeletal muscle pathology,* ed 2, Edinburgh, 1992, Churchill Livingstone.
132. Penn AS: Myoglobulinuria. In Engel AG, Banker BQ, editors: *Myology: basic and clinical,* vol 2, New York, 1986, McGraw-Hill.
133. Tonin P, Lewis P, Servidei S, DiMauro S: Metabolic causes of myoglobinuria, *Ann Neurol* 27:181, 1990.
134. Gabow PA, Kaehny WD, Kelleher SP: The spectrum of rhabdomyolysis, *Medicine* 61:141, 1982.
135. Caccamo DV, Keene CY, Durham J, Peven D: Fulminant rhabdomyolysis in a patient with dermatomyositis, *Neurology* 43:844, 1993.
136. Charness ME, Simon RP, Greenberg DA: Ethanol and the nervous system, *N Engl J Med* 321:442, 1989.
137. Neville HE, Manuder-Sewry CA, McDougall J et al: Chloroquine-induced cytosomes with curvilinear profiles in muscle, *Muscle Nerve* 2:376, 1979.
138. Kuncl RW, Duncan G, Watson D et al: Colchicine myopathy and neuropathy, *N Engl J Med* 316:1562, 1987.
139. Simpson DM, Citak KA, Godfrey E et al: Myopathies associated with human immunodeficiency virus and zidovudine: can their effects be distinguished? *Neurology* 43:971, 1993.
140. Pezeshkpour G, Illa I, Dalakas MC: Ultrastructural characteristics and DNA immunocytochemistry in human immunodeficiency virus and zidovudine-associated myopathies, *Hum Pathol* 22:1281, 1991.
141. Chariot P, Monnet I, Gherardi R: Cytochrome c oxidase reaction improves hitopathological assessment of zidovudine myopathy, *Ann Neurology* 34:561, 1993.

Disorders of the neuromuscular junction

142. Johns TR: Myasthenia gravis, *Semin Neurol* 2:193, 1982.
143. DeBaets MH, Oosterhuis HJGH, editors: *Myasthenia gravis,* Ann Arbor, Mich., 1993, CRC Press.

144. Engel AG, Lambert EH, Howard FM: Immune complexes (IgG and C3) at the motor end-plate in myasthenia gravis: ultrastructural and light microscopic localization and electrophysiologic correlations, *Mayo Clin Proc* 52:267, 1977.
145. Horton RM, Manfredi AA, Conti-Tronconi BM: The 'embryonic' gamma subunit of the nicotinic acetylcholine receptor is expressed in adult extraocular muscle, *Neurology* 43:983, 1993.
146. Santa T, Engel AG, Lambert EH: Histometric study of neuromuscular junction ultrastructure. I. Myasthenia gravis, *Neurology* 22:71, 1972.
147. Toyka KV, Drachman DB, Griffin DE et al: Myasthenia gravis: study of humoral immune mechanisms by transfer to mice, *N Engl J Med* 296:125, 1977.
148. Richman DP, Gomez CM, Berman PW et al: Monoclonal anti-acetylcholine receptor antibody can cause experimental myasthenia, *Nature* 286:738, 1980.
149. Martino G, DuPont BL, Wollmann RL et al: The human-severe combined immunodeficiency myasthenia mouse model: a new approach for the study of myasthenia gravis, *Ann Neurol* 34:48, 1993.
150. Nakano S, Engel AG: Myasthenia gravis: quantitative immunocytochemical analysis of inflammatory cells and detection of complement membrane attack complex at the end-plate in 30 patients, *Neurology* 43:1167, 1993.
151. Eaton LM, Lambert EH: Electromyography and electrical stimulation of nerves in diseases of the motor unit: observations on a myasthenic syndrome associated with malignant tumors, *JAMA* 163:1117, 1957.
152. Nagel A, Engel Ag, Lang B et al: Lambert-Eaton myasthenic syndrome IgG depletes presynaptic membrane active zone particles by antigenic modulation, *Ann Neurol* 24:552, 1988.
153. Engel AG, Uchitel OD, Walls TJ et al: Newly recognized congenital myasthenic syndrome associated with high conductance and fast closure of the acetylcholine receptor channel, *Ann Neurol* 34:38, 1993.
154. Wokke JHJ, Jennekens FGI, Molenaar PC et al: Congenital paucity of secondary synaptic clefts (CPSC) syndrome in 2 adult sibs, *Neurology* 39:648, 1989.
155. Smit LME, Hageman G, Veldman H et al: A myasthenic syndrome with congenital paucity of secondary synaptic clefts: CPSC syndrome, *Muscle Nerve* 11:337, 1988.
156. Engel AG, Lambert EH, Mulder DM et al: A newly recognized congenital myasthenic syndrome attributed to a prolonged open time of the acetylcholine-induced ion channel, *Ann Neurol* 11:553, 1982.
157. Engel AG: Myasthenia gravis and myasthenic syndromes, *Ann Neurol Surg* 16:519, 1984.

Denervating diseases

158. Armbrustmacher VW: Skeletal muscle in denervation, *Pathol Annu* 13:1, 1978.
159. Karpati G, Engel WK: "Type grouping" in skeletal muscles after experimental reinnervation, *Neurology* 18:447, 1968.
160. Engel WK: Muscle target fibers, a newly recognized sign of denervation, *Nature* 191:389, 1961.

Part Nine

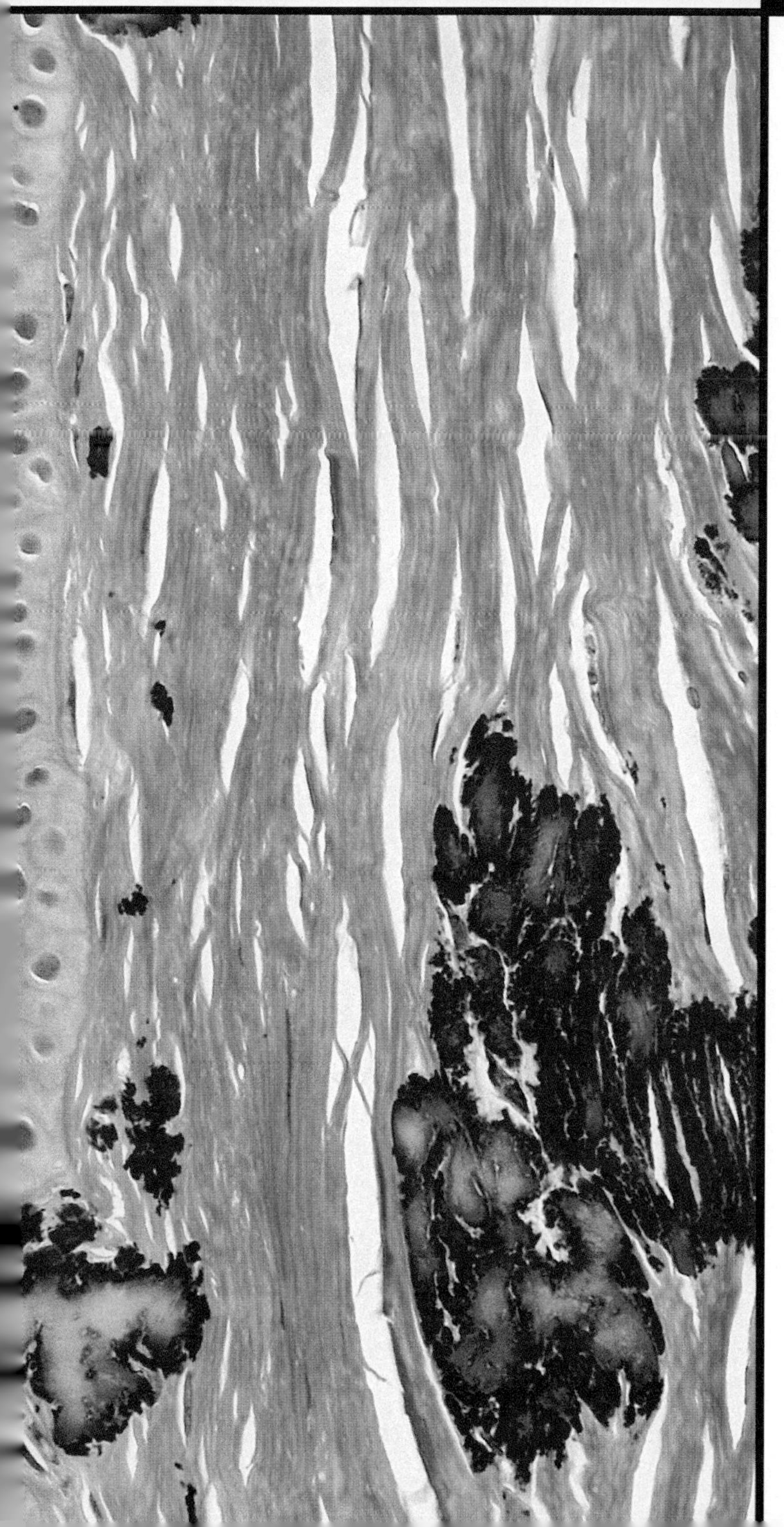

DISEASES OF THE NERVOUS SYSTEM AND SENSORY ORGANS

77 Central Nervous System

James M. Powers
Dikran S. Horoupian

GENERAL CONSIDERATIONS

Central nervous system (CNS) diseases traditionally are divided into broad etiologic categories: vascular, infectious, traumatic, degenerative, neoplastic, developmental, demyelinative-dysmyelinative, and metabolic-toxic.[1-11] Of these, some have no legitimate systemic counterpart: degenerative and demyelinative. The others usually follow the same basic principles as systemic diseases, even though they include entities unique to the CNS: infectious (prion diseases), vascular (hypertensive encephalopathy), neoplastic (gliomas), metabolic (Wernicke's encephalopathy), and developmental (neural tube defects). Many of the degenerative and metabolic diseases have familial patterns; a large number of these have been linked to specific chromosomal loci, and relevant genes have been cloned.[12,13]

The CNS differs from most organs because of the diversity of its cell types (neurons, astrocytes, oligodendrocytes and myelin, microglia and endothelium) and because of its disparate neuronal populations with inherent differences in susceptibility to disease-producing agents or defects (selective vulnerability).[14-16] This, in part, results in different patterns of disease: diffuse, multifocal, focal, or those restricted to specific groups of neurons and axons (system degenerations). Although these selective vulnerabilities and patterns are poorly understood, they often provide excellent pathologic correlations for clinical deficits. Because of morphologic similarities between cell types that are intricately interwoven with each other, special stains often have been needed for adequate evaluation of neuropathologic specimens. The hematoxylin and eosin–stained paraffin section is the current routine preparation; but neuronal (cresyl violet and other Nissl), myelin (Luxol fast blue, Heidenhain, Weil, Loyez, and others), axonal (Bodian, Bielschowsky, Gallyas, and others), and astrocytic (phosphotungstic acid–hematoxylin, Holzer, gold sublimate) stains also are routine in many laboratories.[4,6,8,9] Immunostains with antibodies to neuronal proteins (neurofilament, synaptophysin, synapsin), astrocytic proteins (glial fibrillary acidic protein, vimentin, S-100), oligodendrocyte membrane glycolipids or proteins (galactocerebroside, carbonic anhydrase, Leu-7) and microglia (CLA, HAM-56), and lectin histochemical techniques for microglia (*Ricinus communis* agglutinin) have facilitated the recognition of specific cell types.[10] However, cross reactions between some cells with these techniques (such as microglia and endothelial cells) and the lack of specific and practical markers for other cells (such as ependymal and oligodendroglial) limit their utility. In situ hybridization techniques, often coupled with polymerase chain reaction (PCR) or other amplification methods, hold great promise for more specific and sensitive recognition markers.[7] Electron microscopy has played an important role in the elucidation of several neuropathologic entities, particularly congenital myopathies, peripheral nerve lesions, metabolic diseases, neoplasms, and some degenerative diseases, but its utility at present is limited.

In view of the diversity of neuronal populations with disparate functions, a basic knowledge of neuroanatomy[14,15] and an accurate history are needed to properly evaluate CNS specimens at autopsy.[4] Surgical margins rarely are a consideration in neurosurgical specimens, but considerable discretion must be exercised when one is handling minuscule or stereotactic specimens. Cytologic preparations, in place of or with frozen sections, often provide significant independent or complementary data, particularly in noncohesive cellular lesions such as pituitary adenomas and lymphomas.

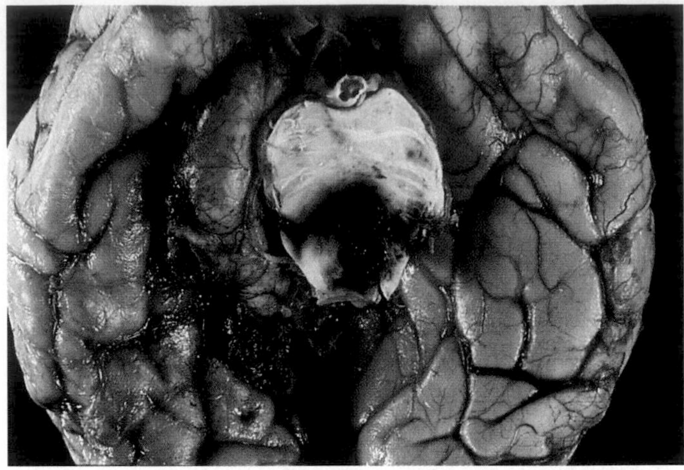

Fig. 77-1 Unilateral herniation of parahippocampal gyrus with secondary brainstem hemorrhages.

Neuroanatomic considerations and constraints: herniations

The CNS also differs from most other organs because its major cell, the neuron, is irreplaceable if lost and regeneration of its processes generally is ineffective. On the other hand, the CNS has considerable redundancy and plasticity, at least in the young,[14] and clinically silent areas do exist. Some areas (such as the spinal cord, brainstem, dentate nucleus, posterior limb of internal capsule, and motor cortex) usually are unforgiving of even slight lesions, but others (such as the cerebellar cortex, frontal lobe, nondominant parietal and temporal lobes, and anterior limb of internal capsule) can sustain lesions without displaying significant clinical deficits.

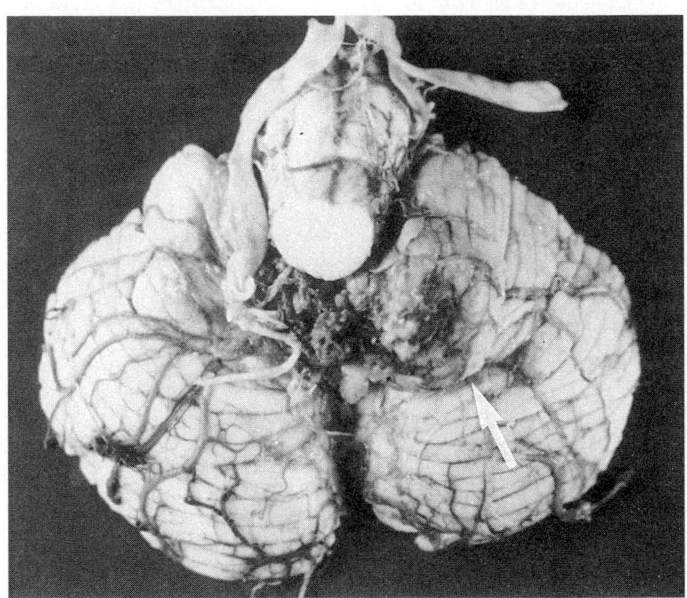

Fig. 77-2 Unilateral tonsillar herniation *(arrow)*.

The fibrous and rigid dura mater and skull (or vertebrae) protect the soft CNS from trauma and physical compression or distortion but exact a high price for this protection in that they render the brain (and to a lesser extent the spinal cord) a closed box. Space is at a premium within the skull, and space-occupying lesions generally will displace brain parenchyma. Such displacements, usually referred to as *herniations,* have limited options: down into the floor of the anterior fossa, over the sphenoid wing, under the falx cerebri, into the tentorial notch, into bony orifices, into the sella turcica (empty sella syndrome), down into the foramen magnum, or through a calvarial defect (fungus cerebri).[17,18] The two most clinically relevant herniations are those involving the tentorial notch (transtentorial, uncal, tentorial, parahippocampal) (Fig. 77-1) and foramen magnum (tonsillar) (Fig. 77-2) because the displaced medial temporal lobe or cerebellar tonsil impinges on vital centers in the midbrain and medulla, respectively. Subfalcial (subfalcine, cingulate), upward herniation of the superior cerebellum through the tentorial notch and orbital and sphenoid wing herniations are usually clinically silent. Rarely upward herniation of cerebellum caused by posterior fossa mass lesions or too rapid decompression of increased intracranial pressure (ICP) in the supratentorial compartment may cause ocular findings, alterations in consciousness, or even death.[18] Subfalcial herniation even more rarely may compress the anterior cerebral artery causing infarction in its distribution.[17] Focal hemispheric masses (such as neoplastic, infectious, traumatic, or vascular causes) in the temporal lobe or cerebellum can produce unilateral medial temporal or tonsillar herniations, respectively. Diffuse mass lesions (such as brain swelling, leptomeningitis, subarachnoid hemorrhage), which raise ICP in either the supratentorial or infratentorial compartments, can produce the same herniations but usually bilaterally. Central (transtentorial) herniation, manifesting as a downward displacement of the diencephalon and rostral brainstem, also may develop from supratentorial increased (↑) ICP. It has a typical clinical progression of postural, reflex, and breathing abnormalities; infarcts in the hypothalamus and thalamus may be seen.[17] Clinical signs of supratentorial ↑ ICP with unilateral transtentorial herniation include: (1) ipsilateral pupillary dilatation caused by physical interference with the cholinergic parasympathetic portion of the oculomotor (III) nerve; (2) ipsilateral (a false localizing sign) hemiparesis caused by compression of the contralateral cerebral peduncle against the free edge of the tentorium with focal hemorrhage and necrosis of the peduncle (so-called Kernohan's notch); (3) contralateral hemiparesis caused by compression of the ipsilateral peduncle against the clivus; (4) variable visual field defects, usually asymptomatic, caused by compression of the ipsilateral posterior cerebral artery; and (5) most significantly, alterations in consciousness, abnormal breathing patterns, coma, or death caused by distortion of the midbrain reticular activating system.[10] Signs of tonsillar herniation with medullary compression caused by ↑ ICP in the infratentorial compartment (posterior fossa) are less well characterized but may include head tilt, paresthesias, stiff neck, and arching of the neck in chronic cases and coma, respiratory arrest, and death in acute cases. If these clinical signs of herniation are present in the patient at the time of death, it is safe to conclude that medial temporal or tonsillar herniations encountered at autopsy were significant in the fatal outcome. If such clinical information is not available or absent, one can safely rely on two grossly detectable lesions to ascribe a lethal effect to the herniations: multiple, linear, usually midline hemorrhages in the midbrain and upper pons (secondary hemorrhages of Duret) (Fig. 77-3) with transtentorial herniation, or acute hemorrhages or hemorrhagic necrosis in the cerebellar tonsils with tonsillar herniation. In the absence of either clinical or gross neuropathologic correlates, the significance of medial temporal lobe or tonsillar prominence ("herniations") is problematic, especially in respect to their lethality. Deleterious repercussions from these herniations are dependent on the rapidity with which ↑ ICP occurs and the herniation develops, as well as the anatomic capacity of the tentorial notch and foramen magnum.[17] For example, cerebellar tonsils may be chronically herniated into the cervical spinal canal in Arnold-Chiari malformations without any or only mild manifestations referable to that site.[19] The term *herniation* often has a fatal connotation; for this reason, other ambiguous terms (notching, grooving, or coning) are used by some, when its significance is unclear or until additional information is obtained. The inexperienced should be wary of overinterpreting prominent, even asymmetric, medial temporal lobes or cerebellar tonsils.

Before discussing the issue of *brain edema* (Fig. 77-4), we need to make one other point about ↑ ICP. After the cranial sutures fuse and the brain is confined in a closed space, a characteristic volume-to-pressure relationship is established. This relationship is exponential, not linear.[17] For example, the addition or subtraction of a few milliliters of CSF at normal intracranial pressure (less than 200 mm H_2O when horizontal) will have little or no effect, but at elevated pressure levels (around 600 mm H_2O) the same manipulations can dramatically raise or lower intracranial pressure. Therefore a person may have a sizable mass lesion for some time without symptoms, particularly in a "silent" area, until it reaches a critical size; at that point the patient may present catastrophically because of a rapid rise in ICP.

Brain swelling and edema

A swollen brain may be caused by an increase in the volume of any of its compartments: intravascular, intraventricular, or intraparenchymal. The term *brain swelling* generally indicates an increase in the intravascular compartment, whereas *brain edema* is used to denote a volumetric increase in the water content of its parenchymal compartment: interstitial, cellular, or both.[17]

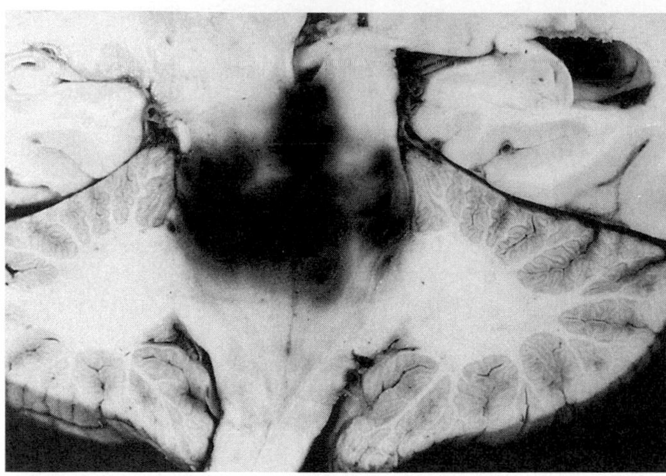

Fig. 77-3 Secondary brainstem hemorrhages of Duret caused by hypertensive hemorrhage in basal ganglia.

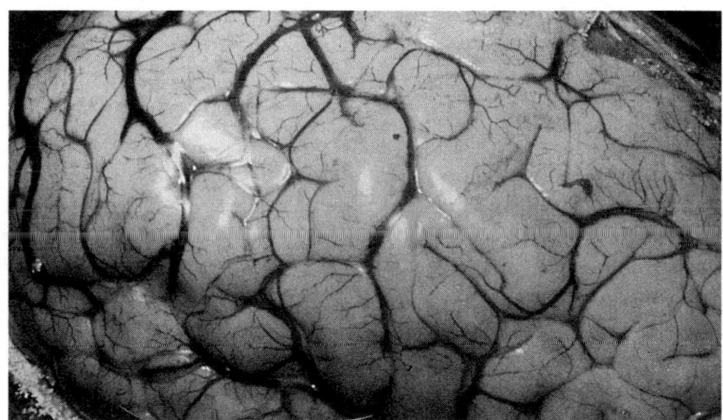

Fig. 77-4 Cerebral edema. Flattened gyri and narrowed sulci.

The brain's limited options for expansion and lack of classical lymphatics to facilitate removal of fluids necessitate other mechanisms to counteract harmful increases in ICP. Alternatively, since neurons are so dependent on oxygen and glucose to perform and survive,[19] vascular perfusion pressures in the CNS must be insulated to some extent from systemic hypotension. Autoregulation of intracranial vascular tone, through local vasoconstriction or vasodilatation, particularly of leptomeningeal arterioles,[20] provides fairly constant perfusion pressures in brain despite mild to moderate elevations or reductions in systemic blood pressures. Additionally, the production of CSF is reduced with ↑ ICP. Thus physiologic mechanisms exist in two of the three intracranial compartments (intravascular and intraventricular) to control ICP. The blood-brain barrier (BBB), mediated primarily by specific characteristics of brain capillary endothelium (no fenestrations, tight junctions with high resistance, and low pinocytotic and endocytotic activity), and the blood-CSF barrier, located at the tight junctions of choroid plexus cells,[18] are critical for maintaining the interstitial microenvironment needed for neurons to function properly. The BBB also plays a major role in preventing the egress of intravascular fluids into (and out of) the interstitial space. This function is best appreciated when the BBB is damaged, resulting in an excess of plasma filtrate within the interstitium and cells of the brain, *vasogenic edema* (Fig. 77-5). This type of edema may be conspicuous in neoplastic, infectious, toxic, and vascular conditions; it has great clinical significance because it can produce either focal or diffuse mass effect and ↑ ICP. This edema is predominantly interstitial and in white matter. The second major type of edema is referred to as *cytotoxic;* the excessive fluid, consisting predominantly of water and sodium, is found within cells (astrocytes, neurons, and endothelium) of both gray and white matter. This is seen most commonly in hypoxia, early ischemia, or trauma or in a variety of metabolic and toxic conditions. In the latter conditions the excessive fluid may be largely confined within myelin sheaths and has been designated *intramyelinic edema.* The third type of edema is referred to as *interstitial* and was defined in the context of obstructive hydrocephalus. The fluid is largely CSF and is located in the interstitial space around the lateral ventricles.[17,18] Since vasogenic edema also is predominantly interstitial, this modifier was ill chosen.

Common artifacts

The CNS may display a variety of artifactual alterations,[21,22] which can confuse or at least distract the novice. A brief depiction of the commonest ones is offered to minimize the distraction. The *"Swiss cheese" brain* refers to grossly obvious and sharply defined spherical holes, simulating cystic infarcts or cysticercosis, within the parenchyma of inadequately fixed or autolyzed brain, usually deep in cerebral and cerebellar hemispheres (Fig. 77-6); it is caused by the proliferation of gas-forming bacteria (such as clostridia and lactobacilli) between death and adequate fixation. Microscopically, one may find bacilli within the holes or adjacent to them in poorly stained parenchyma without any cellular reaction. The "toothpaste" artifact, noted in spinal cords that have been handled too roughly or kinked, has been so designated because the soft and distorted spinal cord has the appearance of a strip of toothpaste atop a toothbrush; it can mimic an intra-axial neoplasm, developmental anomaly, or infarction. Gyri can be artifactually flattened, resembling cerebral swelling or edema, when one improperly allows the surface of the brain to rest on the bottom or side of the fixation container. Inadequate fixation may result in pink discoloration of deep cerebral or cerebellar white matter; this also can involve the central pons when the ventral surface of the brainstem is suspended too close to the surface of the fixative.[21] Prolonged fixation can produce a grayish-yellow, firm peripheral rim a few millimeters thick. The cut surface of cerebellar cortex can display a bluish-gray discoloration (conglutination artifact, *état glacé*) because of autolysis of the internal granular layer. Rough handling is not tolerated by many organs, especially brain and spinal cord where the Stryker saw can produce cuts resembling infarcts. The gross distribution, lack of microscopic changes, and presence of bone dust should reveal its artifactual nature.

The term *respirator brain*[20] is a misnomer in that one might assume that its congested, gray, swollen, and soft to liquid state (Fig. 77-7), even after an adequate period of fixation, is attributable to respirator therapy. Actually the brain is severely autolyzed because, after a lethal insult to the brain (usually global hypoxia-ischemia), the comatose and brain-dead patient was maintained for some time on a mechanical respirator—allowing the brain time to autolyze. A minimum of about 12 hours is necessary to produce a typical example, which is most prominent in cerebellum. Diffuse neuronal eosinophilia, congestion, edema, and sometimes petechial hemorrhages without significant inflammatory response are typical histopathologic

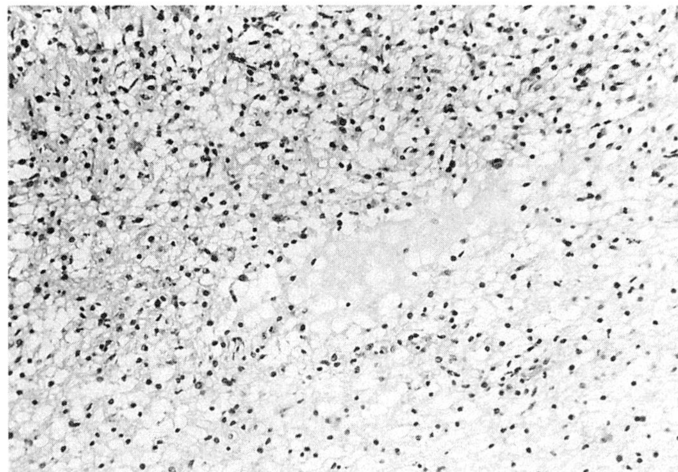

Fig. 77-5 Pronounced vasogenic edema. Proteinaceous pools of fluid and vacuolation of white matter.

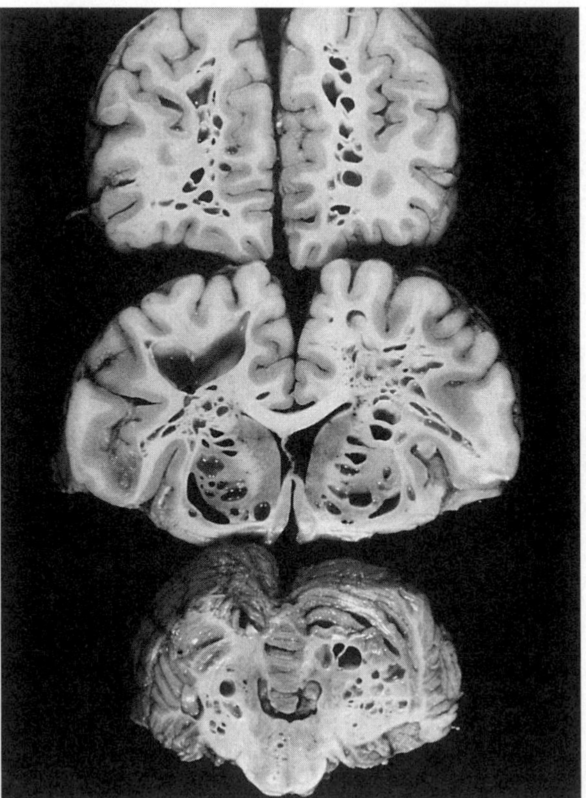

Fig. 77-6 Severe "Swiss-cheese" artifact.

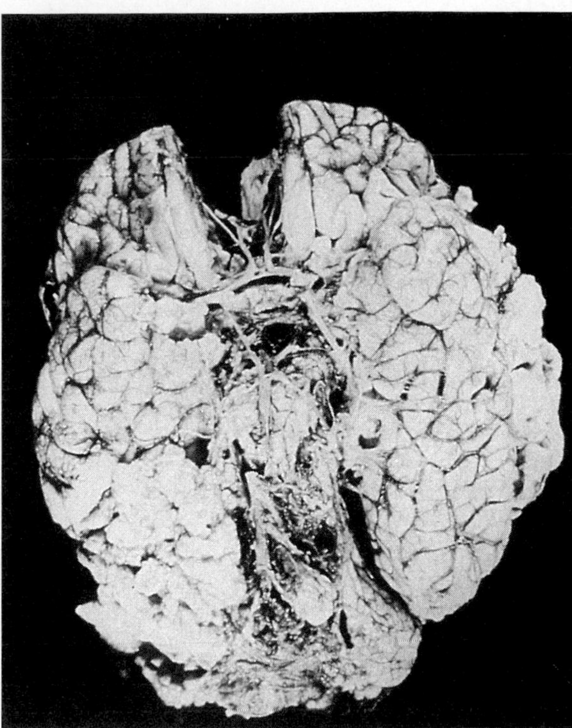

Fig. 77-7 Respirator brain (ventral view).

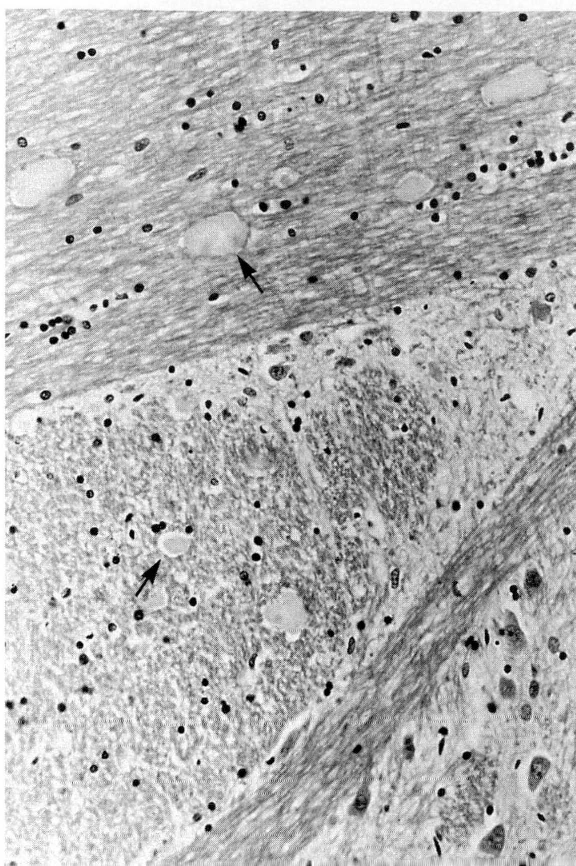

Fig. 77-8 Buscaino bodies *(arrows)* in white matter.

findings. Fragments of autolyzed cerebellum may be found in spinal subarachnoid space and simulate a neoplastic or infectious process. These changes also can involve the upper cervical cord causing it to swell and, especially when hemorrhagic, to mimic a physically induced cord injury. Clots in the major venous sinuses are common. This phenomenon is much less common now that criteria for brain death have been established.

Microscopic artifacts,[21,22] characterized as elsewhere by a lack of cellular reaction, include a variety of *vacuoles* and *spongy change* (perineuronal, perivascular, Purkinje cell layer, and periphery of spinal cord). These may be difficult to distinguish from genuine vacuoles of vasogenic and cytotoxic (including intramyelinic) edema, axonal degeneration, and rarefaction. Oligodendrocytes typically display artifactual cytoplasmic swelling at autopsy, often of great assistance in their identification, but this change may be exaggerated by agonal or postmortem factors and may be minimal or absent in well-fixed surgical specimens. Weakly hematoxylinophilic material may fill completely or partially irregular vacuoles of variable sizes (up to 200 μm) in myelinated areas, or they may be empty. It has been debated whether these vacuoles, referred to as "Buscaino bodies" (Fig. 77-8), have a relationship to "mucoid degeneration" of oligodendroglia.[23] They appear to be derived from myelin sheaths, probably because of exposure to alcohol-containing solutions. The "dark neuron" has a shrunken, irregular hematoxylinophilic and argyrophilic nucleus and cytoplasm, often with a corkscrew apical dendrite and perineuronal swelling (Fig. 77-9). It is most common in brain biopsy specimens, since it results from handling before adequate fixation;[23] it should not be confused with neurofibrillary degeneration. Poor fixation or excessive washing can produce *myelin pallor* and *pale swollen neurons,* as in the central pons where it can superficially resemble central pontine myelinolysis. Improper freezing-thawing can produce multiple cavities. A peculiar linear hematoxylinophilia of superficial cortex resembling pseudolaminar calcification or ferrugination[22] may be seen, perhaps related to improperly buffered formaldehyde solutions.

Nonspecific pathologic findings

A large variety of mild abnormalities in the CNS, particularly in the aging brain, usually or at present lack clinical significance. Gross examples include meningeal calcification or ossification (such as falx); leptomeningeal fibrosis in the absence of hydrocephalus and usually in the presence of cerebral atrophy; small cysts, calcification, xanthoma, and xanthogranuloma of the choroid plexus; and small cysts and calcifications of the pineal gland. Microscopic examples include corpora amylacea (Fig. 77-10), subpial (marginal sclerosis), and subependymal astrogliosis; irregular clusters of ependymal cells around ventricles and in the central spinal cord; lipofuscin in neurons, glia, and perivascular cells; mild to moderate siderocalcinosis of blood vessels in globus pallidus (Fig. 77-11), dentate nucleus and hippocampal sulcus; dystrophic axonal spheroids in the nucleus gracilis and the cuneatus (Fig. 77-12); mild pallor of myelin of the centrum semiovale or the cord periphery; mild neuronal loss (such as

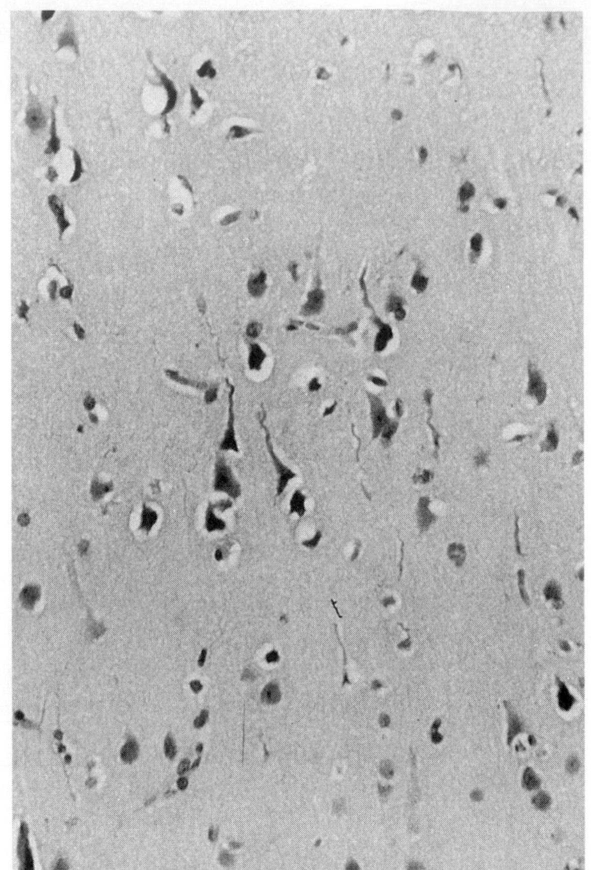

Fig. 77-9 Dark neurons in cerebral neocortex.

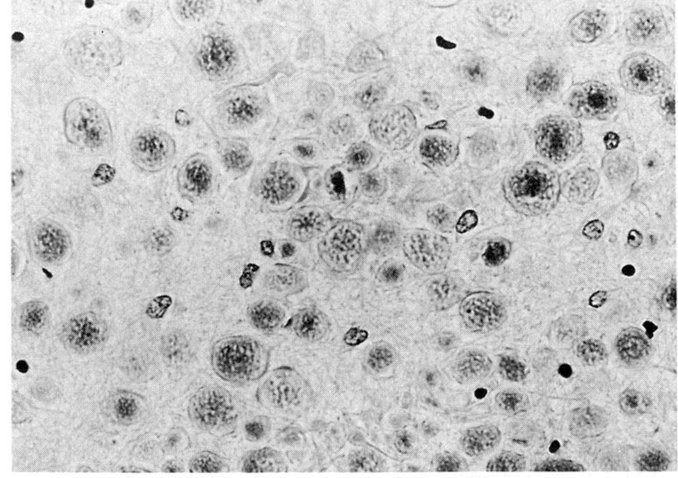

Fig. 77-10 Corpora amylacea in subependymal area.

Purkinje cells), argyrophilic bodies in anterior horns; calcification, fibrosis, and clusters of arachnoid cells in the stroma of the choroid plexus; calcification, gliosis or fibrosis, and cysts of the pineal gland; and proliferations (caps) of the arachnoid cells[24,25] (Fig. 77-13).

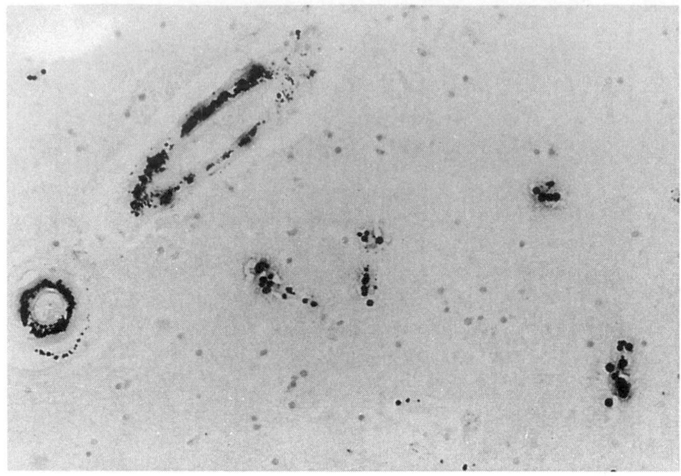

Fig. 77-11 Siderocalcinosis of blood vessels in globus pallidus.

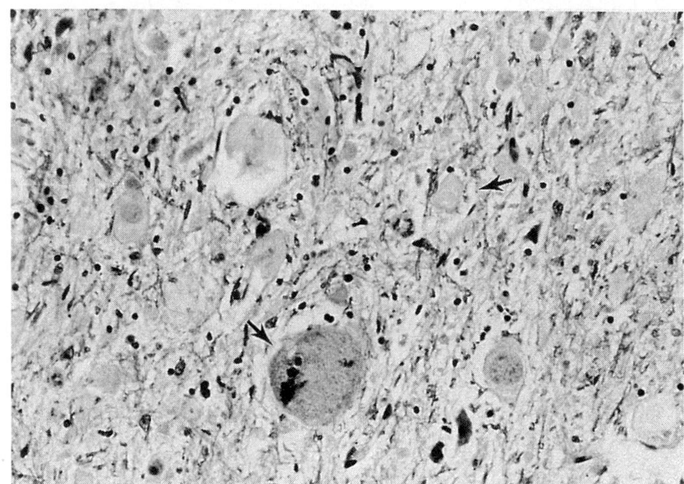

Fig. 77-12 Dystrophic spheroids *(arrows)* in nucleus gracilis.

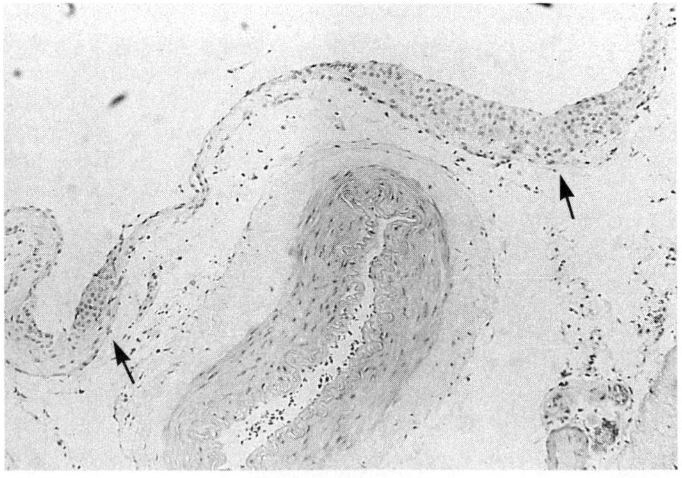

Fig. 77-13 Arachnoid caps *(arrows)*.

MAJOR RESPONSES OF CENTRAL NEURAL CELLS TO INJURY

Neurons. The normal neuron consists of a perinuclear cell body called the "perikaryon" and cytoplasmic processes, dendrites, and axons. The most prominent lesions in these postmitotic cells are those that involve the perikaryon.[23,24,26] *Eosinophilia* (pink or red neuron, hypoxic or ischemic change) of the cytoplasm refers to excessive eosinophilic staining of contracted neuronal cytoplasm, usually with pyknotic nuclei (Fig. 77-14). It is a common alteration, most frequently caused by hypoxia or hypoxia-ischemia, and may be recognizable about 6 to 8 hours after the insult. In view of the associated nuclear change, neuronal eosinophilia is presumably irreversible and thus represents acute neuronal necrosis.

Neuronal *atrophy* is the noneosinophilic shrinkage of the cell body with nuclear hyperchromasia or pyknosis; it may be produced by direct (simple) or indirect (transsynaptic) mechanisms. *Simple atrophy,* often with excessive lipofuscin, is common in many degenerative diseases. *Transsynaptic* or *transneuronal atrophy,* unique to the nervous system, may be either retrograde (interference with efferent or axonal transmission) or anterograde (interference with afferent or dendritic transmission). Both of these changes depend on the type and location of the neuron, the age of the patient, and probably the amount of synaptic loss. For example, neurons of the lateral geniculate body can undergo anterograde transsynaptic atrophy after loss of an eye (or retinal-optic damage), but only specific geniculate neurons atrophy: those of layers 1, 4, and 6 of the contralateral body and layers 2, 3, and 5 of the ipilateral body. On the other hand, when neurons of the inferior olivary nucleus are deafferented because of lesions of the contralateral dentate nucleus or its projections, they undergo an initial phase of hypertrophy as a result of vacuolization and neurofilamentous proliferation before becoming atrophic. This peculiar reaction seems unique to olivary neurons. Diffuse atrophy of lateral geniculate neurons secondary to damage to calcarine cortex or optic radiations is an example of retrograde degeneration. If the optic nerve also is atrophic, retrograde transsynaptic degeneration has occurred. Transsynaptic degeneration probably is responsible for much of the neuronal atrophy seen in the system degenerations.[6]

Chromatolysis, often spoken about but seldom encountered in routine surgical or autopsy samples, may be either central or peripheral. Chromatolytic neurons are enlarged (hypertrophic) and rounded with peripheral displacement of the nucleus and enlargement of its nucleolus; the cytoplasm acquires a homogeneous granular appearance because of the dispersion of its Nissl substance. The neuron undergoing peripheral chromatolysis, a rare event, displays absence of peripheral, and the presence of central, Nissl substance; this is presumed to represent early recovery from central chromatolysis. *Central chromatolysis* (Fig. 77-15), which includes the sparing of a peripheral rim of Nissl substance, generally is a regenerative response to axonal damage (axonal reaction) in that these neurons have increased free polysomes and an upregulation of neuronal proteins (e.g., neurofilament). However, chromatolysis of central neurons also may occur in the absence of an identifiable axonal lesion (such as pellagra). Numerous factors influence the development and the fate of chromatolytic neurons. If the axonal damage occurs close to the cell body or to neurons whose axons are confined within the CNS, the lesion can be lethal. On the other hand, if the lesion occurs distal to the cell body and especially on central neurons with a peripheral nervous system projection, regeneration is more likely to be successful. Some neurons within the central nervous system normally appear to exhibit central chromatolysis: the mesencephalic nucleus of V, dorsal nucleus of Clarke, among others. Perikaryal swelling caused by *storage* (Fig. 77-16) of a large variety of metabolites (lipids, carbohydrates, mucosubstances, lipopigments, glycoproteins) should not be confused with chromatolysis; this neuron usually displays no or dispersed Nissl substance, the cytoplasm may be foamy or irregularly stained, and the nucleus may not be displaced to the periphery. The storage-induced change tends to involve many neurons and is diffuse or multifocal. However, special stains to demonstrate the abnormal cytoplasmic storage occasionally may be necessary.

Mineralization (ferrugination) (Fig. 77-17) of neurons and astrocytes is attributable to the deposition of iron and calcium

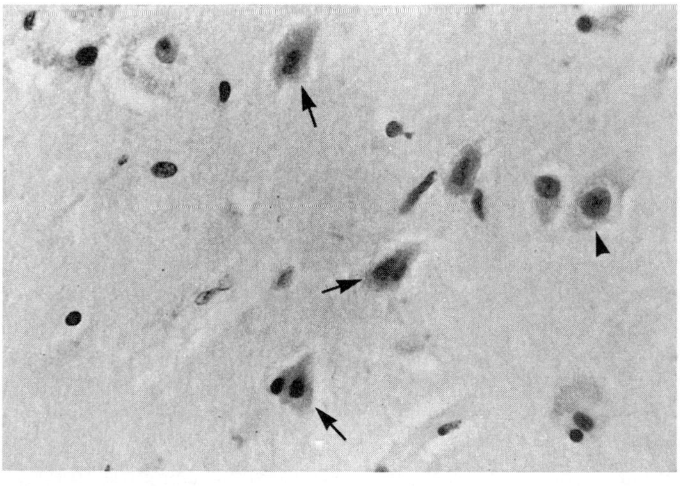

Fig. 77-14 Eosinophilic *(arrows)* and normal neurons *(arrowhead).*

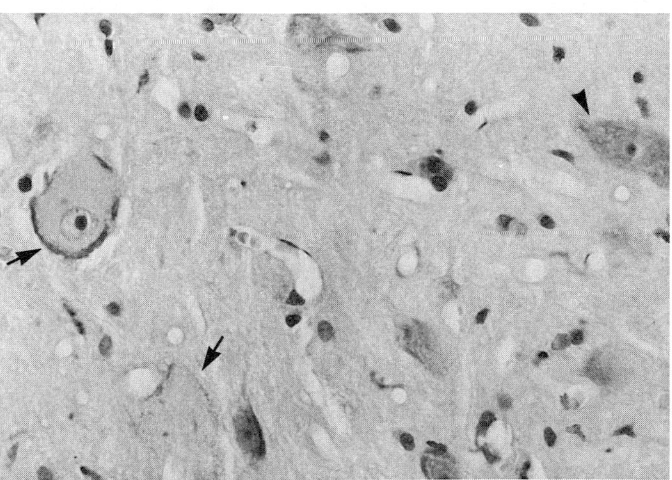

Fig. 77-15 Two neurons undergoing central chromatolysis *(arrows)* and normal neuron *(arrowhead).*

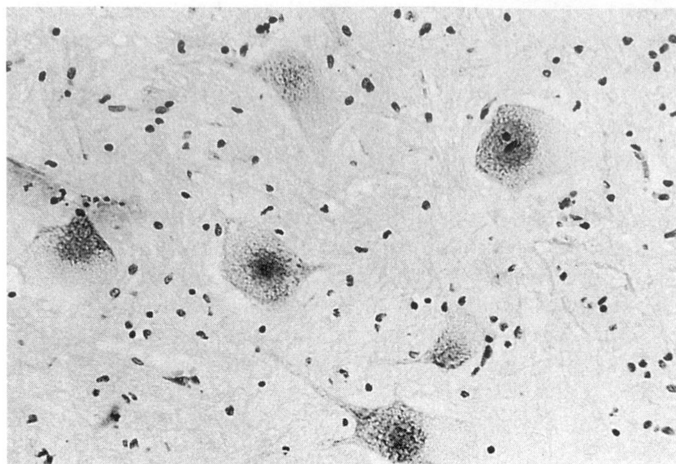

Fig. 77-16 Neuronal storage in Pompe's disease.

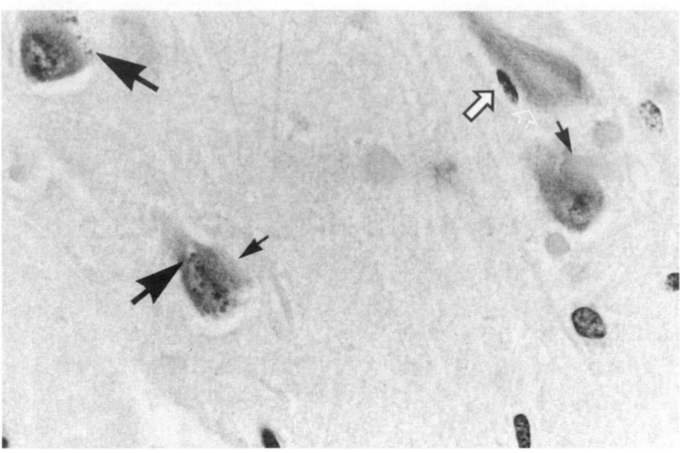

Fig. 77-18 Granulovacuolar degeneration *(large arrows),* Hirano rodlike bodies *(small arrows)* and neurofibrillary tangle *(open arrow)* in hippocampus.

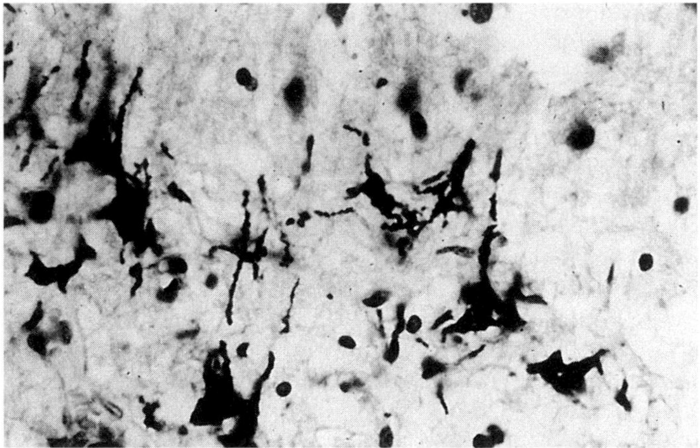

Fig. 77-17 Ferrugination.

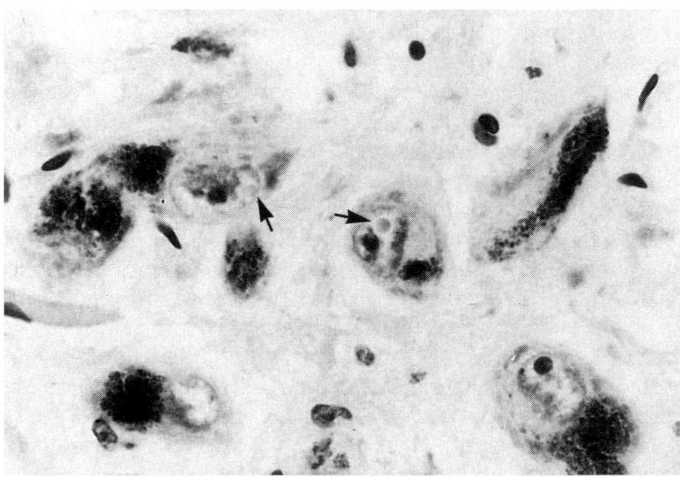

Fig. 77-19 Marinesco bodies *(arrows)* in neuromelanin-containing neurons of substantia nigra.

on cells near necrotic foci, particularly hemorrhagic infarcts or contusions.

Neurons probably are best known for an often bewildering array of eponymic *inclusions,*[26] mostly cytoplasmic, which may be diagnostic of specific diseases. Many of these are described under their respective, usually degenerative, diseases: *neurofibrillary tangles* in Alzheimer's disease, progressive supranuclear palsy and postencephalitic Parkinson's disease; *Pick bodies* in Pick's disease; *granulovacuolar degeneration* (Fig. 77-18) and *Hirano bodies* in Alzheimer's disease; *Bunina bodies* in amyotrophic lateral sclerosis; the *Lewy body* in idiopathic Parkinson's disease and diffuse Lewy body disease, *Lafora bodies* in Lafora body disease and adult polyglucosan body disease; intranuclear *viral inclusions* in measles encephalitis, subacute sclerosing panencephalitis, herpes simplex I and II, herpes zoster-varicella and cytomegalovirus (owl's eye); intracytoplasmic viral *Negri* and *Lyssa bodies* in rabies; and intracytoplasmic viral bodies in cytomegalovirus. Eosinophilic intranuclear inclusions in substantia nigra and other pigmented neurons, referred to as "Marinesco bodies" (Fig. 77-19), seem to have no pathologic significance. They should not be confused with viral intranuclear inclusions, *neuronal intranuclear hyaline inclusion disease,* or with the cytoplasmic Lewy body. Other cytoplasmic inclusions of little to no diagnostic import are hyaline inclusions in hypoglossal and anterior horn neurons, eosinophilic rodlike inclusions in neurons of the caudate nucleus, and eosinophilic inclusions in thalamic neurons.[26]

Although neuronal necrosis and loss is the result of a large number of disease processes, phagocytosis of dead neurons (*neuronophagia*) is usually conspicuoous only in hypoxic-ischemic lesions and viral diseases. The predominant phagocyte is the microglial cell or monocyte.

Axon. Wallerian-like tract degeneration, the CNS counterpart of true degeneration of Waller (PNS), is a common lesion of central axons; it usually occurs after infarcts or traumatic lesions (contusions, lacerations) have destroyed groups of neuronal perikarya or their axonal projections (Fig. 77-20). Axons fragment in a proximodistal gradient from the site of damage and usually one internode back toward the perikaryon. As the axon fragments, its myelin sheath breaks up into myelin ovoids, large vacuoles containing compact balls of myelin and some axonal debris. Macrophages and to some extent astrocytes phagocytose the debris, with the reaction being most intense

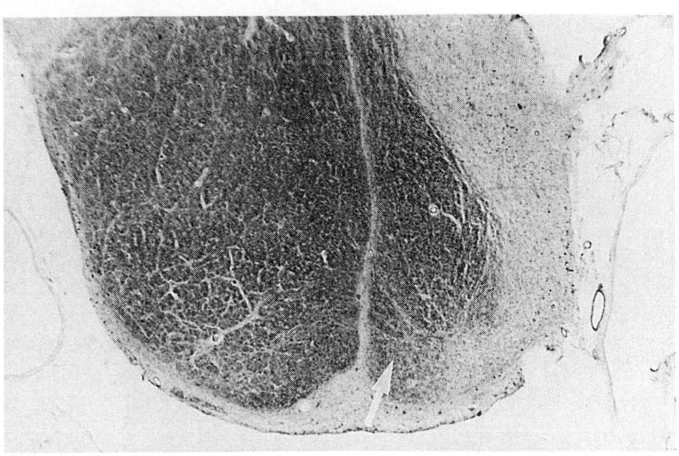

Fig. 77-20 Secondary (Wallerian-like) degeneration of one fornix *(arrow)* caused by old and severe trauma to ipsilateral hippocampus.

nearest the lesion. The rate at which this axonal degeneration occurs depends on the size of the axons (larger, faster), the age of the patient (younger, faster), and the location (PNS, faster). *Dying-back degeneration* of the axon refers to a withering loss of the distal axon (and myelin sheath) followed by progressive loss of more proximal segments in a distoproximal gradient. This lesion primarily affects the peripheral nervous system in a metabolic-toxic setting, but a central component may coexist (central-peripheral distal axonopathy); several CNS degenerative diseases, especially the system degenerations, also may display this phenomenon. *Axonal atrophy,* attributable in some cases to loss of neurofilaments, is a subtle morphologic lesion seen in chronic degenerative and metabolic-toxic diseases, often as part of the dying-back phenomenon. *Spheroids* (axonal swellings) are focal enlargements of axons usually caused by traumatic, ischemic, or metabolic-toxic insults. Ultrastructural studies have delineated two major types: the common *reactive,* which may exhibit proliferations of normal organelles (retraction balls), or lysosomes (degenerative), or neurofilaments and mitochondria (regenerative); and the *dystrophic,* which additionally contains smooth membranous and vesicular proliferations with electron-dense material of obscure origin. The former usually results from local damage to the axon either by traumatic shearing forces or by focal infarction (such as adjacency to a lacune). The latter is a common change in the aged but in a highly localized pattern: nucleus gracilis, nucleus cuneatus, substantia nigra, and globus pallidus (Fig. 77-12); they seem to lack clinical significance. Symptomatic dystrophic spheroids in a diffuse pattern are characteristic of the rare metabolic or degenerative diseases, *neuroaxonal dystrophies* (Seitelberger's disease, or infantile neuroaxonal dystrophy, and Hallervorden-Spatz disease). "Torpedoes" are reactive spheroids of Purkinje cell axons, composed largely of neurofilaments and located in the internal granular layer. This is a nonspecific finding in many degenerative and metabolic-toxic diseases. Distention of axons (and dendrites) by abnormal storage material also may be seen in neuronal *storage* diseases.

Myelin. Two major lesions affect myelin sheaths: primary demyelination and spongy degeneration or change. In primary demyelination the myelin sheath (and usually oligodendrocyte) is lost with relative preservation of its axon, (as in multiple sclerosis). Spongy degeneration of myelin (status spongiosus of white matter, spongy myelinopathy) usually reflects intramyelinic edema and is seen in numerous metabolic-toxic diseases. A variety of nonspecific and apparently minor disturbances, such as blebs or pallor, also may involve myelin sheaths. The interpretation (and significance) of myelin pallor, however, can be as problematic as the issue of vacuolation in the CNS.

Dendrite. Few dendritic lesions are apparent in a light microscopic assessment of a routinely stained section. Swelling or vacuolation can be appreciated, especially with the electron microscope, in seizures, storage diseases, and cytotoxic edema. Excitotoxic amino acids (such as glutamate and aspartate) can induce dendritic swelling in an experimental setting. Hypoplasia in congenital hypothyroidism (cretinism), or atrophy in aging and some degenerative diseases, can be recognized in thick sections stained with a Golgi technique.

Neuropil. The neuropil is the intervening feltwork that fills the spaces between cell bodies of gray matter; it contains small, usually unmyelinated, axons, dendrites, synapses, and glial processes. Several lesions are readily appreciated in routine preparations: (1) neuritic plaques containing amyloid, degenerating and regenerating axons, and dendrites; (2) spongy change (status spongiosus of gray matter) caused by neuronal loss, resorption of spheroids, cytotoxic and vasogenic edema, or the spongiform change of prion diseases (such as Creutzfeldt-Jakob); (3) dystrophic spheroids of infantile neuroaxonal dystrophy; and (4) polyglucosan bodies. The spongy and spongiform changes are caused, in part, by neuritic (dendrite and axon) and astrocytic swelling. Spongy change of gray matter invokes a more limited differential than its white matter counterpart.

Astrocytes. In striking contrast to neurons, astrocytes have great regenerative potential, even though they seldom display mitotic figures in normal or reactive human material. Traditionally, morphologic distinctions have been made between protoplasmic astrocytes of gray matter with their short, complex branching processes in gold sublimate preparations and the *fibrous* astrocytes of white matter and adjacent to blood or CSF interfaces (perivascular, subpial, subependymal) with their longer and sparsely branched processes. Both display ovoid to round nuclei, measuring about 10 μm in diameter, without visible cytoplasm or processes in routine stains. Generally, only the resting fibrous astrocyte contains enough intermediate cytofilaments to be recognized with the phosphotungstic acid–hematoxylin (PTAH) and Holzer stains and with antibodies to glial fibrillary acidic protein (GFAP). Both types, however, readily and commonly undergo hyperplasia and hypertrophy. The term *astrocytosis* is appropriate for both and may be subdivided into *protoplasmic*, or *metabolic*, since this change usually accompanies systemic metabolic-toxic imbalances, and *fibrous*. The term *gliosis* usually refers to astrocytic proliferations (astrogliosis) and has been used for either cell type and in either acute or chronic situations. Some use the modifier "reactive" *(reactive gliosis* or *astrocytosis)* for acute situations in which the cytoplasm exhibits a prominent hyaline, eosinophilic, $PTAH^+$, and $GFAP^+$ enlargement (gemistocyte) (Fig. 77-21). The nuclei may be atypical or multiple. The term *fibrillary gliosis* would then be restricted to the chronic form, where the cytoplasmic enlargement subsides, leaving behind a variably dense fibrillary background of its cytoplasmic processes. If the fibrils are

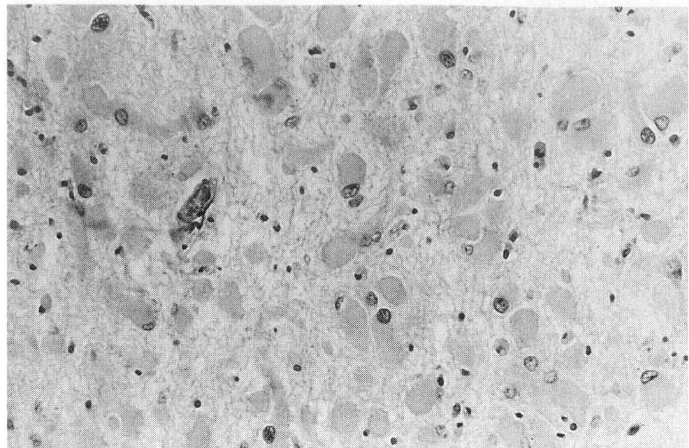

Fig. 77-21 Reactive (hypertrophic and hyperplastic) astrocytes.

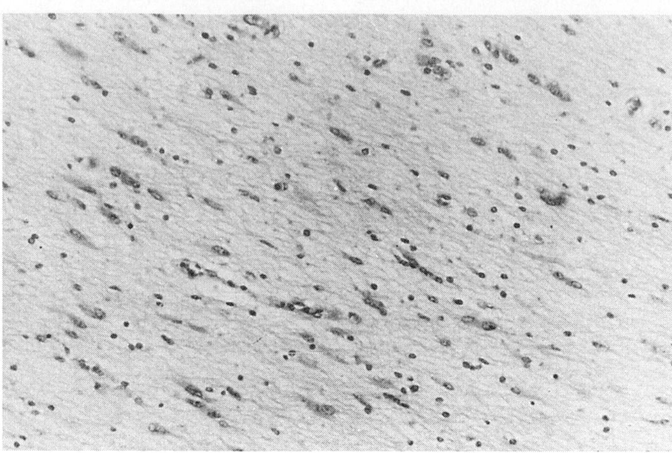

Fig. 77-22 Isomorphic fibrillary gliosis in chronic inactive lesion of multiple sclerosis.

haphazardly arranged the term *anisomorphic (fibrillary) gliosis* is used; if they run parallel to each other, usually within a tract of myelinated fibers, it is referred to as *isomorphic (fibrillary) gliosis* (Fig. 77-22). At this stage the GFAP immunostain may be less successful in labeling the cells than the traditional special stains. The protoplasmic astrocyte also responds frequently to systemic metabolic imbalances, correlating especially well with the hyperammonemia of hepatic disease, by a hydropic enlargement (about 15 to 20 μm) and lobulation of its nucleus. This change is most easily appreciated in globus pallidus, caudate nucleus, and dentate nucleus. When such astrocytic nuclei are about 20 μm with distinct lobulations and often containing eosinophilic granules (glycogen), they are referred to as *Alzheimer type II glia.* Some limit this designation only to hepatic encephalopathy, Wilsonian or nonwilsonian. *Alzheimer type I glia,* consisting of enlarged, hyperchromatic, and atypical to bizarre nuclei with eosinophilic cytoplasm, are seen rarely in hepatic encephalopathy (usually of Wilson's disease) or progressive multifocal leukoencephalopathy. Astrocytic hypertrophy and hyperplasia are among the commonest pathologic reactions in CNS but are also among the least specific.

Reactive astrocytosis generally indicates an active irritation or destruction, whereas fibrillary gliosis (chronic) indicates that the major process may have subsided or equilibrated with its environment. Several practical points should be mentioned. Reactive, often atypical, astrocytes may be difficult to distinguish from neoplastic gemistocytic astrocytes, especially when both are associated with a mass effect and contrast enhancement. Reactive astrocytosis is more often associated with macrophages and parenchymal necrosis, whereas in gemistocytic astrocytoma the cells are more monomorphous with few or no macrophages. Additional differential features are considered in the section dealing with astrocytic neoplasms. Chronic fibrillary gliosis, also often atypical, may be difficult to distinguish from low-grade fibrillary astrocytoma. In this instance the clinical history and the imaging studies can be decisive. If the lesion has a mass effect or contrast enhancement, a neoplasm should be strongly considered; chronic fibrillary gliosis usually is associated with a long-standing, often characteristic clinical course and atrophy of neural parenchyma.

Only two characteristic inclusions occur in astrocytes, except for the common accumulations of lipofuscin: *corpora amylacea* and *Rosenthal fibers.* The former are spherical, hematoxylinophilic, often laminated polyglucosan accumulations within the cytoplasmic processes of fibrous astrocytes. They are extremely common in the aging brain and most conspicuous in subpial, subependymal, and perivascular areas. They can be labeled nonspecifically with many special stains and immunostains. They average about 20 to 30 μm in diameter and are PAS positive (diastase resistant) because of their carbohydrate nature, which approximates the plant starch amylopectin more than glycogen. They also are alcianophilic and metachromatic because of their high content of phosphate and sulfate groups. Ultrastructurally they consist of 6- to 8-μm filaments. They may be useful diagnostically in establishing fibrillary gliosis or neuronal loss, since their presence in an atypical location generally signifies a chronic astrocytic reaction. Biochemically and ultrastructurally similar to identical material with different light microscopic features can be seen in neurons, hepatic cells, myocardium, and skeletal and smooth muscle in a rare group of metabolic diseases (polyglucosan body diseases). *Rosenthal fibers* are inclusions of astrocytes with the same topographic distribution as that of corpora amylacea. It consists of deeply eosinophilic, elongated, irregular, often seemingly refractile, intracytoplasmic accumulations of proteins (Fig. 77-23), predominantly α-B crystalline (a lens protein). It stains well with PTAH and usually poorly with anti-GFAP antibodies; intermediate filaments with electron-dense granular material are seen under the electron microscope (Fig. 77-24). It is the hallmark of low-grade, particularly the juvenile pilocytic, astrocytoma and the rare Alexander's disease. Its detection, especially in frozen sections of mass lesions, is of great aid in the identification of a low-grade astrocytic neoplasm, but they can also be seen in reactive settings, notably around infiltrating craniopharyngioma, some lacunes, a syrinx, spinal ependymomas, and pineal cysts. Infrequently, astrocytes may contain iron that has been phagocytosed. In *storage* diseases astrocytes commonly display material that is similar but not identical to that in neurons. In some situations this probably reflects *phagocytosis* of debris from dead neurons. Even though microglia-monocytes are the major phagocytes in CNS, astrocytes frequently perform this function (facultative phagocyte).

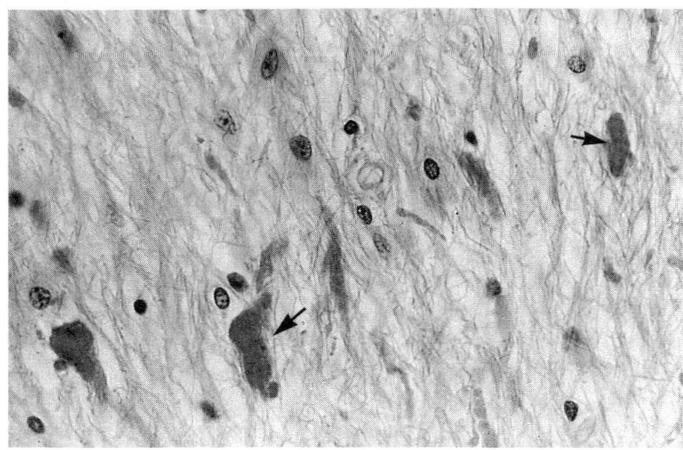

Fig. 77-23 Rosenthal fibers *(arrows)* among astrocytic fibrils.

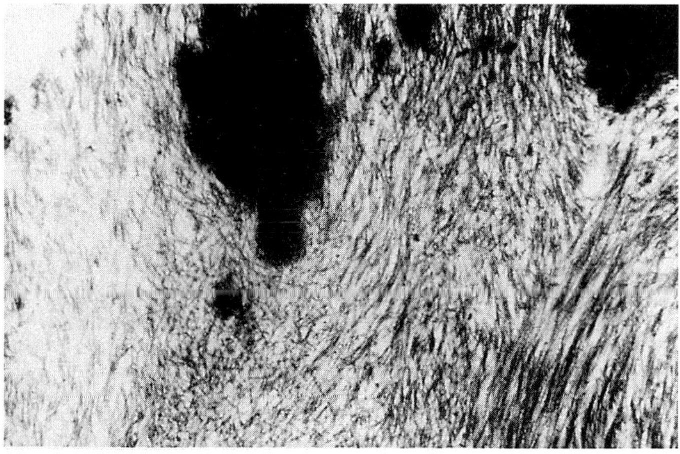

Fig. 77-24 Fine structure of Rosenthal fibers. Electron-dense granular material admixed with intermediate cytofilaments.

Astrocytes do not succumb to the many lethal insults that affect neurons, but they do undergo necrosis within infarcts. In this setting their cell bodies vacuolate, their processes disintegrate (clasmatodendrosis), and their nuclei become pyknotic. They also may display swollen, glassy to foamy cytoplasm in edematous situations. Finally, the astrocyte is the preeminent cell involved in CNS neoplasms.[22-24,26]

Oligodendrocytes. Oligodendrocytes have a limited regenerative capacity when compared with astrocytes or their peripheral counterparts, Schwann cells. Although Schwann cells readily display mitotic activity and *hyperplasia,* oligodendrocytes do so only rarely, adjacent to and within demyelinative plaques or near necrotic lesions. This is one reason for the poor remyelinative (and regenerative) potential of the CNS. One should recall that oligodendrocytes myelinate longer internodes of many axons, whereas Schwann cells myelinate only one shorter internode of one axon. Oligodendrocytes also lack the extracellular support and guidance of a basement membrane and collagenous framework. Nevertheless, the oligodendrocyte is quite capable of *neoplastic transformation.*

Their other major reaction is that of necrosis or loss. Specific toxins (such as psychosine), viruses (such as papova

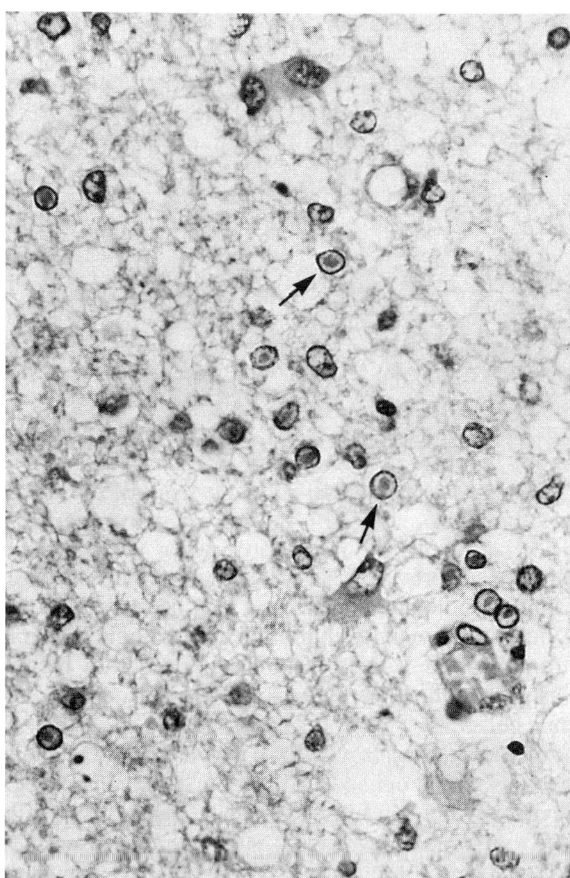

Fig. 77-25 Oligodendroglial inclusions *(arrows)* in subacute sclerosing panencephalitis.

JC, measles) or immune-mediated diseases (such as multiple sclerosis) can destroy oligodendrocytes (Fig. 77-25). Hypoxia-ischemia also can kill them, but their sensitivity is much less than that of neurons and greater than that of astrocytes. Oligodendrocytes predominantly occupy white matter but also are found in gray matter, where they typically surround neurons (as astrocytes and microglia do), so-called satellitosis. This has no pathologic significance and may be more prominent in some areas (such as amygdala), where it should not be misinterpreted as neoplastic satellitosis of infiltrating oligodendroglioma.[22-24,26]

Ependyma and choroid plexus. Their pathologic repertoire is even less exciting than that of oligodendrocytes. They too have limited regenerative potential, even though *neoplastic transformation* occurs readily in ependymal cells. Many noxious stimuli, such as hydrocephalus, hemoventricle, or ventriculitis attributable to infectious agents (notably cytomegalovirus), can destroy ependymal cells. This results in their loss, creating gaps with variable proliferations of subependymal astrocytic processes *(granular ependymitis, ependymal granulations)* (Fig. 77-26).

Choroidal epithelium is quite resilient and has a low potential for neoplastic transformation; it rarely may show subtle cytoplasmic changes, such as congophilic Biondi rings in the aged, oncocytic change in mitochondrial diseases, iron in hemochromatosis-hemosiderosis, or storage in mucolipidosis IV. A variety of nonspecific and inconsequential stromal

event. All major cerebral arteries emanating from the circle of Willis give rise to deep (penetrating) branches and superficial (cortical) branches. The deep branches such as the lenticulostriate arteries, which arise from the middle cerebral arteries and supply the striatum and posterior limb of the internal capsule, are essentially end arteries. Their occlusion results in infarctions roughly corresponding to the area supplied by the occluded artery. The superficial branches anastomose freely over the surface of the brain and provide overlapping collateral circulation between the terminal ramifications of contiguous vessels. The areas between two contiguous fields of blood supply, such as those between anterior and middle or middle and posterior cerebral arteries, are known as "watershed areas," or "border zones."[20,29,30] After occlusion of a superficial cerebral artery, the collateral anastomoses may be sufficient for the survival of a considerable amount of tissue in the border zone originally supplied by the occluded artery. On the other hand, a sudden drop of perfusion pressure within these anastomotic vessels, such as that caused by a cardiac arrythmia, makes the border zones between anterior and middle cerebral arteries most vulnerable to ischemia and results in *watershed,* or *border (boundary) zone, infarctions* (Fig. 77-30). Border zones may exist between the deep and superficial divisions and explain some of the deep intracerebral infarcts that occur outside the territories normally served by these vessels.[31] One of the two major extracranial collateral anastomoses between the internal and external carotid arteries is via the ophthalmic artery, a branch of the internal carotid that enlarges after occlusion of the internal carotid artery. Ipsilateral occlusion of the external carotid artery in such a patient, therefore, seriously jeopardizes cerebral circulation. The second important anastomosis is between the branches of the vertebral and brachial arteries; occlusion of the subclavian artery proximal to the origin of the vertebral artery causes retrograde flow of blood from the posterior cerebral circulation into the arm. Vigorous exercise of that arm leads to "stealing" of blood from the cerebral circulation into the arm and may precipitate signs of cerebral ischemia. "Subclavian steal syndrome," as it is called, illustrates how occlusion of a vessel remote from the brain can affect cerebral circulation and underscores the necessity of a thorough examination of the cardiovascular system, including the extracranial portions of the carotids and vertebrals, in all patients with CVD.[32]

Cerebrovascular disease can be classified into three categories: occlusive, hemorrhagic, and hypotensive (border zone infarcts).

Occlusive cerebrovascular diseases

Occlusive cerebrovascular diseases are usually attributable to atherosclerosis, thrombosis, or embolism. Less frequent causes include vasculitides, trauma, vasospasm, and hematologic disorders.

Atherosclerosis (arteriosclerosis) is the most common cause of CVD, and, as elsewhere in the body, hypertension and diabetes are major predisposing factors of significant atherogenesis in cerebral arteries. Certain sites are at great risk for developing atheromatous plaques: the ostia of vertebral arteries, the proximal and distal segments of the basilar artery, and the internal carotid arteries at their origin, syphon, and supraclinoid segment.[29] As plaques gradually enlarge or become ulcerated and acquire mural thrombi, they cause stenosis. It is generally assumed that cerebral blood flow

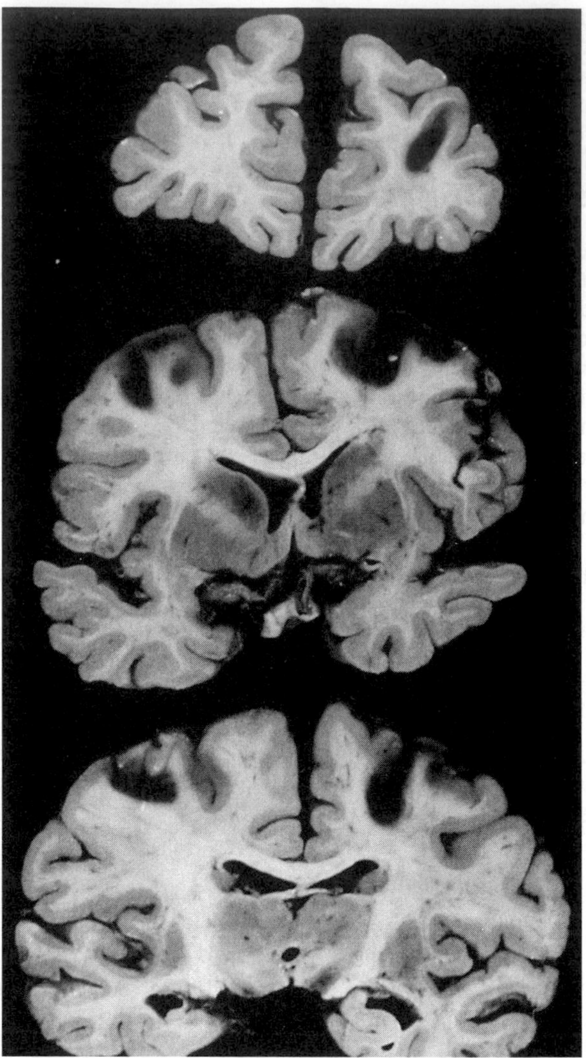

Fig. 77-30 Border zone infarcts, excessively hemorrhagic because of superimposed bleeding diathesis.

becomes impaired when the atheromatous plaque or the grafted mural thrombus reduces the lumen by at least 80%. The reduction in blood flow in turn predisposes to complete thrombotic occlusion of the arterial lumen that is often accompanied by anterograde extension of the blood clot (red or stagnation thrombus) downstream to the first major collateral branch. In large vessels such as the internal carotid artery, a mural thrombus also becomes a source of emboli. If small pieces are detached from the clot, they may be responsible for brief episodes of neurologic deficits, *transient ischemic attacks* (TIA). TIA last no more than 24 hours, after which the patients fully recover. They are harbingers of more serious cerebrovascular events.[33] *Emboli* are most common in the distribution of the middle cerebral artery where they tend to lodge at its origin or trifurcation. A frequent source of emboli other than mural thrombi of ulcerated atheromatous plaques in large vessels is the heart. Thromboemboli originate from atrial clots, especially in patients with atrial fibrillation, from mural thrombi developing on endomyocardial infarctions, or from valvular and prosthetic vegetations.[34] Thromboemboli are largely made up of laminated or partially organizing blood clots, but occasionally atheromatous material forms the main bulk of the clot, *atheromatous* or *cholesterol emboli*. Cholesterol emboli usually complicate vigorous manipulations of an atheromatous aorta during surgery or occur after invasive neuroradiologic procedures or anticoagulant therapy in patients with advanced atherosclerosis. Cholesterol emboli have a predilection to become impacted in the cortical branches of the cerebral arteries, usually in a border zone distribution. In situ thrombi associated with ulcerated plaques are usually converted to a fibrous plug with variable degrees of recanalization, whereas thromboemboli often fragment or lyse without leaving any trace. With septic emboli, often lodged in peripheral arterial branches, inflammation spreads and destroys the vessel wall resulting in aneurysmal dilatation (mycotic aneurysm) with its inherent risk of hemorrhagic rupture. Small emboli such as *fat, air,* and *foreign bodies* occlude the cerebral microvasculature. Fat embolism is typically characterized by widespread petechiae in the white matter (Fig. 77-31).

Infectious and *noninfectious vasculitides* are less frequent causes of obstruction of cerebral vessels. *Endarteritis* typically occurs in syphilitic vasculitis; however, a similar intimal response complicates tuberculous meningitis and certain parasitic diseases. Occasionally, infarctions may also complicate vasculitis associated with CNS-limited or *systemic collagen vascular diseases*.

Trauma to either the carotid or vertebral arteries attributable to blunt neck injury or puncture during angiographic procedures may induce focal or dissecting aneurysms, arteriovenous fistulas, or local thrombosis.[35] Dissection and thrombosis typically cause stenosis or total occlusion of the vessel. Dissection of the vertebral arteries has been associated with vigorous rotation of the neck, such as that during overzealous chiropractic manipulations and wrestling. *Spasm* of cerebral arteries occurs in patients with subarachnoid hemorrhage caused by rupture of berry aneurysms and less frequently as a complication of head injury or severe migraine.[36]

Occlusion of vessels may occur in the absence of primary vascular disease caused by hypercoagulable disorders, such as polycythemia rubra vera and Waldenström macroglobulinemia. Sickle cell disease can cause either sludging of the microcirculation with perivascular hemorrhages or actual thrombosis of larger arteries, including the carotid syphons.[37] Veins and sinuses, particularly the sagittal, also may become occluded in dehydrated "marasmic" children, occasionally in women using contraceptive pills high in estrogen content, during pregnancy, in the puerperium, and in other hypercoagulable states (such as malignancy) leading to *hemorrhagic infarctions* (Fig. 77-32).

Occlusion of an artery for a sufficient period of time, most commonly as a result of thromboemboli, causes cerebral infarction that develops into an area of softening, hence the antiquated term "encephalomalacia." The extent of an infarct can best be appreciated after formalin fixation; the infarcted tissue remains soft while the rest of the brain becomes firm. Infarcts are either "pale" (Fig. 77-33, *A*) or "hemorrhagic" (Fig. 77-33, *B*) depending on whether the vascular occlusion was a gradual process as in local thrombosis or abrupt as in embolism, respectively. The often hemorrhagic nature of embolic infarcts is attributed to lysis of the clot exposing the infarcted tissue and its permeable capillary bed to recirculating blood. The proclivity of the superimposed hemorrhagic component to be restricted to gray matter is largely attributable to its profuse capillary supply. In hemorrhagic infarcts caused by venous thromboses, the hemorrhagic element is more extensive and also involves the infarcted white matter. Sometimes hemorrhagic stippling of the cortex is seen also at margins of pale infarcts. Swelling is an early feature of a cerebral infarct and is more pronounced in the white matter. It is frequently associated with edema of surrounding brain parenchyma, and the true extent of an infarct may be difficult to ascertain in early lesions. Infarcted gray matter is dusky, and its junction with white matter is blurred. An infarct undergoes sequential microscopic changes reflecting its age; however, the precise timing of these changes varies from series to series.[38] One of the earliest changes is loss of affinity of myelin and neuropil for stains, which may be seen within 6 to 8 hours (Fig. 77-34). In the meantime, in the gray matter neurons undergo acute

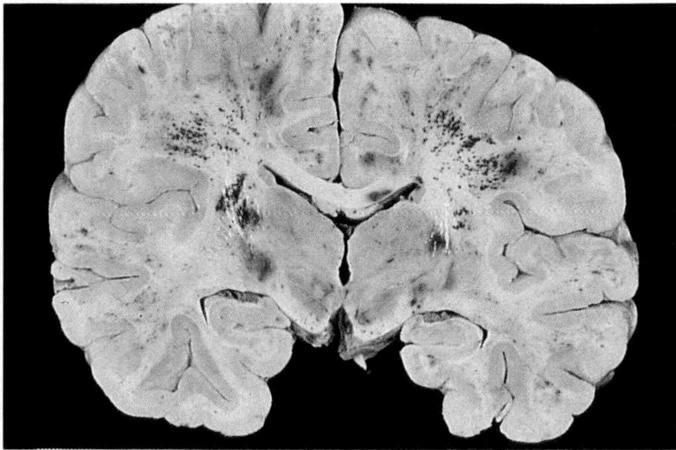

Fig. 77-31 Fat embolism. Multiple petechiae especially in white matter.

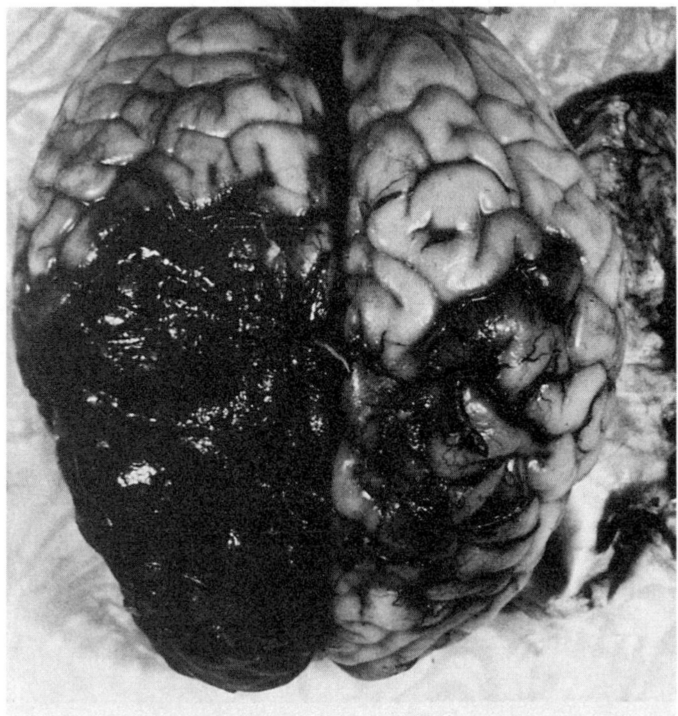

Fig. 77-32 Hemorrhagic infarction. Thrombosis of superior sagittal sinus and cortical veins in a dehydrated child.

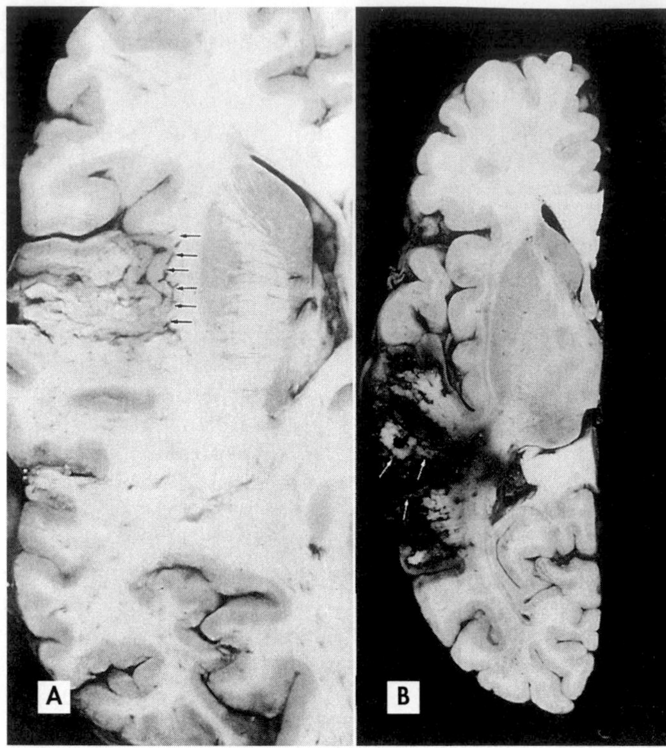

Fig. 77-33 **A,** Pale infarct (about 2 weeks in duration) with "cracks" *(arrows)* demarcating intact from infarcted tissue. **B,** Hemorrhagic infarct also in middle cerebral artery distribution and containing necrotic brain tissue *(arrows).*

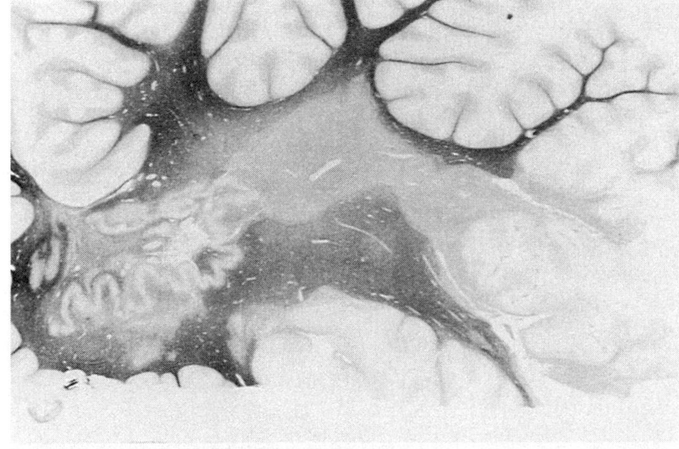

Fig. 77-34 Acute cerebellar infarct. Band of pallor involving gray and white matter.

eosinophilic degeneration, and the neuropil becomes vacuolated, especially around capillaries (Fig. 77-35). Neutrophils, usually in small numbers, and erythrocytes in embolic infarcts permeate the vessel walls during the first 24 to 48 hours; they are soon followed by mononuclear phagocytes. By the fourth day reactive astrocytes, macrophages, and capillary prominence and proliferation begin to appear, and their numbers continue to increase with time. Phagocytes are gradually converted into foamy macrophages (lipophages, gitter cells) by

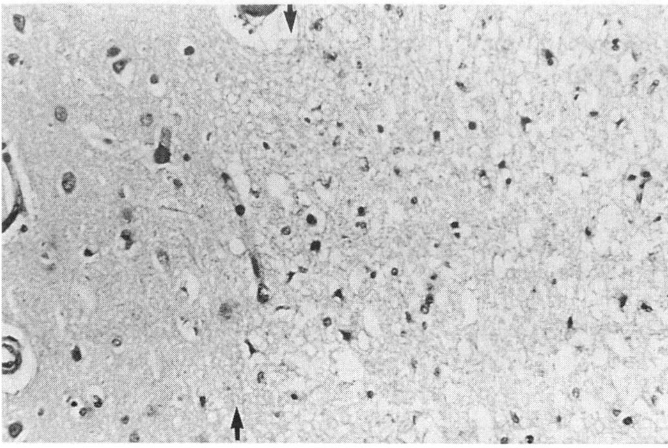

Fig. 77-35 Acute pale infarct. Shrunken neurons with vacuolation of neuropil *(right)* and relatively well-preserved gray matter *(left of arrows).*

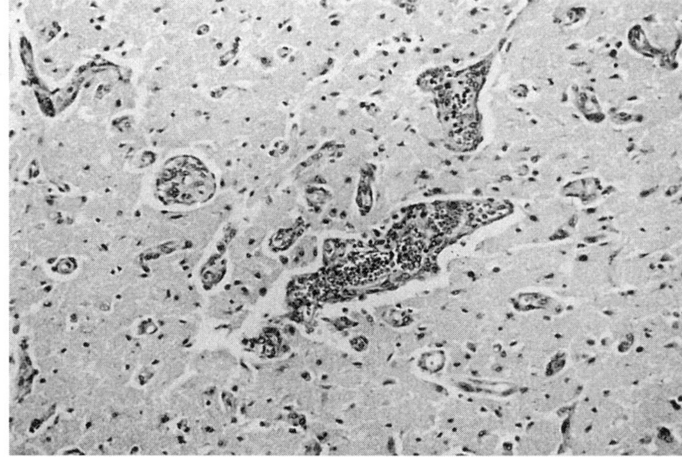

Fig. 77-36 Edge of 2-week-old infarct displaying capillary proliferation.

ingestion and conversion of lipid breakdown products (Fig. 77-28) or hemosiderin-laden macrophages (siderophages). By the tenth day the infarcted area is largely occupied by foamy macrophages with variable numbers of reactive astrocytes and hyperplastic capillaries that are particularly prominent around the margins of the infarct (Fig. 77-36). Tissue lysis and phagocytosis continue to break down the necrotic coagulum, and the infarcted area is gradually converted into cystic spaces filled with serous fluid (Fig. 77-37); the bigger the infarct, the longer the resorption process. Reactive astrocytes are eventually transformed into fibrous astrocytes that line the cyst walls and extend along the adjacent degenerating tracts in parallel bundles, isomorphic gliosis. They also ensheath the fine cobweb-like vascular network that bridges the cysts. A variable number of foamy macrophages may remain in the cavities for extended periods of time, especially in large infarcts.[20,29,30]

Occlusive CVD exhibiting special features

Special occlusive CVD include lacunes, multi-infarct state, granular atrophy of cortex, and subcortical arteriosclerotic leukoencephalopathy.

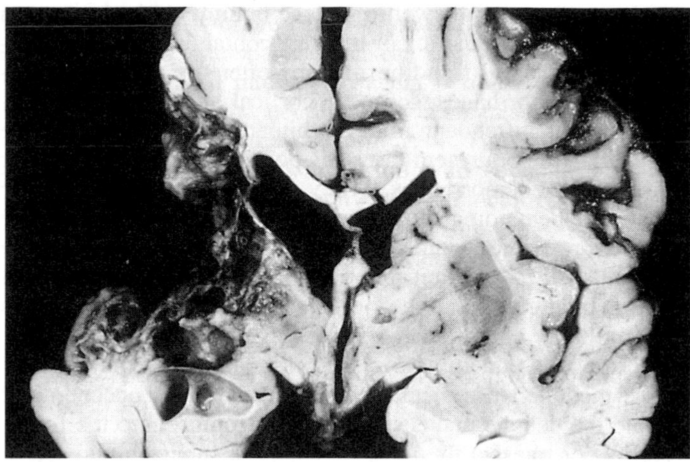

Fig. 77-37 Old cystic infarct in the left middle cerebral artery distribution.

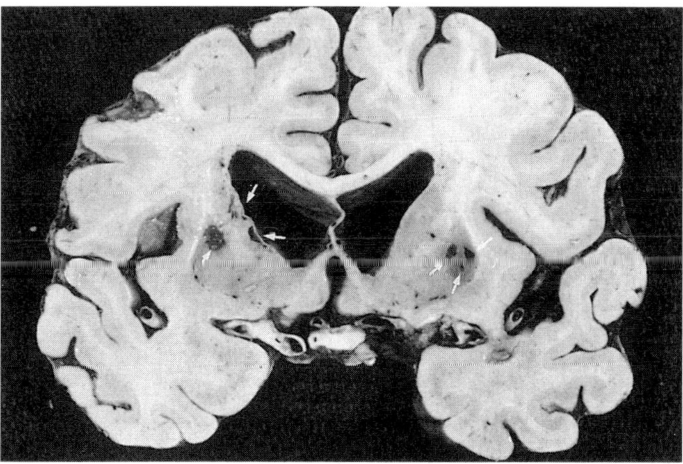

Fig. 77-38 Multiple lacunes *(état lacunaire)* in basal ganglia *(arrows)*.

Lacunes. Lacunes[39-41] are small cavities about 0.5 to 1.5 cm in diameter usually seen in older hypertensive patients and diabetics. They preferentially occur in basal ganglia, internal capsule, basis pontis, and hemispheric white matter. If multiple, which is often the case, the condition is known as *état lacunaire* (Fig. 77-38). Many represent old infarcts as manifested by their gliotic walls and the occasional residual foamy macrophages in their cavities. They are the result of segmental obliteration of perforating arteries by a variety of degenerative vascular lesions, including so-called lipohyalinosis. Others are considered to be resolved old hemorrhagic infarcts or hemorrhages, as indicated by their yellow-tinged walls, and the source of hemorrhage in the latter is assumed to be the hypertensive microaneurysms of Charcot and Bouchard. A few of the lacunes, however, are simply dilatations of the perivascular spaces caused by the tortuosity and spiraling of the perforating arteries—the effects of sustained arterial hypertension. Characteristically the thickened vessels are seen in the center of these cavities and are surrounded by loose connective tissue containing scant hemosiderin granules. Neurologic symptoms or signs are usually associated with the former two types of lacunes.[29]

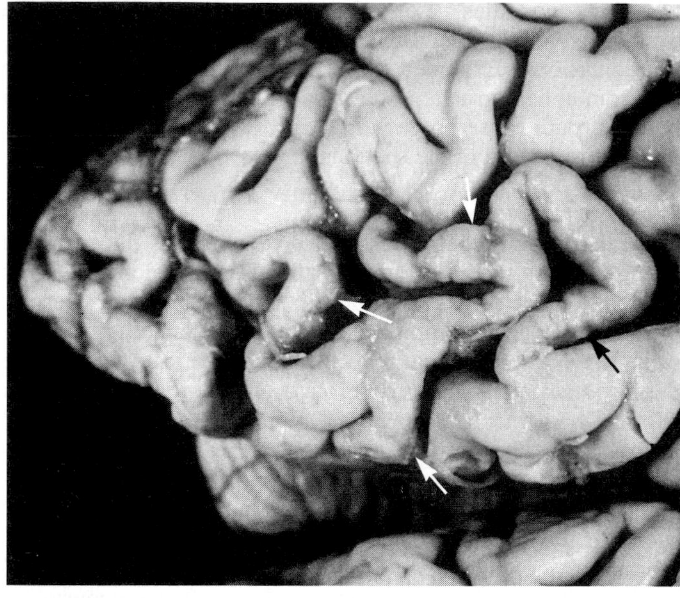

Fig. 77-39 Granular atrophy of the cortex *(arrows)* with border zone distribution.

Multi-infarct state. Infarcts of variable sizes and widely scattered throughout the brain account for most cases of vascular dementia, multi-infarct dementia, and sometimes are associated with normal-pressure hydrocephalus.

Granular atrophy of cortex. Granular atrophy of the cortex superficially resembles the granular cortex of nephrosclerotic kidneys. The surface of the affected gyri is studded with irregular shallow depressions imparting a granular appearance to the cortex. The depressions are the result of gliotic scarring of numerous wedge or stellate intracortical infarcts. Their distribution is roughly bandlike and corresponds to watershed zones (Fig. 77-39). The gyri in the affected regions are thinned, and the overlying cortical vessels are often thickened and stenotic. These microinfarcts may arise from microemboli or circulatory stasis in stenotic vessels of the border zones. The condition is sometimes associated with lacunes, multiple infarcts, or both.

Subcortical arteriosclerotic leukoencephalopathy. Subcortical arteriosclerotic leukoencephalopathy (Binswanger's disease) (Fig. 77-40) is a rare cause of vascular dementia characterized by multicentric or diffuse degeneration of white matter; in neuroimaging studies it is one explanation for abnormal densities and signals—leukoaraiosis (rarefied white matter, Greek 'white' and 'slight').[42,43] Microscopically, myelin destruction and loss are associated with gliosis and scattered foamy macrophages. The intraparenchymal vessels are thickened and hyalinized, and the perivascular spaces are dilated. The arcuate fibers are typically spared. Its pathogenesis is attributed to the combined effects of ischemia and persistent increase in vascular permeability because of sustained arterial hypertension.[29,30,43] An autosomal dominant variant, CADASIL, produces such lesions in the absence of hypertension and in association with a distinctive medial degeneration. It has been mapped to chromosome 19.[44]

Hemorrhagic cerebrovascular disease

Hemorrhagic cerebrovascular diseases are most commonly attributable to hypertensive vascular disease or secondary to

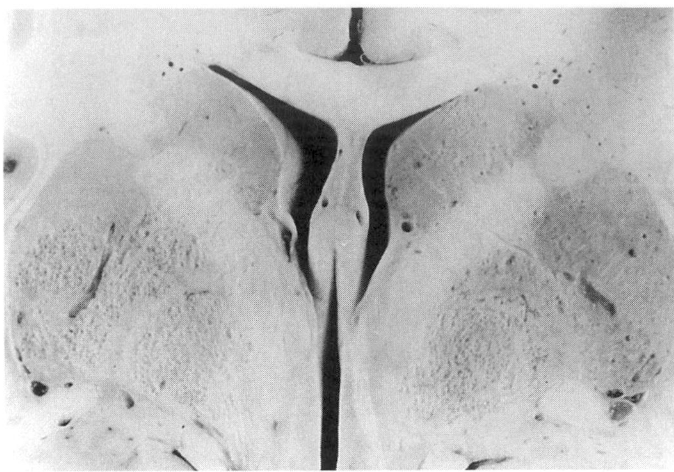

Fig. 77-62 Cryptococcosis with "spongy" basal ganglia caused by perivascular distention by encapsulated cryptococci.

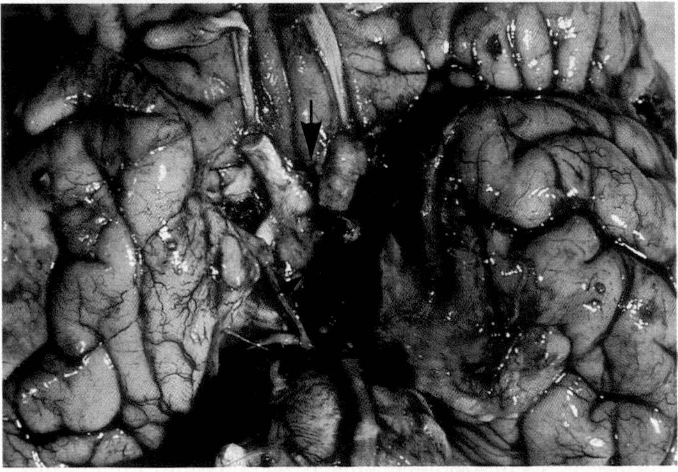

Fig. 77-63 Rhinocerebral mucormycosis. Necrosis of medial temporal lobe simulating a contusion or HSV I but also necrosis of ipsilateral optic nerve *(large arrow)* and occlusion of internal carotid artery *(small arrow)* by fungus.

form. Fungi colonize nasal mucosa, destroy adjacent bones, and extend into the cranium through the blood vessels. Hematogenous spread from pulmonary or cutaneous infections also occurs, especially in leukemic patients, intravenous drug abusers, and individuals with burns. Large areas of necrosis, predominantly basilar, microscopically display a blend of hemorrhagic infarction and acute neutrophilic cerebritis caused by the intravascular growth of fungi (Fig. 77-63). Some patients have recovered after débridement, antimycotic therapy, and, most of all, correction of ketoacidosis in diabetic patients.

Parasitic infections

The influx of immigrants from countries where parasitic diseases are endemic and the expansion of international air travel to many remote places where sanitary conditions are unsatisfactory have resulted in an increase in parasitic infections of the CNS, previously rare in the United States and Western countries. The size of the parasite, to some degree, determines the brain lesions. Small protozoa like *Plasmodium* organisms cause sludging of the microcirculation, and larger ones such as *Toxoplasma* organisms and amebas result in cerebritis or brain abscesses. Larvae of metazoans and ova of trematode parasites tend to lodge in larger vessels, penetrate them, and settle in neural parenchyma. Sometimes larvae grow and present as space-occupying lesions. Migrating parasites may give rise to eosinophilic meningitis. Only the CNS manifestations are covered here. General morphologic features are discussed in Chapters 38 and 39.

Protozoal infections

Amebiasis is either a primary infestation by free-living amebas or secondary from a liver infection with the intestinal parasite *Entamoeba histolytica.* The free-living amebas, *Naegleria fowleri, Acanthamoeba,* and most recently those of the Leptomyxid order, account for the *primary amebic meningoencephalitides* (PAM).[84] In *Naegleria PAM* the infection is acquired by swimming and diving, usually in brackish, warm waters or in swimming pools inadequately sanitized. The amebas penetrate the nasal mucosa and probably reach the CNS via the olfactory nerves through the cribriform plate. Exposure of these healthy children and young adults commonly occurs in the summer and fall. The fulminating and rapidly fatal meningoencephalitis is necrotizing and often hemorrhagic; it is associated with focal areas of softening, usually basilar and including the olfactory bulbs, and brain swelling. The exudate contains neutrophils, lymphocytes, and macrophages, and the adjacent vessels are often necrotic. Amebas are present in large numbers in the exudate and Virchow-Robin spaces and may be mistaken for macrophages or degenerating neurons (Fig. 77-64). Fluorescent antibodies can be used for positive identification of amebas. The 10 to 20 μm trophozoites have distinct nuclear membranes and prominent nucleoli (karyosomes). In *Acanthamoeba PAM* the portal of entry and mode of infection are not fully understood, but the disorder occurs mostly in debilitated or immunocompromised persons.[85,86] The subacute clinical course is characterized by foci of granulomatous meningoencephalitis. Trophozoites with an even more prominent nucleolus and 15 μm cysts are present. Amphotericin B, often combined with other drugs, may be helpful, but the disease is usually fatal. Cerebral *amebic abscess* is rare and elicits a neutrophilic response and poor encapsulation. Cerebral *malaria* caused by severe infection with *Plasmodium falciparum,* usually affects children in endemic areas and unprotected visitors. Pronounced congestion and petechial hemorrhages are associated with capillaries clogged with schizont-bearing erythrocytes in direct contact with the endothelium.[87] In "blackwater fever," malarial pigment produces a slate-gray discoloration of brain. *Babesiosis* causes similar brain lesions. *Toxoplasmosis,* caused by infection with *Toxoplasma gondii,* is acquired by eating poorly cooked infected meat or food contaminated with feline feces. Toxoplasmosis in humans occurs in two forms; congenital or acquired. In *congenital toxoplasmosis,* the organism is transmitted to the fetus through the placenta when maternal infection occurs during pregnancy. The incidence of clinical cases shows geographical variations, such as 1 out of 4000 births in the United States compared with 1 out of 100 in France.[88] Affected children classically display the tetrad of convulsions,

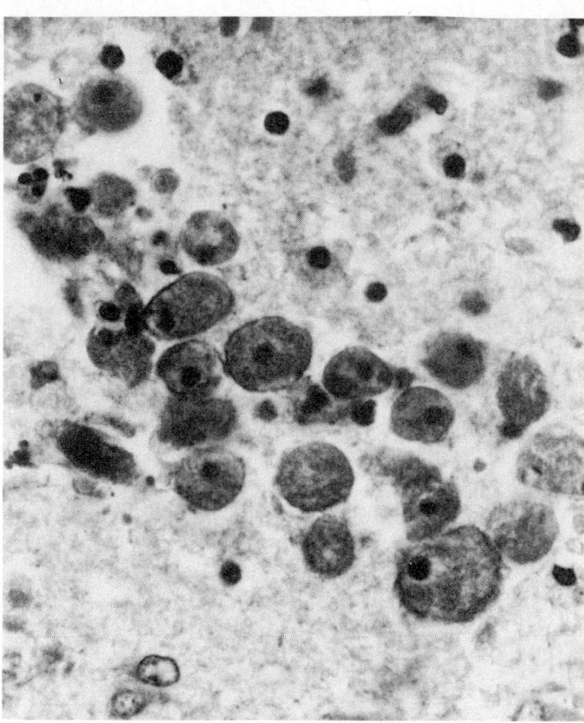

Fig. 77-64 *Naegleria* meningoencephalitis. Large numbers of trophozoites within necrotic brain.

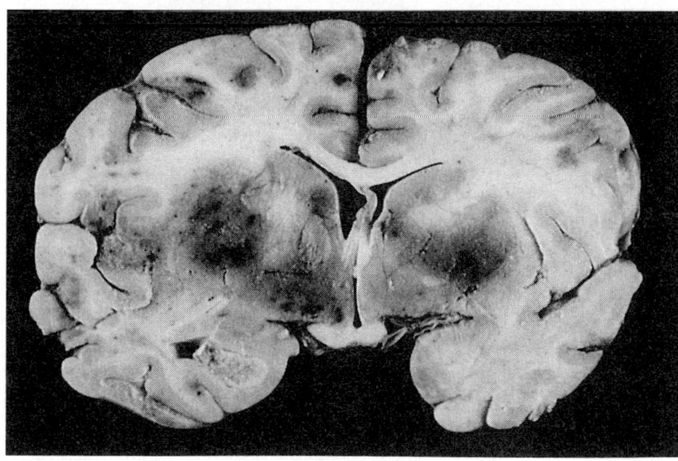

Fig. 77-65 Toxoplasmic encephalitis. Necrotizing lesions prominent in deep gray matter.

chorioretinitis, hydrocephalus, and cerebral calcifications. The brains are often micrencephalic. Diffuse leptomeningitis, ependymitis, focal areas of cerebritis, and calcifications are widely distributed. Subependymal mixed inflammatory exudates and gliosis often cause aqueductal obstruction and hydrocephalus. Both tachyzoites and encapsulated forms are present in the lesions and leptomeninges. *Acquired toxoplasmosis* rarely causes cerebral symptoms in healthy subjects. CNS toxoplasmosis has become the commonest opportunistic infection in CNS in adults with AIDS,[89,90] especially in France and certain regions of the United States such as New York and Florida, accounting for 10% to 30% of these infections.[67] Corticosteroid therapy also can reactivate latent *Toxoplasma*

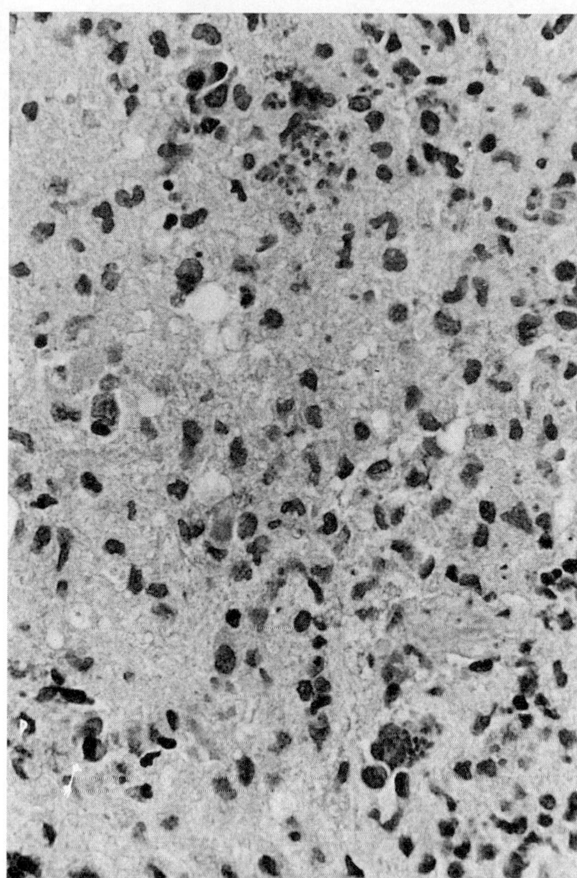

Fig. 77-66 Toxoplasmic encephalitis. Mixed inflammatory exudate, tachyozoites, and a cyst releasing tachyzoites.

organisms in brain. Areas of necrotizing cerebritis evolve into chronic abscesses, which tend to prefer deep gray matter (Fig. 77-65) and corticosubcortical junctions, usually accompanied by severe edema. Irregular patches of necrosis are surrounded by a zone of considerable vascular congestion, intense mixed inflammatory exudate, reactive astrocytes, macrophages, and variable numbers of dormant cysts or pseudocysts and extracellular tachyzoites (Fig. 77-66). Fibrinoid necrosis of hyperplastic vessels with a peculiar sclerosing endovasculitis and fibrin thrombi is common[91] (Fig. 77-67). Cortical abscesses tend to rupture into subarachnoid space, a feature rarely observed with pyogenic abscesses. In treated cases, both tachyzoites and encysted forms may be demonstrable only by immunocytochemical testing. Diffuse encephalitis with microglial nodules containing cysts may be seen.[92] In *African trypanosomiasis, T. gambiense* infection has a protracted course lasting several months, and meningoencephalitis occurs late. Increasing somnolence ("sleeping sickness") is associated with gait disturbances, masklike facies, tremors, restlessness, convulsions, and paralysis. Microscopically, trypanosomes are not seen in neural parenchyma. Lymphoplasmacytic infiltrates, particularly around vessels and displaying Russell bodies, gliosis, and siderophages are widely distributed. In *T. rhodesiense,* the disease has a shorter duration, more severe inflammation, slight neuronal loss, occasional demyelination, and lymphophagocytosis by histiocytes. *South American trypanosomiasis (Chagas's disease),* caused by *T. cruzi,* may

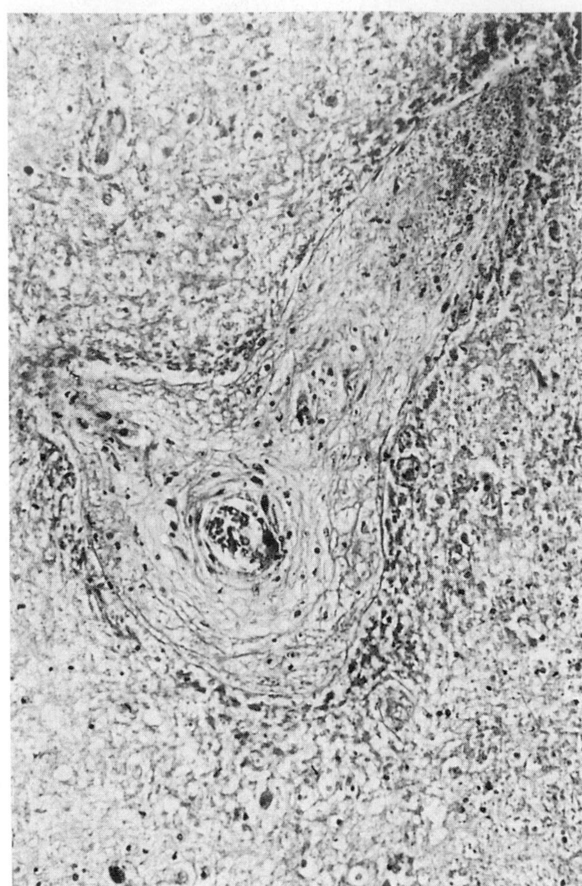

Fig. 77-67 Toxoplasmic encephalitis. Ghosts of enlarged vessels showing fibrinoid necrosis and sclerosing endovasculitis in an area of coagulative necrosis.

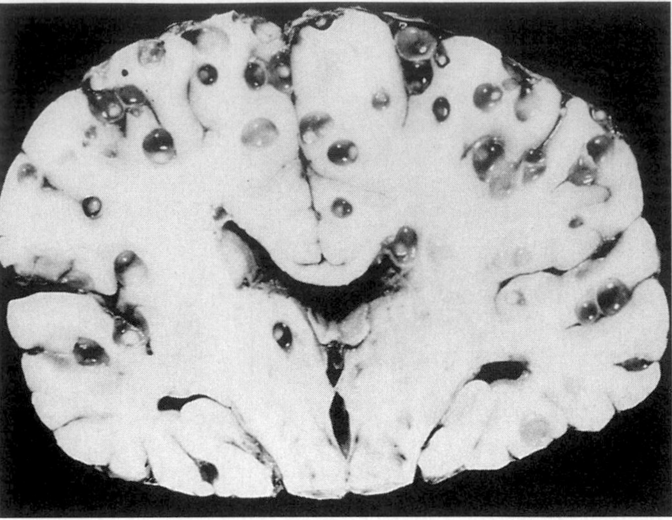

Fig. 77-68 Cysticercosis. Several cysts mostly at gray-white junctions.

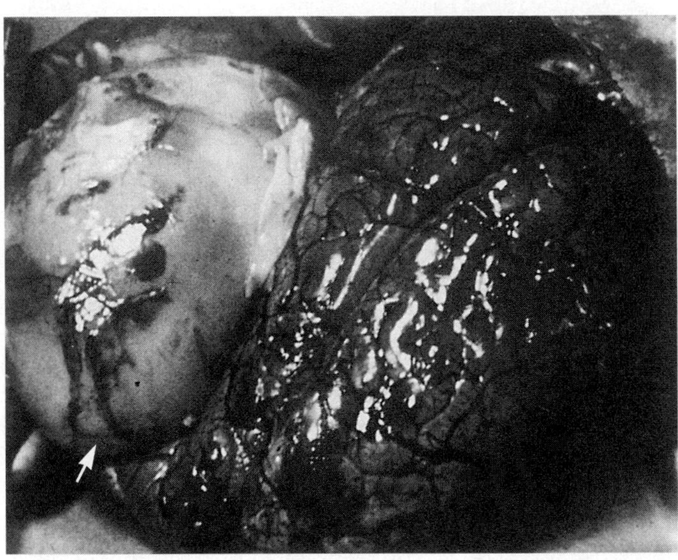

Fig. 77-69 Hydatid cyst *(arrow)* compressing and displacing the brain.

have an acute or chronic course. CNS changes are seen mainly in acutely infected children with acute myocarditis. The brain is edematous, and petechiae are widespread. Glial nodules usually related to small vessels are seen throughout the neuraxis and occasional leishmanial forms are encountered within glial cells. Chronic perivasculitis with some neutrophils are present both in meninges and parenchyma. Inflammatory lesions of the autonomic ganglia also have been described.[93]

Metazoal infections

Cestodes. Cerebral *cysticercosis* is produced by the larvae of the pork tapeworm, *Taenia solium,* cysticercus cellulosae. The larvae settle in brain parenchyma, sometimes in the meninges and ventricles, and develop a cyst wall.[68] Their number varies from a few to several hundred (Fig. 77-68). Many cysts remain small and calcify, but a few may enlarge to form larger, tense cysts containing a mural nodule representing the embryo. The cyst wall has three histologically distinct layers: a corrugated cuticular layer with hairlike protrusions (microtrichia) in contact with host tissue, a thin middle cellular layer, and a thick inner layer containing a loosely packed network of small canaliculi. The larva has a perioral double row of hooklets. Little tissue reaction is seen around the cyst unless the larva dies, in which case the cyst wall becomes permeable producing a severe acute inflammatory reaction sometimes associated with foreign-body giant cells.

If the larvae settle in the subarachnoid space or ventricles, the cysticercus becomes multilocular and spreads over a wide area. These *racemose* cysts often cause hydrocephalus and cranial nerve palsies. Small cerebral and meningeal vessels adjacent to the cysts often display peculiar intimal thickening and sclerosis, cysticercus endarteritis.[94] The most frequent clinical presentations of cerebral cysticercosis are seizures, hydrocephalus, focal neurologic deficits, cranial nerve palsies, and dementia. CNS *echinococcosis (hydatid disease),* caused by the larva of the tapeworm *Echinococcus granulosus,* is seen most frequently in the sheep-raising countries in Australia, New Zealand, South America, and the Mediterranean basin. CNS hydatid cysts are usually solitary and unilocular (Fig. 77-69). The clinical presentations include seizures, focal neurologic deficits, and spinal cord compression, the last being observed mainly in adults. Symptomatic cysts are large, at least 6 cm in diameter, and contain clear fluid in which daughter cysts and scoleces are present. The cyst is thin and consists of three layers: an outer fibrous layer of host origin, a middle cuticular layer, and an inner germinal layer to which are attached brood capsules and scoleces. As in cysticercosis, inflammation in the surrounding host tissue occurs only if the larva dies.[95] a similar but rarer condition in humans is *coenurosis* produced by *Coenurus cerebralis,* the larvae of the dog tapeworm, *Multiceps multiceps. Sparganosis,* caused by the larva (sparganum) of the feline and canine tapeworms, *Spirometra* spp., is acquired by drinking contaminated water or direct invasion with poultices of infected raw frog meat. It is relatively common in Asia. Single or multiple nodular hemorrhagic lesions contain a thin, solid, white larva devoid of a bladder wall and hooked scoleces.[96] It produces a severe mixed inflammatory reaction and occasionally subarachnoid hemorrhage.

Trematodes. Infection with trematodes, such as *paragonimiasis,* is endemic in the Orient, Africa, and Latin America. *Schistosomiasis,* caused by *Schistosoma mansoni* in South America, the Caribbean islands, the Middle East, and Africa, or *S. haematobium* in the Middle East and Africa, has a predilection for spinal cord; whereas that caused by *S. japonicum* in the Far East involves the brain. The ova elicit a granulomatous reaction with radially arranged fibroblasts. Ova of *S. japonicum* and *S. haematobium* have a single polar spine, whereas in *S. mansoni* the spine is laterally placed.

Nematodes. The granulomatous lesion of *trichinosis* is caused by consumption of poorly cooked pork containing encysted larvae of *Trichinella spiralis.* Serious neurologic complications often resolve gradually, especially with anthelmintic medication. *Toxocara canis* or *T. cati* and other ascarids, which cause visceral larva migrans, occasionally induce eosinophilic meningoencephalitis that is rarely fatal.

Viral infections

It has been traditional to classify viral infections, including the meningoencephalitides, according to their nucleic acid composition, family, or epidemiologic characteristics[97] (Table 77-2). From the pathologic perspective one can gain much by dividing them according to their clinical course and tissue reaction: acute, latent, subacute-chronic, or allergic, and by subdividing the acute infections by anatomic distribution: meningitic, encephalitic, myelitic, ganglioradiculitic, meningoencephalitic, or diffuse (meningoencephalomyelitic).[98] General virologic principles are applicable to acute and latent infections of the central nervous system (CNS). Viruses are obligate intracellular organisms possessing either DNA or RNA surrounded by protein (nucleocapsid), which may be enclosed by an envelope of protein-glycoprotein-lipid derived in part from host membranes. Cell targeting or tropism appears to be effected largely by complementary host membrane ligands or receptors.[97]

Most neurotropic viral infections are acute. Herpesviruses (I, II, varicella-zoster, CMV) are latent prototypes that, when activated, produce the expected acute reaction.[99] The "slow viruses" (of JC papova, measles, rubella, and "prions") are distinctly uncommon and characteristically encephalitic with a predilection for gray matter (prions), white matter (JC papova), or both (panencephalitic—measles and rubella). Several typically acute viruses, especially exanthematous (measles before vaccination, varicella, rubella, pox), have been associated with a monophasic neurologic illness beginning about 3 to 5 days after systemic viral symptoms; the brain exhibits foci of perivenous inflammation and demyelination in white matter throughout the neuraxis (acute disseminated leukoencephalitis). This entity usually is referred to as "allergic" because its pathogenesis is believed to be immune mediated rather than the result of direct viral infection of the CNS. It is discussed more fully with the myelin diseases.

Acute viral infections may be limited, especially clinically, to the meninges (meningitis), brain parenchyma (encephalitis), or spinal cord (myelitis), or they may transgress these anatomic boundaries, especially pathologically. Neurotropic viruses generally arrive in the CNS by way of a peripheral portal and a viremic phase, but a few can travel by peripheral nerves (rabies) or olfactory-trigeminal cranial nerves (herpes). To establish a specific causative agent, one traditionally had to resort to correlative serum or CSF antibody titers or tissue culture isolation of virus from parenchymal or CSF samples. Immunostaining of frozen or paraffin tissue sections using antibodies to specific viral proteins and the demonstration of virus-specific segments of either RNA or DNA in tissue sections or CSF by in situ hybridization or PCR–in situ hybridization have provided a more direct confirmation.[100] The same result can be achieved by identification of specific viral proteins or nucleic acids in tissue or CSF samples through appropriate blotting techniques, often enhanced by PCR.[101] All these techniques have their limitations, as did electron microscopy, which was used extensively before the advent of immunostains. The ultrastructural characteristics of some viruses are so distinctive (such as rabies) that when taken in concert with other morphologic or epidemiologic data a specific diagnosis can be established.[97] However, one can recognize only the family (such as Herpesviridae), not the particular genus (such as *Simplexvirus* versus *Varicellavirus*). This limitation, complicated by inevitable sampling problems, has presently diminished the use of electron microscopy in this diagnostic area.

Table 77-2 Major neurotropic viruses

RNA-containing viruses
- Picorna virus (enteroviruses): polio, coxsackievirus, echovirus
- Togavirus (arboviruses): equine (eastern, western, Venezuela, Borna); rubella
- Flavivirus (arboviruses): St. Louis, Japanese B, Russian, spring-summer
- Bunyavirus (arbovirus): California
- Rhabdovirus: rabies
- Paramyxovirus: measles, mumps
- Arenavirus: lymphocytic choriomeningitis
- Retrovirus: HTLV-I and HTLV-III (HIV)

DNA-containing viruses
- Herpes: herpes simplex I and II, varicella-zoster, cytomegalovirus (Epstein-Barr)
- Papova

Acute viral meningitis and encephalitis

Viruses that induce acute (lymphocytic, aseptic) meningitis, as mumps, coxsackievirus B, echovirus, poliovirus, Epstein-Barr, herpes, and lymphocytic choriomeningitis usually produce a self-limiting disease characterized by headaches, stiff neck, and fever. Pathologists' major encounter with meningitis is through the cytologic evaluation of CSF, or incidentally at autopsy where a minimal to modest lymphocytic infiltration of the subarachnoid space may be evident.

An acute viral infection of neural parenchyma (encephalitis, myelitis, encephalomyelitis), or of both coverings and parenchyma (meningoencephalitis), is of more practical importance to pathologists because of their increased morbidity and mortality and the need for biopsy or autopsy evaluations. Alterations in consciousness, seizures, and often focal neurologic deficits may be reflected by the nonspecific gross findings of edema, vascular congestion, and perhaps petechial hemorrhages and microscopically by diffuse but often subtle involvement of the neuraxis. Although a few viruses inflict a distinctive topographic or histopathologic lesion (such as herpes simplex I), most evoke a rather stereotypic response. This usually manifests as lesions with (1) diffuse or multifocal distributions; (2) predominant involvement of neurons (gray matter) in the form of neuronal degeneration (eosinophilia, atrophy) or death with neuronophagia; (3) hyperplasia and hypertrophy of microglia-macrophages, including glial nodules or shrubs (Fig. 77-70), and astrocytes; and (4) perivascular cuffs of mononuclear cells. Initially the inflammatory reaction may be neutrophilic and later plasmacytic, but the major inflammatory cell is the lymphocyte.[98] Unless otherwise specified, this is the standard histopathologic lesion of acute viral encephalitis. It is noteworthy that the tissue reaction often is disproportionately modest in comparison to clinical severity. Occasionally a virus may induce a characteristic inclusion body (such as Cowdry type A intranuclear eosinophilic) or inflict a distinctive necrotic or demyelinitive lesion to warrant an appropriate diagnosis.

Poliomyelitis. In addition to producing aseptic meningitis and nonspecific encephalitis, the enteroviruses (particularly the Brunhilde, or type 2, poliovirus, coxsackieviruses A and B, and echoviruses) have an affinity for infecting large motor neurons of anterior horns (spinal or paralytic form) and of brainstem, including the reticular formation (bulbar form). Neurons in other sites, such as hypothalamus and posterior horns, are commonly infected. Localized neuronal necrosis with neuronophagia is associated with neutrophils (during the first 24 to 48 hours) and macrophages, in addition to lymphocytes. Neuronal loss and astrogliosis (Fig. 77-71) result in a commensurate loss of gray matter, motor nerve roots, and innervated muscle bulk (neurogenic atrophy). As in the arbovirus infections, no distinctive intracellular inclusions are noted, but characteristically small (25 nm) naked virions may be seen in the cytoplasm of infected neurons under the electron microscope.[97] A progressive amyotrophic lateral sclerosis–like illness is seen in some who suffered from acute anterior poliomyelitis many years earlier (postpoliomyelitis syndrome).

Arbovirus (arthropod-borne) encephalitis. The transmitting vector (mosquitos, ticks, and so forth), natural reservoir or host, and geographic or climatic pattern are more distinctive than the nonspecific and diffuse morphologic involvement of neuraxis (Fig. 77-72) produced by several families of RNA viruses (Togaviridae, Flaviviridae, Bunyaviridae, and Reoviridae). The uncommon eastern equine and common Japanese (Japanese B) types are noteworthy for their high mortality in the very young and aged; corresponding widespread necrosis,

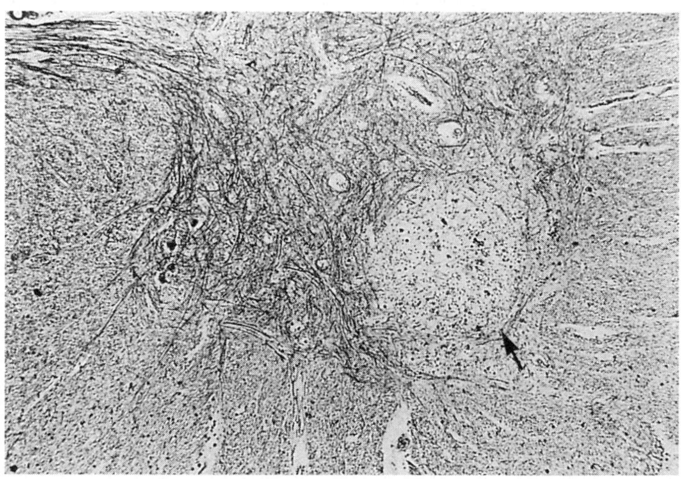

Fig. 77-71 Remote poliomyelitis. Neuronal loss and astrocytosis *(arrow)*.

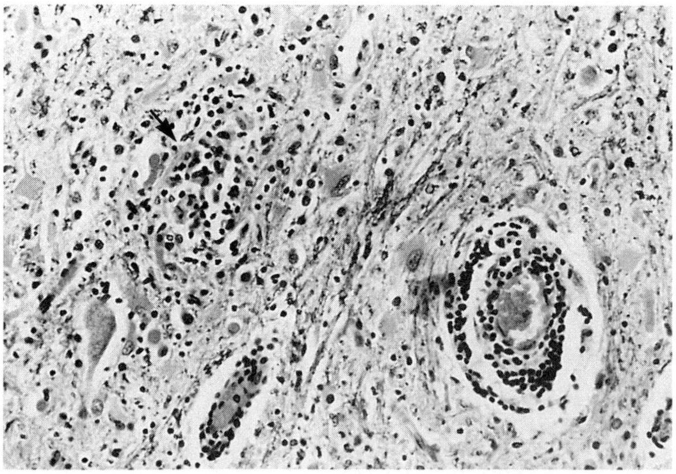

Fig. 77-70 Acute viral encephalitis. Neuronal necrosis and neuronophagia *(arrow)*, astrocytic and microglial proliferation, chronic perivasculitis.

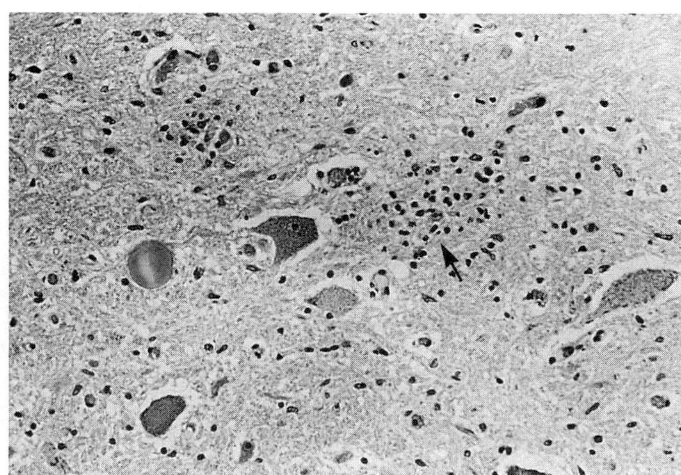

Fig. 77-72 Acute viral encephalitis. Nonspecific glial nodule *(arrow)* and minimal chronic perivasculitis.

appreciated grossly, of cerebral gray and white matter including blood vessels and with a prominent polymorphonuclear cell reaction is seen. St. Louis, probably the commonest type of viral encephalitis in the United States, California (La Crosse), western equine, and Venezuela equine usually have lower morbidity and mortality.

Rabies. Once symptomatic, this universal disease is almost invariably fatal. It is known by various names, and is transmitted to humans almost always by the bite of a rabid mammal (dog, fox, coyote, raccoon, skunk, bat). Retrograde axonal transport of virus through peripheral nerves eventuates in a predominantly lower brainstem or spinal (paralytic form) localization. Distinctive bullet-shaped virions are noted under the electron microscope; eosinophilic (with hematoxylinophilic core) intracytoplasmic inclusions (Negri bodies with core but Lyssa without) in hippocampal pyramidal neurons and Purkinje cells are diagnostically useful.

Measles (rubeola). Before the advent of the vaccine, this was the major cause of allergic (postinfectious) or perivenous encephalomyelitis. Its second major CNS form, subacute sclerosing panencephalitis, also has been strongly influenced by the vaccine and is discussed below. Most recently measles encephalitis or panencephalitis, with minimal inflammation but with intranuclear and intracytoplasmic inclusions, has been reported in some immunosuppressed individuals. One should also recall that measles virus has garnished most of the blame, still unsubstantiated, for multiple sclerosis.

Herpesvirus. The herpes family, including *herpes simplex viruses (HSV) I and II, varicella-zoster virus (VZV), cytomegalovirus (CMV)* and *Epstein-Barr virus (EBV),* is one of the most prominent and destructive in the field of neuropathology. Each shows a strong topographic predilection, except for Epstein-Barr virus. *EBV* rarely infects the CNS, usually in severe cases of infectious mononucleosis, but has become notorious for its role in CNS non-Hodgkin's lymphoma, particularly in HIV-infected patients. HSV II is best known for aseptic meningitis in adults but can wreak havoc in the newborn brain, usually seen with active genital herpes at the time of vaginal delivery. The necrosis of brain may be so severe as to eventuate in a multicystic encephalopathy if the infant survives for some time. *CMV* may cause multifocal but usually less extensive areas of brain necrosis, especially ependymal and subependymal, because of intrauterine infection. This can result in spontaneous abortion, stillbirth, prematurity, micrencephaly, polymicrogyria, hydrocephalus, and intracranial calcifications. Characteristic hematoxylinophilic to amphophilic owl's-eye intranuclear (also Cowdry type A) and less apparent amphophilic intracytoplasmic inclusions distinguish congenital CMV from others, such as rubella with its characteristic vascular calcifications. CMV encephalitis also is seen in immunocompromised adults, usually as nonspecific and widespread glial nodules with only a rare diagnostic inclusion-bearing cell; immunostaining or serial sections of several lesions may be necessary to identify the agent. Prominent ependymitis with numerous inclusions, transverse myelitis, or radiculitis with vasculitis also are seen in this setting (Fig. 77-73). Finally, CMV has been implicated but not confirmed in Rasmussen's encephalitis, a rare form of chronic encephalitis with intractable seizures.[102]

VZV typically restricts itself to a latent stage in cranial sensory (such as trigeminal) or dorsal root ganglia until it is "activated" as "shingles" with its painful and vesicular lesions in a radicular or cranial nerve distribution. Necrotizing, often hemorrhagic, inflammation in these ganglia are associated with many intranuclear eosinophilic inclusions. A milder reaction can spread to the segmental nerve, local spinal meninges, and even cord. VZV also can produce meningoencephalitis, transverse myelitis, Landry-Guillain-Barré syndrome, and some cases of granulomatous angiitis (isolated angiitis of the CNS). A vasculitic lesion of ipsilateral cranial arteries in herpes zoster ophthalmicus may produce contralateral hemiplegia. Rarely it may present like congenital CMV, or as a demyelinative disease with oligodendroglial inclusions in the immunocompromised simulating PML.

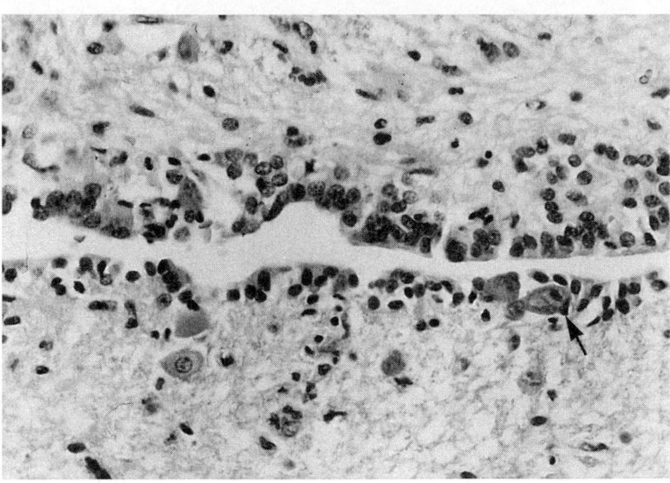

Fig. 77-73 Cytomegaloviral ependymitis with owl's eye inclusion *(arrow).*

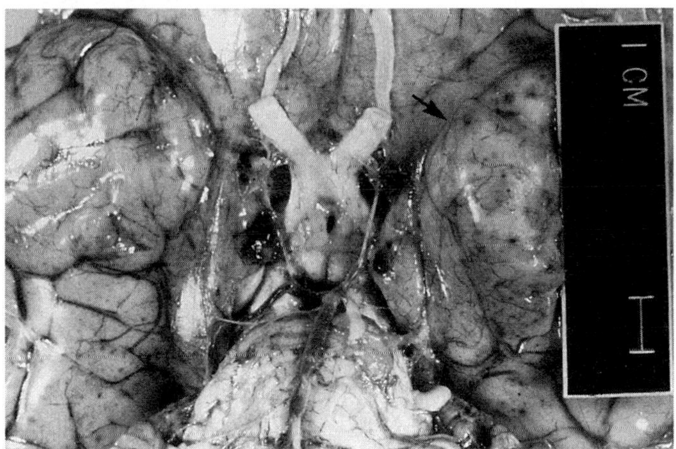

Fig. 77-74 Herpes simplex virus (HSV) I encephalitis. Petechial hemorrhages and necrosis of medial temporal lobe *(arrows).*

HSV I, usually latent in trigeminal ganglia, is the most infamous member of the family because it is the commonest cause of severe, sporadic encephalitis. It characteristically produces a necrotizing, often hemorrhagic, meningoencephalitis with a predilection for the limbic areas of brain (orbitofrontal, insula, cingulate gyrus, amygdala, hippocampus), particularly the mesial temporal lobes (Fig. 77-74). Although neurons are its primary target, all cell types can be infected and destroyed, resulting in large areas of gross tissue necrosis (Fig. 77-75).

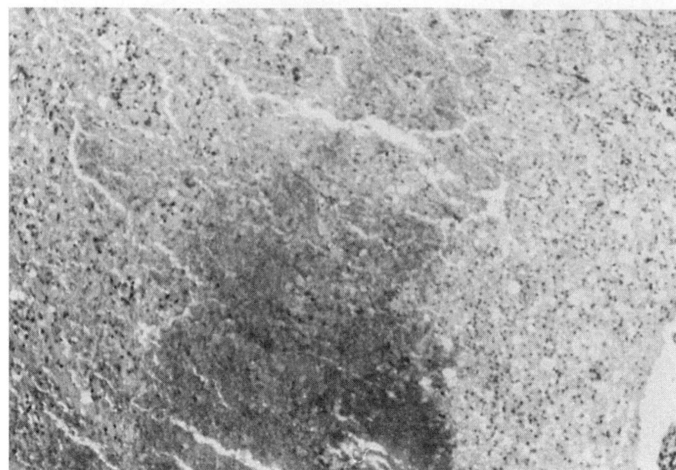

Fig. 77-75 HSV I encephalitis. Widespread cortical necrosis with acute hemorrhage.

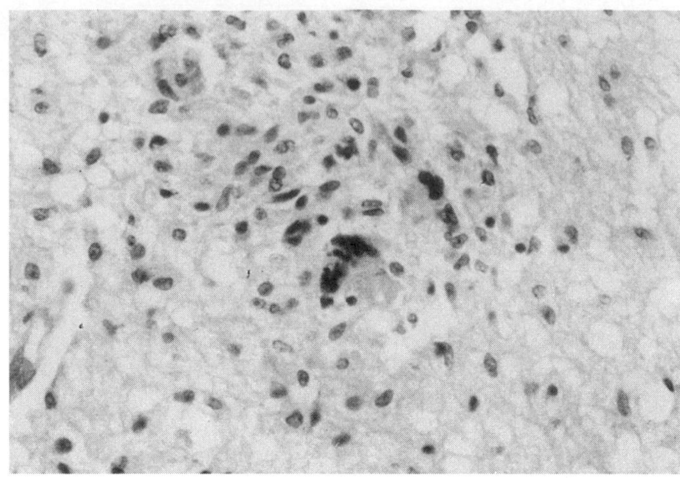

Fig. 77-77 Human immunodeficiency virus (HIV) subacute encephalitis. Perivascular multinucleated giant cells and microglia.

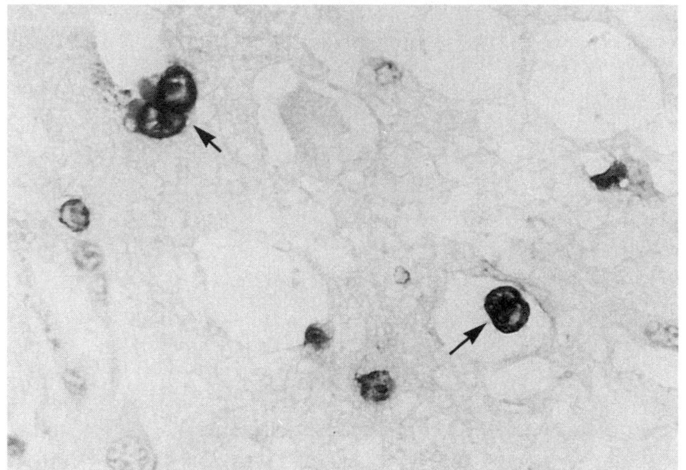

Fig. 77-76 HSV I encephalitis. Immunoreactive intranuclear viral protein *(arrows)*.

Intranuclear eosinophilic inclusions are seldom seen after the first week or so, and electron microscopic identification of targetlike virions usually is more rewarding, but immunostaining for HSV proteins (Fig. 77-76) or in situ hybridization are most effective. HSV I, may produce an ascending myelitis and recurrent (Mollaret) meningitis. Brain biopsy for diagnosis is still debatable. A combination of magnetic resonance imaging, displaying the characteristic location and nature of herpetic lesions, and the identification of specific viral proteins or genome in CSF, with appropriate blotting and PCR techniques, seems likely to replace the diagnostic brain biopsy required by some for treatment with acyclovir.

Retroviral infections

The main CNS offender in this family is HTLV-III or HIV-1 (human T-cell lymphotrophic virus, human immunodeficiency virus), a member of the lentivirus subfamily. Numerous and often multiple opportunistic agents, particularly *Toxoplasma,* CMV, and *Cryptococcus,* infect the brains of adults with HIV. Primary CNS lymphoma is seen in about 5% of the same population. Both toxoplasmosis and lymphoma can present as mass lesions, especially in deep white and gray matter; this differential may be resolved only with a surgical biopsy and pathologic examination. Embolic strokes caused by nonbacterial thrombotic endocarditis, subarachnoid and intraparenchymal hemorrhages caused by thrombocytopenia, and angiitis caused by herpes zoster or fungi (especially *Aspergillus*) also may be seen.[67,90]

On the other hand, HIV often affects the brain more directly, primarily by infecting macrophages (monocytes and microglia) but also endothelium, astrocytes, and probably neurons; the last two may be a nonproductive infection. The Trojan horse analogy, in which HIV is carried in monocytes that invade the CNS, is commonly invoked as a unique portal of entry; this entry is gained early in the disease, perhaps during an asymptomatic meningitic phase. The consequences of this invasion include HIV encephalitis, HIV-associated leukoencephalopathy, and vacuolar myelopathy; much less frequently multifocal vacuolar leukoencephalopathy of the brain, neocortical neuronal loss and astrocytosis (diffuse poliodystrophy), synaptic loss and dendritic abnormalities in cerebral neocortex, central spinal myelinolysis, and gracile tract degeneration have been reported. The major neurologic manifestation of HIV infection of brain, which occurs late in the disease, is that of the AIDS-dementia complex (ADC, also referred to as "HIV-1–associated cognitive-motor disorder"). This complex includes impairments of cognition, behavior, and motor function with a variable degree of progression to dementia, psychosis, and quadriplegia. The pathologic substrate of ADC appears to be HIV encephalitis and HIV-associated leukoencephalopathy. Although "HIV encephalitis" is the recommended term for the former condition, the lesion is panencephalitic (involving both gray and white matter) and involves all levels of the neuraxis. Therefore, the term encephalomyelitis is more appropriate. Unlike most viral encephalitides, HIV does not seem to blatantly infect neurons, and chronic perivasculitis usually is inconspicuous. Characteristic multinucleated giant cells of macrophage origin (Fig. 77-77) are seen in the deep white matter of frontal and temporal lobes and deep gray matter, particularly in perivascular locations. These cells may be associated with glial nodules or scattered macrophages. The multinucleated giant cell encephalomyelitis is so typical as to be virtually diagnostic of HIV (except for immunodeficient measles encephalitis), even in the absence of supporting immunologic or ultrastructural data. It is also common to observe nonspecific glial nodules, which most frequently contain HIV epitopes and less commonly CMV. HIV-associated leukoencephalopathy manifests as diffuse white matter pallor and astrocytosis with or without focal necrosis and multinucleated cell-macrophage clusters. The pathogenesis of ADC is unknown. Some believe that one of the external glycoproteins of HIV, gp120, may inhibit neuronal function because of its homology to a neuronal growth factor, neuroleukin. Others suspect an undetected and nonproductive neuronal infection or release of toxic cytokines by infected macrophages or astrocytes. The cause of HIV-associated leukoencephalopathy is even more uncertain, but some propose a breakdown of the blood-brain barrier with chronic vasogenic edema and demyelination. In addition to HIV encephalo-myelitis of the spinal cord (often asymptomatic) and transverse myelitis caused by CMV, HSV, or VZV, a vacuolar myelopathy is seen in about 17% to 30% of AIDS patients. This noninflammatory vacuolation of myelinated fibers (spongy myelin, intramyelinic edema) has a propensity to involve the posterior and posterolateral columns of thoracic cord and is highly reminiscent of subacute combined degeneration of vitamin B_{12} or folic acid deficiency. Lipophages are detected within some vacuoles, but macrophage and astrocyte responses are mild. Vacuolar myelopathy does not appear to be related to HIV infection of spinal cord, since an association with multinucleated giant cells or HIV epitopes in spinal cord rarely has been found. Nor does it appear to be attributable to HIV infection per se, since it has been described in HIV-negative, severely immunocompromised patients.[67,89]

Children with HIV encephalopathy may exhibit micrencephaly, extensive vascular mineralization of basal ganglia and deep white matter, and a severe leukoencephalopathy. Opportunistic infections and vacuolar myelopathy are uncommon. Treatment with zidovudine (AZT) may decrease HIV encephalitis in adults and particularly children. Another retrovirus, HTLV-1, is responsible for a chronic inflammatory myelopathy referred to as tropical spastic paraparesis (TSP) in the Caribbean or HTLV-1-associated myelopathy (HAM) in Japan.[101,104]

Slow viral infections

In addition to the subacute to chronic encephalitis of Rasmussen alluded to earlier, and those attributable to retroviral infections, a small group of uniquely encephalopathic to encephalitic diseases has a prolonged clinical course. These were originally designated as "slow viruses" because of their atypically prolonged clinical courses; they were divided into unconventional and conventional types. The previously classified unconventional types are covered in detail under Chapter 36. Here we need only mention that the brain lesions of kuru, Creutzfeldt-Jakob disease, and Gerstmann-Sträussler disease consist of a noninflammatory spongy alteration of gray matter, non-Alzheimer amyloid plaques, neuronal loss, and reactive astrocytosis.

There are three conventional types of slow viral infection: *subacute sclerosing panencephalitis (SSPE), progressive multifocal leukoencephalopathy (PML),* and *progressive rubella encephalitis. SSPE* has been shown morphologically and by other techniques to be attributable to measles, which lacks a membrane (M) protein, resulting in incomplete assembly of the virus and persistence of virus in infected cells. This disease of children or young adults develops several to many years after an infantile exposure to measles and then runs a course of behavioral problems, myoclonus, seizures, motor impairment, and coma over months to years. This illness, as PML, is almost invariably fatal; but stabilization and even remissions have been reported. Gross atrophy and firmness of gray matter reflect significant neuronal loss and astrocytosis with variable degrees of perivascular inflammation and numbers of intranuclear neuronal inclusions. Destruction of white matter, also apparent grossly, is attributable to severe perivascular and interstitial inflammation with lymphocytes and plasma cells, microgliosis and reactive astrocytosis, oligodendroglial inclusions (Fig. 77-25), demyelination, and axonal loss (Fig. 77-78). Intranuclear inclusions in neurons and oligodendrocytes consist of masses of smooth tubular (18 to 20 nm in diameter) nucleocapsids identical to paramyxoviruses (Fig. 77-79), such as measles. The relative degree of cerebral gray and white matter involvement may vary widely. The basal ganglia, thalamus, and even brainstem may be involved.

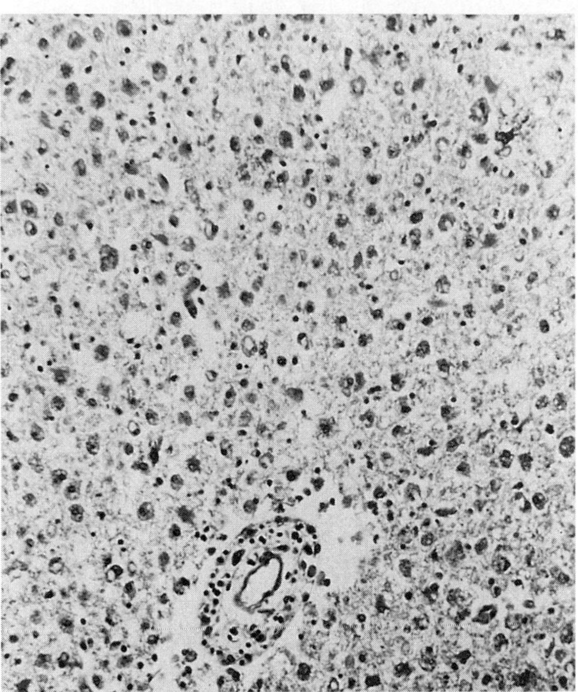

Fig. 77-78 Subacute sclerosing panencephalitis (SSPE). Chronic inflammation and demyelination of white matter.

Progressive multifocal leukoencephalopathy (PML), though similar to SSPE in the duration and outcome of its clinical course, is seen almost always in immunocompromised patients, including those with HIV. All cases of PML are now believed to be caused by the JC (the initials of the first patient from whom virus was isolated and not to be confused with "CJ," or Creutzfeldt-Jakob disease) strain of papova virus group B. The pathogenesis of PML involves a latent state (purportedly renal), direct infection and lysis of oligodendrocytes, expression of T-antigen, and demyelination. Focal neurologic findings of hemiparesis to hemiplegia, visual deficits, and aphasia usually are the presenting features. Grossly evident areas of asymmetric and multifocal white matter destruction, especially subcortical and deep cortical of the parieto-occipital

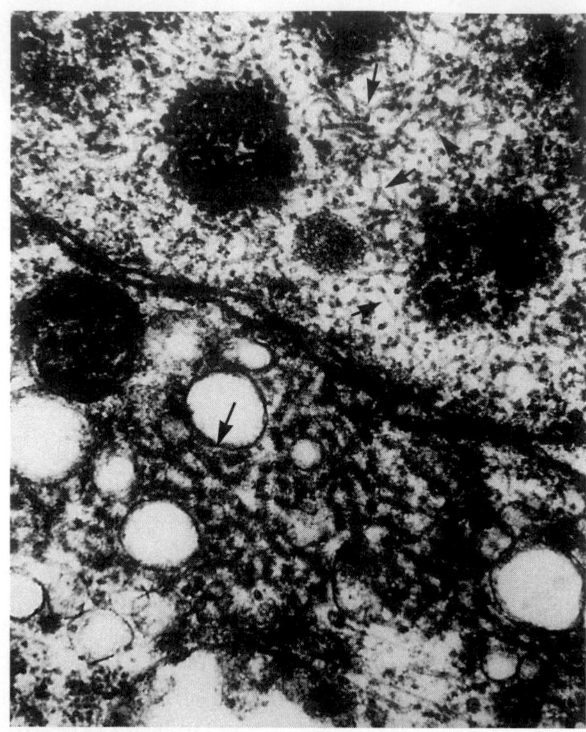

Fig. 77-79 SSPE. Fine structure of naked intranuclear *(small arrows)* and coated intracytoplasmic *(arrow)* nucleocapsids.

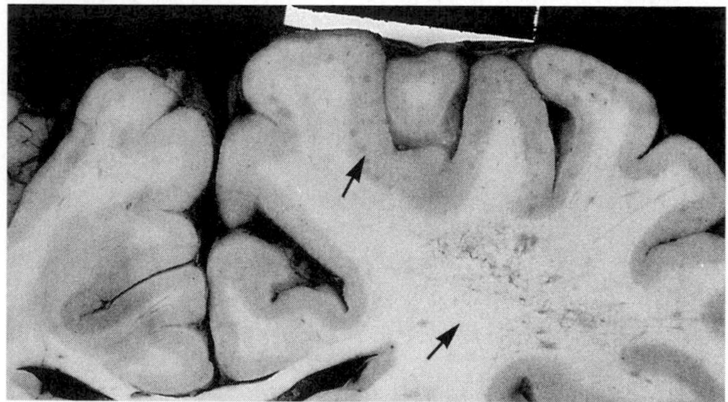

Fig. 77-80 Progressive multifocal leukoencephalopathy (PML). Granular, soft lesions in white matter and in deep cortex *(arrows)*.

areas (Fig. 77-80), may reflect a microscopic lesion so distinctive as to be almost diagnostic with routine hematoxylin and eosin staining. Lipophages, bizarre hypertrophic (Alzheimer type I) astrocytes, demyelinated axons, and enlarged oligodendrocytic nuclei with amphophilic inclusions are seen (Fig. 77-81). The latter cells are most diagnostic and may be restricted to the lesion's periphery; the inclusions are often poorly defined. Confirmatory immunohistochemical or molecular identification of papova virus probably will supersede the ultrastructural search for paracrystalline arrays of electron-dense, naked virions around 50 nm in diameter. Inflammatory reaction usually is minimal but infrequently is abundant and lymphoplasmacytic.

Progressive rubella encephalitis is rare and simulates SSPE, except for the absence of viral inclusions and the presence of

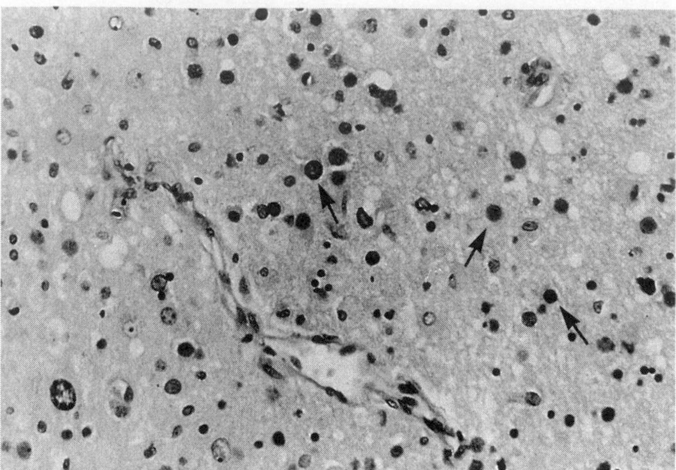

Fig. 77-81 PML. Lipophages, atypical astrocytes, and oligodendroglial inclusions *(arrows)* in demyelinated area.

vascular calcifications (like rubella embryopathy) and fibrinoid necrosis.

TRAUMA

In the United States and other industrialized nations, accidents are the leading cause of deaths under 45 years of age and the fourth most common cause of deaths for individuals of all ages. In the United States, the incidence of patients hospitalized for craniocerebral injuries is about 200 per 100,000 population with a mortality estimated at 31.4 per 100,000 from all accidents, with vehicular injuries accounting for 16.3 per 100,000. Sixty-five percent of brain injuries caused by traffic accidents occur in occupants of cars and 12% involve pedestrians. Males between 15 and 35 years and driving under the influence of alcohol or drugs are high-risk factors. Other causes of craniocerebral injuries include accidental falls, particularly frequent in young children and the elderly; sports, especially boxing; recreational activities such as bicycle riding; and assaults, particularly in socioeconomically depressed areas.[105] In vehicular accidents the brain sustains injuries at the time of impact and after ejection. Therefore, different mechanical forces are involved and include acceleration-deceleration movements, linear or rotational impacts, fractures of skull, and others, making it difficult to single out a specific mechanism as being the most damaging.

Craniofacial injuries

For practical purposes craniofacial injuries have been classified into *closed* and *open.* Closed injuries are further divided into *focal* and *diffuse.* In open injuries, the skull is fractured, and communication is established between the external environment and the intracranial cavity, as in compound fractures or penetrating wounds of the skull.

Closed injuries

Focal injuries. Focal injuries include fractures of the skull, brain contusions and lacerations, and intracranial hemorrhages.

Skull fractures. Fractures of the skull display specific patterns depending on the type, severity, and direction of the mechanical force applied to the skull as well as the site and surface area subjected to that force. Several forms are recognized, and only the following are considered: linear (fissure), compound, depressed, comminuted, hinge, diastatic, and ring fractures.[106] Skull fractures are present in about 80% of fatal head injuries; however, death from severe brain injuries can occur in their absence. Therefore, fractures attest to a violent impact to the head and constitute a warning for possible major intracranial injury. *Linear* fractures result when the head strikes a large immobile surface, such as a fall on a hard floor. The bony ridges that buttress the base of the skull deflect the fracture lines, causing them to pursue certain predictable directions. Those involving the cranial vault may cause tears of meningeal vessels or extend into the base of the skull, causing lacerations of cranial nerves. When the overlying scalp is lacerated and the dura is torn, they are converted to *compound fractures*. Fractures of the anterior fossa may involve the ethmoid sinus, and those of the middle fossa may communicate with the external ear, causing CSF leakage, rhinorrhea, and otorrhea, respectively. These carry the risk of ascending intracranial infections. *Depressed fractures* result from low-velocity impact to a limited surface area and, if the bone is shattered, are referred to as *comminuted,* as after a blow with a hammer. In these cases, the bone fragments become detached from the rest of the skull and may be driven into the brain. Sometimes this may cause massive brain destruction that may heal with an extensive fibrous scar, predisposing to posttraumatic seizures. *Ring fractures* are a form of depressed fracture around the foramen magnum caused by impaction of the cervical spine as in violent falls on the buttocks. *Diastatic* fractures manifest as separation of skull bones at their sutures and are occasionally seen in children. In adults they are associated with *hinge* fractures in which separation takes place at the dorsum sellae and petrosquamous fissures bilaterally, causing the base of the skull to move like a hinge. Hinge fractures occur when the head is run over by heavy vehicles.

Brain contusions and lacerations. *Contusions* are bruises in which extravasation of blood occurs while tissue integrity is retained, whereas in lacerations there is also detachment or loss of tissue. The anatomic features of contusions and lacerations largely depends on whether the head is stationary or in motion at the time of head injury. A direct blow to a resting but mobile head causes deformation and inbending of the skull bone and produces maximal contusions at the site of cranial impact—*coup contusions* (Fig. 77-82). If the head is in motion (acceleration), as in a fall, and comes to an abrupt standstill (deceleration), the lagging brain is flung back and forth against the temporarily deformed skull, resulting in major contusions on the surface of the brain diametrically opposite to the site of cranial impact—*contrecoup contusions* (Fig. 77-83). Contrecoup contusions to the inferior frontal and anterior temporal lobes, however, occur more frequently during severe angular acceleration-deceleration movement of the head, and cranial impact is not necessary. The angular motion causes the brain to swirl in the cranial cavity, and during this process the orbital surfaces of the frontal lobes and the temporal poles are rubbed against the irregular bony projections of the base of the skull, resulting in contusions and lacerations at these sites (Fig. 77-84). *Herniation* contusions occur when the brain is jolted by a severe blow causing the hippocampi, cerebellar tonsils, or both, to be impacted and bruised by the free edge of the tentorium and the foramen magnum, respectively. *Gliding,*

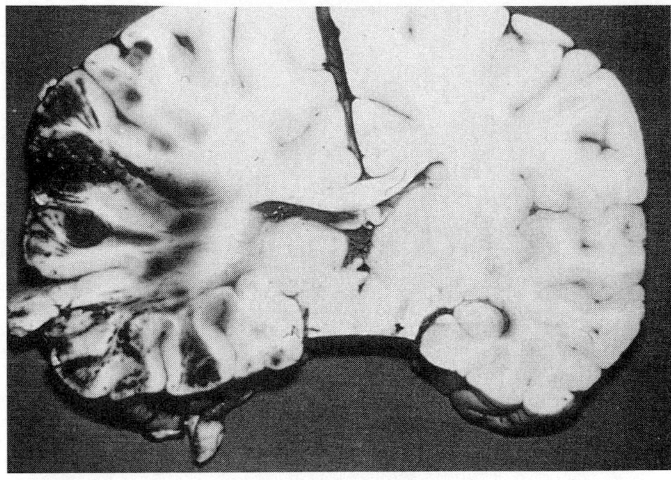

Fig. 77-82 Coup contusion with hemorrhages perpendicular to surface caused by direct blow with a blunt object.

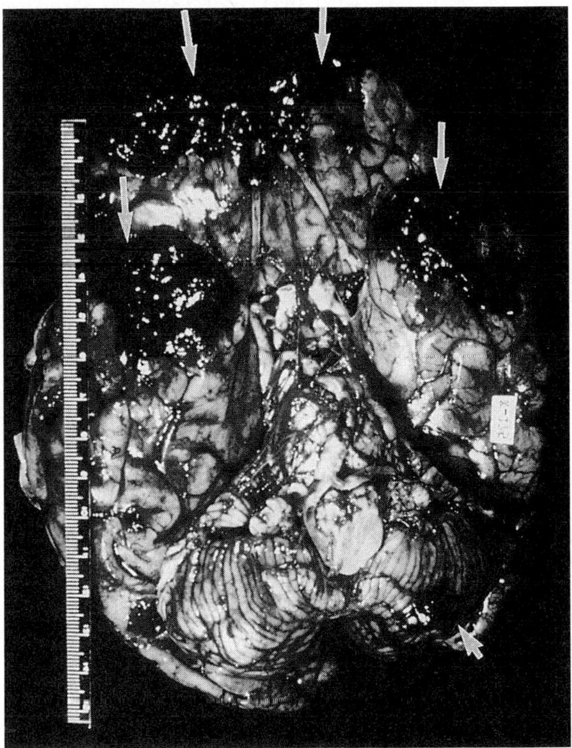

Fig. 77-83 Contrecoup contusions of frontal and temporal poles *(arrows)*; a small coup lesion over cerebellum *(small arrow)*.

or *parasagittal, contusions* represent bilateral, often symmetrical, hemorrhagic disruption involving mostly white matter. They occur along the superior margins of the cerebral hemispheres and are caused by shearing forces brought about by the interference of the dura with rotational movement of the brain. *Intermediary* contusions are hemorrhagic lesions with a tendency to involve midline structures such as the walls of the third ventricle, corpus callosum, and basal ganglia. Both gliding and intermediary contusions are different from the conventional surface contusions in that they are related to diffuse brain damage.[107]

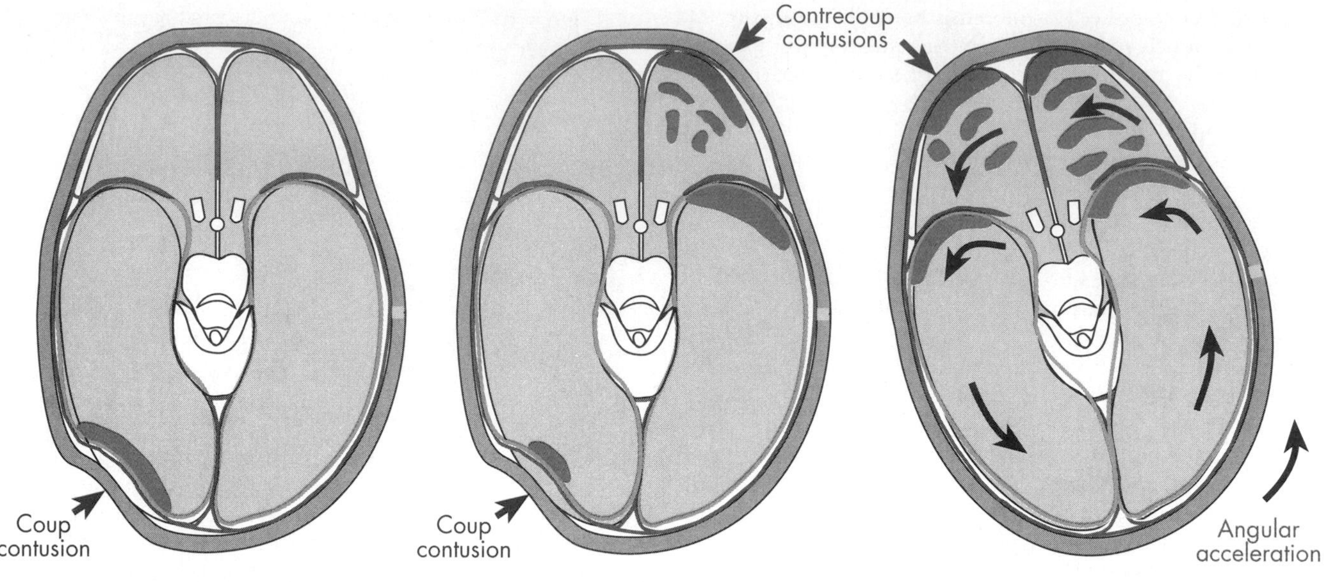

Fig. 77-84 Diagrams comparing impact and nonimpact injuries. **A,** Coup contusions *(c)* at impact site. **B,** Contrecoup *(cc)* contusions diametrically opposite impact site. **C,** Nonimpact contrecoup contusions caused by sudden angular acceleration *(aa)* of the head.

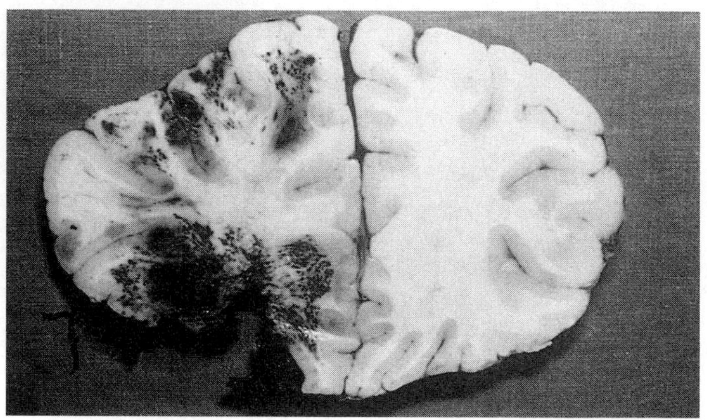

Fig. 77-85 Cerebral laceration. Hemorrhages and tissue loss.

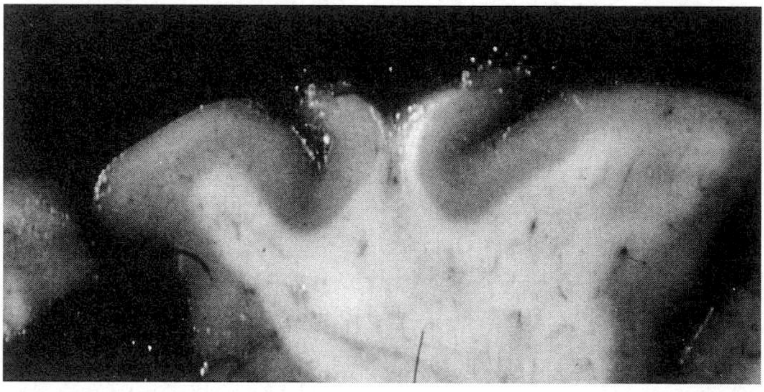

Fig. 77-86 Healed contusion. Saucer-shaped loss of surface tissue involving cortical crest and subjacent white matter.

Lacerations occur in the same locations as contusions, at sites of depressed fractures, and with penetrating or perforating head injuries (Fig. 77-85). Lacerations at the pontomedullary junction and tears of cerebral peduncles have been described in severe hyperextension of the neck accompanied by basal fractures of the posterior fossa.

Cortical contusions and lacerations are conical or wedge shaped and involve the crests of the gyri, causing greater destruction of the superficial cortex and overlying leptomeninges (Fig. 77-86). Splinter-shaped hemorrhages are arranged perpendicularly to the surface of the brain, and ball-and-ring hemorrhages are present around blood vessels (Fig. 77-87). Resorption of blood and necrotic material results in saucer-shaped depressions with variable deposition of hemosiderin over the surface of the affected gyri. *Plaques jaunes* (Fig. 77-88) refer to old contusions or lacerations; they are most frequent on the orbital surfaces of the frontal lobes and olfactory bulbs and are usually seen in repeated head injuries, as in those sustained by alcoholics.

Intracranial hemorrhages. Bleeding from craniocerebral trauma may take place in one or more of the potential spaces surrounding the brain; namely, epidural (extradural), subdural, and subarachnoid spaces as well as in brain parenchyma. They are often associated with high mortality.

In *epidural hemorrhage* bleeding occurs between the skull and the dura. As blood accumulates in the space, it gradually strips the dura off the skull and develops into a pancake-like hematoma that frequently occupies the temporoparietal region (Fig. 77-89). It usually is associated with linear fracture of the thin squamous portion of the temporal bone containing the anterior division of the middle meningeal artery. In children, tears of the artery may occur in the absence of fractures. In 95% of cases epidural hematomas are unilateral; most are associated with a posttraumatic lucid interval. It is

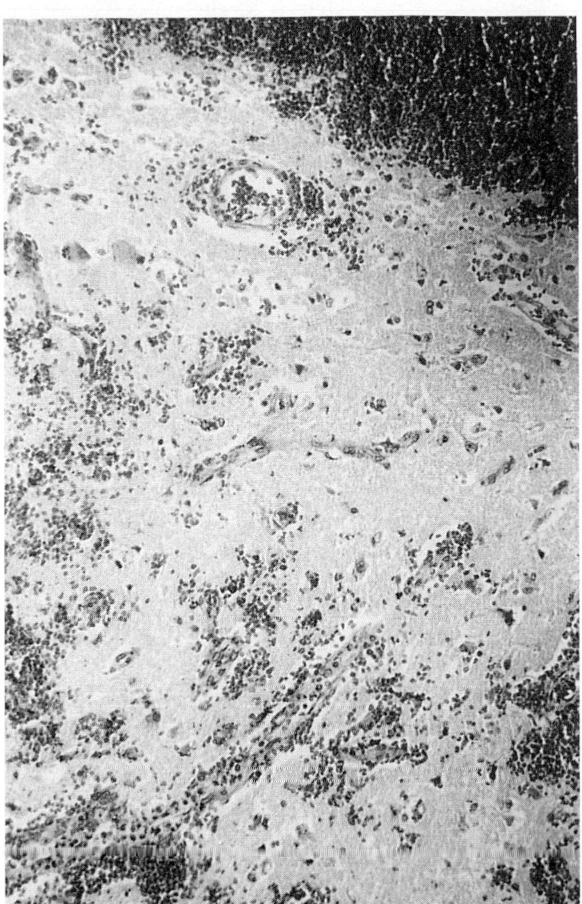

Fig. 77-87 Early contusion with ball-and-ring hemorrhages around blood vessels.

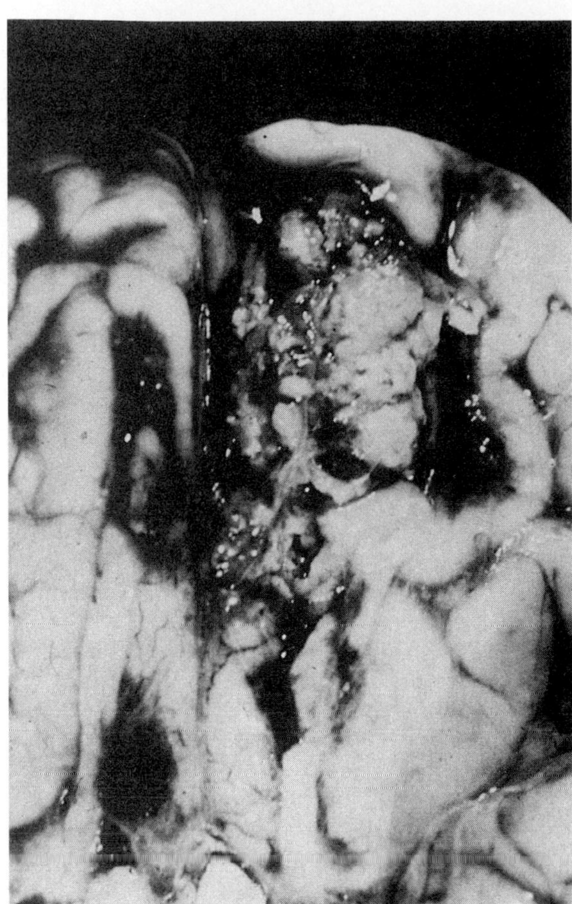

Fig. 77-88 *Plaque jaune.* Old contusion of orbital surface of left frontal lobe with destruction of olfactory bulb and nerve.

seen in about 2% of head injuries and 15% in fatal cases. Being arterial in origin, the hematomas develop and expand rapidly, and their risk of causing early brain displacement and herniation makes them a neurosurgical emergency. It has been estimated that 50 to 75 ml of blood is lethal. CT studies have shown that most epidural hematomas develop within 2 to 3 hours after head injury.[108] Infratentorial epidural hemorrhages are commonly caused by basilar skull fractures, which usually lacerate a dural sinus. Being venous in origin, the clinical course is less acute but still can result in cerebellar and brainstem compression with the ultimate risk of tonsillar herniation. Smaller epidural blood clots can organize by forming granulation tissue, which often tends to ossify. The mortality of epidural hemorrhages has been substantially reduced during the past decade because of improved neuroimaging techniques, early detection, and prompt surgical intervention.[109]

In *subdural hematoma* bleeding takes place between the dura and the outer surface of the arachnoid membrane (Fig. 77-90). Two main types are distinguished: *early* (acute or subacute) and *late* (chronic) subdural hematomas. *Acute* hematomas are often associated with severe head injuries and may be bilateral in 20% of cases. The source of bleeding may be arterial or venous, especially the "bridging" veins that drain cortical veins into the superior sagittal sinus. Over the cortex, these veins are tethered down by the arachnoid membrane, but during their brief course in the subdural space they are unprotected and liable to tear when subjected to shearing forces. Especially in fatal cases, an acute subdural hematoma may be associated with underlying cerebral contusion, hemorrhage, or both—a condition referred to as "burst lobe." Acute subdural hematomas (Fig. 77-91) also necessitate emergency neurosurgical care; accumulations of 100 ml of blood are often fatal if not evacuated. Unlike epidural hemorrhages, 30% to 35% of cases are not associated with skull fractures. In *chronic* subdural hematomas, a history of trauma is often trivial or long forgotten. The condition is seen in elderly patients in whom cerebral atrophy causes widening of the subdural space thus exposing the bridging veins to a greater risk of rupture when subjected to angular shearing forces. Oozing of blood is usually gradual and spreads over a large area of the surface of the brain and may extend in the interhemispheric fissure along the falx cerebri. Several hundred milliliters of blood may accumulate gradually in this space without causing symptoms, at least initially. Subdural hematomas evoke a peculiar reaction largely derived from the inner surface of the dura and results in granulation tissue, referred to as "neomembranes," that encircle the hematoma (Fig. 77-92). The neomembrane facing the dura (outer membrane) may attain the thickness of the overlying dura in about 4 weeks and initially is highly vascular. That facing and sometimes adherent to the arachnoid (inner membrane) remains thin and relatively avascular. The blood in the center liquefies and is

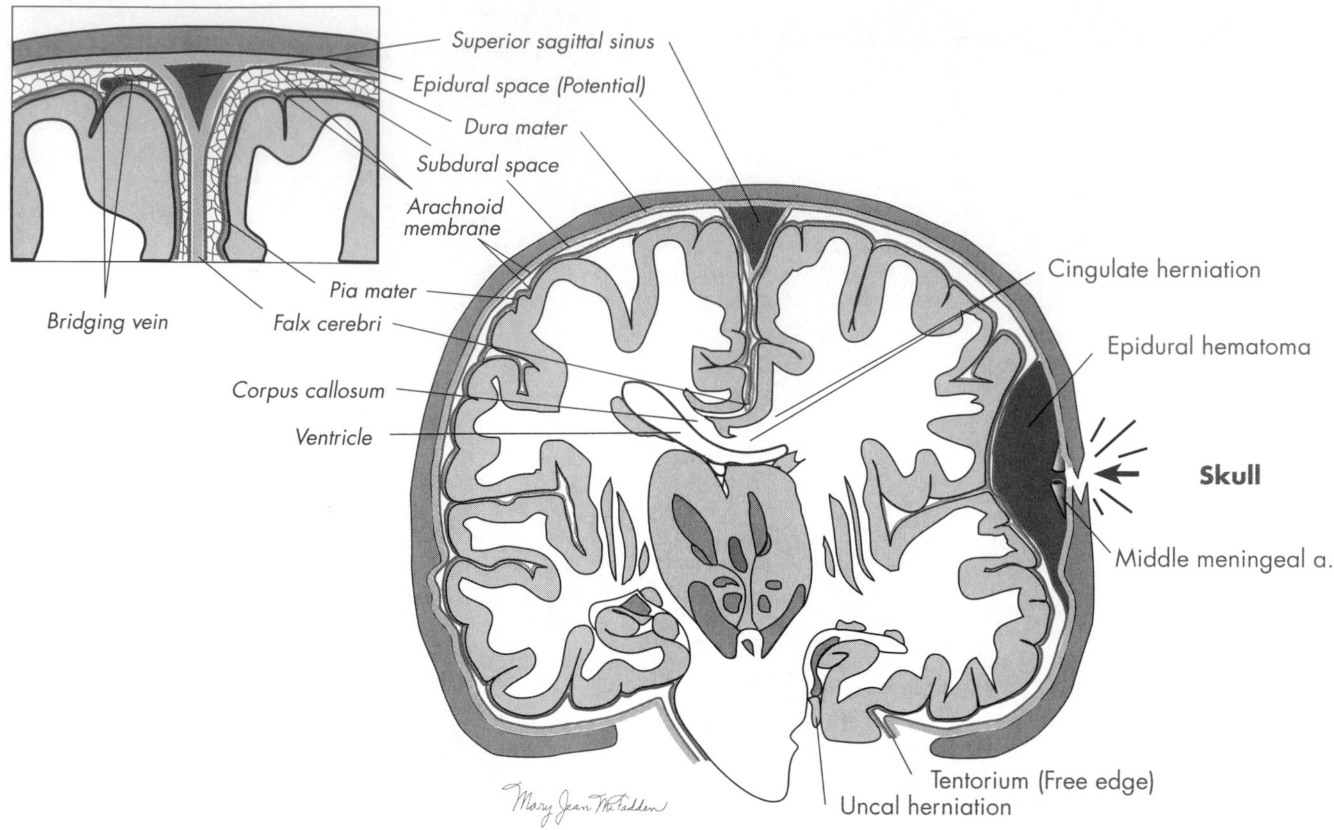

Fig. 77-89 Epidural hemorrhage. Torn middle meningeal artery at skull fracture *(arrow)* with accumulation of blood in epidural space causing midline shift with uncal and incipient cingulate herniations.

resorbed. Bleeding from poorly supported capillaries of the neomembranes into the cavity accounts for progressive enlargement of the hematoma, which may lead to seizures and focal neurologic deficits. Sometimes the loculated fluid is totally absorbed, and the two membranes fuse. Bilateral subdural hematomas, more common in children, may impede the free flow of CSF in the subarachnoid space and can cause hydrocephalus and dementia. Histologic studies of multiple segments of the neomembranes can be used to determine the age of a hematoma.[106] *Subdural hygroma* usually results from tears of the arachnoid with leakage and entrapment of CSF in the subdural space caused by head trauma or occurrence after bacterial meningitis. The hygromas are often distended with clear, hemorrhagic, or xanthochromic fluid. Their walls vary in thickness; if rusty brown, their origin from subdural hematoma is suspected. They may occur bilaterally and become symptomatic if fluid accumulation is considerable.

Subarachnoid hemorrhage occurs in any craniocerebral injury of some magnitude (Fig. 77-93). It is secondary to superficial contusions or lacerations of the brain releasing blood in the subarachnoid space. Small amounts of blood are readily disposed of by the arachnoid granulations; however, massive or repeated subarachnoid hemorrhages may cause fibrosis of arachnoid and its granulations, hindering CSF flow and absorption, respectively and may result in normal-pressure hydrocephalus.

Intracerebral hematomas may be solitary or multiple. Solitary hematomas tend to occur in the temporal or frontal lobe (Fig. 77-94), whereas multiple large hemorrhages often are seen in fatal head injuries and are usually associated with severe contrecoup lesions. They may extend into the ventricles and cause hemoventricle. Smaller hemorrhages usually in the parasagittal plane and the "gliding" contusions previously described occur in diffuse brain injury. Widespread petechial hemorrhages in the white matter are highly suspicious of fat embolism. Delayed post traumatic hematoma, "Bollinger's traumatische Spätapoplexie," is a relatively uncommon condition in which intracerebral hemorrhage suddenly develops days to weeks after head injury.

Diffuse injuries. Diffuse injuries result from severe head trauma and include diffuse axonal injury, brain swelling, and diffuse hypoxic encephalopathy.

Diffuse axonal injury (DAI)[110] is another term for what has been known previously as "shearing injury," "diffuse damage of white matter of immediate impact," and "white matter shearing injury," emphasizing the widespread *tearing of axons,* primarily in white matter. It is produced by angular acceleration or deceleration of the head during vehicular accidents or falls from considerable heights. Impact is not necessary. Primate experiments have replicated these injuries when the heads were rotated at right angle to the midline and were subjected to sudden nonimpact acceleration forces. Patients with DAI are comatose immediately after injury and, should they survive, most are demented or live in apallic (vegetative) states with variable degrees of brainstem activities. Grossly the brain may display hemorrhages in the corpus callosum, usually sparing the midline (Fig. 77-95), walls of the third ventricle, and dorsolateral upper brain stem, especially the

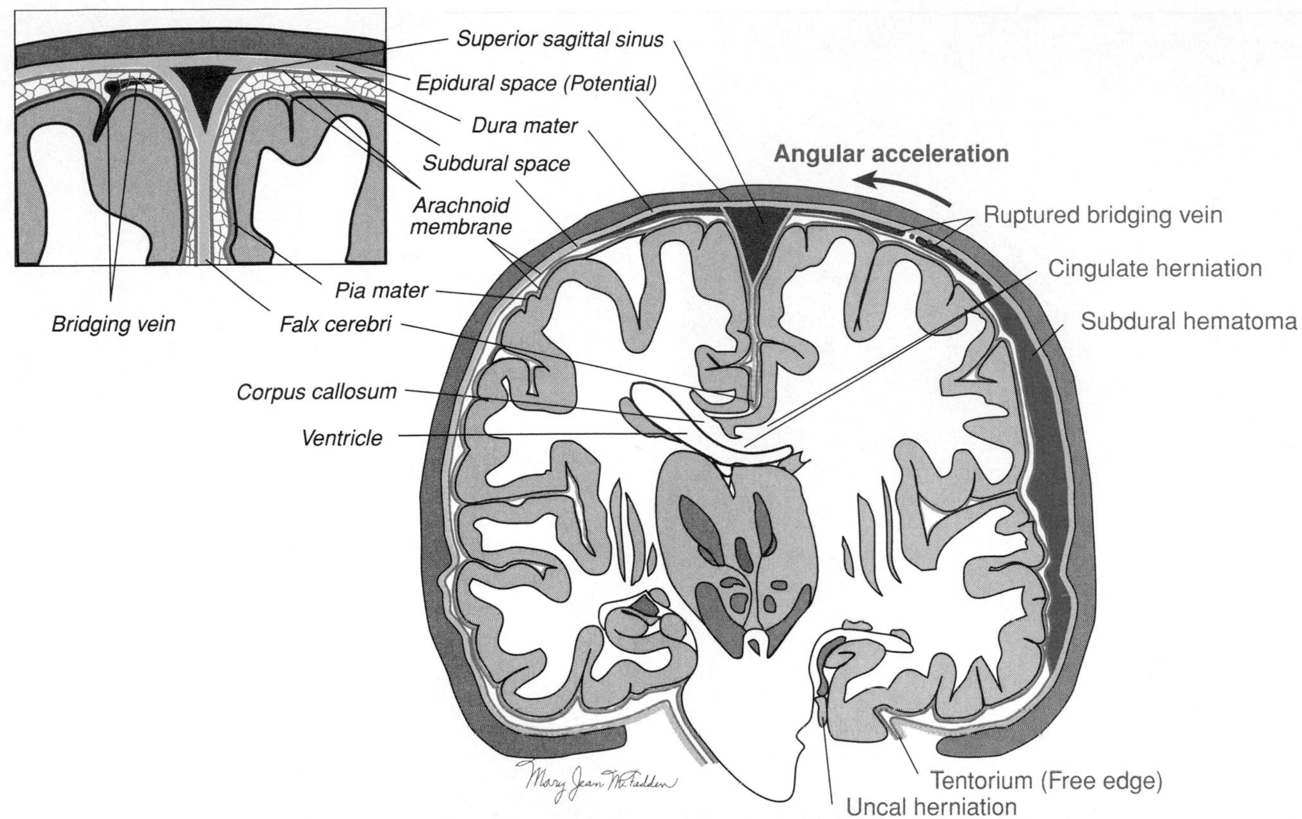

Fig. 77-90 Chronic subdural hematoma. Ruptured bridging vein secondary to angular acceleration with accumulation of blood in the subdural space, midline shift with uncal and incipient cingulate herniations.

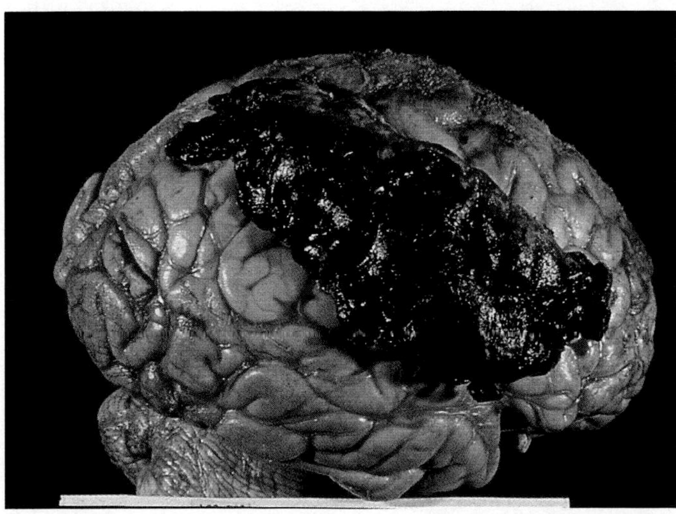

Fig. 77-91 Acute subdural hematoma (dura removed) with intact leptomeninges.

superior cerebellar peduncles (Fig. 77-96). The hemorrhagic lesions are caused by rupture of small blood vessels by the same shearing forces that damage axons. Microscopically the edges of torn axons develop over many hours (about 12 to 15) to a few days into pear-shaped or circular eosinophilic profiles best demonstrated in silver preparations as dark "retraction balls." Axonal swellings or spheroids predominate in these hemorrhagic lesions, subcortical parasagittal white matter, internal capsule, and cerebellar white matter. Microglial nodules develop in a few weeks at these damaged sites and persist for prolonged periods. Atrophy of corpus callosum and cavitation of white matter may result from wallerian-like degeneration of affected axons.

The pathogenesis of *cerebral swelling,* a relatively common complication of severe head injury, is poorly understood, despite being a major cause of fatal increased intracranial pressure. Swelling of one hemisphere may accompany ipsilateral acute subdural hematoma. In children and adolescents, especially, this can have grave consequences and has been attributed to loss of normal cerebral vasoregulation causing the blood to pool, increasing the total volume of brain.

Diffuse hypoxic encephalopathy also is common in patients dying as a result of nonimpact head injury and is related to a variable combination of arterial spasm, hypotension, systemic hypoxia and other factors. Hypoxic-ischemic changes are often seen in the arterial boundary zones.

Open injuries

Open injuries usually are caused by gunshot wounds (GSW). The extent of brain damage along the trajectory of a bullet is dependent on many factors, and the most popularly cited are the speed and weight of the bullet. A low-velocity bullet causes much greater damage at the site of entry and may become arrested halfway through its course in the intracranial cavity. Its track is roughly conical in shape and contains pulped brain tissue, blood clots, pieces of scalp, bone debris,

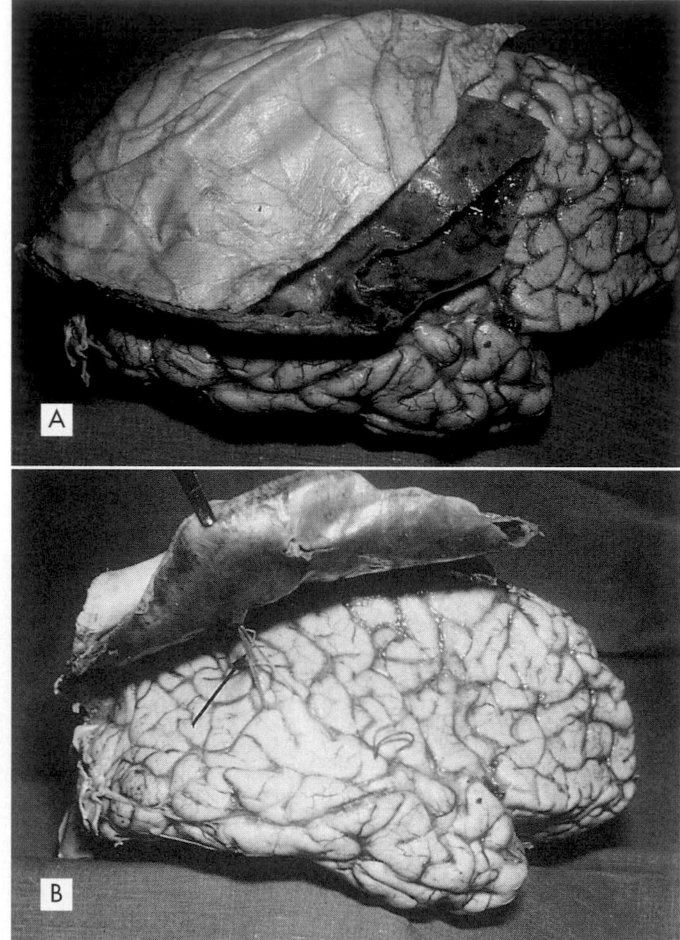

Fig. 77-92 Chronic subdural hematoma. **A,** Reflected dura revealing outer membrane and resected anterior segment of the hematoma exposing cavity and inner membrane. **B,** Lifted inner membrane exposing compressed but intact cerebrum and leptomeninges and torn bridging vein *(arrow)*.

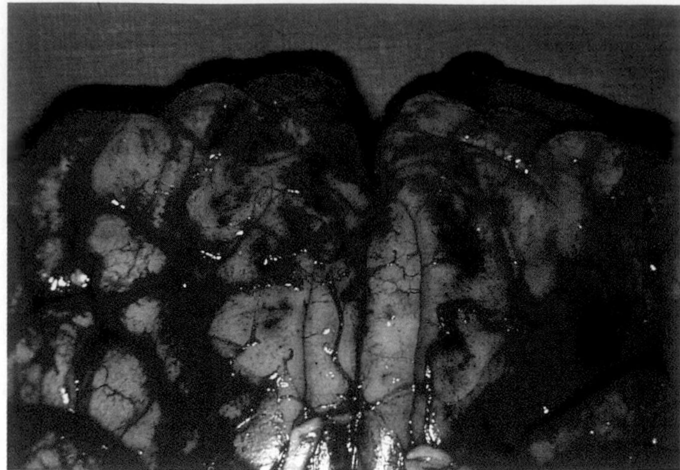

Fig. 77-93 Acute subarachnoid hemorrhage with focal accentuation over superficial cortical contusions.

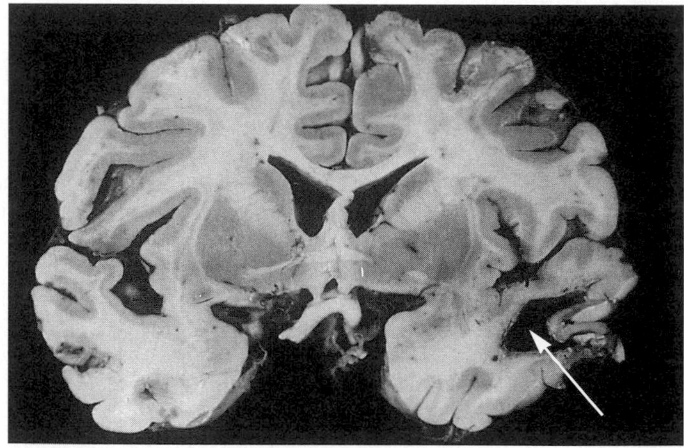

Fig. 77-94 Solitary intracerebral hematoma, old, in the right temporal lobe *(arrow)*.

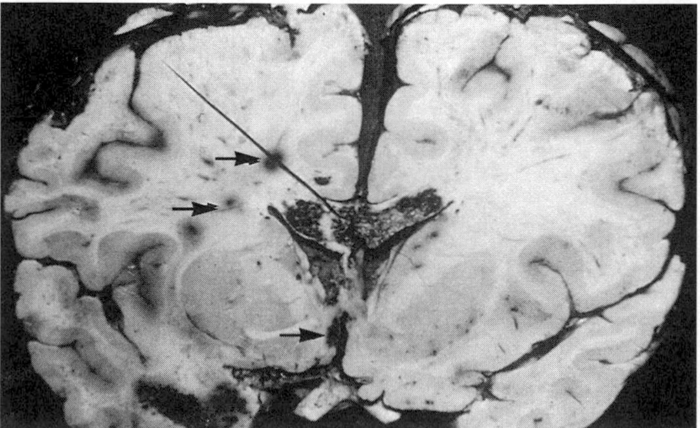

Fig. 77-95 Diffuse axonal injury. Extensive necrosis of the corpus callosum (at medial end of incision) caused by massive tearing of axons and capillaries; intermediary contusions *(arrows)*.

or cloth. With a slightly higher velocity, the bullet reaches the opposite side of the skull and may become fragmented, and the bullet or its fragments may richochet once or more, causing extensive brain damage. These types of GSW are called "penetrating" in contrast to "perforating," in which the bullet traverses the cranial cavity and leaves through the skull. A high-velocity bullet causes a hemorrhagic tunnel in the brain and generates sufficient pressure to cause tentorial and tonsillar herniations. With high-velocity rifles the resulting intracranial pressure may cause an explosive outward bursting of the skull. If the victim survives, neurologic deficits, seizures, and secondary infections are common.[111]

Spinal cord injuries

Spinal cord injuries often accompany closed-head injuries. Approximately 40% of all cord injuries are attributable to motor vehicle accidents; falls, GSW, and penetrating wounds by sharp objects account for the rest. In closed injuries excessive angulation of the vertebral column by either hyperflexion or hyperextension tears the spinal ligaments, causing subluxation and fractures of vertebrae; in extreme cases it may produce fracture-dislocation of the bony spine. In hyperflexion

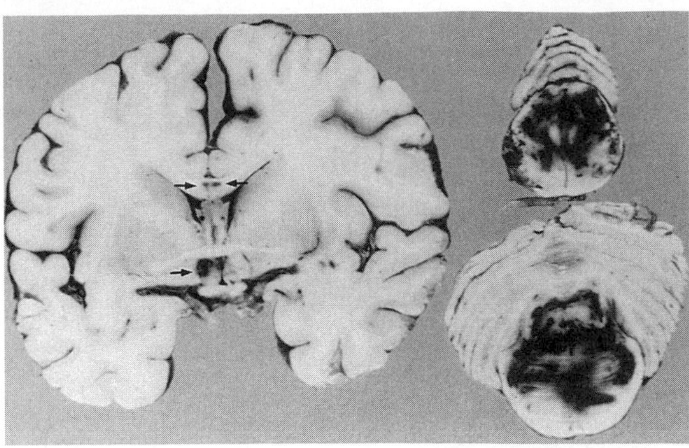

Fig. 77-96 Brainstem contusions in closed head injury associated with smaller lesions in corpus callosum and third ventricle *(arrows).*

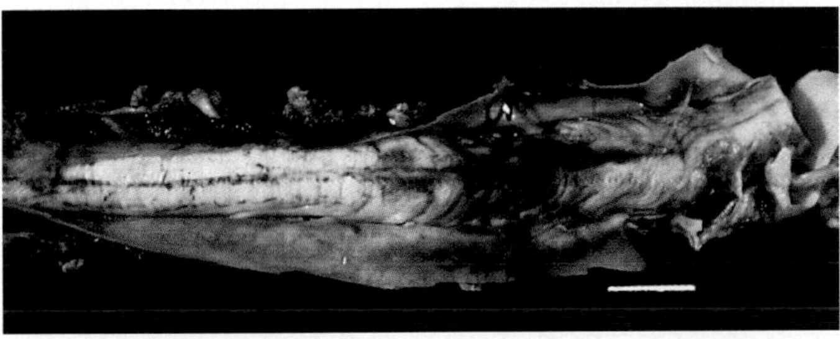

Fig. 77-97 Spinal cord contusion caused by fracture dislocation of spine.

injuries the ventral aspect of the spinal cord is most vulnerable, whereas in hyperextension injuries the dorsal aspect suffers most. In fracture-dislocation or in penetrating injuries, the spinal cord may display contusions, lacerations, or complete transections at the site of maximal injury (Fig. 77-97). Furthermore, ischemic softening (myelomalacia cordis) beyond the traumatized area may develop from damage to the vascular supply of the spinal cord, especially the anterior spinal artery. As in the cranial cavity, hematomas may be present in the epidural, subdural, and subarachnoid spaces as well as in the cord itself (hematomyelia). At the site of damage, gliosis, traumatic "neuromas," and cavitation can develop. Posttraumatic syringomyelia is seen in about 2% of patients who survive traumatic paraplegia and also as a late complication of adhesive spinal arachnoiditis resulting from the trauma. Wallerian-like degeneration is seen in the dorsal columns and lateral spinothalamic and spinocerebellar tracts above the transection and descending corticospinal tracts below the lesion.

DEGENERATIVE DISEASES

Degenerative diseases constitute a heterogeneous group of diseases primarily germane to the CNS. They share in common a gradual, idiopathic, and symmetrical loss of specific neurons, groups of neurons, and nerve fiber tracts that are often functionally related *(multisystem degenerations).* In some diseases, such as Alzheimer's disease, the process is less selective and more widespread. In most multisystem degenerations the affected group of neurons shrink (simple atrophy) or vanish; in some, disorganization of neuronal cytoskeleton or the appearance of abnormal inclusions precedes cell death; and in a few the neurons appear morphologically intact, but their distal axonal segments undergo centripetal degeneration, the "dying-back" phenomenon. The affected regions collapse and become gliotic, and inflammatory reaction is inconspicuous, at best. The factors responsible for these changes are not yet known. It is postulated that in susceptible individuals certain groups of cells are programmed to degenerate prematurely (Gower's concept of *abiotrophy*). This concept has diminished over time, since diseases previously believed to be degenerative, such as subacute combined degeneration and Leber's optic atrophy, have been shown to result from specific causes. It is likely that in the future metabolic or genetic causations for most of these diseases will be elucidated. Since their causes are unknown, the classification of neurodegenerative diseases is difficult and somewhat arbitrary. One approach is to divide them according to their predominant anatomic sites and consequent clinical presentation (Table 77-3) with the understanding that other sites can be affected.

Degenerative diseases of cortex

Cortical degenerative diseases are responsible for most cases of organic dementia, with Alzheimer's disease accounting for at least 80% to 85% of the cases.

Alzheimer's disease (AD)/senile dementia, Alzheimer type (SDAT), was formerly restricted to a dementia occurring before 65 years of age and having the same histologic features as originally described by Alzheimer; however, now AD and SDAT are used interchangeably for this common neurodegenerative malady. Brains of nondemented elderly patients may display changes of SDAT, but the extent and distribution of the lesions are quite limited when compared with that of SDAT. This finding has led some authors to propose that SDAT results from acceleration of the normal cerebral ageing process, whereas others espouse a threshold-effect theory. The cause of SDAT, however, remains obscure. The premature development of AD in Down syndrome (trisomy 21) and the localization of the gene responsible for some autosomal dominant forms of AD to the long arm of chromosome 21[112] led to cloning the gene for beta-amyloid precursor protein (APP), but this was found to be at a locus different from that of familial AD on chromosome 21. This finding nonetheless has raised speculation that aberrant regulation in APP processing plays a major role in the pathogenesis of AD. Other etiologic factors proposed in AD have included *aluminum, trauma, slow virus infection,* and a *disorder of cortical cholinergic innervation* analogous to the disturbance of the dopaminergic system in idiopathic parkinsonism.[25] A highly significant association of late-onset familial and sporadic AD with the apolipoprotein E4 allele (chromosome 19) also has been reported.[113] Impaired communication among neurons caused by loss of synapses has been proposed by some to explain the dementia.[114] The cerebrum shows moderate-to-severe atrophy, particularly in the presenile group, and a variable decrease in brain weight. Atrophy of the gyri and widening of the sulci may be diffuse or most prominent in the frontal and temporal lobes, notably the hippocampi (Fig 77-98). The white matter and head of the caudate nuclei may be attenuated, resulting in hydrocephalus ex vacuo. During the course of normal aging, there is signifi-

Table 77-3 Neurodegenerative diseases

Cortical
1. **Alzheimer's disease**
2. **Pick's disease**
3. Nonspecific lobar atrophies
4. Cortical or diffuse Lewy body disease

Subcortical nuclei
1. **Huntington's disease**
2. **Parkinsonian syndromes**
   a. **Idiopathic. Diffuse Lewy body disease**
   b. **Progressive supranuclear palsy**
   c. **Multisystem atrophy**
      (1) Striatonigral degeneration
      (2) Olivopontocerebellar atrophy
      (3) Shy-Drager syndrome
   d. Acquired: postencephalitic, drugs, trauma

Cerebellar, brainstem, and spinal cord
1. Cerebello-olivary degeneration
2. Olivopontocerebellar atrophy
3. Spinocerebellar syndromes:
   a. **Friedreich's ataxia**
   b. Hereditary spastic paraplegia
   c. Machado-Joseph disease

Motor neurons
1. **Amyotrophic lateral sclerosis**
   a. Variants
   b. Secondary
      (1) Toxic/metabolic
      (2) Paraneoplastic
      (3) Post poliomyelitic, etc.
2. Heredofamilial spinal muscular atrophies
   a. **Infantile (Werdnig-Hoffmann)**
   b. Juvenile (Kugelberg-Welander)
   c. Adult form

Diseases shown in boldface type are the best characterized.

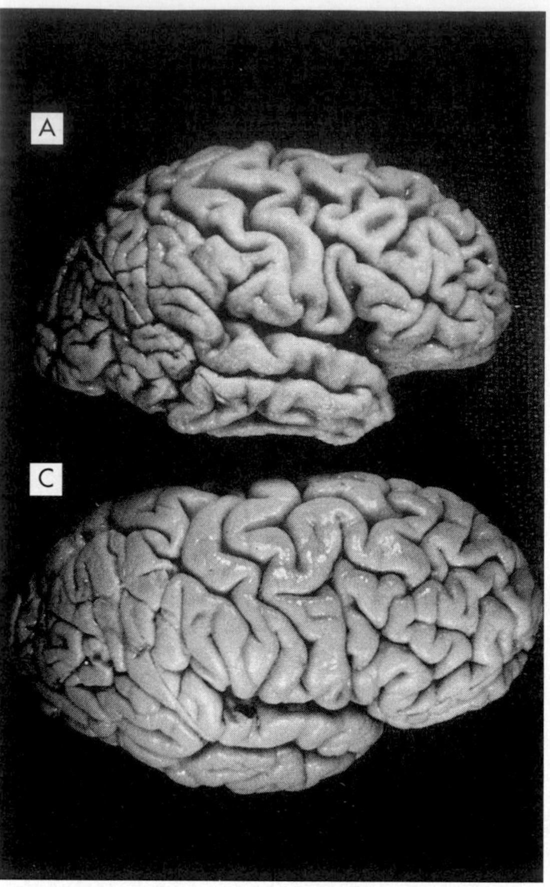

Fig. 77-98 Alzheimer's disease *A* compared to age, sex-matched control *C*: reduced size, narrow gyri, and wide sulci, notably in frontal and temporal lobes.

cant loss of neurons from the cortex, and this loss shows regional variation. In AD, the loss is greatest among large neocortical pyramidal neurons and is also present in the basal nucleus of Meynert (nbM), a major source of cholinergic input to the cortex. Fibrous astrocytes are increased in the cortex and sponginess of the upper layers may occur. Additionally, a peculiar vacuolation reminiscent of spongiform encephalopathy (Creutzfeldt-Jakob disease) but usually restricted to the medial temporal cortex and amygdala may be present in some cases. In addition to these general features, two distinct changes constitute the hallmarks of AD: *neurofibrillary tangles* (degeneration) and *senile plaques*. Although these occur to some degree in the hippocampi of aged brains, their presense in large numbers, particularly tangles in the neocortex, correlates highly with dementia.

Neurofibrillary tangles (NFT) appear as intracytoplasmic masses of coarse linear fibrils displacing the nucleus and other organelles. Their configurations depend on their stages of development and the shape of affected neurons. They are *flame shaped* in pyramidal neurons of hippocampus, *coil-like* in medium-sized cortical neurons, and ball-like, or *globose,* in brainstem neurons (Fig. 77-99). They are faintly hematoxylinophilic when stained with hematoxylin and eosin, but the true extent of NFTs can be appreciated only with special preparations such as the modified Bielschowsky and Gallyas argyrophilic methods. Like amyloid they are congophilic and birefringent and fluoresce with thioflavin S stain. Extracellular tangles representing "tombstones" of effete tangle-bearing neurons tend to be eosinophilic, stain brown in silver preparations, and fail to express most of the antigenic properties normally displayed by intracellular tangles. Ultrastructurally, the tangles are formed of 10 nm tightly packed pairs of filaments, wound in a double helix, hence the designation *paired-helical filaments* (PHF). The spiral winding produces constrictions of about 10 nm at 80 nm intervals, and the widest distance between the paired filaments is 20 to 22 nm (Fig. 77-100). Tau, a microtubule-associated protein (MAP), is hyperphosphorylated in AD and is a major immunoreactive constituent of PHF. In addition, NFTs are variably immunoreactive for ubiquitin, neurofilaments, and microtubules.[115] These immunocytochemical studies support the view that NFTs result from disorders of assembly and disassembly of cytoskeletal proteins, including hyper-phosphorylation of tau.[116] NFTs also are present in dendrites, axons, and synaptic terminals as threadlike argyrophilic or PHF-immunoreactive profiles, referred to as *neuritic,* or *neuropil, threads* (NTs).[117] NFTs can be found in small numbers in most individuals past 50 years of age usually confined to the amygdala, parahippocampal gyrus, and subiculum complex but not in the neocortex. In SDAT, NFTs are far more widespread in the hippocampal formation and are seen in neocortical neu-

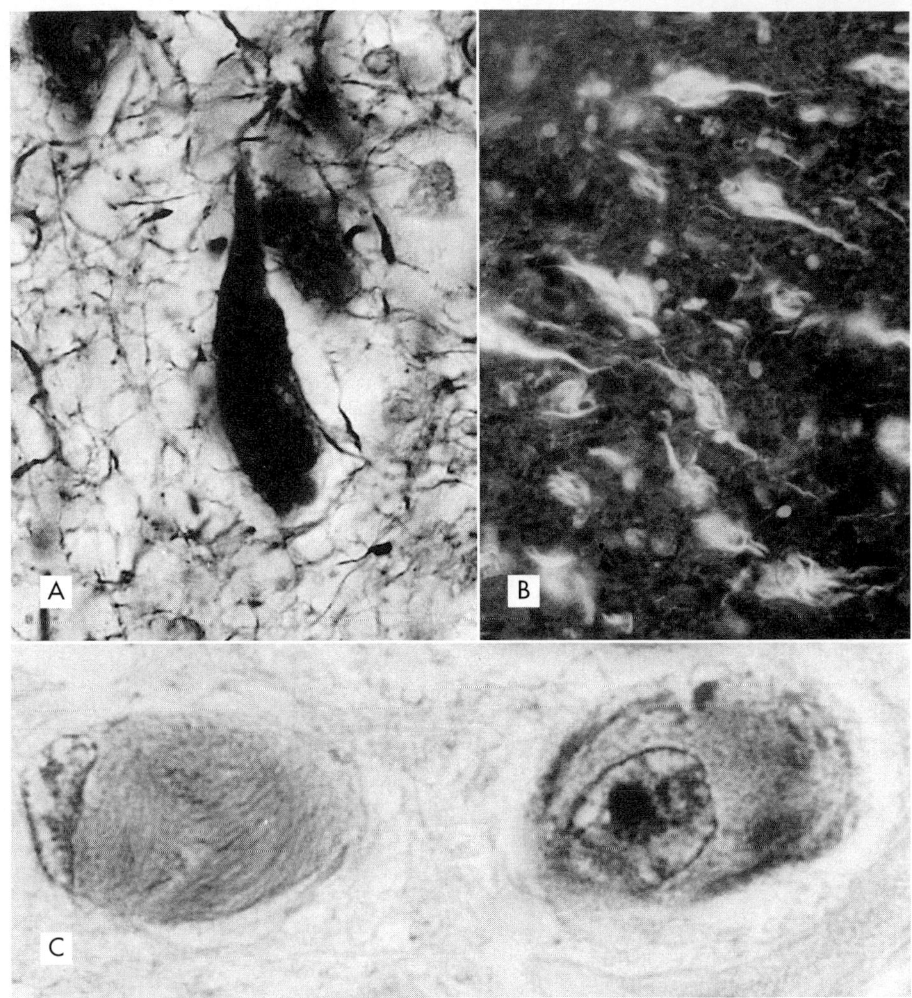

Fig. 77-99 Neurofibrillary tangles in Alzheimer's disease *(AD).* **A,** Argyrophilic flame-shaped in pyramidal neuron. **B,** Fluorescent coil-like in cortical neurons. **C,** Striated globose in median raphe neuron next to normal neuron.

rons. In severe SDAT, NFTs are present in the striatum and brainstem, particularly in the periaqueductal gray matter and median raphe. NFTs also have been seen around focal lesions such as vascular malformations and meningioangiomatosis[118] and in a variety of other disorders.

Senile plaques also are known as *neuritic, dendritic,* and *amyloid* plaques, each emphasizing a particular aspect of the plaque. They have been classified as *immature* (primitive), *mature* (classical), and *burned out* (compact), depending on the concentrations of individual components, purportedly reflecting the various stages of plaque development. They are difficult to see in sections stained with hematoxylin and eosin but are readily demonstrable in the Bielschowsky preparation and with thioflavin S (Fig. 77-101). Plaques are spherical and range from 50 to 100 μm in diameter, often near a capillary. A *mature* plaque has an amyloid core surrounded by a ring of radiating bulbous irregular neurites and processes of microglia and reactive astrocytes (Fig. 77-102). Ultrastructurally the amyloid core is extracellular, and the neuritic processes may contain PHF, lysosomes, neurofilaments, and altered mitochondria.[119] Some of the neurites represent axon terminals, but a few are abnormal dendrites arising from adjacent tangle-bearing neurons. An *immature plaque* is supposed to be formed exclusively of abnormal neurites, whereas a *burned-out plaque* consists of a dense globule of amyloid surrounded by a clear rim with few or no detectable neurites. A plaque, unassociated with dystrophic neurites or fibrillar amyloid and detected by the Bielschowsky method or by its immunoreactivity for beta (A_4) amyloid, is called *diffuse,* or *very immature, plaque.* The relevance and significance of diffuse plaques are uncertain at present.[120] The pathogenesis of plaque formation is a matter of heated debate as to whether the neuritic changes precede or follow deposition of amyloid.[121] Frequent senile plaques are more characteristic of SDAT than of NFT, and their quantitation has been used to establish histologic criteria for the diagnosis of SDAT. For practical purposes, the neuritic and mature plaques have been used for counting. The provisional criteria outlined by Khachaturian are reproducible and relatively easy to apply.[122] A guide for practicing pathologists using the criteria of CERAD (Consortium to Establish a Registry for Alzheimer's Disease) is also useful for that purpose.[123] In general, many neuritic plaques and at least some tangles in the neocortex of a demented patient (in the absence of other lesions) warrant a diagnosis of probable AD. Most cases at autopsy are of this type. A small percentage may need closer scrutiny and quantitative analysis.

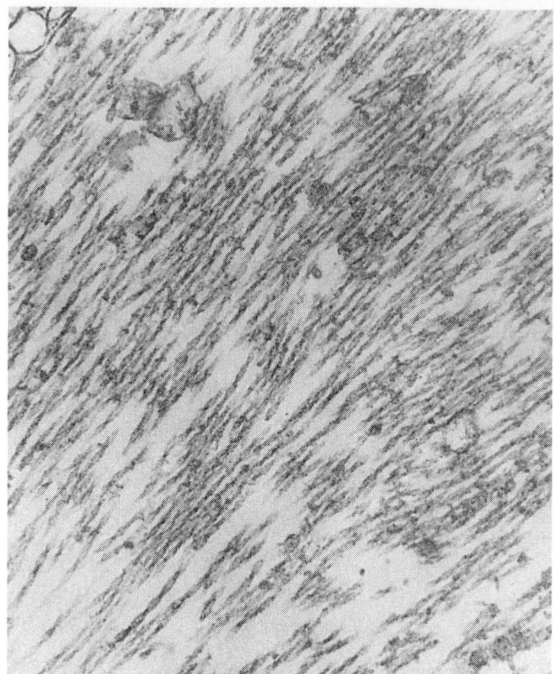

Fig. 77-100 Alzheimer's disease. NFT formed of paired helical filaments.

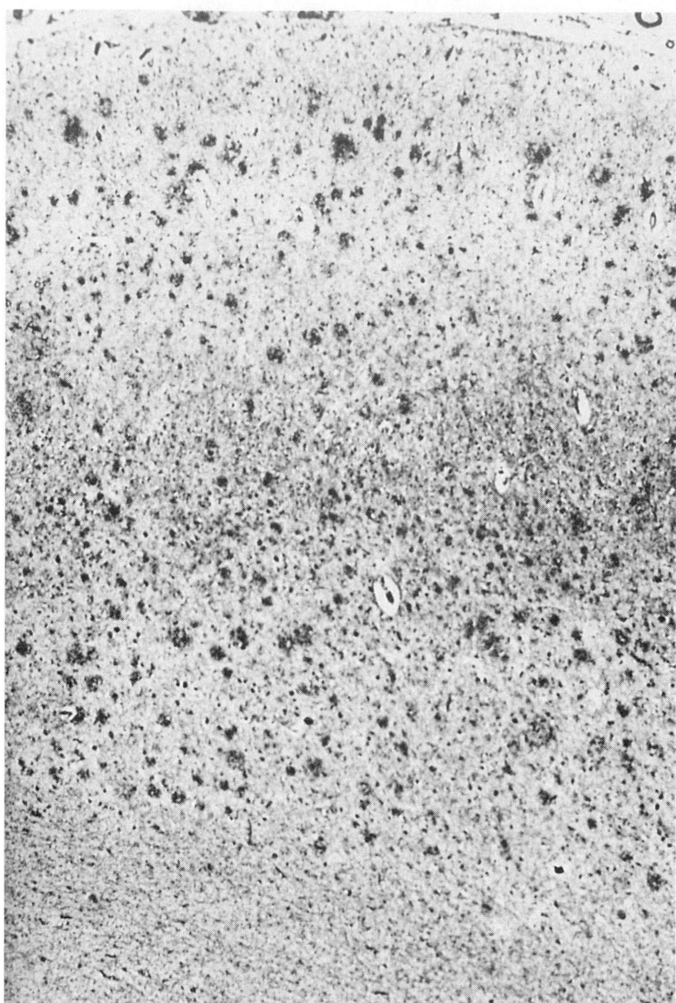

Fig. 77-101 Alzheimer's disease. Numerous punctate "senile" plaques in cortex.

Additional findings, often present in aged brains and increased in SDAT include *granulovacuolar degeneration* (GVD) (Fig. 77-18) and eosinophilic rods or Hirano bodies in the pyramidal neurons of hippocampus, cerebral amyloid (congophilic) angiopathy (CAA), and the accumulation of lipofuscin. *GVD* consists of several small, clear, membrane-bound intracytoplasmic vacuoles containing a coarse hematoxyphilic granule having strong affinity for silver stains and reactive for several cytoskeletal proteins. *Eosinophilic rods* (Hirano bodies), though most often seen in Ammon's horn of elderly patients and in SDAT, have been described in a variety of other diseases and locations. They are refractile hyaline profiles measuring 10 to 30 μm in length and 8 μm across; ultrastructurally they are formed of parallel filaments probably derived from cytoskeletal proteins, primarily actin. *CAA* is present in about 85% of patients with SDAT and is commonly but not invariably associated with neuritic plaques.

Pick's disease is a rare dementing illness in comparison to AD, and most cases are sporadic. Macroscopically, severe brain atrophy classically involves the orbitofrontal and anterior temporal regions *(lobar sclerosis)* (Fig. 77-103). The corresponding white matter is greatly attenuated and firm resulting in hydrocephalus ex vacuo. Atrophy of the caudate nucleus often simulates that of Huntington's chorea, and the substantia nigra is frequently depigmented. Microscopically the affected gyri show considerable neuronal loss, robust astrogliosis, "ballooned" neurons *(Pick cells),* and intracytoplasmic globular argyrophilic masses *(Pick bodies)* (Fig. 77-104). Pick bodies are most prevalent in neurons of Ammon's horn, fascia dentata, and subiculum. Ultrastructurally, Pick bodies are non–membrane bound conglomerations of haphazardly arranged filaments of variable appearance and diameters; they share many antigenic determinants with PHFs.[124] Some do not require the presence of Pick cells or bodies for diagnosis and are satisfied with the severe selective lobar atrophy to establish the diagnosis of Pick's disease.[125] *Progressive subcortical gliosis* may be a form of Pick's disease without Pick bodies. Occasionally, Pick's disease and Alzheimer's may coexist. Comparison of hippocampal changes in these two diseases are illustrated schematically (Fig. 77-105).

Dementing illnesses with "nonspecific" neuronal loss and gliosis manifest in less than 5% of cases of dementia without distinctive histologic markers.[126] The frontal lobes, temporal lobes, or both, may be involved. *Progressive dysphasic dementia* (atrophy of the left perisylvian region) may be considered in this group.

Degenerative diseases of subcortical nuclei

The subcortical nuclei are a collection of nuclei comprising the basal ganglia which in their broadest context include the striatum (caudate-putamen), globus pallidus, amygdala, septal nuclei, nucleus basalis of Meynert (nbM), subthalamic and red nuclei, substantia nigra, locus ceruleus, and certain nuclei of the thalamus. These nuclei integrate and modulate the various inputs from the motor cortex and cerebellum. Diseases affecting this circuitry (extrapyramidal system) result in disturbances of movement and posture, the clinical manifestations

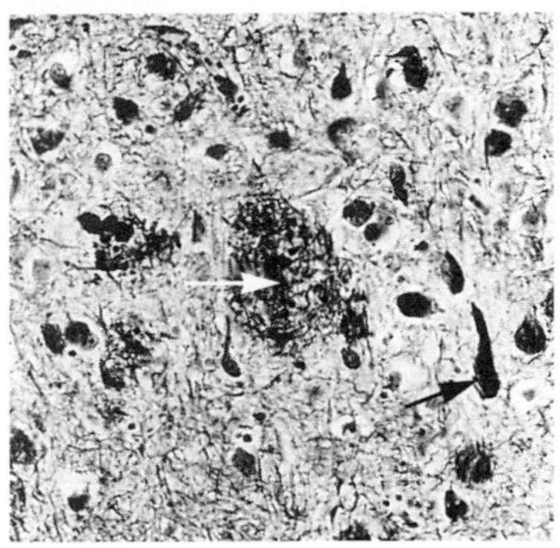

Fig. 77-102 Alzheimer's disease. A neuritic (mature) plaque with central amyloid core *(white arrow)* next to a neurofibrillary tangle *(black arrow)*.

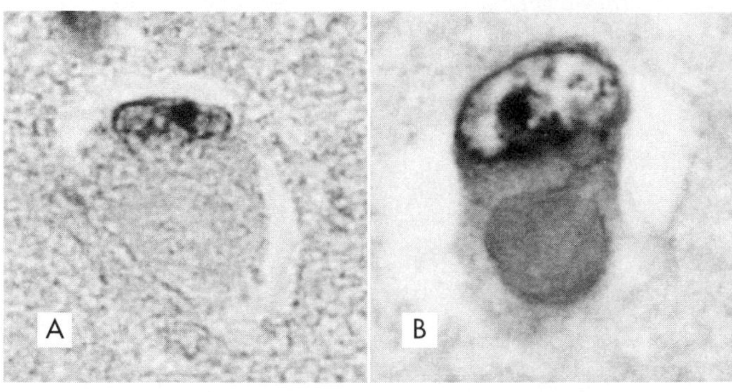

Fig. 77-104 Pick's disease. **A,** Pick cell showing ballooned neuron with eccentric nucleus. **B,** Pick body consisting of hematoxylinophilic discrete globule in perikaryon.

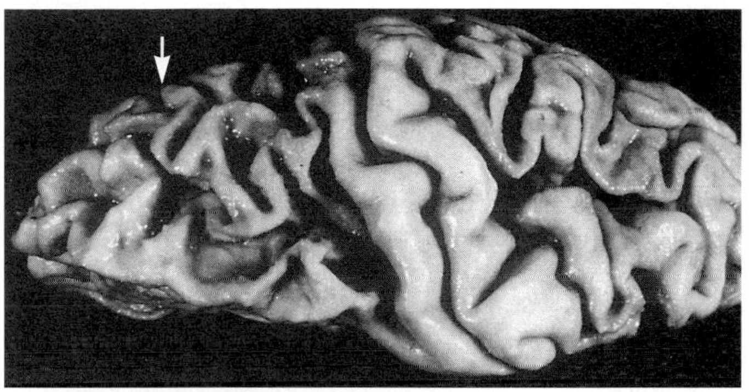

Fig. 77-103 Pick's disease. Severe lobar atrophy with "knife-edge" frontal gyri (arrow).

of which depend on the location of the lesions. Although dementia and paralysis are not essential features of these disorders, dementia of the "subcortical type" may be present to a variable extent in some.

Huntington's disease is an autosomal dominant condition with a high degree of penetrance; the gene is located on the short arm of chromosome 4. The HD gene contains an unstable trinucleotide repeat $(CAG)^n$, which is expanded in patients with the disease.[127] Occasionally, spontaneous mutation may account for sporadic cases. It usually becomes symptomatic during the fourth decade, whereas in the *juvenile form* the manifestations begin before 20 years of age. Emotional disturbances, chorea, and dementia form the classic clinical triad but any one of them may precede, follow, or dominate the picture. In the juvenile form, chorea is often absent and dementia with dystonia is more common. Usually, gyral atrophy is not pronounced, and if present the frontal and parietal lobes are affected. The caudate nucleus may be grossly normal (grade 0) or atrophic (grades I to IV) and may be reduced to a thin concave strip of tissue (grade IV) resulting in enlargement of the anterior horns of the lateral ventricles (Fig. 77-106). Atrophy also affects the putamen. There is preferential loss of small to medium neurons, mostly the gamma-aminobutyric acid (GABA) spiny type. Large and most medium-sized neurons are relatively spared, especially in the rigid variant. Neuronal loss is accompanied by fibrous astrocytosis. The occurrence of some cell loss and gliosis in other nuclei is inconstant. Cortical neuronal loss has likewise varied in severity and distribution in demented patients.

Parkinsonian syndromes are characterized by rigidity, akinesia, and resting tremors. Pharmacologically their common denominator is failure of the nigrostriatal dopaminergic system because of a variety of pathologic conditions.

Idiopathic parkinsonism (Parkinson's disease, paralysis agitans) is a relatively common neurodegenerative disease with a prevalence rate estimated between 73 and 79 per 100,000. It usually becomes symptomatic during the sixth or seventh decade, the course is progressively incapacitating, and death occurs in about 10 years. It is usually sporadic, and search for an environmental toxin, such as MPTP (1-methyl-4-phenyl-1,2,3,6-tetrahydropyridine), has been unsuccessful. In about 10% to 15% of cases, however, there is a family history and the mode of inheritance may be either autosomal dominant or recessive.[128] Gyral atrophy may be present if the patient has concomitant SDAT. The substantia nigra and locus ceruleus are pale because of destruction of their neuromelanin-containing neurons (Fig. 77-107). Nigral cell loss and gliosis are particularly prominent in the zona compacta, and the released pigment is often engulfed by macrophages. The tyrosine hydroxylase–containing neurons are particularly affected, accounting for the dopamine depletion in the striatum to which these neurons project. Some of the surviving neurons are slightly enlarged and pale, and others display the diagnostic intracytoplasmic eosinophilic and spherical inclusions, Lewy bodies (LBs)[129] (Fig. 77-108). LBs have a central dense core, sometimes laminated, surrounded by a clear halo. They immunoreact for neurofilament and microtubule but not tau. Their intense reaction for ubiquitin has become valuable in screening and determining the extent and distribution of LBs.[130] Ultrastructurally, the central core consists of dense granular material from which radiate tightly packed 7 to 8 nm filaments that gradually become looser at the periphery and corresponds to the halo seen in hematoxylin and eosin stain. Cell loss, gliosis, and LBs are found in other pigmented nuclei, such as the locus ceruleus and dorsal nucleus of the vagus, and in nonpigmented nuclei, particularly the nbM where LBs were first described. LBs with different morphologies also have been described in autonomic and myenteric neurons. Rare LBs occur in 4% of "normal" brains. LBs are more widespread in *diffuse Lewy body disease* (DLBD) with numerous

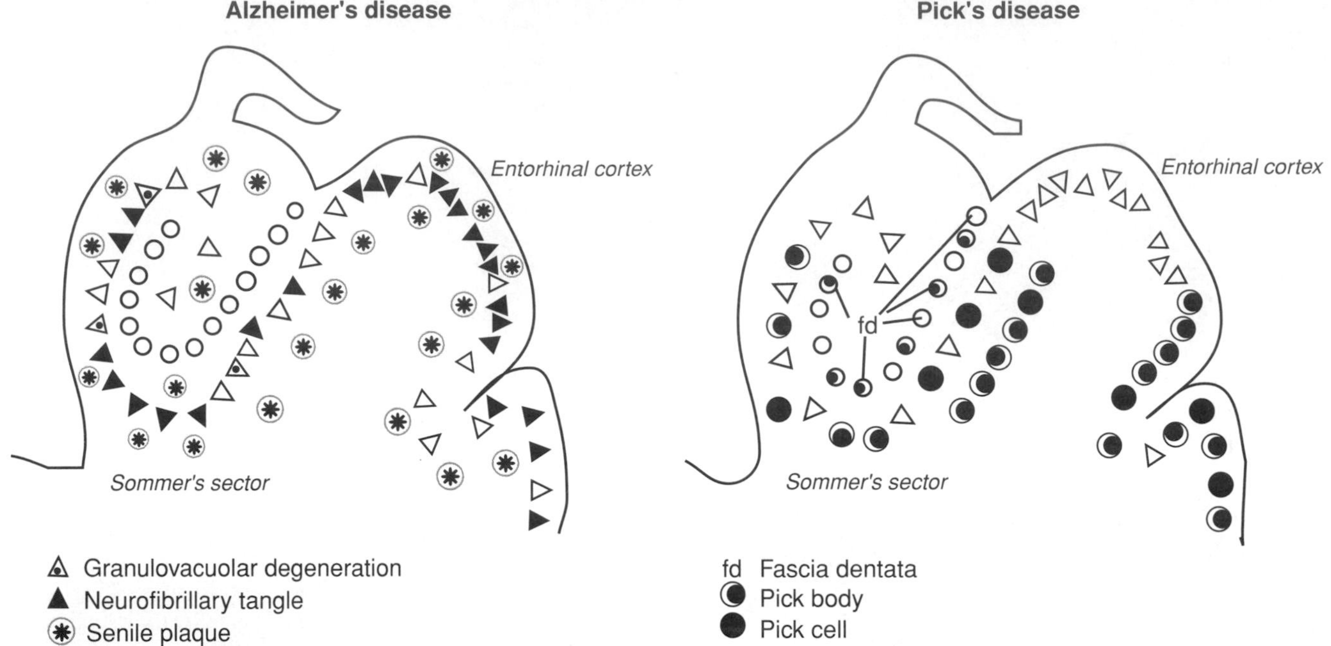

Fig. 77-105 Comparison between hippocampal lesions in Alzheimer's disease and Pick's disease in silver preparations. (Modified from Constantinidis J: *Interdiscipl Topics Gerontol* 19:72, 1985).

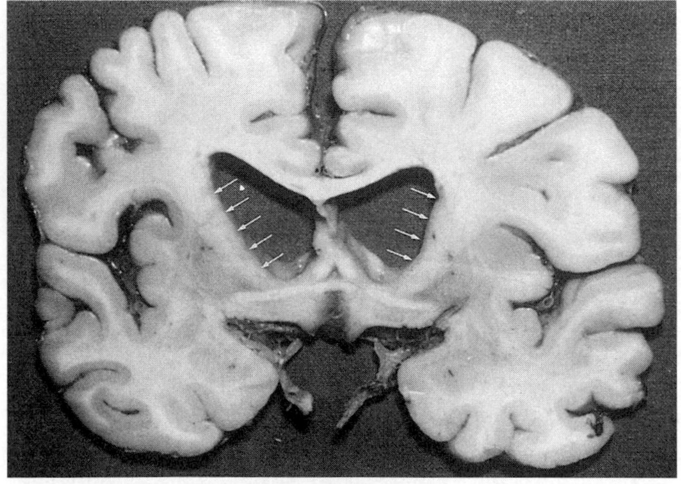

Fig. 77-106 Huntington's disease. Atrophic caudate nuclei with concave *(arrows)* configuration (grade IV).

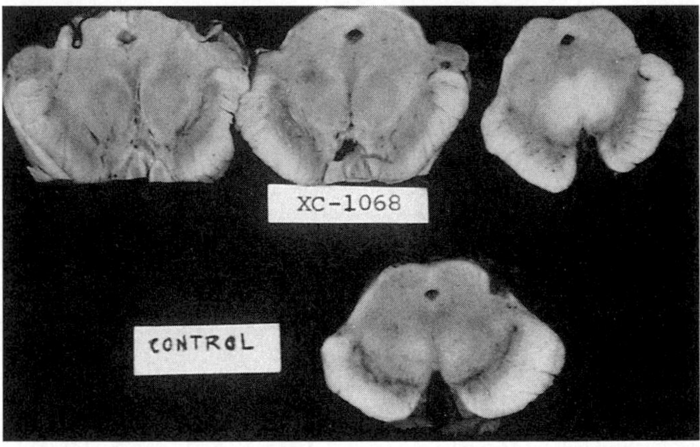

Fig. 77-107 *Top,* Three consecutive levels of greatly depigmented substantia nigra of idiopathic parkinsonism compared with control.

LBs also in the cerebral cortex, particularly in the parahippocampal and cingulate gyri. Patients with DLBD often present with dementing illness and psychotic behavior with little or no extrapyramidal symptoms.[131] *Dementia associated with Parkinson's disease* is estimated to occur in about 15% of patients, much more than in age-matched controls. The large majority of cases show changes indistingishable from those occurring in SDAT. Some have DLBD and others DLBD with tangles and neuritic plaques, the "Lewy body variant of Alzheimer disease." Most cases of "plaque-only Alzheimer disease" also are included in the Lewy body variant.[132] *Parkinsonism-dementia complex of Guam* (Lytico-Bodig) is a condition confined to Guam, Kii peninsula, Japan, and certain regions of West New Guinea and accounts for about 10% of adult deaths in Guam. Parkinsonism and dementia are complicated by degeneration of motor neurons and an ALS-like syndrome. The brains are atrophic and exhibit widespread neurofibrillary tangles, especially in the hippocampi; senile plaques are virtually absent. Ingestion of cycad seeds is suspected in its pathogenesis.

Progressive supranuclear palsy (PSP), Steele-Richardson-Olszewski syndrome may account for 4% to 7% of patients with Parkinsonism.[132a] It is a sporadic disease usually presenting around 60 years of age and characterized by akinesia

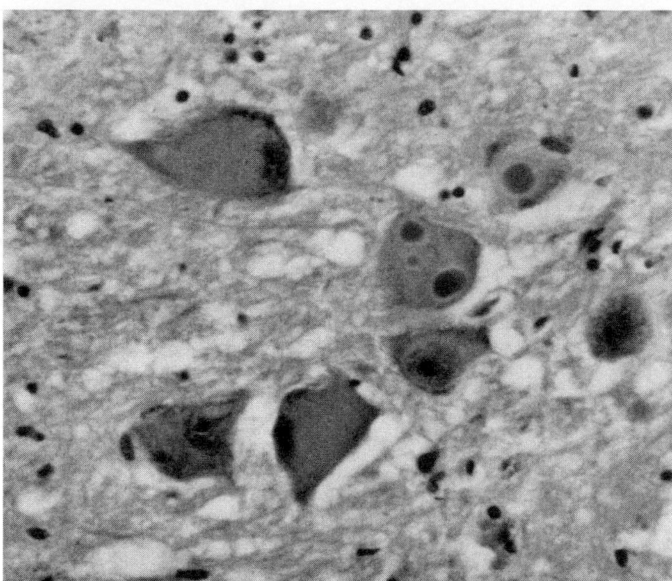

Fig. 77-108 Lewy bodies in pigmented neurons of locus ceruleus.

and axial rigidity, notably nuchal with negligible tremors. Impaired vertical eye movements, which are considered the hallmark of this disease, may be absent in atypical cases. In some patients dementia may occur late in the course of the disease. Death usually occurs within 10 years. Grossly the subthalamic nucleus, and the globus pallidus are shrunken. The tectum, especially the superior colliculi, and the tegmentum of the brainstem are atrophic, causing widening of the aqueduct of Sylvius. The substantia nigra is depigmented. Microscopically, cell loss, gliosis, neurofibrillary tangles, and neuritic threads are most prominent in the subthalamic nucleus, globus pallidus, substantia nigra, basis pontis, dentate nucleus, and inferior olivary nucleus. NFTs of PSP share many epitopes with SDAT tangles, but ultrastructurally they differ in that they are largely made up of 15 nm straight filaments. *Corticobasal degeneration* shares some features with PSP, especially the presence of neurofibrillary changes in the substantia nigra, "corticobasal inclusions"; its main features, however, are neuronal loss, gliosis, and ballooned (achromatic or Pick-like) neurons, chiefly in posterior frontal–anterior parietal areas.[133]

Multisystem atrophy (MSA) is to be distinguished from multisystem degeneration, which is a generic term encompassing many of the neurodegenerative diseases. MSA refers to three clinicopathologic entities, either occurring singly or with variable degrees of overlap: *striatonigral degeneration (SND), olivopontocerebellar atrophy (OPCA),* and *Shy-Drager syndrome (SDS).* MSA is a sporadic disease with its onset between the fourth and sixth decades. Clinically parkinsonism, cerebellar, and autonomic dysfunctions are seen. A recently discovered histologic hallmark is the widespread occurrence of cytoplasmic argyrophilic inclusions in oligodendroglia in all three entities[134] and Pick-like inclusions in neurons, notably in the basis pontis of patients with OPCA.[135] The concomitant occurrence of these fibrillar inclusions in oligodendroglia and neurons is suggestive of a disorder of cytoskeletal protein common to both cells.[136] In *striatonigral degeneration* there is shrinkage and brownish discoloration of the putamen because of deposition of abundant intracellular and extracellular brownish pigment of uncertain derivation and pallor of the substantia nigra because of cell loss and gliosis. Unlike idiopathic parkinsonism, SND is refractory to L-dopa treatment. In *olivopontocerebellar atrophy* there is atrophy of basis pontis, middle cerebellar peduncles,

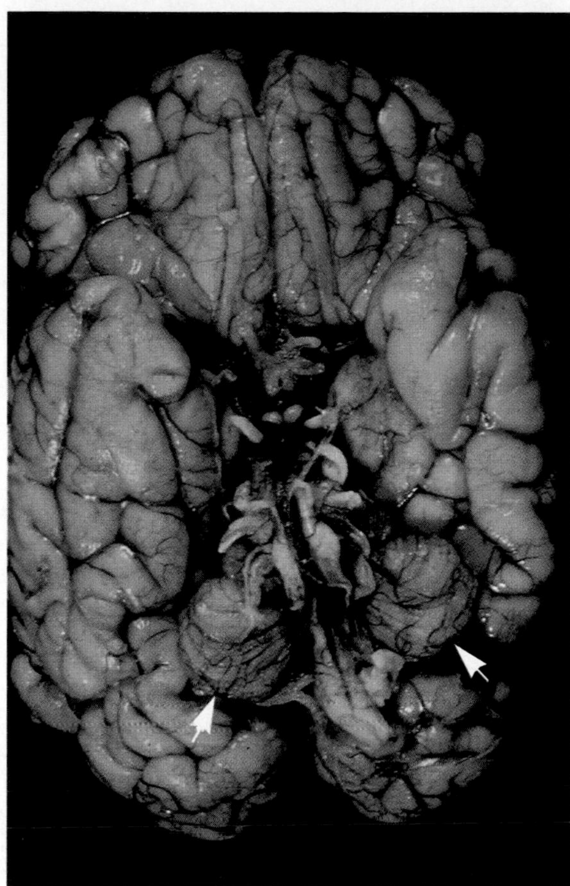

Fig. 77-109 Olivopontocerebellar atrophy (OPCA) with disproportionately small cerebellar hemispheres *(arrows)* and flattening of pontine bulge.

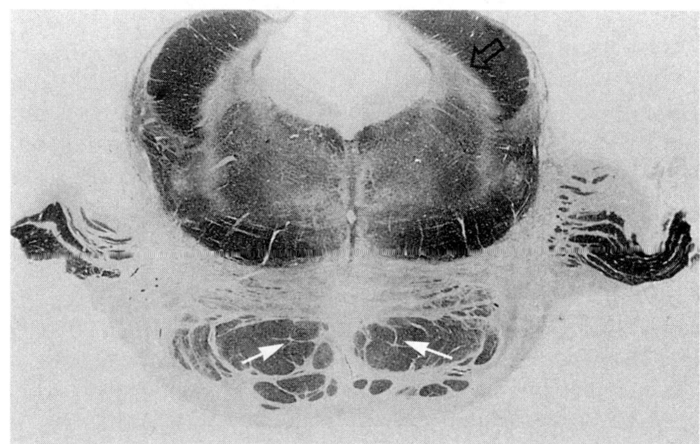

Fig. 77-110 OPCA. Shrinkage of the basis pontis caused by loss of pontine nuclei and transverse tracts; preservation of vertical descending tracts *(arrows)* and superior cerebellar peduncle *(open arrow).*

cerebellar folia (except for vermis and flocculi), and inferior olives (Fig. 77-109). Microscopically there is near total loss of pontine transverse myelinated fibers with preservation of pyramidal fibers (Fig. 77-110), loss of neurons in basis pontis, moderate loss of Purkinje cells, and loss of olivary neurons. Cerebellar white matter is greatly reduced and partially gliotic. In *Shy-Drager syndrome* orthostatic hypotension and other features of autonomic dysfunction dominate the clinical picture.[137] Microscopically, neuronal loss may occur in the intermediolateral horns of the thoracic cord and occasionally in sympathetic ganglia. It occurs in two distinct settings: MSA and idiopathic Parkinsonism.

There are several *acquired (non–Lewy body) parkinsonian syndromes.* In *postencephalitic parkinsonism* a virus, presumably influenzal that caused the pandemic of encephalitis lethargica, is believed responsible for cell loss, gliosis, and globose tangles in the diencephalon and brainstem, especially substantia nigra.[138] The most frequent cause of secondary parkinsonism now is prolonged use of *antipsychotic medications,* especially chlorpromazine. An outbreak of parkinsonism occurred after the use of methyl phenyltetrahydropyridine *(MPTP)* attributable to selective destruction of nigral cells. *Trauma* may result in parkinsonism, especially in boxers and usually in the context of *dementia pugilistica* in which there is thinning and fenestration of the septum pellucidum, atrophy of the fornix, and old contusions. NFTs are present in the neocortex but mainly in the hippocampus and substantia nigra. Neuritic plaques are negligible in number, but diffuse plaques often are detectable by A4 amyloid immunoreactivity.[139] The Parkinsonian syndromes in both *manganese* and *carbon monoxide poisoning* are largely caused by destruction of the globus pallidus.

Degenerative diseases of cerebellum, brainstem, and spinal cord

Many of the degenerative brain diseases present with ataxia, abnormal muscle tone, movement incoordination, tremors, speech disturbances, nystagmus, and sensory changes as a result of progressive degeneration of the cerebellum, brainstem nuclei, and different tracts in the spinal cord.[137] Depending on the topographic distribution of the lesions several syndromes have been identified. Most of them are hereditary, and although the clinicopathologic findings in a given family may be similar, variations between families are frequent resulting in a bewildering array of transitional forms. *Olivopontocerebellar atrophy* (OPCA) in its sporadic form (Dejerine-Thomas type) belongs to the complex picture of MSA (Figs. 77-109 and 77-110), whereas its autosomal variant (Menzel type) has features that overlap with Friedreich's ataxia, and in some the gene has been localized to the short arm of chromosome 6 (spinal cerebellar ataxia 1).

Friedreich's ataxia is the best characterized of the *hereditary degenerative spinocerebellar syndromes.* It is usually autosomal recessive, and the gene has been localized to chromosome 9. The onset of the disease begins during the second decade; most patients are wheelchair bound within 5 years and dead by the end of the third decade. Unlike in most neurodegenerative diseases organs other than the CNS are affected, notably the heart. It shows concentric hypertrophic cardiomyopathy and accounts for 50% of deaths. Mixed cerebellar and sensory ataxia caused by peripheral neuropathy dominate the clinical picture. Optic atrophy and sensorineuronal hearing loss are common but not constant. The spinal cord is thin because of loss of ascending and descending myelinated fiber tracts and their replacement by fibrous astrocytes (Fig. 77-111). The neurons in Clarke's columns and dorsal root ganglia are reduced in number. In the cerebellum, the dentate nucleus and superior cerebellar tracts are invariably involved.[137] *Hereditary spastic paraplegia*[140] and *Machado-Joseph disease* are rare multisystem degenerations.[141] A small number of multisystem degenerations may be associated with inherited metabolic disorders, such as *low-density lipoprotein deficiency* (abetalipoproteinemia or Bassen-Kornzweig syndrome) and *ataxia-telangiectasia* (Louis-Bar syndrome).

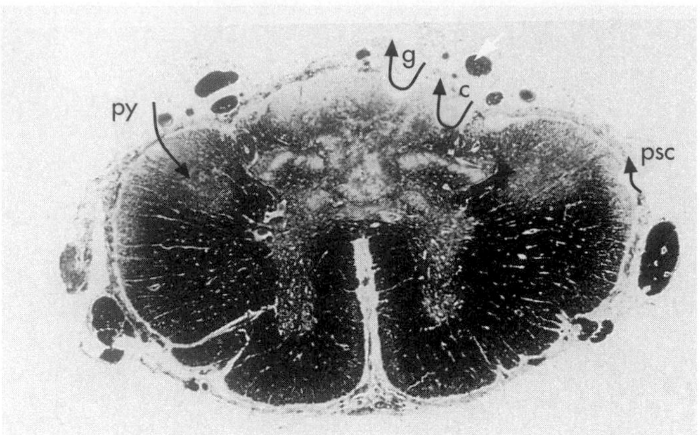

Fig. 77-111 Friedreich's ataxia. Attenuation and flattening of dorsal spinal cord caused by nerve fiber loss in ascending tracts (c, Cuneate; g, gracile; *psc,* posterior spinocerebellar) and descending pyramidal (*py*) tracts.

Degenerative diseases of motor neurons

Motor neurons (MNs) are distributed in the motor cortex (upper MNs), certain brainstem nuclei (bulbar lower MNs) and anterior horns of the spinal cord (lower MNs). The axons of upper MNs course in the internal capsule, in the middle third of the basis pedunculi, and in the medullary pyramids, at the lower end of which 90% decussate. When they reach the spinal cord, the decussating fibers form the large lateral corticospinal tract located in the lateral funiculus, whereas the smaller bundle of uncrossed fibers form the anterior corticospinal tract, which descends in the anterior funiculus along the anterior median fissure. The corticospinal fibers terminate in the spinal gray matter where they relay with the internuncial neurons, which in turn are connected to the motor anterior horn cells. Paralysis caused by diseases of upper MNs are characterized by spasticity, hyperactive tendon reflexes, and extensor plantar response (Babinski sign). In lower MN diseases the paralysis is associated with flaccidity, fasciculations, twitching and severe atrophy of the denervated muscles, and abnormal nerve conduction studies; the Babinski sign is absent.

Progressive degeneration of motor neurons results in heterogeneous disorders, depending on the groups of MNs that are maximally involved. However, a certain degree of overlap exists between these disorders, and depending on the age of onset and the pattern of inheritance, several individualized syndromes are identified.

Amyotrophic lateral sclerosis (ALS) and *motor neuron disease (MND)* are two terms used interchangeably, with MND

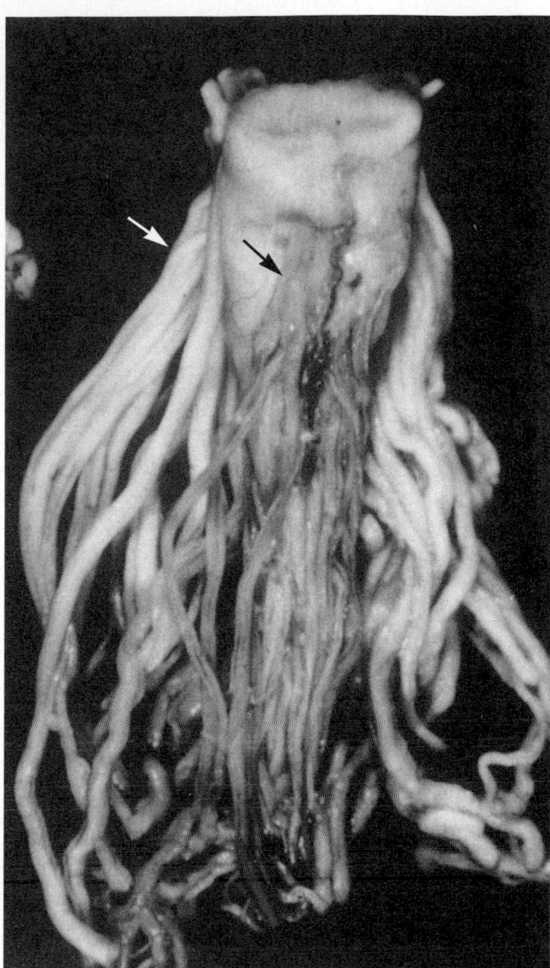

Fig. 77-112 Amyotrophic lateral sclerosis (ALS). Atrophic and gray anterior roots of cauda equina *(black arrow)* in contrast to normal posterior roots *(white arrow).*

being preferred in Britain and ALS, or Lou Gehrig's disease, being preferred in the United States. It is the most frequent form of MND, and its annual incidence is about 1.5 per 100,000 population with a male-to-female ratio of 1.5 : 1. The mean age at onset is 55 years, and the course of the disease ranges from 2 to 6 years. It is invariably fatal, and death is often attributable to failure of respiratory muscles. The majority of cases occur sporadically, though about 10% of cases are inherited usually as an autosomal dominant trait. In some families, mutations in the Cu/Zn superoxide dismutase gene on chromosome 21 have been reported, fueling the speculation about a potential role for free radical toxicity in this disorder.[142] However, the selective damage of MNs remains to be resolved. The incidence of ALS is severalfold higher in Guam than anywhere else in the world, notably in the context of the *ALS-Parkinsonism-dementia complex.*

In ALS both upper and lower MNs are involved. The patients present with fasciculations and atrophy of muscles beginning in the hands and progressively involving the arms. Spasticity of legs, generalized hyperreflexia, and Babinski signs are present. Variable bulbar nuclear involvement leads to dysarthria, dysphagia, and a tendency for aspiration. The brain is usually normal, and visible atrophy of the precentral gyrus

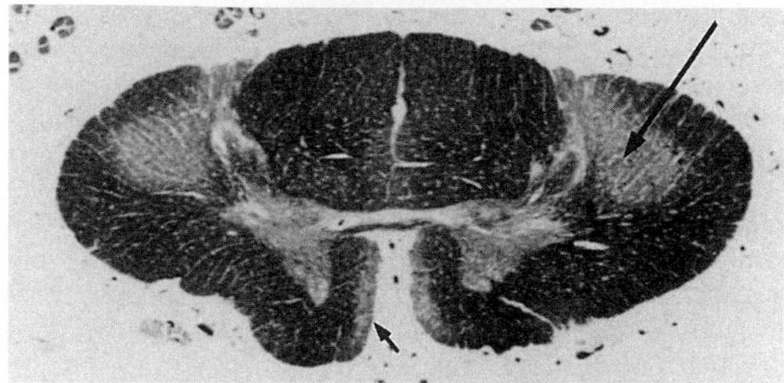

Fig. 77-113 ALS. Pale crossed *(long arrow)* and uncrossed *(short arrow)* pyramidal tracts.

(motor cortex) is exceptional. The pyramids are flattened. The anterior spinal roots are atrophic and gray (Fig. 77-112). Microscopically, loss of MNs and gliosis are best appreciated in the hypoglossal nuclei and the anterior horns of the cervical and lumbosacral enlargements. In the motor cortex, Betz cells are reduced, both in number and size. The nuclei of the extraocular muscles are spared. *Bunina bodies,* which are eosinophilic cytoplasmic inclusions of uncertain derivation, are inconsistently found in surviving anterior horn cells, whereas ubiquinated skeinlike inclusions are.[143] Gliosis and pallor caused by loss of myelinated fibers are particularly prominent in the lateral corticospinal tracts (Fig. 77-113), but some degeneration also occurs in other spinal tracts.[144] The posterior funiculi are intact except in *familial ALS.*

Other variants of MND include *primary lateral sclerosis* in which degeneration remains confined to the corticospinal tracts, *progressive bulbar palsy* when the weakness and wasting preferentially involves the muscles of the face, tongue, jaw, pharynx, and larynx, and *progressive spinal atrophy* when lower MN symptoms dominate the clinical picture without signs of corticospinal tract dysfunction.

Secondary ALS-like syndromes have been described in association with lead and mercury poisoning, remote effects of carcinoma-lymphoma, paraproteinemia, antiganglioside antibodies, postpoliomyelitis syndrome, physical trauma, and so forth. These findings led to speculations about the possible role of environmental toxins or minerals, viral or immunologic factors, and the release of excitotoxic neurotransmitters in the pathogenesis of ALS.

Heredofamilial spinal muscular atrophies are usually inherited as autosomal recessive traits, and the degeneration is largely limited to the MNs of the spinal cord. The severity and progress of the disease usually depend on the age of onset (the earlier, the worse).

In *infantile spinal muscular atrophy* or *Werdnig-Hoffmann disease (WHD),* the infant is noted to be "floppy" at or shortly after birth. The generalized muscle weakness and wasting causes the infant to acquire a "frog-leg" posture. Motor milestones are not achieved, and as the intercostal muscles become involved, the chest wall collapses. Death usually occurs by 2 years of age and is attributable to respiratory failure. The gene for WHD was localized to chromosome 5q near the gene that regulates the hexosaminidase B subunit, a deficiency of which has been associated with a few cases of childhood and adult-onset spinal muscular atrophy. Pathologic changes in the spinal cord manifest as atrophy of anterior spinal roots and considerable loss of MNs in the anterior horns and to a lesser extent in lower brainstem nuclei, particularly the hypoglossal. Surviving motor neurons show various degenerative features.[145] The MNs of the phrenic nerve and those in Onuf's nucleus are relatively unaffected, explaining the preservation of the diaphragmatic and sphincteric muscle functions, respectively. Some neuronal loss occurs in nonmotor systems, such as the thalamus, as well as degeneration of peripheral sensory nerves, but upper motor neurons are spared. A possible variant with more widespread neuronal changes has been termed "infantile neuronal degeneration."[146]

NEOPLASMS

The incidence of intracranial (IC) tumors depends on the sources and methods used to collect the data and whether conditions such as tuberculomas, parasitic cysts, and vascular malformations are included. The general consensus is that the annual incidence rate of primary intracranial neoplams is between 10 and 12 per 100,000, and these constitute approximately 9% of all primary cancers.[10] These figures, however, may have to be revised upwards with the increasing cases of primary CNS lymphomas in recent years, primarily as a result of the AIDS pandemic. The pathogenesis of spontaneously occurring CNS neoplasms in man remains unknown. There is little evidence to suggest that environmental carcinogens, viruses, or trauma are involved, since the CNS is well-shielded from extraneous factors. Infrequently, ionizing radiation can trigger the formation of meningiomas, sarcomas, and rarely gliomas. This observation and the occurrence of primary CNS neoplasms in some inherited disorders, such as von Recklinghausen's disease, led to the identification of mutations of the p53 tumor-suppressor gene and deletions of chromosome 10 in glioblastomas,[147,148] loss of heterozygosity on chromosome 17p in astrocytomas, and loss of heterozygosity on 19q in anaplastic astrocytomas.[149] Like neoplasms elsewhere, those in the CNS seem to require several small mutations to produce new clones of increasingly aggressive cells. This phenomenon helps to explain why a relatively benign astrocytoma may exhibit increasing degrees of anaplasia when it recurs. Other studies have focused on oncogenes, which, when activated, act as powerful mitogens. Many oncogenes exhibit sequence homologies with genes encoding growth factors and their receptors. Their gene products act as transducers of growth signals between the cell surface and nucleus, resulting in increased levels of mRNA transcripts. An aberrant loop of autocrine stimulation that can promote and perpetuate the growth of tumor cells is thus created. Examples of oncogenes found to be amplified and overexpressed include N-*myc* gene in neuroblastomas and the EGR-R proto-oncogene (*erb*-B_1) in some cases of glioblastoma. Although gene amplification is demonstrated in slightly less than half of malignant gliomas, its exact relationship to neoplastic transformation remains a complex subject that is beyond the scope of this text.[150,151]

In children, because a large pool of undifferentiated cells is still present, primitive CNS neoplasms are common. In adults with a low reserve of such cells and with only glial cells, particularly astrocytes, capable of replicating, glial neoplasms are more frequent. Pediatric CNS neoplasms tend to be infratentorial, whereas in adults they are mainly supratentorial. In general, gliomas are twice as common in men than in women, whereas meningiomas and acoustic schwannomas are more frequent in women. Glial neoplasms are not encapsulated. More differentiated gliomas, especially astrocytomas, have ill-defined borders and ultimately kill the patient because their infiltrative behavior eludes radical excision or their growth in vital areas makes them inaccessible to surgery. Histologically benign CNS neoplasms in strategic locations can be as life threatening as histologically malignant ones. Highly anaplastic neoplasms with deceptively sharp margins also respond poorly to combined surgical ablation and radiotherapy. This also may be attributed to a wide field of progressive neoplastic transformation (Willis's field theory), which could explain the rare gliomatosis cerebri and multicentric glioblastomas seen in about 6% of cases. In addition to infiltrating adjacent brain tissue, gliomas invade meninges, sometimes inciting a severe desmoplastic reaction, creating difficulties in diagnosis. Gliomas also have the propensity to disseminate in, "metastasize," or seed CSF pathways. This feature is not restricted to malignant neoplasms but is also shared infrequently by "benign" tumors such as choroid plexus papilloma. CNS tumors rarely metastasize outside the cranial cavity because the CNS lacks traditional lymphatics, and more anaplastic CNS tumors often kill patients from increased intracranial pressure before visceral metastases have time to develop. When a glial neoplasm invades extracranial tissues after craniotomy or a diversionary shunting procedure, the lung, cervical lymph nodes, and coelomic cavities are frequent sites.

CNS tumors are classified into glial (and pineal) and nonglial neoplasms.[2,10]

Glial neoplasms

By definition gliomas should include only tumors of glial origin, but it has become a generic term encompassing all intrinsic neuroectodermal tumors, including those that are poorly differentiated, such as primitive neuroectodermal tumors (PNET). The first comprehensive classification of CNS tumors was achieved by Bailey and Cushing, who compared cytologic features of gliomas with those of normal-developing neural cells at various stages of differentiation and categorized 14 different types of gliomas. Most modern classifications are based on the same principles; a modification of the latest version of *WHO* classification of brain tumors is illustrated in Table 77-4.[152] A grading system for gliomas was introduced by Kernohan and Sayre, with grade 1 being the most differentiated and grade 4 the least, which also included glioblastoma multiforme. Although this scheme gained popularity among general pathologists because of its simplicity, it has been largely abandoned by many neuropathologists because of its shortcomings. It is paramount that any morphologic classification and hence prognostic implication should take into account clinical parameters such as the location of the tumor and age of patient (Fig. 77-114). For example, vascular proliferation in juvenile pilocytic astrocytoma does not have the same ominous implication as it does in a cerebral fibrillary astrocytoma of an adult.

Astrocytic neoplasms

Astrocytomas along with *glioblastoma multiforme* constitute about 70% of all gliomas. Astrocytomas include diverse subsets with distinct clinicopathologic features. The most common is the group of diffuse (fibrillary) astrocytomas, which account for 90% of all astrocytic neoplasms of the adult cere-

Table 77-4 Classification of CNS tumors

I. *GLIAL NEOPLASMS*
  A. *Astrocytoma*
    1. Diffuse astrocytoma
      a. Differentiated: fibrillary, protoplasmic, gemistocytic
      b. Poorly differentiated: anaplastic (malignant) astrocytoma, glioblastoma multiforme and variants, gliomatosis cerebri
    2. Localized astrocytoma: pilocytic, pleomorphic xanthoastrocytoma, subependymal giant cell astrocytoma, astroblastoma, polar spongioblastoma
  B. *Oligodendroglioma:* oligodendroglioma, "gliofibrillary," anaplastic (malignant)
  C. *Mixed glioma:* oligoastrocytoma, malignant mixed glioma
  D. *Ependymoma:* cellular, fibrillary, clear cell, anaplastic (malignant)
    Variants: ependymoblastoma, myxopapillary ependymoma, subependymoma
  E. *Choroid plexus papilloma, carcinoma*

II. *NEURONAL, MIXED NEURONAL-GLIAL, AND NEUROENDOCRINE NEOPLASMS*
  A. *Primitive:* medulloepithelioma, medulloblastoma and variants, neuroblastoma and variants, primitive neuroectodermal tumors (PNET)
  B. *Differentiating:* central neurocytoma, ganglioglioma/gangliocytoma and variants, dysembryoplastic neuroepithelial tumor (DNET)
  C. *Paraganglioma*
  D. *Esthesioneuroblastoma*

III. *PINEAL NEOPLASMS*
  A. *Parenchymal:* pineoblastoma, pineocytoma, mixed pineocytoma/pineoblastoma
  B. *Germ cell neoplasms and teratomas*
  C. *Glial neoplasms* including glioblastoma multiforme

IV. *SPINAL CORD NEOPLASMS*

V. *MENINGEAL AND MELANOCYTIC NEOPLASMS*
  A. *Meningioma*
    1. Syncytial (meningothelial), fibroblastic, transitional, psammomatous, angiomatous; angioblastic; degenerative and metaplastic change
    2. Malignant—papillary; atypical
  B. *Meningeal sarcoma:* fibrosarcoma, mesenchymal chondrosarcoma, and others
  C. *Melanocytic neoplasms:* melanocytoma, malignant melanoma, melanotic neuroectodermal tumor

VI. *VASCULAR NEOPLASMS:* hemangioblastoma, hemangiopericytoma.

VII. *NERVE SHEATH NEOPLASMS:* schwannoma, neurofibroma

VIII. *HEMATOPOIETIC NEOPLASMS:* non-Hodgkin's lymphoma and others

IX. *GERM CELL NEOPLASMS AND TERATOMAS*

X. *MALFORMATIVE AND NONNEOPLASTIC MASS LESIONS:* craniopharyngioma; epidermoid and dermoid cysts (benign cystic teratoma); arachnoid cyst; colloid cyst of third ventricle; lipoma; pineal cyst.

XI. *SECONDARY NEOPLASMS*
  A. Locally invasive; chordoma
  B. Metastatic

XII. *REMOTE EFFECTS OF SYSTEMIC MALIGNANCIES (PARANEOPLASTIC SYNDROMES)*

XIII. *THERAPEUTIC COMPLICATIONS OF NERVOUS SYSTEM NEOPLASMS*
  A. Radionecrosis
  B. Radiation-induced neoplasms
  C. Adverse drug reactions

brum. Currently, this group is graded into a three-tiered system that is based on the principles of the Ringertz classification.[153] It identifies astrocytomas, anaplastic (malignant) astrocytomas, and glioblastoma multiforme. The histologic criteria include increasing degrees of cellularity, nuclear and cytoplasmic pleomorphism, mitotic activity, endothelial prominence and proliferation, and necrosis. Foci of tumor necrosis (not individual cell necrosis) in an otherwise typical anaplastic astrocytoma justifies the diagnosis of glioblastoma and its correspondingly grim prognosis. A recent four-tiered numerical grading (St. Anne—Mayo) was introduced; it recognizes four histologic variables: nuclear atypia, mitoses, endothelial proliferation, and necrosis, each of which is weighted on the scale of one. According to this scheme 0 variable = grade 1, 1 variable = grade 2, 2 variables = grade 3, and 3 or 4 variables = grade 4. The system seems to be easily reproducible and effective in predicting outcome; the higher the scores, the worse is the prognosis.[154] All grading systems have proved to be suc-

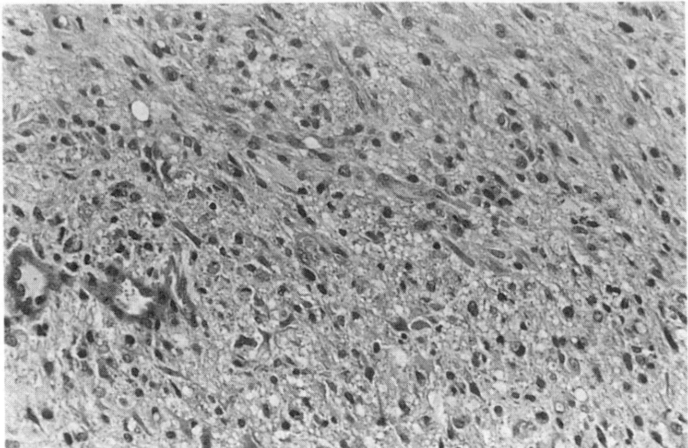

Fig. 77-119 Anaplastic astrocytoma. Moderate anaplasia and prominent endothelial cells.

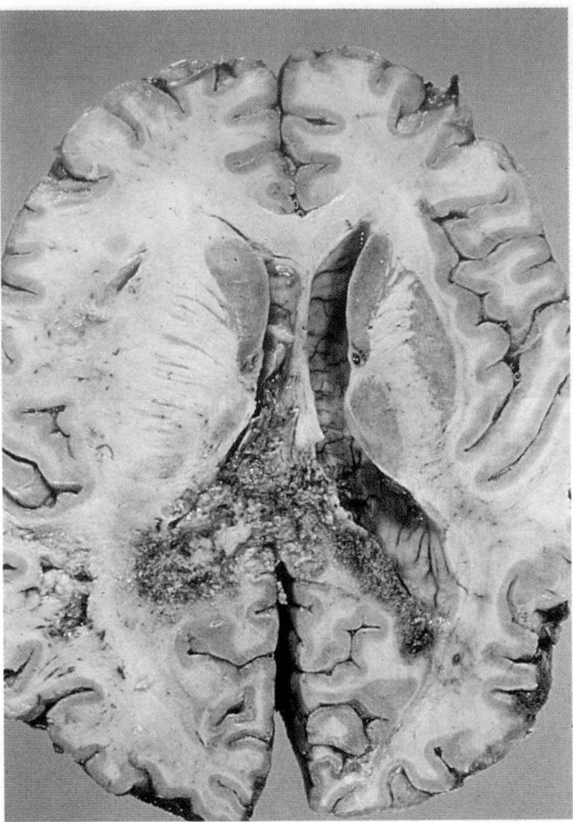

Fig. 77-120 Glioblastoma multiforme involving the splenium of corpus callosum and spreading into adjacent hemisphere.

years after the diagnosis. *Anaplastic (malignant) astrocytomas* arise usually in the fourth or fifth decade of life in diffuse astrocytomas. Recent neuroimaging techniques may detect such transformation when foci of contrast enhancement begin to appear in previously nonenhancing astrocytomas. At autopsy these foci correspond to patchy areas of necrosis and vascular proliferation, which may be multifocal or restricted to one region of the tumor. The cut surface is more granular and friable, and the border is better demarcated than that in astrocytomas. Microscopically, these tumors are moderately to highly cellular. The degree of anaplasia is moderate to severe, and, accordingly, nuclear pleomorphism and the nuclear-to-cytoplasmic ratio vary considerably (Fig. 77-119). Mitoses, including abnormal forms, may be present. The cytoplasm may be scant or abundant, and occasional giant cells may be seen. They usually retain the fibrillated background characteristic of all astrocytomas. The tumor is vascular, and a variable degree of endothelial prominence and proliferation may be seen. Only necrosis separates the very anaplastic astrocytomas from glioblastoma multiforme. The indices of cell replication and cycling, such as BrdU, Ki-67, and proliferating cell nuclear antigen expression (PCNA), are increased.[158] *Secondary structures of Scherer,* which consist of collections of neoplastic cells around neurons and blood vessels and especially in the subpial zone are commonly observed, sometimes beyond the margin of the anaplastic astrocytoma. The prognosis of malignant astrocytomas is grave but slightly better than that of glioblastoma. Postoperative survival rates range between 1½ to 3 years.

Glioblastoma multiforme accounts for 10% to 20% of all intracranial neoplasms and are most commonly seen in the fifth and sixth decades. Like anaplastic astrocytomas they are said to occur *de novo* or arise within astrocytomas; in about 6% of cases they are multicentric.[159] The cerebral hemispheres are the most frequent sites, but in infants and adolescents in whom glioblastomas are rare, they tend to occur in the brainstem. The neoplasm expands the involved region and often extends across the corpus callosum to the opposite hemisphere, assuming the classic "butterfly" distribution (Fig. 77-120). Hemorrhages and necrosis are common and account for its variegated colors. Microscopically the tumor cells exhibit uniform or diverse cytologic features with a wide range of anaplasia. The neoplastic cells may be small and spindly, the "microcellular variant," or large, bizarre, and multinucleated, the "monstruocellular

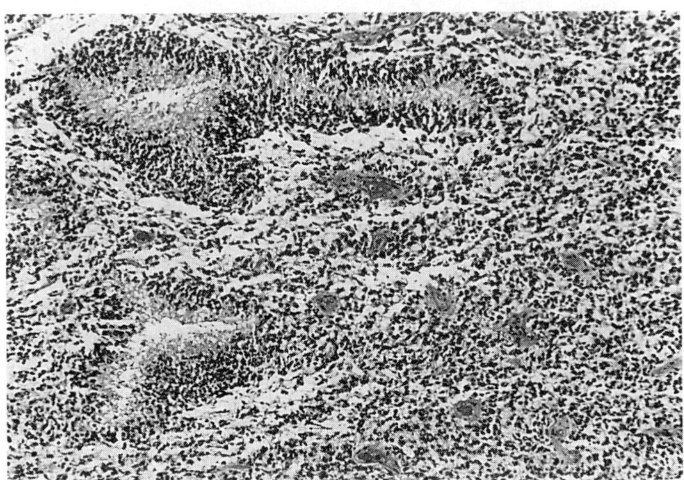

Fig. 77-121 Glioblastoma multiforme, microcellular variant. Neoplastic primitive cells palisading around necrotic foci and admixed with hyperplastic tufted vessels.

variant." More often the tumor is made up of heterogeneous anaplastic glial cells, many resembing astrocytes, and others reminiscent of oligodendrocytes and ependymal cells. Necrosis and vascular proliferation are the hallmarks of glioblastoma. Tumor necrosis ranges from minute foci to large geographic areas, and the viable primitive cells are often positioned perpendicularly to these foci, pseudopalisading or palisading (Fig. 77-121). The vascular changes manifest as hypertrophy and hyperplasia of the endothelial cells of capillaries, forming

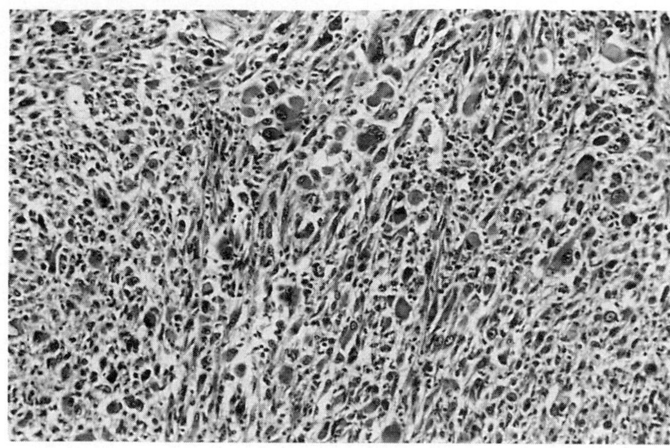

Fig. 77-122 Gliosarcoma. Pleomorphic spindle cells (fibrosarcoma).

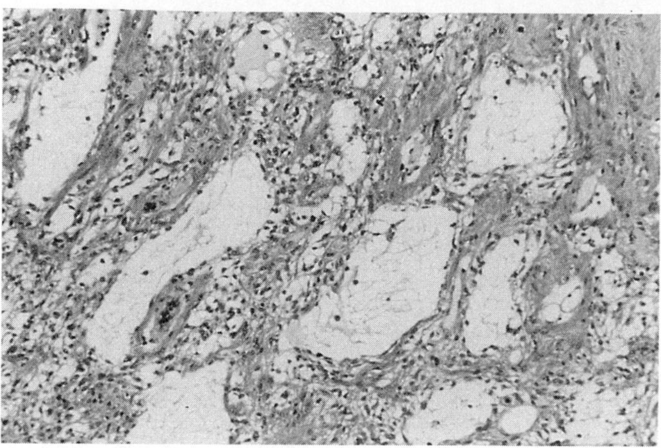

Fig. 77-124 Juvenile pilocytic astrocytoma. Loosely arranged stellate cells alternating with densely packed elongated (pilocytic) cells.

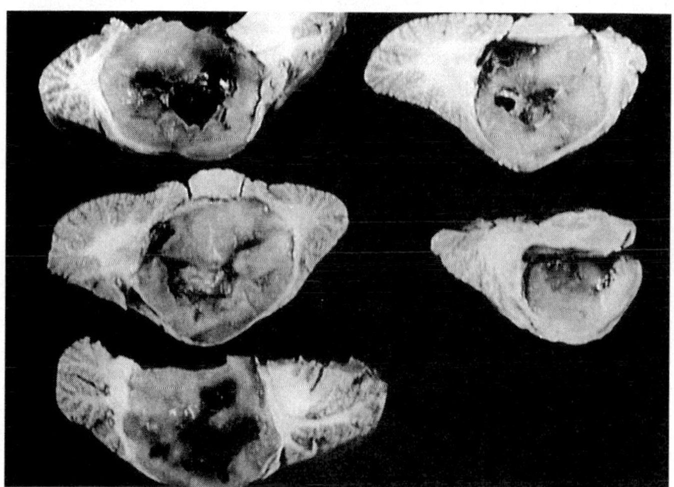

Fig. 77-123 Cystic cerebellar astrocytoma originating in the hemisphere and partially filling the fourth ventricle.

masses resembling glomerular tufts. Sometimes pronounced proliferation of large blood vessel walls is observed, many of which contain fibrin thrombi. The mechanism that leads to this exuberant neovascularization in glioblastomas remains unknown, but several endothelial growth factors with angiogenic activity, such as vascular endothelial growth factor, have been suggested to play a major role.[160] In some glioblastomas the adventitial fibroblasts (or smooth muscle cells) of vessels acquire malignant potential, and the tumor is converted to a mixed glioma and sarcoma, a "gliosarcoma." The glial component is sometimes overshadowed by the sarcomatous element (Fig. 77-122), and staining for GFAP may be necessary to demonstrate residual neoplastic glial cells. Gliosarcoma has a predilection for the temporal lobe and appears as a firm, lobulated mass. When attached to the dura, it may be mistaken for meningioma or meningeal sarcoma; when intraaxial it can mimic a metastatic neoplasm. The prognosis for glioblastomas and gliosarcoma is dismal; survival rates range from 6 to 18 months.

Gliomatosis cerebri is a diffuse neoplastic transformation of usually poorly differentiated astrocytes over wide fields.[161] The process predominantly involves hemispheric white matter causing minimal destruction to neural parenchyma. The condition may occur at any age and is fatal.

Astrocytic neoplasms, mostly circumscribed and occurring in younger age groups. Pilocytic astrocytomas usually occur in children and young adults and are most frequently seen in the cerebellum and midline structures, namely, the optic nerve and chiasm (optic gliomas), the walls of the third ventricle (infundibuloma), and less frequently in brainstem and spinal cord. Their occurrence in the cerebral hemispheres, notably in the temporal lobes, is more common in young adults. They are fairly well localized and lobulated. Cyst formation is especially common in cerebellar tumors (Fig. 77-123). The cyst may replace most of the vermis or hemisphere, and the tumor is often relegated to a small mural nodule. Two subsets are distinguished: the circumscribed "juvenile" form and a less discrete "adult" form. Juvenile pilocytic astrocytomas are characterized by areas of tightly packed pilocytic astrocytes alternating with areas of loosely arranged stellate cells (Fig. 77-124). The pilocytic astrocytes are fusiform with elongated processes that immunoreact for GFAP, whereas the stellate cells show variable reactivity. Microcysts coalescing into large cysts are common. Mitoses are usually absent, and any nuclear pleomorphism or multinucleation is regarded as degenerative. In childhood cerebellar astrocytomas, clusters of cells reminiscent of oligodendrocytes and fibrillary astrocytomatous areas can be seen. Vascular proliferation with tufting and localized leptomeningeal spread may be present, but contrary to diffuse astrocytomas these have no prognostic significance. A striking feature is the presence of granular eosinophilic bodies and Rosenthal fibers, which are intensely eosinophilic sausage-shaped profiles. Rosenthal fibers, however, also may be seen in reactive gliosis. The prognosis of juvenile pilocytic astrocytomas, especially of cerebellum, is excellent. Most patients survive 20 years or longer. Adult pilocytic astrocytomas are formed of delicate elongated nuclei with thin bipolar hairlike fibrillar processes usually arranged in a fascicular pattern. Microcysts and Rosenthal fibers are usually absent. They have a less favorable prognosis than the juvenile type because they tend to infiltrate adjacent brain and hence occupy an intermediate position between juvenile pilocytic and adult diffuse astrocytomas.[2] *Pleomorphic xanthoastrocytomas (PXA)* usually occur in young subjects with a long history of seizures and have a predilection for the temporal lobes. They are

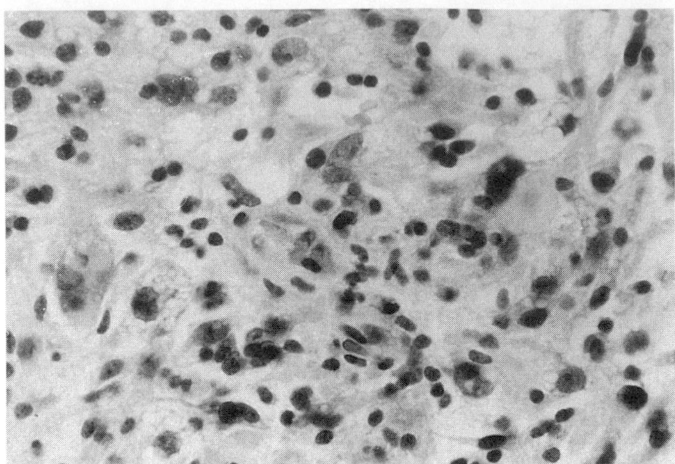

Fig. 77-125 Pleomorphic xanthoastrocytoma.

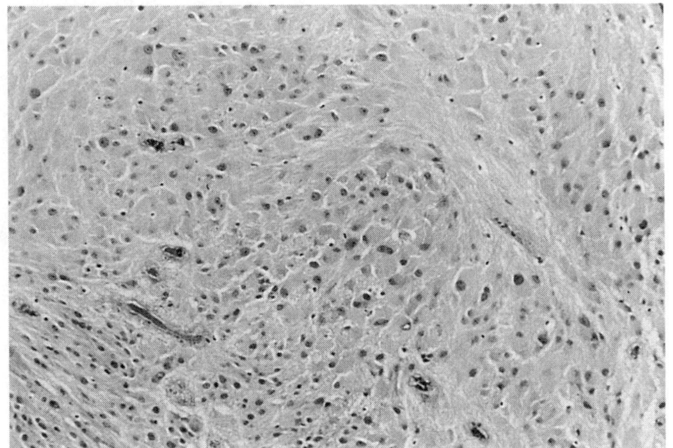

Fig. 77-126 Subependymal giant cell astrocytoma.

superficially located with involvement of both cortex and overlying pia-arachnoid, often are associated with cysts, and typically are yellow and firm. Microscopically, the tumor is densely cellular and, as the name implies is formed of pleomorphic cells that range from large globoid to spindle shaped with a variable number of lipidized cells (Fig. 77-125). The tumor is rich in reticulin that invests individual cells or nests of cells. Perivascular focal collections of lymphocytes are common. The large cells often display hyperchromatic bizarre nuclei or are multinucleated.[162] Mitoses and necrosis are rare and, if both are conspicuous, may indicate an unfavorable outcome in this otherwise relatively slow-growing neoplasm. It has been proposed that this tumor is derived from subpial astrocytes, which normally are covered by basal lamina, explaining the abundance of reticulin. GFAP immunoreactivity of the neoplastic cells is variable. *Subependymal giant cell astrocytomas* usually are seen during the first two decades of life in association with tuberous sclerosis. Occasionally they can occur in the absence of obvious stigmas of the disease. They seem to originate from the nodular lesions, candle gutterings, of the lateral ventricles and often obstruct the foramen of Monro. Histologically they are vascular, and focal calcifications are common. They are formed of large fusiform or strap-shaped cells with abundant hyaline eosinophilic cytoplasm. Broad processes emerge from the cells and produce a coarsely fibrillated background. The cells are usually arranged in pseudorosettes around vessel walls (Fig. 77-126). The nuclei are often eccentric and moderately pleomorphic, and rare mitoses may be present. The tumor cells may or may not express GFAP immunoreactivity, and hence their astrocytic derivation remains a matter of debate. They are relatively benign, but their presentation is often sudden because of obstruction of CSF; only a few recur after resection.[163] *Astroblastoma*[164] is a rare tumor usually occurring in the cerebral hemispheres during the first three decades. Microscopically it forms a discrete mass and is characterized by club-shaped cells with short, thick processes loosely arranged around hyalinized blood vessels. The nuclei are often angulated and hyperchromatic, and such features help distinguish astroblastomas from ependymomas with their characteristically uniform oval nuclei. The tumor cell processes are strongly immunopositive for GFAP. In its pure form the prognosis may be more favorable than diffuse astrocytomas. *Polar spongioblastoma*[165] is a rare childhood neoplasm with a predilection for the walls of the third and fourth ventricles. The neoplastic cells are finely fibrillated with their nuclei closely apposed and arranged in palisades. Usually the cell processes do not stain for GFAP. Because of the rarity of this tumor, the biologic behavior is unsettled.

Other glial neoplasms

Oligodendrogliomas account for approximately 10% of all gliomas. They are tumors of middle age and are found most commonly in the deep frontotemporal white matter. They tend to grow toward the surface and infiltrate the cortex. They are relatively well defined, gelatinous, and grayish and may display cysts, focal mineralization, necrosis, and hemorrhages. Microscopically the tumor is made up of sheets of round cells with closely apposed, well-defined cell borders imparting a "honeycomb" appearance to the tumor. Typically the nuclei are round and have delicate chromatin and small nucleoli. The cytoplasm is often clear if the tissue is not promptly fixed producing the characteristic perinuclear haloes, "fried-egg cells" (Fig. 77-127). In less typical cases, cytologic variations such as elongation of cells, nucleomegaly, nuclear palisading, and mucoid degeneration may

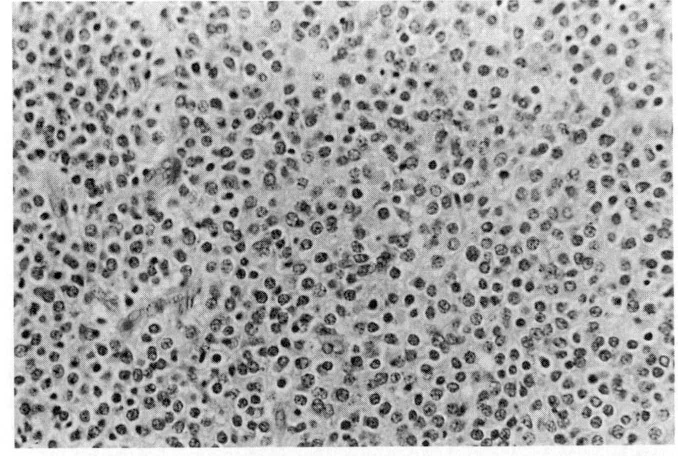

Fig. 77-127 Oligodendroglioma with round nuclei, perinuclear halos, and delicate capillaries.

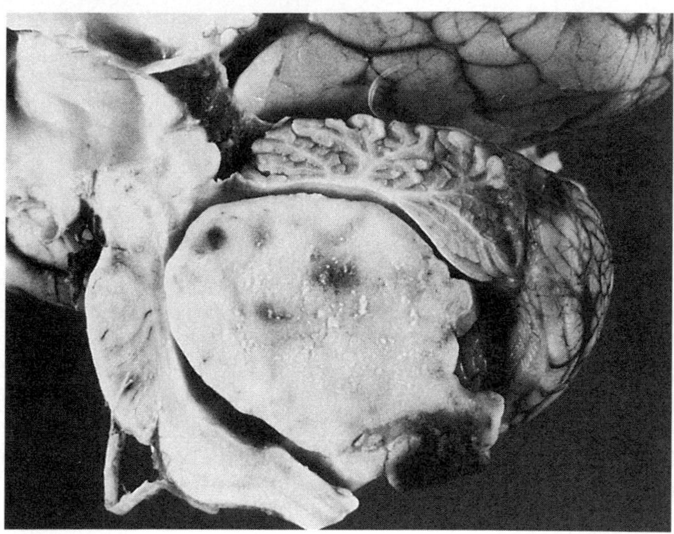

Fig. 77-128 Ependymoma of the fourth ventricle.

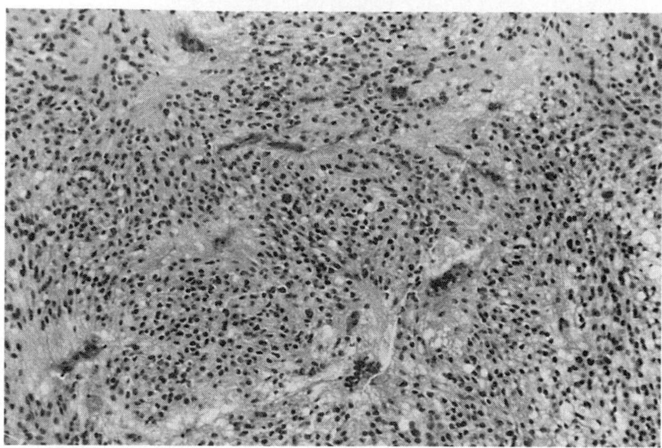

Fig. 77-129 Cellular ependymoma. Nuclei arranged equidistant from the vessels with intervening fibrillary zones.

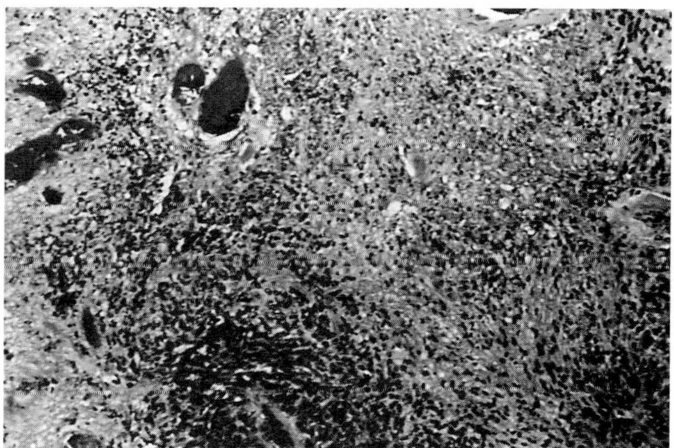

Fig. 77-130 Malignant ependymoma. The tumor is hypercellular and hemorrhagic and contains foci of early necrosis.

cause difficulties in establishing the diagnosis of oligodendroglioma.[10] Typically the tumor cells do not stain for GFAP; however, in a subset, the "gliofibrillary oligodendroglioma," they do display strong GFAP immunoreactivity of both cytoplasm and their sparse, diminutive processes.[166] These cells should be distinguished from reactive astrocytes, which have extensive long processes and are often seen scattered in an oligodendroglioma. Gliofibrillary oligodendrogliomas should also be separated from mixed glioma, "oligoastrocytomas," in which two distinct populations of oligodendroglioma and astrocytoma, often gemistocytic, are found in juxtaposition. Secondary structures of Scherer, particularly satellitosis, are common. A delicate "chicken-wire" network of capillaries intersects and divides the tumor into vague lobules. Endothelial proliferation, if present, is not necessarily a feature of malignancy as in diffuse cerebral astrocytomas. Occasionally, a prominent vascular element may account for spontaneous massive hemorrhage in the tumor, a complication that is infrequently observed in other gliomas. Calcospherites and calcifications of the blood vessels occur in 90% of cases and appear in plain x-ray films of the skull in 40% of patients. Sometimes, calcification is so dense that it partially obliterates the tumor. In neuroimaging studies, oligodendrogliomas usually appear as well-demarcated hypodense areas and show enhancement only if vascular proliferation is present. Grading of oligodendroglioma has proponents as well as detractors. One classification that assigned four grades, *A* to *D*, according to the severity of pleomorphism and cell density, has shown a significant correlation between grades and patient survivals. The mean survival rate of patients in category *A* was 94 months, whereas that in *D* was 17 months, approximating that of glioblastoma multiforme.[167] Others have identified mitoses, necrosis, and vascular proliferation as unfavorable histologic features associated with shorter survival.[2] *Anaplastic (malignant) oligodendroglioma* exhibit many or all of the abovementioned findings,[2,168] and the most malignant is often indistinguishable from glioblastoma multiforme.

Ependymomas constitute 4% to 6% of gliomas at all ages and about 10% of those occurring in childhood and adolescence. They occur anywhere along the ventricular lining; 60% to 70% are infratentorial. The fourth ventricle is a favorite site where it usually arises from the floor as a globular to lobulated exophytic mass. It may protrude from the roof foramina and partially encircle the brainstem (Fig. 77-128). Supratentorial ependymomas, however, tend to expand within adjacent brain rather than grow in the ventricles. Less common sites are the cerebellopontine angle, posterior third ventricle, and aqueduct. Ependymomas are the most common intraspinal tumors. Ependymomas differ from astrocytomas in that they are better demarcated from surrounding neural tissue, a feature that lends to better surgical eradication. Hence this diagnostic distinction, especially in the spinal cord, usually will dictate the extent of the neurosurgical resection. Histologically the most common variant is the "cellular" type, which consists of sheets of unvarying neoplastic cells that align themselves around blood vessels, forming "perivascular pseudorosettes" (Fig. 77-129). The nuclei lie equidistant from the vessel, and fibrillated processes occupy the intervening zones. Sometimes the fibrillation may be very pronounced (tanycytic) and mimic pilocytic astrocytomas, which can make their intraoperative recognition extremely difficult for the pathologist. In a smaller number of cases, certain populations of the neoplastic cells have epithelial features and display prominent blepharoplasts and line canaliculi or cleftlike spaces—"ependymal rosettes." Occasionally, the tumor acquires papillary features, "papillary ependymoma," or the cells display perinuclear halos, the "clear cell" type, which mimics oligodendroglioma. The nuclei of ependymomas are round to ovoid and contain abundant chromatin; in well-differentiated ependymomas they display little pleomorphism and infrequent mitoses. In *anaplastic (malignant) ependymomas,* however, cellular density, pleomorphism, and mitotic activity are increased; the tumor displays vascular proliferation and areas of necrosis (Fig. 77-130). Metaplastic areas of cartilage and bone are sometimes observed in ependymomas. Immunoperoxidase studies have shown that about 60% to 70% of ependymomas are GFAP positive, and a smaller percentage express vimentin and S-100. The epithelial areas may be immunoreactive for EMA (epithelial membrane antigen). Electron microscopy of the ependymal rosettes show microvilli and cilia occupying the central space and zipper-like (zonulae adherentes) junctional complexes joining the neoplastic cells. The prognosis of ependymomas is difficult to predict, except to say that long-term survival is better in "noninvasive tumors" when completely excised and in adolescents than in infants.[169] For example, spinal forms do well with complete removal, whereas those in the fourth ventricle of infants do poorly. Some authors have found no correlation between the histologic features of increased anaplasia and length of postoperative survivals,[170] whereas others have reported significant differences in survivals between low-grade and high-grade tumors. The role of radiotherapy in improving life-span after surgery and in prevention of CSF dissemination of the ependymoma is controversial. *Subependymomas* usually are small asymptomatic nodules in the fourth and lateral ventricles incidentally found at autopsy, usually in older patients. They are sharply demarcated, lobulated and sessile, or pedunculated tumors. Sometimes they are multiple. Depending on their location and size, they become symptomatic by obstructing CSF fluid and causing hydrocephalus. The tumor consists of nests of uniform ependyma-like to astrocyte-like cells separated by a dense and relatively anuclear glial meshwork; in some cases microcysts dominate the tumor (Fig. 77-131). Transitional forms bridging features of subependymoma and ependymoma are uncommon except in some symptomatic cases.[171] *Myxopapillary ependymoma* is a distinct subset that almost exclusively occurs in the filum terminale and may secondarily involve the conus medullaris and the nerve roots of the cauda equina. It is usually seen in the third and fourth decade. It forms a large nodular sausage-like midline mass that insinuates and surrounds the nerve roots. The histologic appearance of the tumor can be quite variable. Classically the neoplastic ependymal cells are often cuboidal and circumferentially arranged around a hyaline to myxoid acellular matrix that contains a vessel at its center. The number of fibrillated processes is variable (Fig. 77-132). Occasionally, segments of the tumor are replaced by mucin or collagen. The prognosis after total resection of the tumor is excellent. Recurrences or remote metastases develop when the tumor is incompletely excised or when bone is eroded.[2] *Ependymoblastoma* should be distinguished from anaplastic ependymomas. They are bulky, embryonal, primitive tumors almost exclusively occurring in childhood. Although fairly well demarcated macroscopically, they notoriously invade surrounding tissues and disseminate along CSF pathways. Histologically this cellular tumor has well-formed canals, clefts, and rosettes lined by

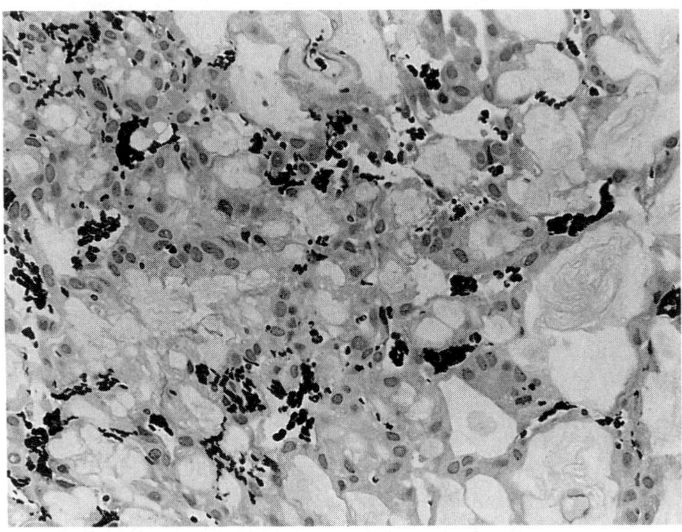

Fig. 77-132 Myxopapillary ependymoma with perivascular mucinous spaces partially bordered by tumor cells.

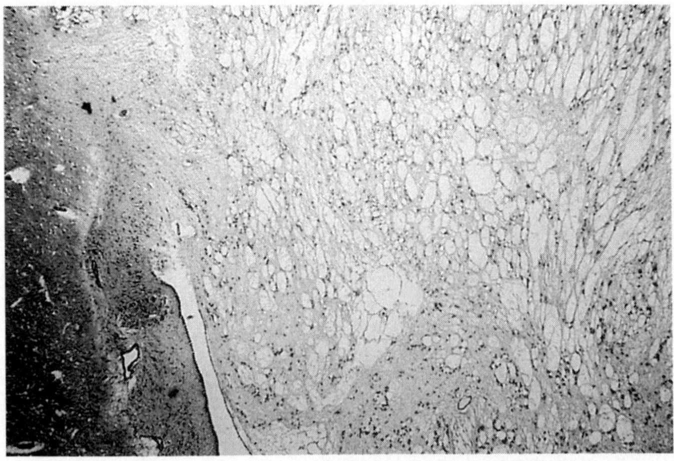

Fig. 77-131 Subependymoma. Sharp demarcation, exophytic growth into ventricle, and unusually prominent microcysts.

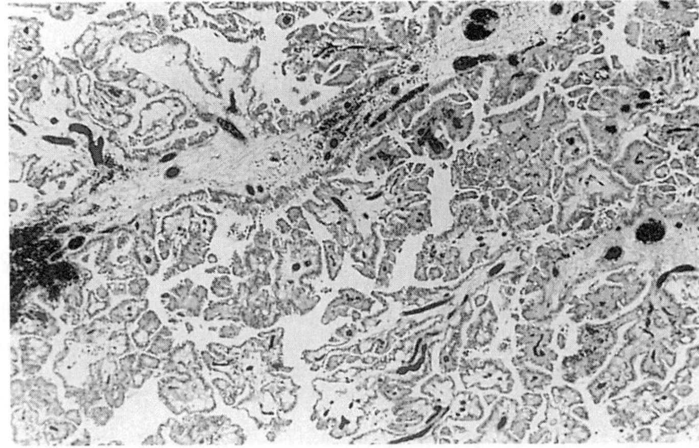

Fig. 77-133 Choroid plexus papilloma.

ependymal cells that are multilayered with many mitotically active cells. Unlike anaplastic ependymomas, the interstitial cells in ependymoblastomas are made up of primitive undifferentiated small cells, and ependymal pseudorosettes are often absent. Most patients die within a year.[10]

Choroid plexus papillomas and carcinomas are rare neoplasms accounting for less than 1% of all glial tumors. They have a predilection for the lateral ventricles in children and the fourth ventricle in adults. Hydrocephalus is the most frequent presenting manifestation because of either hypersecretion or obstruction of CSF pathways by the tumor. The tumor has a granular surface, "cauliflower-like," and expands the cavity that it occupies. Histologically it recapitulates the features of the choroid plexus, except that the cells lining the fronds are crowded and mildly pleomorphic (Fig. 77-133). The choroid plexus frond has a fibrovascular core that distinguishes it from the glial core of papillary ependymoma. The epithelial cells usually show the presence of cytokeratin, transthyretin, and S-100, and infrequently they may exhibit focal GFAP immunoreactivity. When the cells lining the fronds acquire increasing anaplastic features and mitotic activity, the tumor is called "choroid plexus carcinoma." Sometimes a poorly differentiated plexus carcinoma is difficult to distinguish from metastatic papillary carcinoma. Transthyretin expression and the demonstration of cilia with 9 + 0 pattern by electron microscopy may help in identifying choroid plexus tumors. The prognosis for resected choroid plexus papilloma is excellent, whereas that of choroid carcinoma is guarded.[172]

Differential diagnosis. Classic presentations of common glial neoplasms pose few diagnostic problems; however, the histologic features may not be fully expressed in some cases, especially if the specimen is small or the tumor is hypercellular and patternless. Nuclear morphology, tumor background, and vascular arrangement and thickness can, in such cases, offer some clues in the distinction between various glial neoplasms. In astrocytomas, the nuclei are angulated with focal coarse chromatin, the background is a feltwork of fibrillary processes, and the vascular thickening and hyperplasia is commensurate with the degree of hypercellularity of the tumor. In ependymomas, the nuclei are round or oval with fine, evenly distributed chromatin. The background is also fibrillated, but, unlike astrocytomas, the cell processes are aligned more regularly and retain their polarity for blood vessels. In oligodendrogliomas, differentiated and well-fixed nuclei are round with delicate chromatin, the background is less fibrillated and may display segments of myelinated fibers, and the vessels usually retain their reticular pattern irrespective of the hypercellularity of the tumor. Immunocytochemistry, however, has become a necessary tool in the identification of more difficult cases, but specific markers for ependymal or oligodendroglial cells still are unavailable. In most astrocytomas, GFAP immunoreactivity is consistently expressed by the neoplastic cells, whereas this feature is present in only 60% of ependymomas and exceptionally in oligodendroglioma (gliofibrillary variant). EMA is expressed only in a small percentage of ependymomas but not in astrocytomas or oligodendrogliomas. Electron microscopy is only occasionally used for further characterization of a glial tumor. For example, demonstration of cilia and zipper-like intercellular junctions distinguishes a clear cell ependymoma from an oligodendroglioma, and the presence of secretory granules and synaptic junctions help separate cerebral neurocytomas from oligodendrogliomas. Sometimes a glial neoplasm exhibits more than one cell type, a "mixed glioma" such as oligoastrocytoma. Especially in "mixed malignant gliomas" the composition may be more varied.[173]

Occasionally anaplastic glial tumors, notably glioblastoma multiforme, have to be distinguished from metastatic anaplastic carcinomas and CNS lymphomas. The sharp demarcation between tumor and surrounding neural tissue; the cohesive epithelial character of the tumor cells; the absence of fibrillary background, vascular proliferation, and pseudopalisading of neoplastic cells around necrotic foci; and the expression of EMA and cytokeratin markers, but not GFAP, are features that characterize metastatic carcinoma. CNS lymphomas are distinguished by the angiocentric distribution of neoplastic cells associated with strands of reticulin in the Virchow-Robin spaces and by the expression of leukocyte common antigen and other lymphoid markers (especially B cells). Acute demyelinating lesions with exuberant and often atypical astrogliosis may be confused with anaplastic astrocytomas but are characterized by lipophages, relative preservation of axons, and almost total absence of myelin.

Neuronal, mixed neuronal-glial, and neuroendocrine neoplasms

Medulloepithelioma, medulloblastoma, and *neuroblastoma* are designated in the WHO classification as embryonal and cytologically pleuripotential tumors. However, they are discussed here because neuroblastic differentiation is frequently observed in these tumors. *Medulloepitheliomas* are rare childhood tumors recapitulating the embryonic medullary epithelium. The tumor cells are aligned on a basement lamina forming bands, cords, or vague tubular elements. The cells have hyperchromatic nuclei and numerous mitoses. Divergent lines of differentiation, including neuroblastic and ependymoblastic, may be present.[174] *Medulloblastomas*[2,10] account for 7% to 8% of all gliomas and have two peaks of incidence, one at 10 and the other around 22 years of age. Of the pediatric primary intracranial neoplasms, medulloblastomas are second only in frequency to cerebellar astrocytomas. It usually arises in the vermis as a well-demarcated mass that is grayish, granular, and, depending on the extent of necrosis, friable and hemorrhagic (Fig. 77-134). They protrude into the fourth ventricle, infiltrate its floor,

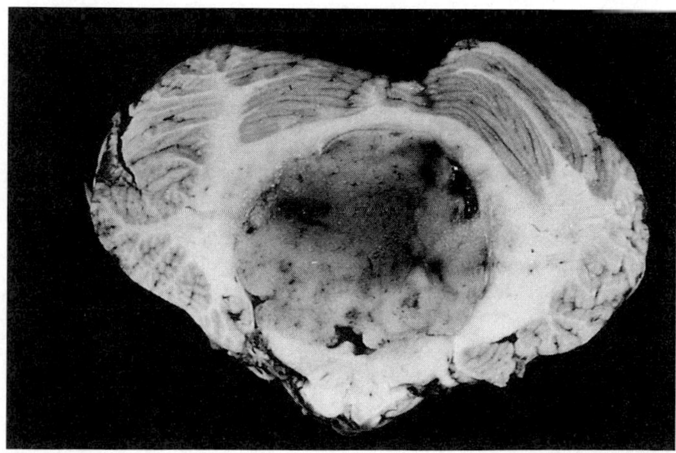

Fig. 77-134 Medulloblastoma with necrotic areas filling the fourth ventricle.

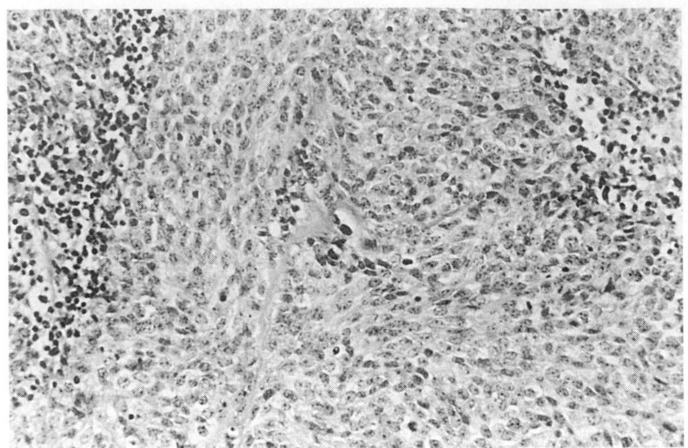

Fig. 77-135 Medulloblastoma. Primitive carrot-shaped cells without visible cytoplasm.

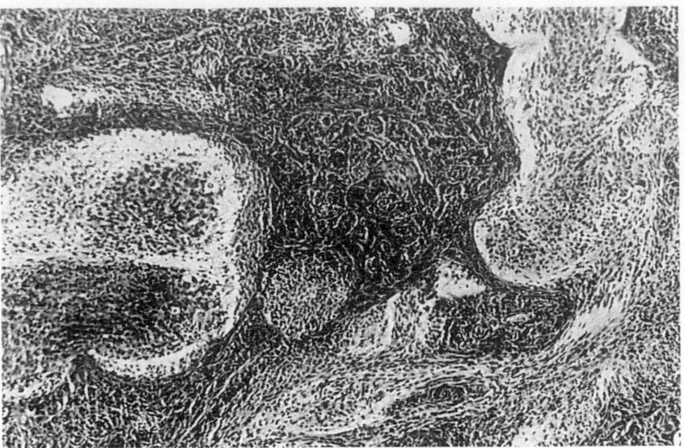

Fig. 77-136 Desmoplastic medulloblastoma. Lobules of densely packed cells alternating with more loosely arranged and better differentiated cells.

and extend into the cerebellar peduncles. In older patients, the tumor tends to be laterally placed in the cerebellar hemisphere and forms a discrete firm mass blending with the overlying leptomeninges. Microscopically, medulloblastomas exhibit highly variable histologic features, most frequently appearing as an infiltrative, extremely undifferentiated, cellular neoplasm. The cells have carrot-shaped or ovoid nuclei with coarse dark chromatin and scant or no visible cytoplasm (Fig. 77-135). Mitoses and necrosis are highly variable. Homer-Wright rosettes, the core of which is formed of tenuous fibrillated processes, may be present. Exceptionally, neurons in various stages of maturation are observed. When numerous, these tumors may be referred to as "cerebellar ganglioneuroblastoma"; when they form a lobulated pattern with cells streaming in a fine fibrillated background, they are designated "cerebellar neuroblastoma." Laterally placed tumors, often exhibit a nodular pattern with reticulin-free islands bordered by reticulin-rich trabeculas, "desmoplastic medulloblastoma" (Fig. 77-136). In a minority of cases "glial (spongioblastic) differentiation" takes place, and the fibrillated areas are immunoreactive for GFAP. Rarely, when undifferentiated myoblasts (strap cells) or darkly pigmented, melanin-containing cells with melanosomes are present, they are referred to as "medullomyoblastoma" and "melanocytic medulloblastoma" respectively. Although positive immunostaining for GFAP is demonstrated in a limited number of medulloblastomas, others show variable or inconclusive immunoreactivity for synaptophysin, neurofilament, S-100 protein, and retinal S-antigen. Irrespective of their patterns and various lines or stages of differentiation, medulloblastomas are highly malignant neoplasms. In recent years, surgical ablation followed by radiotherapy and chemotherapy has improved the length of survival; 75% of patients are reported to be alive 5 to 10 years later.[175] *Cerebral neuroblastomas* are rare tumors of early childhood, often arising in the cerebral hemispheres and growing to large sizes. Histologically, immunohistochemically, and ultrastructurally they can be indistinguishable from medulloblastomas. Despite their high malignant potentials and propensity for CSF dissemination, one large series has reported 5-year survivals in about a third of their cases. *Central neurocytomas*[176,177] are better differentiated yet immature neuroblastic tumors with distinct clinicopathologic findings. They usually occur in the second or third decades and arise from the ventricular wall around the foramen of Monro, septum pellucidum, or corpus callosum. They grow as an exophytic mass into the ventricle causing hydrocephalus. They are formed of uniform cells arranged in a fine fibrillated background, some mimicking oligodendrogliomas and others ependymomas, because they often display perinuclear halos or vascular pseudorosettes respectively (Fig. 77-137). The nuclei are uniformly round with finely dispersed, salt-and-pepper chromatin. Mitoses are rare.

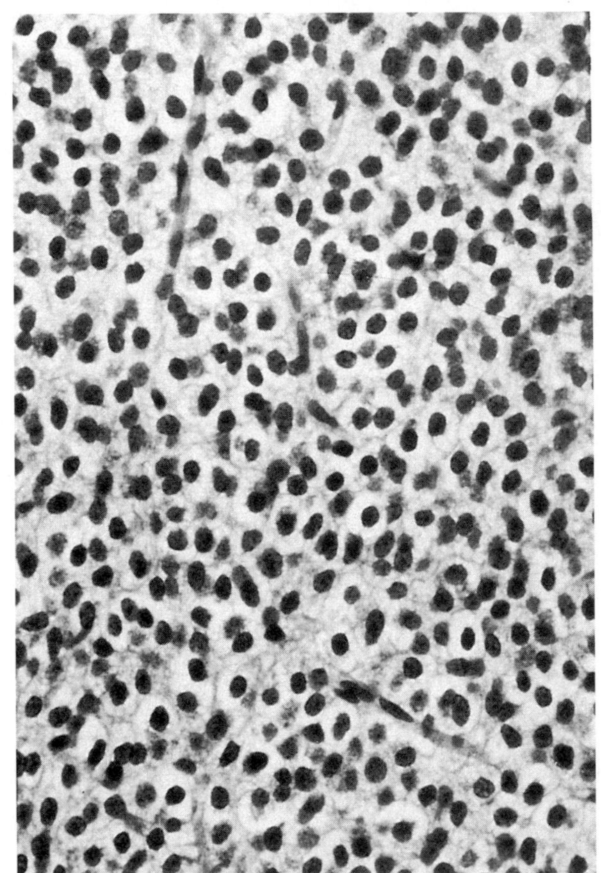

Fig. 77-137 Neurocytoma.

They stain most commonly for synaptophysin and sometimes for neurofilaments.[177] Ultrastructurally the cells and their processes display neurosecretory granules, microtubules, and synapses. Infiltration of the brain at the base of the tumor is limited, and their rate of growth is slow, which accounts for the relatively good prognosis. Those few cases that have exhibited mitoses and features of poor differentiation have behaved like neuroblastomas.

Gangliocytomas (ganglioneuromas) and gangliogliomas are neoplasms containing mature neurons. The term *gangliocytoma* is applied to tumors that are predominantly neuronal with negligible glial component and *ganglioglioma* to those in which glial cells occupy a significant portion of the tumor. The topography of both types is similar, with a predeliction for the temporal lobes, third ventricular region, and frontal lobes. Less frequent sites are the cerebellum and spinal cord. Eighty percent of the cases occur during the first three decades of life; a long-standing history of seizures is a common complaint. Macroscopically they are usually well demarcated, gritty, and cystic. The ganglion cells are of variable size and shape and may have more than one nucleus. They are either clustered or diffusely scattered in an eosinophilic fibrillary matrix. Their perikarya typically show strong synaptophysin and neurofilament immunoreactivity. Ultrastructurally, neurosecretory granules are demonstrated in perikarya and neurites. Gangliocytoma in the hypothalamic region of children often presents with precocious puberty, whereas in adults they frequently are associated with a secretory pituitary adenoma that produces acromegaly, galactorrhea, or both. Dysplastic gangliocytoma (Lhermite-Duclos disease) of cerebellum usually occurs in young adults, mostly males, and is characterized by localized thickening of the folia. Microscopically, the affected folia show some stratification, which includes a superficial layer with parallel myelinated fibers and an intermediate zone of radially arranged fibers associated with abnormal neurons that are most numerous in deeper layers. The abnormal neurons seem to represent either dysplastic granule cells or Purkinje cells.[178] In *ganglioglioma* the variable but significant glial component usually consists of pilocytic astrocytes with mild nuclear pleomorphism, but gemistocytes and cells resembling oligodendrocytes can be encountered. Both gangliocytomas and gangliogliomas display a patchy reticulin network, thick hyalinized vessels, focal lymphocytic infiltrates, particularly around blood vessels, and variable calcifications (Fig. 77-138). Ganglioglioma should be distinguishable from a fibrillary astrocytoma infiltrating indigenous neurons by multinucleation, lack of satellites, and disorientation of the tumor ganglion cells. The prognosis is excellent for gangliocytomas even if partially resected. For gangliogliomas, the prognosis depends on the extent of resection and behavior of the glial element, but prolonged survival is expected.[179] Malignant transformation of the glial element, such as to frank anaplastic astrocytoma, is uncommon. A rare cerebral variant, the *"desmoplastic infantile ganglioglioma,"*[180] occurs in the very young age group and characteristically reaches massive dimensions. It is superficially located and contains small ganglion cells and glia enmeshed in a matrix rich in reticulin and connective tissue.

Dysembryoplastic neuroepithelial tumors (DNET) are lesions first described in resected specimens for epilepsy and usually occur during the first two decades of life. A long-standing history of partial complex seizures is the main complaint. Neuroimaging demonstrates a nonenhancing lesion expanding the cortex without surrounding edema. Microscopically it is formed of nests of loosely arranged small cells resembling oligodendrocytes with occasional randomly scattered neurons in pools of faintly hematoxylinophilic material. DNETs have an excellent prognosis[181] (Fig. 77-139). *Primitive neuroectodermal tumors (PNET)* encompass all poorly differentiated neuroepithelial tumors irrespective of anatomic sites. The term has gained some advocates, but many still prefer to identify these tumors according to their locations and retain such terms as medulloblastomas, neuroblastomas, pineoblastomas. PNET is then restricted to describe primitive neural tumors in unusual sites.

Tumors closely allied to ganglionic neoplasms are the *paragangliomas* and *esthesioneuroblastomas. Paragangliomas (glomus tumors, chemodectomas)* originating in the neuraxis are rare and occur almost exclusively in the filum terminale. Intracranial paragangliomas are usually extensions from paragangliomas arising at the base of the skull from the glomus jugulare, glomus tympanicum, and vagal bodies, usually of middle-aged women. Microscopically the tumor cells

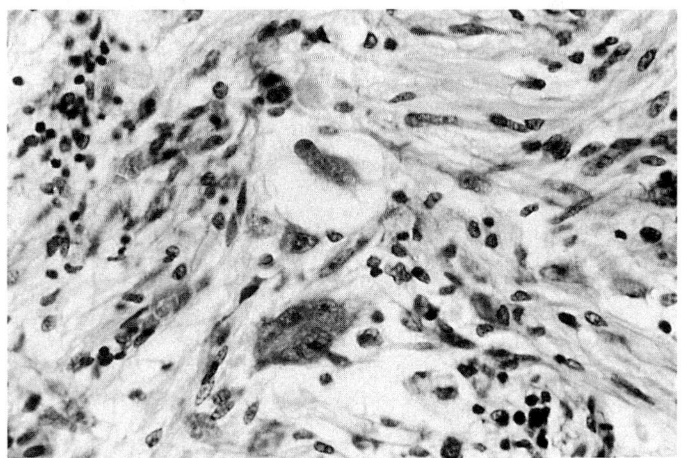

Fig. 77-138 Ganglioglioma. A mixture of randomly arranged, sometimes multinucleated ganglion cells and spindle-shaped astrocytes.

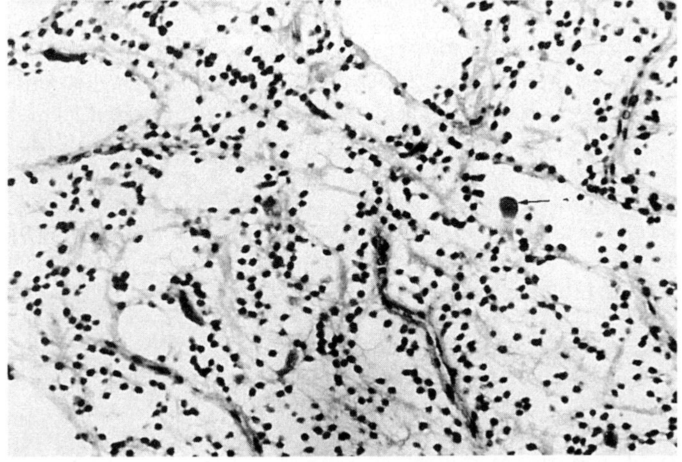

Fig. 77-139 Dysembryoplastic neuroepithelial tumor. Loosely arranged small cells of glioneuronal origin with a mature neuron *(arrow)*.

are arranged in nests separated by delicate capillaries that are readily outlined in reticulin stain (*Zellballen* pattern). Occasionally, this nesting pattern is inconspicuous. The cells are monomorphous and have round-to-oval nuclei with stippled chromatin. Nucleomegaly, pleomorphism, and occasional mitoses do not signify malignancy. Argyrophilic granules and synaptic epitopes (synaptophysin, chromogranin) are easily demonstrated. By electron microscopy, neurosecretory granules are identified in the chief cells but not in the less frequent S-100 positive sustentacular cells. They respond favorably to total surgical ablation, but local recurrences may occur in up to 50% of cases, especially with glomus jugulare tumors, and distant metastases are rare.

Paragangliomas of the cauda equina are often mistaken for an ependymoma because of their location, encapsulation, and perivascular arrangement of the cells. They usually originate from the filum terminale. They are histologically and ultrastructurally similar to their counterparts elsewhere; however, ganglionic and schwannian differentiation are more frequent. *Esthesioneuroblastomas (olfactory neuroblastomas, neuroendocrine carcinoma)* occasionally grow upwards with involvement of the extradural space and eventually the base of the brain. They form lobules or sheets separated by fibrovascular stroma, occasional Homer-Wright rosettes, and rarely Flexner-Wintersteiner rosettes may be identified. They are associated with a fine fibrillated background that may be argyrophilic and display synaptophysin immunoreactivity. Neurosecretory granules can be demonstrated by argyrophilic stains (Grimelius) and by electron microscopy.[182] Esthesioneuroblastomas have a bimodal age distribution with peaks at 20 and 50 years of age. They are slow growing, highly radiosensitive tumors. Total excision of the tumor is associated with longer than 5-year survivals in 50% of patients, and local recurrences respond readily to radiotherapy. Distant metastases do occur in about 20% of cases, but dissemination by the CSF pathways is uncommon. Some cases are difficult to distinguish from nasopharyngeal or metastatic carcinomas.

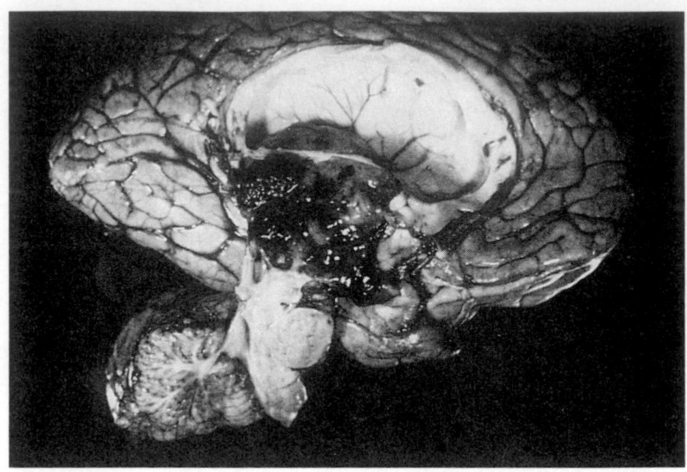

Fig. 77-140 Pineoblastoma. Sagittal section. A large necrotic mass extending from the pineal region into the diencephalon.

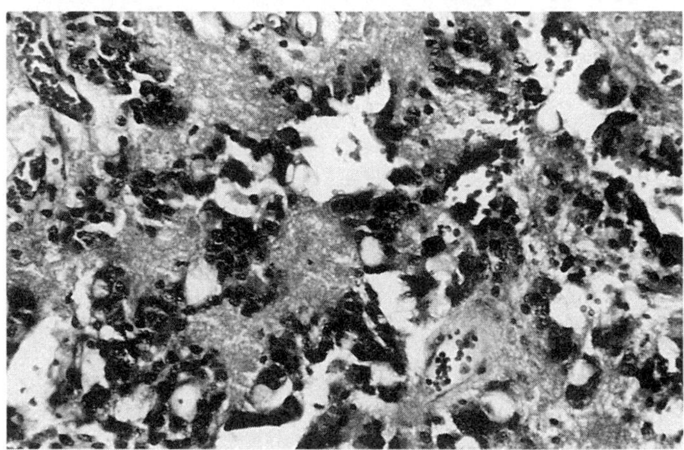

Fig. 77-141 Pineocytoma. Pineocytes forming vague and large rosettes.

Pineal neoplasms

Most of the tumors in the pineal region originate from misplaced germ cells, a few from pineal parenchymal cells, and some from glia. Symptomatic cysts, metastases, meningiomas, primary melanomas, and other rare curiosities may involve the pineal gland.

Being histologically identical to those occurring in gonads, the histologic features of germ cell tumors in the pineal region will not be considered further in this chapter. Suffice it to say, germinomas usually occur during the first three decades of life, mainly in males in the region of the pineal gland, but are equally distributed between sexes in the suprasellar region (ectopic pinealoma). An associated granulomatous response in the former and a mixed lymphocytic-plasmacytic infiltrate in the latter may overshadow the malignant epithelial component. Germinomas are exquisitely radiosensitive, if not associated with more recalcitrant germ cell elements such as embryonal carcinoma, endodermal sinus (yolk sac) tumor, or choriocarcinoma.

Parenchymal tumors traditionally include pineoblastomas and pineocytomas.[147,161] However, the histologic criteria and the biologic behavior of these two tumors are still poorly defined because of their rarity, limited sampling at surgery, and overlapping or mixed histologic findings.[183] Furthermore, individual variations in normal pineal histologic features because of sex and age pose serious difficulties in distinguishing normal pineal from a low-grade parenchymal or astrocytic neoplasm. *Pineoblastomas* usually occur in children and young adults (Fig. 77-140). Such tumors are composed of poorly differentiated cells having the cytologic and histologic features of a medulloblastoma. Homer-Wright rosettes may be identified in some and Flexner-Wintersteiner rosettes indicating retinoblastomatous differentiation in others. Rarely, "fleurettes" recapitulating photoreceptors and melanocytic cells may be present. Although they are extremely radiosensitive, the prognosis is poor on account of recurrences and propensity to seed the subarachnoid space. *Pineocytomas* tend to be more localized and slower-growing than pineoblastomas. They are formed of relatively mature uniform cells. The cells are arranged in sheetlike or lobular patterns with intervening paucicellular fibrillated zones forming large rosettes (Fig. 77-141). Neuronal or glial differentiation may be seen in exceptional cases, and the tumor therefore acquires features of a ganglioglioma. The prognosis is variable but considered more favorable than that of pineoblastomas.[183,184]

Spinal cord neoplasms

Intrinsic (intramedullary) spinal tumors account for about 20% of all spinal tumors and are mostly gliomas, especially ependymomas and astrocytomas; glioblastomas and oligodendrogliomas are uncommon. The incidence of ependymomas is higher than astrocytomas, particularly if myxopapillary ependymomas of the filum terminale are included. In children, however, astrocytoma is more frequent.[185] *Intraspinal astrocytomas* are classified and graded like their counterparts in the brain.[186] They can occur anywhere along the length of the cord, but the thoracic segment is the most frequent site. They diffusely infiltrate the parenchyma, resulting in fusiform enlargement of the cord. Occasionally, they are associated with secondary syringomyelia, especially if they are low grade. The median survival is about 2 years for the well-differentiated tumors and less than a year for glioblastomas. *Primary leptomeningeal astrocytomas* are exceptionally rare and are assumed to arise, like their counterparts in the intracranial cavity, from heterotopic glial nests in the leptomeninges. *Intraspinal ependymoma,* excluding the myxopapillary variant, are mostly fibrillary. They frequently involve the dorsal columns, extend over several segments of the cord, and are well demarcated from surrounding tissues. It is therefore critical at frozen section to distinguish between ependymoma and astrocytoma, since this may determine whether the neurosurgeon will proceed with total excision of the ependymoma or terminate the operation of an astrocytoma. Syrinx formation proximal and distal to the tumor is common and may be lined by pilocytic astrocytes with Rosenthal fibers. Occasionally intraspinal ependymomas are multifocal, especially in patients with von Recklinghausen's disease.

Nonglial neoplasms and nonneoplastic mass lesions

Except for germ cell tumors and teratomas, most primary types are predominantly extra-axial neoplasms of adults. The commonest are the meningioma (15% of intracranial tumors and 25% of intraspinal tumors) and schwannoma (about 8% to 10% of intracranial tumors and 30% of intraspinal tumors).[10]

Meningeal and melanocytic neoplasms

Meningioma[2,10,187] is a neoplasm of middle-aged adults; the much less common (about 8% to 10%) spinal examples display a pronounced female predominance (10:1). There may be an increased association with breast cancer, and hormone (particularly progesterone) receptors have been identified. The latter may explain why meningiomas occasionally have growth spurts during pregnancy. About half of the cases show a characteristic monosomy 22, which they share with schwannoma. The central form of neurofibromatosis (NF type 2) shows genetic linkage to chromosome 22; meningiomas and schwannomas (often multiple) are the most common types of CNS tumors in this disease. Recent genetic mapping studies indicate a linkage to the NF type 2 locus for sporadic meningiomas.[188] Trauma, in particular from previous radiation therapy, also has been implicated in their causation.

Meningiomas arise from leptomeningeal arachnoid cells, which are most concentrated in the parasagittal arachnoid (pacchionian) granulations and dural sleeves of the spinal canal. In addition to these two dural sites, the sphenoid wing (often flattened or en plaque), tuberculum sellae (suprasellar and intrasellar), olfactory groove, optic nerve, tentorium cerebelli, falx, and especially the convexity of the cerebral hemispheres are common sites for these discrete, dura-based, firm growths (Fig. 77-142). The thoracic region is the commonest spinal location, and lumbosacral examples are distinctly uncommon. Intraventricular (tela choroidea), intraosseous and even extracranial or extraspinal examples are rare. The common histologic subtypes: syncytial (sheets of cells), fibroblastic (spindle cells in a fascicular or storiform pattern), and transitional (syncytial and fibroblastic with whorls and psammoma bodies) (Fig. 77-143) often are admixed and of no prognostic significance. A predominant psammomatous pattern may be more common in the spinal canal; the fibroblastic type may be difficult to distinguish from schwannoma, pilocytic astrocytoma, or fibrous histiocytoma. The classical histologic pattern manifests as cells with ovoid, large (in comparison to astrocytes) pale nuclei, with vacuoles or cytoplasmic invaginations (often propitiously exaggerated in frozen sections), and inconspicuous cytoplasmic borders; the cells are arranged concentrically (whorls) around calcified blood vessels or connective tissue (psammoma bodies). They typically display scant mitotic activity and atypia without necrosis; vascularity may be conspicuous in the angiomatous type or the disputable "angioblastic" variant (see the discussion of vascular neoplasms below). They are indolent in their growth but commonly invade dura, bone, or dural sinuses. Although the last does not herald metastatic potential, it is responsible for most of the recurrences (about 15% in 5 years) after surgery because of incomplete resection. Meningiomas usually contain little stromal reticulin, except in fibroblastic areas; most meningiomas are immunoreactive for vimentin and epithelial membrane antigen (EMA) and less commonly for cytokeratin and S-100 protein.[189] Ultrastructurally, meningioma cells have abundant intermediate filaments (vimentin and cytokeratin), some glycogen, desmosomal attachments and interdigitating cytoplasmic processes with focal external laminae (basement membranes).

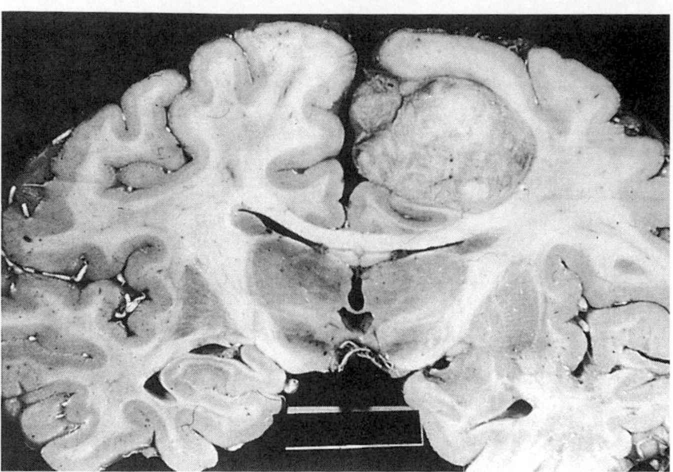

Fig. 77-142 Meningioma of falx (not shown).

Several degenerative, reactive, or metaplastic changes may complicate the recognition of its meningeal origin: myxomatous, xanthomatous, lipoblastic, osteoblastic, chondroid, chordoid, microcystic, secretory, and inflammatory (lymphoplasmacytic).[187]

Malignant meningioma. The criteria for histologic malignancy in meningiomas are imprecise, but hypercellularity, high

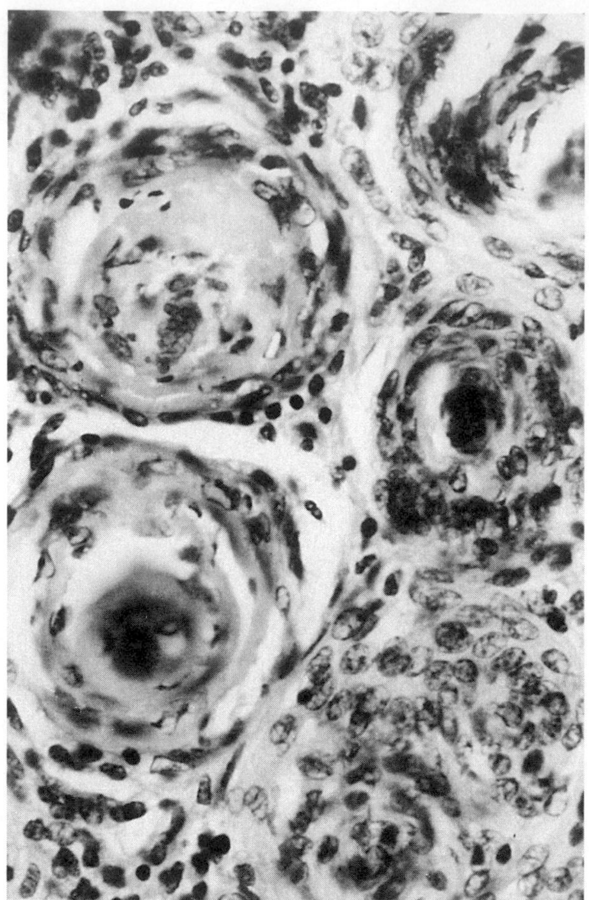

Fig. 77-143 Meningioma. Whorls and psammoma bodies.

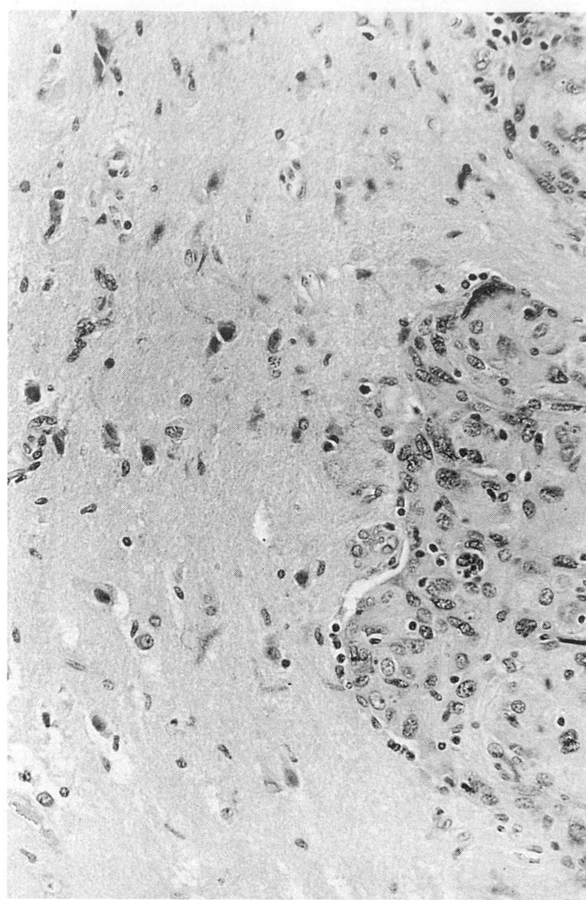

Fig. 77-144 Malignant meningioma invading brain parenchyma.

mitotic activity, tumor necrosis, and especially invasion of pristine brain parenchyma warrant this appellation (Fig. 77-144), which predicts early recurrence and rarely CSF seeding or distant metastases.[2,10,161,187] The papillary and hemangiopericytic patterns have been added to these criteria.[152] The qualifier of "atypical" or "aggressive" meningioma is used even more subjectively but usually when only one or two of these general criteria are encountered.

Meningeal sarcoma. The term *meningeal sarcoma* is usually restricted to the rare fibrosarcoma or pleomorphic (polymorphic) sarcoma arising in meninges but not from a preexisting meningioma; they tend to occur in infants and young children and disseminate widely by means of the CSF.[147] Mesenchymal chondrosarcoma, with its distinctive admixture of atypical chondroid and undifferentiated cellular areas, occasionally arises in the cranial or spinal dura of children or young adults. Both meningeal fibrosarcoma and mesenchymal chondrosarcoma have been reported after irradiation.

Melanocytic neoplasms. Melanocytic neoplasms include the continuum of better differentiated and behaved melanocytoma (many of which have been referred to as "melanotic meningioma") and primary malignant melanoma of the leptomeninges.[10] These may occur in association with pigmented skin lesions, usually in children (neurocutaneous melanosis), or isolated in the central nervous system. Pigmented or melanotic schwannoma, neurofibroma, ependymoma, choroid plexus papilloma, and medulloblastoma have been reported. The pigmented or melanotic neuroectodermal tumor of infancy (melanotic prognoma, retinal anlage tumor), most commonly seen in the jaw, may involve the cranial vault or rarely the brain parenchyma. It approximates the melanotic medulloblastoma histologically but has a more benign biologic behavior than medulloblastoma.

Vascular neoplasms

Hemangiopericytoma and hemangioblastoma are the common types, but angiosarcoma and epithelioid hemangioma rarely involve the CNS or its coverings.[2,10] *Hemangioblastoma* or *capillary hemangioblastoma* occurs most frequently as an intra-axial lesion of cerebellum or brainstem (representing about 10% of posterior fossa neoplasms) and spinal cord in young adults (20 to 50 years). They may be multiple in patients with Lindau's disease or associated with the same lesion in retina (von Hippel's disease). The autosomal dominant (chromosome 3) von Hippel-Lindau disease also includes nonneoplastic cysts of kidney, liver, and pancreas, pheochromocytoma, and renal cell adenoma or carcinoma. Renal cell carcinoma histologically mimics hemangioblastoma, sometimes necessitating immunohistochemical (low molecular weight cytokeratins or epithelial membrane antigen, EMA) or ultrastructural assistance, especially in these patients. Grossly, hemangioblastoma usually is well demarcated and both cystic and solid; many consist of a solid yellow to red mural nodule in a cyst of yellow to brown fluid. The solid component or mural nodule (known for its contrast enhancing quality on CT or MRI and rich vascularity on angiogram) consists of hypercellular endothelium-lined

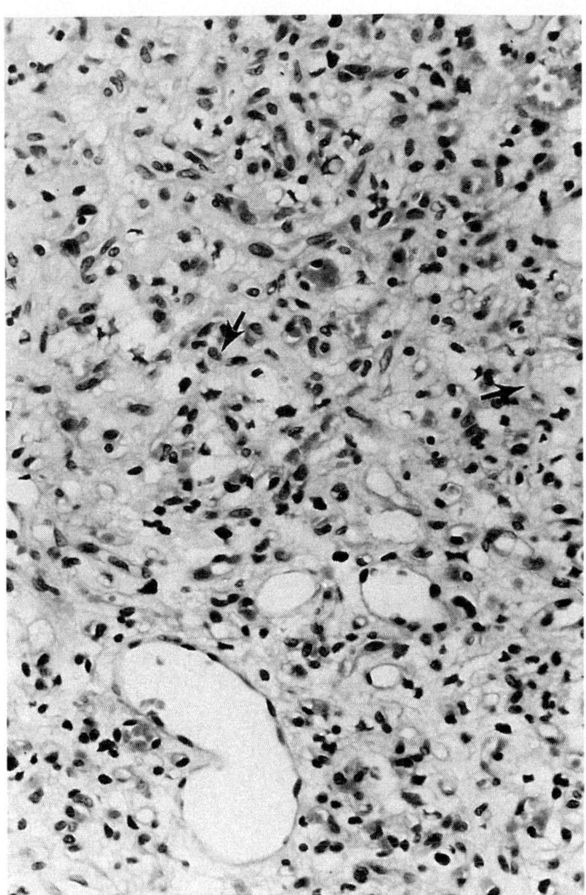

Fig. 77-145 Hemangioblastoma with multiple small blood vessels and vacuolated stromal cells *(arrows).*

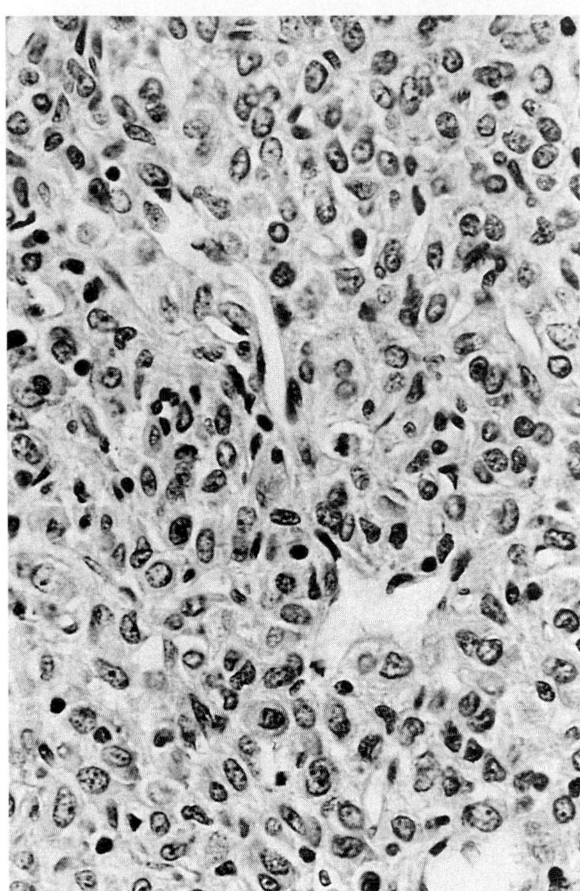

Fig. 77-146 Hemangiopericytoma with monomorphic elongated nuclei and dilated vascular spaces.

small to dilated vascular channels (difficult to appreciate on frozen section), pericytes, and variable numbers of stromal cells (Fig. 77-145). The origin of the stromal cells is still unsettled, but their cytoplasm contains variable amounts of neutral or sudanophilic lipid, scant glycogen, and intermediate filaments recognized by antibodies to vimentin and occasionally to GFAP.[2] They are not immunoreactive for EMA or factor VIII. Stromal cells are not mitotically active, but many display considerable pleomorphism. The cyst wall is lined by indolent to exuberant astroglial cells, often with Rosenthal fibers, which may simulate low-grade astrocytoma. Variable numbers of GFAP positive-reactive astrocytes may be found at the edge of or within the neoplasm. Extramedullary hematopoiesis and erythropoietin production occasionally may be present. Supratentorial examples, which may be attached to dura, generally occur in patients with von Hippel-Lindau disease. Hemangioblastomas infiltrate parenchyma to some degree and recur after incomplete surgical removal. Isolated supratentorial, usually dura-based, lesions have been considered by some to be variants of the angioblastic meningioma as originally described by Cushing and Eisenhardt.[10]

Hemangiopericytoma. Even more controversy has existed over the relationship of this lesion to another variant of angioblastic meningioma (hemangiopericytic) as originally described by Bailey, Cushing, and Eisenhardt.[10] Current opinion favors its separation,[2,152,190,191] but one should recall that several neoplasms can display hemangiopericytoma-like areas.[192] Regardless of their nosologic placement, all agree that these are aggressive neoplasms with high recurrence rates (averaging about 50% in 5 years) and even metastases (about 20%). Most are intracranial and occur in adults (30 to 50 years). Although their sites of occurrence are the same as those of meningioma, their histologic, immunohistochemical, and ultrastructural features are more similar to the soft-tissue hemangiopericytoma (reticulin rich; immunoreactive for vimentin but not EMA or cytokeratins;[191] lacking desmosomes and gap junctions). Grossly, these are firm and vascular, usually attached to dura; microscopically they are cellular neoplasms with variable mitotic activity and prominent "staghorn" sinusoids or perivascular fibrosis (Fig. 77-146). There is some evidence that increased anaplasia allows one to predict increased aggressivity (median survivals of 62 months versus 144).[190] As in hemangioblastoma, the vascular channels may be inapparent in frozen sections.

Nerve sheath neoplasms

The *schwannoma,* usually of the vestibular branch of the acoustic (VIII) nerve (acoustic schwannoma, acoustic neuroma) or the trigeminal (V) nerve, constitutes about 8% to 10% of intracranial tumors; those arising on spinal (usually sensory or posterior) roots are responsible for about 30% of spinal tumors. Multiple central schwannomas, including bilateral acoustic, are diagnostic of neurofibromatosis type 2. Intracranial *neurofibromas* are rare. Full coverage of this topic is provided in Chapter

78. A practical consideration is that the acoustic schwannoma often exhibits a predominance of the Antoni type B pattern, mimicking glioma, whereas the spinal forms have more Antoni type A, simulating fibroblastic and transitional meningioma or pilocytic astrocytoma. Schwannoma also can occur within brain parenchyma and resemble an adult pilocytic astrocytoma.[193] Cytic degeneration and hemorrhages are common. Dorsal root ganglia, located in the dural sleeves at intervertebral foramina, should not be confused with neoplastic processes.

Hematopoietic neoplasms

Hodgkin's disease, solitary plasmacytoma, multiple myeloma, Waldenström's macroglobulinemia, plasma cell granuloma or pseudotumor, Langerhans' cell histiocytoses, hemophagocytic lymphohistiocytosis, and sinus histiocytosis with massive lymphadenopathy (Rosai-Dorfman disease) uncommonly involve the CNS or more frequently the meninges.[2,10] Leukemias, particularly acute lymphocytic or lymphoblastic, commonly involve the nervous system as infiltrations (usually leptomeningeal), as hemorrhages (all compartments) and rarely as a solid mass or chloroma.[10] Meningeal relapse has been greatly reduced by prophylactic CNS irradiation and chemotherapy. The major hematopoietic lesion to involve the CNS is *primary non-Hodgkin's malignant lymphoma* (perithelial sarcoma, microglioma, reticulum cell sarcoma), particularly in the setting of HIV infection and AIDS, where Epstein-Barr virus has been pathogenetically implicated.[194] Primary CNS lymphomas usually are of B-cell phenotype, diffuse large cell (intermediate grade) or immunoblastic (high grade), and involve brain parenchyma, primarily cerebral periventricular and deep gray structures (Fig. 77-147). Its histologic hallmark is thick perivascular cuffs of monomorphous neoplastic lymphoid cells with concentric layers of reticulin admixed with variable numbers of macrophages, plasma cells, reactive lymphocytes, reactive to atypical astrocytes, and elongated microglial cells; this results in a polymorphous lesion. They are often multifocal (almost invariably in AIDS) and highly infiltrative like astrocytoma, including corpus callosum. A peripheral sample may simulate an inflammatory process or an astrocytic neoplasm, particularly in frozen sections. Touch or smear preparations may be of great assistance at this time. Prolonged preoperative corticosteroid therapy may eradicate the neoplastic cells, leaving only the reactive elements behind for misinterpretation. Immunohistochemical reagents suitable for formalin-fixed, wax-embedded specimens has facilitated diagnostic accuracy, even on necrotic specimens. Intravascular lymphoma, previously known as *malignant hemangioendotheliosis,* where the infiltrate is confined to vascular lumens and usually generalized, commonly produces CNS signs or symptoms as a result of multiple small hemorrhages or infarcts. Secondary or generalized malignant lymphoma, other than the intravascular type, tends to involve leptomeninges more than the parenchyma.

Germ cell neoplasms and teratomas

Germ cell neoplasms and teratomas are rare and usually found in the midline (pineal gland, tuberculum sellae, or sacrococcygeal region) of young males. They may occur with or without teratomatous elements, which may be cystic or solid, mature or immature, benign or malignant.[2,10]

Malformative and nonneoplastic mass lesions

Craniopharyngioma has been considered the most common (about 3% to 4% of primary intracranial tumors) example of

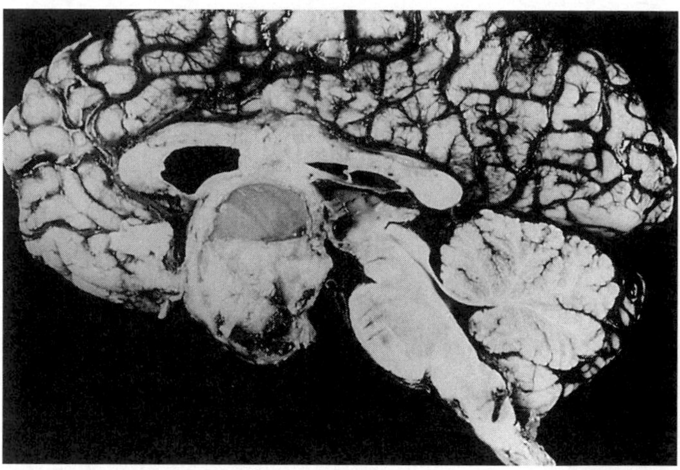

Fig. 77-148 Craniopharyngioma with cystic and solid components.

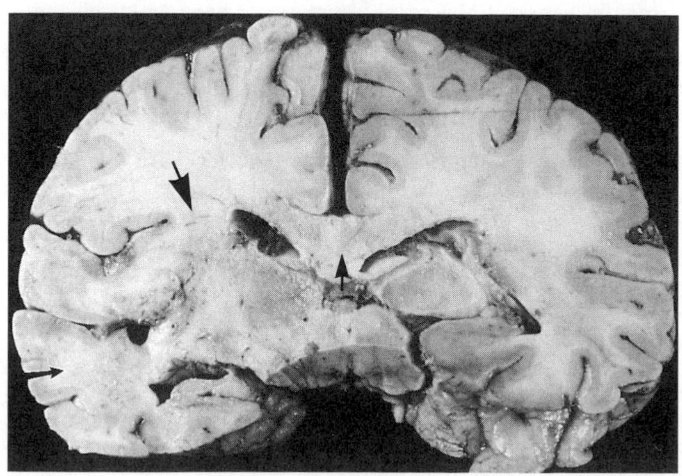

Fig. 77-147 Primary CNS lymphoma *(large arrow)* with involvement of corpus callosum *(small arrow).*

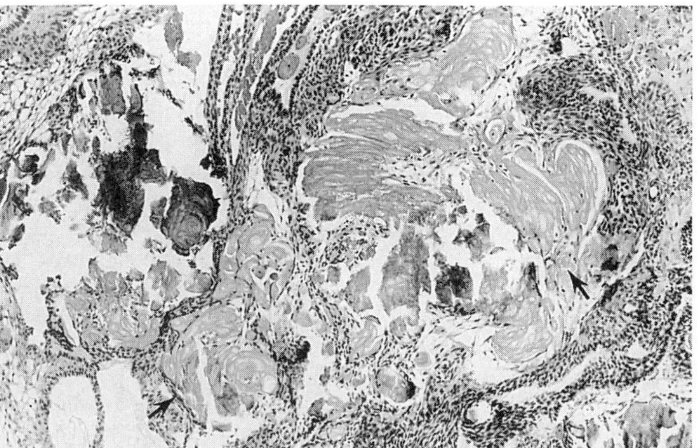

Fig. 77-149 Craniopharyngioma with keratinaceous bodies *(arrows),* calcification, basaloid epithelium, and mesenchymal stroma.

this category;[147] however, it looks and behaves as a neoplasm, and malignant transformation has been reported once.[195] This encapsulated or at least well-demarcated neoplasm is almost restricted to the sellar region (suprasellar and intrasellar) and may be cystic (resembling motor oil fluid) or more commonly cystic and solid (Fig. 77-148). The cell of origin is still unsettled, but most consider a remnant of Rathke's duct or primitive oral stomatodeum as a likely ancestor.[10] The most common type, seen in children and calcified, is referred to as *adamantinomatous;* it has a histologic similarity to adamantinoma of the jaw and to another odontogenic tumor, the keratinizing and calcifying odontogenic cyst.[2] This type of craniopharyngioma is a cellular neoplasm with a columnar to basaloid cell layer, which often palisades on a collagenous stroma of stellate cells, and keratinaceous ghosts (Fig. 77-149). The epithelium of this type typically insinuates itself into the floor of the third ventricle, where it elicits a peculiar astrocytic response rich in Rosenthal fibers simulating a pilocytic astrocytoma (Fig. 77-23). This involvement of the base of the brain may lead to incomplete removal and recurrence, which has been greatly reduced since the advent of the operating microscope. Although some of the clinical manifestations may be attributable to this "infiltration," most are compressive in origin. Multiple layers of loosely stratified squamous epithelium abut the other side of the basaloid cells. In the cystic areas only a thin layer of stratified squamous epithelium is noted, as in the epidermoid cyst. Both the cystic type[196] and a more solid papillary variant are more typical of adults, calcify infrequently, and recur much less commonly. The rare papillary variant[2] *(suprasellar papillary squamous eptihelioma)* appears to arise within the third ventricle and is composed of well-differentiated stratified squamous epithelium lacking the histologic features of the adamantinomatous type; it may contain foci of columnar epithelium and goblet cells reminiscent of a *Rathke's cleft cyst* (Fig. 77-150). Thus craniopharyngioma may be difficult to distinguish from epidermoid or Rathke cleft cysts in small biopsy specimens. The motor-oil quality of the adamantinomatous craniopharyngioma contrasts with the pearly-white fluid of the epidermoid cyst. The lining and contents of the Rathke cleft cyst more closely approximate the colloid cyst of the third ventricle, though squamous metaplasia of the former may occur.

In addition to a suprasellar location, *epidermoid cysts* more commonly are found off the midline, as in the cerebellopontine angle or diploë of the skull; they uncommonly occur in the spine. *Dermoid cysts* tend to be midline in the cerebellum, the fourth ventricle, or more commonly intraspinal, usually in the lumbosacral region. Both are encapsulated and believed attributable to the inclusion of ectoderm during the closure of the neural tube. Dermoids may be associated with a dermal sinus, and some epidermoids have been caused by the mechanical injection of skin epithelium, as during a spinal tap. The pearly-white and glistening contents of the epidermoid differ from the cheesy to hairy contents of the dermoid, since the dermoid has hair follicles, sweat glands, and sebaceous glands in addition to the simple to stratified squamous epithelial lining. Both usually produce symptoms by compression and displacement, but malignant change rarely has been reported. The spillage of the contents of epidermoids, dermoids, or craniopharyngioma can provoke a chemical granulomatous meningitis.[10]

Another compressive to incidental nonneoplastic lesion is the *arachnoid cyst.* Like dermoids they may be recognized in children or adults but are predominantly intracranial, extra-axial collections of CSF lined by arachnoid cells on a thin collagenous wall (Fig. 77-13). Some restrict this term to congenital malformations of the leptomeninges and do not include posttraumatic or postinflammatory loculations. Of the congenital type, the parasylvian area is the most common site, commonly in association with atrophic or hypoplastic brain, but the cerebellopontine angle and cisterna magna also are common locations. The latter must be differentiated from cystic dilatation of the fourth ventricle (Dandy-Walker malformation).

The *colloid cyst* in the anterior roof of the third ventricle (Fig. 77-151) also is a congenital lesion but derived from misplaced endoderm; it enlarges over time because of the sloughing and secretion of its ciliated to goblet cell–rich pseudostratified columnar lining, which rests on a collagenous capsule. The colloidal contents may contain degenerate hyphae-like structures. Colloid cysts can be small and incidental or highly symptomatic because of blockage of CSF flow and even sudden death. The discussion of rare cysts, such as spinal *enterogenous* and *perineurial cysts* and cranial *ependymal* or *neuroepithelial cysts,* is beyond the scope of this chapter.[2,10]

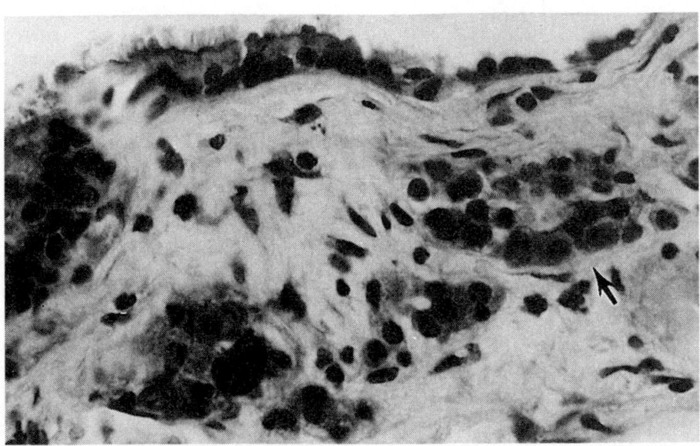

Fig. 77-150 Rathke's cleft-cyst epithelium with ciliated cells; adenohypophyseal cells *(arrow)* in collagenous wall.

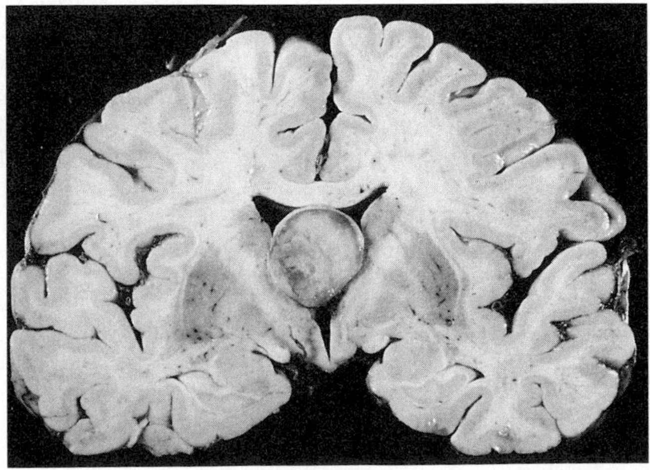

Fig. 77-151 Colloid cyst of third ventricle.

Lipoma, or *lipomatous hamartoma,* is also believed to be attributable to the inclusion of ectopic elements that increase in size slowly over time. Mature fat is the predominant component with variable degrees of fibrovascular tissue; rarely elements of muscle, cartilage, or bone can be seen. They are usually midline, such as those above the corpus callosum (often in association with agenesis) or above the quadrigeminal plate, but they also may be lateral in the cerebellopontine angle or sylvian fissure. Most appear to be incidental, but intraspinal lipomas may be symptomatic when they extend into cord parenchyma.

Secondary neoplasms

Secondary neoplasms may be either locally invasive, such as chordoma, chondrosarcoma, osteosarcoma, paraganglioma, nasopharyngeal carcinoma and esthesioneuroblastoma, or metastases. Of the locally invasive neoplasms only the chordoma is discussed.

Chordoma is a midline, extradural neoplasm of the axial skeleton most common in the clivus (40%) or lumbosacral spinal region. They grow slowly and inexorably, destroy bone, recur, and can metastasize—in about 30% of cases usually after many years. Their gross characteristics range from a firm lobulated and translucent tumor to a mucinous infiltrate. Microscopically the pattern is usually epithelial manifesting as lobules of cells with abundant eosinophilic cytoplasm, often vacuolated because of intracellular (intracisternal) mucin. When the cells are loaded with mucinous vacuoles, the characteristic physaliphorous (bubbly) cells are of great diagnostic utility. When they are not present and the cells are arranged in a trabecular pattern with a prominent myxoid stroma (chondroid), their immunoreactivity with both epithelial (EMA, cytokeratin) and mesenchymal (vimentin) markers helps to distinguish it from myxomatous chondrosarcoma that lacks epithelial epitopes. Both are S-100 positive. Ultrastructural features of epithelial differentiation, such as desmosomes, also are characteristic of chordoma. Malignant "degeneration" usually resembles malignant fibrous histiocytoma.

Metastatic neoplasms to the CNS are hematogenous, often multiple, and predominantly arise from carcinomas of the lung, gastrointestinal tract (particularly colon), breast, kidney, and prostate or from a malignant melanoma. The incidence and prevalence of parenchymal metastases are variable and depend primarily on the nature of the sample (autopsy versus surgical biopsy) and the sex and age of the patient population. All compartments of the CNS and its coverings may be involved; both the location and gross characteristics may help to identify the primary site. In bone and dural metastasis, one should suspect breast, lung, and prostate. Epidural spinal metastasis is suggestive of a lung, breast, prostate, lymphoma, melanoma, renal cell, or myeloma origin. Intraspinal metastases are rare, but lung, breast, renal cell, and melanoma should be considered. Leptomeningeal deposits (meningeal carcinomatosis, carcinomatous meningitis) should prompt a search for a lung, breast, melanoma, or gastric origin. Lung primaries are frequently occult at the time of neurosurgical exploration. Hemorrhagic metastases are characteristic of lung, melanoma, renal cell, and choriocarcinoma, whereas necrotic, particularly umbilicated, metastases are suggestive of a lung, colon, and breast origin.

Parenchymal metastases often are multiple and cerebral, most commonly at the junctions of cortex and white matter in the middle cerebral artery distribution; intraspinal metastases usually involve thoracic cord. Both locations represent the largest area or volume of parenchyma intracranially or intraspinally, respectively. Brain metastases tend to globular and well demarcated with variable degrees of tumor necrosis and hemorrhage (Fig. 77-152); the surrounding brain often displays a pronounced degree of vasogenic edema, neovascularity, and reactive to atypical astrocytosis. The edematous rim may exert greater mass effect than the metastasis itself, but it usually can be effectively treated with drugs, particularly corticosteroids. In contrast to gliomas, mitotic figures are numerous, and large geographic areas of necrosis with perivascular sparing may be conspicuous. The microscopic recognition of their metastatic nature usually is not difficult, but identification of the primary source may be problematic. In such cases, or when the neoplasm is highly undifferentiated, or when a glioblastoma displays prominent epithelial differentiation, immunohistochemical and less commonly ultrastructural evaluation can be of considerable value. Consultation with well-informed clinicians may facilitate and shorten this morphologic search.

Remote effects of systemic malignancies (paraneoplastic syndromes)

A variety of neurologic manifestations may occur rarely in patients with a systemic malignancy, which are not attributable to metastasis, direct infiltration, or compression by the neoplasm.[197] Paraneoplastic syndromes are seen most commonly in association with undifferentiated carcinoma of the lung and ovarian carcinoma. Any area of the neuraxis or neuromuscular system may be affected. The lesions may be inflammatory or noninflammatory with selective neuronal involvement. Suspected pathogenetic mechanisms have included toxic metabolites produced by tumor cells, activation of latent viruses, and immune mechanisms. Most recent evidence indicates that some are caused by host antibodies to tumor antigens that cross react with epitopes on CNS cells, usually neurons, or elements of the neuromuscular system. For example, in a cerebellar degeneration where Purkinje cells are selectively destroyed, antibodies that react with both ovarian carcinoma and Purkinje cells have been identified (anti-Yo) in the serum of some patients.[198]

Therapeutic complications of nervous system neoplasms

In addition to the morbidity and mortality of neurosurgical intervention, chemotherapy and radiotherapy may aggravate

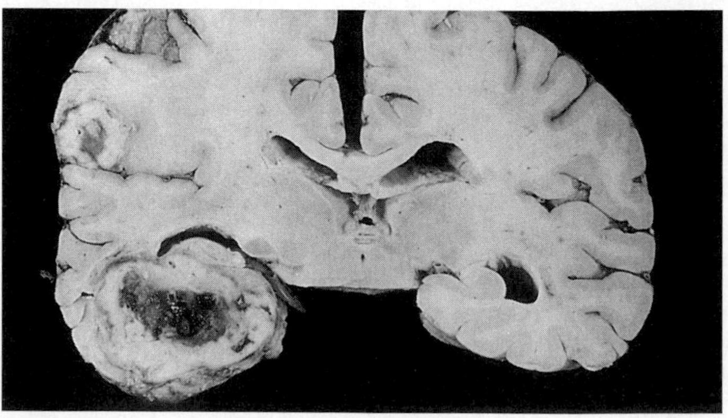

Fig. 77-152 Metastatic carcinoma. Multiple well-demarcated nodules at gray-white junctions.

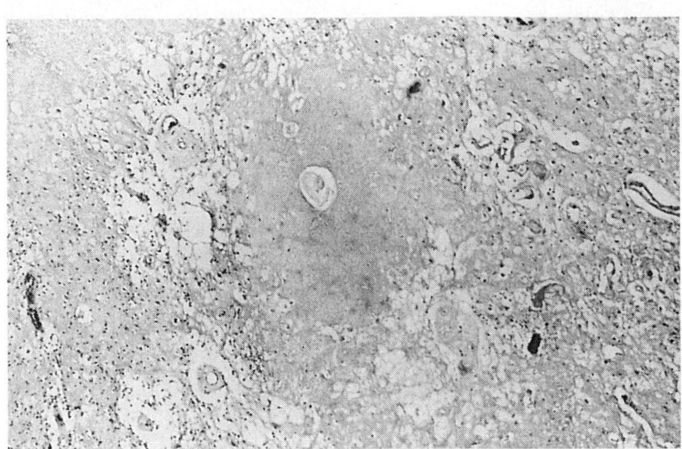

Fig. 77-153 Late delayed radionecrosis. Hyalinized vessels, eosinophilic coagulum, and cystic necrosis of white matter.

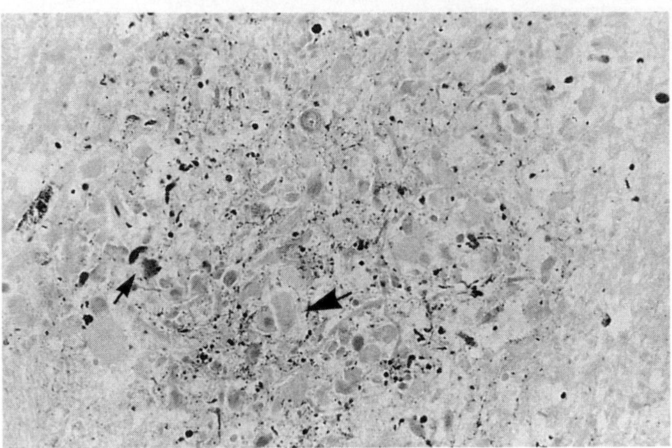

Fig. 77-154 Methotrexate toxicity. Coagulation necrosis of white matter, reactive spheroids (*large arrow*), and mineralizations (*small arrow*).

the patient's tumor-induced disability and mimic a recurrence or extension of the neoplasm.

Adverse morphologic effects of radiotherapy in the nervous system are usually divided into two types: early delayed (about 2 weeks to 3 months after irradiation) and late delayed (about 6 months to several years). In general the PNS is more resistant than the CNS. The destructive dosage depends on a variety of factors, but the approximate permissible dose is 6000 rad for brain and 5000 rad for spinal cord. Early delayed radiation injury is predominantly directed at the myelin, and the CNS lesions are similar to the demyelinative plaques of multiple sclerosis. Late delayed effects are largely directed at CNS blood vessels and result in radionecrosis, or radiation necrosis, of brain parenchyma (Fig. 77-153); the term does not include tumor necrosis, the goal of the radiotherapy. Hyalinization, fibrosis, thrombosis, lipohyalinosis of vessels, and leakage of serum proteins and blood cells are associated with coagulative necrosis (presumably ischemic) of CNS parenchyma. Its major clinical importance lies in the mass effect that this lesion may produce, which simulates a recurrence or increased growth of the neoplasm. Recent imaging techniques, especially positron-emission tomography (PET), may be able to resolve this differential, but at present biopsy and histologic examination usually are necessary.[10]

Radiation-induced neoplasms are the second major adverse reaction to radiotherapy of brain tumors. Rarely, radiotherapy may induce glial neoplasms; more commonly but still infrequently, meningioma, fibrosarcoma, mesenchymal chondrosarcoma, malignant fibrous histiocytoma, and osteogenic sarcoma have been reported. For example, intracranial meningiomas occur in young adults who have been treated with radiation for tinea capitis as children. Generally, low doses have induced benign, whereas high doses have resulted in malignant, neoplasms. Specific criteria for inclusion in this group are that the neoplasm must be (1) within the radiated field, (2) absent before the radiation exposure, (3) confirmed histologically, (4) of a different histologic type, and (5) detected after a latent period of several years (usually 2 to 20).[199]

Adverse neurologic complications of neoplastic drugs are common and include peripheral axonopathies, brain swelling, intracranial bleeds, and so forth. The only one to be discussed here is that classically reported after treatment with methotrexate, with or without radiotherapy of the neuraxis. A well-defined neurologic syndrome of seizures, ataxia, paraplegia, spasticity, dementia, coma, and even death has been related to multifocal areas of white matter necrosis in cerebrum, brainstem, and spinal cord. These foci are characterized by coagulative necrosis of axons, myelin, and oligodendrocytes (Fig. 77-154). Axonal swellings (spheroids), often mineralized, are diagnostic in this setting. This lesion, disseminated necrotizing leukoencephalopathy, may mimic progressive multifocal leukoencephalopathy, lymphoma, or other entities.[10]

DEVELOPMENTAL DISORDERS

The brain is one of the fastest growing organs in the fetus, and its rate of growth is especially rapid during the first semester[200-202] (Table 77-6). Postnatally the increase in size persists at a relatively fast pace, and the brain weight doubles by 9 months. It should be noted, however, that the range in weight at any specific gestational age is wide and altered by factors such as formalin fixation (gaining about 30%), maternal and gestational influences, and intrauterine growth retardation.[203] Adult weights and proportions are reached by the twelfth year.

Embryology. The CNS develops from the midline neural plate on the dorsal surface of the embryo. By the end of the fourth week of gestation, the neural plate is transformed into a tube through growth and fusion of its lateral folds. Closure of the tube follows a rostrocaudal direction. At about 5 weeks, the prechordal mesenchyme induces cleavage of the neural tube into paired telencephalic vesicles, precursors of the cerebral hemispheres. The growth of brain and subsequent increase in weight are accomplished through the rapid division, migration, and maturation of the primitive cells that line the ventricles, the periventricular germinal layer (matrix), and through myelination of white matter. The surface of the immature brain is smooth, but as migrating waves of immature cells reach the cortex, indentations begin to appear on the surface (sulci) and define the future cortical convolutions (gyri). The chronology and pattern of the major fissures and sulci are faithfully maintained throughout the various stages of brain development, and the gestational age of a baby can be accurately determined when one counts the number of gyri or com-

Table 77-6 Brain weights from the twentieth gestational week till birth

Gestational age (weeks)	Brain weight (g)	Body weight (g)	Body length: crown-heel (cm)
20	53 ± 25	380	26
22	73 ± 25	475	29
24	92 ± 30	630	31
26	111 ± 40	800	34
28	139 ± 48	1100	36
30	166 ± 55	1230	38
32	209 ± 45	1750	43
34	246 ± 60	2200	46
36	288 ± 60	2820	48
38	340 ± 50	3100	50
40	380 ± 50	3400	51

These figures represent averages compiled from various sources.[5,200-202]

pares their chronologic appearance to reference charts.[204,205] While the subcortical nuclei are being formed, waves of neuroblasts guided by radial glia reach the cortex and pass by their predecessors, and so the last neuroblasts to reach the cortex will settle nearest the surface. By the fifth month a superficial paucicellular molecular layer and a deeper densely packed cellular layer (plate) are recognized. A month later the six-layered neocortex with differentiating deep pyramidal neurons is established. Myelination begins, proceeding caudorostrally in the spinal cord, with different fiber tracts myelinating at different stages of neural development.[206] In the cerebrum myelination starts soon after birth and the centrum semiovale is well myelinated by the end of the second year.[207] The growth of the cerebellum lags behind that of the cerebrum until the fifth month of gestation after which it is accelerated, and the adult proportion of 10% to 12% of the total brain weight is reached at 18 months postnatally.[208] Foliation begins at about the fourteenth gestational week and rapidly increases in number. The external granule cells, which become discernible about the twenty-fifth week, migrate inwards and develop into internal granule cells. The cells migrating from the germinal matrix lining the rhombencephalon form the cerebellar nuclei and Purkinje cells.

A variety of factors, such as intrinsic germ cell disorders, infections, and environmental teratogens (that is, "stimulus nonspecific") can perturb any of the above stages of development (that is, "time specific"), seriously interfering with subsequent stages of growth and maturation of the CNS and resulting in characteristic developmental anomalies.[209] Furthermore, during the first 6 months of gestation, the immature CNS tends to react swiftly to injury with modest macrophage response and little or no glial proliferation in comparison to the mature brain. Therefore, healing may take place with limited or no glial scarring, depending on the age of the fetus. For the above two reasons, classification of developmental anomalies into congenital and acquired are often unwarranted, since factors as widely disparate as abnormal genetic programming and in utero infection can lead to the same anomaly. For example, aqueductal stenosis in its X-linked inherited form is histologically indistinguishable from that attributable to early intrauterine viral infection. The causes and types of CNS malformations are extensive; only a few of the more common anomalies will be considered.[5,210,211]

Chromosomal disorders

Chromosomal aberrations, particularly trisomies, may be associated with abnormal brains. In *Down syndrome* (trisomy 21 (92%), translocation 14 or 22, or mosaic) the brain is usually small and pear shaped when viewed from the top because of truncated frontal lobes with upward slanting orbital surfaces and flattened occipital poles. The superior temporal gyri are narrow, a characteristic that partially accounts for the nonoperculization of the insulae. The cerebellum is disproportionately smaller than the cerebrum (Fig. 77-155). The microscopic findings are nonspecific, but morphometric studies have demonstrated fewer cortical neurons and in Golgi preparations simplification and reduction of dendritic arbors.[212] Myelination is delayed, particularly when Down syndrome is complicated by congenital heart diseases.[213] Senile changes of Alzheimer type are seen even before 40 years of age. In *Patau's syndrome* (trisomy 13 more than 80% or translocation 14 or mosaic) holoprosencephaly occurs in about two thirds of the cases. In *Edward's syndrome* (trisomy 18 more than 90% or mosaic) CNS anomalies are variable.

Neural tube defects

These malformations are attributed to failure of fusion of the lateral folds of the neural plate *(dysraphism)* or to rupture of a previously closed tube *(neuroschisis)* resulting in secondary maldevelopment of mesodermal structures destined to surround the CNS. However, some have proposed that these disorders result from primary mesodermal failure.[214] The type and extent of the defect are dictated by the stage at which the event takes place.

Anencephaly is the most rostral example of these defects and develops about the twentieth day of gestation, at a time when the neural tube begins to close in a rostrocaudal direction. It is a common anomaly, and its incidence is higher in female than in male fetuses. Its relatively high frequency in Ireland and Wales is suggestive, as in other forms of neural tube defects, of an interplay of poorly defined environmental factors and genetic predis-

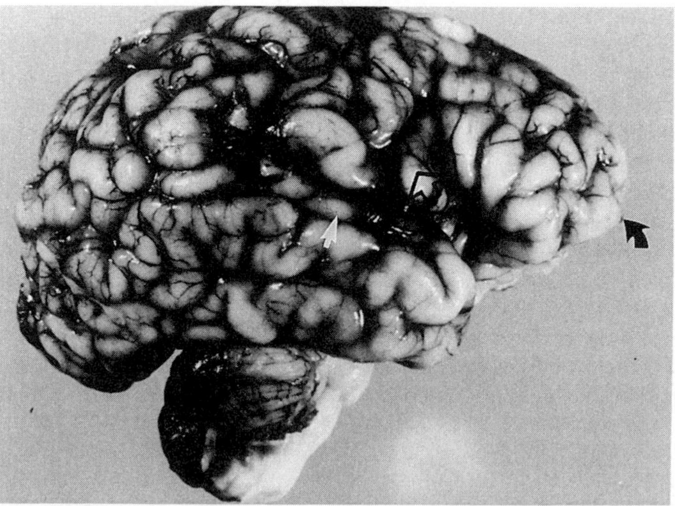

Fig. 77-155 An infant with Down syndrome: narrow superior temporal gyrus *(white arrow)*, exposed insula *(open arrow)*, foreshortened frontal lobe *(curved arrow)*, and disproportionately small cerebellum.

position. Vitamin and folic acid supplementation before conception have reduced its recurrence rate in mothers with a previous history of such defects. Polyhydramnios coexists in 50% of cases. The bony cranial vault is missing *(holoacrania)* or rudimentary *(meroacrania)*, and a reddish spongy mass (area cerebrovasculosa) covered by a thin membrane occupies the gap in the skull (Fig. 77-156). The area cerebrovaculosa consists of thin-walled vessels mixed with variable amounts of glial tissue, ependyma-lined cavities, and tufts of choroid plexus. Disorganized rudimentary cerebellar folia, trigeminal ganglia, and some caudal cranial nerves are often identified, particularly in meroanencephaly. The optic nerves end blindly in the orbit. The base of the skull is deformed and thick with a shallow pituitary fossa containing a hypoplastic anterior and no posterior pituitary tissue. Various dysraphic conditions of the spine and anomalies of the spinal cord may be present. In *craniorachischisis*, an extreme example, the open cranial defect extends along the whole length of the vertebral column, and both brain and spinal cord may be absent. A range of malformations in other organs, such as heterotopic glial tissue in lungs, may be present. Measurement of alpha-fetoprotein or specific isoenzymes of amniotic fluid acetylcholinesterase and ultrasonography allow early prenatal detection of most neural tube defects.

Encephaloceles and cranial meningoceles are frequently located in the occipital region and consist of cranial defects associated with displaced cerebral tissue in the former and meninges in the latter. Frontal (anterior) encephaloceles are more common in Southeast Asia and occur at the bridge of the nose, in the ethmoid or sphenoid sinus, and less frequently between the frontal bones. The cerebral tissue may exhibit disorganization or recent to remote infarctions.

Spina bifida, meningocele, and meningomyelocele (Fig. 77-157), like anencephaly, are defects that are time specific and occur before 26 days of gestation. The vertebral anomaly ranges from nonfusion to total absence of the vertebral arches with lateral displacement of the pedicles and widening of the spinal canal. Additional bony vertebral anomalies and skeletal

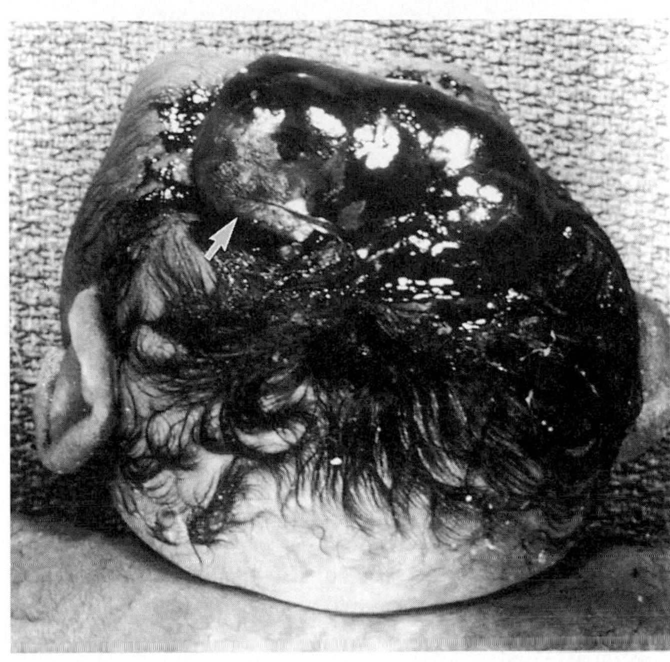

Fig. 77-156 Area cerebrovasculosa *(arrow)* in anencephaly.

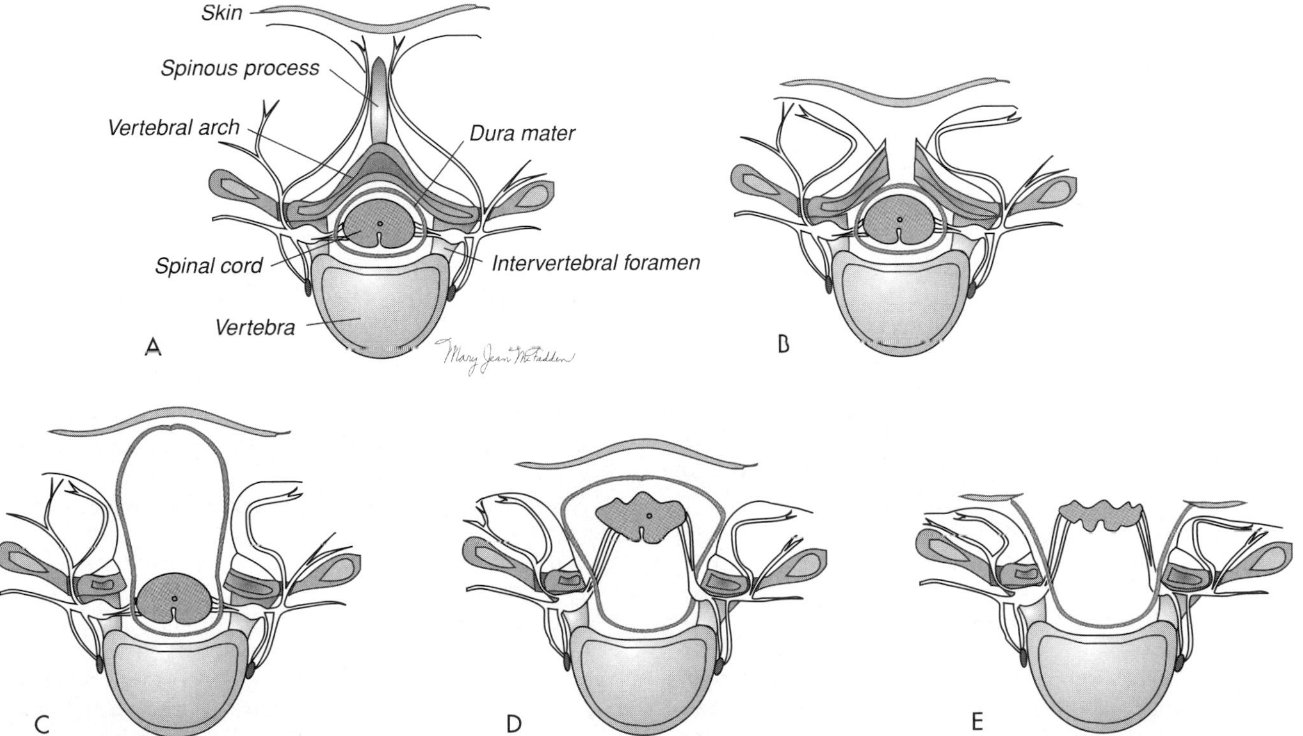

Fig. 77-157 Schema of spinal dysraphism; **A,** Normal. **B,** Spina bifida occulta. The median segment of vertebral bony arch is missing and covered by skin. **C,** Meningocele. The arch is mostly absent and dura is bulging, but spinal cord is in vertebral canal. **D,** Myelomeningocele with deformed spinal cord within the protruding dural sac. **E,** Myelocele; "area medullovasculosa" totally exposed.

deformities are common. *Spina bifida occulta* is the mildest form. The defect occurs in L5-S1, is not associated with protrusion of any of the contents of the spinal canal, and is usually asymptomatic. Symptomatic cases may be associated with a median bony spur, diastematomyelia, and hamartomas or lipomas of the filum terminale. In *spina bifida cystica,* which also has a predilection for the lumbosacral spine, the vertebral defect is associated with a cystic mass. In 15% of cases the cyst contains dura and arachnoid, a *meningocele.* The skin overlying the mass is thin, with atrophic rete pegs and absent appendages. In 85% of the cases, however, a portion of spinal cord and spinal roots accompany the herniated meninges, a *myelomeningocele.* In severe cases the spinal cord may form a flat vascular discoidal mass (area medullovasculosa) at the site of the bony defect, *myelocele.* Microscopically the mass displays highly vascularized arachnoid, neural tissue containing mature neurons, ependyma-lined cavities, and spinal ganglia and roots. Other anomalies of the cord rostral to these defects and hydrocephalus are common.[215] Surgical intervention prevents secondary infection, but the prognosis for future neurologic development in myelomeningoceles remains guarded.[216]

Miscellaneous disorders

Diastematomyelia refers to separation and rotation of the spinal cord into two segments by a bony or fibrous spur protruding from the dorsal surface of a vertebral body. *Hydromyelia* is usually an asymptomatic distention of the central canal of the cord found incidentally at autopsy. *Syringomyelia* manifests as a tubular cavity in the spinal cord readily detectable by neuroimaging. Typically, it involves the cervical spinal cord, often sparing its first segment, and extends into the upper thoracic cord. The lumbosacral enlargement is rarely affected.[217] The cavity or *syrinx* is circular when distended and collapses into a slitlike space when ruptured. Classically in cross sections, the cavity stretches from the posterior aspect of the anterior horns on one side to the contralateral posterior horns, sometimes reaching the pial surface (Fig. 77-158, *A*). The motor neurons anterior to the cavity and the contiguous white matter display variable degrees of degeneration depending on the duration, size, and location of the syrinx. In late stages, fibrous astrocytes line a thin glial wall, perhaps admixed with scant collagen. More exceptionally, a few reactive hypertrophic astrocytes may be detected outside the wall, or the astrocytic wall may be sufficiently cellular (occasionally with Rosenthal fibers) to mimic an astrocytoma. The central canal with its ependymal lining may be incorporated in the cavity, especially in the cervical region. If the syrinx occurs primarily in the medulla, the condition is known as *syringobulbia*[211] (Fig. 77-158, *B*). The slitlike cavity interrupts or destroys various fiber tracts and cranial nerve nuclei resulting in an array of neurologic impairments. The cause of syringomyelia remains controversial. One theory suggests that transmission of increased CSF pressure in the fourth ventricle to the cervical central canal causes its distention (hydromyelia), rupture, and extension into the spinal cord parenchyma (syrinx).[218] Another theory proposes the confluence of minute traumatic tears from repeated torsional forces during rotation and flexion of the neck.

Hydrocephalus

Anatomic note. CSF is produced by the choroid plexus at the rate of 20 ml/hour: first, by passive filtration through its fenestrated capillaries and then by active secretion by the choroid epithelium into the ventricles. From the lateral ventricles, CSF traverses the foramina of Monro into the third ventricle, passes through the aqueduct of Sylvius into the fourth ventricle, and leaves the latter through its foramina (Magendie and Luschka) into the subarachnoid space of both brain and spinal cord. In a normal adult, the total volume of CSF in these compartments is about 140 ml. CSF is absorbed largely in the arachnoid granulations of the large intracranial venous sinuses, and about 10% drains into the small veins of the dural sleeves lining the intervertebral foramina. In obstructive hydrocephalus, some CSF diffuses transependymally into the intercellular compartment of the brain parenchyma (interstitial edema).

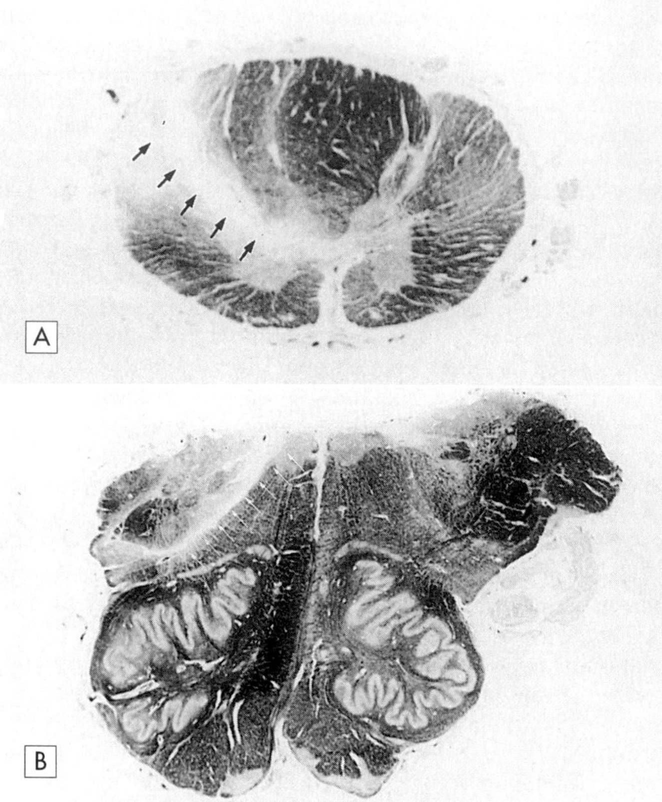

Fig. 77-158 A, Syringomyelia. Syrinx *(arrows)* surrounded by edema and tract degeneration. **B,** Syringobulbia. Syrinx extending from the floor of the fourth ventricle almost to the dorsal surface of the inferior olivary nucleus.

Hydrocephalus means distention of the ventricular system, the subarachnoid space, or both, by CSF. Usually it is caused by mechanical obstruction of the CSF pathway (obstructive hydrocephalus) and rarely is attributable to overproduction of CSF by choroid plexus neoplasms (nonobstructive). In both conditions the intraventricular pressure is increased. Obstructive hydrocephalus traditionally is divided into noncommunicating (lack of communication between the internal or ventricular and the external or subarachnoid compartments) and communicating types. In some patients, CSF pressure may be within the physiologic range because a pressure gradient between ventricular cavity and CNS parenchyma has been established. Such patients may present with the triad of dementia, ataxia, and urinary incontinence—*normal pressure hydrocephalus (NPH);* it usually is attributable to arachnoidal obstruction. *Compensatory hydrocephalus ("ex vacuo")* may be focal or diffuse and refers to dilatation of ventricles secondary to loss of parenchymal tissue. If obstructive hydrocephalus occurs before the sutures are closed, the head enlarges, the fontanelles are widened, and the skull bones are thinned. The cerebral hemispheres are distended, and the gyri may be flattened or abnormally convoluted, sometimes erroneously interpreted as polymicrogyria. The small gyri actually represent outwardly displaced intrasulcal cortex (redundant gyration).[5] The ventricles are enlarged, the corpus callosum is attenuated, and the septum pellucidum is thinned or fenestrated. The ependymal lining over large areas is denuded and covered by thickened, astroglial tissue. In severe hydrocephalus the hemispheric wall may be reduced to a few millimeters in thickness, and, if untreated, permanent tissue damage ensues, especially of white matter. Developmental conditions and perinatal complications that cause obstructive hydrocephalus are many, but only a few are discussed. Excluded from this section are tumors causing hydrocephalus.

Disorders of the aqueduct of Sylvius account for about 20% of the cases.[211] Normally the aqueduct is an irregular short tube and, depending on the level at which it is cross-sectioned, is triangular or ovoid in shape. The lumen at its narrowest segment is about 0.5 mm^2 in children and variable in adults (0.4 to 1.5 mm^2). Hydrocephalus may occur when the lumen is reduced to 0.15 mm.[2] Two main types of congenital, or in utero acquired, aqueductal obstructions are recognized: (1) "atresia" in which randomly dispersed ependymal cells or irregular canaliculi replace the aqueduct (Fig. 77-159) and (2) "stenosis" in which the aqueduct is partially preserved but compromised by either astroglial tissue (aqueductal gliosis) or a histologically unremarkable small lumen. Obstruction of the aqueduct also may occur after inflammatory conditions of the ventricular lining, ventricular shunting procedures, and compression by neoplasm. Obstructive hydrocephalus is frequently associated with other developmental anomalies, such as Arnold-Chiari and Dandy-Walker malformations.

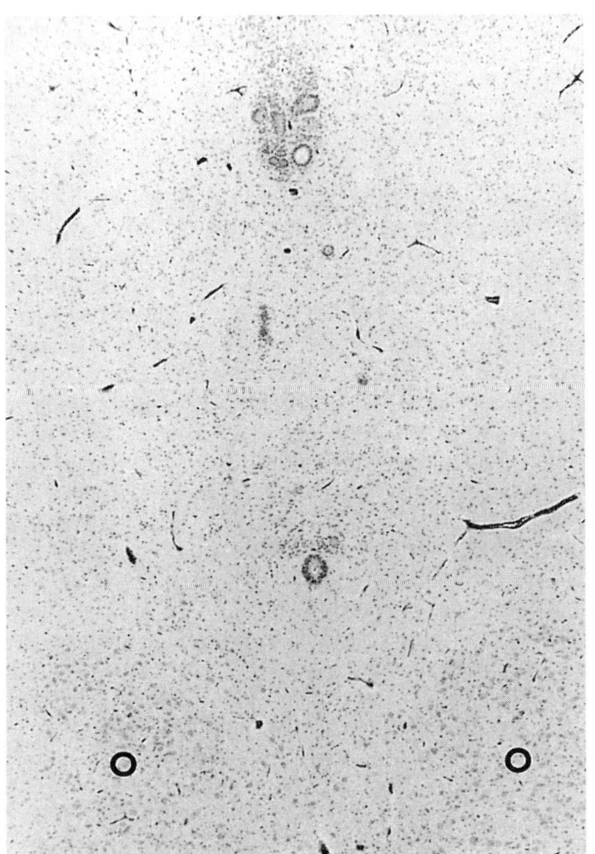

Fig. 77-159 Aqueductal "atresia." Dispersed ependymal cells and irregular calaniculi in the midline. *O,* Oculomotor nuclei.

Arnold-Chiari malformation (ACM) comprises three recognized types; I, II, and III. ACM II is the classic type.[5,219] In its most extreme form it is characterized by a shallow posterior fossa with low insertion of tentorium cerebelli, crowding of hindbrain structures, and downward displacement of medulla and dorsal cerebellum (vermis and others) through a funnel-shaped foramen magnum into the cervical canal. The elongated medulla acquires an S-shaped curvature ending in a bump that overrides the dorsal cerivcal cord, and the fourth ventricle is greatly compressed. The inferior vermis extends like a tongue over the surface of the medulla and cord to which it is tethered by fibrous meningeal adhesions (Fig 77-160). The cervical nerve roots that normally course downward, project upward. The quadrigeminal plate is "beaked." A lumbosacral myelomeningocele is invariably present, and other spinal cord malformations may coexist.[220] Hydrocephalus from associated aqueductal stenosis or resulting from impaction of the hindbrain structures in the posterior fossa also is common. In ACM I, "chronic tonsillar herniation," only the cerebellar tonsis are displaced caudally, but the brainstem is not elongated, and spina bifida is not a feature. However, craniocervical anomalies such as occipital dysplasia and platybasia are common. In ACM III, posterior encephalocele, the cerebellum herniates through a bony defect in the occipito-cervical region. The pathogenesis of ACM II is controversial;[221] theories have included (1) traction of the hindbrain by the myelomeningocele tethering the spinal cord, (2) downward pressure of hindbrain by hydrocephalus, and (3), most popularly, dyssynchronous growth between hindbrain neuroectoderm and the posterior fossa mesoderm resulting in an inadequate posterior fossa.

Dandy-Walker malformation (DWM) (Fig. 77-161) is characterized by hypoplasia of the vermis, cystic dilatation of fourth ventricle, and enlargement of the posterior fossa with upward displacement of tentorium and torcula. Hydrocephalus, usually milder than that in ACM II, occurs in 80% of patients. The edge of the residual cerebellum merges into the ependymal cyst wall that forms the roof of a greatly dilated fourth ventricle. Midline cranial malformations, such as agenesis of corpus callosum, and systemic anomalies are common. The inferior olivary nuclei are invariably dysplastic, and since these nuclei and vermis are derivatives of the rhombic lips, DWM is believed to result from a disturbance of hindbrain development. The foramina of the fourth ventricle are usually patent. True *atresia of the foramina* is a rare cause of hydrocephalus and is distinguished from DWM by the absence of dysplastic nuclei in the brainstem. *Retrocerebellar arachnoid cysts* can lead to enlargement of the posterior fossa; the cerebellum is compressed but not hypoplastic, a difficult gross differential.

Disorders of forebrain (anterior) induction

Arrhinencephaly is a generic term that includes a range of malformations of variable severity. The common denominator is *olfactory aplasia,* which may occur as an incidental isolated

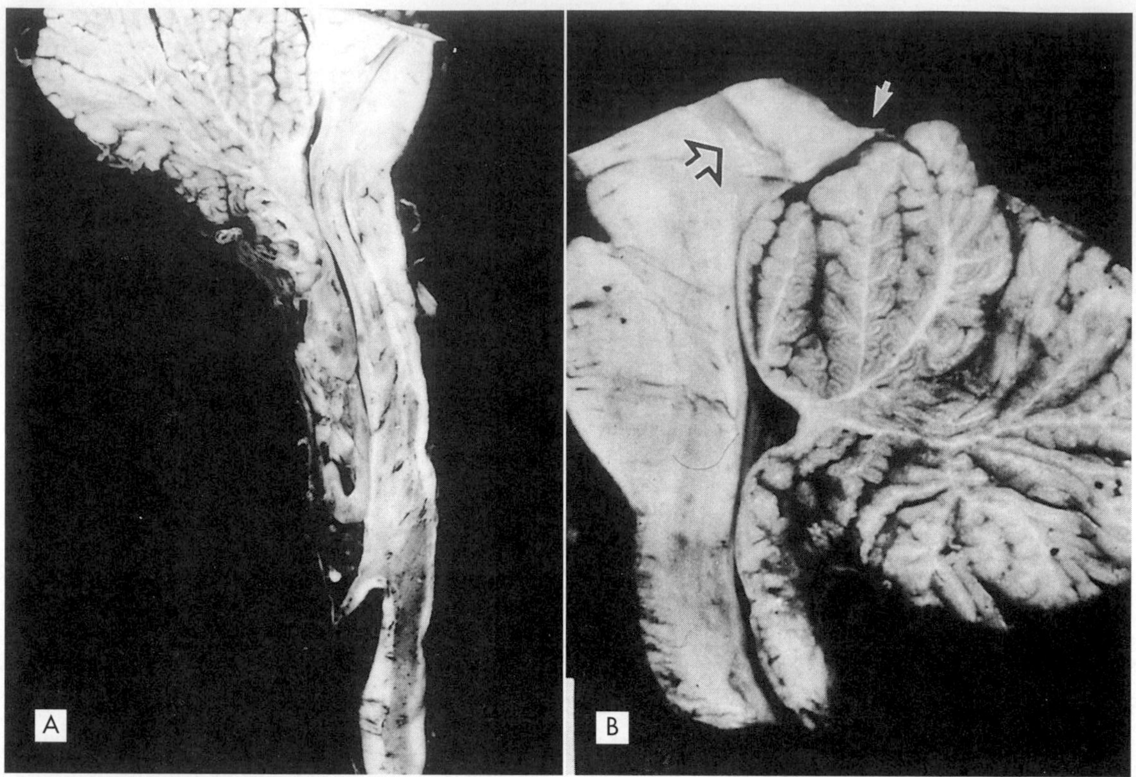

Fig. 77-160 Two different cases of Arnold-Chiari malformation. **A,** Severe elongation of the medulla and vermis. **B,** "Beaking" of the tectum *(white arrow)* and dilatation of the aqueduct *(open arrow)* caused by compression of the fourth ventricle.

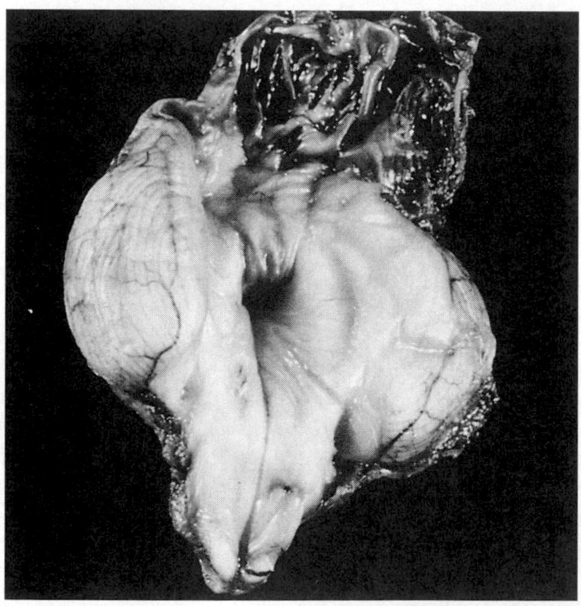

Fig. 77-161 Dandy-Walker malformation. Hypoplastic vermis and cyst reflected to expose a dilated fourth ventricle.

finding, or may be associated with varying degrees of incomplete separation of the cerebral hemispheres *(holoprosencephaly). Alobar* holoprosencephaly is the severest form. The undivided cerebral hemispheres surround a single large ventricle (holosphere), whereas in the *lobar* form there is a variable separation of the brain into two hemispheres (Fig. 77-162, *A*). In the alobar type, the brain is small and has an abnormal gyral pattern. A cyst continuous with the unicameral ventricle and representing the roof of the third ventricle projects from its caudal aspect (Fig. 77-162, *B*). The basal ganglia and thalami are fused in the midline, and the hippocampi form an arch beneath the attachment of the roof membrane to the holosphere.[210] Abnormalities of facial structures include cyclopia, cebocephaly, cleft palate and lip, and frontonasal dysplasias.

Agenesis of corpus callosum may occur as an isolated finding and be manifested externally by hypertelorism, but more often it is associated with other cerebral malformations, mental retardation, and certain congenital neurologic syndromes. Agenesis may be partial or complete; usually a thin fibrous membrane, or rarely a lipoma, replaces the absent corpus callosum. Radial arrangement of gyri around the ventricle on the medial surface of the hemispheres and the upward projection of the angles of the lateral ventricles (bat-wing ventricles) on coronal sections are the gross hallmarks of callosal agenesis (Fig. 77-163).

Malformations of septum pellucidum also occur. An absent septum may be seen in the former two malformations as well as in other developmental syndromes such as those in *septo-optic dysplasia* and porencephaly. *Persistence of cavum septi pellucidi* is a common asymptomatic finding that rarely enlarges to cause obstruction of the foramina of Monro and hydrocephalus.

Disorders of neuronal migration

Agyria-pachygyria. In agyria *(lissencephaly)* the brain has a smooth surface and resembles that of an immature fetus,

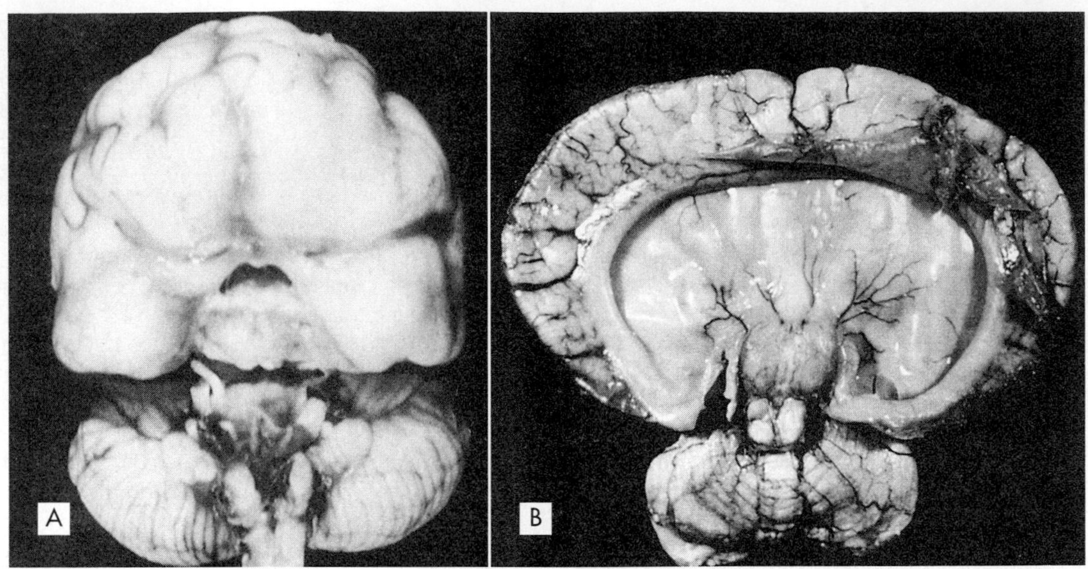

Fig. 77-162 Holoprosencephaly. **A,** Frontobasal view showing almost total fusion of frontal lobes, absence of olfactory bulbs and nerves, and abnormal gyral pattern. **B,** Posterodorsal view showing the reflected cyst wall communicating with a unicameral ventricle.

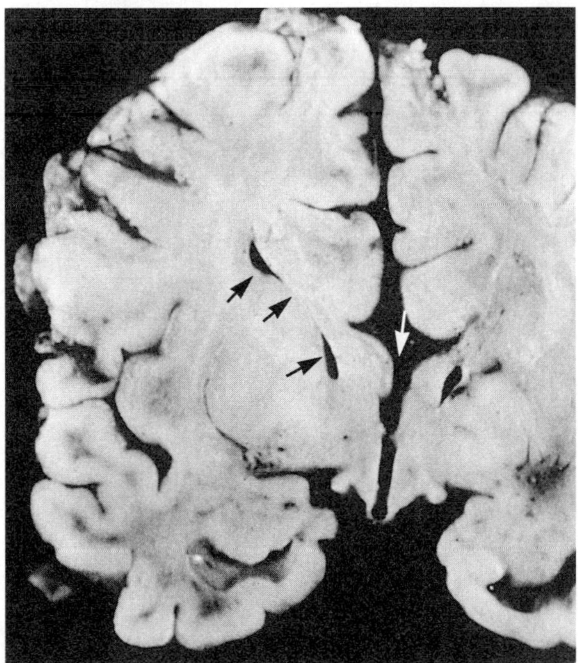

Fig. 77-163 Agenesis of corpus callosum *(white arrow)* and bat wing–like lateral ventricle outlined by black arrows.

whereas in pachygyria *(macrogyria)* the brain exhibits a few broad convolutions with shallow sulci (Fig. 77-164, *A*). Agyria or pachygyria results from interruption of succeeding waves of neuroblasts from reaching the cortex at about the twelfth week of gestation. The cortex is greatly thickened and the white matter reduced (Fig. 77-164, *B*). Instead of the normal six layers, a pachygyric cortex exhibits four layers; a superficial molecular layer, a narrow neuronal cell layer, a paucicellular plexiform layer formed of myelinated fibers, and a deep

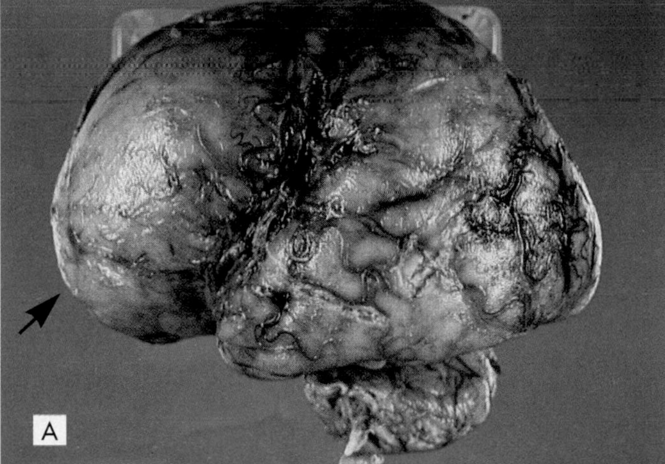

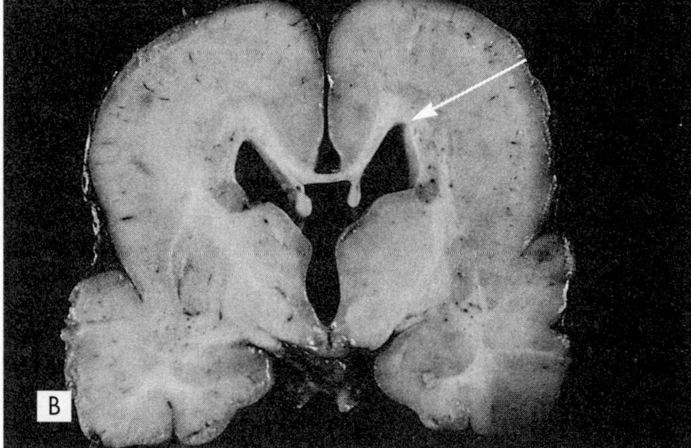

Fig. 77-164 Agyria-pachygyria complex in Miller-Dieker syndrome. **A,** Absent gyri (frontal lobe, *arrow*) and broad gyri with shallow sulci (rest of the brain); **B,** Coronal section showing thick cortex *(length of arrow)* and attenuated white matter *(tip of the arrow)*.

heterotopic, thick cell layer with disorderly arranged neurons. Associated CNS anomalies are common, particularly dysplasia of inferior olivary nuclei. Agyria or pachygyria can be sporadic or familial and seen in a variety of syndromes, such as Miller-Dieker (17p chromosomal deletion), Fukuyama congenital muscular dystrophy, and Zellweger (peroxisomal disorder) syndrome,[222] or may be associated with in-utero infections such as congenital cytomegalovirus.[223]

Polymicrogyria. The brain surface exhibits numerous small, irregular gyri and has been likened to morocco leather or a chestnut kernel (Fig. 77-165, *A*). The anomaly may be focal or widespread involving one or both hemispheres. Its distribution often corresponds to the territory of a major artery, especially the middle cerebral or surrounds the orifice of porencephalic defects[5,224] (Fig. 77-165, *B*). Polymicrogyria manifests as fused, abortive gyri and histologically displays a thin, two-layered cortex (superficial molecular and deeper neuronal layer) arranged in a complex, undulating pattern (unlayered polymicrogyria). Sometimes a four-layered cortex thinner and distinct from that of pachygyria is encountered. The anomaly may result from interruption of late neuroblast migration or by a postmigrational destructive lesion around the sixth month of gestation. Severe forms of polymicrogyria are associated with psychomotor retardation.

Heterotopias. Gray-matter heterotopias are irregular nodules or symmetrical layers (laminar) closely related to the ventricles and are often associated with an abnormal gyral pattern, especially polymicrogyria and other CNS malformations (Fig. 77-166). Mental retardation and seizures are common.

Dysplasia (microdysgenesis). Dysplasia refers to a disorderly arrangement of neurons focally in the cortex, nuclei, or both. Since neurons are postmitotic cells, the term in this setting does not connote the potential for excessive mitotic activity as in the area of carcinogenesis. Dysplasia may be a minor incidental finding or may be part of a more profound developmental disorder. In the dentate or inferior olivary nuclei, dysplasia is manifested by loss of their normal undulating pattern or by a discontinuous arrangement of islands of gray matter while retaining the original outline of the nucleus (Fig. 77-167).

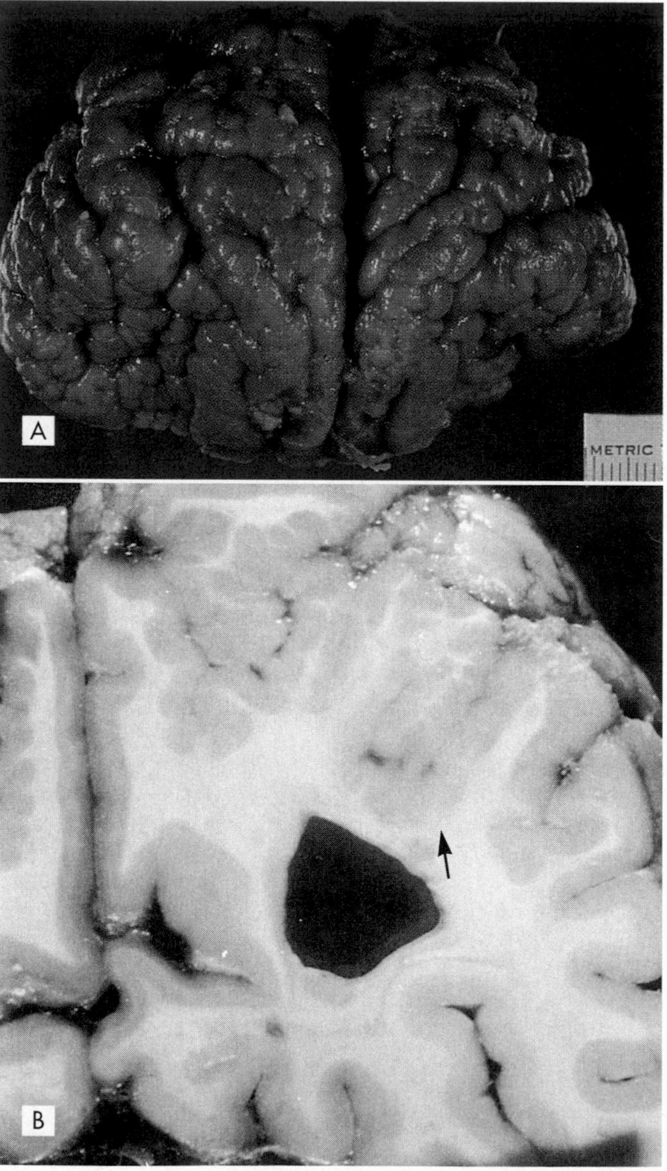

Fig. 77-165 Polymicrogyria. **A,** Puckered, "morocco leather" surface. **B,** Undulating crowded gyri *(arrow)* in middle cerebral artery distribution contrasting with contiguous normal-appearing cortex.

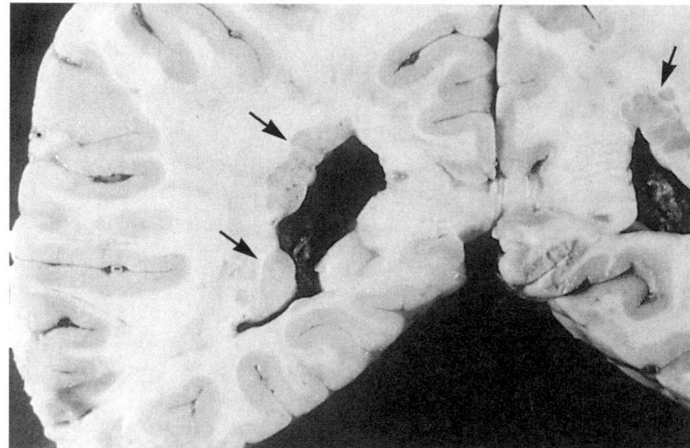

Fig. 77-166 Nodular gray matter heterotopias *(arrows).*

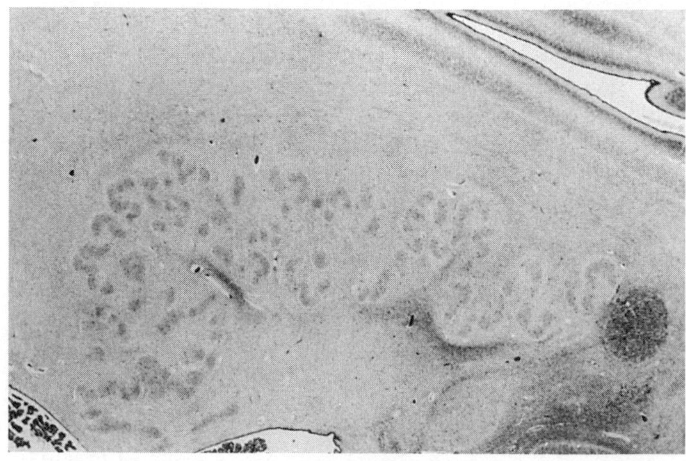

Fig. 77-167 Dysplastic dentate nucleus.

Ectopic neurons. Ectopic neurons in the molecular layer representing persistence of the horizontal cells of Cajal-Retzius sometimes are observed in malformed brains. Scattered neurons in subcortical white matter are of questionable clinical significance and are frequent in young patients, especially epileptics.

Disorders of growth

Aplasia and hypoplasia are attributable to complete or partial agenesis of certain regions of the brain (Fig. 77-168). It often coexists with other CNS anomalies such as the hypoplastic cerebellar vermis in Dandy-Walker malformation. Aplasia may be limited to certain groups of neurons, such as the granular layer of cerebellum.

Although the terms *microcephaly* and *micrencephaly* are used interchangeably, microcephaly indicates a small cranium, which is often secondary to micrencephaly, meaning a 'small brain.' In the adult brain weights below 900 g may be considered abnormal; in the infant and child the weight should exceed 3 standard deviations. Micrencephaly may be sporadic or familial and is seen in diverse, rare, dysgenetic syndromes and the fetal alcohol syndrome. In its extreme forms, the cerebral hemispheres are greatly reduced in size and the convolutions are simplified. Both cortex and white matter are attenuated, but the basal ganglia and the cerebellum are often unaffected.[210,211]

Megalencephaly (macrocephaly, or *cerebral gigantism)* refers to any abnormally heavy brain, with the upper range of normal being debatable, but a brain weighing above 1800 g may be considered abnormal. Megalencephaly is a feature of some storage diseases (such as Tay-Sachs) and certain phakomatoses (such as tuberous sclerosis). It should not be confused with *primary diffuse megalencephaly,* which is seen in rare inherited disorders such as achondroplasia or multiple angiomatoses. In *hemimegalencephaly* (one cerebral hemisphere) an increased number and size of gyri is attributable to a disturbance in the cortical cytoarchitecture with bizarre neurons and astrocytes, simulating ganglioglioma.

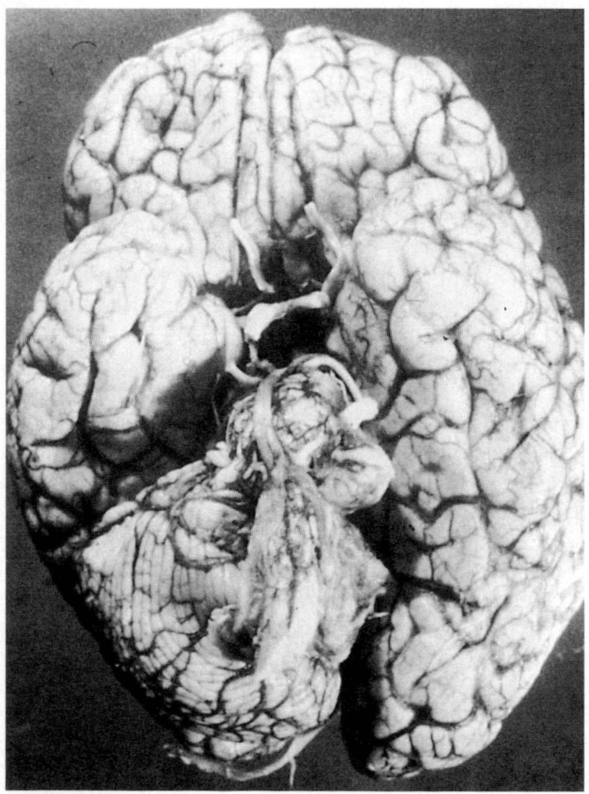

Fig. 77-168 Congenital aplasia of left cerebellar hemisphere.

Neurocutaneous syndromes (phakomatoses)

Neurofibromatosis is an autosomal dominant disorder with a high degree of penetrance. The spontaneous mutation rate is high. The most common form is von Recklinghausen's disease, frequently known as "neurofibromatosis 1," or NF-1. Its gene has been localized to chromosome 17q11-12. It afflicts about 1 in 4000 individuals and is characterized clinically by multiple areas of hyperpigmentation (café-au-lait spots), multiple neurofibromas, Lisch nodules (pigmented iris hamartomas), and rarely CNS astrocytoma. The second form previously known as central neurofibromatosis and now designated "neurofibromatosis 2," or NF-2, has its gene locus on chromosome 22q12. It is less common than NF-1 and occurs in about 1 in 135,000 individuals. It is characterized by bilateral acoustic schwannomas, but other intracranial and intraspinal tumors can be present.[225] Given the numerous hyperplastic and frank neoplastic lesions of neural crest derivatives, neurofibromatosis has been considered a "neurocristopathy." In addition to schwannomas and neurofibromas, which are covered in Chapter 78, these patients are prone to develop particular glial neoplasms: optic gliomas, pilocytic astrocytomas of the third ventricle, and spinal cord and cerebral gliomas, including ependymomas and glioblastoma multiforme. Meningiomas also are common. Nonneural malignancies occurring with relatively high frequency in patients with neurofibromatosis include leukemia and Wilms' tumor.[10]

Tuberous sclerosis (Bourneville's disease, epiloia) is an autosomal dominant disorder with variable penetrance.[226] Spontaneous mutations may account for some of the sporadic cases. *Formes frustes* are relatively common. Its prevalence varies from series to series; 1 in 20,000 may be a fair estimate. Although it is a complex disorder involving neuroectodermal and mesodermal tissues, the brain is the most frequently affected organ. The characteristic lesions are cortical tubers, subependymal nodules, and retinal hamartomas (phakomas). Typically the cortical tubers appear as pale, firm nodules projecting slightly above the surface (Fig. 77-169, *A*). They vary in size from a few millimeters to 3 cm in diameter and may number up to 40 or more. Histologically the disturbed laminations and gliosis result in expansion of the tuberous cortex and blurring of its margins. Multinucleated, hypertrophic astrocytes and clusters of giant bizarre neuron-like cells with disorderly, stout processes are often present. Neurofibrillary tangles and granulovacuolar degeneration have been described in the latter. The hamartomatous subependymal nodules can occur anywhere in the ventricles but most often are seen along the sulcus terminalis partially embedded in the caudate nucleus, thalamus, or both (Fig. 77-169, *B*). When present in rows, they form what has been termed "candle gutterings." They tend to calcify and become readily detectable on plain films of the skull. Microscopically they resemble the glial retinal hamartomas (phakomas) and are formed of a mixture of hyperplastic fibrillary astrocytes and large, atypical cells of undetermined neural derivation. These nodules may evolve into subependy-

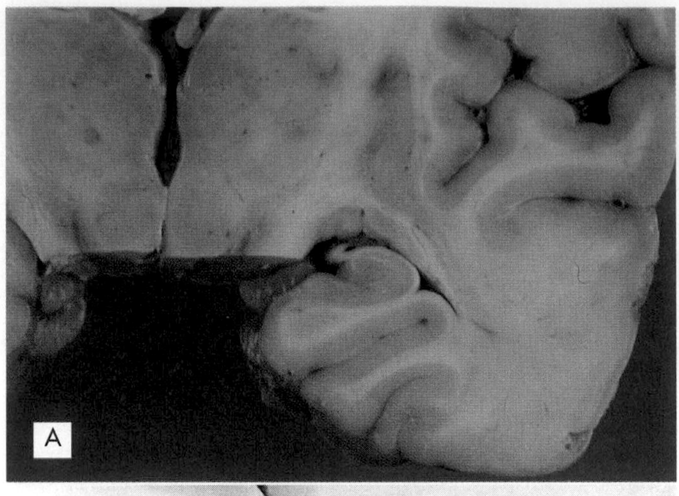

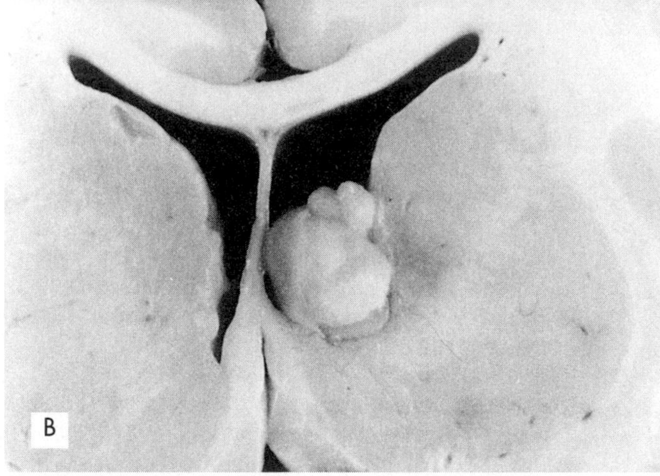

Fig. 77-169 Tuberous sclerosis. **A,** Pale, cortical tuber replacing normal cortex. **B,** Subependymal nodule embedded in the head of the caudate nucleus.

mal giant cell tumors (astrocytomas). The subependymal nodules or tumors can obstruct the CSF pathways, especially at the foramen of Monro, and account for considerable morbidity and mortality in these patients.

Seizures, behavioral problems, and mental retardation are common presenting symptoms, but skin manifestations may be the earliest clinical findings; these include hypomelanotic macules (1 to 3 cm in diameter), facial angiofibromas (erroneously termed "adenoma sebaceum"), subungual fibromas, and shagreen patches. Mesenchymal tumors often coexist and include cardiac rhabdomyoma, renal angiomyolipomas, and pulmonary lymphangiomyomatosis.[227]

Encephalofacial angiomatosis (Sturge-Weber syndrome) is a rare, nonfamilial disorder characterized by port-wine angioma in the distribution of one or more of the sensory divisions of the trigeminal nerve; ocular and leptomeningeal angioma tend to coexist. Ocular angiomas cause buphthalmos. Leptomeningeal angiomatosis, composed of anomalous thin-walled pial vessels, usually involves the parieto-occipital region (Fig. 77-170). It may extend into the underlying brain and often develops with variable degrees of calcification of cortical vessels and parenchyma producing the classic radiologic pattern called "railroad tracking." Laminar necrosis of the involved

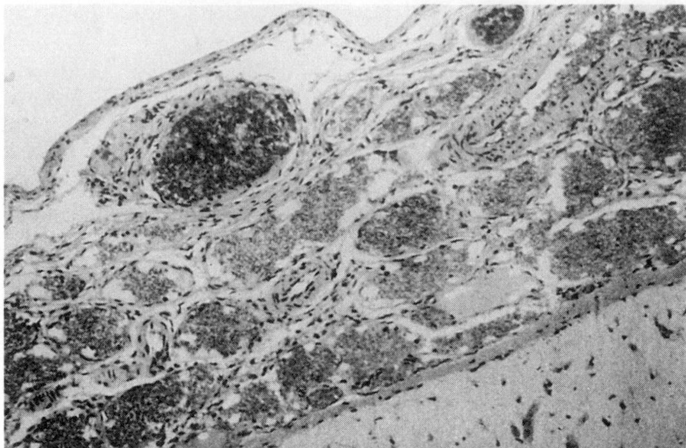

Fig. 77-170 Sturge-Weber syndrome. Closely apposed and dilated pial vessels.

cortex or atrophy of the affected cerebral hemisphere are present in severe cases. Seizures, hemiplegia, and mental retardation are the main neurologic manifestations.

Perinatal birth lesions

This area of neuropathology traditionally has been inappropriately designated as "birth injuries." Since most of these lesions are nontraumatic in origin and it is difficult at best to specify exactly when in the perinatal period such lesions occur, the unrestricted usage of this term should be strongly discouraged. Premature infants are highly susceptible to developing intracranial hemorrhages; the lower their birth weight, the greater the risk. Their occurrence in stillborns and in infants born by cesarean section indicates that they can result from complex hemodynamic disturbances in cerebral circulation, usually brought about by in utero fetal hypoxia-ischemia. In mature infants, these hemorrhagic lesions may be directly linked to mechanical trauma to the head, such as that after excessive head molding or forceps extraction.[5,228,229]

Intradural hematomas occur in the loose connective tissue between the two leaves of the falx cerebri or tentorium cerebelli. They appear as smooth swellings up to several millimeters in thickness. They are usually asymptomatic and resorb without leaving a trace. *Lacerations of tentorium and falx* are seen in serious mechanical birth injuries. They may occur at the free edge or at the base, in which case rupture of major dural venous sinuses lead to *subdural hematomas*. Rarely the vein of Galen may be torn. Their frequency increases with advanced gestational ages and greater birth weights. *Epidural hemorrhages* are extremely rare and usually complicate depressed skull fractures. *Subarachnoid hemorrhages* may be diffuse or patchy. Sometimes the hemorrhage, especially over the ventral aspect of the temporal lobes, results in thick, sharply demarcated hematomas. Subarachnoid hemorrhages are invariably present in premature infants dying from cardiorespiratory failure. Massive clots in the basal cisterns and cisterna magna usually are the result of subarachnoid extension of intraventricular hemorrhages. *Subpial hemorrhages* occurring in the cerebellar folia may result in hematomas that expand the involved folia.

Subependymal and intraventricular hemorrhages are the most common major intracranial complications found in premature infants. Their incidence varies, but it is definitely higher in premature infants weighing less than 1500 g or whose gestational ages are less than 34 weeks. Although they can occur anytime in the immediate perinatal period, they frequently develop a few hours after delivery. The condition is associated with a high mortality, but infants may survive the event with or without developing neurologic sequelae. The subependymal hemorrhages originate anywhere in the germinal layer, but they usually occur near the sulcus terminalis just posterior to the foramen of Monro (ganglionic eminence) (Fig. 77-171). The hemorrhages are often bilateral and vary in size from focal patchy extravasation of blood (ultrasound grade I) to large hematomas that rupture into the lateral ventricle (grade II) (Fig. 77-172), to those that fill the ventricle (grade III) and eventually extend into the third and fourth ventricles and perhaps the basal subarachnoid space, and to those that infiltrate adjacent brain parenchyma. The intraventricular hemorrhage causes acute hydrocephalus. If the infants survive, resorption and organization of the blood clot takes place; some infants may be left with either asymptomatic residual subependymal cysts or may develop more serious complications such as posthemorrhagic hydrocephalus. The pathogenesis of subependymal hemorrhages remains controversial. They seem to be related to structural peculiarities of the germinal matrix and its delicate vascular bed, which may be unduly susceptible to physiologic, hemodynamic, and iatrogenic stresses.[230] *Choroid plexus hemorrhages* are usually seen in term infants and can cause intraventricular hemorrhages. *Parenchymal hemorrhages* in immature infants are rare, and those occurring in term infants are multifactorial. Those related to mechanical birth trauma classically occur in the parasagittal subcortical white matter.

Periventricular leukomalacia (PVLM) manifests as multiple, irregular yellowish or chalky white lesions in the white matter adjacent to the lateral ventricles, particularly in rostral frontal lobes and parieto-occipital regions (Fig. 77-173). Microscopically, they display a few foamy macrophages, some reactive astrocytes, and irregularly swollen axons that mineralize with longer survival. PVLM is more frequent in premature than in mature infants and is often associated with other CNS lesions, such as subependymal or intraventricular hemorrhages. It may occur in utero.[231] The pathogenesis of PVLM is a subject of debate. One theory proposes that these are borderzone infarcts between the ventriculofugal and ventriculopetal arteries resulting from shock attributable to either primary circulatory failure or sepsis. If the infants survive, these lesions are transformed into uniloculated or multiloculated cysts. The white matter of the centrum semiovale and corpus callosum is reduced in thickness, and the reduction is commensurate with the degree of tissue destruction. In extreme cases, the entire white matter is replaced by cavities, one of the many causes of *multicystic encephalopathy,* and rarely it may be represented by a thin white strip with remarkable preservation of cortical mantle, "hypoplasia of white matter."

Telencephalic leukoencephalopathy[232] is characterized by hypertrophic astrocytes, pyknotic degenerating glial cells, and amphophilic globular bodies diffusely distributed throughout the white matter of the cerebrum. Foci of necrosis are sometimes present. The lesion is best appreciated with an immunostain for glial fibrillary acidic protein. The condition is associated with diverse maternal and fetal risk factors, notably maternal endotoxemia and urinary tract infections.

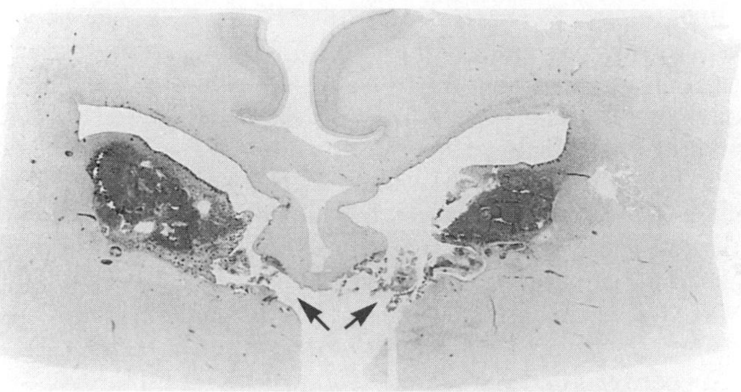

Fig. 77-171 Bilateral germinal matrix hemorrhages in the ganglionic eminence at foramen of Monro *(arrows).*

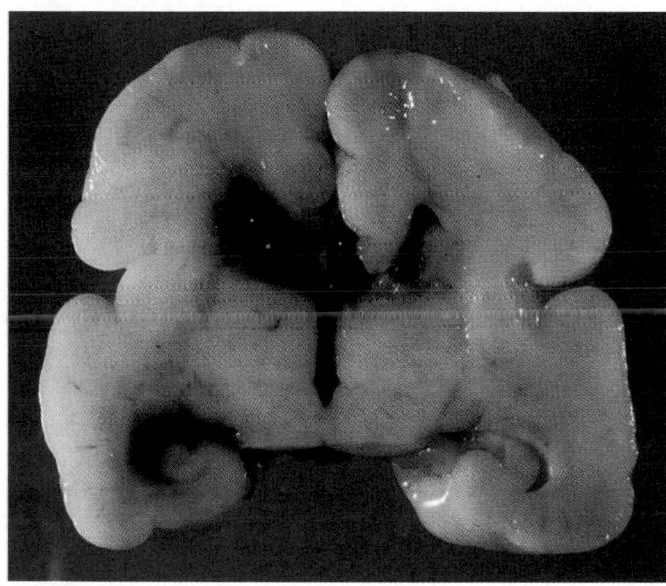

Fig. 77-172 Left germinal matrix hemorrhage extending into ventricles.

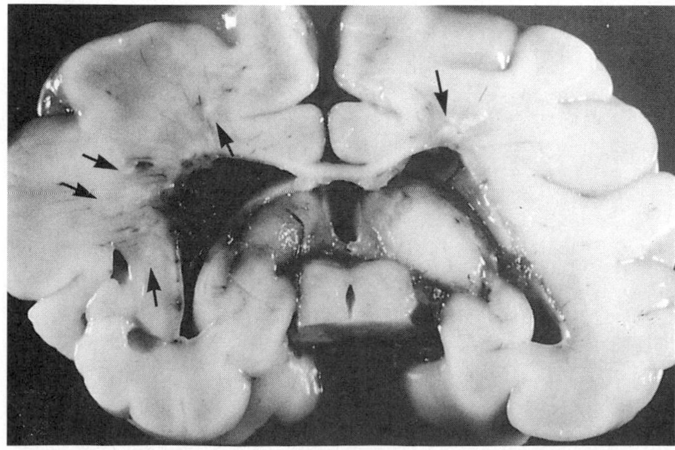

Fig. 77-173 Periventricular leukomalacia showing irregular chalky white lesions *(arrows).*

Infarctions often occur in the distribution of a major cerebral artery or vein, either in utero from thromboemboli originating in the placenta, or postnatally from in situ thrombosis complicating congenital heart diseases and hypercoagulable conditions, such as dehydration and sepsis. Hemorrhagic infarcts and hemorrhages also are seen in infants treated with extracorporeal membrane oxygenation (ECMO).[233] *Ulegyria* is an ischemic lesion resulting in one to several mushroom-shaped gyri (Fig. 77-174). The cortex in the depths of sulci is reduced to a glial scar, whereas the crest remains relatively intact. Ulegyria is often seen in arterial border zones, especially between the anterior and middle cerebral arteries, and is usually bilateral. "Mushroom" folia in the border zones of cerebellar arteries may coexist.[5]

Status marmoratus refers to a "marbled" appearance of the basal ganglia, thalamus, or both. It is caused by a hypoxic-ischemic insult resulting in glial scarring and aberrant myelination. It is usually seen in term infants who are the products of complicated deliveries. The basal ganglia is more frequently involved. Mineralized neurons and Lafora body–like inclusions also may be seen. Ulegyria and thalamic gliosis with mineralized neurons are common companions. In *symmetrical thalamic sclerosis* the thalami may bear the brunt of the insult. Clinically, status marmoratus is manifested by choreoathetosis, and symmetrical thalamic sclerosis is manifested by profound psychomotor retardation.

Pontosubicular neuronal necrosis is characterized by neuronal necrosis predominantly in the basis pontis and subiculum. Karyorrhexis and acute eosinophilic degeneration of neurons are the main histologic hallmarks. The condition, however, may be associated with other CNS lesions complicating respiratory distress syndromes. It occurs mostly in premature infants from 30 weeks of gestation up to 2 months of age. Hypoxia, hyperoxygenation, or both, have been implicated in its pathogenesis.[234] *Hypotensive (cardiac arrest) brain stem necrosis* is characterized by symmetrical neuronal death and gliosis affecting the motor cranial nerve nuclei; in severe cases, the whole tegmentum, colliculi, and the anterior horns of the spinal cord may be involved. The condition complicates cardiac arrest or sudden acute hypotension, especially in neonates. Usually these infants remain comatose and die. Some may survive and present with the neuropathic variant of *arthrogryposis multiplex congenita*[235] (a syndrome of nonprogressive multiple joint contractures present at birth) or *Moebius syndrome* (nonprogressive facial diplegia and ophthalmoplegia).

Porencephaly and *hydranencephaly* represent sequelae of major destructive brain lesions usually occurring during the first 6 months of fetal life before the immature brain is able to mount sufficient glial reaction to injury.[236] *Porencephaly* refers to linear or funnel-shaped defects of variable sizes involving the whole thickness of the cerebral hemispheres (Fig. 77-175). The defect or porus often communicates with the ventricular cavity, but sometimes a thin membranous diaphragm, usually made up of arachnoid, seals it from the ventricle. The porus may be surrounded by polymicrogyria, nodular heterotopias, or radially arranged gyri, which histologically exhibit abnormal cortical laminations.[211] In *hydranencephaly* (literally [6]'water-no-brain', thus "bubble brain") the cerebral hemispheres are converted into thin-walled, fluid-filled vesicles. The walls consist of leptomeninges and islets of glial tissue with no trace of ependymal lining.[5] The occipital and inferior temporal lobes, especially the hippocampi, may be partially preserved, an indication of probable perfusion failure in the anterior and middle cerebral arterial circulations. Grossly, the brainstem and the cerebellum appear relatively intact. In *multicystic encephalopathy,* the cerebral hemispheres are transformed to multiloculated cavities separated by gliovascular trabeculas (Fig. 77-176). The condition, unlike the previous two, occurs at later stages of gestation and in the postnatal period. The causes of multicystic encephalopathy include anoxia, necrotizing viral encephalitides, most notably herpes simplex,[237] and neonatal meningitides.

Miscellaneous disorders

Sudden infant death syndrome (SIDS), or "crib death," occurs in infants that show no significant abnormalities, and the pathogenesis of the death remains a mystery. The main neu-

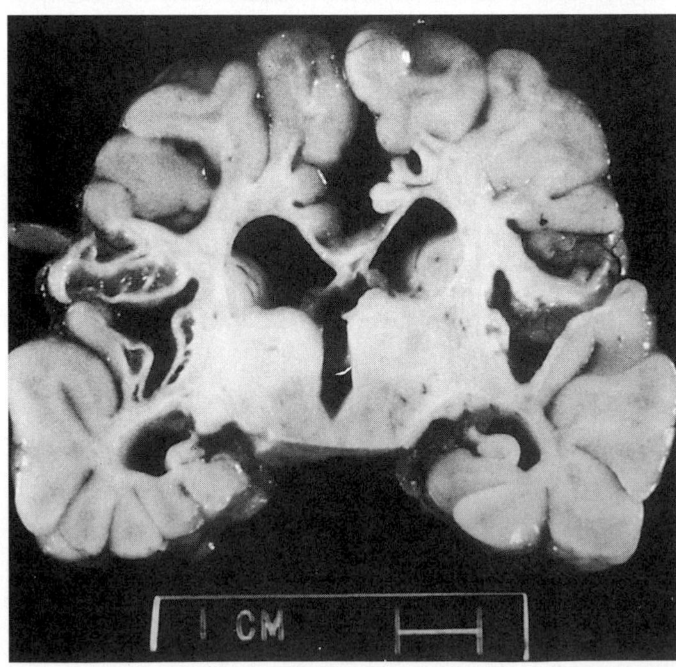

Fig. 77-174 Ulegyria.

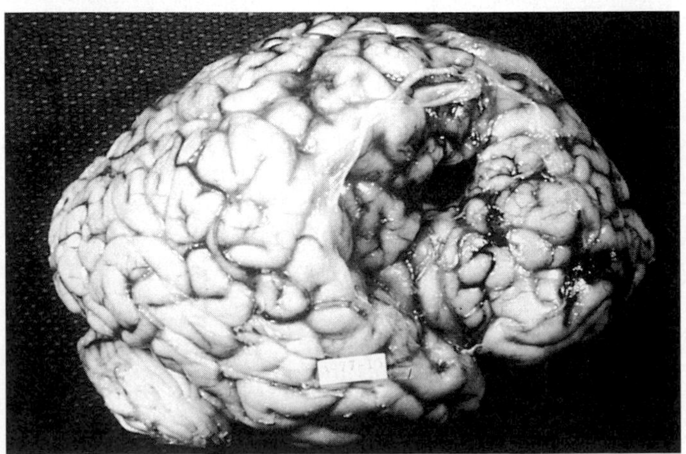

Fig. 77-175 Porencephaly. Funnel-shaped defect (porus) bordered by polymicrogyria.

ropathologic focus has been on possible abnormalities in the brainstem.[238]

Perinatal maternal infections can spread to the fetus and result in fetal encephalitis, cerebritis, or meningitis, which may lead to destructive or malformative lesions. In *rubella embryopathy* maternal infection usually occurs during the first month of gestation. The brain may be micrencephalic and show mild-to-moderate chronic lymphoplasmacytic meningitis and mineralization of blood vessels. In *generalized cytomegalovirus infection* of the neonate, the brain is often involved, especially if infection occurs during the first trimester.[239]

In *epilepsy,* seizures are common manifestations or sequelae of many of the above-mentioned developmental disorders and some of the metabolic diseases that are discussed later. In some infants, however, seizures may be unassociated with overt lesions and are said to be *idiopathic*. Idiopathic epilepsy has a strong genetic basis. Data obtained from modern neuroimaging studies and surgically resected temporal lobes for complex partial seizures have shown that more than half of these epileptic patients have changes in the hippocampus and a few have minor dysgenetic lesions.[240] The hippocampus, including its uncinate process, is often atrophic, *mesial temporal sclerosis,* with neuronal loss and gliosis being most severe in Sommer's sector. The pathogenesis of mesial temporal sclerosis is still debated as to whether it is the result or the cause of seizures.[241] Unrecognized intrauterine hypoxia or hypoxia occurring after prolonged febrile convulsions in infancy may initiate these changes. Like a glial scar elsewhere in the cortex, it may evolve into a permanent epileptogenic focus. Associated changes, especially in long-standing and poorly controlled cases, include subpial gliosis (Chaslin's marginal sclerosis), atrophy of cerebellar folia with loss of Purkinje cells and Bergmann gliosis, patchy neuronal loss in the cortex and thalami, and exceptionally atrophy of the hemisphere. Small low-grade neoplasms, vascular malformations, hamartomas, and dysgenetic lesions may be seen in temporal lobes with or without hippocampal sclerosis. In about 1% to 2% of resected temporal lobes, changes suggestive of enceph-alitis may be encountered as part of *Rasmussen's chronic encephalitis*.[242] The nature of the causative agent is not known, but cytomegalovirus genomic material was recovered in some of the patients.[102,243]

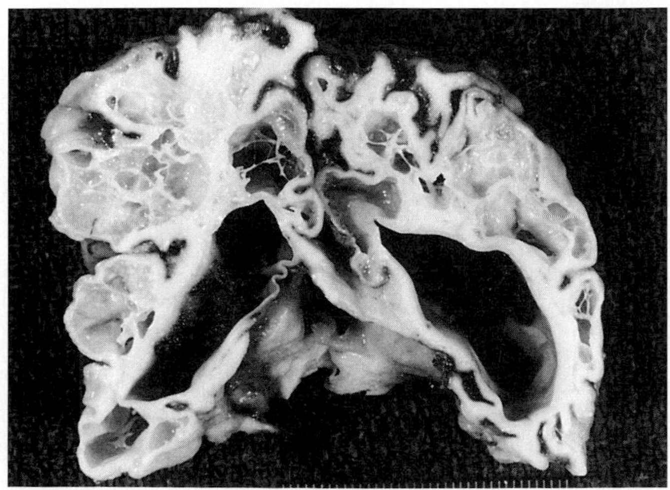

Fig. 77-176 Multicystic encephalopathy.

DISEASES OF MYELIN

The heterogeneous diseases of myelin may include autoimmune, infectious, genetic, and metabolic-toxic causes. Myelin, a biochemically modified plasmalemma of oligodendrocytes or Schwann cells, is a highly specialized membrane unique in many ways and limited to nervous tissue.[16] Hence, signs and symptoms of these diseases are primarily if not exclusively referrable to nervous tissue. Subtle biochemical and ultrastructural differences between central and peripheral myelin are observed, but significant antigenic differences exist.[16,244] The degradation of biochemically normal myelin proceeds to a catabolic endpoint of neutral lipid (predominantly cholesterol esters), sudanophilic breakdown products. These are phagocytosed primarily by macrophages and removed from the damaged area. The degradation of biochemically "abnormal" myelin, such as that in the leukodystrophies with their inherent catabolic enzyme deficiencies, usually results in the accumulation of nonsudanophilic intermediate breakdown products, often demonstrable with other special stains such as periodic acid–Schiff (carbohydrates) or acid cresyl violet (metachromasia).[245]

Controversy exists over the definition of "demyelination" and the nosology of myelin diseases.[246,247] A prerequisite for inclusion should be the primary involvement of myelin sheaths (or their oligodendrocytes/Schwann cells) with relative preservation of axons. "Secondary demyelination" consequent to primary or concomitant axonal loss because of neuronal degeneration, hypoxia-ischemia, trauma, edema, or infection should not be included. Diseases of myelin may be divided into three major categories: demyelinating (myelinoclastic diseases), dysmyelinating (leukodystrophies), and myelinolytic (spongy myelinopathies). Demyelinating diseases are inflammatory, usually sporadic, and characterized by the immune or infectious destruction of biochemically normal myelin or its supporting cell; axons are generally spared. The target usually is either central (as in multiple sclerosis) or peripheral (as in idiopathic polyneuritis) myelin, reflecting their significant antigenic (protein) differences. Dysmyelinating diseases (leukodystrophies) are generally noninflammatory, familial, and characterized by the confluent destruction of (presumably) biochemically abnormal myelin or its supporting cells; axonal loss is more prevalent than in demyelinating or myelinolytic types. Simultaneous involvement of central (especially cerebral) and peripheral myelin is characteristic, reflecting their biochemical (lipid) similarities. Myelinolytic diseases are noninflammatory, either sporadic or familial, and characterized by spongy change (intramyelinic edema) of chemically "normal" myelin. Supporting cells and axons are spared, at least in the early stages. Central involvement is more common. The origin of intramyelinic edema may be either at the major dense line (intracellular) or intraperiod line (extracellular). A list of representative diseases from each category is offered in Table 77-7; several diseases may be validly categorized in some other classification scheme. For example, metachromatic leukodystrophy also is a storage or metabolic disease, progressive multifocal leukoencephalopathy is a viral disease, and so forth.

Demyelinating diseases

Multiple sclerosis (MS).[246-248] The prevalence of multiple sclerosis, the common and prototypic myelin disease of young adults (20 to 40 years of age), correlates directly with certain latitudes (such as northern) and genetic background (such as Caucasian). The commonest form is chronic remitting (remissions and exacerbations) or chronic progressive. The documentation of variably aged lesions at several sites in the neuraxis (time and space) is necessary for a definite diagnosis. There are no definite laboratory tests; however, visualization of lesions with modern imaging techniques, notably magnetic resonance imaging (MRI), and the demonstration of oligoclonal bands in CSF containing excessive protein (including IgG and myelin basic protein) are considered highly consistent with the disease. This usually obviates the need for biopsy. Signs and symptoms correlate with distribution of lesions and are therefore protean, but sometimes incidental lesions are found without the patient having had overt clinical manifestations. The pathogenesis of MS is believed to be related in part to an early (before 15 years) exposure to an environmental factor (purportedly infectious and viral, perhaps measles or perhaps HTLV I) combined with a genetically determined (A3, B7, D2, Dw2, DRw2 haplotypes in whites) immune response entailing humoral (IgG) and cellular factors, cytokines (including tumor necrosis factor), and interleukins.

The pathologic hallmark of classical MS, the demyelinative plaque (Fig. 77-177), is a sharply demarcated lesion devoid of myelin staining, which is usually focal, asymmetrical if bilateral, and disrespectful of anatomic boundaries (such as tracts or gray-white junctions). Sites of predilection include the pial surface of optic nerves and optic chiasm, basis pontis, and spinal cord and the periventricular white matter, that is, white matter close to the cerebrospinal fluid and deep cerebral veins. Shadow plaques, displaying partial myelin staining, reflect ineffectual remyelination (Fig. 77-178). Acute lesions are grossly pink to chalky white and soft; microscopically, vari-

Table 77-7 Diseases of myelin

I. DEMYELINATING DISEASES
  A. Multiple (disseminated) sclerosis
    1. Chronic
      a. Classical (Charcot)
      b. Diffuse cerebral variant (Schilder)
    2. Acute variants
      a. Disseminated (Marburg)
      b. Concentric sclerosis (Balo)
      c. Neuromyelitis optica (Devic)
  B. Acute disseminated encephalomyelitis
    1. Classical
      a. Postinfectious encephalomyelitis
      b. Postvaccinal encephalomyelitis
    2. Hyperacute
      Acute hemorrhagic leukoencephalitis (Hurst)
  C. Focal inflammatory demyelinating lesions with mass effect (Pseudotumor)
  D. Infectious
    1. Progressive multifocal leukoencephalopathy (PML)
    2. Subacute sclerosing panencephalitis (SSPE)
II. DYSMYELINATING DISEASES
  A. Adrenoleukodystrophy. Adrenomyeloneuropathy (X-linked)
  B. Metachromatic leukodystrophy
  C. Globoid cell leukodystrophy (Krabbe's disease)
  D. Sudanophilic leukodystrophies (not otherwise classified)
  E. Pelizaeus-Merzbacher disease (X-linked)
  F. Alexander's disease
III. MYELINOLYTIC DISEASES
  A. Spongy degeneration of infancy and childhood (Canavan or van Bogaert-Bertrand disease)
  B. Central pontine myelinolysis
  C. Aminoacidurias
  D. Vitamin B_{12} deficiency and HIV vacuolar myelopathy
  E. Hexachlorophene and triethyl tin toxicity

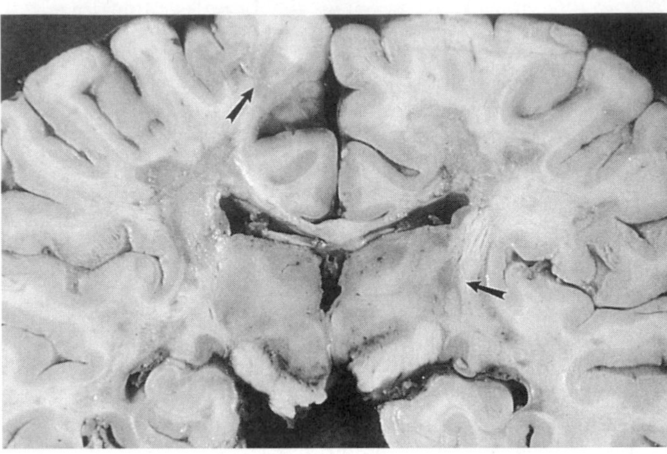

Fig. 77-177 Chronic multiple sclerosis. Periventricular demyelinative plaques and others *(arrows)*.

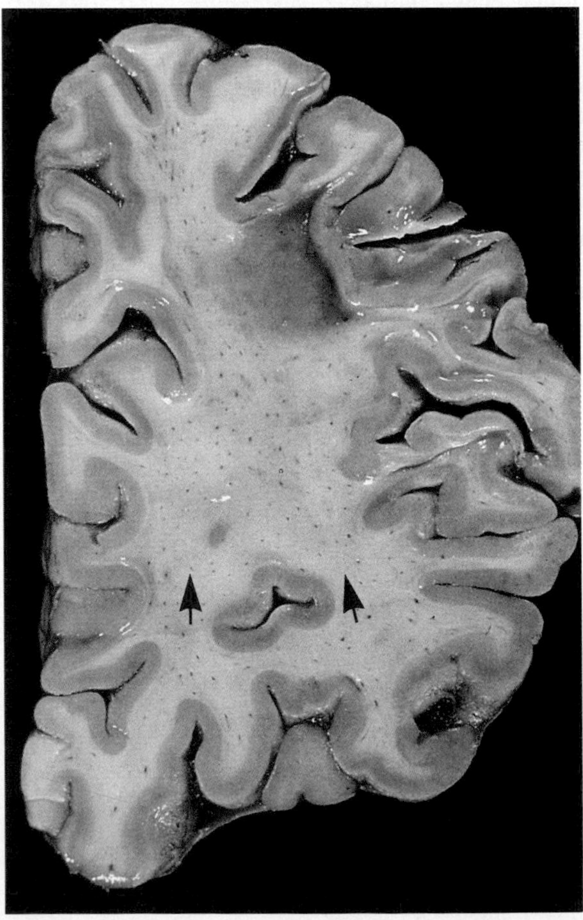

Fig. 77-178 Chronic multiple sclerosis. Demyelinative plaque at gray-white junction and adjacent partially remyelinated shadow plaque *(arrows)*.

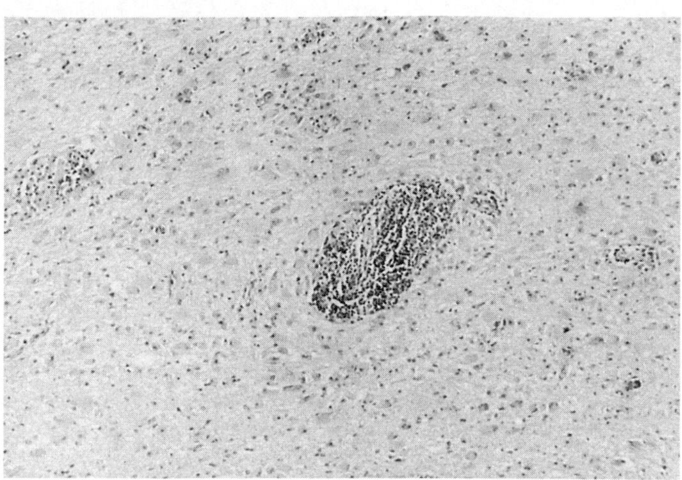

Fig. 77-179 Chronic multiple sclerosis. Active demyelinative plaque with perivascular and interstitial lymphocytes, reactive astrocytes, and lipophages.

able numbers of perivascular and interstitial lymphocytes (CD4 and CD8), plasma cells (often containing IgG), and class II–positive macrophages are associated with loss of myelin and relative preservation of axons (Fig. 77-179). Oligodendrocytic loss and reactive astrocytosis seem to follow. Ultrastructurally, perivenular myelinated axons are in immediate physical contact with macrophages, which appear to cause separation and thinning of myelin sheaths and to peel off peripheral lamellae. Phagocytosis and removal of myelin debris, primarily by macrophages, and ultimately chronic astrogliosis (isomorphic and anisomorphic) eventuate in a firm, gray atrophic lesion. The PNS is spared, except for rare cases in which polyneuritis or hypertrophic neuropathy have been reported,[246] but their relation to MS remains contentious. Acute forms of MS tend to be clinically more catastrophic and more necrotizing with comparable losses of axons and robust astrocytosis that may mimic gliomas. The concentric sclerosis variant (of Balo) is more of a subacute form of the disease characterized by demyelinating lesions alternating with bands of relatively intact white matter; it seems to be relatively common in Southeast Asia. Devic's disease is more prevalent in Japan; the demyelinating process occurs at about the same time in both optic nerves and the spinal cord.

Acute disseminated (allergic) encephalomyelitis (ADE).[246,247,249] Acute disseminated encephalomyelitis is an uncommon, usually monophasic, illness that occurs after either an infection, usually viral, or vaccination. The postvaccinal form tends to be more severe. Both types are believed to be mediated by a misdirected cellular immune response in which some myelin protein is mistaken for a homologous viral protein. Viral invasion of CNS does not appear to be necessary. Experimental allergic encephalomyelitis (EAE), which is produced by the systemic injection of white matter or myelin proteins, is an excellent experimental model. Chronic forms of EAE, developed in particular strains of experimental animals, resemble chronic multiple sclerosis. All areas of the neuraxis may be affected in ADE and feature perivascular lymphocytic cuffs and demyelination. The lesions are histologically comparable (the same age) and usually diffuse, but a confluence of lesions simulating demyelinative plaques may occur. Acute hemorrhagic leukoencephalitis (of Hurst) is believed to be a hyperacute form of ADE with a dramatic, often focal presentation and asymmetric cerebral localization. Fibrinoid necrosis of blood vessels, considerable fibrinous exudate, and neutrophils distinguish it from ADE.

Focal inflammatory demyelinative lesions with mass effect. This recently publicized pseudotumor, more closely related to ADE than to MS,[250] can be treacherous. Focal neurologic signs and symptoms, occurring at any age in association with significant mass effect, so strongly simulate a neoplasm that preoperative radiologic, intraoperative neurosurgical and pathologic, and even postoperative pathologic diagnostic difficulties occur. Pathologically the usually intense lymphocytic inflammation and atypical astrocytosis may be confused with non-Hodgkin's lymphoma, or alternatively with anaplastic astrocytoma, particularly if previously treated with steroids. The most reliable histologic discriminator is the lipophage, usually numerous and containing myelin debris; however, their prominence or presence may be difficult to appreciate in frozen sections (Fig. 77-180). A myelin stain showing diffuse loss of myelin, in conjunction with an axonal stain demonstrating axonal preservation, can help in the differential diagnosis. Caution is indicated if one suspects this lesion, for inappropriate radiotherapy can be catastrophic for the patient.[251]

Dysmyelinating diseases (leukodystrophies)

Most are autosomal recessive diseases of infancy or childhood, but rare adolescent and adult presentations occur in all. Age of onset differs between the major types, but all pursue a progressive downhill course combining ataxia, spasticity, blindness, deafness, psychomotor retardation, or motor deficits with death usually supervening in 6 months to 3 years. Most demonstrate diffuse, confluent dysmyelination, and atrophy of cerebral and cerebellar white matter (Fig. 77-181) with significant axonal loss and relative sparing of arcuate (subcortical U) fibers. In addition to the common features of myelin and oligodendrocyte loss, myelin breakdown products, and acute (reactive)-to-chronic astrogliosis, each type has characteristic light and electron microscopic features. The peripheral nervous system is commonly involved, at least pathologically, except in classical Pelizaeus-Merzbacher and Alexander's disease.[5,12,13,16,246,252]

Adrenoleukodystrophy (ALD) is an X-linked disease, usually of young boys, has a characteristic posterior cerebral distribution, and can include adrenal (glucocorticoid) failure.[253]

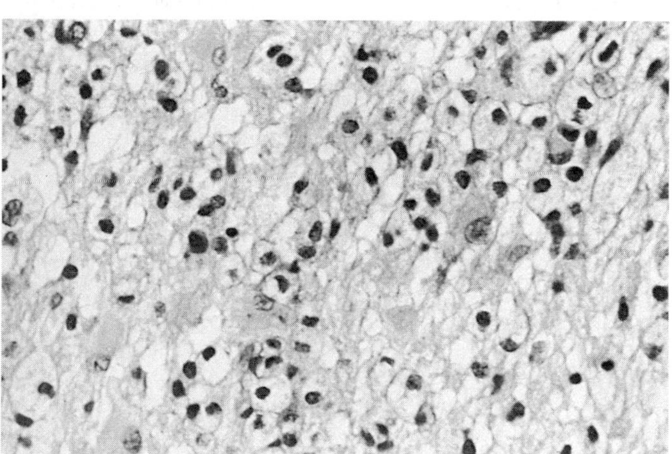

Fig. 77-180 Demyelinating pseudotumor. Prominent lipophages and reactive astrocytes.

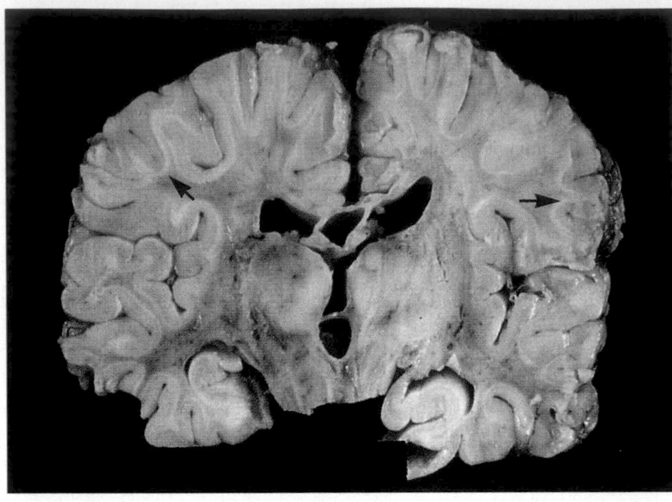

Fig. 77-181 Leukodystrophy (globoid cell). Confluent demyelination with relative sparing of arcuate fibers *(arrows).*

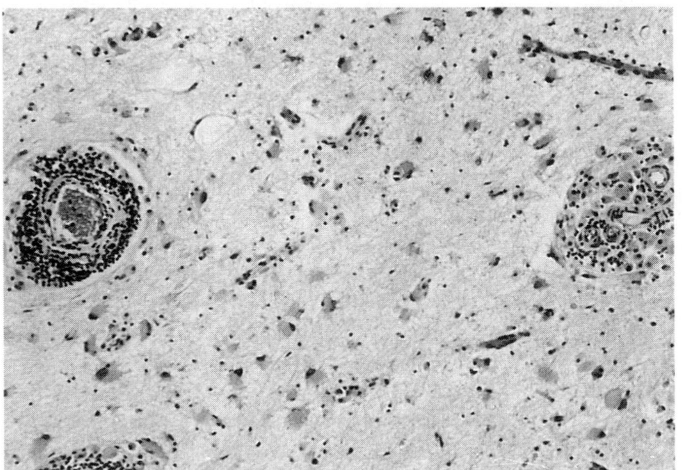

Fig. 77-182 Adrenoleukodystrophy (ALD). Inflammatory (atypical for leukodystrophy) demyelination similar to multiple sclerosis.

In contrast to other leukodystrophies, the demyelination of ALD shows pronounced lymphocytic infiltrates (Fig. 77-182) and sudanophilia. Cytokines, particularly tumor necrosis factor–alpha, also have been identified in the brain lesions.[254] Ultrastructurally, characteristic lamellar and crystalloid inclusions are observed in striated ballooned adrenocortical cells, faintly striated Leydig cells, nonstriated Schwann cells, brain macrophages, and probably in oligodendrocytes. The deficiency of a peroxisomal enzyme, very long chain fatty acid (VLCFA) acyl CoA synthetase (lignoceroyl CoA ligase), is believed to impair the entrance of very long chain (more than 22 carbons) fatty acids to the degradative beta-oxidation system of the peroxisome; there also appears to be increased microsomal elongation. These two defects result in the accumulation of saturated VLCFA in several lipids and proteolipid protein. The putative gene at Xq28 has been cloned, and its predicted gene product has the properties of a membrane protein of the ABC (ATP-binding cassette) transporter family.[255] Both point mutations and deletions in this gene have been identified. The pathogenesis of adrenal atrophy and testicular insufficiency (in

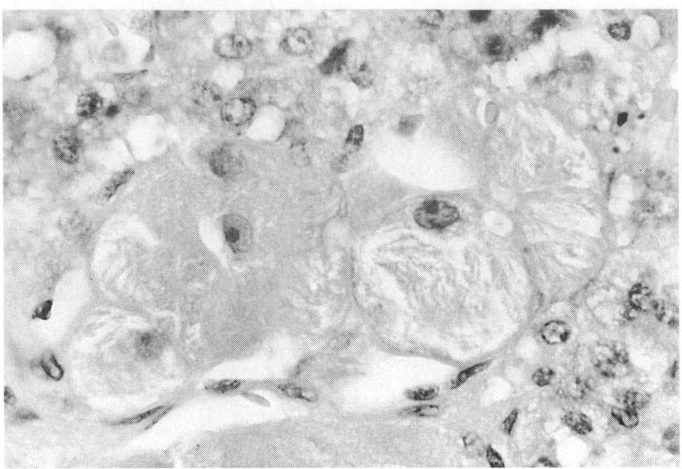

Fig. 77-183 ALD. Ballooned, striated adrenocortical cells.

adults) is believed to be attributable to cytoplasmic accumulations or storage of toxic free saturated fatty acids.[256] CNS demyelination probably results more from myelin instability because of the buildup of VLCFA in myelin lipids and proteolipid protein combined with a prominent cytokine-immune mediated reaction.[254] PAS-positive macrophages, occasionally multinucleated, might simulate Krabbe's disease. However, other morphologic findings, including adrenocortical striations (Fig. 77-183), the family history, and age of onset (3 to 10 years) help to distinguish these two conditions. Adult presentations, especially adrenomyeloneurop-athy with its predominant noninflammatory myelopathy and variable peripheral neuropathy,[253,256] do occur.

Metachromatic leukodystrophy (MLD) in its classic form with a late infantile presentation is attributable to a lack of arylsulfatase A, resulting in the accumulation of metachromatic sulfatide in myelin but predominantly in macrophages; it most commonly is attributable to a splice-site, single-base mutation in chromosome 22q.[12,13] The pathogenesis of the myelin defect appears related to the myelin instability caused by excess sulfatide in myelin. The metachromatic stains toluidine blue and acid cresyl violet (Hirsch-Pfeiffer) color the excess sulfatide red to brown, which is found within the characteristic eosinophilic, granular macrophages of CNS (Fig. 77-184) and in endoneurial macrophages. Ultrastructurally, diagnostic prismatic structures in macrophages and tuffstone bodies in Schwann cells exhibit a lamellar substructure with a 5 to 6 nm periodicity. Although ALD has its distinctive concomitant adrenal involvement, MLD is unique in that it also is a systemic (especially gallbladder and kidney) and neuronal (Fig. 77-185) (CNS and PNS) lipidosis.

Globoid cell leukodystrophy (GLD, Krabbe's disease), usually of infants, lacks systemic features and is attributable to a deficiency of beta-galactocerebrosidase (galactosyl ceramide-β-galactosidase), which has been localized to chromosome 14.[12,13] This results in the accumulation of the usually inconspicuous side-chain reaction product psychosine (galactosyl sphingosine). Psychosine is toxic to oligodendrocytes and myelin sheaths in experimental animals.[252] The distinguishing histologic feature of GLD is the presence of large uninucleated epithelioid and multinucleated globoid cells (Fig. 77-186), which are PAS positive. Ultrastructurally, crystalloid multan-

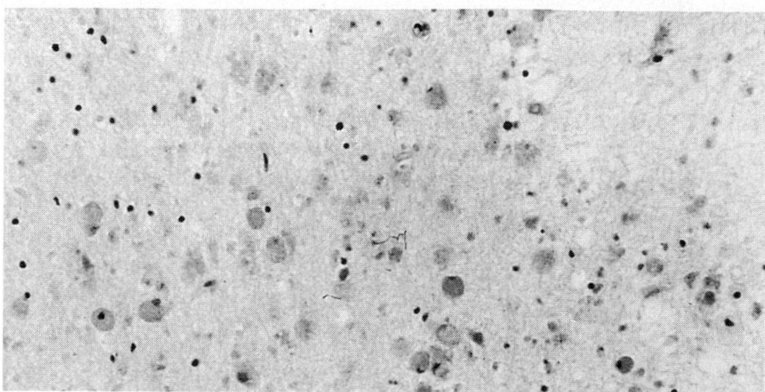

Fig. 77-184 Metachromatic leukodystrophy (MLD). Eosinophilic granular macrophages especially prominent in areas undergoing active demyelination.

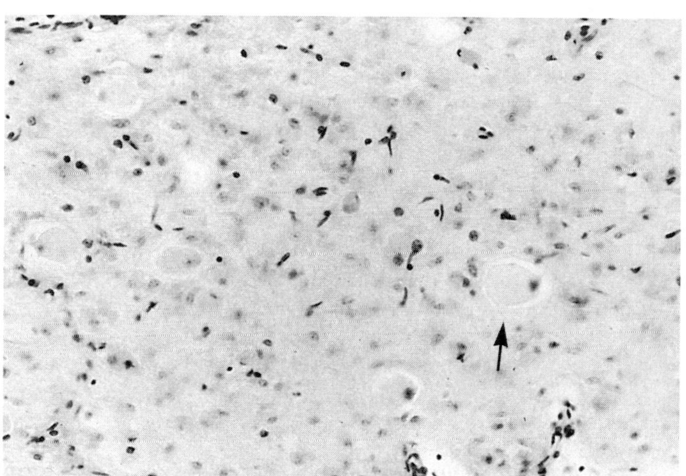

Fig. 77-185 MLD. Neuronal storage *(arrow)* in dentate nucleus.

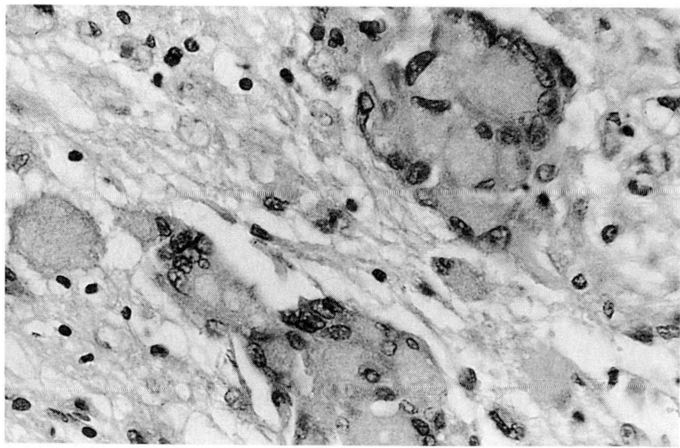

Fig. 77-186 Globoid cell leukodystrophy (GLD). Multinucleated globoid cells.

gular inclusions are characteristic. The twitcher mouse mutant is an excellent animal model.

Pelizaeus-Merzbacher disease (a hypomyelinative leukodystrophy) manifests in several known types, all rare. The classical X-linked infantile form is known for its tigroid CNS

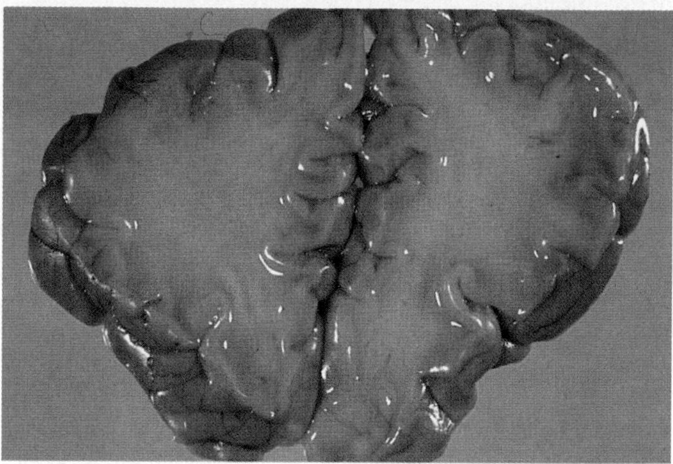

Fig. 77-187 Canavan's disease. Confluent gelatinous transformation of white matter most noticeable at arcuate fibres.

demyelination in which there is a paucity of myelin debris and perivascular sparing of myelin. This form has been shown to have a selective deficiency of the CNS-restricted myelin proteolipid protein (PLP) because of a variety of point mutations in the gene located at Xq22.[12,13,252] Several animal models, including the jimpy mouse mutant, are known.

Alexander's disease is an exceptionally rare and apparently genetic infantile white matter disease characterized by numerous Rosenthal fibers (Fig. 77-23) in fibrous astrocytes (subpial, perivascular, subependymal) and a paucity of central myelin. More rarely, adult variants and localized forms (formes frustes) have been reported.[5,246,252]

Myelinolytic diseases (spongy myelinopathies)

A variety of metabolic and toxic conditions, often uncommon, display the histopathologic lesions of spongy myelin (intramyelinic edema). Amino and organic acidurias, mitochondrial encephalopathies, iatrogenic intoxication with hexachlorophene, commercial intoxication with triethyl tin, subacute combined degeneration of the spinal cord from a deficiency of Vitamin B_{12}, and others. Hence, most of these diseases also are classified as metabolic or toxic and are mentioned in that section. Only two are discussed here: Canavan's disease (simulating a leukodystrophy) and central pontine myelinolysis (a primary demyelinating lesion).

Spongy degeneration of the CNS in infancy (Canavan's, van Bogaert-Bertrand disease)[5,246,252] is an autosomal recessive disease, primarily affecting infants of Ashkenazi Jews, usually presents at 2 to 6 months, and behaves clinically as a leukodystrophy. As in Alexander's disease and the late stages of Tay-Sachs disease, megalencephaly (increased brain weight) and peripheral nerve sparing are typical. Many features justify its inclusion in the leukodystrophies (Fig. 77-187), but its histopathologic hallmark of spongy (vacuolar) myelinopathy, initially and consistently of subcortical (arcuate) white matter and deep cortex (Fig. 77-188) with a paucity of myelin breakdown products and macrophages, and a grossly detectable gelatinous to aqueous transformation of cerebral and cerebellar white matter set it apart. The vacuoles reflect intramyelinic edema predominantly arising between major dense lines (that is, within the intraperiod line or extracellular) (Fig. 77-189), but swollen astrocytic cytoplasm contributes to the vacuolation of white matter and particularly gray matter. Hydropic astrocytic nuclei in deep cortex, resembling Alzheimer II glia of hepatic encephalopathy, and abnormal mitochondria in these astrocytes are also characteristic. A deficiency of *N*-acetylaspartase (aspartoacylase) leading to accumulations of *N*-acetylaspartate has been documented.[257] The astrocyte may play a significant pathogenetic role, as it may in Alexander's disease.

Central pontine myelinolysis (CPM),[246,258] a modern disease, manifests with clinical effects varying from none to coma and quadriplegia. Primary demyelination caused by intramyelinic edema, apparently arising at the intraperiod line (extracellular), classically affects middorsal crossing fibers of the pons (Fig. 77-190). Axonal loss, spheroids, lipophages, and conspicuous to atypical reactive astrocytes often are observed (Fig. 77-191). In severe cases, the pontine lesions are more extensive, and extrapontine lesions commonly occur. Risk factors of alcoholism, liver disease, malnutrition, and chronic hyponatremia have been identified, but excessive swings in serum osmolality now seem the more likely pathogenetic common denominator.[258] Overzealous correction of chronic hyponatremia, facilitated by the advent of intravenous lines at the time of this disease's birth, is believed to result in extravascular fluid accumulations most pronounced in areas with intimate admixtures of gray and white matter: basis pontis, lateral geniculate body, thalamus, and so forth. *Marchiafava-Bignami* disease, another rare disease of chronic alcoholics, shares some of the demyelinative features of CPM, but primarily affects the corpus callosum.[259] Another lesion that shows a topographic similarity to CPM, but histologic features like disseminated necrotizing leukoencephalopathy, recently has been reported as "multifocal necrotizing leukoencephalopathy with pontine predilection." Immunosuppression appears to be a common denominator among these patients.[260]

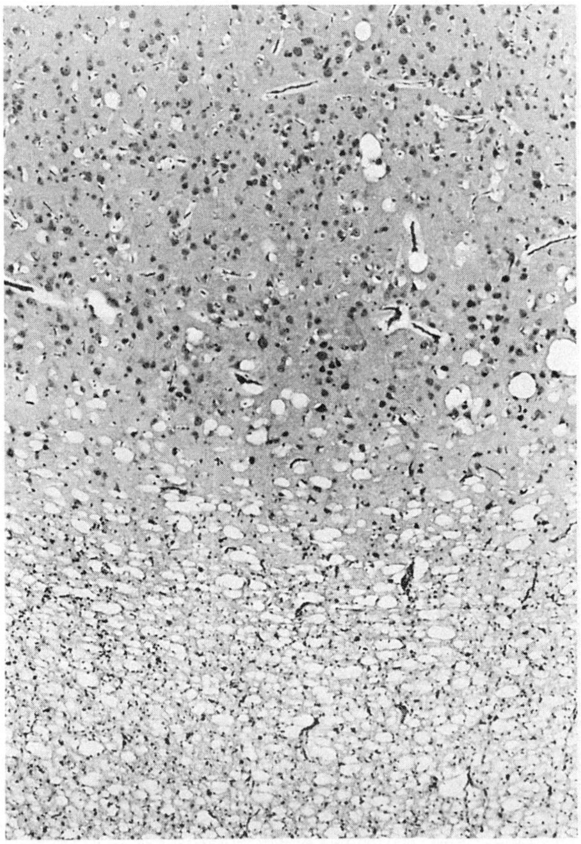

Fig. 77-188 Canavan's disease. Spongy myelinopathy of myelinated fibers and hydropic astrocytes in deep cortex.

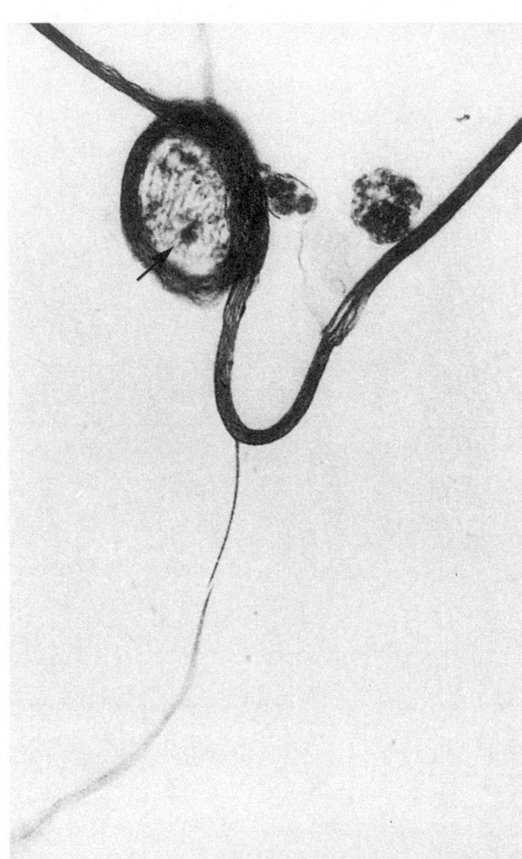

Fig. 77-189 Canavan's disease. Intramyelinic edema with intact axon *(arrow)*.

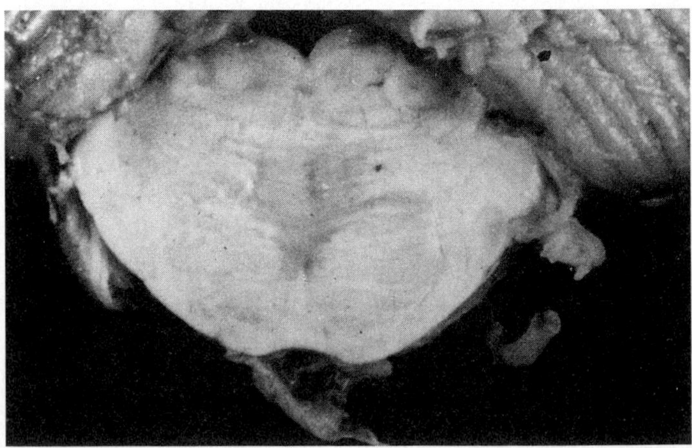

Fig. 77-190 Central pontine myelinolysis (CPM). Sharply circumscribed demyelination in central pons.

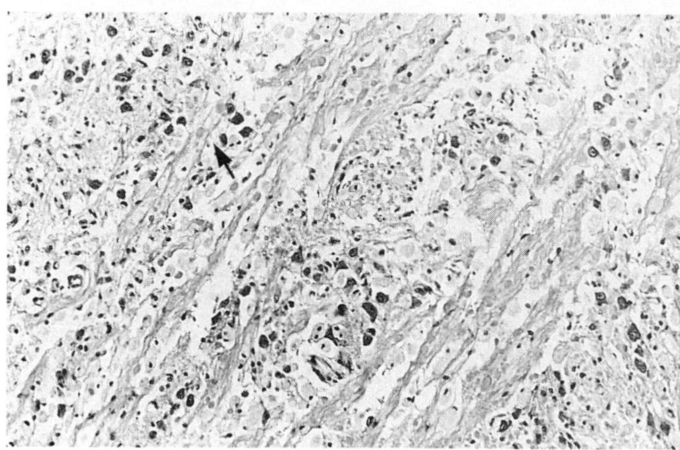

Fig. 77-191 CPM. Demyelination, lipophages, reactive astrocytes, neuronal sparing, and some reactive spheroids *(arrow)*.

METABOLIC AND TOXIC DISEASES

Central to understanding the pathophysiology and distribution of metabolic and toxic diseases is the concept of selective vulnerability, which states that specific cell types or populations are more susceptible to a particular insult than others.[20,259] If the insult is lethal and the neuron is susceptible, one should recall that neurons are postmitotic cells and irreplaceable. The following abridged classification (Table 77-8) is offered to facilitate the management of this myriad of diseases.

Table 77-8 Metabolic and toxic diseases

1. Deficiency of metabolic substrate or cofactor (acquired, sporadic):
   Hypoxia, hypoglycemia, hypovitaminosis
2. Deficiency of enzyme (usually catabolic and lysosomal) with or without excess (storage) of normal or toxic substrates (congenital, familial):
   Mitochondrial, peroxisomal, lysosomal
   Ceroid-lipofuscinoses
   Amino and organic acidurias, urea cycle defects
   Spongy degeneration of the CNS in infancy (Canavan's disease)
   Neuroaxonal dystrophy–Hallervorden-Spatz disease.
3. Excess of endogenous toxic metabolite (familial or sporadic):
   Copper (Wilson's disease, Menkes' syndrome)
   Iron (hemochromatosis, hemosiderosis)
   Bilirubin (kernicterus)
   Systemic encephalopathies
4. Excess of exogenous toxic metabolites (toxins) (sporadic):
   Natural, industrial, therapeutic

Substrate or cofactor deficiency

Hypoxia and *hypoglycemia*[20] can be considered together, since neurons require both oxygen and glucose, and deprivation from either results in similar pathologic effects. Most clinical examples of hypoxia are oligemic or ischemic; thus impaired delivery of nutrients is associated with accumulation of deleterious metabolites. The hallmark of this hypoxia (or hypoglycemia) is individual neuronal necrosis, acutely manifest (around 6 hours) as cytoplasmic eosinophilia (ischemic or hypoxic cell change; pink, red, or eosinophilic neurons) (Fig. 77-4) and ultimately as neuronal loss. The release of excitotoxic amino acid neurotransmitters (such as glutamate) from damaged neurons results in an acute influx of sodium with intracellular (cytoxic) edema and a delayed lethal influx of calcium. If, as often happens, blood flow is severely compromised, widespread cytoxic edema evident as pallor and microvacuolization of neuropil and damage to other cells (such as astrocytes and endothelial cells) occurs; this may be followed 6 to 8 hours later by vasogenic edema, and infarction may occur. The distribution of "hypoxic" neuronal necrosis is highly variable, but favored sites in the child and adult include pyramidal neurons of Sommer's sector (CA1, h1) and end plate (CA3-4, h4-5) of the hippocampus, Purkinje cells of the cerebellum, large neurons of the inner globus pallidus, and neocortical pyramidal neurons of layer III, especially in border zones and at the depth of parieto-occipital sulci (Fig. 77-192). In the neonate and infant favored sites include the subiculum of hippocampus and brainstem nuclei, such as inferior colliculi and vestibular nuclei. Sometimes the major lesions are localized to white matter with relative preservation of gray matter; this seems to occur when hypoxia is associated with acidosis or chronic edema and when oligodendrocytes are myelinating.

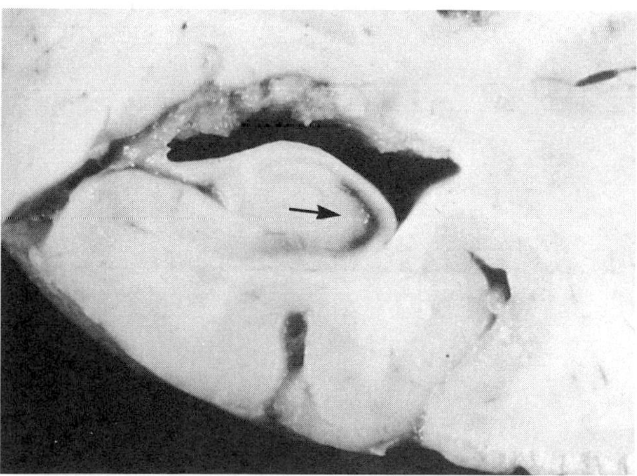

Fig. 77-192 Remote hypoxic damage to Sommer's sector of hippocampus *(arrow)*.

Acute Wernicke's disease, most commonly encountered in chronic alcoholics but attributable to thiamine deficiency (vitamin B_1), is characterized by confusion, ocular disturbances, and ataxia; it usually is reversible if treated early with thiamine.[259,261] Gross changes may be inapparent or appear as petechial to more extensive hemorrhages, the latter being seen with concomitant hepatic insufficiency and clotting problems. Histologically, endothelial swelling and proliferation, sponginess of the neuropil, and astrocytosis with neuronal preservation (Fig. 77-193) are noted bilaterally and symmetrically in mammillary bodies, medial dorsal nuclei of the thalamus and other nuclei around the third and fourth ventricles. *Chronic Wernicke's disease* displays atrophy and tan discoloration of the same areas because of neuronal shrinkage and loss with astrogliosis and hemosiderin deposits (Fig. 77-194); this explains its irreversibility and prominent amnestic component (*Wernicke-Korsakoff disease* or psychosis), since the mammillary bodies are relay nuclei of the Papez circuit. Bilateral interruption of this "limbic circuit" is believed responsible for the amnestic Korsakoff component, and hence other pathophysiologic processes can produce this clinical disability (such as bilateral destruction of temporal lobes). Chronic Wernicke patients often have peripheral neuropathy, as does the classical thiamine dietary deficiency of beriberi, but only a few have a concomitant cardiomyopathy.[261]

Subacute combined degeneration of the spinal cord, caused by a chronic deficiency of cobalamin (vitamin B_{12}), most commonly results from the malabsorption syndrome of pernicious anemia. Pathologic changes affect optic nerve, brain, spinal cord, and peripheral nerve. The classical myelopathy manifests as an initial spongy change of myelin caused by intramyelinic edema, followed by axonal and oligodendrocytic loss, astrocytosis and a macrophage response. The localization of these lesions to the posterior and posterolateral columns (Fig. 77-195), particularly of the upper thoracic cord, their asymmetry, and their transgression of tract boundaries are characteristic. White matter changes also are detected elsewhere.[261]

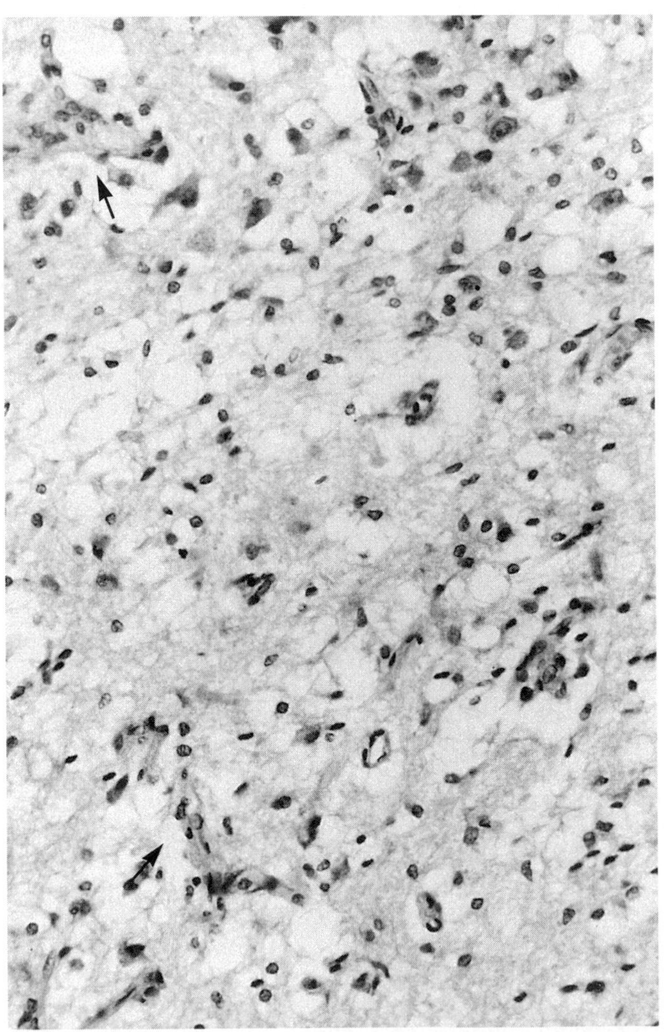

Fig. 77-193 Acute Wernicke's disease. Rarefaction and capillary prominence *(arrows).*

Enzyme deficiency

Mitochondrial disorders

Mitochondrial disorders are rare systemic diseases, often characterized by chronic lactic acidemia, in which involvement of

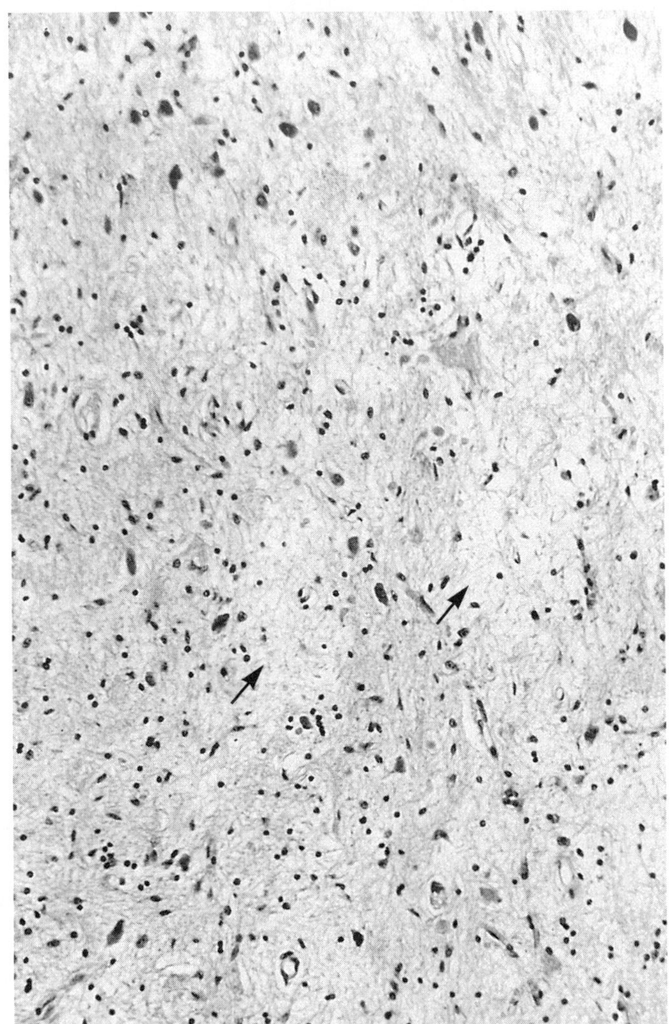

Fig. 77-194 Chronic Wernicke's disease. Neuronal loss and fibrillary gliosis *(arrows).*

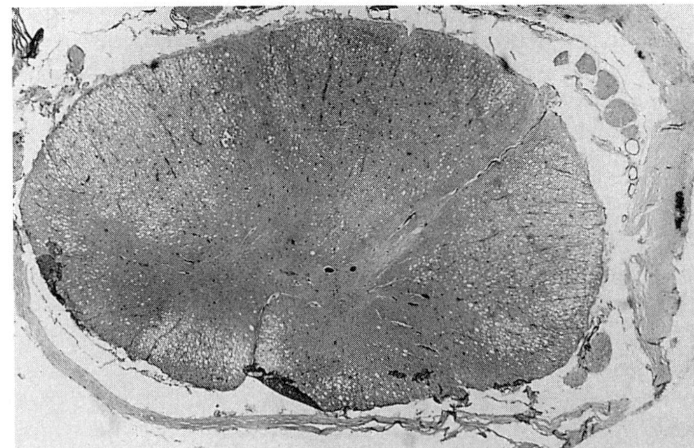

Fig. 77-195 Subacute combined degeneration. Spongy change of thoracic lateral, posterior, and even anterior columns.

Table 77-9 Mitochondrial disorders

Disease or enzyme deficiency	Systemic lesion	CNS site	CNS lesion
Luft's disease	Ragged red fibers (muscle)	—	—
Leigh's disease	—	Deep and periventricular gray matter	Spongy change; Vascular proliferation
Pyruvate dehydrogenase complex:			
Pyruvate decarboxylase	—	Cerebrum; deep and periventricular gray matter	Cystic lesions in white > gray; Leigh's disease
Pyruvate carboxylase	Hepatic steatosis	Cerebral white matter; neocortex	Paucity of myelin; neuronal loss
Glioneuronal dystrophy (some Alper's disease)	Hepatic fibrosis	Neocortex	Spongy change and neuronal loss
Respiratory chain enzymes:			
Menkes' syndrome	Pili torti (hair)	Neocortex; cerebellum	Neuronal loss; Purkinje dysmorphism
Biotin dependent enzymes:			
Biotinidase	Skin rash; alopecia	Insufficient data	
Carnitine deficiency	Lipid myopathy	—	—
Carnitine palmityl transferase	Rhabdomyolysis	—	—
Ragged red fiber–related diseases:			
Kearns-Sayre disease	Ragged red fibers	Brainstem, cerebellar white	Spongy change
MERRF	Ragged red fibers	Dentate nucleus; brainstem	Neuronal loss; tract degeneration
MELAS	Ragged red fibers	Neocortex	Microinfarcts

—, None reported; *MELAS*, Mitochondrial encephalomyopathy, lactic acidosis, and strokelike episodes; *MERRF*, Myoclonic epilepsy with ragged red fibers.

skeletal muscle and CNS predominates (Table 77-9). Since mitochondria are regulated by both nuclear DNA and their own mitochondrial (mt) DNA, genetic mitochondrial diseases may be transmitted by mendelian or maternal (nonmendelian) inheritance, respectively. The high phenotypic variability of diseases associated with mutations in mtDNA is believed attributable to heteroplasmy (mixture of wild and mutant mt DNA in the same cell), replicative segregation (random partitioning of mt DNA into daughter cells), and a threshold effect (mutant mt DNA must reach a certain relative proportion).[262] Pathologic data for the rare types should be viewed as provisional. Discussion will be restricted to subacute necrotizing encephalomyelopathy of Leigh (nuclear DNA) and ragged red fiber disorders (mt DNA) that include *Kearns-Sayre syndrome, MERRF (myoclonic epilepsy, ragged red fibers),* and *MELAS (mitochondrial encephalomyopathy, lactic acidosis, strokelike episodes).*[12,16,262,263]

Subacute necrotizing encephalomyelopathy (SNE, Leigh's disease) usually presents within the first few years as failure to thrive, psychomotor retardation, hypotonia, nystagmus, deafness, and seizures. Family history is often positive, and juvenile and adult onsets (simulating acute Wernicke's disease) are known. At least four metabolic defects have been reported, the commonest being a deficiency of cytochrome *c* oxidase (COX), but most cases are idiopathic. The histopathologic lesions are similar to those of acute Wernicke's disease, but there is a greater tendency for the rarefied spongy microcystic lesions of the neuropil to proceed to cavitary necrosis. Bilateral and symmetric involvement of the diencephalon (especially putamen and thalamus), brainstem (especially the substantia nigra), cerebral and cerebellar white matter, dentate nuclei, spinal gray matter, and optic system with sparing of the mammillary bodies are characteristic (Fig. 77-196).[261]

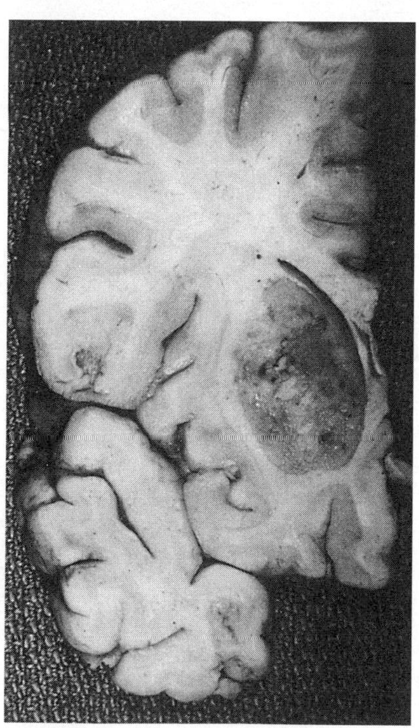

Fig. 77-196 Subacute necrotizing encephalomyelopathy (Leigh's disease). Necrotic lesions in caudate and putamen.

Ragged red (skeletal muscle) fibers, named for their light microscopic displays of abnormal mitochondria with a rapid modified Gomori trichrome stain, are seen in association with a variety of CNS lesions. Kearns-Sayre (ophthalmoplegia plus) syndrome, a sporadic disease caused by large deletions in mt DNA, is characterized by status spongiosus of brainstem gray matter and spongy myelinopathy of cerebral and cerebellar white matter. Familial MERRF and MELAS, caused by different point mutations in tRNA mitochondrial genes, exhibit respectively neuronal loss (particularly of the dentate nucleus) with tract degeneration and microinfarcts (particularly of the neocortex) with mineralization of basal ganglia[263] (Fig. 77-197).

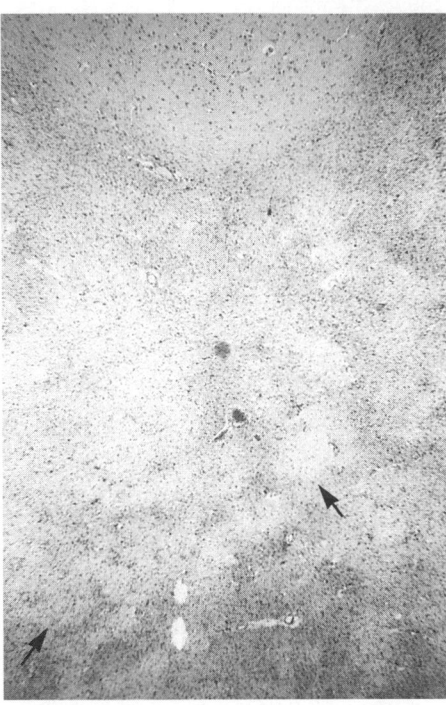

Fig. 77-197 Kearns-Sayre disease. Spongy change in subcortical cerebral white matter *(arrows)*.

Peroxisomal disorders

Peroxisomal disorders also are rare systemic, multiorgan diseases with prominent involvement of the nervous system (Table 77-10). Peroxisomes, formerly called "microbodies," now are known to contain approximately 50 enzymes, which are responsible for much more than catalase-mediated removal of hydrogen peroxide: catabolism of very long chain fatty acids (VLCFA) and pipecolic acid, synthesis of ether lipids and bile acids, and others. Pathologic data for the rare types should be viewed as provisional. Some patients display an "absence" of peroxisomes (as in the Zellweger syndrome), whereas others lack a specific enzyme (as in ALD; see discussion of myelin diseases).[253,264-266]

Cerebrohepatorenal (Zellweger) syndrome (CHRS) is the prototype of a rare group of fatal infantile diseases with dysmorphic facies and the neonatal onset of profound hypotonia and seizures. CHRS is caused by heterogeneous genetic abnormalities (such as a microdeletion or inversion on chromosome 7p) with the identification of multiple complementation groups; these molecular aberrations eventuate in a targeting failure of peroxisomal matrix proteins. The molecular defect takes the morphologic appearance of peroxisomal "ghosts" with a biochemical deficiency of multiple enzyme systems, particularly those that catabolize VLCFA and synthesize plasmalogens.[253,265] Centrosylvian polymicrogyria and pachygyria are most characteristic in the CNS (Fig. 77-198), whereas renal cysts, hepatic fibrosis, and adrenocortical striated cells are seen systemically.[266]

Lysosomal disorders

Although still rare, this diverse group is the most established and includes the classical storage diseases, such as lipidoses and neuronal storage diseases (Table 77-11). The deficiency of a catabolic enzyme in these autosomal-recessive diseases results in the accumulation, or storage, of substrates and intermediates proximal to the affected enzymatic step. There are four major types of lysosomal storage diseases with

Table 77-10 **Peroxisomal disorders**

Disease or enzyme deficiency	Systemic lesion	CNS site and lesion
I. Peroxisomes numerically reduced; multiple enzymes deficient		
Cerebrohepatorenal (Zellweger) syndrome	Renal cysts to microcysts; hepatic fibrosis to cirrhosis; calcific stippling of patellae	Polymicrogyria-pachygyria; abnormal white matter
Neonatal adrenoleukodystrophy (NALD)	Adrenal atrophy; PAS+ macrophages	Demyelination; polymicrogyria
Infantile Refsum disease	Hepatic PAS+ macrophages with angulate lysosomes	Cerebellar atrophy*
Hyperpipecolic acidemia	Micronodular cirrhosis	Demyelination*
II. Peroxisomes numerically normal; multiple enzymes deficient		
Rhizomelic chondrodysplasia punctata	Shortened long bones; stippled calcifications	Conflicting data*
III. Peroxisomes numerically normal; single enzyme deficient		
Adrenoleukodystrophy	Adrenal atrophy	Inflammatory demyelination
Adrenomyeloneuropathy	Adrenal atrophy	Spinal tract degeneration
Acyl CoA oxidase (pseudo-NALD)	Hepatic fibrosis; adrenal atrophy	Demyelination* (CT only)
Bifunctional enzyme	Hepatic fibrosis; renal microcysts; adrenal atrophy	Polymicrogyria*
Thiolase (pseudo-Zellweger)	Renal microcysts; adrenal atrophy	Demyelination*, polymicrogyria
Primary hyperoxaluria I	Renal calculi	—

*Insufficient data; —, none reported.

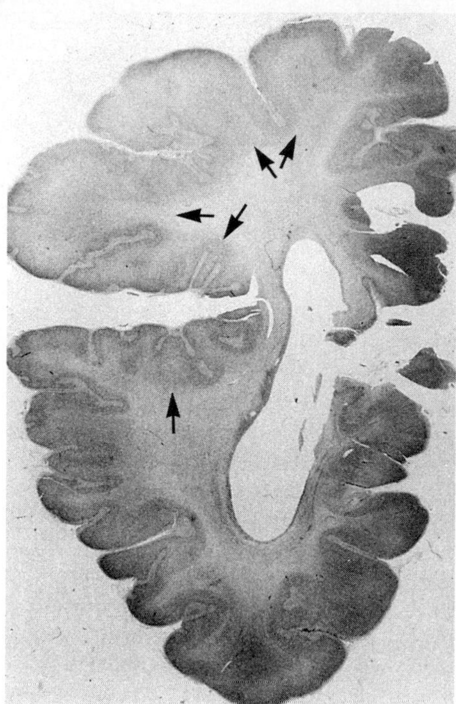

Fig. 77-198 Cerebrohepatorenal (Zellweger) syndrome. Pachygyria with heterotopias in superficial white matter *(arrows)* and lateral polymicrogyria. (Courtesy S. Duckett, editor: *Pediatric neuropathology,* 1995, Williams and Wilkins.)

prominent involvement of the CNS: (1) sphingolipidoses: gangliosides G_{M2}- *(Tay-Sachs)* and G_{M1}-, glucocerebroside *(Gaucher),* sulfatide *(metachromatic leukodystrophy),* sphingomyelin *(Niemann-Pick),* ceramide *(Fabry)* (2) glycosaminoglycanoses (mucopolysaccharidoses, MPS): *Hurler, Hunter, San Filippo;* (3) the confusing sialidoses, mucolipidoses, and glycoproteinoses including mannosidosis and fucosidosis;[12,252,264] and (4) glycogenoses: *Pompe's* disease, Andersen's disease, galactosemia, polyglucosan body disease. Specific details of these classical diseases and their many permutations are available elsewhere. It should be emphasized that the distribution, histochemical staining properties, and ultrastructural appearance of storage material is highly characteristic of specific diseases or groups of diseases. Pathologic data traditionally have played a major role in the diagnostic evaluation of such patients. However, the morphologic assessment of a biochemical defect has inherent limitations, and consequently has been superseded by more direct biochemical methodologies: isolation of the storage material or more recently documentation of a specific enzyme deficiency in serum, white cells, or fibroblasts. The enzyme deficiency may be related to a failure of synthesis of the enzyme, the synthesis of a biochemically defective enzyme, the absence of an activator or protective system needed by the enzyme, the failure to direct the enzyme to a conducive environment (organelle), and other cellular or molecular defects. The traditional morphologic evaluation, particularly electron microscopy, still can limit nosologic possibilities and direct diagnostic evaluation options.[12,13,16,252,264]

In *G_{M2} gangliosidosis (Tay-Sachs)* a deficiency of hexosaminidase A (an alpha/beta heterodimer encoded on chromosomes 15 and 5) prevents the removal of the terminal *N*-acetylgalactosamine and results in the storage of G_{M2} (and other lipids) in central, retinal (cherry-red spot) and peripheral (including autonomic) neurons of infants, usually Ashkenazi Jewish. These infants manifest severe psychomotor retardation with myoclonic seizures and die within a few years. The most characteristic pathologic feature is a swollen or ballooned neuron (Fig. 77-17) filled with membranous cytoplasmic bodies (MCB) at the electron microscopic level (Fig. 77-199), which generally stains strongly with lipid dyes and weakly with PAS in paraffin sections. The brain may be large in the late stages (megalencephaly), normal, or atrophic. Pallor to cavitation of cerebral and cerebellar white matter reflect axonal loss and gliosis. In addition to perikaryal swelling, dendrites, proximal axons (meganeurites), and even glial cells accumulate abnormal storage material. The MCB is round or ovoid, varies from 0.5 to 2 μm in diameter, and consists of concentric alternating electron-dense and electron-lucent lines with a 5 to 6 nm period. MCBs consist of ganglioside (G_{M2} forms about 50% of total lipid in this gangliosidosis), cholesterol, phosphatides, and glycolipids. Adult and juvenile variants generally show less storage, neuronal loss, and gliosis with greater variability in the fine structure of cytosomes and distribution of lesions. G_{M1} gangliosidosis is a generalized disorder that more closely approximates MPS, but the CNS lesions are similar to those of G_{M2} gangliosidosis.

Hurler's disease (MPS IH), a prototypic autosomal recessive disease of glycosaminoglycans (GAGS), is attributable to a deficiency of alpha-L-iduronidase. Since GAGS or mucopolysaccharides (MPS) are constituents of many organs, the disorder is systemic and manifests as hepatomegaly, splenomegaly, joint and bone deformities, opacities of lens and cornea, connective tissue abnormalities, and neuronal storage. Ultrastructurally in mesenchymal cells, including the meninges, the stored material (GAGS) consists of 1 to 2 μm clear vacuoles, whereas storage in neurons is similar (Zebra bodies) or identical to MCB of gangliosidoses. The leptomeningeal (mesenchymal) storage of poorly stainable, metachromatic, and water-soluble GAGS can lead to obstructive communicating hydrocephalus and greatly widened perivascular spaces in white matter (Fig. 77-200).

Pompe's disease, because of a deficiency of alpha-1,4-glucosidase and resulting in membrane-bound (lysosomal) glycogen storage, is a generalized disorder involving all cell types in the nervous system simultaneously. Involvement of fibrous astrocytes and large motor neurons, such as those in anterior horns, is most impressive. The glycogen is normal and hence is unstained in hematoxylin and eosin and its PAS positivity is sensitive to diastase pretreatment. This stands in striking contrast to a family of diseases referred to as "polyglucosan body diseases," in which astrocytes, neurons, or both types, may accumulate a weakly hematoxylinophilic, PAS-positive, relatively diastase-resistant, amylopectin-like polysaccharide along with restricted systemic deposits in heart (basophilic degeneration), liver, and skeletal or smooth muscle. The infantile member of this family is glycogen storage disease type IV *(Andersen's disease),* which is characterized by fatal cirrhosis and accumulations of polyglucosan in fibrous astrocytes and neurons because of a deficiency, probably generalized, of the branching enzyme. The juvenile form, with normal branching activity in brain and muscle, typically has myoclonic epilepsy with perikaryal inclusions *(Lafora bodies)* (Fig. 77-201). Adults have a motor neuron disorder and dementia with wide-

Table 77-11 CNS lysosomal disorders

Disease	Deficiency	Lesion site	CNS lesion
Lipidoses			
G_{M2}-Gangliosidosis			
Infantile (Tay-Sachs)	Hexosaminidase A	CNS and PNS neurons, diffuse	Swollen neurons (PAS±, SB+; MCB)
AB variant	Activator protein	CNS and PNS neurons, diffuse	
Sandhoff's disease	Hexosaminidase A and B	CNS and PNS neurons, diffuse; visceral storage	
G_{M1}-gangliosidosis	β-Galactosidase	CNS and PNS neurons, diffuse; visceral storage	
Niemann-Pick disease			
Infantile (type A)	Sphingomyelinase	CNS and PNS neurons, diffuse; visceral storage	Swollen neurons (PAS+, SB+; loose MCB to complex MCB)
Types C and D	Cholesterol esterification	CNS and PNS neurons, diffuse to localized; visceral storage	
Gaucher's disease			
Infantile (type 2)	Glucocerebrosidase	CNS macrophages and neurons; visceral storage	Neuronal loss; distended macrophages (PAS+, SB+; tubules)
Fabry's disease	α-Galactosidase	CNS blood vessels and autonomic neurons, PNS perineurial cells; visceral storage	Swollen neurons (PAS+, SB+; pleomorphic MCB)
Metachromatic leukodystrophy	Arylsulfatase A or activator protein	CNS, PNS myelin, diffuse; neurons, localized; visceral storage	Demyelination with metachromatic debris and lamellar stacks; neuronal pleomorphic MCB)
Mucosulfatidosis (Austin's variant)	Multiple sulfatases	Leukodystrophy and neuronal storage of ganglioside (like MLD), and MPS in viscera	
Krabbe's (globoid cell) leukodystrophy	Galactocerebrosidase	CNS and PNS myelin	Demyelination with PAS+ globoid cells; multangular bodies
Farber's disease	Acid ceramidase	CNS and PNS neurons, localized to diffuse; visceral storage	Swollen neurons (PAS+, SB±; zebra bodies)
Wolman's disease	Cholesterol ester hydrolase	PNS neurons, perineurial, endoneurial, and Schwann cells; visceral storage	Swollen neurons (SB+, Schultz cholesterol +; electron-lucent globules)
Disease	**Enzyme deficiency**	**Sites and lesions**	
Mucopolysaccharidoses			
Hurler's (MPSIH) Hurler-Scheie	α-L-Iduronidase	CNS and PNS neurons* and mesenchyme,† diffuse; systemic lesions	
Scheie's (MPSIS, formerly V)		Compressive myelopathy†	
Hunter's (MPSII) (X-linked)	Iduronosulfate sulfatase	CNS and PNS neurons and mesenchyme, diffuse; systemic lesions	
Sanfilippo's (MPSIII)	Heparan sulfatase (type A)	CNS and PNS neurons and mesenchyme, diffuse; mild systemic lesions	
Morquio's A (MPS IV)	Acetylgalactosamine-4-sulfate sulfatase	Compressive myelopathy†	
Sly (MPSVII)	β-Glucuronidase	Hurler-like	
Sialidoses, mucolipidoses, and glycoproteinoses			
Neuraminidase deficiency	Neuraminidase (sialidase)	Rare diseases of unsettled nosology with clinical resemblance to MPS and pathologic findings similar to those of gangliosidoses and MPS	
Sialidosis type I (cherry-red spot/myoclonus syndrome)			
Sialidosis type II—dysmorphic (mucolipidosis I, lipomucopolysaccharidosis, Goldberg syndrome)			
Galactosialidosis	Neuraminidase/β-Galactosidase		
Mucolipidosis II (I-cell disease)	*N*-Acetylglucosamine-1-phosphotransferase		
Mucolipidosis III	*N*-Acetylglucosamine-1-phosphotransferase		
Fucosidosis	α-L-Fucosidase		
Mannosidosis	α-Mannosidase, β-Mannosidase		
Aspartylglycosaminuria	Aspartylglucosaminidase		
Salla's disease	Normal; ?↑sialidase		
Infantile sialic acid storage disease	Normal; ?↑sialidase		

MCB, membranous cytoplasmic bodies; *PAS*, periodic acid–Schiff stain; *SB*, sudan black; *Swollen neurons (PAS+, SB+; zebra bodies and MCB); †Mesenchymal cells—metachromasia in frozen sections; ‡Fine structure of systemic inclusions. Clear membrane-bound vacuoles in MPS, clear to granulo-filamentous to MCB to lipofuscin in sialidoses, mucolipidoses, and glycoproteinoses.

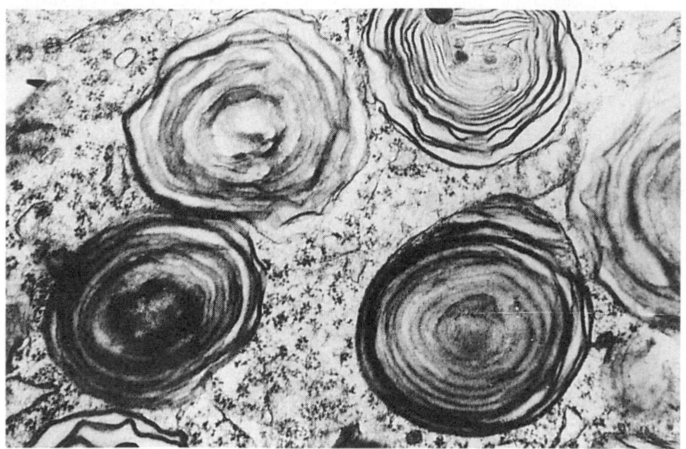

Fig. 77-199 Membranous cytoplasmic bodies typical of sphingolipidoses, especially gangliosidoses.

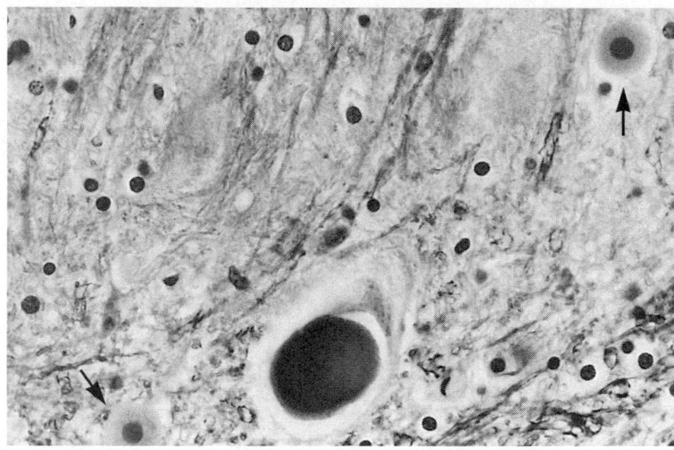

Fig. 77-201 Lafora body disease with large perikaryal hematoxylinophilic (type III) and cored inclusions (type II) *(arrows)*.

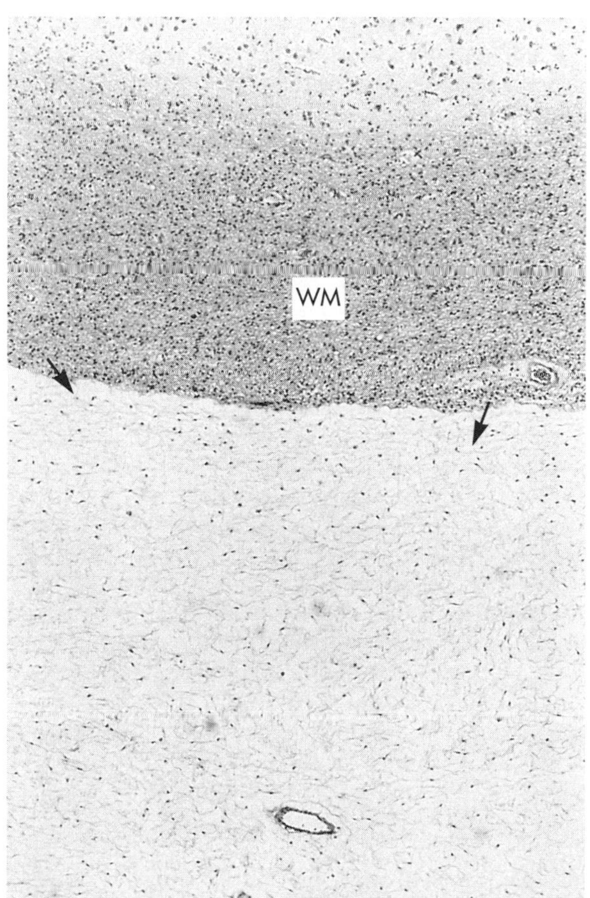

Fig. 77-200 Hurler's disease. Massively widened perivascular spaces *(arrow)* in white matter *(WM)* caused by mesenchymal storage of MPS.

spread small polyglucosan inclusions in neuronal perikarya, axons, and astrocytes. Branching enzyme activity in the adult type is variable. Although Lafora bodies are easily recognized as large (10 to 40 μm), hematoxylinophilic and often cored inclusions, the smaller ones in neuropil (1 to 5 μm) can be difficult to identify without the PAS stain. Ultrastructurally, polyglucosan bodies consist of 6 to 8 nm filaments. Their fine structure and chemical properties are identical or highly similar to corpora amylacea.[12,144]

Ceroid lipofuscinoses (Batten disease)

This group has three main variants: late *infantile (Jansky-Bielschowsky), juvenile (Spielmeyer-Sjögren-Vogt; Batten),* and an atypical and variable *adult (Kufs).* An *infantile* form *(Santavuori-Haltia)* also has been accepted after initial reservations. The infantile form has been linked with chromosome 1 and the juvenile with chromosome 16.[12] All but the adult form also have pigmentary degeneration of the retina and blindness. Neuronal loss is prominent as in most lysosomal disorders, and cerebral and cerebellar atrophy is expected in the late stages[5,252] (Fig. 77-202).

Morphologically, all display distention of neurons by a yellow-brown autofluorescent, PAS-positive, diastase-resistant, sudanophilic pigment. Each form has a characteristic ultrastructural inclusion: infantile (electron-dense granular), late infantile (curvilinear), juvenile (fingerprint) (Fig. 77-203), and adult (granular to granular with electron-lucent vacuoles). Although most of this pigment had been thought to be lipid, the storage material has been found to consist primarily of a protein, subunit c of mitochondrial ATP synthase. Since neither an enzymatic defect has been identified, nor are probes currently available, the diagnosis of this storage disease rests primarily on the demonstration of autofluorescent (yellow green to brown peaking at 460 nm with a 360 nm excitatory wavelength) inclusions with the typical fine structure in neurons, muscle, nerve, skin, or white cells.

Amino and organic acidurias and urea cycle defects

Any discussion of these topics must be sought elsewhere. The major disorders of amino acid catabolism that affect CNS are *maple syrup urine disease, phenylketonuria* (greatly reduced in incidence since routine natal testing and dietary restriction of phenylalanine), *nonketotic hyperglycinemia,* and *homocystinuria.* Generally, these diseases are associated with myelin lesions: spongy myelin (intramyelinic blebs) in the younger patients and myelin loss or deficiency in the older ones. Homocystinuria is also associated with arterial thrombosis and multiple cerebral infarcts. The organic acidurias (such

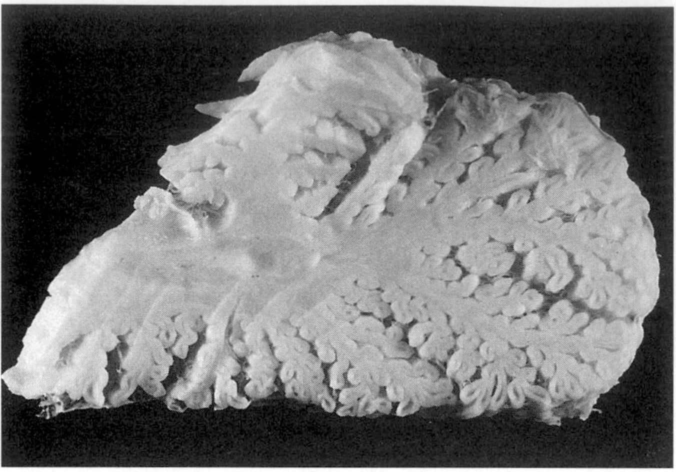

Fig. 77-202 Ceroid lipofuscinosis (juvenile). Cerebellar atrophy caused by severe neuronal loss.

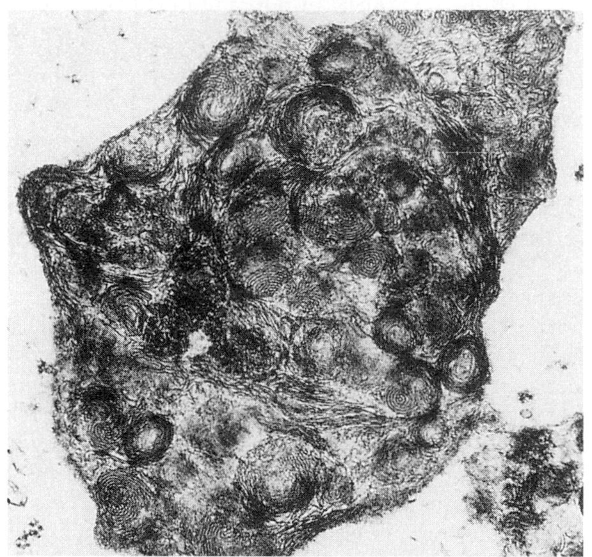

Fig. 77-203 Ceroid lipofuscinosis (juvenile). Membrane-bound fingerprint bodies.

as, *propionic, isovaleric,* and *methylmalonic acidemia*) are usually severe infantile diseases with vomiting, seizures, and coma. Myelin changes are similar to those in the aminoacidurias. The urea cycle defects (such as *carbamyl phosphate synthetase* and *ornithine transcarbamylase [X-linked] deficiencies)* are manifest clinically by hyperammonemia and coma. Neuropathologic lesions include Alzheimer type II gliosis and neuronal loss to necrosis of cerebral cortex, white matter, and basal ganglia.[12,13,16,252]

Neuroaxonal dystrophy (NAD) and Hallervorden-Spatz disease (HSD)

NAD and HSD are considered by some to be infantile and juvenile variants of a range of familial diseases characterized by widespread to localized axonal swellings or dystrophic spheroids respectively (see Fig. 77-12). Dystrophic spheroids, varying from about 10 to 125 μm, have variable histologic and histochemical staining properties and differ ultrastructurally somewhat from reactive axonal swellings by their smooth membranous proliferations, electron-dense material, and tubulovesicular profiles. In addition to the more localized distribution of dystrophic spheroids in Hallervorden-Spatz to globus pallidus and substantia nigra, these same areas display a rusty-brown discoloration caused by the deposition of brown-yellow pigment in neurons, astrocytes, macrophages and extracellularly. This pigment is usually positive for iron, lipid, and carbohydrate. An *adult* form of HSD is characterized by concomitant neurofibrillary tangles, comparable to what has been reported in cases of *Niemann-Pick disease, type C*. One family with infantile NAD has been found to have a deficiency of the lysosomal enzyme alpha-*N*-acetylgalactosaminidase (Schindler disease).[267] A family with Hallervorden-Spatz disease has been reported to display a deficiency of cysteine dioxygenase in globus pallidus.[5,144,261]

Endogenous toxins

Wilson's disease (hepatolenticular degeneration),[268] presenting usually as an extrapyramidial syndrome or hepatic failure in a young adult, is characterized by Kayser-Fleischer corneal rings (copper granules in Descemet's membrane), micronodular cirrhosis, and rarefactive spongy change (Fig. 77-204) to cavitary necrosis (Fig. 77-205) with astrocytosis primarily in putamen and rarely in neocortical layers V and V1. Severe white matter degeneration may be seen in some untreated cases. Both the liver and brain have high concentrations of copper; serum ceruloplasmin (a copper-binding protein encoded by chromosome 3) is low. An enzymatic defect has not been identified in this autosomal recessive disease, but the gene has been linked to an esterase locus on chromosome 13q.[12] *Menkes', or Kinky hair, disease* (trichopoliodystrophy) is an X-linked disorder of copper metabolism caused by impaired intestinal absorption and secondary mitochondrial dysfunction. Diffuse and severe cerebral and cerebellar atrophy and Purkinje cell dendritic "cacti" are typical.[5] The brindled mouse mutant is an animal model.

Kernicterus, also referred to as "nuclear jaundice" because of the yellow staining of specific neuronal groups, was most commonly found in newborn premature infants with maternal-fetal blood incompatibilities. Clinically these infants present with feeding difficulties, a high-pitched cry, and hypertonicity.

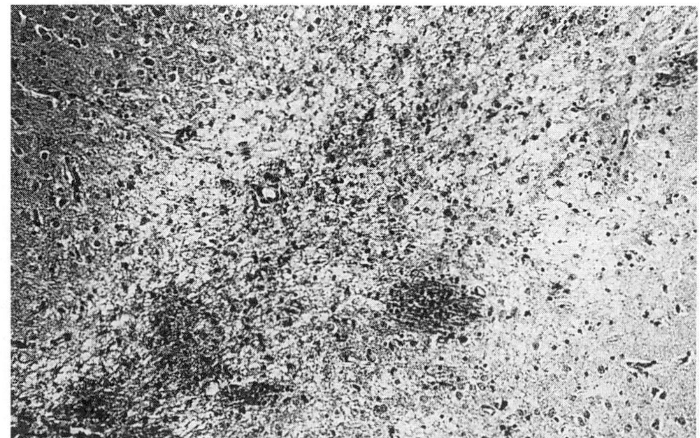

Fig. 77-204 Wilson's disease. Rarefaction of the putamen and neuronal loss with sparing of upper left corner.

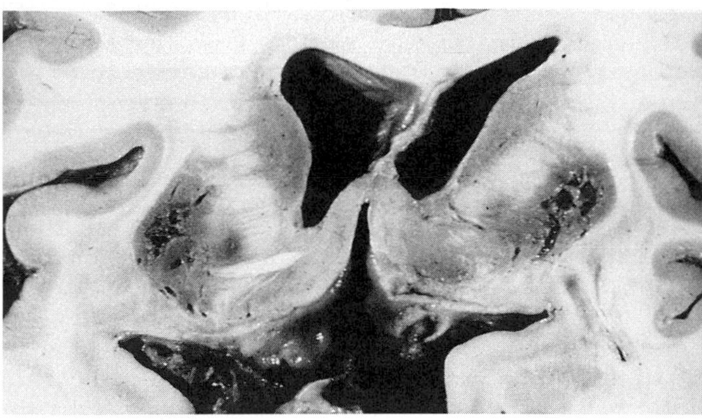

Fig. 77-205 Wilson's disease. Cavitary necrosis of the putamen.

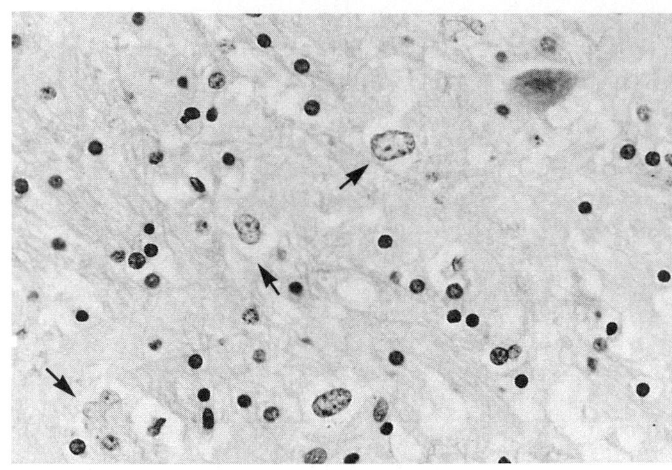

Fig. 77-206 Hepatic encephalopathy. Alzheimer type II glia *(arrows)*.

This incompatibility and consequent hemolysis results in the presentation of excessive bilirubin to immature hepatic cells lacking sufficient glucuronyltransferase activity for conjugation. Therefore large amounts of indirect or unconjugated bilirubin accumulate in blood. Its incidence has been reduced dramatically because of the decrease in hemolytic jaundice of the newborn. Gross abnormalities consist of yellow discoloration of specific nuclei: globus pallidus, subthalamic nucleus, hippocampus, superior and inferior colliculi, vestibular nuclei, inferior olives, and dentate nucleus. This is best appreciated in the fresh state. These infants also have superimposed anemic and oligemic hypoxia because of hemolysis and problems with cardiac function. Consequently, the observed lesion is believed to result from both unconjugated hyperbilirubinemia and hypoxic-ischemic damage to "old" neuronal groups, which are active metabolically at birth. The pigment is lethal to neurons. Surviving the kernicteric episode leads to the classical triad of opisthotonus, sensorineural deafness, and defective ocular supraversion (upward gaze).

Hepatic encephalopathy, whether sporadic or wilsonian, is characterized by Alzheimer's type II astrocytosis (Fig. 77-206) in gray matter, particularly of globus pallidus, caudate nucleus, and dentate nucleus. Their polyploid nuclei undergo hypertrophy, vesiculation, and lobulation (though artifactual in part), which are fairly specific for this entity and correlate best with hyperammonemia; less impressive but similar changes can be seen in uremia and other conditions.[258]

Reye's syndrome is an acute hepatoencephalopathy of children who have had an influenza or varicella infection and were usually treated with aspirin. Neuropathologic lesions include cerebral swelling, eosinophilic neurons, vascular congestion, intramyelinic edema, lipid droplets in astrocytes, and abnormal mitochondria in neurons (and hepatocytes). A dramatic decline in incidence has occurred after avoidance of aspirin in this setting was recommended.[258]

Exogenous toxins

A large number of substances are toxic to the nervous system. Some are natural, others are industrial, and many are prescription or illicit drugs. Some affect the CNS; others affect the PNS; some attack neuronal elements; others destroy myelin or endothelial cells. A comprehensive list or discussion of such toxins is beyond the scope of this introductory material. Those interested in more detailed coverage should consult the references listed at the end.[259,269] We will emphasize the more common substances with their classic presentations and established neuropathologic lesions (Table 77-12).

Lead. Acute lead intoxication is rare today but may be seen in infants who eat old paints containing inorganic lead. Severe cerebral edema with uncal or tonsillar herniations are attributable to capillary damage with perivascular hemorrhages, proteinaceous fluid, protein droplets, and necrosis. This is believed to be attributable to a direct effect of lead on the energy metabolism of endothelial cells.

Ethanol abuse. The pathophysiology of the lesions in ethanol abuse probably is attributable to a combination of direct toxic effects of ethanol or other substances and the *almost invariant element of malnutrition.* Traumatic, PNS, and skeletal muscle lesions associated with ethanol abuse are considered elsewhere. Acute ethanol intoxication, delirium tremens, or withdrawal seizures (rum fits) are not associated with specific neuropathologic lesions. Chronic ethanol abuse is associated with at least two "metabolic-toxic" CNS lesions. A characteristic atrophy of the anterosuperior cerebellar vermis caused by loss of Purkinje and granular cells correlates with truncal ataxia. Alcoholic cerebral atrophy is more variable, initially affecting the dorsolateral aspects of frontal lobes, particularly the white matter. There is evidence that this dementing lesion is reversible to some degree with abstinence, at least in the early stages.[25] Exposure of the fetal central nervous system to alcohol through maternal abuse results in nonspecific but fairly consistent lesions of micrencephaly, neuroglial heterotopia of leptomeninges or ventricles, compensatory hydrocephalus, and atrophy or hypoplasia of centrum semiovale and cerebellum.[256]

ACKNOWLEDGMENTS

The authors wish to acknowledge that some of the illustrative material used in this chapter was derived from the teaching collections of our former affiliations: The Health Science Center, Winnipeg, Canada; The Medical University of South Carolina; Columbia University College of Physicians and Surgeons; and especially Albert Einstein College of Medicine. We also thank Linda Crandall and Barbara Rockafellow for their secretarial expertise and Phil Verzola for photographic assistance.

Table 77-12 Toxic diseases

Toxins	Lesion site	Lesion
Natural toxins		
Mushrooms (mycetism)		
Amanita muscaria (acute)	CNS	Nonspecific agonal
Amanita phalloides (delayed)	CNS	Alzheimer II gliosis, edema
Buckthorn		
Karwinskia lumboldtiana	PNS (motor)	Segmental demyelination
Lathyrism		
Lathyrus sativus (β-*N*-oxalylamino-L-alanine)	CNS (spinal cord)	Corticospinal tract degeneration
Cycas circinalis		
(β-*N*-methylamino-L-alanine)	CNS	Chromatolysis of motor neurons *(macaques)*
Industrial toxins		
Metals		
Lead		
1. Inorganic		
a. Acute	CNS (cortex)	Edema, capillary damage
b. Chronic	PNS (motor)	Axonal degeneration, segmental demyelination
2. Organic		
a. Acute	CNS (cortex)	Edema
b. Chronic	CNS (reticular)	Purkinje loss and chromatolysis
Mercury		
1. Inorganic	CNS (cerebellum)	Granular cell loss
2. Organic	CNS (cerebellum and calcarine)	Granular cell loss, neuronal loss (II-III)
Arsenic		
1. Acute	CNS (brainstem)	Hemorrhages and necrosis
2. Chronic	PNS	Axonal degeneration
Thallium	PNS	Axonal degeneration (vacuolated mitochondria)
Tin	CNS (centrum semiovale)	Intramyelinic edema
Manganese	CNS (basal ganglia)	Neuronal loss
Aluminum		
Dialysis	CNS (cortex)	Nonspecific astrocytosis, microgliosis, spongiosus (II and III)
Dementia		
Chemicals		
Hexacarbons (*n*-hexane; methyl *n*-butylketone)	PNS, CNS	Distal axonopathy (giant swellings)
Acrylamide	PNS, CNS	Distal axonopathy
Organophosphates	PNS, CNS	Distal axonopathy, edema and periventricular hemorrhagic necrosis
Methanol	CNS (cortex; visual; putamen)	Edema; retinal ganglion loss, optic atrophy, chromatolysis; hemorrhagic necrosis
Ethanol		
1. Adult	CNS (cerebellum)	Neuronal loss
	PNS	Axonal degeneration
2. Fetal	CNS	Micrencephaly, neuroglial heterotopia
Drugs		
Illicit		
1. Opiates	CNS (diffuse; spinal)	Hypoxic-ischemic neuronal loss and necrosis
2. Amphetamines	CNS	Hemorrhages (necrotizing vasculitis)
3. Cocaine, phencyclidine	CNS	Edema, hemorrhages (hypertension)
4. MPTP (1-methyl-4-phenyl-1,2,3,6-tetrahydropyridine)	CNS (substantia nigra)	Neuronal loss
Therapeutic		
1. Psychotropic		
a. Phenothiazines or haloperidol	CNS (basal ganglia)	Neuronal loss and lipofuscin
2. Antineoplastic		Necrotizing leukoencephalopathy
a. Methotrexate	CNS (multifocal)	Axonal degeneration
b. Vincristine	PNS	

(continued)

Table 77-12 Toxic diseases—cont'd

Toxins	Lesion site	Lesion
3. Anti-infectious		
a. Isoniazid	PNS	Axonal degeneration
b. Chloroquine	PNS; skeletal muscle	Axonal degeneration; schwann cell
c. Hexachlorophene	CNS	Intramyelinic edema
d. Clioquinol	CNS (spinal), PNS	Distal axonopathy
e. Gentamicin	CNS (brainstem),	Necrotizing leukoencephalopathy
	PNS (VIII)	Neurosensory cell loss
4. Miscellaneous		
a. Diphenylhydantoin	CNS (cerebellum)	Purkinje cell loss
b. Metrizamide	CNS (periventricular)	Perivascular cuffs
c. Perhexilene	PNS	Segmental demyelination; cytoplasmic inclusions

REFERENCES

General neuropathology texts

1. Adams JH, Duchen LW, editors: *Greenfield's neuropathology,* ed 5, New York, 1992, Oxford University Press.
2. Burger PC, Scheithauer BW, Vogel FS: *Surgical pathology of the nervous system and its coverings,* ed 3, New York, 1991, Churchill Livingstone.

2a. Burger PC, Scheithauer: *Tumors of the central nervous system*, 3rd series, Washington, 1994, Armed Forces of Pathology.

3. Davis RL, Robertson DM, editors: *Textbook of neuropathology,* ed 2, Baltimore, 1991, Williams & Wilkins.
4. Esiri MM, Oppenheimer DR: *Diagnostic neuropathology,* Boston, 1989, Blackwell Scientific Publications.
5. Friede RL: *Developmental neuropathology,* ed 2, New York, 1989, Springer-Verlag.

5a. Duckett S, editor: *Pediatric neuropathology*, Baltimore, 1995, Williams and Wilkins.

5b. Norman MG, McGillivray BC, Kalousek DK et al: *Congenital malformations of the brain,* New York, 1995, Oxford University Press.

6. Haymaker W, Adams RD: *Histology and histopathology of the nervous system,* Springfield, Ill, 1982, Charles C Thomas.
7. Nelson JS, Parisi JE, Schochet SS et al: *Principles and practice of neuropathology,* St. Louis, 1993, Mosby.
8. Okazaki H: *Fundamentals of neuropathology,* ed 2, New York, 1989, Igaku-Shoin.
9. Poirier J, Gray F, Escourolle R: *Manual of basic neuropathology,* ed 3, Philadelphia, 1990, Saunders.
10. Russell DS, Rubinstein LJ: *Pathology of tumors of the nervous system,* ed 5, Baltimore, 1989, Williams & Wilkins.
11. Vinken PJ, Bruyn GW, Klawans HL: *Handbook of clinical neurology,* New York, 1994, volume 64, Elsevier.

Clinical neuroscience and molecular neurogenetics

12. Rosenberg RN, Prusiner SB, DiMauro S et al: *The molecular and genetic basis of neurological disease,* Boston, 1993, Butterworth-Heinemann.
13. Scriver CR, Beaudet AL, Sly WS, Valle D, editors: *The metabolic and molecular bases of inherited disease,* ed 7, vol 1, 2, and 3, New York, 1995, McGraw-Hill.

Neuroscience and molecular neurobiology

14. Kandel ER, Schwartz JH, Jessell TM, editors: *Principles of neural science,* ed 3, New York, 1991, Elsevier.
15. Martin JH: *Neuroanatomy, text and atlas,* New York, 1989, Elsevier.
16. Siegel GJ, Agranoff BW, Albers RW, Molinoff PB: *Basic neurochemistry,* ed 5, New York, 1994, Raven Press.

General considerations

17. Miller JD, Adams JH: The pathophysiology of raised intracranial pressure. In Adams JH, Duchen LW, editors: *Greenfield's neuropathology,* ed 5, New York, 1992, Oxford University Press.
18. McComb JG, Davis RL: Choroid plexus, cerebrospinal fluid, hydrocephalus, cerebral edema, and herniation phenomena. In Davis RL, Robertson DM, editors: *Textbook of neuropathology,* ed 2, Baltimore, 1991, Williams & Wilkins.
19. Friede RL, Roessmann U: Chronic tonsillar herniation: an attempt at clarifying chronic herniations at the foramen magnum, *Acta Neuropathol* 34:219, 1986.
20. Graham DI: Hypoxia and vascular disorders. In Adams JH, Duchen LW, editors: *Greenfield's neuropathology,* ed 5, New York, 1992, Oxford University Press.
21. Esiri MM, Oppenheimer DR: *Diagnostic neuropathology,* Boston, 1989, Blackwell Scientific Publications.
22. Poirier J, Gray F, Escourolle R: *Manual of basic neuropathology,* ed 3, Philadelphia, 1990, Saunders.
23. Duchen LW: General pathology of neurons and neuroglia. In Adams JH, Duchen LW, editors: *Greenfield's neuropathology,* ed 5, New York, 1992, Oxford University Press.
24. Okazaki H: *Fundamentals of neuropathology,* ed 2, New York, 1989, Igaku-Shoin.
25. Tomlinson BE: Ageing and the dementias. In Adams JH, Duchen LW, editors: *Greenfield's neuropathology,* ed 5, New York, 1992, Oxford University Press.
26. Hirano A: Neurons and astrocytes. In Davis RL, Robertson DM, editors: *Textbook of neuropathology,* ed 2, Baltimore, 1991, Williams & Wilkins.
27. Dolman CL: Microglia. In Davis RL, Robertson DM, editors: *Textbook of neuropathology,* ed 2, Baltimore, 1991, Williams & Wilkins.

Vascular diseases

28. Carpenter MB: *Core text of neuroanatomy,* ed 3, Baltimore, 1985, Williams & Wilkins.
29. Poirier J, Gray F, Escourolle R: *Manual of basic neuropathology,* ed 3, Philadelphia, 1990, Saunders, p 65.
30. Garcia JH, Anderson ML: Circulatory disorders and their effects on the brain. In Davis RL, Robertson DM, editors: *Textbook of neuropathology,* ed 2, Baltimore, 1991, Williams & Wilkins.
31. Waterston JA, Brown MM, Butler P, Swash M: Small deep cerebral infarcts associated with occlusive internal carotid artery disease. A hemodynamic phenomenon? *Arch Neurol* 47:953, 1990.
32. Caplan LR: Vertebrobasilar system syndromes. In Toole JF: *Handbook of clinical neurology,* vol 53, *Vascular diseases,* part I, Amsterdam, 1988, Elsevier, p 371.
33. Hennerici MG: Atherosclerotic and hypertensive vascular disease. In Asbury AK, McKhann GM, McDonald WI, editors: *Diseases of the nervous system, clinical neurobiology,* ed 2, vol 2, Philadelphia, 1992, Saunders.
34. Timsit SG, Sacco RL, Mohr JP et al: Brain infarction severity differs according to cardiac or arterial embolic source, *Neurology* 43:728, 1993.
35. Hart RG, Easton JD: Dissections and trauma of cervico-cerebral arteries. In Barnett HJM, Mohr JP, Stein BM, Yatsu FM, editors: *Stroke,* vol 2, Edinburgh, 1986, Churchill Livingstone.

36. Tatemichi TK, Mohr, JP: Migraine and stroke. In Barnett HJM, Mohr JP, Stein BM, Yatsu FM, editors: *Stroke: pathophysiology, diagnosis and management,* vol 2, Edinburgh, 1986, Churchill Livingstone.
37. Rothman SM, Fulling KH, Nelson JS: Sickle cell anemia and central nervous system infarction: a neuropathological study, *Ann Neurol* 20:684, 1986.
38. Chuaqui R, Tapia J: Histologic assessment of the age of recent brain infarcts in man, *J Neuropathol Exp Neurol* 52:481, 1993.
39. Orgogozo JM, Bogousslavsky J: Lacunar syndromes. In Toole JF, editor: *Handbook of clinical neurology,* vol 54, *Vascular diseases,* part II, Amsterdam, 1989, Elsevier, p 235.
40. Horowitz DR, Tuhrim S, Weinberger JM et al: Mechanisms in lacunar infarctions, *Stroke* 23:325, 1992.
41. Tuszynski MH, Petito CK, Levy DL: Risk factors and clinical manifestations of pathologically verified lacunar infarction, *Stroke* 20:900, 1989.
42. Hijdra A, Verbeeten B Jr: Leukoaraiosis and ventricular enlargement in patients with ischemic strokes, *Stroke* 22:447, 1991.
43. Babikian V, Ropper AH: Binswanger's disease: a review, *Stroke* 18:2, 1987.
44. Tournier-Lasserve E, Joutel A, Melki J et al: Cerebral autosomal dominant arteriopathy with subcortical infarcts and leukoencephalopathy maps to chromosome 19q12, *Nat Genet* 3:256, 1993.
45. Weller RO: Spontaneous intracranial hemorrhage. In Adams JH, Duchen LW, editors: *Greenfield's neuropathology,* ed 5, New York, 1992, Oxford University Press.
46. Stehbens WE: Etiology of intracranial berry aneurysms, *J Neurosurg* 70:823, 1989.
47. Atkinson JLD, Sundt TM, Houser OW, Whisnant JP: Angiographic frequency of anterior circulation intracranial aneurysms, *J Neurosurg* 70:551, 1989.
48. Rodda R: The necropsy demonstration of cerebral aneurysms by intra-arterial injection, *Proc Austr Assoc Neurol* 7:115, 1967.
49. Brust JCM, Dickinson PCT, Hughes JEO, Holtzman RNN: The diagnosis and treatment of cerebral mycotic aneurysms, *Ann Neurol* 27:238, 1990.
50. Gueguen B, Merland JJ, Riche MC, Rey A: Vascular malformation of the spinal cord: intrathecal perimedullary arteriovenous fistulas fed by medullary arteries, *Neurol* 37:969, 1987.
51. Rigamonti D, Hadley MN, Drayer BP et al: Cerebral cavernous malformations: incidence and familial occurrence, *N Engl J Med* 319:343, 1988.
51a. Kattapong VJ, Hart BL, Davis LE: Familial cerebral cavernous angiomas: clinical and radiologic studies, *Neurology* 45:492, 1995.
52. Dobyns WB, Michels VV, Groover RV et al: Familial cavernous malformations of the central nervous system and retina, *Ann Neurol* 21:578, 1987.
53. Barnwell SL, Dowd CF, Davis RL et al: Cryptic vascular malformations of the spinal cord: diagnosis by magnetic resonance imaging and outcome of surgery, *J Neurosurg* 72:403, 1990.
54. Allen NB: Miscellaneous vasculitic syndromes including Behçwet's disease and central nervous system vasculitis, *Curr Opin Rheumatol* 5:51, 1993.
55. Brown MM, Swash M: Polyarteritis nodosa and other systemic vasculitides. In Toole JF, editor: *Handbook of clinical neurology,* vol 55, *Vascular diseases,* part III, Amsterdam, 1989, Elsevier.
56. Chang Y, Kargas SA, Goates JJ, Horoupian DS: Intraventricular and subarachnoid hemorrhage resulting from necrotizing vasculitis of the choroid plexus in a patient with Churg-Strauss syndrome, *Clin Neuropathol* 12:84, 1993.
57. Huston KA, Hunder GG: Giant cell (cranial) arteritis: a clinical review, *N Engl J Med* 323:699, 1990.
58. Devinsky O, Petito CK, Alonso DR: Clinical and neuropathological findings in systemic lupus erythematosus. The role of vasculitis, heart emboli and thrombotic thrombocytopenic purpura, *Ann Neurol* 23:380, 1988.
59. Levine SR, Deegan MJ, Futrell N, Welch KMA: Cerebrovascular and neurologic disease associated with antiphospholipid antibodies: 48 cases, *Neurology* 40:1181, 1990.
60. Mandybur TJ: Cerebral amyloid angiopathy: the vascular pathology and complications, *J Neuropathol Exp Neurol* 45:79, 1986.
61. Gray F, Dubas F Roullet E, Escourolle R: Leukoencephalopathy in diffuse hemorrhagic cerebral amyloid angiopathy, *Ann Neurol* 18:54, 1985.
62. Jensson O, Gudmundson G, Arnason A et al: Hereditary cystatin C (gamma-trace) amyloid of the CNS causing cerebral hemorrhage, *Acta Neurol Scand* 76:102, 1987.
63. Haan J, Algra PR, Ross RAC: Hereditary cerebral hemorrhage with amyloidosis-Dutch type: clinical and computed tomographic analysis of 24 cases, *Arch Neurol* 47:649, 1990.
64. Lie JT: Primary (granulomatous) angiitis of the central nervous system: a clinicopathologic analysis of 15 new cases and a review of the literature, *Hum Pathol* 23:164, 1992.

Infections

65. Reid H, Fallon RJ: Bacterial infections: In Adams JH, Duchen LW, editors: *Greenfield's neuropathology,* ed 5, New York, 1992, Oxford University Press.
66. Tunkel AR, Scheld WM: Pathogenesis and pathophysiology of bacterial infection of the central nervous system. In Scheld WM, Whitley RJ, Durack DT, editors: *Infections of the central nervous system,* New York, 1991, Raven Press.
67. Petito CK: Neuropathology of acquired immunodeficiency syndrome: In Nelson JS, Parisi JE, Schochet SS et al, editors: *Principles and practice of neuropathology,* St. Louis, 1993, Mosby.
68. Kirkpatrick JB: Neurologic infections due to bacteria, fungi, and parasites. In Davis RL, Robertson DM, editors: *Textbook of neuropathology,* ed 2, Baltimore, 1991, Williams & Wilkins.
69. Pfister HW, Feiden W, Einhäupl KM: Spectrum of complications during bacterial meningitis in adults: results of a prospective clinical study, *Arch Neurol* 50:575, 1993.
70. Roos KL, Tunkel AR, Scheld MW: Acute bacterial meningitis in children and adults. In Scheld WM, Whitley RJ, Durack DT, editors: *Infections of the central nervous system,* New York, 1991, Raven Press.
71. Leiguarda R, Berthier M, Starkstein S et al: Ischemic infarction in 25 children with tuberculous meningitis, *Stroke* 19:200, 1988.
72. Stern BJ, Krumholz A, Johns C et al: Sarcoidosis and its neurological manifestations, *Arch Neurol* 42:909, 1985.
73. Clark CW, Acker JD, Dohan FC Jr, Robertson JH: Presentation of central nervous system sarcoidosis as intracranial tumors, *J Neurosurg* 63:851, 1985.
74. Terunuma H, Konno H, Iizuka H et al: Sarcoidosis presenting as progressive myelopathy, *Clin Neuropathol* 7:77, 1988.
75. Kelley RE, Bell L, Kelley SE, Lee SC: Syphilitic detection in cerebrovascular disease, *Stroke* 20:230, 1989.
76. Morgello S, Laufer H: Quaternary neurosyphilis in a Haitian man with human immunodeficiency virus infection, *Hum Pathol* 20:808, 1989.
77. Finkel MJ, Halperin JJ: Nervous system Lyme borreliosis—revisited, *Arch Neurol* 49:102, 1992.
78. Wroe SJ, Pires M, Harding B et al: Whipple's disease confined to the CNS presenting with multiple intracerebral lesions, *J Neurol Neurosurg Psychiatr* 54:989, 1991.
79. Powers JM, Rawe SF: A neuropathologic study of Whipple's disease, *Acta Neuropathol* 48:223, 1979.
80. Katz DA, Dworzack DL, Horowitz EA, Bogard PJ: Encephalitis associated with Rocky Mountain spotted fever, *Arch Pathol Lab Med* 109:777, 1985.
81. Pendleburry WW, Perl DP, Mũnoz DG: Multiple micro-abscesses in the central nervous system: a clinicopathologic study, *J Neuropathol Exp Neurol* 48:290, 1989.
82. Torre-Cisneros J, López OL, Kusne S et al: CNS aspergillosis in organ transplantation: a clinicopathological study, *J Neurol Neurosurg Psychiatr* 56:188, 1993.
83. Fetter BF, Klintworth GK, Hendry WS: *Mycoses of the central nervous system,* Baltimore, 1967, Williams & Wilkins.
84. Martinez AJ: Infection of the central nervous system due to *Acanthamoeba, Rev Infect Dis* 13(suppl 5):S399, 1991.
85. Duma RJ: Primary amebic meningoencephalitis. In Warren KS, Mahmoud AAF, editors: *Tropical and geographical medicine,* ed 2, New York, 1990, McGraw-Hill.

86. Anzil AP, Rao C, Wrzolek A et al: Acanthamebic meningoencephalitis in an AIDS patient: an autopsy report, *J Neuropathol Exp Neurol* 48:313, 1989.
87. Oo MM, Aikawa M, Than T et al: Human cerebral malaria, *J Neuropathol Exp Neurol* 46:223, 1987.
88. Larroche JC: Developmental pathology of the neonate, Amsterdam, 1977, *Excerpta* Medica.
89. Henin D, Smith TW, DeGirolami U et al: Neuropathology of the spinal cord in the acquired immunodeficiency syndrome, *Hum Pathol* 23:1106, 1992.
90. Gray F, Gherardi R, Scaravilli F: The neuropathology of the acquired immune deficiency syndrome (AIDS): a review, *Brain* 111:245, 1988.
91. Huang TE, Chou SM: Occlusive hypertrophic arteritis as the cause of discrete necrosis in CNS toxoplasmosis in the acquired immunodeficiency syndrome, *Hum Pathol* 19:1210, 1988.
92. Gray F, Gherardi R, Wingate E et al: Diffuse "encephalitis" cerebral toxoplasmosis in AIDS: report of four cases, *J Neurol* 236:273, 1989.
93. Cegielski JP, Durack DT: Protozoal infections of the central nervous system. In Scheld WM, Whitley RJ, Durack DT, editors: *Infections of the central nervous system,* New York, 1991, Raven Press.
94. Davis LE, Kornfeld M: Neurocysticercosis: neurologic, pathogenic, diagnostic and therapeutic aspects, *Eur Neurol* 31:229, 1991.
95. Scaravilli F: Parasitic and fungal infections. In Adams JR, Duchen LW, editors: *Greenfield's neuropathology,* ed 5, New York, 1992, Oxford University Press.
96. Holodniy M, Almenoff J, Loutit J, Steinberg GK: Cerebral sparganosis: case report and review, *Rev Infect Dis* 13:155, 1991.
97. Leestma JE: Viral infections of the nervous system. In Davis RL, Robertson DM, editors: *Textbook of neuropathology,* ed 2, Baltimore, 1991, Williams & Wilkins.
98. Esiri MM, Kennedy PGE: Viral diseases. In Adams JH, Duchen LW, editors: *Greenfield's neuropathology,* ed 5, New York, 1992, Oxford University Press.
99. Ho DY: Herpes simplex latency: molecular aspects, *Prog Med Virol* 39:76, 1992.
100. Nuovo GJ, Gallery F, MacConnell P et al: In situ detection of polymerase chain reaction-amplified HIV-1 nucleic acids and tumor necrosis factor-α RNA in the central nervous system, *Am J Pathol* 144:659, 1994.
101. Rosenblum MK, Brew BJ, Hahn B et al: Human T-lymphotropic virus type I–associated myelopathy in patients with the acquired immunodeficiency syndrome, *Hum Pathol* 23:513, 1992.
102. Vinters HV, Wang R, Wiley CA: Herpes viruses in chronic encephalitis associated with intractable childhood epilepsy, *Hum Pathol* 24:871, 1993.
103. Rhodes RH: Histopathologic features in the central nervous system of 400 acquired immunodeficiency syndrome cases: implications of rates of occurrence, *Hum Pathol* 24:1189, 1993.
104. Iwasaki Y: Pathology of chronic myelopathy associated with HTLV-I infection (HAM/TSP), *J Neurol Sci* 96:103, 1990.

Trauma

105. Jennett B, Frankowski RF: The epidemiology of head injuries. In Vinken PJ, Bruyn GW, Klawans HL, editors: *Handbook of clinical neurology,* vol 57, *Head injury,* Amsterdam, 1990, Elsevier.
106. Hardman JM: Cerebrospinal trauma. In Davis RL, Robertson DM, editors: *Textbook of neuropathology,* ed 2, Baltimore, 1991, Williams & Wilkins.
107. Adams JH: Head injury. In Adams JH, Duchen LW, editors: *Greenfield's Neuropathology,* ed 5, New York, 1992, Oxford University Press.
108. Frowein RA, Firsching R: Classification of head injury. In Vinken PJ, Bruyn GW, Klawans HL, editors: *Handbook of clinical neurology,* vol 57, *Head injury.* Amsterdam, 1990, Elsevier.
109. Baykaner K, Alp H, Ceviker N et al: Observation of 95 patients with extradural hematoma and review of the literature, *Surg Neurol* 30:339, 1988.
110. Adams JH, Graham DI, Murray LS, Scott G: Diffuse axonal injury due to nonmissile head injury in humans: an analysis of 45 cases, *Ann Neurol* 12:557, 1982.
111. Leestma JE: *Forensic neuropathology,* New York, 1988, Raven Press.

Degenerative diseases

112. Lai F, Williams RS: A prospective study of Alzheimer disease in Down syndrome, *Arch Neurol* 46:849, 1989.
113. Saunders AM, Strittmatter WJ, Schmechel D et al: Association of apolipoprotein E allele e4 with late-onset familial and sporadic Alzheimer's disease, *Neurology* 43:1467, 1993.
114. Masliah E, Mallory M, Hansen L et al: Quantitative synaptic alterations in the human neocortex during normal aging, *Neurology* 43:192, 1993.
115. Yen SH, Dickson DW, Crowe A et al: Alzheimer's neurofibrillary tangles contain unique epitopes and epitopes in common with heat stable microtubule-associated proteins tau and MAP_2, *Am J Pathol* 126:81, 1987.
116. Shankar SS, Yanagihara R, Garruto RM et al: Immunocytochemical characterization of neurofibrillary tangles in amyotrophic lateral sclerosis and parkinsonism-dementia of Guam, *Ann Neurol* 25:146, 1989.
117. Braak H, Braak E, Grundke-Igbal I, Igbal K: Occurrence of neuropil threads in the senile human brain and in Alzheimer's disease: a third location of paired helical filaments outside of neurofibrillary tangles and neuritic plaques, *Neurosci Lett* 65:351, 1986.
118. Goates JJ, Dickson DW, Horoupian DS: Meningioangiomatosis: immunocytochemical study, *Acta Neuropathol* 82:527, 1991.
119. Wisniewski HM, Bancher C, Barcikowska M et al: Spectrum of morphological appearance of amyloid deposits in Alzheimer's disease, *Acta Neuropathol* 78:337, 1989.
120. McKee AC, Kosik KS, Kowall NW: Neuritic pathology and dementia in Alzheimer's disease, *Ann Neurol* 30:156, 1991.
121. Glenner GG, Murphy MA: Amyloidosis of the nervous system, *J Neurol Sci* 94:1, 1989.
122. Khachaturian ZS: Diagnosis of Alzheimer's disease, *Arch Neurol* 42:1097, 1985.
123. Mirra SS, Hart MN, Terry RD: Making the diagnosis of Alzheimer's disease: a primer for practicing pathologists, *Arch Pathol Lab Med* 117:132, 1993.
124. Murayama S, Mori H, Ihara Y, Tomonaga M: Immunocytochemical and ultrastructural studies of Pick's disease, *Ann Neurol* 27:394, 1990.
125. Constantinidis J: Pick dementia: anatomoclinical correlations and pathophysiological considerations, *Interdiscipl Topics Gerontol* 19:72, 1985.
126. Giannakopoulos P, Hof PR, Bouras C: Dementia lacking distinctive histopathology: Clinicopathological evaluation of 32 cases, *Acta Neuropathol* 89:346, 1995.
127. The Huntington's disease collaborative research group: a novel gene containing a trinucleotide repeat that is expanded and unstable on Huntington's disease chromosomes, *Cell* 72:971, 1993.
128. Golbe LI, Di Iorio G, Bonavita V et al: A large kindred with autosomal dominant Parkinson's disease, *Ann Neurol* 27:276, 1990.
129. Pollanen MS, Dickson DW, Bergeron C: Pathology and biology of the Lewy body, *J Neuropathol Exp Neurol* 52:183, 1993.
130. Lennox G, Lowe J, Morrell, K et al: Anti-ubiquitin immunocytochemistry is more sensitive than conventional techniques in the detection of diffuse Lewy body disease, *J Neurol Neurosurg Psychiatr* 52:67, 1989.
131. Kosaka K: Dementia and neuropathology in Lewy body disease, *Adv Neurol* 60:456, 1993.
132. Hansen LA, Masliah E, Galasko D, Terry RD: Plaque-only Alzheimer disease is usually the Lewy body variant, and vice versa, *J Neuropathol Exp Neurol* 52:648, 1993.
132a. Litvan J, Agid Y, editors: *Progressive supranuclear palsy, clinical and research approaches,* New York, 1992, Oxford University press.
133. Wakabayashi K, Oyanagi K, Makifuchi T et al: Corticobasal degeneration: etiopathological significance of the cytoskeletal alterations, *Acta Neuropathol* 87:545, 1994.
134. Papp MI, Kahn JE, Lantos PL: Glial cytoplasmic inclusions in the CNS of patients with multisystem atrophy (striatonigral degeneration, olivopontocerebellar atrophy and Shy-Drager syndrome), *J Neurol Sci* 94:79, 1989.
135. Kato S, Nakamura H: Cytoplasmic argyrophilic inclusions in neurons of pontine nuclei with olivopontocerebellar atrophy: immunohistochemical and ultrastructural status, *Acta Neuropathol* 79:584, 1990.
136. Horoupian DS: Oligodendroglial and neuronal cytoplasmic inclusions in multisystem atrophy, *Prog Brain Res* 94:423, 1992.

137. Oppenheimer DR, Esiri MM: Diseases of the basal ganglia, cerebellum and motor neurons. In Adams JH, Duchen LW, editors: *Greenfield's neuropathology,* ed 5, New York, 1992, Oxford University Press.
138. Geddes JR, Hughes AJ, Lees AJ, Daniel SE: Pathological overlap in cases of parkinsonism associated with neurofibrillary tangles: a study of recent cases of postencephalitic parkinsonism and comparison with progressive supranuclear palsy and Guamanian parkinsonism-dementia complex, *Brain* 116:281, 1993.
139. Roberts GW, Allsop D, Bruton C: The occult aftermath of boxing, *J Neurol Neurosurg Psychiatry* 53:373, 1990.
140. Bruyn RP: The neuropathology of hereditary spastic paraparesis, *Clin Neurol Neurosurg* 94(suppl S):16, 1992.
141. Rosenberg RN: Machado-Joseph disease: an autosomal dominant motor system degeneration, *Mov Disord* 7:193, 1992.
142. Rosen DR, Siddique T, Patterson D et al: Mutations in Cu/Zn superoxide dismutase gene are associated with familial amyotrophic lateral sclerosis, *Nature* 362:59, 1993.
143. Matsumoto S, Goto S, Kusaka H et al: Ubiquitin-positive inclusions in anterior horn cells in subgroups of motor neuron diseases: a comparative study of adult-onset amyotrophic lateral sclerosis, juvenile amyotrophic lateral sclerosis and Werdnig-Hoffmann disease, *J Neurol Sci* 115:208, 1993.
144. Rewcastle NB: Degenerative diseases of the central nervous system In Davis RL, Robertson DM, editors: *Textbook of neuropathology,* ed 2, Baltimore, 1991, Williams & Wilkins.
145. Murayama S, Bouldin TW, Suzuki K: Immunocytochemical and ultrastructural studies of Werdnig-Hoffmann disease, *Acta Neuropathol* 81:408, 1991.
146. Steiman GS, Rorke LB, Brown MJ: Infantile neuronal degeneration masquerading as Werdnig-Hoffmann disease, *Ann Neurol* 8:317, 1980.

Neoplasms

147. Louis DN, von Deimling A, Chung RY et al: Comparative study of p53 gene and protein alterations in human astrocytic tumors, *J Neuropathol Exp Neurol* 51:31, 1993.
148. Leon SP, Zhu J, Black P: Genetic alterations in human brain tumors, *Neurosurgery* 34:708, 1994.
149. von Deimling, Louis DN, von Ammon K et al: Evidence for a tumor suppressor gene on chromosome 19q associated with astrocytomas, oligodendrogliomas and mixed gliomas, *Cancer Res* 52:4277, 1992.
150. Batra SK, Ahmed Rasheed BK, Bigner SH et al: Biology of disease: oncogenes and anti-oncogenes in human central nervous system tumors, *Lab Invest* 71:621, 1994.
151. Levine AJ, Schmidek HH: *Molecular genetics of nervous system tumors,* New York, 1993, Wiley-Liss.
152. Kleihues P, Burger PC, Scheithauer B: *Histological typing of tumors of the central nervous system,* World Health Organization, International classification of tumours, Berlin, 1993, Springer-Verlag.
153. Ringertz N: Grading of gliomas, *Acta Pathol Microbiol Scand* 27:51, 1950.
154. Daumas-Duport C, Sheithauer B, O'Fallon J, Kelly P: Grading of astrocytomas: a simple and reproducible method, *Cancer* 62:2152, 1988.
155. Louis DN, Meehan SM, Ferrante RJ, Hedley-White ET: Use of the silver nucleolar organizer region (AgNOR) technique in the differential diagnosis of central nervous system neoplasia, *J Neuropathol Exp Neurol* 51:150, 1992.
156. Vertosick FT, Selker RG, Arena VC: Survival of patients with well-differentiated astrocytomas diagnosed in the era of computed tomography, *Neurosurgery* 28:496, 1991.
157. Krouwer HGJ, Davis RL, Silver P, Prados M: Gemistocytic astrocytomas: a reappraisal, *J Neurosurg* 74:399, 1991.
158. Allegranza A, Girlando S, Arrigoni GL et al: Proliferating cell nuclear antigen expression in central nervous system neoplasms, *Virchows Arch [A] (Pathol Anat Histopathol)* 419:417, 1991.
159. Barnard RO, Geddes JF: The incidence of multifocal cerebral gliomas: a histologic study of large hemisphere sections, *Cancer* 60:1519, 1987.
160. Plate KH, Brier G, Weich HA, Risau W: Vascular endothelial growth factor is a potential tumor angiogenesis factor in human gliomas in vivo, *Nature* 359:845, 1992.
161. Kandler, RH, Smith CM, Broome JC, Davies-Jones GA: Gliomatosis cerebri: a clinical, radiological and pathological report of four cases, *Br J Neurosurg* 5:187, 1991.
162. Kepes JJ: Pleomorphic xanthoastrocytoma: the birth of a diagnosis and a concept, *Brain Pathol* 3:269, 1993.
163. Shepherd CW, Scheithauer BW, Gómez MR et al: Subependymal giant cell astrocytoma: a clnical, pathological and flow cytometric study, *Neurosurgery* 28:864, 1991.
164. Bonnin JM, Rubinstein LJ: Astroblastomas: a pathological study of 23 tumors with a postoperative follow up in 13 patients, *Neurosurgery* 25:6, 1989.
165. Schiffer D, Cravioto H, Giordana MT et al: Is polar spongioblastoma a tumor entity? *J Neurosurg* 78:587, 1993.
166. Herpers MJHM, Budka H: Glial fibrillary acidic protein (GFAP) in oligodendroglial tumors: gliofibrillary oligodendroglioma and transitional oligoastrocytoma as subtypes of oligodendroglioma, *Acta Neuropathol* 64:265, 1984.
167. Smith MT, Ludwig CL, Godfrey AD, Armbrustmacher VM: Grading of oligodendrogliomas, *Cancer* 52:2107, 1983.
168. Burger PC, Rawlings CE, Cox EB et al: Clinicopathologic correlations in the oligodendroglioma, *Cancer* 59:1345, 1987.
169. Nazar GB, Hoffman HJ, Becker LE et al: Infratentorial ependymomas in childhood: prognostic factors and treatment, *J Neurosurg* 72:408, 1990.
170. Ross GW, Rubinstein LJ: Lack of histopathologic correlation of malignant ependymomas with postoperative survival, *J Neurosurg* 70:31, 1989.
171. Lombardi D, Scheithauer BW, Meyer FB et al: Symptomatic subependymoma: a clinicopathological and flow cytometric study, *J Neurosurg* 75:583, 1991.
172. Paulus W, Janisch W: Clinicopathologic correlations in epithelial choroid plexus neoplasms: a study of 52 cases, *Acta Neuropathol* 80:635, 1990.
173. Hart MN, Petito CK, Earle KM: Mixed gliomas, *Cancer* 33:134, 1974.
174. Caccamo DV, Herman MM, Rubinstein LF: An immunohistochemical study of the primitive and maturing elements of human cerebral medulloepitheliomas, *Acta Neuropathol* 79:248, 1989.
175. Leibel SA, Sheline GE: Radiation therapy for neoplasms of the brain, *J Neurosurg* 66:1, 1987.
176. Figarella-Branger D, Pellissier JF, Daumas-Duport C et al: Central neurocytomas: critical evaluation of a small-cell neuronal tumor, *Am J Surg Pathol* 16:97, 1992.
177. Hassoun J, Soylemezoglu F, Gambarelli D et al: Central neurocytoma: a synopsis of clinical and histological features, *Brain Pathol* 3:297, 1993.
178. Hair LS, Symmans F, Powers JM, Carmel P: Immunohistochemistry and proliferative activity in Lhermitte-Duclos disease, *Acta Neuropathol* 84:570, 1992.
179. Diepholder HM, Schwechheimer K, Mohadjer M: A clinicopathologic and immunomorphologic study of 13 cases of ganglioglioma, *Cancer* 68:2192, 1991.
180. VandenBerg SR: Desmoplastic infantile ganglioglioma and desmoplastic cerebral astrocytoma of infancy, *Brain Pathol* 3:275, 1993.
181. Daumas-Duport C: Dysembryoplastic neuroepithelial tumors, *Brain Pathol* 3:283, 1993.
182. Taxy JB, Bharani NK, Mills SE et al: The spectrum of olfactory neural tumors: a light microscopic, immunohistochemical and ultrastructural analysis, *Am J Surg Pathol* 10:687, 1986.
183. Schild SE, Scheithauer BW, Schomberg PJ et al: Pineal parenchymal tumors: clinical, pathologic and therapeutic aspects, *Cancer* 72:870, 1993.
184. Disclafani A, Hudgins RJ, Edwards MSB et al: Pineocytomas, *Cancer* 63:302, 1989.
185. Slooff JL, Kernohan JW, MacCarty CS: *Primary intramedullary tumors of the spinal cord and filum terminale,* Philadelphia, 1964, Saunders.
186. Cohen AR, Wisoff JH, Allen JC, Epstein F: Malignant astrocytomas of the spinal cord, *J Neurosurg* 70:50, 1989.
187. Kepes JJ: *Meningiomas: biology, pathology, and differential diagnosis,* New York, 1982, Masson.
188. von Diemling A, Kraus JA, Stangl AP: Evidence for subarachnoid spread in the development of multiple meningiomas, *Brain Pathol* 5:11, 1995.
189. Artlich A, Schmidt D: Immunohistochemical profile of meningiomas and their histological subtypes, *Hum Pathol* 21:843, 1990.
190. Mena H, Ribas JL, Pezeshkpour GH et al: Hemangiopericytoma of the central nervous system: a review of 94 cases, *Hum Pathol* 22:84, 1991.

191. Winek RR, Scheithauer BW, Wick MR: Meningioma, meningeal hemangiopericytoma (angioblastic meningioma), peripheral hemangiopericytoma, and acoustic schwannoma: a comparative immunohistochemical study, *Am J Surg Pathol* 13:251, 1989.
192. Enzinger FM, Weiss SW: *Soft tissue tumors,* ed 3, St. Louis, 1995, Mosby.
193. Ezura M, Ikeda H, Ogawa A, Yoshimoto T: Intracerebral schwannoma: case report, *Neurosurgery* 30:97, 1992.
194. Chang KL, Flavis N, Hickey WF et al: Brain lymphomas of immunocompetent and immunocompromised patients: study of the association with Epstein-Barr virus, *Mod Pathol* 6:427, 1993.
195. Nelson GA, Bastian FO, Schlitt M, White RL: Malignant transformation in craniopharyngioma, *Neurosurgery* 22:427, 1988.
196. Kahn EA, Gosch HH, Seeger JF, Hicks SP: Forty-five years experience with craniopharyngiomas, *Surg Neurol* 1:5, 1973.
197. Rosenblum M: Paraneoplasia and autoimmunologic injury of the nervous system: the anti-Hu syndrome: a review, *Brain Pathol* 3:199, 1993.
198. Peterson K, Rosenblum MK, Kotanides H, Posner JB: Paraneoplastic cerebellar degeneration. I. A clinical analysis of 55 anti-Yo antibody positive patients, *Neurology* 42:1931, 1992.
199. Hardman JM: Non-glial tumors of the nervous system. In *The clinical neurosciences,* vol 3, New York, 1983, Churchill Livingstone.

Developmental diseases

200. Gilles FH, Leviton A, Dooling EC: The developing human brain. In *Growth and epidemiologic neuropathology,* Boston, 1983, John Wright PSG.
201. Lemire RJ, Loeser JD, Leech RW, Alvord EC Jr: *Normal and abnormal development of the human nervous system,* Hagerstown, Md., 1975, Harper & Row.
202. Encha-Razavi F: Fetal neuropathology. In Duckett S, editors: *Pediatric neuropathology,* Baltimore, 1995, Williams and Wilkins
203. Dimmick JE, Kalousek DK, editors: *Developmental pathology of the embryo and fetus,* New York, 1992, Lippincott.
204. Dorovini-Zis K, Dolman CL: Gestational development of brain, *Arch Pathol Lab Med* 101:192, 1977.
205. Fees-Higgins A, Larroche J-C: *Development of the human foetal brain, an anatomical atlas,* Paris, 1987, INSERM CNRS, Masson.
206. Riggs HE, Rorke LB: *Myelination of the brain in the newborn,* Philadelphia, 1969, Lippincott.
207. Yakovlev PI, Lecours A-R: The myelogenetic cycles of regional maturation of the human brain. In *Regional development of the brain in early life,* Oxford, 1967, Blackwell Scientific Publications.
208. Dobbing J, Sands J: Quantitative growth and development of human brain, *Arch Dis Child* 48:757, 1973.
209. Menkes JH: *Textbook of child neurology,* ed 5, Philadelphia, 1995, Lea & Febiger.
210. Norman MG, Ludwin SK: Congenital malformations of the nervous system. In Davis RL, Robertson DM, editors: *Textbook of neuropathology,* ed 2, Baltimore, 1991, Williams & Wilkins.
211. Harding BN: Malformations. In Adams JH, Duchen LW, editors: *Greenfield's neuropathology,* ed 5, New York, 1992, Oxford University Press.
212. Ferrer I, Gullotta F: Down's syndrome and Alzheimer's disease: dendritic spine counts in the hippocampus, *Acta Neuropathol* (Berl) 79:680, 1990.
213. Wisniewski KE, Schmidt-Sidar B: Postnatal delay of myelin formation in brains from Down syndrome infants and children, *Clin Neuropathol* 8:55, 1989.
214. Marin-Padilla M: Cephalic axial skeletal-neural dysraphic disorders: embryology and pathology, *Can J Neurol Sci* 18:153, 1991.
215. Azimullah PC, Smit LM, Rietveld-Knol E, Valk J: Malformations of the spinal cord in 53 patients with spina bifida studied by magnetic resonance imaging, *Childs Nerv System* 7:63, 1991.
216. Volpe JJ: *Neurology of the newborn,* Philadelphia, 1995, WB Saunders.
217. Barnett HJM, Foster JB, Hudgson P: *Syringomyelia Major problems in neurology,* vol 1, London, 1973, Saunders.
218. Milhorat TH, Capocelli AL, Anzil AP et al: Pathological basis of spinal cord cavitation in syringomyelia: analysis of 100 autopsy cases, *J Neurosurg* 82:802, 1995.
219. Gilbert JN, Jones KL, Rorke LB et al: Central nervous system anomalies associated with meningocele, hydrocephalus, and the Arnold-Chiari malformations: reappraisal of theories regarding the pathogenesis of posterior neural tube defects, *Neurosurgery* 18:559, 1986.
220. Ruge JR, Masciopinto J, Storrs BB, McLone DG: Anatomical progression of the Chiari II malformation, *Childs Nerv System* 8:86, 1992.
221. Padget DH: Development of so-called dysraphism; with embryologic evidence of clinical Arnold-Chiari and Dandy-Walker malformations, *Johns Hopkins Med J* 130:127, 1972.
222. Aicardi J: The agyria-pachygyria complex: a spectrum of cortical malformations, *Brain Dev* 13:1, 1991.
223. Hayward JC, Titelbaum DC, Clancy RR, Zimmerman RA: Lissencephaly-pachygyria associated with congenital cytomegalovirus infection, *J Child Neurol* 6:109, 1991.
224. Ferrer I, Catala I: Unlayered polymicrogyria: structural and developmental aspects, *Anat Embryol* 184:517, 1991.
225. Martuza RL, Eldridge R: Neurofibromatosis 2 (bilateral acoustic neurofibromatosis), *N Engl J Med* 318:684, 1988.
226. Gómez MR: *Tuberous sclerosis,* ed 2, New York, 1988, Raven Press.
227. Lie JT: Cardiac, pulmonary and vascular involvement in tuberous sclerosis, *Ann NY Acad Sci* 615:58, 1991.
228. Rorke LB: Perinatal brain damage. In Adams JH, Duchen LW, editors: *Greenfield's neuropathology,* ed 5, New York, 1992, Oxford University Press.
229. Gilles FH: Perinatal neuropathology. In Davis RL, Robertson DM, editors: *Textbook of neuropathology,* ed 2, Baltimore, 1991, Williams & Wilkins.
230. Volpe JJ: Intraventricular hemorrhage in the premature infant: current concepts, part I, *Ann Neurol* 25:3, 1989.
231. Iada K, Takashima S, Takeuchi Y et al: Neuropathologic study of newborns with prenatal onset leukomalacia, *Pediatr Neurol* 9:45, 1993.
232. Gilles FH, Murphy SF: Perinatal telencephalic leucoencephalopathy, *J Neurol Neurosurg Psychiatry* 32:404, 1969.
233. Schumacher RE, Barks JDE, Johnston MV et al: Right-sided brain lesions in infants following extracorporeal membrane oxygenation, *Pediatrics* 82:155, 1988.
234. Ahdab-Barmada M, Moossy J, Nemato EM, Lin MR: Hyperoxia produces neuronal necrosis in the rat, *J Neuropathol Exp Neurol* 45:233, 1986.
235. Horoupian DS, Yoon JJ: Neuropathic arthrogryposis multiplex congenita and intrauterine ischemia of anterior horn cells: a hypothesis, *Clin Neuropathol* 7:258, 1988.
236. Friede RL, Mikolasek J: Postencephalitic porencephaly, hydranencephaly or polymicrogyria: a review, *Acta Neuropathol* 43:161, 1978.
237. Chang Y, Soffer D, Horoupian DS, Weiss L: Evolution of postnatal herpes virus encephalitis to multicystic encephalopathy, *Acta Neuropathol* 80:668, 1990.
238. Kinney HC, Filiano JJ, Harper RM: The neuropathology of the sudden infant death syndrome: a review, *J Neuropathol Exp Neurol* 51:115, 1992.
239. Perlman JM, Argyle C: Lethal cytomegalovirus infection in preterm infants: clinical, radiological and neuropathological findings, *Ann Neurol* 31:64, 1992.
240. Meldrum BS, Bruton CJ: Epilepsy. In Adams JH, Duchen LW, editors: *Greenfield's neuropathology,* ed 5, New York, 1992, Oxford University Press.
241. Armstrong DD: The neuropathology of temporal lobe epilepsy, *J Neuropathol Exp Neurol* 52:433, 1993.
242. Rasmussen T: Further observations on the syndrome of chronic encephalitis and epilepsy, *Appl Neurophysiol* 41:1, 1978.
243. Jay V, Becker LE, Otsubo IH et al: Chronic encephalitis and epilepsy (Rasmussen's encephalitis): detection of cytomegalovirus and herpes simplex I by polymerase chain reaction and in-situ hybridization, *Neurol* 45:108, 1995.

Diseases of myelin

244. Raine CS: Oligodendrocytes and central nervous system myelin. In Davis RL, Robertson DM, editors: *Textbook of neuropathology,* ed 2, Baltimore, 1991, Williams & Wilkins.
245. Poirier J, Gray F, Escourolle R: *Manual of basic neuropathology,* ed 3, Philadelphia, 1990, Saunders.

246. Allen IV, Kirk J: Demyelinating diseases. In Adams JH, Duchen LW, editors: *Greenfield's neuropathology,* ed 5, New York, 1992, Oxford University Press.
247. Raine CS: Demyelinating diseases. In Davis RL, Robertson DM, editors: *Textbook of neuropathology,* ed 2, Baltimore, 1991, Williams & Wilkins.
248. Prineas JW: The neuropathology of multiple sclerosis. In Vinken PJ, Bruyn GW, Klawans HL, editors: *Handbook of clinical neurology,* vol 47, Amsterdam, 1985, Elsevier.
249. Alvord EC: Disseminated encephalomyelitis: its variations in form and their relationships to other diseases of the nervous system, In Vinken PJ, Bruyn GW, Klawans HL, editors: *Handbook of clinical neurology,* vol 47, Amsterdam, 1985, Elsevier.
250. Kepes JJ: Large focal tumor-like demyelinating lesions of the brain: intermediate entity between multiple sclerosis and acute disseminated encephalomyelitis? A study of 31 patients, *Ann Neurol* 33:18, 1993.
251. Peterson K, Rosenblum MK, Powers JM et al: Effect of brain irradiation on demyelinating lesions, *Neurology* 43:2105, 1993.
252. Becker LE, Yates AJ: Inherited metabolic disease. In Davis RL, Robertson DM: *Textbook of neuropathology,* ed 2, Baltimore, 1991, Williams & Wilkins.
253. Moser HW: Peroxisomal disorders. In Rosenberg RN, Prusiner SB, DiMauro S, et al, editors: *The molecular and genetic basis of neurological disease,* Boston, 1993, Butterworth-Heinemann.
254. Powers JM, Liu Y, Moser AB, Moser HW: The inflammatory myelinopathy of adreno-leukodystrophy: cells, effector molecules, and pathogenetic implications, *J Neuropathol Exp Neurol* 51:630, 1992.
255. Mosser J, Douar AM, Sarde CO et al: Putative X-linked adrenoleukodystrophy gene shows unexpected homology with ABC transporters, *Nature* 361:736, 1993.
256. Powers JM: Adreno-leukodystrophy (adreno-testiculo-leukomyeloneuropathic complex): a review, *Clin Neuropathol* 4:181, 1985.
257. Matalon R, Kaul R, Michals K: Canavan disease. In Rosenberg RN, Prusiner SB, DiMauro S et al, editors: *The molecular and genetic basis of neurological disease,* Boston, 1993, Butterworth-Heinemann.
258. Norenberg MD, Bruce-Gregorios J: Nervous system manifestations of systemic disease. In Davis RL, Robertson DM, editors: *Textbook of neuropathology,* ed 2, Baltimore, 1991, Williams & Wilkins.
259. Schochet SS, Nelson J: Exogenous toxic-metabolic diseases, including vitamin deficiency. In Davis RL, Robertson DM, editors: *Textbook of neuropathology,* ed 2, Baltimore, 1991, Williams & Wilkins.
260. Anders KH, Becker PS, Holden JK et al: Multifocal necrotizing leukoencephalopathy with pontine predilection in immunosuppressed patients: a clinicopathologic review of 16 cases, *Hum Pathol* 24:897, 1993.

Metabolic and toxic diseases

261. Duchen LW, Jacobs JM: Nutritional deficiencies and metabolic disorders. In Adams JH, Duchen LW, editors: *Greenfield's neuropathology,* ed 5, New York, 1992, Oxford University Press.
262. DiMauro S: Mitochondrial encephalomyopathies. In Rosenberg RN, Prusiner SB, DiMauro S et al, editors: *The molecular and genetic basis of neurological disease,* Boston, 1993, Butterworth-Heinemann.
263. Sparaco M, Bonilla E, DiMauro S, Powers JM: Neuropathology of mitochondrial encephalopathies due to mitochondrial defects, *J Neuropathol Exp Neurol* 52:1, 1993.
264. Lake BD: Lysosomal and peroxisomal disorders. In Adams JH, Duchen LW, editors: *Greenfield's neuropathology,* ed 5, New York, 1992, Oxford University Press.
265. Lazarow P, Moser HW: Disorders of peroxisome biogenesis. In Scriver CR, Beaudet AL, Sly WS, Valle D, editors: *The metabolic basis of inherited disease,* ed 7, vol 2, New York, 1995, McGraw-Hill.
266. Dimmick JE, Applegarth DA: Pathology of peroxisomal disorders, *Perspect Pediatr Pathol* 17:45, 1993.
267. Desnick RJ, Wang AM: Schindler disease: deficient alpha-*N*-acetylgalactosaminidase activity. In Rosenberg RN, Prusiner SB, DiMauro S, et al, editors: *The molecular and genetic basis of neurological disease,* Boston, 1993, Butterworth-Heinemann.
268. Menkes JH: Disorders of copper metabolism. In Rosenberg RN, Prusiner SB, DiMauro S, et al, editors: *The molecular and genetic basis of neurological disease,* Boston, 1993, Butterworth-Heinemann.
269. Jacobs JM, LeQuesne PM: Toxic disorders. In Adams JH, Duchen LW, editors: *Greenfield's neuropathology,* ed 5, New York, 1992, Oxford University Press.

78 Peripheral Nervous System

Douglas C. Anthony
F. Stephen Vogel

NORMAL PERIPHERAL NERVES AND THEIR RESPONSE TO INJURY

Normal anatomy and physiology. The boundary between the central and peripheral nervous systems is marked by the transition from oligodendroglial myelin enveloping axons to Schwann cell myelin. The dorsal spinal roots are attached to the spinal cord by a series of small rootlets that enter dorsally just lateral to the dorsal horns in a region known as the dorsal root entry zone. In a similar manner, each ventral root is attached to the spinal cord by a series of rootlets that emerge from the anterior horn cells just lateral to the ventral sulcus of the spinal cord. The interface between myelination by oligodendrocytes and Schwann cells (Obersteiner-Redlich zone) is less than 2 mm distal from the point of entry of the roots into the spinal cord. The exception to this is the transition zone of the eighth cranial nerve, which is at the level of the internal auditory meatus, 8 to 10 mm from the nerve's exit from the medulla. Interestingly, this transition zone is the site of origin of many schwannomas.[1]

Peripheral nerves transmit sensory, motor, and autonomic impulses. Sensory endings of peripheral nerves reach the receptors in an anatomic distribution known as dermatomes (Fig. 78-1); each dermatome is innervated by the sensory endings of a single ganglion. Similarly, a myotome includes muscle groups that are innervated by motor neurons within a single segment of the spinal cord. At the level of the dorsal ganglion, however, fibers of the motor and sensory system merge to form the mixed sensorimotor peripheral nerves. As a result, the neurologic examination is quite precise in localizing symptoms to a spinal root (radiculopathy), as opposed to a single nerve (mononeuropathy), because the functional distribution of mixed nerves is different from the dermatomal distribution of the spinal cord segments and roots.

The motor function of peripheral nerve and corresponding muscles is evaluated physiologically by electromyography (EMG).[2] Four features of the EMG are particularly informative in determining whether weakness is of neurogenic or muscular origin: (1) insertional activity; (2) spontaneous activity or fibrillations; (3) the amplitude, duration, and phase number of motor unit potentials; and (4) the recruitment pattern of simultaneously occurring discharges during effort.[3]

Fibrillations and positive sharp waves may result from insertional excitation of individual muscle fibers, but this insertional activity is short lived in normal muscle, which rapidly becomes electrically silent (that is, no spontaneous activity). Normal insertional activity is also seen in weak

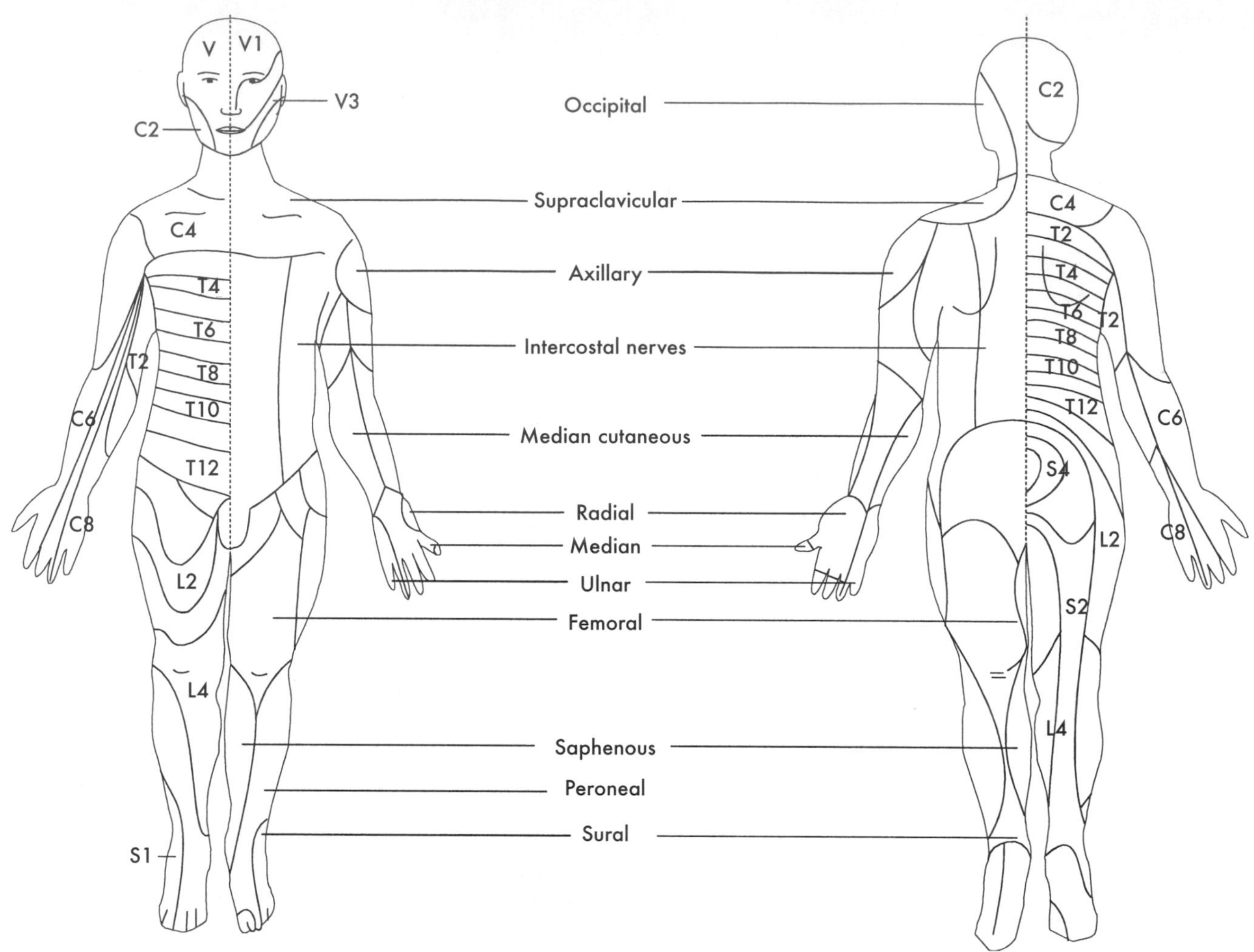

Fig. 78-1 Schema of dermatomes and peripheral nerve innervation. The trigeminal nerve (cranial nerve, *V*) provides cutaneous sensation over the face. Cervical spinal roots (*C*) supply most of the dermatomes of the neck and arm, thoracic (*T*) spinal roots the chest and abdomen, and lumbar (*L*) and sacral (*S*) spinal roots the lower extremities and perineum.

patients with upper motor neuron lesions. When myopathy has led to fibrosis of muscle, there may be decreased insertional activity and inflammatory myopathies often show increased insertional activity (Table 78-1). On the other hand, patients with peripheral neuropathies or other disorders of the lower motor neuron show increased insertional activity, including spontaneous fibrillations. Fibrillations may also occur as a component of inflammatory myopathies.

Analysis of the motor unit potential, particularly determination of mean motor unit duration, is helpful in distinguishing peripheral neuropathy (long duration) from myopathy (short duration). Recruitment refers to the increased participation of additional motor units with increased muscle force. In normal individuals, with increasing effort, previously inactive motor units are recruited and units that are already active fire more rapidly. In disorders of the lower motor neuron and peripheral nerve, larger motor units are formed by collateral sprouting and reinnervation of denervated muscle fibers. As a result, motor unit potentials are larger (higher amplitudes, longer duration, more phases), and recruitment is reduced. In contrast, myopathic processes tend to have smaller motor units with early recruitment. With maximal effort, interference patterns tend to be diminished in patients with peripheral neuropathies and upper motor neuron disease but are normal in most myopathic disorders.

Nerve conduction studies are performed by recording responses after direct stimulation of nerve. In addition, late responses, such as F wave and H-reflex, are physiologic measures that allow assessment of conduction through spinal roots. Nerve conduction studies provide measurements of the amplitude of impulses conducted along the nerve, and the delay (latency) between the time of stimulation and the recorded impulse, allowing calculation of the conduction velocity through a given nerve segment.

In general, myelin serves to increase conduction velocity; therefore, demyelination of peripheral nerve leads to diminished velocities and prolonged latencies. On the other hand, overt degeneration of axons has a lesser effect on velocity, but it frequently results in reduced amplitude without conduction block because of the diminished number of axons conducting the impulse.[3]

Histology. Peripheral nerves contain axons ensheathed and supported by Schwann cells, residing within a connective tissue matrix. The epineurium, an outer sheath of dense connec-

Table 78-1 Electromyography in peripheral neuropathy

EMG findings	Myopathy	Peripheral neuropathy	Upper motor neuron disease
Insertional activity	N,↓,↑*	↑	N
Spontaneous activity	N,↑	↑(+fibrillations)	N
Motor unit potential duration	↓	↑	N
Recruitment	↑	↓	N
Interference pattern	N	↓	↓

N, normal; ↑, increased; ↓, decreased.
*Increased insertional activity often occurs in polymyositis.

tive tissue, maintains the structural integrity of the entire nerve. The perineurium compartmentalizes individual fascicles, forming a physiologic barrier that regulates the environment of the endoneurial space. The endoneurium surrounds the axons and their supporting Schwann cells, forming the interstitium of each fascicle. The fascicles of peripheral nerve roots are less well defined because of the absence of epineurium or perineurium.

Cross section of a peripheral nerve stained with hematoxylin and eosin permits the recognition of each of the major structural components of peripheral nerve. Three separate histologic compartments of nerve are recognized: epineurium, perineurium, and endoneurium (Fig. 78-2). The epineurium is composed of dense collagen, fibroblasts, and blood vessels. The perineurium is composed of spindle-shaped cells that surround fascicles, forming concentrically arranged layers that delimit the lightly stained subjacent area known as the subperineurial space. Within the fascicles, the endoneurial space contains blood vessels, collagen, and multiple circular clear structures, which represent extracted myelin around axons. At high magnification, it is often possible to resolve individual large myelinated axons as eosinophilic structures located within the extracted myelin layer. At times, Schwann cell nuclei may be identified at the periphery of the myelin layer.

Small myelinated axons are poorly resolved in routine histologic sections. They may be resolved by embedding osmicated nerve in a plastic resin and examining sections 1 to 2 μm in thickness. In these sections, perineurial cells are recognized by their faint blue cytoplasm with interlacing rings of smooth collagen bundles (Fig. 78-3). Within the endoneurium, myelinated axons have varying diameters, ranging from 2 to 12 μm, with an apparent bimodal distribution of axonal diameters.[4] Large-caliber myelinated axons range from 6 to 12 μm in diameter and have a proportionally thick myelin sheath.[5] Small-caliber myelinated axons range from 2 to 6 μm with a thin myelin sheath. The relationship between axonal diameter and myelin thickness is relatively constant; the G ratio (axonal diameter/fiber diameter) is 0.5 to 0.7 over a large range of axonal diameters.[6] Overall, the small-caliber fibers occupy a smaller area but are numerically more abundant than axons of larger caliber.

Two types of Schwann cells are recognized: those that surround myelinated fibers and those that surround unmyelinated fibers. For those surrounding myelinated fibers, most nuclei do not appear in the plane of section; however, when visible, they are crescent shaped and located lateral to the myelin sheath. Unmyelinated fibers are not seen clearly by light microscopy

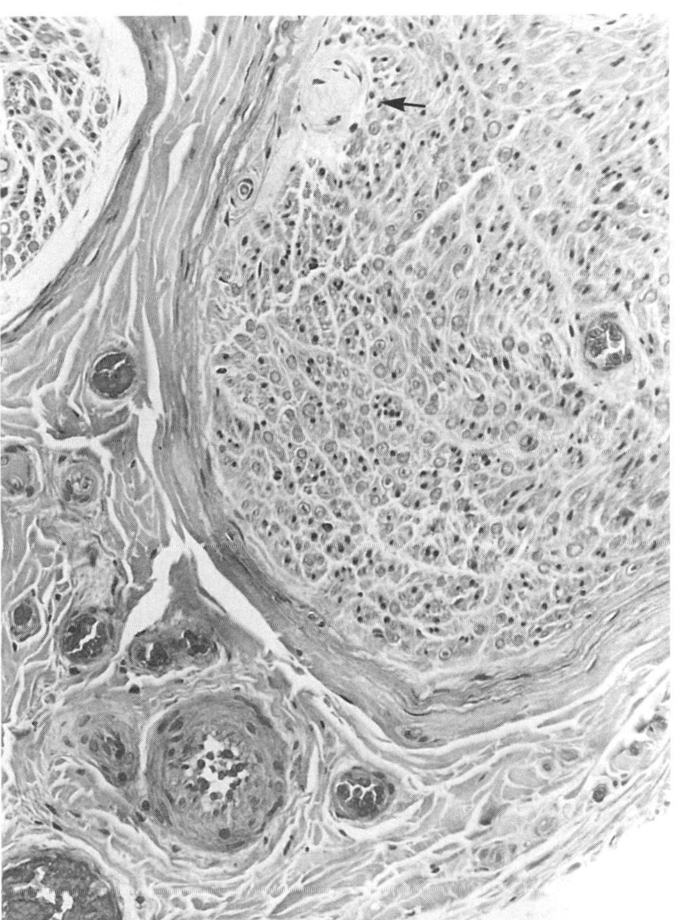

Fig. 78-2 Normal nerve, including perineurial-based Renaut bodies (*arrow*).

but may be recognized by their association with the Schwann cells that support them. These Schwann cells, or Remak cells, are recognized by their pale cytoplasm, which encases pale axonal profiles 1 to 2 μm in diameter. In contrast, fibroblasts have oval nuclei and spindle-shaped cytoplasm located within the connective tissue. Their lack of association with the perineurium or with axons distinguishes them from perineurial cells and Schwann cells. Also within the endoneurial space are scattered mast cells, which are readily visible in toluidine blue–stained sections, because of their dark cytoplasmic granules. Macrophages, derived from bone marrow,[7] are also normal residents of the endoneurial space; they are best recog-

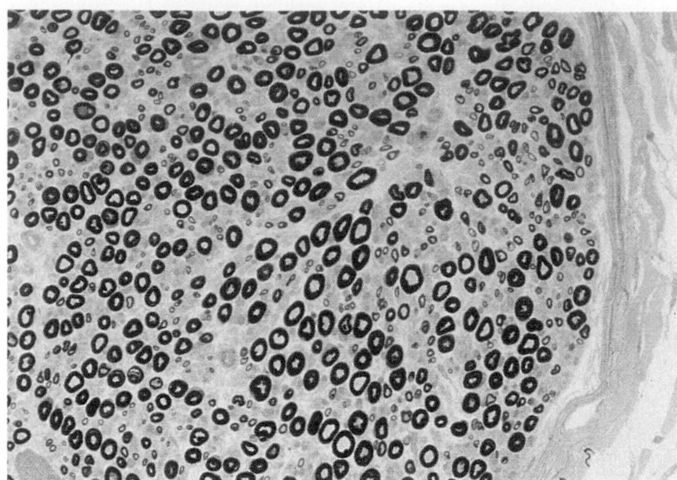

Fig. 78-3 Normal nerve. Individual myelinated axons are highlighted by the surrounding circular profile of the myelin layer. Perineurium is at right. (Epoxy resin section, toluidine blue stain.)

nized immunohistochemically with antibodies to their cell surface markers.

Electron microscopy. Ultrastructural features of normal nerves have been studied extensively.[8] The axons have a lucent cytoplasm that contains microtubules and neurofilaments. Neurofilaments, unlike intermediate filaments in other cell types, are oriented along the long axis of the axon and are evenly spaced throughout the axoplasm with perpendicular side arms. In myelinated nerves, the outer surface of the axonal plasma membrane is immediately adjacent to the innermost membrane layer of Schwann cells, with multiple concentric layers of membrane forming myelin (Fig. 78-4). Small portions of Schwann cell cytoplasm, known as Schmidt-Lanterman incisures, are sequestered between the layers of myelin. The outermost layer of myelin is continuous with the external plasma membrane of the Schwann cell. The cytoplasm of Schwann cells contains intermediate filaments, microtubules, mitochondria, and occasional multilayered membranous structures (pi granules). The entire external surface of the Schwann cell is surrounded by a condensation of extracellular matrix, the external lamina.

Unmyelinated fibers are of small caliber (0.2 to 2.0 μm) but are otherwise similar in ultrastructure to that of large-caliber myelinated fibers; however, they are surrounded by processes of Schwann cell cytoplasm with a single cell membrane, rather than the compacted, multilayered membranes of myelin. Several unmyelinated axons are surrounded by the same Remak cell and are also encased by an external lamina.

Perineurial cells form concentric layers at the periphery of the fascicle. Thin cytoplasmic processes form continuous layers, separated from one another by adjacent lamellae of thick collagen fibrils. The cytoplasm of the perineurial cells frequently contains multiple pinocytotic vesicles and may have a reticular appearance created by interspersed collagen pockets. An external lamina is also apparent surrounding each perineurial cell.

Teased-fiber preparations. Precise longitudinal sections of peripheral nerve are difficult to prepare because the plane of section is usually not perfectly parallel to the long axis of the axons. As a result, it is difficult to gather information concerning the distribution of myelin along the length of a single fiber. To circumvent this problem, one may use teased-fiber preparations. To this end, the peripheral nerve is fixed in glutaraldehyde and osmicated, and the perineurial sheath is removed under a dissecting microscope. Individual large-caliber axons are then dissected in bundles until a small number of fibers can be isolated and individual fibers teased apart from this bundle. Examination of teased fibers reveals darkly stained myelin sheaths and pale, or indiscernible, axons. The myelin sheath is usually smooth or slightly corrugated on its external contour. The region of the Schwann cell nucleus can be localized by its approximation to the osmophilic pi granules in the cytoplasm. Nodes of Ranvier appear as gaps in the myelin layer (Fig. 78-5), and although internodal lengths are variable in accord with fiber size, in large-caliber fibers they are uniform and approximately 1 mm in length. These internodes represent the portion of the axon that is myelinated by a single Schwann cell. In general, the internodal length and myelin thickness are constant along the length of a single fiber.

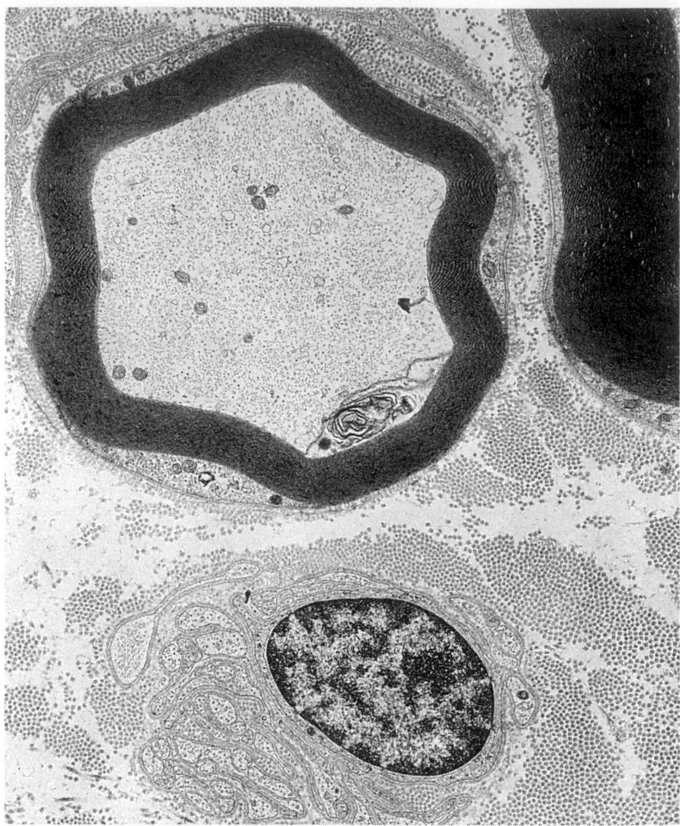

Fig. 78-4 Normal small myelinated axon ensheathed by a single Schwann cell, and unmyelinated axons surrounded by the processes of a single Schwann cell (Remak cell). Basal laminae surround each type of Schwann cell. Collagen fibrils are arranged parallel to the axons and are seen here in cross section.

Morphometric methods have provided quantitative data concerning the density of axons of all sizes within human sural nerve,[4,9] the nerve most commonly biopsied for diagnostic purposes. Histograms reveal a bimodal distribution of myelinated fibers (Fig. 78-6), with an overall density of 7000 to 20,000 myelinated axons/mm^2 in the sural nerve. Of these, there are two to four times as many small myelinated fibers as large myelinated fibers. The density of myelinated fibers and

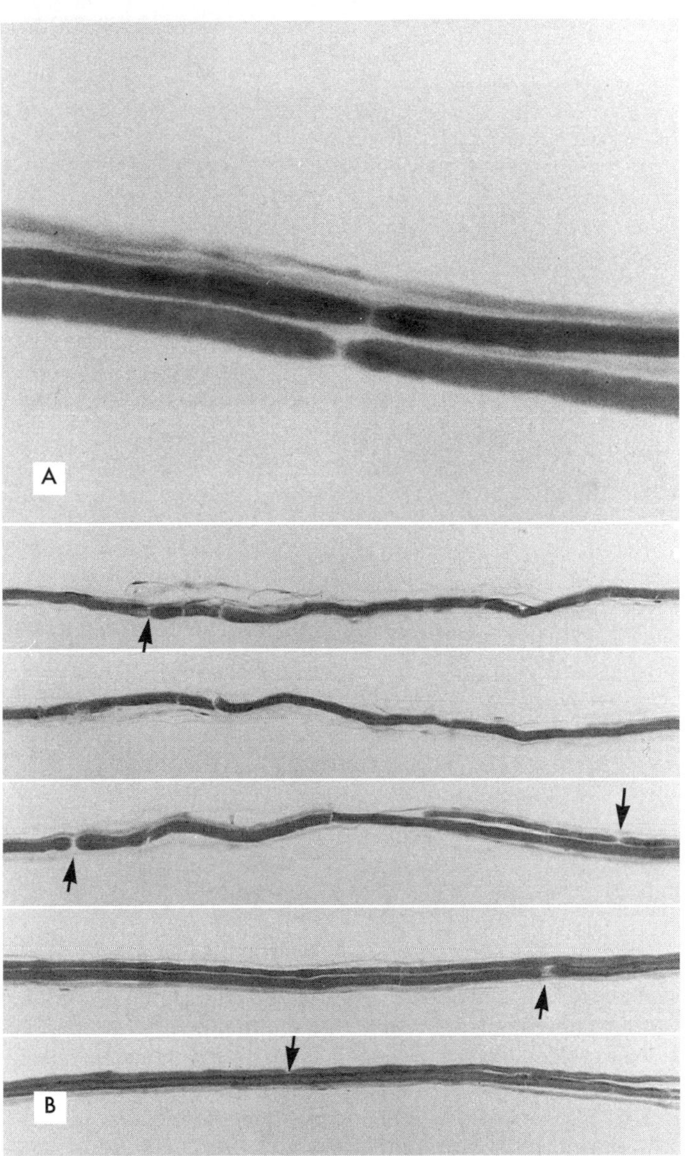

Fig. 78-5 Teased-fiber preparations. **A,** Nodes of Ranvier are detected as a gap in myelin between internodes with smooth contours of myelin approaching the node. **B,** Sequential regions of a teased-fiber preparation. Fractures of the fiber appear as sharp breaks in the myelin, and the myelin tapers at nodes of Ranvier (*arrows*).

the thickness of myelin decrease slightly with increasing age.[10] In infants, myelin sheaths appear thin compared with those of young adults (Fig. 78-7).

Ganglia. The ganglia of the peripheral nervous system may be divided into two broad categories: dorsal root and autonomic ganglia.[11] The dorsal root (spinal) ganglia are located along the spinal column at an outpouching of the dural sac, where they are palpable at postmortem examination as firm nodules. Histologically, they contain large neurons ranging up to 100 μm in size. These cells contain a single large nucleus with vesicular chromatin and a prominent nucleolus. A single axon emanates from each neuron; it branches and sends one process centrally and the other peripherally. Each ganglion cell is surrounded by a ring of small satellite cells whose cytoplasm forms a continuous halo around each ganglion cell. Bundles of axons course through the ganglion, partially segregated by collagenous stroma from the ganglion cell bodies and their satellite cells. In contrast, the autonomic ganglion cells are intermingled with axons throughout the ganglion. These neurons are somewhat smaller in size, ranging up to 60 μm, and the nucleus is located eccentrically within the cytoplasm. As in the dorsal root ganglia, the neurons of autonomic ganglia are ensheathed by satellite cells.

Reaction to injury

Axonal degeneration

Cytoplasmic disintegration induced by injury of the distal axon (that is, that portion of the axon furthest from the neuronal cell body) is called "axonal degeneration" (Fig. 78-8). Degeneration begins at a single point within the axon and progresses to involve more distal segments. Within a few days after the injury, all portions of the distal axon begin the process of disintegration.[12] Neurofilaments and microtubules are no longer discernible within the cytoplasm and are replaced by an amorphous cytoplasmic granular material. Concurrently, the axolemma becomes discontinuous, and electrical propagation is interrupted.[13] The myelin sheath disintegrates, and the axon fragments into small oval segments at all points distal to the site of injury. Because these fragments contain prominent myelin debris in addition to the axonal remnants, they are often termed "myelin ovoids." If the injury is in the immediate proximity of the neuronal cell body, the latter degenerates. Otherwise, the cell body enlarges, with a central eosinophilic region and displacement of the Nissl substance to the periphery of the cell, termed "chromatolysis," or "axonal reaction."

Schwann cells actively participate in the process of axonal degeneration and regeneration.[14] Shortly after the onset of disintegration of the axonal cylinder, Schwann cells proliferate and encircle the axonal remnants. Macrophages are recruited to the site of axonal degeneration and adhere to the outer surface of the fiber.[15] They insert cytoplasm beneath the external lamina of the Schwann cell and insinuate beneath the Schwann cell cytoplasm to participate in phagocytosis of myelin and axonal debris. The debris is removed over a period of weeks as foamy macrophages migrate toward vascular spaces.[16] If axonal regeneration is incomplete, the space previously occupied by the axon is filled by collagen.

Fast axonal transport has been implicated in the process of axonal degeneration. In fact, the anterograde degeneration of the axon after transection was the first evidence of axonal transport. Anterograde axonal transport has been extensively studied, and multiple components are currently recognized.[17] The most rapid movement (fast axonal transport) concerns materials that are largely contained within membrane-delimited vesicles, propelled in an anterograde direction by a microtubule-associated ATPase (or ATPases) known as kinesin.[18] Kinesin binds both axonal vesicles and microtubules and can reconstitute movement of vesicles along microtubules in vitro. Evidence implicating fast axonal transport in the process of axonal degeneration includes the fact that long axons degenerate more slowly than short axons, implying that material (perhaps vesicles) is depleted more rapidly in shorter axons. In addition, vesicles that appear to be rapidly transported accumulate on the proximal side of the axonal transection. Finally, the onset of axonal degeneration begins within 1 to 4 days after transection, a time frame in

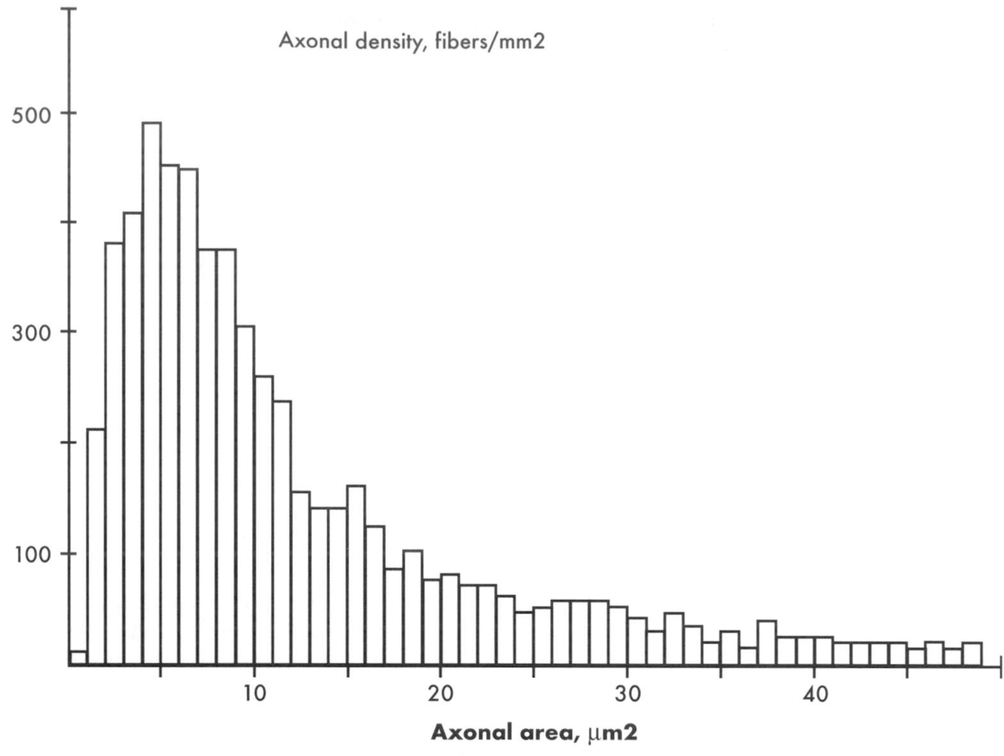

Fig. 78-6 Morphometric analysis of normal sural nerve.

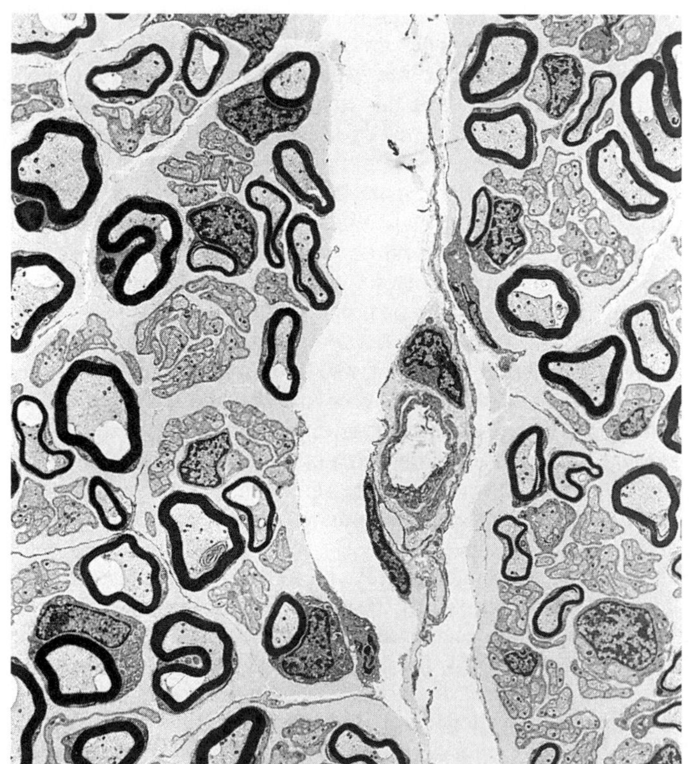

Fig. 78-7 Normal nerve biopsy, 1-year-old infant. The clear spaces in some fibers represent retraction of the axon from the myelin sheath and are a common artifact.

which fast axonal transport is the principal wave of molecular movement.

Axonal degeneration is a frequent finding in biopsies from patients with peripheral neuropathy. In hematoxylin and eosin–stained sections, it is best identified in longitudinal sections as linear arrays of "myelin ovoids," which appear as vacuolated spaces and eosinophilic material arranged in a linear chain. The adjacent Schwann cell nucleus may be indented, and, at times, the Schwann cell cytoplasm may be seen encircling the vacuolated debris. In plastic-embedded sections, degenerating axons are vacuolated, with an ill-defined cytoplasm devoid of the normal particulate structures. In early stages, material derived from the myelin sheath is arranged as irregular clusters within the diameter of the original axon (Fig. 78-9). In later stages, the debris may appear as small clear vacuoles within phagocytes. In teased fibers, linear chains of myelin ovoids are readily visualized. In the early stages of axonal degeneration, the myelin ovoids are nearly continuous along the length of the fiber; however, with time, the ovoids become dispersed at increasingly greater distances.

The interval from injury to total axonal fragmentation is generally less than 2 weeks. Thus, an acute axonopathy is characterized by abundant degenerating fibers (Fig. 78-9), while a chronic axonopathy features fiber loss. Therefore, in chronic axonopathies, the number of axons per cross-sectional diameter is diminished, and the endoneurial space is increased as collagen gradually replaces the lost axons (Fig. 78-10).

The peripheral nervous system, however, has a large capacity for regeneration if the injurious agent is eliminated. There are two patterns of axonal sprouting and regrowth. The first and most rapid is sprouting of intact axons contiguous to sites

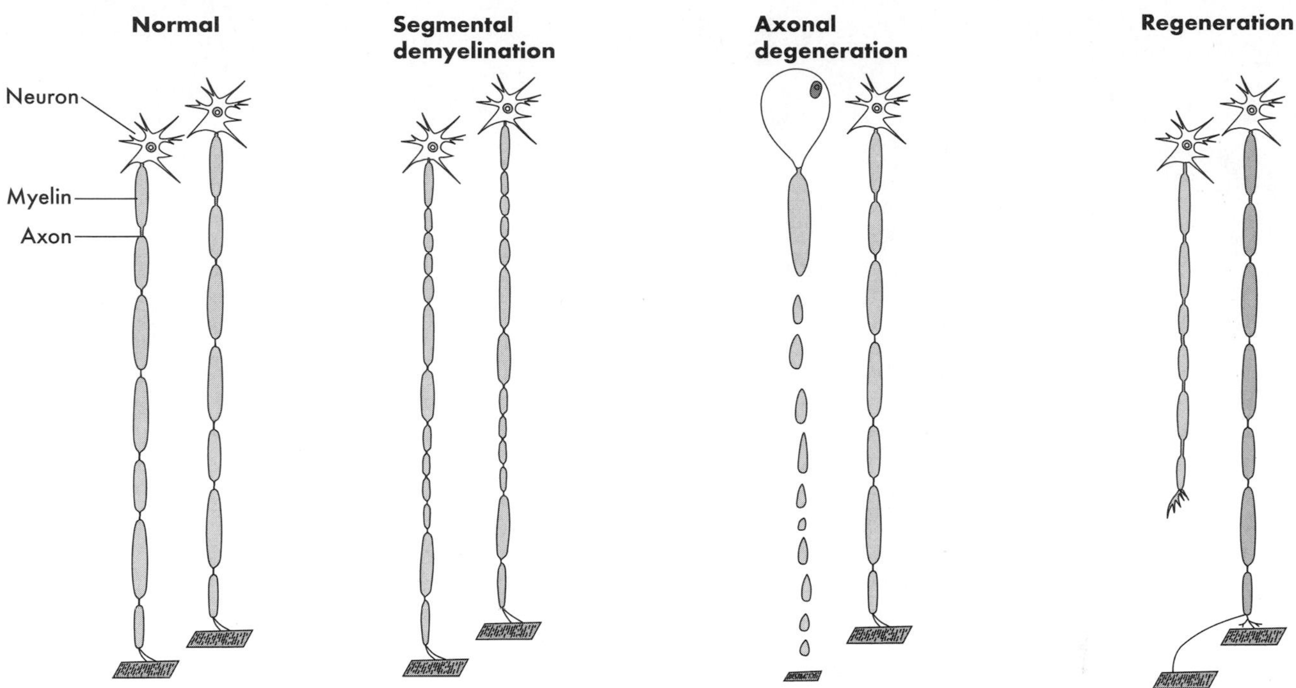

Fig. 78-8 Schema of elementary lesions of peripheral nerve. During the process of segmental demyelination, axonal continuity is maintained but irregular internodes are created during remyelination of the demyelinated segment. The entire axon disintegrates in axonal degeneration, beginning at one point and including all points distal. Reinnervation occurs both by sprouting and regrowth from the distal stump of degenerated axons and by collateral sprouting of surviving axons.

of denervation. This process is well documented in skeletal muscle, where sprouting of terminal axons reinnervates atrophic muscle fibers.

The second type of sprouting occurs at the distal stump of the injured axon and results in the formation of growth cones. Several factors play roles in the efficiency of growth cone extension and axonal growth. These growth cones contain a specialized cytoskeleton rich in actin and have unique vesicle and membrane characteristics that include elevated levels of the growth-associated protein GAP-43.[19] Other growth factors, including nerve growth factor (NGF), facilitate axonal regeneration. Schwann cells that have been "denervated" express increased levels of NGF receptor,[20] an increase, which suggests that NGF plays a dual role in axonal regeneration, interacting with both axonal growth cones and Schwann cells. Schwann cells appear to assist the guidance of growth cones to their appropriate end organ. For example, one membrane protein (L2) is expressed only on Schwann cells that ensheathe motor axons.[21] Because the expression of L2 is governed by Schwann cells during axonal regeneration, it and other pathway-specific molecules seemingly facilitate the directional regrowth of axons toward their targets.

Axonal regeneration is not readily identified in hematoxylin and eosin–stained sections; however, regenerating axons can be readily recognized with the greater resolution provided by plastic-embedded cross sections as diminutive, thinly myelinated axons clustered closely together (Fig. 78-11). When viewed by electron microscopy, they are surrounded by a band of Büngner.[8] Regeneration is also evident on teased-fiber preparations; the internodal lengths of regenerated axons appear uniformly shorter than normal.

Wallerian degeneration may be viewed as a type of axonal degeneration. It is defined as degeneration of axons distal to a point of cutting injury. The events of axonal degeneration and regeneration appear to be equivalent after cutting injuries; however, because transection injuries destroy the continuity of the nerve, regeneration is impaired by the misalignment of the growth cones with their distal segments. This misalignment may diminish the efficacy of axonal regeneration and lead to the formation of traumatic neuromas.

Segmental demyelination

Demyelination refers to pathologic processes that selectively interfere with the ability of the Schwann cell to maintain myelin (Fig. 78-8). Because each Schwann cell myelinates the segment of the axon between two nodes of Ranvier (internode), injury to individual Schwann cells leads to a loss of myelin over a segment of the axon. This process is heralded by a disintegration of myelin with preservation of the companion axon. Schwann cells proliferate to ensheathe the denuded axon, first forming a cytoplasmic coat and only later the full complement of myelin.

The phases of remyelination appear to be regulated by separate molecular signals. In cell culture, axonal integral membrane proteins stimulate resting Schwann cells to divide. When regenerating axons are grafted to a chronically denervated nerve, Schwann cells are also stimulated to proliferate. However, because Schwann cell proliferation occurs after crush injuries before the arrival of axonal sprouts, axonal disintegration is also believed to yield Schwann cell mitogens. Although not fully characterized, partially digested myelin proteins appear to be mitogenic for Schwann cells.[22] Myelin is

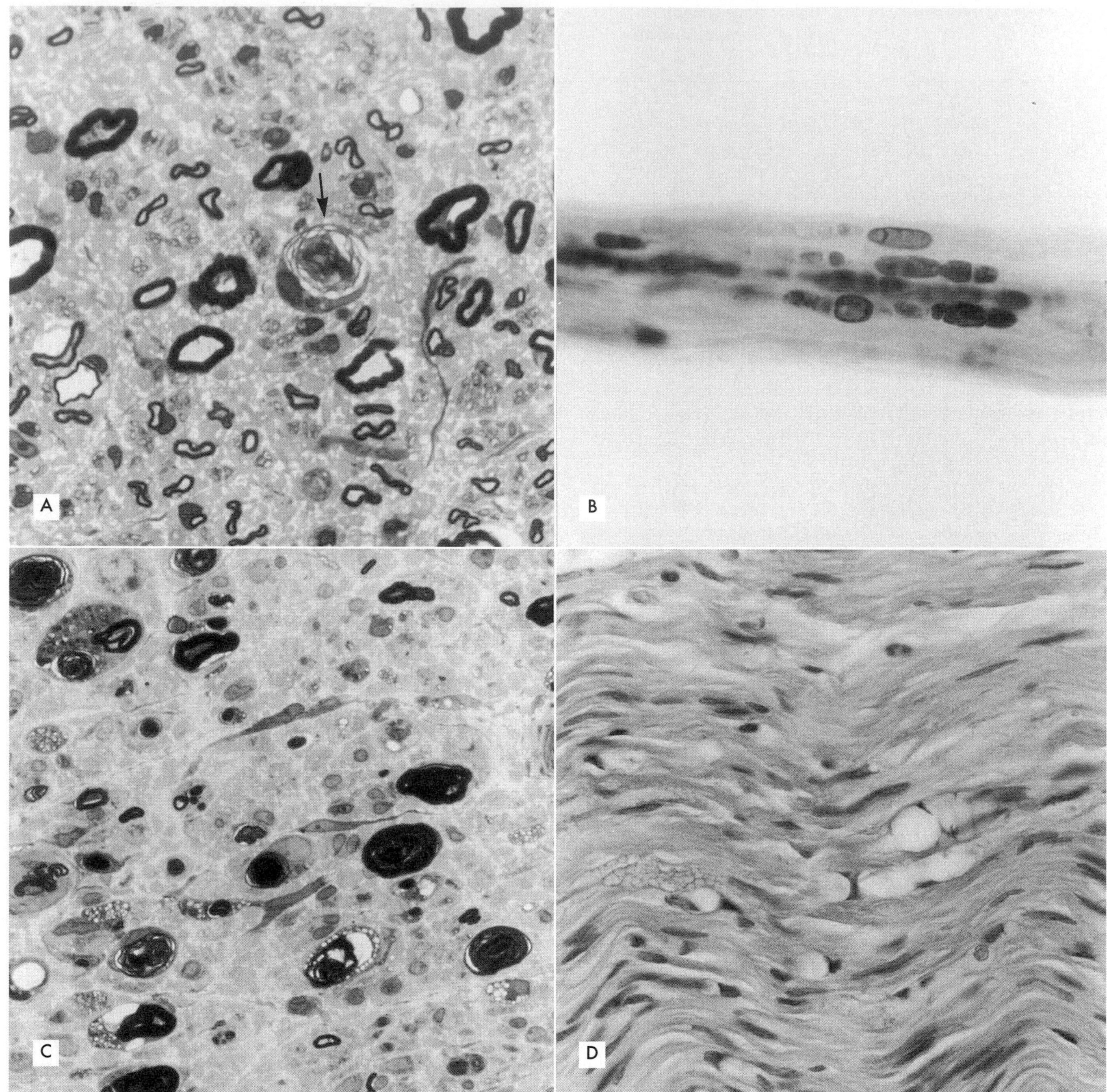

Fig. 78-9 Acute axonopathy. **A,** Degenerating axon (*arrow*) with myelin debris completely replacing the axonal profile. (Epoxy resin section, toluidine blue stain.) **B,** Linear arrangement of "myelin ovoids" characteristic of degenerating axons. (teased-fiber preparation.) **C,** Because most axons are in acute stages of axonal degeneration, this biopsy represents an acute axonopathy. (Epoxy resin section, toluidine blue stain.) **D,** When severe, axonal degeneration with linear "myelin ovoids" and encircling Schwann cell cytoplasm may be evident by routine histologic examination.

not produced during the initial Schwann cell proliferation; however, a second phase of repair of the demyelinated segment involves the elaboration of myelin. Myelin protein expression is regulated at the level of transcription, and mRNA for myelin proteins is expressed in Schwann cells only on axonal contact.[23]

Segmental demyelination cannot be assessed using paraffin-embedded sections; however, the process is readily identified using plastic-embedded sections and teased-fiber preparations. In the early phases of the process, the microscopic appearance is that of denuded axons and retraction of myelin from the node on teased fibers. More frequently, there are large-caliber axons with thin myelin sheaths (Fig. 78-12). This variability in myelin thickness on plastic-embedded cross sections is a hallmark of a demyelinating neuropathy. Teased-fiber analysis is even more sensitive in detecting segmental demyelination

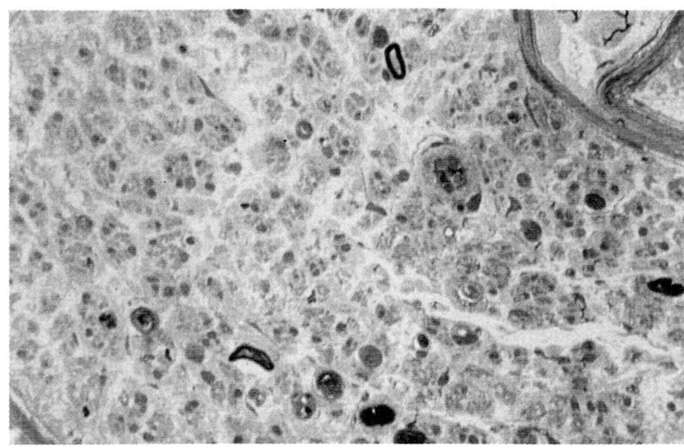

Fig. 78-10 Chronic axonopathy, characterized by severe loss of axons. (Epoxy resin section, toluidine blue stain.)

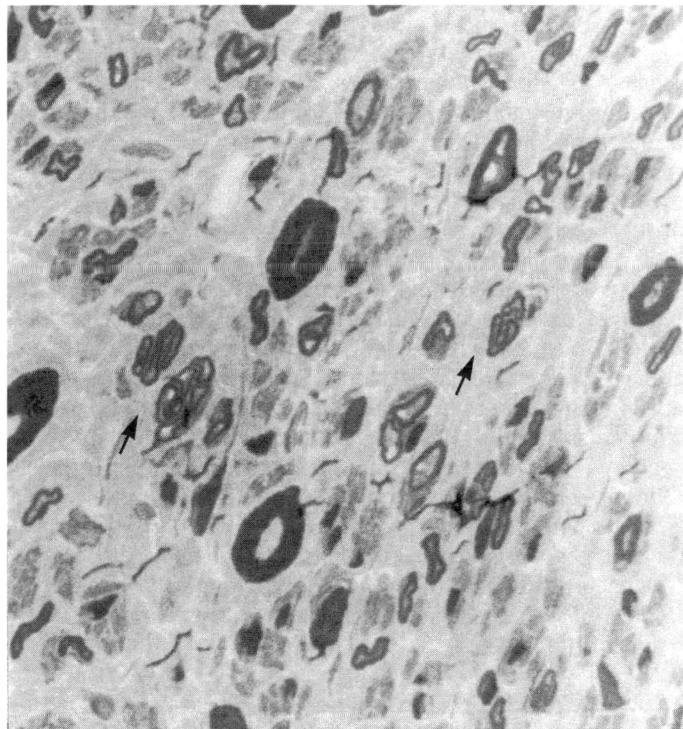

Fig. 78-11 Axonal regeneration, evident in the clusters of regenerating axonal sprouts (*arrows*). (Epoxy resin section, toluidine blue stain.)

because the longitudinal orientation of fibers allows the identification of segments of the axon that have been remyelinated. Remyelinated internodes are short in length and, when the full complement of myelin has not been restored, are also of diminished thickness. Therefore, after demyelination, the internodes are of variable length and myelin thickness along the length of a single fiber (Fig. 78-13).

Repetitive episodes of demyelination may involve the same internode. When this occurs, proliferation of Schwann cells creates additional concentrically-oriented layers of Schwann cell processes. These layers of Schwann cell processes, when few in number, are referred to as "Schwann cell hyperplasia"[8]

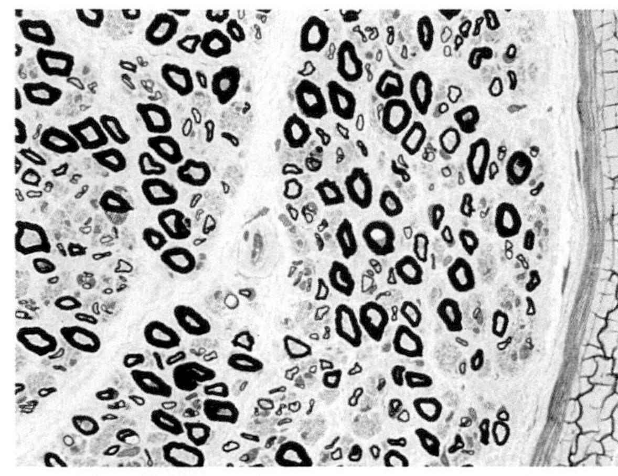

Fig. 78-12 Segmental demyelination may be inferred from the variability in myelin thickness for axons of similar caliber. Compare the axonal diameters and myelin thickness. (Epoxy resin section, toluidine blue stain.)

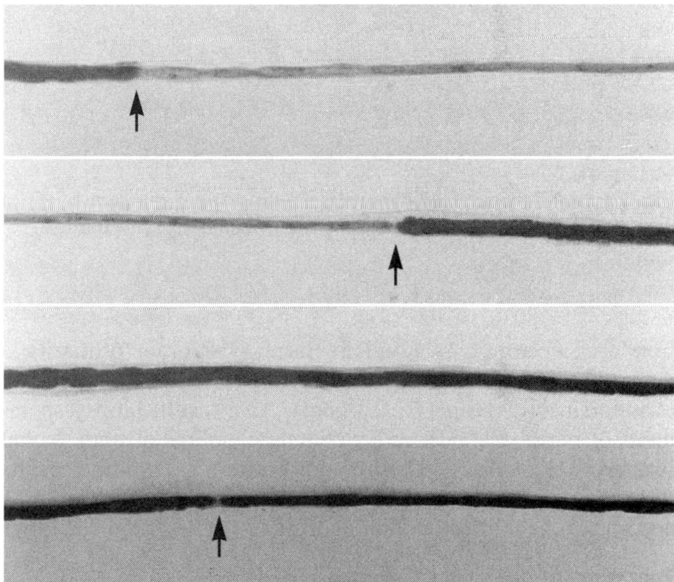

Fig. 78-13 Segmental demyelination. The demyelinated segment (*between upper arrows*) has a thinner myelin layer and is shorter than the adjacent internodes. (teased-fiber preparation.)

(Fig. 78-14) and are suggestive of repetitive demyelination and remyelination within the same internode. As this process continues, multiple concentric layers of Schwann cells are formed, which on cross section are similar in appearance to an onion bulb. Scattered fibers with onion bulbs may be seen in a variety of chronic demyelinating neuropathies; however, their abundance encircling the majority of axons is characteristic of the hereditary "onion bulb neuropathies."

Long-standing peripheral nerve disease, regardless of cause, may lead to pathologic changes that are indistinguishable one from another. Axonopathies are associated with "secondary" demyelination, and demyelinating disease may result in axonal loss. In uremic neuropathy, for example, although the initial changes are those of an axonopathy with axonal degeneration and progressive fiber loss, segmental demyelina-

Table 78-3 Evaluation of a peripheral nerve biopsy

Clinical diagnosis	Paraffin embedding	Plastic embedding	Frozen	Teased fiber	Electron microscopy
Normal nerve (e.g., vagotomy)	+	–	–	–	–
Nerve tumor	+	+/–	–	–	+/–
Acute ascending neuropathy	+/–	+	+/–	+	+/–
Subacute symmetric neuropathy	+	+	+/–	+/–	–
Subacute asymmetric neuropathy	+	+	+/–	+/–	–
Chronic progressive neuropathy	+	+	+/–	+	+/–
Hereditary neuropathy	+/–	+	+/–	+/–	+
Chronic relapsing neuropathy	+	+	+/–	+	+/–
Mononeuropathy or multineuropathy	+	+	+/–	+	+/–

Symbols: +, routinely used for diagnostic evaluation; +/–, may be necessary for diagnosis in some cases; –, not generally necessary for diagnosis.

materials. It is therefore essential in the evaluation of autonomic neuropathies and, particularly, hereditary neuropathies of childhood.

HEREDITARY NEUROPATHIES

Significant regional differences in the prevalence of hereditary neuropathies have been reported in different series. In Norway, the prevalence of Charcot-Marie-Tooth disease is as high as 1 out of 2400 population;[30] in the United Kingdom, the prevalence is 1 out of 5000;[31] and in the United States, the prevalence is 1 out of 3500.[2] However, prevalence rates are difficult to determine because of the variability in the severity of hereditary neuropathies among involved patients. Some individuals do not seek medical assistance, and among those who do, the methods of detection vary greatly in accuracy. In fact, the designation of unclassified peripheral neuropathy often includes examples of hereditary neuropathies in which other family members have not complained of their symptoms.[32]

The most widely used classification of hereditary neuropathies, proposed by Dyck, uses a numerical approach.[2] Hereditary motor and sensory neuropathies (HMSN) and hereditary sensory and autonomic neuropathies (HSAN) are the two major categories of hereditary neuropathy, each of which embraces characteristic subtypes (Table 78-4).[33]

Charcot-Marie-Tooth disease (HMSN I and HMSN II)

Charcot-Marie-Tooth disease (CMT) is a slowly progressive distal, symmetric neuropathy, the first symptoms of which appear in late childhood or early adulthood. The term *peroneal muscular atrophy* is used as a synonym because of pronounced atrophy of calf muscles. In addition to motor symptoms, there are sensory deficits and secondary complications such as pes cavus or neurogenic ulcers. The disease typically affects several members of a family in an autosomal-dominant pattern. Two major forms of the clinical syndrome have been recognized, designated type I hypertrophic form (also known as hereditary motor and sensory neuropathy, type I) and type II neuronal form (HMSN II). Type I is more common and is a demyelinating neuropathy, both by nerve conduction velocity studies and pathologically.[34,35] Type II neuronal form of CMT is an axonal neuropathy. Although less prevalent, type II CMT may account for up to 25% of the total number of cases of Charcot-Marie-Tooth disease.

The majority of type I CMT pedigrees are designated type 1A and show linkage to markers on chromosome 17, in the pericentric region of the short arm.[36] Additional kindreds of CMT have been reported, with linkage of the disease to the region of Duffy blood group proteins on chromosome 1 (type 1B) and an X-linked pattern of inheritance and linkage to the q13-q21 region of the X chromosome. There are, therefore, at least three separate genes, located on chromosomes 1, 17, and X, which can induce the phenotype of the hypertrophic form of CMT disease.[37,38]

The gene products have only recently been identified in CMT type I. Type IA usually involves a duplication of a region of 17p,[39,40] including peripheral myelin protein (PMP-22), but it may also result from a point mutation in PMP-22.[41] An identical point mutation in the analogous PMP gene in mice results in the mutant strain *Trembler,*[42] which has thinly myelinated axons with some Schwann cell hyperplasia, a morphologic finding similar to type I CMT disease. The genes on chromosomes 1 and X also appear to involve Schwann cell proteins, P_0 myelin protein (type IB CMT),[43,44] and connexin-32 (type IX CMT).[45] One genetic locus (chromosome 1p) for type II CMT disease has been identified,[46] but it does not map near any of the chromosomal regions established for type I CMT.[47]

Type I CMT disease evolves as repetitive episodes of demyelination and remyelination. Schwann cell proliferation and onion bulb formation lead to a progressive enlargement of the nerve, which may become palpable. This enlargement forms a cordlike structure that has been descriptively designated "hypertrophic" neuropathy. In contrast, type II CMT disease is characterized by an insidiously progressive distal axonopathy without nerve enlargement.

Microscopically, type I CMT disease is characterized by a moderate loss of large-caliber axons and prominent onion bulb formation. Although the onion bulbs may be difficult to identify in hematoxylin and eosin–stained sections (Fig. 78-15), they are prominent in plastic-embedded sections and, by electron microscopy, often surround most axons in distal nerves. Onion bulb formations are often less frequent in specimens of proximal nerve and in childhood. Many axons show a diminished amount of myelin surrounding large-caliber fibers, and

Table 78-4 Hereditary peripheral neuropathies

Motor and sensory (Dyck HMSN classification)	Inheritance	Clinical syndrome	Eponym	Onion bulbs	Dystrophic axons
I	AD, X	Peroneal muscular atrophy, hypertrophic	Charcot-Marie-Tooth disease, hypertrophic	++	–
II	AD	Peroneal muscular atrophy, neuronal	Charcot-Marie-Tooth disease, neuronal	–	+/–
III	AR	Infantile hypertrophic neuropathy	Dejerine-Sottas disease	+++	–
IV	AR	Phytanic acid storage disease	Refsum disease	+++	–
	AR	Giant axonal neuropathy		+	++
	AR	Neuroaxonal dystrophy	Seitelberger	+/–	++
	AD	Tomaculous neuropathy		+/–	–
	AD	Porphyrias		–	–

Sensory and autonomic (Dyck HSAN classification)	Inheritance	Clinical syndrome	Eponym	Large fiber	Small fiber	Unmyelinated fiber
I	AD	Ulcerative and mutilating acropathy	Morvan	++	+	+/–
II	AR	Congenital sensory neuropathy	Giaccai	++	++	+
III	AR	Familial dysautonomia	Riley-Day	+/–	+/–	++
	AD	Hereditary amyloid neuropathy		+	+	++

Metabolic disorders with peripheral neuropathy	Inheritance	Clinical syndrome	Eponym	Ultrastructural inclusions	Histochemical biochemical
	AR	Metachromatic leukodystrophy		Prismatic inclusions and zebra bodies	Metachromasia, arylsulfatase A
	X	Adrenoleukodystrophy/ adrenomyeloneuropathy	Schaumburg	Platelike inclusions ("leaflets")	Very long chain (>C24) fatty acids
	AR	Globoid cell leukodystrophy	Krabbe	Platelike inclusions ("tubular")	Galactocerebrosidase
	X	Angiokeratoma corporis diffusum	Fabry	Endothelial zebra (lamellated) bodies	Birefringent lipid (frozen), Oil red O (+), PAS (+) Ceramide-trihexosidase
	AR	Abetalipoproteinemia	Bassen-Kornzweig	—	Apolipoprotein B deficiency
	AR	Familial HDL deficiency	Tangier	Clear, spherical vacuoles	Oil red O (+) HDL deficiency

AD, autosomal dominant; *AR,* autosomal recessive; *C24,* 24-carbon-length fatty acid; *HDL,* high-density lipoprotein; *PAS,* Periodic acid–Schiff; *X,* X-linked; +/– — +++, severity of pathologic abnormality.

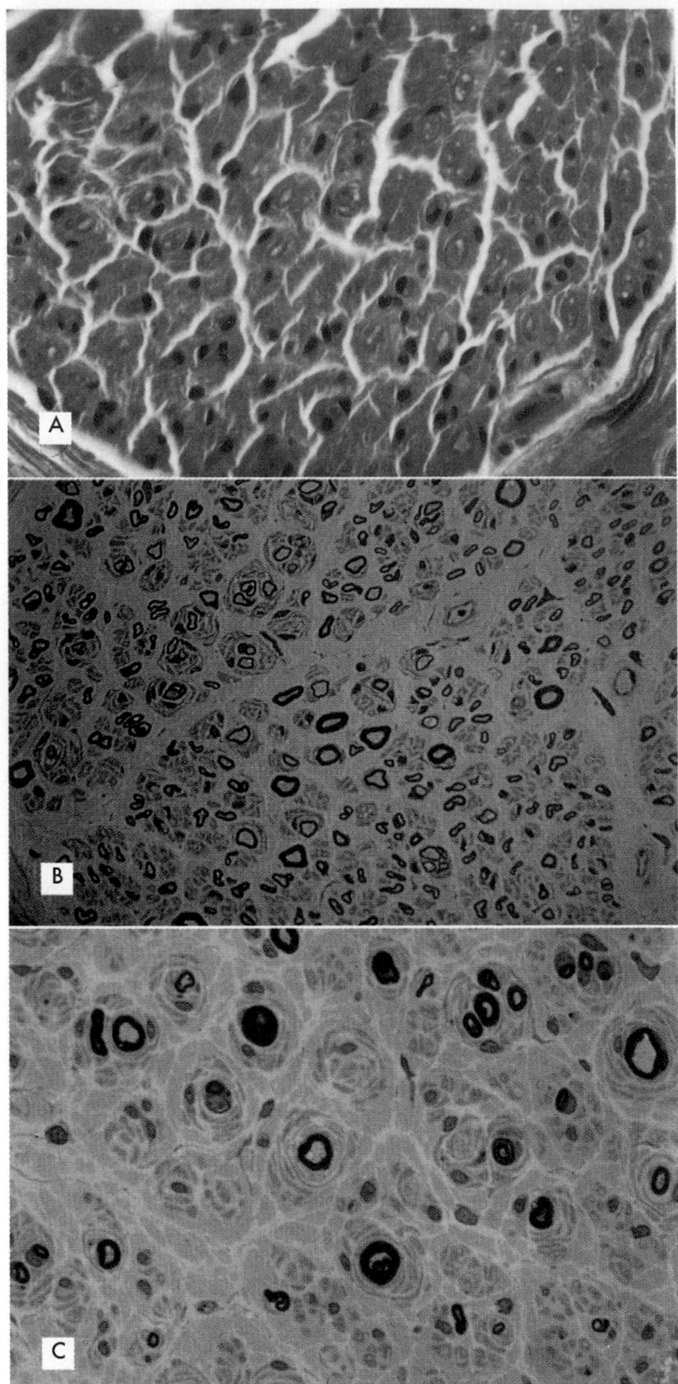

Fig. 78-15 Type I Charcot-Marie-Tooth disease, hypertrophic form (HMSN I). **A**, Onion bulbs may be difficult to identify by routine histology, with ill-defined layers of Schwann cell processes and the occasional presence of two Schwann cell nuclei adjacent to a single fiber. **B**, In the same case, prominent onion bulb formations are readily identified surrounding most of the fibers in plastic-embedded sections. **C**, Onion bulbs are composed of concentric layers of Schwann cell cytoplasm, with only occasional Schwann cell nuclei identifiable. (**B** and **C** Epoxy resin section, toluidine blue stain.)

teased-fiber preparations reveal a variability in both internodal length and myelin thickness along single fibers. The segmental demyelination may be more prominent on some fibers than on others; however, many fibers are affected in the later stages of the disease. Type II CMT disease, in contrast, shows a loss of large-caliber and small-caliber myelinated axons. Onion bulbs, if present, are infrequent.[48] Axonal loss may be difficult to identify in hematoxylin and eosin–stained sections; however, it is often prominent in plastic-embedded sections, where it can be quantitated by morphometry.

Nerve conduction velocity has been useful in classifying patients with CMT. Slowing of nerve conduction velocity has been associated with the demyelinating or hypertrophic form of disease (type I), is often dramatic (<30 m/s), and shows a strong relationship with clinical severity within a single subtype.[49] In contrast, the conduction velocity is usually normal (>45 m/s) in patients with type II CMT disease. In type I CMT disease, symptoms appear in the second decade, slightly earlier than in type II. In both types, the clinical course is slowly progressive. Progressive sensory deficits and muscular atrophy impede ambulation and cause foot deformities but do not shorten the life span.

Dejerine-Sottas disease (HMSN III)

Dejerine-Sottas disease, a hereditary neuropathy of childhood, also known as hypertrophic neuropathy of infancy, is inherited as an autosomal-recessive trait.[50] The disease commonly occurs between 5 and 15 years of age; however, delayed motor skills may be evident earlier in life, with delay in the onset of walking and difficulty with running and jumping. Nerve conduction is slow,[51] and there may be palpable enlargement of peripheral nerves. Clubfoot, kyphoscoliosis, and muscular atrophy are common.

Microscopically, nerves show prominent onion bulb formation, which is usually readily apparent on hematoxylin and eosin–stained sections (Fig. 78-16) and corresponds to clinically evident nerve enlargement. In the early stages of this disease, the layering of Schwann cells and formation of onion bulbs is the most dramatic finding, often surrounding thinly myelinated axons. In later stages of the disease, however, the axons may have degenerated, leaving only the onion bulbs as

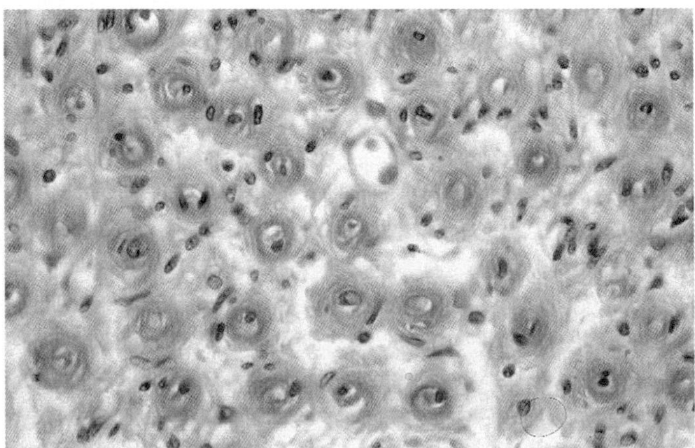

Fig. 78-16 Dejerine-Sottas disease with prominent onion bulb formations.

markers. Teased fibers generally show variability in internodal lengths and myelin thicknesses and may contain long regions that are completely devoid of myelin.

The clinical features are those of a severe, chronically progressive symmetric peripheral neuropathy. Patients are often weak and areflexic, with a delay in the onset of motor skills. The parents are typically unaffected. The gradual progression of the disease may lead to wheelchair confinement in young adult life.

Refsum disease (HMSN IV)

Refsum disease is a hereditary neuropathy often combined with pigmentary retinopathy and cerebellar ataxia. It results from a selective impairment in the peroxisomal α-oxidation of phytanic acid,[52] leading to elevated serum levels. Because catabolism of phytanic acid occurs within peroxisomes, serum levels of phytanic acids are also elevated in more global disorders of peroxisome genesis, such as neonatal adrenoleukodystrophy, infantile Refsum's disease, and Zellweger disease.

Peripheral nerves show a severe onion bulb neuropathy that resembles Dejerine-Sottas disease. In addition, there is involvement of the olivocerebellar tract and atrophy of the inferior olive.

Some patients present primarily with the pigmentary retinopathy, others with cerebellar ataxia, and still others with the peripheral neuropathy. Those presenting primarily with peripheral neuropathy may be confused with Dejerine-Sottas disease or with early onset CMT; however, elevation of serum phytanic acid resolves this difficulty.

Giant axonal neuropathy of childhood

Giant axonal neuropathy is an uncommon peripheral neuropathy of childhood, inherited in an autosomal-recessive pattern.[53] The pathogenesis appears to involve the assembly and processing of intermediate filaments within the cytoplasm. Accumulation of neurofilaments within the axon is the diagnostic hallmark of giant axonal neuropathy; however, intermediate filament aggregates also occur in other cell types, including glia, Schwann cells, and fibroblasts. Cultured fibroblasts from affected children accumulate vimentin filaments in a perinuclear distribution. Because each of the intermediate filament proteins are encoded at separate genetic foci, it is widely suspected that giant axonal neuropathy represents a disorder of a conserved mechanism of intermediate filament processing.

Microscopically, the disorder is characterized by the presence of greatly enlarged axons that appear in routine sections as homogeneous eosinophilic spheroids (Fig. 78-17). In plastic-embedded sections, greatly enlarged axons have homogeneous, smooth axoplasm. The myelin surrounding the giant axons is extremely thin and may be surrounded by Schwann cell hyperplasia, indicative of secondary demyelination. Teased fibers show a fusiform enlargement of axons, which are distended by disorganized interlacing fascicles of intermediate filaments by electron microscopy.

Clinically, the children become symptomatic from 5 to 10 years of age with a gradually progressive peripheral neuropathy. Symptoms include weakness, diminished sensation, and absent reflexes. Nerve conduction studies usually show diminished amplitudes but may also show diminished velocity caused by the secondary demyelination. Interestingly, many children with the disorder have abnormally coiled hair, which may reflect aberrant processing of hair keratins.

Neuroaxonal dystrophy

The progressive neurologic disorder neuroaxonal dystrophy is characterized by dystrophic enlargement of CNS and PNS axons. The cause of neuroaxonal dystrophy is unknown; in some cases there has been a deficiency of the enzyme α-*N*-acetylgalactosaminidase.[54] Paraffin-embedded nerve biopsy specimens may not show any diagnostic features, but plastic-embedded sections reveal axons with greatly distended contours. The axoplasm is often granular, in contrast to the more homogeneous appearance of giant axonal neuropathy. As with giant axonal neuropathy, secondary demyelination may occur around the distended axons.

Electron microscopy is required to identify the diagnostic intra-axonal membranous structures. These tubulovesicular structures may have a vesicular appearance in some axons; in

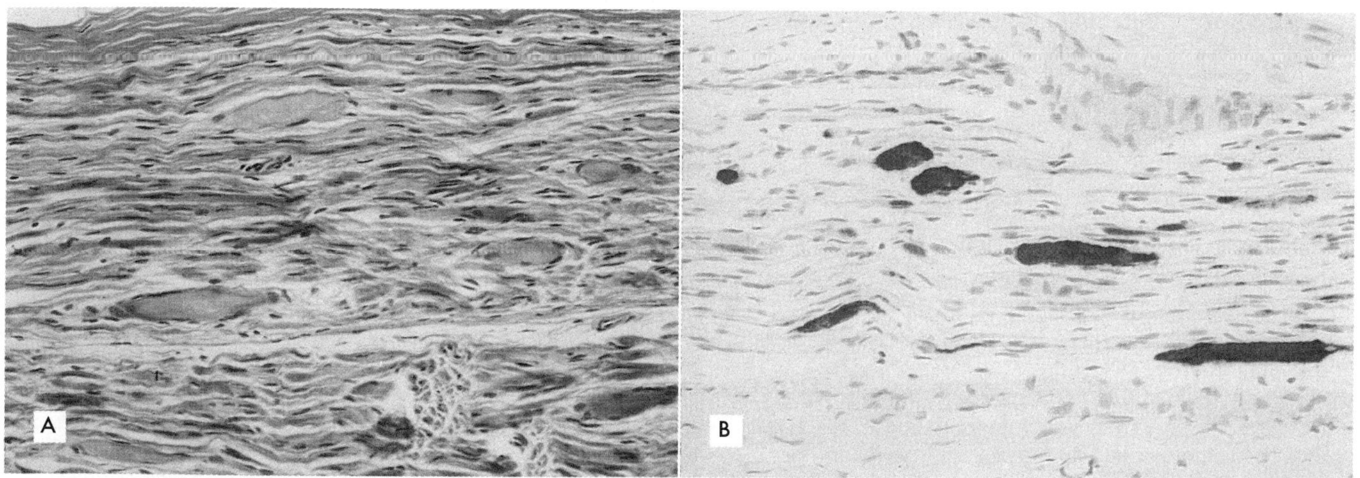

Fig. 78-17 Giant axonal neuropathy. **A**, Prominent eosinophilic enlarged axons are identified. Some are surrounded with rings of Schwann cells representing Schwann cell hyperplasia. **B**, Neurofilament immunohistochemistry accentuates the enlarged axons filled with neurofilaments. (Immunohistochemistry with anti-NFP.)

others, tubular or longitudinally oriented membranous structures may predominate. The cytoskeletal elements, including filaments and microtubules, and mitochondria are displaced to one side of the tubulovesicular aggregates. The dystrophic axons may be detected in skin biopsy specimens,[55] and similar dystrophic axons are present throughout the brain.

Children with neuroaxonal dystrophy develop neurologic symptoms in the first 2 years of life, after a normal birth and early development. Progressive involvement of the central nervous system is usually the dominant clinical problem, usually resulting in death during childhood.

Tomaculous neuropathy

The term *tomaculous neuropathy* has been used to convey two meanings: a pathologic finding or a clinical disorder. The clinical disorder is an autosomal-dominant hereditary neuropathy characterized by a tendency to develop compression neuropathy, also known as "inherited liability to pressure palsies" or "hereditary neuropathy with pressure palsies." As a pathologic term, *tomaculous neuropathy* refers to the presence of focal hypermyelination, usually involving a large percentage of internodes.[56] Recent linkage studies suggest that the disorder results from the heterozygous deletion of a region of chromosome 17p, including the gene for PMP 22.[40]

Microscopically the focal hypermyelination is not readily detected on hematoxylin and eosin–stained slides. Plastic-embedded sections show a few fibers with excessively thick myelin sheaths (Fig. 78-18). The hypermyelination may be concentric around the axon or may show eccentric folds of myelin. Teased-fiber preparations reveal fusiform, well-defined areas of thickened myelin (Fig. 78-18), which have been likened to a sausage (Latin: *tomaculum*). By electron microscopy, the hypermyelination consists of concentric hypermyelination of some fibers, or eccentric inner or outer layers of myelin that have a redundant folded pattern. In addition to focal hypermyelination, there is also extensive segmental demyelination and Schwann cell hyperplasia.[57]

Although patients may have a demyelinating neuropathy, they are more often identified during the evaluation of recurrent pressure palsies. Nerve conduction studies may reveal a diffuse slowing that is most likely caused by the severe segmental demyelination. A related disorder is hereditary brachial plexopathy, an autosomal-dominant disorder with a tendency to develop brachial plexus neuropathy. Nerve biopsy specimens from these patients have also revealed the pathologic findings of tomaculous neuropathy.

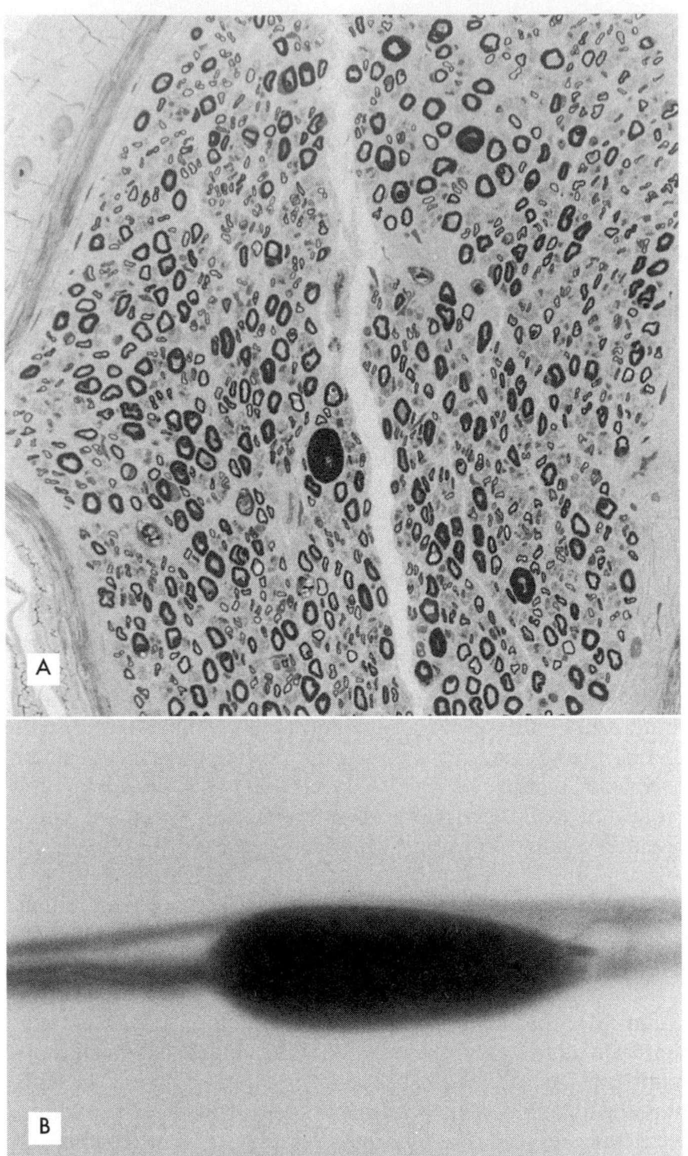

Fig. 78-18 Tomaculous neuropathy. **A**, Cross-sections reveal the occasional "hypermyelinated" axons with thickened myelin sheaths. (Epoxy resin section, toluidine blue stain, **B**, The focal regions of myelin thickening are identified on at least 25% of the individual fibers. (Teased-fiber preparation.)

Sensorimotor neuropathies associated with hereditary metabolic disease

Several hereditary metabolic diseases, most notably the group of leukodystrophies, may be associated with a peripheral neuropathy (Table 78-4). Although central nervous system (CNS) symptoms are often the dominant clinical feature, peripheral neuropathy may be the initial complaint or may be a prominent component of the disorder.

Krabbe disease (globoid cell leukodystrophy), caused by a deficiency of the enzyme galactocerebrosidase, is characterized by cerebral leukoencephalopathy and peripheral neuropathy. The peripheral nervous system is devoid of globoid cells, which are the hallmark of the disease in the CNS. Instead, a demyelinating neuropathy is detectable in plastic-embedded sections with variability in myelin thickness and occasional Schwann cell hyperplasia. Schwann cells contain storage material appearing as platelike electron-lucent areas in the cytoplasm that may aggregate to form prisms of electron lucency.

Adrenoleukodystrophy is an X-linked disorder resulting from impaired peroxisomal catabolism of very long chain (>24 carbon) fatty acids.[58] Demyelination in the CNS, which usually begins between 5 and 15 years of age, is accompanied by a prominent inflammatory infiltrate oriented along fiber pathways.[59] Unlike the central nervous system, demyelination in the peripheral nervous system occurs without an inflammatory component. Usually undetectable on routine sections, the neuropathy is characterized by segmental demyelination with variable myelin thickness and occasional Schwann cell hyperplasia. A characteristic ultrastructural feature in Schwann cells is the presence of needle-shaped electron-lucent inclusions bounded by leaflets.

Although peripheral nerve involvement may occur in young males with the hemizygous (X-linked) disease, their clinical course is more often related to progressive leukoencephalopathy. However, peripheral neuropathy may be the initial symptom in older hemizygous males or heterozygous females. These patients have a diffuse peripheral neuropathy ("adrenomyeloneuropathy"), with spasticity of the lower limbs related to involvement of the long tracts of the spinal cord, adrenal insufficiency, and elevated serum levels of very long chain fatty acids.

Metachromatic leukodystrophy is inherited in an autosomal-recessive pattern and results from deficiency of arylsulfatase A activity. In most patients, this is the result of the deficiency of the arylsulfatase enzyme; however, a rare variant (AB variant) is related to a deficiency of an activator protein.[60] A deficiency of arylsulfatase A activity results in the accumulation of sulfated sphingolipids (sulfatides), which are metachromatic when they bind to certain dyes.

In the central nervous system, there is severe involvement of the white matter, which shows diffuse demyelination. In the peripheral nervous system, there is often a demyelinating peripheral neuropathy, which may be the initial symptom in the juvenile or adult forms. Paraffin-embedded sections may reveal macrophages within nerve; however, the metabolic product is partially removed during the dehydration for paraffin embedding, and so metachromasia is more difficult to identify in these sections. Plastic-embedded sections reveal the thin myelin sheath surrounding many fibers and the proliferation of Schwann cells characteristic of a chronic demyelinating neuropathy. At times, the degree of demyelination with onion bulb formation may raise the possibility of a hereditary "onion-bulb" neuropathy. The demonstration of metachromasia in macrophages is most reliably performed on frozen sections and is diagnostic of metachromatic leukodystrophy. In addition, the metachromatic granules have characteristic prismatic and zebra body shapes by electron microscopy.

Progressive neurologic deterioration occurs with weakness, hypotonia, unsteady gait, and eventual difficulty walking. This subsequent clinical course, however, is related to the age of onset, with a more rapid course in patients who develop symptoms in infancy.

Hereditary sensory and autonomic neuropathies

The hereditary sensory and autonomic neuropathies have been classified by Dyck into three major types; however, some less common hereditary sensory and autonomic neuropathies are also described. The disorders differ in the degree of involvement of the sensory and autonomic modalities and in the age of onset.

The microscopic appearance in each of the hereditary sensory and autonomic neuropathies parallels the clinical symptoms (Table 78-4). Type I HSAN, clinically dominated by numbness, involves large myelinated fibers. There is a degeneration of dorsal root ganglion cells with a proliferation of satellite cells. Degenerating axons and axonal loss are found in peripheral nerve and in the posterior columns of the spinal cord. Type II HSAN, a congenital neuropathy with a more severe sensory deficit, is characterized by a complete absence of large and small myelinated fibers. In type III HSAN, autonomic symptoms predominate, and there is a loss of neurons and neuronophagia involving the autonomic ganglia. Peripheral nerve shows a dramatic loss of unmyelinated fibers, with a relative preservation of myelinated fibers.

The prognosis is different in the three types of HSAN. Type I HSAN shows a slow progression of sensory deficits, but with a persistently greater involvement of the lower extremities. Ulcers of the feet may develop, complicated by osteomyelitis and thrombophlebitis. Type II HSAN often shows progressive involvement of the upper and lower extremities with suppurative lesions developing in the insensitive limbs, but it may be nonprogressive.[61] Treatment is directed toward avoidance of injuries to the hands and feet. In type III HSAN, the dysautonomia is progressive, and death often occurs in infancy.

Hereditary amyloid neuropathy

Hereditary amyloid neuropathy is characterized by endoneurial deposits of amyloid, most often derived from transthyretin. A point mutation in the transthyretin gene, located on chromosome 18q, has been found in most affected families. Although described independently in different regions of the world, many of these different forms have shown the same mutation or mutations at different sites in the same gene. The Portuguese, Japanese, and Swedish kindreds all show a mutation at amino acid 30 with a substitution of methionine for valine (MET 30).[62] Other mutations include those of the Jewish kindred (ILE 33), West Virginia kindred (VAL 55), Illinois-German kindred (TYR 77), Indiana (SER 84), and German type (HIS 58).[33]

As in other forms of amyloidosis, there is an interstitial deposition of smooth eosinophilic material (Fig. 78-19). The amyloid material is located predominantly within the endoneurial space and in the walls of small endoneurial blood vessels. Congo red staining shows the typical congophilic properties of amyloid. In plastic sections, there is a greater loss of small myelinated fibers than large myelinated fibers, and electron microscopy identifies a large depletion of unmyelinated fibers and masses of unbranching extracellular amyloid fibrils, 7 to 9 nm in diameter. Immunohistochemistry may be used to differentiate the transthyretin-derived amyloid from light-chain deposits in immunocyte-derived amyloid.[63]

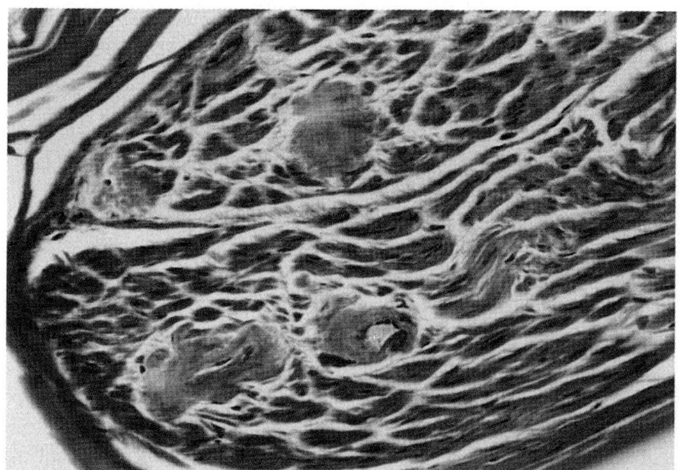

Fig. 78-19 Familial amyloid neuropathy. Smooth eosinophilic deposits are present in the endoneurium and around blood vessels.

The set of symptoms reflects the relative involvement of small myelinated and unmyelinated fibers and includes impairment of pain and temperature sensations followed by touch and vibration. Autonomic symptoms are often prominent and include nausea, vomiting, other gastrointestinal symptoms, incontinence, impotence, and hypotension. In Portuguese and Japanese kindreds, the onset is between 20 and 40 years of age,[64] and in Swedish kindreds it occurs at an average age of 55 years. The course is progressive, and death usually ensues within 10 years of onset of symptoms, though clinical improvement after liver transplantation has been reported.[65]

ISCHEMIC NEUROPATHIES

The peripheral nervous system is relatively resistant to ischemia; however, large vessel occlusions of the limb may lead to infarction of soft tissue, including peripheral nerve. In addition, vascular disease affecting smaller-caliber arteries can lead to ischemic injury of nerve, which most often occurs as single nerve involvement or involvement of multiple nerves (Fig. 78-20).

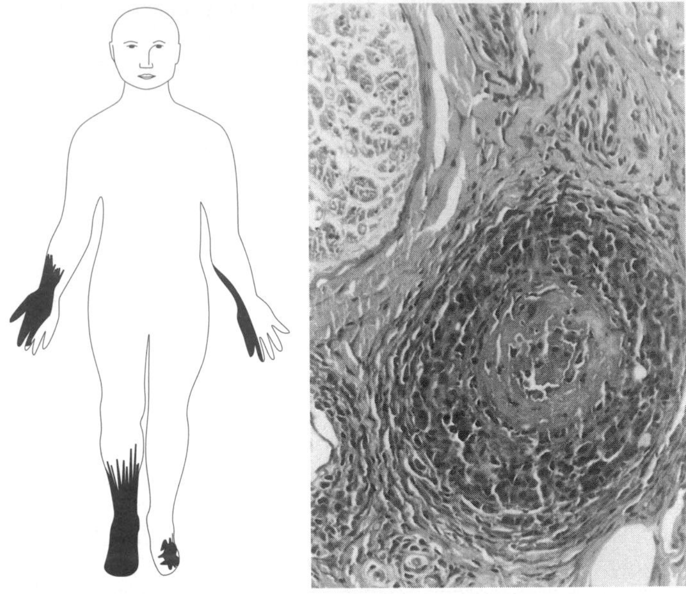

Fig. 78-20 Asymmetric neuropathy. **A**, When the asymmetry includes involvement of multiple individual nerves, the term *mononeuritis multiplex* is often used. **B**, Polyarteritis nodosa, with a dense inflammatory infiltrate extending through the vessel wall, accompanied by fibrinoid necrosis. There is endoneurial edema of the adjacent fascicle.

Vasculitis

The vasculitides are a group of inflammatory diseases of blood vessels that often affect peripheral nerves. Based on the caliber of the involved vessels and the distribution of involvement, three major categories of vasculitides affect peripheral nerves: polyarteritis nodosa, Churg-Strauss disease, and hypersensitivity vasculitis.

Polyarteritis nodosa and *Churg-Strauss disease,* which could be considered a variant of polyarteritis,[66] are characterized by inflammation of medium or small arteries. The onset of neuropathy in these diseases is often subacute and is typically asymmetric. The asymmetry may be so pronounced that multiple single nerves appear to be involved (mononeuritis multiplex).

Hypersensitivity vasculitis, characterized by inflammation of capillaries and venules, is an allergic reaction that may be precipitated by drugs, bacterial infections, or heterologous proteins. On occasion, this type of small vessel vasculitis may be limited to peripheral nerves and has been referred to as nonsystemic vasculitic neuropathy.[67] Although each of these vasculitides has distinct clinical and pathologic characteristics, they share certain features: asymmetric polyneuropathy, abrupt onset and rapid progression, inflammatory destruction of blood vessels, injury to peripheral nerves by ischemia, and therapeutic response to immunosuppression.

Ischemic axonal degeneration is often recognizable in hematoxylin and eosin–stained sections. On cross section, the endoneurium may show large fibers replaced by axonal and myelin debris. In longitudinal sections, these tissue products form eosinophilic ovoids separated by clear vacuoles, typical of acute axonal degeneration. Although the presence of focal regions of acute axonal degeneration is suggestive of an ischemic cause, the definitive diagnostic criteria for vasculitis remains the identification of inflammatory and destructive lesions of blood vessels (Fig. 78-20). In plastic-embedded sections, each of the vasculitides reveals axonal degeneration involving both large-caliber and small-caliber myelinated fibers, with degenerating axons often clustered within individual fascicles (Fig. 78-21). There may also be chronic axonal loss in some areas of the fascicle, reflecting the random distribution of the vascular lesions over time. Teased-fiber analysis often shows varying stages of degeneration, again with linear arrays of myelin ovoids. The relationship of vasculitis to clinically similar cases in which necrotizing vasculitis is not identified on biopsy remains uncertain, though the latter patients also respond to steroid therapy.[68]

Atherosclerosis

Peripheral vascular disease affects nerves unpredictably, and many individuals with severe atherosclerosis show no signs of peripheral neuropathy. Infarction of peripheral nerve is exceedingly uncommon and most often is associated with diabetes mellitus. On the other hand, claudication (pain initiated by arterial insufficiency in an extremity during physical exertion) is quite common and is attributed to ischemia of nerve fibers. Severe atherosclerosis may exist without detectable nerve involvement; however, physiologic testing of patients admitted for surgical therapy of limb ischemia has revealed 88% with signs of peripheral neuropathy.[69] Nerve biopsies performed on limbs amputated for ischemia have shown chronic axonal loss involving both large-caliber and small-caliber myelinated axons.

Critical illness neuropathy

Polyneuropathy is a common complication in patients maintained in intensive care units for greater than 30 days ("intensive care neuropathy"). In this setting, up to 50% of patients who have been septic for greater than 2 weeks develop a peripheral neuropathy that, at times, requires prolonged rehabilitation.[70] The neuropathy that complicates complex medical problems, including sepsis and multiple organ failure, usually is not discovered until the patient is removed from ventilator support. Because the severity of the underlying illness may

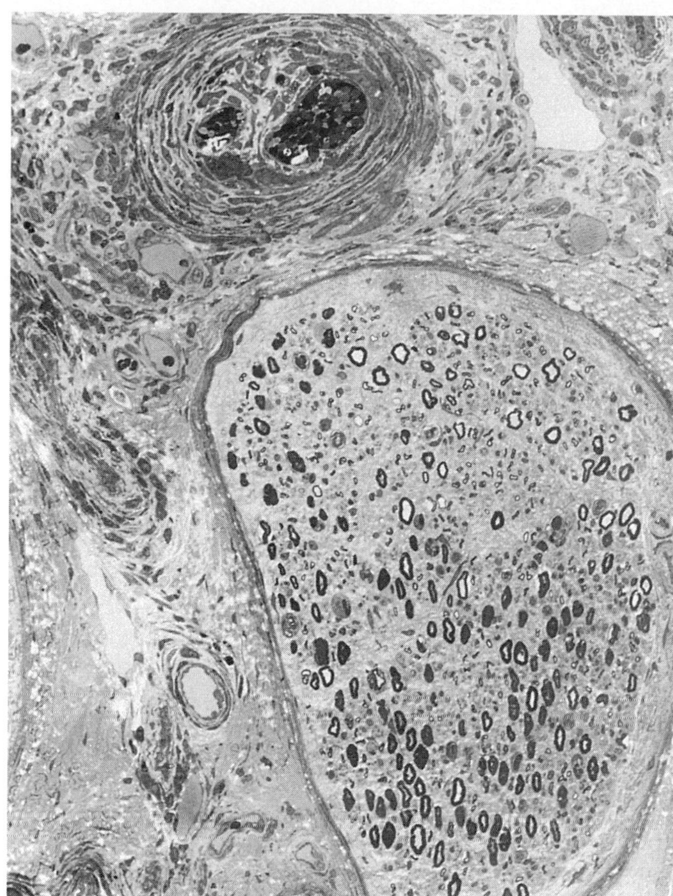

Fig. 78-21 Ischemic neuropathy. An inflammatory infiltrate permeates the arterial wall, with thrombosis and recanalization. The adjacent fascicle shows both axonal loss and acutely degenerating axons, most prominent near the affected blood vessel (Epoxy resin section, toluidine blue stain.)

overshadow the onset of peripheral neuropathy, these patients may be detected by electrophysiologic methods.[71]

The neuropathy is characterized by normal conduction velocity and a sharp decrease in amplitude, suggestive of axonal neuropathy. Pathologic studies in these patients have been limited because of the recent awareness of the occurrence of critical care neuropathy; however, muscle biopsy specimens have shown denervation, and nerve biopsy specimens have revealed an axonal degeneration that is most severe in distal nerves.

TOXIC NEUROPATHIES

Many metals and organic compounds are known to cause toxic peripheral neuropathy (Table 78-5). In general, toxic peripheral neuropathies are dose related and most often characterized by axonal degeneration. Nerve conduction is usually decreased in amplitude with relative sparing of velocity. Most toxic neuropathies show a distal symmetric pattern of sensorimotor involvement (Fig. 78-22). This "stocking-glove" distribution is typical at the onset, with sensory deficits over the toes and feet; however, continued exposure to the toxic compound extends the deficit to the lower calves and hands.

Table 78-5 Toxic peripheral neuropathies

Industrial	Therapeutic
Acrylamide	Almitrine
Allyl chloride	Aminoglycosides
Arsenic	Amiodarone
Carbon disulfide	Amitryptyline
Chlorphos	Chloramphenicol
Dimethylaminopropionitrile	Chloroquine
Ethylene oxide	Clioquinol
Hexacarbons (hexane)	Colchicine
Kepone	Dapsone
Lead	Disulfiram
Leptophos	Doxorubicin
Mercury	Glutethimide
Methyl bromide	Gold
Mipafox	Hexachlorophene
Polychlorinated biphenyls	Hydralazine
Thallium	Isoniazid
Trichlorfon	Metronidazole
Trichloroethylene	Nitrofurantoin
Tri-*ortho*-cresyl phosphate	Perhexilene
Vacor	Phenytoin
	Platinum
	Sodium cyanate
	Vincristine

Arsenic toxicity

Chronic exposure to arsenic occurs in industrial workers employed in smelting or handling arsenical pesticides. Most poisonings are caused by food contamination or homicidal or suicidal attempts. Acute poisoning may lead to cerebral edema and is often fatal; peripheral neuropathy more commonly occurs in chronic arsenic intoxication and is accompanied by gastrointestinal complaints and linear discolorations of the nails (Mees lines). The peripheral neuropathy is axonal in type and diffuse in distribution, with arsenic demonstrable within nerve.[72] Sensory involvement predominates over motor; however, distal weakness may develop.

The elimination of absorbed arsenic may be facilitated by administration of BAL or D-penicillamine.[73] Recovery of sensory deficits may occur, but slowly, over months or years.

Hexacarbon neuropathy

Although initially identified and characterized as *n*-hexane neuropathy, the subsequent recognition that methyl *n*-butyl ketone (2-hexanone) induces an identical neuropathy has led to the designation of "hexacarbon" neuropathy. Industrial epidemics have been reported among people working in poorly ventilated spaces, and sporadic cases have resulted from glue sniffing for the euphoric effect of the solvent. The development of neuropathy results from long-term, low-dose exposure. The neuropathy requires metabolic activation of hexane or methyl *n*-butyl ketone to the toxic six-carbon compound 2,5-hexanedione, and several experimental studies indicate that this toxic metabolite is capable of alkylating and cross-linking a variety of proteins.[74] In peripheral nerve, neurofilaments aggregate as a result of abnormalities in the slow component of axonal transport.[75] The aggregation of neurofilaments is associated with axonal enlargement, most

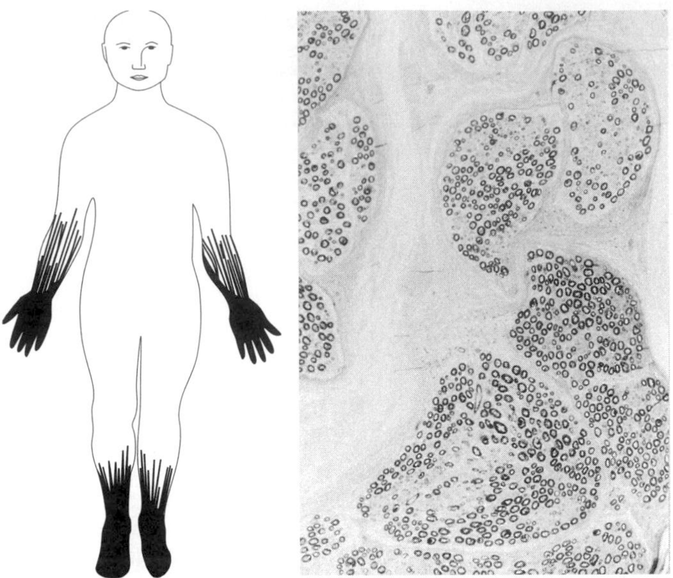

Fig. 78-22 Distal symmetric neuropathy. **A**, The distribution of numbness and paresthesias is typically in a "stocking-glove" distribution. **B**, In this case, there is a mild degree of axonal loss throughout each of the individual fascicles. (Epoxy resin section, toluidine blue stain.)

common in distal peripheral nerves. Axonal degeneration frequently accompanies the axonal enlargement.

Chronic exposure to hexane leads to a distal symmetric peripheral neuropathy with diminished amplitude on nerve conduction studies. Numbness is the most common initial complaint, with position sense and motor functions being frequently spared in the early stages. With severe neuropathy, motor weakness occurs, and involvement of the long spinal tracts may initiate spasticity. Symptoms often progress for a period after cessation of exposure, a phenomenon termed "coasting."

Vincristine toxicity

All vinca alkaloids, used for their antimitotic effects in cancer chemotherapy, impair microtubule function and axonal transport. The most characteristic pathologic features induced by vincristine are found in the perikarya of neurons in the anterior spinal horns and dorsal root ganglia, where eosinophilic protein aggregates develop into well-defined cytoplasmic inclusions.[76] Axons of both the peripheral nervous system and the long tracks of the spinal cord may also be affected. In peripheral nerves axonal degeneration is most pronounced distally.

Alcohol (ethanol) neuropathy

There is a regional variability in the incidence of peripheral neuropathy associated with alcoholism, being estimated at approximately 9% of alcoholics in inner cities.[77] Although this higher incidence in inner cities indicates that diet may play a role, no individual nutritional deficiencies have been identified. In addition, alcohol may have direct effects on the central nervous system; these effects have been implicated in the cerebellar degeneration.[78]

The peripheral neuropathy is characterized by axonal degeneration. Its distribution is predominantly distal and symmetric, with a greater involvement of sensory modalities than motor and diminished amplitudes in nerve conduction.

METABOLIC NEUROPATHIES

Nutritional deficiencies

Vitamin B_1 (thiamine) deficiency causes beriberi. The peripheral neuropathy that typically occurs in so-called dry beriberi is chronic and symmetric, where it is the predominant symptom. In addition to sensory loss, there may be weakness of the tongue, larynx, and facial muscles. Axonal degeneration is seen in both peripheral nerves and the posterior columns of the spinal cord and, analogous to pellagra, may be accompanied by a striking chromatolysis. Peripheral neuropathy coexists in some patients with Wernicke's encephalopathy; however, the two clinical syndromes, both of which result from thiamine deficiency, frequently occur in isolation.

Vitamin B_{12} deficiency is characterized by megaloblastic anemia, often associated with progressive sensory and motor dysfunction. The onset of neurologic symptoms is often abrupt and dominated by involvement of the spinal cord, where a degeneration involves both ascending and descending tracts, predominantly in the thoracic spinal cord. Peripheral nerves show segmental demyelination and axonal degeneration, with distal accentuation. Therapy, aimed at vitamin replacement, may lead to complete resolution of symptoms.

Endocrine disorders with peripheral neuropathy

Peripheral neuropathy occurs in both type I and type II diabetes mellitus.[79] The reported prevalence of neuropathy in patients with diabetes mellitus varies from 10% to 60% as assessed by clinical criteria and up to 100% when evaluated by nerve conduction studies.[80] The prevalence also depends on the duration of the disease; in a recent series, 7% of patients with diabetes mellitus had clinical peripheral neuropathy at the time of diagnosis, and 50% of diabetics had peripheral neuropathy 25 years after diagnosis.[81] Approximately 17 million people with diabetes in the United States and Europe suffer from peripheral neuropathy.[82]

Although the generic term *diabetic neuropathy* is used widely in the literature, it encompasses several distinct clinicopathologic disorders that occur in diabetes mellitus, often with overlapping features.[83] Common to all types are vascular changes, evidenced by thickening of the walls of capillaries.[84] In peripheral nerve biopsy specimens, this vasculopathy appears as a prominent reduplication of the basal lamina that surrounds the endoneurial capillaries.[85]

Diabetic symmetric sensorimotor neuropathy is the most common form of peripheral neuropathy in diabetes mellitus. It is distal in location, symmetric in distribution, and sensorimotor in composition. Cutaneous ulceration and mild weakness may complicate its late course. Alternatively, the neuropathy may be symmetric, proximal, and motor, with involvement of the lower extremities predominating. In both of these manifestations of neuropathy, there is axonal loss that affects large-diameter and small-diameter myelinated axons, commonly accompanied by segmental demyelination.

Diabetic asymmetric sensorimotor neuropathy is a distinct second type of diabetic peripheral neuropathy that differs by the asymmetric involvement. It often occurs in a subacute manner, with muscle weakness and pain that is exaggerated at night. It occurs most frequently in patients over 50 but may affect younger patients as well. The asymmetry and subacute expression of the axonal degeneration are suggestive of an ischemic cause.

Diabetic autonomic neuropathy targets the autonomic nervous system. It is symmetric and almost always includes some sensory involvement. Patients may experience gastrointestinal symptoms and have gastric atony, as well as symmetric anhydrosis, orthostatic hypotension, impotence, and bladder dysfunction. Small myelinated and unmyelinated fibers may be severely affected.[86] Enlargement of sympathetic ganglion cells has been reported in association with PAS-positive deposits, and autonomic ganglia have been demonstrated by electron microscopy and Bielschowsky stains to contain dystrophic neuritic processes with abundant disorganized neurofilaments.[87]

Diabetic mononeuropathy may occur abruptly. The oculomotor nerve (III) is commonly involved with a tendency to affect extraocular motor activity while sparing pupillary function. A peripheral nerve infarction, sparing the peripheral pupillary fibers of the oculomotor nerve, has been implicated in diabetic oculomotor palsy. Mononeuropathy may involve the abducens (VI) nerve, or a single nerve of the extremities, notably the radial, median, ulnar, or common peroneal. These peripheral mononeuropathies in diabetes share anatomic sites with entrapment neuropathies in nondiabetic patients, and suggesting an increased susceptibility to compression neuropathy in diabetic patients.[88]

Hyperglycemia induces two biochemical processes that may be relevant to the pathogenesis of diabetic neuropathies. The first involves upregulation in the expression of the enzyme aldose reductase, which activates the polyol metabolic pathway. Increased polyol metabolites (sorbitol and fructose) have been demonstrated in a variety of tissues, including peripheral nerve. The accumulation of intracellular sorbitol is associated with a decrease of intracellular myoinositol and subsequent impairment in the phosphoinositide pathway. In addition, aldose reductase may compete with nitric oxide synthase, leading to impaired synthesis of the vasodilator nitric oxide.[89] A second biochemical event is the nonenzymatic glycation of proteins, which occurs in a variety of cellular proteins. Although initially reversible, glycation may be followed by the Amadori rearrangement, which leads to irreversible alkylation and cross-linking of proteins. Glycation and Amadori products are present in hemoglobin of diabetic patients and have been a useful measure of the level of control of hyperglycemia.[90]

Hypothyroidism may also be accompanied by peripheral neuropathy. Carpal tunnel syndrome is common and is believed to result from myxedema of the tendon sheaths. Mononeuropathies may also include isolated deafness or hoarseness. The prolongation of deep tendon reflex relaxation is a common clinical sign, and distal paresthesias have been noted in up to 60% of patients with hypothyroidism.[91] Histologically, nerves from patients with distal symmetric polyneuropathy show a decreased number of large myelinated fibers, with lesser involvement of small myelinated fibers. There are also descriptions of an increased frequency of Renaut bodies, the focal subperineurial deposits (Fig. 78-2).

Organ failure and peripheral neuropathy

Peripheral neuropathy is commonly seen with organ failure (Table 78-6). Uremia, regardless of cause, is frequently associated with peripheral neuropathy. Approximately 60% of patients with chronic renal failure have symptoms of uremic neuropathy at the onset of dialysis.[92] Expressed as pain and paresthesia, both sensory and motor functions are vulnerable, with lower extremities preferentially involved. The distribution of symptoms suggests a slow "dying-back" progression in upper and lower limbs. Axonal degeneration predominates in distal nerve specimens. Generally, dialysis may improve symptoms; however, the neuropathy may persist or even progress during dialysis. The results of renal transplantation are usually more dramatic, though there is less success with diabetic patients, perhaps because of concomitant diabetic neuropathy.

Table 78-6 Peripheral neuropathy in acquired metabolic disease

Vitamin deficiencies
Beriberi (thiamine deficiency)
Pellagra
Pyridoxine (B_6) deficiency
Vitamin B_{12} deficiency
Vitamin E deficiency
Endocrine disorders
Acromegaly
Diabetes mellitus
Hyperthyroidism
Hypoglycemia
Hypothyroidism
Organ dysfunction
Chronic respiratory failure
Hepatic failure
Uremia
Wilson disease

INFECTIOUS NEUROPATHIES

Herpes infections

Three members of the herpes virus family may infect the peripheral nervous system: herpes varicella-zoster, herpes simplex, and cytomegalovirus. *Varicella-zoster virus (VZV)* causes chickenpox in childhood and shingles in adults. After an acute infection, VZV can reside latently in ganglia and become reactivated at a later time. The predominance of zoster within dermatomes of the face and chest, areas most involved in varicella eruptions, indicates that ganglia with the highest initial infection may be more susceptible to reactivation. The incidence of shingles, which overall is 1 out of 1000 per year, is higher in patients with malignancy, especially lymphomas and leukemias, as well as AIDS. Although usually limited to a single dermatome, in 2% to 10% of cases it is disseminated, especially in patients who are immunocompromised.[93]

Herpes simplex is characterized by recurrent vesicular eruptions of the oral or genital mucosa. Latency of type 1 HSV has been documented within trigeminal ganglia in 50% of individuals at autopsy. In experimental models, reactivation of latent virus is enhanced by nerve injury.

Cytomegalovirus (CMV) is a widespread DNA virus of the herpes family. The most common expression of nerve involvement is a polyradiculoneuropathy in AIDS.[94] This disorder mimics a cauda equina syndrome with asymmetric weakness and sensory deficits of the lower extremities. Low back pain with radiation into the leg and disturbances in bladder and bowel functions are common. In addition, CMV is one of the more common viral infections occurring before the onset of Guillain-Barré syndrome.

All herpes virus infections are characterized by inflammation of ganglia and nerves with axonal degeneration distally. The ganglionic inflammatory lesions may be intense, with prominent lymphocytic infiltration and proliferation of satellite cells. Necrosis of individual ganglion cells is common and may be accompanied by hemorrhage. Typical intranuclear rounded and eosinophilic inclusions (Cowdry type A) may be difficult to find, though immunohistochemistry may be helpful in identifying viral antigen. Axonal degeneration occurs peripherally, sometimes in the presence of lymphocytic infiltrates, but inclusions are usually not identified in distal segments of the affected nerve. By electron microscopy, members of the herpesvirus family share the morphology of an encapsulated virus with a core 70 nm in diameter, surrounded by a lucent rim and a 100 nm electron-dense capsid.

Leprosy

Neuropathy caused by the acid fast bacillus *Mycobacterium leprae* is the most common infectious neuropathy worldwide. This mycobacterium has a diameter of 0.5 μm and a length of 1 to 8 μm and is best demonstrated in tissue sections by the Fite stain. The occurrence of leprosy varies greatly throughout the world, with an incidence in certain areas of Southeast Asia as high as 6 out of 1000 population.[95]

Three forms of leprosy reflect the continuum of the host-mediated response to the organism, and nerve involvement may occur in each form.[96] The *tuberculoid form* is characterized by a vigorous cell-mediated immune response and a positive lepromin test. The hallmark of nerve involvement is well-formed granulomas with centrally placed epithelioid macrophages and peripheral rims of lymphocytes. In contrast, the *lepromatous form* develops in patients with a negative lepromin test and represents a minimal immune response to the organism. It is characterized by intense infiltration of nerves by vacuolated macrophages, infiltrating in rows and sheets and often clustered throughout the perineurium and subperineurial regions. In the tuberculoid form, few organisms can be demonstrated; however, in the lepromatous form, the foamy macrophages are often replete with acid-fast bacilli.[97] They are encountered within macrophages, Schwann cells, and perineurial cells as electron-dense rod-shaped organisms within cytoplasmic vacuoles. An *intermediate form,* borderline leprosy, is characterized by intermediate numbers of bacilli and by granulomatous inflammation with ill-defined tubercles (Fig. 78-23).

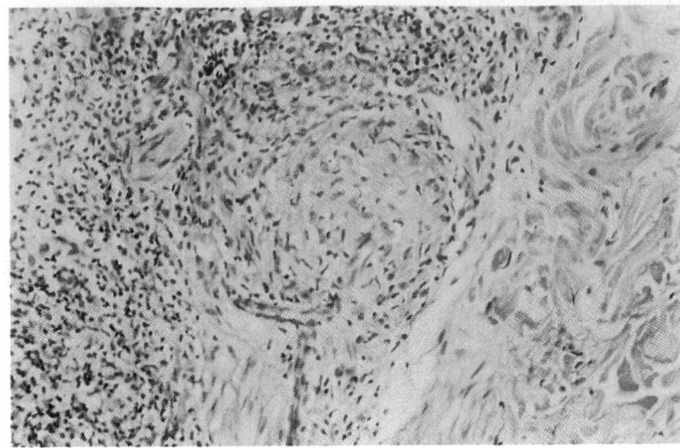

Fig. 78-23 Leprosy, with granulomatous inflammation involving a cutaneous nerve.

Lepromatous neuropathy involves both sensory and motor modalities; however, the distributions of these functional deficits do not always coincide geographically. Cutaneous sensory deficits tend to be superficial and focal, lacking correspondence to nerve or root distribution. This sensory loss may be accompanied by motor weakness, which more often has the distribution of a mononeuropathy or multiple neuropathy, as related to involvement of major nerves.

Combined therapy with dapson and rifampin renders the patient noninfectious but may be complicated by "reversal reaction" as bactericidal activity produces a more vigorous inflammatory response with brief exacerbations of skin lesions and progression of the neuropathy.[98]

Lyme disease

Lyme disease is caused by infection with the spirochete *Borrelia burgdorferi,* which is transmitted by the deer tick species *Ixodes* and is most common in the northeastern United States, northern Europe, China, and Japan. As many as 80% of the ticks in endemic areas of the United States harbor *B. burgdorferi.*[99]

The initial lesion, a red macule that surrounds the tick bite, is followed by systemic symptoms of malaise, fever, chills, and headache. As spirochetes disseminate, meningism may occur as a component of meningoencephalitis and may be accompanied by focal neurologic deficits. Up to 50% of the patients with meningoencephalitis have neurologic deficits that relate to cranial nerves, among which the facial nerve is frequently targeted, with abrupt symptoms suggestive of Bell's palsy. Other patients develop radicular pain and sensory dysfunctions. The pain usually begins acutely or subacutely. Approximately 4 weeks thereafter motor weakness may become evident in a radicular distribution. Still later, a diffuse, distal neuropathy may develop, producing sensory symptoms predominantly in a "stocking-and-glove" distribution.

The most characteristic histologic associate of diffuse neuropathy is a perivascular lymphocytic infiltrate into a nerve.[100] This may extend into the vessel walls and cause thrombosis; however, fibrinoid necrosis is not expected. Axonal degeneration occurs with a predilection for distal large fibers. The cranial nerve and radicular involvement is seemingly caused by direct invasion by the spirochete. However, the inability to identify the organism in peripheral nerve and the presence of a shared antigenic determinant by the organism and peripheral nerve[101] have led to the suggestion that the peripheral neuropathy may be immune mediated.

AIDS neuropathy

Thirty percent of patients with AIDS have symptoms of peripheral neuropathy, and electrophysiologic studies document nerve involvement in 70% to 90%.[102] At autopsy, the incidence approaches 100% regardless of risk factors. There are at least four distinct neuropathies associated with AIDS.[103]

A *demyelinating peripheral neuropathy* occurs either acutely, simulating Guillain-Barré syndrome, or chronically as an immune-mediated demyelinating polyneuropathy (CIDP). Both disorders closely simulate the immune-mediated demyelinating polyneuropathies that occur in immunocompetent patients, though the incidence is higher in AIDS.

A *vasculitic neuropathy* occurs as mononeuritis multiplex and shows the typical histologic features of vasculitis. This neuropathy also simulates that in non-AIDS patients.

A *caudal equina syndrome,* caused by CMV infection, occurs.

A *distal symmetric axonal neuropathy* is the most common neuropathy syndrome in AIDS.[104] Sensory symptoms begin with pain in the soles of the feet; the pain then spreads to involve the ankles. Deep tendon reflexes are often diminished, especially at the ankles. The pain may be severe enough to create difficulty in walking. Although the pain is frequently limited to the legs, nerve conduction is diminished in amplitude and velocity in a wide distribution. In contrast to the severe sensory symptoms, motor weakness may be minimal. Sural nerve biopsy specimens have revealed a loss of large-caliber myelinated fibers in the early stages of the disease. At autopsy, there is often axonal degeneration with severe distal axonal loss. In distal sites, there may be few remaining myelinated fibers, and the residual often show active axonal degeneration. Neurons of the dorsal root ganglia may show some degeneration, but it is generally less severe than in the distal axonopathy.[105]

IDIOPATHIC NEUROPATHIES

Paraneoplastic neuropathy

Cancer patients may have neurologic symptoms caused by direct infiltration of individual nerves or plexuses ("metastatic neuropathy"). In addition, some patients develop symmetric paraneoplastic neuropathy. Symptomatic peripheral neuropathy develops in up to 5% of patients with lung carcinoma, and nerve conduction studies expand this figure to 20% to 40%.[106] Less commonly, paraneoplastic neuropathy complicates carcinomas of stomach, colon, and other sites. Two major types of paraneoplastic neuropathy, sensory paraneoplastic neuropathy and sensorimotor paraneoplastic neuropathy, are recognized.

Sensory paraneoplastic neuropathy usually begins with numbness and pain without clinical weakness or muscle atrophy. The numbness and pain may be associated with loss of position and vibration sensations. Nerve conduction studies document an absent or diminished amplitude in sensory nerves, with normal or only mildly affected motor nerve conduction. The onset of the neuropathy is typically subacute and may precede the recognition of carcinoma by 6 months to 1 year. The majority of patients have oat cell carcinoma of the lung;[107] most patients have circulating anti-Hu antibodies that recognize a 35 kD protein expressed in both the tumor and in the brain.[108]

Histologically the neuropathy is characterized by severe neuronal loss in dorsal root ganglia with a prominent proliferation of satellite cells and an inflammatory infiltration by lymphocytes and plasma cells. Most dorsal roots are atrophic and show a prominent loss of axons. The posterior columns of the spinal cord may be depleted of ascending posterior column fibers and consequently stain poorly for myelin. The peripheral projections of the dorsal root ganglionic neurons are similarly affected. Sural nerve biopsies show severe axonal loss, but mixed sensorimotor nerves are somewhat spared. Sensory paraneoplastic neuropathy is most likely caused by an immune response to the tumor antigen (Hu), with immunoglobulins entering the dorsal root ganglia across the incomplete blood-nerve barrier to cross-react with neuronal antigens.

The sensorimotor paraneoplastic neuropathies are less well characterized. They may occur as an acute demyelinating peripheral neuropathy that resembles Guillain-Barré syndrome, or subacutely or chronically with a progressive or intermittent course. These sensorimotor paraneoplastic neuropathies are more common than the pure sensory neuropathy. Although the most frequent association is with lung carcinoma, they may also be seen in conjunction with carcinomas of the stomach, breast, gastrointestinal tract, and elsewhere. Histologically the number of large and small myelinated fibers is decreased.

Sarcoidosis

Up to 4% of patients with sarcoidosis develop peripheral neuropathy, with facial nerve involvement being particularly common.[109] More generalized involvement of the peripheral nervous system may occur before other manifestations of the disease ("neurosarcoid") and presents as a chronic, asymmetric, sensorimotor neuropathy. The diagnosis is made by demonstration of noncaseating granulomas dispersed through the epineurium, perineurium, and endoneurium of nerve (Fig. 78-24). As in other sites, the granulomas are discrete and have prominent, centrally placed mononuclear and multinucleated epithelioid histiocytes, which are rimmed by lymphocytes. Plastic-embedded sections disclose axonal degeneration in the vicinity of the granulomas.

The clinical course is variable. Cranial neuropathies generally resolve without therapy. The course of the chronic sensorimotor neuropathy is less predictable.

Sensory perineuritis

The uncommon disorder sensory perineuritis has been viewed as a clinicopathologic entity because of its distinctive pathologic findings. The initial descriptions are those of a chronic, painful, asymmetric, sensory neuropathy. More recently, patients have been identified with similar perineurial involvement but with symptoms that include motor functions.[110] In these patients, the disorder has followed a chronic or subacute progressive course with a predominantly distal distribution.

Intense granulomatous inflammation largely restricted to the perineurium is the unique histologic finding in all cases (Fig. 78-25). Macrophages are embedded between layers of greatly thickened perineurium. Endoneurial and epineurial granulomas are typically absent though perivascular inflammation may highlight the patchy distribution of perineuritis. The prominence of macrophages mimics lepromatous leprosy; however, these cells do not permeate the endoneurium, organisms are not demonstrated with the Fite stain, and cutaneous lesions do not occur. In contrast to sarcoidosis, there are no discrete granulomas.

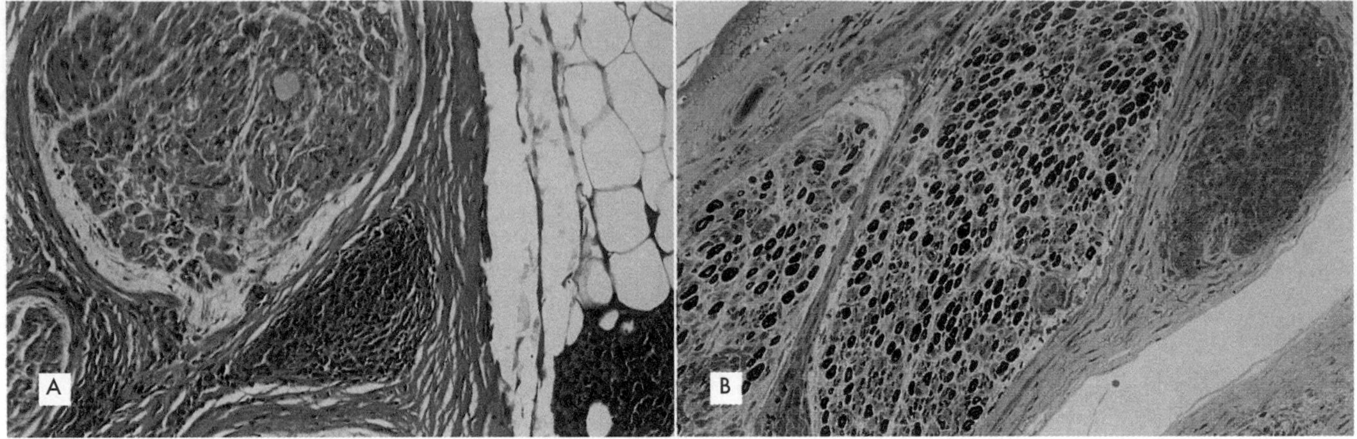

Fig. 78-24 Sarcoidosis. **A**, Prominent epineurial noncaseating granulomas in sarcoidosis, presenting with peripheral neuropathy. **B**, The epineurial granulomas are seen to extend into the perineurial layer, and the axonal loss in this region is minimal. (Epoxy resin section, toluidine blue stain.)

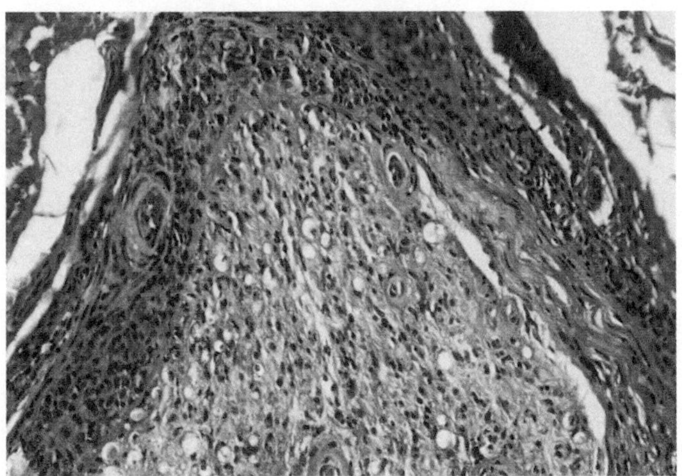

Fig. 78-25 Perineuritis, with dense granulomatous inflammation restricted to the perineurial layers.

IMMUNE-MEDIATED NEUROPATHIES

Guillain-Barré syndrome

Guillain-Barré syndrome is an acute or subacute demyelinating peripheral neuropathy, also known as acute inflammatory demyelinating polyradiculoneuropathy (AIDP) or Landry-Guillain-Barré-Strohl syndrome. It occurs worldwide and has an annual incidence in the United States of 1 to 2 out of 100,000.[111] Most patients have a history of a self-limited viral syndrome that has antedated the neuropathy by 1 week to 1 month. Some of the recognized viral prodromes include cytomegalovirus, Epstein-Barr virus (mononucleosis), vaccinia, variola, varicella-zoster, and measles. Guillain-Barré syndrome may occur after *Campylobacter* infections,[112] may occur after surgery or vaccination, and has been reported with increased frequency in AIDS.

Pathogenesis. There is abundant evidence that Guillain-Barré syndrome is mediated by an immune response to peripheral nerve myelin. Sera from patients with Guillain-Barré syndrome may initiate the breakdown of myelin in cell cultures, and an immunoglobulin has been identified in serum that reacts with peripheral nerve antigens. In addition to these findings, which are suggestive of a role for humoral immune responses, the similarities of Guillain-Barré syndrome to experimental allergic neuritis (EAN) are suggestive of a major role for T-cells. In experimental animals, an acute demyelinating peripheral neuropathy may be induced by the inoculation of a 20–amino acid neuritogenic portion of P_2 myelin protein.[113] T-cells infiltrate the nerve 10 to 12 days after the inoculation and before the onset of symptoms. There follows an acute demyelinating peripheral neuropathy with a variable degree of axonal degeneration. The intensity of the immune response and demyelination are proportional to the dose of P_2 protein, and axonal degeneration may be seen with high doses.[114] In further support of the concept that the disorder is mediated by a T-cell immune response, an abortive neuropathy may be induced in naïve animals by transfer of sensitized T-cells.

The pathologic findings in peripheral nerves of patients with Guillain-Barré syndrome are similar to those of EAN; the cardinal feature is demyelination. Although frequently widespread, it is characteristically most severe in spinal roots. Denuded axons in acute stages of demyelination (Fig. 78-26) are often but not always surrounded by inflammatory infiltrates of varying intensities and distribution patterns. Fatal and other severe cases may show a substantial amount of axonal degeneration. T-cells may be identified, with CD4 helper cells outnumbering CD8 cells.[115]

Respiratory paralysis is a common complication and was often fatal in the absence of ventilator support. Today, survival occurs in more than 95% of cases, and complete recovery is the usual outcome. However, 15% of patients may have permanent residual neurologic deficits. The risk of permanent neurologic deficits parallels the rapidity of onset and the severity of symptoms, including evidence of axonal damage such as early recruitment and diminished amplitudes on EMG. Plasmapheresis has been shown to be an effective therapy.

Chronic inflammatory demyelinating polyneuropathy (CIDP)

The disorder chronic imflammatory demyelinating polyradiculo-neuropathy bears a relationship to Guillain-Barré syndrome in its immune-mediated pathogenesis and targeted

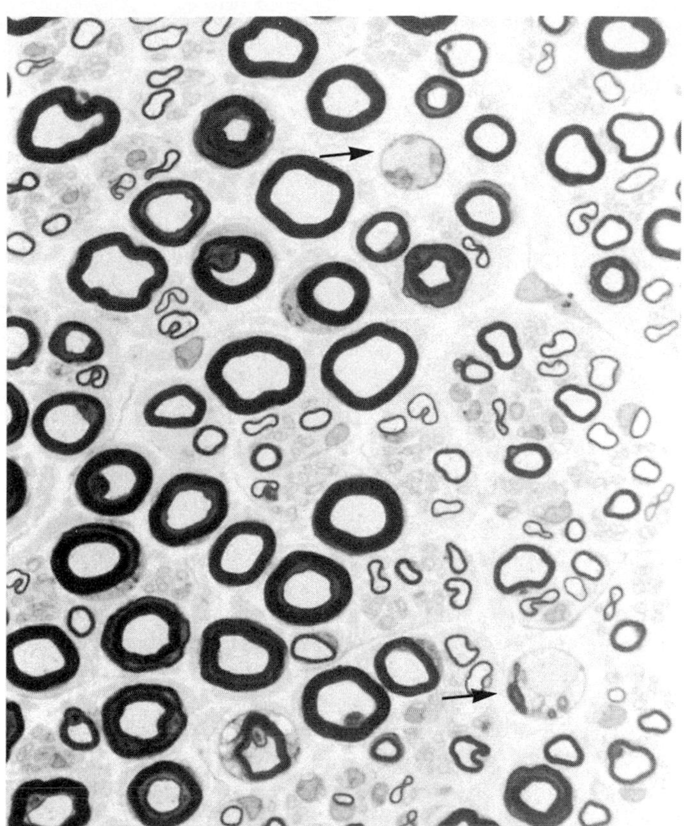

Fig. 78-26 Guillain-Barré syndrome. Demyelinated axons (*arrows*) are evident, in addition to variability of the myelin thickness among the large-caliber axons. (Epoxy resin section, toluidine blue stain.)

demyelination; however, it is distinguished by an insidious onset, progressive course, and variable response to therapy.[116] Perhaps analogously, some animals with experimentally induced EAN express a chronic relapsing course.[117] CIDP is characterized by a symmetric sensorimotor neuropathy with weakness and areflexia in the lower and upper extremities that is progressive for months. The clinical course may be unremitting or relapsing with stepwise progression. Typically, nerve conduction velocities are dramatically slowed, and CSF protein is usually elevated above 0.45 g/L.

Biopsy specimens of sural nerve show a chronic demyelinating neuropathy (Fig. 78-27). In plastic-embedded sections, myelin sheaths appear to have variable thicknesses, and Schwann cells show hyperplasia with the formation of occasional onion bulbs. Inflammatory infiltrates may occupy the endoneurial or epineurial spaces, often in a perivascular distribution. Teased fiber preparations reveal chronic segmental demyelination.[118] Steroid therapy has been used with some success, but clinical response is not universal. Additional immunosuppressive measures, notably plasma exchange and intravenous immunoglobulin therapy, have been instituted in refractory cases.

Peripheral neuropathy and systemic immune-mediated disorders

Peripheral neuropathy may occur in patients with rheumatoid arthritis, systemic lupus erythematosus, or Sjögren's syndrome. A vasculitis may accompany rheumatoid arthritis and

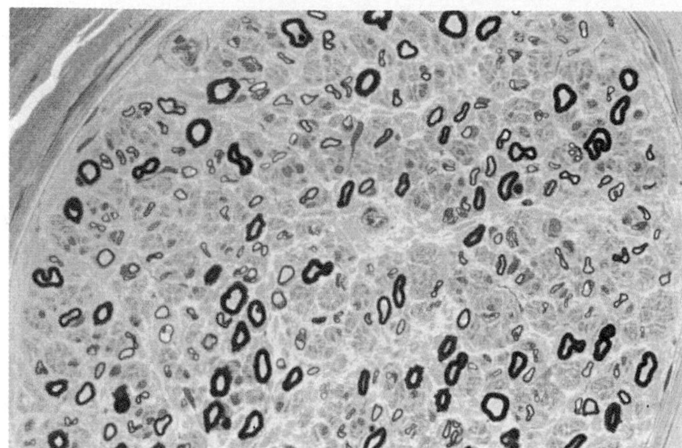

Fig. 78-27 Chronic inflammatory demyelinating polyradiculoneuropathy, with variability in myelin thickness and axonal loss. (Epoxy resin section, toluidine blue stain.)

has the histologic features of polyarteritis nodosa. Although systemic amyloidosis also occurs in 8% to 25% of patients with rheumatoid arthritis,[119,120] this reactive systemic amyloidosis rarely involves peripheral nerves. In Sjögren's syndrome, peripheral neuropathy may assume two forms: (1) a distal sensorimotor disorder, generally caused by inflammation of small arteries and venules; or (2) a pure sensory neuropathy resulting from inflammation in the dorsal root ganglia. Systemic lupus erythematosus (SLE) bears the complications of three apparently distinct peripheral neuropathies. The first is a distal, symmetric, sensorimotor neuropathy of unknown cause. Second, patients with SLE may develop a mononeuritis multiplex as an expression of vasculitis. Third, an ascending motor neuropathy clinically and pathologically indistinguishable from typical Guillain-Barré syndrome occurs with increased frequency in patients with SLE.

The vasculitides that complicate rheumatoid arthritis, Sjögren's syndrome, and SLE are generally characterized by intense inflammatory infiltrates in association with fibrinoid necrosis and regional areas of abrupt onset of axonal degeneration. The acute ascending paralysis that occurs with SLE has the pathologic features of Guillain-Barré syndrome. Teased-fiber studies reveal segmental demyelination with a propensity for involvement of the spinal roots. In severe cases, segmental demyelination is accompanied by axonal degeneration. The ganglionopathy that is associated with Sjögren's syndrome is distinctively characterized by an inflammatory infiltrate of dorsal root ganglia accompanied by a loss of neurons. Sensory symptoms predominate and include hyperalgesia and sensory ataxia.

Monoclonal gammopathy

Peripheral neuropathies may complicate monoclonal gammopathies of unknown significance (MGUS), multiple myeloma, or B-cell lymphoma. The process is best characterized in the IgM monoclonal gammopathies in which IgM can be demonstrated in peripheral nerve and is predominantly located within the myelin sheath. In up to 50% of these cases, the IgM reacts with the myelin-associated glycoprotein (MAG), a 100 kD glycoprotein.[121] Because complement proteins may also be detected within myelin sheaths, it has been suggested that the deposition of monoclonal immunoglobulins may initiate complement-mediated demyelination. Similar myelin specificity has not been demonstrated in monoclonal gammopathies associated with IgG or IgA.

Sural nerve biopsy specimens from patients with B-cell malignancies or MGUS may reveal axonal loss and segmental demyelination, and Schwann cell hyperplasia is sometimes evident. Teased fibers disclose segmental demyelination. Deposits of IgM may be demonstrated in myelin sheaths by immunofluorescence in frozen cross sections of nerve, and myelin lamellae in the outer layers of myelin sheaths are characteristically widened by electron microscopy.[8] The IgG- and IgA-associated monoclonal gammopathies may also be accompanied by demyelination; however, the immunoglobulin is infrequently demonstrable within myelin sheaths.

Amyloidosis associated with monoclonal gammopathy (AL amyloidosis) occurs with an incidence of 5% to 15% of patients with multiple myeloma and is characterized histologically by nodular, smooth eosinophilic deposits in the endoneurium and in the region of blood vessels. The deposits bind Congo red dye and show characteristic green birefringence under polarized light. A severe axonal loss accompanies the amyloid deposits.

Therapy for the peripheral neuropathies associated with monoclonal gammopathy is directed toward the B-cell dyscrasia. Treatment of multiple myeloma and Waldenström macroglobulinemia improves the peripheral neuropathy, and patients with MGUS and peripheral neuropathy have responded favorably to chemotherapy and plasma exchange.

NEOPLASMS OF PERIPHERAL NERVE

Schwannoma

The schwannoma (neurilemoma) is the most common tumor of peripheral nerve, accounting for 8% of all primary intracranial tumors and 80% to 90% of those in the cerebellopontine angle.[122] The peak incidence is in the third to sixth decades, with a slight female predominance. Although all the cranial nerves or spinal roots are vulnerable, there is a striking predilection for sensory nerves, especially the vestibular branch of the eighth nerve. Rarely, schwannomas occur intraparenchymally within the brain, cerebellum, or spinal cord; in such rare instances they presumably arise from Schwann cells that accompany blood vessels. In extradural locations, schwannomas arise in mixed motor and sensory peripheral nerves, particularly those of the limbs or intercostal spaces.

The great majority of schwannomas create a solitary, discrete mass. However, bilateral acoustic schwannomas, as well as multiple meningiomas, occur in the setting of type 2 neurofibromatosis (NF2), an autosomal-dominant disorder. The NF2 gene, located on the long arm of chromosome 22, encodes an ezrin-like protein termed "schwannomin."[123] Ostensibly, this protein represents a new type of tumor-suppressor agent because it resembles a cytoskeletal protein that is involved in membrane interactions.

Grossly, schwannomas are firm, encapsulated tumors (Fig. 78-28) whose cut surface is tan and translucent, often speckled yellow and red, as reflective of xanthomatous degeneration and hemorrhage. When they take origin from a peripheral nerve, they generally grow centrifugally and assume a spherical contour, but they may seemingly divest themselves from

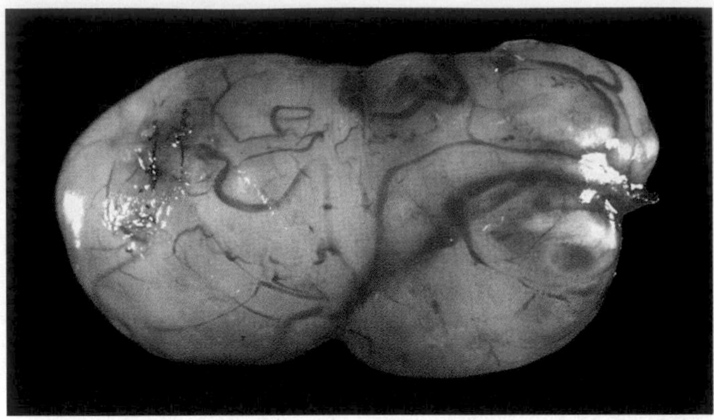

Fig. 78-28 Schwannoma. The encapsulation creates a smooth contour with blood vessels splayed over the tumor.

the nerve of origin. Restrained by a capsule, they compress and displace adjacent tissues without infiltration. With origin in the eighth cranial nerve, characteristically at the interface between oligodendroglial and Schwann cell stroma, they expand the internal auditory meatus and produce a mass in the cerebellopontine angle.

Histologically, the schwannoma is composed of a uniform population of cells that express the phenotype of Schwann cells. The tumor cells are spindle shaped and have pale eosinophilic cytoplasm that merges imperceptibly with adjacent collagen bundles. The nuclei are elongated with tapering ends. In parallel alignment, they form interwoven fascicles. When compact, this configuration is termed "Antoni A"; when areolar or myxomatous, it is termed "Antoni B" (Fig. 78-29). Palisading tumor cells, arranged in military battle lines with an intermediary anuclear zone, constitute the hallmark Verocay body (Fig. 78-29). Areas of degeneration are marked by hemosiderin or xanthomatous macrophages. Mitoses are few, except in the cellular variant, where there are often as many as 4 out of 10 HPF.[124,125] Pleomorphism of an occasional nucleus is not indicative of anaplasia but has been viewed as a degenerative event.

Schwannomas rich in Antoni B tissue may be confused with neurofibromas. The presence of axons, as demonstrated by silver stains, confirms the diagnosis of neurofibroma, but their absence or paucity is less helpful. Typically, Schwann cells uniformly express S-100 protein and, as detected by electron microscopy, have prominent external laminae and produce collagen with a long-spacing (120 to 150 nm) pattern (Luse bodies).

Schwannomas are benign, with an indolent growth that induces symptoms of mass effect. Those in the cerebellopontine angle cause tinnitus, hearing loss, and headaches. When they take origin from the dorsal roots of the spinal cord, they compress the cord and produce long tract signs. Subcutaneous schwannomas create a nodule that may be painful. Schwannomas and neurofibromas share their origin from and association with nerves; however, the former grows largely as an exophytic mass and for this reason is usually amenable to total surgical resection without loss of nerve function.

Neurofibroma

Neurofibromas, in contrast to schwannomas, are composed of tumor cells with a polymorphic cellular phenotype. Some of

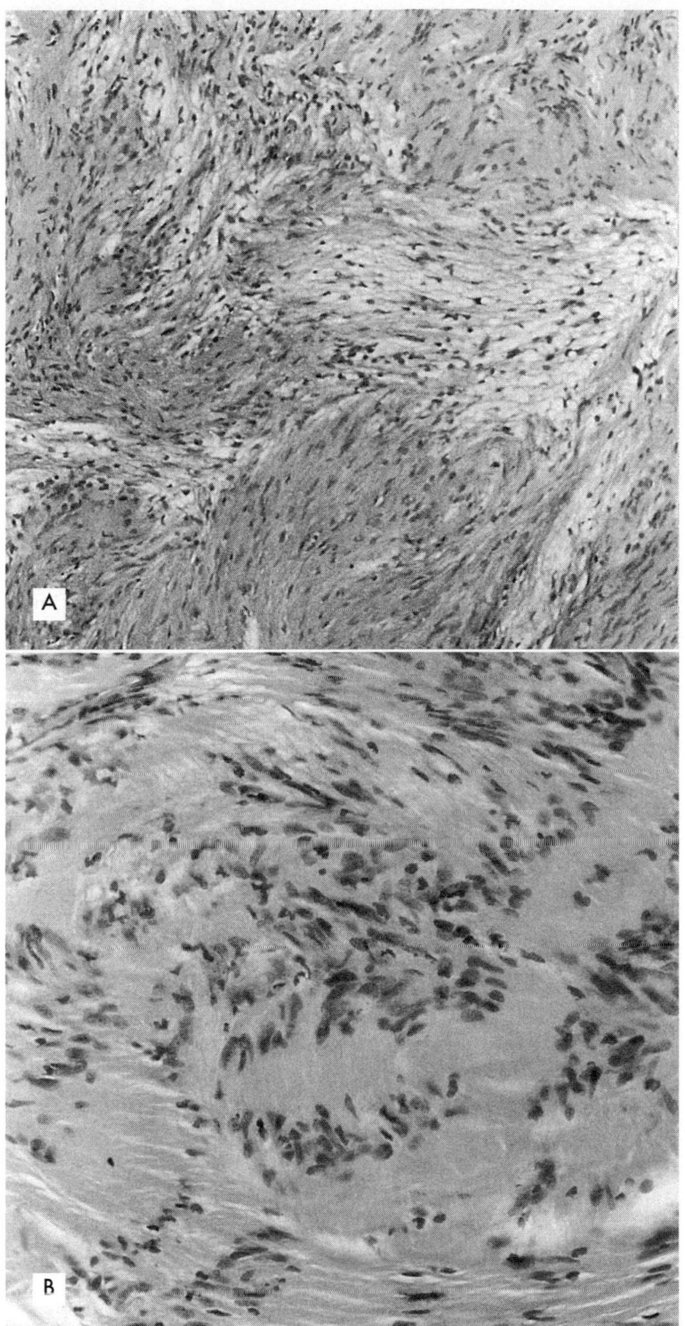

Fig. 78-29 Schwannoma. **A,** Interwoven dense (Antoni A) and myxomatous (Antoni B) areas are characteristic. **B,** Verocay body, with alignment of the nuclei around anuclear zones.

the cells express the phenotype of Schwann cells, some express the phenotype of perineurial cells, and others are negative for these markers and are considered, therefore, to be endoneurial fibroblasts.

Neurofibromas have two distinctive presentations: (1) as a solitary lesion, either within the skin (dermal neurofibroma) or, less commonly, along a nerve trunk (solitary neurofibroma); or (2) as a fusiform, ropelike expansion of a nerve (plexiform neurofibroma). Although they may arise spontaneously and are then usually solitary, their occurrence in multiplicity is largely enhanced by association with neurofibromatosis type 1 (NF1, von Recklinghausen's disease). NF1 is an autosomal-dominant disorder with a prevalence of 1 out of 3000[122] and an origin in the mutation of a tumor-suppressor gene on chromosome 17. The gene product, neurofibromin, is homologous to GTPase-activating proteins and is capable of downregulating the growth promoter, p21*ras*.[126,127] Normally expressed in Schwann cells,[128] somatic mutations in neurofibromin have also been detected in colon carcinomas and anaplastic astrocytomas,[129] as well as the germ line mutation in NF1. Although the disorder is dominantly inherited, the expression of the disease is quite variable. It may initiate abundant, disfiguring neurofibromas of the skin and nerves with numerous café-au-lait spots or, at the other extreme, have few signs. In addition to neurofibromas, NF1 is also associated with Lisch nodules (hamartomas) of the iris, with gliomas, particularly of the optic nerve and hypothalamus, and with an increased incidence of meningiomas, pheochromocytomas, and medullary thyroid carcinomas. Schwannomas may also occur in NF1, but when they do, they are usually solitary, in contrast to the bilateral acoustic schwannomas that are commonly seen in NF2.

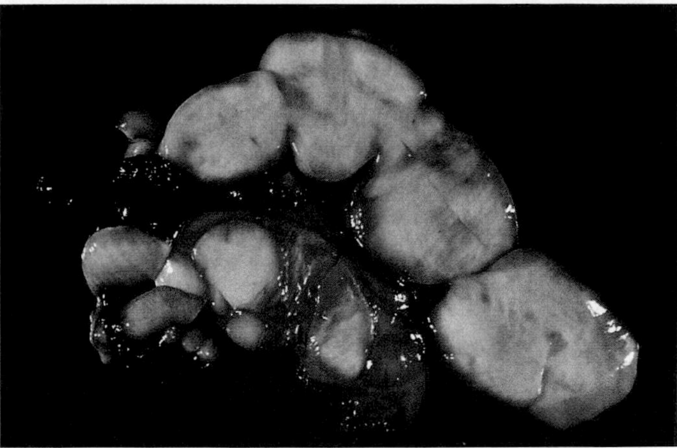

Fig. 78-30 Neurofibroma. The tumor is lobulated as it follows the course of a nerve.

Grossly, neurofibromas are soft and malleable, with a mucoid or translucent cut surface (Fig. 78-30). They are usually unencapsulated and blend indistinctly with adjacent connective tissue or peripheral nerve. The *plexiform neurofibroma* is a variant form that diffusely intermingles with a peripheral nerve or nerve trunk, occasionally causing grotesque disfigurement. The histologic appearance of neurofibromas may simulate Antoni B tissue of schwannomas and thus create diagnostic difficulties.

In general, three features distinguish the neurofibroma from the schwannoma: the extracellular matrix, the interface between the tumor and peripheral nerve, and the cellular composition. The neurofibroma is generally characterized by a more abundant extracellular matrix composed of both dense collagen fibers and extracellular mucoid material. The latter stains positively for acid mucopolysaccharides. Neurofibromas also infiltrate peripheral nerve more than schwannomas. As a result, neurofibromas typically contain entrapped axons that can be disclosed by silver stains, whereas schwannomas are typically encapsulated along the edge of a nerve. Because they have this aggressive property, neurofibromas may be mistaken for ganglioneuromas when they infiltrate ganglia (Fig. 78-31).

Immunohistochemistry reveals the cellular polymorphism within neurofibromas. Some tumor cells elaborate S-100 protein, as normal Schwann cells do; others express epithelial membrane antigen (EMA), as normal perineurial cells do. This mixed cellular composition is also evident by electron microscopy; some cells create an external lamina, and others cannot be distinguished from fibroblasts. In contrast, schwannomas are of a more uniform Schwann-cell phenotype.

Solitary neurofibromas may be resected but often with difficulty because the tumor frequently incorporates the nerve. Plexiform neurofibromas are rarely amenable to surgery. Their course is characterized by gradual enlargement and a propensity for malignant transformation.

Malignant peripheral nerve sheath tumors

Malignant peripheral nerve sheath tumors (MPNST) arise from peripheral mixed motor and sensory nerves and only rarely from cranial nerves or spinal roots. Although they may appear de novo, nearly half of cases are associated with NF1, where they take origin in a preexisting neurofibroma, generally at an early age (20 to 40 years as compared with 40 to 50 years in sporadic cases).[130,131] The malignant transformation is usually heralded by rapid enlargement and pain. MPNSTs almost never arise within a benign schwannoma; for this reason, the synonymous term *malignant schwannoma* may be misleading.

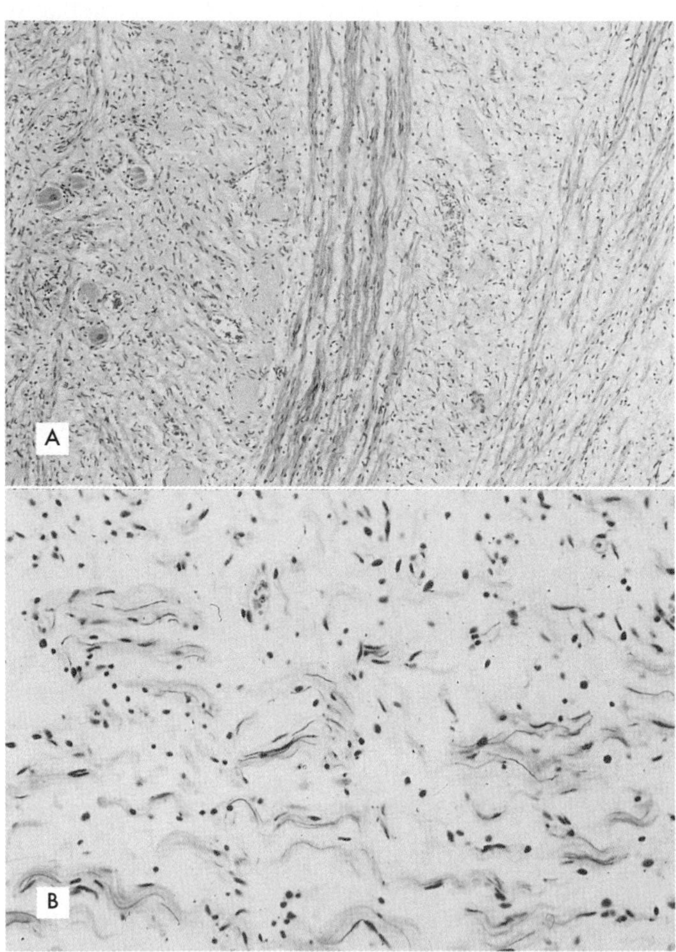

Fig. 78-31 Neurofibroma. **A,** Infiltration of a ganglion by neurofibroma is evident by the localization of ganglion cells and the presence of a rim of satellite cells that surround each of the entrapped ganglion cells. **B,** Silver stains for axons accentuate the infiltration of the nerve. (Bielschowsky silver stain.)

On gross examination, the lesions of MPNST are large and fleshy and most have an obvious, intimate association with a nerve. The tissue may be homogeneously gray and translucent, but characteristically there is necrosis and hemorrhage (Fig. 78-32). The rare lesion lacks a clear relationship to a nerve and instead appears as an ill-defined, fleshy mass.

Tumor cells infiltrate peripheral nerve and adjacent connective tissue. They may form tight fascicles with interwoven herringbone patterns reminiscent of fibrosarcomas. Other areas have a more areolar composition, but distinctively these lesions are highly cellular with numerous mitoses, usually more than 10 per 10 HPF, associated with pleomorphism and necrosis. In the majority of cases, the tumor cells show the presence of S-100 and, by electron microscopy, show focal external membrane material. The distinction of MPNST from cellular schwannomas may be difficult. Although cellularity and pleomorphism may be observed in both tumors, these features are generally more exaggerated in MPNST, as the presence of mitoses and necrosis is. Degeneration of cellular schwannomas accompanied by the formation of xanthoma cells should not be misinterpreted as evidence of malignancy.

The prognosis for MPNST is poor.[132] The 5-year survival in NF1 is approximately 15% to 30%.[131] Recurrence is often local in the nerve of origin; metastases generally involve lung and liver.

Granular cell tumor

The granular cell tumor (granular cell myoblastoma) is a distinctive peripheral nerve tumor that occurs in the skin,

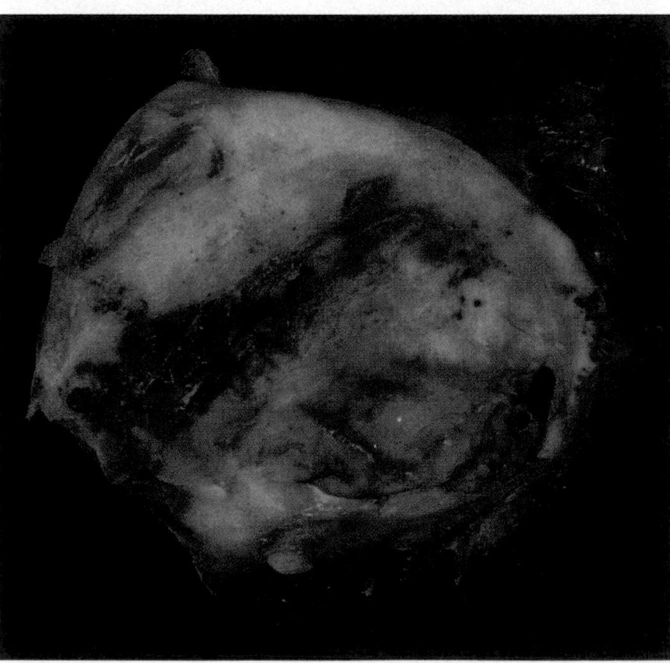

Fig. 78-32 Malignant peripheral nerve sheath tumor arising in a patient with neurofibromatosis type 1. The large fleshy mass has a yellow color with regions of hemorrhage and necrosis scattered through the tumor.

tongue, submucosal regions of the gastrointestinal tract, and peripheral nerves. Originally believed to arise from muscle cells, it is now recognized that the lesion consists of cells that have markers of a Schwann cell. Characteristically the lesion is a firm, pea-sized mass, composed of a uniform population of cells with small regular nuclei and abundant granular eosinophilic cytoplasm (Fig. 78-33). Most lesions lack a capsule and show infiltration into the adjacent connective tissue. The cytoplasmic granules stain with PAS and often for S-100 protein. Electron microscopy reveals the granular appearance of the cytoplasm to be caused by lysosomal vacuoles that contain membranous material. Basal membranes may also be present around clusters of cells. The tumor is benign and rarely recurs after resection.

Other tumors of the peripheral nervous system

Perineurioma is a localized mass that occupies a single nerve and expands each of its fascicles. The lesion commonly creates a mononeuropathy predominantly with motor symptoms. The predilection of this tumor for sites shared with entrapment neuropathies has led to the suggestion that it may be a reactive process;[133] however, the presence of a single cell constituency and the proliferative nature of the lesion support a neoplastic process of perineurial cells.[134] Each individual fascicle is enlarged and is hypercellular with a single cell species. The tumor cells lie concentric to the perineurial sheath or concentrically around individual nerve fibers (Fig. 78-34). This latter pattern is reminiscent of the onion bulbs in the hereditary hypertrophic neuropathies and has led to the synonymous term *localized hypertrophic neuropathy*. However, the onion bulbs of perineurioma are formed by perineurial cells rather than Schwann cells and therefore do not express S-100 protein, but do express EMA. The tumor cells have the ultrastructural characteristics of perineurial cells, including external laminae, prominent collagen pockets, and a concentric arrangement around groups of nerve fibers.[135] Like the neurofibroma, the perineurioma may occur as either an intraneural plexiform tumor or a solitary extraneural tumor (intramuscular perineurioma).

Ganglioneuromas most often arise in association with sympathetic ganglia and create slow-growing masses. They may occur in adulthood but more commonly appear during childhood, with 60% of patients being below 20 years of age.[136] The posterior mediastinum and the lumbar and sacral plexuses are preferred sites of origin. The lesions create large, lobulated, circumscribed, but nonencapsulated masses of firm, pale-gray tissue. The spindle cells form a prominent fascicular pattern that resembles the pattern seen in neurofibromas. However, the presence of neoplastic ganglion cells, often binucleate, distinguishes this tumor (Fig. 78-35). These ganglion cells are scattered throughout the neoplasm and are devoid of satellite cells.

Traumatic neuroma is a painful mass created by sprouting axons at the site of previous peripheral nerve injury. They are often superficial, subcutaneous masses that are tender to the touch. The identity of the lesion is revealed by its association with a peripheral nerve at a point of previous trauma. Histologically, axons abound in a matrix of dense connective tissue (Fig. 78-36).

Morton's neuroma (perineural fibrosis) is a painful enlargement of an interdigital plantar nerve. It occurs most often in females, usually between the third and fourth metatarsals. A

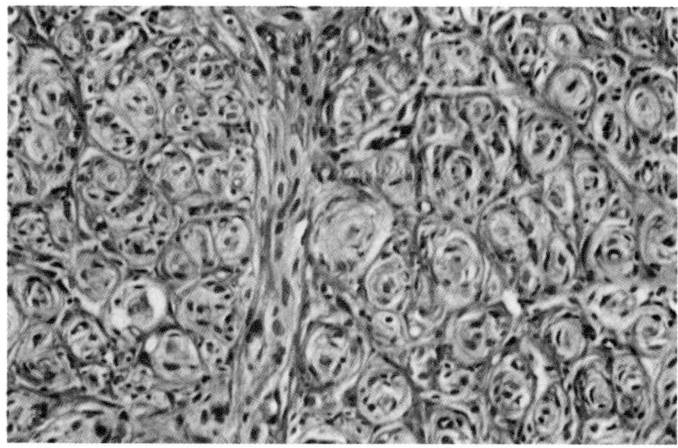

Fig. 78-34 Perineurioma. Concentrically oriented cells create a hypercellular endoneurium.

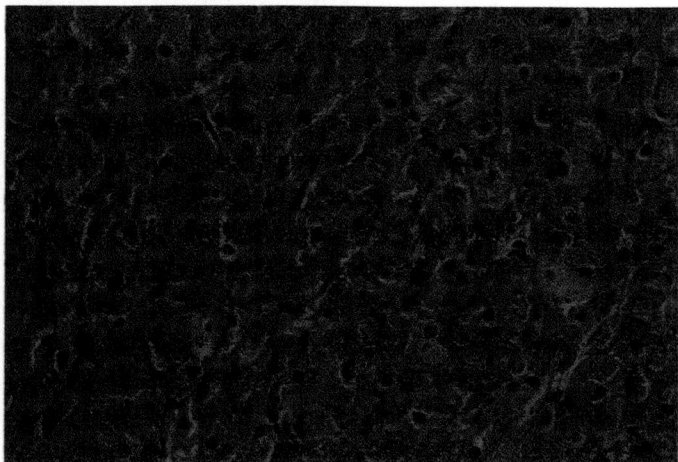

Fig. 78-33 Granular cell tumor. The tumor cells are uniform, with abundant granular cytoplasm.

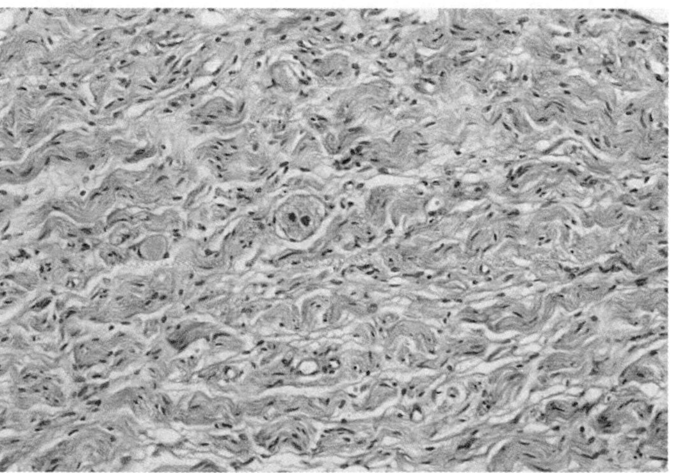

Fig. 78-35 Ganglioneuroma, with a biphasic composition of spindle-shaped Schwann cells and neoplastic ganglion cells. Binucleate forms devoid of satellite cells aid in the recognition of the neoplastic ganglion cell.

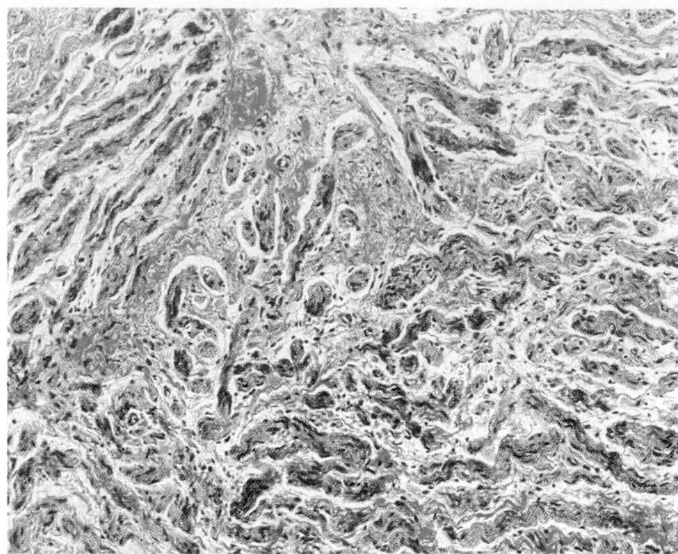

Fig. 78-36 Traumatic neuroma. Interwoven organoid fascicles characterize the mass and are highlighted by connective tissue stains. (Masson trichrome.)

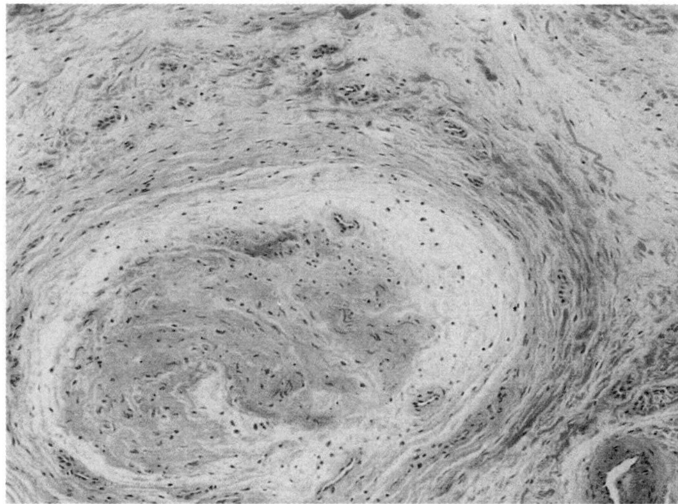

Fig. 78-37 Morton's neuroma, with fibrosis and proliferation of the perineurial layer.

focal segment of the nerve is enlarged by gray tissue that represents thickened perineurium with fibrosis (Fig. 78-37), with an often severe loss of axons.

Compression neuropathy refers to any mononeuropathy caused by compression of a peripheral nerve trunk. Carpal tunnel syndrome is the most common expression of entrapment neuropathy. The median nerve is compressed within the carpal tunnel and is further traumatized with repetitive wrist movements. Interestingly, it is associated with pregnancy, hypothyroidism, amyloidosis, and diabetes mellitus, and often it is bilateral. Females are affected more commonly than males. The condition causes pain in the wrist and hand, with numbness and tingling in the distribution of the median nerve. Electrophysiologically, the conduction abnormality is localized to the region of the carpal tunnel. Immobilization of the wrist may lead to improvement and is particularly useful therapy in cases associated with pregnancy. Persistent symptoms may be relieved with surgical release of the carpal ligament.

Metastatic neuropathy is most often a mononeuropathy or plexopathy. Examples include involvement of the brachial plexus by carcinoma in the apex of the lung and cauda equina syndrome that develops in association with carcinomatosis of the spinal meninges. Although nerve compression and infiltration may occur with any type of carcinoma, infiltration along peripheral nerves, often in the subperineurial space, is particularly characteristic of adenoid cystic carcinoma.

REFERENCES

Normal peripheral nerves and their response to injury

1. Burger PC, Scheithauer BW, Vogel FS: *Surgical pathology of the nervous system and its coverings,* ed 3, New York, 1991, Churchill Livingstone.
2. Dyck PJ, Thomas PK, Griffin JW et al, editors: *Peripheral neuropathy,* ed 3, Philadelphia, 1993, Saunders.
3. Kimura J: *Electrodiagnosis in diseases of nerve and muscle: principles and practice,* ed 2, Philadelphia, 1989, Davis.
4. Dyck PJ, Karnes J, Sparks M et al: The morphometric composition of myelinated fibers by nerve, level, and species related to nerve microenvironment and ischaemia, *Electroencephalogr Clin Neurophysiol Suppl* 36:39, 1982.
5. Smith KJ, Blakemore WF, Murray JA et al: Internodal myelin volume and axon surface area: a relationship determining myelin thickness? *J Neurol Sci* 55:231, 1982.
6. Friede RL, Beuche W: A new approach toward analyzing peripheral nerve fiber populations. I. Variance in sheath thickness corresponds to different geometric proportions of the internodes, *J Neuropathol Exp Neurol* 44:60, 1985.
7. Vass K, Hickey WF, Schmidt RE et al: Bone marrow–derived elements in the peripheral nervous system: an immunohistochemical and ultrastructural investigation in chimeric rats, *Lab Invest* 69:275, 1993.
8. Vital C, Vallat JM: *Ultrastructural study of the human diseased peripheral nerve,* ed 2, New York, 1987, Elsevier.
9. Usson Y, Torch S, Saxod R: Morphometry of human nerve biopsies by means of automated cytometry: assessment with reference to ultrastructural analysis, *Anal Cell Pathol* 3:91, 1991.
10. Vital A, Vital C, Rigal B et al: Morphological study of the aging human peripheral nerve, *Clin Neuropathol* 9:10, 1990.
11. Carpenter MB, Sutin J: *Human neuroanatomy,* ed 8, Baltimore, 1983, Williams & Wilkins.
12. Chaudhry V, Glass JD, Griffin JW: Wallerian degeneration in peripheral nerve disease, *Neurol Clin* 10:613, 1992.
13. Chaudhry V, Cornblath DR: Wallerian degeneration in human nerves: serial electrophysiological studies, *Muscle Nerve* 15:687, 1992.
14. Azzarelli B, Woodburn R, Olivelle S et al: The A-1 antigen: a novel marker in experimental peripheral nerve injury, *J Comp Neurol* 337:353, 1993.
15. Griffin JW, George R, Lobato C et al: Macrophage responses and myelin clearance during Wallerian degeneration: relevance to immune-mediated demyelination, *J Neuroimmunol* 40:153, 1992.
16. Goodrum JF, Earnhardt T, Goines N et al: Fate of myelin lipids during degeneration and regeneration of peripheral nerve: an autoradiographic study, *J Neurosci* 14:357, 1994.
17. Grafstein B, Forman DS: Intracellular transport in neurons, *Physiol Rev* 60:1167, 1980.
18. Vale RD, Schnapp BJ, Mitchison T et al: Different axoplasmic proteins generate movement in opposite directions along microtubules in vitro, *Cell* 43:623, 1985.
19. Skene JH, Jacobson RD, Snipes GJ et al: A protein induced during nerve growth (GAP-43) is a major component of growth-cone membranes, *Science* 233:783, 1986.
20. Taniuchi M, Clark HB, Schweitzer JB et al: Expression of nerve growth factor receptors by Schwann cells of axotomized peripheral nerves:

ultrastructural location, suppression by axonal contact, and binding properties, *J Neurosci* 8:664, 1988.
21. Martini R, Bollensen E, Schachner M: Immunocytochemical localization of the major peripheral nervous system glycoprotein P_0 and the L2/HNK-1 and L3 carbohydrate structures in developing and adult mouse sciatic nerve, *Dev Biol* 129:330, 1988.
22. Bigbee JW, Yoshino JE, DeVries GH: Morphological and proliferative responses of cultured Schwann cells following rapid phagocytosis of a myelin-enriched fraction, *J Neurocytol* 16:487, 1987.
23. LeBlanc AC, Poduslo JF: Axonal modulation of myelin gene expression in the peripheral nerve, *J Neurosci Res* 26:317, 1990.
24. Dyck PJ, Johnson WJ, Lambert EH et al: Segmental demyelination secondary to axonal degeneration in uremic neuropathy, *Mayo Clin Proc* 46:400, 1971.
25. Adams RD, Victor M: *Principles of neurology,* ed 5, New York, 1993, McGraw-Hill.
26. Rappaport WD, Valente J, Hunter GC et al: Clinical utilization and complications of sural nerve biopsy, *Am J Surg* 166:252, 1993.
27. Dyck PJ: Invited review: limitations in predicting pathologic abnormality of nerves from the EMG examination, *Muscle Nerve* 13:371, 1990.
28. Argov Z, Steiner I, Soffer D: The yield of sural nerve biopsy in the evaluation of peripheral neuropathies, *Acta Neurol Scand* 79:243, 1989.
29. Neundorfer B, Grahmann F, Engelhardt A et al: Postoperative effects and value of sural nerve biopsies: a retrospective study, *Eur Neurol* 30:350, 1990.

Hereditary neuropathies

30. Brust JC, Lovelace RE, Devi S: Clinical and electrodiagnostic features of Charcot-Marie-Tooth syndrome, *Acta Neurol Scand* 68 (suppl):1, 1978.
31. Thomas PK, Harding AE: Inherited neuropathies: the interface between molecular genetics and pathology, *Brain Pathol* 3:129, 1993.
32. Dyck PJ, Oviatt KF, Lambert EH: Intensive evaluation of referred unclassified neuropathies yields improved diagnosis, *Ann Neurol* 10:222, 1981.
33. Anthony DA, Hevner RF: Advances in the molecular genetics of hereditary peripheral neuropathies, *Adv Anat Pathol,* 1995. (In press.)
34. Berciano J, Combarros O, Calleja J et al: The application of nerve conduction and clinical studies to genetic counseling in hereditary motor and sensory neuropathy type I, *Muscle Nerve* 12:302, 1989.
35. Gabreels-Festen AA, Joosten EM, Gabreels FJ et al: Early morphological features in dominantly inherited demyelinating motor and sensory neuropathy (HMSN type I), *J Neurol Sci* 107:145, 1992.
36. Vance JM, Barker D, Yamaoka LH et al: Localization of Charcot-Marie-Tooth disease type 1a (CMT1A) to chromosome 17p11.2, *Genomics* 9:623, 1991.
37. Chance PF, Pleasure D: Charcot-Marie-Tooth syndrome, *Arch Neurol* 50:1180, 1993.
38. Defesche JC, Hoogendijk JE, de Visser M et al: Genetic linkage of hereditary motor and sensory neuropathy type I (Charcot-Marie-Tooth disease) to markers of chromosomes 1 and 17, *Neurology* 40:1450, 1990.
39. Lupski JR, de O, Luna RM et al: DNA duplication associated with Charcot-Marie-Tooth disease type 1A, *Cell* 66:219, 1991.
40. Lupski JR, Chance PF, Garcia CA: Inherited primary peripheral neuropathies: molecular genetics and clinical implications of CMT1A and HNPP, *JAMA* 270:2326, 1993.
41. Roa BB, Garcia CA, Suter U et al: Charcot-Marie-Tooth disease type 1A: association with a spontaneous point mutation in the PMP22 gene, *N Engl J Med* 329:96, 1993.
42. Valentijn LJ, Baas F, Wolterman RA et al: Identical point mutations of PMP-22 in Trembler-J mouse and Charcot-Marie-Tooth disease type 1A, *Nat Genet* 2:288, 1992.
43. Hayasaka K, Himoro M, Sato W et al: Charcot-Marie-Tooth neuropathy type 1B is associated with mutations of the myelin P_0 gene, *Nat Genet* 5:31, 1993.
44. Kulkens T, Bolhuis PA, Wolterman RA et al: Deletion of the serine 34 codon from the major peripheral myelin protein P_0 gene in Charcot-Marie-Tooth disease type 1B, *Nat Genet* 5:35, 1993.
45. Bergoffen J, Scherer SS, Wang S et al: Connexin mutations in X-linked Charcot-Marie-Tooth disease, *Science* 262:2039, 1993.
46. Ben Othmane K, Middleton LT, Loprest LJ et al: Localization of a gene (CMT2A) for autosomal dominant Charcot-Marie-Tooth disease type 2 to chromosome 1p and evidence of genetic heterogeneity, *Genomics* 17:370, 1993.
47. Hentati A, Lamy C, Melki J et al: Clinical and genetic heterogeneity of Charcot-Marie-Tooth disease, *Genomics* 12:155, 1992.
48. Hahn AF: Hereditary motor and sensory neuropathy: HMSN type II (neuronal type) and X-linked HMSN, *Brain Pathol* 3:147, 1993.
49. Hoogendijk JE, de Visser M, Bolhuis PA et al: Hereditary motor and sensory neuropathy type I: clinical and neurographical features of the 17p duplication subtype, *Muscle Nerve* 17:85, 1994.
50. Ouvrier RA, McLeod JF, Conchin TE: The hypertrophic forms of hereditary motor and sensory neuropathy: a study of hypertrophic Charcot-Marie-Tooth disease (HMSN I) and Dejerine-Sottas disease (HMSN II) in childhood, *Brain* 110:121, 1987.
51. Benstead TJ, Kuntz NL, Miller RG et al: The electrophysiologic profile of Dejerine-Sottas disease (HMSN III), *Muscle Nerve* 13:586, 1990.
52. Singh I, Pahan K, Singh AK et al: Refsum disease: a defect in the alpha-oxidation of phytanic acid in peroxisomes, *J Lipid Res* 34:1755, 1993.
53. Ouvrier RA: Giant axonal neuropathy: a review, *Brain Dev* 11:207, 1989.
54. Desnick RJ, Wang AM: Schindler disease: an inherited neuroaxonal dystrophy due to alpha-N-acetylgalactosaminidase deficiency, *J Inherit Metab Dis* 13:549, 1990.
55. Ozmen M, Caliçlskan M, Goebel HH, Apak S: Infantile neuroaxonal dystrophy: diagnosis by skin biopsy, *Brain Dev* 13:256, 1991.
56. Madrid R, Bradley WG: The pathology of neuropathies with focal thickening of the myelin sheath (tomaculous neuropathy), *J Neurol Sci* 25:45, 1975.
57. Barbieri F, Santangelo R, Crisci C et al: A family with tomaculous neuropathy mimicking Charcot-Marie-Tooth disease, *Clin Neurol Neurosurg* 92:289, 1990.
58. Mosser J, Douar AM, Sarde CO et al: Putative X-linked adrenoleukodystrophy gene shares unexpected homology with ABC transporters, *Nature* 361:726, 1993.
59. Powers JM, Liu Y, Moser AB et al: The inflammatory myelinopathy of adrenoleukodystrophy: cells, effector molecules, and pathogenetic implications, *J Neuropathol Exp Neurol* 51:630, 1992.
60. Kolodny EH: Metachromatic leukodystrophy and multiple sulfatase deficiency: sulfatide lipidosis. In Scriver CR, Beaudet AL, Sly WS, editors: *The metabolic basis of inherited disease,* New York, 1989, McGraw-Hill.
61. Ferriere G, Guzzetta F, Kulakowski S et al: Nonprogressive type II hereditary sensory autonomic neuropathy: a homogeneous clinicopathologic entity, *J Child Neurol* 7:364, 1992.
62. Holmgren G, Bergström S, Drugge U et al: Homozygosity for the transthyretin-Met30-gene in seven individuals with familial amyloidosis with polyneuropathy detected by restriction enzyme analysis of amplified genomic DNA sequences, *Clin Genet* 41:39, 1992.
63. Li K, Kyle RA, Dyck PJ: Immunohistochemical characterization of amyloid proteins in sural nerves and clinical associations in amyloid neuropathy, *Am J Pathol* 141:217, 1992.
64. Ikeda S, Hanyu N, Hongo M et al: Hereditary generalized amyloidosis with polyneuropathy: clinicopathological study of 65 Japanese patients, *Brain* 110:315, 1987.
65. Holmgren G, Ericzon BG, Groth CG et al: Clinical improvement and amyloid regression after liver transplantation in hereditary transthyretin amyloidosis, *Lancet* 341:1113, 1993.

Ischemic neuropathies

66. Chumbley LC, Harrison EG, DeRemee RA: Allergic granulomatosis and angiitis (Churg-Strauss syndrome): report and analysis of 30 cases, *Mayo Clin Proc* 52:477, 1977.
67. Dyck PJ, Benstead TJ, Conn DL et al: Nonsystemic vasculitic neuropathy, *Brain* 110:843, 1987.
68. Logigian EL, Shefner JM, Frosch MP et al: Nonvasculitic, steroid-responsive mononeuritis multiplex, *Neurology* 43:879, 1993.

69. Eames RA, Lange LS: Clinical and pathological study of ischaemic neuropathy, *J Neurol Neurosurg Psychiatr* 30:215, 1967.
70. Bolton CF: Electrophysiological studies of critically ill patients, *Muscle Nerve* 10:129, 1987.
71. Lopez Messa JB, Garcia A: Acute polyneuropathy in critically ill patients, *Intensive Care Med* 16:159, 1990.

Toxic neuropathies

72. Goebel HH, Schmidt PF, Bohl J et al: Polyneuropathy due to acute arsenic intoxication: biopsy studies, *J Neuropathol Exp Neurol* 49:137, 1990.
73. Chhuttani PN, Chawla LS, Sharma TD: Arsenical neuropathy, *Neurology* 17:269, 1967.
74. Graham DG, Amarnath V, Valentine WM et al: Pathogenetic studies of hexane and carbon disulfide neurotoxicity, *Crit Rev Toxicol* 25:91, 1995.
75. Griffin JW, Anthony DC, Fahnestock KE et al: 3,4-Dimethyl-2,5-hexanedione impairs the axonal transport of neurofilament proteins, *J Neurosci* 4:1516, 1984.
76. Schochet SS, Lampert PW, Earle KM: Neuronal changes induced by intrathecal vincristine sulfate, *J Neuropathol Exp Neurol* 27:645, 1968.
77. Victor M: The effect of alcohol on the nervous system, *Res Publ Assoc Res Nerv Ment Dis* 32:526, 1963.
78. Goodlett CR, Thomas JD, West JR: Long-term deficits in cerebellar growth and rotarod performance of rats following "binge-like" alcohol exposure during the neonatal brain growth spurt, *Neurotoxicol Teratol* 13:69, 1991.

Metabolic neuropathies

79. Hendriksen PH, Oey PL, Wieneke GH et al: Subclinical diabetic neuropathy: similarities between electrophysiological results of patients with type 1 (insulin-dependent) and type 2 (non-insulin-dependent) diabetes mellitus, *Diabetologia* 35:690, 1992.
80. Bruyn GW, Garland H: Neuropathies of endocrine origin. In Vinken PJ, Bruyn GW, editors: *Handbook of clinical neurology,* Amsterdam, 1970, North-Holland.
81. Pirart J: Diabetes mellitus and its degenerative complications: a prospective study of 4,400 patients observed between 1947 and 1973, *Diabète Metab* 3:97, 1977.
82. Sima AAF: Diabetic neuropathy: the presence and future of a common but silent disorder, *Mod Pathol* 6:399, 1993.
83. Anonymous: Proceedings of a consensus development conference on standardized measures in diabetic neuropathy: morphological and biochemical measures, *Neurology* 42:1825, 1992.
84. Britland ST, Young RJ, Sharma AK et al: Relationship of endoneurial capillary abnormalities to type and severity of diabetic polyneuropathy, *Diabetes* 39:909, 1990.
85. King RH, Llewelyn JG, Thomas PK et al: Diabetic neuropathy: abnormalities of Schwann cell and perineurial basal laminae: implications for diabetic vasculopathy, *Neuropathol Appl Neurobiol* 15:339, 1989.
86. Llewelyn JG, Gilbey SG, Thomas PK et al: Sural nerve morphometry in diabetic autonomic and painful sensory neuropathy: a clinicopathological study, *Brain* 114:867, 1991.
87. Schmidt RE, Plurad SB, Parvin CA et al: Effect of diabetes and aging on human sympathetic autonomic ganglia, *Am J Pathol* 143:143, 1993.
88. Mulder DW, Lambert EH, Bastron JA et al: The neuropathies associated with diabetes mellitus: a clinical and electromyographic study of 103 unselected diabetic patients, *Neurology* 11:275, 1961.
89. Cameron NE, Cotter MA: Contraction and relaxation of aortas from galactosaemic rats and the effects of aldose reductase inhibition, *Eur J Pharmacol* 243:47, 1993.
90. Makita Z, Vlassara H, Rayfield E et al: Hemoglobin-AGE: a circulating marker of advanced glycosylation, *Science* 258:651, 1992.
91. Nickel SN, Frame B: Nervous and muscular systems in myxedema, *J Chronic Dis* 14:570, 1961.
92. Bolton CF: Peripheral neuropathies associated with chronic renal failure, *Can J Neurol Sci* 7:89, 1980.

Infectious neuropathies

93. Balfour HH, Bean B, Laskin OL et al: Acyclovir halts progression of herpes zoster in immunocompromised patients, *N Engl J Med* 308:1448, 1983.
94. Miller RG, Storey JR, Greco CM: Ganciclovir in the treatment of progressive AIDS-related polyradiculopathy, *Neurology* 40:569, 1990.
95. World Health Organization: *A guide to leprosy control*, ed 2, Geneva, 1988, World Health Organization.
96. Kaur G, Girdhar BK, Girdhar A et al: A clinical, immunological, and histological study of neuritic leprosy patients, *Int J Lepr Other Mycobact Dis* 59:385, 1991.
97. Kumar V, Katoch K, Katoch VM et al: A preliminary study of correlation of immuno-histological and ultrastructural characteristics of neural granuloma in leprosy patients, *Acta Lepr* 8:87, 1992.
98. Lockwood DN, Vinayakumar S, Stanley JN et al: Clinical features and outcome of reversal (type 1) reactions in Hyderabad, India, *Int J Lepr Other Mycobact Dis* 61:8, 1993.
99. Johnson SE, Klein GC, Schmid GP et al: Lyme disease: a selective medium for isolation of the suspected etiological agent, a spirochete, *J Clin Microbiol* 19:81, 1984.
100. Meier C, Grahmann F, Engelhardt A et al: Peripheral nerve disorders in Lyme-borreliosis: nerve biopsy studies from eight cases, *Acta Neuropathol* 79:271, 1989.
101. Sigal LH: Cross-reactivity between *Borrelia burgdorferi* flagellin and a human axonal 64,000 molecular weight protein, *J Infect Dis* 167:1372, 1993.
102. Cruz Martinez A, Villoslada C: Electrophysiologic study in peripheral neuropathy associated with HIV infection, *Electromyogr Clin Neurophysiol* 31:407, 1991.
103. Chaunu MP, Ratinahirana H, Raphaël M et al: The spectrum of changes on 20 nerve biopsies in patients with HIV infection, *Muscle Nerve* 12:452, 1989.
104. Cornblath DR, McArthur JC, Parry GJG et al: Peripheral neuropathies in human immunodeficiency virus infection. In Dyck PJ, Thomas PK, Griffin, JW, et al, editors: *Peripheral neuropathy,* Philadelphia, 1993, Saunders.
105. Bacellar H, Munoz A, Miller EN et al: Temporal trends in the incidence of HIV-1-related neurologic diseases: multicenter AIDS cohort study, 1985-1992, *Neurology* 44:1892, 1994.

Idiopathic neuropathies

106. Trojaborg W, Frantzen E, Andersen I: Peripheral neuropathy and myopathy associated with carcinoma of the lung, *Brain* 92:71, 1969.
107. Dalmau J, Graus F, Rosenblum MK et al: Anti-Hu–associated paraneoplastic encephalomyelitis/sensory neuronopathy: a clinical study of 71 patients, *Medicine* 71:59, 1992.
108. Graus F, Elkon KB, Cordon-Cardo C et al: Sensory neuronopathy and small cell lung cancer: antineuronal antibody that also reacts with the tumor, *Am J Med* 80:45, 1986.
109. Stern BJ, Krumholz A, Johns C et al: Sarcoidosis and its neurological manifestations, *Arch Neurol* 42:909, 1985.
110. Simmons Z, Albers JW, Sima AA: Case-of-the-month: perineuritis presenting as mononeuritis multiplex, *Muscle Nerve* 15:630, 1992.

Immune-mediated neuropathies

111. Riggs JE, Gutmann L, Whited JD: Guillain-Barré syndrome (GBS): another immune-mediated neurologic disease with a predilection for young women? *W V Med J* 85:382, 1989.
112. Feasby TE: Inflammatory-demyelinating polyneuropathies, *Neurol Clin* 10:651, 1992.
113. Olee T, Powers JM, Brostoff SW: A T-cell epitope for experimental allergic neuritis, *J Neuroimmunol* 19:167, 1988.
114. Hahn AF, Feasby TE, Steele A et al: Demyelination and axonal degeneration in Lewis rat experimental allergic neuritis depend on the myelin dosage, *Lab Invest* 59:115, 1988.
115. Honavar M, Tharakan KJ, Hughes RAC et al: A clinicopathological study of Guillain-Barré syndrome, *Brain* 114:1245, 1991.

116. Barohn RJ, Kissel JT, Warmolts JR et al: Chronic inflammatory demyelinating polyradiculoneuropathy: clinical characteristics, course, and recommendations for diagnostic criteria, *Arch Neurol* 46:878, 1989.
117. Harvey GK, Pollard JD, Schindhelm K et al: Chronic experimental allergic neuritis: an electrophysiological and histological study in the rabbit, *J Neurol Sci* 81:215, 1987.
118. Krendel DA, Parks HP, Anthony DC et al: Sural nerve biopsy in chronic inflammatory demyelinating polyradiculoneuropathy, *Muscle Nerve* 12:257, 1989.
119. Pai S, Helin H, Isomaki H: Frequency of amyloidosis in Estonian patients with rheumatoid arthritis, *Scand J Rheumatol* 22:248, 1993.
120. Tiitinen S, Kaarela K, Helin H et al: Amyloidosis—incidence and early risk factors in patients with rheumatoid arthritis, *Scand J Rheumatol* 22:158, 1993.
121. Latov N, Hays AP, Sherman WH: Peripheral neuropathy and anti-MAG antibodies, *Crit Rev Neurobiol* 3:301, 1988.

Neoplasms of peripheral nerve

122. Russell DS, Rubinstein LJ: *Pathology of tumours of the nervous system,* ed 5, Baltimore, 1989, Williams & Wilkins.
123. Trofatter JA, MacCollin MM, Rutter JL et al: A novel moesin-, ezrin-, radixin-like gene is a candidate for the neurofibromatosis-2 tumor suppressor, *Cell* 72:791, 1993.
124. White W, Shiu MH, Rosenblum MK et al: Cellular schwannoma: a clinicopathologic study of 57 patients and 58 tumors, *Cancer* 66:1266, 1990.
125. Deruaz JP, Janzer RC, Costa J: Cellular schwannomas of the intracranial and intraspinal compartment: morphological and immunological characteristics compared with classical benign schwannomas, *J Neuropathol Exp Neurol* 52:114, 1993.
126. Viskochil D, White R, Cawthon R: The neurofibromatosis type 1 gene, *Annu Rev Neurosci* 16:183, 1993.
127. Andersen LB, Ballester R, Marchuk DA et al: A conserved alternative splice in the von Recklinghausen neurofibromatosis (NF1) gene produces two neurofibromin isoforms, both of which have GTPase-activating protein activity, *Mol Cell Biol* 13:487, 1993.
128. Daston MM, Scrable H, Nordlund M et al: The protein product of the neurofibromatosis type 1 gene is expressed at highest abundance in neurons, Schwann cells, and oligodendrocytes, *Neuron* 8:415, 1992.
129. Li Y, Bollag G, Clark R et al: Somatic mutations in the neurofibromatosis 1 gene in human tumors, *Cell* 69:275, 1992.
130. Enzinger FM, Weiss SW: *Soft tissue tumors,* ed 2, St Louis, 1995, Mosby.
131. Ducatman BS, Scheithauer BW, Piepgras DG et al: Malignant peripheral nerve sheath tumors: a clinicopathological study of 120 cases, *Cancer* 57:2006, 1986.
132. Wanebo JE, Malik JM, VandenBerg SR et al: Malignant peripheral nerve sheath tumors: a clinicopathologic study of 28 cases, *Cancer* 71:1247, 1993.
133. Mitsumoto H, Estes ML, Wilbourn AJ et al: Perineurial cell hypertrophic mononeuropathy manifesting as carpal tunnel syndrome, *Muscle Nerve* 15:1364, 1992.
134. Bilbao JM, Khoury NJ, Hudson AR et al: Perineurioma (localized hypertrophic neuropathy), *Arch Pathol Lab Med* 108:557, 1984.
135. Erlandson RA: The enigmatic perineurial cell and its participation in tumors and in tumorlike entities, *Ultrastruct Pathol* 15:335, 1991.
136. Stout AP: Ganglioneuroma of the sympathetic nervous system, *Surg Gynecol Obstet* 84:101, 1947.

79 Eye and Ocular Adnexa

Gordon K. Klintworth
Ralph C. Eagle, Jr.

The causes and reactions of the eye to injurious agents are basically identical to those in other parts of the body, but some components of this organ manifest disorders peculiar to specific parts. The unprotected superficial location of the eye exposes it to a myriad of microorganisms, antigens, and toxic chemicals, as well as to solar radiation, adverse climatic conditions, and physical injuries.

NORMAL EYE

The normal anatomy of the eye is detailed in specialized textbooks;[1,2] only the salient features are reviewed here. The eye consists of several distinct tissues. These include the conjunctiva, which has a nonkeratinizing stratified squamous epithelium with goblet cells and contains lymphatics, blood vessels, lymphocytes, and melanocytes. The caruncle is a fleshy nodular island of skin in the nasal portion of the interpalpebral fissure surrounded by conjunctiva. Its surface is lined by keratinized epithelium with cutaneous adnexal structures.

The cornea is the eye's major refractive element. A monolayer of endothelial cells with little or no regenerative capability covers the posterior surface of this largely collagenous structure and helps maintain corneal hydration and transparency. With aging, the endothelial cells diminish in number and Descemet's membrane thickens.

The retina is composed of cells arranged in distinct layers (Fig. 79-1). The nuclear layers contain the cell nuclei, whereas the plexiform layers consist of axons and dendrites. The axons of ganglion cells in the inner retina form the nerve fiber layer that passes through a sievelike area in the posterior sclera called the lamina cribrosa. Surrounding the fovea, the retinal ganglion cell layer is five or more layers thick. At the center of the fovea, where visual acuity is greatest, the retina is only two layers thick, and a high concentration of cones rests on the retinal pigment epithelium. The external part of the outer plexiform layer is composed of photoreceptor axons (Henle's fibers) arranged in parallel rows. The inner retina is supplied by capillaries derived from the central retinal artery that penetrate the retina to the level of the middle limiting membrane. The external avascular retina derives oxygen and nutrients from choroidal vessels.

During ocular development a space between the sensory retina and the retinal pigment epithelium is obliterated when these two layers become apposed. Loss of retinal neurons accounts for visual loss in such varied conditions as glaucoma, retinitis pigmentosa, retinal detachment, and macular degeneration.

The transparent crystalline lens grows slowly throughout life as older fibers in the lens nucleus become buried by new ones, which continually form in the lens periphery. The anterior subcapsular epithelial monolayer normally terminates at the lens equator. The lens capsule is thicker anteriorly than posteriorly. The primary optical function of the lens is accommodation. This ability to focus on both far and near objects is achieved because the lens is anchored to the ciliary body by

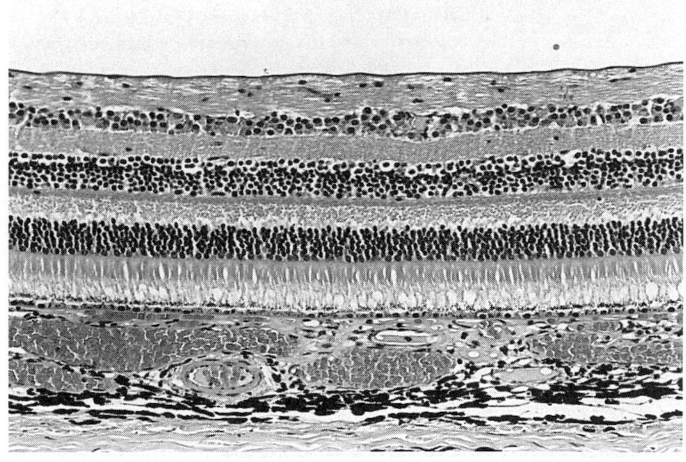

Fig. 79-1 Normal retina. Thickness of ganglion cell layer indicates perifoveal location of specimen. Healthy outer and inner nuclear layers are approximately equal in caliber. The retina has 10 layers including the retinal pigment epithelium.

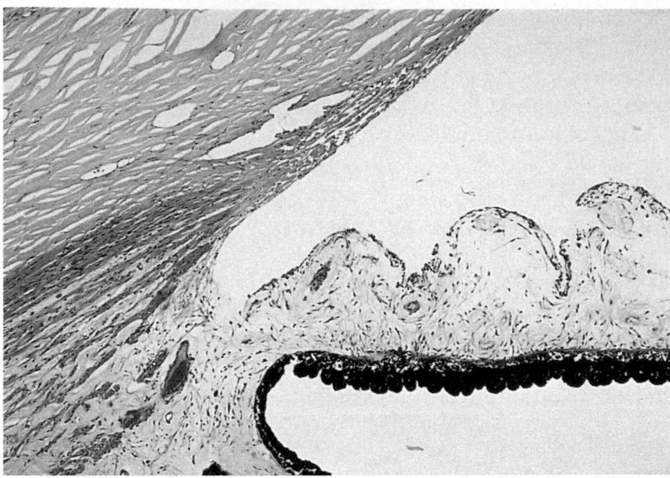

Fig. 79-2 Normal iridocorneal angle. The canal of Schlemm and the trabecular meshwork are located in the anterior chamber angle formed by the cornea and the iris. The longitudinal fibers of the ciliary muscle insert on the posterior aspect of the scleral spur directly behind the canal and meshwork.

zonular fibers composed of elastic microfibrils. During accommodation, contraction of the ciliary muscle decreases tension on the zonule, allowing the lens to assume a more spherical shape with greater refractive power.

The vitreous is the most delicate connective tissue in the body. Its major constituents are water, hyaluronic acid, and delicate, unbranched, randomly oriented type II collagen fibrils. The vitreous adheres to the internal limiting membrane of the retina, to the margin of the optic disk, and particularly firmly to a narrow zone straddling the ora serrata (vitreous base). The tenuous attachment of the vitreous to the retina posteriorly becomes broken in 60% of individuals over 70 years of age, leading to posterior vitreous detachment.

The pigmented part of the eye (uvea) consists of the iris, ciliary body, and choroid. Aqueous is secreted by the ciliary body and flows through the pupil into the anterior chamber, where it drains mainly through the iridocorneal angle via the trabecular meshwork and Schlemm's canal (Fig. 79-2). A delicate balance between aqueous production and its egress from the eye maintains intraocular pressure within its physiologic range (10 to 20 mm Hg). Obstruction of aqueous outflow causes elevated intraocular pressure, and this generally occurs in the vicinity of the trabecular meshwork (see the discussion of glaucoma later in this chapter). A small fragment of the trabecular meshwork is often excised (trabeculectomy) to decrease intraocular pressure in glaucoma by enhancing aqueous drainage from the eye. Under certain circumstances, as with some intraocular tumors, the aqueous is aspirated for cytologic evaluation.

In addition to the eye, the orbital cavity contains the optic nerve, smooth and striated muscle, adipose tissue, blood vessels, nerves, fibrous tissue, cartilage (the trochlea), and the lacrimal gland. Located in a bony fossa behind the superotemporal orbital rim, the lacrimal gland is the only epithelial structure of the normal orbit. Occasional lymphocytes and plasma cells are interspersed among its acini. The orbit communicates with the intracranial cavity through fissures and foramina. Anteriorly the orbital contents are limited by a fibrous tissue septum and protected by the eyelids.

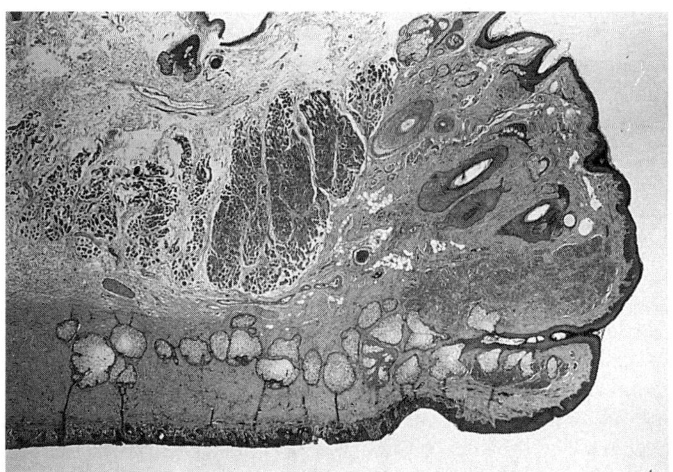

Fig. 79-3 Upper eyelid. Lined posteriorly by palpebral conjunctiva, tarsal plate *(below)* contains sebaceous meibomian glands. Transversely sectioned bundles of orbicularis muscle are seen anterior to tarsus. Lid margin contains mucocutaneous junction and lash follicles. Long tarsal plate and roughly rectangular configuration indicates that specimen is an upper eyelid.

The lacrimal drainage apparatus (the puncta, canaliculi, lacrimal sac, and nasolacrimal duct) transports tears to the nose. Most pathologic processes involving the lacrimal drainage apparatus are inflammatory in nature.

Intraocular tumors and chorioretinal inflammatory conditions occasionally are examined through biopsy. Sometimes the cornea and intraocular contents are removed with retention of the scleral shell (ocular evisceration). Especially when the orbit harbors a malignant neoplasm, the entire orbital contents, globe, eyelids, and periosteum, are excised (orbital exenteration).

Aside from tumors, surgically excised eyelid specimens include relatively normal tissues (Fig. 79-3) obtained during cosmetic blepharoplasty to alleviate blepharoptosis, entropion, or ectropion. Cutaneous disorders affecting the eyelid are identical to those elsewhere in the skin (see Chapter 71).

Because a detailed discussion of the pathology of the ocular tissues is beyond the scope of this survey, refer elsewhere for additional information.[3-9]

DEVELOPMENTAL ANOMALIES

Anomalous development of the eye results in a variety of malformations that involve the entire globe or specific parts of it (Table 79-1). The causes of many developmental anomalies are unknown, but some are genetically determined or are caused by chromosomal abnormalities, viruses, or drugs, such as cyclophosphamide and 13-*cis*-retinoic acid.

Table 79-1 Developmental anomalies of the eye

Anomalies of whole eye
Anencephaly
Anophthalmia
Microphthalmos
Nanophthalmos
Coloboma
Cystic coloboma
Coloboma and abnormal intraocular tissue
Atypical coloboma
Cystic eye
Anomalies of cornea, sclera, and conjunctiva
Microcornea
Megalocornea
Sclerocornea
Cornea plana
Posterior ulcer of von Hippel
Peters' anomaly
Axenfeld-Rieger syndrome
Limbal choristoma (dermoid, dermolipoma, complex choristoma)
Posterior keratoconus
Episcleral osseous choristoma
Anomalies of uvea
Aniridia
Hypoplasia of iris
Hyperplasia of iris
Hamartoma of iris
Polycoria
Corectopia
Microcoria
Persistent pupillary membrane
Anomalies of anterior chamber
Axenfeld-Rieger anomaly
Peters' anomaly
Prominent Schwalbe's ring
Anomalies of lens
Aphakia
Ectopia lentis
Biphakia
Microphakia (spherophakia)
Lenticonus, anterior
Lenticonus, posterior
Cataracts, congenital
Coloboma, lens
Anomalies of vitreous
Persistent hyperplastic primary vitreous
Persistent remnant of hyaloid artery
Anomalies of retina
Retinal aplasia
Retinal hypoplasia
Retinal dysgenesis (retinal dysplasia)
Retinoschisis
Astrocytic hamartoma
Vascular anomalies of retina
Ectopic retinal tissue
Congenital retinal detachment
Retinal folds
Anomalies of retinal pigment epithelium
Anomalies of optic nerve
Optic nerve aplasia
Optic nerve hypoplasia
Optic disk coloboma
Optic pit

INFLAMMATION AND IMMUNOLOGIC DISORDERS

Inflammation may be limited to the conjunctiva (conjunctivitis), cornea (keratitis), cornea and conjunctiva (keratoconjunctivitis), corneal stroma (interstitial keratitis), episclera (episcleritis),[10] sclera (scleritis),[10,11] orbital connective tissue (orbital cellulitis), uvea (uveitis), iris (iritis), ciliary body (cyclitis), choroid (choroiditis), iris and ciliary body (iridocyclitis), retina (retinitis), optic nerve (optic neuritis), eyelid (blepharitis), choroid and retina (chorioretinitis), vitreous (vitritis), pars plana of ciliary body (pars planitis), lacrimal gland (dacryoadenitis), the intraocular contents with sparing of the sclera and orbit (endophthalmitis), or the ocular contents and cornea or sclera (panophthalmitis).

The more common specific entities worth mentioning include the following:

Blepharitis and hordeolum. Blepharitis and acute suppurative inflammation of the sebaceous glands or follicles of the eyelid (hordeolum) are common. Hordeolums (styes) are divided into internal and external varieties. *Internal hordeolums* affect the meibomian glands, whereas *external hordeolums* involve the glands of Moll or Zeis or the adjacent hair follicles and eyelashes (cilia). Hordeolums are usually caused by *Staphylococcus.*

Conjunctivitis. Conjunctivitis is classified according to the nature of the inflammatory reaction (acute conjunctivitis, chronic conjunctivitis, granulomatous conjunctivitis,[12] inclusion conjunctivitis, ligneous conjunctivitis, membranous conjunctivitis, pseudomembranous conjunctivitis, chronic follicular conjunctivitis, giant papillary conjunctivitis, vernal conjunctivitis) or the etiologic agent (bacterial conjunctivitis, viral conjunctivitis, allergic conjunctivitis, trachoma). Causes of giant papillary conjunctivitis include vernal conjunctivitis and contact lens wearing. In contrast to sarcoidosis the granulomatous inflammation in tuberculosis, cat-scratch fever, and tularemia is characterized by extensive necrosis.

A severe, acute, purulent conjunctivitis with a copious purulent discharge may develop in the neonate (ophthalmia neonatorum) after exposure during natural childbirth to *Chlamydia trachomatis* (serotypes D to K, also known as *Chlamydia oculogenitalis*), *Neisseria gonorrhoeae,* other pyogenic bacteria in an infected mother, or even after the silver nitrate administered to the conjunctiva to prevent gonococcal conjunctivitis. This common cause of blindness in some parts

Table 79-1 Developmental anomalies of the eye—cont'd

Craniofacio-ocular anomalies
Cyclopia
Synophthalmia
Diophthalmos
Cryptophthalmos
Eyelid anomalies
Coloboma of eyelid
Congenital symblepharon
Microblepharon
Euryblepharon
Epicanthus
Congenital of eyelashes
Anomalies of lacrimal gland sac and duct
Agenesis of lacrimal gland
Ectopic lacrimal gland
Congenital atresia of nasolacrimal duct
Anomalies of extraocular muscles
Absence of extraocular muscle

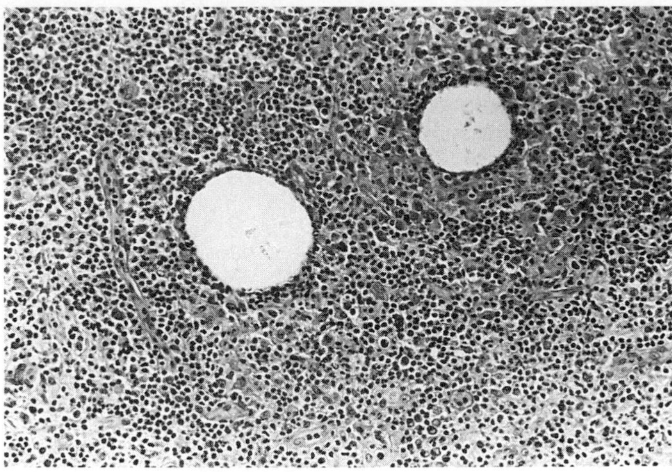

Fig. 79-4 Chalazion. Epithelioid cells surround empty lipid vacuoles in lipogranulomatous inflammatory infiltrate centered in the tarsal plate of posterior eyelid.

of the world is complicated by corneal ulceration, perforation and scarring, and panophthalmitis. The intracytoplasmic inclusion bodies of inclusion conjunctivitis are indistinguishable from those of trachoma, but in contrast to trachoma the lower tarsal conjunctiva is involved, scarring and necrosis do not develop, and keratitis is rare and mild.

Cicatricial pemphigoid. The chronic cicatrizing disorder known as "cicatricial pemphigoid" (mucous membrane pemphigoid, or ocular pemphigoid) affects the ocular mucous membrane, other mucosae, and the skin.[13] This type II hypersensitivity reaction with a genetic predisposition usually involves the conjunctiva, and the cicatrizing process causes a dry eye with symblepharon and shortening of the ocular fornix. Most patients (>90%) have immunoglobulin and complement in the conjunctival basement membrane, and the substantia propria contains many CD4 + T-lymphocytes (helper T-cells).[14-16]

Chalazion. After an obstruction from inspissated secretions, infections, neoplasms, or other conditions, the ducts draining the sebaceous glands (meibomian or zeis glands) within the eyelid may rupture, releasing material that incites a lipogranulomatous reaction. Curettings or biopsies of discrete chalazia are characterized by a chronic lipogranulomatous reaction (Fig. 79-4). Microscopically, chalazia resemble granulomatous inflammation from other causes, such as sarcoidosis, tuberculosis, or fungal infections. Special stains for microorganisms usually are unrevealing and unnecessary in the typical case, which has empty lipid vacuoles. More importantly, sebaceous carcinoma of the eyelid can mimic chalazia clinically and can even be associated with contiguous chronic granulomatosis inflammation. This most commonly excised, sometimes encapsulated, eyelid lesion consists of a mixed inflammatory cell infiltrate composed of polymorphonuclear leukocytes, lymphocytes, plasma cells, macrophages, epithelioid histiocytes, and, often, multinucleated giant cells.

Endophthalmitis and panophthalmitis. Endophthalmitis and panophthalmitis are divided into endogenous and exogenous types depending on the source of the etiologic agent and can also be classified according to the pathogen (bacterial, fungal).[17] Both endophthalmitis and panophthalmitis may occur after penetrating ocular trauma or surgery, infected corneal ulcers that perforate, or infection of filtering blebs after fistulization surgery for glaucoma. The organisms may be introduced by penetrating injuries or contaminated intraocular foreign bodies. They may also result from the hematogenous dissemination of bacteria or fungi, as in septicemia or infected emboli, as in subacute bacterial endocarditis, or systemic fungal infections in immune-compromised patients. The most commonly implicated organisms are listed in Table 79-2.

In both acute purulent endophthalmitis and panophthalmitis, a profuse, intense polymorphonuclear leukocytic infiltration is present, but natural barriers, such as Bruch's membrane, often confine the cellular infiltrate. Inflammatory cells often collect in the inferior portion of the anterior chamber (hypopyon). In endogenous infections, the ocular posterior segment may harbor the bulk of the inflammatory process. The involved tissues are usually necrotic and disorganized, and the causal bacteria or fungus may be identified with special stains, but extensive dispersion of ocular pigment may hinder identification of bacteria.

Sequelae of endophthalmitis include corneal scarring and vascularization, band keratopathy, cataract, and secondary glaucoma. Secondary glaucoma often occurs after adhesions between the iris and lens (posterior synechiae). The organization of inflammatory debris produces intraocular fibrosis and membranes. A membrane may stretch across the globe, linking different parts of the ciliary body from organization of the vitreous (cyclitic membrane). Inflammatory membranes contract and detach the ciliary body or retina. After the disorganization and destruction of ocular structures the eye becomes hypotonic and atrophic.

Sympathetic uveitis (sympathetic ophthalmia). Sympathetic uveitis is a rare, but extremely important, bilateral granulomatous inflammation of the uvea that occurs after unilateral perforating ocular injury or surgery, usually complicated by the incarceration of uveal tissue in the wound[18,19] (Fig. 79-5). It also rarely occurs after evisceration and intraocular melanomas. This uveitis develops in the originally injured eye ("exciting eye") after a latent period of at least 5 days (usually about 8 weeks, rarely as long as 12 years). The condition is believed to be an autoimmune response after sensitization to released ocular isoantigens. The relevant antigen has not been identified, but recent studies indicate that it may be retinal "S-antigen" (arestin), interphotoreceptor retinoid binding protein, or another retinal photoreceptor antigen. Enucleation of an eye within 7 to 14 days of injury usually prevents sympathetic uveitis. Surgical removal of the inciting eye may decrease the severity of the inflammation in the sympathizing eye after bilateral uveitis develops.

Phacoantigenic endophthalmitis. Phacoantigenic endophthalmitis (inappropriately designated "phacoanaphylactic endophthalmitis") is a granulomatous response around or within the lens (or its remains) in an eye with a traumatized or

Table 79-2 Common infections and inflammations of the eye and its adnexa

Organism/disease	Lesions
Viruses	
Cytomegalovirus	Necrotizing retinitis
Rubella	Congenital cataracts
Herpes simplex	Keratitis
	Follicular conjunctivitis
	Acute retinal necrosis
	Eyelid vesicles
Herpes zoster	Keratitis
	Acute retinal necrosis
	Eyelid vesicles
Adenovirus	Pseudomembranous conjunctivitis
Molluscum contagiosum	Molluscum contagiosum of eyelid
	Follicular conjunctivitis
Measles virus	Macular degeneration
Verruca vulgaris	Verruca vulgaris of eyelid
Bacteria	
Bacillus sp.	Endophthalmitis
Clostridium perfringens	Endophthalmitis
Corynebacterium diphtheriae	Pseudomembranous conjunctivitis
Escherichia coli	Keratitis
	Endophthalmitis
Haemophilus influenzae	Keratitis
	Endophthalmitis
	Orbital cellulitis
Klebsiella sp.	Keratitis
	Endophthalmitis
Listeria monocytogenes	Endophthalmitis
Mycobacterium sp.	Keratitis
	Endophthalmitis
Mycobacterium leprae	Keratitis
	Fibrohistiocytic keratitis
	Granulomatous uveitis
Mycobacterium tuberculosis	Granulomatous endophthalmitis
	Granulomatous uveitis
Neisseria gonorrhoeae	Keratitis
	Ophthalmia neonatorum
Neisseria meningitidis	Endophthalmitis
Nocardia asteroides	Keratitis
	Endophthalmitis
Proprionibacterium acnes	Endophthalmitis
Proteus sp.	Keratitis
	Endophthalmitis
Pseudomonas aeruginosa	Keratitis
Pseudomonas sp.	Endophthalmitis
Salmonella typhimurium	Endophthalmitis
Serratia marcescens	Endophthalmitis
Staphylococcus sp.	Pseudomembranous conjunctivitis
	Hordeolum
Staphylococcus aureus	Keratitis
	Endophthalmitis
Staphylococcus epidermidis	Keratitis
	Endophthalmitis

Table 79-2 Common infections and inflammation of the eye and its adnexa—cont'd

Organism/disease	Lesions
Bacteria *(continued)*	
Streptococcus pneumoniae	Keratitis
Streptococcus sp.	Keratitis
	Endophthalmitis
Streptococcus viridans	Infectious pseudocrystalline keratopathy
Treponema pallidum	Parinaud's oculoglandular syndrome
	Keratitis
	Granulomatous endophthalmitis
	Granulomatous uveitis
Afipia felis	Parinaud's oculoglandular syndrome
Fungi	
Aspergillus sp.	Keratitis
	Granulomatous endophthalmitis
	Orbital cellulitis
Blastomyces dermatitidis	Granulomatous endophthalmitis
	Granulomatous uveitis
Candida sp.	Keratitis
	Granulomatous endophthalmitis
	Granulomatous uveitis
Cladosporium sp.	Keratitis
Coccidioides immitis	Granulomatous endophthalmitis
	Granulomatous uveitis
Curvularia sp.	Keratitis
Fusarium sp.	Keratitis
Histoplasma capsulatum	Granulomatous endophthalmitis
	Granulomatous uveitis
Mucor sp.	Orbital cellulitis
Myrathecium sp.	Keratitis
Paecilomyces sp.	Keratitis
Petriellidium boydii	Keratitis
Phialophora sp.	Keratitis
Rhizopus sp.	Orbital cellulitis
Sporotrichum schenckii	Granulomatous endophthalmitis
	Granulomatous uveitis
Protozoa	
Acanthamoeba	Keratitis
Nosema	Keratitis
Parasites	
Taenia solium (as larva; cysticercus cellulosae)	Granulomatous inflammation
Toxocara canis	Granulomatous inflammation
Idiopathic	
Sarcoidosis	Granulomatous conjunctivitis
	Dacryoadenitis
	Uveitis
	Retinitis
Vogt-Koyanagi-Harada syndrome	Granulomatous endophthalmitis
Chlamydia sp.	Parinaud's oculoglandular syndrome
	Trachoma
	Inclusion body conjunctivitis
Chlamydia trachomatis	Trachoma
	Ophthalmia neonatorum
Immunologic disorders	
Juvenile rheumatoid arthritis	Granulomatous scleritis
	Uveitis
Sympathetic uveitis	Granulomatous uveitis
Rheumatoid arthritis	Peripheral corneal ulceration
	Scleritis
	Scleromalacia perforans
Systemic lupus erythematosus	Peripheral corneal ulceration
	Scleritis
Polyarteritis nodosa	Peripheral corneal ulceration

(continued)

Table 79-2 Common infections and inflammation of the eye and its adnexa—cont'd

Organism/disease	Lesions
Immunologic disorders	
Wegener's granulomatosis	Peripheral corneal ulceration Scleritis
Relapsing polychondritis	Peripheral corneal ulceration Scleritis
Ankylosing spondylitis	Uveitis
Reiter's syndrome	Uveitis
Ulcerative colitis	Uveitis
Regional enteritis	Uveitis
Behçet's disease	Uveitis

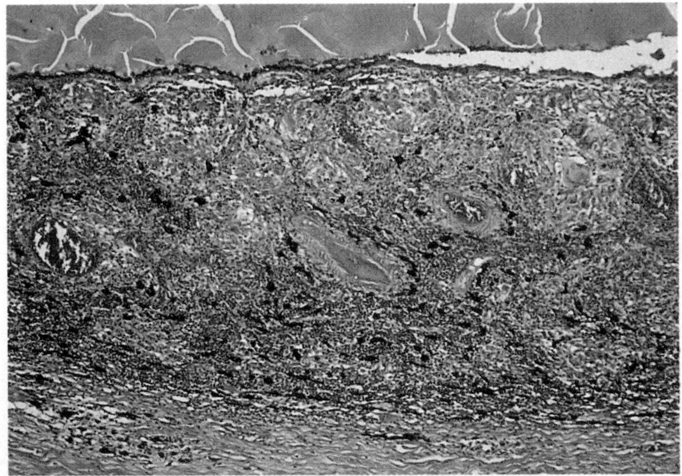

Fig. 79-5 Sympathetic uveitis. The choroid is massively thickened by a diffuse chronic inflammatory infiltrate composed of epithelioid histiocytes and lymphocytes. The choriocapillaris is visible ("spared"). The retina is detached.

cataractous lens, or after the surgical removal of a cataractous lens. A similar reaction may occur spontaneously in the contralateral eye months or years later. It can be provoked experimentally by immunization with autologous lens material in conjunction with Freund's adjuvant and was once considered to be an autoimmune response to immunologically sequestered lens-specific proteins that led to sensitization after lens disruption. Phacoanaphylactic endophthalmitis is now believed to be caused by loss of immune tolerance.[20]

Idiopathic orbital inflammatory pseudotumor. Orbital inflammatory pseudotumors are frequently examined through biopsy. They typically consist of a mixed inflammatory cell infiltrate of lymphocytes, plasma cells, eosinophils, and, occasionally, epithelioid cells. Lymphoid follicles and germinal centers are found in some cases, and varying degrees of fibrosis are usually present. Extensive sclerosis often characterizes chronic lesions. Some inflammatory pseudotumors are composed predominantly of lymphocytes.

Idiopathic orbital inflammatory pseudotumor is a diagnosis of exclusion, both clinically and histopathologically.[21,22] Pathogens, such as bacteria and fungi, need to be ruled out. Some pseudotumors need to be differentiated from reactive and atypical lymphoid hyperplasias, polyarteritis nodosa and other systemic vasculitides, limited and systemic forms of Wegener's granulomatosis,[23-26] sarcoidosis, Kimura's disease, midline lethal granuloma, necrobiotic xanthogranuloma, Erdheim-Chester disease, multiple myeloma, lymphoplasmacytoid tumors, Burkitt's lymphoma, and mycosis fungoides. Because biopsies provide a limited amount of material for histopathologic evaluation, inflammatory reactions around other lesions, such as a pleomorphic adenoma of the lacrimal gland or ruptured dermoid cyst, may be mistaken for an inflammatory pseudotumor.

Iritis. As a sequel to iritis, adhesions develop between the iris and the lens (posterior synechiae) or between the peripheral iris and the anterior chamber angle (peripheral anterior synechiae), causing glaucoma.

INFECTIOUS AND PARASITIC DISEASES

Microorganisms lodging on the surface of the eye frequently cause conjunctivitis, keratitis, or corneal ulcers. The eye may also become infected by hematogenous spread from a focus of infection elsewhere. Ocular infections occasionally complicate surgical procedures, such as cataract extractions, corneal grafts,[27] and the implantation of ocular prosthetic lenses.[28,29] Adenoviruses and other pathogens may be introduced into the eye by infected eyedrops or by ophthalmologists using a contaminated tonometer (an instrument used to measure intraocular pressure). Common microorganisms affecting the eye and its adnexa are summarized in Table 79-2. Specific infections affecting the eye include measles,[30] AIDS[31-33] (including *Pneumocystis carinii*[34] infection and microsporidiosis[35,36]), rubella,[37] syphilis,[38] cat-scratch disease,[39] phycomycosis (mucormycosis),[40,41] and numerous other viral[42] and parasitic[43] diseases. *Mycobacterium tuberculosis* and some other organisms can enter the body by way of the ocular mucous membranes to cause localized or systemic disease.

Infectious keratitis. The histopathologic features of acute bacterial ulcerative keratitis include destruction of the corneal epithelium, Bowman's layer, and stroma with necrosis and a prominent polymorphonuclear leukocytic infiltrate. With corneal perforation inflammatory debris adheres to the posterior surface of the cornea. Fungi can infiltrate through the corneal stroma and Descemet's membrane and invade the anterior chamber. Colonies of *Streptococcus viridans* and some other bacteria may produce crystalline-like stromal opacities in the absence of an inflammatory cell infiltrate ("infectious pseudocrystalline keratopathy").[27]

Onchocerciasis. Onchocerciasis is by far the most important helminthic disease of the eye. The nematode *Onchocerca volvulus* is transmitted by bites-of infected black simuliid flies (*Simulium* sp.), which breed in swift-running streams in parts of tropical West Africa, South America, Guatemala, and Mexico. Five to 6 years after the appearance of subcutaneous nodules (cercomas), microfilaria spawned by fertilized adult female *Onchocerca* migrate into the superficial cornea, bulbar conjunctiva, aqueous, and other ocular tissues. The demise of intracorneal microfilaria produces keratitis, corneal opacification, pannus formation, anterior uveitis, secondary glaucoma, and visual impairment ("river blindness"). Less frequently, endophthalmitis, chorioretinitis, and optic atrophy occur.

Toxoplasmosis. Ocular toxoplasmosis can be congenital or acquired, and the lesion is a retinochoroiditis. Encysted organisms in the margins of congenital chorioretinal scars are believed to be responsible for recrudescent infection in adults. Histologically, free and encysted *Toxoplasma* are found in a sharply demarcated zone of retinal necrosis overlying a focal granulomatous choroidal infiltrate. Necrotizing retinitides that need to be differentiated from toxoplasmosis include cytomegalovirus retinitis and the acute retinal necrosis syndrome, which is caused by *Herpes simplex* or *varicella-zoster* virus.

Cytomegalovirus retinitis. Infection with cytomegalovirus commonly involves the retina, particularly in immunosuppressed individuals such as renal graft recipients and persons with AIDS.[44] A necrotizing retinitis accompanied by hemorrhage, vasculitis, and devastating visual consequences is the usual lesion, and infections may be congenital or acquired.

Herpes simplex keratitis and retinal necrosis. Herpesvirus has a predilection for the corneal epithelium, but it can invade the corneal stroma and occasionally other ocular tissues. The histopathologic features of long-standing keratitis caused by *herpes simplex virus* are nonspecific. Frequently the epithelium is irregular in thickness, Bowman's layer is disrupted, and pannus is present (Fig. 79-6). Herpes simplex may incite a hypersensitivity reaction, which causes most of the tissue damage in chronic herpetic keratitis. Neovascularization and an infiltrate of lymphocytes, plasma cells and other mononuclear cells may be present in the corneal stroma. The corneal stroma may become greatly thinned, and Descemet's membrane may bulge into it (descemetocele). Corneal perforation can also occur. Recurrent *Herpes simplex* corneal ulcers may be precipitated by trauma, menstruation, emotional and physical stress, exposure to bright or ultraviolet light, vaccination, and other factors. In chronic or recurrent *Herpes simplex* keratitis, the virus is usually not isolated in culture, and viral inclusions are rarely identified in tissue sections. Transmission electron microscopy, immunocytochemistry, in situ hybridization, and the polymerase chain reaction may be helpful in establishing the diagnosis in some cases. Acute retinal necrosis is sometimes caused by herpes simplex, but it may also be caused by varicella-zoster and perhaps other viruses.[45-47]

Amebic keratitis. Wearers of soft contact lens are particularly susceptible to keratitis caused by acanthamebas *(Acanthamoeba castellani, A. polyphaga, A. culbertsoni,* or *A. rhysodes),* especially if they improperly clean their lenses, use homemade saline solutions, or swim while wearing the lenses.[48] Amebic trophozoites, which resemble macrophages, and more readily apparent encysted organisms are found in the mildly inflamed corneal stroma. Both the trophozoites and encysted organisms are most often found near areas of stromal necrosis. This protozoon can be recognized in hematoxylin and eosin–stained sections, but special stains (calcofluor white, periodic acid–Schiff, methenamine silver, Giemsa), immunofluorescent techniques, and transmission electron microscopy have been advocated in the diagnosis of amebic keratitis. In the absence of specific stains, differentiation of trophozoites from reactive corneal fibroblasts may be difficult.

Toxocariasis. Ocular toxocariasis is characterized by eosinophilic abscess formation incited by dead larvae of the nematode *Toxocara canis* or *Toxocara cati.* Serial sectioning is frequently necessary to disclose the worm, but it occasionally fails to demonstrate a parasite in an eye with an eosinophilic abscess.

Demodicosis. Acarine mites are commonly found within the eyelid hair follicles *(Demodex folliculorum)* or sebaceous glands *(Demodex brevis).* These mites may incite inflammation but are often evident in eyelid tissue excised for unrelated reasons from individuals without blepharitis. *Demodex folliculorum* is found with increasing incidence with age and is present in virtually all eyelid specimens from individuals older than 70 yearsof age.

Trachoma. Trachoma caused by *Chlamydia trachomatis* is a major cause of blindness in many countries. The disease affects the conjunctivae, corneas, and eyelids. The conjunctiva contains glycogen-rich intracytoplasmic inclusion bodies within epithelial cells, and macrophages possess nuclear fragments (Leber cells). In the conjunctiva a predominantly lymphocytic infiltrate accumulates together with follicles that develop necrotic germinal centers. Lymphocytes and blood vessels eventually invade the superior cornea between its epithelium and Bowman's zone (trachomatous pannus), impairing vision. Scarring of the conjunctivae and eyelids distorts the eyelids.

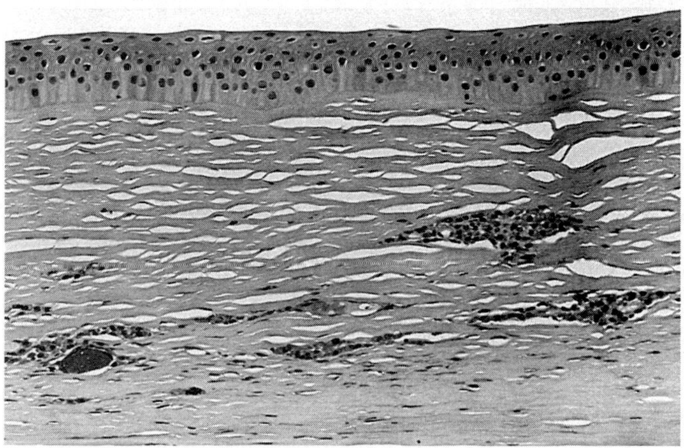

Fig. 79-6 Chronic *Herpes simplex* keratitis. The scarred and vascularized corneal stroma contains chronic inflammatory cells. Bowman's layer has been destroyed. The epithelium is mildly thickened and irregular in caliber.

NEOPLASMS AND RELATED MASSES

A wide variety of cell types in and around the eye spawn benign and malignant neoplasms (Table 79-3), and the frequency with which the different cell types become neoplastic varies immensely. An intraocular neoplasm of the human lens epithelium has not been documented, but a phakomatous choristoma of the lenticular anlage rarely arises in the lower eyelid.[49] Although the retinal pigment epithelium often undergoes reactive proliferation, it seldom becomes neoplastic. Pigmented melanocytic lesions of the conjunctiva and uvea may be benign, premalignant, or malignant. The histopathologic features of most tumors in and around the eye are identical to those found elsewhere, and only a few salient points relevant to them are presented here.

The most common primary intraocular neoplasms are uveal melanoma and choroidal hemangioma in adults, and retinoblastoma and medulloepithelioma in children. Other childhood neural tumors include plexiform neurofibromas and juvenile pilocytic astrocytomas (optic nerve gliomas) found in von Recklinghausen's neurofibromatosis type I.

The lymphoid tissue of the conjunctiva and arguably of the orbit forms part of the mucosa-associated lymphoid tissue (MALT). Lymphoid hyperplasia and lymphomas are common in the conjunctiva, orbit, and lacrimal gland but are less frequent in the intraocular tissues. Ocular lymphoid lesions include polyclonal reactive lymphoid hyperplasias, cytologically indeterminate atypical lymphoid hyperplasias, and malignant lymphomas composed of monoclonal cytologically atypical cells.

Tumors of conjunctiva, caruncle, and cornea

Tumors of the conjunctiva, caruncle, and cornea are classified according to the cell of origin (Table 79-3). Tumors of the cornea are rare and almost invariably represent direct spread of squamous cell carcinoma or melanoma from the conjunctiva or eyelid. Primary neoplasms seldom arise in the caruncle, but conjunctival tumors may extend into this specialized structure.

The cause of most tumors of the conjunctiva, caruncle and cornea is unknown, but human papillomavirus (types 6, 6a, 16, and 18) accounts for at least some conjunctival papillomas and intraepithelial neoplasms.[50] Some tumors accompany the phakomatoses.[51]

Conjunctival lymphoid tumors. Lymphoid tumors of the conjunctiva appear as a salmon-colored mass within the fornix or on the surface of the globe. The conjunctiva of apparently healthy persons always contains lymphocytes, but when present in large number, especially when arranged in lymphoid follicles with germinal centers, reactive lymphoid hyperplasia (as in acute follicular conjunctivitis) needs to be considered in the differential diagnosis of lesions obtained at biopsy. Lymphoid tumors include reactive lymphoid hyperplasia, atypical lymphoid hyperplasia, and malignant lymphomas.[52-54] Most lymphomas of the conjunctiva are well-differentiated, small-cell lymphocytic lymphomas. The classification of ocular lymphoid lesions as benign or malignant and as monoclonal or polyclonal immunophenotypically does not appear to be a useful predictor of the predisposition to extraocular lymphoma or of other aspects of biologic behavior. Most lymphoid tumors remain localized, but sometimes a systemic lymphoma is found at the initial ocular presentation or on subsequent follow-up study. Their malignant potential is often difficult if not impossible to predict using conventional light microscopy, immunohistochemicals analysis, and even molecular biologic studies for immunoglobulin and T-cell receptor gene rearrangements.

Squamous papilloma. Squamous papillomas arise from the conjunctival epithelium in diverse clinical settings. In children, they are often bilateral and recur after excision ("recurrent juvenile conjunctival papillomatosis"). In adults, papillomas are usually solitary and unilateral. Some conjunctival intraepithelial neoplasms appear papillomatous clinically. Inverted papillomas of the conjunctiva are rare.

Dysplasia and intraepithelial neoplasia. Conjunctival dysplasia and carcinoma in situ resemble comparable lesions of the uterine cervix morphologically but pursue a more benign course than cervical lesions. Conjunctival dysplasia arises in the basal germinative layer, and atypical cells replace part or all of the epithelium. When the epithelium is totally replaced by the cytologic atypia, the diagnosis of carcinoma in situ is warranted. Because dysplasia and intraepithelial carcinoma represent a continuum of change, the nature of which depends on tissue sampling these lesions are often designated "intraepithelial neoplasia"[55] (Fig. 79-7).

Squamous cell carcinoma. Conjunctival squamous cell carcinoma usually grows as a papillary exophytic mass. Cellular atypia occurs throughout the entire epithelial thickness, and neoplastic cells extend into the underlying stroma either individually or in nests. The epithelium is sometimes keratinized. The adjacent conjunctival epithelium frequently has an intraepithelial neoplasm. Occasionally the globe or orbit are invaded,[56] but metastases or death are rarely attributable to the tumor. Epibulbar pigmented squamous cell carcinomas are jet black and mimic a melanoma clinically, but in contrast to malignant melanocytic neoplasms they occur in heavily pigmented individuals.

Mucoepidermoid carcinoma. Mucoepidermoid carcinoma of the conjunctiva resembles the more common squamous cell carcinoma but contains mucus-secreting cells and intraepithelial mucin.[57] The mucin may not be readily apparent without special stains, such as Alcian blue, Hale's colloidal iron technique, or mucicarmine. These tumors behave more aggressively than the usual squamous cell carcinomas, with early invasion of the eye and orbit and frequent recurrences.

Spindle cell carcinoma. Spindle cell carcinoma rarely arises in the conjunctiva, but it pursues a more aggressive clinical course than the usual well-differentiated conjunctival squamous carcinoma.[58] Immunohistocytochemical analysis and transmission electron microscopy are useful in differentiating the tumor from sarcomas. The tumor cells possess immunohistochemically detectable intracytoplasmic cytokeratin and epithelial ultrastructural features such as desmosomes and tonofibrils.

Nevocellular nevus. The most commonly excised melanocytic lesion of the conjunctiva is the compound nevus of adolescents or young adults.[59,60] It is frequently pigmented but not invariably so. Increase in pigmentation or size during puberty or pregnancy often prompts excision. Conjunctival compound and subepithelial nevi typically contain cystic or solid rests of surface epithelium (Fig. 79-8). The epithelial hyperplasia associated with conjunctival nevi has been confused with invasive squamous cell carcinoma. Unlike nevi of the skin, a substantial mononuclear inflammatory infiltrate is

Table 79-3 Common tumors, cysts, and related lesions of the eye and its adnexa

Retina and neural ectoderm
Glial
Benign
- Astrocytoma
- Astrocytic hamartoma
- "Massive retinal gliosis"

Neuronal
Benign
- Retinocytoma
- Medulloepithelioma
- Medulloepithelioma, teratoid
- Glioneuroma

Malignant
- Retinoblastoma
- Medulloepithelioma, malignant
- Medulloepithelioma, malignant teratoid

Neural ectoderm
Benign
- Adenoma of pigment epithelium

Vascular
Benign
- Hemangioma (capillary, cavernous, and racemose)

Lymphoid
Malignant
- Intraocular B-cell lymphoma (formerly called "reticulum cell sarcoma")

Ciliary body
Ciliary epithelium
Benign
- Adenoma, pigmented epithelium
- Adenoma, nonpigmented epithelium

Malignant
- Adenocarcinoma

Vascular
Benign
- Hemangioma

Smooth muscle
Benign
- Leiomyoma
- Mesectodermal leiomyoma

Neural
Benign
- Neurofibroma
- Schwannoma
- Neurofibroma

Melanocytic
Benign
- Nevi

Malignant
- Malignant melanoma

Mesenchymal
Malignant
- Rhabdomyosarcoma

Lymphoid
- Lymphoma

Choroid
Vascular
Benign
- Hemangioma (cavernous)
- Inflammatory pseudotumor (reactive lymphoid hypoplasia)

Smooth muscle
Benign
- Leiomyoma
- Neurofibroma

Table 79-3 Common tumors, cysts, and related lesions of the eye and its adnexa—cont'd

Melanocytic
Benign
- Nevi

Malignant
- Malignant melanoma

Mesenchymal
Benign
- Osteoma

Neural
Benign
- Ganglioneuroma
- Schwannoma

Iris
Iris pigment epithelium
Benign
- Adenoma of pigment epithelium

Cysts
- Pigment epithelial
- Stromal
- Epithelial, traumatic (epithelial, implantation)

Vascular
Benign
- Hemangioma

Mesenchymal
Malignant
- Rhabdomyosarcoma

Histiocytic
Benign
- Juvenile xanthogranuloma

Smooth muscle
Benign
- Xanthoma
- Leiomyoma

Neural
- Neurofibroma
- Granular cell tumor

Melanocytic
Benign
- Nevi

Malignant
- Melanoma

Conjunctiva
Epithelial
Benign
- Squamous papilloma
- Recurrent juvenile papillomatosis
- Hereditary benign intraepithelial dyskeratosis

Premalignant and early malignant
- Intraepithelial neoplasm
- Dysplasia
  - Epidermoid variant
  - Spindle cell variant
- Carcinoma in situ

Lymphoid
- Lymphoid hyperplasia

Melanocytic
Premalignant and early malignant
- Primary acquired melanosis

Malignant
- Carcinoma, squamous cell
- Carcinoma, spindle cell
- Carcinoma, mucoepidermoid
- Carcinoma, pigmented squamous cell

(continued)

Table 79-3 Common tumors, cysts, and related lesions of the eye and its adnexa—cont'd

Malignant
  Malignant melanoma
Mesenchymal
Malignant
  Rhabdomyosarcoma (botryoid)
Smooth muscle
Malignant
  Leiomyosarcoma
Neural
Benign
  Neurofibroma
Lymphoid
Benign
  Lymphoid hyperplasia
Malignant
  Lymphoma
Vascular
Malignant
  Kaposi sarcoma
Cornea
Benign
  Benign hereditary intraepithelial dyskeratosis
Premalignant and early malignant
  Dysplasia
  Intraepithelial neoplasm
  Carcinoma in situ
Malignant
  Melanoma
  Carcinoma, squamous cell
Caruncle
Benign
  Oncocytoma
  Sebaceous gland hyperplasia
Malignant
  Sebaceous carcinoma
  Melanoma
Eyelid
Epithelial
Benign
  Benign keratoses
  Papilloma, squamous cell
  Keratoacanthoma
  Seborrheic keratosis
  Inverted folliculoma (inverted follicular keratosis)
  Skin tags
  Calcifying epithelioma of Malherbe
  Carcinoma
    Basal cell
    Sebaceous cell (meibomian gland carcinoma)
    Squamous cell
Melanocytic
Benign
  Nevocellular nevi
Malignant
  Malignant melanoma
Vascular
Benign
  Hemangioma
    Capillary
    Cavernous
  Glomus tumor
  Lymphangioma

Table 79-3 Common tumors, cysts, and related lesions of the eye and its adnexa—cont'd

Malignant
  Angiosarcoma
  Kaposi's sarcoma
Adnexal
Benign
  Apocrine gland adenoma (Moll's glands)
  Eccrine acrospiroma
  Pilomatrixoma
  Pleomorphic adenoma
  Syringoma
  Trichoepithelioma
  Trichofolliculoma
  Trichilemmoma
  Adenoma of sebaceous glands (meibomian glands)
  Adenoma of Krause's accessory lacrimal gland
  Adenoma of sweat glands
Malignant
  Carcinoma
    Apocrine gland
    Eccrine sweat gland (sweat gland adenocarcinoma)
    Mucinous sweat gland
Developmental
  Phakomatous choristoma
Cysts
  Dermoid
  Epidermal inclusion
  Sudoriferous (apocrine and eccrine hidrocystomas)
Mesenchymal
  Fibrous histiocytoma
  Myxoma
  Leiomyoma
Neural
  Neurofibroma
  Schwannoma
  Granular cell tumor
Nonneoplastic masses
  Xanthelasma
  Extramammary Paget's disease
Lymphoid
Malignant
  Mycosis fungoides
  Lymphoma
  Merkel cell tumor
  Metastatic
    Carcinoma
    Melanoma
Orbit
Developmental masses
  Teratoma
  Meningocele
  Meningoencephalocele
  Microphthalmos with cyst
  Prominent palpebral lobe of lacrimal gland
  Ectopic brain tissue
  Dermoid cysts
  Arteriovenous malformations
  Lymphangioma
Tumors of blood vessels
Benign
  Hemangioma
    Capillary
    Cavernous
  Vascular malformation
  Hemangiopericytoma

Table 79-3 Common tumors, cysts, and related lesions of the eye and its adnexa—cont'd

Hemangioendothelioma
Varices
Glomus tumors
Intravascular papillary endothelial hyperplasia
Malignant
Malignant hemangiopericytoma
Malignant hemangioendothelioma
Angiosarcoma
Tumors of muscle
Benign
Leiomyoma
Vascular leiomyoma
Malignant
Rhabdomyosarcoma
Secondary tumors
Direct extension from:
Intraocular tumors
Retinoblastoma
Melanoma
Medulloepithelioma
Other
Tumors of periocular skin
Paranasal sinuses
Intracranial cavity
Metastases
Miscellaneous
Mucocele
Cholesterol granuloma
Others
Pseudotumor, inflammatory
Lymphoma
Leukemia
Sarcoma, undifferentiated
Epithelial or "sebaceous" cysts
Pseudotumor, noninflammatory
Epibulbar, eyelid, and orbital osseous choristoma
Dermolipoma
Lacrimal gland duct cyst
Neurosarcoma
Embryonal sarcoma, metastatic
Benign adenomatous epithelial hyperplasia of sweat/lacrimal gland
Amyloidosis
Malignant teratoid medulloepithelioma of optic nerve
"Metastatic" astrocytoma
Cyst, posttraumatic hemorrhagic
Myxosarcoma
Tumors of bone
Benign
Aneurysmal bone cyst
Benign osteoblastoma
Giant cell tumor
Eosinophilic granuloma
Fibrous dysplasia
Osteoma
Giant cell reparative granuloma
Brown tumor of hyperparathyroidism
Malignant
Osteogenic sarcoma
Tumors of cartilage
Benign
Chondroma
Malignant

Table 79-3 Common tumors, cysts, and related lesions of the eye and its adnexa—cont'd

Chondrosarcoma
Mesenchymal chondrosarcoma
Tumors of germ cell origin
Malignant
Endodermal sinus tumor
Malignant rhabdoid tumor
Tumors of lacrimal gland
Benign
Pleomorphic adenoma
Oncocytoma
Malignant
Carcinoma, adenoid cystic
Carcinoma, mucoepidermoid
Adenocarcinoma
Tumors of peripheral nerves
Benign
Schwannoma
Neurofibroma
Granular cell tumor
Paraganglioma
Traumatic neuroma
Malignant
Neurofibrosarcoma
Alveolar soft-part sarcoma
Tumors of adipose tissue
Benign
Lipoma
Prolapsed orbital fat
Malignant
Liposarcoma
Tumors of fibrous tissue
Benign
Fibrous histiocytoma (benign)
Juvenile fibromatosis
Fibrous xanthoma
Fibroma
Myxoma
Juvenile psammomatoid ossifying fibroma
Malignant
Fibrous histiocytoma (malignant)
Fibrosarcoma
Malignant fibrous histiocytoma
Inflammatory masses
Sarcoidosis
Nodular fasciitis
Mucoceles secondary to sinusitis
Histiocytic tumors
Benign
Eosinophilic granulomas
Xanthogranuloma
Malignant
Histiocytosis X (Langerhans' cell histiocytosis)
Lymphoid tumors
Benign
Lymphoid hyperplasia
Indeterminate
Plasma cell myeloma
Malignant
Lymphoma (non-Hodgkin)
Tumors of melanogenic system
Malignant
Primary melanoma

(continued)

Table 79-3 Common tumors, cysts, and related lesions of the eye and its adnexa—cont'd

Optic nerve
Benign
- Astrocytoma, pilocytic
- Glioneuroma
- Drusen
- Medulloepithelioma, benign
- Melanocytoma
- Meningioma

Malignant
- Medulloepithelioma, malignant
- Anaplastic astrocytoma

Miscellaneous tumors
- Carcinoid tumor
- Retinal anlage tumor
- Neuroepithelioma
- Ectomesenchyma

Lacrimal sac
Benign
Inflammatory tumors
- Granuloma
- Pseudotumor

Epithelial tumors
- Papilloma, squamous cell
- Papilloma, transitional cell
- Papilloma, mixed squamous and transitional cell

Tumors of fibrous tissue
- Fibrous histiocytoma

Tumors of peripheral nerves
- Schwannoma

Miscellaneous tumors
- Oncocytoma

Malignant
- Malignant oncocytic tumor

Vascular tumors
- Angiosarcoma

Carcinomas
- Squamous cell
- Transitional cell
- Adenocarcinomas
- Mucoepidermoid

Lymphoid tumors
- Lymphoma

Melanocytic tumors
- Melanoma

Malignant tumors from adjacent structures

Miscellaneous intraocular tumors
Developmental masses
- Ectopic lacrimal gland

Malignant
- Schwannoma, malignant
- Neurofibroma, malignant
- Peripheral nerve sheath tumor, malignant

often present. Junctional nevi are rare and are almost always found in children.

Ephelis (freckle). Congenital pigmentation of the conjunctival epithelium (ephelis, or freckle) is a pigmentary lesion similar to those on the skin. It does not evolve into a melanoma.

Congenital ocular and oculodermal melanocytosis (nevus of Ota). In congenital ocular or oculodermal melanocytosis the epibulbar pigmentation is slate gray in color. Dendritic

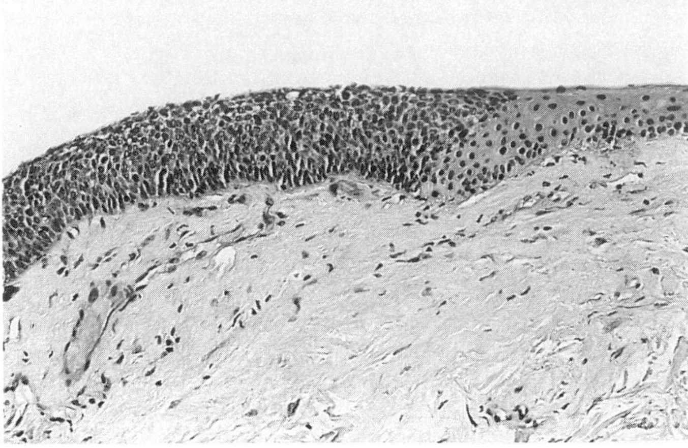

Fig. 79-7 Conjunctival intraepithelial neoplasia. Limbal epithelium at left is totally replaced by densely cellular infiltrate of atypical cells, which remain confined by epithelial basement membrane. Totality of epithelial replacement warrants diagnosis of carcinoma in situ. Transition from tumor to normal epithelium is characteristically abrupt.

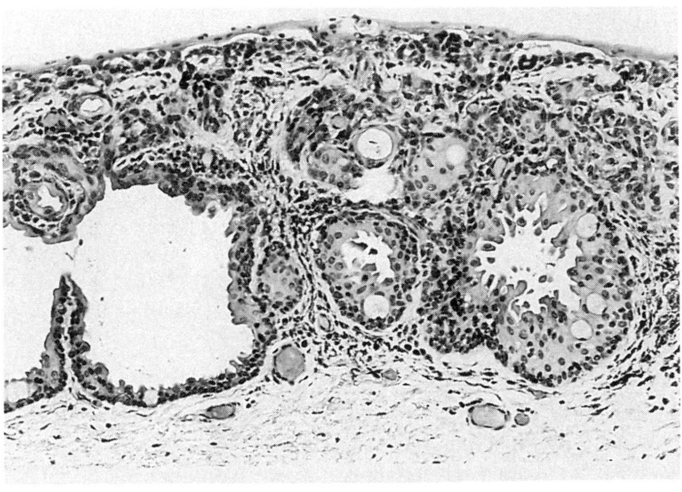

Fig. 79-8 Cystic compound nevus in conjunctiva. The substantia propria in many conjunctival nevi contains solid and cystic rests of surface epithelium. Persistent junctional activity indicates that the patient is young.

melanocytes are located deep in the conjunctival substantia propria and episcleral tissues. Patients with Ota's nevus have an associated blue nevus of the periocular skin. Heterochromia iridum (involved eye darker) reflects an associated diffuse nevus of the uvea that can give rise to a uveal malignant melanoma.

Primary acquired melanosis. One or more irregular areas of pigmentation may appear spontaneously in a nonpigmented portion of the conjunctiva of one eye. This condition, called "primary acquired melanosis" (PAM), usually affects middle-aged to elderly whites (mostly about 40 to 50 years of age) in whom the patchy epithelial pigmentation tends to wax and wane. PAM can be amelanotic and rarely occurs in blacks. Atypical melanocytic hyperplasia is initially seen in the basal epithelium, but it can involve the full thickness in PAM with

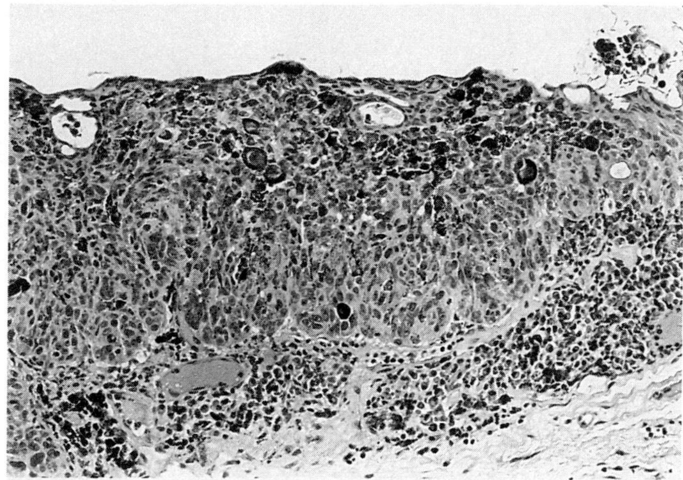

Fig. 79-9 Primary acquired melanosis with atypia in conjunctiva. Conjunctival epithelium is massively thickened by atypical melanocytes, including epithelioid cells. Substantia propria contains lymphocytes and plasma cells. Invasive malignant melanoma was found nearby.

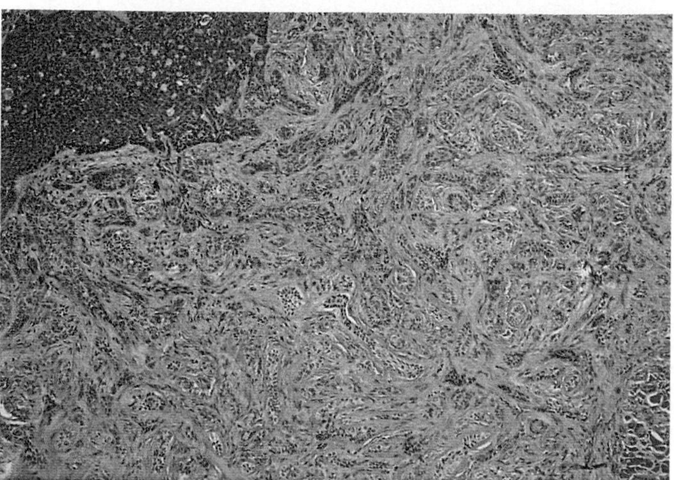

Fig. 79-10 Morphealike basal cell carcinoma. Slender tendrils of tumor cells deeply infiltrate substance of lower eyelid. A focus of more differentiated tumor is seen directly beneath the epidermis.

atypia (Fig. 79-9), which often progresses to invasive malignant melanoma. Different parts of the same conjunctiva manifest different stages of the disorder. Patients should be followed carefully with photographic documentation and biopsies of thickened areas.

Secondary acquired melanosis. Conjunctival melanosis may be secondary to inflammation, a conjunctival neoplasm, a metabolic disease (such as Addison's disease) or chemicals (such as thorazine).

Malignant melanoma. Relatively rare, conjunctival melanomas may be pigmented or amelanotic.[61-63] They are one tenth as common as uveal melanomas. Malignant melanomas of the conjunctiva may be preceded by PAM, a nevocellular nevus, or no overt antecedent lesion. Others represent extraocular extension of a uveal melanoma. In about two thirds of cases histologic evidence of preexisting PAM is found. Conjunctival melanomas are often apparently multicentric, especially when preceded by PAM. Lymphatic spread to the preauricular and intraparotid nodes is common. The nature of the initial lesion is of no apparent prognostic importance. The behavior of conjunctival melanomas is unpredictable, but in a series of 131 patients with this tumor followed for a median period of at least 8 years, about 25% of the individuals died from metastases.[61]

Kaposi's sarcoma. Kaposi's sarcoma of the conjunctiva most often develops in patients with AIDS.[64]

Tumors of eyelid

Actinic keratoses and intraepithelial squamous cell carcinoma of the eyelid occasionally evolve into invasive squamous cell carcinoma.[65] Risk factors for basal cell and squamous cell carcinomas of the eyelid include excessive chronic solar irradiation and prior radiotherapy to the eyelid, as in the treatment of paranasal sinus malignant neoplasms. Xeroderma pigmentosum also predisposes to basal cell carcinoma, squamous cell carcinoma, and malignant melanoma of the eyelid. Kaposi's sarcoma of the eyelid mainly occurs in persons with AIDS.

Basal cell carcinoma. Basal cell carcinoma accounts for about 90% of all eyelid malignancies in the United States, where it is 16 times more common than sebaceous carcinoma, the second most common eyelid malignancy, and 18.5 times more common than squamous cell carcinoma.[3] The lower eyelid is most frequently affected, followed by the upper eyelid and the inner and outer canthi[66,67] (Fig. 79-10). Basal cell carcinomas may be ulcerated, pigmented, superficial, or sclerosing. Many have elevated, pearly margins and ulcerated centers. Neglected tumors ("rodent ulcers") can extensively destroy facial structures producing ghastly disfigurement. The morphea variant of basal cell carcinoma is particularly aggressive and tends to infiltrate diffusely and invade the eyelid and orbit. During the excision of basal cell carcinomas the surgical margins of resection should be evaluated under frozen section control because this significantly reduces the incidence of tumor recurrence.[66]

Squamous cell carcinoma. Squamous cell carcinoma of the eyelid usually arises in elderly fair-skinned individuals. In the Western Hemisphere this tumor accounts for 9% of eyelid malignancies. The lower eyelid margin is most often involved, but the upper eyelid and lateral canthus are affected more often than with basal cell carcinoma. Especially if it arises from actinic keratosis, squamous cell carcinoma rarely invades the eye or orbit. Metastases are also rare.

Sebaceous carcinoma. Sebaceous carcinoma is an important neoplasm of the eyelid, where it accounts for about 1% to 3% of malignant epithelial tumors in the United States and is encountered almost as often as squamous cell carcinoma.[3] Rare before 40 years of age, sebaceous carcinoma is more common in females and Asians. This neoplasm may originate from the sebaceous glands of the tarsal plate (meibomian glands), eyelash follicles (glands of Zeis), or the caruncle. Two thirds of cases arise from the upper eyelid.

The sebaceous carcinoma often resembles a chalazion, but it may produce loss of eyelashes (madarosis). It can also present as a cutaneous horn or "cyst." Extensive pagetoid spread in the conjunctival epithelium may produce a clinical picture of unilateral chronic blepharoconjunctivitis ("masquerade syndrome").[68]

Sebaceous carcinomas manifest varying degrees of differentiation. Mitotic figures may be sparse in well-differentiated tumors, which contain lobules of cells with abundant, lipid-laden, finely vacuolated cytoplasm and well-defined cellular borders (Fig. 79-11). Such sebaceous differentiation tends to be most conspicuous in the center of the neoplastic lobules. As cellular differentiation decreases, the tumor cells manifest pronounced pleomorphism, prominent nucleoli, and numerous mitoses. Nuclei are hyperchromatic and pleomorphic, and peripheral palisading is absent.

Sebaceous carcinoma commonly invades adjacent conjunctival and cutaneous epithelium and spreads intraepithelially in a manner reminescent of the pagetoid spread of breast carcinoma in the skin of the nipple.[69] Individual or small clusters of intraepithelial neoplastic cells contain a vacuolated, foamy, lipid-containing cytoplasm.

Sebaceous carcinoma spreads locally by direct extension and commonly metastasizes to regional lymph node and to distant sites.[69] Indicators of a poor prognosis include origin from the meibomian glands or upper eyelid, prediagnostic symptoms for longer than 6 months, a tumor diameter of greater than 10 mm, an infiltrative growth pattern, poor sebaceous differentiation, pagetoid spread, and lymphatic, vascular, or orbital invasion. The overall mortality from eyelid sebaceous carcinoma is approximately 15%.

Melanoma. Primary melanomas of the eyelid are rare and account for less than 1% of all eyelid malignancies, with most having a nodular pattern.

Capillary hemangioma. Capillary hemangiomas of the eyelid are common in childhood and cause a strawberry-colored cutaneous mass. Although they involute spontaneously, capillary hemangiomas can be a major cosmetic blemish and frequently produce visual loss (amblyopia) by inducing astigmatism or occluding the pupil. The cellularity and mitotic activity in capillary hemangiomas may lead to undue concern about malignant potential.

Other tumors. Myxomas of the eyelid and conjunctiva are rare but may be part of Carney's syndrome (spotty pigmentation of the skin, overactivity of endocrine glands, and myxoma of the heart). The correct diagnosis may permit a life-threatening disorder to be treated.[70]

A plexiform neurofibroma of the eyelid often produces an S configuration of the ipsilateral upper eyelid fissure. On palpation this mass of enlarged nerves feels like a "bag of worms."

Uncommon eyelid neoplasms include the Merkel cell-tumor,[71] mucinous sweat gland carcinoma,[72] and sebaceous adenoma–related tumors in the Muir-Torre syndrome (multiple cutaneous keratoacanthomas or sebaceous tumors with visceral malignancies).[73]

Tumors of uvea

Melanoma. Uveal malignant melanoma is the most common primary intraocular tumor of adults in Europe and the United States, but it is rare— only about 1500 new tumors are diagnosed in the United States yearly. Intraocular malignant melanomas arise from melanocytes in the iris, ciliary body, and choroid and are usually solitary and unilateral. These tumors range from totally amelanotic white lesions to jet-black masses, and parts of individual tumors often vary greatly in pigment content.

Uveal melanomas are classified according to their site of origin (iris, choroid, or ciliary body) and are further subdivided into spindle, epithelioid and mixed-cell tumors (modified Callender classification).[74]

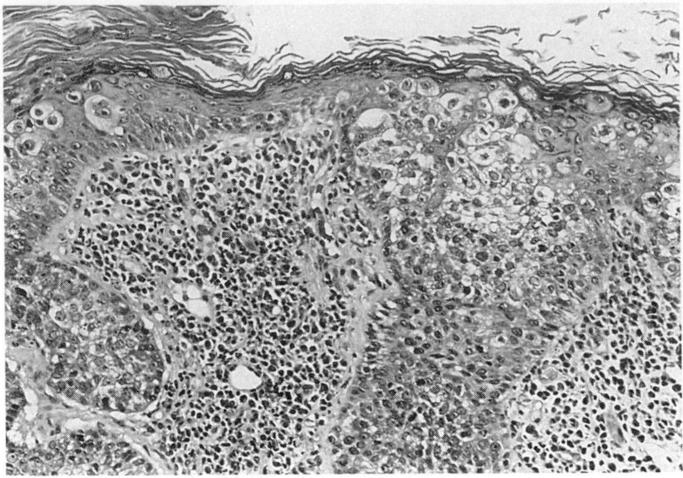

Fig. 79-11 Sebaceous gland carcinoma in eyelid. Tumor cells with foamy lipidized cytoplasm infiltrate epidermis in pagetoid fashion. Tumor arose from the meibomian glands. Pagetoid involvement of epidermis can be confused with an actinic keratosis histopathologically.

Uveal melanomas develop mainly in adulthood; the median age at diagnosis is 53 years. Only 1.6% of cases occur before 20 years of age. Melanomas involving the iris occur 1 to 2 decades earlier than those in the choroid and ciliary body, perhaps because they are more easily seen.

Race is a major risk factor for uveal melanomas and there is a propensity for white, blue-eyed individuals. This tumor is the commonest primary intraocular malignant neoplasm in whites, but, like cutaneous melanomas, it is rare in Asians and other pigmented races in Africa and Latin America. In the United States it occurs 8.5 to 15 times more often in whites than in blacks.

Lesions believed to predispose to uveal melanomas include uveal nevi, neurofibromatosis type I, the dysplastic nevus syndrome and the extensive diffuse melanocytosis of congenital ocular or oculodermal melanocytosis (nevus of Ota). The estimated rate of malignant transformation from choroidal nevi is 1 out of 10,000 to 15,000 per year. Frequent involvement of the exposed inferior part of the iris is suggestive that light may be a prediposing factor.

Most posterior uveal melanomas become symptomatic with visual loss because of retinal detachment, physical obscuration, or foveal edema. Infrequently, they present with a unilateral glaucoma or cataract, vitreous hemorrhage, or inflammatory manifestations secondary to tumor necrosis. Asymptomatic melanomas are occasionally discovered during a routine eye examination. A diffuse choroidal melanoma either causes a gradual visual deterioration over many years or becomes apparent only after extraocular or distant dissemination. A malignant iris melanoma can be heralded by an enlarging pigmented blemish, a change in eye color (iris heterochromia), and unilateral glaucoma.

The clinical differential diagnosis of uveal malignant melanoma includes benign nevi, hemangiomas, metastases from distant nonocular primary neoplasms, and other rare primary intraocular tumors (choroidal schwannomas and leiomyomas, adenomas and adenocarcinomas of the retinal or ciliary pigment epithelium, and choroidal osteomas), as well as non-neoplastic lesions such as posterior scleritis and age-related macular degeneration.[75]

Complications of intraocular melanomas include hemorrhage, cataract, glaucoma, retinal detachment, and inflammation. Blind, painful eyes with opaque media, glaucoma, or total retinal detachment sometimes harbor unsuspected melanomas when examined pathologically.

Initially, melanomas of the choroid or ciliary body are ovoid but choroidal tumors often rupture through Bruch's membrane and proliferate in the subretinal space, and so a characteristic mushroom or "collar button" configuration is assumed. A flat, diffuse, or multinodular growth pattern occasionally occurs but is more typical of metastatic carcinoma.

Spindle-shaped melanoma cells grow in a cohesive manner, forming a syncytium. Some spindle cells have slender nuclei (occasionally with a prominent longitudinal fold in the nuclear membrane) but without nucleoli (spindle A cells) (Fig. 79-12). Other spindle-shaped cells have plumper nuclei with small distinct nucleoli (spindle B-cells) (Fig. 79-13). Less-differentiated epithelioid cells are larger, polygonal, and are poorly cohesive with distinct cytoplasmic margins. Epithelioid cell nuclei are round or oval and have one or more prominent nucleoli, and their chromatin clumps along the nuclear membrane (Fig. 79-14).

Most primary uveal melanomas contain variable numbers of spindle A and B-cells and epithelioid cells (mixed cell melanomas) (Fig. 79-15). Poorly differentiated melanomas sometimes contain abundant cytoplasmic lipid ("balloon cell degeneration") or bizarre giant cells. Necrosis is common in uveal melanomas.

An exudative retinal detachment commonly accompanies a choroidal melanoma. The retina overlying the tumor is often atrophic, and the subretinal space contains protein-rich fluid. The detached part of the retina shows photoreceptor degeneration and, occasionally, microcystoid degeneration. Retinal pigment epithelial proliferation with the formation of drusen and

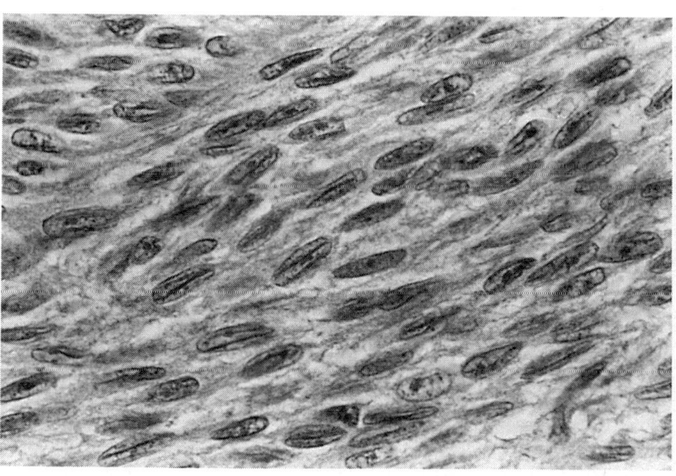

Fig. 79-12 Spindle A cell uveal melanoma, low-grade. Longitudinal chromatin stripes reflect folds in membrane of cigar-shaped nuclei of spindle A melanoma cells.

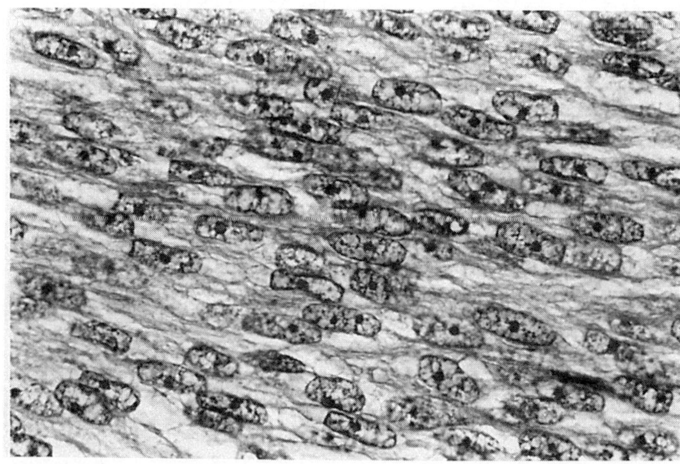

Fig. 79-13 Spindle B cell uveal melanoma. Spindle B-cells have plump oval nuclei and a distinct nucleolus compared to the low-grade type. Spindle melanoma cells form a syncytium.

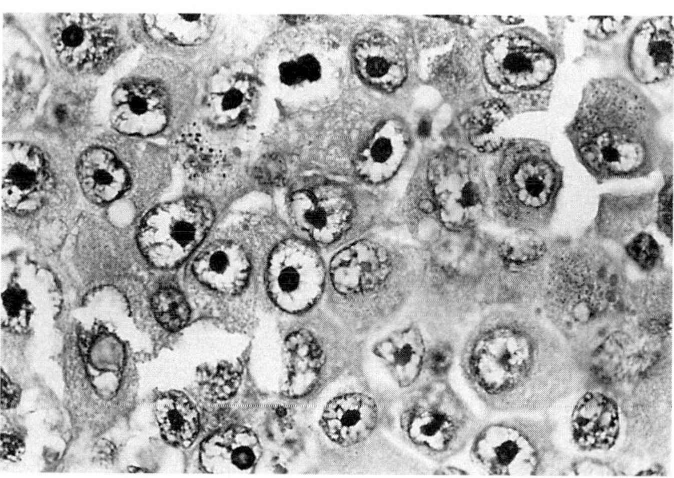

Fig. 79-14 Epithelioid cells, uveal malignant melanoma. Epithelioid melanoma cells are poorly cohesive and have distinct cytoplasmic margins. Epithelioid cell nuclei are large and round and have prominent nucleoli. The chromatin is often clumped along the inside of the nuclear membrane (peripheral margination of chromatin). Tumors with epithelioid cells have a poorer prognosis.

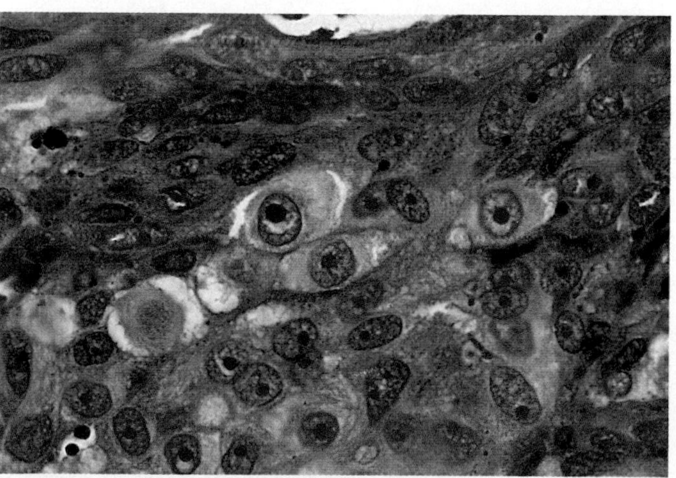

Fig. 79-15 Uveal malignant melanoma, mixed epithelioid and spindle cell type. Mixed cell tumors are fairly common. This field contains a clone of epithelioid cells.

other types of extracellular matrix material is often observed on the surface of the tumor. Highly elevated mushroom-shaped tumors occasionally infiltrate or even erode through the overlying retina, causing vitreous hemorrhage and epiretinal tumor seeding in exceptional cases. Histopathologic examination discloses that the clumps of orange pigment seen on the surface of actively growing tumors are clumps of macrophages laden with lipofuscin pigment from the disrupted retinal pigment epithelium.

Uveal melanomas commonly spread to the orbital tissues by traversing the sclera, especially through the emissarial canals of blood vessels and nerves, and form epibulbar nodules or an orbital mass. Such extraocular extension predisposes to tumor recurrence in the orbit after enucleation. Optic nerve invasion by melanomas occurs almost exclusively in blind glaucomatous eyes, and spread into the subarachnoid space is rare. Because the eye lacks lymphatics, uveal melanomas do not spread by this route. Metastases are almost never clinically evident when a uveal melanoma is first detected, but hepatic metastases are the most common first evidence of systemic spread. Approximately 50% of patients with uveal malignant melanomas die from widespread hematogenous metastases, and the liver is eventually involved in more than 90% of cases.

Tumor size and cell type are the most important prognostic factors.[76-78] Survival is poorer if uveal melanomas contain epithelioid cells (melanomas of the epithelioid or mixed epithelioid–spindle cell type). With uveal epithelioid melanomas the mortality after enucleation is 42% at 5 years and 63% at 15 years. Spindle cell tumors have a much better prognosis; survival is 90% at 5 years and 72% at 15 years. Although rare, fatal spindle A melanomas are recognized, but these have usually contained epithelioid cells on closer scrutiny and the melanomas have had several mitoses per high-power field.[79] Most tumors composed entirely of spindle A cells are now considered to be benign spindle cell nevi (Fig. 79-16). Most melanocytic tumors of the iris are nevi or low-grade spindle melanomas with an excellent prognosis. The 5-year survival of diffuse melanomas, which are usually of mixed-cell type, is 27%, probably reflecting delayed diagnosis. Totally necrotic melanomas have the same prognosis as those of mixed-cell type.

Large tumors (which are more likely to contain epithelioid cells) fare worse than small or medium-sized melanomas. The 5-year survival of small (<10 mm), medium (10 to 15 mm), and large (>15 mm) melanomas are 86%, 66%, and 56% respectively. These survival rates drop to 76%, 51%, and 41% at 10 years and 70%, 43%, and 35% at 15 years.

Less important prognostic factors according to multivariant statistical analysis include mitotic activity, the presence of extraocular extension, necrosis, pigmentation, anterior location, and lymphocytic infiltration.[80] Mitoses are uncommon in most tumors, and mitotic activity seems to be a better predictor in spindle cell tumors. Patients whose tumors contain certain microcirculatory patterns, such as vascular loops, are also more likely to die from metastatic melanoma.[81] T-lymphocytic infiltration of the tumor seems to affect survival adversely.[82]

Osteoma. Choroidal osteomas (osseous choristomas) are rare tumors that chiefly affect young women. They are often bilateral, peripapillary in location, and yellow-orange in color, and they have characteristic scalloped margins. Ultrasonography or computerized tomography scans readily establish the diagnosis clinically. A choroidal osteoma needs to be distinguished from the intraocular ossification of phthisis bulbi, but the bone is situated in choroid, not on its inner surface (unlike the bone produced by osseous metaplasia of the retinal pigment epithelium in phthisical eyes).

Hemangioma. Diffuse hemangiomas of the choroid occur chiefly in the Sturge-Weber syndrome.[83] They can also appear sporadically, usually as discrete, localized orange-red tumefactions. Cystoid degeneration of the retina and exudative retinal detachment commonly complicate choroidal hemangiomas. Choroidal hemangiomas in individuals with the Sturge-Weber syndrome obscure normal choroidal landmarks on ophthalmoscopy and impart a "tomato-ketchup" appearance to the fundus. The diffuse choroidal hemangioma is ipsilateral to the facial port-wine stain, and the affected eye is often glaucomatous. Most of these diffuse lesions have an associated exudative retinal detachment, and this or secondary glaucoma can lead to the loss of chronically affected eyes. The clinical appearance, intravenous fluorescein angiographic characteristics, and ultrasonographic characteristics of choroidal hemangiomas distinguish them from melanomas.[84]

Nevi. Most pigmented lesions of the iris are nevi.[85] Most choroidal nevi appear as flat patches of increased choroidal pigmentation 1 to 2 mm in diameter. Choroidal nevi are relatively common, and larger lesions may be extremely difficult

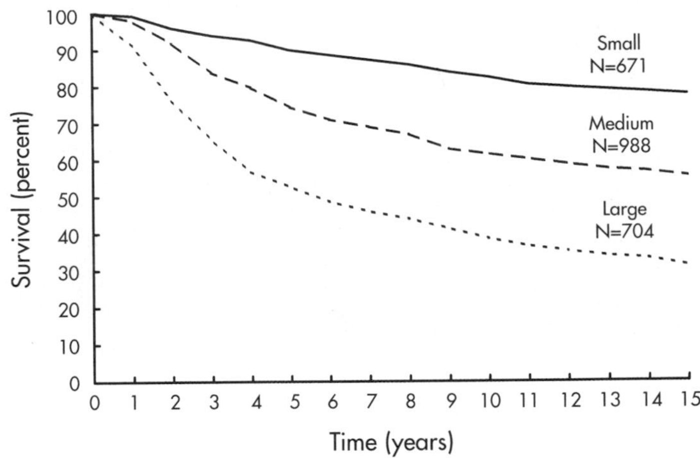

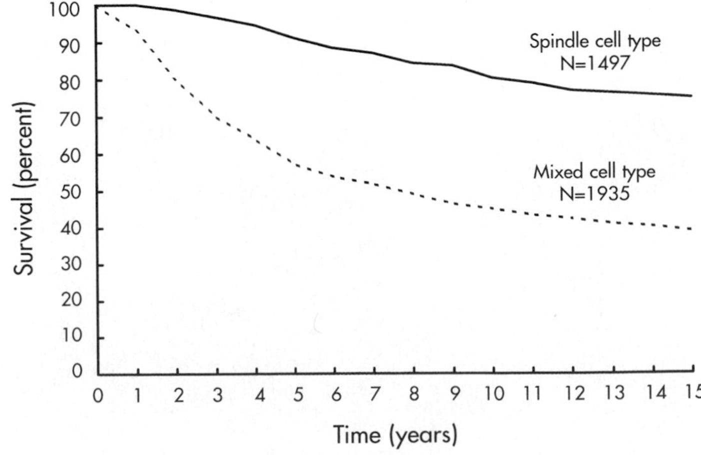

Fig. 79-16 Uveal malignant melanoma. Survival based on tumor size **A,** and cell type, **B.** (Modified from McLean IW, Foster WD, Zimmerman LE: *Hum Pathol* 113:123, 1982.)

to distinguish clinically from small malignant melanomas. Large choroidal nevi occasionally cause retinal pigment epithelial changes, focal visual field loss, and localized retinal detachment, and eyes containing them are, on rare occasions, enucleated because of suspected melanomas.

A specific type of nevus designated a melanocytoma *(magnocellular nevus)* can occur anywhere in the uveal tract but is most common in the optic nerve head. Bleached tissue sections disclose cells with bland nuclei and a low nuclear/cytoplasmic ratio. About 15% of these lesions enlarge on continued observation, but malignant transformation is rare.

Peripheral nerve tumors. Schwannomas and isolated neurofibromas rarely arise intraocularly, but a diffuse thickening of the choroid by hamartomatous tissue is prevalent in patients with von Recklinghausen's neurofibromatosis type 1 (NF1). Ovoid bodies that resemble tactile corpuscles, nevi, and increased numbers of ganglion cells may be observed in the hamartomatous uveal infiltrate of NF1 (Fig. 79-17).

Leiomyoma. Ocular leiomyomas are rare and found mainly in young women. Most are situated in the suprauveal space external to the stroma of the ciliary body or anterior choroid. Fibrillar eosinophilic cytoplasm and positive immunoreactivity for muscle markers distinguish these mildly cellular tumors from melanomas and neurogenic tumors. A variant of the leiomyoma called "mesectodermal leiomyoma" has a distinctly neural light microscopic appearance.

Lymphoid hyperplasia. In constrast to the conjunctiva and orbit, a benign reactive lymphoid hyperplasia involves the uvea in rare cases.

Tumors of retina and neural ectoderm

Retinoblastoma. Retinoblastoma is the most common primary intraocular tumor of childhood. In parts of the world where uveal melanoma is rare, it is probably the most frequent primary intraocular malignancy.[86] An immense preponderance of cases are diagnosed before 2 years of age; only about 8% of cases occur after 5 years of age.[87]

Most retinoblastomas (about 85% to 95%) develop sporadically, but some (5% to 10%) are inherited as an autosomal-recessive trait at the molecular level, even though pedigrees

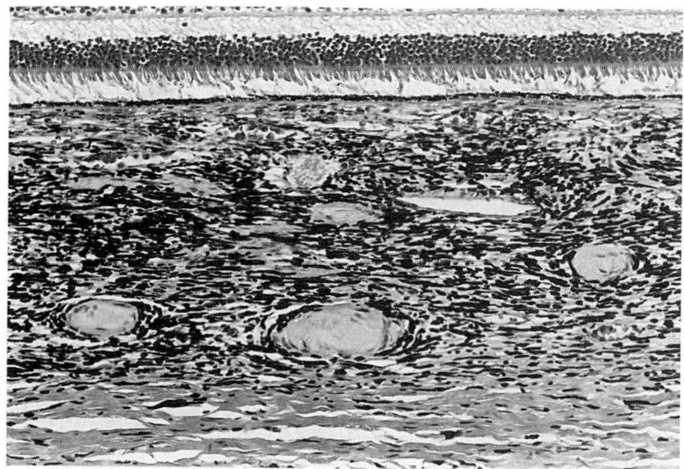

Fig. 79-17 Neurofibromatosis type I in choroidal infiltrate showing ovoid bodies. Ovoid bodies found in hamartomatously thickened choroid have been likened to tactile corpuscles. They are composed of concentric lamellae of Schwann cell processes.

once were suggestive of an autosomal-dominant mode of inheritance. Before an understanding of the molecular biology of retinoblastoma Knudson and colleagues[88] predicted that two mutations were needed, the first being either germinal or somatic and the second always somatic. The presence of bilateral retinoblastoma implies that the individual has a germline mutation and will transmit the retinoblastoma susceptibility gene (Rb) to 50% of the offspring, but the converse is not true. Germline mutations can result in unilateral sporadic tumors. About 25% of sporadic retinoblastomas result from new germinal mutations, and survivors of such tumors transmit retinoblastomas to their offspring, who are especially prone to bilateral neoplasms.

Although less than 5% of retinoblastomas are found in patients having obvious deletions in the long arm of chromosome 13 ($13q^-$ syndrome), the association of this syndrome with retinoblastoma led to the eventual mapping of the Rb gene on chromosome 13. The Rb-susceptibility gene is located on the long arm of chromosome 13 (13q14) at the Rb-1 locus in proximity to the gene for esterase D.[89] The Rb gene, which has been cloned and sequenced, has 27 exons and spans almost 200 kilo–base pairs of DNA.[90] It encodes the synthesis of a set of 105 kD nuclear phosphoproteins with DNA binding activity that act in the nucleus to modulate cell proliferation and prevent malignant transformation.[91] Rb protein is believed to bind directly to at least two other nuclear transcription factors that promote the expression of genes involved in cell growth, including the protein encoded by the *myc* proto-oncogene. A deletion or mutation in the Rb gene is insufficient to induce a retinoblastoma by itself. All retinoblastomas have chromosomal changes in addition to a homozygous loss of the gene.[92] A recent hypothesis indicates that the Rb gene normally may regulate a set of proto-oncogenes and that when both alleles of this gene are lost or inactivated the structural transforming gene (which may be an oncogene) is expressed. In common with neuroblastoma the oncogene MYCN (formerly called "N-*myc*") is amplified 10 to 200 times in some retinoblastomas and may play a role in their tumorigenesis. Certain tumor viruses, including human papillomavirus, adenovirus, and simian virus 40, apparently cause cancer by producing oncoproteins that bind to and inactivate Rb protein.

Retinoblastoma develops in carriers of familial (constitutional) retinoblastoma, who are hemizygous for the mutant Rb gene, if the single remaining functional copy of the gene is lost or inactivated in a retinal cell (usually during cellular division). Because the number of mitotic cell divisions occurring in each retina during development exceeds the spontaneous mutation rate of the Rb gene, the probability that one or more more retinal tumors will arise in each eye of persons hemizygous for the Rb gene is high.

Retinoblastomas arise from and focally destroy the retina, producing a cream-colored mass with scattered chalky white calcified flecks within yellowish necrotic regions. The retina often contains several distinct foci of tumor in the same eye, some of which represent different points of origin; others may reflect tumor implantations from intravitreal dissemination. Retinoblastomas may be endophytic, or exophytic, or have a mixed endophytic and exophytic growth pattern. A diffuse infiltrative retinoblastoma is rare.[93] Large retinoblastomas fill the eye, totally disrupting its internal architecture.

Retinoblastomas vary in their degree of differentiation. Some tumors are intensely cellular and composed of densely packed, poorly differentiated, round neuroblastic cells with hyperchromatic nuclei, scant cytoplasm, and abundant mitoses. Flexner-Wintersteiner rosettes (Fig. 79-18), delineated by a distinct circular lumen, are common in differentiated retinoblastomas.[94] The cells forming the rosette are joined by a series of zonulae adherentes analogous to the outer limiting membrane of the normal retina. The nuclei of the neoplastic cells are displaced away from the lumen because they differentiate toward photoreceptors. The most differentiated tumors contain bouquet like aggregates of relatively bland neoplastic photoreceptors called "fleurettes," which are composed of bulbous eosinophilic cell processes that correspond to photoreceptor inner segments.[95] Usually such differentiation is found in an area of tumor that appears relatively eosinophilic at low magnification (Fig. 79-19). Less frequently, the cells in retinoblastomas form rosettes that lack a central lumen (Homer Wright rosettes). Viable tumor cells cuffing blood vessels (pseudorosettes) frequently impart a multilobulated appearance to the tumor, and necrotic areas with calcification are seen a short distance from the vascularized regions (Fig. 79-20). DNA released from necrotic cells may precipitate and adhere to intraocular blood vessels, the iris, the trabecular meshwork, the lens capsule, and other ocular basement membranes.[96] Iris neovascularization is common and can cause peripheral anterior synechias and neovascular glaucoma.

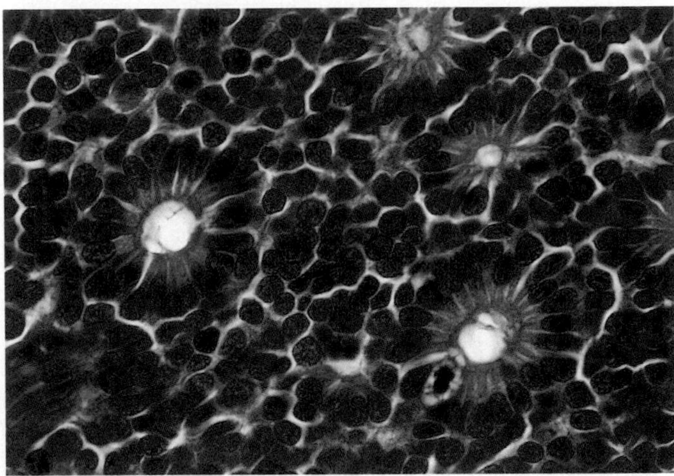

Fig. 79-18 Retinoblastoma with Flexner-Wintersteiner rosettes. The cells forming the rosettes are joined near their apices by a band of intercellular junctions analogous to the retinal external limiting membrane. The lumen corresponds to the subretinal space.

Retinoblastomas frequently spread intraocularly, producing multiple macroscopic retinal and vitreous seedings, and occasionally reach the anterior segment. They also have a propensity for optic nerve invasion and extend by this route toward the brain, seeding neoplastic cells into the cerebrospinal fluid (hence the importance of evaluation of the surgical margin of resection of the optic nerve in eyes enucleated with retinoblastomas). Retinoblastomas also invade the highly vascular choroid. The bone marrow is a common site of blood-borne metastases,[97] but surprisingly the lung is rarely involved. Retinoblastomas with extensive involvement of the anterior orbit and conjunctiva can spread through the lymphatics to cervical and preauricular lymph nodes. Infrequently, retinoblastomas spread extraocularly by scleral channels that contain blood vessels and nerves (emissarial canals). Neglected tumors fill the eye, totally disrupting its internal architecture, and then grow extraocularly, forming an orbital mass. Tumors that have extended into the orbit can invade the intracranial cavity through the orbital bones or foramina. Late metastases are rare; they usually occur within 1 to 2 years of diagnosis.

Favorable prognostic indicators include the presence of abundant fleurettes or Flexner-Wintersteiner rosettes. Ominous prognostic signs are optic nerve, choroidal, and orbital invasion. The degree of optic nerve invasion correlates with prognosis (no invasion, 8% mortality; invasion to lamina cribrosa, 15%; invasion posterior to lamina cribrosa, 44%; and invasion to line of transection or posterior to point of exit of central retinal vessels, 65%). Mortality is greater in eyes with massive choroidal invasion than in eyes with slight or no invasion.

The survival rate for retinoblastoma is usually good in developed countries (about 90%) because of early diagnosis and modern therapy, but fatalities are the rule in the absence of

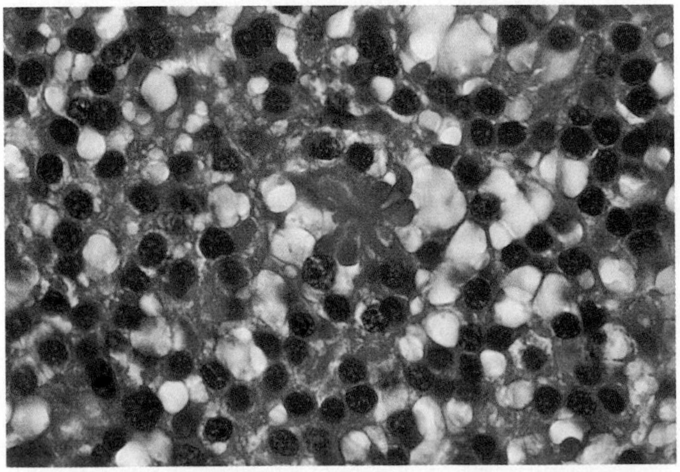

Fig. 79-19 Retinoblastoma with photoreceptor differentiation. Groups of bulbous abortive photoreceptor inner segments are called "fleurettes."

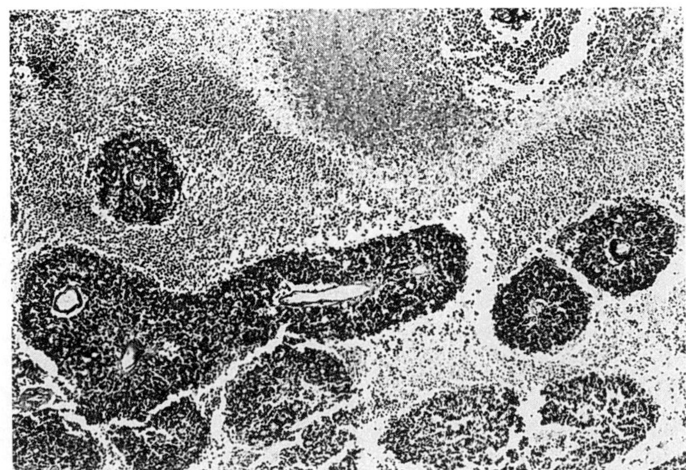

Fig. 79-20 Retinoblastoma. Cuffs of viable tumor cells about 100 μm in width encompass vessels in extensively necrotic tumor. A focus of dystrophic calcification is seen above.

treatment. Exceptionally, retinoblastomas regress spontaneously, causing a focal necrotic calcified mass mixed with scar tissue, often in a blind phthisical eye. An immunologic mechanism probably does not cause the regression because it can occur unilaterally in individuals with bilateral retinoblastomas.

Patients with germline deletions of the Rb gene sometimes develop a benign counterpart of retinoblastoma. This tumor is composed almost entirely of fleurettes and has been designated a retinocytoma (retinoma).[98-100] These retinomas may progress to malignancy,[92,101] and such progression indicates that other factors may be involved in malignant transformation.[102] Hemizygous carriers of a mutant Rb gene are at risk for numerous nonocular tumors,[103,104] including osteosarcoma, small cell lung, and breast carcinoma; about 16% of individuals with retinoblastomas develop another nonocular tumor within 20 years.[105] Aside from retinoblastoma the Rb gene predisposes to the development of several malignant neoplasms, particularly osteogenic sarcoma, Ewing's sarcoma, and pineal or suprasellar pineoblastoma ("trilateral retinoblastoma").[106,107] An independent primary intracranial neoplasm is found in about 3% of patients with bilateral retinoblastoma,[108] and this is usually diagnosed several years after the intraocular neoplasm.[106]

Medulloepithelioma. Medulloepitheliomas are composed of cords and sheets of polarized neuroepithelial cells that form elongated tubules and cystic structures in an abundant loose mesenchymal stroma rich in hyaluronic acid (analogous to primitive vitreous).[109,110] These rare pediatric tumors usually arise from the neuroectoderm on the surface of the ciliary body, but they rarely involve the optic nerve. Teratoid medulloepitheliomas contain heteroplastic elements such as hyaline cartilage, rhabdomyoblasts or striated muscle, and brain. Parts of malignant medulloepitheliomas resemble retinoblastoma and can contain Flexner-Wintersteiner rosettes. After orbital invasion intracranial extension can be fatal.

Intraocular large B-cell lymphoma. Systemic lymphomas that involve the eye secondarily usually infiltrate the uveal tract. Bilateral ocular involvement can occur in primary lymphomas of the central nervous system or as a primary intraocular lymphoma. Such large cell lymphomas opacify the vitreous (Fig. 79-21). The lymphoma cells can infiltrate the retina and typically accumulate between the retinal pigment epithelium and Bruch's membrane, forming characteristic yellowish plaques but sparing the choroid.[111]

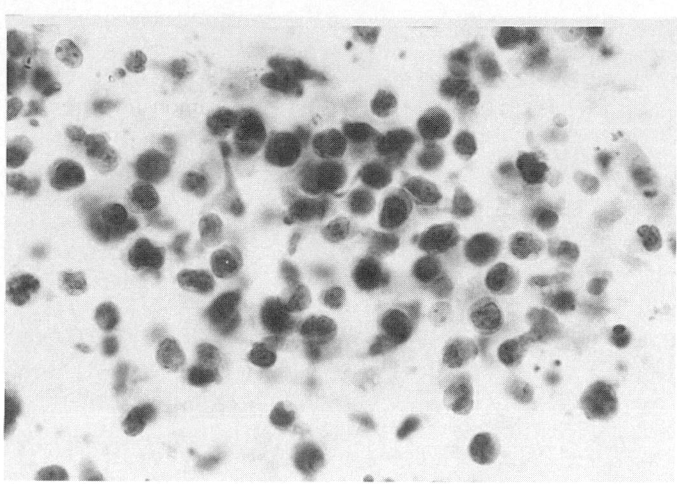

Fig. 79-21 Primary lymphoma of the central nervous system and retina. Lymphoma cells are seen in Millipore filter preparation of vitreous fluid. Bilateral vitreous opacification by lymphoma cells causes visual loss in elderly patients who are at risk for central nervous system lymphoma.

Tumors of orbit

The most frequently encountered orbital masses are inflammatory in nature and not neoplasms[112-117] (Figs. 79-22 and 79-23). The cause of most orbital tumors is unknown, but some (including osteosarcoma, chondrosarcoma, and leiomyosarcoma) have followed radiation to eyes with retinoblastoma. Orbital tumors commonly cause proptosis, and several potentially blinding complications, such as as corneal exposure with subsequent ulceration, secondary glaucoma, and optic nerve compression, may ensue.

Lymphoid tumors. Orbital lymphoid tumors are soft, friable, tan or salmon-colored masses that lack a connective tissue stroma.[52-54] They are pliable and mold to the globe and other orbital structures. Orbital lymphoid tumors typically occur as an insidious, painless, well-tolerated proptosis in older patients (average age at diagnosis 60 years). Sometimes an orbital tumor occurs as a conjunctival lymphoid mass. Orbital tumors are often sharply delimited by tissue planes that form linear margins, which are evident on imaging studies. In contrast to spherical epithelial neoplasms of the lacrimal gland, lymphomas diffusely infiltrate and thicken the gland. Ninety percent of orbital lymphomas involve the superior orbit behind the orbital septum, and more than 40% involve the lacrimal gland, especially the palpebral lobe. Bone destruction is rare except in multiple myeloma. Only a single extraocular muscle usually is affected, and ocular motility remains normal.

Although polyclonal reactive or atypical lymphoid hyperplasias occur, about two thirds are diffuse low-grade lymphomas composed of well-differentiated monoclonal B-lymphocytes. Some polyclonal reactive B-lymphocyte hyperplasias express immunoglobulin gene rearrangements using molecular genetic analysis. Although monoclonal lymphomatous orbital masses are regarded as neoplastic, many, such as those in the conjunctiva, do not progress to systemic disease. In common with mucosa-associated lymphoid tissue (MALT)–derived lymphomas they remain localized for a long time and are often preceded by an apparent reactive inflammatory stage. Most ocular and adnexal lymphomas are diffuse non-Hodgkin's lymphomas. Less than 15% are follicular or nodular lymphomas. T-cell lymphomas and Hodgkin's disease rarely involve the orbit. Many patients with orbital atypical lymphoid hyperplasia are preceded by or followed within 5 years by an extraorbital lymphoma. Histopathologic features of reactive lymphoid hyperplasia include germinal centers, plump hyperplastic vascular endothelial cells, and a polymorphous infiltrate of well-differentiated polyclonal lymphocytes with occasional plasma cells, macrophages, eosinophils, and reactive germinal follicles. These follicles are often irregular in shape and distribution, within a stroma containing scant fibrous tissue, and they often contain tingible body macrophages and significant mitoses.

Orbital lymphoid tumors need to be distinguished from the lymphocytic infiltration of Graves' disease. In Graves' disease a focal lymphocytic infiltrate is virtually limited to the extraocular muscles and spares the muscle tendon.

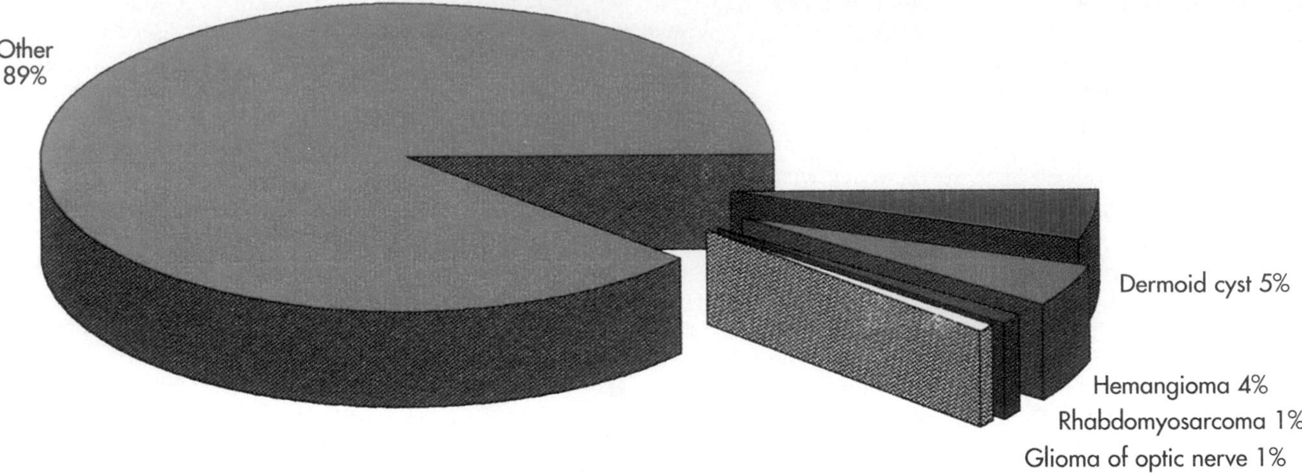

Fig. 79-22 Relative incidence of orbital masses in adults. (Based on series of 820 cases of Kennedy RE: *Trans Am Ophthalmol Soc* 82:134, 1984.)

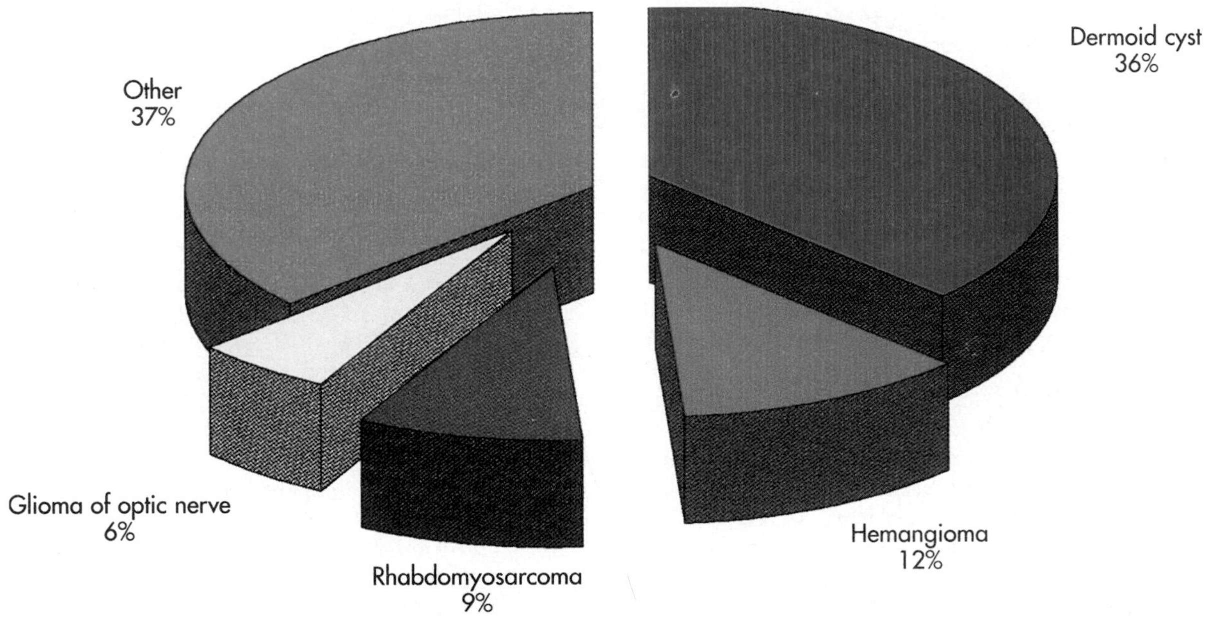

Fig. 79-23 Relative incidence of orbital masses in childhood. (Based on series of 358 cases reviewed by Iliff WJ, Green WR: Orbital tumors in children. In Jakobiec FA, editor: *Ocular and adnexal tumors,* Birmingham, Ala, 1978, Aesculapius.)

Tumors of nerves. Patients with NF1 are prone to juvenile pilocytic astrocytomas of the optic nerve, meningiomas, neurofibromas, schwannomas, and malignant peripheral nerve sheath tumors in the orbit and in other sites.[118]

Rhabdomyosarcoma. Orbital rhabdomyosarcoma is the most common orbital malignant neoplasm in childhood and embryonal, alveolar, botryoid and pleomorphic (differentiated) variants are recognized[119,120] (Fig. 79-24). Rhabdomyosarcoma must be excluded in any child who has orbital disease. The tumor usually does not arise from extraocular muscles and is hence believed to be spawned from pluripotential mesenchymal cells rather than from dedifferentiated striated muscle. The rapid growth of orbital rhabdomyosarcomas occasionally mimics inflammatory disease in this location. An embryonal rhabdomyosarcoma needs to be suspected when a malignant spindle cell tumor with prominent cytoplasmic eosinophilia is encountered in the orbit.

Fibrous histiocytoma. Fibrous histiocytoma, the most common mesenchymal tumor of the orbit in adults, has an apparent predilection for this site.[121] Aside from the benign variant, rare malignant fibrous histiocytomas and an intermediate locally aggressive form of the tumor are recognized. Benign and locally aggressive fibrous histiocytomas recur if incompletely excised and may undergo malignant transformation.

Hemangiopericytoma. Distant metastases develop in 15% of patients with orbital hemangiopericytomas,[122] but it is impossible to predict metastatic potential from histopathologic characteristics; benign-appearing tumors occasionally spawn metastases.

Cavernous hemangioma. Cavernous hemangioma is the commonest primary orbital tumor in adults. This benign, discrete, well-circumscribed, encapsulated, dusky red or purplish blue vascular mass (Fig. 79-25) typically causes a slowly progressive, relatively asymptomatic mild proptosis, especially in middle-aged women.[123] The mass is usually well tolerated, sparing vision and ocular motility. In computed tomographic studies radiographic contrast material may not be initially obvious because of the sluggish internal circulation of the lesion. The latter feature distinguishes cavernous hemangioma from the rarer highly vascular hemangiopericytoma, which contrast-enhances vividly.

Meningioma. Orbital meningiomas may arise from the optic nerve meninges or, rarely, from ectopic arachnoidal rests, but most represent an extension of an intracranial meningioma. Individuals with von Recklinghausen's neurofibromatosis are at risk for meningiomas, and a meningioma-suppressor gene is located on the long arm of chromosome 22.[124] Primary orbital meningiomas occur in adults and children and cause optic atrophy and visual loss by optic nerve compression. Most orbital meningiomas are meningothelial or transitional in type. Dilated blood vessels (retinal choroidal venous collaterals previously called "optociliary shunts") are often observed ophthalmoscopically on the optic disk. In contrast to gliomas, meningiomas frequently transgress the meninges surrounding the optic nerve and invade the orbital soft tissues. Orbital meningiomas need to be differentiated from psammatoid ossifying fibromas.[125]

Histiocytosis X. The orbit may be involved in Langerhans' cell histiocytosis (histiocytosis X), especially the eosinophilic granuloma variant.[126] Typically a cystic or erosive lesion develops in the supratemporal orbital bone.

Granulocytic sarcoma. Orbital lymphomas are extremely rare in childhood. If an apparent orbital lymphoma is encountered in this age group, acute lymphoblastic and myelogenous leukemia need to be ruled out. Granulocytic sarcoma (myeloid sarcoma, chloroma) may have a greenish hue caused by myeloperoxidase, and the Leder esterase stain is useful in establishing a diagnosis. Infiltration of the orbital tissues by leukemic cells may antedate the blood leukocytosis or even bone marrow involvement by months.[127]

Schwannoma. Orbital schwannomas are encapsulated, well-circumscribed tumors that can be confused with cavernous hemangiomas clinically. Because of their close relationship to peripheral nerves, schwannomas are often painful.

Lymphangioma. In childhood, orbital lymphangiomas may enlarge during upper respiratory infections, presumably because of hyperplasia of associated lymphoid tissue.[128] Rapid enlargement may result from hemorrhage into these progressive lesions, which may lead to the formation of a "chocolate cyst." The infiltrative nature of lymphangiomas makes them difficult to extirpate. Focal lymphoid infiltrates in the contiguous stroma, which may include germinal centers, serve to differentiate lymphangiomas from cavernous hemangiomas, particularly if there has been secondary intraluminal hemorrhage.

Tumors of lacrimal gland and lacrimal drainage apparatus

In nonreferral clinical practice inflammatory and lymphoid lesions of the lacrimal gland are encountered at least five times more often than primary epithelial tumors.[129] Most lesions of this modified salivary gland prompting biopsy or excision are lymphoid or inflammatory masses. Tumors of the lacrimal gland constitute only 10% to 15% of orbital lesions. Compared to the major salivary glands the lacrimal gland spawns a limited variety of primary epithelial tumors, but a greater proportion of them are malignant. About one half of epithelial tumors of the lacrimal gland are benign mixed tumors (pleomorphic adenomas) and half are malignant.[130] Lacrimal gland malignancies include adenoid cystic carcinomas, malignant mixed tumors derived from pleomorphic adenomas, and adenocarcinomas that arise *de novo*.[131]

Neoplasms of the lacrimal drainage apparatus are uncommon and include primary tumors, which are mainly epithelial in origin, and secondary lesions arising in the adjacent eyelid, nose, paranasal sinuses, and orbit (Table 79-3).

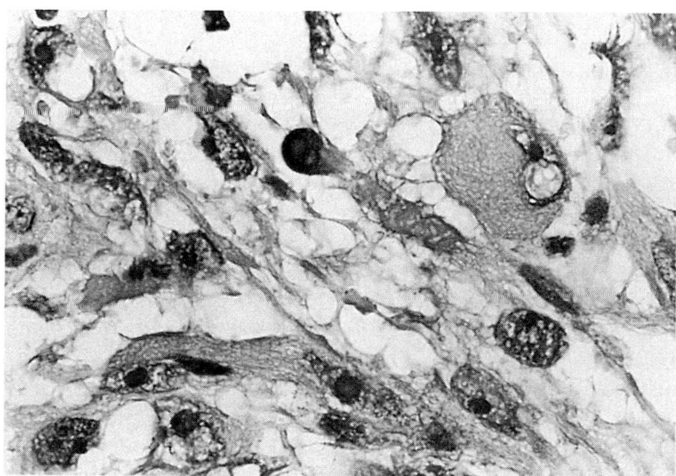

Fig. 79-24 Rhabdomyosarcoma. This orbital rhabdomyosarcoma contains cross striationa and rhabdomyoblasts. Many orbital rhabdomyosarcomas are embryonal and lack cross striations. The patient was 8 years old, the mean age for orbital rhabdomyosarcoma.

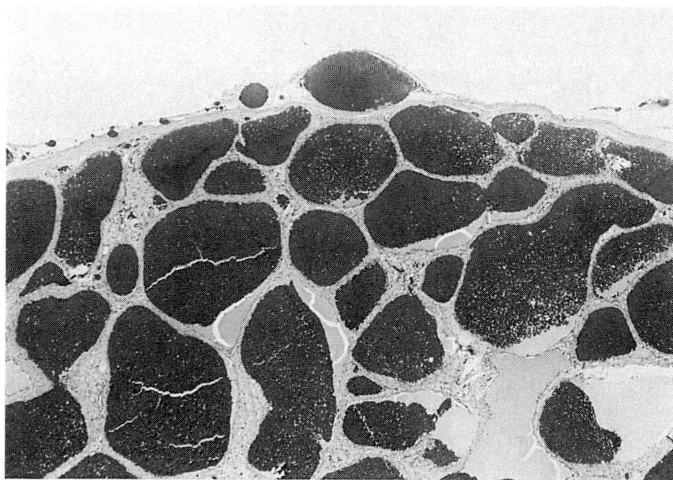

Fig. 79-25 Cavernous hemangioma in orbit. Encapsulated vascular tumor is composed of large blood-filled, endothelium-lined vascular spaces separated by fibrous septae.

Pleomorphic adenoma. Pleomorphic adenomas account for half of the lacrimal gland epithelial tumors. They resemble histologically the salivary gland tumor and contain a mixture of epithelial and mesenchymal elements.

Adenoid cystic carcinoma. Adenoid cystic carcinoma is the commonest malignant tumor of the lacrimal gland.[132,133] Despite its highly aggressive behavior, the individual neoplastic cells often possess a surprisingly bland cytologic appearance (Fig. 79-26). Perineural invasion is common and signifies the route of spread toward the brain. Tumors with foci of basaloid differentiation behave particularly aggressively.

Mucoepidermoid carcinoma. Rare in the lacrimal gland, mucoepidermoid carcinoma has a more favorable prognosis than other epithelial malignancies arising from this structure have.

Malignant mixed tumor. Malignant mixed tumors and adenocarcinomas that arise de novo are mostly encountered in older men and have an extremely poor prognosis. Affected individuals are generally older than those with benign mixed tumors. Patients usually die within 3 years with lung metastases and evidence of lymphatic spread. Malignant mixed tumors have features of a pleomorphic adenoma combined with malignant foci, especially of adenocarcinoma. Less often, foci of adenoid cystic, squamous cell, sebaceous, or undifferentiated carcinoma or sarcoma are identified.

Lacrimal sac tumors. Exophytic and inverted papillomas can arise from the transitional epithelial lining of the lacrimal-sac.[134] Lacrimal sac carcinomas are composed of either atypical transitional epithelial or squamous cells. Many arise from inverted papillomas. Other tumors occasionally involve the lacrimal sac (Table 79-3).

Tumors of optic nerve

Tumors of the optic nerve are uncommon and include gliomas, meningiomas, medulloepitheliomas, and metastatic and secondary neoplasms. Tumors, such as retinoblastomas, that spread into the optic nerve from the globe are more common than primary optic nerve neoplasms.

Optic nerve astrocytoma. Optic nerve pilocytic astrocytomas most often affect children (2 to 6 years of age) and diffusely enlarge the optic nerve. They typically have unilateral visual loss and painless axial proptosis. Optic atrophy or papilledema are usually present. Strabismus and an afferent pupillary defect are common. Computerized tomography discloses a fusiform swelling of the optic nerve and enlargement of the ipsilateral optic canal. Most optic nerve gliomas are juvenile pilocytic astrocytomas,[135] but, rarely, a glioblastoma multiforme (malignant glioma) arises in adults.[136] Rosenthal fibers are found in some tumors. In a small biopsy specimen a meningothelial proliferation surrounding an optic nerve glioma needs to be differentiated from a meningioma.[137] Optic nerve astrocytomas are frequently (as many as 50%) associated with NF1. When this occurs, the tumor cells often infiltrate the subarachnoid space around the nerve, forming a prominent thickened mantle, but the tumor remains confined by the nerve's dural sheath and does not invade the adjacent orbital tissues.

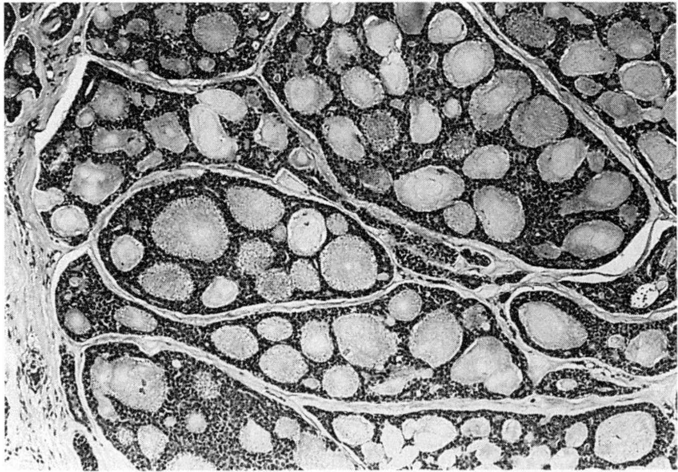

Fig. 79-26 Adenoid cystic carcinoma in lacrimal gland. Cribriform, or "Swiss cheese," pattern. Adenoid cystic carcinoma is the most common malignant epithelial tumor of the lacrimal gland.

Metastatic and secondary tumors

Blood-borne metastatic tumors to the eye and its adnexa are common and consist mostly of carcinomas and leukemias.[138,139] Sometimes the distant primary malignant neoplasm is a skin melanoma, and rarely a sarcoma. Although any carcinoma may, in theory, metastasize to the ocular tissues, carcinomas of the breast and lung account for most cases. Other, less common, primary sites include the kidney, gastrointestine, prostate, and testicle. Neuroblastoma frequently metastasizes to the orbit in infancy and childhood.

Direct invasion of the eye from contiguous structures also occurs. Neoplasms of the eyelid (basal cell, squamous cell, and sebaceous gland carcinomas and malignant melanomas), conjunctiva (squamous cell and mucoepidermoid carcinomas and malignant melanomas), globe (retinoblastoma and melanoma), paranasal sinuses, lacrimal sac, nose, pharynx, and intracranial cavity occasionally invade the orbit. Secondary orbital invasion by intracranial meningioma is more common than primary optic nerve meningiomas.

Eye. Although metastatic neoplasms in the eye are more common than primary tumors, many are not detected clinically. They may be bilateral and multiple. Any part of the uvea can be affected, but metastases usually involve the posterior choroid, which has the richest blood supply.[139] Metastases diffusely infiltrate the choroid and usually appear as relatively flat amelanotic masses with a secondary exudative retinal detachment. Because Bruch's membrane remains intact, choroidal metastases almost never assume the characteristic mushroom configuration that typifies many uveal melanomas. Metastases to the retina are rare. Metastatic skin melanoma often causes vitreous seeding by pigmented tumor cells. Systemic lymphomas preferentially infiltrate the uvea rather than the retina. Metastatic neoplasms from distant tissues rarely metastasize to the optic nerve.

Orbit. In children most orbital metastases stem from neuroblastoma or Ewing's sarcoma. Metastatic orbital neuroblastoma occurs in the late stages of the disease in children known to have had a neuroblastoma. Orbital metastases from neuroblastoma are often hemorrhagic and cause periocular ecchymoses ("raccoon eyes").

Eyelid. Metastases to the eyelid are rare but occasionally become evident before the primary neoplasm is recognized.[140] Sometimes they are the first detectable metastasis. Metastatic breast carcinoma in the eyelid is occasionally composed of individual cells with a histiocytoid appearance suggestive of macrophages.

Nonneoplastic masses

Epibulbar limbal choristoma. Dense fibrocollagenous tissue containing sebaceous glands, hair follicles, and sweat glands and covered by epidermis is frequently located in the inferotemporal conjunctiva at the corneoscleral junction (solid epibulbar dermoid). Adipose tissue may be a major component (dermolipoma). Sometimes this congenital choristomatous mass contains varying amounts of cartilage, lacrimal tissue, smooth muscle, adipose tissue. and even neural tissue (complex choristoma).

Epibulbar dermoids are usually isolated choristomas, but sometimes colobomas of the eyelid, Goldenhar syndrome (pretragal auricular appendages, blind-ended preauricular fistulas, vertebral anomalies) or the organoid nevus syndrome (linear nevus sebaceus of Jadassohn, Solomon syndrome) are associated.

Pinguecula. A focal yellowish white mound located adjacent to the corneoscleral limbus (pinguecula) is the commonest conjunctival lump.[141] Cosmesis is a rare indication for surgical removal. Despite its yellowish appearance, the lesion contains no fat but consists of sun-damaged connective tissue identical to that found in similarly injured skin ("actinic elastosis").[60,141,142] A prominent foreign-body giant cell reaction sometimes surrounds and incorporates the elastotic material. Most pingueculae are located nasal to the corneoscleral limbus.

Pterygium. A pterygium is a triangular fold of vascularized conjunctival tissue that invades the peripheral cornea.[141,142] It is probably caused by chronic solar ultraviolet radiation exposure or other environmental irritants, but a genetic predisposition also seems to exist. In most parts of the world pterygia are almost always associated with foci of actinic elastosis in the conjunctival connective tissue with basophilia, hyalinization, and vermiform collagen fibrils identical to the alterations that characterize pingueculae. In the cornea Bowman's layer may be focally destroyed, and the contiguous epithelium may be atrophic or thickened and dysplastic. The conjunctival epithelium frequently contains more mucus-secreting goblet cells than normal, and in keeping with its actinic basis the epithelium is occasionally dysplastic or has intraepithelial carcinoma. Pterygia frequently recur after excision.

Xanthelasma. Often seen in the elderly, xanthelasmas appear as soft, flat or slightly elevated, yellowish plaques on the skin of the inner canthi of the eyelids. These lesions are composed of lipid-laden macrophages (xanthoma cells), and although hyperlipidemia is sometimes associated, two thirds of affected individuals have normal serum lipid levels. Xanthelasmas need to be distinguished from necrobiotic xanthogranuloma, Erdheim-Chester disease, and lepromatous leprosy.

Cysts

Cysts of the eyelids and periocular skin include epidermal inclusion cysts, milia, eccrine and apocrine hidrocystomas (sudoriferous cysts, or sweat ductal retention cysts), and dermoid cysts. In the eyelid, conjunctiva, anterior chamber, or cornea, epithelial inclusion cysts may develop spontaneously or follow trauma or surgery.

The eccrine hidrocystoma is lined by a dual layer of ductal epithelium but lacks papillary infoldings. In tissue sections its multilocular lumen is empty or contains sparse granular eosinophilic material. The lining of the apocrine hidrocystoma consists of a double layer of columnar cells with eosinophilic cytoplasm and apical snouts and often manifests prominent papillary projections. Apocrine hidrocystomas often contain pigmented fluid that leads to the clinical suspicion of melanocytic lesions. Some regard this cyst as a variant of the papillary cystadenoma as opposed to a true retention cyst.

Dermoid cysts may occur in the eyelids, but they are much more common in the orbit. This congenital lesion results from the entrapment of skin in developing facial bony sutures. It frequently develops within the bones or soft tissue of the orbit, most commonly in the superotemporal quadrant of the anterior orbit, where it is often affixed to the underlying periosteum. A pronounced granulomatous inflammatory reaction with multinucleated giant cells replaces part of the lining if the cyst ruptures, and this may be the only component in tissue obtained at biopsy. Choristomatous cysts sometimes form in the orbit and carcinoma rarely arises from them.[143]

Mucoceles of the frontal and ethmoid sinuses occasionally extend into the orbit. These benign cystic lesions are lined by a ciliated pseudostratified columnar epithelium typical of respiratory mucosa and have an abundant mononuclear inflammatory cell infiltrate in the adjacent connective tissue.

VASCULAR DISORDERS

Hyperemia

In conjunctivitis, irrespective of cause, a diffuse hyperemia of the conjunctival vessels occurs, with the engorged vessels tapering toward the corneoscleral limbus. Another variety of pericorneal hyperemia (called "ciliary flush" by ophthalmologists) is associated with iritis and corneal epithelial defects and is caused by a reflex dilatation of deep vessels penetrating the interior of the globe.

Hemorrhage

Conjunctiva. Conjunctival hemorrhage may occur after blunt trauma, anoxia, or severe bouts of coughing, but it sometimes occurs spontaneously, often first being noted on arising after sleep. Conjunctival hemorrhages do not extend into the cornea because of the barrier imposed by the close apposition of the corneal epithelium to the underlying substantia propria.

Retina. Retinal hemorrhages are a feature of many disorders, including hypertension, diabetes mellitus, trauma, and central retinal vein occlusion. Based on their location, retinal hemorrhages have various shapes. Hemorrhage in the nerve fiber layer spreads between axons and causes a flame-shaped or splinter appearance on funduscopy, whereas deep retinal hemorrhages tend to be round. When located between the retinal pigment epithelium and Bruch's membrane, blood appears as a dark mass and clinically resembles a melanoma.

Choroid. Sudden decompression of the globe during accidental or surgical perforation may rupture a choroidal blood vessel and cause hemorrhagic detachment of the choroid. The enlarging suprachoroidal hematoma can displace the retina, vitreous, and other intraocular structures anteriorly, extruding them through the open wound (expulsive choroidal hemorrhage).

Anterior chamber. Most anterior chamber hemorrhages (hyphemas) in adults are caused by trauma and iris neovascularization; in children important causes of spontaneous hyphema include retinoblastoma and juvenile xanthogranuloma.[144] Blood in the anterior chamber gravitates to the most dependent part, forming a horizontal line of demarcation from the clear aqueous. Complications of hyphema include blood staining of the corneal stroma and glaucoma.

Vitreous. Vitreous hemorrhage may occur after vitreoretinal neovascularization (as in proliferative diabetic retinopathy, central or branch retinal vein occlusion, and sickle cell retinopathy), trauma, retinal tears, age-related macular degeneration, and, rarely, intraocular tumors. Chronic vitreous hemorrhage contains numerous erythrocyte ghost cells (erythroclasts), hemoglobin spherules, and macrophages laden with hemosiderin and other blood-breakdown products. Degenerated blood in chronic vitreous hemorrhage is yellow-ochre in color.

Ischemia

Retina. Hallmarks of retinal ischemia include cotton-wool spots, microaneurysms, capillary dropout, and neovascularization. Superficial white patches with fluffy margins that resemble cotton (cotton-wool spots) appear in the superficial retina in patients with hypertension, diabetic retinopathy, and central retinal vein occlusion, as well as in persons with AIDS and systemic lupus erythematosus in whom antigen-antibody complexes cause precapillary arteriolar occlusion. Caused by focal ischemic blockage of axoplasmic flow, cotton-wool spots consist of aggregates of swollen axons in the retinal nerve fiber layer. Some swollen axons are termed "cytoid bodies" because they resemble cells and contain eosinophilic nucleoids of dammed mitochondria and other cellular organelles. These cotton-wool spots portend the development of neovascularization in preproliferative diabetic retinopathy and central retinal vein occlusion.

Hard exudates, a clinical marker of retinal vascular incompetence, are pools of lipoproteinaceous material in the retinal outer plexiform layer, which is the watershed zone between the inner part of the retina supplied by the central retinal artery and the outer part nourished by the choroid.

Neovascularization

Ocular angiogenesis is believed to result from angiogenic factors produced by ischemic retina, intraocular tumors, or inflammatory reactions.[145] Neovascularization is a prominent feature of proliferative diabetic retinopathy, central retinal vascular occlusion, sickle cell retinopathy,[146] the retinopathy of prematurity, and other retinopathies associated with retinal ischemia caused by extensive nonperfusion of the retinal capillary bed. Chronic retinal hypoxia presumably provokes the liberation of a diffusible angiogenic factor.

Iris ("rubeosis iridis"). In iris neovascularization a fibrovascular layer extends along the normally avascular anterior surface of the iris, flattening it. The fibrovascular membrane contains myofibroblasts and blood vessels and extends into the anterior chamber angle, causing adhesions between the iris and the cornea (peripheral anterior synechiae) that block the trabecular meshwork. Myofibroblasts in the fibrovascular membrane are involved in synechia formation and exert traction, which draws the iris pigment epithelium around the pupillary margin (ectropion uveae).[147] The friable new vessels on the iris lack the thick collagenous mantle that distinguishes normal iris vessels and sometimes occlude the pupil. The vessels readily bleed, causing hyphema. In long-standing iris neovascularization corneal endothelial cells sometimes migrate onto the iris and elaborate a hyaline membrane. Most examples of iris neovascularization accompany retinal neovascularization and retinoblastoma. Iris neovascularization frequently develops or worsens in diabetics after cataract extraction, which removes a physical barrier to the anterior diffusion of angiogenic factor. Less common causes include chronic retinal detachment, intraocular tumors, chronic intraocular inflammation, and carotid artery occlusion.

Vitreoretinal. Vitreoretinal neovascularization is the dominant pathologic feature in proliferative diabetic retinopathy. The neovascularization begins within the retina and then breaches the retinal internal limiting membrane. The new vessels grow on the inner retina and the posterior surface of the vitreous after it has detached, fortifying residual vitreoretinal attachments to the optic disk and vessels. Neovascularization may erupt from the surface of the optic disk or the retina.

Occlusovascular diseases

Causes of ocular occlusovascular disease include thrombosis (as in atherosclerosis and giant cell arteritis[148,149]), embolism, stenosis (as in atherosclerosis), vascular compression, intravascular sludging or coagulation, and vasoconstriction (as in hypertensive retinopathy and migraine).

Central retinal artery occlusion. Most central retinal artery occlusions result from thrombosis or emboli. Affected elderly patients usually suffer from atherosclerosis, hypertension, diabetes mellitus, or giant cell arteritis (which may cause bilateral occlusion). Younger patients often have a cardiac myxoma, vasculitis, or anticardiolipin antibodies. Thrombosis usually relates to atherosclerosis in the central retinal artery posterior to the lamina cribrosa in the optic nerve head. Uncommon causes of central retinal artery occlusion include collagen vascular disease, aortic arch syndromes, homocystinuria, and other vasculitides.

The effect of vascular occlusion depends on the size of the vessel involved, the degree of resultant ischemia, and the nature of the embolus. Neurons of the retina, like those in the rest of the nervous system, are extremely susceptible to hypoxia. Coagulative necrosis of the inner retinal layers (supplied by the central retinal artery) often follows acute central retinal artery occlusion. In its acute stages, intracellular edema, manifested by retinal pallor, is prominent, especially in the macula (where the ganglion cells are most numerous). Cellular dissolution and nuclear pyknosis of the affected retinal layers are common. Chronic cases have ischemic atrophy of the inner retinal layers (the nerve fiber, ganglion cell, inner plexiform, and inner portion of the inner nuclear layers) supplied by the central retinal artery (Fig. 79-27).

Thrombosed vessels are found, and the inner retinal layers appear glassy and hyalinized. Because astrocytes and accessory glial cells perish in the retinal ictus, reactive gliosis does not occur. Retinal hemorrhages are usually absent because the intravascular pressure within the ischemic tissue is low.

Central retinal vein occlusion. Causes of central retinal vein occlusion include primary open-angle glaucoma, diabetes mellitus, polycythemia vera, mediastinal syndromes with increased venous pressure, dysproteinemias, and collagen vascular disease.[150,151] Occlusion of the central retinal vein or its branches often results when sclerotic arterioles impinge on neighboring veins within a common adventitial sheath, induc-

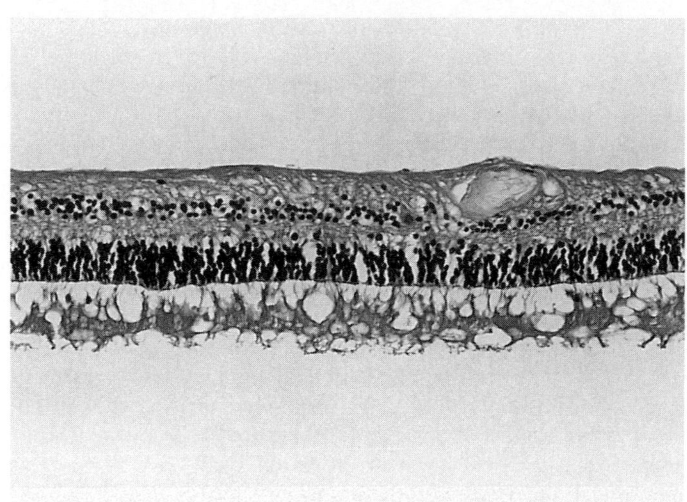

Fig. 79-27 Inner ischemic retinal atrophy caused by central retinal artery occlusion. A thrombosed retinal vessel is seen at right. All retinal layers supplied by the central retinal artery are atrophic. The outer nuclear and plexiform layers are normal. The retina is artifactitiously detached.

ing intravascular turbulence and thrombosis. Diabetic men over 50 years of age with hypertension and arteriosclerosis are especially at risk. Other predisposing conditions include drusen or edema of the optic nerve head. Arteriosclerosis of the central retinal artery is believed to promote venous occlusion by impinging on the neighboring central retinal vein within their shared adventitial sheath in the anterior part of the optic nerve. Central retinal vein occlusion after Waldenström's macroglobulinemia has been attributed to the associated hyperviscosity of the blood.

Retinal venous occlusion produces hemorrhagic infarction of the retina. Numerous deep and superficial retinal hemorrhages are caused by the high intravascular pressure, which dilates the veins and their collateral vessels. An impaired absorption of interstitial fluid produces edema of the optic nerve head and retina.

Most venous occlusions involve a branch of the central retinal vein, especially the superotemporal venule. Occlusion of the central retinal vein or a major branch produces a hemorrhagic infarction of retinal tissue. Early lesions are characterized by retinal edema, macular cystoid edema, numerous retinal and preretinal hemorrhages, shallow serous retinal detachment, and optic disk edema. Focal retinal necrosis and cytoid bodies occur with capillary nonperfusion in cases with retinal ischemia. Rarely, hemorrhage extends subretinally, causing hemorrhagic retinal detachment. Features of late lesions in enucleated eyes include disrupted retinal architecture with gliosis and hemosiderin-laden macrophages, thick-walled retinal vessels, and neovascularization of the retina, optic nerve head, and iris. The central retinal vein may be recanalized with endothelial proliferation and foci of chronic inflammation in its wall. Central retinal vein occlusion is divided into ischemic and nonischemic variants, depending on the degree of associated ischemia. In cases with retinal ischemia, neovascular glaucoma commonly ensues 2 to 3 months after central retinal vein occlusion ("100-day glaucoma," "thrombotic glaucoma") (see the discussion of glaucoma later in this chapter).

TRAUMA

Trauma to the eye commonly occurs in recreational, domestic, and occupational injuries, as well as in violence, automobile accidents, and child abuse.[152] The eye is frequently injured by a variety of household and industrial chemicals that enter it accidentally or maliciously. A seemingly infinite variety of foreign materials commonly injure the eye. Small particles commonly lodge in the superficial ocular tissues, but some penetrate into or through the eye. When the eye is ruptured or lacerated, the pressure of eyelid closure and surrounding orbital tissues tends to expel the intraocular contents. Structures including retina, uvea, and vitreous are frequently lost or incarcerated in the wound.

Blunt trauma

Physical injury to the eye commonly causes ecchymosis of the highly vascular eyelids ("black eye"), and when this occurs, other parts of the eye may also be injured. Superficial disruptions of the corneal epithelium occur after traumatic abrasions, prolonged wearing of a contact lens, foreign bodies on the eye, exposure to ultraviolet rays, and chemical exposure. Blunt trauma increases the intraorbital pressure momentarily, sometimes causing the bones in the floor of the orbit to fracture into the maxillary sinus ("blowout fracture"). Enophthalmos and diminished motility caused by entrapment of the inferior rectus muscle often result. Blunt trauma to the eye may rupture the eyeball, especially at the corneoscleral junction or where the sclera is thinnest immediately behind the insertion of the rectus muscles. After perforating ocular trauma, fibroblasts and vessels can invade the vitreous along tracks of hemorrhage and cause connective tissue bands.

Intraocular foreign bodies

A variety of foreign bodies may accompany sharp objects that perforate the globe or enter it as projectiles. Some foreign bodies incite an inflammatory reaction, which may be granulomatous. Sterile foreign objects may not evoke inflammation or other adverse effects. Iron-containing foreign bodies are especially toxic to the retina and aqueous outflow pathways and may discolor the ocular tissue (siderosis bulbi). In siderosis, iron deposits in epithelial or neuroectodermal derivatives (epithelia of cornea, lens, and ciliary body; iris musculature, retina; and retinal pigment epithelium). A similar deposition of iron may occur after intraocular hemorrhage (ocular hemosiderosis). Foreign bodies containing more than 90% copper incite a prominent sterile purulent reaction. Brass or bronze alloys that contain 70% to 90% copper can produce chalcosis, which is characterized by the deposition of copper in Descemet's membrane and the lens capsule. Lead, zinc, nickel, aluminum, and mercury may also evoke intraocular inflammation. Energy-dispersive x-ray microanalysis is often helpful in identifying the composition of intraocular foreign bodies.[153]

Intraoperative vitreous loss and incarceration predispose to infection, retinal detachment, and defective wound healing. Incarcerated vitreous can serve as a scaffold for fibroblastic proliferation in the anterior chamber (fibrous ingrowth). Rarely, corneal or conjunctival epithelium enters the eye through inadequately apposed surgical wounds or intraoperative seeding. An intraocular surface epithelial proliferation

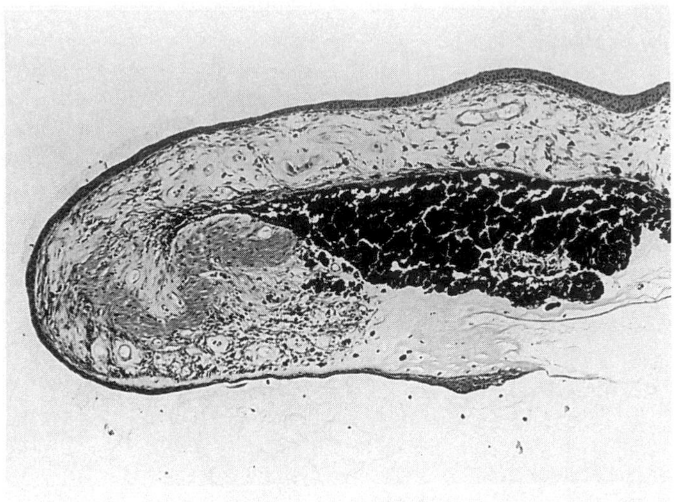

Fig. 79-28 Epithelial downgrowth. Sheet of proliferating ocular surface epithelium flattens anterior surface of the iris and extends around distorted pupil onto its posterior surface. The epithelium gained access to the interior of the eye through a poorly apposed surgical wound.

(epithelial downgrowth) (Fig. 79-28) causes intractable secondary glaucoma.

THE EYE IN SYSTEMIC DISEASE

The eye is involved in numerous systemic diseases[154] (Table 79-4).

Arteriolosclerosis

Chronic hypertension and probably aging induce onionskin perivascular fibrosis in the normally transparent walls of retinal arterioles. Thickening of the arteriolar media and adventitia and subintimal hyaline deposition gradually opacifies the vessel walls, widening the vascular light reflex, and obscuring the column of blood. The vessels first appear orange on ophthalmoscopic examination ("copper wiring"), but in advanced cases the intra-arteriolar blood becomes totally hidden by fibrosis and the sclerotic vessels appear as white threads ("silver wiring"). The thickened retinal arterioles become attenuated, increasingly tortuous, and of irregular caliber, and where they cross venules the latter are partly hidden and may appear kinked (arteriovenous nicking). Thickening of the venular wall rather than an impediment to blood flow caused by compression produces this effect; the column of blood proximal to the compression is not wider than the part distal to the crossing. Small superficial or deep retina hemorrhages often accompany retinal arteriolosclerosis.

Hypertension

Hypertensive retinopathy. Severe systemic hypertension produces a characteristic retinopathy that reflects vascular incompetence and disruption of the blood-retinal barrier. Retinal arteriolar narrowing and focal vasospasm is caused by acute, severe elevations of the blood pressure. Prolonged persistent vasospasm produces necrosis of retinal muscular and endothelial cells. Cotton-wool spots ("cytoid bodies") and areas of retinal infarction result from occlusion of small damaged vessels. Vascular incompetence caused by endothelial damage leads to hemorrhage, exudation, retinal edema, and even exudative serous retinal detachment. Arteriolosclerosis accompanies long-standing hypertension and commonly affects the retinal and choroidal vessels.

Hypertension commonly affects the retina, causing abnormalities that are readily seen with the ophthalmoscope and that relate to the severity of the hypertension. Hypertensive retinopathy has been classified according to severity as grades 1 through 4, with the higher numbers having more serious changes and a poorer prognosis than the lower ones. Features of hypertensive retinopathy include focal spasm, variable degrees of arteriolar narrowing, hemorrhages in the retinal nerve fiber layer ("flame-shaped hemorrhages"), and microaneurysms. In cases of severe hypertension, the retinal arterioles are much narrower than normal, and exudative retinal detachment and edema of the optic nerve head ensue. The latter serves as a clinical marker for malignant hypertension and impending hypertensive encephalopathy. Focal areas of choroidal infarction with secondary pigmentation (Elschnig spots and Seegrist streaks) are found in some patients with malignant hypertension. Electron microscopy of retinal vessels in severe hypertension discloses endothelial degeneration, necrosis of vascular smooth muscle, and insudation of fibrin-rich plasma in the vessel wall. In malignant hypertension, a necrotizing arteriolitis occurs, with fibrinoid necrosis and thrombosis of the precapillary retinal and choroidal arterioles. The retinal exudates frequently are arranged in a stellate configuration around the fovea ("macular star"), reflecting the orientation of axons in the perifoveal outer plexiform layer (nerve fibers of Henle).

Diabetes mellitus

Ocular symptoms occur in 20% to 40% of diabetics at the clinical onset of this common cause of blindness.[155] Visual loss, attributable largely to diabetic retinopathy, complicates the latter stages of the disease and usually takes years to develop. The retinopathy, which is divided into background (nonproliferative), preproliferative, and proliferative types, is not related to the cause of the diabetes, but, like other delayed lesions in diabetes mellitus, it is an outcome of diabetic microangiopathy. Retinal edema, exudation, and hemorrhages result from leakage of incompetent blood vessels. A preferential loss of pericytes in the capillaries in the early stages of diabetic retinopathy is believed to contribute to a breakdown in the blood-retinal barrier and vascular incompetence. Diabetic retinal microangiography correlates directly with diabetic glomerulosclerosis, and the risk of diabetic retinopathy decreases with better control of the hyperglycemia.[155]

Diabetic retinopathy is typified histopathologically by a characteristic microangiopathy that is readily detected in trypsin-digested retinal flat preparations.[156,157] Prominent leaky capillary microaneurysms (50 to 100 μm in diameter) are present (mainly in the posterior retina). In contrast to normal retinal capillaries, which have equal numbers of endothelial cells and pericytes, pericytes are lost, and the endothelial cell to pericyte ratio is greater than 1. Parts of the retinal capillary network become obliterated. Trypsin retinal digestions reveal totally acellular and occluded vessels in these areas of capillary nonperfusion. "Blot-and-dot" hemorrhages occur mostly in the inner nuclear and outer plexiform layers of the

Table 79-4 Noninherited systemic disease with ocular involvement

Cardiovascular disease	**Chromosomal disorders**
Aortic arch syndrome (Takayasu's disease, pulseless disease)	Deletion of short arm of chromosome 5 (5p-)
Atherosclerosis	Deletion of long arm of chromosome 13 (13q-)
Atrial myxoma	Deletion of short arm of chomosome 18 (18p-)
Bacterial endocarditis	Disseminated intravascular coagulation
Calcified cardiac valves	Down syndrome
Cardiac mural thrombi	**Fractures**
Carotid cavernous fistula	Fractures of long bones
Carotid ischemia	**Endocrine disorders**
Giant cell arteritis	Hyperparathyroidism
Hypertension	Hyperthyroidism
Malignant hypertension	Jaundice
Nutritional disorders	Liver disease
Avitaminosis A	Macroglobulinemia
Vitamin D toxication	Multiple myeloma
Diseases caused by organisms	**Renal disorders**
Behçet's disease	Nephroblastoma (Wilms tumor)
Cytomegalovirus	Severe renal disease
Measles	**Bone disorders**
Rubella	Paget's disease of bone
Toxoplasmosis	Pernicious anemia
Typhoid fever	Collagen disease
Syphilis	Systemic lupus erythematosus
Onchocerciasis	Systemic sclerosis
Benign monoclonal hypergammopathies	Polyarteritis nodosa
Benign mucous membrane pemphigoid	Psoriatic arthritis
Drugs	Retinopathy of prematurity
Chloroquine	**Autoimmune diseases**
Chlorpromazine	Rheumatoid arthritis
Intravenous drug addiction	Sjögren's syndrome
Quinacrine hydrochloride (atabrine)	Smallpox vaccination
Metabolic diseases	Stevens-Johnson syndrome
Cretinism	Still's disease
Diabetes mellitus	**Idiopathic disorders and syndromes**
Hypocalcemia	Sarcoidosis
de Lange syndrome	Sturge-Weber syndrome
	Sudden barometric decompression
	Surgical procedures or accidental injuries to neck or thorax

retina. Retinal exudates are rich in lipid (because of the hyperlipoproteinemia of diabetics).

In proliferative diabetic retinopathy an extensive network of delicate newly formed blood vessels surrounded by fibrous and glial tissue invade the vitreous from the region of the optic disk or the inner retina (Fig. 79-29). The neovascularization is associated with a proliferation and migration of astrocytes, which grow around the new vessels to form delicate white veils (gliosis).

Retinal ischemia, which can account for most features of diabetic retinopathy, including the cotton-wool spots and retinal neovascularization, may result from narrowing or occlusion of retinal arterioles (as from arteriolosclerosis or platelet and lipid thrombi), or from atheromatosis of the central retinal or ophthalmic arteries.

The neovascularization of the retina and iris in diabetes is believed to follow the release of angiogenic factors from ischemic parts of the retina. Fragile new vessels arising from the retina break through the retinal internal limiting membrane and grow on the inner retina and posterior surface of the detached vitreous. They rupture, producing vitreous hemorrhage and progressive vitreoretinal neovascularization, and fibrosis results in tractional detachment of the macula and

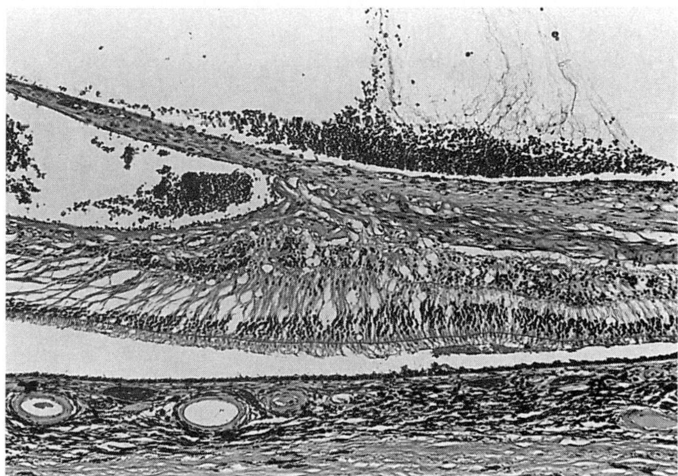

Fig. 79-29 Proliferative diabetic retinopathy. Neovascularization grows on anterior surface of retina and extends onto the posterior face of the detached vitreous. Hemorrhage is present in the vitreous and the subhyaloid space. The vitreoretinal membrane is beginning to cause a tractional retinal detachment.

other parts of the retina. The end stage of proliferative diabetic retinopathy is known as "retinitis proliferans."

The progression of proliferative diabetic retinopathy is retarded by treatment of the retina in multiple sites by laser photocoagulation (panretinal photocoagulation). This is believed to be accomplished by destruction of photoreceptors, which consume a considerable amount of oxygen, or by enabling more oxygen to reach the retina from the highly vascular choroid.

Thyroid eye disease

Graves' disease is a disorder that affects the thyroid gland and orbital structures, especially the extraocular muscle.[158,159] Forward protrusion of the eyeball from the orbit (exophthalmos) results from an increase in the volume of orbital tissue produced by imbibed water caused by the osmotic pressure of excessive orbital glycosaminoglycans and enlargement of extraocular muscles infiltrated with lymphocytes and other mononuclear cells.

The enlarged extraocular muscles contain patchy infiltrates of lymphocytes and plasma cells, progressive endomysial fibrosis, and an accumulation of glycosaminoglycans (Figs. 79-30 and 79-31). The inflammation characteristically spares the muscle tendon and the orbital fat.

Although usually bilateral, one side may be involved earlier or more extensively than the other. Other ocular manifestations of hyperthyroidism include retraction of the upper eyelid (because of increased sympathetic tone) and a characteristic stare caused by exposure of the conjunctiva above the corneoscleral limbus. Exophthalmos caused by thyroid disease usually occurs in early adult life, especially in women, who are affected more often than men (about 4 to 1). It may be severe and progressive, particularly in middle life, when the exophthalmos no longer correlates well with the state of the thyroid function. Edema of the eyelid and conjunctiva and limited ocular motility may be associated.

The pathogenesis of dysthyroid exophthalmos remains uncertain, but affected individuals appear to develop autoimmunity to several antigens, including thyroglobulin, thyroid microsomes (thyroid peroxisomes), and the receptor for thyroid-stimulating hormone on the thyroid cell surface. Most of these immunoglobulins do not seem to cause dysthyroid exophthalmos. Because portions of thyroglobulin and acetylcholine possess identical amino acid sequences, a shared epitope is possible, but this would not account for the predilection for the extraocular muscles. An autoimmune reaction involving sensitized lymphocytes presumably takes place on the surface of extraocular muscles and in other orbital tissues.[160,161] Thyroglobulin-antithyroglobulin complexes bind with greater affinity to extraocular muscle membranes than to other tissue membranes.

Exophthalmos-producing substances have been identified in pituitary extracts, in sera of patients with Graves' disease, and in digests of thyroid-stimulating hormone, but the significance of these substances in the pathogenesis of dysthyroid exophthalmos remains uncertain.

Sarcoidosis

Although any ocular and orbital tissue may be involved in sarcoidosis, this granulomatous disease has a predilection for the anterior segment of the eye.[162] Ocular involvement is usually bilateral and is most often a granulomatous uveitis. Other ocular manifestations include band keratopathy, cataracts, retinal vascularization, vitreous hemorrhage, Mikulicz's syndrome, and granulomatous dacryoadenitis (sometimes bilateral). Because of their common involvement in sarcoidosis, the conjunctiva[163] and lacrimal gland are frequently biopsied in suspected sarcoidosis. Light microscopy reveals the typical non necrotizing granulomatous inflammation in the absence of stainable microorganisms. Because the granulomatous inflammation may be focal, step sections through the entire biopsy specimen is often indicated in clinically suspected sarcoidosis.

Rheumatoid arthritis

The cornea and sclera are frequently affected in rheumatoid arthritis. Individuals with rheumatoid arthritis are susceptible to scleritis and spontaneous thinning of the corneal stroma.[164] Stromal tissue is often lost without an associated inflammatory

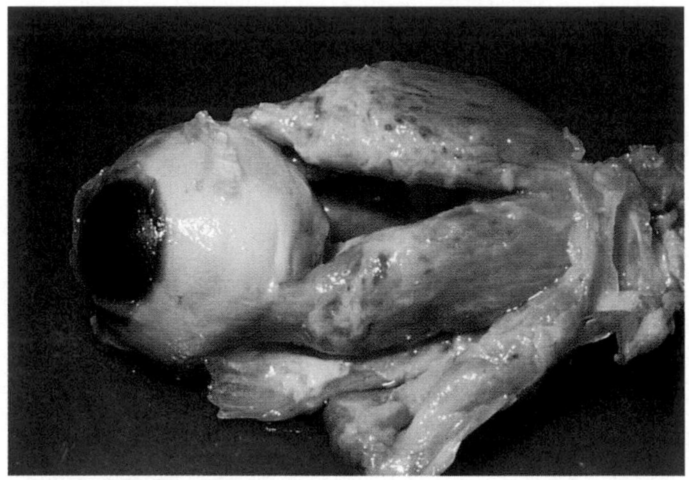

Fig. 79-30 Graves' orbitopathy. Postmortem exenteration specimen showing massive enlargement of extraocular muscles. (From Hufnagel TJ, Hickey WF, Cobbs WH et al: *Ophthalmology* 91:1411, 1984.)

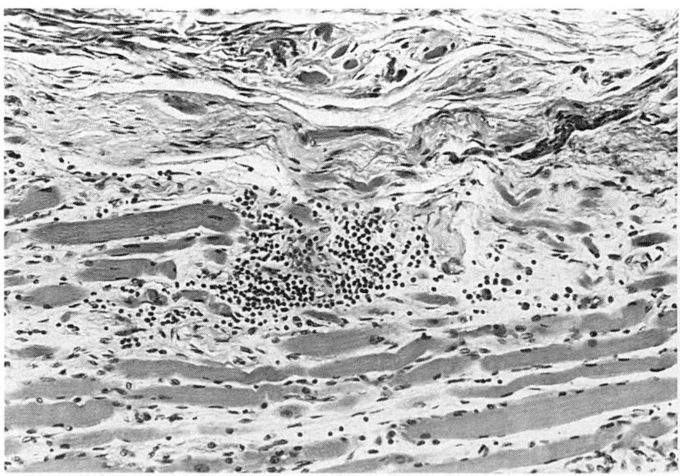

Fig. 79-31 Graves' orbitopathy. Extraocular muscle contains patchy foci of chronic inflammation. Fibrosis separates myofibers. Chronic inflammation in Graves' disease typically spares extraocular muscle tendon and orbital fat.

infiltrate in the keratopathy of rheumatoid arthritis. The peripheral cornea becomes thin more often than the central cornea, but the latter more frequently leads to perforation. In some instances a full-thickness perforation develops, whereas in others the stromal tissue is lost but Descemet's membrane remains intact (descemetocele).

SPECIFIC OCULAR DISORDERS

Glaucoma

Glaucoma is a group of disorders that share the common denominator of an optic neuropathy associated with a characteristic excavation of the optic disk and a progressive loss of visual field sensitivity. In most cases the intraocular pressure is elevated. The condition may develop in a person without an apparent antecedent underlying ocular disease (primary glaucomas), or it may follow or occur concomitantly with a known ocular disorder (secondary glaucomas). Primary and secondary glaucomas are subdivided into open-angle and closed-angle types, depending on whether the iridocorneal angle appears open or closed. Glaucoma can also be subdivided into congenital (developmental) or acquired types, depending on the time of onset.

Glaucoma almost always follows a congenital or acquired lesion of the anterior segment of the eye that mechanically obstructs the outflow of aqueous. Glaucoma resulting from a hypersecretion of aqueous is extremely rare. Individuals vary in their ability to tolerate elevated intraocular pressure. Some do not develop visual field loss or optic atrophy after having ocular hypertension for many years; others suffer damage at normal levels of intraocular pressure. In adults prolonged ocular hypertension usually leads to a characteristic cupped excavation of the optic disk (glaucomatous cupping) and a nasalward displacement of the retinal blood vessels (Fig. 79-32). Cupping of the optic disk is less prominent in infants. The ganglion cell layer of the retina degenerates, and optic atrophy, with a loss of axons, gliosis, and thickening of the pial septa, follows the retinal degeneration and damage to the nerve fibers at the optic disk. The outer retina remains intact (Fig. 79-33). Glaucomatous eyes rarely enlarge after 3 years of age because the sclera becomes rigid.

Chronically elevated intraocular pressure probably destroys retinal ganglion cells by compressing their axons as they exit the eye through pores of the specialized area of the sclera (lamina cribrosa) to form the optic nerve.[165-167] Cupping of the optic disk in glaucoma indicates that elevation of intraocular pressure may be involved in the pathogenesis of axonal loss. A pressure gradient across the lamina cribrosa induced by high intraocular pressure bows the lamina cribrosa posteriorly, distorting its pores and compressing the axons. Experimental tracer studies indicate that axonal compression in the lamina cribrosa greatly impedes orthograde and retrograde axoplasmic transport.

Histopathologic studies on eyes with glaucoma discloses abnormalities relevant to the effects of elevated intraocular pressure, such as a loss of ganglion cells and axons in the retinal nerve fiber layer, posterior bowing of the lamina cribrosa, excavation of the optic nerve head ("glaucomatous cupping"), and optic atrophy. Sometimes the latter is accompanied by an accumulation of hyaluronic acid within the optic nerve (Schnabel's cavernous atrophy). With long-standing glaucoma the corneal endothelium may be deficient, and the cornea may have features of a bullous keratopathy. Most enucleated blind glaucomatous eyes have secondary closed-angle glaucoma. Pathologic alterations relevant to the cause of the glaucoma may also be apparent. These abnormalities include the presence of epithelium on the surface of the iris and even in the vitreous (epithelial downgrowth). Iris neovascularization is found in cases of neovascular glaucoma, the most common and clinically significant form of secondary closed-angle glaucoma.

Primary open-angle glaucoma. Primary open-angle glaucoma, the commonest type of glaucoma, is a major blinding disorder in the United States and some other countries. In the United States it affects 1% to 3% of the population over 40 years of age and occurs principally in the sixth decade. A frequent positive family history points to an inherited predisposition, and at least some cases are caused by a gene on chromo-

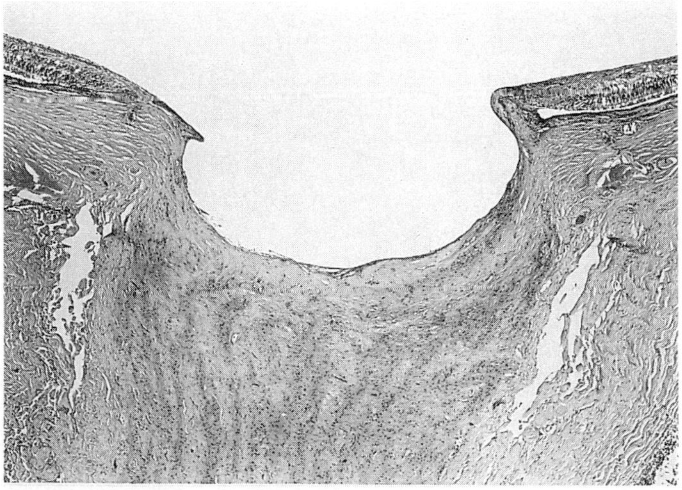

Fig. 79-32 Glaucomatous optic atrophy in optic disk. The optic disk has been massively excavated and the lamina cribrosa bowed posteriorly by chronically elevated intraocular pressure. The nerve fiber layer of the peripapillary retina is greatly atrophic.

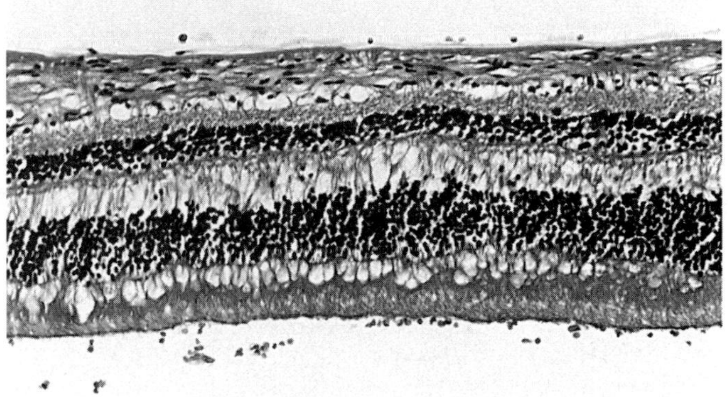

Fig. 79-33 Glaucomatous retinal atrophy in posterior area of retina. Atrophy of inner retina is confined to ganglion cells and their axons, which constitute the nerve fiber layer. Spindle cells in nerve fiber layer are glial cells. The retina is detached artifactitiously.

some 1 (1q21-q31).[168] The intraocular pressure increases insidiously and asymptomatically, and although the disease is almost always bilateral, one eye may be affected more severely than the other. The angle of the anterior chamber is open and appears normal on gonioscopy, but an increased resistance to the outflow of the aqueous is present within the vicinity of Schlemm's canal.[169] The cause of this resistance remains uncertain. With time, damage to the retina and optic nerve causes an irreversible loss of peripheral vision, which is usually unnoticed by the affected individual in the early stages of the disease. Central visual acuity is affected late in the course of the disease. The glaucoma is often diagnosed only when elevated intraocular pressure and glaucomatous cupping of the optic disk are detected during a routine ophthalmologic examination.

Primary closed-angle glaucoma (acute angle–closure glaucoma, primary narrow-angle glaucoma). Primary closed-angle glaucoma affects both eyes but may become apparent in one eye 2 to 5 years before becoming apparent in the other. The intraocular pressure is normal between attacks. Primary narrow-angle glaucoma almost always becomes manifest after 40 years of age in individuals who have small hyperopic eyes that have a shallow anterior chamber and an abnormally narrow angle. Acute symptoms from elevated intraocular pressure are caused by sudden blockage of the trabecular meshwork by an anteriorly displaced peripheral iris. These episodes are often precipitated by pupillary dilatation or a functional pupillary block. With pupillary dilatation the iris tissue may not only block the narrow anterior chamber, but also impair flow of aqueous through the pupil, which contributes to angle blockage by elevating the pressure in the posterior chamber, which, in turn, bows the peripheral iris forward. Sudden intraocular pressure elevation causes severe ocular pain and headache, corneal edema evident as halos around lights, and, occasionally, gastrointestinal symptoms (including nausea and vomiting related to a vagal oculogastric reflex). The affected eye is red, with a fixed dilated pupil, and vision is diminished by corneal epithelial edema or posterior segment ischemia. The iridocorneal angle is "closed" gonioscopically. After many episodes of intraocular hypertension, adhesions form between the iris and the trabecular meshwork and cornea (peripheral anterior synechiae) and accentuate the block to the outflow of the aqueous. Segmental iris atrophy and pupillary dilatation caused by ischemic necrosis are late stigmas of acute closed-angle glaucoma.

Secondary glaucoma. Glaucoma secondary to some ocular pathologic process can occur in eyes with open or closed angles. Because the underlying disorder is usually limited to one eye, secondary glaucomas are usually unilateral. Causes of secondary open-angle glaucoma include developmental anomalies, injuries, inflammatory reactions, and neoplasms[170-172] (Fig. 79-34). Anterior uveitis can cause secondary glaucoma by producing posterior synechiae, which partially or completely occlude the pupil (pupillary block). Scarring induced by chronic inflammation or repeated anterior chamber hemorrhages can impede aqueous outflow. An ocular contusional injury often tears the ciliary body between its longitudinal and radial muscles and disrupts the greater arterial circle of the iris, causing hyphema. After healing a significant number of patients with postcontusion angle recession develop unilateral glaucoma (Fig. 79-35). Such eyes often have a new layer of Descemet's membrane on the inner surface of the trabecular meshwork, which may cause the glaucoma.

In secondary closed-angle glaucoma the anterior chamber angle is obstructed by adhesions between the iris and the posterior surface of the cornea (peripheral anterior synechiae) caused by a fibrovascular membrane on the anterior iris (neovascular glaucoma) (Fig. 79-36) or an intraocular proliferation of corneal or conjunctival epithelium after intraocular surgery or perforating trauma (epithelial downgrowth).[173] In the iridocorneal endothelial (ICE) syndrome, abnormal corneal endothelial cells proliferate, causing unilateral closed-angle glaucoma and a characteristic variety of iris abnormalities, including full-thickness holes.[174] Eyes with advanced posterior segment tumors may cause secondary angle-closure glaucoma by iris neovascularization or pupillary block.[170]

The aqueous-outflow and trabecular meshwork can be occluded by a variety of cells and debris[175,176] (Fig. 79-37). These include blood and macrophages that have ingested

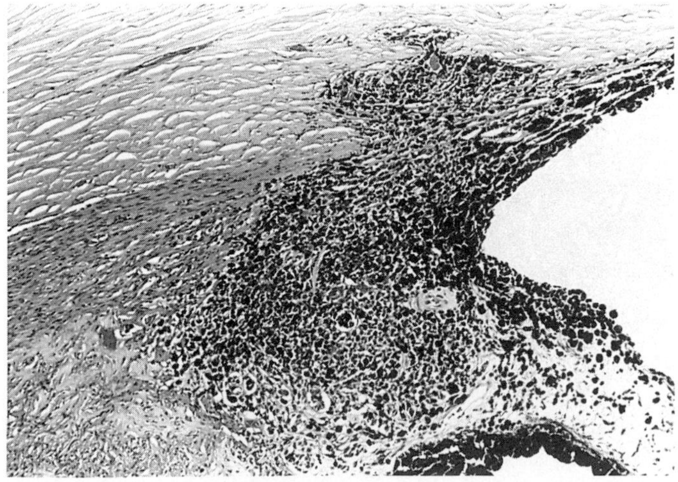

Fig. 79-34 Iridociliary malignant melanoma with secondary glaucoma. Tumor cells infiltrate the anterior part of the ciliary body and the trabecular meshwork and Schlemm's canal.

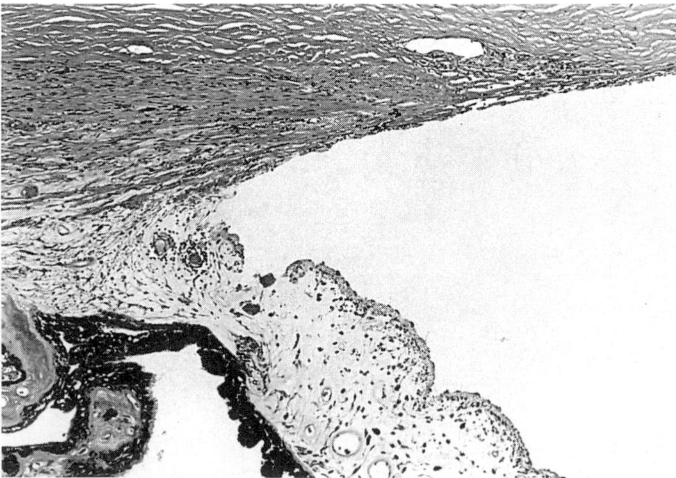

Fig. 79-35 Postcontusion angle recession. The root of the iris and first ciliary process are displaced posteriorly. The ciliary muscle has a fusiform configuration caused by atrophy of its circumferential component.

degenerated lens material, blood-breakdown products, or melanosomes from necrotic tumors. Melanin released from the iris pigment epithelium by zonular abrasion accumulates in the trabecular meshwork in the pigment-dispersion syndrome.[177] Anterior segment tumors can cause glaucoma by directly infiltrating or seeding the trabecular meshwork. Pseudoexfoliation of the lens capsule is a relatively common cause of secondary open-angle glaucoma in elderly patients.

Developmental glaucoma. Sometimes developmental anomalies that are usually bilateral produce glaucoma by blocking aqueous drainage. This form of glaucoma is much more common in boys. Excessive tearing, photophobia, and blepharospasm in infancy or childhood often herald glaucoma. Many cases are present at birth (40%) (congenital glaucoma), and most become evident during the first year of life (80%) (infantile glaucoma). A variety of other ocular malformations and systemic syndromes may be associated (including Lowe's syndrome, Peters' anomaly, aniridia, Axenfeld's syndrome, Rieger's syndrome, NF1, and Sturge-Weber syndrome).

When intraocular pressure becomes elevated before 3 years of age, the eye often enlarges (buphthalmos) from stretching of the cornea and adjacent limbal tissues, which become ectatic. As the cornea stretches and enlarges, Descemet's membrane and the endothelium often rupture, causing stromal edema and clouding.

Low tension glaucoma. The characteristic visual-field defect and all the ophthalmoscopic features of chronic open-angle glaucoma can occur without an elevation in intraocular pressure. Some of these eyes may be hypersensitive to normal intraocular pressure; others are caused by an infarction of the optic nerve head.

Phthisis bulbi

In a disorganized atrophic blind hypotonous eye, the sclera is usually thickened and folded, and the intraocular contents are greatly disorganized, with chronic retinal detachment (phthisis bulbi). A diaphragm caused by fibrosis of the vitreous often extends circumferentially from the ciliary body behind the lens (cyclitic membrane). Phthisical eyes almost always contain radiographically detectable lamellar bone, and decalcification is usually required before the globe can be processed for light microscopy. Derived from osseous metaplasia of the retinal pigment epithelium, the bone usually contains a marrow with adipose tissue and blood vessels. Occasionally, megakaryocytes, as well as erythrocytic and myelocytic lineage precursors, are present. Histologic examination of phthisical eyes usually fails to disclose evidence of the initial condition that led to phthisis. Rarely, phthisical eyes contain an unsuspected intraocular melanoma or lymphoma.

Diseases of cornea

Bullous keratopathy. In numerous disorders of the corneal endothelium the corneal stroma and epithelium become edematous, and bullae form between the epithelium and Bowman's layer. This common entity, designated "bullous keratopathy," is classified according to the cause of the endothelial loss: cataract extraction (aphakic bullous keratopathy), cataract extraction combined with the implantation of a prosthetic intraocular lens (pseudophakic bullous keratopathy), and Fuchs' corneal dystrophy. The corneal endothelium may also be lost by immunologic mechanisms in corneal graft rejection. In addition to intraepithelial vesicles and subepithelial bullae, the endothelial cells are often atrophic or absent in corneal tissue with bullous keratopathy (Fig. 79-38). Ectopic intraepithelial basement membrane may be present. A thickened, edematous stroma possesses an appearance reminiscent of cotton candy, and artifactual clefts between the collagen lamellae are diminished or absent. A thin layer of connective tissue frequently becomes interposed between the epithelium and Bowman's layer (degenerative pannus).

Calcific band keratopathy. Calcium sometimes deposits as a band across the exposed, interpalpebral part of the cornea. In its early stages, delicate basophilic calcified granules stipple Bowman's layer. In advanced cases, the entire thickness of Bowman's layer and sometimes the adjacent corneal stroma are involved.

Corneal dystrophies. The corneal dystrophies are a heterogeneous group of rare noninflammatory bilateral corneal-

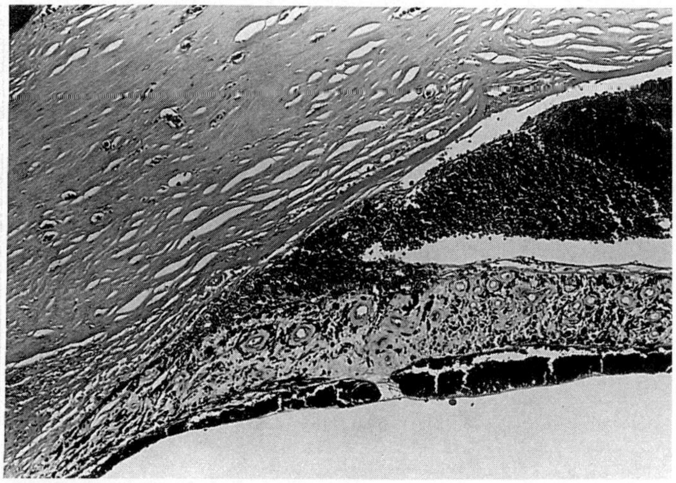

Fig. 79-36 Neovascular glaucoma with hyphema. The anterior chamber angle is occluded by a peripheral anterior synechia. A florid neovascular membrane flattens the anterior iridic surface. The inferior anterior chamber contains blood.

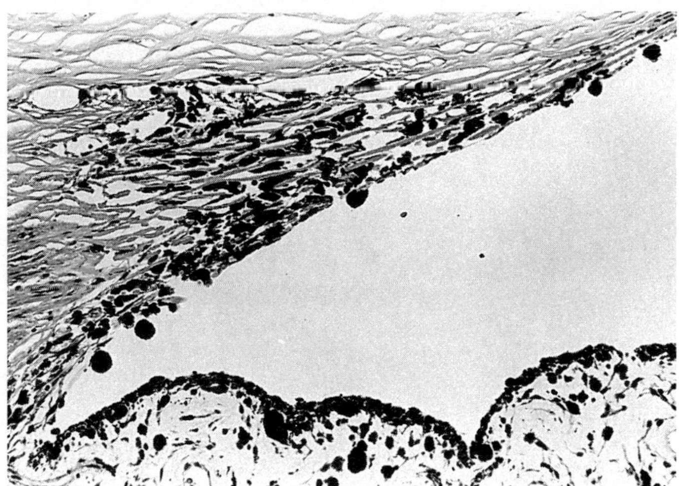

Fig. 79-37 Melanocytomalytic glaucoma. Pigment-laden macrophages infiltrate trabecular meshwork, blocking outflow of aqueous humor. Melanin pigment was released from necrotic iris melanocytoma.

disorders.[178-180] Most of them are inherited. Some have an autosomal dominant or autosomal-recessive mode of inheritance; a few have an X-linked recessive inheritance. The prevalence of each specific corneal dystrophy varies in different communities. The abnormalities in the epithelial dystrophies include microcysts or intracytoplasmic accumulations of anomalous material, defects in the epithelial basement membrane, and the deposition of finely fibrillar substance in Bowman's layer. In the stromal dystrophies different substances, including amyloid, glycosaminoglycans,[181] unidentified proteins[182] (Fig. 79-39), and lipids, accumulate within the corneal stroma because of an inherited metabolic disorder. Although the clinical manifestations may be limited to the cornea, other tissues are involved in some dystrophies. Several endothelial dystrophies are accompanied by abnormalities in Descemet's membrane, the basement membrane of the corneal endothelium.

Fuchs' endothelial dystrophy. Fuchs' endothelial dystrophy, which accounts for many corneal specimens submitted for pathologic examination in the United States, is characterized by multiple centrally located wartlike excrescences (corneal guttae) on a thickened Descemet's membrane in addition to features of bullous keratopathy (Fig. 79-40). Corneal guttae, which are synthesized by the corneal endothelium, are identical to warts that form on the peripheral Descemet's membrane with aging (Hassall-Henle bodies). They are also found in macular corneal dystrophy and in some cases of interstitial keratitis. The presence of inconspicuous "ghost" vessels in the posterior corneal stroma distinguishes interstitial keratitis from Fuchs' corneal dystrophy.

Lattice dystrophies. The inherited lattice corneal dystrophies are characterized by irregular linear opacities caused by stromal amyloid deposition in corneas with an unremarkable Descemet's membrane and endothelium[182] (Fig. 79-41). In most types of lattice corneal dystrophy (types I, III, IIIA) amyloid is apparently localized to the cornea, but in type II it is a manifestation of familial amyloid polyneuropathy type IV (Finnish or Meretoja type).[183] In most corneal amyloidoses the amyloid has not been identified, but in lattice corneal dystrophy type II it is derived from a mutant fragment of gelsolin. The gene for lattice corneal dystrophy type I appears to be closely linked to, or identical with, the gene for granular corneal dystrophy.[184]

Macular dystrophies. Corneas with the macular corneal dystrophies accumulate a keratan sulfate–related glycosaminoglycan within both the fibroblasts, in the endothelium of the cornea, among the collagen lamellae, and in Descemet's membrane [178,181,185] (Fig. 79-42). Hale's colloidal iron technique and the Alcian blue stain are particularly useful in coloring the abnormal accumulations. Macular corneal dystrophy type I involves cartilage asymptomatically.

Keratoconus. Keratoconus is a common progressive thinning of the central corneal stroma that causes a conical cornea in the absence of inflammation or vascularization.[141] This poorly understood disorder is sometimes familial and may

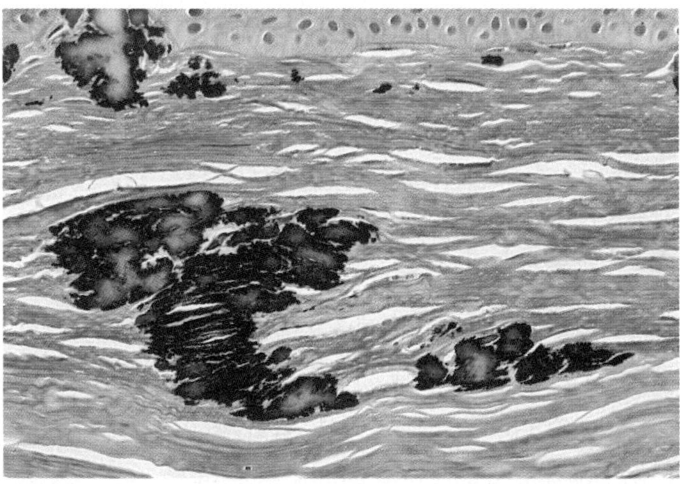

Fig. 79-39 Granular corneal dystrophy. Stroma contains aggregates of intensely eosinophilic crystalloids with "rock-candy" appearance. Material stains intensely with Luxol fast blue and shows acid fuchsinophilia (red staining) with Masson trichrome.

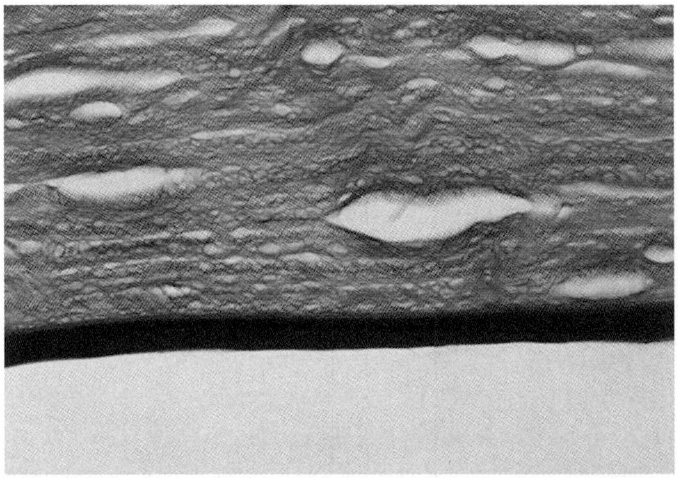

Fig. 79-38 Pseudophakic bullous keratopathy. Descemet's membrane is normal. The endothelial cells are absent, and the stroma is edematous. Endothelial damage caused by cataract surgery and prosthetic intraocular lens implantation is the most common indication for corneal transplantation.

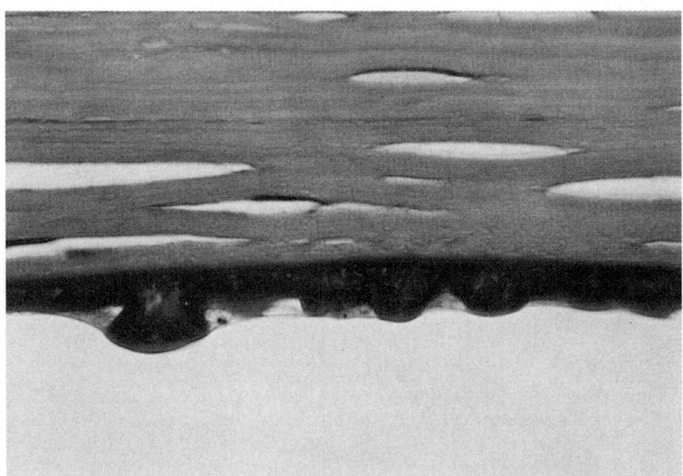

Fig. 79-40 Fuchs' corneal dystrophy. Guttate excrescences of abnormal basement membrane material stud posterior surface of thickened Descemet's membrane. Some residual endothelial cells contain granules of melanin pigment from iris. Stroma has edematous "cotton-candy" appearance.

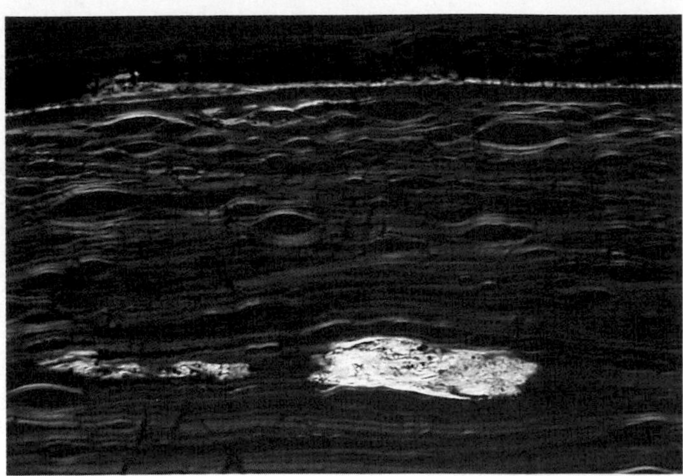

Fig. 79-41 Lattice corneal dystrophy. Smudgy oval deposit of stromal amyloid stained positively with Congo red and showed apple-green birefringence and dichroism on polarization microscopy.

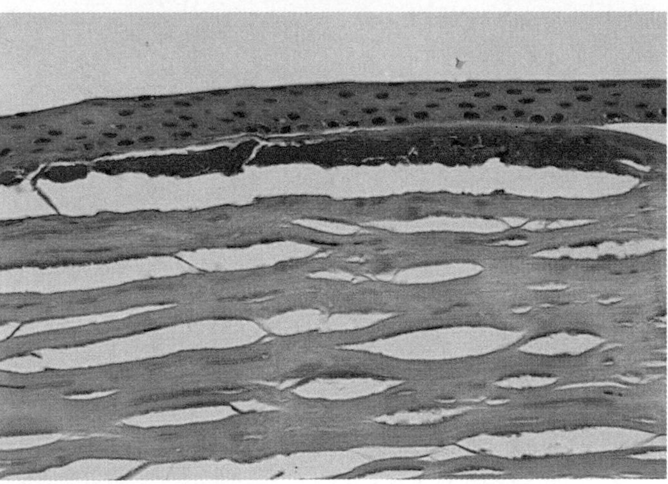

Fig. 79-42 Macular corneal dystrophy. Deposits of lucent, finely granular storage material (abnormal nonsulfated keratan sulfate) are seen in anterior interlamellar spaces. Alcian blue and colloidal iron stains confirmed presence of mucopolysaccharide material.

have a multifactorial mode of inheritance. It is associated with atopic dermatitis and trisomy 21, and rare cases have accompanied disorders of collagen metabolism and Ehlers-Danlos and Marfan syndromes. Excessive eye rubbing is common in persons with keratoconus and may precede the formation of a conical cornea. The epithelium frequently contains a ring of stainable iron surrounding the cone (Fleischer's ring). Numerous focal dehiscences in Bowman's layer associated with thinning of the central corneal stroma occur in advanced cases (Fig. 79-43). The endothelium in corneas with keratoconus is usually unremarkable, but endothelial cell loss may accompany ruptures of Descemet's membrane ("acute corneal hydrops").

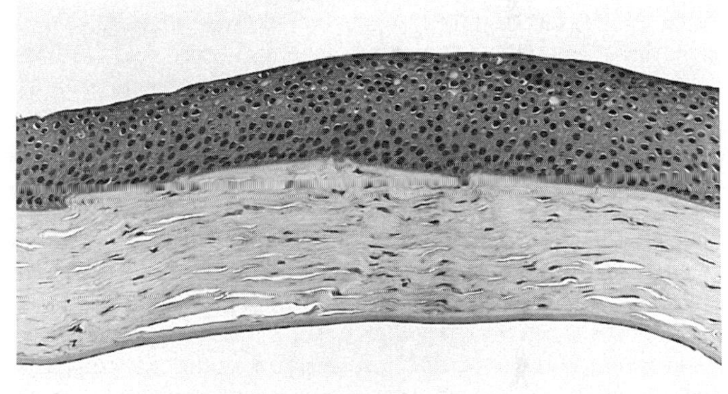

Fig. 79-43 Keratoconus. The corneal stroma is greatly ectatic. Bowman's layer contains characteristic dehiscences. The epithelium has undergone compensatory hyperplasia. Descemet's membrane is thin, and the endothelium is well preserved.

Diseases of retina

Retinal diseases include many hereditary disorders and numerous degenerations secondary to vascular, systemic, or idiopathic conditions. Several genetically determined retinal disorders have been mapped to specific chromosomes. The X chromosome carries the genes for retinoschisis, choroideremia, Norrie's disease, red-green color blindness, and at least two varieties of retinitis pigmentosa.

Retinal detachment. Retinal detachment is a common cause of visual impairment and blindness. Factors predisposing to retinal detachment include retinal holes (from trauma or certain retinal degenerations) and vitreoretinal traction. A collection of fluid (liquid vitreous, hemorrhage, or exudate) separates the photoreceptors from the retinal pigment epithelium (Fig. 79-44). This disruption of normal anatomic relationship deprives the outer retina of oxygen and nutrients and prevents vital cellular interactions between the retinal pigment epithelium and photoreceptors.

A hole, break, or tear in the retina may give vitreous fluid access to the subretinal space (rhegmatogenous retinal detachment). Some retinal detachments are caused by an accumulation of fluid between the sensory retina and the retinal pigment epithelium (exudative retinal detachment). Causes include toxemia of pregnancy, malignant hypertension, severe choroiditis (as in sympathetic uveitis or Vogt-Koyanagi-Harada disease), retinal diseases with increased vascular permeability (such as Coats' disease, the hemangioblastomas of von Hippel-Lindau's disease, and the damaged vessels of radiation retinopathy). Choroidal neoplasms, including melanomas, metastatic carcinomas, and hemangiomas, also commonly cause exudative retinal detachment.

Rhegmatogenous retinal detachment, the commonest form of retinal detachment, is often associated with degenerative changes in the vitreous or peripheral retina. Causes of retinal breaks include vitreoretinal traction, trauma, lattice degeneration of the retina, high myopia with vitreous degeneration, and intracapsular cataract extraction. Disorders of the vitreous (vitreous detachment and mobility, syneresis, and vitreoretinal adhesions and traction) contribute to retinal tears and breaks. Full-thickness holes in the retina are not complicated by retinal detachment unless liquid vitreous gains access to the potential space between the sensory retina and the retinal pigment epithe-

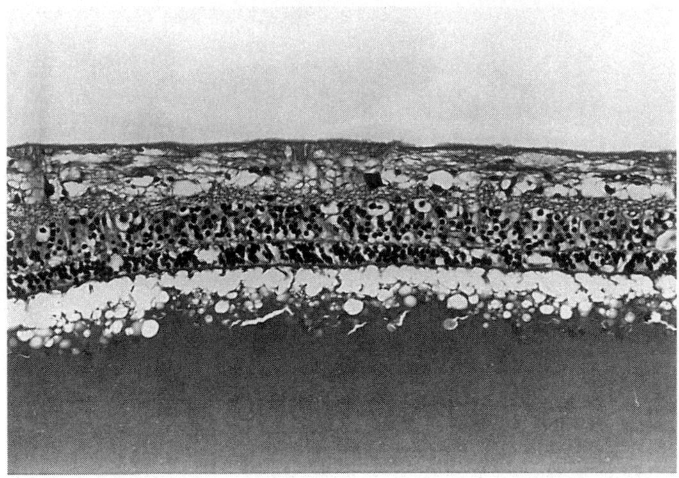

Fig. 79-44 Outer retinal atrophy as a result of chronic retinal detachment. Loss of photoreceptors and proteinaceous exudate in the subretinal space indicate that retinal detachment is real. The outer nuclear layer is thinned.

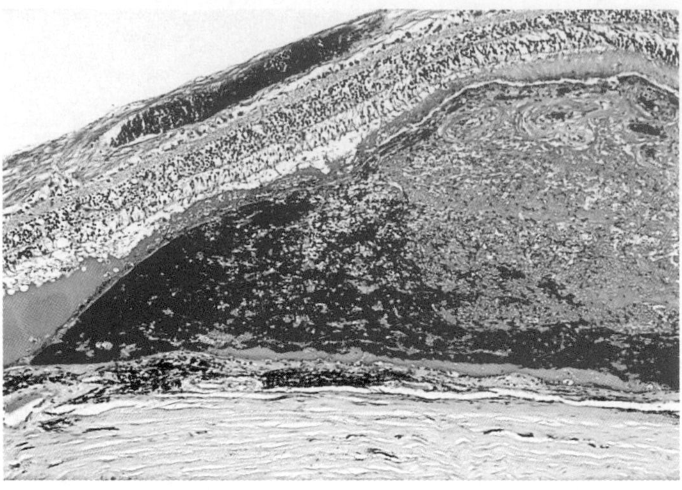

Fig. 79-45 Age-related macular degeneration. A hemorrhagic RPE detachment of the retinal pigment epithelium is undergoing organization into a collagenous disciform scar. The retina is shallowly detached by serous fluid.

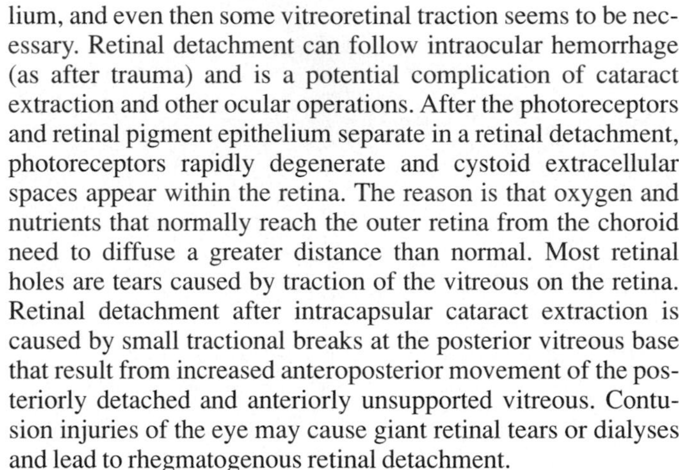

lium, and even then some vitreoretinal traction seems to be necessary. Retinal detachment can follow intraocular hemorrhage (as after trauma) and is a potential complication of cataract extraction and other ocular operations. After the photoreceptors and retinal pigment epithelium separate in a retinal detachment, photoreceptors rapidly degenerate and cystoid extracellular spaces appear within the retina. The reason is that oxygen and nutrients that normally reach the outer retina from the choroid need to diffuse a greater distance than normal. Most retinal holes are tears caused by traction of the vitreous on the retina. Retinal detachment after intracapsular cataract extraction is caused by small tractional breaks at the posterior vitreous base that result from increased anteroposterior movement of the posteriorly detached and anteriorly unsupported vitreous. Contusion injuries of the eye may cause giant retinal tears or dialyses and lead to rhegmatogenous retinal detachment.

Contracting fibrous or fibrovascular membranes in the vitreous can pull the sensory retina from the retinal pigment epithelium. Such tractional retinal detachment is an important complication of proliferative diabetic retinopathy, retinopathy of prematurity, organized vitreous hemorrhage, and ocular trauma or inflammation. In diabetics, contraction of organized vitreous exerts traction on areas of vitreoretinal adhesion, causing tractional detachment of the retina.

Cherry-red spot at the macula. Causes of a cherry-red spot at the macula include central retinal artery occlusion and a variety of lysosomal storage diseases, such as G_{M2}-gangliosidosis type II variant B (Tay-Sachs disease), G_{M1}-gangliosidosis type I, G_{M2}-gangliosidosis type II variant O (Sandhoff), mucolipidosis type I, and Niemann-Pick disease. The lysosomal storage of gangliosides or other substances within the multilayered retinal ganglion cells in the perifoveal retina opacifies the affected retina, making the foveola, which lacks ganglion cells, appear red. After central retinal artery occlusion, the retinal pigment epithelium and highly vascular choroid beneath the thin foveal floor stand out in sharp contrast to the pale sensory retina.

Macular degenerations. With aging, in certain drug toxicities (such as that of chloroquine), and in several inherited disorders, the macula degenerates as central vision becomes impaired. There are numerous causes for macular degeneration, and the proper diagnosis can be established when one takes into account the clinical manifestations and histopathologic features. Age-related macular degeneration is an extremely common blinding disease caused by degeneration of the outer retina and retinal pigment epithelium of the macula as individuals age[186,187] (Fig. 79-45). Loss of retinal pigment epithelium and subretinal neovascularization causes degeneration of the adjacent photoreceptors. The new vessels leak serous fluid and often bleed, causing hemorrhagic detachment of the retinal pigment epithelium. Organization of such hemorrhages results in the formation of a collagenous disciform scar.

Pigmentary retinopathies. The generic misnomer "retinitis pigmentosa" is applied to a large group of noninflammatory, bilateral progressive, degenerative pigmentary retinopathies that are characterized by loss of retinal photoreceptors (rods and cones) and by perivascular pigment accumulation within the retina[188] (Fig. 79-46). Multiple genetic mutations cause retinitis pigmentosa (Table 79-5). Most cases occur sporadically, but others have autosomal-dominant, autosomal-recessive, or X-linked recessive modes of inheritance. Some pigmentary retinopathies are associated with neurologic or systemic disorders. Single amino acid substitutions in the rod photopigment rhodopsin account for some autosomal dominant pigmentary retinopathies.[188] In 12% of cases with autosomal-dominant retinitis pigmentosa, histidine replaces proline at position 23 of the opsin molecule. This substitution corresponds to a single nucleotide transversion (C to A) in the rhodopsin gene. Numerous other mutations in different parts of the opsin molecule also cause retinitis pigmentosa and so do inherited abnormalities in other photoreceptor proteins (peripherin, cGMP phosphodiesterase). The diagnosis of a pigmentary retinopathy necessitates the identification of the type and cause (Table 79-6).

Retinopathy of prematurity. Retinopathy of prematurity is characterized by vitreoretinal neovascular proliferation and retinal detachment. Organization of the vitreous is responsible for secondary tractional retinal detachment. Vascular prolifera-

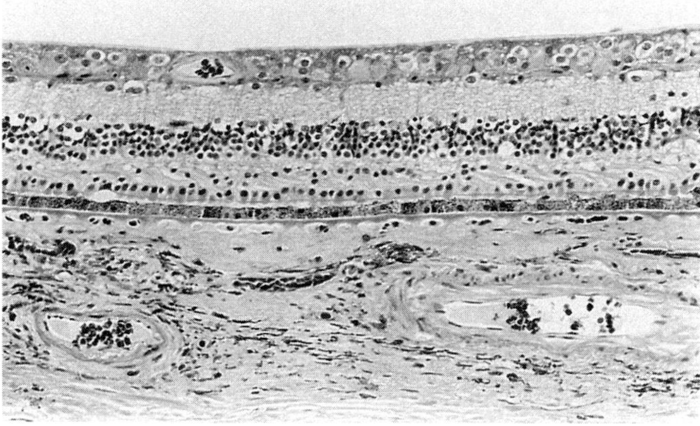

Fig. 79-46 Retinitis pigmentosa. Outer nuclear layer of posterior retina is reduced to single interrupted layer of cone nuclei that lack inner and outer segments. The retinal pigment epithelium and the inner retinal layers are intact. Peripherally the retinal pigment epithelium had invaded the perivascular spaces of the atrophic retina, forming bone spicule pigmentation.

tion and vitreous fibrosis are believed to result from the effect of increased oxygen levels on the immature, incompletely vascularized peripheral retina. This retinopathy occurs almost exclusively in premature infants and is caused by the administration of high concentrations of oxygen. After exposure to high levels of ambient oxygen, as in an incubator, the developing blood vessels in the peripheral retina becomes obliterated and the peripheral retina, which does not normally vascularize until the end of fetal life, remains avascular. When the premature infant eventually returns to room air, an intense proliferation of vascular endothelium and glial cells begins at the junction of the avascular and vascularized portions of the retina. Usually apparent 5 to 10 weeks after removal from the incubator, this neovascularization is believed to result from the liberation of a putative angiogenic factor. About 25% of infants with retinopathy of prematurity progress to a cicatricial phase, characterized by retinal detachment and a retrolental, fibrovascular mass.

Angioid streaks. In a variety of systemic conditions, including Ehlers-Danlos syndrome, Gardner's syndrome, Paget's disease of bone, pseudoxanthoma elasticum, and sickle cell disease,[154] Bruchs' membrane calcifies and fractures, producing irregular lines vaguely resembling blood vessels that radiate beneath the retina from the optic nerve head.

Coats' disease. One of the entities that can mimic retinoblastoma clinically is an exudative retinal detachment known as Coats' disease. Two thirds of individuals with this usually unilateral disorder are boys in their first decade of life. The condition is characterized by a massive exudative retinal detachment caused by leakage from abnormal telangiectatic retinal vessels. The outer layers of the detached retina are greatly thickened by exudates, and the lipid-rich subretinal fluid contains cholesterol clefts and foamy macrophages (Fig. 79-47).

Norrie's disease. Patients with Norrie's disease, an X-linked recessive hereditary disorder, usually develop mental retardation, deafness, and bilateral blindness caused by masses of malformed detached retina.[189]

Table 79-5 Inherited diseases involving the ocular tissues

Abetalipoproteinemia (Bassen-Kornzweig syndrome)
Alkaptonuria (ochronosis)
Alport's syndrome
Ataxia telangiectasia (Louis-Bar syndrome)
Chédiak-Higashi syndrome
Cockayne's syndrome
Congenital ichthyosis
Cystinosis
Ehlers-Danlos syndrome
Fabry's disease
Familial dysautonomia (Riley-Day syndrome)
Familial high-density lipoprotein deficiency (Tangier disease)
Familial lecithin cholesterol acyltransferase deficiency
Farber's disease
Galactosemia
Gaucher's disease type II (infantile, acute neuronopathic)
Globoid cell leukodystrophy (Krabbe disease)
G_{M1} gangliosidosis type I
G_{M2} gangliosidosis type II (Sandhoff)
G_{M2} gangliosidosis type II (Tay-Sachs)
G_{M2} gangliosidosis type III
Hallervorden-Spatz syndrome
Hallgren syndrome
Hepatolenticular degeneration (Wilson disease)
Hidrotic ectodermal dysplasia (Marshall type)
Homocystinuria
Hyperlipoproteinemia type I
Hyperlipoproteinemia type II
Hyperlipoproteinemia type III
Hyperlipoproteinemia type IV
Hyperlipoproteinemia type V
Hyperornithinemia (chorioretinal gyrate atrophy)
Incontinentia pigmenti
Familial amyloid polyneuropathy type IV (Meretoja)
Kearns-Sayre syndrome
Klinefelter's syndrome (45X and mosaic variants)
Laurence-Moon-Biedl syndrome
Lowe's oculocerebrorenal syndrome
Mannosidosis
Marfan syndrome
Marie-Strumpell disease
Marinesco-Sjögren syndrome
Metachromatic leukodystrophy variant
Mucolipidosis type I
Mucopolysaccharidosis type I-H (Hurler)
Mucopolysaccharidosis type I-S (Scheie)
Mucopolysaccharidosis type II (Hunter)
Mucopolysaccharidosis type IIIA and IIIB (Sanfilippo)
Multiple endocrine neoplasia syndrome type II B
Myotonic dystrophy
Neuronal ceroid lipofuscinosis
Neuronal ceroid lipofuscinosis type I (infantile, Hagberg-Haltia-Santavuon)
Niemann-Pick disease
Norrie's disease
Oculocutaneous albinism (various types)
Osteogenesis imperfecta
Pelizaeus-Merzbacher syndrome
Phytanic acid storage disease (Refsum syndrome)
Pierre Robin syndrome
Pseudoxanthoma elasticum
Rothmund-Thomson syndrome
Rubinstein-Taybi syndrome
Sickle cell disease

(continued)

Table 79-5 Inherited diseases involving the ocular tissues—cont'd

Sickle cell hemoglobin C disease
Stickler's progressive arthro-ophthalmopathy
Sulfatide lipidosis (metachromatic leukodystrophy)
Trisomy 13
Tuberous sclerosis
Turner's syndrome (XXY, XXXY, XXXXY)
Type II late infantile (Janský-Bielschowsky)
Type III juvenile (Spielmeyer-Sjögren-Batten)
Tyrosinemia
Usher's syndrome
Various forms of oculocutaneous albinism
von Hippel-Lindau disease
Waardenburg-Klein syndrome
X-linked copper malabsorption syndrome (Menke's disease)

Diseases of the vitreous

Cells, amyloid, and other vitreal opacities are sometimes removed by specialized mechanized cutting and aspiration instruments.[190] Fibrocellular and neovascular vitreoretinal bands and membranes that cause retinal detachment are also often excised (pars plana vitrectomy).

Vitreous opacification. Opacification of the vitreous occurs in several pathologic conditions when the vitreous serves as a repository for blood, inflammatory cells, tumor cells, and other debris. Remnants of the embryonic hyaloid vascular system and degeneration of the vitreous in myopes cause innocuous opacities (floaters). In asteroid hyalosis, which affects about 1% of the population, tiny white spherules composed of calcium soaps are attached to the vitreous framework and move with the syneretic vitreous (Fig. 79-48). They appear gray in hematoxylin and eosin–stained preparations, are moderately periodic acid–Schiff positive, and show a vivid Maltese-cross pattern of birefringence on polarization microscopy. Cholesterol crystals may also accumulate in the vitreous (synchysis scintillans). In many of the familial amyloidoses caused by single amino substitutions in transthyretin, amyloid accumulates in the vitreous.

Proliferative vitreoretinopathy. In eyes with retinal and vitreous detachment, the retinal pigment epithelium and glial cells and myofibroblasts grow on the inner and newly exposed outer surface of the retina, forming membranes that exert traction on or weld together adjacent parts of the retina.

Persistent hyperplastic primary vitreous. Persistent hyperplastic primary vitreous (PHPV) is a congenital retrolenticular mass of fibrovascular tissue derived from the embryonic primary vitreous which often is supplied by a patent hyaloid artery. PHPV is usually found at birth in microphthalmic eyes and may be confused clinically with retinoblastoma. The retrolental fibrocellular plaque typically draws the tips of the ciliary process centrally into the pupillary aperture.

Diseases of the crystalline lens

Cataract. A cataract is an opacity in the lens usually severe enough to impair visual acuity. Lens opacification has numerous causes, and each type of cataract differs in its pathogenesis[191,192] (Table 79-7). Most cataracts in the United States are associated with aging. Four basic types of cataract are recognized histopathologically: cortical, nuclear, anterior

Table 79-6 Some conditions associated with a pigmentary retinopathy

Condition	Chromosome location
Inherited diseases	
Retinitis pigmentosa, autosomal recessive	(3q21-q24)
Retinitis pigmentosa, peripherin related	(6q21 cen)
Retinitis pigmentosa—1	(8p11-q21)
Retinitis pigmentosa—2	(Xp11-3
Retinitis pigmentosa—3	(Xp21.1
Retinitis pigmentosa—4	(3q21-q24)
Retinitis pigmentosa—5 (opsin gene)	(3q)
Retinitis pigmentosa—6	(Xp21.3-q21.2)
Retinitis pigmentosa—9	(7p15.1-p13)
Retinitis pigmentosa—10	(7q)
Retinitis pigmentosa—chromosome 1	(1q32)
Retinitis pigmentosa—cGMP phosphodiesterase gene	
Postinflammatory and degenerative	
Syphilis	
Typhoid fever	
Rubella	
Measles	
Smallpox vaccination	
Behçet's disease	
Cytomegalic inclusion disease	
Toxoplasmosis	
Onchocerciasis	
Drugs	
Phenothiazine: chlorpromazine, iminophenoxine	
Antimalarials: chloroquine, atrabrine	
Antimetabolites: iodoacetate, sodium fluoride	
Disorders of lipid and mucopolysaccharide metabolism	
Neuronal ceroid lipofuscinosis	
Bassen-Kornzweig (abetalipoproteinemia)	
Refsum syndrome	
Niemann-Pick disease	
Hurler syndrome (MPS I-H)	
Scheie syndrome (MPS I-S)	
Hunter syndrome (MPS II)	
Sanfilippo syndromes A and B (MPS III)	
Miscellaneous syndromes	
Kearn-Sayre	
Usher syndrome type 1A	(14q32)
Usher syndrome type 1B	(11q13.5)
Usher syndrome type 1C	(11p)
Usher syndrome type 2	(1q32)
Cockayne	
Laurence-Moon	
Bardet-Biedl	
Pelizaeus-Merzbacher	
Hallervorden-Spatz	
Siderosis bulbi	
Congenital ichthyosis	
Hallgren	
Vitamin A deficiency	

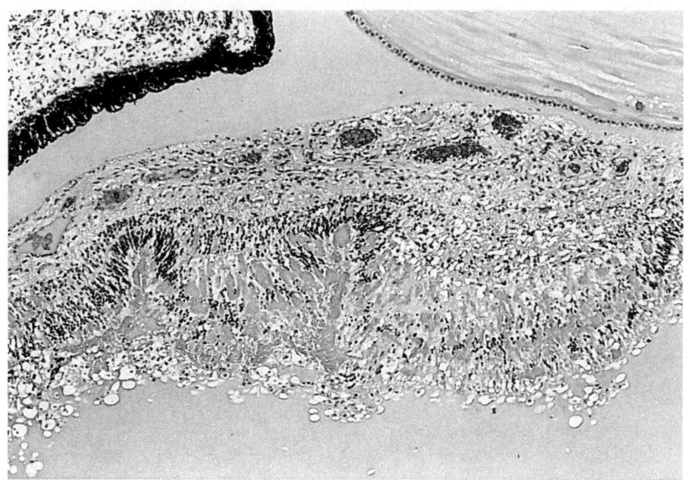

Fig. 79-47 Coats's disease. Leakage from abnormal retinal vessels has caused a bullous exudative retinal detachment. Proteinaceous exudates thicken outer retina. Subretinal fluid contains lipid histiocytes.

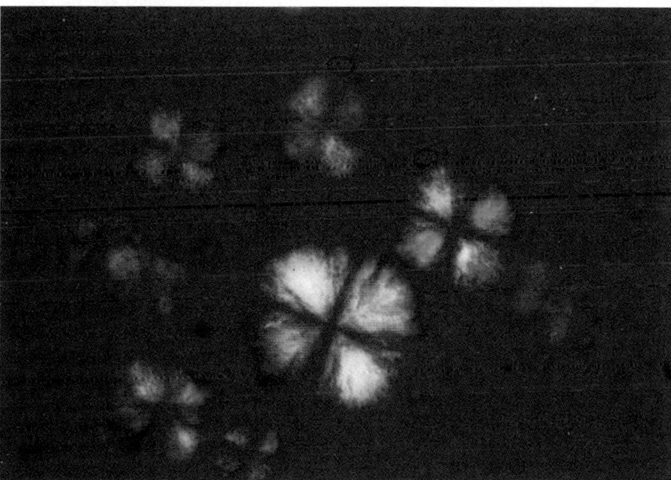

Fig. 79-48 Asteroid hyalosis. Spherules of calcium soap attached to vitreous framework in vitrectomy specimen show vivid "Maltese cross" birefringence to plane polarized light. (Millipore filter preparation, polarization microscopy.)

subcapsular, and posterior subcapsular. The cataract of congenital rubella is characterized by the nonspecific persistence of lens epithelial nuclei within the lens fibers.

Nuclear cataract. In the nuclear sclerotic cataract the hardened central lens nucleus appears yellowish or brown, reflecting the accumulation of the photo-oxidation pigment urochrome. The colored lens absorbs blue light, distorting color vision. Increase in the lens's index of refraction causes lenticular myopia. Nuclear sclerosis is characterized microscopically by an increased eosinophilia and homogeneity of the lens nucleus, which lacks the artifactitious clefts observed in a normal lens cortex (Fig. 79-49). Nuclear cataracts occasionally contain oval birefringent crystals of calcium oxalate.

Cortical cataract. A cortical (soft) cataract results from degeneration of the lens cells or fibers and is characterized by

Table 79-7 Conditions associated with cataracts

Disorders of carbohydrate metabolism
Diabetes mellitus
Galactosemia
Deficiency states
Riboflavin
Tryptophan
Genetic disorders
Myotonic dystrophy
Wilson's disease (hepatolenticular degeneration)
Fabry's disease
Lowe's syndrome
Toxins
Dinitrophenol
Naphthalene
Ergot
Mercury
Drugs
Phospholine iodide (topical)
Corticosteroids (systemic)
Phenothiazines
Anticholinesterases
Triparanol
Chronic miotic therapy
Physical agents
Heat
Electromagnetic radiation
Ultraviolet radiation
Microwaves
Trauma
Intraocular surgery
Ultrasound
Electric shock
Ocular diseases
Intraocular neoplasms
Ciliary body tumors
Glaucoma
Retinitis pigmentosa
Sensory retinal detachment
Chronic uveitis
Sarcoidosis
Rheumatoid arthritis (pauciarticular, seronegative, juvenile)
Fuchs' heterochromic cyclitis
Viruses
Rubella virus
Aging
Skin diseases
Atopic dermatitis
Scleroderma
Acrodermatitis enteropathica
Werner's and Rothmund's ectodermal dysplasia syndromes
Systemic diseases
Inborn errors of metabolism
Down syndrome

fractures, degeneration, and liquefaction of the fiber cells of the lens cortex (Fig. 79-50). Its incipient stage is characterized by the formation of vacuoles or clefts in the lens cortex. Interrupted and folded lens fibers and cortical clefts are filled with morgagnian globules. The sclerotic nucleus usually resists liquefaction. The osmotic effect of the degenerated cortex causes the lens to imbibe aqueous and swell. Total cortical liquefaction may eventually ensue (morgagnian cataract).

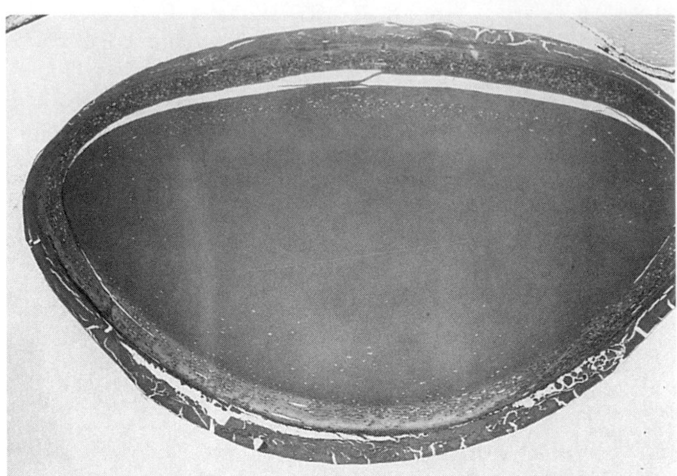

Fig. 79-49 Nuclear sclerotic cataract. Artifactitious cleft separated dense sclerotic nucleus from degenerated cortex. Nucleus shows intense homogeneous staining and lacks artifactitiously intercellular clefts seen in cortex.

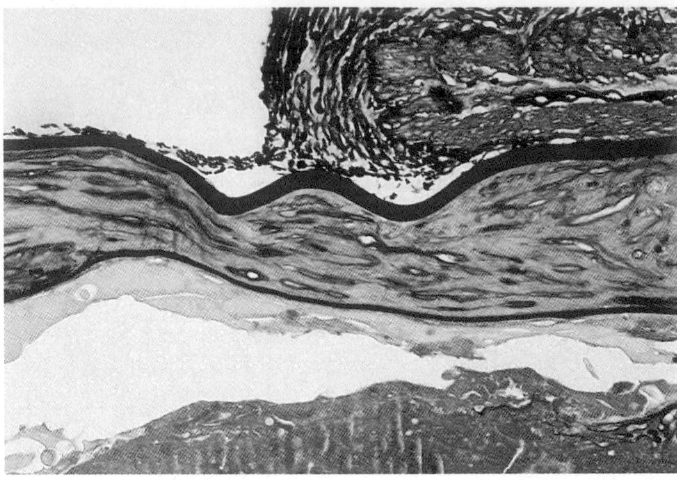

Fig. 79-51 Anterior subcapsular cataract. Collagenous plaque made by distressed lens epithelial cells is seen beneath folded anterior lens capsule. Basement membrane capsules surround residual lens epithelial cells within plaque. A fibrous pupillary membrane rests on anterior surface of this cataract.

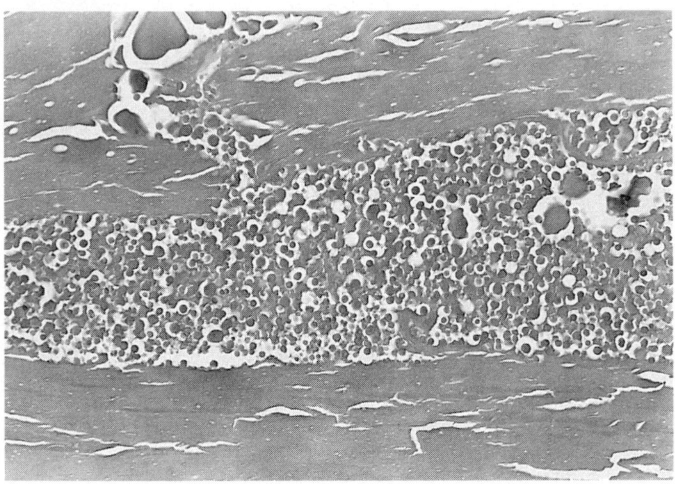

Fig. 79-50 Cortical cataract. Morgagnian globules of degenerated lens protein fill cleft in lens cortex.

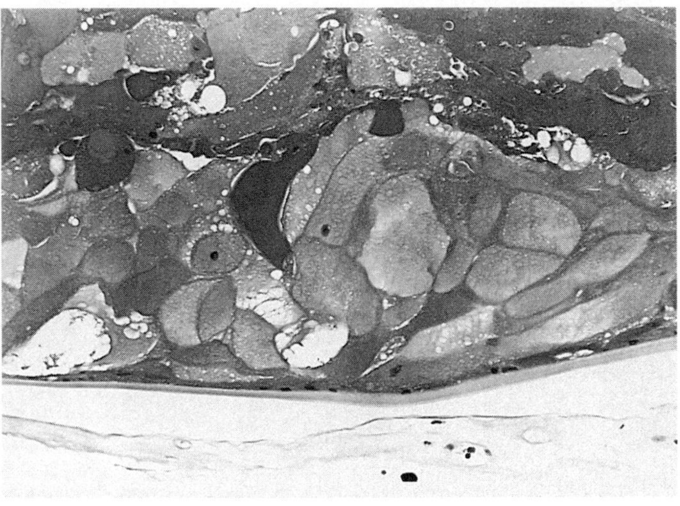

Fig. 79-52 Posterior subcapsular cataract with Wedl cells. An aggregate of Wedl, or bladder, cells formed by posterior migration of the lens epithelium is seen next to thin posterior lens capsule. Wedl cells represent abortive attempts by lens epithelial cells to form new lens fibers.

Anterior subcapsular cataract. Inflammation, adhesions between the iris and lens (posterior synechiae), and other factors occasionally stimulate the anterior subcapsular monolayer of cuboidal lens epithelium to proliferate, undergo metaplasia, or migrate posteriorly. The proliferating lens epithelial cells synthesize a thick plaque of collagen beneath a sinuously folded anterior lens capsule (Fig. 79-51). Within the plaque, the cells are surrounded by basement membrane material that is periodic acid–Schiff positive, bearing testimony to the lens epithelial lineage of the cells. Proliferation and fibrous transformation of residual lens epithelial cells is a major cause of posterior capsular fibrosis after extracapsular cataract extraction.

Posterior subcapsular cataract. The posterior subcapsular cataract results from the migration of lens epithelial cells posterior to the normal termination of the epithelium at the lens equator. Situated abnormally, the cells retain their nuclei and form large aberrant globular lens fibers called "bladder," or "Wedl," cells (Fig. 79-52). Globular transparent aggregates of lens cortical material called "Elschnig's pearls," which occasionally develop after extracapsular surgery, reflect an identical proliferation of residual lens epithelial cells.

Pseudophakos. Lens capsule and cortical remnants are found in the posterior chamber after extracapsular cataract extraction. Usually in sectioning eyes, prosthetic intraocular lenses (pseudophakos) become lost during processing. With whole-mounted specimens, however, multinucleated giant cells, mononuclear and other inflammatory cells, fragments of lens capsule, and melanin granules (which may be within macrophages) are often adherent to prosthetic intraocular lenses. Sometimes they injure the corneal endothelium, causing bullous keratopathy, damage the iris, or provoke an inflammatory response.[193]

Anterior lenticonus. In anterior lenticonus the anterior lens surface has a conical configuration caused by focal thinning of the lens capsule.

Pseudoexfoliation syndrome. Bushlike deposits of eosinophilic material are found on the anterior lens capsule in the pseudoexfoliation syndrome.[191,194-196] Coarser clumps adhere to zonules, ciliary processes, and the iris pigment epithelium, which shows coarsening and coalescence of its circumferential ridges. Pseudoexfoliation material has also been identified in the conjunctiva, around orbital vessels, in eyelid and buttock skin, and in the lung, liver, and heart.[194,195] In extraocular loci the material is always associated with elastic tissue and reacts with antibodies against elastic microfibrils.

Diseases of optic nerve

The optic nerve is affected by many of the same conditions as the central nervous system, as one might expect from its structure. Edema of the optic nerve head (papilledema) occurs with increased intracranial pressure and other conditions.[196,197] Optic atrophy occurs after loss of axons and their myelin sheaths within the nerve.[198] This may follow degenerative disorders of the retina or central nervous system proximal to the globe. One variety of optic neuropathy results from mutations in the mitochondrial genome (Leber's hereditary optic neuropathy).[199]

Diseases of lacrimal drainage system

Lacrimal obstruction. Obstruction of the lacrimal drainage apparatus causes epiphora (tearing) and results from congenital abnormalities, trauma, chronic dacryocystitis, epithelial hyperplasia secondary to topical medications, and tumors. Surgical specimens obtained during dacryocystorhinostomy contain chronic inflammation, inflamed segments of pseudostratified columnar epithelium, and occasional intraluminal casts or concretions formed by colonies of anaerobic actinomycetes *(Actinomyces israeli)* or *Arachnia (Actinomyces) propionica.*[200]

REFERENCES

Normal eye

1. Jakobiec FA, editor: *Ocular anatomy, embryology and teratology,* New York, 1982, Harper & Row.
2. Scroggs MW, Klintworth GK: Normal eye and ocular adnexa. In Sternberg SS, editor: *Histology for pathologists,* New York, 1992, Raven Press.

General texts on ocular pathology

3. Eagle RC Jr: The eye. In Silverberg SG, editor: *Principles and practices of surgical pathology,* ed 2, New York, 1990, Churchill Livingstone.
4. Garner A, Klintworth GK: *Pathobiology of ocular disease: a dynamic approach,* ed 2, New York, 1994, Marcel Dekker.
5. Merin S: *Inherited eye diseases: diagnosis and clinical management,* New York, 1991, Marcel Dekker.
6. Naumann GOH, Apple DJ: *Pathology of the eye,* New York, 1986, Springer-Verlag.
7. Scroggs MW, Klintworth GK: The eye and ocular adnexa. In Sternberg SS, editor: *Diagnostic surgical pathology,* ed 2, New York, 1994, Raven Press.
8. Shields JA, Shields CL: *Intraocular tumors, a text and atlas,* Philadelphia, 1992, Saunders.
9. Spencer WH: *Ophthalmic pathology: an atlas and textbook,* ed 3, Philadelphia, 1985, Saunders.

Inflammation and immunologic reactions

10. Watson PG, Hayreh SS: Scleritis and episcleritis, *Br J Ophthalmol* 60:163, 1994.
11. Rao NA, Marak GE, Hidayat AA: Necrotizing scleritis: a clinicopathologic study of 41 cases, *Ophthalmology* 92:1542, 1985.
12. Weinberg JC, Eagle RC Jr, Font RL et al: Conjunctival synthetic fiber granuloma: a lesion that resembles conjunctivitis nodosa, *Ophthalmology* 91:867, 1984.
13. Foster CS: Cicatricial pemphigoid, *Trans Am Ophthalmol Soc* 84:527, 1986.
14. Ahmed AR, Foster CS, Zaltas M et al: Association of DQW7 (DQB1*0301) with ocular cicatricial pemphigoid, *Proc Natl Acad Sci USA* 88:11579, 1992.
15. Mondino BJ, Ross AN, Rabin BS: Autoimmune phenomena in ocular cicatricial pemphigoid, *Am J Ophthalmol* 83:443, 1977.
16. Sacks EH, Jakobiec FA, Wieczorek R et al: Immunophenotypic analysis of the inflammatory infiltrate in ocular cicatricial pemphigoid: further evidence for a T cell–mediated disease. *Ophthalmology* 96:236, 1989.
17. Meisler DM, Zakov AN, Bruner WE et al: Endophthalmitis associated with sequestered intraocular *Propionibacterium acnes, Am J Ophthalmol* 104:428, 1987.
18. Jakobiec FA, Marboe CC, Knowles DM II et al: Human sympathetic ophthalmia: an analysis of the inflammatory infiltrate by hybridoma-monoclonal antibodies, immunochemistry, and correlative electron microscopy, *Ophthalmology* 90:76, 1983.
19. Lubin JR, Albert DM, Weinstein M: Sixty-five years of sympathetic ophthalmia: a clinicopathologic review of 105 cases (1913-1978), *Ophthalmology* 87:109, 1980.
20. Marak GE Jr: Phacoanaphylactic endophthalmitis, *Surv Ophthalmol* 36:325, 1992.
21. Kennerdell JS, Dresner SC: The nonspecific orbital inflammatory syndromes, *Surv Ophthalmol* 29:93, 1994.
22. Mottow-Lippa L, Jakobiec FA: Idiopathic inflammatory orbital pseudotumor in childhood, *Arch Ophthalmol* 96:1410, 1978.
23. Bullen CL, Liesegang TJ, McDonald TJ: Ocular complications of Wegener's granulomatosis, *Ophthalmology* 90:279, 1983.
24. Kalina PH, Lie JT, Campbell RJ, Garrity JA: Diagnostic value and limitations of orbital biopsy in Wegener's granulomatosis, *Ophthalmology* 99:120, 1994.
25. Koyama T, Matsuo N, Watanabe Y et al: Wegener's granulomatosis with destructive ocular manifestations, *Am J Ophthalmol* 98:736, 1994.
26. Bulen CI, Liesegang TJ, McDonald TJ, DeRemee RA: Ocular complications of Wegener's granulomatosis, *Ophthalmology* 90:279, 1993.

Infectious and parasitic diseases

27. Gorovoy MS, Stern GA, Hood CI, Allen C: Intrastromal noninflammatory bacterial colonization of a corneal graft, *Arch Ophthalmol* 101:1749, 1983.
28. Weber DJ, Hoffman KL, Thoft R, Baker A. Endophthalmitis following intraocular lens implantation: report of 30 cases and review of the literature, *Rev Infect Dis* 8:12, 1986.
29. Meisler DM, Palestine AG, Vastine DW, et al: Chronic *Propionibacterium* endophthalmitis after extracapsular cataract extraction and intraocular lens implantation, *Am J Ophthalmol* 102:733, 1986.
30. Dekkers NW: The cornea in measles, *Documenta Opthalmologica* 52:1, 1981.
31. Pepose JS, Holland GN, Nestor MS et al: Acquired immune deficiency syndrome; pathogenic mechanisms of ocular disease, *Ophthalmology* 92:472, 1985.
32. Schuman JS, Orellana J, Friedman AH et al: Acquired immunodeficiency syndrome (AIDS), *Surv Ophthalmol* 31:384, 1987.
33. Jabs DA, Green WR, Fox R et al: Ocular manifestations of acquired immune deficiency syndrome, *Ophthalmology* 96:1092, 1989.
34. Dugel PU, Rao NA, Forster DJ et al: *Pneumocystitis carinii* choroiditis after long-term aerosolized pentamidine therapy, *Am J Ophthalmol* 110:113, 1990.
35. Davis RM, Font RL, Keisler MS, Shadduck JA: Corneal microsporidiosis: a case report including ultrastructural observations, *Ophthalmology* 7:953, 1990.

36. Schwartz DA, Visvesvara GS, Diesenhouse MC et al: Pathologic features and immunofluorescent antibody demonstration of ocular microsporidiosis *(Encephalitozoon hellem)* in seven patents with acquired immunodeficiency syndrome, *Am J Ophthalmol* 115:285, 1993.
37. Freij BJ, South MA, Sever JL: Maternal rubella and the congenital rubella syndrome, *Clin Perinatol* 15:247, 1988.
38. Margo CE, Hamel Al: Ocular syphilis, *Surv Ophthalmol* 37:203, 1992.
39. Wear DJ, Raga HM, Zimmerman LE et al: Cat scratch disease bacilli in the conjunctiva of patients with Paranaud's oculoglandular syndrome, *Ophthalmology* 92:1282, 1985.
40. Parfrey N: Improved diagnosis and prognosis of mucormycosis, *Medicine* 65:113, 1986.
41. Schwartz JN, Donnelly EH, Klintworth GK: Ocular and orbital phycomycosis, *Surv Ophthalmol* 22:3, 1977.
42. Easty DL: *Virus disease of the eye,* London, 1985, Lloyd-Luke.
43. Kean BH, Sun T, Elsworth RM: *Color atlas/text on ophthalmic parasitology,* New York, 1991, Igaku-Shoin.
44. Hennis HL, Scott HL, Apple DJ: Cytomegalovirus retinitis, *Surv Ophthalmol* 34:193, 1989.
45. Culbertson WW, Blumenkranz MS, Haines H et al: The acute retinal necrosis syndrome. Part 2: Histopathology and etiology, *Ophthalmology* 89:1317, 1982.
46. Fisher JP, Lewis ML, Blumenkranz M et al: The acute retinal necrosis syndrome. Part 1: clinical manifestations, *Ophthalmology* 89:1309, 1982.
47. Gartry DS, Spalton DJ, Tilzey A, Hykin PG: Acute retinal necrosis syndrome, *Br J Ophthalmol* 75:292, 1991.
48. *Auran DJ, Starr MB, Jakobiec FA:* Acanthamoeba keratitis: a review of the literature, *Cornea* 62:2, 1987.

Neoplasms and related masses

49. Phakomatous choristoma (Zimmerman's tumor): immunohistochemical confirmation of lens-specific proteins. *Ophthalmology* 100:955, 1993.

Tumors of conjunctiva, caruncle, and cornea

50. Odrich MG, Jakobiec FA, Lancaster WD et al: A spectrum of bilateral squamous conjunctival tumors associated with human papillomavirus type 16, *Ophthalmology* 98:628, 1991.
51. Ferry AP, Font RL: The phakomatoses, *Int Ophthalmol Clin* 12:1, 1972.
52. Ellis JH, Banks PM, Campbell RJ, Liesegang TJ: Lymphoid tumors of the ocular adnexa, *Ophthalmology* 92:1311, 1895.
53. Knowles DM, Jakobiec FA, McNally L, Burke JS: Lymphoid hyperplasia and malignant lymphoma occurring in the ocular adnexa (orbit, conjunctiva, and eyelids): a prospective multiparametric analysis of 108 cases during 1977 to 1987, *Hum Pathol* 21:959, 1990.
54. Jakobiec FA, Knowles DM: An overview of ocular lymphoid tumors, *Trans Am Ophthalmol Soc* 87:420, 1990.
55. Erie JC, Liesegang TJ, Campbell RJ: Conjunctival and corneal intraepithelial neoplasia: experience at the Mayo clinic, *Ophthalmology* 93:176, 1986.
56. Illif WF, Marbeck R, Green WR: Invasive squamous cell carcinoma of the conjunctiva, *Arch Ophthalmol* 93:119, 1975.
57. Gamel JW, Eiferman RA, Guibor P: Mucoepidermoid carcinoma of the conjunctiva, *Arch Ophthalmol* 102:730, 1984.
58. Huntington AC, Langloss JM, Hidayat AA: Spindle cell carcinoma of the conjunctiva: an immunohistochemical and ultrastructural study of six cases, *Ophthalmology* 97:711, 1990.
59. Folberg R, Jakobiec FA, Bernardino VB, Iwamoto T: Benign conjunctival melanocytic lesions: clinicopathologic features, *Ophthalmology* 96:436, 1989.
60. Grossniklaus HE, Green WR, Luckenbach M, Chan C: Conjunctival lesions in adults: a clinical and histopathologic review, *Cornea* 6:78, 1987.
61. Folberg R, McLean IW, Zimmerman LE: Malignant melanoma of the conjunctiva, *Hum Pathol* 16:136, 1985.
62. Jakobiec FA, Folberg R, Iwamoto T: Clinicopathologic characteristics of premalignant melanocytic lesions of the conjunctiva, *Ophthalmology* 96:147, 1989.
63. Jakobiec FA: The ultrastructure of conjunctival melanocytic tumors, *Trans Am Ophthalmol Soc* 82:599, 1984.
64. Machar AM, Palestine A, Masur H et al: Multicentric Kaposi's sarcoma of the conjunctiva in a male homosexual with the acquired immunodeficiency syndrome, *Ophthalmology* 90:879, 1983.

Tumors of eyelid

65. Font RL: Eyelids and lacrimal drainage system. In Spencer WH, editor: *Ophthalmic pathology: an atlas and textbook,* ed 3, Philadelphia, 1986, Saunders.
66. Doxanas MT, Green WR, Iliff CE: Factors in the successful surgical management of basal cell carcinoma of the eyelid, *Am J Ophthalmol* 91:726, 1981.
67. Einaugler RB, Henkind P: Basal cell carcinoma of the eyelid: apparent incomplete removal, *Am J Ophthalmol* 413, 1969.
68. Wolfe JT III, Yeatts RP, Wick MR et al: Sebaceous carcinoma of the eyelid: errors in clinical and pathological diagnosis, *Am J Surg Pathol* 8:597, 1984.
69. Rao NA, Hidayat AA, McLean IW, Zimmerman LE: Sebaceous gland carcinoma of the ocular adnexa: a clinicopathologic study of 104 cases with five year follow-up data, *Hum Pathol* 13:113, 1982.
70. Kennedy RH, Flanagan JC, Eagle RC Jr, Carney JA: The Carney complex with ocular signs suggestive of cardiac myxoma, *Am J Ophthalmol* 111:699, 1991.
71. Kivelä T, Tarkkanen A: The Merkel cell and associated neoplasm in the eyelids and periocular region, *Surv Ophthalmol* 35:171, 1990.
72. Wright JD, Font RL: Mucinous sweat gland carcinoma of the eyelid: a clinicopathologic study of 21 cases with histochemical and electron microscopic observations, *Cancer* 44:1757, 1979.
73. Jakobiec FA, Zimmerman LE, La Piana F et al: Unusual eyelid tumors with sebaceous differentiation in the Muir-Torre syndrome. rapid clinical regrowth and frank squamous transformation after biopsy, *Ophthalmology* 95:1543, 1988.

Tumors of uvea

74. McLean IW, Foster WD, Zimmerman LE: Modifications of Callender's classification of uveal melanoma at the Armed Forces Institute of Pathology, *Am J Ophthalmol* 96:502, 1983.
75. Shields JA, Zimmerman LE: Lesions simulating malignant melanoma of the posterior uvea, *Arch Ophthalmol* 89:466, 1973.
76. McLean IW, Foster WD, Zimmerman LE: Prognostic factors in small malignant melanomas of the choroid and ciliary body, *Arch Ophthalmol* 95:48, 1977.
77. McLean IW, Foster WD, Zimmerman LE: Uveal melanoma: location, size, cell type, and enucleation as risk factors in metastasis, *Hum Pathol* 13:123, 1982.
78. Zimmerman LE, McLean IW: The Montgomery lecture, 1975: changing concepts of the prognosis and management of small malignant melanomas of the choroid, *Trans Ophthalmol Soc UK* 95:487, 1975.
79. McLean IW, Zimmerman LE, Evans RM: Reappraisal of Callender's spindle A type of malignant melanoma of choroid and ciliary body, *Am J Ophthalmol* 86:557, 1978.
80. Gamel JW, McLean IW: Modern developments in histopathologic asssessment of uveal melanomas, *Ophthalmology* 91:679, 1984.
81. Folberg R, Rummelt V, Parys-Van Ginderdeuren R, et al: The prognostic value of tumor blood vessel morphology in primary uveal melanoma, *Ophthalmology* 100:1389, 1993.
82. Whelchel JC, Farah SE, McLean IW, Burnier MN: Immunohistochemistry of infiltrating lymphocytes in uveal malignant melanoma, *Invest Ophthalmol Vis Sci* 34:2603, 1993.
83. Witschel H, Font RL: Hemangioma of the choroid: a clinicopathologic study of 71 cases and a review of the literature, *Surv Ophthalmol* 20:415, 1976.
84. Shields JA, Stephen RF, Eagle RC Jr et al: Progressive enlargement of a circumscribed choroidal hemangioma: a clinicopathological correlation, *Arch Ophthalmol* 110:1276, 1992.
85. Jakobiec FA, Silbert G: Are most iris "melanomas" really nevi? *Arch Ophthalmol* 99:2117, 1981.

Tumors of retina and neural ectoderm

86. Zimmerman LE: Retinoblastoma and retinocytoma. In Spencer WH, editor: *Ophthalmic pathology: an atlas and textbook,* ed 3, Philadelphia, 1985, Saunders.
87. Shields CL, Shields JA, Shah P: Retinoblastoma in older children, *Ophthalmology* 98:395, 1991.

88. Knudson AG Jr, Hethcote HW, Brown BW: Mutation and childhood cancer: a probabilistic model for the incidence or retinoblastoma, *Proc Natl Acad Sci USA* 72:5116, 1975.
89. Cavenee WK, Dryja TP, Phillips RA et al: Expression of recessive alleles by chromosomal mechanisms in retinoblastoma, *Nature* 305:779, 1983.
90. Sopta M, Gallie BL, Gill RM et al: The retinoblastoma protein and the cell cycle, *Semin Cancer Biol* 3:107, 1992.
91. Horowitz JM, Yandell DW, Park SH, et al: Point mutational: inactivation of the retinoblastoma antioncogene, *Science* 243:937, 1989.
92. Gallie BL, Squire JA, Goddard A et al: Mechanisms of oncogenesis in retinoblastoma: review, *Lab Invest* 62:394, 1990.
93. Mansour AM, Greenwald MJ, O'Grady R: Diffuse infiltrating retinoblastoma, *J Pediatr Ophthalmol Strabismus* 26:152, 1989.
94. Tso MOM, Fine BS, Zimmerman LE: The Flexner-Wintersteiner rosettes in retinoblastoma, *Arch Pathol* 88:665, 1969.
95. Tso MOM, Zimmerman LE, Fine BS: The nature of retinoblastoma. Photoreceptor differentiation: a clinical and histopathological study, *Am J Ophthalmol* 69:339, 1970.
96. Mullaney J: DNA in retinoblastoma, *Lancet* 2:918, 1968.
97. MacKay CJ, Abrahamson DH, Ellsworth RM: Metastatic patterns of retinoblastoma, *Arch Ophthalmol* 102:391, 1984.
98. Gallie BL, Ellsworth RM, Abramson DH, Phillips RA: Retinoma: spontaneous regression of retinoblastoma or benign manifestion of the mutation? *Br J Cancer* 45:513, 1982.
99. Margo C, Hidayat A, Kopelman J, Zimmerman LE: Retinocytoma: a benign variant of retinoblastoma, *Arch Ophthalmol* 101:1519, 1983.
100. Abramson DH: Retinoma, retinocytoma, and the retinoblastoma gene, *Arch Ophthalmol* 101:1517, 1983.
101. Eagle RC Jr, Shields JA, Donoso L et al: Malignant transformation of spontaneously regressed retinoblastoma, retinoma/retinocytoma variant, *Ophthalmology* 96:1389, 1989.
102. Gallie BL, Dunn JM, Chan HS et al: The genetics of retinoblastoma: relevance to the patient, *Pediatr Clin North Am* 38:299, 1991.
103. Roarty JD, McLean IW, Zimmerman LE: Incidence of second neoplasms in patients with bilateral retinoblastoma, *Ophthalmology* 95:1583, 1988.
104. Abramson DH, Ellsworth RM, Zimmerman LE: Nonocular cancer in retinoblastoma survivors, *Trans Am Acad Ophthalmol Otolaryngol* 81:454, 1976.
105. Anonymous: Survival rate and risk factors for patients with retinoblastoma in Japan: the committee for the National Registry of Retinoblastoma, *Jpn J Ophthalmol* 36:121, 1992.
106. Holladay DA, Holladay A, Montebello JF, Redmond KP: Clinical presentation, treatment, and outcome of trilateral retinoblastoma, *Cancer* 67:710, 1991.
107. Bader JL, Meadows AT, Zimmerman LE et al: Bilateral retinoblastoma with ectopic intracranial retinoblastoma: trilateral retinoblastoma, *Cancer Genet Cytogenet* 5:203, 1982.
108. Pesin SR, Shields JA: Seven cases of trilateral retinoblastoma, *Am J Ophthalmol* 107:121, 1989.
109. Broughton WL, Zimmerman LE: A clinicopathologic study of 56 cases of intraocular medulloblastoma, *Am J Ophthalmol* 85:407, 1978.
110. Canning CR, McCartney ACE, Hungerford JL: Medulloepithelioma (diktyoma), *Br J Ophthalmol* 72:764, 1988.
111. Freeman LM, Schachat AP, Knox DL et al: Clinical features, laboratory investigation, and survival in ocular reticulum cell sarcoma, *Ophthalmology* 94:1631, 1987.

Tumors of orbit

112. Iliff WJ: Orbital tumors in children. In Jakobiec FA, editor: *Ocular and adnexal tumors,* Birmingham, Ala, 1978, Aesculapius.
113. Jakobiec FA, Font RL: Orbit. In Spencer WH, editor: *Ophthalmic pathology: an atlas and textbook,* ed 3, Philadelphia, 1986, Saunders.
114. Kennedy RE: An evaluation of 820 orbital cases, *Trans Am Ophthalmol Soc* 82:134, 1984.
115. Rootman J: *Diseases of the orbit,* Philadelphia, 1988, Lippincott.
116. Shields JA: *Diagnosis and management of orbital tumors,* Philadelphia, 1989, Saunders.
117. Shields JA, Bakewell B, Augsburger JJ et al: Space-occupying orbital masses in children: a review of 250 consecutive biopsies, *Ophthalmology* 93:379, 1986.
118. Kobrin JL, Blodi FC, Weingeist TA: Ocular and orbital manifestations of neurofibromatosis, *Surv Ophthalmol* 24:45, 1979.
119. Newton WA, Soule EH, Hamoudi AB et al: Histopathology of childhood sarcomas, intergroup rhabdomyosarcoma studies I and II: clinicopathologic correlation, *J Clin Oncol* 6:67, 1988.
120. Porterfield JF, Zimmerman LE: Rhabdomyosarcoma of the orbit: a clinicopathologic study of 55 cases, *Virchows Arch [A]* 335:329, 1962.
121. Font RL, Hidayat AA: Fibrous histiocytoma of the orbit, *Hum Pathol* 13:199, 1982.
122. Croxatto O, Font RL: Hemangiopericytoma of the orbit: a clinicopathologic study of 30 cases, *Hum Pathol* 13:210, 1982.
123. Iwamoto T, Jakobiec FA: Ultrastructural comparison of capillary and cavernous hemangiomas of the orbit, *Arch Ophthalmol* 97:1144, 1979.
124. Collins VP, Nordenskjöld M, Dumanski JP: The molecular genetics of meningiomas, *Brain Pathol* 1:19, 1990.
125. Margo CE, Ragsdale B, Purman K et al: Psammotoid (juvenile) ossifying fibroma of the orbit, *Ophthalmology* 92:150, 1985.
126. Feldman RB, Moore RB, Hood CI et al: Solitary eosinophilic granuloma of the lateral orbital wall, *Am J Ophthalmol* 100:318, 1985.
127. Davis JL, Parke DW II, Font RL: Granulocytic sarcoma of the orbit: a clinicopathologic study, *Ophthalmology* 92:1758, 1985.
128. Iliff WJ, Green WR: Orbital lymphangiomas, *Ophthalmology* 86:914, 1979.

Tumors of lacrimal gland and lacrimal drainage apparatus

129. Shields CL, Shields JA: Lacrimal gland tumors, *Int Ophthalmol Clin* 33:181, 1993.
130. Font RL, Gamel JW: Epithelial tumors of the lacrimal gland: an analysis of 256 cases. In Jakobiec FA, editor: *Ocular and adnexal tumors,* Birmingham, Ala, 1978, Aesculapius.
131. Wright JE, Rose GE: Primary malignant neoplasms of the lacrimal gland, *Br J Ophthalmol* 76:401, 1992.
132. Gamel JW, Font RL: Adenoid cystic carcinoma of the lacrimal gland: the clinical significance of a basaloid histologic pattern, *Hum Pathol* 13:219, 1982.
133. Lee DA, Campbell RJ, Waller RR, Ilstrup DM: A clinicopathologic study of primary adenoid cystic carcinoma of the lacrimal gland, *Ophthalmology* 92:128, 1985.
134. Ni C, D'Amico DJ, Fan CQ, Kuo P-K: Tumors of the lacrimal sac: a clinicopathological analysis of 82 cases, *Int Ophthalmol Clin* 22:121, 1982.

Tumors of optic nerve

135. Rush JA, Younge BR, Campbell RJ, McCarthy CS: Optic glioma: long-term follow-up of 85 histopathologically verified cases, *Ophthalmology* 289:1213, 1982.
136. Manor RS, Israeli J, Sandbank U: Malignant optic glioma in a 70 year old patient, *Arch Ophthalmol* 94:1142, 1976.
137. Marquardt MD, Zimmerman LE: Histopathology of meningiomas and gliomas of the optic nerve, *Hum Pathol* 13:226, 1982.

Metastatic and secondary tumors

138. Leonardy NJ, Rupani M, Dent G, Klintworth GK: Analysis of 135 eyes for ocular involvement in leukemia, *Am J Ophthalmol* 109:436, 1990.
139. Nelson CC, Herzberg BS, Klintworth GK: A histopathologic study of 716 unselected eyes in patients with cancer at the time of death, *Am J Ophthalmol* 95:788, 1983.
140. Arnold AC, Bullock AC, Foos RY: Metastatic eyelid carcinoma, *Ophthalmology* 92:114, 1985.

Non-neoplastic masses

141. Klintworth GK: Degenerations, depositions, and miscellaneous reactions of the ocular anterior segment. In Garner A, Klintworth GK, editors: *Pathobiology of ocular disease: a dynamic approach,* ed 2, New York, 1994, Marcel Dekker.
142. Austin P, Jakobiec FA, Iwamoto T: Elastodysplasia and elastodystrophy as the pathologic bases of ocular pterygia and pinguecula, *Ophthalmology* 90:96, 1983.

143. Holds JB, Anderson RI, Mamalis N et al: Invasive squamous cell carcinoma arising from asymptomatic choristomatous cysts of the orbit: two cases and a review of the literature. *Ophthalmology* 100:1244, 1993.

Vascular diseases

144. Zimmerman LE: Ocular lesions of juvenile xanthogranuloma, nevoxanthoendothelioma, *Trans Am Acad Ophthalmol Otolaryngol* 69:412, 1965.
145. Klintworth GK: *Corneal angiogenesis: a comprehensive critical review,* New York, 1991, Springer-Verlag.
146. Goldberg MF: Retinal neovascularization in sickle cell retinopathy, *Trans Am Acad Ophthalmol Otolaryngol* 83:OP409, 1977.
147. John TJ, Sassani JW, Eagle RC Jr: The myofibroblastic component of rubeosis iridis, *Ophthalmology* 90:721, 1983.
148. Chess J, Albert DM, Bhan AK: Serologic and immunopathologic findings in temporal arteritis, *Am J Ophthalmol* 96:283, 1983.
149. McDonnell PJ, Moore GW, Miller NR et al: Temporal arteritis: a clinicopathological study, *Ophthalmology* 93:518, 1986.
150. Green WR, Chan CC, Hutchins GM, Terry JM: Central retinal vein occlusion: a prospective histopathologic study of 29 eyes in 28 cases, *Trans Am Ophthalmol Soc* 79:371, 1981.
151. Hayreh SS: Pathogenesis of occlusion of the central retinal vessels, *Am J Ophthalmol* 72:998, 1971.

Trauma

152. Riffenburgh RS, Sathyavagiswaran L: Ocular findings at autopsy of child abuse victims, *Ophthalmology* 98:1519, 1991.
153. Klintworth GK, Streeten BM, Eagle RC Jr: Applications of energy dispersive microprobe analysis in ophthalmic pathology. In Ingram P, Shelburne JD, Roggli VI, editors: *Microprobe analysis in medicine,* New York, 1989, Hemisphere.

Eye in systemic disease

154. Gold DH, Weingeist TA, editors: *The eye in systemic disease,* Philadelphia, 1990, Lippincott.

Diabetes mellitus

155. Caird FI, Pirie A, Ramsell TG: *Diabetes and the eye,* Oxford, 1994, Blackwell.
156. Cogan DG, Touissant D, Kuwabara T: Retinal vascular patterns. IV. Diabetic retinopathy, *Arch Ophthalmol* 66:366, 1961.
157. Yanoff M: Ocular pathology of diabetes mellitus, *Am J Ophthalmol* 67:21, 1969.

Thyroid eye disease

158. Werner WC: Modification of the classification of the eye changes of Graves' disease, *Am J Ophthalmol* 83:725, 1977.
159. Char DH: The ophthalmopathy of Graves' disease, *Med Clin North Am* 70:97, 1991.
160. Hufnagel TJ, Hickey WF, Cobbs WH et al: Immunohistochemical and ultrastructural studies on the exenterated orbital tissues of a patient with Graves' disease, *Ophthalmology* 91:1411, 1984.
161. van der Gaag R, Vernimmen R, Fiebelkorn N et al: Graves' ophthalmopathy: what is the evidence for extraocular muscle specific autoantibodies, *Int Ophthalmol* 14:25, 1990.

Sarcoidosis

162. Obenauf CD, Sydnor CF, Klintworth GK: Sarcoidosis and its ophthalmic manifestations, *Am J Ophthalmol* 86:648, 1978.
163. Nichols CW, Eagle RC Jr, Yanoff M, Menocal NG: Conjunctival biopsy as an aid in the evaluation of the patient with suspected sarcoidosis, *Ophthalmology* 87:287, 1980.

Rheumatoid arthritis

164. Foster CS, Forstot SL, Wilson LA: Mortality rate in rheumatoid arthritis patients developing necrotizing scleritis peripheral ulcerative keratitis: effects of systemic immunosuppression, *Ophthalmology* 91:1253, 1984.

Specific ocular disorders

Glaucoma

165. Quigley HA, Addicks EM, Green WR, Maumenee AE: Optic nerve damage in human glaucoma. II. The site of injury and susceptibility to damage, *Arch Ophthalmol* 99:635, 1981.
166. Quigley HA: Optic nerve damage in human glaucoma. III. Quantitative correlation of nerve fiber loss and visual field defect in glaucoma, ischemic optic neuropathy, papilledema and toxic neuropathy, *Arch Ophthalmol* 100:135, 1982.
167. Quigley HA, Green WR: The histology of human glaucoma and nerve damage: clinicopathologic correlation in 21 eyes. *Ophthalmology* 86:1803, 1979.
168. Sheffield VC, Stone EM, Alward WL et al: Genetic linkage of familial open angle glaucoma to chromosome 1q21-q31, *Nat Genet* 4:47, 1993.
169. Alvarado JA, Murphy CG, Juster R: Trabecular meshwork cellularity in primary open-angle glaucoma and nonglaucomatous normals, *Ophthalmology* 91:564, 1984.
170. Shields CL, Shields JA, Shields MB, Augsburger JJ: Prevalence and mechanisms of secondary intraocular pressure elevation in eyes with intraocular tumors, *Ophthalmology* 94:839, 1987.
171. Yanoff M, Scheie HG: Melanomalytic glaucoma, *Arch Ophthalmol* 84:471, 1970.
172. Murphy CG, Johnson M, Alvarado JA: Juxtacanalicular tissue in pigmentary and open angle glaucoma: the hydrodynamic role of pigment and other constituents, *Arch Ophthalmol* 110:1779, 1992.
173. Bernardino VB Jr, Kim JC, Smith TR: Epithelialization of the anterior chamber after cataract surgery, *Arch Ophthalmol* 82:742, 1969.
174. Eagle RC Jr, Font RL, Yanoff M, Fine BS: Proliferative endotheliopathy with iris abnormalities: the iridocorneal endothelial syndrome, *Arch Ophthalmol* 97:2104, 1979.
175. Alvarado JA, Murphy CG: Outflow obstruction in pigmentary and primary open angle glaucoma, *Arch Ophthalmol* 110:1769, 1992.
176. Flocks M, Littwin CS, Zimmerman LE: Phakolytic glaucoma: a clinicopathologic study of 138 cases of glaucoma associated with hypermature cataract, *Am J Ophthalmol* 54:37, 1955.
177. Campbell DG: Pigmentary dispersion and glaucoma: a new theory, *Arch Ophthalmol* 97:1667, 1979.

Diseases of cornea

178. Klintworth GK: Corneal dystrophies, *Curr Opin Ophthalmol* 2:382, 1991.
179. Starck T, Hersh PS, Kenyon KR: Corneal dysgeneses, dystrophies and degenerations. In Albert DM, Jakobiec FA, editors: *Principles and practice of ophthalmology, clinical practice,* Philadelphia, 1993, Saunders.
180. Klintworth GK: Corneal dystrophies. In Nicholson DH, editor: *Ocular pathology update,* New York, 1980, Masson.
181. Klintworth GK: Disorders of glycosaminoglycans (mucopolysaccharides) and proteoglycans. In Garner A, Klintworth GK, editors: *Pathobiology of ocular disease: a dynamic approach,* ed 2, New York, 1994, Marcel Dekker.
182. Klintworth GK: Proteins in ocular disease. In Garner A, Klintworth GK, editors: *Pathobiology of ocular disease: a dynamic approach,* ed 2, New York, 1994, Marcel Dekker.
183. Klintworth GK: Lattice corneal dystrophy: an inherited variety of amyloidosis restricted to the cornea, *Am J Pathol* 50:371, 1967.
184. Stone EM, Mathers WD, Rossenwasser GOD, et al: Three autosomal dominant corneal dystrophies map to chromosome 5q, *Nat Genet* 6:47, 1994.
185. Edward DP, Thonar EJ, Srinivasan M et al: Macular dystrophy of the cornea: a systemic disorder of keratan sulfate metabolism, *Ophthalmology* 97:1194, 1990.

Diseases of retina

186. Green WR, Enger C: Age-related macular degeneration histopathologic studies: the 1992 Lorenz E. Zimmerman lecture. *Ophthalmology* 100:1519, 1993.
187. van der Schaft TL, de Bruijn WC, Mooy CM et al: Is basal laminar deposit unique for age-related macular degeneration? *Arch Ophthalmol* 109:420, 1991.
188. Bird A, Jay B, Hussain AA, Marshall J: Retinal photoreceptor disorders. In Garner A, Klintworth GK, editors: *Pathobiology of ocular disease: a dynamic approach,* ed 2, New York, 1994, Marcel Dekker.
189. Meindl A, Berger W, Meitinger T et al: Norrie disease is caused by mutations in an extracellular protein resembling C-terminal globular domain of mucins, *Nat Genet* 2:139, 1992.

Diseases of the vitreous

190. Engel HM, Green WR, Michels RG, et al: Diagnostic vitrectomy, *Retina* 1:121, 1981.

Diseases of crystalline lens

191. Streeten BW: Pseudoexfoliation syndrome. In Garner A, Klintworth GK, editors: *Pathobiology of ocular disease: a dynamic approach,* ed 2, New York, 1994, Marcel Dekker.
192. Klintworth GK, Garner A: The causes, types, and morphology of cataracts. In Garner A, Klintworth GK, editors: *Pathobiology of ocular disease: a dynamic approach,* ed 2, New York, 1994, Marcel Dekker.
193. Apple DJ, Mamilis N, Loftfield K et al: Complications of intraocular lenses: a historical and histochemical review, *Surv Ophthalmol* 29:1, 1984.
194. Streeten BW: Pseudoexfoliative fibrillopathy in visceral organs of a patient with pseudoexfoliation syndrome, *Arch Ophthalmol* 110:1757, 1992.
195. Schlotzer-Schredhardt UM, Koca MR, Naumann GOH, Volkholz H: Pseudoexfoliation syndrome: ocular manifestations of a systemic disorder? *Arch Ophthalmol* 110:1752, 1992.

Diseases of optic nerve

196. Tso MOM, Fine BS: Electron microscopic study of papilledema in man, *Am J Ophthalmol* 82:424, 1976.
197. Tso MOM, Hayreh SS: Optic disc edema in raised intracranial pressures. IV. Axoplasmic transport in experimental papilledema, *Arch Ophthalmol* 95:1458, 1977.
198. Andersen DR: Ascending and descending optic atrophy produced experimentally in squirrel monkeys, *Am J Ophthalmol* 76:693, 1973.
199. Brown MD, Voljavec AS, Lott MT et al: Leber's hereditary optic neuropathy: a model for mitochondrial neurodegenerative diseases, *FASEB J* 6:2791, 1992.

Diseases of lacrimal drainage apparatus

200. Seal DV, McGill J, Flanagan O, Purrier B: Lacrimal canaliculitis due to *Arachnia (Actinomyces) propionica, Br J Ophthalmol* 65:10, 1981.

80 Ear

Leslie Michaels

NORMAL ANATOMY AND HISTOLOGY

The ear is divided into external, middle and inner parts, and its structure (Fig. 80-1) may be considered from the standpoint of its functions in hearing and balance. The pinna and external canal conduct sound waves in air to the tympanic membrane. The middle ear enhances the transmission of sound energy to the fluids of the inner ear by conveying vibrations from the larger area of the tympanic membrane through the ossicular chain, comprising the malleus, incus, and stapes, to the much smaller area of the footplate of the stapes, which lies in the oval window of the vestibule in contact with perilymph. The air space of the middle ear cavity is magnified by the mastoid air cells which are complex expansions into the mastoid bone. The middle ear space is connected with the nasopharynx and hence with the external air through the eustachian tube, by which air pressure can be adjusted.

From the vestibular perilymph, vibrations derived from sound waves pass directly into the spirally coiled perilymphatic spaces of the cochlea, where an upper compartment, the scala vestibuli, ascending from the vestibule and oval window, and a lower compartment, the scala tympani, are located. The latter descends to a connective tissue disk, the round window membrane, which separates the perilymph compartment from the middle ear. Between the scalae vestibuli and tympani there is an endolymph-containing, coiled middle compartment, the cochlear duct (scala media), which houses the sensory organ of sound reception, the organ of Corti. The cochlear duct communicates with the vestibular endolymph-containing sacs by means of two fine canals, such that the endolymphatic system of the cochlea and vestibule is continuous like the perilymphatic one. Waves of vibration are conveyed from the perilymph to the walls of the scala media, from which they are conveyed to the organ of Corti through the endolymph.

Gravitational acceleration of the head is detected by a sensory organ arranged within endolymph-containing sacs in the vestibule (the utricle and saccule), and angular acceleration is detected by tubes emanating in three dimensions from the utricle (the lateral, posterior, and superior semicircular canals). The sensory cells are located as a thickened portion of epithelium, the macula, in the saccule and utricle and a raised prominence of epithelium, the crista, in expansions of each semicircular canal, the ampullae. The vestibular aqueduct contains the endolymphatic duct and sac, which form a blind offshoot of the endolymphatic system, probably functioning in the absorption of endolymph. The cochlear aqueduct serves as a communication between the cerebrospinal fluid (CSF) in the subarachnoid space and the perilymph of the scala tympani near the round window. The cochlea, vestibule, and semicircular canals are surrounded by very dense bone, the otic capsule.

The cochlear and vestibular sensory structures are supplied by a double nerve, the audiovestibular nerve, or eighth cranial nerve, which enters the temporal bone through the internal auditory canal. The facial nerve, or seventh cranial nerve, enters the temporal bone through the same canal and, after making a right-angled bend in the genu, where the geniculate ganglion is located, reaches the posterior wall of the middle ear, from which it passes down through the mastoid to emerge in the region of the parotid gland.

The histologic features of ear and temporal bone structures are summarized in Table 80-1.[1]

EXTERNAL EAR

Malformations

Malformations of the external ear include:

1. Partial or complete absence and abnormalities in the shape and size of the auricle.

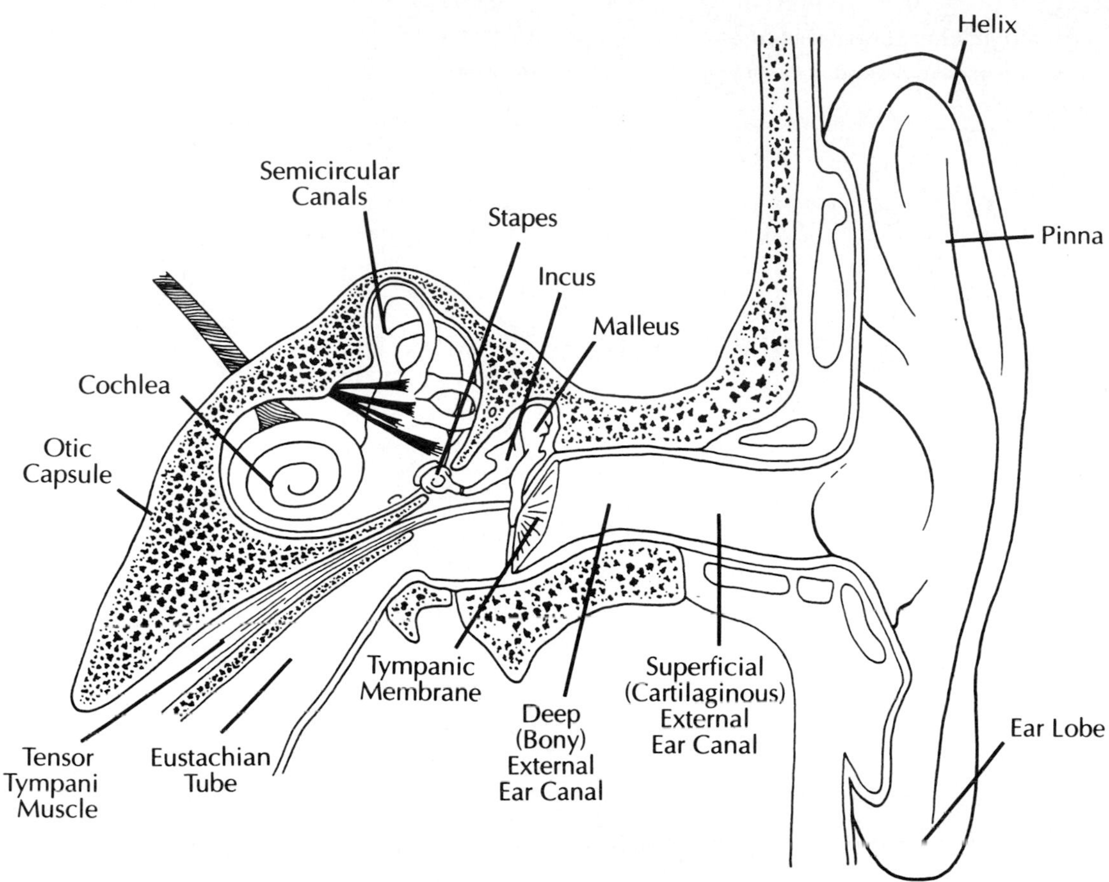

Fig. 80-1 Anatomy of the ear.

2. Accessory auricles.
3. Preauricular sinus, which usually has a squamous epithelial lining (occasionally respiratory) and elastic cartilage in the wall.
4. Atresia of the external auditory meatus, which may be a blind protrusion or may be completely absent. The middle ear is usually normal.

Diagonal earlobe crease

A crease in the earlobe has been reliably associated with heart disease, especially that resulting from coronary artery ischemia.[2] Earlobes may be normally free or attached, with the "soldered" form being an extreme version of the latter.[3] Creases occur in all three forms of earlobes and run diagonally backward and downward across the lateral surface of the earlobe from the external meatus. A cardiovascular cause of death was found in 73% of patients with creases and 45% of patients without creases.[4] Most of the cardiovascular deaths resulted from ischemic or hypertensive disease, or both, with aneurysms, valvular disease, cor pulmonale, and cardiomyopathy accounting for the remainder.

Inflammatory lesions

Diffuse external otitis

Diffuse external otitis is common in the external auditory meatus. Several different species of organisms, but most commonly *Pseudomonas aeruginosa,* have been recovered from the inflammatory exudate, but a hot, humid environment and local trauma to the external canal are also important causes.[5] Superficial fungi, including aspergilli, may cause external otitis. In this setting the skin of the external canal is erythematous, edematous and discharging. Histologic examination reveals the presence of pronounced acanthosis, hyperkeratosis, and an acute inflammatory exudate in the dermis, particularly around apocrine glands.

Malignant otitis externa

Malignant otitis externa, with "malignant" referring to the severity of the lesion and not to a neoplastic process, was first reported as a severe infection of the external auditory canal that usually affects elderly diabetic patients and is caused by *P. aeruginosa.*[6] The condition frequently progresses, with ninth, tenth, eleventh, and twelfth cranial nerve palsies, meningitis, and death ensuing. At autopsy, severe otitis media, involvement of the jugular foramen by the inflammatory process, and thrombophlebitis of the jugular bulb were found in the temporal bone of all of four patients.[7] It seems likely that the advanced manifestations of malignant otitis externa result from the spread of inflammation from the *middle ear* to the petrous apex, and the reduced tissue immunity to infection that occurs in diabetic patients makes them particularly prone to this infection. Tissue changes include necrosis of external canal bone, osteomyelitis and osteogenesis.

Pneumocystis carinii *infection*

Pneumocystis carinii infection may develop in the external ear[9,10] and the middle ear of patients with the acquired immun-

Table 80-1 Histologic characteristics of ear and temporal bone structures

Structures	Features
Pinna	Cartilage, skin with appendages
External auditory canal	
Superficial	Cartilage, skin with appendages, and ceruminal glands
Deep	Lamellar bone, thick stratified squamous epithelium (migrating); no appendages
Tympanic membrane	
Pars flaccida	External: thick stratified squamous epithelium (migrating); *middle:* nonstructured connective tissue; internal cuboidal epithelium
Pars tensa	External: thin stratified squamous epithelium (migrating); *middle:* structured collagen; internal: cuboidal epithelium
Middle ear cavity and mastoid air cells	Lamellar bony wall, cuboidal epithelium
Ossicles (malleus, incus, and stapes superstructure)	Periosteal and endochondral bone, cuboidal epithelium
Stapes footplate	Endochondral bone on tympanic surface, cartilage on vestibular surface
Eustachian tube	
Nasopharyngeal part	Cartilaginous framework, pseudostratified respiratory epithelium, seromucinous glands
Middle ear part	Bony framework (thin), pseudostratified respiratory epithelium
Otic capsule (surrounding cochlea, vestibule, and semicircular canals)	Dense cortical bone with globuli ossei
Cochlea	Three spiral compartments: *upper*, scala vestibuli (perilymph); *middle,* scala media (endolymph); *lower,* scala tympani (perilymph)
Scala media	Triangular compartment bounded by Reissner's membrane, basilar membrane with sensory organ of Corti, and stria vascularis (endolymph secretion)
Vestibule (perilymph)	
Saccule (endolymph)	Sensory macula with otolithic membrane and nonsensory flat
Utricle (endolymph)	Sensory macula with otolithic membrane and nonsensory flat epithelium
Semicircular canals: lateral, posterior and superior (perilymph)	
Ampullae (endolymph)	Sensory cristae with mucoproteinous cupulae
Semicircular ducts (endolymph)	Flat epithelium
Vestibular aqueduct	Lamellar bone
Endolymphatic duct	Cuboidal epithelium
Endolymphatic sac	Papillary columnar epithelium (endolymph absorption)
Cochlear aqueduct (cerebrospinal fluid—perilymph)	From subarachnoid space to scala tympani—flat epithelium
Audiovestibular nerve (eighth cranial nerve)	Myelinated; neurilemmal-glial junction in internal auditory canal
Vestibular branch	Vestibular ganglion (sensory) in internal auditory canal
Auditory branch	Spiral ganglion (sensory) in modiolus of cochlea
Facial nerve (seventh cranial nerve)	Geniculate ganglion (sensory fibers of taste from palate) in genu of fallopian canal; nerve often dehiscent in middle ear portion of fallopian canal
Paraganglia	
Tympanic	*Zellballen,* blood vessels, and nerves
Jugular	*Zellballen,* blood vessels, and nerves

odeficiency syndrome (AIDS); in the latter instance aural polyps containing the organism also develop.[11-13] On histologic examination, lakes of foamy eosinophilic material are seen beneath the epithelium, accompanied by a mixed inflammatory exudate and surrounded by fibrovascular proliferation. Methenamine silver staining reveals the existence of dark-rimmed spherical and cup-shaped organisms characteristic of *P. carinii*. The ear lesion may precede involvement of the lungs, but the latter eventually show the changes characteristics of pneumonia resulting from this organism.

Viral infections

Both types 1 and 2 herpes simplex virus may cause blisters to form in the external canal. Histologically these lesions are intraepidermal vesicles produced by acantholysis of epidermal cells. Cells in the epidermis surrounding the vesicle exhibit ballooning degeneration and intranuclear eosinophilic inclusions surrounded by a halo (see Chapter 36).

Herpes zoster is caused by the varicella-zoster virus, which travels from the nerve ganglia, where it has been in a latent state, along nerves to the skin. When the geniculate ganglion is affected there results a vesicular eruption that involves the pinna, external canal, postauricular skin, uvula, palate, and anterior portion of the tongue. When this is combined with disturbances of hearing and balance resulting from involvement of the ganglia of the eighth cranial nerve, the condition is termed the "Ramsay Hunt syndrome." The skin lesions are histologically similar to those of herpes simplex. Specific varicella-zoster virus antigens can be demonstrated by immunofluorescence.

Granulomatous inflammation

Granulomatous inflammation that arises in reaction to the starch granules used as a vehicle in antibiotics occurs in the external and middle ear. Microscopically there is an exudate of lymphocytes and histiocytes containing granules of starch; these granules are spherical or polyhedral basophilic bodies with a diameter of 10 to 20 μm and a Maltese cross birefringence that become a brilliant red after staining with periodic acid–Schiff (PAS) reagent.[15]

Another type of granulomatous reaction is the hair granuloma. Histologically the foreign-body type giant cells are seen surrounding and engulfing hair shafts. The hairs in the granulomas are derived from those of the patient, possibly by ingrowth from the orifice of the canal, in the same fashion as occurs in the setting of a pilonidal sinus of the sacroiliac skin. In some instances the lesion may arise after haircutting.

Relapsing polychondritis

Relapsing polychondritis is characterized by recurring bouts of inflammation affecting cartilaginous structures and the eye and heart. Although the cartilage of the external ear is most frequently involved, it is the inflammation with attendant destruction of the cartilages of the larynx that threatens life by causing respiratory obstruction.[16]

The earlobe is usually normal (Fig. 80-2). In the acute stage the auricle is hot and erythematous. Later the anterior surface may have a cobblestone appearance, and the auricle may eventually become atrophic. Microscopy reveals that the ground substance of the cartilage becomes acidophilic and is more deeply stained by the PAS stain. Granulation tissue with inflammatory cells composed of neutrophils in the early stages and plasma cells and lymphocytes in the later stages invades the cartilage from the perichondrium (Fig. 80-3). Fibroblasts multiply, and eventually a dense, poorly cellular scar forms.

The significance of the antibodies to type II collagen in the blood[17] and of immunoglobulin and the C3 component of complement in the affected tissues of patients with relapsing polychondritis[18] still remains doubtful.

Other disorders

In *keratosis obturans* the keratin produced by exfoliation from the skin of the tympanic membrane and external canal is retained on the epithelial surface and forms a solid plug filling the whole canal. This enlarges and may cause erosion of the bony wall of the ear canal. Patients with this lesion are reputed to suffer more frequently from chronic sinusitis or bronchiectasis.

Keratosis obturans may represent an advanced stage of the recently described "keratosis of the tympanic membrane and deep external canal," in which keratin deposits form on the tympanic membrane as a result of a defect in auditory epithelial migration.[19]

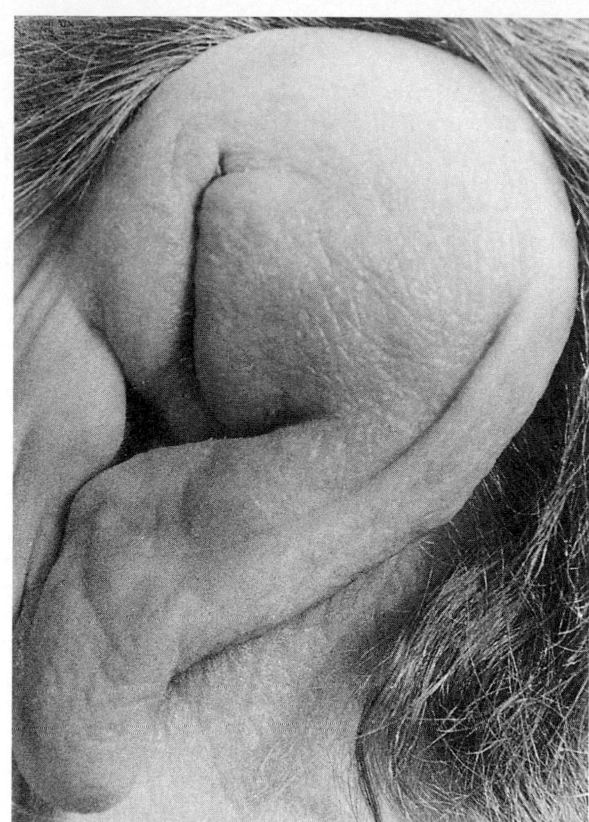

Fig. 80-2 Relapsing polychondritis showing a distorted pinna in the cartilaginous region but with a normal earlobe. (From Michaels L. *Ear, nose and throat histopathology,* London, 1987, Springer-Verlag.)

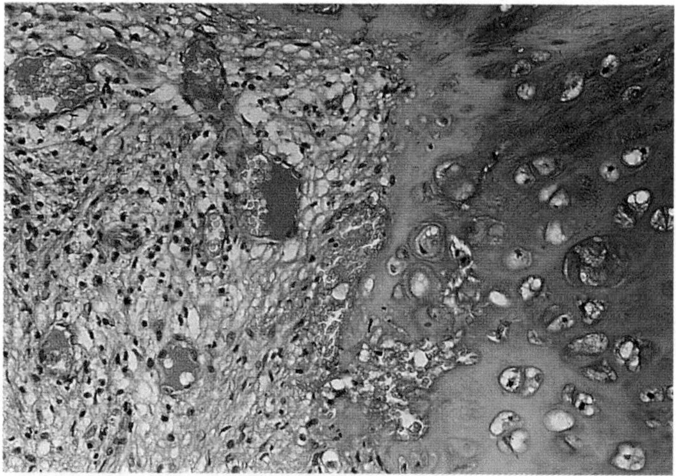

Fig. 80-3 Relapsing polychondritis of cricoid cartilage showing inflammatory granulation tissue eroding the edge of the cartilage.

Cholesteatoma of the external canal has been identified as a process in which the inferior and posterior ear canal wall is eroded in localized fashion by a squamous epithelium-lined sac derived focally from the epidermis of the canal.[20]

In *keratin implantation granuloma* a granulomatous process may occur in the external canal in reaction to the implantation of keratin squames into the deeper tissues after traumatic laceration.[21]

Metabolic conditions

Gout

The external ear is one of the most frequent sites of urate deposition in the setting of gout (tophi); this occurs in the helix and antihelix. These deposits may ulcerate, discharging a creamy white material containing sodium urate crystals. Histologically the gouty tophus is composed of basophilic masses of amorphous material surrounded by foreign-body giant cells and histiocytes accompanied by birefringent sodium urate crystals, particularly if the tissue is fixed in alcohol to preserve the latter.

Ochronosis

In ochronosis (alkaptonuria) there may be one or both of two alterations in the external ear: (1) darkly colored wax and (2) darkly colored aural cartilage resulting from the binding of the homogentisic acid to the cartilage ground substance.[22] The former may be the first manifestation of the disease in children.

Xanthoma associated with hyperlipoproteinemia

Some inherited hyperlipoproteinemic conditions are associated with the development of cutaneous and tendinous xanthomas and severe atherosclerotic coronary artery disease. Deposits of lipid with an associated histiocytic reaction are found in the temporal bone in occasional patients.[23,24] (Fig. 80-4).

Lesions simulating neoplasms

Malakoplakia

Malakoplakia (see Chapter 66) is rare in the ear, but it has been found in both the external and the middle ear.[25-27] The lesion is characterized by macrophages with an abundant cytoplasm containing diastase-resistant, PAS-positive granules. Lamellated, calcified (Michaelis-Gutmann) bodies can be seen within macrophages.

Chondrodermatitis nodularis chronica helicis

In chondrodermatitis nodularis chronica helicis (Winkler's disease),[2] a small, painful nodule forms on the auricle, usually in the superior portion of the helix. Histologically the nodule usually shows ulceration with pronounced irregular acanthosis at its margins. The collagen in its center show increased eosinophilia, is often degenerated, and is surrounded by chronic inflammatory granulation tissue. The perichondrium adjacent to the lesion is usually involved by the inflammatory tissue (Fig. 80-5), and the nearby elastic cartilage is also often degenerated.[29]

Spectacle-frame acanthoma (granuloma fissuratum)

Spectacle-frame acanthoma arises behind the ear in the region of the postauricular groove and results from irritation caused by the bow of spectacle frames. Clinically, it is commonly mistaken for basal cell carcinoma. Grossly there is a raised pink nodule with a linear depression running through its center. The bow of the spectacle frame usually fits exactly into the depression when in its usual position.[30] Histologically there is acanthosis and chronic inflammation of the dermis. A shallow sulcus containing keratin and parakeratotic material may be seen in the epidermis.

Epithelioid hemangioma

Epithelioid hemangioma (benign angiomatous nodules, angiolymphoid hyperplasia, and atypical pyogenic granuloma) is a skin lesion with a particular predilection for the pinna and external auditory canal.[31] Grossly there are sessile or plaque-like, red or reddish blue lesions from 2 to 10 mm in diameter that may coalesce to form larger plaques that obstruct the external canal. Microscopically the dermis or subcutaneous tissue contains a mixture of proliferated capillary blood vessels that are lined by plump, sometimes multilayered endothelial cells, associated with lymphoid tissue mixed with eosinophils, mast cells, and macrophages (Fig. 80-6).

It is not certain whether this lesion is neoplastic or reactive. Surgical excision is recommended because spontaneous regression is rare. Kimura's disease lacking the vascular proliferation is probably a different entity.[31]

Idiopathic cystic chondromalacia

Idiopathic cystic chondromalacia (pseudocysts) is an unusual lesion of the cartilage of the auricle.[32,33] It occurs mainly in

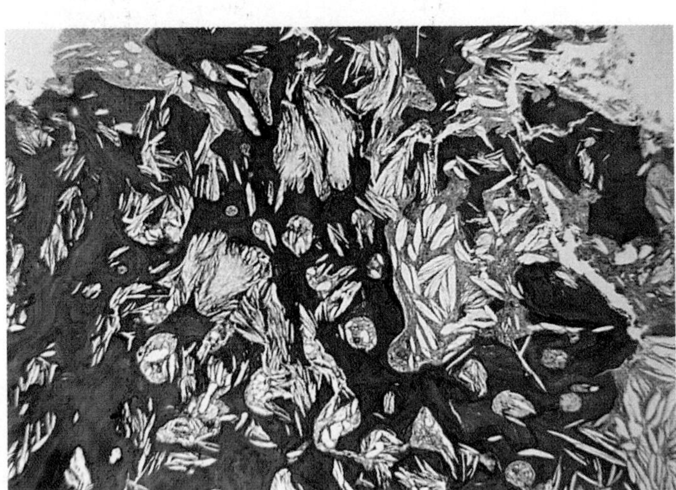

Fig. 80-4 Mastoid bone in type V hyperlipoproteinemia. Marrow spaces, air cells, and bony trabeculas are infiltrated by clefts of cholesterol crystals.

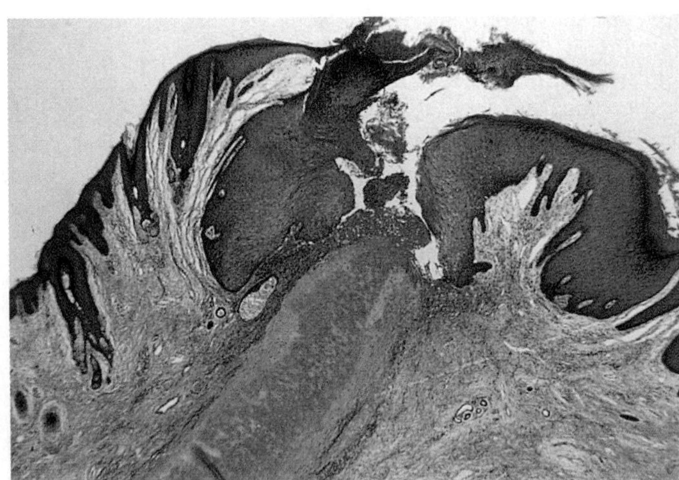

Fig. 80-5 Chondrodermatitis nodularis chronica helicis. There is an ulcer extending down to the cartilage of the pinna and severe acanthosis.

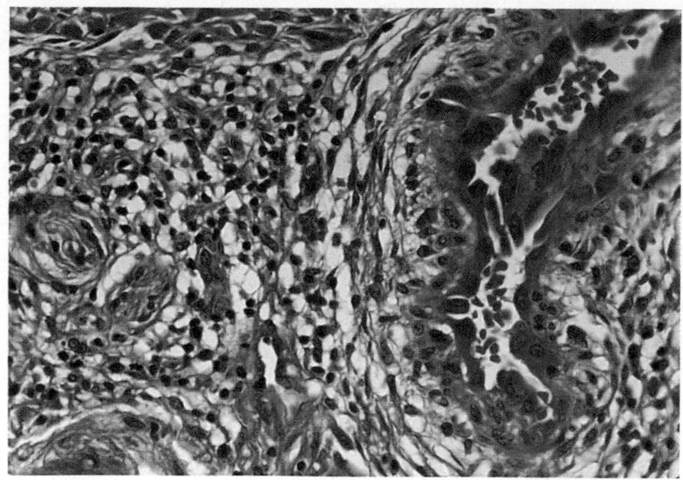

Fig. 80-6 Epithelioid hemangioma of the pinna showing capillaries with plump endothelial cells and lymphoid tissue with eosinophils.

young and middle-aged persons. Grossly there is a localized swelling of the auricular cartilage. Cut-surface shows a well-defined cystic cavity in the cartilage, which is distended with yellowish, watery fluid. Microscopically the cyst is a simple space lined with normal cartilage.[34] Its association with severe atopic eczema in four children[35] indicates that minor trauma resulting from repeated rubbing of the auricle may play a part. Simple curettage eliminates the lesion.

Keloid

Keloid, a common benign skin lesion, occurs after an injury to the skin of the ear, often after the earlobe has been pierced for an earring, and is more common in black people. Grossly there is a lobulated swelling covered by normal skin, most often on the back of the lobe.[36] Microscopically the dermis is enlarged by deposits of eosinophilic, poorly cellular collagen (see Chapter 71).

Neoplasms

Basal cell carcinoma

Most malignant epithelial neoplasms of the external ear are basal cell carcinomas; only a small number are squamous cell carcinomas.[37] The paucity of basal cell carcinomas arising deeply in the external canal and their predominant occurrence on the pinna are in keeping with the accepted view of the causal role of sunlight.

This is not an aggressive neoplasm; and in at least 90% of patients a 3-year cure can easily be achieved by surgical excision.[38] In a few cases, however, these are repeated recurrences, with deep extension to the middle ear, mastoid, and even cranial cavity.[39] Metastasis is rare.

Squamous cell carcinoma

Squamous cell carcinoma of the external ear accounts for 7% of all squamous cell carcinomas of the head and neck.[40] The gross appearances of the lesion are similar to those of such tumors elsewhere in the skin. In those tumors arising deeply within the external canal, there is usually a concomitant origin from middle ear epithelium and dissolution of the tympanic membrane (see later discussion). An adenoid (pseudoglandular) pattern is not uncommonly seen in this neoplasm, and such tumors are said to have a better prognosis than those with the more usual structure.[41] Metastasis from squamous cell carcinoma of the pinna and external auditory meatus takes place in about 8% of cases.[38] The prognosis in patients with tumors confined to the external ear is usually good after they have undergone surgical therapy.

Verrucous squamous cell carcinoma

A verrucous form of squamous cell carcinoma has been seen in the external canal.[42-45] As happens in patients with such tumors at other sites, the diagnosis may be delayed pending the results of several biopsy studies because of the close histologic resemblance of the neoplasm to benign squamous cell papilloma or squamous cell hyperplasia secondary to inflammation. In doubtful cases at their initial presentation, measurement of the mean cell area in the malpighian cell region of the lesion (or, more simply, the mean cell diameter using an eyepiece micrometer) is a useful diagnostic aid. The mean cell area of verrucous squamous cell carcinomas is greater than 300 μm^2; that of benign squamous cell lesions is less than 250 μm.[2,46]

Benign ceruminous gland tumors

Most ceruminous gland tumors are benign; malignant tumors are less common. *Ceruminoma adenomas* usually present with a blockage of the lateral part of the external auditory canal, often associated with deafness and discharge. An important part of the clinical investigation of all glandular neoplasms of the external canal is to exclude parotid gland or middle ear origin of the tumor. Grossly the lesion is a superficial gray mass that is covered by skin. Microscopically, although benign, this neoplasm lacks a definite capsule. It is composed of regular glands, often with intraluminal epithelial cell projections. The glandular epithelium is distinctly bilayered, the layer farthest from the epithelium being myoepithelial (Fig. 80-7), but this may not be obvious in all parts of the neoplasm. The glands are often arranged in groups surrounded by fibrous tissue. The tumor-cells of some ceruminomas contain acid-fast fluorescent pigment similar to that found in normal ceruminous glands.[47,48]

Syringocystadenoma papilliferum, a benign lesion of apocrine cell origin, occasionally occurs in the external auditory

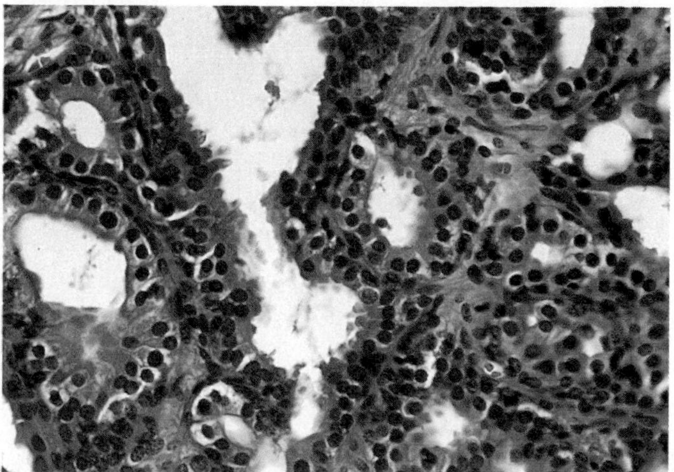

Fig. 80-7 Ceruminal adenoma showing an apocrine type of secretion in the inner layer of glands and myoepithelial cells making up the outer layer.

canal. Histologically it is identical to skin syringocystadenomas in other sites.

Cylindroma is a benign tumor that may occur in the external canal. It is important not to confuse it with primary adenoid cystic carcinoma of this location (see later discussion). Grossly, it is a dome-shaped, smooth swelling that usually develops in the scalp. When there are multiple growths in the scalp, it is usually referred to as a "turban tumor." The tumor may be present on the pinna or in the external canal. Histologically it appears in the dermis and is composed of rounded masses of small, darkly staining cells in masses that seem to fit together in a jigsaw-like pattern and are surrounded by pink-staining hyaline material (Fig. 80-8, *A*). Hyaline globules are often present in the cellular masses, and these are also larger cells with vesicular nuclei (Fig. 80-8, *B*). The tumor differs from adenoid cystic carcinoma in that it has no cribriform structure and has the larger cells.[49]

Malignant ceruminous gland tumors

Malignant ceruminous gland tumors are similar to their counterparts in the salivary gland. They are sometimes seen in the external canal. The most common of these is adenoid cystic carcinoma, and it has the gross and microscopic features of the corresponding major or minor salivary gland neoplasm, including its tendency to invade along nerve sheaths. It may sometimes be mistaken for cylindroma (see earlier discussion). Relentless recurrence over years and eventual hematogenous metastasis to the lungs is a feature of adenoid cystic carcinomas of the external canal, as it is with those arising from salivary glands. Primary mucoepidermoid carcinoma of the external canal has been described.[50] A malignant glandular neoplasm without an adenoid cystic or mucoepidermoid structure may also arise in the external canal.

Melanocytic tumors

Nevi are occasionaly seen in the external canal but are distinctly rare on the pinna. Malignant melanotic neoplasms are uncommon in any part of the external ear. When they do occur in the ear, they usually arise on the pinna; in one third of the patients metastatic lesions in the regional lymph nodes are found at presentation.[51]

Tumors of connective tissue and bone

Skin myxomas that occur with myxoma of the left or right cardiac atrium constitute a rare syndrome that also includes endocrine overactivity and skin lentigines.[52] The skin myxomas most often occur on the lower eyelid, but the pinna and external auditory canal have been involved in some cases. Histologically the myxomas of the ear consist of an accumulation of basophilic ground substance in the dermis containing spindle-shaped mesenchymal cells that stain negatively for S-100 protein.

Benign fibro-osseous lesions, also known as "monostotic fibrous dysplasia or ossifying fibroma," may cause constriction of the external canal and may involve the temporal bone.[53] Grossly benign fibro-osseous lesions of the temporal bone are yellowish white patches of calcified tissue. Microscopically, irregular trabeculas of woven bone are embedded in a connective tissue stroma. Squamous epithelium-lined inclusions may also be found in the tumor.

Osteoma and exostosis

Two types of benign bony enlargement of the deeper bony portion of the external auditory meatus are recognized: osteoma and exostosis.[54,55] *Osteoma* is a spherical mass that projects into the external ear and has a distinct bony pedicle. Microscopically the osteoma is composed of lamellar bone and is covered by the normal stratified squamous epithelium of the external canal. Rarely, osteomas occur in the temporal bone apart from the external canal.[56,57]

Exostosis is a broad-based lesion that is often bilateral and symmetrical.[54] It is usually situated deeper in the ear canal than an osteoma. There are no adnexal structures in the bony portion of the normal external auditory canal, and the distance between the epidermal surface and underlying bone is consequently small.[1] This explains why exostoses of the tympanic bone develop in this region in those who swim frequently in cold water; this probably exerts a cooling effect on the nearby periosteum, stimulating new bone production.

Histiocytic neoplasms and lymphomas

Langerhans' cell histiocytosis (histiocytosis X, eosinophilic granuloma, and Hand-Schüller-Christian disease) frequently

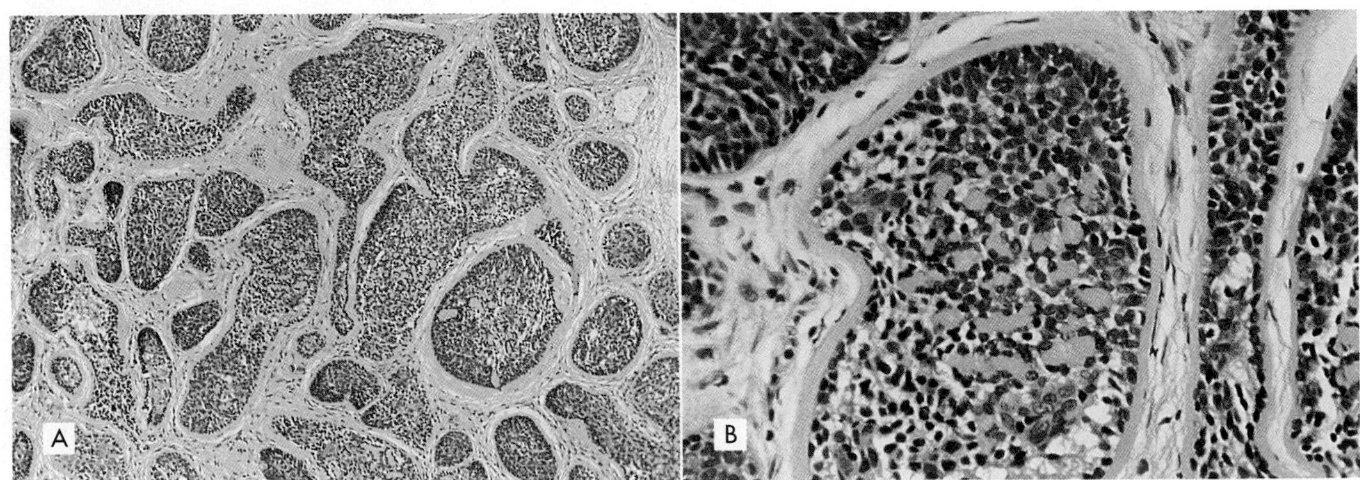

Fig. 80-8 Cylindroma of external canal. **A,** Jigsaw puzzle–like arrangement of tumor cell masses. **B,** Hyaline material around and within tumor masses.

affects bone. In the temporal bone, which sometimes is the first site affected, the disease is usually manifested as a bony lesion of the medial part of the external auditory meatus; it typically occurs in children.[58,59] In patients younger than 3 years of age, the disease process is more likely to be multifocal in the skull and the prognosis is worse.

Malignant lymphoma may appear in the external ear as part of a generalized process. Occasionally it is primary in this setting, presenting as a B- or T-cell lymphoma of the skin of the pinna. In some cases there is a striking symmetry in the deposition of the lymphoid neoplasia, each earlobe or both earlobes and helices on each side being similarly affected.[60]

MIDDLE EAR

Bacterial otitis media

Children are more often affected by acute otitis media than adults are. The causative organisms are most frequently *Streptococcus pneumoniae* and *Haemophilus influenzae*. The mucosa of the middle ear, including that of the mastoid air cells, is congested and edematous. Hemorrhage may be severe, and the mucosa and mastoid air cells are filled with neutrophils that then fill the middle ear cavity. There is also osteoclastic destruction of the mastoid bone. At the same time, new bone forms, commencing as osteoid and later becoming woven and finally lamellar. Fibrosis may also be active even in the acute stage. The tympanic membrane shows much congestion, with the dilated vessels distending the connective tissue layer. The acute inflammation may spread deeply into the temporal bone (see below).

The chronic form of otitis media frequently develops without a preceding acute phase. The causative organisms are most frequently gram-negative bacilli such as *Proteus species* and *Pseudomonas aeruginosa*. Clinically a discharging perforation of the tympanic membrane is frequently but not always present.

Grossly there is a considerable variation in the degree and extent of the inflammation. The tubotympanic region and mastoid air cells are the most frequently involved. The mucosa is thickened, and congestion may be severe. Granulation tissue formation may be extensive, showing as a red mucosal thickening, particularly on the promontory, and this may be sufficiently thick to protrude through the perforation in the tympanic membrane. Such a lesion is the common aural polyp that is detected clinically in the external canal. A variable degree of ossicular bone may be lost, particularly in the long process of the incus. Cholesterol granulomas and cholesteatomas are frequently present in association with chronic otitis media (see later discussion).

Microscopically, aural polyps are composed of chronic inflammatory cells and granulation tissue. Their surface is covered with columnar epithelium, which is often ciliated or stratified squamous epithelium. The presence of a foreign-body giant cell reaction to keratin squames in an aural polyp has been held to be indicative of cholesteatoma in the middle ear,[61] but this has been disputed.[62,63]

Unlike other parts of the respiratory tract, including the cartilaginous portion of the eustachian tube, where tubuloalveolar glands containing mucous and serous elements are normally present, the middle ear contains few glands. Under pathologic conditions, however, the epithelium of the middle ear comes to resemble the rest of the respiratory tract by the appearance of many glands consisting of simple cylinders of mucus-producing cells (Fig. 80-9).

Repair processes are evident in many cases. The mastoid air cells and tympanic cavity may show fibrosis and thickened bony walls. Cement lines in the lamellar bone are numerous and irregular, forming a mosaic pattern, and the haversian systems of mastoid bone exhibit an irregular pattern when viewed in polarized light. A cholesteatoma often accompanies chronic otitis media and, when present, exacerbates the inflammation.

Cholesterol granuloma

Yellow nodules are often found in the tympanic cavity and mastoid in chronic otitis media. Microscopically these are composed of cholesterol crystals (dissolved away to leave empty clefts in paraffin-embedded histologic sections) that are surrounded by foreign-body giant cells and other chronic inflammatory cells. Such cholesterol granulomas are almost always found in the midst of hemorrhagic material and hemosiderin-containing macrophages in the middle ear mucosa, indicating that the process is a consequence of hemorrhage.

Tympanosclerosis

Tympanosclerosis is a special form of fibrosis that is often encountered in chronic otitis media. It is characterized by aggregates of diffuse hyalinized collagen laid down in the middle ear mucosa, especially on the tympanic membrane and on the crura of the stapes. Deposits of calcium salts, appearing as a basophilic dusting, are irregularly distributed throughout the collagen. A lamellated structure is frequently observed. Bone is also often present in tympanosclerotic plaques (Fig. 80-10). There may be an autoimmune factor in the development of tympanosclerosis, and this is possibly enhanced by trauma, such as that produced by ventilating tubes.[64]

Otitis media with effusion

Synonyms for otitis media with effusion (OME) are "serous otitis media," "catarrhal otitis media," "tubotympanitis," and "glue ear." It is a very common cause of hearing loss in children and is characterized by an effusion behind a nonperforated eardrum in the absence of frank symptoms of acute infection.[65] The findings from only a few pathologic studies of

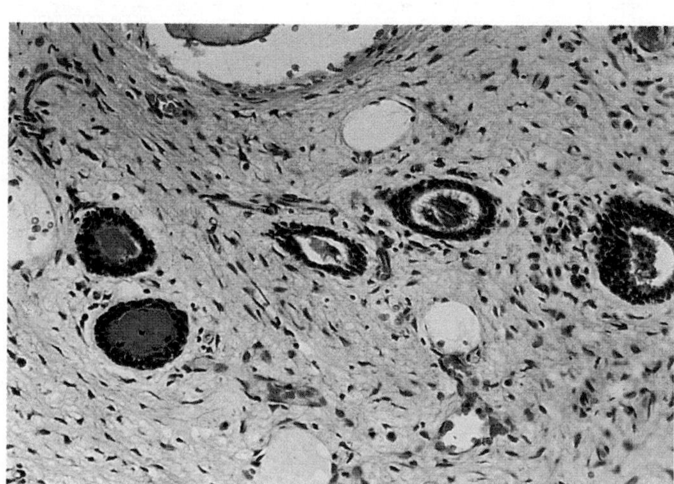

Fig. 80-9 Glandular metaplasia of the middle ear mucosa.

temporal bone have been described. All the features of chronic otitis may be present, including cholesterol granulomas, chronic inflammatory granulation tissue, ossicular destruction, and tympanosclerosis. The most prominent histopathologic feature of childhood OME seems to be new formation of glands in the middle ear mucosa.[66]

OME occurs also in adults, often in association with neoplasms of the nasopharynx, which may occlude the distal orifice of the eustachian tube.[67]

Granulomatous otitis media and related conditions

Tuberculous otitis media is an unusual form of chronic otitis media and is generally associated with active pulmonary tuberculosis. Complications, especially involvement of the facial nerve, are more frequent than they are in the more common form of chronic otitis media.[6] Histologically the inflammation is characterized by the formation of typical caseating granulomas or a mixture of epithelioid cells and nonspecific granulation tissue (Fig. 80-11). There is often prominent bone destruction. Acid-fast bacilli may be hard to find, but there are also exceptional cases in which there are numerous mycobacteria.[69] Some of these patients have been otherwise healthy men who have little or no evidence of tuberculosis of the lung or other internal organs. It must be distinguished from sarcoidosis, which is very rare in the middle ear.

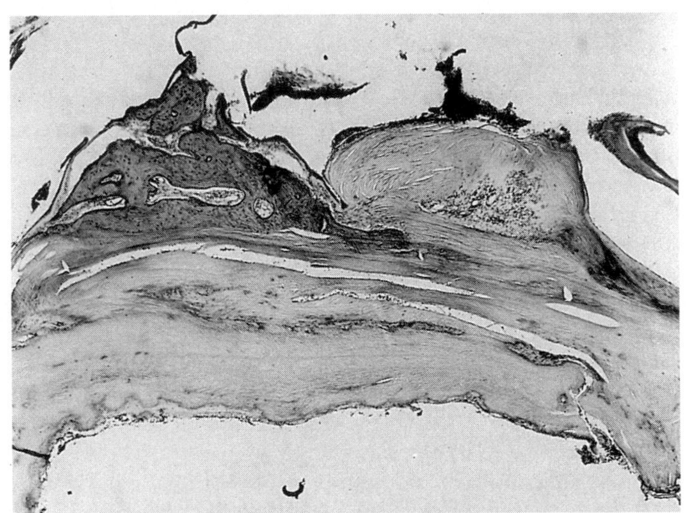

Fig. 80-10 Tympanosclerosis of the middle ear mucosa with ossification. (From Michaels L: *Ear, nose and throat histopathology,* London, 1987, Springer-Verlag.)

Actinomycosis of the middle ear, an uncommon infection caused by the anaerobic organism *Actinomyces israelii,* cannot usually be identified except during open operation on the middle ear.[70,71]

Wegener's granulomatosis can also affect the middle ear, but its incidence is not known. Some case of otitis media without renal or pulmonary manifestations, and even without histologic evidence of Wegener's granulomatous such as angiitis, have been deemed Wegener's granulomatosis only on the basis of a positive c-ANCA test result and apparent success in treating the condition with cyclophosphamide.[72] Pathologists should be cautious about interpreting such cases as a "locoregional" form of Wegener's granulomatosis.[73]

AIDS otitis media

In a postmortem study of patients with AIDS, OME was found in 60% of 49 temporal bones.[74] This was characterized by the extensive exudation of fibrin into the middle ear spaces, as well as by the features of OME already mentioned above (Fig. 80-12 and 80-13). Cytomegalovirus infection was present in the middle ear mucosa of one patient. Changes characteristic of a more active otitis media that included suppuration in the middle ear cleft were identified in 23%, a much higher percentage than that found in a large clinical study carried out concomitantly. This indicates that severe otitis media may occur frequently in the terminally sick patient with AIDS, perhaps at the site of a middle ear mucosa already weakened by OME.

Hemorrhage in drowning

Hemorrhage into the cavity of the middle ear has long been regarded as a finding supporting drowning as a cause of death.[75] This occurs only when the tympanic membrane is intact because the blood vessels will rupture only if there is sufficient negative pressure. Congestive swelling of the

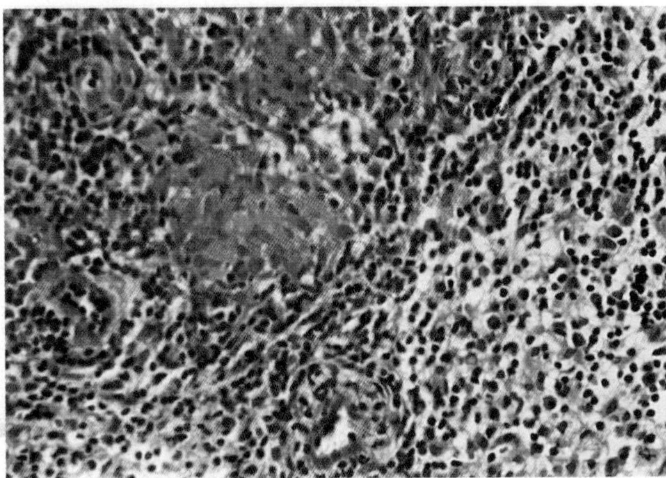

Fig. 80-11 Tuberculosis of the middle ear showing a tuberculoid granulomatous infiltrate accompanied by nonspecific chronic inflammatory granulation tissue.

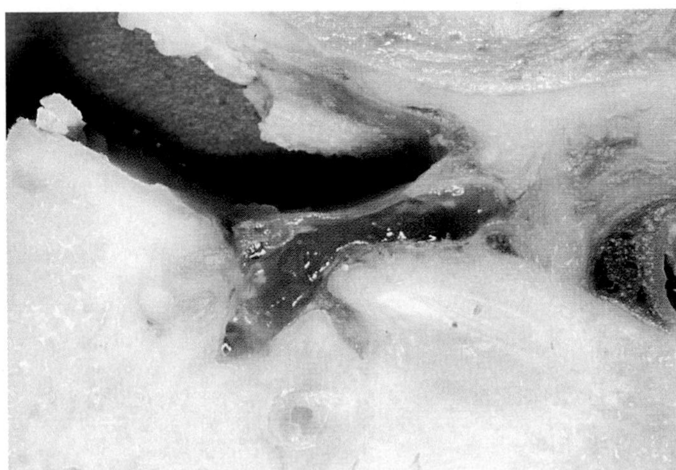

Fig. 80-12 Microslice preparation showing a gelatinous exudate in the middle ear cavity in a patient with the serous otitis media of AIDS.

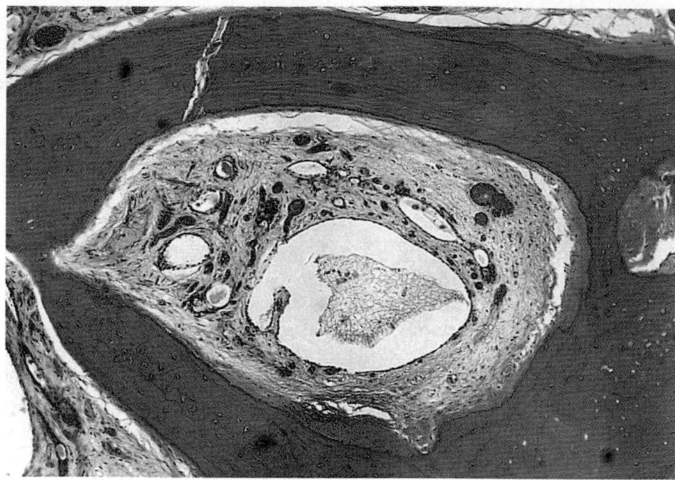

Fig. 80-13 Low-grade otitis media in a patient with AIDS. There is glandular metaplasia of the mastoid air cell mucosa with a fibrin exudate in the lumen.

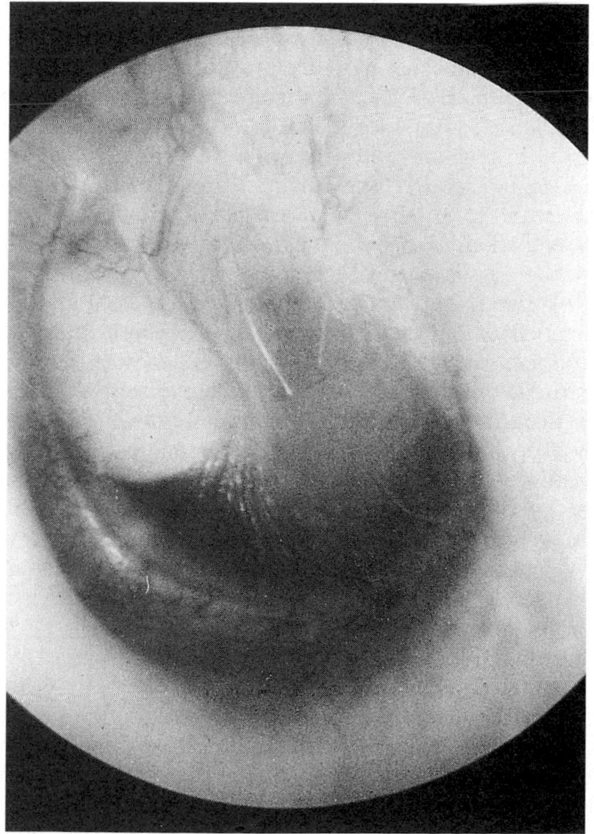

Fig. 80-14 Endoscopic photograph of the tympanic membrane in a patient with a congenital cholesteatoma that is in the anterosuperior part of the middle ear cleft (that is, it appears anterior to the handle of the malleus and superior to the cone of light). (Courtesy Mark Levenson, M.D., New York, N.Y.)

mucosa covering the periosteum in the middle ear is also a feature in drowning victims.[76]

Neoplasms and similar lesions

Cholesteatomas

In cholesteatoma, stratified squamous epithelium, which is actively growing and desquamating, is found within the middle

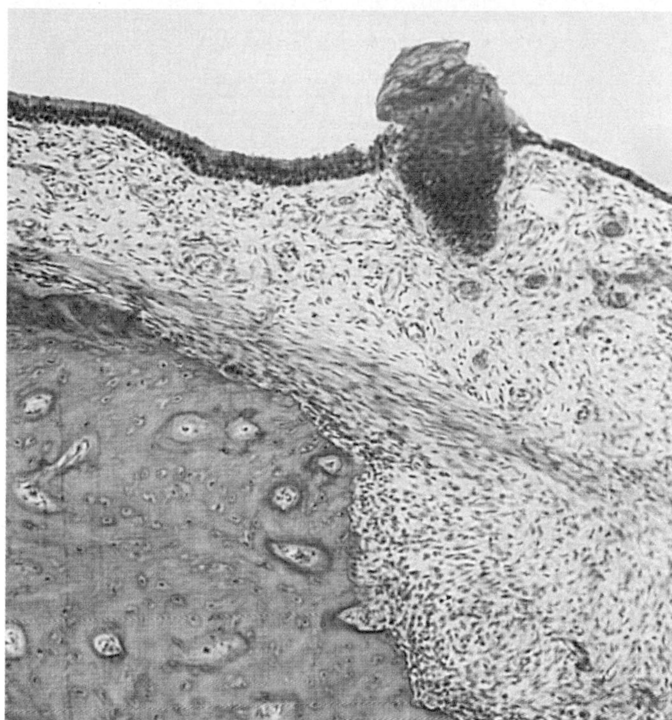

Fig. 80-15 Epidermoid formation in a fetal ear at 32 weeks of gestation.

ear cavity. It is not a neoplasm, nor is it a typical epidermoid cyst, but it has a locally aggressive behavior suggestive of a kinship to neoplasia. It is far more frequent than true middle ear neoplasms are. It may be "closed" in the sense that it contains a cystic squamous mass, or it may be "open" such that the keratin squames are shed directly into the middle ear cavity.[77] Cholesteatomas are classified as congenital or acquired.

In most cases *congenital cholesteatoma* is situated in the upper anterior middle ear (Fig. 80-14). It occurs in young children.[7] Microscopically it is usually, but not always, a closed epidermoid cyst. The growing epithelium makes up only the outer layers (matrix); the rest of the cyst is composed of dead keratin squames.[79,80]

Most congenital cholesteatomas almost certainly arise from a cell rest in the developing middle ear.[81] This is seen in most fetal ears before term, after which it disappears. It is always found in the same position, in the epithelium of the middle ear at its junction with that of the eustachian tube, adjacent to the anterior limb of the osseous tympanic ring. This is also the site of most congenital cholesteatomas. The cell rest is a collection of epidermoid cells that often has a keratin cap, sometimes with rete ridges (Figs. 80-15 and 80-16).

Acquired cholesteatoma appears grossly as a pearly gray or yellow structure, often with corrugations. It commences in the upper posterior part of the middle ear but eventually fills most of the middle ear cavity. It discharges through a perforation in the pars flaccida of the tympanic membrane usually posteriorly. The cholesteatoma may extend into the mastoid air cells, and in most cases at least one ossicle is seriously damaged.

The matrix of the acquired cholesteatoma is similar to that of the congenital variety, except that the acquired variety is more often "open" and thicker.[79] Furrows frequently form in it, and they may separate the cholesteatoma into lobules. Tongues of epidermoid basal cells often penetrate into the

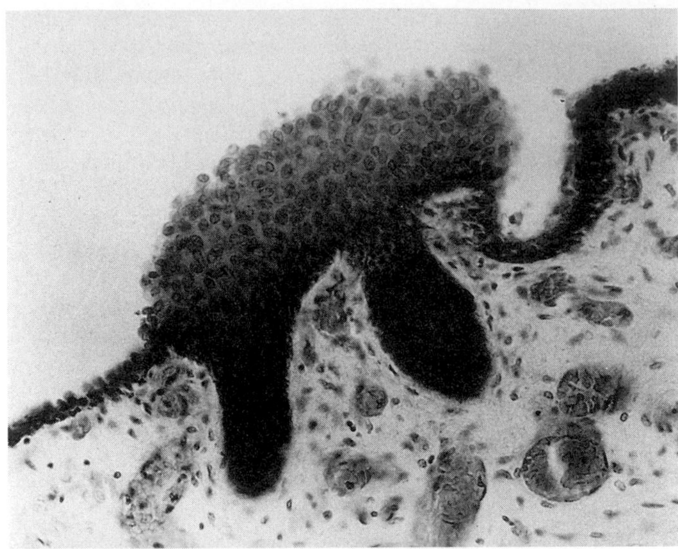

Fig. 80-16 Epidermoid formation in a fetal ear at 38 weeks of gestation that has two rete ridges. The structure lies at the junction of the epithelium of the eustachian tube with that of the middle ear.

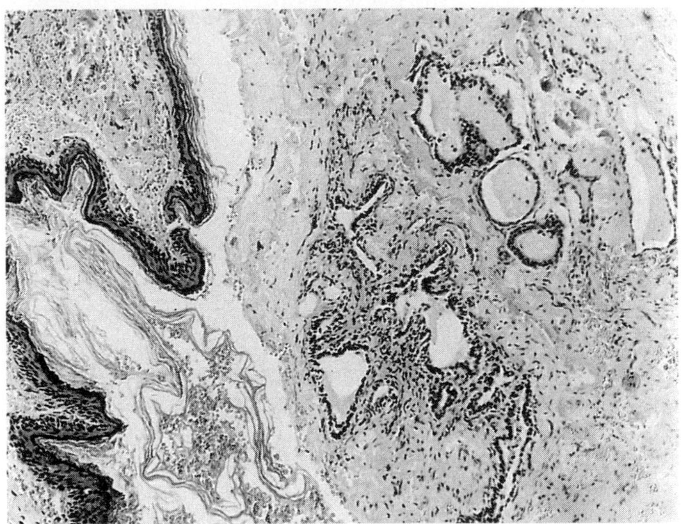

Fig. 80-17 Acquired cholesteatoma accompanied by glandular metaplasia of the middle ear.

surrounding tissue from the basal layer of the cholesteatoma. Cytologic studies of the stratified squamous epithelical lining of cholesteatoma has not revealed any significant difference between it and the normal epithelium of the deep external auditory meatus (Figs. 80-17 and 80-18). The eroded ossicles that are frequently present in a cholesteatoma may be invested by the squamous epithelial wall of the sac. An acquired cholesteatoma is always associated with severe chronic otitis media.

Acquired cholesteatoma most likely arises from the stratified squamous epithelium covering the *external* surface of the tympanic memberane as the result of a pathologic aberration in the normal physiologic process of auditory epithelial migration. A detailed study of the pathways and embryologic basis of the migration of stratified squamons epithelium on the tympanic membrane has recently been reported on, [82-85] but the

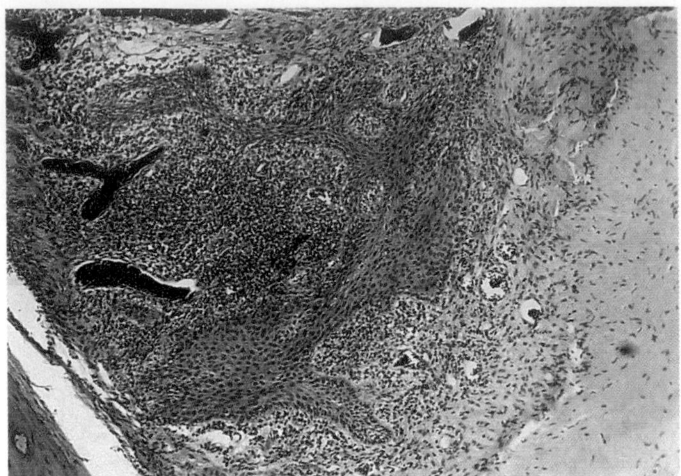

Fig. 80-18 Acquired cholesteatoma showing downgrowths of stratified squamous epithelium.

findings have not yet helped to clarify the problem. Some evidence in support of an origin of acquired cholesteatoma from the stratified squamous epithelium of the tympanic membrane and deep external canal has been provided by the finding that, although both cho-lesteatoma and these epithelia express cytokeratins 5, 10, 14, and 16, cytokeratin 16 is rarely expressed in skin epithelium elsewhere.[86]

A *retraction pocket* is an invagination of part of the tympanic membrane, usually the pars flaccida, into the middle ear cavity as a result of chronic otitis media (Fig. 80-19). Retraction pockets have been observed as a phase in the development of some, perhaps most, cholesteatomas.[87] Histologic examination of 12 retraction pockets in temporal bones done post mortem revealed no evidence either of cholesteatoma or of obstruction of the mouth of a retraction pocket, which could lead to the development of cholesteatoma. In two of the retraction pockets, however, small keratinizing epidermoid foci that were connected to the squamous epithelium of the retraction pocket by a band of nonkeratinizing squamous epithelium were seen on the malleus and incus within the middle ear (Fig. 80-20). If a retraction pocket gives rise to a cholesteatoma, it may do so because of such an invasive activity rather than because of any failure in its drainage process.[89]

A distinct type of cholesteatoma is that arising in the petrous apex.[90] *Cholesteatoma of the petrous apex* is found mainly in middle-aged patients and often is manifested by mandibular nerve pain and blurring of vision and syncope related to compression of the fifth cranial nerve and internal carotid artery respectively.[91] These cholesteatomas are actually epidermoid cysts and are probably congential in origin, but the embryonic source must differ from the source of the middle ear variety.[92]

Developmental tumorlike anomalies

Choristomas are occasionally seen in the middle ear. Three varieties have been observed: salivary gland, glial tissue, and sebaceous. Salivary gland choristomas consist as a rule of mixed mucous and serous elements like the histologic composition of the normal submandibular or sublingual gland, but unlike that of the parotid gland[93] (Fig. 80-21). Glial masses are composed largely of astrocytic cells the identity of which may be confirmed by immunochemical staining for glial acidic fibrillary protein. When such masses are identified in biopsy material from the middle ear, a bony deficit with consequent herniation of brain tissue into the middle ear should also be considered.[94] A sebaceous choristoma that presented as a mass in the hypotympanum has been reported.[95]

Adenoma

A benign glandular neoplasm confined to the middle ear and originating from its epithelium was not recognized until 1976.[96,97] Glands easily form in the epithelium of the middle ear, though it is normally nonglandular and adenoma would seem to represent a benign neoplastic transformation of this epithelium that occurs along the same lines.

The tympanic membrane is usually intact, and the neoplasm is confined to the middle ear. Sometimes it extends to the mastoid spaces, either through a perforation into the external canal[96] or through an apparently intact tympanic membrane.[98] The neoplasm has recurred in a few cases,[99,100] but metastasis has not been reported.

The neoplasm appears white, gray, or reddish brown at operation and, unlike paraganglioma, is not vascular. It seems to peel away easily from the walls of the surrounding middle ear, though ossicles may sometimes be entrapped in the tumor mass and may even show destruction.

Microscopically adenoma appears to be formed by closely apposed, small glands with a back-to-back appearance (Fig. 80-22). A solid or trabecular arrangement may result in apparent loss of the glandular pattern. This may be artifactual and produced by biopsy-related trauma that has disrupted the delicate structure of this neoplasm. The cells are regular, cuboidal, or columnar and may enclose a luminal secretion. No myoepithelial layer is seen.

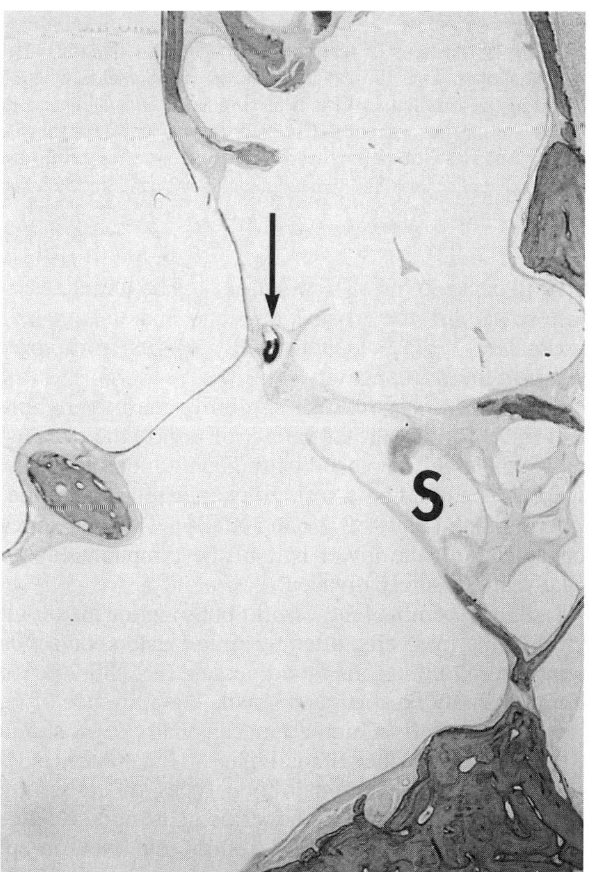

Fig. 80-19 Retraction pocket characteristic of the pars flaccida of the tympanic membrane attached to the stapes *(S)* by a fibrous band. Notice the keratin cyst *(arrow)* within the band. (From Michaels L: *Ear, nose and throat histopathology,* London, 1987, Springer-Verlag.)

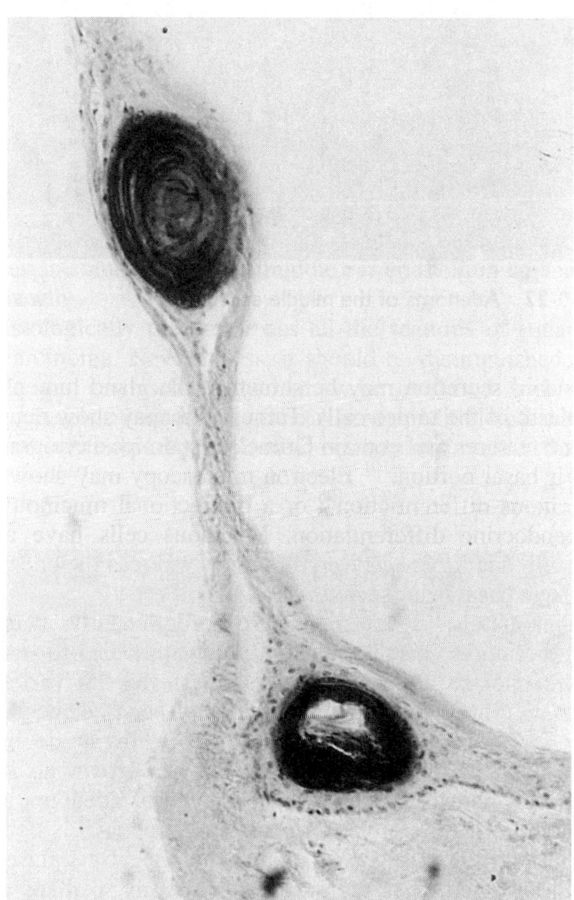

Fig. 80-20 Keratin cysts and a ribbon of stratified squamous epithelium extends in the middle ear from a retraction pocket above. (From Michaels L: *Ear, nose and throat histopathology,* London, 1987, Springer-Verlag.)

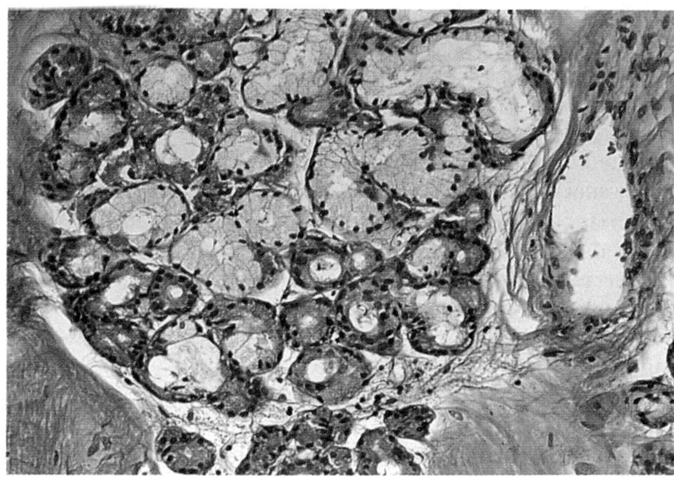

Fig. 80-21 Salivary gland choristoma of the middle ear.

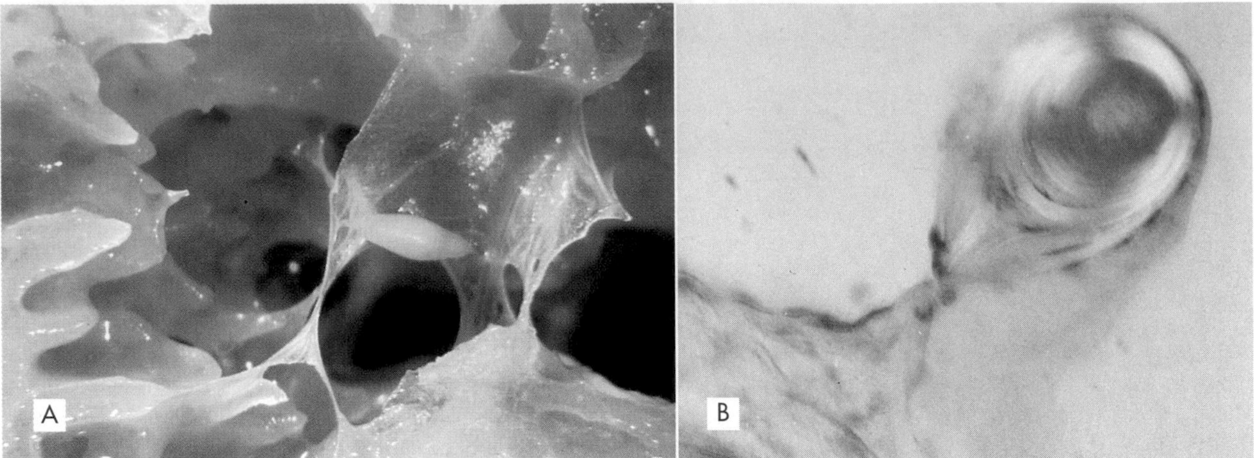

Fig. 80-26 **A,** Middle ear corpuscle arising from a fibrous band of the mastoid antrum. **B,** Histologically the middle ear corpuscle shows concentric, alternating light and dark layers under polarized light.

normally found in the middle ear of aging persons. They are composed largely of collagen and sometimes form in considerable numbers in bone-free mastoid air cell septa in the mastoid antrum[111] (Fig. 80-26).

The carcinoma spreads widely, tending to grow into and eroding the thin bony plate into the carotid canal.[1] It may spread along the dura mater of the posterior surface of the temporal bone into the internal auditory meatus. It causes death by direct intracranial extension.[112,113] Lymph node metastasis is unusual, and hematogenous spread is even more so.

Papillary adenocarcinoma

A primary papillary glandular neoplasm of the middle ear has been described.[114] This may be the same entity as low-grade adenocarcinoma of endolymphatic sac origin (see later discussion). A primary papillary adenocarcinoma of the nasopharynx may spread to the middle ear cavity by way of the eustachian tube.

Other middle ear neoplasm

Primary tumors originating from the connective tissue or nerves of the middle ear are rare. A *schwannoma* of the facial nerve in its tympanic or extratympanic (descending) portion is occasionally seen. Histologically the features are those of the typical neurilemoma.

Hemangioma of the middle ear is rare but has been found filling the middle ear,[115] and arising from the region of the facial nerve or the eustachian tube.

Rhabdomyosarcoma, usually of the embryonal type, is seen occasionally in the middle and external ear of young children; in this site it forms a lobulated, dark red, hemorrhagic mass. It is highly malignant and spreads extensively into the cranial cavity, externally to the skin or internally to the pharyngeal region. Lymph node and hematogenous metastasis frequently occurs.

Meningiomas may arise from several regions within the temporal bone itself, most commonly the middle ear cleft,[116] but imaging studies have revealed that they usually arise from outside the petrous bone, which the tumor infiltrates until it reaches the middle ear. Microscopically and immunohistochemically the tumor is identical to other intracranial meningiomas[117] (Fig. 80-27).

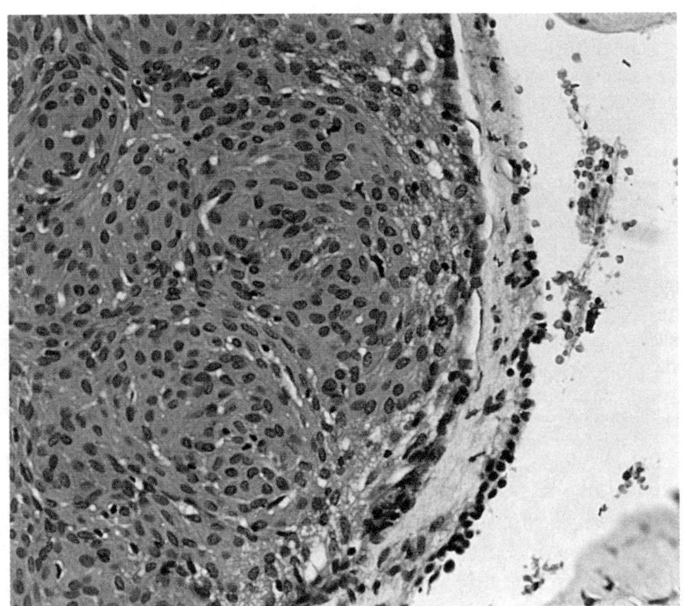

Fig. 80-27 Meningioma in the middle ear mucosa.

Metastasis of malignant neoplasms to the middle ear region of the temporal bone is not uncommon. Breasts, lung, kidney, stomach, and larynx are possible primary sources of metastatic tumors,[118] as is malignant melanoma.[119]

INNER EAR

Malformations

Four types of malformation of the inner ear have been delineated[120]:

1. *Michel type:* complete absence of development.
2. *Mondini type:* cochlea and vestibule represented by only a single curved tube.

3. *Bing-Siebenmann type:* underdevelopment of the membranous labyrinth, particularly its sense organ, with a well-formed bony labyrinth.

4. *Scheibe type:* absence of development confined to the organ of Corti and the saccular neuroepithelium.

Findings yielded by computerized tomography, have allowed a milder malformation of the coiling of the cochlea—the Mondini defect—in which some hearing function is retained (Fig. 80-28), to be distinguished from a severe dysplasia of the whole inner ear, in which no cochlear or vestibular structures develop in the single tube and there is no hearing. In the latter there is a deficiency of bone between the internal auditory canal and primitive tube, and there may also be a deficiency in the footplate of the stapes. A communication may thus arise between the middle ear and the subarachnoid space in the internal auditory canal, resulting in meningitis.[121]

The Mondini and severe dysplasia malformations of the otic capsule may be regarded as morphogenetic defects. Most patients with congenital hearing loss do not have a morphogenetic defect, but their inner ear abnormalities are confined to the membranous labyrinth. The nonmorphogenetic defects that occur in genetically deaf mice have been classified into neuroepithelial and cochleosaccular malformations.[122] A similar grouping of nonmorphogenetic malformations has been detected in human beings.[123] In the neuroepithelial forms, first the organ of Corti and later the spiral ganglion cells and spiral laminar nerve fibers atrophy. In the cochleosaccular form it is the stria vascularis and sometimes the saccular macula that are defective.

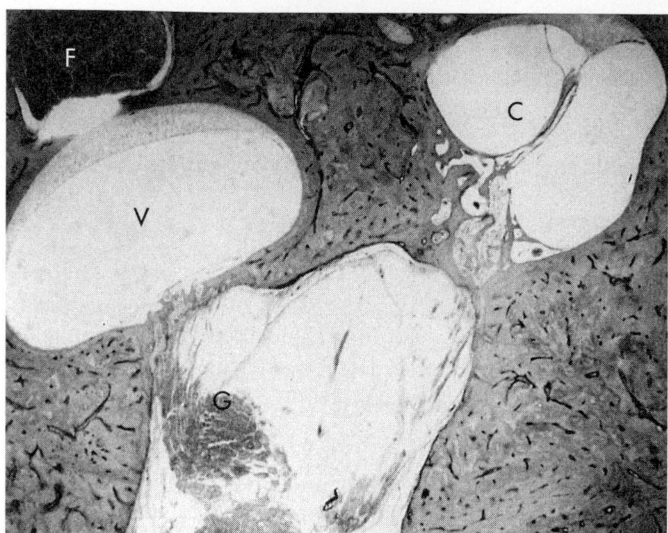

Fig. 80-28 Mondini type of malformation of the middle ear. The cochlea *(C)* consists of a single tube. The vestibule *(V)* does not contain an utricle or a saccule. Notice the anomalous position of the facial nerve *(F)*. *G,* Vestibular ganglion. (From Michaels L: *Ear, nose and throat histopathology,* London, 1987, Springer-Verlag.)

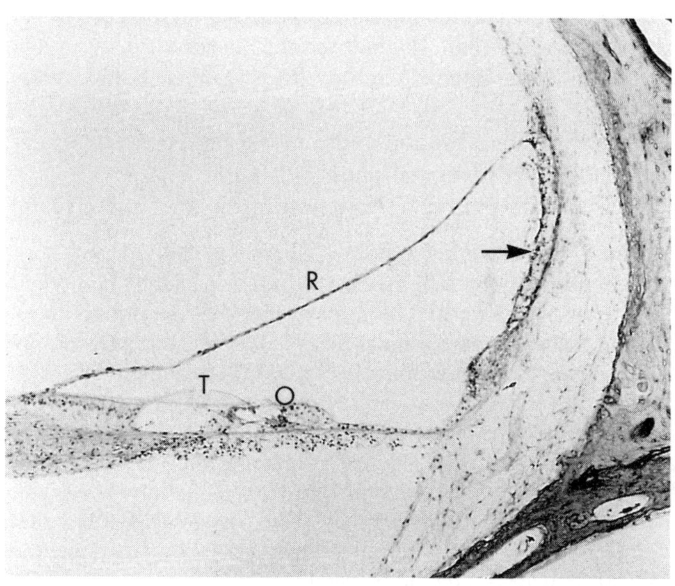

Fig. 80-29 Cochlea of a 7-year-old boy who died of multiple metastatic lesions of neuroblastoma, treated by *cis*-platinum (cisplatin). There is cystic degeneration of the stria vascularis *(arrow)* and an absence of inner and outer hair cells in the organ of Corti *(O)*. *R,* Reissner's membrane; *T,* tectorial membrane. (From Michaels L: *Ear, nose and throat histopathology,* London, 1987, Springer-Verlag.)

Ototoxic conditions

Ototoxic injury to the inner ear results from a variety of drugs. The five major classes of such substances frequently used in clinical practice are (1) aminoglycoside antibiotics, (2) loop diuretics, (3) salicylates, (4) quinine, and (5) cytotoxic drugs used in the treatment of malignant disease. The structures in the inner ear that are particularly susceptible to damage by such drugs are the stria vascularis, the outer hair cells of the cochlea, and the maculae and cristae of the vestibule. An example is *cis*-platinum (cisplatin) a cytotoxic drug frequently used to treat malignancy (Fig. 80-29).

Infections

Viral diseases

Infecting viruses reach the inner ear by way of the bloodstream and the nerves. Little is known about the acute histopathologic effects of the four viral infections derived from the bloodstream: cytomegalovirus (CMV) infection, measles, mumps, and rubella. Although changes in many of the membranous structures of the inner ear have been observed, these are usually late sequelae of the viral damage.

The developing ear is particularly susceptible to infection in the setting of CMV disease.[124] The virus is an important cause of congenital hearing loss,[125] the endolabyrith in particular showing inclusions of this virus at autopsy.[126] In the setting of congenital rubella there is a general retardation in the development of the parts of the membranous labyrith as well as a variety of malformations of these structures.

The passage of the varicella virus along the seventh and eight cranial nerves to reach the inner ear produces *herpes zoster otitis,* or the *Ramsay Hunt syndrome,* in which vesicles of herpes zoster appear on the skin of the pinna and mucosa of the pharynx, occurring at the same time as the facial palsy and hearing loss.

Bell's palsy may result from a viral infection in the inner ear, possibly herpes simplex. Clinically it presents as a lower motor neuron facial paralysis. Although the temporal bones from several patients with Bell's palsy have been studied, the nature of the disease remains enigmatic. Inflammation of the nerve and its compression in its bony canal may cause it to degenerate more distally.[127] Herpes simplex virus DNA has been isolated from the temporal bone containing the inflamed facial nerve, supporting the concept that this virus may be the etiologic agent in Bell's palsy.[128]

Bacterial diseases

Bacterial infections may cause petrositis or labyrinthitis, or both. Baterial infection of the petrous bone is always derived by extension from middle ear infection by means of neighboring infected air cells, by direct spread of the inflammation through necrotic bone (osteitis), by extension though the bone marrow of the petrous bone (osteomyelitis), and along vessels and nerves.

Petrositis takes the form of three main changes in the bone tissue, all of which can occur simultaneously. There are bone necrosis, bone erosion, and new bone formation. Petrositis may cause serious damage to the following adjacent structures:

1. Membranous labyrinth (labyrinthitis) with destruction of the organs of hearing and balance
2. Cranial nerves in the vicinity of the temporal bone, leading to several clinical syndromes: a. Facial nerve (facial palsy) b. Trigeminal ganglion and sixth cranial nerve (Gradenigo's syndrome) c. Ninth, tenth, and eleventh cranial nerves in the jugular foramen region (jugular foramen syndrome)
3. Wall of the internal carotid artery, leading to thrombosis within
4. Lateral sinus, leading to thrombosis and possibly extension to the superior sagittal sinus
5. Meninges and brain, leading to meningitis and cerebral abscess formation

Infections of the labyrith are in most instances complications of otitis media. Infection may enter the labyrinth by penetrating the oval or the round window. An infected air cell may rupture into the labyrinthine system. Occasionally, damage to bone by the inflammation causes a fistula to form between the middle ear and the labyrinth, usually in the lateral semicircular canal because this is the nearest vulnerable site the middle ear. Meningitis is another source of infection of the labyrinth, with the infection being conveyed by ways of the two tubes that join the membranous labyrinth to the subarachnoid space, the cochlear aqueduct, and the internal auditory meatus.

In suppurative labyrinthitis the perilymph spaces usually contain a considerable amount of exudate of neutrophils, and this may spread to the endolymphatic spaces and result in irreparable damage to the sensory epithelia (Fig. 80-30). Healing is at first by fibrosis and later by osseous repair, leading to *labyrinthitis ossificans* (Fig. 80-31). This is one of the most common indications for the performance of cochlear implantation, which is the electrical stimulation of spiral ganglion cells in the cochlea. This can restore a degree of hearing.

Fungal diseases

Fungal infections of the inner ear are rare. The most common is caused by *Cryptococcus neoformans,* which involves the inner ear in cases of meningitis, the organism entering the cochlea and vestibule by way of the corresponding nerves. This occurs mainly in the context of cryptococcal meningitis associated with AIDS[72] (Fig. 80-32).

Ménière's disease

Ménière's disease is an affliction of both the hearing and balance organs of the inner ear, and episodes of vertigo, hearing loss, and tinnitus are the presenting symptoms. Its pathologic basis is hydrops (that is, distention of the endolymphatic spaces) of the labyrinth.[129] The cause of the hydrops in

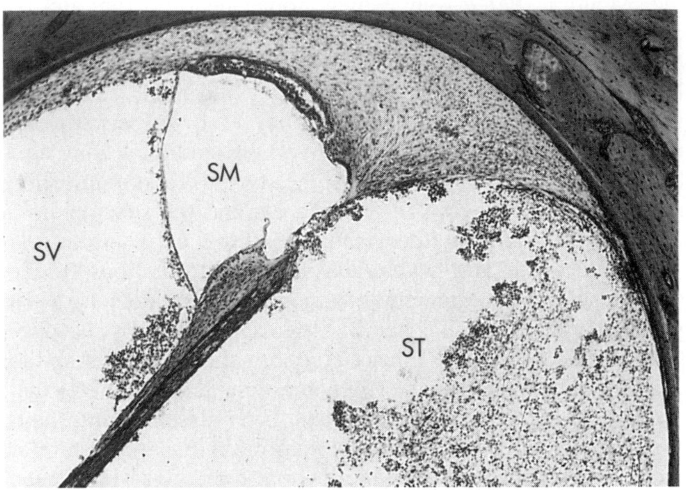

Fig. 80-30 Suppurative labyrinthitis. The scala vestibuli *(SV)* and scala tympani *(ST)* contain numerous pus cells. *SM,* scala media (From Michaels L: London, 1987, Springer-Verlag.)

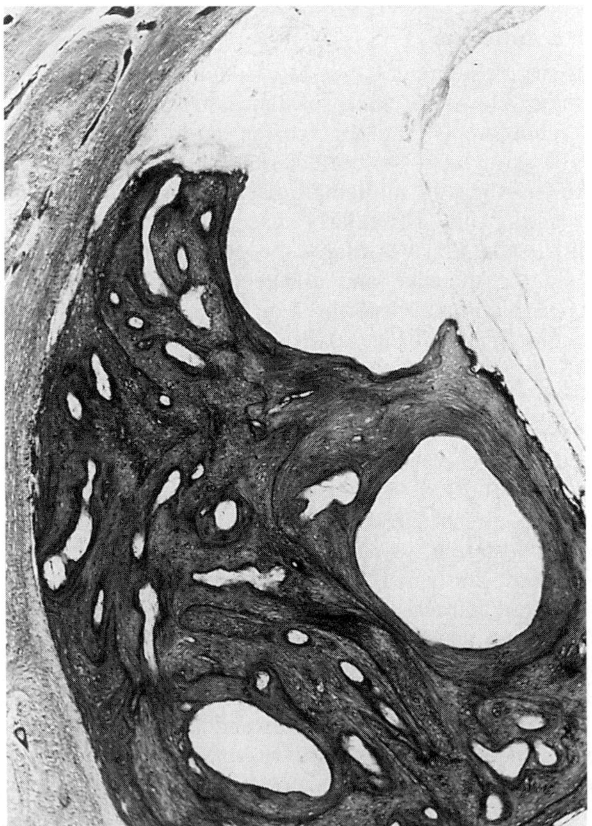

Fig. 80-31 Labyrinthitis ossificans. The scala tympani is occupied by new bone. (From Michaels L: *Ear, nose and throat histopathology,* London, 1987, Springer-Verlag.)

Ménière's disease is unknown. Hydrops may also, however, be a complication of inflammation or neoplastic involvement of the perilymphatic spaces.

In hydrops the cochlear duct and saccule are involved, but the utricle and semicircular ducts usually are not. Reissner's membrane, which is elastic, shows a variable degree of bulging. In the most severe cases the membrane reaches the top of the scala vestibuli and may be in contact with a wide area of the cochlear wall (Fig. 80-33). The saccule swells up from its position on the medial wall of the vestibule and frequently touches the vestibular surface of the footplate of the stapes, often compressing the utricle. Patients with the symptoms of Ménière's disease show the more severe changes characteristic of hydrops, including ruptures of the labyrinthine membranes; those without such symptoms do not show these severe changes.[130] It has been suggested that the hydrops that occurs in the setting of Ménière's disease is caused by obstruction to the drainage of endolymph resulting from pathologic changes around the endolymphatic duct and sac.

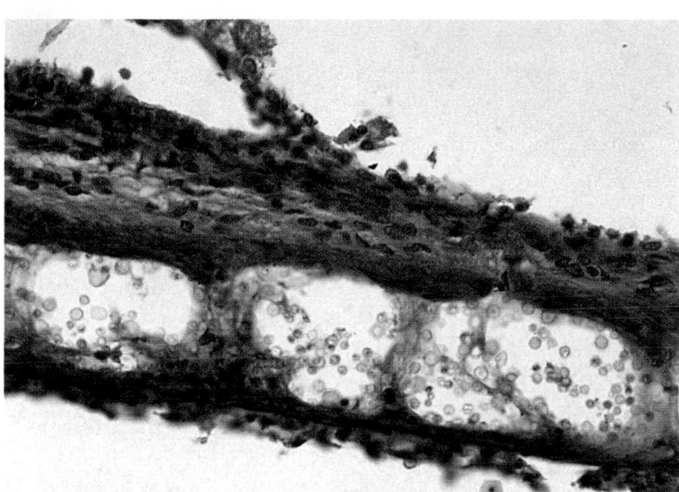

Fig. 80-32 Cryptococcois of the cochlea in AIDS. The cryptococci fill spaces in the basilar membrane normally occupied by nerve fibers.

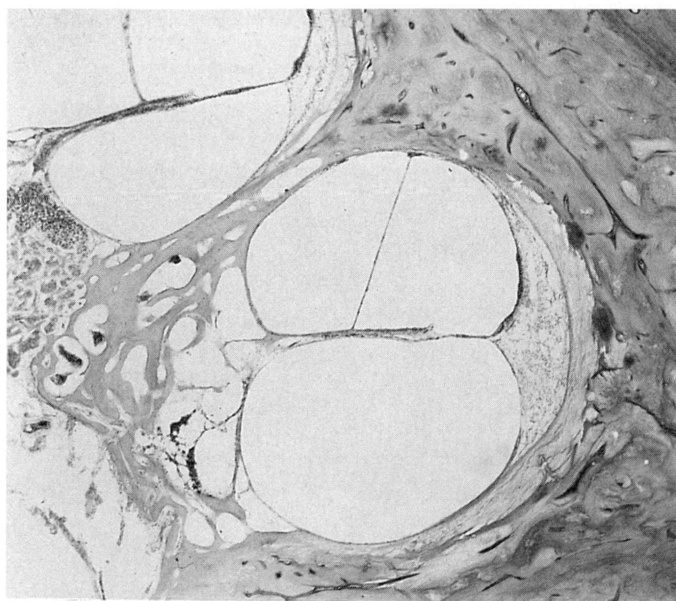

Fig. 80-33 Cochlear hydrops in Ménière's disease. The distended Reissner's membrane reaches the top of the scala vestibuli. (From Michaels L: *Ear, nose and throat histopathology,* Springer-Verlag.)

Presbycusis

Presbycusis (presbyacusis) is the hearing loss that occurs in aged persons that cannot be ascribed to any cause other than old age. Degenerative changes in at least four different sites in the cochlea have been incriminated as the pathologic basis for this hearing loss. These sites are the hair cells, spiral ganglion cells, stria vascularis and basilar membrane.[131] Findings from other studies have pointed toward a loss of hair cells as the sole cause of the disorder.[132]

Surface preparations of perfused cochleas stained for light microscopy[1] show considerable losses in the outer hair cells. A degree of loss of outer hair cells is present in all cochlea cells of all elderly persons. In addition, there is a complete loss of all hair cells of all rows, both inner and outer, at the extreme lower end of the basal coil in the cochleas of all elderly subjects (Fig. 80-34). The cochleas of all elderly persons also show enormously lengthened and thickened stereocilia emanating from some surviving outer hair cells (Fig. 80-35), which may represent a stage in the dissolution of these cells. The numbers of spiral ganglion cells are also reduced in a certain proportion of patients with presbycusis, but this appears to be a late change, possibly secondary to the primary atrophy of hair cells.[132]

Bony abnormalities

Bony abnormalities include (1) congenital disorders, such as osteogenesis imperfecta and osteopetrosis; (2) systemic disease of bones, such as Paget's disease; and (3) specific diseases of the auditory apparatus.

Osteogenesis imperfecta

In osteogenesis imperfecta the bony labyrith is sometimes deficient,[133] but the membranous structures of the inner ear are usually normal. The stapes footplate is frequently fixed by new bone at the same site as it occurs in otosclerosis. Some claim

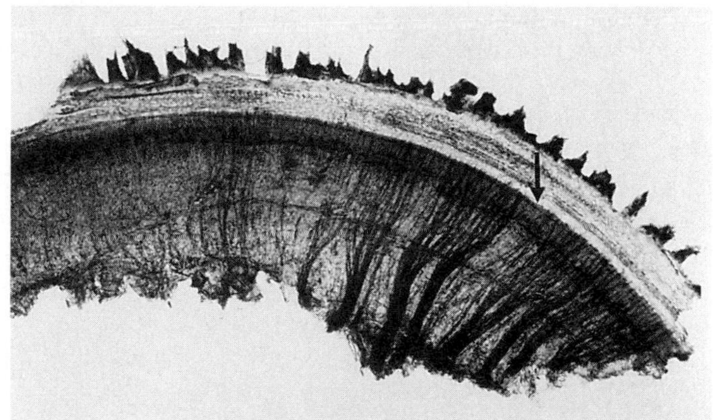

Fig. 80-34 Surface preparation of the basal coil of a cochlea in presbycusis. There is atrophy of the nerve fibers and of the inner and outer rows of hair cells at the extreme basal end *(left)*. Another zone of atrophy higher up the basal coil is marked by an arrow. (Osmic acid, alcian blue, phloxine stain.)

that it is conventional otosclerotis bone; others claim that it is the product of a bone reaction specific to osteogenesis imperfecta.[134]

Otosclerosis

In the benign dominant form of osteopetrosis (marble bone disease), often prominent otologic symptoms are the presenting features; these include sensorineural and conductive hearing loss and facial palsy.[135] Grossly the bone is abnormally hard and dense, and this condition has caused the internal auditory meatus and eustachian tube to narrow. Microscopically the intermediate endochondral portion of the otic capsule is swollen and the number of globuli ossei is greatly increased (Fig. 80-36). The ossicles are expanded such that they have a fetal shape and are filled with unabsorbed, calcified cartilage.[136,137]

Paget's disease

In patients with Paget's disease of bone, which often affects the temporal bone, the periosteal part of the bony labyrinth is the first to undergo changes, and this progresses to involve the endochondral layer. Patients with Paget's disease more frequently have small fissure fractures in the temporal bone, probably occurring during life. A spindle cell sarcoma of the temporal bone was found in one such patient, and this is consistent with the notion that Paget's disease is a known predisposing factor for the formation of bone neoplasms.[138]

Otosclerosis

Otosclerosis is a common focal lesion of the otic capsule of unknown cause and is found principally in relation to the cochlea and footplate of the stapes. Otosclerotic deposits not associated with hearing loss have been noted at autopsy in 10% to 12.75% of the temporal bones of adult white people in the United States.[139,140] These are found mainly in the otic capsule bone anterior to the oval window (footplate of the stapes). Conductive deafness occurs in a smaller number of such persons as the result of extension of this otosclerotic lesion to involve the stapes footplate. This causes the stapes to be fixed and unable to transmit sound vibrations.

In patients with prominent otosclerotic involvement of the otic capsule and conductive deafness, the lesion may be seen at operation on the middle ear as a pink swelling of the promontory, and this may sometimes even be detected clinically through a particularly transparent tympanic membrane. When manipulated at operation; the stapes is found to be rigidly fixed and clearly unable to vibrate. At autopsy the focus appears well demarcated and pink. Blood vessels are prominent and evenly distributed (Fig. 80-37).

The surgical treatment of otosclerosis is stapedectomy with replacement of the natural stapes by a prosthesis to restore the continuity of the ossicular chain. The stapedectomy may be partial, such that only the head or crura are removed, or total, in which case the footplate is also removed. Because the otosclerotic process involves only the footplate and not the crura, when only the latter are available

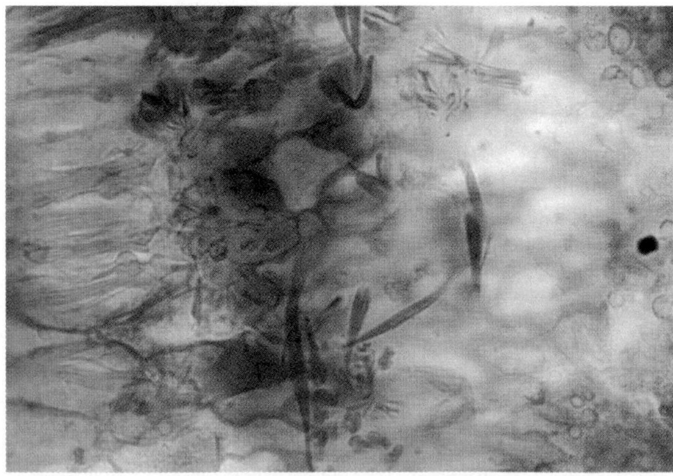

Fig. 80-35 Surface preparation of the middle coil of a cochlea in presbycusis. There is a pronounced diminution in the number of outer hair cells and giant stereociliary degeneration. (Osmic acid, alcian blue, phloxine stain.)

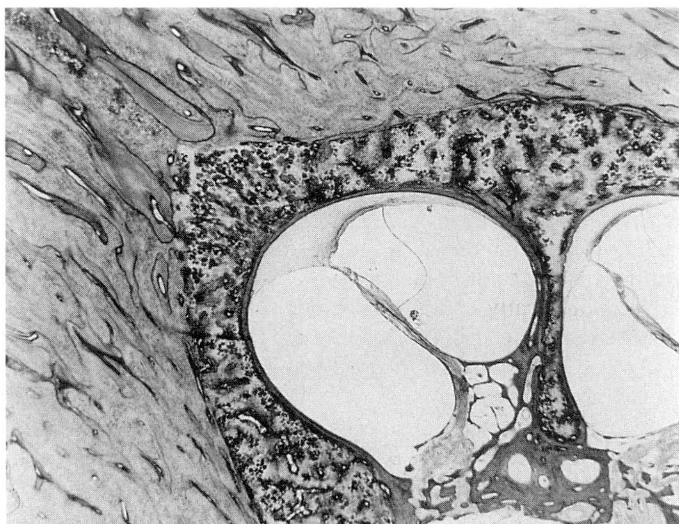

Fig. 80-36 Osteopetrosis involving the bony cochlea. The endochondral layer is enlarged and the globuli ossei (calcified cartilage cells) are excessively basophilic. (Courtesy Vince Hyams, MD, Washington, D.C.; from Michaels L: *Ear, nose and throat histopathology,* London, 1987, Springer-Verlag.)

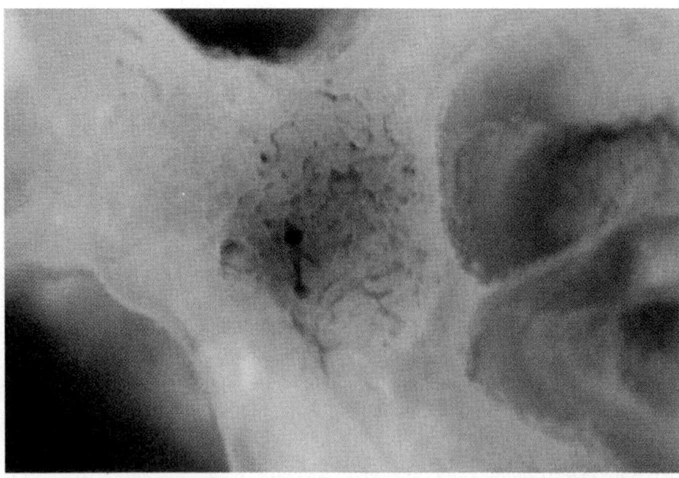

Fig. 80-37 Microslice of temporal bone showing a focus of otosclerosis adjacent to the cochlea.

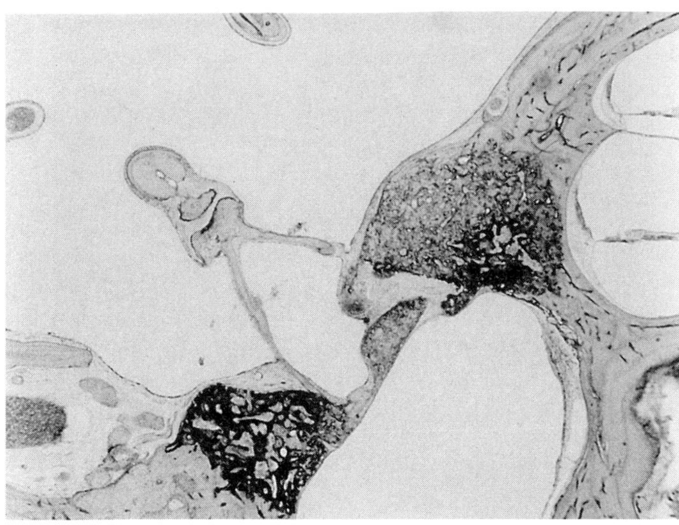

Fig. 80-38 Otosclerotic foci anterior and posterior to the footplate of the stapes. The former extends toward the center of the footplate.

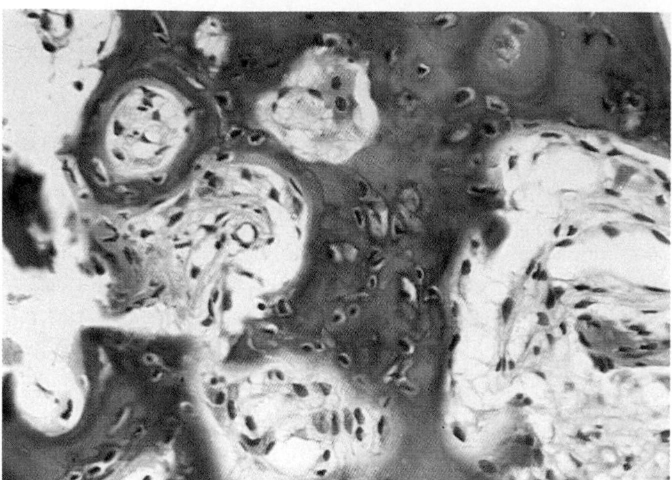

Fig. 80-39 Otosclerotic focus showing vascular woven bone.

for histologic examination, as is usually the case, no otosclerosis is seen in the specimen. In the unusual event that the whole stapes is removed, the otosclerotis process is found only in the footplate.

Histologically otosclerostic foci are made up of trabeculae of woven bone with abundant osteoblasts (Figs. 80-38 and 80-39). Osteoclasts may be present, and this is accompanied by evidence of bone resorption. Blood vessels are always numerous and prominent. This irregular cellular and vascular new-tissue formation is in contrast to the normal pattern of bone and cartilage in the normal footplate.[1] Lamellar bone may appear later in otosclerosis.

Because histologically otosclerosis is some what similar to Paget's disease of bone and there is mounting evidence of a viral cause in Paget's disease,[141] a possible viral cause of otosclerosis has also been investigated. Transmission electron microscopy of surgically removed fragments of a stapes footplate with active otosclerosis has revealed the presence of structures in osteoblasts, that are morphologically identical to the measles virus nucleocapsid, and immunocytochemical studies of the same material have shown that the same nucleocapsid antigen exists in active lesions.[142,143] A deposit of lamellar bone in the scala tympani near the round window membrane has been invoked as an indication of an autoimmune process,[144] and the finding of similar bony deposits in the setting of otosclerosis indicates that this reaction may be provoked by the measles virus antigen.[145]

Congenital stapes fixation: "gushers" and "oozers" of CSF

Fixation of the footplate to the surrounding otic capsule bone may occur as a congenital condition. In such cases a prosthesis may be inserted surgically to restore ossicular vibration. In some cases there is an associated congenital communication of the vestibule with the subarachnoid space, and as soon as the stapes is released surgically from the oval window, a strong flow of CSF occurs ("gushers"); sometimes there may be only a relentless slow ooze ("oozers").[146,147]

A communication between CSF and the middle ear associated with meningitis may form spontaneously in the absence of stapedectomy in patients with a congenitally defective labyrinth. The stapes in such patients and in those with the spontaneous "gushers" and "oozers" shows a central defect in the footplate. This would normally be covered by the mucosa of the middle ear and by the lining of the vestibule. In the presence of otitis media, however, these coverings may rupture, thus causing a direct connection to form between the subarachnoid space and the middle ear.[121]

Neoplasms

Acoustic neuroma

Acoustic neuroma or schwannoma of the eight cranial nerve is a benign tumor that because of its location, may nevertheless cause death. It is usually unilateral, but 9% of the tumors are bilateral[148] (that is, a manifestation of neurofibromatosis 2). The neoplasm may grow for years without causing symptoms and may be diagnosed only postmortem, as shown by the fact that it has been found at autopsy in about one in 220 consecutive adults who showed no symptoms of the tumor.[149]

The neoplasm is stated to arise most commonly at the glial-neurilemmal junction of the eighth nerve, which is usually within the internal auditory meatus.[1] In most cases it arises from the vestibular division of the nerve. Growth takes place from its point of origin, both centrally into the cerebellopontine angle and peripherally along the canal. An acoustic neuroma may rarely arise from the intravestibular portion of the nerve[150] or even in the cochlea, the bony capsule of which has been affected by Paget's disease of bone.[7,133]

The neoplasm varies in size and is round or oval. The larger tumors often have a mushroom shape, which has two components: the stalk (an elongated intratemporal part) and an expanded extratympanic part. The bone of the internal auditory meatus is often widened funnelwise as the result of the slow growth of the neoplasm. The tumor surface is smooth and lobulated. The cut surface is yellowish and often shows areas of hemorrhage. The vestibular division of the eighth nerve may be identified on the surface of the tumor (Fig. 80-40).

Histologically, acoustic neuromas possess the features typical of schwannomas in other sites, showing Antoni A and

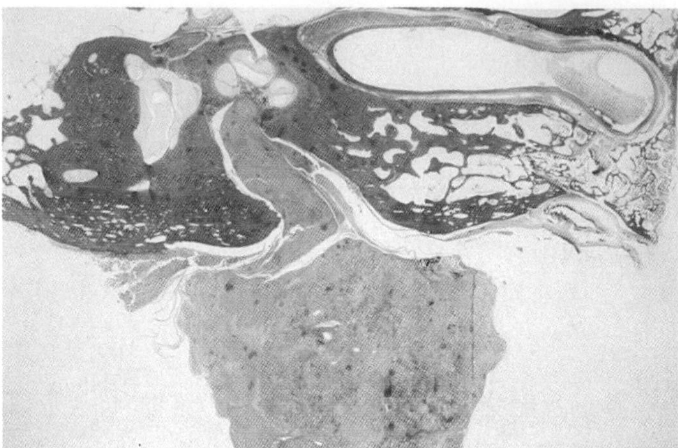

Fig. 80-40 Acoustic neuroma inside and outside the internal canal.

Antoni B type of areas. Antoni A areas are composed of spindle cells that are often moderately pleomorphic. Mitotic figures are rare, and the presence of pleomorphism should not be interpreted as evidence of malignancy. Antoni B areas are rarely prominent. Thrombosis and necrosis may be present in some parts of the neoplasm.

A granular or homogeneous fluid exudate is usually present in the perilymphatic spaces of the cochlea and vestibule. This may arise as a result of pressure by the neoplasm on veins in the internal auditory meatus.

Bilateral acoustic neuromas are a feature of neurofibromatosis 2, which, unlike neurofibromatosis 1, is not assocated with large numbers of cutaneous neurofibromas and café au lait spots. The temporal bone location of the neural tumor and its bilaterality are inherited as an autosomal dominant trait encoded by a gene localizing near the center of the long arm of chromosome 22.[151,152] Autopsy studies have shown that patients with neurofibromatosis 2 not only have bilateral eighth nerve tumors but also have small neuromas, schwannomas, and neurofibromas of other cranial nerves as well as meningiomas in the vicinity of the acoustic neuromas and sometimes even intermixed with them microscopically. The neuromas are histologically identical to those of the single acoustic tumors but are more invasive in their behavior, tending to infiltrate into the cochlea and vestibule.[153]

Low-grade adenocarcinoma of probable endolymphatic sac origin

A rare epithelial neoplasm presumably originating from the endolymphatic sac[7,154-157] has been described as a "low-grade adenocarcinoma of probable endolymphatic sac origin."[157] Two patients have been found to have bilateral neoplasms of the same type, and some tumors have also been associated with von Hippel-Lindau disease.[158]

The tumor may grow for many years before causing symptoms. Tinnitus or vertigo is the presenting symptom in about a third of the patients each, presumably resulting from early obstruction of the endolymphatic sac. Imaging studies show a lytic temporal bone lesion that appears to originate from the region between the internal auditory canal and sigmoid sinus, which is the approximate postion of the endolymphatic sac. There is usually prominent extension into the posterior cranial cavity and invasion of the middle ear (Fig. 80-41).

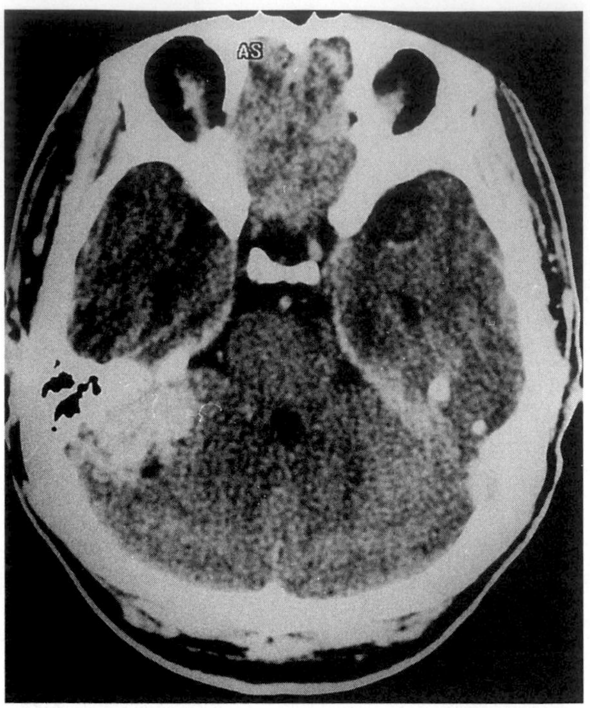

Fig. 80-41 Computerized tomographic scan of low-grade adenocarcinoma of the endolymphatic sac with prominent extension into the posterior cranial cavity and invasion of temporal bone.

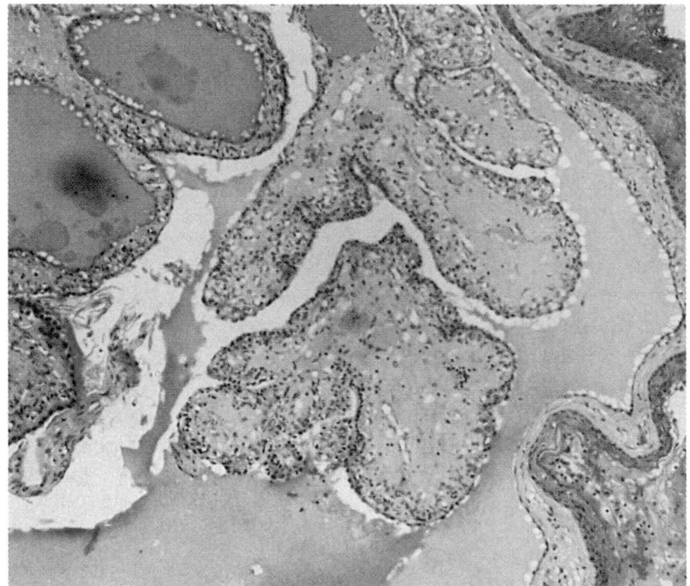

Fig. 80-42 Low-grade adenocarcinoma of the endolymphatic sac showing a papillary adenocarcinomatous appearance.

In most cases the tumor has the character of a papillary-glandular structure, with the papillae being composed of single rows of low cuboidal cells (Fig. 80-42), and a vascular core that is reminiscent of those in choroid plexus papillomas. Secretory material similar to thyroid colloid accumulates in some tumors, and under these circumstances the lesion may resemble papillary adenocarcinoma of the thyroid (Fig. 80-43). Immunohistochemical analysis of this colloid

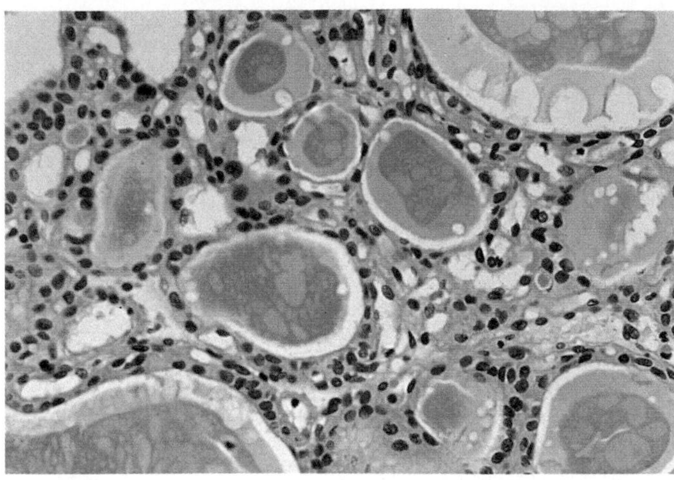

Fig. 80-43 Low-grade adenocarcinoma of the endolymphatic sac showing glands and secretion forming a thyroidlike area.

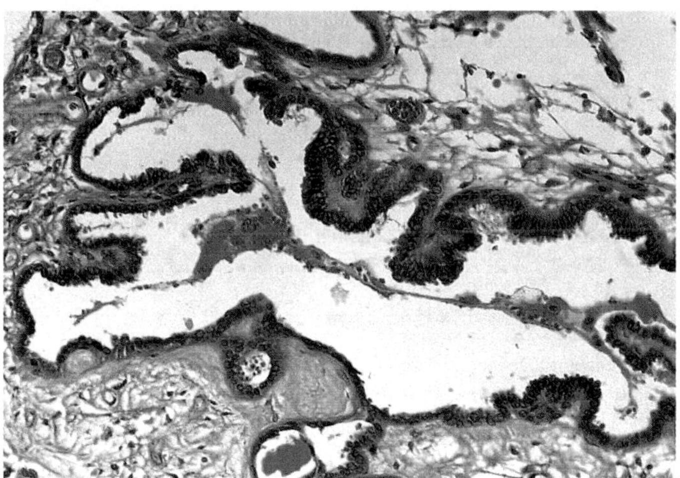

Fig. 80-44 Normal endolymphatic sac showing papillary lining.

has shown that it contains no thyroid hormones. A few lesions show a predominance of clear cells and resemble carcinoma of the kidney.[147]

It seems possible that the so-called aggressive papillary middle ear tumor[114] is a low-grade adenocarcinoma of the endolymphatic sac (see earlier discussion) that has extended into the middle ear.

The histologic appearances of low-grade adenocarcinomas of probable endolymphatic sac origin are in keeping with the normal histologic structure of the endolymphatic sac, which is lined by a papillary columnar epithelium (Fig. 80-44). During the development of the endolymphatic sac, there is a stage in which the epithelium is closely associated with a network of capillaries that give rise to the "endolymphatic glomerulus."[159,160] This may explain why some of the low-grade adenocarcinomas of the endolymphatic sac have an appearance similar to that of choroid plexus papillomas.

Secondary tumors

There are two routes by which tumors invading from outside can reach the inner ear. In the first route the tumor invades directly through the petrous bone, but the otic capsule seems

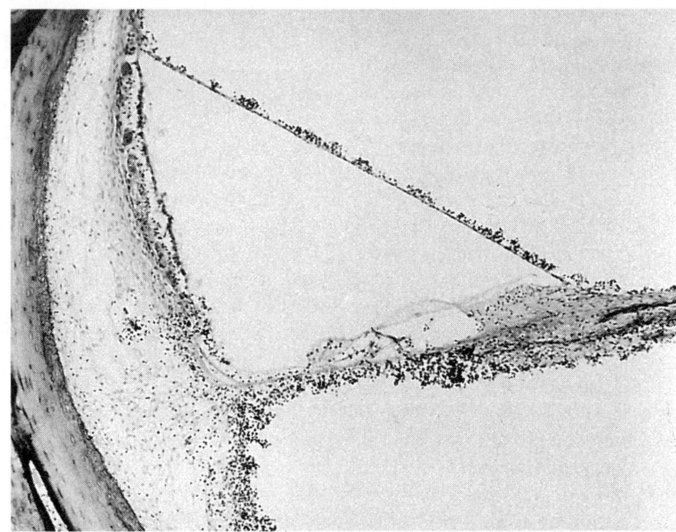

Fig. 80-45 Cochlea in chronic lymphatic leukemia. Numerous lymphoid cells are present in the scala vestibuli adjacent to Reissner's membrane, in the scala tympani adjacent to the basilar membrane, and in the spiral ligament. (From Michaels L: *Ear, nose and throat histopathology,* London, 1987, Springer-Verlag.)

to provide a particularly strong barrier against such invasion.[112] In the other route, the tumor invades the internal auditory canal, entering the foramina in the modiolus alongside the filaments of the cochlear nerves and progressing as far as the spiral lamina.[112]

The temporal bone is frequently the site of blood-borne metastasis of carcinomas originating in the breast, kidney, lung, stomach, larynx, prostate, and thyroid. The internal auditory meatus is a common location for such growth. Once deposited, further spread into the cochlea may take place by the route just described.[161]

Kaposi's sarcoma may be found in many parts of the body in patients with AIDS, most commonly in the lungs and skin, including that of the external ear.[162] A patient with Kaposi's sarcoma of the eighth nerve in the internal auditory meatus has been reported.[74]

Leukemia may involve the inner ear, by causing hemorrhage into the membranous spaces or by leukemic infiltration of the perilymphatic spaces of the cochlea (Fig. 80-45). The leukemic cells are probably conveyed from the CSF by means of the cochlear aqueduct. Extensive fibrosis and new bone formation in labyrinthine spaces, probably resulting from the resolution of leukemic deposits with treatment, have been noted in a patient suffering from deafness associated with chronic myeloid leukemia.[163] Inner ear hemorrhage is a well-known complication of leukemia.

REFERENCES

Normal anatomy and histology

1. Michaels L: The ear. In Sternberg S, editor: *Histology for pathologists,* New York, 1992, Raven Press.

External ear

Diagonal earlobe crease

2. Elliot WJ, Karrison T: Increased all-cause and cardiac morbidity and mortality associated with the diagonal earlobe crease: a prospective cohort study, *Am J Med* 91:247, 1991.

3. Overfield T, Call EB: Earlobe type, race and age: effects on earlobe creasing, *Am J Geriatr Soc* 31:479, 1983.
4. Kirkham N, Murrels T, Melcher DH, Morrison EA: Diagonal earlobe creases and fatal cardiovascular disease: a necropsy study, *Br Heart J* 61:361, 1989.

Inflammatory lesions

5. Senturia BH, Marcus MD, Lucente FE: *Diseases of the external ear: an otologic-dermatologic manual,* New York, 1980, Grune & Stratton.
6. Chandler JR: Malignant external otitis, Laryngoscope 7:1257, 1968.
7. Michaels L: *Ear, nose and throat histopathology,* London, 1987, Springer-Verlag
8. Ostfeld E, Segal M, Czernobilsky B: External otitis: early histopathologic changes and pathogenic mechanism, *Laryngoscope* 91:965, 1982.
9. Williams M: Head and neck findings in pediatric acquired immune deficiency syndrome, *Laryngoscope* 97:713, 1987.
10. Schinella RA, Breda SD, Hammerschlag PE: Otic infection due to Pneumocystis carinii in an apparently healthy man with antibody to the human immunodeficiency virus, *Ann Intern Med* 106:399, 1987.
11. Gherman CR, Ward RR, Bassis ML: *Pneumocystis carinii* otitis media and mastoiditis as the initial manifestation of the acquired immunodeficiency syndrome, *Am J Med* 5:250, 1988.
12. Smith MA, Hirschfield LS, Zahtz G, Siegal FP: *Pneumocystis carinii* otitis media, *Am J Med* 5:745, 1988.
13. Sandler ED, Sandler JM, LeBoit PE et al: *Pneumocystis carinii* otitis media in AIDS: a case report and review of the literature regarding extrapulmonary pneumocystosis, *Otolaryngol Head Neck Surg* 103:817, 1990.
14. Fujiwara N, Kurata T: Middle ear mucosa in Ramsay Hunt syndrome, *Ann Otol Rhinol Laryngol* 99:359, 1990.
15. Michaels L, Shah N: Dangers of corn starch powder [letter], *Br Med J* 2:714, 1973.
16. Hughes RA, Berry CL, Seifert M et al: Relapsing polychondritis. Three cases with a clinicopathological study and literature review, *Q J Med* 41:363, 1972.
17. Foidart JM, Abe S, Martin GR et al: Antibodies to type II collagen in relapsing polychondritis, *N Engl J Med* 299:1203, 1978.
18. Valenzuela R, Cooperrider PA, Gogate P et al: Relapsing polychondritis: immunomicroscopic findings in cartilage of ear biopsy specimens, *Hum Pathol* 11:19, 1980
19. Soucek S, Michaels L: Keratosis of the tympanic membrane and deep external canal: a defect of auditory epithelial migration, *Eur Arch Otorhinolaryngol* 250:140, 1993.
20. Piepergerdes JC, Kramer BM, Behnke EE: Keratosis obturans and external auditory canal cholesteatoma, *Laryngoscope* 90:383, 1980.
21. Hawke M, Jahn AF: Keratin implantation granuloma in external ear canal, *Arch Otolaryngol* 100:317, 1974.

Metabolic conditions

22. Gaines JJ Jr: The pathology of alkaptonuric ochronosis, *Hum Pathol* 20:40, 1989.
23. Koch HJ, Lewis JJ: Hyperlipemic xanthomatosis with associated osseous granulomas: a clinical report, *N Engl J Med* 255:387, 1956.
24. Emery PS, Gore M: An extensive solitary xanthoma of the temporal bone associated with hyperlipoproteinaemia, *J Laryngol Otol* 96:451, 1982.

Lesions simulating neoplasms

25. Azadeh B, Ardehali S: Malakoplakia of middle ear: a case report, *Histopathology* 7:129, 1983.
26. Azadeh B, Dabiri S, Moshfegh I: Malakoplakia of the middle ear, *Histopathology* 19:276, 1991.
27. Nayar RC, Garg I, Alapath JJ: Malakoplakia of the temporal bone in a nine-month-old infant, *J Laryngol Otol* 105:568, 1991.
28. Winkler M: Knötchenförmige Erkrankung am Helix (Chondrodermatitis nodularis chronica helicis), *Arch Dermatol Syph* 12:278, 1915.
29. Metzger SA, Goodman ML: Chondrodermatitis helicis: a clinical re-evaluation and pathological review, *Laryngoscope* 86:1402, 1976.
30. Barnes HM, Calman CD, Sarkany I: Spectacle frame acanthoma (granuloma fissuratum), *Trans St. John Hosp Dermatol Soc* 60:99, 1974.
31. Enzinger FM, Weiss SW: *Soft tissue tumors,* ed 3, St. Louis, 1995, Mosby.
32. Hansen JE: Pseudocysts of the auricle in Caucasians, *Arch Otolaryngol* 5:13, 1967.
33. Santos VB, Pilisar IA, Ruffy ML: Bilateral pseudocysts in a female, *Ann Otol Rhinol Laryngol* 83:9, 1974.
34. Heffner DK, Hyams VJ: Cystic chondromalacia (enchondral pseudocysts of the auricle, *Arch Pathol Lab Med* 110:740, 1986.
35. Devlin J, Harrison CJ, Whitby DJ, David T: Cartilaginous pseudocyst of the external auricle in children with atopic eczema, *Br J Dermatol* 122:699, 1990.
36. Slobodkin D: Why more keloids on the back than on the front of the earlobe [letter], *Lancet* 335:923, 1990.

Neoplasms

37. Bailin PH, Levine HL, Wood BG et al: Cutaneous carcinoma of the auricular and preauricular region, *Arch Otolaryngol* 106:692, 1980.
38. Metcalf PB Jr: Carcinoma of the pinna, *N Engl J Med* 251:91, 1954.
39. Goodwin WC, Jesse RH: Malignant neoplasms of the external auditory canal and temporal bone, *Arch Otolaryngol* 106:675, 1980.
40. Lewis JS: Squamous carcinoma of the ear, *Arch Otolaryngol* 97:49, 1973.
41. Johnson WC, Helwig EB: Adenoid squamous carcinoma (adenoacanthoma): a clinicopathologic study of 155 patients, *Cancer* 19:1639, 1966.
42. Woodson GE, Jurco S III, Alford BR, McGavran MH: Verrucous carcinoma of the middle ear, *Arch Otolaryngol* 107:63, 1981.
43. Proops DW, Hawke WM, Van Nostrand AWP et al: Verrucous carcinoma of the ear: case report, *Ann Otol Rhinol Laryngol* 93: 385, 1984.
44. Edelstein DR, Smouha E, Sacks SH et al: Verrucous carcinoma of the temporal bone, *Ann Otol Rhinol Laryngol* 95: 447, 1986.
45. Stafford ND, Frootko NJ: Verrucous carcinoma in the external auditory canal, *Am J Otol* 7:443, 1986.
46. Cooper JR, Hellquist HB, Michaels L: Image analysis in the discrimination of verrucous carcinoma and squamous papilloma, *J Pathol* 166:383, 1992.
47. Cankar V, Crowley H: Tumors of ceruminous glands: a clinicopathological study of seven cases, *Cancer* 17:67, 1964.
48. Wetli CV, Pardo V, Millard M et al: Tumors of ceruminous glands, *Cancer* 29:1169, 1972.
49. Wilson RS, Johnson JT: Benign eccrine cylindroma of the external auditory canal, *Laryngoscope* 90:379, 1980.
50. Pulec JL: Glandular tumors of the external auditory canal, *Laryngoscope* 7:1601, 1977.
51. Pack GT, Conley J, Oropega R: Melanoma of the external ear, *Arch Otolaryngol* 92:106, 1970.
52. Carney JA, Gordon H, Carpenter PC et al: The complex of myxomas, spotty pigmentation and endocrine overactivity, *Medicine* 64:270, 1985.
53. Nager GT, Kennedy DW, Kopstein E: Fibrous dysplasia: a review of the disease and its manifestations in the temporal bone, *Ann Otol Rhinol Laryngol* 92:Suppl:1, 1982.
54. Sheehey JH: Diffuse exostosis and osteomata of the external auditory canal: a report of 100 operations, *Otolaryngol Head Neck Surg* 90:337, 1982.
55. Graham M: Osteomas and exostosis of the external auditory canal: a clinical, histopathological and scanning electron microscopic study, *Ann Otol Rhinol Laryngol* 88:566, 1979.
56. Milroy CM, Phelps PD, Michaels L, Grant H: Osteoma of the incus, *J Otolaryngol* 18:226, 1989.
57. Silver FM, Orobello PW Jr, Mangal A, Pensak ML: Asymptomatic osteomas of the middle ear, *Am J Otol* 14:189, 1993.
58. Tos M: A survey of Hand-Schüller-Christian's disease in otolaryngology, *Acta Otolaryngol (Stockh)* 62:217, 1966.
59. Quesada P, Navarrete ML, Perrello E: Eosinophilic granuloma of the temporal bone, *Eur Arch Otorhinolaryngol* 247:194, 1990.
60. Goudie RB, Soukop M, Dagg JH, Lee FD: Hypothesis: symmetrical cutaneous lymphoma, *Lancet* 1:316, 1990.

Middle ear

Bacterial otitis media

61. Milroy CM, Slack RWT, Maw AR Bradfield JWB: Aural polyps as predictors of underlying cholesteatoma, *J Clin Pathol* 42:460, 1989.

62. Hussain SSM: Histology of aural polyp as a predictor of middle ear disease activity, *J Laryngol Otol* 105:268, 1991.
63. Gliklich RE, Cunningham MJ, Eavey RD: The cause of aural polyps in children, *Arch Otolaryngol Head Neck Surg* 119:669, 1993.
64. Poliquin JF, Catanzaro A, Robb J et al: Adaptive immunity of the tympanic membrane, *Am J Otolaryngol* 2:94, 1981.
65. Sade J: The biopathology of secretory otitis media, *Ann Otol Rhinol Laryngol* 83(suppl 11):59, 1974.
66. Tos M.: Pathogenesis and pathology of chronic secretory otitis media, *Ann Otol Laryngol* 89(suppl 68):91, 1980.
67. Ishii T, Toriyama M, Suzuki J-I: Histopathological study of otitis media with effusion, *Ann Otol Rhinol Laryngol* 89(suppl 68):83, 1980.
68. Ramages LJ, Gertler R: Aural tuberculosis: a series of 25 patients, *J Laryngol Otol* 99:1073, 1985.
69. Buchanan G, Rainer EH: Tuberculous mastoiditis, *J Laryngol Otol* 102:440, 1988.
70. Olsen TS, Seid AB, Pransky SM: Actinomycosis of the middle ear, *Int J Pediatr Otorhinolaryngol* 17:51, 1989.
71. Tarabichi M: Actinomycosis otomycosis, *Arch Otolaryngol Head Neck Surg* 119:561, 1993.
72. Macias JD, Wackym PA, McCabe BF: Early diagnosis of otologic Wegener's granulomatosis using the serologic marker C-ANCA, *Ann Otol Rhino Laryngol* 102:337, 1993.
73. Fauci AS, Wolff SM: Wegener's granulomatosis: studies in eighteen patients with a review of the literature, *Medicine* (Baltimore) 52:535, 1973.
74. Michaels L, Soucek S, Liang J: The ear in the acquired immunodeficiency syndrome. I. Temporal bone histopathologic study, *Am J Otol* 15:515, 1994.

Hemorrhage in drowning

75. Babin R, Graves N, Rose E: Temporal bone pathology in drowning, *Am J Otolaryngol* 3:168, 1982.
76. Robbins RD, Sekhar CS, Siveris V: Temporal bone histopathologic findings in drowning victims, *Arch Otolaryngol Head Neck Surg* 114:1020, 1988.

Neoplasma and similar lesions

77. Politzer A: Das Cholesteatom des Gehörorgans von anatomische und klinische Standpunkten, *Wien Med Wochenschr* 8:331, 1981.
78. Levenson MJ, Parisier SC, Chute P et al: A review of twenty congenital cholesteatomas of the middle ear in children, *Otolaryngol Head Neck Surg* 94:560, 1986.
79. Michaels L: Origin of congenital cholesteatoma from a normally occurring epidermoid rest in the developing middle ear, *Int J Pediath Otolaryngol* 15:51, 1988.
80. Levenson MJ, Michaels L, Parisier SC: Congenital cholesteatomas of the middle ear in children: origin and management, *Otolaryngol Clin North Am* 22:941, 1989.
81. Michaels L: An epidermoid formation in the developing middle ear: possible source of cholesteatoma, *J Otolaryngol* 15:169, 1986.
82. Michaels L, Soucek S: Development of the stratified squamous epithelium of the human tympanic membrane and external canal: the origin of auditory epithelial migration, *Am J Anat* 184:334, 1989.
83. Michaels L, Soucek S: Auditory epithelial migration. II. The existence of two discrete pathways and their embryologic correlates, *Am J Anat* 189:189, 1990.
84. Michaels L, Soucek S: Auditory epithelial migration. III. Development of the stratified squamous epithelium of the tympanic membrane and external canal in the mouse, *Am J Anat* 191:280, 1991.
85. Michaels L, Soucek S: Stratified squamous epithelium in relation to the tympanic membrane: its development and kinetics, *Inter J Pediatr Otolaryngol* 22:135, 1991.
86. Broekaert D, Couke P, Ramaekers F et al: Immunohistochemical analysis of the cytokeratin expression in middle ear cholesteatoma and related epithelial tissues, *Ann Otol Rhinol Laryngol* 101:931, 1992.
87. Tos M: Atelectasis, retraction pockets and cholesteatoma, *Ann Otol Rhinol Laryngol* 94(suppl 120):49, 1985.
88. Wells MD, Michaels L: Role of retraction pockets in cholesteatoma formation, *Clin Otolaryngol* 8:39, 1983.
89. Wells MD, Michaels L: Mode of growth of acquired cholesteatoma, *J Laryngol Otol* 105:261, 1991.
90. Valvassori GE: Benign tumors of the temporal bone, *Radiol Clin North Am* 12:533, 1974.
91. Paparella MM, Rybak L: Congenital cholesteatoma, *Otolaryngol Clin North Am* 11:113, 1978.
92. Gacek RR: Diagnosis and management of primary tumors of the petrous apex, *Ann Otol Rhinol Laryngol* 84(suppl 19):1, 1975.
93. Kartush JM, Graham MD: Salivary gland choristoma of the middle ear: a case report and review of the literature, *Laryngoscope* 94:228, 1984.
94. Kamerer DB, Caparosa RJ: Temporal bone encephalocele—diagnosis and treatment, *Laryngoscope* 92:878, 1982.
95. Nelson EG, Kratz RC: Sebaceous choristoma of the middle ear, *Otolaryngol Head Neck Surg* 108:372, 1993.
96. Hyams VJ, Michaels L: Benign adenomatous neoplasms (adenoma) of the middle ear, *Clin Otolaryngol* 1:17, 1976.
97. Derlacki EL, Barney PL: Adenomatous tumors of the middle ear and mastoid, *Laryngoscope* 86:1123, 1976.
98. Jahrdoerfer RA, Fechner RE, Selman JW et al: Adenoma of the middle ear, *Laryngoscope* 93:1041, 1983.
99. Mills SE, Fechner RE: Middle ear adenoma: a cytologically uniform neoplasm displaying a variety of architectural patterns, *Am J Surg Pathol* 8:677, 1984.
100. Stanley MW, Horwitz J, Levinson RM, Sibley RK: Carcinoid tumors of the middle ear, *Am J Clin Pathol* 87:592, 1987.
101. Hale RJ, McMahon RF, Whittaker JS: Middle ear adenoma: tumour of mixed mucinous and neuroendocrine differentiation, *J Clin Pathol* 44:652, 1991.
102. Wassef M, Panagiotis K, Polivka M et al: Middle ear adenoma: a tumor displaying mucinous and neuroendocrine differentiation, *Am J Surg Pathol* 13:838, 1989.
103. Polak JM, Bloom SR: *Endocrine tumours,* Edinburgh, 1959, Churchill Livingstone.
104. Krouse JH, Nadol JB, Goodman ML: Carcinoid tumors of the middle ear, *Ann Otol Rhinol Laryngol* 99:547, 1990.
105. Alford BR, Guilford FR: A comprehensive study of tumors of the glomus jugulare, *Laryngoscope* 72:765, 1962.
106. Bartels LJ, Pennington J, Kamerer DB, Browarsky I: Primary fallopian canal glomus tumors, *Otolaryngol Head Neck Surg* 102:85, 1990.
107. Kliewer KE, Duan-Ren W, Pasquale A, Cochrane AJ: Paragangliomas: assessment of prognosis by histologic, immunohistochemical and ultrastructural techniques, *Hum Pathol* 20:29, 1989.
108. Rosenwasser H: Long-term results of therapy of glomus jugulare tumors, *Arch Otolaryngol* 97:49, 1973.
109. DeLillis RA, Roth JA: Norepinephrine in a glomus jugulare tumor, *Arch Pathol* 92:73, 1971.
110. Ostfeld E, Segal M, Czernobilsky B: External otitis: early histopathologic changes and pathogenic mechanism, *Laryngoscope* 91:965, 1982.
111. Michaels L, Liang J: Origin and structure of middle ear corpuscles, *Clin Otolaryngol* 18:257, 1993.
112. Michaels L, Wells M: Squamous cell carcinoma of the middle ear, *Clin Otolaryngol* 5:235, 1980.
113. Phelps PD, Lloyd GA: The radiology of carcinoma of the ear, *Br J Radiol* 54:103, 1981.
114. Gaffey MJ, Mills ES, Fechner RE et al: Aggressive papillary middle-ear tumors: a clinico-pathologic entity distinct from middle-ear adenoma, *Am J Surg Pathol* 12:790, 1988.
115. Jackson CG, Levine SC, McKennan KX: Hemangioma of the middle ear, *Am J Otol* 8:131, 1987.
116. Nager GT: *Meningiomas involving the temporal bone,* Springfield, Ill., 1963, Charles C Thomas.
117. Shanmugaratnam K, editor: *Histological typing of upper respiratory tract tumours,* ed 2, Berlin, 1991, Springer-Verlag.
118. Hill BA, Kohut RI: Metastatic adenocarcinomas of the temporal bone, *Arch Otolaryngol* 102:568, 1976.
119. Jahn AF, Farkashidy J, Berman JM: Metastatic tumors in the temporal bone—a pathophysiologic study, *J Otolaryngol* 8:85, 1979.

Table 1 —cont'd

Organ	Weight in grams	Measurements in centimeters	
Endocrines:			
Pituitary:		2.1 by 1.4 by 0.5	
10–20 years	Average 0.56		
20–70 years	Average 0.61		
Pregnancy	0.84–1.06 (average 0.95)		
Thyroid	30–70 (average 40)	5–7 by 3–4 by 1.5–2.5	
Testis:			
Newborn		1 by 0.5 by 0.4	
Puberty		3 by 2 by 1.6	
Adult	20–27 (average 25)	4–5 by 2.5–3.5 by 2–2.7	
Ovary:			
Virgin		4.1–5.2 by 2–2.7 by 1–1.1	
After pregnancy	Average 7	2.7–4.1 by 1.5 by 0.8	
Adrenal	Average 6	4.5 by 2.5–3.5 by 0.5	
Parathyroids	0.12–0.18	0.3–0.6 by 0.2–0.4 by 0.05–0.2 (each)	
Thymus:			
Newborn	6.05–25.88 (average 13.98)		
1–9 months	6.74–34.10 (average 20.14)		
9–24 months	19.97–37.72 (average 26.60)		
6–25 years	Average 25		
26–35 years	Average 20		
36–65 years	Average 16		
65 years and over	Average 6		
Gastrointestinal tract:			
Esophagus		25	
Duodenum		30	
Small intestine		550–650	
Colon		150–170	
Brain:			
Male	1100–1700 (average 1400)	Sagittal diameter 15–17	
Female	1050–1550 (average 1275)	Vertical diameter 12.5	
Spinal cord:	Average 27	Length, 45	
		Frontal	**Sagittal**
Cervical		1.3–1.4	Average 0.9
Thoracic		Average 1	Average 0.8
Lumbar		Average 1.2	Average 0.9
Pineal gland	Average 0.2		

Table 2 Size (cm), body weight (kg) and organ weight (gm) as a function of age and sex

Age	Height		Body Weight		Heart		Lungs*		Liver		Kidneys		Spleen		Adrenal Glands		Testes	Ovar-ies	Brain	
	♂	♀	♂	♀	♂	♀	♂	♀	♂	♀	♂	♀	♂	♀	♂	♀	♂	♀	♂	♀
Birth	50.6	50.2	3.4	3.3	23	21	50	47	135	134	24	23	11	10	6.2	5.2	1.1	0.25	385	365
6 mo	66.4	65.2	7.5	7.26	28	25	60	60	160	140	31	28	14	12	3.2	2.0	1.5	0.3	300	360
1 yr	75.2	74.2	10.0	9.7	60	55	170	170	380	330	70	60	30	25	5.6	5.4	1.9	1.0	960	960
2 yr	87.5	86.6	12.5	12.2	65	58	190	180	420	350	77	72	35	30	6.0	5.5	2.0	1.0	970	950
5 yr	111.3	109.7	19.4	18.7	100	90	270	266	600	450	105	105	55	52	6.6	6.0	2.8	1.8	1200	1050
10 yr	140.3	138.6	32.6	31.8	130	120	360	310	950	800	150	125	80	70	9.0	8.0	4.0	4.0	1250	1230
15 yr	167.8	161.1	54.8	51.4	240	200	550	500	1270	930	200	185	120	110	13.0	11.0	20.0	8.0	1340	1260
20 yr	170.0	165.0	62.0	56.2	280	260	700	620	1560	1370	270	240	155	130	13.5	12.0	42.0	9.5	1400	1260
25 yr	170.0	165.0	65.0	56.6	310	265	770	620	1580	1370	280	260	170	130	14.0	13.0	45.0	11.0	1400	1250
30 yr	170.0	165.0	68.0	58.5	315	270	800	620	1580	1370	285	240	170	130	14.0	13.0	42.0	11.0	1390	1250
40 yr	170.0	165.0	71.0	61.2	320	285	800	660	1590	1400	275	240	150	130	14.0	13.5	40.0	9.0	1380	1250
50 yr	170.0	165.0	72.0	64.8	340	305	800	620	1600	1430	270	235	145	115	13.0	12.5	35.0	6.0	1340	1240
60 yr	170.0	165.0	73.0	67.1	330	310	800	620	1520	1380	270	235	130	105	13.0	12.0	33.0	4.5	1300	1200
70 yr	170.0	165.0	72.0	67.5	320	300	770	620	1400	1250	260	220	110	90	12.5	12.0	30.0	4.0	1250	1150

From Sandritter W, Thomas C, Kirsten W H: *Color atlas and textbook of macropathology*, St. Louis, 1972, Mosby.
*Lung weights are falsified by pulmonary edema. In cases of acute electric death (e.g., execution), the lung weight is said to be 200 gm.

Table 3 Weights and lengths of newborn infants and their organs related to body weight and gestational age

Body weight (g)	Number of cases	Body length (cm)	Heart (g)	Lungs combined (g)	Spleen (g)	Liver (g)	Adrenals combined (g)	Kidneys combined (g)	Thymus (g)	Brain (g)	Gestational age	
											Weeks	Days
500	317	29.4	5.0	12	1.3	26	2.6	5.4	2.2	70	23	5
		±2.5	±1.6	±5	±0.8	±10	±1.7	±2.1	±0.8	±18	±2	3
750	311	32.9	6.3	19	2.0	39	3.2	7.8	2.8	107	26	0
		±3.0	±1.8	±6	±1.2	±12	±1.5	±2.6	±1.3	±27	±2	6
1000	295	35.6	7.7	24	2.6	47	3.5	10.4	3.7	143	27	5
		±3.1	±2.0	±8	±1.5	±12	±1.6	±3.4	±2.0	±34	±3	1
1250	217	38.4	9.6	30	3.4	56	4.0	12.9	4.9	174	29	0
		±3.0	±3.3	±9	±1.8	±21	±1.7	±3.9	±2.1	±38	±3	0
1500	167	41.0	11.5	34	4.3	65	4.5	14.9	6.1	219	31	3
		±2.7	±3.3	±11	±2.0	±18	±1.8	±4.2	±2.7	±52	±2	3
1750	148	42.6	12.8	40	5.0	74	5.3	17.4	6.8	247	32	4
		±3.1	±3.2	±13	±2.5	±20	±2.0	±4.7	±3.0	±51	±2	6
2000	140	44.9	14.9	44	6.0	82	5.3	18.8	7.9	281	34	6
		±2.8	±4.2	±13	±2.7	±23	±2.0	±5.0	±3.4	±56	±3	2
2250	124	46.3	16.0	48	7.0	88	6.0	20.2	8.2	308	36	4
		±2.9	±4.3	±15	±3.3	±24	±2.3	±4.9	±3.4	±49	±3	0
2500	120	47.3	17.7	48	8.5	105	7.1	22.6	8.3	339	38	0
		±2.3	±4.2	±14	±3.5	±21	±2.8	±5.5	±4.4	±50	±3	2
2750	138	48.7	19.1	51	9.1	117	7.5	24.0	9.6	362	39	2
		±2.9	±3.8	±15	±3.6	±26	±2.7	±5.4	±3.8	±48	±2	2
3000	144	50.0	20.7	53	10.1	127	8.3	24.7	10.2	380	40	0
		±2.9	±5.3	±13	±3.3	±30	±2.9	±5.3	±4.3	±55	±2	1
3250	133	50.7	21.5	59	11.0	145	9.2	27.3	11.6	395	40	4
		±2.6	±4.3	±18	±4.0	±33	±3.4	±6.6	±4.4	±53	±1	6
3500	106	51.8	22.8	63	11.3	153	9.8	28.0	12.8	411	40	4
		±3.0	±5.9	±17	±3.6	±33	±3.5	±6.5	±5.1	±55	±1	5
3750	57	52.1	23.8	65	12.5	159	10.2	29.5	13.0	413	40	6
		±2.3	±5.1	±15	±4.1	±40	±3.3	±6.8	±4.8	±55	±2	3
4000	31	52.4	25.8	67	14.1	180	10.8	30.2	11.4	420	41	4
		±2.7	±5.3	±20	±4.0	±39	±3.4	±6.2	±3.2	±62	±1	3
4250	15	53.2	26.5	68	13.0	197	12.0	30.7	11.7	415	41	2
		±2.5	±5.3	±16	±2.5	±42	±3.7	±5.8	±3.7	±38	±2	1

From Reed GB, Claireaux AE, Bain AD, editors: Diseases of the fetus and newborn: pathology, radiology, genetics, St. Louis, 1989, Mosby. Data from Gruenwald P, Minh H: Evaluation of body and organ weights in perinatal pathology. I. Normal standard derived from autopsies, *Am J Clin Pathol* 34:247, 1960.

Table 4 **Weights of organs of male infants**

Age (mo)	Cases		Body length (cm)	Brain (gm)	Thymus (gm)	Heart (gm)	Lungs combined (gm)	Liver (gm)	Spleen (gm)	Pancreas (gm)	Adrenals combined (gm)	Kidneys combined (gm)
1	56	M*	51.4	460	7.8	23	64	140	12	6.2	5.1	34
		SD*	3.2	47	5.3	7	21	40	4	3.6	1.7	9
		SE*	0.4	10	0.9	1.3	5.3	5.5	0.6	0.5	0.3	1.3
2	53	M	54.0	506	9.4	27	74	160	15	7.2	5.0	39
		SD	2.9	67	4.4	7	26	46	5	4.4	1.6	9
		SE	0.5	16	0.8	1.2	5.4	6.5	0.7	0.8	0.3	1.4
3	43	M	57.7	567	10	30	89	179	16	7.7	5.0	45
		SD	2.9	81	5	7	23	41	5	3.1	1.3	10
		SE	0.5	20	1.0	1.4	4.5	6.3	0.8	0.6	0.2	1.6
4	42	M	60.4	620	10	31	96	195	17	11	4.9	47
		SD	4.1	71	6	7	27	41	5	5	2.0	12
		SE	0.6	18	1.0	1.4	6.0	6.6	0.8	0.9	0.3	2.1
5	40	M	62.0	746	12	35	93	228	18	11	5.3	54
		SD	3.1	91	7	5	18	47	7	4	1.9	11
		SE	0.5	21	1.3	0.9	4.4	7.6	1.2	0.7	0.3	1.9
6	47	M	64.2	762	10	40	115	259	20	11	5.2	62
		SD	3.9	73	6	8	31	58	7	5	2.0	14
		SE	0.6	20	1.1	1.4	6.5	8.7	1.1	0.9	0.3	2.2
7	27	M	66.7	767	12	43	118	276	23	12	5.5	69
		SD	5.0	32	9	8	33	54	10	6	2.1	14
		SE	1.0	11	2.2	1.9	7.8	10	2.1	1.5	0.4	2.7
8	27	M	68.2	774	10	44	104	285	20	13	5.4	66
		SD	3.4	95	6	8	32	57	7	7	2.3	14
		SE	0.8	30	1.7	1.8	7.8	12	1.5	1.8	0.6	2.8
9	25	M	69.4	820	10	45	109	288	22	16	5.4	67
		SD	4.2	49	4	7	33	47	5	7	2.0	16
		SE	0.9	19	1.1	1.7	9.2	11	1.1	1.5	0.5	3.5
10	20	M	69.7	850	9	46	110	300	24	14	5.7	72
		SD	3.9	96	5	6	34	69	11	6	2.1	17
		SE	0.9	32	1.4	1.6	11	16	2.7	1.5	0.5	3.8
11	16	M	70.5	875	19	48	130	305	28	16	6.1	76
		SD	4.3	89	4	7	31	81	10	3	1.8	19
		SE	1.1	28	1.8	1.9	10	20	2.7	0.9	0.5	5.0
12	19	M	73.8	954	12	50	116	325	28	14	6.3	76
		SD	4.1	35	5	6	23	39	7	6	2.2	13
		SE	0.9	13	1.4	1.7	7.2	9.8	1.7	1.6	0.7	3.1

From Schulz DM, Giordano D A, Schulz D H: Weights of organs of fetuses and infants, *Arch Pathol* 74:244, 1962.
*M indicates the mean; *SD*, the standard deviation; and *SE*, the standard error of the mean.

Table 5 **Weights of organs of female infants**

Age (mo)	Cases		Body length (cm)	Brain (gm)	Thymus (gm)	Heart (gm)	Lungs combined (gm)	Liver (gm)	Spleen (gm)	Pancreas (gm)	Adrenals combined (gm)	Kidneys combined (gm)
1	28	M**	51.9	433	6.6	21	64	139	11	5.0	4.8	31
		SD**	4.5	59	4.9	5	27	31	4	1.8	1.9	8
		SE**	0.9	19	1.3	1.2	6.6	5.9	0.8	0.4	0.4	1.5
2	39	M	54.0	490	5.8	26	74	159	14	7.1	4.7	36
		SD	3.7	51	4.7	6	23	31	5	2.9	1.4	10
		SE	0.7	14	0.9	1.1	4.8	5.1	0.8	0.6	0.2	1.8
3	36	M	57.0	525	9.7	28	81	183	15	8.5	4.8	42
		SD	3.7	89	6.9	4	14	39	5	3.2	1.4	12
		SE	0.6	22	1.4	0.8	3.0	6.8	0.9	0.6	0.3	2.1
4	29	M	59.0	595	9.0	30	91	204	17	9.0	4.6	50
		SD	3.7	80	7.3	6	24	49	5	3.0	2.1	11
		SE	0.7	20	2.0	1.3	6.2	9.2	1.0	0.7	0.4	2.2
5	24	M	62.2	725	13	36	102	227	19	11	4.8	52
		SD	3.3	62	5	5	22	38	5	3	2.2	13
		SE	0.7	19	1.4	1.3	6.9	8.1	1.1	0.7	0.6	3.5
6	23	M	63.0	730	10	37	111	242	18	11	4.6	58
		SD	3.0	85	6	7	30	58	8	4	1.5	20
		SE	0.6	28	1.4	1.6	8.1	13	1.9	1.1	0.4	4.4
7	21	M	65.4	750	10	40	111	272	22	10	5.5	65
		SD	4.2	92	8	9	38	51	8	3	2.2	14
		SE	0.9	31	2.0	2.2	11	11	1.8	0.7	0.5	3.3
8	24	M	66.5	770	8	41	109	276	20	11	5.3	60
		SD	4.5	96	5	7	35	54	9	5	2.3	13
		SE	1.0	28	1.3	1.5	9	13	2.2	1.2	0.6	2.8
9	15	M	68.3	810	9	41	105	288	18	14	5.4	62
		SD	4.7	82	5	5	28	67	6	5	1.5	10
		SE	1.2	25	2.2	1.6	8.5	19	1.9	1.7	0.5	2.7
10	14	M	67.5	830	12	43	105	284	25	13	5.7	66
		SD	4.2	117	7	7	21	48	11	6	1.7	10
		SE	1.2	35	2.9	2.4	8.1	15	3.3	2.3	0.5	2.7
11	18	M	70.5	875	15	44	125	292	23	14	6.2	68
		SD	3.1	64	8	8	31	36	9	7	2.0	14
		SE	0.8	20	2.7	2.0	9.7	9.7	2.3	2.0	0.6	3.9
12	15	M	71.5	886	11	49	115	315	27	15	6.0	72
		SD	4.7	64	8	6	34	38	9	8	1.4	19
		SE	1.3	23	3.6	1.8	11	9.7	2.6	2.7	0.4	4.7

From Schulz DM, Giordano D A, Schulz D H: Weights of organs of fetuses and infants, *Arch Pathol* 74:244, 1962.
**M* indicates the mean; *SD*, the standard deviation; and *SE*, the standard error of the mean.

Index

Page numbers in *italics* indicate illustrations. Page numbers followed by a t indicate tables.

B

D

H

J

K

L

P

Q

R

S

T

V

Y

Z